MW01057004

Clinical Cardiac Pacing, Defibrillation, and Resynchronization Therapy

Clinical Cardiac Pacing, Defibrillation, and Resynchronization Therapy

THIRD EDITION

Kenneth A. Ellenbogen, MD
Kontos Professor of Cardiology
Clinical Assistant Professor of Surgery
Director, Clinical Electrophysiology Laboratory
Medical College of Virginia
Richmond, Virginia

G. Neal Kay, MD
Professor of Medicine
Division of Cardiovascular Disease
Director, Clinical Electrophysiology Section
The University of Alabama at Birmingham
Birmingham, Alabama

Chu-Pak Lau, MD
William M. W. Mong Professor in Cardiology
Department of Medicine
The University of Hong Kong
Queen Mary Hospital
Hong Kong

Bruce L. Wilkoff, MD
Professor of Medicine
Cleveland Clinic Lerner College of Medicine of Case Western Reserve University
Director, Cardiac Pacing and Tachyarrhythmia Devices
Department of Cardiovascular Medicine
Cleveland Clinic
Cleveland, Ohio

SAUNDERS

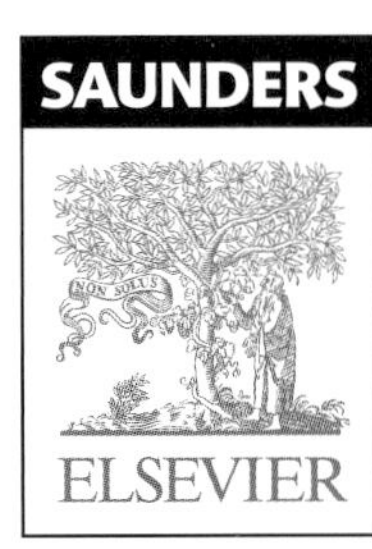

ELSEVIER

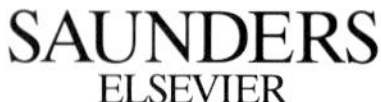

SAUNDERS
ELSEVIER

1600 John F. Kennedy Blvd.
Suite 1800
Philadelphia, PA 19103-2899

CLINICAL CARDIAC PACING, DEFIBRILLATION, AND RESYNCHRONIZATION THERAPY
ISBN-13: 978-1-4160-2536-8
ISBN-10: 1-4160-2536-7

Copyright © 2007 by Saunders, an imprint of Elsevier Inc.

All rights reserved. No part of this publication may be reproduced or transmitted in any form or by any means, electronic or mechanical, including photocopying, recording, or any information storage and retrieval system, without permission in writing from the publisher. Permissions may be sought directly from Elsevier's Health Sciences Rights Department in Philadelphia, PA, USA: phone: (+1) 215 239 3804, fax: (+1) 215 239 3805, e-mail: healthpermissions@elsevier.com. You may also complete your request on-line via the Elsevier homepage (http://www.elsevier.com), by selecting "Customer Support" and then "Obtaining Permissions".

Notice

Knowledge and best practice in this field are constantly changing. As new research and experience broaden our knowledge, changes in practice, treatment, and drug therapy may become necessary or appropriate. Readers are advised to check the most current information provided (i) on procedures featured or (ii) by the manufacturer of each product to be administered, to verify the recommended dose or formula, the method and duration of administration, and contraindications. It is the responsibility of the practitioner, relying on their own experience and knowledge of the patient, to make diagnoses, to determine dosages and the best treatment for each individual patient, and to take all appropriate safety precautions. To the fullest extent of the law, neither the Publisher nor the Editors assume any liability for any injury and/or damage to persons or property arising out of or related to any use of the material contained in this book.

The Publisher

Previous editions copyrighted 2000, 1995

Library of Congress Cataloging-in-Publication Data

Clinical cardiac pacing, defibrillation, and resynchronization therapy / [edited by]
Kenneth A. Ellenbogen, G. Neal Kay, Chu-Pak Lau.—3rd ed.
p. ; cm.
Includes bibliographical references and index.
ISBN-13: 978-1-4160-2536-8 ISBN-10: 1-4160-2536-7
1. Cardiac pacing. 2. Defibrillators. I. Ellenbogen, Kenneth A. II. Kay, G. Neal.
III. Lau, Chu-Pak.
[DNLM: 1. Cardiac Pacing, Artificial. 2. Defibrillators, Implantable. 3. Pacemaker, Artificial. WG 168 C6413 2007]
RC684.P3C54 2006
617.4′120645—dc22

2006040047

Executive Publisher: Natasha Andjelkovic
Editorial Assistant: Katie Davenport
Publishing Services Manager: Frank Polizzano
Project Manager: Michael H. Goldberg
Design Direction: Ellen Zanolle
Multimedia Producer: Bruce Robison
Marketing Manager: Dana Butler

ISBN-13: 978-1-4160-2536-8
ISBN-10: 1-4160-2536-7

Printed in China

Last digit is the print number: 9 8 7 6 5 4 3 2

Working together to grow
libraries in developing countries

www.elsevier.com | www.bookaid.org | www.sabre.org

ELSEVIER BOOK AID International Sabre Foundation

To my wife and family, Phyllis, Michael, Amy, and Bethany,
for their patience, support, and love.
To my parents, Roslyn and Leon,
who instilled in me a thirst for learning.
To my students, teachers, and colleagues, who make each day an absolute delight.

KAE

To my teachers, colleagues, and students,
who have taught me about cardiac pacing.
I am also indebted to the many members of the industry who have dedicated their
professional careers to the design and improvement of pacing technology.
These individuals have greatly improved the therapy that clinicians can offer
to their patients, undoubtedly resulting in an improvement in their lives.
Perhaps most important, this book is dedicated to my wife, Linda,
for her patience and understanding during its preparation.

GNK

To my wife and family, Carven, Yuk-Fai, and Yuk-Ming, for their understanding, support, and love.
To my teachers, patients, and colleagues, who are my source of inspiration and encouragement.

CPL

To my wife, Ellyn,
and children Jacob, Benjamin, Kara, and Ephram
for their godly and inspirational patience and support.
To my granddaughter, Isabelle, for life, hope, and love.
To my parents, Harvey and Glenna, for their unconditional love and insights.
To Yeshua, the Messiah, for His salvation,
and His sustaining covenant love.
And for the inspiration of His words in Proverbs 15:2:
"The tongue of the wise makes knowledge acceptable."
May the words of this book prove to be wise and useful to the student of cardiac pacing,
defibrillation, and heart failure device therapy.

BLW

Contributors

Amin Al-Ahmad, MD
Assistant Professor of Medicine, Stanford University School of Medicine; Associate Director, Stanford Hospital and Clinics, Stanford, California
Timing Cycles of Implantable Devices

Angelo Auricchio, MD, PhD
Fondazione Cardiocentro Ticino, Lugano, Switzerland
Basic Physiology and Hemodynamics of Cardiac Pacing

Peter H. Belott, MD, FACC, FHRS
Director, Electrophysiology, Sharp Grossmont Hospital, La Mesa, California
Permanent Pacemaker and Implantable Cardioverter-Defibrillator Implantation

Alan D. Bernstein, MD
Division of Surgical Research, New Jersey Pacemaker and Defibrillator Evaluation Center, Newark Beth Israel Medical Center, Newark, New Jersey
Pacemaker, Defibrillator, and Lead Codes

Charles L. Byrd, MD
Director of Electrophysiology Institute, Broward General Medical Center, Fort Lauderdale, Florida
Managing Device-Related Complications and Transvenous Lead Extractions

Henry Chen, MD
Cardiac Electrophysiology Fellow, Stanford University School of Medicine and Stanford Hospital and Clinics, Stanford, California
Timing Cycles of Implantable Devices

Mina K. Chung, MD
Associate Professor, Cleveland Clinic College of Medicine of Case Western Reserve University; Attending Physician, Cleveland Clinic, Cleveland, Ohio
Imaging in Pacing and Defibrillation

Stuart J. Connolly, MD
Professor, Faculty of Health Sciences, McMaster University; Chief of Cardiology, Hamilton Health Sciences, Hamilton, Ontario, Canada
Clinical Trials of Pacing Modes

Ann M. Crespi, PhD
Medtronic, Inc., Minneapolis, Minnesota
Power Systems for Implantable Pacemakers, Cardioverters, and Defibrillators

Teresa De Marco, MD
Professor of Medicine, University of California, San Francisco, School of Medicine; Director of Heart Failure and Pulmonary Hypertension Program and Medical Director of Heart Transplantation, UCSF Medical Center, San Francisco, California
Clinical Trials of Cardiac Resynchronization Therapy: Pacemakers and Defibrillators

Kenneth A. Ellenbogen, MD
Kontos Professor of Cardiology, Virginia Commonwealth University School of Medicine; Director, Electrophysiology and Pacing Laboratory, Medical College of Virginia and McGuire Veterans Affairs Medical Center, Richmond, Virginia
Clinical Trials of Cardiac Resynchronization Therapy: Pacemakers and Defibrillators; Pacing for Atrioventricular Conduction System Disease

Andrew E. Epstein, MD
Professor of Medicine, Division of Cardiovascular Disease, Department of Medicine, University of Alabama at Birmingham, Birmingham, Alabama
Troubleshooting of Implantable Cardioverter-Defibrillators

Derek V. Exner, MD, MPH, FRCPC
Assistant Professor, Faculty of Medicine, University of Calgary;
Libin Cardiovascular Institute of Alberta, Calgary, Alberta, Canada
Clinical Trials of Defibrillator Therapy

Jeffrey M. Gillberg, MS
Senior Staff Scientist, Medtronic, Inc., Minneapolis, Minnesota
Sensing and Detection

Anne M. Gillis, MD, FRCPC
Professor of Medicine, Faculty of Medicine, University of Calgary; Medical Director, Pacing and Electrophysiology, Calgary Health Region, Calgary, Alberta, Canada
Pacing for Sinus Node Disease: Indications, Techniques, and Clinical Trials

Lorne J. Gula, MD, FRCPC
Assistant Professor of Medicine, University of Western Ontario Faculty of Medicine and Dentistry; Electrophysiologist, Arrhythmia Service, London Health Sciences Centre, London, Ontario, Canada
Follow-up and Interpretation of Implantable Syncope Monitors

Jeff S. Healey, MD, MSc
Assistant Professor, Faculty of Health Sciences, McMaster University; Cardiologist and Electrophysiologist, Hamilton Health Sciences, Hamilton, Ontario, Canada
Clinical Trials of Pacing Modes

Ahmad Hersi, MD
Cardiac Electrophysiology Fellow, Faculty of Medicine, University of Calgary, Calgary, Alberta, Canada
Evolving Indications for Pacing: Hypertrophic Cardiomyopathy, Sleep Apnea, Long QT Syndromes, and Neurally Mediated Syncope Syndromes

Henry H. Hsia, MD

Associate Director, Stanford University School of Medicine; Associate Director, Cardiac Electrophysiology Laboratory, Stanford Hospital and Clinics, Stanford, California

Timing Cycles of Implantable Devices

Raymond E. Ideker, MD, PhD

Professor, Division of Cardiology, Department of Medicine, University of Alabama at Birmingham, Birmingham, Alabama

Principles of Defibrillation: From Cellular Physiology to Fields and Waveforms

Bharat K. Kantharia, MD, FRCP, FACC, FESC

Associate Professor, Department of Internal Medicine, Division of Cardiology, The Ohio State University; Director, Cardiac Electrophysiology Laboratories, The Ohio State University Medical Center, Columbus, Ohio

Approach to Generator Change

G. Neal Kay, MD

Professor of Medicine, Division of Cardiovascular Disease, and Director of Clinical Electrophysiology Section, University of Alabama at Birmingham, Birmingham, Alabama

Cardiac Electrical Stimulation; Sensor Driven Pacing: Device Specifics

George J. Klein, MD, FRCPC, FACC

Professor of Medicine, University of Western Ontario Faculty of Medicine and Dentistry; Chief, Division of Cardiology, London Health Sciences Centre, London, Ontario, Canada

Follow-up and Interpretation of Implantable Syncope Monitors

Andrew D. Krahn, MD, FRCPC, FACC

Professor of Medicine, University of Western Ontario Faculty of Medicine and Dentistry; Director of Education, Division of Cardiology, London Health Sciences Centre, London, Ontario, Canada

Follow-up and Interpretation of Implantable Syncope Monitors

Mark W. Kroll, PhD

Adjunct Professor of Biomedical Engineering, California Polytechnic State University, San Luis Obispo, California, and University of Minnesota, Minneapolis, Minnesota

Pacemaker and Implantable Cardioverter-Defibrillator Circuitry; Testing and Programming of Implantable Defibrillator Functions at Implantation

Steven P. Kutalek, MD

Associate Professor of Medicine and Pharmacology, Drexel University College of Medicine; Director of Clinical Cardiac Electrophysiology and Associate Chief of Division of Cardiology, Hahnemann University Hospital, Philadelphia, Pennsylvania

Approach to Generator Change

Dhanunjaya R. Lakkireddy, MD

Clinical Assistant Professor, Kansas University Medical Center; Staff Electrophysiologist, Mid America Cardiology at Kansas University Medical Center, Kansas City, Kansas

Imaging in Pacing and Defibrillation

Chu-Pak Lau, MD

William M. W. Mong Professor in Cardiology, Cardiology Division (Chief), The University of Hong Kong; Chief, Cardiology Division, Queen Mary Hospital, Hong Kong

Sensors for Implantable Devices: Ideal Characteristics, Sensor Combination, and Automaticity; Sensor Driven Pacing: Device Specifics

Sarah S. LeRoy, MSN

Pediatric Nurse Practitioner, University of Michigan Congenital Heart Center, University of Michigan Health System, Ann Arbor, Michigan

Pediatric Pacing and Defibrillator Use

Paul A. Levine, MD

Vice President, Medical Services of the Cardiac Rhythm Management Division, St. Jude Medical, Inc., St. Paul, Minnesota

Pacemaker and Implantable Cardioverter-Defibrillator Circuitry

Charles J. Love, MD

Professor of Clinical Medicine, The Ohio State University College of Medicine, Columbus, Ohio

Pacemaker Troubleshooting and Follow-up

J. March Maquilan, MD, FACS

Clinical Senior Instructor, Hahnemann University Hospital, Philadelphia; Attending Cardiothoracic Surgeon, St. Mary Medical Center, Langhorne, Pennsylvania

Approach to Generator Change

Francis E. Marchlinksi, MD

Professor of Medicine, University of Pennsylvania School of Medicine; Director of Electrophysiology, University of Pennsylvania Health System, Philadelphia, Pennsylvania

Engineering and Construction of Pacemaker and Implantable Cardioverter-Defibrillator Leads

Carlos A. Morillo, MD

Professor, Faculty of Health Sciences, McMaster University; Cardiologist and Electrophysiologist, Hamilton Health Sciences, Hamilton, Ontario, Canada

Clinical Trials of Pacing Modes

Hideo Okamura, MD

Research Associate, Division of Cardiology, Department of Internal Medicine, National Cardiovascular Center, Suita, Osaka, Japan

Timing Cycles of Implantable Devices

Walter H. Olson, MD

Senior Research Fellow, Bakken Foundation, Tachyarrhythmia Research, Medtronic, Inc., Minneapolis, Minnesota

Sensing and Detection

Victor Parsonnet, MD

Medical Director, New Jersey Pacemaker and Defibrillator Evaluation Center; Director of Surgical Research, Newark Beth Israel Medical Center, Newark, New Jersey

Pacemaker, Defibrillator, and Lead Codes

Sergio L. Pinski, MD

Clinical Associate Professor of Medicine, University of South Florida College of Medicine, Tampa; Head, Section of Cardiac Pacing and Electrophysiology, Cleveland Clinic Florida, Weston, Florida

Electromagnetic Interference and Implantable Devices

Frits Prinzen, PhD

Associate Professor of Physiology, Maastricht University, Maastricht, The Netherlands

Basic Physiology and Hemodynamics of Cardiac Pacing

Shahbudin H. Rahimtoola, MD

Distinguished Professor and GC Griffith Professor of Cardiology; Chairman, Griffith Center, University of Southern California, Los Angeles, California

Pacing for Atrioventricular Conduction System Disease

Dwight W. Reynolds, MD

Professor and Chief, Cardiovascular Section, The University of Oklahoma Health Sciences Center, Oklahoma City, Oklahoma

Permanent Pacemaker and Implantable Cardioverter-Defibrillator Implantation

Anthony Rorvick

Medtronic, Inc., Minneapolis, Minnesota

Power Systems for Implantable Pacemakers, Cardioverters, and Defibrillators

Andrea M. Russo, MD

Clinical Associate Professor of Medicine, University of Pennsylvania School of Medicine; Director, Electrophysiology Laboratory, Penn-Presbyterian Medical Center, University of Pennsylvania Health System, Philadelphia, Pennsylvania

Engineering and Construction of Pacemaker and Implantable Cardioverter-Defibrillator Leads

Elizabeth Saarel, MD

Assistant Professor of Pediatric Cardiology, University of Utah School of Medicine; Attending Physician, Pediatric Cardiology, Primary Children's Medical Center, Salt Lake City, Utah

Imaging in Pacing and Defibrillation

Leslie A. Saxon, MD

Professor of Medicine (Clinical Scholar), University of Southern California Keck School of Medicine; Director, Cardiac Electrophysiology, USC University Hospital, Los Angeles, California

Clinical Trials of Cardiac Resynchronization Therapy: Pacemakers and Defibrillators

Craig L. Schmidt, PhD

Medtronic, Inc., Minneapolis, Minnesota

Power Systems for Implantable Pacemakers, Cardioverters, and Defibrillators

Gerald A. Serwer, MD

Professor, University of Michigan Medical School; Director of Pacing Services, University of Michigan Congenital Heart Center, University of Michigan Health System, Ann Arbor, Michigan

Pediatric Pacing and Defibrillator Use

Robert S. Sheldon, MD, PhD

Professor of Cardiac Sciences and Associate Dean for Clinical Research, Libin Cardiovascular Institute of Alberta, University of Calgary, Calgary, Alberta, Canada

Evolving Indications for Pacing: Hypertrophic Cardiomyopathy, Sleep Apnea, Long QT Syndromes, and Neurally Mediated Syncope Syndromes

Richard B. Shepard, MD

Emeritus Professor, Division of Cardiothoracic Surgery, University of Alabama at Birmingham, Birmingham, Alabama

Cardiac Electrical Stimulation

Allan C. Skanes, MD, FRCPC

Assistant Professor of Medicine, University of Western Ontario Faculty of Medicine and Dentistry; Director, Electrophysiology Laboratory, Arrhythmia Service, London Health Sciences Centre, London, Ontario, Canada

Follow-up and Interpretation of Implantable Syncope Monitors

Paul M. Skarstad, PhD

Medtronic, Inc., Minneapolis, Minnesota

Power Systems for Implantable Pacemakers, Cardioverters, and Defibrillators

Julio C. Spinelli, PhD

Guidant Corporation, St. Paul, Minnesota

Basic Physiology and Hemodynamics of Cardiac Pacing

Bruce S. Stambler, MD

Professor of Medicine, Case Western Reserve University School of Medicine; Attending Physician, University Hospitals of Cleveland, Cleveland, Ohio

Pacing for Atrioventricular Conduction System Disease

Michael O. Sweeney, MD

Assistant Professor, Harvard Medical School; Attending Physician, Cardiac Arrhythmia Service, Brigham and Women's Hospital, Boston, Massachusetts

Programming and Follow-up of Cardiac Resynchronization Devices

Charles D. Swerdlow, MD

Clinical Professor, Division of Cardiology, Department of Medicine, University of California, Los Angeles, School of Medicine; Division of Cardiology, Department of Medicine, Cedars-Sinai Medical Center, Los Angeles, California

Sensing and Detection

Patrick J. Tchou, MD

Attending Physician, Department of Cardiovascular Medicine, Cardiac Electrophysiology and Pacing Section, Cleveland Clinic, Cleveland, Ohio

Testing and Programming of Implantable Defibrillator Functions at Implantation

Hung-Fat Tse, MD

Professor of Medicine, Cardiology Division, University of Hong Kong and Queen Mary Hospital, Hong Kong

Sensors for Implantable Devices: Ideal Characteristics, Sensor Combination, and Automaticity; Sensor Driven Pacing: Device Specifics

Darrel F. Untereker, PhD

Senior Director of Research and Technology, Medtronic, Inc., Minneapolis, Minnesota

Power Systems for Implantable Pacemakers, Cardioverters, and Defibrillators

Gregory P. Walcott, MD

Assistant Professor, Division of Cardiology, Department of Medicine, University of Alabama at Birmingham, Birmingham, Alabama

Principles of Defibrillation: From Cellular Physiology to Fields and Waveforms

Paul J. Wang, MD

Professor of Medicine, Stanford University School of Medicine; Director, Cardiac Arrhythmia Service and Cardiac Electrophysiology Laboratory, Stanford Hospital and Clinics, Stanford, California

Timing Cycles of Implantable Devices

Seth Worley, MD, FACC, FHRS

Medical Director, Lancaster Heart and Stroke Foundation, Lancaster General Hospital, Lancaster, Pennsylvania

Left Ventricular Lead Implantation

Raymond Yee, MD

Professor of Medicine, University of Western Ontario Faculty of Medicine and Dentistry; Director, Arrhythmia Service, London Health Sciences Centre, London, Ontario, Canada

Follow-up and Interpretation of Implantable Syncope Monitors

Preface

Cardiac pacing and implantable defibrillators have had a great impact on the treatment of patients with cardiac arrhythmias. The first pacing system was implanted in 1958, but the transformation of the technology, indications, and supporting clinical data in the almost five subsequent decades has been impressive. Particularly remarkable have been the recent technological developments and the growth in pacemaker and defibrillator implantation volume in the United States and around the world. It is hard to believe that six years have gone by since the second edition. With our third edition, the field of cardiac resynchronization therapy has added new complexity and understanding to the science and practice of device therapy. A great deal of effort has been expended to include new information on implantation, troubleshooting, physiology, clinical trials, and engineering of this new therapy.

There are many consumers of pacemakers and defibrillator technology besides the patient. There are numerous physicians, including cardiologists, surgeons, internists, and emergency and family physicians, who care for these patients and need to evaluate the impact of this therapy on various medical conditions and treatments. In addition, nurses, engineers from pacemaker companies, and technical and sales representatives from these companies also interact with physicians and patients.

Our philosophy in putting together the third edition remains the same as that of our first and second efforts. We have planned this book to emphasize the science of cardiac pacing and defibrillation and to underline the importance of the fact that it is an interdisciplinary field. Physicians are part of a web of health professionals who need increasing amounts of information about implantable devices. We have included a DVD with this edition that includes figures and movies not included in the paper version of our text, as well as much additional material. All of the figures from the text are included with this DVD.

The evolution of cardiac pacing has inspired the publication of subspecialty journals, including *Heart Rhythm, PACE, StimuCoeur, Journal of Cardiovascular Electrophysiology, Journal of Interventional Cardiac Electrophysiology, Cardiac Electrophysiology Review,* and *Europace,* as well as monographs and a number of new books on implantable devices. Several national and international conferences on pacing and defibrillation take place every year.

We have sought to meet the needs of many with this textbook. Clinicians, scientists, nurses, technicians, and engineers will find the information in these pages practical, authoritative, and helpful in better understanding this therapy. We are excited about the opportunity to present this material in a comprehensive scientific manner.

We gratefully acknowledge the invaluable assistance and encouragement of Susan Pioli and Natasha Andjelkovic of the Health Sciences Division of Elsevier for all their help in keeping the third edition on track. We owe a great debt of gratitude to our colleagues from the Medical College of Virginia and the McGuire Veterans Affairs Medical Center, the University of Alabama, The University of Hong Kong and Queen Mary Hospital, and the Cleveland Clinic for their patience and support in shouldering the extra workload that allowed us to finish our chapters and editing on time.

Most important, we cannot thank enough our many contributors and their colleagues, who labored extensively, often taking time from family and other projects to finish their chapters. This large group of individuals deserves all the credit and thanks for making the third edition possible.

Our wonderful secretaries, Vera Wilkerson (Virginia Commonwealth University/ Medical College of Virginia), Julie Griffis (Cleveland Clinic), Eleanor Lee (The University of Hong Kong), and Dorothy Welch (University of Alabama) were invaluable for their contributions to help complete this project.

This textbook is designed to be a functional tool and reference, helping clinicians, scientists, and engineers make the decisions that improve patients' lives. It is our desire that this book serve as a valuable resource to all of these people for many years to come.

Kenneth A. Ellenbogen, MD
G. Neal Kay, MD
Chu-Pak Lau, MD
Bruce L. Wilkoff, MD

Contents

DVD Contents

BRUCE L. WILKOFF, MD

Section One

Basic Principles of Device Therapy

Chapter 1

Cardiac Electrical Stimulation

G. NEAL KAY • RICHARD B. SHEPARD

Electrical stimulation is the fundamental principle supporting artificial cardiac pacing. An electrical stimulus interacts with myocardium through one or more electrodes. It produces a flow of electric current within the myocardium and blood pool. If the stimulus has the necessary characteristics, local action potentials occur. For the stimulus application to result in pumping of blood, the stimulus must start a local membrane depolarization process that becomes a self-propagating wavefront of myocyte contraction.

Clinical application of cardiac pacing involves the placing of electrical stimulus sites and the timing of stimulus firings so that an efficient mechanical contraction sequence occurs. Each of these aspects of pacing must be managed to obtain hemodynamic and energy efficiency.

This chapter is designed to introduce readers to fundamental concepts relevant to artificial electrical cardiac stimulation.

Concepts Related to Electrical Stimulation of the Heart

Myocardial stimulation by means of pacemaker or defibrillator electrodes is a complex electrical, biophysical, and biochemical process. Brief definitions of some of the terms used are given below.

Stimulation

For the purposes of this chapter, the term *stimulation* is defined as the initiation of a self-propagating wave of myocardial depolarization and contraction. An electrical stimulus that stimulates myocardium is often said to "capture" the chamber to which it is applied.

Anisotropy

Anisotropy is the existence of unequal physical properties along different axes. In the heart, myocardial conduction velocity is greater in the direction parallel to the long axis of myocardial fibers than along the transverse axis.

Electric Circuit

An *electric circuit* is an electrical charge–conducting pathway that ends at its beginning. Electric circuits involved in myocardial stimulation by pacemakers or implantable cardioverter-defibrillators (ICDs) include the pulse generator and its leads, electrodes, extracellular electrolytes, cell membranes with highly regulated transmission of charged ions in both directions through the membrane, and intracellular ions and charged molecules.*

*Björn Nordenstrom, who was Professor of Diagnostic Radiology at Karolinska Institute, found much evidence for many usually unrecognized electric circuits in the body. See Nordenstrom BEJ: Biologically Closed Electric Circuits: Clinical, Experimental and Theoretical Evidence for an Additional Circulatory System. Stockholm, Nordic Medical Publications, 1983.

Series Circuit

In a series circuit, or circuit module, the elements are connected one after another. Therefore, current must flow sequentially through each element in the circuit, one after another. The current flow through all elements is the same.

Parallel Circuit

In a parallel circuit, two or more elements are joined at each end to a common conductor. Therefore, current may flow from one of the common conductors to the other through any or all of the elements. The degree of current flow in each element is roughly inverse to the factors opposing the flow of electrical charge in that element.

Most biologic circuits are made of various combinations of series and parallel modules or subcircuits. For example, because of electrochemical effects, an electrode placed in the heart may act like a capacitor in parallel with a resistor, both in series with the lead joining the pulse generator to the electrode.

Electric Current

An applied electric field gradient induces a net directional movement of electrical charge. In ordinary terminology, current is said to flow from positive to negative, as from the positive terminal of a battery through an external circuit to the negative terminal. However, electrons in the circuit external to the battery actually move from the negative terminal of the battery to the positive terminal. For clarity in this chapter, current is often stated in terms of electron or ion motion.

Electrode Polarity

All defibrillator and pacemaker electric circuits have, during a stimulation pulse, both a positively charged electrode and a negatively charged electrode in contact with tissue. The negatively charged electrode (the catheter tip electrode in a bipolar pacing catheter) is a cathode. It receives electrons from the pulse generator and furnishes electrons to the electrode-tissue interface.

Electrodes in a battery were named *anode* (electron sink) and *cathode* (electron source) by Michael Faraday after he received suggestions from a philologist friend.[1] In a battery by Faraday's definition, the electrode at which oxidation occurs (e.g., oxidation of Li to yield Li^+ and an electron) is an anode. The anode, by continuing oxidation, furnishes electrons to the circuit external to it. Therefore, the negative terminal of the battery is the anode. From there, electrons go through the circuitry and eventually enter the pacemaker electrode that touches myocardium. This electrode, receiving electrons from the pulse generator and furnishing electrons to the tissue, is a cathode. The return electrode in the heart is an anode. It collects electrons from the tissue and returns them through the pulse generator circuitry to the positive electrode of the battery. There, reduction occurs (e.g., $I_2 + 2e^-$ yields $2I^-$); this electrode is a cathode. The consistency in the terminology is that, when oxidation occurs, it occurs at an anode, and in the circuitry an anode connects to a cathode that subsequently connects to another anode, and so on.

Unipolar pacing is not to be confused with uniphasic pacing. In unipolar pacing, a single electrode (a cathode) is in contact with the heart. The anode is the pulse generator metal case or some other electrode away from the heart.

Bipolar pacing is pacing with the cathode in contact with the myocardium and with the anode also in contact with the heart or blood within the heart.

Uniphasic (monophasic) pacing is pacing with an electrical waveshape that, as measured at the pulse generator *during* the pulse, is entirely either positive or negative relative to zero current and voltage.

Biphasic pacing has a waveshape that is initially either positive or negative and then reverses polarity during the final portion of the pulse.

Capacitor

A capacitor is an object that stores energy in an electric field by holding positive charges apart from closely approximated negative charges (unlike a battery, which stores energy in chemical form). The normally nonconducting material or space between the layers of negative and positive charges is the *dielectric*. A cell membrane acts as a leaky capacitor. Cell membranes have very high capacitance per unit area of cell membrane.

Electrode-electrolyte interfaces act in part as capacitors. *Helmholtz capacitor* and *Helmholtz capacitance* are the terms used in this chapter for capacitor-like effects that occur at pacemaker and defibrillator electrode-electrolyte interfaces.

Capacitance

Capacitance (C) is the term that specifies, *for a given voltage* applied across a capacitor, how much electrical charge (Q) can be stored by the capacitor. If V represents a steady voltage applied across the capacitor, then $Q = CV$. (If E is used instead of V as the symbol for electrical potential, then the relationship may be expressed as $Q = CE$.) The unit for capacitance is the farad. A farad is the capacitance of a capacitor that on being charged to 1 volt will have stored 1 coulomb of charge. A coulomb is the amount of charge delivered by 1 ampere flowing for 1 second. Coulombs delivered can be expressed as

$$Q_t = \int_0^t i_t dt$$

in which Q_t is the total charge delivered between time 0 and time t, i_t is the instantaneous current at each tiny time segment between time 0 and time t, and the integral $\int_0^t i_t dt$ is the net area under the instantaneous current versus time plot.

Inductor

When electric current flows through a wire, a magnetic field surrounding the wire is induced. An *inductor* is an object that stores or releases energy in or from a changing magnetic field. The voltage difference across an inductor is proportional to the rate of change of current flowing through the inductor. Energy is stored during the formation of the magnetic field and is released when the magnetic field decreases or disappears. No energy is lost in a perfect inductor.

Inductance

Inductance is the term that specifies the relationship between the voltage across an inductor and the rate of change of current traversing the inductor. The magnitude of the inductance can be represented by the symbol L. If V_t represents the instantaneous voltage across the inductor and i_L represents the instantaneous current flowing through the inductor, the relationship is given by the equation

$$v_t = L\frac{di_L}{dt} \quad \text{or} \quad i_L = \frac{1}{L}\int_0^t v_t dt$$

Note that the voltage across the inductor is directly proportional to the rate of change of current flowing through the inductor.

Cell membrane currents have some of the current- and voltage-versus-time characteristics of an inductance in parallel with a capacitance.[2] This inductance-like effect is related to timing and magnitude of potassium movement into and out of the cell.[3]

Reactance

When a changing electric potential is applied across a physical or biologic circuit, some of the opposition to current flow can occur because energy is being stored in an electric field or in a changing magnetic field. This opposition that represents energy storage is termed *reactance* (symbol X). Reactance and resistance are determining factors in impedance (see later discussion). For reactive elements connected in series, net reactance is the scalar sum of inductive reactance (positive in the mathematical complex plane) and capacitive reactance (negative in the mathematical complex plane). Pure reactance values are dependent on the rates of change of current and voltage, whereas pure resistance values are not.

Ohm's law–type calculations involving the relationships between current, voltage, and power dissipation in various portions of circuits that contain reactive components are more complicated than calculations for circuits involving resistance alone. For example, the peak voltages across individual reactive components in a series circuit may, if added in the ordinary arithmetical way, give a sum that is greater than the peak voltage driving the circuit. Phenomena of this type are caused by differences in the timing of the peaks (phase angles) of the voltages or currents in the various reactive components. These reactive effects can be important in biventricular pacing threshold measurements (see the discussion of biventricular pacing later in this chapter).

Both pacing electrodes and cell membranes have reactance qualities, predominately capacitive. Although all physical and biologic electric circuits in principle exhibit all three qualities (resistance, capacitance, and inductance), one or more of the qualities is often so small as to be insignificant. For example, the cardiac action potential spreading throughout the heart generates a changing magnetic field, and a very small amount of energy is transiently stored in the magnetic field. However, the changing magnetic field generated by spread of the action potential is so small that it is not clinically significant except in the research setting.[4]

Resistance and Impedance

Electrical resistance is the type of opposition to current flow in which energy is lost as heat. The instantaneous voltage developed across a perfect resistor is linearly proportional to the instantaneous current flow through the resistor. If a steady voltage across the resistor is represented by *V*, the current by *I*, and an unchanging resistance by *R*, then the relationship is $V = IR$ (Ohm's law). In reality, cardiac pacing is much more complex and involves many factors, including capacitance, resistance, and stop and start currents. For calculations involving pulsed (e.g., pacemaker stimulus) or alternating current (AC) circuits that contain reactive elements (e.g., electrodes in electrolytes), *impedance* (Z), a vector sum of resistance R and reactance X, must for accuracy be used in place of resistance.

Impedance

Impedance is a concept used to calculate the combined effects of resistance, capacitance, and inductance in opposition to current flow. Impedance comes into play when an applied current and/or voltage starts, stops, or changes over the duration of the stimulus. Both pacemaker pulses and defibrillator shocks start from zero current and voltage and go back to zero current and voltage, typically within a few milliseconds or less. At a pacemaker electrode in the heart, capacitance and resistance are major factors in impedance. Within the heart, inductance effects on pacemaker stimuli are too small to be important to clinicians.

For circuits with resistance R, capacitance C, and inductance L in *series*, where q_t represents the charge accumulated across the capacitance at any time t, and where the current through the group at time t is i_t, the voltage V_t across the whole group at time t is described by the equation

$$v_t = i_t R + \frac{q_t}{C} + L\frac{di}{dt} \quad \text{or} \quad v_t = i_t R + \frac{\int_0^t idt}{C} + L\frac{di}{dt}$$

$\left(\text{remembering that } q_t = \int_0^t i_t dt \text{ and that the voltage across a capacitor at time t is } \frac{q_t}{C}\right).$

These equations indicate that, for an instantaneous current i_t, the instantaneous voltage across the series circuit is the sum of the *effects at that instant in time* of the resistance, capacitance, and inductance of the circuit. Note especially that *the instantaneous effects are highly related to what has already happened*, for example to the net amount of charge, $\left(q_t = \int_0^t i_t dt\right)$, that has accumulated in the capacitor from time 0 to the instantaneous time t. The equations show that the capacitance effect on a series circuit voltage magnitude decreases as the capacitance increases. This has clinical relevance in that, for example, the polarization voltage that interferes with autosensing pulse generators decreases as the electrode capacitance increases.

That portion of a pulse generator circuit from the output connector through the lead and electrode into the tissue and then back to the pulse generator represents a set of series and series-parallel connections. For accuracy, this circuit must be viewed as an impedance, not just a resistance. The Helmholtz double-layer capacitance at the electrode-electrolyte junction, together with an ion diffusional effect (the Warburg impedance, described later), makes this necessary.

When right ventricular (RV) and left ventricular (LV) pacing leads are connected to a pulse generator through a single ventricular output connector, the RV electrode and the LV electrode combinations are impedances in *parallel*. One possible effect of biventricular lead connections in parallel is a deceptive (if obtained in the ordinary way) set of threshold measurements.[5] This is discussed further in the section on biventricular pacing.

Electrolyte

In this chapter, *electrolyte* is used as a generic term for the extracellular and intracellular electrically conductive fluids near pacemaker or defibrillator electrodes and elsewhere in the heart. The electrolyte conducts ions but not electrons.

Cellular Aspects of Myocardial Stimulation

The Phospholipid Bimembrane

Living cells maintain or regenerate a difference in electric potential across the cell membrane. Excitable tissues such as myocardium respond to electrical stimulation of one or more cells with a wave of electrical depolarization, a transient reversal of the voltage gradient across the membrane, that can propagate from cell to cell. Excitable cells respond to a relatively small applied change in electric potential difference across the cell membrane by triggering a series of biochemical/biophysical events (described later). These depolarization events result in myocyte contraction. Depolarization propagates along excitable cell membranes, as in the transmission of an action potential along a squid axon, and from myocyte to myocyte through gap junctions.

Cell Membrane Characteristics

Cell membrane characteristics are major determinants of tissue excitability. The membrane of the cardiac myocyte is composed principally of phospholipids, cholesterol, and proteins.[6] The membrane phospholipids have a charged polar headgroup and two long hydrocarbon chains arranged as shown in Figure 1-1. The cell membrane comprises two layers of phospholipids with their hydrophobic aliphatic chains oriented toward the central portion of the bilayer membrane and their polar headgroup regions toward the outside boundaries of the membrane. Because the membrane is composed of two layers of phospholipids, the polar regions of the phospholipid molecules interface with the aqueous environments inside and outside the cell. The lipid-soluble hydrocarbon chains are forced away from the aqueous phase to form a nonpolar interior.

Determinants of the Resting Transmembrane Potential

Relatively large gradients of individual ion concentrations exist across the cardiac cell membrane.[7] The gradient of sodium (Na^+) ions across the membrane is approximately 145 mmol/L (outside) to 10 mmol/L (inside). In contrast, the potassium (K^+) ion concentration outside the cell is approximately 4.5 mmol/L, whereas the inside concentration is 140 mmol/L. In the absence of a cell membrane, both Na^+ and K^+ would rapidly move in a direction determined by the concentration gradient. The diffusion force tending to move K^+ out of and Na^+ into the cell is proportional to the concentration gradients of those ions. The potential energy attributable to the diffusion force (PE_d) tending to move K^+ out of the cell is given by the following equation:

$$PE_d = RT\left(\ln\left(\frac{[K^+]_i}{[K^+]_o}\right)\right) \tag{1-1}$$

where R is the gas constant, T is the absolute temperature, ln is the natural logarithm operator, $[K^+]_i$ is the concentration of potassium ion inside the cell, and $[K^+]_o$ is the concentration of potassium ion outside the cell. If the ratio of $[K^+]_i$ to $[K^+]_o$ is large, the potential energy across the membrane is large. For each ion species, the difference in concentration between the inside and the outside of the cell results in that ion's contribution to the difference in electric potential across the cell membrane.

In resting cardiac cells, the intracellular cytoplasm has a measured potential of about −90 mV, relative to the extracellular fluid. This electric force tends to move positively charged ions such as K^+ and Na^+ to the inside of the cell and negatively charged ions such as chloride (Cl^-) to the outside of the cell in proportion to the potential gradient. The potential energy attributable to the electric force (PE_e) tending to move K^+ into the cell is expressed as follows:

$$PE_e = zFV_m \tag{1-2}$$

where z here is the valence (the number of positive or negative electrical charges) of the ion, F is the Faraday constant (96,500 coulombs/equivalent), and V_m is the

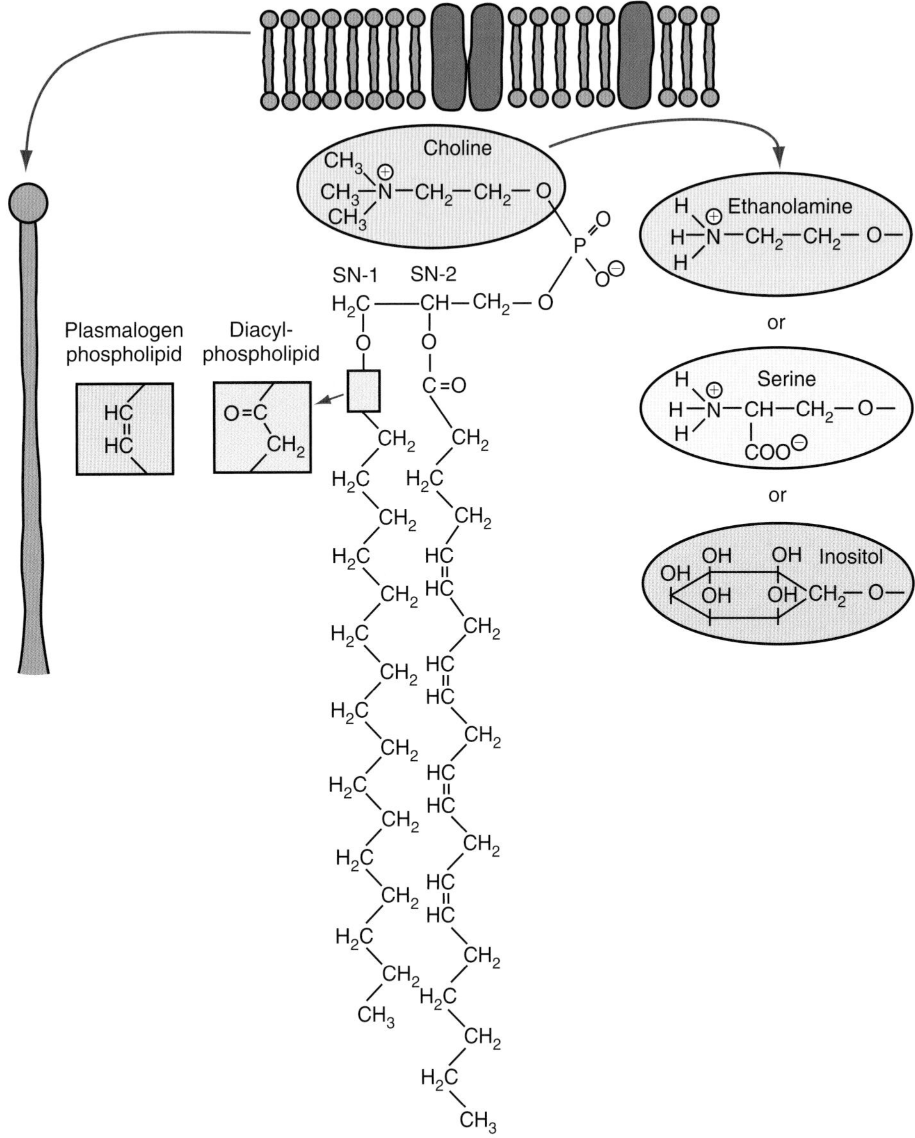

Figure 1-1. Sarcolemmal structure and phospholipid composition. The lipid bilayer containing two membrane proteins is shown at the top of the figure. The detailed structure of the phospholipids is shown below. All of the aliphatic hydrocarbon groups on the sn-2 position are fatty acids that are covalently bound in the form of esters. The aliphatic hydrocarbon groups at the sn-1 position include O-acyl esters and vinyl ethers. (From Creer MH, Dabmeyer DJ, Corr PB: Amphipathic lipid metabolites and arrhythmias during myocardial ischemia. In Zipes DP, Jalife J [eds]: Cardiac Electrophysiology: From Cell to Bedside. Philadelphia, WB Saunders, 1990, pp 417-432.)

transmembrane potential difference (measured in millivolts). During equilibrium, the total of the potential energies due to diffusion and electric forces is zero, and no net ionic movement occurs. Therefore, the sum of Equation 1-1 and Equation 1-2 may be set to zero. This yields the Nernst equation, which describes in measurable electrical units the potential that must exist for a single ionic species, here K^+, to be in equilibrium across the membrane of a resting cardiac cell:

$$V_m(K^+) = -26.7\ln\left(\frac{[K^+]_i}{[K^+]_o}\right) \tag{1-3}$$

or, in log base 10 terms, $V_m(K^+) = -61.5\log\left(\frac{[K^+]_i}{[K^+]_o}\right)$.

Using known values for extracellular K^+, $V_m(K^+)$ = 90 mV. When Equation 1-3 is solved using Na^+ concentrations, a $V_m(Na^+)$ of +50 mV is obtained. Therefore, it is the equilibrium potential for potassium ion (not sodium ion) that is the major factor responsible for the resting transmembrane potential. This suggests that the resting membrane is more permeable to K^+ than to Na^+.

To calculate the transmembrane potential when multiple ionic species exist in different concentrations across the membrane, the Goldman constant field equation (modified by Hodgkin and Katz[8]) is used:

$$V_m = \left(\frac{-RT}{F}\right)\ln\left(\frac{P_k^+[K^+]_i + P_{Na}^+[Na^+]_i + P_{Cl}^-[Cl^-]_o + \ldots}{P_k^+[K^+]_o + P_{Na}^+[Na^+]_o + P_{Cl}^-[Cl^-]_i + \ldots}\right) \tag{1-4}$$

where P_{K^+}, P_{Na^+}, and P_{Cl^-} are the cell membrane permeabilities for the respective ions. At physiologic concentrations, this equation yields a transmembrane potential of –90 mV (the equilibrium potential for K^+). Equation 1-4 describes how resting potentials vary as sodium and potassium ion concentrations are changed. Because there is a passive leak of charged ions through the membrane, the resting potential would not exist at the 90 mV level unless it were actively maintained. This is accomplished by two active transport mechanisms that exchange Na^+ ions for K^+ and Ca^{2+} ions.

One might ask whether, with all the potassium ions and other positively charged ions in the cell, and with a relatively small amount of negatively charged chloride ions in the cell, how can the interior of the cell be negative with respect to the outside? The answer is that an array of intracellular organic and inorganic anions inside the cell, molecules that do not cross the membrane, carry net negative charges sufficient to make the overall balance of charge negative.

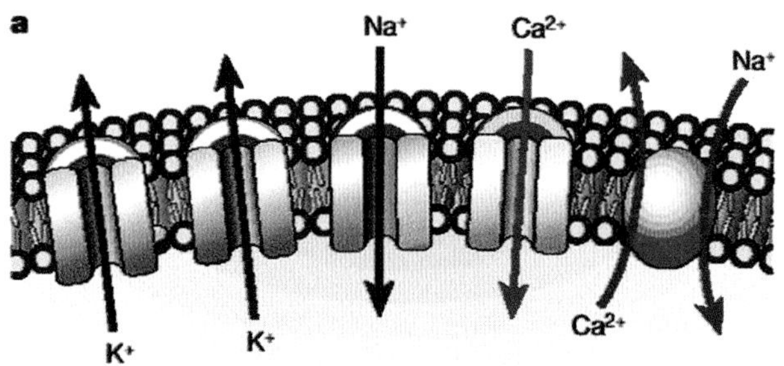

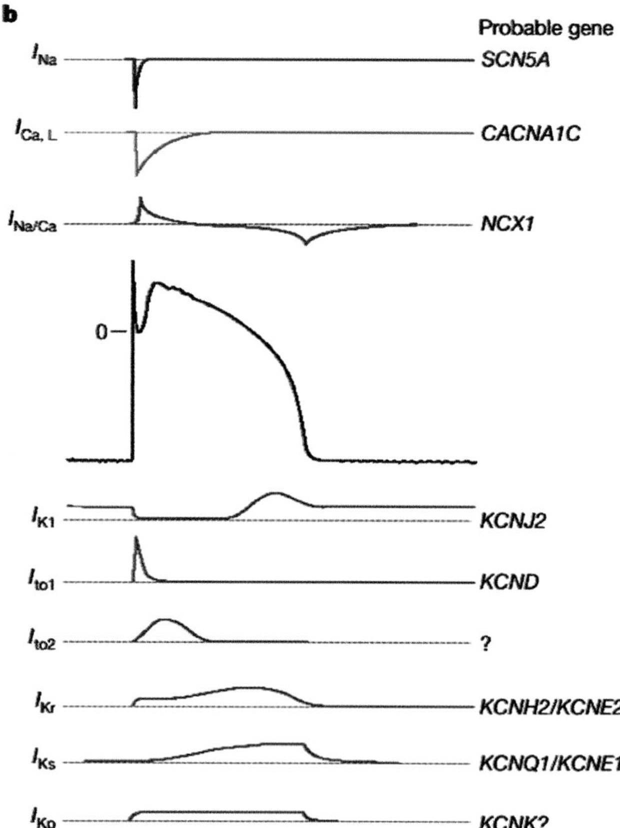

Figure 1-2. Ion channels underlie cardiac excitability. ***a,*** *The key ion channels (and an electrogenic transporter) in cardiac cells. K^+ channels* (green) *mediate K^+ efflux from the cell; Na^+ channels* (purple) *and Ca^{2+} channels* (yellow) *mediate Na^+ and Ca^{2+} influx, respectively. The Na^+/Ca^{2+} exchanger* (red) *is electrogenic, because it transports three Na^+ ions for each Ca^{2+} ion across the surface membrane.* ***b,*** *Ionic currents and genes underlying the cardiac action potential.* Top, *depolarizing currents as functions of time, and their corresponding genes.* Center, *a ventricular action potential.* Bottom, *repolarizing currents and their corresponding genes. (From Marban E: Cardiac channelopathies. Nature 415:213-218, 2002, with permission. ©Nature Publishing Group, http://www.nature.com)*

Ion Channels

Protein molecules embedded within the cell membrane have numerous functions, including those of being ion channels (Fig. 1-2) and signal transducers. The concept of ion channels was proposed in the 1950s by Hodgkin and Huxley.[9] However, it was not until the introduction of the patch clamp technique by Neher and Sakmann in 1976 that the properties of these channels could be directly studied.[10,11] There are two basic types of ion channels, distinguished by the factors that control opening and closing of the channel. Ion channels at muscle fiber end plates are *chemically* gated by specific transmitters. The opening of these channels is triggered by the binding of acetylcholine, and their closing is induced by its unbinding. In neuronal axons, conduction is mediated by faster, *voltage*-gated channels. These channels respond to differences in electric potential between the inside and outside of the cell, across the membrane. Voltage-gated channels for sodium, potassium, and calcium appear to operate in similar ways, sharing many of the same structural features. In addition, each type of channel can be subdivided into several subtypes with different conductance or gating properties.

Voltage-gated Channels

Voltage-gated channels open in response to an applied electric potential. The source of this voltage can be an action potential propagated from an adjacent cell or the electric field of an artificial pacemaker electrode. If depolarization of the membrane exceeds a threshold voltage, an action potential is triggered, resulting in a complex cascade of ionic currents flowing across the membrane into and out of the cell. As a result of this flow of charge across the membrane, the potential gradient across the membrane (Fig. 1-3) changes in a characteristic pattern of events that produce the cardiac action potential.

Selective membrane-bound proteins (ion channels) determine the passive transmembrane flux of an individual ion species. The transmembrane currents determine or influence cellular polarization at rest, action potential depolarization and repolarization, conduction, excitation-contraction coupling, and myofibril contraction. The channels that regulate transmembrane conductance of Na^+ and Ca^{2+} are voltage gated. The sodium channel is a large protein molecule composed of approximately 1830 amino acids.[12] It contains four internally homologous repeating domains. These are believed to be arranged around a central water-filled pore that is lined with hydrophilic amino acids. It is estimated that there are 5 to 10 Na^+ channels per square micrometer of cell membrane. When an alteration changes the membrane potential to about −70 to −60 mV (the threshold potential), four to six positively charged amino acids move across the membrane in response to the change in electric field. This causes a change in the conformations of the channel proteins, resulting in opening of the channel. After a single

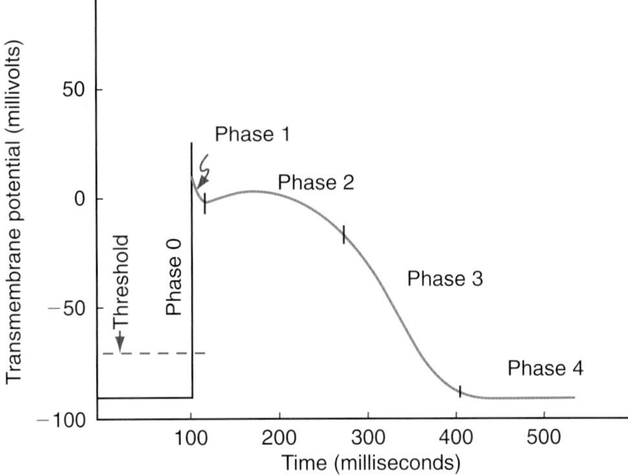

Figure 1-3. A typical action potential, showing the various phases of depolarization and repolarization. In phase 0 (depolarization), sodium ions (Na^+) rapidly enters the cell through fast channels. In phase 1, the initial repolarization is primarily the result of activation of a transient outward potassium ion (K^+) current and inactivation of the fast Na^+ current. In phase 2 (plateau), the net current is very small, although the individual Na^+, Ca^{2+}, and K^+ currents are about an order of magnitude larger. Phase 3 (final repolarization) completes the cycle, with the Na^+-K^+ pump bringing the membrane potential to a stable point at which inward and outward currents are again in balance. During phase 4 the cell is polarized and gradually undergoes slow depolarization. (From Stokes K, Bornzin G: The electrode-biointerface [stimulation]. In Barold SS [ed]: Modern Cardiac Pacing. Mt. Kisco, NY, Futura, 1985, pp 33-78.)

Na^+ channel changes to the open conformation, about 10^4 Na^+ ions enter the cell. On depolarization of the membrane, the Na^+ channels remain open for less than 1 msec. After rapid depolarization of the membrane, the Na^+ channel again changes to the closed conformation. In addition to the Na^+ channel, specialized proteins are suspended in the cell membrane that have differential selectivity for K^+, Ca^{2+}, and Cl^- ions, with markedly different time constants for activation and inactivation.

Atrioventricular Node Cells

In contrast to Purkinje fibers, sinus and atrioventricular (AV) nodal cells are characterized by action potentials with slower rates of depolarization. In these structures, depolarization is primarily mediated by inward Ca^{2+} conductance through specialized Ca^{2+} channels. There are two types of Ca^{2+} channel in the mammalian heart: the L type and the T type. The L-type channels are the major voltage-gated pathway for entry of Ca^{2+} into the myocyte, and they are heavily modulated by catecholamines.[13] The T-type channels contribute to spontaneous depolarization of the cell associated with automaticity (pacemaker currents). The pore of the Ca^{2+} channel has a functional diameter of about 0.6 nm, larger than that of the Na^+ channels (0.3 to 0.5 nm).[14] The selectivity for Ca^{2+} is high, up to 10,000-fold greater than that for Na^+ or K^+. The key elements are high-affinity binding sites for Ca^{2+}, positioned along a single file pore. "Elution" of a Ca^{2+} ion occurs when another Ca^{2+} ion enters and is selectively bound.

Maintenance of Resting Membrane Potential

The resting membrane potential is maintained by the pumping of Na^+ ions out of the cell and K^+ ions into the cell. The Na^+,K^+-ATPase pump moves three Na^+ ions out of the cell in exchange for two K^+ ions moved into the cell.[15-17] The basic unit of the Na^+,K^+-ATPase protein (pump) consists of one α- and one β-subunit. The β-subunit is large (1016 amino acids) and spans the entire membrane, whereas the β-subunit is a smaller glycoprotein. There appear to be about 1000 pump sites per square micrometer of cardiac cell membrane. The fully activated pump cycles about 50 to 70 times per second (an interval of 15 to 20 msec/cycle). Similarly, the Na^+-Ca^{2+} pump moves three Na^+ ions out of the cell in exchange for one Ca^{2+} ion.[18,19] Therefore, both transport mechanisms result in the *net* movement of one positive charge out of the cell, polarizing the membrane and maintaining a negatively charged interior. The function of both exchange mechanisms is dependent on the expenditure of energy in the form of high-energy phosphates and is susceptible to interruptions in aerobic cellular metabolism (e.g., during ischemia).

The Cardiac Action Potential

When the voltage gradient across the membrane of a myocyte decreases so that the inside of the cell becomes less negatively charged with respect to the outside of the cell, a critical transmembrane voltage difference is reached (the *threshold voltage*). At threshold, the cell membrane suddenly undergoes a further depolarization that is out of proportion to the intensity of the applied stimulus. This abrupt change in the potential across the membrane is the start of a cascade of inward and outward currents that together are known as an *action potential*.[20]

The cardiac action potential is an enormously complex event and consists of five phases:[21] phase 0, the upstroke phase of rapid depolarization; phase 1, the overshoot phase of initial rapid repolarization; phase 2, the plateau phase; phase 3, the rapid repolarization phase (see Fig. 1-3); and phase 4, which in cells with spontaneous pacemaker activity is characterized by a slow, spontaneous depolarization of the membrane until the threshold potential is again reached and a new action potential is generated.

Phase 0: Rapid Depolarization

The upstroke of the action potential is triggered by a decrease in the potential gradient across the membrane to the threshold potential of −70 to −60 mV. On depolarization of the membrane to the less negative threshold voltage, the Na^+ channels open, resulting in an influx of positively charged ions (the inward Na^+ current) and rapid reversal of membrane polarity. The rate of depolarization in phase 0 ranges from 800 V/sec in Purkinje cells to 200 to 500 V/sec in atrial and ventricular myocytes. In these cells, the inward Na^+ current is primarily responsible for phase 0 of the action potential. In sinoatrial and AV nodal cells, where the inward Ca^{2+} current predominates, the upstroke velocity of phase 0 is much lower (20 to 50 V/sec).

Phase 1: Initial Repolarization

After voltage-dependent activation of the Na^+ current in phase 0, the membrane potential rapidly changes from negative to positive. The increased conductance of Na^+ is rapidly followed by voltage-dependent inactivation. Phase 1 is characterized by the transient outward K^+ current (I_{Kto}). The outward movement of K^+ is a major contributor to the various repolarization phases. It is complex and has a number of discrete pathways.[22,23] Most K^+ currents demonstrate *rectification,* that is, decreased K^+ conductance with depolarization. The K^+ currents include the instantaneous inward rectifier K^+ current, the outward (delayed) rectifier K^+ current, the transient outward currents, and ATP-, Na^+-, and acetylcholine-regulated K^+ currents. The initial repolarization, however, is mainly the result of activation of a transient outward K^+ current and inactivation of the fast inward Na^+ current. The transient outward K^+ current has two components, one voltage gated and the other activated by a local rise in Ca^{2+}.[24]

Phase 2: Plateau

The net current during the plateau phase is apparently small, although the individual currents (inward Na^+ and Ca^{2+} and outward K^+) are each about an order of magnitude larger.[25] Among the inward currents are the slowly activating Na^+ current, a Ca^{2+} current, and an Na^+-Ca^{2+} exchange current. Outward currents include a slowly activating K^+ current (I_{Ks}), a Cl^- current, a more rapidly activating K^+ current (I_{Kr}), an ultra-rapidly activating K^+ current (I_{Kur}), and the Na^+-K^+ electrogenic pump. During phase 2 of the action potential (the *absolute refractory period*), the cardiac cell cannot be excited by an electrical stimulus, regardless of its intensity.

Phase 3: Final Repolarization

Deactivation of inward Na^+ and Ca^{2+} currents occurs earlier than for the K^+ currents, favoring net repolarization of the membrane. When the membrane is sufficiently repolarized, an inward K^+ rectifier current is progressively activated, resulting in a regenerative increase in outward currents and an increasing rate of repolarization. Repolarization is also accomplished by the function of the Na^+,K^+-ATPase pump. The membrane potential eventually becomes stable, so that inward and outward currents are again in balance and the resting potential reestablished. Between the end of the plateau phase and full repolarization, the cell is partially refractory to electrical stimulation. During this period (the *relative refractory period*), a greater stimulus intensity is required to generate an action potential than is required after full recovery of the resting membrane potential. For clinical measurement of myocardial refractoriness (the *effective refractory period*), stimulation of the heart is usually performed at twice the threshold current as determined during late diastole.

Phase 4: Automaticity and the Conduction System

Automaticity is the property of certain cells by which they are able to initiate an action potential spontaneously. It has been known for centuries that the heart can exhibit spontaneous contraction even when completely denervated. Leonardo da Vinci observed that the heart could "move by itself."[26] William Harvey reported that pieces of the heart could "contract and relax" separately.[27] Many cells within the specialized conduction system have the potential for automaticity.

Not all parts of the heart, however, possess this property. In fact, cells in different areas of the heart have different transmembrane potentials, thresholds, and action potentials. Fast responses are characteristic of ordinary working ventricular muscle cells and His-Purkinje fibers (resting membrane potentials of −70 to −90 mV, rapid conduction velocities). Normal sinus and AV nodal cells have slow responses, with resting potentials of −40 to −70 mV and slow conduction velocities. Those cells, or group of cells, with the fastest rate of spontaneous membrane depolarization during phase 4 are the first to reach threshold potential and initiate a propagated impulse. Therefore, cells with the steepest slope in phase 4 become the heart's natural pacemaker. Ordinary working myocardial cells usually are not automatic.

Normally, depolarization is initiated at the sinoatrial node (Fig. 1-4).[28,29] Action potentials from an isolated sinoatrial node cell are shown in Figure 1-5.[30] Rather than maintaining a stable resting membrane potential,

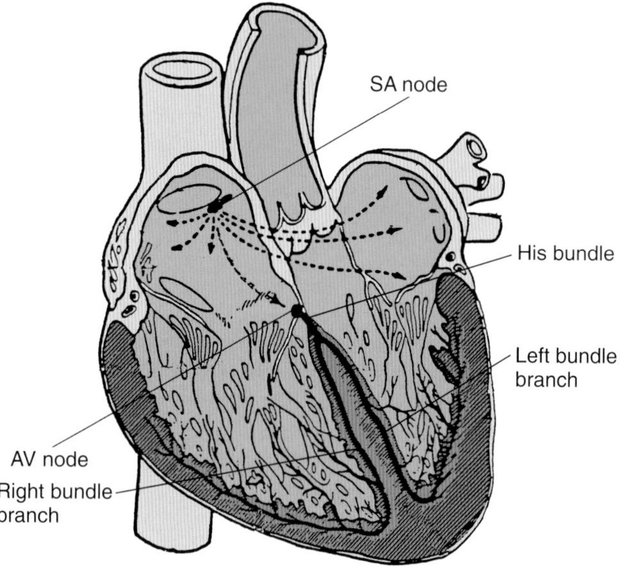

Figure 1-4. Schematic representation of the normal conduction system of the heart. The cycle begins at the sinoatrial (SA) node, propagating a wave of depolarization across the atrium. As the stimulus enters the atrioventricular (AV) node, its conduction slows. This allows complete contraction of the atria before the impulse reaches the ventricles. As the impulse enters the His bundle, conduction velocity increases. The impulse is then transmitted through the left and right bundle branches and the Purkinje fibers throughout the right and left ventricular endocardial shells.

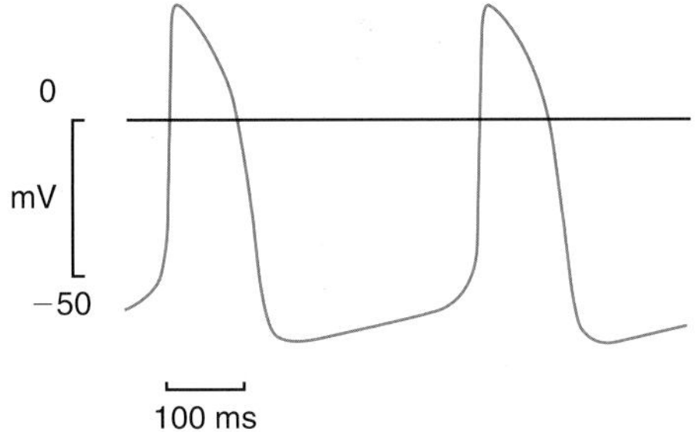

Figure 1-5. Spontaneous activity recorded in a single sinoatrial myocyte. The slow diastolic "pacemaker" depolarization extends from the maximum diastolic potential of −71 mV to the threshold for action potential onset, about −54 mV. (From DiFrancesco D: The hyperpolarization-activated current, I_f, and cardiac pacemaking. In Rosen MR, Jause ML, Wit AL [eds]: Cardiac Electrophysiology: A Textbook. Mt. Kisco, NY, Futura, 1990, pp 117-132.)

the repolarization of the action potential is followed by a slow depolarization from about −71 to −54 mV, the threshold required to initiate another action potential. This slow, spontaneous depolarization drives cardiac automaticity and is related to a specialized current (the funny current, I_f). In the case of AV nodal cells, the fast upstroke is carried predominantly by an inward Ca^{2+} current. Repolarization is caused by delayed activation of the K^+ current. The balance of inward and outward currents determines the net "pacemaker" current and is finely regulated by both adrenergic and cholinergic neurotransmitters. In the presence of AV block or abnormal sinoatrial nodal function, AV junctional cells in the region of the proximal penetrating bundle usually assume the role of pacemaker at rates slower than that of the sinus node. In the absence of disease in the AV junction, the escape rhythm occurs with a frequency that is about 67% of the sinus rate.[31]

Artificial Electrical Stimulation of Cardiac Tissue

Artificial lipid membranes in their pure form are electrical insulators. The myocyte cell membrane (sarcolemma) is much more complicated. Specialized protein molecules in the membrane allow it to be conductive.[32,33] These proteins, either singly or in certain groupings, form channels that open and close for transport of specific ions through the membrane in response to particular stimuli. The channel proteins are the end stages of processes that provides both active and passive transport of ions and molecules through the membrane.

When application of a pacemaker or defibrillator pulse produces a local electric field gradient, ion drift in the extracellular fluid at that site, as well as ion flow within the cell and within the membrane, are affected by the field. The field-induced ion drift cannot be uniform within and outside the cell because of the different drift properties of different ion types, different ion and protein concentrations within and without the cell, and the barrier impedance effect of connections between cells.

The effect of the stimulus is to change the transmembrane voltage of nearby myocytes sufficiently so that depolarization begins in and spreads from those myocyte membranes. Propagation of the stimulus to nearby myocytes occurs because the local transmembrane depolarization changes the voltage gradient across adjacent membranes sufficiently to trigger depolarization of those membranes. The result is a self-regenerating action potential that progresses in a wavelike, relatively slow, manner beyond the local effect of the pacemaker stimulus. Away from immediate vicinity of the electrode, transmission of depolarization and its velocity are in part dependent on the resistance and capacitance properties of the membrane, on the opening and closing of ion channels, and on ion flows through the sarcolemma.

Myocardial Cell Electrical Properties

A single Purkinje fiber typically has an internal resistance that is two to three times greater than that of blood. The specific membrane resistance of a Purkinje fiber is on the order of 10^4 Ω-cm^2. The time constant of the surface membrane is on the order of 10 msec, and the membrane capacity is about 1 μF/cm^2. *Gap junctions* are intercellular channels that provide a pathway for electrical communication between myocytes. Their diameter is about 2 nm, and their length about 12 nm. Gap conductance is voltage sensitive.[34] Under pathologic conditions such as severe hypoxia or ischemia, gap junctions will not function normally.

Cable-like Properties in Depolarization

Transmission of electric pulses can be thought of as occurring by two broad mechanisms. One is a regenerative mechanism, like the spread of depolarization over the heart by depolarization from cell to cell. The other is a nonregenerative mechanism. In this, the amplitude of the stimulation pulse decreases with distance from its origin and is not regenerated; this is *electrotonic* propagation.[35] Transmission along a cable is nonregenerative transmission.

The manner in which a voltage pulse travels along a Purkinje fiber is somewhat similar to transmission of a voltage pulse along a coaxial cable (Fig. 1-6).[36] Propagation amplitude and velocity of a voltage pulse applied to the beginning of the cable are dependent on cable properties. These include the unit-length capacitance between the center wire and the shield, the resistance along the wire, and the nature of the insulation between the center wire and the shield. In a cable, the signal amplitude gradually decreases with distance from the source.

Cable theory applied to a squid axon or a very long cell equates the bathing solution to ground (the shield of the cable) and the electrolyte inside the cell to the center wire of the cable. The cell membrane is assumed to be analogous to the insulating material—the dielectric

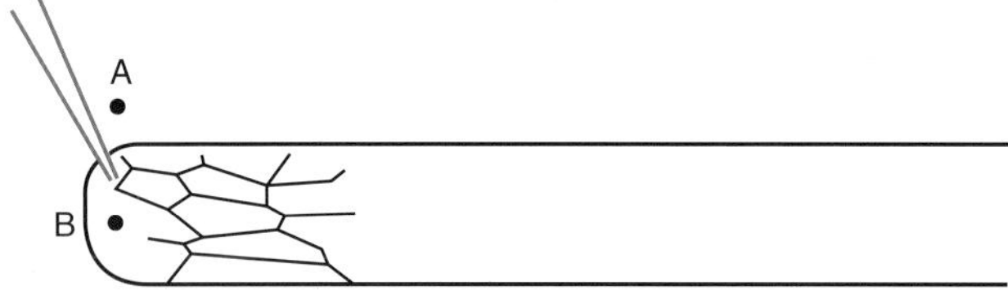

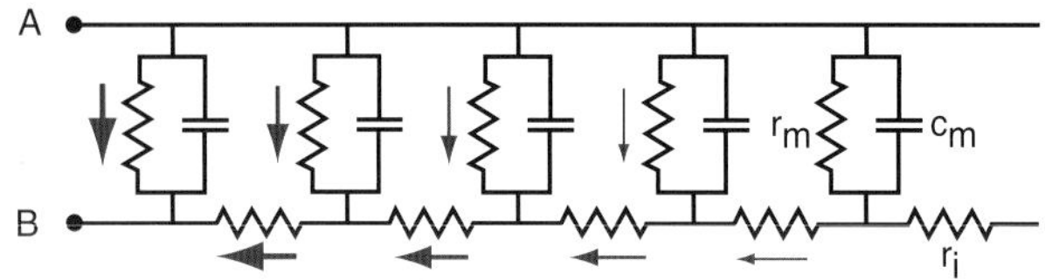

Figure 1-6. Equivalent circuit for a single fiber composed of electrically coupled single cells placed in an electrically conductive medium. A constant current is made to flow from A to B through the surface membrane and along the fiber core. Small voltage changes are produced to ensure constant values of the resistors. c_m, capacitance across the membrane; r_i, resistance in the intercellular space; r_m resistance across the membrane. (From Weidmann S: Passive properties of cardiac fibers. In Rosen MR, Jause MJ, Wit AL [eds]: Cardiac Electrophysiology: A Textbook. Mt. Kisco, NY, Futura, 1990, p 30.)

substance—between the center wire and the shield of the cable. The cell membrane acts as an electrically leaky dielectric substance between two conductors, the electrolyte inside and that outside the cell.

The membrane of a Purkinje fiber modeled as a cable (see Fig. 1-6) can be viewed as a series of modules placed sequentially.[36] One end of each module is connected to the interstitial fluid, which is viewed as having negligible resistance. The other end of each module is connected to the interior of the cell. The electrolyte within the cell and junctions between cells are viewed as having resistance. Between the outside and inside of the cell is the sarcolemma, which is viewed as a series of modules connected in parallel between interstitial fluid and the cell interior. Each module spanning the membrane is made of a resistor and a parallel capacitor. In this schematic representation, the electric pulse being transmitted along the fiber is not regenerated. The electric pulse gradually dies away with distance from its origin at the beginning end of the fiber, as in a coaxial cable lacking booster amplifiers.

Cable Theory Applied to Isolated Cardiac Fibers Is Useful But for the Whole Heart Is Inadequate

One can immediately see that cable theory applied to the whole heart would be an oversimplification. Applied to isolated fibers, it is conceptually and experimentally useful. Knisley (paraphrasing Weidmann[37]) pointed out that, *in isolated cardiac fibers*, intracellular microelectrode techniques demonstrated a distribution of transmembrane voltage that agreed with cable model predictions. Transmembrane voltage differences induced by a negative-going stimulus decreased in an exponential manner with distance from the electrode. However, Knisley[38] found that, in perfused rabbit hearts, polarization was not that predicted by cable theory. He found that, in regions distant from the stimulating electrode in a direction parallel to the fibers, polarization changed sign, and in dog bone–shaped regions perpendicular to the fibers, no polarization sign change occurred.

This and similar studies have demonstrated that cable theory is inadequate for predicting how depolarization spreads in a three-dimensional heart. A three-dimensional heart not only has three dimensions but also has extracellular and intracellular electrical domains, each of which is anisotropic.

Factors Determining Capture by an Electrical Stimulus

In order for an electrical stimulus to stimulate (capture) myocardium, it must be applied with sufficient amplitude, for a sufficient duration (measured in milliseconds), at a time when the myocardium is electrically excitable. There are a great many clinical factors that determine whether a stimulus of a given amplitude will result in capture, including proximity of the electrode to the myocardium, pathology of the underlying cardiac tissue, size and shape of the electrode, and effects of drugs and hormones, as well as electrolytes. For routine clinical practice, the most important factor is that the lead must be positioned in close proximity to well-functioning myocardium in a secure manner. (It is also important that the lead does not stimulate the diaphragm or the phrenic nerve, that it is at a site that results in good hemodynamic function, and that the location does not allow the electrode to bump other electrodes.) After adequate lead positioning, the strength-duration relation is the next most important consideration.

Current Density, Electric Field Gradient, and Propagation of Depolarization

There are two approaches to thinking about how an electrical stimulus induces a self-propagating wavefront of depolarization within myocardium. The *current density* approach considers the magnitude of current flowing through a given mass of myocardium between the stimulating electrodes and finds this to be the critical factor required to induce a regenerative wavefront of depolarization. From this point of view, the stimulation threshold is a function of current density (amperes/cm^2) in the excitable myocardium underlying the electrode.[39-42] The *electric field* approach holds that the critical factor affecting myocardial depolarization is the magnitude of the electric field gradient (volts/cm in viable tissue) that is induced in the myocardium beneath the stimulating electrode.[43,44] These approaches are fundamentally the same in that there is a mathematical relationship between the electric field gradient and the current density at the stimulating electrode.

Because reactance as well as resistance are present, Ohm's law in this context must be stated in terms of impedance, z:

$$v = iz \tag{1-5}$$

where v is the stimulus voltage, i is the current, and z is the impedance to current flow. Note that each of these is a vector. Also note that z varies with current density at the electrode (because of interface properties), with direction of current flow (anisotropy), and with domain (extracellular or intracellular).

The total energy of the pacing stimulus is determined by the applied voltage, the current, and the duration of the stimulus:

$$J_t = \int_0^t v_t i_t dt$$

where J_t is the energy delivered (expressed in joules) from time zero to time t during the pulse, v_t is the voltage, and i_t is the current at the electrode at instantaneous time (t) during the pulse. This equation indicates that the total energy delivered during the pulse is proportional to the area under a curve. The curve is formed in the vertical dimension by the instantaneous product of voltage and current applied to the electrode, and in the horizontal dimension by the time elapsing during the pulse. When the time t reaches the programmed pulse duration, the pulse ends. The area under the curve then represents the electrical energy transferred during the time span of the pulse. The equation can easily be solved in real time with a small digital computer, provided that continuous phasic measurements of the voltage and current in the wire going to the electrode are available. (Note that this equation has blood flow and pressure energy analogs.[45])

For pacemakers in almost all clinical situations, it is more practical and very reasonable to calculate the energy delivered by a constant-voltage pulse through a pacemaker electrode by means of an approximation. The assumptions are (1) that the voltage during the pulse really is constant and (2) that the current flowing is linearly related to the voltage. Because neither of these is quite true, the questions become whether the information obtained proves useful and to what degree it can be misleading. If the assumptions are not too far from being correct, then the equation $J = VIt = V\frac{V}{R}t = \frac{V^2}{R}t$, in which J is the energy delivered, V is the "constant" voltage, I is the current, R is the resistance, and t is the stimulus duration, can be approximately correct and useful. This equation indicates that the total energy delivered can be estimated by multiplying the voltage reading displayed on the pacing systems analyzer (PSA) by the current reading on the PSA and multiplying that product by the stimulus duration. Alternatively, the voltage reading can be squared, then divided by the resistance reading, and the quotient multiplied by the stimulus duration. The virtue in this calculation is that ordinary equipment can provide a quick, approximate determination of the total energy delivered per stimulus. In clinical practice, however, the usual range of good or acceptable values for pacing threshold current and voltage is known, and there is rarely a need to calculate the delivered energy.

The stimulation threshold of isolated cardiac myocytes has been shown to depend on their orientation within an electric field. The threshold is lowest when the myocytes are oriented parallel to the field and highest when the axis of the myocytes is perpendicular to the field.[46] It is clear that myocardial stimulation may be induced with anodal or cathodal stimulation, or both, although with somewhat different characteristics. Various investigators have used several different parameters to express stimulation threshold, including current (mA), potential (V), energy (J), charge (Q), pulse width (t, msec), and voltage multiplied by stimulus duration (V-sec).[47-53] For the purposes of this chapter, the myocardial stimulation threshold for pacing is defined as *the minimum stimulus amplitude at any given pulse width required to consistently achieve myocardial depolarization outside the heart's refractory period*.[54] Stimulation thresholds measured with a constant-voltage (CV) generator are stated in volts, and those of a constant-current generator (CI) are stated in milliamperes. Note that a true constant-voltage generator may yield a slightly different stimulation threshold than the pseudoconstant-voltage generators in ordinary use.

Why must an electrical pacing stimulus rely on propagation in myocardium rather than directly exciting the entire heart? With the magnitude of a stimulus generated by a pacemaker pulse generator, the electric field gradient and ion current density near the electrode are great enough to trigger an action potential only very near the electrode. Unless propagation of the local depolarization occurs, no cardiac contraction will result.

In contrast to cardiac pacing with direct production of only local depolarization and dependence on self-propagation of depolarization, defibrillation involves direct depolarization or hyperpolarization of a large portion of the heart. This is necessary to provide at least the minimum local voltage gradient required to produce depolarization over major portions of the myocardium. To do so requires a stimulus intensity that is very much greater than that required for pacing[55] (see Chapter 2 for a thorough discussion of the principles underlying defibrillation).

Electric Potential Gradients for Stimulation and Defibrillation

When the electric field exceeds approximately 1 V/cm in the extracellular space during diastole, myocardial stimulation (capture) results. When the electric field strength is increased to 6 V/cm, ventricular fibrillation may occur if the stimulus is applied during the vulnerable period (approximately the peak of the T wave). This same field strength (6 V/cm) is also required to interrupt ventricular fibrillation (defibrillation). However, defibrillation requires the minimum field intensity to be approximately 6 V/cm *at almost all points* in the myocardium. In order to achieve this minimum electric field gradient at the same instant over the entire heart, a very large shock current must be applied. This current is thousands of times greater than the current required for pacing.[55]

When a pacemaker pulse is applied, electrically excitable myocytes respond with a wave of *depolarization followed by repolarization* in the myocardium. Depolarization of a small local group of myocytes begins the self-propagating process. The initial depolarization adjacent to the electrode produces a potential gradient great enough at neighboring myocytes to result in their depolarization. The process is a self-regenerating mechanism that requires time to spread, and, once established, it is largely independent of the distance from the stimulating electrode.

Defibrillation is largely accomplished by providing a very large potential gradient between the defibrillation electrodes. This produces, at one instant within local myocardium everywhere in the heart, at least a 6 V/cm gradient. In contrast, pacing is accomplished by providing a gradient of approximately 1 V/cm or less at a local site and relies on self-propagation to spread the depolarization process throughout the myocardium.

The Virtual Electrode Effect

Virtual electrodes are important because they can serve as sites that initiate or prevent depolarization of myocytes.[56] Newton and Knisley defined virtual electrodes as "experimentally observed regions of large delta Vm that arise distant from the stimulating electrode."[57] "Delta Vm" (ΔVm) here represents the change in voltage difference across the myocyte membrane during application of the stimulation current.

A virtual electrode can be described as a collection of charge predominately of one sign at a site away from a regular electrode. If, in an electrically neutral solution, ions of one charge sign are moved away by an electric field, a relative excess of ions of the other charge sign will be left or will move in the opposite direction. For example, if the regular electrode is paced with a negative-going stimulus, a site elsewhere in the tissue (i.e., not at this physical electrode) may become transiently positive and alter the transmembrane potentials of cells at that site.[58-61] In cardiac tissue, a virtual electrode can occur as an effect of anisotropy after a defibrillation shock and can initiate refibrillation. A virtual electrode can also occur as a result of ion redistribution patterns in a nonanisotropic medium. In anisotropic tissue, charge redistribution produced by a physical electrode can have a dog bone shape.[62]

The virtual electrodes occur at sites where ions flow into or out of cells by crossing the cell membrane. An applied unipolar stimulation current flows into some cells while simultaneously flowing out of others, thus producing negative and positive virtual electrodes at different locations. In an anisotropic medium, a cathodal pulse produces a virtual electrode with a dog bone shape oriented perpendicular to cardiac fibers and containing a large ΔVm, and a pair of virtual electrodes containing negative ΔVm at locations along the fibers. Theoretical models have shown that this effect can be attributed to unequal tissue anisotropy in the intracellular and extracellular spaces; that is, intracellular current at a given location favors the longitudinal direction 10 to 1, whereas extracellular current favors the longitudinal direction only 3 to 1 (Dr. S. B. Knisley, personal communication, July 2005). Knisley and Pollard[63] studied the effects of electrode-myocardial separation on cardiac stimulation of rabbit hearts in conductive solution. The electrode-myocardial separation altered the spatial distribution of ΔVm and increased the pacing threshold.

In regard to electrode-myocardial tissue separation, Shepard and colleagues,[64] during 1980s transthoracic defibrillator implantation procedures, sewed the electrodes used for rate sensing onto the outer surface of the pericardium. Sensing voltages were normal. Pacing thresholds of these electrodes measured were high (3.7 ± 1.9 mA and 4.5 ± 2.19 V at 0.5 msec stimulus duration), as would be expected both from current density considerations and from Knisley's findings. The initial impedance was 1209 ± 383 Ω, and the chronic impedance was 1550 ± 358 Ω at a median follow-up time of 964 days. The thresholds had by then decreased to 3.8 ± 2.07 V and 2.7 ± 1.8 mA. The transpericardial distance from underlying myocardium did result in high initial pacing thresholds (and in the special distribution of ΔVm near the electrodes). However the long-term tissue reaction of pericardium and underlying myocardium to the presence of these electrodes was not detrimental in terms of threshold evolution.

Virtual electrodes normally exist near an electrode when a pacing pulse is applied. Nikolski and Sambelashvili,[65] studying Langendorff-perfused rabbit hearts, found that stimuli of magnitude five times threshold produced "make" or stimulus-onset excitation from virtual cathodes, whereas near-threshold stimuli produced "break" or stimulus-termination excitation from virtual anodes.

In studying how cardiac tissue damage at an electrode results in a pacing threshold increase, Sambelashvili and associates[66] found that the virtual electrode effect was destroyed by very strong (40 mA, 4 msec, biphasic, rate 240/minute) pacing pulses applied for 5 minutes. Fluorescent optical mapping showed that decrease or loss of the virtual electrode polarization was associated with pacing threshold increase. Propidium iodide staining showed tissue damage within an area of about 1 mm diameter surrounding the electrode.

Another possible way of looking at the effect of very strong stimuli as described in the previous paragraph is to note that local tissue damage at a pacing electrode increases the distance from the electrode to normal myocytes. Because electric field strength and current density decrease with distance from the electrode, an increase in pacing stimulus amplitude applied to the electrode is necessary to restore the stimulus current density to the pacing threshold level of myocytes at the outer edge of the damaged tissue.

Strength-Duration Relationships

Chronaxie, Rheobase, Energy, and Pulse Duration Thresholds

The intensity of an electrical stimulus (measured in volts or milliamperes) that is required to capture the atrial or ventricular myocardium depends on the duration of the stimulus.[67,68] The historical background and the relations between the various electrical factors have been reviewed, further studied, and very clearly stated by Blair,[69] and by Geddes for electrode-electrolyte interface function and models.[70]

The interaction of stimulus amplitude and stimulus duration (pulse width) defines the strength-duration curve (Fig. 1-7). The voltage or current amplitude required for endocardial stimulation has an exponential relation to the pulse duration, with a relatively flat curve at durations of longer than 1 msec and a rapidly rising curve at durations of less than 0.25 msec. Because of this fundamental property, a stimulus of short pulse duration must be of much greater intensity to capture the myocardium than a longer-duration pulse. Conversely, increasing the pulse width to longer than 1 msec has little influence on the intensity of the stimulus required for capture. Therefore, if one defines the stimulation threshold in terms of pulse amplitude without also specifying the pulse duration, important information is neglected. Similarly, specifying the capture threshold in terms of pulse duration can be misleading if the stimulus amplitude setting is omitted or unknown.

Hoorweg,[71] in 1892, used a voltage source, a galvanometer, and low-leakage capacitors to conduct quantitative stimulation studies. He found that the voltage at which a capacitor must be charged to cause depolarization of nerves and muscles is an inverse function of the capacitance of the capacitor, as follows:

$$V_C = aR + b/C \qquad (1\text{-}6)$$

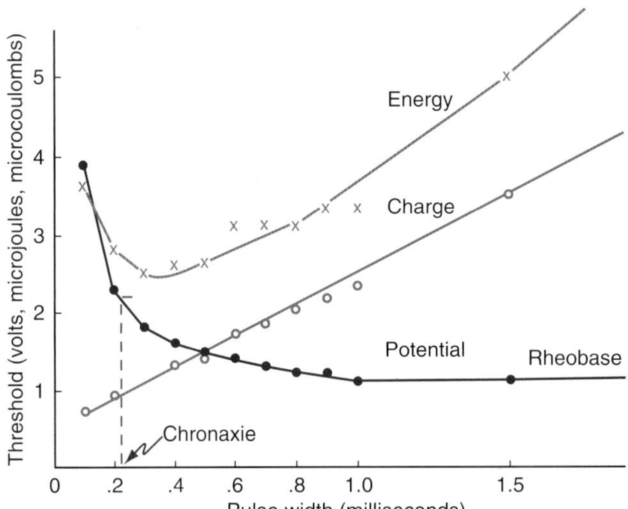

Figure 1-7. Relationships between chronic ventricular canine constant-voltage strength-duration curves expressed in terms of potential (V), charge (μC), and energy (μJ) for a tined unipolar lead with an 8-mm² polished ring-tip electrode. Thresholds are measured at the point of gain of capture. Rheobase is the current or voltage threshold to the right that is independent of pulse width. Chronaxie is the pulse width at twice the rheobase. (From Stokes K, Bornzin G: The electrode-biointerface [stimulation]. In Barold SS [ed]: Modern Cardiac Pacing. Mt. Kisco, NY, Futura, 1985, pp 33-78.)

In this experimentally determined equation, V_c is the threshold voltage to which a capacitor of capacitance C must be charged to produce stimulation on discharge. R is the resistance of the circuit through which the capacitor is discharged, and a and b are coefficients that vary with the specimen (tissue) tested. Here, the experimentally determined constant a has the dimension amperes and the constant b has the dimension ampere-seconds. (The capacitance can be derived from the equation

$$C = \frac{Q}{V}$$

where C is the capacitance, Q is the charge on either conductor, and V is the magnitude of the potential difference across the capacitor; the capacitance has the dimension ampere-seconds [or coulombs] per volt; 1 coulomb per volt = 1 farad). Hoorweg determined that there was only one specific capacitance value for which the threshold charge was a minimum. He also determined that the threshold charge was a linear function of the stimulus duration, "intersecting the y-axis above zero." However, Hoorweg did not have the capability to measure thresholds at very short pulse durations. In reality, the threshold charge increases toward infinity as the pulse duration approaches zero.

In 1901, Weiss[72] reported that the threshold charge required for stimulation increases linearly with stimulus duration. He called this relationship the "formule fondamentale." If I represents the magnitude of the current, t is the stimulus duration, and a and b are constants determined by analyzing the data, Weiss found that

$$\int_0^t I dt = at + b \qquad (1\text{-}7)$$

or, because $\int_0^t i dt = Q$, the charge in the capacitor at threshold stimulus duration t, $Q = at + b$. For a constant-current stimulus, this can be stated in words as *threshold charge requirement = a amperes times t seconds + b*, where b is a constant with dimensional units of ampere-seconds. The values of the constants a and b vary with the tissue tested.

The left-hand side of Equation 1-7 indicates that the charge delivered into the electrode is, for a constant current, the magnitude of the current multiplied by the duration of the current. The right-hand side says that the charge required to stimulate at threshold is a minimum of b ampere-seconds plus the product of the current level (a) and the stimulus duration (t). Weiss[72] noted that, for various stimulus durations tested, the quantity of charge required to initiate depolarization remained constant.

The statement that the threshold charge requirement does not change with stimulus duration is true only within a limited range. The limitation leads to the concept of *rheobase,* as stated in 1909 by Lapique.[73] He pointed out that when pulse duration is increased beyond a limited range, the current requirement does not decrease further. The charge delivered continues to increase as pulse duration is increased. Lapique called this minimum current the *rheobase*. Rheobase can be defined as *the lowest stimulus current that continues to capture the heart when the stimulus duration is made very long.* In this situation, further increases in stimulus duration no longer reduce the magnitude of current required to stimulate the heart.

Note from Equation 1-7 that the ratio a/b has the dimensions amperes divided by (ampere-seconds); this expression reduces in dimensions to the reciprocal of the stimulus duration. Lapique called the time seen in the a/b ratio the *chronaxie*, specified in seconds. Chronaxie time experimentally turns out to be approximately *the threshold pulse duration at twice rheobase amplitude*, and it has become defined as such. This is illustrated in Figure 1-7. *Note again that rheobase is specified in terms of current, and chronaxie is specified in terms of time.*

Lapique redefined the Weiss equation (Equation 1-7) as follows. The stimulation threshold charge Q in the capacitor at stimulation time t is equal to $at + b$, in which a and b are constants determined from threshold measurements. Then, because $Q = It$, $It = at + b$. Dividing both sides of the latter equation by t yields

$$I_t = a + \frac{b}{t}. \qquad (1\text{-}8)$$

The constant a has the same dimension as current, and the constant b has the same dimension as current × time, or charge. If the constant magnitude a is named the rheobase, the equation can be restated as

$$I_t = I_{rheobase} + \left(\frac{I_{rheobase} \times t_{chronaxie}}{t_{stimulusduration}} \right)$$

in which the product $I_{rheobase} \times t_{chronaxie}$ has the numerical value of the constant b. Therefore,

$$I_t = a + \frac{b}{t} = I_{rheobase}\left(1 + \frac{t_{chronaxie}}{t}\right)$$

where I_t is the current during the pulse duration t. This new equation specifies the threshold constant-current stimulus amplitude in terms of chronaxie time, stimulus duration, and rheobase current. If, for reasons discussed later, one moves the $I_{rheobase}$ term inside the parentheses, the equation becomes

$$I_t = a + \frac{b}{t} = \left(I_{rheobase} + \frac{I_{rheobase} \times t_{chronaxie}}{t} \right)$$

Next, if both sides of this threshold current equation are multiplied by the stimulus duration, the equation becomes one of the charge delivered at that pulse duration:

$$Q = It = (t_{stimulusduration} \times I_{rheobase}) + t_{stimulusduration} \times (I_{rheobase} \times t_{chronaxie} / t_{stimulusduration})$$

In the term on the right, the stimulus duration cancels out, and this equation becomes

$$Q = (t_{stimulusduration} \times I_{rheobase}) + (I_{rheobase} \times t_{chronaxie})$$

At very short stimulus durations, the product in the left-hand set of parentheses (stimulus duration times rheobase current) approaches zero. Therefore, when the stimulus duration is very short, the charge quantity represented by Equation 1-9 approaches the limit of chronaxie time multiplied by rheobase current.

$$Q = It = (I_{rheobase} \times t_{chronaxie}) \qquad (1\text{-}9)$$

The lower this product, the lower the charge necessary to stimulate the heart. Lapique[74] also determined that stimulation at the chronaxie pulse width approaches the minimum threshold energy. This is a very useful clinical concept.

Therefore, the two most important reference points on a current or voltage strength-duration curve are rheobase and chronaxie. Obtaining a true rheobase typically requires pulse widths of 10 msec or greater. For clinical purposes, rheobase can be approximately measured at pulse widths of 1.5 to 2 msec. The value obtained may be slightly greater than the true rheobase. Therefore, the chronaxie stimulus duration obtained by setting the stimulus current at twice the approximate rheobase current and then finding the minimum stimulus duration that will result in capture is slightly low. In a time-saving, useful, and reasonable clinical sense, one may empirically set the stimulus duration at a value determined from experience, such as 0.4 to 0.5 msec and then determine the current and voltage thresholds. Safety factor allowances of current and voltage are then added or subtracted based on the patient's current and projected clinical status (see later discussion).

The goal is to find the combination of pacing threshold stimulus current, voltage, and pulse width that results in minimal charge drain from the pulse generator battery at normal pulse rates. Figure 1-7 shows that, for capture to be accomplished, the least charge was required at the shortest pulse duration (0.1 msec in the figure), but the least energy was required at about 0.3 msec stimulus duration. A very short pulse duration puts thresholds close to the steeply ascending limb of the voltage or current curve, where slight fluctuations can risk loss of capture. For this reason, Irnich[75,76] recommended that chronaxie, or the pulse duration slightly to the left of chronaxie, is the most efficient pulse duration for both pacing and defibrillation. In most cases, the pulse duration at chronaxie or slightly greater appears to represent the best overall compromise between adequate safety and generator longevity. One also considers the expected stability or instability of the patient's status, patient compliance, and follow-up arrangements both short and long term.

Pacing thresholds can also be specified in terms of only energy (microjoules) or only pulse duration (milliseconds). However, reliance on specifications in either of these units alone can be misleading. Doing so disregards the fact that, regardless of the pulse duration or energy used, the heart cannot be stimulated unless the stimulus *amplitude* exceeds the rheobase current.[77]

For example, if rheobase is achieved with a pulse amplitude of 0.5 V and 10 msec, the pulse at this point on the strength-duration curve will have 5 μJ of energy (current × voltage × time) with a 500-Ω lead (1 mA × 0.5 V × 10 msec = 5 μJ). A 0.4-V, 20-msec pulse on a 500-Ω lead has 6.4 μJ energy (28% greater than the "threshold" energy at 10 msec) but will not result in cardiac capture. Increasing the pulse duration to 100-msec at 0.4 V results in 32 μJ energy (540% greater than "threshold" energy at 10 msec) but will still not capture the heart, for the same reason. No matter how far the pulse duration is extended (with increased energy), the myocardium will not be captured unless the stimulus amplitude is at least as great as the rheobase value. Therefore, calculation of the energy threshold at very long pulse durations does not provide clinically useful information.[78]

Coates and Thwaites[79] studied the strength-duration curve in 229 patients with 325 leads. The mean atrial chronaxie (n = 101) was 0.24 ± 0.07 msec, and the mean ventricular chronaxie (n = 224) was 0.25 ± 0.07 msec. Mean atrial and ventricular rheobase values were 0.51 ± 0.2 V and 0.35 ± 0.14 V, respectively. Because the pulse generators were set at factory-nominal pulse durations of 0.45 to 0.50 msec, the authors concluded that pacing was suboptimal from the efficiency point of view. They pointed out that battery drain would be reduced by programming pulse duration to the chronaxie value and then programming the voltage to double the chronaxie value. In a study of excitability of rat atria during postnatal development up to 120 days, de Godoy and associates[80] found that atrial rheobase decreased with animal age and was altered by electric field orientation. Atrial chronaxie increased only with age. The clinician might keep in mind that the chronaxie is influenced by not only electrode material, size, and stimulation mode but also by clinically varying biochemical factors. Certainly, marked variations in pacing threshold, either up or down, do occur months and years after implantation in some children and adults.[81]

As stated earlier, on the left side of the chronaxie point of the strength-duration curve the current and voltage rise rapidly as stimulus duration decreases. At pulse durations greater than chronaxie, the slope of the strength-duration curve gradually flattens. Small changes in stimulus amplitude are then less likely to result in loss of capture, especially if the threshold has increased for any one of several pathophysiologic reasons. This increased safety comes at the cost of some decrease in battery life.

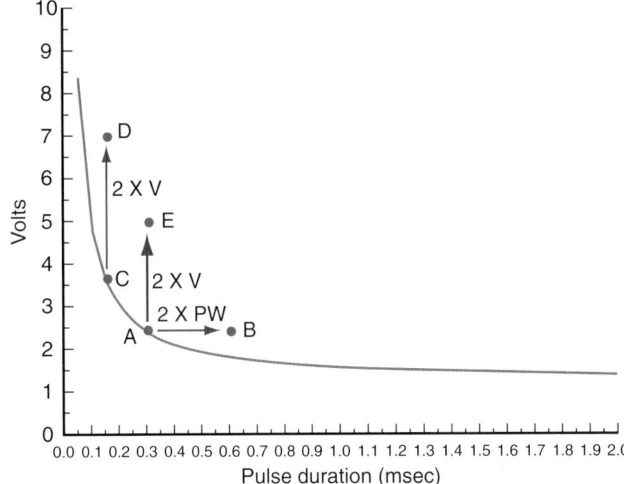

Figure 1-8. Programming of pulse amplitude and pulse duration based on analysis of the strength-duration curve in a patient evaluated at the time of pulse generator replacement (6 years after lead implantation). The rheobase voltage was 1.4 V, and the chronaxie pulse width (PW) was 0.30 msec. Note that the stimulation threshold, determined by decreasing the stimulus amplitude at a constant pulse duration of 0.5 msec, was about 2 V (point A). Doubling of the PW on the relatively flat portion of the strength-duration curve (point B) provides little safety margin for ventricular capture. In contrast, consider a threshold value on the steeply ascending portion of the strength-duration curve (point C). Doubling of the pulse amplitude doubles the safety margin on this portion of the curve, but it lies very close to the curve (point D). An appropriate setting for the chronic pacing pulse might be achieved by doubling the pulse amplitude from point A to point E. Also note that a similar programmed setting would have been obtained had the pulse duration been tripled from point C. Thus, the shape of the strength-duration curve has an important influence on the choice of the amplitude and duration of the pacing pulse.

Practical Application of the Strength-Duration Relationship to Threshold Measurement

Determination of the strength-duration relationship requires that the clinician measure the stimulation threshold at specific amplitudes and pulse durations. However, the result obtained varies somewhat with the manner in which the threshold is measured.

Usually, the threshold measured at a specific stimulus duration (e.g., 0.5 msec) will be slightly higher when the stimulus amplitude is gradually being increased than when it is gradually being decreased. The threshold can also in a sense be measured by holding the output voltage constant and changing the stimulus duration. The stimulation threshold then is defined as the lowest amplitude pulse duration that results in consistent capture of the myocardium. Threshold measured only in this way can be clinically useful, as noted earlier. It also can be deceptive, because the strength duration curve is not linear.

For example, if the pulse duration threshold is 0.5 msec at an amplitude of 2 V, reprogramming the pacemaker stimulus to a pulse duration of 1 or even 1.5 msec would provide a very small margin of safety (Fig. 1-8). Instead, doubling the stimulus amplitude to 4 V at a pulse duration of 0.5 msec would provide an adequate margin of safety. In contrast, consider that, in this same patient, the pulse duration threshold is 0.15 msec at a pulse amplitude of 3.5 V. Increasing the pulse width to 0.45 msec would also provide an adequate safety margin. The reason that a threefold increase in pulse width is not adequate in the first example but is acceptable in the second relates to the location of the threshold stimulus on the strength-duration curve.

Thinking about programming the pulse generator to twice the voltage threshold found at the chronaxie pulse duration is only a starting point. In deciding how much safety margin is necessary for any particular patient, several physiologic factors come into play. These are discussed in the following paragraphs.

Capture Hysteresis (Wedensky Effect)

The threshold stimulus amplitude that is measured by decreasing the voltage or current until loss of capture occurs is sometimes less than that determined by

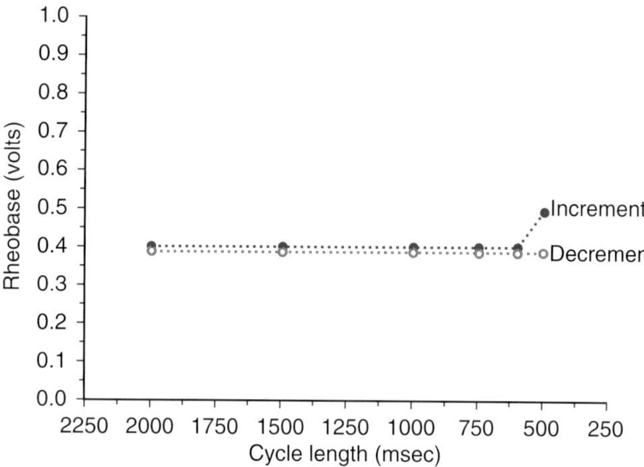

Figure 1-9. Pacing thresholds determined by gradually incrementing and decrementing the pulse amplitude until gain and loss of capture, respectively, are demonstrated in a patient with complete atrioventricular block. The pacing threshold was determined at cycle lengths of 2000, 1500, 1000, 750, and 500 msec and with a constant pulse duration of 2.0 msec. To prevent variation in cycle length during incrementing and decrementing pulse amplitudes, a backup pulse was delivered at 25 msec. Note that the threshold values determined in this manner, with increments and decrements of the stimulus amplitude, are similar. Therefore, the Wedensky effect may be marginal when the pacing cycle length is maintained at a constant value.

increasing the stimulus intensity from below threshold until gain of capture occurs. This hysteresis-like phenomenon is the *Wedensky effect*.[82] It is the effect of subthreshold stimulation on the subsequent suprathreshold stimulation when the stimulus amplitude is being increased. Figure 1-9 shows the Wedensky effect.

Langberg and colleagues[83] observed that there was no demonstrable capture hysteresis at pacing cycle lengths greater than 400 msec. They concluded that the Wedensky effect was related to asynchronous pacing in the relative refractory period when incrementing the stimulus intensity, as compared with synchronous late diastolic stimulation when decrementing the stimulus amplitude until loss of capture.

Swerdlow and associates[84] showed in a study of 40 patients that cardiovascular collapse occurs at AC current levels less than the ventricular fibrillation current threshold. They noted that the continuous capture threshold for AC current is less than the capture threshold for a single ordinary pacing stimulus. They suggested that continuous capture at low levels of AC current requires a cumulative effect of subthreshold stimuli. This is a variety of the Wedensky effect. They stated that the safety standard for 60-Hz leakage current lasting longer than 5 seconds should be 20 μA or less to avoid intermittent capture.

Effect of Pacing Rate on Stimulation Threshold

Hook and coworkers[85] reported a significant increase in ventricular pacing threshold in 10 of 16 patients at 400 msec and in 15 of 16 at 300 msec (relative to a pacing cycle length of 600 msec). The phenomenon was not observed at every trial (e.g., 12 of 72 trials at 400 msec). The patients were all candidates for ICDs, and 9 of 12 were receiving antiarrhythmic drugs. The leads were bipolar (a pair of epicardial corkscrews in 11 patients, an endocardial screw-in lead in 5 patients).

The atrial stimulation threshold has also been shown to vary as a function of pacing rate.[86,87] Katsumoto and associates[88] reported that 29 of 36 patients exhibited constant-current atrial pacing threshold energy and current variations as a function of pacing rate in the range of 60 to 120 beats per minute (bpm). The pacing was done with activated vitreous carbon electrodes.

Also, Kay and colleagues[89] found significant human atrial threshold changes as a function of pacing rate (between 125 and 300 bpm) using constant-voltage stimulation. They found a significant increase in rheobase voltage, chronaxie, and minimum threshold energy at pacing rates greater than 225 bpm using platinized (low-polarizing) unipolar electrodes. They also determined strength-interval curves and found no correlation between atrial effective refractory period and rheobase voltage, chronaxie, or rate-dependent changes in either of these values. They concluded that the phenomenon is probably related to the "opposing effects of decreasing cycle length on the action potential duration and the slope of the strength-interval curve. Thus, if the pacing interval shortens to a greater extent than the refractory period and pacing stimuli are delivered during the ascending limb of the strength-interval curve (the relative refractory period), the diastolic threshold will increase."[89]

The increase in stimulation threshold with increasing stimulation rate probably has minimal implications for bradycardia pacing. It is important for antitachycardia pacing, however, because threshold must be measured at rates required to interrupt the arrhythmia. In addition, the safety factors used with antitachycardia pacemakers must be based on thresholds measured at the clinically appropriate rates, rather than during pacing at resting rates.

Strength-Interval Relationships

Voltage and current stimulation thresholds vary as a function of the coupling interval of the stimulus to prior beats and to the stimulation frequency used for the basic drive train. A typical ventricular constant-current strength-interval curve is shown in Figure 1-10. At relatively long extrastimulus coupling intervals (>270 msec), the intensity of the extrastimulus required for ventricular capture is relatively constant, approaching the rheobase value. At shorter extrastimulus coupling intervals (<250 msec), the intensity of the extrastimulus must be increased for it to elicit myocardial capture.

The exponential rise in amplitude required for capture at short coupling intervals is the result of encroachment into the refractory period of the myocardium. During the *relative* refractory period (corresponding to the repolarization phase of the action potential), the myocardium can be induced to generate

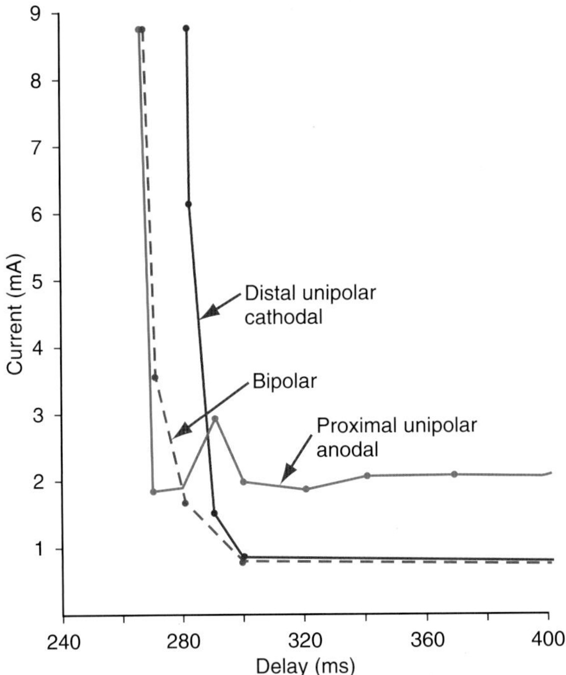

Figure 1-10. Strength-interval curves. Unipolar distal cathodal, unipolar proximal anodal, and bipolar strength-interval curves during an acute study in a patient with a temporary bipolar lead (equal-sized cathode and anode). The bipolar and unipolar anodal refractory periods are equal and are shorter than the unipolar cathodal refractory period. (From Mehra R, Furman S: Comparison of cathodal, anodal, and bipolar strength-interval curves with temporary and permanent pacing electrodes. Br Heart J 41:468, 1979.)

a new action potential if the stimulus has sufficient intensity. During the *absolute* refractory period (corresponding to the plateau phase of the action potential), no depolarization can be effected, regardless of the stimulus intensity. The strength-interval curve of atrial and ventricular myocardium is shifted to the left at shorter basic drive cycle lengths. Therefore, the effective refractory period, which is usually measured at a pulse duration of 2 msec and an amplitude that is twice that of the late diastolic threshold, decreases as a function of the pacing cycle length. At relatively slow pacing rates (<200 bpm), there is relatively little interaction of the strength-duration and strength-interval curves. As discussed previously, however, at rapid pacing rates (>225 bpm), pacing stimuli during the basic drive may encounter the relative refractory period. If the stimulus amplitude becomes subthreshold, 2:1 capture of the myocardium results.

Factors Opposing Pacemaker Current Flow

When an electrical stimulus is applied to a pacing lead in contact with the heart, factors opposing current flow include the electrical resistance of the pacemaker lead wires, the impedance of the electrode-tissue interface, and characteristics of ion movement in the myocardium. All of these are important to both the efficiency of stimulation and the longevity of a pacemaker or ICD battery.

Conductor Resistance and Conduction Losses

Energy dissipation in the lead from the pulse generator to the electrode is proportional to the square of the current. To minimize charge drain from the battery, low lead resistance and low current are desirable. Because the purpose of a pacing stimulus is to produce high current density at the electrode-electrolyte interface in the heart, the ideal situation is to deliver a low current from a very small surface area of electrode. If high current density (current magnitude divided by the plane area of the myocardium touched by the electrode) can be obtained with a small, high-impedance electrode, the current drained from the battery will be less than with a lower impedance.

At pacing threshold, a certain current density exists. If the interface area is made smaller, the current can be reduced equivalently and the same current density maintained. To minimize the current required for stimulation, an optimal combination of interface area, current density, surface material and structure of the electrode, and impedance increase brought about by making the electrode interface area smaller must be found.

The important point is that an increase in impedance made to reduce current drain from the battery should be accomplished by making changes in the electrode, not by increasing the resistance of the wires to and from the pacemaker.

Opposition to Stimulus Current Flow

The resistance of the wire leading from the pulse generator to the stimulating electrode—the cathode—is typically in the range of 50 to 150 Ω. The resistance of the pathway leading to the anode may be in the 50- to 150-Ω range, or it may be lower, as in some unipolar pacing systems. For some practical purposes, one can usefully consider the electrode and the tissue to act as resistances rather than having a combination of reactive and resistive elements (i.e., impedance). By measuring the ratio of peak or average voltage to peak or average current when a pulse is applied, useful information about load on the pulse generator and expected battery life can be obtained.

An increase in resistance calculated from voltage/current ratios may indicate a lead fracture, poor lead contact in the connector block, or an electrode that is not in good contact with tissue or blood. Very low impedance values may indicate an insulation defect. The absence of gross change from normal lead resistance does not rule out a broken lead or an insulation defect. An insulation defect can act as a shunt to ground. Its effect depends on its magnitude and location.

A broken wire can separate markedly and produce a very high measured lead resistance (e.g., 1800 Ω). However, the broken ends may remain in contact or in intermittent contact. If the ends are in continuous contact, lead resistance may not increase significantly. If the ends contact intermittently, erratic pacing, sensing, or lead resistance measurements can occur.

Impedance at the Electrode-Tissue Interface

The resistance (ohmic polarization) of the stimulating electrode is inversely and exponentially proportional to the size of the electrode and the temperature and conductivity of the tissue.[90,91] For practical purposes, in vivo temperature and conductivity are essentially constant. Decreasing the geometric surface area of the electrode, as illustrated in Figure 1-11, is a way to increase the current density at the electrode for any given level of output current from the pulse generator.

Size reduction alone, however, has the negative effect of increasing polarization impedance. In effect, the Helmholtz capacitance at the interface is decreased by reducing the area of the electrode. One remembers from the equation

$$v_t = \frac{1}{C}\int_0^t i_t dt$$

that the voltage v_t across the Helmholtz capacitance at the electrode is proportional to the accumulated charge and inversely proportional to the capacitance. If the electrode contact area with the tissue is made smaller to increase the current density and nothing else is changed, the capacitance will be decreased. For a given applied charge, that action will increase the Helmholtz capacitance voltage, because of the inverse relationship between the voltage and the capacitance.

For a given electrode material (as a first approximation), capacitance (C) is a function of the interfacial surface area (A_i):

$$C = eA_t/d \qquad (1\text{-}10)$$

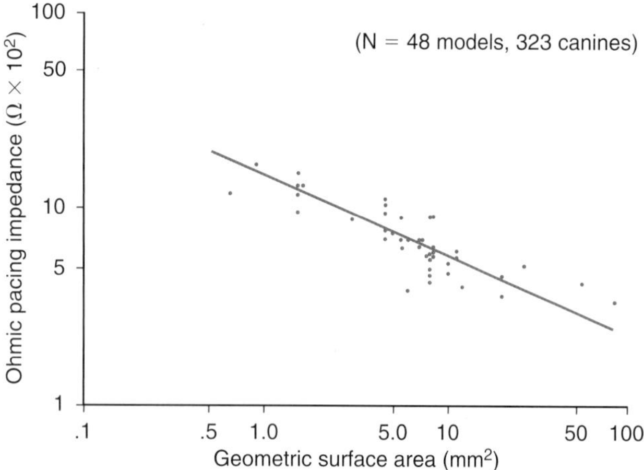

Figure 1-11. Leading-edge ohmic polarization or electrode resistance of chronic canine ventricular leads (12 weeks after implantation) measured with a Medtronic Model 5311 pacing systems analyzer as a function of the unipolar cathode's geometric surface area. Each data point was obtained from a population of animals testing one lead design. The study included 323 animals and 48 lead models.

where e is the dielectric constant of the Helmholtz double layer and d is its thickness. Because e and d are essentially constants in vivo, the capacitance of the electrode varies as a function of the interface surface area A_t.

How does one obtain a very large surface area to contact the tissue and at the same time not require a large-diameter electrode? Initially this was accomplished by making the electrodes porous.[92-94] Microporous electrodes, such as activated carbon or platinized platinum, have a higher real surface area.[95,96] The capacitance of microporous surfaces is greater than that of porous surfaces and still greater than that of polished surfaces. Fractal-surface electrodes have turned out to be best at meeting the requirements of very small geometric areas and large Helmholtz interface areas at the same time.

Another approach to the problem of decreasing polarization is to use a material that supplies its own majority charge carriers. An example is the silver–silver chloride (Ag/AgCl) electrode in chloride solution. The majority carrier, in this case Cl^-, cannot be depleted: Cl^- evolves at the cathode and is formed at the anode. Therefore, voltage across the electrode interface has a waveshape essentially identical to that of the applied constant current, and the electrode is said to be nonpolarizing. Unfortunately, there does not appear to be a clinically usable, nonpolarizing (charge-carrier supplying) electrode material available for permanent implantation. Ag/AgCl electrodes, for example, are not used for permanent pacing because the anode erodes and the AgCl eventually dissolves from the cathode.[97,98]

The ideal, practical stimulating electrode is made of a corrosion-resistant, biocompatible material with small geometric size and very high interfacial surface area, which gives it the characteristics of very high capacitance and a lower polarization voltage.

Impedance

Impedance can be defined as the vector sum of all forces opposing the flow of current in an electric circuit. Pure inductors and pure capacitors have no energy losses. They store or release energy in or from an electric field (capacitor) or a magnetic field (inductor). They also change the time relationships between varying voltage and current. The effects can be quantified in terms of reactance. Capacitive and inductive reactances oppose each other. If a sine wave voltage is applied to a pure capacitance, the current peaks occur 90 degrees earlier than the voltage peaks. If a sine wave voltage is applied to a pure inductance, the current peaks occur 90 degrees later than the voltage peaks.

The total reactance in a simple series circuit is the scalar sum of the inductive and capacitive reactances. Each of these varies with the frequency content of the applied signal. Impedance also varies with signal frequency content. It is the vector sum of reactance and resistance. Impedance has a magnitude and a phase angle, both dependent on the rates of change of the applied voltage. The phase angle represents the difference in timing of sinusoidal current flow peaks as compared with sinusoidal voltage peaks when a sinusoidal voltage is applied to a circuit. A voltage or current pulse of any shape can be broken down mathematically into combinations of sinusoidal components.

In a simple series circuit, where R is the resistance and X is the sum of the capacitive and inductive reactances, the magnitude of impedance Z is defined as follows:

$$Z = \sqrt{R^2 + X^2} \tag{1-11}$$

for a single R-X series combination. For various combinations of reactance and resistive elements in parallel and in parallel-series combinations, each component of impedance (Z_1, Z_2, Z_3, and so on) used in determining the total impedance must be treated as a vector quantity. Serial and parallel connection calculations using such vector components cannot be accurately performed by ordinary scalar, algebraic, Ohm's law manipulations.[99]

RV and coronary sinus catheters connected to a single pulse generator output socket represent impedances in parallel.

Reactance is positive for inductance (i.e., when a sine wave voltage is applied, the voltage leads the current, as seen on an oscilloscope screen) and negative for capacitance (when a sine wave voltage is applied, the voltage lags the current).

Reactance and Charge Movement at the Electrode-Electrolyte Interface

The electrode and the tissue act not as pure resistances but as reactances that change the time relationships between voltage and current when a pacemaker or defibrillator pulse is applied. The only elements of almost pure resistance in the pacemaker circuit external to the pulse generator are the lead wires.

When the pacing pulse begins, several events occur almost immediately. Electron motion in the lead wires and electrodes must result in ion motion in the interstitial fluid. The electric field between the electrodes results in (1) reversible or irreversible oxidation-reduction processes occurring at the interface between the electrode and the electrolyte, and/or (2) the electrode-tissue interface's acceptance of current without charge crossing the interface. In the latter case, the interface acts as a capacitor. The result is the sequence of events shown in Figure 1-12. The leading-edge voltage/current ratio is referred to as *ohmic polarization*. The increasing charge on the Helmholtz capacitor results in increasing opposition to further current inflow. The figure shows this as polarization overvoltage. The rates of voltage and current change are dependent on rates of ion movement within the electrolyte. These in turn are dependent on the mass and charge of ion species, species interactions and concentrations, and the applied electric field. The result is that lead wire current and voltage are not linearly related. The circuit is reactive. The vector combination of this reactance and the resistive elements (e.g., lead wires) make up the impedance faced by the pulse generator output.

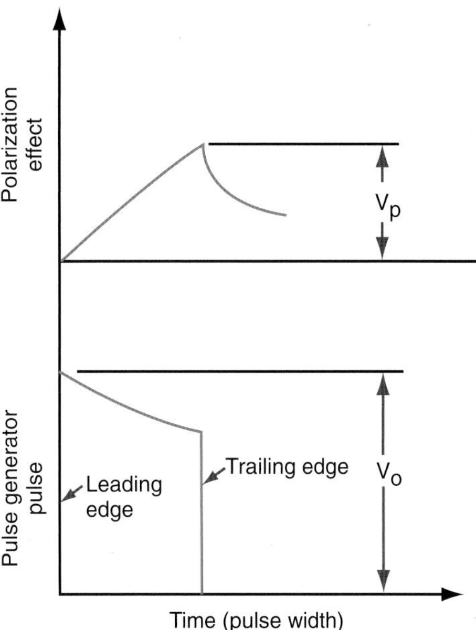

Figure 1-12. The effect of polarization (upper diagram) *has been separated from the capacitively coupled constant-voltage pacing pulse* (lower diagram) *to help clarify the electrical manifestation of electrode polarization. At the leading edge of the pulse, polarization is essentially zero. With time* (pulse duration), *the voltage resulting from polarization (sometimes called* polarization overvoltage, *V_p) increases. When the pacing pulse is shut off, polarization overvoltage decays exponentially as a result of diffusion. (From Stokes K, Bornzin G: The electrode-biointerface [stimulation]. In Barold SS [ed]: Modern Cardiac Pacing. Mt. Kisco, NY, Futura, pp 33-78.)*

Charge Conduction and Transmembrane Potential Changes in Cardiac Pacing and Defibrillation

The directed motion of electrical charge is the result of electric field gradients. Currents at pacemaker or defibrillator electrodes and within the heart can be considered in several categories. Two of these categories are (1) ion movement currents external to cells, within cells, and across cell membranes and (2) charge separation currents that bring opposing charges to the electrode-electrolyte interface and membrane intracellular-extracellular interfaces, *without charge actually crossing the interface*. The latter currents are capacitive; they charge the Helmholtz capacitor at the electrode and change the voltage difference across the cell membrane before it depolarizes.

Otto Schmidt in 1969 described biologic information processing using the concept of "interpenetrating domains."[100] In the heart, two domains of charge flow exist: extracellular and intracellular. The two domain pathways are different in their anisotropic characteristics, and they are interwoven. Current passes from one domain to the other through cell membranes. Bidomain theory and studies are based on the concept that at every point in the heart there are two electric potential vectors, one intracellular and one extracellular. Mathematically, each domain is continuous and occupies the entire domain. Membrane current leaves one domain and enters the other at the same coordinates. Much analytical mathematical and laboratory experimental work has proceeded from these concepts. Insight about depolarization wavefront passage over the myocardium, current flow directions in relation to wavefront direction, and virtual electrode formation have come from such studies.[101-104]

Roth[104] pointed out that stimulation of myocytes by application of a defibrillation shock can result in transmembrane voltage changes by four mechanisms: (1) direct polarization of the tissue, as described by cable theory (see later discussion); (2) production of virtual anodes and cathodes, as described by bidomain models with unequal anisotropy ratios of the intracellular and extracellular spaces; (3) polarization of the tissue secondary to change in orientation of cardiac fibers (curving); and, possibly, (4) polarization of individual cells or groups of cells because of a sawtooth electric potential effect. Sawtooth alterations of potential may occur because of resistive discontinuities introduced by intercellular gap junctions. Plonsey and Barr[105] predicted the occurrence of sawtooth effects in 1986. Under what circumstances and to what degree, if any, the sawtooth effect might become important in fibrillation or defibrillation is uncertain.[106-108]

Electrical Charge Movement in Wires and in Tissue

Whether contraction of a myocyte occurs when a pacemaker pulse is applied is a function several factors: (1) the amplitude, waveform, and duration of ion flow in the extracellular tissue resulting from the electric field gradient produced by the pulse; (2) the state of the preexisting voltage difference from the outside to the inside of the cell (degree of *polarization* or *depolarization* of the cell membrane); and (3) the biochemical state of the cell.

Irnich 1990 discussed fundamental laws of electrostimulation,[109] and in 2002 he discussed three myocardial stimulation theorems introduced by George Weiss 100 years earlier.[110] The three theorems are as follows: (1) the pacing threshold, as measured by the voltage-time product of the stimulus, is a linear function of the pulse duration; (2) there is a minimum of the delivered threshold energy requirement that is dependent on the pulse duration; and (3) pulse shape plays no role in electrostimulation. That pulse shape plays no role in electrostimulation is a concept with clinically apparent limitations and requires some interpretation.[111,112] Some of the factors involved are discussed in a later section.

Electron Flow Versus Ion Flow

An *interface* between ion drift current and electron drift current occurs at the electrode-electrolyte interface. In pacemaker and defibrillator leads and electrodes connected to the negative output socket of the pulse generator, current flow consists of a net drift of *electrons* through the negative lead toward the electrode surface. In contrast, in the extracellular fluid the current flow is *ion* drift.

The motion of an individual ion is that of random motion, with the drift imposed by the electric field superimposed on the random motion. Drift velocity is proportional to the magnitude of charge on the ion, the mean time between collisions with other ions divided by the mass of the ion, and the electric field strength and direction. In addition, ions interact with each other. For a pacemaker electrode in the heart, all of these properties, together with the Helmholtz double-layer capacitance effect, mean that current flow in the lead wires going to the electrodes does not vary instantaneously in proportion to the applied voltage.

Capacitance and Polarization

When an electric field is applied to an electrode, the interface with the surrounding tissue stores electrical charge separated by charge sign. It thereby is acting as a capacitor. A capacitor requires a finite amount of time to charge or discharge to any specified voltage. The relationship between the voltage across a pure capacitor at any time t, when i represents the instantaneous current flow and the capacitance has magnitude C (measured in farads), is

$$v_t = \frac{1}{C}\int_0^t i_t dt$$

and the instantaneous current i entering or leaving the capacitor is

$$i_t = C\frac{dv}{dt}$$

where dv/dt represents the rate of change of the voltage across the capacitor. The amount of charge stored, $\int_0^t i_t dt$, is directly proportional to the net area under the curve of instantaneous current entering and leaving the capacitor plotted against time. Note also that, for a given amount of charge, the voltage across the capacitor is inversely proportional to the capacitance. A perfect capacitor with no energy loss in storage or discharge is described by these equations.

Neither cell membranes nor manmade capacitors are perfect capacitors. In nonperfect capacitors, some energy is dissipated in the capacitor during storage or discharge. Pacemaker and defibrillator electrodes act as imperfect capacitors by means of the Helmholtz double-layer effect (described later).

The capacitance of canine myocytes in isosmotic solution is about 175 picofarads (pF). Cell membrane capacitance is about 0.01 microfarad (μF) per square millimeter of membrane surface area.[113] The capacitance of pacemaker electrodes has been reported to range from 0.2 μF/mm^2 (smooth surface) to 40 μF/mm^2 (fractal-surface electrode). The area of pacemaker tip electrodes is usually in the range of 4 to 10 mm^2. Therefore, the capacitance might be 200 μF or more. The time constant for a 200-μF capacitor C discharging through a 500-Ω resistor R is R × C, or 100 msec. This means that the voltage across the capacitor, or across an ideal electrode-electrolyte interface, if the capacitance were a truly constant 200 μF and the interface impedance

500 Ω, would on discharge decrease from its maximum level to 37% of its maximum level in 100 msec.

Figure 1-13 shows measurements of current in a bipolar cardiac pacing catheter. The catheter is applying a constant-current pulse into a fibroblast cell culture dish. The current waveshape at its onset is almost straight up to its programmed magnitude, after which it remains unchanged for the duration of the pulse. The current charges the electrode-electrolyte interface Helmholtz capacitor (see later discussion).

When the pulse stops, what happens to the current and voltage measurements at the pulse generator terminals depends in part on the pulse generator circuitry. In this case, the laboratory pulse generator internally, in effect, connects its negative and positive output sockets, and the voltage difference between the output sockets goes to almost zero. The Helmholtz capacitor discharges in part within the electrolyte (equivalent circuit shown in Fig. 1-14). It also discharges in part by reverse current flow back through the catheter wires, which now act as a short circuit around the Helmholtz capacitor. The reverse current flow is shown in Figure 1-13. Figure 1-15A shows both the constant-current pulse and the voltage response to the pulse into the fibroblast cell culture. The voltage measured between the tip and ring electrode wires rises almost straight up for only part of the way to its final value. The voltage then rises slowly until the current pulse stops. This is the effect of polarization at the electrode-electrolyte interface—the Helmholtz capacitor effect.

If the impedance between the positive and negative sockets of the pulse generator were made to go to very high rather than very low when the pacemaker pulse ends, almost no current would flow in the bipolar

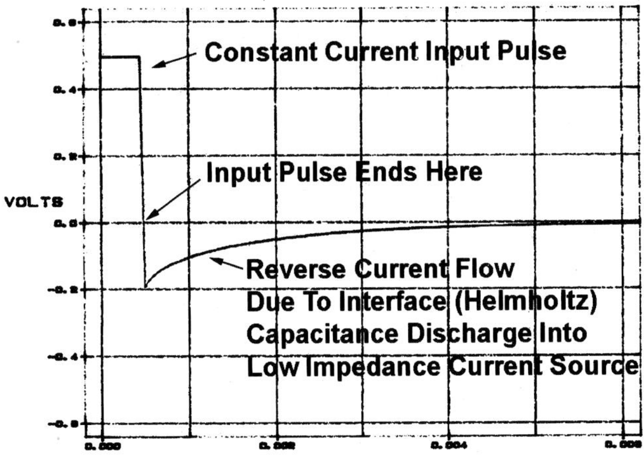

Figure 1-13. Stimulus current waveshape in a bipolar catheter lead, showing reverse current flow after the stimulus ends. A constant-current pulse generator is applying a negative-going pulse into a fibroblast cell culture. The recording terminals are reversed to show the pulse upright. The shape of the pulse at its onset is almost straight up to the programmed magnitude. Then it remains flat for the duration of the 0.5-msec pulse. During this time, the current charges the electrode-electrolyte interface capacitor (Helmholtz capacitance effect—see text). When the stimulus ends, the laboratory pulse generator in effect shorts its output terminals between pulses, thereby connecting the anodal and cathodal leads together at the pulse generator. When the pulse stops, the ions in the electrolyte rearrange themselves, producing transient ionic current flow in the electrolyte, and also in the catheter, leading the reverse-direction current flow shown in the plot. (The current was measured by the voltage drop across a 100-Ω resistor; this does increase the decay current time constant.)

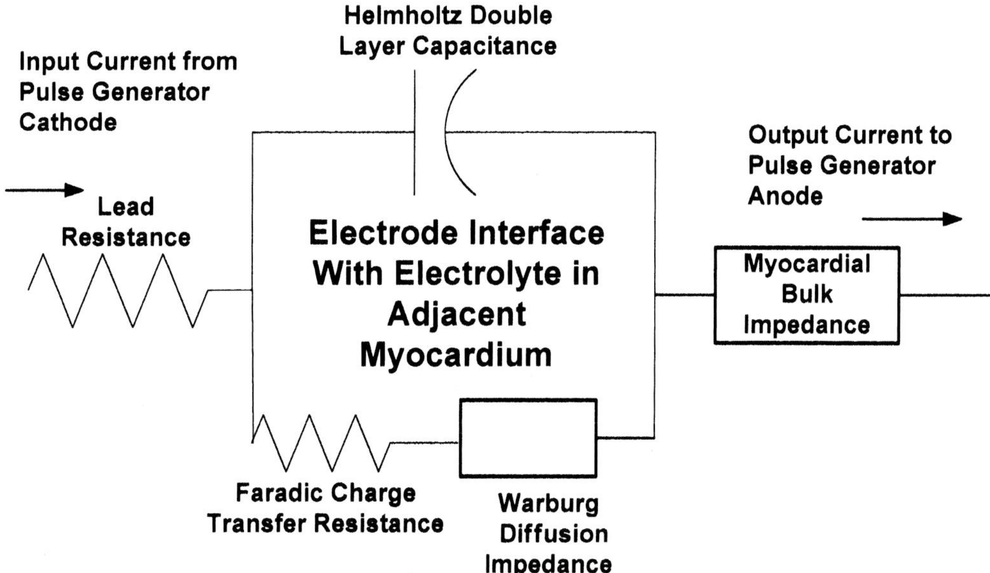

Figure 1-14. Equivalent circuit representation of an electrode-electrolyte interface, including the Helmholtz capacitance and the Warburg impedance. (Modified from Rodman JE: Solution, Surface and Solid State Assembly of Porphyrins [PhD thesis]. Cambridge, University of Cambridge, 2000, Fig. 4.6.)

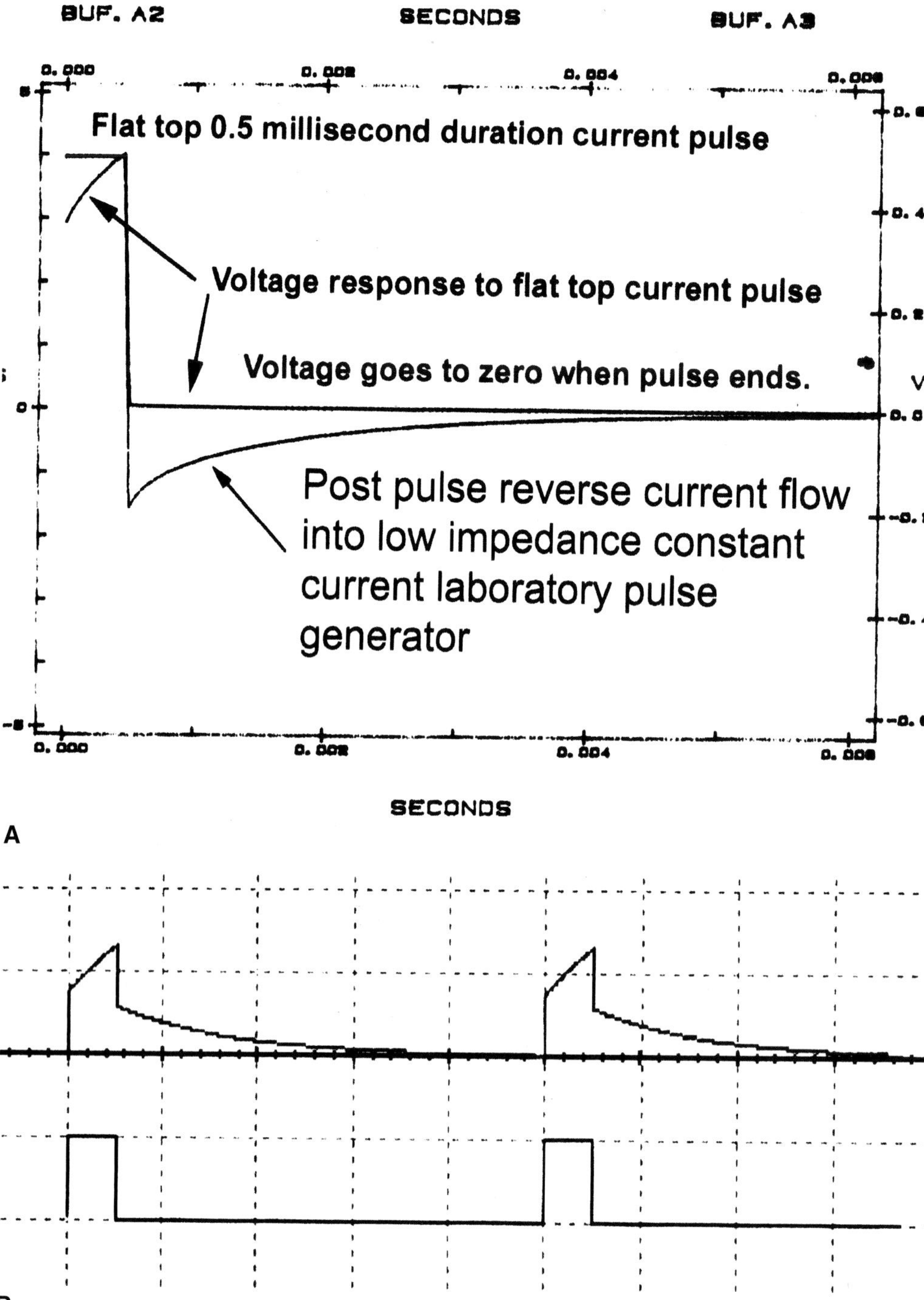

Figure 1-15. ***A,*** *Current and voltage response when a constant-current pacing stimulus was applied to an MC3T3 cell culture. This is the same as Figure 1-13 except that both the current and the voltage response are plotted. Note that, while the constant current is at its programmed level, the voltage between the leads rises slowly after an initial rapid rise. This and the reverse current flow when the pulse ends are effects of polarization at the electrodes. (The voltage as measured between the leads at the laboratory pulse generator goes to approximately zero immediately at the end of the pulse, because the pulse generator connects the leads together between pulses. This is in contrast to clinical pulse generators, which maintain a high impedance to facilitate sensing between pulses.)* ***B,*** *Electronic circuit simulation of constant-current pulse applied to an electrode-electrolyte interface. The top trace is the voltage response to the current shown in the bottom trace. Here, in contrast to Figures 1-13 and 1-15A, the pulse generator between pulses goes to high impedance between its terminals. The voltage across the simulated interface when the pulse ends at first falls rapidly, but then slowly, as the simulated Helmholtz interface capacitor discharges into the simulated electrolyte.*

catheter wires between pulses. The Helmholtz capacitor at the electrode would discharge mainly through resistive components in the electrode-electrolyte interface (see Fig. 1-14). In that case, when the constant-current stimulus stops, the voltage measured across the catheter pins would keep the same polarity and would decay slowly rather than go to zero precipitously. This decay is illustrated by an electronic circuit simulation in Figure 1-15B.

This situation is illustrated during pacing of a fibroblast cell culture through a bipolar cardiac pacing catheter in Figure 1-16. The top trace shows a biphasic constant-current pulse with 1.5 msec between the end of the initial, negative phase and the beginning of the positive phase. The duration of each phase is 0.5 msec. The pulse generator circuit here goes to a high impedance rather than a low impedance when each phase ends. The bottom trace shows the voltage response. At the end of each phase, the voltage measured at the pulse generator terminals initially goes rapidly toward zero but, part of the way toward zero, it begins to change only slowly. This is the effect of the Helmholtz capacitor's discharging into the surrounding electrolyte, and it is a function of the rates of ion movement at that time during the discharge cycle.

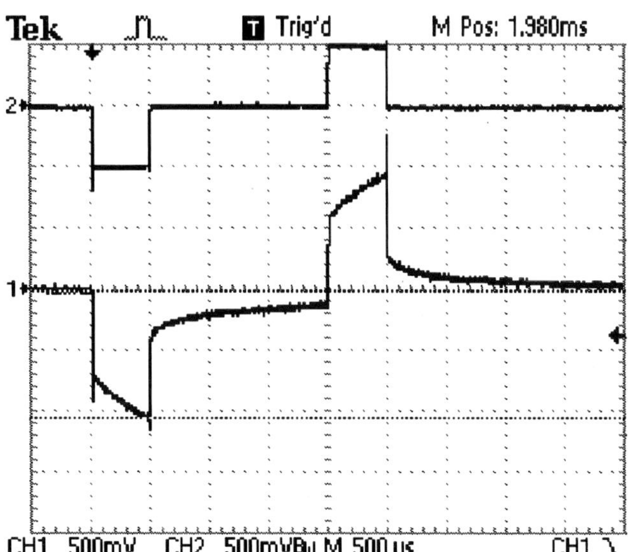

Figure 1-16. Slow decay of pacing catheter lead voltage between biphasic stimulus phases. The plot shows voltages occurring during biphasic pacing of a fibroblast cell culture through a bipolar cardiac pacing catheter. The top trace shows a biphasic constant-current pulse with 1.5 msec between the end of the initial, negative phase and the beginning of the positive phase. The duration of each phase is 0.5 msec. The pulse generator circuit here goes to a high impedance rather than a low impedance when each phase ends. The bottom trace shows the voltage response. At the end of each phase, the voltage measured at the pulse generator terminals initially goes rapidly toward zero but then, partway toward zero, it begins to change only slowly. This is the effect of discharge of the Helmholtz capacitor into the surrounding electrolyte. This voltage response between phases is a function of the rates of ion movement in the electrolyte.

Biphasic Stimulus Effect

Of great interest is the effect of decreasing the delay time between the end of the first and the beginning of the second phase. Compare Figure 1-16 with Figure 1-17. When the stimulus is biphasic with almost no delay (here about 10 μsec) between phases, the slow decay of voltage at the end of the first phase is aborted by the beginning of the second, opposite-polarity phase. The amplitude and duration of the voltage decay after the second phase are each less when the second phase occurs immediately rather than being delayed by 1.5 msec.

Figure 1-18 shows the electrode and Helmholtz capacitance voltage response to a pacing-level, negative-going, constant-current stimulus applied across defibrillator epicardial patch electrodes in saline. The electrodes were in a foot-long plastic basin. The pulse amplitude was 5 mA, and the duration was 0.5 msec. The baseline before the pulse begins is flat. When the pulse begins, the trace initially goes straight down about 500 mV. Then it decreases its rate of change—the downward slanted line—until the pulse stops 0.5 msec after it began. This is the polarization effect. When the pulse stops, the voltage starts back up toward zero in a straight upward line for about 500 mV, after which it very gradually slopes upward toward the baseline. This represents the very slow decay of the Helmholtz capacitance voltage. Eight milliseconds after the stimulus ends, the decay voltage existing between the patch electrodes is still 20% of its maximum below-baseline value. In considering possible causes of refibrillation, one wonders how large and persistent the Helmholtz decay voltage and current would be if a defibrillator-level shock rather than a pacemaker-stimulus-level pulse were applied.

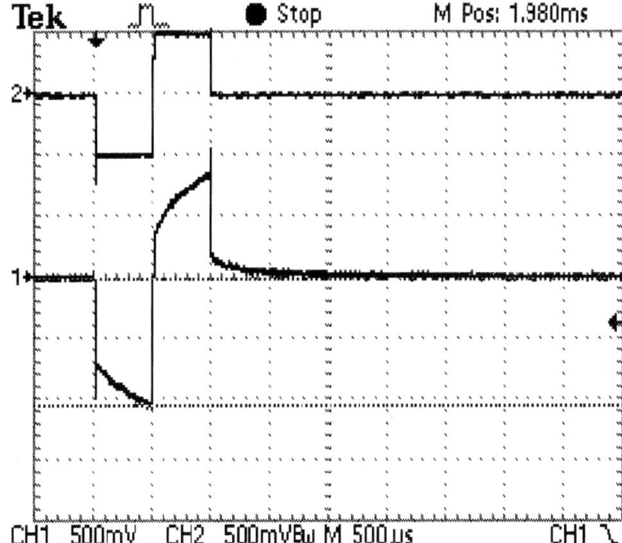

Figure 1-17. Effect of near-zero delay between phases on voltage response to biphasic constant-current pulse. This plot was made under the same conditions as Figure 1-16, except that the delay between phases was decreased from 1.5 msec to approximately 10 msec. When the stimulus is biphasic with almost no delay between phases, the slow decay of voltage at the end of the first phase is aborted by the beginning of the second, opposite-polarity, phase.

Constant 5 Ma, ½ Msec, Monophasic Pulse

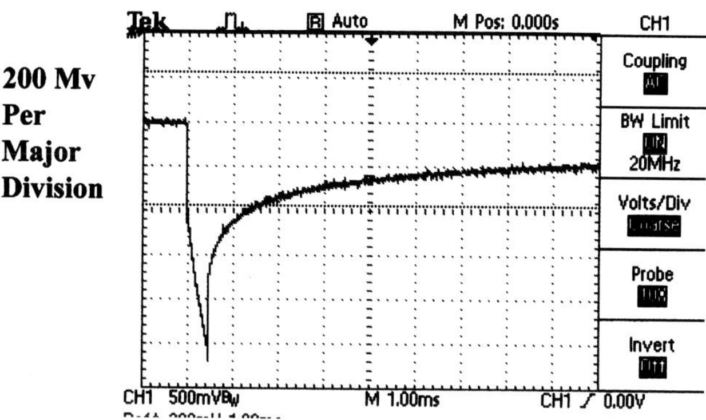

Figure 1-18. Voltage response to uniphasic constant-current pulse applied across defibrillator epicardial patch electrodes in saline. Here, one large and one small epicardial patch electrode were placed at opposite ends of a foot-long plastic basin filled with normal saline. The pulse amplitude was 5 mA, and the duration was 0.5 msec. The baseline before the pulse begins is flat. When the negative-going constant-current pulse begins, the trace initially goes straight down about 500 mV. It then decreases its rate of change—the downward slanted line—until the pulse stops 0.5 msec after it began. The slant is a polarization effect, caused by the charging of the Helmholtz capacitor at each electrode-electrolyte interface. When the pulse stops, the voltage starts back up toward zero in a straight upward line for about 500 mV, after which it very gradually slopes upward toward the baseline. Note how gradually the postpulse voltage decay persists.

When a *biphasic* constant-current pacemaker magnitude pulse with a 10-μsec delay between phases is used with the defibrillator patch electrodes under the same conditions, the voltage returns almost immediately to baseline (Fig. 1-19). The lack of a slow Helmholtz capacitance voltage decay suggests (but does not prove) possible partial causes for two physiologic observations. The first was Lilly's observation that biphasic (compared with uniphasic) stimulation resulted in electrodes functioning longer for chronic stimulation of monkey brains.[114] Lilly attributed this finding to second-phase high-speed reversal of undesirable electrochemical reactions begun by the first phase. The second observation is familiar to all. It is that defibrillation thresholds are lower with biphasic shocks than with uniphasic shocks.

The practical point is that, because of Helmholtz effects, electrical activity continues to occur at and near the electrode after the stimulating pulse stops. Details of the activity depend on whether the stimulus has been uniphasic or biphasic, what the delay time between phases is, what the characteristics of each phase are, and what the pulse generator output circuit does when the stimulus stops (i.e., does it go to high impedance, go to low impedance, or emit a recharge pulse). The electrical activity also depends on the characteristics of the electrode (e.g., geometric versus electrical surface area) the ionic solution, and the tissue.

VOLTAGE RESPONSE VERSUS TIME

DEFIBRILLATOR PATCH ELECTRODES in SALINE

Constant 5 Ma, Biphasic ½ Msec per Phase, Pulse

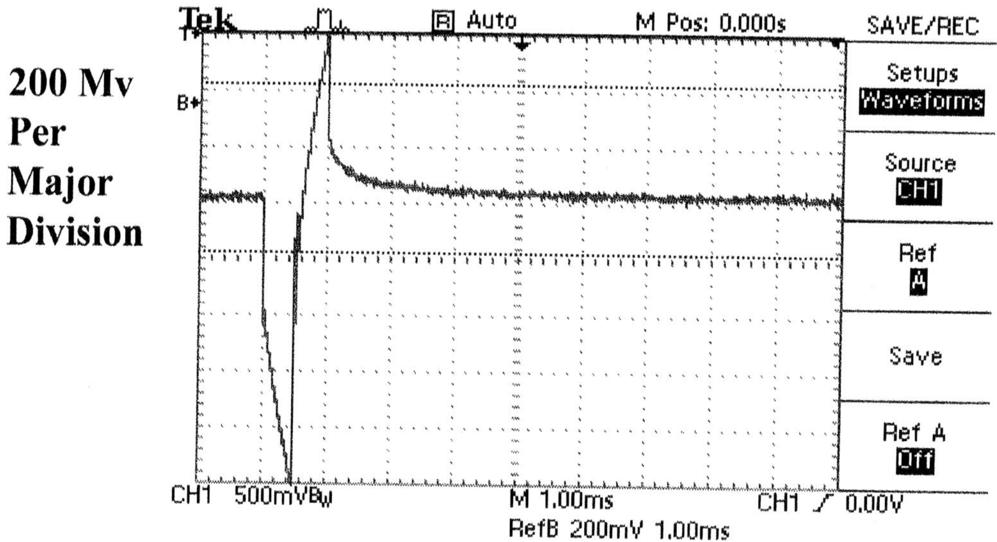

1.0 Msec per Major Division

Figure 1-19. Effect of changing from a uniphasic to a biphasic pulse applied to defibrillator electrodes in saline. Here the conditions are the same as described for Figure 1-18, except that the biphasic constant-current pulse now has only approximately 10 msec between phases. With this minimal time between phases, the postpulse Helmholtz capacitance decay voltage is almost eliminated.

Capacitance, Polarization, and True Impedance

When using an ordinary PSA, one thinks of impedance as a voltage/current ratio. If reactance is present, as it is at a pacemaker or defibrillator electrode because of the Helmholtz capacitance effect, the voltage/current ratio as seen on the PSA can be deceptive (see the section on biventricular pacing). Because of the charging and discharging of the Helmholtz capacitor at the electrode-electrolyte interface, the applied voltage and resultant current are not linearly related. Therefore, the circuit is reactive, and impedance rather than resistance is the correct measure of opposition to current flow (see earlier discussion).

There are practical problems in easily measuring true impedance during implantation procedures. In most clinical circumstances, however, the voltage/current ratio provides a reasonable estimate of the load into which the pulse generator is working, which is one of the major factors determining current drawn from the battery.

Charge Grouping and Polarization

When an electrical stimulus is applied to the heart, the negatively charged cathode in contact with the myocardium attracts positively charged ions in the extracellular space. Likewise, the positively charged anode attracts negatively charged ions. This grouping phenomenon is known as *polarization.* The word *polarization* in this chapter has several meanings:

1. The grouping and subgrouping by charge sign of electrons in the metal, and of ions in the electrolyte, at and near pacemaker or defibrillator electrodes, resulting in the formation of two or more electrical charge layers and voltage gradients during the application of a pacemaker or defibrillator stimulus, and their subsequent decline after cessation of the stimulus.
2. The charge separation across a cell membrane, measurable as a voltage gradient between the inside and the outside of the cell.
3. The opposition to current flow within a battery, which results, when current is being drawn from the battery, in a decrease in the voltage available at its terminals.

The Capacitance Effect of the Helmholtz Double Layer

About 1879, Helmholtz suggested that a layer of ions (the inner Helmholtz layer) is attracted to the surface of a charged electrode and also that this layer is bounded on its nonelectrode side by a layer of oppositely charged ions (the outer Helmholtz layer) in the solution.[115] This interface acts as a capacitor. Helmholtz assumed for this model that no electron transfer reactions occur at the electrode and that the electrode environment is only an electrolyte. These (and more complicated charge redistributions) occur because of attraction and repulsion interactions between an electrode held at a given electric potential (e.g., 2 V negative during a 0.5-msec pacemaker pulse) and the ions and charged molecules in the interstitial fluid. The charge placed on the electrode forces, by electrostatic attraction, the accumulation of a polarized water layer and a second layer of hydrated, oppositely charged ions adjacent to the electrode surface. The oppositely charged ions come from the electrolyte. The interface at the electrode becomes an electrical double layer. This is in effect a charged capacitor.[116]

However, the actual interface is not a simple double layer. The Helmholtz model does not take into account other factors, such as absorption on the surface, thermal buffeting, and interaction between solvent dipole moments and the electrode. Models more complicated than the Helmholtz one include the Gouy-Chapman and the Gouy-Chapman-Stern.[117] These models have dissimilar shapes for the plot of electric potential variation with distance from the electrode. The layers have relatively high dielectric constants and form an interface that behaves electrically like a capacitor (C_c and C_a in Fig. 1-20). In a semiconductor or in localized regions of an electrolyte, an excess of positive or of negative charge may be present. If the excess is of positive charge carriers, the positive carriers are the majority carriers and the negative charge carriers are the minority carriers. If the excess is of negative charge carriers, then they are the majority carriers, and the positive charge carriers are the minority carriers.

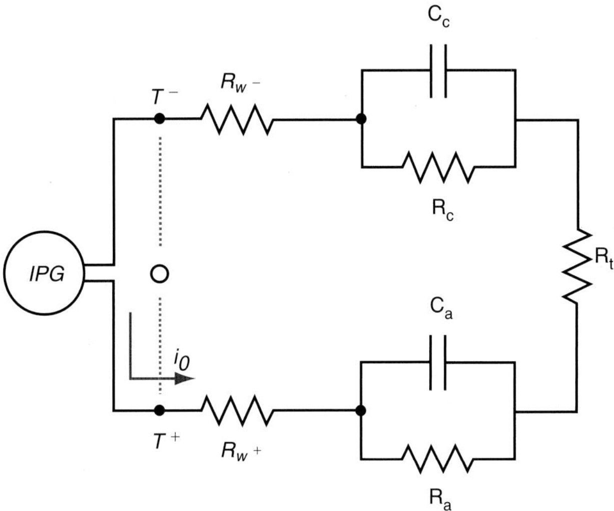

Figure 1-20. A simplified equivalent circuit for a cardiac pacemaker. T^- and T^+ are, respectively, the negative (cathode) and positive (anode) terminals of the pulse generator (in a unipolar device, T^+ is inside the can). R_W^- is the resistance of the conductor wire leading to the distal tip of the lead (cathode), whereas R_W^+ is that of the wire leading to the bipolar lead's proximal ring electrode or the unipolar pulse generator's can. R_t is the resistance of the tissue between the bipolar lead's two electrodes, or the lead tip to the pulse generator can in a unipolar system. R_c is the ohmic polarization of the cathode, whereas R_a is that of the bipolar anode or unipolar generator can. C_c is the capacitance of the cathode, and C_a is that of the anode (can). The equivalent circuit is the same for unipolar and bipolar systems, but the values for some of the components differ.

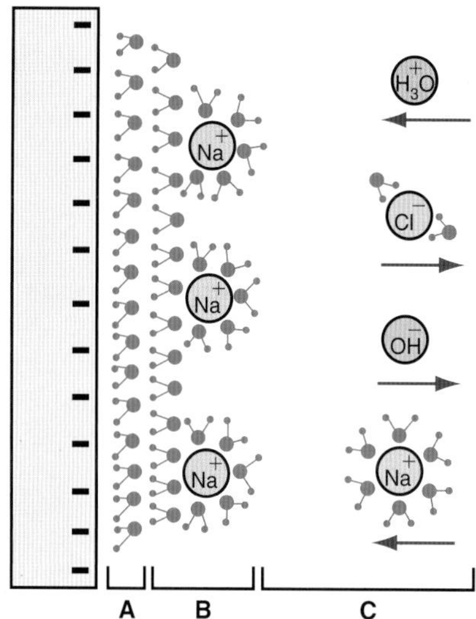

Figure 1-21. Hypothesized structure of the Helmholtz double layer. At the left is an uncharged cathodic electrode interface. When the electrode is charged, a layer of surface hydration develops (Region A). Region B contains a second, more loosely held hydration layer with hydrated ions. Based on electrostatic considerations, layer B has a high dielectric constant, approaching that of pure water. It has a thickness of less than 10 Å. Region C represents bulk solution. (From Stokes K, Bornzin G: The electrode-biointerface [stimulation]. In Barold SS [ed]: Modern Cardiac Pacing. Mt. Kisco, NY, Futura, p 63.)

The second layer of the double layer is formed of hydrated ions and more water (Fig.1-21). In physiologic electrolytes, the ions include Na^+ and Cl^- in major concentrations (majority carriers). Other ions present in lower concentrations (minority carriers) include hydronium (H_3O^+), hydroxyl (OH^-), and phosphate (HPO_4^{2-}).

The ions attracted to or repelled from the electrode during the electrical stimulation pulse make up a separation of charge in the tissue electrolyte. When the pacemaker pulse is applied as a negative voltage to the electrode, electrons accumulate in the electrode. Reversible reactions may form metal-oxide complexes on the surface of the electrode. A primary water layer forms on the electrode. Positive ions surrounded by water molecules—a water shell—make a secondary water layer. This accumulation of positive ions in the electrolyte near the electrode unbalances local electrolyte charge neutrality. Secondary ion rearrangements occur in great complexity, with several names for the various processes.

When the pacemaker pulse stops, the ions, being no longer attracted to or repelled from the electrode (depending on the polarity of the electrode and of the ions), are forced by their charges to rearrange themselves back toward their original, more electrically neutral positions (determined by random motion) in the electrolyte near the electrode. Ion rearrangement is not as fast as the transmission of an electric potential in a wire. The result is that, after a pacemaker or defibrillator pulse stops, the Helmholtz capacitor acts as if it were a temporary battery of declining voltage discharging itself into the tissue. (If, between pulses, the impedance across the output terminals of the pulse generator is low, the Helmholtz capacitor will also in part discharge back through the leads, as shown in Fig. 1-13.) The decaying voltage gradient in the tissue persists long enough to be detected by a pacemaker or defibrillator and may be great enough to interfere with sensing in autocapture devices in some situations. Other things being equal, the voltage decay duration is greater and the polarization voltage is less when the electrode surface area is great versus small.

Electrode-Electrolyte Interface Processes

At equilibrium, an electrode in a solution will have, relative to a reference electrode, a potential that depends on the composition of the electrode, the composition of the solution, and other factors such as temperature.[118] When a pacemaker pulse is applied, the electrode is forced to a different electric potential. This new potential forces ion flow to occur in the vicinity of the electrode. Ion secondary rearrangements occur distally. The net ion drift near the electrode is in a direction that will produce a new equilibrium, a balance of charge across the interface.

At least two types of processes involving ion flow occur at the interface between a pacemaker or defibrillator electrode and tissue. One is oxidation-reduction reactions, which can be reversible or irreversible. They involve electron movement across the interface and constitute faradic current. The second process, nonfaradic current, occurs without transfer of electrons across the interface. It consists of electron flow in or out of the electrode itself and a flow of ions in various layers or "clouds" toward or away from the interface. This nonfaradic process is similar to charging or discharging an electrical capacitor, but at an electrode in electrolyte there is directed electron drift in or out of the electrode and directed ion drift within the electrolyte. The ion flow and the electron flow each constitute an electric current, yet no charge crosses the interface.

Away from the electrode in the body of the electrolyte, the electric potential gradient causes ions to move away from or toward the electrode region, depending on their charge. Ion mobility characteristics, concentration gradients, and temperature gradients also affect ion movement. In the heart the process is more complicated than in an electrolyte solution alone, because of the anisotropic properties of the extracellular and intracellular domains.

Faradic Current Flow

Faradic current is so named because Michael Faraday (1791-1867) quantitatively described the effects of electric current through an electrolyte in 1834, stating that "the chemical decomposing action of a current is constant for a constant quantity of electricity, notwithstanding the greatest variations in its sources, in its intensity, in the size of the electrodes used, in the nature of the conductors (or nonconductors) through which it is passed, or in other circumstances."[119]

If one thinks of an electrode-electrolyte interface as resembling a variable resistor and variable capacitor in parallel, faradic current flow would be flow—electron transfer—through the resistor. Whether electron transfer across the interface occurs depends on the properties of the electrode and the electrolyte and on the applied electric pulse characteristics. The current crossing the interface when one is charging a battery is faradic current produced by oxidation-reduction reactions.

Capacitive Current Flow

This mechanism is not a transfer of electrons in one direction or the other across the electrode-electrolyte interface. It is the accumulation of charge on the electrode at the interface balanced by a corresponding accumulation of charge of net opposite sign in the electrolyte adjacent to the interface. Charge flows in the lead, and in the electrolyte, but not across the interface. The flow of charge into the capacitor is measurable current in a pacemaker lead, even though in a perfect capacitor no charge crosses the interface.

The resulting arrangement of ion groupings at and near the electrode-electrolyte interface can be very complicated.[120] The accumulation of charge separated by charge sign at the interface defines the Helmholtz double-layer capacitance.[121] Energy is stored as an electrostatic field that exists between the positive and negative charge layers.

When a pacemaker pulse is applied to an electrode in the heart, the charge movement into or out of the Helmholtz capacitance—both electrons in the electrode and ions in the electrolyte—is an electric current even though no charged particle necessarily crosses the interface. (See Fig. 1-13 and the previous discussion of capacitance and polarization.)

At a pacemaker electrode, the capacitance is not constant. It is dependent on current density, electrolyte composition, and the area and other surface characteristics (e.g., fractal surface) of the electrode material.[122]

Because of the minute distances separating positive and negative charge layers at an electrode in electrolyte, the capacitance is high, ranging from about 0.2 to 40 mF/mm^2 of geometric area of the electrode.[123] The fractal-surface electrode has a much higher capacitance than a smooth-surface electrode.

The equation $i_t = C\dfrac{dv}{dt}$ states that the current i entering or leaving a capacitor at time t varies directly as the magnitude of the capacitance (C, measured in farads) multiplied by the rate of change of the voltage difference across the capacitor. Because a constant-voltage pulse is nominally a rectangular wave, its rate of change is small except when the pulse is being turned on or off. Therefore, current flow into the capacitor (i.e., into the pacemaker electrode-electrolyte interface Helmholtz capacitance) occurs very rapidly during the leading edge of a nominal constant-voltage pacemaker pulse. Then, as charge accumulates at the electrode-electrolyte interface, the accumulating negative charge collection at the electrode surface slows the rate of further accumulation. It does so because the accumulating negative charge opposes the inflow of additional negative charge. Finally, unless the pacemaker output voltage were to be raised during the pulse, no further accumulation can occur. The voltage across the capacitor becomes equal and opposite to the constant-voltage pulse that had been driving current flow into the lead. Note that the Helmholtz capacitance is influenced by the current density at the electrode, the types and numbers of ions in the electrolyte, the material and surface of the electrode, the temperature, and other factors.

Relation of Electrode-Tissue Interface Capacitance to Polarization Voltage

Note that in the expression $v_t = \dfrac{1}{C}\int_0^t i_t dt$, describing the voltage that occurs across a capacitor when current flows into it, the developed voltage varies inversely as the capacitance (C, measured in farads). If both sides of this equation are multiplied by C, the equation becomes $Cv_t = \int_0^t i_t dt$. The amount Q_t of stored charge at any time t is $\int_0^t i_t dt$. Therefore, $Cv_t = Q_t$, and $v_t = Q_t/C$. That is, for a given amount of charge put into the defibrillator or pacemaker electrode, the voltage across the interface will be decreased if the surface area of the electrode (and therefore the capacitance) is increased. This voltage is the polarization voltage. During its decay time after the stimulation pulse has ended, the polarization voltage can interfere with autosensing of capture.

For a given stimulus voltage, the greater the polarization voltage at the electrode-tissue interface, the lesser the voltage gradient elsewhere in the tissue between the cathode and the anode. A fractal-surface electrode, with its high capacitance,[123] has, for the same charge flow in and out, a lesser potential difference across the electrode-electrolyte interface than a smooth electrode does. Therefore, the fractal surface is preferred.

No electrode is completely free of charge transfer across the interface between its surface and the electrolyte. Some current flow across the interface does occur by means of electron transfer through oxidation-reduction reactions. At a pacemaker electrode, these reactions, if reversible, may be desirable. Irreversible charge transfer results either in corrosion or in electrochemical reactions in the tissue.

For present-day implantable pacemaker electrodes, if the pulse duration is short, or if the pulse is biphasic with a sufficiently short time between balanced phases, the charge transfer reactions do not normally result in gross corrosion or gross tissue changes. Therefore, those reactions that do occur must be largely reversible. John Lilly, working in Britton Chance's laboratory at the Johnson Foundation of the University of Pennsylvania, used electrodes embedded in monkeys' brains for chronic stimulation studies. The electrodes functioned much longer when the stimulation waveform was biphasic than when it was uniphasic.[114] Lilly attributed this improvement to immediate reversal of electrolytic reactions at the tissue-electrode interface by the second phase of each biphasic pulse. He made biphasic pulses simply by differentiating monophasic rectangular wave pulses.

Ideal and Non-Ideal Electrodes

To avoid corrosion and deposition of toxic products in the adjacent tissue, electrodes that undergo irreversible reactions only minutely are highly desirable for pacemakers and defibrillators.

Michael Faraday worked out the quantitative relationship between electrode-electrolyte chemical changes and the total amount of charge passed through the electrode into the electrolyte.[124,*] Electrodes that under the conditions of use produce irreversible electrochemical reactions by means of these faradic currents entering or leaving the electrolyte are *non-ideal* electrodes.

Equal back-and-forth transfer of electrons from an inert electrode to an electrolyte occurs naturally and is an equilibrium situation. When an external voltage is applied, electrodes that then do not produce irreversible chemical reactions are so-called *ideal electrodes*. Although metal oxide films form on the electrodes, occurrence of other oxidation-reduction reactions and corresponding electron transfer through the interface do not occur or are minimal in ideal electrodes. In this sense, no real electrode can be completely ideal in all circumstances. If the magnitude and duration of polarization secondary to occurrence of the electric pulse is brief, electrochemical reactions occurring at the electrode may reverse. If the charge redistribution time is long, the effects of charge redistribution on the electrode and on the tissue may become irreversible.

When biphasic pulses are used, minimal postpulse polarization persists, provided the time between phases is in the microsecond range. If the time between phases is increased into the millisecond range, the duration and amplitude of persisting polarization increases (see Figures 1-16 through 1-19).

Electrode Polarization in More Detail

When a negative-going pacemaker pulse is turned on, electrons are forced into the electrode. Then, in response to the electric field, nearby positive ions rapidly collect near the electrode surface. The number of positive ions nearby is insufficient to neutralize the charge. Nearby negatively charged ions are forced away from the electrode. Because the approach of nearby positive ions and the repulsion of nearby negative ions are insufficient to balance the electrons accumulating on the electrode, more positive ions diffuse into the region from relatively remote areas,[125] and more remote negative ions are pushed away. As time during the pulse increases, electrons already at the interface become balanced by the net positive charge of nearby ions collecting at the interface. A greater negative voltage on the electrode is then necessary to force more electrons into the electrode. Because the voltage rise is dependent on the concentration of majority and minority carriers, this phenomenon is known as concentration polarization (CP).[126]

A pacemaker catheter pacing a fibroblast cell culture shows this effect (see Figures 1-13 and 1-15). The plots show the time course of a constant-current pulse introduced through a permanent pacing catheter into a fibroblast cell culture. Figure 1-15A shows that, when the 0.5-msec constant-current pulse is stopped and the connections at the pulse generator are electronically shorted, the voltage between the lead wires go to zero. However, current (as in Fig. 1-13) began flowing in the reverse direction. This is the effect of the ions rearranging themselves back to electrical neutrality when the pulse is turned off. The effect is that of a capacitor—the Helmholtz capacitance—discharging partially back into the circuit that charged it. The magnitude and duration of the reverse current flow are impressive.

The pacemaker pulse generator, in its sensing, looks at the voltage between bipolar electrodes or between a unipolar electrode and the pulse generator surface. When the pulse stops, the Helmholtz capacitance begins to discharge. For current and voltage in the leads during this pulse generator "diastole," at least three situations could exist. In the first situation, the pulse generator has a very high impedance between its two output poles during the time between pulses. In that case, most of the Helmholtz capacitance charge dissipates within the electrolyte and at the electrode-electrolyte interface through reversible oxidation-reduction reactions. The second situation is that the pulse generator has a very low impedance during the time between pulses. In that case, the Helmholtz capacitance charge dissipates in part by forcing current flow in the reverse direction through the leads. The third situation is that, when the pacemaker negative-going pulse stops, the pulse generator within microseconds emits a second pulse of polarity opposite to the first. This actively discharges the Helmholtz capacitance, and undesirable electrochemical reactions occurring at the electrode and in the tissue may be aborted or reversed.

If biphasic pacing were to be used chronically as a possible means of reducing electrochemical problems at the electrodes, there would be a practical problem of higher threshold energy requirements. Thresholds are greater with biphasic than with uniphasic pacing at normal stimulus durations.[127] The stimulus duration for biphasic pacing is here defined as the sum of the equal durations of the negative and positive phases. If one defines the stimulus duration as the duration of only the first phase, the biphasic pacing threshold in isolated, perfused rabbit hearts is approximately the same as it is for uniphasic pacing (Benser M, Shepard

*Racker states that when Gladstone, on seeing Faraday demonstrate his experiments, asked Faraday what electricity was good for, Faraday replied, "One day, sir, you may tax it." (Racker E: A New Look at Mechanisms in Bioenergetics. New York, Academic Press, 1976, Preface.)

RB, unpublished data, personal communication, May 1999.) If biphasic pacing were to be used with non-steroid-eluting electrodes, as Lilly did to reduce electrode problems, the battery life of the implanted pulse generator would be shortened because of the increase in energy requirements necessary for stimulation.

Concentration Polarization and Ohmic Polarization

As a result of the electric potential gradients produced by the pulse near the electrode, local accumulations and depletions of ionic species occur. In a manner dependent on elapsed time, ion charge, ion mass, and other factors, ions in an electrolyte subject to an electric field become grouped by charge sign. This grouping by charge sign is concentration polarization. Concentration polarization disappears as a slow decay of the potential difference between the charge grouping sites. This decay is illustrated in Figure 1-22. A biphasic constant-current pulse of 5-mA, with a duration of 0.5 msec per phase, is applied between two electrodes in cell culture solution. When the first phase ends, the slowness of the voltage decay back toward the zero level is a result of the time required for diffusion of the ion groupings by charge (concentration polarization) back toward a less-grouped, average electroneutral state. The second phase of the biphasic pulse abolishes in its upstroke this polarization voltage that has been decaying during the time between phases (see also Figures 1-18 and 1-19).

Ohmic polarization, on the other hand, is a potential difference between two sites that is associated with energy loss in current flow between the sites. A constant-current pulse that is producing charge movement in the interstitial fluid is producing ohmic polarization. In ordinary electrical parlance, there is a voltage difference between the ends of the path *during current flow* because of path resistance.

Demonstration of Polarization at a Pacing Catheter Electrode

A culture of fibroblast cells was paced through a clinical cardiac bipolar pacing catheter (fibroblast cell culture pacing in transplantation biochemistry laboratory courtesy of J. A. Thompson, Department of Surgery, University of Alabama at Birmingham). The laboratory pulse generator was set to produce constant-current pulses of 0.5-msec duration. The current and the resultant voltage waveforms are shown in Figure 1-15A. When the pulse starts, the current rises immediately to its set level. It then remains at that level for the duration of the pulse. The voltage response, as measured between the laboratory pulse generator output sockets (which internally connect after each biphasic pulse), is at first a rapid rise (ohmic polarization) followed by a slow, curved-slope rise due to opposite charge accumulations on each side of the electrode-electrolyte interface. This slow voltage increase represents charging of the electrode-electrolyte interface Helmholtz capacitor.

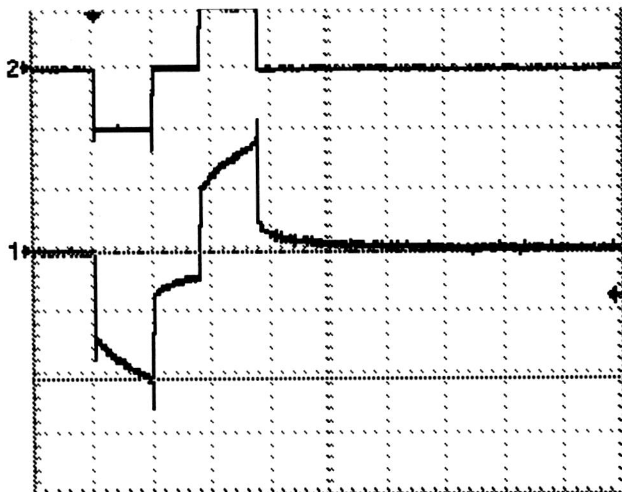

Figure 1-22. Application of a bipolar cardiac pacing catheter constant-current biphasic stimulus, showing the voltage response when the pulse generator has high impedance between phases. This is the same as Figure 1-17, except that the time between phases has been increased from about 10 msec to almost 500 msec. The consequence is that, at the end of the first phase, the voltage goes rapidly only about 65% of the way back to baseline and then begins a slow decline. That decline is interrupted by the 0.5-msec second phase. When the second phase ends, the Helmholtz capacitance effect is minimal with this combination of patches, electrolyte, and time between phases.

Energy Dissipation When a Pacemaker Pulse Is Applied

One way of looking at energy requirements for cardiac pacing is to calculate the energy dissipated from the beginning of one stimulus to the beginning of the next. Reactive components shift the timing between applied voltage and current flow so that current magnitude is no longer necessarily directly proportional to the voltage magnitude at that instant. If v is the instantaneous voltage across the electrode-electrolyte interface at time t during the course of the stimulus and i is the instantaneous current passing into the interface at the same time t, then the energy dissipation at the interface by time t in the stimulus cycle is $W_t = \int_0^t vidt$.

Tracking the voltage and current waveforms exactly across the interface itself is neither clinically practical nor necessary. More obtainable and useful is the energy dissipation around the whole circuit external to the pulse generator. The same equation applies, except that v is now the instantaneous voltage between the leads at the pulse generator, i is the current in the leads, and t begins with pulse onset and ends at the onset of the next pulse. Then W_t represents, over one stimulus cycle, the total energy dissipation around the whole circuit external to the pulse generator.

A question of interest is how much the energy dissipation obtained in this computationally accurate way, by using voltage and current waveforms, differs in various clinical situations from that obtained by using the PSA. The readout values of voltage, current, and stimulus duration can be multiplied to approximate the energy dissipation per pulse. In most situations, except during some biventricular pacing procedures (see later discussion), the differences are highly likely to be insignificant compared with other factors involved in choosing lead locations and pulse generator settings.

Optimizing Impedance for Minimum Battery Consumption

The effects of high impedance on the pacing system vary with the cause and location. The way in which the resistance is distributed in the system can produce markedly different effects, increasing or decreasing the efficiency of the stimulating pulse. To clarify these issues, one needs to examine the leads and the electrode-tissue interface impedance and conduction losses.

What is desirable for clinical use is an electrode that does not waste energy in mini-heat production or in undesirable chemical reactions and also has a low pacing threshold. This means that the electrode should have minimal energy loss in the lead wires, minimal energy loss in moving ions in the electrolyte during charge and discharge of the Helmholtz capacitance, and high current density at the electrode, so that depolarization of the membranes of nearby myocytes can be accomplished with less lead current than otherwise.

All of these factors influence the impedance as seen at the pulse generator. Note that fibrous tissue formation around an electrode does not necessarily increase the impedance but does increase the pacing threshold. (For further discussion of these issues, see the section on clinical aspects of pacing.)

Impedance in the Extracellular Electrolyte

Warburg Impedance

In 1899, Warburg described as an impedance one of the effects of ion motion brought on by a voltage difference between two electrodes placed in an electrolyte. The *Warburg impedance* is an effect of ion diffusion activity under the influence of the potential gradient at the interface between electrode and electrolyte. It is said that "a Warburg impedance can be difficult to recognize because it is nearly always associated with a charge transfer resistance and a double layer capacitance."[128] The Helmholtz capacitance concept is based on the separation of charges in the electrode from charges in the electrolyte at angstrom-dimension levels. Warburg developed his impedance concept to model the effects of diffusion. When a sine-wave voltage is applied across an electrolyte, this impedance manifests itself as a 45-degree phase shift between the voltage and the current if the current density is infinitely low. The Warburg impedance magnitude becomes small compared with other impedances at the electrode-electrolyte interface as the electrolyte concentration is made greater and as the stimulation frequency increases.[129]

Ovadia and Zavitz[130] made an impedance spectroscopy study of the interface between a platinum electrode and a metabolically active perfused living heart. Three impedance spectral components were found: the Warburg impedance, a thin-film impedance, and a single high-angle constant-phase impedance. The impedance spectrum was not single-valued and was not stable in time. A drawing (modified from Rodman[131]) showing one equivalent circuit representation of an electrode-electrolyte interface, including the Helmholtz capacitance and the Warburg impedance, is shown in Figure 1-14.

The Helmholtz capacitance–Warburg impedance effects can become especially important in explaining some of the threshold measurements and seeming contradictions that can be found during biventricular pacing procedures.[5,132] This is discussed further in the section on biventricular pacing.

Capacitance and Electric Potential Gradients Related to Membrane Depolarization in Pacing and Defibrillation

The cell membrane does charge and discharge somewhat like a nonlinear capacitor. Ions under both electric gradient and biochemical-signaling control traverse the membrane as if it were both a variable and a highly ion species–selective resistor connected in parallel with a variable capacitor. When a negative-going pacemaker stimulus reaches the membrane, the stimulus reverses the voltage gradient across the membrane, beginning processes that in effect discharge the capacitor. Krassowska and Neu[133] pointed out that the response of the cell to an external field is a two-stage process. The initial polarization proceeds with the cellular time constant (magnitude <1 μsec). The actual change of physiologic state proceeds with the membrane time constant (several milliseconds).[133] The membrane resistance changes as ion channels open and close (see Fig. 1-2). The membrane capacitance may vary with ion concentrations and with stimulating voltage and frequency.[134] Membrane capacitance and resistance determine the membrane time constant.

An ordinary pacemaker stimulus can reverse the membrane potential to threshold levels only locally. The voltage gradient produced in the tissue by a pacemaker electrode decreases to below-threshold values with distance from the electrode. In order to depolarize much more myocardium at once than a pacemaker does, a defibrillator electrode must have a much greater voltage gradient between its electrodes. To initiate fibrillation during the vulnerable period or to defibrillate, an extracellular electric field of approximately 6 V/cm in a large volume of tissue is required, whereas for pacing a local electric field of only about 1 V/cm in a small volume is necessary. Ideker and coworkers[55] noted that, because the potential gradient decreases rapidly with distance from the stimulating electrode, a current about 40 times greater than the diastolic pacing threshold is required to generate an electric field of 6 V/cm approximately 1 cm from the stimulating electrode. To generate the 6 V/cm field over the entire ventricular myocardium, a current thousands of times greater than the low milliampere level necessary for pacing is required.

In thinking of the difference in voltage and current requirements for pacing and for defibrillation, one can use a lumped and distributed systems analogy. A line of cars is stopped at a traffic light. When the light changes from red to green, the front car moves. That prompts the next car to move. The motion propagates back down the line of cars in the manner of a string of myocytes undergoing sequential depolarization, or like a line of upright dominos falling over one after the other, each domino pushing over the next one. That is an analogy for pacing. Defibrillation is like having all the cars connected by a big iron rod. Much force would be required to move the whole string of cars at once, even though the force required for each individual car is relatively little. Similarly, to depolarize most of the ventricles at once, a very large voltage is needed to obtain the small transmembrane voltage gradient reversal that is required at each distant myocyte.

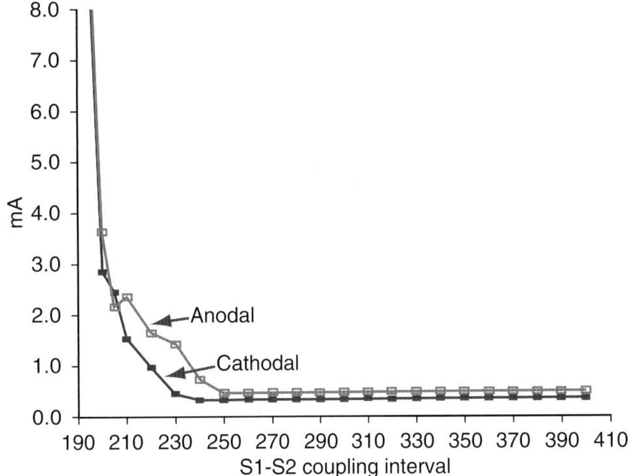

Figure 1-23. Anodal and cathodal ventricular strength-interval curves are demonstrated in a patient with atrioventricular block, using unipolar constant-current stimuli. The anodal threshold is slightly higher than the cathodal threshold at coupling intervals greater than 250 msec. At coupling intervals of less than 210 msec, the anodal threshold is about equal to the cathodal threshold. In some patients, the anodal threshold may not decrease ("dip") to a value that is lower than the cathodal threshold.

Cathodal and Anodal Stimulation, Constant Voltage, Constant Current, Monophasic and Biphasic Stimulation

Anodal and Cathodal Stimulation

Generally speaking, anodal stimulation is associated with properties that are less desirable than those of cathodal stimulation. If the stimulating electrode is a unipolar cathode, the strength-interval curve has a shape that is similar to a strength-duration curve. The shape of the typical anodal strength-interval curve is somewhat different from that of a cathodal curve (Fig. 1-23). Given equal-sized electrodes, the anodal stimulation threshold is generally somewhat greater than that for cathodal stimulation at long coupling intervals. With progressively more premature coupling intervals, there is a dip in the anodal curve to threshold values lower than those of the cathodal curve. At still more premature coupling intervals, the anodal curve rises steeply (as observed with cathodal stimulation).[135] The "dip" phenomenon is not always seen.[136] If the electrodes of a bipolar lead are of equal size, or if the anode is smaller than the cathode, it is possible to stimulate earlier in the cardiac cycle (in the relative refractory period) than with unipolar cathodal stimulation. This may occur because the threshold for anodal stimulation with electrodes of equal size is lower than that for cathodal stimulation in the strength-interval curve at shorter pulse widths.[135,136]

That anodal stimulation can generate tachyarrhythmias in ischemic or electrolyte unbalanced hearts is well documented.[137-140] This is one of several reasons that implantable bipolar leads are designed with considerably larger anodes than cathodes. In fact, it is commonly believed that the bipolar anode needs to be large enough that anodal stimulation is prevented. It is unlikely that this actually prevents anodal stimulation, however, because most pulse generators are set at outputs much higher than threshold. Even a 50-mm^2 anode probably can reach threshold at a stimulus intensity well below 5 V and 0.5 msec. It is likely that delivery of the stimulation pulse with many bipolar leads at times actually results in capture of the myocardium at both the cathode and the anode. Therefore, there is probably more to the size relationship between cathode and anode than is known. Many newer bipolar leads have smaller anodes because the cathodes are smaller. The anode/cathode ratio should be maintained, and the designs should be supported with strength-interval tests.

Bipolar pacing with equal-sized electrodes has been common in temporary pacing and in implanted epicardial systems (in which two unipolar leads are often used for bipolar pacing). The clinician should keep in mind the arrhythmogenic possibilities of such combinations in addition to their occasional advantages. For example, if two epicardial leads have been used in the past for bipolar pacing, with one electrode on the right ventricle and the other at an easily available site on the left, the hemodynamic result compared with unipolar pacing could have been better or worse. The sequences of contraction of the left ventricle periphery, septum, and right ventricle are hemodynamically important.

Another reason that anodes should be relatively large is to preclude unacceptable corrosion rates. Platinum, for example, does not corrode under the cathodic current densities used in pacing, but anodic potentials can cause corrosion. To preclude significant corrosion, the proximal electrode (anode) of a transvenous bipolar pacing lead is made large enough to ensure that current density is low in that electrode. Careful examinations of explanted platinum polished distal tips (cathodes) have often revealed rough surfaces that are the result of corrosion.

One explanation for the occurrence of corrosion at that the distal tip electrode is that it is a cathode only during the *stimulation* pulse. Some pulse generators also have a fast recharge pulse immediately after the stimulus to neutralize the afterpotential. Because the polarity of the fast recharge is then reversed, this portion of the pulse is actually anodal. Therefore, as "cathode" size decreases, current density increases and corrosion can rise to eventually unacceptable levels. Nonetheless, excellent canine performance has been reported with electrodes as small as 0.6 mm^2 in geometric surface area.[141] If the electrode is porous or fractal, the surface area of the electrolyte interface is actually large despite the small volume encompassed by the geometric surface. This can reduce current density and interface voltage at the electrode-electrolyte interface to a level below that required for corrosion by the fast-recharge pulse.

Unipolar and Bipolar Stimulation

All pacing systems require both a cathodal and an anodal electrode to complete the electric circuit from the pulse generator to, through, and from the myocardium back to the pulse generator. Therefore, all pacemakers are bipolar with respect to the body but not with respect to the heart. Ordinary terminology defines a bipolar system as one that has two electrodes in contact with myocardium. A unipolar system has only one electrode in contact with myocardium. The effects of unipolar and bipolar configurations on sensing are profound and are covered in Chapter 2. The engineering aspects are equally important and are discussed in Chapter 3.

In an ordinary unipolar pacing system, one electrode—the cathode—is in contact with myocardium. The metal case of the pulse generator is the anode. Bipolar leads may have higher stimulation thresholds than unipolar leads if the two electrodes are of equal size. In this case, the output voltage delivered by the pulse generator is divided equally between the two electrodes, causing the measured threshold to be higher. The voltage required to force threshold current through two small electrodes is greater than that required for one small electrode. By making the cathode relatively small and the anode relatively large, the overall impedance can be kept at about the same value as for the cathode alone. The threshold current can be delivered with little increase in the driving voltage. Making the anode large makes it a relatively poor stimulating electrode, thereby reducing the arrhythmogenic potential of anodal stimulation, compared with a bipolar lead with equal-sized electrodes.

To produce bipolar thresholds that are statistically equivalent to unipolar leads, the anode must be at least three times larger than the cathode.[142] It has become standard practice in the design of pacing leads to ensure that the anode area is at least 4.5 times larger than the geometric surface area of the cathode.

Bipolar electrode spacing can also be important, especially for sensing (see Chapter 2). It is generally accepted, for example, that as the electrodes are moved closer together, the signal-to-noise ratio, resistance to crosstalk, and median frequency of the sensed signal increase, whereas signal amplitude may decrease. If the spacing is too close, transvenous electrode pairs can have high stimulation thresholds, because current can be shunted between the two electrodes, producing a partial short circuit. In his classic thesis, De Caprio[143] determined that the optimal bipolar spacing (for sensing) was about 8 mm.

Constant-Current Versus Constant-Voltage Stimulation

A constant-current generator delivers a current pulse that is rectangular in shape. That is, the trailing edge (I_{te}) of the pulse equals the leading-edge (I_{le}) current in amplitude and the pulse is flat on top. The current delivered by a constant-current pulse generator is independent of pacing impedance to the limits of the power source (Fig. 1-24). If impedance decreases, the pulse generator output voltage automatically decreases to keep the

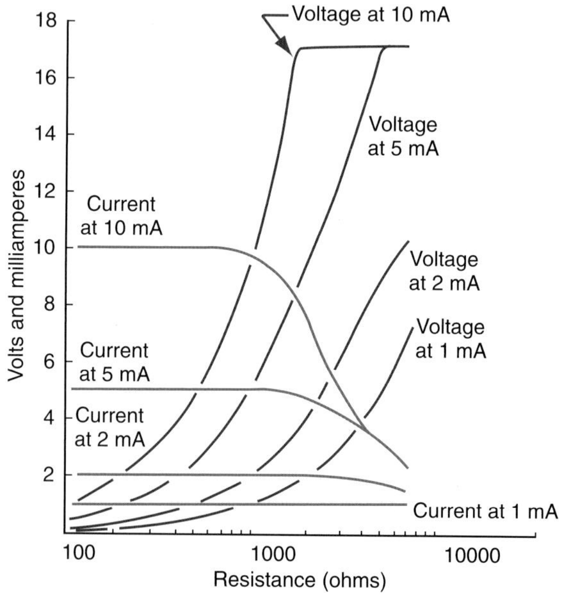

Figure 1-24. The effects of pacing impedance on constant-current leading-edge waveform amplitudes using a Medtronic Model 5880A external pulse generator. Current is independent of impedance until the battery is "saturated." This occurs when the voltage cannot increase any more to keep the current constant. (From Barold SS, Winner JA: Techniques and significance of threshold measurement for cardiac pacing. Chest 70:760, 1976.)

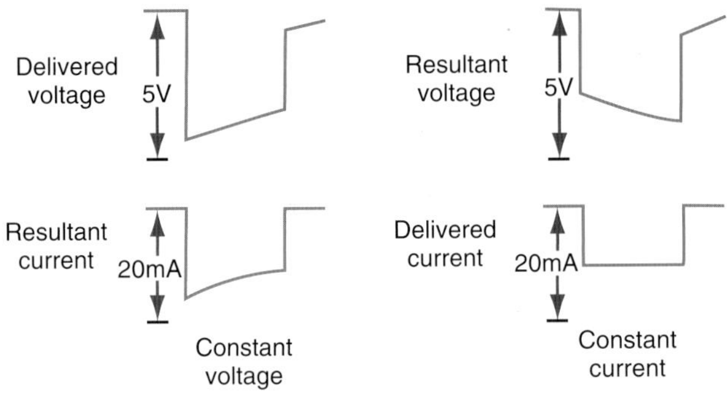

Figure 1-25. Voltage and current waveforms from a capacitively coupled, constant-voltage implantable pulse generator, the Medtronic Model 7000A (left), *and the constant-current mode output of an external research stimulator, Medtronic Model 1356* (right). *A unipolar lead with a polished platinum, 8-mm² ring-tip is used in conjunction with a 900-mm² titanium anode in 0.18% NaCl solution. The voltage across the lead is measured against a 100-mm² Ag/AgCl electrode to eliminate the anode's polarization from the waveform. (From Stokes K, Bornzin G: The electrode-biointerface [stimulation]. In Barold SS [ed]: Modern Cardiac Pacing. Mt. Kisco, NY, Futura 1985, pp 33-78.)*

current constant. In the presence of a high-resistance circuit, such as one with a lead partial fracture, the limits of the power source can be reached. In this instance, the pulse generator does not generate enough voltage to maintain a preset level of current. The result is delivery of a lower current than is programmed.

Although, under normal operating conditions, the current waveform of a constant-current pulse generator is rectangular, the resultant voltage waveform is not. It would be rectangular if the circuit beyond the pulse generator were purely resistive. However, because of the reactance in the circuit, capacitive in nature at the electrode-electrolyte interface, the initial leading-edge voltage (V_{le}) rises rapidly then rises more slowly to a larger trailing-edge voltage (V_{te}), as shown in Figure 1-25. At the end of the pulse, an immediate drop in voltage equal to V_{le} is observed, followed by an exponential decay back to baseline. The voltage rise during the pulse (called the *overvoltage*) is caused by an increase in pacing impedance due to electrode polarization, and the afterpotential is caused by the gradual dissipation of that polarization.

Today, probably all implantable pulse generators are capacitively coupled devices of approximately constant voltage. Because the pulse generator output comes from a capacitor, the voltage delivered decreases as charge is delivered from the capacitor to the electrode in the heart. The fully charged capacitor in the output circuit of the pulse generator delivers a set leading-edge voltage (Fig. 1-26). This results in continuing charge transfer from the capacitor to the heart during the duration of the pulse. The difference in voltage at the beginning and end of the pulse is directly proportional to the amount of charge transferred out of the capacitor: $V_{le} - V_{te} = Q^*/C_{pg}$, in which V_{le} is the leading-edge voltage of the pulse, V_{te} is the trailing-edge voltage, Q^* is the amount of charge removed from the capacitor (measured in coulombs), and C_{pg} is the capacitance of the

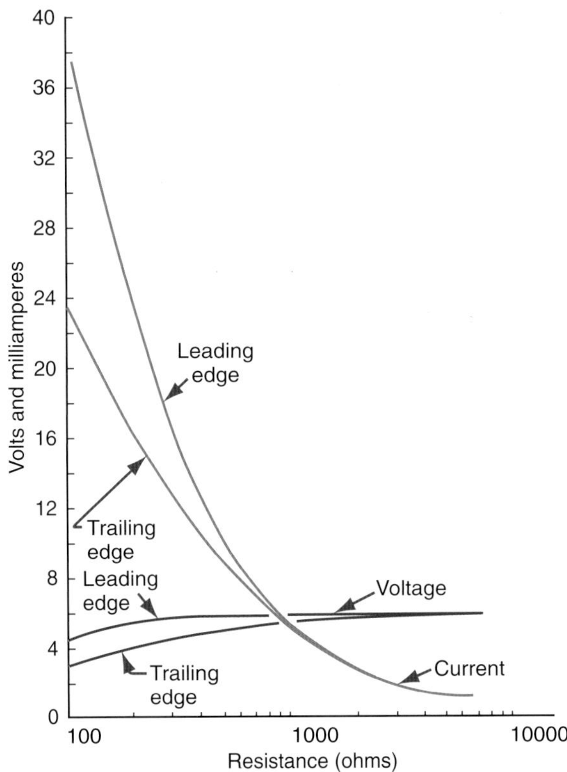

Figure 1-26. The effect of pacing impedance on capacitively coupled constant-voltage leading- and trailing-edge waveform amplitudes of a Medtronic Model 5950 pulse generator. The leading-edge voltage remains constant as a function of pacing impedance at values of 200 Ω or greater. The trailing edge of the voltage waveform changes slightly with impedance up to about 1000 Ω. Current falls significantly with increasing impedance. Any constant-voltage source may no longer be constant at very low pacing impedances, because the battery becomes unable to supply enough current to maintain a steady voltage. These very low impedance values are not likely to be encountered clinically in a properly functioning pacing system. (From Barold SS, Winner JA: Techniques and significance of threshold measurements for cardiac pacing. Chest 70:760, 1976.)

capacitor (measured in farads). Obviously, what is delivered through the lead wire to the pulse generator is not truly a constant-voltage pulse. The change in voltage over the pulse duration ("droop") is directly proportional to the total charge delivered (Q^*) during the pulse. For a given leading-edge voltage, the charge delivered will be less for a high-impedance lead than for a low-impedance lead. Also, the rate of charge delivery decreases as the pulse generator capacitor output voltage decreases. This means that the voltage droop line is not a straight line, although it may appear to be one when the impedance is very high.

The output voltage pulse becomes almost rectangular (i.e., $V_{le} - V_{te}$ is very small) when the impedance of the lead-heart-lead circuit into which the pulse generator capacitor is discharging is very high. If the impedance is low, the pulse waveform droop is steeper. If it is very low (<200 Ω), the capacitor may not be able to maintain even an approximate constant voltage.

Constant-current thresholds are related to constant-voltage thresholds by impedance. However, impedance is not constant during the pulse. It increases with polarization. Therefore, constant-current strength-duration curves can have slightly different shapes than constant-voltage curves. Most modern endocardial leads (such as those with iridium oxide, fractal, platinized platinum, or "activated" carbon surfaces) have relatively low-polarizing electrodes. These tend to have a lower-voltage rheobase and a somewhat higher chronaxie than highly-polarizing electrodes (Figs. 1-27 and 1-28).[144] In fact, a nonpolarizing electrode made from Ag/AgCl has the same shape strength-duration curve for constant-voltage stimulation as for constant-current stimulation (see Fig. 1-28). Therefore, polarization affects the value of the constant-voltage stimulus chronaxie. This accounts for most of the differences in shape between constant-voltage and constant-current strength-duration curves.

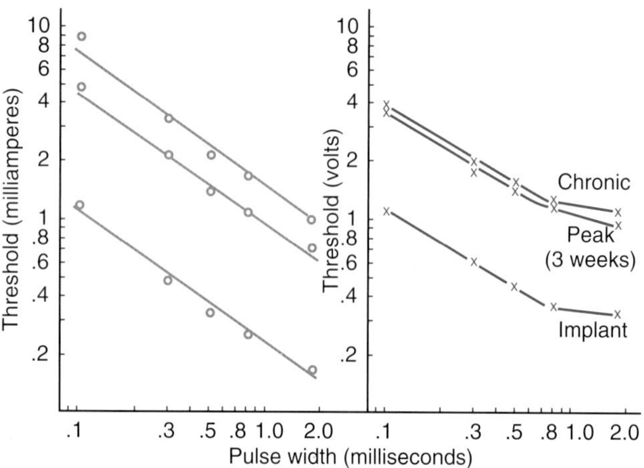

Figure 1-27. Logarithmic plots of canine ventricular constant-current (left) *and* constant-voltage (right) *strength-duration curves for a passively fixed, atraumatic, unipolar lead with an 8-mm² polished platinum ring-tip at various times after implementation (three different animals). (From Stokes K, Bornzin G: The electrode-biointerface [stimulation]. In Barold SS [ed]: Modern Cardiac Pacing. Mt. Kisco, NY, Futura 1985, p 41.)*

Monophasic and Biphasic Waveforms

A biphasic defibrillator stimulus, compared with a monophasic stimulus, has a lower voltage threshold for atrial and ventricular defibrillation.[145] Knisley and colleagues[127] studied the effect of biphasic and monophasic stimuli on excitation thresholds in rabbit and frog ventricles (Fig. 1-29). At very long pulse durations (20 msec), there was no difference in the stimulation threshold for monophasic versus biphasic waveforms. Therefore, reversal of waveform polarity during a long stimulus did not affect rheobase voltage. At shorter pulse durations (2.5 msec), the threshold voltage was significantly greater for biphasic than for monophasic waveforms. Therefore, the chronaxie pulse duration was significantly increased by an intrastimulus polarity reversal during shorter stimuli.

The energy requirements for pacing and defibrillation are different for monophasic stimuli compared with biphasic stimuli. The energy requirement for pacing is greater with biphasic stimuli. For defibrillation, however, biphasic stimuli decrease the energy requirements required.

Overlapping biphasic waveforms for pacing the atria in single-lead DDD pacing have been studied. One object was the reduction of atrial pacing thresholds and, consequently, reduction of the incidence of diaphragmatic stimulation compared with monophasic pacing under the same conditions.[146] This configuration uses unipolar anodal and cathodal pulses delivered to two closely spaced, floating atrial electrodes so that the

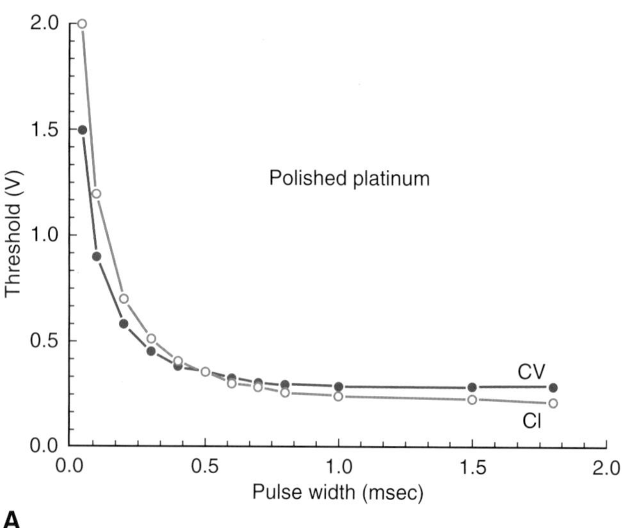

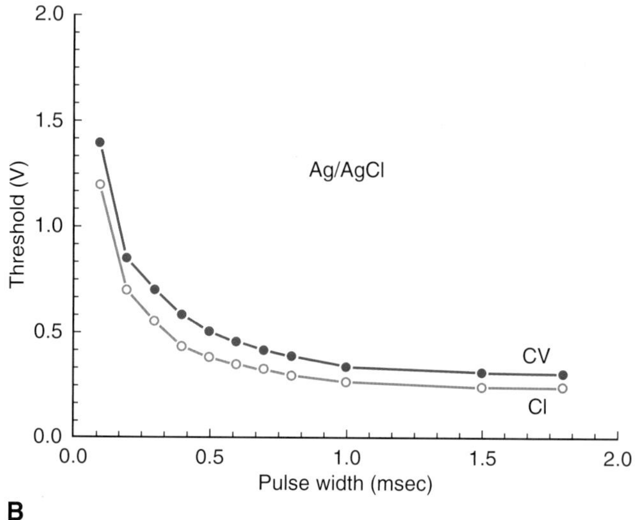

Figure 1-28. Constant-current (CI) compared with constant-voltage (CV) canine ventricular strength-duration curves for passively fixed, atraumatic electrodes. ***A,*** *Polarizing, 8-mm², polished ring-tip electrode.* ***B,*** *Nonpolarizing, Ag/AgCl, 8-mm² electrode.*

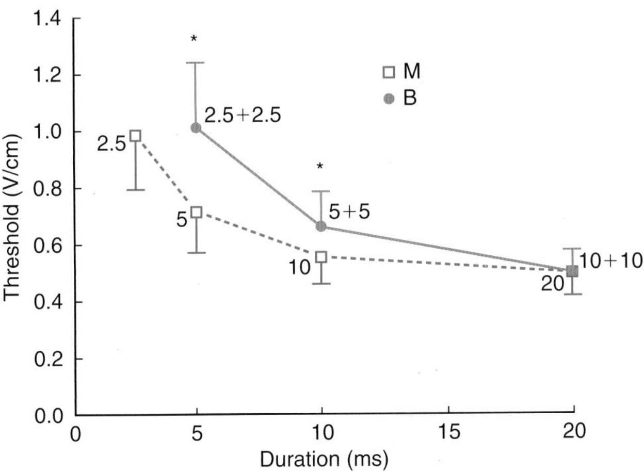

Figure 1-29. Monophasic (M) and biphasic (B) strength-duration curves obtained in strips of frog ventricular myocardium superfused with a solution containing 3 mmol/L of potassium. At a pulse duration of 20 msec, there is no significant difference in the rheobase threshold. Note that the M waveform produces a lower threshold than the B waveform at pulse durations of 5 msec and less. Therefore, although the M and B waveforms have a similar rheobase, chronaxie is less with M than with B stimuli. ms, millisecond. (From Knisley SB, Smith WM, Ideker RE: Effect of intrastimulus polarity reversal on electric field stimulation thresholds in frog and rabbit myocardium. J Cardiovasc Electrophysiol 3:239, 1992.)

pulses of opposite polarity overlap. Phrenic stimulation remains a problem.[147]

Design Features of Pacing Electrodes That Affect Performance

The performance of any pacing electrode is one of the major determinants of the pacing threshold. Stimulation characteristics of the electrode, together with the present and future states of the myocardium, determine the pacing margin of safety. This margin is the difference between the stimulus magnitude delivered by the pulse generator and the magnitude, now and in the future, required for myocardial stimulation. The electrodes normally are the major factor in determining the impedance into which the pulse generator delivers its stimuli. In addition, the electrodes, along with the pulse generator circuitry, determine the sensing characteristics of the pacing system.[148] Size, material, surface structure, and biologic response of the tissue to the particular electrode material are critical factors in electrode design. These factors are reviewed in the following sections, along with some effects of shape, spacing, fixation methods, and material.

Size of the Stimulating Electrode (Geometric Surface Area)

Stimulation threshold varies as an inverse function of the size or geometric surface area of the stimulating electrode.[43,149-151] Irnich[44] stated that, in theory, the chronic stimulation threshold of a spherical electrode should decrease as its radius (geometric surface area) decreases to a certain value. With further decreases below that value, the chronic threshold should begin to increase. Therefore, the electric field strength (E) necessary for stimulation is a nonlinear function of the electrode radius r and of the potential (V) applied to a spherical electrode.

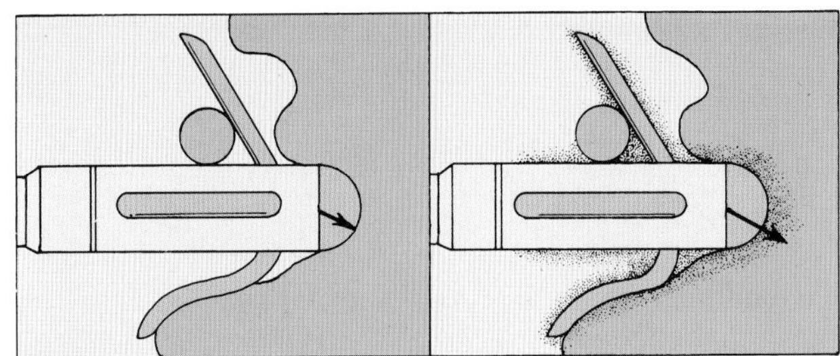

Figure 1-30. Schematic representation of a simple collagenous capsule around an electrode, which separates it from excitable tissue. The length of the arrow in the left panel indicates the radius (r) of the spherical electrode. In effect, the fibrous tissue becomes a "virtual electrode" with radius r + d (arrow in right panel), *where d is the thickness of the fibrous tissue (stippled area). (From Stokes K, Bornzin G: The electrode-biointerface [stimulation]. In Barold SS [ed]: Modern Cardiac Pacing. Mt. Kisco, NY, Futura, 1985, pp 33-78.)*

Stimulation threshold increases during the first several weeks after lead implantation. This increase in threshold is related to the development of a conductive but nonexcitable fibrotic capsule that forms around the electrode and separates it from normal, excitable myocardium (Fig. 1-30) [43,44,152,153] The fibrous capsule is a biologic response to the presence of a foreign body, in this case the electrode. With perhaps rare exceptions, the fibrous capsule is not a response to the electrical stimulus.[154] In reality, if r is the electrode radius and d is the approximate mean thickness of the fibrotic capsule, $r + d$ describes the dimensions of the effective or "virtual electrode," as defined by Furman and associates.[155] If the stimulus voltage is held constant, the field strength varies as a function of the thickness of the inexcitable capsule. Higher voltages must be applied to maintain the intensity of the field at the interface of the virtual electrode and the excitable myocardium. Therefore, chronic thresholds (for steroid-free electrodes) must be higher than the values at implantation. This theory was modeled by Irinch,[43,148] as follows:

$$E = \frac{V}{r}\left[\frac{r}{(r+d)}\right]^2 \tag{1-12}$$

Equation 1-12 is lacking a crucial parameter, stimulus duration, that is required by the strength-duration relationship. According to Irnich, the equation is based on measurements taken at a pulse duration of 1 msec. Holding everything else constant, the capsule thickness is the same for a large electrode radius as for a small one. If, for example, two electrodes of different radii

(0.5 mm and 5 mm) develop a 1-mm thick capsule (d), the electrode with the smaller actual radius will be associated with a greater percentage increase (r + d versus r) with the formation of the virtual electrode (300% versus 20%, respectively). This helps to explain the observation that smaller electrodes have lower acute thresholds but develop a greater rise in threshold over time.[91,94] There is a point (r = d) at which chronic threshold reaches a minimum. According to Equation 1-12, when d is greater than r, thresholds increase. Therefore, there is a theoretical minimum spherical electrode radius at which thresholds must reach their minimum value. Irnich found this to be 0.72 mm for polished electrodes. In reality, because currently used electrodes are not polished and are not spherical, the relationship between stimulation threshold and electrode radius is more complex. Electrode size is more meaningful when it is discussed not only in terms of geometric surface area but also in terms of electrical surface area; the latter can be vastly increased by having a fractal surface.

Effects of Maximizing Electrode Surface Area

Maximizing the electrical surface area of the electrode has the effect of increasing the Helmholtz capacitance. For a given stimulus amplitude expressed in terms of charge delivered, the voltage across the capacitance will decrease as the magnitude of the capacitance increases($V = Q/C$; see earlier discussion). This means that increasing the Helmholtz capacitance decreases the polarization voltage, provided the delivered charge is kept the same. A very small-diameter electrode with a large surface area (due to its fractal structure) can have a high Helmholtz capacitance and a high current density at the electrode-tissue interface. The result is an electrode with high impedance and a lower threshold current requirement. Sensing performance may be good or not so good, depending on the electrode and pulse generator design (see later discussion).

Electrode Surface Structure (Interfacial Surface Area)

Based on animal studies, it has been stated that electrodes with pores that allow tissue ingrowth have thinner fibrous capsules and somewhat lower chronic thresholds than do those with solid or polished surfaces.[156-159] These claims have been somewhat controversial when applied to humans.[160-163] Pore structures of certain dimensions are known to promote rapid tissue ingrowth (Fig. 1-31).[164] Activated carbon electrodes are reported to have porosity on the order of 10 nm.[165] It has been argued that microporosity provides rapid stability of the electrode at its interface with the myocardium and prevents electrode motion that otherwise may result in tissue irritation and high chronic stimulation thresholds. The importance of microporosity among the many other factors involved in electrode mechanical stability is uncertain.

Relationship of Electrode Size and Sensing Performance

The amplitude of the electrogram sensed by the amplifier of the pulse generator is less than the amplitude of the available signal in the myocardium. The attenuation of the signal is related to the ratio of the source impedance (of the electrode-myocardial interface) and the input impedance of the sensing amplifier. The higher the source impedance, the more the signal amplitude is attenuated for a given input impedance. Signal attenuation can be greatly minimized by increasing the input impedance of the sense amplifier, so that the ratio of input impedance to source impedance is very large.

Clinical Aspects of Myocardial Stimulation by Pacemakers

Stability of Strength-Duration Curves and the Distorting Effect of Polarization

None of the relationships published in the last 100 years has exactly duplicated the capacitively coupled, constant-voltage strength-duration curves that have been measured empirically with various types of electrodes. This may be due, in part, to the confounding effect of polarization, which varies significantly with electrode size, shape, surface finish, material, and so forth. Another problem, however, is that the voltage and current strength-duration relationships, typically plotted on linear coordinates, are really logarithmic (see Fig. 1-27).[166] When plotted in this manner, the strength-duration curve for constant-current stimuli is now seen to be a straight line up to rheobase, whereas the constant-voltage line turns upward, as seen at stimulus duration 2 msec in Figure 1-27. The effect of polarization on reducing current flow in constant-voltage pacing does not occur with constant-current pacing; because with the latter the pulse generator develops whatever voltage is necessary to force the set level of current into the circuit.

The slope of the strength-duration curves for passively fixed, atraumatic leads does not change with time after implantation (see Fig. 1-27). The acute, peak, and chronic mean thresholds of five ventricular and three atrial passively fixed, atraumatic leads in 77 canines had a ($\log_{10}$) slope of about 0.60 ± 0.07 V/msec.[166] The correlation coefficient for these relationships was typically more than 0.99 at pulse durations of less than 0.5 msec for polished electrodes and at durations of less than 1.0 msec for low-polarizing designs. Traumatic electrodes (such as those with active fixation) in this canine experience typically had a lower slope immediately after implantation, which shifted to about the same 0.60V/msec value within days as the acute trauma to the electrode-tissue interface healed.

Because strength-duration curves are typically plotted on linear rather than logarithmic coordinates, changes in voltage and current threshold after implantation are

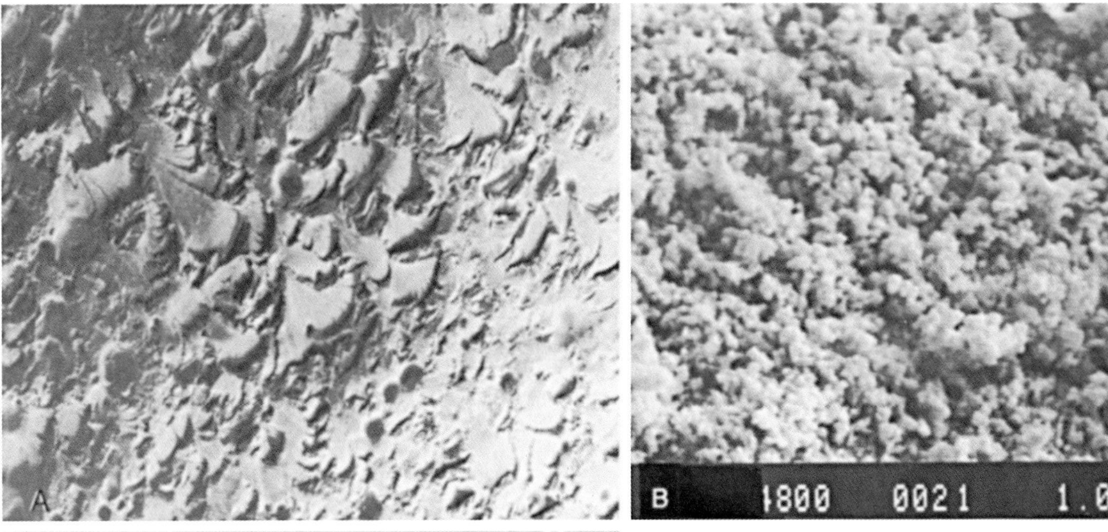

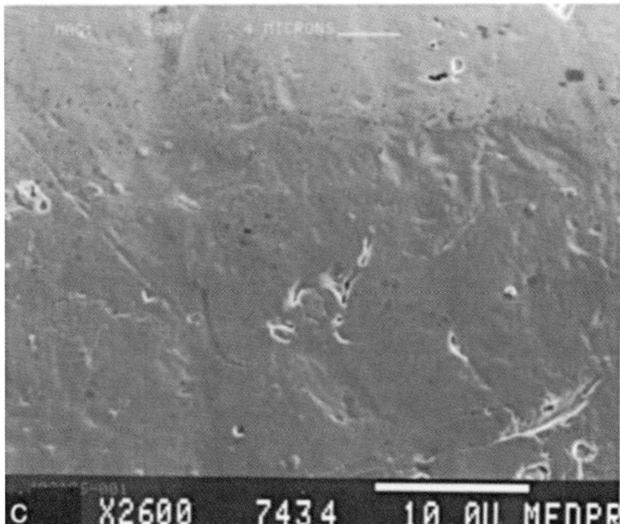

Figure 1-31. Electron micrographs of microporous electrode surfaces. ***A,*** *Activated carbon surface of Siemans Model 412S/60 electrode at about ×8000 magnification.* ***B,*** *Medtronic Model 4011 platinized surface at ×6900 magnification.* ***C,*** *Polished platinum surface of Medtronic Model 6971 at ×7000 magnification. The polished platinum surface has little microstructure. Its actual microscopic surface area is similar to its apparent or geometric surface area (8 mm^2). The platinized platinum surface (**B**) is composed of particles so small that they absorb visible light, and the surface appears black. The true surface area of the interface is many orders of magnitude greater than the geometric surface area. (From Seeger W: A scanning electron microscopic study on explanted electrode tips. In Aubert AE, Ector H [eds]: Pacemaker Leads. Amsterdam, Elsevier Science Publishers, 1985, pp 417-432.)*

usually seen as a shift upward and to the right. In most cases, chronaxie, being related to the slope of the curve (the tissue's time constant), does not change significantly with time. However, Cornacchia and colleagues,[167] showed that the administration of propafenone shifted both the strength-duration curve and the chronaxie to the right. The pacing threshold also increased.

Some older pulse generator designs attempted to compensate for the gradual decline in stimulus voltage that occurs as a consequence of battery depletion by automatic "stretching" of the pulse duration to maintain the stimulus energy at an almost constant value. Although this feature was designed to prevent loss of capture, increasing the pulse duration from a programmed value of 0.5 msec adds little to the pacing safety margin, because it approaches an essentially flat portion of the strength-duration curve. In fact, although this automatic increase in pulse duration was added in the name of safety, it is a wasteful use of battery energy. Preventing the decrease in output voltage of the pulse generator, while at the same time giving adequate warning of the depleted state of the battery, is a better solution. The pulse-duration increase method did temporarily prolong pacing capture, although inefficiently. This was valuable for patients who were far away from medical care for a short time. It did also provide a warning in that both transtelephonic checking devices and clinical devices measure the actual pulse width. Newer pulse generators have abandoned this approach to compensating for battery depletion in favor of automatic regulation of stimulus voltage. They maintain constant stimulus amplitude despite declining battery voltage.

Threshold Changes as a Function of Time after Lead Implantation

It is well known that stimulation thresholds change as a function of time after implantation, typically rising to a peak value after several weeks.[168-171] With older polished electrodes, some patients had thresholds that evolved over longer periods (as long as 6 months).[172] Luceri and colleagues[173] observed that, after the acute rise in stimulation threshold, 43% of 120 patients had stable chronic thresholds for up to 8 years; 17% had chronic thresholds that decreased at a rate of 5% per year, and 19% had thresholds that rose at a rate of 14% per year. Twenty percent of the patients had thresholds that varied widely around a stable mean.

Modern pacing electrodes have a porous or microporous surface structure. Most also elute a glucocorticosteroid. As shown in Figure 1-32, the technological progression from polished to porous to microporous to steroid-eluting electrodes has significantly reduced the evolution of stimulation threshold as a function of time after implantation.[174] In fact, as can be determined from the follow-up data available, the thresholds of porous and microporous steroid-eluting leads do not change significantly with increasing time after implantation.[175-178] The reasons for threshold changes as a function of time and electrode design are to be found in the foreign body response to the electrodes.

The Electrode-Tissue Interface and the Foreign Body Response

The body's response to an implanted device has been relatively well characterized.[179] Figure 1-33 shows schematically what ordinarily happens at an implantation site as a function of time. If one analyzes the tissues adjacent to canine ventricular endocardial atraumatic electrodes as a function of time after implantation, the evolution depicted in Figure 1-33 is typically observed (with one exception). In the first 1 to 3 days, there is no evidence of cellular inflammation, and thresholds do not change significantly. This lack of a cellular response in the first few days is an exception to the classic view of surgical wound inflammation. In a surgical wound, polymorphonuclear leukocytes normally are present during this period to scavenge necrotic debris and bacteria.

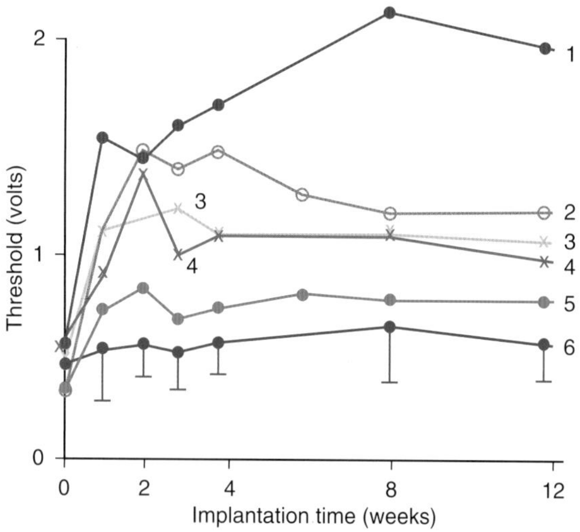

Figure 1-32. Canine ventricular voltage thresholds at 0.5 msec for 8-mm² unipolar, transvenous, tined leads as a function of time after implantation. 1, Polished platinum ring-tip (manufacturer A); 2, polished platinum ring-tip (manufacturer B); 3, porous-surface platinum hemisphere (manufacturer C); 4, porous-surface titanium hemisphere (manufacturer B); 5, platinized Target Tip (manufacturer B); 6, steroid-eluting titanium porous-surface electrode (manufacturer B).

The classic view of inflammation holds that the initial event is dilation of blood vessels and alteration in the vascular endothelium resulting in increased permeability. This increased perfusion and permeability of the blood vessel walls allows plasma to leak into the surrounding tissue, producing edema. Because plasma and serum are more conductive than myocardium, pacing impedance decreases almost immediately after lead implantation. After 2 to 3 days, a mixed cellular inflammation begins to appear in the tissues surrounding the electrode, and the stimulation threshold begins to rise. Tissue inflammation reaches its peak in about 1 week, with clearly evident interstitial edema and cellular necrosis. Pacing impedance typically reaches its minimum value at the inflammatory peak (about 1 week after implantation), after which it increases as the edema resolves. The stimulation threshold may or may not reach its peak at the same time as the nadir of pacing impedance.

After the early, mixed cellular reaction, the inflammatory response is characterized by a gradual accumulation of macrophages that reach the electrode surface, adhere, and become activated. The major function of the macrophage is to dispose of dead or foreign cells and particles by the process of endocytosis (Fig. 1-34).[122,180] In the case of a large foreign object, such as a pacing electrode, the process of endocytosis is impos-

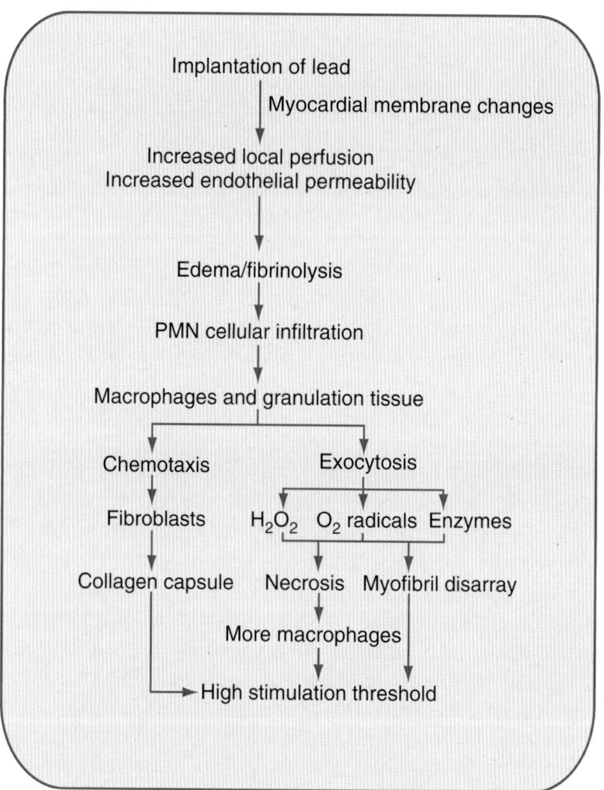

Figure 1-33. Schematic representation of the inflammatory process and foreign body response to lead implantation. This has been correlated approximately with time after implantation of a cardiac pacemaker lead, based on histologic studies of canine electrode-tissue sites. PMN, polymorphonuclear neutrophils.

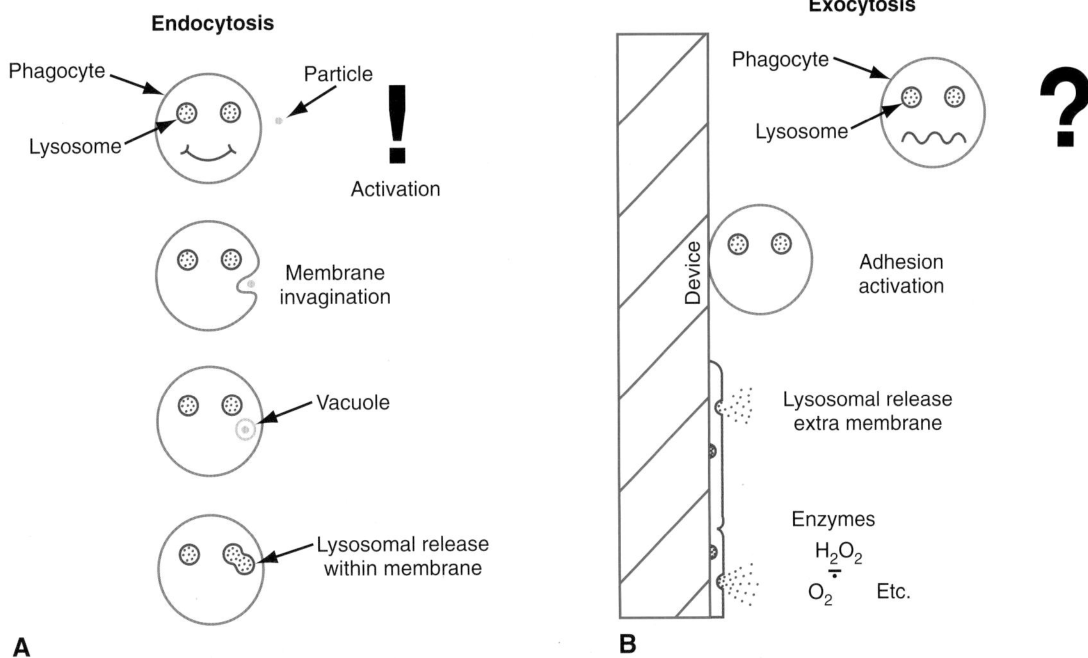

Figure 1-34. ***A,*** *Schematic representation of phagocytosis by endocytosis. A small particle attaches to the macrophage's membrane. The membrane invaginates, encapsulating the particle in a membrane-lined vacuole. The vacuole and lysosome migrate toward each other, and their membranes fuse. The particle is then destroyed by lysosomal enzymes and oxidants.* ***B,*** *Schematic representation of the process of "frustrated phagocytosis" by exocytosis, or the acute foreign body response on the device surface, which results in lysosomal release of inflammatory mediators on the device surface and into the adjacent tissue.*

sible. In this case, the macrophage tries to destroy the large foreign body by the process of exocytosis, the extracellular release of enzymes and oxidants. Macrophages spread over the electrode surface, often differentiating into foreign body giant cells. Their lysosomes migrate to the membrane surface, releasing hydrolytic enzymes and oxidants into the surrounding tissue and onto the electrode surface. Additional macrophages settle on the foreign body giant cells and are activated. Myocytes adjacent to the electrode-tissue interface are bathed in a "soup" of inflammatory mediators resulting from exocytosis. These mediators of the inflammatory response dissolve the subcellular collagen beams, struts, and nets that hold the myocytes in the normal orderly array of myocardium.[181]

After 3 to 4 weeks (for a stable, biocompatible device), the more global inflammatory response has essentially resolved with the development of a collagenous capsule surrounding the electrode. If the electrode is biocompatible and stable relative to the myocardium, there are few further significant visible histologic changes in the adjacent tissues after this period. Thresholds may subsequently decrease, remain stable, or increase, depending on the intensity of the chronic foreign body response at the electrode-tissue interface.

Chronic atraumatic polished electrodes (Fig. 1-35A) typically have a layer of foreign body giant cells on their surface. These are covered by a layer (or layers) of macrophages that can be surprisingly thick. This cellular component of the capsule is not an acute, transient phenomenon but has been observed on electrodes up to 13 years after implantation in Stoke's canine studies. These cells are covered by a layer of collagen that is oriented along the surface of the electrode. The myocytes adjacent to the collagen layers are disarrayed and are interspersed with collagen fibers that are radially oriented with respect to the surface of the electrode. There may also be circular "holes" in this layer of disoriented myocytes, which appear to be infiltrated with fatty material. Groups of macrophages with fused membranes (foreign body giant cells) enveloping bundles of myocardial fibers adjacent to the electrode were observed 1 to 4 weeks after implantation. The presence of this fatty infiltration, its location, and its severity depend on the stability, myocardial location, and shape of the electrode relative to the vector of myocardial contraction. Outside the disarrayed myofiber zone, one finds normally oriented myocardium. Therefore, it is clear that the concept of a simple fibrous capsule (Irnich's "d") separating the electrode surface from viable myocardium does not completely describe this complex biologic response and its effect on pacing.

Passively Fixed Leads with Porous and Microporous Electrodes

Electrodes with pores on the order of 10 to 100 μm in diameter allow the formation of collagen as a result of chronic inflammation. Therefore, in a sense, macroporous electrodes promote inflammation. In addition, the chronic capsule surrounding porous electrodes can be associated with significant myofibrillar disarray (see

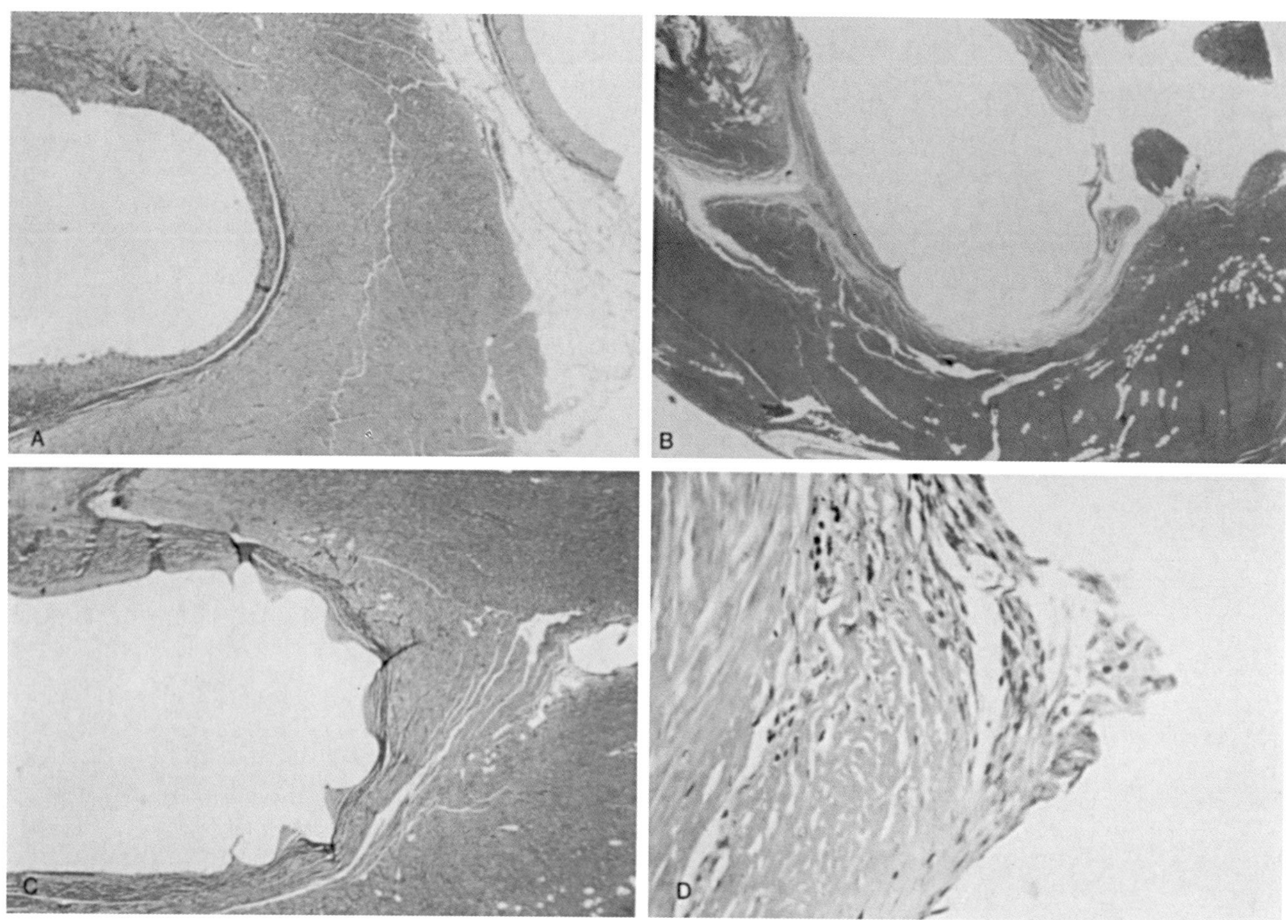

Figure 1-35. Optical micrographs of chronic electrode-tissue interfaces. ***A,*** *The capsule surrounding a polished electrode* (upper left) *has a relatively thick layer of activated phagocytic cells, including foreign body giant cells on the surface and macrophages further out. Collagenous material encapsulates these cells, with fibrous stringers extending outward into the myocardium.* ***B,*** *Myofibrillar disarray is seen between the collagenous capsule and normal myocardium. The capsule surrounding a porous electrode* (upper right) *appears to be thinner. However, the active cellular component of the capsule and some of the collagen have been removed with the electrode to facilitate trimming of the tissues.* ***C,*** *A microporous (Target Tip) electrode-tissue interface is shown in the lower left section of the micrograph. Note the thin fibrous capsule over the external surfaces and at the ridges.* ***D,*** *Some macrophages are seen deep in the Target Tip electrode's grooves at higher magnification.*

Fig. 1-35B). Despite these factors, porous electrodes are associated with a relatively thin collagenous capsule. Histologic study of the chronic tissue reaction surrounding porous electrodes has shown that inflammatory cells are usually not found on the surface of the electrode. Rather, the active cellular component of the fibrous capsule is located *within* the pores. Similarly, microporous electrodes tend to have few cells on their surfaces with well-healed interfaces (see Fig. 1-35C). Target Tip design electrodes showed an active cellular component deep in the grooves of the electrode (see Fig. 1-35D). The smooth outer surface interfaced directly with collagen.

Passively Fixed Leads with Steroid-Eluting Electrodes

It has long been recognized that systemically administered glucocorticosteroids decrease both acute and chronic stimulation thresholds. During the early days of cardiac pacing, it sometimes happened that one or more of the several mercury cells in the pulse generators would internally short and fail suddenly, causing loss of capture. In these cases, intravenous administration of hydrocortisone was sometimes an effective emergency measure for temporarily regaining and maintaining capture on the way to the operating room. Initially, it was believed that the threshold-lowering effect of systemic glucocorticoid therapy was due to effects on the myocyte membrane and sodium and potassium "retention."[182] Steroid-eluting leads, in which dexamethasone sodium phosphate or acetate is gradually released from a reservoir within or around the electrode, have become standard for permanent pacing. It has been conclusively demonstrated that steroid elution decreases chronic thresholds. Despite the clear clinical benefits of steroid elution on the evolution of stimulation thresholds, the mechanism of this effect is not well understood.[183] Although steroid-eluting, porous electrodes tend to have thinner capsules than polished platinum electrodes, these capsule surrounding steroid-eluting leads can be difficult to differentiate from those steroid-free electrodes in blind analyses. The capsule surrounding a steroid-eluting lead is characterized by minimal cellularity between the collagen and the electrode surface and minimal myofibrillar disarray.

Effect of Glucocorticoids on the Evolution of Pacing Thresholds

Glucocorticosteroids are known to stabilize the membranes of phagocytes, such as the macrophage, through interaction with surface receptors, inhibiting release of lysosomal contents.[184] It has been shown, however, that dexamethasone and its derivatives have no significant electrical effects on myocyte membranes.[185,186] It is probable that the salutary effect of systemic glucocorticoids on stimulation threshold is the result of inhibition of the release of inflammatory mediators from the cellular components of the fibrous capsule. When steroid therapy is discontinued, the release of inflammatory mediators resumes and stimulation thresholds once again increase. The same phenomenon minimizes inflammation (foreign body response) on and adjacent to the surface of a steroid-eluting electrode. Acute stabilization of macrophage membranes on the electrode surface reduces or minimizes lysosomal release, thereby minimizing myofibrillar disarray and myocyte membrane damage. Chronic steroid elution suppresses the slow, insidious leakage of inflammatory mediators, thereby preventing threshold increase, without the risk of systemic side effects.

Pathologic Changes due to Mechanical Instability at the Myocardium-Electrode Interface

Mechanically unstable electrodes can provoke a significant pathologic response in the myocardium. Consider, for example, a transvenous corkscrew electrode that "rocks" at the interface with the endocardium because the lead behind it is too stiff. In some cases, large pockets of activated macrophages may develop on either side of the helix, resulting in the formation of a "preabscess." In other cases, thick collagenous capsules form and then differentiate into cartilage and, if the instability is severe enough, into bone. Because active-fixation myocardial electrodes interfere with the contractile motion of the adjacent myofibers, myocardial degeneration with fatty infiltration may result in patterns that are clearly related to this mechanical interference. For example, the center of a myocardial helix may fill in with fatty "cells." A myocardial pin may also provoke myocardial degeneration and fatty infiltration. Therefore, mechanical instability at the electrode-myocardium interface can produce marked histologic and physiologic effects that result in deterioration of the stimulation threshold. A particularly notable example of a lead with a high potential for exit block was an active-fixation lead that used an electrically inactive helix and a platinum-iridium electrode. The presence of a stiff, metal, J-shaped retention wire increased the stiffness effect of this lead. It had an exit block rate of about 10%.

Some Second-Order Effects of Electrode Design

Spatial and Size Relationships between Electrode Pairs

It was established previously that, within clinically relevant limits, porous and microporous electrode size and shape per se have no significant effects on the chronic stimulation thresholds (at least with steroid-free electrodes). Nonetheless, the size and shape of the electrode can still be important factors under certain circumstances. For example, a small displacement can affect the performance of a smaller electrode because its high-density field influences relatively few cells.[187,188] A larger electrode is not as threshold efficient, but perforation is less likely, and small displacements have less effect on lead performance. The ring-tip electrode design is essentially a small electrode made into a large shape.[189] This allows high electric field strength coverage of a larger number of myocardial cells, while affording a lower probability of perforation than a lead with a smaller tip. Although myocardial screws, barbs, hooks, and so forth are traumatic to the underlying myocardium, these electrodes all have points that serve as sources of high field strength. Therefore, myocardial electrodes of this design can still have good chronic performance, assuming that the lead is not so stiff as to apply undue force on the electrode-myocardium interface.

Electrode Fixation

The most efficient electrode design has poor long-term performance if it is mechanically unstable, resulting in both high stimulation thresholds and histopathologic evidence of excessive trauma. For chronically stable, steroid-free electrodes in canines, however, there was no correlation between the mechanism of fixation and the chronic stimulation threshold (Table 1-1). Given similar geometric surface areas, there were comparable chronic canine ventricular thresholds with tined, flanged, screw-in, and hook-in polished electrodes, whether endocardial or myocardial. These results were confirmed by human studies in both the atrium and ventricle.[190-192] Therefore, the hypothesis that fixation remote from the electrode stimulation site is necessary for low chronic thresholds does not appear to be valid.[193,194] It has not been established whether this is also true for steroid-eluting electrodes. However, a variety of leads are available that combine active fixation and steroid elution. The long-term pacing thresholds of these leads are much lower than those for similar models without steroid elution.

Electrode Materials

To minimize inflammation and its subsequent effects on stimulation threshold, electrodes for permanent pacing should be biocompatible and resistant to chemical degradation. Many materials, such as platinum, titanium, titanium oxide, titanium nitride, carbon, tantalum pentoxide, iridium, and iridium oxide, have been shown to be acceptable for use as pacing electrodes.[195-197] Even silver, which is toxic in neurologic tissue and is certainly not corrosion resistant, has been used successfully in the heart as an electrode.[190] Titanium and tantalum have been known to acquire a surface coating of oxides, which, it has been argued, may impede charge transfer at the electrode interface. To prevent this, titanium has been coated with platinized platinum or vitreous carbon. Others accept the concept that the oxide layer acts as the dielectric of a capacitor, so that no charge is transferred across the dielectric during stimulation. In that situation, current continues to enter and leave each side of the capacitor (see earlier discussion of Helmholtz capacitance). In any case, titanium oxide electrodes are highly corrosion resistant, and these combinations have been found to have excellent long-term performance as pacing electrodes.[198-202]

Some theories have held that the foreign body reaction is a response to the electrode material per se.[203,204] As a result, many attempts have been made to improve thresholds through the use of more biocompatible materials. For example, it has been claimed that pyrolytic carbons are more biocompatible and produce lower chronic thresholds than platinum.[99,205-207] Besides having a different composition, these electrodes are also microporous. When similar electrodes are polished, we have found that the chronic canine thresholds are not significantly different from those observed with polished platinum electrodes. There can be no doubt that proper electrode material selection is necessary to prevent unacceptable toxic responses or corrosion. At this point, however, there does not appear to be a biocompatible electrode composition that significantly improves thresholds.

Of course, not all conductive materials are suitable for use as electrodes. Certain materials, such as zinc, copper, mercury, nickel, and lead, are associated with toxic reactions in the myocardium and are unsuitable for use in permanent pacing leads.[190] Stainless steel materials are highly varying in composition and microstructure, with great variation between production lots. Electrodes made from one lot may be acceptable, whereas those made from another lot may corrode unacceptably. Because some of the corrosion products may be inflammatory or toxic, high thresholds occasionally occur with these materials. Therefore, stainless steel materials are no longer used for implantable electrodes. The polarity of the electrode may also have an important influence on its chemical stability. For example, Elgiloy (Elgiloy Limited Partnership, Elgin, Ill.), a non-noble and highly polarizing metal alloy, was used in the past as a cathode. It could not be used as an anode because it is susceptible to a significant degree of corrosion. Although Elgiloy had other excellent qualities, it is not used as pacemaker electrode today.

The materials presently used for permanent pacing electrodes include platinum-iridium, titanium (oxide), platinum- or carbon-coated titanium, platinized platinum, vitreous carbon, and iridium oxide. The platinized platinum, "activated" carbon, and iridium oxide electrodes are associated with a reduced degree of polarization. A negligible degree of corrosion occurs with these materials. The vitreous carbon electrodes have been improved by roughening the surface, a process known as activation that increases the surface area of the interface, thereby reducing polarization. Fractal coating of the distal electrode also has been introduced as a method for reducing electrode polarization. This technique involves coating the distal electrode with a microscopic granular structure that produces a complex surface.

Electrode Location (Epicardial, Endocardial, Intramyocardial)

As shown previously in canine ventricles for electrodes without steroid elution, the type of fixation (as opposed to the location of the electrode) has no effect on stimulation thresholds, in that epicardially applied corkscrews, transvenous corkscrews, and passively fixed endocardial electrodes all tend to have about the same chronic thresholds in canines (see Table 1-4). Most epicardial or myocardial pacing leads are used in pediatric patients, in whom threshold complications are relatively frequent.[208,209] It is generally perceived that epicardial and myocardial electrodes without steroid elution have less desirable threshold performance than endocardial leads. One reason that the performance of epicardial and myocardial leads has lagged behind that of endocardial passively fixed leads is the mechanical limitations involved. Epicardial and transvenous active-fixation leads are significantly more complex and are more difficult to design with all the attributes necessary for low chronic stimulation thresholds. Nonetheless, there is no inherent reason that transvenous active-fixation or myocardial electrodes should not perform as well as or better than endocardial systems.

The first transvenous steroid-eluting active-fixation lead (Medtronic Model 5078, Medtronic, Inc., Minneapolis, Minn.) was bipolar, with an electrically inactive fixed helix surrounding a 5.8-mm^2 porous, platinized cathode. This lead had excellent electrical performance in both the atrium and the ventricle.[210-213] There were some difficulties with helix distortion and entrapment in some cases, however, resulting in the abandonment of the design. Active-fixation steroid-eluting leads provide significantly reduced pacing thresholds compared with standard active-fixation leads. Active-fixation electrode thresholds tend to be slightly higher than those of passive-fixation steroid-eluting electrodes.[214] Steroid elution has also been applied to epicardial leads; with a significant reduction in long-term pacing threshold compared with steroid-free leads.[215]

Pharmacologic Effects on Cardiac Stimulation

Antiarrhythmic Drugs

Several types of antiarrhythmic drugs have been demonstrated to increase stimulation thresholds in both humans and animals. Type 1 drugs decrease Na^+ conductance and decrease the rate of rise of the action potential. Therefore, it should be no surprise that these agents can increase the threshold for pacing. Type 1A drugs, such as quinidine[216] and procainamide,[217] may result in increased thresholds, especially when administered in high doses.[218] Type 1C drugs, such as encainide, flecainide, and propafenone, have been associated with increased pacing thresholds.[219-223] The increase in stimulation threshold with these drugs has been demonstrated to correlate with the change in QRS duration. In addition to the type 1 agents, propranolol has been demonstrated to result in an increase in pacing threshold when administered intravenously.[224] Amiodarone, lidocaine, tocainide, and verapamil have been reported to have minimal effects on pacing threshold, although we have seen one patient with congenital heart disease in whom amiodarone reproducibly increased the pacing threshold to the point of exit block.[225]

Metabolic Effects on Cardiac Stimulation

Stimulation Thresholds

Stimulation thresholds may rise during sleeping or eating, factors associated with withdrawal of sympathetic tone and increased vagal tone.[226,227] In contrast, factors associated with increased sympathetic tone, such as exercise or assumption of the upright posture, are associated with a decrease in threshold. The myocardial stimulation threshold is increased by several metabolic abnormalities, including hypoxemia, hypercarbia, metabolic alkalosis, and metabolic acidosis. In the presence of respiratory or cardiac arrest, the pacing threshold may increase by well over 100%, resulting in loss of capture despite the use of a conventional safety margin. Because of this observation, antitachycardia pacing devices, such as pacemakers and ICDs, are often designed to deliver high-intensity stimuli during antitachycardia pacing or after a high-energy shock. In patients undergoing implantation of an ICD, Khastgir and colleagues[228] were unable to demonstrate an increase in pacing threshold 10 and 60 seconds after defibrillation. Ventricular fibrillation was electrically induced, however, and defibrillation was promptly performed under controlled circumstances in this study.

Physiologic and Pharmacologic Effects on Pacing

In the presence of a primary respiratory arrest, pacing stimuli may not capture the myocardium until adequate ventilation and pH balance are restored. Therefore, careful attention to respiration and pH must be maintained during anesthesia in patients with implanted pacemakers to ensure continued myocardial capture. Ischemia produces variable effects on stimulation threshold, depending on the location of the pacing electrode relative to the ischemic myocardium. In the presence of acute myocardial ischemia, the resting membrane potential decreases (cells become partially depolarized), the action potential upstroke velocity decreases, and the action potential duration dramatically shortens. In the presence of metabolic blockade with 2,4-dinitrophenol, Delmar[229] noted an upward shift in the strength-duration curve, indicating an increase in the current required for capture at all pulse durations. Therefore, if the stimulating electrode is located in an ischemic region, the stimulation threshold would be expected to increase. With further ischemia and infarction, the myocardial threshold may rise dramatically. This may be seen clinically in patients who develop an acute inferior myocardial infarction with RV infarction; in such patients, a previously implanted pacemaker may suddenly lose capture. However, if the stimulating electrode is located in a nonischemic region (e.g., right ventricle), activation of the sympathetic nervous system may reduce the pacing threshold.

Hyperkalemia has been shown to increase the stimulation threshold when the serum K^+ concentration exceeds 7 mEq/L.[230,231] In contrast, in the presence of hypokalemia, intravenous K^+ may decrease the pacing threshold and restore capture of a subthreshold pulse.[232] In addition, the reduced excitability during hyperkalemia can be corrected by the intravenous administration of calcium.[233] Hyperglycemia in the range of 600 mg/dL may increase stimulation thresholds by as much as 60%.[234] Therefore, patients who have diabetes or renal failure, conditions associated with the potential for altered glucose metabolism and electrolyte abnormalities, may need a larger safety margin than other patients. Hypothyroidism has also been demonstrated to increase pacing thresholds, an effect that is reversible with thyroxine replacement.[235,236] As stated previously, glucocorticosteroids decrease stimulation thresholds and have been used to treat exit block both acutely and chronically.[237] Endogenous and synthetic catecholamines are effective in lowering pacing thresholds.[238,239] The effect of intravenous epinephrine or isoproterenol is to decrease the stimulation threshold initially, followed by an increase. Intravenous or sublingual isoproterenol has been demonstrated to reverse high pacing thresholds related to antiarrhythmic drug toxicity.[240]

Biventricular Pacing

Optimal clinical outcomes with permanent pacing require that the hemodynamic effects of the pacing site and the timing of atrial and ventricular contraction be carefully considered. As a result, cardiac resynchronization pacemakers and ICDs typically use electrodes in the coronary venous system to allow LV stimulation. Implantation of permanent pacing leads in the cardiac veins is the predominant method for chronic LV stimulation.[241] Although epicardial LV pacing using standard myocardial leads has been studied as a method for biventricular pacing for the treatment of congestive heart failure, it requires a more extensive operation than a transvenous approach. Transvenous stimulation of the left ventricle requires placement of the lead into

TABLE 1-1. **Chronic (12-Week) Unipolar Canine (Constant-Voltage) Thresholds of Polished Platinum Electrodes at 0.5 msec versus Fixation Mechanism**

Model No.	Insertion Fixation	Electrode Location and Shape	Surface Area (mm^2)	Stimulation Threshold (V)	*n*	*P* vs Model 6971*
6901	Endocardial flange	Endocardial cylinder	11	1.9 ± .77	11	.2
6950	Endocardial long tines	Endocardial cylinder	11	1.6 ± .48	4	>.5
6961	Endocardial short tines	Endocardial ring	8	1.8 ± .69	9	.35
6971	Endocardial medium tines	Endocardial ring	8	1.5 ± .57	8	—
4016	Endocardial helix	Myocardial helix	10	1.1 ± .30	6	.1
6959	Endocardial helix	Endocardial ring	13	1.3 ± .42	8	.4
6955	Endocardial helix	Myocardial helix	10	1.6 ± .51	10	>.5
4951	Epicardial hook	Myocardial hook	10	1.5 ± .44	10	>.5
6917	Epicardial helix	Myocardial helix	12	1.4 ± .53	17	>.5

*$P < .05$ considered statistically significant.
From Stokes K, Bornzin G: The electrode-biointerface (stimulation). In Barold SS (ed): Modern Cardiac Pacing. Mt. Kisco, NY, Futura, 1985, p 40.

a branch of the cardiac venous circulation, usually the anterior interventricular or posterolateral vein. The electrical properties of chronic stimulation of both the right and left ventricles are complex. The complexity of dual ventricular stimulation has been reported in canine studies.[242]

In canine studies, bipolar leads were placed transvenously into a distal epicardial ventricular branch of the great cardiac vein. The distal electrode was a 5.8-mm^2 porous, platinized hemisphere with a steroid coating. A transvenous lead was also placed at the RV apex. Two varieties of RV apex electrodes were used, one with a 4-mm^2 platinized Target Tip and the other with a 1.2-mm^2 steroid-eluting tip. Several modes of stimulation were compared (Tables 1-2, 1-3, and 1-4). One configuration (ventricular split bipole) used two unipolar leads and an adapter such that the electrode in one chamber was the cathode and the electrode in the other chamber served as the anode. The second configuration (dual-cathode) joined the LV and RV electrodes in parallel as a common cathode; the anode was the pulse generator can. The thresholds as a function of time after implantation are shown in Figure 1-36. The single-chamber chronic coronary venous LV thresholds were two to three times higher than the RV single-chamber values. The threshold for simultaneous capture of both the right and left ventricles was similar to the unipolar LV threshold. Similar findings were observed regardless of whether the anode was the pulse generator can or a ring electrode in the right ventricle. In contrast, with the ventricular split bipole configuration, the threshold for combined capture of both ventricles was much higher, leading to exit block (>5 V) in many cases.

The pacing impedance with the dual-cathode configuration was 43% lower than the average of the two single-chamber values. When a small electrode with high impedance (1.2 mm^2) was paired with a larger

TABLE 1-2. **Canine Thresholds (V) at 0.5 msec 12 Weeks after Implantation (n = 13)**

Chambers Paced	Unipolar LV	Unipolar RV	Unipolar DCO
1	1.8 ± 1.2	0.9 ± 0.2	0.9 ± 0.2
2			2.0 ± 1.4
1	2.6 ± 1.9	0.9 ± 0.5	1.1 ± 0.6
2			3.3 ± 2.0
	Bipolar RV–, LV+	**Bipolar LV–, RV+**	**Bipolar DCO–, RV Ring+**
1	1.4 ± 0.5	2.0 ± 0.9	1.0 ± 0.4
2	7.2 ± 3.5	3.5 ± 1.0	1.7 ± 0.9
1	1.4 ± 1.0	3.0 ± 1.6	NA
2	8.5 ± 3.0	4.6 ± 2.3	NA

DCO, dual cathodal output; LV, left ventricular coronary vein; NA, not applicable; RV, right ventricular apex.

electrode (4 mm^2), the dual-cathode impedance was 51% lower than the average of the two unipolar impedances values. Pacing impedance in the ventricular split bipole configuration was markedly higher than that for either electrode alone.

The first generation of cardiac resynchronization therapy (CRT) devices used a bipolar RV pacing or ICD lead and a unipolar coronary venous lead with the ventricular output pulse delivered to both the coronary venous tip and the RV tip electrodes in a split-cathodal configuration. The anode was programmable to be either the pulse generator casing (unipolar split-cathodal configuration) or the ring electrode on the RV lead (bipolar split-cathodal configuration). As a result of splitting the

TABLE 1-3. Canine Pacing Impedance (Ω) at 2.5V and 0.5 msec, 12 Weeks after Implantation

Unipolar LV	Unipolar RV	Unipolar DCO
790 ± 118	734 ± 190	433 ± 68
829 ± 642	1193 ± 297	488 ± 157
Bipolar RV–, LV+	**Bipolar LV–, RV+**	**Bipolar DCO–, RV Ring+**
1193 ± 186	1014 ± 157	410 ± 64
1863 ± 745	1216 ± 806	NA

DCO, dual cathodal output; LV, left ventricular coronary vein; NA, not applicable; RV, right ventricular apex.

TABLE 1-4. Canine R-Wave Amplitudes (mV) 12 Weeks after Implantation

Unipolar LV	Unipolar RV	Unipolar DCO
13 ± 4	26 ± 4	14 ± 2
13 ± 4	26 ± 4	14 ± 7
Bipolar RV–, LV+	**Bipolar LV–, RV+**	**Bipolar DCO–, RV Ring+**
29 ± 4	35 ± 7	NA
29 ± 4	29 ± 4	NA

DCO, dual cathodal output; LV, left ventricular coronary vein; NA, not applicable; RV, right ventricular apex.

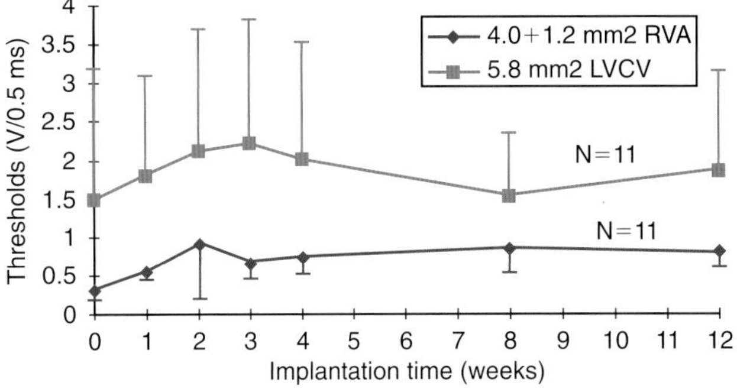

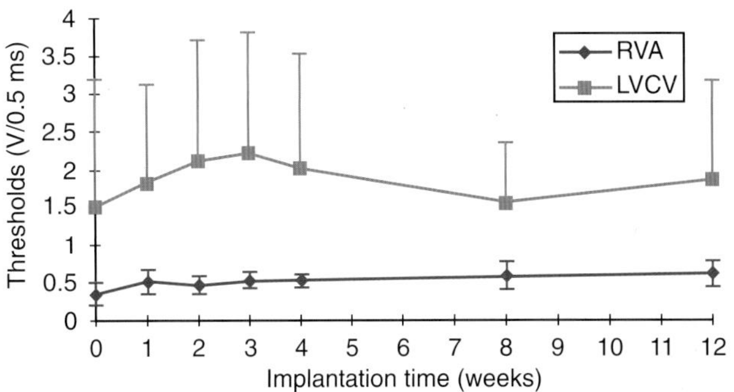

Figure 1-36. Unipolar canine right ventricular apex (RVA) and left cardiac vein ventricular (LVCV) thresholds as functions of time after implantation. In the upper panel, the leads are paired in each animal with a 5.8-mm² LV lead, and pooled data are shown in the RV from 1.2- and 4.0-mm² electrodes. Pooling was allowed because there was no statistically significant difference in threshold between the two electrodes (P < .5). In the lower panel, the LV lead is compared with one of the same design in different animals. In both cases, the LV thresholds are about twice those of the right-sided leads.

pacing current between two cathodal electrodes, the current was delivered in parallel to both the right and left ventricles. The magnitude of the current flowing to either ventricular electrode was determined by the impedance of the two leads. The apparent pacing threshold in the left ventricle was dramatically affected by this split-cathodal configuration. For example, Mayhew and coworkers[5] found that, when the unipolar LV (coronary venous) threshold was measured using the coronary venous tip electrode as the cathode and the pulse generator casing as the anode, the mean threshold was 0.7 ± 0.5 V at 0.5-msec pulse duration. Splitting the cathode between the LV tip and the RV tip electrodes increased the apparent LV threshold to 1.0 ± 0.8 V. When the anode was changed from the pulse generator casing to the RV ring electrode, the apparent LV threshold further increased to 1.3 ± 0.9 V. Therefore, a split-cathodal configuration markedly increased the apparent pacing threshold, compared with pacing the coronary venous lead alone.

A further observation with the split-cathodal pacing configuration is that the impedance measured with a PSA does not behave as predicted by the simple application of Ohm's law. For example, when the bipolar pacing configuration was used with the RV ring electrode as the anode,[5] the pacing impedance was measured to be 705 Ω in the right ventricle and 874 Ω in the left ventricle. Using a split-cathodal bipolar configuration, the measured impedance was 516 Ω, higher than would be predicted by Ohm's law with both ventricles stimulated in parallel (390 Ω). The higher than predicted impedance is explained by the fact that the size and shape of the combined cathodes are different from those for either electrode alone. The combined cathodal configuration results in a Warburg resistance and capacitance. Combining electrodes of similar size essentially doubles the cathodal surface area. Because the electrode resistance of a hemispherical electrode is roughly proportional to the square root of the electrode surface area, doubling the size of the cathode by combining the RV and LV electrodes decreases the Warburg resistance by a factor of $1/\sqrt{2}$. This helps to explain why the measured impedance using a split-cathodal configuration is not halved, as would be predicted by doubling the size of electrodes joined in parallel. Combining electrodes in parallel also increases the voltage droop during a constant-voltage pulse. Coronary venous pacing leads tend to result in higher impedance compared with endocardial RV leads (based on a lower volume of blood surrounding the electrode), and this further tends to shunt current from the higher-impedance electrode to the lower-impedance electrode when both ventricles are stimulated in parallel. This factor serves to increase the apparent LV threshold with the split-cathodal configuration.

These undesirable effects of a split-cathodal pacing configuration have largely been overcome by the addition of independent output circuits in newer CRT devices. However, because of the additional output circuit, there is additional battery drain with these devices. Another feature of CRT devices concerns the use of bipolar coronary venous leads. These leads differ from traditional right atrial or RV leads in that the surface area of the two coronary venous electrodes is quite similar. Therefore, when they are programmed to the bipolar pacing configuration, the impedance is much higher than with unipolar pacing, because current flows between two small electrodes rather than between one small and one large electrode. In addition, the bipolar pacing threshold is often considerably higher than the unipolar configuration. Bipolar leads have the advantage of offering the possibility of LV stimulation from either electrode, however. When combined with pulse generators capable of stimulating either of the two electrodes in a unipolar configuration, there may be a better chance of finding a coronary venous site that offers a low stimulation threshold. Another feature of bipolar coronary venous leads is that left phrenic nerve stimulation may be reduced if either electrode can be selected for unipolar pacing. However, when the electrodes are programmed to the bipolar configuration, the chances of left phrenic nerve stimulation may actually increase with a bipolar coronary venous lead, because there are two chances for an electrode to stimulate the phrenic nerve (one anodally and the other cathodally). Therefore, the chief advantage of the use of bipolar coronary venous leads in regard to stimulation is that there are two electrodes from which to choose for unipolar stimulation. Another advantage is that bipolar coronary venous stimulation avoids the chances of anodal RV stimulation when the RV ring electrode is used as the anode. The greatest advantages of bipolar leads in the coronary venous circulation relate to improved LV sensing.

Automated Capture Features

In order to ensure ventricular capture and to allow programming of a low margin of safety, newer pacemakers use algorithms that automatically detect ventricular capture. Based on the measured stimulation threshold, the amplitude of the pacing stimulus is automatically adjusted to provide a programmed margin of safety. The Autocapture feature of St. Jude Medical (St. Paul, Minn.) pacemakers automatically adjusts the amplitude of the stimulation pulse by detecting capture in the ventricle from the evoked ventricular electrogram (the evoked response). The St. Jude Medical pacemakers require a bipolar ventricular pacing lead with low polarization properties for the distal electrode. The presence or absence of ventricular capture is determined by sensing of the evoked response (ER) from the ring electrode. These devices automatically determine the evoked response gain and sensitivity levels by delivering five paired ventricular pulses of 4.5 V at a minimum pulse duration of 0.5 msec or the programmed value. The first of the paired pulses measures the evoked response, and the second pulse is delivered within 100 msec after the first (i.e., during the physiologic refractory period of the myocardium) to determine the level of polarization. If the amplitude of the evoked response is greater than 2.5 mV, the measured lead polarization is less than 4.0 mV, and the ratio of the evoked response to evoked response sensitivity is greater than 1.8 : 1, the device will automatically determine that the safety margin is acceptable and recommend Autocapture as a programmed feature. The Autocapture feature uses unipolar pacing from the tip electrode and determines capture on a beat-to-beat basis. If a ventricular stimulus is not followed by a detectable evoked response, a second test pulse is given at a value equal to 0.25 V greater than the last threshold measurement (a value known as the Automatic Pulse Amplitude, or APA). If a pulse is not followed by detectable capture, a backup pulse is delivered within 80 to 100 msec at an amplitude of 4.5 V. If two consecutive APA pulses are not followed by an evoked response, the threshold is measured to determine whether the APA needs adjustment. Specifically, the pulse is incremented 0.25 V above the last APA. If capture is not confirmed, the APA is repeated in 0.125 V increments until two consecutive captured events occur. For these devices, all loss-of-capture pulses are immediately followed by a backup pulse. A potential complicating factor with detection of the evoked response is differentiating fusion from capture. In the DDD(R) pacing mode, precisely timed intrinsic conduction can result in false detection of loss of capture. To differentiate true loss of capture from fusion, the AV delay is incremented by 100 msec after two consecutive loss-of-capture events to search for intrinsic conduction. If intrinsic conduction is indeed present during this extension of the AV delay, the backup pulse is eliminated. On the other hand, if subsequent backup pulses or APA increments are required due to loss of capture, the AV/PV delay is shortened to 50/25 msec. This sequence can introduce confusion into the interpretation of electrocardiographic tracings with irregular AV delays. However, knowledge of the function of the Autocapture algorithm allows recognition that this is a normal phenomenon.

Automatic capture algorithms have also been applied to unipolar leads. The ELA Symphony pacemakers (ELA Medical, Sorin Group, Milan, Italy) detect the evoked response on the tip electrode of a unipolar lead, provided that the polarization properties of the electrode are favorable. Guidant (Boston Scientific, Natick, Mass.) pacemakers use a lower-capacitance output capacitor to minimize the afterpotentials on the ventricular lead as a method for improving detection of the evoked response. The smaller-output capacitor increases the droop of the pacing pulse, but the afterpotential is reduced. The smaller-output capacitor may have the effect of slightly increasing the apparent stimulation threshold, an effect that is measurable only when the pacing threshold exceeds 2.5 V.

Other manufacturers offer variants of the automatic capture algorithm that do not deliver backup pulses on a beat-to-beat basis but provide automatic determination of pacing threshold at programmed intervals during the day. These devices determine the pacing threshold and adjust the pacing amplitude to provide a programmed margin of safety. In general, automatic capture algorithms function quite effectively and may reduce the risk of loss of capture due to fluctuations in pacing threshold caused by drugs, metabolic derangement, or lead dislodgment. The capability for reducing the programmed margin of safety is effective for prolonging battery life and may reduce the frequency of clinic follow-up visits. The Medtronic Ventricular Capture Management feature determines a strength-duration threshold at a programmable interval (nominally, once per day). After the amplitude threshold is determined at a pulse duration of 0.4 msec, the pulse amplitude is doubled and a pulse duration threshold is measured. The permanent ventricular stimulation amplitude is then automatically reprogrammed using a programmable amplitude safety margin (usually twice the threshold) or a programmable minimum amplitude, whichever is higher. The nominal values for ventricular capture management are a safety margin of twice the threshold with a pulse duration of 0.4 msec and a minimum ventricular amplitude of 2.5 V. During measurement of the pacing threshold, each test pulse is followed by a backup pulse 110 msec later to ensure that a pacing pause does not occur. If the automatically measured ventricular stimulation threshold is greater than 2.5 V at 0.4 msec, the ventricular output is automatically programmed to 5.0 V and 1.0 msec.

The Medtronic Atrial Capture Management feature is designed to periodically measure the atrial stimulation threshold and adapt the atrial output to a programmable amplitude safety margin. This feature does not use the evoked potential to determine the presence or absence of atrial capture. Rather, the pacemaker searches for evidence that atrial test pulses reset the sinus node (Atrial Chamber Reset Method) or observes the ventricular response to determine whether a captured atrial test pulse is conducted to the ventricles through the AV conduction system. The Atrial Capture Management feature performs an atrial amplitude threshold at 0.4-msec pulse duration and after loss of capture is detected (defined as two of three test pulses indicating loss of capture); the amplitude setting is increased until atrial capture is confirmed. Because this feature does not rely on detection of the evoked response, there is no restriction on the type of atrial lead that can be used. This feature will not measure thresholds if the sinus rate is consistently faster than 87 bpm.

Adequate Margin of Safety

A pacemaker must be programmed with a safety factor that allows for changes in pacing threshold. One needs to know how much thresholds actually change in the acute to chronic period as well as chronically on an hour-to-hour and day-to-day basis. Settings as low as 2.5 V and 0.5 msec at implantation appear to ensure capture for most adult patients with modern microporous, steroid-eluting leads. Higher values should be used with older technology leads. Some patients have large variations in threshold. The factors involved in estimating how great a margin of safety to allow in programming are the presently measured threshold, the probability of a catastrophe if pacing ceases, the ability of the patient to recognize intermittent loss of capture if it is occurring, the pharmacologic milieu, and how often the pacing threshold will be checked. In most patients, a ratio of output voltage (V_o) to threshold voltage (V_{thr}), or output current to threshold current, that is 1.5 : 1 or 2 : 1 provides a reasonable safety factor. The balance over years is that of safety factor beyond threshold versus how long the pulse generator can be used. Again, clinical factors and patient reliability in checking have to be considered.

Children may experience a higher rate of exit block because of their active inflammatory responses. In all patients, but especially children, use of steroid-eluting electrodes is wise whenever possible.[243-245] In a study reporting on 4953 threshold measurements made up to 20 years after implantation, long-term thresholds and threshold variations of non–steroid-eluting electrodes were found to be greater in children than in adults.[81]

The safety factors provided during the peak threshold phase are highest for steroid-eluting porous electrodes and lower for (in descending order) microporous electrodes, porous electrodes, and polished-tip electrodes, based on data represented in Figure 1-32. There may also be situations in which the patient's pacemaker must be set at the maximum output at implantation (e.g., if the patient will not be available for follow-up). In these cases, an acceptable balance of safety margin and battery longevity might be obtained with a setting of 2.5 V and 0.5 msec for a steroid-eluting electrode, or a setting of up to 5 V and 0.5 msec with other leads. These numbers are at best only general guides. It is far better to arrange, by whatever means possible, for actual follow-up threshold measurements, both acutely and chronically.

Modern perception of the range of chronic circadian threshold variation is based mainly on the work of Sowton and Norman[246] (published in the mid-1960s), Preston and coworkers[247] (in the late 1960s), and Westerholm[248] (in 1971). The first two studies used constant-current generators and reported thresholds in terms of energy. Because the computed energy "thresholds" could have been a reflection of changes in impedance, the actual variation in voltage threshold cannot be determined from these studies. Westerholm, who reported both voltage and energy data, noted substantial circadian variations in both parameters. In all of these studies, the leads were primarily epicardial/myocardial with polished electrodes. These human data, however, may be of marginal relevance to modern constant-voltage generators and porous, steroid-eluting electrodes.

Long-Term and Diurnal Variations in Pacing Threshold

McVenes and associates,[249] in 1992, found no significant threshold changes in adult canines using then-modern chronic atrial or ventricular leads as a function of eating, sleeping, or exercise. This finding is supported by Kadish and coauthors,[250] who found no changes in chronic human pacing thresholds during a 24-hour period in four of five patients studied. Although in one patient the threshold at 0.6 msec changed from 1 to 1.5 V between 3:00 and 6:00 PM, these investigators concluded that "ventricular pacing thresholds do not show substantial diurnal variability."[250] Grendahl and Schaanning also found minimal variation in pacing threshold during the day, after meals, or during sleeping or physical activity.[192,251]

Shepard and associates[81] reviewed 4942 pacing threshold measurements they made in 257 patients with 312 non–steroid-eluting leads at up to 295 months after implantation. The median in-use time was 17 months. Of the measurements, 1053 were in children younger than 12 years of age. At stimulus durations of 0.5 ± 0.04 msec, for thresholds measured 1 month or more after implantation, the mean threshold was 1.2 ± 0.66 V for endocardial electrodes and 2.8 ± 1.39 V for epicardially applied electrodes. Highest mean thresholds were in the 6- to 12-year-old age group. In patients with five or more measurements after 3 months use, an increase in pacing threshold occurred after 3 months in 24%. An additional 21% had at least one threshold that exceeded the post-3-months individual patient mean by three standard deviations. Among other clinical events possibly related to threshold increases, one was the occurrence in a child of doubling of the threshold during two successive summers, at the times when symptoms resembling a mild cold began.

The effects of various drugs on thresholds have been reported, but neither the test protocols nor the results have been consistent.[252] Therefore, there appears to be little in the literature to support the statistical validity of any particular safety factor.

On the basis of the earlier report of Preston and colleagues,[247] Barold and associates[253] suggested that V_o/V_{thr} must be at least 1.75 to ensure an adequate safety margin, assuming a 50% increase in energy at threshold throughout the day. Ohm and colleagues[178,254] studied threshold evolution as a function of implant duration for an 8-mm^2 polished platinum ring electrode and found that this lead had a peak threshold of 2.2 ± 0.75 V at a pulse duration of 0.5 msec measured 2 weeks after implantation. Assuming an output setting of 5 V and 0.5 msec pulse duration, the average patient had a V_o/V_{thr} of 2.3 : 1 during the peak threshold time. The 98th percentile patient (mean ± 2 standard deviations) had a V_o of 5 V and a V_{thr} of 2.2 ± 0.75 V, or a safety margin of about 1.35 : 1 at peak threshold. Unpredictable or unusual situations (e.g., myxedema) may occur that justify greater safety factor ratios.[255] The important clinical point is that, for patients who are always or intermittently dependent on pacing to stay alive, a much greater pacing safety factor reduces the risk of otherwise unexplained sudden death.

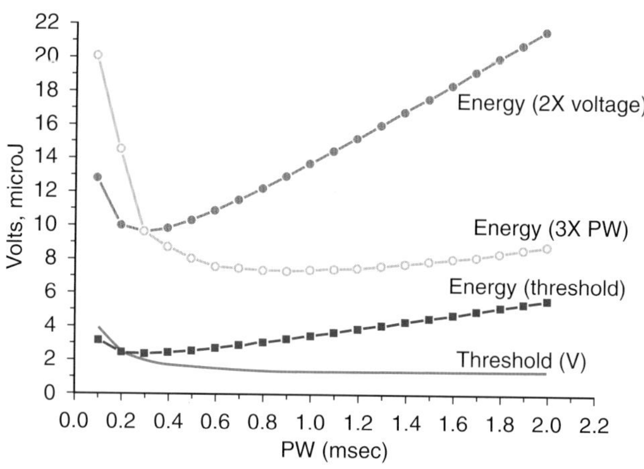

Figure 1-37. Effect on current drain and safety margin of programming the stimulus voltage to twice the threshold (at a constant pulse duration) or programming the pulse width (PW) to three times the threshold value (at the threshold voltage). See text for discussion.

Programming Voltage Versus Pulse Width for Maximum Pulse Generator Longevity

A common clinical concern for programming of the pulse generator to optimize battery longevity relates to whether it is more useful to program the amplitude or the duration of the output pulse. Based on examination of the strength-duration relationship, it is more efficient to reduce the V_o of the pulse, because the current drain varies as the square of voltage. Figure 1-37 illustrates the effect of doubling the V_{thr} (at a constant pulse width) or tripling the threshold pulse width (without changing voltage) on current drain. In this example, the rheobase voltage was determined to be 1 V and the chronaxie duration was 0.3 msec. The stimulation threshold was 4 V at a pulse duration of 0.1 msec or 2 V at 0.3 msec. Tripling the pulse duration at 4 V to 0.3 msec provided an adequate (2 : 1) safety margin with a current of 8 mA per pulse (4.8 μA continuous current) and a stimulus energy of 9.6 μJ. Similarly, doubling the V_{thr} at a pulse duration of 0.3 msec from 2 to 4 V yielded an identical current drain (8 mA/pulse, or 4.8 μA) and safety factor. If the patient had a higher threshold, for example 2 V at 1 msec, doubling of the voltage or tripling of the pulse width would still give the same current drain (12 μA), but the safety factor would be significantly different. Tripling the pulse width would provide a marginal (at best) safety margin, because threshold is approaching rheobase on the flat portion of the strength-duration curve. It would be necessary to double the voltage in this case to ensure a 2 : 1 safety margin. The foremost consideration for programming voltage and pulse duration is patient safety.

Summary

Myocardial stimulation is the fundamental principle underlying artificial cardiac pacing. Perhaps the most important concept for programming of an implantable pacing system is a thorough understanding of the strength-duration relationship. Pulse generators allow the clinician to program both the pulse amplitude (in volts) and the pulse duration (in milliseconds). The stimulation threshold is a function of both of these parameters. The exponential shape of the strength-duration curve must always be considered when programming the output pulse to ensure an adequate margin of safety between the delivered stimulus and the capture threshold.

For example, pulse durations of 1 msec and greater are located on the flat portion of the strength-duration curve, whereas pulse durations of less than 0.15 msec are on the steeply rising portion of the curve. The practical importance of these facts can be appreciated by considering two points on the strength-duration curve shown in Figure 1-8. If the clinician determines the threshold to occur at point A (2 V and 0.5 msec) by decrementing the stimulus voltage at a constant pulse duration, programming of the pulse duration to 1 msec (point B) would provide very little margin of safety. Similarly, if the threshold is measured to be at point C (3.5 V and 0.15 msec) by decrementing the pulse duration at a constant voltage, doubling of the stimulation voltage to 7 V (point D) also would provide a poor safety margin. When one considers the shape of the strength-duration curve, a more appropriate programmed setting would be provided by doubling the threshold voltage at a pulse duration of 0.5 msec (point E, 4 V and 0.5 msec). As a general rule, if the threshold is determined by decrementing the stimulus voltage, an adequate margin of safety can be assumed by doubling the voltage if the pulse duration used was greater than 0.3 msec.

The two most important points on the strength-duration curve (rheobase and chronaxie) are easily estimated with modern pulse generators (see Fig. 1-8). Rheobase can be estimated by decrementing the output voltage at a pulse duration of 1.5 to 2 msec. Chronaxie can then be estimated by determining the threshold pulse duration at twice the rheobase voltage.

If instead the threshold is determined by decrementing the pulse duration, an adequate safety margin can be assumed by tripling the pulse duration only if the threshold is 0.15 msec or less. If the rheobase and chronaxie are measured, doubling of the threshold voltage at the chronaxie pulse duration provides an excellent method for programming a pacing system. However, in most circumstances, experienced clinicians will measure the pacing threshold at an initial stimulus duration of 0.4 or 0.5 msec and then make decisions based on their knowledge of the patient's problems and medicines.

What constitutes an adequate safety factor depends on knowledge of the patient's status. How dependent on the pacemaker is the patient? How medically stable is the patient? What medicines that can influence the pacing threshold is this patient taking? Have important threshold variations been seen or are they anticipated in this patient after the initial stabilization period? Are there problems with the leads? How old is the pulse generator, and what is the known history of this pulse generator and of the leads attached to it in other patients? These are important factors that move clinical judgment in regard to voltage or current safety factors, how often pacing and medical status will be checked, and whether there should be early or late replacement of the pulse generator and/or leads. The rules described in the previous paragraph are only a guide. Added to this must be clinical knowledge of the patient and of the particular pacing system.

When programming the pulse generator at the time of implantation, the clinician must also consider the acute to chronic evolution of the stimulation threshold. Because there is typically an acute rise in threshold during the first several weeks after lead implantation, the voltage and pulse duration may need to be programmed to higher values than would be needed for chronic pacing. The physician is wise to re-evaluate the stimulation threshold after the acute rise (and sometimes subsequent fall) that may occur after implantation. For most patients, the pacing system can be programmed to chronic output settings at a follow-up evaluation about 6 weeks after lead implantation. Although these recommendations may not be as applicable to patients receiving a steroid-eluting lead, caution is still warranted.

The importance of drug and electrolyte effects on the strength-duration curve should also be appreciated. For patients requiring antiarrhythmic drug therapy, the stimulation threshold should be measured a number of times after drug initiation to ensure an adequate margin of safety for pacing. Similarly, patients who are more likely to experience alterations in electrolyte concentration (e.g., patients with renal failure, patients taking potassium-wasting diuretics) may need their pacemakers to be programmed with a greater margin of safety.

Perhaps most important, the degree to which the heart is dependent on pacing to sustain life or to prevent severe symptoms must be factored into the choice of a programmed margin of safety. For pacemaker-dependent patients, a pacing pulse that is at least 2.5 times the chronic capture threshold is usually recommended. In contrast, patients who are unlikely to experience severe symptoms should failure to capture occur may have their pacemaker programmed to a lower margin of safety (perhaps 2 times the threshold). The effect of pacing rate on the stimulation threshold should also be considered for patients who require antitachycardia pacing. The pacing threshold should be measured at all rates likely to be used for antitachycardia pacing.

In the presence of high impedance due to lead fracture, the current output of a constant-voltage pulse generator decreases. Loss of capture can occur. If lead insulation failure occurs, the impedance as seen by the pulse generator may decrease because of current shunting to noncardiac tissue. This results in an increase in the current from the pulse generator without a change in the nominal output voltage. This change may not be detected early on if threshold is determined only by the voltage required for pacing capture. Of course, if one

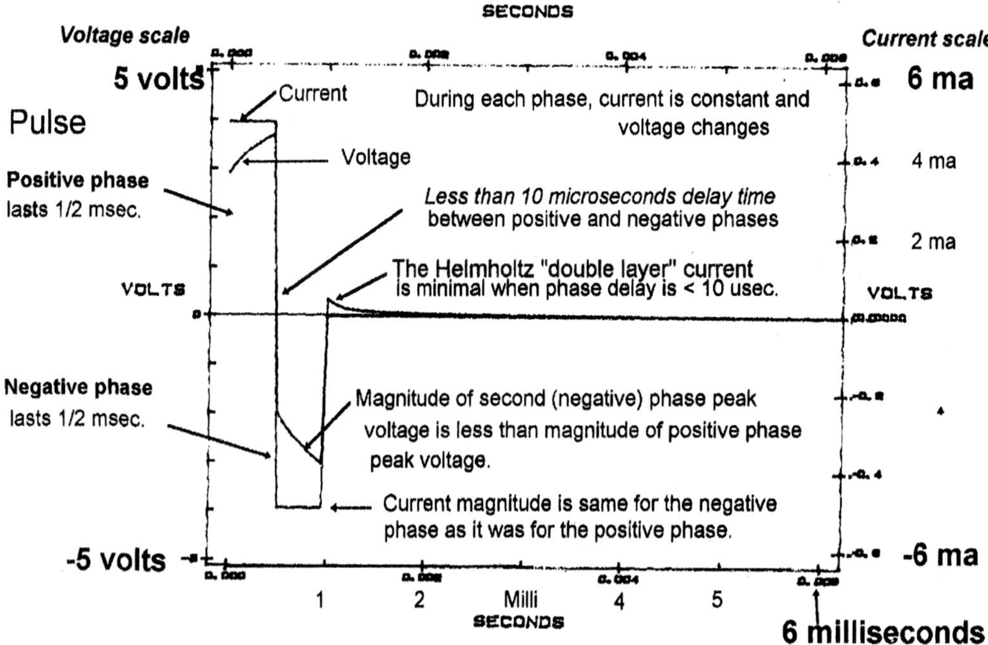

Figure 1-38. Effects of bipolar constant–current pacing on voltage response and on after–current.

measures the voltage/current ratio, the nominal impedance and alterations in lead insulation or in wire continuity may be detectable. Because some wire fractures intermittently make and break contact, a normal impedance measurement does not always ensure that the lead is intact.

Pacing impedance is determined by four factors: (1) resistance in the conductor wire pathways, (2) polarization at the electrode-tissue interfaces, (3) resistance (small geometric size for high resistance) at the electrode-tissue interface, and (4) impedance/resistance of the tissues between the electrodes. The first two of these factors are energy inefficient, decreasing the current available for stimulation, whereas the third factor decreases current drain without decreasing the efficiency of stimulation. An ideal electrode would have, among other attributes, high resistance and high capacitance (low polarization voltage) at the electrode-tissue interface.

Pacing with a monophasic stimulus is more energy efficient than pacing with a bipolar stimulus. One reason is that the pacing threshold is greater at normal stimulus durations for biphasic stimuli compared with uniphasic stimuli with the same total duration. For successful defibrillation, biphasic stimuli are more energy efficient.

Figure 1-38 shows the relationships between a constant-current biphasic stimulus with microsecond-level delay between the phases and the electrode-electrolyte interface effects on voltage during the stimulus and on current flow after the stimulus stops. A biphasic stimulus with proper characteristics reduces the postpulse ion rearrangements. Biphasic stimuli also may reverse some otherwise continuing local and undesirable chemical processes at the electrode.

Electrical stimulation, not only of the heart but also of other kinds of tissue (e.g., brain), is being used clinically more and more. Increasing knowledge of fundamental factors in electrical stimulation and of what can be useful and practical or developed for particular clinical circumstances is desirable. Such knowledge will help cardiologists, as well as physicians and surgeons of other disciplines, make good decisions and expand the range of patient care.

REFERENCES

1. Bockris JO'M, Reddy AKN, Gamboa-Aldeco M: Modern Electrochemistry 2A: Fundamentals of Electrodics, 2nd ed. New York, Kluwer Academic/Plenum Publishers, 2000, p 1050.
2. Huxley Sir AH: Regarding Kenneth Stewart Cole, July 10, 1900-April 18, 1984. In Huxley Sir AH: Biographical Memoirs). Washington, DC, National Academies Press, 1996, pp 24-45. Available at http://books.nap.edu/html/biomems/kcole.html
3. Cole KS: Membranes, Ions and Impulses: A Chapter of Classical Biophysics. Berkeley, University of California Press, 1968, p 173, figure 2:50, and chapter beginning on p 204.
4. Koch H: Recent advances in magnetocardiography. J Electrocardiol 37(Suppl):117-122, 2004.
5. Mayhew M, Johnson P, Slabaugh J, et al: Electrical characteristics of a split cathodal pacing configuration. PACE 26:2264-2271, 2003.
6. Corr PB: Contribution of lipid metabolites to arrhythmogenesis during early myocardial ischemia. In Rosen MR, Janse MJ, Wit AL (eds): Cardiac Electrophysiology: A Textbook. Mt. Kisco, NY, Futura, 1990, pp 720-722.

7. Kleber AG: Sodium-potassium pumping. In Rosen MR, Janse MJ, Wit AL (eds): Cardiac Electrophysiology: A Textbook. Mt. Kisco, NY, Futura, 1990, pp 37-54.
8. Hodgkin AL, Katz B: The effect of sodium ions on the electrical activity of the giant axon of the squid. J Physiol (Lond) 108:37, 1949.
9. Hodgkin AL, Huxley AF: A quantitative description of membrane current and its application to conduction and excitation in nerve. J Physiol (Lond) 117:500-544, 1952.
10. Neher E, Sakmann B, Steinbach JH: The extracellular patch clamp: Method for resolving currents through individual open channels in biological membranes. Plugers Arch Eur J Physiol 375:219, 1978.
11. Neher E, Sakmann B: The patch clamp technique. Sci Am 266: 44-51, 1992.
12. Ebihara L: The sodium current. In Rosen MR, Janse MJ, Wit AL (eds): Cardiac Electrophysiology: A Textbook. Mt. Kisco, NY, Futura, 1990, pp 63-74.
13. Hartel HC, Duchatelle-Gourdon I: Structure and neural modulation of cardiac calcium channels. J Cardiovasc Electrophysiol 3:567-578, 1992.
14. Tsien RW: Calcium channels in the cardiovascular system. In Rosen MR, Janse MJ, Wit AL (eds): Cardiac Electrophysiology: A Textbook. Mt. Kisco, NY, Futura, 1990, pp 75-89.
15. Thomas RC: Electrogenic sodium pump in nerve and muscle cells. Physiol Rev 52:563-594, 1972.
16. Glitsch HG: Electrogenic Na pumping in the heart. Annu Rev Physiol 44:389-400, 1982.
17. Gadsky DC: The Na/K pump of cardiac cells. Annu Rev Biophys Bioeng 13:373-398, 1984.
18. Mullins IJ: The generation of electric currents in cardiac fibers by Na/Ca exchange. Am J Physiol 236:C103-C110, 1979.
19. Hilgemann DW: Numerical approximations of sodium-calcium exchange. Prog Biophys Mol Biol 51:1-45, 1988.
20. Carmeliet E: The cardiac action potential. In Rosen MR, Janse MJ, Wit AL (eds): Cardiac Electrophysiology: A Textbook. Mt. Kisco, NY, Futura, 1990, pp 55-62.
21. Hoffman BF, Cranefield PF: Electrophysiology of the Heart. New York, McGraw-Hill, 1960.
22. Binah O: The transient outward current in the mammalian heart. In Rosen MR, Janse MJ, Wit AL (eds): Cardiac Electrophysiology: A Textbook. Mt. Kisco, NY, Futura, 1990, pp 93-106.
23. Joho RH: Toward a molecular understanding of voltage-gated potassium channels. J Cardiovasc Electrophysiol 3:589-601, 1992.
24. Coraboeuf E, Carmeliet E: Existence of two transient outward currents in sheep cardiac Purkinje fibers. Pflugers Arch 392:352-359, 1982.
25. Cohen IS, Datyner N: Repolarizing membrane currents. In Rosen MR, Janse MJ, Wit AL (eds): Cardiac Electrophysiology: A Textbook. Mt. Kisco, NY, Futura, 1990, pp 107-116.
26. Bottazzi F: Leonardo as physiologist. In Bottazzi F, Leonardo da Vinci. London, Leisure Arts, 1964, pp 373-387.
27. Harvey W: De Motu Cordis. [The Movement of the Heart and Blood]. Translated by D. Whiteridge. Oxford, Blackwell, 1976, 1628.
28. Keith A, Flack M: The form and nature of the muscular connections between the primary divisions of the vertebrate heart. J Anat Physiol 41:172-189, 1907.
29. Irisawa H: Comparative physiology of the cardiac pacemaker mechanism. Physiol Rev 58:461-498, 1978.
30. DiFrancesco D: The hyperpolarization-activated current, If, and cardiac pacemaking. In Rosen, MR, Janse ML, Wit AL (eds): Cardiac Electrophysiology: A Textbook. Mt. Kisco, NY, Futura, 1990, pp 117-132.
31. Urthaler F, Isobe JH, James TN: Comparative effects of glucagon on automaticity of the sinus node and atrioventricular junction. Am J Physiol 227:1415-1421, 1974.
32. Bean RC: Protein-mediated mechanisms of variable ion conductance in thin lipid membranes. Membranes 2:409-477, 1973.
33. Haydon DA, Hladky SB: Ion transport across thin lipid membranes: A critical discussion of mechanisms in selected systems. Q Rev Biophys 5:187-282, 1972.
34. Jongsma HJ, Rook MB: Biophysics of cardiac gap junction channels. In Zipes DP, Jalif J (eds): Cardiac Electrophysiology: From Cell to Bedside, 3rd ed. Philadelphia, WB Saunders, 2000, pp 119-125.
35. Bény J-L: Information networks in the arterial wall. News Physiol Sci 14:68-73, 1999.
36. Weidmann S: Passive properties of cardiac fibers. In Rosen MR, Janse MJ, Wit AL (eds): Cardiac Electrophysiology: A Textbook. Mt. Kisco, NY, Futura, 1990, 29-35.
37. Weidmann, S: Electrical constants of trabecular muscle from mammalian heart. J Physiol (Lond) 210:1041-1054, 1970.
38. Knisley SB: Transmembrane voltage changes during unipolar stimulation of rabbit ventricle. Circ Res 77:1229-1239, 1995.
39. Furman S, Parker B, Escher DJW: Decreasing electrode size and increasing efficiency of cardiac stimulation. J Surg Res 11:105, 1971.
40. Furman S, Hurzler P, Parker B: Clinical thresholds of endocardial cardiac stimulation: A long-term study. J Surg Res 19:149, 1975.
41. Angello DA, McAnulty JH, Dobbs J: Characterization of chronically implanted ventricular endocardial pacing leads. Am Heart J 107:1142-1145, 1984.
42. Geddes LA, Bourland JD: The strength-duration curve. IEEE Trans Biomed Eng BME-32:458-459, 1985.
43. Irnich W: Considerations in electrode design for permanent pacing. In Thalen HJT (ed): Cardiac Pacing. Proceedings of the IVth International Symposium on Cardiac Pacing. Assen, The Netherlands, Van Gorcum, 1973, p 268.
44. Irnich W: Engineering concepts of pacemaker electrodes. In Schaldach M, Furman S (eds): Advances in Pacemaker Technology. New York, Springer-Verlag, 1975, p 241.
45. Shepard RB: Invited letter concerning: The effect of extraanatomic bypass on aortic root impedance in open chest dogs: Should the vascular prosthesis be compliant to unload the left ventricle? J Thorac Cardiovasc Surg 104:1175-1177, 1992.
46. Bardou AL, Chenais J-M, Birkui PJ, et al: Directional variability of stimulation threshold measurements in isolated guinea pig cardiomyocytes: Relationship with orthogonal sequential defibrillating pulses. PACE 13:1590-1595, 1990.
47. Preston TA, Fletcher RD, Lucchesi BR, Judge RD: Changes in myocardial thresholds: Physiologic and pharmacologic factors in patients with implanted pacemakers. Am Heart J 74:235-242, 1967.
48. Katsumoto K, Niibori I, Takamatsu T, Kaibara M: Development of glassy carbon electrode (Dead Sea scroll) for low energy cardiac pacing. PACE 9(6 Pt 2):1220-1224, 1986.
49. Mond H, Stokes KB, Helland J, et al: The porous titanium steroid eluting electrode: A double blind study assessing the stimulation threshold effects of steroid. PACE 11:214-219, 1988.
50. Hill WE, Murray A, Bourks JP, et al: Minimum energy for cardiac pacing. Clin Phys Physiol Meas 9:41-46, 1988.
51. Breivik K, Ohm O-J, Engedal H: Acute and chronic pulse-width thresholds in solid versus porous tip electrodes. PACE 5:650-657, 1982.
52. Irnich W: The chronaxie time and its practical importance. PACE 3:292-301, 1980.
53. Barold SS, Stokes KB, Byrd CL, McVenes R: Energy parameters in cardiac pacing should be abandoned. PACE 20:112-121, 1996.
54. Furman S, Hurzler P, Parker B: Clinical thresholds of endocardial cardiac stimulation: A long-term study. J Surg Res 19:149, 1975.
55. Ideker RE, Zhou X, Knisley SB: Correlation among fibrillation, defibrillation, and cardiac pacing. PACE 18:512-525, 1995.
56. Roth BJ: Virtual electrodes made simple: A cellular excitable medium modified for strong electrical stimuli. Rochester, MI,

Department of Physics, Oakland University, 2002. Available at http://sprojects.mmi.mcgill.ca/heart/pages/rot/rothom.html
57. Newton JC, Knisley SB: Review of mechanisms by which electrical stimulation alters the transmembrane potential. J Cardiovasc Electrophysiol 10:234-243, 1999.
58. Knisley SB: Transmembrane voltage changes during unipolar stimulation of rabbit ventricle. Circ Res 77:1229-1239, 1995.
59. Srinivasan R, Roth BJ: A mathematical model for electrical stimulation of a monolayer of cardiac cells. Biomed Eng Online 3:1, 2004.
60. Wikswo JP Jr, Lin SF, Abbas RA: Virtual electrodes in cardiac tissue: A common mechanism for anodal and cathodal stimulation. Biophys J 69:2195-2210, 1995.
61. Efimove IR, Gray RA, Roth BJ: Virtual electrodes and deexcitation: New insights into fibrillation induction and defibrillation. J Cardiovasc Electrophysiol 11:339-353, 2000.
62. Knisley SB, Pollard AE, Fast VG: Effects of electrode-myocardial separation on cardiac stimulation in conductive solution. J Cardiovasc Electrophysiol 11:1132-1143, 2000.
63. Knisley SB, Pollard AE: Effects of electrode-myocardial separation on cardiac stimulation in conductive solution. J Cardiovasc Electrophysiol 11:1132-1143, 2000.
64. Shepard RB, Epstein AE, Kirklin JK, et al: Use of epipericardial rate-sensing/pacing electrodes in defibrillator implantation (avoid intra-pericardial scarring pretransplantation). PACE 15:575, 1992.
65. Nikolski VP, Sambelashvili AT: Mechanisms of make and break excitation revisited: Paradoxical break excitation during diastolic stimulation. Am J Physiol Heart Circ Physiol 282:H565-H575, 2002.
66. Sambelashvili AT, Nikolski VP, Efimov IR: Virtual electrode theory explains pacing threshold increase caused by cardiac tissue damage. Am J Physiol Heart Circ Physiol 286:H2183-H2194, 2004.
67. Dressler L, Gruse G, von Knorre GH, et al: The optimization of the pulse delivered by the pacemaker. PACE 2:282, 1979.
68. Chaptal AP, Ribot A: Statistical survey of strength-duration threshold curves with endocardial electrodes and long-term behavior of these electrodes. In Meere C (ed): Proceedings of the VI World Symposium on Cardiac Pacing. Montreal: PACESYMP 1979, pp 21-22.
69. Blair HA: On the quantity of electricity and the energy in electrical stimulation. J Gen Physiol 19:951-964, 1936.
70. Geddes LA: Historical evolution of circuit models for the electrode-electrolyte interface. Ann Biomed Eng 25:1-14, 1997.
71. Hoorweg JL: Condensatorentladung und auseinandersetzung mit du Bois-Reymond. Pflugers Arch 52:87-108, 1892.
72. Weiss G: Sur la possibilité de render comparable entre les appareils cervant à l'excitation électrique. Arch Ital Biol 35:413, 1901.
73. Lapique L: Definition experimentale de l'excitabilité. C R Soc Bil 67:280, 1909.
74. Lapique L: La chronaxie et ses applications physiologiques. Paris, Hermann et Cie, 1938.
75. Irnich W: Elektrotherapie des herzens. Berlin, Fachverlag Schiele & Schon, 1976.
76. Irnich W: The chronaxie time and its practical importance. PACE 3:292, 1980.
77. Bernstein AD, Parsonnet V: Implications of constant energy pacing. PACE 6:1229-1233, 1983.
78. Barold SS, Stokes KB, Byrd CL, McVenes R: Energy parameters in cardiac pacing should be abandoned. PACE 20:112-121, 1996.
79. Coates S, Thwaites B: The strength-duration curve and its importance in pacing efficiency. PACE 23:1273-1277, 2000.
80. Gurjao de Goday CM, de Magalhaes Galvao K, de Almeida Bacarin T, Franco GR: The effects of electrode position on the excitability of rat atria during postnatal development. Physiol Meas 23:649-659, 2002.
81. Shepard RB, Kim J, Colvin EC, et al: Pacing threshold spikes months and years after implant. PACE 14:1835-1841, 1991.
82. Wedensky NE: Uber die Beziehungzwischen Reizung und erregung im Tetanus. St. Petersburg, Ber Akad Wiss, 54:96, 1887.
83. Langberg JJ, Sousa J, El-Atassi R, et al: The mechanism of pacing capture hysteresis in humans [abstract]. PACE 15:577, 1992.
84. Swerdlow CD, Olson WH, O'Connor ME, et al: Cardiovascular collapse caused by electrocardiographically silent 60-Hz intracardiac leakage current. Circulation 99:2559-2564, 1999.
85. Hook BC, Perlman RL, Callans JD, et al: Acute and chronic cycle length dependent increase in ventricular pacing threshold. PACE 15:1437-1444, 1992.
86. Plumb VJ, Karp RB, James TN, Waldo AL: Atrial excitability and conduction during rapid atrial pacing. Circulation 63:1140-1149, 1981.
87. Buxton AE, Marchlinski FE, Miller JM, et al: The human atrial strength-interval relation: Influence of cycle length and procainamide. Circulation 79:271-280, 1989.
88. Katsumoto K, Niibori T, Watanabe Y: Rate dependent threshold changes during atrial pacing: Clinical and experimental studies. PACE 13:1009-1019, 1990.
89. Kay GN, Mulholland DH, Epstein AE, Plumb VJ: Effect of pacing rate on human atrial strength-duration curves. J Am Coll Cardiol 15:1618-1623, 1990.
90. Lindemans FW, Denier van der Gon JJ: Current thresholds and luminal size in excitation of heart muscle. Cardiovasc Res 12:477, 1977.
91. Irnich W, Gebhardt U: The pacemaker-electrode combination and its relationship to service life. In Thalen HJTh (ed): To Pace or Not to Pace: Controversial Subjects in Cardiac Pacing. The Hague, Martin Nijhoff, 1978, p 209.
92. Parsonnet V, Zucker IR, Kannerstein ML: The fate of permanent intracardiac electrodes. J Surg Res 6:285, 1966.
93. Thalen HJTh, Van den Berg JW: Threshold measurements and electrodes of the cardiac pacemaker. Acta Pharmacol Nederl 14:227, 1966.
94. Akyurekli Y, Taichman GC, White DL, et al: Myocardial responses to sutureless epicardial lead pacing. In Meere C (ed): Proceedings of the VI World Symposium on Cardiac Pacing. Montreal: PACESYMP 1979.
95. Stokes K, Bornzin G: The electrode-biointerface (stimulation). In Barold SS (ed): Modern Cardiac Pacing. Mt. Kisco, NY, Futura, 1985, pp 33-78.
96. Amundson DC, McArthur W, Moshaffafa M: The porous endocardial electrode. PACE 2:40, 1979.
97. Stokes KB, Frohlig G, Bird T, et al.: A new bipolar low threshold steroid eluting screw-in lead [abstract]. Eur JCPE 2:A89, 1992.
98. Greatbatch W: Metal electrodes in bioengineering. CRC Crit Rev Bioeng 5:1, 1981.
99. Horowitz P, Hill W: Section 1.18: Frequency analysis of reactive circuits. In Horowitz P, Hill W: The Art of Electronics. Cambridge, Cambridge University Press, 1980, pp 25-29.
100. Schmitt OH: Biological information processing using the concept of interpenetrating domains. In Leibovic KN (ed): Information Processing in the Nervous System. New York, Springer-Verlag, 1969, pp 325-331.
101. Geselowitz DB, Miller WT 3rd: A bidomain model for anisotropic cardiac muscle. Ann Biomed Eng.11:191-206, 1983.
102. Sepulveda NG, Roth BJ, Wikswo JP Jr: Current injection into a two-dimensional anisotropic bidomain. Biophys J 55:987-999, 1989.
103. Ashihara T, Trayanova NA: Asymmetry in membrane responses to electric shocks: Insights from bidomain simulations. Biophys J 87:2271-2282, 2004.
104. Roth BJ: The bidomain model: Two dimensional propagation in cardiac muscle. In Zipes DP, Jalife J (eds): Cardiac Electrophysiology: From Cell to Bedside, 3rd ed. Philadelphia, WB Saunders, 2000, pp 268-270.

105. Plonsey R, Barr RC: Inclusion of junction elements in a linear cardiac model through secondary sources: Application to defibrillation. Med Biol Eng Comput 24:137-144, 1986.
106. Roth BJ, Krassowska W: The induction of reentry in cardiac tissue. The missing link: How electric fields alter the transmembrane potential. Chaos 8:204-220, 1998.
107. Sharma V, Tung T: Theoretical and experimental study of sawtooth effect in isolated cardiac cell-pairs. J Cardiovasc Electrophysiol 12:1164-1173, 2001.
108. Sharma V, Tung L: Spatial heterogeneity of transmembrane potential responses of single guinea-pig cardiac cells during electric field stimulation. J Physiol 542:477-492, 2002.
109. Irnich W: The fundamental law of electrostimulation and its application to defibrillation. PACE 13(11 Pt 1):1433-1447, 1990.
110. Irnich W: George Weiss' fundamental law of electrostimulation is 100 years old. PACE 25:245-248, 2002.
111. Thakor NV, Ranjan MS, Rajasekhar MS, et al: Effect of varying pacing waveform shapes on propagation and hemodynamics in the rabbit heart. Am J Cardiol 79:36-43, 1997.
112. Huang J, Ken-Knight BH, Walcott GP, et al: Effects of transvenous electrode polarity and waveform duration on the relationship between defibrillation threshold and upper limit of vulnerability. Circulation 96:1351-1359, 1997.
113. Wagner B: Electrodes, leads, and biocompatibility. In Webster J (ed): Design of Cardiac Pacemakers. Piscataway, NJ, IEEE Press, 1995, p 138.
114. Lilly JC, Hughes JR, Ellsworth CA, et al: Noninjurious electric waveform for stimulation of the brain. Science 121:468, 1955.
115. Moor WJ: Physical Chemistry. Englewood Cliffs, NJ, Prentice-Hall, 1972, p 510.
116. von Helmholtz H: The modern development of Faraday's conception of electricity, delivered before the Fellows of the Chemical Society in London on April 5, 1881.
117. Bockris J O'M, Reddy AKN, Gamboa-Aldeco M: Modern Electrochemistry 2A: Fundamentals of Electrodics, 2nd ed. New York, Kluwer Academic/Plenum Publishers, 2000, p 885.
118. Bockris J O'M, Reddy AKN, Gamboa-Aldeco M: Modern Electrochemistry 2A: Fundamentals of Electrodics, 2nd ed. New York, Kluwer Academic/Plenum Publishers, 2000, pp 1047-1049, 1122-1123.
119. Faraday M: On Electrical Decomposition. Philosophical Transactions of the Royal Society, 1834.
120. Bockris J O'M, Reddy AKN, Gamboa-Aldeco M: Modern Electrochemistry 2A: Fundamentals of Electrodics, 2nd ed. New York, Kluwer Academic/Plenum Publishers, 2000, pp 771-1033.
121. Bockris J O'M, Reddy AKN, Gamboa-Aldeco M: Modern Electrochemistry 2A: Fundamentals of Electrodics, 2nd ed. New York, Kluwer Academic/Plenum Publishers, 2000, pp 873-882.
122. Ragheb T, Geddes LA: Electrical properties of metallic electrodes. Biol Eng Comput 28:182-186, 1990.
123. Wagner B: Electrodes, leads, and biocompatibility. In Webster J (ed): Design of Cardiac Pacemakers. Piscataway, NJ, IEEE Press, 1995, p 138.
124. Bockris JO'M, Reddy AKN, Gamboa-Aldeco M: Modern Electrochemistry 2A: Fundamentals of Electrodics, 2nd ed. New York, Kluwer Academic/Plenum, 2000, p 1455.
125. Kahn A, Greatbatch W: Physiologic electrodes. In Ray C (ed): Medical Engineering. Chicago, Year Book Medical, 1974, p 1073.
126. Mindt W, Schaldach M: Electrochemical aspects of pacing electrodes. In Schaldach M, Furman S (eds): Advances in Pacemaker Technology. New York, Springer-Verlag, 1975, p 297.
127. Knisley SB, Smith WM, Ideker RE: Effect of intrastimulus polarity reversal on electric field stimulation thresholds in frog and rabbit myocardium. J Cardiovasc Electrophysiol 3:239-254, 1992.
128. Recognizing a Warburg impedance. Research Solutions & Resources (Dr. Bob Rodgers). Available at http://www.consultrsr.com/resources/eis/warburg1.htm
129. Bockris JO'M, Reddy AKN, Gamboa-Aldeco M: Modern Electrochemistry 2A: Fundamentals of Electrodics, 2nd ed. New York, Kluwer Academic/Plenum Publishers, 2000, p 1133.
130. Ovadia M, Zavitz DH: Impedance spectroscopy of the electrode-tissue interface of living heart with isoosmotic conductivity perturbation. Chem Phys Lett 390:445-453, 2004.
131. Rodman JE: Solution, Surface and Solid State Assembly of Porphyrins [PhD thesis]. Cambridge, University of Cambridge, 2000, Fig. 4.6.
132. Rho RW, Patel VV, Gerstenfeld EP, et al: Elevations in ventricular pacing threshold with the use of the Y Adapter: Implications for biventricular pacing. PACE 26:747-751, 2003.
133. Krassowska W, Neu JC: Response of a single cell to an external electric field. Biophys J 66:1768-1776, 1994.
134. Lu C-C, Kabakov A, Maarkin V: Membrane transport mechanisms probed by capacitance measurements with megahertz voltage clamp. Proc Natl Acad Sci U S A 92:11220-11224, 1995.
135. Mehra R, Furman S: Comparison of cathodal, anodal, and bipolar strength-interval curves with temporary and permanent pacing electrodes. Br Heart J 41:468-476, 1979.
136. Kay GN: Basic aspects of cardiac pacing. In Ellenbogen KA (ed): Cardiac Pacing. Cambridge, MA, Blackwell Scientific, 1992.
137. Preston TA: Anodal stimulation as a cause of pacemaker-induced ventricular fibrillation. Am Heart J 86:366-372, 1973.
138. Wiggers CJ, Wegria R, Pinera B: Effects of myocardial ischemia on fibrillation threshold: Mechanism of spontaneous ventricular fibrillation following coronary occlusion. Am J Physiol 131:309-316, 1940.
139. Mehra R, Furman S, Crump JF: Vulnerability of the mildly ischemic ventricle to cathodal, anodal and bipolar stimulation. Circ Res 41:159-166, 1977.
140. Bilitch M, Cosby RS, Cafferry EA: Ventricular fibrillation and competitive pacing. N Engl J Med 276:598-604, 1967.
141. Stokes K, Bird T, Taepke R: A new low threshold, high impedance microelectrode. In Antonioli GE, Reufeut AE, Ector H (eds): Pacemaker Leads. Amsterdam, Elsevier, 1991, pp 543-548.
142. Bird T, Stokes KB: Ventricular electrode spacing and anode size [abstract 205]. Revue Europeene De Technologie Biomedicale 3:63, 1990.
143. De Caprio V: Endocardial Electrograms from Transvenous Pacemaker Electrodes [PhD thesis in biomedical engineering.] New York, Polytechnic Institute of New York, 1977.
144. Garberoglio B, Inguaggiato B, Chinaglia B, Cerise O: Initial results with an activated pyrolytic carbon tip electrode. PACE 6:440, 1982.
145. Jones JL, Jones RE, Balasky G: Improved cardiac cell excitation with symmetrical biphasic defibrillation waveforms. Am J Physiol 253:H1418-H1424, 1987.
146. Tse HF, Lau CP, Leung SK, et al: Single lead DDD system: A comparative evaluation of unipolar, bipolar and overlapping biphasic stimulation and the effects of right atrial floating electrode location on atrial pacing and sensing thresholds: PACE 19:1758-1763, 1996.
147. Izquierdo R, Rodrigo G, Pelegrin J, et al: Single lead DDD pacing using electrodes with longitudinal and diagonal atrial floating dipoles. PACE 25:1692-1698, 2002.
148. Ripart A, Fletcher R: Sensing. In Ellenbogen KA, Kay GN, Wilkoff B (eds): Clinical Cardiac Pacing. Philadelphia, WB Saunders, 1992.
149. Barold SS, Ong LS, Heinle RA: Stimulation and sensing thresholds for cardiac pacing: Electrophysiologic and technical aspects. Prog Cardiovasc Dis 24:1, 1981.
150. Barold SS, Ong LS, Heinle RA: Stimulation and sensing thresholds for cardiac pacing: Electrophysiologic and technical aspects. Prog Cardiovasc Dis 24:1, 1981.
151. Smyth NPD, Tarjan PP, Chernoff E, et al: The significance of electrode surface area and stimulating thresholds in permanent cardiac pacing. J Thorac Cardiovasc Surg 71:559, 1976.

152. Parsonnet V, Zucker IR, Kannerstein ML: The fate of permanent intracardiac electrodes. J Surg Res 6:285, 1966.
153. Thalen HJTh, Van den Berg JW: Threshold measurements and electrodes of the cardiac pacemaker. Acta Pharmacol Nederl 14:227, 1966.
154. Akyurekli Y, Taichman GC, White DL, et al: Myocardial responses to sutureless epicardial lead pacing. In Meere C (ed): Proceedings of the VI World Symposium on Cardiac Pacing. Montreal: PACESYMP 1979.
155. Furman S, Hurzler P, Parker B: Clinical thresholds of endocardial cardiac stimulation: A long-term study. J Surg Res 19:149, 1975.
156. Wilson GJ, MacGregor DC, Bobyn JD, et al: Tissue response to porous-surface electrodes: basis for a new atrial lead design. In Moore C (ed): Proceedings of the VI World Symposium on Cardiac Pacing: PACESYMP 1979.
157. Amundson D, McArthur W, MacCarter D, et al: Porous electrode-tissue interface. In Moore C (ed): Proceedings of the VI World Symposium on Cardiac Pacing: PACESYMP 1979.
158. Amundson DC, McArthur W, Moshaffafa M: The porous endocardial electrode. PACE 2:40, 1979.
159. MacGregor DC, Wilson GJ, Lixfeld W, et al: The porous surface electrode: A new concept in pacemaker lead design. J Thorac Cardiovasc Surg 78:281, 1979.
160. Breivik K, Ohm O-J, Engedahl H: Acute and chronic pulse-width thresholds in solid versus porous tip electrodes. PACE 5:650, 1982.
161. Berman ND, Dickson SE, Lipton IM: Acute and chronic clinical performance comparison of porous and solid electrode design. PACE 5:67, 1982.
162. Freud GE, Chinaglia B: Sintered platinum for cardiac pacing. Int J Artif Organs 4:238, 1981.
163. MacCarter DM, Lundberg KM, Corstjens JP: Porous electrodes: Concept, technology and results. PACE 6:427, 1983.
164. MacGregor DC, Pilliar RM, Wilson GJ, et al: Porous metal surfaces: A radical new concept in prosthetic heart valve design. Trans Am Soc Artif Intern Organs 22:646, 1976.
165. Elmqvist H, Schuller H, Richter G: The carbon tip electrode. PACE 6:436, 1983.
166. Stokes KB, Bornzin G: The electrode-biointerface (stimulation). In Barold SS (ed): Modern Cardiac Pacing. Mt. Kisco, NY, Futura, 1985, pp 33-78.
167. Cornacchia O, Maresta A, Nigro P, et al: Effect of propafenone on chronic ventricular pacing threshold in patients with steroid-eluting (capture) and conventional leads. Eur J Cardiac Pacing Electrophysiol 2:A88, 1992.
168. Pearce JA, Bourland JD, Neilsen W, et al: Myocardial stimulation with ultrashort duration current pulses. PACE 5:52-58, 1982.
169. Meyers GH, Parsonnet V: Engineering in the Heart and Blood Vessels. New York, Wiley-Interscience, 1989.
170. Hurzeler P, Furman S, Escher DJW: Cardiac pacemaker current thresholds versus pulse duration. In Silverman HT, Miller IF, Salkind AJ (eds): Electrochemical Bioscience and Bioengineering. Princeton, NJ, Electrochemical Society, 1973, p 124.
171. Barold SS, Winner JA: Techniques and significance of threshold measurement for cardiac pacing. Chest 70:760, 1976.
172. Brownlee WC, Hirst R: Six years experience with atrial leads. PACE 9(6 Pt 2):1239-1242, 1989.
173. Luceri RM, Furman S, Hurzeler P, et al: Threshold behavior of electrodes in long-term ventricular pacing. Am J Cardiol 40:184, 1977.
174. Bornzin GA, Stokes KB, Wiebusch WA: A low-threshold, low-polarization platinized endocardial electrode [abstract]. PACE 6:A-70, 1983.
175. Elmqvist H, Schuller H, Richter G: The carbon tip electrode. PACE 6:436, 1983.
176. Mond H, Stokes KB: The electrode-tissue interface: The revolutionary role of steroid elution. PACE 15:95-107, 1992.
177. Ohm O-J, Breivik K: Pacing leads. In Gomez FP (ed): Cardiac Pacing, Electrophysiology, Tachyarrhythmias. Madrid, Editorial Group, 1985, pp 971-985.
178. Hoff PI, Breivik K, Tronstad A, et al: A new steroid-eluting electrode for low-threshold pacing. In Gomez FP (ed): Cardiac Pacing, Electrophysiology, Tachyarrhythmias. Mt. Kisco, NY, Futura, 1985, pp 1014-1019.
179. Anderson JM: Inflammatory response to implants. ASAIO Trans 34:101-107, 1988.
180. Henson PM: Mechanisms of exocytosis in phagocytic inflammatory cells. Am J Pathol 101:494-514, 1980.
181. Robinson TF, Cohen-Gould L, Factor SM: Skeletal framewok of mammalian heart muscle: Arrangement of inter- and pericellular connective tissue structures. Lab Invest 29:482-498, 1983.
182. Preston TA, Judge RD: Alteration of pacemaker threshold by drug and physiologic factors. Ann N Y Acad Sci 167:686-692, 1969.
183. Stokes KB, Anderson J: Low threshold leads: The effect of steroid elution. In Antonioli GE (ed): Pacemaker Leads. Amsterdam, Elsevier, 1991, pp 537-542.
184. Sibille Y, Reynolds HY: Macrophages and polymorphonuclear neutrophils in lung defense and injury. Am Rev Respir Dis 141:471-502, 1990.
185. Benditt DG, Kriett JS, Ryberg C, et al: Cellular electrophysiologic effects of dexamethasone sodium phosphate: Implications for cardiac stimulation with steroid-eluting electrodes. Int J Cardiol 22:67-73, 1989.
186. Stokes KB, Kriett JM, Gornick CA, et al: Low-threshold cardiac pacing electrodes. In Frontiers of Engineering in Health Care, 1983: Proceedings of the Fifth Annual Conference IEEE Engineering in Medicine and Biology Society, 1983.
187. Irnich W: Considerations in electrode design for permanent pacing. In Thalen HJT (ed): Cardiac Pacing. Proceedings of the IVth International Symposium on Cardiac Pacing. Assen, The Netherlands, Van Gorcum, 1973, p 268.
188. Irnich W: Engineering concepts of pacemaker electrodes. In Schaldach M, Furman S (eds): Advances in Pacemaker Technology. New York, Springer-Verlag, 1975, p 241.
189. Mond H, Sloman JG, Cowling R, et al: The small tined pacemaker lead: Absence of displacement. In Meere C (ed): Proceedings of the VI World Symposium on Cardiac Pacing, Montreal: PACESYMP 1979, pp 29-35.
190. Baker JH, Shepard RB, Plimb VJ, Kay GN: Effects of fixation mechanism and electrode material on atrial stimulation threshold: Long-term evaluation in 338 patients [abstract]. PACE 15:54, 1992.
191. Cornacchia D, Jacopi F, Fabbri M, et al: Comparison between active screw-in and passive leads for permanent transvenous ventricular pacing [abstract]. PACE 6:A56, 1983.
192. El Gamal M, Van Gelder L, Bonnier J, et al: Comparison of transvenous atrial electrodes employing active (helicoidal) and passive (tined J-lead) fixation in 116 patients [abstract]. PACE 6:205, 1983.
193. Kay GN, Anderson K, Epstein AE, Plumb VJ: Active fixation atrial leads: Randomized comparison of two lead designs. PACE 12:1355-1361, 1989.
194. Rasor NS, Spickler JW, Clabaugh JW: Comparison of power sources for advanced pacemaker applications. In Proceedings of the 7th Intersociety Energy Conversion Engineering Conference, Washington, DC, American Chemical Society, 1972, p 752.
195. Hirshorn MS, Holley LK, Hales JR, et al: Screening of solid and porous materials for pacemaker electrodes. PACE 4:380, 1981.
196. Schaldah M: New pacemaker electrodes. Trans Am Soc Artif Intern Organs 17:29, 1971.
197. Helland J, Stokes KB: Nonfibrosing cardiac pacing electrode. U.S. Patent No. 4033357. February 17, 1976.
198. Elmqvist H, Schuller H, Richter G: The carbon tip electrode. PACE 6:436, 1983.

199. Thuesen L, Jensen PJ, Vejby-Christensen H, et al: Lower chronic stimulation threshold in the carbon-tip than in the platinum-tip endocardial electrode: A randomized study. PACE 12:1592-1599, 1989.
200. Bornzin GA, Stokes KB, Wiebush WA: A low threshold, low polarization, platonized endocardial electrode. PACE 6:A-70, 1983.
201. Mugica J, Duconge B, Henry L, et al: Clinical experience with new leads. PACE 11:1745-1752, 1988.
202. Djordjevic M, Stojanov P, Velimirovic D, et al: Target lead-low threshold electrode. PACE 9:1206-1210, 1986.
203. Amundson DC, McArthur W, Moshaffafa M: The porous endocardial electrode. PACE 2:40, 1979.
204. Timmis GC, Helland J, Westveer DC, et al: The evolution of low threshold leads. Clin Prog Pacing Electrophysiol 1:313, 1983.
205. Berman ND, Dickson SE, Lipton IM: Acute and chronic clinical performance comparison of porous and solid electrode design. PACE 5:67, 1982.
206. Freud GE, Chinaglia B: Sintered platinum for cardiac pacing. Int J Artif Organs 4:238, 1981.
207. Kay GN, Anderson K, Epstein AE, Plumb VJ: Active fixation atrial leads: Randomized comparison of two lead designs. PACE 12:1355-1361, 1989.
208. Stokes KB: Preliminary studies on a new steroid eluting epicardial electrode. PACE 11:1797-1803, 1988.
209. Hamilton R, Gow R, Bahoric B, et al: Steroid-eluting epicardial leads in pediatrics: Improve epicardial thresholds in the first year. PACE 14:2066, 1991.
210. Stokes KB, Frohling G, Bird T, et al: A new bipolar low threshold steroid eluting screw-in lead. Eur J Cardiac Pacing Electrophysiol 2:A89, 1992.
211. Schwaab B, Frohling G, Schwerdt H, et al: Long-term follow-up of a bipolar steroid eluting pacing lead with active and passive fixation. In Antoniolo GE (ed): Pacemaker Leads 1997. Bologna, Monduzzi Editore, 1997, pp 361-364.
212. Schwaab B, Frohling G, Schwerdt H, et al: Long-term follow-up of three microporous active fixation leads in atrial position. In Antoniolo GE (ed): Pacemaker Leads 1997. Bologna, Monduzzi Editore, 1997, pp 365-368.
213. Schwaab B, Frohling G, Schwerdt H, et al: Atrial and ventricular pacing characteristics of a steroid eluting screw-in lead. In Antoniolo GE (ed): Pacemaker Leads 1997. Bologna, Monduzzi Editore, 1997, pp 383-388.
214. Menozzi C: Comparison between latest generation steroid-eluting screw-in and tined leads: Long term follow-up. In Antoniolo GE (ed): Pacemaker Leads 1997. Bologna, Monduzzi Editore, 1997, pp 389-394.
215. Nurnberg JH, Schopper H, Busscher U, et al: Retrospective comparison of epicardial steroid-eluting and conventional leads for pacing after corrective surgery in congenital heart disease. PACE 20:1193, 1997.
216. Wallace AG, Cline RE, Sealy WC, et al: Electrophysiologic effects of quinidine. Circ Res 19:960-969, 1966.
217. Gay RJ, Brown DF: Pacemaker failure due to procainamide toxicity. Am J Cardiol 34:728-731, 1974.
218. Moss AJ, Goldstein S: Clinical and pharmacological factors associated with pacemaker latency and incomplete pacemaker capture. Br Heart J 31:112, 1969.
219. Hellestrand KJ, Burnett PJ, Milne JR, et al: Effect of the antiarrhythmic agent flecainide acetate on acute and chronic pacing thresholds. PACE 6:892, 1983.
220. Salel AF, Seagren SC, Pool PE: Effects on encainide on the function of implanted pacemakers. PACE 12:1439, 1989.
221. Montefoschi N, Boccadamo R: Propafenone induced acute variation of chronic atrial pacing threshold: A case report. PACE 13:480-483, 1990.
222. Huang SK, Hedberg PS, Marcus FI: Effects of antiarrhythmic drugs on the chronic pacing threshold and the endocardial R wave amplitude in the conscious dog. PACE 9:660, 1986.
223. Bianconi L, Boccadamo R, Toscano S, et al: Effects of oral propafenone therapy on chronic myocardial pacing threshold. PACE 15:148-154, 1992.
224. Kubler W, Sowton E: Influence of beta-blockade on myocardial threshold in patients with pacemakers. Lancet 2:67, 1970.
225. Irnich W, Gebhardt U: The pacemaker-electrode combination and its relationship to service life. In Thalen HJTh (ed): To Pace or Not to Pace: Controversial Subjects in Cardiac Pacing. The Hague, Martin Nijhoff, 1978, p 209.
226. Gay RJ, Brown DF: Pacemaker failure due to procainamide toxicity. Am J Cardiol 34:728-731, 1974.
227. Preston TA, Fletcher RD, Lucchesi BR, Judge RD: Changes in myocardial threshold: Physiologic and pharmacologic factors in patients with implanted pacemakers. Am Heart J 74:235, 1967.
228. Khastgir T, Lattuca J, Aarons D, et al: Ventricular pacing threshold and time to capture postdefibrillation in patients undergoing implantable cardioverter-defibrillator implantation. PACE 14:768-772, 1991.
229. Delmar M: Role of potassium currents on cell excitability in cardiac ventricular myocytes. J Cardiovasc Electrophysiol 3:474-486, 1992.
230. Gettes LS, Shabetai R, Downs TA, et al: Effect of changes in potassium and calcium concentrations on diastolic threshold and strength-interval relationships of the human heart. Ann N Y Acad Sci 167:693-705, 1969.
231. Lee D, Greenspan K, Edmands RE, et al: The effect of electrolyte alteration on stimulus requirement of cardiac pacemakers. Circulation 38:124, 1968.
232. Walker WJ, Elkins JT, Wood LW, et al: Effect of potassium in restoring myocardial response to a subthreshold cardiac pacemaker. N Engl J Med 271:597, 1964.
233. Surawicz B, Chelbus H, Reeves JT, et al: Increase of ventricular excitability threshold by hyperpotassemia. JAMA 191:71-76, 1965.
234. Westerholm CJ: Threshold studies in transvenous cardiac pacemaker treatment. Scand J Thorac Cardiovasc Surg 8(Suppl):1, 1971.
235. Schlesinger Z, Rosenberg T, Stryjer D, et al: Exit block in myxedema, treated effectively by thyroid hormone replacement. PACE 3:737-739, 1980.
236. Basu D, Chatterjee K: Unusually high pacemaker threshold in severe myedema: Decrease with thyroid hormone therapy. Chest 70:677-679, 1976.
237. Nagatomo Y, Ogawa T, Kumagae H, et al: Pacing failure due to markedly increased stimulation threshold 2 years after implantation: Successful management with oral prednisolone. A case report. PACE 12:1034-1037, 1989.
238. Haywood J, Wyman MG: Effects of isoproterenol, ephedrine, and potassium on artificial pacemaker failure. Circulation 32(Suppl II):110, 1965.
239. Katz A, Knilans TK, Evans JJ, Prystowsky EN: The effects of isoproterenol on excitability, supranormal excitability and conduction in the human ventricle [abstract]. PACE 14:710, 1991.
240. Levick CE, Mizgala HF, Kerr CR: Failure to pace following high dose anti-arrhythmic therapy: Reversal with isoproterenol. PACE 7:252-256, 1984.
241. Daubert C, Ritter P, Cazeau S, et al: Permanent biventricular pacing in dilated cardiomyopathy: Is a totally endocardial approach technically feasible? PACE 19:699, 1996.
242. McVenes R, Stokes K: Alternative pacing sites: How the modern technology deals with this new challenge. In Antonioli GE (ed): Pacemaker Leads 1997. Bologna, Monduzi Editore, 1997, pp 223-228.
243. Hurzeler P, Furman S, Escher DJW: Cardiac pacemaker current thresholds versus pulse duration. In Silverman HT, Miller IF, Salkind AJ (eds): Electrochemical Bioscience and Bioengineering. Princeton, NJ, Electrochemical Society, 1973, p 124.
244. Stokes KB, Church T: The elimination of exit block as a pacing complication using a transvenous steroid-eluting lead. Proceed-

ings of the VIII World Symposium on Cardiac Pacing and Electrophysiology, Jerusalem, 1987. [abstract 475] PACE 10(3 Pt 2):748, 1987.

245. Till JA, Jones S, Rowland E, et al: Clinical experience with a steroid eluting lead in children [abstract]. Circulation 80:389, 1989.
246. Sowton E, Norman J: Variations in cardiac stimulation thresholds in patients with pacing electrodes. Digest of the 7th International Conference on Medical and Biological Engineering, Stockholm, 1967.
247. Preston TA, Fletcher RD, Luchesi BR, et al: Changes in myocardial threshold: Physiologic and pharmacologic factors in patients with implanted pacemakers. Am Heart J 74:235-242, 1967.
248. Westerholm C-J: Threshold studies in transvenous cardiac pacemaker treatment. Scand J Thorac Surg Suppl 8 (Suppl):1-35, 1971.
249. McVenes R, Lahtinen S, Hansen N, Stokes K: Physiologic and drug induced changes in cardiac pacing and sensing parameters [abstract 324]. Eur JCPE 2:A86, 1992.
250. Kadish A, Kong T, Goldberger J: Diurnal variability in ventricular stimulation threshold and electrogram amplitude [abstract]. Eur JCPE 2:A86, 1992.
251. Grendahl H, Schaanning CG: Variations in pacing threshold. Acta Med Scand 187:75-78, 1970.
252. Barold S: Effect of drugs on pacing thresholds. In Antonioli GE, Aubert AE, Ector H (eds): Pacemaker Leads 1991. New York, Elsevier, 1991, pp 73-86.
253. Barold SS, Ong LS, Heinle RA: Stimulation and sensing thresholds for cardiac pacing: Electrophysiologic and technical aspects. Prog Cardiovasc Dis. 24:1, 1981.
254. Ohm O-J, Breivik K: Pacing leads. In Gomez FP (ed): Cardiac Pacing, Electrophysiology, Tachyarrhythmias. Madrid, Editorial Group, 1985, pp 971-985.
255. Basu D, Chatterjee K: Unusually high pacemaker threshold in severe myedema: Decrease with thyroid hormone therapy. Chest 70:677-679, 1976.

Chapter 2

Principles of Defibrillation: From Cellular Physiology to Fields and Waveforms

GREGORY P. WALCOTT • RAYMOND E. IDEKER

Electrical defibrillation is the only practical means for halting ventricular fibrillation (VF). Although it has been known for more than a century that application of an electric shock directly to the myocardium causes VF and that the heart can be returned to normal rhythm by subsequent application of a shock of greater magnitude,[1-3] knowledge of the mechanisms underlying the process of defibrillation was slow in developing. It was only with the relatively recent introduction of novel techniques for the analysis of action potentials and activation sequences[4-8] that greater insight into the physiology of both fibrillation and defibrillation has been achieved. It is hoped that this insight will result in a higher success rate for external defibrillation and improved design of implantable cardioverter-defibrillators (ICDs).

A large part of current research is dedicated to determining the underlying reason for the success or failure of a defibrillating shock. VF is maintained by multiple activation fronts that are constantly moving in a pattern of reentry. Characteristics of the activation pattern and action potential are believed to be important determinants of whether a shock will successfully defibrillate the heart. A successful defibrillating shock is believed to extinguish most of these activation fronts, permitting the resumption of coordinated responsiveness.[9-13] For the defibrillating shock to be completely successful, this must be accomplished without creating an environment that promotes susceptibility to reinitiation of fibrillation.[12,13] It has been established that adequate *distribution* of the potential gradient (an estimate of local current flow) created by the shock throughout the ventricular myocardium is required for successful defibrillation.[14-16]

Fundamentally, defibrillation is believed to be realized through an electrical pulse that causes an alteration in the transmembrane potential of the myocyte. It most likely requires a rapid induction of changes in the transmembrane potential of the myocytes in a critical mass of myocardium (75% to 90% of the myocardium in dogs).[11,14,16] Because this represents a large mass of tissue, depolarization must be achieved at a considerable distance from the stimulating electrode. To gain an understanding of this complex far-field process, various mathematical models have been generated, and the predictions of computer simulations have been compared with physiologic findings. Both discontinuities in the anisotropic properties of the extracellular and intracellular domains, as described by the bidomain model,[17,18] and highly resistive discontinuities in the intracellular space (e.g., collagenous septa), as described in the secondary source model,[19-21] may contribute to the far-field changes in the potential gradient that halt the activation fronts of fibrillation.

The mechanisms underlying degeneration into fibrillation in failed shocks remain incompletely understood. Residual wandering wavelets,[22] nonuniform refractoriness,[23] and areas of low potential gradient in which critical points (centers of reentrant circuits) form[15] may be the sources of propagating wavefronts that can result in fibrillation through reentry. Centrifugal propagation from ectopic foci induced by the defibrillation shock may also play a role, especially in the atrium.[13]

This chapter expands on the subjects mentioned previously. Some of the characteristics of VF that are believed to be important to understanding defibrillation and some of the characteristics of shock that lead to successful defibrillation, such as waveform shape and electrode configuration, are discussed. Then, a shock is traced from its origin at the defibrillation electrodes to its distribution through the heart with a discussion of its affect on the transmembrane potential and how it leads to the successful cessation of fibrillation.

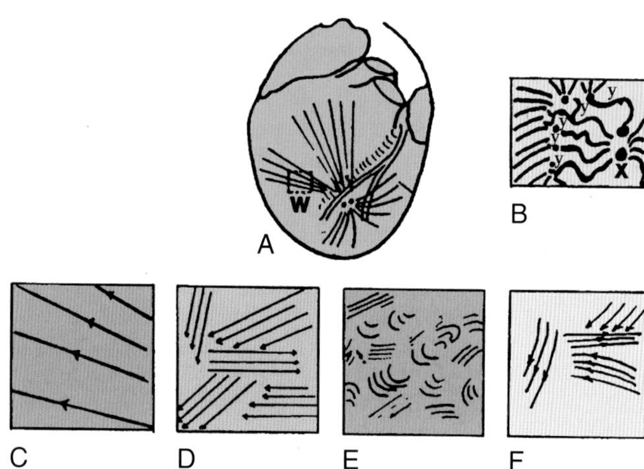

Figure 2-1. Diagrams indicating the spread of waves observed in the analysis of motion pictures obtained during the four stages of fibrillation described by Wiggers. ***A,*** *Spread of wavefront during initial, undulatory stage.* ***B,*** *Theoretical passage of impulses from point x to form a wavefront at y. Panels* ***C*** *through* ***F*** *show the appearance of contraction waves in the small rectangular area W from panel* ***A,*** *magnified.* ***C,*** *Undulatory stage.* ***D,*** *Convulsive stage.* ***E,*** *Tremulous stage.* ***F,*** *Atonic stage. (From Wiggers CJ: Studies of ventricular fibrillation caused by electric shock. Cinematographic and electrocardiographic observations of the natural process in the dog's heart: Its inhibition by potassium and the revival of coordinated beats by calcium. Am Heart J 5:351-365, 1930.)*

Fibrillation

To understand defibrillation, it is necessary to have an understanding of fibrillation. Knowing the basic characteristics of VF and whether it is maintained by reentrant or focal activity, as well as the characteristics of the action potential and the excitability of the fibrillating tissue, helps to define the therapy that will be successful in stopping the arrhythmia.

VF has been characterized as progressing through four stages based on high-speed cinematography of electrically induced fibrillation in dog hearts (Fig. 2-1).[24] A brief *undulatory*, or tachysystolic, stage lasting only 1 to 2 seconds occurs first. It is characterized by three to six undulatory contractions that resemble a series of closely occurring systoles and involve the sequential contraction of large areas of the myocardium. This is followed by a second stage of *convulsive* incoordination, in which more frequent waves of contraction sweep over smaller regions of the myocardium. Because the contractions in each region are not in phase, the ventricles are pulled in a convulsive manner. It is during this stage of fibrillation that the ICD shocks are given—10 to 20 seconds after the onset of fibrillation. In the third stage of *tremulous* incoordination, the independently contracting areas of the ventricular surface become even smaller, giving the heart a tremulous appearance. Tremulous incoordination lasts for 2 to 4 minutes before the fourth and final stage of *atonic* fibrillation occurs. Atonic fibrillation develops within 2 to 5 minutes after the onset of fibrillation and is characterized by the slow passage of feeble contraction wavelets over short distances. With time, the number of quiescent areas increases. Ischemia plays a role in the development of the third and fourth stages, because the fibrillating heart remains in the second stage if the coronary arteries are perfused with oxygenated blood.[25,26]

Driving the mechanical activity of the heart during fibrillation is the electrical activity of the myocardium. The electrical activity of the heart during fibrillation has been studied using both extracellular and optical recordings. Several groups have suggested that fibrillation is maintained by reentry. In most cases, reentry appears to be caused by "wandering wavelets" of activation, activation fronts that follow continually changing pathways from cycle to cycle. In some studies, the activation sequence appears moderately repeatable from cycle to cycle, following approximately the same pathway.[27-29] Occasionally, a spiraling pattern of functional reentry emanates from the same region for several cycles. Sometimes, the central core of these spiral waves meanders across the heart.[8] At other times, new reentrant activation fronts are generated when one front interacts with another during its vulnerable period.

Study of VF has suggested that there is a level of organization to the seemingly random patterns of wandering wavelets. Two competing hypotheses have been proposed to explain this organization. The "mother rotor" hypothesis was first proposed by Sir Thomas Lewis in 1925[30] and was recently revived by Jalife and colleagues.[33] This hypothesis proposes that a single stationary reentrant circuit or mother rotor, located in the fastest-activating region of the heart, "drives" VF by giving rise to activation fronts that propagate throughout the remainder of the myocardium.[29] These wavefronts propagate away from this fast-activating region, encounter areas of unidirectional block, and break up into smaller, slower-moving waveforms that resemble Wiggers' wandering wavelets. Experiments that have best demonstrated the mother rotor have been performed in small hearts, from guinea pigs or rabbits. Studies of larger hearts have shown areas of faster and slower activation across the heart, but the existence of a single reentrant rotor that drives fibrillation has not been clearly demonstrated.[31,32]

In contrast to the mother rotor hypothesis is the "restitution" hypothesis. Restitution properties of the heart have been recognized for many years. *Restitution* in the heart refers to the relationship between the duration of an action potential in a particular cell and the duration of the previous diastolic or resting interval. If the previous diastolic interval (DI) is short, the current action potential duration (APD) will also be short. If the previous DI is long, then the current APD will be long. For a regular rhythm, the preceding DI is constant and, therefore, so is the duration of the subsequent APD. The relationship between an APD and the previous DI is often described graphically as a plot of APD_n versus DI_{n-1} (Fig. 2-2). The steepness of the restitution curve is an important characteristic of this curve, especially at short DIs. If this slope is greater than 1, then, at a constant cycle length, a single perturbation in DI will cause the ensuing APDs and DIs to oscillate, with the oscillations progressively increasing until the site is refractory at the time of the next cycle, causing conduction block and VF initiation. And during VF, it is hypothesized that, when the slope of the restitution curve is greater than 1, oscillations in DI and APD increase until block occurs and wavefronts break up. Figure 2-2 shows an example of a restitution curve recorded from the right ventricle of a pig. The relationship between a DI and the subsequent APD is well defined during paced rhythm but less well defined during VF.

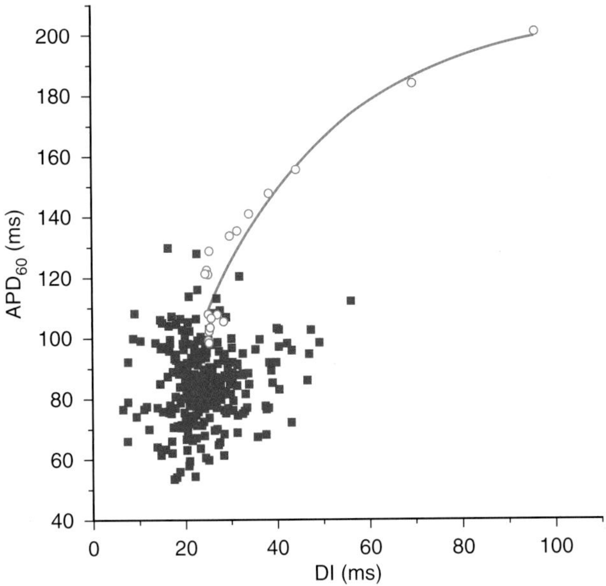

Figure 2-2. Dynamic action potential duration APD_{60} restitution relationship during pacing and ventricular fibrillation (VF) in one animal. (APD_{60} is the action potential duration at 60% of return to resting membrane voltage.) Open circles represent data from pacing, and solid squares represent data throughout 60 seconds of VF. Data were recorded from the anterior right ventricle using a floating microelectrode. The heart was stimulated using decremental pacing at an initial pacing rate of 1 pulse every 450 msec. The stimulus-to-stimulus interval was progressively shortened until either the heart was refractory to the stimulation or VF was induced. Note that the open circles form an exponential relationship between the diastolic interval (DI) and APD_{60}, whereas the relationship between DI and APD_{60} is not well defined during VF. (From Huang J, Zhou X, Smith WM, Ideker RE: Restitution properties during ventricular fibrillation in the in situ swine heart. Circulation 110:3161-3167, 2004.)

Understanding how VF is maintained may help develop new therapies that will make fibrillation easier to stop. If VF is maintained by a mother rotor, then targeting of electrical therapy, either shocks or pacing, to the region that contains the dominant reentrant circuit may be successful in halting VF. If VF is started and maintained primarily due to the DI restitution properties of the heart, then drugs that decrease the slope of the restitution curve, especially at short coupling intervals, may be successful in halting VF.

The Cellular Action Potential and the Excitable Gap During Fibrillation

In the past few years, knowledge of the characteristics of the action potentials during fibrillation has increased greatly. This is a direct result of the introduction of techniques for recording action potentials in whole hearts, either in vivo or in perfused, isolated hearts.[4-6,8,33] During fibrillation, the action potentials are altered; the APD is decreased, the action potential upstroke is slowed (decreased first-order derivative, dV/dt) and of decreased magnitude, the plateau phase is abbreviated, and DIs are abbreviated or absent (Fig. 2-3). During the first few seconds of VF or of atrial fibrillation, the activation rate is quite rapid; the mean cycle length of VF in patients undergoing defibrillator implantation was measured to be 213 ± 27 msec.[6] DIs are rarely seen during early fibrillation, and the upstroke of most action potentials occurs before the transmembrane potential has returned to baseline from the previous action potential. The demonstration of an *excitable gap* in fibrillating atrial tissue[34] and evidence of an excitable gap in fibrillating ventricular tissue[35] suggest that there are periods late in the action potential in the fibrillating myocardium during which an electrical stimulus can capture a portion of the fibrillating myocardium. Knowing that there is an excitable gap suggests that there is an opportunity to stimulate the tissue just in front of a fibrillating wavefront, to cause wavefront block.

As described in Chapter 1, the electrical activity of the heart is controlled ultimately by ion channels located in the cell membrane of the myocyte. It has been established that both the voltage-gated fast channels (sodium [Na^+]) and slow channels (Na^+ and calcium [Ca^{2+}]) are active during the first few seconds of VF.[5] The fast channel activity is indicated by the rapidity of

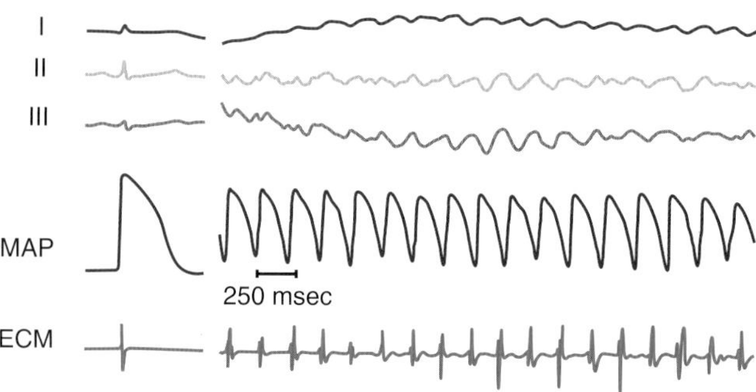

Figure 2-3. Recording taken during ventricular fibrillation in a human. Leads I, II, and III are body surface electrocardiograms. Note that there is no period of diastole between action potentials. MAP, right ventricular monophasic action potentials; ECM, local bipolar electrogram. (From Swartz JF, Jones JL, Fletcher RD: Characterization of ventricular fibrillation based on monophasic action potential morphology in the human heart. Circulation 87:1907-1914, 1993.)

the upstroke of the action potential (phase 0) during early fibrillation and its sensitivity to administration of the Na^+ channel blocker, tetrodotoxin. As fibrillation proceeds, the upstrokes of the action potentials become increasingly slower, with a decreased dV/dt_{max}, but the action potentials remain sensitive to tetrodotoxin until 1 to 5 minutes after initiation of fibrillation. A transition then occurs in which the action potential upstrokes become insensitive to tetrodotoxin. This suggests that the propagation of the action potential is no longer mediated primarily by the fast voltage-gated Na^+ channels and may be mediated by slow voltage-gated Ca^{2+} channel activity in the later stages of fibrillation.[4] The activation complexes recorded from the ventricular myocardium remain active only as long as the coronary arteries are perfused with oxygenated blood, suggesting that ischemia may be responsible for the loss of fast channel activation during prolonged VF.[25]

Defibrillation

Successful defibrillation can reflect either the immediate cessation of all activation fronts or the cessation of activation fronts after two to three cycles,[10,36] followed by coordinated beating of the heart. Unsuccessful defibrillation can reflect a failure to inhibit the fibrillating activation fronts or the resumption of fibrillating activation fronts after their initial inhibition. As previously mentioned, application of a powerful electrical shock to the heart is the only reliable means of stopping fibrillation.

Waveforms, Current Strength, and Distribution during Defibrillation

The two most common waveform shapes used clinically are the *monophasic* and *biphasic* waveforms. In monophasic waveforms, the polarity of the shock is unchanged at each electrode for the entire duration of the electrical shock. In biphasic waveforms, the polarity of the shock reverses at each electrode partway through the defibrillation waveform. Many studies, in both animals and humans, have shown that biphasic waveforms can defibrillate with less current and energy than monophasic waveforms, in both internal and transthoracic defibrillation configurations.[37-40] Within each type, waveforms can be described as truncated exponential or damped sinusoidal shapes. ICDs use truncated exponential biphasic waveforms. Until recently, most external defibrillators used damped sinusoidal waveforms. Because of the inductor necessary to shape the damped sinusoidal monophasic waveform, these defibrillators tend to be large and heavy. More recently, smaller, lighter external defibrillators have been developed that use truncated exponential biphasic waveforms similar to those used in ICDs. Damped sinusoidal biphasic waveforms are used in external defibrillators in Russia; similar to truncated exponential biphasic waveforms, they have been shown to have an improved efficacy over monophasic waveforms.[41,42]

Not all biphasic waveforms are superior to monophasic waveforms, however. For example, if the second phase of the biphasic waveform becomes much longer than the first phase, then the energy required for defibrillation increases and can eventually rise to a level greater than the energy required to defibrillate with a monophasic waveform with duration equal to the first phase of the biphasic waveform.[40,43,44] The optimum duration of the two phases of the biphasic waveform depends on the electrode impedance and the defibrillator capacitance.[45-48]

Several groups have shown that defibrillation efficacy for square waveforms follows a strength-duration relationship similar to that for cardiac stimulation[49,50]; as the waveform gets longer, the average current at the 50% success point (the current when one half of delivered shocks will succeed) becomes progressively less, approaching an asymptote called the *rheobase*.[51] On the basis of this observation, several groups have suggested that cardiac defibrillation can be mathematically modeled using a resistor-capacitor (RC) network to represent the heart (Fig. 2-4).[46,52-54] Empirically, it has been determined that the time constant for the parallel RC network is in the range of 2.5 to 5 msec.[46,47,53] In one version of the model,[53] a current waveform is applied to the RC network. The voltage across the network is then calculated for each time point during the defibrillation pulse. The relative efficacies of different waveform shapes and durations can be compared by determining the current strength that is necessary to make the voltage across the RC network reach a particular value, called the *defibrillation threshold.*

Several observations can be made from this model. First, for square waves, as the waveform duration gets longer, the voltage across the network increases, approaching an asymptote or rheobase. For truncated exponential waveforms, however, the model voltage rises, reaches a peak, and then, if the waveform is long enough, begins to decrease (see Fig. 2-4). Therefore, the model predicts that monophasic exponential waveforms should be truncated at a time when the peak voltage across the RC network is reached. Current or

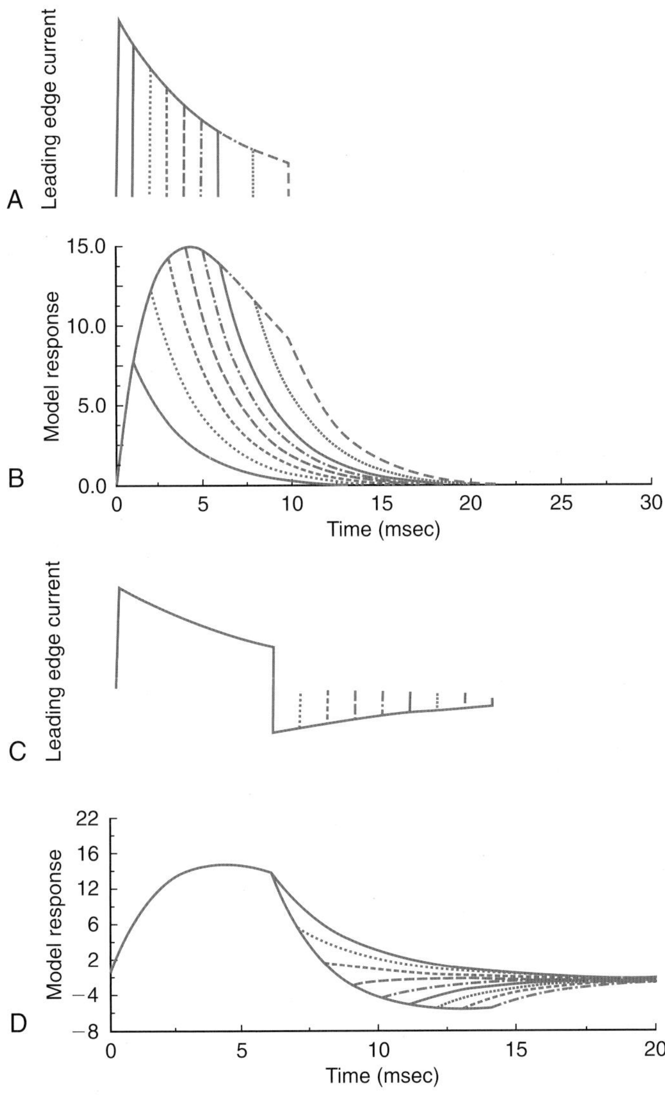

Figure 2-4. The response of a parallel resistor-capacitor network representation of the heart to monophasic and biphasic truncated exponential waveforms with a time constant of 7 msec. The parallel resistor-capacitor network has a time constant of 2.8 msec. ***A,*** *The input monophasic waveforms. The leading-edge current of the input waveform was 10 A. The waveforms were truncated at 1, 2, 3, 4, 5, 6, 8, and 10 msec.* ***B,*** *The model response, V(t). Initially, as the waveform gets longer, V(t) increases until it reaches a maximum at about 4 msec, after which it begins to decrease.* ***C,*** *The input biphasic waveforms. The leading-edge current was 10 A. Phase 1 was truncated at 6 msec. Phase 2 was truncated after 1, 2, 3, 4, 5, 6, 7, and 8 msec.* ***D,*** *The model response does not change polarity until the phase 2 duration is longer than 2 msec. (From Walcott GP, Walker RG, Cates AW, et al: Choosing the optimal monophasic and biphasic waveforms for ventricular defibrillation. J Cardiovasc Electrophysiol 6:737-750, 1995.)*

energy delivered after that point is wasted. In supporting this prediction, strength-duration relationships measured in both animals[53] and humans[55] do not approach an asymptote but rather reach a minimum and remain constant as the waveform gets longer. This minimum occurs over a range of waveform durations and does not extend indefinitely. Schuder and colleagues[56] showed that, if the duration of a waveform gets too long, defibrillation efficacy decreases.

Second, the model predicts that the heart acts as a low-pass filter.[54] Therefore, waveforms that rise gradually should have better efficacy than waveforms that turn on immediately. This prediction has been shown to hold true for external defibrillation,[57] internal atrial defibrillation,[58] and internal ventricular defibrillation.[59] Ascending ramps defibrillate with a greater efficacy than do descending ramps.[59,60]

Third, several groups have suggested that the optimal first phase of a biphasic waveform is the optimal monophasic waveform.[45,48] If this is true, then what does the model predict as the "best" second phase of a biphasic waveform? Empirically, it appears that the role of the second phase is to return the model voltage response back to zero as quickly as possible, to maximize the increased efficacy of the biphasic waveform over that of the monophasic waveform with the same duration as phase 1 of the biphasic waveform. If the network voltage does not reach zero or if it overshoots zero, efficacy is lost.[45,53] Swerdlow and colleagues[47] showed in humans that the "best" second phase of a biphasic waveform is one that returns the model response close to zero.

Together, these ideas allow the clinician to choose optimal capacitor sizes and phase durations for truncated exponential biphasic waveforms, the waveforms most commonly used in ICDs. The capacitor must be large enough to be able to raise the network voltage to its threshold value and still hold enough charge to drive the network voltage back to zero. For a 40-Ω interelectrode impedance and a network time constant of 2.8 msec, the minimum capacitor that can accomplish this has a capacitance of 75 microfarads (μF).

The location of the defibrillation electrodes affects the magnitude of the shock necessary to defibrillate the heart. Typically, 200 to 360 J of energy are necessary for successful defibrillation with the defibrillation electrodes located on the body surface, during transthoracic defibrillation with a damped sinusoidal monophasic waveform. Less energy is required for a truncated exponential biphasic waveform.[61] However, only about 4% to 20% of the current that is delivered to transthoracic defibrillation electrodes ever reaches the heart.[62,63] Indeed, when the defibrillation electrodes are placed in the heart itself, usually only 20 to 34 J of energy are required, and the requirement may be as low as only a few joules when very large, contoured epicardial electrodes are used.[40,64] The strength of the shock also varies for different locations on or in the heart; epicardial patches defibrillate with a lower shock energy than do transvenous electrode configurations.[65]

Although defibrillation efficacy is usually described by some measure of defibrillation shock strength (energy, voltage, or current), little insight into the mechanisms of defibrillation can be obtained from these measures. Knowing how the current (or voltage) of a defibrillation shock is distributed over the heart allows a much deeper understanding of how defibrillation occurs. Several studies have been performed that measure the potential gradient distribution throughout the heart during a defibrillation shock.[14,66,67] The *potential gradient* is a measure of the spatial variation of shock voltage across the heart. The potential gradient is measured in volts per centimeter of tissue. In a region with a high potential gradient, the difference in voltage between a given point and an area 1 cm distant from that point is high. Regions of low potential gradient have a measured voltage that is similar to that of nearby points.

These studies show, for most electrode configurations, an uneven distribution, with areas of high potential gradient near the defibrillation electrodes and areas of low potential gradient in regions distant from the defibrillating electrodes. It has been hypothesized that a minimum potential gradient must be attained for successful defibrillation to occur and that this requirement is independent of the current applied or the electrode configuration.[15,16] After a shock that fails to defibrillate VF, the site of earliest activation immediately after the shock can be mapped and related to the electric field that was produced by the shock. For shocks near the defibrillation threshold, the sites of earliest activation after a failed shock occur in the areas of lowest potential gradient.[15,16]

The minimum potential gradient required for defibrillation is lower for biphasic than for monophasic waveforms (4 versus 6 V/cm).[16] A minimum potential gradient of 6 V/cm was required for successful defibrillation using a 10-msec truncated exponential monophasic waveform in the open-chest dog model.[16] Similar findings were observed using a 14-msec truncated exponential monophasic waveform and multiple electrode configurations.[15] In contrast, a minimum potential gradient of 4 V/cm was required for successful defibrillation using a truncated exponential biphasic waveform. Because higher shock strengths are required to induce a higher potential gradient, biphasic shocks successfully defibrillate with lower energy than monophasic shocks (i.e., a lower-voltage gradient is required).

The requirement for a minimum potential gradient may reflect the need for a shock to prevent the generation of new activation fronts that can result in reinitiation of fibrillation.[68] Examination of activation patterns after failed defibrillation for progressively larger shock strengths indicate that postshock activation occurs at numerous sites throughout the ventricle, and reentry is common when the shock strength is much lower than that needed for defibrillation (Fig. 2-5).[69] At shock strengths just lower than those required for defibrillation, postshock activation arises in a limited number of myocardial regions. The activation fronts then propagate to activate other regions of the myocardium for a few cycles before reentry occurs, activation becomes disorganized, and fibrillation is reinitiated. Although postshock activation sites can still arise in regions of lowest potential gradient after a shock slightly greater than that required for defibrillation, the cycles of activation that originate from these sites are slower. These activations terminate after a few cycles without reinitiating fibrillation.[68-70]

So far, we have discussed how defibrillation can fail because a shock is of insufficient strength. What happens if a defibrillation shock gets very large? At high shock strengths, the probability of defibrillation success begins to decrease again. It is believed that, at large strengths, defibrillation shocks can have detrimental effects on the heart. Increasing the shock strength to very high levels (>1000 V with transvenous electrodes) can result in activation fronts arising from regions of high potential gradient that reinduce VF.[71] Cates and coworkers[72] showed that, for both monophasic and biphasic shocks, increasing shock strength does not always improve the probability of successful defib-

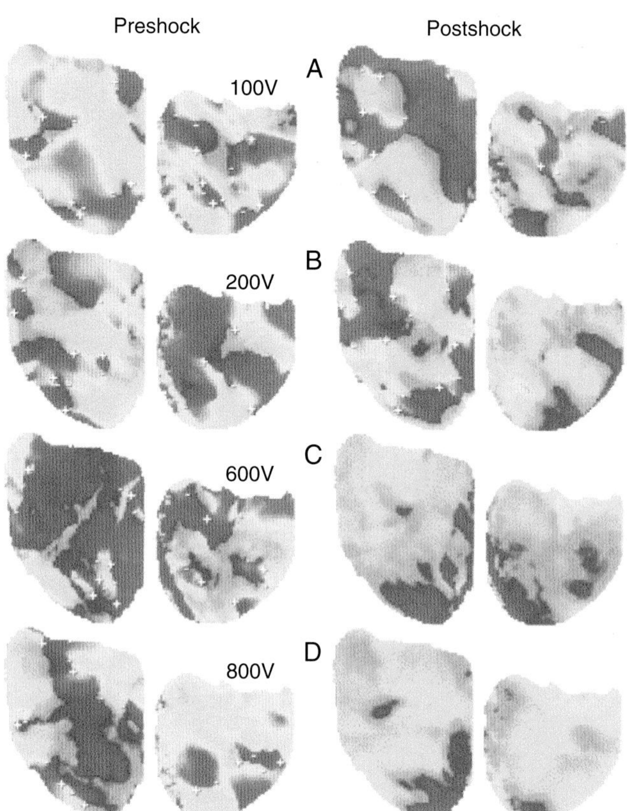

Figure 2-5. Phase maps of a single rabbit heart showing the last cycle before (left panel) and the first cycle after (right panel) a shock of 100 V ***(A)****, 200 V* ***(B)****, 600 V* ***(C)****, and 800 V* ***(D)*** *that failed to defibrillate. The defibrillation threshold was 800 ± 200 V in this series. Colors represent* phase, *and the symbols + and – indicate phase singularities or centers of reentrant circuits of opposite direction. Phase singularities as a marker of reentry were observed during ventricular fibrillation just before the shock in all cases.* ***A*** *and* ***B,*** *Postshock phase singularities were observed after failed 100- and 200-V shocks. Visual analysis of animations of the optical recordings indicated that many of the phase singularities represented reentrant activations occurring immediately after the shock, so that the postshock interval was 0 msec.* ***C*** *and* ***D,*** *No phase singularities were observed after the 600- and 800-V shocks. For the 600-V shock, activation propagated away in all directions from two early sites, one at the apex and the other at the lateral base of the left ventricle, both of which appeared after a postshock interval of 42 msec. For the 800-V shock, a single wavefront of activation appeared at the apex and propagated away in all directions in a focal pattern after a postshock interval of 72 msec. (From Chattipakorn N, Banville I, Gray RA, Ideker RE. Effects of shock strengths on ventricular defibrillation failure. Cardiovasc Res 61:39-44, 2004.)*

rillation and may in fact increase the incidence of postshock arrhythmias. Chapman and associates[73] showed in dogs that the time required for the heart to recover hemodynamically after a defibrillation episode was shorter for biphasic than for monophasic shocks. Further, they showed that hemodynamic recovery took longer after high-energy shocks than after low-energy shocks. Reddy and colleagues[74] showed that transthoracic defibrillation with biphasic shocks resulted in less postshock electrocardiographic evidence of myocardial dysfunction (injury or ischemia), than did standard monophasic damped sinusoidal waveforms, and without compromise of defibrillation efficacy.

One mechanism that has been implicated in the means by which shocks cause damage to the myocardium is *electroporation*, the formation of holes or pores in the cell membrane. Electroporation may occur in regions in which the shock potential gradient is high (>50 to 70 V/cm) and may even occur in regions where the potential gradient is much less than 50 V/cm.[75] The very high voltage can result in disruption of the phospholipid membrane bilayer and in the formation of pores that permit the free influx and efflux of ions and micromolecules. Electroporation can cause the transmembrane potential to change temporarily to a value almost equal to that of the plateau of the action potential. At this transmembrane potential, the cell is paralyzed electrically, being both unresponsive and unable to conduct an action potential. Exposure of the myocardium to yet higher potential gradients, probably greater than 150 V/cm, results in arrhythmic beating, and at very high potential gradients, necrosis may occur.[76]

The shape of the waveform alters the strength of the shock at which these detrimental effects occur. Use of a 10-msec truncated exponential monophasic waveform for VF in dogs resulted in conduction block in regions where the potential gradient was greater than 64 ± 4 V/cm.[77] Shocks that created even higher potential gradients in the myocardium (71 ± 6 V/cm) were required for conduction block when a 5-msec/5-msec truncated exponential biphasic shock was used. Adding a second phase to a monophasic waveform, thereby making it a biphasic waveform, reduced the damage sustained by cultured chick myocytes compared with that induced by the monophasic waveform alone.[78] Therefore, biphasic waveforms are less apt to cause damage or dysfunction in high-gradient regions than monophasic waveforms.

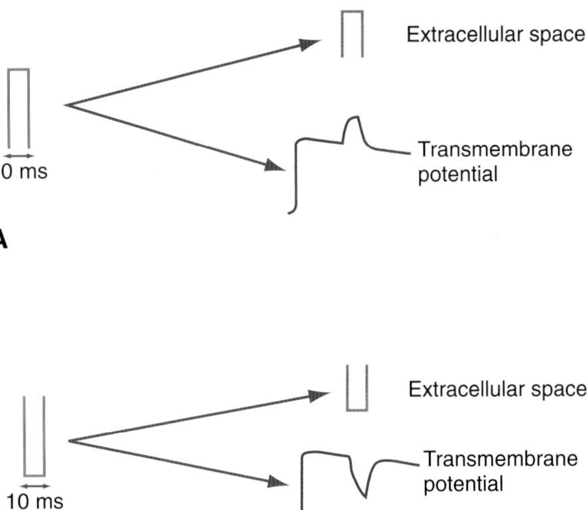

Figure 2-6. The effect of a square-wave shock on the extracellular potential and on the transmembrane potential. The square-wave shock appears immediately as a relatively undistorted square wave in the extracellular space. It appears as an exponentially increasing change in the transmembrane potential. When a shock of a given polarity is delivered during the action potential plateau ***(A)****, the depolarization obtained is different in magnitude and time course from the hyperpolarization obtained with a shock of the opposite polarity* ***(B)****. (From Walcott GP, Knisley SB, Zhou X, et al: On the mechanism of ventricular defibrillation. PACE 20:422-431, 1997.)*

Models Proposed to Explain the Induction of Changes in the Transmembrane Potential throughout the Heart during a Defibrillation Shock

A shock in the form of a square wave given across the defibrillation electrodes appears almost immediately as a square wave in the extracellular space of the heart. There is no significant distortion, because the extracellular space throughout the body is primarily resistive, with little reactive component. Phase delays and alterations of the appearance of the shock wave occur in the transmembrane potential, however, owing to the capacitance and ion channels of the membrane of the myocyte.[79] Consequently, a square wave shock can elicit an exponential change with time in the transmembrane potential (Fig. 2-6).

The nonlinear behavior of the membrane caused by the ion channels also affects the outcome of reversing the polarity of the defibrillation shock. Reversing the polarity may reverse the sign of the change in the transmembrane potential in some regions of the myocardium, and the nonlinear behavior of the membrane can alter the magnitude and the time course of this change. As discussed previously, reversing the polarity of the shock may not reverse the sign of the change in the transmembrane potential in all regions of the heart; some areas may be hyperpolarized with both shock polarities.[80] This may reflect the nonlinear behavior of the membrane ion channels.

Several models have been formulated in an attempt to explain the mechanisms by which the defibrillation shock is distributed throughout the myocardium to effectively restore coordinated, effective action potentials. As yet, none of the models adequately describes all of the experimental findings regarding the changes in the action potential that occur during defibrillation. It is well established experimentally that changes occur many centimeters from the defibrillating shock electrodes. These changes in transmembrane potential can result in new action potentials or prolongation of the action potential as described previously.[23,81] Direct excitation can be observed[23] even at great distances from the electrode (>30 mm)[82] or across the entire heart.[83]

Although the one-dimensional cable model described in Chapter 1 adequately describes the generation of self-propagating action potentials close to an electrode as required for pacing, it fails to account for the far-field changes observed during defibrillation. During stimulation or defibrillation, this model predicts that the tissue near the anode should be hyperpolarized, whereas the tissue near the cathode should be depolarized.[84] The magnitude of the hyperpolarization or depolarization decreases exponentially with the distance from the electrodes according to the membrane space constant (the distance at which the hyperpolarization or depolarization has decreased by 63%). For cardiac tissue, the space constant is only 0.5 to 1 mm.[84,85] Therefore, the one-dimensional cable equations predict that tissue more than 10 space constants (about 1 cm) distant from the defibrillation electrodes should not directly undergo changes in transmembrane potential because of the shock field. That is, new action potentials should not arise by direct excitation at distances greater than 1 cm from the electrodes. This model fails to describe the experimentally observed global distribution of action potentials during defibrillation.

Therefore, several additional mathematical formulations have been proposed, including the sawtooth model,[20,86-88] the bidomain model,[89] and the formation of secondary sources at barriers in the myocardium,[19,90] to explain how a defibrillation shock affects the transmembrane potential a long distance away from the shocking electrodes. In the simplest formulation of these models, the extracellular and intracellular spaces are considered to be low-resistance media and the membrane to be a high-resistance medium in parallel with capacitance. The simple case models incorporate only passive myocardial properties. The models have been rendered more realistic by the addition of active components to represent the ion channels in the membrane, gap junctions, and membrane discontinuities.[91,92] By convention, the current is defined as the flow of positive ions from the anode to the cathode.

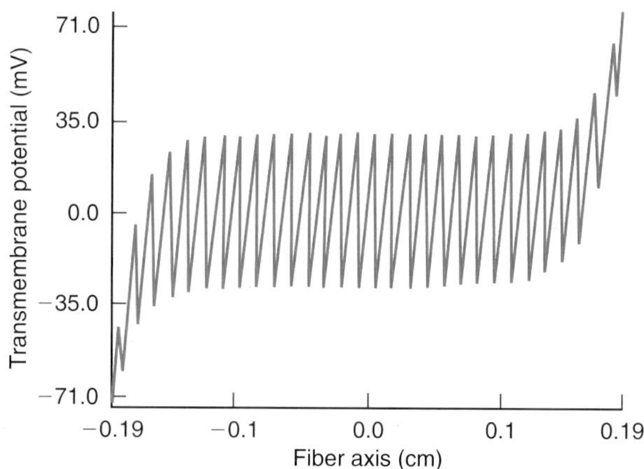

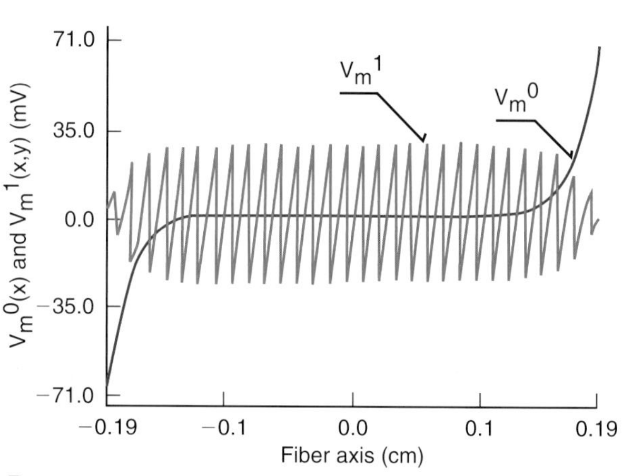

Figure 2-7. The transmembrane potential during a shock, according to the sawtooth model. ***A,*** *The transmembrane potential shown is a summation of the membrane potential profile of the cable model and the periodicity arising from the periodic changes in intracellular resistance. The anode is to the left and the cathode is to the right in this one-dimensional model. The fiber is divided into 31 cells of equal length separated by junctions of high resistance. In the figure, the junctional resistance is shown much greater than is believed to occur in cardiac fibers, to allow the sawtooth pattern to be seen.* ***B,*** *The two parts of the summation shown in panel* ***A*** *are shown. V_m^0, the transmembrane potential profile of the cable model; V_m^1, the periodicity arising from the periodic changes in intracellular resistance. (Adapted from Krassowska W, Pilkington TC, Ideker RE: Periodic conductivity as a mechanism for cardiac stimulation and defibrillation. IEEE Trans Biomed Eng 34:555-560, 1987.)*

The Sawtooth Model

The one-dimensional cable model posits two low-resistance continuous spaces that conduct current from the shock, the intracellular and the extracellular spaces, separated by a high-resistance cell membrane. In the sawtooth model, the intracellular space is divided by a series of high-resistance barriers, the gap junctions. Because of these high-resistance barriers, current moving in the intracellular space is forced to exit into the extracellular space and reenter the cell on the other side of the barrier. Exit and reentry of the current from the intracellular domain results in hyperpolarization near the end of the cell closest to the anode and depolarization near the end of the cell closest to the cathode. A tracing of the changes in transmembrane potential along a fiber during the shock should, therefore, resemble the teeth of a saw, with each tooth corresponding to an individual cell (Fig. 2-7).[20,86-88] Increases in the junctional resistances are predicted to increase the magnitude of the potential changes at the ends of the cell.[20] Although gap junctions are of low resistivity, they can present significant junctional resistance under certain conditions, such as hypoxia[93,94] and calcium depletion.[95] As the resistance of the gap junctions increases, it is predicted that a greater fraction of current passes preferentially across the cell membrane rather than along the cell.

The sawtooth model adequately describes the requirement for a minimum potential gradient, because the magnitude of the hyperpolarization and polarization at the ends of the cells is directly proportional to the strength of the stimulus. It also adequately describes the generation of action potentials at a distance from the electrodes and the differences in threshold stimuli between cathodal and anodal stimulation. Sawtooth changes in transmembrane potential have been observed in preparations of isolated cardiomyocytes[96,97]; however, such a pattern in isolated cells would be consistent with the cable model. This pattern has not been observed in a syncytium of cardiac cells.[19,98,99]

Although the resistivity of the gap junctions at the boundaries between the cells may not adequately explain the physiologic effects of defibrillation, the resistivity of other intracellular discontinuities and interruptions may well play a role. Most theories concerning the generation of action potentials and their propagation across the ventricle, such as the bidomain theory described later, consider the myocardium to be a uniform electrical continuum. This assumption does not take into account the discontinuities of the intracellular domain, where the myocardium is interrupted by barriers such as connective tissue septa, blood vessels, and scar tissue. As described previously for the sawtooth model, the intracellular current, on encountering such a barrier, must leave the intracellular space, cross the barrier, and reenter the intracellular domain on the other side. Depolarization should occur on one side of the barrier and hyperpolarization on the other side. Therefore, the barrier acts as a set of electrodes during the shock, becoming a secondary source of action potentials (Fig. 2-8). These secondary sources are important causes of depolarization and hyperpolarization throughout the myocardial tissues during a shock.[19] The resistive barriers act in a manner similar to that described for the sawtooth model. In this case, however, the resistive barriers represent larger discontinuities, which tend to increase with age and cardiac hypertrophy.[100]

Computer simulations have shown that the cathodal stimulation delivered to the myocardium near the oval scar results in three distinct activation fronts: the primary activation front and secondary fronts at the distal and proximal edges, which are generated by the exit and reentry of current from the intracellular and extracellular spaces (see Fig. 2-8).[101] Optical recording techniques have been used to directly record changes in transmembrane potentials throughout a monolayer of ventricular myocytes.[19] Localized regions of depolarization and hyperpolarization were observed that coincided with discontinuities in the monolayer that resulted in slow conductance. Microscopic regions of depolarization and hyperpolarization have also been observed in isolated slabs of left ventricle, although their correlation with anatomic structures was not possible using optical mapping techniques due to the light scattering properties of myocardium.[102] The significance of secondary sources was demonstrated in whole hearts by mapping of potentials and determination of shock thresholds before and after the generation of a transmural lesion in the myocardial walls of dogs.[90] Generation of the lesion resulted in the development of a region of direct activation in the area of the lesion, in addition to the region of direct activation resulting

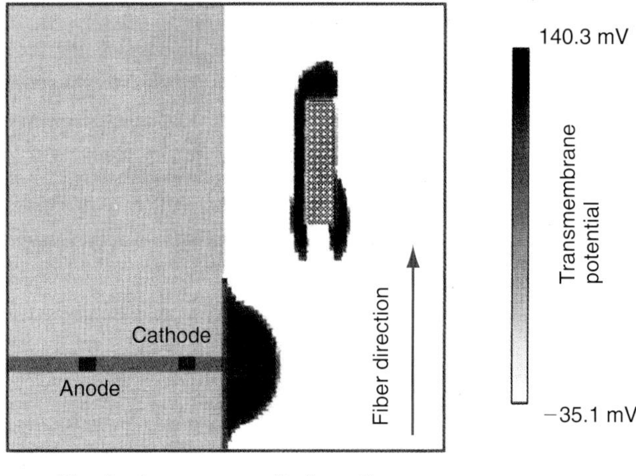

Figure 2-8. Secondary sources adjacent to a scar elicited by a single large pacing pulse, as seen in a computer model. The area to the right represents myocardium that contains a rectangular scar (stippled region). *To the left is the blood pool with a pacing catheter in it. Notice that a pacing pulse depolarizes not only the tissue near the cathode but also that near the scar. (From Street AM: Effects of Connective Tissue Embedded in Viable Cardiac Tissue on Propagation and Pacing: Implications for Arrhythmias. Durham, NC, Duke University, Department of Biomedical Engineering, 1996, p 134.)*

from the stimulating electrode observed before the lesion. Furthermore, the strength of the shock required to cause direct activation in the area of the lesion was less than one half of that required before generation of the lesion (Fig. 2-9).

The effects of secondary sources obviously have major implications for the probability of successful defibrillation at different shock strengths in individual patients, particularly elderly patients, as well as the potential for reentry. Furthermore, the size and placement of operative lesions may play significant roles in the success of subsequent defibrillation.

The Bidomain Model

The bidomain model is an extension of the one-dimensional cable model into two or three dimensions. That is, the extracellular and intracellular spaces are represented as single, continuous domains that extend in two or three dimensions and are separated by the highly resistive cell membrane (Fig. 2-10).[89] If the conductivities of the intracellular and extracellular spaces are constant in all directions, then the model collapses to the one-dimensional cable model. *Anisotropy* refers to the manner in which conductivities change with the direction of myocardial fiber orientation. Clerc[103] showed that conductivity is higher in the direction parallel to the long axis of myocardial fibers (longitudinal) than in the direction perpendicular to the fibers (transverse) for both the intracellular and extracellular spaces. If conductivities change with direction but change the same for the intracellular and extracellular spaces, the bidomain model collapses to the one-dimensional cable model.

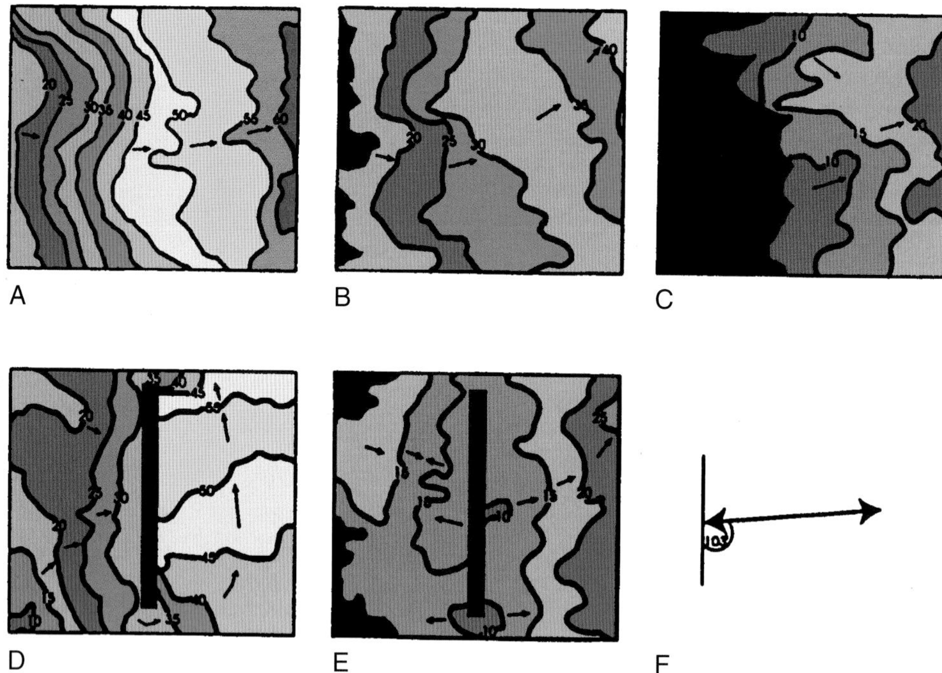

Figure 2-9. Isochronal activation maps obtained after cathodal stimulation before and after creation of a transmural incision that caused secondary sources adjacent to the lesion. Isochrones are drawn at 5-msec intervals, timed from the onset of the S1 or S2 stimulus. Arrows represent direction of activation. Darkened regions represent areas directly activated by the stimulus. Black vertical bars represent the approximate location of the transmural incision. ***A,*** *S1 stimulus delivered before incision.* ***B,*** *75-mA S2 stimulus delivered before incision.* ***C,*** *250-mA S2 stimulus delivered before incision.* ***D,*** *S1 stimulus delivered after incision.* ***E,*** *75-mA S2 stimulus delivered after incision.* ***F,*** *Orientation of the long axis of myocardial fibers. (From White JB, Walcott GP, Pollard AE, et al: Myocardial discontinuities: A substrate for producing virtual electrodes to increase directly excited areas of the myocardium by shocks. Circulation 97:1738-1745, 1998.)*

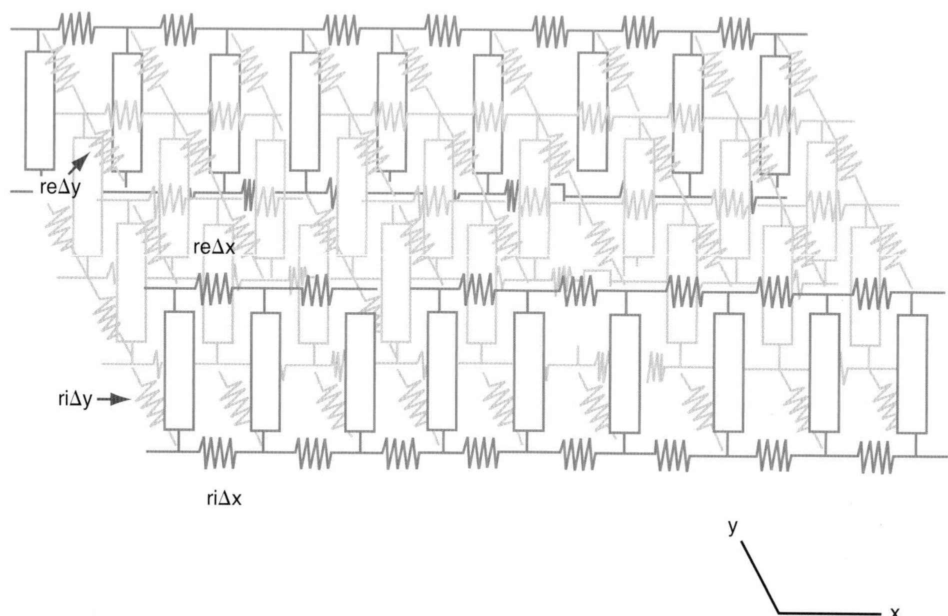

Figure 2-10. A circuit diagram of a two-dimensional bidomain model. The top of the resistor network represents the extracellular space, and the bottom of the network represents the intracellular space. The symbol reΔx represents the extracellular resistivity in the x direction; reΔY represents the extracellular resistivity in the y direction; riΔx and riΔy represent the intracellular resistivities in the x and y directions. The rectangles represent the cell membrane. For a passive model, the rectangle would be replaced by a parallel resistor-capacitor network. For an active model, the rectangle would be replaced by a membrane ion model.

Studies have shown that the anisotropy ratio is about 3:1 in the extracellular space and 10:1 in the intracellular space. When anisotropy ratios are used, the bidomain model begins to give new insights into how shocks change the transmembrane potential. Similar to the one-dimensional cable model, the bidomain model predicts that hyperpolarization occurs in tissue that lies under the extracellular anodal electrode. Likewise, depolarization occurs in tissue under the extracellular cathodal electrode. Unlike the one-dimensional cable model, the bidomain model also predicts that depolarization occurs along the long axis of the myocardial fibers at distances just a few millimeters from the anode. A similar effect is predicted to occur at the cathode, with hyperpolarization at distances of a few millimeters.[104,105] Therefore, the effect on the transmembrane potential near the shocking electrode is predicted to be much more complicated by the bidomain model than by the one-dimensional cable model.

The power of the bidomain model, however, is that it hypothesizes that there should be changes in the transmembrane potential, either hyperpolarization or depolarization, across the entire heart. In this model, the change in transmembrane potential elicited by the shock depends on the distribution of intracellular and extracellular current, which is affected by the change in potential gradient with distance, the distance from the electrode, and the orientation of the myocardial fibers. Experimental studies have shown that there is a complex pattern of transmembrane potential changes during the delivery of a defibrillation shock, similar to those predicted by the bidomain model.[80,106,107]

The transmembrane potential changes that occur during the delivery of a defibrillation shock can lead to the initiation of reentry and subsequent reinitiation of fibrillation after the shock. Reentrant circuits can be described by the mathematical concept of a phase singularity.[108] Phase can be used to describe the cardiac action potential, with 0 phase assigned to the upstroke of the action potential and 2Π phase assigned to the end of the action potential. A reentrant circuit can be thought of as a circle of phase starting at 0 (excitation) and continuing to 2Π (recovery). The reentrant circuit moves around a central point, called a *phase singularity.* Efimov and colleagues[106] showed that a defibrillation shock can impose changes on the transmembrane potential extending from 0 phase through 2Π phase (Fig. 2-11). Thus, a reentrant circuit is generated and

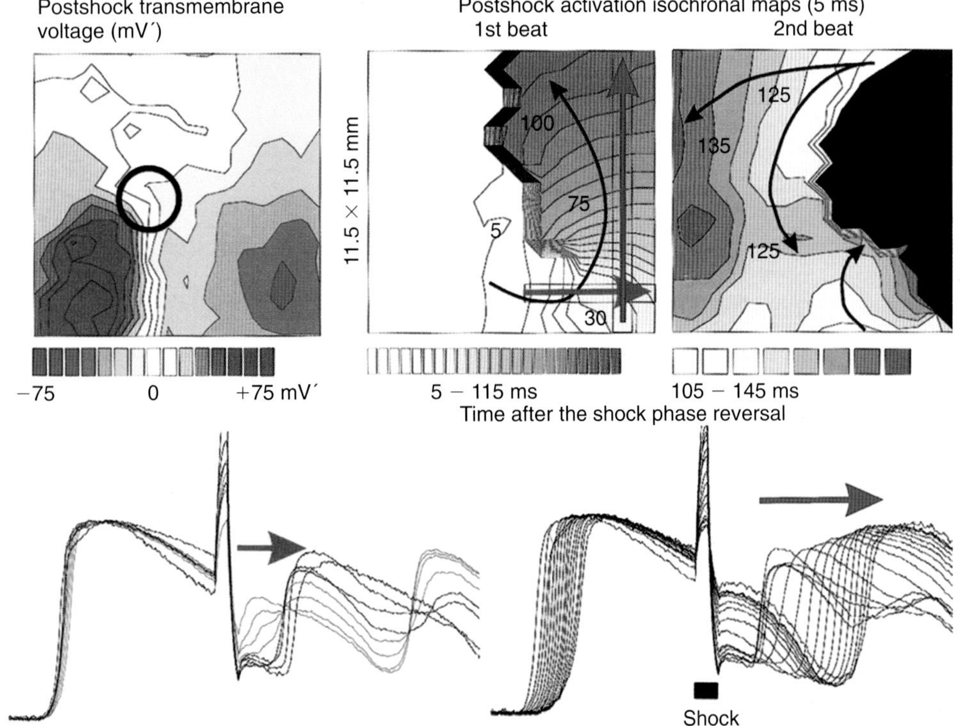

Figure 2-11. Creation of a shock-induced phase singularity. The upper left panel shows the change in transmembrane potential at the end of a +100/−200 V biphasic shock (i.e., at the 15th msec of a 16-msec shock), which resulted in a single extra beat. The scale is shown in millivolts, calibrated to a control 100-mV action potential. The point of phase singularity is indicated by the black circle. The upper middle panel shows a 5-msec isochronal map that depicts the initiation of the postshock spread of activation. The map starts at the onset of the 8-msec second phase of the shock (polarity reversal). The lower left and lower right panels show optical recordings from several recording sites used to reconstruct the activation maps. The upper right panel shows a continuation of the reentrant activation shown in the middle panel. Reentrant activity self-terminates after encountering refractory tissue in the lower right corner of the field of view (see traces in lower right panel). (From Efimov IR, Cheng Y, Van Wagoner DR, et al: Virtual electrode-induced phase singularity: A basic mechanism of defibrillation failure. Circ Res 82:918-925, 1998.)

fibrillation is induced. These same authors suggested that induced reentrant circuits may be one way that defibrillation shocks can fail.

The secondary source and bidomain models may not be mutually exclusive; rather, both may contribute to the changes in transmembrane potential. The exact mechanism by which an electrical pulse results in defibrillation remains incompletely understood at the level of the cell membrane and the ion channels. As the transmembrane potential attains values closer to the typical resting transmembrane potential than the usual minimum of −65 mV observed in fibrillating myocytes, this may allow the voltage-gated Na^+ channels to recover sufficiently and the myocytes to regain full excitability.

The Effect of the Defibrillating Shock Field on the Cellular Action Potential

The final common pathway of changes in the transmembrane potential caused by a defibrillation shock involves affects on the shape and duration of the cellular action potential. The shock can have one of three effects on the myocardium, depending on the local strength of the shock and its timing with respect to the local action potential. If the shock is delivered during the early plateau, there will be little or no prolongation of the action potential. If the shock is strong enough and is delivered relatively late during the action potential, it will initiate a new action potential. A shock that is strong enough but is delivered during early phase 3 of the action potential will modify and prolong an ongoing action potential without initiating an entirely new action potential (Fig. 2-12).

A defibrillating shock must do two things to defibrillate the heart successfully. First, it must stop most or all activation wavefronts on the heart. Second, it must not reinitiate fibrillation. The *extension of refractoriness hypothesis* helps to explain how a shock can stop fibrillation. A shock can prolong the refractory period of an action potential without triggering a new action potential if it is of sufficient strength and is delivered at an appropriate interval with respect to the upstroke.[23,109] If the first activation front that forms after a defibrillation shock encounters tissue with an extended refractory period, the front will be stopped because it cannot propagate into the region of refractory tissue.

Also, a defibrillation shock must not restart fibrillation. If only part of the front encounters tissue with an

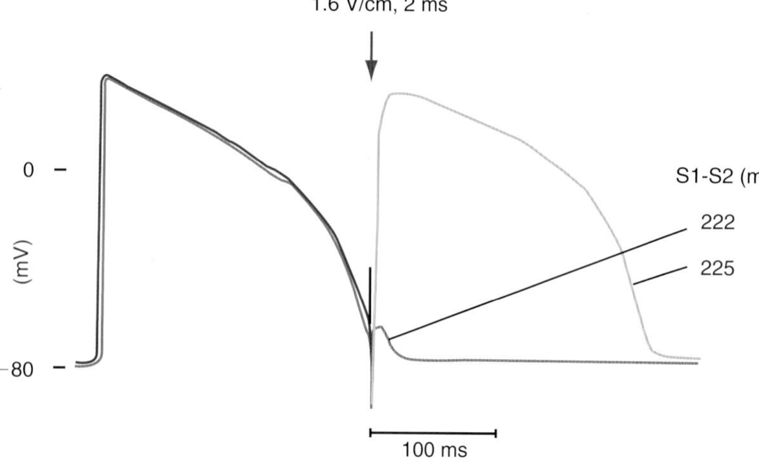

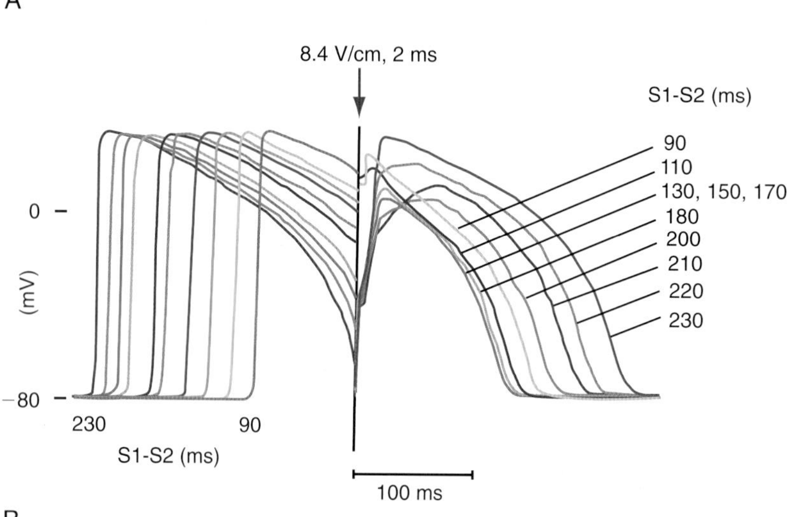

Figure 2-12. Transmembrane recordings from a guinea pig papillary muscle showing an all-or-none response to a weak field stimulus and action potential prolongation in response to a larger stimulus. ***A,*** *Recordings that illustrate the response to an S2 stimulus of 1.6 V/cm oriented along the fibers. The S1-S2 stimulus interval for each response (milliseconds) is indicated to the right of the recordings. The responses are markedly different even though the change in S2 timing was only 3 msec. An S1-S2 interval of 222 msec caused almost no response, whereas an interval of 225 msec produced a new action potential.* ***B,*** *A range of action potential extensions produced by an S2 stimulus generating a potential gradient of 8.4 V/cm oriented along the long axis of the myofibers. The recordings were obtained from the same cell as in panel* ***A.*** *The action potential recordings, obtained from one cellular impairment, are aligned with the S2 time. An S1 stimulus was applied 3 msec before phase 0 of each recording. The longest and shortest S1-S2 intervals tested (230 and 90 msec, respectively) are indicated beneath their respective phase 0 depolarizations. The S1-S2 interval for each response is indicated to the right. (From Knisley SB, Smith WM, Ideker RE: Effect of field stimulation on cellular repolarization in rabbit myocardium: Implications for reentry induction. Circ Res 70:707-715, 1992.)*

extended refractory period, only part of the front will be halted. The rest of the activation front will propagate forward and will eventually move into the area that could not be stimulated or that would not allow propagation (unidirectional block). This process of stimulating some tissue and creating unidirectional block in adjacent regions creates a reentrant circuit that eventually breaks down into fibrillation. The *critical point* is that point at which a critical shock strength intersects a critical level of refractoriness, leading to the formation of a reentrant circuit.[110-112]

To understand better how reentrant circuits and critical points are formed after a defibrillation shock, studies have examined the behavior of the heart after delivery of a shock during a paced ventricular rhythm.[111] Shocks were used to initiate VF during the vulnerable period of the paced rhythm. A large premature S2 stimulus was delivered through a long, narrow electrode oriented perpendicular to an activation front arising from an S1 stimulus (Fig. 2-13). S2 shocks were given to scan the vulnerable period after the last S1 stimulus. At an appropriate S1-to-S2 coupling interval, a reentrant circuit formed and continued for several cycles before breaking down into fibrillation. The initial postshock activation front circled a point at which a shock potential gradient field of 5 to 6 V/cm for a 10-msec monophasic shock intersected tissue that

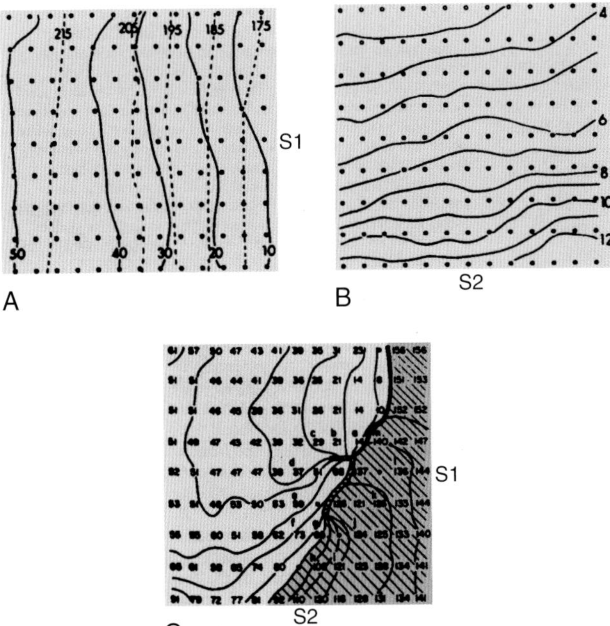

Figure 2-13. Initiation of reentry and ventricular fibrillation after orthogonal interaction of myocardial refractoriness and the potential gradient field created by a large stimulus. ***A,*** *Distribution of activation times during the last S1 beat (solid lines) and recovery times in relation to a local 2-mA stimulus (dashed lines) in milliseconds after this activation.* ***B,*** *S2 stimulus field (V/cm).* ***C,*** *Initial activation pattern just after the S2 stimulus. The hatched region is believed to be directly excited by the S2 stimulus field. (From Frazier DW, Wolf PD, Wharton JM, et al: Stimulus-induced critical point: Mechanism for electrical initiation of reentry in normal canine myocardium. J Clin Invest 83:1039-1052, 1989.)*

was just passing out of its refractory period to a 2-mA local stimulus. This intersection formed a critical point.

The intersection of a particular potential gradient level with a particular refractory state divides the tissue into four regions centered on the critical point (see Fig. 2-13C). The region to the left of the critical point was still in its refractory period and was not directly excited by the shock. The region to the right of the critical point had recovered enough to be directly excited by the S2 stimulus. Above the critical point, the shock had no effect on the refractory period of the tissue, whereas below the critical point, the shock prolonged the refractory period of the tissue. Therefore, an excitation wavefront propagated from the upper right quadrant of the mapped region across the top half of the plaque. Because of the prolongation of refractoriness in the tissue below the critical point, the excitation wavefront was unable to propagate across the bottom half of the plaque directly. As this tissue recovered, the excitation wavefront from the top half of the plaque entered the area at the bottom half and re-excited the tissue, creating a reentrant circuit around the critical point.

Recent studies provide some insight into why the activation pattern observed in Figure 2-13 occurs. When the myocardium is stimulated with a shock field whose potential gradient is less than the critical value for that waveform, an all-or-none response is observed (see Fig. 2-11). If the stimulus is applied with a coupling interval greater than the refractory period, a new action potential is generated. If the coupling interval is shorter than the refractory period, almost no response is seen. When the shock field strength is greater than a critical value, a whole gradation of responses is observed, depending on the coupling interval. As the coupling interval is made shorter, a smaller response occurs. However, even these smaller responses prolong refractoriness. It is this prolongation of refractoriness adjacent to directly stimulated myocardium that leads to unidirectional block and ultimately to the formation of critical points and functional reentrant circuits. If fibrillation is initiated by the reentrant pathway formed whenever a critical point is created within the myocardium, then, to be successful, the strength of a defibrillation shock should be greater than that at which no critical points are formed.

Ideker and associates[113] examined the potential gradient and degree of refractoriness at the critical point for a series of monophasic and biphasic waveforms and compared these values with the defibrillation threshold. Monophasic waveforms lasting 1, 2, 3, 8, and 16 msec were delivered, as were biphasic waveforms in which both phases were of equal duration, the two phases totaling 2, 4, 8, and 16 msec. The defibrillation threshold decreased as the degree of refractoriness at the critical point decreased. The waveform that induced a critical point located where both the potential gradient and the degree of refractoriness were lowest (i.e., the 4/4-msec biphasic waveform) had the lowest defibrillation threshold. This observation may explain why some waveforms defibrillate at lower voltages than others.

The mechanisms for the formation of critical points described here may be too simplistic in light of the complex ways in which a shock can affect the transmembrane potential. Furthermore, the requirement that no critical point be formed for a shock to succeed may be too stringent. Several studies have shown that a defibrillation shock can still be successful even if it creates rapid postshock activation for one or two cycles, suggesting that it may not be necessary to prevent the creation of critical points and reentry. Rather, it is only necessary that the reentrant circuits die out in one or two cycles before secondary reentry occurs. Further research is necessary to understand these phenomena more completely.

Acknowledgment

This work was supported in part by National Institutes of Health grant HL-42760.

REFERENCES

1. Prevost JL, Battelli F: Sur quelques effets des décharges électriques sur le coeur des Mammifères. CRSAS 129:1267-1268, 1899.
2. Beck CS, Pritchard WH, Feil HS: Ventricular fibrillation of long duration abolished by electric shock. JAMA 135:985-986, 1947.
3. Zoll PM, Linenthal AJ, Gibson W, et al: Termination of ventricular fibrillation in man by externally applied electric countershock. N Engl J Med 254:727-732, 1956.
4. Akiyama T: Intracellular recording of in situ ventricular cells during ventricular fibrillation. Am J Physiol 240:H465-H471, 1981.
5. Zhou X, Guse P, Wolf PD, et al: Existence of both fast and slow channel activity during the early stage of ventricular fibrillation. Circ Res 70:773-786, 1992.
6. Swartz JF, Jones JL, Fletcher RD: Characterization of ventricular fibrillation based on monophasic action potential morphology in the human heart. Circulation 87:1907-1914, 1993.
7. Witkowski FX, Penkoske PS, Kavanagh KM: Activation patterns during ventricular fibrillation. In Zipes DP, Jalife J (eds): Cardiac Electrophysiology: From Cell to Bedside, 2nd ed. Philadelphia: WB Saunders, 1995, pp 539-544.
8. Gray RA, Jalife J, Panfilov AV, et al: Mechanisms of cardiac fibrillation: Drifting rotors as a mechanism of cardiac fibrillation. Science 270:1222-1225, 1995.
9. Wiggers CJ: The physiologic basis for cardiac resuscitation from ventricular fibrillation: Method for serial defibrillation. Am Heart J 20:413-422, 1940.
10. Mower MM, Mirowski M, Spear JF, Moore EN: Patterns of ventricular activity during catheter defibrillation. Circulation 49:858-861, 1974.
11. Zipes DP, Fischer J, King RM, et al: Termination of ventricular fibrillation in dogs by depolarizing a critical amount of myocardium. Am J Cardiol 36:37-44, 1975.
12. Chen P-S, Shibata N, Wolf PD, et al: Epicardial activation during successful and unsuccessful ventricular defibrillation in open chest dogs. Cardiovasc Rev Rep 7:625-648, 1986.
13. Gray RA, Ayers G, Jalife J: Video imaging of atrial defibrillation in the sheep heart. Circulation 95:1038-1047, 1997.
14. Chen P-S, Wolf PD, Claydon FJ III, et al: The potential gradient field created by epicardial defibrillation electrodes in dogs. Circulation 74:626-636, 1986.
15. Wharton JM, Wolf PD, Smith WM, et al: Cardiac potential and potential gradient fields generated by single, combined, and sequential shocks during ventricular defibrillation. Circulation 85:1510-1523, 1992.
16. Zhou X, Daubert JP, Wolf PD, et al: Epicardial mapping of ventricular defibrillation with monophasic and biphasic shocks in dogs. Circ Res 72:145-160, 1993.
17. Henriquez CS: Simulating the electrical behavior of cardiac muscle using the bidomain model. Crit Rev Biomed Eng 21:1-77, 1993.
18. Fishler MG, Sobie EA, Thakor NV, Tung L: Mechanisms of cardiac cell excitation with premature monophasic and biphasic field stimuli: A model study. Biophys J 70:1347-1362, 1996.
19. Gillis AM, Fast VG, Rohr S, Kléber AG: Spatial changes in transmembrane potential during extracellular electrical shocks in cultured monolayers of neonatal rat ventricular myocytes. Circ Res 79:676-690, 1996.
20. Plonsey R, Barr RC: Inclusion of junction elements in a linear cardiac model through secondary sources: Application to defibrillation. Med Biol Eng Comput 24:137-144, 1986.
21. Fast VG, Rohr S, Gillis AM, Kléber AG: Activation of cardiac tissue by extracellular electrical shocks: Formation of "secondary sources" at intercellular clefts in monolayers of cultured myocytes. Circ Res 82:375-385, 1998.
22. Moe GK, Abildskov JA, Han J: Factors responsible for the initiation and maintenance of ventricular fibrillation. In Surawicz B, Pellegrino ED (eds): Sudden Cardiac Death. New York: Grune & Stratton, 1964.
23. Dillon SM, Mehra R: Prolongation of ventricular refractoriness by defibrillation shocks may be due to additional depolarization of the action potential. J Cardiovasc Electrophysiol 3:442-456, 1992.
24. Wiggers CJ: Studies of ventricular fibrillation caused by electric shock. Cinematographic and electrocardiographic observations of the natural process in the dog's heart: Its inhibition by potassium and the revival of coordinated beats by calcium. Am Heart J 5:351-365, 1930.
25. Worley SJ, Swain JL, Colavita PG, et al: Development of an endocardial-epicardial gradient of activation rate during electrically induced, sustained ventricular fibrillation in the dog. Am J Cardiol 55:813-820, 1985.
26. Opthof T, Ramdat Misier AR, Coronel R, et al: Dispersion of refractoriness in canine ventricular myocardium: Effects of sympathetic stimulation. Circ Res 68:1204-1215, 1991.
27. Ideker RE, Klein GJ, Harrison L, et al: Epicardial mapping of the initiation of ventricular fibrillation induced by reperfusion following acute ischemia. Circulation 58:II-64, 1978.
28. Rogers J, Usui M, KenKnight B, et al: Recurrent wavefront morphologies: A method for quantifying the complexity of epicardial activation patterns. Ann Biomed Eng 25:761-768, 1997.
29. Samie FH, Berenfeld O, Anumonwo J, et al: Rectification of the background potassium current: A determinant of rotor dynamics in ventricular fibrillation. Circ Res 89:1216-1223, 2001.
30. Lewis T: The Mechanism and Registration of the Heart Beat. London, Shaw and Sons, 1925.
31. Newton JC, Evans FG, Chattipakorn N, et al: Peak frequency distribution across the whole fibrillating heart. PACE 23:617, 2000.
32. Newton JC, Ideker RE: Estimated global transmural distribution of activation rate and conduction block during porcine and canine ventricular fibrillation. Circ Res 94:836-842, 2004.
33. Gray RA, Jalife J: Self-organized drifting spiral waves as a mechanism for atrial fibrillation. Circulation 94:I-94, 1996.
34. Allessie M, Kirchhof C, Scheffer GJ, et al: Regional control of atrial fibrillation by rapid pacing in concious dogs. Circulation 84:1689-1697, 1991.
35. Ken-Knight BH, Bayly PV, Gerstle RJ, et al: Regional capture of fibrillating ventricular myocardium: Evidence of an excitable gap. Circ Res 77:849-855, 1995.
36. Witkowski FX, Penkoske PA, Plonsey R: Mechanism of cardiac defibrillation in open-chest dogs with unipolar DC-coupled simultaneous activation and shock potential recordings. Circulation 82:244-260, 1990.

37. Bardy GH, Ivey TD, Allen MD, et al: A prospective randomized evaluation of biphasic versus monophasic waveform pulses on defibrillation efficacy in humans. J Am Coll Cardiol 14:728-733, 1989.
38. Block M, Hammel D, Böcker D, et al: A prospective randomized cross-over comparison on mono- and biphasic defibrillation using nonthoracotomy lead configurations in humans. J Cardiovasc Electrophysiol 5:581-590, 1994.
39. Chapman PD, Vetter JW, Souza JJ, et al: Comparison of monophasic with single and dual capacitor biphasic waveforms for nonthoracotomy canine internal defibrillation. J Am Coll Cardiol 14:242-245, 1989.
40. Dixon EG, Tang ASL, Wolf PD, et al: Improved defibrillation thresholds with large contoured epicardial electrodes and biphasic waveforms. Circulation 76:1176-1184, 1987.
41. Gurvich NL, Markarychev VA: Defibrillation of the heart with biphasic electrical impulses. Kardiologiia 7:109-112, 1967.
42. Walcott GP, Melnick SB, Chapman FW, et al: Comparison of monophasic and biphasic waveforms for external defibrillation in an animal model of cardiac arrest and resuscitation. J Am Coll Cardiol 25:405A, 1995.
43. Tang ASL, Yabe S, Wharton JM, et al: Ventricular defibrillation using biphasic waveforms: The importance of phasic duration. J Am Coll Cardiol 13:207-214, 1989.
44. Feeser SA, Tang ASL, Kavanagh KM, et al: Strength-duration and probability of success curves for defibrillation with biphasic waveforms. Circulation 82:2128-2141, 1990.
45. Kroll MW: A minimal model of the single capacitor biphasic defibrillation waveform. PACE 17:1782-1792, 1994.
46. Kroll MW: A minimal model of the monophasic defibrillation pulse. PACE 16:769-777, 1993.
47. Swerdlow CD, Fan W, Brewer JE: Charge-burping theory correctly predicts optimal ratios of phase duration for biphasic defibrillation waveforms. Circulation 94:2278-2284, 1996.
48. Walcott GP, Walker RG, Krassowska W, et al: Choosing the optimum monophasic and biphasic waveforms for defibrillation. PACE 17:789, 1994.
49. Blair HA: On the intensity-time relations for stimulation by electric currents: II. JGENPH 15:731-755, 1932.
50. Lapicque L: L'Excitabilite en Fonction du Temps. Paris, Libraire J. Gilbert, 1926.
51. Mouchawar GA, Geddes LA, Bourland JD, Pearce JA: Ability of the Lapicque and Blair strength-duration curves to fit experimentally obtained data from the dog heart. IEEE Trans Biomed Eng 36:971-974, 1989.
52. Irnich W: The fundamental law of electrostimulation and its application to defibrillation. PACE 13:1433-1447, 1990.
53. Walcott GP, Walker RG, Cates AW, et al: Choosing the optimal monophasic and biphasic waveforms for ventricular defibrillation. J Cardiovasc Electrophysiol 6:737-750, 1995.
54. Sweeney RJ, Gill RM, Jones JL, Reid PR: Defibrillation using a high-frequency series of monophasic rectangular pulses: Observations and model predictions. J Cardiovasc Electrophysiol 7:134-143, 1996.
55. Gold MR, Shorofsky SR: Strength-duration relationship for human transvenous defibrillation. Circulation 96:3517-3520, 1997.
56. Schuder JC, Stoeckle H, West JA, Keskar PY: Transthoracic ventricular defibrillation in the dog with truncated and untruncated exponential stimuli. IEEE Trans Biomed Eng 18:410-415, 1971.
57. Walcott GP, Melnick SB, Chapman FW, et al: Comparison of damped sinusoidal and truncated exponential waveforms for external defibrillation. J Am Coll Cardiol 27:237A, 1996.
58. Harbinson MT, Allen JD, Imam Z, et al: Rounded biphasic waveform reduces energy requirements for transvenous catheter cardioversion of atrial fibrillation and flutter. PACE 20:226-229, 1997.
59. Hillsley RE, Walker RG, Swanson DK, et al: Is the second phase of a biphasic defibrillation waveform the defibrillating phase? PACE 16:1401-1411, 1993.
60. Schuder JC, Rahmoeller GA, Stoeckle H: Transthoracic ventricular defibrillation with triangular and trapezoidal waveforms. Circ Res 19:689-694, 1966.
61. Bardy GH, Marchlinski FE, Sharma AD, et al: Multicenter comparison of truncated biphasic shocks and standard damped sine wave monophasic shocks for transthoracic ventricular defibrillation. Transthoracic Investigators. Circulation 94:2507-2514, 1996.
62. Camacho MA, Lehr JL, Eisenberg SR: A three-dimensional finite element model of human transthoracic defibrillation: Paddle placement and size. IEEE Transact Biomed Eng 42:572-578, 1995.
63. Deale OC, Lerman BB: Intrathoracic current flow during transthoracic defibrillation in dogs: Transcardiac current fraction. Circ Res 67:1405-1419, 1990.
64. Karlon WJ, Eisenberg SR, Lehr JL: Effects of paddle placement and size on defibrillation current distribution: A three-dimensional finite element model. IEEE Trans Biomed Eng 40:246-255, 1993.
65. Block M, Hammel D, Isburch F, et al: Results and realistic expectations with transvenous lead systems. PACE 15:665-670, 1992.
66. Tang ASL, Wolf PD, Claydon FJ III, et al: Measurement of defibrillation shock potential distributions and activation sequences of the heart in three-dimensions. Proc IEEE 76:1176-1186, 1988.
67. Tang ASL, Wolf PD, Afework Y, et al: Three-dimensional potential gradient fields generated by intracardiac catheter and cutaneous patch electrodes. Circulation 85:1857-1864, 1992.
68. Chen P-S, Wolf PD, Melnick SD, et al: Comparison of activation during ventricular fibrillation and following unsuccessful defibrillation shocks in open chest dogs. Circ Res 66:1544-1560, 1990.
69. Chattipakorn N, Banville I, Gray RA, Ideker RE: Effects of shock strengths on ventricular defibrillation failure. Cardiovasc Res 61:39-44, 2004.
70. Shibata N, Chen P-S, Dixon EG, et al: Epicardial activation following unsuccessful defibrillation shocks in dogs. Am J Physiol 255:H902-H909, 1988.
71. Walker RG, Walcott GP, Smith WM, Ideker RE: Sites of earliest activation following transvenous defibrillation. Circulation 90:I-447, 1994.
72. Cates AW, Wolf PD, Hillsley RE, et al: The probability of defibrillation success and the incidence of postshock arrhythmia as a function of shock strength. PACE 17:1208-1217, 1994.
73. Chapman FW, El-Abbady TZ, Walcott GP, et al: Dysfunction following transthoracic defibrillation shocks in dogs. PACE 20:1128, 1997.
74. Reddy RK, Gleva MJ, Gliner BE, et al: Biphasic transthoracic defibrillation causes fewer ECG ST-segment changes after shock. Ann Emerg Med 30:127-134, 1997.
75. DeBruin KA, Krassowska W: Electroporation and shock-induced transmembrane potential in a cardiac fiber during defibrillation strength shocks. Ann Biomed Eng 26:584-596, 1998.
76. Schuder JC, Gold JH, Stoeckle H, et al: Transthoracic ventricular defibrillation in the 100 kg calf with symmetrical one-cycle bidirectional rectangular wave stimuli. IEEE Trans Biomed Eng 30:415-422, 1983.
77. Yabe S, Smith WM, Daubert JP, et al: Conduction disturbances caused by high current density electric fields. Circ Res 66:1190-1203, 1990.
78. Jones JL, Jones RE: Decreased defibrillator-induced dysfunction with biphasic rectangular waveforms. An J Physiol 247:H792-H796, 1984.
79. Walcott GP, Knisley SB, Zhou X, et al: On the mechanism of ventricular defibrillation. PACE 20:422-431, 1997.

80. Clark DM, Rogers JM, Ideker RE, Knisley SB: Intracardiac defibrillation-strength shocks produce large regions of hyperpolarization and depolarization. J Am Coll Cardiol 27:147A, 1996.
81. Zhou X, Wolf PD, Rollins DL, et al: Effects of monophasic and biphasic shocks on action potentials during ventricular fibrillation in dogs. Circ Res 73:325-334, 1993.
82. Daubert JP, Frazier DW, Wolf PD, et al: Response of relatively refractory canine myocardium to monophasic and biphasic shocks. Circulation 84:2522-2538, 1991.
83. Colavita PG, Wolf PD, Smith WM, et al: Determination of effects of internal countershock by direct cardiac recordings during normal rhythm. Am J Physiol 250:H736-H740, 1986.
84. Weidmann S: Electrical constants of trabecular muscle from mammalian heart. J Physiol 210:1041-1054, 1970.
85. Kléber AG, Riegger CB: Electrical constants of arterially perfused rabbit papillary muscle. J Physiol 385:307-324, 1987.
86. Plonsey R, Barr RC: Effect of microscopic and macroscopic discontinuities on the response of cardiac tissue to defibrillating (stimulating) currents. Med Biol Eng Comput 24:130-136, 1986.
87. Krassowska W, Frazier DW, Pilkington TC, Ideker RE: Potential distribution in three-dimensional periodic myocardium: Part II. Application to extracellular stimulation. IEEE Trans Biomed Eng 37:267-284, 1990.
88. Krassowska W, Pilkington TC, Ideker RE: Potential distribution in three-dimensional periodic myocardium: Part I. Solution with two-scale asymptotic analysis. IEEE Trans Biomed Eng 37:252-266, 1990.
89. Tung L: A Bidomain Nodel for Describing Ischemic Myocardial DC Potentials. Cambridge, MA, Massechusetts Institute of Technology, 1978.
90. White JB, Walcott GP, Pollard AE, Ideker RE: Myocardial discontinuities: A substrate for producing virtual electrodes to increase directly excited areas of the myocardium by shocks. Circulation 97:1738-1745, 1998.
91. Trayanova N: Discrete versus syncytial tissue behavior in a model of cardiac stimulation. I: Mathematical formulation. IEEE Trans Biomed Eng 43:1129-1140, 1996.
92. Trayanova N: Discrete versus syncytial tissue behavior in a model of cardiac stimulation. II: Results of simulation. IEEE Trans Biomed Eng 43:1141-1150, 1996.
93. Kieval RS, Spear JF, Moore EN: Gap junctional conductance in ventricular myocyte pairs isolated from postischemic rabbit myocardium. Circ Res 71:127-136, 1992.
94. Shaw RM, Rudy Y: Electrophysiologic effects of acute myocardial ischemia: A mechanistic investigation of action potential conduction and conduction failure. Circ Res 80:124-138, 1997.
95. Shaw RM, Rudy Y: Ionic mechanisms of propagation in cardiac tissue: Roles of the sodium and L-type calcium currents during reduced excitability and decreased gap junction coupling. Circ Res 81:727-741, 1997.
96. Knisley SB, Blitchington TF, Hill BC, et al: Optical measurements of transmembrane potential changes during electric field stimulation of ventricular cells. Circ Res 72:255-270, 1993.
97. Windisch H, Ahammer H, Schaffer P, et al: Optical multisite monitoring of cell excitation phenomenon in isolated cardiomyocytes. Pflugers Arch 430:508-518, 1995.
98. Zhou X, Ideker RE, Blitchington TF, et al: Optical transmembrane potential measurements during defibrillation-strength shocks in perfused rabbit hearts. Circ Res 77:593-602, 1995.
99. Wikswo JP Jr, Lin S-F, Abbas RA: Virtual electrodes in cardiac tissue: A common mechanism for anodal and cathodal stimulation. Biophys J 69:2195-2210, 1995.
100. Sommer JR, Scherer B: Geometry of cell and bundle appositions in cardiac muscle: Light microscopy. Am J Physiol 248:H792-H803, 1985.
101. Street AM, Plonsey R: Activation fronts elicited remote to the pacing site due to the presence of scar tissue. In Proceedings of the 18th Annual International Conference, IEEE Engineering Medical Biological Society. Amsterdam, The Netherlands, Institute of Electrical and Electronics Engineers. Available on CD-ROM (Piscataway, NJ, 1996, p 358).
102. Sharifov OF, Ideker RE, Fast VG: High-resolution optical mapping of intramural virtual electrodes in porcine left ventricular wall. Cardiovasc Res 64:448-456, 2004.
103. Clerc L: Directional differences of impulse spread in trabecular muscle from mammalian heart. J Physiol 255:335-346, 1976.
104. Wikswo JP Jr: Tissue anisotropy, the cardiac bidomain, and the virtual cathode effect. In Zipes DP, Jalife J (eds): Cardiac Electrophysiology: From Cell to Bedside, 2nd ed. Philadelphia: WB Saunders, 1995, pp 348-362.
105. Knisley SB: Transmembrane voltage changes during unipolar stimulation of rabbit ventricle. Circ Res 77:1229-1239, 1995.
106. Efimov IR, Cheng Y, Van Wagoner DR, et al: Virtual electrode-induced phase singularity: A basic mechanism of defibrillation failure. Circ Res 82:918-925, 1998.
107. Efimov IR, Cheng YN, Biermann M, et al: Transmembrane voltage changes produced by real and virtual electrodes during monophasic defibrillation shocks delivered by an implantable electrode. J Cardiovasc Electrophysiol 8:1031-1045, 1997.
108. Iyer AN, Gray RA:. An experimentalist's approach to accurate localization of phase singularities during reentry. Ann Biomed Eng 29:47-59, 2001.
109. Knisley SB, Smith WM, Ideker RE: Effect of field stimulation on cellular repolarization in rabbit myocardium: Implications for reentry induction. Circ Res 70:707-715, 1992.
110. Winfree AT: When Time Breaks Down: The Three-dimensional Dynamics of Electrochemical Waves and Cardiac Arrhythmias. Princeton, NJ: Princeton University Press; 1987.
111. Frazier DW, Wolf PD, Wharton JM, et al: Stimulus-induced critical point: Mechanism for electrical initiation of reentry in normal canine myocardium. J Clin Invest 83:1039-1052, 1989.
112. Chen P-S, Wolf PD, Dixon EG, et al: Mechanism of ventricular vulnerability to single premature stimuli in open-chest dogs. Circ Res 62:1191-1209, 1988.
113. Ideker RE, Alferness C, Hagler J, et al: Rotor site correlates with defibrillation waveform efficacy. Circulation 84:II-499, 1991.

Chapter 3

Sensing and Detection

CHARLES D. SWERDLOW • JEFFREY M. GILLBERG • WALTER H. OLSON

The electrical therapies of pacemakers and implantable cardioverter-defibrillators (ICDs) are controlled by *sensing* of cardiac depolarizations and *detection* of arrhythmias by analysis of the timing and morphology of sensed events. When a wavefront of depolarization passes the tip electrode of an intracardiac lead, a deflection in the continuous *electrogram* (EGM) signal travels instantaneously up the lead wire to the pacemaker or ICD. There, the signal is amplified, filtered, digitized, and processed by the sensing electronics. A *sensed event* is an instant in time when a pacemaker or ICD determines that an atrial or ventricular depolarization has occurred based on processing of the continuous EGM signal. Dual-chamber pacemakers and ICDs have separate sensing systems for the atrium and ventricle.

Appropriate sensing results in one sensed event for each activation wavefront in the corresponding chamber. Failure to sense activation wavefronts results in *undersensing*, which can cause inappropriate pacing, failure to switch modes, or failure to detect a tachyarrhythmia. Undersensing occurs if the depolarization signal has insufficient amplitude or frequency content to be recognized as a sensed event or if a *blanking* period disables the sensing amplifier at the time of the event. *Oversensing* occurs when nonphysiologic signals are recorded or when physiologic signals that do not reflect local myocardial depolarization are recognized inappropriately as sensed events. Oversensing can cause inappropriate inhibition of pacing, inappropriate tracking, or inappropriate ICD therapy.

Detection algorithms process sensed events to classify the atrial or ventricular rhythm. This classification is used to control beat-by-beat paced events, to change the pacing mode, to store data regarding untreated tachyarrhythmias, and to terminate sustained tachyarrhythmias with antitachycardia pacing (ATP) or shocks.

Intracardiac Electrograms

Surface Electrocardiogram Versus Intracardiac Electrogram

An EGM is a graphic display of the potential difference between two points in space over time. The myocardium is composed of cells that maintain a resting potential across the membrane (i.e., the cell is polarized) such that the inside of the cell is electrically negative with respect to the outside of the cell. During the upstroke of the action potential, the inside of the cell abruptly changes from a negative potential (with respect to the outside of the cell) to a neutral or slightly positive potential. After a period of 300 to 400 msec, the cell membrane is then repolarized, with the inside of the cell returning to its resting, negatively charged state. Figure 3-1 illustrates how an EGM is recorded between two electrodes in contact with the myocardium.

The electrocardiogram (ECG) is recorded from two electrodes on the surface of the body at some distance from the heart. The typical amplitude of its QRS complex is about 1 mV. The locations of the two electrodes determine the vectorial "viewpoint" from which the electrical activity of the entire heart is observed from the body surface. In contrast, the ventricular endocardial unipolar EGM typically is 5 to 20 mV in amplitude when recorded from a small electrode on the tip of a lead placed in direct contact with the apex of the right ventricle (Fig. 3-2). The second electrode needed to record this unipolar EGM is the pacemaker or ICD metal can, which is located some distance from the heart. The location of this distant second electrode, sometimes called the indifferent electrode, has a much smaller effect on the signal's properties, although it may record noncardiac electrical potentials (e.g., from the pectoral muscle). The ECG records electrical activity from the entire heart, whereas the EGM records only the local wavefronts of depolarization and repolarization that pass the tip electrode. The EGM depends on the viability of approximately 1 or 2 cm^3 of myocardium immediately under the tip electrode,[1,2] as depicted in Figure 3-2.

Electrode Systems: Unipolar, Bipolar, Integrated Bipolar, Epicardial

Figure 3-3 contrasts endocardial *unipolar* (tip-to-can), *bipolar* (tip-to-ring), and *integrated bipolar* (tip-to-coil) electrode systems, and Figure 3-4 shows representative examples. Epicardial electrode systems may be either unipolar (tip-to-can) or bipolar (tip-to-tip). These different electrode configurations have EGMs with similar R-wave amplitudes and slew rates, provided that the interelectrode spacing is at least 10 mm, as is true of almost all commercial pacemaker and defibrillator leads. Because unipolar electrode systems are more likely to oversense than are bipolar EGMs, they are contraindicated for ICDs and are used infrequently for modern pacemakers. Integrated bipolar electrodes used in ICDs have sensing characteristics that are more similar to the bipolar than the unipolar configuration. They are more likely to oversense, compared with true bipolar electrodes.[3,4] In one study, oversensing occurred in 40% of patients with integrated bipolar sensing, compared with 8% of patients with true bipolar systems.[4]

Amplitude, Slew Rate, and Waveshape of Electrograms

The largest and steepest deflection on the local EGM, called the *intrinsic deflection,* occurs when the wavefront of depolarization passes the small-tip electrode. The *EGM amplitude* traditionally is defined as the peak-to-peak amplitude, measured in millivolts, of the intrinsic deflection, as shown in Figure 3-5. The duration of a ventricular EGM usually is less than that of the QRS of the surface ECG, because the EGM is a local signal. The amplitude of an atrial or ventricular EGM is determined primarily by the excitable tissue near the tip electrode and therefore is usually similar for unipolar and bipolar signals. Typical amplitudes are 5 to 30 mV for ventricular EGMs and 1.5 to 6 mV for atrial EGMs.[1,2]

Increasing the size of the tip electrode in the range of 2 to 10 mm has minimal effect on atrial EGM amplitude but does increase EGM duration (Fig. 3-6). For short ventricular bipolar interelectrode spacing of 5 mm or less, the R-wave amplitude decreases, because the difference between the two unipolar EGMs from each electrode causes cancellation in the net bipolar signal.

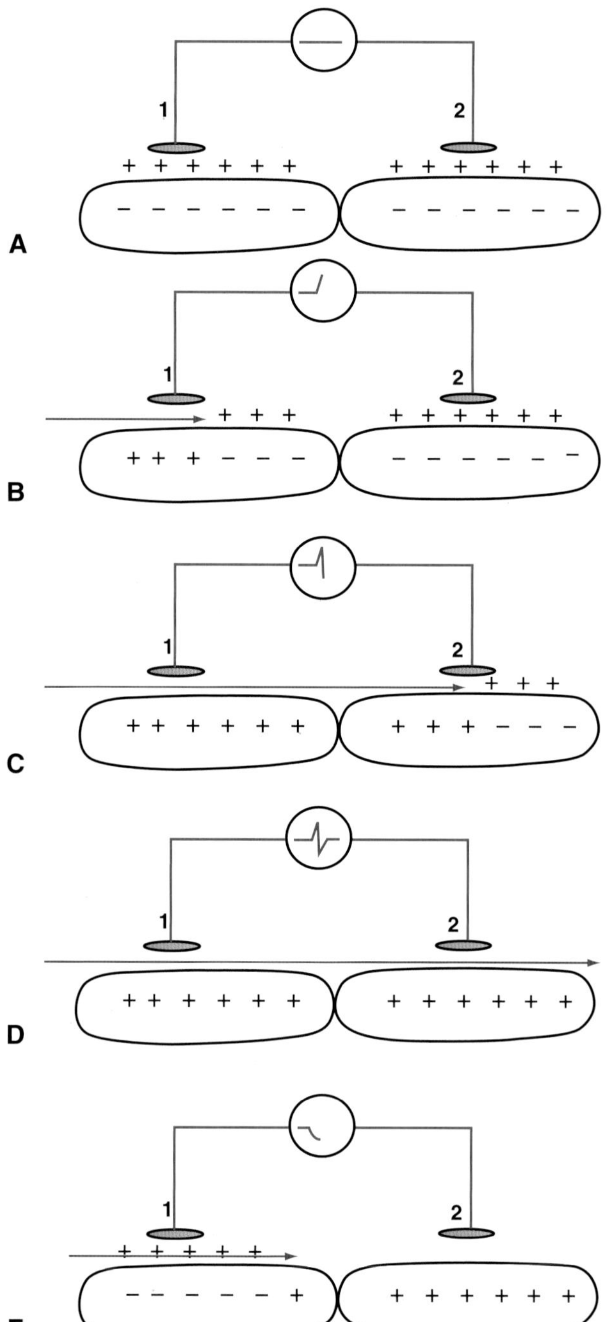

Figure 3-1. Illustration of how an EGM is recorded between two electrodes that are in contact with the myocardium. ***A,*** *At rest, both electrodes record a similar charge, with no potential difference between them.* ***B*** *and* ***C,*** *As a wavefront of depolarization moves under electrode 1, a difference in electrical charge is generated such that electrode 1 becomes electrically negative with respect to electrode 2.* ***D,*** *As the wavefront propagates under electrode 2, no potential difference between the two electrodes is recorded.* ***E,*** *The depolarization wavefront is followed by a wavefront of repolarization, during which a potential difference of opposite polarity is recorded. Because the EGM is determined by the instantaneous potential difference between the electrodes, the amplitude and shape of the recorded signal are determined by the direction from which the wavefront approaches the electrodes. For example, if a wavefront of depolarization reached both electrodes at the same time, there would be no potential difference between the electrodes, and an EGM would not be inscribed.*

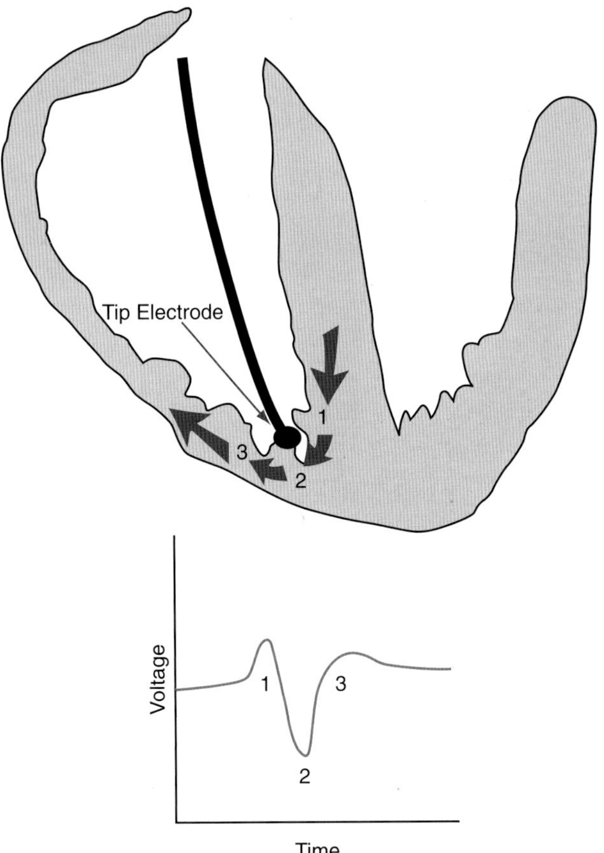

Figure 3-2. *This concept drawing indicates the spatial and temporal relationships for a unipolar endocardial EGM. The upper panel shows an anatomic drawing, and the lower panel shows the EGM recorded from a small-surface-area electrode at the tip of a pacemaker or defibrillator lead that makes direct contact with the endocardium in the right ventricular (RV) apex. The second electrode required to record an EGM is not shown, because it is a distant and indifferent electrode, usually the metal can of the pulse generator, and its location is not important provided that it is a substantial distance from the tip electrode. During a ventricular depolarization, the depolarization wavefront propagates from the septum, around the RV apex, and up the RV free wall* (arrows). *When the wavefront of depolarization arrives at location 1, just as it approaches the electrode, the initial positive deflection of the EGM occurs, at time 1. When the wavefront passes closest to the tip electrode at location 2, the major negative deflection on the EGM occurs, labeled as time 2. As the wavefront recedes from the electrode at location 3, the final portion of the EGM is inscribed at time 3. This local EGM is not affected by the depolarization wavefront as it travels further from the electrode. Therefore, the local EGM is shorter in duration than the surface electrocardiographic QRS complex.*

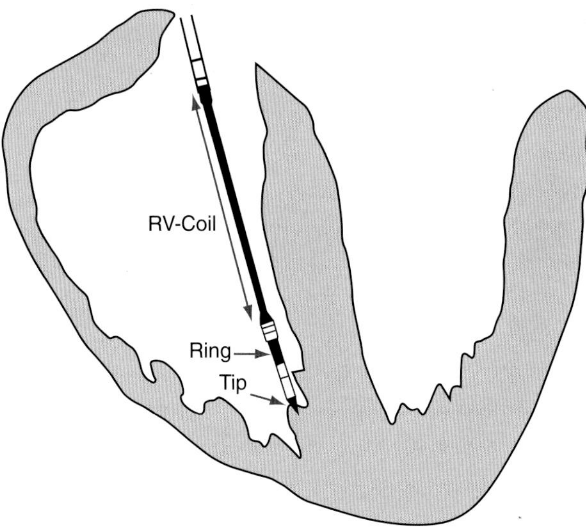

Figure 3-3. *The three practical endocardial electrode configurations used by most pacemakers and ICDs can be described with this figure. The distant indifferent or can electrode is not shown, because it is out of the field of view. The unipolar configuration used in Figure 3-1 to explain EGM formation simply records the signal between the tip electrode and the can. The tip electrode can be an active-fix screw or a small-surface-area tip electrode with various geometries. This unipolar configuration is subject to considerable noise and interference signals and is not suitable for ICDs. The* bipolar *configuration uses the Tip and Ring electrodes shown in the figure. The interelectrode spacing is typically 12 to 15 mm, and the ring electrode may or may not make contact with the endocardium. The* integrated bipolar *configuration uses the Tip and RV-Coil electrodes shown in the figure. EGMs recorded from bipolar and integrated bipolar configurations are very similar, and one less conductor is needed for the integrated bipolar configuration. The main disadvantages of the integrated bipolar configuration are susceptibility to diaphragmatic myopotentials, undesired atrial EGMs in small hearts, and slower post-shock recovery times due to electrode polarization. RV, right ventricular.*

The slew rate increases, because the time between arrival of the wavefront at the two electrodes decreases more than the EGM amplitude does. When two electrodes are widely separated, as in early Y-adapted cardiac resynchronization electrode systems, two distinct intrinsic deflections may be recorded on the EGM—one representing right ventricular (RV) activation and the other representing left ventricular (LV) activation. The interval between these deflections is determined by the conduction delay between the ventricles near the two electrodes.

The waveshapes of EGMs are quite variable (Fig. 3-7), probably because of the complex geometry of the trabecular endocardium adjacent to the tip electrode. In one study done at pacemaker lead implantation, 58% of unipolar EGMs were biphasic, with an initial upstroke followed by a roughly equal downstroke; 30% were predominantly monophasic negative, and 12% were predominantly monophasic positive.[1]

The maximum slope of the intrinsic deflection is the *slew rate,* measured in volts per second. It represents the maximum sustained rate of change of the EGM voltage. Mathematically, the slew rate is the first derivative of the voltage, dV/dt, so it depends on both the amplitude and the duration of the EGM. It is a crude representation of the frequency content of the EGM. The frequency content of ventricular and atrial EGMs is similar and in the range of 5 to 50 Hz. T waves and far-field R waves have lower frequency content, whereas most myopotentials and electromagnetic interference (EMI) have higher frequency content (Fig. 3-8).

Typical values for slew rates are 2 to 3 V/sec for ventricular EGMs and 1 to 2 V/sec for atrial EGMs.[1,2] Usually, an EGM with acceptable amplitude also has an

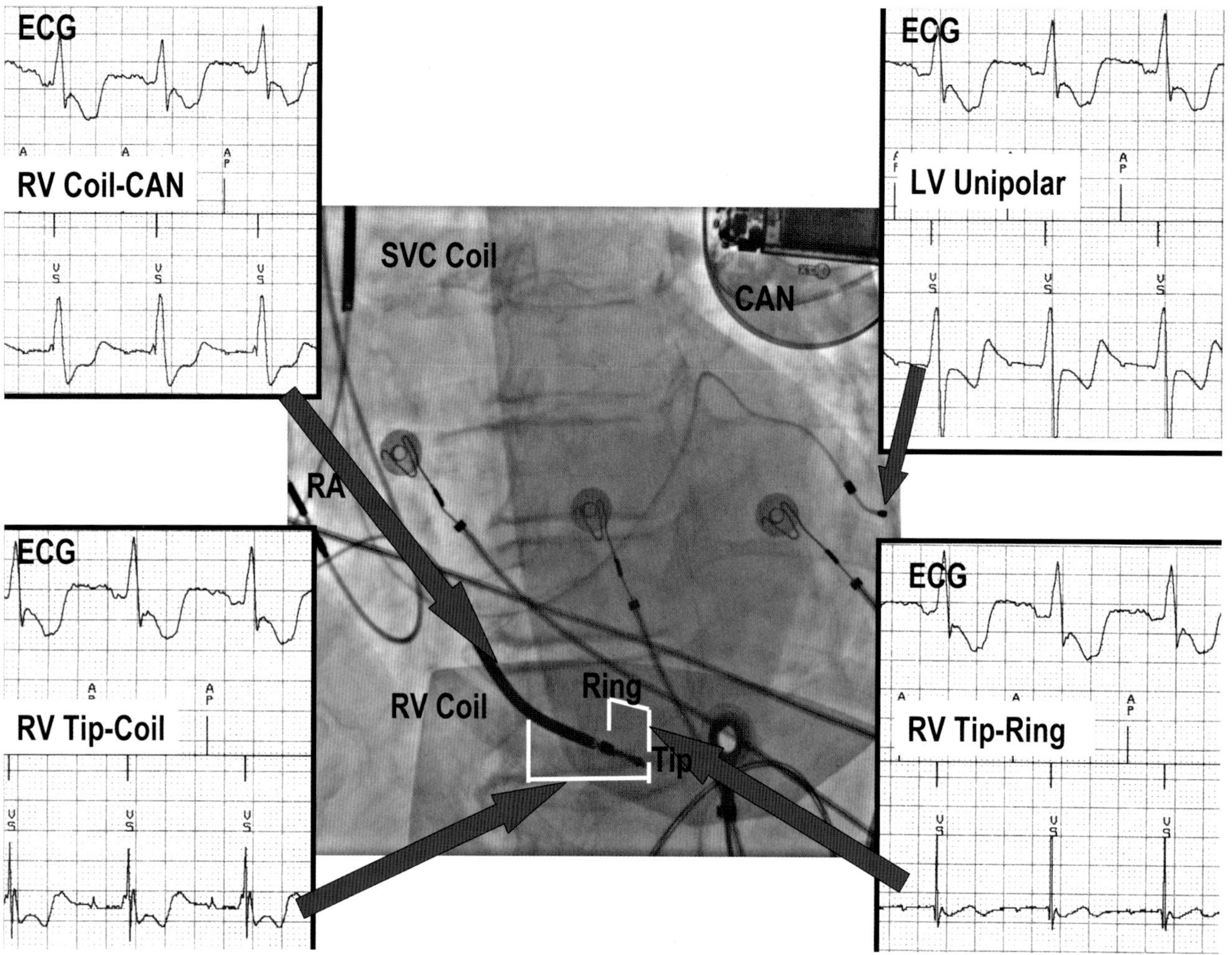

Figure 3-4. Ventricular electrocardiograms (ECGs) recorded from different electrode configurations in a single patient. The central panel shows a left anterior oblique radiograph of a cardiac resynchronization ICD system. Each of the four tracings shows surface ECG lead II, EGM markers, and one ventricular EGM during atrial pacing at a rate of 75 bpm. Top left, *far-field EGM recorded between the right ventricular (RV) coil electrode and the electrically active ICD housing (CAN).* Lower left, *Integrated bipolar EGM recorded between RV tip and RV coil electrodes.* Lower right, *True bipolar EGM recorded between the RV tip and ring electrodes.* Top right, *Left ventricular (LV) unipolar EGM recorded between the LV tip electrode and CAN. EGM scale is 0.5 mV/mm, except for the LV unipolar EGM, which has a scale of 2 mV/mm. The downward EGM ventricular sense (VS) markers correspond to the time at which the true bipolar RV tip-ring EGM crosses the sensing threshold. Because the "field of view" of this EGM is local, its duration is short. It occurs early in the QRS complex of this patient with left bundle branch block. The integrated bipolar tip-coil EGM has a peak-to-peak amplitude and slew rate similar to those of the true bipolar EGM. However, its field of view is larger due to the size of the RV coil, and therefore the T wave is larger. Low-amplitude atrial EGMs are visible because of the proximity of the coil to the tricuspid annulus. Both the RV coil-CAN and the LV unipolar EGM are widely spaced, between an intracardiac electrode and the extracardiac CAN. Their duration is closer to that of the QRS complex. The intrinsicoid deflection of the LV unipolar electrode is late in the QRS complex, corresponding to late activation of the lateral LV. The greater amplitude of the LV unipolar EGM reflects the greater muscle mass of the LV. EGMs recorded from the superior vena cava (SVC) coil and from the atrial bipole (RA) are not shown. Radiograph and EGMs are from different patients. Radiograph is for illustrative purposes only.*

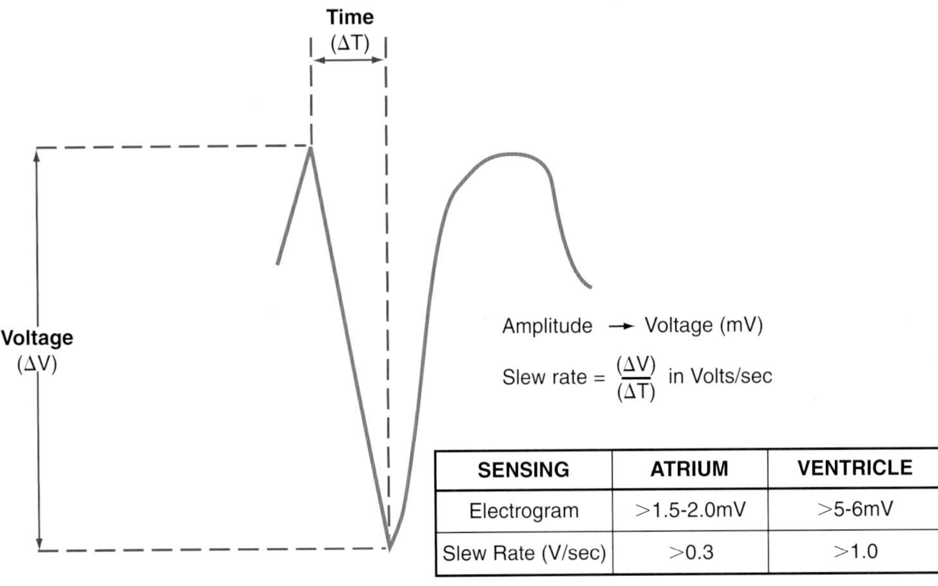

SENSING	ATRIUM	VENTRICLE
Electrogram	>1.5-2.0mV	>5-6mV
Slew Rate (V/sec)	>0.3	>1.0

Figure 3-5. The major clinical descriptors of an intracardiac EGM are illustrated. The peak-to-peak amplitude of the EGM is the difference in voltage recorded between two electrodes and is measured in millivolts (mV). The slew rate is equal to the first derivative of the EGM (dV/dt) and is a measure of the sharpness of the EGM and therefore its frequency content. Slew rate is measured in volts per second (V/sec). Usually, the amplitude of the EGM should be greater than 1.5 to 2.0 mV in the atrium and at least 5 to 6 mV in the ventricle at the time of lead implantation, to ensure adequate sensing. The slew rate should be at least 0.3 V/sec in the atrium and at least 1 V/sec in the ventricle.

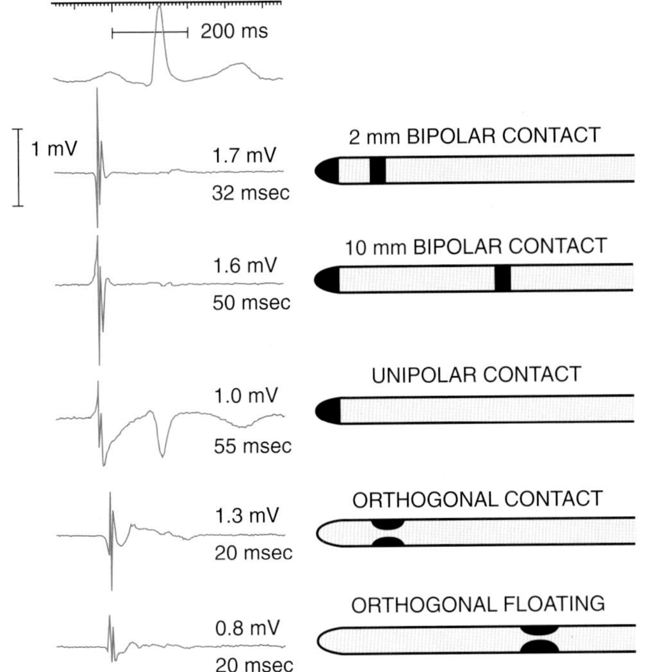

Figure 3-6. Effects of electrode configurations on the atrial endocardial EGM. The EGMs were obtained from a single patient with two catheters placed simultaneously in the right atrial appendage. One catheter had 2-mm ring electrodes (top three tracings), *and the other catheter had 1-mm orthogonal electrodes. The surface electrocardiogram tracing is shown at the top of the figure. Time and voltage amplitude scales are shown. For each electrode configuration* (right), *the corresponding EGM is shown* (left), *with the peak-to-peak amplitude and EGM duration labeled. "Contact" refers to electrodes in contact with the atrial tissue. "Floating" refers to noncontact electrodes in the atrial chamber. Note that greater ring electrode spacing, from 2 to 10 mm, prolongs EGM duration without altering the amplitude. The unipolar EGM shows a wider and diminished atrial EGM and a prominent far-field ventricular EGM as well. The orthogonal electrode configurations provide EGMs of lesser amplitude and shorter duration, compared with the ring electrodes.*

acceptable minimum slew rate (>1 V/sec for ventricular EGMs, >0.3 V/sec for atrial EGMs). EGMs with very low amplitude will not be sensed regardless of the slew rate.

The ventricular depolarization recorded on the atrial electrode is referred to as the *far-field R wave* (FFRW). Oversensing of the FFRW confounds interpretation of the atrial rhythm. The amplitude of the FFRW depends strongly on the location of the atrial electrode. It is greatest near the septum, intermediate in the right atrial appendage, and least on the right atrial free wall. Even if the FFRW has comparable amplitude to the P wave, its slew rate usually is much lower. In one series, the mean slew rate was 1.2 V/sec for atrial EGMs and 0.13 V/sec for FFRWs.[1]

If an active-fixation, screw-in tip electrode is successfully attached to the myocardium, the acute ventricular EGM has a *current of injury,* with an elevated ST segment (Fig. 3-9) that is usually markedly reduced within 10 minutes after fixation. During the 10-minute period after electrode fixation, the EGM amplitude and slew rate usually do not change despite changes in waveshape, but the pacing threshold decreases by an average of 40% for EGMs.[2]

Acute to Chronic Electrogram Changes, Fixation Mechanism, and Steroid Elution

The amplitude and slew rate of intracardiac EGMs typically decline during the first several days to weeks after lead implantation and then increase to chronic values that are slightly lower than those measured at implantation.[5] The initial decrease in EGM amplitude is caused by the inflammatory response and edema at the electrode-tissue interface. This gradually resolves and is followed by the development of a small, inexcitable fibrotic zone surrounding the electrode tip (Fig. 3-10). This inflammation and fibrotic tissue effectively increases the distance between the surface of the electrode and the excitable myocardium that generates the EGM signal. Although

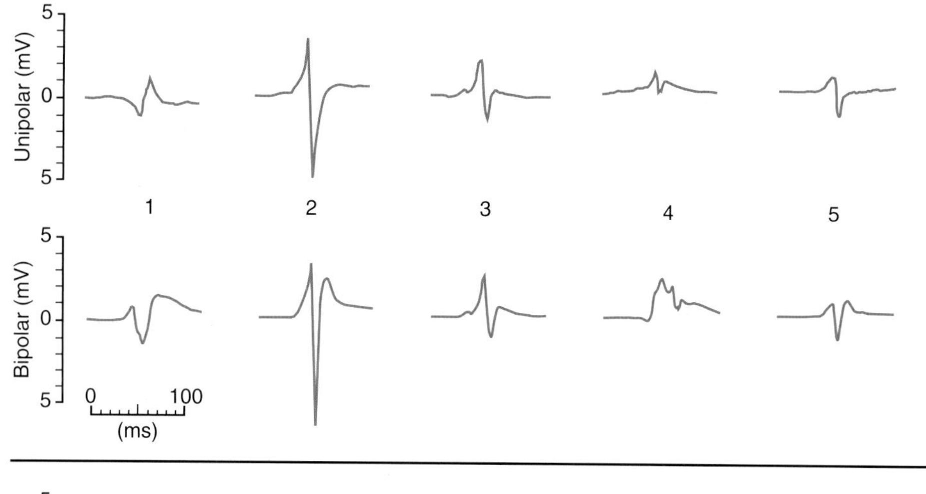

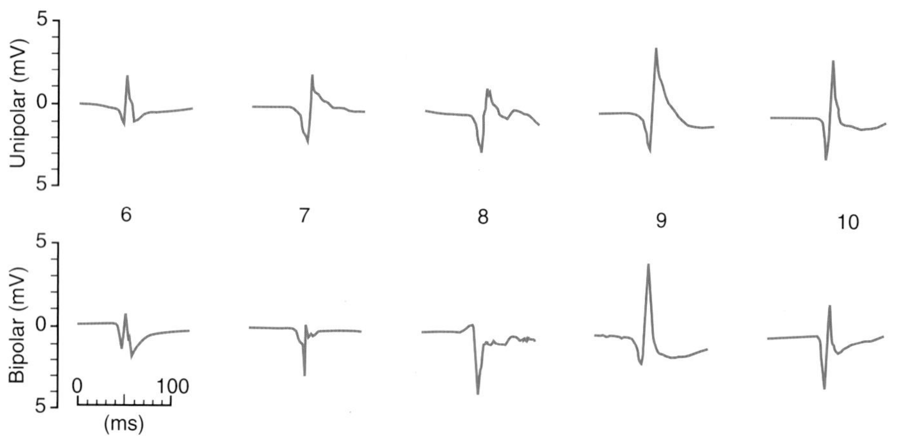

Figure 3-7. Similarities of unipolar and bipolar EGMs are shown by these examples recorded from a lead placed in the right atrial appendage in 10 patients. Note that the amplitudes of unipolar and bipolar EGMs are similar for each patient. The waveshapes of unipolar and bipolar EGMs for a given patient may be quite similar (patient 3) or quite different (patient 8), although these differences can be attributed to the relative size of the major inflections. Some of these differences may depend on whether the ring electrode for the bipolar recording makes contact with the myocardium. On the whole, intrapatient differences between unipolar and bipolar recordings appear to be less than interpatient differences.

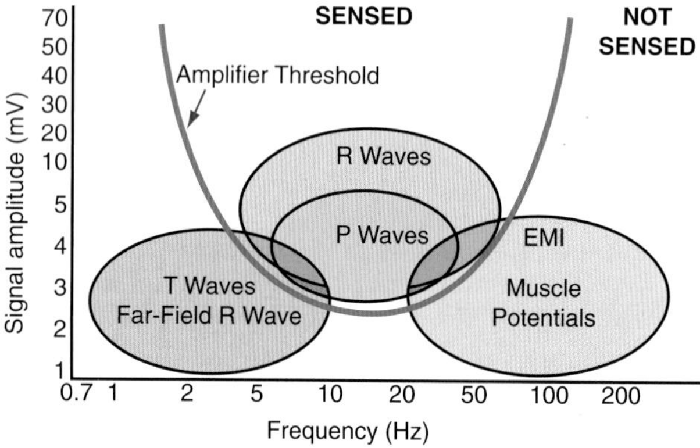

Figure 3-8. This plot of signal amplitude versus frequency shows the approximate characteristics of the P and R waves that pacemakers and ICDs are intended to sense and the approximate characteristics of the electromagnetic interference (EMI, muscle potentials), T waves, and far-field R waves that they are intended not to sense. The sense amplifier's filters are designed to sense signals that are above the U-shaped amplifier threshold curve and to reject signals that are below the curve. P waves and R waves have similar frequency characteristics, but usually R waves have higher dominant frequency than P waves. Muscle potentials usually have higher-frequency components than intracardiac signals. T waves and far-field R waves have lower frequencies. As shown, there are some overlaps in these amplitude-frequency characteristics that cause oversensing or undersensing in particular situations. The ellipses representing the amplitude-frequency characteristics in this figure are conceptual and are not based on quantitative measurements.

chronic EGM amplitudes usually are reduced by less than 10% compared with acute amplitudes, chronic slew rates are reduced by 30% to 40%.[6]

The acute reduction in EGM amplitude is often greater with active-fixation leads than with passive-fixation leads. Atrial undersensing can occur during the acute phase despite adequate EGM amplitudes at implantation. To account for these time-related changes in EGM amplitude, the filtered EGM recorded at lead implantation should be at least twice the sensitivity threshold that will be programmed in the pulse generator. Greater sensing safety margins are preferred for active-fixation leads.

The method of lead tip stabilization, active screw-in or passive tines, has had no significant effect on sensing characteristics in most studies.[7,8] Steroid-eluting electrodes reduce chronic pacing thresholds substantially but have no clinically significant effects on the sensing characteristics of endocardial leads.[9-12]

Metabolic, Ischemic, Aging, and Drug Effects on Electrograms

The effects of metabolic abnormalities and drugs on pacing thresholds are well described. Much less information is available concerning their effects on EGMs and sensing functions of implantable pacemakers and ICDs. Factors that reduce EGM amplitude, slow con-

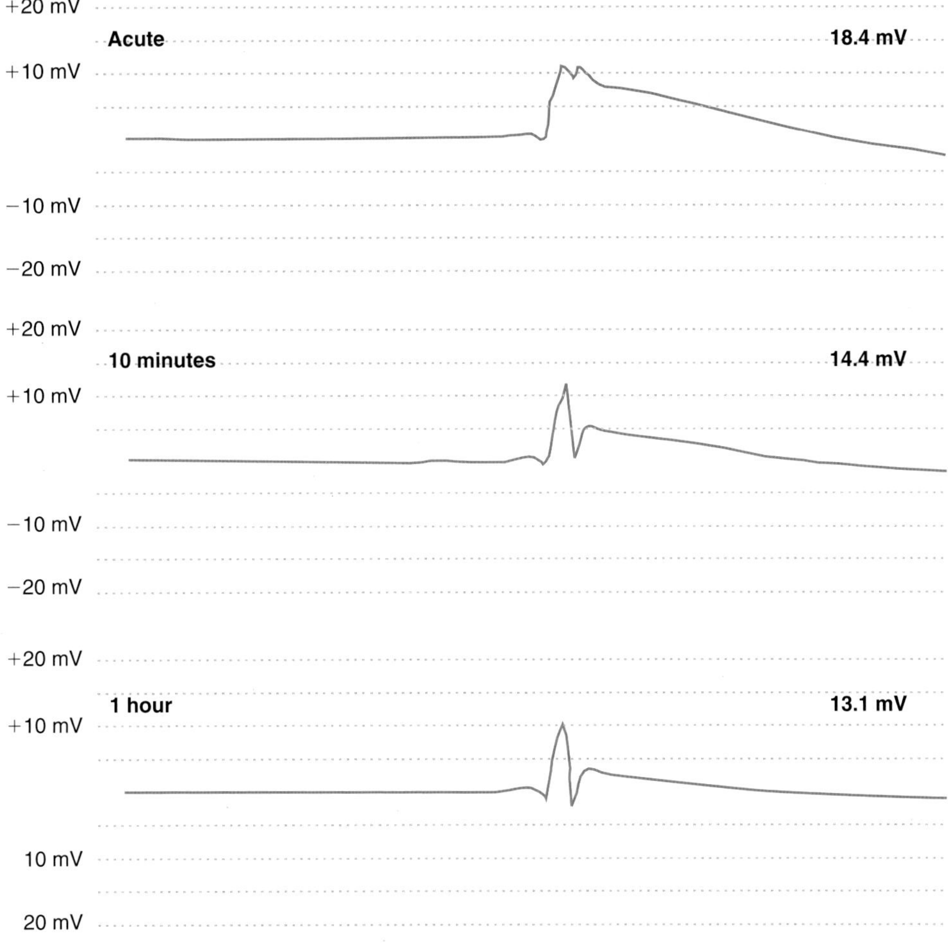

Figure 3-9. Acute current of injury at implantation. Top panel, *High-resolution recording shows marked ST-segment elevation, indicating the current of injury when an active fixation screw-in tip electrode is extended into the endocardium.* Middle panel, *After only 10 minutes, most of the ST-segment elevation in the signal has disappeared.* Bottom panel, *The EGM is not appreciably different at 1 hour after implantation.*

duction velocity, or diminish slew rate may produce either oversensing or undersensing. By prolonging the intracardiac EGM duration beyond blanking periods, ischemia or antiarrhythmic drugs can produce double-counting of the QRS complex.[13] Similarly, drugs that prolong the PR or QT interval beyond the refractory period may result in oversensing.[14,15]

Undersensing may result from reduction in EGM amplitude or slew rate after myocardial infarction at the electrode-tissue interface, from drug and electrolyte effects,[14,15] or from progression of conduction system disease. Acute ischemia causes ST-segment changes that can be detected on ventricular EGMs. Monitoring of EGM ST-segment shifts has been proposed as a method for monitoring ischemia for pacemakers and ICDs.[16] The likelihood of recording abnormal atrial EGMs (defined as ≥100 msec in duration or having ≥8 fragmented deflections) correlates with age of the patient ($r = 0.34$; $P < .0005$).[17]

Exercise, Respiratory, and Postural Effects on Electrograms

The effect of exercise on the atrial EGM amplitude and slew rate is variable. Some studies have reported statistically significant decreases in amplitude that average 10% to 20% but may reach 40% in some patients.[18,19] Other studies did not find significant changes between rest and exercise.[20,21] Decreases in atrial EGM amplitude were not caused by atrial rate alone or by β-blockade.[22] VDD/R lead studies with "floating" atrial electrodes showed particularly large decreases with exercise.[23,24] These large decreases in atrial EGM amplitude for some patients support the value of programming a large safety margin for sensing at implantation when combined with the effects of lead maturation.

P-wave amplitude increases significantly during full inspiration, during full expiration, and with erect posture.[21] Substantial respiratory variations in the amplitude of the ventricular intrinsic deflection and slew rate are illustrated in Figure 3-11. Respiratory variation averaged 9.7% for unipolar atrial EGMs and 11.5% for bipolar atrial EGMs.[24,25] The effect of respiration on ventricular EGMs was less, especially with the unipolar configuration.[25]

Ventricular Electrograms during Premature Ventricular Complexes, Ventricular Tachycardia, and Ventricular Fibrillation

Premature ventricular complexes (PVCs) may have lower-amplitude R waves than sinus-rhythm R waves, as shown in Figure 3-12, but the reverse may also be

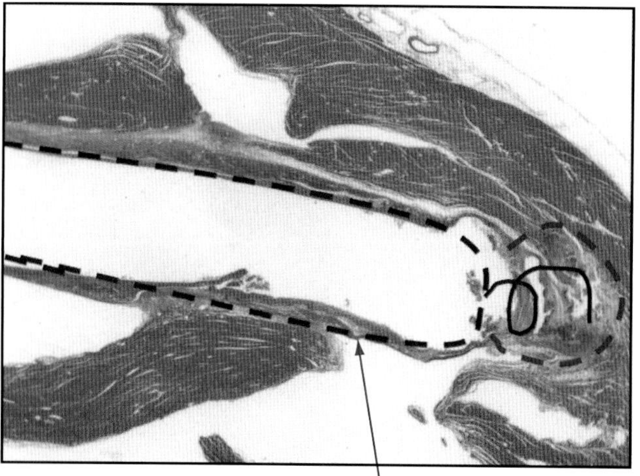

Figure 3-10. The myocardium remaining after removal of an endocardial active-fixation screw lead is shown on this gross microscopic slide. The large dotted line shows where the lead body was located, and the colored staining shows a thin fibrotic sheath around the lead body. The approximate location of the helical screw-tip electrode is shown by the solid coiled line. The oval shape (dotted line) *shows the size of the fibrotic capsule that formed around the helical extended-tip electrode. Most of the tissue outside the dotted lines stained red, indicating that it was active myocardium capable of conducting depolarizations. The tip region of this electrode is similar to that of the tip electrode in Figure 3-1, so propagation of depolarization wavefronts must travel around the tip electrode, in tissue largely out of the field of view on the right side of this figure.*

true. For monomorphic ventricular tachycardia (VT), mean amplitude decreased only slightly from values in sinus rhythm—14% for epicardial EGMs and 5% endocardial EGMs.[26] In contrast, EGM amplitudes during ventricular fibrillation (VF) decreased by 25% for epicardial and 41% for endocardial EGMs. More importantly, EGMs in VF often have low, highly variable, and rapidly changing amplitudes and slew rates. Figure 3-13 shows endocardial spontaneous VF EGMs from different patients, illustrating variability in intrinsic deflections, amplitudes, slew rates, and morphologies. In a study of induced VF reproducibility, 50% of the variability was due to interpatient differences and the other 50% was due to repeated episodes in the same patient.[27] In another study, the ventricular EGM amplitude in VF was 1 mV or less in at least one VF episode in 29% of patients.[26] When analyzing the sensed EGMs during induced VF at ICD implantation, care should be paid to variability in the beat-to-beat amplitude. If this variability in EGM amplitude is large, undersensing of VF may occur. Undersensing in VF may necessitate lead repositioning or insertion of another sensing lead despite an adequate EGM in sinus rhythm. See "Undersensing." If VF persists for several minutes, the amplitude and slew rate of the EGMs deteriorate as shown in Figure 3-14.

Atrial Electrograms during Rhythms Other Than Sinus

Compared with sinus rhythm, atrial activation from ectopic sites or atrial arrhythmias can alter the ampli-

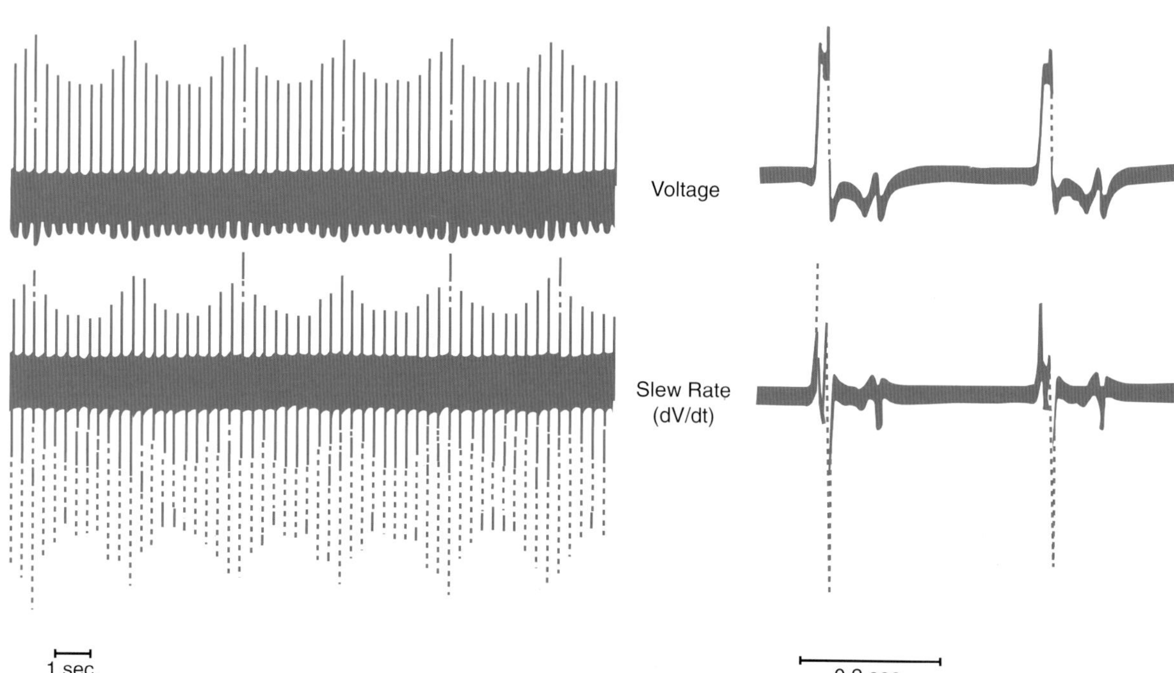

Figure 3-11. Respiratory variations of intracardiac EGM amplitude and slew rate (dV/dt) are typically about 10% for the atrium and ventricle. These variations result from beat-to-beat changes in stroke volume caused by respiration or movement at the electrode-tissue interface. (From Furman S, Hurzeler P, De Caprio V: Cardiac pacing and pacemaker. III. Sensing the cardiac electrogram. Am Heart J 93:794-801, 1977, with permission.)

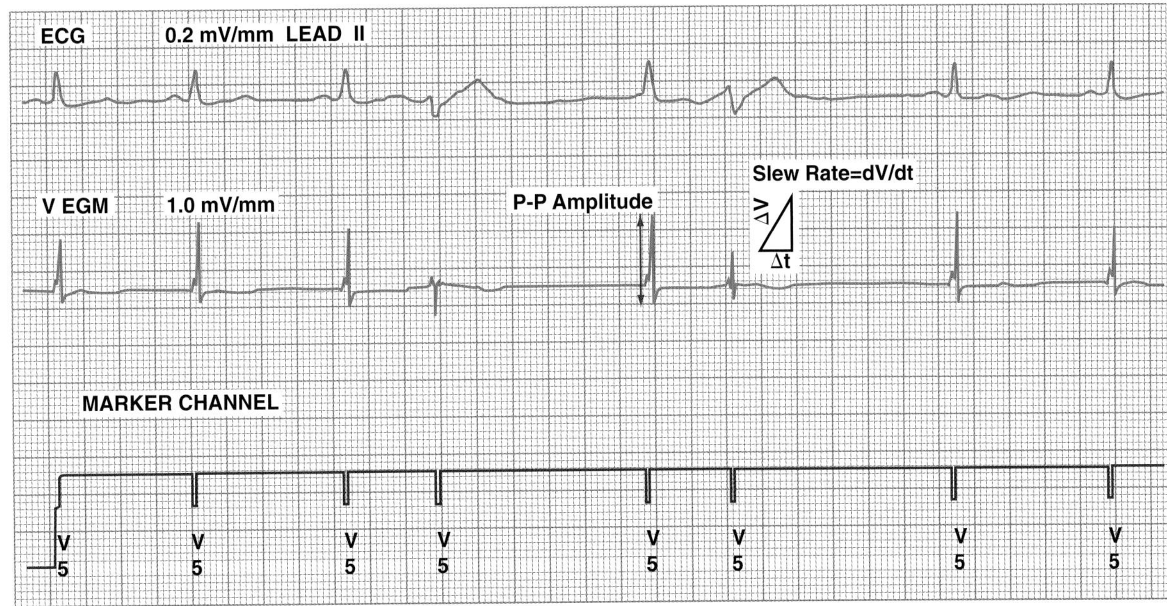

Figure 3-12. A surface electrocardiogram (ECG) lead II, a bipolar right ventricular (V) EGM, and event markers with downward pulses that show when sensing occurred. The QRS amplitude on the ECG is about 1 mV, which is typical. The peak-to-peak amplitude of the sinus R waves is about 10 to 12 mV, which is also typical. The slew rate is the maximum slope (dV/dt) of the EGM intrinsic deflection; it is difficult to measure with a paper speed this slow. The two premature ventricular complexes (PVCs) (fourth and sixth) have different amplitudes and shapes on both the ECG and the EGM. The sinus beat in the center, between the two PVCs, has its main intrinsic deflection during the last part of the ECG QRS complex. The left edge of the sense marker indicates the instant that sensing by the device occurred. Therefore, the EGM morphology and timing of the sense marker may not correspond to the start of the QRS on the ECG as electrocardiographers expect. Each R wave was sensed only once because sensing is blanked by the device for 120 msec after each ventricular sense (VS).

tude, frequency content, slew rate, and morphology of the atrial EGM. Retrograde atrial activation during ventricular pacing reduces atrial EGM amplitude and slew rate by up to 50%.[28] These EGM changes are more pronounced in the high right atrium than in the right atrial appendage or low right atrium.[29] The frequency content of the atrial EGM is not significantly altered by retrograde atrial activation.[30] Analysis of EGM turning-point morphology or the first-differential coefficient of slew rate has been used to discriminate sinus EGMs from those recorded during retrograde and ectopic atrial activation in small groups of patients.[31] Less sophisticated visual morphologic analysis did not effectively discriminate sinus from ectopic atrial electrical activity.[28]

Atrial EGMs during atrial fibrillation (AF) are characterized by extreme temporal and spatial variability. EGMs tend to be most organized in the trabeculated right atrial appendage and more disorganized in the smooth right atrium or coronary sinus.[32-34] The amplitude, width, and morphology of atrial EGMs during AF vary markedly at various anatomic locations. The amplitude of chronic, unipolar pacemaker EGMs in AF was decreased by 40%, compared with sinus rhythm.[35] The spectral components of EGMs from two separate atrial (or ventricular) sites show greatly reduced spectral coherence during fibrillation, as opposed to an atrial rhythm other than AF.[36]

A comparison of atrial EGM amplitudes in sinus rhythm, AF, and atrial flutter with temporary pacing catheters in the high right atrium or right atrial appendage showed that the mean sinus-rhythm EGM amplitude decreased only slightly in atrial flutter but decreased by about 50% in AF.[34] The mean EGM amplitudes in both AF and atrial flutter were highly correlated to the amplitudes in sinus rhythm. The coefficient of variance of EGM amplitude was similar for sinus rhythm (19%) and atrial flutter (22%) but markedly increased for AF (42%, $P < .0001$ versus sinus). The likelihood of any patient demonstrating very-low-amplitude atrial EGMs (<0.3 mV) during AF or atrial flutter correlated with the mean sinus EGM amplitude.

Electrode spacing and the positioning of atrial leads have dramatic effects on the characteristics of the recorded AF EGMs[36-38] and can result in inconsistent diagnosis of AF based on rate criteria. By reducing atrial rate, median frequency, and EGM amplitude, antiarrhythmic drugs may also interfere with the detection of AF.[39]

Sensing

The methods and technology of sensing and detection in ICDs and pacemakers share many features. One

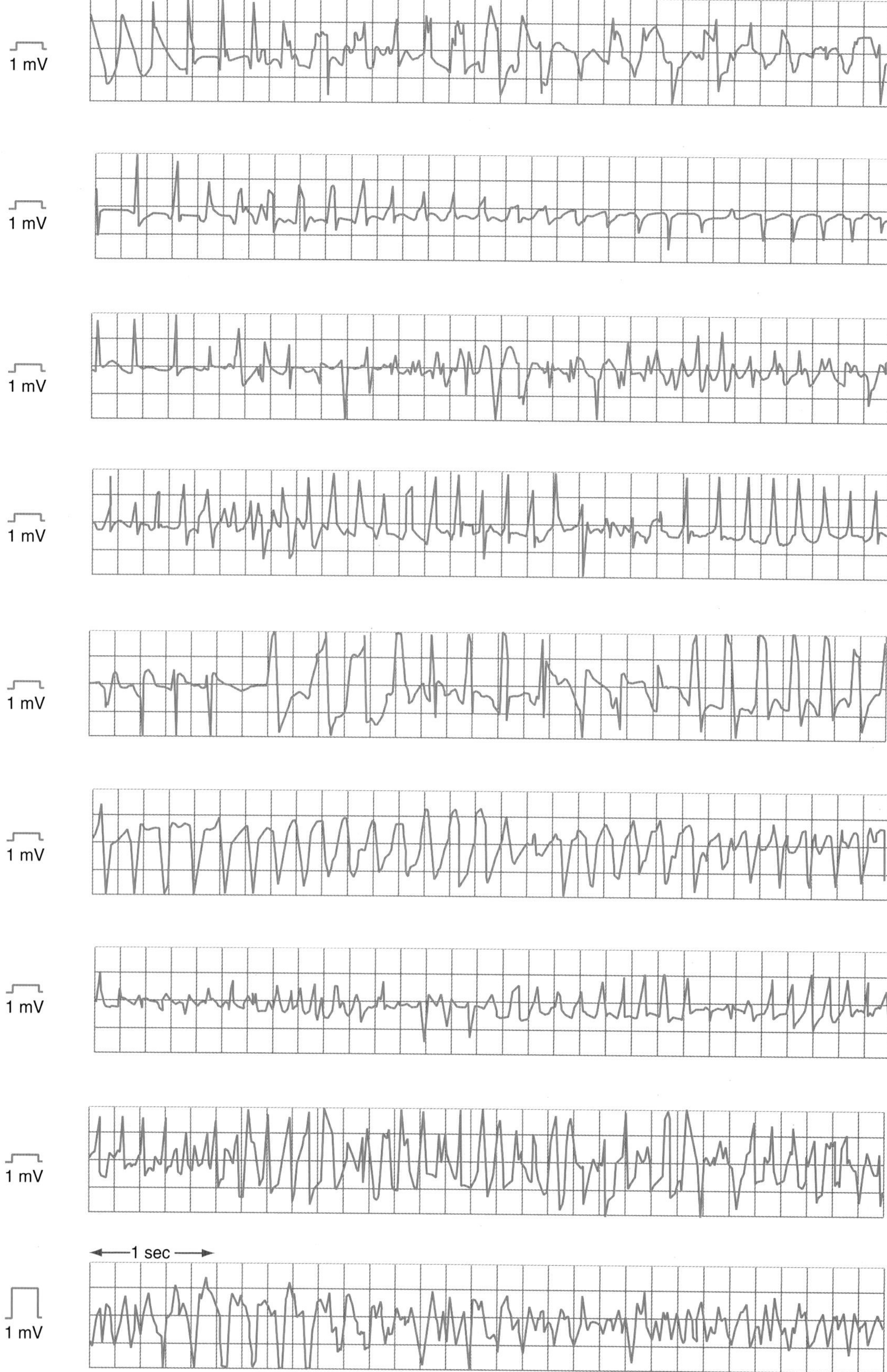

Figure 3-13. *Spontaneous bipolar EGMs recorded during ventricular fibrillation (VF) detection and charging by Medtronic Gem ICDs are shown for nine patients. Note that the 1-mV calibration markers are the same except for the bottom tracing, where the calibration pulse is about three times larger, meaning that the ventricular EGM for this patient was three times smaller than for the other eight patients. Also note that rapid intrinsic deflections are visible on all tracings, although some substantial beat-to-beat variations in amplitude occurred. The abbreviated sense markers are shown at the bottom edge of each stored EGM strip. The sense amplifier blanking period was 120 msec, and the programmed sensitivity in each case was 0.3 mV, except in the sixth tracing from the top, which had 0.6 mV sensitivity. Note that there was slight VF undersensing on the bottom tracing when large EGMs were followed by smaller EGMs.*

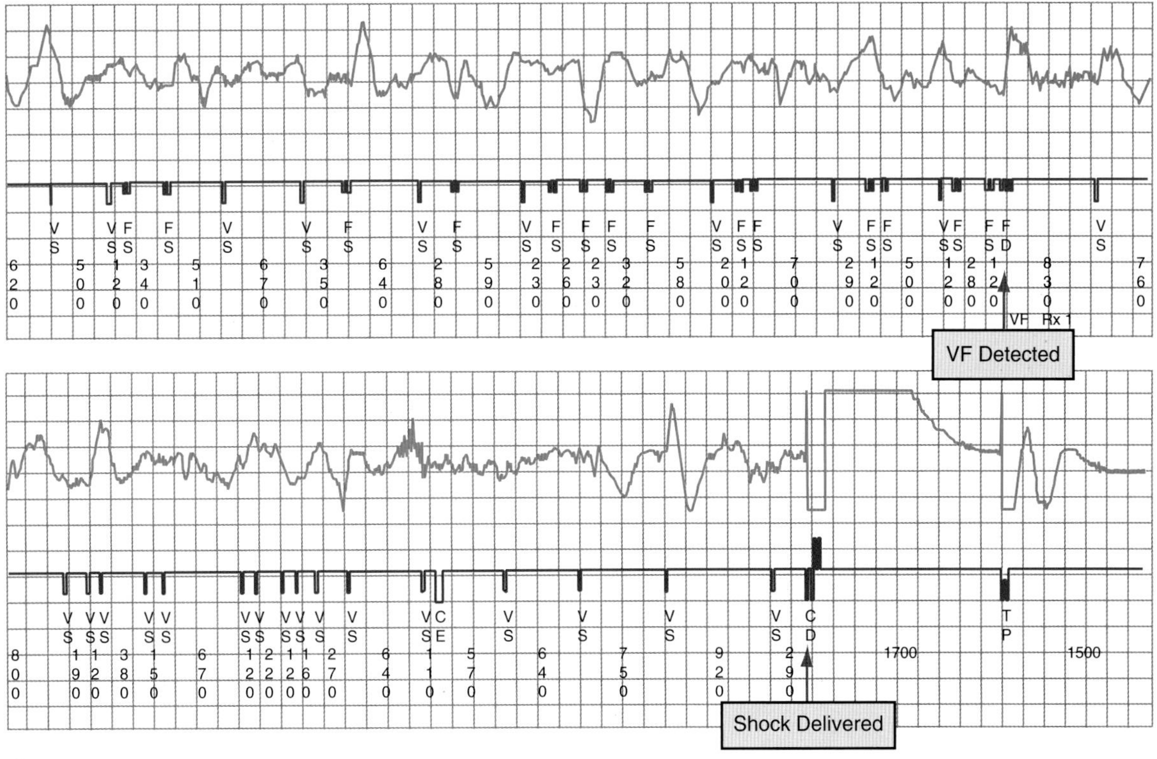

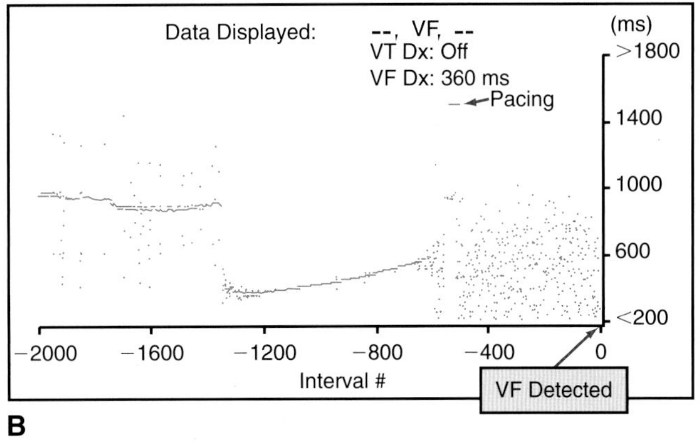

Figure 3-14. Effect of ischemia on EGMs. ***A,*** *A right ventricular (RV) coil-to-can EGM that was stored approximately 9 minutes after the onset of a rapid tachyarrhythmia, probably ventricular tachycardia (VT) that degenerated to ventricular fibrillation (VF). The amplitude calibration was 0.1 mV/mm, and the sensitivity was programmed to the nominal value of 0.3 mV. The EGM has low slew-rate irregular deflections that do not align well with the sense markers. This is consistent with poor EGM sensing due to ischemia, but in this case the bipolar tip-to-ring EGM was not stored. The defibrillation shock appears to have been effective.* ***B,*** *Flashback diagram of 2000 R-R intervals before the detection of ventricular fibrillation (VF) shown in* ***A.*** *The programmed interval for detection was 360 msec. The onset of the tachyarrhythmia was not detected as far back as about 1350 R-R intervals before VF detection. Note that, until about 600 R-R intervals before detection, the sensing was good although the R-R intervals were lengthening, which, based on animal data, is again at least consistent with ischemia. Note that there was some low-rate (1500 msec) pacing followed by erratic ventricular sensing and oversensing at 120 msec for the last 600 R-R intervals. In retrospect, it is unfortunate that empirical fast VT detection and therapy were programmed off. See Figure 3-82 for a similar, shorter Flashback example with about 500 R-R intervals before a VF detection.*

major difference is that ICDs need reliable sensing and detection during VF, but pacemakers do not. A second difference relates to sensing dipoles: Pacemakers may use unipolar or bipolar sensing, whereas ICDs always use bipolar sensing. Some RV ICD leads are designed for integrated bipolar sensing in which one sensing electrode is the RV high-voltage coil.

General Concepts: Electrodes, Filter, Rectification, Threshold, Blanking

The primary functional operations within the sensing system of a pacemaker or ICD are shown in Figure 3-15. The raw signal passes from the leads to the connector, through hermetic feedthroughs with high-frequency filters, and encounters high-voltage protection circuitry before reaching the sensing amplifier. After amplification, the EGM signal is processed by a band-pass filter to reduce T waves, myopotentials, and EMI. Then it is rectified to nullify effects of signal polarity. Finally, it is compared with the sensing threshold voltage. At the instant the processed signal exceeds the sensing threshold voltage, a sensed event is declared to the timing circuits and is indicated by a marker pulse on the programmer ECG. The sense amplifier in the same chamber is turned off or "blanked" for a short *blanking period* (20 to 250 msec) after each spontaneous depolarization or paced event, to prevent multiple sensed events from being recorded during a single depolarization. In contrast, during the *refractory period* that follows the blanking period, the sense amplifier remains enabled because amplifier saturation is not expected to occur. However, the pulse generator will not alter pacemaker function in response to signals that exceed the programmed sensitivity threshold during the refractory period. Events during the refractory period may be sensed for tachyarrhythmia detection algorithms but generally do not alter pacemaker timing cycles.

Blanking and Refractory Periods

Blanking periods and refractory periods are used to prevent undesirable behavior caused by oversensing or double-counting of cardiac activity (Figs. 3-16 and 3-17). The specifications of blanking/refractory periods have substantial impact on device sensing and pacing functions (Fig. 3-18). *Same-chamber blanking/refractory periods* after sensed events reduce double-counting of intrinsic cardiac depolarizations that may result in escape pacing at a rate slower than the programmed lower rate in pacemakers or inappropriate detection of VT/VF in ICDs. After paced events, the same-chamber blanking/refractory periods are typically longer and prevent oversensing of the pacing artifact and the evoked response. The blanking/refractory periods in the ventricle after atrial sensed or paced events and in the atrium after ventricular sensed or paced events are called *cross-chamber blanking/refractory periods*. Cross-chamber blanking periods help to prevent oversensing of the pacing artifact after a paced event in the opposite chamber. The atrial blanking period after ventricular events (postventricular atrial blanking, or PVAB) is designed to avoid oversensing of ventricular pacing stimuli and FFRWs. Longer postventricular atrial refractory periods (PVARP) prevent oversensing of retro-

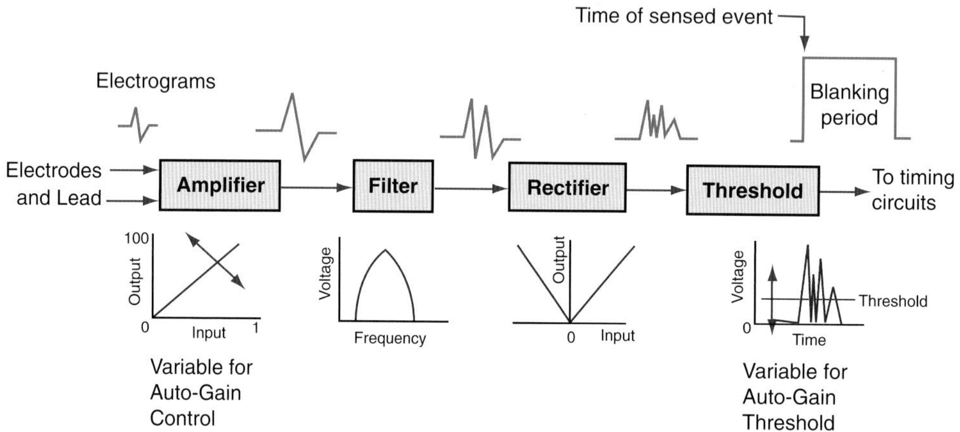

Figure 3-15. A functional block diagram for a pacemaker or ICD sense amplifier. The EGM signal from the two implanted electrodes is first amplified for subsequent processing. Bandpass filtering reduces the amplitude of lower-frequency signals such as T waves and far-field R waves and higher-frequency signals such as myopotentials and electromagnetic interference. After bandpass filtering, the signal is rectified to make polarity unimportant. The thresholding operation compares the amplified, filtered, and rectified signals with the sensing threshold voltage. At the instant the processed signal exceeds the sensing threshold voltage, the sense amplifier is blanked (turned off) for a short period (20 to 120 msec), so that each depolarization is sensed only once, and a sensed event is declared to pacemaker or ICD timing circuits. For pacemakers, the programmed sensitivity controls the constant sensing threshold voltage. For ICDs, the amplifier gain may be controlled by the input EGM amplitude. The programmable sensing threshold for ICDs controls the high and low limits on the sensing threshold, which automatically adjusts on a beat-by-beat basis (see text discussion). In actual circuits, some functions such as amplification and filtering may be integrated.

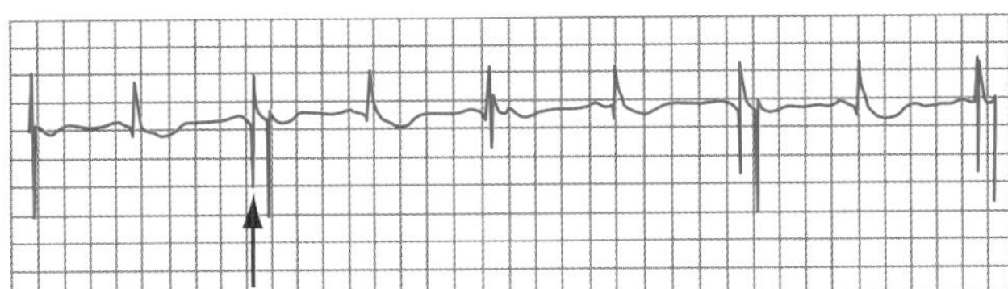

Figure 3-16. Loss of atrial sensing with apparent ventricular undersensing and ventricular pacing. In the second complex, an atrial pacing stimulus follows the P wave because of undersensing in the atrium. The atrial pacing stimulus occurs at the start of the ventricular QRS complex. The ventricular EGM is not sensed because of blanking in the ventricular sensing amplifier immediately after the atrial pacing stimulus. This sequence is repeated in the fourth, sixth, and eighth complexes. Atrial undersensing may lead to apparent ventricular undersensing because the ventricular blanking period does not permit sensing of electrical signals for a period of 10 to 40 msec after an atrial output pulse.

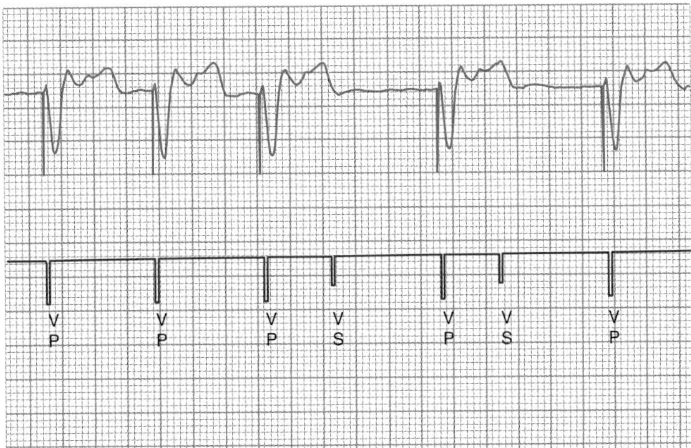

Figure 3-17. Oversensing of T waves causing interruptions in VVI pacemaker timing. The surface electrocardiogram (top tracing) *and pacemaker marker channel* (bottom tracing) *show ventricular oversensing of T waves. The first three complexes show ventricular pacing (VP) with capture. The pauses after the third and fourth complexes result from T-wave oversensing (VS), demonstrated by the marker channel.*

gradely conducted atrial activation that may occur after ventricular activation or ventricular premature depolarizations. Cross-chamber blanking in the atrium after a ventricular event must be minimized in devices with tachyarrhythmia detection (ICDs or atrial therapy devices) to avoid undersensing the atrial rhythm, particularly during high ventricular rates. Long atrial cross-blanking periods would preclude reliable sensing of most atrial rhythms, especially atrial tachycardias (AT). However, short atrial cross-blanking periods may result in atrial sensing of far-field ventricular depolarizations (FFRWs).

Devices that incorporate tachyarrhythmia detection, such as ICDs and atrial therapy devices, typically have shorter blanking and refractory periods than standard pacemakers, so that short cardiac cycles can be sensed reliably (compare top and bottom panels of Figure 3-18). As shown in the bottom panel of Figure 3-18, blanking periods may be adaptively extended based on noise-sampling windows (30-60 msec) if suprathreshold activity (due to cardiac or extracardiac sources such as EMI) is seen on the EGM immediately after a sensed event. If noise is seen in consecutive windows after a sensed event, the blanking period is "retriggered" for that beat to avoid double-counting or continuous oversensing. This operation may also result in paradoxical undersensing when more sensitive sensing levels are programmed.[40,41]

The duration of the total atrial refractory period (TARP, equal to the atrioventricular [AV] delay plus the PVARP) in DDD pacing modes limits atrial tracking of the atrium at high sinus rates without affecting atrial sensing, as shown in Figure 3-19. Because the AV delay of most dual-chamber pacemakers shortens in response to increasing atrial rates or sensor input, the TARP also shortens. Several manufacturers now offer dual-chamber pacemakers that also shorten the PVARP with increasing atrial or sensor-indicated rates, further reducing the TARP during exercise. The result of these newer algorithms is that the programmed upper tracking rate can be safely increased while providing protection at lower heart rates from initiation of pacemaker-mediated tachycardia caused by retrograde conduction.

Sensing Thresholds in Pacemakers

Sensing thresholds in most pacemakers are programmable to a constant value. Ventricular sensing channels in pacemakers typically operate at sensing thresholds of 2.5 to 3.5 mV, about 10 times smaller than those in ICDs. Therefore, pacemakers may undersense VF. Atrial sensitivity thresholds are typically 0.3 to 0.6 mV, to allow sensing of small-amplitude atrial EGMs during AF and to improve the accuracy of atrial tachyarrhythmia diagnostics.

Unipolar sensing thresholds are typically set higher (less sensitive) than bipolar sensing thresholds to reduce oversensing of far-field cardiac and extracardiac signals that can lead to inappropriate pacemaker inhibition or tracking. Newer pacemakers automatically adjust the sensitivity setting to adapt to changes in EGM amplitude over time. Typically, these functions operate to modify sensing thresholds based on a series of 10 to 20 ventricular beats. One such algorithm employs two simultaneous sensing levels: the programmed sensitivity (inner target) and a value twice the programmed value (outer target) (Fig. 3-20).[42] Sensed EGMs exceeding both target values decrease the sensitivity. Signals exceeding only the inner target increase the sensitivity. In this manner, a 2:1 sensing margin is maintained. Although this is clinically equivalent to manual sensitivity adjustment, faster sensitivity adjustments may be desired when EGM amplitudes can be expected to change over a brief period (e.g., beat-to-beat variations due to respiration, body position changes, or fluctuating EGM morphologies during AF).[43]

FFRW oversensing can be minimized by selecting an atrial lead with a closely spaced bipolar electrode pair (≤10 mm), choosing an implantation location that yields a FFRW-to-P wave ratio of less than 0.5,[44] or by titrating programmed sensitivity to reject FFRWs without undersensing P waves and low-amplitude AF.

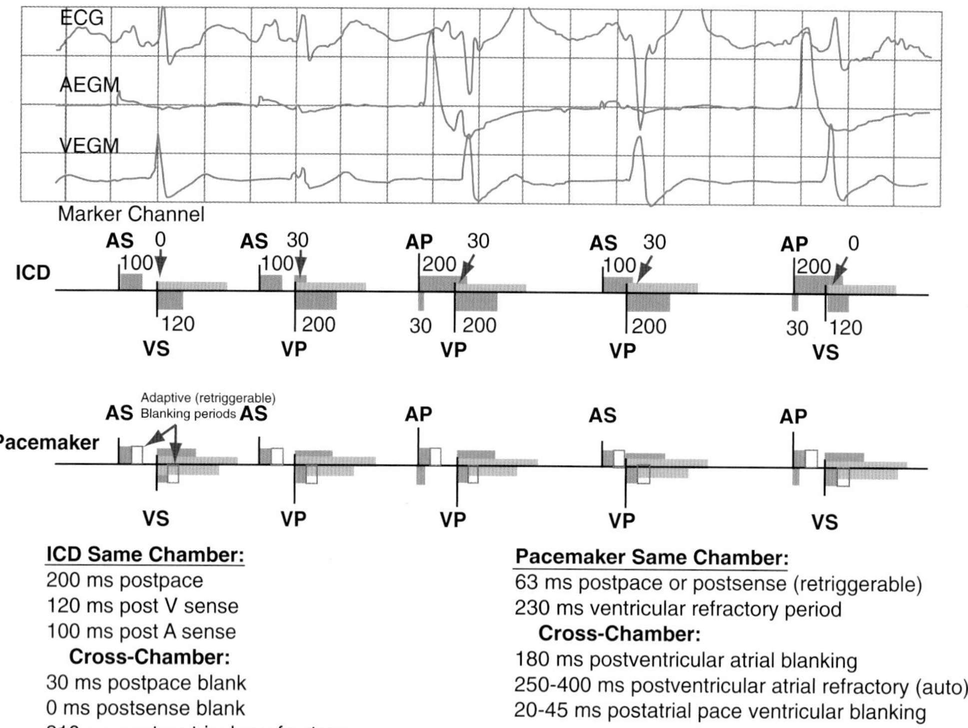

Figure 3-18. *The basic blanking and refractory periods for DDDR mode are shown for the Marquis DR ICD and EnPulse DR pacemakers (Medtronic, Inc., Minneapolis, Minn.). The top tracings show the surface electrocardiogram (ECG), atrial electrogram (AEGM), and ventricular electrogram (VEGM) signals. The bottom two marker diagrams illustrate atrial or ventricular pacing (AP, VP), atrial or ventricular sensing (AS, VS), blanking periods* (purple), *and refractory periods* (blue). *Blanking periods in ICDs are usually of fixed duration, whereas same-chamber blanking in pacemakers is generally adaptive, with short (30-50 msec) blanking periods that "retrigger" when suprathreshold signals are present during the blanking period. Adaptive blanking periods can extend indefinitely, resulting in activation of noise-reversion asynchronous pacing. Note the considerably shorter blanking periods on the atrial channel in the ICD; this allows more accurate sensing of atrial depolarizations during high ventricular rates, which is critical for tachyarrhythmia detection and discrimination algorithms. Also note the lack of ventricular refractory periods in ICDs; this allows inhibition of pacing when high rates are sensed. Ventricular blanking periods in pacemakers may be shorter than in ICDs, due to the approximately 10-fold less sensitive sensing threshold in pacemakers compared with ICDs.*

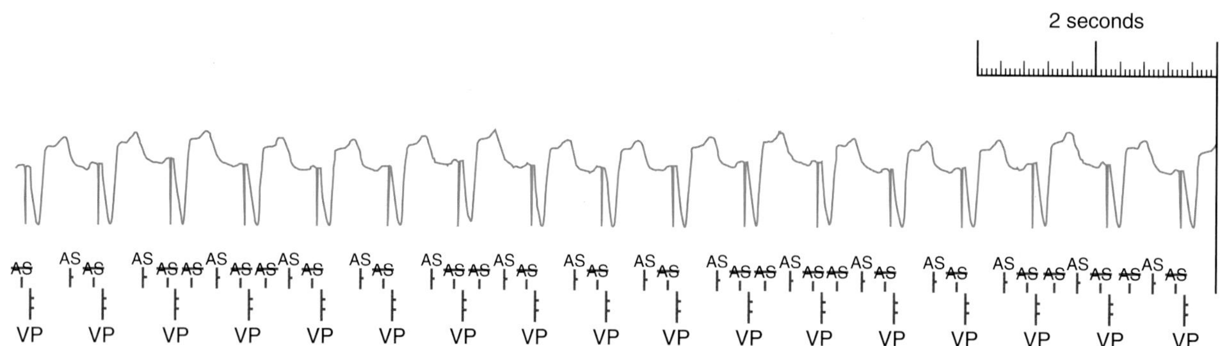

Figure 3-19. *Intracardiac marker channels in a patient with a DDD pacemaker identify atrial events within postventricular atrial refractory periods (PVARPs) that are sensed but not tracked. The surface electrocardiogram* (top tracing) *demonstrates ventricular pacing at the upper rate limit during atrial flutter. The atrial marker channel demonstrates atrial events that were sensed within PVARP (-AS-) and atrial events sensed outside PVARP (AS). After a ventricular pacing stimulus (VP), some atrial EGMs are not sensed, resulting in apparent EGM dropout because the atrium is blanked for a period after delivery of a VP. Only atrial signals recorded outside PVARP (AS) are tracked.*

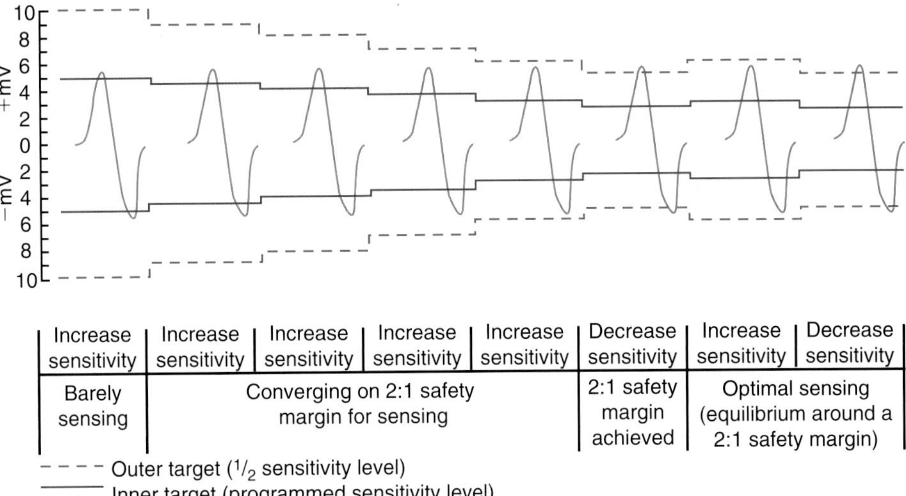

Figure 3-20. Autosensing algorithm to maintain a 2:1 sensing safety margin. See text for details. (From Castro A, Liebold A, Vincente J, et al: Evaluation of autosensing as an automatic means of maintaining a 2:1 sensing safety margin in an implanted pacemaker. Autosensing Investigation Team. PACE 19[11 Pt 2]: 1708-1713, 1996, with permission.)

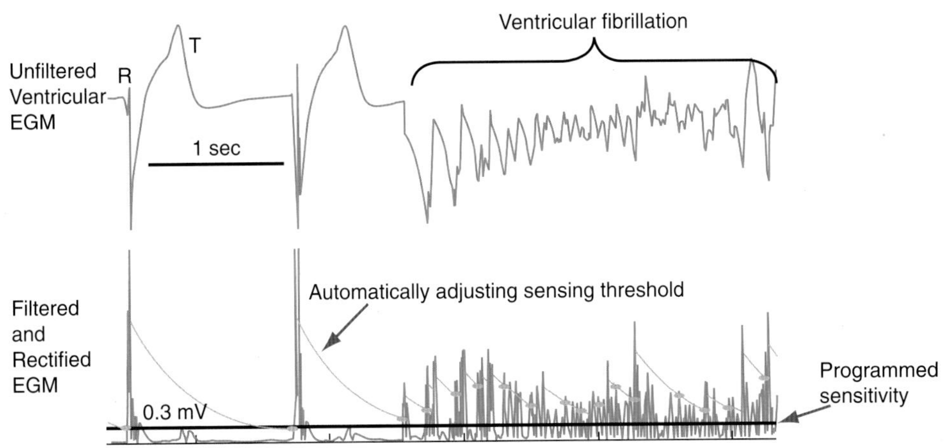

Figure 3-21. Automatic adjustment of sensitivity. ICDs adjust sensitivity in relation to the amplitude of each sensed R wave. The goal of this feature is to permit sensing of low-amplitude and varying-amplitude EGMs while minimizing T-wave oversensing. The figure shows two sinus beats followed by the onset of ventricular fibrillation (VF). The upper panel shows the unfiltered ventricular EGM. The lower panel shows the corresponding filtered and rectified EGM. After each sensed ventricular event, the sensing threshold is set to a predetermined fraction of the R-wave amplitude. For large R waves, the initial sensing threshold may have a maximum value. The threshold then decreases with time until it reaches a minimum value equal to the programmed sensitivity, which is nominally about 0.3 mV. For sinus beats, the threshold is larger than the T waves, preventing oversensing. When VF begins, the smaller R waves keep the threshold at a lower value, which allows sensing of R waves that are even smaller than the T waves in sinus rhythm.

Ventricular Sensing in Ventricular ICDs

The guiding design principle is that sensing of VF and polymorphic VT should be sufficiently reliable that clinically significant delays in detection do not occur. Although high sensitivity is required to ensure reliable sensing in VF, continuous high sensitivity may result in oversensing of cardiac or extracardiac signals during regular rhythm. Inappropriate detection of VT or VF may result from oversensing. Therefore, the tradeoff is to minimize both undersensing during VF and oversensing during regular rhythms. To achieve this goal, ICDs use feedback mechanisms based on R-wave amplitude to adjust the sensing threshold dynamically. To maximize the likelihood of detecting VF, blanking periods are kept short.

Automatic Adjustment of Sensitivity

Adjustment of Sensitivity in Normal Rhythm. ICDs automatically adjust sensitivity in relation to the amplitude of each sensed R wave (Fig. 3-21). At the end of the blanking period after each sensed ventricular event, the sensing threshold is set to a high value. It then decreases with time until a minimum value is reached. In comparison with a fixed sensing threshold, automatic adjustment of sensitivity increases the likelihood of sensing low-amplitude and varying EGMs, while minimizing the likelihood of T-wave oversensing. This feature is referred to as Auto-adjusting Sensitivity (Medtronic, Inc., Minneapolis, Minn.), Automatic Sensitivity Control (St. Jude Medical, St. Paul, Minn.), or fast Automatic Gain Control (Guidant, Boston Scientific,

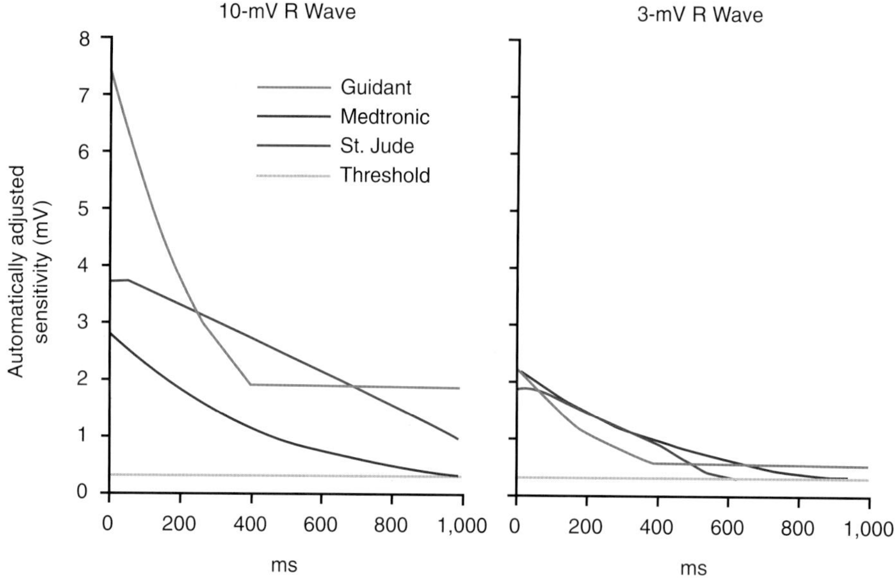

Figure 3-22. Comparison of automatically adjusted sensitivity after sensed ventricular events for three manufacturers of ICDs. Left panel shows markedly different performances after large (10 mV) R wave. Right panel shows similar performances after small (3 mV) R wave. The nominal sensing threshold is approximately 0.3 mV. After sensed ventricular events, Medtronic ICDs reset the sensing threshold to 8 to 10 times the time programmed sensitivity, up to a maximum of 75% of the sensed R wave. The value of Auto-Adjusting Sensitivity then decays exponentially from the end of the (sense) blanking period, with a time constant of 450 msec, until it reaches the programmed (maximum) sensitivity. At the nominal sensitivity of 0.3 mV, there is little difference between the sensitivity curves of Medtronic ICDs after large and small spontaneous R waves. If the R wave is big, the entire Auto-Adjusting Sensitivity curve can be altered substantially by changing the programmed value of maximum sensitivity (Figure 3-23). At nominal settings, the St. Jude Threshold Start begins at 62.5% of the measured R wave for values between 3 and 6 mV. If the R-wave amplitude is greater than 6 mV or less than 3 mV, the Threshold Start is set to 62.5% of these values (3.75 mV and 1.875 mV, respectively). The sensing threshold remains constant for a Decay Delay period of 60 msec and then decays linearly with a slope of 3 mV/sec. Both the Threshold Start percent and the Decay Delay are programmable, over the range of 50% to 75% and 0 to 220 msec, respectively (Fig. 3-21). Guidant ICDs set the starting threshold to 75% of the sensed R wave. Sensitivity ("fast" Automatic Gain Control) then decays with a half-time of 200 msec (time constant of 289 msec) to a minimum value that depends on the dynamic range of the sensing amplifier. "Slow" Automatic Gain Control adjusts the maximum value of this dynamic range to 150% of the value of the average R wave (see Fig. 3-24.) The minimum value of the dynamic range is one eighth of the maximum value. This is equivalent to three sixteenths (18.75%) of the amplitude of the average R wave. After a paced ventricular event, all ICDs also adjust sensitivity dynamically, starting at the end of the (pace) blanking period, but the threshold starts at a more sensitive setting. (From Swerdlow C, Friedman P: Advanced ICD troubleshooting: Part I. PACE 28:1322-1346, 2005, with permission.)

Natick, Mass.; note that "fast" Automatic Gain Control adjusts sensitivity, not gain.) The specific behavior of this adjustment depends on the manufacturer (Fig. 3-22). In Medtronic and St. Jude ICDs, this minimum value is the programmed sensitivity. In Guidant ICDs, the minimum value depends both on programmed sensitivity and "slow" Automatic Gain Control (see later discussion).

Figure 3-22 shows that the methods of the different manufacturers for automatic adjustment of sensitivity perform similarly after small R waves but differently after large R waves. By increasing the sensing floor during normal rhythm, "Slow" Automatic Gain Control in Guidant ICDs prevents T-wave oversensing after large R waves.

Postpacing Automatic Adjustment of Sensitivity. After ventricular pacing, all ICDs set ventricular sensitivity to a highly sensitive value to prevent pacing during VF. The sensitivity threshold then decays to the programmed sensitivity level (Fig. 3-23). Because the automatic adjustment of sensitivity after a pacing stimulus is very sensitive, ICDs are especially vulnerable to oversensing of low-amplitude signals late in diastole during pacing when the amplifier sensitivity or gain is maximal. Clinically, the most important manifestation is the oversensing of diaphragmatic myopotentials.[3]

Automatic Gain Control. Early Ventritex ICDs (St. Jude Medical) used automatic step adjustments of gain as a primary means for avoiding T-wave oversensing and ensuring detection of low-amplitude VF EGMs. Because this resulted in sensing errors when EGM amplitude changed abruptly,[45-47] automatic control of sensitivity, rather than gain, became the primary method of beat-to-beat adjustment in St. Jude ICDs.

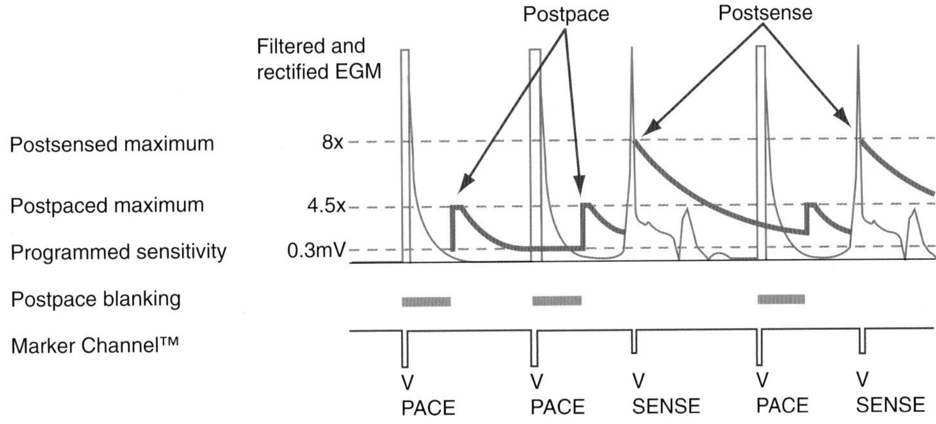

Figure 3-23. Comparison of automatic adjustment of sensitivity after paced and sensed ventricular events. The figure shows the filtered and rectified ventricular EGM, the corresponding sensing threshold, and ventricular event markers. Horizontal bars denote postpacing blanking periods. The blanking periods after paced events are longer than those after sensed events (approximately 250-350 msec versus 120-140 msec), and the initial values of sensitivity are less. In this example taken from a Medtronic ICD, the initial sensing threshold after sensed events is eight times the minimum programmed sensitivity of 0.3 mV, whereas the initial threshold after paced events is 4.5 times that value. The goal of a lower initial postpacing threshold is to prevent pacing into ventricular fibrillation. It compensates in part for the longer postpacing blanking period. V pace, ventricular pacing; V sense, ventricular sensing.

As used presently in Guidant ICDs, "slow" Automatic Gain Control adjusts the dynamic gain of the sensing amplifier slowly in response to temporal changes in R-wave amplitude. This ensures that the peak of the sensed R wave reaches about 75% of the amplifier gain and that the sensing EGM is not truncated or "clipped." Slow Automatic Gain Control also increases the minimum value of amplifier range (i.e., reduces sensitivity) as R-wave amplitude increases (Fig. 3-24), preventing T-wave oversensing in the setting of large R waves. It may increase the risk of undersensing during rare episodes of VF with large variability in the EGM amplitude.[48]

Ventricular Blanking Periods

Ventricular blanking periods prevent ventricular oversensing of same-chamber EGMs (R-wave double-counting) and cross-chamber signals (atrial pacing pulses and P waves) in regular rhythms. Because the likelihood of sensing VF is increased when blanking periods are minimized, blanking periods in ICDs are short and may occasionally be insufficient.

Short Same-Chamber Blanking Periods and R-wave Double-Counting. In adults who are not taking antiarrhythmic drugs, inter-EGM intervals in VF vary from about 130 to 300 msec, with a peak near 200 msec (Fig. 3-25). For this reason, fixed or nominal blanking ICD periods after ventricular sensed events range from 120 to 135 msec. R-wave double-counting occurs if the duration of the sensing EGM exceeds the ventricular blanking period.

Cross-Chamber Blanking Periods and Undersensing of Ventricular Tachycardia/Fibrillation. Under most conditions, ICDs apply only the minimum cross-chamber ventricular blanking required to prevent crosstalk resulting from an atrial pacing stimulus.

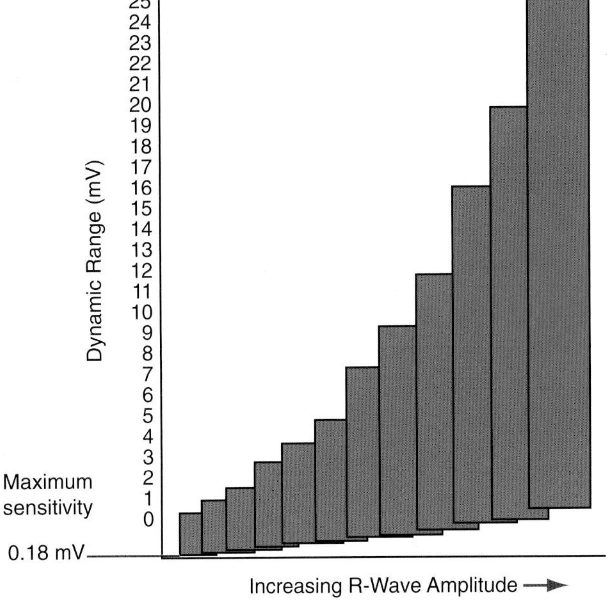

Figure 3-24. Slow automatic gain control. In Guidant ICDs, this feature scales dynamic range depending on the value of the sensed R wave. The maximum value is 150% of the amplitude of the average R wave, and the minimum value is one eighth of the maximum value. The feature reduces the possibility of T-wave oversensing in the setting of large R waves.

During high-rate atrial or dual-chamber pacing, ventricular sensing may be restricted to short periods of the cardiac cycle because of the combined effects of ventricular blanking after ventricular events and cross-chamber ventricular blanking after atrial pacing. If a

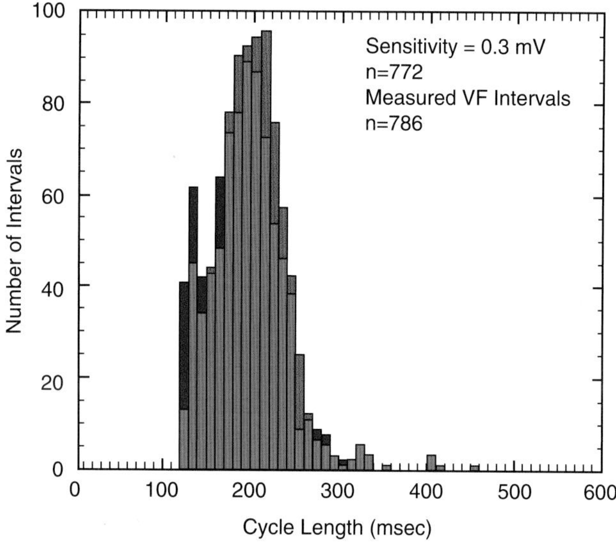

Figure 3-25. Sensed cycle lengths of human ventricular fibrillation (VF) EGMs by an ICD sensing system are compared with manual cycle length measurements of the same signals from many patients. Two histograms are superimposed. The red and orange vertical bars show the manually measured cycle lengths during VF (786 intervals); the blue bars show the intervals sensed by the ICD (772 intervals). Intervals of less than 120 msec, the blanking period, were not permitted. Note that there was some oversensing for intervals shorter than 180 msec, a slight amount of undersensing for intervals between 180 and 280 msec, and a small number of long intervals greater than 280 msec, which represent undersensing during VF. The peak in the histograms occurs at about 220 msec.

sufficient fraction of the cardiac cycle is blanked, systematic undersensing of VT or VF may occur. When pacing and blanking events occur at intervals that are multiples of a VT cycle length, ventricular complexes may be repeatedly undersensed, delaying or preventing detection.[49-51] This occurs most commonly with rate-smoothing algorithms.

"Sensing" the High-Voltage Electrogram

ICDs do not use EGMs from the shocking channel for rate counting. However, some manufacturers (Guidant and Medtronic) use morphologic characteristics of high-voltage EGMs for discrimination of supraventricular tachycardia (SVT) from VT. Pectoral myopotentials are more prominent on EGMs that include the ICD can as an electrode than on the local RV rate-sensing bipole. Oversensing of pectoral myopotentials may prevent SVT-VT discrimination during exercise-induced sinus tachycardia.

Evaluating Sensing of Ventricular Fibrillation at Implantation

Historically, the primary reason for inducing VF at ICD implantation was assessment of defibrillation efficacy. Recently, increasing interest in implanting ICDs without assessing defibrillation efficacy has focused attention on the extent to which adequacy of VF sensing can be determined from EGMs recorded in baseline rhythm. Although the statistical correlation between R-wave amplitude in VF and baseline rhythm is weak,[52,53] two studies reported that sensing of VF is adequate with nominal sensitivities near 0.3 mV if the baseline R wave is sufficiently large (≥5 mV or ≥7 mV[54]). Rarely, clinically significant undersensing of VF may occur despite adequate sinus rhythm R waves.[48] In these instances, undersensing occurs because R-wave amplitude varies faster than the automatic adjustment of sensitivity can react, not because of consistently low-amplitude R waves. The reproducibility of this phenomenon is unknown, as is the extent to which it can be predicted at implantation. Therefore, it is uncertain whether any clinically appropriate testing at implantation can detect this rare cause of undersensing. Reliable sensing of VF cannot be predicted from baseline EGMs if the baseline ventricular rhythm is paced, if sensitivity is programmed to a less sensitive value than nominal (e.g., to avoid T-wave oversensing), or if patients have other implanted electronic devices, such as pacemakers or transcutaneous electrical nerve stimulation (TENS) units, that could cause device-device interactions.

Postshock Sensing

Postshock sensing is critical for redetection of VF after unsuccessful shocks and for accurate detection of episode termination. Postshock signal distortion was a major problem for the first implantable defibrillators, which used a single electrode pair for sensing and shocking. *Electroporation*, the process by which strong electric fields create microscopic holes in the cardiac cell membranes, has been proposed as the mechanism for postshock distortion of EGMs recorded from high-voltage electrodes.[55] Separate, dedicated bipolar sensing electrodes have EGMs that are minimally affected by shocks[56] and became standard for early epicardial ICDs. As for transvenous ICDs, postshock sensing recovers more rapidly with dedicated (true) bipolar sensing configurations than with integrated bipolar sensing configurations. This difference was significant clinically for early-model integrated bipolar electrodes, in which the pacing tip electrode and distal coil were separated by only 6 mm (Guidant Endotak 60 series).[57,58] It is a minor issue for present integrated bipolar leads, in which the spacing is approximately 12 mm.[59]

Both Medtronic and Guidant ICDs analyze the morphology of high-voltage EGMs to discriminate VT from SVT. Because postshock distortion of high-voltage EGM morphology persists for 30 seconds to several minutes,[60] no SVT-VT discrimination algorithm uses EGM morphology after shock. ICD detection algorithms use rate alone to reclassify the rhythm as sinus and revert to their initial detection mode within a few seconds after a shock. If this occurs, an SVT that begins a few seconds to a few minutes after shock will be analyzed by the initial morphology-based detection algorithm and may be classified incorrectly as VT until postshock EGM distortion dissipates.[60] Therefore, distortion of the EGM after a shock could potentially lead to a repetitive sequence of inappropriate shocks in which each shock perpetuates postshock EGM changes in SVT, resulting in inappropriate classification of SVT as VT.

Atrial Sensing in Dual-Chamber ICDs and Atrial ICDs

Accurate sensing of atrial EGMs is essential for accurate discrimination between VT/VF and rapidly-conducted SVTs that satisfy ventricular rate criteria in dual-chamber devices. Rapid discrimination is essential to ensure prompt delivery of ventricular therapy while minimizing inappropriate shocks. Some inappropriate detection of AT/AF is an acceptable consequence for maintaining high sensitivity for detecting VT/VF.

Atrial lead dislodgment, oversensing of FFRWs, or undersensing due to low-amplitude atrial EGMs or atrial blanking periods can cause inaccurate identification of atrial EGMs. These errors in sensing may result in misclassification of VT as SVT or of SVT as VT. Ideally, the atrial lead should have an interelectrode spacing of about 10 mm and should be positioned at implantation to minimize FFRWs.

Postventricular Atrial Blanking and Rejection of Far-Field R Waves

To prevent oversensing of FFRWs, older dual-chamber ICDs had fixed PVAB periods, similar to those in pacemakers (Fig. 3-26). Because the blanking period is fixed, the blanked fraction of the cardiac cycle increases as the ventricular rate increases. Atrial undersensing caused by PVAB can cause underestimation of the atrial rate during rapidly conducted atrial flutter or AF, resulting in inappropriate detection of VT (see Fig. 3-26, lower panel).[61] However, without PVAB, atrial oversensing of FFRWs could cause overestimation of the atrial rate during tachycardias with a 1:1 AV relationship.[62] This could cause either inappropriate rejection of VT as SVT, if FFRWs are consistently counted as atrial EGMs, or inappropriate detection of SVT as VT, if FFRWs are inconsistently counted.[63]

Until recently, Medtronic ICDs provided no atrial blanking after sensed ventricular events, to ensure reliable sensing of atrial EGMs during AF and atrial flutter. Instead, they rejected FFRWs algorithmically by identifying a specific pattern of atrial and ventricular events that fulfill specific criteria (Fig. 3-27). Intermittent sensing of FFRWs or frequent premature atrial events may disrupt this pattern, resulting in misclassification of a tachycardia. Therefore, it is preferable to reject FFRWs after sensed ventricular events by decreasing atrial sensitivity, if this can be done without undersensing of AF. Atrial sensitivity can be reduced to 0.45 mV with a low risk of undersensing AF. Less sensitive values should be programmed only if the likelihood of

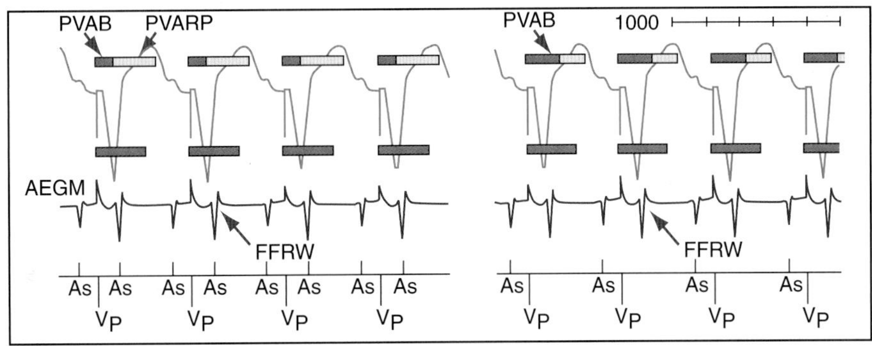

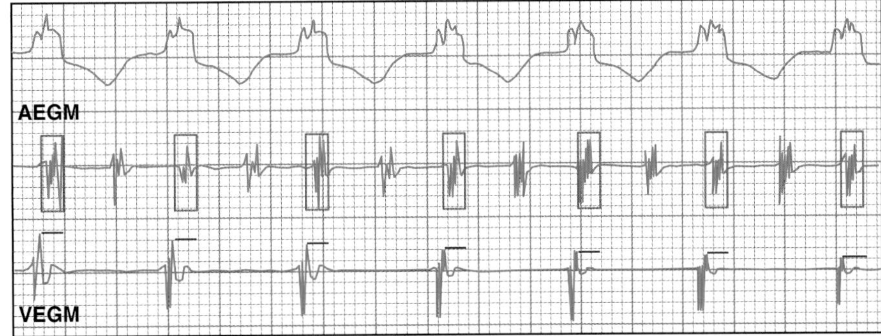

Figure 3-26. Effect of postventricular atrial blanking (PVAB) on atrial sensing. Upper panel shows the surface electrocardiogram (ECG), atrial electrogram (AEGM), and event markers during atrial sensed (As)–ventricular paced (Vp) rhythm. The first segment of each upper horizontal bar denotes the period of PVAB; the second segment denotes the postventricular atrial refractory period (PVARP); FFRW denotes a far-field R wave on the atrial channel. The lower horizontal bars denote the post-pacing ventricular blanking periods. With a short PVAB (left), *the FFRWs are oversensed. A longer PVABP* (right) *prevents oversensing of FFRWs. The lower panel shows the ECG, AEGM, and ventricular electrogram (V-EGM) tracings from a patient with atrial flutter with 2:1 atrioventricular (AV) conduction. The thin horizontal bars on the ventricular channel denote the periods of PVAB, which resulted in atrial undersensing of alternate atrial flutter EGMs (in boxes). The resultant incorrect calculation of atrial rate resulted in inappropriate ventricular therapy for atrial flutter (not shown), because the ICD did not classify the ventricular rate as less than the atrial rate.*

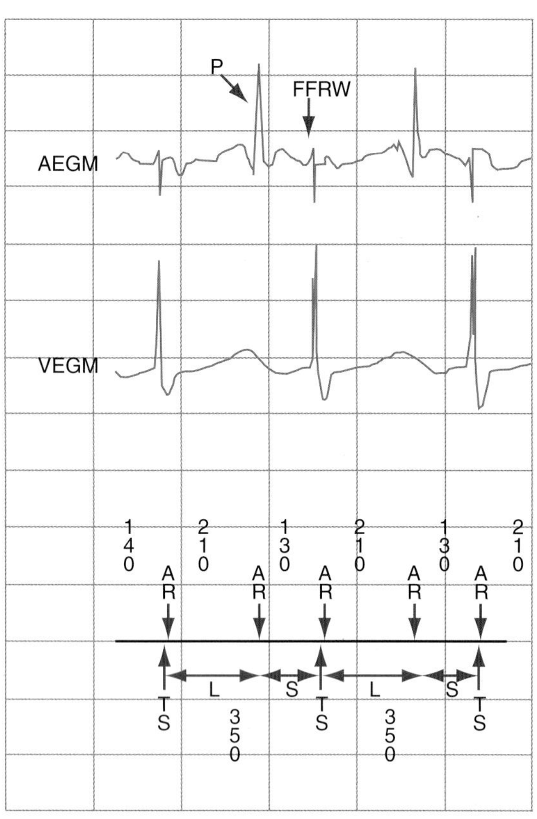

A

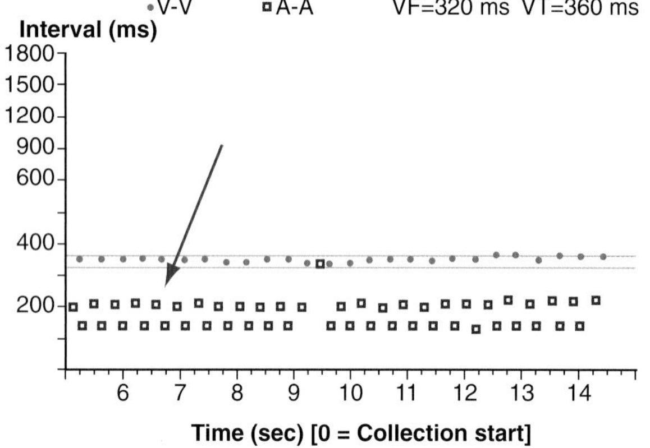

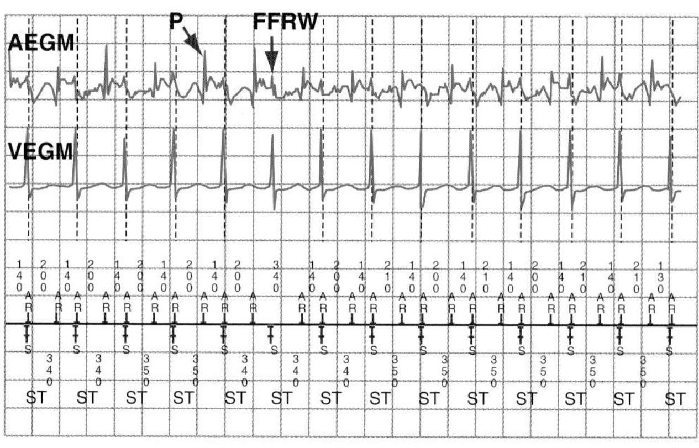

B

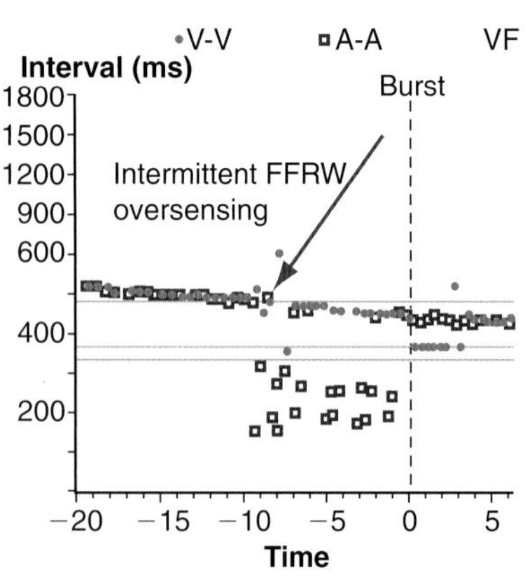

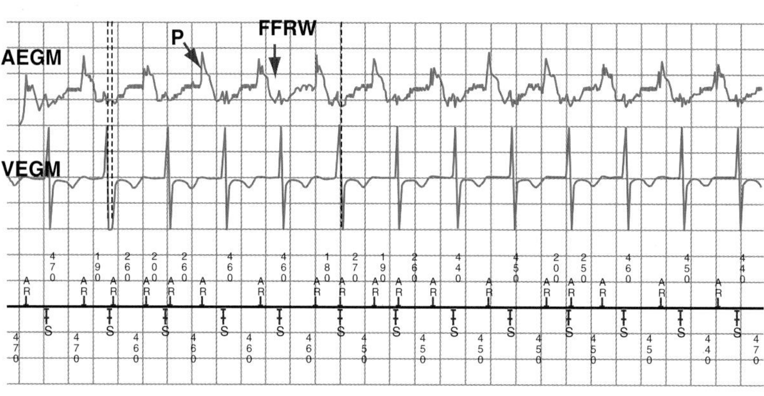

C

Figure 3-27. *Algorithmic rejection of far-field R waves (FFRW) by pattern analysis. ICDs with minimum cross-chamber blanking (Medtronic) reject FFRWs by the timing pattern of atrial and ventricular intervals. Atrial events are classified as FFRWs if all of the following criteria are met: (1) there are exactly two atrial events for each V-V interval; (2) the timing of one P wave is consistent with a FFRW (R-P interval <160 msec); (3) there is a stable interval between the FFRW and the ventricular electrogram (VEGM); (4) there is a short-long pattern of P-P intervals (to distinguish FFRW oversensing from atrial flutter); and (5) the pattern occurs frequently (4 of 12 intervals).* ***A,*** *Atrial electrogram (AEGM), VEGM, and dual-chamber event markers are shown. All five criteria for FFRWs are fulfilled. Horizontal double-ended arrows below event markers denote alternation of long (L) and short (S) atrial intervals. AR, atrial refractory event; P, P wave; TS, ventricular event in ventricular tachycardia (VT) zone.* ***B,*** *Interval plot* (left) *and stored EGM* (right) *from episode of sinus tachycardia with consistent FFRW oversensing that is classified correctly. On the interval plot, open squares denote A-A interval and closed circles denote V-V interval. Horizontal lines denote VT and ventricular fibrillation (VF) detection intervals of 400 and 320 msec, respectively. Alternating A-A intervals whose sum equals that of the V-V intervals produce a characteristic "railroad track" appearance* (arrow). *The algorithm rejects FFRWs despite the fact that FFRW oversensing does not occur for one V-V interval between seconds 9 and 10.* ***C,*** *Interval plot* (left) *and stored EGM* (right) *from episode of sinus tachycardia with consistent FFRW oversensing that was detected inappropriately as VT. Intermittent oversensing of FFRWs occurs as sinus tachycardia accelerates gradually across the VT detection interval of 480 msec* (arrow), *resulting in inappropriate therapy ("Burst" antitachycardia pacing marker on interval plot, VT marker on EGM event markers).*

rapidly-conducted AF is low. FFRW oversensing that occurs only after paced ventricular events (when auto-adjusting atrial sensitivity is maximal) need not be eliminated to prevent inappropriate detection of SVT as VT, but it may cause inappropriate mode switching and can contribute to inappropriate detection of AF or atrial flutter by atrial antiarrhythmic pacemakers and ICDs.

Medtronic ICDs (starting with Entrust) and Guidant ICDs (starting with Vitality) may use brief atrial blanking or a period of reduced, automatically adjusting sensitivity (or both) to reject FFRWs without preventing detection of AF (Fig. 3-28). Older Guidant ICDs have obligatory blanking periods after atrial sensed events, which often caused the atrial rate to be underestimated during AF and atrial flutter.[61]

St. Jude ICDs and Medtronic ICDs starting with the Entrust family provide programmable atrial blanking after sensed ventricular events to individualize the tradeoff between oversensing of FFRWs and undersensing of atrial EGMs in AF. St. Jude ICDs also provide programmable atrial sensing Threshold Start and Decay Delay, corresponding to the same features in the ventricular channel.

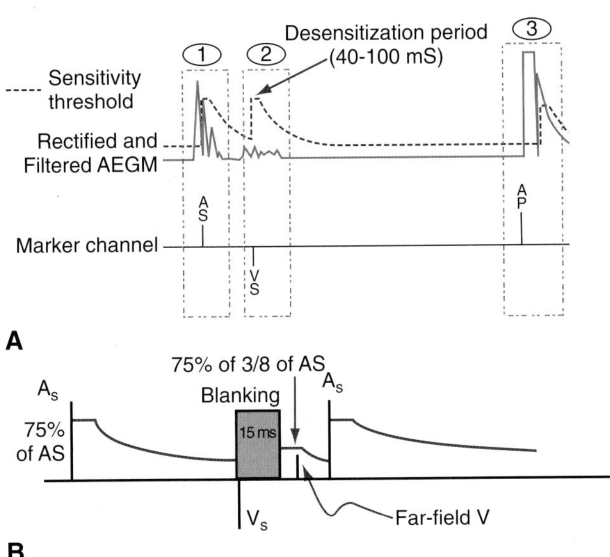

Figure 3-28. Atrial sensing features intended to prevent far-field R-wave (FFRW) oversensing while still permitting detection of atrial fibrillation. These features, which combine limited atrial blanking with automatic adjustment of atrial sensitivity are less strict than conventional blanking periods. ***A,*** *Medtronic ICDs, starting with Entrust, have an optional "Partial +" postventricular atrial blanking period (PVAB) setting that increases the sensing threshold for a programmable duration (40-100 msec) after a ventricular event (2). Entrust operation after ventricular sensed events nominally has no absolute blanking or sensitivity changes. With Partial + PVAB enabled, the sensing threshold is raised to 75% of the prior sensed atrial electrogram (AEGM) amplitude to reduce the likelihood of sensing FFRWs. "Absolute" PVAB, another selectable option, blanks all atrial sensed events within the programmable PVAB interval. Because significant atrial undersensing can occur, this method is recommended only for addressing complications not addressed by the Partial + PVAB method. Partial + or Absolute PVAB does not affect atrial sensing operation after sensed events (1) or after atrial paced events (3). AS, atrial sensed event; AP, atrial paced event; mS, microseconds; VS, ventricular sensed event.* ***B,*** *Guidant ICDs, starting with Vitality, introduce a brief (15-msec) blanking period after each sensed ventricular event, followed by a decrease in atrial sensitivity to three eighths of the mean P-wave amplitude. This is sufficient to prevent oversensing of FFRWs, provided that the amplitude of the AEGM is at least eight thirds that of the FFRW.*

Sensing in Cardiac Resynchronization ICDs

Few special considerations apply to present cardiac resynchronization ICDs that use RV sensing to define timing cycles for bradycardia pacing and detection of tachyarrhythmias. Additional periods may be present in systems with programmable offsets for LV and RV pace timing. These blanking periods may affect both atrial and ventricular sensing, as shown in Figure 3-29. Guidant cardiac resynchronization ICDs also sense in

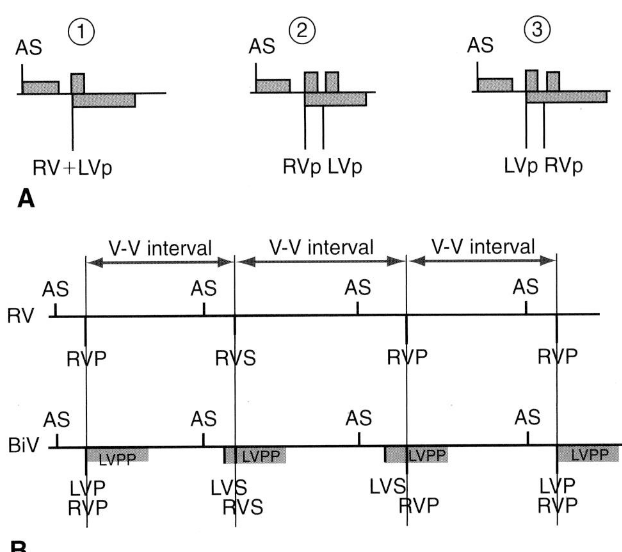

Figure 3-29. Event markers illustrate blanking periods in cardiac resynchronization ICDs. ***A,*** *Blanking periods in Medtronic Marquis Insync III ICD. In condition 1, there is simultaneous right ventricular and left ventricular pacing (RV+LVp). There is a single cross-chamber blanking period (approximately 30 msec in duration) on the atrial channel. In condition 2, RVp first with LVp delayed (up to 80 msec), and in condition 3, LVp first with RVp delayed, there are two cross-chamber blanking periods on the atrial channel, one for each ventricular paced event. In both cases, ventricular blanking is timed from the RVp event, resulting in a postpace ventricular blanking period that is longer by the V-V pacing delay (up to 80 msec). These additional blanking periods increase the risk of undersensing in both chambers. To date, there are no reports of undetected ventricular tachycardia (VT) caused by offsets in timing of V-V pacing.* ***B,*** *Left ventricular protection period (LVPP) of the Guidant Renewal ICD. This ICD has RV timing and independent RV and LV stimulation channels without a programmable RV-LV delay. The LVPP allows LV sensing to occur with inhibition of the LV stimulus for a period that is programmable to prevent pacing into the vulnerable period of the LV. Therefore, this feature allows biventricular sensing but RV-based timing. AS, atrial sensed; BIV, biventricular; LVP, left-ventricular paced; LVS, left-ventricular sensed; RVP, right-ventricular sensed. (Courtesy of Guidant Corporation, Indianapolis, Ind.) (**B,** From Kay G: Troubleshooting and programming of cardiac resynchronization therapy. In Ellenbogen K, Kay G, Wilkoff B [eds]: Device Therapy for Congestive Heart Failure. Philadelphia, Elsevier, 2004, pp 232-293, with permission.)*

the left ventricle for the purpose of preventing pacing into the LV vulnerable period. A sensed LV event initiates a programmable LV protection period of 300 to 500 msec (see Fig. 3-29B). R-wave double-counting associated with older cardiac resynchronization devices integrating the RV and LV tip electrodes as a composite ventricular EGM is discussed later.

Ventricular Oversensing: Recognition and Troubleshooting

Oversensing is defined as sensing of unintended nonphysiologic signals or of physiologic signals that do not accurately reflect local depolarization. Nonphysiologic signals usually arise from extracardiac EMI (e.g., ungrounded electrical equipment, anti-theft detectors). Electrical artifacts are a common cause of oversensing from leads with insulation failure or intermittent fracture resulting in "make-break" potentials. Rarely, these electrical artifacts arise from retained fragments of abandoned intracardiac leads. Physiologic signals may be intracardiac (P, R, or T waves) or extracardiac (myopotentials). Oversensing often results in characteristic patterns of stored EGMs and associated markers (Fig. 3-30).[64,65] In pacemakers, oversensing may manifest as either failure to deliver an expected pacing stimulus or inappropriate tracking of artifactual signals in the atrial channel of a dual-chamber device. In ICDs, it usually manifests as inappropriate detection of VT or VF. This section focuses on oversensing in ICDs.

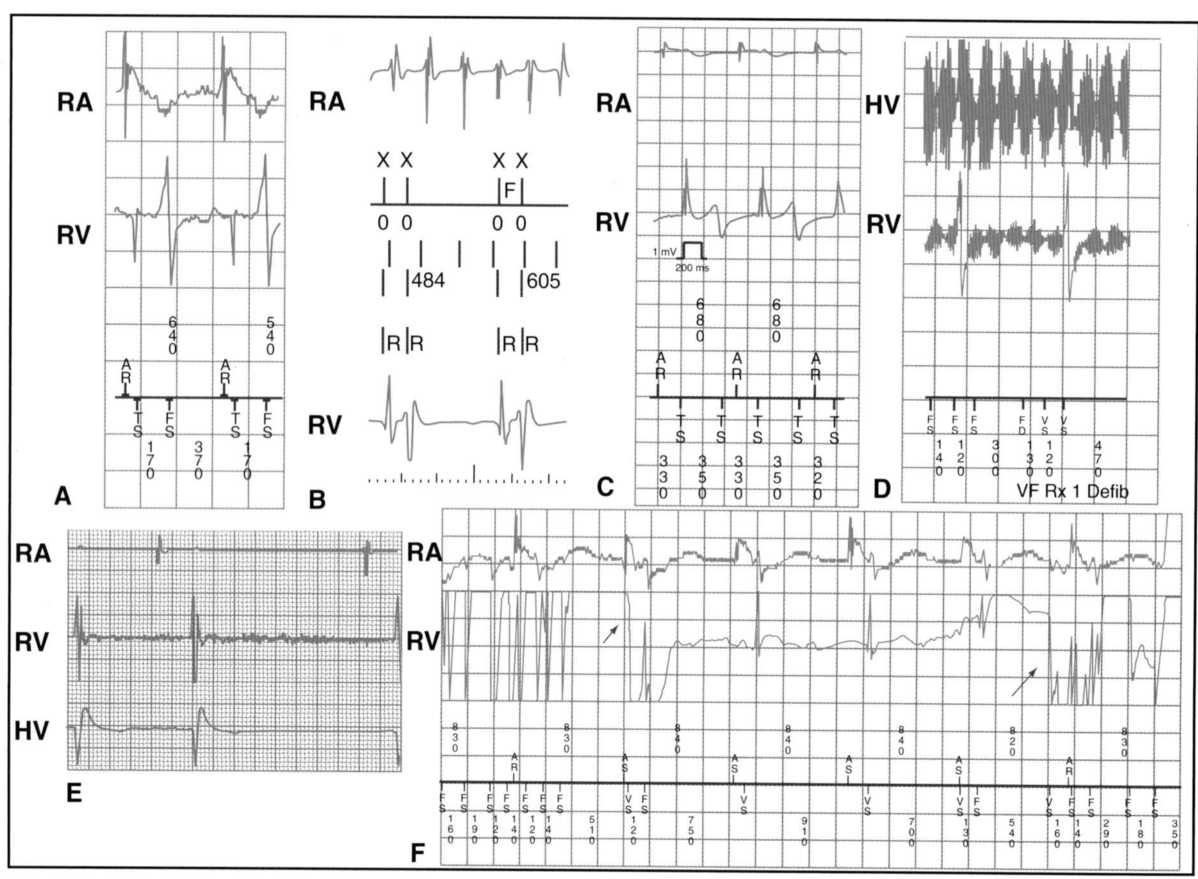

Figure 3-30. Types of oversensing resulting in inappropriate detection of ventricular tachycardia/fibrillation (VT/VF). ***A** through **C**, oversensing of physiologic intracardiac signals.* ***D** through **F**, oversensing of extracardiac signals.* ***A**, P-wave oversensing in sinus rhythm from an integrated bipolar lead with distal coil near the tricuspid valve.* ***B**, R-wave double-counting during conducted atrial fibrillation (AF) in a biventricular-sensing ICD.* ***C**, T-wave oversensing in a patient with low-amplitude R wave (note millivolt calibration marker).* ***D**, Electromagnetic interference from a power drill has higher amplitude on widely-spaced high-voltage EGM than on closely-spaced true bipolar-sensing EGM.* ***E**, Diaphragmatic myopotential oversensing in a patient with an integrated bipolar lead at the right ventricular apex. Note that the noise level is constant, but oversensing does not occur until automatic gain control increases the gain sufficiently, about 600 msec after the sensed R waves.* ***F**, Lead fracture noise results in intermittent saturation of amplifier range, denoted by arrows. RA, right atrium; RV, right-ventricular sensing EGM; HV, high-voltage EGM. (From Swerdlow C, Shivkumar K: Implantable cardioverter defibrillators: Clinical aspects. In Zipes DP, Jalife J [eds]: Cardiac Electrophysiology: From Cell to Bedside, 4th ed. Philadelphia, WB Saunders, 2004, pp 980-993, with permission.)*

Recognition of Oversensing

Intracardiac Signals

Ventricular oversensing of physiologic intracardiac signals results in two or more sensed ventricular events for each cardiac cycle. This may result in inappropriate detection of VT or VF.

T-wave Oversensing. Oversensing of spontaneous T waves may cause inappropriate detection of either VT or VF, depending on the sensed R wave–to–T wave interval and the programmed VF detection interval. T-wave oversensing is typically identified by alternating EGM morphologies.[64] R-R intervals usually alternate, but the amount of alternation may be small.

R-wave Double-Counting. R-wave double-counting is the penalty for short ventricular blanking periods. It occurs if the duration of the sensed EGM exceeds the ventricular blanking period of 120 to 135 msec. On rare occasions, R-wave double-counting may occur as a result of local ventricular delays in the baseline state or of use-dependent effects of sodium channel blocking antiarrhythmic drugs or hyperkalemia, both of which slow ventricular conduction. R-wave double-counting was a common problem in cardiac resynchronization ICDs that used Y-adapted or extended bipolar sensing between RV and LV electrodes.[66] In this case, the composite ventricular EGM included deflections from the RV and the LV, both of which could be counted as separate R waves if the interventricular conduction delay exceeded the ventricular blanking period.

If R-wave double-counting results in alternation of ventricular cycle lengths with an isoelectric interval between sensed events, a characteristic "railroad track" pattern of ventricular intervals is recorded (Fig. 3-31).

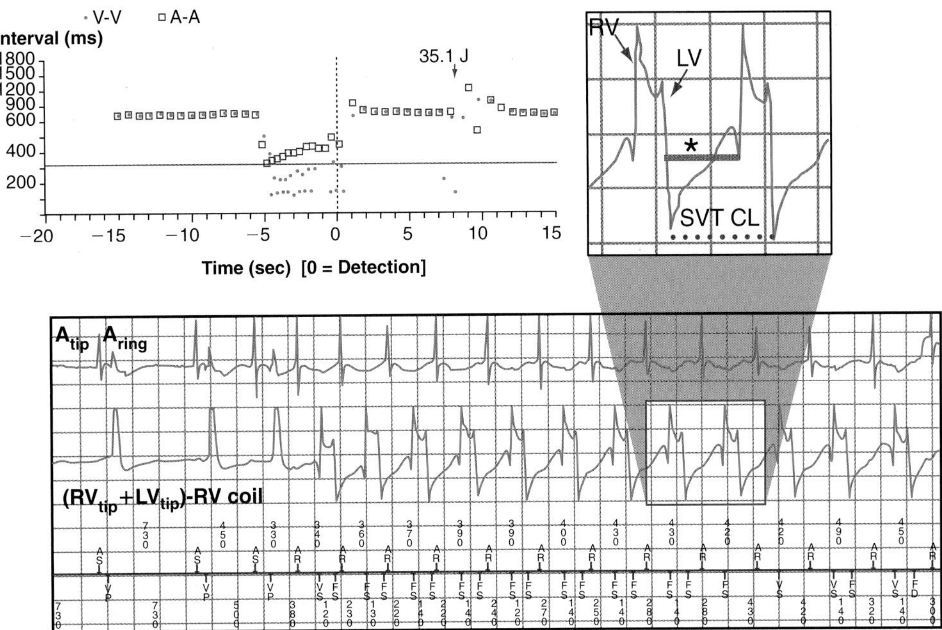

Figure 3-31. R-wave double-counting in a patient with a Y-adapted cardiac resynchronization ICD and left bundle branch block. The main panel shows the atrial (A_{tip}-A_{ring}) EGM, the extended bipolar ventricular ([RV_{tip}+LV_{tip}]–RV coil) EGM, and event markers. The first two complexes show atrial-sensed, ventricular-paced rhythm. The third atrial complex is premature and initiates supraventricular tachycardia (SVT) faster than the programmed upper tracking limit, resulting in intermittent R-wave double-counting. The insert shows that the first component of the ventricular EGM represents right ventricular (RV) activation, and the second component represents left ventricular (LV) activation. The insert also illustrates conditions for inappropriate detection of SVT. The double-counted RV-LV interval measures within 20 msec of the ventricular blanking period of 120 msec (see event markers) and is always classified in the ventricular fibrillation (VF) zone. Inappropriate detection occurs when the interval represented by the solid line segment (asterisk) *in the insert is less than the ventricular tachycardia (VT) detection interval. This interval represents the difference between the true SVT cycle length (CL,* dotted line in insert*) and the double-counted RV-LV interval. For example, if the VT detection interval is 400 msec and the double-counted RV-LV interval is 140 msec, inappropriate detection occurs for any tachycardia CL shorter than 540 msec. AS, sensed atrial interval; AR, atrial interval in postventricular atrial refractory period; VS, interval in sinus zone; FS, interval in VF zone. The plot in the upper left panel shows atrial intervals as open squares and ventricular intervals as closed circles. The initial rhythm is atrial sensed, ventricular paced with a cycle length of approximately 700 msec. At the onset of SVT, there is an abrupt decrease in atrial intervals. Sensed "ventricular intervals" alternate. Their sum equals the atrial interval. This "railroad track" pattern of ventricular intervals also occurs with P-wave oversensing and may occur with T-wave oversensing. A corresponding "railroad track" pattern of atrial intervals occurs with far-field R-wave oversensing on the atrial channel. Compare Figure 3-27. (From Swerdlow C, Friedman P: Advanced ICD troubleshooting: Part I. PACE 28:1322-1346, 2005, with permission.)*

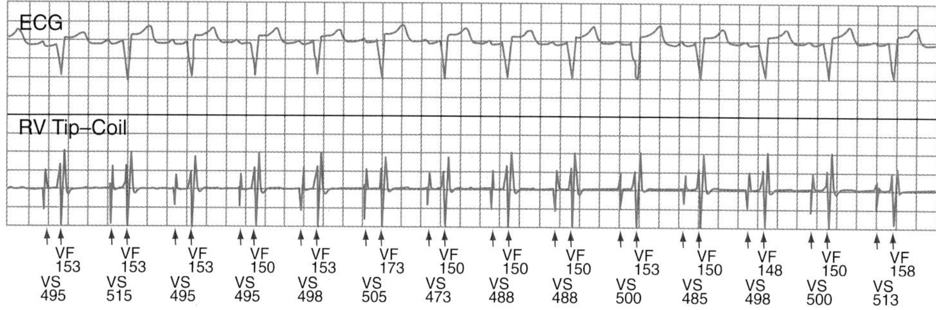

Figure 3-32. P-wave oversensing. The surface electrocardiographic (ECG) lead, integrated bipolar right ventricular electrogram (RV Tip-Coil), and ventricular event markers are shown. P-wave oversensing caused by the proximity of the RV coil to the right atrium results in ICD sensing of alternating sinus (ventricular-sensed, VS) and ventricular fibrillation (VF) intervals, the latter corresponding to the P-R interval. The sum of the VS and VF intervals equals the true R-R interval.

Because the second component of the R wave is sensed as soon as the blanking period terminates, the double-counted RV-RV or RV-LV interval measures within 20 msec of the ventricular blanking period and is always classified in the VF zone. Inappropriate detection may occur despite a true ventricular rate below the VT detection interval, and most of these inappropriate detections are in the VF zone. R-wave double-counting is almost eliminated by true bipolar sensing.

P-wave Oversensing. P-wave oversensing may occur if the distal coil of an integrated bipolar lead is close to the tricuspid valve and the sensed P-R interval exceeds the ventricular blanking period[4] (Fig. 3-32). It is rare in adults with ventricular sensing electrodes near the RV apex, but it may occur in children or in adults if the RV electrode dislodges or is positioned in the proximal septum or inflow portion of the RV. If P-wave oversensing occurs during a 1:1 rhythm, the pattern is similar to that of R-wave double-counting, provided that the sensed P-R or R-P interval is less than the VF detection interval. However, oversensing of P waves as R waves can cause inappropriate detection of VF during AF or atrial flutter, independent of the ventricular rate.

Far-Field R-wave Oversensing. FFRW oversensing on the atrial channel, the inverse of P-wave oversensing on the ventricular channel, shows a pattern of alternating atrial cycle lengths with one sense marker timed close to the ventricular EGM. If rate and duration criteria for VT are fulfilled, FFRW oversensing may confound dual-chamber SVT-VT discrimination. However, such oversensing in the atrium does not cause inappropriate detection of VT if the ventricular rate is in the sinus zone. It may also cause inappropriate mode switching.

Extracardiac Signals

The distinctive feature of oversensing of extracardiac signals is replacement of the isoelectric baseline with high-frequency noise that does not have a constant relationship to the cardiac cycle.[64,67]

External Electromagnetic Interference. With oversensing of external electromagnetic interference,[64,67] signal amplitude is greater on the high-voltage EGM recorded from widely-spaced electrodes than on the sensing EGM recorded from closely-spaced electrodes. Although the interference signal may be continuous, oversensing is often intermittent due to autoadjusting sensitivity. Clinical data may suggest a specific identifiable cause (Fig. 3-33).

Lead/Connector Problems. Oversensing caused by lead or connector (header, adapter, or set-screw) problems is usually intermittent. It may occur only during a small fraction (<10%) of the cardiac cycle, and it often saturates the amplifier (Figs. 3-34 through 3-37). It may be limited to the sensing EGM and may be associated with postural changes. Often, the pacing-lead impedance is abnormal, indicating complete or partial interruption of the pace-sense circuit. However, abnormal impedance measurements may be intermittent. Metal ion oxidation of the middle insulation layer is a common failure mode for older coaxial leads. In this case, abnormal impedance may be measured only in the ring-to-coil pathway, which may not be reported on the programmer. Early signs include frequent sensing of 120- to 130-msec nonphysiologic V-V intervals and an increase in frequency of detected nonsustained "VT" with intervals shorter than 200 msec (Fig. 3-38). A "signature" presentation of this type of lead failure is oversensing of electrical noise after shocks (Fig. 3-39).[68]

Myopotential Oversensing. Myopotential oversensing may persist for variable fractions of the cardiac cycle. Diaphragmatic myopotentials are most prominent on the sensing EGM. Oversensing usually occurs after long diastolic intervals or after ventricular paced events when amplifier sensitivity or gain is maximal. It often ends with a sensed R wave, which abruptly reduces sensitivity. In pacemaker-dependent patients, diaphragmatic oversensing causes inhibition of pacing, resulting in persistent oversensing and inappropriate detection of VF (Fig. 3-40). Clinically, this may manifest as syncope due to inhibition of pacing followed by an inappropriate shock. This is an exception to the clinical rule that antecedent syncope usually indicates an appropriate shock. A short time constant for automatic adjustment

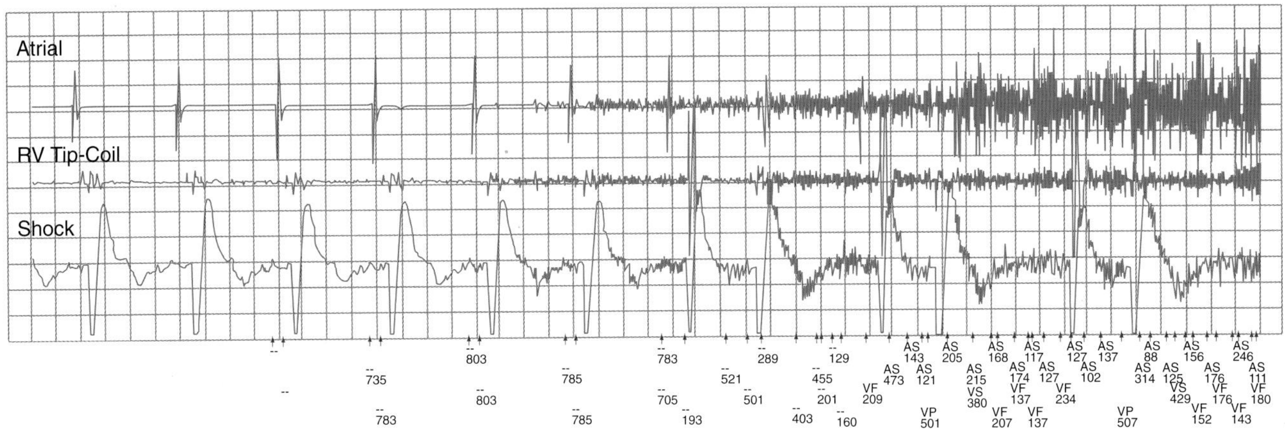

Figure 3-33. External electromagnetic interference caused by an electric drill. Atrial, integrated bipolar (RV Tip-Coil), and high-voltage (Shock) EGMs are shown, together with a dual-chamber channel showing event markers. Electromagnetic interference is continuous. Oversensing occurs first on the atrial channel, which has a higher sensitivity setting (and gain) than the ventricular sensing channel. Although the amplitude of external electromagnetic interference is typically less on true bipolar sensing electrodes than on shocking electrodes, it may be similar on integrated bipolar and shocking electrodes.

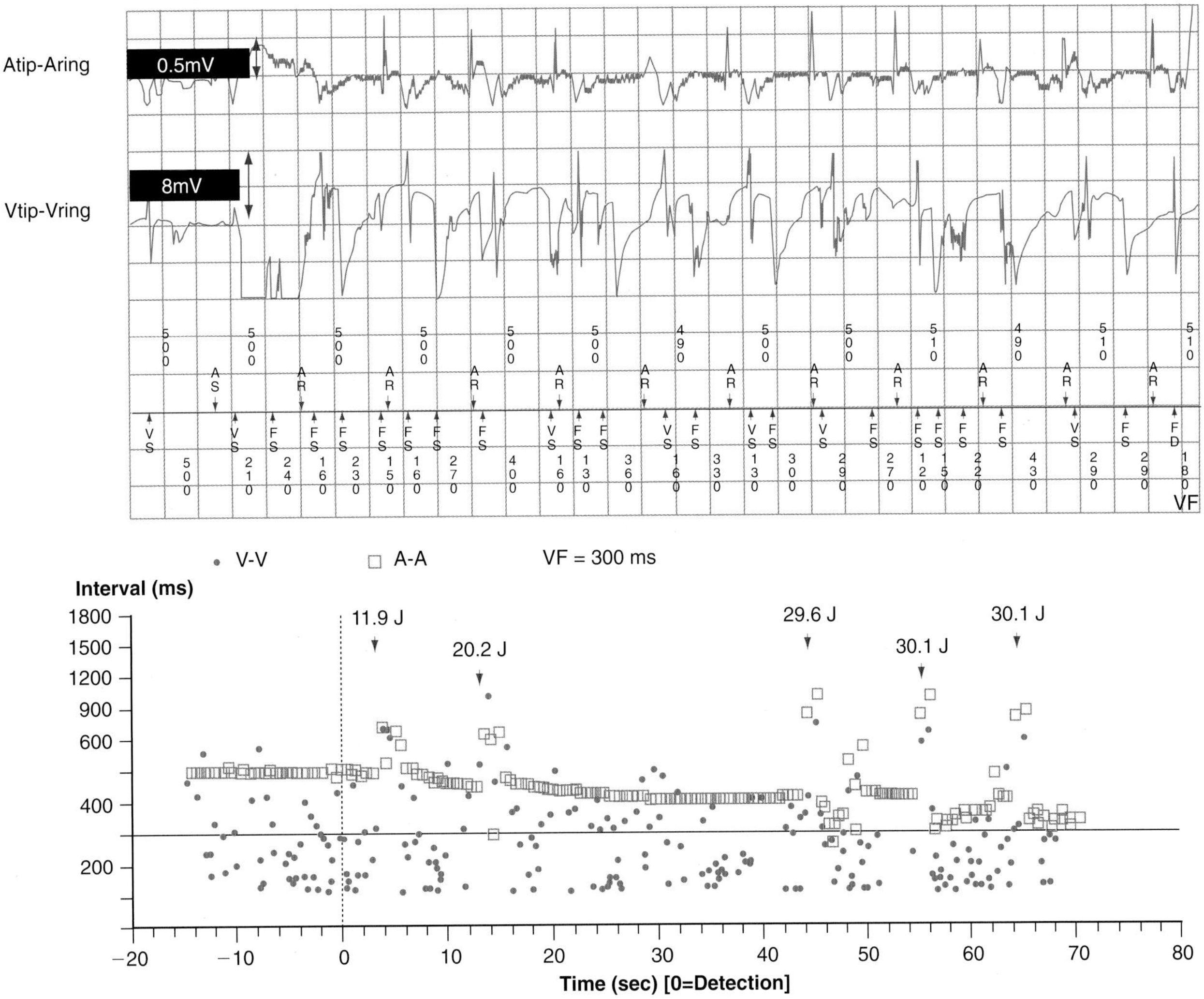

Figure 3-34. Oversensing caused by lead insulation failure. The top panel shows the atrial (Atip-Aring) EGM, the ventricular true bipolar (Vtip-Vring) EGM, and event markers. The bottom panel shows the interval plot. In the ventricular channel, there are intermittent, erratic signals that saturate the sensing amplifier. The interval plot highlights the wide range of sensed intervals, including many "short" intervals close to the ventricular blanking period of 120 msec. Arrows denote five inappropriate shocks.

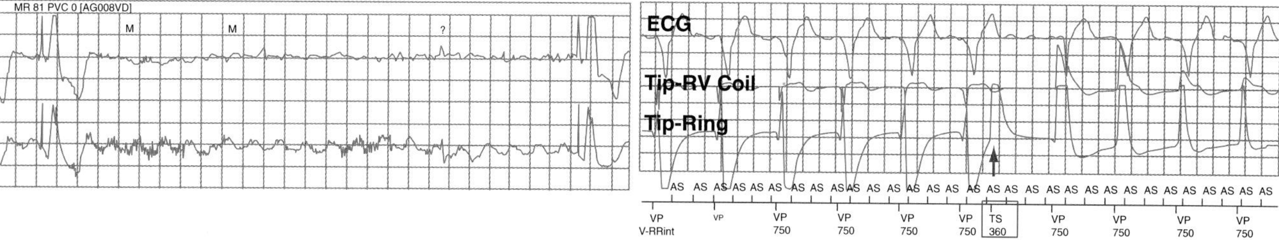

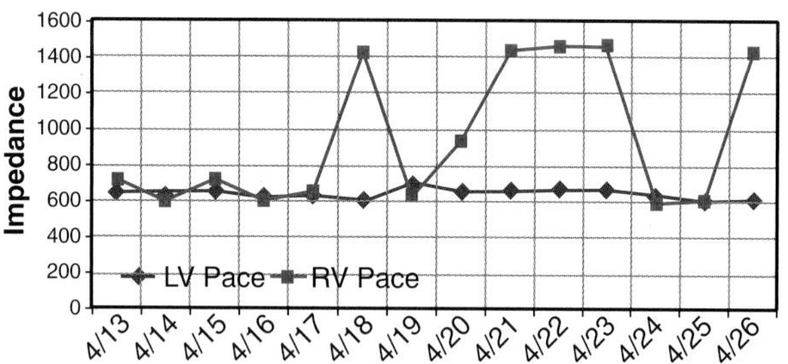

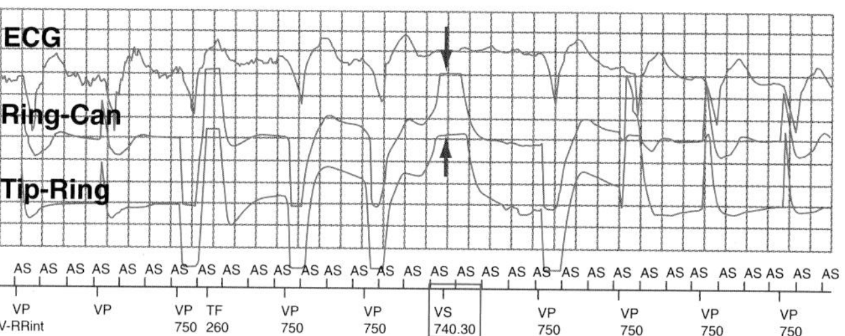

Figure 3-35. Ventricular oversensing leads to inhibition of pacing in a pacemaker-dependent patient 2 weeks after replacement of an ICD pulse generator. Top left, *in-hospital electrocardiogram (ECG) monitoring strip with 4.46-sec pause in paced ventricular rhythm. The atrial rhythm is atrial fibrillation.* Bottom left, *marked variability in right ventricular (RV) pacing impedance with constant impedance in left ventricular (LV) lead. The two right panels show telemetry Holter recordings, including one ECG channel, two ventricular EGMs, and event markers.* Top right, *oversensing on Tip-Ring EGM* (arrow, box) *but not on Tip-RV Coil EGM. Oversensing is intermittent and saturates the amplifier.* Bottom right, *oversensing on both Tip-Ring and Ring-Can EGMs, localizing the oversensing problem to connections related to the ring EGM* (box). *AS, atrial sense; VP, ventricular pace; TS, ventricular interval in ventricular tachycardia (VT) zone.*

Before Revision

After Revision

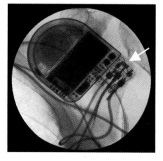

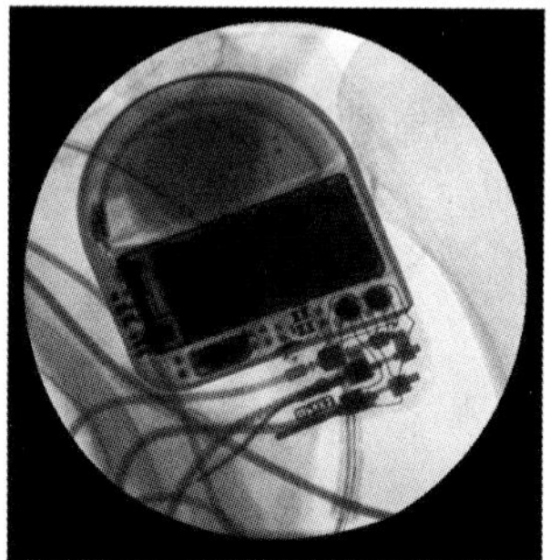

Figure 3-36. Intraoperative fluoroscopic images corresponding to the data presented in Figure 3-35. The ICD has been removed from the pocket to enhance image quality. Before revision, the lead connector pin was not advanced completely into the header (arrow). *The proximal connection between the ring electrode and the header was intermittent, accounting for the high impedance and oversensing illustrated in Figure 3-35. After revision, the ventricular electrode is advanced completely into the header.*

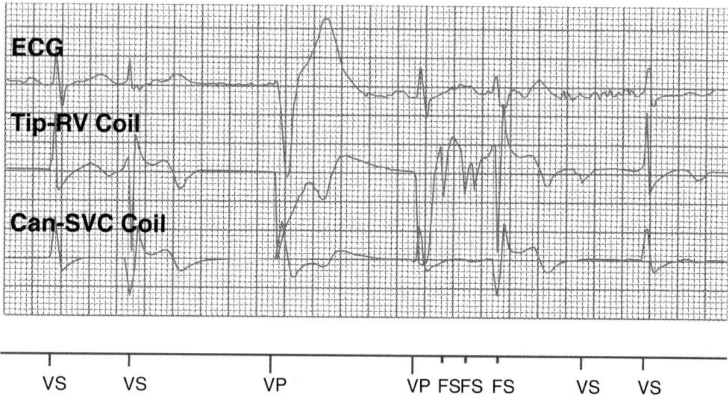

Figure 3-37. Oversensing caused by contact between active electrode and retained lead. The surface electrocardiogram (ECG), integrated bipolar (Tip-RV Coil) and Can–superior vena cava (SVC) coil EGMs are shown with ventricular event markers. Oversensing is intermittent. Abnormal signals are recorded only on the sensing channel. In this case, a retained, inactive coronary sinus defibrillation lead made intermittent mechanical contact with the distal coil of an integrated bipolar right ventricular (RV) electrode. VS, ventricular sense; VP, ventricular pace; FS, ventricular interval in ventricular fibrillation (VF) zone.

Sensing Integrity Counter

Since Sep 18, 2004 19:50:36
120-130 ms V-V intervals 2333
(if >300 counts, check for sensing issues)

VT/VF Episodes

ID#	Date/Time	Type	V.Cycle	Last Rx	Success	Duration
	(No data since last session.)					
	Last Session (Sep 15, 2004)					
	(Data prior to last session has not been interrogated.)					

SVT/NST Episodes

ID#	Date/Time	V.Cycle	Duration	Reason
12	Jan 09 00:54:31	150 ms	5 beats	Nonsustained
11	Jan 08 00:33:42	160 ms	5 beats	Nonsustained
10	Jan 06 13:40:28	220 ms	7 beats	Nonsustained
9	Jan 04 18:40:31	160 ms	5 beats	Nonsustained
8	Dec 31 18:41:20	200 ms	5 beats	Nonsustained
7	Dec 05 10:34:13	200 ms	5 beats	Nonsustained
6	Dec 04 12:21:58	210 ms	5 beats	Nonsustained
5	Dec 04 11:41:08	180 ms	7 beats	Nonsustained
4	Nov 16 20:42:51	140 ms	5 beats	Nonsustained
	Last Session (Sep 15, 2004)			

Lead Performance	Venricular
Pacing Impedance	444 ohms
Defibrillation (HVB) Impedance	20 ohms

Figure 3-38. Asymptomatic malfunction in coaxial defibrillation lead (Medtronic Model 6936) detected by Internet-based, remote patient monitoring (Medtronic CareLink). The Sensing Integrity Counter provides a cumulative count of nonphysiologic short intervals caused by oversensing. Multiple episodes of nonsustained ventricular tachycardia (VT) with cycle lengths of 140 to 210 msec also suggest oversensing. In the absence of exposure to electromagnetic interference, the combination of frequent short intervals and detected nonsustained VT is highly suggestive of an inner-insulation failure. The pacing and defibrillation lead impedances are insensitive to early insulation failure. Analysis of ring-coil impedance from the programmer "Save to Disk" file is often diagnostic. HVB, high voltage distal coil; SVT/NST, supraventricular tachycardia/nonsustained ventricular tachycardia; VF, ventricular fibrillation. (From Swerdlow CD, Friedman PA. Advanced ICD troubleshooting: Part II. PACE 29:70-96, 2006, with permission.)

of sensitivity increases the probability of this type of oversensing. It is most common in male patients who have integrated bipolar leads in the RV apex.[3,4]

Pectoral myopotentials are more prominent on a far-field EGM that includes the ICD can rather than the near-field EGM. Because ICDs do not use this EGM for rate-counting, oversensing of pectoral myopotentials does not cause inappropriate detection unless the far-field EGM is used for SVT-VT morphology discrimination during exercise-induced sinus tachycardia. Pectoral myopotentials are a major cause of oversensing in unipolar pacemakers and may result in either inhibition of ventricular pacing (if sensed by the ventricular channel) or rapid ventricular pacing (if sensed and tracked by the atrial channel). Myopotential oversensing may be suspected if symptoms occur during arm motion and can often be demonstrated in the clinic by having the patient forcefully press his or her hands together while the intracardiac EGM is monitored.

Troubleshooting for Oversensing

Troubleshooting of oversensing is reviewed in detail and summarized below.[69]

P-wave Oversensing

Consistent oversensing of spontaneous P waves often requires lead revision. One amelioration strategy is to force atrial pacing using DDDR or Dynamic Overdrive modes. This shortens the ventricular cycle length, to prevent ventricular sensitivity from reaching its minimum value, and introduces cross-chamber ventricular blanking after each atrial event, to avoid the oversensing of P waves.

R-wave Double-Counting

In St. Jude ICDs and newer Medtronic ICDs (Entrust family), this may be overcome by increasing the ventricular blanking period from the nominal value (120-125 msec) to values closer to 150 to 160 msec. In Guidant ICDs and older Medtronic ICDs, it usually requires lead revision. Occasionally, reducing ventricular sensitivity can avoid it; but ventricular sensitivity should not be reduced unless reliable sensing of VF is confirmed at the reduced level of sensitivity. This typically requires reinduction of VF with assessment of ventricular sensing at the higher programmed sensitivity threshold.

T-wave Oversensing

T-wave oversensing may be divided into three classes: postpacing, large R wave (>3 mV) in spontaneous rhythm, and small R wave (<3 mV) in spontaneous rhythm (Fig. 3-41). Postpacing T-wave oversensing can cause inappropriate inhibition of bradycardia pacing[45,70] or delivery of ATP at the wrong rate.[45] It does not cause inappropriate detection of VT, but it may increment VT or VF counters and thereby increase the likelihood that

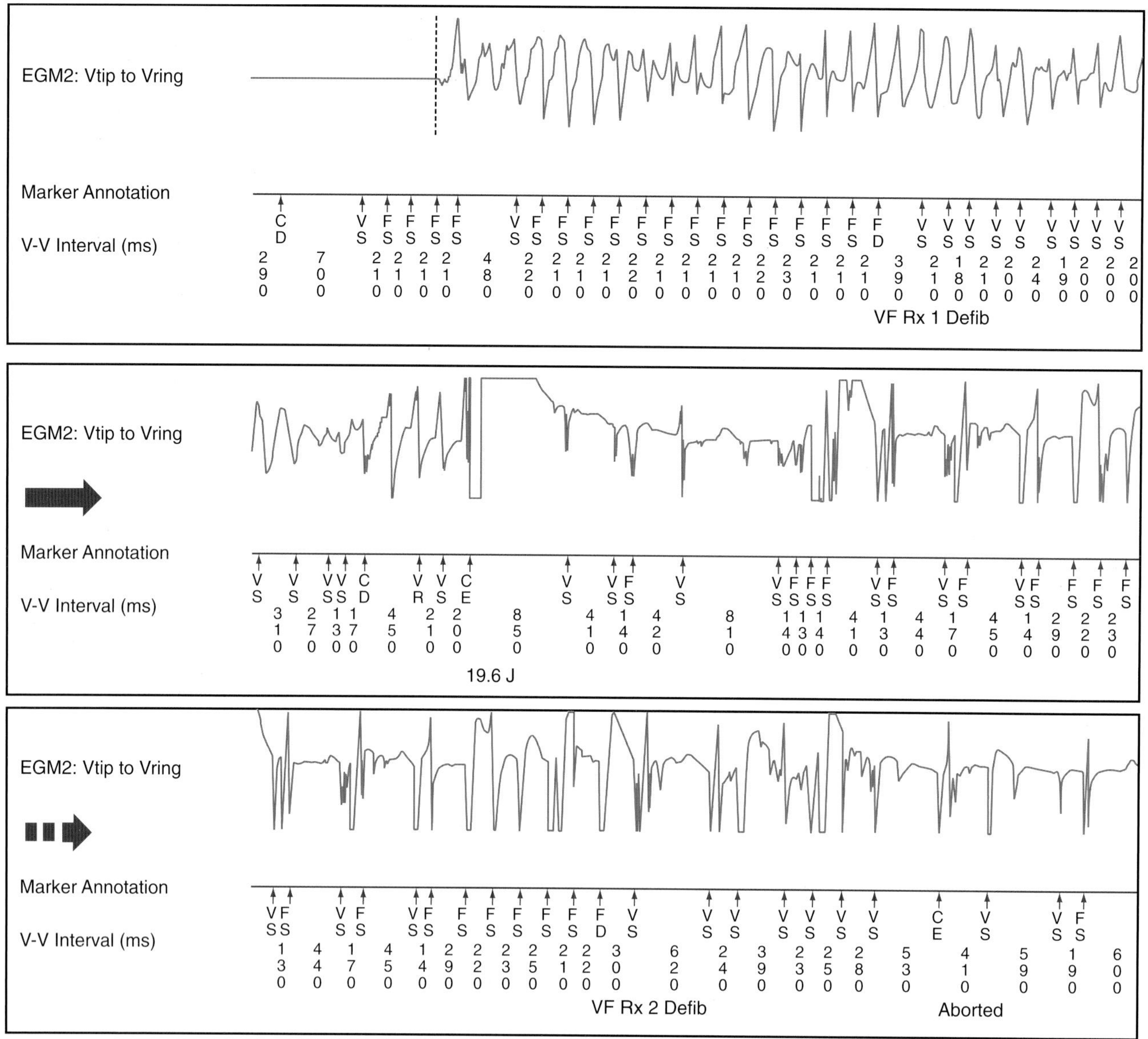

Figure 3-39. Postshock oversensing. Panels show recordings of true bipolar sensing and event markers during ventricular fibrillation (VF) induced at replacement of an ICD pulse generator attached to a chronically implanted Medtronic Model 6936 Transvenous, coaxial defibrillation electrode. The top and middle panels are continuous. At left of top panel, T-wave shock (CD) induces VF, which is reliably sensed, detected, and terminated by a programmed 20-J shock (CD 19.6 J) in the middle of the middle panel. Postshock intermittent oversensing saturates EGM signals, resulting in failure to identify sinus rhythm and repetitive inappropriate redetection of VF, with multiple aborted shocks. The lower panel is not continuous and shows one aborted shock with detection of VF (FD). The short charge time between FD and CE markers is caused by a high residual voltage output capacitor after previous aborted shocks. Postshock oversensing is the typical early sign of inner insulation failure in this coaxial defibrillation electrode. FS, fibrillation zone sensing; VS, ventricular sensing; VR, ventricular refractory event. (From Swerdlow CD, Friedman PA. Advanced ICD troubleshooting: Part II. PACE 29:70-96, 2006, with permission.)

nonsustained VT will be detected. It is corrected by increasing the postpacing ventricular blanking period.

Oversensing of spontaneous T waves often occurs in the setting of low-amplitude R waves, because the sensitivity of the sensing threshold is not adequately raised due to the low-amplitude preceding R wave.[71] Further, patients with low-amplitude R waves may require lower minimum sensing thresholds to ensure reliable sensing of VF. T-wave oversensing in this setting is a warning that detection of VF may be unreliable. The ventricular lead should be revised if the safety margin for sensing of VF is insufficient.

Specific programming features may be used to reduce T-wave oversensing if the R-wave amplitude is low, provided that detection of VF is reliable. (1) St. Jude ICDs provide a programmable "Threshold Start" and "Decay Delay," which are designed to reduce oversensing of spontaneous T waves. These features may

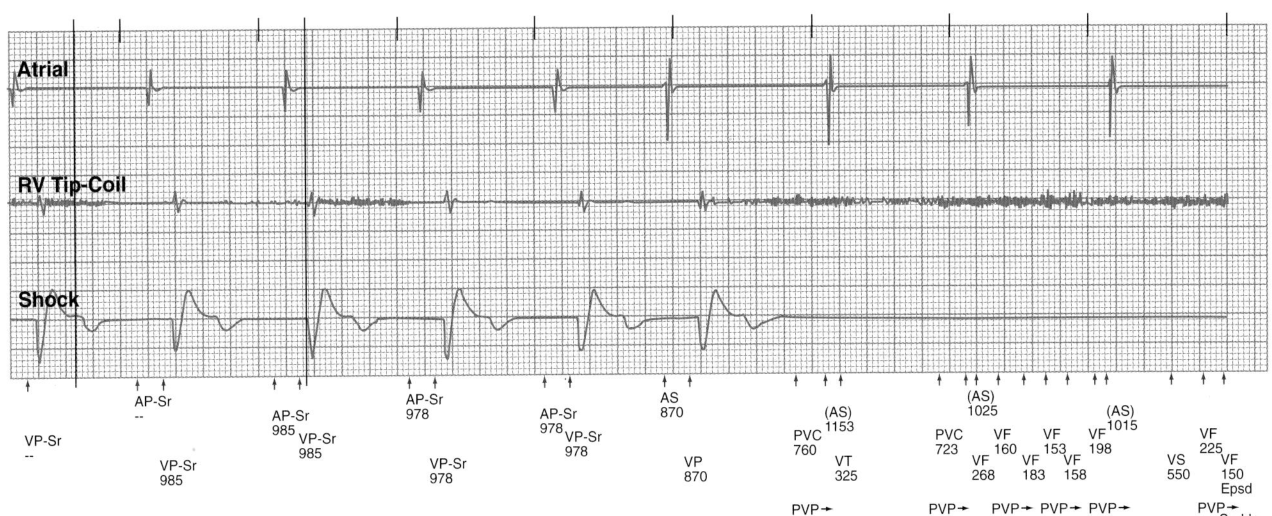

Figure 3-40. Oversensing of diaphragmatic myopotentials. Atrial EGM, integrated right ventricular (RV) Tip-Coil bipolar sensing EGM, high-voltage (Shock) EGM, and marker channels from a Guidant Prizm II ICD in a patient with complete heart block are shown. Low-amplitude, high-frequency signals are recorded on the integrated bipolar channel, inhibiting pacing and resulting in inappropriate detection of ventricular fibrillation (VF) at right (labeled Epsd, for episode start/end). Oversensing of diaphragmatic myopotentials usually occurs after long diastolic intervals or after ventricular-paced events when amplifier sensitivity or gain is maximal. Repositioning of the lead eliminated the problem. AS, atrial-sensed event; AP, atrial-paced event; VP, ventricular-paced event; PVC, premature ventricular complex; PVP→ = extension of postventricular atrial refractory period (PVARP); Sr, sensed refractory event.

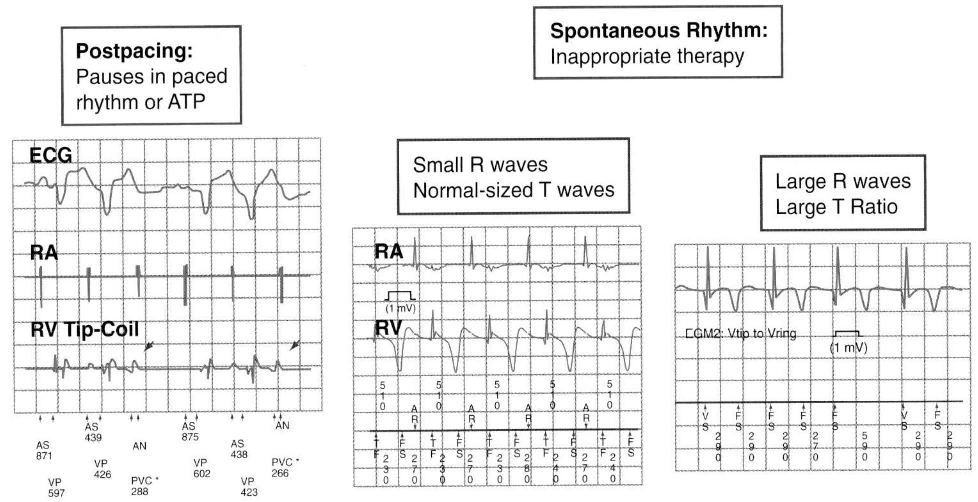

Figure 3-41. Classification of T-wave oversensing. Left panel, *Postpacing oversensing results in inhibition of pacing. Inhibition of antitachycardia pacing may also occur.* Middle and right panels, *T-wave oversensing in spontaneous rhythm can result in inappropriate detection of ventricular tachycardia or ventricular fibrillation. Management often depends on whether the R waves are small* (middle panel) *or large* (right panel). *See text for details.*

be helpful even if the R wave is small (Fig. 3-42). (2) The apparent alternation of ventricular EGM morphologies caused by T-wave oversensing may be exploited to prevent inappropriate detection of VT. The SVT-VT morphology discriminator may be programmed "on" to classify alternate EGMs as "sinus" and thereby withhold inappropriate detection. The long-term reliability of this approach is not established; but it may be sufficient to prevent inappropriate therapy due to rare episodes of T-wave oversensing. (3) Occasionally, the R-T and T-R intervals differ sufficiently that the stability algorithm may be used to reject T-wave oversensing, but this is rare in sinus tachycardia. (4) Rarely, T-wave oversensing can be eliminated by forcing ventricular pacing. This alters the sequence of repolarization and may reduce T-wave amplitude. However, unnecessary ventricular pacing may result in adverse, desynchronizing hemodynamic effects.[72,73] Often, lead revision or

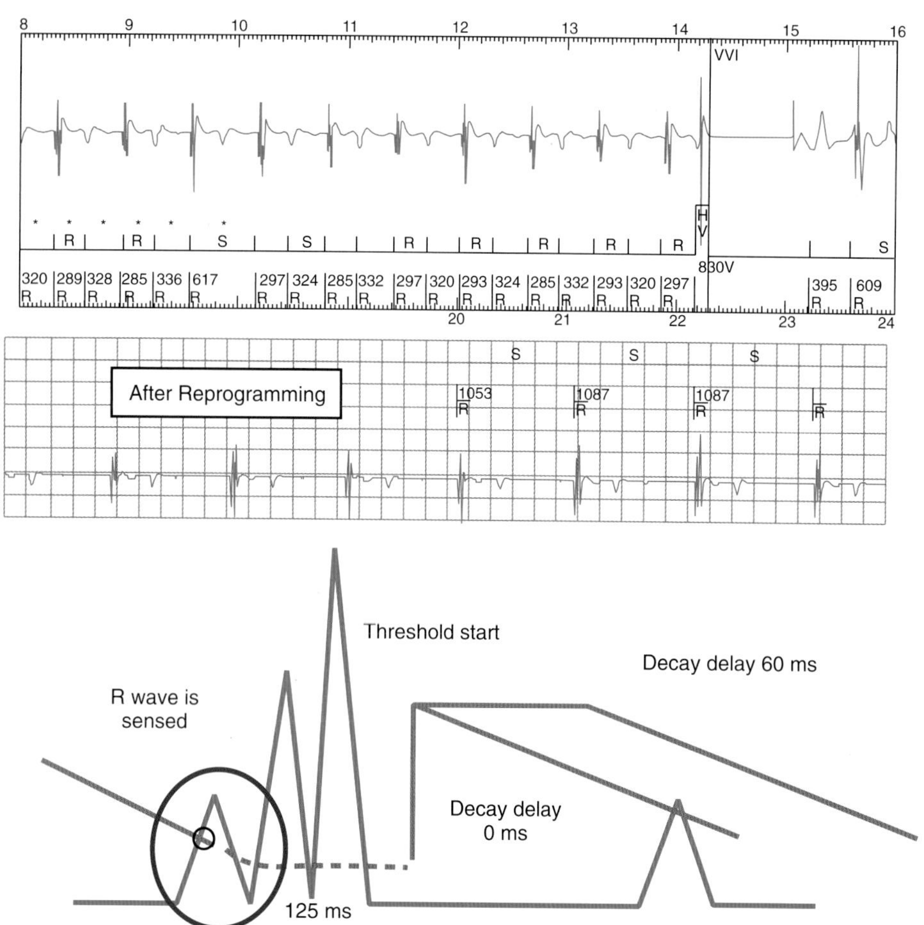

Figure 3-42. Specific programmable features to correct T-wave oversensing. Upper panel, *Stored EGM from a St. Jude ICD showing inappropriate shock for sinus tachycardia with T-wave oversensing. The lower strip was recorded from the programmer after reprogramming of the Decay Delay from 0 to 220 msec.* Lower panel, *Diagram of programmable features to avoid and correct T-wave oversensing in St. Jude ICDs. Automatic Sensitivity Control begins to adjust sensing at the end of the 125-msec ventricular blanking period. Both the initial sensitivity (Threshold Start as percentage of R-wave amplitude) and the time delay before onset of linear decrease in sensing threshold (increase in sensitivity) are programmable parameters. (From Swerdlow CD, Friedman PA: Advanced ICD troubleshooting: Part I. PACE 28:1322-1346, 2005, with permission.)*

the addition of a separate pace/sense lead is necessary to ensure detection of VF without T-wave oversensing. If the defibrillation lead is replaced, a true bipolar lead may be preferred, because T-wave oversensing with true bipolar leads is less frequent than with integrated bipolar leads.[4]

The methods used to avoid T-wave oversensing in the presence of small R waves are as effective or more effective in the presence of large R waves. In Medtronic ICDs, a small decrease in programmed sensitivity (i.e., an increase in the programmed sensitivity threshold value) may prevent T-wave oversensing by the implicit effect on the starting value for threshold decay. "Slow" Automatic Gain Control in Guidant ICDs is particularly effective for reducing the likelihood of T-wave oversensing after large R waves.

In many cases, *oversensing of diaphragmatic myopotentials* may be corrected by reducing ventricular sensitivity, provided that VF sensing and detection are reliable at the reduced level of sensitivity. Occasionally, correction of diaphragmatic oversensing requires insertion of a new rate-sensing electrode.

Automatic Optimization of Pacemaker Function

Pacemakers and ICDs incorporate special algorithms to prevent serious errors in pacemaker function such as inhibition during oversensing, inappropriately high pacing rates due to tracking of atrial tachyarrhythmias, unnecessary ventricular pacing in patients with intact AV conduction, and loss of pacemaker capture. *Ventricular safety pacing* prevents inappropriate pacemaker inhibition caused by ventricular oversensing of atrial pacing stimuli (crosstalk). *Noise reversion* to fixed-rate pacing prevents pacemaker inhibition during continuous ventricular oversensing. *Automatic mode switching* in dual-chamber pacing systems helps avoid inappropriate tracking of high atrial rates during atrial tachyarrhythmias.

Ventricular Safety Pacing and Noise Reversion

Ventricular safety pacing prevents inappropriate inhibition of ventricular pacing after atrial paced events. This feature augments the protection provided by cross-chamber blanking after atrial pacing stimuli. If a ventricular event is sensed after the delivery of an atrial pacing stimulus in a "nonphysiologic" period (10-100 msec) during the AV delay, a ventricular pacing stimulus is delivered at the end of the nonphysiologic time period (usually 110 msec). This prevents pacemaker crosstalk from causing inhibition of ventricular pacing output, but it may also result in (noncaptured) ventricular pacing immediately after true ventricular events that occur during the AV delay. Because the ven-

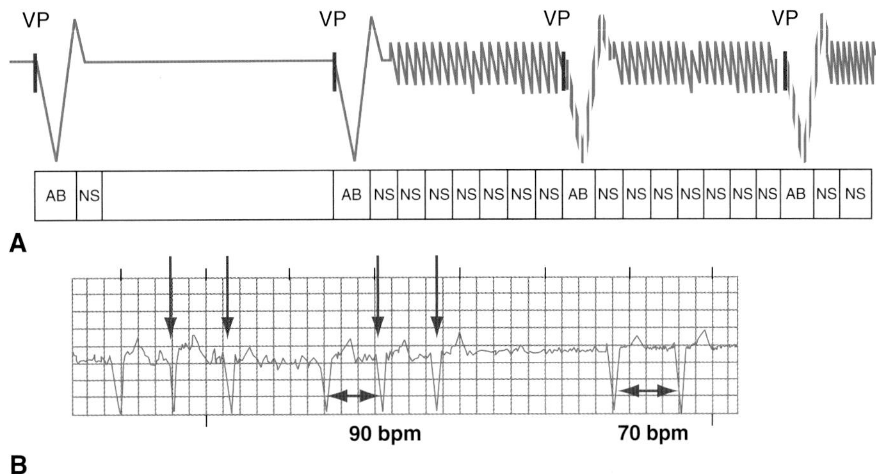

Figure 3-43. ***A,*** *Extension of refractory period due to detection of noise during the noise-sampling (NS) portion of the ventricular refractory period. The first portion of the ventricular refractory period is absolute (AB). When suprathreshold signals are seen during the NS portion of the ventricular refractory period, a new NS window is initiated, "retriggering" the ventricular refractory period by a duration equal to the NS window. Continuous extension of the ventricular refractory period invokes noise reversion pacing at the programmed reversion rate.* ***A,*** *Normal VVI pacing at 60 bpm on the left. When electromagnetic interference begins, the ventricular refractory period is continuously retriggered, and noise reversion pacing starts at 90 bpm.* ***B,*** *Combination of ventricular inhibition and noise reversion. The noise reversion rate of this VVI pacemaker is 90 bpm, and the base rate is programmed at 70 bpm. Beats with arrows indicate noise reversion pacing caused by continuous retriggering of the ventricular refractory period, as in* ***A.*** *Some beats are slower than 70 bpm due to intermittent (not continuous) oversensing of noise such that ventricular refractory periods are not continuously retriggered. (****B,*** *Adapted from Sweesy MW, Holland JL, Smith KW: Electromagnetic interference in cardiac rhythm management devices. AACN Clin Issues 15:391-403, 2004.)*

tricular pacing stimulus is delivered only 110 msec after the atrial stimulus, such safety paces often are delivered at a time when the ventricle is refractory. Ventricular safety pacing is especially likely to occur during atrial undersensing, during AF, or during a junctional rhythm.

Pacemakers also contain algorithms to protect against prolonged inhibition of ventricular pacing due to oversensing. Noise sampling windows (30-60 msec in duration) are used during the blanking periods to identify spurious signals and cause the device to change to an asynchronous "reversion" pacing mode, to ensure ventricular backup pacing.[74] Noise reversion operation is particularly important for unipolar sensing, which is more likely than bipolar sensing to exhibit oversensing of extracardiac signals (Fig. 3-43).[75]

Automatic Mode Switching to Avoid Ventricular Tracking of Atrial Tachyarrhythmias

Pacemakers programmed to dual-chamber synchronous pacing modes may use automatic algorithms to initiate a temporary change to a nontracking pacing mode during paroxysmal atrial tachyarrhythmias, to avoid inappropriately high ventricular pacing rates. Different methods of detecting atrial tachyarrhythmias are employed by different devices.[76,77] These methods can be classified into five different categories (Table 3-1 and Fig. 3-44); their performance characteristics have been reviewed.[77] Accurate atrial sensing is critical to appropriate mode switching, because all methods depend on measurement of atrial rate or A:V patterns or both. The atrial sensing configuration (unipolar versus bipolar), programmed atrial sensitivity, and atrial blanking periods influence the methods used by the various manufacturers and their performance for detection of atrial tachyarrhythmias. Algorithms to recognize repetitive blanking of atrial events during atrial flutter allow mode switching to occur more rapidly when this condition is confirmed (Fig. 3-45). No matter what method is employed, poor atrial sensing will degrade atrial tachyarrhythmia detection performance.[76-79]

Mode-switching algorithms and their diagnostics have been used as a surrogate marker for atrial tachyarrhythmia detection in patients with dual-chamber pacemakers.[80,81] A Holter monitoring study of 40 patients with bipolar pacemakers demonstrated that mode-switching diagnostics appropriately identified 53 of 54 (98.1%) true atrial tachyarrhythmias with only one short (13-second) false mode-switching episode.[81] Other studies have reviewed stored pacemaker EGMs and found high percentages of inappropriate mode switching due to atrial oversensing.[82,83] Care must be taken when relying on mode-switching diagnostics before concluding that atrial tachyarrhythmias actually are occurring. Major clinical decisions, such as starting anticoagulation, should be based on analysis of stored intracardiac atrial EGMs whenever possible. Devices with long PVAB periods or low atrial sensitivity may fail to switch modes if a substantial fraction of atrial events are undersensed. Oversensing of FFRWs or of

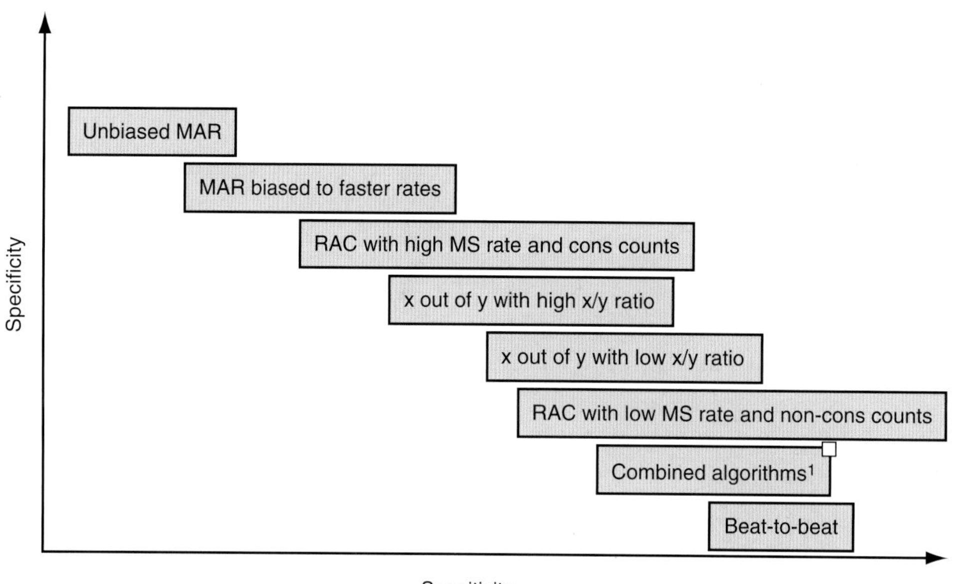

Figure 3-44. Sensitivity and specificity of automatic mode-switching (MS) algorithms for atrial tachyarrhythmia detection. Relative performances of the five different classes of algorithms (see Table 3-1) are shown; performance of the mean atrial rate (MAR), rate and count (RAC), and x out of y algorithms are shown twice to emphasize performance variability with specific parameter selections. Algorithms that use MAR calculation favor specificity over sensitivity but are generally slower-acting than algorithms that favor sensitivity (e.g., beat-to-beat). Atrial events with short and long atrial cycle lengths equally affect atrial rate estimation in "unbiased" MAR algorithms; long atrial cycle lengths have less impact on atrial rate estimation in "biased" MAR calculations, to reduce the impact of atrial undersensing. Cons, consecutive; non-cons, nonconsecutive. (From Israel CW: Analysis of mode switching algorithms in dual chamber pacemakers. PACE 25:380-393, 2002, with permission.)

TABLE 3-1. Algorithms for Detecting Atrial Tachyarrhythmias for Automatic Pacemaker Mode Switching

Algorithm Type	Pacemaker System	Algorithm Description
Mean atrial rate (MAR)	Medtronic Thera/Kappa 400 St. Jude-Pacesetter Trilogy DR St. Jude-Pacesetter Affinity DR	Identifies atrial tachyarrhythmia when MAR exceeds programmed threshold. Estimate of MAR is increased by 8-25 msec on short atrial intervals and decreased by 23-39 msec on long atrial intervals
"Rate and count" (RAC)	Guidant-CPI Vigor Guidant-CPI Pulsar/Discovery Intermedics Marathon Medtronic AT 500 model 7253 Sorin MiniSwing Sorin Living Teletronics Meta 1254 Teletronics Meta 1256	Identifies atrial tachyarrhythmias when a preset number of atrial beats (5-11 beats, sometimes programmable) exceeds a programmable rate threshold. May or may not require confirmation for a certain number of beats for mode switch to occur
"X out of Y"	Biotronik Inos Biotronik Logos ELA Chorus/Talent	Identifies atrial tachyarrhythmias when X out of Y atrial beats have a rate faster than the rate threshold or have short V-A intervals
Beat-to-beat	Biotronik Actros/Kairos Teletronics Meta 1250 Vitatron Diamond/Clarity	Switches mode based on single short atrial interval or short V-A interval
Combined algorithms	Guidant-CPI Pulsar/Discovery Medtronic Kappa 700	Combination of RAC or X out of Y and beat-to-beat modes for special cases

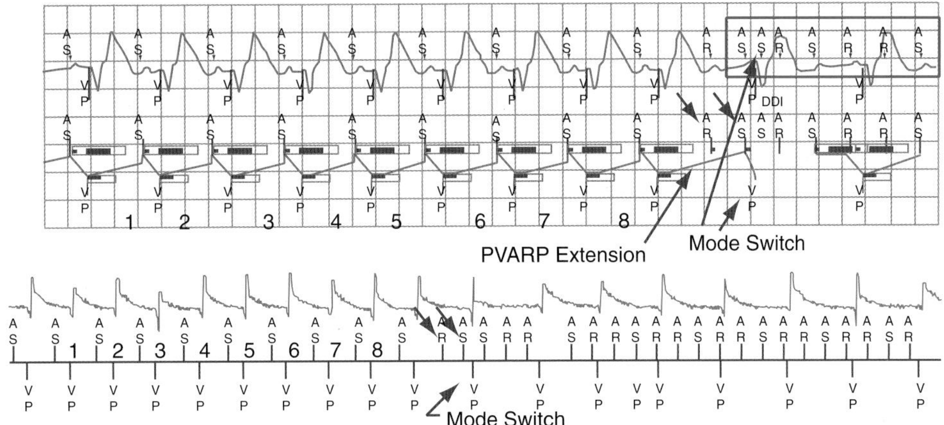

Figure 3-45. Algorithm to prevent upper rate limit tracking of alternate atrial EGMs during atrial flutter (Blanked Flutter Search) even if EGMs are recorded in the postventricular atrial blanking period (PVAB), when sensing cannot occur. Upper panel shows simulated electrocardiogram (ECG) and ladder diagram. Black horizontal bars denote blanking periods, and white bars denote refractory periods for atrium (upper bars) and ventricle (lower bars). Lower panel shows stored ventricular EGM and dual-chamber EGM markers from a clinical event. Upper panel, The intention of this algorithm is to infer that alternate atrial EGMs are "hiding" in the PVAB. To determine whether this is occurring, the algorithm transiently interrupts atrial tracking to assess the atrial rhythm when it is likely that alternate atrial intervals are occurring in the PVAB. The specific criterion is that the measured A-A interval is both less than twice the sum of the sensed AV interval and the PVAB and less than the mode switch interval for 8 beats. When this occurs, the algorithm extends the postventricular atrial refractory period (PVARP extension). The next atrial EGM that would have been tracked is now in the PVARP (AR marker, first arrow) and is not tracked. The next atrial flutter EGM is sensed because it no longer times in the PVAB (AS marker, second arrow).The pacemaker then switches mode rapidly (DDI). Lower panel, In this stored clinical EGM, ventricular intervals are numbered to correspond to those in the simulation in the upper panel. As in the upper panel, the first arrow (AR) corresponds to PVARP extension, and the second arrow (AS) corresponds to a sensed atrial flutter EGM that would have been blanked in tracking mode. Mode switching follows immediately. VP, ventricular paced event.

EMI or noise in unipolar atrial sensing systems can also cause false-positive mode switching.

Algorithms to Reduce Ventricular Pacing

Conventional DDDR pacing often results in an unnecessarily high percentage of ventricular pacing. Studies have shown that unnecessary ventricular pacing contributes to adverse clinical outcomes (e.g., heart failure hospitalizations) and increased risk of AF.[72,73] Algorithms to adaptively lengthen AV intervals to promote intrinsic conduction (and reduce ventricular pacing) are available, and studies have demonstrated some reduction of ventricular pacing.[84-87] Medtronic and ELA Medical (Sorin Group, Munich, Germany) have developed new pacing modes (MVP and AAIRsafe) that may surpass the performance of automatic AV search algorithms by operating in AAIR mode during normal operation, with mode switching to DDDR to prevent ventricular asystole if AV block occurs.[88,89] Single beats of AV conduction failure are allowed by both algorithms, with switching to DDD mode occurring only with higher levels of AV conduction block. Once switched to DDD mode, both algorithms test for AV conduction periodically, in order to avoid unnecessary ventricular pacing for transient AV block that spontaneously resolves. Clinical studies have demonstrated impressive reductions in cumulative percent ventricular pacing with these new methods, compared with DDD pacing modes (73% versus 0.2% and 81% versus 4%).[88,89]

Automatic Assessment of Pacemaker Capture

Automatic sensing of the evoked response (local myocardial depolarization) that results from a pacing stimulus allows for verification of myocardial capture. However, sensing of the evoked response is obscured by the decaying polarization afterpotential that follows the pacing stimulus.[90] This polarization artifact can be attenuated by use of high-capacitance, low-polarization leads or by use of multiphasic pacing impulses to neutralize the postpacing polarization capacitance. Figure 3-46 shows an example of the evoked response signal combined with polarization artifact after a pacing stimulus.[90] To minimize the afterpotential from ventricular pacing stimuli and improve detection of the evoked response, some manufacturers use a smaller-output capacitor. This approach further enhances the accuracy of evoked response detection.

Ventricular capture verification has not yet been incorporated into commercially released ICDs, but not because of technical limitations. One study has shown that the polarization artifact that challenges evoked response detection in bipolar pacing leads is eliminated or reduced by use of the RV coil-to-can EGM available in ICD systems.[91]

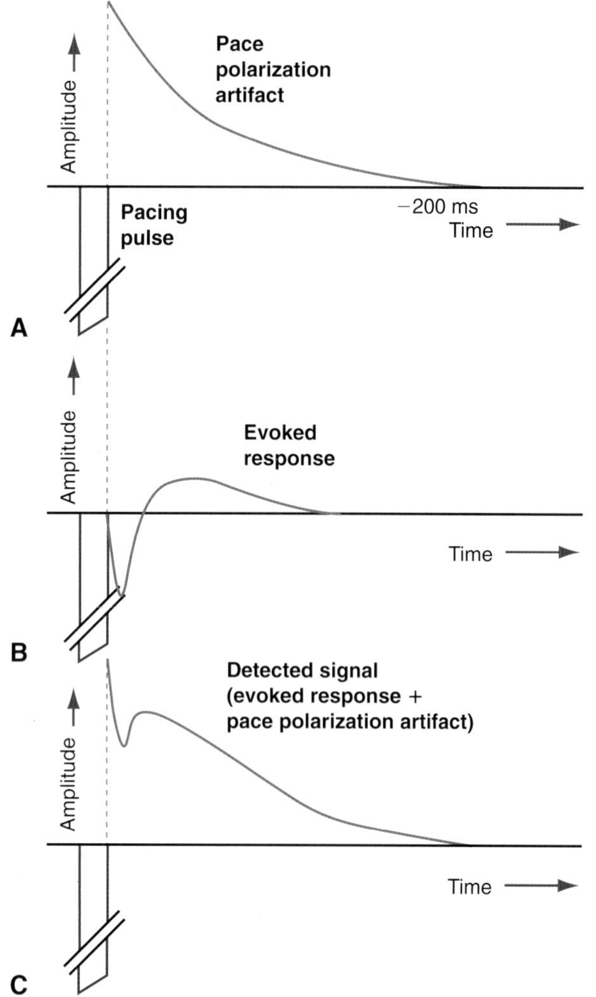

Figure 3-46. Local myocardial depolarization (evoked response) is obscured by the postpacing polarization artifact. ***A,*** *The pace polarization artifact is observed as a positive deflection that generally decreases toward the initial cell potential within about 200 msec after the pacing pulse.* ***B,*** *The evoked response is present immediately after the pacing pulse and shows an initial negative deflection.* ***C,*** *The signal sensed by the pacemaker is the summation of the pace polarization artifact and the evoked response. (From de Voogt WG, Vonk BF, Albers BA, et al: Understanding capture detection. Europace 6:561-569, 2004, with permission.)*

There are two different ventricular capture verification schemes in today's pacemakers: beat-to-beat approaches that monitor capture almost continuously, and daily measurements that test pacing thresholds intermittently, for example, once every several hours. Algorithms that perform periodic capture threshold algorithms typically set the pacing output at twice the threshold to avoid transient loss of capture until the next test. Beat-to-beat capture management algorithms can adjust pacing outputs to values that are just above pacing thresholds. More high-output backup pacing stimuli may be delivered with transient loss of capture.[92]

Atrial capture detection using the evoked response is much more dependent on the use of low-polarization electrodes than is ventricular capture detection.[93] The atrial evoked response is much smaller than the ventricular evoked response, and reliable detection is a major barrier to widespread clinical use. An alternative method has been proposed that relies on critical timing of atrial and/or ventricular response to atrial pacing stimuli during normal sinus rhythm (Fig. 3-47). In ambulatory patients, this method has been reported to perform comparably with manual atrial pacing threshold measurements without causing atrial proarrhythmia.[94]

Basics of Detection of Ventricular Tachycardia/Fibrillation

Figure 3-48 provides an overview of the structure of VT/VF detection algorithms. Presently, initial detection of tachycardia is based on rate and duration. The minimum duration of tachycardia required for detection is programmable, either directly (in seconds) or indirectly by setting the number of ventricular intervals required for detection. A tachycardia *episode* begins when the minimum rate and duration criteria are satisfied. During detection, more computationally intensive features of detection algorithms, such as morphology analysis, are activated so the power required to operate them does not deplete the battery of the ICD.

Ventricular Tachycardia and Ventricular Fibrillation Rate Detection Zones

Tiered-therapy ICDs have up to three ventricular rate detection zones that permit programming of zone-specific therapies and SVT-VT discriminators (Fig. 3-49). The duration of a rapid ventricular rate required for detection is programmable independently in at least the slowest and fastest zone (see "Zones and Zone Boundaries"). The two slower zones are classified as VT zones, and the fastest one as a VF zone. Counters in each zone may be independent, or sensed events in one zone may increment counters in all slower zones. The latter approach minimizes the risk of prolonged detection times if successive VT intervals are classified in different zones. An alternative method for classifying rhythms that straddle zone boundaries is a combined-count (summation) criterion, which is satisfied if a sufficient fraction of intervals is in either zone.[95] Some ICDs also use regularity of the ventricular rhythm to discriminate between VT and VF in the two fastest rate zones.

Ventricular Rate and Counting Methods

The specific methods used to count ventricular intervals vary and influence the sensitivity and specificity of VT detection. Initial detection in the VF zone must be tolerant of undersensing for low-amplitude VF EGMs. Detection usually occurs when a certain percentage (typically 70% to 80%) of intervals in a sliding window (usually 10 to 24 intervals) fulfill the programmed rate criterion. Most ICD manufacturers also use this "X out of Y" counting in the slower (VT) zones, but one manufacturer (Medtronic) requires that all

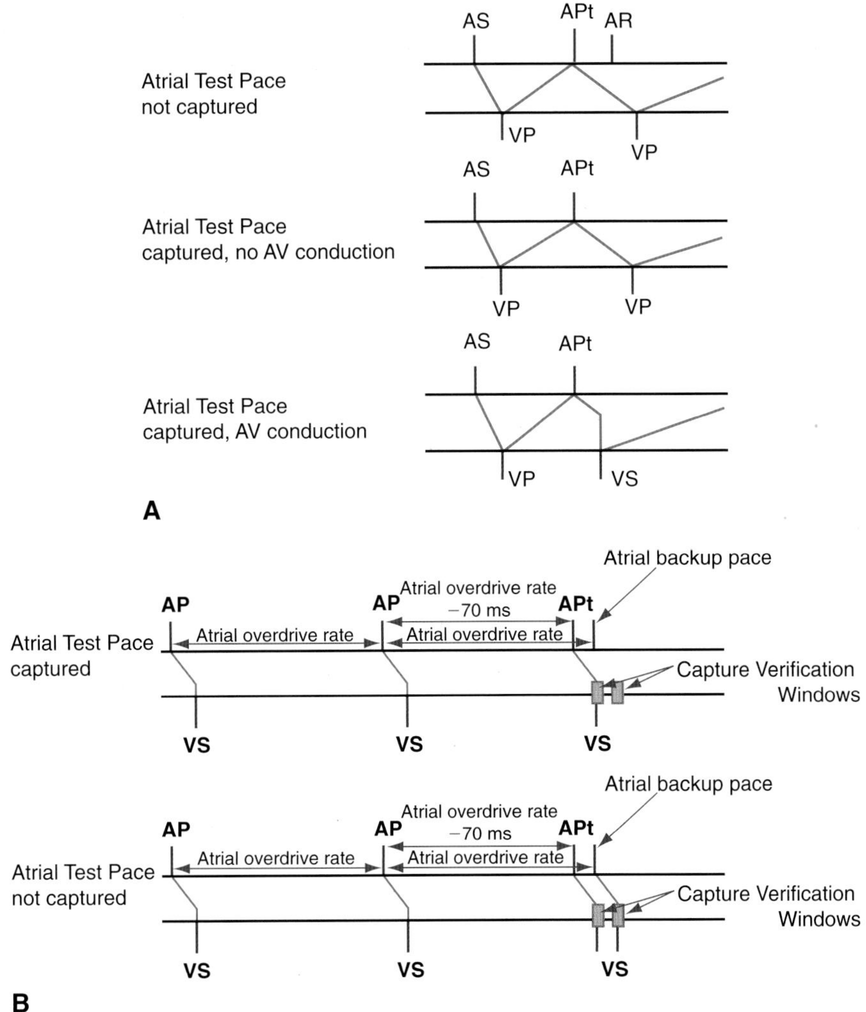

Figure 3-47. Atrial capture verification method that relies on atrial or ventricular responses to atrial pacing. A high-level control algorithm determines which of two timing assessment methods should be used, based on the recent history of atrial pacing, atrial sensing, and atrioventricular (AV) conduction. At least two test paces are required to verify capture or loss of capture. Failed, inconclusive, or aborted threshold tests are repeated after a delay. This method cannot measure atrial capture during atrial-paced–ventricular-paced rhythms or rhythms with irregular atrial or ventricular cycle lengths. ***A,*** *The Atrial Chamber Reset method is used if recent history indicates primarily atrial sensed events. A premature atrial test pace (APt) is delivered, and the resulting atrial timing is observed. An atrial refractory event within 10 bpm after the prior intrinsic atrial rate suggests loss of capture* (top panel). *The lack of an atrial refractory event in this time period suggests resetting of the atrial timing and atrial capture* (middle and bottom panels). ***B,*** *The AV conduction check method is used if the recent history indicates that AV conduction is present. The average AV conduction time is measured before delivery of the APt. A backup atrial pace at the operating atrial output is also delivered 70 msec after the APt. The algorithm looks for ventricular sensed events in one of two capture verification windows (40 msec in duration) that are placed relative to the APt and the backup atrial-paced events based on the average AV conduction time. A ventricular event sensed in the first capture verification window suggests capture by the APt* (top panel). *Lack of a sensed ventricular event in the first capture verification window and presence of a ventricular event in the second window is evidence of noncapture by the APt* (bottom panel).

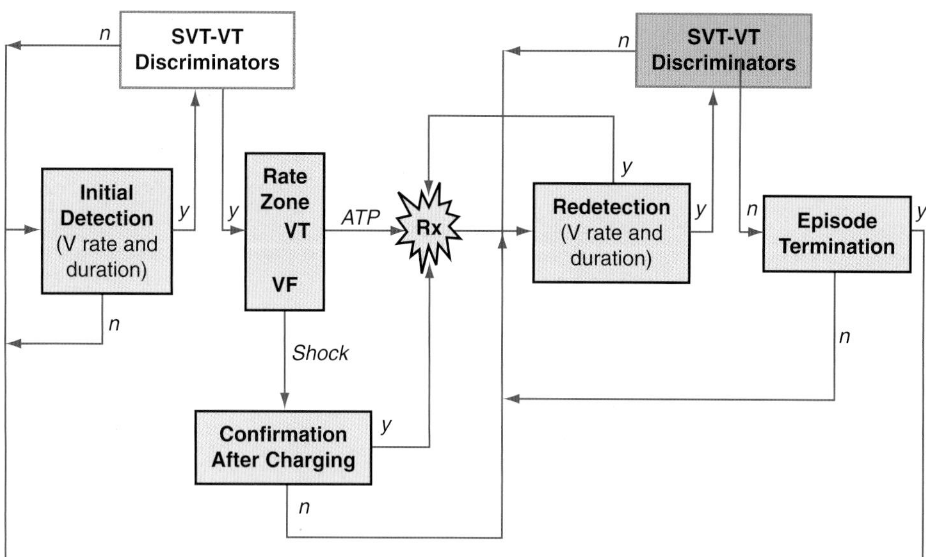

Figure 3-48. Overview of ICD detection algorithm. See text for details. Algorithms apply varying degrees of SVT-VT discrimination to redetection. n, no; y, yes; ATP, antitachycardia pacing; Rx, antitachycardia therapy; SVT, supraventricular tachycardia; V, ventricular; VF, ventricular fibrillation; VT, ventricular tachycardia.

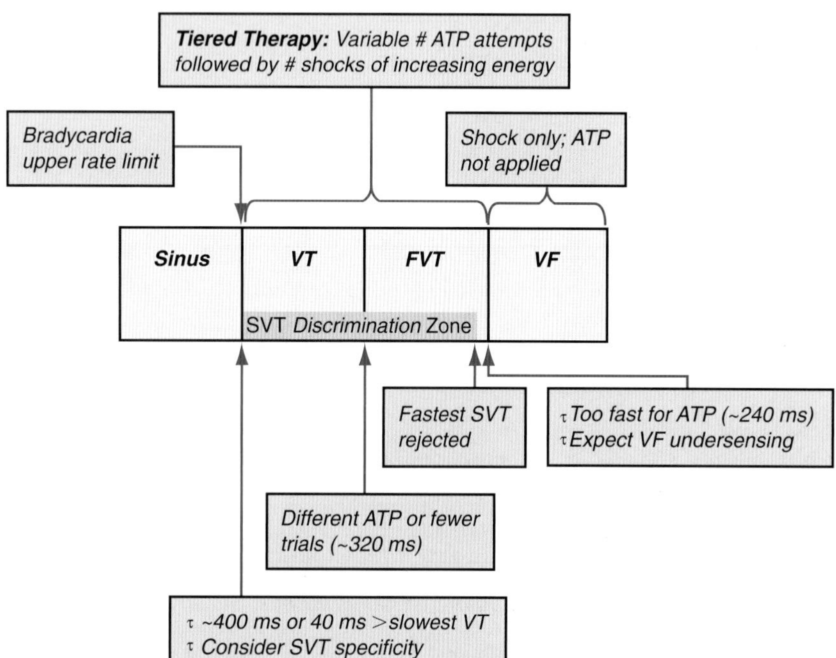

Figure 3-49. ICD rate detection zones. See text for details. Some ICDs permit programming of an additional monitor-only zone. ATP, antitachycardia pacing; FVT, fast VT; SVT, supraventricular tachycardia; VF, ventricular fibrillation; VT, ventricular tachycardia.

intervals exceed the rate criterion to detect slow VT. This consecutive-interval method diminishes inappropriate detection of AF without compromising sensitivity for detection of regular, monomorphic VT.[95-97] St. Jude ICDs classify intervals based both on the last interval and on the average of the last four intervals (Figs. 3-50 and 3-51). A potential advantage of this method is that averaging minimizes the effects of intermittent undersensing.[95]

SVT-VT Discriminators

SVT-VT discriminators are a programmable subset of an ICD's detection algorithm for VT/VF. They withhold ventricular ATP or shocks for SVT to improve specificity of therapy. Usually, they differ from the SVT detection algorithms used to switch modes during bradycardia pacing or to deliver atrial therapy for AF or atrial flutter.

Confirmation, Redetection, and Episode Termination

Once a tachycardia has been classified as ventricular in origin, the therapy that is appropriate for the zone is delivered. ATP is delivered immediately, but shocks require capacitor charging, which takes 6 to 15 seconds for maximum-energy shocks. The first shock in a shock sequence is "noncommitted," meaning that it may be aborted during charging if the detection algorithm iden-

Figure 3-50. Interval classification based on current interval and average interval (St. Jude). The table shows classification of ventricular intervals by St. Jude ICDs based on both the value of the current interval and the average of the current interval with the preceding three intervals (average interval). Detection zones from slowest to fastest are Sinus, Tach A (slower ventricular tachycardia [VT] zone), Tach B (faster VT zone), and Fib (ventricular fibrillation [VF]). If both the current and the average interval are in the same zone, the current interval is classified in that zone. If they are in different VT or VF zones, the current interval is classified in the faster zone. If one interval is in the sinus zone and the other is in a VT or VF zone, the current interval is not classified (not binned).

		Current Interval				
		Fib	Tach B	Tach A	Tach	Sinus
Average Interval	Fib	Fib	Fib	Fib	Fib	Not Binned
	Tach B	Fib	Tach B	Tach B	N/A	Not Binned
	Tach A	Fib	Tach B	Tach A	N/A	Not Binned
	Tach	Fib	N/A	N/A	Tach	Not Binned
	Sinus	Not Binned	Not Binned	Not Binned	Not Binned	Sinus

tifies termination of the arrhythmia during or immediately after charging of the high-energy capacitors (Fig. 3-52). *Confirmation or reconfirmation* is the brief process that occurs after charging by which ICDs determine whether to deliver or abort the first shock in a sequence. In all ICDs, the confirmation algorithm delivers the stored shock if a few intervals immediately after charge completion are shorter than the programmed VT interval (St. Jude and Guidant) or are 60 msec longer than the VT interval (Medtronic) (Fig. 3-53). Therefore, the first VF shock is effectively "committed" if the VT interval (or, in some ICDs, the Monitor-Only interval) is programmed to a long cycle length.[98,99] Depending on the manufacturer and the programming, each shock after the first shock may be "committed," meaning that it is always delivered if the capacitor charges. A shock is also committed if VT or VF is detected after a diverted shock and before episode termination.[74]

Redetection is the process by which ICDs determine whether VT or VF detection criteria remain satisfied after therapy is delivered. Typically, the duration for redetection is less than that for initial detection and is independently programmable. Episodes continue after each tiered therapy until either a tachyarrhythmia is redetected to initiate the next therapy or the rhythm is classified as normal ("sinus"), resulting in *episode termination*. Episode termination is based on (slow) rate and duration. Atrial tachyarrhythmia episodes in atrial antiarrhythmic pacemakers and ICDs are based on similar criteria corresponding to AF or AT/atrial flutter.

SVT-VT Discrimination in Ventricular ICDs

Building Blocks for SVT-VT Discrimination

ICDs analyze information derived from a sequence of sensed atrial and ventricular EGMs to detect VT/VF and discriminate ventricular arrhythmias from SVT. These algorithms operate in a stepwise manner, using a series of physiologically relevant logical "building blocks" based on the timing relationships and morphology of sensed EGMs. The focus here is on the tool kit provided by these building blocks rather than on the specific details of proprietary algorithms, which have been reported and reviewed elsewhere in detail.[100]

Table 3-2 presents a list of the building blocks, which may also be used by pacemakers and atrial antitachycardia pacemakers or atrial ICDs. Detection algorithms combine complementary building blocks to form the final detection decision. Each building block has advantages and limitations. Some are redundant, and some interact. The interactions vary depending on the order in which they are applied. Clinicians and algorithm designers must consider these issues to understand tradeoffs in clinical performance.

Single-Chamber Ventricular Building Blocks

The first five building blocks in Table 3-2 apply to single-chamber ICDs or the ventricular component of dual-chamber ICDs. The *R-R interval+duration* analysis building block classifies ventricular intervals into zones by programmable cycle length (or rate) thresholds. All single- and dual-chamber devices use cycle length or rate in combination with tachyarrhythmia *duration* as the most basic method of detection. When used alone, R-R interval+duration analysis provides the highest sensitivity for detection of VT or VF but cannot discriminate ventricular arrhythmias from SVT. The *R-R regularity* building block is used to discriminate between regular ventricular intervals due to monomorphic VT and irregular ventricular intervals due to rapidly conducted AF. The *R-R onset* building block is used to discriminate sudden-onset VT from gradual-onset sinus tachycardia. The ventricular EGM *(VEGM) morphology* building block classifies tachyarrhythmias as SVT if morphologic characteristics of the ventricular EGM are similar to those of beats of known

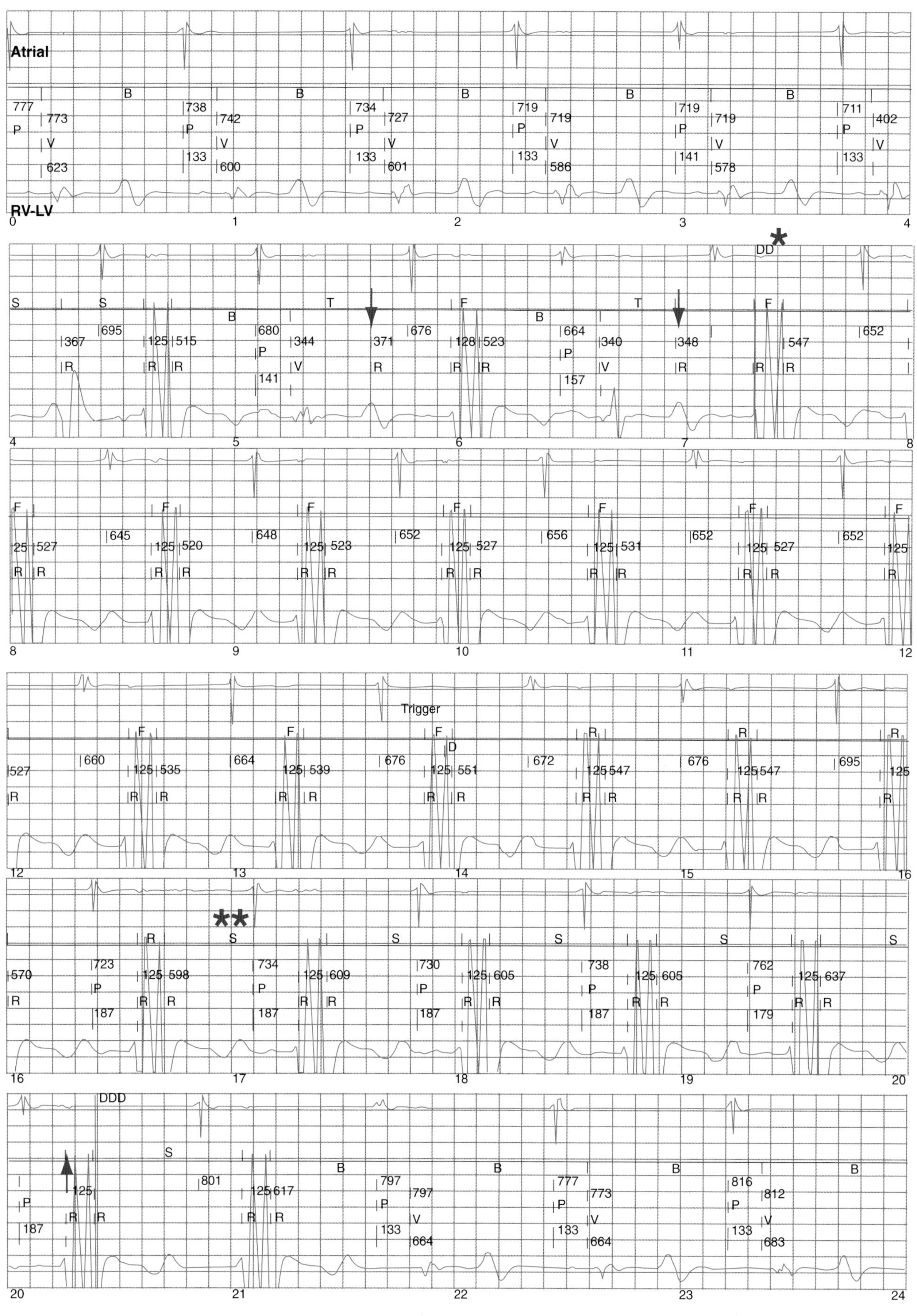
Atrial
RV-LV
DD
Trigger
DDD

Figure 3-51. Illustration of interval classification based on current interval and average interval. T-wave oversensing initiates R-wave double-counting in a St. Jude ICD. The figure shows continuous recording of atrial EGM, event markers, and extended bipolar ventricular EGM (between Y-adapted left ventricular [LV] and right ventricular [RV] tip electrodes). The ICD is programmed with a single ventricular tachycardia (Tach) zone at 345 msec and a ventricular fibrillation (Fib) zone at 290 msec. The top panel shows atrial-sensed, ventricular-paced rhythm. In the second panel, the first ventricular EGM is an interpolated premature ventricular complex (PVC). Ventricular pacing is inhibited after the next P wave because the resultant PVC-V paced interval would have been less than the interval corresponding to the programmed upper rate limit (approximately 450 msec). This results in a conducted R wave that is double-counted at the ventricular blanking period of 125 msec, but this interval is not classified in the VF zone because the interval average of (719 + 402 + 367 + 125)/4 = 403 msec exceeds the Tach detection interval. The third and fifth beats show postpacing T-wave oversensing (down arrows). *The interval ending with the first oversensed T wave is classified in the Tach zone because the interval average is less than 345 msec: (367 + 125 + 516 + 344)/4 = 338 msec. The next ventricular interval, corresponding to the subsequent double-counted R wave, is classified in the Fib zone because the interval average is in the Tach zone ([516 + 344 + 371 + 125]/4 = 339 msec) but the current interval is in the Fib zone. Mode switching to the DDI pacing mode occurs after the counter of Tach + Fib beats equal 4 (DDI,* asterisk*). The third and fourth panels show conducted sinus rhythm after mode switching, with alternate intervals classified in the Fib zone. VF is detected when the Fib counter reaches 12. This counter increments for each interval classified in the Fib zone and is reset to zero by five consecutive sinus intervals. The count of Fib intervals reaches 12 after the third interval in the fourth panel, and Fib is detected (Trigger, D marker), resulting in capacitor charging. However, sinus slowing results in an increase in the average interval, so that the interval average is no longer in the Tach zone. This occurs at the second R wave in the fifth panel (S marker,* double asterisk; *interval average = [125 + 570 + 125 + 596]/4 = 354 msec). Once this occurs, alternate detected intervals are classified as "Sinus" or "Not Binned." The shock is aborted when the count of consecutive binned Sinus intervals reaches 5 at the beginning of the bottom panel (RS = return to sinus,* up arrow*), and this is followed by mode switch to DDD pacing. Note that St. Jude ICDs have a "Bigeminal Avoidance" counter that prevents bigeminal rhythms from being classified as Tach. This counter does not apply in the Fib zone. R, ventricular sensed event; V, ventricular paced event.*

supraventricular origin. Otherwise, it classifies the rhythm as VT. The postpacing interval after *burst ventricular pacing* has been proposed as a method for discriminating between SVT and VT.[101]

Dual-Chamber Building Block: Atrial versus Ventricular Rate

Direct or indirect comparison of atrial and ventricular rates is the cornerstone of most dual-chamber algorithms. The ventricular rate exceeds the atrial rate in more than 80% of VTs in the VT zone of dual-chamber ICDs in most studies.[62,102] Therefore, algorithms that compare atrial and ventricular rates as their first step (Guidant Rhythm ID, St. Jude, and Biotronik [Biotronik GmbH & Co., Berlin]) apply SVT discriminators to fewer than 20% of VTs; this reduces the risk that they will misclassify VT as SVT, provided that the atrial rate is measured correctly. The Medtronic PR Logic indirectly applies a comparison of atrial rate versus ventricular rate by using dual-chamber pattern analysis as the first step to achieve the same result.

Dual-Chamber Building Blocks

The next four building blocks in Table 3-2 are based on combinations of atrial and ventricular information. Their primary role is to discriminate VT with 1:1 V-A conduction from SVT. Their secondary roles are to classify rhythms with stable N:1 AV relationships (stable ratio of N atrial events for each ventricular event) as SVT and to classify isorhythmic tachycardias (with AV dissociation and similar ventricular rate) as VT. The *P-R dissociation* building block can detect the presence of VT during SVT. The *P-R patterns/relationships* building block applies to stable associations of atrial and ventricular events. For tachycardias with 1:1 AV relationships, it analyzes the relative timing of P-R and R-P intervals to classify the rhythm as SVT or VT. It

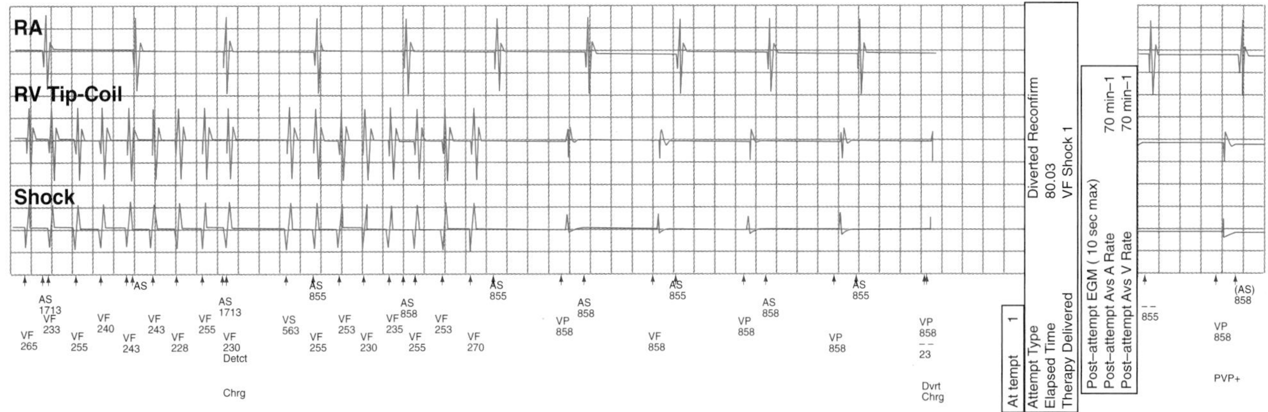

Figure 3-52. Confirmation ("reconfirmation") and aborted shock. Ventricular tachycardia (VT) in the ventricular fibrillation (VF) detection zone is detected and initiates capacitor charging (Chrg) before it terminates spontaneously. The noncommitted shock is diverted (Dvrt Chrg). AS, atrial sensed event; VP, ventricular paced event.

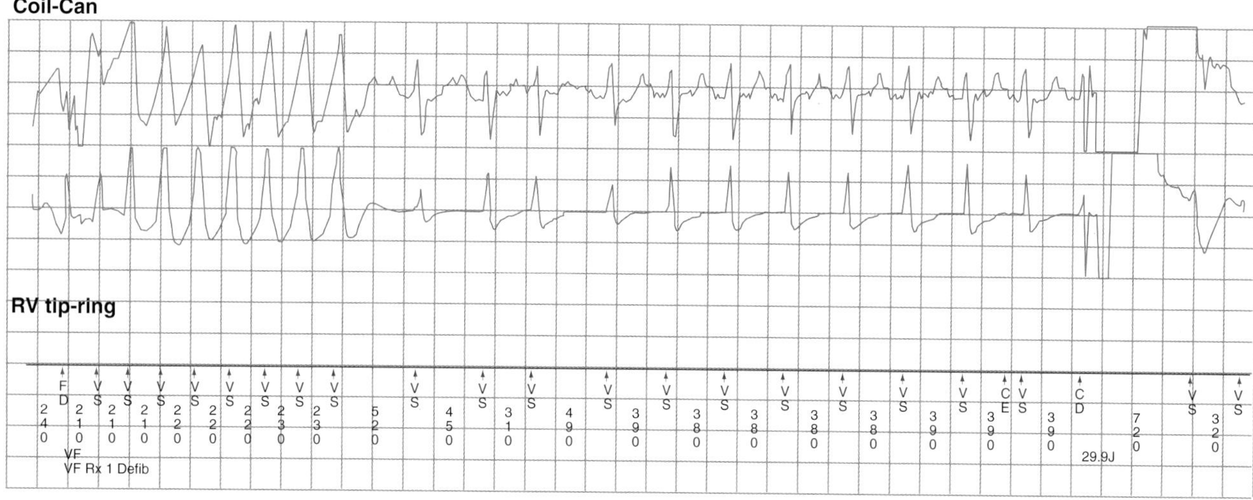

Figure 3-53. Confirmation failure. Two ventricular EGMs and event markers are shown from a single-chamber ICD. The programmed ventricular tachycardia (VT) and ventricular fibrillation (VF) detection intervals are 380 and 320 msec, respectively. Detection of rapid VT as VF results in capacitor charging (VF Rx 1 Defib). After the charging cycle ends (CE), Medtronic ICDs deliver the shock (CD) if the ventricular cycle length after charging is less than the programmed VT interval + 60 msec. In St. Jude and Guidant ICDs, shocks for VF are confirmed if the ventricular cycle length is less than the VT interval. RV, right ventricular. (From Swerdlow CD, Friedman PA: Advanced ICD troubleshooting: Part II. PACE 29:70-96, 2006, with permission.)

also identifies consistent N:1 AV patterns that occur primarily during atrial flutter. The *chamber of origin* building block discriminates between VT and SVT with 1:1 P-R association by identifying whether the tachycardia originates in the atrium or in the ventricle. Usually, at the start of an SVT, there is an intrinsic atrial event in the interval between the last ventricular event in the sinus rate zone and the first ventricular event in the VT zone. Conversely, at the start of spontaneous VT, there is usually no atrial event in this interval. The *response of the opposite chamber to atrial or ventricular pacing* has long been a critical tool in the electrophysiology laboratory for diagnosing tachycardias with 1:1 AV relationship. It has been proposed for use in ICDs.

Single-Chamber Atrial Building Blocks

The final four detection building blocks are the atrial correlates of the single-chamber ventricular building blocks: *P-P interval* (atrial cycle length), *P-P regularity, P-P onset,* and atrial EGM *(AEGM) morphology*. Their primary role is to assist in discriminating rapidly conducted atrial arrhythmias from double tachycardias (simultaneous atrial and ventricular tachyarrhythmias). To date, atrial EGM morphology has not been applied in ICDs to discriminate between antegrade and retrograde conduction.

SVT-VT Discrimination in Single-Chamber ICDs

R-R Interval Regularity

Measures of R-R interval regularity usually are referred to as measures of R-R interval stability or "stability algorithms." Technical details and optimal programmed values differ among manufacturers. Further, specific measures of R-R regularity interact with the method of counting R-R intervals and the duration required for detection. Requiring consecutive R-R intervals or a higher number of intervals to fulfill the rate and regularity criteria improves rejection of AF and increases the risk that detection of VT will be delayed.[96,97,103-107]

Regularity criteria usually reject AF with ventricular rates slower than 170 bpm in the absence of antiarrhythmic drugs; at faster rates, however, they cannot discriminate AF from VT reliably, because R-R intervals in AF are more regular.[103,107] They may prevent detection of VT in the presence of amiodarone or type IC antiarrhythmic drugs.[104,106] These drugs may cause regular VT to become irregular, or they may cause rapid polymorphic VT to slow from the VF zone, where discriminators do not apply, to the VT zone, where regularity discriminators do apply.

R-R regularity may also be used to select the first VT therapy: ATP for regular VT and shock for irregular and presumed VF or polymorphic VT.

Sudden Onset

Measures of abruptness of onset of a tachycardia have high specificity for rejecting sinus tachycardia[103,105-107] but may prevent detection of VT that originates during SVT or VT that starts abruptly with an initial rate below the VT detection limit. In the latter case, the ICD misclassifies the "onset" of the arrhythmia as the gradual acceleration of the VT rate across the VT rate boundary. This criterion does not prevent SVT with sudden onset (e.g., AT) from being treated inappropriately.

Ventricular EGM Morphology

Analysis of ventricular EGM morphology,[60,102,108-110] alone or in combination with stability, probably provides the

TABLE 3-2. **Tachyarrhythmia Detection Building Blocks**

Tachyarrhythmia Detection Building Blocks	Purpose/Information	Potential Weaknesses
Single-chamber ventricular building blocks		
R-R interval+duration	Identifies sustained high ventricular rates	SVT with high ventricular rates that overlap with VT/VF rates
R-R regularity	Discrimination of monomorphic VT (regular cycle lengths) from rapid AF (irregular cycle lengths)	May lose effectiveness as ventricular rates during AF increase; 2:1 atrial flutter has regular R-R intervals; may cause underdetection of VT with irregular R-R intervals
R-R onset	Identifies sudden ventricular rate changes	Not specific for atrial or ventricular tachyarrhythmias; may miss VT arising during sinus tachycardia
VEGM morphology	Abnormal VEGM morphology may indicate ventricular tachyarrhythmias	Confounded by conduction aberrancy or changes in "normal" VEGM morphology
Burst ventricular pacing	Intervals after entrainment of VT by burst pacing are less variable than intervals after burst pacing during SVT	Sensitive to single interval measurement, potential detection time delay, and potential proarrhythmia
Key dual-chamber building block		
Comparison of atrial vs ventricular rate	VT diagnosed if atrial rate is less than ventricular rate	Confounded by atrial undersensing or far-field R-wave oversensing
Dual-chamber building blocks		
P-R dissociation	P-R dissociation usually indicates VT	AV reentrant tachycardia; VT with 1:1 retrograde conduction; AF that conducts rapidly with apparent P-R dissociation
P-R patterns/relationships	Consistent P-R patterns/relationships usually indicate SVT	AV reentrant tachycardia and VT with 1:1 retrograde conduction
Chamber of acceleration	Identifies whether tachycardia initiates in atrium or ventricle	A single oversensed/undersensed event may result in misclassification
Atrial or ventricular pacing, response in opposite chamber	Discrimination of 1:1 rhythms using ventricular response to atrial extrastimuli	Primarily aids diagnosis for 1:1 rhythms; concerns for VT detection delay and proarrhythmia
Single-chamber atrial building blocks		
P-P intervals	Identifies high atrial rates	High atrial rates may be present during true VT/VF
P-P regularity	Regular atrial rate indicates organized atrial activity	Little benefit for ventricular tachyarrhythmia characterization
P-P onset	Identifies sudden atrial rate changes	Not specific for atrial or ventricular tachyarrhythmias (e.g., VT with 1:1 retrograde association)
AEGM morphology	Identifies atrial tachyarrhythmias and/or retrograde conduction	Confounded by far-field R waves and changes in "normal" AEGM morphology

AEGM, atrial electrogram; AF, atrial fibrillation; AV, atrioventricular; SVT, supraventricular tachycardia; VEGM, ventricular electrogram; VF, ventricular fibrillation; VT, ventricular tachycardia.

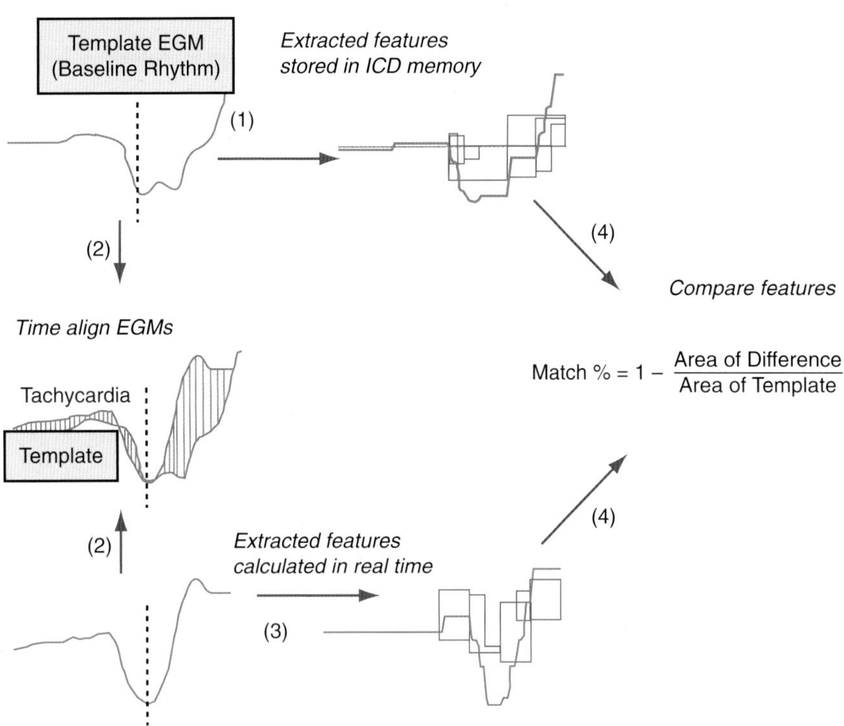

Figure 3-54. Steps in morphology algorithm. See text for details.

best single-chamber SVT-VT discrimination for initial detection of VT.[102] The morphology building block is the key element of newer single-chamber algorithms. Similarly, it is the central single-chamber component of dual-chamber algorithms with this feature. For this reason, a more detailed analysis is provided in the following section.

Ventricular EGM Morphology for SVT-VT Discrimination

General

EGM morphology algorithms are the most complex and effective building blocks in single-chamber detection algorithms. All morphology algorithms share common steps (Fig. 3-54): (1) record a template EGM of baseline rhythm; (2) construct and store a quantitative representation of this template; (3) record EGMs from an unknown tachycardia; (4) time-align the template and tachycardia EGMs; (5) construct a quantitative, normalized representation of each tachycardia EGM; (6) compare the representation of each tachycardia EGM with that of the template to determine its degree of morphologic similarity; (7) classify each tachycardia EGM as a morphology match or nonmatch with the template; (8) classify the tachycardia rhythm as VT or SVT based on the fraction of EGMs that match the template. Steps 3 through 8 are performed in real time. Morphology algorithms differ according to EGM source or sources, methods of filtering and alignment, and details of quantitative representations. The features of specific algorithms are described in Figure 3-55.

Limitations of Morphology Algorithms

Morphology algorithms share common failure modes for inappropriate detection of SVT as VT: (1) inaccurate template, (2) EGM truncation, (3) alignment errors, (4) oversensing of pectoral myopotentials, (5) rate-related aberrancy, (6) SVT soon after shocks, and (7) inappropriate classification of VT as SVT.

Inaccurate Template. The template may be inaccurate because the baseline EGM has changed (e.g., postimplantation lead maturation, intermittent bundle branch block) or because the template was recorded from an abnormal rhythm (e.g., idioventricular or bigeminal PVCs). Accurate SVT-VT discrimination requires periodic automatic or manual template updates. If automatic updates are not available, the morphology algorithm should not be programmed "On" until a chronic EGM is present. However, the template cannot be updated without intrinsic AV conduction. If software permits (Medtronic and St. Jude ICDs), the template match should be verified initially and during follow-up.

Electrogram Truncation. EGM truncation ("clipping") occurs when the recorded EGM signal amplitude exceeds the range of the EGM amplifier so that the maximum or minimum portion of the EGM is clipped. This both removes EGM features for analysis and alters the timing of the tallest peak, which can affect alignment. The amplitude scale in Medtronic and St. Jude ICDs should be adjusted so that the EGM used for morphology analysis is 25% to 75% of the dynamic range (Fig. 3-56).

Alignment Errors. Alignment errors prevent match between a tachycardia EGM and a morphologically similar stored EGM. Mechanisms depend on the method used for EGM alignment (Fig. 3-57). Accurate

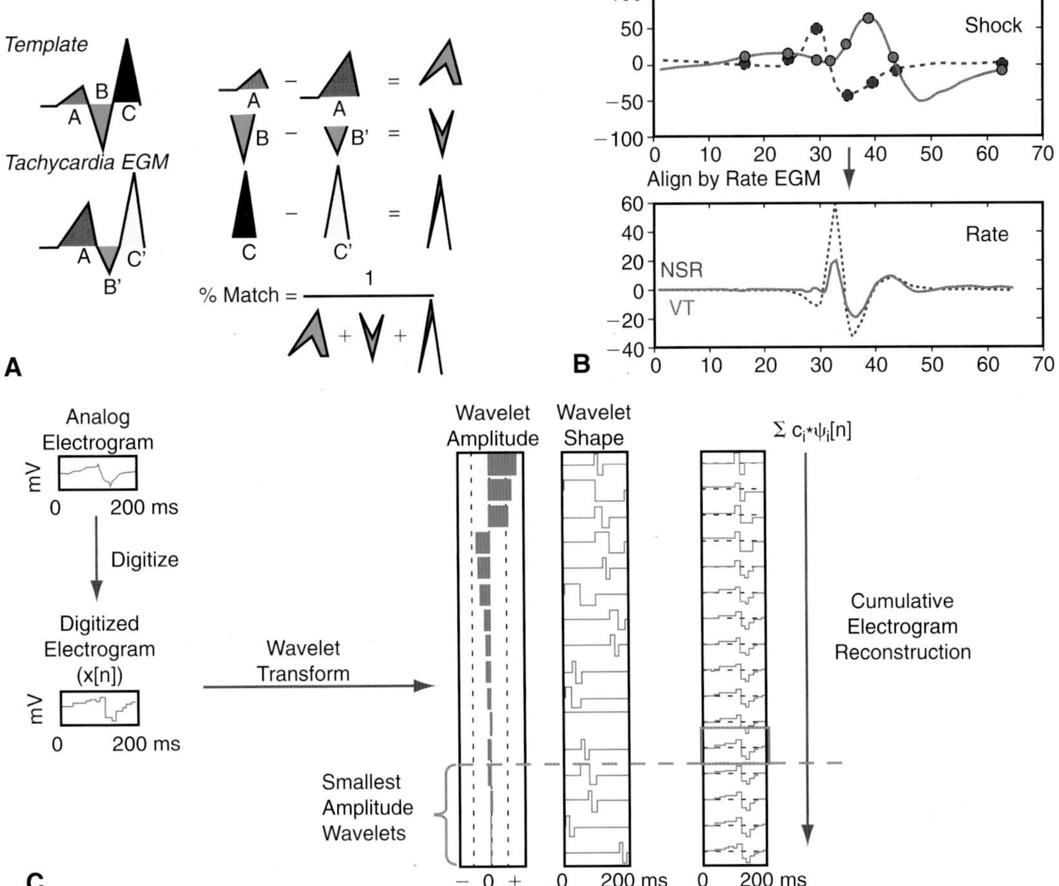

Figure 3-55. Specific morphology algorithms. ***A,*** *St. Jude MD algorithm. The positive and negative deflections in the sensing EGM are normalized and modeled as a series of three polygons (A, B and C in the template EGM; A′, B′, and C′ in the tachycardia EGM). The normalized areas of these polygons are then computed. Each tachycardia EGM is compared with the template EGM in three steps. First, the difference in area of corresponding polygons is computed. Second, the absolute values of these differences are summed. Third, a match score is constructed to be inversely proportional to the sum of these differences. If a programmable number (= 4) of 8 complexes in a sliding window exceed the programmable threshold (nominally 60%), the rhythm is classified as supraventricular tachycardia (SVT). If not, it is classified as ventricular tachycardia (VT).* ***B,*** *Guidant Vector Timing and Correlation (VTC) algorithm. This algorithm aligns shocking EGMs of the tachycardia and template based on the peak of the rate-sensing EGM. This method takes advantage of spatiotemporal differences between activation sequences in VT and baseline rhythm that cannot be detected from a single EGM. In this example, the peak of the shock EGM has similar timing to the peak of the rate-sensing EGM in sinus rhythm, but much later timing in VT. The amplitude of the shocking EGM* (upper panel) *is computed at each of 8 points selected on the basis of their timing relative to the peak of the sensing EGM* (lower panel) *and extracted as an eight-element "feature set," corresponding to an eight-dimensional vector. Feature sets of each tachycardia EGM are compared with the template EGM by computing the product-moment correlation coefficient between the two feature sets. This value, named the feature correlation coefficient (FCC), is a measure of mean spatiotemporal difference in ventricular activation between tachycardia and baseline rhythm. A threshold value for the feature correlation coefficient was selected to optimize SVT-VT discrimination on a test data set. This value is neither published nor programmable. If at least 3 of 10 complexes in a sliding window exceed the threshold, the rhythm is classified as SVT; if not, it is classified as VT.* ***C,*** *Medtronic Wavelet algorithm. The algorithm expresses the morphology of ventricular EGMs using the wavelet-transform. Wavelets[175] are functions of constant shape and limited time duration. They form the basis of a mathematical transformation that represents signals efficiently if they are both highly localized in time and preceded and followed by isoelectric intervals. They are therefore well-suited for representing transient biomedical signals such as ventricular EGMs. The algorithm compares the morphology of ventricular EGMs during a tachycardia with a template recorded during baseline rhythm. This comparison is expressed as a percent-match score that describes the degree of morphologic similarity of the baseline and tachycardia EGMs using a programmable source. In general, the EGM recorded between right-ventricular and superior vena cava coils is preferred as a default. This signal combines far-field sensitivity to morphology differences between VT and SVT with resistance to pectoral myopotentials. The algorithm begins processing when a tachycardia fulfills the programmed rate criterion for detection of VT and 8 beats remain to fulfill the programmed duration criterion for detection of VT. Percent-match scores are calculated for each of the last 8 beats before detection. Beats with match scores less than a programmable threshold (nominally 70%) are classified as ventricular. Nominally, a tachycardia is classified as VT if 6 or more of the 8 analyzed EGMs are classified as ventricular. Otherwise, it is classified initially as SVT. If the tachycardia is classified as SVT, the algorithm is applied to each successive 8-beat sliding window until the rate criterion for VT is no longer fulfilled.*

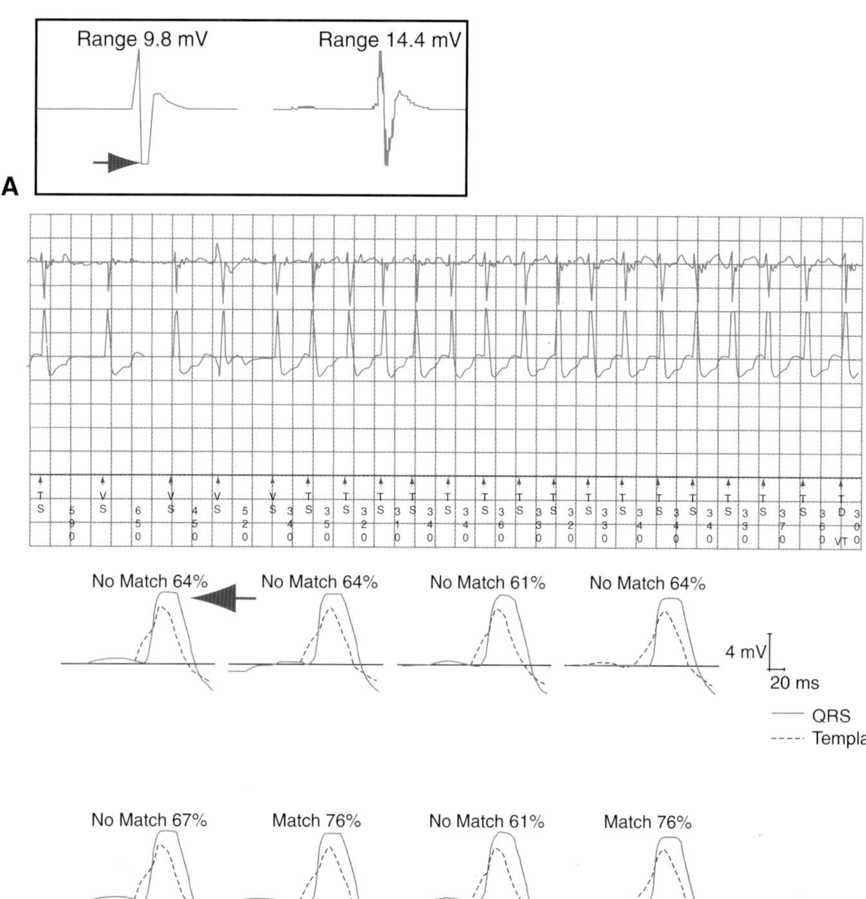

Figure 3-56. EGM truncation as a source of error for morphology algorithms. **A,** St. Jude MD template EGM is truncated (arrow) with an amplifier range of 9.8 mV. Truncation was corrected by increasing the range to 14.4 mV. Inconsistent truncation may prevent supraventricular tachycardia (SVT) morphology from matching the template. **B,** Medtronic Wavelet algorithm. EGMs in rapidly conducted atrial fibrillation exceed the maximum amplitude range of 8 mV, resulting in varying degrees of truncation ("clipping") of the right ventricular (RV) Coil-to-Can + superior vena cava (SVC) signal compared with the template. Inappropriate detection of ventricular tachycardia (VT) occurs at right. Complexes below show the last eight EGMs before detection at higher resolution. These tachycardia EGMs are clipped (arrow) so that the peaks are cut off. The rhythm is classified as VT because six of the last eight EGMs have <70% match. This problem was corrected by expanding the EGM scale ±16 mV. AS, atrial sensed event; VP, ventricular paced event.

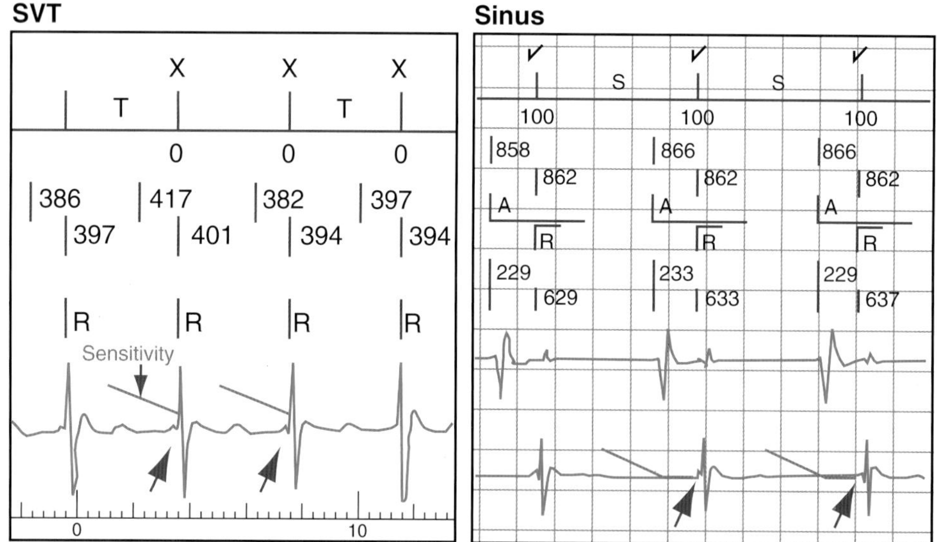

Figure 3-57. Alignment error in morphology algorithm. Interaction of Automatic Sensitivity Control and morphology analysis in St. Jude MD algorithm. Left panel, stored EGM of supraventricular tachycardia (SVT) inappropriately detected as ventricular tachycardia (VT). Right panel, programmer strip of validated template in sinus rhythm. Despite identical ventricular EGMs, morphology match scores are 0% in SVT and 100% in sinus rhythm. Slanted line denotes slope of Automatic Sensitivity Control. In sinus rhythm, Automatic Sensitivity Control reaches minimum value before the next ventricular EGM, so that the small peak at onset of EGM (arrows) is used for alignment. In SVT, Automatic Sensitivity Control does not reach minimum, and the small peak is not used for alignment.

alignment in the St. Jude algorithm is sensitive to the value of the sensing threshold at the onset of the ventricular EGM, as determined by Automatic Sensitivity Control. If a template EGM is acquired at the most sensitive setting of Automatic Sensitivity Control (either because of a slow sinus rate or after a ventricular paced beat), a low-amplitude peak at the onset of the ventricular EGM may be used for alignment. An identical tachycardia EGM may be acquired at a sufficiently fast rate that Automatic Sensitivity Control does not reach its most sensitive value at the onset of the R wave. If this occurs, the low-amplitude peak at the onset of the ventricular EGM may not be used for alignment. If identical template and tachycardia EGMs are then compared, their representations in the morphology algorithm may not match. Usually, they are assigned morphology match scores of either 0% or 100% (see Fig. 3-57). In patients who have dual-chamber ICDs and intact AV conduction, the template should be acquired or verified during atrial pacing at a rate close to the VT rate. In single-chamber ICDs, solutions to alignment problems may include altering the minimum sensitivity, Threshold Start, or Threshold Delay.

Medtronic ICDs align EGMs based on their tallest (positive or negative) peaks. If an EGM has two peaks of almost equal amplitude, or if such peaks are caused artificially by truncation of large EGMs that exceed the programmed dynamic range, minor variations in their relative amplitudes may result in an alignment error.[60] An alternative source EGM should be selected.

The Guidant morphology algorithm[110] aligns high-voltage EGMs based on the peak of the rate-sensing EGM. "Slow" automatic gain control (see "Ventricular Sensing in Ventricular ICDs") adjusts the dynamic range based on the amplitude of the sensed R wave, to minimize alignment errors caused by truncation. Presently, data regarding errors with this algorithm are limited.

Oversensing of Pectoral Myopotentials. In Medtronic ICDs, oversensing of pectoral myopotentials may prevent an SVT from matching the sinus template if the RV coil-to-can EGM is used for morphology analysis and the R-wave amplitude is small. The effect of myopotentials on match percent can be tested by pectoral muscle exercise. Select an alternative source EGM (e.g., distal coil to proximal coil) to prevent such oversensing. Pectoral myopotentials also pose a source of error in Guidant ICDs, which necessarily incorporate the high-voltage EGM in morphology analysis. Oversensing of pectoral myopotentials is not a problem for St. Jude ICDs, which use near-field EGMs for morphology analysis.

Rate-Related Aberrancy. If complete bundle branch aberrancy occurs reproducibly, the template may be recorded during rapid atrial pacing (Fig. 3-58). However, subtle and varying aberrancy confounds morphology algorithms (Fig. 3-59). Automatic template updating should then be deactivated to prevent subsequent automatic acquisition of a slow baseline template without aberrancy. During rapidly conducted AF, subtle degrees of aberration commonly distort the terminal portion of the EGM sufficiently that the percent match is less than the nominal threshold. In St. Jude ICDs, reducing the fraction of EGMs required to exceed the match threshold from 5 of 8 beats to 4 of 8 beats may reduce this problem without compromising detection of monomorphic VT. Reducing the match percent required to exceed the match threshold may also prevent misclassification of aberrantly conducted SVT as VT, but it results in a greater chance of misclassifying VT as SVT than does reducing the fraction of EGMs.

Supraventricular Tachycardia Occurring Soon after a Shock. After a shock, ICD detection algorithms reclassify the rhythm as sinus and revert to their initial detection mode within a few seconds, but postshock distortion of EGM morphology may persist for 30 seconds to several minutes.[60] If postshock SVT starts after the rhythm has been classified as sinus but before postshock EGM distortion dissipates, any morphology algorithm may misclassify SVT as VT. One appropriate (or inappropriate) shock may be followed by a repetitive sequence of inappropriate shocks in which each shock perpetuates postshock EGM changes in SVT, resulting in inappropriate detection of VT and the next inappropriate shock.

Inappropriate Classification of Ventricular Tachycardia as Supraventricular. The St. Jude morphology algorithm, which analyzes only the rate-sensing electrode, continuously misclassifies 5% to 10% of monomorphic VTs as SVT (Fig. 3-60). But, if it is restricted to tachycardias with the ventricular rate less than or equal to the atrial rate in dual-chamber ICDs, only 2% of VTs are misclassified.[102] The Medtronic morphology algorithm, which usually analyzes high-voltage EGMs, misclassifies 1% to 2% of VTs as SVTs.[111] If misclassification occurs, an alternative EGM source may provide adequate discrimination. Limited data indicate that the corresponding error rate for the Guidant algorithm is comparable or lower. When used as part of a dual-chamber algorithm, inappropriate shocks for the Guidant and St. Jude algorithms decrease by an order of magnitude, because at least 90% of VTs in ICD patients have AV dissociation. For this reason, the morphology algorithm is not needed. When the St. Jude morphology algorithm is used in a single-chamber ICD, the sustained-duration time out (Maximum Time to Diagnosis, Section V.F) should be programmed unless the algorithm is known to classify all clinical VTs correctly. Opinions differ about whether comparable features are required for the Medtronic and Guidant algorithms.

SVT-VT Discrimination in Dual-Chamber and Cardiac Resynchronization ICDs

The integration of dual-chamber building blocks into detection algorithms may be considered in terms of the relative rates of the atrium and ventricle (Fig. 3-61).

Operation for Atrial Rate Less Than Ventricular Rate

All dual-chamber detection algorithms revert to single-chamber operation when the atrial rate is slower than

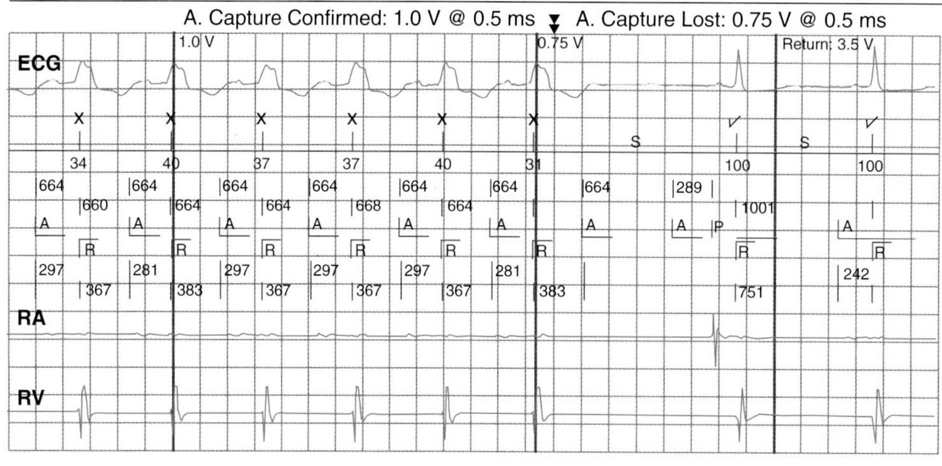

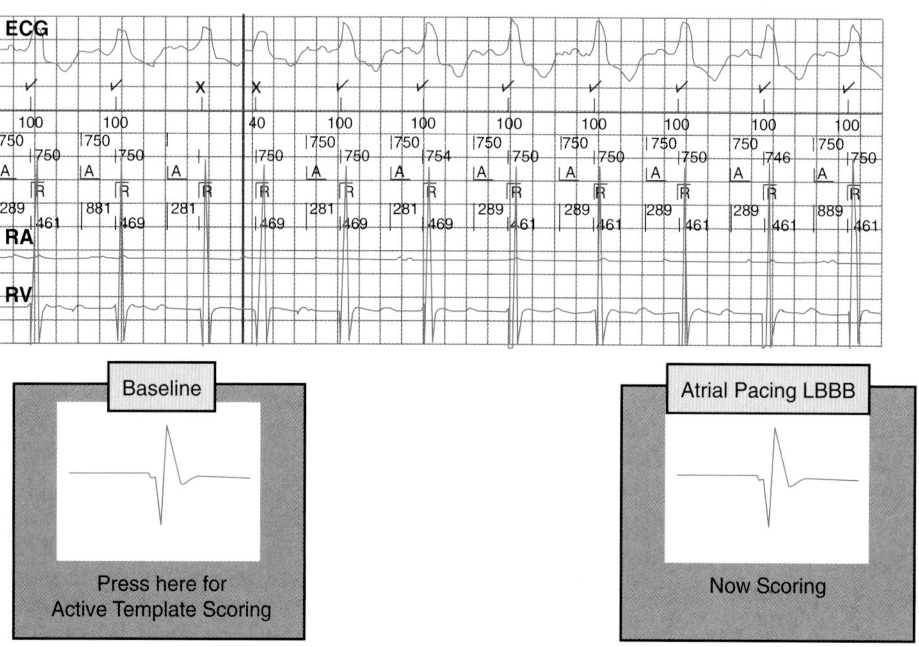

Figure 3-58. Left bundle branch aberrancy error in morphology algorithm. Programmer strips show electrocardiogram (ECG), event markers, right atrial EGM, and right ventricular (RV) true bipolar EGM. Top panel, *Measurement of atrial pacing threshold. Captured beats are conducted with rate-related left bundle branch aberrancy resulting in failure of morphology to match template collected in sinus rhythm. The last two ventricular EGMs at the slower sinus rate show 100% template match. A new template was acquired during atrial pacing.* Middle panel, *Near 100% morphology match to new template during conduction with left bundle branch aberrancy.* Bottom panel, *EGM morphology templates recorded during baseline sinus rhythm* (left) *and atrial pacing* (right). *LBBB, left bundle branch block; RA, right atrium.*

the ventricular rate. Guidant, St. Jude, and Biotronik ICDs do not apply any single-chamber discriminators when the atrial rate is slower than the ventricular rate. Medtronic ICDs optionally apply the single-chamber R-R stability criterion or the R-R onset criterion, or both, to allow discrimination of VT from rapidly-conducted AF or sinus tachycardia that is severely undersensed on the atrial channel. The risk of this approach is that there may be failure to detect an irregular or gradual-onset VT.

Operation for Atrial Rate Equal to Ventricular Rate

The vast majority of tachycardias with 1:1 AV relationship are SVT, primarily sinus tachycardia. VT with 1:1 VA conduction accounts for less than 5% of VTs detected by ICDs. The building blocks used by each manufacturer for distinguishing 1:1 AV conduction of SVT from 1:1 VA conduction are summarized in Table 3-3. A dual-chamber onset rule that evaluates

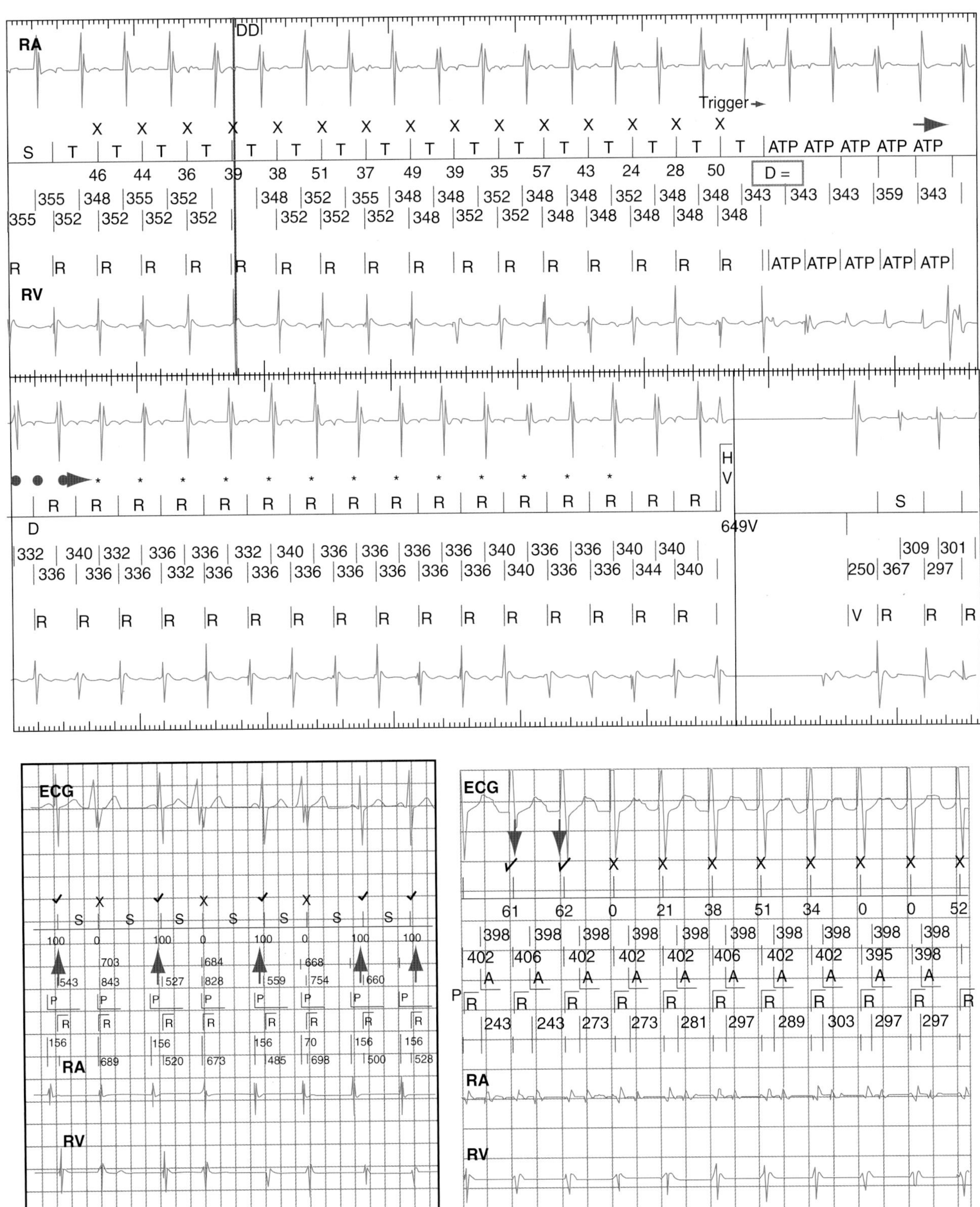

Figure 3-59. Error in morphology algorithm due to subtle rate-related aberrancy. Top and middle panels, *Dual-chamber stored EGM from inappropriately treated sinus tachycardia. Right atrial (RA) EGMs, event markers, and true bipolar right ventricular (RV) EGMs are shown. Values immediately below event markers—corresponding to EGMs in ventricular tachycardia (VT) zone (labeled "T")—indicate the percent match between EGM morphology in VT and sinus morphology (seen in lower left panel). Corresponding "X" labels above event markers indicate that the morphology algorithm classifies the beat as VT because the match is less than 60%. Burst antitachycardia pacing (ATP) is delivered at the right of the first panel. Dotted arrow indicates that panels are not continuous. After several trials of ATP (not shown), a shock is delivered toward the end of the second panel (HV). "Trigger" at right of upper panel indicates (inappropriate) detection of VT. "D =" at right of upper panel indicates that the atrial rate is equal to the ventricular rate. S denotes intervals in the Sinus zone above the VT detection interval of 360 msec. Time line is in seconds. Bottom panels show real-time programmer strips.* Bottom left panel, *100% template match in sinus rhythm* (arrows) *and 0% match on premature ventricular complexes (PVCs). However, the* bottom right panel, *recorded during atrial pacing at a cycle length of 400 msec, shows only two EGMs with adequate match (check marks, arrows). Note that the surface electrocardiogram (ECG) does not show identifiable aberrancy despite sufficient changes in EGM to prevent template match.*

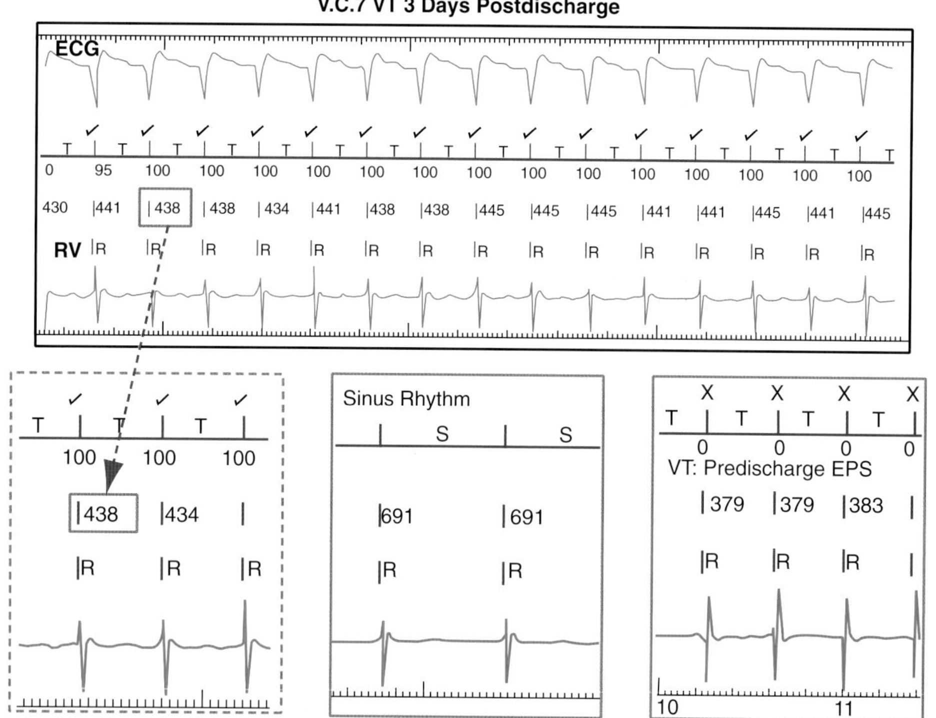

Figure 3-60. Failure to detect ventricular tachycardia (VT) due to inappropriate classification of VT as supraventricular tachycardia (SVT) by morphology algorithm (St. Jude MD). Upper panel, *programmer strip from symptomatic tachycardia classified as SVT 3 days after implantation. Electrocardiogram (ECG), event markers, and right ventricular (RV) true bipolar EGM are displayed. Morphology match is 100% on most beats. The 12-lead ECG showed a left bundle branch block–type pattern, a broad R wave in V1 (distinctly different from conducted sinus QRS complexes), and atrioventricular (AV) dissociation.* Lower panel, *event markers and RV EGM during tachycardia* (left), *sinus rhythm after manually delivered antitachycardia pacing* (center), *and induced VT at predischarge electrophysiologic study (EPS)* (right). *EGM morphology during spontaneous VT and sinus rhythm are similar and distinct from induced VT at predischarge EPS. True bipolar EGMs fail to distinguish VT from SVT in 5% to 10% of VTs.*

TABLE 3-3. Discrimination of Tachycardias with Atrial Rate Equal to Ventricular Rate

Building Blocks	GDT Rhythm ID	MDT PR Logic	St. Jude Rate Branch	ELA PARAD+	Biotronik SMART
Single-chamber					
R-R stability				X	
P-P stability		X			X
Sudden onset		[X]	X		X
VEGM morphology	X		X		
Dual-chamber					
A rate vs V rate	X	(X)	X		X
P-R patterns		X			
AV association		(X)	X	X	X
Chamber of acceleration		[X]		X	

A, atrial; AV, atrioventricular; GDT, Guidant; MDT, Medtronic; V, ventricular; VEGM, ventricular electrogram; X, algorithm uses this building block; [X], new PR Logic ST rule (Entrust) uses sudden R-R and P-R onsets; (X), "implicit" use of these building blocks via pattern analysis.

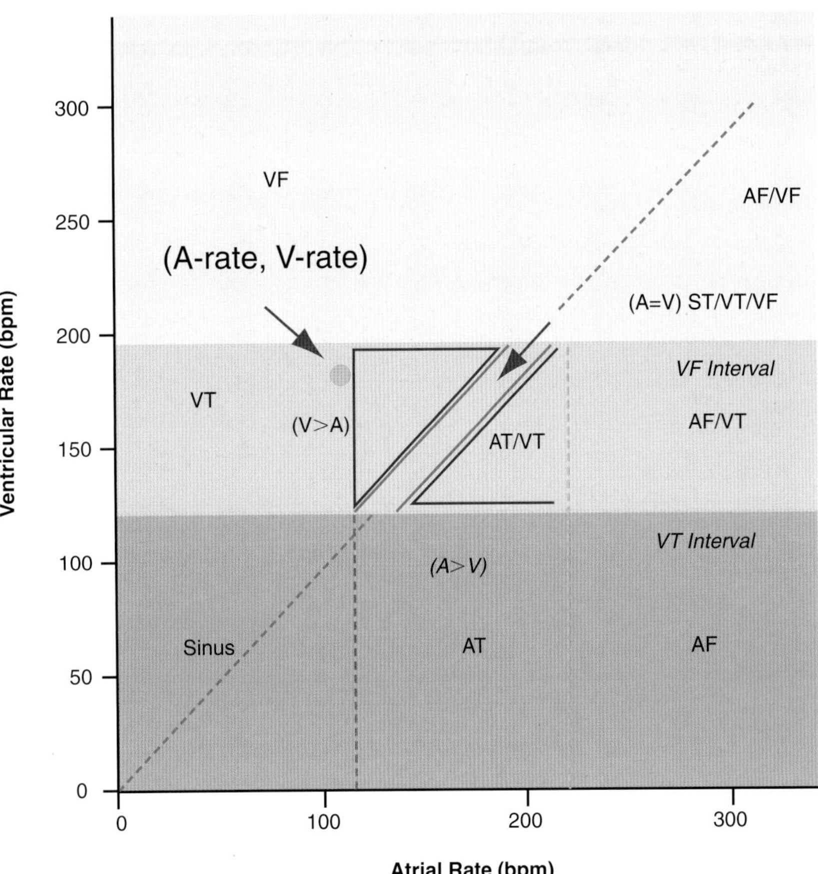

Figure 3-61. Dual-chamber "rate plane" highlights power of atrial versus ventricular rate. Dual-chamber rhythm classification can be visualized as a graph that plots atrial rate (A-rate) on the abscissa and ventricular rate (V-rate) on the ordinate. All points above the horizontal line representing the ventricular tachycardia (VT) intervals will be detected as VT or ventricular fibrillation (VF) on the basis of ventricular rate alone. Points that are both above this line and above and to the left of the line of identity are VT, and no additional discriminators need to be applied in this region, provided that atrial sensing is reliable. These discriminators can be restricted to rhythms with 1:1 atrioventricular (AV) relationship on the line of identity and those in which the atrial rate exceeds the ventricular rate in the region below and to the right of the line of identity. AF, atrial fibrillation; AT, atrial tachycardia; ST, sinus tachycardia. (Modified from Morris M, Marcovecchio A, KenKnight B, et al: Retrospective evaluation of detection enhancements in a dual-chamber implantable cardioverter defibrillator: Implications for device programming [abstract]. PACE 22(4 Part II):849, 1999, with permission.)

both P-R and R-R interval onset improves specificity of R-R interval onset-type building blocks for sinus tachycardia with minimal loss of sensitivity for VT.[112] Individual examples are shown in Figures 3-62 to 3-65.

Operation for Atrial Rate Greater Than Ventricular Rate

The building blocks used by each manufacturer for distinguishing rapidly conducted AF and atrial flutter from VT during atrial arrhythmias are summarized in Table 3-4. Although various combinations of these building blocks successfully discriminate VT from SVT in VT zones, most VT during AF is sufficiently rapid to be detected in the VF zone,[113] where discriminators lose reliability or may not be applied at all. For example, R-R regularity cannot be applied in the VF zone because polymorphic VT has irregular R-R intervals, and undersensing of VF exaggerates the irregularity of measured R-R intervals. AV dissociation is uniformly detected during rapidly conducted AF,[62] and morphology templates acquired during sinus rhythm often misclassify aberrantly conducted beats. Individual examples are shown in Figures 3-66 to 3-68.

Specific Algorithms

Figures 3-69 to 3-73 show block diagrams of the principal dual-chamber detection algorithms in clinical use today. Legends identify unique features of each algorithm.

Single-Chamber Versus Dual-Chamber Discriminators

Nominal programming of dual-chamber algorithms is safe.[114,115] Because SVT-VT discriminators are nominally "ON" in some dual-chamber ICDs but "OFF" in all single-chamber ICDs, use of discriminators may be greater in dual-chamber ICDs. Dual-chamber stored EGMs provide higher diagnostic accuracy for troubleshooting than single-chamber stored EGMs. However, dual-chamber discriminators incur disadvantages: They cannot be implemented without the complications inherent with atrial leads, and dual-chamber ICDs introduce unique risks for underdetection of VT due to cross-chamber ventricular blanking after atrial pacing (see "Intradevice Interactions"). Early dual-chamber algorithms had additional limitations: Optimal values of programmable parameters were not known; initial approaches to the problem of atrial blanking versus FFRW oversensing had limited success; and atrial sensing problems and specific design flaws degraded performance. Not surprisingly, clinical studies of early dual-chamber algorithms reported no benefit over single-chamber algorithms.[61,62,116,117] More recent large, randomized, prospective studies of the

Text continued on p. 131

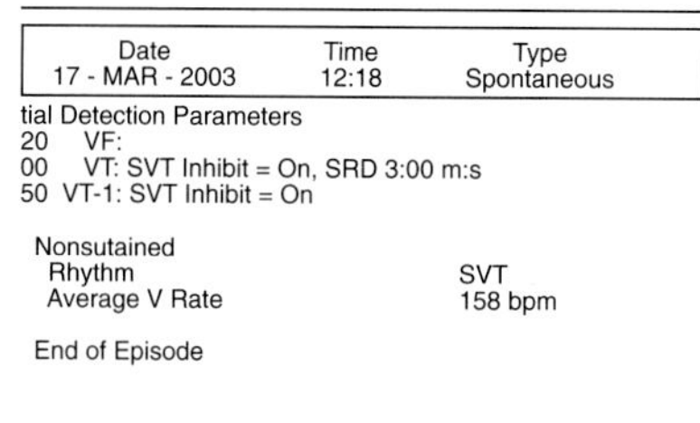

Date	Time	Type
17 - MAR - 2003	12:18	Spontaneous

tial Detection Parameters
20 VF:
00 VT: SVT Inhibit = On, SRD 3:00 m:s
50 VT-1: SVT Inhibit = On

Nonsutained
Rhythm SVT
Average V Rate 158 bpm

End of Episode

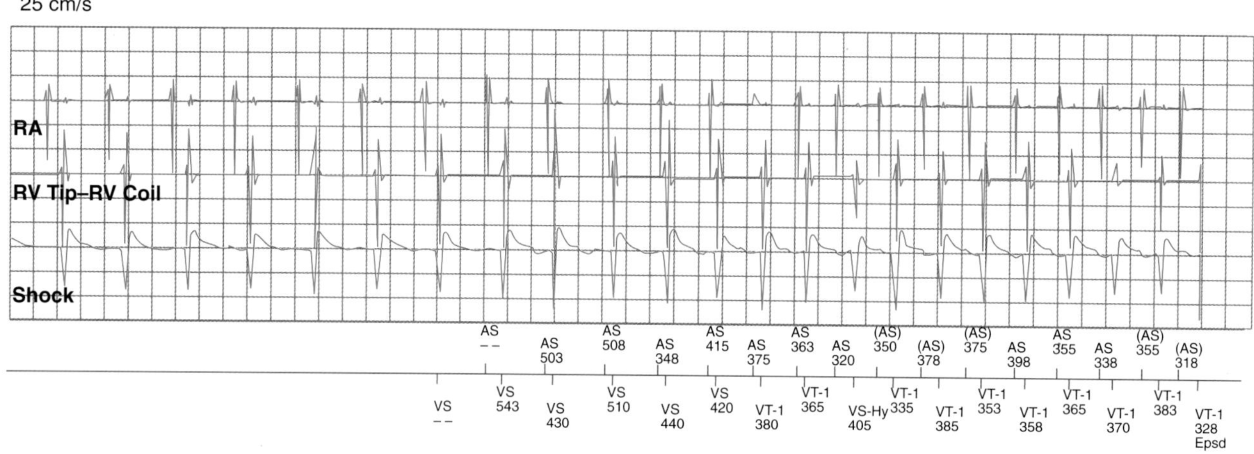

Figure 3-62. Appropriate rejection of supraventricular tachycardia (SVT) with 1:1 atrioventricular (AV) conduction by AV relationship and morphology algorithm. Right atrial (RA), right ventricular (RV) rate-sensing, and Shock EGMs are shown in order with dual-chamber event markers. SVT begins with gradual warm-up, accelerating from a cycle length of approximately 540 msec to 380 msec in 3 seconds. The Guidant Rhythm ID algorithm classifies morphology as SVT based on 1:1 AV association combined with constant shock morphology and constant timing relationship between peaks of two ventricular EGMs. The label ATR at bottom of event markers indicates that the rhythm is classified as SVT. Upper panel shows episode summary classifying rhythm as SVT.

TABLE 3-4. Discrimination of Tachycardias with Atrial Rate Greater Than Ventricular Rate

Building Blocks	GDT Rhythm ID	MDT PR Logic	St. Jude Rate Branch	ELA PARAD+	Biotronik SMART
Single-chamber					
R-R stability	X	X	X	X	X
P-P stability		X			X
VEGM morphology	X		X		
Dual-chamber					
A rate vs V rate	X	X	X		X
P-R patterns		X			
AV association		X	X	X	X

A, atrial; AV, atrioventricular; GDT, Guidant; MDT, Medtronic; V, ventricular; VEGM, ventricular electrogram; X, algorithm uses this building block; X = algorithm uses this building block.

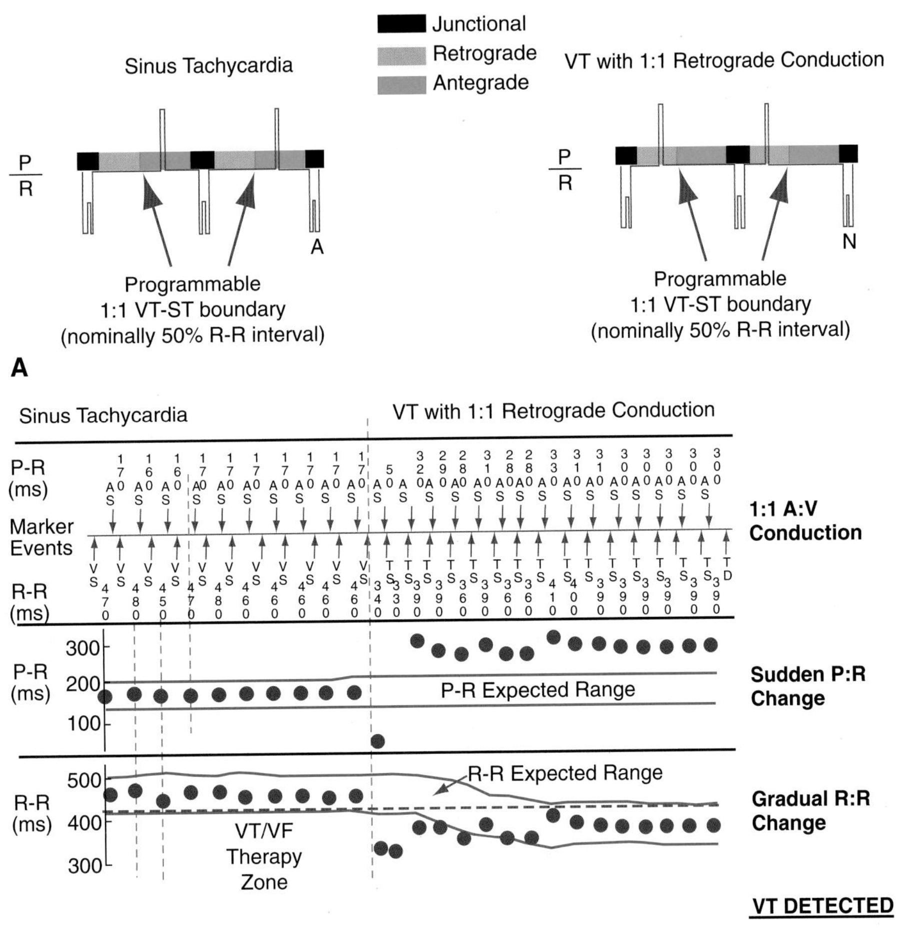

Figure 3-63. ***A,*** *Discrimination of 1:1 tachycardias by P-R pattern using the original sinus tachycardia criterion in Medtronic PR Logic (GEM III, Marquis, Maximo, InSync Marquis, InSync Maximo) ICDs. PR Logic uses patterns of A-V, V-A, V-V, and A-A intervals from consecutive ventricular events to form couple codes describing supraventricular tachycardias (SVTs). These couple codes are based on the number of atrial (A) events within the ventricular (V) interval and their relative timing. Discrimination of sinus tachycardia from ventricular tachycardia (VT) with 1:1 retrograde conduction is critically dependent on the programmable 1:1 VT-Sinus Tachycardia (ST) boundary, which is defined nominally as 50% of the current R-R interval (with optional values of 35%, 66%, 75%, and 85%). P-R intervals less than the defined percentage of the current R-R interval and greater than 70 msec are considered antegrade* (left panel), *and P-R intervals that are equal to or greater than that percentage of the R-R interval and also greater than 40 msec are considered retrograde* (right panel). *Rhythms in the detection zone with 1:1 pattern and antegrade P-R intervals are classified as ST, and therapies are withheld. Rhythms with 1:1 pattern and retrograde P-R intervals are classified as VT.* ***B,*** *The new adaptive ST rule in PR Logic (Medtronic Entrust DR ICD) no longer uses the 1:1 VT-ST boundary to discriminate ST from VT with 1:1 retrograde conduction; rather, it uses a combination of pattern, sudden R-R onset, and sudden P-R onset. The operation of the new adaptive ST criterion is illustrated by this example of a spontaneous episode of ST that converted into VT with 1:1 retrograde conduction. During the ST, the R-R and P-R intervals occurred within their expected ranges. After initiation of VT, the R-R and P-R intervals occurred outside their expected ranges. Evidence of ST was lost by the third beat of VT. The sudden change in R-R intervals was small (460-msec), so that the R-R intervals during the VT occurred within twice the R-R interval expected range, and adaptation of the R-R interval expected range continued. Eventually, the R-R interval expected range adapts to accept the R-R intervals of the VT. Conversely, the P-R intervals occurred outside of twice the P-R expected range, and adaptation was inhibited. VT is appropriately detected after 16 consecutive R-R intervals in the VT detection zone despite gradual R-R onset of a 1:1 rhythm, because the P-R intervals had sudden onset and were no longer within the expected P-R interval range. VF, Ventricular fibrillation. (From Stadler RW, Gunderson BD, Gillberg JM: An adaptive interval-based algorithm for withholding ICD therapy during sinus tachycardia. PACE 26:1189-1201, 2003, with permission.)*

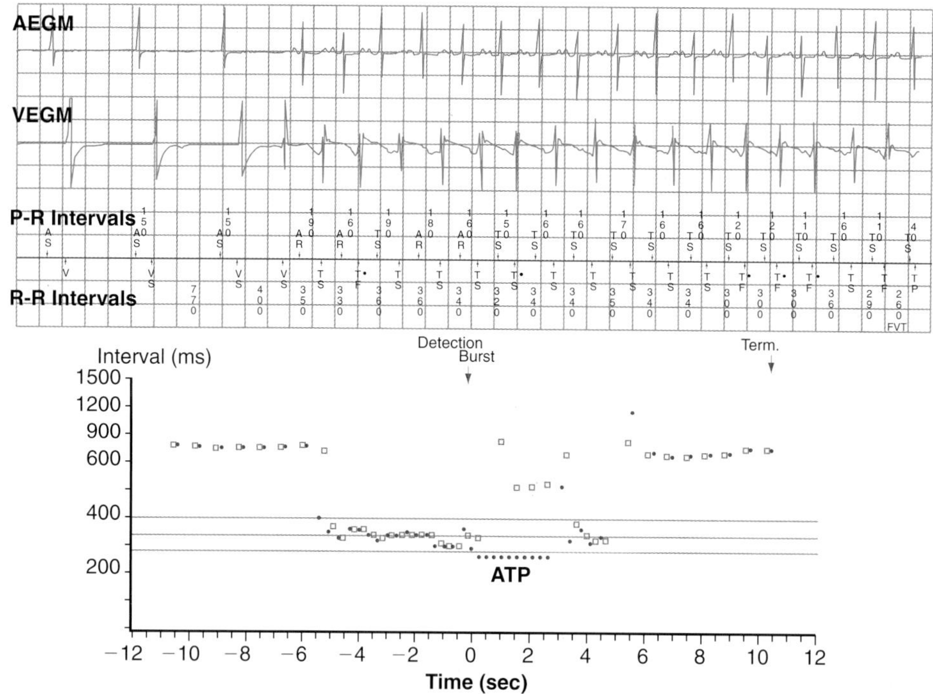

Figure 3-64. Appropriate detection of ventricular tachycardia (VT) with 1:1 ventricular-atrial (VA) conduction by abrupt change in P-R pattern and ventricular rate. Upper panel *shows dual-chamber stored EGMs and dual-chamber EGM markers. Note that upper numerical values indicate P-R interval, not P-P interval.* Lower panel *shows interval plot. VT starts in the ventricle with a premature ventricular complex, followed by abrupt change in ventricular rate, ventricular EGM morphology, and the PR-RR relationship (Medtronic PR Logic). Fast VT (FVT) detection at right of EGM is followed by burst antitachycardia pacing (VT Rx 1 Burst), designated by ATP on interval plot. This results in abrupt termination of VT. Note that older versions of this algorithm, which discriminated VT from SVT based only on the PR-RP percentage, may have classified this long-RP tachycardia incorrectly as SVT. AEGM, atrial EGM; TF, interval in FVT zone; TS, interval in VT zone; VEGM, true bipolar EGM; VS, ventricular sense.*

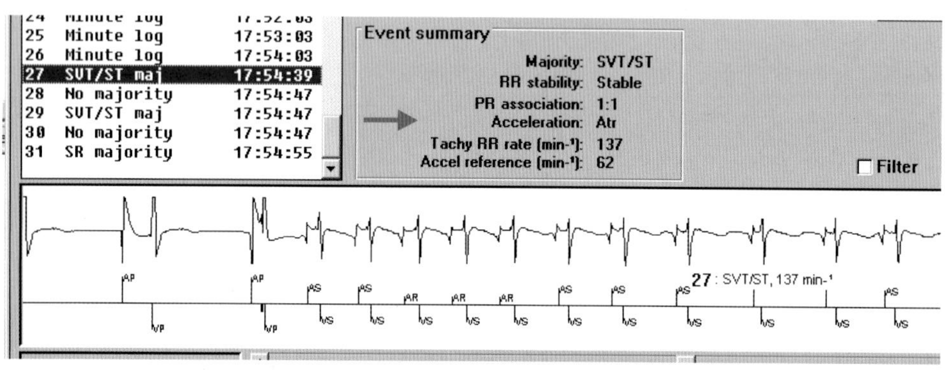

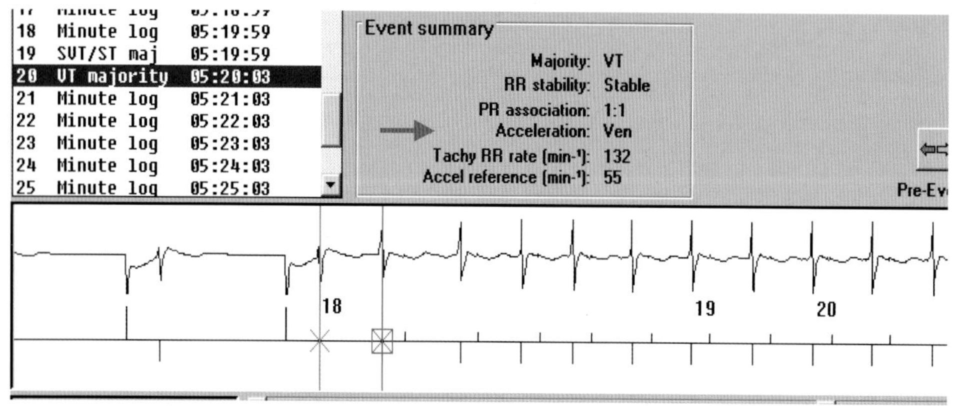

Figure 3-65. Classification of 1:1 tachycardias by chamber of origin. The ELA Parad algorithm classifies 1:1 tachycardias by chamber of onset. Stored ventricular EGM is shown with dual-chamber event markers (atrial on top, ventricular on bottom). Event log and Event summary are shown above each stored EGM. Upper panel, *supraventricular tachycardia (SVT) is diagnosed by atrial onset.* Lower panel, *ventricular tachycardia (VT) is diagnosed by ventricular onset.*

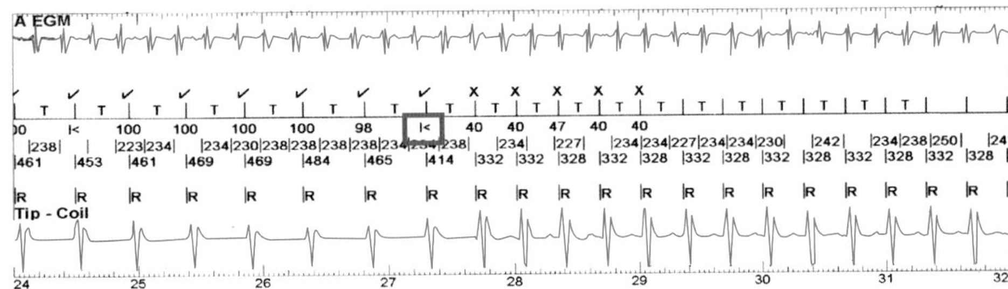

Figure 3-66. Ventricular tachycardia (VT) during rapidly conducted atrial flutter discriminated by morphology of the ventricular EGM. VT occurs during atrial flutter with 2:1 atrioventricular (AV) conduction. Time line marks indicate that the ventricular rate had been in the VT zone for 24 seconds at the beginning of the panel. VT therapy is withheld because of both the 2:1 AV relationship and morphology match of ventricular EGMs to baseline sinus-rhythm EGMs (not shown). Numbers below event markers indicate 98% to 100% morphology match in atrial flutter, compared with 40% to 47% match in VT. "<" (box) marks indicate that ventricular rate is less than atrial rate. VT is detected by AV dissociation and morphology match percentage less than the threshold value of 60%. Morphology classification of each beat as SVT (check marks) or VT ("X" marks) is indicated above event markers. (From Swerdlow C, Shivkumar K: Implantable cardioverter defibrillators: Clinical aspects. In Zipes DP, Jalife J (eds): Cardiac Electrophysiology: From Cell to Bedside, 4th ed. Philadelphia, WB Saunders, 2004, pp 980-993, with permission.)

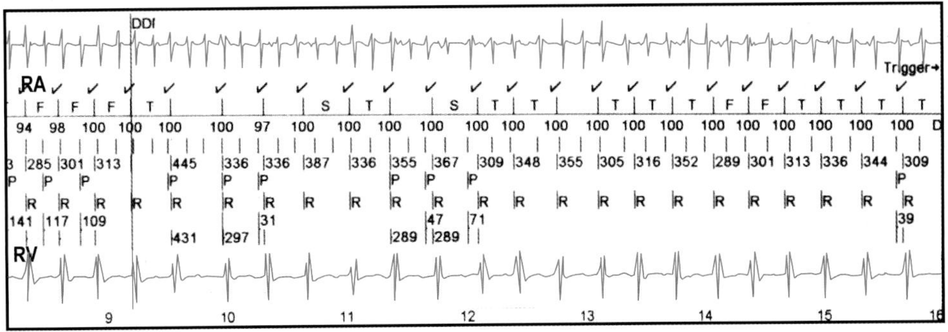

Figure 3-67. Inappropriate detection of rapidly conducted atrial fibrillation (AF) despite rejection by morphology. Right atrial (RA) EGM, event markers, and true bipolar right ventricular (RV) EGM are shown. Values immediately below event markers corresponding to EGMs in ventricular tachycardia (VT) zone (marked T) indicate the percent match between EGM morphology in tachycardia and sinus morphology. Corresponding check marks above event markers indicate that the morphology algorithm classifies the beats as supraventricular tachycardia (SVT) because the match is greater than 60%. Stability and morphology algorithms are combined with "AND" logic in this St. Jude ICD, so that VT is diagnosed if either discriminator classifies the rhythm as VT. The stability algorithm incorrectly classifies the rhythm because the ventricular cycle lengths regularize. The rhythm would have been classified correctly if the morphology discriminator alone had been programmed. F markers indicate ventricular intervals in ventricular fibrillation ("Fib") zone. S denotes intervals in the "Sinus" zone above the VT detection interval. T denotes intervals in VT zone. DDI, mode switch to DDI pacing. (From Swerdlow CD, Friedman PA: Advanced ICD Troubleshooting: Part I. PACE 28:1322-1346, 2005, with permission.)

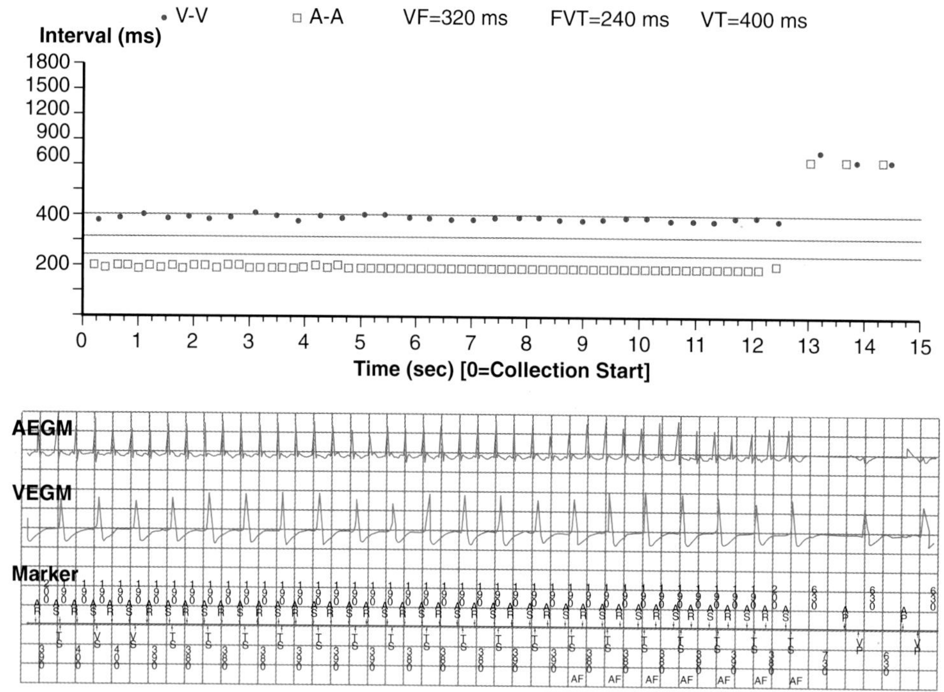

Figure 3-68. Appropriate rejection of rapidly conducted atrial flutter by pattern analysis. Interval plot (upper panel) and dual-chamber stored EGM with event markers (lower panel) are shown. Atrial flutter is identified by the consistent 2:1 P-R association of the regular atrial and ventricular rhythms. AF annotations indicate that the number of intervals in the ventricular tachycardia (VT) rate zone required for detection (16) has been reached, but that therapy is withheld because atrial flutter is diagnosed. Interval plot displays 2:1 atrioventricular (AV) association until termination of atrial flutter after 12 seconds. AR denotes atrial intervals in pacing refractory period. TS denotes ventricular intervals in VT zone.

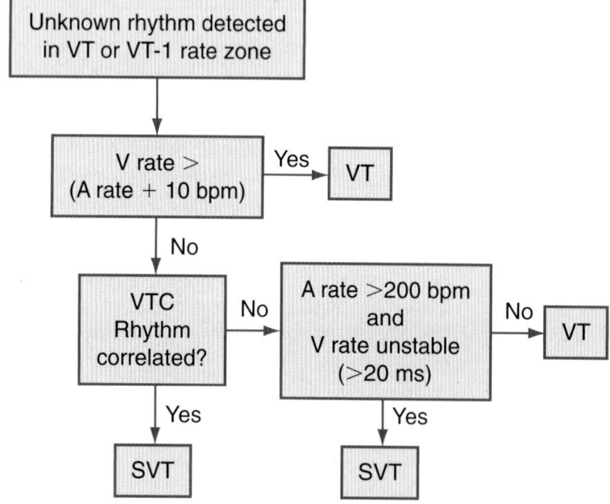

Figure 3-69. Guidant Rhythm ID algorithm. The central features of this algorithm are comparison of atrial (A) and ventricular (V) rates (first step) and analysis of ventricular EGM morphology (Vector Timing and Correlation, or VTC). If the V rate exceeds the A rate by at least 10 bpm, the rhythm is classified as ventricular tachycardia (VT). If at least 3 of the last 10 beats are classified as supraventricular by morphology analysis, the rhythm is classified as supraventricular tachycardia (SVT). If morphology analysis does not classify the rhythm as SVT, the A rate and the regularity of the V rate are evaluated. The rhythm is classified as SVT if the A rate exceeds 200 bpm and the ventricular rhythm is irregular (measured ventricular interval stability >20 msec). Otherwise, it is classified as a VT.

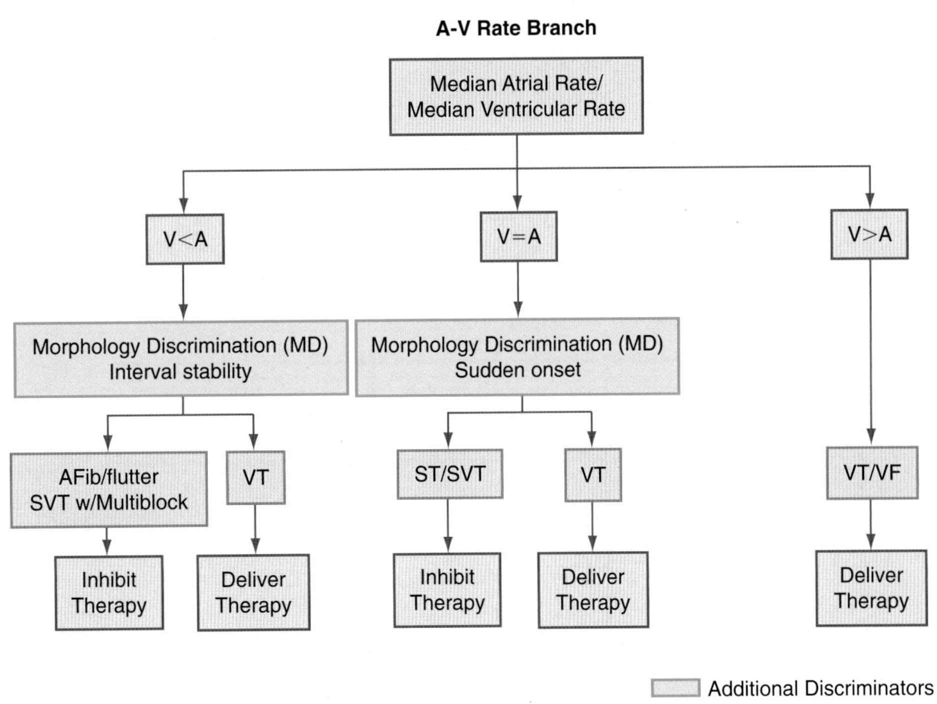

Figure 3-70. St. Jude A-V Rate Branch + Morphology Discrimination (MD) algorithm. Similar to the Rhythm ID, the central features of this algorithm are a comparison of the atrial (A) and ventricular (V) rates (first step) and analysis of ventricular EGM morphology (MD). Rhythms are classified into three Rate Branches: ventricular rate less than atrial rate (V < A), ventricular rate equal to atrial rate (V = A), and ventricular rate greater than atrial rate (V > A). If V < A, the algorithm applies morphology discrimination (and/or both interval stability and N:1 AV association). If V = A, it applies morphology discrimination (and/or sudden onset). All rhythms in the V > A rate branch are treated as ventricular tachycardia (VT). ST, sinus tachycardia; SVT, supraventricular tachycardia; VF, ventricular fibrillation.

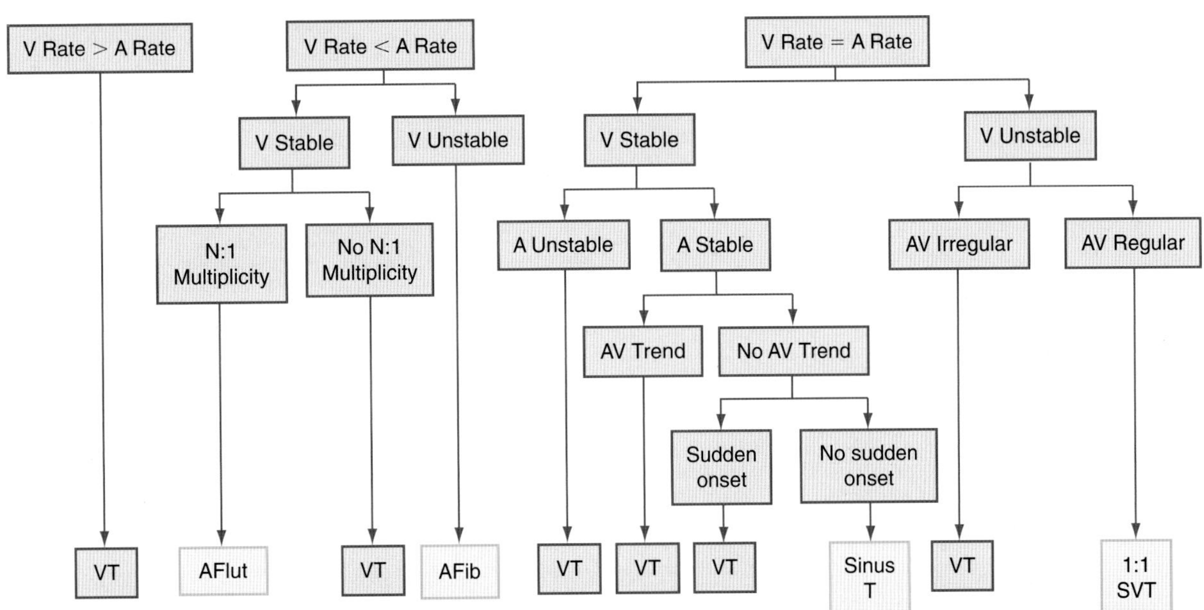

Figure 3-71. Biotronik SMART algorithm. The high-level structure of this algorithm is similar to that of the St. Jude ICD. SMART first compares atrial (A) and ventricular (V) rates. If the V rate is faster, ventricular tachycardia (VT) is diagnosed. If the V rate is slower, ventricular interval stability and A:V ratio analysis results in discrimination of atrial fibrillation (AFib; unstable ventricular rhythm), atrial flutter (AFlut; stable rhythm, N:1 association), and VT (stable rhythm, AV dissociated). If the A rate and V rate are equal, SMART analyzes the interval stability. If the R-R interval is stable and the P-P interval is unstable, VT is diagnosed. If the P-P interval is stable, the algorithm sequentially analyzes AV association ("AV Trend") and sudden onset as discriminators. Sinus T, sinus tachycardia; SVT, supraventricular tachycardia.

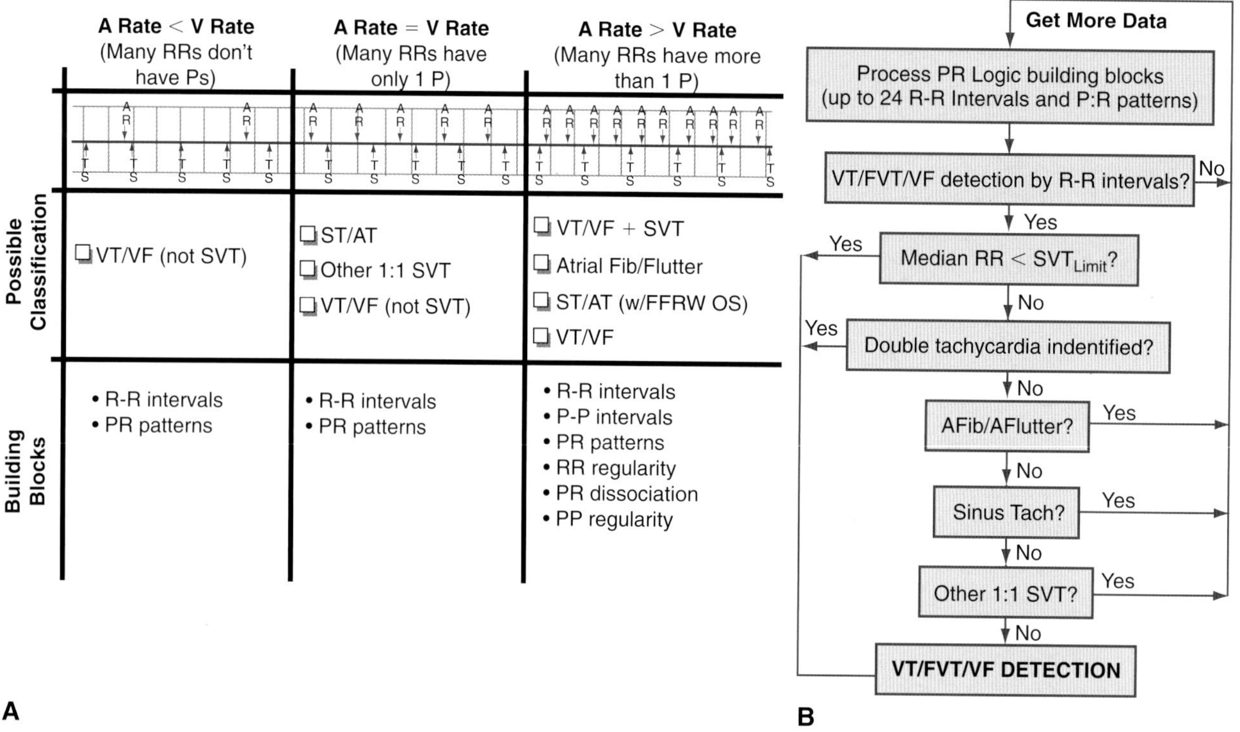

Figure 3-72. Medtronic PR Logic algorithm. ***A,*** *The clinical decision process. The rhythm types are represented using P-R marker diagram examples* (top), *from least complex* (left) *to most complex* (right). *A list of possible PR Logic decisions and the building blocks used are shown in the middle and on the bottom, respectively, for each of the rhythm types. Note that PR Logic implicitly employs a ventricular (V) rate > atrial (A) rate override (first column), because all rhythms with A rate < V rate and V rate in one of the detection zones are classified as ventricular tachycardia/fibrillation (VT/VF). For tachycardias with A rate = V rate (i.e., 1:1 tachycardias, center column), the original PR Logic uses P-R patterns and discriminates 1:1 rhythms with critical P-R interval timing zones (see Fig. 3-63A). The new sinus tachycardia (ST) criterion in PR Logic (Entrust and later) uses the P-R pattern along with P-R and R-R sudden-onset criteria (see Fig. 3-63B). For rhythms with A rate > V rate, PR Logic uses P-R patterns along with R-R regularity, P-R dissociation, and P-P regularity to ensure detection of double tachycardia (VT or VF during atrial fibrillation [AFib]) and to withhold therapy for 2:1 atrial flutter (AFlutter), rapid AFib, and ST with far-field R wave (FFRW) os.* ***B,*** *PR Logic computational flow diagram. On each ventricular event, PR Logic processes the new P-R, R-P, P-P, and R-R patterns and timing information for the building blocks. If VT/fast VT (FVT) or VF rate detection criteria are satisfied, the ventricular rate override criterion is checked first. If the median R-R interval is less than the supraventricular tachycardia (SVT) limit, detection occurs via the single-chamber detection criteria without considering the PR Logic discrimination algorithm. If the median R-R interval is greater than the SVT limit and double tachycardia (VT/FVT/VF + SVT) is not detected, then the three PR Logic criteria for identifying SVTs are tested in the order shown. If any one of the PR Logic SVT criteria is satisfied, inappropriate detection is avoided. If an SVT is not positively identified, VT/FVT/VF is detected when the R-R interval–based criterion is satisfied. If SVT is identified, the entire process repeats itself on each ventricular event until VT/FVT or VF is detected or the rhythm slows out of the ventricular rate detection zones.*

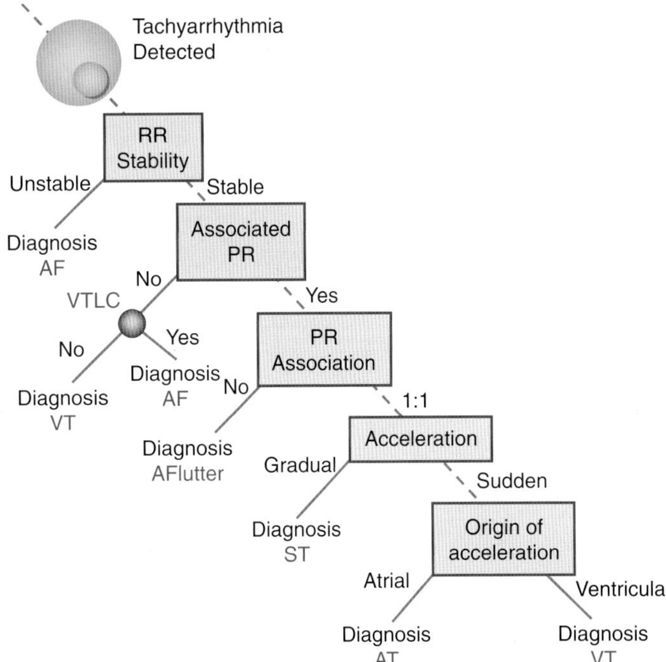

Figure 3-73. *ELA PARAD+ algorithm. If most of the detected R-R intervals are in the ventricular tachycardia (VT) zone, ventricular interval stability is analyzed in a first step, using a histogram of R-R intervals. If the rhythm is irregular, atrial fibrillation (AF) is diagnosed and therapy is withheld. If the rhythm is regular, the atrioventricular (AV) association is assessed by comparing peak amplitudes of R-R and P-R interval histograms. If the rhythm is AV dissociated, VT is diagnosed, unless the Long Cycle Search is activated, which inhibits therapy if a long ventricular cycle (VTLC; characteristic of AF) is identified. If N:1 P-R association is identified, the rhythm is classified as supraventricular tachycardia (SVT). In the presence of 1:1 P-R association, the PARAD+ evaluates the rate of acceleration of the ventricular rate. If acceleration is gradual, sinus tachycardia (ST) is diagnosed. If acceleration is sudden, PARAD+ identifies the chamber of origin and withholds therapy if it is the atrium. AFlutter, atrial flutter; AT, atrial tachycardia.*

ELA[118] and St. Jude[119] algorithms demonstrated moderate superiority in SVT-VT discrimination for dual-chamber algorithms.

Active Discrimination

Pacing maneuvers were not incorporated into early detection algorithms for many reasons, including concerns regarding proarrhythmia and the complexity of interpreting responses (Fig. 3-74). It is now recognized that conservative burst ventricular pacing at approximately 90% of the tachycardia cycle length has a low (1% to 2%) risk of proarrhythmia and that active discrimination provides unique advantages. In addition to terminating most monomorphic VTs, burst ventricular pacing terminates more than 50% of inappropriately detected pathologic SVTs with a 1:1 AV relationship.[120] During other SVTs, concealed retrograde conduction of ventricular ATP may slow the ventricular response by causing AV conduction delay or block. Active discrimination represents a paradigm shift in the design of detection algorithms, from "diagnose before intervening" to "treat first; analyze only those tachycardias that persist after treatment." To date, active discrimination methods have not been implemented in an ICD.

Single-Chamber Analysis

The number of pulses required for entrainment of a reentrant tachycardia is related to the conduction time from the pacing site to the tachycardia circuit. If the VT circuit is entrained, the first postpacing interval is independent of the number of pacing pulses delivered. There is a high probability of entraining reentrant VT with only a few pacing pulses. In contrast, nonreentrant SVT cannot be entrained, and reentrant SVT usually requires about 10 ventricular pacing pulses for entrainment.[101] Therefore, the difference between first postpacing intervals after the entrainment of VT by two sets of pacing bursts with different numbers of intervals is less than the comparable difference in postpacing intervals for bursts delivered during SVT. A limitation of this method is delay in detection of VT required to deliver and analyze the outcome of at least two sequences of burst pacing.

Dual-Chamber Analysis

In dual-chamber algorithms, the principal value of active discrimination applies to tachycardias with 1:1 AV association. Pacing is performed in one chamber with analysis in the opposite chamber. If the atrial cycle length is unchanged by ventricular burst pacing, the atrial rhythm does not depend on retrograde conduction, and the diagnosis is SVT. This feature has been tested but not yet implemented in an ICD.

If the atrial rate accelerates to the ventricular rate during ventricular burst pacing, the response at the termination of unsuccessful pacing may be helpful: Two atrial events followed by a ventricular event (A-A-V response) is quite suggestive of AT[121] (Fig. 3-75), although a slowly conducting retrograde accessory pathway or the slow AV nodal pathway may give the same result. Rarely, the pattern of two ventricular events followed by an atrial event (V-V-A response) is diagnostic of VT. But a ventricular event followed by an atrial event followed by another ventricular event (V-A-V response) indicates VT if AV nodal and AV reentrant SVT are excluded (Fig. 3-76).

Atrial extrastimuli or overdrive pacing may also discriminate between SVT and VT with 1:1 association. One method is to deliver a single atrial extrastimulus

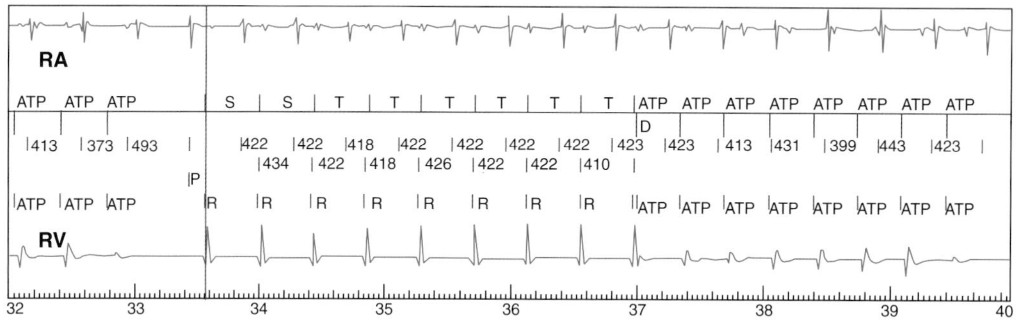

Proarrhythmia ATP in 1:1 SVT (rapidly conducted AF)

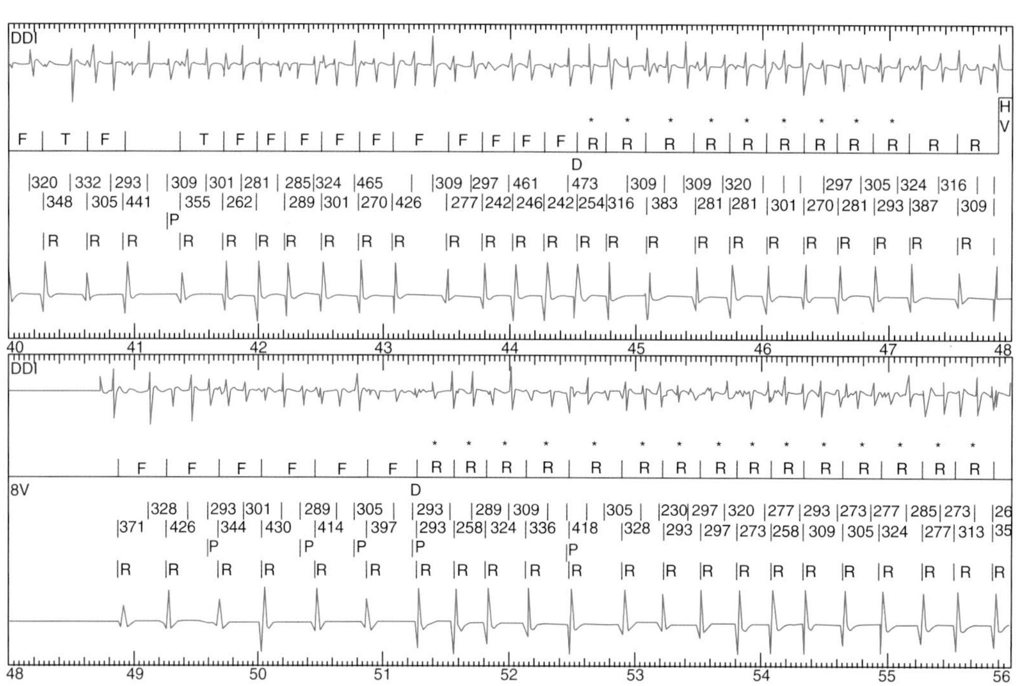

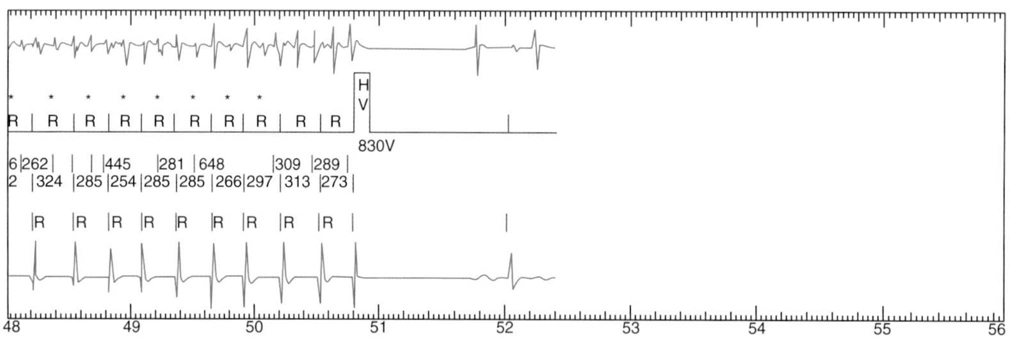

Figure 3-74. Atrial proarrhythmia caused by ventricular antitachycardia pacing in 1:1 supraventricular tachycardia (SVT). Continuous stored EGM shows right atrial (RA) EGM, event markers, and true bipolar right ventricular (RV) EGM. In the top panel, antitachycardia pacing (ATP) is delivered after rate-only, inappropriate detection of sinus tachycardia as ventricular tachycardia. Ventricular-atrial conduction occurs, initiating atrial fibrillation (AF), which is detected as ventricular fibrillation and requires two shocks (HV) before termination. The first shock is delivered at the end of the middle panel and the second in the middle of the lower panel. Recording is suspended for approximately 1 second after each shock.

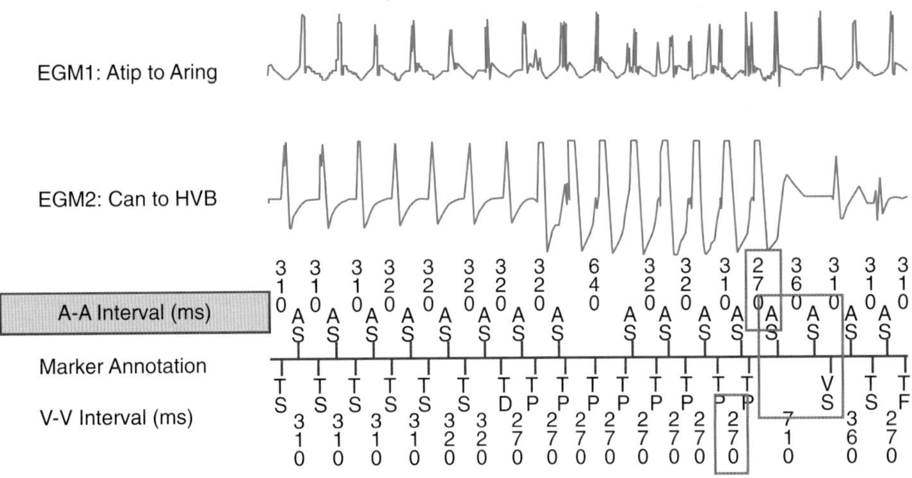

Figure 3-75. Effect of ventricular antitachycardia pacing on supraventricular tachycardia (SVT) with 1:1 atrioventricular (AV) relationship. Atrial EGM (Atip to Aring), high-voltage ventricular EGM (Can to HVB), and dual-chamber event markers are shown. Burst ventricular antitachycardia pacing at cycle length 270 msec is applied to SVTs with cycle lengths of 310 to 320 msec. The atrial interval after the last paced beat is accelerated to the pacing rate, probably indicating entrainment of the atrium. The A-A-V response at termination of pacing is diagnostic of atrial tachycardia.

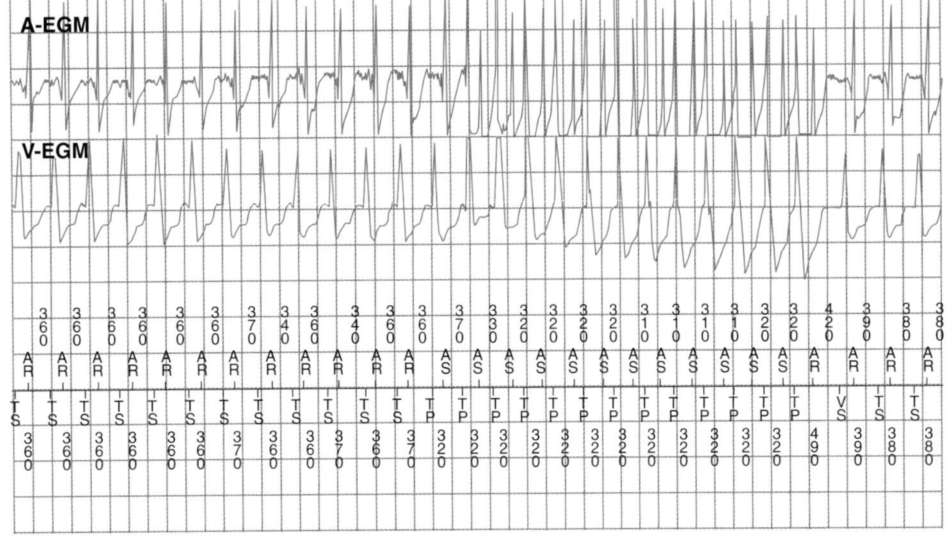

Figure 3-76. Atrial response to ventricular antitachycardia pacing during ventricular tachycardia (VT) with 1:1 ventricular-atrial (VA) conduction. Stored atrial (A) and ventricular (V) EGMs are shown with event markers. During antitachycardia pacing, atrial rate accelerates to ventricular rate. The V-A-V response at termination of pacing is characteristic of VT, although atrioventricular (AV) nodal and AV reciprocating tachycardias cannot be excluded.

and analyze the timing of the next ventricular event. Another is to deliver a train of atrial pacing and evaluate the ventricular response. Atrial extrastimuli usually shorten the next R-R interval in SVT, and atrial overdrive pacing usually accelerates the ventricular rate during SVT. This method may classify the rhythm incorrectly if the atrial stimuli block in the AV conduction system or conduct with too much decrement. It may also misclassify VT if ventricular capture occurs, usually in slower VTs. Atrial pacing may be proarrhythmic for either the atrium or the ventricle.[122]

Duration-Based "Safety-Net" Features to Override Discriminators

These programmable features deliver therapy if an arrhythmia satisfies the ventricular rate criterion for a sufficiently long duration even if discriminators indicate SVT (Guidant Sustained-Duration Override, Medtronic High Rate Timeout, St. Jude Maximum Time to Diagnosis). The premise is that VT will continue to satisfy the rate criterion for the programmed duration, whereas the ventricular rate during transient sinus tachycardia or AF will decrease below the VT rate boundary before the duration is exceeded. The limitation is delivery of inappropriate therapy when SVT exceeds the programmed duration, which occurs in approximately 10% of SVTs at 1 minute and 3% of SVTs at 3 minutes.[103,111] The decision to use a discriminator override should be based on clinical factors, including the probability that discriminators will prevent detection of VT, the likely consequences of failure to detect VT, and the likelihood that SVT in the VT rate zone will persist long enough to trigger inappropriate therapy because of the override. For example, override features may be considered whenever a morphology algorithm is programmed without inducing VT at electrophysiologic study. The programmed duration in the Guidant Atrial View and St. Jude algorithms should be increased from the nominal value of 30 seconds to reduce inappropriate therapies. In most patients, a duration of 2 to 5 minutes is appropriate.

SVT-VT Discriminators in Redetection

SVT-VT discrimination during redetection serves two purposes: (1) to prevent inappropriate therapy for SVT after appropriate therapy for VT (Fig. 3-77) and (2) to provide a second chance for the algorithm to classify SVT correctly after inappropriate therapy. Biotronik ICDs (Fig. 3-78) and ELA ICDs provide essentially equivalent SVT-VT discrimination in initial detection and redetection, except that algorithm building blocks related to tachycardia onset are disabled. Guidant algorithms permit programming discriminators after shocks, but not after ATP. In Medtronic ICDs, the single-chamber stability discriminator applies to redetection if it is ON for initial detection, but dual-chamber discrimination is not applied. St. Jude devices do not

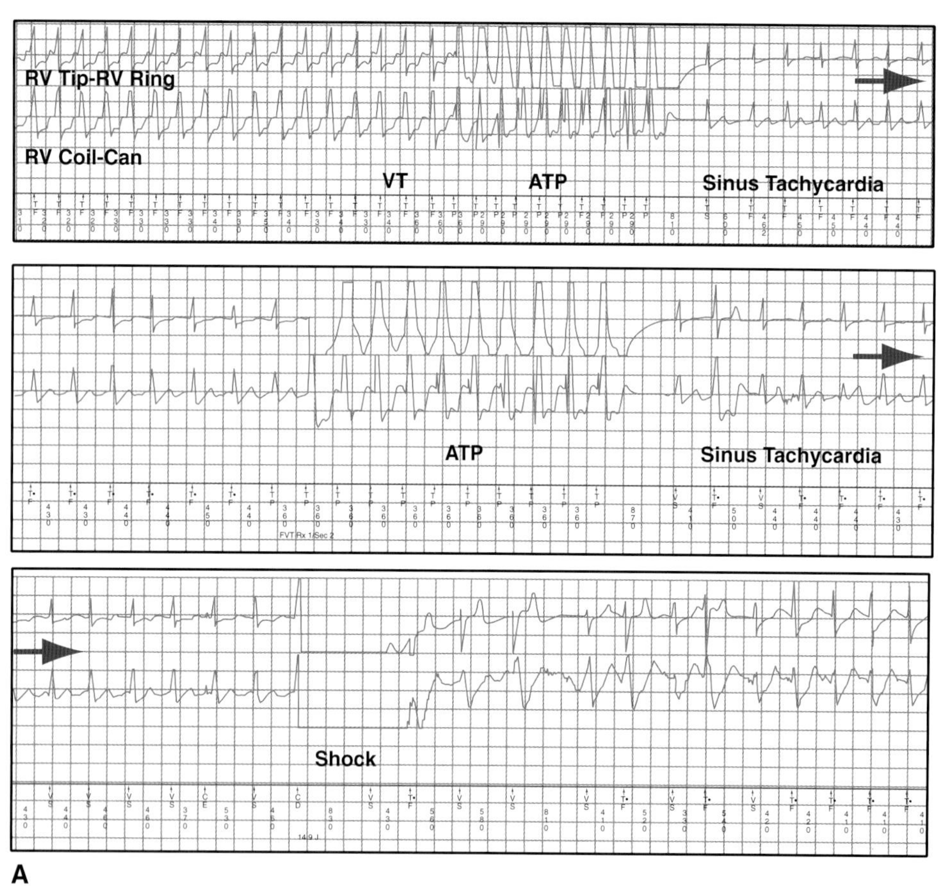

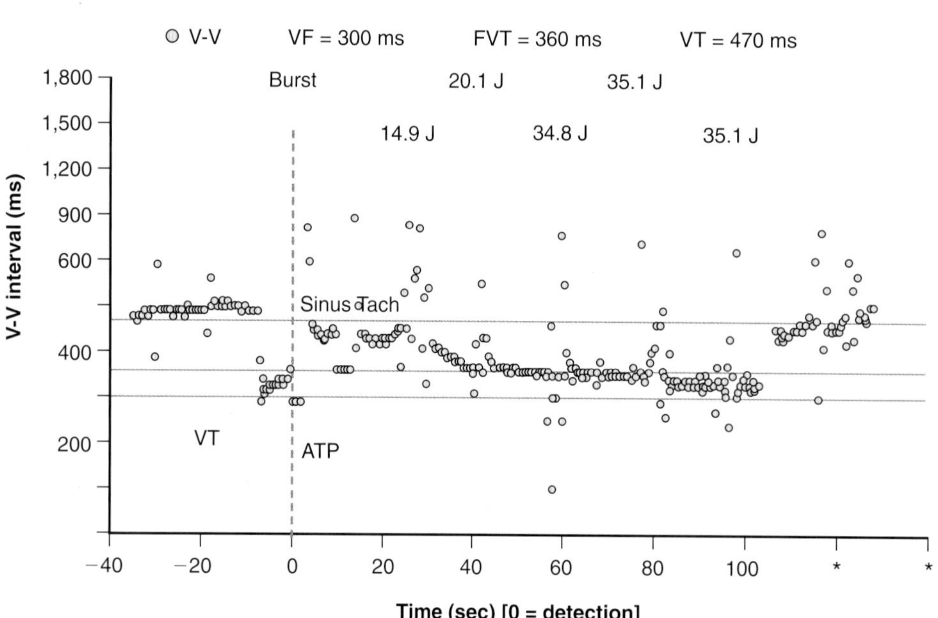

Figure 3-77. *Redetection. Inappropriate therapy of sinus tachycardia after appropriate therapy for ventricular tachycardia (VT) in a single-chamber ICD. Ventricular sensing and high-voltage leads are shown with event markers.* ***A,*** *Continuous stored EGM strips after detection of VT. The top strip shows successful antitachycardia pacing (ATP) of VT followed by sinus tachycardia in the Fast VT (FVT) zone (TF on event markers). The second strip shows the first inappropriate sequence of ATP. The third strip shows the first of five shocks delivered after ATP.* ***B,*** *Interval plot shows the entire episode. No U.S. ICD manufacturer provides for VT-supraventricular tachycardia (SVT) discrimination after ATP. (From Swerdlow CD, Friedman PA: Advanced ICD Troubleshooting: Part II. PACE 29: 70-96, 2006, with permission.) RV, right ventricular; VF, ventricular fibrillation.*

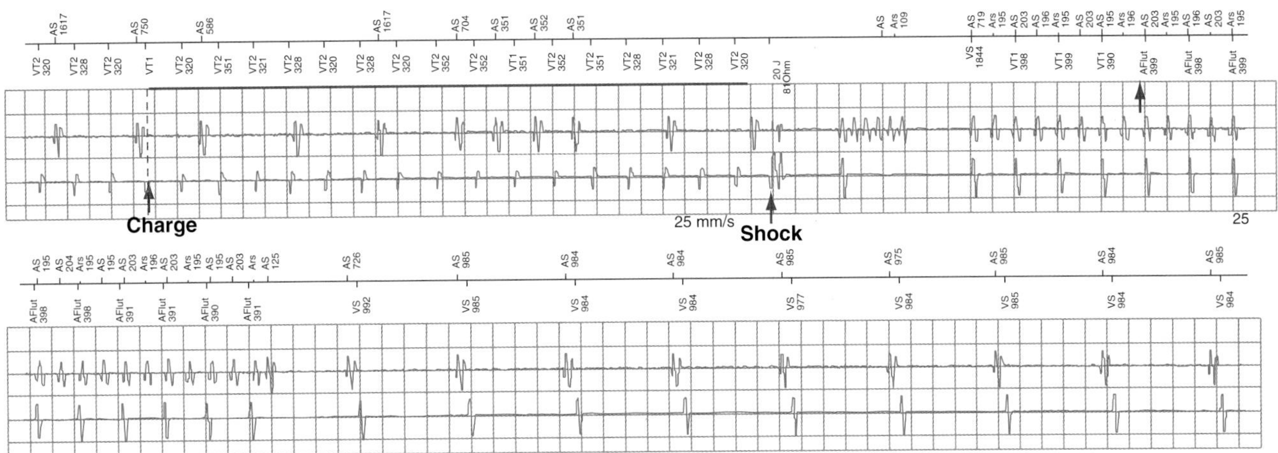

Figure 3-78. Supraventricular tachycardia/ventricular tachycardia (SVT-VT) discrimination in redetection. Dual-chamber EGM markers, atrial EGM, and true bipolar EGM are shown in this continuous strip from a Biotronik Lexos ICD, Model 347000. Rhythm at beginning of upper panel is VT with ventricular-atrial (VA) dissociation. Vertical dotted line indicates detection and start of capacitor charging (Charge). Black horizontal line indicates period of capacitor charging followed by successful shock. Postshock nonsustained atrial flutter begins toward right side of upper panel, continues into lower panel, and shows transient atrial flutter followed by conversion to sinus rhythm. Ventricular rhythm is classified by the lower row of markers as VT2 (faster VT zone) before shock, VT1 (slower VT zone) for the first four ventricular EGMs of atrial flutter, and conducted atrial flutter (Aflut) beginning at the fifth conducted ventricular EGM during atrial flutter (arrowhead). *Without SVT-VT discrimination in redetection, VT would have been redetected after 10 intervals.*

apply discriminators to redetection. Therefore, neither Medtronic nor St. Jude ICDs provide any single- or dual-chamber discriminators to reject sinus tachycardia after therapy.

Measuring Performance of SVT-VT Discrimination Algorithms

A comprehensive assessment requires analysis of all tachycardia episodes, including those that are not stored in ICD memory and those in the VF zone to which discriminators may not apply.[62,63,114] Programmed detection parameters may influence reported algorithm performance.[63] In most studies, a few patients contribute a large number of SVT or VT episodes. Therefore, statistical methods such as the generalized estimating equation (GEE)[123] should be used to remove bias in raw performance measures introduced by these unusual patients. Although there are valid reasons to focus analysis on a limited class of tachycardias to evaluate the differential performance of specific algorithm building blocks, overall performance across the patient population must always be considered.

Quantitative Considerations

All detection algorithms must maintain almost 100% sensitivity for detection of VT. If patient populations and programmed detection boundaries are equivalent, *positive predictive accuracy* may be the most useful statistical measure of algorithm performance.[62] It is highly dependent on the ratio of SVT to VT episodes and therefore on the programmed detection rate and patient population (prevalence of SVT and VT). Nevertheless, it is usually preferable to specificity, an commonly used alternative measure. Regardless of what specific performance measure is employed, it is almost impossible to obtain clinically meaningful insights into the performance of two different detection algorithms based only on their performance numbers on different sets of data. Consider the following two examples.

In the first example, the distribution of SVT versus VT and the distribution of “easy” versus “difficult” arrhythmias (e.g., AF with a highly irregular ventricular rate versus AF with a faster, regular ventricular rate) presented to an algorithm influences its performance.[124,125] For instance, an algorithm that uses consecutive-interval counting rejects “easy” AF with highly irregular ventricular rate at the level of rate counting and does not store the episode in ICD memory. Only “difficult” AF with a more regular ventricular rhythm is presented to the discriminator and stored in the ICD. In contrast, algorithms that use X out of Y counting or interval averaging present most AF episodes with highly irregular ventricular rhythms to the discriminator for storage in ICD memory.[96,126] However, if both ICDs delivered eight appropriate therapies for VT and two inappropriate therapies for AF, they would have the same positive predictive value, 80%.

In the second example, single clinical SVTs frequently are counted as multiple SVT episodes in ICD data logs, because the ventricular rate varies spontaneously around the VT rate threshold. This is especially true of AF. Consider one clinical episode of AF that is rejected correctly nine times within a few minutes and then treated inappropriately with a shock that terminates it. By analysis of the ICD data log for ICD episodes, the specificity is 90%. By the patient’s reckoning, the inappropriate shock is the same whenever it happens, during the episode of AF or not. On the other hand, credit is rarely assigned to algorithms for "partial success" or for success despite compromised sensing. An algorithm that detects VT inappropriately after 10 minutes of SVT has performed better than one that detects inappropriately after 10 seconds of the same SVT. An algorithm that classifies the atrial rhythm correctly with low-amplitude atrial EGMs and large FFRWs is more robust than one that makes the same classification from an exemplary atrial signal.

Inappropriate Detection Versus Inappropriate Therapy

ATP is delivered immediately after detection. Therefore, the numbers of detections and therapies are equivalent. In contrast, shock delivery requires capacitor charging, during which therapy may be aborted. However, delivery of an inappropriate shock results in a more adverse clinical outcome than delivery of inappropriate ATP.

Active discrimination blurs the distinction between detection and therapy, introducing new complexity into the evaluation of algorithm performance. With active discrimination, only tachycardias that persist immediately after diagnostic pacing are classified. Further, concealed conduction into the AV node may cause transient slowing of the ventricular rate during atrial arrhythmias, resulting in repetitive ICD-defined detections and terminations of a single SVT episode.

Comment

Valid assessments and comparisons of algorithm performance require consideration of multiple device-related and clinical factors. In isolation, statistical measures are rarely informative.

Is Ventricular Therapy for Supraventricular Tachycardia Always Inappropriate?

Persistent, rapidly-conducted atrial arrhythmias can cause hemodynamic compromise in patients with LV dysfunction or ischemia in patients with severe coronary artery disease. Because ventricular shocks often terminate AF and ventricular ATP often terminates 1:1 AT, algorithmically inappropriate ventricular therapy may fortuitously terminate clinically significant SVT.

However, inappropriate ventricular therapy for SVT can have serious consequences. ATP may be proarrhythmic,[127] and shocks for rapidly conducted AF have multiple drawbacks. First, AF in patients with ICDs is often paroxysmal, rapid conduction is often transient, and symptoms are usually mild, but ventricular shocks delivered shortly after detection do not permit spontaneous termination of AF or slowing of the ventricular rate. Therefore, they will be delivered for AF that would either have terminated spontaneously or have had only transient, rapid conduction. Second, detection algorithms in ventricular ICDs cannot use the total duration of (slowly conducted) AF to withhold shocks. Therefore, inappropriate shocks for AF may place patients at risk for thromboembolism if they are not anticoagulated. Finally, early recurrence is common after transvenous cardioversion of AF.[128]

Experts differ about whether algorithmically inappropriate ventricular therapy of SVT may be clinically appropriate in specific clinical situations. ICDs designed to deliver both atrial and ventricular therapies may be implanted in patients who are likely to benefit from device-based therapy of SVT.

Detection: Programming and Troubleshooting

Present ICDs have multiple programmable parameters that affect detection directly or indirectly. They provide opportunity both for customizing detection and for operator error. The trend of the 1990s for maximizing flexibility has been replaced by one to simplify the user interface while minimizing loss of automatic or operator-programmed versatility to address a wide range of clinical situations. A recent prospective study reported that empirical programming of dual-chamber ICDs provided comparable performance to individualized programming.[115] Even if nearly universal nominal programming may soon be possible, it is important to understand the many tradeoffs and compromises inherent in programming and troubleshooting ICD detection.

Detection Zones and Duration

Zones and Zone Boundaries

Typical values for rate zone boundaries are 500 to 360 msec for slower VT, 360 to 300 msec for faster VT, and 300 to 240 msec for VF. Two- or three-zone programming is preferred in most patients, even those undergoing implantation for secondary prevention and those whose only clinical arrhythmia is VF, because most spontaneous VF begins with rapid VT, and most rapid VT can be terminated by ATP.[129-131] Three zones permit different ATP therapies for two distinct rates of VT, as well as ATP for monomorphic VT that overlaps in rate with polymorphic VT. Other experts recommend two rate zones, with the slowest at a cycle length of 340 to 320 msec, for primary prevention patients[132] and those whose only spontaneous arrhythmia is VF. This approach lowers the risk of inappropriate therapy but increases the risk of not treating VT. In the largest primary prevention trial,[132] ICDs were programmed to a single detection zone at a cycle length of 320 msec, without SVT-VT discriminators. Approximately one third of shocks were inappropriate; the incidence of sudden death from undetected VT was not reported.

The sinus-VT rate boundary should be slow enough to ensure detection of all hemodynamically compromising VTs. To prevent underdetection of irregular VT, the VT detection interval should be set with a safety margin at least 40 to 50 msec longer than the slowest predicted VT for consecutive-interval counting and 30 to 40 msec longer for X out of Y or interval+interval-average counting.[118] This safety margin should be a longer cycle length if rapidly conducted SVT is unlikely or SVT-VT discrimination is reliable at long cycle lengths (ELA ICDs).

The boundary between the two VT zones should be based on the cycle length at which different types or fewer trials of ATP are preferred. The VT-VF rate boundary is based on the cycle length below which ATP should not be delivered. In Medtronic ICDs, which use consecutive interval counting above the VF interval and X out of Y counting below it, this boundary should be set to prevent underdetection of irregular, polymorphic VT by consecutive interval counting.

Monitor-only Zones

If therapy is not programmed "on" for slow VT, the slowest rate zone may be programmed as a "monitor-only" zone, with detection "on" and therapies "off." However, in Guidant, St. Jude, and older Medtronic ICDs (before Marquis), interactions between the counters in the monitor-only zone and the next zone may restrict use of SVT-VT discriminators or decrease the number of intervals required for detection in the therapy zone. Newer Medtronic ICDs (Marquis and later) provide independent monitor-only zones that avoid these limitations: because events in the "monitor" zone do not increment the detection counter, tachycardias in the monitor-only zone do not accelerate therapy even if a few intervals cross into the slowest therapy zone. The associated risk is delay in VT therapy if the VT cycle length fluctuates around the border between the monitor-only and therapy zones.

Duration for Detection of Ventricular Tachycardia

Detection duration before ATP should not be decreased from nominal values, because therapy is immediate after detection, and undersensing of monomorphic VT is rare. It should be increased in patients who have long episodes of nonsustained VT (e.g., long QT syndrome). Substantial increases in duration for detection of VT probably are safe in St. Jude and Guidant ICDs, which use counting methods that are insensitive to occasional long ventricular intervals or undersensing. In contrast, consecutive-interval counting used by Medtronic ICDs in the VT zone may underdetect VT if occasional long ventricular intervals or undersensing occurs.[106] Unless VT is known to be highly regular, the number of intervals to detect VT probably should not be more than 50% greater than the nominal value in Medtronic ICDs.

Duration for Detection of Ventricular Fibrillation

Because the confirmation process is necessarily "trigger happy," the first line of defense against inappropriate therapy for nonsustained VT or SVT in the VF zone is an appropriately long detection duration. Nominal values should be increased in patients who have long episodes of nonsustained device-detected VF (e.g., long QT syndrome). In Medtronic ICDs, nominal programming of the number of intervals for initial detection of VF (18 of 24) substantially reduces inappropriate therapies without significantly delaying detection, compared with 12 of 16 intervals,[130,133] another commonly used setting. Comparable settings for number of intervals or duration are available in ICDs from other manufacturers also. Duration for detection of VF should not be reduced from nominal if there is any alternative method to ensure reliable detection.

Duration for Redetection

Inappropriate therapy for nonsustained VT or SVT may be delivered after appropriate or inappropriate ATP or shocks (see Fig. 3-77). Increasing the duration for redetection may prevent inappropriate redetection of delayed termination of VT (type II break) or postshock nonsustained VT. However, excessive delays in detection or redetection may result in syncope, increase in defibrillation threshold, or undersensing caused by reduced amplitude and frequency of the sensed ventricular EGM. Fortunately, these adverse effects are rare for VF durations shorter than 30 seconds.[134]

ICDs misclassify effective therapy as ineffective if VT/VF recurs before the ICD identifies episode termination and reclassifies the post-therapy rhythm as sinus (Fig. 3-79). Misclassification may also occur due to limited SVT-VT discrimination during redetection if therapy successfully terminates VT during a double tachycardia (simultaneous SVT and VT) or if SVT begins after successful VT therapy but before episode termination because of frequent premature beats or nonsustained tachycardia. Decreasing the duration for redetection of sinus rhythm (St. Jude) may correct this classification error. However, this type of misclassification often does not constitute a clinical problem, whereas postshock detection of nonsustained VT does. An exception occurs when one iteration of ATP is programmed for the first therapy and a shock for the second. If ATP terminates VT, but it recurs before the rhythm is classified as sinus, the recurrent VT will receive a shock instead of a second potentially effective burst of ATP.

Range of Cycle Lengths to which SVT-VT Discriminators Apply

SVT-VT discriminators apply in a range of cycle lengths bounded on the slower end by the VT detection interval and on the faster end by a minimum cycle length that varies among manufacturers (see Fig. 3-49). Usually, SVT-VT discriminators will not withhold inappropriate therapy for SVT if the majority of ventricular intervals (typically 70% to 80%) are shorter than the SVT limit. Therefore, rapidly conducted AF may be classified as VT even if the mean cycle length is 20 to 40 msec longer than the SVT limit. Programming a sufficiently short minimum cycle length for SVT-VT discrimination is critical to reliable rejection of SVT. When discriminators are programmed, approximately 25% of inappropriate therapy is caused by SVT with ventricular cycle lengths shorter than that minimum cycle length.[62,135]

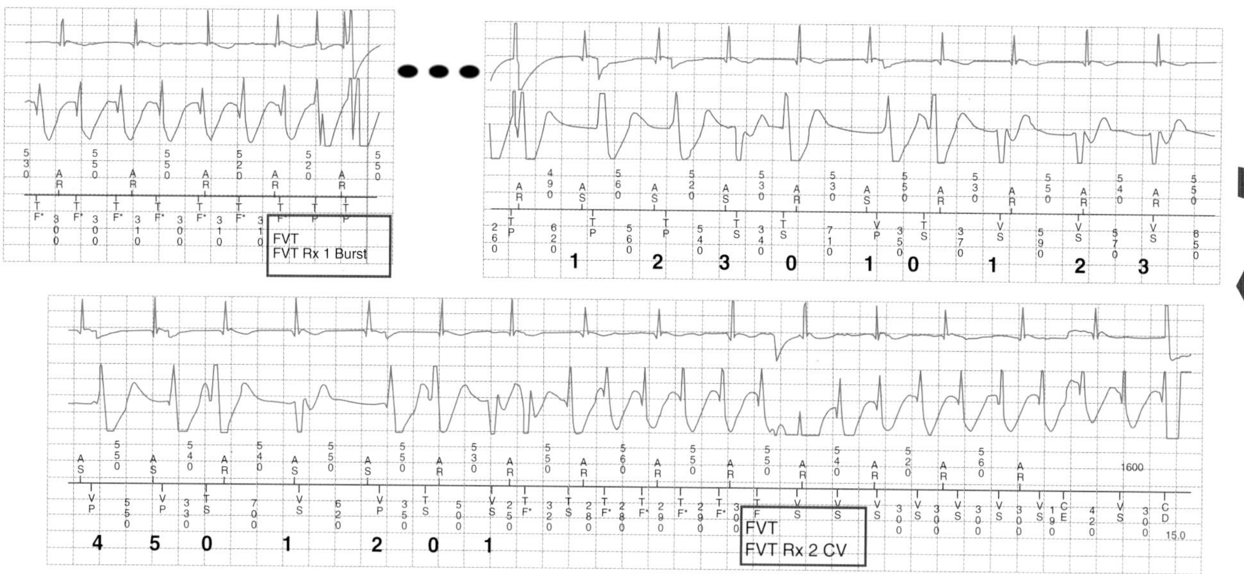

Figure 3-79. Failure to identify post-therapy sinus rhythm due to rapid reinitiation of ventricular tachycardia (VT) after successful therapy. Atrial EGM, ventricular true bipolar EGM, and EGM markers classify the rhythm as sinus (8 consecutive intervals). Therefore, VT is inappropriately redetected instead of being detected de novo for the second time. This results in delivery of the second programmed Fast VT (FVT) therapy, cardioversion, rather than repeat delivery of the previously successful antitachycardia pacing (ATP) stimulus, which is both painless and more energy efficient. Redetection marker (FV Rx 2 CV) indicates onset of capacitor charging for the second VT therapy. Shock is not shown. Large numbers below right side of upper panel and left side of lower panel show value of sinus rhythm counter, which increments for each interval in the sinus zone (VS) and is reset to zero by premature ventricular complexes (PVCs) with a coupling interval of less than the VT detection interval of 400 msec (TS). VS markers indicate unclassified ventricular intervals during capacitor charging. AS, atrial sense; AR, atrial intervals in pacing refractory period.

The performance of SVT-VT discriminators is linked explicitly or implicitly to boundaries between detection zones for ventricular arrhythmias. In Guidant ICDs, the link is explicit. Starting with the Vitality models (2004), SVT-VT discriminators are programmable to the entirety of either or both VT zones; previously, they were limited to the slower VT zone. In St. Jude ICDs, SVT-VT discriminators are programmable independently within the two VT zones but cannot be programmed in the VF zone. In Medtronic ICDs, the SVT Limit is programmable independently of VT/VF zone boundaries. However, the performance of the SVT rejection algorithm changes at the programmed VF detection interval, so that SVT with AV dissociation (AF) is not classified as SVT because it cannot be distinguished from VF. Further, Medtronic ICDs use consecutive-interval counting and other measures of R-R interval regularity to withhold inappropriate therapy for AF for rhythms with cycle length equal to or greater than the V-F interval. To ensure reliable detection of VF, they are not applied in the VF zone. Therefore, in the portion of the VF zone in which discriminators are applied, sinus tachycardia, AT, and 2:1 atrial flutter are rejected, but conducted AF is not. In nominal programming of Medtronic ICDs, the "VF Detection Interval" forms the boundary between the VT and Fast VT zones. Therefore, this degradation in discrimination of VT from rapidly conducted AF usually occurs between the VT and Fast VT zones. Conducted AF in the Fast VT zone may be classified correctly by programming "Fast VT via VT" rather than the nominal "Fast VT via VF." The risk is delay in detection of unusual, markedly irregular fast VT with occasional cycle lengths in the sinus zone.

Programming of SVT-VT Discriminators

Single-Chamber SVT-VT Discriminators

Technical details vary among manufacturers, as do corresponding recommended programmed values, which are summarized in Table 3-5. See "Ventricular EGM Morphology for SVT-VT Discrimination" for programming and troubleshooting of morphology algorithms.

Dual-Chamber SVT-VT Discriminators

Dual-chamber algorithms should be programmed ON in any patient with intact AV conduction and a functioning atrial lead. Specific considerations for each manufacturer are summarized in Table 3-6. In Medtronic and Guidant algorithms, incremental addition of discriminators increases the likelihood that SVT will be classified correctly (specificity) but decreases the likelihood that VT will be classified correctly (sensitivity). In St. Jude ICDs, discriminators may be combined using either the "ANY" or "ALL" operators. Using ANY, the algorithm detects VT if any discriminator classifies the tachycardia as VT, resulting in higher sensitivity and lower specificity. Conversely, using ALL, the algorithm detects VT only if all discriminators classify the tachy-

TABLE 3-5. Recommended Programming of SVT-VT Discriminators in Single-Chamber ICDs

	Medtronic	Guidant	St. Jude
Stability*	40-50 msec, NID = 16	24-40 msec, duration 2.5 sec	80 msec
Onset	84-88%	9%	150 msec
Morphology	3 of 8 electrograms ≥70% match	Not programmable†	5 of 8 electrograms ≥60% match

*Less strict values are required for patients taking type I or III antiarrhythmic drugs.
†3 of 10 electrograms with Feature Correlation Coefficient greater than threshold.
NID, number of intervals to detect VT.

TABLE 3-6. Recommended Programming of SVT-VT Discriminators in Dual-Chamber ICDs

	Guidant		
Medtronic PR Logic	Atrial View	Rhythm ID	St. Jude Rate Branch
AFib/AFlutter ON	AFib Rate Threshold	ON	Rate Branch ON
Sinus Tach ON	200 bpm		A = V Branch: Morphology
Other 1:1 SVTs	Onset 9%		A > V Branch Morphology; may combine Stability† with "ANY" logic
OFF 1:1 VT-ST	Inhibit If unstable 10%		
Boundary 66%*	V rate > A rate ON Sustained Rate Duration 3 min		

*Older models before Entrust (Model D153DRG).
†Stability at 80 msec with AV Association of 60 msec.

cardia as VT, resulting in lower sensitivity and higher specificity. The ALL operator corresponds to addition of discriminators in other algorithms.

St. Jude Rate Branch. Morphology should be programmed in both the V = A and V < A rate branches. Recommended programming adds the stability discriminator in the V < A branch using the ANY operator. This results in a minor increase in sensitivity for detection of VT (98% to 99%) and a similarly minor decrease in specificity (82% to 79%).[102] Addition of the stability discriminator using the ALL operator reduces inappropriate detection of aberrantly conducted AF but may also reduce sensitivity for detection of VT.[102]

Guidant Rhythm ID. This algorithm uses atrial versus ventricular rate, EGM morphology, and interval stability to discriminate VT from SVT,[110] the same three general features used by the St. Jude algorithm. It has no programmable features. The benefit of this algorithm's design is that it requires no custom programming; the limitation is that troubleshooting is not possible.

Guidant Atrial View. A major limitation of this earlier algorithm, inappropriate detection of rapidly conducted AF[61,135,136] due to obligatory PVAB, may be ameliorated by programming the PVAB period to the minimum value of 45 msec, the "AFib Rate" to the minimum value of 200 bpm, and the "Stability" feature to the highly specific value of 10%. This programming takes advantage of the fact that VT during AF or atrial flutter usually is highly regular and often is more regular than conducted 2:1 atrial flutter. However, highly regular 2:1 conduction of atrial flutter will be misclassified as VT, and slightly irregular VT that occurs during AF will be misclassified as SVT—especially in the setting of antiarrhythmic drugs.[106,137] There are no programming solutions for inability to detect VT with both 1:1 VA conduction and a gradual onset or for inability to reject 1:1 AT with abrupt onset.

Medtronic PR Logic. At implantation, rejection rules should be programmed "ON" for Sinus Tachycardia and Atrial Fibrillation/Flutter. The 1:1 SVT rejection rule should not be programmed until the atrial lead is stable, because its dislodgment to the ventricle may result in misclassification of VT as a 1:1 SVT. (This potential problem also applies to the St. Jude Rate Branch algorithm without additional discriminators.) PR Logic uses the patterns and rates of A-A, V-V, A-V, and V-A intervals to discriminate VT from SVT. This dependence, combined with the absence of atrial blanking periods after sensed ventricular events, made several generations of this algorithm susceptible to errors based on intermittent oversensing of FFRWs. These versions of PR Logic (still in use in cardiac resynchronization ICDs) also discriminate VT with 1:1 VA conduction from SVT, based on the ratio of P-R to R-R intervals. Increasing the value from the nominal setting of 50% to 66% reduces inappropriate therapy for 1:1 SVT with long P-R intervals without significantly increasing the risk of failing to detect VT with 1:1 VA conduction.[138] The present generation of Medtronic ICDs includes a new algorithm for identifying sinus tachycardia that reduces inappropriate detection of VT due to FFRWs and long P-R intervals in sinus tachycardia. It also reduces misclassification of VT with 1:1 VA conduction and a long R-P interval as sinus tachycardia.[112]

Undersensing and Underdetection

Undersensing and underdetection may be caused by ICD system performance, programmed values (including human error), or a combination of the two. They result in failure to delivery therapy or delay in therapy.

Undersensing

VF may be undersensed due to combinations of programming (sensitivity, rate, or duration), low-amplitude EGMs, rapidly varying EGM amplitude, drug effects, and postshock tissue changes. Clinically significant undersensing of VF is rare in modern ICD systems if the baseline R-wave amplitude is 5 to 7 mV or higher.[54] Postshock undersensing was an important clinical problem in older ICD systems that used integrated bipolar leads with closely spaced electrodes.[139] Presently, the most common causes of VF undersensing are drug or hyperkalemic effects that slow VF into the VT zone, ischemia, and rapidly varying EGM amplitude (Fig. 3-80).[48,65] ICDs that adjust dynamic range based on the amplitude of the sensed R wave (Guidant) may be the most vulnerable to the extremely rare problem of rapidly varying EGM amplitude[48] (Fig. 3-81). Prolonged ischemia from sustained VT slower than the VT detection interval may cause deterioration of signal quality, resulting in undersensing of VF. Lead, connector, or generator problems may also manifest as undersensing.

ICD Inactivation

If detection is programmed OFF for surgery using electrocautery, reprogramming must be performed at the end of the procedure, a fact that is easily forgotten, especially without patient surgery. One study reported an unexplained 11% annual incidence of transient suspension of detection.[140] This unfortunate problem is addressed in Medtronic Marquis and subsequent ICDs with an audible patient alert that sounds if programmed detection or therapy is "OFF" for longer than 6 hours.

Ventricular Tachycardia Slower than the Programmed Detection Interval

In most ICD patients, VT with cycle lengths greater than 400 to 450 msec are tolerated well, but repeated inappropriate therapies are not. However, slow VT can be catastrophic in patients with severe LV dysfunction or ischemia.[141] All SVT-VT discrimination algorithms (except those in ELA models[65,118,142]) deliver fewer inappropriate therapies if the VT detection interval is programmed to a shorter cycle length, simply because fewer SVTs are evaluated. A long VT detection interval is important in patients with advanced heart failure, in whom slow VT can be catastrophic[141] (Fig. 3-82; see Fig. 3-14). The VT detection interval should be increased if antiarrhythmic drug therapy is initiated, particularly with amiodarone or a sodium-channel blocking (type 1A or 1C) drug.[14,143] It may be prudent to measure the cycle length of induced VT at electrophysiologic testing after initiation of drug therapy.[143] However, spontaneous VT often is slower than induced VT.[144]

SVT-VT Discriminators

SVT-VT discriminators may prevent or delay therapy if they misclassify VT or VF as SVT.[102,103,106,145] Discriminators that re-evaluate the rhythm diagnosis during an ongoing tachycardia (e.g., stability, most dual-chamber algorithms) reduce the risk of underdetection of VT compared with discriminators that withhold therapy if the rhythm is not classified correctly by the initial evaluation (e.g., onset, chamber of origin algorithms). The minimum cycle length for SVT-VT discrimination should be set to prevent clinically significant delay in detection of hemodynamically unstable VT. See earlier discussions of discriminators and programming.

Pacemaker-ICD Interactions

Although interactions between ICDs and separate pacemakers have become rare since ICDs incorporated dual-chamber bradycardia pacing in the late 1990s, some combined systems have not been revised due to vascular access problems or other reasons. The multiple potential interactions have been reviewed, and testing protocols to detect them have been developed.[146-148] The principal interaction that may delay or prevent ICD therapy is oversensing of high-amplitude pacemaker stimulus artifacts. If this occurs during VF, repetitive automatic adjustment of sensing threshold and/or gain may prevent detection of VF.

Intradevice Interactions

Presently, intradevice interactions, in which bradycardia pacing features of dual-chamber ICDs interact with and impair detection of VT or VF, pose a greater challenge than pacemaker-ICD interactions between separate devices.[51] During high-rate, atrial or dual-chamber pacing, sensing may be restricted to short periods of the cardiac cycle because of the combined effects of ventricular blanking after ventricular pacing and cross-chamber ventricular blanking after atrial pacing, which is needed to avoid crosstalk. If a sufficient fraction of the cardiac cycle is blanked, systematic undersensing of VT or VF may occur. When pacing and blanking

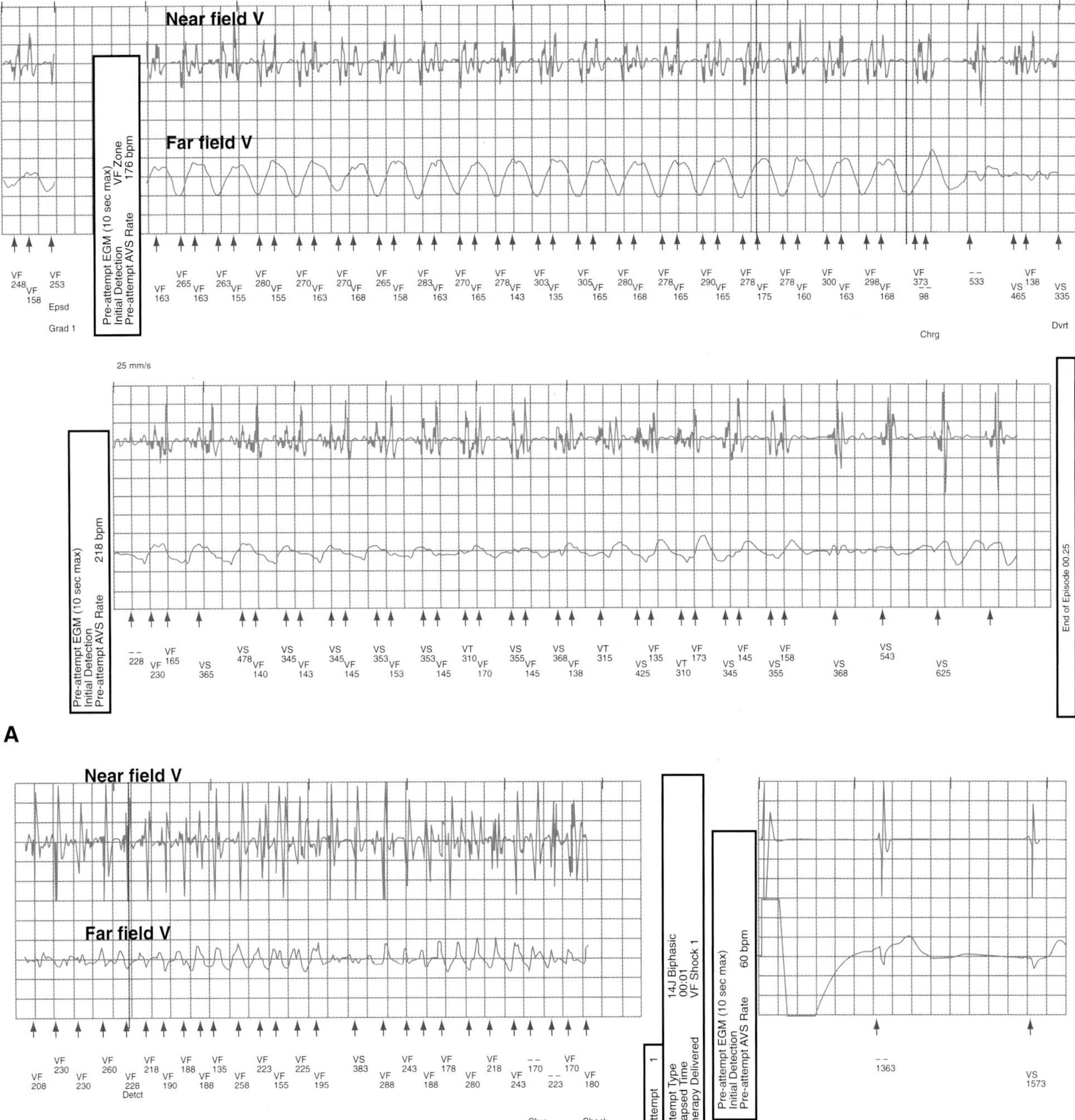

Figure 3-80. *Underdetection of ventricular fibrillation (VF) caused by hyperkalemia (potassium level, 6.7 mg/dL) in the setting of chronic amiodarone therapy.* ***A,*** *Near-field and far-field ventricular (V) EGM and event markers of a Guidant Prizm VR ICD are shown. The top panel shows a sine-wave ventricular tachycardia (VT) in the far-field channel, which is detected as VF because local EGMs on the near-field channel are double-counted. At right of upper panel, four intervals greater than the programmed VF detection interval of 316 msec (190 bpm) result in an aborted shock. The lower panel shows persistence of VF after the shock is aborted. Too few intervals are sensed in the VF zone to permit detection of VF. The patient was resuscitated by external shock.* ***B,*** *ICD system testing after correction of hyperkalemia. Induced VF is sensed reliably and is terminated by an ICD shock. The near-field EGM is narrow, indicating that double EGMs present during the clinical arrhythmia were caused by functional conduction block. (Courtesy of Dr. Felix Schnoell.)*

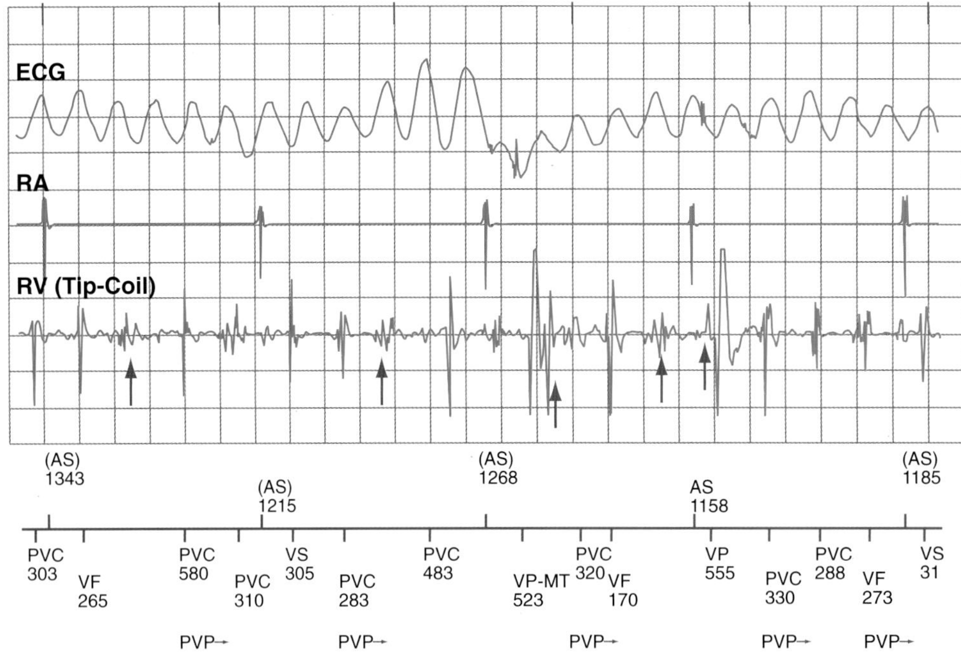

Figure 3-81. Undersensing of ventricular fibrillation (VF) despite normal R wave in sinus rhythm (18.5 mV). Programmer strip recorded at implantation testing of a Guidant Prizm ICD shows electrocardiogram (ECG), right atrial (RA) EGM, and integrated bipolar ventricular sensing EGM (RV Tip-Coil) during implantation testing. The VF EGMs have highly variable amplitudes, resulting in undersensing of low-amplitude EGMs immediately after high-amplitude ones (arrows). *Intermittent ventricular pacing (VP) introduces postpacing blanking periods. Slow Automatic Gain Control may contribute to this type of undersensing. AS, atrial sensed event; PVC, premature ventricular complex; PVP→, extension of postventricular atrial refractory period (PVARP); VP, ventricular paced event. (Modified from Dekker LR, Schrama TA, Steinmetz FH, et al: Undersensing of VF in a patient with optimal R wave sensing during sinus rhythm. PACE 27(6 Pt 1):833-834, 2004, with permission.)*

events occur at intervals that are multiples of a VT/VF cycle length, ventricular complexes are repeatedly undersensed, delaying or preventing detection (Fig. 3-83).[49-51]

Although intradevice interactions are uncommon, they have been reported most frequently with the use of the Rate Smoothing algorithm in ICDs.[49-51] This algorithm is intended to prevent VT/VF initiated by sudden changes in ventricular rate.[149] It prevents sudden changes in ventricular rate by pacing both the atrium and the ventricle at intervals based on the preceding (baseline) R-R interval. As an unintended consequence, it may prevent sensing of VT/VF in some patients, because it introduces repetitive postpacing blanking periods. The algorithm applies rate smoothing to baseline intervals independent of their cycle length, including intervals in the VT or VF zones. Intradevice interactions that result in delayed or absent detection of VT/VF are most common and most dangerous when VT is fast. The parameter interrelationships that result in delayed or absent detection of VT/VF are complex and difficult to predict, but they usually elicit a programmer warning. Generally, aggressive rate smoothing (a small allowable percentage change in R-R intervals), a high upper pacing rate, and a long and fixed AV interval favor undersensing and should be avoided. If rate smoothing is required, the AV delay should be dynamic, the upper rates should be 125 bpm or less, and parameter combinations that result in warnings should be avoided. This programming reduces, but does not eliminate, the risk of undersensing.[49-51,150]

Detection of SVT and VT as a Diagnostic Tool and as a Basis for Atrial Antitachycardia Pacemakers and Atrial ICDs

Detection of SVT and VT provides diagnostics that are useful for pacemaker management.[80] Atrial ATP and atrial shocks provide a therapeutic option for some patients with paroxysmal atrial tachyarrhythmias. Appropriate delivery of this therapy requires accurate detection and discrimination of atrial tachycardia/flutter (AT) and AF.

Pacemaker Diagnostics

Monitoring for Ventricular Tachycardia

Some pacemakers have ventricular high-rate diagnostics that trigger EGM and/or marker storage of nonpaced rhythms that are faster than a specific rate. Triggers based on ventricular rate alone store episodes

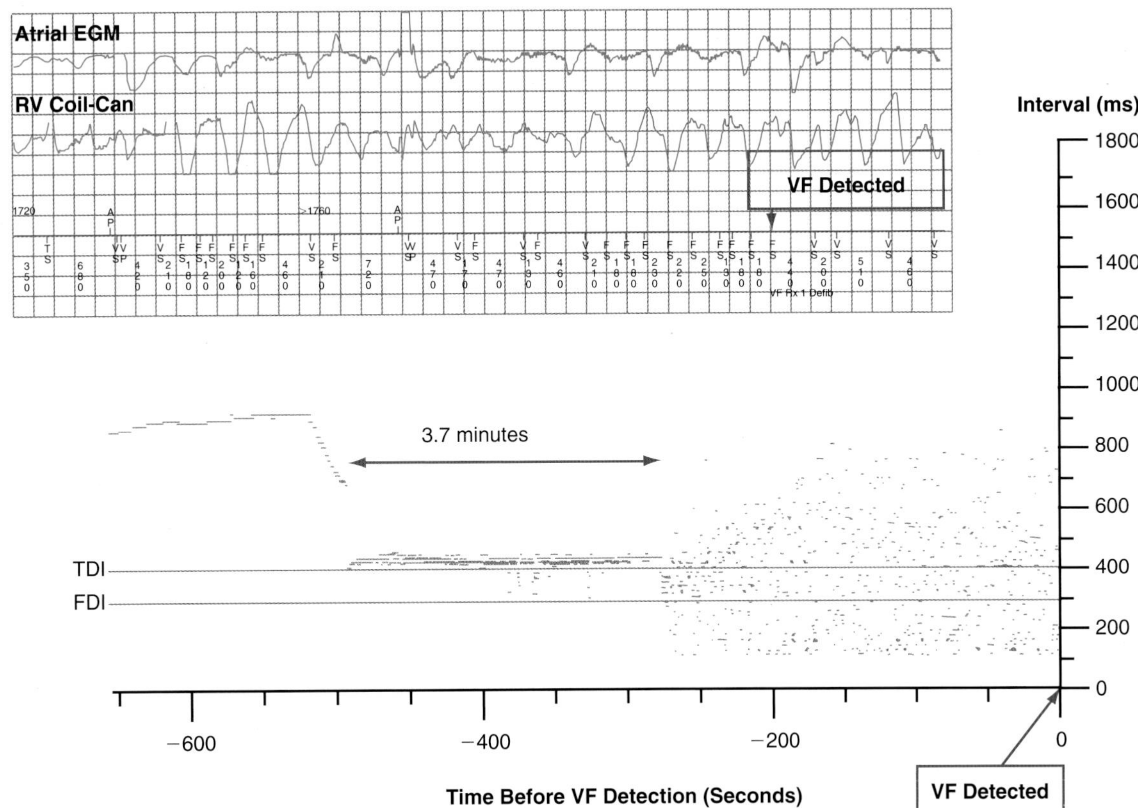

Figure 3-82. Ventricular tachycardia (VT) slower than the programmed detection interval. The lower panel is a "Flashback Interval" plot of R-R interval cycle lengths before detection of ventricular fibrillation (VF), which occurs at the right side of each panel. The interval number before detection is plotted on the abscissa, and the corresponding interval is plotted on the ordinate. Horizontal lines indicate the VT detection interval (TDI) of 400 msec and the VF detection interval (FDI) of 320 msec. Shortly after the 500th interval preceding detection, regular tachycardia begins abruptly. The constant cycle length indicates reliable ventricular sensing. Atrial flashback intervals (not shown) demonstrated atrioventricular (AV) dissociation. This VT is not detected despite reliable sensing, because the cycle length is greater than the programmed TDI. VT persists for 3.7 minutes until approximately interval 280 before detection, when sensed intervals become highly variable. This indicates degeneration of the rhythm to VF with undersensing that delays detection. During VT and VF, atrial Flashback Intervals (not shown) indicated lower rate limit bradycardia pacing at 40 bpm (1500 msec). The upper panel shows stored atrial and far-field ventricular EGMs immediately before detection with atrial and ventricular channel showing event markers. Specific undersensed EGMs cannot be identified because the rate-sensing EGM was not recorded. However, long sensed R-R intervals ending with VS (ventricular sense) markers indicate undersensing and correspond to long intervals in the upper panel. "VF Therapy 1 Defib" at lower right (arrow) *denotes detection of VF. AP, atrial pace; FD, VF detected; FS, intervals in VF zone. (From Swerdlow C, Friedman P: Advanced ICD Troubleshooting: Part I. PACE 28:1322-1346, 2005, with permission.)*

that may be rapidly conducted SVT, ventricular oversensing, or VT. Studies of these diagnostics demonstrate the importance of stored EGMs to confirm the diagnosis, because the false-positive detection rate is high.[82,151] Newer dual-chamber pacemakers and antitachycardia pacemakers incorporate tachyarrhythmia detection algorithms that are identical or substantially identical to those in dual-chamber ICDs (Fig. 3-84). The performance of these algorithms may be influenced by differences in pacemaker and ICD atrial sensing characteristics (fixed atrial sensitivity, automatically adjusting sensitivity, or an intermediate case) and atrial blanking periods (Figs. 3-85 and 3-86). Even with accurate atrial sensing, Bayes theorem predicts that the fraction of false-positive VT detections in patients with pacemakers is large, because the incidence of true VT is low compared with most ICD patient groups.

Monitoring for Atrial Tachycardia and Atrial Fibrillation

Traditional pacemaker diagnostics for atrial high-rate episodes and automatic mode switches have been validated as a means of monitoring AT/AF.[81,152] Diagnostic accuracy of these methods depends on the specific detection algorithm used and the accuracy of atrial sensing. Detection algorithms for atrial antiarrhythmic pacemakers and ICDs provide substantial additional information, including atrial EGMs, classification of AT

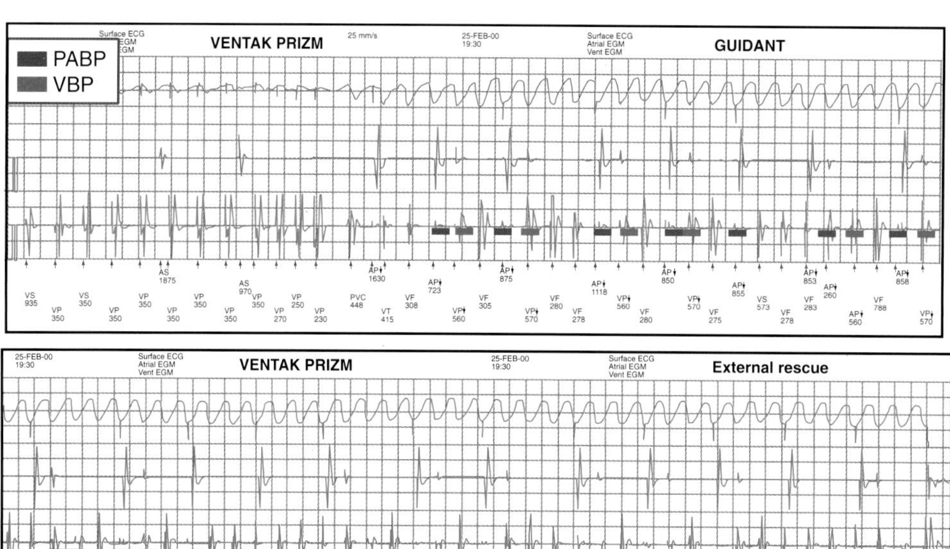

Figure 3-83. Failure to detect ventricular tachycardia (VT) due to an intradevice interaction. The rate-smoothing algorithm introduced atrial and ventricular pacing complexes with associated blanking periods that prevented detection of VT during postimplantation testing. An external rescue shock was required. Shown from top to bottom are the surface electrocardiogram (ECG), atrial EGM, ventricular EGM, and event markers. At top, VT is induced by programmed electrical stimulation with a drive cycle length of 350 msec and premature stimuli at 270, 250, and 230 msec (intervals labeled next to event markers). The first sensed ventricular event occurs 448 msec after the pacing drive (PVC 448). The rate-smoothing algorithm drives pacing to prevent a pause after the premature ventricular complex (PVC), labeled AP↓1638. A ventricular paced event does not follow the first AP↓ because a ventricular event is sensed (VT 415). Subsequent rate smoothing generated atrial and ventricular pacing pulses (indicated by AP↓ and VP↓ markers, respectively). The resultant postpacing blanking periods are shown on the figure as horizontal bars. PABP denotes cross-chamber (postatrial pacing) ventricular blanking period. VBP denotes same-chamber (postventricular pacing) blanking period. Together, they prevent approximately four of every six VT complexes from being sensed. Because the VT counter must accumulate 8 out of 10 consecutive complexes in the VT zone for detection of VT to occur, VT is not detected. (From Swerdlow C, Friedman P: Advanced ICD Troubleshooting: Part II. PACE 29:70-96, 2006, with permission.)

versus AF, and integrated displays of data from multiple episodes. These include histograms of episode duration and ventricular rate during AT/AF that may be of value in managing atrial antiarrhythmic drugs and AV nodal blocking drugs (Fig. 3-87). The former histogram, combined with patient-activated device interrogations (Fig. 3-88), may permit discontinuation of anticoagulation in some patients.

Detection of Atrial Tachycardia and Atrial Fibrillation

Principles

Bradycardia pacemakers must detect AT/AF rapidly so that mode switching will avoid uncomfortable pacing at the upper rate limit. To determine the atrial rate and rhythm accurately, atrial blanking must be minimized. As long as the atrial rate exceeds the upper tracking limit, accurate determination of atrial rate and rhythm is not important. Ventricular ICDs must discriminate VT from rapidly conducted AF quickly, to permit rapid detection of hemodynamically compromising VT. Discrimination of AT versus AF is less important and less urgent. In contrast, atrial antiarrhythmic pacemakers and ICDs must detect AF with high specificity to minimize painful and potentially proarrhythmic therapy. Rapid detection is not important, because AF usually is clinically stable and may terminate spontaneously after hours to days. Therefore, atrial antiarrhythmic devices should be capable of permitting therapy for long-duration AT/AF while withholding therapy from self-terminating AT/AF. To achieve this goal, they must be capable of detecting AF continuously for extended periods, in order to discriminate between repetitive self-terminating episodes and persistent episodes. Because atrial EGMs in AF have low and variable amplitudes and slew rates, antiarrhythmic devices must have high (automatically adjusting) atrial sensitivity and apply algorithms that are tolerant of some atrial undersensing. They must also discriminate between AT and AF to deliver ATP for AT.

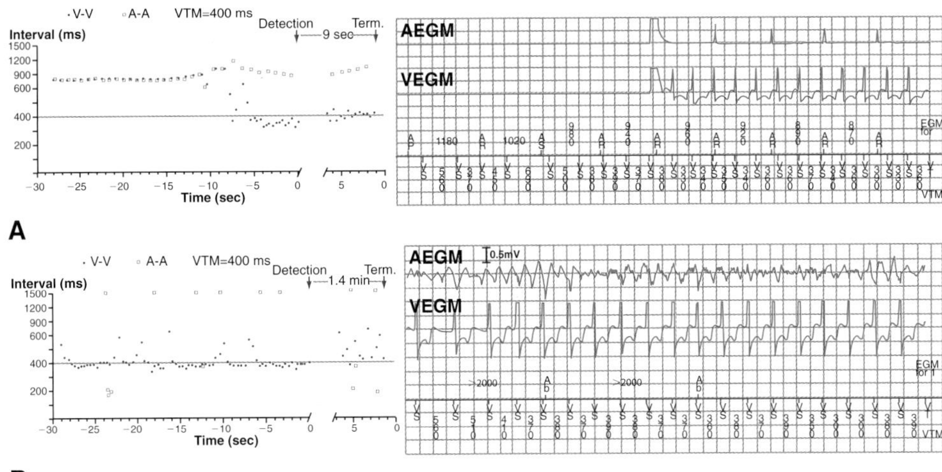

Figure 3-84. Pacemaker diagnostics for monitoring of ventricular tachycardia (VT), showing stored intervals, atrial EGM (AEGM), ventricular EGM (VEGM), and markers from a patient with a Medtronic EnRhythm DR pacemaker. The left panels show the A-A and V-V intervals plotted against time before VT detection, which requires 16 consecutive intervals at less than the VT monitoring interval of 400 msec (horizontal line). *The right panels show dual-chamber EGM and markers.* ***A,*** *Onset of spontaneous VT occurs with several premature ventricular complexes (PVCs) and sudden acceleration of ventricular rate with little or no change in A-A intervals* (left panel). *The VT cycle length is initially 340 msec and progressively lengthens to greater than 400 msec after several seconds. After 8 consecutive intervals of 400 msec or longer, the device declares the episode to be "terminated" despite clear atrioventricular (AV) dissociation and ongoing VT (right-hand side of interval plot). The duration of VT is reported as 9 seconds, representing the time that the R-R intervals remained less than 400 msec after initial detection. Dual-chamber EGM and markers leading up to detection of VT indicate appropriate sensing in both chambers and AV dissociation* (right panel). ***B,*** *Rapidly conducted atrial fibrillation with severe atrial undersensing reported as VT. The interval plot shows fast and irregular R-R intervals and long A-A intervals (1500 msec), with sporadic A-A intervals shorter than 200 msec. Dual-chamber EGMs indicate appropriate ventricular sensing but severe atrial undersensing of small-amplitude atrial fibrillation, resulting in false-positive detection of VT. AB, atrial sense in postventricular atrial blanking period; AR, atrial refractory sense; AS, atrial sense; VS, ventricular sense; VT, VT detected.*

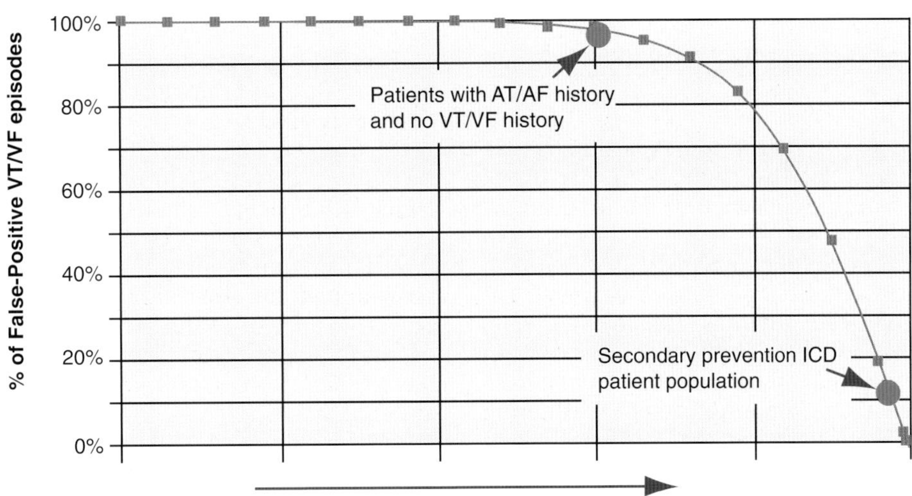

Figure 3-85. Rate of inappropriate ventricular tachycardia/fibrillation (VT/VF) detection depends on the patient population. Bayes theorem predicts that patients with a higher incidence of true VT/VF relative to supraventricular tachycardia (SVT) will have fewer inappropriate detections than patients with a lower incidence of VT/VF. The receiver operator curve shows the Bayes theorem prediction of detection performance of an algorithm with a fixed sensitivity and specificity. The curve plots percentage of false-positive detections of VT/VF on the ordinate and estimated incidence of true VT/VF on abscissa. Two data points are plotted from clinical studies of two different patient populations with implanted devices running the same VT/SVT discrimination algorithm (Medtronic GEM DR[62] and AT500 devices[177] with PR Logic).

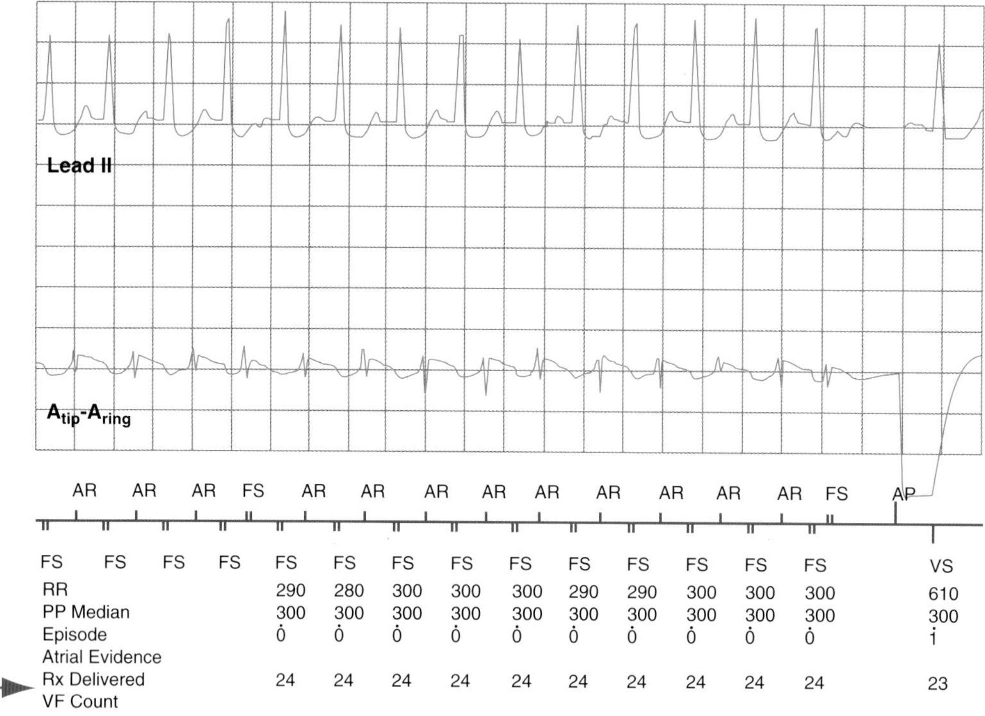

Figure 3-86. Transient short ventricular cycle lengths before spontaneous termination of rapidly conducted atrial tachycardia/fibrillation (AT/AF). Telemetry Holter monitor shows electrocardiographic (ECG) lead II, atrial EGM, and dual-chamber markers along with multiple channels indicating rhythm classification and status of Medtronic Jewel AF Model 7250 atrial/ventricular ICD. Conduction of this AT episode was 1:1, driving ventricular rates up to 200 bpm before spontaneous termination. Most atrial antiarrhythmic devices detect atrial arrhythmias only if the atrial rate exceeds the ventricular rate. Therefore, tachycardias with 1:1 AV relationship are classified as ventricular in origin. In this patient, the ventricular fibrillation (VF) detection interval was programmed to 320 msec with VF therapies OFF. This rhythm was classified as VF, as indicated by the values of the Atrial Evidence Counter (zero), and the VF Count (24, maximum value). AR, atrial refractory event; FS, event in fibrillation zone of either channel; VS, ventricular sensed event.

Detection of Atrial Tachycardia/Fibrillation for Atrial Therapy

High specificity in AT/AF detection has been achieved by multistep methods for detection of AT/AF. Initial detection is based on the presence of an atrial tachyarrhythmia and absence of VT. This is achieved by a measure of atrial rate combined with either comparison of atrial and ventricular rates (Guidant)[153] or use of A:V patterns to identify N:1 rhythms (Medtronic) (Fig. 3-89). The tradeoff between atrial undersensing and oversensing of FFRWs that applies to dual-chamber ICD algorithms is even more important when considering detection of AT/AF for atrial therapy. Minimization of atrial blanking is important to prevent undersensing of AF, and rejection of FFRWs is important to prevent inappropriate detection of AT/AF. (See "Atrial Sensing in Dual-Chamber ICDs and Atrial ICDs.")

Once initial detection occurs (Fig. 3-90), the episode timer begins, initiating a sustained-detection mode in which AT/AF remains detected despite a moderate degree of undersensing (Fig. 3-91). When this timer expires, atrial therapy is delivered if AT/AF still persists (Fig. 3-92). Atrial episodes must be interrupted if true VT occurs (Fig. 3-93).

The final step in detection is discrimination of AT from AF or, alternatively, determining whether the rhythm is likely to respond to atrial ATP. Typically, there may be one timer for ATP and one for shock therapy. In newer Medtronic ICDs, the "reactive antitachycardia pacing" algorithm resets the ATP timer to permit repeat attempts at ATP if changes in atrial rate or atrial rhythm regularity are detected, or after a preprogrammed duration of sustained AT/AF. Changes in rate or regularity of the atrial rhythm are classified as a shift to a new rhythm, which may be more susceptible to ATP termination (Fig. 3-94). Additional ATP attempts hours after failed ATP may be more successful due to shifts in the patient's autonomic tone or physiologic changes that render the rhythm more likely to be terminated with ATP.

As shown in Figure 3-89, Medtronic atrial ICDs discriminate between AT and AF based on the median rate and regularity of the atrial rhythm. Guidant atrial ICDs use a more complex scheme based on maximum rate, standard deviation, and range of the 12 most recent atrial cycle lengths to plot a point in a three-dimensional space. A decision boundary divides the space into two regions: faster/irregular atrial cycle lengths (AF) and

Text continued on p. 152

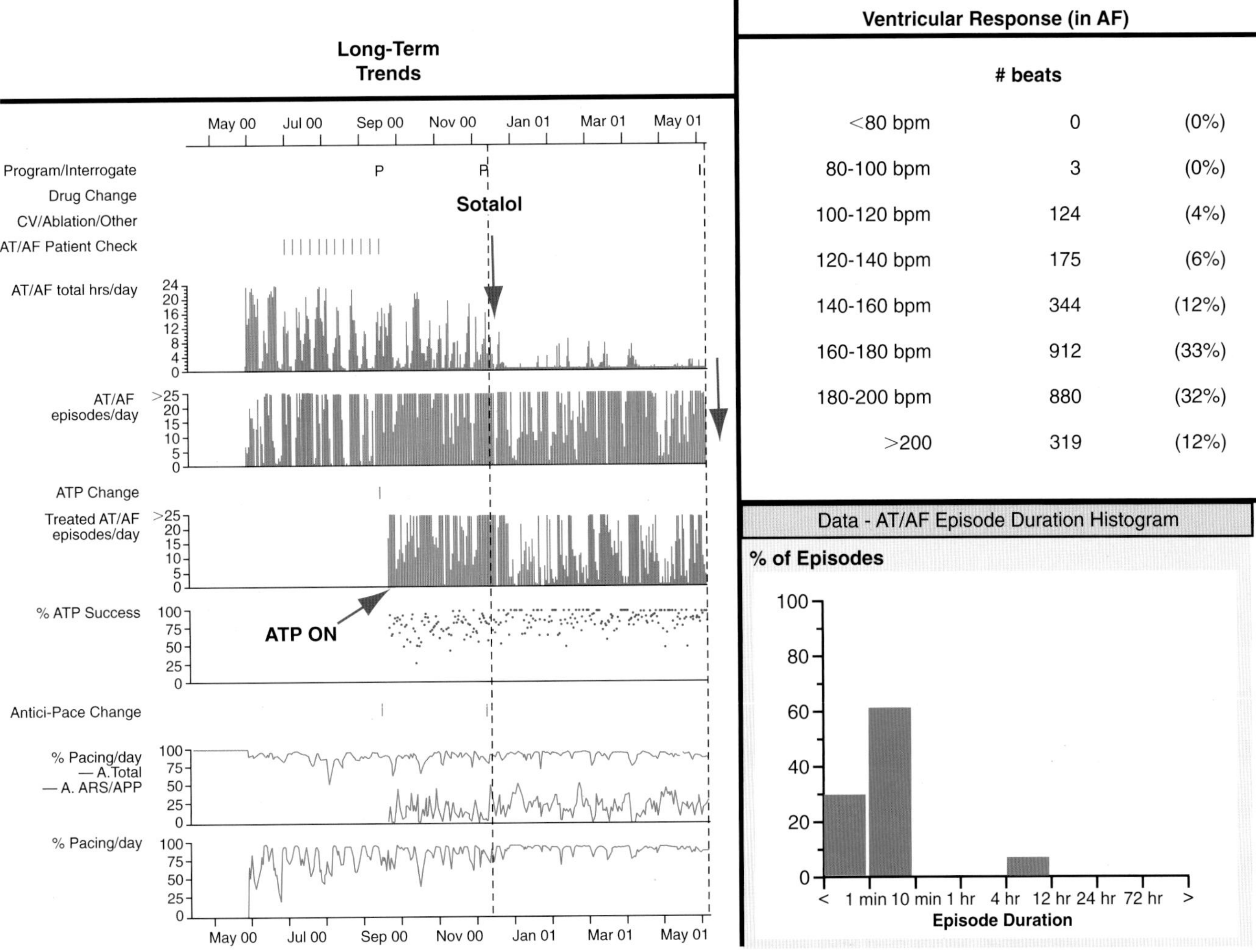

Figure 3-87. *Diagnostic data stored in atrial antiarrhythmic pacemakers and ICDs assist medical management of atrial arrhythmias. Data are taken from three patients with Medtronic AT500 pacemakers.* Left panels, *Long-term trend data over 1 year. Panels from top to bottom show total hours per day in atrial tachycardia/flutter (AT) or atrial fibrillation (AF), total AT/AF device-detected episodes per day, number of daily episodes treated by antitachycardia pacing (ATP), percentage of ATP therapies classified as "successful" by the device, percent atrial pacing, and percent ventricular pacing. ATP ON denotes activation of atrial ATP. Note that, although the many episodes of AT/AF are treated and this treatment is usually classified as successful, there is no detectable change in the number of hours per day of AT/AF until sotalol therapy is initiated. Sotalol decreases the total hourly "burden" of AT/AF more by shortening episodes rather than by preventing them. Percent ventricular pacing is high throughout but increases after sotalol treatment to almost 100%.* Top right panel, *Ventricular rate during AT/AF as percentage of time spent in AT/AF. Seventy-seven percent of intervals are shorter than intervals corresponding to 160 bpm, and 12% are shorter than intervals corresponding to 200 bpm, indicating inadequate control of ventricular rate.* Lower right panel, *Histogram of durations of AT/AF episodes since the last follow-up visit. This patient had 10 episodes of AF since the last visit, but only 1 episode lasted longer than 10 minutes.*

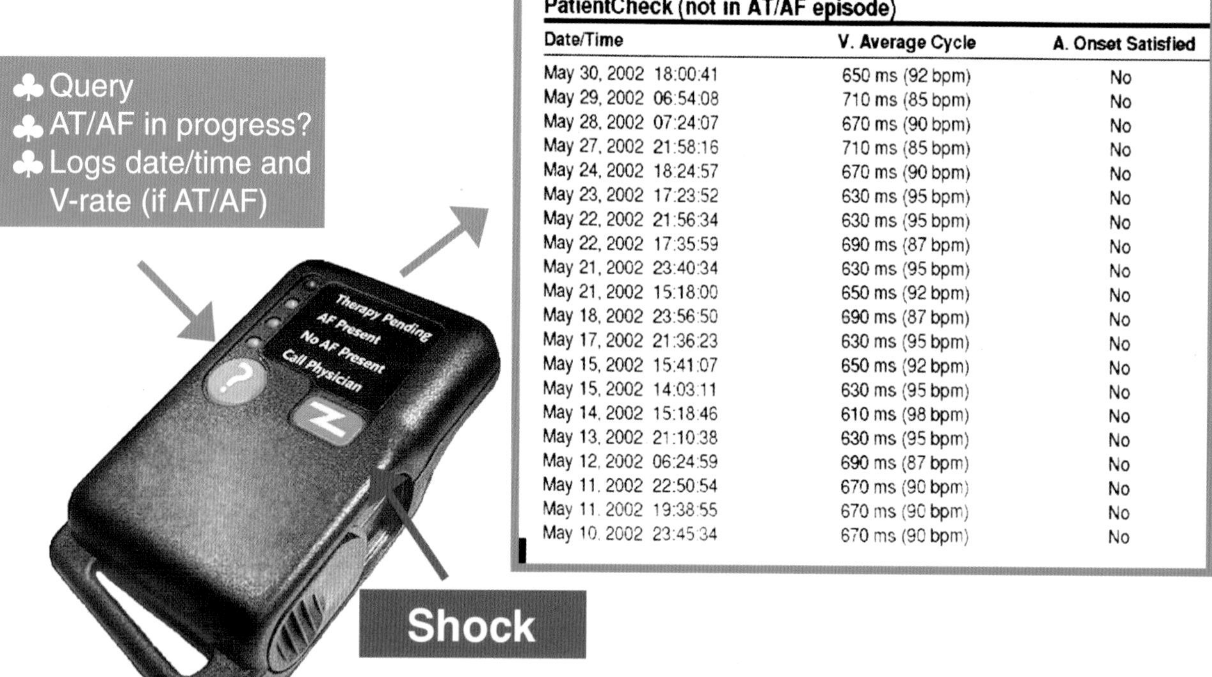

PatientCheck (not in AT/AF episode)

Date/Time	V. Average Cycle	A. Onset Satisfied
May 30, 2002 18:00:41	650 ms (92 bpm)	No
May 29, 2002 06:54:08	710 ms (85 bpm)	No
May 28, 2002 07:24:07	670 ms (90 bpm)	No
May 27, 2002 21:58:16	710 ms (85 bpm)	No
May 24, 2002 18:24:57	670 ms (90 bpm)	No
May 23, 2002 17:23:52	630 ms (95 bpm)	No
May 22, 2002 21:56:34	630 ms (95 bpm)	No
May 22, 2002 17:35:59	690 ms (87 bpm)	No
May 21, 2002 23:40:34	630 ms (95 bpm)	No
May 21, 2002 15:18:00	650 ms (92 bpm)	No
May 18, 2002 23:56:50	690 ms (87 bpm)	No
May 17, 2002 21:36:23	630 ms (95 bpm)	No
May 15, 2002 15:41:07	650 ms (92 bpm)	No
May 15, 2002 14:03:11	630 ms (95 bpm)	No
May 14, 2002 15:18:46	610 ms (98 bpm)	No
May 13, 2002 21:10:38	630 ms (95 bpm)	No
May 12, 2002 06:24:59	690 ms (87 bpm)	No
May 11, 2002 22:50:54	670 ms (90 bpm)	No
May 11, 2002 19:38:55	670 ms (90 bpm)	No
May 10, 2002 23:45:34	670 ms (90 bpm)	No

Figure 3-88. Handheld devices used by patients with combined atrial/ventricular ICDs communicates with the ICD via telemetry. They permit patients both to determine their atrial rhythm diagnosis and to deliver atrial shocks. To use this device in conjunction with the Medtronic GEM III AT ICD, the patient initiates an interrogation by pushing the blue query ("?") button. The ICD responds by illuminating one of four colored light-emitting diodes (LEDs): Therapy Pending, AF present, No AF present, or Call Physician. On interrogation of the ICD with the standard programmer, a date/time log of patient queries is available to help correlate symptoms and rhythm. The log at right shows date/time of patient queries in the left column, ventricular rate in the center column, and presence or absence of an AT/AF episode in the right column. This patient, who was not anticoagulated, queried his ICD once or twice on most days.

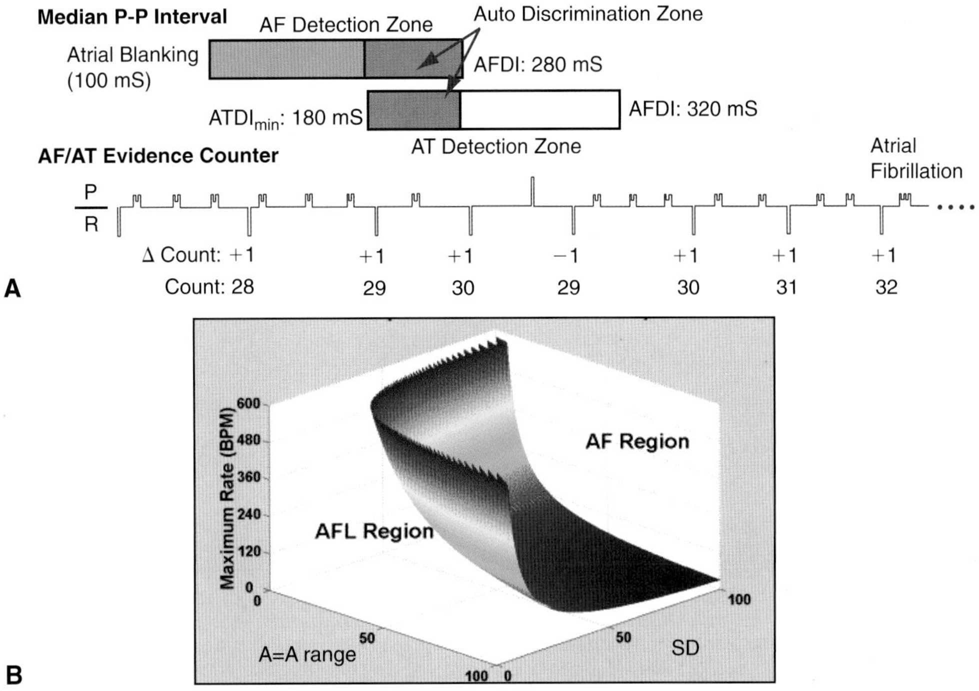

Figure 3-89. Criteria for detection of atrial tachyarrhythmias. ***A,*** *Medtronic atrial therapy devices (Jewel AF, GEM III AT, AT500, and EnRhythm DR) use a combination of atrial cycle length and atrial/ventricular (A:V) patterns to detect atrial fibrillation and atrial flutter. The atrial tachycardia (AT) and atrial fibrillation (AF) detection zones are based on median atrial cycle length (12 P-P intervals) and may overlap. The overlap region is the "autodiscrimination" zone, where regularity of the P-P intervals determines whether rhythm classification is AT (regular P-P intervals) or AF (irregular P-P intervals). Detection of AT or AF requires (1) that the median P-P interval is in one of the detection zones AND (2) that the rhythm is N:1 as determined by the AF/AT evidence counter. The AF/AT evidence counter is an up-down counter (minimum value, 0; maximum value of detection threshold, +15). The counter increments by 1 on each ventricular event if there are two or more atrial events and there is no pattern-based evidence of far-field R-wave oversensing on the atrial channel (see Fig. 3-27A), and it decrements by 1 if there is strong evidence of lack of N:1 rhythm (e.g., two consecutive 1:1 beats). Isolated 1:1 beats contribute AF/AT evidence if they are preceded by a confirmed N:1 beat. The AF/AT counter detection threshold is between 24 and 32, depending on the specific device. AFDI, atrial fibrillation detection interval; mS, msec.* ***B,*** *The Atrial Rhythm Classification (ARC) algorithm (Guidant) discriminates AF from atrial flutter (AFL) based on the atrial rate and two measurements of variability of atrial rate: the range of the atrial intervals (i.e., the difference between the longest and shortest A-A intervals [A-A range]) and the standard deviation of A-A intervals (SD). The values of these three variables define a point in a three-dimensional space. A curved surface separates the AF region from the AFL region. Points in the AF region have higher atrial rates, a higher range of A-A intervals, and a greater standard deviation of A-A intervals. (From Morris MM, KenKnight BH, Lang DJ: Detection of atrial arrhythmia for cardiac rhythm management by implantable devices. J Electrocardiol 33(Suppl):133-139, 2000, with permission.)*

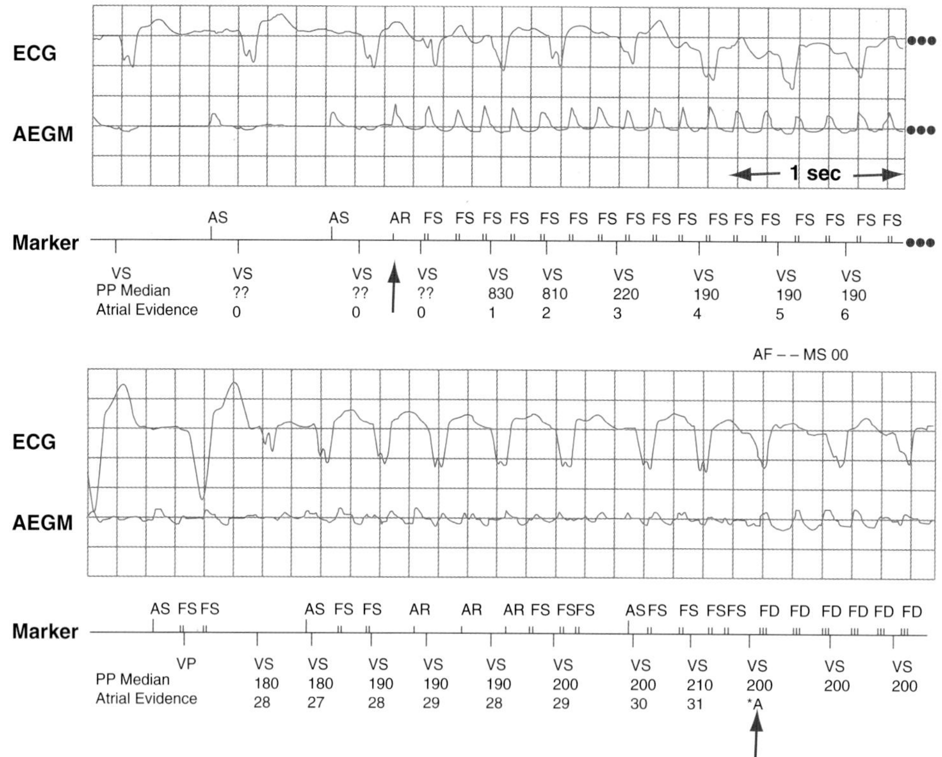

Figure 3-90. Holter recording shows detection of spontaneous atrial fibrillation (AF). Electrocardiogram (ECG), telemetered atrial EGM (AEGM), and event markers are shown. The two lines below the event markers indicate the median P-P interval for the last 12 atrial events and the value of atrial tachycardia/fibrillation (AT/AF) evidence counter. Top panel shows onset of AF (arrow), *and bottom panel shows AF detection* (arrow). *Panels are not continuous; bottom panel begins 10 seconds after top panel ends. Intermediate-height atrial markers (AS) correspond to sensed sinus P waves. Short markers (AR) indicate atrial events in the postventricular atrial refractory period for pacing. Short double markers (FS) indicate intervals below the programmed AF detection interval of 270 msec. Intermediate-height ventricular markers (VS) correspond to sensed R waves; tall ventricular markers (VP) correspond to ventricular paced events. Sinus rhythm is present at the beginning of the top panel. The AEGM shows a low-amplitude far-field R wave that is not sensed. The AT/AF evidence counter remains at 0 for the first four QRS complexes because a single atrial event exists in the preceding R-R interval. There are three atrial events in the R-R interval between the fourth and fifth complexes, and the counter first creates increments on the fifth complex. Absence of postventricular atrial blanking permits sensing of the first AF EGM, which follows the sensed ventricular event by only 30 msec. Intermittent undersensing occurs at the beginning of the bottom panel. The counter creates decrements from 28 to 27 on the fourth QRS complex and from 29 to 28 on the seventh complex. Detection of AF occurs when the count reaches 32* (arrow) *and the P-P median is less than the AF detection interval. This starts the AT/AF duration timer and begins the atrial episode designated by *A. Short triple atrial markers indicate an ongoing AT/AF episode. (From Swerdlow CD, Schsls W, Dijkman B, et al: Detection of atrial fibrillation and flutter by a dual-chamber implantable cardioverter-defibrillator. For the Worldwide Jewel AF Investigators. Circulation 101:878-885, 2000, with permission.)*

Figure 3-91. *Holter recording illustrates continuous detection of atrial fibrillation (AF).* ***A,*** *Onset of AF and initial detection of AF after 32 ventricular events* (arrow). *Double atrial markers (FS) change to triple markers (FD), and the symbol *A appears on the atrial evidence channel to indicate AF episode in progress.* ***B,*** *Rhythms after 5 hours of continuous recording. AP, atrial-paced event; VP, ventricular-paced event; VS, sensed R wave. (From Swerdlow CD, Schsls W, Dijkman B, et al: Detection of atrial fibrillation and flutter by a dual-chamber implantable cardioverter-defibrillator. For the Worldwide Jewel AF Investigators. Circulation 101:878-885, with permission.)*

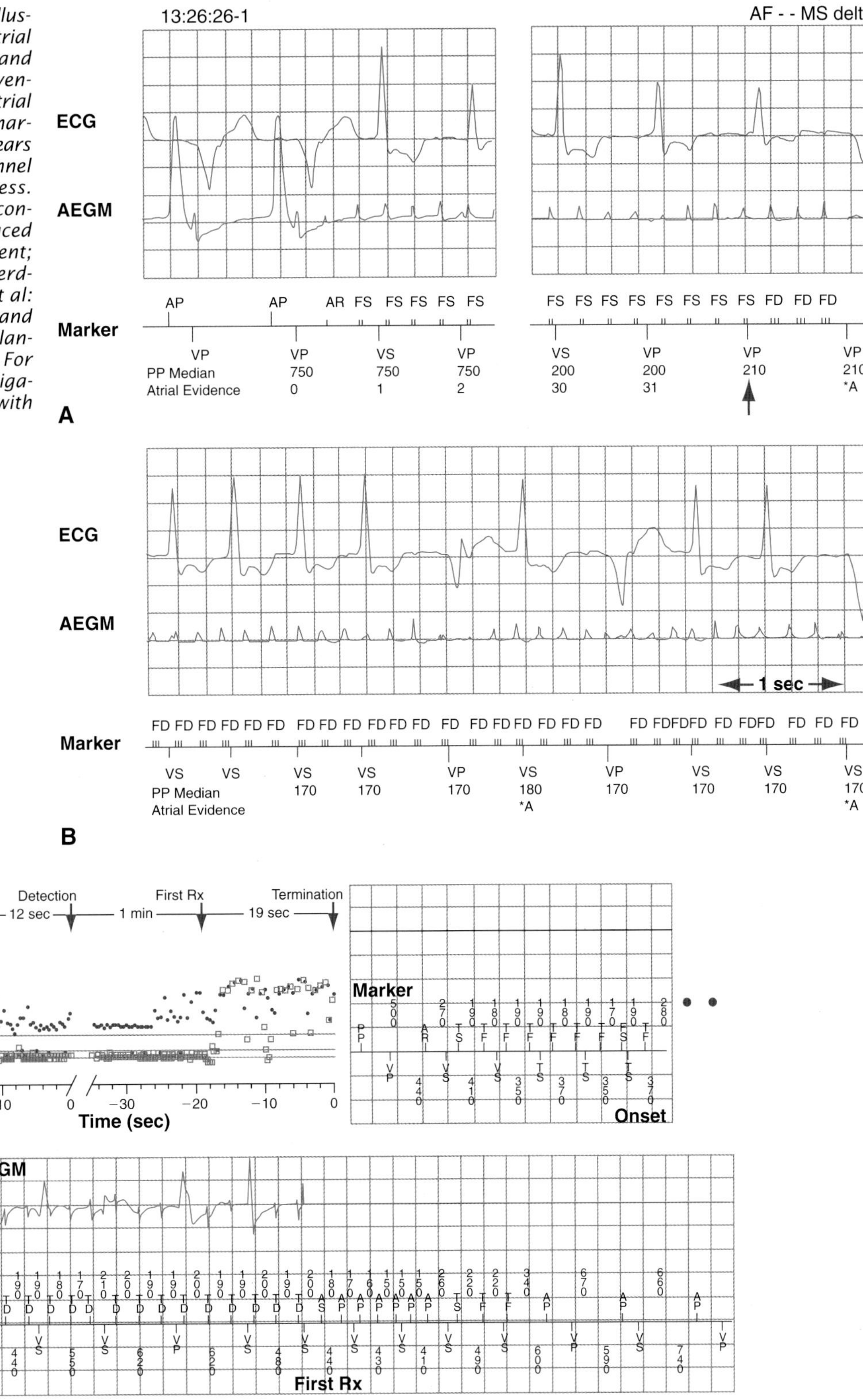

Figure 3-92. *Atrial tachycardia (AT) detection and therapy after 1 minute of sustained detection. Spontaneous episode of AT from a Medtronic GEM III AT device.* Upper left panel, *P-P intervals* (open squares) *and R-R intervals* (closed circles) *for this episode. Onset of the AT episode is labeled on the interval plot and on the stored marker channel* (top right). *The interval plot also labels the initial detection of AT (Detection), delivery of the first therapy (First ATP Rx), and device recognition of episode termination (Termination). In this case, therapies were programmed to begin 1 minute after initial detection.* Top right panel, *Dual-chamber EGM markers preceding detection of AT. Dots indicate discontinuous recording between top and bottom panels.* Bottom panel, *Composite EGM recorded between the atrial tip electrode (Atip) and the ventricular ring electrode (Vring) and dual-chamber EGM markers immediately preceding delivery of successful antitachycardia pacing (First Rx, fast AP events). TS, FS, and TF events refer to atrial intervals in the AT, atrial fibrillation (AF), and overlap zones, respectively. TD (atrial marker), atrial tachycardia detected; VP, ventricular paced event; VS, ventricular sensed event.*

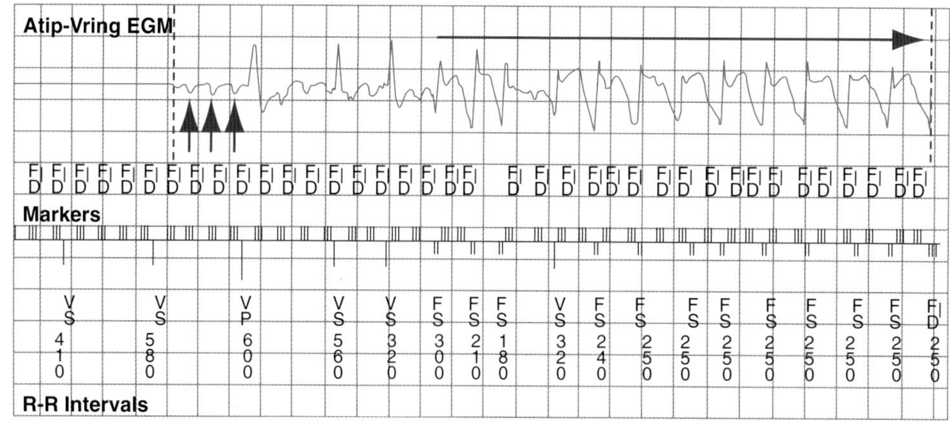

Figure 3-93. Spontaneous rapid ventricular tachycardia (VT) detected in the ventricular fibrillation (VF) zone during ongoing atrial fibrillation (AF) in this Medtronic Jewel AF Model 7250 atrial/ventricular ICD. Tracing shows composite EGM recorded between atrial tip electrode (Atip) and ventricular ring electrode (Vring), with dual-chamber EGM markers. Vertical arrows on left point to atrial component of the composite atrioventricular (AV) EGM. Horizontal arrow overlies the VT portion of the tracing. FD on atrial markers indicates ongoing AF episode. FD at right of tracing on ventricular channel indicates detection of VF. VS and FS are ventricular intervals in the sinus and VF zones, respectively. VP, ventricular paced interval.

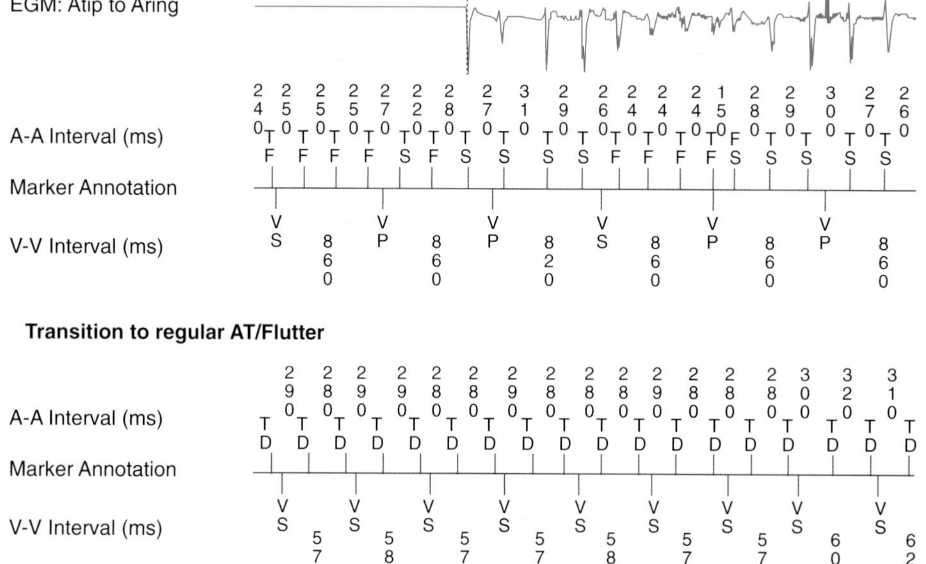

Figure 3-94. Atrial arrhythmia episode begins as atrial fibrillation (AF) (upper panel) *but 1 hour later shows organization of local right atrial EGMs* (lower panel), *possibly indicating global transition to atrial flutter. One therapeutic strategy is to withhold antitachycardia pacing (ATP) until slowing and regularity of atrial sensed EGM indicates a high probability that it will be effective. This example is from a Medtronic AT500 pacemaker. Aring, atrial ring electrode; Atip, atrial tip electrode; TD, atrial tachycardia detected; VP, ventricular paced event; VS, ventricular sensed event.*

slower/regular cycle lengths (AT). Classifications are made on a sliding window of 12 consecutive cycles until the end of the episode is reached.[153,154]

Detection Considerations for Atrial Shocks

In addition to permitting therapy after hours of continuous AF, atrial ICDs may withhold therapy if the episode duration is sufficiently long that patients may be at risk for thromboembolism if they are not adequately anticoagulated, typically 24 hours. R-wave synchronized atrial shock therapy is restricted to R-R intervals greater than 400 to 500 msec. This minimizes the risk that a therapeutic atrial shock can be delivered into the vulnerable period of the preceding cardiac cycle, but it may prevent shock therapy for rapidly conducted AF. Early or immediate recurrence of AF after shock is an important clinical problem in patients with atrial ICDs.[128] Early recurrence of AF before postshock redetection of sinus rhythm will result in incorrect classification of shock success (Fig. 3-95).

Subcutaneous Electrocardiography

The subcutaneous ECG is similar to the surface ECG because the two subcutaneous electrodes are suffi-

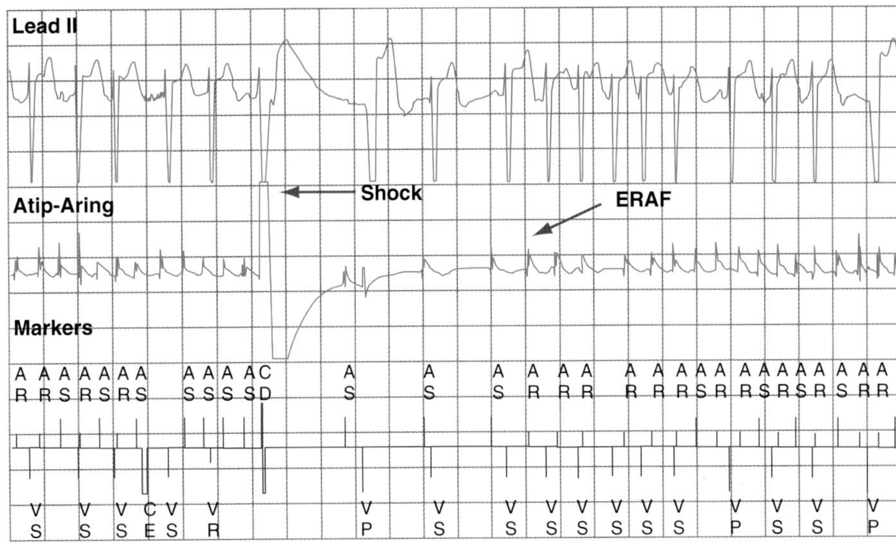

Figure 3-95. Postshock ERAF recorded at implantation occurs three R-R intervals after shock. Because the ICD requires five consecutive postshock beats of sinus or atrial-paced rhythm to detect termination of atrial fibrillation (AF) and store intervals, no data were stored for this clinically unsuccessful shock. Lead II of the surface electrocardiogram, the atrial EGM, and the atrial and ventricular channels with event markers are shown. AR, atrial refractory event; AS, atrial sensed event; CD, charge delivered; CE, charge end; ERAF, early recurrence of atrial fibrillation; VP, ventricular paced event, VS, ventricular sensed event. (From Swerdlow CD, Schwartzman D, Hoyt R, et al: Determinants of first-shock success for atrial implantable cardioverter defibrillators. J Cardiovasc Electrophysiol 13:347-354, 2002, with permission.)

ciently distant from the heart that they record electrical activity from the entire heart. Clinically, subcutaneous ECGs are used to detect arrhythmias in an implantable syncope monitor, to obviate the need for surface ECG electrodes during follow-up of pacemakers and ICDs, and to detect VT/VF in a subcutaneous ICD.

Like the surface ECG, the amplitude of subcutaneous ECG signals usually is 1 mV or less. During development of an implantable syncope monitor (Medtronic Reveal), subcutaneous ECG signals with typical amplitudes of 0.25 mV were recorded between two electrodes separated by 3.2 cm on the surface of a pacemaker-sized device placed under the skin or muscle in the left pectoral region.[53] Unlike EGMs, the amplitude of these subcutaneous ECGs increases over time to 0.30 mV at 2 to 3 months, and 0.35 mV at 4 to 6 months, and then remains stable.[155]

Practical implantation considerations usually limit the subcutaneous electrode separation distance to 4 to 8 cm, compared with the typical surface ECG limb lead electrode separation of 40 to 60 cm. The orientation of the two subcutaneous electrodes relative to the heart can affect the amplitude of the signal recorded. Mapping studies on the chest skin with the 4-cm electrode spacing of the implantable syncope monitor show larger intrinsic QRS amplitudes of 0.5 ± 0.1 mV for vertical orientation in the left parasternal zone and for horizontal orientation near the apex of the heart.[156] These two locations had comparable amplitudes of subcutaneous ECGs. No significant differences were found for patients placed in five body positions (supine, left, right, sitting, and standing). Undersensing of intrinsic rhythm due to abrupt unexplained decreases in QRS amplitude, transient loss of signal, or baseline drift causes inappropriate detection of bradycardia by implantable syncope monitors. However, signal quality is usually sufficient to be diagnostic. Figures 3-96 to 3-98 show examples of rhythms recorded by implantable monitors, including bradycardia, VT, and skeletal myopotentials.

An intraoperative study using three "button" electrodes mounted on an ICD can placed in the left infraclavicular region showed that electrode orientation had little effect. But P-wave amplitudes were only about 0.02 mV, and the ratio of P to QRS amplitude was about one half that of surface ECGs.[157] Subcutaneous ECGs recorded between a defibrillation coil in the superior vena cava and the ICD can are a programmable option in some ICDs (Medtronic Marquis). These subcutaneous ECGs have properties similar to those of the syncope monitor. They are used to store an ECG-like signal during ICD episodes and in lieu of surface electrodes during ICD follow-up. Usable P waves are visible in about 80% of these patients.[157]

Future Directions

Subcutaneous ICDs

Subcutaneous ICDs with no transvenous or epicardial leads are undergoing early trials. They must rely on subcutaneous ECGs for sensing and detection of VF[158] (Fig. 3-99). In one version, correlation waveform analysis using two different channels of subcutaneous ECG is employed to detect fast-VT/VF and to avoid inappropriate detection of myopotential noise and EMI.[159] There are no published data on sensing and detection performance.

Hemodynamic Sensors for ICDs

Despite the substantial changes in ICD technology since the late 1980s, modern ICDs do not differentiate directly between hemodynamically stable and unstable tachycardias. Historically, detection durations and therapy sequences have been programmed aggressively to minimize the potential for syncope, but this results in more shocks being delivered than are necessary. Reduction of morbidity associated with

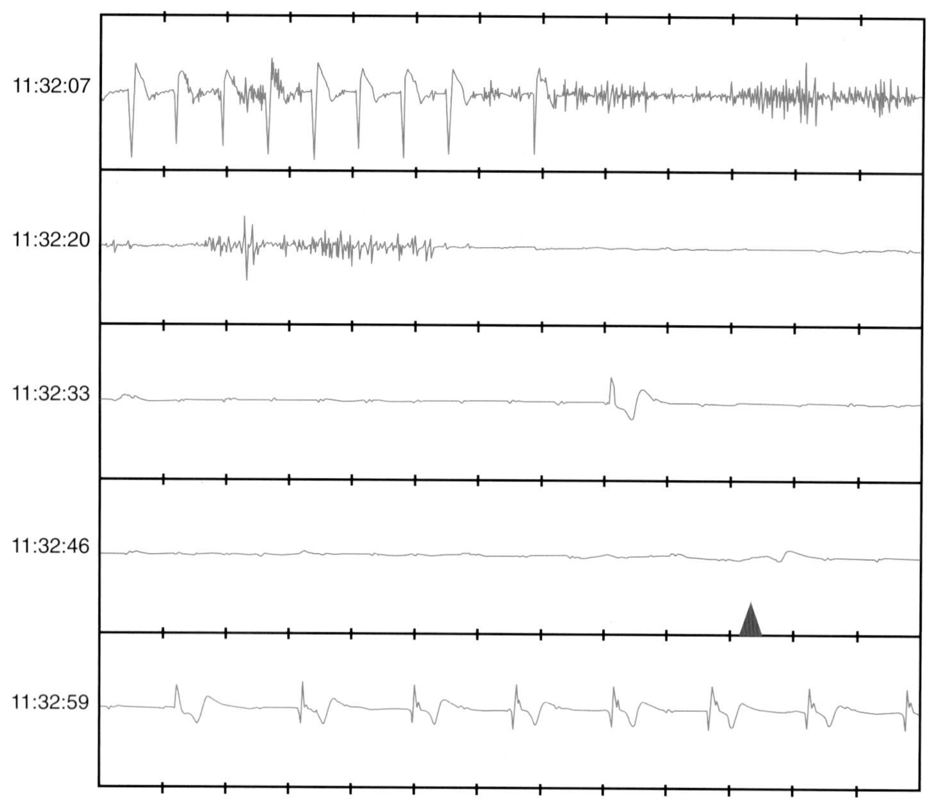

Figure 3-96. Stored EGM recorded by an implantable loop recorder (Reveal, Medtronic) shows about 45 seconds of asystole, some myopotentials, perhaps one depolarization in the middle of the asystole, very small deflections throughout that are probably P waves, and relative bradycardia on the bottom panel. The amplitude of the subcutaneous electrocardiogram is approximately 0.25 mV.

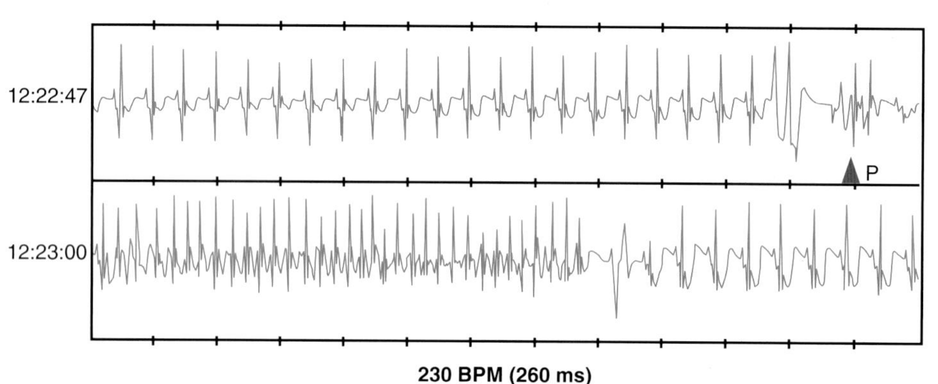

Figure 3-97. Stored EGM recorded by an implantable loop recorder (Reveal, Medtronic) shows nonsustained tachycardia at about 230 bpm with a duration of 8 seconds. The underlying rhythm is reset by the high-rate segment. The patient did activate this stored strip, as indicated by the dark triangle and the "P" marker.

unnecessary shocks for hemodynamically stable VT and for repetitive shocks due to SVT may be achieved through the use of implantable hemodynamic sensors integrated with the detection and therapy decision process. Mixed venous oxygen saturation, right atrial pressure, RV pressure, subcutaneous photoplethysmography, endocardial accelerometers, and impedance measurements have been proposed as methods of discriminating between hemodynamically stable and unstable tachycardias.[52,160-168] Subcutaneous photoplethysmography technology has been described and tested in acute and chronic animal models. These studies have found a good correlation between mean arterial pressure and photoplethysmography pulse amplitude and have demonstrated the feasibility of discriminating perfusing (stable) from nonperfusing (unstable) tachycardias.[169,170] Implantable systems for ambulatory hemodynamic monitoring using RV pressure and mixed venous oxygen sensors has been described.[171]

A recent prospective clinical study with RV pressure monitoring using the Medtronic Chronicle B reported the usefulness of the sensor for heart failure monitoring.[172] This device has the capability of recording RV pressure waveforms during tachycardias detected using rate + interval analysis. Episodes of recorded spontaneous VF demonstrate substantial changes in RV pressure waveforms (Fig. 3-100). Many factors influence the hemodynamic stability of a tachyarrhythmia. Developing reliable metrics that discriminate stable versus unstable tachyarrhythmias for integration into ICD algorithms remains a major challenge.

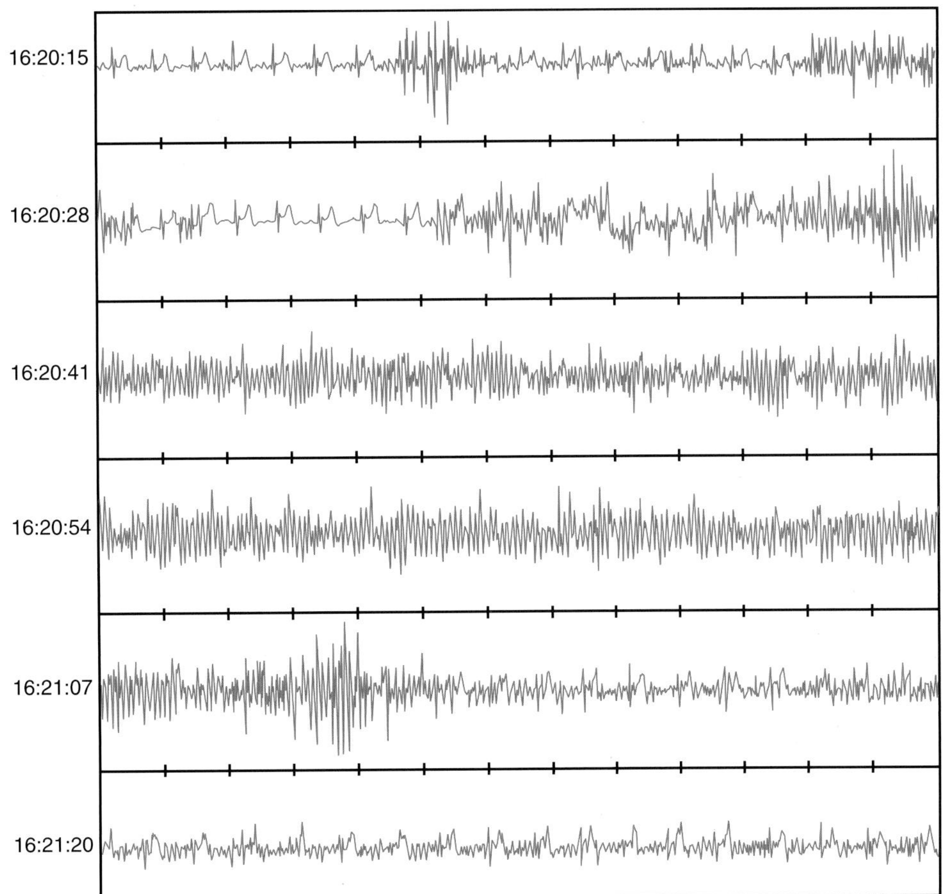

Figure 3-98. Stored EGM recorded by an implantable loop recorder (Reveal, Medtronic) shows high-frequency electrical activity at a rate of about 800 bpm, probably myopotential artifacts. The rate is too fast to represent cardiac ventricular activation, and in some portions the underlying cardiac rhythm can be seen to be "marching through" the recording. Many artifacts are recorded by subcutaneous implantable loop recorders because the subcutaneous electrodes are closely spaced, greater than normal ECG amplification is required, and the frequency contents of myopotentials and electrocardiograms overlap extensively, so that filtering is of limited value in rejecting noise.

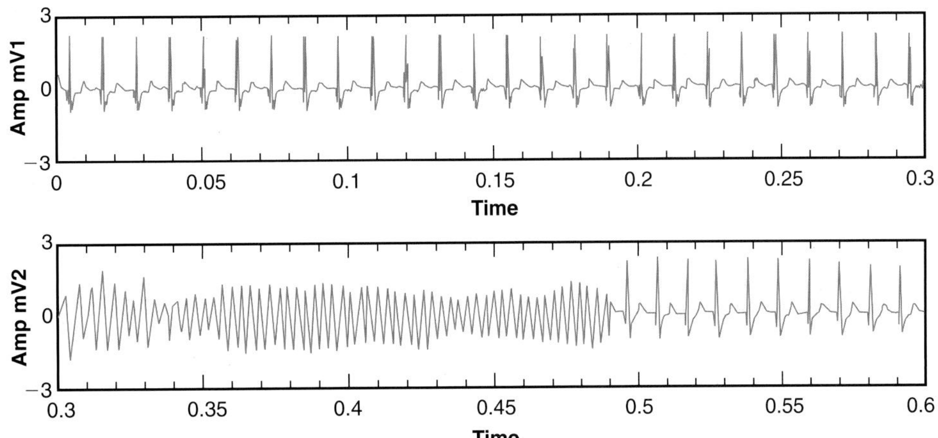

Figure 3-99. Ventricular fibrillation (VF) recorded from sensing electrodes of an investigational subcutaneous ICD (AXIOM Model 1010, Cameron Health, Inc., San Clemente, Calif.). Sensing occurs between a parasternal electrode and the implantable device placed in the left midaxillary region. VF is induced by DC stimulation and terminated by a shock. Shock artifact is not seen well in this tracing.

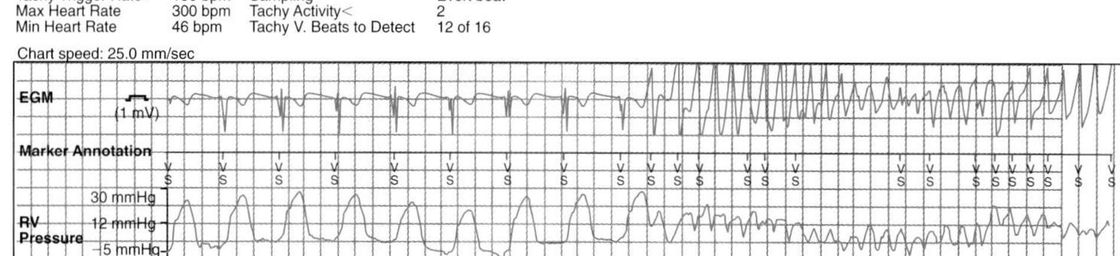

Figure 3-100. Spontaneous ventricular fibrillation (VF) recording from an implanted Chronicle B hemodynamic monitoring system (Medtronic). The criterion to trigger diagnostic storage for tachycardia episodes is 12 of 16 beats faster than 150 bpm in this example. The tracings shown are (from top to bottom) unipolar ventricular EGM, ventricular markers, and right ventricular (RV) pressure as measured from the chronic pressure sensor. Note the dramatic decrease in RV pulse pressure immediately after onset of VF. Undersensing of VF occurs due to fixed threshold sensing with a programmed sensitivity of 2.0 mV. VS, ventricular sensed event.

REFERENCES

1. Parsonnet V, Myers GH, Kresh YM: Characteristics of intracardiac electrograms II: Atrial endocardial electrograms. PACE 3:406-417, 1980.
2. Saxonhouse SJ, Conti JB, Curtis AB: Current of injury predicts adequate active lead fixation in permanent pacemaker/defibrillation leads. J Am Coll Cardiol 45:412-417, 2005.
3. Sweeney MO, Ellison KE, Shea JB, et al: Provoked and spontaneous high-frequency, low-amplitude, respirophasic noise transients in patients with implantable cardioverter defibrillators. J Cardiovasc Electrophysiol 12:402-410, 2001.
4. Weretka S, Michaelsen J, Becker R, et al: Ventricular oversensing: A study of 101 patients implanted with dual chamber defibrillators and two different lead systems. PACE 26(1 Pt 1):65-70, 2003.
5. Platia EV, Brinker JA: Time course of transvenous pacemaker stimulation impedance, capture threshold, and electrogram amplitude. PACE 9:620-625, 1986.
6. DeCaprio V, Hurzeler P, Furman S: A comparison of unipolar and bipolar electrograms for cardiac pacemaker sensing. Circulation 56:750-755, 1977.
7. Cornacchia D, Jacopi F, Fabbri M, et al: [Comparison between active screw type and passive electrodes in permanent intraventricular pacing]. Minerva Cardioangiol 32:101-103, 1984.
8. Ceviz N, Celiker A, Kucukosmanoglu O, et al: Comparison of mid-term clinical experience with steroid-eluting active and passive fixation ventricular electrodes in children. PACE 23:1245-1249, 2000.
9. Danilovic D, Ohm OJ: Pacing impedance variability in tined steroid eluting leads. PACE 21:1356-1363, 1998.
10. Hua W, Mond HG, Strathmore N: Chronic steroid-eluting lead performance: A comparison of atrial and ventricular pacing. PACE 20(1 Pt 1):17-24, 1997.
11. Crossley GH, Brinker JA, Reynolds D, et al: Steroid elution improves the stimulation threshold in an active-fixation atrial permanent pacing lead: A randomized, controlled study. Model 4068 Investigators. Circulation 92:2935-2939, 1995.
12. Wish M, Swartz J, Cohen A, et al: Steroid-tipped leads versus porous platinum permanent pacemaker leads: A controlled study. PACE 13(12 Pt 2):1887-1890, 1990.
13. Ellenbogen KA, Wood MA, Gilligan DM: Evaluation of "inappropriate" ICD shocks in an asymptomatic patient following myocardial infarction. PACE 19:254-255, 1996.
14. Goldschlager N, Epstein A, Friedman P, et al: Environmental and drug effects on patients with pacemakers and implantable cardioverter/defibrillators: A practical guide to patient treatment. Arch Intern Med 161:649-655, 2001.
15. Rajawat YS, Patel VV, Gerstenfeld EP, et al: Advantages and pitfalls of combining device-based and pharmacologic therapies for the treatment of ventricular arrhythmias. PACE 27:1670-1681, 2004.
16. Theres H, Stadler RW, Stylos L, et al: Comparison of electrocardiogram and intrathoracic electrogram signals for detection of ischemic ST segment changes during normal sinus and ventricular paced rhythms. J Cardiovasc Electrophysiol 13:990-995, 2002.
17. Centurion OA, Isomoto S, Shimizu A, et al: The effects of aging on atrial endocardial electrograms in patients with paroxysmal atrial fibrillation. Clin Cardiol 26:435-438, 2003.
18. Frohlig G, Schwerdt H, Schieffer H, et al: Atrial signal variations and pacemaker malsensing during exercise: A study in the time and frequency domain. J Am Coll Cardiol 11:806-813, 1988.
19. Ross BA, Zeigler V, Zinner A, et al: The effect of exercise on the atrial electrogram voltage in young patients. PACE 14:2092-2097, 1991.
20. Schuchert A, Kuck KH, Bleifeld W: Stability of pacing threshold, impedance, and R wave amplitude at rest and during exercise. PACE 13(12 Pt 1):1602-1608, 1990.
21. Shandling AH, Florio J, Castellanet MJ, et al: Physical determinants of the endocardial P wave. PACE 13(12 Pt 1):1585-1589, 1990.
22. Rosenheck S, Schmaltz S, Kadish AH, et al: Effect of rate augmentation and isoproterenol on the amplitude of atrial and ventricular electrograms. Am J Cardiol 66:101-102, 1990.
23. Varriale P, Chryssos BE: Atrial sensing performance of the single-lead VDD pacemaker during exercise. J Am Coll Cardiol 22:1854-1857, 1993.
24. Chan CC, Lau CP, Leung SK, et al: Comparative evaluation of bipolar atrial electrogram amplitude during everyday activities: Atrial active fixation versus two types of single pass VDD/R leads. PACE 17(11 Pt 2):1873-1877, 1994.
25. Furman S, Hurzeler P, De Caprio V: Cardiac pacing and pacemaker. III. Sensing the cardiac electrogram. Am Heart J 93:794-801, 1997.
26. Ellenbogen KA, Wood MA, Stambler BS, et al: Measurement of ventricular electrogram amplitude during intraoperative induction of ventricular tachyarrhythmias. Am J Cardiol 70:1017-1022, 1992.
27. Taneja T, Goldberger J, Parker MA, et al: Reproducibility of ventricular fibrillation characteristics in patients undergoing implantable cardioverter defibrillator implantation. J Cardiovasc Electrophysiol 8:1209-1217, 1997.
28. McAlister HF, Klementowicz PT, Calderon EM, et al: Atrial electrogram analysis: Antegrade versus retrograde. PACE 11(11 Pt 2):1703-1707, 1988.
29. Wainwright R, Davies W, Tooley M: Ideal atrial lead positioning to detect retrograde atrial depolarization by digitization and slope analysis of the atrial electrogram. PACE 7(6 Pt 2):1152-1158, 1984.

30. Timmis GC, Westveer DC, Bakalyar DM, et al: Discrimination of anterograde from retrograde atrial electrograms for physiologic pacing. PACE 11:130-140, 1988.
31. Davies DW, Wainwright RJ, Tooley MA, et al: Detection of pathological tachycardia by analysis of electrogram morphology. PACE 9:200-208, 1986.
32. Roithinger FX, SippensGroenewegen A, Karch MR, et al: Organized activation during atrial fibrillation in man: Endocardial and electrocardiographic manifestations. J Cardiovasc Electrophysiol 9:451-461, 1998.
33. Konings KT, Smeets JL, Penn OC, et al: Configuration of unipolar atrial electrograms during electrically induced atrial fibrillation in humans. Circulation 95:1231-1241, 1997.
34. Wood M, Moskovljevic P, Stambler B, et al: Comparison of bipolar atrial electrogram amplitude in sinus rhythm, atrial fibrillation, and atrial flutter. PACE 19:150-156, 1996.
35. Lewalter T, Schimpf R, Kulik D, et al: Comparison of spontaneous atrial fibrillation electrogram potentials with the P-wave electrogram amplitude in dual chamber pacing with unipolar atrial sensing. Europace 2:136-140, 2000.
36. Ropella KM, Sahakian AV, Baerman JM, et al: The coherence spectrum: A quantitative discriminator of fibrillatory and nonfibrillatory cardiac rhythms. Circulation 80:112-119, 1989.
37. Baerman JM, Ropella KM, Sahakian AV, et al: Effect of bipole configuration on atrial electrograms during atrial fibrillation. PACE 13:78-87, 1990.
38. Karagueuzian HS, Khan SS, Peters W, et al: Nonhomogeneous local atrial activity during acute atrial fibrillation: Spectral and dynamic analysis. PACE 13(12 Pt 2):1937-1942, 1990.
39. Ropella KM, Sahakian AV, Baerman JM, et al: Effects of procainamide on intra-atrial [corrected] electrograms during atrial fibrillation: Implications [corrected] for detection algorithms. Circulation 77:1047-1054, 1988.
40. Beeman AL, Deutsch G, Rea RF: Paradoxical undersensing due to quiet timer blanking. Heart Rhythm 1:345-347, 2004.
41. Willems R, Holemans P, Ector H, et al: Paradoxical undersensing at a high sensitivity in dual chamber pacemakers. PACE 24:308-315, 2001.
42. Castro A, Liebold A, Vincente J, et al: Evaluation of autosensing as an automatic means of maintaining a 2:1 sensing safety margin in an implanted pacemaker. Autosensing Investigation Team. PACE 19(11 Pt 2):1708-1713, 1996.
43. Nowak B, Kampmann C, Schmid FX, et al: Pacemaker therapy in premature children with high degree AV block. PACE 21:2695-2698, 1998.
44. Inama G, Santini M, Padeletti L, et al: Far-field R wave oversensing in dual chamber pacemakers designed for atrial arrhythmia management: Effect of pacing site and lead tip to ring distance. PACE 27:1221-1230, 2004.
45. Callans DJ, Hook BG, Kleiman RB, et al: Unique sensing errors in third-generation implantable cardioverter-defibrillators. J Am Coll Cardiol 22:1135-1140, 1993.
46. Callans DJ, Hook BG, Marchlinski FE: Paced beats following single nonsensed complexes in a "codependent" cardioverter defibrillator and bradycardia pacing system: Potential for ventricular tachycardia induction. PACE 14:1281-1287, 1991.
47. Callans DJ, Hook BG, Marchlinski FE: Effect of rate and coupling interval on endocardial R wave amplitude variability in permanent ventricular sensing lead systems. J Am Coll Cardiol 22:746-750, 1993.
48. Dekker LR, Schrama TA, Steinmetz FH, et al: Undersensing of VF in a patient with optimal R wave sensing during sinus rhythm. PACE 27(6 Pt 1):833-834, 2004.
49. Glikson M, Beeman AL, Luria DM, et al: Impaired detection of ventricular tachyarrhythmias by a rate-smoothing algorithm in dual-chamber implantable defibrillators: Intradevice interactions. J Cardiovasc Electrophysiol 13:312-318, 2002.
50. Cooper JM, Sauer W, Verdino R: Absent ventricular tachycardia detection in a biventricular implantable cardioverter-defibrillator due to intradevice interaction with a rate smoothing pacing algorithm. Heart Rhythm 1:728-731, 2004.
51. Shivkumar K, Feliciano Z, Boyle NG, et al: Intradevice interaction in a dual chamber implantable cardioverter defibrillator preventing ventricular tachyarrhythmia detection. J Cardiovasc Electrophysiol 11:1285-1288, 2000.
52. Ellenbogen KA, Wood MA, Kapadia K, et al: Short-term reproducibility over time of right ventricular pulse pressure as a potential hemodynamic sensor for ventricular tachyarrhythmias. PACE 15:971-974, 1992.
53. Leitch J, Klein G, Yee R, et al: Feasibility of an implantable arrhythmia monitor. PACE 15:2232-2235, 1992.
54. Swerdlow CD: Implantation of cardioverter defibrillators without induction of ventricular fibrillation. Circulation 103:2159-2164, 2001.
55. Tung L, Tovar O, Neunlist M, et al: Effects of strong electrical shock on cardiac muscle tissue. Ann N Y Acad Sci 720:160-175, 1994.
56. Winkle RA, Bach SM Jr, Echt DS, et al: The automatic implantable defibrillator: Local ventricular bipolar sensing to detect ventricular tachycardia and fibrillation. Am J Cardiol 52:265-270, 1983.
57. Goldberger JJ, Horvath G, Donovan D, et al: Detection of ventricular fibrillation by transvenous defibrillating leads: Integrated versus dedicated bipolar sensing. J Cardiovasc Electrophysiol 9:677-688, 1998.
58. Yee R, Jones D, Jarvis E, et al: Changes in pacing threshold and R wave amplitude after transvenous catheter countershock. J Am Coll Cardiol 4:543-549, 1984.
59. Jung W, Manz M, Moosdorf R, et al: Changes in the amplitude of endocardial electrograms following defibrillator discharge: Comparison of two lead systems. PACE 18(12 Pt 1):2163-2172, 1995.
60. Swerdlow CD, Brown ML, Lurie K, et al: Discrimination of ventricular tachycardia from supraventricular tachycardia by a downloaded wavelet-transform morphology algorithm: A paradigm for development of implantable cardioverter defibrillator detection algorithms. J Cardiovasc Electrophysiol 13:432-441, 2002.
61. Kuhlkamp V, Dornberger V, Mewis C, et al: Clinical experience with the new detection algorithms for atrial fibrillation of a defibrillator with dual chamber sensing and pacing. J Cardiovasc Electrophysiol 10:905-915, 1999.
62. Wilkoff BL, Kuhlkamp V, Volosin K, et al: Critical analysis of dual-chamber implantable cardioverter-defibrillator arrhythmia detection: Results and technical considerations. Circulation 103:381-386, 2001.
63. Swerdlow CD: Supraventricular tachycardia-ventricular tachycardia discrimination algorithms in implantable cardioverter defibrillators: State-of-the-art review. J Cardiovasc Electrophysiol 12:606-612, 2001.
64. Gunderson B, Patel A, Bounds C: Automatic identification of implantable cardioverter-defibrillator lead problems using intracardiac electrograms. Comput Cardiol 29:121-124, 2002.
65. Swerdlow C, Shivkumar K: Implantable cardioverter defibrillators: Clinical aspects. In Zipes DP, Jalife J (eds): Cardiac Electrophysiology: From Cell to Bedside, 4th ed. Philadephia, WB Saunders, 2004, pp 980-993.
66. Garcia-Moran E, Mont L, Brugada J: Inappropriate tachycardia detection by a biventricular implantable cardioverter defibrillator. PACE 25:123-124, 2002.
67. Lloyd M, Hayes D, Friedman P: Troubleshooting. In Hayes D, Lloyd M, Friedman P (eds): Cardiac Pacing and Defibrillation: A Clinical Approach. Armonk, NY, Futura, 2000, pp 347-452.
68. Ellenbogen KA, Wood MA, Shepard RK, et al: Detection and management of an implantable cardioverter defibrillator lead

failure: Incidence and clinical implications. J Am Coll Cardiol 41:73-80, 2003.
69. Swerdlow C, Friedman P: Advanced ICD troubleshooting: Part I. PACE 28:1322-1346, 2005.
70. Pinski SL: 2:1 Tracking of sinus rhythm in a patient with a dual-chamber implantable cardioverter defibrillator: What is the mechanism? J Cardiovasc Electrophysiol 12:503-504, 2001.
71. Hsu SS, Mohib S, Schroeder A, et al: T wave oversensing in implantable cardioverter defibrillators. J Interv Card Electrophysiol 11:67-72, 2004.
72. Sweeney MO, Hellkamp AS, Ellenbogen KA, et al: Adverse effect of ventricular pacing on heart failure and atrial fibrillation among patients with normal baseline QRS duration in a clinical trial of pacemaker therapy for sinus node dysfunction. Circulation 107:2932-2937, 2003.
73. Wilkoff BL, Cook JR, Epstein AE, et al: Dual-chamber pacing or ventricular backup pacing in patients with an implantable defibrillator: The Dual Chamber and VVI Implantable Defibrillator (DAVID) Trial [see comment]. JAMA 288:3115-3123, 2002.
74. Pinski S, Egula L, Sgarbossa E, et al: Incidence and causes of commlted shocks in noncommited implantable defibrillators [abstract]. J Am Coll Cardiol 39:93A, 2002.
75. Sweesy MW, Holland JL, Smith KW: Electromagnetic interference in cardiac rhythm management devices. AACN Clin Issues 15:391-403, 2004.
76. Lau CP, Leung SK, Tse HF, et al: Automatic mode switching of implantable pacemakers: II. Clinical performance of current algorithms and their programming. PACE 25:1094-1113, 2002.
77. Israel CW: Analysis of mode switching algorithms in dual chamber pacemakers. PACE 25:380-393, 2002.
78. Lam CT, Lau CP, Leung SK, et al: Improved efficacy of mode switching during atrial fibrillation using automatic atrial sensitivity adjustment. PACE 22(1 Pt 1):17-25, 1999.
79. Leung SK, Lau CP, Lam C, et al: Programmed atrial sensitivity: A critical determinant in atrial fibrillation detection and optimal automatic mode switching. PACE 21(11 Pt 2):2214-2219, 1998.
80. Pollak WM, Simmons JD, Interian A Jr, et al: Pacemaker diagnostics: A critical appraisal of current technology. PACE 26(1 Pt 1):76-98, 2003.
81. Passman RS, Weinberg KM, Freher M, et al: Accuracy of mode switch algorithms for detection of atrial tachyarrhythmias. J Cardiovasc Electrophysiol 15:773-777, 2004.
82. Hammel E, Hudelo C, Mailland L, et al: Appropriate detection of Guidant pacemaker stored electrograms assessed by centralized arrhythmia workstation [abstract]. PACE 23:680, 2000.
83. Israel CW, Gascon D, Nowak B, et al: Diagnostic value of stored electrograms in single-lead VDD systems. PACE 23(11 Pt 2): 1801-1803, 2000.
84. Melzer C, Sowelam S, Sheldon TJ, et al: Reduction of right ventricular pacing in patients with sinus node dysfunction using an enhanced search AV algorithm. PACE 28:521-527, 2005.
85. Sweeney M, Nsah E, McGrew F, et al: Reduction in ventricular pacing and its long term clinical outcomes: Preliminary results of the Save Pace Trial [abstract]. Heart Rhythm 2(Suppl):S322, 2005.
86. Olshansky B, Day J, McGuire M, et al: Inhibition of unnecessary RV pacing with AV search hysteresis in ICDs (INTRINSIC RV): Design and clinical protocol. PACE 28:62-66, 2005.
87. Deering T, Wilensky M, Tondato F, et al: Auto intrinsic conduction search algorithm: A prospective analysis [abstract 606]. PACE 26:1080, 2003.
88. Savoure A, Frohlig G, Galley D, et al: A new dual-chamber pacing mode to minimize ventricular pacing. PACE 28(Suppl 1):S43-S46, 2005.
89. Sweeney MO, Shea JB, Fox V, et al: Randomized pilot study of a new atrial-based minimal ventricular pacing mode in dual-chamber implantable cardioverter-defibrillators. Heart Rhythm 1:160-167, 2004.
90. de Voogt WG, Vonk BF, Albers BA, et al: Understanding capture detection. Europace 6:561-569, 2004.
91. Splett V, Trusty JM, Hayes DL, et al: Determination of pacing capture in implantable defibrillators: Benefit of evoked response detection using RV coil to can vector. PACE 23(11 Pt 1):1645-1650, 2000.
92. Schuchert A, Frese J, Stammwitz E, et al: Low settings of the ventricular pacing output in patients dependent on a pacemaker: Are they really safe? Am Heart J 143:1009-1011, 2002.
93. Sperzel J, Binner L, Boriani G, et al: Evaluation of the atrial evoked response for capture detection with high-polarization leads. PACE 28(Suppl 1):S57-S62, 2005.
94. Sperzel J, Compton S, et al: Automatic measurement of atrial pacing thresholds in dual chamber pacemakers: Atrial Capture Management [abstract]. Heart Rhythm 1:S118, 2004.
95. Olson W: Safety margins for sensing and detection: Programming tradeoffs. In Kroll M, Lehmann M (eds): Implantable Cardioverter Defibrillator Therapy: The Engineering-Clinical Interface. Norwell, MA, Kluwer Academic Publishers, 1996, pp 389-420.
96. Anderson MH, Murgatroyd FD, Hnatkova K, et al: Performance of basic ventricular tachycardia detection algorithms in implantable cardioverter defibrillators: Implications for device programming. PACE 20(12 Pt 1):2975-2983, 1997.
97. Murgatroyd F, Anderson M, Hnatkova K, et al: Comparison of misdiagnosis of atrial fibrillation as ventricular tachycardia by algorithms employed in current implantable cardioverter-defibrillators. Circulation 88:I-353, 1993.
98. Grimm W, Menz V, Hoffmann J, et al: Failure of third-generation implantable cardioverter defibrillators to abort shock therapy for nonsustained ventricular tachycardia due to shortcomings of the VF confirmation algorithm. PACE 21(4 Pt 1):722-727, 1998.
99. Raedle-Hurst TM, Wiecha J, Schwab JO, et al: Clinical performance of a specific algorithm to reconfirm self-terminating ventricular arrhythmias in current implantable cardioverter-defibrillators. Am J Cardiol 88:744-749, 2001.
100. Gillberg J, Olson W (eds): Dual-chamber sensing and detection for implantable cardioverter-defibrillators. In Singer I (ed): Interventional Electrophysiology. Philadelphia, Lippincott Williams & Wilkins, 2001.
101. Arenal A, Almendral J, Villacastin J, et al: First postpacing interval variability during right ventricular stimulation: A single algorithm for the differential diagnosis of regular tachycardias. Circulation 98:671-677, 1998.
102. Glikson M, Swerdlow CD, Gurevitz OT, et al: Optimal combination of discriminators for differentiating ventricular from supraventricular tachycardia by dual-chamber defibrillators. J Cardiovasc Electrophysiol 16:732-739, 2005.
103. Brugada J, Mont L, Figueiredo M, et al: Enhanced detection criteria in implantable defibrillators. J Cardiovasc Electrophysiol 9:261-268, 1998.
104. Le Franc P, Kus T, Vinet A, et al: Underdetection of ventricular tachycardia using a 40 ms stability criterion: Effect of antiarrythmic therapy. PACE 20:2882-2892, 1997.
105. Neuzner J, Pitschner HF, Schlepper M: Programmable VT detection enhancements in implantable cardioverter defibrillator therapy. PACE 18(3 Pt 2):539-547, 1995.
106. Swerdlow CD, Ahern T, Chen PS, et al: Underdetection of ventricular tachycardia by algorithms to enhance specificity in a tiered-therapy cardioverter-defibrillator. J Am Coll Cardiol 24:416-424, 1994.
107. Swerdlow CD, Chen PS, Kass RM, et al: Discrimination of ventricular tachycardia from sinus tachycardia and atrial fibrillation in a tiered-therapy cardioverter-defibrillator. J Am Coll Cardiol 23:1342-1355, 1994.
108. Gronefeld GC, Schulte B, Hohnloser SH, et al: Morphology discrimination: A beat-to-beat algorithm for the discrimination of

ventricular from supraventricular tachycardia by implantable cardioverter defibrillators. PACE 24:1519-1524, 2001.
109. Boriani G, Biffi M, Frabetti L, et al: Clinical evaluation of morphology discrimination: An algorithm for rhythm discrimination in cardioverter defibrillators. PACE 24:994-1001, 2001.
110. Gold MR, Shorofsky SR, Thompson JA, et al: Advanced rhythm discrimination for implantable cardioverter defibrillators using electrogram vector timing and correlation. J Cardiovasc Electrophysiol 13:1092-1097, 2002.
111. Klein G, Manolis A, Viskin S, et al: Clinical performance of Wavelet™ morphology discrimination algorithm in a worldwide single chamber ICD population [abstract]. Circulation 110:III-345, 2003.
112. Stadler RW, Gunderson BD, Gillberg JM: An adaptive interval-based algorithm for withholding ICD therapy during sinus tachycardia. PACE 26:1189-1201, 2003.
113. Stein KM, Euler DE, Mehra R, et al: Do atrial tachyarrhythmias beget ventricular tachyarrhythmias in defibrillator recipients? J Am Coll Cardiol 40:335-340, 2002.
114. Aliot E, Nitzsche R, Ripart A: Arrhythmia detection by dual-chamber implantable cardioverter defibrillators: A review of current algorithms. Europace 6:273-286, 2004.
115. Wilkoff B, Sterns L, Morgan JM, et al: Preventing shocks after ICD implantation: Can a strategy of standardized ICD programming match physician tailored? Heart Rhythm 2:1034, 2005.
116. Deisenhofer I, Kolb C, Ndrepepa G, et al: Do current dual chamber cardioverter defibrillators have advantages over conventional single chamber cardioverter defibrillators in reducing inappropriate therapies? A randomized, prospective study. J Cardiovasc Electrophysiol 12:134-142, 2001.
117. Theuns DA, Klootwijk AP, Goedhart DM, et al: Prevention of inappropriate therapy in implantable cardioverter-defibrillators: Results of a prospective, randomized study of tachyarrhythmia detection algorithms. J Am Coll Cardiol 44:2362-2367, 2004.
118. Bansch D, Steffgen F, Gronefeld G, et al: The 1+1 trial: A prospective trial of a dual- versus a single-chamber implantable defibrillator in patients with slow ventricular tachycardias. Circulation 110:1022-1029, 2004.
119. Friedman PA, McClelland RL, Bamlet WR, et al: Dual chamber versus single chamber detection enhancements for implantable defibrillator rhythm diagnosis: The detect supraventricular tachycardia study. Circulation 113:2871-2879, 2006.
120. Wathen MS, Volosin KJ, Sweeney MO, et al: Ventricular antitachycardia pacing by implantable cardioverter defibrillators reduces shocks for inappropriately detected supraventricular tachycardia [abstract]. Heart Rhythm 1:S148, 2004.
121. Knight BP, Zivin A, Souza J, et al: A technique for the rapid diagnosis of atrial tachycardia in the electrophysiology laboratory. J Am Coll Cardiol 33:775-781, 1999.
122. Paz O, Birgersdotter-Green U, Swerdlow C: Acceleration of ventricular rate following atrial antitachycardia pacing: What is the mechanism? J Cardiovasc Electrophysiol 14:1382-1384, 2003.
123. Zeger SL, Liang KY, Albert PS: Models for longitudinal data: A generalized estimating equation approach. Biometrics 44:1049-1060, 1998.
124. Hall GH: The clinical application of Bayes' theorem. Lancet 2:555-557, 1967.
125. Malik M: Pitfalls of the concept of incremental specificity used in comparisons of dual chamber VT/VF detection algorithms. PACE 23:1166-1170, 2000.
126. Olson W, Gunderson BD, Fang-Yen M, et al: Properties and peformance of rate detection algorithms in three implantable cardioverter defibrillators. Comput Cardiol 65-68, 1994.
127. Birgersdotter-Green U, Rosenqvist M, Lindemans FW, et al: Holter documented sudden death in a patient with an implanted defibrillator. PACE 15:1008-1014, 1991.
128. Schwartzman D, Musley SK, Swerdlow C, et al: Early recurrence of atrial fibrillation after ambulatory shock conversion. J Am Coll Cardiol 40:93-99, 2002.
129. Schaumann A, von zur Muhlen F, Herse B, et al: Empirical versus tested antitachycardia pacing in implantable cardioverter defibrillators: A prospective study including 200 patients. Circulation 97:66-74, 1998.
130. Wathen MS, Sweeney MO, DeGroot PJ, et al: Shock reduction using antitachycardia pacing for spontaneous rapid ventricular tachycardia in patients with coronary artery disease. Circulation 104:796-801, 2001.
131. Wathen MS, DeGroot PJ, Sweeney MO, et al: Prospective randomized multicenter trial of empirical antitachycardia pacing versus shocks for spontaneous rapid ventricular tachycardia in patients with implantable cardioverter-defibrillators: Pacing Fast Ventricular Tachycardia Reduces Shock Therapies (PainFREE Rx II) trial results. Circulation 110:2591-2596, 2004.
132. Bardy GH, Lee KL, Mark DB, et al: Amiodarone or an implantable cardioverter-defibrillator for congestive heart failure. N Engl J Med 352:225-237, 2005.
133. Gunderson BD, Gillberg JM, Olson WH, et al: Effect of programmed number of intervals to detect ventricular fibrillation on implantable cardioverter defibrillator longevity and unnecessary shocks [abstract]. Circulation 106:322, 2002.
134. Aminoff MJ, Scheinman MM, Griffin JC, et al: Electrocerebral accompaniments of syncope associated with malignant ventricular arrhythmias. Ann Intern Med 108:791-796, 1988.
135. Daubert JP, Wojciech Z, Cannom DC, et al: Frequency and mechanisms of inappropriate ICD therapy in MADIT II [abstract]. J Am Coll Cardiol 43:132A, 2004.
136. Kouakam C, Kacet S, Hazard JR, et al: Performance of a dual-chamber implantable defibrillator algorithm for discrimination of ventricular from supraventricular tachycardia. Europace 6:32-42, 2004.
137. Frang P, Kus T, Vinet A, et al: Underdetection of ventricular tachycardia using 40 ms stability criterion: Effect of antiarrhythmic thearpy. PACE 20:2882-2892, 1997.
138. Morgan JM, Sterns LD, Hanson JL, et al: A trial design for evaluation of empiric programming of implantable cardioverter defibrillators to improve patient management. Curr Control Trials Cardiovasc Med 5:12, 2004.
139. Panotopoulos P, Krum D, Axtell K, et al: Ventricular fibrillation sensing and detection by implantable defibrillators: Is one better than the others? A prospective, comparative study. J Cardiovasc Electrophysiol 12:445-452, 2001.
140. Kolb C, Deisenhofer I, Weyerbrock S, et al: Incidence of antitachycardia therapy suspension due to magnet reversion in implantable cardioverter defibrillators. PACE 27:221-223, 2004.
141. Bansch D, Castrucci M, Bocker D, et al: Ventricular tachycardias above the initially programmed tachycardia detection interval in patients with implantable cardioverter-defibrillators: Incidence, prediction and significance. J Am Coll Cardiol 36:557-565, 2000.
142. Shukla HH, Flaker GC, Jayam V, et al: High defibrillation thresholds in transvenous biphasic implantable defibrillators: Clinical predictors and prognostic implications. PACE 26(1 Pt 1):44-48, 2003.
143. Brode SE, Schwartzman D, Callans DJ, et al: ICD-antiarrhythmic drug and ICD-pacemaker interactions. J Cardiovasc Electrophysiol 8:830-842, 1997.
144. Monahan KM, Hadjis T, Hallett N, et al: Relation of induced to spontaneous ventricular tachycardia from analysis of stored far-field implantable defibrillator electrograms. Am J Cardiol 83:349-353, 1999.
145. Weber M, Bocker D, Bansch D, et al: Efficacy and safety of the initial use of stability and onset criteria in implantable cardioverter defibrillators. J Cardiovasc Electrophysiol 10:145-153, 1999.

146. Cohen AI, Wish MH, Fletcher RD, et al: The use and interaction of permanent pacemakers and the automatic implantable cardioverter defibrillator. PACE 11(6 Pt 1):704-711, 1988.
147. Geiger MJ, O'Neill P, Sharma A, et al: Interactions between transvenous nonthoracotomy cardioverter defibrillator systems and permanent transvenous endocardial pacemakers. PACE 20(3 Pt 1):624-630, 1997.
148. Glikson M, Trusty JM, Grice SK, et al: A stepwise testing protocol for modern implantable cardioverter-defibrillator systems to prevent pacemaker-implantable cardioverter-defibrillator interactions. Am J Cardiol 83:360-366, 1999.
149. Wietholt D, Kuehlkamp V, Meisel E, et al: Prevention of sustained ventricular tachyarrhythmias in patients with implantable cardioverter-defibrillators: The PREVENT study. J Interv Card Electrophysiol 9:383-389, 2003.
150. Shalaby AA: Delayed detection of ventricular tachycardia in a dual chamber rate adaptive pacing implantable cardioverter defibrillator: A case of intradevice interaction. PACE 2004;27: 1164-1166, 2004.
151. Pascal D, Hazard J, Besson B, et al: Contribution of pacemaker stored electrograms to patient management [abstract]. PACE 23(Part II):681, 2000.
152. Seidl K, Meisel E, VanAgt E, et al: Is the atrial high rate episode diagnostic feature reliable in detecting paroxysmal episodes of atrial tachyarrhythmias? PACE 21(4 Pt 1):694-700, 1998.
153. Morris MM, KenKnight BH, Lang DJ: Detection of atrial arrhythmia for cardiac rhythm management by implantable devices. J Electrocardiol 33(Suppl):133-139, 2000.
154. Schuchert A, Boriani G, Wollmann C, et al: Implantable dual-chamber defibrillator for the selective treatment of spontaneous atrial and ventricular arrhythmias: Arrhythmia incidence and device performance. J Interv Card Electrophysiol 12:149-156, 2005.
155. Krahn AD, Klein GJ, Yee R, et al: Maturation of the sensed electrogram amplitude over time in a new subcutaneous implantable loop recorder. PACE 20:1686-1690, 1997.
156. Chrysostomakis SI, Klapsinos NC, Simantirakis EN, et al: Sensing issues related to the clinical use of implantable loop recorders. Europace 5:143-148, 2003.
157. Mazur A, Wang L, Anderson ME, et al: Functional similarity between electrograms recorded from an implantable cardioverter defibrillator emulator and the surface electrocardiogram. PACE 24:34-40, 2001.
158. Bardy G, Cappato R, Smith WM, et al: The totally subcutaneous ICD system (the S-ICD) [abstract]. PACE 25:222, 2002.
159. Bardy G: Subcutaneous implantable defibrillator. In Malik M (ed): Dynamic Electrocardiography. Armonk, NY, Futura, 2004.
160. Bordachar P, Garrigue S, Reuter S, et al: Hemodynamic assessment of right, left, and biventricular pacing by peak endocardial acceleration and echocardiography in patients with end-stage heart failure. PACE 23(11 Pt 2):1726-1730, 2000.
161. Hegbom F, Hoff PI, Oie B, et al: RV function in stable and unstable VT: Is there a need for hemodynamic monitoring in future defibrillators? PACE 24:172-182, 2001.
162. Kaye G, Astridge P, Perrins J: Tachycardia recognition and diagnosis from changes in right atrial pressure waveform: A feasibility study. PACE 14:1384-1392, 1991.
163. Khoury D, McAlister H, Wilkoff B, et al: Continuous right ventricular volume assessment by catheter measurement of impedance for antitachycardia system control. PACE 12:1918-1926, 1989.
164. Sharma AD, Bennett TD, Erickson M, et al: Right ventricular pressure during ventricular arrhythmias in humans: Potential implications for implantable antitachycardia devices. J Am Coll Cardiol 15:648-655, 1990.
165. Wood M, Ellenbogen KA, Lu B, et al: A prospective study of right ventricular pulse pressure and dP/dt to discriminant-induced ventricular tachycardia from supraventricular and sinus tachycardia in man. PACE 13:1148-1157, 1990.
166. Ellenbogen KA, Lu B, Kapadia K, et al: Usefulness of right ventricular pulse pressure as a potential sensor for hemodynamically unstable ventricular tachycardia. Am J Cardiol 65: 1105-1111, 1990.
167. Plicchi G, Marcelli E, Marini S: An endocardial acceleration sensor for sustained ventricular tachycardia detection [abstract]. Europace Suppl 3:96, 2002.
168. Whitman T, Sheldon T, McFadden S: Endocardial acceleration measurements in tachycardia induced heart failure in canines [abstract]. PACE 24:569, 2002.
169. Nabutovsky Y, Pavek T, Wright G, Turcott R: Chronic performance of a subcutaneous photoplethysmography sensor [abstract]. Heart Rhythm 1:476, 2004.
170. Turcott R: Detection of hemodynamically unstable arrhythmias using subcutaneous photoplethysmography [abstract]. Heart Rhythm 2:S83, 2005.
171. Bennett T, Kjellstrom B, Taepke R, et al: Development of implantable devices for continuous ambulatory monitoring of central hemodynamic values in heart failure patients. PACE 28:573-584, 2005.
172. Cleland JG, Coletta AP, Freemantle N, et al: Clinical trials update from the American College of Cardiology meeting: CARE-HF and the Remission of Heart Failure, Women's Health Study, TNT, COMPASS-HF, VERITAS, CANPAP, PEECH and PREMIER. Eur J Heart Fail 7:931-936, 2005.
173. Kay G: Troubleshooting and programming of cardiac resynchronization therapy. In Ellenbogen KA, Kay G, Wilkoff B (eds): Device Therapy for Congestive Heart Failure. Philadelphia, Elsevier, 2004, pp 232-293.
174. Swerdlow C, Friedman P: Advanced ICD troubleshooting: Part II. PACE 29:70-96, 2006.
175. Meyer Y: Wavelets: Algorithms and Applications. Philadelphia, Society for Industrial and Applied Mathematics, 1993.
176. Morris M, Marcovecchio A, KenKnight B, et al: Retrospective evaluation of detection enhancements in a dual-chamber implantable cardioverter defibrillator: Implications for device programming [abstract]. PACE 22(4 Part II):849, 1999.
177. Willems R, Morck ML, Exner DV, et al: Ventricular high-rate episodes in pacemaker diagnostics identify a high-risk subgroup of patients with tachy-brady syndrome. Heart Rhythm 1:414-421, 2004.
178. Swerdlow CD, Schsls W, Dijkman B, et al: Detection of atrial fibrillation and flutter by a dual-chamber implantable cardioverter-defibrillator. For the Worldwide Jewel AF Investigators. Circulation 101:878-885, 2000.
179. Swerdlow CD, Schwartzman D, Hoyt R, et al: Determinants of first-shock success for atrial implantable cardioverter defibrillators. J Cardiovasc Electrophysiol 13:347-354, 2002.

Chapter 4

Engineering and Construction of Pacemaker and Implantable Cardioverter-Defibrillator Leads

ANDREA M. RUSSO • FRANCIS E. MARCHLINSKI

The role of the implantable cardioverter-defibrillator (ICD) in both primary and secondary prevention is now well established.[1-5] ICD lead and device technology, as well as implantation approach, have changed substantially since approval of the first ICD system in 1985. Lead technology has had a significant impact on the sensing characteristics and defibrillation performance of ICD systems. This chapter describes the design and characteristics of ICD leads, focusing on the evolution of lead technology and implantation methods occurring over the past two decades. In addition, newer technology related to left ventricular (LV) pacing leads, designed for coronary sinus pacing and cardiac resynchronization therapy (CRT), is also discussed.

IMPLANTABLE CARDIOVERTER-DEFIBRILLATOR LEADS

The lead is an essential part of the defibrillation system that conducts electrical impulses between the pulse generator and the patient. It is composed of one or more electrodes, conductors, insulation, connectors, and a fixation mechanism. The electrode is the portion of the lead that is responsible for sensing, pacing, and defibrillation. Lead locations may be epicardial, endocardial, or extrathoracic, or they may include a combination of these systems. Epicardial systems were the first systems studied clinically, and they are only briefly discussed here, because they have been supplanted by less invasive endocardial systems. Current technology using endocardial lead systems is the main focus of this chapter.

Epicardial ICD Lead Systems: Historical Perspective

Since the pioneering work of Michel Mirowski in the 1970s, rapid advancements in lead technology have occurred. With epicardial systems, the surgical procedures included median sternotomy, lateral thoracotomy, subxiphoid, and subcostal approaches, and transvenous access also was used for placement of an additional shocking lead in the superior vena cava (SVC) or an endocardial sensing lead in the right ventricle (RV). The first human implants used a titanium spring electrode positioned in the SVC and an epicardial patch.[6,7] Initially, sensing was performed using the high-voltage electrodes, but this resulted in sensing problems, leading to the use of separate epicardial or endocardial rate sensing leads to address this problem.[8] Complications of the initially implanted defibrillation lead systems included migration of the SVC coil,[9] which could have an impact on defibrillator function. The SVC electrode/epicardial patch electrode configuration was supplanted by the epicardial patch/patch electrode configuration, which demonstrated better defibrillation efficacy and avoided the problem of SVC lead migration.[10] Figure 4-1 illustrates a fully epicardial patch lead system, including epicardial rate sensing leads.

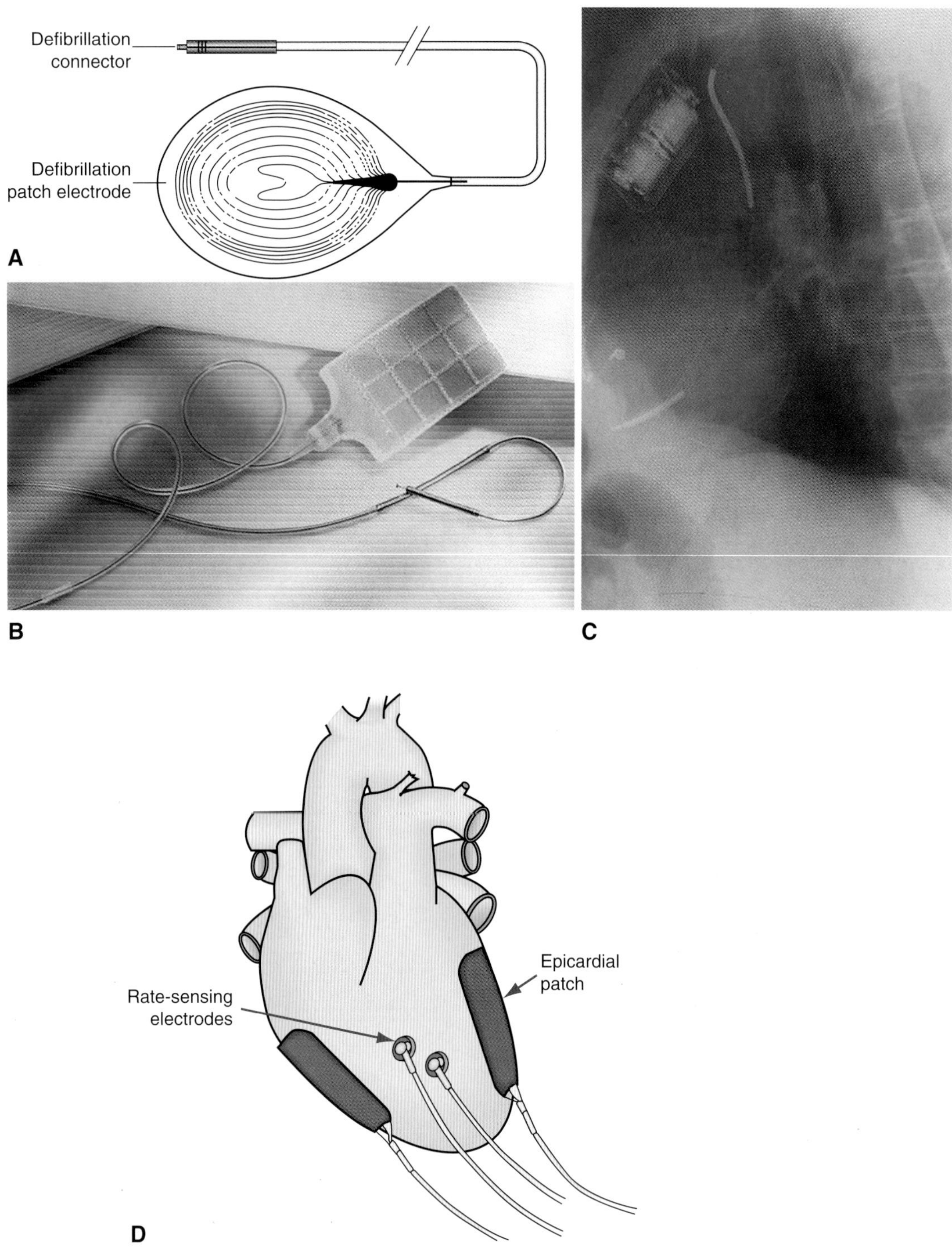

Figure 4-1. Epicardial patch lead systems. ***A,*** *Schematic illustration of an oval-shaped epicardial patch electrode (St. Jude/Ventritex, Sunnyvale, Calif.).* ***B,*** *Photograph of a rectangular-shaped patch (Guidant/CPI).* ***C,*** *Lateral radiograph demonstrating epicardial defibrillation patches.* ***D,*** *Schematic drawing showing epicardial defibrillation patches and epicardial sensing leads. (From Accorti PR: Leads technology. In Singer I [ed]: Implantable Cardioverter Defibrillator. Armonk, NY, Futura, 1994, with permission.)*

Epicardial lead implantation requires a thoracotomy and is associated with significant morbidity and mortality. The perioperative surgical mortality rate has been reported to be as high as 5%.[11-16] Some of this mortality may be seen in patients undergoing other concomitant cardiac surgery at the time of patch lead placement. Other concerns include bacterial infections, which can spread directly from the pocket to leads on the heart, and subsequent difficulty removing epicardial patch leads due to fibrosis after long-term implantation. Later cardiac surgery, such as bypass graft surgery or valve replacement, may also be increasingly difficult if patches were placed directly on the heart, as opposed to outside the pericardium. In addition, patients with epicardial patches in place may be resistant to external defibrillation due to an increase in transthoracic impedance.

A high rate of lead malfunction was identified with epicardial patch leads.[17-19] Some patch leads had a failure rate of 28% at 4 years in one study.[17] Many patients with fractured leads were asymptomatic and were identified during routine surveillance radiography and formal lead testing; they were most frequently detected more than 2 years after implantation.[17] This finding highlighted the importance of regular lead testing in patients with epicardial systems. In addition to lead failures with identification of obvious fractures, fluid may sometimes be apparent within the lead insulation. The insulation of leads manufactured from silicone is permeable to serous fluid under normal circumstances.[17] However, large elements such as cells or blood should not permeate silicone; if they do, it suggests the presence of a breach of insulation or leakage through the vulnerable parts of the leads, such as the joints or connector ends. If the electrical performance of the lead is normal, the clinical significance of the finding of blood or fluid beneath the lead is unclear as to whether this small breach could eventually result in lead dysfunction.[17] Although no deaths were directly attributed to lead malfunction in two studies, unsuccessful defibrillation due to epicardial patch fracture can require external defibrillation.[17,20] Symptomatic pericardial constriction may also be seen as a complication of epicardial patch placement.[21]

Malfunctions of epicardial pace/sense leads are common, occurring in 3.4% to 15.4% of patients,[18-20,22,23] and they often manifest with inappropriate ICD discharges due to oversensing.[17,23] This is frequently related to lead fracture, which may be detected by abnormally high impedance values, oversensing with delivery of inappropriate therapy, high pacing thresholds, or direct visualization.[18,23] The presence of an adapter increases the risk of sensing lead problems in epicardial systems.[22,24,25] There is also a high incidence of elevated pacing thresholds or complete loss of capture with epicardial pacing.[26]

Endocardial ICD Lead Systems

Although the concept of transvenous defibrillation was first developed by the pioneering work of Michel Mirowski[27] and early studies established the feasibility of successful defibrillation using endocardial leads,[28,29] widespread application was limited because of high defibrillation energy requirements and lead complications. These problems were later addressed by further advances in lead and especially device technology. The development of a lead that incorporates both shock and sensing functions permitted widespread use of transvenous systems. Initially, subcutaneous patches were routinely used as part of the defibrillation system. After lead design advances and improvements in defibrillation energy requirements with biphasic shocks became available, implantation of complete transvenous systems became more common.

There are several potential advantages to an endocardial system. A transvenous or nonthoracotomy lead system obviates the need for a thoracotomy procedure and reduces morbidity and mortality associated with the procedure. Elimination of the need for a thoracotomy shortens hospital stay and makes convalescence easier, with reduced patient discomfort. Comparisons of epicardial and endocardial lead systems have demonstrated that endocardial systems are as effective as epicardial systems with respect to successful termination of spontaneous ventricular tachyarrhythmias.[30,31] Although lead dislodgment and pocket infection were more frequent with endocardial systems, perioperative mortality was higher with epicardial systems.[30] Endocardial systems can be implanted with a mortality rate of less than or equal to 1.0%,[32-34] whereas the perioperative mortality rate with epicardial leads can be 2 to 5 times greater.[12-16,26,34]

General Description of ICD Lead Technology

In addition to sensing and pacing, ICD leads have the function of delivering high-voltage shocks for defibrillation therapy. Despite some similarities, ICD leads must be designed somewhat differently from pacemaker leads. Like pacemaker leads, ICD leads are composed of electrodes, conductors, insulation, connectors, and a fixation mechanism.

The initial endocardial leads were large in caliber,[35] measuring 12F, and were subsequently reduced to 6.6F to 8.2F in size. One of the earliest endocardial leads was produced by Intec/CPI (Pittsburgh) and was tested in the 1980s.[36] The Intec endovascular lead had a 16-mm^2 distal platinum-iridium tip used for pacing and sensing functions. Distal 4.3-cm^2 and proximal 8.5-cm^2 platinum electrodes with helically wound coils were used for defibrillation, and this lead was the predecessor of the Endotak endocardial lead manufactured by Guidant/CPI (Boston Scientific, Natick, Mass.). Since the first implantations in 1988 and its approval in 1993, the Endotak lead has undergone several modifications. The current lead specifications are outlined in Table 4-1A. Early endocardial leads from three different manufacturers are demonstrated in Figure 4-2.

Other manufacturers—including Medtronic, Inc. (Minneapolis, Minn.); St. Jude Medical (St. Paul, Minn.); Telectronics (now a division of St. Jude Medical,

TABLE 4-1A. **Specifications of Guidant/CPI Defibrillation Leads**

Features	Endotak 60 0060/62/64	Endotak 70 0070/72/74	Endotak 0073/75 0113/15	Endotak DSP 90 0092/93/95	Endotak DSP 120 0123/25	Endotak Endurance 0134/35/36	Endotak Endurance Rx 0144/45/46	Endotak Endurance EZ 0154/55/56
Defibrillation coils	RV/SVC	RV/SVC	RV/SVC	RV/SVC	RV/SVC	RV/SVC	RV/SVC	RV/SVC
Fixation mechanism	Tines	Tines	Tines	Tines	Tines	Tines	Tines	Screw
Sensing	Integ bipolar	Integ bipolar	Integ bipolar	Integ bipolar	Integ bipolar	Integ bipolar	Integ bipolar	Integ bipolar
Tip electrode mm^2	9	9	9	8	8	2	2	6
Steroid	No	No	No	No	No	No	Yes	Yes
Insulation	Silicone	Silicone	Silicone	Silicone	Silicone	Silicone	Silicone	Silicone
Coil electrode coating	NA	NA	NA	NA	NA	NA	NA	NA
Lead lengths (cm)	100	100	100, 70	100	70	64, 70, 100	64, 70, 100	64, 70, 100
Lead body diameter (F)	9.7/12	9.7/12	9.7/12	8.2/10	8.2/10	8.2/10	8.2/10	8.2/10
Tube design	Coaxial	Coaxial	Coaxial	Multilumen	Multilumen	Multilumen	Multilumen	Multilumen
Connector terminal								
Pace/sense	4.75 mm	4.75 mm	4.75 mm	IS-1	IS-1	IS-1	IS-1	IS-1
High voltage	6.1 mm	6.1 mm	6.1 mm	DF-1	DF-1	DF-1	DF-1	DF-1
Interelectrode spacing								
Tip-Ring	NA	NA	NA	NA	NA	NA	NA	NA
Tip-RV coil (mm)	6	12	12	12	12	12	12	12
Tip-SVC coil (cm)	10/13/16	12/15/18	15/18	18	18	18	18	18
Electrode surface area								
RV (mm^2)	295	379	379	450	450	450	450	450
SVC (mm^2)	617	617	617	660	660	660	660	660

Integ, integrated; NA, not applicable; ePTFE, an expanded polytetrafluoroethylene polymer; RV, right ventricle; SVC, superior vena cava.

Sylmar, Calif.); Intermedics, Inc. (Boston Scientific, Natick, Mass.); and Biotronik GmbH & Co. (Berlin, Germany)—have also developed endocardial leads demonstrating defibrillation efficacy. The characteristics of these endocardial leads are summarized in Tables 4-1B through 4-1D. In addition to the Guidant/CPI Endotak lead, which is a single lead composed of two separate endocardial defibrillation coils and was the first nonthoracotomy lead approved in the United States, the use of two separate catheter endocardial braided defibrillation electrodes, one positioned at the RV apex and the other in the SVC or high right atrium also demonstrated defibrillation efficacy (Telectronics). These leads were used in conjunction with a subcutaneous patch electrode positioned on the left lateral thorax at the midclavicular to midaxillary line in the second to sixth intercostal spaces.[37] Other manufacturers, including Medtronic and St. Jude, have also marketed defibrillation systems with separate endocardial RV and SVC coils (see Table 4-1).

Since the early 1990s, ICDs have been implanted like pacemakers in the infraclavicular position.[38,39] This was the result of development of the transvenous lead system, as well as improvements in ICD technology that allowed a reduction in pulse generator size. Initially, ICDs were used as a therapy of last resort, but they are now considered the therapy of choice for treatment of life-threatening sustained ventricular arrhythmias, as well as in the prevention of sudden cardiac death in high-risk populations with underlying struc-

Endotak Reliance G 0174/75/76/77	Endotak Reliance G 0164/65/66	Endotak Reliance SG 0170/71/72	Endotak Reliance G 0160/61	Endotak Reliance 0157/58/59	Endotak Reliance S 0137/38	Endotak Reliance G 0184/85,86,87	Endotak Reliance SG 0180,81,82
RV/SVC	RV/SVC	RV	RV	RV/SVC	RV	RV/SVC	RV
Tines	Screw	Tines	Screw	Screw	Screw	Screw	Screw
Integ bipolar	Integ bipolar	Integ bipolar	Integ bipolar	Integ bipolar	Integ bipolar	Integ bipolar	Integ bipolar
2	5.7	2	5.7	5.7	5.7	5.7	5.7
Yes	Yes	Yes	Yes	Yes	Yes	Yes	Yes
Silicone	Silicone	Silicone	Silicone	Silicone	Silicone	Silicone	Silicone
ePTFE	ePTFE	ePTFE	ePTFE	ePTFE	ePTFE	ePTFE	ePTFE
59, 64, 70, 90	59, 64, 70	59, 64, 70	59, 64	59, 64, 90	59, 64	59, 64, 70, 90	59, 64, 70
8.2	8.2	8.2	8.2	8.2	8.2	8.2	8.2
Multilumen	Multilumen	Multilumen	Multilumen	Multilumen	Multilumen	Multilumen	Multilumen
IS-1	IS-1	IS-1	IS-1	IS-1	IS-1	IS-1	IS-1
DF-1	DF-1	DF-1	DF-1	DF-1	DF-1	DF-1	DF-1
NA	NA	NA	NA	NA	NA	NA	NA
12	12	12	12	12	12	12	12
18	18	NA	NA	18	NA	18	NA
450	450	450	450	450	450	450	450
660	660	NA	NA	660	NA	660	NA

tural heart disease.[40] The transvenous lead technology has had a major impact on this development.

Integrated Bipolar Versus Dedicated Bipolar Leads

The two types of endocardial defibrillation leads are true bipolar leads and integrated bipolar leads. ICD leads that have true bipolar sensing and pacing capabilities have separate tip and ring electrodes designed for sensing and pacing purposes, similar to permanent pacemaker leads. They have the best sensing and pacing performances and are less likely to manifest sensing errors. However, true bipolar leads have a longer distance from the tip to the distal defibrillation coil in the RV, compared with integrated leads. ICD leads with integrated sensing and pacing capabilities have only a single tip electrode, and the distal defibrillation coil is used as the anode for sensing and pacing functions. The electrograms (EGMs) obtained from an integrated bipolar lead have a more "unipolar" appearance than those recorded from a dedicated bipolar lead. One advantage of ICD leads with integrated bipolar sensing and pacing functions is that there is a shorter tip-to-defibrillation coil distance. The placement of the defibrillation coil closer to the myocardium of the right ventricle and septum may represent an advantage with respect to defibrillation success. However, integrated bipolar leads are more susceptible to sensing problems.[41]

Text continued on p. 170

TABLE 4-1B. Specifications of Medtronic Defibrillation Leads

Features	Sprint Fidelis 6930	Sprint Fidelis 6931	Sprint Fidelis 6948	Sprint Fidelis 6949	Sprint Quattro 6944	Sprint Quattro Secure 6947	Transvene 6936
Defibrillation coils	RV	RV	RV/SVC	RV/SVC	RV/SVC	RV/SVC	RV
Fixation mechanism	Tines	Screw	Tines	Screw	Tines	Screw	Screw
Sensing	True bipolar	True bipolar	True bipolar	True bipolar	True bipolar	True bipolar	True bipolar
Tip electrode (mm^2)	2.5	4.2	2.5	4.2	1.6	5.7	10
Steroid	Yes	Yes	Yes	Yes	Yes	Yes	—
Insulation	Polyurethane	Polyurethane	Polyurethane	Polyurethane	Polyurethane	Polyurethane	Polyurethane
Coil electrode coating	Silicone	Silicone	Silicone	Silicone	Silicone	Silicone	None
Lead lengths (cm)	58, 65, 75, 100	58, 65, 75, 100	58, 65, 75, 100	58, 65, 75, 100	58, 65, 75, 100	58, 65, 75, 100	65, 75, 110
Lead body diameter (F)	6.6	6.6	6.6	6.6	8.2	8.6	10.5
Tube design	Multilumen	Multilumen	Multilumen	Multilumen	Multilumen	Multilumen	Coaxial
Connector terminal							
Pace/sense	IS-1	IS-1	IS-1	IS-1	IS-1	IS-1	IS-1
High voltage	DF-1	DF-1	DF-1	DF-1	DF-1	DF-1	DF-1
Interelectrode spacing							
Tip-Ring (mm)	8	8	8	8	8	8	12
Tip-RV coil (mm)	12	12	12	12	12	12	25
Tip-SVC coil (cm)	NA	NA	18	18	18	18	NA
Electrode surface area							
RV (mm^2)	513	513	513	513	585	614	426
SVC (mm^2)	NA	NA	663	663	819	860	NA

NA, not applicable; RV, right ventricle; SVC, superior vena cava.

TABLE 4-1C. **Specifications of St. Jude/Ventritex Defibrillation Leads**

Features	**Riata 1570/71**	**Riata 1572**	**Riata 1580/81**	**Riata 1582**	**Riata i 1560/61**	**Riata i 1562**	**Riata i 1590/91**	**Riata i 1592**	**TVL RV02**	**TVL RV01/1101**	**SPL SP01/SP02**
Defibrillation coils	RV/SVC	RV	RV/SVC	RV	RV/SVC	RV	RV/SVC	RV	RV	RV	RV/SVC
Fixation mechanism	Tines	Tines	Screw	Screw	Tines	Tines	Screw	Screw	Tines	Screw	Tines
Sensing	True bipolar	True bipolar	True bipolar	True bipolar	Integ bipolar	Integ bipolar	Integ bipolar	Integ bipolar	Integ bipolar	Integ bipolar	Integ bipolar
Tip electrode (mm^2)	5	5	8	8	5	5	8	8	6	6	6
Steroid	Yes	Yes	Yes	Yes	Yes	Yes	Yes	Yes	No	No	No
Insulation	Silicone	Silicone	Silicone	Silicone	Silicone	Silicone	Silicone	Silicone	Silicone	Silicone	Silicone
Coil electrode coating	None	None	None	None	None	None	None	None	None	None	None
Lead lengths (cm)	65	60, 65	60, 65, 75	60, 65, 75	60, 65, 75	60, 65, 75	60, 65, 75	60, 65, 75	67	110	70
Lead body diameter (F)	6.7	6.7	7.6	7.6	6.7	6.7	6.7	6.7	10.5	10.5	6.7
Tube design	Multilumen	Multilumen	Multilumen	Multilumen	Multilumen	Multilumen	Multilumen	Multilumen	Coaxial	Coaxial	Multilumen
Connector terminal											
Pace/sense	IS-1	IS-1	IS-1	IS-1	IS-1	IS-1	IS-1	IS-1	IS-1	IS-1	IS-1
High voltage	DF-1	DF-1	DF-1	DF-1	DF-1	DF-1	DF-1	DF-1	DF-1	DF-1	DF-1
Interelectrode spacing											
Tip-Ring (mm)	11	11	11	11	NA	NA	NA	NA	NA	NA	NA
Tip-RV coil (mm)	17	17	17	17	11	11	11	11	11	11	11
Tip-SVC coil (cm)	1570:17 1571:21	NA	1580:17 1581:21	NA	1560:17 1561:21	NA	1590:17 1591:21	NA	NA	NA	21
Electrode surface area											
RV (mm^2)	414	414	414	414	414	414	414	414	470	470	480
SVC (mm^2)	663	NA	663	NA	663	NA	663	NA	NA	NA	671

Integ, integrated; NA, not applicable; RV, right ventricle, SVC, superior vena cava.

TABLE 4-1D. **Specifications of Biotronik and Intermedics Defibrillation Leads**

Features	Biotronik Kainox SL 217,8,38,9,40	Biotronik Kainox RV 124-005	Biotronik Kainox RV-S 124-574	Biotronik Kentrox RV 348090,91	Biotronik Kentrox SL 7351-4,9,50	Biotronik Kentrox RV-S 343080	Biotronik Kentrox SL-S 345988,9	Intermedics 497-05/06	Intermedics 497-19/20	Intermedics 497-23/24
Defibrillation coils	RV/SVC	RV	RV	RV	RV/SVC	RV	RV/SVC	RV	RV	RV
Fixation mechanism	Tines	Tines	Screw	Tines	Tines	Screw	Screw	Screw	Screw	Screw
Sensing	True bipolar	True bipolar	True bipolar	True bipolar	True bipolar	True bipolar	True bipolar	—	—	—
Tip electrode (mm^2)	6	5	5.3	1.8	1.8	8.2	8.2	10	8	8
Steroid	No	No	No	Yes	Yes	Yes	Yes	—	—	—
Insulation	Silicone	Silicone	Silicone	Silicone	Silicone	Silicone	Silicone	Silicone	Silicone	Silicone
Coil electrode coating	None	None	None	Yes	Yes	Yes	Yes	None	IROX	IROX
Lead lengths (cm)	75, 100	75	74	65, 75	65, 75, 100	65	65	100	—	60, 70, 100
Lead body diameter (F)	10.5	8.7	10.5	9.3	9.3	9.3	9.3	11	11	11
Tube design	Multilumen	Multilumen	Multilumen	Multilumen	Multilumen	Multilumen	Multilumen	—	—	—
Connector terminal										
Pace/sense	IS-1	IS-1	IS-1	IS-1	IS-1	IS-1	IS-1	2 mm	IS-1	IS-1
High voltage	DF-1	DF-1	DF-1	DF-1	DF-1	DF-1	DF-1	4.0 mm	DF-1	DF-1
Interelectrode spacing										
Tip-Ring (mm)	9	9	14	9	9	11.5	11.5	—	—	—
Tip-RV coil (mm)	17	15	21	16	16	18.5	18.5	6 mm	—	8 mm/6 mm
Tip-SVC coil (cm)	13, 16, 18	NA	NA	NA	16, 18	NA	16, 18	—	—	—
Electrode surface area										
RV (mm^2)	320	300	300	310	310	310	310	440/880	440	440
SVC (mm^2)	600	NA	NA	NA	480	NA	480	NA	NA	NA

IROX, iridium oxide; NA, not applicable; RV, right ventricle; SVC, superior vena cava.

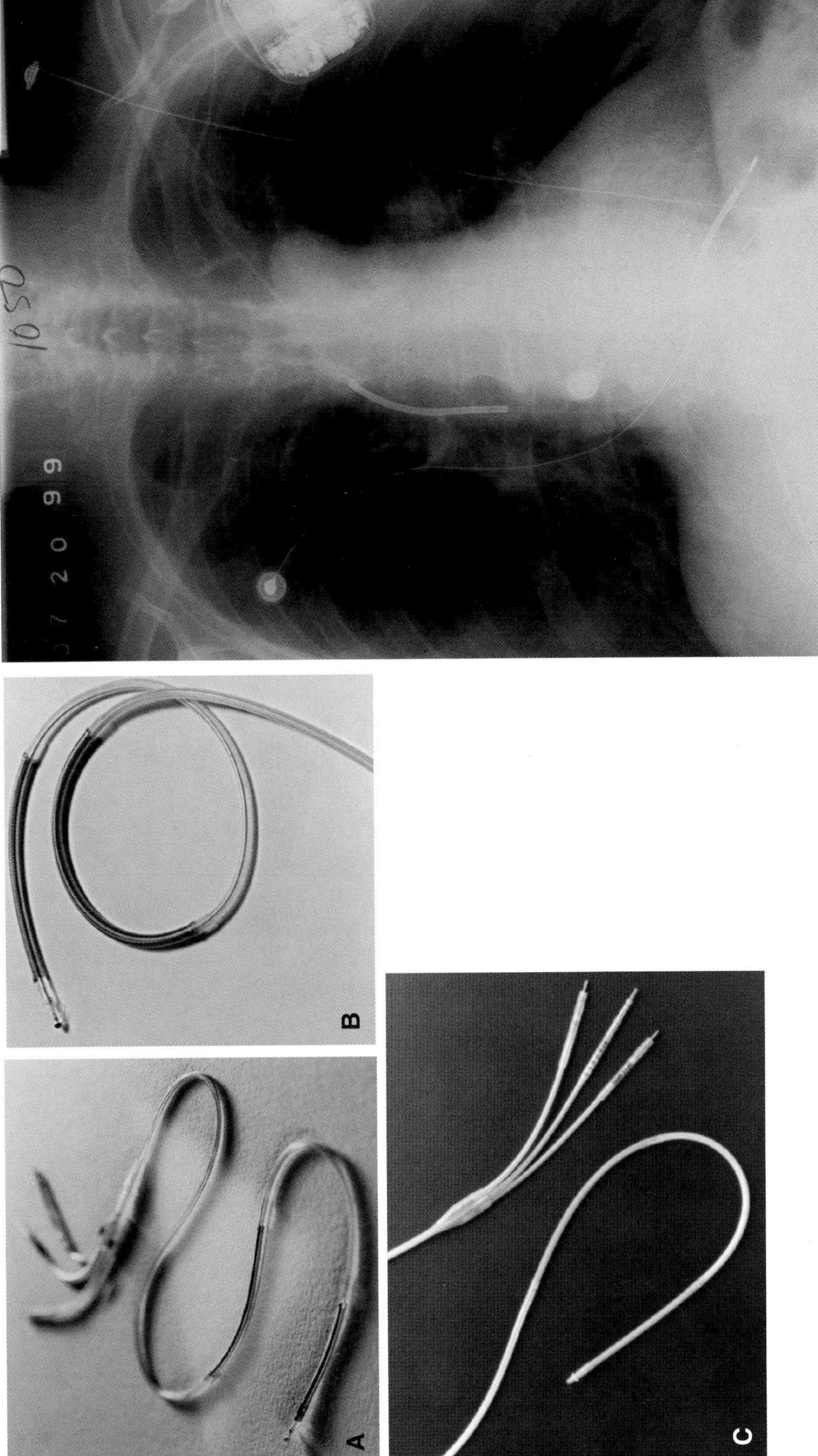

Figure 4-2. Photographs and a radiograph of several early transvenous ICD leads from various manufacturers. **A,** Endotak DSP lead. (Courtesy of Guidant/CPI, Boston Scientific, Natick, Mass.) **B,** Sprint 6942 lead. (Courtesy of Medtronic, Inc., Minneapolis, Minn.) **C,** SPL lead. (Courtesy of St. Jude/Ventritex, Sunnyvale, Calif.) **D,** Chest radiograph demonstrating the appearance of a dual-coil Guidant transvenous lead in a patient requiring ICD implantation.

Previous investigation demonstrated that the ranges of EGM amplitudes recorded in sinus rhythm and ventricular arrhythmias were not significantly different with true bipolar versus integrated bipolar leads.[42] Filtering of the postshock EGM results in a dramatic reduction of R-wave amplitudes, whereas unfiltered amplitudes are similar to the preshock values. In contrast to integrated bipolar sensing, this effect is minimized for true bipolar sensing.[42] Proximity of the defibrillation electrode to the sensing tip of the lead may result in conduction block during shock delivery.[42,43] This could effect postshock sensing of ventricular fibrillation (VF).[44] Delay with capture has also been a concern after shock delivery, because of a temporary increase in pacing threshold. Devices can now be programmed to higher pacing outputs after shock delivery to compensate for this effect.

Single- and Dual-Coil Defibrillation Leads

Single-coil defibrillation leads have one coil that lies in the right ventricle, which typically is used as the defibrillation cathode. When used in conjunction with an active or "hot" can defibrillator, the shell of the device is typically the defibrillation anode. However, polarity can be reversed noninvasively in the newer-generation ICDs. Dual-coil defibrillation leads have an additional proximal coil that typically lies within the junction of the high right atrium and the SVC. The proximal coil can be used alone as the defibrillation anode, or it can be combined with an active can as a combined defibrillation anode. One advantage of dual-coil systems may be an improvement in defibrillation threshold (DFT) compared with single-coil systems.

Steroid-Eluting Leads

The benefits of steroid-eluting leads have been demonstrated for permanent pacemaker leads.[45-48] Steroid (e.g., dexamethasone sodium phosphate) elution at the electrode-tissue interface has helped maintain chronically low stimulation thresholds.[45,47,48] This allows programmed devices to be set at a low pacing output, which has potential implications for device longevity.[46] Steroid-eluting leads appear to reduce the inflammatory response and attenuate the connective tissue reaction at the tip of the lead, resulting in a decrease in the pacing threshold peak.[45,49] In contrast to pacing threshold, steroid-eluting leads were not found to influence chronic ventricular EGM amplitude, compared with leads without steroid elution.[50] Defibrillation lead systems now incorporate steroid elution.

Sensing

Oversensing and Undersensing

In addition to the defibrillation function of ICD leads, it is equally important for the lead to provide reliable sensing of intracardiac signals, in order to detect and differentiate ventricular tachyarrhythmias from sinus rhythm. At the time of implantation, initial R-wave testing in sinus rhythm is performed, aiming for an R-wave amplitude of 5 mV or greater in most instances. A significant relationship has been demonstrated between the ventricular EGM amplitude in sinus rhythm and the amplitude in VF.[51] During epicardial device implantation, one study suggested that up to a fourfold decrease may be seen in mean ventricular EGM amplitude during VF compared with sinus rhythm, although a wide variation among individuals was seen.[51] This may be useful in the initial assessment of sensing lead function at the time of implantation testing, and it has implications with respect to programming device sensitivity for detection of VF.

The sensing issues related to defibrillation leads have been the focus of several papers.[52-54] In addition to sensing issues related to lead problems, undersensing of ventricular tachycardia in one report[53] was related to the ICD generator itself, with use of fixed-gain sensing. The system's ability to sense depends on the quality of the EGM; the input amplifier, including filtering and gain; and the detection algorithm.[42] Although it is crucial to sense small-amplitude signals during VF, it is also important for the defibrillator system to avoid oversensing of other intracardiac signals (e.g., T waves) or extracardiac signals (e.g., noise, myopotentials) during sinus rhythm. Although the role of the device amplifiers and detection algorithms is clearly crucial for appropriate sensing, high-quality lead performance and stability of the EGM are also essential.

Endocardial leads may be associated with fibrotic reactions within the endocardium.[55,56] This may result in a deterioration of the intracardiac EGMs. In addition, fibrotic reactions associated with endocardial leads and cumulative acute damage produced by defibrillator discharges may lead to new arrhythmogenic foci, changes in pacing threshold or DFTs, or future difficulty with lead extraction.[55,56]

An Internet-based registry of pacemaker and ICD pulse generators and leads revealed that disrupted insulation accounted for 29% of ICD lead failures.[57] Failures of the conductor, electrode, fixation mechanism, or pin were identified as other causes of lead failure. Oversensing with delivery of inappropriate shocks was the most frequent consequence of ICD lead failure. Other signs and symptoms of lead failure included high or low impedance, noncapture, undersensing, and failure to defibrillate.[57] Routine follow-up to document impedance and sense/pace functions may detect many unexpected lead failures before they are manifested clinically.

One concern related to endocardial lead systems was the potential failure to redetect VF after an appropriately delivered but unsuccessful first shock.[44,58-61] Redetection of VF after a failed first shock demonstrates longer redetection times with integrated lead sensing than with dedicated bipolar leads. This is probably due to the high-voltage field that results in local myocardial stunning, which is most apparent immediately after a shock.[62] One study demonstrated that there are voltage- and time-dependent reductions in postshock R-wave amplitude and that integrated bipolar systems appear to be more affected than true bipolar systems in this regard. This may be a consequence of lead design, specifically the distance of the distal defibrillating coil from the rate-sensing cathode, with the distal defibrillating coil used as the rate-sensing anode.[63] Rather than a uniform reduction of intracardiac EGM amplitude, other investigations have demonstrated that a rapid and repetitive change in amplitude occurred after a shock, resulting in failure to redetect VF.[44,59,60] The problem appeared to improve when the spacing between the rate-sensing tip of the electrode and the distal coil was increased.[44,59,62] The redetection malfunction was never seen in patients with integrated bipolar systems when the distal coil-to-ring electrode distance was greater than 6 mm.[59] It should be noted that the distal end of the coil is separated from the tip electrode by only 6 mm in the Guidant Endotak C 60 series, by 12 mm in the Endotak 70 series, and by 11 mm in the Ventritex RV-1101 lead.

The sensing algorithm in specific devices may also contribute to sensing problems, with marked variation of signal amplitude leading to inappropriate redetection of sinus rhythm in a device with an amplifier that has automatic gain control.[60] The amplifier may be adjusted for optimal sensing of the predominate signal amplitude, and these large-amplitude signals may prevent the automatic gain amplifier from increasing the gain to a setting necessary to detect the low-amplitude signals, leading to signal dropout and failure to redetect VF after an unsuccessful first shock. Newer leads and detection algorithms may now reduce the chance of postshock undersensing.

Early Detection of Sensing Problems

The newer generation of ICDs may have several features designed to detect and alert the patient and physician to early lead problems. The use of short interval counters to monitor nonphysiologic R-R intervals (<140 msec) may be useful in detecting potential sensing problems.[64] Most devices now have not only the ability to measure pacing lead impedance at the time of device interrogation but also the capability to measure impedance between the shocking portions of the system, including coils and the can in some instances. In one study involving measurement of ring-to-coil impedance, a decrease in the impedance predicted early lead failures in some patients.[64] Some devices have "patient alerts," which emit a tone from the device when high or low pacing or shock impedances are detected. For example, the device may be programmed to emit the alert when the pacing lead impedance is less than 200 or greater than 3000 ohms (Ω). Alerts may also be programmed to be emitted if defibrillation lead impedance values are out of range (e.g., <20 or >200 Ω). With the availability of stored and real-time intracardiac EGMs, "noise" may also be visualized in the setting of an insulation defect or lead fracture. Even if patients do not receive ICD therapy, outpatient ICD follow-up remains crucial, particularly to allow early detection of lead problems, which is now feasible with the availability of this noninvasive monitoring at the time of interrogation.

Endocardial ICD Lead Composition

The lead is composed of connectors, conductors, insulation, electrodes, and a fixation mechanism. Important considerations in the design and manufacturing of endocardial defibrillation leads include biocompatibility, biostability, and durability. Lead materials must be inert and durable in the body. There are strict U.S. Food and Drug Administration (FDA) requirements with respect to testing for biocompatibility for devices that will have contact with the blood. Current leads use technology that has already undergone rigorous biocompatibility testing. Although the choices for materials may be somewhat limited, based on previous long-term testing in the body, design issues vary among manufacturers. The insulation and the conductors of the lead are major design factors influencing reliability.

Insulation

The most frequently used insulation materials are silicone, polyurethane, and fluoropolymers. Electrical insulation is used between conductors within the lead, as well as between the conductors and the body. Design considerations include tensile strength, wear, dielectric properties, and stiffness.[42]

Silicone is also often used as an insulator for endocardial leads, because it is biostable, biocompatible, flexible, inert, and a good insulator.[42] The main advantage of silicone rubber is provision of an insulation barrier without any known long-term degradation.[65] The main disadvantage of silicone is its softness, which makes it prone to damage during implantation.[41] Another disadvantage is that it may abrade when in constant contact with the edge of a pulse generator, with eventual wear through the insulation to the conductor.[41,65] Silicone has a poor resistance to tearing, and the tear strength of polyurethane is much better in comparison. To counteract this deficiency of silicone, leads made with silicone tend to have a larger diameter than those made of polyurethane, due to the lower tensile strength of the former.[42,65] In addition, silicone leads have a higher coefficient of friction.[42] Therefore, two silicone leads tend to stick together, leading to difficulty passing one lead next to another, which could be a potential technical concern when implantation involves passing more than one lead through a single venous stick. Coatings have been useful in this regard, allowing more easy passage of silicone leads side-by-side.[65]

Polyurethane is also frequently used as an insulation material for defibrillation and pacemaker leads. It has a high tear strength, high elasticity, and a low coefficient of friction.[42] Because of the higher tear strength, the leads can be made with a smaller diameter. Because of the lower coefficient of friction, two polyurethane leads placed next to each other remain slippery and are potentially easier to manipulate through a single venous access site.[65] The main disadvantages of polyurethane include environmental stress cracking and metal ion oxidation, which affect reliability.[41] Concerns have been raised about polyurethane in some pacemaker leads, with reports of a high rate of failure due to insulation problems.[66] There may be an increased long-term failure rate (with degradation factors for Pellathane 80A), including metal ion oxidation and environmental stress cracking. In contrast, another polyurethane (55D) is stiffer and has a good reliability.[65] Coating of the conductor with a fluoropolymer layer can prevent metal oxidation, but fluoropolymer use may be limited by the stiffness of the material.[41]

Based on these concerns, the current ICD leads use several insulating materials. The insulating body is usually made of silicone. This is supplemented by an outside polyurethane layer to reduce the coefficient of friction and reduce scar formation while protecting against abrasion.[41] Because the polyurethane is not in direct contact with the conductors, metal ion oxidation is avoided.[41] The polyurethane is also pretreated in an inert gas for protection against environmental stress cracking. The conductors are often insulated with an extra layer of a fluoropolymer, resulting in a complex lead that has coiled and straight conductors inside several insulation layers.[41] Figure 4-3 depicts a schematic cross-section of defibrillation leads and cross-sectional photographs of leads from three different manufacturers, demonstrating the various thicknesses

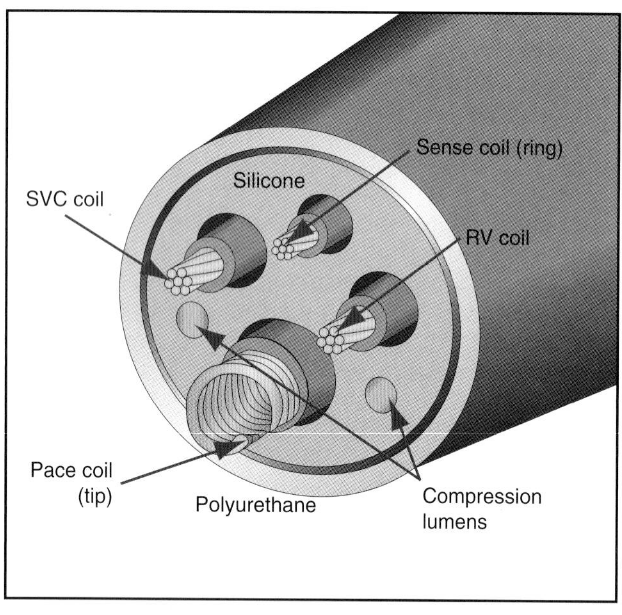

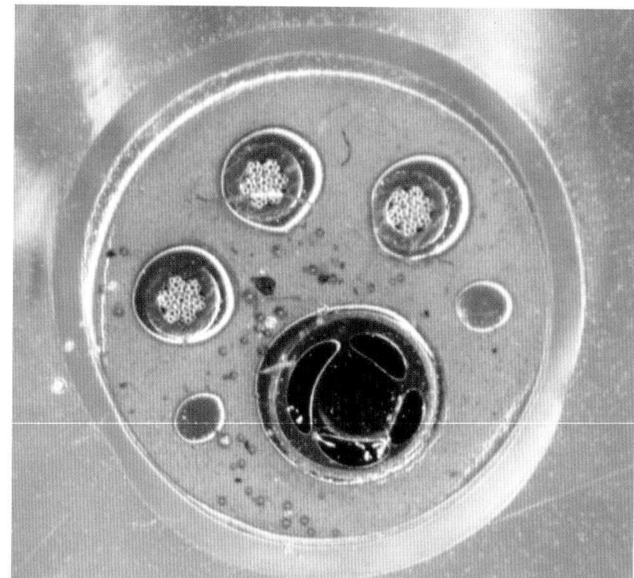

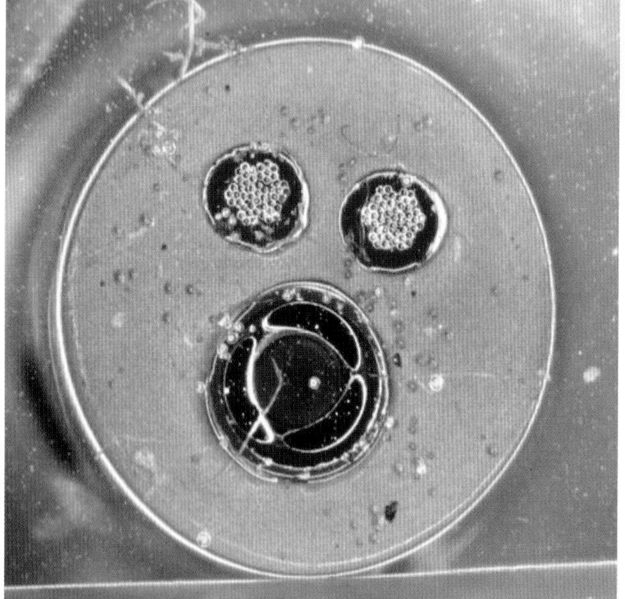

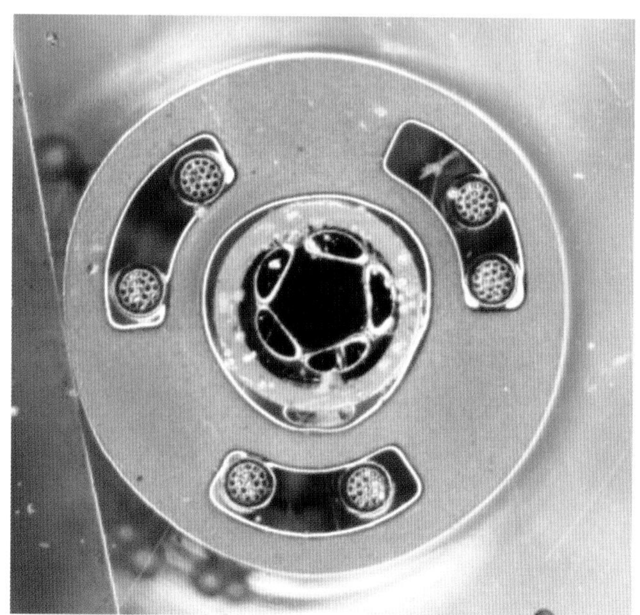

Figure 4-3. Defibrillation lead insulation. ***A,*** *Schematic view of a Medtronic lead that uses both silicone as an inner insulation and polyurethane as an outer insulation. (Courtesy of Medtronic, Inc., Minneapolis, Minn.) Cross-sectional views show the insulation in a Guidant Endotak Reliance lead (**B**), a Medtronic Sprint Quattro Secure lead (**C**), and a St. Jude Riata lead (**D**). (Cross-sectional views courtesy of Guidant, Boston Scientific, Natick, Mass.).*

of insulation incorporating both silicone and polyurethane insulation materials.

Defibrillation Conductors and Electrodes

To deliver current efficiently, conductors with a low resistance must be used to minimize voltage losses. This has been achieved by using a composite wire of Drawn Brazed Strand (DBS) or Drawn Filled Tube (DFT) construction (Fig. 4-4). These wires combine low-resistance metals such as silver with stainless steel, MP35N (an alloy of nickel, cobalt, chromium, and molybdenum), titanium, or another high-strength metal to obtain a strong and low-resistance wire.[65] Figure 4-4A demonstrates a DBS wire conductor, which is composed of six wires combined with a single strand of a relatively soft and low-resistance metal. The strands are drawn through a series of dies to force the silver between and around the other strands, resulting in a single composite strand of wire having low resistance with high strength and fatigue life.[65] DFT wire is made from a high-strength shell such as stainless steel, MP35N, or titanium that is filled with a low-resistance metal and drawn through a series of dies in a similar manner to make a composite. A third outer layer, such as platinum or platinum-iridium, may also be added (see Fig. 4-4B). The wires can then be formed into coils (for DFT) or twisted into cables (for DSB wire).[65] Coils can provide a lumen for passage of a stylet.

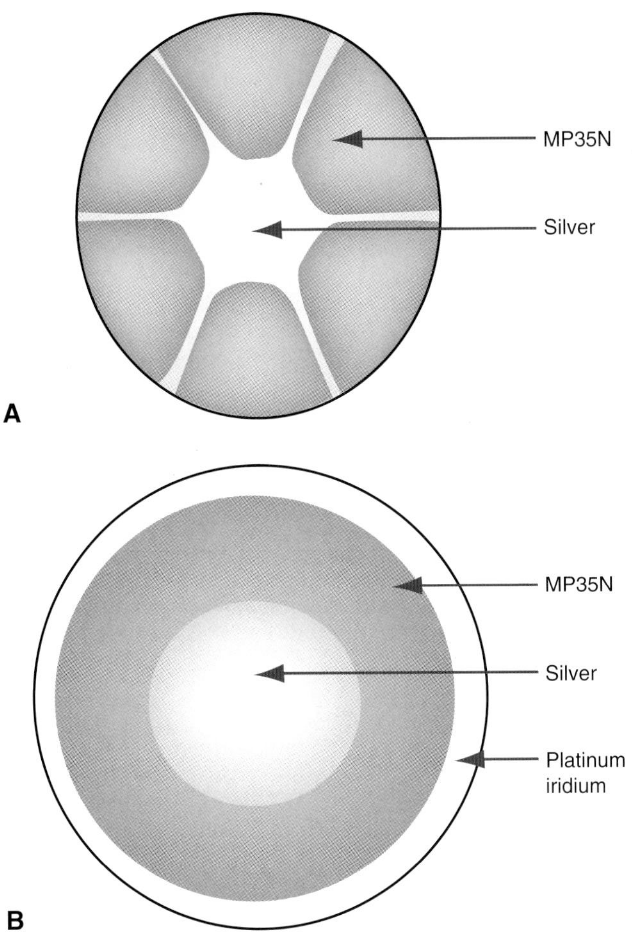

*Figure 4-4. Defibrillator conductors. **A,** Cross-sectional photograph of Drawn Brazed Strand (DBS) composite wire showing six stainless steel strands and silver in the center, between the strands, and on the outer surface. The low-resistance silver is typically drawn between and around the high-strength MP35N, an alloy of nickel, cobalt, chromium, and molybdenum. **B,** Cross-sectional photograph of Drawn Filled Tube (DFT) composite wire showing the low-resistance inner conductor (silver), high-strength shell (MP35N), and metal outer layer (platinum-iridium) for use as an electrode. (From Nelson RS, Gilman BL, Shapland JE, Lehmann MH: Leads for the ICD. In Kroll MW, Lehmann MH [eds]: Implantable Cardioverter Defibrillator Therapy. Norwell, Mass., Kluwer Academic Publishers, 1996, with permission.)*

The coils can be arranged concentrically or in parallel to combine the wires needed for defibrillation, sensing, and pacing (Fig. 4-5). Parallel pathways are now more frequently used. This prevents the lead body from becoming too large or stiff.[65]

Although the electrode design for defibrillation leads varies among manufacturers, the choice for materials is somewhat standard. The material used for the electrodes is limited to high-conducting, low-corrosion, materials that are biocompatible and biostable.[42] Most electrodes are therefore composed of platinum, platinum alloy (such as platinum-iridium), or titanium.[42,65] Platinum is very resistant to corrosion in the body and is very conductive, with long-term reliability proved in pacemaker leads composed of platinum-iridium composition.[42] Investigation of other metals for use in defibrillation systems, such as carbon electrodes, has been promising.[67,68]

When a charge is passed through an electrode, complex electrochemical reactions occur at the metal-solution interface. The area of transition between the electrode and the insulation results in a phenomenon called an "edge effect," with high current densities at the edge of the electrode.[42] These high current densities may result in less efficient energy delivery and possible tissue damage near the electrode.[43] It is also possible that high current densities located near the sensing tip of the electrode may result in postshock sensing abnormalities, with a reduction of postshock R-wave amplitude in integrated bipolar sensing systems,

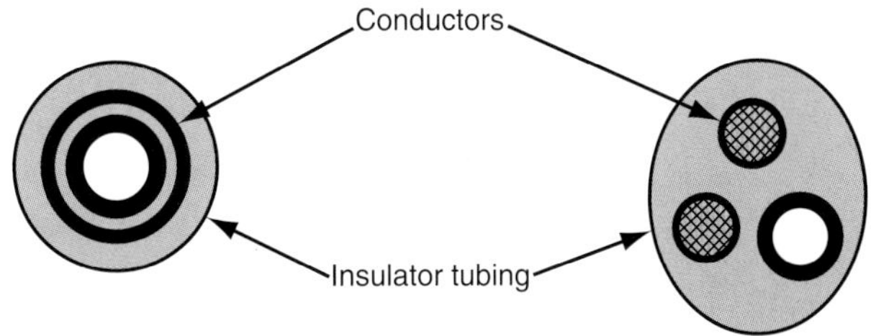

Figure 4-5. Potential lead construction configurations. The left figure demonstrates a concentric two-conductor configuration, and the right figure demonstrates the parallel construction of two Drawn Brazed Strand (DBS) cables and a Drawn Filled Tube (DFT) coil. The DFT coil contains a center lumen for a stylet. (From Nelson RS, Gilman BL, Shapland JE, Lehmann MH: Leads for the ICD. In Kroll MW, Lehmann MH [eds]: Implantable Cardioverter Defibrillator Therapy. Norwell, Mass., Kluwer Academic Publishers, 1996, with permission.)

as previously discussed. These EGM changes and abnormalities in sensing were seen with the Endotak C lead, which has a close proximity between the distal defibrillation coil and the sense/pace tip (6 mm); and may be minimized if the defibrillation electrode is moved further away from the sensing tip.[44,58,59]

Electrode designs are unique and vary among manufacturers, including single-wire coil, multiwire braid, and ribbon designs. Lead design and material limitations include issues regarding impedance, fatigue life, stiffness, and corrosion, which are common concerns for all manufacturers.[42] It may be argued that one of the most important concerns is fatigue performance, because the lead should be built to outlive the pulse generator, withstanding multiple generator replacements throughout the years.[42]

For defibrillation, conductors with low resistance and high fatigue life are required. In addition to fatigue, sources of physical stress on the conductor of the defibrillation lead include the potential for compression or fracture at the junction of the clavicle and first rib and kinking of the lead within the defibrillator pocket.[69,70] Leads may pass through the subclavius muscle or costoclavicular ligament before entering the subclavian vein, leading to soft tissue entrapment and potential lead damage related to repeated flexure at these potential points of entrapment. Autopsy data have confirmed the significant increase in pressures generated at the costoclavicular angle for medial subclavian puncture, compared with a more lateral percutaneous subclavian puncture or, especially, a cephalic vein cutdown approach.[69] The cephalic vein approach may be preferable for lead longevity by minimizing the chance of lead fracture from subclavian crush injury.

High-voltage defibrillation systems may have impedance measures ranging from 20 to less than 100 Ω. Epicardial patches demonstrate impedance values at the lower end of this range, whereas transvenous systems are usually in the 40- to 80-Ω range. If impedance values are outside this range, a problem with the lead system is likely.[65]

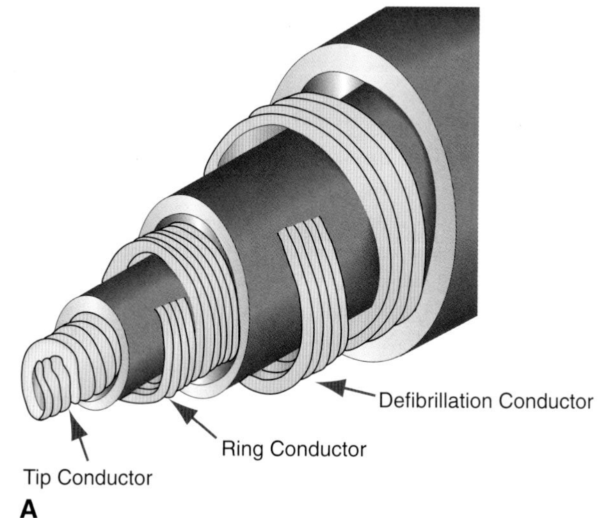

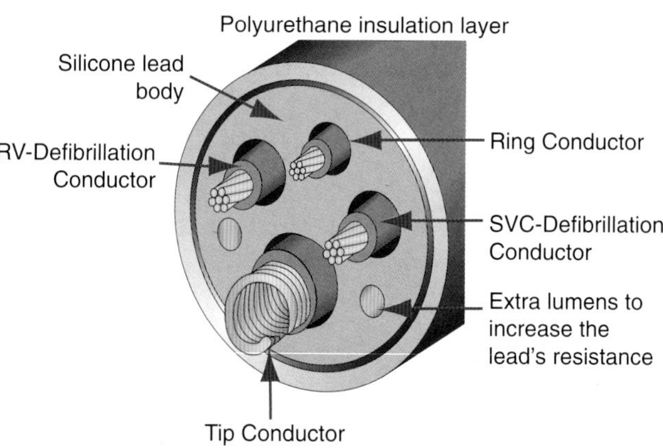

Figure 4-6. ICD lead design. ***A,*** *Coaxial lead construction demonstrating a single-coil defibrillation lead with true bipolar sensing and pacing. The tip and ring conductors are responsible for sensing and pacing, and the defibrillation conductor is responsible for conducting current for defibrillation.* ***B,*** *Multilumen lead construction of a dual-coil defibrillation lead with true bipolar sensing and pacing. The tip and ring conductor are responsible for sensing and pacing, whereas the right ventricular (RV) defibrillation conductor is the conductor for the distal defibrillation coil in the RV and the superior vena cava (SVC) defibrillation conductor is the proximal defibrillation coil in the SVC. (From Gradaus R, Breithardt G, Bocker D: ICD leads: Design and chronic dysfunctions. PACE 26:649-657, 2003, with permission.)*

ICD Lead Design

ICD leads may have a coaxial construction or multilumen lead construction (Fig. 4-6). The coaxial construction is characterized by a coiled conductor with an outside insulation layer, both of which are surrounded by another conductor. The lead body has a layered design with an insulating layer between each of the conductors. During implantation, a stylet is inserted through a channel inside the innermost conductor. Examples of leads with this type of construction include the earlier Transvene Medtronic leads and the TVL Ventritex (St. Jude) leads.[41]

In the mid 1990s, the multilumen construction became favored (see Fig. 4-6B). This design has coiled and straight conductors running in parallel through a single insulating body, with an additional insulating layer covering each conductor. This design also includes extra lumens inside the multilumen body, to increase the lead's resistance to compression. During implantation, a stylet is inserted through a coiled conductor to the lead tip. Examples of this type of design include the Endotak 60, Endotak 70, Endotak-DSP, Endurance, and Reliance leads from Guidant, Medtronic's Sprint lead family, and the St. Jude Medical/Ventritex SPL and Riata lead families. The advantage of multilumen leads is the smaller size, because more conductors can fit into a smaller lead.[41] The details regarding design of specific leads from different manufacturers are summarized in Table 4-1.

Connectors/Terminators

The connectors must ensure that the lead is secured to the pulse generator. In endocardial systems, one of the connectors has a lumen through which a stylet is passed, enabling placement of the lead in the heart. The current standard for connectors includes a DF-1 connection for the high-voltage portion and an IS-1 connection (6-mm termination) for the pace/sense portion of the lead. This allows different leads to be exchanged with various pulse generators made by different manufacturers. The standard IS-1 and DF-1 terminals are shown in Figure 4-7.

In more recent years, there has been a call for standardization of the connection between the pacemaker or ICD lead and the pulse generator. Incompatibility of the lead connector with the pulse generator requires the use of adapters, which may reduce reliability of the system. The design of the connector should contribute to the overall reliability of the lead and pulse generator system.[71] The lead connector must fit into the pulse generator header and be secured by set-screws. During implantation, the pin of the lead connector should extend past the inner connector block and should be clearly visualized by the implanting physician before the set-screw is tightened.

At the present time, the proximal end of the lead is composed of three connections, which are inserted separately into the header of pulse generator. A new connector, the IS-4 terminal, may soon replace the current standard in defibrillation systems. This single connector includes both defibrillation and pacing elements and is connected to the pulse generator as a single unit, reducing the bulk of leads in the generator pocket. One potential disadvantage of this new system may be the inability to easily "cap" the proximal defibrillation coil, if a high DFT is noted and alternative configurations for DFT testing are necessary. However, it is anticipated that future pulse generators will incorporate the noninvasive capability of "eliminating" the proximal coil from the defibrillation system, obviating this potential problem.

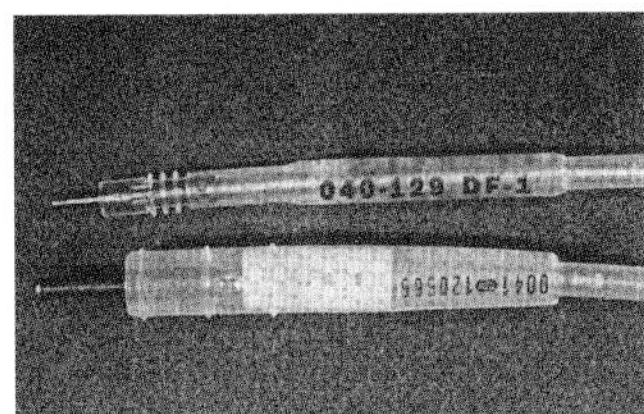

Figure 4-7. Connectors. A comparison of the DF-1 defibrillation terminal (top) and the standard 6-mm connector (IS-1 pace/sense connector). (From Accorti PR: Leads technology. In Singer I [ed]: Implantable Cardioverter Defibrillator. Armonk, NY, Futura, 1994, with permission.)

Adapters and Extenders

The adapter, when used, is an important part of the defibrillation system, because failure of the adapter will result in failure of the defibrillator system. An example of one adapter previously used to connect two unipolar 6-mm pace/sense electrodes to a VS-1 bipolar connector is shown in Figure 4-8. Adapters (and extenders) may be needed to mate replacement pulse generators to preexisting leads or to tie electrode combinations (e.g., SVC and subcutaneous patch) together to work as a common electrode.[65] Extenders may be used if the additional length is needed to match the two components. These adapters and extenders must be reliable, with performance characteristics similar to those present in leads. Older adapters used medical adhesive to seal the set-screw, whereas the newer adapters use a set-screw seal, similar to that present in the pulse generator connection.[65]

Endocardial Lead Fixation Mechanisms

Similar to pacemaker leads, the distal tip of the defibrillation lead is fixed within the heart. Defibrillation leads have either passive fixation tines or active fixation screws to ensure lead stability (Fig. 4-9). The main disadvantage of tined leads is the inability to position the lead in multiple locations, which usually limits positioning to the RV apex. For active fixation leads, a helical screw mechanism is usually present, and these leads have the advantage of offering positioning in areas other than the RV apex. In addition, active-fixation leads may offer some advantage with respect to easier removal at a later date with extraction systems, compared with passive leads.[42]

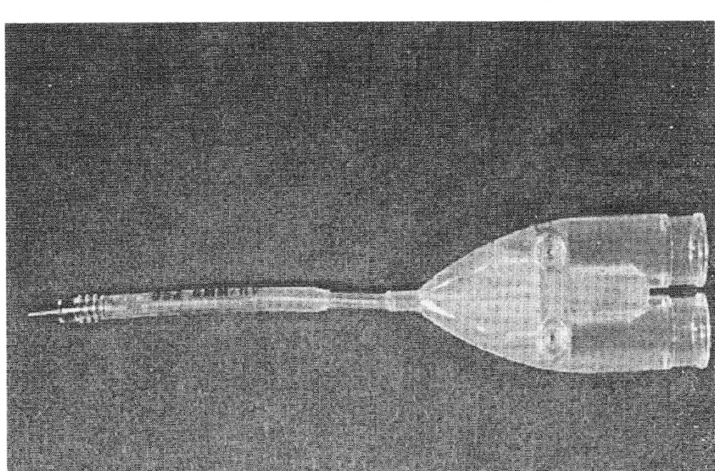

Figure 4-8. Lead adapter. A 6-mm unipolar to VS-1 bipolar adapter was necessary for some ICD generator replacements. (From Accorti PR: Leads technology. In Singer I [ed]: Implantable Cardioverter Defibrillator. Armonk, NY, Futura, 1994, with permission.)

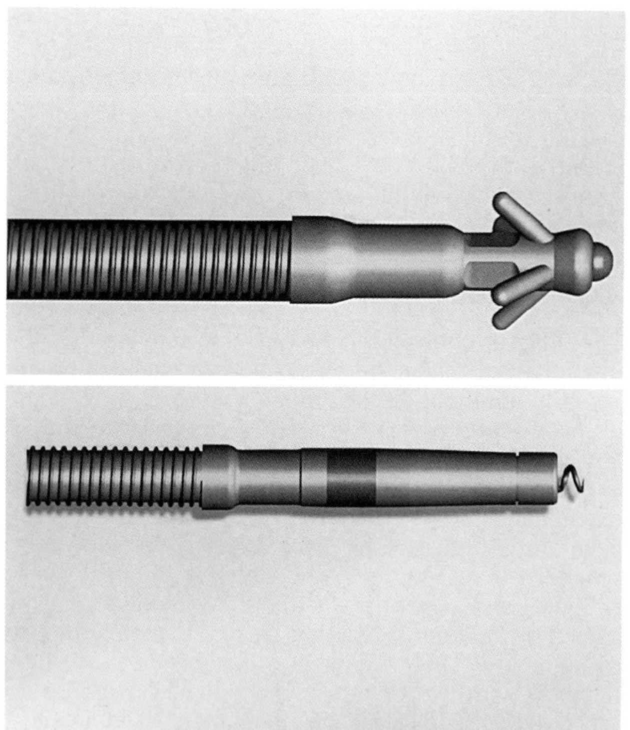

Figure 4-9. Fixation mechanisms for transvenous ICD leads. The top figure illustrates a passive fixation or tined lead system. The bottom figure shows an active fixation or screw-in lead system. (Courtesy of Medtronic, Inc., Minneapolis, Minn.)

Leads should also be anchored at the venous puncture site to reduce migration or lead dislodgment. Suture sleeves should be used to avoid placing sutures directly on the lead itself, because this could lead to insulation problems. In addition, care should be taken to avoid excessive kinking of the leads in the pocket, to reduce insulation problems or connector fracture.[42]

Dual-Chamber Sensing and Pacing

As with permanent pacing systems, atrial leads can be implanted separately for sensing and pacing capabilities in currently available dual-chamber ICD systems. The use of an atrial lead may give additional diagnostic information, in addition to the ability to sense and pace in the atrium. The availability of enhanced diagnostic features that discriminate supraventricular tachyarrhythmias from ventricular tachyarrhythmias may also be useful to reduce the risk of inappropriate ICD therapies.[72] There is no longer the need to implant a separate permanent pacemaker system in patients who require dual-chamber pacing.

Similar to VDD leads used in bradycardia pacing, a prototype for a single-pass dual-chamber passive fixation lead was developed and tested for dual-chamber ICDs.[73] The prototype was a modification of the Guidant/CPI Endotak DSP lead, which used an additional atrial ring electrode. In most instances, adequate sensing and pacing parameters were demonstrated in sinus rhythm, with reasonable sensing also noted during atrial arrhythmias.[73] This single-pass lead might offer an alternative for dual-chamber ICD systems in the future.

Extrathoracic Defibrillation Electrodes

Subcutaneous Patch

Subcutaneous patches have been used with endocardial defibrillation lead systems to lower the DFT. The patch is typically implanted subcutaneously in the axillary region of the left chest, although other positions have been investigated. The axillary location of the subcutaneous patch was notably more efficacious than apical or pectoral position in reducing DFT in one study.[74] In another study, Bardy and colleagues[33] found a potential DFT advantage when the patch was positioned in a high chest position beneath the left clavicle, compared with lower axillary placement.

Subcutaneous Array

Use of the subcutaneous array lead (CPI/Guidant) has demonstrated improved defibrillation performance using three electrodes placed subcutaneously.[75] This lead is composed of three electrically common multifilar lead elements joined to a silicone yoke that attaches to a lead body and ends in a single 6.1-mm titanium terminal pin. Each lead element is 25 mm long, has a 6F diameter, and is tunneled subcutaneously in the left lateral chest using a tear-away sheath. The pin is connected to the proximal coil of the endocardial lead using a Y adapter. The addition of the subcutaneous array significantly lowered the monophasic DFT by an average of 10 joules in one study.[75] The chest radiographic appearance of the array is shown in Figure 4-10.

Other Defibrillator Electrode Configurations

Successful implantation of a nonthoracotomy system using a coronary sinus (CS) defibrillation lead has also been demonstrated.[76] A 7F monopolar defibrillation lead (Medtronic Model 6881) with a 50-mm coil electrode having a 90-mm^2 surface area was used for insertion in the CS or SVC. Successful and safe implantation of a transvenous lead system that incorporates leads in the RV apex, SVC, and CS, or a combination of leads in the RV apex, CS, and subcutaneous patch, have been shown to have adequate DFTs at implantation.[76] Despite the absence of any mechanism for active or passive fixation on this CS lead, dislodgment did not appear to be a significant issue in one study.[76] Defibrillation using the CS defibrillation coil does not appear to have complications related to CS perforation. Pathol-

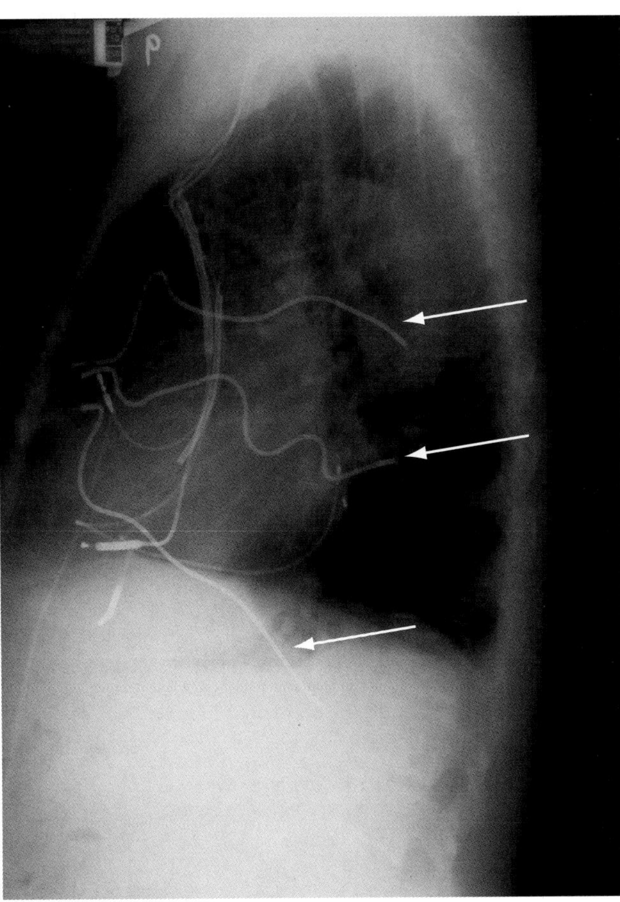

Figure 4-10. Subcutaneous array. Lateral chest radiograph demonstrates the appearance of the Guidant subcutaneous array. Three finger-like projections (arrows) are noted, extending out from a yolk, with each electrode tunneled subcutaneously along the lateral chest.

ogy data suggested no evidence of damage to the circumflex artery, and, although there may have been some evidence for thrombus formation in the CS, complete occlusion was not seen.[76] Overall, implantation of a nonthoracotomy system that incorporates a CS lead was found to be safe and effective.

Lead Determinants of Defibrillation Threshold

Endocardial defibrillation lead systems were investigated very early in the development of ICDs,[28,29] but efficacy of defibrillation was limited when using monophasic devices in conjunction with endocardial defibrillation. An increase in DFT during follow-up was also seen with monophasic devices.[77] Reversal of lead polarity may result in a significant reduction in DFT.[78] Improvements in device technology, such as the use of biphasic waveforms[37,79-85] and active can technology[86,87] have resulted in a decrease in DFT, improved efficacy, and increased ease of nonthoracotomy system implantation. These developments in technology have virtually eliminated the need for implantation of a thoracotomy system.

Although advancements in device technology have clearly made a major impact on reduction of defibrillation requirements, the performance of the ICD system still depends in part on lead performance. Engineering tradeoffs are made in designing leads to optimize performance characteristics such as lead handling, fatigue life, size, and optimal therapy delivery.[88] Lead design characteristics, including conductor materials, wire thickness, lead body diameter, and lead construction technique, determine efficacy of the lead. The goal is to produce a lead that has low DFTs through a more uniform current distribution to the heart or a higher efficiency in delivering current. As shock distribution becomes nonuniform, DFTs increase. If a lead is less efficient, DFTs will also be higher, because a portion of the energy intended for delivery to the heart is lost near the surface of the defibrillation electrodes or inside the lead itself.[88] Four basic design rules should be followed to enhance energy delivery through the lead:[88] (1) minimize electrode pullback, (2) deliver current to the apex, (3) minimize energy loss within the lead, and (4) use of efficient electrodes.

Electrode Pullback

The term "pullback" is used to describe the distance between the lower active edge of the RV defibrillation electrode and the RV apex. In dedicated bipolar leads, sensing and pacing are performed through a pair of electrodes, separate from the defibrillation electrode (Fig. 4-11). Sensing is accomplished by using an electrode at the tip of the lead and a ring electrode 1 to 2 cm proximal from the tip. The shocking electrode is proximal to these dedicated sensing and pacing electrodes. One ICD lead system that uses dedicated bipolar sensing is the Medtronic Model 6936 lead. In contrast, in an integrated bipolar lead, rate sensing is accomplished between the catheter tip electrode and the RV defibrillation electrode. Therefore, the RV defibrillation electrode is typically closer to the tip of the lead, because the separate rate sensing ring is not required (see Fig. 4-11). Most of the current leads now incorporate this integrated bipolar strategy, including the CPI (Guidant) endocardial leads (60, 70, and 90 series models), the Telectronics lead (Model 040-068), the Intermedics (Guidant) lead (Model 497-05), and the St. Jude/Ventritex lead (Model RV-1101 and Riata i series). As noted in Table 4-2, endocardial leads with dedicated bipolar sensing must use a larger pullback (2.5 cm) to provide space for the sensing ring between the tip of the lead and the RV defibrillation coil. Even these small differences in pullback may be important with respect to the DFT.

Location of Current Delivery

The goal in lead design is to deliver current as deep into the apex of the heart as possible. Not only does electrode pullback play a role, but the current distribution as it leaves the RV electrode is also important.[88] Design characteristics can affect the distribution of current from the

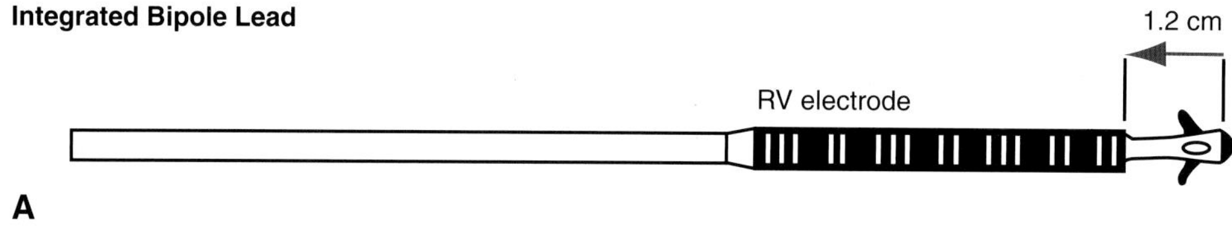

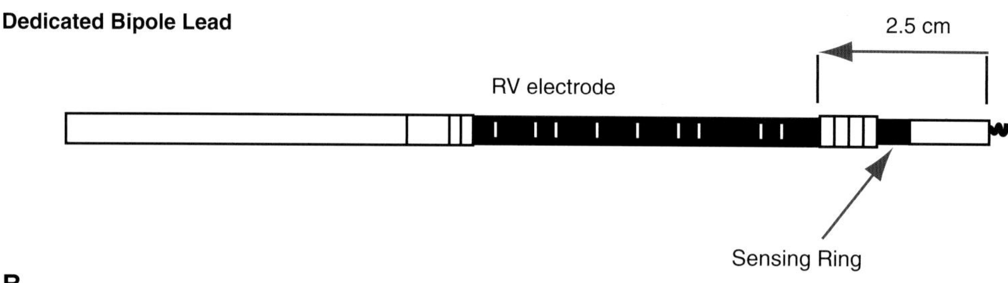

Figure 4-11. Design pullback. "Pullback" refers to the distance between the lower active edge of the right ventricular (RV) defibrillation electrode and the RV apex. Design pullback should be minimized for lower defibrillation thresholds. The diagrams show the impact of sensing methods on catheter design and the magnitude of the RV electrode pullback. ***A,*** *Leads using integrated bipolar sensing/pacing methods (from the tip to the RV defibrillation electrode) typically have a shorter pullback distance (e.g., 1.2 cm here).* ***B,*** *Leads using dedicated bipolar sensing/pacing methods have larger distances from the catheter tip to the active RV defibrillation electrode due to the presence of the sensing ring (e.g., 2.5 cm here). (From Lang DJ, Heil JE, Hahn SJ, et al: Implantable cardioverter defibrillator lead technology: Improved performance and lower defibrillation thresholds. PACE 18:548-559, 1995, with permission.)*

TABLE 4-2. **Design Pullback of Right Ventricular Electrode**

Manufacturer	Model Numbers	Design Pullback (cm)
CPI/Guidant	60 series 70 series 90 series	0.5 1.2 1.2
Medtronic	Transvene series Sprint series	2.5 1.2
Telectronics	040-068 and 040-069	1.8
Ventritex	TVL series Riata series Riata i series	1.1 1.7 1.1

RV defibrillation electrode; such characteristics include the termination method, by which the internal lead conductor is connected to the RV electrode, and the resistance of the material from which the RV electrode is composed. Almost all endocardial defibrillation leads are constructed with the proximal termination technique, which connects the high-voltage conductor inside the lead body to the proximal end of the RV defibrillation electrode (Fig. 4-12). To optimize current distribution from the RV defibrillation electrode, defibrillation leads (e.g., Guidant/CPI 60 and 70 series) also incorporate an internal shunting wire to connect the proximal and distal ends of the RV electrode, making the delivery of current balanced from both ends (see Fig. 4-12A). If the conductor terminates in the distal end, the defibrillation current is strongest at the terminal point (see Fig. 4-12C).

Energy Loss within the Lead

To design an efficient lead, energy loss inside the lead during defibrillation should be minimized.[88] During shock delivery, some energy is dissipated as heat inside the conductors of the lead and never reaches the heart. A lead with high performance would be one with a low-resistance lead body. This reduces energy loss inside the lead by minimizing the resistance of the conductors in the lead, enhancing efficiency and resulting in a lower DFT.[88]

Efficiency of Electrodes

An additional goal for designing a high-performance lead is to use large, efficient electrodes. If the surface area of the defibrillation electrodes is too small, the ability to deliver current to the patient is limited.[88] An inefficient lead has a high resistance. Energy may be lost within a few centimeters of the electrode-heart interface. Design factors that influence electrode efficiency include the electrode material, the electrode's dimensions (length and diameter), and the construction technique.[88] Increasing the length of the electrode may improve efficiency, but the length of the RV defib-

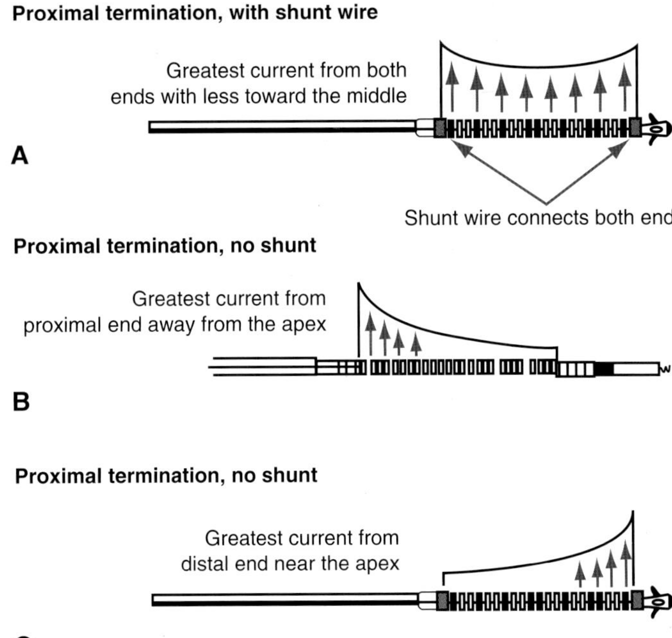

Figure 4-12. Distribution of defibrillation current along the defibrillation electrode for three methods of terminating the lead conductor to the right ventricular electrode. The distribution of current from the electrode to the heart may influence the defibrillation threshold for the particular lead. **A,** The lead with the conductor terminated at the proximal end of the defibrillation electrode and a shunt wire connecting the proximal and distal electrode ends results in current delivery that is balanced from both ends of the electrode. **B,** A lead with the conductor terminated at the proximal end of the electrode and no shunt wire results in current delivery that is highest near the termination point at the proximal end and weakest at the distal end, near the apex of the heart. **C,** A lead with the conductor terminated at the distal end only, with no shunt wire, results in a defibrillation current that is strongest at the termination point at the distal end, near the cardiac apex. (From Lang DJ, Heil JE, Hahn SJ, et al: Implantable cardioverter defibrillator lead technology: Improved performance and lower defibrillation thresholds. PACE 18:548-559, 1995, with permission.)

rillation electrode is limited due to the presence of the tricuspid valve and potential damage. The SVC electrode does not have this limitation, and there appears to be a minimum SVC surface area needed to maintain defibrillation performance.[88]

Lead Coating

Iridium oxide (IROX) can be used as a coating on ICD leads and results in a reduction in shock-induced polarization, compared with an otherwise identical uncoated lead.[89,90] It has been demonstrated in animal studies that nonthoracotomy leads with an IROX coating (Model 497-20 Sulzer Intermedics, now owned by Guidant) exhibit lower DFTs than do uncoated leads (Model 497-06, Sulzer Intermedics/Guidant).[89,90] IROX coating applied to the surface of electrodes increases the microscopic surface area and reduces “crowding” of ions at the electrode-tissue interface by spreading out the charge, reducing the biphasic DFT.[89] However, these results could not be reproduced in humans.[91] Increasing the electrically active surface of an endocardial tripolar ICD lead by iridium coating (Biotronik, SPS 75 UP/BP) did not lead to a significant reduction in DFT in one study.[91] The discrepancy between this study and previous animal data may be due to the small number of patients evaluated or limitations with DFT testing in humans in this investigation.

Implantation Techniques

Access

The implantation technique for insertion of transvenous defibrillation systems is similar to that of permanent pacing systems. To avoid risks of pneumothorax and crush injury at the costochondral junction, the cephalic vein cutdown approach is preferred. However, a small vein may not accommodate more than one lead. Puncture of the subclavian or axillary vein may be performed by Seldinger’s technique. The lead is introduced into the heart with use of a peel-away sheath.

Sensing and Pacing Parameters

Once the lead is positioned in the correct chamber, sensing and pacing parameters are evaluated. An R-wave amplitude of 5 mV or larger is typically sought. A correlation between R-wave amplitude in sinus rhythm and amplitude during ventricular tachyarrhythmias has been identified.[51] A pacing threshold of 1.5 V or less measured at 0.5 msec is also sought for active fixation leads, with a threshold of less than 1 V at 0.5 msec for passive leads. Evaluation for diaphragmatic pacing with a maximum output in the RV (10 V) should also be performed. The pacing impedance at 5 V should measure between 400 to 1200 Ω. An insulation break is suspected if the impedance is lower or coil fracture if the impedance is higher. Alternatively, poor tissue contact or perforation may lead to abnormally low or high pacing impedance values.

Shock Impedance/Test Shocks

A shock system integrity test is also routinely performed after the lead is connected to the pulse generator, to ensure appropriate connections. Previously, sedation was required to deliver a 1- to 2-J high-voltage synchronized test shock. The current generation of ICDs has a built-in integrity test, in which 10 V is delivered through various components of the high-voltage system, resulting in a measured impedance. The shocking or high-voltage impedance should measure 35 to 70 Ω. It should be noted that lead impedance values are manufacturer specific, so awareness of the appropriate values for the specific system is needed. After appropriate connections are confirmed, a DFT evaluation is performed. If the DFT is too high, configurations of the implanted system can be altered, or a subcutaneous patch or array lead may be added.

Complications of Nonthoracotomy ICD Leads

Types of complications and the frequency of nonthoracotomy lead complications are outlined in Tables 4-3 and 4-4. The frequency of mechanical lead problems, such as lead dislodgment, perforation, subclavian crush, insulation breaks, or loose set-screws, has been reported

TABLE 4-3. Nonthoracotomy Lead Complications

I. Sensing lead problems
   - Lead fracture
   - Insulation break
   - Dislodgment
   - Poor connection to header

II. Endocardial defibrillation lead problem
   - Lead fracture
   - Insulation break
   - Dislodgment

III. Subcutaneous patch problem
   - Lead fracture
   - Crimping
   - Lead migration

IV. Adapter problems
   - Poor connection
   - Adapter failure

TABLE 4-4. Nonthoracotomy ICD Complication Rate*

Authors and Year (Ref. No.)	Complication Rate (%)	Lead Complication Detected (mo)
Tullo et al. 1990 (106)**	56	13 ± 9
Mattke et al. 1995 (20)	5.0	14 ± 10
Korte et al. 1995 (19)	10.1	13 ± 6
Stambler et al. 1994 (22)	7.7	~13 ± 7
Schwartzman et al. 1995 (100)	15.9	17 ± 12
Lawton et al. 1996 (115)	2.8	15 ± 11
Mehta et al. 1998 (98)	13.0	32
Grimm et al. 1999 (96)	4.0	21 ± 15
Dorwarth et al. 2003 (99)	12.0	48 ± 31
Kron et al. 2001 (93)	4.3	27 ± 13
Degeratu et al. 2000 (94)†		29 ± 15
CPI, Endotak	4.3	
CPI BT-10	17.8	
Ellenbogen et al. 2003 (64)‡	19	69 ± 8
Gold et al. 1997 (95)	2.1	634 pt-yr (65% > 6 mo)
Brooks et al. 1993 (101)	10	12 ± 8
Raviele et al. 1995 (103)	7.3	14 ± 10
Bardy et al. 1993 (33)	20	11 ± 7
Thakur et al. 1995 (39)	0	15 ± 6
Jones et al. 1995 (104)	15	21 ± 10

*Specific lead complications typically include endocardial lead dislodgment, right ventricular perforation, insulation break, electrode/conductor fracture, connector failure or loose set-screw, adapter failure, patch migration, crinkled patch, and venous thrombosis.

**High complication rates with old CPI Endotak C and SQ patch.

†Compares abdominal implantation sites using integrated bipolar CPI Endotak lead ($N = 140$) for sensing and defibrillation with CPI BT-10 ($N = 107$) sensing lead, both tunneled to the abdomen.

‡High failure rate refers to Medtronic 6936 coaxial, true bipolar, polyurethane active-fixation lead.

to be 2% to 4% in some large series.[92-96] A higher complication rate of 7% to 16% involving endocardial leads or patches has also been reported in other studies.[18,22,97-105] An exceptionally high complication rate of 56% was seen in a single study in which Endotak C leads were used in conjunction with subcutaneous patch electrodes.[106] The reported incidence of lead-related complications varies widely and may be related to patient selection, lead used, mode of implantation, and particularly duration of follow-up. The risk of failure tended to increase over time[93,99] and appeared to be particularly high during the first year after reoperation for battery depletion.[99] Problems appeared to be more frequent when adapters between the pulse generator and the lead or extenders were used.[22] Other factors potentially related to lead failure may include lead design, venous approach, type of insulation, abdominal location, and size of the pulse generator.

Routine screening radiography appears to have a limited role in the diagnosis of lead complications after the first postimplantation month, and most complications are diagnosed clinically.[97] It should also be noted that insulation failure may be associated with normal values of impedance, sensing, and pacing threshold at the time when lead failure is diagnosed.[99] One study suggested that visible insulation breaks on silicone sensing leads may be repaired with the use of silicone sleeves and adhesive, demonstrating that there was no difference in subsequent lead survival in patients with lead repair compared with those who underwent insertion of new sensing leads.[107]

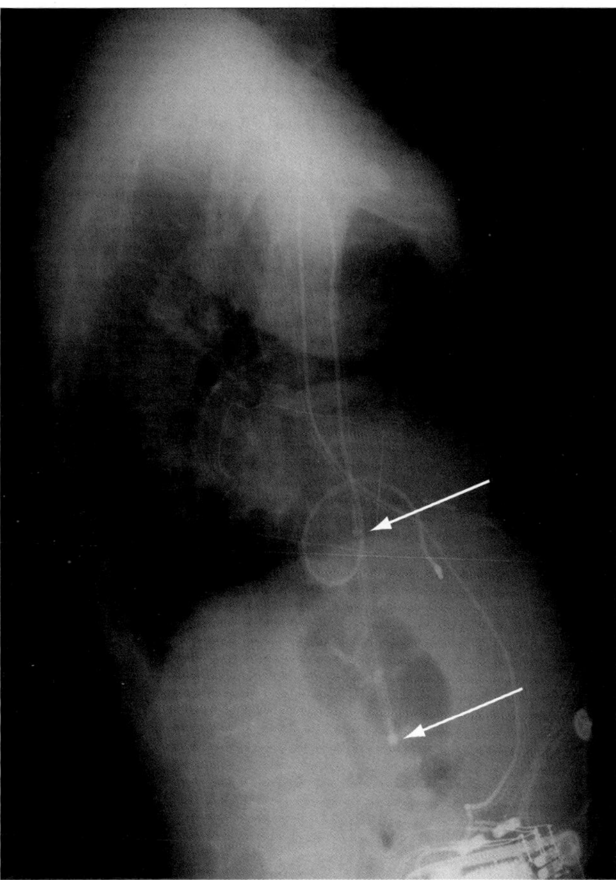

Figure 4-13. Radiograph demonstrating superior vena cava (SVC) lead dislodgment. The tip of the SVC and the proximal portion of the SVC coil are marked by arrows. The lead has dislodged into the inferior vena cava in this "hybrid" nonthoracotomy lead system, with a right ventricular (RV) sensing lead and subcutaneous patch also visualized on this radiograph.

Acute Lead Failures

Acute lead failures may involve lead dislodgment or high stimulation thresholds, often requiring surgical intervention to correct the problem. A higher dislodgment rate may be seen with transvenous systems that use a separate SVC coil, because these defibrillation coils do not incorporate a fixation mechanism.[19] Dislodgment of the SVC lead may lead to an increase in the DFT[19] or may be asymptomatic and detectable by routine radiography (Fig. 4-13). Earlier investigations reported lead migration or dislodgment occurring in 10% of cases.[33] The incidence of lead dislodgment in patients who underwent implantation later in the study improved (3%), reflecting improved implantation technique and more experience with anchoring methods.[33] A high incidence of lead dislodgment may be seen with defibrillation leads placed in the CS.[33,108,109] Lead dislodgment may be asymptomatic, or it may result in oversensing or undersensing, as well as ineffective defibrillation.

Acute lead failure may also be caused by cardiac perforation. In addition to symptoms of pain, which is often pleuritic, patients with perforation may develop high pacing thresholds or noncapture, undersensing, diaphragmatic pacing, or tamponade. Oversensing of noise may be seen with loose set-screws or loose connectors[103] and may occur early after implantation. These problems can be easily treated and corrected, if detected early.

Chronic Lead Failures

Chronic lead failure is most often a result of insulation defects or fractured conductors. Signs and symptoms of lead failure are outlined in Table 4-5. Conductor fractures can lead to an increase in pacing impedance, intermittent loss of sensing or pacing, complete failure to sense or pace, or oversensing. Insulation defects can also lead to oversensing or undersensing problems. If the insulation defect involves the outer insulation and the stress point is located at an extracardiac site, stimulation of the pectoral muscle or diaphragm may also be seen. If the inner insulation is also involved, intermittent or complete loss of pacing may also occur.[41] Due to similar clinical manifestations in some cases of lead and insulation problems, the exact cause of lead failure may not always be apparent, particularly before surgical intervention.

Polyurethane leads with a coaxial design are susceptible to inner insulation failure and shorts between the conductors, often caused by metal ion oxidation.[41] Silicone-coated leads with multilumen design are prone to erosions of the insulation, particularly in abdominal locations with larger devices. Friction of the lead due

TABLE 4-5. Symptoms and Signs of Lead Problems

I. Sensing lead problems
   A. Oversensing (most common) due to detection of noise
      Inappropriate shocks
      Inappropriate aborted shocks
      Inhibition of pacing
      Change in pacing impedance
      Prolonged oversensing immediately after shock delivery
   B. Undersensing in SR
   C. Undersensing or nonsensing of VT/VF, with failure to deliver therapy
   D. Elevated pacing thresholds or noncapture
II. Defibrillation lead problems
   A. Ineffective defibrillation
   B. Change in high voltage impedance
   C. Sudden death

to contact with the ICD generator itself can result in abrasion of the insulation.[41] Continuous or forceful traction of the lead may also result in thinning of the insulation and potential tearing of the insulation,[41] emphasizing the importance of correct lead handling and the potential contribution of certain daily strenuous activities on lead reliability. Lead compression under the clavicle may result in conductor failure as well as damage to the insulation. A lateral or cephalic vein access approach may help reduce subclavian crush injuries or lead fractures.[41,110,111]

Data regarding the long-term reliability of multilumen defibrillator leads are limited, because these leads have been in use for less than 10 years. Previous reports regarding polyurethane coaxial leads with subpectoral ICDs showed an increase in failure rates after 4 to 5 years.[99,112] The Medtronic Transvene single-coil, coaxial polyurethane leads (model numbers 6936/6966) comprised 54% of ICD lead failures detected by the multicenter registry published by Hauser and colleagues.[112] The mean time to failure for these leads was 4.8 ± 2.1 years.[112] Lead survival analysis of the Medtronic polyurethane coaxial 6963 lead revealed a cumulative failure probability of 37% at a mean follow-up of 69 months in another study.[64] Insulation defects, pace/sense conductor fractures, or high-voltage coil fracture may be involved in the structural failure of these particular leads.[112] (The middle insulation layer of the 6936 lead is 80A polyurethane, which is the same polyurethane used to manufacture Medtronic 4004 and 4012 leads, and insulation degradation presumably occurs over time in high-stress areas.)

The incidence of lead failure increased over time with Medtronic coaxial polyurethane leads,[99,112,64] with the risk of lead failure being particularly high during the first year after generator replacement due to battery depletion in one study.[99]

One study compared the incidence of structural failure in a dedicated bipolar sensing lead (CPI BT-10) with that in an integrated lead (CPI Endotak) in 247 patients undergoing abdominal ICD implantation.[94] Over a mean follow-up of 29 ± 15 months, there were 17.8% lead failures with the BT-10 lead (occurring 261 to 1505 days after implantation) but only 4.3% with the Endotak lead (occurring 410 to 1211 days after implantation; $P < .01$).[94] Lead failure was believed to be related to insulation defects in all cases, with the problem occurring in the proximal portion of the lead within the generator pocket in all but one case. The BT-10 lead is a standard silicone lead that is almost identical to those used in permanent pacing systems for years. Lead failure with the BT-10 lead continued to occur as long as 4 years after implantation, suggesting that the problem with lead failure may be progressive and that higher failure rates may be seen with longer follow-up. It should be noted that all implants were abdominal, and the tunneling technique was the same for both leads. One possible reason for lead failure is the mechanical force of the heavy pulse generator against a nonreinforced lead, resulting in insulation wear; a lower rate of problems is seen with the more reinforced, larger Endotak lead.

Abdominal ICD implantations appear to have a higher associated lead failure rate, and the rate increases progressively from the time of implantation.[41,113] Mechanical stresses placed on the lead from tunneling to the abdomen and wear on the lead from a heavy pulse generator may contribute to insulation problems.[62,94,98] Other studies also demonstrated a higher failure rate in abdominal devices, with lead complications occurring in 15% to 16% of abdominal devices[100,104] and 4% of pectoral devices,[96] with higher rates of lead complications in devices with dual-chamber pacing capabilities, during a mean follow-up period of only 21 months.

The first-generation endocardial defibrillation lead system (CPI Endotak-C), often used in conjunction with a subcutaneous patch, was associated with an extremely high rate of complications.[106] During a follow-up period of only 51 ± 36 weeks, 56% (5 of 9) patients developed lead-related complications. These complications included conductor fractures, leading to sudden death in one patient. Patch electrode conductor fractures were also observed. Because of an unacceptable incidence of lead fracture in the earlier versions of endocardial leads,[106] the high-energy conductor was changed from a coiled wire to Teflon-coated braided flexible cable, which appeared to solve this problem.[114]

The management of sensing lead failure in patients with Endotak integrated bipolar endocardial defibrillator leads remains controversial. In one study, a new sensing lead alone was placed in 9 of 10 patients, assuming the "independent" function of the sensing component in the circuit based on lead design.[115] However, failure of defibrillation occurred in one patient 3 years later, raising concern about the long-term reliability of defibrillation once a sensing lead problem is diagnosed in patients with integrated bipolar leads.

Sensing lead complications may manifest with inappropriate shock therapy or aborted shocks due to sensing of noise, complete loss of pacing, or asynchronous pacing with undersensing during sinus rhythm, or they may be initially asymptomatic and detected at the time of generator replacement or chest radiography.[19,20,22,52,64,92,94,98,99,103,106,110-112,115] In extreme cases, complete loss of sensing may lead to nondetection of ventricular arrhythmias, requiring resuscitation and external defibrillation or sudden cardiac death.[20,106] One study also described prolonged oversensing of electrical noise immediately after shock delivery.[64] Defects with the defibrillation portion of the lead may result in failure to defibrillate ventricular arrhythmias.[99] The true incidence of endocardial defibrillation lead failure will require continued follow-up, because more lead problems are likely to be detected over time. This emphasizes the need for continued close follow-up of patients with endocardial systems.

Lead failure may result from conductor and/or insulation damage just beyond the stiff terminal ring of the IS-1 rate-sensing terminal connector of one particular Guidant Endotak lead (DSP model 0125).[116] Lead failure occurred in 3.5% of patients who underwent pectoral ICD implantation using a submuscular approach, after a mean follow-up of only 16 ± 11 months.[116] This was related to extension of the metal terminal ring beyond the header when a smaller pulse generator was used, creating a rigid fulcrum in this area. Flexing of the lead in this region could create sufficient stress to disrupt insulation or conductors at this point. Lead problems manifested with asymptomatic oversensing or inappropriate shocks in these patients. This lead was placed on advisory with a technical memorandum reporting the potential problems with the long IS-1 terminal pin connector in 1999.

Other complications of endocardial lead systems include infections, with a reported incidence of up to 5%.[20,34,93,97,98,100-102,108,117,118] Subclavian venous thrombosis or obstruction remains a potential long-term problem, particularly in patients who have multiple leads in place. Complications may also be seen with subcutaneous patches, including fractures, dislodgment, crinkling, erosion, and hematomas.[19,20,30,100,101,109,117,118] Fractures of patch leads may be initially asymptomatic and may be detectable by chest radiography.[19]

Despite improvements in ICD lead technology, it is anticipated that the lead failure rate will progressively increase over time. As more patients have ICDs implanted for primary as well as secondary prevention, the need for lead removal will probably also increase over time.

Reporting of Lead Failure

At present, there are inadequate reporting mechanisms to identify lead failure in the ICD industry. Device manufacturers currently provide product performance reports that are designed to supply information to physicians regarding device system survivability and to alert clinicians to particular devices that may be failing at a higher rate than expected, perhaps warranting closer follow-up. Returned product analysis (RPA) provides a means for manufacturers to examine products that have been explanted and returned to the manufacturer to determine the mechanism of failure. However, most leads that have failed are not explanted, so reports of failure will be grossly underestimated by this reporting mechanism.[119] An ongoing prospective study, the Tachyarrhythmia Chronic System Study (TCSS) is being conducted at 11 medical centers in the United States, and specific follow-up findings and reports are required at 6-month intervals. Centers provide information regarding clinical observations related to the lead, as well as clinical responses, including whether the lead was explanted, abandoned, or replaced, or whether reprogramming was performed to rectify the problem. This study does not require return of the lead for analysis to be counted as a "failing lead." The proportion of nonperforming leads detected by the RPA was 0.5%, compared with 2.2% in the TCSS ($P < .001$).[119] The prospective follow-up of chronic leads by the TCSS, which includes identification of clinical performance at the time of follow-up, provides a more accurate basis for determination of ICD lead failure than the RPA reports do.

Biventricular Pacing: Cardiac Resynchronization Therapy Leads

Multiple clinical trials have demonstrated the benefit of CRT in the treatment of patients with congestive heart failure, LV dysfunction, and a wide QRS, with and without ICD backup.[120-127] Hemodynamics and heart failure symptoms are improved with CRT in patients with class III or IV heart failure and an ejection fraction of 35% or less. The branches of the CS are typically visualized through CS angiography, with contrast dye injected through a balloon-tipped catheter or specially designed guiding sheath (Fig. 4-14). LV leads are placed through the CS into venous branches to pace the LV and resynchronize myocardial contraction. The site of LV pacing may play an important role in the efficacy of CRT.[128,129] Therefore, it is important to be able to direct these leads into specific branches. This can be accomplished by using leads that have a variety of shapes, which can be altered by use of a stylet-driven lead system. An example of a Medtronic unipolar LV lead with a preshaped distal curve to increase stability in the CS is shown in Figure 4-15. An over-the-wire lead system can be used.[130,131] When the stylet is inserted into the distal tip of the lead, the lead is straightened. As the stylet is withdrawn, the lead assumes its shape with a curve on the end. Some leads have a combination of stylet-driven and over-the-wire capabilities. Table 4-6 outlines the currently available LV leads. It should be noted that LV leads may have a higher rate of lead dislodgment than RV or RA leads. This is probably related to the absence of any "active" fixation mechanism. Some LV leads do have "tines" (Fig. 4-16), but the absence of trabeculation within the venous branches may still limit stability of these leads, compared with RV leads. The size of the venous branch may also affect lead stability. In addition to 7F and 6F leads, some LV leads are now available in 4F to accommodate smaller venous branches. More recently

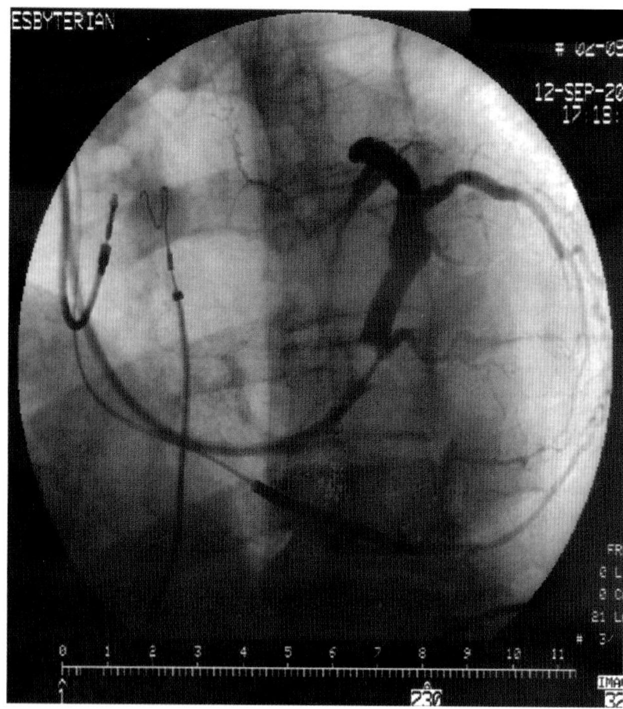

Figure 4-14. Coronary sinus angiography. Contrast dye is injected through a balloon-tipped catheter to enable visualization of the venous branches of the coronary sinus, to help guide left ventricular lead placement.

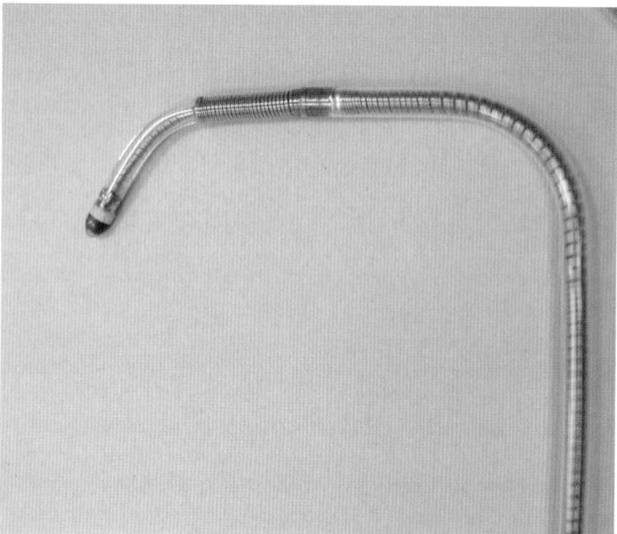

Figure 4-15. Over-the-wire left ventricular lead (Attain OTW 4194). The preshaped distal curve is constructed to increase stability. When a stylet is introduced into the lead, the lead is straightened. As the stylet is withdrawn, the lead assumes its shape with the curve on the end. (Courtesy of Medtronic, Inc., Minneapolis, Minn.)

designed leads assume a variety of shapes after the stylet is removed, which may help with lead stability. Figure 4-16 demonstrates the variety of different lead shapes available from various manufacturers.

In addition to lead dislodgment, another complication of LV lead placement is diaphragmatic pacing. This

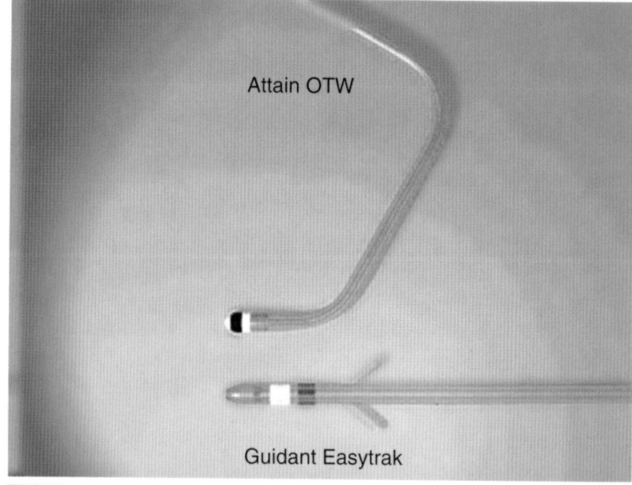

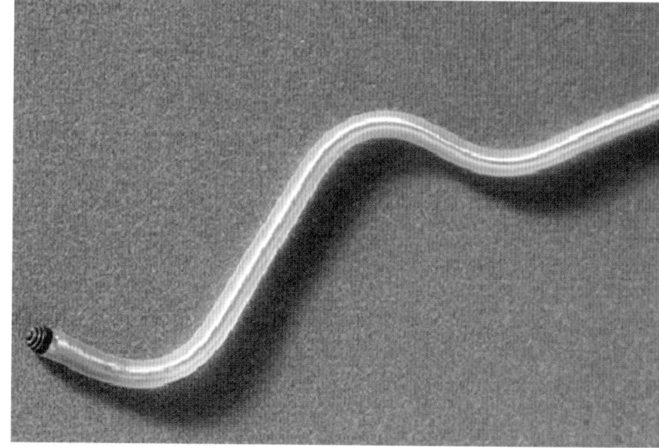

*Figure 4-16. Comparison of left ventricular leads from various manufacturers. **A,** The Medtronic Attain over-the-wire lead is shown on top of the Guidant Easytrak lead. This particular Guidant lead is straight and has "tines" for stability. **B,** The St. Jude Aescula 1055K lead has a multicurved or "S" shape to help with lead stability in the coronary sinus. (Courtesy of Medtronic, Inc., Minneapolis, Minn.)*

is related to stimulation of the phrenic nerve, which may be in close proximity to the more lateral venous branches. The newer, smaller-caliber leads tend to have lower pacing thresholds, and therefore the pacing output may be minimized, often reducing or eliminating diaphragmatic pacing. The initial LV leads were unipolar, with one electrode on the distal tip of the lead. Pacing occurred between the LV tip and the RV coil. This sometimes resulted in anodal capture. Newer LV lead technology includes bipolar LV pacing capabilities, with a more proximal ring electrode on the LV lead. This allows multiple pacing configurations, which can be programmed noninvasively through the newer ICDs with CRT capabilities, leaving additional options in an attempt to reduce diaphragmatic pacing or improve LV pacing thresholds (Fig. 4-17).

Because some earlier ICDs did not have the availability of separate RV sensing, or an external adapter was used to connect RV and LV leads for pacing, the sensing circuit included both RV and LV EGMs. This could lead to "double-counting" of the RV and LV EGMs, with inappropriate shock delivery for sinus

TABLE 4-6. **Specifications of Left Ventricular Pacing Leads**

Features	Guidant Easy Trak 4510/11/12/13/37/38	Guidant Easy Trak 2 4515/17/18/20/42/43/44	Guidant Easy Trak 3 4522/24/25/27/48/49/50	Medtronic Attain 2187	Medtronic Attain 4193	Medtronic Attain 4194	St. Jude Aescula 1055 K	St. Jude QuickSite 1056 K
Delivery	OTW	OTW	OTW	Stylet	OTW and Stylet	OTW and Stylet	Stylet	OTW and Stylet
Proximal lead body diameter (F)	6	6	6.3	6	4	6.2	4.7	5
Distal lead body diameter (F)	4.8	5.4	5.7	—	5.4	5.4	4.5	5.6
Distal shape	Straight	Straight	Spiral	Curved	Angled	Angled	S curved	S curved
Fixation	Tines	Tines	3D spiral	Curved	Angled	Angled	Curved	Curved
Electrode configuration/polarity	Unipolar	Bipolar	Bipolar	Unipolar	Unipolar	Bipolar	Unipolar	Unipolar
Connector terminal	LV-1 (10-13) IS-1 (37, 38)	LV-1 (15-20) IS-1 (42-44)	LV-1 (22-27) IS-1 (48-50)	IS-1	IS-1	IS-1	IS-1	IS-1
Insulation	Silicone with poly	Silicone with eTFE/poly	Silicone with eTFE/poly	Poly 55D	Poly 55D	Poly 55D	Silicone	Silicone with poly
Tip seal	No	No	No	NA	Yes	Yes	NA	No
Steroid	Yes	Yes	Yes	No	Yes	Yes	No	Yes
Lead lengths (cm)	65, 72, 80, 90	65, 80, 90, 100	65, 80, 90, 100	58, 65, 75	78, 88, 103	78, 88	75	75, 86
Electrode surface area (mm^2)	3.5	4.2 (proximal) 4 (distal)	9 (proximal) 8.5 (distal)	5.8	5.8	5.8 (proximal) 38 (distal)	6.8	4.8
Electrode spacing (mm)	NA	11	11	NA	NA	11	NA	NA
Tip electrode material	Platinum iridium	Platinum iridium	Platinum iridium	Platinum	Platinum	Platinum	TiN	Pt/Ir,TiN

eTFE, expanded tetrafluoroethylene; NA, not applicable; OTW, over the wire; poly, polyurethane; Pt/Ir, platinum-iridium; TiN, titanium nitride fractal coating.

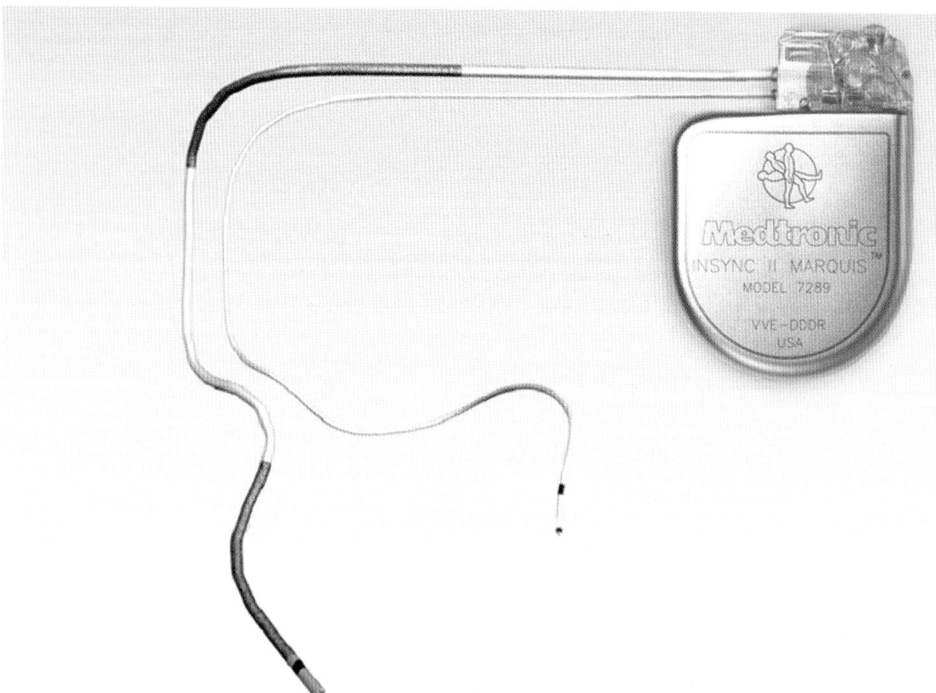

Figure 4-17. Bipolar left ventricular (LV) lead. The availability of the more proximal ring on the LV lead (Attain 4194) allows a variety of pacing options using enhanced programmability within the InSync pulse generator. Pacing may still be performed between the LV tip and the right ventricular coil. In addition, pacing can be performed from the LV tip to the LV ring. (Courtesy of Medtronic, Inc., Minneapolis, Minn.)

tachycardia or atrial arrhythmias (Fig. 4-18). With the current generation of CRT devices, separate RV sensing has eliminated this problem.

As noted earlier, steroid elution is frequently used with permanent pacing leads and with ICD leads. Steroid-eluting CS leads are also available. Satisfactory pacing and sensing parameters have been demonstrated acutely and during follow-up with these leads. The pacing threshold stabilized 2 weeks after implantation, and the sensing threshold remained stable from implantation to 4-month follow-up in these patients.[132]

Lead Follow-up

Regular outpatient follow-up is necessary to identify and anticipate potential problems with ICD leads. Routine follow-up every 3 to 4 months is recommended, with additional follow-up as needed if ICD therapy is delivered or if symptoms, such as syncope or presyncope, develop in the interim. Interrogation reveals pacing lead impedance values, and pacing threshold and sensing can be evaluated. Current devices also have the ability to perform a lead integrity test to measure the impedance within the high-voltage lead system. High-voltage values greater than 100 Ω suggest conductor fracture, and values lower than 20 Ω suggest insulation failure. In addition, after shock delivery, a large disparity between the programmed energy and the delivered energy suggests lead conductor failure.

The current generation of devices also has the availability of intracardiac EGMs that can be reviewed in real time to exclude evidence for "noise," which may be apparent in patients with insulation breaks or conductor fracture (Fig. 4-19). Chest radiographs, although they may play a limited role, can be used to exclude lead dislodgment, in the event that a significant change in sensing or pacing parameters is noted. Follow-up DFT testing may also be considered in patients who are found to have significant changes from baseline in certain lead parameters, such as sensing and impedance values, to confirm lead integrity and appropriate sensing of ventricular tachyarrhythmias.

Lead Extraction

With the increasing numbers of ICDs implanted, it is anticipated that there will be an increasing need for ICD lead extraction. ICD lead extraction may be more complex than pacemaker lead extraction, because ICD leads are bulkier and shocking electrodes may uncoil with extraction techniques.[133] There may also be a greater fibrotic reaction around the shocking coils, due to the irregularity of the coils, leaving more space for inflammation and fibrous tissue ingrowth (Fig. 4-20A). Effective lead extraction has been demonstrated with a variety of extraction systems, including intravascular traction techniques[133,134] and laser extraction.[134,135] Improvements in lead technology may also play a role in lead extraction. It is believed that the ease of extraction may be improved with new Gore (expanded polytetrafluoroethylene [ePTFE]–coated leads, due to the reduction in the degree of fibrous ingrowth (see Fig. 4-20B). This lead has a coating of ePTFE, an expanded polytetrafluoroethylene polymer, which is electrically inert without having any effect on DFTs. This coating prevents tissue ingrowth at the shocking electrode surfaces. This is evident by the absence of fibroblastic growth in the outer coil filars during preclinical studies (see Fig. 4-20B).

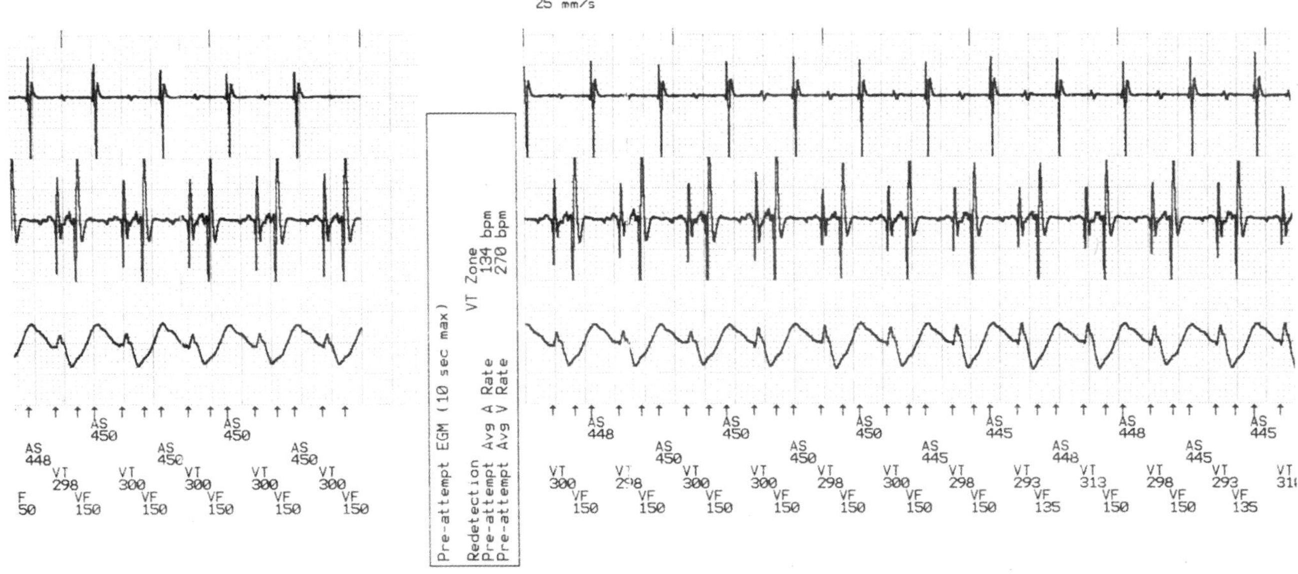

Figure 4-18. Double-counting of the ventricular EGM during sinus tachycardia. The earlier ICDs did not have separate right ventricular (RV) sensing, or an external adapter was sometimes used to connect the RV and left ventricular (LV) leads for pacing. This could lead to "double-counting" of the RV and LV EGMs, with inappropriate shock delivery for sinus tachycardia. With the current cardiac resynchronization therapy (CRT) devices, separate RV sensing is available, eliminating this problem. AS, atrial sensed event; VF, ventricular fibrillation zone sensed event; VT, ventricular tachycardia zone sensed event.

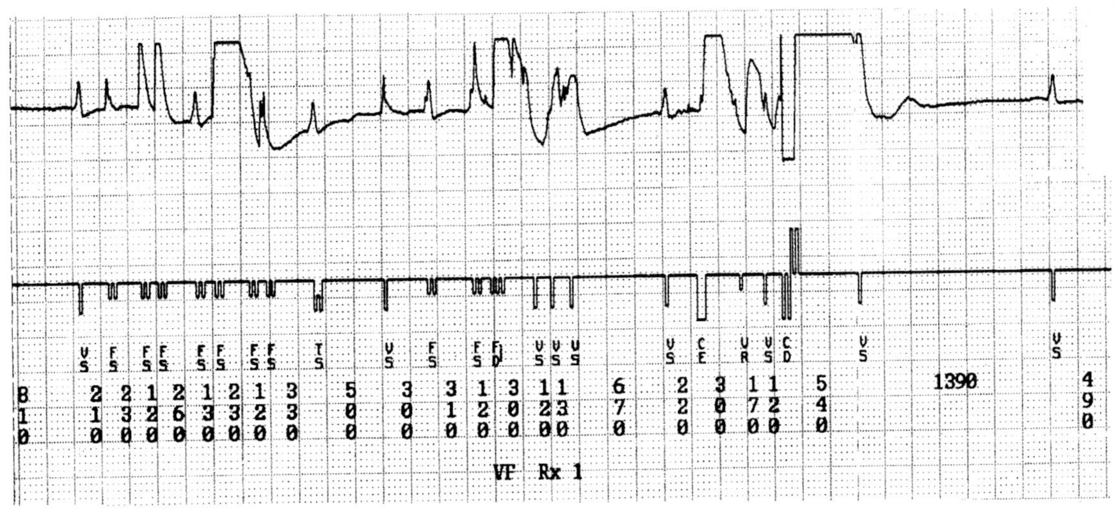

Figure 4-19. Intracardiac EGMs with electrical noise. Very short R-R intervals with electrical noise, shown on the stored intracardiac EGMs, demonstrate evidence for a lead integrity problem (e.g., lead fracture) resulting in ICD shock delivery. CD, charge delivered; CE, charge ended; FD, fibrillation detection; FS, fibrillation zone sensed event; TS, ventricular tachycardia zone sensed event; VS, ventricular sensed event.

Future Advances

Lead development has focused on new materials and designs, size reductions, improved steering and handling, and maintenance of long-term reliability. The IS-1 pacing and DF-1 shocking standards for the lead/device interface may be updated to an IS-4 terminal, to allow a reduction in connector/header size. Newer leads have high-impedance electrode technology, which may help to maximize the longevity of ICD generators.[136] Additional investigation should help determine ways to further increase the long-term reliability of endocardial leads, and newer designs may aid in easier lead extraction.

Summary

Over the past decade, ICDs have become the treatment of choice for patients with sustained ventricular

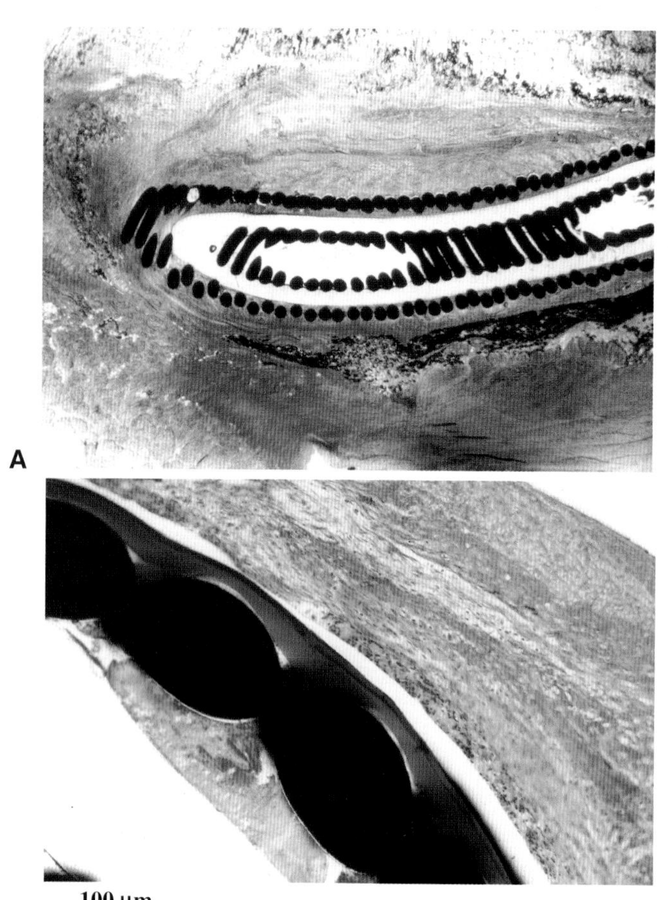

*Figure 4-20. Fibrous ingrowth and lead histology. **A,** There appears to be a marked fibrous reaction around the shocking coils of defibrillation leads. The irregularity of the shocking coils leaves more space for inflammation and fibrous tissue ingrowth. **B,** The new Gore-coated (ePTFE) defibrillation lead (Guidant) appears to have less fibrous ingrowth, which may enhance the ease of lead extraction. (Courtesy of Guidant, Boston Scientific, Natick, Mass.)*

tachyarrhythmias, in addition to playing a very important role in the primary prevention of sudden cardiac death. Technological advances in ICD therapy, including the development and refinement of ICD lead technology, have been largely responsible for these changes in the treatment of ventricular arrhythmias. However, lead failures are still an important complication of ICD therapy, despite technological advances. Insulation defects and fractured conductors or electrodes are common lead complications that have important clinical implications with respect to ICD efficacy as well as patient comfort and quality of life. The high failure rate of endocardial leads adds greatly to follow-up costs, including costs related to rehospitalization and reoperation. Although advancements have been made in the field of lead extraction, removal of any chronically implanted lead still carries a risk of significant complications. Additional advancements in lead technology are still needed, especially because many devices are implanted prophylactically, and more patients receiving devices are younger and will require multiple generator replacements throughout their lifetime.

One possible solution to this problem is development of a leadless ICD system. A prototype of this system (Cameron Health, Inc., San Clemente, Calif.) is currently undergoing investigational studies abroad and should be available for investigational use soon in the United States.[137] Alternatively, development of lead systems with better durability and greater resistance to damage is needed. This subchapter highlights the need for close clinical follow-up of all current ICD systems and the importance of follow-up performed by skilled personnel who have extensive training to ensure early detection of lead problems. This may affect not only patient quality of life but also long-term morbidity and mortality in the ICD population.

PERMANENT PACEMAKER LEADS: GENERAL CONCEPTS

Pacemaker lead development and advances in technology preceded the development of ICD leads by many years, setting the stage for current advances with the more complex ICD leads, which require defibrillation circuits in addition to bradycardia stimulation. Both permanent pacing systems and defibrillation lead systems need to offer reliable sensing and pacing.

A variety of factors influence lead performance and pacing threshold. In addition to lead and electrode factors, myocardial factors (e.g., fibrosis, infarction), drugs, and electrolytes can influence pacing thresholds. Lead and electrode factors to be considered include the time since the electrode was implanted, unipolar versus bipolar electrode, electrode surface area and shape, electrode material, lead insulation, lead fixation, and steroid elution. Lead and electrode factors are discussed in more detail in the following sections.

Lead Polarity: Unipolar Versus Bipolar Electrodes

According to strict definition, all pacemaker circuits are bipolar, and electrons flow from the cathode to the anode. In reference to pacemaker leads, the terms "unipolar" and "bipolar" refer to the number of electrodes that have contact within the heart.[138] Figure 4-21 demonstrates that a unipolar lead has one electrode at the tip of the lead (the cathode or negatively charged end), which is in contact with the heart muscle. The pulse generator serves as the anode (or positively charged end). Current flows from the negatively charged tip of the lead to the heart muscle and then to the positively charged pulse generator, completing the circuit. Figure 4-21 also demonstrates a bipolar pacemaker lead, in which both electrodes are in the heart. The tip electrode is the negatively charged cathode. A proximal electrode ring, which is a short distance from the tip electrode, serves as the positively charged anode.

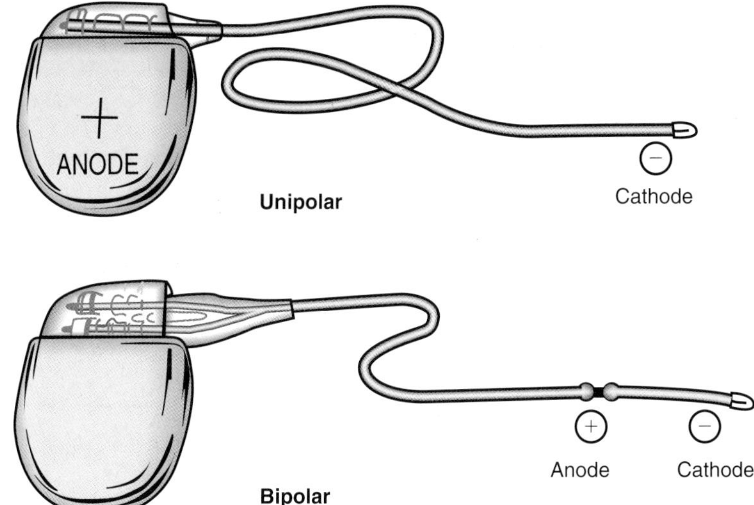

Figure 4-21. Unipolar and bipolar pacemaker leads. A unipolar lead has only one electrode, the cathode, at the tip of the lead, which lies within the heart. The anode lies on the surface of the pulse generator. A bipolar lead has both poles on the end of the lead, located close to each other. In this diagram, the cathode is at the tip of the lead, and the anode is slightly proximal to the cathode. (From Mond HG: Unipolar versus bipolar pacing: Poles apart. PACE 14:1411, 1991, with permission.)

There has been a continued trend toward use of bipolar pacing leads in the United States. Initially, bipolar leads were large, stiff, and difficult to implant. However, with advances in technology, bipolar leads are now smaller and easier to implant, similar to unipolar leads.[138] Both types of leads have demonstrated reliability with pacing and low pacing thresholds.[139] With modern pacemaker systems, similar ventricular EGM amplitudes have been seen with unipolar and bipolar sensing configurations.[139,140] Bipolar sensing has been shown to be similar to unipolar R-wave sensing during acute testing or at follow-up in most patients.[140]

The unipolar system has a larger interelectrode distance, which is the distance between the distal tip electrode and the pulse generator. For this reason, the unipolar sensing system will "see" more of the heart to detect the intracardiac signal. Unipolar systems are more susceptible to crosstalk, such as inappropriate sensing of the atrial stimulus artifact by the ventricular channel in a dual-chamber pacing system, which can result in the inhibition of the ventricular output. In a pacemaker-dependent patient, this could be life-threatening.[138] Crosstalk is less common with bipolar systems because of the smaller amplitude of the pacing stimulus.[138] Unipolar pacing systems are also more likely than bipolar systems to result in oversensing of skeletal muscle myopotentials, resulting in inhibition of pacing.[139-143] A bipolar lead, with its more closely spaced electrodes, is less likely to record far-field electrical signals than a unipolar lead. For example, a bipolar lead is less likely to oversense ventricular EGMs in the atrial channel. These sensed far-field electrical signals may result in inappropriate mode switching with current pacemaker algorithms. Because of the proximity of skeletal muscle to the pulse generator in a unipolar pacing system, skeletal muscle stimulation can occur during unipolar pacing, especially at high outputs, which is not typically seen with bipolar pacing systems.[138,139]

It is particularly important for ICD systems, which now have complete bradycardia sensing and pacing capabilities, to be bipolar. This minimizes inappropriate oversensing of far-field intracardiac or extracardiac signals in order to prevent inappropriate defibrillator therapy. Previously, a separate pacemaker was implanted with an ICD to provide bradycardia backup pacing. This required special testing at the time of implantation to evaluate for interactions between the ICD and the permanent pacemaker, to assure the absence of oversensing of pacemaker spikes, which could lead to the withholding of defibrillator therapy during VF. After delivery of an ICD shock, some permanent pacemaker pulse generators revert to unipolar pacing. Therefore, only dedicated bipolar pulse generators were recommended for use in the patient who has an implanted defibrillator.

A unipolar pacing stimulus artifact is much larger than a bipolar pacing artifact on surface electrocardiography, as shown in Figure 4-22. At times, the bipolar pacing stimulus may be difficult to see on the surface 12-lead ECG (see Fig. 4-22B). The bipolar pacing stimulus may be particularly difficult to see on transtelephonic monitoring performed for pacemaker follow-up, because usually only one surface lead recording is available, and the paced beats are sometimes difficult to distinguish from underlying conducted beats with a wide QRS.

Electrode Size

The earlier pacemaker lead electrodes had a large surface area in contact with the endocardium, resulting in a low pacing lead impedance and high current drain. The current was distributed over a large surface area, often resulting in a higher pacing threshold. With the goal of increasing pulse generator longevity, the cathodal surface area was reduced in size. As the cathodal surface area was reduced, higher current densities resulted, and a lower pacing threshold was obtained with a higher impedance (400-800 Ω) at the electrode-tissue interface.[144-146] Subsequently, leads with smaller distal electrodes (4-6 mm^2) and higher impedance values were developed.[147-148] Eventually, distal electrodes with very small surface areas (1.2 mm^2) and even higher impedance values (>1000 Ω) were developed.[149-151] (Reducing the size of the electrode results in an increased pacing impedance. A decrease in current is predicted, as predicted by Ohm's law, I = V/R.) These newer, high-impedance leads also had very low pacing thresholds and resulted in less current drain (Fig. 4-23),[149,150,152,153] which was expected to lead to better pacemaker generator longevity.

The improved pacemaker battery longevity with high-impedance leads, compared with standard impedance leads, has been confirmed.[152] Sensing characteristics of these high-impedance leads are similar to those of standard pacing leads.[149,152,153] A relatively low dislodgment rate of the small-surface (1.2 mm^2), high-impedance pacing lead was reported in one investigation in which careful lead positioning and securing techniques were used.[151]

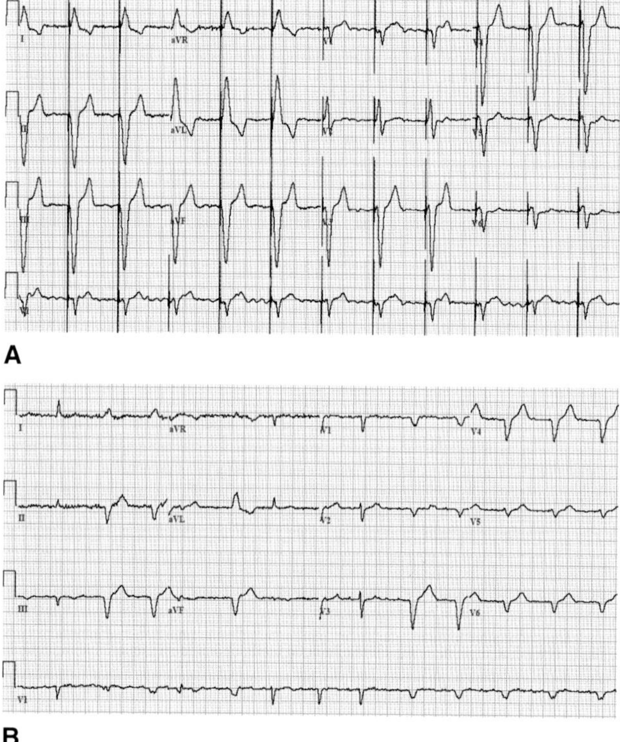

Figure 4-22. Unipolar and bipolar pacing stimuli. ***A,*** *A large pacing artifact is visualized on 12-lead electrocardiography in a unipolar pacing system.* ***B,*** *Small pacing artifacts are seen in bipolar pacing systems.*

Polarization

Polarization refers to the electrochemical impedance generated at the electrode-tissue interface. The ideal lead has a low polarization, in addition to a high electrode impedance and low resistance of the conductor.[154] The polarization effect increases as the electrode surface area is reduced. The accumulation of ions in the myocardium gives rise to an afterpotential, and this is recorded after a pacing stimulus.[154]

Polarization occurs at the electrode-myocardium interface due to the electrical current from the tip of the electrode to the tissue. After the stimulus is delivered, electrical signals are generated due to ion movement in the extracellular spaces around the electrodes. Certain pacemaker pulse generators have a function called AutoCapture, which allows automatic measurement of pacing thresholds. A low-amplitude pacing stimulus (just above the pacing threshold) is delivered while the device assesses whether the stimulus has captured the myocardium. By maintaining a stimulus amplitude that is only 0.5 to 0.7 V above threshold, the

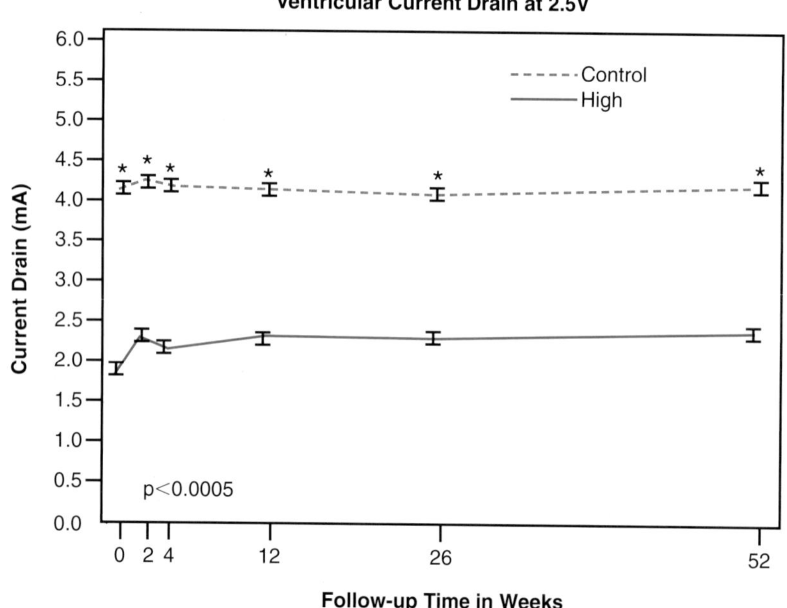

*Figure 4-23. Ventricular current drain at 2.5 V, comparing a high-impedance lead (solid line) with a standard lead (dashed line). A higher current drain was demonstrated at each follow-up visit up to 1 year in control leads having a larger (5.8 mm^2) distal electrode, compared with the high-impedance lead with a smaller (1.2 mm^2) distal electrode. *P < .001. (From Ellenbogen KA, Wood MA, Gilliagan DM, et al, and the Capsure Z Investigators: Steroid-eluting high-impedance pacing leads decrease short and long-term current drain: Results from a multicenter clinical trial. PACE 22:39-48, 1999, with permission.)*

longevity of the pacemaker generator is increased. To allow a reliable determination of capture, the device must be able to distinguish the myocardial depolarization-evoked response (ER) from the electrode polarization signal (PS). The polarization signal (PS) could be detected by the pacemaker and confused with myocardial depolarization, leading to pacing at an output below the true threshold. Autocapture is most reliable when low-polarization leads are used. Use of non–low-polarization leads can lead to incorrect threshold determination and noncapture,[155] which could be a serious problem in pacemaker-dependent patients. An additional schema that has been used to reduce the polarization artifact is to reduce the capacitance of the stimulus output capacitor, thereby improving the signal-to-noise ratio between the evoked response and the polarization artifact.

Electrode Design

Porous electrodes were designed to help reduce lead dislodgment and to reduce excessive threshold rises compared with standard smooth-tip electrodes. An electrode with a porous electrode tip, composed of sintered platinum-iridium fibers having a 20-μm diameter with hemispherical shape, was examined in dogs and compared with a standard solid electrode of similar size.[156] Porous electrodes, which have this complex surface structure, have low-polarization properties.[156] Histologic examination demonstrated tissue ingrowth throughout the electrode interior and a fibrotic capsule that was about one half the thickness of the capsule seen with solid electrodes. R-wave stability and improved anchoring were also seen in dogs with the porous electrode.[156] This design allows the geometric area to be small, with a large total electrode surface area that includes the internal spaces within the electrode pores (Fig. 4-24).[157] Electrodes with porous designs have been shown to have better stimulation thresholds in humans.[158] Active-fixation leads may also include a porous electrode used as a surface cathode. The screw is used as the fixation mechanism, but it may be either electrically active or inert, being used or not used for sensing or pacing.[159]

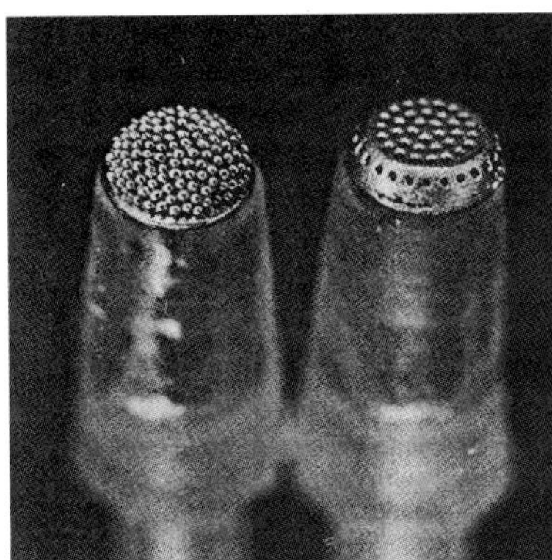

Figure 4-24. The sintered porous electrode (left) and the laser porous electrode (right). (From Hirshorn MS, Holley LK, Skalsky M, et al: Characteristics of advanced porous and textured surface pacemaker electrodes. PACE 6:525-536, 1983, with permission.)

Porous electrode tips can also be created by fabricating a laser-drilled platinum cap, which is treated to increase the external surface area, as shown in Figure 4-24. Lead tips are texturized or etched to enlarge the active surface area and reduce polarization properties.[157] The laser porous electrode demonstrated improved fixation by tissue ingrowth, when compared with smooth electrodes, in sheep.[157]

Electrode Material

The choice of metals used for electrodes is important in terms of long-term function, including minimizing corrosion and avoiding an excessive foreign-body reaction and excessive fibrosis. Platinum and platinum-iridium electrodes have been used. An alloy of cobalt, iron, chromium, molybdenum, nickel, and manganese (Elgiloy) has been used for cathodes. Microscopic corrosion has been noted with platinum-iridium and Elgiloy electrodes, but no consistent clinical adverse effects were observed.[160] Corrosion was directly related to the duration of implantation of the electrode.[160] Carbon has also been used for cathodes.[161] Vitreous carbon has excellent mechanical strength and biocompatibility, and is inert in body tissues.[161] Carbon-tipped electrodes resulted in lower chronic stimulation thresholds when compared with platinum or Elgiloy.[161,162] Excellent stimulation thresholds have been achieved with carbon electrodes.[163,164]

Lead Conductors

The conductor of the lead is a wire that conducts electrical current from the pacemaker generator to the tip electrode to allow pacing. Unipolar leads have one conductor, and bipolar leads have two. Details regarding conductor materials and standard design were discussed in the ICD section.

Bipolar leads require two conductors. The original design used a parallel arrangement; subsequent advancements in technology included the coaxial design. The coaxial design allowed introduction of a stylet which is passed through the inner lumen (Fig. 4-25). A more recent development of coated wire technology has allowed the development of "thin bipolar leads." The thin lead has an outside diameter similar to that of a unipolar lead. This is possible because the single strands of conductor wire are coated with a thin layer of ethylene tetrafluoroethylene (ETFE) insulation. Therefore, two or more conductors can be placed into a single coil to form the lead body[165,166] (see Fig. 4-25). Excellent acute and chronic stimulation thresholds at follow-up are obtained, with a relatively low short-term failure rate.[166]

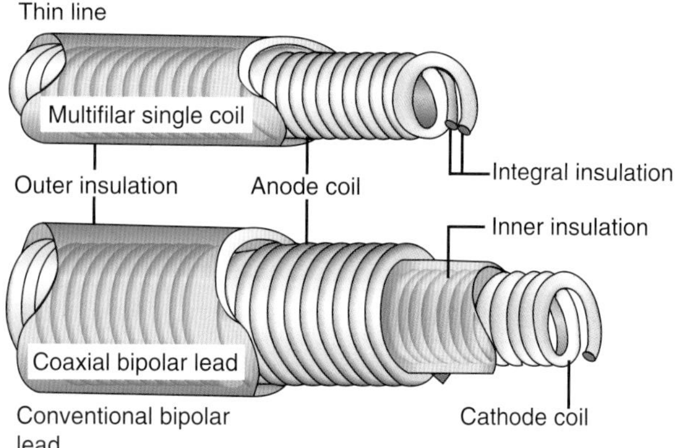

Figure 4-25. Multifilar, single-coil, coated lead (top) and conventional bipolar lead (bottom). (From Mond HG, Grenz D: Implantable transvenous pacing leads: The shape of things to come. PACE 27:887-893, 2004, with permission.)

Insulation

Insulation material extends from the tip of the lead to the lead connector. As with defibrillator leads, pacemaker leads are composed of polyurethane or silicone. Silicone was used for pacemaker leads in the 1960s, and polyurethane was introduced in 1979.[167]

Silicone Rubber

Silicone has a high biocompatibility and biostability but a relatively low tear strength.[154] Therefore, it can easily be damaged during implantation, especially by sharp tools or tight sutures. Therefore, a thick layer of silicone is necessary, making the lead diameter much larger than leads composed of polyethylene.[167] Silicone also has a high coefficient of friction, making it difficult to pass one lead next to another during implantation from a single subclavian stick with the original version of the silicone lead.[167] To overcome this, leads can be coated with a more lubricious material to allow easier handling. A stronger silicone was manufactured in later years, allowing silicone leads to be thinner than originally constructed.

Polyurethanes

Polyurethanes have an excellent biocompatibility and were initially believed to have a good biostability.[167] However, leads with polyurethane insulation are stiff. Polyurethane has high tensile and tear strengths, making it possible to construct leads of smaller diameter than silicone leads.[167] Unlike silicone, polyurethane also has a high flexibility and a low coefficient of friction,[154,168] so that two leads can be passed more easily side-by-side during implantation.

A poor long-term performance has been noted with some chemical varieties of polyurethane, whereas excellent long-term reliability has been observed with other forms.[168-173] The probability of failure of one Medtronic bipolar polyurethane ventricular lead (Model 4012 insulated with Pellethane 80A) was 20.9% at 6 years after implantation by Kaplan-Meier analysis.[171] Surface cracking and insulation failure have been noted. Clinically, insulation failure may manifest with muscle stimulation, oversensing, undersensing, loss of capture, reduced lead impedance, or premature battery depletion.[169,172-174] An early sign of diminishing EGM amplitude predicted lead failure several months before clinical manifestations.[174]

Leads composed of Pellethane 80A, a polyurethane insulation material, were shown to have insulation degradation, or environmental stress cracking, when explanted.[169] Environmental stress cracking is caused by the tendency of soft and hard segments of the lead to separate, causing damage to the surface.[167] More severe damage may occur in areas of the lead that are exposed to stress or strain, such as the region near the lead connector or the site of the ligature.[175] Another area of stress is the region between the clavicle and the first rib, when a subclavian puncture is used for access.[176] Leads with Pellethane 80A insulation are more prone to insulation failure when the subclavian venous approach is used, rather than the cephalic vein approach.[177] It was suggested that pacemaker-dependent patients with earlier implanted polyurethane leads should be given consideration for prophylactic replacement because of the high failure rate.[171,172]

Metal-induced oxidation is another mechanism of failure for polyurethane leads. An adverse chemical reaction may occur when the conductor produces corrosion products, which can lead to oxidative degradation of polyurethane insulation.[154] These adverse reactions appear to be design and model specific; they are not generic to all polyurethane leads.[178] This can be minimized by coating the conductor.[154]

Current polyurethane leads now typically use Pellethane 55D for insulation, which is stiffer and harder than Pellethane 80A. Long-term studies of leads using Pellethane 55D have shown better performance compared with Pellethane 80A.[154,179] The newer leads appear to be less susceptible to environmental stress cracking.[167] However, because of the stiffness of Pellethane 55D leads, they may be more prone to RV perforation.[179] Leads may now also have a combination of silicone and polyurethane insulation materials. To avoid excessive stiffness at the tip of the lead, the distal end of the lead may include silicone for insulation. In addition, silicone may be placed between the conductor and the polyurethane, in an attempt to minimize metal-induced oxidation.[154]

Subsequent studies suggested improved reliability for other leads made from polyurethane insulation.[180] It has been suggested that the early failure rate was related to the design of particular leads, rather than the insulation material itself.[180,181] Low-stress designs using noncorrosive coil wire have a good reported clinical history, without the high failure rate of designs in which tensile stress was not minimized.[181] Nevertheless, the preponderance of data suggests that Pellethane 80A is an unacceptable insulation material for pacing and ICD leads.

A clinically significant difference related to lead insulation is the response of the lead to electrocautery.

Silicone rubber is very resistant to the thermal effects of electrocautery, a major advantage at the time of pulse generator replacement. In contrast, polyurethane may melt when exposed to electrocautery, and great care must be taken at the time of operation to minimize heating of the insulation, to avoid insulation breakdown.

Fixation Mechanisms

Endocardial leads may have active- or passive-fixation mechanisms to allow attachment of the lead to the endocardial surface. The current passive-fixation leads typically use tines, located immediately behind the electrode, to allow attachment to the endocardium. The tines are extensions of the insulation material; they protrude backward just proximal to the tip and are designed to become entrapped within the trabeculae in the heart (Fig. 4-26). In addition to tines, other passive-fixation mechanisms tried in the past included wedge tips or flanges, wings, and fins.[154,167] Tined leads have a low rate of lead dislodgment.[182] Compared with older-style wedge-tip leads, tined ventricular leads were superior with respect to a significantly lower dislodgment rate and fewer reoperations.[183]

Active-fixation leads have a screw at the distal end. The screw in these leads may or may not be an electrically active component of the lead. The original screws were fixed and unprotected, placing venous and endocardial structures at risk of damage as the lead was passed through the vasculature and heart. To minimize this hazard, a mannitol covering over the screw was used by one manufacturer, which was designed to dissolve within 5 minutes. After the capsule dissolves, the screw on the tip of the lead can be fixed in the atrium or ventricle by rotating the lead over the stylet.[184,185] The rate of dissolution varied as a function of flow, taking approximately 3 minutes to dissolve in high-flow areas and up to 10 minutes in the case of stagnant flow.[185] The more common active-fixation mechanism now involves a retractable screw[184,186] (Fig. 4-27). A clothes-pin-type instrument is used to extend and retract the screw during implantation by turning the connector pin. All active-fixation leads result in some trauma to the endocardium and myocardium, and steroid elution at the base of the screw has resulted in significantly improved stimulation thresholds in active-fixation leads,[187,188] similar to the improvement seen with passive-fixation leads.

Advantages of active-fixation leads include the ability to place the lead at various sites in the ventricle or atrium and a low dislodgment rate.[167,188] Active-fixation leads are also easier to extract than passive-fixation leads. However, both types perform well, with low rates of dislodgment with current systems. The selection of an active or passive mechanism is now largely based on physician preference.

Electrode-Tissue Interface

A normal rise in stimulation threshold occurs after lead implantation. This is caused by an inflammatory response at the electrode-tissue interface.[189] A higher stimulus output may be programmed within the first 3 months after implantation to allow an acceptable safety margin for pacing in case an excessive increase in stimulation threshold is noted. A fibrous capsule forms at the electrode-tissue interface, and the stimulation threshold eventually falls, but typically it remains at a level higher than the implantation value.

The design of the pacemaker lead is one important factor in determining the amount of inflammatory response at the electrode-tissue interface. It is important that the electrode be in a stable position against the tissue surface to avoid excessive irritation, which should help to minimize the inflammatory response. A smaller distal tip of the lead is also important in reducing the inflammatory response. Bipolar leads are stiffer than unipolar leads, and bipolar leads made with polyurethane insulation are much stiffer than bipolar leads made from silicone rubber.[179] The stiffer the distal segment of the lead, the greater the force on the endocardium, which may increase the risk of perforation.[179] Softer insulation materials at the tip of the lead might also help to reduce trauma and therefore reduce the inflammatory response. Steroid-eluting electrodes have been effective in reducing inflammation and reducing the peak and chronic stimulation thresholds.

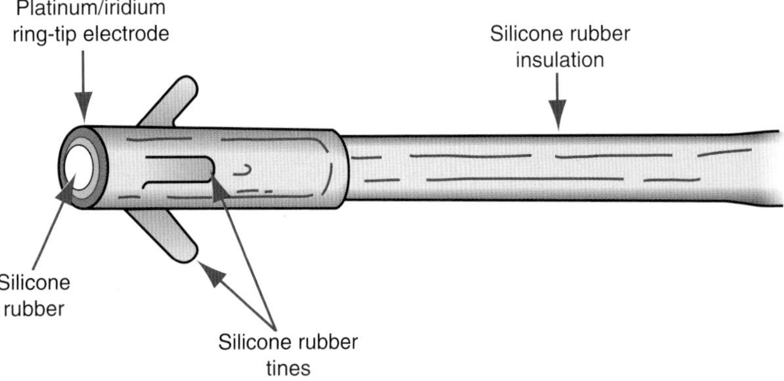

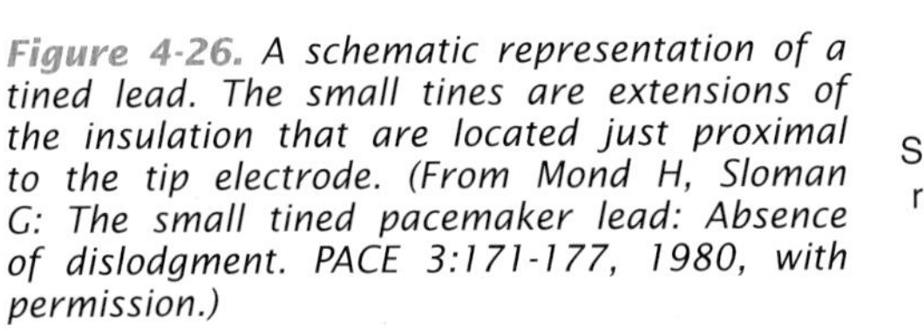
Figure 4-26. A schematic representation of a tined lead. The small tines are extensions of the insulation that are located just proximal to the tip electrode. (From Mond H, Sloman G: The small tined pacemaker lead: Absence of dislodgment. PACE 3:171-177, 1980, with permission.)

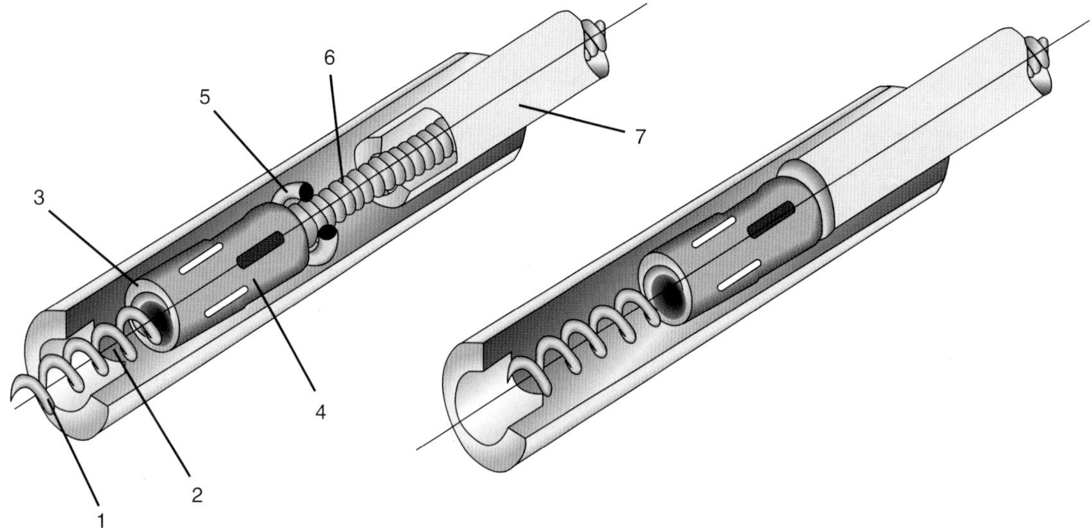

Figure 4-27. A schematic representation of a retractable screw-in lead. On the left portion of the diagram the tip is protracted, and on the right it is retracted. 1, helical electrode; 2, front section; 3, radiopaque ring; 4, crimp bus; 5, sealing ring; 6, conductor coil; 7, insulation tubing. (From Bisping HJ, Kreuzer J, Birkenheier H: Three year clinical experience with a new endocardial screw-in lead with introduction protection for use in the atrium and ventricle. PACE 3:424-435, 1980, with permission.)

Steroid-Eluting Leads

Steroid-eluting leads were designed to reduce or eliminate the early and late rises in pacing threshold that were seen with permanent pacemaker leads. Dexamethasone sodium phosphate has been used in the steroid-eluting electrode systems.[189,190] Multiple studies have demonstrated the effectiveness of steroid elution in obtaining very low acute and chronic stimulation thresholds in the atrium and ventricle, with near-elimination of the acute rise in stimulation threshold early after implantation.[187,190-192] The steroid effect is believed to result from a reduction in the inflammatory response at the electrode tip.

Both passive- and active-fixation leads may incorporate steroid elution.[187,193] A passive-fixation lead (Medtronic CapSure SP) with steroid elution demonstrated a much improved and "flat" response with respect to pacing threshold during 18 months of follow-up, when compared with another passive-fixation, non–steroid-eluting lead (Telectronics Encor) and with active-fixation leads (Medtronic Bisping, electrically active; Telectronics Accufix, electrically inactive, non–steroid-eluting)[159] (Fig. 4-28). The ability to pace at low outputs chronically has clear ramifications with respect to current drain and pulse generator longevity. Excellent sensing characteristics have also been noted with steroid-eluting leads.[192-194]

Lead Recalls: Accufix Issues

In November of 1994, a Telectronics atrial lead was recalled because of reported fractures noted in the J-shaped retention wire used in Accufix leads (Model 330-801 and 329-701). The electrically inactive J-retention wire lies beneath the outer insulation; it is welded at the distal end to the anode and is free at its proximal end. If a fracture occurs, the lead typically functions normally. However, the retention wire may protrude through the lead insulation and may cause damage to cardiac or other vascular structures. In addition, this wire may embolize to the lung vasculature. Cardiac or other vascular tears have led to deaths related to this lead. Periodic fluoroscopy was recommended to evaluate the lead and exclude protrusion of the retention wire.[195-196]

Clinical manifestations of retention wire fracture included pericardial effusion, tamponade, intracardiac thrombosis, pulmonary embolism, tricuspid valve laceration, aortic erosion, and migration of the fractured retention wire to the lungs.[197-199] It has been suggested that the shape of the Accufix lead after implantation is a strong predictor of fracture, and that a lower threshold for lead extraction is indicated in patients with non–J-shaped leads.[196,200,201] It has also been suggested that leads with retention-wire fracture should be extracted, with continued regular fluoroscopic screening for those leads that demonstrated a normal fluoroscopic appearance.[202] One study reported that the incidence of retention-wire fracture in the Accufix 330-801 lead was 25.6%.[202] It was initially suggested that many of these leads should be extracted, particularly in younger patients and in those with a more open appearance of the J wire.[203]

The Multicenter Clinical Study of patients with Accufix leads was designed to determine the rate of injury due to the J retention wire and the outcome of lead extraction. In this study of 2589 patients with Accufix atrial leads who were monitored by cinefluo-

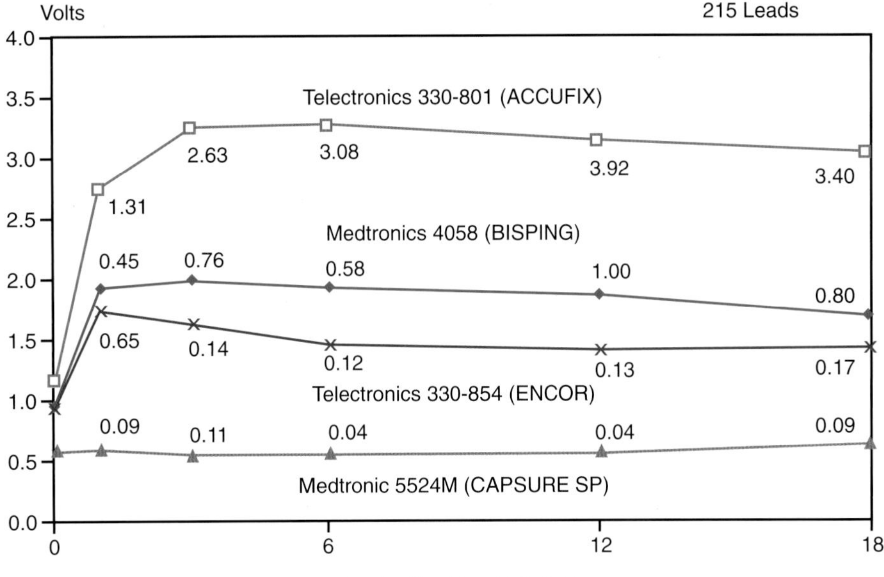

Figure 4-28. Bipolar stimulation thresholds for specific active- and passive-fixation leads. The Medtronic CapSure SP lead (passive fixation, steroid-eluting) had better pacing thresholds ($P < .05$) after implantation at all periods of follow-up, compared with another passive, non–steroid-eluting lead (Telectronics Encor) and with active fixation leads (Medtronic Bisping and Telectronics Accufix). (From Mond H, Hua W, Wang CC: Atrial pacing leads: The clinical contribution of steroid elution. PACE 18:1601, 1995, with permission.)

roscopic imaging, the risk of J-wire fracture was approximately 5.6% per year at 5 years and 4.7% per year at 10 years after implantation. Lead extraction was found to carry higher risks, suggesting that a conservative approach is indicated for most patients.[195] The overall advantage of a more conservative approach was confirmed in another study.[196] The hazard of J-wire fracture decreased over time after implantation.[201]

Telectronics Encor leads also have J-shaped retention wires. However, the wires are located deeper, within the cathode conductor, as opposed to the wire of the Accufix leads, which lies just beneath the outer insulation.[154] Fracture and protrusion of the wire in the Encor leads appear to have been related to the way the lead was implanted, with trauma during implantation potentially leading to deformity of the lead. Fluoroscopy was recommended on at least one occasion for these leads.[203]

Conclusions

Considerable advances have been made in the construction and design of permanent pacemaker leads. Improvements include the development of small, porous, steroid-eluting leads, which result in better long-term pacing thresholds, as well as leads with better reliability and long-term safety. Future advances may include additional improvements in lead insulation and advances that enhance the ease of lead extraction for older leads that are no longer functional. Continued improvements in lead technology are still warranted to further increase the reliability and long-term durability of endocardial leads, particularly for leads implanted in younger patients, who will require multiple generator replacements throughout their lifetime.

REFERENCES

1. Moss AJ, Hall WJ, Cannom DS, et al: Improved survival with an implanted defibrillator in patients with coronary disease at high risk for ventricular arrhythmia. N Engl J Med 335:1933-1940, 1996.
2. Buxton AE, Lee KL, Fisher JD, et al., and the Multicenter Unsustained Tachycardia Trial Investigators: A randomized study of the prevention of sudden death in patients with coronary artery disease. N Engl J Med 341:1882-1890, 1999.
3. Moss AJ, Zareba W, Hall J, et al: Prophylactic implantation of a defibrillator in patients with myocardial infarction and reduced ejection fraction (The Multicenter Automatic Defibrillator Implantation Trial II). N Engl J Med 346:877-883, 2002.
4. Antiarrhythmics Versus Implantable Defibrillator (AVID) Investigators: A comparison of antiarrhythmic drug therapy with implantable defibrillators in patients resuscitated from near fatal ventricular arrhythmias. N Engl J Med 337:1576-1583, 1997.
5. Connolly SJ, Hallstrom AP, Cappato R, et al: Meta-analysis of the implantable cardioverter defibrillator secondary prevention trials. AVID, CASH and CIDS studies. Antiarrhythmics Versus Implantable Defibrillator study. Cardiac Arrest Study Hamburg. Canadian Implantable Defibrillator Study. Eur Heart J 21:2071-2078, 2000.
6. Mirowski M, Mower MM, Reid PR, Watkins L Jr: Implantable automatic defibrillators: Their potential in prevention of sudden coronary death. Ann N Y Acad Sci 382:371-380, 1982.
7. Mirowski M, Reid PR, Mower MM, et al: Termination of malignant ventricular arrhythmias with an implanted automatic defibrillator in human beings. N Engl J Med 303:322-324, 1980.
8. Reid PR, Mirowski M, Mower MM, et al: Clinical evaluation of the internal automatic cardioverter defibrillator in survivors of sudden cardiac death. Am J Cardiol 51:1608-1613, 1983.
9. Marchlinski FE, Flores BT, Buxton AE, et al: Automatic implantable cardioverter defibrillator: Efficacy, complicationas and device failures. Ann Intern Med 104:481, 1986.
10. Troup PJ, Chapman PD, Olinger GN, Kleinman LH: The implanted defibrillator: Relation of defibrillating lead configuration and clinical variables to defibrillation threshold. J Am Coll Cardiol 6:1315-1321, 1985.
11. Mirowski M: The automatic implantable cardioverter defibrillator: An overview. J Am Coll Cardiol 6:461-466, 1985.
12. Kelly PA, Cannom DS, Garan H, et al: The automatic implantable cardioverter defibrillator: Efficacy, complications and

survival in patients with malignant ventricular arrhythmias. J Am Coll Cardiol 11:1278-1286, 1988.
13. Gartman DM, Bardy GH, Allen MD, et al: Short-term morbidity and mortality of implantation of automatic implantable cardioverter defibrillator. J Thorac Cardiovasc Surg 100:353-359, 1990.
14. Echt DS, Armstrong K, Schmidt P, et al: Clinical experience, complications and survival in 70 patients with the automatic implantable cardioverter defibrillator. Circulation 71:289-296, 1985.
15. Fromer M, Brachmann J, Block M, et al: Efficacy of automatic multimodal device therapy for ventricular tachyarrhythmias as delivered by a new implantable pacing cardioverter defibrillator: Results of a European multicenter study of 102 implants. Circulation 86:363-374, 1992.
16. Saksena S: Defibrillation threshold and perioperative mortality associated with either endocardial and epicardial defibrillation lead systems. The PCD Investigators and participating institutions. PACE 16:202-207, 1993.
17. Brady PA, Friedman PA, Trusty JM, et al: High failure rate of epicardial implantable cardioverter defibrillator lead: Implications for long-term follow-up of patients with an implantable cardioverter defibrillator. J Am Coll Cardiol 31:616-622, 1998.
18. Almassi GH, Olinger GN, Wetherbee JN, Fehl G: Long-term complications of implantable cardioverter defibrillator lead systems. Ann Thorac Surg 55:888-892, 1993.
19. Korte T, Jung W, Spehl S, et al: Incidence of ICD lead related complications during long-term follow-up: Comparison of epicardial and endocardial electrode systems. PACE 18:2053-2061, 1995.
20. Mattke S, Muller D, Markewitz A, et al: Failures of epicardial and transvenous leads for implantable cardioverter defibrilators. Am Heart J 130:1040-1044, 1995.
21. Chevalier P, Mancada E, Canu G, et al: Symptomatic pericardial disease associated with patch electrodes of automatic implantable cardioverter defibrillator: An underestimated complication? PACE 19:2150-2152, 1996.
22. Stambler BS, Wood MA, Damiano RJ, et al: Sensing/pacing lead complications with a newer generation implantable cardioverter defibrillator: Worldwide experience from the Guardian ATP 4210 clinical trial. J Am Coll Cardiol 23:123-132, 1994.
23. Daoud EG, Kirsh MM, Bolling SF, et al: Incidence, presentation, diagnosis, and management of malfunctioning implantable cardioverter defibrillator rate sensing leads. Am Heart J 128:892-895, 1994.
24. Grimm W, Flores BF, Marchlinski FE: Complications of implantable cardioverter defibrillator therapy: Follow-up of 241 patients. PACE 16:218-222, 1993.
25. Sgarbossa EB, Shewchik J, Pinski SL: Performance of implantable defibrillator pacing/sensing lead adapters. PACE 19:811-814, 1996.
26. Saksena S, Poczobutt-Johanos M, Castle LW, et al, for the Guardian Multicenter Investigators Group. Long-term multicenter experience with second generation implantable pacemaker defibrillator in patients with malignant ventricular tachyarrhythmias. J Am Coll Cardiol 19:490-499, 1992.
27. Kastor JS: Michel Mirowski and the automatic implantable defibrillator. Am J Cardiol 63:1121-1126, 1989.
28. Mirowski M, Mower MM, Gott VL, Brawley RK: Feasibility and effectiveness of low energy catheter defibrillation in man. Circulation 47:79-85, 1973.
29. Zipes DP, Jackman WM, Heger JJ, et al: Clinical transvenous cardioversion of recurrent life-threatening tachyarrhythmias: Low energy synchronized cardioversion of ventricular tachycardia and termination of ventricular fibrillation in patients using a catheter electrode. Am Heart J 103:789-794, 1982.
30. Zipes DP, Roberts D, for the Pacemaker Cardioverter-Defibrillator Investigators. Results of the international study of the implantable pacemaker cardioverter defibrillator: A comparison of epicardial and endocardial lead systems. Circulation 92:59-65, 1995.
31. Trappe HJ, Fieguth HG, Pfitzner P, et al: Epicardial and nonthoracotomy lead systems combined with a cardioverter defibrillator. PACE 18:127-132, 1995.
32. Bocker D, Block M, Isbruch F, et al: Do patients with an implantable defibrillator live longer? J Am Coll Cardiol 21:1638-1644, 1993.
33. Bardy GH, Hofer B, Johnson G, et al: Implantable transvenous cardioverter defibrillators. Circulation 87:1152-1168, 1993.
34. Hauser RG, Kurschinski DT, McVeigh K, et al: Clinical results with nonthoracotomy ICD systems. PACE 16:141-148, 1993.
35. Saksena S, An H: Clinical efficacy of dual electrode systems for endocardial cardioversion of ventricular tachycardia: A prospective randomized crossover trial. Am Heart J 119:15-22, 1990.
36. Winkle RA, Bach SM, Mead RH, et al: Comparison of defibrillation efficacy in humans using a new catheter and superior vena cava spring left ventricular patch electrode. J Am Coll Cardiol 11;365-370, 1988.
37. Saksena S, Luceri R, Krol RB, et al: Endocardial pacing, cardioversion and defibrillation using a braided endocardial lead system. Am J Cardiol 71:834-841, 1993.
38. Hammel D, Block M, Borggrefe M, et al: Implantation of a cardioverter/defibrillator in the subpectoral region combined with a nonthoracotomy lead system. PACE 15:367-368, 1992.
39. Thakur RK, Ip JH, Mehta D, et al: Subpectoral implantation of ICD generators: Long-term follow-up. PACE 18:159-162, 1995.
40. Gregoratos G, Cheitlin MD, Conill A, et al: ACC/AHA guidelines for implantation of cardiac pacemakers and antiarrhythmia devices: A report of the American College of Cardiology/American Heart Association Task Force on Practice Guidelyines (Committee on Pacemaker Implantation). J Am Coll Cardiol 31:1175-1209, 1998.
41. Gradaus R, Breithardt G, Bocker D: ICD leads: Design and chronic dysfunctions. PACE 26:649-657, 2003.
42. Accorti PR: Leads technology. In Singer I (ed): Implantable Cardioverter Defibrillator. Armonk NY, Futura, 1994.
43. Yabe S, Smith WM, Daubert JP, et al: Conduction disturbances caused by high current density electric fields. Circ Res 66:1190-1203, 1990.
44. Callans DJ, Swarna US, Schwartzman D, et al: Postshock sensing performance in transvenous defibrillation lead systems: Analysis of detection and redetection of ventricular fibrillation. J Cardiovasc Electrophysiol 6:604-612, 1995.
45. Mond H, Stokes K: The electrode-tissue interface: The revolutionary role of steroid elution. PACE 15:95-107, 1992.
46. Stamato N, O'Toole MF, Fetter JG, Enger EL: The safety and efficacy of chronic ventricular pacing at 1.6 volts using a steroid eluting lead. PACE 15:248-251, 1992.
47. Mond H, Stokes K, Helland J, et al: The porous titanium steroid eluting electrode: A double blind study assessing the stimulation threshold effects of steroid. PACE 11:214-219, 1988.
48. Kruse M: Long-term performance of endocardial leads with steroid-eluting electrodes. PACE 9:1217-1219, 1986.
49. Radovsky AS, van Vleet JF, Stokes KB, Tacker WA Jr: Paired comparisons of steroid-eluting and nonsteriod endocardial pacemaker leads in dogs: Electrical performance and morphologic alterations. PACE 11:1085-1094, 1988.
50. Schuchert A, Hopf M, Kuck KH, Bleifeld W: Chronic ventricular electrograms: Do steroid-eluting leads differ from conventional leads? PACE 13:1879-1882, 1990.
51. Leitch JW, Yee R, Klein GJ, et al: Correlation between the ventricular electrogram amplitude in sinus rhythm and in ventricular fibrillation. PACE 13:1105-1109, 1990.
52. Almeida HF, Buckingham TA: Inappropriate implantable cardioverter defibrillator shocks secondary to sensing lead failure: Utility of stored electrograms. PACE 16:407-410, 1993.

53. Sperry RE, Ellenbogen KA, Wood MA, et al: Failure of a second and third generation implantable cardioverter defibrillator to sense ventricular tachycardia: Implications for fixed-gain sensing devices. PACE 15:749-755, 1992.
54. Callans DJ, Hook BG, Kleiman RB, et al: Unique sensing errors in third-generation implantable cardioverter defibrillators. J Am Coll Cardiol 22:1135-1140, 1993.
55. Epstein AE, Kay GN, Plumb VJ, et al: Gross and microscopic pathological changes associated with nonthoracotomy implantable defibrillator leads. Circulation 98:1517-1524, 1998.
56. Epstein A, Anderson P, Kay GN, et al: Gross and microscopic changes associated with a nonthoracotomy implantable cardioverter defibrillators. PACE 15:382-386, 1992.
57. Hauser R, Hayes D, Parsonnet V, et al: Feasibility and initial results of an Internet-based pacemaker and ICD pulse generator and lead registry. PACE 24:82-87, 2001.
58. Jung W, Manz M, Moosdorf R, Luderitz B: Failure of an implantable cardioverter defibrillator to redetect ventricular fibrillation in patients with a nonthoracotomy lead system. Circulation 86:1217-1222, 1992.
59. Natale A, Sra J, Axtell K, et al: Undetected ventricular fibrillation in transvenous implantable cardioverter defibrillators: Prosepective comparison of different lead system-device combinations. Circulation 93:91-98, 1996.
60. Berul CI, Callans DJ, Schwartzman DS, et al: Comparison of initial detection and redetection of ventricular fibrillation in a transvenous defibrillator system with automatic gain control. J Am Coll Cardiol 25:431-436, 1995.
61. Goldberger JJ, Horvath G, Donovan D, et al: Detection of ventricular fibrillation by transvenous defibrillating leads: Integrated versus dedicated bipolar sensing. J Cardiovasc Electrophysiol 9:677-688, 1998.
62. Gold MR, Shorofsky SR: Transvenous defibrillation lead systems. J Cardiovasc Electrophysiol 7:570-580, 1996.
63. Gottlieb CD, Schwartzman DS, Callans DJ, et al: Effects of high and low shock energies on sinus electrograms recorded via integrated and true bipolar nonthoracotomy lead systems. J Cardiovasc Electrophysiol 7:189-196, 1996.
64. Ellenbogen KA, Wood MA, Shepard RK, et al: Detection and management of an implantable cardioverter defibrillator lead failure: Incidence and clinical implications. J Am Coll Cardiol 41:73-80, 2003.
65. Nelson RS, Gilman BL, Shapland JE, Lehmann MH: Leads for the ICD. In Kroll MW, Lehmann MH (eds): Implantable Cardioverter Defibrillator Therapy. Norwell, Mass., Kluwer Academic, 1996.
66. Hayes DL, Graham KJ, Irwin M, et al: A multicenter experience with a bipolar tined polyurethane ventricular lead. PACE 15:1033-1039, 1992.
67. Fotuhi P, Alt E, Callihan R, et al: Endocardial carbon braid electrodes: New approach to lowering defibrillation thresholds. PACE 16:1919A, 1993.
68. Alt E, Theres H, Heinz M, et al: A new approach towards defibrillation electrodes: Highly conductive isotropic carbon fibers. PACE 14:1923-1928, 1991.
69. Jacobs DM, Fink AS, Miller RP, et al: Anatomical and morphological evaluation of pacemaker lead compression. PACE 16:434-444, 1993.
70. Magney JE, Flynn DM, Parsons JA, et al: Anatomical mechnaisms explaining damage to pacemaker leads, defibrillator leads, and failure of central venous catheters adjacent to the sternoclavicular joint. PACE 16:445-457, 1993.
71. Doring J, Flink R: The impact of pending technologies on a universal connector standard. PACE 9:1186-1190, 1986.
72. Schaumann A, von zur Muhlen F, Gonska BD, Kreuzer H: Enhanced detection criteria in implantable cardioverter-defibrillators to avoid inappropriate therapy. Am J Cardiol 78:42-50, 1996.
73. Butter C, Auricchio A, Schwarz T, et al: Clinical evaluation of a prototype passive fixation dual chamber single pass lead for dual chamber ICD systems. PACE 22:169-173, 1999.
74. Saksena S, DeGroot P, Krol RB, et al: Low energy endocardial defibrillation using an axillary or a pectoral thoracic electrode location. Circulation 88:2655-2660, 1993.
75. Higgins SL, Alexander DC, Kuypers CJ, Brewster SA: The subcutaneous array: A new lead adjunct for the transvenous ICD to lower defibrillation thresholds. PACE 18:1540-1548, 1995.
76. Yee R, Klein GJ, Leitch JW, et al: A permanent transvenous lead system for an implantable pacemaker cardioverter defibrillator: Nonthoracotomy approach to implantation. Circulation 85:196-204, 1992.
77. Venditti FJ, Martin DT, Vassolas G, Bowen S: Rise in chronic defibrillation thresholds in nonthroacotomy implantable defibrillators. Circulation 89:216-223, 1994.
78. Strickberger SA, Hummel JD, Horwood LE, et al: Effect of shock polarity on ventricular defibrillation threshold using a transvenous lead system. J Am Coll Cardiol 24:1069-1072, 1994.
79. Natale A, Sra J, Axtell K, et al: Preliminary experience with a hybrid nonthoracotomy defibrillating system that includes a biphasic device: Comparison with a standard monophasic device using the same lead system. J Am Coll Cardiol 24:406-412, 1994.
80. Bardy GH, Ivey TD, Allen MD, et al: A prospective randomized evaluation of biphasic versus monophasic waveform pulses on defibrillation efficacy in humans. J Am Coll Cardiol 14:728-733, 1989.
81. Block M, Hammel D, Bocker D, et al: A prospective randomized cross-over comparison of mono- and biphasic defibrillation using nonthoracotomy lead configurations in humans. J Cardiovasc Electrophysiol 5:581-590, 1994.
82. Natale A, Sra J, Krum D, et al: Comparsion of biphasic and monophasic pulses: Does the advantage of biphasic shocks depend on the waveshape? PACE 18:1354-1361, 1995.
83. Saksena S, An H, Mehara R, et al: Prospective comparison of biphasic and monophasic shocks for implantable cardioverter defibrillators using endocardial leads. Am J Cardiol 70:304-310, 1992.
84. Saksena S, Scott SE, Accorti PR, et al: Efficacy and safety of monophasic and biphasic waveform shocks using a braided endocardial defibrillation lead system. Am Heart J 20:1342-1347, 1990.
85. Neuzner J, Pitschner HF, Huth C, Schlepper M: Effect of biphasic waveform pulse on endocardial defibrillation efficacy in humans. PACE 17:207-212, 1994.
86. Bardy GH, Johnson G, Poole JE, et al: A simplified, single-lead unipolar transvenous cardioversion defibrillation system. Circulation 88:543-547, 1993.
87. Mattke S, Fiek M, Markewitz A, et al: Comparison of a unipolar defibrillation system with a dual lead system using an enlarged defibrillation anode. PACE 19:2083-2088, 1996.
88. Lang DJ, Heil JE, Hahn SJ, et al: Implantable cardioverter defibrillator lead technology: Improved performance and lower defibrillation thresholds. PACE 18:548-559, 1995.
89. Niebauer MJ, Yamanouchi Y, Hills D, et al: Voltage dependence of ICD lead polarization and the effect of iridium oxide coating. PACE 23:818-823, 2000.
90. Niebauer MJ, Wilkoff B, Yamanouchi Y, et al: Iridium oxide-coated defibrillation electrode: Reduced shock polarization and improved defibrillation efficacy. Circulation 96:3732-3736, 1997.
91. Gradaus R, Bocker D, Dorszewski A, et al: Fractally coated defibrillation electrodes: Is an improvement in defibrillation threshold possible? Europace 2:154-159, 2000.
92. Peters RW, Foster AH, Shorofsky SR, et al: Spurious discharges due to late insulation break in endocardial sensing leads for cardioverter defibrillators. PACE 18:478-481, 1995.

93. Kron J, Herre J, Renfroe EG, et al., and the AVID Investigators. Lead and device-related complications in the Antiarrhythmics Versus Implantable Defibrillators Trial. Am Heart J 141:92-98, 2001.
94. Degeratu FT, Khalighi K, Peters RW, et al: Sensing lead failure in implantable defibrillators: A comparison of two commonly used leads. J Cardiovasc Electrophysiol 11:21-24, 2000.
95. Gold MR, Peters RW, Johnson JW, Shorofsky SR: Complications associated with pctoral implantation of cardioverter defibrillators. World-Wide Jewel Investigators. PACE 20:208-211, 1997.
96. Grimm W, Menz J, Hoffmann J, et al: Complications of third-generation implantable cardioverter defibrillator therapy. PACE 22:206-211, 1999.
97. Gupta A, Zegel HG, Dravid VS, et al: Value of radiography in diagnosing complications of cardioverter defibrillators implanted without thoracotomy in 437 patients. Am J Radiol 168:105-108, 1997.
98. Mehta D, Nayak HM, Signson M, et al: Late complications in patients with pectoral defibrillator implants with transvenous defibrillator lead systems: High incidence of insulation breakdown. PACE 21:1893-1900, 1998.
99. Dorwarth U, Frey B, Dugas M, et al: Transvenous defibrillatin leads: High incidence of failure during long-term follow-up. J Cardiovasc Electrophysiol 14:38-43, 2003.
100. Schwartzman D, Nallamouthu N, Callans DJ, et al: Postoperative lead-related complications in patients with nonthoracotomy defibrillator lead systems. J Am Coll Cardiol 26:776-786, 1995.
101. Brooks R, Garan H, Torchiana D, et al: Determinants of successful nonthoracotomy cardioverter defibrillator implantation: Experience in 101 patients using two different lead systems. J Am Coll Cardiol 22:1835-1842m 1993.
102. Zipes DP, Roberts D: Results of the international study of the implantable pacemaker cardioverter defibrillator: Intention-to-treat comparison of lnical outcomes. Circulation 92:59-65, 1995.
103. Raviele A, Gasparini G, for the Italian Endotak Investigator Group. Italian multicenter clinical experience with endocardial defibrillation: Acute and long-term results in 307 patients. PACE 18:599-608, 1995.
104. Jones GK, Bardy GH, Kudenchuk PJ, et al: Mechanical complications after implantation of multiple lead nonthoracotomy defibrillator system: Implications for management and future system design. Am Heart J 130:327-333, 1995.
105. Lawton JS, Wood MA, Gilligan DM, et al: Implantable transvenous cardioverter defibrillator leads: The dark side. PACE 19:1273-1278, 1996.
106. Tullo NG, Saksena S, Krol RB, et al: Management of complications associated with a first-generation endocardial defibrillation lead system for implantable cardioverter defibrillators. Am J Cardiol 66:411-415, 1990.
107. Mahapatra S, Homound MK, Wang PJ, et al: Durability of repaired sensing leads equivalent to that of new leads in implantable cardioverter defibrillator patients with sensing abnormalities. PACE 26:2225-2229, 2003.
108. Sra JS, Natale A, Axtell K, et al: Experience with two different nonthoracotomy systems for implantable defibrillators in 170 patients. PACE 17:1741-1750, 1994.
109. Fahy GJ, Kleman JM, Wilkoff BL, et al: Low incidence of lead related complications associated with nonthoracotomy implantable cardioverter defibrillator systems. PACE 18:172-178, 1995.
110. Roelke M, O'Nunain SS, Osswald S, et al: Subclavian crush syndrome complicationg transvenous caredioverter defibrillator systems. PACE 18:973-979, 1995.
111. Gallik DKM, Ben-zur UM, Gross JN, Furman S: Lead fracture in cephalic versus subclavian approach with transvenous implantable cardioverter defibrillator systems. PACE 19:1089-1094, 1996.
112. Hauser RG, Cannom D, Hayes DL, et al: Long-term structural failure of coaxial polyurethane implantable cardioverter defibrillator leads. PACE 25:879-882, 2002.
113. Peralta AO, John RM, Martin DT, Venditti FJ: Long term performance of the Endotak C defibrillator lead [abstract] Circulation 98:1-787, 1998.
114. Moore SL, Maloney JD, Edel TB, et al: Implantable cardioverter defibrillator implanted by nonthoracotomy approach: Initial clinical experience with the redesigned transvenous lead system. PACE 14:1865-1869, 1991.
115. Lawton JS, Ellenbogen KA, Wood MA, et al: Sensing lead-related complications in patients with transvenous implantable cardioverter defibrillators. Am J Cardiol 78:647-651, 1996.
116. Mera F, Delurgio DB, Langberg JJ, et al: Transvenous cardioverter defibrillator lead malfunction due to terminal connector damage in pectoral implants. PACE 22:1797-1801, 1999.
117. Block M, Hammel D, Isbruch F, et al: Results and realistic expectations with transvenous lead systems. PACE 15:665-670, 1992.
118. Schwartzman D, Nallamothu N, Callans DJ, et al: Postoperative lead-related complications in patients with nonthoractomy defibrillation lead systems. J Am Coll Cardiol 26:776-786, 1995.
119. Pratt TR, Pulling CC, Stanton MS: Prospective postmarket device studies versus returned product analysis as a predictor of system survival. PACE 23:1150-1155, 2000.
120. Gras D, Leclereq C, Tang AS, et al: Cardiac resynchronization therapy in advanced heart failure: The multicenter InSync clinical study. Eur J Heart Fail 4:311-320, 2002.
121. Auricchio A, Stellbrink C, Sack S, et al., and the Pacing Therapies in Congestive Heart Failure (PATH-CHF) Study Group. Long-term clinical effect of hemodynamically optimized cardiac resychronization therapy in patients with heart failure and ventricular conduction delay. J Am Coll Card 39:2026-2033, 2002.
122. Cazeau S, Leclercq C, Lavergne T, et al., and the Multisite Stimulation in Cardiomyopathies (MUSTIC) Study Investigators. Effects of multisite biventricular pacing in patients with heart failure and intraventricular conduction delay. N Engl J Med 344:873-880, 2001.
123. Linde C, Leclercq C, Rex S, et al: Long-term benefits of biventricular pacing in congestive heart failure: Results from the Multisite stimulation in caredioomyopathy (MUSTIC) study. J Am Coll Card 40:111-118, 2002.
124. Abraham WT, Fisher WG, Smith AL, et al, and the MIRACLE Study Group Multicenter InSync Randomized Clinical Evaluation. Cardiac resynchronization in chronic heart failure. N Engl J Med 346:1845-1853, 2002.
125. Blanc JJ, Etienne Y, Giloard M, et al: Evaluation of different ventricular pacing sites in patients with severe heart failure: Results of an acute hemodynamic study. Circulation 96:3273-3277, 1997.
126. Young JB, Abraham WT, Smith AL, et al., and the Multicenter InSync ICD Randomized Clinical Evaluation (MIRACLE ICD) Trial Investigators. Combined cardiac resynchronization and implantable cardioversion defibrillation in advanced chronic heart failure: The MIRACLE ICD Trial. JAMA 289:2685-2694, 2003.
127. Bristow MR, Saxon LA, Boehmeer J, et al., and the Comparison of Medical Therapy, Pacing and Defibrillation in Heart Failure (COMPANION) Investigators. N Engl J Med 350:2140-2150, 2004.
128. Rossillo A, Verma A, Saad EB, et al: Impact of coronary sinus lead position on biventricular pacing: Mortality and echocardiographic evaluation during long-term follow-up. J Cardiovasc Electrophysiol 15:1120-1125, 2004.
129. Butter C, Auricchio A, Stellbrink C, et al: Should stimulation site be tailored in the individual heart failure patient? Am J Cardiol 86:144K-151K, 2000.
130. Purerfellner H, Nesser HJ, Winter S, et al., for the EASYTRAK Clinical Investigation Study Group and the European EASY-

TRAK Registry. Transvenous left venticular lead implantation with the EASYTRAK lead system: The European experience. Am J Cardiol 86:157K-164K, 2000.

131. Sack S, Heinzel F, Dagres N, et al: Stimulation of the left ventricle through the coronary sinus with a newly developed "over the wire" lead system: Early experiences with lead handling and positioning. Europace 3:317-323, 2001.
132. Achtelik M, Bocchiardo M, Trappe HJ, et al., on behalf of the Ventak CHF/Contak CD Clinical Investigation Study Group. Performance of a new steroid-eluting coronary sinus lead designed for lefter ventricular pacing. PACE 23:1741-1743, 2000.
133. Kantharia BK, Padder FA, Pennington JC, et al: Feasibility, safety, and determinants of extraction time of percutaneous extraction of endocardial implantable cardioverter defibrillator leads by intravascular countertraction method. Am J Cardiol 85:593-597, 2000.
134. Saad EB, Saliba WI, Schweikert RA, et al: Nonthoracotomy implantable defibrillator lead extraction: Results and comparison with extraction of pacemaker leads. Pacing Clin Electrophysiol 26:1944-1950, 2003.
135. Parsonnet V, Roelke M, Trivedi A, et al: Laser extraction of entrapped leads. PACE 24:329-332, 2001.
136. Morris MM, KenKnight BH, Warren JA, Lang DJ: A preview of implantable cardioverter derfibrillator systems in the next millennium: An integrative cardiac rhythm management approach. Am J Cardiol 83:48D-54D, 1999.
137. Bardy GH, Cappato R, Smith WM, et al: The totally subcutaneous ICD system (the S-ICD) [abstract]. PACE 24:578, 2002.
138. Mond HG: Unipolar versus bipolar pacing: Poles apart. PACE 14:1411, 1991.
139. Wiegand UK, Bode F, Bonnemeier H, et al: Incidence and predictors of pacemaker dysfunction with unipolar ventricular lead configuration: Can we identify patients who benefit from bipolar electrodes? PACE 24:1383-1388, 2001.
140. Breivik K, Ohm OJ, Engedal H: Long-term comparison of unipolar and bipolar pacing and sensing, using a new multiprogrammable pacemaker system. PACE 6:592-600, 1983.
141. Secemsky SI, Hauser RG, Denes P, Edwards LM: Unipolar sensing abnormalities: Incidence and clinical significance of skeletal muscle interference and undersensing in 228 patients. PACE 5:10-19, 1982.
142. Echeverria HJ, Luceri RM, Thurber RJ, Castellanos A: Myopotential inhibition of unipolar AV sequential (DVI) pacemaker. PACE 5:20-22, 1982.
143. Zimmern SH, Clark MF, Austin WK, et al: Characteristics and clinical effects of myopotential signals in a unipolar DDD pacemaker population. PACE 9:1019, 1986.
144. Smyth NP, Tarjan PP, Chernoff E, Baker N: The significance of electrode surface area and stimulation thresholds in permanent cardiac pacing. J Thorac Cardiovasc Surg 71:559-65, 1976.
145. Furman S, Garvey J, Hurzeler P: Pulse duration variation and electrode size as factors in pacemaker longevity. J Thorac Cardiovasc Surg 69:382-389, 1975.
146. Barold SS, Ong LS, Heinle RA: Stimulation and sensing thresholds for cardiac pacing: Electrophysiologic and technical aspects. Prog Cardiovasc Dis 1981;24:1-24.
147. Mond H, Holley L, Hirshorn M: The high impedance dish electrode: Clinical experience with a new tined lead. PACE 5:529-534, 1982.
148. Schuchert A, Kuch KH: Benefits of smaller electrode surface area (4 mm^2) on steroid-eluting leads. PACE 14:2098-2104, 1991.
149. Ellenbogen KA, Wood MA, Gilliagan DM, et al, and the CapSure Z Investigators. Steroid-eluting high-impedance pacing leads decrease short and long-term current drain: Results from a multicenter clinical trial. PACE 22:39-48, 1999.
150. Moracchini PV, Cornacchia D, Bernasconi M, et al: High impedance low energy pacing leads: Long-term results with a very small surface area, steroid-eluting lead compared to three conventional electrodes. PACE 22:326-334, 1999.
151. Deshmukh P, Casavant D, Anderson K, Romanyshyn M: Stable electrical performance of high efficiency pacing leads having small surface, steroid-eluting pacing electrodes. PACE 22:1599-1603, 1999.
152. Berger T, Roithinger FX, Antretter H, et al: The influence of high versus normal impedance ventricular leads on pacemaker generator longevity. PACE 26:2116-2120, 2003.
153. Scherer M, Ezziddin K, Klesius A, et al: Extension of generator longevity by use of high impedance ventricular leads. PACE 24:206-211, 2001.
154. Mond HG. Engineering and clinical aspects of pacing leads. In Ellenbogen K, Kay G, Wilkoff B (eds.): Clincial Cardiac Pacing and Defibrillation, 2nd ed. Philadelphia, WB Saunders, 2000.
155. Luria D, Gurevitz O, Bar Lev D, et al: Use of automatic threshold tracking function with non-low polarization leads. PACE 27:453-459, 2004.
156. Amundson DC, McArthur W, Mosharrafa M: The porous endocardial electrode. PACE 2:40-50, 1979.
157. Hirshorn MS, Holley LK, Skalsky M, et al: Characteristics of advanced porous and textured surface pacemaker electrodes. PACE 6:525-536, 1983.
158. Djordjevic M, Stojanov P, Velimirovic D: Target lead: Low threshold electrode. PACE 9:1206, 1986.
159. Mond H, Hua W, Wang CC: Atrial pacing leads: The clinical contribution of steroid elution. PACE 18:1601, 1995.
160. Parsonnet V, Villaneuva A, Driller J, Bernstein AD: Corrosion of pacemaker electrodes. PACE 4:289-296, 1981.
161. Elmqvist H, Schueller H, Richter G: The carbon tip electrode. PACE 6:436-439, 1983.
162. Mugica J, Henry L, Attuel P, et al: Clinical experience with 910 carbon tip leads: Comparison with polished platinum leads. PACE 9:1230-1238, 1986.
163. Gargeroglio B, Inguaggiato B, Chinaglia B, Cerise O: Initial results with an activated carbon tip electrode. PACE 6:440-448, 1983.
164. Pioger G, Ripart A: Clinical results of low energy unipolar or bipolar activated carbon tip leads. PACE 9:1243-1248, 1986.
165. Mond HG, Grenz D: Implantable transvenous pacing leads: The shape of things to come. PACE 27:887-893, 2004.
166. Breivik K, Danilovic D, Ohm OJ, et al: Clinical evaluation of thin bipolar pacing lead. PACE 20:637-646, 1997.
167. Crossley GH: Cardiac pacing leads. Cardiol Clin 18:95-112, 2000.
168. Scheuer-Lesser M, Irnich W, Kreuzer J: Polyurethane leads: Facts and controversy. PACE 6:454-458, 1983.
169. Byrd CL, McArthur W, Stokes K, et al: Implant experience with unipolar polyurethane pacing leads. PACE 6:868-882, 1983.
170. Woscoboinik JR, Maloney JD, Helguera ME, et al: Pacing lead survival: Performance of different models. PACE 15:1991-1995, 1992.
171. Hayes DL, Graham KJ, Irwin M, et al: A multicenter experience with a bipolar tined polyurethane ventricular lead. PACE 15:1033-1039, 1992.
172. Sweesy MW, Forney CC, Hayes DL, et al: Evaluation of an in-line bipolar polyurethane ventricular pacing lead. PACE 15:1982-1985, 1992.
173. Hayes DL, Graham KJ, Irwin M, et al: Multicenter experience with a bipolar tined polyurethane ventricular lead. PACE 18:999-1004, 1995.
174. Van Beek GJ, Den Dulk K, Lindemans FW, et al: Detection of insulation failure by gradual reduction in noninvasively measured electrogram amplitudes. PACE 9:772-775, 1986.
175. Pirzada FA, Seltzer JP, Blair-Saletin D, Killian M: Five-year performance of the Medtronic 6971 polyurethane endocardial electrode. PACE 9:1173-1180, 1986.
176. Stokes KB, Church T: Ten-year experience with implanted polyurethane lead insulation. PACE 9:1160-1164, 1986.

177. Antonelli D, Rosenfeld T, Freedberg NA, et al: Insulation lead failure: Is it a matter of insulation coating, venous approach, or both? PACE 21:418-421, 1998.
178. Philips R, Frey M, Martin RO: Long-term performance of polyurethane pacing leads: Mechanisms of design-related failures. PACE 9:1166-1172, 1986.
179. Cameron J, Mond H, Ciddor G, et al: Stiffness of the distal tip of bipolar pacemaker leads. PACE 13:1915-1920, 1990.
180. Mugica J, Daubert JC, Lazarus B, et al: Is polyurethane lead insulation still controversial? PACE 15:1967-1970, 1992.
181. Phillips R, Frey M, Martin RO: Long-term performance of polyurethane pacing leads: Mechanisms of design-related failures. PACE 9:1166-1172, 1986.
182. Mond H, Sloman G: The small tined pacemaker lead: Absence of dislodgement. PACE 3:171-177, 1980.
183. Kertes P, Mond H, Sloman G, et al: Comparison of lead complications with polyurethane tined, silicone rubber tined, and wedge tip leads: Clinical experience with 822 ventricular endocardial leads. PACE 6:957-962, 1983.
184. Stokes KB: Recent advances in lead technology. In Barold SS, Mugica J (eds): New Perspectives in Cardiac Pacing. Mount Kisco, NY, Futura, 1988, pp 217-227.
185. Ormerod D, Walgren S, Berglund J, Heil R: Design and evaluation of a low threshold porous tip lead with a mannitol coated screw-in tip ("Sweet Tip"). PACE 11:1784-1790, 1988.
186. Bisping HJ, Kreuzer J, Birkenheier H: Three year clinical experience with a new endocardial screw-in lead with introduction protection for use in the atrium and ventricle. PACE 3:424-435, 1980.
187. Crossley GH, Brinkler JA, Reynolds D, et al: Steroid elution improves the stimulation threshold in an active-fixation atrial permanent pacing lead. Circulation 92:2935-2939, 1995.
188. Hidden-Lucet F, Halimi F, Gallais Y, et al: Low chronic pacing thresholds of steroid-eluting active-fixation ventricular pacemaker leads: A useful alternative to passive-fixation leads. PACE 23:1798-1800, 2000.
189. Mond H, Stokes KB: The electrode-tissue interface: The revolutionary role of steroid elution. PACE 15:95-107, 1992.
190. Mond H, Stokes K, Helland J, et al: The porous titanium steroid eluting electrode: A double blind study assessing the stimulation threshold effects of steroid. PACE 11:214-219, 1988.
191. Mond H, Stokes KB: The steroid-eluting electrode: A 10 year experience. PACE 19:1016-1020, 1997.
192. Kruse IM: Long-term performance of endocardial leads with steroid-eluting electrodes. PACE 9:1217-1219, 1986.
193. Hua W, Mond H, Sparks P: The clinical performance of three designs of atrial pacing leads from a single manufacturer: The value of steroid elution. Eur J Cardiac Pacing Electrophysiol 6:99-103, 1996.
194. Schuchert A, Hopf M, Kuck KH, et al: Chronic ventricular electrograms: Do steroid eluting leads differ from conventional leads? PACE 13:1879, 1990.
195. Kay GN, Brinker JA, Kawanishi DT, et al: Risks of spontaneous injury and extraction of an active fixation pacemaker lead: report of the Accufix Multicenter Clinical Study and Worldwide Registry. Circulation 100:2344-2352, 1999.
196. Parsonnet V, Roelke M, Bernstein AD, Stern M: Reduced frequency of retention wire fractures suggests that elective explantation of affected atrial leads is no longer indicated. PACE 23:380-383, 2000.
197. Lau C, Nishimura SC, Oxorn D, Goldman BS: Is this the natural history of the retention wire? A case report. PACE 20:1373-1376, 1997.
198. Kao HL, Wang SS, Chen WJ, et al: Migration of a fractured retention wire in the pulmonary artery from an active fixation atrial lead. PACE 18:1966, 1995.
199. Tatou E, Lefex C, Reybet-Degat O, et al: Intrapulmonary artery and intrabronchial migration and extraction of a fragment of J-shaped atrial pacing catheter. PACE 22:1829-1830, 1999.
200. Saliba BC, Ardesia RJ, John RM, et al: Predictors of fracture in the Accufix atrial "J" lead. Am J Cardiol 80:229-231, 1997.
201. Kawanishi DT, Brinker JA, Reeves R, et al: Cumulative hazard analysis of J-wire fracture in the Accufix series of atrial permanent pacemaker leads. PACE 21:2322-2326, 1998.
202. Lloyd MA, Hayes D, Holmes DR Jr: Atrial J-pacing lead retention wire fracture: Radiographic assessment, incidence of fracture and clinical management. PACE 18:958-964, 1995.
203. Important Information about Telectronics Accufix and Encor Atrial "J" Leads. Accufix Research Institute, April 2005.

Chapter 5

Sensors for Implantable Devices: Ideal Characteristics, Sensor Combinations, and Automaticity

HUNG-FAT TSE • CHU PAK LAU

Physiologic pacing aims to restore the rate and sequence of cardiac activation in the presence of abnormal cardiac automaticity and conduction. The atrial electrogram can be used for rate control if sinus node (SN) function is adequate. However, a high proportion of pacemaker recipients have abnormal SN function, either at rest or during exercise. Such chronotropic incompetence may be the result of medications or intrinsically abnormal SN function. In addition, in patients whose atrium is unreliable for sensing or pacing (e.g., during atrial fibrillation), an alternative means to simulate SN responsiveness is required.

These problems with the pacemaker function of the SN prompted the development of artificial implantable sensors for cardiac pacing. Although the optimal rate adaptation in a pacemaker recipient may be different from that of a healthy subject, it is assumed that these sensors should mimic the behavior of the healthy SN response to exercise and nonexercise needs. In addition, atrioventricular (AV) conduction is normally under the control of the autonomic nervous system, and a sensor may also contribute to adapting the AV interval to changes in atrial rate. The role of sensors has also been expanded to include functions other than rate augmentation—such as detection of ventricular capture and monitoring for heart failure, sleep apnea, and hemodynamic status. In this chapter, the basic principles and the clinical applications of sensors in implantable devices are reviewed.

Historical Landmarks of Rate-Adaptive Pacing

The limitations of dual-chamber pacing in the setting of SN dysfunction led to the development of nonatrial sensors. This development was possible because of the recognition that during exercise an increase in heart rate (HR), rather than the maintenance of AV synchrony, is the main determinant of increases in cardiac output.[1] Therefore, a single-chamber rate-adaptive pacemaker that varies the pacing rate with exercise according to a nonatrial sensor can achieve near-normal exercise physiology in patients with bradycardia.

Cammilli and associates[2,3] implanted the first rate-variable single-chamber pacemaker, which sensed changes in blood pH during exercise. In 1981, a "physiologically adaptive" cardiac pacemaker responding to changes in the QT interval during exercise was described by Rickards and Norman.[4] In the same year, Wirtzfeld and coworkers[5] reported the use of central venous oxygen saturation ($S\bar{v}O_2$) for the control of automatic rate-responsive pacing. Despite the fact that respiratory changes during exercise were proposed as a physiologic parameter to be sensed by a rate-adaptive pacemaker as early as 1975,[6] a rate-adaptive pacemaker capable of detecting the respiratory rate was introduced by Rossi and colleagues[7] only in 1982. With continuing research, the number of sensors available for rate-adaptive pacing steadily increased. In particular, activity sensors[8] and minute ventilation sensors[9,10] have been used with extensive clinical application.

Although single-chamber ventricular rate-adaptive pacing was originally meant to replace dual-chamber pacing, the additional benefits of atrial sensing and pacing became well recognized. Dual-chamber rate-adaptive pacing became available as early as 1986.[11] Since then, virtually all pacemaker companies have introduced their own versions of rate-adaptive dual-chamber devices. Technical improvement in the sensing of atrial electrograms with "floating," diagonally opposed atrial electrodes or closely spaced rings has enabled the use of a single-pass lead for VDD pacing. When combined with a rate-adaptive sensor, VDDR pacing with a single-pass lead has become a possibility.[12]

With the proliferation of sensor technology, it soon became apparent that none of the sensors could simulate the normal SN function in all aspects,[13] although different sensors were better in some areas of performance. Therefore, it was logical to combine sensors for optimal rate adaptation. Although this idea was not new, investigational units became available only in 1988,[14] first in the form of combined activity and QT-interval sensing, and later with combined activity and minute-ventilation sensors.[15] The increasing sophistication of sensors and their combinations prompted the use of automatic sensor calibration for optimal programming.[16-18]

Currently, rate-adaptive pacing has become a standard component of implantable devices and was incorporated into the pacing code after the joint effort between the North American Society of Pacing and Electrophysiology Mode Code Committee and the British Pacing and Electrophysiology Group. The original three-letter code for pacemaker mode proposed in 1974 was revised to the five-letter pacing code, and the rate-adaptive function is now denoted by the use of the letter *R* in the fourth position.[19-21]

Normal Heart Rate and Respiratory Responses to Exercise and Nonexercise Needs

Cardiac output is the product of HR and stroke volume. Stroke volume is enhanced during exercise when venous return increases cardiac filling, and cardiac contractility is augmented in response to sympathetic stimulation and a more vigorous pumping action of the skeletal muscles. Because of the difference in venous return, the changes in HR and cardiac hemodynamics are highly influenced by whether the exercise is carried out in the upright or supine posture.

Normal Heart Rate Response during Exercise

An anticipatory response of the HR occurs in many patients before exercise. With both supine and upright isotonic exercise, HR and cardiac output increase within 10 seconds after the onset of exercise.[22-24] This initial increase in HR is mediated by parasympathetic withdrawal rather than sympathetic stimulation. The cardiac output may increase by as much as 40% within three heartbeats after the onset of vigorous muscular exercise. Both cardiac output and sinus rate increase exponentially, with a half-time that ranges from 10 to 45 seconds (Fig. 5-1A), the rate of rise being proportional to the intensity of work (see Fig. 5-1B).[22] At the termination of upright exercise, there is a delay of about 5 to 10 seconds before cardiac output starts to decrease, followed by an exponential fall with a half-time of 25 to 60 seconds. The recovery time is related to age, work intensity, total work performed, and physical condition of the patient.[25] Although the optimal rate onset and decay kinetics for patients with pacemakers have not been firmly established, artificial sensors for rate-adaptive pacing should probably simulate the onset and recovery kinetics of the normal SN as the ideal physiologic standard.

Respiratory Changes during Exercise

The change in HR during muscular exercise is linearly related to oxygen consumption and workload. Because of the relationship between oxygen uptake and ventilatory volume during aerobic metabolism, minute ventilation is closely related to HR during exercise. At rest, the respiratory rate is typically between 10 and 20 breaths/min. During low-intensity exercise, an increase in tidal volume is the primary respiratory adaptation.[26] At higher work levels, a further increase in tidal volume of up to 50% of the vital capacity occurs, together with an increase in breathing frequency. The relationship between breathing rate and tidal volume varies considerably among individuals. In addition, the breathing rate is often synchronized with the work rhythm (e.g., the walking pace). However, because respiration is carefully controlled to maintain the concentration of arterial carbon dioxide within a narrow physiologic range, compensatory adjustments in tidal volume ensure an appropriate minute ventilation and gas exchange.

Minute ventilation (the product of breathing rate and tidal volume) is linearly related to the rate of carbon dioxide production. At low- and medium-intensity workloads, minute ventilation is also linearly related to oxygen consumption during incremental exercise.

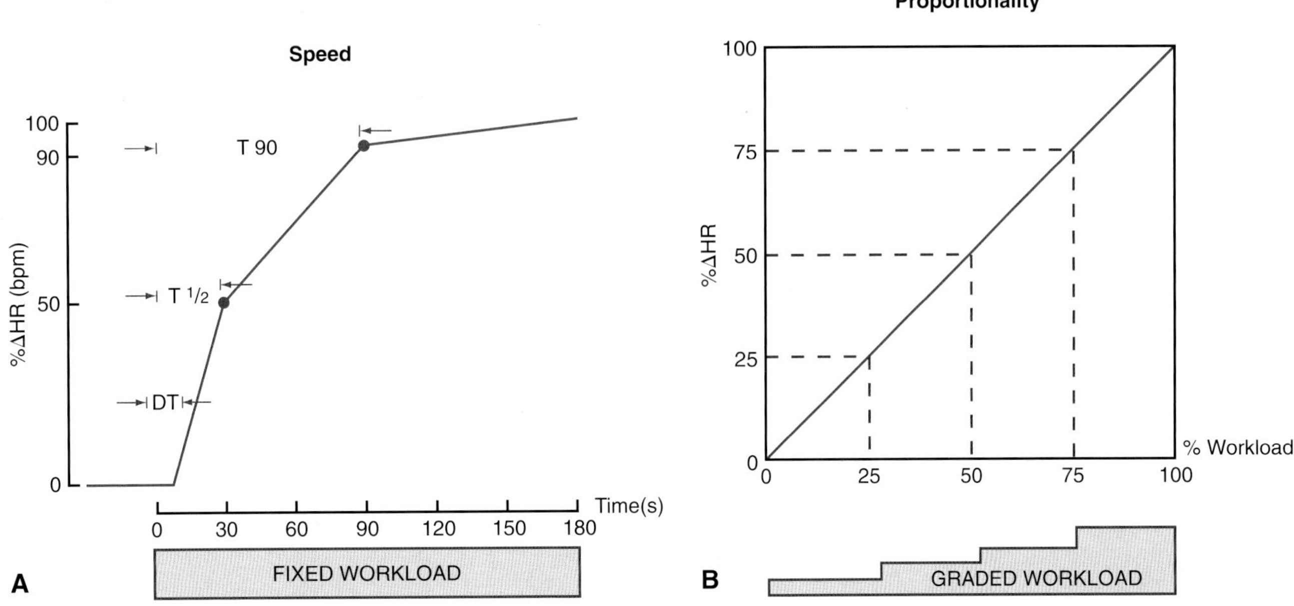

Figure 5-1. Quantification of sensor response: speed and proportionality. ***A,*** *The heart rate (HR) changes at the onset of exercise. The normal sinus rate responds almost immediately; one half of the change is achieved in less than 30 seconds, and most of the change is achieved within 1 minute. This speed of response was quantified by the response times; DT is the delay time, and T½ and T90 represent times needed to reach 50% and 90% of maximum HR, respectively. %ΔHR is the change in HR expressed as a percentage of the maximum increase in HR.* ***B,*** *Relationship between exercise workload and the HR increase during incremental exercise. The workload is expressed as a percentage of the maximum workload (% workload) at each quartile of exercise. The %ΔHR is linearly related to % workload, with a slope that is almost 1.*

Resting values for minute ventilation are about 6 L/min and can increase to 100 L/min during exercise for normal men and up to 200 L/min for trained athletes. Tidal volume may rise from a resting value of 0.5 L/min to 3 L/min at maximal exercise in normal individuals. The breathing rate may increase from a resting value of 12 to 16 breaths/min to 40 to 50 breaths/min during peak exercise. In normal children and some adults with restrictive lung disease, the respiratory rate may exceed 60 breaths/min.

At about 70% of the maximum oxygen uptake, the rate of tissue metabolism outstrips the rate of tissue oxygen delivery. Anaerobic metabolism of carbohydrate, fat, and protein is accelerated, resulting in an accumulation of lactic acid, the so-called anaerobic threshold. Acidosis is initially prevented by plasma buffers, but continuous lactate production eventually leads to excess production of carbon dioxide from plasma bicarbonate. This excess carbon dioxide stimulates the respiratory center, leading to respiratory compensation (increased minute ventilation). Hence, carbon dioxide production and minute ventilation increase in a manner that is disproportionate to the increase in oxygen consumption at workloads that surpass the anaerobic threshold. The anaerobic threshold is defined more clearly using a protocol in which the work intensity is increased more rapidly than with a gradual exercise protocol.

It has been customary to use the slope of the curve of HR versus minute ventilation as a measure of the appropriateness of rate adaptation by an artificial sensor, with the regression line at 1 to 2 bpm/L. In addition, this slope is said to be relatively independent of the functional class or the degree of left ventricular dysfunction.[27] At workloads that surpass the anaerobic threshold, however, oxygen consumption asymptotically reaches its maximum value, whereas carbon dioxide production and minute ventilation increase disproportionately to oxygen consumption. Because of the disproportionate increase in minute ventilation above the anaerobic threshold, the HR/minute ventilation slope is reduced. The reduction in the HR/minute ventilation slope above the anaerobic threshold, compared with below it, is an average of 29% for women and 26% for men.[28] This fact may be important, both in assessment of rate adaptation and in the design of the minute ventilation–sensing algorithms.

Oxygen Uptake Kinetics

In healthy subjects, exercise-induced cardiac and respiratory changes occur simultaneously to provide blood flow commensurate with the increase in oxygen consumption in the skeletal muscles. Figure 5-2 shows the oxygen uptake curve during exercise at a constant workload. When exercise begins, oxygen uptake increases gradually, following an exponential time course because of the slow adjustment of respiration and circulation, until it reaches a steady state at which oxygen uptake corresponds to the demands of the

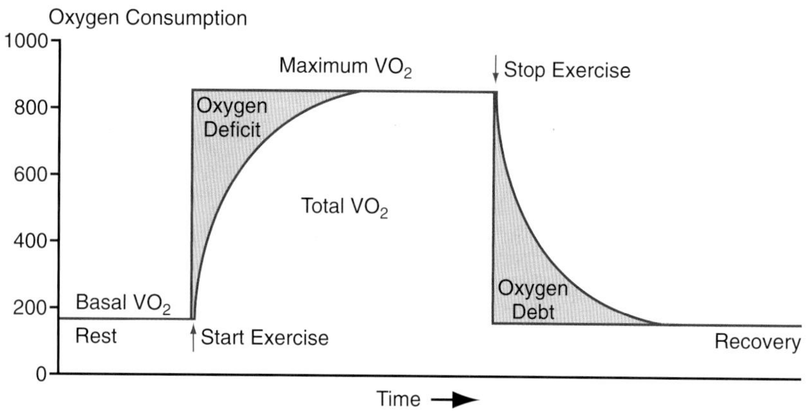

Figure 5-2. Oxygen kinetics during a steady-state exercise test. An oxygen deficit is incurred as the subject increases oxygen consumption (Vo_2) to the steady state, which usually takes 3 to 5 minutes. The incurred deficit is repaid at the termination of exercise as the oxygen debt. The oxygen deficit is closely related to the alactic oxygen debt; therefore, the oxygen debt, which includes the fast alactic and the slower lactic oxygen debt, is a better measurement of oxygen kinetics. (From Leung SK, Lau CP, Wu CW, et al: Quantitative comparison of rate response and oxygen uptake kinetics between different sensor modes in multisensor rate adaptive pacing. PACE 17:1920-1927, 1994).

tissues. Because oxygen uptake does not reach the required steady state immediately, the inadequate supply of energy from aerobic sources during the first 2 to 3 minutes must be met largely by use of creatine phosphate high-energy stores.[29] This inadequacy of oxygen use at the onset of exercise is described as the *oxygen deficit*. After exercise stops, replenishment of energy stores requires oxygen consumption in excess of the baseline recovery conditions before the oxygen uptake gradually decreases to the resting level. This elevated postexercise oxygen uptake repays the initial deficit and is described as repaying the "oxygen debt."[30]

The oxygen debt includes a fast alactic phase during moderate exercise. The magnitude of the oxygen deficit is usually found to be about equivalent to that of the oxygen debt in submaximal exercise before the anaerobic threshold is reached.[31] If the level of exertion remains relatively modest, the oxygen deficit may be paid back during exercise, so that the debt measured after exercise is actually less than the deficit at the onset. In contrast, during more strenuous exercise, the oxygen debt has both a fast alactic phase and a slower lactic phase, and the oxygen debt exceeds the size of the deficit.[32] The rate-limiting step for the increase in oxygen uptake at the onset of exercise is the rate of oxygen transport; this is primarily a cardiac function that is dependent on the change in pulmonary blood flow.[33,34] Therefore, an appropriate rate response behavior is the best way to ensure optimal oxygen delivery with either submaximal or maximal exercise. Because the oxygen debt may require a long period for repayment and may be affected by postexercise oxygen consumption for processes other than the simple deficit repayment,[35] and because of variability in recovery of the baseline oxygen consumption,[36] the oxygen deficit is used to assess the contribution of rate response to oxygen transport.

By artificially increasing the rate response of a sensor beyond that expected of the SN, it was shown that oxygen deficit was reduced, compared with an optimal sensor setting. The dependence on a quick initial response to minimize oxygen debt was demonstrated in studies of minute ventilation and activity and dP/dt sensors,[37,38] and oxygen uptake kinetics is often used as a sensitive indicator of appropriate rate-adaptive response at the submaximal workload.

Heart Rate Response during Exercise in Patients with Heart Disease

In patients with significant heart disease (e.g., heart failure, ischemic heart disease), pharmacologic treatment with β-blockers[39] and/or coexisting chronotropic incompetence[40-43] frequently limits the increase in HR during exercise, which may have a negative effect on exercise capacity. In patients with heart failure, the ability to augment left ventricular stroke volume and ventricular filling without a concomitant increase in left atrial pressure during exercise may be lost. Because the left atrial pressure is already high, the atrial contribution to left ventricular stroke volume is small. In addition, maintaining left ventricular stroke volume during exercise by increasing myocardial contractility is also markedly attenuated in patients with heart disease. HR augmentation is therefore a major determinant of cardiac output during exercise. Appropriate rate adaptation during exercise may provide incremental benefit to patients with heart disease. Conversely, inappropriate use of rate-adaptive pacing with excessive tachycardia in patients with heart disease may lead to an adverse outcome.[44]

Heart Rate Modulation for Nonexercise Needs

Exercise is but one of the many physiologic requirements for variation in HR (Table 5-1). Emotions such as anxiety may trigger a substantial change in HR. The sinus rate is higher when a person moves from the supine to the upright posture, and cardiac output decreases. Isometric exercise also results in an increase in cardiac output and HR.[45] An appropriate compensatory HR response is especially important in pathologic conditions such as anemia, acute blood loss, or other causes of hypovolemia.

The normal resting HR peaks during the day and reaches a trough in the early morning hours during sleep. A sensor that is responsive only to exercise will increase the pacing rate during periods of physiologic stress, but the lower rate remains fixed at the programmed base rate. This faster programmed lower rate, which is normal for the day, may be too rapid during periods of rest. The lack of an ability to decrease the

TABLE 5-1. Some Physiologic Factors that Affect the Responses of the Sinus Node to Body Requirements

Exercise—isotonic and isometric, during and after exercise
Postural changes
Anxiety and stress
Postprandial changes
Vagal maneuvers
Circadian changes
Fever

pacing rate in patients with VVI pacemakers during sleep may result in palpitations and sleep disturbances.[46] By means of sensors that are always active in monitoring the level of metabolic demand, the appropriate lower rate can be calculated and adapted to individual need (see later discussion). HR increases during febrile episodes may be detected by a sensor that measures the central venous temperature.[47]

Components of a Rate-Adaptive Pacing System

At least three aspects of a rate-adaptive pacing system influence its rate-modulating characteristics (Fig. 5-3). First, a sensor (or a combination of sensors) must detect a physical or physiologic parameter that is either directly or indirectly related to metabolic demand. Second, the rate-modulating circuit in the pulse generator must have an algorithm that relates changes in the sensed parameter to a change in pacing rate. The design of the rate-control algorithm can have a profound impact on the overall rate-response characteristics of a pacing system. Third, because the magnitude of the physical or physiologic changes that are monitored by a sensor differs among patients, physician input is usually necessary to adjust the algorithm (usually by programming one or more rate-responsive variables) to achieve the clinically desired rate response.[48]

Classification of Sensors

Physiologic Classification

A *primary* sensor is defined as one that detects the *physiologic factors* that control the normal SN during varying metabolic needs.[49] Primary sensed parameters include circulating catecholamines and autonomic nervous system activities. Although these parameters may be the most physiologically accurate indicators for use by a rate-adaptive pacing system, technical realization of a rate-adaptive pacemaker that uses a primary sensor has yet to be achieved.

The bulk of rate-adaptive sensors that have been proposed belong to the class of *secondary* sensors, those that detect physiologic parameters that are a *consequence* of exercise. Some of these parameters, such as the QT interval,[4] respiratory rate or minute ventilation,[9,10,50-52] average atrial rate,[53] central venous temperature,[47,54,55] venous blood pH,[2,3] right ventricular stroke volume,[56] pre-ejection interval[57] or pressure,[58] $S\bar{v}O_2$,[5,59] and ventricular inotropic indices (ventricular inotropic parameter[60,61] and peak endocardial acceleration[62,63]) have been developed for either clinical or investigational pacing systems. Each of these physiologic variables responds to the onset of exercise with its own

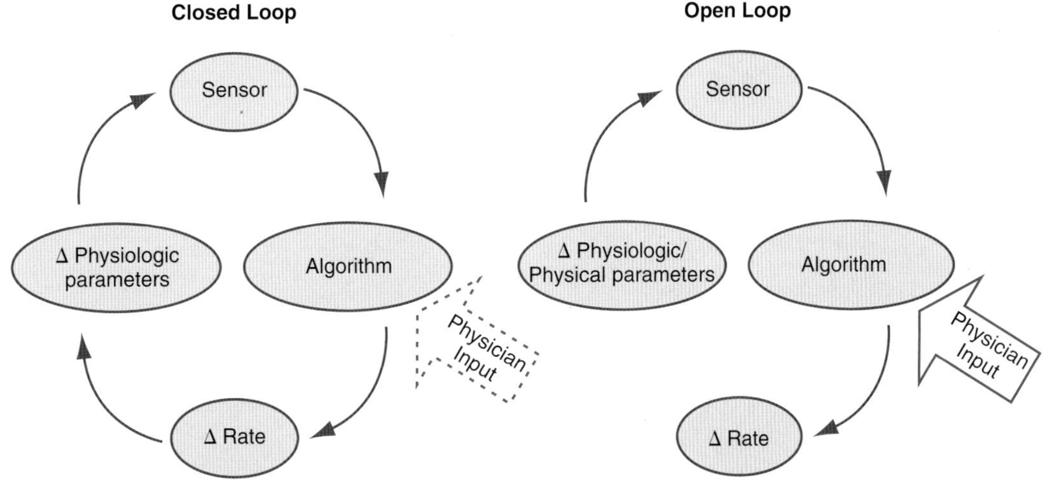

Figure 5-3. Design of a rate-adaptive system. Open loop: The physiologic or physical change detected by the sensor is converted to a change in rate using an algorithm. The resultant rate change does not have a negative feedback effect on the physiologic/physical parameter. Closed loop: The physiologic change detected by the sensor is converted to a change in rate using an algorithm. The resultant rate change induces a change in the physiologic parameter in the opposite direction, thereby establishing a negative feedback loop.

kinetics and has a different proportionality to exercise workload.

The *tertiary* sensors detect *external changes* that result from exercise. An example of a tertiary sensed parameter is body movement.[64] As expected, the relationship between exercise workload and these tertiary variables is less tightly linked, and there is often greater susceptibility to environmental influences, such as vibration. Other measures, such as the use of a 24-hour clock to vary the lower pacing rate, can be considered tertiary sensors. Likewise, in the most primitive rate-adaptive pacemaker, the pacing rate was changed by the patient, using a hand-held programmer, before beginning exercise.[65]

Technical Classification

Although conceptually attractive, the physiologic classification does not adequately separate the bulk of the so-called secondary sensors. A more practical classification is to categorize sensors according to the technical methods that are used to measure the sensed parameter (Table 5-2). During isotonic exercise, body movements (especially those produced by heel strike during walking) result in changes in acceleration forces that are transmitted to the pacemaker. Sensors that are capable of measuring the acceleration or vibration forces in the pulse generator are broadly referred to as activity sensors. The sensing of *body vibrations* is therefore a simple way to indicate the onset of exercise. Technically, detection of body movement can be achieved with the use of a piezoelectric crystal, an accelerometer, a tilt switch, or an inductive sensor. Each of these devices transduces motion of the sensor, either directly into voltage, or indirectly into measurable changes in the electrical resistance of a piezoresistive crystal. Although activity sensing is a tertiary sensor, it is the most widely used control parameter in rate-adaptive pacing because of its ease of implementation and its compatibility with all standard unipolar and bipolar pacing leads.

Impedance is a measure of all factors that oppose the flow of electric current and is derived by measuring resistivity to an injected electric current across a tissue. The impedance principle has been used extensively for measuring respiratory parameters[66,67] and parameters associated with right ventricular contractility, such as relative stroke volume or the pre-ejection interval,[68] in situations involving invasive monitoring. The elegant simplicity of impedance has enabled it to be used with implantable pacing leads, including both standard pacing leads and specialized multielectrode catheters. The pulse generator casing has been used as one electrode for the measurement of impedance in most of these pacing systems. Impedance can be used to detect relative changes in ventilatory mechanics, right ventricular mechanical function, or the combination of these parameters. Relative motions between electrodes for impedance sensing also lead to changes in imped-

TABLE 5-2. Major Classes of Sensors Used in Rate-Adaptive Pacing, Classified According to Method of Technical Realization

Methods	Physiologic Parameter	Models	Manufacturers*
Vibration sensing	Body movement	Sigma, Kappa, Enpulse	Medtronic
		Diamond, Clarity, Selection AF	Vitatron
		Talent	ELA Medical
		Miniswing, Neway	Sorin Biomedica
		Insignia, Pulsar Max, Discovery	Guidant
		Actros, Protos, Philos	Biotronik
		Identity, Integrity, Affinity	St. Jude Medical
Impedance sensing	Minute ventilation	Kappa	Medtronic
		Talent	ELA Medical
		Insignia, Pulsar Max	Guidant
	Ventricular inotropic parameter	Protos, Inos	Biotronik
	Pre-ejection interval	Precept†	Guidant
	Lung fluid status	InSync Sentry	Medtronic
Ventricular evoked response	Evoked QT interval	Diamond, Clarity, Selection AF	Vitatron
Special sensors on pacing electrode	**Physical parameters**		
	Central venous temperature	Thermos†	Biotronik
	dP/dt	Deltatrax†	Medtronic
	Right ventricular pressure	Chronicle‡	Medtronic
	Pulmonary arterial pressure	—	—
	Peak endocardial acceleration	Best-Living system	Sorin Biomedica
	Chemical parameters		
	pH	—	—
	Mixed venous oxygen saturation	OxyElite†	Medtronic
	Catecholamine	—	—

*Biotronik GmbH & Co., Berlin; Guidant, Boston Scientific, Natick, Mass.; ELA Medical, Sorin Group, Milan; Medtronic, Inc., Minneapolis, Minn.; Sorin Biomedica, Sorin Group, Milan; Vitatron, Dieren, the Netherlands.

†Not commercially available.

‡Investigational device.

ance, and this is inversely related to the number of electrodes used to measure impedance.[69] In rate-adaptive pacemakers, motion artifacts are usually the result of arm movements that cause the pulse generator to move within the prepectoral pocket,[70,71] thereby changing the relative electrode separation between the pacemaker and the intracardiac electrodes. Because arm movement accompanies normal walking, these artifacts in the impedance signal occur with both walking and upper limb exercises.

The *intracardiac ventricular electrograms* resulting from a suprathreshold pacing stimulus have been used to provide several parameters that can guide rate modulation. The area under the curve inscribed by the depolarization phase of the paced ventricular electrogram (the intracardiac R wave) has been termed the *ventricular depolarization gradient* or *paced depolarization integral* (PDI).[72] In addition to depolarization, the total duration of depolarization and repolarization can be estimated by the interval from the pacing stimulus to the intracardiac T wave (the QT or stimulus-to-T interval). Both of these parameters are sensitive to changes in HR and circulating catecholamines and can be derived from the paced intracardiac electrogram with conventional pacing electrodes. Because a large polarization effect occurs after a pacing stimulus, a modified waveform of the output pulse that compensates for afterpotentials is needed to eliminate this effect, so that these parameters can be accurately measured. The interaction of the "square wave" output pulse with the endocardium of a ventricular pacemaker leads to a distortion of the pacing waveform,[73,74] and the "shape" of the resultant output pulse has been proposed to be useful in estimating intracardiac volume.

The last group of sensors are those that are incorporated into a specialized pacing lead. Examples of these leads include thermistors (used to measure blood temperature), piezoelectric crystals (used to measure right ventricular pressure), optical sensors (used to measure $S\bar{v}O_2$), and accelerometers at the tip of pacing leads. Some of these sensors measure highly physiologic parameters. For example, $S\bar{v}O_2$ is closely related to oxygen consumption during exercise. Physical activities increase cardiac output and oxygen extraction from the blood, and a widening of the tissue arteriovenous oxygen difference occurs during exercise.[59,75,76] However, $S\bar{v}O_2$ is not linearly related to the workload, and most of the drop in $S\bar{v}O_2$ occurs during the first minute of exercise, with less decrease in $S\bar{v}O_2$ with increased workload. The preliminary clinical experience with implanted $S\bar{v}O_2$ sensors showed a rate response proportional to exercise level.[77-80] In one study, the rate response of an $S\bar{v}O_2$ sensor (OxyElite, Medtronic, Inc., Minneapolis, Minn.) was compared with that of a conventional piezoelectric activity sensor during activities of daily living (ADLs) and non–exercise-related physiologic changes. The $S\bar{v}O_2$ sensor showed a better proportionality of rate response than the activity sensor and occurred at a comparable speed of onset.[78,79] The main concern with the $S\bar{v}O_2$ sensor is its long-term stability, which may be affected by fibrin coating on the sensor. Although to a certain extent this instability is reduced by using two different wavelengths for $S\bar{v}O_2$ measurements, the sensor's ability to function in the long term remains an issue.[79]

Right ventricular pressure can be detected by a hermetically sealed pressure sensor containing a piezoelectric crystal and electronic circuitry incorporated into a pacing lead. The first derivative of the right ventricular pressure (dP/dt) is influenced by the contractile state of the heart, the ventricular filling pressure, and the HR, with a positive correlation between maximum dP/dt and sinus rate in healthy subjects.[80] The change in the maximum value of dP/dt is a sensitive indicator of the change in right ventricular contractility and is directly proportional to change in sympathetic tone.[81,82] The dP/dt sensing principle is highly proportional to workload, as shown in a limited number of investigational implants (Deltatrax, DPDT, Medtronic). The pacing rate achieved with the dP/dt sensor was reported to correlate well with estimated oxygen consumption during exercise ($r = 0.93$).[13,83,84] The increases in pacing rate paralleled the HR that was expected from the metabolic reserve during treadmill testing in the VVIR mode. Exercise time was significantly prolonged in the VVIR mode compared with the VVI mode during paired exercise testing.[85]

An accelerometer incorporated at the tip of a unipolar ventricular electrode can be used to assess the contractile state indirectly from the endocardial vibration generated during isovolumic contraction of the heart, a parameter known as *peak endocardial acceleration* (PEA).[86,87] Such a microaccelerometer has been developed by Sorin Biomedica (Saluggia, Italy) and has a frequency response of up to 1 kHz and a sensitivity of 5 mV/G (1 G = 9.8 m/sec). In preliminary experience in sheep under basal conditions using an external system and an implantable radiotelemetry system, the PEA was not affected by HR but was significantly increased by emotional stress, exercise, and natural inotropic stimulation.[86] This parameter follows the changes in the maximum left ventricular dP/dt and apparently measures the global left ventricular contractile performance rather than the regional mechanical function of the right ventricle.[88,89] In preliminary studies on the PEA-driven rate-adaptive pacemaker, there was a good correlation between the sinus rate and the PEA-indicated rate during ADLs and a submaximal stress test.[90,91] A potential role of the PEA is its ability to optimize the A-V interval automatically. Limitations with this sensor system are several. First, the effects of the relative contributions of valvular movement and change in preload to the myocardial vibrations and the measured PEA are uncertain. Second, this system requires a dedicated lead with unproved long-term reliability and stability, although an initial study on sheep showed acceptable medium-term results.[87]

Closed-loop versus Open-loop Sensors

A rate-adaptive pacing system can operate in either a *closed-loop* or an *open-loop* manner. In a completely closed-loop system (see Fig. 5-3), the physiologic parameter that is monitored is used to effect a change in the pacing rate. Changes in pacing rate in turn induce a physiologic change in the sensed parameter in the opposite direction. Therefore, closed-loop pacing systems have *negative feedback,* such that the sensed physiologic variable tends to return toward its baseline value in the presence of an appropriately modulated pacing rate. A partial degree of closed-loop negative feedback control is observed with pacemakers that use $S\bar{v}O_2$ as the rate-control parameter.[59,75,76] Exercise in the absence of adequate cardiac output (as in a patient with a fixed-rate pacemaker) increases tissue oxygen extraction from arterial blood, thereby decreasing the content of oxygen in the returning venous blood. This decrease in $S\bar{v}O_2$ can be measured and used to increase the pacing rate, thereby increasing the cardiac output to a value that is optimal for the level of exercise workload, resulting in improved oxygen delivery to the tissues. Under conditions of equilibrium, the pacing rate is adjusted to maintain the maximum possible $S\bar{v}O_2$ for any level of metabolic demand. The PDI has also been advocated as a closed-loop sensed parameter.[72] An increase in sympathetic activity decreases the PDI, whereas an increase in HR increases it, thereby establishing a negative feedback loop that tends to maintain the sensed parameter at a relatively constant value during exercise. However, true closed-loop performance was not achieved in clinical trials with this sensor. Theoretically, the physician input required for a closed-loop system should be minimal, because the system is designed to be fully automatic. In practice, a rate-adaptive algorithm is still necessary, because the available pacing systems provide only partial closed-loop negative feedback. In an ideal closed-loop system, the sensor automatically takes into account any changes in the patient's cardiovascular condition. Apart from setting the lower and upper rate limits, the physician can indirectly control the rate changes in a closed-loop system by determining the speed at which the pacing rate adjusts to return the sensed parameter to its baseline value.

Although a closed-loop sensor is theoretically attractive, the practical application of this concept has been less than ideal. Normal control of HR involves multiple parameters and feedback measures, and it is unlikely that a single sensor can accurately control HR in all clinical circumstances. In addition, a closed-loop sensor involved in rate control may be affected by factors other than metabolic demand. Therefore, at present, the potential of closed-loop sensors remains unrealized.

Open-loop logic is employed in most available sensors that measure either physiologic or biophysical parameters (see Fig. 5-3). In such open-loop systems, a change in the HR does not result in a negative feedback effect on the physiologic or physical parameter used to modulate the pacing rate. Therefore, open-loop algorithms require the physician to prescribe the relationship between the parameter monitored by the sensors and the desired change in pacing rate. An example of this is an activity-sensing pacing system that detects body movements. Physical exercise results in acceleration forces on the pulse generator that can be used to increase the pacing rate.[8,64] The resultant increases in pacing rate usually have minimal effects on body movement.

In the extreme case, a positive feedback of HR on the rate-control parameter might occur, as exemplified by the old version of the QT interval sensing pacemaker. The QT interval shortens during exercise. However, an increase in the pacing rate itself induces further shortening of the QT interval, especially if a linear slope is used to relate changes in the QT interval to changes in pacing rate. Increases in pacing rate during exercise could shorten the QT interval excessively, leading to an excessive increase in rate.[92] This type of "sensor feedback tachycardia"[93] has also been described with rate-adaptive pacemakers that detect minute ventilation[94] or body activity.[95] The mixed venous oxygen sensor also has the potential for positive feedback during exercise-induced myocardial ischemia. For example, the $S\bar{v}O_2$ decreases in response to either reduced cardiac output (e.g., during ischemia) or increased oxygen consumption. If exercise-induced ischemia is the cause, the resultant decrease in $S\bar{v}O_2$ might trigger a further increase in pacing rate, which may further exacerbate myocardial ischemia. Such a scenario has been observed with this sensor.

Rate-Control Algorithms and Rate-Response Curves

The term *algorithm* refers to the way in which the raw sensor data are converted to a change in pacing rate. Typically, sensor data are first filtered to exclude unwanted signals (e.g., signals outside the frequency range of the rate-control parameter). The changes in the sensor signal over an averaged baseline (or, on rare occasions, the absolute sensor signals) are used for further processing. The filtered signals are appropriately modified through rectification and gain control (Fig. 5-4). The processed signals are then used to modulate pacing rate through the application of a rate-control algorithm. The physician must determine the ultimate rate response that will be observed by choosing the lower pacing rate, the upper pacing rate, and a rate-response curve that determines the slope of the sensor-pacing rate relationship. In some pacemakers, the physician can also modify the rate response by changing the "filter" used to process the raw sensor signal. An example of such filtering is the threshold feature of activity-sensing pacemakers. The relationship between the processed signals and pacing rate can be linear, curvilinear, or a more complex function (see Fig. 5-4).

An example of an even more complex rate-response curve is the biphasic pattern of response of a more recent minute ventilation sensor. This algorithm provides a steeper slope of the pacing rate–minute ventilation relationship at the beginning of exercise than at the end of the exercise. The initial aggressive slope is made possible by a separately programmable "rate augmentation factor," so that different slopes control

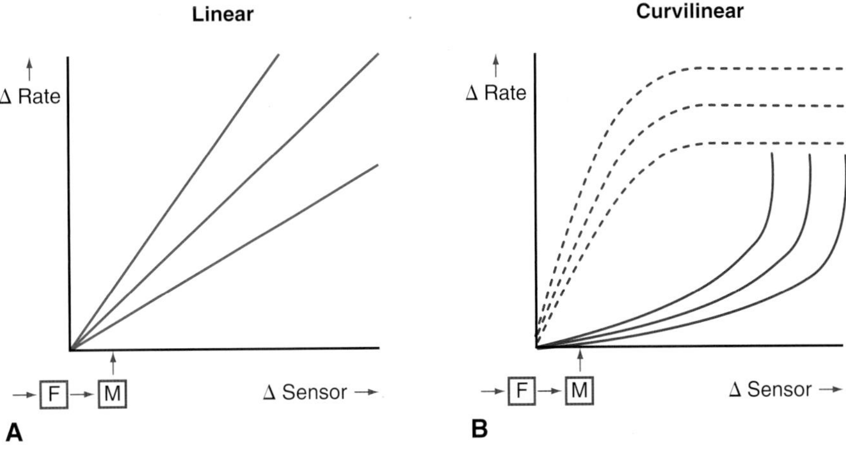

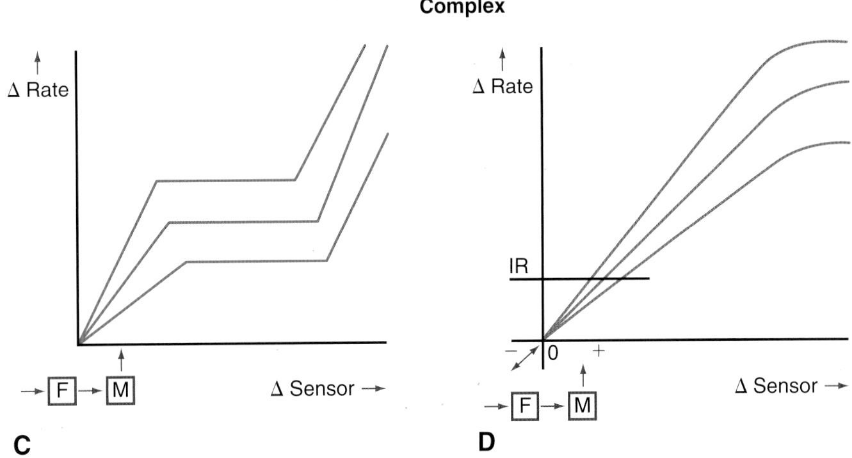

*Figure 5-4. Types of rate-responsive curves used in rate-adaptive pacemakers employing a single sensed parameter (sensor level). An appropriate filter (F) eliminates unwanted raw signals (e.g., high- or low-pass frequency filters and thresholds). The filtered signals are then appropriately modified (M) (e.g., with gains and rectification) before being converted to a rate change. The curves can be linear (**A**), curvilinear (**B**), or complex (**C** and **D**). The physician can select an appropriate rate-responsive slope from a family of curves. See text for further discussion. IR, interim rate.*

the first and second halves of the pacing range. Furthermore, a linear relationship is maintained within the aerobic range of exercise but a less aggressive slope is used above the anaerobic threshold, where minute ventilation increases disproportionately to the HR change.

Perhaps the most sophisticated rate-response curves are those proposed for temperature sensing (see Fig. 5-4D). In one algorithm, a curvilinear relation is employed when the temperature increases. Because a temperature "dip" characteristically occurs at the beginning of exercise, this algorithm responds to a rapid decline in temperature with a rapid increase in the pacing rate to an interim value. Subsequent increases in temperature are used to modulate further increases in pacing rate. In addition to programming the rate-response curve, temperature-sensing pacing systems provide for a gradual decrease in the lower pacing rate in response to diurnal variation in blood temperature (*bidirectional arrow* in Fig 5-4D). Thus, the rate of change in the rate-control parameter (in this case, a slow decrease in temperature within predefined limits during periods of rest) is used to vary the lower rate limit. Although the rate-response curves discussed previously define the relationship between sensor output and increases in pacing rate during exercise, many rate-adaptive pacemakers use a different set of curves to control decreases in pacing rate during the recovery phase.

Note that the rate-response curves that have been discussed relate changes in the sensed parameter to changes in the *desired* pacing rate. In addition to these sensor-desired, pacing rate-response curves, other factors control the speed (or time constant) with which the sensor-indicated desired pacing rate is translated into a change in the *actual* pacing rate. Obviously, an abrupt change in the sensed parameter must be translated into a gradual increase (or decrease) in the pacing rate. For example, if the activity signals of a pacemaker were to double abruptly, the rate-response curve might indicate that the pacing rate should be increased from 70 to 100 bpm. The interval required for the pacing rate to increase from 70 to 100 bpm is a programmable feature in some rate-adaptive pacing systems and has a fixed time constant in others. Similarly, if the sensor indicates that the pacing rate should be decreased from 100 bpm to 70 bpm, a time constant is required to translate this desired change into an actual decline in pacing rate. These "attack" and "decay" constants can have a major effect on the chronotropic response characteristics of rate-adaptive pacemakers.

Characteristics of an Ideal Rate-Adaptive Pacing System

The normal human SN increases the rate of its spontaneous depolarization during exercise in a manner that is linearly related to Vo_2. Because this response undoubtedly has evolutionary advantages, the goal of rate-adaptive pacemakers that modulate pacing rate by artificial sensors has been to simulate the chronotropic characteristics of the SN. It is uncertain, however, whether the SN provides the ideal rate response in patients who require permanent pacemakers. Nevertheless, until there is evidence indicating otherwise, rate-adaptive pacemakers will strive to reproduce this physiologic standard. Keeping these uncertainties in mind, the ideal rate-adaptive pacing system should provide pacing rates that are *proportional* to the level of metabolic demand. In addition, the change in pacing rate should occur with kinetics (or *speed of response*) similar to those of the SN. The artificial sensor should be *sensitive* enough to detect both exercise and non-exercise needs for changes in HR and yet be *specific* enough not to be affected by unrelated signals arising from both the internal and the external environments. Although the ideal sensor should provide these functional characteristics, it must also be technically feasible to implement with a reliability that is acceptable with modern implantable pacemakers (Table 5-3).[96]

TABLE 5-3. Characteristics of an Ideal Sensor for Rate-Adaptive Pacing

Considerations	Examples and Remarks
Sensor consideration	
Proportionality	Oxygen saturation sensing has good proportionality
Speed of response	Activity sensing has the best speed of response
Sensitivity	QT sensing can detect non–exercise-related changes, such as anxiety reaction
Specificity	Activity sensing is affected by environmental vibration
	Respiratory sensing is affected by voluntary hyperventilation
Technical consideration	
Stability	Stability of early pH sensor was a problem
Size	Large size or requirement for additional electrodes may be a problem
	Energy consumption must not harm pacemaker longevity unduly
Biocompatibility	Important for sensor in direct contact with the bloodstream
Ease of programming	Difficult programming in early QT-sensing pacemakers

Principles Used for Comparing and Evaluating Rate-Adaptive Systems

Proportionality of Rate Response

One of the best indicators of sensor proportionality is the correlation between the sensor-indicated pacing rate and the level of oxygen consumption during exercise.[13] In general, parameters such as minute ventilation and the paced QT interval are proportional sensors. Some sensors for which specialized pacing leads are used are also highly proportional. For example, $S\bar{v}o_2$ is closely related to oxygen consumption during exercise.

To assess the proportionality of chronotropic response during exertion, the exercise workload should be increased gradually. Traditional treadmill exercise protocols used to evaluate coronary artery disease usually aim to reach maximum HR rapidly and tend to skip the lower workloads (3-5 Mets) that are performed normally by pacemaker recipients in their daily lives. Exercise protocols with gradually increasing workloads, such as the Chronotropic Assessment Exercise Protocol, are probably more appropriate for assessing the rate response of a pacemaker over the wider range of workloads (and oxygen consumption) that are relevant to these patients.[97] Graded exercise testing to maximal tolerated workload may be impractical for some patients for assessing the function of a rate-adaptive pacemaker. Brief, submaximal ramp exercise tests are especially valuable for assessing the proportionality of current rate-adaptive pacing systems.[13] These tests can be "informal," such as asking the patient to walk at varying speeds or to ascend and descend stairs. In addition, monitoring of pacemaker function during ADLs may provide the most clinically relevant method of evaluating an elderly patient. Alternatively, submaximal exercises, such as treadmill tests at a low speed and grade, may be performed to assess the sensor response. These tests show that walking at a faster speed increases the pacing rate of most rate-adaptive pacemakers. However, the rate is not necessarily increased by walking up a slope in patients with activity-sensing pacemakers, which respond according to the pattern of body motion or vibration associated with each type of activity. For example, with many activity-sensing pacemakers, ascending stairs is associated with a lower pacing rate than is descending stairs, because the intensity of the heel strike is less walking upstairs than downstairs. These findings suggest that there is only a moderate correlation between the rate achieved by activity-sensing pacemakers and exercise workload.

These differences in chronotropic response may not be detected with graded treadmill exercise. Ambulatory electrocardiographic (ECG) monitoring, rate histograms, or stored rate trends may provide useful methods for evaluating the chronotropic response of rate-adaptive pacing systems in patients who are less active or who cannot exercise. Furthermore, very few patients with pacemakers (or, indeed, in the general population) exercise to maximal levels of workload on a regular basis. Therefore, formal exercise testing may have little clinical relevance in these patients.

Speed of Onset of Rate Response and Recovery from Exercise

An appropriate speed of response of the pacing rate to the onset of and recovery from exercise is an essential feature of a rate-adaptive pacing system. The onset kinetics are best assessed during treadmill exercise, such as walking at a fixed speed on the treadmill. From ECG monitoring, the *delay time* for the onset of rate response, the time required to reach one half of the maximum change in pacing rate during exercise (half-time), and the time required to reach 90% of the maximum response can be derived and used as a basis for comparison. The exercise responses of six different types of rate-adaptive pacemakers (with sensors for activity, QT interval, respiratory rate, minute ventilation, and right ventricular dP/dt) were compared with normal sinus rate in one study.[13] The results demonstrated that the activity-sensing pacemakers best simulated the normal speed of rate response at the start of exercise. The rate response of activity sensors is usually immediate (no delay time), and the half-time was within 45 seconds from the onset of exercise. The maximum change in pacing rate was reached within 2 minutes after beginning an ordinary activity, such as walking. The respiratory rate and the right ventricular dP/dt sensors had a longer delay time (about 30 seconds) and half-time (1 to 2 minutes), although the maximum change in rate was still attained within 2 to 3 minutes after beginning exercise. The slowest sensor to respond to exercise was an early version of the QT-sensing pacemaker, which required up to 1 minute to initiate a rate response, and the maximum change in pacing rate was attained only in the recovery period after a short duration of exercise. The onset of rate response and proportionality to workload of the QT-sensing pacemaker was in sharp contrast to those of activity-sensing pacemakers.

The speed of onset of the newer generation of QT-sensing pacemakers has been significantly improved by the use of a linear (rather than curvilinear) rate-response slope that produces a larger change in pacing rate per unit change in QT interval at the onset of exercise (slow HRs) than at higher workloads.[98] These minute ventilation–sensing pacemakers produce an increase in pacing rate that is linearly related to minute ventilation throughout exercise, providing the effect of shortening the rate-response half-time. Furthermore, the speed of onset of rate response is programmable in these newer generations of minute ventilation sensors.

After termination of exercise, body movement decreases, and the pacing rate of an activity-sensing pacemaker returns toward the resting level based on an arbitrary rate-decay curve.[99] If the rate decay is faster than is physiologically appropriate, adverse hemodynamic consequences may occur in the presence of a substantial decrease in HR. In one study in which pacing rate was reduced either abruptly or gradually after identical exercise, it was shown that an appropriately modulated rate recovery was associated with a higher cardiac output, lower sinus rate, and faster lactate clearance, compared with a nonphysiologic rate-recovery pattern.[100] Appropriate adjustment of the rate-recovery curve is important to enhance recovery from exercise.

Sensitivity of a Rate-Adaptive Pacing System to Changes in Exercise Workload and Other Physiologic Stresses

Table 5-4 shows the factors to which some rate-adaptive pacemakers are sensitive. Rate-adaptive pacemakers that are controlled by ventricular-evoked response and intracardiac hemodynamic parameters are able to respond to emotional stresses. A reverse rate response has been observed during the Valsalva maneuver in patients with respiratory sensing pacing systems and some dP/dt sensing pacemakers. None of the available pacemakers reliably detects changes in posture, although several sensors, such as intracardiac impedance or accelerometer designs, have the potential to do so (Fig. 5-5).[79,101,102] A paradoxical decrease in HR may be observed during movement to the upright position with pacemakers that sense the ventricular depolarization gradient.[103] A varying postural drop in HR has also been reported with a rate-adaptive pacemaker that detects the dP/dt.[89,90] A diurnal rate variation is possible with temperature-sensing and QT-sensing pacemakers. The clinical implication of some of these rate changes to nonexercise stimuli remains to be determined.

Specificity of Rate-Adaptive Pacing Systems

One of the main limitations of activity-sensing pacemakers is their susceptibility to extraneous vibrations. This typically occurs during various forms of transport. The degree of susceptibility to extraneous vibrations may vary with different types of activity sensors. For example, an accelerometer using a tilt switch (Swing, Sorin Biomedica) may be one of the most susceptible types. The QT interval and the PDI may be significantly affected by such factors as cardioactive medications and myocardial ischemia. Ischemia may result in shortening of the QT interval, leading to an increase in pacing rate and further myocardial ischemia.[104,105] Sensors that use impedance to measure respiratory mechanics or the right ventricular pre-ejection interval are susceptible to artifacts produced by arm movement, hyperventilation, and speech.[70,71,106] Electric diathermy is likely to cause inappropriate changes in pacing rate in pacemakers that

TABLE 5-4. **Physiologic Sensitivity of Some Currently Available Rate-Adaptive Pacemakers**

Physiologic Measure	Exercise		Emotion	Valsalva Maneuver	Posture	Diurnal Variation
	Isotonic	Isometric				
Sinus	+	+	+	+	+	+
Activity	+					
Respiration	+			R		
QT interval	+		+			+
Gradient	+	+	+		R	
Temperature	+		±			+
PEI	+	+	+		V	
dP/dt	+	+	+	V	V	
$S\bar{v}O_2$	+	+				
PEA	+		+		+	
VIP	+		+			

dP/dt, maximum first derivation of right ventricular pressure; PEA, peak endocardial acceleration; PEI, pre-ejection interval; R, reversed response; $S\bar{v}O_2$, mixed venous oxygen saturation; V, variable; VIP, ventricular inotropic parameter.

measure impedance.[107] The same problem may be expected to occur during radiofrequency ablation in impedance-sensing pacemakers. In addition, external temperature change can significantly affect the pacing rate of temperature-sensing pacemakers.

Clinical Contraindications to Specific Rate-Adaptive Sensors

A number of clinical factors may preclude the use of some sensors for an individual patient (Table 5-5). When a parameter can be detected only at the ventricular level, the sensor cannot be used in an AAIR pacing system. The use of antiarrhythmic medications, the use of β-blockers, and the presence of myocardial ischemia may interfere with the detection of the QT and affect its duration. The QT system is sensitive to adrenergic stimulation and response to emotional stress.[108,109] In patients with ischemic heart disease, this response to psychological stress may occasionally be excessive, with an undesirable rate increase, thereby precipitating angina. Excessive adrenergic tone may cause a QT pacemaker to pace at the upper rate limit in the setting of acute myocardial infarction, creating an undesirable and potentially harmful response.[104,105] On the other hand, the dP/dt sensor does not appear to be adversely affected by myocardial ischemia.[110] The clinical impact of ischemia in patients with rate-adaptive pacemakers controlled by oxygen saturation remains to be determined.[78]

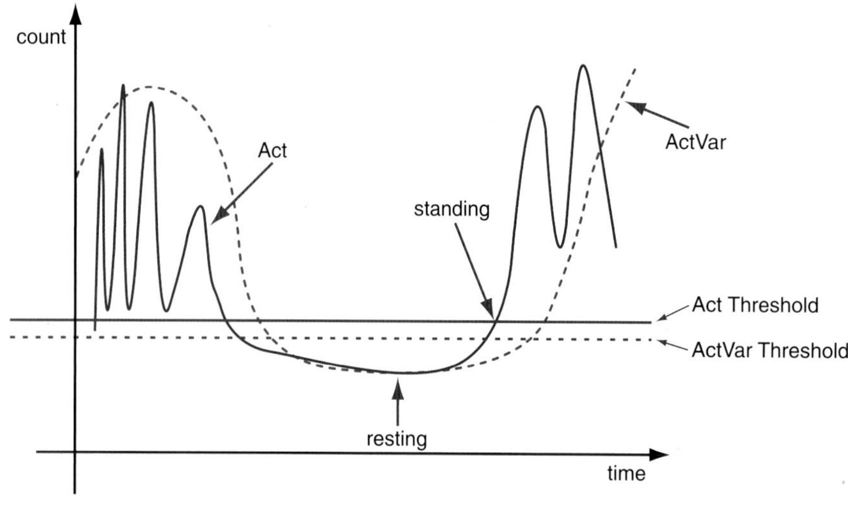

Figure 5-5. Schematic representation of the Orthostatic Response (OSR) algorithm for detection of posture change. The accelerometer sensor provides two outputs: the instantaneous activity level (Act, solid line) and the moving average of the absolute difference between Act levels (ActVar, dotted line). If both signals are lower than the corresponding threshold (horizontal lines), prolonged rest is detected. With changes in posture, the Act rises above the Act threshold, ActVar remains below ActVar threshold, and OSR pacing is triggered. (From Tse HF, Siu CW, Tsang V, et al: Blood pressure response to transition from supine to standing posture using an orthostatic response algorithm. PACE 28:S242-S245, 2005.)

TABLE 5-5. Clinical Factors Contraindicating Use of Some Currently Available Rate-Adaptive Pacemakers

Factor	Atrial Pacing	Antiarrhythmic Drugs	Myocardial Ischemia	Young Children or Respiratory Disease	Standard Unipolar Lead	Exposure to High-Vibration Environment
Activity						—
Respiration				—	—	
QT interval	—	—	—			
Gradient	—	—	—		—	
Temperature	±				—	
PEI	—	—	—		—	
dP/dt	—	±	—		—	
$S\bar{v}O_2$	±			—	—	
PEA	—	±	±		—	±
VIP	—	±	—			

dP/dt, maximum first derivation of right ventricular pressure; PEA, peak endocardial acceleration; PEI, pre-ejection interval; $S\bar{v}O_2$, mixed venous oxygen saturation; VIP, ventricular inotropic parameter; —, unsuitable; ±, feasibility remains to be validated.

The minute ventilation–sensing pacemakers are best avoided in young children, who may have very rapid respiratory rates during exercise that exceed the range detected by the pacemaker. Inappropriate tachycardia may occur in patients with advanced heart failure and the rapid breathing phase of Cheyne-Stokes dyspnea.[94] During cesarean section[111] and general anesthesia,[112] passive hyperventilation may induce pacemaker tachycardia; hence, a non–rate-adaptive mode is preferred when these patients undergo general anesthesia. Electrocautery in the thoracic area may affect impedance-sensing pacemakers and may lead to upper rate pacing; therefore, it is preferable to program the pacemaker to the non–rate-adaptive mode when electrocautery or radiofrequency ablation is used.[107]

Occupations associated with exposure to vibrations in the environment, such as horseback riding,[113] and various types of transportation that may cause rate acceleration are a relative contraindication to the use of an activity sensor. In patients with heart failure, the use of temperature sensors tends to be difficult because a prolonged temperature fall occurs at the onset of exercise in some of these patients.[114] In addition, replacing or upgrading a pulse generator requires that the new sensor be compatible with the existing pacing lead, unless a new lead is contemplated. Therefore, if a unipolar ventricular pacing lead is to be used, a minute-ventilation pacemaker that requires a bipolar lead in the ventricle is not feasible.

Sensor Combinations

The only sensors that are presently in clinical use are those that can be used with a standard lead. The instability of sensors requiring a special lead prevents their widespread use for rate adaptation. The surviving sensors include activity, minute ventilation, intracardiac impedance, and QT sensors (used only in combinations). Combining artificial sensors is feasible and may be superior to rate adaptation with a single sensor. In addition, automatic programming of sensors is feasible and effective, making the complexity of multisensor pacemaker programming an insignificant issue.

Justification for Sensor Combinations

There has been significant improvement in instrumentation, and rate-adaptive algorithms have been incorporated in the "clinical sensors" to address the issues of speed of onset, proportionality, specificity, and sensitivity of sensor response. For example, piezoelectric crystals for activity sensing using a "peak counting" algorithm are limited by the relatively poor ability of the sensor to differentiate between different levels of workload[99] and their susceptibility to external vibration. Some of these aspects are improved by the use of an accelerometer and an algorithm that integrates the activity signals to determine the sensor-indicated rate.[115-117] Because body movement has no direct relationship to metabolic requirement, however, this sensor remains inadequate to detect isometric exercise, nonexercise needs, and exercises that do not result in significant vibration (e.g., bicycle riding).

Minute ventilation as measured by impedance delivers appropriate rate-adaptive therapy that is proportional to workload.[9,10] Criticism has centered on the slower HR response of minute ventilation sensors to the

TABLE 5-6. **Components of a Multisensor System for Rate-Adaptive Pacing**

Speed of Response	Proportionality	Sensitivity	Specificity	"Energy Saver"
Activity	Minute ventilation	Diurnal variation: 24-hour clock Diurnal activity change Diurnal minute ventilation change	Minute ventilation	Detection of capture: Evoked QRS Stroke volume
	QT	Emotional response: QT PEA	QT	Rate reduction during sleep
	PEA		Activity	Minimize myocardial oxygen consumption

PEA, peak endocardial acceleration.

onset of exercise, as compared with activity sensors, with a 30-second delay when compared with the response of the SN.[118] This response is also potentially influenced by conditions that may not be directly relevant to cardiac output, such as talking or voluntary respiration.[119] New, faster algorithms with a programmable rate augmentation factor and speed of response have improved this slow response during the early stages of exercise.[120] This, however, leads to a more rapid recovery, with a significantly shortened recovery time at the end of exercise.

The main limitation of the QT sensor is the relatively slow speed of onset of the rate response[121] and the susceptibility of the QT interval to drugs and ischemia. With the use of curvilinear rate-response curves that have a higher slope at the onset of exercise, the lag in the onset of rate response is reduced,[98] but the speed of rate response is still too slow during brief periods of exercise.[122] Therefore, the new generation of clinical sensors remains imperfect, even when only speed and proportionality of rate response are considered. In addition, apart from the QT and the ventricular impedance sensors, which react to emotional changes,[123] none of the other clinical sensors is sensitive to nonexercise needs such as changes induced by postural, postprandial, and vagal maneuvers; fever; and circadian variations.

These limitations of the available sensors mean that none of them is suitable for every patient under all circumstances. Despite the fact that the response of a sensor can be significantly enhanced by fine-tuning the characteristics of the sensor and the algorithms used to translate sensor output into modulation of pacing rate, the "clinical" sensors are mainly limited because a fast-responding sensor is not proportional, whereas a proportional sensor is relatively slow (Table 5-6). In addition, an activity sensor is relatively insensitive to nonexercise stress and is nonspecific and liable to external interference.

Dual sensor combinations are aimed to create an integrated sensor that simulates the SN response of healthy individuals by combining the strong points and eliminating the weak points of the individual sensors (Table 5-7). The sensor combination aims to improve the speed of rate response, proportionality to workload, sensitivity to physiologic changes induced by exercise and nonexercise requirements, and specificity in rate adaptation (Fig. 5-6). A sensor that is more specific to the onset of exercise can be used to prevent false-positive rate acceleration caused by a more sensitive yet relatively nonspecific sensor. In the absence of the specific sensor indicating that exercise is occurring, the HR response of the other sensor can either be nullified or restrained.

Multisensor pacing may also offer the possibility of selecting an alternative sensor should one sensor fail or become inappropriate for an individual patient. In addition, an appropriate rate of recovery can shorten

TABLE 5-7. **Relative Advantages of Clinically Used Sensors**

	Speed	Proportionality	Specificity	Sensitivity
Activity	High	Low	Low	Low
Minute ventilation	Moderate	High	Moderate	Low
QT interval	Low	Moderate	High	Moderate
PEA	Moderate	Moderate	Moderate	High
VIP	Moderate	Moderate	Moderate	High

PEA, peak endocardial acceleration; VIP, ventricular inotropic parameter.

repayment of oxygen debt and promote lactate clearance.[100] The potential for combining sensors for purposes other than rate modulation during exercise is a strong incentive for the development of multisensor pacemakers.

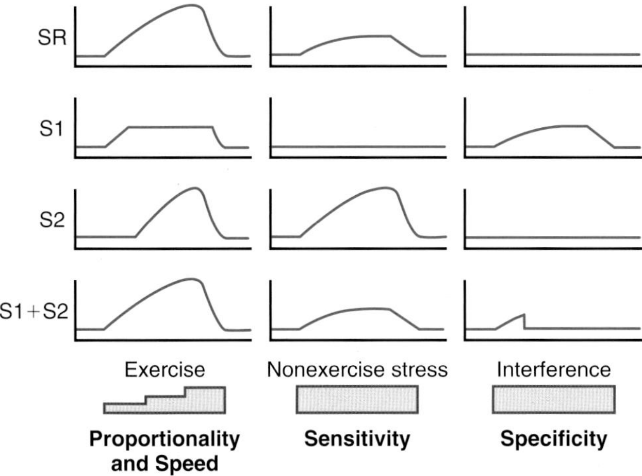

Figure 5-6. Algorithms for sensor combinations needed to achieve better (1) proportionality and speed of response, (2) sensitivity, and (3) specificity. The graphs (top to bottom) depict the responses of the sinus node (SR), sensor 1 (S1), sensor 2 (S2), and combined rate profile of S1 and S2. SR shows ideal proportionality, speed of rate response, and freedom from interference. S1 is a rapidly responding sensor, although it is neither proportional nor sensitive and is susceptible to interference. S2 is a proportional and sensitive sensor, although it has a slow response. It is also specific to exercise. Note the improved ability of the combined sensor approach in simulating the sinus rate under different conditions.

Principles for Integrating Rate-Adaptive Sensors

Algorithms for Combining Rate-Adaptive Sensors

Two basic methods for combining sensors to control chronotropic response during exercise have been used. The types of sensor combination can be "faster-win" or "blending" (Fig. 5-7A and B). In the faster-win form, the inputs from two sensors are compared, and the sensor indicating the faster rate is chosen to regulate the pacing rate. A differential combination (blending) combines the input of two sensors, either as a fixed ratio of one sensor to the other or as a variable ratio that changes in relation to the HR. For example, a fast-responding sensor (such as an activity sensor) can be used to modulate pacing rate at the onset of exercise, with a second sensor (such as a minute ventilation or QT sensor) to modulate the pacing rate during more prolonged exercise. The pacing rate may increase to an "interim" or intermediate value when the faster sensor detects the onset of exercise; a more proportional rate increase will occur when the slower, more proportional sensor "catches up." A variation of this approach is to calculate the output of each sensor in a relative proportion, so that the ultimate rate profile is a blend of both.

The pacing rate can be controlled by two sensors that have different sensitivities to exercise and nonexercise physiologic stresses, so that the system can respond to both exertional and emotional needs. It is conceivable that separate rate-adaptive slopes (or different upper and lower rates) can be programmed for modulation of rate in response to exertional versus

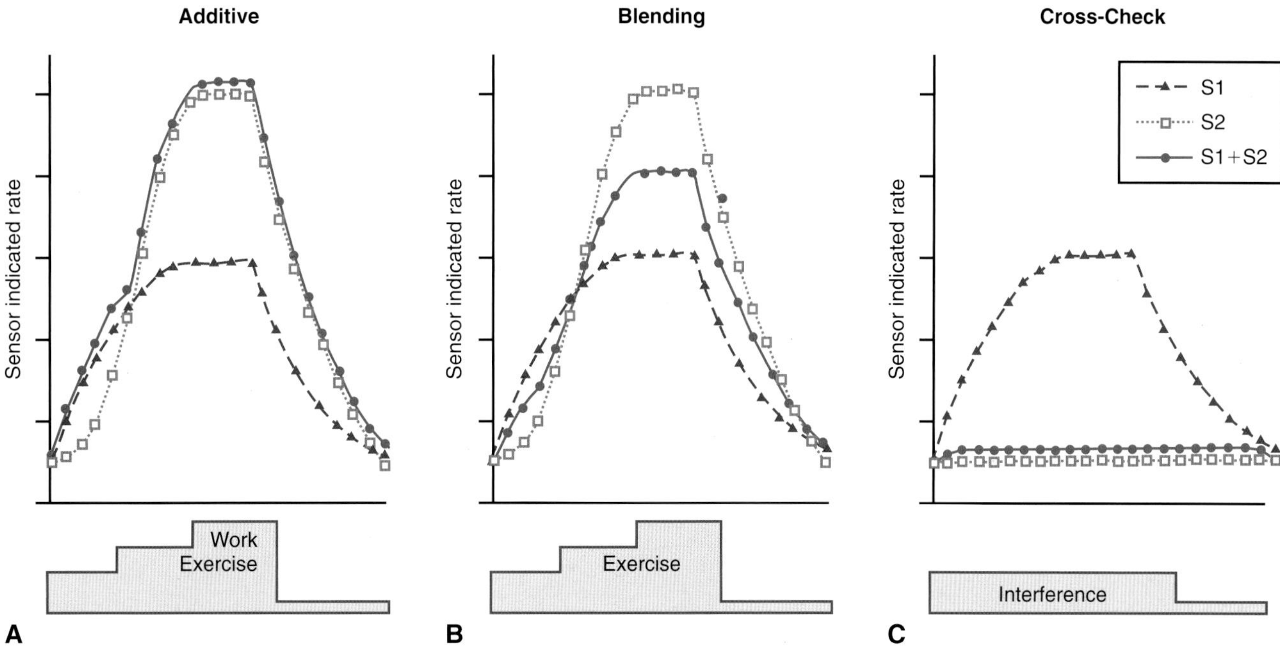

*Figure 5-7. Algorithms to combine sensors. **A,** In the faster-win algorithm, the faster rate, from either sensor 1 (S1) or sensor 2 (S2), is chosen. **B,** In the blending algorithm, the sensor rate responses from S1 and S2 are blended to give an intermediate rate. **C,** In the sensor cross-checking algorithm, the more specific sensor S2 cross-checks the less specific fast sensor S1 when S2 does not indicate the presence of exercise.*

emotional needs. The algorithm can be designed to weigh the input of both sensors to diagnose a nonexercise physiologic stress and provide a different pattern of rate adaptation.

Sensor Cross-Checking Algorithms for Enhancing Specificity

The response of one sensor can also be checked against the output from another sensor to improve the specificity of the chronotropic response (see Fig. 5-7C). A more specific sensor may be used to cross-check a nonspecific sensor, thereby avoiding inappropriate rate acceleration. In this instrumentation, the rate adaptation of a less specific sensor is allowed to increase the pacing rate only over a restricted range of HRs and for a limited duration. In the absence of a determination of exercise by the other sensor, the diagnosis of false-positive rate acceleration with the first sensor is made, and the pacing rate returns to the baseline, so that prolonged high rate pacing is avoided. Such sensor cross-checking can be reciprocal between the two sensors, so that either sensor may limit the chronotropic response that results from the other. In practice, cross-checking is usually applied to limit the less specific of the two sensors.

Possible Sensor Combinations

A number of possible sensor combinations have been suggested (see Table 5-6). One of the simplest is a 24-hour clock that is used to vary the lower pacing rate. The normal diurnal variation in HR is well recognized, and an automatic decrease in the lower rate during the hours of sleep is physiologically appropriate. Battery consumption can also be reduced by this reduction in average pacing rate. Because of its simplicity, reliability, and compatibility with any pacing lead, an activity sensor that has a fast onset of response to exercise may be used as one sensor in combination with another sensor that provides a more proportional response to workload. An activity sensor can be easily added to the pulse generator. It requires minimal energy consumption to operate and is compatible with other sensors. Activity has been combined with central venous temperature,[124] a parameter that is more proportional to metabolic need during prolonged exertion than is activity. Similarly, the combination of QT interval and activity sensing (e.g., Diamond, Vitatron B.V., Arnhem, The Netherlands) enhances the speed of response compared with a QT sensor alone.[14,125-127] An activity sensor has been combined with a minute ventilation sensor in single- and dual-chamber pacemakers (e.g., Kappa 400, Medtronic; Pulsar Max and Insignia, Guidant, Boston Scientific, Natick, Mass.; Symphony and Talent, ELA Medical, Sorin Group, Milan).

The sensing of intracardiac impedance is one of the simplest ways to combine sensors. Despite the many possible sensor combinations, only three clinical sensors have been used clinically in sensor combination (activity, minute ventilation, and QT).

Dual-sensor Rate-adaptive Pacemakers

QT and Activity

In the Topaz and Diamond pacemakers (Vitatron), a piezoelectric sensor is used for activity sensing. The algorithms for combining the activity and QT sensors are both blending and cross-checking. Activity and QT input can be programmed at different contribution levels: activity < QT, activity = QT, or activity > QT, representing ratios of 30:70, 50:50, and 70:30, respectively. To avoid false rate acceleration by the activity sensor, the pacemaker allows activity rate response for only a short duration unless confirmed by changes in QT sensor (sensor cross-checking).

The blending of the QT and activity sensors shows a quick rate response at exercise onset and a more proportional rate response during the latter part of exercise and during the recovery period.[125] The fast rate-adaptive response during the first stage of exercise is due primarily to the activity sensing, with a high correlation between the activity sensor counts and the mean pacing rate (r = 0.94). The QT sensor predominates during higher levels of exertion, with a low correlation between activity sensor counts and the pacing rate (r = 0.14).[125] In a multicenter study of 79 patients with the Topaz pacemaker, exercise in the dual-sensor mode produced a more gradual rate response than it did with the activity mode alone. The rate profile during treadmill exercise testing with dual-sensor pacing was improved over that of single-sensor pacing.[38,126] In one study, simultaneous recording and comparison of combined sensor pacing and the sinus rate during ADLs and standardized exercise testing were performed in 12 patients. There was an improved correlation between the dual-sensor-indicated rate and the sinus rate with the combination, compared with either individual sensor alone (Fig. 5-8).[127] Furthermore, an inappropriate high rate response from the activity sensor caused by external vibrations could be limited by sensor blending and cross-checking (Fig. 5-9).[128,129] With a too-sensitive activity sensor setting, however, activity counts may be registered at rest when the QT sensor is inactive. This may result in cross-checking of the activity sensor by the QT sensor, which could delay the speed of the dual-sensor rate response when exercise begins.[129]

Minute Ventilation and Activity

A piezoelectric activity sensor has been combined with a minute ventilation sensor to improve the initial response time while allowing a proportional rate response to higher workload. In the Kappa 400 pacemaker (Medtronic), the pacing rate is determined by automatic blending of the activity and minute ventilation sensors, using daily activities as a guide. Both sensors in the Kappa 400 contribute to the sensor-indicated rate between the lower and an interim rate limit, the so-called ADL rate.[130] The influence of the activity sensor diminishes and shifts toward the minute ventilation sensor as the integrated sensor-indicated rate increases toward the ADL rate. At HRs greater than

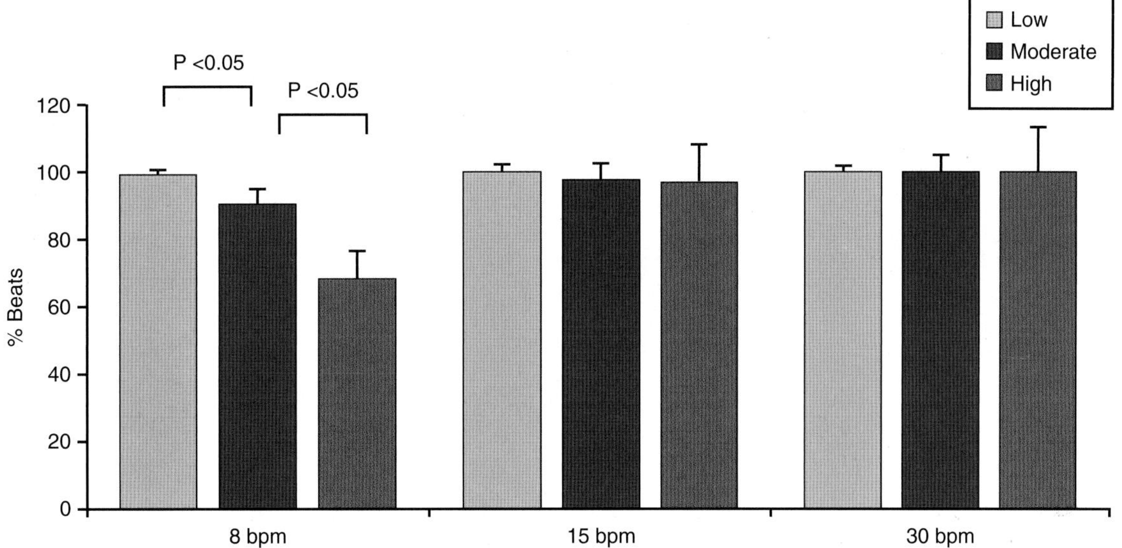

Figure 5-8. Differences between sinus and sensor-indicated rates from 12 patients during daily activities. At a low level of exercise, most of the sensor-indicated rates were within 8 bpm of the sinus rate; at higher exercise workloads, the sinus-sensor differences increased. The difference between the sensor-indicated rate and the sinus rate was almost always within 15 bpm at all rate ranges. The difference between the sinus and sensor-indicated rate was almost always less than 30 bpm even at high exercise workloads. (From Lau CP, Leung SK, Guerola M, et al: Efficacy of automatically optimized rate adaptive dual sensor to simulate sinus rhythm: Evaluation by continuous recording of sinus and sensor rates during exercise testing and daily activities. PACE 19:1672-1677, 1996.)

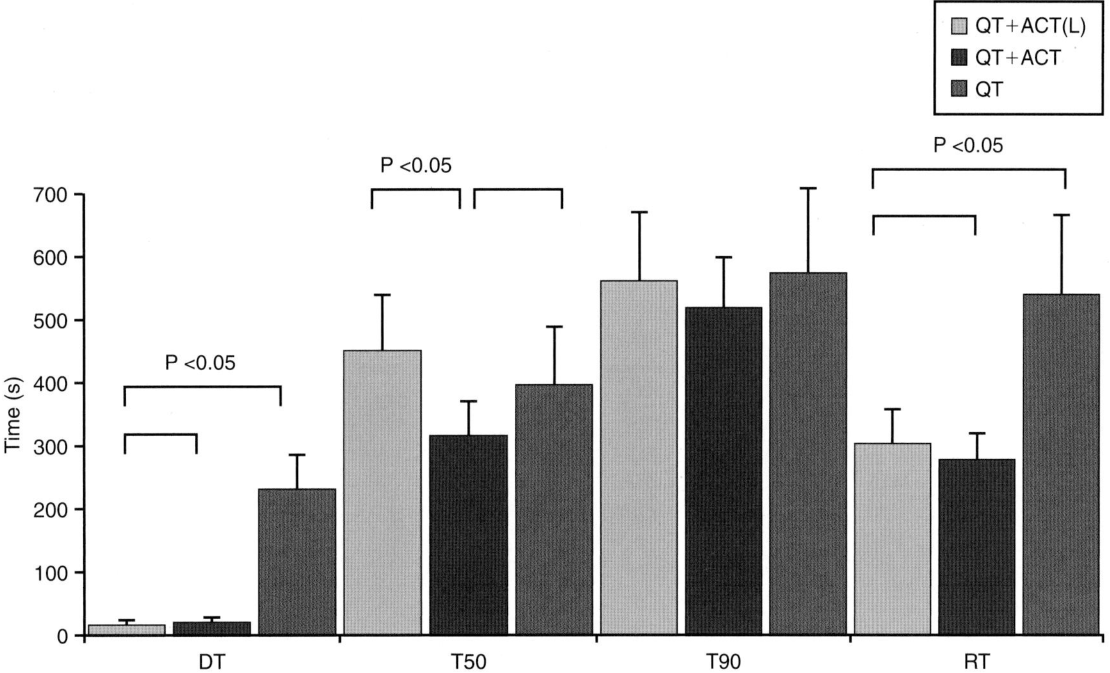

Figure 5-9. Rate-response kinetics of dual-sensor modes compared with QT-only VVIR pacing. DT, delay time; RT, recovery time; T50 and T90, time to reach 50% and 90% of rate response, respectively; QT + ACT, dual-sensor VVIR mode with optimally programmed activity sensor; QT + ACT (L), dual-sensor VVIR mode with an overprogrammed activity sensor (lowest threshold). (From Lau CP, Leung SK, Lee SFI: Delayed exercise rate response kinetics due to sensor cross-checking in a dual sensor rate adaptive pacing system: The importance of individual sensor programming. PACE 19:1021-1025, 1996.)

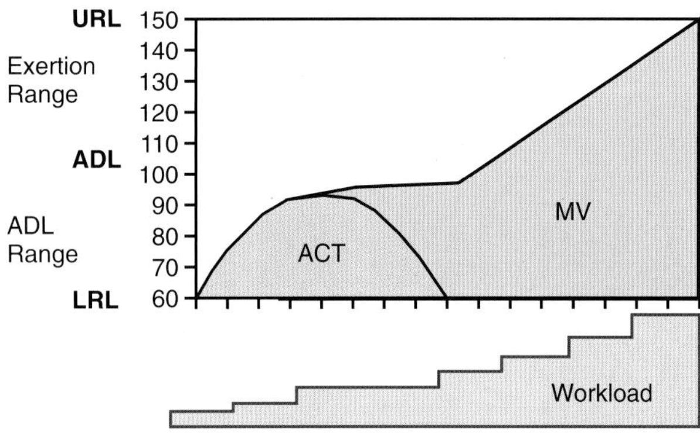

Figure 5-10. Sensor integration algorithm used by Kappa 400 (Medtronic) combined minute ventilation (MV) + activity sensor (ACT) pacemaker. ACT contributes to the integrated sensor-indicated rate between the lower rate limit (LRL) and activity of daily living (ADL) rate. The influence shifts toward the MV sensor until the ADL rate is achieved; thereafter, MV determines the exertional rate up to the upper rate limit (URL). (From Leung SK, Lau CP, Tang MO, et al: New integrated sensor pacemaker: Comparison of rate responses between an integrated minute ventilation and activity sensor and single sensor modes during exercise and daily activities and nonphysiological interference. PACE 19:1664-1671, 1996.)

the ADL rate, the pacing rate is controlled by the minute ventilation sensor alone (Fig. 5-10).[130] The activity sensor also cross-checks against high minute ventilation–indicated pacing rates. Such cross-checking is activated if the activity sensor counts are low, and the increase in the minute ventilation-indicated rate is limited. This minimizes the influence of nonphysiologic minute ventilation signals associated with upper body motion (e.g., arm movement) or during hyperventilation.[130]

During treadmill exercise and stair climbing, the combined sensor mode was shown to be more proportional to low and high workload activities than the activity VVIR sensor mode but similar to the minute ventilation VVIR sensor mode.[15,131] There was a faster speed of rate response with a shorter delay time, time to reach 50% of the overall rate response, and time to reach 90% of the rate response in the Kappa 400 pacemaker, compared with the minute ventilation sensor alone during submaximal exercise and ADLs. Although the sensor rate kinetics between the activity sensor and the combined minute ventilation and activity sensor were similar,[131] the average maximal sensor rate was significantly higher for the dual-sensor mode than for either the activity or minute ventilation mode alone during ADLs (Fig. 5-11).

Automaticity

An appropriate rate-control algorithm or careful programming can overcome some intrinsic limitations of many sensors. In contrast, inappropriate programming of a pacing system can distort the chronotropic response of an otherwise ideal sensor. In addition, programming of rate-adaptive sensors is often time-consuming for clinicians. It may involve repeated exercise testing. The use of a dual-sensor pacemaker can more than double the effort required for appropriate programming. There is no simple standard for programming one sensor, and often the sensor is programmed to achieve an output based on the physician's "assessment" of the patient's overall physical state and activity level. For the patient, apart from the inconvenience of repeated reprogramming, the appropriate rate response may change over time as cardiac conditions change. Therefore, the ability of a sensor to adjust itself automatically is not only a convenience for patients and physicians but also a clinical necessity. Automaticity can be achieved using a closed-loop sensor (theoretical only), semiautomatic adjustment, or autoprogramming.

Semiautomatic Programming

To simplify programming, many rate-adaptive pacemakers automatically determine the sensor output during a given workload and suggest the sensor threshold or slope settings that will provide a prescribed pacing rate. In the Sensolog and Synchrony activity-sensing pacemakers (Siemens-Elema AB, Solna, Sweden), sensor data were collected during casual and brisk walking to define two levels of exercise workload. The appropriate rate-adaptive parameters were then derived automatically to achieve the desired HR response.[132-134] The advantage of programming the activity sensor using walking as opposed to treadmill exercise testing is that the rate-response parameters determined by treadmill exercise tend to result in a higher than expected rate during ADLs and are highly dependent on the type of footwear worn.[132,134,135] In the accelerometer-based pacemakers (Discovery, Guidant), acceleration data are collected during a 1- to 3-minute exercise test and automatically coupled to a programmable rate response, a feature known as "tailor to patient." This is useful to achieve an appropriate rate response sufficient for most patients during ADLs. However, because the rate-adaptive slope uses a triphasic curve, which has a more aggressive slope at the lower and higher levels of exercise, a formal exercise test may still be needed to assess the rate-response characteristics at the higher workloads.

Autoprogrammability

There are currently two methods of automatic programming for open-loop sensors: one using sensor matching at upper and lower rate limits, and the other using a target rate distribution approach.

Automatic Rate Adaptation by Matching Sensor Output at Upper and Lower Pacing Rate Limits

An automatic slope adaptation mechanism has been incorporated in the new version of the QT-sensing pacemaker (Rythmx, Vitatron)[16] and in combined QT- and activity-sensing pacemakers (Topaz VVIR and Diamond DDDR, Vitatron). This algorithm involves two different

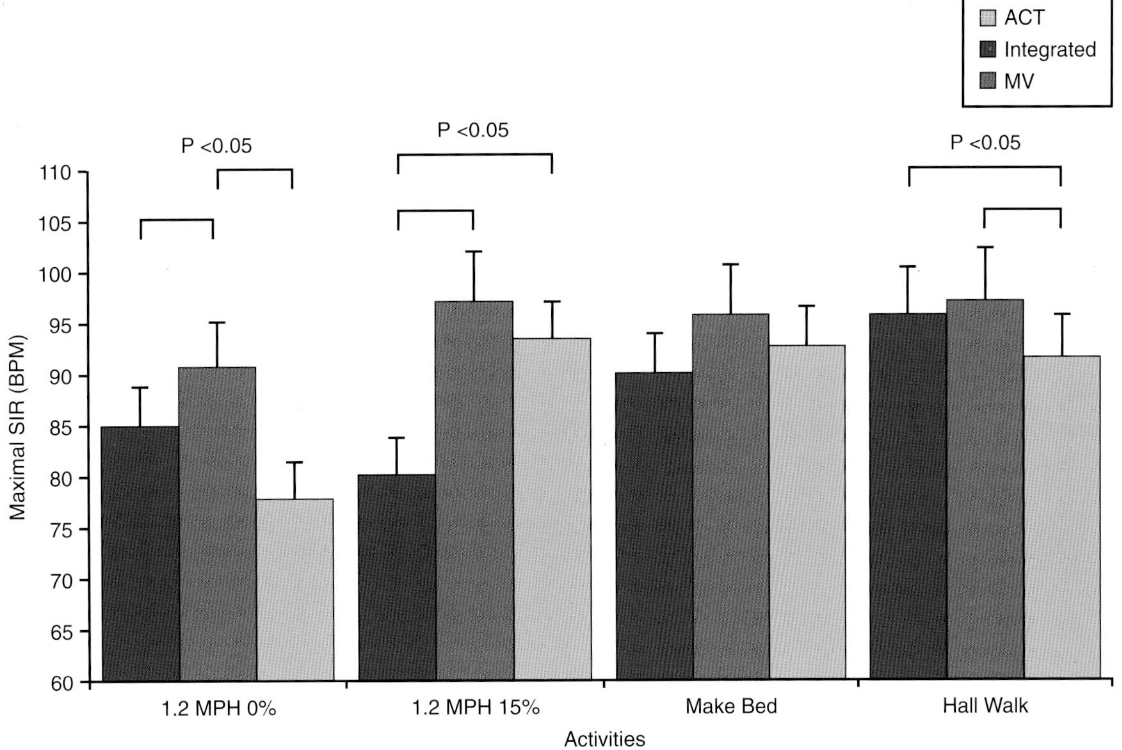

Figure 5-11. Comparison of the average maximal sensor-indicated rate (SIR) during submaximal exercise and activity of daily living (ADL). The minute ventilation (MV) + activity sensor (ACT) mode gave a better average maximal sensor rate during the submaximal exercise and hall walk than did the MV or ACT sensor mode alone. (From Leung SK, Lau CP, Tang MO, et al: New integrated sensor pacemaker: Comparison of rate responses between an integrated minute ventilation and activity sensor and single sensor modes during exercise and daily activities and nonphysiological interference. PACE 19:1664-1671, 1996.)

rate-adaptive slopes, one designed for low exercise workloads and the other for higher workloads. The QT and activity slopes at the upper and lower rate limits are automatically adjusted by a daily learning process. The pacemaker monitors the dynamics of the QT interval and activity counts and continuously updates its maximum and minimum sensor values.[17] This self-learning process adjusts the rate-response slope at the upper and lower rate limits (Fig. 5-12). Each time the pacemaker reaches the upper rate limit, it continues to monitor the QT interval and the activity counts. Further shortening of the QT interval or increase in activity counts while pacing at the upper rate limit indicates that the upper limit has been reached too soon, and the rate-response slope at the upper rate is automatically decreased by one step, which gives a more gradual approach to the upper rate limit in future. On the other hand, if the upper rate limit has not been reached for more than 8 days, its rate-response slope is automatically increased by one step. Similarly, the QT interval is measured regularly at the lower rate interval, with the patient presumably at rest. If the QT interval continues to lengthen at rest, this suggests that the lower rate limit is reached too quickly, and the slope for the lower rate limit is decreased.

The changes of the QT and activity slopes from factory settings have been reported.[17] Most of the

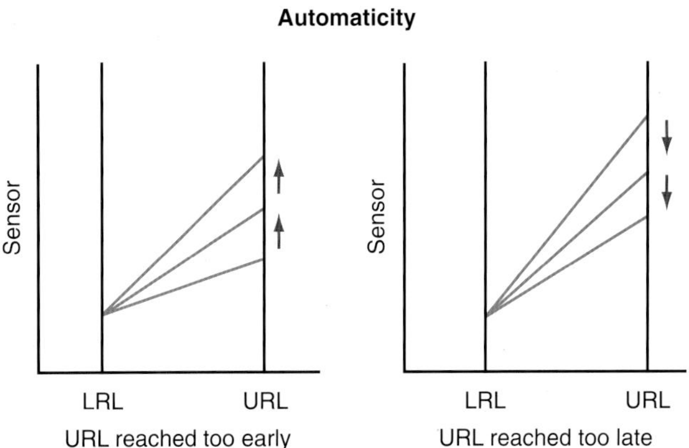

Figure 5-12. Automatic adjustment of the QT rate-response slope aims to pace at the lower rate limit (LRL) when the QT interval indicates no physical or mental stress and to pace at the upper rate limit (URL) when the QT interval indicates maximum workload. At the LRL, the QT-rate relationship is assessed once every night, and the slope is adjusted automatically one step in the direction of change. During maximum exercise at the URL, if further QT shortening occurs, the slope declining factor is advanced one step further, so that the URL will be attained after a longer interval in a repeat exercise (left panel). Conversely, if the upper rate is not attained in 8 days, the slope declining factor is reduced by one step (right panel).

changes occurred within the first 2 weeks and stabilized within a 6-week time frame. Starting at a lower rate of 60 or 70 bpm, the combined sensor reached the programmed maximum rate of 110 or 120 bpm after 2 to 5 weeks (mean, 19 days).

The clinical efficacy of self-learning automatic programming has been shown to result in pacing rates close to the sinus rate for ADLs (see Fig. 5-11).[127] A prospective comparative study on the efficacy of self-learning versus manual programming was conducted in 12 patients with complete heart block and normal SN function who received a combined activity- and QT interval–sensing DDDR pacemaker (Model 800, Diamond, Vitatron). Patients underwent treadmill exercise and 12 ADLs in the VDD mode. Sensor-indicated rates during these activities, as derived from automatic programming and from manual optimization using a submaximal treadmill exercise, were compared. The sensor rate determined by either method was close to sinus rhythm, although the rate-response profile and rate kinetics could be further improved by manual optimization.[136]

A similar automatic rate-adaptation algorithm matching sensor output at upper and lower pacing rate limits was also used by the minute ventilation–sensing pacemaker and the combined accelerometer and minute ventilation–sensing DDDR pacemakers (Talent DR 213, ELA Medical). The pacemaker constantly monitors the minute ventilation signal at the upper and lower rates. The slope of the minute-ventilation rate response was decreased by one step for every eight pacing cycles if the minute ventilation signals continue to rise while the pacemaker was pacing at the upper rate. The slope was increased by 3% per day if the upper pacing rate was not reached in 24 hours. This automatic algorithm stabilized the rate response slope with the first month.[137] The pacing response by combining the acceleration sensor with the automatically calibrated minute ventilation sensor was shown to provide a good correlation to sinus rate during exercise.[133]

The main limitation of these self-learning approaches is that the algorithms assume that every patient will exercise up to the programmed upper rate during their spontaneous activities. In practice, the automatic optimization may overadjust the rate-response slope at the upper rate range in patients who perform maximum exertion infrequently or who have been confined to bed, resulting in inappropriately fast pacing rates when the patient resumes usual ADLs.

Automatic Rate Optimization by Target Rate Distribution

In healthy subjects, a characteristic rate distribution occurs over 24 hours, depending on the subject's sex, age, activity, and fitness level.[139,140] HR profiles were recorded during 48-hour ambulatory ECG monitoring in healthy subjects performing regular ADLs and seven upper- and lower-extremity exercises. In this study, the distribution of daily HRs was mainly submaximal, but some transient HR increases exceeded 55% of the HR reserve.[141] The less physically fit subjects had greater increases in HR and used greater HR reserve during ADLs than did the average and the more physically fit subjects. Patients who were older than 65 years of age also had a longer duration of HR increase to greater than 110 bpm during normal activities. Based on these data, a "nominal" target rate profile that resembles the normal rate profile for the population, with different physical fitness levels as determined by age, sex, and activity, was derived and used to adjust the desired distribution of pacing rate for an individual patient, using the following two approaches.

Automatic Slope Optimization by Target Distribution of Heart Rate Reserve. In this approach to automatic rate-response adjustment, it is assumed that the HR of most individuals exceeds the 23rd percentile of the HR reserve during only 1% of the day. The Triology DR+ (St. Jude Medical, St. Paul, Minn.) activity-sensing pacemaker maintains a 7-day histogram of the sensor level and automatically adjusts the sensor slope once every 7 days, so that 99% of the sensor activity is within the initial 23% of the HR reserve (Fig. 5-13). The maximum adjustment is limited to two slopes, and the slope changes are not made if the patient is inactive (as defined by absence of activity sensor activities). In addition, offsets from −1 to +3 are available for fine titration of sensor response in individual patients. Positive offsets increase and negative offsets decrease the functional slope.

In 93 patients with the Pacesetter Trilogy DR + pacemaker, the sensor-indicated rate during a brisk walk after automatic slope optimization was compared with a desired sensor rate selected by the clinician. The automatic slope optimization provided the desired sensor rate in 75.6% of patients.[18] The rate modulation provided by the automatic slope optimization was appropriate in 76.3% of patients during follow-up. Despite the use of automatic slope optimization, about one half of the patients required further programming of the slope offset to titrate the sensor rate response. Some of this reprogramming was necessary because of the relatively conservative upper rate programming used in this study. In this study, the desired sensor rate and the appropriateness of the rate modulation were decided subjectively at the discretion of the clinician rather than objectively evaluated.

Rate Profile Optimization by Target Rate Histogram. Based on the nominal rate histogram, another device was introduced to adjust the sensor setting automatically to match this target rate histogram. This device, the Kappa 400, is a combined activity- and minute ventilation–sensing DDDR pacemaker. In addition to sensor autoprogramming, the device initiates implant detection through the detection of lead impedance (Fig. 5-14) and lead polarity recognition.[141] After confirming implantation by measuring stable lead impedance for 6 hours, the device is automatically programmed to the DDDR mode, and the baseline minute ventilation is automatically measured.[131] An optimal HR profile based on the patient's activity level and frequency of exercise is programmed as the target rate histogram (Fig. 5-15). This template is used to adjust the submaximal rate response during both ADLs and more vigorous exer-

Sensor-Indicated Rate Histogram

Mode...DDDR
Sensor..On
Base Rate...50 ppm
Max Sensor Rate.......................................110 ppm
Threshold.....................................Auto (+0.0)
Measured Average Sensor.....................2.9
Slope... Auto (+0)
Measured Average Sensor........................4
Reaction Time...Fast
Recovery Time..................................Medium

Note: The above values were obtained when the histogram was interrogated.

Date Read: ....26 Jan 2005 10:25 am
Total Time Sampled: 55d 23h 19m 58s
Date Last Cleared: ....1 Dec 2004 10:57 am

Bin Number	Range (ppm)	Time	Sample Counts
1	45 – <60	50d 9h 49m 44s	2,177,692
2	60 – <75	5d 8h 43m 52s	231,716
3	75 – <90	0d 4h 34m 50s	8,245
4	90 – <105	0d 0h 11m 12s	336
5	105 – <120	0d 0h 0m 20s	10
6	120 – <135	0d 0h 0m 0s	0
7	135 – <150	0d 0h 0m 0s	0
8	150 – <165	0d 0h 0m 0s	0
9	165 – 187	0d 0h 0m 0s	0
		Total:	2,417,999

Percent Counts
90
10
<1 <1 <1 0 0 0 0
45 60 75 90 105 120 135 150 165 187
Rate (ppm)

Figure 5-13. An illustration of the distribution of heart rate frequency on which the automatic rate adaptive algorithm of the Integrity DR (St. Jude) was based.

cise. Once each day, the pacemaker evaluates the percentage of time spent pacing in both the submaximal and maximal rate ranges by comparing the sensor rate profile with the target rate histogram. From this comparison, the pacemaker automatically controls how rapidly the sensor-indicated rate increases and decreases in these ranges.

The reliability of implant management in providing automatic detection of lead polarity and sensor initiation has been reported.[131] The efficacy of automatic optimization of the rate response was compared with that of manual programming in a prospective study measuring rate kinetics during ADLs and maximal and submaximal treadmill exercise in seven patients who received this device. The rate changes derived by automatic programming and by manual adjustment were compared. After automatic rate profile optimization, the pacing rate during a hall walk increased from 78 ± 3 bpm at predischarge to 90 ± 5 bpm at 2 weeks and 98 ± 3 bpm at 3 months' follow-up (Fig. 5-16). The pacing rate during maximal treadmill exercise increased from 89 ± 6 bpm to 115 ± 5 at 3 months after implantation, with a significant increase in exercise duration from 7.2 ± 1.0 minute to 9.6 ± 2.0 minutes. The accuracy of automatic programming versus manual programming was reassessed at 1 month, and the average maximal pacing rates attained and the speed of rate response for the dual-sensor mode after automatic and manual optimization did not differ significantly during maximal exercise, submaximal exercise, and ADLs between the two methods of programming (Fig. 5-17).[142]

The main limitation of the automatic rate optimization by the target rate distribution approach is that a

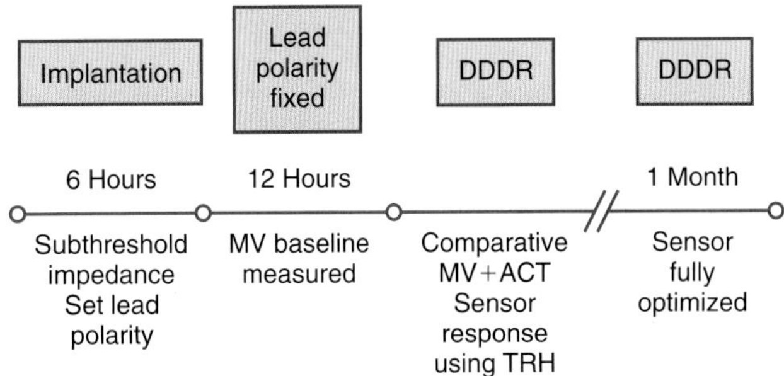

Figure 5-14. Automatic implant detection and sensor initiation algorithm used by Kappa 400 combined minute ventilation (MV) and activity (ACT) DDDR pacemaker. The first step is to detect lead implantation by continuous subthreshold current injection and impedance measurement by the pacemaker atrial and ventricular ports in the unipolar and bipolar fashions. On connection of the lead to the pacemaker port, the circuit is closed, and detection of implant and lead configuration and lead polarity are set automatically. After stable lead impedance is measured for 6 hours, the MV and ACT sensors are initialized automatically, and operating baselines for the MV and ACT sensors are determined automatically by collection of MV and ACT sensor data while pacing at the programmed lower rate. After an additional 6 hours, the pacemaker automatically begins dual-sensor DDDR pacing, self-optimizing to achieve the programmed target rate histogram (TRH). (From Leung SK, Lau CP, Tang MO, et al: An integrated dual sensor system automatically optimized by target rate histogram. PACE 21:1559-1566, 1998.)

nominal population standard for an individual patient still must be programmed, and a wider patient population is necessary to ascertain the safety of this approach. An inherent risk of using a histogram as the target for sensor setting is the uncertainty about whether the rate response that is recorded actually occurred at the appropriate time, because only the rate distribution, rather than the rate profile, is used as the template. In addition, the onset and recovery patterns, which are important characteristics of the sensor rate response, are not addressed by the histogram approach.

Maximum and Minimum Sensor-Indicated Rates and Automaticity

In a rate-adaptive pacing system, apart from the sensitivity of the sensor and the rate-response slopes, a minimum and maximum pacing rate must also be programmed. In a VVI pacemaker, a lower rate was programmed that was also the "average" pacing rate, which in most cases was arbitrarily programmed at about 60 to 80 bpm. Some authors have suggested that the optimum lower pacing rate can be adjusted to achieve the minimum atrial rate in patients who have complete AV block.[143] Unlike the VVI pacing mode, in which a single, fixed pacing rate must be programmed to accommodate both rest and exercise, higher rates can be achieved during exercise by sensors in rate-adaptive pacemakers. Hence, the lower rate limit should be less crucial. Although the programmed lower rate does not affect the maximal pacing rate during exercise, it influences the rate response at submaximal exercise levels.[144] In addition, it is clinically useful to program a lower pacing rate that is physiologically appropriate for the hours of sleep.[145] The lower resting HRs also serve to improve the longevity of the pulse generator. On the other hand, in elderly patients who are generally limited in their ability to perform certain types of activities, a faster lower pacing rate could benefit quality of life more than a lower HR.[146]

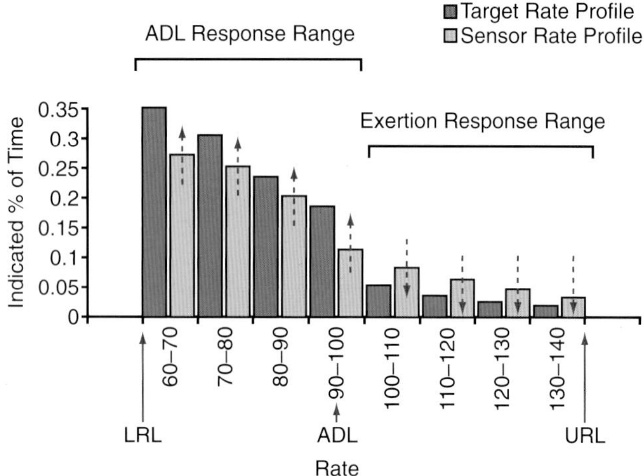

Figure 5-15. Optimization using target rate histogram. An illustration of the sensor rate profile matched against a target rate profile. The activity of daily living (ADL) range includes moderate pacing rates between the lower rate limit (LRL) and the ADL rate. The exertion rates range from the ADL rate to the upper rate limit (URL). By comparing the sensor rate profile with the target rate profile once each day, the pacemaker automatically controls how rapidly the sensor-indicated rate increases and decreases in these ranges. (From Leung SK, Lau CP, Tang MO, et al: An integrated dual sensor system automatically optimized by target rate histogram. PACE 21:1559-1566, 1998.)

The variability of the lower and upper rate parameters is best addressed using automatic programming. The simplest of these programs uses a 24-hour clock to reduce the lower rate during sleep. This becomes difficult, however, when the patient changes sleeping hours or travels to a different time zone. Hence, it is beneficial to have a sensor that varies the lower rate according to the patient's need by directly monitoring the metabolic demand. This may also simulate the spontaneous circadian rhythm of the resting rate in healthy subjects. By using special software to memorize the 24-hour minute ventilation data, a minute ventilation–driven DDDR pacemaker (Chorus RM, ELA Medical) allows the continuous recording and analysis of the circadian variations in minute ventilation, which correlate well with the metabolic demand. This could be used to modify the minimum pacing rate automatically.[147,148] Currently, however, full automaticity in lower rate programming

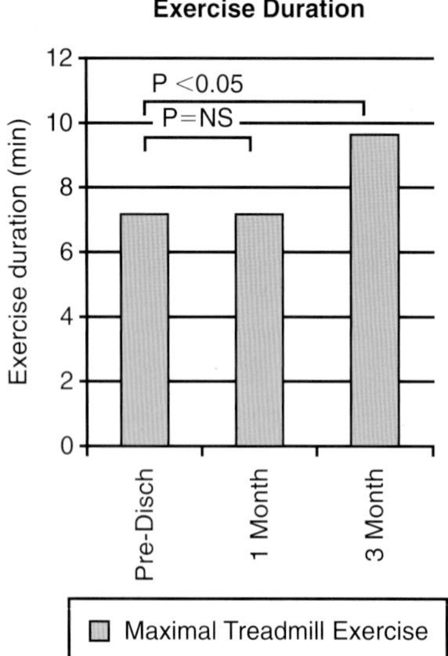

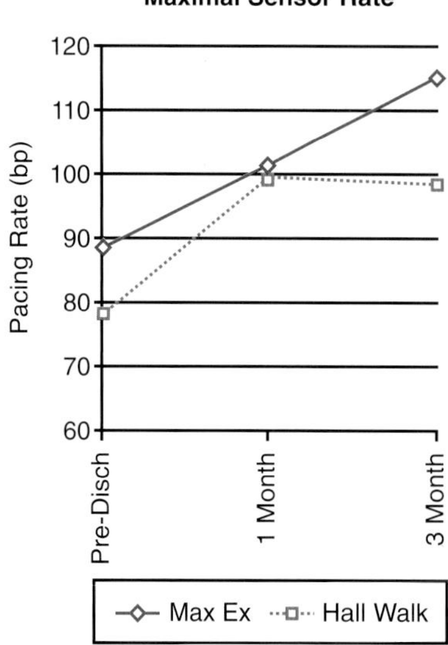

Figure 5-16. Left, Changes in the exercise duration during maximum exercise, by time since implantation. There is an increase in exercise duration at 3 months, compared with a predischarged (Pre-Disch) exercise test with automatic rate optimization. The exercise duration at 1 month did not differ significantly from the predischarge exercise duration. Right, Changes in sensor rate responses to hall walk and maximal treadmill exercise by time since implantation. The daily activity range optimized by 1 month, but continuous adaptation of the sensor to achieve a higher rate response occurred for up to 3 months after implantation. (From Leung SK, Lau CP, Tang MO, et al: An integrated dual sensor system automatically optimized by target rate histogram. PACE 21:1559-1566, 1998.)

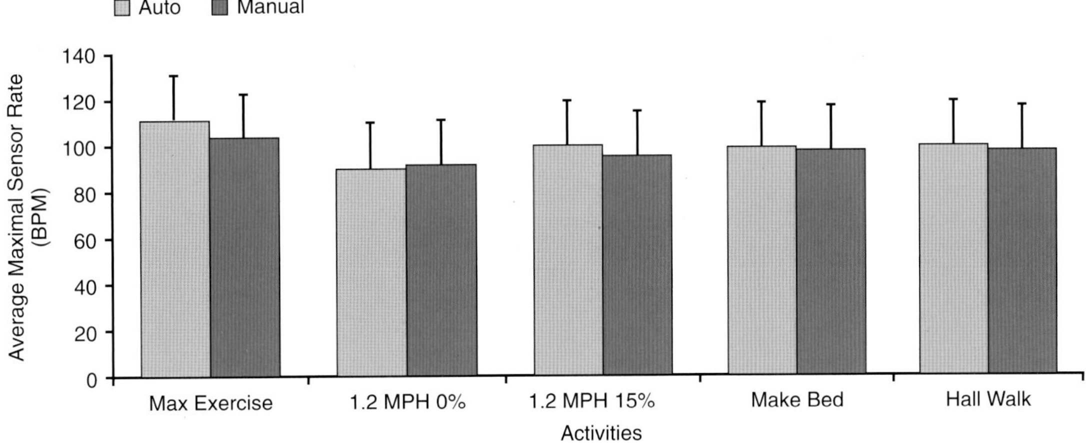

Figure 5-17. Comparison of the sensor rate responses during hall walk, submaximal exercise, and maximal exercise between manual and automatic rate optimization at 1 month. There was no significant difference in the average maximal sensor rate obtained after manual versus automatic programming of the rate-adaptive response. 1.2 mph 0%, submaximal exercise at 1.2 miles per hour at 0% gradient; 1.2 mph 15%, submaximal exercise at 1.2 miles per hour at 15% gradient; BPM, beats per minute. (From Leung SK, Lau CP, Tang MO, et al: New integrated sensor pacemaker: Comparison of rate responses between an integrated minute ventilation and activity sensor and single sensor modes during exercise and daily activities and nonphysiological interference. PACE 19:1664-1671, 1996.)

still cannot be achieved because the "rate band" for the lower rate—the base rate and rest rate—needs to be programmed at the discretion of the physician.

Diurnal variation is also theoretically possible for the temperature-,[149] pressure-,[150] and QT-sensing devices.[151] The QT signal showed a good correlation with the circadian sinus rate, with a correlation coefficient of more than 0.87.[152] The daily activity and HR trends showed a relatively high variation in the activity signals when awake and active and low variability during sleep. By measuring the variation of the activity signal (activity variance) with an activity-sensing pacemaker, the pacemaker can automatically adjust the lower rate during rest and sleep.[153] This circadian modulation based on accelerometer sensor signals was shown to match the normal sinus rate histogram.[154]

An appropriately programmed upper rate limit is important, because it determines the hemodynamics at high exercise levels. The patient's age and activity level and the presence of structural heart disease should be taken into account when choosing the maximum sensor-driven rate. In general, a higher upper rate may benefit a young patient. In a review of nine studies of physiologic pacemakers, Nordlander and colleagues[155] found that the percentage of improvement in maximum exercise capacity was linearly related to the maximum HR achieved. An overly aggressive rate response was associated with improved exercise performance compared with no rate response, but it produced the worst sense of well-being,[156] a larger oxygen deficit, a worsened level of perceived exertion,[157] and deteriorations in cardiac output and exercise performance.[158]

The proportion of time spent by these patients with HRs near the upper rate limit must also be considered. A study using Holter monitor recordings of 44 patients with complete heart block who were treated with VDD pacemakers showed that only 5 of 39 patients with an upper rate of 150 bpm ever reached this limit during recording. The typical pacemaker recipient in this study (mean age, 68 years; range, 18 to 84 years) achieved a rate of 150 bpm for less than 0.5% of the day.[159] Using 12-minute walking distance as a measure of submaximal exercise capacity, the distance covered was longest in patients with an upper rate limit of 125 bpm and in those with a limit of 150 bpm (Fig. 5-18).[160] The exercise capacity was significantly reduced when the programmed rates were either higher or lower than these "optimal" rates. Therefore, it appears that an upper rate of between 125 and 150 bpm can be chosen for most patients, except for young or athletic patients.

The effect of the upper programmed rate during submaximal exercise workloads and maximum exercise performance was assessed by oxygen kinetics in 11 patients with VVIR pacemakers implanted after AV nodal ablation for refractory atrial fibrillation.[161] By programming the upper rate limit of the VVIR pacemakers to either the maximum age-predicted HR or the nominal upper rate limit of 120 bpm, the patients were subjected to symptom-limited treadmill exercise. The exercise duration and maximum oxygen uptake during submaximal and maximal exercise were improved with an age-predicted upper rate. The oxygen deficit was also significantly lower during submaximal exercise with an age-predicted upper rate compared with the nominal upper rate. The mean Borg score was lower during both maximal and submaximal exercise with a higher upper rate. Although the results of this study may not be generally applied because of the younger age of the subjects and the use of only VVIR pacing, they do suggest the importance of upper rate adjustment, not only for exercise capacity but also for avoiding myocardial ischemia.

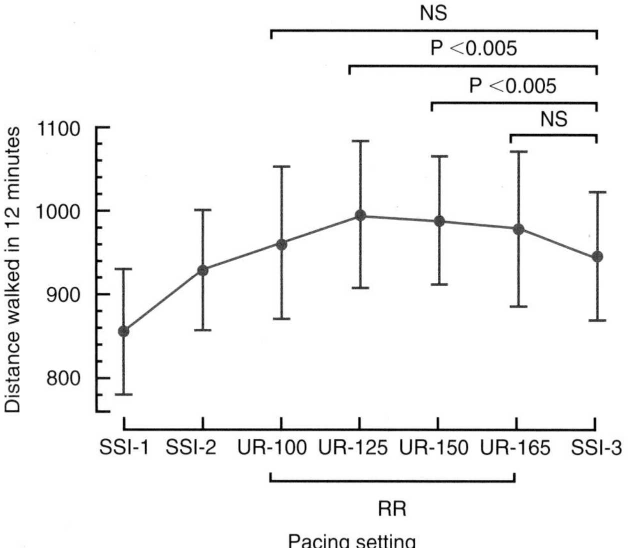

Figure 5-18. Distances covered in 12 minutes by patients with rate-adaptive pacemakers at different programmed settings. SSI-1 to SSI-3 represent repeated walking tests performed at a fixed rate, and SSI-3 is the distance covered after the "learning" effect resulting from SSI-1 and SSI-2. UR-100 to UR-165 represent the rate-adaptive pacing rates achieved during walking. The longest distance was covered with a maximum rate of 125 to 150 bpm. (From Lau CP, Leung WH, Wong CK, et al: Adaptive rate pacing at submaximal exercise: The importance of the programmed upper rate. J Electrophysiol 3:283-288, 1989.)

Is Ideal Behavior Necessary?

This question can be addressed in terms of the need for rate response, accuracy of rate adaptation, physiologic benefit, and clinical benefit.[162]

The Need for Rate Response

In the broadest sense, a rate-adaptive pacemaker should be considered for any patient who requires pacing. For patients with complete AV block, the VDD and DDD pacing modes provide both rate modulation and AV synchrony in the presence of normal SN function. Therefore, an artificial sensor is not a requirement for rate-adaptive pacing. On the other hand, chronic atrial fibrillation or flutter with AV block cannot be managed with these dual-chamber pacing modes and are ideal candidates for VVIR pacing, especially if the ventricular rate is inappropriately slow during exercise. For patients in whom SN disease is the primary indication for pacing, the need for rate-adaptive pacing is more variable. Some patients with SN dysfunction demonstrate normal chronotropic response to exercise and require AAI pacing only to prevent sinus pauses. In contrast, others with SN dysfunction have little or no chronotropic response to exercise and are ideal candidates for AAIR or DDDR pacemakers, depending on the status of AV conduction.

The overall pattern of chronotropic response in an individual patient varies and may evolve over time. Chronotropic incompetence tends to develop in patients with sick sinus syndrome; it may be provoked by disease such as heart failure, cardiomyopathy, and ischemic heart disease; or it may be induced by drugs. These conditions make predictions unreliable regarding the ultimate need for rate-adaptive pacing. Furthermore, the frequency of chronotropic incompetence depends on the method of assessment and the definition that is chosen. In general, rate modulation and AV synchrony are provided whenever possible to all patients who require permanent pacemakers. The SN is given priority as the primary modulator of HR if its function is unimpaired. For patients with paroxysmal or chronic atrial arrhythmias, a rate-adaptive pacing system that incorporates an artificial sensor is usually preferred, and the choice of single- or dual-chamber pacing is dependent on the status of AV conduction and the frequency of atrial tachyarrhythmias.

Accuracy of Rate Adaptation

When programming in patients with rate-adaptive pacemakers is either above or below the optimal values, subjective well-being may be adversely affected.[163] Among 10 patients with activity-sensing, rate-adaptive pacemakers who were randomly programmed to the VVI mode, the VVIR mode with standard slope, or the VVIR mode with an excessively sensitive rate-adaptive slope, many requested early crossover from the VVI and the over-programmed VVIR modes. Objective treadmill exercise tolerance was lowest in the VVI mode but there was no difference between the two VVIR modes. A similar decrease in general well-being was observed with the dual-chamber rate-adaptive modes, although objective differences in exercise tolerance were similar among DDD, DDDR, and over-programmed DDDR modes.

So far, none of the single sensors available has demonstrated ideal rate-response characteristics. Dual sensors show a more accurate rate response than do single sensors, especially activity sensors. For example, in the combined activity and minute ventilation sensor mode, the correlations between pacing rate and externally measured oxygen uptake for treadmill testing and bicycle testing were $r = 0.837$ and $r = 0.733$, respectively, compared with $r = 0.620$ and $r = 0.643$ for the activity sensor alone.[131] There was no significant difference when the combined mode was compared with the minute ventilation sensor mode. In the combined QT and activity pacemakers, the activity sensor overpaced, the QT sensor underpaced, and the combination worked significantly better than either of the individual sensors.[38,164] The effect of automaticity on fine tuning of sensors remains to be addressed. Therefore, as far as proportionality and speed of rate response are concerned, the current sensor combinations represent an improvement over single-sensor pacing.

Optimal programming of the upper rate limit during rate-adaptive pacing needs to be individualized. Other than the use of exercise testing, there is as yet no algorithm to vary the upper rate limit automatically. Furthermore, in patients with impaired cardiac function, the optimal upper rate limit during exercise was significantly lower than in patients with normal left ventricular function. Patients with impaired cardiac function cannot increase left ventricular stroke volume and oxygen uptake despite ongoing exercise with increasing workloads and increasing pacing rate.[165] Therefore, inappropriate increase in HR during exercise with rate-adaptive pacing can be potentially harmful.

Physiologic Benefits

Accurate rate adaptation may lead to better cardiopulmonary physiology. At higher levels of exertion, the ability to increase rate is the most important determinant of cardiac output and exercise capacity. In pooled data, a positive linear correlation between improvement of exercise capacity and HR was also observed.[155] However, because exercise capacity is a relatively insensitive measurement of functional benefit,[166] total exercise duration and maximal exercise workload usually do not differ among the different sensors or for the dual-sensor versus single-sensor rate-adaptive modes.[38,164] Therefore, the use of more sensitive and perhaps multiple indicators, such as cardiac output and respiratory gas exchanges, may be necessary to unmask sensor mode differences.

Application of oxygen kinetics to measure oxygen deficit at the onset of exercise may be an alternative indicator of an appropriate speed of rate response. When a minute ventilation–sensing pacemaker was programmed to two different rate-response slopes,[167] the anaerobic threshold was significantly enhanced by the higher slope (i.e., oxygen consumption at anaerobic threshold improved from 10.6 to 11.6 mL/kg per minute), with normalization of the minute ventilation-to-HR ratio compared with controls. Although both rate-adaptive settings were superior to fixed-rate pacing during exercise, the slight change in the rate-response slope significantly improved anaerobic threshold and chronotropic competence during submaximal exercise.

The HR-V_{O_2} relationship was examined for dual-sensor and single-sensor modes in a combined minute ventilation and activity VVIR pacemaker.[15] The dual-sensor mode behaved similarly to the minute ventilation mode, and both were superior to activity sensor mode alone. Anaerobic threshold and maximum exercise performance were also similar in the single-sensor mode compared with the dual-sensor mode.[15]

In the combined QT and activity pacemakers, it was found that the activity sensor overpaced, the QT sensor underpaced, and the combined QT and activity sensors paced at an in-between rate. The activity sensor improved oxygen uptake kinetics compared with the QT sensor, and the dual-sensor device functioned at an intermediate level (Fig. 5-19).[38] Despite the marked difference in pacing rate response among the three sensor modes, sensor response was not well reflected in the maximal oxygen uptake, total exercise duration, or anaerobic threshold. A similar finding was reported from the addition of an activity sensor to a minute ventilation sensor.[37]

It appears that sensor combination with an activity sensor to give a quick initial response significantly improves oxygen transport during ADLs in patients with rate-adaptive pacemakers. The performance of single-sensor and combined QT and activity dual-sensor VVIR modes during submaximal and maximal treadmill exercise was compared using exercise cardiac output by carbon dioxide rebreathing method in eight patients.[165] Compared with the pacing rate response based on the change in metabolic workload, the activity-sensor mode overpaced, the QT-sensor mode underpaced, and the dual-sensor achieved the best approximation to normal. The increase in cardiac output at 1 minute after the exercise onset was higher in the activity-sensor mode and in the dual-sensor mode than in the QT-sensor mode (Fig. 5-20). The underpaced QT sensor mode uses the contractility reserve to compensate for the slower rate increase with a compensatory increase in stroke volume during submaximal exercise. The more rapid rate-dependent increase in cardiac output at the beginning of exercise may be related to the physiologic changes associated with the better HR and workload relationship in the dual-sensor pacing mode.

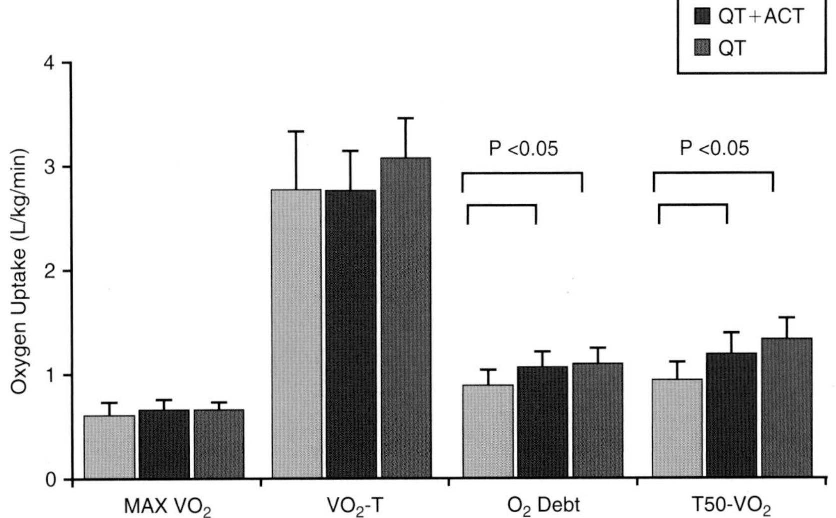

Figure 5-19. Oxygen kinetics in different VVIR sensor modes during constant submaximal exercise. Because the activity sensor (ACT) is the fastest to respond, it incurs the minimum oxygen debt and time to achieve 50% of maximal oxygen uptake (T50-VO_2). There was no statistically significant difference in oxygen debt and T50-VO_2 between the combined sensor mode and the QT sensor mode. The steady-state oxygen uptake (maximum VO_2) and the total oxygen uptake (VO_2-T) were similar among the three sensor modes. (From Leung SK, Lau CP, Wu CW, et al: Quantitative comparison of rate response and oxygen uptake kinetics between different sensor modes in multi-sensor rate adaptive pacing. PACE 17:1920-1927, 1994.)

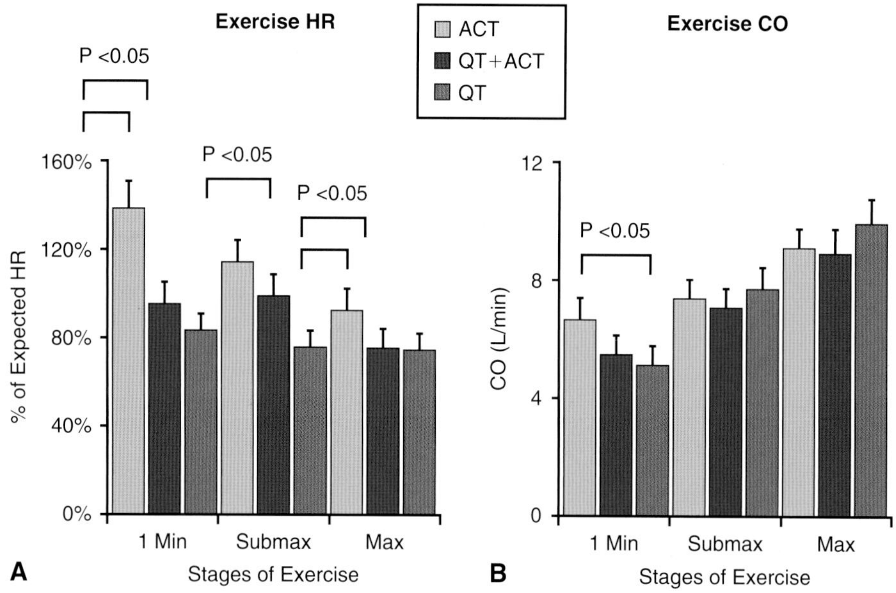

Figure 5-20. Heart rate (HR) and cardiac output (CO) in dual-sensor pacing. ***A,*** *Exercise HR response in the activity sensor (ACT), QT + ACT, and QT VVIR modes expressed as a percentage of the HR predicted according to the metabolic workload. Overpacing is defined as actual HR ≥120% of the expected HR and underpacing as HR ≤80% of expected at each quartile of exercise. The ACT overpaced, especially in the first minute of exercise, whereas the QT sensor underpaced throughout exercise. The QT + ACT sensor gave a rate response close to the expected rate.* ***B,*** *Exercise CO in the ACT, QT + ACT, and QT VVIR modes. The ACT VVIR sensor mode gave a significantly higher CO at 1 minute after exercise began than did the QT VVIR sensor mode. The QT + ACT VVIR sensor mode resulted in an intermediate response. There was no statistically significant difference in CO among the three sensor modes at the submaximal and maximal exercise levels. (From Leung SK, Lau CP, Tang MO, et al: Cardiac output is a sensitive indicator of difference in exercise performance between single and dual sensor pacemakers. PACE 21:35-41, 1998.)*

Clinical Benefit

The ultimate goal of pacemaker therapy is to improve symptoms and thus patient quality of life, and this has been used as a basis for comparing pacing modes. In terms of symptom improvement, VVIR pacing is superior to VVI pacing. However, the overall contribution of improved control of symptoms to enhanced quality of life is probably small in the typical pacemaker recipient, in whom quality of life is already close to that of age-matched healthy subjects.[168] There is still no comparative study of different sensors in regard to their effect on symptoms or quality of life.

A randomized, double-blind crossover study was done on 10 patients using the combined activity and minute ventilation dual-sensor VVIR pacemaker for high-grade AV block and chronic or persistent paroxysmal atrial fibrillation. These patients performed 2 weeks of out-of-hospital activity in the activity-only, minute ventilation–only, or dual-sensor VVIR and VVI modes.[169] Patients were assessed according to their perceived general well-being using the visual analog scale and the Specific Activities Scale functional status questionnaire, and on their objective improvement by standardized ADL protocols and graded treadmill testing. Subjective perception of exercise capacity and functional status was significantly reduced in the VVI mode compared with the VVIR modes. However, there was no clear advantage of dual-sensor VVIR pacing over activity-sensor pacing. Four of the 10 patients preferred the activity VVIR mode, 3 preferred the dual-sensor mode, and 3 had no preference. Three patients found dual-sensor VVIR least acceptable, 3 patients found minute ventilation least acceptable, and 1 patient found both dual-sensor and minute ventilation–sensor pacing unacceptable. There was no significant difference in objective performance among the three VVIR modes. These not unexpected results suggest that there are no major differences between sensors and combinations of sensors in gross clinical terms.

The overall number of patients studied has been small, however, and does not have sufficient statistical power to unveil less than major differences, which may be important for the long-term effects of a pacing mode. In addition, the difficulty of multiple comparisons and the order of pacing modes studied are limitations. Lukl and colleagues[170] assessed patient quality of life with regard to cardiovascular symptoms, physical activity, psychosocial and emotional functioning, and self-perceived health during DDD and dual-sensor VVIR pacing. Significant improvement during DDD pacing was demonstrated in all subgroups of patients (patients with sick sinus syndrome, chronotropically competent and incompetent patients, and patients with high-degree AV block). The overall result showed that DDD pacing offers better quality of life than dual-sensor VVIR pacing. Therefore, dual-sensor VVIR pacing cannot compensate for the lack of AV synchrony.

Rate-adaptive Pacing in Patients with Structural Heart Disease

Ischemic Heart Disease

Previous studies demonstrated that a significant proportion of patients receiving pacemaker implantation for conventional indications have significant coronary artery disease.[171] Furthermore, an increasing number of patients with ischemic heart disease and poor left ventricular function have received an implantable defibrillator for prevention of sudden cardiac death and treatment of ventricular arrhythmias. Although an increase in HR during exercise might increase myocardial oxygen demand in patients with ischemic heart disease, rate-adaptive pacing can counteract this potential deleterious effect by decreasing ventricular volume and wall stress during exercise. In fact, in patients with ischemic heart disease, atrial synchronous ventricular pacing may improve exercise tolerance compared with VVI pacing.[172] Furthermore, there was no significant difference in the extent and severity of myocardial ischemia, as determined by thallium exercise scintigraphy, during pacing with or without sensor-based rate modulation.[173] Nevertheless, an aggressively programmed rate-adaptive pacemaker may induce angina in some patients. Therefore, patients with angina pectoris may benefit from exercise testing to determine whether an appropriate chronotropic response can improve exercise capacity without exacerbating anginal symptoms.[171,174,175] A full clinical evaluation is required, because myocardial ischemia is often subclinical. Provided that the upper rate is judiciously chosen, rate-adaptive pacing enhances cardiac efficiency compared with VVI pacing. Furthermore, preliminary observation has suggested that dual-sensor might be better than single-sensor pacing in patients with ischemic heart disease.[128] The cross-checking function of dual-sensor pacing can prevent an inappropriately high rate response from the activity sensor as a result of external noise sensing.

Congestive Heart Failure

In patients with heart failure, chronotropic incompetence is frequently observed and potentially contributes to the impairment of exercise capacity.[41-43] Previous studies demonstrated that rate-adaptive pacing improves cardiac performance and exercise capacity in patients with impaired left ventricular systolic function.[176,177] However, an increased percentage of right ventricular apical pacing in these patients might lead to worsening of cardiac function and increased mortality.[178,179] Rate-adaptive pacing increases the percentage of ventricular pacing over VVI pacing, but the increase is likely to be small, because the sensor is active only during exercise. It is unknown whether rate-adaptive ventricular pacing will worsen left ventricular function. The use of cardiac resynchronization therapy (CRT) in patients with heart failure may provide an opportunity to use appropriate rate adaptation to further improve exercise capacity for these patients.[180] Currently, there are very limited data on the use of rate-adaptive pacing during CRT. A recent study[181] investigated the use of rate-adaptive pacing during CRT in patients with heart failure and chronotropic incompetence. In this study, chronotropic incompetence was defined as failure to achieve 85% of age-predicted HR. In patients with severe chronotropic incompetence (<70% of age-predicted HR) during exercise, rate adaptation during CRT significantly increased peak exercise HR and exercise capacity (Fig. 5-21). Conversely, in patients who reached more than 70% of age-predicted HR, exercise capacity was either reduced or remained unchanged with rate-adaptive pacing during exercise. In patients with heart failure, the changes in HR during exercise significantly correlated with exercise capacity as determined by Vo_{2max}. Therefore, patients receiving pacemaker implantation with CRT should undergo exercise testing to assess the HR response and determine the need for rate adaptation. In patients with severe chronotropic incompetence, as defined by failure to achieve 70% of age-predicted HR, appropriate use of rate-adaptive pacing with CRT provides an incremental benefit in exercise capacity.

Sensors for Purposes Other Than Rate Modulation

Sensors may also be used for purposes other than modulation of pacing rate (Table 5-8). Several of the available sensors can be used to automate other diagnostic and therapeutic pacemaker functions. For example, the

TABLE 5-8. Utility of Sensors for Purposes Other Than Rate Modulation

Functions	Examples
Pacing lead	Sensing and pacing in atrium and ventricle (may extend to the left side of the heart) Automatic switchable polarity
Basic pacemaker parameters	Autosensing and capture Automatic atrioventricular interval and PVARP Interference protection Upper rate behavior
Mode variability	Spontaneous mode changes
Tachycardia management	Pacemaker-mediated tachycardias Diagnosis and action (in conjunction with antitachycardia devices)
Diagnosis and monitoring	Rate Hemodynamics Hormonal and metabolic profiles Myocardial function Myocardial ischemia Postural detection Sleep apnea Lung fluid status

PVARP, postventricular atrial refractory period.

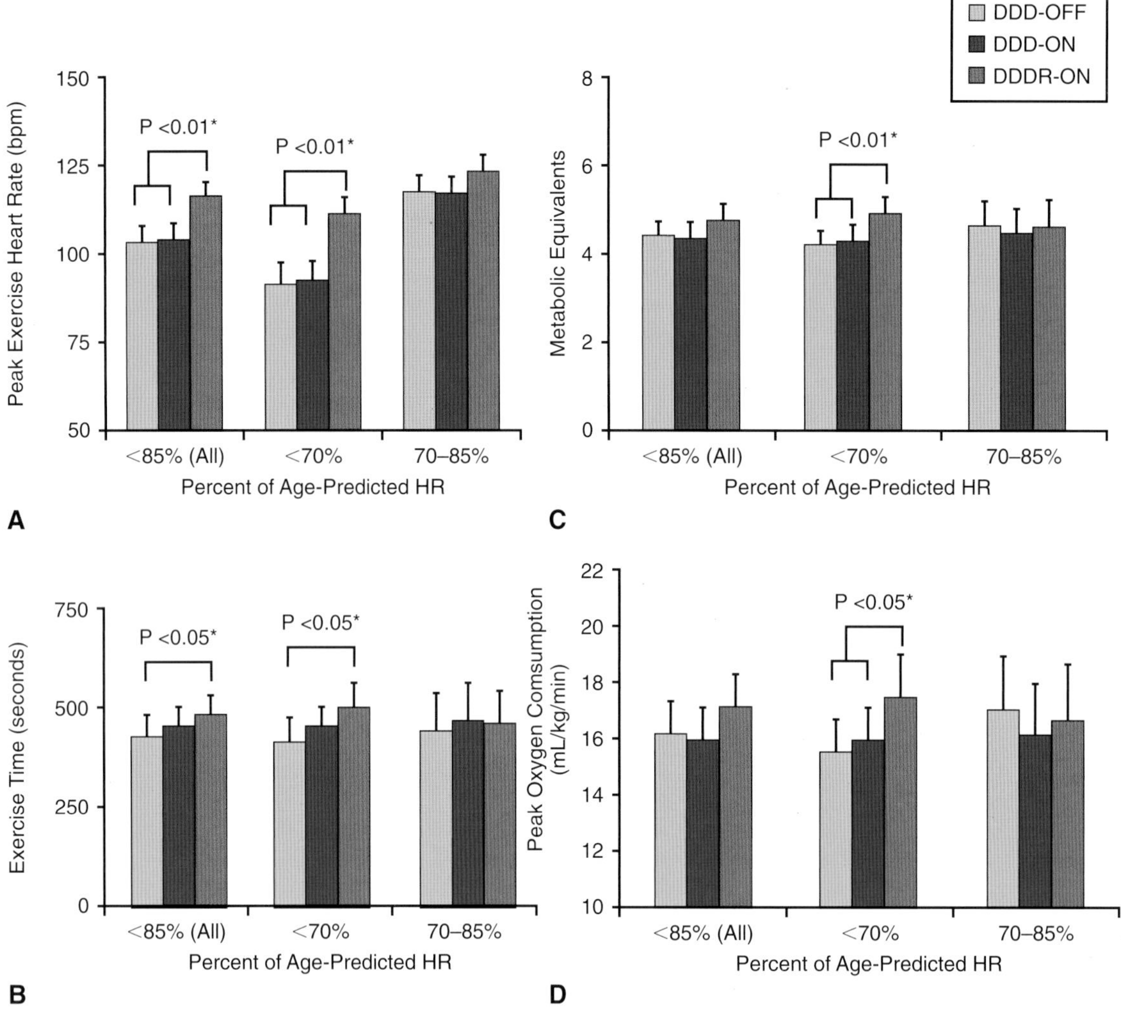

*Figure 5-21. Changes in peak exercise heart rate (**A**), exercise time (**B**), metabolic equivalents (**C**), and peak oxygen consumption (**D**) during DDD-OFF, DDD-ON, and DDDR-ON modes in patients who achieved less than 85% (All patients, n = 20), less than 70% (n = 11), and 70% to 85% (n = 9) of age-predicted heart rate (HR) during exercise in DDD-OFF mode. See text for details. (From Tse HF, Siu CW, Lee KLF, et al: The incremental benefit of rate-adaptive pacing on exercise performance during cardiac resynchronization therapy. J Am Coll Cardiol 46:2292-2297, 2005.)*

ability to detect the evoked intracardiac R wave may provide a means for capture detection and allow automatic regulation of the stimulus amplitude based on threshold measurements. In a DDDR pacemaker, sensors have been used to adapt the AV interval and the postventricular atrial refractory period (PVARP).[182] A sensor can be used to monitor the atrial rate. A disproportionate increase in the atrial rate compared with the sensor-indicated rate is interpreted by the pacemaker as an atrial tachyarrhythmia, which triggers a change in the pacing mode from DDDR to a nontracking mode. In this way, a rapid-paced ventricular response during atrial fibrillation can be avoided by an appropriate algorithm.[183]

AV-interval optimization using PEA,[184] a stroke volume sensor, and an oxygen saturation sensor has also been proposed. These sensors may also extend the use of sensor-driven automatic features in implantable devices other than pacemakers. An intrathoracic impedance sensor has been incorporated into an implantable cardioverter-defibrillator (InSync Sentry, Medtronic) to monitor fluid status in patients with heart failure, potentially allowing early detection and treatment of worsening heart failure.[185] Furthermore, the use of an implantable right ventricular pressure sensor (Chronicle IHM, Medtronic) for regular hemodynamic monitoring in patients with advanced heart failure has been shown to reduce hospitalization and worsening of heart failure.[186] Finally, minute ventilation sensors of pacemakers that measure ventilation by means of transthoracic impedance changes have been used for diagnosis and monitoring of sleep-related disorders.[187,188]

Summary

Because of the simplicity and proven clinical efficacy of rate-adaptive pacing to improve cardiac output and exercise capacity over fixed-rate ventricular pacing, these devices are now the standard of practice in cardiac pacing. Dual-sensor pacemakers seek to exploit the advantages of each sensor, to provide chronotropic modulation that more closely emulates that of the normal SN. The clinical benefits of dual-sensor pacemakers have yet to be proved in randomized trials. Nevertheless, the potential for automating rate response is an important advantage of combining rate-adaptive sensors. Increasing numbers of patients with ischemic heart disease and/or heart failure are receiving device therapies for the prevention of sudden death and CRT. The optimal use of sensors in these patient populations requires future investigations. Finally, in addition to rate modulation, the potential applications of sensors in implantable devices have been extended to other indications, including monitoring for heart failure.

REFERENCES

1. Karlof I: Haemodynamic effect of atrial triggered versus fixed rate pacing at rest and during exercise in complete heart block. Acta Med Scand 197:195-206, 1975.
2. Cammilli L, Alcidi L, Papeschi G: A new pacemaker autoregulating the rate of pacing in relation to metabolic needs. In Watanabe Y (ed): Proceedings of the Fifth International Symposium, Tokyo. Amsterdam, Excerpta Medica, 1976, pp 414-419.
3. Cammilli L: Initial use of a PH triggered pacemaker. PACE 12:1000-1007, 1989.
4. Rickards AF, Norman J: Relation between QT interval and heart rate: New design of physiologically adaptive cardiac pacemaker. Br Heart J 45:56-61, 1981.
5. Wirtzfeld AL, Goedel-Meinen L, Bock T, et al: Central venous oxygen saturation for the control of automatic rate responsive pacing [abstract]. Circulation 64(Suppl IV):299, 1981.
6. Funke HD: Ein Herschrittmacher mit belastung sabhangiger Frequenzregulation. Biomed Tech 20:225-228, 1975.
7. Rossi P: The birth of the respiratory pacemaker. PACE 13:812-815, 1990.
8. Anderson KM, Moore AA: Sensors in pacing. PACE 9:954-959, 1986.
9. Lau CP, Antoniou A, Ward DE, Camm AJ: Initial clinical experience with a minute ventilation-sensing rate modulated pacemaker: Improvements in exercise capacity and symptomatology. PACE 11:1815-1822, 1988.
10. Mond H, Strathmore N, Kertes P, et al: Rate responsive pacing using a minute ventilation sensor. PACE 11:1866-1874, 1988.
11. Kappenberger LJ, Herpers L: Rate responsive dual chamber pacing. PACE 9:987-991, 1986.
12. Lau CP, Tai YT, Li JPS, et al: Initial clinical experience with a single pass VDDR pacing system. PACE 15:1504-1514, 1992.
13. Lau CP, Butrous GS, Ward DE, et al: Comparison of exercise performance of six rate-adaptive right ventricular cardiac pacemakers. Am J Cardiol 63:833-838, 1989.
14. Landman MAJ, Senden PJ, van Pooijen, et al: Initial clinical experience with rate-adaptive cardiac pacing using two sensors simultaneously. PACE 13:1615-1622, 1990.
15. Ovsyshcher I, Guldal M, Karazguz R, et al: Evaluation of a new rate adaptive ventricular pacemaker controlled by double sensors. PACE 18:386-390, 1995.
16. Baig MW, Boute W, Begeman M, Perrins EJ: One-year follow-up of automatic adaptation of the rate response algorithm of the QT sensing, rate-adaptive pacemaker. PACE 14:1598-1605, 1991.
17. van Krieken FM, Perrins JP, Sigmund M: Clinical results of automatic slope adaptation in a dual sensor VVIR pacemaker. PACE 15:1815-1820, 1992.
18. Gentzler RD, Lucus E, and the North American Trilogy DR+ Phase I Clinical Investigators: Automatic sensor adjustment in a rate modulated pacemaker. PACE 19:1809-1812, 1996.
19. Bernstein AD, Camm AJ, Fletcher RD, et al: NAPSE/BPEG generic pacemaker code for antibradyarrhythmia and adaptive-rate pacing and antitachyarrhythmia devices. PACE 10:794-799, 1987.
20. Parsonnet V, Furman S, Smyth NP: Implantable cardiac pacemakers status report and resource guideline. Pacemaker Study Group. Circulation 50:A21-A35, 1974.
21. Parsonnet V, Furman S, Smyth NP: Revised code for pacemaker identification. PACE 4:400-403, 1981.
22. Loeppky JA, Greene ER, Hoekenga DE, et al: Beat-by-beat stroke volume assessment by pulsed Doppler in upright and supine exercise. J Appl Physiol 50:1173-1182, 1981.
23. Miyamoto Y: Transient changes in ventilation and cardiac output at the start and end of exercise. Jpn J Physiol 31:149-164, 1981.
24. Higginbotham MB, Morris KG, Williams RS, et al: Regulation of stroke volume during submaximal and maximal upright exercise in normal man. Circ Res 58:281-291, 1986.
25. Cardus D, Spenser WA: Recovery time of heart frequency in healthy men: Its relations to age and physical condition. Arch Phys Med 48:71-77, 1967.
26. Astrand P, Rodahl K: Textbook of Work Physiology: Physiological Basis of Exercise, 3rd ed. New York, McGraw-Hill, 1986, pp 260-261.
27. McElroy PA, Janicki JS, Weber KT: Physiological correlates of the heart rate response to upright isotonic exercise: Relevance to rate-responsive pacemakers. J Am Coll Cardiol 11:94-99, 1988.
28. Lewalter T, MacCarter D, Jung W, et al: The low intensity treadmill exercise protocol for appropriate rate adaptive programming of minute ventilation controlled pacemakers. PACE 18: 1374-1387, 1995.
29. Margarta R, Edwards HT, Dill DB: The possible mechanism of contracting and paying the oxygen debt and the role of lactic acid in muscular contraction. Am J Physiol 106:689-714, 1933.
30. Astrand P, Rodahl K: Textbook of Work Physiology: Physiological Basis of Exercise, 3rd ed. New York, McGraw-Hill, pp 295-353.
31. Linnarsson D: Dynamics of pulmonary gas exchange and heart rate changes at start and end of exercise. Acta Physiol Scand 415(Suppl):1-68, 1974.
32. Cerretelli P, Rennie DW, Pendergast DP: Kinetics of metabolic transients during exercise. Int J Sports Med 1:171-180, 1980.
33. Jones PW: Ventilatory response to cardiac output changes in patients with pacemakers. J Appl Physiol 51:1103-1107, 1981.
34. Casaburi R, Spitzer S, Haskell R, et al: Effect of altering heart rate on oxygen uptake at exercise onset. Chest 95:6-12, 1989.
35. Brooks GA, Hittelman KJ, Faulkner JA, et al: Temperature, skeletal muscle mitochondrial functions and oxygen debt. Am J Physiol 220:1053-1059, 1971.
36. Stainsby WN, Barclay JK: Exercise metabolism: O_2 steady level O_2 uptake and O_2 uptake for recovery. Med Sci Sports 2:177-181, 1970.
37. Kay GN, Ashar MS, Bubien R, et al: Relationship between heart rate and oxygen kinetics during constant workload exercise. PACE 18:1853-1860, 1995.
38. Leung SK, Lau CP, Wu CW, et al: Quantitative comparison of rate response and oxygen uptake kinetics between different sensor modes in multisensor rate adaptive pacing. PACE 17:1920-1927, 1994.
39. Gauri AJ, Raxwal VK, Roux L, et al: Effects of chronotropic incompetence and beta-blocker use on the exercise treadmill test in men. Am Heart J 142:136-141, 2001.
40. Higginbotham MB, Morris KG, Conn EH, et al: Determinants of variable exercise performance among patients with severe left ventricular dysfunction. Am J Cardiol 51:52-60, 1983.

41. Colucci WS, Ribeiro JP, Rocco MB, et al: Impaired chronotropic response to exercise in patients with congestive heart failure: Role of postsynaptic beta-adrenergic desensitization. Circulation 80:314-323, 1989.
42. Sullivan MJ, Knight JD, Higginbotham MB, Cobb FR: Relation between central and peripheral hemodynamics during exercise in patients with chronic heart failure: Muscle blood flow is reduced with maintenance of arterial perfusion pressure. Circulation 80:769-781, 1989.
43. Lauer MS, Larson MG, Evans JC, Levy D: Association of left ventricular dilatation and hypertrophy with chronotropic incompetence in the Framingham Heart Study. Am Heart J 137:903-909, 1999.
44. Kjekshus J, Gullestad L: Heart rate as a therapeutic target in heart failure. Eur Heart J 1(Suppl):64-69, 1999.
45. Longhurst JC, Kelley AR, Gonyea WJ, et al: Cardiovascular responses to static exercise in distance runners and weight lifters. J Appl Physiol 49:676-683, 1980.
46. Neumann G, Grube E, Leschhorn JE, et al: Symptoms control and psychosocial rehabilitation of chronic pacemaker patients with different pacing modes. In Steinback K, Glogar D, Laczkovics A (eds): Cardiac Pacing, Proceedings of the Seventh World Symposium on Cardiac Pacing. Darmstadt, Steinkopff Verlag, 1983, pp 455-461.
47. Alt E, Hirgstetter C, Heinz M, et al: Rate control of physiologic pacemakers by central venous blood temperature. Circulation 73:1206-1212, 1986.
48. Lau CP: The range of sensors and algorithms used in rate adaptive pacing. PACE 15:1177-1211, 1992.
49. Rickards AF, Donaldson RM: Rate-responsive pacing. Clin Prog Pacing Electrophysiol 1:12-19, 1983.
50. Rossi P, Plicchi G, Canducci G, et al: Respiratory rate as a determinant of optimal pacing rate. PACE 6:502-510, 1983.
51. Rossi P, Plicchi G, Canducci G, et al: Respiration as a reliable physiological sensor for the control of cardiac pacing rate. Br Heart J 51:7-14, 1984.
52. Nappholtz T, Valenta H, Maloney J, et al: Electrode configurations for respiratory impedance measurement suitable for rate-responsive pacing. PACE 9:960-964, 1986.
53. Goldreyer BN, Olive AL, Leslie J, et al: A new orthogonal lead for P synchronous pacing. PACE 4:638-644, 1981.
54. Griffin JC, Jutzy KR, Claude JP, et al: Central body temperature as a guide to optimal heart rate. PACE 6:498-501, 1983.
55. Fearnot NE, Smith HJ, Sellers D, et al: Evaluation of the temperature response to exercise testing in patients with single-chamber, rate-adaptive pacemakers: A multicentre study. PACE 12:1806-1815, 1989.
56. Salo RW, Pederson BD, Olive AL, et al: Continuous ventricular volume assessment for diagnosis and pacemaker control. PACE 7:1267-1272, 1984.
57. Chirife R: Physiological principles of a new method for rate responsive pacing using the presystolic interval. PACE 11:1545-1554, 1988.
58. Anderson KM, Moore AA: Sensors in pacing. PACE 9:954-959, 1986.
59. Wirtzfeld AL, Goedel-Meinen L, Bock T, et al: Central venous oxygen saturation for the control of automatic rate responsive pacing. PACE 5:829-835, 1982.
60. Schaldach M, Hutten H: Intracardiac impedance to determine sympathetic activity in rate responsive pacing. PACE 15:1778-1786, 1992.
61. Pichlmaier AM, Braile D, Ebner E, et al: Autonomic nervous system controlled closed loop cardiac pacing. PACE 15:1787-1791, 1992.
62. Occhetta E, Perucca A, Rognoni G, et al: Experience with a new myocardial acceleration sensor during dobutamine infusion and exercise test. Eur J Cardiac Pacing Electrophysiol 5:204-209, 1995.
63. Rickards AF, Bombardini T, Corbucci G, et al: An implantable intracardiac accelerometer for monitoring myocardial contractility. PACE 19:2066-2071, 1996.
64. Humen DP, Kostuk WJ, Klein GJ: Activity-sensing, rate-responsive pacing: Improvement in myocardial performance with exercise. PACE 8:52-59, 1985.
65. Palmer G, de Bellis F, Solinas A, et al: Sensor-free physiological pacing. In Behrenbeck DW, Sowton E, Fontaine G, Winter UJ (eds): Cardiac Pacemakers. Darmstadt, Steinkopff Verlag, 1985, pp 781-785.
66. Pacela AF: Impedance pneumography: A survey of instrumentation technique. Med Biol Eng 4:1-15, 1965.
67. Van de Water JM, Mount B, Barela JR, et al: Monitoring the chest with impedance. Chest 64:597-603, 1973.
68. Rushmer RF, Crystal DK, Wagner C, et al: Intracardiac impedance plethysmography. Am J Physiol 174:171-174, 1953.
69. Sahakian AV, Tompkins WJ, Webster JG: Electrode motion artifacts in electrical impedance pneumography. IEEE Trans Bio Med Eng 32:448-451, 1985.
70. Lau CP, Ritchie D, Butrous GS, et al: Rate modulation by arm movements of the respiratory-dependent rate-responsive pacemaker. PACE 11:744-752, 1988.
71. Webb SC, Lewis LM, Morris-Thurgood JA, et al: Respiratory-dependent pacing: A dual response from a single sensor. PACE 11:730-735, 1988.
72. Callaghan F, Vollmann W, Livingston A, et al: The ventricular depolarization gradient: Effects of exercise, pacing rate, epinephrine, and intrinsic heart rate control on the right ventricular evoked response. PACE 12:1115-1130, 1990.
73. Chirife R: Acquisition of hemodynamic data and sensor signals for rate control from standard pacing electrodes. PACE 14:1563-1565, 1991.
74. Chirife R: Sensor for right ventricular volumes using the trailing edge voltage of a pulse generator output. PACE 14:1821-1827, 1991.
75. Wirtzfeld A, Heinze R, Liess HD, et al: An active optical sensor for monitoring mixed venous oxygen-saturation for an implantable rate-regulating pacing system. PACE 6:494-497, 1983.
76. Casaburi R, Daly J, Hansen JE, et al: Abrupt changes in mixed venous blood gas composition after the onset of exercise. J Appl Physiol 67:1106-1112, 1989.
77. Stangl K, Wirtzfeld A, Heinze R, et al: First clinical experience with an oxygen saturation controlled pacemaker in man. PACE 11:1882-1887, 1988.
78. Farerestrand S, Ohm OJ, Stangl K, et al: Long-term clinical performance of a central venous oxygen saturation sensor for rate adaptive cardiac pacing. PACE 17:1355-1372, 1994.
79. Lau CP, Tai YT, Leung WH, et al: Rate adaptive cardiac pacing using right ventricular venous oxygen saturation: Quantification of chronotropic behavior during daily activities and maximal exercise. PACE 17:2236-2246, 1994.
80. Stangl K, Wirtzfeld A, Heinze R, et al: A new multisensor pacing system using stroke volume, respiratory rate, mixed venous oxygen saturation and temperature, right atrial pressure, right ventricular pressure, and dP/dt. PACE 11:712-724, 1988.
81. Mason DT: Usefulness and limitations of the rate of rise of intraventricular pressure (dP/dt) in the evaluation of myocardial contractility in man. Am J Cardiol 23:516-527, 1969.
82. Gleason WL, Braunwald E: Studies of the first derivative of the ventricular pressure pulse in man. J Clin Invest 41:80-91, 1962.
83. Bennett T, Sharma A, Sutton R, et al: Development of a rate adaptive pacemaker based on the maximum rate of rise of right ventricular pressure (RV dP/dt max). PACE 15:219-234, 1992.
84. Ovsyshcher I, Guetta V, Bondy C, et al: First derivative of right ventricular pressure, dP/dt, as a sensor for a rate adaptive VVI pacemaker: Initial experience. PACE 15:211-218, 1992.
85. Kay GN, Philippon F, Bubien RS, et al: Rate modulated pacing based on right ventricular dP/dt: Quantitative analysis of chronotropic response. PACE 17:1344-1354, 1994.
86. Occhetta E, Perucca A, Rognoni G, et al: Experience with a new myocardial acceleration sensor during dobutamine infusion and

exercise test. Eur J Cardiac Pacing Electrophysiol 5:204-209, 1995.
87. Rickards AF, Bombardini T, Corbucci G, et al: An implantable intracardiac accelerometer for monitoring myocardial contractility. PACE 19:2066-2071, 1996.
88. Wood JC, Fensten MP, Lim MJ, et al: Regional effects of myocardial ischemia on epicardially recorded canine first heart sound. J Appl Physiol 76:291-302, 1994.
89. Soldati E, Bongiorni MG, Arena G, et al: Endocardial acceleration signals detected by a transvenous pacing lead: Do they reflect local contractility? [abstract] PACE 19:659, 1996.
90. Clementy J, Renesto F, Gillo L, et al: Stress test and 24 h Holter analysis of 79 patients implanted with a peak endocardial acceleration (PEA) based DDDR pacemaker (Living 1) [abstract]. PACE 20:1591, 1997.
91. Binner L, for the European PEA Clinical Investigation Group: One year follow-up of a new DDDR pacemaker based on contractility: A multicentric European study on peak endocardial acceleration (PEA) [abstract]. PACE 21:894, 1998.
92. Winter UJ, Behrenbeck DW, Candelon B, et al: Problems with the slope adjustment and rate adaptation in rate-responsive pacemakers: Oscillation phenomena and sudden rate jumps. In Behrenbeck DW, Sowton E, Fontaine G, Winter UJ (eds): Cardiac Pacemakers. Darmstadt, Steinkopff Verlag, 1985, pp 107-112.
93. Lau CP: Sensors and pacemaker mediated tachycardias. PACE 14:495-498, 1991.
94. Scanu P, Guilleman D, Grollier G, et al: Inappropriate rate response of the minute ventilation rate-responsive pacemaker in a patient with Cheyne-Stokes dyspnea [letter]. PACE 12:1963, 1989.
95. Lau CP, Tai YT, Fong PC, et al: Pacemaker-mediated tachycardias in rate-responsive pacemaker. PACE 13:1575-1579, 1990.
96. Wen HK: A review of implantable sensors. PACE 6:482-487, 1998.
97. Wilkoff BL, Covey J, Blackburn G: A mathematical model of the cardiac chronotropic response to exercise. J Electrophysiol 3:176-180, 1989.
98. Baig MW, Wilson J, Boute W, et al: Improved pattern of rate responsiveness with dynamic slope setting for the QT sensing pacemaker. PACE 12:311-320, 1989.
99. Lau CP, Mehtha D, Toff W, et al: Limitations of rate response of activity sensing rate responsive pacing to different forms of activity. PACE 11:141-150, 1988.
100. Lau CP, Wong CK, Cheng CH, et al: Importance of heart rate modulation on cardiac hemodynamics during post-exercise recovery. PACE 13:1277-1285, 1990.
101. Alt E, Matula M, Thilo R, et al: A new mechanical sensor for detecting body activity and posture, suitable for rate-responsive pacing. PACE 11:1875-1881, 1988.
102. Tse HF, Siu CW, Tsang V, et al: Blood pressure response to transition from supine to standing posture using an orthostatic response algorithm. PACE 28:S242-S245, 2005.
103. Paul V, Garrett C, Ward DE, et al: Closed-loop control of rate-adaptive pacing: Clinical assessment of a system analysing the ventricular depolarization gradient. PACE 12:1896-1902, 1989.
104. Edelstam C, Hedman A, Nordlander R, Pehrsson SK: QT-sensing rate-responsive pacing and myocardial infarction. PACE 12:502-504, 1989.
105. Robbens EJ, Clement DL, Jordaens LJ: QT related rate-responsive pacing during acute myocardial infarction. PACE 11:339-342, 1988.
106. Lau CP, Ward DE, Camm AJ: Single-chamber cardiac pacing with two forms of respiration-controlled rate-responsive pacemakers. Chest 95:352-358, 1989.
107. Von Hemel NM, Hamerlijnck RPHM, Pronk KJ, et al: Upper limit ventricular stimulation in respiratory rate responsive pacing due to electrocautery. PACE 12:1720-1723, 1989.
108. Jordeans L, Backers J, Moerman E, et al: Catecholamine levels and pacing behavior of QT driven pacemakers during exercise. PACE 13:603-607, 1990.
109. Frais MA, Dowie A, McEwen B, et al: Response of the QT-sensing rate-adaptive ventricular pacemaker to mental stress. Am Heart J 126:1219-1222, 1993.
110. Candinas R, Mayer IV, Heywood JT, et al: Influence of exercise induced myocardial ischemia on right ventricular dP/dt: Potential implications for rate-responsive pacing. PACE 18:2121-2127, 1995.
111. Lau CP, Lee CP, Wong CK, et al: Rate responsive pacing with a minute ventilation sensing pacemaker during pregnancy and delivery. PACE 13:158-163, 1990.
112. Madsen GM, Anderson C: Pacemaker-induced tachycardia during general anaesthesia: A case report. Br J Anaesth 63:300-361, 1989.
113. Lamas GA, Keefe JM: The effects of equitation (horseback riding) on a motion responsive DDDR pacemaker. PACE 13: 1371-1373, 1990.
114. Shellock FG, Rubin SA, Ellrodt AG, et al: Unusual core temperature decrease in exercising heart-failure patients. J Appl Physiol 52:544-550, 1983.
115. Lau CP, Stott JRR, Toff W, et al: Selective vibration sensing: A new concept for activity sensing rate responsive pacing. PACE 11:1299-1309, 1988.
116. Lau CP, Tai YT, Fong PC, et al: Clinical experience with an accelerometer based activity sensing dual chamber rate adaptive pacemaker. PACE 15:334-343, 1992.
117. Greenhut SE, Shreve EA, Lau CP: A comparative analysis of signal processing methods for motion-based rate responsive pacing. PACE 19:1230-1247, 1996.
118. Lau CP, Wong CK, Leung WH, et al: A comparative evaluation of a minute ventilation sensing and activity sensing adaptive-rate pacemakers during daily activities. PACE 12:1514-1521, 1989.
119. Lau CP, Antoniou A, Ward DE, et al: Reliablity of minute ventilation as a parameter for rate responsive pacing. PACE 12:321-330, 1989.
120. Slade AKB, Pee S, Jones S, et al: New algorithms to increase the initial rate response in a minute volume rate adaptive pacemaker. PACE 17:1960-1965, 1994.
121. Metha D, Lau CP, Ward DE, et al: Comparative evaluation of chronotropic response of activity sensing and QT sensing rate responsive pacemakers to different activities. PACE 11:1405-1414, 1988.
122. Roberts DH, Bellamy M, Hughes, et al: Limitations of rate response of new generation QT sensing (Rhythmx) pacemaker [abstract]. PACE 13:1208, 1990.
123. Hedman A, Nordlander R: Changes in QT and Q-Ta intervals induced by mental and physical stress with fixed rate and atrial triggered ventricular inhibited cardiac pacing. PACE 11:1405-1414, 1988.
124. Alt E, Theres H, Heinz M, et al: A new rate-modulated pacemaker system optimized by combination of two sensors. PACE 11:1119-1129, 1988.
125. Provenier F, van Acker R, Backers J, et al: Clinical observations with a dual sensor rate adaptive single chamber pacemaker. PACE 15:1821-1825, 1992.
126. Connell DT, and the Topaz Study Group: Initial experience with a new single chamber dual sensor rate responsive pacemaker. PACE 16:1833-1841, 1993.
127. Lau CP, Leung SK, Guerola M, et al: Efficacy of automatically optimized rate adaptive dual sensor to simulate sinus rhythm: Evaluation by continuous recording of sinus and sensor rates during exercise testing and daily activities. PACE 19:1672-1677, 1996.
128. Cowell R, Morris-Thurgood J, Paul V, et al: Are we being driven to two sensors? Clinical benefits of sensor cross checking. PACE 16:1441-1444, 1993.

129. Lau CP, Leung SK, Lee SFI: Delayed exercise rate response kinetics due to sensor cross-checking in a dual sensor rate adaptive pacing system: The importance of individual sensor programming. PACE 19:1021-1025, 1996.
130. Leung SK, Lau CP, Tang MO, et al: New integrated sensor pacemaker: Comparison of rate responses between an integrated minute ventilation and activity sensor and single sensor modes during exercise and daily activities and nonphysiological interference. PACE 19:1664-1671, 1996.
131. Alt E, Combs W, Fotuhi P, et al: Initial clinical experience with a new dual sensor SSIR pacemaker controlled by body activity and minute ventilation. PACE 18:1487-1495, 1995.
132. Lau CP, Tse WS, Camm AJ: Clinical experience with Sensolog 703: A new activity-sensing, rate-responsive pacemaker. PACE 11:1444-1455, 1988.
133. Hayds DL, Higano ST: Utility of rate histograms in programming and follow up of a DDDR pacemaker. Mayo Clin Proc 64:495-502, 1989.
134. Mahaux V, Waleffe A, Kulbertus HE: Clinical experience with a new activity-sensing, rate-modulated pacemaker using autoprogrammability. PACE 12:1362-1368, 1989.
135. Lau CP: Sensolog 703 (Siemens-Elema, Solna, Sweden) activity-sensing rate-responsive pacing [letter]. PACE 3:819-820, 1990.
136. Leung SK, Lau CP, Tang MO: Appropriateness of automatic versus manual optimization in a dual sensor rate response pacemaker [abstract]. Eur J Cardiac Pacing Electrophysiol 6:168, 1996.
137. Ritter P, Anselme F, Bonnet JL, et al: Clinical evaluation of an automatic slope calibration function in a minute ventilation controlled DDDR pacemaker [abstract]. PACE 20:1173, 1997.
138. Geroux L, Bonnet JL, Cazeau, et al: Evaluation of a new principle of dual sensor. Arch Mal Coeur Vaiss 91(Suppl III):40, 1998.
139. Mianulli M, Birchfield D, Yakimow K, et al: The relationship between fitness level and daily heart rate behavior in normal adults: Implication for rate-adaptive pacing [abstract]. PACE 18:870, 1995.
140. Mianulli M, Birchfield D, Yakimow K, et al: Do elderly pacemaker patients need rate adaptation? Implications of daily heart rate behavior in normal adults [abstract]. Eur J Card Pacing Electrophysiol 6:182, 1996.
141. Lau CP, Pietersen A, Ohm O, et al: Automatic implant detection for initiating lead polarity programming and rate adaptive sensors: Multicentre study [abstract]. PACE 19:592, 1996.
142. Leung SK, Lau CP, Tang MO, et al: An integrated dual sensor system automatically optimized by target rate histogram. PACE 21:1559-1566, 1998.
143. Mitsui T, Hori M, Suma K, Saigusa M: Optimal heart rate in cardiac pacing in coronary sclerosis and non-sclerosis. Ann N Y Acad Sci 167:745, 1969.
144. Leung SK, Lau CP, Choi YC, et al: Does the programmed lower rate affect the rate response in rate adaptive pacemakers? [abstract] PACE 15:579, 1992.
145. Swinehart JM, Recker RR: Tachycardia and nightmares. Nebr Med J 58:314-315, 1973.
146. Zimerman L, Newby KH, Barold H, et al: Effects of the lower pacing rate on quality of life of elderly patients with a VVIR pacemaker implanted following AV node ablation for chronic atrial fibrillation [abstract]. PACE 20:1191, 1997.
147. Morris-Thurgood, J, Chiang CM, Rochelle J, et al: A rate responsive pacemaker that physiologically reduces pacing rates at rest. PACE 17:1928-1932, 1994.
148. Bonnet JL, Vai F, Pioger G, et al: Circadian variations in minute ventilation can be reproduced by a pacemaker sensor. PACE 21:701-703, 1998.
149. Devyagina GP, Kraerskii YM: Circadian rhythm of body temperature, blood pressure and heart rate. Hum Physiol 9:133-140, 1983.
150. Jones RI, Cashman PMM, Hornung RS, et al: Ambulatory blood pressure and assessment of pacemaker function. Br Heart J 55:462-468, 1986.
151. Djordjevic M, Kocovic D, Pavlovic S, et al: Circadian variations of heart rate and stim-T interval: Adaptation for nighttime pacing. PACE 12:1757-1762, 1989.
152. Kocovic D, Velimirovic D, Djordjevic M, et al: Circadian variations of stim-T interval and their correlation with sinus rhythm [abstract]. PACE 10:700, 1987.
153. Bornzin GA, Arambula ER, Florio J, et al: Adjusting heart rate during sleep using activity variance. PACE 17:1933-1938, 1994.
154. Park E, Gibb WJ, Bornzin GA, et al: Activity controlled circadian base rate. Arch Mal Coeur Vaiss 91(Suppl III):144, 1998.
155. Nordlander R, Hedman A, Pehrsson JK: Rate-responsive pacing and exercise capacity [editorial]. PACE 12:749-751, 1989.
156. Sulke N, Dritsas A, Chambers J, et al: Is accurate rate response programming necessary? PACE 13:1031-1044, 1990.
157. Kay GN, Bubien RS, Epstein AE, et al: Rate modulated pacing based on transthoracic impedance measurements of minute ventilation: Correlation with exercise gas exchange. J Am Coll Cardiol 15:1283-1288, 1989.
158. Payne G, Spinelli J, Garratt CJ, et al: The optimal pacing rate: An unpredictable parameter. PACE 20:866-873, 1997.
159. Kristensson B, Karlsson O, Ryden L: Holter-monitored heart rhythm during atrioventricular synchronous and fixed-rate ventricular pacing. PACE 9:511-518, 1986.
160. Lau CP, Leung WH, Wong CK, et al: Adaptive rate pacing at submaximal exercise: The importance of the programmed upper rate. J Electrophysiol 3:283-288, 1989.
161. Carmouche DG, Bubien RS, Neal Kay G: The effect of maximum heart rate on oxygen kinetics and exercise performance at low and high workload. PACE 21:679-686, 1998.
162. Lau CP, Leung SK: Clinical usefulness of rate adaptive pacing systems; What should we assess? PACE 17:2233-2235, 1994.
163. Sulke N, Dritsas A, Chambers J, et al: Is accurate rate response programming necessary? PACE 13:1031-1044, 1990.
164. Leung SK, Lau CP, Tang MO, et al: Cardiac output is a sensitive indicator of difference in exercise performance between single and dual sensor pacemakers. PACE 21:35-41, 1998.
165. Kindermann M, Schwaab B, Finkler N, et al: Defining the optimum upper heart rate limit during exercise: A study in pacemaker patients with heart failure. Eur Heart J. 23:1301-1308, 2003.
166. Jutzy RV, Florio J, Isaeff DM, et al: Comparative evaluation of rate modulated dual chamber and VVIR pacing. PACE 13:1838-1846, 1990.
167. Brachmann J, MacCarter DJ, Frees U, et al: The effects of pacemaker slope programming on chronotropic function and aerobic capacity [abstract]. Circulation 84(III):158, 1990.
168. Lau CP, Rushby J, Leigh-Jones M, et al: Symptomatology and quality of life in patients with rate-responsive pacemakers: A double-blind crossover study. Clin Cardiol 12:505-512, 1989.
169. Sulke N, Tan K, Kamalvand K, et al: Dual sensor VVIR mode pacing: Is it worth it? PACE 19:1560-1567, 1996.
170. Lukl J, Doupal V, Heinc P: Quality of life during DDD and dual sensor VVIR pacing. PACE 17:1844-1848, 1994.
171. Mosseri M, Izak T, Rosenheck S, et al: Coronary angiographic characteristics of patients with permanent artificial pacemakers. Circulation 96:809-815, 1997.
172. Kristensson BE, Arnman K, Ryden L: Atrial synchronous ventricular pacing in ischaemic heart disease. Eur Heart J 4:668-673, 1983.
173. van Campen LC, De Cock CC, Visser FC, Visser CA: The effect of rate responsive pacing in patients with angina pectoris on the extent of ischemia on 201-thallium exercise scintigraphy. PACE 25:430-434, 2002.
174. De Cock CC, Panis JHC, Van Eenigl MJ, et al: Efficacy and safety of rate-responsive pacing in patients with coronary artery disease and angina pectoris. PACE 12:1405-1411, 1989.

175. Kenny RA, Ingram A, Mitsuoka T, et al: Optimum pacing mode for patients with angina. Br Heart J 56:463-468, 1986.
176. Buckingham TA, Woodruff RC, Pennington DG, et al: Effect of ventricular function on the exercise hemodynamics of variable rate pacing. J Am Coll Cardiol 11:1269-1277, 1988.
177. Lau CP, Camm AJ: Role of left ventricular function and Doppler-derived variables in predicting hemodynamic benefits of rate-responsive pacing. Am J Cardiol 62:906-911, 1988.
178. Tse HF, Yu C, Wong KK, et al: Functional abnormalities in patients with permanent right ventricular pacing: The effect of sites of electrical stimulation. J Am Coll Cardiol. 40:1451-1458, 2002.
179. Wilkoff BL, Cook JR, Epstein AE, et al: Dual-chamber pacing or ventricular backup pacing in patients with an implantable defibrillator: The Dual Chamber and VVI Implantable Defibrillator (DAVID) Trial. JAMA 288:3115-3123, 2002.
180. Cleland JG, Daubert JC, Erdmann E, et al: The effect of cardiac resynchronization on morbidity and mortality in heart dailure. N Engl J Med 352:1539-1549, 2005.
181. Tse HF, Siu CW, Lee KLF, et al: The incremental benefit of rate-adaptive pacing on exercise performance during cardiac resynchronization therapy. J Am Coll Cardiol 46:2292-2297, 2005.
182. Lau CP, Tai YT, Fong PC, et al: Atrial arrhythmia management with sensor controlled atrial refractory period and automatic mode switching in patients with minute ventilation-sensing, dual-chamber, rate-adaptive pacemakers. PACE 15:1504-1514, 1992.
183. Lau CP, Tai YT, Fong PC, et al: The use of implantable sensors for the control of pacemaker-mediated tachycardias: A comparative evaluation between minute ventilation-sensing and acceleration-sensing dual-chamber rate-adaptive pacemakers. PACE 15:34-44, 1992.
184. Leung SK, Lau CP, Lam CT, et al: Automatic optimization of resting and exercise atrioventricular interval using a peak endocardial acceleration sensor: Validation with Doppler echocardiography and direct cardiac output measurements. PACE 23:1762-1766, 2000.
185. Yu CM, Wang L, Stadler RW, et al: Impedance measurements from implanted devices provide automated prediction of CHF hospitalization [abstract]. Eur Heart J 25:27, 2004.
186. Bourge RC, Abraham WT, Aaron MF, et al, for the COMPASS-HF Investigators and Coordinators. Chronicle Offers Management to Patients with Advanced Signs and Symptoms of Heart Failure (COMPASS-HF): Ambulatory hemodynamic guided management of heart failure. Program and abstracts of the American College of Cardiology Annual Scientific Session 2005, Orlando, Florida, March 6-9, 2005. Late Breaking Clinical Trials II.
187. Defaye P, Pepin JL, Poezevara Y, et al: Automatic recognition of abnormal respiratory events during sleep by a pacemaker transthoracic impedance sensor. J Cardiovasc Electrophysiol 15:1034-1040, 2004.
188. Scharf C, Cho YK, Bloch KE, et al: Diagnosis of sleep-related breathing disorders by visual analysis of transthoracic impedance signals in pacemakers. Circulation 110:2562-2567, 2004.

Chapter 6

Power Systems for Implantable Pacemakers, Cardioverters, and Defibrillators

DARREL F. UNTEREKER • ANN M. CRESPI • ANTHONY RORVICK • CRAIG L. SCHMIDT • PAUL M. SKARSTAD

This chapter provides the clinician with information about power systems (batteries and capacitors) used in implantable pacemakers and defibrillators. Batteries are active devices that convert chemical energy into electrical energy, whereas capacitors are passive devices that temporarily store energy, often to increase the available power (rate of energy delivery) in an electric circuit. The purpose of this chapter is to communicate useful information that will aid clinical management for patients who have implanted medical devices.

The battery is conceptually different from the other components of an implantable pacing or defibrillator system. In principle, the other components of pacing systems are designed to last indefinitely. However, the available chemical energy of the battery is consumed during its normal use. Therefore, the battery has a finite service life, because it contains a fixed amount of the active materials that furnish its energy. Eventually, as the device is used, the output of the battery becomes insufficient to operate the device. Unless the battery can be recharged, it is no longer useful and must be replaced. At present, most implantable device batteries are not rechargeable, and the entire pulse generator must be replaced to renew the battery. Pulse generators in the future may well use rechargeable batteries so that the energy powering the device can be renewed.

Whereas batteries transform chemical energy into electrical energy, capacitors are energy storage devices. The use of capacitors to intermittently boost the power capability of electronic circuits is of principal interest here. The large capacitors in an implantable cardioverter-defibrillator (ICD) allow the device to deliver a therapeutic, high-voltage, high-energy shock to the heart in a few milliseconds, something the battery could not do by itself.

We believe that understanding of the major properties and limitations of the batteries used to power implantable devices will lead to a better understanding of the devices themselves and of how best to manage them in clinical use. This understanding is one facet of optimal patient management.

Definitions

Some basic terminology relating to batteries and capacitors is given here. The reader may wish to refer to these definitions when needed.

Oxidation and Reduction: Oxidation (the loss of electrons) and reduction (the gain of electrons) are the fundamental electrochemical processes that allow a battery to operate.

Anions and Cations: Anions are negatively charged ions, and cations are positively charged ions. Anions and cations are the carriers of electrical charge in solutions.

Conduction: There are two fundamental forms of conduction: electronic, in which electrons are the charge carriers, and ionic, in which charged chemical species, or ions, are the charge carriers. Conductivity in electrolytic solutions is due to movement of ions, whereas conductivity in metals is due to electrons.

Anode: The anode is the electrode in a battery at which oxidation occurs; the anode furnishes electrons to the external circuit and therefore is the negative terminal of the battery. In a capacitor, the anode is the plate that loses electrons and has a positive charge.

Cathode: The cathode is the electrode in a battery at which reduction occurs; it is the positive terminal. In a capacitor, the cathode is the plate that has a net negative charge.

Battery: A battery is an electrochemical cell that can convert the free energy of a chemical reaction into electricity, or a group of such cells connected in a series or parallel configuration. It is also called a galvanic cell.

Capacitor: A capacitor is a passive device that stores energy by separating charge across a dielectric (insulating) medium.

Rate Capability: The ability of a battery to deliver a sustained current. This should not be confused with pacing rate.

Capacity: The amount of charge stored in a battery, usually expressed in ampere-hours (A-hr).

Energy: The ability to do work; for batteries, usually expressed in units of watt-hours (W-hr).

Energy Density: The energy content of a battery or capacitor based on volume or mass. For a battery, energy density is usually expressed in units of watt-hours per cubic centimeter ($W\text{-}hr/cm^3$) or watt-hours per gram (W-hr/g).

Power: The rate at which energy is made available from a battery or capacitor.

Batteries

Basic Function and Electrochemistry of Batteries

Energy Storage in Batteries

A battery converts chemical energy into electrical energy. The source of this energy is the electrochemical reactions that occur within the battery. The type and amount of materials participating in these reactions determine the deliverable energy of a battery.

Chemical Reactions

During a spontaneous chemical reaction, substances interact to form reaction products that are more stable than the starting materials. For example, during burning, a fuel combines with oxygen from the air to form products such as water, carbon dioxide, and other molecules. The fuel is oxidized during this process. Oxygen from the air is reduced. The exact amounts of each are determined by the *stoichiometry* of the reaction. Equations 6-1 through 6-4 are examples of types of reactions in which oxidation and reduction occur. They are called *redox reactions,* and they show an exact or stoichiometric relationship between the reactants and the products.

Formation of water:

$$2H_2 + O_2 \rightarrow 2H_2O \qquad (6\text{-}1)$$

Burning of benzene:

$$2C_6H_6 + 15O_2 \rightarrow 12CO_2 + 6H_2O \qquad (6\text{-}2)$$

Rusting of iron:

$$4Fe + 3O_2 \rightarrow 2Fe_2O_3 \qquad (6\text{-}3)$$

Discharge of a lithium/iodine (Li/I_2) pacemaker battery:

$$2Li + I_2 \rightarrow 2LiI \qquad (6\text{-}4)$$

Chemical reactions like these occur spontaneously because the products are in a lower energy state than the reactants. The difference in energy appears as heat in the case of combustion or rusting. A battery or galvanic cell is designed to convert much of this energy difference into electrical energy rather than heat. A battery operates because the electrons transferred during a redox reaction are channeled from one terminal of the battery through the external circuit and back to the battery through its other terminal. The maximum work these electrons can do outside the battery is related to the difference in a thermodynamic quantity called the *free energy* of the reactions.

Major Components of Batteries

Figure 6-1 schematically shows a simple battery. The major parts of a battery are the anode, the cathode, and the electrolyte. The anode and cathode must be physically separated, and both must be in contact with the electrolyte, which is often a solution.

Anode and Cathode

The two major battery components involved in the electrochemical reaction during discharge of a galvanic cell are the anode and the cathode. The anode, which is often a metallic substance, furnishes electrons to the external circuit, whereas the cathode, which is usually not a metal, receives them.

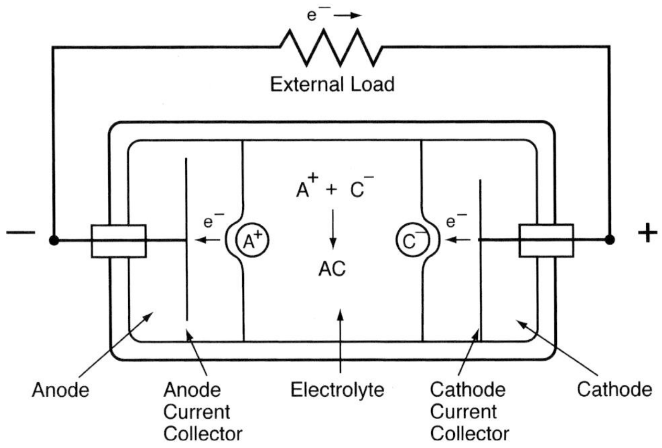

Figure 6-1. Schematic representation of a sealed battery. The anode material is on the left, the cathode material on the right, and the electrolyte in the middle of the cell. The discharge reaction is $A + C \rightarrow AC$. In this example, both A^+ and C^- are mobile ions, and the discharge product, AC, is insoluble and precipitates in the electrolyte solution. In this figure, connections to the interior of the cell are made via feedthroughs. e^-, electron.

The anode in a battery is the negative electrode, and the cathode is the positive electrode. This can be confusing, because the pacing stimulus occurs at the cathode tip of the lead and is a negative pulse. However, the terminology is not inconsistent. Oxidation always occurs at an anode and reduction at a cathode. In a battery, oxidation at the anode delivers electrons to the external circuit, and the anode is therefore negative. These electrons cause electrochemical reduction to occur in the solution surrounding the pacing lead tip (cathode).

Electrolyte

The anode and the cathode are separated by the electrolyte, which is a necessary component of the battery. As the battery discharges, it furnishes electrons at one terminal, pushes them through an external circuit, and receives them at a second terminal. If this were all that happened, the discharge process would not occur for very long, because a large positive charge would quickly develop near the anode-electrode interface, and an equally large negative charge would develop on the cathode side. The buildup of these charges would suppress further reaction. It is the electrolyte that prevents this from happening, by allowing the accumulating opposite charges at the two electrodes to migrate and neutralize each other. The requirement for an electrolyte is that it conducts ions but not electrons. If the electrolyte conducted electrons as well as ions, the battery would be internally shorted, just as it would if a wire directly connected the positive and negative terminals.

A broad distinction between types of batteries is based on the choice of the electrolyte solvent. Batteries with aqueous electrolytes include many systems using zinc, lead, cadmium, aluminum, or magnesium anodes. Water is an excellent solvent for salts and forms electrolyte solutions with excellent ionic conductivity. However, water cannot be used as a component of long-lived, high-energy-density batteries employing lithium anodes, because this very active metal undergoes a rapid reaction with water to form hydrogen gas and lithium hydroxide. Lithium metal anode batteries use nonaqueous solvents that react minimally with lithium. Most lithium-based batteries employ a mixture of organic ethers and esters as solvents for the electrolyte. For example, lithium/manganese dioxide batteries, which are widely used to power automatic cameras, use mixtures containing the ether dimethoxyethane and the ester propylene carbonate, in which the salt lithium perchlorate is dissolved, as the electrolyte.

Separator

The separator is a structural member of the cell that keeps anode and cathode materials apart, thus preventing shorting of the cell. The separator should not be confused with the electrolyte. The electrolyte is the medium that conducts ions within the battery, including across the separator. All batteries need an electrolyte, but not all batteries require a separator. A separator is usually needed in batteries that contain liquid electrolytes. Without a separator in these batteries, there would be little to stop the anode from shorting to the cathode if the cell were squeezed or if there were any internal movement of the electrodes during use, which could result from volume changes during discharge. The separator is made of a material that has a porous structure so that the electrolyte solution can fill the pores and ions can move between the anode and cathode sides of the battery. Medical batteries with liquid electrolytes use porous polymer films that do not react with other components of the battery system. To increase safety, these batteries often use a separator that melts and loses its porosity in case the battery becomes shorted.

Current Collector

The current collector makes the connection between the positive or negative terminal of the battery and its respective active electrode material inside the cell. A current collector is usually a wire connected to a screen or grid that is embedded in the anode or cathode material. The current collector may also serve as a structural member of the battery to provide physical integrity and strength to that electrode. Some medical batteries use the case of the cell as the current collector for the cathode.

Hermetic Seal

Most batteries need to be sealed, but few batteries other than those used for implantable medical devices and aerospace applications need to be so well sealed that they are truly hermetic (i.e., gas tight). Hermeticity implies the use of welded construction and glass or similar feedthroughs to make electrical connections between the inside and the outside of the battery. This is necessary to prevent slow interchanges of materials between the battery and its surroundings. Batteries using lithium anodes must be sealed to prevent water from entering the case. In addition, some of the components used inside medical lithium batteries are volatile and could be corrosive or damaging if they leaked out. Medical batteries are typically considered hermetically sealed if the leak rate out of the battery for a test gas, usually helium, is less than 1×10^{-7} cm^3/sec at 1 atmosphere pressure difference between the inside and the outside of the cell.

Classification of Batteries

Batteries can be classified in many ways, such as by application, functional characteristics, chemistry, or the physical state of some component. One fundamental distinction is between primary and secondary batteries.

Primary Batteries

Primary batteries can only be used once. They are not designed to be recharged, and in fact it is dangerous to attempt to recharge them. A familiar example of a primary battery is the alkaline zinc/manganese dioxide flashlight battery. Most modern implantable medical devices are powered by primary batteries with lithium anodes because of their very high energy densities.

Secondary Batteries

Secondary batteries are designed to be repetitively discharged and recharged. Familiar examples of secondary batteries include the lead-acid batteries used in automobiles and the cadmium/nickel oxide ("NiCad") and metal hydride/nickel oxide (NiMH) batteries, which are widely used in portable home appliances and power tools. Rechargeable NiCad batteries were used to power some cardiac pacemakers built in the 1970s, but this battery system has not been used in implantable pacemakers for several decades.

The barrier to using secondary batteries for implantable medical applications has been technological: until recently, rechargeable batteries did not have high enough energy density, and they had to be recharged too frequently to compete with primary lithium anode batteries. However, over the past 15 years, a new rechargeable battery system called the lithium-ion battery has come into widespread use in portable consumer electronics. Lithium-ion batteries have high energy density and excellent charge retention, which is the ability to deliver the same amount of capacity cycle after cycle. These characteristics make the system a good candidate for powering implantable devices that require relatively high, sustained currents. Recently, neurologic stimulators powered by lithium-ion batteries have been implanted. In the future, this battery system may find many more applications in implantable medical devices. Lithium-ion batteries are discussed in more detail later in this chapter.

Functional Characteristics of Batteries

Capacity

The fundamental unit of battery capacity is the coulomb (6.2×10^{18} electrons), which is the amount of charge delivered by 1 ampere (A) of current in 1 second. In the context of implantable devices, a more practical unit of capacity is the ampere-hour (A-hr), which represents the charge carried by a current of 1 ampere flowing for 1 hour. An ampere-hour represents 3600 coulombs. A battery for an implantable medical device usually has a capacity rating of between 0.5 and 2.0 A-hr. Many papers have been written about the proper way of determining and specifying the capacity of a medical battery.[1-3] No single method is uniquely correct. Various methods produce numbers ranging from theoretical values that can never be achieved in the field to very realistic values that are based on detailed models or accelerated testing. Because most batteries are not able to use up all of their active components before they cease to function, the actual capacity of a battery is often less than that predicted from theoretical calculations. In addition, the load-circuit voltage generally decreases as the battery is used. Because the electronic circuits of a pulse generator can operate only above a specified minimum voltage, the cell capacity that is generated below this voltage is not usable and should not be counted. Self-discharge and other parasitic chemical reactions further reduce the amount of energy a battery will deliver, so the deliverable capacity may also depend on the time it takes to discharge a battery.

The time frame for the operation of most implantable medical devices is so long (5-10 years) that real-time measurements of battery capacity are not practical. Therefore, accelerated tests and models are typically used to estimate the amount of deliverable capacity in these batteries. Technology in this area has improved a great deal, and it is now possible to make quite accurate projections of battery capacity.[4-6]

Energy and Energy Density

The fundamental unit of energy is the joule (J), which represents the energy given to 1 coulomb of charge that is accelerated by a difference in potential of 1 volt. One joule is also the energy transferred by 1 watt (W) of power in 1 second. Just as battery capacity is often measured in ampere-hours, battery energy is often expressed in watt-hours (W-hr) instead of joules.

A battery parameter that is important in the design of an implantable device is energy density, a quantity that can be expressed on either a mass or a volume basis. For medical applications, volume is usually more important than mass, so ratings based on volumetric energy density are most commonly used. The time integral of the product of voltage and current divided by the total volume of the battery is its energy density. Modern batteries for implantable devices have energy densities as high as 1 W-hr/cm^3, including the case.

Stoichiometry and Cell Balance

The specific ratio of the anode and cathode materials that will react is determined by the stoichiometry of the cell reaction. A cell that contains exactly the required ratio of anode and cathode materials is said to be a balanced cell. However, most medical batteries are not designed with exactly the stoichiometric ratio of the active cathode and anode in order to provide predictable end-of-service (EOS) characteristics.

Cell Voltage and Current

The voltage of a single cell can be calculated from fundamental thermodynamic quantities. The *theoretical* voltage is calculated from the free energy for the discharge reaction. This is the voltage that is measured when there are no kinetic limitations, a condition that occurs only when an insignificant amount of current is being drawn from the battery. The terminology for this is *open-circuit* voltage. In practice, the open-circuit voltage can be measured using a high-impedance voltmeter that draws almost no current from the battery during the measurement process. With the onset of current flow, the voltage at the battery terminals will be less than the open-circuit value. Both chemistry and battery design determine the relationship between voltage and current drawn from the battery. A typical current-voltage relationship is shown in Figure 6-2.

In Figure 6-2, the load voltage approaches the open-circuit voltage as the current approaches zero. At the other extreme, the maximum (short-circuit) current is observed when the load voltage approaches zero.

Internal Impedance

Electrical impedance and resistance are important battery properties that play a crucial role in the clinical performance of many implantable devices. The terms *impedance* and *resistance* are often used interchangeably, but they are not precisely the same. For most simple electric circuit elements, Ohm's law, $\Delta V = IR$, accurately describes a linear relationship between voltage drop (ΔV) and current (I), with resistance (R) as the proportionality constant. However, a battery is a complex electrochemical device with several nonlinear processes operating in series. Different processes may dominate at different current levels, depths of discharge, and time. Consequently, the relationship between current and voltage for a battery is, in general, nonlinear, even at very low currents.

Non-ideal Battery Behavior

The previous discussion has focused on the principles and nomenclature of battery operation. It is also important to understand some of the things that limit a battery's ability to power an implantable device. Several important non-ideal processes are discussed in the following paragraphs.

Polarization. Polarization is any process that causes the voltage at the terminals of a battery to drop below its open-circuit value when it is providing current. Internal impedance is one important cause. This is well illustrated in Figure 6-3 for the Li/I_2 battery, but it is true for all batteries to some degree.

This figure shows the curve of discharge voltage versus capacity at four rates of constant-current discharge. The differences among these curves are mainly due to the voltage drop associated with internal resistance of the battery, according to Ohm's law.

Another cause of polarization is the development of a concentration gradient within the battery. As a battery discharges, the ions in the electrolyte must move to maintain electrical neutrality. If they cannot

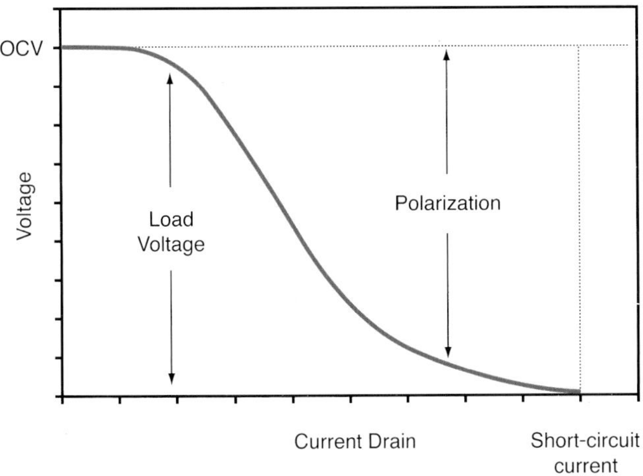

Figure 6-2. Typical load voltage versus current drain plot for a battery. The load voltage is always less than the open-circuit voltage (OCV). Current drain increases toward the right. The maximum cell voltage is obtained at zero current, and the maximum current drain occurs at zero load voltage. The exact shape of the plot depends on the chemistry and design of the battery.

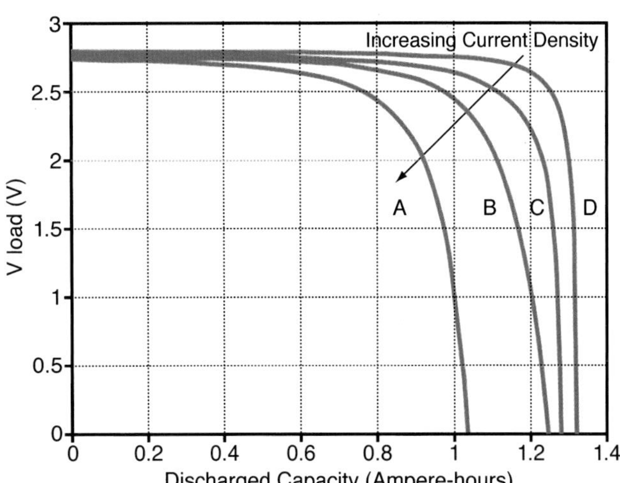

Figure 6-3. Load voltage versus capacity plot for a lithium/iodine battery discharged at four magnitudes of constant current: curve A = 40 $\mu A/cm^2$; curve B = 20 $\mu A/cm^2$; curve C = 10 $\mu A/cm^2$; and curve D = 2 $\mu A/cm^2$. The deliverable capacity decreases with increasing current in this current range because of increasing effects of polarization.

move quickly enough, concentration gradients develop within the battery. A concentration gradient lowers the cell's load voltage.

Similarly, the electron transfer rate may not be able to occur as rapidly as the external demand requires. In such cases, the maximum rate of discharge of the battery becomes governed by the rates at which the battery reactions can occur. When current is drawn from a battery, all of these processes occur to some extent. The net effect of these kinetic limitations is always observed as a decrease in voltage at the terminals of the battery. In general, neither concentration polarization nor electron-transfer polarization conforms to Ohm's law.

Self-discharge. Self-discharge is the spontaneous discharge of a cell or battery by an internal chemical reaction rather than through useful electrochemical discharge. A typical example is a reaction between the anode and the electrolyte solvent to form a passive film or a gas. These parasitic reactions are usually very slow, but because medical batteries are expected to operate for many years, their accumulated effects can be appreciable.[7,8]

Use of Batteries in Implantable Devices

Implantable Battery Design Requirements

The main requirement in battery selection for implantable devices is high reliability. Other significant factors include the desired longevity of the device (which is directly related to battery energy density, circuit design, and allowable device size) and an appropriate indication of impending battery depletion (EOS warning). The basic considerations when designing a battery for an implantable medical device include the voltage and current variations that will be required by the circuit, therapy, and the individual patient. Once these application requirements are formulated, the current, voltage, and capacity requirements of the battery can be determined. An important limitation is the physical space, both volume and shape, within the device that can be allotted to the battery.

Battery Chemistry

Primary batteries used in modern implantable devices use lithium anodes, but the cathode material can vary. Voltage, energy density, and inherent current capability are all primarily functions of the battery chemistry. The chemistry of the battery must be chosen to match the needs of the application. These considerations are discussed with specific examples later in this chapter.

Power Requirements

The peak power requirement differs markedly for pacemakers and defibrillators. Pacemakers use very small amounts of energy with each stimulus, on the order of 15 μJ. Defibrillators, on the other hand, deliver as much as 40 J. A battery optimized for a pacemaker could never come close to supplying energy at the rate required to power a defibrillator. Likewise, a defibrillator battery is not an optimal choice to power a pacemaker, although it could easily supply the current needed. The high-power design of a defibrillator battery has a significantly lower energy density than that of a pacemaker battery, by a factor of two to three. Therefore, if a defibrillator battery were used primarily for pacing, and everything else were equal, it would need to be three times larger than an optimized pacemaker battery to obtain the same longevity. Additionally, a high-current cell poses more inherent safety risks (e.g., gross overheating from a short) than a low-current cell, another reason for matching the battery to the application. How to optimize a battery for longevity and power becomes more complicated when a device performs multiple functions such as both pacing and defibrillation.

Up to now, the Li/I_2 battery has been the dominant power source for implantable cardiac pacemakers, which typically have peak power demands on the order of 100 to 200 μW. Under these conditions, the Li/I_2 battery can maintain an adequate voltage even when its internal resistance reaches several thousand ohms. On the other hand, ICDs have peak power requirements approximately 10,000 times greater than those of a pacemaker, and a Li/I_2 battery is incapable of meeting these requirements. In the past few years, the power and current demands for bradycardia pacemakers have been increasing due to more use of telemetry and features such as multisite pacing. This is causing pacemaker designers to consider chemistries other than Li/I_2 as power sources for new products. These new chemistries are discussed later in this chapter.

Average Versus Instantaneous Current Drain

Implantable medical devices are often characterized by their average current drain. However, therapy delivery and telemetry may require temporary current excursions that can be very different from the average value. Often, the effect of the instantaneous current demand is mitigated by the use of a capacitor that buffers the battery to allow short bursts of power that may be more than two orders of magnitude greater than it could deliver directly. This allows the use of battery designs with reduced anode and cathode surface areas and improved volumetric efficiency. The same principle applies to the use of batteries to charge the large capacitors used to deliver the defibrillation therapy to the heart from an ICD, even though the magnitudes of the current and voltage are much greater.

Shape, Size, and Mass Constraints

Finally, all of these requirements (e.g., longevity, EOS indication, peak power) must be balanced against size, shape, and mass constraints. In the case of ICDs, improvements in packaging and circuit technology have dramatically reduced their size. The ratio of volume to surface area in the battery is an important factor. The performance of a battery of fixed volume can vary substantially depending on its electrode surface area-to-volume ratios. The operating current and longevity demanded of the battery determine both the minimum areas and the amounts of anode and cathode needed.

Relationship between Size, Energy Density, and Current Drain

The relationship between battery size and average current is not one of direct proportionality. For example, decreasing the average current by 50% will not permit a 50% reduction in battery size without compromising longevity because of the inactive materials in a battery (e.g., case, electrolyte, current collectors). Likewise, the usable energy density is also a function of the current demand on the cell. This is particularly true for a battery like the Li/I_2 battery, which has inherently high internal impedance. As the current from the cell is increased, the resulting voltage drops significantly (see Fig. 6-3) and reduces the length of time during which the cell can provide current at or above the minimum voltage necessary to operate the electronic circuits. The useable energy density, which is directly proportional to the area under the discharge (voltage versus capacity) curve, is also reduced. For higher-rate batteries like those used to power ICDs, this is not as big an issue, because the internal resistance of these batteries is very low.

Medical Battery Design and Management Issues

The Battery and Longevity of the Pulse Generator

Longevity is typically defined as the interval between implantation of the device and detection of the EOS indicator. Because longevity can vary dramatically among patients, the longevity requirement is typically linked to a specified set of nominal conditions and programmed parameters. The minimum battery capacity required to achieve the specified longevity can be calculated from the average current needed for this nominal set of conditions. The following equation relates the longevity of the pulse generator (L, in years) to the deliverable capacity of the battery (Q_{del}, in milliampere-hours), and the average pacing current (I, in milliamperes):

$$L = Q_{del}/8766 \cdot I \qquad (6\text{-}5)$$

The conversion factor, 8766 (365.25 days per year × 24 hours per day), is needed because longevity is expressed in years, not hours.

The actual capacity that is built into the battery must be larger than Q_{del}. Additional capacity is needed to account for self-discharge and other parasitic losses of capacity (Q_{sd}). More capacity must also be included to allow for an interval between the occurrence of the EOS indicator and the time when the battery can no longer power the device (Q_{EOL}). The total capacity (Q_{Total}) is defined as follows:

$$Q_{Total} = Q_{del} + Q_{sd} + Q_{EOL} \qquad (6\text{-}6)$$

The average current drain (I in Eq. 6-5) depends on the characteristic of the pulse generator and the patient's requirements for therapy. It has two main components: the static current drain, which powers the electronic components even when no therapy is delivered, and the therapeutic current. Because of better pacing electrodes and better electronic circuits, the average current drain for bradycardia devices has decreased substantially during the past decade.

Effect of Pulse Width on Pacing Current

Increasing the pacing rate, pulse width, or pulse amplitude increases the average pacing current. However, some of these relationships are highly nonlinear. For example, as shown in the following discussion, doubling of the pacing stimulus voltage quadruples the current drain on the battery.

The average pacing current, excluding overhead current, is directly proportional to the pacing rate. However, the effect of pulse width on the average pacing current is not linear. Recall that the pacing pulse results from discharge of a capacitor through the electrode-heart interface. This capacitor produces a pulse in which the current decays exponentially with time, as shown for two different pulse widths in Figure 6-4.

The time-dependent behavior of the current during the pacing pulse is given by the following equation:

$$I = (V_A/R_H)\, e^{-t/R_H C} \qquad (6\text{-}7)$$

where V_A is the amplitude at the beginning of the pacing pulse, R_H is the resistance of the heart, C is the value of the capacitor that delivers the pacing pulse, and t is the time since the beginning of the pacing pulse. In Figures 6-4A and B, the pulse widths are t_w and $t_{w/2}$, respectively. The area under each current-time curve gives the total charge delivered during the pulse. Although the width of the pulse in Figure 6-4B is one half that of the pulse in Figure 6-4A, the charge delivered is considerably more than one half that of the longer pulse. The exact ratio of the charge delivered in the two cases depends on the values of the resistance and capacitance. Nevertheless, reducing the pulse width by a given fraction will always reduce the average pacing current by a substantially smaller fraction because of the exponentially decaying shape of the pacing stimulus current curve.

Effect of Pulse Amplitude on Pacing Current

The definition of pacing pulse amplitude varies somewhat among manufacturers of implantable pulse generators. For the purposes of this chapter, pulse amplitude is defined as the voltage delivered to the heart at the beginning of the pacing pulse (leading edge voltage). As stated earlier, the area under the current-time curve gives the charge delivered per pulse. Doubling of the amplitude doubles both the current and the total charge delivered to the heart. It might seem that, because the charge per pulse is doubled, the average pacing current drawn from the battery would also be doubled. However, the impact on the pacing current is

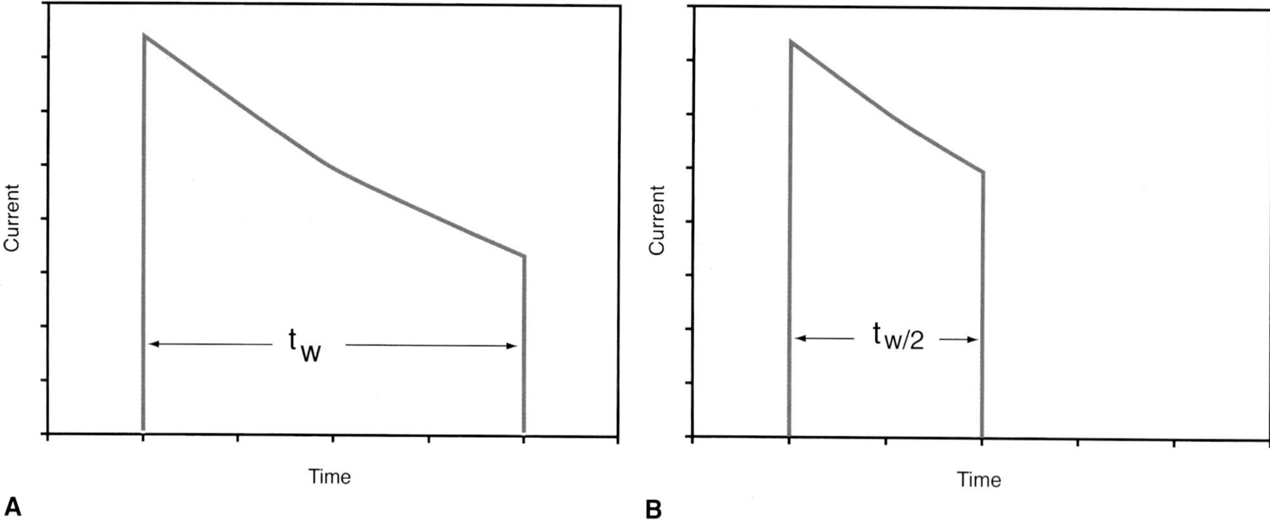

*Figure 6-4. Comparison of charge delivered to the heart as the pacing pulse width is shortened. The two cases in (**A**) and (**B**) assume a discharge into the same patient. The pulse width, t_w, is typically between 0.2 and 1.5 msec, and the maximum current is between 2 and 15 mA, depending on the pulse generator output voltage and the lead-heart interface resistance. In **B**, the pulse width ($t_{w/2}$) is one half that in **A**, but the charge delivered to the heart is substantially greater than one half of that delivered in **A**.*

much larger than that, as seen from the following argument. The energy per pacing pulse is defined by the equation

$$E = V_A \cdot I_A \cdot t_w \quad (6\text{-}8)$$

In this equation, V_A is the average pacing stimulus output voltage of the pulse generator, I_A is the average pacing current delivered to the heart, and t_w is the pulse width. If the lead-electrode-heart interface is considered to be mainly resistive, Ohm's law ($I = V/R$) can be substituted in Equation 6-8, making it

$$E = (V_A^2/R_H)t_w \quad (6\text{-}9)$$

Here, R_H is the effective ohmic load of the heart and lead. From this equation, it is readily apparent that energy consumption increases with the square of the output voltage. In fact, this is the best situation; additional energy losses occur when the stimulus voltage is programmed to a higher level, because the electronic processes for increasing the stimulus voltage are not 100% efficient.

Effect of Lead Impedance on Pacing Current

Finally, it is important to consider the effect of the lead impedance, R_H, on the average pacing current. In a sense, the term *lead impedance* is really a misnomer. The resistance of the lead itself is relatively small (50-100 Ω), and most of the impedance actually arises at the electrode-tissue interface (500-1000 Ω or more). The factors affecting the impedance of this interface are discussed in Chapter 1. In general, the average pacing current is approximately inversely proportional to the sum of the actual lead and tissue interface resistances. Therefore, there is a substantial interest in lead technologies that can increase the impedance of the electrode-tissue interface (without increasing the lead conductor resistance), thereby decreasing the pacing current, while at the same time maintaining a constant or even a reduced pacing threshold voltage.

Summary of Programming Effects on Longevity of Bradycardia Pulse Generators

In summary, the wide range of pacing parameters that can be selected can have a dramatic effect on current drain from the battery in an implanted pulse generator. For example, in the same patient, a bradycardia pulse generator with a 6-year longevity under nominal pacing parameters may reach its replacement time in 2 years at one extreme or after more than 10 years at the other extreme, emphasizing the importance of considering battery longevity when programming pacemakers and ICDs.

Considerations for Longevity of ICDs

ICDs are much more complicated than typical pacemakers, so it is not as easy to generalize about the effects of different factors on their longevity. In general, the two biggest factors to consider are the frequency of tachyarrhythmia therapies and the percentage of time spent pacing the heart. It is possible for the longevity to vary by a factor of 2 to 3 due to these issues alone (see later discussion).

Battery End-of-Service Indication

EOS requirements result from the need to indicate impending battery depletion in both pacemakers and defibrillators in a manner that allows the patient and physician adequate time to replace the device. In general, this requires a battery to have some measurable characteristic, such as voltage or impedance, that can be related to its state of discharge. The pulse generator EOS indication must occur well before the battery voltage falls to a value that cannot sustain cardiac pacing or perform defibrillation.

Elective Replacement Indicator

All modern implantable pulse generators have an elective replacement indicator (ERI), also referred to as the recommended replacement time (RRT) or the EOS point. As a general rule, this indicator is designed to occur at least 3 months before the battery voltage drops to a level at which erratic pacing or loss of capture results.

Battery Voltage. The most common method for monitoring battery function measures battery voltage. Historically, this was accomplished by comparing the battery voltage with a diode reference voltage generated by the pacemaker circuitry. The ERI was triggered when the battery voltage dropped below the reference level. Most modern devices incorporate a voltage measurement circuit in the form of an analog-to-digital converter. The digitized battery voltage can be compared with a value stored in a nonvolatile memory to trigger the ERI, or it can be telemetered to the programmer where the comparison is made.

For Li/I_2 batteries, the battery voltage remains relatively constant throughout most of its discharge under low load conditions. This is shown in the voltage-versus-capacity curve in Figure 6-5. This figure also shows the resistance of the battery as it discharges. Notice that the resistance changes from a modest value at the beginning of service to a large value when the battery is almost depleted.

Because the battery voltage is relatively constant for much of the pulse generator's useful life, the telemetered voltage may not be particularly useful for estimating its remaining service life until the EOS time draws near. On the other hand, the measured voltage may be useful for determining the battery's ability to remain above the ERI voltage after reprogramming to a higher current.

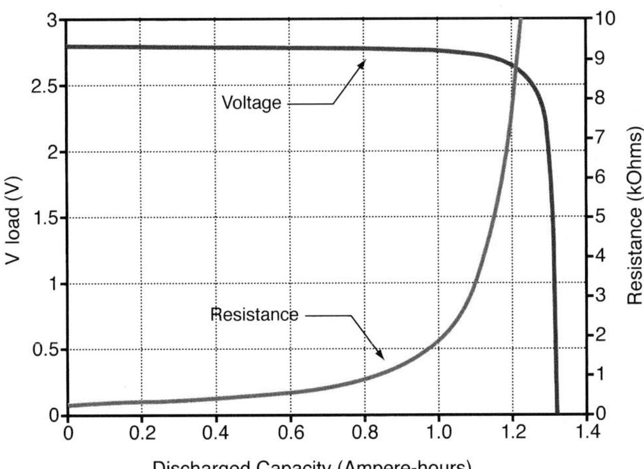

Figure 6-5. Relationships between voltage, resistance, and delivered capacity of a lithium/iodine battery. The voltage remains reasonably constant through the service life of the battery, whereas the resistance steadily builds up with discharge. Note the sudden fall-off in voltage as the resistance rapidly increases near the end-of-service life.

Voltage characteristics differ for different battery chemistries. For example, the Li/I_2 battery has a fairly flat discharge curve throughout most of its life at pacing currents. Its ERI is chosen somewhere on the "knee" of the discharge curve. The exact voltage chosen depends on the expected average drain current for that particular device at the end of the implant's service life. The lithium/silver vanadium oxide (Li/SVO) battery used in ICDs has two very distinct voltage regions before the typical ERI voltage. The region after the second plateau is sloped. The switch from the second plateau to the sloped discharge region is used as the ERI trigger in some devices using this battery chemistry. This voltage is much less sensitive to current variances than is the voltage chosen for a Li/I_2 battery, because the internal resistance of this battery is much lower than that of the Li/I_2 battery.

Battery Impedance. Battery impedance, another parameter used to signal the elective replacement point, is usually much less dependent on current than is battery voltage. Although the voltage of a Li/I_2 battery remains relatively constant through most of its discharge, its impedance increases continuously, and it increases especially rapidly as the battery approaches depletion (see Fig. 6-5). At depletion, battery impedance is useful not only for signaling the elective replacement point but also for providing an estimate of remaining service life. Battery impedance is usually determined from the open- and load-circuit voltages of the battery, by measuring the voltage drop across a known resistor within the pulse generator and then assuming that Ohm's law can be applied.

Consumed Charge. A final method used to indicate remaining battery life has been to measure the cumulative sum of the charge removed from the battery. This is accomplished by monitoring the current drawn from the battery or the current and voltage (i.e., energy) delivered to the heart. This method requires an accurate knowledge of the original deliverable capacity of the battery, because the technique actually measures the capacity already used, and the amount left must be calculated by subtracting the amount used from the initial capacity. This method is sometimes referred to as the "gas gauge." "Gas gauge" indicators of remaining longevity have been implemented in some devices. The inherent variability of the battery system in pacemakers powered by Li/I_2 batteries limits the accuracy of the "gas gauge" significantly. However, in some devices powered by newer battery systems, such as those discussed later, robust and accurate "gas gauges" are possible.

Elective Replacement Indicator Triggering

The relatively high resistance of power sources such as the Li/I_2 battery results in a battery voltage that is highly dependent on current. Therefore, large changes in average battery current in pulse generators that use battery voltage to indicate the elective replacement point (even if temporary) may drop the battery voltage below the ERI trigger value. Such changes in current can occur, for example, as a result of rate-responsive pacing, magnet-rate pacing, or telemetry. They could also occur during electrophysiologic studies with noninvasively programmed stimulation (NIPS), in which the pacemaker is used to interrupt an episode of tachycardia by delivering short bursts of pacing at a very high rate. Because the ERI is usually latched (stored) when it is triggered, these temporary increases in current can cause a premature appearance of the ERI. The amount of service life lost to these premature triggers is typically small. In most cases, devices are designed to make it possible to reset an ERI that has been prematurely triggered. In some devices, the ERI is inhibited during temporary high-current events to circumvent some of the issues just described.

In ICDs, the ERI is usually based on the battery voltage or on the time required to charge the capacitor. Typically, the battery voltage is measured during normal sensing and pacing operations and not during defibrillation therapy, when the battery voltage is much lower. Because of the very low internal resistance of ICD batteries, there is little effect of pacing parameters on triggering of the ERI. Alternatively, some ICDs base their ERI determination on the time required to charge the output capacitor. This approach is possible because some Li/SVO battery designs have a reduced power capability as they approach depletion.

Clinical Indicators of the Battery Replacement Time

The clinical indicators of battery depletion vary widely among manufacturers of pulse generators and even among the models of a single manufacturer. Some of the more common indicators are listed here.

1. Stepwise change in pacing rate. Elective replacement time is indicated by a change in the pacing rate to a predetermined fixed rate (e.g., 65 bpm) or a fractional change in rate (e.g., a 10% decrease from the programmed rate).
2. Stepwise change in magnet rate. The magnet-pacing rate decreases in a stepwise fashion that is related to remaining battery life.
3. Pacing mode change. DDD and DDDR pulse generators may automatically revert to another mode, such as VVI or VOO, to reduce current drain and extend battery life.
4. Telemetered battery voltage or impedance. This information is used to estimate remaining battery service life or to indicate an imminent ERI by algorithms performed outside the pulse generator.

All manufacturers provide technical manuals containing tables or graphs that indicate the relationship between battery voltage or impedance and the estimated remaining service life of the device. This estimated time differs for different loads on the battery and is influenced by pacing rates and stimulus currents, as discussed previously.

The Elective Replacement Indicator in Practice

The object of having an ERI is to allow the use of the pulse generator as long as safely possible. Several questions must be addressed when considering elective pulse generator replacement based on the ERI. First, how does the ERI for this particular pulse generator manifest itself? Second, because the goal is to replace the pulse generator not too long before its continued use becomes unsafe, what is the definition of "safe" in terms of pacing loss for the patient in question? Third, what factors other than the need for pacing, such as the temporary presence of pneumonia, must be considered in making a decision about the timing of pulse generator replacement in this patient?

Concerns for the Patient if Pacing Ceases. A small percentage of patients with pacemakers are extremely likely to develop fatal asystole if pacing capture is lost. Another fraction will be asystolic for a few seconds and then will develop an escape rhythm at very slow rates. A third group will develop transient presyncope or lightheadedness but will then be able to function reasonably normally. A fourth, and probably the largest, group of patients will slowly develop symptoms such as reduced exercise tolerance but otherwise will be at least temporarily asymptomatic. The fifth and last group will not even know that the pacemaker has stopped working unless an Adams-Stokes attack occurs at some time in the future. Therefore, the consequences of loss of pacing vary tremendously, and for these reasons the time relationship between the appearance of the ERI and the loss of capture is much more important for some patients than for others.

Effects of High Current Drains In or Near the Elective Replacement Indicator. If the pacing threshold is very high, the output voltage of the pulse generator may decrease below the level necessary for capture before the ERI appears or reaches its nominal value. For example, the output voltage of some pulse generators starts to decrease when the magnet rate begins to decrease (but before ERI). If the stimulus voltage approaches the actual pacing threshold, capture may be lost. It is worth noting that reprogramming the pulse generator to a higher output voltage near the end of its expected service life will have an especially large effect on reducing the remaining service life of the pulse generator if it is powered by a Li/I_2 battery. The result of increasing the output is both an increase in current drain, due to the higher output, and a large increase in polarization voltage, because of the high internal resistance. These two effects combine to shorten the remaining service life more than might be expected.

Pacing Output Voltage Near the Elective Replacement Indicator. The pulse generator output voltage decreases more rapidly when the cell is nearing or in the ERI phase than it does earlier in its service life. When the magnet rate is changing because ERI has been detected in pulse generators that feature a gradual rate change, the output voltage decreases faster at high-output voltages than it does for normal output settings. This should be expected because of the high current drain on the battery.

Common Sense Clinical Guidelines Regarding the Elective Replacement Indicator. These points translate into two clinical guidelines regarding the status of the patient and the status of the pulse generator battery at ERI: (1) The physician should replace the pulse generator sooner than he or she otherwise would if the patient is highly pacemaker dependent; (2) If the patient is pacemaker dependent, the pulse generator (or the pulse generator and lead) should be replaced even sooner if the pacing threshold is high.

Battery Chemistries Used in Implantable Cardiac Rhythm Management Devices

Lithium Cells

Lithium was chosen as the anode material in pacemakers for several reasons. First, it has a very high capacity density, 2.06 A-hr/cm^3. Lithium also forms many electrochemical couples that have appropriate stability, adequately fast discharge kinetics, and high energy density. Several lithium anode battery chemistries were developed for implantation. These included three chemistries with liquid organic electrolytes—lithium/silver chromate, lithium/cupric sulfide, and lithium/manganese dioxide; one chemistry with a liquid cathode component—lithium/thionyl chloride; and one chemistry that behaved almost like a solid state battery—Li/I_2.[9] Although none of the several varieties of lithium batteries developed for implantable medical use proved to be inherently unreliable, only the Li/I_2 system has remained in widespread use for cardiac pacing, although that is again changing today.

The lithium/cupric sulfide and lithium/silver chromate batteries had some very attractive features, although they are no longer used today. The type of lithium/manganese dioxide cells used in the late 1970s is also no longer made; however, newer versions of this system are beginning to be used again to power some implantable cardiac pacemakers and defibrillators.

Today, two chemical systems are used to power the overwhelming majority of implantable cardiac rhythm management devices. Most implantable pacemakers are powered by the Li/I_2 battery, and ICDs are powered by Li/SVO batteries.

The Lithium/Iodine Battery

The Li/I_2 battery is probably the most well-known implantable battery because it has been used in the vast majority of cardiac pacemakers. The first implantation of a pacemaker powered by a Li/I_2 battery occurred in 1972.[5,6,10] About 10 million Li/I_2-powered pacemakers have now been implanted. There are many factors favoring the use of this battery system. When the current demand is low, it is hard to beat the Li/I_2 battery. It has a high energy density and a low rate of self-discharge, resulting in good longevity and small size. The inherently high impedance of the Li/I_2 battery has not been a large disadvantage up to now, because the current required by modern pacemaker circuits is so low, typically about 10 μA. The much greater stimulation current is drawn from a capacitor, which can charge for a very long time between pacing pulses compared with its discharge time. The voltage and impedance characteristics of the Li/I_2 cell also allow the clinician to monitor the approaching EOS indication. This battery system is simple, elegant in concept, and inherently resistant to many common modes of failure (discussed later). As a result, Li/I_2 batteries have attained a record of reliability unsurpassed among electrochemical power sources.

Lithium/Iodine Cell Structure. Most Li/I_2 batteries consist of an anode of lithium coated with a thin film of poly-2-vinylpyridine (P2VP) and a cathode composed of a thermally reacted mixture of iodine and P2VP.

Figure 6-6 shows a cutaway view of a typical Li/I_2 battery. In general, Li/I_2 batteries have a single, central anode that is surrounded by cathode material. Such a battery has a fairly small electrode area, and therefore a rather modest current-delivering capability, but small currents are all that have been needed for bradycardia pacemakers in the past. Visible in this figure are the central anode, with an embedded current collector wire, and the iodine cathode that fills much of the volume inside the battery. This figure also shows several other important structures. One of these is the electrical feedthrough that connects the anode to the outside of the cell. The case serves as the site of the electrical connection to the cathode, which is in direct contact with the inside of the container. Another visible feature is the fillport. The fillport is the means

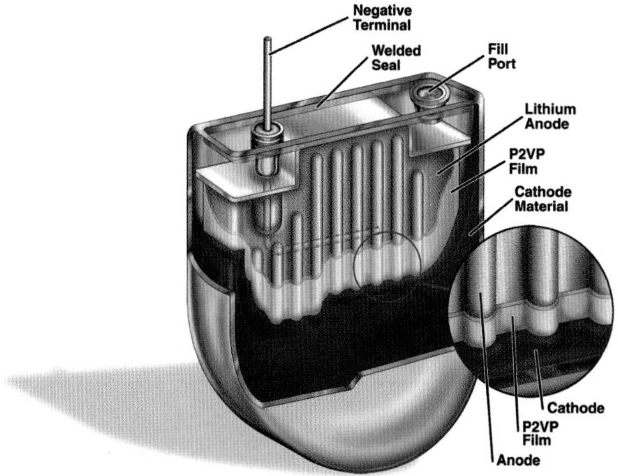

Figure 6-6. Cutaway view of a typical lithium/iodine battery, showing its internal construction. Easily identifiable interior parts include the anode feedthrough, the anode current collector (wire), the cathode, the P2VP film on the anode, and the fill port where the cathode material is poured into the cell. The connection to the cathode is via the battery case.

by which the cathode mixture is introduced into the cell. The fillport is welded shut after the cathode is put in the cell.

Electrochemical Properties of Lithium/Iodine Cells. When Li/I_2 batteries are manufactured, the iodine initially reaching the surface of lithium reacts directly with the lithium, yielding lithium iodide. This reaction needs to proceed only to a small extent before the surface of the lithium is covered by lithium iodide, after which the reaction rate slows greatly. The voltage of the cell rises quickly to 2.8 V as this layer forms; 2.8 V is characteristic of the Li/I_2 couple. Lithium iodide is an electronic insulator with a high enough lithium-ion conductivity to act as a solid electrolyte in the cell. It accumulates near the surface of the anode because it is not soluble in the cathode mixture. Because the product of the direct reaction of the anode and cathode is also the electrolyte, a breach of the electrolyte layer in a cell simply results in the creation of more electrolyte. Therefore, the electrolyte is said to be self-healing. This characteristic contributes to the high reliability of this battery.

As iodine is removed, the resistivity of the remaining material increases by several orders of magnitude before the cell is completely discharged. This effect is primarily responsible for the battery's high resistance in the latter part of its service life. This is a fundamental characteristic of this battery system that limits its application to uses that do not require very high or very frequent bursts of current, especially toward the end of its service life.

Discharge Curve for the Lithium/Iodine Battery. Figure 6-7 shows the characteristic shapes of the voltage and resistance curves as a function of discharge for a typical Li/I_2 battery. The most salient characteristic of these curves is the initial slow change of each parameter followed by a rapid change near the end of discharge. The point at which the resistance curve becomes noticeably steeper corresponds to the point in the discharge at which the crystalline iodine becomes depleted from the two-phase cathode mixture. Before this point, the resistance change is dominated by the growing electrolyte. Beyond it, the cathode rapidly dominates the resistance of the cell, as the cathode becomes lower in iodine content. The region of discharge dominated by cathode resistance is used to signal the approaching EOS for most pacemakers.[11]

Effects of Current Drain on Deliverable Capacity of Lithium/Iodine Cells. The high energy density of the Li/I_2 battery may be negated if the application requires frequent periods of high current drain. This is because there is an optimum average current for the operation of this (or any) battery. Figure 6-8 shows a plot of the deliverable capacity versus the log of average current drain for a typical Li/I_2 battery.

If currents higher than the optimum are drawn from any battery, polarization lowers the deliverable capacity. For currents lower than the optimum, self-discharge uses up capacity increasingly faster than the application current, resulting in a reduced deliverable capacity. For applications that require an average current drain that is significantly different from the optimum, a different battery system may result in more favorable deliverable capacity and longevity. Comparisons of these curves for different battery systems and even for different sizes and designs of a single type of battery can help a device designer choose the best power source. Consider the following example. In the typical

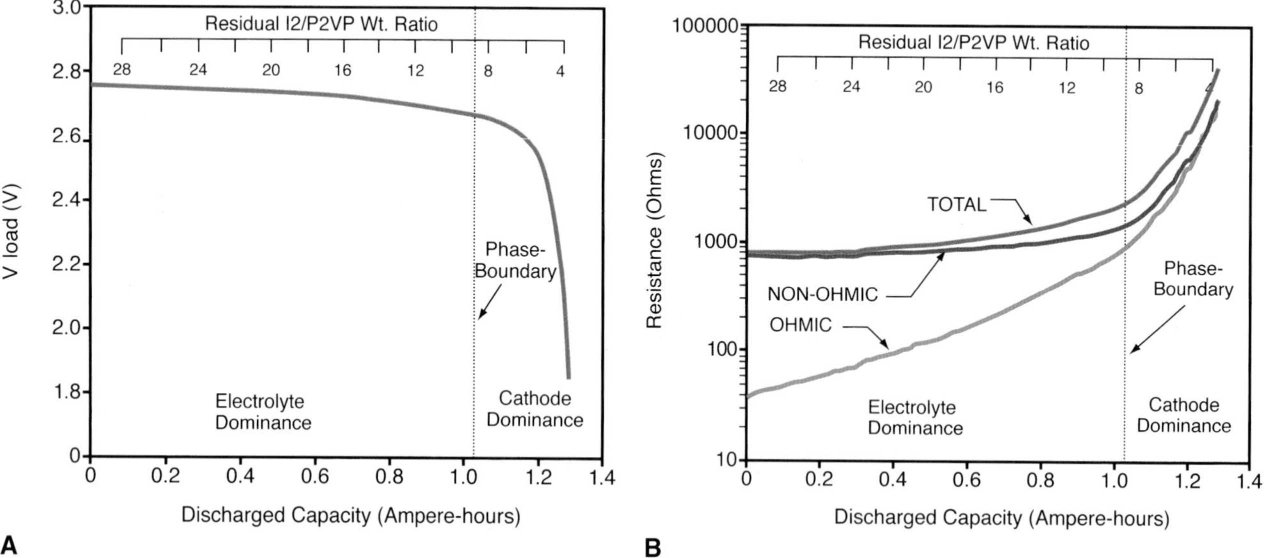

Figure 6-7. ***A,*** *Voltage-capacity plot for a lithium/iodine (Li/I_2) battery during discharge. The superimposed scale shows the residual I_2/P2VP weight ratio (starting at 50:1). The vertical line defines the boundary between the two-phase and the single-phase cathode regions, where the electrolyte and cathode, respectively, dominate the internal resistance.* ***B,*** *Resistance-capacity plot analogous to the voltage-capacity plot in* ***A****. The ohmic and non-ohmic contributions to the internal resistance are shown along with their sums.*

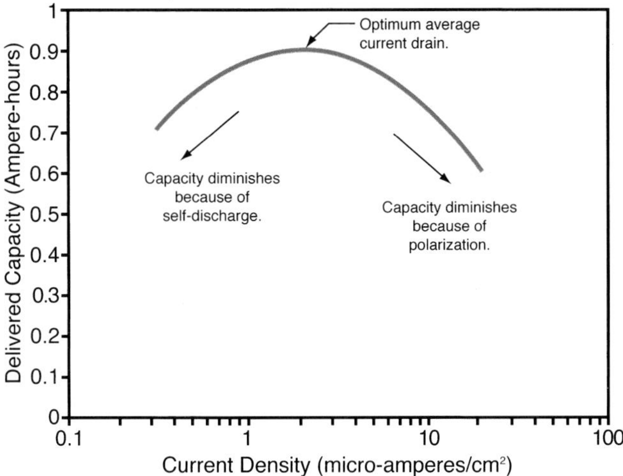

Figure 6-8. Graph of capacity versus log current drain for a typical lithium/iodine medical battery, showing that deliverable battery capacity has a maximum value due to the competing effects of self-discharge and polarization.

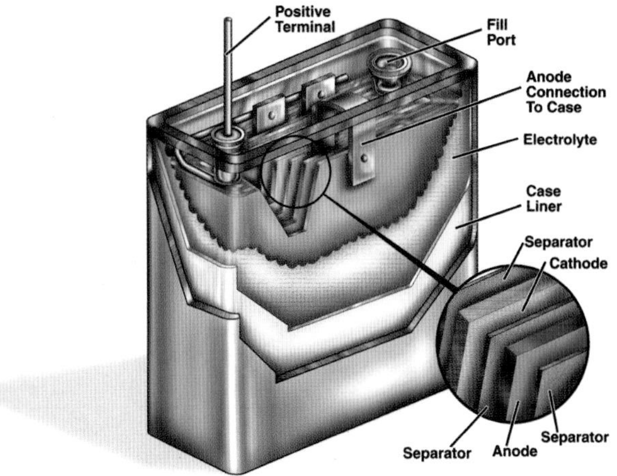

Figure 6-9. Cutaway view of a typical high-rate defibrillator battery, showing a wound construction in which a sandwich of anode, separator, and cathode are rolled, flattened, and fit inside the battery case. This battery uses a liquid electrolyte to ensure high internal conductivity. In the battery shown here, the anode is connected to the case and the cathode is connected to the feedthrough. Notice the multiple connections to the cathode to ensure low internal resistance.

conditions encountered in an implanted cardiac pacemaker, a lithium/manganese dioxide battery has a volumetric energy density about 80% that of a Li/I_2 battery. However, if the application requires frequent current pulses at a 10-fold increase in magnitude, the overall deliverable energy density of the lithium/manganese dioxide battery may become greater than that of the Li/I_2 battery.

Comparison of Pacemaker and Defibrillator Batteries

Implantable defibrillators are designed to deliver a shock within 10 seconds after the fibrillation or tachycardia is detected. When the ICD determines that a shock may be required, it begins to charge a high-voltage capacitor. The time needed to charge the capacitor before the shock is delivered depends on the ability of the battery to sustain a very high current during this period, while maintaining a high voltage. Therefore, the implantable defibrillator requires a battery with high peak power, where power is the product of current and voltage ($P = I \cdot V$).

The high power required of defibrillator batteries dictates a design that is quite different from that of a bradycardia battery. Figure 6-6, discussed earlier, shows a cutaway view of a typical battery used to power a pacemaker. This battery has small and rather thick electrodes. Contrast this figure with Figure 6-9, which shows an analogous cutaway for a defibrillator battery.

The defibrillator battery has very different construction. Instead of a single central anode, it has wound layers of anode and cathode material separated by a thin porous film. Both the anode and cathode layers are very thin. The electrolyte in the defibrillator battery is a highly conductive solution of a lithium salt in organic solvents. The design of the defibrillator battery, with large thin electrodes and liquid electrolyte, gives this battery the high power needed to quickly charge the high-voltage capacitors in the defibrillator.

The Lithium/Silver Vanadium Oxide Battery

The first implantable defibrillators were powered by batteries having a lithium anode and a vanadium oxide cathode.[12,13] However, these batteries had some limitations in terms of reproducible discharge characteristics and a higher than desirable rate of self-discharge. Today, lithium batteries having an SVO cathode, chemically $Ag_2V_4O_{11}$, power almost all ICDs.[14-16] The SVO cathode provides a reasonable balance between good energy density, high power, and a gradual decrease in voltage as the cathode is depleted. Although alternative cathode materials are likely to be developed and implemented in future devices, it is worthwhile to consider the discharge characteristics of the Li/SVO battery.

Typical discharge behavior for the Li/SVO battery is shown in Figure 6-10. The uppermost curve in each graph represents the battery voltage during normal sensing and bradycardia pacing operations. This is sometimes referred to as the "background" voltage. It is this background voltage that is typically monitored by the ICD and reported via telemetry. Its fall below a specified value may also be used as an ERI, as is sometimes done in a bradycardia pacemaker. Because of the high power capability (i.e., low internal resistance) of these batteries, there is relatively little dependence of the background voltage on pulse generator settings. This is in sharp contrast to the behavior described for the Li/I_2 batteries used to power bradycardia pacemakers.

The background voltage for the Li/SVO battery is relatively independent of ICD model and manufacturer. The voltage slopes gently from about 3.25 V at the beginning of service life to about 3.15 V at about 30%

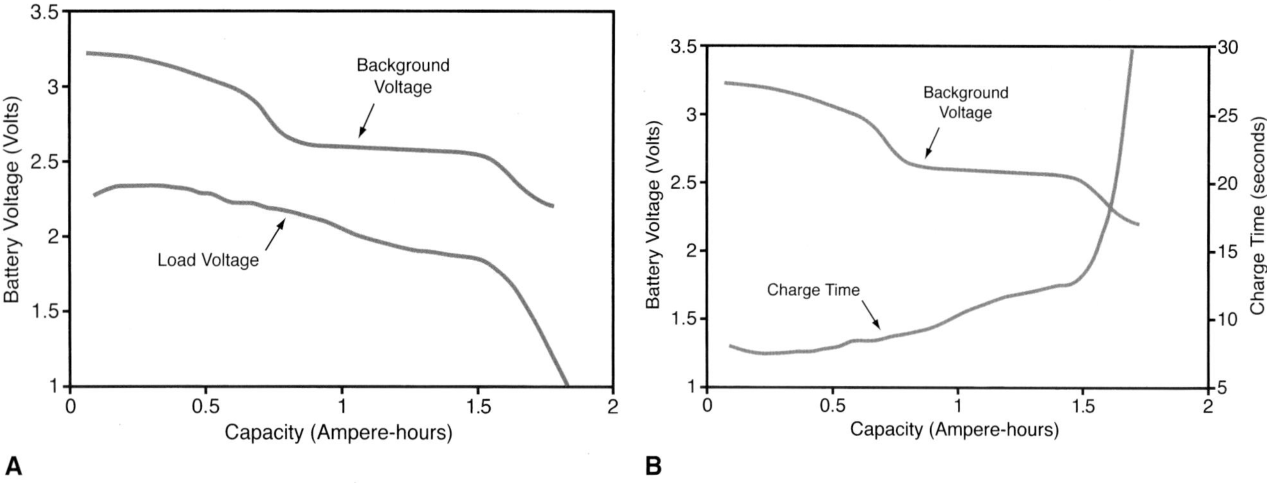

Figure 6-10. ***A,*** *Typical voltage-capacity plot for a lithium/silver vanadium oxide single-cell battery. The upper curve represents the battery voltage during monitoring and pacing activities. The lower curve represents the battery voltage whenever capacitor charging is occurring.* ***B,*** *Similar plot to* ***A,*** *except that the lower curve represents the time required to charge the capacitor at various states of battery discharge.*

depth of discharge. This is followed by a region of more rapidly declining voltage, which levels off at a value of about 2.6 V at approximately 50% depth of discharge. This 2.6 V region is very flat, sloping less than 0.1 V until about 85% depth of discharge. After this point, the background voltage resumes a more rapid decline throughout the remainder of useful battery life.

The battery voltage during the period when the output capacitor is being charged is much lower than the background voltage. This is shown in Figure 6-11, which presents the typical voltage of a Li/SVO battery before, during, and after the charging of a defibrillator capacitor. This is often referred to as the "pulse" voltage or "load" voltage of the battery. The lower curve on Figure 6-10A depicts the typical load voltage as a function of discharge capacity. The actual value of the load voltage is highly dependent on the ICD design and programmed parameters. However, the general trend of a gradually decreasing load voltage throughout the life of the battery is typical of all Li/SVO batteries (and most other battery chemistries as well). As the battery approaches the end of its useful life, the loss of load voltage becomes much more rapid.

The declining load voltage is associated with both declining background voltage and slightly increasing internal resistance of the battery. The decline in load voltage is indicative of reduced battery power and is accompanied by a corresponding increase in the time required to charge the output capacitor. Typical charge time behavior is shown in the lower curve of Figure 6-10B. Again, the specific charge time values vary significantly from one ICD model and manufacturer to another. However, the general trend of a gradually increasing charge time throughout device life is typical. Most significant is the rapid increase in charge time as the battery reaches the end of its useful life.

Elective replacement of the ICD is typically indicated by either the background voltage or the charge time. In the case of an ERI based on background voltage, it is important to be aware of the long voltage plateau in the region of 2.6 V. The elective replacement voltage is normally set just below this value, in the region of 2.55 V to 2.45 V. There has been some tendency for ICDs to be prematurely explanted due to concern about the remaining longevity when the telemetered battery voltage is close to the ERI voltage. However, inspection of Figures 6-10A and B shows that the device continues to perform well throughout this entire region of discharge. Therefore, the fact that the telemetered voltage is "close" to the ERI value should not normally be of

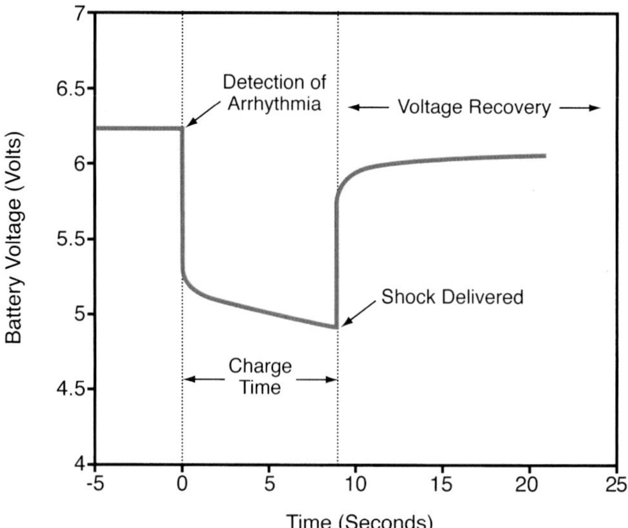

Figure 6-11. Typical voltage-time curve showing defibrillator battery voltage during the course of delivery of a defibrillator shock. The voltage is shown before and during detection (left), *during charging of the high-voltage capacitor* (middle), *and after delivery of the defibrillation shock* (right).

concern. However, as explained in the next section, in some cases the internal impedance of the battery increases beyond the desired value while the voltage is on the 2.6V plateau. For this reason, manufacturers may recommend monitoring the charge time as well as the battery voltage to determine when the ICD should be replaced.

Long-Term Performance of Lithium/Silver Vanadium Oxide Batteries. After many years of laboratory testing and experience in the field with Li/SVO batteries, it is apparent that the performance of these batteries depends on how rapidly the battery is depleted. When the battery is depleted over a longer period of time, the internal impedance of the battery is higher in the latter half of the discharge curve. This phenomenon is illustrated in Figure 6-12.

This figure shows the background voltage and internal impedance of Li/SVO batteries discharged over 3, 5, and 7 years. The internal impedance is unaffected by the discharge rate until midway through discharge. After that point, there is a larger increase in internal impedance for batteries discharged over a longer period. The higher internal resistance results in longer charge times.[17]

Two manufacturers make Li/SVO batteries for ICDs, and they use slightly different versions of SVO. The earlier form of SVO, used by one manufacturer, is made at a low temperature using decomposable starting materials; it is called DSVO, for *d*ecomposition *s*ilver *v*anadium *o*xide. A newer material, made by the other manufacturer, is made at a higher temperature using simple silver and vanadium oxides; it is called CSVO, for *c*ombination *s*ilver *v*anadium *o*xide.[18] The increase in resistance shown in Figure 6-13 occurs two to three times faster for DSVO compared with CSVO. As a result, ICDs with DSVO batteries can reach an undesirably long charge time before the ERI voltage is reached. Figure 6-13 compares actual longevities of the two types of SVO in one model of ICD.

Clearly, the devices with the CSVO batteries lasted longer. Sixty percent of the ICDs powered by DSVO batteries lasted 60 months, whereas 60% of CSVO batteries lasted longer than 90 months, an improvement of about 50% in longevity.[19]

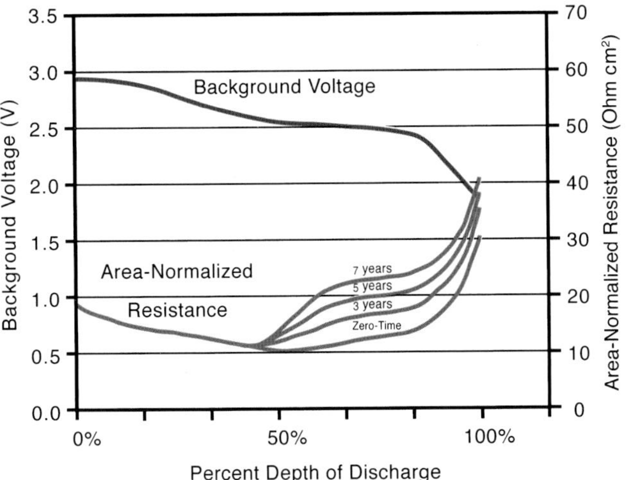

Figure 6-12. Comparison of the area-normalized resistance of a lithium/silver vanadium oxide battery for various battery longevities. The area-normalized resistance is the internal impedance of the battery, calculated from the drop in voltage (V) during the pulse, the current (I), and the area (A) of the cathode: Area-normalized resistance = $A_{cathode} \cdot (V_{background} - V_{pulse})/I_{pulse}$.

Charge Time-Optimized ICD Batteries. Although ICD batteries made with CSVO cathodes maintain low charge time better than DSVO batteries do, the charge time still increases as the battery approaches ERI (see Fig. 6-10B). One manufacturer solved this problem simply by changing the ratio of anode to cathode material in the battery. All of the batteries discussed so far have been cathode limited; the amount of charge in the anode exceeds the amount in the cathode by a small amount, to ensure that all of the cathode can be discharged. Cathode limitation is the most efficient battery design if the goal is to optimize energy density. If the goal is to maintain a low charge time, it makes sense to use only part of the cathode capacity, ending the discharge a short way onto the 2.6-volt plateau. The amount of anode in the battery is reduced, and the amount of SVO is increased. As a result, the battery always remains in the region where internal impedance is low and charge times are short.

Figure 6-14 compares the voltage and charge time of conventional ICD batteries with charge time-optimized batteries that occupy the same volume in an ICD. The charge time-optimized battery maintains a much lower charge time in the latter half of ICD life, without sacrificing longevity.[20]

Safety. Safety is a concern with high-power batteries because they contain a large amount of energy and are designed to deliver it quickly. If an internal short circuit occurs, the relatively large current traveling through the short can heat the cell contents, and could, under some rare circumstances, initiate a violent chemical reaction. Batteries for implantable defibrillators are designed and

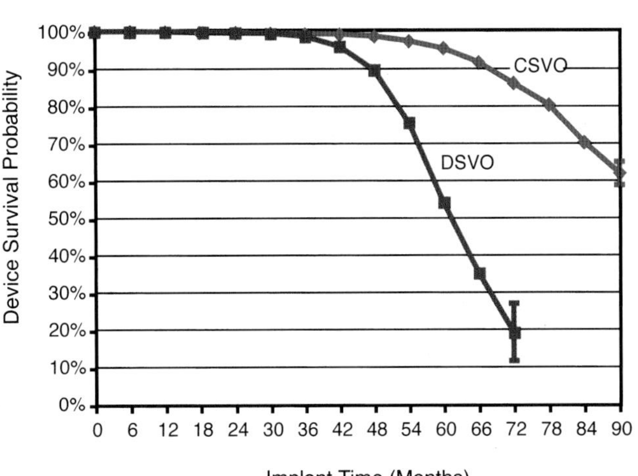

Figure 6-13. Comparison of ICD longevity of DSVO and CSVO batteries in one model of ICD. See text for details.

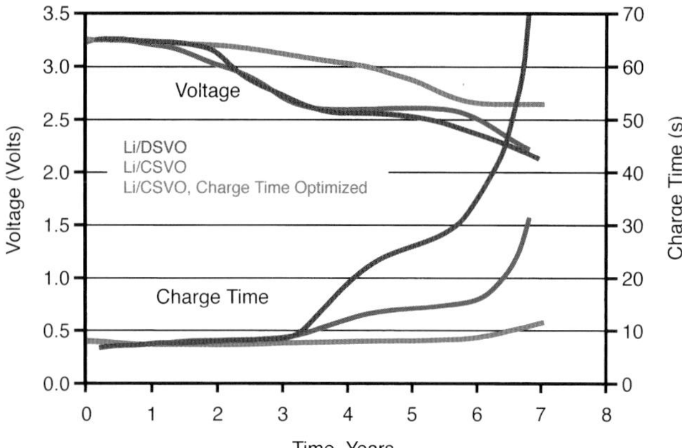

Figure 6-14. Comparison of the performance of charge time-optimized batteries with conventionally balanced DSVO and CSVO batteries as a function of time. All batteries occupy the same volume in the ICD.

constructed with great care to ensure that the occurrence of such a hazardous condition is almost impossible. For example, two layers of separator material are typically used in these batteries, whereas consumer lithium batteries of similar power capability may use only one. The polymeric separator materials chosen for this application are designed to melt at a relatively low temperature. This is very useful if either an external or an internal short develops in the battery. If a short occurs, the battery heats up, the separator melts, and the porous structure of the separator is lost. The dense polymer sheet that results from melting will not allow ions to pass through it, and the electrochemical reaction is stopped.

Emerging Power Sources

Hybrid Cathode Batteries

In the late 1990s, several changes in implantable cardiac devices occurred that increased peak power requirements beyond the capability of Li/I_2 batteries. These included increased use of addressable memory in implantable pulse generators (IPGs) to capture and store information about the electrical activity of the heart, the need for faster and longer-range telemetry to transmit this information outside the body, new physiologic sensors and new therapies with higher power requirements, such as cardiac resynchronization and treatment of atrial fibrillation. The peak power requirements for these features are well outside the range of efficient discharge for Li/I_2 batteries, as discussed previously.

Several existing implantable battery chemistries could meet the need for higher power better than Li/I_2 systems can, but until recently this always involved a compromise of energy density or inadequate EOS warning. A new lithium battery chemistry with a cathode consisting of a mixture of SVO and carbon monofluoride (CF_x) has been developed to meet the needs of implantable devices with higher-rate therapies and features.[21,22] CF_x is a commercial cathode material with modest power capability and abrupt EOS characteristics but a very high energy density. The blend of the two cathode materials, called a hybrid cathode, yields a primary battery that has an energy density equal to that of a Li/I_2 battery, with 40 to 50 times the power; enough to support the new features. Hybrid cathode batteries have been used in implantable cardiac devices since 1999. Cumulative implants of these devices through 2004 total about 100,000.

Plots of voltage versus percentage of discharged capacity for SVO and CF_x batteries are shown in Figure 6-15A and B. The voltage curve of a hybrid cathode behaves like a superposition of the two types in proportion to the starting composition of the mixture. An example is shown in Figure 6-15C.

The composition of the hybrid can be chosen based on the application, enhancing the capacity with a greater proportion of CF_x or enhancing the power capability and EOS characteristics with more SVO. For low- and medium-rate applications, the composition can be chosen so that 85% to 90% of the battery capacity comes from CF_x. In this composition range, efficiently designed medium-rate hybrid cathode batteries can match Li/I_2 batteries in energy density, at about 1 $W\text{-}hr/cm^3$.

Hybrid cathode batteries may be specifically adapted for ICD applications as an alternative battery chemistry. Although no ICDs powered by hybrid cathode batteries had been implanted by the end of 2004, this system is likely to allow significant size reduction in ICD batteries in the future.

For ICD applications, a higher proportion of SVO is required to provide adequate power. High-rate ICD batteries designed with hybrid cathodes maintain almost uniform power capability throughout the discharge lifetime of the battery. This means that charge times for ICDs remain constant and low, similar to charge-time optimized SVO batteries, but with significantly higher energy density.

Rechargeable Lithium-ion Batteries

Rechargeable lithium-ion cells were introduced to the consumer market by the Sony Corporation in 1992. Since that time, lithium-ion technology has been the major focus of research and development investment by many leading battery manufacturers. Lithium-ion technology exhibits several characteristics that make it highly suitable for implantable medical applications, including the following.

1. High energy density. Although lithium-ion batteries have only about one half the energy density of a typical ICD battery, they have double the energy density of older rechargeable batteries such as the NiCad battery. For applications that have a high average power requirement, lithium-ion batteries can provide both small size and excellent longevity.
2. No memory effect. NiCad batteries require complete discharge and complete recharge to maintain the full

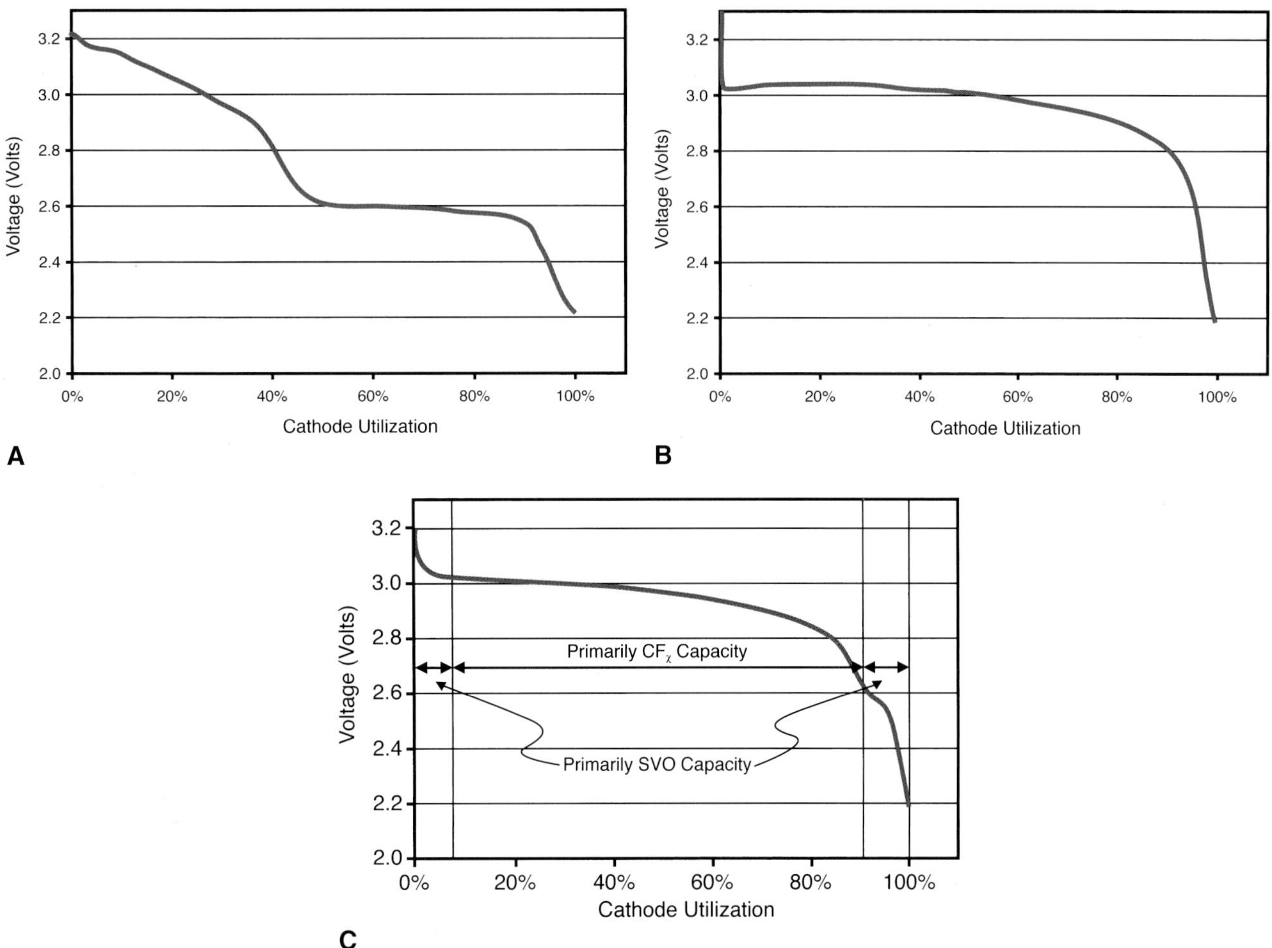

Figure 6-15. ***A,*** *Typical discharge of a lithium/silver vanadium oxide (Li/SVO) battery.* ***B,*** *Typical discharge curve of a lithium/carbon monofluoride (Li/CF_x) battery.* ***C,*** *Typical discharge curve of a CF_x/SVO hybrid cathode battery.*

battery capacity. Lithium-ion batteries can be partially charged or discharged with no deleterious effects. Therefore, the patient is free to develop a recharge schedule that is convenient.

3. High voltage. Lithium-ion batteries typically operate in the 3- to 4-V range and are generally compatible with electronics for implantable devices that have historically used 3-V primary lithium batteries.
4. Low self-discharge. Lithium-ion batteries can be designed to have self-discharge rates of less than 1% per month. This is at least an order of magnitude better than typical with NiCad technology. Furthermore, the self-discharged capacity is almost fully recoverable on subsequent recharge.
5. High cycle life. Several thousand charge/discharge cycles can be completed with well over 50% capacity retention. This far exceeds the demands of most anticipated implantable applications.
6. Long calendar life. The best lithium-ion batteries maintain more than 50% of initial capacity after 10 years of use. The only effect of capacity loss to the patient is reduced time between required recharges.

It is not yet clear what future applications will emerge for rechargeable batteries in the cardiac rhythm management arena, but some applications are likely, and substantial patent activity is already occurring. By the end of 2004, neurologic stimulators powered by rechargeable lithium-ion batteries had been implanted by two different device manufacturers. Lithium-ion batteries are also used to provide temporary power for some left-ventricular assist devices (e.g., while the patient is bathing). In many applications, the time between recharges could be as long as weeks or months.

Possible modes of application include the following.

1. Supporting relatively high-power, non–life-support features of a device (e.g., long-distance telemetry, various types of physiologic sensors). In this case, a primary battery is still used to provide life-sustaining therapy.
2. Using a high-power rechargeable battery to charge the capacitor of an ICD while incorporating a low-power, high-energy density primary battery to provide the recharge energy. In some cases, this may be accomplished by placing the two cells in parallel.

3. Providing excellent longevity (perhaps as long as 20 years) with small devices. In this case, the rechargeable battery would serve as the major power source. Presumably, such devices would be limited to patients who are physically and mentally capable of managing the recharge requirements.

Principles of Operation. The defining feature of a lithium-ion battery is that it contains no metallic lithium. Instead, lithium ions are shuttled back and forth between the positive and negative electrodes during charge and discharge (Fig. 6-16).

The most common materials are cobalt oxide (CoO_2) for the positive cathode material and a graphitic carbon to contain the intercalated lithium for the negative anode material. The general cell construction is similar to that shown for the Li/SVO battery. However, lithium-ion batteries are manufactured in their discharged state (using lithium cobalt oxide and graphite) and then charged ("formed") after the cell is fully assembled.

Method of Recharge. To date, all of the implantable applications for rechargeable batteries involve recharge by transcutaneous electromagnetic induction. The implanted device incorporates a wound-wire coil that acts as the secondary to an externally located primary coil, which is placed adjacent to the implanted device. Typical lithium-ion batteries are capable of accepting a full charge in 2 hours or less. Actual recharge time in an implanted device depends on a number of factors in addition to the capacity of the battery, including the relative positions of the primary and secondary coils, the depth of the implant, and the maximum power that can be transmitted while limiting heating of either the primary coil or the implanted device.

End-of-Service Life Indication. Lithium-ion batteries typically exhibit a gradually declining voltage during discharge that can be used as a "gas gauge" to tell the state of -discharge at a given time. The discharge curve for a lithium-ion battery is shown in Figure 6-17.

Information about the voltage can be telemetered to a patient controller or some monitor so that the patient is made aware of the need to recharge the battery. However, the EOS for a device powered by a lithium-ion battery is not as readily apparent as for a device powered by a primary battery. Because the lithium-ion battery slowly loses capacity as a function of both time and the total number of charge/discharge cycles, the patient will eventually experience a reduced time interval between recharge sessions. Therefore, the eventual EOS may be determined by the lifetime of some other component of the implanted device or by a recharge interval that becomes too short to be acceptable to the patient.

Capacitors

ICDs defibrillate the heart by delivering one or more high-energy, high-voltage shocks. The power capability and voltage of the battery alone are not sufficient to accomplish this. High-voltage capacitors are necessary to store and deliver the energy required for these shocks. The use of capacitors has important clinical implications. High-voltage capacitors are the largest and thickest component in an ICD. They are largely responsible for the larger size and thickness of ICDs relative to cardiac pacemakers. Capacitor performance

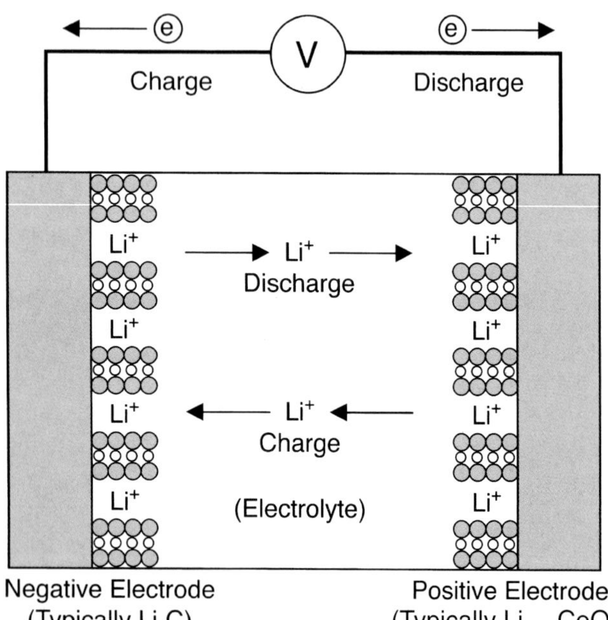

Figure 6-16. Schematic diagram of a lithium-ion battery showing lithium ions and electrons shuttling between the positive and negative electrodes as the battery is charged and discharged.

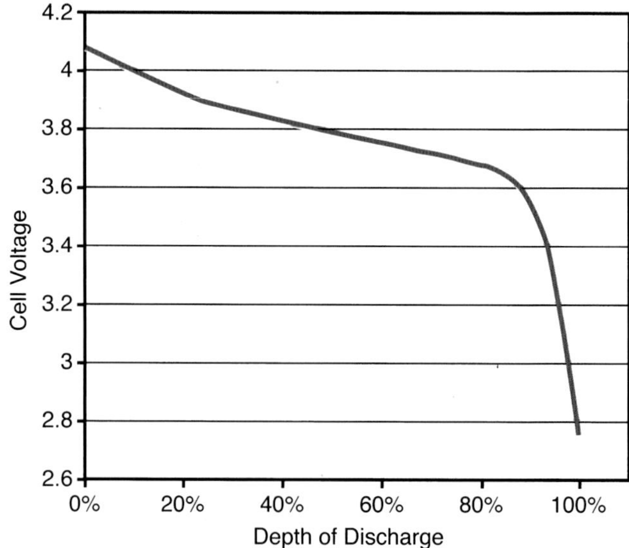

Figure 6-17. The monotonic discharge curve of a lithium-ion battery shows how it can be used as a "gas gauge" for determining the remaining capacity in the battery.

characteristics can also significantly affect important device characteristics such charge time, delivered energy, and longevity.

Basic Capacitor Concepts

Capacitance

In its simplest form, a capacitor consists of two conductors that are separated in space and electrically insulated from each other. The Leyden Jar of Benjamin Franklin's famous kite experiment was an early example of a capacitor conforming to this description. When the conductors are charged, each carries an equal and opposite amount of charge. In an ideal capacitor, the amount of charge (Q) on each conductor is proportional to the difference in voltage (V) between the two conductors. The proportionality constant, C, is called the capacitance.

$$Q = C \cdot V \tag{6-10}$$

The simplest model of a capacitor is shown in Figure 6-18A. The conductors (or electrodes) consist of two parallel plates of area *A*, separated by a distance, *d*. Figure 6-18A shows the plates separated in a vacuum.

The capacitance, or ability to store charge as a function of voltage, is equal to A/d multiplied by a fundamental constant, ε_0, the permittivity of free space, which is a measure of the ability of a vacuum to separate charge. The value of the capacitance can be increased by inserting insulating materials, known as dielectrics, between the electrodes instead of a vacuum. The factor by which these materials increase the capacitance is called the dielectric constant, κ, which is the ratio of the permittivity of the material to the permittivity of free space: $\varepsilon/\varepsilon_0$. A simple capacitor containing a dielectric material is shown in Figure 6-18B. A wide variety of materials are used as dielectrics. The properties of the dielectric largely determine the properties of the capacitor (see later discussion).

Energy Storage

In an ICD, the capacitor or capacitors are required to deliver a high-voltage, high-energy electrical shock through the lead system to the heart. Capacitors are passive devices and therefore must store energy before it can be delivered. The process of storing energy in a capacitor is called charging. For a capacitor to be charged, both terminals must be connected to a charging circuit that includes a transformer, and to a voltage source such as a battery. The transformer converts the low-voltage energy supplied by the battery into the high-voltage energy stored by the capacitor. The opposite terminals of the capacitor take on equal and opposite charges. The amount of energy stored on the capacitor is proportional to the square of the voltage in the capacitor:

$$E = \tfrac{1}{2} C \cdot V^2 \tag{6-11}$$

Energy Delivery

During defibrillation, the energy stored in the capacitor is discharged (delivered to the heart) through leads that connect the heart in an electrical path between the opposing electrodes of the capacitor. This connection allows the separated charge to recombine by traveling through the leads and the heart.

When an ideal capacitor is discharged through a constant resistance, R, the voltage decays with time in an exponential manner, as seen in Figure 6-19.

The shape of the exponential decay depends on the capacitance, C, and the resistance of the electrical path between the terminals of the capacitor, R. The exponential decay is characterized by a time constant, τ, which is simply R times C. After the capacitor has discharged for a period of time equal to τ, the voltage will have decayed to 37% (100%) of its initial value.

Parallel Plate Capacitor

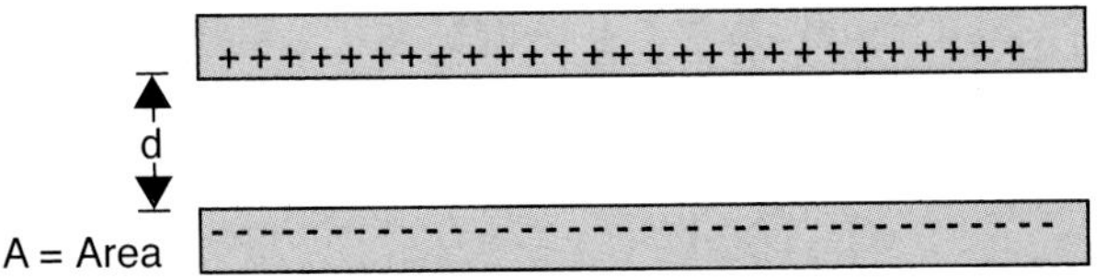

$$C_0 = \text{Capacitance} = \frac{\text{Charge}}{\text{Voltage}} = \frac{Q}{V} = \frac{\varepsilon_0 A}{d}$$

A

Parallel Plate Capacitor with Dielectric

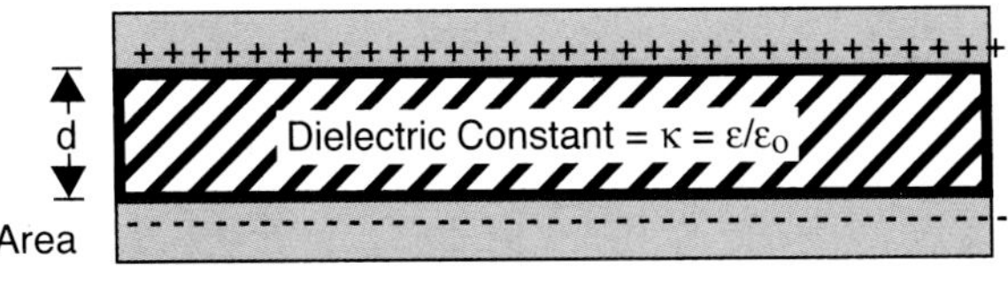

$$C = \text{Capacitance} = \frac{\text{Charge}}{\text{Voltage}} = \frac{Q}{V} = \frac{\kappa\varepsilon_0 A}{d}$$

B

*Figure 6-18. Schematic representation of a parallel plate capacitor with a vacuum (**A**) and one with a dielectric between the capacitor plates (**B**). The capacitance is directly proportional to the area of the plates (A), and inversely proportional to the distance between the plates (d). The insertion of a dielectric material between the plates increases the capacitance by a factor of κ, the dielectric constant, which is a characteristic of the particular insulating material. ε_0 is the permittivity of a vacuum.*

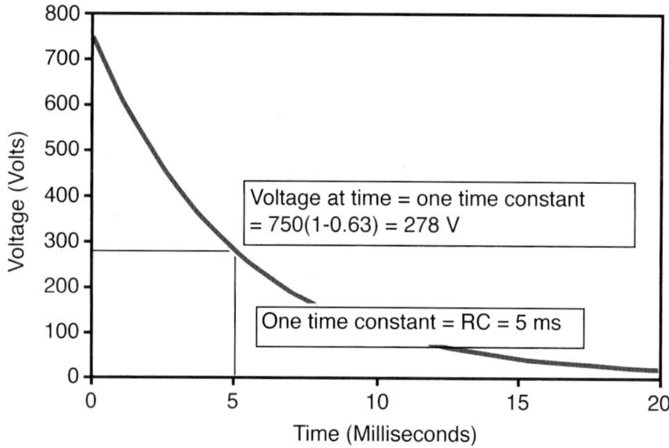

Figure 6-19. Waveform for the discharge of an ideal 100-microfarad (μF) capacitor, charged to 750 V, into a 50-Ω load. After one time constant (5 msec in this case), the voltage in the capacitor has been reduced to 37% of its initial value. These parameters approximate those for an implantable defibrillator in use. C, capacitance; R, resistance.

For an ideal capacitor discharged to zero volts, the delivered energy is equal to the stored energy. In real ICDs, the amount of energy delivered from the capacitor is less than the amount stored. Circuit- and therapy-related losses reduce delivered energy. The most significant loss is truncation of the discharge waveform during defibrillation, before the voltage on the capacitor reaches zero. A truncated waveform is used because it defibrillates the heart more effectively than a waveform that is allowed to decay to zero volts, despite the fact that less energy is delivered to the heart.

Energy Density

Energy density is an important parameter for capacitors as well as batteries. Capacitor energy density is typically expressed in terms of volume, in units of joules per cubic centimeter (J/cm^3). The most energy-dense modern defibrillation capacitors have energy densities in excess of 5 J/cm^3. Recall, in the discussion of batteries, that the highest energy density seen for implantable batteries is about 1 W-hr/cm^3, which is the same as 3600 J/cm^3, or more than 500 times as high as the best defibrillation capacitor. Why, then, use capacitors at all? The reasons are voltage and power. Defibrillation therapy requires the energy to be delivered rapidly at about 1000 W of power and starting at a voltage of 750 to 800 V. ICD batteries are designed to deliver the needed energy to the circuit at about 10 W of power with voltage between 2.5 V and 3 V. An 800-V battery capable of 1000 W could be designed in principle, but it would have very low energy density and would be impractical in other ways. However, reasonably sized high-voltage capacitors designed to operate at this power and voltage are very practical. Consequently, the ICD is designed with the battery as a large energy reservoir, analogous to the gas tank of an automobile, and the capacitor as the delivery system, capable of administering the defibrillation energy in pulses at high voltage and high power, analogous to the fuel injector of an automobile. Nevertheless, it is important for the capacitors to have the highest practicable energy density in order to minimize the overall volume of the ICD.

Types of Capacitors

Electrostatic Capacitors

Electrostatic capacitors are conceptually the simplest capacitors, and they most closely resemble the idealized drawing in Figure 6-18B. They consist of thin sheets of dielectric material separating opposing metal electrodes. Typical dielectric materials used in these capacitors are polymer films and ceramics.

Film capacitors use a wide range of polymeric materials as the dielectric. They can be constructed either by coating a thin polymer film with a metallic electrode material or by using a discrete metal foil as the electrode. The film and electrode are usually wound into a cylindrical package, but they can also be fashioned into a flat stack cut from a large roll or sheet. Polymer films typically have high dielectric strength, but their dielectric constant is typically low, which results in an energy density (≈1 J/cm^3) that is too low for use in ICDs. They are, however, used in many external defibrillators, where low cost and near-ideal performance are more important than small size.

A second type of electrostatic capacitor uses a ceramic material as the capacitor dielectric. There are many possible ceramic dielectric materials. Ceramic capacitors are constructed as stacked, alternating layers of the ceramic dielectric and metal electrode material. In contrast to polymer films, ceramic dielectrics typically have a high dielectric constant but a low dielectric strength, and their performance is significantly non-ideal. The capacitance of many ceramic capacitors actually decreases as the applied voltage is increased. Ceramic capacitors today do not have energy densities high enough to warrant their use in ICDs.

Electrolytic Capacitors

Electrolytic capacitors are the only type of capacitor that has been used in ICDs. They are most commonly based on either aluminum or tantalum electrode materials. The metal electrode materials are processed so that they have a very high surface area, which results in a high capacitance. In the case of aluminum electrolytic capacitors, the positive electrode (anode in a capacitor) starts as a thin foil that has been etched to create a large number of tunnels.

Figure 6-20 shows a scanning electron micrograph of a replica made from a cross-section of a highly etched anode foil. The long, tubular structures are microscopic tunnels that have been etched into (and in some cases through) the aluminum from each side of the foil. There are well over 1 million tunnels per square centimeter in this foil, and they are responsible for the large surface area and high capacitance of this type of capacitor. For tantalum electrolytic capacitors,

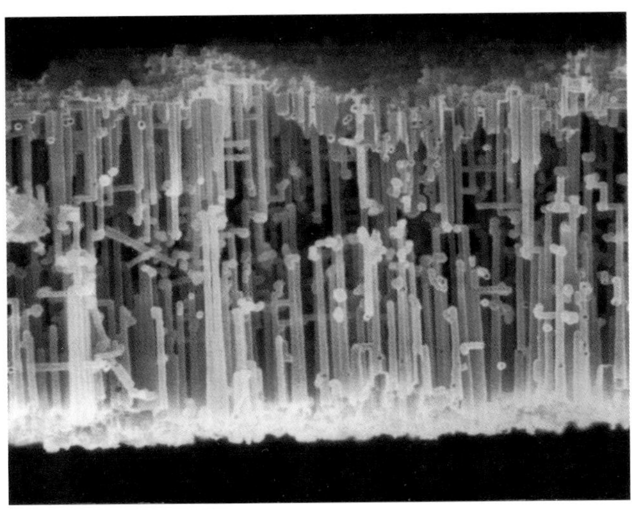

Figure 6-20. Photomicrograph of a replica made from the etched anode foil used in aluminum electrolytic capacitors. The long, linear structures are tunnels etched into the aluminum foil. In this example, some of the tunnels are etched completely through the foil to provide an electrical connection between the two sides. Magnification, approximately 800×.

the anode is made from tantalum metal powder that is pressed into a porous pellet and heated to a high enough temperature to make the metal particles bond to one another (sintering) while remaining porous. For either material, an oxide film is electrochemically grown on the exposed surfaces of the metal electrode. The oxide serves as the capacitor dielectric. During the formation process, a voltage is applied to the electrode, and the oxide grows to a thickness that is proportional to the voltage. Thicker oxides have lower capacitance but can support higher voltage. Oxides formed by electrolysis are relatively free of defects and have high dielectric strength. If defects occur, the oxide is automatically regrown in situ the next time the capacitor is charged, and the defect is healed. Aluminum anodes are typically formed to support charging to about 400 V. Two capacitors are connected in series in the ICD to provide sufficient voltage for defibrillation. Tantalum anodes are typically formed to support charging to 175 to 250 V. Three or four capacitors are connected in series in the ICD to provide sufficient voltage for defibrillation.

The dielectric oxide that coats the irregular anode surface needs to maintain ionic contact with the opposing electrode in the capacitor, the cathode. Contact with the cathode is made via the electrolyte, just as in batteries. The electrolyte is usually an organic solvent with dissolved salts to make it conductive. The capacitances of the anode and cathode are in series in electrolytic capacitors, so the capacitance of the whole capacitor is calculated by adding the reciprocals of their individual capacitances. Electrolytic capacitors are designed so that the capacitance of the cathode ($C_{cathode}$) is much larger than that of the anode (C_{anode}). The overall capacitance (C_{total}) is therefore a close approximation to the capacitance of the anode alone.

$$1/C_{total} = 1/C_{anode} + 1/C_{cathode} \cong 1/C_{anode} \qquad (6\text{-}12)$$

The voltage on the capacitor is divided between the anode and the cathode such that the product of voltage and capacitance, which is the charge, is equal on each electrode. Because the anode has a much smaller capacitance than the cathode, most of the voltage is on the anode.

$$C_{anode} \cdot V_{anode} = C_{cathode} \cdot V_{cathode} \qquad (6\text{-}13)$$

The high capacitance, high voltage and relatively low resistance of aluminum and tantalum electrolytic capacitors give them the high energy density (2.5-5 J/cm^3) and quick, efficient energy delivery that make them the capacitors of choice for ICDs.

ICD Capacitor Construction

Early ICD devices used commercially produced, cylindrically wound, aluminum electrolytic capacitors developed for flash photography applications. The need for smaller, thinner capacitors and specialized shapes led ICD manufacturers to develop stacked-plate aluminum electrolytic capacitors and, more recently, custom tantalum electrolytic capacitors.[23,24] Capacitors used in ICDs come in three basic varieties: cylindrically wound aluminum electrolytic capacitors, custom stacked-plate aluminum electrolytic capacitors, and tantalum electrolytic capacitors.

Aluminum Electrolytic Capacitor Components

All aluminum electrolytic capacitors are produced using the same basic materials of construction. Cylindrical and stacked-plate designs both incorporate an anode, a cathode, an electrolyte, and separator material between the anode and cathode. The anode and cathode are aluminum foils that have been etched and formed, as described earlier. The electrolyte typically consists of ethylene glycol with dissolved salts that usually have a large organic cation or anion (or both) to provide conductivity. The electrolyte composition can vary widely, depending on the manufacturer. In a practical capacitor, the anode and cathode must be mechanically separated from each other to prevent a short circuit, just as with a battery. The dielectric material alone is not sufficient to keep the electrodes apart, because it might easily wear through, resulting in direct metal-to-metal contact between the anode and cathode. Whereas the lithium batteries that power ICDs use a porous polymer as a separator material, aluminum electrolytic capacitors generally use porous Kraft paper as a separator. The porosity of the paper allows the electrolyte to pass through but does not allow the electrodes to directly touch each other.

Cylindrical Aluminum Electrolytic Construction

Most commercially produced aluminum electrolytic capacitors employ wound electrodes in a cylindrical shape. Strips of anode and cathode foils, spaced apart by a paper separator, are wound into a coil. Two layers of anode foil are used for each layer of cathode foil. Figure 6-21 shows a cutaway view of an aluminum elec-

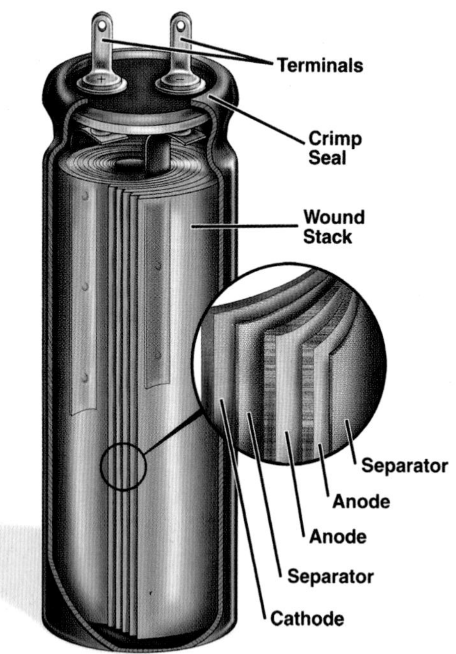

Figure 6-21. Cutaway view of a wound aluminum electrolytic capacitor used in early implantable defibrillators. In this capacitor, the anode and cathode connections are brought out of the capacitor using feedthroughs. The capacitor is closed with a crimp seal. Notice that two layers of anode material are used for each layer of cathode material. The entire wound capacitor coil is saturated with electrolyte (not shown).

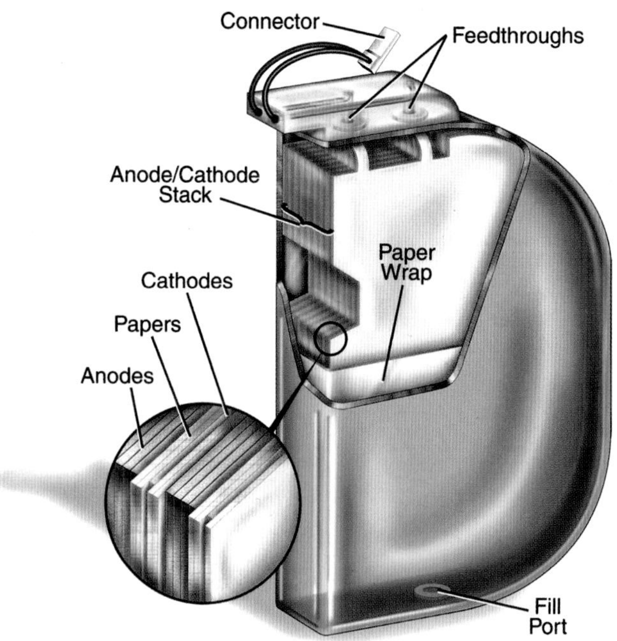

Figure 6-22. Cutaway view of a stacked-plate aluminum electrolytic capacitor presently used in implantable defibrillators. Anode and cathode layers are cut to a specific geometry and are stacked on one another. Anode and cathode terminals exit the welded capacitor housing through feedthroughs. The capacitor encasement is laser welded. Notice that four layers of anode material are used for each layer of cathode material (some designs use up to five layers). The entire capacitor stack is saturated with electrolyte (not shown).

trolytic photoflash capacitor of the type commonly used in the first few generations of ICDs.

Stacked-plate Aluminum Electrolytic Construction

ICD manufacturers have developed stacked-plate aluminum electrolytic capacitor technology to improve the energy density, minimize the thickness, and allow a variety of shapes, compared with cylindrically wound capacitors. The details of construction vary among manufacturers, but several design themes are common. In the case of stacked-plate capacitors, foils and separators are cut to a specific geometry and are layered so that each anode is sandwiched between two separators and two cathodes. The geometry of the plates is selected so that the finished capacitor fits efficiently in the ICD. Electrolyte is introduced into the capacitor through a hole under vacuum to remove entrapped air bubbles. The hole, or fillport, is sealed by welding.

Stacked-plate capacitors have three primary advantages over cylindrical designs. Rather than two layers of anode foil per cathode, as many as five layers are employed in stacked designs. This maximizes the relative fraction of anode in the capacitor and increases the energy density. Because anode foils are not bent in stacked capacitors, it is possible to use more brittle and highly etched anode foils that have higher capacitance than the foils used for cylindrical capacitors. The energy density of stacked-plate capacitors can approach 4 J/cm^3, resulting in a capacitor of approximately 9 cm^3 for a 35-J device. Figure 6-22 shows a cutaway view of a stacked-plate aluminum electrolytic capacitor similar to those used in current ICDs.

Tantalum Electrolytic Capacitor Construction

Tantalum electrolytic capacitors have the same basic elements as aluminum electrolytic capacitors. Each incorporates an anode, a cathode, an electrolyte, and separator material between the anode and cathode. In the case of tantalum capacitors, the anode is made using pressed, sintered, and formed tantalum powder, as described earlier. The cathode in a tantalum capacitor is typically deposited directly on the inside of the capacitor case, making it the negative terminal of the capacitor. The planar surface area of the case is small compared with the multiple foils used in aluminum electrolytic capacitors. High capacitance is derived from the use of materials with high microscopic surface area that operate on the same principle as double-layer capacitors.[25] The composition of the electrolyte is similar to that of aluminum electrolytic capacitors. The separator used to mechanically space the anode and cathode in tantalum capacitors is a microporous polymer material almost identical to that used in batteries.

Tantalum capacitors have benefits similar to those of stacked-plate aluminum capacitors: higher energy density, thinner profile, and more flexible shapes.

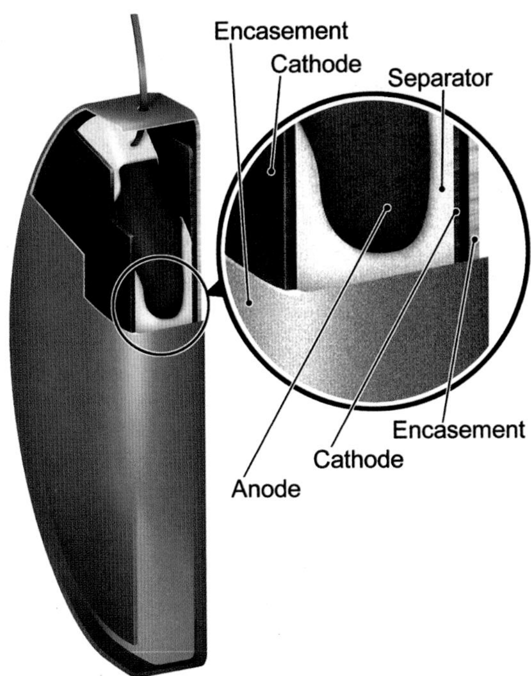

Figure 6-23. Cutaway view of a tantalum electrolytic capacitor presently used in implantable defibrillators. The design incorporates a single tantalum anode pellet pressed from tantalum powder. A tantalum lead wire exits the welded housing through a feedthrough. High-capacitance cathode material is deposited directly on the case. The entire electrode assembly is saturated with electrolyte (not shown).

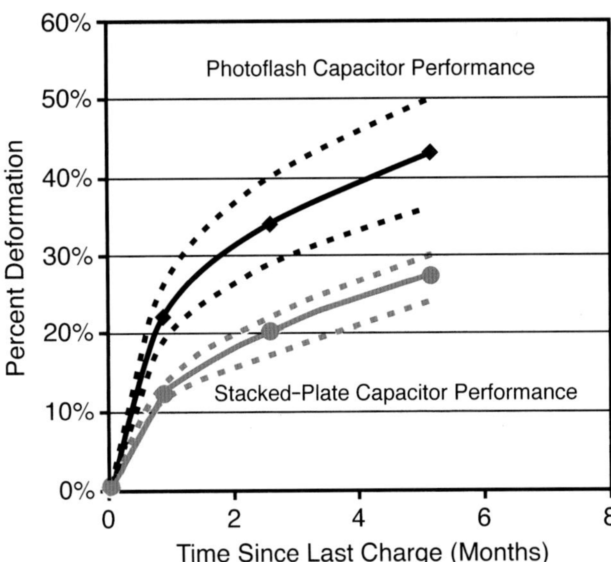

Figure 6-24. Percent deformation for typical photoflash capacitor used in early ICDs and typical stacked-plate performance. Percent deformation is the percentage of additional energy required to charge a capacitor after some period at open-circuit voltage.

Tantalum capacitors tend to have simpler construction than aluminum capacitors. The layered anode foils in the aluminum electrolytic capacitors are replaced with a single pressed anode pellet that is sealed in a polymer separator envelope. The sealed anode pellet is inserted into a titanium case, which is welded closed. Electrolyte is introduced through a fillport hole using vacuum to remove entrapped air bubbles, as described earlier for aluminum electrolytic capacitors.

Tantalum capacitors have one advantage and one drawback when compared with cylindrical and stacked-plate aluminum electrolytic capacitors. The simple and efficient construction of tantalum capacitors minimizes the volume of materials that do not contribute to energy storage (cathode, separator, encasement), thereby maximizing energy density. Tantalum capacitors used in current ICDs have an energy density of 5 J/cm^3 or higher. The drawback of tantalum capacitors is their mass. Tantalum is substantially denser than aluminum, and, although their size for a given energy level is likely to be smaller than that of an aluminum capacitor, their mass is likely to be about 50% greater. Figure 6-23 shows a cutaway view of a tantalum electrolytic capacitor similar to those used in current ICDs.

Non-ideal Behavior in Capacitors

In an ideal capacitor, the amount of energy needed to charge the capacitor would be exactly equal to the energy delivered from the capacitor when it is discharged. Some types of capacitors (e.g., polymer film) more closely approximate this ideal performance than others. Although the electrolytic capacitors used in ICDs have performance characteristics well suited to the ICD application, their performance does deviate from ideal in ways that are sometimes clinically significant.

Deformation

The non-ideal process that is most apparent is called deformation. As explained earlier, the dielectric material in electrolytic capacitors is created using an electrolytic process known as forming. Immediately after forming, the dielectric is almost free of defects. However, over time, the chemical environment within the capacitors causes very small cracks or other imperfections in the oxide film on the anode. When the capacitor is charged to a high voltage after a long period of disuse, additional energy is required to regrow oxide in these areas and heal the defects.[26] This process is known as reformation. The additional energy needed to reform the dielectric is apparent because a deformed capacitor takes longer to charge than a capacitor that has been recently reformed. This energy is not recovered when the capacitor is discharged. In a typical cylindrical aluminum capacitor, 40% or more additional energy (and time) may be required to charge the capacitor if it has been a long time since the capacitor was last charged. The amount of additional energy drops to about 20% if the time since the last charge is on the order of 1 month. Capacitor deformation performance for cylindrical and stacked capacitors is shown for various charging intervals in Figure 6-24.

To minimize the clinical effect of deformation, ICDs today incorporate a programmable maintenance routine that automatically charges the capacitor to high voltage to heal the dielectric at intervals of 1, 3, or 6 months.

Leakage Current

Leakage current is another non-ideal process that occurs to some extent in all capacitors. After a capacitor is charged, some of the energy "leaks" off the capacitor, and the voltage decreases with time. Aluminum and tantalum electrolytic capacitors tend to have relatively high leakage current compared with other types of capacitors. The voltage of an aluminum electrolytic capacitor will decay to a low level, relative to its maximum charging voltage, within several minutes due to leakage current. In the ICD application, the defibrillation therapy is delivered quickly after charging, so insignificant charge is lost before delivery of the high-voltage shock. Leakage current is the major reason why ICDs are only charged just before a shock is to be delivered.

Internal Resistance

The final important non-ideality is internal resistance. All capacitor types have some level of internal resistance, just as batteries do. For capacitors, this resistance is often referred to as equivalent series resistance (ESR). Electrolytic capacitors used in ICDs typically have an ESR of about 2 to 4 Ω. This resistance leads to energy loss when the capacitor is discharged. For example, if the energy from a capacitor with an ESR of 3 Ω were delivered into a lead system with an impedance of 50 Ω, slightly more than 5% of the energy stored on the capacitor would be lost as heat during discharge. ESR is factored into the design of the capacitor and ICD so that appropriate energy will be delivered during defibrillation therapy.

Effects of Batteries and Capacitors on Defibrillation Performance

Energy Losses in Defibrillators

The processes of charging the capacitors and discharging the energy through the leads of a cardiac defibrillator have numerous inefficiencies which result in a substantial disparity between the chemical energy consumed in the battery and the electrical energy delivered to the heart. The charging circuit has a finite level of resistance and other voltage losses inherent to the operation of certain components (e.g., diodes). These translate into energy lost to heat as the capacitor is charged and later discharged. Similarly, a small amount of energy is lost in the leads as the discharge occurs, as a result of their finite resistance.

The large defibrillation capacitors themselves contribute to some energy losses in the device. Energy losses can vary from about 5% to more than 40% in an aluminum electrolytic capacitor that has not been formed in many months.

The most significant loss of energy is associated with the battery. Batteries in ICDs are designed to be as small as possible, which means that they tend to be operated near their maximum power capability. An ideal power source operates at maximum power when the load placed on the power source matches the internal resistance of the power source. This well-known concept is often referred to as "impedance matching." In terms of energy efficiency, it means that, when a power source is operating at maximum power, only one half of the total energy consumed is delivered to the external load. The remainder of the energy is dissipated as heat inside the ICD. Considering all of these contributions, the overall efficiency of the battery/charging-circuit/capacitor/lead system is, at best, only about 35%. In many instances, the overall efficiency is less than 25%. The energy content of a typical ICD battery is on the order of 20,000 J. When the ICD delivers a 35-J shock, a system operating at 25% efficiency would consume 140 J, or about 0.7% of the total battery energy. To put this energy consumption in a clinical perspective, an ICD that would last 7 years if no defibrillation shocks were delivered will have its longevity reduced by 15 to 20 days for each shock delivered.

Clinical Implications of Battery and Capacitor Design for Defibrillation Therapy

Four principal characteristics of an ICD are interrelated, primarily due to the battery and the defibrillation capacitors: size, longevity, charge time, and the maximum energy of a defibrillation shock. Smaller ICDs may be desirable, but, all else being equal, small size trades off longevity, charge time, and/or maximum shock energy. Higher maximum shock energy results primarily in higher charge time, and also lower longevity, depending on how many shocks are delivered. The only exceptions occur when new technologies are introduced, such as charge time-optimized batteries, tantalum capacitors, or more efficient or smaller electronic components. It is the job of the ICD manufacturer to strike an appropriate balance between ICD volume and clinically important parameters such as longevity, charge time, and maximum shock energy.

The clinician should also be aware that charge times are generally quoted for formed capacitors. Charge times for capacitors that have not been recently formed can be up to 40% longer for the first pulse. Also, a low charge time at the time of implantation does not necessarily mean that charge times will remain low through ERI. As discussed in the section on ICD batteries, the charge time depends on battery design and manufacture.

As discussed previously, the energy removed from the battery during each charge of the output capacitor represents a significant fraction of its total energy (on the order of 0.5% to 1.0%). Hence, the longevity of a defibrillator is strongly dependent on the frequency of the shock therapy. The situation is further complicated in modern ICDs that routinely perform other functions, such as bradycardia pacing, in addition to providing defibrillation shocks. As an example, the manual of one device estimates longevity as about 6 years if the device is used only as a defibrillator and is required to deliver very few high-voltage shocks. However, the longevity estimate for this same device is only about $3^1/_2$ years if it is implanted in a patient who requires 100% pacing at nominal conditions and also undergoes a shock about once a month. This difference of a factor of 2 could be even greater if the patient required more tachyarrhythmia shocks or more extreme pacing parameters.

REFERENCES

1. Brennen KR, Fester KE, Owens BB, Untereker DF: Pacemaker battery capacity: A consideration of the manufacturer's problem. Proceedings of the Sixth World Symposium on Cardiac Pacing, Montreal, Pacesymp, 1979.
2. Brennen KR, Fester KE, Owens, BB, Untereker DF: A capacity rating system for cardiac pacemaker batteries. J Power Sources 5:25, 1980.
3. Broadhead J: Electrochemical principles and reactions. In Linden D (ed): Handbook of Batteries and Fuel Cells, 2nd ed. New York, McGraw-Hill, 1994, Chapter 2.
4. Visbisky M, Stinebring RC, Holmes CF: An approach to the reliability of implantable lithium batteries. J Power Sources 26:185, 1989.
5. Schmidt CL, Skarstad PM: Impedance behavior in lithium-iodine batteries. In Abraham KM, Solomon M (eds): Proceedings of the Symposium on Primary and Secondary Lithium Batteries. The Electrochemical Society, PV91-3, pp 75-85, 1991.
6. Schmidt CL, Skarstad PM: Development of a physically based model for the lithium-iodine battery. In Keily T, Baxter BW (eds): Power Sources 13. Leatherhead, England, International Power Sources Committee, 1991, pp 347-361.
7. Untereker DF, Owens BB: Microcalorimetry: A tool for the assessment of self-discharge processes in batteries. Reliability Technology for Cardiac Pacemakers II. Gaithersburg, Md., National Bureau of Standards Workshop, October, 1977.
8. Untereker DF: The use of a microcalorimeter for analysis of load-dependent processes occurring in a primary battery. J Electrochem Soc 125:1907, 1978.
9. Owens BB (ed): Batteries for Implantable Biomedical Devices. New York, Plenum Press, 1986.
10. Antonioli G, Baggioni F, Consiglio F, et al: Stimulatore cardiaco implantible con nuova battaria a sato solido al litio. Minerva Med 64:2298, 1973.
11. Schmidt CL, Skarstad PM: Modeling the discharge behavior of the lithium-iodine battery. J Power Sources 43(1B3):111, 1993.
12. Walk CR: Lithium-vanadium pentoxide cells. In Gabano JP (ed): Lithium Batteries. London, Academic Press, 1983, pp 265-280.
13. Gabano JP, Broussely M, Grimm M: Lithium solid cathode batteries for biomedical implantable applications. In Owens BB (ed): Batteries for Implantable Biomedical Devices. New York, Plenum, 1986, pp 181-213.
14. Takeuchi ES, Quattrini JP: Batteries for implantable defibrillators. Med Electronics 119:114-117, 1989.
15. Liang CC, Bolster E, Murphy RM: Metal oxide cathode material for high energy density batteries. U.S. Patents 4,310,609 (1982) and 4,391,729 (1983).
16. Holmes CF, Keister P, Takeuchi E: High rate lithium solid cathode battery for implantable medical devices. Prog Batteries Solar Cells 6:64, 1987.
17. Crespi AM, Schmidt C, Norton J, et al: Modeling and characteristics of the resistance of lithium/SVO batteries for implantable cardioverter defibrillators. J Electrochem Soc 148:A30-A37, 2001.
18. Crespi AM: Silver vanadium oxide cathode material and method of preparation. U.S. Patent 5,221,453. September 27, 1990.
19. Tachyarrhythmia products. In Medtronic Product Performance Report, 2nd ed., vol. 14. Minneapolis, Minn., Medtronics, Inc., 2003, p 11.
20. Marquis ICD battery technology. In Medtronic Tachyarrhythmia Technical Concept Paper, vol. V, no. 1.
21. Weiss DJ, Cretzmeyer JW, Crespi AM, et al: Electrochemical cells with end-of-service indicator. U. S. Patent 5,180,642 (1993).
22. Schmidt CL, Skarstad PM: The future of lithium and lithium-ion batteries in implantable medical devices. J Power Sources 97-98 (2001) 742-746.
23. Strange TF, Graham TV: Proceedings of the 20th Capacitor and Resistor Technology Symposium CARTS 2000, Huntington Beach, Calif., 2000, pp. 16-21.
24. Breyen MD, Rorvick AW, Skarstad PM: Proceedings of the 22nd Capacitor and Resistor Technology Symposium CARTS 2002, New Orleans, 2002, pp. 197-202.
25. Evans DA: Proceedings of the 14th Capacitor and Resistor Technology Symposium CARTS 1994, Jupiter, Fla, 1994.
26. Norton J, Anderson C: Proceedings of the 23rd Capacitor and Resistor Technology Symposium CARTS 2003, Scottsdale, Ariz., 2003, pp. 269-277.

Chapter 7

Pacemaker and Implantable Cardioverter-Defibrillator Circuitry

MARK W. KROLL • PAUL A. LEVINE

The technology used in pacemakers and implantable cardioverter-defibrillators (ICDs) has made impressive advances since the first pacemaker was implanted in 1959. These enhancements have provided benefits for both patients and clinicians. For the patient, size reduction, improved longevity, noninvasive programmability, and improved therapy in the form of dual-chamber and rate-adaptive pacing are just a few of the benefits. For the clinician, enhanced therapies have improved patient outcomes, resulting in more effective care, and better diagnostics have led to more insight into the clinical condition of patients. The efficient delivery of care is particularly important for containing health care costs.

Design considerations play a fundamental role in device performance and operation, and device performance in turn plays an important role in clinical practice. For this reason, it is important for physicians and engineers to develop a common understanding of the role each plays in patient treatment. Engineers must understand the needs of the patient and the factors that drive clinical decisions in the care of patients. Physicians benefit from an understanding of the fundamentals of device technology and, with this knowledge, are able to make decisions that optimize device performance given inherent technical characteristics. Additionally, an understanding of device design allows the clinician to more accurately match the appropriate device to each patient.

The objective of this chapter is to provide an overview of the major technical issues that drive pacemaker and ICD performance. The major functional blocks of a typical implantable device are reviewed. A discussion of pacemaker technology is followed by an overview of the unique technological challenges faced in the design of ICDs. The chapter concludes with a discussion of the impact of future technology on implantable devices.

The emphasis throughout this chapter is on highlighting the specific areas in which technology affects clinical performance and on providing guidance as to how best to manage that impact. Rather than discussing the specifics of early device designs, the discussion focuses on how recent advances have altered and improved implantable device performance.

Functional Design Elements of Pacemakers

The major physical elements of a typical modern pacemaker are shown in Figure 7-1A and an older device

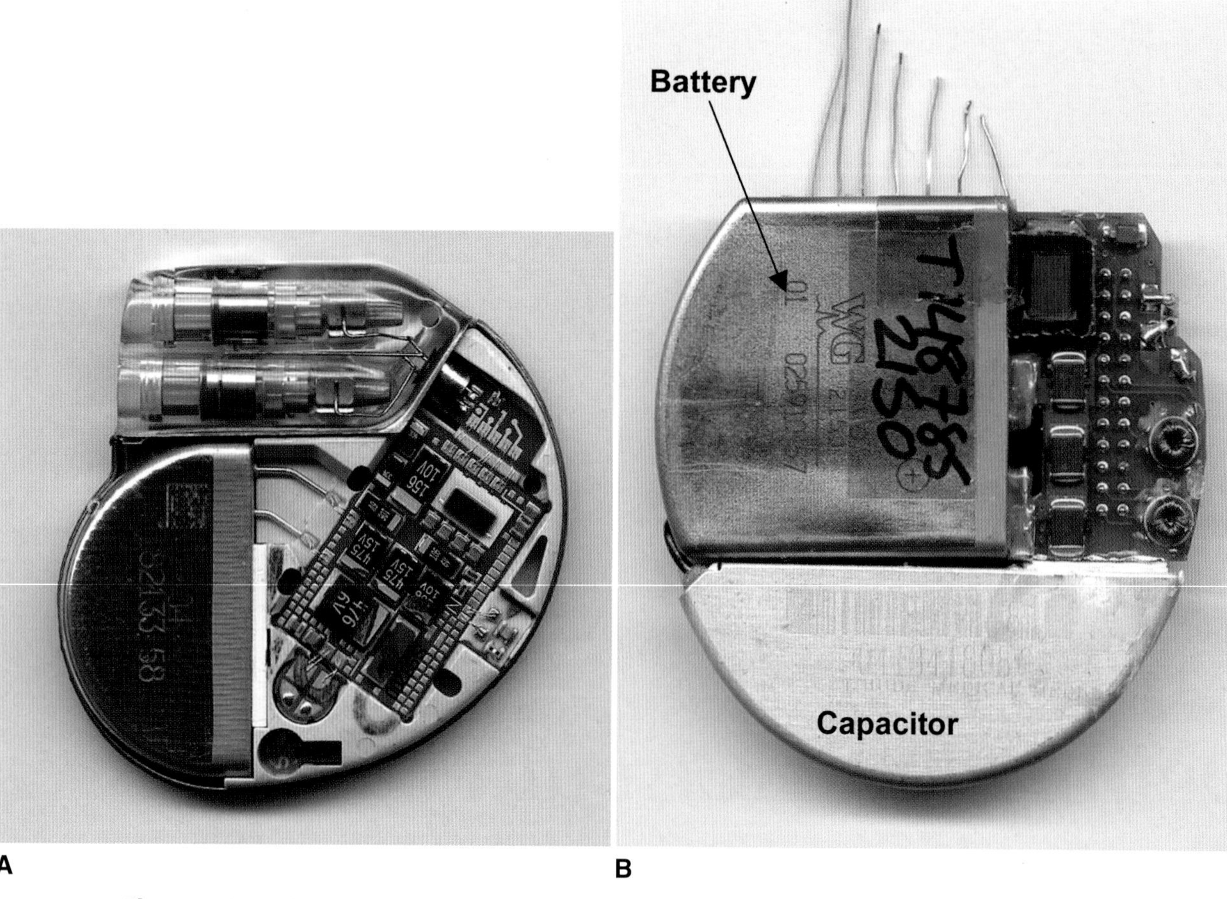

Figure 7-1. ***A,*** *Cutaway view of DDDR pacemaker showing the battery alongside the hybrid that contains integrated B circuits, accelerometer sensor, and electronic components.* ***B,*** *Cutaway view of a VVED defibrillator showing the significantly larger battery and capacitor. Electronic circuitry is to the right. The wires on the top go to the connector block.*

in Figure 7-1B. This photograph shows the pacemaker can and header. Within the can, the lithium iodine battery can be seen next to the hybrid substrate that carries the electronic components. Despite important advances in circuit design that have increased circuit density while reducing current drain, the ratio of battery volume to circuit board volume has remained relatively constant since the mid-1980s. The potential for size reduction of pacemaker circuitry and batteries has been offset by a corresponding increase in pacemaker capability. This increased functionality translates into increased circuit complexity while maintaining power requirements similar to the less capable devices of the past.

Major subsystems of the implanted pulse generator are shown in Figure 7-2. Functions of the various blocks are described briefly here.

Pace control: sense amplifiers, pacing output, and timing circuits to deliver pacing pulses to the heart when required; also tracks cardiac activity during arrhythmias.

Rate-adaptive circuitry: amplifiers, filters, and current sources for various types of sensors; this circuitry may be significantly different for each particular type of sensor.

Microprocessor: controls overall system functions; an 8-bit design is sufficient for most systems; use of an industry standard design (e.g., 6502, 8852, Z80) allows the use of standard development languages and tools and also facilitates integrated circuit implementation with a "megacell" or VHDL model.

ROM: sufficient nonvolatile memory is available for system start-up tasks and some program space; program space requirements can be as large as 32 kilobytes (Kb) in a pacemaker.

RAM: used for additional program space, storage of operating parameters, and storage of lead electrogram (EGM) data; storage of several minutes of EGMs requires a RAM of 16 to 512 Kb, depending on bandwidth, type of data compression used, and number of channels stored.

Telemetry control: dedicated circuitry to control the specifics of communications protocol and telemetry schema.

System control: contains support circuitry for the microprocessor, including the telemetry interface, typically implemented with a universal-asynchronous, receiver-transmitter (UART)-like interface, several general-purpose timers, and sleep-wake control.

Voltage supply: supplies various current and voltage sources to the system. Digital circuits operate from

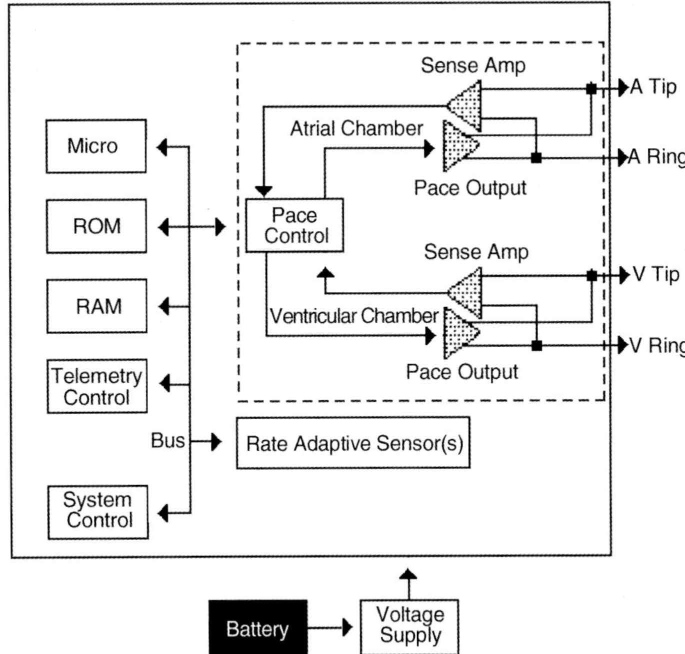

Figure 7-2. Block diagram of a DDDR pacemaker showing main functional elements.

2.2 V or lower supplies; analog circuits typically require precision nanoampere current source inputs.

Battery: one lithium iodine battery supplies an open-circuit voltage of 2.8 V throughout battery life; high-energy density makes this chemistry appropriate for pacemaker applications; low-power density, acceptable in a pacing application, makes this chemistry inappropriate for defibrillation applications (see Chapter 6).

Pacing Output

The function of the output circuit is to translate the lithium iodine battery voltage of 2.8 V into a programmable selection of pacing voltages that range from 0.1 V to more than 7 V. In the most simple situation, the output pulse is programmed to be identical to the voltage of the battery, 2.8 V for a lithium iodine battery at beginning of life (BOL). In this case, the battery is used to charge a pacing capacitor, which itself is then discharged for a duration (t) to the myocardium, where t is the pulse duration. Modern pacemakers, however, offer a variety of programmable stimulus amplitudes ranging from less than 2.8 V to more than 7.5 V. Increasing the stimulus amplitude to a value greater than the battery voltage requires that more than one capacitor be charged in parallel from the battery and then discharged in series to the myocardium.

In order to increase the amplitude of stimulus above the battery voltage, older pulse generators used a capacitive voltage doubler circuit. A capacitive voltage doubler consists of a specific arrangement of switches and capacitors and operates in two distinct phases: one set of switches is closed during the first phase, and a second set of switches closes during the second phase. This clock circuit controls the two phases that are designed to be nonoverlapping, meaning that the switches controlled by each phase are never closed at the same time. Voltage doublers work by charging to capacitors during this first phase (capacitors C1 and C2, connected in parallel with the battery), so that they charge to the battery voltage. In the second phase, these two capacitors are reconnected in series, and their combined voltage is delivered to the heart. The effect of this second phase is that the battery voltage is multiplied (in this case by a factor of 2), and the charge is transferred to the heart. In a similar manner, the stimulus voltage can be tripled by using three charging capacitors rather than two.

A limitation of this technique is that the voltage output is limited to three settings, 1×, 2×, and 3×, corresponding to pacing voltages of 2.8, 5.6, and 8.4 V, respectively. The result is that the current drain caused by a particular pacing output selection is often higher than necessary given the actual pacing threshold. For example, consider a patient with a pacing threshold of 1.5 V. Providing for a pacing safety margin of 2:1 would require an output voltage selection of 3 V. Given 2.8, 5.6, and 8.4 V as the only choices, 5.6 V becomes the only reasonable selection. This 5.6 V selection results in substantially more current required from the pacing circuitry and an attendant reduction in longevity of the pulse generator.

Modern pacemakers overcome this limitation by adding additional circuitry that adds a voltage comparator and an output capacitor to the pacing output circuit. This circuit works in a like manner to the voltage doubler circuit, except that during phase two, the smaller doubler capacitors are reconnected in series and placed across a larger pacing output capacitor. Because the doubler capacitors in this configuration are smaller than the output capacitor, it takes a number of cycles of charging in parallel and then discharging in series to fill the output capacitor completely. This action is sometimes called a charge pump, because charge is being transferred in discrete amounts from the battery, through the small capacitors, to the larger output capacitor. Additionally, a comparator circuit interrupts the charge transfer process when the output capacitor reaches a programmed value. This enhancement allows for finer resolution in pacing output voltage. Using the patient data from the previous example, the voltage output setting of a modern pacemaker given a 1.5-V threshold and using a 2:1 safety margin could be reduced from 5.6 to 3 V. The benefit of this pacing output reduction can be translated into an improvement in longevity by decreasing the current requirements. The equation that approximates average pacing current is as follows:

$$I_p = (V_p \times PW)(V_x/V_{bat})/(P_{Interval})R_l \qquad (7\text{-}1)$$

where I_p is the pacing current, V_p is pacing amplitude, R_l is lead impedance, PW is pulse width, $P_{Interval}$ is the pacing interval, V_x is the pacing multiple (1×, 2×, or 3×), and V_{bat} is battery voltage.

A couple of points are worth noting in this equation. First, voltage appears twice in the numerator, as pacing voltage V_p and as a voltage multiplier V_x. As a result, increasing the pacing voltage has a squared effect on pacing current. The second point to note is that pacing is affected by lead impedance. This effect is reflected in the R_l variable in the pacing equation. This helps explain the benefit of the new generation of high-impedance pacing leads.

Continuing with the 2× pacing example, current drains for the 5.6 V (2×) and 3 V outputs are calculated as 8.6 and 4.8 μA, respectively. These values are based on nominal values of 0.4 msec for PW, 500 Ω for R_l, 1000 msec for the interval (60 ppm or pulses per minute), and 2 for V_x. Assuming a quiescent current of 11 μA for a typical VVIR (the quiescent current is the current required to power the device electronics that are needed to perform "housekeeping" tasks), and with an available battery capacity of 1.2 ampere-hours (A hr), the pacemaker longevity can be calculated as follows:

$$L = C_a \times K/I_e \qquad (7\text{-}2)$$

where L is the longevity of the pacemaker under nominal conditions measured in years; C_a (measured in ampere-hours) is the capacity available in a particular battery cell after subtracting reductions to theoretical capacity, as noted previously; K is a constant that converts hours to years; I_e is the average current drain for pacing, sensing, and circuit function; and I_e is current drain by the pacemaker from the battery.

The resultant longevity is 7 years for the 5.6 V setting and 8.7 years for the 3 V setting. An improvement of 1.7 years in longevity is achieved with the addition of the more flexible pacing output voltage settings. A more detailed discussion of longevity is provided in the section on power requirements of pulse generator circuits and in Chapter 6.

Automatic Capture

A potentially important advance in pacing output circuitry is the concept of automatic capture (or autocapture) verification and threshold tracking.[1] Capture verification refers to the ability of a pacemaker to automatically detect when a pacing stimulus captures the chamber being paced. Threshold tracking uses capture verification as a means to adjust the pacing pulse amplitude automatically to guarantee capture. For example, if capture is verified, the pacing stimulus amplitude remains unchanged. If capture is lost, however, a large-amplitude backup pacing stimulus is delivered (typically within 100 msec) to ensure capture of the heart, and the amplitude of subsequent pacing stimuli is increased. This basic technique can be modified to track the pacing threshold continuously by algorithmically iterating the output to adjust the stimulus output to a level slightly higher than what is necessary for capture. Paradoxically, continuously adjusting the pacing output to a level that is too close to threshold can actually result in increased energy demand from the battery. For each missed beat, the device delivers a large-amplitude pacing stimulus closely coupled to the ineffective stimulus, and this high-output backup pacing pulse can consume as much as 25 times more energy than a stimulus at threshold.

A number of manufacturers have developed pacemakers with autocapture verification. These attempts have proved that capture detection is possible, although with several limitations. The most common technique used to accomplish autocapture is to measure the evoked response. The evoked response is the local intracardiac signal that occurs in response to the pacing stimulus when capture is achieved. In other words, if capture occurs, an evoked response will arise and can be detected. If capture does not occur, there will be no evoked response.

There are a number of technical challenges facing designers in the implementation of autocapture verification and threshold tracking. The primary technical challenge involves the accurate assessment of the evoked response. This challenge can be appreciated by considering that the pacing stimulus may be 350 times greater than the signal to be measured (3.5 V for pacing versus 10 mV for a ventricular-evoked response). Remnants of the stimulus afterpotential (known as polarization) remain long after the pacing pulse is complete, owing to the capacitance at the lead-tissue interface (see Chapter 1). These stimulus remnants have forced some designs to require leads with low polarization characteristics to allow correct operation. When combined with a low-polarization lead, autocapture detection has been proved possible for most patients. The afterpotential must be removed within 50 to 100 msec to delineate the evoked response accurately. The difficulty in distinguishing the evoked response, combined with the fact that the evoked response of the atrial chamber is smaller in magnitude, has limited the introduction of this feature to the ventricular chamber.

An additional challenge in the implementation of autocapture is the accurate assessment of capture in the presence of fusion and pseudofusion beats.[2] Fusion beats can confuse the autocapture algorithm and produce false-negative results, such that a stimulus is determined to be subthreshold when in fact capture has occurred. False-negative results with fusion beats occasionally occur when the intrinsic cardiac signal obscures the evoked response, causing the evoked potential to go undetected. In contrast, pseudofusion beats can result in a false-positive classification. Pseudofusion occurs when a pacing stimulus occurs coincident with the intrinsic depolarization. With pseudofusion, however, the pacing pulse does not capture the heart but is detected as capture. A false-positive classification can occur when the intrinsic waveform is incorrectly classified as an evoked response.

The impact of inaccurately classified events on a threshold-tracking algorithm can be serious. For example, a false-positive classification might promote loss of capture as the algorithm mistakenly assumes that capture has occurred and reduces the amplitude of the pacing stimulus. After a sequence of these misclassified events, the pacing output might be reduced to a dangerously low level. A false-negative classification would result in high-output pacing, as the algorithm increases pacing stimulus amplitude to guarantee capture. This would result in a measurable decrease in device longevity because of the elevated pacing current. A number of approaches have been developed to minimize the impact of fusion and pseudofusion beats. Most of these approaches involve controlling the pacing rate to prevent the possibility of fusion events. As an example, the pacing rate can be automatically increased during a threshold test, so that intrinsic activity is overdriven.

Sense Amplifiers

A dual-chamber pacemaker has two separate sensing channels: one for the atrium and one for the ventricle. Each sense amplifier has five primary attributes: gain, dynamic range, sensitivity, signal-to-noise ratio, and filtering capability. Each of these characteristics is discussed in this section. To begin the discussion, a block diagram of a typical atrial or ventricular sense amplifier is shown in Figure 7-3.

Connection to the input of the amplifier is made to both the lead tip electrode and the device can for unipolar sensing and to the lead tip and ring electrodes for bipolar sensing. Each connection from the patient to the sense amplifier is made through a capacitor and resistor network. This network acts as a prefilter to reduce baseline wander, which results from variations at the electrode-tissue interface. This prefilter also eliminates high-frequency noise, which would cause signal distortion (known as aliasing) if not removed before the signal enters the sense amplifier.

Sense amplifier gain is defined as follows:

$$V_{out} = A \times V_{in} \tag{7-3}$$

where V_{out} is the amplifier output, V_{in} is the amplifier input, and A is the amplifier gain.

The role of the sense amplifier is to increase the magnitude of the signal originating in the cardiac chamber, which can be as low as 0.25 mV, to a value that is squarely within the range of subsequent analog circuits (which typically have a maximum range of 700 mV). Modern pacemaker sense amplifiers have several programmable gain settings to maximize the effective dynamic range. Dynamic range is the amplitude over which the sense amplifier can faithfully reproduce the input signal.

Filtering presents one of the most complex challenges in sense amplifier design.[3-14] The specific filter characteristics used in pacemaker sense amplifiers are designed to allow signals originating in the heart to be detected while at the same time attenuating unwanted cardiac signals or environmental noise. There are generally four types of unwanted signals that need to be reduced. Cardiac signals that must be attenuated include T waves and far-field signals. Noncardiac physiologic signals that must be attenuated include skeletal myopotentials. A third type of undesirable signal is electrical noise inherent to the pacemaker circuitry itself. A fourth type is environmental noise such as microwave ovens, electrical welding equipment, or cellular telephones.[15-24] Filtering provides the most important, although not the only, method available to pacemaker design engineers to prevent these unwanted signals from causing oversensing by the sense amplifiers. Figure 7-4 shows the effect of amplifier filtering on a typical ventricular endocardial EGM. The top panel shows the unfiltered EGM. Notice the prominent T wave present in this EGM. The bottom panel shows the same EGM after going through a typical pacemaker filter with a pass band of 20 to 80 Hz. Note that the T wave is greatly attenuated by the filter. Except for some attenuation in amplitude and some narrowing of duration, the R wave is not affected.

Figure 7-5 shows the unfiltered spectrum of the EGM. Note that the frequency content ranges from 2 to

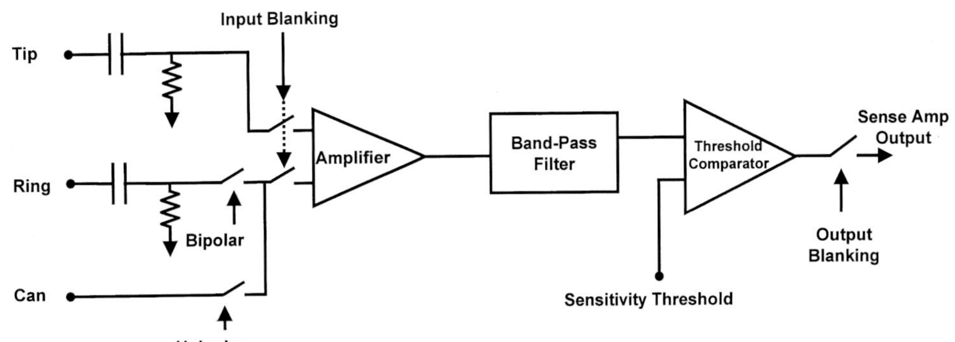

Figure 7-3. Block diagram of a pacemaker sense amplifier showing the main functional elements of a typical atrial or ventricular sense amplifier.

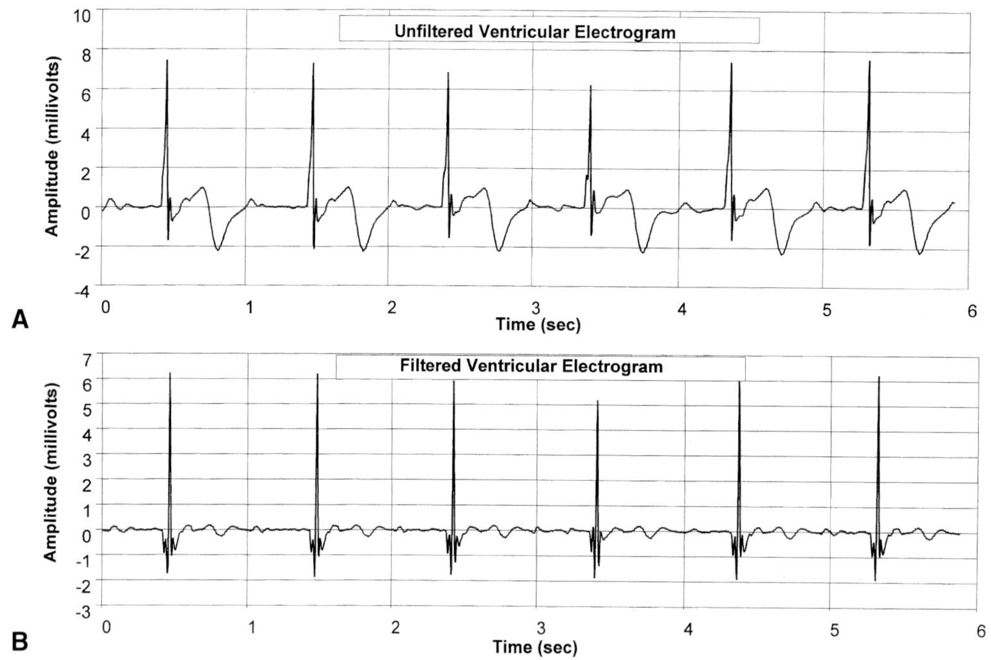

Figure 7-4. ***A,*** *Unfiltered ventricular EGM. Note the prominent T wave.* ***B,*** *The same EGM after filtering by a pacemaker sense amplifier. Filtering has greatly reduced the amplitude of the T wave.*

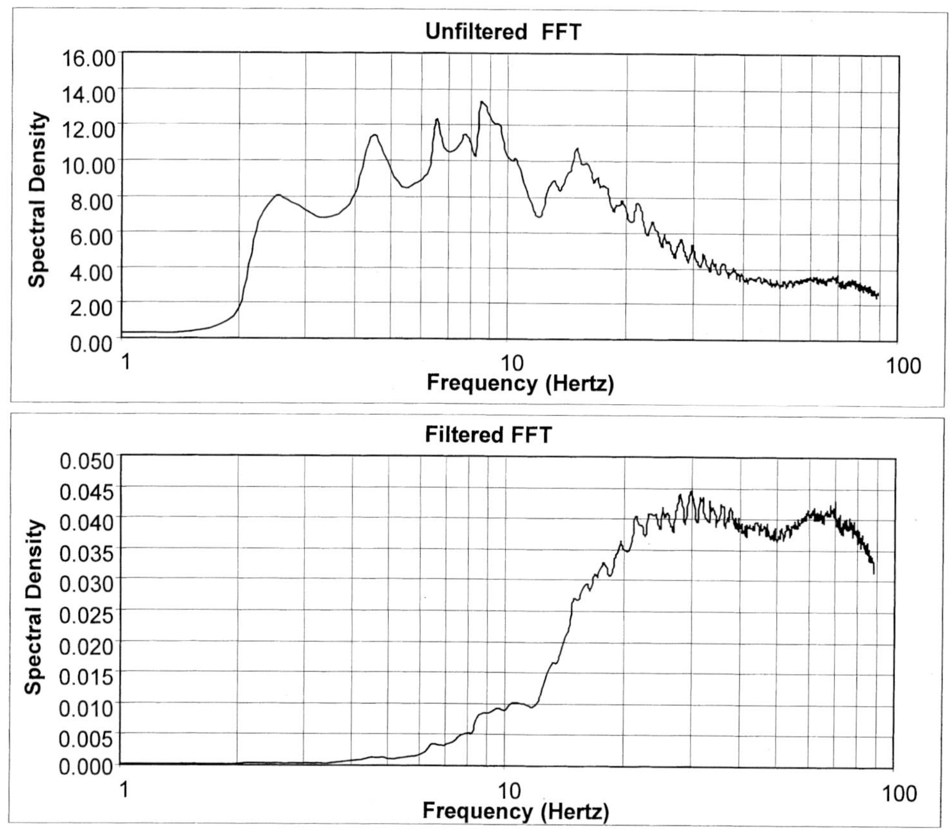

Figure 7-5. Fast Fourier Transforms (FFT) showing frequency content of unfiltered and filtered ventricular EGMs. Top, *Spectrum of an unfiltered EGM. Note the frequency content in the 2 to 10 Hz range, caused by T waves; also note the frequency content between 10 and 40 Hz, caused by R waves.* Bottom, *Spectrum of filtered EGM. The frequency content from 2 to 10 Hz is removed by filtering.*

100 Hz. There is a peak in the range of 6 to 9 Hz that is caused by the T wave. There is a second peak between 10 and 20 Hz, with a gradual decline out to 40 Hz; this is related to the R wave. The lower panel shows the spectrum of the filtered EGM. The filter has significantly reduced most frequency content to less than 10 Hz. Most of the frequency content that remains after filtering is in the 10- to 80-Hz range. Sense amplifier filters make use of the frequency content to distinguish wanted from unwanted signals. Specifically, the filter makes the amplifier most sensitive to frequencies that make up the signal of interest (e.g., R waves) and less sensitive to frequencies that make up unwanted signals, such as T waves.

The last component of the sense amplifier is the threshold comparator. This circuit provides a reference voltage, such that signals above the programmed sensitivity are detected as P waves or R waves, whereas those below this amplitude are not detected. A curve representing how filtering and sensitivity are related is shown in Figure 7-6. This figure shows sensitivity levels on the y-axis and frequency on the x-axis. As noted, signals above the sensitivity level are detected by the sense amplifiers as P waves or R waves. The concave shape of the curve is typical of a bandpass filter. Low-frequency signals require a relatively large amplitude to be detected, because these signals are attenuated by the bandpass filter. Signals in the midband or pass-band region of the filter are detected most easily, because they require the smallest amplitude (i.e., minimal attenuation). As the frequency of the signal increases beyond the pass-band, they become harder to detect because of the higher signal levels required.

Various signals of interest are shown as shaded areas in the figure. The frequency content of typical R waves is shown to be in the range of 25 to 40 Hz. Sense amplifiers are most sensitive to signals in this range and therefore easily detect R waves. T waves, on the other hand, are shown to be lower in frequency (3 to 10 Hz) and are more difficult to detect, as indicated by the fact that the shaded areas lies mostly below the sensitivity line. Similar comments apply to myopotentials, which have a frequency in the 80- to 800-Hz range.

A limitation of sense amplifier filters is apparent from Figure 7-6. As shown in the figure, there is some overlap between unwanted signal frequencies and the sensitivity level corresponding to that frequency. For this reason, filtering alone is not sufficient to reject signals. Additional timing cycles are needed to complete the proper operation of sense amplifiers. The most straightforward example of timing cycles used to reject signals is the ventricular refractory period. The ventricular refractory period rejects T-wave signals that may still be present after filtering. This is accomplished as long as the refractory period covers the timing interval from the R wave to the T wave. Figure 7-7 shows the critical interaction between the amplifier and the comparator.

Power Requirements of Pulse Generator Circuits

The capacity of the battery and the current drain of the pacemaker affect pacemaker longevity. Modern pacemakers use batteries that range in volume from 3.5 to 4.5 mL and have capacities ranging from 1.2 to 1.5 A-hr. The ampere-hour is a unit of measure used by the battery industry to reflect capacity available in the cell. There are two capacity ratings that are of interest in pacemaker design: theoretical capacity and available capacity. Theoretical capacity measures the total capacity of the cell based on the electrochemical content. The available capacity, which is always less than the theoretical capacity, is the capacity that is available after taking into account practical limitations, such as minimum operating voltage of the circuits and reserve capacity needed to manage functions at the end of battery life (EOL).

Pacemaker longevity is calculated as follows:

$$L \cong C_a \times K/I_e \qquad (7\text{-}4)$$

where L is the longevity of the pacemaker under nominal conditions measured in years and C_a is the capacity available in a particular battery cell after subtracting reductions to theoretical capacity. Capacity is measured in units of ampere-hours. I_e is the average current drain for pacing, sensing, and circuit function measured in amperes, and K is a constant that converts hours to years.

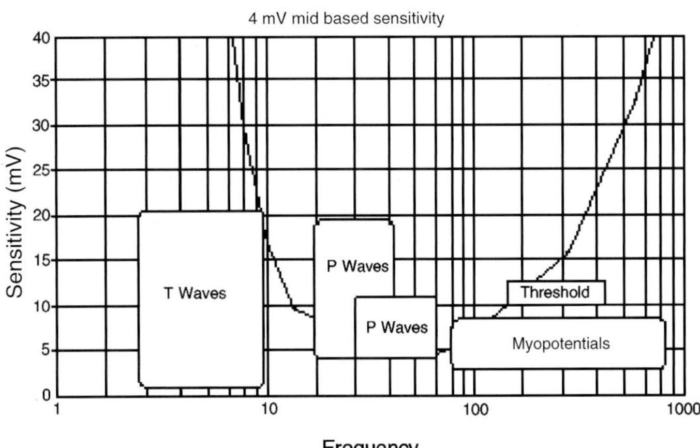

Figure 7-6. Sense amplifier sensitivity versus frequency plot Signals above the threshold (or sensitivity) line are sensed as P waves or R waves. Signals below the sensitivity line are not sensed. Frequencies of typical signals are superimposed on the plot.

TABLE 7-1. **Peak and Average Current Drain Values for Pacemakers**

Function	Peak Current Drain	Average Current Drain (μA)	Average Current Drain as Percentage of Total
Pacing current	17 mA	8	38
Sense amplifiers	2 μA	2	10
Rate-adaptive sensors	2 μA	2	10
Control	16 μA	8	38
Telemetry	60 μA	<1	4
Total	N/A	21	100

Table 7-1 provides a breakdown of pacing current for a typical dual-chamber rate-responsive pacemaker. Pacing current is based on 100% pacing into a 500-Ω lead impedance at programmed settings of 3.5 V, 0.5 msec, and 60 ppm. Pacing current accounts for a significant percentage of the total current drain of the pacemaker. Proper attention to programming of an appropriate pacing amplitude is critical for maximizing pacemaker longevity. Another factor that significantly improves longevity is the use of high-impedance leads. Several companies have developed leads with a pacing impedance of more than 1000 Ω. This results in a substantial reduction in pacing current.

The current drain for both atrial- and ventricular-chamber sense amplifiers is just less than 1 μA each, for a total of 2 μA, as shown in Table 7-1. The current drain represents the energy required for the amplifiers and filters needed in a typical sense amplifier. As noted earlier, low-noise amplifiers needed for more sensitive settings require higher current drain from the battery.

The current drain shown for rate adaptive sensors of 2 μA is typical of an accelerometer-based sensor. The type of sensor incorporated in the pacemaker can have a significant effect on current drain. Sensor current drain can range from less than 1 μA for activity-based sensors that do not use accelerometers to more than 4 μA for some of the physiologic sensors, such as early devices using minute ventilation.

The control current of 8 μA includes the current to run microprocessor circuits as well as the logic that supplements the operation of the microprocessor. The difference between the average current and the peak current for the control circuits results from the fact that, in most pacemakers, the microprocessor "sleeps" when it is not in use. When the microprocessor is placed in stasis, the current drain is virtually zero.

The average telemetry circuit current drain of less than 1 μA reflects the fact that telemetry is used only during implantation and follow-up visits, a small fraction of the total operating life of a pacemaker. When telemetry is not in use, the only current drain required is for the telemetry receiver circuit. This circuit detects the presence of telemetry and powers up the remaining telemetry circuitry.

For pacing and telemetry, the peak current is significantly higher than the average current. This difference has a significant effect on the operation of a lithium iodine battery used in pacemakers.

One of the unique aspects of lithium iodine batteries is the discharge characteristic of the battery chemistry. As cell capacity is depleted, the internal series resistance of the cell increases. This is depicted in Figure 7-8, which shows a simplified model of a battery. As shown in the figure, the series resistance can increase from about 100 Ω at BOL to as high as 10,000 Ω at EOL. This characteristic has significant implications for pacemaker design as well as patient management. The effect on pacemaker design involves constraints that are imposed because of the high series resistance. The high resistance limits the peak current that can be drawn by pacemaker circuits such as telemetry, pacing output, and rate-adaptive sensing. This is seen in Table 7-1 by noting the significant difference in peak versus average current for these functions. For telemetry, the average current is negligible because that function is limited to short periods of time during patient follow-up visits. The peak current, however, is larger than for any other circuit. The peak current, combined with the high series resistance, reduces (according to Ohm's law) the voltage that is available to power the pacemaker electronics. As a result, peak telemetry currents must be limited to values at or below those shown in Table 7-1. This, in turn, limits the telemetry distance and telemetry speed. Greater telemetry distance would increase peak telemetry current because of the higher transmission current pulses needed. Faster telemetry speed would increase peak telemetry current because more pulses would be delivered per second.

The high series resistance of lithium iodine batteries also affects patient management near the end of the pacemaker's useful life (EOL). As the battery depletes and the series resistance increases, the variation in voltage increases. This fluctuation in battery voltage limits the ability of the pacemaker to predict remaining longevity with accuracy. Pacemakers provide a warning of approaching battery depletion. This indicator, known as the Elective Replacement Indicator (ERI), is designed to provide 3 to 6 months' warning before EOL. To preserve remaining capacity and limit voltage variations, most pacemakers limit functionality of the device at ERI by eliminating rate-adaptive features and, in some cases, reverting to VVI mode. Because of the

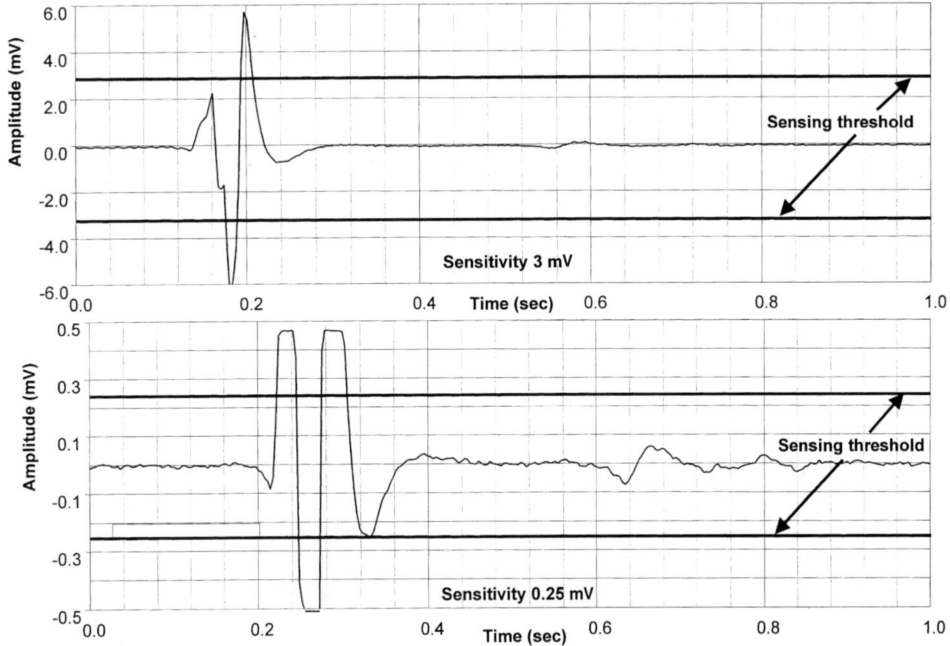

Figure 7-7. Top, *Appropriate sensitivity setting of 3 mV for a 6-mV R wave. This 2:1 sensitivity margin is adequate for the typical variations in R waves.* Bottom, *Effect of setting the sensitivity setting too low (0.25 mV). Note the distortion of the R wave caused by sense amplifier clipping as a result of the increased gain; also note the increased noise.*

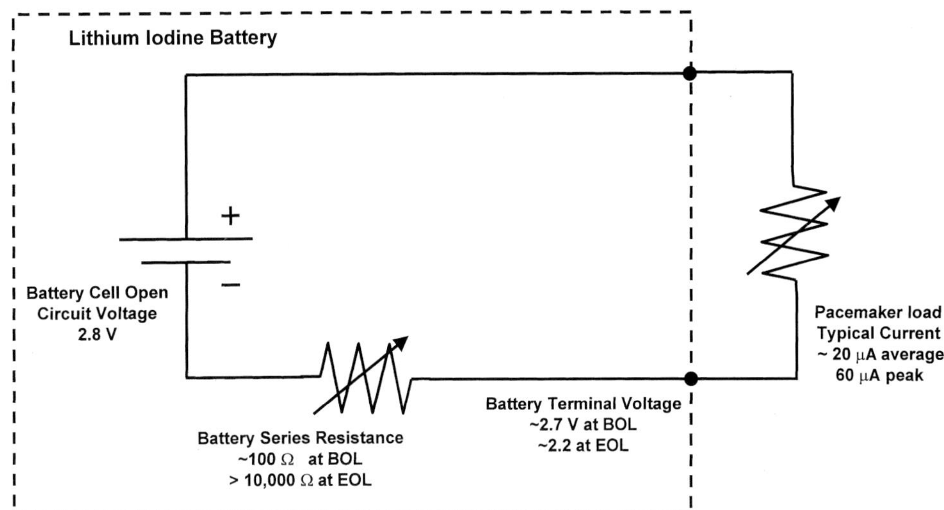

Figure 7-8. Simplified model of a lithium iodine battery. The open-circuit voltage of 2.8 V is characteristic of lithium iodine chemistries. The series resistance increases from 100 Ω at beginning of battery life (BOL) to more than 10,000 Ω at end of life (EOL).

limitations in predicting actual battery EOL, as well as limited device functionality at ERI, it is important to schedule pacemaker replacement as soon as practical after ERI occurs.

Lead Impedance Measurement

Modern pacemakers provide a number of diagnostic measurements that can aid in the evaluation of the pacing system. Measured lead impedance, one of the more clinically useful measurements, can provide important information regarding the integrity of the lead and the lead-pacemaker connection. This information, combined with pacing and sensing thresholds, can assist in troubleshooting lead-related issues.

The first step taken by an implanted device in reporting lead impedance is to measure the leading- and trailing-edge voltages of the pacing pulse, as shown in Figure 7-9. The difference between these two voltages (referred to as "droop" in the pacing pulse) is then used to calculate lead impedance. This impedance calculation is possible because the magnitude of the pacing droop is directly related to the lead impedance. Unfortunately, pacing pulse droop is also affected by components within the pacemaker. As a result of variations in these component values internal to the

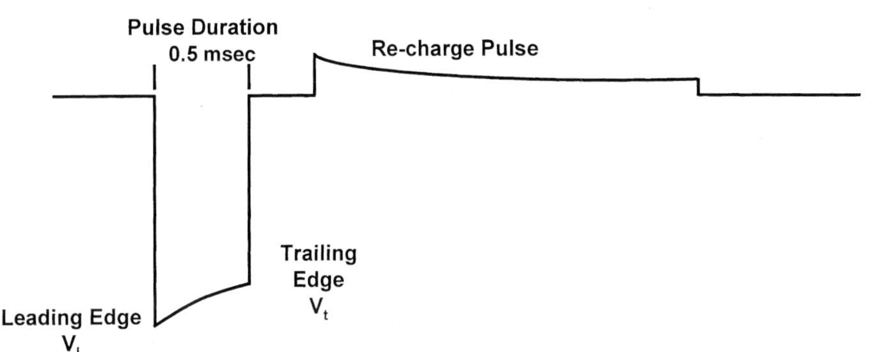

Figure 7-9. Pacemaker output pulse. The decrease in voltage between the leading edge and the trailing edge is measured and used to calculate lead impedance.

implanted device, accuracy of lead impedance measurements is usually ±20%. Although the precision of lead impedance measurements is relatively poor from device to device, the measurements taken from the same device are highly repeatable. Measurements from the same device can be as precise as ±5%. Therefore, it is important to focus on relative trends in lead impedance rather than relying on absolute values when using this measurement for diagnostic purposes.

The method used in pacemakers to measure lead impedance may differ from the measurement method used in a pacing system analyzer (PSA). The different measurement methods may result in differences in measured lead impedance. This difference is important to keep in mind, especially during implantation, when measurements taken from a PSA might differ from measurements of lead impedance taken moments later by the pacemaker.

Lead impedance measurements have traditionally been used only for diagnostic purposes. A relatively new application of lead impedance measurements is the ability of the pacemaker to use them to switch automatically to the appropriate pacing and sensing configuration. If, for example, a conductor within a bipolar pacing lead has fractured, this system could automatically switch to a unipolar configuration, using the remaining intact conductor. This ensures that the patient will continue to receive pacing therapy until appropriate corrective action can be taken.

Another important use of automatic lead configuration switching occurs during device reset. Most pacemakers have a reset mode that is used to ensure proper device operation after disruption from external sources of energy, such as defibrillation shocks, electrocautery, or radiofrequency (RF) ablation. Some modern pacemaker models have incorporated an automatic lead configuration check as part of the reset routine. A lead impedance measurement is taken during rest. If the measurement indicates that a bipolar lead is present, the device will configure pacing and sensing to the bipolar mode. This is an important feature of pacemakers that are implanted in combination with implantable defibrillators, because unipolar pacing markedly interferes with proper defibrillator sensing.

Another enhancement to pacemaker lead impedance measurements is the ability to measure impedance automatically on a periodic basis and store these results for analysis at follow-up. Because trends in lead impedance over time are the most meaningful indicator of lead integrity, this feature provides a valuable troubleshooting tool as well as a time-saving tool during follow-up.

Adaptive Rate Sensors

Although a variety of sensors have been developed for rate-adaptive pacing, those detecting activity, acceleration, or minute ventilation have become dominant. The activity sensor has been the most commonly implanted adaptive rate sensor, and there are two basic types: motion sensors and accelerometers. The primary technical difference between a motion sensor and an accelerometer is that the accelerometer uses an isolated mass (known as a proof mass) as part of the sensor, whereas the motion sensor uses the pacemaker case as the mass. The effective mass that the pacemaker case presents to the sensor can vary considerably from patient to patient. Because force equals mass multiplied by acceleration ($F = ma$), use of the constant mass in accelerometer sensors provides for a precise and repeatable measurement of acceleration.

Two material properties are exploited in the fabricating of activity sensors. Piezoelectric sensors redistribute charge when the material is deflected, and this can be detected and converted to a voltage by the pacemaker circuitry. Piezoresistive sensors change their resistance value when deflected, and this change in resistance is converted to voltage by driving the sensor with a constant current. The piezoelectric activity sensor requires less current than the piezoresistive sensor (about 1.5 versus 3 μA).

Minute ventilation is another important adaptive rate sensor. There are several meaningful improvements that need to be addressed in the next generation of minute ventilation pacemakers. The most important improvement is the reduction of current drain required for measuring minute ventilation, which today ranges from 3 to 5 μA. Other technical issues include increasing the range of respiration rates from the 45 breaths per minute maximum available in some current pacemaker models to rates as high as 60 breaths per minute. The ability to measure higher respiration rates will allow use of the minute ventilation sensor in a wider group of patients (especially children). The key technical challenge in extending the respiration rate will involve better rejection of the cardiac component of the impedance signal used to detect respiration.

The primary technical challenge for designing multisensor pacemakers will be reduction of current drain, so that device size and longevity are not adversely affected. An additional challenge will be integration of the individual sensor algorithms into an appropriate blend.

Microprocessors

The microprocessor has affected the way digital design is accomplished more than any other innovation of the past 25 years. This technology has successfully been applied to the design of implantable devices. During the same period, circuit density has increased by more than 1,000,000 times, whereas the size of the circuitry and the current drain have decreased. These advances in circuit design have allowed implementation of more sophisticated algorithms, including those associated with rate-responsive pacing. These same advances in circuit size and current reduction have allowed greater memory for storing the pacemaker software (sometimes called firmware) used to implement algorithms as well as increased diagnostic data storage. Most early pacemakers were designed with discrete logic.

Memory

With the incorporation of microprocessors into pacemakers comes the requirement to store information in memory. Two types of memory are used in pacemakers. ROM, or read-only memory, is used to store the software programs that the microprocessor uses to control pacemaker function. ROM is a type of nonvolatile memory, which means that, once the memory is written during manufacture, it cannot be changed. This attribute limits the use of ROM to program storage (because diagnostic information changes over the life of the device). It does provide an advantage, however: it is immune to external interference sources, such as electrocautery and other electromagnetic sources, which can disrupt power. For this reason, critical pacemaker codes, such as those used for reset routines, are always stored in ROM.

The other type of memory used in implantable devices is RAM, or random-access memory. The critical attribute of RAM is that the memory contents can be changed throughout the use of the device. RAM is a type of volatile memory. This attribute makes RAM uniquely suited for storing programmable parameters, such as pacing amplitude and diagnostic information.

Some pacemakers have used RAM to store software code as well as diagnostics. The use of RAM to store program code carries with it the potential risk that the code could be corrupted by external interference. This risk increases as memory density becomes greater with advances in digital fabrication technology. The minimum feature size used to manufacture digital circuits, including memory, continues to shrink to as small as 0.35 μm. The smaller feature size makes the circuits more susceptible to interference, such as interruptions in the power supply or interference from subatomic particle radiation from the atmosphere.

One of the important technologies available to help manage this risk is the use of error detection and error correction codes. Error detection codes are algorithms that can automatically detect whether some event has caused a RAM location to be corrupted or changed. Error detection has been used in pacemakers for many years to ensure that data transmitted between the pacemaker and the programmer during telemetry are intact. With increased memory density, these techniques need to be incorporated into the use of RAM as well. The main technique used in error detection is synthetic division, with storage of the result in a different memory location. The division operation is performed using a number that results in a unique solution for each bit pattern being checked. Any result that is different from the stored result confirms an error in the memory. The same principles used for error detection can be extended to provide for error correction. Error correction routines can actually correct the memory location if an error is detected. This is accomplished with algorithms that have more complexity than those used for error detection only.

Error detection and error correction algorithms will become increasingly important as the size and density of memory continue to increase in pacemakers. These algorithms will allow more extensive use of RAM for program information as well as diagnostic storage, which will lead to the capability of pacemaker function to be changed or upgraded after implantation through the use of telemetry. This will some day provide for a functional upgrade years after implantation, with a new algorithm based on research completed during the years following the initial implantation.

The Implantable Cardioverter-Defibrillator

The modern ICD is basically a single- or dual-chamber pacemaker with the additional capability of delivering a high-energy shock from a storage capacitor to the heart for defibrillation. The primary components, in addition to the pacing circuitry, are the battery, charging circuit, capacitor, and output switching circuit. The special battery (technically a single cell) supplies the high current for the charging circuit. This battery must charge the capacitor within a very short period. The battery and capacitor are among the largest components of the ICD (Figure 7-10).

Pulse Generator

The key design constraints of the modern implantable defibrillator are size and power.[27-32] Clinicians expect an

ICD to be small enough for pectoral implantation. To reduce device size, circuitry must be contained in a compact space that is powered by a small battery. Functional requirements include the safe delivery of therapy on demand, a power supply system with a status indicator of the battery, and reliable monitoring of the heart rate. One of the challenges in the design of an implantable defibrillator is the large range of the voltages and currents that are being controlled in a very small physical package. The heart signal being monitored might be as small as 100 μV, whereas the therapeutic shocks approach 750 V, with a leading edge current of 15 A and a pulse termination current spike of 210 A.

Safe delivery of therapy brings special problems to the designer of an implantable defibrillator. Because ICD batteries contain up to 20,000 J, a potential hazard exists if the charging and firing circuits were to "dump" all the energy either thermally or electrically to the patient in a brief time period. An implanted device might reach a temperature in excess of 85°C during a high-current state, such as a direct battery short or a component failure within the high-voltage circuit. Device designers may mitigate this thermal hazard by using both current and thermal fuses in the power supplies. The hazard of overapplication of therapy to a patient is partially mitigated by limiting the specific number of therapeutic shocks during any one episode (usually to a maximum of five or six shocks per arrhythmia).

Capacitor

The capacitor must efficiently store approximately 30 to 40 J and efficiently deliver that energy through the output circuit to the heart. Present capacitor technologies have energy densities on the order of 4 to 5 J/mL and therefore require a minimum volume of 6 to 10 mL just for the capacitor. In spite of the billions of capacitors that are manufactured every year for a myriad of electronic applications, no commercially available capacitor is able to meet the present requirements for an ICD application. Present ICD capacitors are custom-made strictly for use in ICDs. Present ICD capacitor technologies are primarily aluminum sheet and tantalum pellet (some low-cost devices use rolled aluminum capacitors); these are described in more detail in Chapter 6. The critical design choice is the voltage of the capacitor. Obviously, energy alone does not determine the effectiveness of the defibrillation shock. For example, the "DC Fibber" feature, which delivers approximately 10 V for multiple seconds to induce ventricular fibrillation, could be left on and would deliver 30 to 40 J in less than 1 minute. However, that would only succeed in initiating and maintaining fibrillation and would clearly not defibrillate. Defibrillation efficacy is optimized when the shock time constant is close to the cardiac membrane constant. That is because the shock energy is largely delivered during the same time that it takes to charge the cell membrane. Energy delivered much after the cell membrane response peaks is wasted and, in fact, counterproductive (see later discussion on waveform controls in the output circuit).

The typical human membrane time constant during a high voltage shock is 3.5 msec. A low-capacitance capacitor with high voltage can store the same energy as a high-capacitance capacitor with low voltage. Capacitance is the electrical equivalent of hydraulic compliance. An exact analog is the fact that a low-compliance arterial tree requires more pressure to store cardiac output energy than would a high-compliance arterial tree. The formula for the energy storage, based on capacitance (C) and voltage (V), is the well known $E = 0.5\ CV^2$.

The higher the capacitance value, the more time is required to deliver the capacitor charge. This is given by the simple formula for a shock time constant (τ), based on capacitance (C) and resistance (R):

$$\tau = RC$$

This equation gives the amount of time required to deliver 63% of the charge. For a typical patient with a

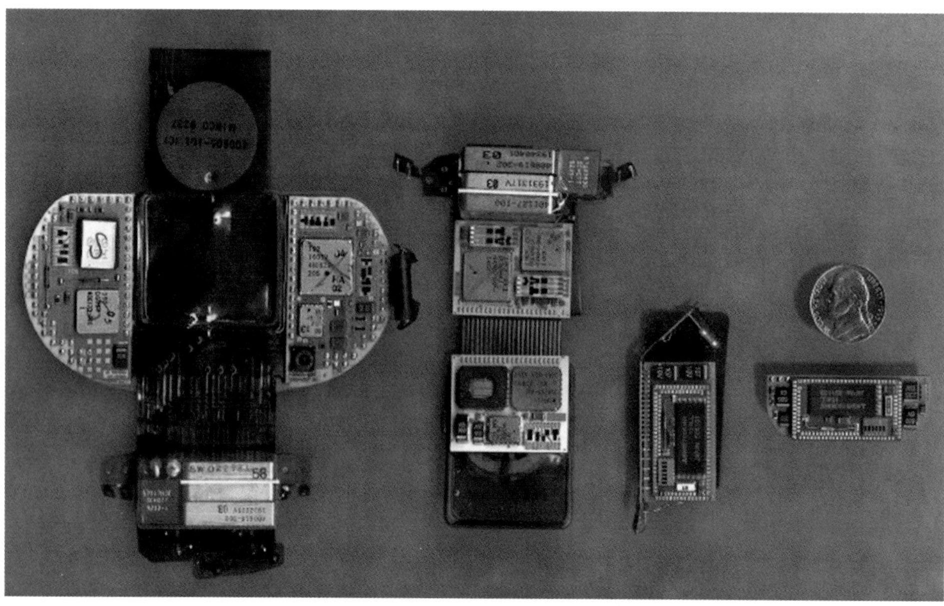

Figure 7-10. Size reduction in electronic defibrillator circuitry.

45-Ω interlead impedance (and a typical membrane time constant of 3.5 msec), the optimal capacitance would be 77 μF in order to match the membrane time constant. Deviations in the capacitance value from this optimum will increase the defibrillation threshold (DFT), as has been demonstrated in numerous animal and human studies. The effect of the changing capacitance on the DFT is shown in Figure 7-16. This effect has also been borne out in larger studies using extremely high capacitance values (approximately 160 μF), which typically lead to high DFTs in 11% to 13% of patients.

However, the voltage is not a trivial choice. For example, using the formula to store 36 J in a 77-μF capacitor, the rising voltage would have to be 967 V. Although this would be a very effective defibrillation shock, at present this level of voltage is limited by capacitor technology. In today's devices, aluminum capacitor energy density is optimized in the range of 400 to 450 V. If two such capacitors were connected in series, the shock would be 800 to 900 V and would still not achieve the required 967 V. With three such capacitors, the voltage would be more than 1200 V. Contrary to a common misunderstanding, there is nothing intrinsically wrong with defibrillating with high voltages. In fact, human hearts have been defibrillated with monophasic catheter-delivered shocks with voltages as high as 1540 V without any ill effects. Therefore, for high-energy devices, some compromises must be made.

The area of capacitor reforming is another one fraught with misunderstanding. The oxide on the capacitor anode degrades with time in the presence of the electrolytic solution. All present ICDs have a feature for automatically "reforming" this oxide by charging the capacitor to a high voltage. It is typically programmed to occur every 1 to 6 months. However, the most advanced aluminum capacitors suffer their degradation in the first week and then no more after that. Therefore, capacitor reformation performed every 2 to 3 days would be very useful to maintain the absolute minimum charge times. However, that would quickly discharge the battery and is not practical. Nevertheless, this calls into question the usefulness of monthly or biannual capacitor reforming.

More advanced methods of reforming are being developed and implemented. One technique is "turbo-forming," in which the capacitor, during reforming, is taken beyond its maximum shock voltage. This yields an oxide layer that lasts much longer and makes reformation practical. A natural question to ask is, if the capacitor is capable of higher voltage, then why would this not be used for every shock? The answer is that more than 30 seconds are required to charge to this higher voltage, and such a delay would not be desirable for therapeutic shocks.

Tantalum capacitors have unique reformation needs and techniques. The future of the tantalum capacitor in the ICD is uncertain as of this writing.

Battery

Lithium silver vanadium oxide (SVO) is the dominant battery chemistry used in commercially available ICDs.

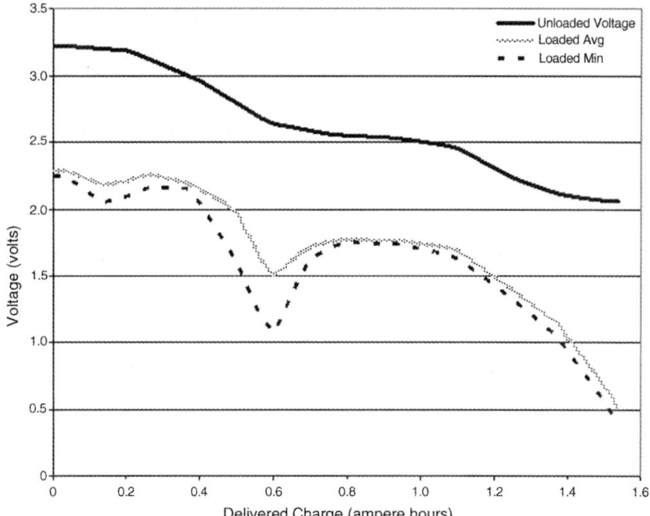

Figure 7-11. Implantable cardioverter-defibrillator voltage under loaded and unloaded conditions. During the shock charging cycle the minimum voltage can be significantly lower than the average.

Unlike the 2.8-V lithium iodine pacemaker cells, which develop high internal impedance as they discharge (up to 20,000 W over their useful lives), SVO cells are characterized by low internal impedance (<1 Ω) over their useful lives. The output voltage is higher than that of lithium iodine, ranging from 3.2 V for a fresh cell to about 2.5 V when the cell is almost depleted. The voltage discharge curve is unusual, having three distinct regions of roughly equal capacity (Fig. 7-11, top tracing). Over the first region of the discharge curve, the voltage is relatively constant at 3.2 to 3.1 V. In the second region, the voltage falls from about 3.1 to 2.6 V. In the final region, the voltage is again relatively constant, falling from 2.6 to 2.5 V. The voltage curves are extended beyond the clinically useful ranges to explain why EOL must occur before an open circuit voltage (OCV) of 2 V.

Although lithium SVO cell chemistry has proved to be as reliable as the lithium iodine technology used in pacemakers, there are a few idiosyncrasies that affect device design. The OCV under a light load is a good indicator of remaining battery capacity, and there is little variation in OCV between SVO cells as a function of capacity delivered. This makes it tempting for the designer to use the OCV exclusively to predict when device replacement is necessary, which would be a good idea if defibrillation therapy were not a factor. More important for the high-voltage circuit designer is the voltage used under the heavy loads typical of DC-to-DC converter operation during charging. This is shown in the lower tracing of Figure 7-11. The battery terminal voltage under this load of several amperes is not well behaved, particularly during the last half of the useful life of the battery. When faced with the requirement of guaranteeing the time to charge for a defibrillation shock, the voltage under load is not the only important factor. Current products rely on a combination of charge time and OCV to predict when replacement is necessary. In defibrillator applications, the load on the battery varies from the continuous monitoring current (typically 15 μA) to the intermittent high-current demands of charging for a high-voltage defibrillation shock (up to 2 to 3 A for 5 to 15 seconds), and therefore the voltage jumps between the two tracings.

SVO cells combine the low self-discharge rate typical of pacemaker cells with the large effective electrode surface area typical of high-current delivery systems. An SVO cell meets the requirements for an implantable defibrillator but requires that high-current pulses be periodically drawn from the cell to maintain its characteristic low impedance. Perhaps the most significant peculiarity of SVO is a characteristic termed voltage delay. This has to do with the instantaneous resistance offered by the cell when switching from low- to high-current demands. Although it is dissipated quickly (≤1 second in most applications), this transient impedance and the attendant droop in terminal voltage can surprise the unwary circuit designer who has made no allowance for the phenomenon. The effects of voltage delay are most pronounced at about the midlife point of the cell, as seen in the lower tracing of Figure 7-11.

Periodic high-current pulsing of the cell is the most effective way to minimize the effects of voltage delay, although making the circuitry tolerant of this aberrant behavior is more energy efficient. Early defibrillators required that this periodic pulsing be accomplished manually by the physician during routine follow-up. Because the electrolytic capacitor used as the storage element for the high-current defibrillation pulse also required reforming periodically (to reform the oxide layer after significant periods without applied voltage), this battery exercising was performed incidentally even though it was usually far more important than the capacitor reforming. Current ICDs have automated this maintenance function by periodically charging and internally dumping the output capacitors. Of course, this comes at the expense of device longevity, with current products sacrificing about 1 to 3 weeks of longevity for each capacitor reforming. During a period of 4 years, about 6 months' worth of energy are consumed to maintain the cells and the capacitors.

The ICD cells are typically tested with a four-shock regimen. Figure 7-11 shows the minimum voltage from the battery during the charging of four maximum-energy shocks. This voltage is significantly lower than the unloaded voltage. This decrease is due to the equivalent series resistance, as shown in Figure 7-8 (in that figure, for a lithium iodine battery). On average, this difference is about 1 V. During the device's "midlife crisis," the resistance is temporarily built up on the anode of the battery, and the voltage momentarily dips to a very low level (e.g., as low as 1 V, as shown in the example in Figure 7-11). However, the battery rather quickly heals itself, and therefore the average voltage during the charging of the four-shock regimen is significantly higher. This significant drop between the loaded average voltage and the loaded minimum voltage is decreased by regular use of the battery. However, that uses precious battery energy. Ironically, the improvement in charge time often seen with "capacitor reforming" is sometimes due mostly to this exercise of the SVO battery.

At the EOL, the voltage has decreased and the internal resistance has increased, so that the loaded voltage of the cell is extremely low and is, in fact, not usable for charging at a reasonable rate. For this reason, the EOL charge times are significantly higher than those at the BOL, because of both the decrease in voltage and the increase in internal resistance. There are some solutions to this problem presently recognized.

The first solution, by Medtronic, is the anode-limited battery. In the traditional SVO cell, the cell has more anode material than is required for optimal charge times. However, this anode material provides an energy storage reserve for a long-term monitoring and pacing. When the cathode is depleted, the ability to provide high currents is limited, and this leads to the typical curve seen in Figure 7-11. This could loosely be described as the battery running out of current before it runs out of energy. In the anode-limited battery, this "dosing" stratagem is reversed. The emphasis is on good charge times throughout the life of the battery, as opposed to long monitoring and pacing times; that is, the emphasis is more on the shock delivery function than on the monitoring and pacing function. This has the advantage of giving more consistent charge times throughout the life of the device. Because this reduces the total energy storage, however, the longevity for pacing and monitoring is reduced. It could be said that this type of battery design runs out of energy before it runs out of current.

Another solution (being introduced by St. Jude Medical) is to have, essentially, a lithium carbon monofluoride battery (CF_X) continuously trickle charge the SVO cell. This both keeps the voltage more stable on the SVO cell and allows delivery of the high currents required to charge the capacitor. In the actual construction, the two chemistries are put together in one case, so that there are alternating cathodes of SVO and CF_X. This battery appears to offer advantages of consistent charge times without sacrifice in total energy storage density.

DC-to-DC Converters

DC-to-DC converters are used in implantable defibrillators to convert the low voltage of the battery to the high voltages required for defibrillation. A number of unique issues confront the ICD designer: the sheer magnitude of the conversion from 3 to 750 V; the intermittent nature of the charging operation; the need to make the converter as small and lightweight as possible; the high efficiency demanded; and the need to integrate the converter on a hybrid with circuitry that must sense intracardiac signals of 100 μV.

The basic configuration, shown in Figure 7-12, includes a low-voltage, high-current switch (S) and flyback transformer (T), a diode (D), a battery (B), and storage capacitor elements (C1 and C2). Charging of the capacitors before a defibrillation shock requires closure of the low-voltage switch, which causes a linear increase in primary current.

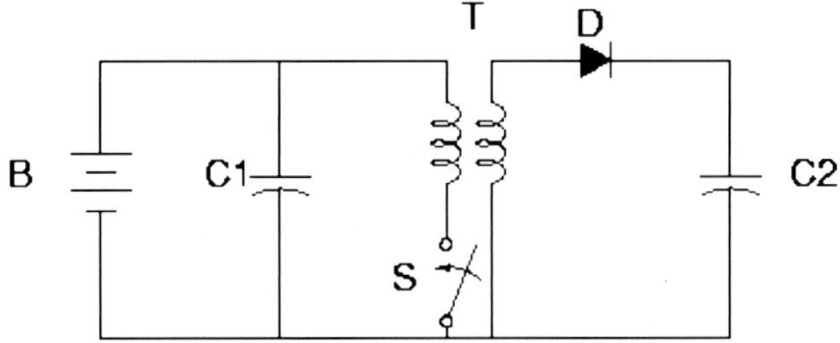

Figure 7-12. DC-DC converter simplified schematic. B, battery; C, capacitor; D, diode; S, switch; T, transformer.

The terms DC-to-DC converter, inverter, and charging circuit are all used interchangeably in the ICD engineering world. The function of the DC-to-DC converter in Figure 7-12 is as follows. The transformer T consists of two coils of wire wound around shared magnetic material. In the beginning of the operation, switch S is turned on, and a current begins to flow through the first coil in the transformer. The energy in a coil is related to the current (i.e., proportional to the square of the current); as the energy from the battery B begins to be stored in the transformer coil, this current continues to increase. At a certain point, a maximum amount of energy is stored in the coil. This typically takes 5 to 10 μsec. At that point, the switch S is opened. This presents a quandary to the transformer. Energy in the coil is proportional to the current squared, yet there is now no path for the current. However, due to energy conservation, the energy stored in the magnetic field must manifest itself as an electrical current. Because it cannot travel back through the first coil (because S has been opened), it finds a new path through the second coil and the diode D, into the storage capacitor C2. As soon as that energy is dumped into the C2, the cycle continues. The ability of this "fly-back" transformer charging system to generate very high voltages is based on the fact that the coil will generate whatever voltage is necessary to deliver its current as required by energy conservation. Therefore, even if C2 is already charged to 800 V and the transformer is charged by a current from a battery of only 3 V, the only path to deliver the stored energy is into the 800-V capacitor, and the transformer will generate enough voltage to "climb above" the capacitor voltage and deliver that energy into the capacitor in order to complete its current path and deliver its energy. The battery energy is thus cycled off and on, at a roughly 50% duty cycle. The function of the capacitor C1 is to prevent the minimum battery voltage from dipping down below a level at which the rest of the circuits can function. The battery keeps the small capacitor C1 charged to approximately 2 to 3 V. Specifically, when the transformer switch S is open, then the battery B is recharging the capacitor C1. When the transformer switch is on, capacitor C1 is providing the primary current to the transformer.

Defibrillator DC-to-DC converters are operated at as high a frequency as is practical to facilitate the use of the smallest possible core—typically, 30 to 60 kHz. The design constraints are preventing core saturation, overheating the core during the typical 10 to 15 seconds of operation, and hysteresis losses in the core itself. Efficiency rates on the order of 50% are typical when calculated as a percentage of the energy delivered to the heart versus the energy removed from the battery during charging. Primary currents average 2 A at a terminal voltage of 4 V (in a two-cell system), resulting in an 8 W converter. Considering a typical maximum energy charge (30 to 35 J) over a charging time of 8 seconds, this equates to 40 to 80 J of energy removed from the battery per charge.

Efficiencies are a function of the loaded battery terminal voltage and deteriorate gradually as the cell depletes. Peak primary currents can be 4 to 6 A and are supplied by a battery bypass capacitor (C1) with a capacitance in the range of 50 to 100 μF. The two basic designs used are the fixed-frequency design (mode B), which results in variable average primary current with battery terminal voltage, and the variable frequency design (mode A), which results in constant average primary current with battery voltage decay. The selection of charging circuit mode affects the time required to charge the output capacitors as the battery depletes, as well as the device longevity. In mode B operation, charge time is relatively constant over a wide range of battery voltages. However, maintaining a constant charge time over the entire device lifetime results in reduced longevity. Mode A operation, on the other hand, results in a charge time that is inversely proportional to the battery terminal voltage. Mode A implementations allow the designer to extract the maximum longevity from a battery, at the expense of increasing charge times as the battery is depleted.

Modern ICD charging circuits are tolerant of the midlife crisis. The primary concern is that the voltage not be allowed to dip below approximately 1.5 volts, at which point the control circuitry would fail to perform. This is analogous to maintaining average systemic blood pressure above 60 mm Hg so that the patient does not lose consciousness. The charging of the capacitor, to deliver a shock, places the greatest demand. Therefore, the system must make tradeoffs when the voltage is lowered by the charging activity. Modern ICDs go through an intelligent compromise that increases the charge time when necessary in order to maintain a minimum voltage for the rest of the circuits to operate.

These circuits were sometimes suboptimal in earlier devices, and the electrical power triaging circuits would sometimes overreact. This could result, in one example, in a sudden doubling of charge time, because the voltage briefly dipped too low and the power drawn by the charging circuit was halved. This apparently is not an issue with more modern designs.

Figure 7-13 shows the theoretical versus the actual charging capability performance of such charging circuits coupled to real-life capacitors. Recall that a joule is the same as a watt-second. Therefore, a system that is capable of delivering 6 W should charge a capacitor to 36 J in 6 seconds. This is shown as the BOL theoretical charging curve in Figure 7-13. The actual curve is very consistent for the first 10 J and then begins to fall away. This is due to the fact that the leakage of the capacitor increases with higher voltages. Therefore,

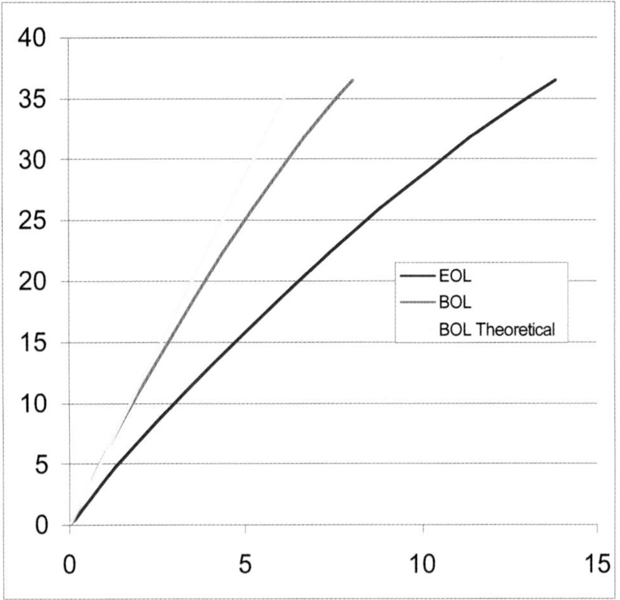

Figure 7-13. Capacitor changing. At EOL more time is required for a given energy.

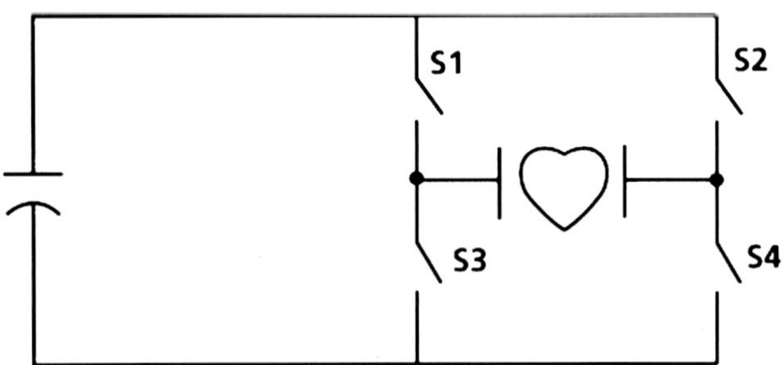

Figure 7-14. Output circuit. See text for description.

although the theoretical charge would have been 6 seconds, the actual time is closer to 7 seconds. For comparison, the EOL charge times are also shown for the same system.

Care must be taken to keep the resistance of all circuit connections to a minimum, because even an additional 0.1 Ω in the primary circuit consumes 4 J of energy in a 10-second charge cycle. Minimizing the resistance of all circuit connections, wire bonds, die bonds, and circuit traces, while also minimizing crosstalk and high-voltage arcing in the secondary circuit, presents a formidable task for the hybrid circuit designer.

Output Switching

Defibrillation efficacy is affected by both the amplitude and the pulse width of the defibrillation shock, and shocks of specific pulse widths are more effective in achieving defibrillation.

To generate multiphasic output pulses, output bridge configurations (Fig. 7-14) with devices capable of turning on and off are required. Because the load resistance associated with defibrillation is in the range of 20 to 50 Ω, peak currents on the order of 40 A are common in output circuits.

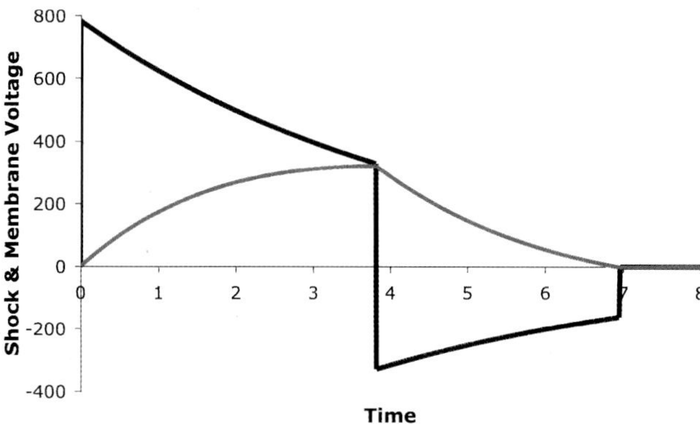

Figure 7-15. Cell charging and burping.

To generate a conventional biphasic waveform, switches S1 and S4 are closed for a predetermined time (see Fig. 7-14). During this phase, S2 and S3 must remain open. To follow phase one, switches S1 and S4 are opened, and S2 and S3 are closed. This second phase remains active until the completion of a certain time period. All switches are then opened. Reversing the order of switch closure reverses the waveform polarity.

Figure 7-15 shows the function of the biphasic waveform. The first phase charges the cell membranes of the majority of the cardiac cells to extend their refractive periods and extinguish wavefronts. The second phase heals the deleterious side effects of the first phase. These deleterious effects are believed to include marginal stimulation in borderline current density areas, electroporation at sites of direct contact of electrodes with the myocardium, and launching of wavefronts from the virtual cathode into the virtual anode. An optimally timed waveform has a first phase that peaks the passive membrane response at the end of the first phase. An optimal second phase is then timed to return the residual membrane back to zero. The optimal times for a typical patient and typical capacitance values are about 4 msec for phase one and 3 msec for phase two.

Figure 7-16 shows the deleterious effects of excessive phase durations. In this case, the first phase is 7 msec in duration. It can be seen that the cell membrane response is peaked at about 4 msec. This immediately suggests that the energy delivered between 4 and 7 msec is wasted. However, it is worse than wasted, because the membrane response is being pulled back, and the excess delivered energy is deleterious. Similarly, as can be seen in the excessively long second phase, the membrane residual charge is not left at a zero potential; rather, it is pulled through zero into a non-zero state.

The most common cause of excessive duration is the use of large capacitance values along with fixed tilt waveforms. The problem with tilt is that the waveform duration is proportional to the resistance and capacitance. This was assumed to be a benefit in the early 1990s, because the amount of energy delivered was independent of the resistance. Then, in fact, clinical data demonstrated significant improvement—especially for high-DFT patients—for the use of fixed-duration pulse widths instead of tilt. A more recent study demonstrated a reduction in the population peak DFT

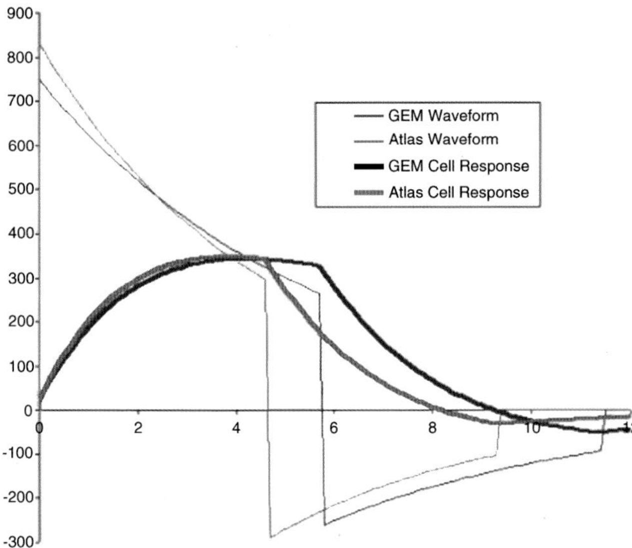

Figure 7-16. Deleterious effects of excessive pulse durations.

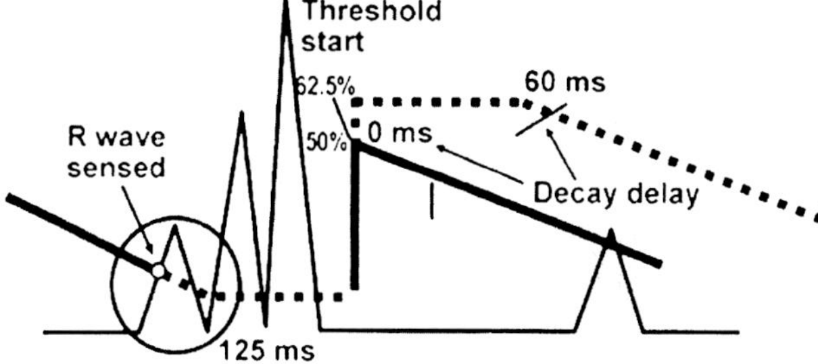

Figure 7-17. General sensing system for a defibrillator.

by 40% simply through use of fixed millisecond durations in place of tilt. Because of the dogmatic acceptance and historical inertia behind tilt, all ICDs continue to offer it, at least as an option. This means that the circuit in Figure 7-14 must sense the capacitor voltage and reverse the switches in the H bridge, so named due to the shape of the switcher, when this voltage has decayed by a certain percentage. Popular tilts (or decay percentage) are 65%, 60%, 50%, and 42% in the first phase, and 65%, 60% 50%, and 42% in the second phase.

Sense Amplifiers

Proper sensing of electrical activity in the heart requires precise sensing and discrimination of each of the components that compose the intracardiac signal. An integrated or dedicated bipolar defibrillation lead in the right ventricular apex of the heart is the typical configuration of current ICD systems. These lead systems present the ICD with a signal that is composed of the near-field electrical events of ventricular depolarization and repolarization as well as the far-field effects of atrial depolarization and repolarization.

As discussed earlier, sensing of ventricular electrical activity to determine heart rate in an implantable pacemaker is performed by the use of a comparator fixed to a given threshold; a detection is issued when the defined amplitude threshold is exceeded. Unfortunately, ventricular electrical activity may be polymorphic (varying in both amplitude and slew rate) in nature during tachyarrhythmia and fibrillation, and the amplitude of electrical activity may be an order of magnitude smaller than during normal sinus rhythm. Accordingly, a more robust sensing algorithm is required.

From an electrical standpoint, the sense amplifier must be able to operate properly over a rate range from 30 to 360 beats per minute or greater. Additionally, the amplifier must be able to respond quickly and accurately to the widely varying intracardiac signals presented during ventricular fibrillation. A number of sensing methods have been used to track these signals.

Sensing systems for defibrillators generally follow the basic configuration shown in Figure 7-17. Signals originating in the ventricles range from 100 μV to more than 20 mV and are amplified and filtered before being processed. The R wave is then sensed by the circuit. This is referred to as autosensing by St. Jude Medical, as autoadjusting sensing by Medtronic, and as "fast AGC" by Guidant. Once an R wave is sensed, the system takes the peak value and resets the threshold to a percentage of that peak. For the device shown in the drawing, this is an adjustable percentage. After an adjustable delay, the threshold is then decreased until it is exceeded by sensed electrical activity. In the example shown, the system was refractory for 125 msec and then went to 50% of the peak value and decayed with no delay. It was then erroneously sensed as a T wave. This problem was fixed by programming the threshold startup to 62.5% (5/8) and setting the decay delay to 60 msec. These sensing algorithms are no longer accomplished with dedicated circuitry but are realized completely in software processing in current devices.

Conclusion

Pacemakers and ICDs include a range of battery, capacitor, and integrated circuit technologies that are specialized for implantable devices with a fixed battery capacity. The remarkable reliability and ever-expanding features offered by implantable medical devices continue to challenge both engineers and the clinicians who implement these therapies.

REFERENCES

1. Sermasi S, Marconi M, Libero L, et al: Italian experience with AutoCapture in conjunction with a membrane lead. Pacesetter Automatic Control of Energy and Membrane Automatic Threshold Evaluation (PACEMATE) Study Group. PACE 19:1799-804, 1996.
2. Levine PA, Brodsky SJ: Fusion, pseudofusion, pseudopseudofusion, and confusion. Clin Prog Pacing Electrophysiol 1:70, 1983.
3. Irnich W: Intracardiac electrograms and sensing test signals: Electrophysiological, physical, and technical considerations. PACE 8:870, 1985.
4. Frohlig G, Schwendt H, Schieffer H, Bette L: Atrial signal variations and pacemaker malsensing during exercise: A study in the time and frequency domain. J Am Coll Cardiol 11:806, 1988.

5. Klitzner TS, Stevenson WG: Effects of filtering on right ventricular electrograms recorded from endocardial catheters in humans. PACE 13:69, 1990.
6. Steinhaus DM, Foley L, Knoll K, Markowitz T: Atrial sensing revisited: Do bandpass filters matter? PACE 16:946, 1993.
7. Fischler H: Polarization properties of small-surface-area pacemaker electrodes: Implications on reliability of sensing and pacing. PACE 2:403, 1979.
8. De Buitleir M, Kou WH, Schmaltz S, et al: Acute changes in pacing threshold and R- or P-wave amplitude during permanent pacemaker implantation. Am J Cardiol 65:999, 1990.
9. Fetter J, Hall DM, Hoff GL, Reeder JT: The effect of myopotential interference on unipolar and bipolar dual-chamber pacemakers in the DDD mode. Clin Prog Electrophysiol Pacing 3:368, 1985.
10. Fetter J, Bobeldyk GL, Engman FJ: The clinical incidence and significance of myopotential sensing with unipolar pacemakers. PACE 7:871, 1984.
11. Lau CP, Linker NJ, Butrous GS, et al: Myopotential interference in unipolar rate-responsive pacemakers. PACE 12:1324, 1989.
12. Kleinert M, Elmqvist H, Strandberg H: Spectral properties of atrial and ventricular endocardial signals. PACE 2:11, 1979.
13. Brandt J, Fahraeus T, Schuller H: Farfield QRS complex sensing via the atrial pacemaker lead. II. Prevalence, clinical significance, and possibility of intraoperative prediction in DDD pacing. PACE 11:1546, 1988.
14. Hauser RG, Susmano A: Afterpotential oversensing by a programmable pulse generator. PACE 4:391, 1981.
15. Hayes DL, Wang PJ, Reynolds DW, et al: Interference with cardiac pacemakers by cellular telephones. N Engl J Med 336:1473-1479, 1997.
16. Joyner KH, Anderson V, Wood MP: Interference and energy deposition rates from digital mobile phones. In Bioelectromagnetics 16th Annual Meeting Abstract Book. Frederick, MD, Bioelectromagnetic Society, 1994, pp 67-68.
17. Hayes DL, Vonfeldt L, Neubauer S, et al: Effect of digital cellular phones on permanent pacemakers [abstract]. PACE 18(Pt 11):863, 1995.
18. Hayes DL, VonFeldt LK, Neubauer SA, et al: Does cellular phone technology cause pacemaker or defibrillator interference? [abstract] PACE 18(Pt 11):842, 1995.
19. Carillo R, Saunkeah B, Pickels M, et al: Preliminary observations on cellular telephones and pacemakers [abstract]. PACE 18(Pt 11):863, 1995.
20. Carillo R, Saunkeah B, Traad E, et al: At what distance do cellular telephones interfere with pacemakers? [abstract]. PACE 18(Pt 11):1777, 1995.
21. Ruggera PS, Witters DM, Bassen HI: In vitro testing of pacemakers for RF interference at fixed distances from U.S. type digital cellular phones. Poster presented at the Annual Electromagnetic Compatibility Forum, Washington, DC, September 11, 1996.
22. Denny HW, Jenkins BM: EMC history of cardiac pacemakers. EMC Test Design 4:33-36, 1993.
23. Ziegler JF, Lanford WA: The effect of sea level cosmic rays on electronic devices. J Appl Physiol 52:4305-4312, 1981.
24. Gossett CA, Hughlock BW, Katoozi M, LaRue GS: Single event phenomena in atmospheric neutron environments. IEEE Trans Nucl Sci 40:1845-1852, 1993.
25. Homing RJ, Rhoback FW: New high rat~lithium/vanadium pentoxide cell for implantable medical devices. Progress in Batteries and Solar Cells 4:97, 1982.
26. Takeuchi ES: Batteries for implantable defibrillators. Proceedings of the 3rd Annual Battery Conference on Applications and Advances Section VI-3. Long Beach, CA, California State University, 1988.
27. Hnatec ER: Design of Solid-State Power Supplies, 2nd ed. New York, Van Nostrand Reinhold, 1981.
28. Schuder JC, Stoeckle H, West JA, et al: Transthoracic ventricular defibrillation in the dog with truncated and untruncated exponential stimuli. IEEE Trans Bio Med Eng 18:410-415, 1971.
29. Bach S: Engineering Aspects of Implantable Defibrillators: Electrical Therapy for Cardiac Arrhythmias. Philadelphia, WB Saunders, 1990.
30. Vittoz E: Micropower Techniques: Design of MIS VLSI Circuits for Telecommunications. New York, Prentice-Hall, 1985.
31. Unbehauen R, Cichocki A: MOS Switched-Capacitor and Continuous Time Integrated Circuits and Systems. New York, Springer-Verlag, 1989.
32. Toumazou C, Hughes JB, Battersby NC (eds): Switched-Currents: An Analog Technique for Digital Technology. London, Peter Peregrinus, 1993.

Chapter 8

Pacemaker, Defibrillator, and Lead Codes

ALAN D. BERNSTEIN • VICTOR PARSONNET

The need for specialized symbols to describe pacemaker function has evolved along with pacemaker technology. Most pacemakers of the 1960s presented no problem in this regard because they were all essentially the same: they paced a single cardiac chamber, had no sensing capability (and therefore no response to sensing that needed to be identified), and had no adjustable characteristics with settings that had to be readily communicated. With the development of atrial and ventricular pacemakers with outputs that were triggered or inhibited by spontaneous cardiac activity, awareness of the pacemaker's configuration and functional design became indispensable for verifying its proper operation or identifying possible problems.

Two separate tasks needed to be addressed in designing a code to describe cardiac-pacemaker function: first, identifying the information that needs to be conveyed and in what circumstances; and second, defining the appropriate symbols and code structure to convey that information. These considerations are central to the design of each of the pacemaker codes described in this chapter.

Pacemaker Codes

Generic Pacemaker Codes: Historical Overview

The Three-Position ICHD Code (1974)

In 1974, the Inter-Society Commission for Heart Disease Resources (ICHD) proposed a three-position "generic" or "conversational" pacemaker code to meet an increasingly apparent need for distinguishing different types of pacemakers according to three fundamental attributes: (1) the chamber or chambers paced, (2) the chamber or chambers in which native cardiac events were sensed, and (3) what the pacemaker did when a spontaneous depolarization was sensed. The 1974 code, which was based on an initial structure suggested several years earlier by Smyth, is summarized in Table 8-1, and the existing pacing modes for which this code was formulated are listed in Table 8-2.[1]

Position I represents the location of pacing (atrium, ventricle, or both); position II shows where spontaneous events are sensed (atrium, ventricle, or both); and position III denotes the pacemaker's response to sensing. For example, a VVI pacemaker stimulates the ventricle (V), and whenever a spontaneous event is sensed in the ventricle (V), the pacemaker inhibits (I) a pending ventricular stimulus.

A certain degree of ambiguity is inherent in position III, although much of that ambiguity may be resolved by the context in which the code is used. For example, a VVT pacemaker is one that paces the ventricle, senses spontaneous ventricular depolarizations, and produces a triggered ventricular output immediately on ventricular sensing. In VAT pacing, on the other hand, triggering means something else: the production of a triggered ventricular output in response to atrial sensing after a delay intended to simulate the normal temporal pattern of atrioventricular (AV) conduction. The delay is assumed implicitly in this use of the code,

TABLE 8-1. The 1974 Three-Position ICHD Code or Three-Letter Identification Code*

First Letter	Second Letter	Third Letter
Chambers paced	Chambers sensed	Mode of response

*Letters used: A, atrium; D, double-chamber; I, inhibited; O, not applicable; T, triggered; V, ventricle.
Adapted from Parsonnet V, Furman S, Smyth NPD: Implantable cardiac pacemakers: Status report and resource guideline. Pacemaker Study Group, Inter-Society Commission for Heart Disease Resources (ICHD). Circulation 50:A-21, 1974. Copyright 1974 American Heart Association.

TABLE 8-2. Pacing Modes Described by the Three-Position ICHD Code

Mode	Description
VOO	Asynchronous ventricular pacing; no sensing function
AOO	Asynchronous atrial pacing; no sensing function
DOO	Dual-chamber (AV-sequential) asynchronous pacing; no sensing function
VVI	Ventricular pacing inhibited by ventricular sensing
VVT	Ventricular pacing triggered instantaneously by ventricular sensing
AAI	Atrial pacing inhibited by atrial sensing
AAT	Atrial pacing triggered instantaneously by atrial sensing
VAT	Ventricular pacing triggered after a delay by atrial sensing
DVI	Dual-chamber (AV-sequential) pacing inhibited by ventricular sensing

AV, atrioventricular.
Modified from Parsonnet V, Furman S, Smyth NPD: Implantable cardiac pacemakers: Status report and resource guidelines. Pacemaker Study Group, Inter-Society Commission for Heart Disease Resources (ICHD). Circulation 50:A21, 1974. Copyright 1974 American Heart Association.

as in other dual-chamber modes, such as DVI, DDD, and DDI.

This was the first of the recognized generic or conversational codes. Its designers' identification of information priorities (the first task referred to previously) was so insightful and its design so convenient (the second task) that the code has been in continuous use worldwide since its publication and has served as the kernel of each of three successive generic codes that superseded it. Its forward compatibility stands as a tribute to its designers, particularly with respect to pacemakers that could sense in both chambers, which had not yet come into existence when the code was formulated.

The Five-Position ICHD Code (1981)

In 1981, a revised code was published by the same designers (Table 8-3).[2] Although it incorporated all of the features of the previous code, it was augmented by two additional positions to allow it to describe two major developments of the intervening 5 years: programmability and antitachyarrhythmia pacing.

With the advent of pacemakers, some of which had operating parameters that could be adjusted noninvasively by means of a programming device, it became important to know that the pacemaker's rate, output amplitude, mode, or timing characteristics could be changed at will so that the reflections of such changes in the electrocardiogram would not be mistaken as evidence of a device malfunction. A fifth position was added to provide information about antitachyarrhythmia pacing functions and the means by which they were activated, whether automatically or by external command using a separate triggering device. The information about antibradycardia pacing modes represented by the five-position code remained in the first three positions and was expressed in the same manner as before, so that compatibility with the previous code was retained. Table 8-4 lists examples of pacing modes described by the five-position ICHD Code that did not exist at the time the original three-position code was designed.

In 1983, this code was amended once again, this time to include the option of the letter C (communi-

TABLE 8-3. The 1981 Five-Position ICHD Code

Position	I (Chambers Paced)	II (Chambers Sensed)	III (Modes of Response)	IV (Programmable Functions)	V (Special Antitachyarrhythmia Functions)
Letters used	V = ventricle A = atrium D = double	V = ventricle A = atrium D = double O = none	T = triggered I = inhibited D = double* O = none R = reverse	P = programmable (rate and/or output) N = normal-rate competition M = multiprogrammable C = communicating O = none	B = bursts S = scanning E = external
Manufacturer's designation only	S = single chamber	S = single chamber	Comma optional here		

*Triggered and inhibited response.
Adapted from Parsonnet V, Furman S, Smyth NPD: Revised code for pacemaker identification. PACE 4:400, 1981.

TABLE 8-4. **Pacing Modes Described by the Five-Position ICHD Code**

Mode	Description
VDD,M (VDDM)	Ventricular antibradycardia pacing inhibited by ventricular sensing, triggered after a delay by atrial sensing. Multiprogrammable device. No antitachyarrhythmia function.
DDD,M (DDDM)	Dual-chamber (AV-sequential) antibradycardia pacing inhibited by sensing in either chamber, with ventricular pacing triggered after a delay by sensing in the atrium after a ventricular event. Multiprogrammable device. No antitachyarrhythmia function.
VVI,MB (VVIMB)	Ventricular antibradycardia pacing inhibited by ventricular sensing. Multiprogrammable device. Pacing bursts for ventricular tachyarrhythmia, means of activation unspecified.
AAR,ON (AARON)	No antibradycardia function. Nonprogrammable device. Normal-rate competition for termination of atrial tachycardia, activated by atrial sensing.
AOO,OE (AOOOE)	Asynchronous atrial antibradycardia pacing. Nonprogrammable device. Externally activated atrial antitachycardia pacing, nature unspecified.

AV, atrioventricular.
Modified from Parsonnet V, Furman S, Smyth NPD: Revised code for pacemaker identification. PACE 4:400, 1981.

cating) in position IV to denote any of three categories of *pacemaker telemetry,* defined as the ability of the implanted device to transmit (1) internally stored information, such as a serial number; (2) device status information, such as the internal resistance of the battery; or (3) physiologic data, such as an intracardiac electrogram signal.[3] The presence of C in position IV of the revised ICHD Code was hierarchical in the sense that it implied that either simple programmability (usually rate and output) or multiprogrammability was present as well. For example, a VVI,C pacemaker would perform ventricular antibradycardia pacing inhibited by ventricular sensing and would be capable of pacemaker telemetry and some degree of programmability.

The NASPE/BPEG Generic (NBG) Pacemaker Code

The pacemaker code in most common use from 1987 to 2000 was introduced by the Mode Code Committee of the North American Society of Pacing and Electrophysiology (NASPE), now known as the Heart Rhythm Society, together with the British Pacing and Electrophysiology Group (BPEG), in response to the continually growing need for a conversational code that could clearly signify the presence of device characteristics beyond basic antibradycardia pacing capabilities.[4] This generic code is summarized in Table 8-5.

The NASPE/BPEG Generic (NBG) Pacemaker Code retains all of the characteristics of the 1974 ICHD Code and some of those of the later five-position codes. To deal with the increasing complexity of later devices, however, it was considered necessary to clarify several features and to define more explicitly how the code was to be used.

The first three positions of the NBG Code are reserved exclusively for antibradycardia-pacing functions. As a result, the R in position III of the 1981 and 1983 ICHD Codes, which denoted reverse pacing, or pacing that was invoked only in the presence of

TABLE 8-5. **The NASPE/BPEG Generic (NBG) Pacemaker Code**

Position*	I (Chambers Paced)	II (Chambers Sensed)	III (Response to Sensing)	IV (Programmability, Rate Modulation)	V (Antitachyarrhythmia Functions)
Letters used	O = none A = atrium V = ventricle D = dual (A + V)	O = none A = atrium V = ventricle D = dual (A + V)	O = none T = triggered I = inhibited D = dual (T + I)	O = none P = simple programmable M = multiprogrammable C = communicating R = rate modulation	O = none P = pacing (antitachyarrhythmia) S = shock D = dual (P + S)
Manufacturer's designation only	S = single (A or V)	S = single (A or V)			

*Positions I to III are used exclusively for antibradyarrhythmia function.
Adapted from Bernstein AD, Camm AJ, Fletcher RD, et al: The NASPE/BPEG Generic Pacemaker Code for antibradyarrhythmia and adaptive-rate pacing and antitachyarrhythmia devices. PACE 10:794, 1987.

tachycardia, is absent. O may be used in all five positions, to accommodate either antibradycardia or antitachycardia pacing without the other, although antibradycardia pacing is the intended focus of the code.

Position IV serves a dual purpose, describing two distinctly different device characteristics: the degree of programmability (P, M, or C), as in the 1983 revised ICHD Code, and the presence or absence of rate modulation (R). Like the C in the revised ICHD Code, the R is hierarchical in that it takes precedence over programmability; it is assumed that adaptive-rate pacemakers are multiprogrammable and usually are capable of some degree of pacemaker telemetry.

Position V indicates the presence of one or more *active* antitachyarrhythmia functions (i.e., excluding normal-rate competition or fixed-rate pacing to suppress a tachyarrhythmia), whether initiated automatically or by external command. A distinction is made between antitachycardia pacing (P) and shock (S) interventions for cardioversion (low energy) or defibrillation (high energy) applied using cardiac electrodes. Position V is thus more general than the corresponding position of the 1981 and 1983 ICHD Codes. In designing the NBG Code, this modification was considered necessary, partly because of the increasing variety of antitachycardia pacing patterns and partly because the B, S, N, and E descriptors of the earlier codes were considered intrinsically restrictive, mixing function (B and N), timing (S), and means of activation (E) in a fashion that allowed only one of the three properties to be represented at a time.[4,5]

To avoid possible confusion, it was also found necessary to identify the possible contexts in which the code could be used: to represent the maximal capabilities of a device (e.g., DDD), the mode to which the device is programmed (e.g., DVI), or the mode in which it is operating at a given moment (e.g., VAT).

The Revised NASPE/BPED (NBG) Generic Pacemaker Code

In light of evolving pacemaker technology and increasing interest in multisite pacing, the 1987 NBG Code was modified by a multinational task force under the chairmanship of David Hayes, MD. The resulting Revised NBG Code was published in 2002.[6]

Three major issues were considered. First, it was recognized that all modern pacemaker pulse generators are capable of extensive bidirectional communication with an external programming device, making them "communicating" pulse generators as defined by the 1987 NBG Code. Second, it was decided that a means of providing basic information regarding the location of multisite pacing would be useful. Third, in view of the extensive antibradycardia-pacing capabilities common in modern implantable cardioverter/defibrillators and the availability of the NASPE/BPEG Defibrillator Code (NBD Code) described later, it was considered unnecessary for the Revised NBG Code to address the presence or absence of antitachycardia features.

Code Structure

The structure of the revised NBG Code is summarized in Table 8-6, and examples of its use are shown in Table 8-7. The Revised NBG Code has five positions, of which the first three are the same as in the previous version. Unlike the previous version, however, all five positions are used exclusively to describe antibradycardia pacing.

Positions I, II, and III indicate the chambers in which pacing and sensing occur and the effect of sensing on the triggering or inhibition of subsequent pacing stimuli. In this context, "sensing" refers specifically to the detection of spontaneous cardiac depolarizations (or spurious interference signals that are interpreted as spontaneous cardiac depolarizations) outside the refractory periods of the pulse generator.

Position IV is used only to indicate the presence (R) or absence (O) of an adaptive-rate mechanism (rate modulation). Unlike the remaining positions, all of which refer to the location of stimulation and spontaneous-depolarization detection and the response to such detection, position IV is unique. It refers to the automatic adjustment of the pacing rate (i.e., the lower rate limit) to compensate for chronotropic incompetence and, in some pulse generators, the simultaneous variation of other timing-related pacing parameters such as refractory periods and AV intervals, under the control of an appropriate measured physiologic variable such as mechanical vibration, acceleration, or minute ventilation. Unlike pacemaker sensing as defined pre-

TABLE 8-6. The Revised NASPE/BPEG Generic Code for Antibradycardia Pacing

Position	I (Chambers Paced)	II (Chambers Sensed)	III (Response to Sensing)	IV (Rate Modulation)	V (Multisite Pacing)
Letters used	O = none A = atrium V = ventricle D = dual (A + V)	O = none A = atrium V = ventricle D = dual (A + V)	O = none T = triggered I = inhibited D = dual (T + I)	O = none R = rate modulation	O = none A = atrium V = ventricle D = dual (A + V)
Manufacturer's designation only	S = single (A or V)	S = single (A or V)			

Modified from Bernstein AD, Daubert J-C, Fletcher RD, et al: The Revised NASPE/BPEG Generic Code for antibradycardia, adaptive-rate, and multisite pacing. PACE 25:260-264, 2000.

TABLE 8-7. **Examples of the Revised NBG Code**

Code	Meaning
VOO, VOOO, or VOOOO	Asynchronous ventricular pacing; no sensing, rate modulation, or multisite pacing.
VVIRV	Ventricular inhibitory pacing with rate modulation and multisite ventricular pacing (i.e., biventricular pacing or more than one pacing site in one ventricle). This mode is often used in patients with heart failure, chronic atrial fibrillation, and intraventricular conduction delay. It was assessed by the atrial-fibrillation group in the "MUSTIC" study.[9]
AAI, AAIO, or AAIOO	Atrial pacing inhibited by sensed spontaneous atrial depolarizations; no rate modulation or multisite pacing.
AAT, AATO, or AATOO	Atrial pacing with atrial outputs elicited without delay on atrial sensing during the alert period outside the pulse generator's refractory period (used primarily as a diagnostic mode to determine exactly when atrial depolarizations are sensed); no rate modulation or multisite pacing.
AATOA	Atrial pacing with atrial outputs elicited without delay on atrial sensing during the alert period outside the pulse generator's refractory period, without rate modulation but with multisite atrial pacing (i.e., biatrial pacing or more than one pacing site in one atrium).[10]
DDD, DDDO, or DDDOO	Dual-chamber pacing (normally inhibited by atrial or ventricular sensing during the alert portion of the VA interval or by ventricular sensing during the alert portion of the AV interval, and with ventricular pacing triggered after a programmed PV interval by atrial sensing during the alert portion of the VA interval); no rate modulation or multisite pacing.
DDI, DDIO, or DDIOO	Dual-chamber pacing without atrium-synchronous ventricular pacing (atrial sensing merely cancels the pending atrial output without affecting escape timing); no rate modulation or multisite pacing.
DDDR or DDDRO	Dual-chamber, adaptive-rate pacing; no multisite pacing.
DDDRA	Dual-chamber, adaptive-rate pacing with multisite atrial pacing (i.e., biatrial pacing or more than one pacing site in one atrium). This mode was assessed in the multicenter "DAPPAF" study.[11]
DDDOV	Dual-chamber pacing without rate modulation but with multisite pacing (i.e., biventricular pacing or more than one pacing site in one ventricle).[12]
DDDRD	Dual-chamber pacing with rate modulation and multisite pacing both in the atrium (i.e., biatrial pacing or pacing in more than one site in one atrium) and in the ventricle (i.e., biventricular pacing or pacing in more than one site in one ventricle).

Adapted from Bernstein AD, Daubert J-C, Fletcher RD, et al: The Revised NASPE/BPEG Generic Code for antibradycardia, adaptive-rate, and multisite pacing. PACE 25:260-264, 2000.

viously (i.e., the detection of spontaneous cardiac depolarizations), position IV addresses a very different process, even though the term "sensor" is often used in this connection.

Position V is used to indicate whether multisite pacing, as described earlier, is present in none of the cardiac chambers (O); in one or both of the atria (A), with stimulation sites in each atrium or more than one stimulation site in either atrium; in one or both of the ventricles (V), with stimulation sites in both ventricles or more than one stimulation site in either ventricle; or in dual chambers (D), in one or both of the atria and in one or both of the ventricles.

Usage Conventions

The Revised NBG Code, like its predecessor, is a resource intended to represent either (1) the maximal capabilities of a device (as in device labeling and record keeping), (2) the mode to which the pulse generator is programmed (as in medical record keeping), or (3) the mode (e.g., VAT in the presence of normal sinus function and complete AV block) in which the device is operating at any particular point in time (as in interpreting paced electrocardiographic rhythm strips).

Although all five positions may be needed for completeness in some circumstances, the first three positions are *always* required. If adaptive-rate pacing and multisite pacing are absent, the first three positions will suffice. If rate modulation is present, position IV is added. Position IV also may be used whenever the *absence* of adaptive-rate pacing requires emphasis. To denote the presence of multisite pacing or to emphasize its absence, all five positions are required even in the absence of rate modulation, in which case position IV serves as a "spacer" so that position V can be used appropriately.

Position I: Chambers Paced. Position I indicates where *antibradycardia* pacing is available, and it is restricted to that purpose. *Antitachycardia* pacing may be addressed more appropriately by means of the NBD Code.

Position II: Chambers Sensed. Position II indicates the chambers in which spontaneous cardiac depolarizations or interference signals may be detected outside the refractory periods of a pulse generator, for the purpose of triggering or inhibiting antibradycardia pacing as indicated in position III. To avoid unnecessary ambiguity, position II specifically excludes the detection of spontaneous depolarizations or other signals for any other purpose, such as the tracking of atrial activity as part of a mode-switching algorithm for use during supraventricular tachycardia.[2,3] As in the previous version of the Code, it indicates nothing about where tachycardia detection takes place.

Position III: Response to Sensing. Position III indicates whether sensing, as defined for position II, *inhibits* pacing (by resetting an escape interval without pacing or, as in DDI, by canceling the next pending atrial stimulus without affecting pacemaker timing) or *triggers* a pacemaker output, either immediately in the same chamber, as in AAT and VVT pacing, or in the ventricle after an appropriate AV interval that begins with a paced or sensed atrial event, as in DDD pacing.

Position IV: Rate Modulation. Position IV indicates only whether adaptive-rate pacing (rate modulation) is present or absent. It is assumed that all contemporary pulse generators are capable of comprehensive noninvasive adjustment and of providing information by telemetry, so the "programmability" hierarchy incorporated in the previous version of the Code is no longer needed.

Position V: Multisite Pacing. The use of position V, as described earlier, reflects the basic design philosophy of a generic code. This position indicates the existence and, to some degree, the location of multisite pacing, but without providing specific details. This area of code design may be revisited as the usefulness of additional or currently unconventional pacing sites becomes more clearly established and accepted patterns for multisite pacing emerge. Simultaneous activation of both atria by pacing at the interatrial septum (to improve left-ventricular hemodynamics by eliminating the interatrial conduction delay associated with right-atrial pacing) is considered multisite pacing, because, although only one electrode is required, it stimulates both atria.[7-12]

Specific Pacemaker Codes

Identifying high-priority information that needs to be conveyed quickly in clinical practice, although a prerequisite for designing a generic code, involves an inherent compromise because some information must be left out if the code is to be of practical value. Because this compromise inevitably generates ambiguity (as in the dual meaning of *triggered*), a need was identified in some situations for summarizing more information than a generic code allows. One such situation is the task of determining whether an electrocardiographic rhythm strip reflects normal or abnormal operation of a complex dual-chamber pacemaker, particularly if instantaneous triggering is present in either chamber, a feature that cannot be conveyed by the NBG Code or its predecessors.

In 1981, a ratio-format code was described that provided separate descriptions of the pacing-mode elements that are operative in the atrial and ventricular channels of the pulse generator.[13] This code, with relatively few modifications, was adopted by NASPE a few years later as the NASPE Specific Code, which is summarized in Table 8-8.[5,14]

Although inappropriate for conversational use, this code provides a means of summarizing pacing-mode characteristics, including antitachyarrhythmia-pacing features, in a concise but accurate manner that is, incidentally, convenient for computer processing. We have found it particularly useful in teaching and as shorthand when notation for an unusual mode is desired.

TABLE 8-8. The NASPE Specific Code[5,14]

Basic structure	Atrial-channel and ventricular-channel functions are described in the numerator and denominator, respectively, of a ratio-format code, or separated by a virgule (slash) or hyphen if restriction to a single line is unavoidable. Example: $\text{DDD} = \frac{\text{PSIaIv}}{\text{PSIvTa}} = \text{PSIaIv/PSIvTa}$		
Antibradycardia-pacing symbols	*Function:* O = none P = pace S = sense	*Pacing type:* T = triggered I = inhibited	*Signal source:* a = atrium v = ventricle
	U = underdrive B = burst R = ramp	X = extrastimulus C = cardioversion D = defibrillation	*Activation:* a = atrial sensing v = ventricular sensing e = external
Antitachycardia-therapy symbols	Antitachycardia-therapy symbols are appended in parentheses as needed. For example, a multiprogrammable DDD pacemaker with atrial-burst capability, either automatically or externally activated, plus automatic defibrillation, would be represented as follows: $\text{DDDMD} = \frac{\text{PSIaIv(BaBe)}}{\text{PSIvTa(DV)}} = \text{PSIaIv(BaBe)/PSIvTa(DV)}$		

Adapted from Bernstein AD, Brownlee RR, Fletcher RD, et al: Report of the NASPE Mode Code Committee. PACE 7:395, 1984, and Bernstein AD, Brownlee RR, Fletcher RD, et al: Pacing mode codes. In Barold SS (ed): Modern Cardiac Pacing. Mt. Kisco, NY, Futura, 1985, pp 307-322.

TABLE 8-9. **The NASPE/BPEG Defibrillator (NBD) Code**

Potential I (Shock Chamber)	Potential II (Antitachycardia-Pacing Chamber)	Potential III (Tachycardia Detection)	Potential IV (Antibradycardia-Pacing Chamber)
O = none	O = none	E = electrogram	O = none
A = atrium	A = atrium	H = hemodynamic	A = atrium
	V = ventricle	V = ventricle	V = ventricle
	D = dual (A + V)	D = dual (A + V)	D = dual (A + V)

Adapted from Bernstein AD, Camm AJ, Fisher JD, et al: The NASPE/BPEG Defibrillator Code. PACE 16:1776, 1993.

For example, it clarifies the basic difference between the DDD and DDI modes:

DDD = PSIaIv/PSIvTa DDI = PSIaIv/PSIv

The difference lies in the ventricular-channel function: Ta is missing from the ventricular-channel descriptor (denominator) of the DDI code. In the DDI mode, ventricular pacing is not triggered by atrial sensing as it is in DDD, but the other functions remain the same. In DDI, therefore, fast atrial rates are not tracked by ventricular pacing but merely inhibit pending atrial outputs, so that AV synchrony is not maintained when the spontaneous atrial rate exceeds the basic pacing rate.

Without the strict constraints on complexity that affect generic codes, the NASPE Specific Code is more amenable to amendment. For example, it has been suggested that adaptive functions, such as rate modulation and AV-interval hysteresis, could be represented by additional symbols appended in square brackets.

The NASPE/BPEG Defibrillator (NBD) Code

On January 23, 1993, the NASPE Board of Trustees approved the adoption of the NASPE/BPEG Defibrillator (NBD) Code, which is summarized in Table 8-9.[15] It was developed by the NASPE Mode Code Committee, composed of members of NASPE and BPEG, and is intended for describing cardiac-defibrillator capabilities and operation in conversation, record keeping, and device labeling. The NBD Code is patterned after the NBG Code and is compatible with it. Like the NBG Code, it is a generic code; but whereas the NBG Code describes antibradycardia pacing functions in detail and indicates the presence of shock capability without providing specific information, the NBD Code gives more information about cardioversion and defibrillation capabilities and indicates the presence of antibradycardia pacing without providing details.

The NBD Code does not indicate shock-energy levels and therefore does not distinguish between cardioversion and defibrillation. Positions I, II, and IV indicate only the location of shock, antitachycardia-pacing functions, and antibradycardia-pacing functions, respectively. Position III indicates the means of tachycardia detection and is hierarchical in the sense that a device that monitors hemodynamic variables is assumed to monitor the intracardiac electrogram signal as well. In this sense, H implies E.

In conversation, at least the first two positions are used, with others added as needed for clarity. In device labeling and record keeping, the first three positions are used, followed by a hyphen and the first four positions of the NBG Code. For example, a ventricular defibrillator with adaptive-rate ventricular antibradycardia pacing would be labeled VOE-VVIR or VOH-VVIR, depending on its tachycardia-detection mechanism.

As an additional means of distinguishing concisely among devices limited to cardioversion or defibrillation and those that incorporate antitachycardia and antibradycardia pacing as well, a short-form code was defined, as summarized in Table 8-10. It is intended only for use in conversation.

The NASPE/BPEG Pacemaker-Lead (NBL) Code

In 1996, the NASPE Board of Trustees voted to adopt a generic code for pacemaker leads, to be known as the NASPE/BPEG Pacemaker-Lead (NBL) Code. The code was approved subsequently by BPEG, and its definition and usage conventions were published as a NASPE Policy Statement.[16]

The NBL Code is a four-position generic code intended for use in conversation, record keeping, writing, and labeling. All four positions, as defined in

TABLE 8-10. **The NASPE/BPEG Defibrillator Code, Short Form**

Code	Meaning
ICD-S	ICD with **s**hock capability only
ICD-B	ICD with **b**radycardia pacing as well as shock
ICD-T	ICD with **t**achycardia (and bradycardia) pacing as well as shock

ICD, implanted cardioverter-defibrillator.
Adapted from Bernstein AD, Camm AJ, Fisher JD, et al: The NASPE/BPEG Defibrillator Code. PACE 16:1776, 1993.

TABLE 8-11. **The NASPE/BPEG Pacemaker-Lead (NBL) Code**

Potential I (Electrode Configuration)	Potential II (Fixation Mechanism)	Potential III (Insulation Material)	Potential IV (Drug Elution)
U = unipolar	A = active	P = polyurethane	S = steroid
B = bipolar	P = passive	S = silicone rubber	N = nonsteroid
M = multipolar	O = none	D = dual (P + S)	O = none

Adapted from Bernstein AD, Parsonnet V: The NASPE/BPEG Pacemaker-Lead Code. PACE 19:1535, 1996.

Table 8-12. **Examples of the NBL Code**

Code	Meaning
UPSO	Unipolar passive-fixation lead with silicone-rubber insulation but without elution of an anti-inflammatory agent
BAPS	Bipolar active-fixation lead with polyurethane insulation and steroid elution

Adapted from Bernstein AD, Parsonnet V: The NASPE/BPEG Pacemaker-Lead Code. PACE 19:1535, 1996.

Table 8-11, are used in every circumstance (unlike the NBG Code, for which only three or four of the five positions is often sufficient).[4,6] Examples of the use of this simple code are shown in Table 8-12.

The NBL Code is designed so that it cannot be confused with the NBG or NBD Codes.[4,6,15] As with those earlier codes, the characteristics considered were chosen in terms of clinical priority to describe characteristics with significant influence on the behavior of the device under consideration. For this reason, features such as connector design were not addressed.

Partly in view of the advent of multisite pacing, electrode location was not addressed by this code. Moreover, until the emergence of clearer patterns in the electrode configurations used for cardioversion and defibrillation, with and without the pulse-generator housing serving as part of the electrode system, it was believed that attempts to design a practical code encompassing leads used for cardioversion and defibrillation as well as pacing would be premature.

Concluding Comments

In the context of clinical pacing, pacing education, and the development of pacing and defibrillator technology, additional symbolic representations not discussed in this chapter have been developed. These potentially useful resources, primarily diagrammatic, include pictorial mode codes,[13,17] mechanisms for annotating electrocardiograms and other records with concise summaries of pacing mode and programmable parameter settings,[18] diagrammatic aids to interpreting paced electrocardiograms,[17,19,20] and state diagrams for illustrating pacemaker-timing design characteristics.[20]

Agreed-on symbols are a basic requirement of successful communication. Not surprisingly, therefore, the search for practical symbols for describing the function of increasingly versatile devices is an ongoing task that will continue as rhythm-management technology continues to evolve.

REFERENCES

1. Parsonnet V, Furman S, Smyth NPD: Implantable cardiac pacemakers: Status report and resource guidelines. Pacemaker Study Group, Inter-Society Commission for Heart Disease Resources (ICHD). Circulation 50:A21, 1974.
2. Parsonnet V, Furman S, Smyth NPD: Revised code for pacemaker identification. PACE 4:400, 1981.
3. Parsonnet V, Furman S, Smyth NPD, Bilitch M: Implantable cardiac pacemakers: Status report and resource guidelines, 1982. Pacemaker Study Group, Inter-Society Commission for Heart Disease Resources (ICHD). Circulation 68:227A, 1983.
4. Bernstein AD, Camm AJ, Fletcher RD, et al: The NASPE/BPEG Generic Pacemaker Code for antibradyarrhythmia and adaptive-rate pacing and antitachyarrhythmia devices. PACE 10:794, 1987.
5. Bernstein AD, Brownlee RR, Fletcher RD, et al: Report of the NASPE Mode Code Committee. PACE 7:395, 1984.
6. Bernstein AD, Daubert J-C, Fletcher RD, et al: The Revised NASPE/BPEG Generic Code for antibradycardia, adaptive-rate, and multisite pacing. PACE 25:260-264, 2000.
7. Bernstein AD: Letter to the Editor. PACE 23:928-929, 2000.
8. Bernstein AD, Camm AJ, Furman S, Parsonnet V: The NASPE/BPEG codes: Use misuse, and evolution. PACE 24:787-788, 2001.
9. Leclercq C, Walker S, Linde C, et al: Comparative effects of permanent biventricular and right-univentricular pacing in heart failure patients with chronic atrial fibrillation. Eur Heart J 23:1780-1787, 2002.
10. Revault d'Allonnes G, Pavin D, Leclercq C, et al: Long-term effects of biatrial synchronous pacing to prevent drug-refractory atrial tachyarrhythmias: A nine-year experience. J Cardiovasc Electrophysiol 11:1081-1091, 2000.
11. Fitts SM, Hill MR, Mehra R, et al: Design and implementation of the Dual Site Atrial Pacing to Prevent Atrial Fibrillation (DAPPAF) clinical trial. J Interv Card Electrophysiol 2:139-144, 1998.
12. Cazeau S, Leclercq C, Lavergne T, et al: Effects of multisite biventricular pacing in patients with heart failure and intraventricular conduction delay. N Engl J Med 344:873-880, 2001.
13. Brownlee RR, Shimmel JB, Del Marco CJ: A new code for pacemaker operating modes. PACE 4:396, 1981.
14. Bernstein AD, Brownlee RR, Fletcher RD, et al: Pacing mode codes. In Barold SS (ed): Modern Cardiac Pacing. Mt. Kisco, NY, Futura, 1985, pp 307-322.
15. Bernstein AD, Camm AJ, Fisher JD, et al: The NASPE/BPEG Defibrillator Code. PACE 16:1776, 1993.
16. Bernstein AD, Parsonnet V: The NASPE/BPEG Pacemaker-Lead Code. PACE 19:1535-1536, 1996.

17. Lindemans F: Diagrammatic representation of pacemaker function. In Barold SS (ed): Modern Cardiac Pacing. Mt. Kisco, NY, Futura, 1985, pp 323-353.
18. Parsonnet V, Bernstein AD: An annotation system for displaying operating-parameter values in dual-chamber pacing. Am Heart J 111:817, 1986.
19. Bernstein AD, Parsonnet V: Notation conventions and overlay diagrams for analysis of paced electrocardiograms. PACE 6:73-80, 1983.
20. Bernstein AD: Visualizing pacing modes. In Course Notebook, Cardiac Pacing 1988. Bethesda, MD, American College of Cardiology, 1988, pp C1-C24.

Section Two

Clinical Concepts

Chapter 9

Basic Physiology and Hemodynamics of Cardiac Pacing

FRITS PRINZEN • JULIO C. SPINELLI • ANGELO AURICCHIO

Cardiac pacing has significantly improved the survival and quality of life in patients with bradycardia. When first introduced, pacemakers were simply lifesaving devices that provided a fixed pacing rate during bradycardia. With advances in technology and in our understanding of cardiac physiology during artificial pacing, devices have been developed that mimic the normal cardiac automaticity and activation sequence. This development has resulted in improved cardiac performance and hemodynamics. Indeed, the latest advances in this field are pacemakers capable of raising the pacing rate with exercise without the need to rely on sinus activity, so-called rate-adaptive pacing, and pacemakers capable of improving the cardiac electromechanical synchrony, so-called cardiac resynchronization devices. The use of cardiac resynchronization therapy (CRT) to treat patients with heart failure has given new impetus to evaluation of the hemodynamic effect of spontaneously occurring or pacing-induced ventricular conduction delay as well as abnormal atrioventricular (AV) timing. In particular, the appreciation that inappropriate right ventricular (RV) pacing not only may have deleterious effects on ventricular mechanics but ultimately may increase morbidity and mortality is rather recent. It is now appreciated that a truly physiologic pacemaker will maintain the normal sequence and timing of atrial and ventricular activation over a wide range of heart rates, vary the heart rate in response to metabolic demands, and preserve the normal rapid, synchronous sequence of ventricular activation when required.

Physiology of Electrical and Mechanical Activation

Electrical Activation during Sinus Rhythm

The cardiac action potential originates from the sinus node, located in the high right atrium (RA) (Fig. 9-1). Its cells depolarize spontaneously and initiate the spontaneous depolarization of action potentials at a regular rate from the sinus node. This rate depends on various conditions, such as atrial stretch and sympathetic activation, but is usually between 60 and 100 beats per minute (bpm) at rest. Myocytes are electrically coupled to each other through gap junctions. These structures consist of connexin molecules and allow direct intercellular communication.[1] Gap junctions do not have a preferential direction of conduction, but because the action potential starts in the sinus node, it spreads from there through the atria. There is evidence for specialized conduction pathways in the atrium, but their (patho)physiologic relevance is still disputed.

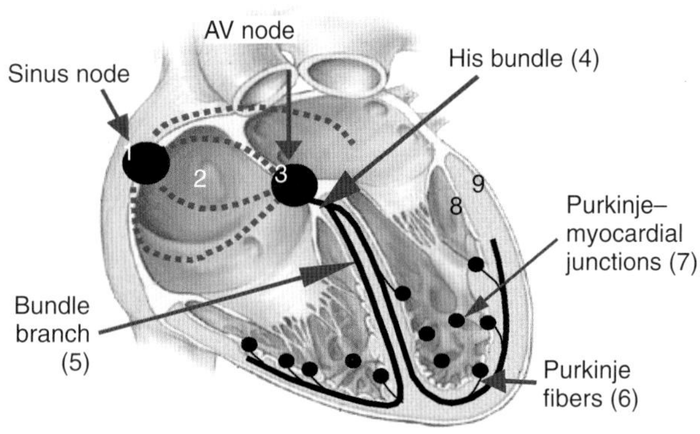

Figure 9-1. Conduction of the impulse in the heart. The impulse originates in the sinus node (1), continues in the atrial wall (2), and is delayed in the atrioventricular (AV) node (3). Conduction within the ventricles is initially rapid within the rapid conduction system: His bundle (4), right and left bundle branches (5), and Purkinje fibers (6). The impulse is transferred from the rapid conduction system to the working myocardium in the Purkinje–myocardial junctions (7), which are located in the endocardium. Within the slowly conducting working myocardium, the impulse is conducted from endocardium to epicardium.

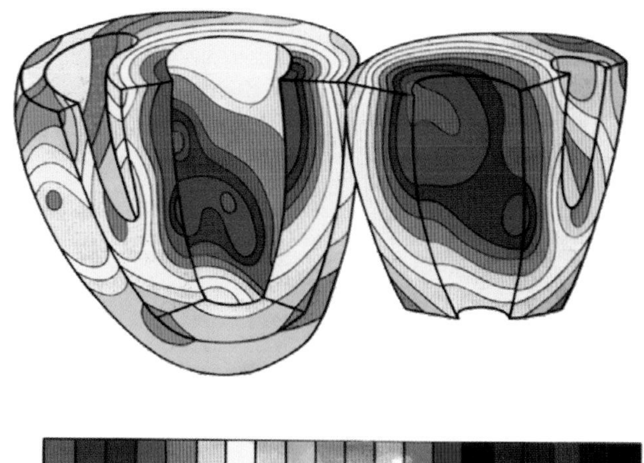

Figure 9-2. Three-dimensional isochronic representation of the electrical activation in an isolated human heart. Shaded scale indicates activation time in milliseconds. (Modified from Durrer D, Dam v. RT, Freud GE, et al: Total excitation of the isolated human heart. Circulation 41:899-912, 1970.)

In the human heart, spreading of the action potential through the atria takes approximately 100 msec, after which the impulse reaches the AV node (see Fig 9-1). In the normal heart the AV node is the only electrical connection between the atria and ventricles, because a fibrous ring (anulus fibrosus) is present between the remaining parts of the atria and ventricles. The AV nodal tissue conducts the electrical impulses very slowly; indeed, it takes approximately 80 msec for these impulses to travel from the atrial side to the ventricular side of the AV node. This delay between atrial activation and ventricular activation has functional importance, because it allows optimal ventricular filling. Its slow conduction renders the AV node sensitive to impaired conduction and even complete conduction block, an important indication for ventricular pacing. Like everywhere else in the heart, conduction in the AV node has no preferential direction. Consequently, impulses can also be conducted retrogradely through the AV node, a condition that can occur when the ventricles are electrically stimulated.

From the AV node, the electrical impulse reaches the His bundle, the first part of the specialized conduction system of the ventricles called the Purkinje system. Within this system the electrical impulse is conducted approximately four times faster (3 to 4 m/sec) than in the working myocardium (0.3 to 1 m/sec).[2,3] This difference is due to the fact that Purkinje cells are longer and have a higher content of gap junctions.[1,4,5]

The intraventricular conduction system can be regarded as a trifascicular conduction system consisting of the right bundle branch (RBB) and two divisions of the left bundle branch (LBB). The RBB proceeds subendocardially along the right side of the interventricular septum until it terminates in the Purkinje plexuses of the right ventricle (RV); the left bundle branch also has a short subendocardial route.

It seems that the bifascicular vision of structure of the LBB is oversimplified.[6] The general picture that now emerges is that the LV Purkinje network is composed of three main, widely interconnected parts, depending on the anterior subdivision, the posterior subdivision, and a centroseptal subdivision of the left main bundle. This third medial or centroseptal division supplies the midseptal area of the left ventricle (LV) and arises from the LBB, from its anterior or posterior subdivision, or both. The fascicles continue in a network of subendocardially located Purkinje fibers.[4,7] In the LV, the Purkinje fibers form a network in the lower third of the septum and free wall, which also covers the papillary muscles.[4,7] In humans the bundles are present only underneath the endocardium, whereas species like ox, sheep, and goat have networks of Purkinje fibers across the entire ventricular wall.[8,9]

It is important to note that the His bundle as well as the right and left bundle branches and their major tributaries are electrically isolated from the adjacent myocardium. The only sites where the Purkinje system and the normal working myocardium are electrically coupled are the Purkinje–myocardial junctions. The exits of the Purkinje system are located in the subendocardium of the anterolateral wall of the RV and the inferolateral LV wall (see Fig. 9-1).[4,10] This area of exit corresponds with the area of the ventricular muscle that is activated earliest.[2-5,11,12] The distribution of the Purkinje–myocardial junctions is spatially inhomogeneous, and the junctions themselves have varying degrees of electrical coupling.[13]

Endocardial activation of the RV starts near the insertion of the anterior papillary muscle 10 msec after onset of LV activation (Fig. 9-2).[11] After activation of the more apical regions, the activation of the ventricular working myocardium occurs predominantly from apex to base, both in the septum and in the LV and RV free wall. Further depolarization occurs centrifugally from endocardium to epicardium as well as tangentially.[11,12] The earliest epicardial breakthrough occurs in the pretrabecular area in the RV, from which there is an overall radial spread toward the apex and base. The last part of the RV that becomes activated is the AV sulcus and pulmonary conus. Overall, the posterobasal area of the LV or an area more lateral is the last part of the heart to be depolarized (see Fig. 9-2).[11]

The time between arrival of the impulse in the His bundle and the first ventricular muscle activation is approximately 20 msec,[4] whereas total ventricular activation lasts 60 to 80 msec, corresponding to a QRS duration of 70 to 80 msec.[11] These numbers illustrate the important role of the Purkinje fiber system in the synchronization of myocardial activity. This role is due to the system's unique propagation properties and its geometrically widespread distribution. During normal orthodromic excitation, fast propagation over long fibers, together with wide distribution of Purkinje–myocardial junctions, induce a high degree of coordination between distant regions of the myocardium.

Mechanical Activation during Sinus Rhythm

As in many other muscle cells, electrical activation leads to contraction in cardiac myocytes, a process referred to as *excitation-contraction* (E-C) *coupling*. In cardiac E-C coupling, the calcium ion (Ca^{2+}) plays a central role (Fig. 9-3).[14] The contraction-relaxation cycle starts when depolarization leads to entry of Ca^{2+} into the cell via voltage-dependent L-type Ca^{2+} channels. This Ca^{2+} entry triggers a much larger amount of Ca^{2+} to be released from the sarcoplasmic reticulum (Ca^{2+}-induced Ca^{2+} release). These processes increase intracellular Ca^{2+} from approximately 10^{-6} M to approximately 10^{-3} M. This high calcium concentration catalyzes the interaction between myosin and actin filaments, leading to contraction. After repolarization, relaxation occurs as Ca^{2+} dissociates from the contractile apparatus and is taken up again by the sarcoplasmic reticulum through the action of sarcoplasmic reticular Ca^{2+} adenosine triphosphatase (SERCA). Intracellular Ca^{2+} homeostasis is also maintained through action of the sodium-calcium (Na^+Ca^{2+}) exchanger (NCX). Normally, this exchanger removes Ca^{2+} from the cell (forward mode). Figure 9-3 also shows that the intracellular Ca^{2+} concentration rises rapidly after the upstroke of the action potential but that there is some delay between the Ca^{2+} increase and the development of force. This delay is the main determinant of the delay between electrical and mechanical activation.

The electromechanical delay—that is, the delay between the depolarization and the onset of force development—amounts to approximately 30 msec.[15,16] On a global basis this delay can be observed as the delay between the R wave of the electrocardiogram (ECG) and the rise in LV pressure (Fig. 9-4). Electromechanical coupling in failing hearts is different from that in normal hearts. A prominent feature of heart failure is that the relation between SERCA and the NCX changes. Often SERCA is downregulated[17] and/or the NCX is upregulated in the heart failure state.[18] On the one hand, the reduced SERCA activity leads to less Ca^{2+} loading of the sarcoplasmic reticulum, resulting in less Ca^{2+} release during the subsequent activation and so a weaker contraction (systolic dysfunction). On the other hand, during diastole, Ca^{2+} removal from the cytosol is slower and incomplete, leading to a slower relaxation and greater diastolic stiffness (diastolic dysfunction). The upregulation of the NCX and the elevated intracellular Na^+ concentrations in failing myocardium[19] may compensate for the SERCA downregulation.[20,21] The high Na^+ concentration facilitates the NCX to work

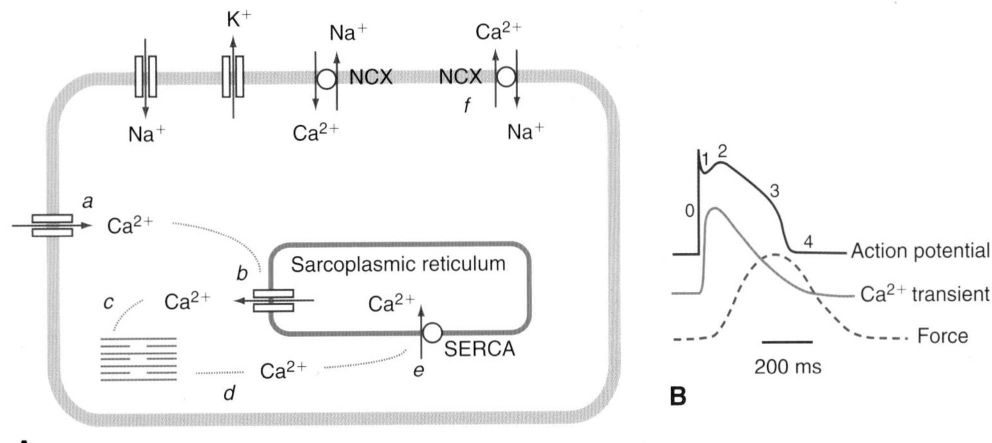

Figure 9-3. Excitation-contraction coupling in the myocardium. ***A,*** *A schematic representation of the major pathways involved in calcium ion (Ca^{2+}) homeostasis in the cardiomyocyte. a, Ca^{2+} entry via L-type Ca^{2+} channel; b, Ca^{2+}-induced Ca^{2+} release from the sarcoplasmic reticulum; c, Ca^{2+}-induced contraction; d, dissociation of Ca^{2+} from the contractile apparatus; e, reuptake of Ca^{2+} via sarcoplasmic reticular Ca^{2+}–adenosine triphosphatase (SERCA); f, Ca^{2+} efflux via the Na^+/Ca^{2+} exchanger (NCX).* ***B,*** *A schematic tracing of a Ca^{2+} transient, an action potential, and contractile force. The numbers indicate the different phases of the action potential: 0, upstroke; 1, fast early depolarization; 2, plateau phase; 3, repolarization phase; 4, resting membrane potential.*

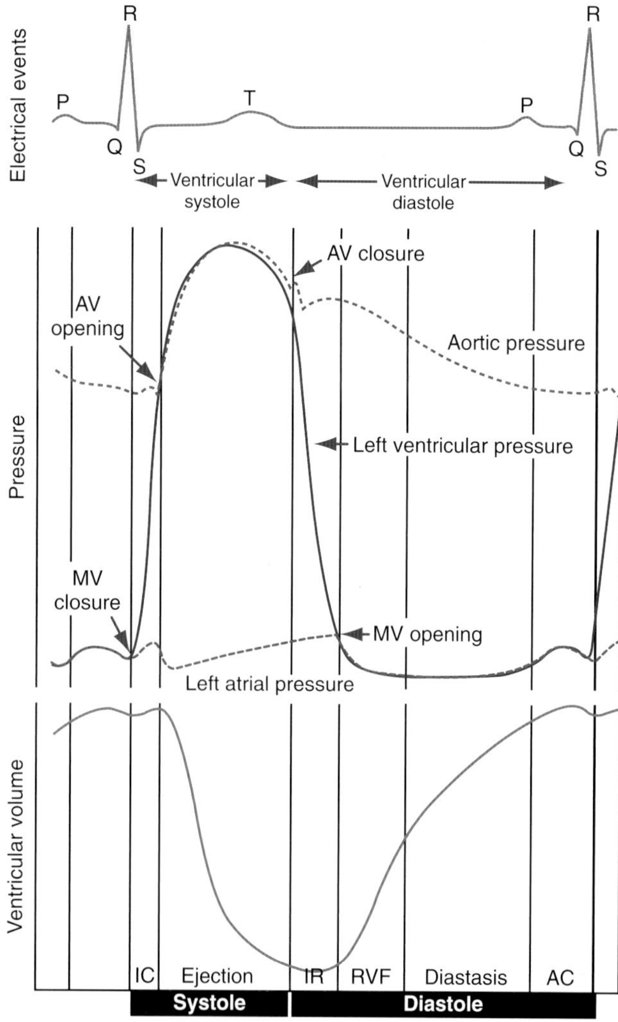

Figure 9-4. Events of the cardiac cycle. Left atrial, aortic, and left ventricular (LV) pressures are correlated with electrical events and LV volume. AC, atrial contraction; AV, aortic valve; IC, isovolumic contraction; IR, isovolumic relaxation; MV, mitral valve; RVF, rapid ventricular filling. See text for description.

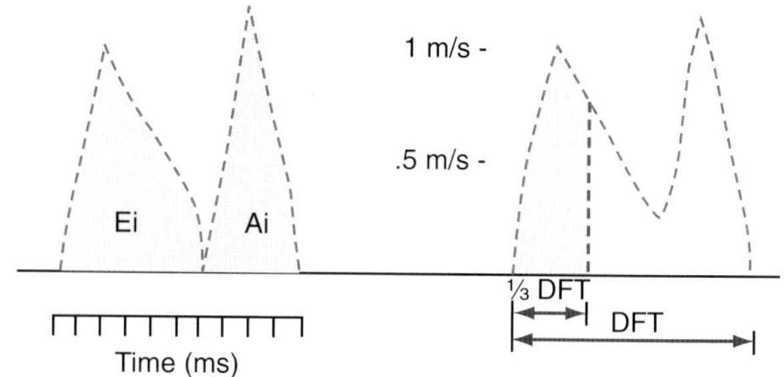

Figure 9-5. Pulsed Doppler recording of transmitral flow, illustrating the technique used to measure various segments of the timed velocity integral and diastolic filling period. The relationship between early diastolic filling and filling associated with atrial systole can be quantitated. Possible measurements include early and atrial velocities, the ratio of early to atrial velocities, the early (Ei) and atrial (Ai) flow-velocity integral (area under the flow-velocity curve), the ratio of early to atrial flow-velocity integrals, and the amount of diastolic filling occurring in the first third of diastole (1/3 DFT [diastolic filling time]). (From Pearson AC, Janosik DL, Redd RM, et al: Doppler echocardiographic assessment of the effect of varying atrioventricular delay and pacemaker mode on left ventricular filling. Am Heart J 115:611, 1988.)

in the "reverse mode," that is, to remove intracellular Na^+ and exchange it for extracellular Ca^{2+}. This additional Ca^{2+} enhances systolic function at least to some extent. Because the SERCA pump is much faster in pumping calcium than the NCX, insufficiencies in contraction and relaxation in failing hearts are most pronounced at higher heart rates. These changes result in decreasing contractile force with increasing heart rate, a negative force-frequency relation.[17] The changes in the failing myocardium lead to the altered expression of other proteins involved in E-C coupling as well as shifts in isoforms of various contractile proteins.[22]

Because of the tight coupling between excitation and contraction, atrial activation is followed by atrial contraction, and ventricular activation by ventricular contraction. Consequently, atrial contraction precedes ventricular contraction, as illustrated in Figure 9-4. Because of this timing, the atrial contraction adds roughly 20% to the volume of the ventricles. This "atrial kick" increases the length of ventricular muscle cells and of their sarcomeres. The sarcomere length is an important determinant of myocardial contractile force. Over the entire physiologic range of sarcomere lengths (1.6 to 2.4 μm), the longer the sarcomeres are, the greater the contractile force. This effect, known as the Frank-Starling relation (Starling's law of the heart), is only partly related to the overlap of actin and myosin, as generally mentioned in textbooks. More important to the Frank-Starling relation is the growing affinity of troponin C for calcium at increasing sarcomere length,[23] although the cause of this greater sensitivity is not completely understood.

Ventricular contraction starts after ventricular depolarization. After a short isovolumic contraction phase, the aortic valve opens, starting the ejection phase. The velocity of emptying of the ventricle is highest in the first half of the ejection phase owing to a higher pressure gradient between the LV and the aorta. In the second half of the ejection phase, LV pressure actually falls below aortic pressure, but the aortic valve stays open because of the inertia of the flowing blood. With increasingly negative LV–aortic pressure gradients, the aortic valve closes and the isovolumic relaxation phase starts, ending with the opening of the mitral valve. Because of the filling of the atrium during ventricular systole, atrial pressure is relatively high. This event, in combination with the rapid fall in LV pressure, causes a positive AV pressure gradient during the early filling phase. Thus, rapid acceleration of blood occurs, contributing to most of the LV filling in the early diastolic phase. This event is also reflected by the large Ei wave on mitral valve Doppler recordings in healthy hearts (Fig. 9-5).

Atrial contraction, after the P wave on the ECG, produces a surge of blood into the ventricle at the end of diastole, causing the final and optimal filling of the ventricle. Reversal of the pressure gradient across the mitral valve, due to atrial relaxation and ventricular contraction, pulls the valve cusps in apposition, facilitating closure of the valve. Therefore, coupling and proper timing of atrial and ventricular contractions are important determinants of ventricular pump function. The loss of atrial systole diminishes effective LV stroke volume by 25% at low heart rates and by almost 50% at higher heart rates. How different modes of pacing influence the atrial contribution to pump function and how this contribution affects pump function in different categories of patients are discussed later in the chapter.

Although both Frank-Starling and force-frequency relations are properties of the myocardium itself, which can regulate cardiac function to an important extent, extrinsic factors also modulate cardiac performance. Many of these factors are related to the autonomic nervous and hormonal systems. The afferent parts of these systems can be divided into low-pressure and high-pressure domains. Low-pressure sensors are present in the atria and pulmonary circulation. Stimulation, from increased pressures and stretch, leads to parasympathetic stimulation and sympathetic withdrawal. Moreover, atrial stretch induces release of atrial natriuretic factor (ANF). This 28–amino acid polypeptide is a potent arterial and venous vasodilator that raises urine production. Effectively, the low-pressure sensors monitor the filling status of the circulation. However, erroneous readings may occur during inadequate AV synchronization, leading to elevated atrial pressures (cannon A waves). Stimulation of the reflexes and ANF production are involved in the so-called pacemaker syndrome (see later).

The high-pressure sensors consist predominantly of the baroreceptors in the arterial system. These sensors feed back to the brainstem through afferent neurons in the vagal and glossopharyngeal nerves. Stimulation of these receptors through a decrease in blood pressure induces sympathetic stimulation and parasympathetic withdrawal. Although reduced parasympathetic activation is the most important factor leading to the increase in heart rate during hypotension, the greater sympathetic stimulation induces arterial and venous vasoconstriction and increases myocardial contractility.

Other pressure sensors are found in the juxtaglomerular apparatus in the kidneys. Their stimulation leads to greater production of renin, angiotensin, and aldosterone, resulting in vasoconstriction as well as water and salt retention. These systems are effective in maintaining equilibrium in blood pressure and cardiac output during short-term variations. However, sustained neurohumoral stimulation is an important factor in the long-term development of hypertrophy and the rise in filling pressure.

Abnormal Activation Sequence during Left Bundle Branch Block and Right Ventricular Pacing

The normal, physiologic, and almost synchronous sequence of electrical activation is lost in diseases affecting the ventricular conduction system, such as block of the left or right bundle branch[24] and the presence of an accessory pathway bypassing the AV node, as in the Wolff-Parkinson-White syndrome.[25] Additionally, ectopic impulse generation, occurring during ventricular pacing and extrasystoles,[26,27] leads to abnormal impulse conduction. Under all of these circumstances, the impulse is conducted primarily through the slowly conducting working myocardium rather than rapidly through the specialized conduction system. As a consequence, under conditions of abnormal activation, the time required for activation of the entire ventricular muscle, expressed as QRS duration, is at least twice as long as that during normal sinus rhythm.

The extent of asynchrony and the sequence of activation during abnormal conduction are determined by at least four myocardial properties, as follows:

1. Conduction through the myocardium is up to four times slower than conduction through the Purkinje system.
2. Conduction is approximately two times faster along the muscle fibers than perpendicular to them.[28] Therefore, in a particular layer, the wavefront around a pacing site has an elliptical shape, especially in the epicardial and midmyocardial layers.[29]
3. Impulses originating from the working myocardium rarely reenter into parts of the rapid conduction system. Early researchers had believed that such reentry was ubiquitous and that the amount of reentry was the main determinant of the total asynchrony of ventricular activation.[30] However, later studies indicated that, although parts of the intact rapid conduction system are often present, ectopically generated impulses appear to couple poorly to the rapidly conducting specialized conduction system.[4,12] Myerburg and colleagues[4] elegantly showed that impulses coming from the normal myocardium can enter the Purkinje system only at the apical part of this system (presumably the Purkinje–myocardial junctions; see Fig. 9-1). This finding implies that the impulse often has traveled already for some time before reaching Purkinje–myocardial junctions. Also, in order to reach remote zones, the impulse has to travel retrogradely through one branch of the system all the way to the proximal part and then descend to another part. Therefore, in most cases, the sequence of activation during ventricular pacing is governed by slow conduction through the normal myocardium, away from the pacing site.[16,26,27,31]
4. Most endocardial fibers, even though not part of the Purkinje system, conduct impulses faster than the fibers in the rest of the LV wall.[32] Moreover, the endocardial circumference is smaller than its epicardial counterpart. Therefore, total time required for electrical activation is shorter for LV endocardial pacing than for LV epicardial pacing.[29] Also, after epicardial stimulation, the fastest way to activate the epicardium in remote regions is through epi-endocardial conduction

close to the pacing site, conduction along the endocardium, and endo-epicardial conduction in the remote zone (epicardial breakthrough).[29]

Detailed studies on the three-dimensional spread of activation during ventricular pacing in canine hearts have been conducted since the 1960s.[12,26] The sequence of electrical activation in LBB block (LBBB) is similar to that during RV apex pacing. This sequence can be derived from the QRS configuration of the surface ECG[27,33,34] and from endocardial activation maps in experimental LBBB and RV pacing.[35] The similarity has lead to the use of AV sequential RV apex pacing as a model for "experimental LBBB."[33,36,37]

Until recently, information on impulse conduction in patients with LBBB was limited to the data reported by Vassallo and associates.[24,27] These investigators mapped LV endocardial activation during RV apex pacing and in LBBB at a limited number of endocardial sites, showing that activation starts at the RV endocardium in both conditions. The first noticeable activation at the LV endocardium after right-to-left (or transseptal) conduction of the impulse occurs at a single breakthrough site, which in nearly all patients is the LV breakthrough time, 50 to 70 msec after the earliest RV activation. The impulse is conducted from the septum toward the distal free wall in a gradual manner, the site of latest activation generally being the inferoposterior wall.[11]

The gradual conduction was also found in later studies using higher-resolution endocardial mapping techniques (Fig. 9-6).[38,39] These studies also showed that activation patterns differ among patients, and this difference may be largely due to differences in the origin of LBBB—either a proximal synaptic barrier at the junction of the right septal and left septal masses[40] or a uniform but slow conduction through the LBB.[41] Although all of these data are derived from endocardial contact mapping measurements, modern noncontact measurements indicate that in approximately one third of patients with heart failure and typical LBBB QRS morphology, transseptal activation time is normal with a slightly prolonged or near-normal LV endocardial activation time. Moreover, in two thirds of patients with LBBB, a functional line of block is present, appearing as a "U-shaped" activation wavefront. The location and length of the line of block are highly variable and are related to the site and time of LV breakthrough. In patients with significant prolongation of the QRS duration (>150 msec), the line of block is consistently located in an anterior position. In contrast, in patients with QRS duration ranging between 120 and 150 msec, the line of block is usually shorter and located either anteriorly, laterally, or posteriorly (Movie 9-1).[39]

Abnormal Contraction Patterns during Left Bundle Branch Block and Right Ventricular Pacing

Given the tight relationship between excitation and contraction in the myocardium, it is not surprising that asynchronous electrical activation also leads to asynchronous contraction. Regions where the impulse arrives first also start to contract first.[42] During LBBB or ventricular pacing, local contraction patterns differ not only in the onset of contraction but also, and more importantly, in the pattern of contraction. These contraction patterns imply that opposing regions of the ventricular wall are out of phase and that energy generated by one region is dissipated in opposite regions.

In patients with LBBB or RV pacing, the early-contracting region is most typically the septum. The

Noncontact mapping

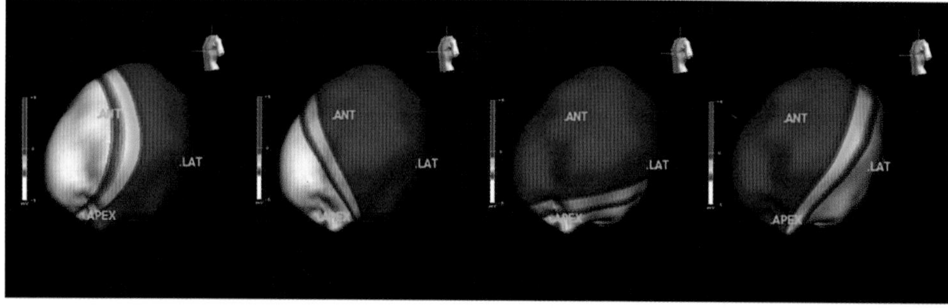

Contact mapping

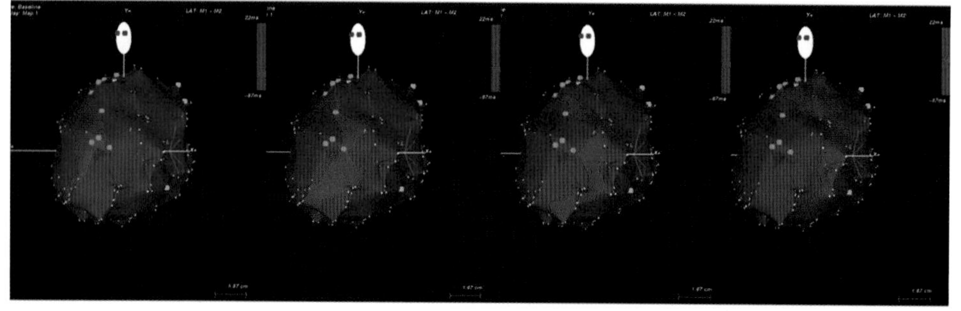

Figure 9-6. Contact and noncontact mapping in patient with left bundle branch block and heart failure. The unipolar isopotential activation sequence (upper panel) *shows a U-shaped activation front that rotated around the apex and activated the lateral wall late, whereas the bipolar propagation map* (lower panel) *shows a longer activation time in the anterior region. LAT, lateral. (Modified from Auricchio A, Fantoni C, Regoli F, et al: Characterization of left ventricular activation in patients with heart failure and left bundle-branch block. Circulation 109:1133-1139, 2004.)*

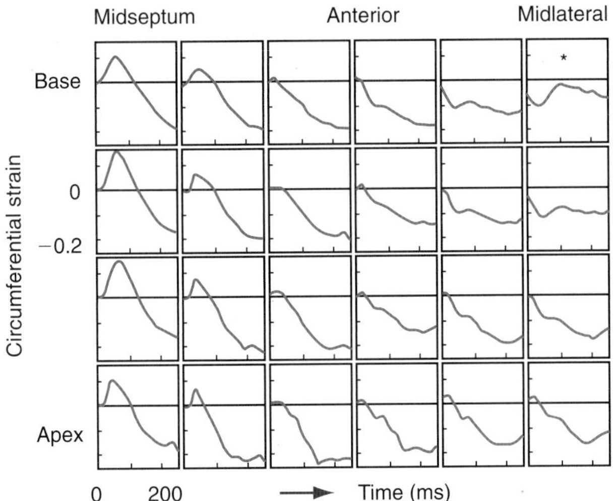

Figure 9-7. Contraction patterns in 24 regions of the anterior septum and anterior left ventricular (LV) free wall during pacing at the LV lateral wall. Each graph in the array represents circumferential strain versus time in a specific region. The LV is displayed as if cut down the septum and folding the surface out onto the page. For the sake of clarity, the posterior half of the LV is not shown, but the distribution of strains in this part of the LV wall is a mirror image of that in the anterior wall. Rows represent different levels from base (top) *to apex* (bottom) *of the LV, and columns are circumferential position from midseptum* (far left) *via the LV anterior wall to the LV lateral wall* (far right). *Tics at the vertical axis denote a strain of 0.1 (≈10% shortening); tics on the horizontal axis denote 100 msec. Please note the early shortening near the pacing site (*) and the prestretch in regions remote from the pacing site. (Modified from Prinzen FW, Peschar M: Relation between the pacing induced sequence of activation and left ventricular pump function in animals. Pacing Clin Electrophysiol 25:484-498, 2002.)*

earliest-contracting fibers can shorten rapidly by up to 10% just during the isovolumic contraction phase; this occurs because the remaining muscle fibers are still in a relaxed state (Movie 9-2). This rapid early shortening is followed by an additional but modest systolic shortening, eventually followed by systolic stretch (due to delayed mechanical contraction of other regions—the lateral wall), and premature relaxation (Fig. 9-7; see Movie 9-2). In late-activated regions, in contrast, the fibers undergo early systolic stretching (by as much as 15%) as a consequence of volume shifted by the early-contracting region. Doubling of net systolic shortening and delayed relaxation occur in late-activated regions (see Fig. 9-7 and Movie 9-2).[31,43] Therefore, pump output and efficiency decrease.

The cause of the regional differences in contraction pattern is most likely related to the local differences in myocardial fiber length during the early systolic phase. This idea is supported by studies using two isolated papillary muscles in series in which asynchronous stimulation caused a downward shift in the force-velocity relation in the earlier-activated muscle and an upward shift in the later-activated one.[44] Furthermore, during ventricular pacing, regional systolic fiber shortening increases with greater isovolumic stretch.[45] Similarly, a close correlation exists between the time of local electrical activation and the extent of systolic fiber shortening.[46] Therefore, the regional differences in contraction pattern during ventricular pacing are most likely caused by regional differences in effective preload and local differences in the contraction force triggered by the Frank-Starling relation.

On M-mode echocardiography, abnormal contraction patterns during RV pacing and LBBB appear as paradoxical septal motion.[47] However, this motion is not actually paradoxical, because it is really the net result of different forces. The motion is caused by the asynchrony between RV and LV, which produces dynamic alterations in transseptal pressure differences,[47,48] and by presystolic shortening of septal muscle fibers.[49] Abnormal septal motion results in a diminished contribution of the interventricular septum to LV ejection.[49]

Effect of Left Bundle Branch Block and Right Ventricular Pacing on Local Energetic Efficiency

The local differences in wall motion and deformation mentioned previously reflect regional differences in myocardial work.[43,50] This relationship was demonstrated by construction of local fiber stress–fiber strain diagrams and calculation of local external and total mechanical work. In regions close to the pacing site (or in the septum in patients with LBBB), shortening occurs at low pressure, whereas these areas are transiently being stretched at higher ventricular pressures. As a consequence, the stress-strain loops have a figure-of-eight–like shape with a low net area, indicating the absence of external work. In regions remote from the pacing site (or in the lateral wall in patients with LBBB), the loops are wide, and external work can be up to twice that during synchronous ventricular activation (Fig. 9-8). Total myocardial work (sum of external work and potential energy) in LBBB and with RV pacing is reduced by 50% in early-activated regions and is increased by 50% in late-activated regions in comparison with atrial pacing.[43,50]

Several studies reported that ventricular pacing and LBBB are associated with regional differences in myocardial blood flow,[31,34,37,49-51] glucose uptake,[37,52] and oxygen consumption.[50,53] During RV apex pacing and LBBB, low values are found in the septum—the early-activated part of the LV. In comparison with sinus rhythm, myocardial blood flow and oxygen consumption are 30% lower in early-activated regions and 30% higher in late-activated regions.[31,50] There is still a controversy regarding the cause of the reduced septal blood flow and glucose uptake in LBBB and RV apex pacing. Various observations, such as close correlations among local myocardial oxygen consumption, work, and blood flow, suggest that the lower blood flow is a physiologic adaptation to the lower demand. However, at higher heart rates, the asynchronous contraction pattern may also impede myocardial perfusion.[37,54]

In isolated, isovolumically beating hearts, ventricular pacing reduces oxygen consumption and pressure development to the same amount, so that total efficiency is not influenced.[55] In a similar preparation, however, Boerth and colleagues[56] found a smaller

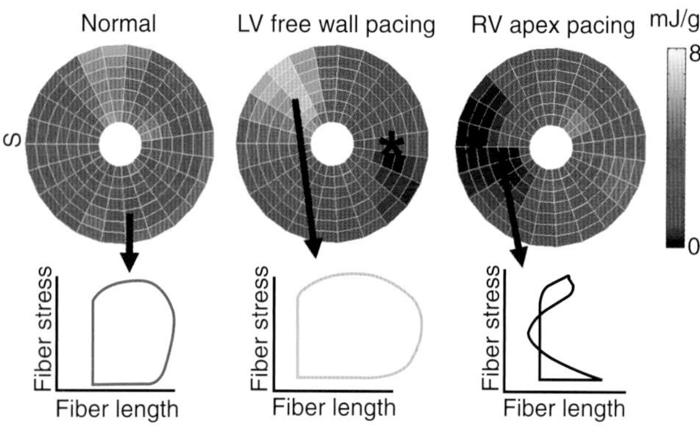

Figure 9-8. Upper panels, *Maps of local external work during right atrial (RA), left ventricle (LV) base, and right ventricle (RV) apex pacing in a dog heart. External work values are presented in grayscale; for values see scale bar. The LV wall is represented as a circle with the base located at the outer contour and the apex in the middle. In the* lower panels, *fiber length–fiber stress diagrams from three regions are displayed, indicating the shape of the diagram in normally activated* (left), *early-activated* (middle), *and late-activated* (right) *regions. The asterisks denote the pacing site. (Modified from Prinzen FW, Hunter WC, Wyman BT, et al: Mapping of regional myocardial strain and work during ventricular pacing: Experimental study using magnetic resonance imaging tagging. J Am Coll Cardiol 33:1735-1742, 1999.)*

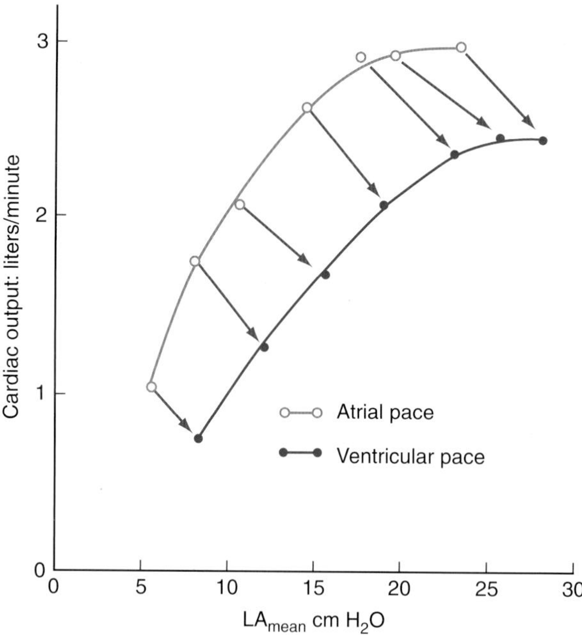

Figure 9-9. Relationship between cardiac output and mean left atrial pressure (LA_{mean}) during atrial pacing (open circles) *compared with ventricular pacing* (solid circles) *in an intact dog model. For any given mean LA pressure, the cardiac output is higher with atrial pacing than with ventricular pacing. (From Mitchell JH, Gilmore JP, Sarnoff SJ: The transport function of the atrium: Factors influencing the relation between mean left atrial pressure and left ventricular end diastolic pressure. Am J Cardiol 9:237, 1962.)*

reduction in oxygen consumption than in pressure development, a combination that resulted in decreased efficiency. In the anesthetized open-chest dog model[57,58] and in conscious dogs,[59] RV apex pacing reduced mechanical output, whereas myocardial oxygen consumption was unchanged or even increased in comparison with atrial pacing; thus, efficiency dropped by 20% to 30% in these studies. The opposite change was found when ventricular activation in patients with preexisting dyssynchrony due to LBBB-like activation was improved by biventricular (BiV) or LV pacing alone. In these patients, BiV pacing improved LV dP/dt_{max} (maximal rate of rise of LV pressure) without increasing myocardial oxygen consumption, indicating improved efficiency.[60] Efficiency of conversion of metabolic energy to pumping energy is of particular interest in patients with compromised coronary circulation, because higher oxygen consumption over longer periods (as in during β-agonist therapy) leads to higher mortality.

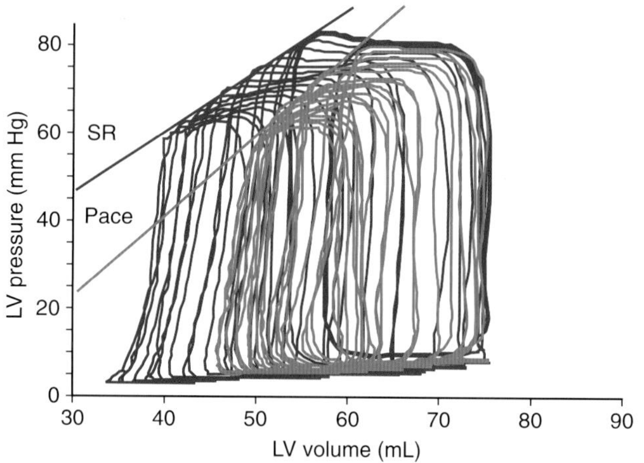

Figure 9-10. Pressure-volume (P-V) diagrams during sinus rhythm (SR) (purple lines) *and ventricular pacing (PACE)* (blue lines) *before and during caval vein occlusion. The end-systolic P-V relation* (straight lines) *shifts rightward during ventricular pacing. These data indicate that the left ventricle (LV) operates at a larger volume under all loading conditions and that at a given LV volume, LV pressure development and stroke volume are reduced. (Modified from Van Oosterhout MFM, Prinzen FW, Arts T, et al: Asynchronous electrical activation induces inhomogeneous hypertrophy of the left ventricular wall. Circulation 98:588-595, 1998.)*

Effect of Asynchronous Activation on Systolic and Diastolic Pump Function

Both RV pacing and LBBB reduce systolic and diastolic functions. These effects are independent of changes in preload and afterload. This conclusion can be reached on the basis of results from studies using preparations in which preload and afterload were controlled[55,56] as well as those in which preload- and afterload-independent indices of ventricular function were determined (Figs. 9-9 and 9-10).[59,61-63] The negative mechanical effect of dys-synchronous activation has been observed under various loading conditions[64] and during exercise.[65] Ventricular pacing also deteriorates pump function in

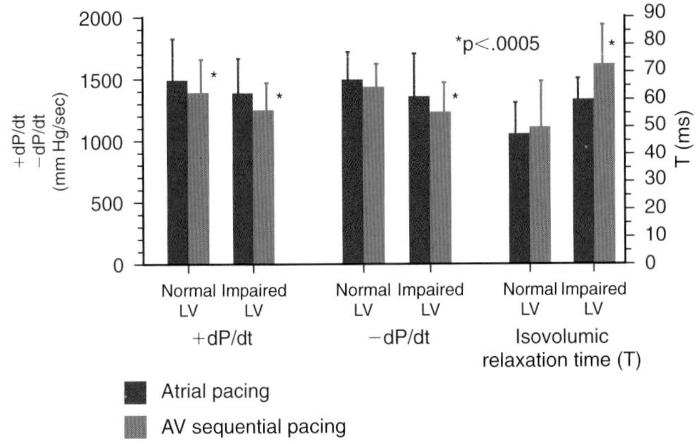

Figure 9-11. Hemodynamic effects of atrial and atrioventricular (AV) sequential pacing in patients with normal and impaired left ventricular (LV) systolic function. Note that +dP/dt (maximal rate of rise in the LV pressure) is significantly lower in both groups of patients with AV sequential pacing than in patients with atrial pacing. However, −dP/dt (maximal rate of decline in LV pressure) is significantly lower, and the isovolumic relaxation time significantly longer, during AV sequential pacing than during atrial pacing only in patients with impaired LV systolic function. (Adapted from Bedotto JB, Grayburn PA, Black WH, et al: Alterations in left ventricular relaxation during atrioventricular pacing in humans. J Am Coll Cardiol 15:658, 1990. Reprinted with permission from the American College of Cardiology.)

patients with coronary artery disease[66] and those with already impaired LV function (Fig. 9-11).[67] Impairments in regional and global cardiac pump function have been observed in patients and animals with LBBB, even if LBBB was not accompanied by other cardiovascular diseases.[48,49] Therefore, it appears that under all circumstances, dyssynchrony is an important, independent determinant of cardiac pump function.

Although LV dP/dt_{max} is a preload-dependent parameter, it is also very sensitive to changes in ventricular activation sequence, as shown both in animal models and in humans (see Fig. 9-11).[33,67-69] Thus, LV dP/dt_{max} appears to be an appropriate marker of dyssynchrony-induced changes in LV global contractile function and its correction by any pacing technique. Additionally, the rate of ventricular relaxation is slower during ventricular pacing, and the detrimental effect of pacing on relaxation is more pronounced, in patients with impaired ventricular function (see Fig. 9-11).[67] Isovolumic relaxation parameters, such as LV dP/dt_{min} and Tau, are strongly influenced by pacing.[69-71] Parameters of auxotonic relaxation (rate of segment lengthening or LV volume increase) are also lower during ventricular pacing than during sinus rhythm, but the difference is less pronounced than for the isovolumic relaxation parameters.[64,69]

As a consequence of the slower contraction and relaxation, isovolumic contraction and relaxation phases last longer, thus leaving less time for ventricular filling and ejection.[48,56,72] Therefore, it is not surprising that cardiac output and systolic arterial and LV pressures are also affected by a dyssynchronous activation. In general, stroke volume is affected more than systolic LV pressure,[63,68] presumably because baroreflex regulatory mechanisms partly compensate the decrease in blood pressure. This idea is supported by the finding of higher catecholamine levels[73] and greater systemic vascular resistance[65] during ventricular pacing. With regard to the changes in stroke volume, it is important to note that ventricular pacing, especially RV apex pacing, can induce mitral regurgitation, as has been demonstrated in animals[74,75] and patients.[76,77] In addition to reduced stroke volume at unchanged preload, ejection fraction is usually found to be depressed during ventricular pacing[65,78] as well as in LBBB.[79] Similarly, ventricular pacing can increase pulmonary wedge pressure.[65] The negative inotropic effect of ventricular pacing under various loading conditions is clearly illustrated by a rightward shift of the LV function curve—that is, the relationship between cardiac output and mean atrial pressure (see Fig. 9-9).[62] Later studies showed a rightward shift of the end-systolic pressure-volume (P-V) relation (see Fig. 9-10), thus suggesting that for each end-systolic pressure, the LV must operate at a larger LV volume.[61,63,80]

Cause of Reduced Pump Function

Mitral valve insufficiency[74,76] obviously diminishes LV pump function directly by reducing the volume ejected into the aorta and indirectly by reducing LV cavity volume. Mitral valve regurgitation during RV apex pacing may be caused by the early activation of the septum, leading to leftward motion of the septum,[47] while the papillary muscles are still passive, because transseptal conduction is slow.[12,27]

An obvious cause of reduced pump function during abnormal electrical activation is the asynchronous contraction of the different parts of the ventricular muscle. This idea has been explored by Suga and coworkers[81] in a mathematical simulation. They divided the LV wall into two elements with similar contractile properties. Contractility of the whole LV decreased considerably when the asynchrony exceeded 100 msec. This concept is supported by experimental observations in dogs with LBBB. In studies using combinations of pacing sites, minimal intra-LV asynchrony, assessed by endocardial electrical activation mapping, consistently led to the highest LV dP/dt_{max}.[35] In addition to intraventricular asynchrony, interventricular asynchrony may affect ventricular pump function. An extensive overview of studies on RV and LV pacing showed that RV pacing consistently reduces LV function more than LV pacing.[82] Even at similar levels of intraventricular asynchrony, LV dP/dt_{max} is lower during RV pacing than during LV pacing.[35] This observation suggests important roles for interventricular asynchrony and, related to it, interventricular mechanical interaction. This ventricular interaction is also expressed by abnormal septal motion in asynchronous ventricles.[47]

Finally, the pathway of activation may be a determinant of ventricular function. The sequence of activation from apex to base appears to be important. As already mentioned, the ventricular myocardium is activated from apex to base during normal sinus rhythm. Among all LV pacing sites, the LV apex appears to keep

LV pump function closest to that seen during atrial pacing.[26,83-85] The observation that the addition of pacing sites during LV apex pacing does not improve and sometimes even reduces LV function emphasizes the importance of a ventricular activation directed from apex to base.[85]

Electrical and Structural Remodeling

Asynchronous electrical activation not only has acute mechanical consequences but also influences cardiac structure and function in the long run. A particular adaptation of the heart to ventricular pacing occurs when the abnormal activation created by pacing is stopped but repolarization remains abnormal, a phenomenon called *cardiac memory*. Several investigators found evidence that, as in the nervous system, short-term cardiac memory (<1 hour) involves changes in ion channels and phosphorylation of target proteins[87] and long-term cardiac memory (≈3 weeks of pacing) involves altered gene programming and protein expression.[86,88] Costard-Jäckle and Franz[89] have demonstrated opposite changes in repolarization in regions remote from and close to a pacing site starting within one hour of ventricular pacing.

The repolarization abnormalities related to cardiac memory also have a mechanical counterpart. During sinus rhythm immediately after a period of ventricular pacing, relaxation is disturbed.[90] Moreover, systolic function deteriorates between 2 hours and 1 week after ventricular pacing has been stopped (Fig. 9-12). After ventricular pacing is stopped for 1 week, it takes $1^1/_2$ days for ejection fraction to return to its prepacing value (see Fig. 9-12).[91] It seems likely that changes in the function of an ion channel, such as the L-type calcium channel,[87] underlie the reduction in ejection fraction during the first week of ventricular pacing. Therefore, electrical and contractile remodeling appears to occur soon after the onset of asynchronous activation.

In addition to the long-term effect on cardiac memory, longer-lasting (>1 month) ventricular pacing and LBBB lead to major structural changes, such as ventricular dilatation and asymmetrical hypertrophy.[49,61,92] The ventricular dilatation appears related to the fact that the LV operates at a larger volume. Global hypertrophy may be induced by this global dilatation as well as by the greater sympathetic stimulation (Fig. 9-13).[73] The asymmetry of hypertrophy appears to be more prominent during LV pacing than during RV pacing and LBBB.[49,61,93] However, regardless of pacing site and underlying conduction disturbance, the asymmetry of hypertrophy is characterized by a more pronounced growth of the late-activated myocardium—that is, the same region that shows enhanced contractile performance due to early systolic prestretch. It has been observed in juvenile canine hearts that ventricular pacing leads to fiber disarray,[94] which potentially is

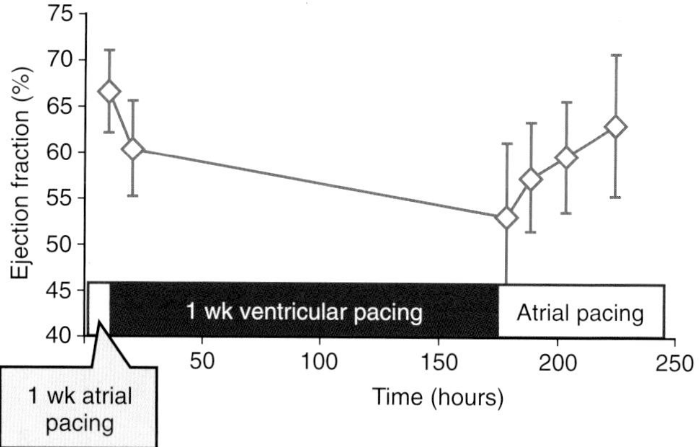

Figure 9-12. Left ventricular (LV) ejection fraction before pacing, during short-term and midterm (1 week) ventricular pacing, and during the first days after restoration of normal sinus rhythm. During the entire experimental period, the heart rate was kept at 80 bpm with the use of fixed-rate pacing at the right atrium and, during the week of ventricular pacing, dual-chamber pacing with an AV interval of 100 msec. (Data derived from Nahlawi M, Waligora M, Spies SM, et al: Left ventricular function during and after right ventricular pacing. J Am Coll Cardiol 44:1883-1888, 2004.)

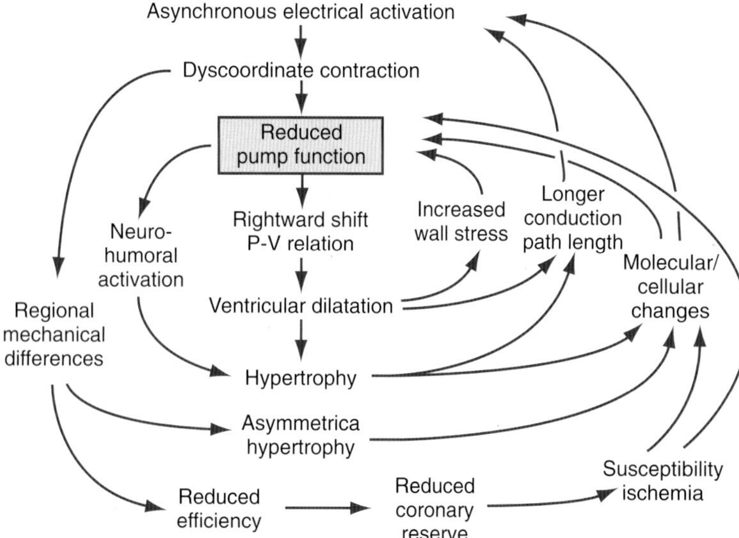

Figure 9-13. Possible relationships among the various consequences of asynchronous activation of the ventricles, owing to ventricular pacing or conduction disturbances, and the deterioration of pump function over time. P-V, pressure-volume. For details, see text.

also the result of the regionally different and abnormal distribution of mechanical work.[31,50,95]

In ventricles undergoing long-term pacing,[61] myocyte diameter is increased in late-activated regions, but the number of capillaries per myocyte is unchanged (MFM van Oosterhout, unpublished data). Therefore, the diffusion distance for oxygen increases, potentially leading to compromised oxygenation—which is known to render hypertrophic myocardium susceptible to ischemia. Resynchronization has been shown to result in improved coronary reserve, suggesting that the structural remodeling at the microvascular level may also be reversible.[96] An alternative explanation is that CRT could be simply decreasing the oxygen demand in the late-activated regions.

In diseases like infarction and hypertension, ventricular remodeling appears, at least initially, to be meant to compensate for the loss of function and the increased load, respectively. However, dilatation and hypertrophy do not reduce the asynchronous activation induced by pacing or LBBB; rather, they increase it.[49,61] The reasons are the longer path length of impulse conduction (dilatation) and the larger muscle mass to be activated (hypertrophy). Moreover, chronic asynchronous activation also reduces expression of gap-junction channels.[97,98] Akar and colleagues[99] have related the reduced expression in nonfailing and failing asynchronous hearts to slower impulse conduction, especially in the late-activated regions.[99] Moreover, they showed that action potential duration increases in the late-activated myocardium. These molecular changes may render the myocardium not only more asynchronous but also more susceptible to arrhythmias.

All of these processes may lead to a vicious circle, in which dilatation and hypertrophy further reduce LV pump function, either directly or by increasing asynchrony of activation (see Fig. 9-13). As is the case after myocardial infarction, initial compensatory hypertrophy may result in heart failure many years later. Clinical evidence for such an important role of asynchronous activation in the development of heart failure is discussed elsewhere in the chapter.

Physiologic Effects of Heart Rate and Atrioventricular Synchrony

Correction of Bradycardia by Pacing

Cardiac pacing is the only effective treatment for symptomatic bradycardia. Permanent pacemakers have been implanted since the early 1960s to prevent death or syncope caused by ventricular asystole. Although asystole is clearly to be prevented, bradycardia does not always immediately lead to pump failure. This fact can be derived from studies on young patients with congenital AV block. As a compensation for the bradycardia, these patients have enlarged hearts and an increased ejection fraction.[100,101] In a 10-year follow-up study, 9 out of 149 patients demonstrated dilated cardiomyopathy.[101]

TABLE 9-1. Hemodynamic Effects of Ventricular Pacing in Complete Heart Block (CHB)

Hemodynamic Parameter	CHB with Slow Ventricular Response	Ventricular Pacing in CHB
Ventricular rate	↓	↑
Cardiac index	↓	↑
Stroke volume	↑	↓
Sympathetic tone	↑	↓
Ventricular contractility	↑	↓
Systemic vascular resistance	↑	↓
Atrial rate	↑	↓

At the onset of acquired complete heart block, cardiac output is smaller than with normal heart rate.[102,103] As a result, compensatory increases in sympathetic tone and end-diastolic ventricular volume occur, leading to higher atrial rates, enhanced ventricular contractility, and augmented stroke volume.[103,104] Over the short term, the canine heart adapts to bradycardia by increasing diastolic volume and neurohumoral activation, which results in BiV hypertrophy (Table 9-1).[103-105] Although these adaptations initially manage to return cardiac output to the level before the onset of AV block, this compensatory effect usually fades after 2 months of heart block. After 4 months, contractility is back to baseline, but LV cavity volume and corrected QT interval (QTc) continue to increase (Fig. 9-14)[103]; the latter increase is associated with an enhanced susceptibility to arrhythmias.[104] If complete AV block persists for more than 4 months, congestive heart failure ensues.[102] It is possible that the development of heart failure originates from the ventricular dilatation and hypertrophy initiated early after the start of heart block.

The importance of the duration of overload is confirmed by the observation that the frequency of congestive heart failure symptoms in patients with complete heart block correlates with the duration of heart block. Congestive heart failure has been described during chronic complete heart block even in patients with normal ventricular function. Brockman and Stoney[106] reported that in two thirds of their patients with complete heart block and congestive heart failure, symptoms were relieved by ventricular pacing alone, and no additional medical therapy was required. Breur and colleagues[107] showed that, in patients with congenital heart block, implantation of a pacemaker resulted in less LV dilatation than in the untreated control group, in which the LV cavity gradually dilated. Similarly, in dogs with AV block, LV dilatation gradually progresses over time (see Fig. 9-14), whereas ventricular pacing readily reverses the LV

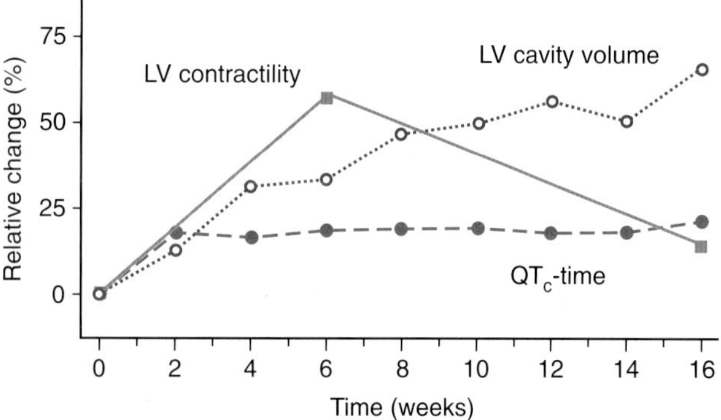

Figure 9-14. Effect of atrioventricular (AV) block on left ventricular (LV) cavity volume (structural remodeling), LV contractility (contractile remodeling), and corrected QT interval (QTc) time (electrical remodeling) in canine hearts, relative to their values before onset of AV block. Note the gradual and continuing increase in LV cavity volume over time, the early-onset and maintained electrical remodeling, and the biphasic contractile remodeling. (Modified from Peschar M, Vernooy K, Cornelussen RN, et al: Structural, electrical and mechanical remodeling of the canine heart in AV-block and LBBB. Eur Heart J 25[Suppl D]:D61-D65, 2004.)

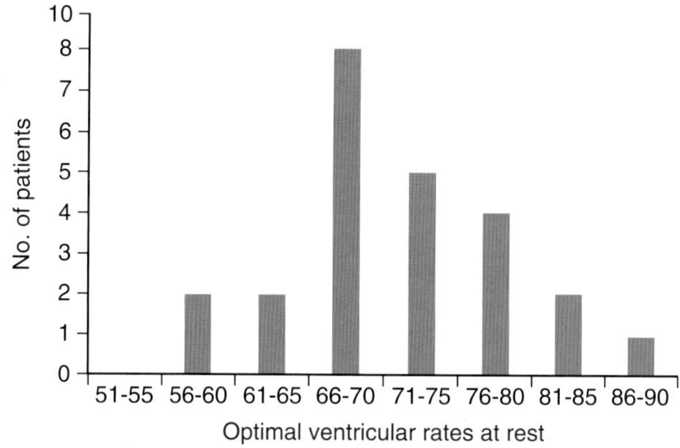

Figure 9-15. Histogram of optimal ventricular pacing rates at rest as defined by cardiac outputs determined by dye dilution in patients with complete heart block. (From Sowton E: Hemodynamic studies in patients with artificial pacemakers. Br Heart J 26:737, 1964.)

dilatation and hypertrophy caused by AV block.[85] However, longer-lasting ventricular pacing in hearts with AV block may lead to LV dilatation and hypertrophy secondary to the effect of asynchronous activation. Two studies on young adults who have received pacing for approximately 10 years showed a high preponderance of heart failure and LV dilatation.[108,109] Moreover, preliminary results in a study on the effect of RV pacing in patients with acquired AV block suggested that RV apex pacing may not decrease but rather may increase dilatation and hypertrophy.[103] These data strongly suggest that in the patient with AV block, the short- and long-term effects of RV pacing are different, indicating that the choice of whether or not to start pacemaker treatment using RV pacing needs to be made carefully.

Early studies suggested that the maximal increase in cardiac output during ventricular pacing at rest occurs at rates between 70 and 90 bpm (Fig. 9-15).[110-112] Further rises in rates result in either no additional increase or a decrease in cardiac output accompanied by greater peripheral vascular resistance. In contrast, there is growing evidence that lower heart rates may be particularly beneficial. Indeed, in animal models it appears that bradycardia promotes angiogenesis.[113-115] Moreover, Lei and associates[116] demonstrated that reducing normal heart rates by 20% to 30% through the continuous infusion of alinidine in a postmyocardial infarction rat model increased basic fibroblast growth factor, its receptor, and expression of related proteins. Bradycardia in this model also increased capillary length density in the border zone of the infarct by 40% and in the remote zone by 14%. It also increased arteriolar density in the septum by 62%. These changes translated to a 23% greater coronary reserve, a smaller increase in left LV volume after myocardial infarction, and a greater preservation of ejection fraction in the bradycardic animals.

Although the relationship between optimal resting ventricular pacing rate and ventricular dysfunction has not been systematically evaluated, it is very likely that different resting ventricular rates are required in patients with systolic and diastolic dysfunction. For example, Ishibashi and coworkers[117] reported that in elderly hypertrophic patients, even 25% increases in heart rate, as induced by atrial pacing, significantly reduced cardiac mechanical efficiency. The investigators went as far as to suggest that coronary perfusion itself in elderly hypertensive hypertrophic patients is negatively affected by an increase in heart rate (Fig. 9-16). They recommended that in the treatment of elderly hypertensive patients, the control of the heart rate in addition to the control of blood pressure might be helpful in minimizing the occurrence of myocardial ischemia and might slow down the subsequent progression to heart failure.[117] Since then, their recommended treatment has become common practice with the use of β-blocker therapy to prevent myocardial infarction and heart failure.

In addition to maintaining resting heart rate in the physiologic range, pacemaker therapy preferably allows the heart rate to rise during exercise. A rise in heart rate with greater workload improves exercise capacity. Over the years a number of sensors have been incorporated into VVIR pacemakers. Many investigators have compared the exercise hemodynamics between sensor-driven VVIR pacing and VVI pacing. The percentage improvements of heart rate and exercise duration during symptoms-limited exercise in the VVIR and VVI pacing modes from a number of larger series for currently available rate-adaptive systems showed variable but consistent increases of 69% in rate and 32% in exercise tolerance when patients received VVIR pacing. Notably, most of the early comparative series of patients given VVI and VVIR pacing are rather small and have mixed patient populations in terms of symptoms of heart failure and degree of ventricular dysfunction. The use of an atrial sensing electrode to synchronize ventricular stimulation with intrinsic sinus node discharge (atrial synchronous ventricular pacing—VAT) allowed the implementation of a more physiologic form of pacing. The addition of ventricular sensing capability to this pacing mode resulted in the development of the VDD mode as a combination of VAT plus VVI. Both VVI and VDD modes of pacing prevent syncope due to bradycardia, but conventional VVI units are unable to respond to exertion by raising the pacing rate to meet the demand for a greater cardiac output.

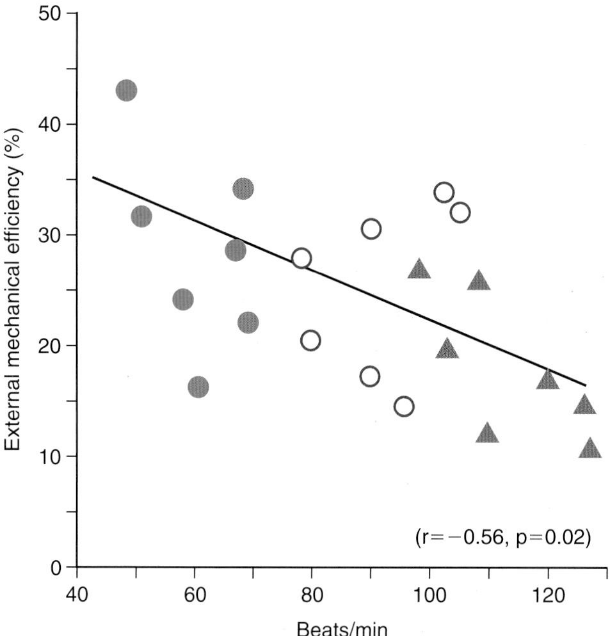

Figure 9-16. The relationship between heart rate and external mechanical efficiency of the heart (measured as left ventricular work divided by myocardial oxygen consumption expressed as energy using a conversion factor of 2.06), for basal condition (closed circles) *and different atrial pacing rates (*open circles, *25% above basal heart rate;* triangles, *50% above basal heart rate) in elderly hypertensive patients.*

The importance of increasing heart rate to augment cardiac output with exercise has been clearly documented in several studies.[118-120] Because the improvement in exercise performance is due predominantly to an increase in heart rate, it is expected that favorable hemodynamic results will be obtained by rate-adaptive systems. Consequently, the modern approach to the management of complete symptomatic heart block involves the use of units that provide not only basic ventricular pacing support but also adaptation of the pacing rate to physiologic needs. Two patterns of hemodynamic response to higher rates of ventricular pacing have been described. In the *flat response,* after an initial increase in heart rate and cardiac output (rate increase from 30 to 60 bpm), cardiac output remains relatively constant as stroke volume decreases with further rises in heart rate (Fig. 9-17). This response occurs most often in individuals with normal cardiac function and indicates that cardiac output is relatively independent of heart rate. In the *peaked response,* cardiac output increases progressively until the optimal pacing rate is achieved, and any further increase in rate results in a diminution in cardiac output (see Fig. 9-17). The peaked response has been more commonly observed in patients with myocardial disease, in whom cardiac output is more sensitive to changes in preload, afterload, myocardial contractility, and distensibility. The major factors limiting the increase in resting cardiac output that can be achieved by pacing rate alone are shortened diastolic filling time, reduced LV compliance at higher rates of ventricular pacing, and increased systemic vascular resistance.[110,111]

Rowe and colleagues[121] found other reasons not to increase pacing rate too much. They examined cardiac output and coronary blood flow at low (47 bpm), intermediate (77 bpm), and high (117 bpm) ventricular

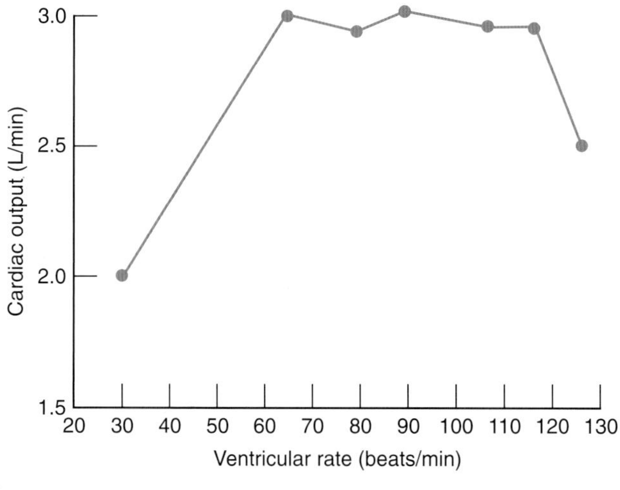

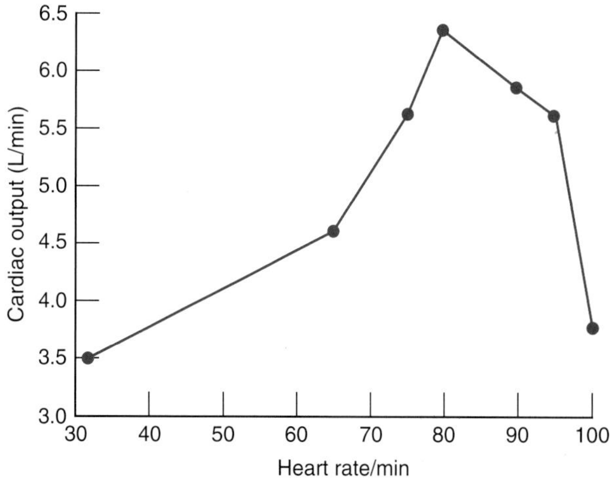

Figure 9-17. ***A,*** *Example of flat response indicating a relatively constant cardiac output over a wide range of ventricular pacing rates.* ***B,*** *Example of a peaked response curve, demonstrating progressive increase in cardiac output with heart rate until an optimal heart rate is achieved. After this optimal heart rate, a further rise in heart rate results in a decrease in cardiac output. (From Sowton E: Hemodynamic studies in patients with artificial pacemakers. Br Heart J 26:737, 1964.)*

pacing rates in subjects with complete heart block. Cardiac output rose with increase from low to intermediate pacing rate but diminished at the higher rate. However, coronary blood flow and cardiac oxygen consumption rose progressively with rising heart rates, thus indicating lower pumping efficiency at the high heart rate.

Significance and Determination of Optimal Atrioventricular Interval

Importance of Atrioventricular Synchronization

Basically, the role of the atrial contraction is to help maintain a laminar flow of blood from the venous system to the ventricles; this role is tightly integrated with the movement of the ventricles to create a smooth motion of blood across the system. To perform its role, the atrium changes its function from that of a conduit during early filling to that of a booster pump during atrial systole, to that of a reservoir during ventricular systole. These changes are closely related to longitudinal displacement of the anulus of the mitral and tricuspid valves along the long axis of the heart. Indeed, the anulus is displaced toward the apex of the ventricles during systole and toward the atria during diastole, thus significantly contributing to the smooth movement of blood from the atria to the ventricles. This displacement keeps the overall volume of the heart nearly constant during systole and diastole.[122]

An optimally timed atrial contraction (before the isovolumic contraction phase) maximizes LV filling and thereby its output by virtue of the Frank-Starling relation. Too early atrial contraction (as in the case of long P-Q times and dual-chamber pacing with long AV intervals) causes a loss of the booster pump function of the atrium. Moreover, early atrial contraction may initiate early mitral valve closure, thereby limiting ventricular diastolic filling time.

This observation can be explained by the importance of three factors collaborating to achieve optimal closure of the AV valves. First, the ending of transvalvular flow at the end of the atrial contraction makes the valvular leaflets approach one another. Second, at the beginning of ventricular contraction, the anulus of the AV valve contracts, and so do the papillary muscles that hold the leaflets. Simultaneously, at the start of the ventricular contraction, ventricular pressure rises above atrial pressure, and the valves close. When these factors are misaligned, an opportunity for diastolic and systolic mitral regurgitation is created.

In the early years of pacing, the electrical stimulus was selectively applied to the ventricle (ventricular single-chamber pacing, or V pacing). With V pacing, the contraction of atria and ventricles is uncoupled, leading to an atrial contribution to LV filling that varies from beat to beat. This also results in large beat-to-beat variations in stroke volume, systolic pressure, and other hemodynamic variables.[123] The introduction of sequential AV pacing resulted in more regular heart beats and improved hemodynamics in both animals[69,124,125] and patients.[126] With advances in pacemaker technology, appreciation of the importance of maintaining AV synchrony has improved, and programming of optimal AV intervals in patients with dual-chamber pacemakers is of great importance.[127]

A summary of the main consequences of an optimal AV timing can be seen in Figure 9-18. Because filling time is limited, especially at high heart rates, the atrial

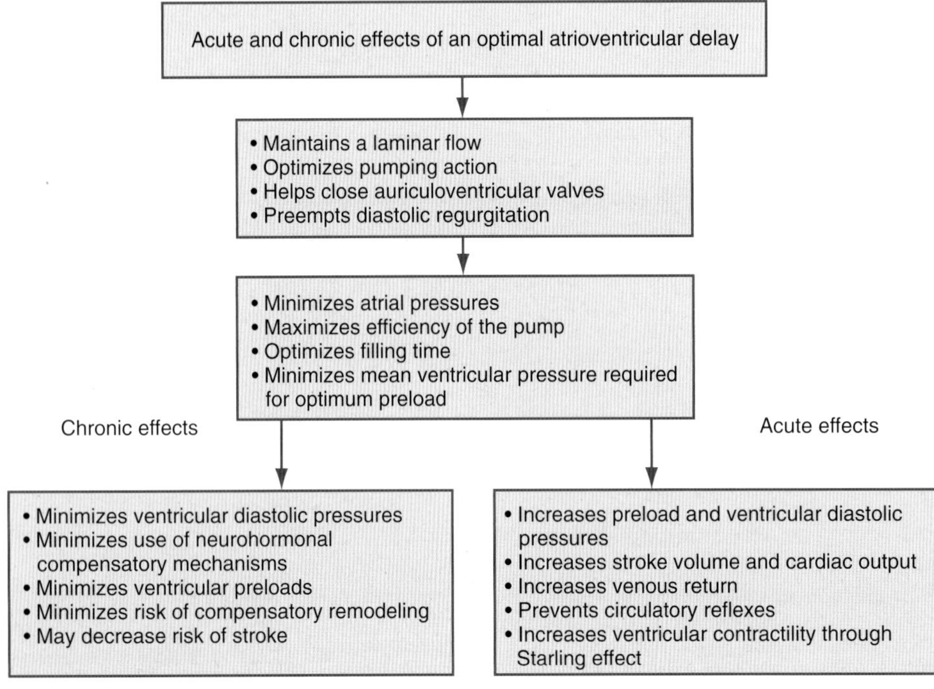

Figure 9-18. The hemodynamic effects of programming an optimal atrioventricular (AV) delay.

contribution to stroke volume is more prominent at high than at low heart rates.[128]

Atrioventricular Optimization in Patients with Normal Left Ventricular Function

The AV interval that maximizes resting cardiac output during dual-chamber pacing varies widely among patients, being reported in most studies to be between 125 and 200 msec. In patients with pacemakers, cardiac output increased by 4% to 20% when the AV interval was lengthened from 0 to between 100 and 130 msec.[126,129-131]

In 1995, Ritter and colleagues[132] proposed a very shrewd algorithm for optimizing the AV interval of patients with complete heart block, although the algorithm is frequently used in patients with different degrees of AV block. The goal of their method was to calculate the optimal AV timing by analyzing filling patterns obtained during only two AV intervals. The principal assumption of the algorithm is that the optimal AV interval for inflow is the AV interval that would start the ventricular contraction right at the end of the deceleration phase of the velocity wave created by the contraction of the atrium (A wave, representing the booster pump action of the atrium). To enable calculation of the optimal AV interval, the method requires the measurement of several intervals of the cardiac cycle (Figs. 9-19 and 9-20) at a short AV interval and then at a long AV interval (see Fig. 9-19, *lower panel*). The optimal AV interval is calculated from the pacemaker spike in the ventricle to the start of the ventricular contraction right at the end of the A-wave deceleration phase. Henceforth, the Ritter method provides a reliable and simple technique for optimizing inflow patterns in patients with complete AV block. This optimal AV interval is the shortest AV interval that does not interrupt atrial filling by making the end of diastolic filling coincide with the beginning of the ventricular systole, resulting in a normal separation of the E and A waves and the maximization of filling time.

Optimal AV interval can be determined in most patients during dual-chamber pacing by means of a variety of invasive and noninvasive measurements. Most commonly, optimal AV interval is assessed by LV outflow recording with Doppler echocardiography (Fig. 9-21). Although not practical or cost-effective for every patient, Doppler-derived cardiac outputs at varying AV intervals can be used to fine-tune the AV interval. In patients with preserved ventricular function, this method is highly reliable, is sensitive to small output changes, and has a low interobserver variability. The optimal AV interval determined with Doppler echocardiography correlates well with the optimal AV interval determined with radionuclide ventriculography. Factors that may influence the optimal AV interval in different patients are summarized in Table 9-2. A few factors in addition to interpatient variability may influence determination of optimal AV interval in the same patient, such as heart rate, paced or sensed atrial event, posture, and drugs.[133-137] Moreover, during the life of a specific patient, there may be situations in which the optimal AV interval is different from the AV interval considered to be physiologic. For example, AV sequential pacing for complete heart block complicating an acute myocardial infarction or after cardiac surgery yields optimal hemodynamics at AV intervals in the range of 80 to 120 msec. This fact may be related to a surge of intrinsic catecholamine levels or to administered inotropic drugs and reduced LV compliance in these acutely stressful situations.

1. Program a short AV delay (i.e. 25% AV interval), forcing the closure of the mitral valve. Measure Qa_{short}

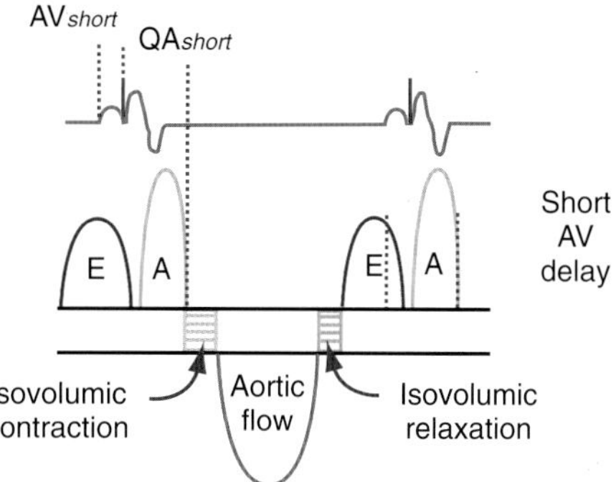

2. Program a long AV delay (i.e. 75% of the AV interval), maintaining capture and allowing the spontaneous closing of the mitral valve. Measure Qa_{long}

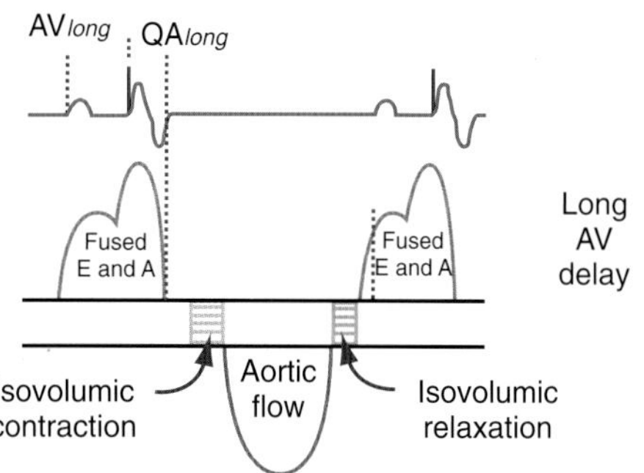

Figure 9-19. *The simultaneous tracings of the Doppler flow velocity profile at the leaflets of the mitral valve (positive E and A waves) and at the leaflets of the aortic valve (negative-going ones marked aortic flow); simultaneously with the surface electrocardiogram. The* top panel *shows the case of a short atrioventricular (AV) interval (AV_{short}) having been programmed such that the contraction of the left ventricle interrupts the deceleration phase of the transmitral velocity profile created by the contraction of the atrium (A wave). The* bottom panel *shows the case of a long AV interval (AV_{long}) being programmed to enable the deceleration phase of the A wave to finish before the start of the ventricular contraction. Having two AV intervals allows the measurement of QA_{short} and QA_{long}, the variables required to calculate the optimal AV interval with the Ritter method.*

- Optimum AV delay is the shortest AV delay that does not interrupt atrial filling
- The end of the diastolic filling matches the start of ventricular systole
- Resulting in:
  - –Separation of E and A waves
  - –Maximizing LV filling time

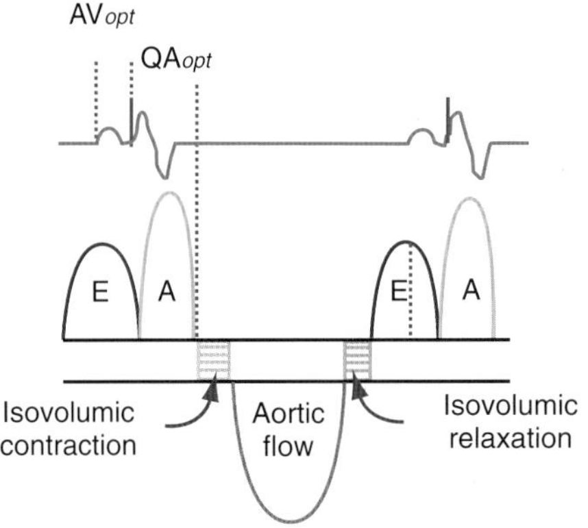

$$AV_{opt} + QA_{short} = AV_{long} + QA_{long}$$

Simplified

$$AV_{opt} = AV_{long} + QA_{long} - QA_{short}$$

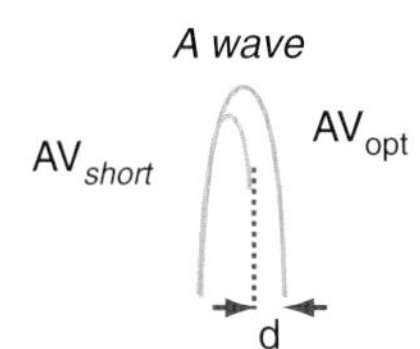

Figure 9-20. The way the E and A waves would look in relationship to the surface electrocardiogram and the aortic velocity wave when the atrioventricular (AV) interval is programmed using the Ritter method. AV_{opt}, optimal AV delay; d, the portion of the A wave finished prematurely by the ventricular contraction with AV_{short}; LV, left ventricular.

The programmed AV interval regulates the timing of right atrial and ventricular conduction, which in a normal heart without significant atrial electrical disease usually coincides with that of left atrium (LA) and LV conduction. From a hemodynamic point of view, LA and LV conduction is most important, followed by the left-sided AV interval. The physiologic left-sided AV interval depends on several parameters, including the programmed AV interval, latency in atrial capture and sensing, interatrial conduction time, latency in ventricular capture, and interventricular conduction time.[138] Because of the complex relationship between these intervals (see Fig. 9-21), significantly different right-sided and left-sided AV intervals in the same patient and in different patients can be recorded. Among these times, the one that most influences the optimal left-sided AV interval is the interatrial conduction time, measured as the time from the atrial pacing spike to the atrial depolarization on the esophageal electrogram or to the A wave on Doppler echocardiography. Patients with near-normal interatrial conduction time (about 90 msec or less) derive the greatest hemodynamic benefit from programmable AV intervals of about 150 msec; in contrast, in those patients presenting with prolonged interatrial conduction time, the AV interval should be set at 200 msec or longer to maximize cardiac output. Of particular note, programming a short AV interval in patients with prolonged interatrial conduction delay may result in depolarization of the LA after LV mechanical activation. This situation may produce hemodynamics equivalent to or worse than those seen in patients with VVI pacing alone. Pacemaker syndrome may also occur under these circumstances.

TABLE 9-2. **Possible Factors Influencing Optimal Atrioventricular Intervals**

Interpatient variables	Atrial capture latency Atrial sensing latency Intra-atrial conduction delay Ventricular capture latency Intraventricular conduction delay Underlying myocardial disease Heart rate Catecholamine levels
Intrapatient variables	Heart rate Paced or sensed atrial event Catecholamine levels Drugs

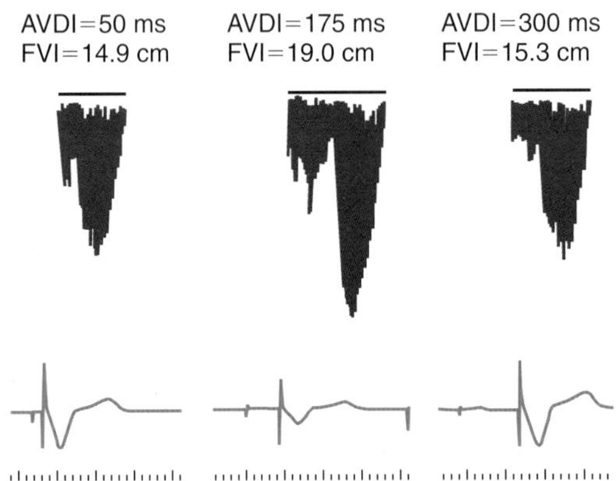

Figure 9-21. Left ventricular outflow recording at atrioventricular delay intervals (AVDIs; also AV intervals) of 50, 175, and 300 msec during AV sequential pacing at identical heart rates in the same patient. The largest flow velocity integral (FVI) reflecting ventricular stroke volume occurs at AVDI 175 msec. Significant decreases are noted in stroke volume at AVDIs 50 and 300 msec. (From Janosik DL, Pearson AC, Buckingham TA, et al: The hemodynamic benefit of differential atrioventricular delay intervals for sensed and paced atrial events during physiologic pacing. J Am Coll Cardiol 14:499, 1989. Reprinted with permission of the American College of Cardiology.)

Latency in atrial capture and sensing may lead to different optimal AV intervals for sensed P waves and paced P waves (Fig. 9-22). The magnitude of atrial

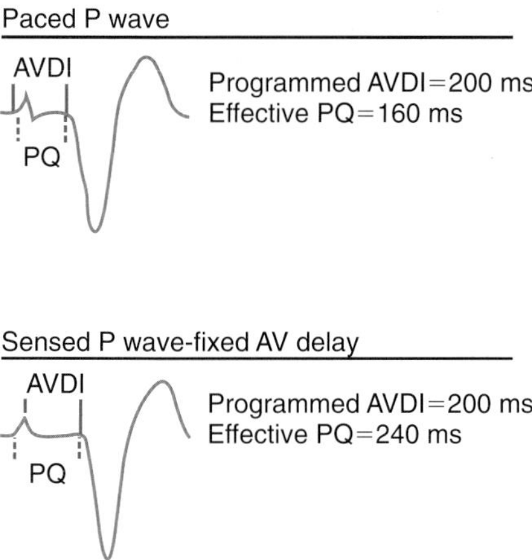

Figure 9-22. Programmed atrioventricular delay intervals (AVDIs; also AV intervals) and effect of P-Q intervals. When a paced P wave occurs (top), *the effective P-Q interval is shorter than the programmed AV delay because of latency in atrial capture. When a sensed P wave occurs* (bottom), *the effective P-Q interval is longer than the programmed AVDI because of latency in atrial sensing. (From Janosik DL, Pearson AC, Buckingham TA, et al: The hemodynamic benefit of differential atrioventricular delay intervals for sensed and paced atrial events during physiologic pacing. J Am Coll Cardiol 14:499, 1989. Reprinted with permission of the American College of Cardiology.)*

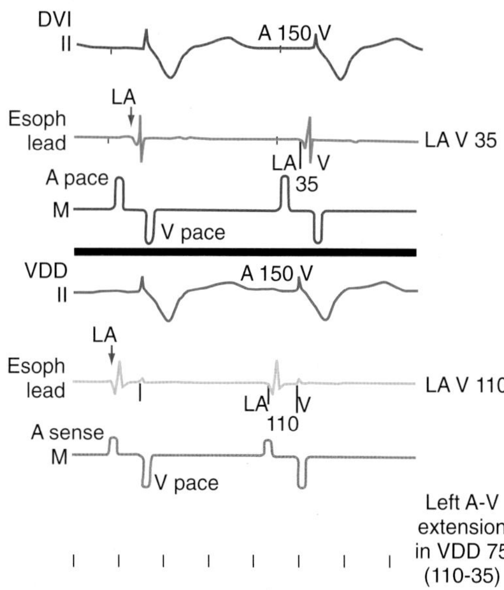

Figure 9-23. Interatrial conduction and change in the timing of left atrial (LA) depolarization with pacing mode change from DDD to VDD. The time delay between right atrial pacing artifact and LA depolarization is 115 msec (top), *resulting in an LA-to-ventricular sequence of only 35 msec. With mode change to VDD* (bottom), *the LA-to-ventricular sequence extends by 75 msec, resulting in an LA-to-ventricular sequence of 110 msec. (From Wish M, Fletcher RD, Gottdiener JS, Cohen AI: Importance of left atrial timing in the programming of dual-chamber pacemakers. Am J Cardiol 60:566, 1987.)*

capture and sensing latencies varies among patients and may be affected by the lead and pacemaker circuitry characteristics, electrode position, tissue interface, amplitude and rate of stimulation, P-wave morphology, myocardial disease, electrolytes and other metabolic factors, and drugs. The optimal AV interval for a sensed P wave is about 30 to 40 msec shorter than the optimal AV interval for a paced P wave followed by a paced QRS at a similar heart rate (Fig. 9-23). However, differences between optimal AV intervals for a paced P wave and a sensed P wave may be as great as 100 msec in some individuals. Some newer dual-chamber pacemakers incorporate programmable features designed to adjust the AV interval automatically in response to paced versus sensed P waves and in response to the atrial rate. It is important to recognize that the physiologic AV interval is never equivalent to the programmed AV interval for either a paced or a sensed atrial event. The physiologic PQ interval begins with the onset of the P wave; however, with a sensed P wave, the programmed AV interval begins when the native P wave is sensed (so with a delay compared with onset of the atrial activation), and with a paced P wave, the programmed AV interval begins with the atrial pacing spike, which is followed by further atrial depolarization.

The importance of variation in AV interval during exercise in patients given physiologic pacing who have normal ventricular function is still controversial. Because the major determinant of augmentation of cardiac output during exercise is heart rate, the contribution of atrial systole and relative timing of the atrial and ventricular contraction may diminish in significance. Studies analyzing the effects of variation in AV interval during exercise have yielded conflicting results.[139-143] There are two major limitations to these studies: the relative small sample size of most of them and the fact that each used a fixed AV interval during each exercise test but a different AV interval between exercise efforts. There is evidence that a rate-adaptive AV interval, which is automatically decremented in response to an increased atrial rate, is beneficial to cardiopulmonary performance during exercise.[144] In patients with chronotropic incompetence and high-level AV block, Sulke and coworkers[145] performed randomized double-blind crossover assessments of rate-adaptive and different fixed AV interval settings during 2 weeks of normal activity and performance on an exercise treadmill in patients undergoing DDDR pacing. There was a subjective improvement in quality of life with rate-adaptive AV intervals compared with fixed AV intervals, and patients preferred the rate-adaptive settings (Fig. 9-24). Notably, the longest AV interval (250 msec) was least preferred by the patients and was associated with the highest symptom prevalence. Moreover, exercise duration was not significantly different in any setting in DDDR mode but was significantly reduced in DDD mode.[145]

AV Interval Optimization in Patients with Depressed Left Ventricular Function

In general, relaxation is slower in failing hearts than in normal hearts. Consequently, less blood enters the ventricles during the rapid filling phase, as can be observed from lower E waves on Doppler echocardiograms. Therefore, failing hearts are more dependent on properly timed atrial contraction than normal hearts. This has been demonstrated in comparisons of patients with decompensated heart failure and compensated nonvalvular heart disease.[110] This knowledge clarifies why optimal timing of atrial and ventricular stimulation in patients with pacemakers is of special interest in patients with heart failure. Some investigators have shown that pacemakers can actually improve the coupling between atria and ventricles over that without pacing. This issue applies to patients with excessively long PQ times. In two studies of subjects with these findings, hemodynamic benefit was achieved with AV-sequential pacing at a physiologic AV interval (Fig. 9-25).[146,147] Reducing the prolonged AV interval increased diastolic filling time and reduced diastolic mitral regurgitation (Fig. 9-26). These beneficial effects are striking, because these studies were performed before the era of resynchronization and the RV apex was used as a ventricular pacing site, presumably the least preferable site from a hemodynamic point of view (see later).

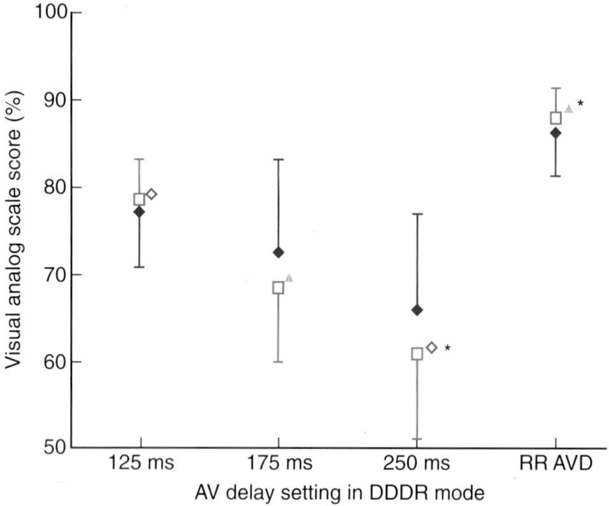

*Figure 9-24. Exercise capacity (◆) and patient's perception of general well-being (□) during everyday activity at fixed arteriovenous (AV) delay settings of 125, 175, and 250 msec and rate-responsive AV delay (RR AVD) settings in DDDR mode. ◇, P < .05; ▲ m, P < .03; *, P < .01. (Adapted from Sulke AN, Chambers JB, Sowton E: The effect of atrioventricular delay programming in patients with DDDR pacemakers. Eur Heart J 13:464, 1992.)*

The actual role of the atrial contraction in patients with dilated ventricles and low ejection fraction varies among individuals (Fig. 9-27). The booster pump action of the LA is noticeable as a "shoulder" in the LV pressure tracing, and the LV does not start contracting immediately after atrial contraction. If this plateau lasts too long, diastolic mitral regurgitation could occur, as is the case in the patient whose electrograms and other data are presented in Figure 9-28, in which a decrease in LV pressure occurs after the atrial contraction. About 20% of the patients in heart failure studies for whom complete hemodynamic data are available show this type of diastolic LV pressure waveform.[148-151] Figure 9-27 shows that using an optimized AV interval, in this case with BiV pacing, results in coincidence of the peak

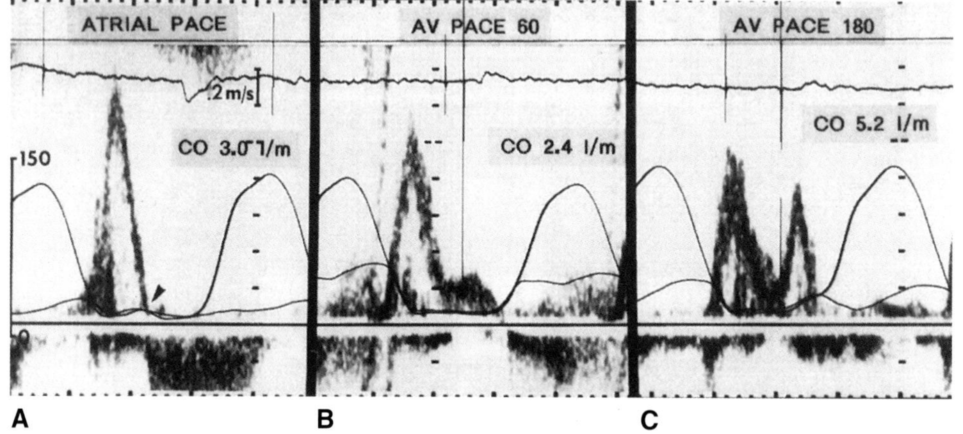

*Figure 9-25. Mitral flow-velocity curve and simultaneous left atrial (LA) and left ventricular (LV) pressure curves in a patient with severe LV dysfunction and long PR interval. **A,** Atrial pacing with antegrade native conduction and long atrioventricular (AV) delay interval (also AV interval). There is an increase in LV pressure above LA pressure during atrial relaxation and mid-diastole* (arrowhead), *resulting in a shortening of diastolic filling time and the onset of diastolic mitral regurgitation. The baseline cardiac output (CO) is 3 L/min. **B,** AV pacing at short AV delay interval of 60 msec. Diastolic filling occurs throughout all of diastole. Atrial contraction occurs simultaneously with LV contraction, resulting in a reduction in cardiac output and an increase in mean LA pressure compared with **A.** **C,** AV pacing at the optimal AV delay interval of 180 msec. There is now an optimal relationship between the mechanical LA and LV contractions, so that diastolic filling period is maximized and the mean LA pressure is maintained at a low level, resulting in a rise in LV diastolic pressure and improvement in CO to 5.2 L/min. (From Nishimura RA, Hayes DL, Holmes DR: Mechanism of hemodynamic improvement by dual chamber pacing for severe left ventricular dysfunction: An acute Doppler and catheterization hemodynamic study. J Am Coll Cardiol 25:281, 1995.)*

of the booster action of the atrial contraction and LV pressure development. Auricchio and colleagues[151] demonstrated that the maximum improvement in aortic pulse pressure, independent of the site being paced, occurs when this coincidence is achieved.[151]

In still another subset of patients with heart failure, no booster pump action from the atrium is present in the ventricular pressure curves. This observation suggests that in such patients, atrial contraction contributes very little to preload (Fig. 9-29). The patient whose data are shown in Figure 9-29 also presents an interesting phenomenon: The RA activation occurs before the end of the LV contraction. This situation is corrected after the application of BiV pacing at an AV interval of 94 msec. In this way, the AV contraction delay is reduced as is the duration of LV systole (see later), thereby increasing diastolic filling time.

Examination and calculation of the cardiac output with Doppler echocardiography, as is easily and frequently performed in patients with dual-chamber pacemakers, is more problematic in patients with depressed ejection fraction. In the latter patients, the value of the effect of pacing may be near the rate of uncertainty in the method.[152] Thus, the number of repetitions required to obtain a clinically meaningful and reproducible approximation of the optimal AV interval makes this method, as single assessment, almost impractical for patients with depressed ejection fraction. Echocardiography-based inflow or preload evaluations are probably the most commonly used methods for optimizing AV interval in patients with heart failure. As emphasized previously, the Ritter method should probably be used with some caution in patients with intact AV conduction. Indeed, in these patients, the electromechanical delay is not constant but varies as a function of the extent of collision between the intrinsically conducted depolarization wavefront and the wavefront generated by the artificial pacing spike. Henceforth, in patients with an intact conduction system, the extent of collision between these two wavefronts will be very different at the long and short AV delay intervals tested in the Ritter method, making the assumption required by the method completely invalid—that is, the electromechanical delay is unchanged at any tested AV delay.

Another important consideration one must take into account when deciding whether to use an inflow-based method for optimization of the AV interval is that, in patients with ventricular conduction delay who have cardiac resynchronization devices, the echocardiographic inflow–based method of optimizing AV delay interval does not optimize the synchrony of the ventricular contraction, nor does it take into consideration

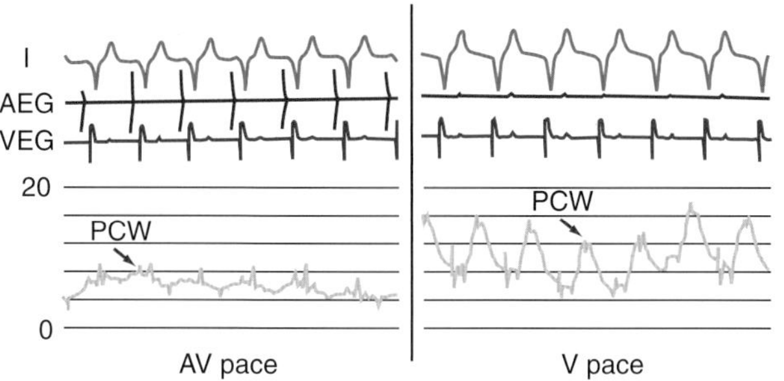

Figure 9-26. Surface electrocardiographic lead I, atrial electrogram (AEG), ventricular electrogram (VEG), and pulmonary capillary wedge pressure (PCW) recordings from a single patient during atrioventricular (AV) pacing (AV Pace) and ventricular pacing (V Pace) at 80 bpm with an A-V interval of 150 msec. The cannon A wave is noted (arrow) *on the PCW tracings. (From Reynolds DW: Hemodynamics of cardiac pacing. In Ellenbogen KA [ed]: Clinical Cardiac Pacing. Cambridge, Blackwell Scientific, 1992, pp 120-161. Reprinted by permission of Blackwell Scientific Publications, Inc.)*

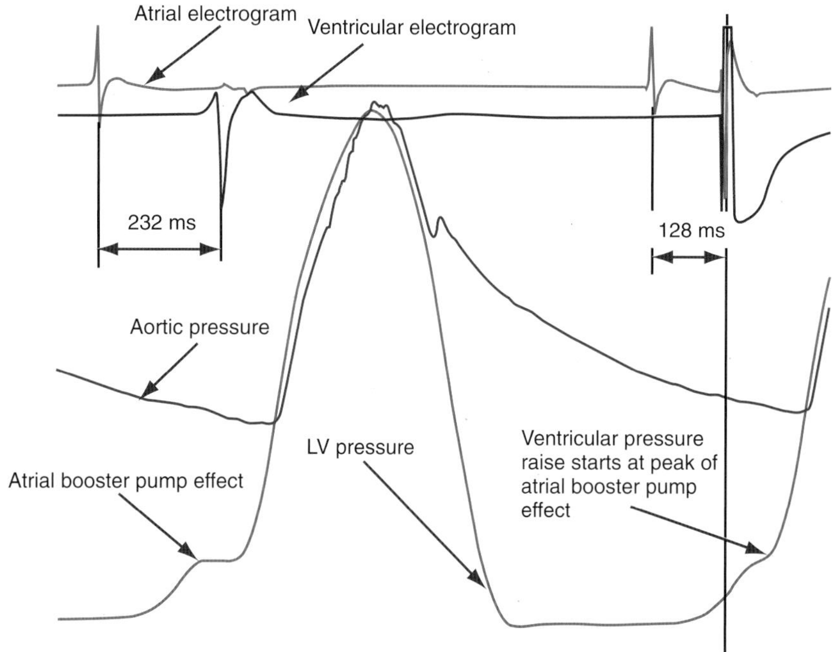

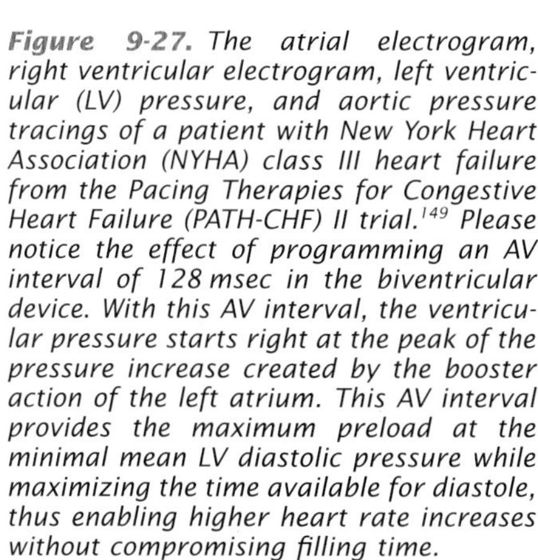

Figure 9-27. The atrial electrogram, right ventricular electrogram, left ventricular (LV) pressure, and aortic pressure tracings of a patient with New York Heart Association (NYHA) class III heart failure from the Pacing Therapies for Congestive Heart Failure (PATH-CHF) II trial.[149] Please notice the effect of programming an AV interval of 128 msec in the biventricular device. With this AV interval, the ventricular pressure starts right at the peak of the pressure increase created by the booster action of the left atrium. This AV interval provides the maximum preload at the minimal mean LV diastolic pressure while maximizing the time available for diastole, thus enabling higher heart rate increases without compromising filling time.

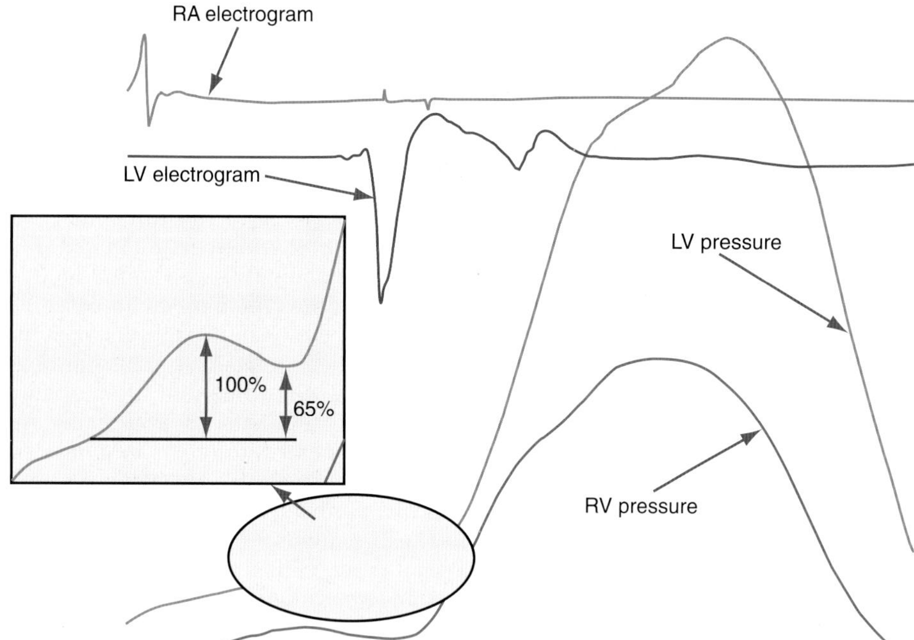

Figure 9-28. Right atrial (RA) and left ventricular (LV) electrograms and LV and right ventricular (RV) pressures from a second patient with New York Heart Association (NYHA) class II heart failure from the Pacing Therapies for Congestive Heart Failure (PATH-CHF) II trial.[149] The booster pump action of the left atrium loses 35% of the increase in LV pressure it created through the delayed start of the ventricular contraction. Most likely this loss is due to diastolic mitral regurgitation. This loss occurred in about 20% of the patients enrolled in the trial.

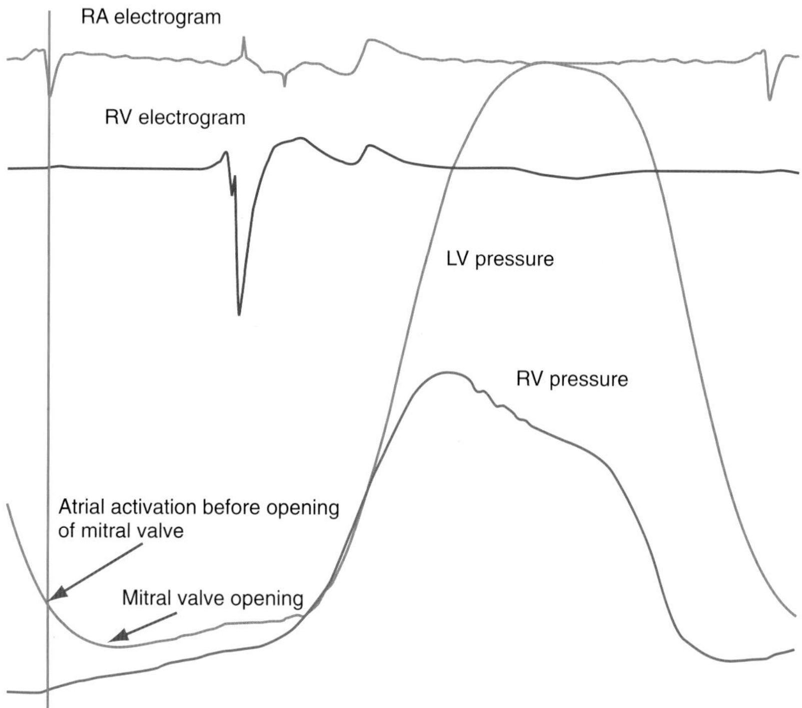

Figure 9-29. Right atrial (RA) and right ventricular (RV) electrograms and right and left ventricular (RV and LV) pressures from a third patient with New York Heart Association (NYHA) class III heart failure from the Pacing Therapies for Congestive Heart Failure (PATH-CHF) II trial.[149] No noticeable atrial booster pump effect can be observed in the ventricular pressure tracings. It is interesting that the RA activation is detected at the RA appendix before the mitral valve has had time to open. Note also the large asynchrony present in this patient at baseline.

how much preexcitation of the late-activated region is required to restore intraventricular synchrony (see later).

Role of Ventricular Synchrony

Abnormal asynchronous activation causes abnormal contraction patterns, inefficient and depressed pump function, and ventricular remodeling. Wiggers[30] recognized the importance of normal electrical activation of the ventricle for optimal pump function in 1925 (Fig. 9-30). However, it took about 70 years for the concept to gained broad interest. Two teams of investigators regarded the abnormal activation as being of little importance, because AV-sequential pacing allowed for significantly better cardiac pump function than V pacing.[123,124] Nevertheless, one group showed better pump function during LV apex pacing than during pacing at RV sites.[124] In the 1960s, Kosowsky and associates[125] compared RV apex pacing with His-bundle

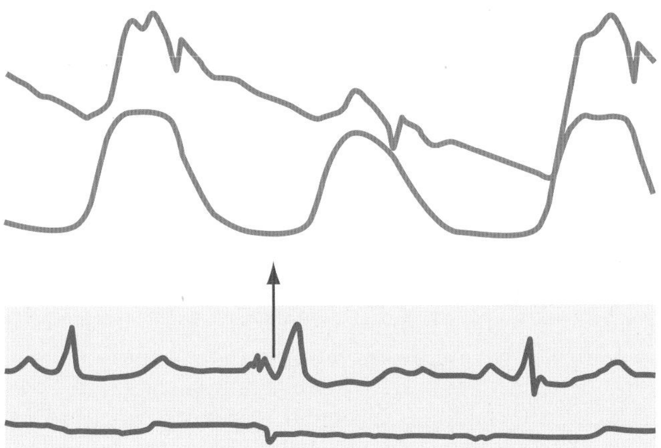

Figure 9-30. Original recording made by Wiggers, showing that in a paced beat (the second; note the widened QRS complex), left ventricular and aortic pressures are lower than in the preceding and sequential beats. (Modified from Wiggers CJ: The muscular reactions of the mammalian ventricles to artificial surface stimuli. Am J Physiol 73:346-378, 1925.)

pacing, the latter maintaining the normal activation but allowing variation of the AV interval. These investigators concluded that AV synchrony and proper sequence of activation are equally important. Their conclusion has been confirmed by later studies in animals and humans.[67,69,130]

Clinical Consequences of Asynchronous Activation

The combination of acute adverse hemodynamic effects and long-term ventricular remodeling (see Fig. 9-13) may explain why abnormal electrical activation and asynchronous electrical activation have major implications for the clinical status of the patient. Several studies have shown that morbidity and mortality are higher in patients with long-term RV apex pacing than with atrial pacing.[131,153-155] In patients with sinus node disease and good ventricular function, the risk for development of heart failure was significantly high after more than 7 years in a comparison of atrial pacing and RV pacing.[155] In a similar population, the risk of hospitalization for heart failure within 3 years increased with the percentage of time the patients underwent pacing at the RV apex.[156] Interestingly, the development of heart failure and atrial fibrillation was more sensitive to the percentage of pacing than to the pacing mode (single- or dual-chamber pacing). In patients who received an implantable cardioverter-defibrillator (ICD), the incidence of heart failure was higher within a year in patients in whom pacing occurred at VVI 70 bpm rather than in the backup mode.[157]

Although pacing and, even more, heart failure started at a later age in the studies just described, RV pacing in children can also induce impaired pump function. Tatengco and coworkers[108] observed such adverse effects after approximately 10 years of pacing.[108] Such dramatic effects of ventricular pacing in otherwise healthy myocardium may be explained by the pronounced structural changes in juvenile hearts.[94,158] The deleterious effect of ventricular pacing is relatively easy to discover because when pacing started is exactly known, but spontaneous evolution in a dilated cardiomyopathy cannot be excluded. Whether adverse effects of asynchronous activation are also applicable to LBBB has been less clear, because LBBB is a silent event that is often accompanied by considerable comorbidity.[159-161]

Longitudinal studies determining cardiovascular mortality and morbidity show that the existence of LBBB always carries a bad prognosis. In a 29-year follow-up study of 3983 pilots, the morbidity and cardiovascular mortality rate among those showing signs of LBBB was 17.2%, and the most common clinical event observed was sudden death without any previous symptoms (17%). These percentages are 10 times higher than those in subjects without LBBB.[162] In the Framingham Study, cumulative cardiovascular mortality over 10 years was approximately five times higher in patients with LBBB than in those without LBBB.[159] In a population of 110,000, the risk for development of cardiovascular diseases was 21% in the 112 patients with LBBB, compared with 11% in age- and sex-matched controls. Moreover, cardiac mortality was strongly increased in the patients with LBBB.

Until recently, the only direct evidence for an effect of LBBB on pump function came from studies in patients with intermittent LBBB.[163,164] Although the reduction in cardiac pump function after onset of LBBB is clear, the interpretation of these data is hampered by the fact that the onset of LBBB usually coincides with an increase in heart rate, elicited by an exercise test. The exercise test itself may confound the LBBB's effect on cardiac function, because it can induce myocardial ischemia.[34] Experimental proof of the negative effect of LBBB on hemodynamics has come from later studies in an animal model of LBBB. LBBB is created by ablation of the proximal part of the LBB.[49,165,166] After ablation of the LBB, the duration of the QRS complex, the asynchrony of contraction between RV and LV, and the asynchrony of electrical activation within the LV all increase significantly; also, relative to normal conduction values in the same species, these increases are similar in degree to the increases seen in patients with LBBB.[24,167] This finding suggests that, although the LBBB in patients may not be exclusively due to proximal lesions, this LBBB model resembles the LBBB in patients quite closely. All studies on this animal model of LBBB so far show that LBBB reduces systolic and diastolic LV function and induces paradoxical septal wall motion.[49,165,166]

Therefore, it appears that both RV apex pacing and LBBB are conditions that increase the risk of heart failure and cardiac death, especially in patients with already compromised function. For this reason, efforts to either prevent RV apex pacing or correct LBBB are rapidly growing. With our knowledge of electrical impulse conduction, it becomes obvious that the best solution may depend on whether the heart has normal or disturbed intrinsic conduction within the ventricles.

In the following discussion, various possible strategies are described, with current and possible future applications. Discrimination is made between strategies meant to maintain synchrony of activation and those meant to restore it.

Strategies to Maintain Ventricular Synchrony

Maintenance of ventricular synchrony has gained increasing attention. Several approaches have been used to achieve or maintain ventricular synchrony, such as atrial pacing and pacing from alternative ventricular sites, including the His bundle. More recently, LV pacing and BiV pacing have been specifically indicated in patients with ventricular conduction disturbance. Both methods are commonly referred as *cardiac resynchronization therapy;* they are discussed separately later in the chapter.

Atrial Pacing

Atrial pacing maintains normal ventricular activation but is obviously limited to patients with intact AV nodal conduction. In a comparison of atrial pacing with RV apex pacing in patients with sinus node disease (e.g., VVI vs. AAI), Andersen and colleagues[155] reported less development of all-cause mortality and cardiovascular death,[155] better maintenance of ventricular function and perfusion,[51] absence of atrial dilatation,[168] and a lower incidence of atrial fibrillation.[155,169] Although older studies compared atrial pacing with single-chamber pacing, later studies in patients with sick sinus syndrome showed a similar disadvantage of ventricular pacing in the dual-chamber mode in comparison with atrial pacing. Because the risk for development of AV block in this patient category (0.6% to 1.7% per year)[170,171] is considerably lower than that for development of heart failure (as high as 12%),[156] atrial pacing is an immediately applicable, easy, and effective way to avoid abnormal ventricular activation.

Alternative-Site Ventricular Pacing

Patients with disturbed AV conduction are pacemaker dependent and require ventricular pacing. In this case, His bundle pacing is obviously the way to maintain physiologic ventricular impulse conduction. Indeed, several animal studies showed QRS duration to be shorter with pacing in the high ventricular septum than with RV apex pacing.[68,158,172] In the 1960s, Scherlag's group showed that His bundle pacing results in the same QRS duration and pressure development as sinus rhythm and atrial pacing and in better hemodynamics than RV apex pacing.[125,173] Deshmukh and colleagues[174] were the first to successfully apply His bundle pacing in patients on a permanent basis.

Nevertheless, because of the relatively difficult positioning of the pacing lead into the His bundle position, pacing in the vicinity of the His bundle is more commonly used. In the literature, this position is referred to as "high RV septal" or "RV outflow tract (RVOT)," but in some studies, *RVOT* appears to imply pacing at the high RV free wall. Pacing in this region leads to abnormal QRS configuration in comparison with atrial pacing. Comparative studies of the acute hemodynamic effects of high septal pacing and RV apex pacing showed a moderate beneficial effect of septal pacing on LV pump function, although several studies did not find a significant difference between high septal and RV apex pacing.[175] Combined RV apex and RVOT pacing in patients resulted in shorter QRS duration than RVOT pacing alone but did not lead to further improvement of cardiac output.[176]

Longer-term studies appear to show a more consistent beneficial effect of high septal pacing. Tse and associates[177] randomly assigned 24 patients to either RV apex or high septal pacing. After 18 months of pacing, perfusion defects and regional wall motion abnormalities were less common and ejection fractions were higher in the high septal pacing group. Preliminary results of a randomized prospective trial reported by Gammage and Marsh,[178] who compared RV apex with high septal pacing in patients with AV block, indicate that after 18 months of pacing, high septal pacing has considerable benefit with regard to ventricular remodeling and neurohumoral activation.[178] The reports by both Tse and associates[177] and Gammage and Marsh[178] explicitly mentioned that the "RVOT" lead was positioned in the interventricular septum. Unfortunately, however, the exact best site at the RV septum is not well known. One animal study showed that the RV site for best hemodynamic function differs for individual hearts.[85]

In contrast, single-site LV pacing often results in better cardiac pump function than RV pacing.[82,179] Turner and colleagues[180] showed that LV pacing may also lead to more synchronous activation, if pacing is performed at longer AV intervals during maintained AV conduction in patients with a relatively narrow QRS complex.[180] Because electrical asynchrony and mechanical asynchrony within the LV wall are similar in RV pacing and LV pacing (Fig. 9-31),[181] the less detrimental hemodynamic effect of LV pacing may be explained by better interventricular coupling. This mechanism may also partially account for the beneficial hemodynamic effects of LV pacing in patients with heart failure and AV node ablation.[182] In these patients, no fusion can occur between the impulse wavefronts from endogenous conduction and LV stimulation. However, long-term comparative data in some subgroups of patients are still missing, so definitive conclusions cannot be drawn.

Animal studies have shown that within the LV, the septum and apex may be ideal pacing sites, because pacing in these sites was associated with LV pump function close to that during normal sinus rhythm, even with pacing at short AV intervals (Table 9-3).[85,183] An acute hemodynamic study in children supports this idea.[84] Experience in and materials for positioning a lead at the LV free wall have improved owing to the greater application of BiV pacing. LV septal pacing is not yet clinically feasible, because positioning a lead in the LV cavity may give rise to risk of embolization and stroke.[184] LV apex pacing would require thoracotomy. It is important to realize that little is known about lead

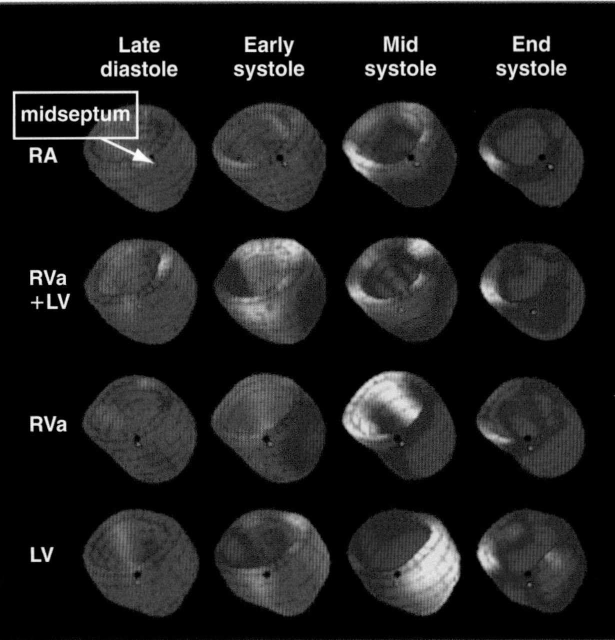

Figure 9-31. Three-dimensional reconstruction of the left ventricular (LV) wall with myocardial strain represented in color. Data were obtained using magnetic resonance tagging in a normal dog heart. Blue *indicates contraction (negative circumferential strain),* red *indicates the reference state (end diastole), and* yellow *indicates stretch (positive circumferential strain). Data are shown for late diastole and early systole, midsystole, and late systole for right atrial (RA), biventricular (RVa+LV), RV apex (RVa), and LV (LV) pacing.* White arrow *points to the midseptum. Note the considerable strain differences during both RVa and LV pacing in early systole and midsystole. RVa + LV pacing reduces these differences, but differences are still more pronounced than during RA pacing. (Modified from Wyman BT, Hunter WC, Prinzen FW, et al: Effects of single- and biventricular pacing on temporal and spatial dynamics of ventricular contraction. Am J Physiol 282:H372-H379, 2002.)*

stability, pacing thresholds, and possible complications associated with long-term LV apex pacing.

The degree of asynchrony induced by single-site ventricular pacing can be reduced by pacing at two or more sites simultaneously, preferably opposite to each other. This "multisite" pacing reduces QRS duration, however, by no more than 20% in comparison with single-site pacing.[45] Animal studies showed that BiV pacing does indeed lead to better LV pump function than RV pacing.[45,85,185] Also, in patients with atrial fibrillation and AV node ablation, hemodynamic performance was better during BiV pacing than during single-site LV or RV pacing.[186]

It is important to note that in patients with normal ventricular conduction, such novel pacing sites (LV apex, RVOT, His bundle, multisite) at best prevented a reduction of pump function compared with atrial pacing or sinus rhythm, but never improved it. Also left intraventricular mechanical asynchrony is only partially normalized despite BiV pacing.[187] This finding may be attributed to the fact that even multisite pacing cannot outmatch the quick impulse conduction and its extensive spread through the network of Purkinje fibers. Therefore, avoiding any kind of ventricular pacing would be preferable in hearts with normal ventricular conduction.

Minimizing Ventricular Pacing

One approach to avoiding any kind of ventricular pacing has been to program fixed long AV intervals; however, this approach resulted in occasional retrograde AV conduction and higher risk of arrhythmias in one third of a selected population.[188] For many years, some pacemakers have incorporated an algorithm based on the programming of two AV delays—a short, physiologic AV delay and a longer AV delay. These devices start pacing with the longer AV delay and continue at this setting if they find intrinsically conducted ventricular beats. If the intrinsic conduction is not present or fails to occur, the devices automatically switch to the shorter and more physiologic AV delay. When these devices function at the shorter AV delay, they periodically extend the AV delay to test for intrinsic conduction at programmable intervals. This type of algorithm is called *AV search hysteresis.*[189,190]

Rather than prolonging the AV delay, an algorithm called *managed ventricular pacing* (MVP) has been implemented in two studies.[191,192] With this algorithm, when intrinsic activity is present, only the atrium is paced; the ventricle is monitored on a beat-to-beat basis to verify intact AV conduction. Only in cases of transient and persistent loss of AV conduction does the MVP algorithm pacemaker switch to the DDDR mode. The mode intermittently tests for return of normal AV conduction. During atrial fibrillation, the device operates in the DDIR mode. With this approach, the cumulative percentage of ventricular pacing was reduced from a mean of 74% to 4%, with 80% of the patients being paced on the ventricle for less than 1% of the time.[191,192] One month follow-up in 181 patients did not find any device-related adverse effects. Because the number of patients who undergo pacing for sinus node disease is considerable, algorithms like AV search hysteresis and MVP appear quite promising for maintenance of ventricular synchrony in patients with predominantly intact AV and intraventricular conduction (Fig. 9-32).

Strategies to Restore Synchrony: Cardiac Resynchronization Therapy

BiV pacing devices, first implanted in March 1993,[193] were approved by the U.S. Food and Drug Administration (FDA) in 2001. The beneficial hemodynamic effects of BiV pacing during that small-scale study have been reproduced many times.[148,194-197] The consistency of the results of small but prospective randomized trials—such as the Pacing Therapies for Congestive Heart Failure (PATH-CHF) study,[149,198] the Multisite Stimulation in Cardiomyopathy (MUSTIC) trial,[199] the CArdiac REsynchronisation in Heart Failure (CARE-HF) study,[201]

TABLE 9-3. **Hemodynamic Parameters during VDD Pacing at Various Ventricular Sites in Dogs***

	Ventricular Site				
Parameter	**RV apex**	**LV lat**	**LV post**	**LV apex**	**LV septum**
Heart rate	1.048†	1.03	1.02	1.03	1.01
Stroke volume	0.930†‡	0.991‡	0.873†‡	1.05	1.03
Stroke work	0.789†‡	0.980‡	0.869‡	1.08	1.00
LV dP/dt_{pos}	0.931†‡	0.926†‡	0.927†‡	0.99	1.00
LV dP/dt_{neg}	0.799†‡	0.840†	0.849†	0.94	0.93
Tau	1.1†	1.189†‡	1.199†‡	1.06	1.04
ESLVP	0.952†	0.978	0.983	0.96	0.99
EDLVP	1.137†	1.231†	1.215	1.3	1.22
QRS duration	1.862†‡	1.997†	1.820†‡	1.940†	1.670†

*All values are expressed relative to the corresponding value during sinus rhythm. For all parameters, values during LV apex and LV septum pacing were not significantly different from those in sinus rhythm, except QRS duration. RV apex pacing leads to the most dramatic reduction in LV systolic and diastolic function.

†$P < .5$ as compared with SR apex pacing.

‡$P < .05$ as compared with LV apex pacing.

Data derived from Peschar M, de Swart H, Michels KJ, et al: Left ventricular septal and apex pacing for optimal pump function in canine hearts. J Am Coll Cardiol 41:1218-1226, 2003.

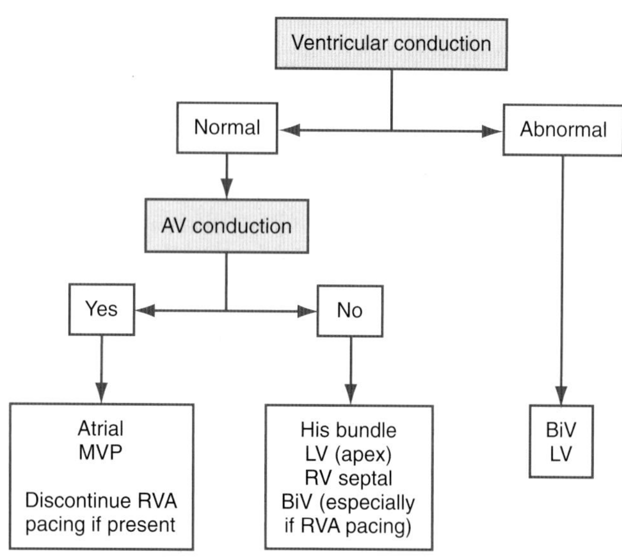

Figure 9-32. Flow diagram showing the most physiologic mode and/or site of pacing. Potential adverse effects of ventricular pacing and conduction disturbance, such as left bundle branch block (LBBB), on cardiac pump function. Ventricular pacing can induce nonphysiologic atrioventricular (AV) as well as interventricular (biventricular [BiV]) and intraventricular asynchrony. Assuming normal PQ times, LBBB causes only abnormal interventricular and intraventricular asynchrony. Effects of AV asynchrony are explained in text. LV, left ventricular; MVP, managed ventricular pacing; RVA, right ventricular apex.

and the Multicenter InSync Randomized Chronic Evaluation (MIRACLE) study[200]—have removed any doubt about the feasibility and clinical efficacy of CRT in highly symptomatic patients with heart failure. Large multicenter, randomized, controlled clinical trials have consistently demonstrated significant reductions in mortality and hospitalization rates for CRT in patients who had moderate to advanced heart failure despite optimal pharmacologic therapy and who presented with ventricular conduction delay, sinus rhythm, and depressed LV ejection fraction.[201]

Physiology of Cardiac Resynchronization Therapy

With the introduction of CRT, the use of cardiac pacemakers has been transformed from "just" artificial maintenance of the heart rhythm to restoration of pump function. Indeed, the restoration of ventricular mechanical synchrony by pacing the LV alone or in combination with the RV also has as its objective the restoration and/or maintenance of the proper timing of the atrial and ventricular contractions as well as RV and LV contractions.

The predominant intraventricular conduction abnormality in about one third of patients with heart failure is LBBB, during which activation spreads from the RBB to the RV wall and, after transseptal conduction, within the LV from the septum to the LV lateral wall (Fig. 9-33). Thus, pacing at the LV lateral wall is used to create an activation wavefront, which moves in the

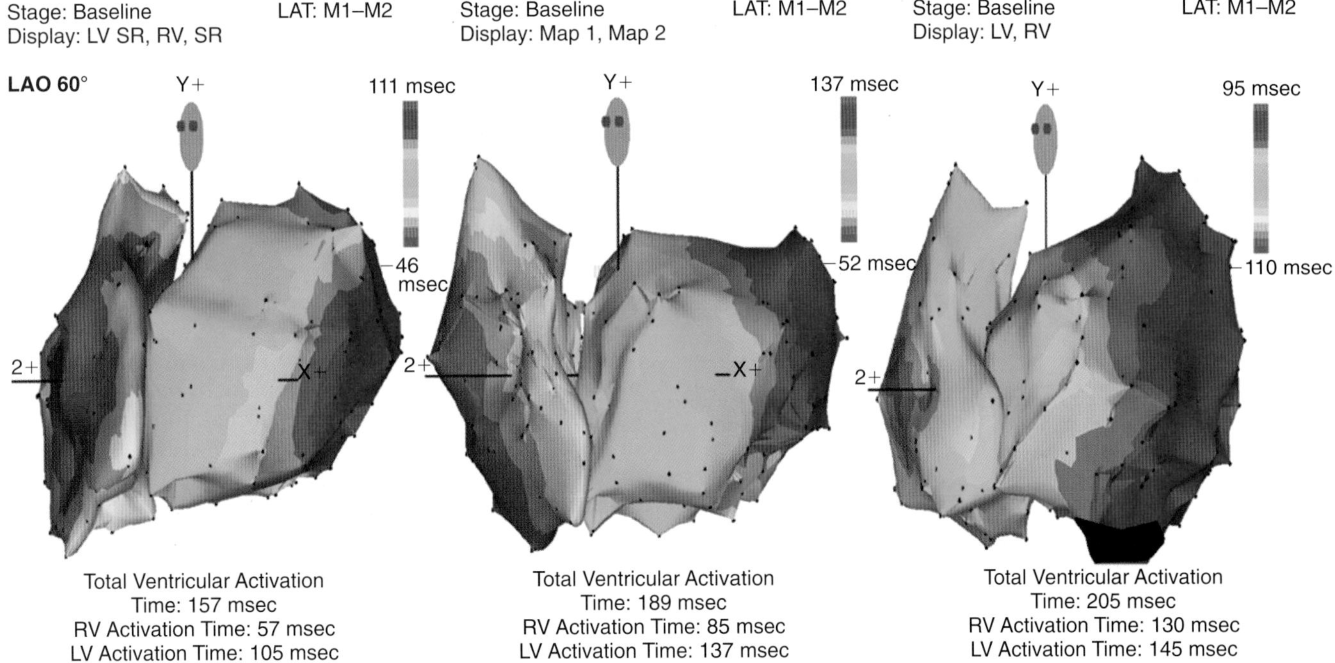

Figure 9-33. *Color-coded electroanatomic isochronal maps of right ventricular (RV) and left ventricular (LV) activation in three patients with heart failure and left bundle branch block. The earliest ventricular activation site is recorded at the RV anterolateral region* (red spot) *in all three cases. After almost 40 to 60 msec, a single LV septal breakthrough site is noted* (not shown). *The latest activated region is the LV posterolateral wall (*blue *to* purple *isochronal lines). The total activation endocardial time as well as the endocardial RV and LV endocardial times are shown for each patient.*

opposite direction from a spontaneously occurring activation wavefront.[16,26,29,31] Consequently, during BiV pacing, two activation wavefronts are generated and merge approximately in the middle.[35] A similar effect is obtained by single-site LV pacing using an AV interval that allows merging of the intrinsic activation originating from the RBB with the wavefront derived from the LV pacing lead. This merging wavefront leads to less electrical asynchrony in comparison with LBBB.[35] Because of the tight E-C coupling in the heart, CRT also improves coordination of contractions between the cardiac chambers and within the LV wall, as has been shown with different imaging techniques (see Fig. 9-31).[202,203] The better synchrony leads to improvement of cardiac pump function, as determined by LV dP/dt_{max}, pulse pressure, cardiac output, and ejection fraction.[35,148,196,197,204,205] Such improved systolic pump function is achieved at unchanged or even lower filling pressures, denoting a true improvement of ventricular contractility through better coordination of contraction. Moreover, Nelson and associates[60] have shown that better coordination of contraction improves mechanical pump function while slightly decreasing myocardial energy consumption. This finding suggests that CRT improves the efficiency of the cardiac pump. Further improvement in pump function is possibly mediated by reduction of mitral regurgitation[203] and prolongation of diastolic filling time.

These beneficial effects occur almost immediately after the start of resynchronization.[35,148] Intriguing data reported by Bleasdale and coworkers[206] suggest still another possible mechanism for LV pacing in patients with heart failure. Pacing the LV at a short AV interval increased LV filling through a mechanism called interventricular coupling or diastolic ventricular interaction. The idea is that early LV contraction also allows early LV filling. In hearts with high central venous pressures, where presumably the RV occupies much of the pericardial space, the early LV activation may allow the LV to fill first, thereby increasing its Frank-Starling relation.[206]

A variety of cardiac and extracardiac processes triggered by CRT are responsible for its long-term beneficial effect. First, the improved pump function reduces neurohumoral activation, an effect evidenced by an increase in heart rate variability and a reduction in plasma brain natriuretic peptide (BNP) levels.[207] Furthermore, the improved contractility and pump efficiency at a smaller end-diastolic volume reduce mechanical ventricular stretch. This latter reduction and the probably associated reduction in neurohumoral activation may well explain the beneficial reverse remodeling effect of CRT.[203,208] As elegantly demonstrated by Yu and colleagues,[203] such reverse remodeling points to structural improvement in the myocardium. These investigators showed the growing reverse remodeling effect of resynchronization over time by measuring the time course of LV cavity volume and LV dP/dt_{max} during the first 3 months after the start of CRT and during 1 month after CRT was temporarily stopped. After CRT was

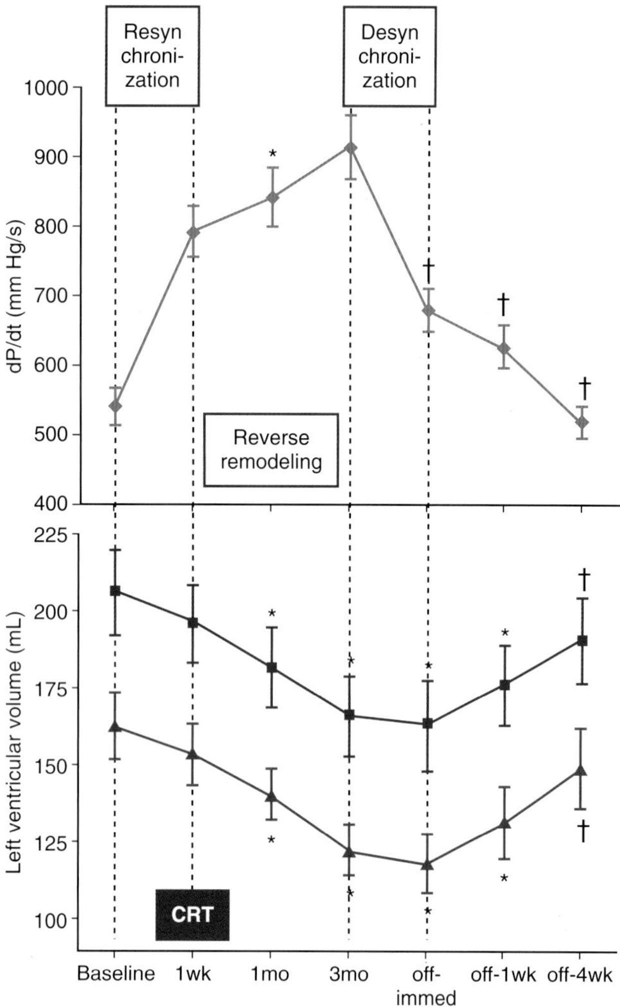

Figure 9-34. Acute hemodynamic and long-term reverse remodeling effects of cardiac resynchronization therapy. (Modified from Yu CM, Chau E, Sanderson JE, et al: Tissue Doppler echocardiographic evidence of reverse remodeling and improved synchronicity by simultaneously delaying regional contraction after biventricular pacing therapy in heart failure. Circulation 105:438-445, 2002.)

halted, some beneficial effect of CRT was still noticeable, pointing to adaptation in the tissue (Fig. 9-34).

Preliminary data from a study in canine LBBB hearts showed that isolated LBBB induces LV dilatation as well as hypertrophy and that these derangements are almost completely reversed by BiV pacing. Interestingly, BiV pacing reversed the hypertrophy in the LV wall, especially in the late-activated LV lateral wall.[49] This reduction in hypertrophy is important because hypertrophy may give rise to various molecular changes,[98] resulting in greater risk for contractile failure and arrhythmias. Notably, both hemodynamic improvement and reverse remodeling have been observed to a similar extent in dogs with LBBB (with and without heart failure)[35,166,209] and in patients with primary and secondary dilated cardiomyopathies. Furthermore, CRT has also been shown to be effective in patients with RBB block QRS morphology and in children with repaired congenital defects who present with right heart failure. Three-dimensional electroanatomic mapping data have provided the rationale for implementing CRT in these latter patient populations.[210]

Determination of Mechanical Asynchrony

The primary goal of CRT is to restore atrioventricular, interventricular, and intraventricular mechanical synchrony. The notion that a correlation between QRS duration and the change in systolic LV function during CRT may[63,158] or may not[85,176] exist has raised concern about whether QRS duration is a useful parameter for selecting candidates for CRT. The quantification of mechanical asynchrony in patients with heart failure is gaining interest. It has been reported that the measurement of mechanical asynchrony is a better predictor of the response to CRT than the duration of the QRS complex.[203,211,212] However, most of the studies evaluating mechanical criteria are small, mostly observational trials. Thus, a large clinical study comparing QRS duration with mechanical criteria is missing. At present, there are many methods for determining mechanical asynchrony; the sensitivity, specificity, and predictive value of each method are unknown.[202,212-221] Generally speaking, a distinction is made between *interventricular asynchrony* (between RV and LV) and *intraventricular asynchrony* (within the LV). Clinically feasible approaches to quantifying mechanical asynchrony have been reviewed.[222]

Interventricular asynchrony can be determined from the time difference between pulmonary and aortic valve openings with conventional echocardiography[167] or from the time to peak velocity in the RV and LV walls on tissue Doppler imaging (TDI). TDI is a relatively new echocardiographic technique that calculates and displays myocardial velocity in real time. It was developed in the early 1990s to quantitatively evaluate wall motion abnormalities in cardiac tissue.[223] Other approaches are determination of the phase difference of RV and LV wall motion using nuclear imaging[48] and use of the time or phase difference in the rise of RV and LV pressures.[165,224] The echocardiographic approach is, for practical reasons, most commonly used.

Intraventricular asynchrony usually requires more sophisticated equipment. The most detailed mechanical activation maps have been obtained through mapping of myocardial shortening (strain) patterns with magnetic resonance imaging tagging (see Fig. 9-7).[43,181,187] These studies have shown that the pattern of deformation gradually changes with increasing distance from the site of earliest activation (*asterisk* in Fig. 9-7). With a less expensive noninvasive method, M-mode echocardiography, the timing difference of maximal inward motion at the septum and posterior wall, or the septal-posterior wall motion delay (SPWMD),[225] can be calculated. The disadvantages of this simple technique are that peaks of septal wall motion are sometimes not precisely defined and that M-mode sections perpendicular to the septum are sometimes hard to acquire.

With color TDI and with pulsed-wave TDI, the time to peak systolic velocity can be measured in different regions of the myocardium.[203,216,226,227] TDI also has several inherent technical limitations. It measures the velocity of displacement of the myocardial segments relative to the ultrasound transducer and in the direction of the ultrasound beam. Likewise, the longitudinal velocity, as usually determined in basal regions, is the sum of all velocities developed in all regions between the transducer and a particular area. Local contraction can be derived only through subtraction of velocities in nearby regions. Such analysis on digitally stored color-coded tissue Doppler images yields myocardial strain and strain rate.[228] Such information is equivalent to that obtained with magnetic resonance imaging tagging, but with the great advantage that TDI can also be employed in the presence of a pacemaker. Strain measurements differentiate better than TDI between active systolic contraction and passive displacement. Likewise, Breithardt and colleagues[228] demonstrated more consistent behavior of strain than of velocity signals. Currently, however, image acquisition and analysis are time-consuming and still operator dependent. Therefore, the clinical applicability of strain-rate imaging is still limited. In a simpler, more user-friendly approach, a display of myocardial displacement called tissue tracking provides rough information about the distribution of regional myocardial motion.[202] This technique has also proved to be helpful in applying CRT.

The Role of the Site of Pacing

From a theoretical point of view, the sites of pacing that may be considered optimal are those that determine the greatest reduction in total activation time—that is, those pacing sites that generate two activation wavefronts starting from exactly opposite positions. Because in LBBB the basal part of the LV posterolateral wall is usually the latest-activated part,[39,38] it is often the preferred LV pacing site. Unfortunately, this site is not always accessible, especially when the transcoronary venous approach is used.

Gasparini and associates[229] showed that placing the LV lead close to the basal portion of the LV led to higher values for LV ejection fraction, quality of life, and distance walked in 6 minutes, similar to those reported for lateral lead placement. Their findings confirm previous observations by Butter and colleagues,[195] who showed that both anterior and lateral wall pacing sites improve LV contractility and pump function. However, pacing from the lateral wall resulted in a significantly larger increase in LV contractility; moreover, in about one third of patients, pacing from the anterior wall significantly depressed LV function. It is important to note that Butter and colleagues[195] paced the LV from a middle-apical position. High-resolution mapping data help explain these apparently discrepant findings (see Fig. 9-33). In patients with LBBB, the basal region of the heart is always the last region to be activated, with minor differences between the superior part of the LV (around the aortic root) and the posterior and posterobasal regions; the latter regions were the pacing sites selected by Gasparini and associates.[229] In contrast, the anterior middle-apical part of the LV is usually early-activated, representing the LV breakthrough site, and activation of the middle-apical part of the lateral wall, one of the pacing sites tested by Butter and colleagues,[195] is significantly delayed.

Finally, findings reported by Ansalone and coworkers,[230] which took into account the differences in activation time in individual patients, further substantiate these points. These investigators used TDI to assess the location of the region with the latest mechanical activation and investigated whether concordance of the position of the LV lead and of the latest-activated region influences the outcome of CRT. Indeed, the largest effect on functional parameters was seen when the LV lead was in the latest-activated region. Although optimization of the pacing site is often difficult when the transcoronary venous access is used, positioning the LV lead through the use of limited thoracotomy may be very helpful. During such a procedure, LV pressure-volume analysis showed the importance of choosing the best position of the LV lead.[204]

Given the electrical similarity of the spontaneously occurring LBBB and the LBBB induced by RV pacing, several centers have explored the feasibility of "upgrading" already implanted RV pacemakers to BiV ones or, in the case of a new implant, to use BiV pacing from the beginning in select patients. The results appear to depend on the clinical setting. In patients with already implanted RV pacing leads, the upgrade leads to improvements in cardiac function and clinical outcome.[231,232] However, the situation is less clear when RV and BiV pacing are compared in patients with atrial fibrillation immediately after AV nodal ablation.[233,234] In these crossover studies, parameters such as quality of life, New York Heart Association (NYHA) diagnostic class, and 6-minute walking distance showed modest differences between RV pacing and BiV pacing. However, echocardiographic measures demonstrated moderate improvements with BiV over RV pacing.[233] These findings are supported by experimental data showing that both RV pacing and BiV DDD pacing are able to completely reverse LV hypertrophy and dilatation as induced by chronic AV nodal ablation in dogs.[85] Altogether, these data suggest that the effects of ventricular pacing should be considered against the background of the disease in which it is used.

Another important issue, yet unresolved, is whether LV pacing alone is sufficient for adequate CRT. In dogs and patients with LBBB, LV pacing improves LV pump function at least as much as BiV pacing.[35,148,196,197] LV pacing has also been shown to lead to clinical improvements at up to 1 year of follow-up.[235,236] The promising effect of pacing at this single site can be explained by the fusion that occurs between the LV pacing–triggered wavefront and the wavefront created by the intrinsic conduction through the RBB.[35] More data on this question will come from the ongoing Device Evaluation of CONTAK RENEWAL 2 and EASYTRAK 2: Assessment of Safety and Effectiveness in Heart Failure (DECREASE HF) Study,[237] in which the effects of BiV and LV pacing in remodeling and exercise capacity are being compared.

Given individual variations in etiology, severity, patterns of delayed ventricular activation, location of regions of scar, and extent of mitral regurgitation in heart failure, it seems unlikely that one pacing site will "fit all." Obviously, even if LV pacing would be sufficient for proper resynchronization, other factors continue to warrant RV lead placement in many patients. In particular, current implantable defibrillator systems require an RV lead for tachyarrhythmia sensing and high-voltage therapies. Moreover, if a patient undergoing CRT also requires optimization of the AV interval owing to prolonged PQ time or backup ventricular pacing, an RV lead would be important to allow pacing in case of dislodgment of the LV lead, a complication that occurs in 5% to 10% of patients.

The Role of Atrial Pacing and Sensing

Given the rationale of CRT, continuous ventricular pacing should be provided to maximize pump function and cardiac efficiency. Many people equivocally equate a pacemaker with a resynchronizer, but even though they are remarkably similar in function and characteristics, the two devices fundamentally differ in one respect. A primary rule of a pacemaker is to restore the rhythm when it is absent; a secondary, less important, and even questionable goal (owing to the extreme difficulty of maintaining the correct sequence of activation in the ventricles during ventricular pacing) is to restore the proper AV timing in patients with first-degree AV block. In contrast, the primary rule of a resynchronizer is to resynchronize all the time, whether intrinsic activation is present or not. This difference creates opposite goals for the two devices in many situations.

For instance, the effect of programming a long postventricular atrial refractory period (PVARP) has manifested itself in the CRT application of BiV pacing with more serious consequences. The issue is triggered by a beat that was supposed to receive BiV pacing but that is skipped by the pacemaker—not paced—owing to either an ectopic beat (or premature ventricular contraction [PVC]) or an atrial sense during PVARP; in both of these cases, an intrinsic beat follows the intrinsic AV interval. In a CRT application, this last intrinsic beat always has a longer AV interval than the programmed AV delay. The intrinsic R wave sensed by the pacemaker triggers a new PVARP, which may block the next P wave even if the heart rate has fallen below the rate defined by the total atrial refractory period (TARP)—which is defined as follows: TARP = PVARP + PR. (The maximal atrial tracking rate [MATR] is equal to 60/TARP; Figs. 9-35 and 9-36.) This occurs at heart rates lower than the MATR, because (1) the TARP after the intrinsic beat (TARPi) is longer than the paced TARP (TARPi = PR + PVARP) and (2) the intrinsic AV interval is longer than the programmed AV interval and higher than MATRi = 60/TARPi. Henceforth, CRT is not restored until the heart rate falls below the new value defined by the TARPi (MATRi = 60/TARPi).

This issue is not important for bradyarrhythmia pacing, because the goal in this method is to restore rhythm, and pacing is not necessary if there is adequate intrinsic activity. The issue becomes critical, however, during CRT, which must be delivered 100% of the time. Some new CRT and CRT-defibrillator (CRT-D) devices have incorporated features that detect this situation; they transiently shorten the PVARP created by ventricular-sensed beats, allowing pacing to be reestablished without increasing the risk of triggering a pacemaker-mediated tachyarrhythmia (PMT). A PVC can also place a pacemaker device into this mode. A novel feature now part of some CRT devices eliminates this problem

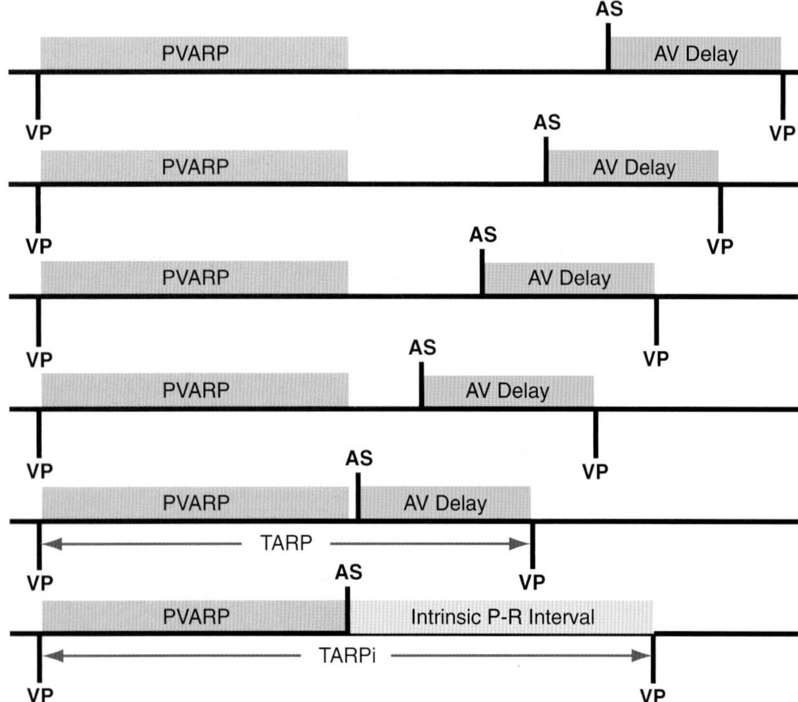

Figure 9-35. The typical findings in a patient undergoing pacing at the sinus rate as this sinus rate increases, approaching the maximum atrial tracking rate (MATR) defined by the TARP (total atrial refractory period = postventricular atrial refractory period + atrioventricular interval). MATR = 60/TARP. In the bottom panel, *when the atrial sense (AS) encroaches into postventricular atrial refractory period (PVARP), the pacemaker, following its logic, will not pace. In a patient with third-degree block, that beat would be kept, but in a typical patient with heart failure who is a candidate for cardiac resynchronization therapy and has intact atrioventricular (AV) conduction, an intrinsic ventricular activation will most likely occur after the PR interval. The intact AV conduction, therefore, leads to a new TARP (TARPi = PVARP + P-R) longer than the previous TARP. VP, ventricular pacing; VS, ventricular sensing.*

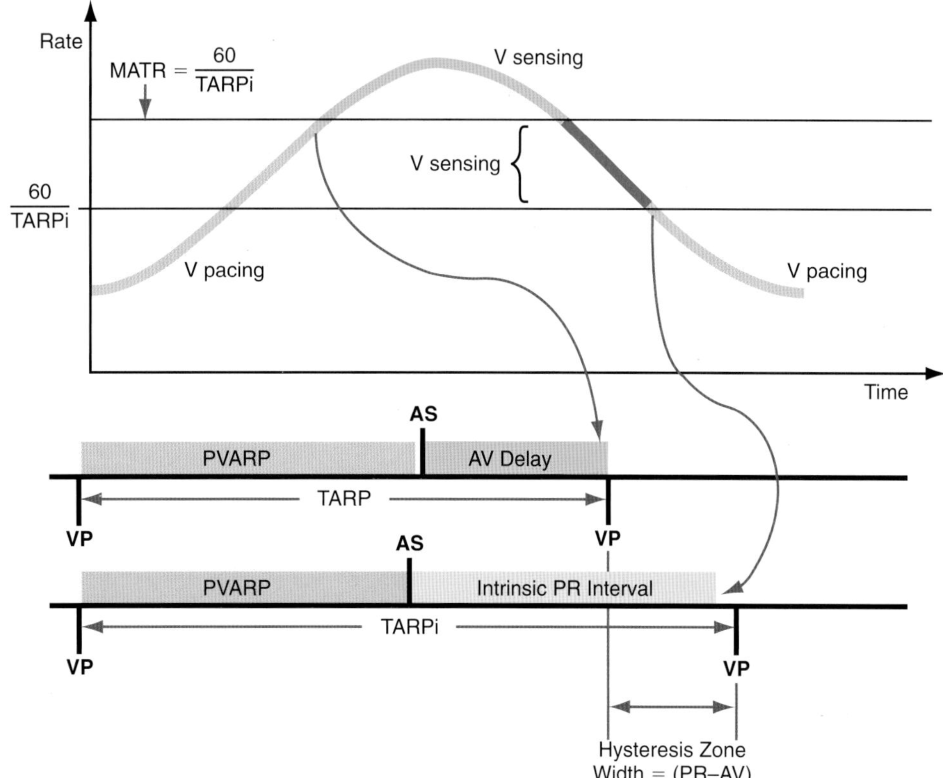

Figure 9-36. Illustration of the fact that after an intrinsic activation of the ventricles has occurred, biventricular pacing will not be resumed even after the atrial rate has fallen below the maximum atrial tracking rate (MATR) (region in red). The sinus rate will need to fall below the new MATR (MATRi = 60/TARPi) for pacing to resume. Creating a region of heart rates between MATRi and MATR, where the patient could be resynchronized or not, depends on the history of the change in heart rate before that region was reached. This effect could be really significant during cardiac resynchronization therapy (CRT), because many patients are programmed with conservatively low MATR and would stop receiving CRT during exercise, when they most need it. AV, atrioventricular; VP, ventricular pacing.

by transiently shortening the PVARP when this condition is detected, thus reestablishing CRT immediately.

A minimum heart rate is required to maintain adequate heart function without triggering heart failure. A minimum heart rate is also required to enable the heart to generate enough cardiac output to sustain the body's metabolic needs. Nevertheless, we now know that the lower the heart rate, the higher the efficiency, even with the lower heart rates favoring angiogenesis. A first attempt to define an adequate heart rate could be taken by stating that given these two opposing driving forces, the optimal heart rate for a given patient would be the lowest rate that creates sufficient cardiac output to satisfy basic metabolic needs in that patient at a given point. For a patient with normal ventricular function and no heart failure, a more aggressive stance could be taken with respect to programming higher parameters for lower rate limit (LRL) and rate response in the presence of sinus bradycardia or chronotropic incompetence. But even for patients with normal ventricular function, the yet-unanswered question is: What are the long-term effects of using higher LRL values than absolutely necessary? In the Dual Chamber and VVI Implantable Defibrillator (DAVID) trial, dual-chamber ICD pacing was programmed to an LRL of 70 bpm and short AV intervals; its results strongly suggest that these settings were worse than a simple setting of the ICD to VVI with an LRL of 40 bpm. Many people now believe that most of the detrimental effects observed in the DDD arm of this trial can be accounted for by the fact that RV pacing creates an asynchronous contraction; one must keep in mind, however, that there was one other difference between the two arms, the higher LRL.[238] The effect seen could have been due to the combination of both an asynchronous contraction and a higher than necessary LRL. The outcome of the DAVID II study should shed some light on this very important issue.

To summarize, the data available strongly suggest that caution is required in programming the pacemaker's LRL to be higher than the sinus rate in patients with heart failure, whether or not they have sick sinus syndrome. Also, acute adverse hemodynamic consequences, such as lower cardiac outputs (see Fig. 9-17) and elevated pulmonary pressures, can occur as a result of LA contraction against a closed mitral valve, triggered by the increase in interatrial conduction time created by atrial pacing (Fig. 9-37). Moreover, higher than necessary heart rates worsen mechanical efficiency (see Fig. 9-16), decrease angiogenesis, exacerbate heart failure, and may even increase mortality (Fig. 9-38). In the case of patients who receive a CRT implant (CRT or CRT-D device) primarily for heart failure indications, a general rule of thumb is to program the lower rate limit (LRL) well below the sinus rate unless a clear clinical need to pace the atrium can be documented; current clinical and scientific evidence strongly suggests that the LRL should not be raised above the sinus rate in patients undergoing CRT.

The Role of Optimizing AV Interval in Cardiac Resynchronization Therapy

As discussed earlier in this chapter, the AV interval strongly influences ventricular preload and thereby stroke volume in patients with reduced ejection fraction. However, during CRT, the AV interval also affects

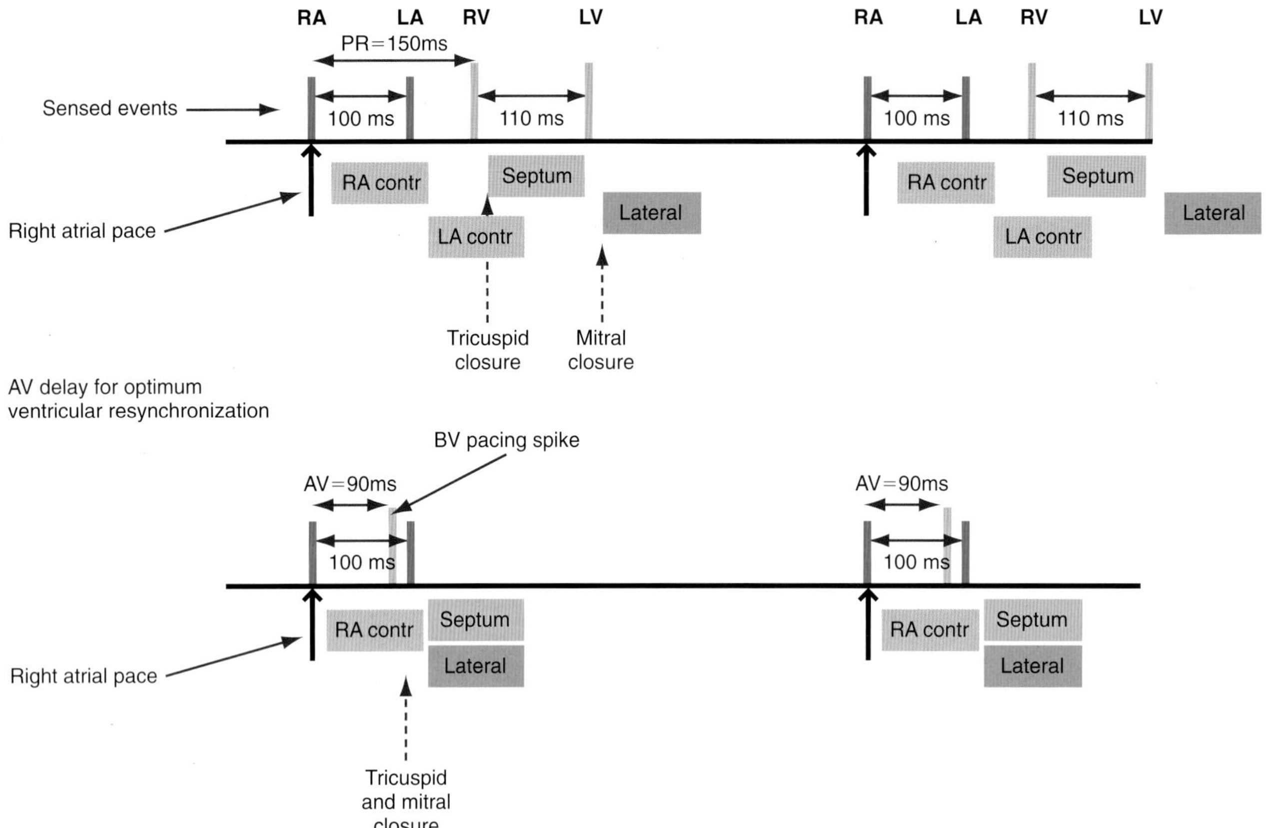

Figure 9-37. *Left atrial (LA) contraction (contr) after mitral valve closure.* Top panel, *Schematic illustration of a patient undergoing atrial pacing, in whom sensing in both ventricles has an interatrial conduction delay of 100 msec and, for the sake of simplicity, an equal mechanical delay. The patient's intrinsic atrioventricular (AV) interval (marked as PR in the figure) is 150 msec. The figure illustrates how after a small electromechanical delay, the right and left atrial (RA and LA) contractions follow their electrical activations. This patient also has an intraventricular conduction defect, which makes the septum (marked as RV) activate 110 msec earlier than the lateral wall of the left ventricle (marked as LV). Similarly, both activations are followed after a small electromechanical delay by the septal and left lateral wall contractions. This figure shows how the mechanical asynchrony of the LV prevents the LA from contracting against a closed mitral valve.* Bottom panel, *What happens when the septum and left lateral wall are resynchronized with the optimum AV interval. Note also the clinically significant increase in filling time created by resynchronization. BV, biventricular.*

ventricular pump function by modifying ventricular asynchrony. At long AV intervals, the impulse conducted through the AV node and RBB spreads into the RV and from there toward the LV. At shorter AV intervals, however, complete capture occurs from the pacing site(s), allowing resynchronization. The largest improvements in dP/dt_{max} have been found to occur at this point of transition from noncapture to complete capture. The best LV pump function is obtained with use of a relatively short AV interval, which allows complete activation of the ventricles from the two pacing sites.[148] This AV interval may be different from the one resulting in optimized preload (Fig. 9-39).[151] In one half of patients, the AV interval for optimal preload is usually longer than the one for optimal synchrony; henceforth, it is no surprise that the mean difference between the two AV intervals is close to zero.[148]

To date, no clinical data are available to help sort through the relative importances of optimizing synchrony and optimizing preload. However, considering that asynchrony is a major cause of depressed pump function in patients with intraventricular conduction abnormalities and that resynchronization has both short- and long-term beneficial effects, the authors of this chapter postulate that the primary target should be resynchronizing the ventricles and that optimizing the ventricular inflow is of secondary importance in the majority of patients, especially when atrial pacing is not used.[239] The importance of restoration of ventricular asynchrony is supported by studies on the beneficial effect of CRT in patients with atrial fibrillation. In these patients, no preload optimization can be performed, and also, any possible beneficial effect on preload through CRT is excluded. Nevertheless, CRT has been shown to be effective in patients with atrial fibrillation and wide QRS complexes, and the extent of improvement appears to be comparable with that seen in patients in sinus rhythm.[240]

Considering that the optimal AV interval is the one that leads to optimal ventricular synchrony, measurements of mechanical asynchrony may be helpful in assessing this interval. In addition, invasive and noninvasive determinations of cardiac contractility and stroke volume may be performed. However, invasive determination is cumbersome and expensive and may carry significant risk for the patient. On the basis of acute hemodynamic data collected in patients with heart failure who were undergoing CRT, a simple and widely applicable formula has been determined.[148,149,151,241] The electrocardiographic formula was based on the observation that the measured intracardiac AV interval was highly correlated with the AV interval that provided the largest improvements in LV dP/dt_{max} over the value seen with intrinsic conduction (Fig. 9-40).

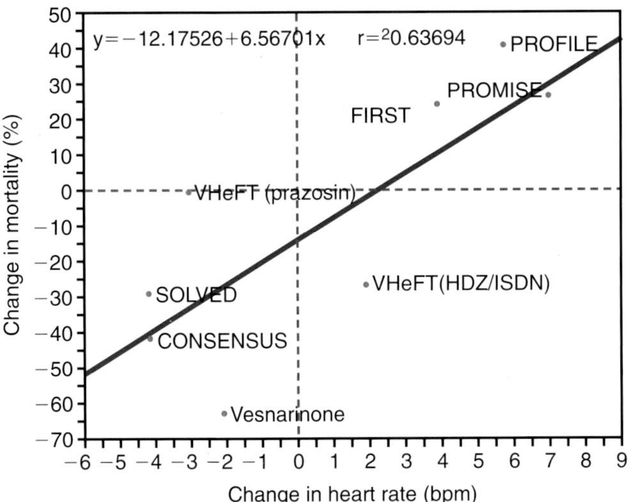

Figure 9-38. The relationship between the chronic changes in heart rate obtained with several drug therapies and their effect on mortality rates in patients with heart failure. Curiously, there is a strong correlation between mortality benefit and the ability of a drug to achieve a reduction in the heart rate of the patients in the active therapy arm of the trial. HDZ/ISDN, hydralazine/isosorbate dinitrate; VHeFT, Veteran Affairs Vasodilator Heart Failure Trial.

An important observation was that the correlation between maximum LV contractility and optimal AV interval varied among patients, but when the patients were grouped according to baseline QRS duration, a consistent relationship was found between intrinsic AV delay and the AV delay that created the highest LV contractility. A cutoff of 150 msec in QRS duration divided patients with heart failure into two groups. The algorithm determines the optimal AV delay interval as time difference from intracardiac atrial deflection (sensed from the RA lead) to the intracardiac RV deflection (sensed by the RV lead) multiplied by a constant factor (0.7). For patients with a QRS width >150 msec, the optimal AV delay interval is:

$$(0.7) \times \text{intrinsic AV delay} - 55 \text{ msec} \qquad (9\text{-}1)$$

For patients with a QRS duration ≤150 msec, the optimal AV delay interval is:

$$(0.7) \times \text{intrinsic AV delay} \qquad (9\text{-}2)$$

However, there are clinical situations in which echocardiographic assessment is also required, especially

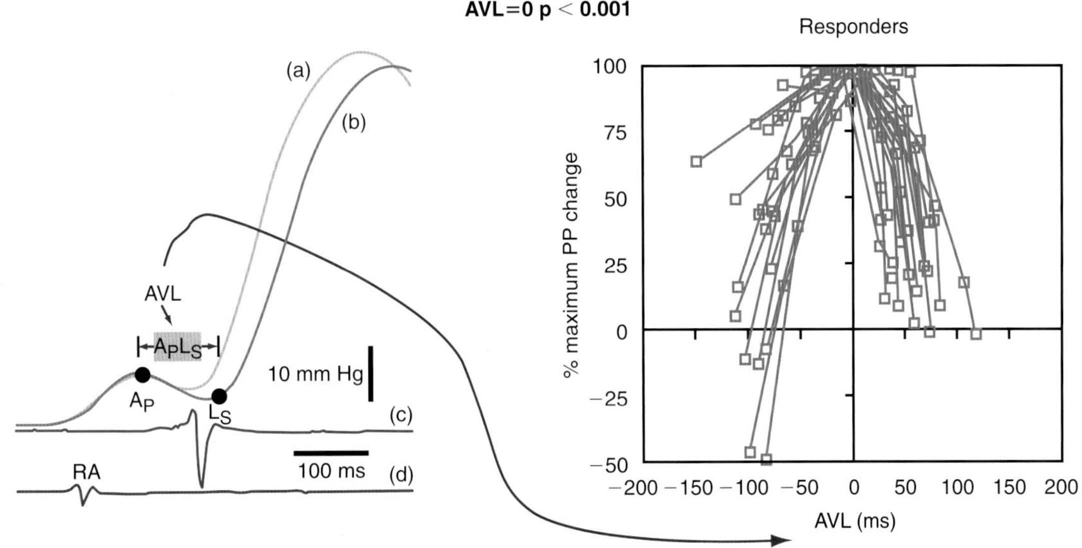

Figure 9-39. Maximum preload is associated with maximum increase in pulse pressure. Left, *The upstroke of the intraventricular pressure waveform in a patient with New York Heart Association (NYHA) class III heart failure from the Pacing Therapies for Congestive Heart Failure (PATH-CHF) I trial.[148] (a), During pacing at an intermediate AV interval; (b), during intrinsic propagation through the AV node of the normal atrial depolarization; (c), the ventricular electrogram during intrinsic activation; (d), the atrial electrogram. AVL is the time from the peak of the intraventricular pressure increase created by the booster pump action of the left atrium (A_p) and the start of the ventricular contraction (L_s). RA, right atrial.* Right, *The relationship between the percentage increase in aortic pulse pressure versus baseline (no pacing) obtained during cardiac resynchronization therapy (CRT) at different atrioventricular (AV) intervals (y-axis) versus the time between A_p and L_s for all the patients in whom hemodynamics improved with CRT in the PATH CHF I trial.*

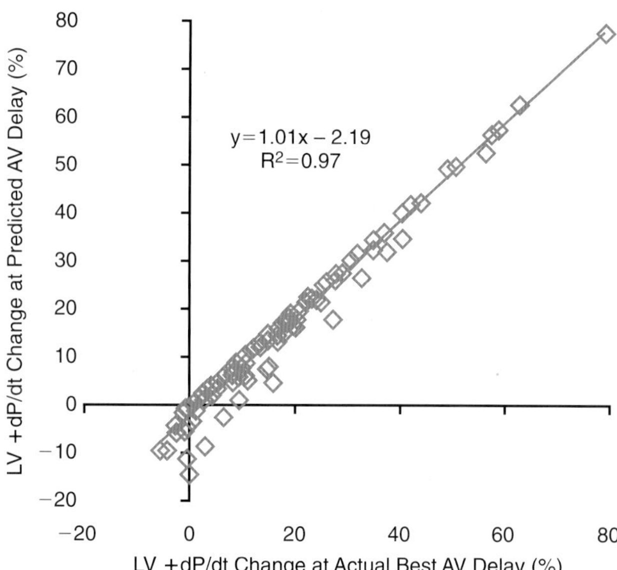

Figure 9-40. The x-axis represents the left ventricular (LV) dP/dt_{max} improvement obtained at the atrioventricular (AV) delay that optimized LV dP/dt_{max} (invasively measured with a Millar Microtip catheter in the Pacing Therapies for Congestive Heart Failure [PATH-CHF] I and II trials). The y-axis represents the LV dP/dt_{max} obtained at the estimated optimal AV delay with the formulas used in the Comparison of Medical Therapy, Pacing, and Defibrillation in Chronic Heart Failure (COMPANION) trial (see text).

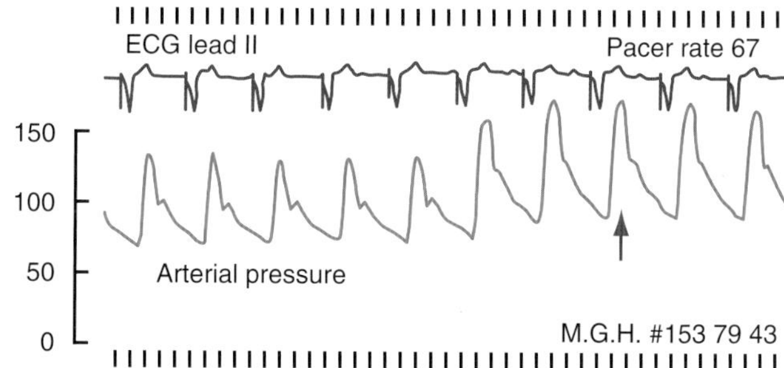

Figure 9-41. Radial artery pressure from a patient with complete atrioventricular (AV) block during fixed-rate ventricular pacing. Peak systolic pressure is seen when the PR interval is 270 msec (arrow).

the patient in whom interatrial block is suspected. A Doppler inflow analysis may be indicated to prevent the increases in pulmonary pressures and hemodynamic decompensation that could be caused by contraction of the LA against a completely closed mitral valve. Another situation that requires the use of Doppler inflow analysis to verify proper timing of the atrial contraction is the presence of high atrial rates. High intrinsic atrial rates are usually associated with short filling times as well as a very narrow range of the optimum AV intervals able to reestablish the proper AV synchrony. For the selected AV interval, the possibility of atrial contraction against a completely closed mitral and/or tricuspid valve should be considered.

Effect of Interventricular Delay

Some of the latest-generation CRT devices offer the possibility of independently programming AV interval and interventricular (VV) interval. A few studies reporting the effect of changing VV intervals during BiV pacing have conflicting results.[186,242-244] In the majority of patients, simultaneous RV-LV activation (0 LV offset) provides the largest increase of LV contractility. However, in a group of patients, preexcitation of the LV 20 to 30 msec before RV pacing may improve LV hemodynamic function.[244]

A positive influence of VV interval is conceivable. According to the current model of how CRT works, the best resynchronization would be achieved by maximizing the synchrony of the activation through manipulation of the three activation wavefronts originating from the RBB, RV, and LV pacing leads. However, this same reasoning also indicates that an optimal VV interval may depend on the AV interval. The previously mentioned studies have not tested all the possible variations. Therefore, differences in optimal VV intervals may, for example, be due to the use of different AV intervals. In clinical practice, testing all the different possible combinations of AV interval and VV interval seems impractical. Thus, optimal use of the extensive possibilities to vary timing of stimulation may be fully applicable only if medical equipment manufacturers provide adequate tools that are specifically designed and validated for the fine-tuning of ventricular synchrony.

Pacemaker Syndrome

When pacemaker syndrome was first described, it was attributed to ventricular pacing and recognized primarily as a problem of single-chamber ventricular pacemakers. However, with the greater use of dual-chamber pacing modes, it has become apparent that pacemaker syndrome is not unique to ventricular pacing but may occur in different pacing modalities.[245-252]

Pacemaker syndrome is an array of cardiovascular and neurologic signs and symptoms resulting from disruption of appropriate AV synchrony (AV dyssynchrony) due to suboptimal pacing, inappropriate programming of pacing parameters, or upper-limit behavior of AV synchronous pacing systems. The pathogenesis of pacemaker syndrome is complex, involving atrial and vascular reflexes and the neurohumoral system as well as the direct hemodynamic consequences of the loss of atrial systole. Patients most prone to the development of pacemaker syndrome are those with 1:1 retrograde ventriculoatrial conduction (Figs. 9-41 and 9-42) and those with lower stroke volume during ventricular pacing than with sinus rhythm or dual-chamber pacing. This syndrome may occur, however, with any mode of pacing that results in permanent or temporary disruption of atrial and ventricular synchronous contraction.

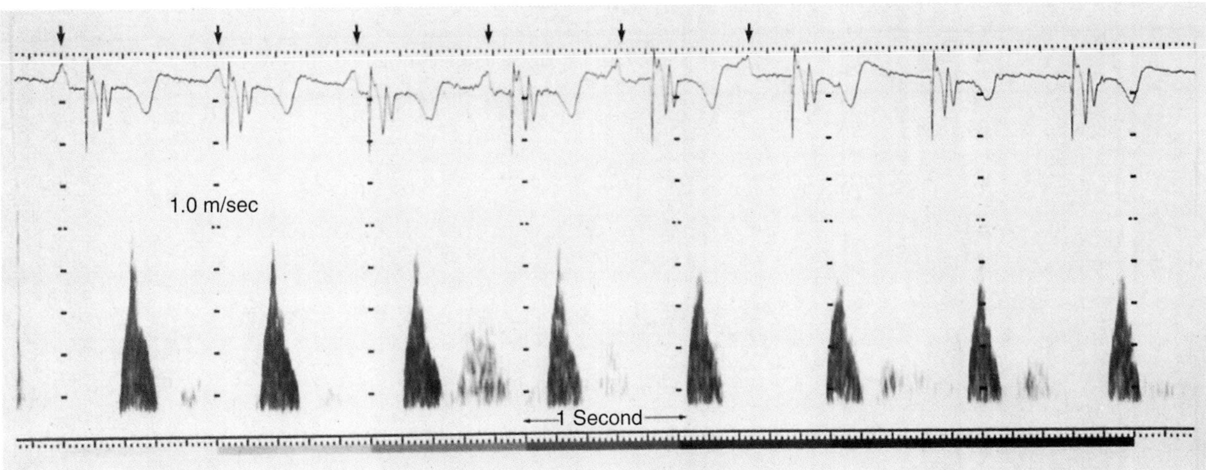

Figure 9-42. Doppler aortic flow-velocity integrals during ventricular pacing in a patient with complete heart block. The effect of fortuitously timed P waves (arrows) *on aortic flow is demonstrated.*

Patients treated with CRT devices may also theoretically demonstrate a pacemaker syndrome owing to inappropriate timing of the LA and LV. Indeed, interatrial conduction time can be significantly prolonged in patients with dilated cardiomyopathy. During CRT, the contraction of the late-activated region (most commonly located in the lateral wall of the LV) is advanced to coincide with the start of the contraction of the early-activated region (most commonly located in the interventricular septum and the RV free wall) to maximize mechanical synchrony and henceforth efficiency.[60,61] In a heart in which the mechanical contraction of the LA has been delayed—because, for instance, of a combination of interatrial block and atrial pacing—it is conceivable that the LA contraction will occur against a closed mitral valve, especially during BiV pacing, in which the contraction of the LV has been advanced with respect to the activation of the atria (Fig. 9-43). This phenomenon has been described for patients with pacemakers, in whom the issue is less likely, because RV pacing normally delays the mechanical contraction of the LV, increasing the time available for the LA to contract before the mitral valve is finally closed by the LV contraction and subsequent pressure increase.[138] In New York Heart Association (NYHA) functional classes III and IV heart failure, occurrence of the LA contraction after the closure of the mitral valve may trigger sudden increases in pulmonary pressures (similar to the cannon A waves seen in pacemaker syndrome, which are usually observable in the jugular veins); the increases could lead to acute decompensation and pulmonary edema in a patient with heart failure. It is also important to realize that this situation could be triggered by atrial pacing because of the increased AV delay that this mode of pacing creates.

Pacemaker syndrome can be treated with an upgrade of the implanted device or with reprogramming of the parameters to achieve the optimal synchrony of atrial and ventricular contraction. Symptoms associated with pacemaker syndrome are variable in severity and onset (Table 9-4). The exact incidence of pacemaker syndrome is unknown. It has been estimated that moderate to severe symptoms of pacemaker syndrome occur in about 5% to 7% of patients in whom the ventricle is mostly paced (see Fig. 9-43) and that a slightly higher percentage of patients (up to 10% of patients undergoing VVI pacing) present with mild symptoms.

TABLE 9-4. Symptoms of Pacemaker Syndrome

Mild	Pulsations in neck, abdomen Palpitations Fatigue, malaise, weakness Cough Apprehension Chest fullness or pain Headache, jaw pain
Moderate	Shortness of breath on exertion Dizziness, tiredness, vertigo Orthopnea, paroxysmal nocturnal dyspnea Choking sensation Confusion or alteration of mental state
Severe	Presyncope Syncope Shortness of breath at rest, pulmonary edema

The pathophysiology of the pacemaker syndrome is rather complex, involving hemodynamic, neurohumoral, and baroreceptor changes. In addition to direct hemodynamic effect of loss of AV synchrony or 1:1 retrograde ventriculoatrial conduction, atrial and vascular reflexes initiated by atrial distention or elevated atrial pressures may also play a role in the pathophysiology of pacemaker syndrome. Atrial receptors and cardiopulmonary reflexes have been the subject of several in-depth reviews.[253,254] Ellenbogen and colleagues[255,256] extensively investigated the role of baroreflex activity

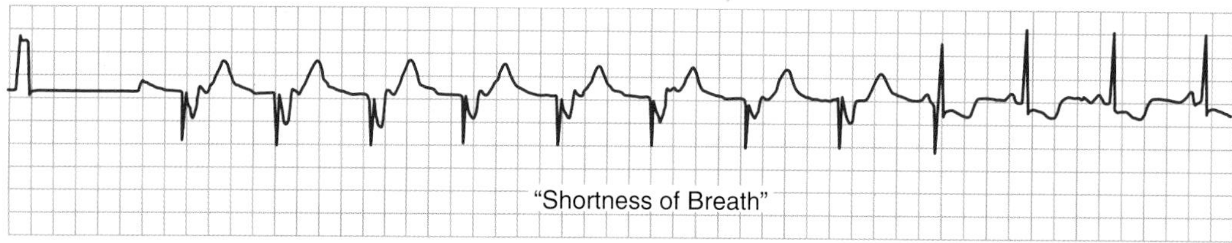

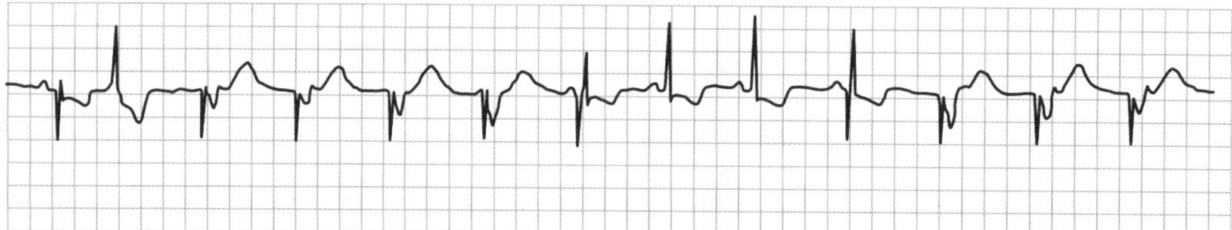

Figure 9-43. Continuous rhythm strips recorded with a transtelephonic cardiac monitor in a 65-year-old farmer with pacemaker syndrome. This patient's underlying rhythm disorder was sick sinus syndrome with sinus bradycardia, and he had experienced multiple episodes of atrial fibrillation 1 year earlier. His sinus bradycardia was exacerbated by treatment with quinidine, verapamil, and digoxin. One month after implantation of a VVIR device, the patient returned to his physician complaining of fatigue, weakness, dizziness, malaise, and shortness of breath. After documentation of this rhythm by a cardiac event monitor, he underwent further testing. During VVI pacing, ventriculoatrial (VA) dissociation occurred. During VVI pacing at 90 bpm, the patient's blood pressure dropped to 90 systolic/68 diastolic mm Hg; during AAI pacing, it was 160/90 mm Hg (at 90 bpm). During sinus rhythm at 58 to 64 bpm, the blood pressure measured 136/70 mm Hg. A DDDR pacemaker was implanted, and within 48 hours, the patient's symptoms were abolished. He returned to his active, vigorous lifestyle and experienced no subsequent episodes of atrial fibrillation for 1 year. (From Ellenbogen KA, Wood MA, Strambler B: Pacemaker syndrome: Clinical, hemodynamic, and neurohumoral features. In Barold SS, Mujica J [eds]: New Perspectives in Cardiac Pacing 3. Mt Kisco, NY, Futura, 1992.)

during pacemaker syndrome provoked by VA pacing, providing evidence that inadequate systemic sympathetic response plays a key role in the onset of pacemaker syndrome (Fig. 9-44). Indeed, when patients assume an upright position, blood is pooled in the lower extremities, and the arterial baroreceptors are activated to compensate for the decrease in cardiac output and systolic blood pressure. In some patients, pacemaker syndrome results from the inability to compensate further for the upright posture and augmentation of autonomic tone. In other patients, pacemaker syndrome may result from modification of these vascular responses through the effects of drugs, such as vasodilators and diuretics. Finally, in still other patients, pacemaker syndrome may result from activation of inhibitory atrial and cardiopulmonary reflexes that counteract the protective vasoconstrictor reflex (see Fig. 9-44). These responses may be further modified by the production of catecholamines and ANF. Circulating levels of ANF are frequently elevated in patients with complete AV block and bradycardia, being reduced within minutes of programming.[257-262]

Pacemaker syndrome during AAI or AAIR pacing has been described and emphasizes the role of AV dyssynchrony in the pathogenesis of the syndrome. Patients originally undergoing pacing for sick sinus syndrome may later demonstrate AV conduction abnormalities, or AV nodal conduction may be impaired by drugs with AV node–blocking properties (digoxin, β-blockers, calcium-channel blockers, antiarrhythmic drugs, etc.), leading to prolonged and hemodynamically unfavorable atrial-R wave (AR) intervals. AV dyssynchrony may also occur in patients with dual AV nodal pathway physiology during a shift in conduction from the fast pathway to the slow pathway with prolonged AV conduction time. Unfavorable sequencing of atrial and ventricular contractions may occur during AAIR pacing at high sensor-driven rates.[248] This situation most often results when the slope determining the sensor-driven rate is programmed too aggressively and out of proportion to the exercise-induced increase in catecholamine levels. As the paced atrial rate progressively increases, the appropriate corresponding decrement in PR interval does not occur, and the interval may even lengthen, eventually resulting in a paced P wave occurring immediately after the preceding R wave (Fig. 9-45). This event most commonly occurs in the earlier stages of exercise and, in some patients, is corrected as the patient continues to exercise.

The VDD pacing mode is very similar to DDD mode but without the capability of atrial pacing. The VDD mode, previously out of favor, has been revived by the development of CRT.[263,264]

AV dyssynchrony and pacemaker syndrome may also occur during dual-chamber pacing as a result of inappropriate programming, prolonged atrial conduction time, or normal upper rate limit behavior.[246,247,252] In AV sequential pacing modes, selection of an inappropriate AV interval may result in an adverse AV sequencing and hemodynamics. Differential AV intervals for paced and sensed atrial events and rate-adaptive AV intervals are useful in some patients for

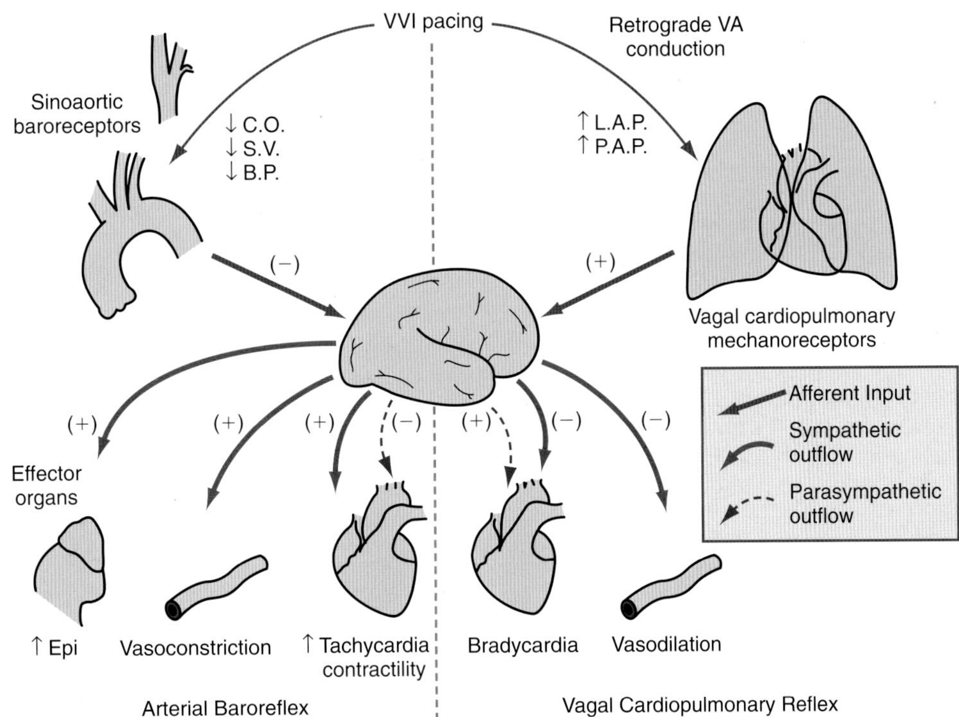

Figure 9-44. Diagrammatic representation of the multiple reflex pathways involved in pacemaker syndrome. See text for discussion. The arterial baroreflexes detect a decrease in stroke volume when atrioventricular (AV) dyssynchrony occurs, leading to sympathetic activation and vasoconstriction. Conversely, AV dyssynchrony results in higher atrial wall tension and activation of reflex pathways, leading to vagally mediated vasodilation as well as release of humoral substances, such as atrial natriuretic peptide (ANP), that further facilitate these reflexes (e.g., counteracting baroreflex-mediated vasoconstriction). BP, blood pressure; CO, cardiac output; EPI, epinephrine; LAP, left atrial pressure; PAP, pulmonary artery pressure; SV, stroke volume.

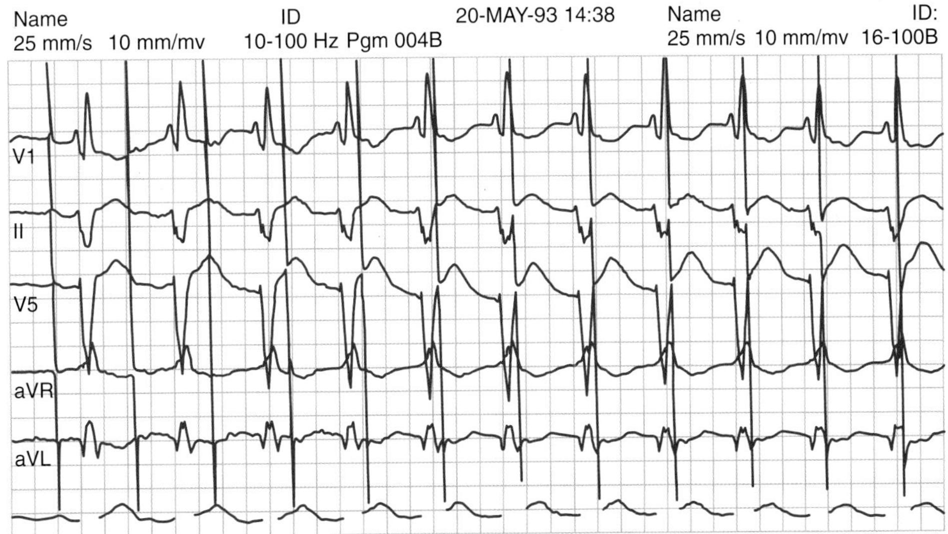

Figure 9-45. AAIR pacemaker recording in a patient receiving β-blockers who experienced pacemaker syndrome while walking. His heart rate increased from 70 to 90 bpm, and his paced atria-sensed QRS (AR) interval increased from 180 msec to more than 500 msec, resulting in shortness of breath. Discontinuing β-blockers and reprogramming the pacemaker to a less "aggressive" slope, resulted in a much shorter prolongation of the AR interval with exercise.

maintaining AV synchrony over a wide range of heart rates at rest and during exercise.

The maximum atrial tracking rate is determined by the TARP, which is composed of the AV interval and PVARP. Long AV intervals or long PVARP intervals are sometimes programmed to avoid pacemaker-mediated tachycardia. When the TARP is too long, the maximal atrial tracking rate is low. Patients may experience symptoms of pacemaker syndrome during exercise when their atrial rate exceeds the MATR, resulting in 2:1 AV block and a sudden, marked decrease in cardiac output in patients with complete heart block or in a lack of ventricular pacing in patients with normal AV conduction (this situation is very important in CRT because therapy would stop). This situation may be improved with reprogramming of shorter AV intervals or PVARP intervals to allow 1:1 ventricular tracking at higher atrial rates.

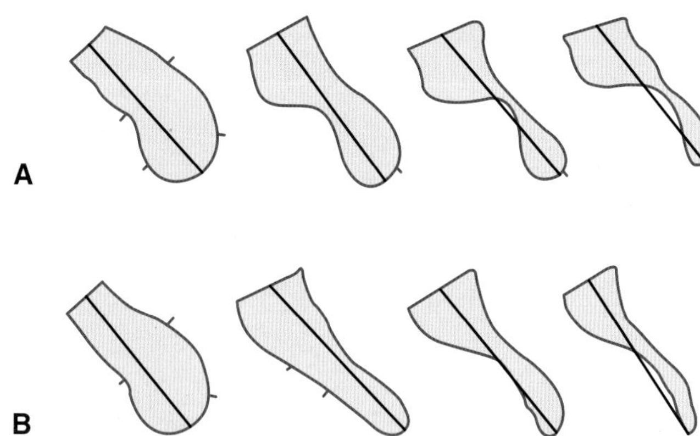

*Figure 9-46. Schematic representation of a monoplane ventriculography in a patient with severe hypertrophic obstructive cardiomyopathy during AAI pacing at a rate of 90 bpm **(A)** and during DDD pacing at a rate of 90 bpm and an atrioventricular (AV) delay interval of 50 msec **(B).** Note that the alteration in ventricular contraction pattern produced by right apical pacing results in less left ventricular outflow tract obstruction during systole. (From Jeanrenaud X, Goy JJ, Kappenberger LK: Effects of dual-chamber pacing in hypertrophic obstructive cardiomyopathy. Lancet 339:1318, 1992. ©by The Lancet Ltd., 1992.)*

Pacing in Specific Conditions

Hypertrophic Obstructive Cardiomyopathy

In patients with hypertrophic obstructive cardiomyopathy (HOCM), systolic anterior motion of the mitral valve toward the intraventricular septum is associated with LV outflow tract obstruction and, often, significant mitral regurgitation. Such patients are extremely sensitive to changes in preload and to conditions that diminish LV filling and result in a decrease in LV cavity size and an increase in intraventricular gradient. Thus, they derive proportionately more benefit from pacing than patients with normal hearts. Indeed, it has long been known that patients with HOCM who require pacing because of bradycardia experience significantly more benefit from pacing modes that preserve AV synchrony than from ventricular pacing.[265,266] Apart from optimization of the AV interval, another mechanism may play a role in the hemodynamic improvement seen in patients with HOCM.

It has been demonstrated that patients with HOCM in the absence of AV or sinus node disease may derive hemodynamic and clinical benefits from the abnormal sequencing of ventricular contraction that is produced by RV apical pacing.[267-271] RV pacing causes the septum to move away from the free wall during systole and, thus, increases the LV outflow tract diameter and reduces the intraventricular outflow gradient (Fig. 9-46). In addition to widening of the LV outflow gradient, apex pacing may also reduce the Venturi effect and diminish systolic anterior motion of the mitral valve. Because of the proposed mechanism of benefit resulting from the altered sequence of a paced ventricular contraction, AV sequential or atrial synchronous pacing must be performed with a short AV interval to ensure ventricular preexcitation (see Fig. 9-46).

Pacing may be indicated in a subset of patients with HOCM, significant intraventricular gradients, and symptoms despite medical therapy. In these patients, implantation of a sequential AV pacemaker results in a significant reduction of outflow ventricular gradient, improvements of New York Heart Association functional class and quality of life, and a reduction in symptoms, including syncope and presyncope. Despite initial enthusiasm regarding the role of pacemaker therapy in patients with HOCM, controversy exists regarding its efficacy and long-term safety, which have not yet been demonstrated in large randomized controlled studies.[272,273] Furthermore, the question whether pacing therapy is as efficacious as transcatheter alcoholic ablation of septal hypertrophy in patients with HOCM has not been addressed yet. Finally, the few existing data suggest that pacing therapy is not beneficial in patients with nonobstructive hypertrophic cardiomyopathy or in those with minimal intraventricular gradients.[274] This topic is discussed in more detail in Chapter 15.

After Cardiac Surgery

Temporary pacing is frequently used during weaning from extracorporeal circulation in patients undergoing cardiac surgery, even in absence of heart block. Immediately after operation, patients require higher pacing rates than usually programmed in patients with pacemakers, to compensate for the somewhat reduced stroke volume and to maintain high cardiac output. In the absence of atrial fibrillation, temporary AAI and DVI pacing is superior to ventricular pacing alone.[275] These patients are particularly sensitive to changes in AV interval, and even small changes in AV interval may significantly change cardiac output. Usually, these patients benefit most from a slightly shorter AV interval than their intrinsic AV intervals. Elevations of catecholamines, impaired diastolic filling, and atrial pacing, which may delay LA contraction and prolong the left AV mechanical interval, may account for this observation.

Acute Aortic Insufficiency

Acute severe aortic insufficiency is associated with a marked elevation in LV diastolic pressure, which may exceed LA pressure and result in mitral valve closure during diastole. Rapid temporary AAI and AV sequential pacing has been reported as a method of stabilizing patients with acute aortic insufficiency until definitive intervention can be performed.[276,277] The mechanism by which rapid pacing improves hemodynamics involves shortening of diastole and, therefore, of regurgitation without significantly altering forward flow.

Acute and Chronic Ischemic Heart Disease

Patients with ischemic heart disease who require pacing, especially those with previous myocardial infarction, benefit significantly more from a mode of pacing that maintains AV synchrony than from VVI pacing alone.[278-285] Similarly, in patients requiring temporary pacing during acute myocardial infarction, physiologic pacing mode is significantly better than VVI pacing alone,[283,286-288] but only if a relatively short AV interval (between 50 and 100 msec) is programmed. Given the current understanding of how AV interval modulates left mechanical function in patients with nearly normal or depressed LV function (see earlier), these data are not surprising.

Congestive Heart Failure in the Absence of Conduction System Disease

Cardiac Contractility Modulation with Nonexcitatory Signal*

The recognition of the limited application of cardiac resynchronization in patients with no electrical ventricular conduction abnormalities and no mechanical dys-synchrony has stimulated research for nonpharmacologic therapy that improves contractility in this group of patients with heart failure. Cardiac contractility modulation (CCM) with a nonexcitatory signal has been proposed as a possible therapy for congestive heart failure in the absence of conduction system disease.

This therapy specifically targets calcium homeostasis of the myocardial cell. In heart failure, reduced amplitude and prolonged duration of the intracellular calcium transient are common defects underlying myocardial contractile dysfunction.[289] In general, these changes in calcium cycling are not primary causes of heart failure but reflect secondary changes in both expression of genes encoding calcium-handling proteins[290] and post-translational modification of these proteins. As mentioned earlier, these changes include downregulation of the sarcoplasmic reticular ATPase-dependent calcium pump (SERCA2a), changes in expression and hypophosphorylation of phospholamban, altered regulation of the NCX, and hyperphosphorylation of the ryanodine release channel.

Early studies of isolated cardiac muscle showed that use of voltage clamping techniques to modulate the amplitude and duration of the action potential could enhance calcium entry and contractility in isolated papillary muscles.[292] Longer duration of depolarization and higher voltage during depolarization have each been associated with increases in the strength of cardiac muscle contraction. A relationship between action potential characteristics and calcium transients was confirmed in myocardium from a rapid-pacing heart failure model in dogs.[293] A later study discovered that similar effects could be achieved with extracellular field stimulation of myocardial tissue.[294] In isovolumically contracting Langendorff-perfused ferret hearts loaded with aequorin, it was shown that the increases in contractility and calcium fluxes caused by these extracellular nonexcitatory stimuli are mediated by greater amplitude and duration of the action potential.[297]

In vivo field stimulation of entire hearts of larger mammals is not feasible because of practical considerations related to power availability and nonspecific stimulation of other tissues in the field (e.g., nerves, skeletal muscles). Therefore, another study examined whether contractile strength of an entire heart could be enhanced by application of nonexcitatory stimulation CCM to a region of the heart of anesthetized dogs. Studies were performed in different laboratories in normal animals[297] and in animals in which heart failure had been introduced by repeated coronary artery microembolizations.[298,299] These studies showed that there was a repeatable significant effect on pressure generation, dP/dt_{max}, ejection fraction, and end-systolic pressure-volume relationship, all indicative of an increase in ventricular contractility that dissipated when the CCM signals delivery was stopped.[298]

One set of studies explored effects of CCM signals on the ventricular end-systolic pressure-volume relationship. Ventricular volume was measured using ultrasonic crystals placed at multiple sites on the heart; volumes were estimated from continuously tracked ventricular dimensions and assuming an ellipsoidal ventricular geometry.[297] These studies showed the upward shift of the end-systolic pressure-volume relationship indicative of the increase in global ventricular contractile strength. In these same experiments, regional myocardial function was assessed with the same crystals through construction of regional pressure-segment length loops. The results showed that contractile performance was enhanced only in the region near the site of stimulation and that there was an accompanying reduction in regional end-diastolic segment length. In remote regions, subtle changes were observed in the shape of the pressure-segment length loop, but there was no effect on contractility. It was further shown that when CCM signals are delivered to two sites, the effects on global function are additive.

In a preliminary report, CCM treatment in dogs with heart failure was associated with no significant change in global myocardial oxygen consumption.[299] However,

*Dr. Julio Spinelli recused himself from participating in the writing and editing of the section on cardiac contractility modulation. Contributors to this section are Dr. Kenneth Ellenbogen, Dr. Frits Prinzen, and Dr. Angelo Auricchio.

in the setting of local application and local mechanical effect (see earlier), it may be difficult to detect regional changes in myocardial oxygen consumption, particularly from the septal wall, from which a significant proportion of venous blood may drain directly into the RV and so may not appear in the coronary sinus. Knowledge of the consequence of CCM for myocardial oxygen consumption is important, because in the past paired pacing, which also increases contractility by manipulating calcium homeostasis, was abandoned because of the rise in myocardial oxygen consumption and the risk of increasing myocardial ischemia. Other approaches to increase contractility through variation in cellular calcium also proved to raise myocardial oxygen consumption (β-adrenergic agonists, phosphodiesterase inhibitors, calcium administration). Long-term administration of inotropic agents such as milrinone to patients with heart failure raises mortality.[300] Conversely, CRT is so far the only nonpharmacologic therapy for patients with heart failure, because it raises contractility without an increase, or even a moderate decrease, in myocardial oxygen consumption.[60] The decrease is associated with lower mortality.[201] These benefits are presumably achieved through improved coordination of contraction. In contrast, CCM exacerbates dyscoordination by selectively increasing contractility around the stimulation site.[297] Thus, in the light of negative outcomes of clinical trials of other inotropic therapies, better insight in the basic mechanisms of CCM seems required before this technique can be used on a large scale in patients. The current status of clinical trials of CCM signals is reviewed in Chapter 12.

REFERENCES

1. Saffitz JE, Davis LM, Darrow BJ, et al: The molecular basis of anisotropy: Role of gap junctions. J Cardiovasc Electrophysiol 6:498-510, 1995.
2. Scher AM, Young AC, Malmgreen AL, et al: Spread of electrical activity through the wall of the ventricle. Circ Res 1:539-547, 1953.
3. Scher AM, Young AC, Malmgreen AL, et al: Activation of the interventricular septum. Circ Res 3:56-64, 1955.
4. Myerburg RJ, Nilsson K, Gelband H: Physiology of canine intraventricular conduction and endocardial excitation. Circ Res 30:217-243, 1972.
5. Hoffman BF, Cranefield PF, Stuckley JH, et al: Direct measurement of conduction velocity in in situ specialized conduction system of mammalian heart. Proc Soc Exp Biol Med 102:55-57, 1959.
6. Kulbertus HE, Demoulin J-C: The left hemiblocks: Significance, prognosis and treatment. Schweiz Med Wochenschr 112:1579-1584, 1982.
7. Uhley HN, Rivkin L: Peripheral distribution of the canine A-V conduction system. Am J Cardiol 5:688-691, 1960.
8. Abramson DI, Margolin SA: Purkinje conduction network in the myocardium of the mammalian ventricles. J Anat 70:251-259, 1936.
9. Truex RC, Copenhaver WM: Histology of the moderator band in man and other mammals with special reference to the conduction system. Am J Anat 80:173-200, 1947.
10. Berenfeld O, Jalife J: Purkinje-muscle reentry as a mechanism of polymorphic ventricular arrhythmias in 3-dimensional model of ventricles. Circ Res 82:1063-1077, 1998.
11. Durrer D, Dam v. RT, Freud GE, et al: Total excitation of the isolated human heart. Circulation 41:899-912, 1970.
12. Spach MS, Barr RC: Analysis of ventricular activation and repolarization from intramural and epicardial potential distributions for ectopic beats in the intact dog. Circ Res 37:830-843, 1975.
13. Rawling DA, Joyner RW, Overholt ED: Variations in the functional electrical coupling between the subendocardial Purkinje and ventricular layers of the canine left ventricle. Circ Res 57:252-261, 1985.
14. Bers DM: Cardiac excitation-contraction coupling. Nature 415:198-205, 2002.
15. Van Heuningen R, Rijnsburger WH, Ter Keurs HEDJ: Sarcomere length control in striated muscle. Am J Physiol 242:H411-H420, 1982.
16. Prinzen FW, Augustijn CH, Allessie MA, et al: The time sequence of electrical and mechanical activation during spontaneous beating and ectopic stimulation. Eur Heart J 13:535-543, 1992.
17. Hasenfuss G, Reinecke H, Studer R: Relation between myocardial function and expression of sarcoplasmic reticulum Ca(2+)-ATPase in failing and non-failing human myocardium. Circ Res 75:434-442, 1994.
18. Studer R, Reinecke H, Bilger J, et al: Gene expression of the cardiac Na(+)-Ca2+ exchanger in end-stage human heart failure. Circ Res 75:443-453, 1994.
19. Verdonck F, Volders PG, Vos MA, et al: Increased Na+ concentration and altered Na/K pump activity in hypertrophied canine ventricular cells. Cardiovasc Res 57:1035-1043, 2003.
20. O'Rourke B, Kass DA, Tomaselli GF, et al: Mechanisms of altered excitation-contraction coupling in canine tachycardia-induced heart failure. Circ Res 84:562-570, 1999.
21. Pogwizd SM, Qi M, Yuan W, et al: Upregulation of Na+/Ca2+ exchanger expression and function in an arrhythmogenic rabbit model of heart failure. Circ Res 85:1009-1019, 1999.
22. Swynghedauw B: Molecular mechanisms of myocardial remodeling: Review. Physiol Rev 79:215-262, 1999.
23. Cooper GI: Load and length regulation of cardiac energetics. Annu Rev Physiol 52:505-522, 1990.
24. Vassallo JA, Cassidy DM, Marchlinski FE, et al: Endocardial activation of left bundle branch block. Circulation 69:914-923, 1984.
25. Durrer D, Roos JP: Epicardial excitation of the ventricles in a patient with a Wolfe-Parkinson-White syndrome (type B). Circulation 35:15-21, 1967.
26. Lister JW, Klotz DH, Jomain SL, et al: Effect of pacemaker site on cardiac output and ventricular activation in dogs with complete heart block. Am J Cardiol 14:494-503, 1964.
27. Vassallo JA, Cassidy DM, Miller JM, et al: Left ventricular endocardial activation during right ventricular pacing: effect of underlying heart disease. J Am Coll Cardiol 7:1228-1233, 1986.
28. Spach MS, Miller WT, Geselowitz DB, et al: The discontinuous nature of propagation in normal canine cardiac muscle: Evidence for recurrent discontinuities of intracellular resistance that affect the membrane currents. Circ Res 48:39-54, 1981.
29. Frazier DW, Krassowska W, Chen P-S, et al: Transmural activations and stimulus potentials in three dimensional anisotropic canine myocardium. Circ Res 63:135-146, 1988.
30. Wiggers CJ: The muscular reactions of the mammalian ventricles to artificial surface stimuli. Am J Physiol 73:346-378, 1925.
31. Prinzen FW, Augustijn CH, Arts T, et al: Redistribution of myocardial fiber strain and blood flow by asynchronous activation. Am J Physiol 259:H300-H308, 1990.
32. Myerburg RJ, Gelband H, Nilsson K, et al: The role of canine superficial ventricular fibers in endocardial impulse conduction. Circ Res 42:27-35, 1978.
33. Askenazi J, Alexander JH, Koenigsberg DI, et al: Alteration of left ventricular performance by left bundle branch block simulated with atrioventricular sequential pacing. Am J Cardiol 53:99-104, 1984.
34. Hirzel HO, Senn M, Nuesch K, et al: Thallium-201 scintigraphy in complete left bundle branch block. Am J Cardiol 53:764-769, 1984.

35. Verbeek X, Vernooy K, Peschar M, et al: Intra-ventricular resynchronization for optimal left ventricular function during pacing in experimental left bundle branch block. J Am Coll Cardiol 42:558-567, 2003.
36. Ono S, Nohara R, Kambara H, et al: Regional myocardial perfusion and glucose metabolism in experimental left bundle branch block. Circulation 85:1125-1131, 1992.
37. Rosenbush SW, Ruggie N, Turner DA, et al: Sequence and timing of ventricular wall motion in patients with bundle branch block. Circulation 66:113-119, 1982.
38. Rodriguez LM, Timmermans C, Nabar A, et al: Variable patterns of septal activation in patients with left bundle branch block and heart failure. J Cardiovasc Electrophysiol 14:135-141, 2003.
39. Auricchio A, Fantoni C, Regoli F, et al: Characterization of left ventricular activation in patients with heart failure and left bundle-branch block. Circulation 109:1133-1139, 2004.
40. Sohi GS, Flowers NC, Horan LG, et al: Comparison of total body surface map depolarization patterns of left bundle branch block and normal axis with left bundle branch block and left-axis deviation. Circulation 67:660-664, 1983.
41. Becker RA, Erickson RV, Scher AM: Ventricular excitation in experimental bundle-branch block. Circ Res 5:5-10, 1957.
42. Badke FR, Boinay P, Covell JW: Effect of ventricular pacing on regional left ventricular performance in the dog. Am J Physiol 238:H858-H867, 1980.
43. Prinzen FW, Hunter WC, Wyman BT, et al: Mapping of regional myocardial strain and work during ventricular pacing: Experimental study using magnetic resonance imaging tagging. J Am Coll Cardiol 33:1735-1742, 1999.
44. Tyberg JV, Parmley WW, Sonnenblick EH: In-vitro studies of myocardial asynchrony and regional hypoxia. Circ Res 25:569-579, 1969.
45. Prinzen FW, van Oosterhout MFM, Vanagt WYR, et al: Optimization of ventricular function by improving the activation sequence during ventricular pacing. Pacing Clin Electrophysiol 21:2256-2260, 1998.
46. Delhaas T, Arts T, Bovendeerd PHM, et al: Subepicardial fiber strain and stress as related to left ventricular pressure and volume. Am J Physiol 264:H1548-H1559, 1993.
47. Little WC, Reeves RC, Arciniegas J, et al: Mechanism of abnormal interventricular septal motion during delayed left ventricular activation. Circ Res 65:1486-1490, 1982.
48. Grines CL, Bashore TM, Boudoulas H, et al: Functional abnormalities in isolated left bundle branch block. Circulation 79:845-853, 1989.
49. Vernooy K, Verbeek XAAM, Peschar M, et al: Left bundle branch block induces ventricular remodeling and functional septal hypoperfusion. Eur Heart J 26:91-98, 2005.
50. Delhaas T, Arts T, Prizen FW, et al: Regional fibre stress-fibre strain area as an estimate of regional blood flow and oxygen demand in the canine heart. J Physiol 477:481-496, 1994.
51. Nielsen JC, Boetcher M, Toftegaard Nielsen T, et al: Regional myocardial blood flow in patients with sick sinus syndrome randomized to long-term single chamber atrial or dual chamber pacing- effect of pacing mode and rate. J Am Coll Cardiol 35:1453-1461, 2000.
52. Nowak B, Sinha AM, Schaefer WM, et al: Cardiac resynchronization therapy homogenizes myocardial glucose metabolism and perfusion in dilated cardiomyopathy and left bundle branch block. J Am Coll Cardiol 41:1523-1528, 2003.
53. Lindner O, Vogt J, Kammeier A, et al: Effect of cardiac resynchronization therapy on global and regional oxygen consumption and myocardial blood flow in patients with non-ischaemic and ischaemic cardiomyopathy. Eur Heart J 26:70-76, 2005.
54. Beppu S, Matsuda H, Shishido T, et al: Functional myocardial perfusion abnormality induced by left ventricular asynchronous contraction: Experimental study using myocardial contrast echocardiography. J Am Coll Cardiol 29:1632-1638, 1997.
55. Burkhoff D, Oikawa RY, Sagawa K: Influence of pacing site on left ventricular contraction. Am J Physiol 251:H428-H435, 1986.
56. Boerth RC, Covell JW: Mechanical performance and efficiency of the left ventricle during ventricular stimulation. Am J Physiol 221:1686-1691, 1971.
57. Baller D, Wolpers HG, Zipfel J, et al: Unfavourable effects of ventricular pacing on myocardial energetic. Basic Res Cardiol 76:115-123, 1981.
58. Baller D, Wolpers H-G, Zipfel J, et al: Comparison of the effects of right atrial, right ventricular apex and atrioventricular sequential pacing on myocardial oxygen consumption and cardiac efficiency: A laboratory investigation. Pacing Clin Electrophysiol 11:394-403, 1988.
59. Owen CH, Esposito DJ, Davis JW, et al: The effects of ventricular pacing on left ventricular geometry, function, myocardial oxygen consumption and efficiency of contraction in conscious dogs. Pacing Clin Electrophysiol 21:1417-1429, 1998.
60. Nelson GS, Berger RD, Fetics BJ, et al: Left ventricular or biventricular pacing improves cardiac function at diminished energy cost in patients with dilated cardiomyopathy and left bundle branch block. Circulation 102:3053-3059, 2000.
61. Van Oosterhout MFM, Prinzen FW, Arts T, et al: Asynchronous electrical activation induces inhomogeneous hypertrophy of the left ventricular wall. Circulation 98:588-595, 1998.
62. Gilmore JP, Sarnoff SJ, Mitchell JH, et al: Synchronicity of ventricular contraction: Observations comparing hæmodynamic effects of atrial and ventricular pacing. Br Heart J 25:299-307, 1963.
63. Park RC, Little WC, O'Rourke RA: Effect of alteration of left ventricular activation sequence on the left ventricular end-systolic pressure-volume relation in closed-chest dogs. Circ Res 57:706-717, 1985.
64. Bahler RC, Martin P: Effects of loading conditions and inotropic state on rapid filling phase of left ventricle. Am J Physiol 248:H523-H533, 1985.
65. Leclercq C, Gras D, Le Helloco A, et al: Hemodynamic importance of preserving the normal sequence of ventricular activation in permanent cardiac pacing. Am Heart J 129:1133-1141, 1995.
66. Betocchi S, Piscione F, Villari B, et al: Effects of induced asynchrony on left ventricular diastolic function in patients with coronary artery disease. J Am Coll Cardiol 21:1124-1131, 1993.
67. Bedotto JB, Grayburn PA, Black WH, et al: Alterations in left ventricular relaxation during atrioventricular pacing in humans. J Am Coll Cardiol 15:658-664, 1990.
68. Rosenqvist M, Bergfeldt L, Haga Y, et al: The effect of ventricular activation sequence on cardiac performance during pacing. Pacing Clin Electrophysiol 19:1279-1287, 1996.
69. Zile MR, Blaustein AS, Shimizu G, et al: Right ventricular pacing reduces the rate of left ventricular relaxation and filling. J Am Coll Cardiol 10:702-709, 1987.
70. Blaustein AS, Gaasch WH: Myocardial relaxation. VI: Effects of beta-adrenergic tone and asynchrony on LV relaxation rate. Am J Physiol 244:H417-H422, 1983.
71. Heyndrickx GR, Vantrimpont PJ, Rousseau MF, et al: Effects of asynchrony on myocardial relaxation at rest and during exercise in conscious dogs. Am J Physiol 254:H817-H822, 1988.
72. Zhou Q, Henein M, Coats A, et al: Different effects of abnormal activation and myocardial disease on left ventricular ejection and filling times. Heart 84:272-276, 2000.
73. Lee MA, Dae MW, Langberg JJ, et al: Effects of long-term right ventricular apical pacing on left ventricular perfusion, innervation, function and histology. J Am Coll Cardiol 24:225-232, 1994.
74. Maurer G, Torres MA, Corday E, et al: Two-dimensional echocardiographic contrast assessment of pacing-induced mitral regurgitation: Relation to altered regional left ventricular function. J Am Coll Cardiol 3:986-991, 1984.

75. Miyazawa K, Shirato K, Haneda T, et al: Effects of varying pacemaker sites on left ventricular performance. Tohoku J Exp Med 120:301-308, 1976.
76. Mark JB, Chetham PM: Ventricular pacing can induce hemodynamically significant mitral valve regurgitation. Anesthesiology 74:375-377, 1991.
77. Twidale N, Manda V, Holliday R, et al: Mitral regurgitation after atrioventricular node catheter ablation for atrial fibrillation and heart failure: Acute hemodynamic features. Am Heart J 138:1166-1175, 1999.
78. Rosenqvist M, Isaaz K, Botvinick EH, et al: Relative importance of activation sequence compared to atrioventricular synchrony in left ventricular function. Am J Cardiol 67:148-156, 1991.
79. Bramlet DA, Morris KG, Coleman RE, et al: Effects of rate-dependent left bundle branch block on global and regional left ventricular function. Circulation 67:1059-1065, 1983.
80. Little WC, Park RC, Freeman GL: Effects of regional ischemia and ventricular pacing on LV dP/dtmax-end-diastolic volume relation. Am J Physiol 252:H933-H940, 1987.
81. Suga H, Goto Y, Yaku H, et al: Simulation of mechanoenergetics of asynchronously contracting ventricle. Am J Physiol 259:R1075-R1082, 1990.
82. Prinzen FW, Peschar M: Relation between the pacing induced sequence of activation and left ventricular pump function in animals. Pacing Clin Electrophysiol 25:484-498, 2002.
83. Klotz DH, Lister JW, Jomain SL, et al: Implantation sites of pacemakers after right ventriculotomy and complete heart block. JAMA 186:929-931, 1963.
84. Vanagt WY, Verbeek XA, Delhaas T, et al: The left ventricular apex is the optimal site for pediatric pacing: Correlation with animal experience. Pacing Clin Electrophysiol 27:837-843, 2004.
85. Peschar M, de Swart H, Michels KJ, et al: Left ventricular septal and apex pacing for optimal pump function in canine hearts. J Am Coll Cardiol 41:1218-1226, 2003.
86. Rosen MR: The heart remembers: Clinical implications. Lancet 357:468-471, 2001.
87. Plotnikov AN, Yu H, Geller JC, et al: Role of L-type calcium channels in pacing-induced short-term and long-term cardiac memory in canine heart. Circulation 107:2844-2849, 2003.
88. Patberg KW, Plotnikov AN, Quamina A, et al: Cardiac memory is associated with decreased levels of the transcriptional factor CREB modulated by angiotensin II and calcium. Circ Res 93:472-478, 2003.
89. Costard-Jäckle A, Franz MR: Slow and long-lasting modulation of myocardial repolarization produced by ectopic activation in isolated rabbit hearts: Evidence for cardiac "memory." Circulation 80:1412-1420, 1989.
90. Alessandrini RS, McPherson DD, Kadish AH, et al: Cardiac memory: A mechanical and electrical phenomenon. Am J Physiol 272:H1952-H1959, 1997.
91. Nahlawi M, Waligora M, Spies SM, et al: Left ventricular function during and after right ventricular pacing. J Am Coll Cardiol 44:1883-1888, 2004.
92. Prinzen FW, Cheriex EM, Delhaas T, et al: Asymmetric thickness of the left ventricular wall resulting from asynchronous electrical activation: A study in patients with left bundle branch block and in dogs with ventricular pacing. Am Heart J 130:1045-1053, 1995.
93. Van Oosterhout MFM, Arts T, Muijtjens AMM, et al: Remodeling by ventricular pacing in hypertrophying dog hearts. Cardiovasc Res 49:771-778, 2001.
94. Karpawich PP, Justice CD, Cavitt DL, et al: Developmental sequelae of fixed-rate ventricular pacing in the immature canine heart: An electrophysiologic, hemodynamic and histopathologic evaluation. Am Heart J 119:1077-1083, 1990.
95. Waldman LK, Covell JW: Effects of ventricular pacing on finite deformation in canine left ventricles. Am J Physiol 252:H1023-H1030, 1987.
96. Knaapen P, van Campen LM, de Cock CC, et al: Effects of cardiac resynchronization therapy on myocardial perfusion reserve. Circulation 110:646-651, 2004.
97. Patel PM, Plotnikov A, Kanagaratnam P, et al: Altering ventricular activation remodels gap junction distribution in canine heart. J Cardiovasc Electrophysiol 12:570-577, 2001.
98. Spragg DD, Leclercq C, Loghmani M, et al: Regional alterations in protein expression in the dyssynchronous failing hearts. Circulation 108:929-932, 2003.
99. Akar FG, Spragg DD, Tunin RS, et al: Mechanisms underlying conduction slowing and arrhythmogenesis in non-ischemic dilated cardiomyopathy. Circ Res 95:717-725, 2004.
100. Kertesz NJ, Fenrich AL, Friedman RA: Congenital complete atrio-ventricular block. Tex Heart Inst J 24:301-307, 1997.
101. Udink ten Cate PE, Breur JM, Cohen MI, et al: Dilated cardiomyopathy in isolated congenital complete atrioventricular block: Early and long-term in children. J Am Coll Cardiol 37:1129-1134, 2001.
102. Brockman SK: Cardiodynamics of complete heart block. Am J Cardiol 16:72-83, 1965.
103. Peschar M, March AM, Verbeek X, et al: Site of right ventricular pacing determines left ventricular remodeling in patients with atrio-ventricular block. Heart Rhythm 1:S245, 2004.
104. Vos MA, de Groot SH, Verduyn SC, et al: Enhanced susceptibility for acquired torsade de pointes arrhythmias in the dog with chronic, complete atrio-ventricular block is related to cardiac hypertrophy and electrical remodeling. Circulation 98:1125-1235, 1998.
105. Katz AM: Pathophysiology of heart failure: Identifying targets for pharmacotherapy. Med Clin North Am 87:303-316, 2003.
106. Brockman SK, Stoney WS: Congestive and heart failure and cardiac output in heart block and during pacing. Ann N Y Acad Sci 167:534-545, 1969.
107. Breur JM, Udink Ten Cate FE, Kapusta L, et al: Pacemaker therapy in isolated congenital complete atrioventricular block. Pacing Clin Electrophysiol 25:1685-1692, 2002.
108. Tantengco MV, Thomas RL, Karpawich PP: Left ventricular dysfunction after long-term right ventricular apical pacing in the young. J Am Coll Cardiol 37:2093-2100, 2001.
109. Thambo JB, Bordachar P, Garrigue S, et al: Detrimental ventricular remodeling in patients with congenital complete heart block and chronic right ventricular apical pacing. Circulation 210:3766-3772, 2004.
110. Benchimol A, Li YB, Dimond EG: Cardiovascular dynamics in complete heart block at various heart rates: Effect of exercise at a fixed heart rate. Circulation 30:542-553, 1964.
111. Sowton E: Haemodynamic studies in patients with artificial pacemakers. Br Heart J 26:737-746, 1964.
112. Karlof I, Bevegard S, Ovenfors CO: Adaptation of the left ventricle to sudden changes in heart rate in patients with artificial pacemakers. Cardiovasc Res 7:322-330, 1973.
113. Wright AJ, Hudlicka O: Capillary growth and changes in heart performance induced by chronic bradycardial pacing in the rabbit. Circ Res 49:469-478, 1981.
114. Brown MD, Davies MK, Hudlicka O: The effect of long-term bradycardia on heart microvascular supply and performance. Cell Mol Biol Res 40:137-142, 1994.
115. Brown MD, Hudlicka O: Protective effects of long-term bradycardial pacing against catecholamine-induced myocardial damage in rabbit hearts. Circ Res 62:965-974, 1988.
116. Lei L, Zhou R, Zheng W, et al: Bradycardia induces angiogenesis in creases coronary reserve and preserves function of the post-infarcted heart. Circulation 110:796-802, 2004.
117. Ishibashi Y, Shimada T, Nosaka S, et al: Effects of heart rate on coronary circulation and external mechanical efficiency in elderly hypertensive patients with left ventricular hypertrophy. Clin Cardiol 19:620-630, 1996.

118. Kristensson B, Arnman K, Ryden L, et al: The haemodynamic importance of atrioventricular synchrony and rate increase at rest and during exercise. Eur Heart J 6:773-778, 1985.
119. Perhsson SK: Influence of heart rate and atrioventricular synchrony on maximal work tolerance in patients treated with artificial pacemakers. Acta Med Scand 214:311-315, 1983.
120. Fananapazir L, Bennett DH, Monks PH: Atrial synchronized pacing: Contribution of the chronotropic response to improved exercise performance. Pacing Clin Electrophysiol 6:601-606, 1983.
121. Rowe GG, Stenlund RR, Thomsen JH, et al: Coronary and systemic hemodynamic effects of cardiac pacing in man with complete heart block. Circulation 40:839-845, 1969.
122. Bowman AW, Kovacs SJ: Left atrial conduit volume is generated by deviation from the constant-volume state of the left heart: A combined MRI-echocardiographic study. Am J Physiol Heart Circ Physiol 286:H2416-H2424, 2004.
123. Samet P, Castillo P, Bernstein WH: Hemodynamic consequences of sequential atrioventricular pacing. Am J Cardiol 21:207-212, 1968.
124. Daggett WM, Bianco JA, Powel WJ, et al: Relative contribution of the atrial systole-ventricular systole interval and of patterns of ventricular activation to ventricular function during electrical pacing of the dog heart. Circ Res 27:69-79, 1970.
125. Kosowsky BD, Scherlag BJ, Damato AN: Re-evaluation of the atrial contribution to ventricular function. Am J Cardiol 21:518-524, 1968.
126. Faerestrand S, Ohm O-J: A time-related study of the hemodynamic benefit of atrioventricular synchronous pacing evaluated by Doppler echocardiography. Pacing Clin Electrophysiol 8:838-848, 1985.
127. Masuyama T, Kodama S, Nakatani S, et al: Effects of atrioventricular interval on left ventricular diastolic filling assessed with pulsed Doppler echocardiography. Cardiovasc Res 23:1034-1042, 1989.
128. Mitchell JH, Gupta DN, Payne RM: Influence of atrial systole on effective ventricular stroke volume. Circ Res 17:11-18, 1965.
129. Mehta D, Gilmour S, Ward DE, et al: Optimal atrioventricular delay at rest and during exercise in patients with dual chamber pacemakers: A non-invasive assessment by continuous wave Doppler. Br Heart J 61:161-166, 1989.
130. Tanabe A, Mohri T, Ohga M, et al: The effects of pacing-induced left bundle branch block on left ventricular systolic and diastolic performances. Jpn Heart J 31:309-317, 1990.
131. Nielsen JC, Andersen HR, Thomsen PEB, et al: Heart failure and echocardiographic changes during long-term follow-up of patients with sick-sinus syndrome randomized to single-chamber atrial or ventricular pacing. Circulation 97:987-995, 1998.
132. Ritter P, Dib JC, Mahaux V, et al: New method for determining the optimal atrio-ventricular delay in patients paced in DDD mode for complete atrioventricular block. Pacing Clin Electrophysiol 18(Part II):237, 1995.
133. Wish M, Fletcher RD, Gottdiener JS, et al: Importance of left atrial timing in the programming of dual-chamber pacemakers. Am J Cardiol 60:566-571, 1987.
134. Janosik DL, Pearson AC, Buckingham TA, et al: The hemodynamic benefit of differential atrioventricular delay intervals for sensed and paced atrial events during physiologic pacing. J Am Coll Cardiol 14:499-507, 1989.
135. Catania SL, Maue-Dickson W: AV delay latency compensation. J Electrophysiol 3:242, 1987.
136. Sutton R: The atrioventricular interval: What considerations influence its programming? Eur J Cardiac Pacing Electrophysiol 3:169, 1992.
137. Alt EU, VonBirbra H, Blömer H: Different beneficial AV intervals with DDD pacing after sensed or paced atrial events. J Electrophysiol 1:250, 1987.
138. Chirife R, Ortega DF, Salazar AI: Nonphysiological left heart AV intervals as a result of DDD and AAI "physiological" pacing. Pacing Clin Electrophysiol 14:1752-1756, 1991.
139. Capucci A, Boriani G, Specchia S, et al: Evaluation by cardiopulmonary exercise test of DDDR versus DDD pacing. Pacing Clin Electrophysiol 15:1908-1913, 1992.
140. Daubert C, Richter P, Mabo P, et al: Physiological relationship between AV interval and heart rate in healthy subjects: Applications to dual chamber pacing. Pacing Clin Electrophysiol 9:1032-1039, 1986.
141. Luceri RM, Brownstein SL, Vardeman L, et al: PR interval behaviour during exercise: Implications for physiological pacemakers. Pacing Clin Electrophysiol 13:1719-1723, 1990.
142. Barbieri D, Percoco GF, Toselli T, et al: AV delay and exercise stress test: Behaviour in normal subjects. Pacing Clin Electrophysiol 13:1724-1727, 1990.
143. Haskell RJ, French WJ: Physiological importance of different atrioventricular intervals to improved exercise performance in patients with dual chamber pacemakers. Br Heart J 61:46-51, 1989.
144. Ritter PH, Vai F, Bonnet JL, et al: Rate-adaptive atrioventricular delay improves cardiopulmonary performance in patients implanted with a dual-chamber pacemaker for complete heart block. Eur J CPE 1:31, 1991.
145. Sulke AN, Chambers JB, Sowton E: The effect of atrio-ventricular delay programming in patients with DDDR pacemakers. Eur Heart J 13:464-472, 1992.
146. Brecker SJ, Xiao HB, Sparrow J, et al: Effects of dual-chamber pacing with short atrioventricular delay in dilated cardiomyopathy. Lancet 340:1308-1312, 1992.
147. Nishimura RA, Hayes DL, Holmes DRJ, et al: Mechanism of hemodynamic improvement by dual-chamber pacing for severe left ventricular dysfunction: An acute Doppler and catheterization hemodynamic study. J Am Coll Cardiol 25:281-288, 1995.
148. Auricchio A, Stellbrink C, Block M, et al: Effect of pacing chamber and atrioventricular delay on acute systolic function of paced patients with congestive heart failure. The Pacing Therapies for Congestive Heart Failure Study Group. The Guidant Congestive Heart Failure Research Group. Circulation 99:2993-3001, 1999.
149. Auricchio A, Stellbrink C, Sack S, et al: Long-term clinical effect of hemodynamically optimized cardiac resynchronization therapy in patients with heart failure and ventricular conduction delay. J Am Coll Cardiol 39:2026-2033, 2002.
150. Stellbrink C, Auricchio A, Butter C, et al: Pacing therapies in congestive heart failure II study. Am J Cardiol 86:K138-K143, 2000.
151. Auricchio A, Ding J, Spinelli JC, et al: Cardiac resynchronization therapy restores optimal atrioventricular mechanical timing in heart failure patients with ventricular conduction delay. J Am Coll Cardiol 39:1163-1169, 2002.
152. Dupont WD, Plummer WD Jr: Power and sample size calculations for studies involving linear regression. Control Clin Trials 19:589-601, 1998.
153. Santini M, Alexidou G, Ansalone G, et al: Relation of prognosis in sick sinus syndrome to age, conduction defects and modes of permanent cardiac pacing. Am J Cardiol 65:729-735, 1990.
154. Rosenqvist M, Brandt J, Schueller H: Atrial versus ventricular pacing in sinus node disease: A treatment comparison study. Am Heart J 111:292-297, 1986.
155. Andersen HR, Nielsen JC, Thomsen PEB, et al: Long-term follow-up of patients from a randomised trial of atrial versus ventricular pacing for sick-sinus syndrome. Lancet 350:1210-1216, 1997.
156. Sweeney MO, Hellkamp AS, Ellenbogen KA, et al: Adverse effect of ventricular pacing on heart failure and atrial fibrillation among patients with normal baseline QRS duration in a clinical trial of pacemaker therapy for sinus node dysfunction. Circulation 107:2932-2937, 2003.
157. Wilkoff BL, Cook JR, Epstein AE, et al: Dual-chamber pacing or ventricular back-up pacing in patients with an implantable defibrillator. JAMA 288:3115-3123, 2002.

158. Karpawich PP, Justice CD, Chang C-H, et al: Septal ventricular pacing in the immature canine heart: A new perspective. Am Heart J 121:827-833, 1991.
159. Schneider JF, Thomas Jr HE, Sorlie P, et al: Comparative features of newly acquired left and right bundle branch block in the general population: The Framingham study. Am J Cardiol 47:931-940, 1981.
160. Freedman RA, Alderman EL, Sheffield LT, et al: Bundle branch block in patients with chronic coronary artery disease: Angiographic correlates and prognostic significance. J Am Coll Cardiol 10:73-80, 1987.
161. Eriksson P, Hansson PO, Eriksson H, et al: Bundle-branch block in a general male population: The study of men born in 1913. Circulation 98:2494-2500, 1998.
162. Rabkin SW, Mathewson FAL, Tate RB: Natural history of left bundle-branch block. Br Heart J 43:164-169, 1980.
163. Takeshita A, Basta LL, Kioschos JM: Effect of intermittent left bundle branch block on left ventricular performance. Am J Med 56:251-255, 1974.
164. De Nardo D, Antolini M, Pitucco G, et al: Effects of left bundle branch block on left ventricular function in apparently normal subjects: Study by equilibrium radionuclide angiocardiography at rest. Cardiology 75:365-371, 1988.
165. Verbeek X, Vernooy K, Peschar M, et al: Quantification of interventricular asynchrony during LBBB and ventricular pacing. Am J Physiol 283:H1370-H1378, 2002.
166. Liu L, Tockman B, Girouard S, et al: Left ventricular resynchronization therapy in a canine model of left bundle branch block. Am J Physiol 282:H2238-H2244, 2002.
167. Rouleau F, Merheb M, Geffroy S, et al: Echocardiographic assessment of the interventricular delay of activation and correlation to the QRS width in dilated cardiomyopathy. Pacing Clin Electrophysiol 24:1500-1506, 2001.
168. Nielsen JC, Kristensen L, Andersen HR, et al: A randomized comparison of atrial and dual-chamber pacing in 177 consecutive patients with sick sinus syndrome: Echocardiographic and clinical outcome. J Am Coll Cardiol 42:614-623, 2003.
169. Kristensen L, Nielsen JC, Mortensen PT, et al: Incidence of atrial fibrillation and thromboembolism in a randomised trial of atrial versus dual chamber pacing in 177 patients with sick sinus syndrome. Heart 90:661-666, 2004.
170. Andersen HR, Nielsen JC, Thomsen PE, et al: Atrioventricular conduction during long-term follow-up of patients with sick sinus syndrome. Circulation 98:1315-1321, 1998.
171. Kristensen L, Nielsen JC, Pedersen AK, et al: AV block and changes in pacing mode during long-term follow-up of 399 consecutive patients with sick sinus syndrome treated with an AAI/AAIR pacemaker. Pacing Clin Electrophysiol. 24:358-365, 2001.
172. Karpawich PP, Gates J, Stokes KB: Septal His-Purkinje ventricular pacing in canines: A new endocardial electrode approach. Pacing Clin Electrophysiol 15:2011-2015, 1992.
173. Scherlag BJ, Kosowsky BD, Damato AN: A technique for ventricular pacing from the His bundle of the intact heart. Am J Physiol 22:584-587, 1967.
174. Deshmukh P, Casavant DA, Romanyshyn M, et al: Permanent, direct His-bundle pacing: A novel approach to cardiac pacing in patients with normal His-Purkinje activation. Circulation 101:869-877, 2000.
175. De Cock CC, Giudici MC, Twisk JW: Comparison of the haemodynamic effects of right ventricular outflow-tract pacing with right ventricular apex pacing: A quantitative review. Europace 5:275-278, 2003.
176. Buckingham TA, Candinas R, Schlapfer J, et al: Acute hemodynamic effects of atrioventricular pacing at different sites in the right ventricle individually and simultaneously. Pacing Clin Electrophysiol 20:909-915, 1997.
177. Tse HF, Yu C, Wong KK, et al: Functional abnormalities in patients with permanent right ventricular pacing: The effect of sites of electrical stimulation. J Am Coll Cardiol 40:1451-1458, 2002.
178. Gammage MD, Marsh AM: Randomized trials for selective site pacing: Do we know where we are going? Pacing Clin Electrophysiol 27:878-882, 2004.
179. Puggioni E, Brignole M, Gammage M, et al: Acute comparative effect of right and left ventricular pacing in patients with permanent atrial fibrillation. J Am Coll Cardiol 21:234-238, 2004.
180. Turner MS, Bleasdale RA, Vinereanu D, et al: Electrical and mechanical components of dyssynchrony in heart failure patients with normal QRS duration and left bundle-branch block, impact of left and biventricular pacing. Circulation 109:2544-2549, 2004.
181. Wyman BT, Hunter WC, Prinzen FW, et al: Mapping propagation of mechanical activation in the paced heart with MRI tagging. Am J Physiol 276:H881-H891, 1999.
182. Etienne Y, Mansourati J, Gilard M, et al: Evaluation of left ventricular based pacing in patients with congestive heart failure and atrial fibrillation. Am J Cardiol 83:1138-1140, 1999.
183. Tyers GFO: Comparison of the effect on cardiac function of single-site and simultaneous multiple site ventricular stimulation after A-V block. J Thor Cardiovasc Surg 59:211-217, 1970.
184. Jais P, Takahashi A, Garrigue S, et al: Mid-term follow-up of endocardial biventricular pacing. Pacing Clin Electrophysiol 23:1744-1747, 2000.
185. Fei L, Wtobleski D, Groh W, et al: Effects of multisite ventricular pacing on cardiac function in normal dogs and dogs with heart failure. J Cardiovasc Electrophysiol 10:935-946, 1999.
186. Hay I, Melenovsky V, Fetics BJ, et al: Short-term effects of right-left heart sequential cardiac resynchronization in patients with heart failure, chronic atrial fibrillation, and atrioventricular nodal block. Circulation 110:3404-3410, 2004.
187. Wyman BT, Hunter WC, Prinzen FW, et al: Effects of single- and biventricular pacing on temporal and spatial dynamics of ventricular contraction. Am J Physiol 282:H372-H379, 2002.
188. Nielsen JC, Pedersen AK, Mortensen PT, et al: Programming a fixed long atrioventricular delay is not effective in preventing ventricular pacing in patients with sick sinus syndrome. Europace 1:113-120, 1999.
189. Stierle U, Kruger D, Vincent AM, et al: An optimized AV delay algorithm for patients with intermittent atrioventricular conduction. Pacing Clin Electrophysiol 21:1035-1043, 1998.
190. Olshansky B, Day J, McGuire M, et al: Inhibition of unnecessary RV pacing with AV search hysteresis in ICDs (INTRINSIC RV): Design and clinical protocol. Pacing Clin Electrophysiol 28:62-66, 2005.
191. Sweeney MO, Shea JB, Fox V, et al: Randomized pilot study of a new atrial-based minimal ventricular pacing mode (MVP) in dual chamber implantable cardioverter-defibrillators. Heart Rhythm 1:160-167, 2004.
192. Sweeney MO, Ellenbogen KA, Casavant D, et al: multicenter, prospective, randomized safety and efficacy study of a new atrial-based managed ventricular pacing mode (MVP) in dual chamber ICDs. J Cardiovasc Electrophys 16:811-817, 2005.
193. Bakker PF, Meijburg HW, de Vries JW, et al: Biventricular pacing in end-stage heart failure improves functional capacity and left ventricular function. J Interv Card Electrophysiol 4:395-404, 2000.
194. Cazeau S, Ritter P, Lazarus A, et al: Multisite pacing for end-stage heart failure: Early experience. Pacing Clin Electrophysiol 19:1748-1757, 1996.
195. Butter C, Auricchio A, Stellbrink C, et al: Effect of resynchronization therapy stimulation site on the systolic function of heart failure patients. Circulation 104:3026-3029, 2001.
196. Blanc JJ, Etienne Y, Gilard M, et al: Evaluation of different ventricular pacing sites in patients with severe heart failure: Results of an acute hemodynamic study. Circulation 96:3273-3277, 1997.

197. Kass DA, Chen CH, Curry C, et al: Improved left ventricular mechanics from acute VDD pacing in patients with dilated cardiomyopathy and ventricular conduction delay. Circulation 99:1567-1573, 1999.
198. Auricchio A, Stellbrink C, Sack S, et al: The Pacing Therapies for Congestive Heart Failure (PATH-CHF) study: Rationale, design, and endpoints of a prospective randomized multicenter study. Am J Cardiol 83:130D-135D, 1999.
199. Cazeau S, Leclercq C, Lavergne T, et al: Multisite Stimulation in Cardiomyopathies (MUSTIC) Study Investigators: Effects of multisite biventricular pacing in patients with heart failure and intraventricular conduction delay. N Engl J Med 344:873-880, 2001.
200. Abraham WT, Fisher WG, Smith AL, et al; MIRACLE Study Group; Multicenter InSync Randomized Clinical Evaluation: Cardiac resynchronization in chronic heart failure. N Engl J Med 346:1845-1853, 2002.
201. Cleland JG, Daubert JC, Erdmann E, et al: The effect of cardiac resynchronization on morbidity and mortality in heart failure. N Engl J Med 352:1539-1549, 2005.
202. Sogaard P, Egeblad H, Kim WY, et al: Tissue Doppler imaging predicts improved systolic performance and reversed left ventricular remodeling during long-term cardiac resynchronization therapy. J Am Coll Cardiol 40:723-730, 2002.
203. Yu CM, Chau E, Sanderson JE, et al: Tissue Doppler echocardiographic evidence of reverse remodeling and improved synchronicity by simultaneously delaying regional contraction after biventricular pacing therapy in heart failure. Circulation 105:438-445, 2002.
204. Dekker AL, Phelps B, Dijkam, et al: Epicardial left ventricular lead placement for cardiac resynchronization therapy: Optimal pace site selection with pressure-volume loops. J Thorac Cardiovasc Surg 127:1642-1647, 2004.
205. Leclercq C, Cazeau S, Le Breton H, et al: Acute hemodynamic effects of biventricular DDD pacing in patients with end-stage heart failure. J Am Coll Cardiol 32:1825-1831, 1998.
206. Bleasdale RA, Turner MS, Mumford CE, et al: Left ventricular pacing minimizes diastolic ventricular interaction, allowing improved preload-dependent systolic performance. Circulation 110:2395-2400, 2004.
207. Adamson PB, Kleckner KJ, VanHout WL, et al: Cardiac resynchronization therapy improves heart rate variability in patients with symptomatic heart failure. Circulation 108:266-269, 2003.
208. St John Sutton MG, Plappert T, Abraham WT, et al: Effect of cardiac resynchronization therapy on left ventricular size and function in chronic heart failure. Circulation 107:1985-1990, 2003.
209. Leclercq C, Faris O, Tunin R, et al: Systolic improvement and mechanical resynchronization does not require electrical synchrony in the dilated failing heart with left bundle-branch block. Circulation 106:1760-1763, 2002.
210. Dubin AM, Feinstein JA, Reddy VM, et al: Electrical resynchronization: A novel therapy for the failing right ventricle. Circulation 107:2287-2289, 2003.
211. Pitzalis MV, Iacoviello M, Romito R, et al: Ventricular asynchrony predicts a better in patients with chronic heart failure receiving cardiac resynchronization therapy. J Am Coll Cardiol 45:65-69, 2005.
212. Penicka M, Bartunek J, De Bruyne B, et al: Improvement of left ventricular function after cardiac resynchronization therapy is predictive by tissue Doppler imaging echocardiography. Circulation 109:978-983, 2004.
213. Ansalone G, Trambaiolo P, Giorda GP, et al: Multisite stimulation in refractory heart failure. G Ital Cardiol 29:451-459, 1999.
214. Faber L, Lamp B, Hering D, et al: [Analysis of inter- and intraventricular asynchrony by tissue Doppler echocardiography]. Z Kardiol 92:994-1002, 2003.
215. Schuster P, Faerestrand S, Ohm OJ: Colour tissue velocity imaging can show resynchronisation of longitudinal left ventricular contraction pattern by biventricular pacing in patients with severe heart failure. Heart 89:859-864, 2003.
216. Bax JJ, Molhoek SG, van Erven L, et al: Usefulness of myocardial tissue Doppler echocardiography to evaluate left ventricular dyssynchrony before and after biventricular pacing in patients with idiopathic dilated cardiomyopathy. Am J Cardiol 91:94-97, 2003.
217. Yu CM, Fung JW, Zhang Q, et al: Tissue Doppler imaging is superior to strain rate imaging and postsystolic shortening on the prediction of reverse remodeling in both ischemic and nonischemic heart failure after cardiac resynchronization therapy. Circulation 110:66-73, 2004.
218. Notabartolo D, Merlino JD, Smith AL, et al: Usefulness of the peak velocity difference by tissue Doppler imaging technique as an effective predictor of response to cardiac resynchronization therapy. Am J Cardiol 94:817-820, 2004.
219. Knebel F, Reibis RK, Bondke HJ, et al: Tissue Doppler echocardiography and biventricular pacing in heart failure: Patient selection, procedural guidance, follow-up, quantification of success. Cardiovasc Ultrasound 2:17, 2004.
220. Sogaard P, Hassager C: Tissue Doppler imaging as a guide to resynchronization therapy in patients with congestive heart failure. Curr Opin Cardiol 19:447-451, 2004.
221. Tada H, Toide H, Naito S, et al: Tissue Doppler imaging and strain Doppler imaging as modalities for predicting clinical improvement in patients receiving biventricular pacing. Circ J 69:194-200, 2005.
222. Bax JJ, Ansalone G, Breithardt OA, et al: Echocardiographic evaluation of cardiac resynchronization therapy: Ready for routine clinical use? A critical appraisal. J Am Coll Cardiol 44: 1-9, 2004.
223. Miyatake K, Yamagishi M, Tanaka N, et al: New method for evaluating left ventricular wall motion by color-coded tissue Doppler imaging: In vitro and in vivo studies. J Am Coll Cardiol 25:717-724, 1995.
224. Yu Y, Kramer A, Spinelli J, et al: Biventricular mechanical asynchrony predicts hemodynamic effects of uni- and biventricular pacing. Am J Physiol Heart Circ Physiol 285:H2788-H2796, 2003.
225. Pitzalis MV, Iacoviello M, Romito R, et al: Cardiac resynchronization therapy tailored by echocardiographic evaluation of ventricular asynchrony. J Am Coll Cardiol 40:1615-1622, 2002.
226. Ansalone G, Giannantoni P, Ricci R, et al: Doppler myocardial imaging in patients with heart failure receiving biventricular pacing treatment. Am Heart J 142:881-896, 2001.
227. Garrigue S, Jais P, Espil G, et al: Comparison of chronic biventricular pacing between epicardial and endocardial left ventricular stimulation using Doppler tissue imaging in patients with heart failure. Am J Cardiol 88:858-862, 2001.
228. Breithardt OA, Stellbrink C, Herbots L, et al: Cardiac resynchronization therapy can reverse abnormal myocardial strain distribution in patients with heart failure and left bundle branch block. J Am Coll Cardiol 42:486-494, 2003.
229. Gasparini M, Mantica M, Galimberti P, et al: Is the left ventricular lateral wall the best lead implantation site for cardiac resynchronisation therapy? Pacing Clin Electrophysiol 26:162-168, 2003.
230. Ansalone G, Giannantoni P, Ricci R, et al: Doppler myocardial imaging to evaluate the effectiveness of pacing site in patients receiving biventricular pacing. J Am Coll Cardiol 39:489-499, 2002.
231. Leon AR, Greenberg JM, Kanuru N, et al: Cardiac resynchronization in patients with congestive heart failure and chronic atrial fibrillation: Effect of upgrading to biventricular pacing after chronic right ventricular pacing. J Am Coll Cardiol 39:1258-1263, 2002.

232. Valls-Bertault V, Fatemi M, Gilard M, et al: Assessment of upgrading to biventricular pacing with right ventricular pacing and congestive heart failure after atrioventricular junction ablation for chronic atrial fibrillation. Europace 6:438-443, 2004.
233. Brignole M, Gammage M, Puggioni E, et al: Comparative assessment of right, left, and biventricular pacing in patients with permanent atrial fibrillation. Eur Heart J 26:712-722, 2005.
234. Leclercq C, Walker S, Linde C, et al: Comparative effects of permanent biventricular and right-univentricular pacing in heart failure patients with chronic atrial fibrillation. Eur Heart J 23:1780-1787, 2002.
235. Touiza A, Etienne Y, Gilard M, et al: Long-term left ventricular pacing: Assessment and comparison with biventricular pacing in patients with severe congestive heart failure. J Am Coll Cardiol 38:1966-1970, 2001.
236. Blanc JJ, Bertault-Valls V, Fatemi M, et al: Midterm benefits of left univentricular pacing in patients with congestive heart failure. Circulation 109:1741-1744, 2003.
237. De Lurgio DB, Foster E, Higginbotham MB, et al: A comparison of cardiac resynchronization by sequential biventricular pacing and left ventricular pacing to simultaneous biventricular pacing: Rationale and design of the DECREASE-HF clinical trial. J Card Fail 11:233-239, 2005.
238. Wilkoff BL, Cook JR, Epstein AE, et al: Dual-chamber pacing or ventricular backup pacing in patients with an implantable defibrillator: The Dual Chamber and VVI Implantable Defibrillator (DAVID) Trial. JAMA 288:3115-3123, 2002.
239. Etienne Y, Mansourati J, Touiza A, et al: Evaluation of left ventricular function and mitral regurgitation during left ventricular-based pacing in patients with heart failure. Eur J Heart Fail 3:441-447, 2001.
240. Molhoek SG, Bax JJ, Bleeker GB, et al: Comparison of response to cardiac resynchronization therapy in patients with sinus rhythm versus chronic atrial fibrillation. Am J Cardiol 94:1506-1509, 2004.
241. Auricchio A, Stellbrink C, Butter C, et al: Clinical efficacy of cardiac resynchronization therapy using left ventricular pacing in heart failure patients stratified by severity of ventricular conduction delay. J Am Coll Cardiol 42:2109-2116, 2003.
242. Riedlbauchova L, Kautzner J, Fridl P: Influence of different atrioventricular and interventricular delays on cardiac output during cardiac resynchronization therapy. Pacing Clin Electrophysiol 28(Suppl 1):S19-S23, 2005.
243. van Gelder BM, Bracke FA, Meijer A, et al: Effect of optimizing the VV interval on left ventricular contractility in cardiac resynchronization therapy. Am J Cardiol 93:1500-1503, 2004.
244. Sogaard P, Egeblad H, Pedersen AK, et al: Sequential versus simultaneous biventricular resynchronization for severe heart failure: Evaluation by tissue Doppler imaging. Circulation 106:2078-2084, 2002.
245. Levine PA, Seltzer JP, Pirzada FA: The "pacemaker syndrome" in a properly functioning physiologic pacing system. Pacing Clin Electrophysiol 6:279-282, 1983.
246. Torresani J, Ebagost A, Alland-Latour G: Pacemaker syndrome with DDD pacing. Pacing Clin Electrophysiol 7:1148-1151, 1984.
247. Pierantozzi A, Bocconcelli P, Syarbi E: DDD pacemaker syndrome and atrial conduction time. Pacing Clin Electrophysiol 17:374-376, 1994.
248. den Dulk K, Lindemans FW, Brugada P, et al: Pacemaker syndrome with AAI rate variable pacing: Importance of atrioventricular conduction properties, medication and pacemaker programmability. Pacing Clin Electrophysiol 11:1226-1233, 1988.
249. Liebert HP, O'Donoghue S, Tullner WF, et al: Pacemaker syndrome in activity-responsive VVI pacing. Am J Cardiol 64:124-126, 1989.
250. Cunningham TM: Pacemaker syndrome due to retrograde conduction in a DDI pacemaker. Am Heart J 115:478-479, 1988.
251. Pitney MR, May CD, Davis MJ: Undesirable mode switching with a dual chamber rate responsive pacemaker. Pacing Clin Electrophysiol 16:729-737, 1993.
252. Pieterse MG, den Dulk K, van Gelder BM, et al: Programming a long pace atrioventricular interval may be risky in DDDR pacing. Pacing Clin Electrophysiol 17:252-257, 1994.
253. Mary DASG: Electrophysiology of atrial receptors. In Hainsworth R, McGregor KH, Mary DASG (eds): Cardiogenic Reflexes. Oxford, Oxford Scientific, 1987, p 3.
254. Hainsworth R: Atrial receptors in reflex control of the circulation. In Zucker IH, Gilmore JP (eds): Reflex Control of the Circulation. Boca Raton, FL, CRC Press, 1991, p 273.
255. Ellenbogen KA, Thames MD, Moharity PK: New insights into pacemaker syndrome gained from hemodynamic, humoral and vascular responses during a ventriculo-atrial pacing. Am J Cardiol 65:53-59, 1990.
256. Ellenbogen KA, Wood MA, Stranbler B: Clinical, hemodynamic and neurohumoral features. In Barold SS, Mugia J (eds): New Perspectives in Cardiac Pacing: 3. Mt Kisco, NY, Futura, 1992.
257. Vardas PE, Travill CM, Williams TDM, et al: Effect of dual chamber pacing on raised plasma atrial natriuretic peptide concentrations in complete atrioventricular block. Br Med J 296:94, 1988.
258. Stangl K, Weil J, Seitz K, et al: Influence of AV synchrony on the plasma levels of atrial natriuretic peptide (ANP) in patients with total AV block. Pacing Clin Electrophysiol 11:1176-1181, 1988.
259. Ellenbogen KA, Kapadia K, Walsh M, et al: Increase in plasma atrial natriuretic factor during ventriculoatrial pacing. Am J Cardiol 64:236-237, 1989.
260. Noll B, Krappe J, Goke B, et al: Influence of pacing mode and rate on peripheral levels of atrial natriuretic peptide (ANP). Pacing Clin Electrophysiol 12:1763-1768, 1989.
261. Barotto MT, Berti S, Clerico A, et al: Atrial natriuretic peptide during different pacing modes in comparison with hemodynamic changes. Pacing Clin Electrophysiol 13:432-442, 1990.
262. Wong CK, Lau CP, Cheng CH, et al: Delayed decline in plasma atrial natriuretic peptide levels after an abrupt reduction in atrial pressures: Observation in patients with dual chamber pacing. Am Heart J 120:882-885, 1990.
263. Bristow MR, Feldman AM, Saxon LA: Heart failure management using implantable devices for ventricular resynchronization: Comparison of Medical Therapy, Pacing, and Defibrillation in Chronic Heart Failure (COMPANION) trial. COMPANION Steering Committee and COMPANION Clinical Investigators. J Card Fail 6:276-285, 2000.
264. Bristow MR, Saxon LA, Boehmer J, et al: Cardiac resynchronization therapy with or without an implantable defibrillator in advanced chronic heart failure. N Engl J Med 350:2140-2150, 2003.
265. Shemin RJ, Scott WC, Kastl DG, et al: Hemodynamic effects of various modes of cardiac pacing after operation for idiopathic hypertrophic subaortic stenosis. Ann Thorac Surg 27:137, 1979.
266. Gross JN, Keltz TN, Cooper JA, et al: Profound "pacemaker syndrome" in hypertrophic cardiomyopathy. Am J Cardiol 70:1507-1511, 1992.
267. Fananapazir L, Cannon RO, Tripodi D, et al: Impact of dual chamber permanent pacing in patients with obstructive hypertrophic cardiomyopathy with symptoms refractory to verapamil and β-adrenergic blocker therapy. Circulation 85:2149-2161, 1992.
268. Jeanrenaud X, Goy JJ, Kappenberger LK: Effects of dual-chamber pacing in hypertrophic obstructive cardiomyopathy. Lancet 339:1318-1323, 1992.
269. Slade AK, Sadoul N, Shapiro L, et al: DDD pacing in hypertrophic cardiomyopathy: A multicenter clinical experience. Heart 75:44-49, 1996.

270. Posma JL, Blanksma PK, van der Wall EE, et al: Effects of permanent dual chamber pacing on myocardial perfusion in symptomatic hypertrophic cardiomyopathy. Heart 76:358-362, 1996.
271. Nishimura RA, Trusty JM, Hayes DL, et al: Dual-chamber pacing for hypertrophic cardiomyopathy: A randomized, double-blind crossover trial. J Am Coll Cardiol 29:435-441, 1997.
272. Nishimura RA, Hayes DL, Ilstrup DM, et al: Effect of dual-chamber pacing on systolic and diastolic function in patients with hypertrophic cardiomyopathy: Acute Doppler echocardiographic and catheterization hemodynamic study. J Am Coll Cardiol 27:421-430, 1996.
273. Maron BJ: Appraisal of dual-chamber pacing therapy in hypertrophic cardiomyopathy: Too soon for a rush to judgment? J Am Coll Cardiol 27:431, 1996.
274. Cannon RO, Tripodi D, Dilsizian V, et al: Results of permanent dual-chamber pacing in symptomatic nonobstructive hypertrophic cardiomyopathy. Am J Cardiol 73:571-576, 1994.
275. Hartzler GO, Maloney JD, Curtis JJ, et al: Hemodynamic benefits of atrioventricular sequential pacing after cardiac surgery. Am J Cardiol 40:232-236, 1977.
276. Laniado S, Yellin EL, Yoran C, et al: Physiologic mechanisms in aortic insufficiency. I: The effect of changing heart rate on flow dynamics. II: Determinants of Austin Flint murmur. Circulation 66:226-235, 1982.
277. Meyer TE, Sareli P, Marcus RH, et al: Beneficial effect of atrial pacing in severe acute aortic regurgitation and role of M-mode echocardiography in determining the optimal pacing interval. Am J Cardiol 67:398-403, 1991.
278. Valero A: Atrial transport dysfunction in acute myocardial infarction. Am J Cardiol 16:22-30, 1965.
279. Cohn JN, Guiha NH, Broder MI, et al: Right ventricular infarction: Clinical and hemodynamic features. Am J Cardiol 33:209-214, 1974.
280. Topol EJ, Goldschlager N, Ports TA, et al: Hemodynamic benefit of atrial pacing in right ventricular myocardial infarction. An Intern Med 96:594-597, 1982.
281. Love JC, Haffajee CI, Gore JM, et al: Reversibility of hypotension and shock by atrial or atrioventricular sequential pacing in patients with right ventricular infarction. Am Heart J 108:5-13, 1984.
282. Matangi MF: Temporary physiologic pacing in inferior wall acute myocardial infarction with right ventricular damage. Am J Cardiol 59:1207-1208, 1987.
283. Murphy P, Morton P, Murtagh JG, et al: Hemodynamic effects of different temporary pacing modes for management of bradycardias complicating acute myocardial infarction. Pacing Clin Electrophysiol 15:391-396, 1992.
284. Shafer A, Rozenman Y, Ben David Y, et al: Left ventricular function during physiological cardiac pacing: Relation to rate, pacing mode and underlying myocardial disease. Pacing Clin Electrophysiol 10:315-325, 1987.
285. Kenny RA, Ingram A, Mitsuoka T, et al: Optimum pacing mode for patients with angina pectoris. Br Heart J 56:463-468, 1986.
286. Chamberlain DA, Leinbach RC, Vassaux CE, et al: Sequential atrio-ventricular pacing in heart block complicating acute myocardial infarction. N Engl J Med 282:577-582, 1970.
287. DiCarlo LA, Morady F, Krol RB, et al: The hemodynamic effects of ventricular pacing with and without atrioventricular synchrony in patients with normal and diminished left ventricular function. Am Heart J 114:746-752, 1987.
288. Peschar M, Vernooy K, Cornelussen RN, et al: Structural, electrical and mechanical remodeling of the canine heart in AV-block and LBBB. Eur Heart J Suppl 6:D61-D65, 2004.
289. Gomez AM, Valdivia HH, Cheng H, et al: Defective excitation—contraction coupling in experimental heart failure. Science 276:800-806, 1976.
290. Fiedler B, Wollert KC: Interference of antihypertrophic molecules and signaling pathways with the Ca2+-calcineurin-NFAT cascase in cardiac myocytes. Cardiovasc Res 63:450-457, 2004.
291. Reiken S, Wehrens XH, Vest JA, et al: Beta-blockers restore calcium release channel function and improve cardiac muscle performance in human heart failure. Circulation 107:2459-2466, 2003.
292. Wood EH, Heppner RL, Weidman S: Inotropic effects of electric currents: 1. Positive and negative effects of constant electric currents or current pulses applied during cardiac action potential. Circ Res 24:409-445, 1969.
293. O'Rourke B, Kass DA, Tomaselli GF, et al: Mechanisms of altered excitation-contraction coupling in canine tachycardia-induced heart failure, I: Experimental studies. Circ Res 84:562-570, 1999.
294. Burkhoff D, Ben Haim SA: Nonexcitatory electrial signals for enhancing ventricular contractility: Rationale and initial investigations of an experimental treatment for heart failure. Am J Physiol Heart Circ Physiol 288:H2550-H2556, 2005.
295. Brunckhorst C, Shemer I, Mika Y, et al: Cardiac contractility modulation by non-excitatory currents: Cellular mechanism in isolated cardiac muscle. Eur J Heart Fail 8:7-15, 2006.
296. Heerdt PM, Holmes JW, Cai B, et al: Chronic unloading by left ventricular assist device reverses contractile dysfunction and alters gene expression in end-stage heart failure. Circulation 102:2713-2719, 2000.
297. Mohri S, He KL, Dickstein M, et al: Cardiac contractility modulation by electric currents applied during the refractory period. Am J Physiol Heart Circ Physiol 282:H1642-H1647, 2002.
298. Morita H, Suzuki G, Haddad W, et al: Cardiac contractility modulation with nonexcitatory electric signals improves left ventricular function in dogs with chronic heart failure. J Card Fail 9:69-75, 2003.
299. Sabbah HN, Imai M, Haddad W, et al: Non-excitatory cardiac contractility modulation electric signals improve left ventricular function in dogs with heart failure without increasing myocardial oxygen consumption [abstract]. Heart Rhythm 1:S181, 2004.
300. Packer M, Carver JR, Rodeheffer RJ, et al: Effect of oral milrinone on mortality in severe chronic heart failure. N Engl J Med 325:1468-1475, 1991.

Chapter 10

Clinical Trials of Pacing Modes

JEFF S. HEALEY • CARLOS A. MORILLO • STUART J. CONNOLLY

History and Rationale for Different Pacing Modes

Since its initial clinical application in the 1950s, the cardiac pacemaker has saved lives and relieved symptoms in patients with bradydysrhythmias.[1,2] Pacemakers have since evolved to become smaller and more reliable and to better approximate normal cardiac physiology. Early devices provided only fixed-rate ventricular pacing, until the development of "demand" pacemakers in the 1960s.[3,4] Before the 1980s, artificial pacemakers could give patients sufficient chronotropic support to maintain life and prevent syncope but could not replicate normal cardiovascular physiology, such as increasing the heart rate in response to exercise and maintaining atrioventricular (AV) synchrony. The subsequent introduction of rate-adaptive pacemakers and dual-chamber pacemakers permitted a closer approximation of this normal cardiac electrical function and led to the concept of the *physiologic pacing*. However, the clinical impact of these enhancements remained undefined.

The use of dual-chamber pacing in patients with AV block or sinus node dysfunction offers several advantages over fixed-rate ventricular pacing, such as the maintenance of AV synchrony, the preservation of sinus node control over heart rate (in patients with AV block), and the maintenance of normal ventricular activation via the His-Purkinje system (in patients with sinus node dysfunction). It was anticipated that this closer approximation of normal physiology would reduce patient morbidity and mortality and improve quality of life (QOL). Given the higher cost, greater complexity, and increased complications of dual-chamber pacemakers, numerous clinical studies were conducted to assess their incremental benefit.

Clinical Outcomes in Nonrandomized Studies of Pacing Mode

Beginning in the late 1980s, several retrospective series examined the effect of pacing mode on clinical outcomes, such as mortality, atrial fibrillation, heart failure, and stroke (Tables 10-1 and 10-2).[5-14] Several overviews of these studies have been published.[15,16] Although limited by their retrospective design and propensity for selection bias, these reports provided the first critical appraisal of pacing mode and laid the groundwork for the clinical trials that followed.

Conservatively treated, complete heart block has a poor prognosis, with 1- and 5-year survival rates of 60% and 30%, respectively. About one third of patients die suddenly, and the prognosis is worse in those who are older, those who have associated cardiac diseases, those with syncope, and those with constant complete heart block. Conservatively treated chronic second-degree AV block, independent of the type of second-degree block, is also associated with a reduced life

TABLE 10-1. **Survival in Sick Sinus Syndrome in Relation to the Mode of Pacing from the Retrospective Observational Studies**

		Physiologic		Ventricular		Death (%/year)		
Study	**Year**	**No.**	**Follow-up (months)**	**No.**	**Follow-up (months)**	**PHYS**	**VENT**	**RRR (%)**
Rosenqvist et al[5]	1988	89	44	79	47	2.1	5.9	−64*
Sasaki et al[6]	1988	19	20	25	35	7.6	8.2	−7
Bianconi et al[7]	1989	153	44	150	59	3.8	6.3	−40
Santini et al[8]	1990	214	61	125	47	2.8	7.7	−64*
Stangl et al[10]	1990	110	52	112	54	4.0	6.2	−35
Zanini et al[88]	1990	53	45	57	40	2.5	5.3	−53
Nurnberg et al[9]	1991	37	41	93	41	7.1	13.8	−49*
Hesselson et al[20]	1992	308	30	193	44	8.3	12.8	−35*
Sgarbossa et al[21]	1993	395	66	112	66	3.9	7.5	−48*
Tung et al[89]	1994	36	44	112	44	8.3	16.5	−50*
Weighted means and totals	—	1414	50	1058	49	4.8	9.4	−49

*$P \leq .05$.
PHYS, Physiologic mode; RRR, relative risk reduction; VENT, ventricular mode.

expectancy, especially when associated with syncope. Nonrandomized data suggest that the use of permanent pacemakers in patients with AV block improves survival[17]; however, retrospective series came to conflicting conclusions regarding the superiority of dual-chamber pacing. Alpert and colleagues[13] found no difference in all-cause mortality rates between 132 patients receiving ventricular pacemakers and 48 patients receiving dual-chamber units (DVI or DDD) for high-grade AV block. Linde-Edelstam and associates[18] also compared survival in 148 patients with AV block (74 receiving VVI pacemakers, and 74 VDD pacemakers) and found no difference in all-cause mortality. However, subsequent, larger studies did appear to suggest a benefit. In a study of 1245 patients (77% with AV block; ventricular pacing in 97% and dual-chamber pacing in only 3%), multivariate analysis demonstrated that survival was related to the mode of pacemaker therapy.[19] In a second report of 391 patients, who underwent pacing for AV block or carotid sinus hypersensitivity,[20] the 7-year survival rate was 54% in the DDD group and 33% in the VVI group ($P < .05$).

Sick sinus syndrome associated with minor symptoms carries a favorable prognosis, and survival of patients with the disorder appears equal to that of the general population. In those with advanced symptoms due to sinus node dysfunction (e.g., syncope), however, survival may be reduced. In patients with sinus node dysfunction, 10 retrospective studies involving more than 1400 patients suggested a 50% reduction in mortality with dual-chamber pacing (see Table 10-1). The studies were unanimous in finding a lower mortality rate in patients receiving physiologically based pacing, and in many of the individual reports, this difference achieved statistical significance.[5,7-10] In one of the larger studies, Sgarbossa and colleagues[21] compared outcomes in 395 patients receiving physiologic pacing and 112 patients receiving VVI pacing who were followed up for a mean of 5.5 years. Univariate analysis showed VVI pacing to be associated with a more than 40% increase in risk of total and cardiovascular mortality; with multivariate analysis, however, ventricular pacing was no longer an independent risk factor, suggesting that ventricular pacing was preferentially used in patients with other baseline characteristics that were associated with a higher risk of death. Ventricular pacing mode was identified as an independent predictor of chronic atrial fibrillation[12] (hazard ratio [HR] = 1.98; $P = .003$) and stroke[12] (HR = 2.61; $P = .008$), but not of congestive heart failure[12] (odds ratio = 0.86; $P = .603$).

Overall, the retrospective studies suggest a large improvement in clinical outcomes with the use of dual-chamber pacemakers—specifically, a 45% relative risk reduction in mortality, a 62% reduction in heart failure, a 66% reduction in stroke, and a 72% reduction in atrial fibrillation (see Table 10-2). However, these data must be interpreted very cautiously, as the retrospective, nonrandomized design of these studies is highly susceptible to selection bias, which would inflate the apparent benefit of dual-chamber pacing. At least one of these studies confirmed that patients given ventricular pacemakers had more comorbidity at baseline,[21] which may have accounted for the higher mortality in patients receiving ventricular pacemakers. Therefore, these retrospective studies should not be used to justify

TABLE 10-2. **Association between Pacing Mode and the Rate of Atrial Fibrillation, Stroke or Embolism, Congestive Heart Failure, and Death in Nonrandomized Observational Studies**

Study	Total Pt-Yrs	Atrial Fibrillation (%/year)			Stroke/Embolism (%/year)			Congestive Heart Failure (%/year)			Death (%/year)		
		PHYS	VENT	RRR	PHYS	VENT	RRR	PHYS	VENT	RRR	PHYS	VENT	RRR
Sutton & Kenny[14]	3239	1.4	6.8	−85*	—	—	—	—	—	—	—	—	—
Markewitz et al[90]	592	3.1	10.0	−69	—	—	—	—	—	—	—	—	—
Ebagosti et al[91]	408	2.0	5.2	−62*	0	1.4	−100	—	—	—	3.5	4.8	−27
Langenfeld et al[92]	1265	0.9	5.4	−83	—	—	—	—	—	—	—	—	—
Rosenqvist et al[5]	636	1.8	12.1	−85*	3.3	3.9	−15	3.9	9.4	−59*	2.1	5.9	−64*
Sasaki et al[6]	112	0	12.3	−100*	0	6.8	−100	2.6	9.6	−73	7.6	8.2	−7
Bianconi et al[7]	1301	4.8	7.9	−39*	1.2	2.1	−43	—	—	—	3.8	6.3	−40
Feuer et al[93]	807	2.5	4.5	−44*	—	—	—	—	—	—	2.2	3.9	−44
Santini et al[8]	1582	1.4	11.8	−88*	0.5	2.6	−81	—	—	—	2.8	7.7	−64*
Stangl et al[10]	981	1.5	4.2	−64	—	—	—	—	—	—	4.0	6.2	−35
Zanini et al[88]	389	1.0	5.3	−81*	0	2.1	−100	0.5	1.6	−69	2.5	5.3	−53
Nurnberg et al[9]	444	4.8	11.0	−56	0	3.1	−100	—	—	—	7.1	13.8	−49*
Hesselson et al[20]	2498	1.4	5.3	−74	—	—	—	—	—	—	9.0	13.6	−34
Linde-Edelstam et al[18]	799	—	—	—	—	—	—	—	—	—	5.8	7.0	−17
Sgarbossa et al[12,21]	2789	—	—	—	—	—	—	—	—	—	3.9	7.5	−48
Tung et al[89]	543	—	—	—	—	—	—	—	—	—	8.3	16.5	−50
Weighted means	18385	1.9	7.0	−72	0.9	2.7	−66	2.6	6.8	−62	4.8	8.9	−45

*$P \leq .05$.
PHYS, Physiologic mode; Pt-Yrs, patient-years of follow-up; RRR, relative risk reduction; VENT, ventricular mode.

one mode of pacing over another but were helpful in the design of subsequent randomized trials that were better suited to determining the relative effectiveness of different pacing modes.

Clinical Outcomes in Randomized Controlled Clinical Trials of Pacing Mode

Although retrospective studies suggest a large benefit of atrial pacing over ventricular pacing, their nonrandomized design makes them susceptible to bias. Physicians tend to offer more complex interventions to younger, healthier patients, so a preferential use of atrial pacemakers in low-risk individuals would inflate their apparent superiority over ventricular pacemakers. By virtue of their size and random treatment allocation, large prospective, randomized controlled trials provide a better estimate of the true incremental effectiveness of atrial pacemakers. In total, eight such studies were completed from 1994 through 2005 (Table 10-3).

Clinical Trials of Atrial Pacing versus Ventricular Pacing

The first prospective, randomized controlled trial of pacing modality was published in 1994 by Andersen and colleagues.[22] This Danish study randomly assigned 225 patients with sinus node dysfunction to receive a single-chamber atrial or ventricular pacemaker. Patients were monitored for a mean of 3.3 years for the outcomes of stroke, atrial fibrillation, and death. The two patient groups were similar at baseline. During follow-up there was no significant difference in the risk of atrial fibrillation or death; however, the risk of stroke was significantly lower with atrial pacing. The Danish study group published a second report when the mean follow-up in these patients was 5.5 years, some patients

TABLE 10-3. **Characteristics of Randomized Controlled Trials of Pacing Mode Selection**

Trial	Year	No. Subjects	Average Follow-up (yrs)	Mean Age (yrs)	Sick Sinus Syndrome (%)	History of Hypertension (%)	Crossover to DDD (%)	Physiologic Mode
Danish[23]	1994	225	5.5	76	100	??	2	AAI
PASE[24]	1998	407	2.5	76	43	52	26	DDD
Mattioli et al[27]	1998	210	2.0	77	52	48	??	Both
CTOPP[28]	2000	2568	6.0	73	42	35	4.3	Both
MOST[35]	2002	2010	4.5	74	100	62	37.6	DDD
PAC-ATACH[45]*	2001	198	2.0	72	100	55	44	DDD
STOP-AF[46]*	2005	350	2.0	>18	100	??	??	Both
UKPACE[48]*	2002	2000	4.0	80	0	34	??	DDD

*Unpublished.

having been monitored for as long as 8 years.[23] At this point, there was a significantly lower risk of atrial fibrillation in the atrial pacing group, with a relative risk reduction of 0.54 (95% confidence interval [CI] = 0.33 to 0.89; P = .012). Thromboembolic events were also reduced by atrial pacing, with a relative risk of 0.47 (95% CI = 0.24 to 0.92; P = .023), as was cardiovascular death, with a relative risk of 0.47 (95% CI = 0.27 to 0.82; P = .0065).

These data would appear to provide strong evidence for a benefit from atrial pacing; however, they must be interpreted cautiously, because the study is small and thus prone to chance variation. Also, all of the statistical power of the trial was attributed to the first analysis in the study, making the second analysis at 5 years exploratory and hypothesis generating rather than definitive. Still, this study supports the concept that specific pacing modalities may improve patient outcomes in particular patient groups.

The Danish study provides important additional information regarding pacing mode selection. The investigators clearly identified a subgroup of patients with sinus node dysfunction and a low risk of development of AV block in whom single-chamber atrial pacing is safe. They excluded patients with bifascicular bundle branch block, those with atrial fibrillation with an R-R interval longer than 3 seconds or a P-Q interval longer than 220 msec (>260 msec in patients >70 years old), and those who could not support 1:1 AV conduction with atrial pacing at a rate of 100 beats per minute (bpm). With adherence to these simple clinical criteria, only four patients receiving atrial pacemakers experienced AV block, corresponding to an incidence of 0.6% per year.[23] The ability to perform physiologic pacing with a single-chamber device is particularly attractive, because atrial pacemakers are no more costly or complex than ventricular pacemakers. Also, atrial pacing seems a more rational choice for the treatment of isolated sinus node dysfunction, in which there is no necessity for ventricular pacing.

Clinical Trials of Dual-Chamber Pacing versus Ventricular Pacing

Pacemaker Selection in the Elderly Study

The next randomized trial of pacemaker mode selection was the Pacemaker Selection in the Elderly (PASE) study, reported in 1998.[24] It was the first randomized controlled trial evaluating the effect of pacing mode on health-related QOL. This multicenter study was performed in 29 American centers, which randomly assigned patients to receive ventricular or dual-chamber pacing (see Table 10-3). All patients received a dual-chamber pacemaker and were then randomly assigned in a single-blind fashion to DDDR or VVIR programming. Initial programming of the devices required the use of rate adaptation. Four hundred and seven patients, with an average age of 76 years, were enrolled and evenly assigned to the two pacing modes. The primary study outcome was QOL as measured by the Medical Outcomes Study 36-Item Short-Form Health Survey (SF-36) and the Specific Activity Scale (SAS), two well-validated measures of health-related QOL.[25,26] Between baseline and 3 months, there was a marked improvement in QOL in all patients enrolled in the study irrespective of pacing mode.[24] There were however, no differences between the two pacing modes in either of the QOL measures. Pacemaker syndrome developed in 26% of patients assigned to VVIR pacing, including 45% of patients with sinus node dysfunction. These symptoms improved with reprogramming to a dual-chamber pacing mode.[24]

There was no significant difference between treatment groups in the risk for atrial fibrillation, stroke, or death (Figs. 10-1 through 10-3). A subgroup analysis did show that patients with sinus node dysfunction, but not those with AV block, exhibited trends toward a lower risk of atrial fibrillation (19% vs. 28%, respectively; P = .06) and death (12% vs. 20%, respectively; P = .09) that did not meet nominal levels of statistical significance.

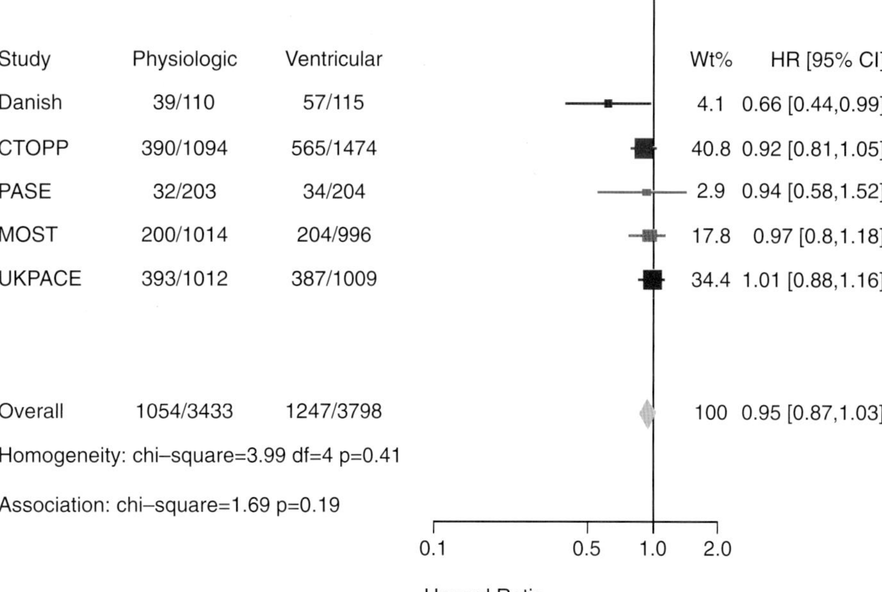

Study Physiologic Ventricular Wt% HR [95% CI]
Danish 39/110 57/115 4.1 0.66 [0.44,0.99]
CTOPP 390/1094 565/1474 40.8 0.92 [0.81,1.05]
PASE 32/203 34/204 2.9 0.94 [0.58,1.52]
MOST 200/1014 204/996 17.8 0.97 [0.8,1.18]
UKPACE 393/1012 387/1009 34.4 1.01 [0.88,1.16]
Overall 1054/3433 1247/3798 100 0.95 [0.87,1.03]
Homogeneity: chi–square=3.99 df=4 p=0.41
Association: chi–square=1.69 p=0.19
0.1 0.5 1.0 2.0
Hazard Ratio

Figure 10-1. Pooled estimate of mortality in randomized trials of pacing mode. CTOPP, Canadian Trial of Physiologic Pacing; Danish, study by Andersen and colleagues[22]; MOST, Mode Selection Trial in Sinus-Node Dysfunction; PASE, Pacemaker Selection in the Elderly; UKPACE, United Kingdom Pacing and Cardiovascular Events.

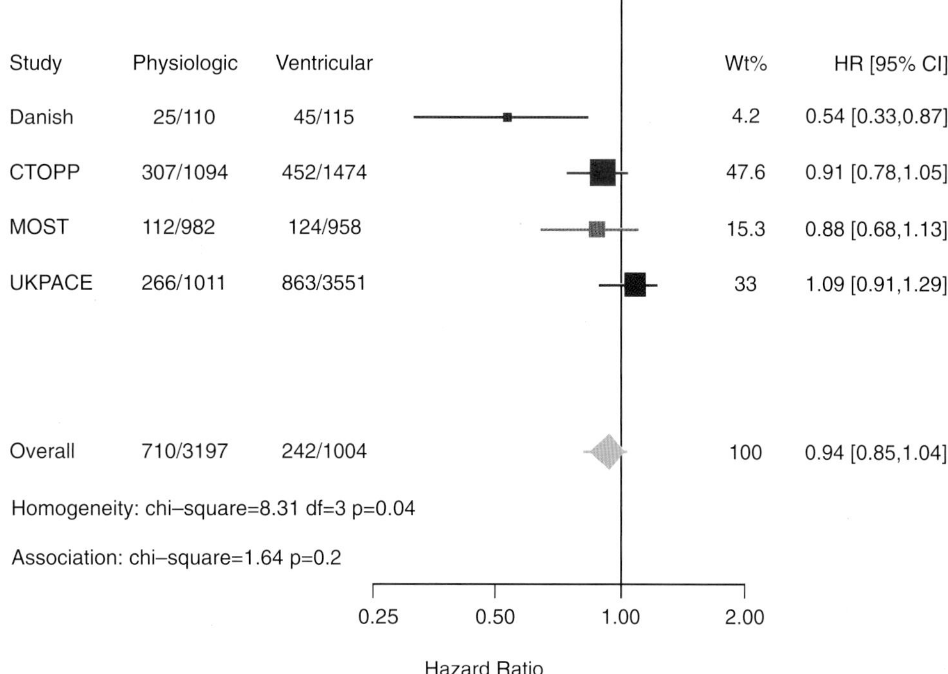

Figure 10-2. Pooled estimate of cardiovascular mortality or stroke. CTOPP, Canadian Trial of Physiologic Pacing; Danish, study by Andersen and colleagues[22]; MOST, Mode Selection Trial in Sinus-Node Dysfunction; UKPACE, United Kingdom Pacing and Cardiovascular Events.

The PASE study concluded that implantation of any kind of permanent pacemaker improves health-related QOL but that QOL does not appear to be affected by pacing mode. Encouraging trends suggested a possible reduction in atrial fibrillation and death in patients with sinus node dysfunction, but results were not conclusive.

Mattioli Study

In 1998, Mattioli and colleagues[27] published the results of a randomized controlled trial comparing ventricular (VVI or VVIR) with physiologic (AAI, DDD, DDDR, VDD) pacing in 210 patients, 110 with sinus node dysfunction and 100 with AV block. Median patient age was 77 years; 26% of the patients had cardiomyopathy and 48% had hypertension. After a maximum follow-up of 5 years, there was no difference in mortality between the treatment groups. Chronic atrial fibrillation was significantly reduced in patients with sinus node dysfunction (28% after pacing vs. 46% before; $P = .02$), but not in patients with AV block. As with the PASE study, only patients with sinus node dysfunction appeared to derive benefit from physiologic pacing.[24]

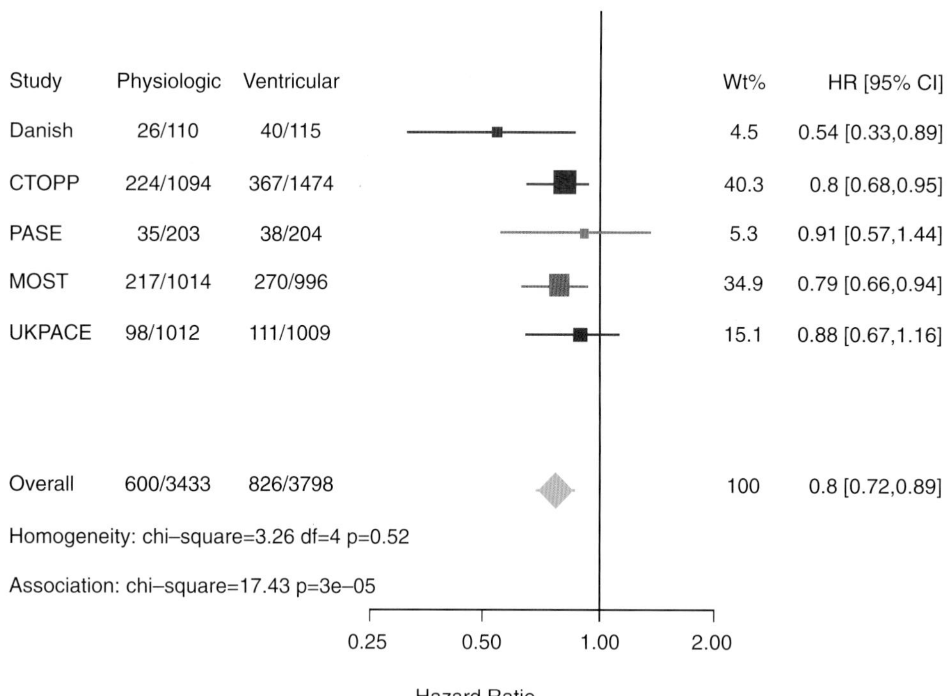

Study Physiologic Ventricular
Wt% HR [95% CI]
Danish 26/110 40/115 4.5 0.54 [0.33,0.89]
CTOPP 224/1094 367/1474 40.3 0.8 [0.68,0.95]
PASE 35/203 38/204 5.3 0.91 [0.57,1.44]
MOST 217/1014 270/996 34.9 0.79 [0.66,0.94]
UKPACE 98/1012 111/1009 15.1 0.88 [0.67,1.16]
Overall 600/3433 826/3798 100 0.8 [0.72,0.89]
Homogeneity: chi–square=3.26 df=4 p=0.52
Association: chi–square=17.43 p=3e–05
0.25
0.50
1.00
2.00
Hazard Ratio

Figure 10-3. *Pooled estimate of atrial fibrillation. CTOPP, Canadian Trial of Physiologic Pacing; Danish, study by Andersen and colleagues[22]; MOST, Mode Selection Trial in Sinus-Node Dysfunction; PASE, Pacemaker Selection in the Elderly; UKPACE, United Kingdom Pacing and Cardiovascular Events.*

The Canadian Trial of Physiologic Pacing

The Canadian Trial of Physiologic Pacing (CTOPP), the largest trial of pacemaker mode selection, was initially reported in 2000.[28] A total of 2568 patients with any standard indications for permanent pacing were randomly assigned to receive ventricular or physiologic (dual-chamber or atrial) pacemakers. Because treatment allocation was asymmetrical and reflective of contemporary Canadian device usage, more patients received ventricular pacemakers (1474 vs. 1094). Only 5.2% of patients assigned to physiologic pacing received single-chamber, atrial pacemakers; the decision to employ such devices was made by the local investigator and was not randomized. Of patients randomly assigned to ventricular pacing, 74.6% received rate-adaptive devices. The majority of patients received their allocated treatment, 99.1% in the ventricular group and 93.5% in the physiologic group. The average age of patients in the CTOPP was 73 years; 34% had sinus node dysfunction, 52% had AV block, and 8% had both.[28] Thirty-five percent of patients had systemic hypertension, and 28% had left ventricular (LV) dysfunction.

Patients were followed up for a mean of 3 years, for the primary outcome of stroke or cardiovascular mortality. There was no significant reduction in stroke or cardiovascular mortality (4.9%/year for physiologic vs. 5.5%/year for ventricular; $P = .33$)[28]; however, progression to chronic atrial fibrillation was significantly reduced with physiologic pacing (2.8%/year for physiologic vs. 3.8%/year for ventricular; $P = .016$).[29] These results were at odds with those of the nonrandomized trials and the results of the smaller Danish study; however, given its high statistical power and methodologic strength, the CTOPP provided the best estimate of the treatment effect of atrial pacing in the general pacemaker population. Unlike the Mattioli study,[27] the CTOPP found no preferential reduction in atrial fibrillation in patients with sinus node dysfunction, nor any particular benefit in patients with hypertension or abnormal ventricular function.[28]

A subsequent report did suggest a reduction in mortality with atrial pacing among patients with an unpaced heart rate of 60 bpm or less[30]; however, this report was a post hoc analysis of a postrandomization variable and must be interpreted with caution. In fact, in the extended follow-up report for the CTOPP, an unpaced heart rate of 60 bpm or less no longer predicted a mortality benefit for physiologic pacing.[31]

Despite the overall negative results of the CTOPP,[28] many authorities believed that the original trial may have been too short and that, with longer follow-up, the reduction in atrial fibrillation would translate into drops in stroke and cardiovascular mortality. However, a subsequent report of the extended follow-up (mean of 6.4 years) of these patients found no reduction in stroke or cardiovascular death.[31] Because the mean age of patients in the CTOPP was 73 years,[28] it is unlikely that additional follow-up would uncover a benefit of physiologic pacing; only 60% of the pacemaker patients were alive more than 6 years after device implantation.[32]

The CTOPP also assessed the rates of hospitalizations for heart failure, which were no different in the two groups (3.5%/year for ventricular vs. 3.1%/year for physiologic).[28] Perioperative complications were higher in patients receiving physiologic pacemakers (9.0% for physiologic vs. 3.8% for ventricular; $P < .001$), resulting from higher rates of inadequate sensing or pacing and lead dislodgment.[28] The rate of crossover from a ventricular to a physiologic mode was only 4.3% at 5 years, suggesting that the rate of pacemaker syndrome was much lower than in the PASE study (26%) or the Mode Selection Trial in Sinus-Node Dysfunction (MOST; see later) (18.3%).[24,28,33] One obvious explanation for the large difference in incidence of pacemaker syndrome between these studies is that in the CTOPP, patients randomly assigned to ventricular pacing received only a ventricular lead, whereas in the other two studies, all patients received both atrial and ventricular leads. Thus, unlike in the PASE study and MOST, patients in the CTOPP required reoperation for crossover to physiologic mode.[28] Accordingly, the relative threshold for diagnosis of pacemaker syndrome may have been higher in the CTOPP. However, overall health-related QOL did not differ between patients receiving ventricular pacemakers and those given physiologic pacemakers in the CTOPP, suggesting that in a general pacemaker population (patients with sinus or AV node disease), ventricular pacing does *not* have a large negative effect on QOL.[34] This substudy used both generic QOL measures and a specifically designed pacemaker syndrome scale.[34] Subanalysis of the QOL instruments did suggest a lower incidence of presyncope, a commonly cited symptom of pacemaker syndrome, with physiologic pacing (31% vs. 38%; $P < .01$)[34]; however, this could simply be the result of the testing of multiple outcomes. It is consistent with the low incidence of pacemaker syndrome seen in the CTOPP.

In summary, the only clear benefit of physiologic pacing observed in the CTOPP was a reduction in atrial fibrillation, which was observed both in patients with sinus node dysfunction and in those with AV block. There were no other benefits of physiologic pacing—specifically, no reduction in the risk of death, stroke, or heart failure was seen. The use of ventricular pacing was associated with a 50% reduction in perioperative complications and a less than 5% incidence of pacemaker syndrome requiring insertion of an atrial lead.[28]

Mode Selection Trial in Sinus-Node Dysfunction

Despite the overall negative results of the PASE study,[24] the subgroup analysis for the study suggested that there might be a benefit of dual-chamber pacing for patients with sinus node dysfunction but that a much larger sample size would be needed to detect such a difference.[24] Accordingly, Lamas and colleagues[35] conducted MOST, which randomly assigned 2010 patients with sinus node dysfunction to either ventricular or dual-chamber pacemakers. As in the PASE study, all patients had rate-adaptive programming. The average age of patients was 74 years; 20% had a history of heart failure and 62% had hypertension. The median follow-up was 2.8 years, at which time there was no difference in the primary outcome of death from any cause or stroke (21.5% for physiologic vs. 23.0% for ventricular; $P = .48$). However, in patients assigned to dual-chamber pacing, the risk of atrial fibrillation was lower (21.4% for physiologic vs. 27.1% for ventricular; $P = .008$). Heart failure scores were also better in patients receiving dual-chamber pacemakers ($P < .001$); however, rates of hospitalization for heart failure were not reduced in unadjusted analyses and had only marginal statistical significance with multivariate analyses. Subgroup analyses based on age, sex, race, and history of supraventricular arrhythmias did not identify any groups deriving particular benefit from dual-chamber pacing.

The power of MOST was compromised by a high rate of crossover from the ventricular pacing mode to a dual-chamber mode, which may have prevented the detection of a significant difference in primary outcome. At the last follow-up visit, 31.4% of patients assigned to ventricular mode had undergone reprogramming to dual-chamber pacing; in 48.9% of these patients, the crossover was made because of pacemaker syndrome. The diagnostic criteria for the pacemaker syndrome were clearly defined in advance, requiring "signs and symptoms of elevated right-sided or left-sided filling pressures or hypotension with ventricular pacing."[35] As well, objective measures of QOL improved after reprogramming to dual-chamber pacing, further supporting the diagnosis of pacemaker syndrome. It is difficult to reconcile the disparate rates of pacemaker syndrome in CTOPP and MOST, particularly because their patient populations differed. However, it is safe to conclude that pacemaker syndrome affects a significant number of patients receiving ventricular pacemakers, perhaps more frequently in those with sinus node dysfunction and a low, unpaced heart rate.[38]

There was also a suggestion, albeit inconsistent, of an improvement in overall health-related QOL in patients receiving dual-chamber pacemakers. Three months after device implantation, both dual-chamber and ventricular pacing groups had significant improvements in SF-36 scores for physical role and physical function. Over 4 years, dual-chamber pacing resulted in greater improvements than ventricular pacing in six of the eight subscales of the SF-36, but not in the Specific Activity Scale.[35]

One important substudy of MOST provides a possible explanation for the modest benefit of dual-chamber pacing in patients with sinus node dysfunction.[36] In 1339 patients enrolled in MOST, who had a baseline QRS duration of less than 120 msec, the cumulative percentage of time they received ventricular pacing was determined and correlated with clinical outcomes. In this subgroup of patients, in whom the baseline electrocardiogram did not identify significant conduction system disease, the cumulative frequency of ventricular pacing was 50% in the VVIR group and 90% in the DDDR group. With the percentage of time with ventricular pacing used as a time-dependent covariate, Cox proportional hazards regression modeling showed a higher risk of hospitalization for heart failure in both DDDR (HR = 2.99; 95% CI = 1.15 to 7.75; for cumulative ventricular pacing >40%) and VVIR (HR = 2.56; 95% CI = 1.48 to 4.43; for cumulative ventricular pacing >80%) modes.[36] The risk of atrial fibrillation also rose in a linear fashion with increasing frequency of ventricular pacing in DDDR (HR = 1.36; 95% CI = 1.09 to 1.69; for each 25% increase in ventricular pacing) and VVIR (HR = 1.21; 95% CI = 1.02 to 1.43; for each 25% increase in ventricular pacing). Thus, the excess risks of heart failure and atrial fibrillation were not due to AV desynchronization because the risks occurred equally with DDDR and VVIR pacing modes.

One likely explanation for the excess risk of heart failure and atrial fibrillation with an increased frequency of ventricular pacing is the induction of ventricular desynchronization with ventricular pacing. Multiple studies in patients with heart failure have shown that electrical dyssynchrony, manifested as a prolonged QRS width, impairs LV contractile function and increases mortality, but that symptoms of heart failure and mortality[37a] can be reduced by biventricular stimulation.[39,40] A detailed discussion of biventricular pacing (cardiac resynchronization) for heart failure is given in Chapter 12. In the opposite fashion, patients in the MOST substudy, who had a normal baseline QRS, were more likely to have a ventricular pacing-induced left bundle branch block when assigned to the dual-chamber mode (90% vs. 50%). Thus, in patients with sinus node dysfunction, dual-chamber pacing created an excess of unnecessary ventricular pacing, owing to conventional programming of the AV delay, and this excess may have led to an adverse hemodynamic situation that then resulted in heart failure and atrial fibrillation. This hypothesis was further confirmed by the Dual-Chamber Pacing or Ventricular Pacing in Defibrillator Patients (DAVID) trial,[41] which compared dual-chamber and ventricular pacing modes in patients with LV dysfunction who received defibrillators (see later).

The excess of ventricular pacing seen in MOST may also explain why a greater benefit from physiologic pacing was seen in the Danish study of patients with sinus node dysfunction than in MOST. The former study employed atrial pacing only in the physiologic pacing arm, which obviously did not result in any unnecessary ventricular pacing. This hypothesis was further explored by the ensuing DANPACE pilot study.[42,43]

United Kingdom Pacing and Cardiovascular Events Trial

The United Kingdom Pacing and Cardiovascular Events (UKPACE) trial was a randomized trial of patients older than 70 years with high-grade AV block. Patients with atrial fibrillation were included only if atrial fibrillation had been present for less than 3 months and sinus rhythm had been restored. Patients were enrolled in one of the following three pacing arms: DDD (50%), VVIR (25%), and VVI (25%). A total of 2021 patients were enrolled, with a mean age of 80 years. Hypertension was present in one third, and a history of heart failure in 16%. After a mean follow-up of 4.6 years, there was no difference in all-cause mortality between the dual-chamber and ventricular pacing groups (7.4%/yr for physiologic vs. 7.2%/yr for ventricular; HR = 1.01; 95% CI = 0.88 to 1.16). There was also no difference in the rate of stroke (1.7%/yr for physiologic vs. 2.1%/yr for ventricular; HR = 0.8; 95% CI = 0.56 to 1.12), atrial fibrillation (2.8%/yr for physiologic vs. 3%/yr for ventricular; HR = 0.88; 95% CI = 0.67 to 1.16), or heart failure hospitalizations (3.3%/yr for physiologic vs. 3.2%/yr for ventricular; HR = 1.04; 95% CI = 0.80 to 1.36).[44]

In summary, the UKPACE trial failed to show any benefit of dual-chamber pacing over ventricular pacing (50% VVI, 50% VVIR). This trial is the largest evaluation of pacing mode in patients with AV block and thus provides the best estimate of treatment effect in this patient population. The results are consistent with those of the CTOPP, which included 1550 patients with AV block and found no reduction in stroke and cardiovascular death with atrial-based pacing. It is also interesting that there was no benefit of dual-chamber pacing even though one half the patients in the ventricular group did not receive rate-adaptive pacing. On the basis of the overall UKPACE results, it is unlikely that the use of non–rate-adaptive pacing in 50% of patients produced any major detriment in the ventricular pacing arm of the study.

Unpublished Randomized, Controlled Trials

Pacemaker Atrial Tachycardia Trial. Wharton and associates[45] presented an abstract in 1998 describing the Pacemaker Atrial Tachycardia (PAC-ATACH) study, their randomized trial comparing DDDR pacing with VVIR pacing in 198 patients with sinus node dysfunction and a history of atrial arrhythmias. The mean age of the patients was 72 years, and 55% had hypertension. Patients were followed up for a median of 2 years, during which time 9% of patients in the DDDR group and 44% of patients in the VVIR group were crossed over to the other pacing mode. At the end of follow-up, there was no difference in rate of recurrent atrial arrhythmia between the groups (DDDR 48%, VVIR 43%; P = .09); however, mortality was lower in the DDDR group (DDDR 3.2%, VVIR 6.8%; P = .007).

Although these results may suggest a specific benefit for dual-chamber pacing in patients with prior atrial arrhythmias, the study is small and thus prone to type I error. The results must also await further scrutiny after publication of the manuscript.

Systematic Trial of Pacing to Prevent Atrial Fibrillation. The Systematic Trial of Pacing to Prevent Atrial Fibrillation (STOP-AF) is a randomized comparison of dual-chamber pacing and ventricular pacing in 350 patients with sick sinus syndrome.[46,47] The primary outcome of the study is chronic atrial fibrillation. Results are anticipated soon.

Systematic Review of Trials Comparing Atrial and Ventricular Pacing

The researchers of the large pacing trials[22,24,28,35,48] collaborated to produce a meta-analysis of the major published trials, using individual patient data on 7231 patients and nearly 35,000 patient-years of follow-up.[48a] A systematic review was performed, using standard database search techniques and a manual search of abstracts, to ensure that all relevant publications were identified. The investigators in all randomized controlled trials comparing any atrial pacing mode with any ventricular pacing mode were contacted and invited to participate. Data from five trials were extracted by means of a common data form and were assembled in a master database.[23,24,28,35,48] Neither patient-level nor summary data were available from one published trial,[27] one unpublished trial,[45] and one trial that had not completed its data collection.[46] In all, data on 95% of the total number of patients in all randomized trials of pacing mode were included in the meta-analysis. There was no significant heterogeneity between trials, so analyses were conducted with use of the fixed effects model.

Overall, there was no significant reduction in mortality with atrial pacing (HR = 0.95; 95% CI = 0.87 to 1.03; $P = .19$) (see Fig.10-1), nor any difference in the composite outcome of stroke or cardiovascular mortality (HR = 0.90; 95% CI = 0.74 to 1.08; $P = .26$) (see Fig. 10-2). There was a significant reduction in atrial fibrillation with atrial pacing (HR = 0.80; 95% CI = 0.72 to 0.89; $P = .00003$) (see Fig.10-3) and a modest reduction in stroke, which were of borderline statistical significance when one considers the many different outcomes that were evaluated (HR = 0.81; 95% CI = 0.67 to 0.99; $P = .038$). A time-dependent analysis of the effect of atrial fibrillation on stroke suggested that the apparent reduction in stroke was not related to the reduction in atrial fibrillation, thus calling into question the plausibility of the borderline reduction in stroke. Finally, the pooled analysis did not demonstrate a reduction in heart failure with atrial pacing (HR = 0.89; 95% CI = 0.77 to 1.03; $P = 0.12$) (Fig.10-4).

One of the main advantages of performing meta-analysis using patient-level data is the ability to perform subgroup analyses. If the cohort is divided according to the presence or absence of sinus node dysfunction, one sees a reduction in the composite of stroke or cardiovascular death in patients with sinus node dysfunction (HR = 0.85; 95% CI = 0.73 to 1.00; $P = .044$) but not in those without it (HR = 1.0; 95% CI = 0.88 to 1.14; $P = .98$) (Fig. 10-5). The reduction in atrial fibrillation was also greater in patients with sinus node dysfunction (HR = 0.76; 95% CI = 0.67 to 0.86; $P = .000016$) and was not seen in those without it (HR = 0.90; 95% CI = 0.74 to 1.09; $P = .27$) (Fig. 10-6). However, the confidence intervals for the two patient groups, for both outcomes, overlapped substantially, so one cannot conclude that there is a benefit of atrial pacing limited to patients with sinus node dysfunction. Rather, these data merely serve to generate hypotheses for further investigation. No other differences in any outcome were observed in subgroups based on age, gender, history of hypertension, LV ejection fraction less than 50%, intrinsic heart rate higher than 60 bpm, history of atrial fibrillation, or history of heart failure.

In summary, this meta-analysis consolidates our current understanding of the role of pacing mode on clinical outcomes. Atrial pacing does not result in lower rates of death or heart failure than ventricular pacing. With nearly 35,000 patient-years of follow-up, this analysis should have detected any clinically meaningful effect of pacing mode. However, the use of atrial pacing does lead to a significant reduction in atrial fibrillation, and possibly in stroke, of approximately 20%. There is a suggestion that the reduction in atrial fibrillation and in the composite outcome of stroke or cardiovascular death is limited to patients with sinus node dysfunction, although this suggestion requires prospective confirmation.

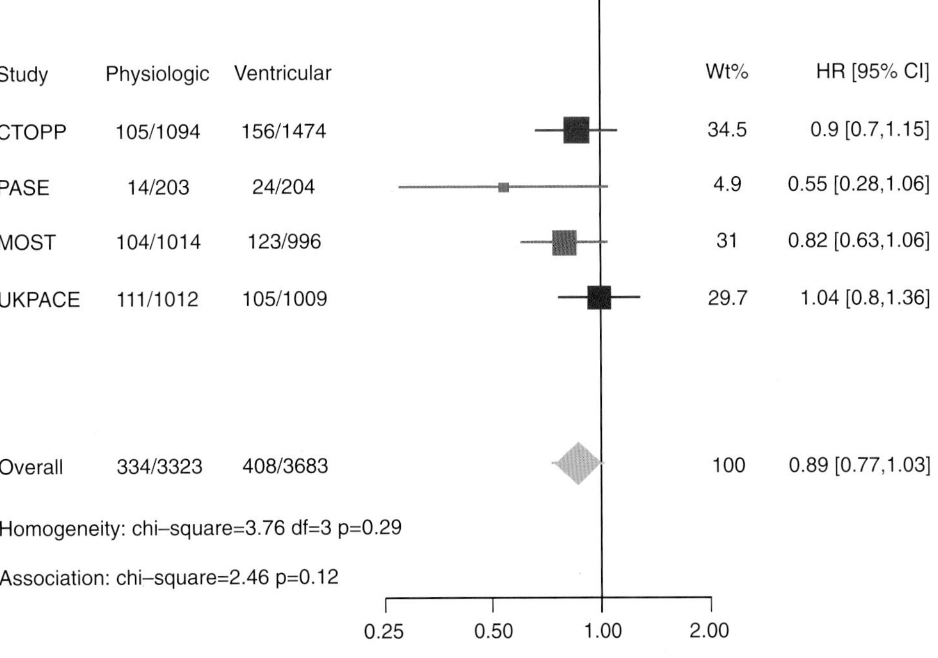

***Figure 10-4.** Pooled estimate of heart failure hospitalization. CTOPP, Canadian Trial of Physiologic Pacing; MOST, Mode Selection Trial in Sinus-Node Dysfunction; PASE, Pacemaker Selection in the Elderly; UKPACE, United Kingdom Pacing and Cardiovascular Events.*

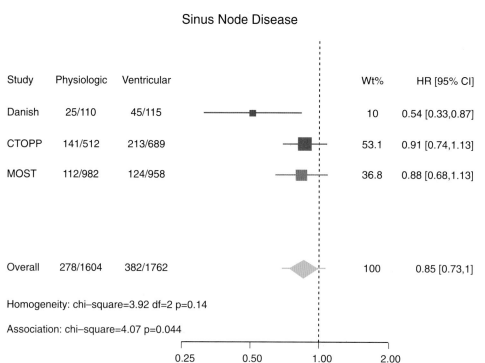

Sinus Node Disease

Study	Physiologic	Ventricular	Wt%	HR [95% CI]
Danish	25/110	45/115	10	0.54 [0.33,0.87]
CTOPP	141/512	213/689	53.1	0.91 [0.74,1.13]
MOST	112/982	124/958	36.8	0.88 [0.68,1.13]
Overall	278/1604	382/1762	100	0.85 [0.73,1]

Homogeneity: chi–square=3.92 df=2 p=0.14

Association: chi–square=4.07 p=0.044

0.25 0.50 1.00 2.00

Hazard Ratio

A

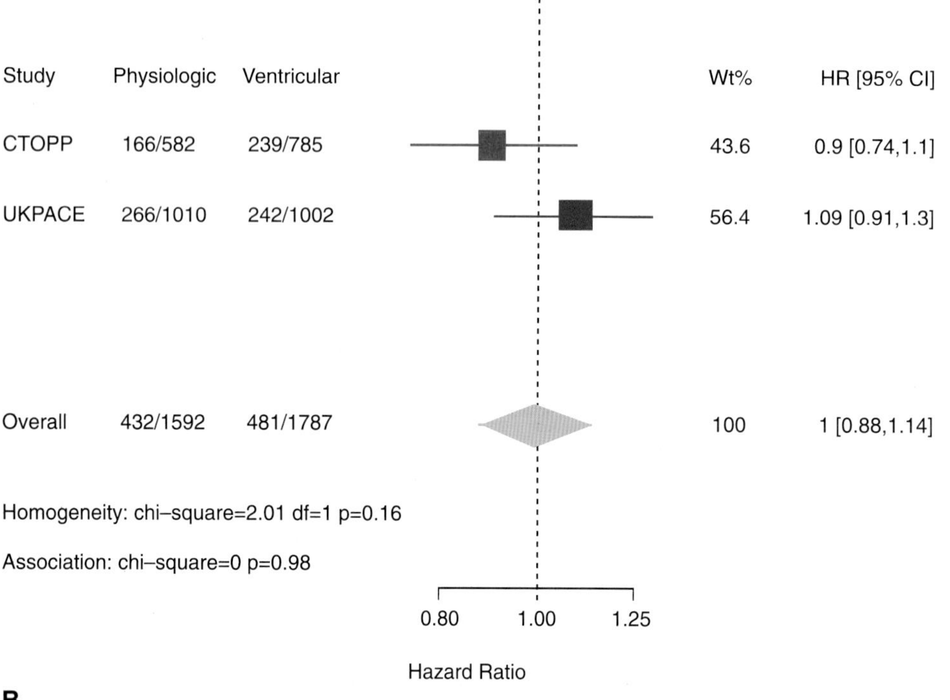

Figure 10-5. Cardiovascular mortality or stroke, based on indication for pacing. ***A,*** *Sinus node disease.* ***B,*** *No sinus node disease. CTOPP, Canadian Trial of Physiologic Pacing; Danish, study by Andersen and colleagues[22]; MOST, Mode Selection Trial in Sinus-Node Dysfunction; UKPACE, United Kingdom Pacing and Cardiovascular Events.*

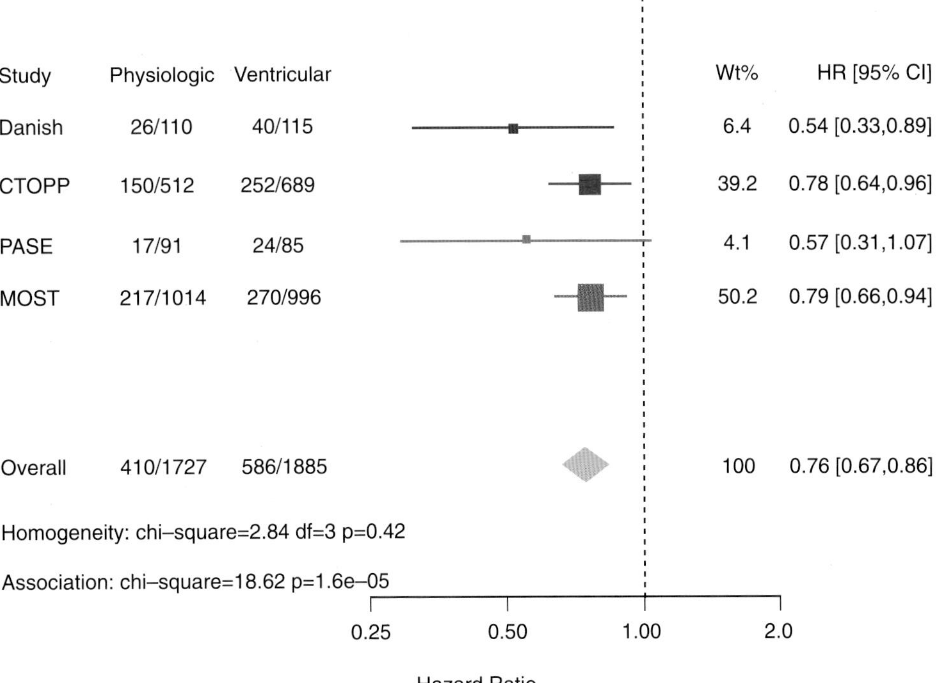

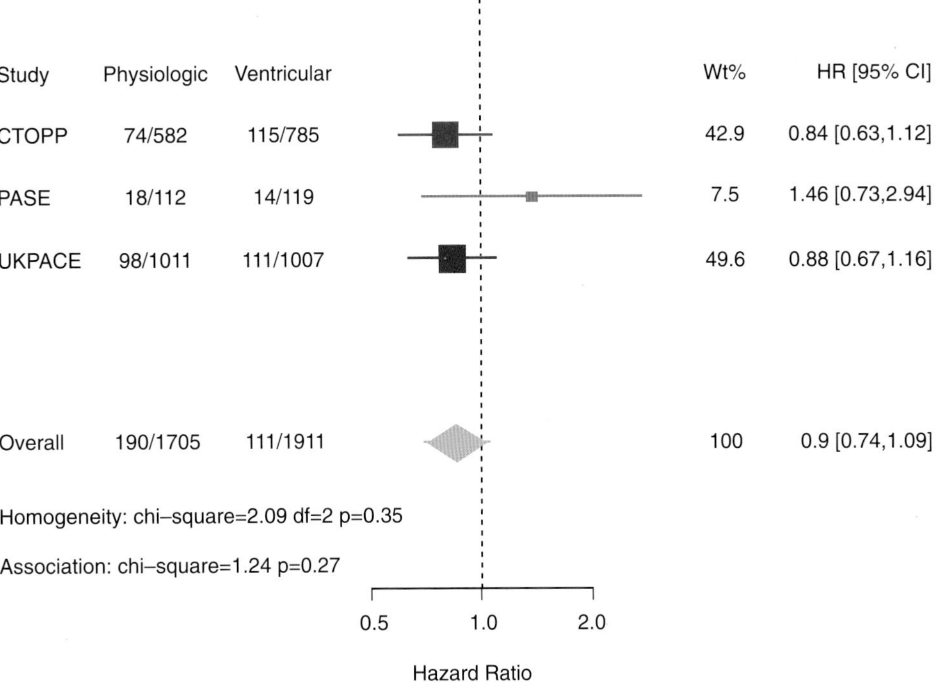

Figure 10-6. *Atrial fibrillation based on indication for pacing.* ***A,*** *Sinus node disease.* ***B,*** *No sinus node disease. CTOPP, Canadian Trial of Physiologic Pacing; Danish, study by Andersen and colleagues[22]; MOST, Mode Selection Trial in Sinus-Node Dysfunction; PASE, Pacemaker Selection in the Elderly; UKPACE, United Kingdom Pacing and Cardiovascular Events.*

Trial of Dual-Chamber Pacing or Ventricular Pacing in Defibrillator Patients

The DAVID trial was the first important trial of pacing mode in patients with implantable cardioverter-defibrillators (ICDs).[41] The hypothesis was that in patients with ICDs, a LV ejection fraction of less than 40%, and no indication for antibradycardia pacing, dual-chamber pacing (DDDR-70) would result in a lower rate of heart failure than ventricular pacing (VVI-40). A total of 506 patients were randomly assigned to one of the two pacing modes and were treated with maximal medical therapy for heart failure. At 1 year, the rate of death or first hospitalization for heart failure was significantly higher in the group receiving DDDR-70 pacing (26.7% for DDDR-70 vs. 16.1% for VVI-40; $P = .03$).

One explanation for this paradoxical increase in mortality is the potentially harmful effect of right ventricular (RV) apex pacing, which occurred more frequently in the DDDR-70 group. MOST had suggested that a higher rate of RV pacing increased the frequency of heart failure and atrial fibrillation.[36] None of the patients enrolled in the DAVID trial had a standard indication for antibradycardia pacing; however, ventricular pacing was performed 3% of the time in patients in the VVI-40 arm and 60% of the time in patients in the DDDR-70 arm. Additionally, poor outcomes in the DDDR-70 group correlated with the level of RV pacing. Thus, in this group of patients with no indication for pacing, dual-chamber pacing was harmful.

It cannot be determined from the DAVID trial whether the harm from DDDR-70 pacing was specifically from increased RV pacing or from increased pacing in general. This issue is currently being explored in DAVID II, which is comparing VVI with AAI pacing.[49] Another study is under way examining the ability of an AV search hysteresis algorithm to reduce ventricular pacing and clinical events.[50] Until the results of these trials are available, only backup pacing should be used in patients with defibrillators who do not have significant bradydysrhythmias.

Trial of Atrial versus Dual-Chamber Pacing

As already described, the Danish study demonstrated a much more impressive improvement in clinical outcomes than any of the other trials comparing ventricular and physiologic pacing.[22,23] One major difference between the Danish study and all the other randomized trials was that the mode of physiologic pacing in the Danish study was always AAI, whereas all other studies used dual-chamber pacing modes in their physiologic groups. The CTOPP did allow AAI(R) pacing; however, patients with such pacing represented only 5% of the trial's physiologic pacing arm.[28]

In the treatment of isolated sinus node dysfunction, the AAI mode may be superior to dual-chamber modes because it completely avoids unnecessary ventricular pacing. Both MOST[36] and the DAVID[41] trial showed that unnecessary ventricular pacing worsens outcomes, so any potential benefits of atrial pacing over ventricular pacing may have been offset, or indeed eliminated, by the harmful effects of unnecessary RV pacing. The DANPACE study and DANPACE pilot study[42,43] were designed to specifically address this issue. The DANPACE pilot study randomly assigned 177 patients with isolated sinus node dysfunction (without any significant AV conduction disturbance) to one of three pacing modes: AAIR, DDDR with a short AV delay (110-150 msec; DDDR-short), and DDDR with a long AV delay (>250 msec; DDDR-long). There were significant differences in the frequency of ventricular pacing between modes—0% for AAIR, 17% for DDDR-long, and 90% for DDDR-short. Increasing frequency of ventricular pacing was associated with higher risk of clinical events. Atrial fibrillation was lowest with atrial pacing; for AAIR, the rate was 3% per year; for DDDR-long, 8.2% per year; and for DDDR-short, 11.7% per year. There was also a trend for fewer thromboembolic events with atrial pacing; for AAIR the rate was 1.9% per year; for DDDR-long, 2.2% per year; and for DDDR-short, 4.0% per year.[43]

In an echocardiographic study of the DANPACE pilot study,[42] Nielsen and colleagues[43] demonstrated that the use of dual-chamber pacing is associated with left atrial enlargement relative to atrial pacing. This finding suggests that one of the deleterious effects of RV pacing may be increased atrial pressure, which in turn induces structural atrial remodeling, which is ultimately responsible for the higher risk of atrial fibrillation with dual-chamber pacing. Similar atrial remodeling also results from the loss of AV synchrony,[51] explaining the 20% increase in atrial fibrillation seen with ventricular pacing in the CTOPP and MOST.[28,35] Thus, the preservation of both AV synchrony and ventricular synchrony appears important in the optimization of pacing mode for patients with sinus node dysfunction.

Trials Evaluating New Modes of Ventricular Pacing

ROVA

With data showing a possible harm from RV apex (RVA) pacing[36,42] and emerging evidence that biventricular pacing reduced heart failure in patients with LV dysfunction and a widened QRS,[39,52] it was timely to consider alternative sites for ventricular pacing in patients who required this therapy. The ROVA[52a] (Right ventricular outflow versus apical) trial randomly assigned 103 patients with chronic atrial fibrillation, an ejection fraction less than 40%, and a standard pacing indication to RVA pacing, RV outflow tract (RVOT) pacing, or both, using a crossover design. Patients were given each pacing mode for 3 months and then underwent QOL assessment, 6-minute hall walk distance testing, and measurement of QRS duration and ejection fraction. Although the QRS duration was shorter with RVOT pacing (167 ± 45 msec) and dual-site pacing (149 ± 19 msec) than with RVA pacing (180 ± 58 msec; $P < .0001$), there was no difference in ejection fraction or hall walk distance. No consistent effect of pacing site on QOL measures was found.

Post AV Nodal Ablation Evaluation

There is mounting evidence that biventricular pacing in patients with heart failure and QRS prolongation improves clinical outcomes.[39,40,54] A detailed review of these data is presented in Chapter 12. Given the benefit in patients with heart failure, it is logical that biventricular stimulation may be superior to RVA pacing in patients who need frequent ventricular pacing. Patients who undergo AV node ablation for chronic atrial fibrillation require 100% ventricular pacing and are thus an ideal population in whom to test this hypothesis. The Post AV Nodal Ablation Evaluation (PAVE) study, which randomly assigned 102 such patients to RVA or biventricular pacing, found improvements in exercise capacity and QOL in the patients with biventricular pacing. The 6-minute hall walk distance at 6 months was longer in the biventricular group (82 m vs. 63 m; $P = .03$). Exercise duration also increased by 41.6 seconds over 6 months in the biventricular group, as did Vo_{2max} (+1.02 mL/kg/min; $P < .01$). The limitations of this study include small sample size, high crossover rate, and the failure to collect complete hemodynamic and echocardiographic data prospectively at baseline and at follow-up.

Trials of Right Atrial Appendage versus Atrial Septal or Biatrial Pacing

Both atrial and dual-chamber pacing have been shown to result in lower rates of atrial fibrillation than ventricular pacing, primarily in patients with sinus node dysfunction.[23,28,35] In this regard, atrial pacing appears to be more effective than dual-chamber pacing.[42] Investigators have examined the role of atrial lead position—right atrial appendage, atrial septum, left atrial, and biatrial[55]—as well as atrial pacing algorithms such as atrial overdrive pacing for the prevention of atrial fibrillation[56] in patients with and without standard bradycardia indications for pacing. This literature is reviewed in detail in Chapter 13. Briefly, the clinical trial evidence is conflicting, and no clear benefit has been established, particularly in patients without bradycardiac indications for pacing.[57]

The Future of Pacing Mode Selection

During the last 10 years, many randomized trials of pacing mode have shaped our current understanding of the role that pacing mode may have on clinical outcomes. It appears that traditional dual-chamber pacing offers a modest clinical advantage over ventricular pacing, perhaps limited to patients with sinus node dysfunction. In these patients, unnecessary RV stimulation may have a deleterious effect and thus should be avoided. The hypothesis that atrial pacing improves outcomes in this group of patients awaits confirmation by the DANPACE study. Newer forms of dual-chamber pacing are now available for patients in whom backup ventricular pacing is desirable. Further evaluation of the site and algorithm of atrial pacing is under way to see whether it can be delivered in a more optimal manner in patients at risk of atrial arrhythmias.

In patients with AV block, in whom ventricular pacing is required, currently available dual-chamber pacing offers no clear advantage over ventricular pacing. Evaluations of biventricular pacing and alternate site right ventricular pacing are ongoing.

In summary, although cardiac pacing can effectively improve survival and palliate symptoms in patients with bradyarrhythmias, it does not perfectly replicate normal physiology. Ten years of clinical trials have taught us that there is more to normal physiology than the AV delay and that other factors, such as ventricular synchrony, are important. With these lessons in mind, one should apply cardiac pacing only where it is needed and, when possible, should address the underlying abnormal physiology. Thus, patients with sinus node dysfunction should be given atrial pacing, with every effort made to minimize ventricular pacing. In patients with conduction disease or AV block, we still need to determine whether therapies that address ventricular dyssynchrony, such as biventricular pacing, can improve patient outcomes. Finally, it is important to realize the important role of randomized clinical trials in the advancement of this field. Careful evaluation in randomized trials has shown that many ideas that made intuitive sense, such as AV sequential pacing for heart block and dual-chamber pacing in LV dysfunction, have no effect or even cause harm. Further progress in the field of pacing modes will be made only through further randomized trials.

Quality of Life, Exercise Tolerance, and Pacemaker Syndrome

When the pacemaker was first introduced in 1960, the focus was on improving survival in patients with complete heart block[4] and Stokes-Adams attacks. With the introduction of newer pacing modalities and features, however, the question has shifted from whether patients with a certain condition should receive a pacemaker to which kind of pacemaker they should receive. Comparisons between physiologic pacing modes and ventricular modes have been the subjects of research. The physiologically based pacing modes have consistently been shown to produce superior central hemodynamic parameters in comparison with the ventricular modes.[58-60] However, the clinical relevance of these findings is questionable. Do differences in central hemodynamics or in exercise capacity translate into a noticeable difference in everyday activities, and do patients *feel* any better? Because most pacemakers are implanted in people who are older[28,35] and more sedentary, any potential hemodynamic benefit may go completely unnoticed. Furthermore, even if an improvement in hemodynamics might make patients feel better, such an effect may be overwhelmed by the effects of other disease processes, which are common in this age group. Thus, in assessment of the overall benefit of any particular pacing mode over another, particularly when one of the modes happens to be more costly[61,62] and complicated[28] (as is the case with dual-chamber pacing), it is not enough to point to an improvement in "laboratory" tests. One must show that the hemodynamic advantage actually translates into a real-life advantage, either making the patient's life more tolerable or preventing a clinically important adverse outcome such as death. Therefore, the assessment of QOL has become an important area in modern pacing research.

QOL as an endpoint in pacing trials has a number of limitations that must be considered. First, many of the early QOL trials are small. The later, large randomized trials have included QOL substudies[28,35]; however, these analyses are among many secondary outcomes evaluated. Only one large trial evaluated QOL as its primary outcome.[24] Second, the trials often contain a mixed group of patients, with AV block, sick sinus syndrome, or both, and these groups may not respond in the same manner to different pacing modes. Third, many of the QOL studies use a crossover design, which has the potential for patient and investigator unblinding. Finally, there is the problem of the QOL instruments themselves. On the one hand, many of the trials have failed to use properly tested and validated instruments. On the other hand, most of the validated instruments have not been specifically designed with pacemaker recipients in mind and thus may be insensitive. Even those measures designed for use in patients with cardiovascular disease, such as the Specific Activity Scale,[25,26] have proved relatively insensitive (at least in the crossover studies). With these limitations in mind, the results of some of the quality-of-life trials are discussed next.

DDD versus VVI

QOL trials have shown a fairly consistent benefit of physiologic pacing over fixed-rate, ventricular-inhibited pacing. Rediker and associates[58] reported on 19 patients in whom DDD pacemakers were implanted for AV block or sick sinus syndrome. The patients had received pacing in the DDD mode for at least 2 months before randomization. Each patient completed a number of questionnaires (which included validated QOL instruments) and an exercise test before randomization and after each of the 6-week pacing periods. During the study, 8 patients requested early crossover from VVI to DDD because of intolerable symptoms, but the other 11 completed the pacing protocols as planned. The group's perception of daily activity performance and health status favored the DDD mode, as did their ratings for fatigue, shortness of breath, and palpitations. This favoring of the DDD mode, however, was accounted for entirely by the 8 patients requesting early crossover; there was no difference in the subjective scores for the two modes in the 11 patients who did not request crossover.

This study is interesting because it demonstrates two distinct responses to VVI pacing. One group was unable to tolerate VVI pacing because of symptoms suggestive of pacemaker syndrome, whereas the other group was apparently able to tolerate the mode. It is not surprising that the patients with pacemaker syndrome showed a significant difference in subjective scores for the two pacing modes. Despite significant improvements in hemodynamic indices and exercise tolerance, however, there was no difference in QOL scores for the second group. When asked to indicate their preferred mode, only four of the latter group chose the DDD mode, the other seven expressing no preference. One other well-designed crossover comparison of these modes also did not show any subjective benefit for the DDD mode.[63]

Sulke and associates,[64] in a study designed to look specifically at patients able to tolerate long-term VVI pacing, did find a significant difference favoring DDD pacing. These researchers evaluated 16 patients in whom VVI pacemakers had been implanted for a long time, who had no symptoms suggestive of pacemaker syndrome, and whose devices were being upgraded to DDD at the time of elective generator replacement. Postoperatively, all pacemakers were programmed to three modes (DDD, DDI, and VVI) in a random sequence. Subjective assessments consisted of three self-administered questionnaires: The first used a visual analog scale (the subjects placed a mark along a 15-cm line) to assess general well-being and exercise capacity; the second assessed functional capacity using the Specific Activity Scale; and the third, using a scale of 0 to 5, assessed specific symptoms suggestive of the pacemaker syndrome or mild cardiac failure. The patients' perceptions of general well-being and exercise capacity were significantly better for the DDD mode than for both the pre-replacement and post-replacement VVI mode. There was no significant difference in the perceived functional status on the Specific Activity Scale. Both subjectively and objectively, the DDI mode was no different from the VVI mode. The researchers proposed a "sub-clinical pacemaker syndrome," even in apparently well patients who appear to tolerate VVI pacing. Thus, on the basis of this study, DDD pacing appears to be subjectively superior to VVI pacing.

VVIR versus VVI

Despite the clear improvement in exercise tolerance with rate-adaptive pacing, the studies comparing VVIR pacing with VVI pacing have not shown a consistent QOL benefit with rate adaptation.[65-69] In the two trials that specifically recorded patient preference, however, patients favored the VVIR mode. Such an unexpectedly modest response to the institution of rate-adaptive pacing may have a number of possible explanations, as follows:

- Most elderly patients with pacemakers are relatively inactive and consequently are likely to derive only a limited benefit from rate adaptation in the first place.
- Those with near-normal cardiac function can presumably increase stroke volume sufficiently to cope

with normal daily activities and thus may notice no benefit.

- The rate-response programming may have been suboptimal.
- Any benefit from the ability to vary the heart rate may have been counterbalanced by the persistence of any negative symptoms accompanying the loss of AV synchrony.

Smedgard and coworkers[68] studied 15 patients in a randomized crossover study consisting of 1 week each of VVI and VVIR pacing. Subjective assessments consisted of questions pertaining to specific symptoms, exercise tolerance, and general feeling of well-being. The total mean symptom score per day was lower (i.e., better) in the VVIR group (165 vs. 194), but the difference was not significant. On the other hand, when questioned about their preferred pacing mode, 13 of the 15 patients indicated a preference for the VVIR mode, and only 2 indicated no preference. This failure of the questionnaires to detect a significant difference between the two modes when most patients appeared to prefer the VVIR mode may indicate a lack of sensitivity of the questionnaires.

Using a QOL instrument designed specifically for patients with pacemakers, Oto and colleagues[66] performed a study in which 11 patients were randomly assigned to either the VVIR or VVI mode of pacing for 3 weeks. At the end of each study period, an exercise test was performed, and QOL was evaluated by means of the Hacettepe Quality-of-Life Questionnaire. In addition to confirming a significant improvement in exercise duration with the VVIR mode, these researchers demonstrated significantly higher QOL scores with this mode.

DDD versus VVIR

On the basis of the studies presented so far, DDD pacing appears clearly superior to VVI pacing, both objectively and subjectively. There is less certainty, however, about whether the DDD mode, which provides AV synchronization and appropriate rate response (in the absence of sinus node disease), is better than the VVIR mode, which allows for appropriate rate response without providing AV synchrony. The studies looking at exercise duration suggest that there is *no* difference between the two modes. As discussed earlier, however, maximum exercise duration may be a poor predictor of overall QOL.

In contrast to studies in which DDD was compared with VVI pacing, virtually all of the studies comparing DDD with VVIR pacing have included validated QOL instruments. Results have varied, however, and may depend in part on the particular instrument chosen. Two studies using the McMaster Health Index showed no difference between these pacing modes.[70,71] Another study (which compared VVIR with VVI), however, showed a significant difference in subjective scores with use of this instrument.[72]

Linde-Edelstam and associates[73] compared QOL in DDD and VVIR pacing modes in 17 patients with high-grade AV block and preserved sinus function. The patients were randomly assigned to each mode for a period of 8 weeks, after which they completed a questionnaire. There was no significant difference in mood, sleep, physical and social ability, or self-perceived health for the two pacing modes. Nine of the patients expressed a preference for the DDD mode, 3 preferred the VVIR mode, and 5 had no preference. One patient insisted on early crossover from the VVIR mode because of shortness of breath.

In a triple crossover study of the DDDR, DDD, and VVIR modes, Lau and colleagues[74] compared QOL in 33 patients with either AV block or sick sinus syndrome. QOL was evaluated using the Specific Activity Scale to assess functional class; no significant difference in the mean functional class for the three pacing modes was found. The overall QOL score was significantly better in the DDD group than in the VVIR group. The remaining three studies comparing DDD with VVIR pacing used questionnaires designed to assess disease-related symptoms; results of all three favored the DDD mode.

DDDR versus VVIR

Only a few studies have reported on the comparison of QOL in DDDR and VVIR pacing. Sulke and associates[75] performed a randomized crossover study of four pacing modes (DDDR, DDIR, DDD, and VVIR) in 22 patients with combined AV block and sick sinus syndrome. They reported significantly lower values for perception of general well-being, exercise tolerance, Specific Activity Scale score, and specific symptom score in the VVIR mode than in the other three modes, among which there was no difference.

Lau and colleagues[76] performed a triple crossover study of three rate-responsive pacing modes (DDDR, AAIR, and VVIR) in 15 patients with sick sinus syndrome. A number of objective assessments were performed along with a QOL assessment. There were no significant differences in any of the specific symptoms assessed by questionnaire, except palpitations, which occurred more frequently with VVIR pacing. There was no difference in overall functional class as assessed by the Specific Activity Scale. Overall QOL scores were no different for the three modes. The only difference was in general well-being, which was rated significantly lower in the VVIR mode than in either the AAIR or DDDR mode.

Large Clinical Trials Evaluating Quality of Life

Pacemaker Selection in the Elderly Study

As already described, the Pacemaker Selection in the Elderly (PASE) study, reported in 1998, was the first randomized controlled trial evaluating the effect of pacing mode on health-related QOL.[24] All patients received a dual-chamber pacemaker and were then randomly assigned in a single-blind fashion to DDDR or VVIR programming. Initial programming of the devices required the use of rate adaptation. Four hundred and seven patients, with an average age of 76 years, were enrolled and evenly randomized to the two pacing modes. The primary study outcome was QOL as measured by the SF-36 and the Specific Activity Scale, two well-validated measures of health-related QOL.[25,26] Between baseline and 3 months, there was a marked improvement in QOL in all patients enrolled in the study, irrespective of pacing mode.[24] There were, however, no differences between the two pacing modes in either of the QOL measures. Pacemaker syndrome developed in 26% of patients assigned to VVIR pacing, including 45% of patients with sinus node dysfunction. These symptoms improved with reprogramming to a dual-chamber pacing mode.[24]

In the subgroup with AV block, there was no difference in overall QOL scores; in the patients with sick sinus syndrome, however, there were modest and statistically significant differences in QOL favoring the DDDR mode, and it is likely that these differences would have been even more impressive had more than 50% of the VVIR group (with sick sinus syndrome) not crossed over to DDDR pacing.

Canadian Trial of Physiologic Pacing

The CTOPP investigators also reported an evaluation of QOL.[34] In this substudy of the overall CTOPP, 983 patients were randomly assigned to ventricular pacing, 457 (46%) with a rate-adaptive sensor; the other 738 patients were randomly assigned to physiologic pacing. QOL was measured using the SF-36, the "Ladder of Life," and the Pacemaker Syndrome Scale, at 6 months after implantation. A more detailed QOL evaluation was conducted at baseline and at 6 months in a subgroup of 269 patients by means of the SF-36, Pacemaker Syndrome Scale, Specific Activity Scale, and a pacemaker-specific scale. Among patients undergoing physiologic pacing in this substudy, 79% received DDD pacing mode, 14% DDD-R, and 7% AAI.

Pacing was associated with a significant unit improvement in all aspects of QOL (SF-36 score 38 ± 9 to 41 ± 11 for physical function, 47 ± 11 to 52 ± 9 for mental function; $P < .001$). However, no significant differences were noted in QOL between assigned physiologic pacing modes. The parent study also failed to demonstrate any significant differences in QOL between pacing modalities. Pacemaker dependency, defined as an unpaced heart rate of less than 50 bpm, did not influence QOL scores in the two assigned pacing modes.

The overall crossover rate from ventricular to physiologic pacing in the CTOPP was only 4.3% at 5 years, suggesting that the rate of pacemaker syndrome was much lower than in the PASE study (26%) or MOST (18.3%).[24,28,33] It is similar to the 3.1% rate of crossover at 4.6 years seen in the UKPACE trial.[44] Furthermore, in the CTOPP QOL substudy, the pacemaker syndrome scale did not reveal any significant differences between pacing modes. There are several explanations for the significant disparity in the incidence of pacemaker syndrome observed in these four major studies. In the CTOPP[28] and UKPACE[44] trial, patients required reoperation to cross over to physiologic pacing, whereas in the PASE[24] study and MOST,[35] only reprogramming was required. Therefore, the threshold for diagnosis of pacemaker syndrome was higher in the former two trials. However, one cannot conclusively determine which estimate of the incidence of pacemaker best approximates the true value. Further complicating matters is the fact that these four trials enrolled different patient populations, and there is a suggestion that pacemaker syndrome may be more common in patients with sinus node dysfunction[24,35] than in patients with AV block.[24,44] Finally, the diagnosis of pacemaker syndrome is quite subjective, because many symptoms of this syndrome are common in elderly patients with pacemakers regardless of pacing mode.[34] Investigators have tried to better quantify pacemaker syndrome through the use of explicit clinical criteria[35] and specifically designed QOL instruments[34]; nevertheless, subjectivity remains.

Exercise tolerance is another potential way to evaluate the QOL impact of different pacing modes. The effects of pacing mode on exercise tolerance in 2568 patients in the CTOPP have been assessed through the use of the 6-minute hall walk distance test; in this trial, 76% of patients completed the test.[76a] At the time of the first postimplantation visit, the mean distance walked was 350 ± 127 meters in the ventricular group and 356 ± 127 meters in the atrial group (P = NS). Similarly, there was no difference in the change in heart rate between the two groups (+17 ± 13 bpm vs. +18 ± 12 bpm, respectively; P = NS). However, among patients with an unpaced heart rate of 60 bpm or less, patients assigned to atrial pacing walked further than those assigned to ventricular pacing (361 ± 127 m vs. 343 ± 121 m, respectively; $P = .04$). This difference was not associated with a difference in heart rate. The use of rate-adaptive pacing, irrespective of the pacing mode, resulted in a greater increase in heart rate with the 6-minute walk test but no increase in the total distance walked. This study concluded that atrial pacemakers did not yield greater exercise capacity, as measured by the 6-minute walk test, than ventricular pacemakers, but that there was a suggestion, albeit borderline in significance, that patients with a low unpaced heart rate derive some benefit from atrial pacing.

Mode Selection Trial in Sinus Node Dysfunction

As previously described, MOST was a randomized study of 2010 patients with sinus node dysfunction who were programmed to ventricular or dual-chamber pacing.[35,38] All patients had rate-adaptive pacing. At the last follow-up visit, 31.4% of patients assigned to the ventricular mode had been reprogrammed to dual-chamber pacing, 48.9% of whom were crossed over because of pacemaker syndrome. The diagnostic criteria for the pacemaker syndrome were clearly defined in advance and required "signs and symptoms of elevated right-sided or left-sided filling pressures or hypotension with ventricular pacing."[35] Also, objective measures of QOL improved after reprogramming to dual-chamber pacing, further supporting the diagnosis of pacemaker syndrome.[38]

There was also a suggestion, albeit inconsistent, of an improvement in overall health-related QOL in patients receiving dual-chamber pacemakers. Three months after device implantation, both the dual-chamber pacing and ventricular pacing groups had significant improvements in SF-36 scores for physical role and physical function. Over 4 years, dual-chamber pacing resulted in greater improvements than ventricular pacing in six of the eight subscales of the SF-36, but not in the Specific Activity Scale.[35]

United Kingdom Pacing and Cardiovascular Events Trial and Systematic Trial of Pacing to Prevent Atrial Fibrillation

Another small trial also assessed QOL in patients randomized to either AAI or VVIR modes.[77] Seventy-three patients recruited in either the UKPACE trial or STOP were included. QOL was assessed, through the use of SF-36 and a modified version of the Karolinska Cardiovascular Symptomatology Questionnaire 24 hours after pacemaker insertion and then 1 month, 1 year, and 2 years later. This study used an individualized assessment of QOL after pacing. Overall, pacing improved QOL, but this improvement was not maintained after 2 years. However, pacemaker mode did not have any influence on QOL.

Effect of Other Pacing Parameters on Quality of Life

A small number of trials have examined the effect of changes in AV delay on QOL. AV delay can be individually optimized to provide the greatest hemodynamic benefit at rest. Studies have shown that this hemodynamic benefit can be maintained during exercise,[78-80] but this benefit does not necessarily translate into an improvement in maximum exercise duration.[81-83] Sulke and coworkers[82] found a significant difference in subjective scores favoring a fixed AV delay of 125 msec and a rate-adaptive AV delay over the longer fixed AV delays of 175 and 250 msec. Linde and colleagues[84] assessed QOL and hemodynamic parameters in 10 patients with severe congestive heart failure who received dual-chamber pacing with individual optimization of AV delay. Despite lack of sustained improvement in hemodynamic parameters over the long term, there was a significant improvement in QOL scores that persisted for the entire 6-month observation period. As the investigators pointed out, however, patients were not blinded as to which AV delay was being used, and a placebo effect could well explain this apparent improvement, especially given the lack of sustained hemodynamic benefit. When one remembers the findings of the DAVID trial,[41] this explanation is almost certainly the case.

The effect of mode switching has also been evaluated in two trials.[85,86] In the first, DDDR with and without mode switching was compared with VVIR mode.[85] DDDR with mode switching resulted in a longer exercise time and better QOL than VVIR. DDDR with mode switching resulted in a better QOL than DDDR without mode switching but no difference in exercise time.[85] In the second study, a substudy of MOST,[86] 202 patients were randomly assigned to mode switch "on" or "off." Although rapid ventricular pacing due to high rate atrial episodes was more common in the mode switch "off" group, these patients experienced no increase in rate of heart failure hospitalizations or any diminution in QOL.[86]

The choice of rate-response sensor has also been shown to affect QOL.[87] In a substudy of MOST,[87] 1245 patients had devices with a piezoelectric sensor, an accelerometer sensor, or a blended sensor. Patient characteristics were similar in the three different sensor groups. QOL assessment found that patients with blended sensors had worse physical function than those with the other types of devices. Although this observation might suggest a detriment for blended sensors, the nonrandomized allocation of sensors may have created a situation whereby sicker patients received blended sensors, thus creating bias.

Summary

In summary, the use of pacemakers to treat sinus node dysfunction and AV block improves overall QOL regardless of the pacing mode employed. However, compared with rate-adaptive ventricular pacemakers, dual-chamber pacing provides little clear improvement in QOL and exercise tolerance. Although small crossover studies appear to suggest a benefit, the large substudies and the major pacing trials do not demonstrate a convincing overall benefit. The PASE study and MOST do suggest an improvement in QOL among patients with sinus node dysfunction, particularly through a reduction in the pacemaker syndrome. However, given the many limitations in the evaluation of QOL in this group of patients as well as the presence of conflicting results, the totality of research to date remains inconclusive.

Cost-Effectiveness of Dual-Chamber Pacing

Two of the large randomized trials of pacing modes conducted concurrent cost-effectiveness studies,[28,35] which have been published. The two analyses are complementary, as they address different facets of the cost-effectiveness question.

The cost-effectiveness substudy of MOST used both trial data and contemporary cost data. Because all patients in MOST received a dual-chamber device, comparative implantation cost data (ventricular vs. dual-chamber) were obtained from a contemporary source. Effectiveness data were collected prospectively during the study.[62] Utility data were derived through the use of a time-tradeoff instrument, administered at baseline, 3 months, and 1 year, and yearly thereafter. Overall, dual-chamber pacing was associated with a cost-effectiveness of $53,000 per quality-adjusted life-year gained. This favorable value was driven by decreased costs in the dual-chamber group associated with atrial fibrillation, heart failure admissions, and pacemaker syndrome. Thus, the routine use of dual-chamber pacemakers appears cost-effective in patients with sinus node dysfunction.

The CTOPP also conducted a prospective cost-effectiveness study at a subset of participating centers.[61] Because the trial included patients with all standard indications for pacing, it is more widely applicable than MOST. The CTOPP also provides a better estimate of the relative implantation-related costs (ventricular vs. physiologic) because these were collected within the study. The CTOPP did not include an evaluation of utilities. Solely on the basis of the effect of physiologic pacing on mortality, the CTOPP found an incremental cost-effectiveness ratio of $297,600 (Canadian) per life-year gained. In the subgroup of patients with an intrinsic heart rate lower than 60 bpm, the incremental cost-effectiveness was $16,343 (Canadian). Although the initial implantation costs were very similar to those in the MOST study, the follow-up costs in the ventricular group were much lower, despite a similar excess of atrial fibrillation with ventricular pacing as seen in MOST. The high rate of pacemaker syndrome was not seen in the CTOPP, which may have accounted for the lower follow-up costs of ventricular pacing and, thus, the higher incremental cost-effectiveness.

Overall, the true cost-effectiveness probably lies somewhere between these two estimates. MOST probably overestimated the cost-effectiveness ratio because of the high costs associated with the pacemaker syndrome and because it applied only to patients with sinus node dysfunction, who may derive greater benefit from dual-chamber pacing. On the other hand, the CTOPP likely underestimated the cost-effectiveness, because it did not capture the effect of pacing on nonlethal events, although all costs were counted and QOL did not differ between groups. Finally, the ultimate cost-effectiveness of atrial pacing has yet to be determined. Newer dual-chamber devices and atrial pacing offer the hope of greater effectiveness, and atrial devices offer this hope at little or no incremental cost. Although still uncertain, it is therefore likely that in a subset of patients, atrial pacing will offer good value for the money.

REFERENCES

1. Zoll PM, Linenthal AJ, Norman LR, et al: Use of external electric pacemaker in cardiac arrest. JAMA 159:1428-1431, 1955.
2. Smith CN (ed): Implantable pacemaker for the heart. In Medical Electronics: Proceedings of the Second International Conference on Medical Electronics. London, 1959.
3. Sowton E, Preston T, Barcelo J, et al: Two years' experience with implanted demand pacemakers. Br Heart J 1969;31:389-390.
4. Sutton R, Chatterjee K, Leatham A: Heart-block following acute myocardial infarction: Treatment with demand and fixed-rate pacemakers. Lancet 2(7569):645-648, 1968.
5. Rosenqvist M, Brandt J, Schuller H: Long-term pacing in sinus node disease: Effects of stimulation mode on cardiovascular morbidity and mortality. Am Heart J 116:16-22, 1988.
6. Sasaki Y, Shimotori M, Akahane K, et al: Long-term follow-up of patients with sick sinus syndrome: A comparison of clinical aspects among unpaced, ventricular inhibited paced, and physiologically paced groups. Pacing Clin Electrophysiol 11:1575-1583, 1988.
7. Bianconi L, Boccademo R, Di Florio A, et al: Atrial versus ventricular stimulation in sick sinus syndrome: Effects on morbidity and mortality. Pacing Clin Electrophysiol 12:1236A, 1989.
8. Santini M, Alexidou G, Ansalone G, et al: Relation of prognosis in sick sinus syndrome to age, conduction defects and mode of permanent cardiac pacing. Am J Cardiol 65:729-735, 1990.
9. Nurnberg M, Frohner K, Podczeck A, et al: Is VVI pacing more dangerous than AV-sequential pacing in patients with sick sinus syndrome? Pacing Clin Electrophysiol 14:674A, 1991.
10. Stangl K, Seitz K, Wirtzfeld A, et al: Differences between atrial single chamber pacing [AAI] and ventricular single chamber pacing [VVI] with respect to prognosis and antiarrhythmic effect in patients with sick sinus syndrome. Pacing Clin Electrophysiol 13:2080-2085, 1990.
11. Sgarbossa EB, Pinski SL, Trohman RG, et al: Single-chamber ventricular pacing is not associated with worsening heart failure in sick sinus syndrome. Am J Cardiol 73:693-697, 1994.
12. Sgarbossa EB, Pinski SL, Maloney JD, et al: Chronic atrial fibrillation and stroke in paced patients with sick sinus syndrome: Relevance of clinical characteristics and pacing modalities. Circulation 88:1045-1053, 1993.
13. Alpert MA, Curtis JJ, Sanfelippo JF, et al: Comparative survival after permanent ventricular and dual chamber pacing for patients with chronic high degree atrioventricular block with and without pre-existing congestive heart failure. J Am Coll Cardiol 7:925-932, 1986.
14. Sutton R, Kenny R-A: The natural history of sick sinus syndrome. Pacing Clin Electrophysiol 9:1114, 1986.
15. Tang CY, Kerr CR, Connolly SJ: Clinical trials of pacing mode selection. Cardiol Clin 18:1-23, 2000.
16. Connolly SJ, Kerr CR, Gent M, et al: Dual-chamber versus ventricular pacing: Critical appraisal of current data. Circulation 94:578-583, 1996.
17. Ohm O-J, Breivik K: Patients with high-grade atrioventricular block treated and not treated with a pacemaker. Acta Med Scand 203:521-528, 1978.
18. Linde-Edelstam C, Gullberg B, Norlander R, et al: Longevity in patients with high degree atrioventricular block paced in the atrial synchronous or the fixed rate ventricular inhibited mode. Pacing Clin Electrophysiol 15:304-313, 1992.
19. Zanini R, Facchinetti AI, Gallo G, et al: Survival rates after pacemaker implantation: A study of patients paced for sick sinus syndrome and atrioventricular block. Pacing Clin Electrophysiol 12:1069, 1989.
20. Hesselson AB, Parsonnet V, Bernstein AD, et al: Deleterious effects of long-term single-chamber ventricular pacing in patients with sick sinus syndrome: The hidden benefits of dual chamber pacing. J Am Coll Cardiol 19:1542-1549, 1992.
21. Sgarbossa EB, Pinski SL, Maloney JD: The role of pacing modality in determining long-term survival in the sick sinus syndrome. Ann Intern Med 119:359-365, 1993.
22. Andersen HR, Thuesen L, Bagger JP, et al: Prospective randomised trial of atrial versus ventricular pacing in sick-sinus syndrome. Lancet 344:1523-1528, 1994.
23. Andersen HR, Nielsen JC, Thomsen PEB, et al: Long-term follow-up of patients from a randomised trial of atrial versus ventricular pacing for sick-sinus syndrome. Lancet 350:1210-1216, 1997.
24. Lamas GA, Orav J, Stambler BS, et al: Quality of life and clinical outcomes in elderly patients treated with ventricular pacing as compared with dual-chamber pacing. N Engl J Med 338:1097-1104, 1998.
25. Ware JE Jr, Sherbourne CD: The MOS 36-item Short-Form Health survey [SF-36]. I: Conceptual framework and item selection. Med Care 30:473-483, 1992.

26. Goldman L, Hashimoto B, Cook EF, et al: Comparative reproducibility and validity of systems for assessing cardiovascular functional class: Advantages of a new Specific Activity Scale. Circulation 64:1227-1234, 1981.
27. Mattioli AV, Vivoli D, Mattioli G: Influence of pacing modalities on the incidence of atrial fibrillation in patients without prior atrial fibrillation. Eur Heart J 19:282-286, 1998.
28. Connolly SJ, Kerr CR, Gent M, et al: Effects of physiologic pacing versus ventricular pacing on the risk of stroke and death due to cardiovascular causes. Canadian Trial of Physiologic Pacing Investigators. N Engl J Med 342:1385-1391, 2000.
29. Skanes AC, Krahn AD, Yee R, et al: Progression to chronic atrial fibrillation after pacing: The Canadian Trial of Physiologic Pacing. J Am Coll Cardiol 38:167-172, 2001.
30. Tang ASL, Roberts RS, Kerr CR, et al: Relationship between pacemaker dependency and the effect of pacing mode on cardiovascular outcomes. Circulation 103:3081-3085, 2001.
31. Kerr CR, Connolly SJ, Abdollah H, et al: Canadian Trial of Physiologic Pacing: Effects of physiologic pacing during long-term follow-up. Circulation 109:357-362, 2004.
32. Gillis AM, MacQuarrie DS, Wilson SL: The impact of pulse generator longevity on the long-term costs of cardiac pacing. Pacing Clin Electrophysiol 19:1459-1468, 1996.
33. Lamassa M, DICarlo A, Pracucci G, et al: Characteristics, outcome, and care of stroke associated with atrial fibrillation in Europe: Data from a multicenter multinational, hospital-based registry (The European Community Stroke Project). Stroke 32:392-398, 2001.
34. Newman D, Lau C, Tang AS, et al: Effect of pacing mode on health-related quality of life in the Canadian Trial of Physiologic Pacing. Am Heart J 145:430-437, 2003.
35. Lamas GA, Lee KL, Sweeny MO, et al: Ventricular pacing or dual-chamber pacing for sinus-node dysfunction. N Engl J Med 346:1854-1862, 2002.
36. Sweeney MO, Hellkamp AS, Ellenbogen KA, et al: Adverse effect of ventricular pacing on heart failure and atrial fibrillation among patients with normal baseline QRS duration in a clinical trial of pacemaker therapy for sinus node dysfunction. Circulation 107:2932-2937, 2003.
37. Glotzer TV, Hellkamp AS, Zimmerman J, et al: Atrial high rate episodes detected by pacemaker diagnostics predict death and stroke: Report of the atrial diagnostics ancillary study of the MOde Selection Trial [MOST]. Circulation 107:1614-1619, 2003.
37a. Cleland JG, Daubert JC, Erdmann E, et al: The effect of cardiac resynchronization on morbidity and mortality in heart failure. N Engl J Med 352:1539-1549, 2005.
38. Link MS, Hellkamp AS, Estes NA 3rd, et al: High incidence of pacemaker syndrome in patients with sinus node dysfunction treated with ventricular-based pacing in the Mode Selection Trial [MOST]. J Am Coll Cardiol 43:2066-2071, 2004.
39. Bradley DJ, Bradley EA, Baughman KL, et al: Cardiac resynchronization and death from progressive heart failure: A meta-analysis of randomized controlled trials. JAMA 289:730-740, 2003.
40. Bristow MR, Saxon LA, Bachmer J, et al: Cardiac resynchronization therapy with or without an implantable defibrillator in advanced chronic heart failure. N Engl J Med 350(21):2140-2150, 2004.
41. Wilkoff BL, Cook JR, Epstein AE, et al; Dual Chamber and VVI Implantable Defibrillator Trial Investigators: Dual-chamber pacing or ventricular backup pacing in patients with an implantable defibrillator: The Dual Chamber and VVI Implantable Defibrillator (DAVID) Trial. JAMA 288:3115-3123, 2002.
42. Kristensen L, Nielsen JC, Mortensen PT, et al: Incidence of atrial fibrillation and thromboembolism in a randomised trial of atrial versus dual chamber pacing in 177 patients with sick sinus syndrome. Heart 90:661-666, 2003.
43. Nielsen JC, Kristensen L, Andersen HR, et al: A randomized comparison of atrial and dual-chamber pacing in 177 consecutive patients with sick sinus syndrome: Echocardiographic and clinical outcome. J Am Coll Cardiol 42:614-623, 2003.
44. Toff WD, Camm AJ, Skehan JD: Single-chamber versus dual-chamber pacing for high-grade atrioventricular block. N Engl J Med 353:202-204, 2005.
45. Wharton JM, Sorrentino RA, Campbell P, et al: Effect of pacing modality on atrial tachyarrhythmia recurrence in the tachycardia-bradycardia syndrome: Preliminary results of the Pacemaker Atrial Tachycardia Trial [abstract]. Circulation 98:I-494, 1998.
46. Charles RG, McComb JM: Systematic Trial of Pacing to Prevent Atrial Fibrillation [STOP-AF]. Heart 78:224-225, 1997.
47. McComb JM, Gribbin GM: Effect of pacing mode on morbidity and mortality: Update of clinical pacing trials. Am J Cardiol. 83:211D-213D, 1999
48. Toff WD, Skehan JD, deBono DP, et al: The United Kingdom Pacing And Cardiovascular Events trial [UK Pacing Clin Electrophysiol]. Heart 78:221-223, 1997.
48a. Healy JS, Toff WD, Lamas GA, et al: Cardiovascular outcomes with atrial-based pacing compared with ventricular pacing: Meta-analysis of randomized trials, using individual patient data. Circulation 114:11-17, 2006.
49. Wilkoff BL: The Dual Chamber And VVI Implantable Defibrillator [DAVID] trial: Rationale, design, results, clinical implications and lessons for future trials. Card Electrophysiol Rev 7:468-472, 2003.
50. Olshansky B, Day J, McGuire M, Pratt T: Inhibition of Unnecessary RV Pacing with AV Search Hysteresis in ICDs (INTRINSIC RV). Pacing Clin Electrophysiol 28:62-66, 2005.
51. Cleland JGF, Daubert J-C, Erdmann E, et al; Cardiac Resynchronization-Heart FAilure [CARE-HF] Study Investigators. N Engl J Med 352: 1539-1549, 2005.
52. Sparks PB, Mond HG, Vohra JK, et al: Mechanical remodeling of the left atrium after loss of atrioventricular synchrony: A long-term study in humans. Circulation 100:1714-1721, 1999.
52a. Stanbler BS, Ellenbogen K, Zhang X, et al: Right ventricular outflow versus apical pacing in pacemaker patients with congestive heart failure and atrial fibrillation. J Cardiovasc Electrophysiol 14:1180-1186, 2003.
53. Bristow MR, Saxon LA, Boehmer J, et al: Cardiac-resynchronization therapy with or without an implantable defibrillator in advanced chronic heart failure. N Engl J Med 350:2140-2150, 2004.
54. Doshi RN, Daoud EG, Fellows C, et al; PAVE Study Group: Left ventricular-based cardiac stimulation Post AV Nodal ablation Evaluation [The PAVE Study]. J Cardiovasc Electrophysiol 16:1-6, 2005.
55. Saksena S, Prakash A, Ziegler P, et al: Improved suppression of recurrent atrial fibrillation with dual-site right atrial pacing and antiarrhythmic drug therapy. J Am Coll Cardiol 40:1140-1150, 2002.
56. Overdrive atrial septum stimulation in patients with paroxysmal atrial fibrillation [AF] and class 1 and 2 pacemaker indication [OASES]. Paper presented at Annual Scientific Sessions of the Heart Rhythm Society, May 17, 2003, Washington, DC.
57. Knight BP, Gersh BJ, Carlson MD, et al: Role of permanent pacing to prevent atrial fibrillation: Science advisory from the American Heart Association Council on Clinical Cardiology and the quality of care and outcomes research interdisciplinary working group, in collaboration with the Heart Rhythm Society. Circulation 111:230-243, 2005.
58. Rediker DE, Eagle KA, Homma S, et al: Clinical and hemodynamic comparison of VVI versus DDD pacing in patients with DDD pacemakers. Am J Cardiol 61:323-329, 1988.
59. Frielingsdorf J, Gerber AE, Hess OM: Importance of maintained atrio-ventricular synchrony in patients with pacemakers. Eur Heart J 15:1431-1440, 1994.

60. Karlof I: Haemodynamic effect of atrial triggered versus fixed rate pacing at rest and during exercise in complete heart block. Acta Med Scand 197:195-206, 1975.
61. O'Brien B, Blackhouse G, Goeree R, et al: Cost-effectiveness of physiologic pacing: Results of the Canadian Health Economic Assessment of Physiologic Pacing. Heart Rhythm 2:270-275, 2005.
62. Rinfret S, Cohen DJ, Lamas GA, et al: Cost-effectiveness of dual-chamber pacing compared with ventricular pacing for sinus node dysfunction. Circulation 111:165-172, 2005.
63. Yee R, Benditt DG, Kostuk WJ, et al: Comparative functional effects of chronic ventricular demand and atrial synchronous ventricular inhibited pacing. Pacing Clin Electrophysiol 8:73-84, 1984.
64. Sulke N, Dristas A, Bostock J, et al: Subclinical pacemaker syndrome: A randomised study of symptom free patients with ventricular demand [VVI] pacemakers upgraded to dual chamber devices. Br Heart J 67:57-64, 1992.
65. Lipkin DP, Buller N, Frenneaux M, et al: Randomised crossover trial of rate responsive Activitrax and conventional fixed rate ventricular pacing. Br Heart J 58:613-616, 1987.
66. Oto MA, Muderrisoglu H, Ozin MB, et al: Quality of life in patients with rate responsive pacemakers: A randomized, crossover study. Pacing Clin Electrophysiol 14:800-806, 1991.
67. Lau CP, Rushby J, Leigh-Jones M, et al: Symptomatology and quality of life in patients with rate-responsive pacemakers: A double-blind, randomized, crossover study. Clin Cardiol 12:505-512, 1989.
68. Smedgard P, Kristensson BE, Kruse I, et al: Rate-responsive pacing by means of activity sensing versus single rate ventricular pacing. Pacing Clin Electrophysiol 10:902-915, 1987.
69. Hedman A, Nordlander R: QT sensing rate responsive pacing compared to fixed rate ventricular inhibited pacing. Pacing Clin Electrophysiol 12:374-385, 1989.
70. Bubien RS, Kay GN: A randomized comparison of quality of life and exercise capacity with DDD and VVIR pacing modes. Pacing Clin Electrophysiol 13:524A, 1990.
71. Oldroyd KG, Rae AP, Carter R, et al: Double blind crossover comparison of the effects of dual chamber pacing [DDD] and ventricular rate adaptive [VVIR] pacing on neuroendocrine variables, exercise performance, and symptoms in complete heart block. Br Heart J 65:188-193, 1991.
72. Benditt DG, Mianulli M, Fetter J, et al: Single-chamber pacing with activity-initiated chronotropic response: Evaluation by cardiopulmonary exercise testing. Circulation 75:184-191, 1987.
73. Linde-Edelstam C, Nordlander R, Unden A-L, et al: Quality of life in patients treated with atrioventricular synchronous pacing compared to rate modulated ventricular pacing: A long-term, double-blind, crossover study. Pacing Clin Electrophysiol 17:1844-1848, 1992.
74. Lau CP, Tai YT, Lee PWH, et al: Quality of life in DDDR pacing: Atrioventricular synchrony of rate adaption. Pacing Clin Electrophysiol 17:1838-1843, 1994.
75. Sulke AN, Chambers J, Dristas A, et al: A randomized double-blind crossover comparison of four rate-responsive pacing modes. J Am Coll Cardiol 17:696-706, 1991.
76. Lau CP, Tai YT, Leung WH, et al: Rate adaptive pacing in sick sinus syndrome: Effects of pacing modes and intrinsic conduction on physiological responses, arrhythmias, symptomatology and quality of life. Eur Heart J 15:1445-1455, 1994.
76a. Baranchuch A, Healy JS, Thorpe KE, et al: The effect of atrial-based pacing on exercise capacity, as measured by the 6-minute walktest: A sub-study of the Canadian Trial of Physiological Pacing (CTOPP). Heart Rhythm [in press].
77. Gribbin GM, Kenny RA, McCue P, et al: Individualised quality of life after pacing: Does mode matter? Europace 6:552-560, 2004.
78. Leman RB, Kratz JM: Radionuclide evaluation of dual chamber pacing: Comparison between variable AV intervals and ventricular pacing. Pacing Clin Electrophysiol 8:408-414, 1985.
79. Mehta D, Gilmour S, Ward DE, et al: Optimal atrioventricular delay at rest and during exercise in patients with dual chamber pacemakers: A non-invasive assessment by continuous wave Doppler. Br Heart J 61:161-166, 1989.
80. Ritter P, Daubert C, Mabo P, et al: Haemodynamic benefit of a rate-adapted A-V delay in dual-chamber pacing. Eur Heart J 10:637-646, 1989.
81. Ryden L, Karlsson O, Kristensson BE: The importance of different atrioventricular intervals for exercise capacity. Pacing Clin Electrophysiol 11:1051-1062, 1988.
82. Sulke AN, Chambers JB, Sowton E: The effect of atrioventricular delay programming in patients with DDDR pacemakers. Eur Heart J 13:464-472, 1992.
83. Haskell RJ, French WJ: Physiological importance of different atrioventricular intervals to improved exercise performance in patients with dual chamber pacemakers. Br Heart J 61:46-51, 1989.
84. Linde C, Gadler F, Edner M, et al: Results of atrioventricular synchronous pacing with optimized delay in patients with severe congestive heart failure. Am J Cardiol 75:919-923, 1995.
85. Kamalvand K, Tan K, Ktsakis A, et al: Is mode switching beneficial? A randomized study in patients with paroxysmal atrial tachyarrhythmias. J Am Coll Cardiol 30:496-504, 1997.
86. Sweeny MO, Hellkamp AS, Ellenbogen KA, et al: Prospective randomized study of mode-switching in a clinical trial of pacemaker therapy for sinus node dysfunction. J Cardiovasc Electrophysiol 15:153-160, 2004.
87. Shukla HH, Flaker GC, Hellkamp AS, et al: Clinical and quality of life comparison of accelerometer, piezoelectric crystal, and blended sensors in DDDR-paced patients sinus node dysfunction in the Mode Selection Trial [MOST]. Pacing Clin Electrophysiol 28:762-770, 2005.
88. Zanini R, Facchinetti AI, Gallo G, et al: Morbidity and mortality of patients with sinus node disease: Comparative effects of atrial and ventricular pacing. Pacing Clin Electrophysiol 13:2079, 1990.
89. Tung RT, Shen W-K, Hayes DL, et al: Long-term survival after permanent pacemaker implantation for sick sinus syndrome. Am J Cardiol 74:1016-1020, 1994.
90. Markewitz A, Schad N, Hemmer W, et al: What is the most appropriate stimulation mode in patients with sinus node dysfunction? Pacing Clin Electrophysiol 9:1115-1120, 1986.
91. Ebagosti A, Guenoun M, Saadjian A, et al: Long-term follow-up of patients treated with VVI pacing and sequential pacing with reference to VA retrograde conduction. Pacing Clin Electrophysiol 11:1929-1934, 1988.
92. Langenfeld H, Schneider B, Grimm W, et al: The six-minute walk: An adequate exercise for pacemaker patients? Pacing Clin Electrophysiol 13:1761-1765, 1990.
93. Feuer JM, Shandling AH, Messenger JC, et al: Influence of cardiac pacing mode on the long-term development of atrial fibrillation. Am J Cardiol 64:1376-1379, 1989.

Chapter 11

Clinical Trials of Defibrillator Therapy

DEREK V. EXNER

In this chapter, the findings from randomized trials of implantable cardioverter-defibrillator (ICD) therapy, current indications for ICD therapy, and ongoing trials are reviewed. Issues related to defining sudden cardiac death, the impact of ICD therapy on quality of life (QOL), the evolution of ICD therapy, and potential limitations of ICD therapy to provide insight into the rationale and direction of past randomized clinical trials and ongoing studies are discussed.

Sudden Cardiac Death: Magnitude, Definition, and Implications for Clinical Trials

Sudden cardiac death is defined as a death attributable to cardiac cause that occurs soon after the onset of symptoms. A 49% reduction in the incidence of sudden death has been documented over the past five decades.[1] A reduction in the incidence of out-of-hospital cardiac arrest from ventricular fibrillation (VF) has also been observed over the past 15 years.[2] These reductions largely appear to be related to better management of coronary heart disease risk factors and prevention strategies that include prophylactic insertion of ICD systems.[3] Despite these advances, sudden death remains a major public health problem. It is estimated that worldwide more than 3 million lives are ended prematurely because of sudden death.[4] Many of these sudden deaths in ambulatory populations are from sustained ventricular tachyarrhythmias,[5] whereas bradyarrhythmic events and electromechanical dissociation may be more common mechanisms in some groups, such as patients with end-stage heart failure.[6]

It is essential to recognize that clinical definitions of sudden death are prone to bias.[7-9] Using a definition of sudden death that includes only those events that occur within 1 hour of symptom onset appears to be more reliable in identifying deaths related to arrhythmias.[10] Definitions of sudden death that incorporate the circumstances surrounding these events may provide additional value in separating arrhythmic from nonarrhythmic causes. These definitions are often used in clinical trials.[11] Despite these refinements, clinical definitions of sudden death do not include all sudden arrhythmic deaths, and these definitions misclassify some deaths from disease processes unrelated to arrhythmias as "sudden arrhythmic."[12-14] Categorizing deaths as either arrhythmic or nonarrhythmic is useful for hypothesis generation and to better define patient groups in whom an ICD may be effective. Because of the inherent problem of defining sudden death, however, the majority of clinical trials evaluating ICD therapy have used *total mortality* as the primary outcome measure.

Evolution of Therapy: Implication for Clinical Trials

The first successful implantation of an automated defibrillator occurred in the late 1970s.[15] Over the past three decades, improvements have been made in device capability and size. The contemporary tiered-therapy ICD is capable of delivering antitachycardia pacing, low-energy cardioversion, and high-energy defibrillation therapy. In addition, it provides backup bradycardia pacing. The ICD effectively terminates the vast majority of sustained ventricular tachyarrhythmias and many bradyarrhythmias.[16] The availability of a device that reliably terminates the vast majority of life-threatening arrhythmias has tremendous clinical appeal.

The ICD has been described as a parachute but has clearly evolved beyond this concept. Improved arrhythmia discrimination,[17] trends toward the use of therapies aimed at reducing the need for painful shocks to terminate life-threatening arrhythmias,[18] the development of algorithms to diminish the burden of atrial tachyarrhythmias,[19,20] and the capacity of these devices to provide advanced patient monitoring[21,22] are some of the important advances. The addition of cardiac resynchronization therapy (CRT) offers the potential to improve left ventricular (LV) function,[23] reduce morbidity, and further decrease mortality[24,25] in select patients with heart failure.

The vast majority of contemporary ICD systems are placed in a subcutaneous or submuscular position in the chest and use the venous anatomy for lead delivery. The risk of death related to placement of nonthoracotomy, transvenous ICD systems approaches 0%. In contrast, earlier ICD systems that required a thoracotomy or sternotomy for lead placement were associated with a 5% risk of death in the first 30 postoperative days.[26,27] The ease of implantation and relatively low risk of surgical morbidity and mortality with contemporary ICD system placement have directly affected the direction of studies examining its efficacy. Although initial trials were limited to patients considered to have a very high risk of cardiac arrest, later trials have included patients at somewhat lower risk.

The results of clinical trials over the past decade have established the ICD as a cornerstone of therapy for patients at high risk for sudden death.[28-30] The number of ICD implantations worldwide now approaches 200,000 per year and is anticipated to rise.[4,31] The exponential increase in the number of ICD systems implanted over the past decade mirrors the quantity of patient data obtained from randomized clinical trials (Fig. 11-1).

Quality of Life

In contrast to antiarrhythmic drugs, which are designed to prevent arrhythmias, the ICD treats arrhythmias that have already developed. Because the ICD prolongs life, patients may experience deterioration in underlying health that might not have occurred otherwise. Stress, anxiety, depression, mood disturbance, sexual dysfunction, and a sense of uncertainty or loss of control have been described in ICD recipients.[32] The ICD also provides a sense of reassurance to some patients, enhancing their QOL. The use of an ICD with cardiac resynchronization may further enhance QOL by reducing heart failure symptoms.[33]

Four randomized trials have published results or preliminary data related to QOL with ICD therapy. They

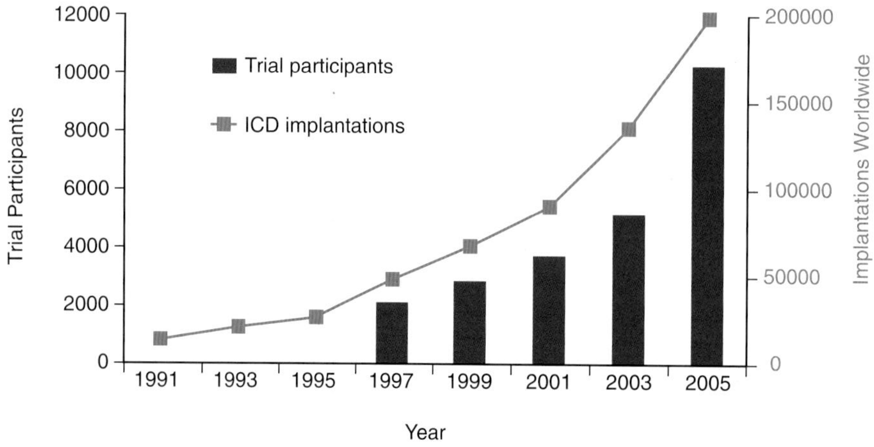

Figure 11-1. Growth of the use of defibrillator system implantations worldwide and of the knowledge from randomized clinical trials of defibrillator therapy. An exponential increase in the number of implantable cardioverter-defibrillator (ICD) systems worldwide has occurred since 1990. This increase is a reflection of the number of patients included in randomized trials evaluating the efficacy of ICD therapy to reduce mortality and sudden death. (Adapted from Josephson M, Wellens HJ: Implantable defibrillators and sudden cardiac death. Circulation 109:2685-2691, 2004; and Hauser RG: The growing mismatch between patient longevity and the service life of implantable cardioverter-defibrillators. J Am Coll Cardiol 45:2022-2025, 2005.)

indicate that ICD therapy and amiodarone are associated with similar alterations in QOL in patients with spontaneous or inducible ventricular arrhythmias.[34,35] Patients who have not experienced a spontaneous sustained ventricular arrhythmia have been shown to have reduced QOL with an ICD in one study[36] and improved QOL in another.[37] Details regarding the influence of ICD therapy on QOL are found in the individual reviews of these four trials (AVID, CIDS, DEFINITE, and CABG Patch; see later). Other trials of ICD therapy have assessed QOL but have not reported results to date. All of the studies assessing QOL data have shown that ICD shocks significantly impair patients' perceptions of well-being. This issue is discussed in the following section.

Limitations of Therapy

Implantable Cardioverter-Defibrillators Shocks

Even sporadic ICD shocks are associated with significant, independent reductions in QOL. Compared with patients who do not experience shocks, patients who experience at least one shock during a year have reduced QOL, independent of ejection fraction values, social circumstances, and medication use.[34] The reduction in QOL associated with shocks was similar in magnitude to clinically important adverse effects from amiodarone. The development of clusters of life-threatening arrhythmias identifies patients at high risk of death in the near term. Patients who experience *electrical storm* (at least three episodes of ventricular tachycardia [VT] or VF in a 24-hour period) have a greater than fivefold higher risk of death in the subsequent 3 months.[38] The majority of these deaths are attributed to progressive heart failure, supporting a link between electrical storm and deteriorating LV function. It is not known whether the development of electrical storm identifies patients with worsening LV function or whether the ICD therapies themselves contribute to progressive LV dysfunction. Evidence links multiple shocks with myocardial injury[39] and fibrosis.[40] There is also evidence in animal models that ICD shocks may be proarrhythmic.[41] Data from human studies support a proarrhythmic effect of some shocks and suggest that multiple shocks can result in myocardial stunning and electromechanical dissociation.[42,43] Strategies to reduce the likelihood of both inappropriate and appropriate shocks, as well as alternative methods to terminate ventricular arrhythmias, are essential areas of research.

Antiarrhythmic drugs can be used to reduce the likelihood of shocks[44,45] but may negatively affect QOL because of adverse effects.[34] Antitachycardia pacing (ATP) therapies painlessly interrupt reentrant ventricular arrhythmias using brief, rapid bursts of pacing. ATP is routinely used to terminate slower ventricular arrhythmias (rates < 188 beats per minute [bpm]) with an efficacy rate of more than 90% and a low (<5%) risk of accelerating these slower arrhythmias to more rapid ones requiring a defibrillation shock. ATP was believed to be of limited value in terminating faster ventricular arrhythmias (188 to 250 bpm) because of an assumed low probability of success and the potential risk of accelerating these arrhythmias or delaying arrhythmia termination with resultant syncope. As a result of these concerns, defibrillation shocks have been primarily used to terminate fast ventricular tachyarrhythmias. The Pain FREE Rx II study evaluated the efficacy of ATP for fast ventricular arrhythmias in 634 patients.[18] Patients were randomly assigned to receive ATP or a shock as the initial therapy for a fast ventricular tachyarrhythmia episode. ATP terminated more than 70% of these tachyarrhythmias without prolonging the time to their termination or increasing either the likelihood of arrhythmia acceleration or the risk of syncope in comparison with shocks. Patients randomly assigned to undergo ATP also had significantly better QOL over time compared with those who underwent shocks. However, these QOL data are based on relatively few patients, because only 15% of subjects randomly assigned had sustained fast ventricular arrhythmias in follow-up. As well, more than one third of the fast ventricular arrhythmias spontaneously terminated before the delivery of a shock in that study arm, suggesting that the true efficacy of ATP for these fast arrhythmias is about 50%. The efficacy and QOL improvements observed with ATP were similar in patients with and without a history of sustained arrhythmias prior to ICD implantation.[46]

Reliability

Despite the intuitive appeal of the ICD, one must recognize that it is an imperfect therapeutic device. Currently, ICD systems have a limited life expectancy and are subject to both complications and unexpected failure over time.[47-51] A growing gap between device longevity and patient survival is evident.[50] The life expectancy of patients receiving ICD systems has improved over time. In one study, the survival of ICD recipients at 5 years was 75%, and at least 40% of ICD recipients lived at least 10 years after ICD placement. Given that contemporary ICD system batteries are designed to last 4 to 7 years, it is clear that patients will require multiple devices in their lifetimes. With the results of trials indicating a survival benefit in patients with less advanced forms of heart disease, this mismatch will continue to grow. Additional research related to assessing reliability and longevity is required.

Cost

Cost efficacy is a vital issue in the setting of limited or restricted health care resources[52] and is particularly relevant as the use of ICDs and resynchronization ICD devices has expanded to include patients sharing only some similarities with populations in which it has been demonstrated to be effective, so-called *indication creep* or indication extrapolation.[53] A major limitation of cost efficacy analyses from randomized trials is that these analyses invariably inflate the cost of ICD therapy and devalue the life-years gained. The estimate of life-years gained from randomized trials depends heavily on the duration of follow-up over which benefit is assessed. The cost of an ICD is heavily front-loaded, yet its benefit accrues over time. Thus, short-term data from randomized trials may artificially underestimate the cost efficacy of this therapy.[54] Cost-effectiveness data are included in the review of individual trials for which these data are available.

Groups at Risk for Sudden Death

The term *primary prevention* has been used to describe the use of ICD therapy in individuals without a history of spontaneous life-threatening arrhythmias. *Secondary prevention* has been used to describe the use of an ICD in a patient with a previously documented life-threatening arrhythmia. This dichotomy is both problematic and inexact, as evidenced by the inclusion criteria and results of completed trials to be discussed. In lieu of these descriptors, the populations studied with ICD therapy will be categorized as belonging to one of the following three groups:

- Spontaneous or inducible ventricular arrhythmias
- Heart failure or LV dysfunction alone
- LV dysfunction in specific circumstances

Identifying Individuals at Risk

A major barrier to preventing sudden death is the lack of accurate and reliable methods of identifying the majority of individuals at risk.[55,56] The majority of persons who experience sudden death can be categorized as belonging to one of the three groups previously listed. Patients with spontaneous or inducible ventricular arrhythmias are known to be at high risk for cardiac arrest but represent only a fraction of those who will experience sudden death (Fig. 11-2).[57,58]

Persons with structural heart disease, notably a previous myocardial infarction (MI) and/or LV dysfunction, represent a significant proportion of those at risk for sudden death and have an intermediate risk of cardiac arrest in the near term. Although individuals with ejection fractions of 0.35 or lower after MI have a higher risk of sudden death, the majority of these patients will *not* experience a cardiac arrest in the near term. Also, most sudden deaths will occur in patients with better-preserved LV function (Fig. 11-3). If an ejection fraction cutoff of 0.35 is used, fewer than 20% of patients who will experience sudden death are identified.[59] In contrast, if an ejection fraction cutoff of 0.50 is used, the majority of patients destined to have a cardiac arrest are identified.[60] The risk of sudden death in patients with ejection fractions of 0.35 or lower will be markedly higher, however, than that in patients with better-preserved LV systolic function. In other words,

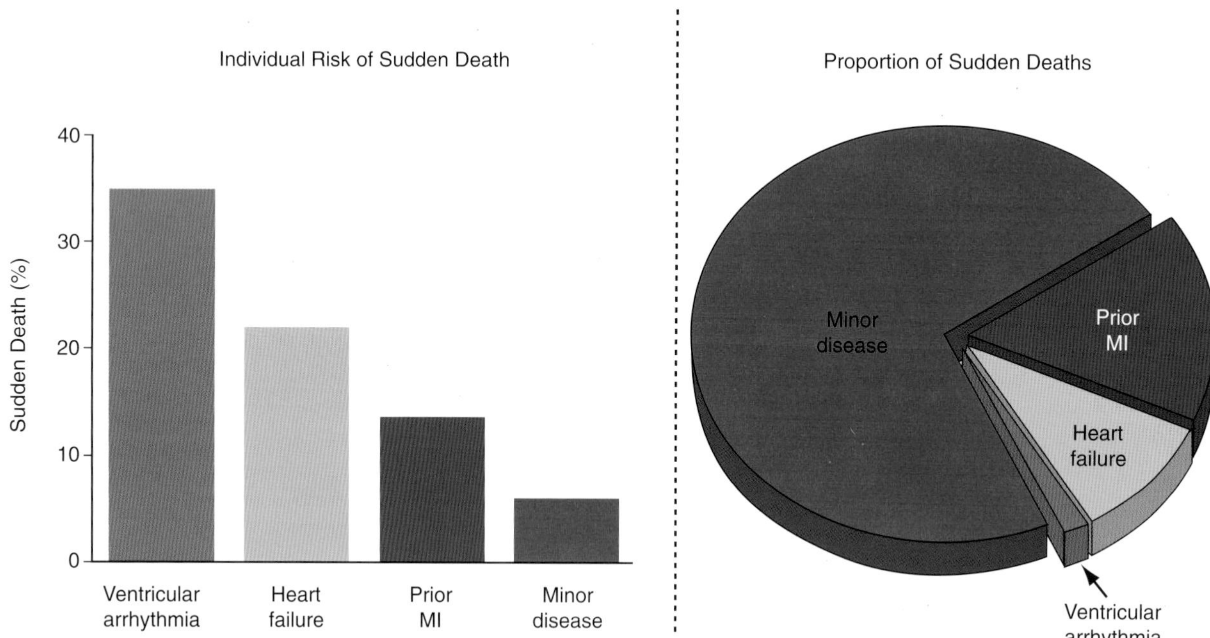

Figure 11-2. Sudden death: individual risk versus population impact. Individuals with spontaneous or inducible sustained ventricular arrhythmias (orange) have a large individual risk of cardiac arrest in the near term. However, only a small number of patients have these ventricular arrhythmias. Thus, the number of sudden deaths in this group is relatively small. Patients with heart failure (yellow) and those with a myocardial infarction (MI) (blue) have an intermediate risk of cardiac arrest in the near term. Because of the large number of patients with these conditions, many more sudden deaths occur in this group. Trials of implantable cardioverter-defibrillator (ICD) therapy in patients with heart failure have been conducted in order to more effectively reduce the burden of sudden death. (Adapted from Rea TD, Pearce RM, Raghunathan TE, et al: Incidence of out-of-hospital cardiac arrest. Am J Cardiol 93:1455-1460, 2004.)

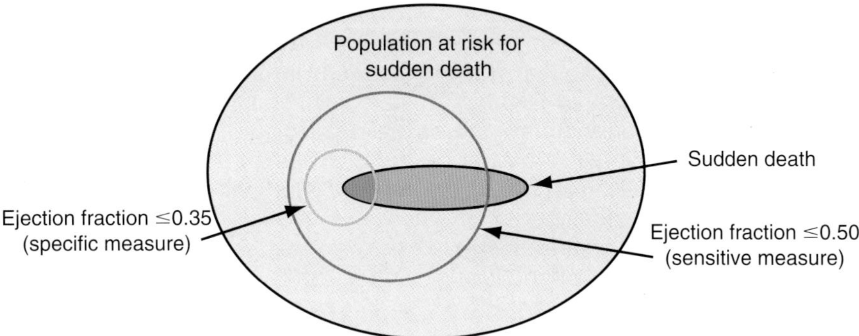

Figure 11-3. Identifying individuals at risk for sudden death, specificity versus sensitivity. Patients with a history of a myocardial infarction (gray) are at risk for sudden death, but only a fraction of these individuals will experience sudden death in the near term (blue). Although patients with severe left ventricular (LV) dysfunction (ejection fraction ≤0.35; yellow circle) have a high risk of death, most of these deaths are not sudden and <20% of all sudden deaths will occur in these patients. Patients with mild LV dysfunction (ejection fraction ≤ 0.50; orange circle) are less likely to die but account for the majority of those who will experience sudden death in the near term. Risk assessment strategies, in addition to the use of ejection fraction, may allow better identification of patients with a history of myocardial infarction who are more likely to benefit from an implantable cardioverter-defibrillator. (Adapted from Gorgels AP, Gijsbers C, de Vreede-Swagemakers J, et al: Baroreflex sensitivity and heart-rate variability in prediction of total cardiac mortality after myocardial infarction. ATRAMI [Autonomic Tone and Reflexes After Myocardial Infarction] Investigators. Lancet 351:478-1484, 1998; and Raviele A, Bongiorni MG, Brignole M, et al: Early EPS/ICD strategy in survivors of acute myocardial infarction with severe left ventricular dysfunction on optimal beta-blocker treatment. The BEta-blocker STrategy plus ICD trial. Europace 7:327-337, 2005.)

an ejection fraction of 0.35 or lower is more *specific* in identifying those at risk for sudden death, whereas an ejection fraction of 0.50 or lower is more *sensitive* in identifying those who will experience sudden death. Additional risk assessment is required to identify the majority of those at risk for sudden death.[61,62]

Individuals with mild or subclinical heart disease account for the majority of sudden deaths,[63] but the likelihood that an individual in this group will experience a cardiac arrest over a decade is very low (see Fig. 11-2). Many of the cardiac arrests in this last group appear to be triggered by unstable coronary artery plaques.[64] Appropriate attention to prophylactic therapy with antiplatelet drugs, statins, fish oils, and other agents may significantly reduce the burden of sudden death.[2,3,65-67] Widespread use of automated external defibrillators may be another effective means of reducing the occurrence of sudden death in the general population, but this possibility requires confirmation.[68] The use of noninvasive risk stratification techniques, such as microvolt T-wave alternans assessment,[69,70] heart rate turbulence,[71,72] other Holter monitor indices,[73-75] imaging methods,[76,77] and genetic assessment in some cases,[78] may help identify a greater proportion of those at risk of sudden death or those at particular risk. The usefulness of these strategies awaits prospective confirmation.

Relative versus Absolute Risk Reduction

When assessing the impact of a therapy, one must understand its relative and absolute benefits. The *absolute risk reduction* is the difference between control and intervention group rates. For example, if a therapy reduces the risk of death from 10% (control) to 6% (intervention), the absolute risk reduction is 4%. The *relative risk reduction* is the percentage reduction in rates with the intervention. For the same example, the relative risk reduction is 40% (4% absolute risk reduction ÷ 10% control rate). It is essential to evaluate both the absolute risk reduction and the relative risk reduction of an intervention. In a second example, an intervention reduces the risk of death from 2% to 1%. Although the relative risk reduction is larger than in the first example (50%), the absolute risk reduction is smaller (1%). The number of patients one needs to treat in order to prevent one event over a specified time is often used to describe the absolute impact of a therapy. The *number needed to treat* (NNT) is the reciprocal of the absolute risk reduction. For the first example, the NNT is 25 (100% ÷ 4%); in the second example, it is 100 (100% ÷ 1%).

Evolution of Implantable Cardioverter-Defibrillator Therapy

Initial observational studies and smaller randomized trials suggested that ICD implantation was associated with a large (>60%) relative reduction in mortality compared with conventional strategies.[79] Owing to limitations in the design of these initial studies, a series of larger, adequately powered, randomized trials were conducted to either confirm or refute these initial observations. Because of the risk of ICD system placement (via thoracotomy or sternotomy) early on, initial randomized trials focused on patients with the highest individual risk for a fatal cardiac arrest, those with a history of spontaneous ventricular arrhythmias (see Fig. 11-2). The next group of studies evaluated patients with an extremely high risk of a fatal cardiac arrest due to a history of a prior MI, severe LV dysfunction, and arrhythmias inducible by invasive programmed electrical stimulation. During this time, studies were also designed to minimize the risk of ICD system implantation by limiting therapy to patients who required a sternotomy for another reason (coronary artery bypass surgery).[80] After the mostly positive results shown in these early trials, studies in populations with lower but significant risk of sudden death were initiated. These trials were mostly limited to patients with heart failure and LV dysfunction.

A number of randomized studies have compared ICD therapy with amiodarone or other medical therapy. The relative benefit values for the ICD are similar in *most* of these studies, but three studies showed no benefit (Fig. 11-4). They included patients with LV dysfunction in specific circumstances. Two studies enrolled patients very early after MI,[81,132] and the other included patients undergoing coronary artery bypass surgery.[80] The lack of ICD efficacy in these populations indicates that coronary artery revascularization and remodeling after an MI dramatically influence ICD efficacy. The results also emphasize the need for randomized trials to definitively assess the efficacy of ICD therapy in specific circumstances and highlight the pitfalls of using a therapy for an indication beyond what has been shown to be efficacious.

Efficacy: A Review of Randomized Trials

Patients with Spontaneous or Inducible Ventricular Arrhythmias

The details of the individual studies involving patients with spontaneous or inducible ventricular arrhythmias

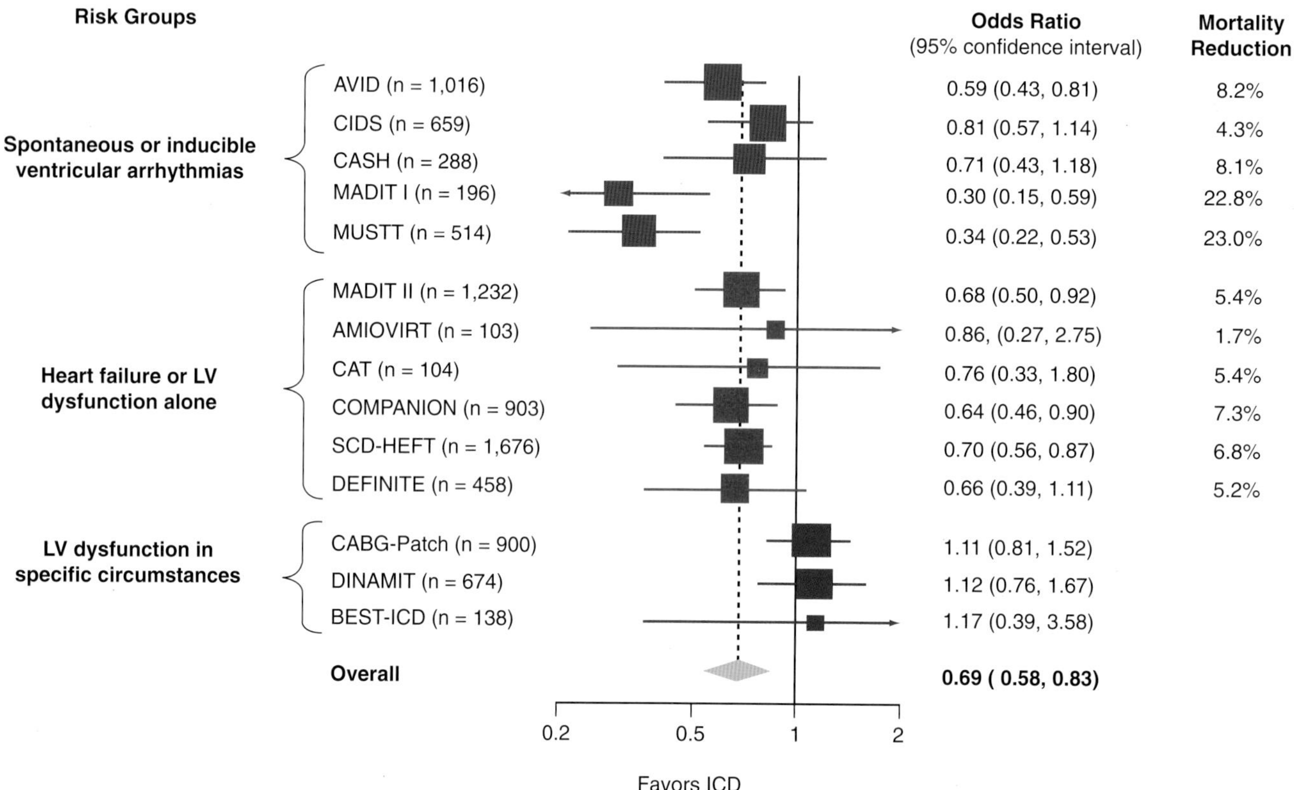

Figure 11-4. Summary of published randomized trials of defibrillator therapy. A large number of randomized trials have evaluated the efficacy of the implantable cardioverter-defibrillator (ICD) versus drug therapy or usual medical care. These patient populations can be separated into those with (1) spontaneous or inducible ventricular arrhythmias, (2) heart failure or left ventricular (LV) dysfunction alone, and (3) LV dysfunction in specific circumstances. The ICD has been proved to reduce mortality in the first two groups but not in the third. The relative benefits (odds ratios) in the first two groups are similar, and the absolute reduction in mortality with ICD therapy is approximately twice as large in patients with spontaneous or inducible ventricular arrhythmias as in patients with heart failure or LV dysfunction alone. AMIOVIRT, Amiodarone Versus Implantable Cardioverter-Defibrillator Trial; AVID, Antiarrhythmics versus Implantable Defibrillators trial; BEST-ICD, BEta-blocker STrategy plus ICD study; CABG-Patch, Coronary Artery Bypass Graft (CABG) Patch trial; CASH, Cardiac Arrest Study Hamburg; CAT, Cardiomyopathy Trial; CIDS, Canadian Implantable Defibrillator Study; COMPANION, Comparison of Medical Therapy, Pacing, and Defibrillation in Heart Failure study; DEFINITE, Defibrillators in Non-Ischemic Cardiomyopathy Treatment Evaluation; DINAMIT, Defibrillators in Acute Myocardial Infarction Trial; MADIT, Multicenter Automatic Defibrillator Implantation Trial; MUSTT, Multicenter Unsustained Tachycardia Trial; SCD-HEFT, Sudden Cardiac Death–Heart Failure Trial.

TABLE 11-1. Clinical Trials of ICD Therapy for Spontaneous or Inducible Ventricular Arrhythmias: Inclusion Criteria, Comparison Groups, and Main Results

Trial (Year)	Inclusion Criteria	Comparison	Primary Endpoint	Main Finding
Antiarrhythmics Versus Implantable Defibrillators (AVID) (1999)	Resuscitated VF, sustained VT and syncope, or sustained VT with EF ≤0.40 and severe symptoms; no reversible cause	ICD vs. antiarrhythmic drugs (amiodarone)	All-cause mortality	31% relative reduction in primary endpoint (*P* < .02) with ICD
Canadian Implantable Defibrillator Study (CIDS) (2000)	Resuscitated VF, sustained VT and syncope, sustained VT and EF ≤ 0.35, or unmonitored syncope with subsequent spontaneous or inducible VT; no reversible cause	ICD vs. amiodarone	All-cause mortality	20% relative reduction in primary endpoint (*P* = .1) with ICD
Cardiac Arrest Study Hamburg (CASH) (2000)	Cardiac arrest secondary to VF or VT not related to a reversible cause	ICD vs. drug therapy (amiodarone, metoprolol)	All-cause mortality	23% relative reduction in primary endpoint (*P* = .2) with ICD
Multicenter Automatic Defibrillator Implantation Trial (MADIT) (1996)	Age 25–80 yrs, NYHA I-III, EF ≤ 0.35, nonrecent MI (>3 wks) or CABG (>3 mos), spontaneous NSVT, and inducible VT	ICD vs. best medical therapy that could include amiodarone	All-cause mortality	56% risk reduction in primary endpoint (*P* = .009) with ICD
Multicenter Unsustained Tachycardia Trial (MUSTT) (1999)*	Age < 80 yrs, NYHA I, II, or III, EF ≤ 0.40, nonrecent MI (≥4 days), spontaneous NSVT, and inducible VT	ICD vs. antiarrhythmic therapy (amiodarone and class I agents)	Cardiac arrest or death from arrhythmia	76% relative reduction in primary endpoint (*P* < .001) with ICD

*Nonrandomized ICD use.

CABG, coronary artery bypass graft; EF, ejection fraction; ICD, implantable cardioverter-defibrillator; MI, myocardial infarction; NSVT, nonsustained ventricular tachycardia; NYHA, New York Heart Association functional class; VF, ventricular fibrillation; VT, ventricular tachycardia.

can be found in Tables 11-1 and 11-2. Table 11-1 summarizes the inclusion criteria, primary endpoints, and main results for each of the five studies. Details of the study populations, the risk of the population untreated (annual control group mortality), and the relative and absolute changes in mortality with ICD therapy are shown in Table 11-2.

Two large[82,83] and one smaller[84] randomized trial provide convincing evidence that ICD therapy is superior to class III antiarrhythmic drugs in reducing mortality among patients with *mostly* spontaneous life-threatening arrhythmias. These studies generally included patients who survived a cardiac arrest due to VT or VT. One large randomized trial comparing ICD therapy with conventional care that generally included amiodarone[85] and another large randomized trial in which ICD therapy was used in a nonrandomized fashion[86] assessed the efficacy of ICD therapy in patients with LV dysfunction and inducible ventricular arrhythmias. They showed a benefit from ICD therapy similar to that in the three studies of patients with spontaneous life-threatening arrhythmias.

Antiarrhythmics versus Implantable Defibrillators Trial

The Antiarrhythmics versus Implantable Defibrillators (AVID) trial was a large (n = 1016) multicenter trial conducted in the United States and Canada. Patients entered into the trial were resuscitated from VT, had sustained VT with syncope, or had sustained VT with an ejection fraction of 0.40 or lower and symptoms suggesting severe hemodynamic compromise (near-syncope, heart failure, and angina).[82] Patients were excluded if the ventricular arrhythmia was attributed to a reversible cause or the episode of VT was categorized as stable. In any patient who underwent revascularization after the index arrhythmia, the ejection fraction had to be 0.40 or lower for inclusion in the study. The primary outcome was all-cause mortality.

The AVID trial began recruitment in mid-1993; it was terminated in 1997, when patients randomly assigned to ICD therapy were found to have a 31% relative reduction in the risk of death compared with patients receiving antiarrhythmic drug therapy, mostly amiodarone (95% confidence interval [CI] = 10% to 52%). This mortality benefit translates into an average life extension of 2.7 months during 18 months of follow-up.[82] The NNT over 36 months is approximately 9 (11.3% absolute risk reduction). The incremental cost of an ICD at 3 years was approximately $67,000 (U.S.) per life-year saved.[87] However, the early termination of the AVID trial has two important implications. First, premature termination may overestimate the magnitude of benefit with ICD therapy compared with amiodarone,[88] and second, the resultant shorter average

TABLE 11-2. **Clinical Trials of ICD Therapy for Spontaneous or Inducible Ventricular Arrhythmias: Population Details and Mortality Results**

							Mortality Results: ICD vs. Other (%)			
Trial	**N**	**Age (yrs)**	**Women (%)**	**NYHA > II (%)**	**Mean Ejection Fraction**	**Mean Follow-up (mos)**	**Annual Rate in Controls**	**Relative Risk Reduction**	**Absolute Risk Reduction**	**Number Needed to Treat (36 mos)**
Antiarrhythmics Versus Implantable Defibrillators (AVID) Trial	1016	65	20	8	0.35	18	12	31	8.2	9
Canadian Implantable Defibrillator Study (CIDS)	659	64	16	11	0.34	36	10	20	4.3	23
Cardiac Arrest Study Hamburg (CASH)	228	58	20	19	0.45	57	9	23	8.1	20
First Multicenter Automatic Defibrillator Implantation Trial (MADIT I)	196	63	8	—	0.26	27	17	54	22.8	3
Multicenter Unsustained Tachycardia Trial (MUSTT)*	704	65	10	24	0.28	39	13	51	23	5

*ICD use was not randomized in MUSTT.
ICD, implantable cardioverter-defibrillator; NYHA, New York Heart Association functional class.

duration of follow-up may lead to underestimation of the true cost-effectiveness of ICD therapy.[89]

Analyses were undertaken to identify groups more likely to benefit from ICD therapy. It was found that the 61% of patients with ejection fraction values lower than 0.35 had a very large (40%) relative reduction in the risk of death with ICD in comparison with drug therapy, whereas patients with higher values did not significantly benefit.[90] The AVID trial included relatively few patients with advanced heart failure, marked reductions in ejection fraction, or advanced age and so has limited power to assess the relative efficacy of ICD in comparison with drug therapy in these and other small subgroups.[91]

As a prespecified secondary endpoint, the investigators also collected QOL data before and at 3, 6, and 12 months after randomization.[34] Data were available for 905 of 1016 (89%) patients enrolled.[34] Of these, 800 patients survived 1 year or longer and composed the QOL study population. Moderate to severe impairment in both physical functioning and mental well-being were evident in both treatment groups at baseline. Patients who had received ICDs had better physical functioning over the subsequent year, but no significant changes were noted in mental well-being. No significant difference in QOL over time was observed between the ICD-treated and amiodarone-treated patients. Adverse symptoms were associated with a decrease in QOL in both groups. As previously discussed, there was an independent association between receipt of a shock and a reduction in QOL. The reduction in QOL associated with experiencing multiple shocks in follow-up was of similar magnitude to that observed in patients with severe adverse symptoms from amiodarone.

One criticism of the AVID results is that an imbalance in β-blocker use between patients randomly assigned to receive an ICD (38% at 1 year) and those receiving amiodarone therapy (11% at 1 year) may have influenced the study results. However, β-blocker use did not alter survival among either ICD-treated or amiodarone-treated patients. In contrast, patients who were eligible for the AVID trial but were not randomly assigned to and did not receive either amiodarone or an ICD had a 53% lower mortality rate with β-blocker than similar patients who did not receive β-blockers.[92] These data suggest that β-blockers appear to reduce mortality in this population primarily through lowering the risk of sudden death. This effect is limited to patients who are not treated with an ICD or amiodarone.

Another intriguing result from the AVID trial is that patients with sustained ventricular arrhythmias due to a reversible cause have a similar, or perhaps higher, risk of death compared with patients in whom the event was considered a primary episode of VT or VT.[93] Likewise, prognosis for patients with *stable* VT was similar to that for patients with unstable VT.[94] These analyses call into question the "dogma" that patients with *stable* VT and those with a potentially reversible cause of sustained ventricular arrhythmia have a good prognosis and are not candidates for an ICD.

Canadian Implantable Defibrillator Study

The Canadian Implantable Defibrillator Study (CIDS) was a large multicenter trial (n = 659) conducted in Canada, Australia, and the United States from 1990 to 1997.[83] Patients were eligible if they had VT, sustained VT causing syncope, sustained VT and an ejection fraction of 0.35 of less, or unmonitored syncope with subsequent spontaneous or inducible ventricular tachyarrhythmia. Patients who had experienced a recent MI (within 72 hours) or had an electrolyte imbalance were excluded. The average follow-up in CIDS (36 months) was twice that in the AVID trial, but the number of deaths was somewhat fewer in CIDS (181) than in AVID (202). The primary outcome in CIDS was all-cause mortality.

CIDS demonstrated a 20% relative (95% CI = 8% increase to 40%) lower risk of death with an ICD than with amiodarone ($P = .14$).[83] On the basis of this 4.3% absolute reduction in mortality, the NNT over 36 months is 23. The incremental cost of an ICD was approximately $150,000 (U.S.) per life-year gained.[95] Patients in CIDS with low ejection fraction values benefited from ICD therapy to a greater extent than those with better-preserved LV function.[96] The selective use of an ICD for patients with ejection fraction values lower than 0.35 lowers the incremental cost of an ICD to less than $70,000 per life-year gained.[95] Another analysis demonstrated that patients with two or more of three characteristics (age ≥ 70 years or less, ejection fraction ≤0.35, and New York Heart Association functional class [NYHA class] III symptoms) benefited from ICD therapy, whereas patients with one or no characteristics did not.[97] However, only a low ejection fraction was found to identify patients more likely to benefit from an ICD in trials that included similar patients.[28,98] In a single center study enrolled 120 patients, treatment strategy was not altered at the end of CIDS unless the initial assigned therapy was ineffective or was associated with side effects. After a mean follow-up of 5.6 ± 2.6 years, there were 28 deaths in the amiodarone group (47%) compared with 16 deaths in the ICD group (27%; $P = .0213$). In the amiodarone group, 49 patients (82% of all patients) experienced side effects related to amiodarone; 30 patients required discontinuation or dose reduction, and 19 crossed over to ICD placement because of amiodarone failure (n = 7) or side effects (n = 12).[148]

QOL was assessed in CIDS.[35] Of the initial 400 enrolled patients, only 178 (45%) provided analyzable QOL data at 1 year. Patients randomly assigned to ICD therapy had significant improvements in several QOL measures over 1 year of follow-up. In patients undergoing amiodarone therapy, these QOL measures either did not improve or deteriorated. Patients with frequent (>5) ICD shocks during follow-up had reduced QOL. Whether ICD therapy truly provides better QOL than amiodarone therapy is uncertain because of the conflicting results from the AVID trial and the methodologic issues related to the CIDS analysis.[99]

Cardiac Arrest Study Hamburg

The Cardiac Arrest Study Hamburg (CASH) was a smaller randomized trial (n = 288) that compared the use of an ICD with drug therapy. Patients were enrolled from 1987 to 1996. Thus, a significant number of patients underwent a thoracotomy or sternotomy for ICD system placement (before July 1991). The study population included patients resuscitated from cardiac arrest secondary to a documented sustained ventricular arrhythmia. Patients were excluded if the cardiac arrest occurred within 72 hours of an MI or cardiac surgery or was related to either an electrolyte abnormality or a proarrhythmic drug. The primary endpoint was all-cause mortality. The average follow-up in CASH (57 months) was substantially longer than that of other trials. However, there were fewer deaths (n = 72) owing to the smaller overall study population. A trend toward a lower risk of death with ICD therapy (23% relative reduction; $P = .16$) was observed.[84] The 8.1% absolute reduction in risk of death over 57 months with ICD therapy is similar to that found in the AVID trial over 18 months and translates into an NNT of 12. Over 36 months, the NNT is 20.

Pooled Analysis of the Three Studies

The combined results of the AVID, CIDS, and CASH[28] data demonstrate that mortality is reduced by 27% (95% CI = 13% to 40%; $P < .001$) with an ICD compared with amiodarone. Death attributed to an arrhythmia was reduced by 51% (95% CI =33% to 64%; $P < .001$). No significant difference between treatment groups in the risk of death from nonarrhythmic causes was evident. This reduction in mortality corresponded to an average extension in life of 2.1 months. The annual mortality with an ICD was 12.3% per year, versus 8.8% per year with amiodarone. The absolute reduction in mortality (10.5%) over 36 months translates into needing to treat fewer than 10 patients in order to prevent one death during this period.

Patients with ejection fraction values of 0.35 or lower benefited from ICD therapy to a greater extent than patients with better-preserved LV systolic function ($P = .01$). Patients who required a thoracotomy or sternotomy for ICD placement (before 1991) did not exhibit any evidence of greater benefit with ICD therapy than with amiodarone, whereas patients who received nonthoracotomy systems did (31% relative reduction; 95% CI = 15% to 44%). A trend toward a greater benefit from ICD therapy than from amiodarone was evident among patients who were treated with β-blockers compared with those who were not ($P = .10$). Patients with a history of coronary artery bypass surgery also tended to benefit from ICD therapy to a greater extent than patients without such a history ($P = .10$). This issue is discussed in greater detail in the later review of the CABG Patch trial.

First Multicenter Automatic Defibrillator Implantation Trial

The First Multicenter Automatic Defibrillator Implantation Trial (MADIT-I) was a small (n = 196) multicenter trial conducted in the United States, Germany, and Italy from December 1990 to March 1996.[86] The first one half of the patients received epicardial ICD systems, and the remaining one half received nonthoracotomy, transvenous systems. ICD therapy was compared with conventional care, mostly empiric amiodarone therapy, in patients with ischemic LV dysfunction, asymptomatic nonsustained VT (NSVT), and inducible, nonsuppressible sustained ventricular arrhythmias during programmed electrical stimulation. Most of the MADIT-I patients (93%) had nonsuppressible, monomorphic VT.

MADIT-I demonstrated a large, 54% (95% CI = 18% to 74%) relative reduction in mortality ($P = .009$). The MADIT-I population has been considered distinct from the patients in the AVID trial, CIDS, and CASH, but the populations are actually quite similar. Both CIDS and the AVID trial included patients with VT unrelated to a cardiac arrest. CIDS also included patients with a history of syncope and a low ejection fraction value with VT inducible at the time of an invasive electrophysiology study. The average extension of life with an ICD was 10 months. This large reduction in mortality (26.2% absolute risk reduction over 27 months) translates into an NNT of 3 over 36 months. ICD therapy costs $27,000 (U.S.) (95% CI = $800 to $68,200) per life-year gained more than conventional care, making ICD very economically attractive.[100]

The annual mortality rate in the MADIT-I control group appears to be somewhat higher than that observed in the three trials evaluating ICD therapy in patients with *mostly* spontaneous sustained ventricular arrhythmias (see Table 11-2). The likely explanation for this observation is that all of the patients in MADIT-I had ejection fractions of 0.35 or lower, whereas ejection fraction was not a primary inclusion criterion in the AVID trial, CIDS, or CASH. If only those patients in the AVID trial, CIDS, and CASH with ejection fraction values of 0.35 or lower are studied, a similar 16% annual mortality rate is observed in patients receiving amiodarone.[28] Moreover, the relative reduction in risk of death with an ICD in comparison with amiodarone among patients with ejection fractions of 0.35 or lower in the AVID trial, CIDS, and CASH (44%; 95% CI = 17% to 47%; $P < .001$) is similar to that found in MADIT-I (54%; 95% CI = 18% to 74% reduction). Thus, patients with spontaneous or inducible sustained ventricular arrhythmias have a similar risk of death and benefit to a similar extent with ICD therapy.

A major limitation of MADIT-I is the lack of information about how many patients with ischemic LV dysfunction and NSVT would have to be screened to identify one patient fulfilling all of the inclusion criteria for this trial. This number is estimated to be large because these criteria are present in very few (<2%) patients after MI.[101] It is also apparent that targeting ICD therapy to only those at highest risk will have a marginal effect on reducing the burden of sudden death (see Fig. 11-2). Another concern regarding MADIT-I is the non–protocol-driven use of antiarrhythmic drugs. For example, 23% of patients assigned to conventional therapy were not receiving antiarrhythmic drug therapy at last follow-up, and only 55% of patients were receiving amiodarone at that time. The significance of this issue is questionable, given the results of the SCD-HeFT (see later), which demonstrate no significant benefit or harm from amiodarone.

First Multicenter Unsustained Tachycardia Trial (MUSTT-I)

The First Multicenter Unsustained Tachycardia Trial (MUSTT-I) was a randomized trial that compared antiarrhythmic therapy with best medical therapy in 704 patients with coronary artery disease, ejection fraction values of 0.40 or lower, NSVT, and inducible sustained ventricular arrhythmias during programmed electrical stimulation.[85] It is important to emphasize that the use or nonuse of ICD therapy in MUSTT-I was not randomly assigned. However, the trial's results are often taken into consideration by anyone interpreting the data from the previously discussed trials of patients with spontaneous or inducible ventricular arrhythmias; therefore, MUSTT-I is reviewed here.

Patients in MUSTT-I were recruited from 85 centers in the United States and Canada from 1990 through 1996. Most (n = 1,435; 65%) of the 2202 patients evaluated did not have inducible ventricular arrhythmias and were not eligible for therapy randomization. Of the 767 eligible patients, only 63 (8%) refused random assignment to therapy arms, strengthening the generalizability of the results. The 351 patients randomly assigned to electrophysiologically guided therapy underwent serial drug testing followed by random assignment to receive antiarrhythmic drugs. ICD therapy could be used only after failure of at least one antiarrhythmic drug, and amiodarone could be tested only after at least two failed drug trials. Similar proportions of patients assigned to this strategy were discharged with drug therapy (n = 158; 45%) versus an ICD (n = 161; 46%). Of the 158 patients discharged with drug therapy, most received a class I agent (26%). Amiodarone (10%) and sotalol (9%) were used in the remaining patients. β-Blockers were less frequently used in patients assigned to electrophysiologically guided therapy (29%) than in those who received no antiarrhythmic therapy (51%).

Over an average follow-up of 39 months, the risk of the primary endpoint—cardiac arrest or death attributed to an arrhythmia—was significantly lower among patients randomly assigned to electrophysiologically guided therapy than in those receiving conventional care (27% relative risk reduction; 95% CI = 1% to 47%; $P = .04$). The absolute risk of death (secondary endpoint) in patients assigned to electrophysiologically guided therapy was 6% over 5 years. However, the benefits in terms of overall survival and the risk of arrhythmic death or cardiac arrest in patients in the electrophysiologically guided therapy group were limited to patients who received an ICD. The risk of death over 5 years was substantially lower in patients discharged with ICDs (24%) than in those discharged with drug therapy (55%), translating into a 49% lower relative risk. This result is very similar to that of MADIT-I and that among patients with low ejection fractions in the AVID trial, CIDS, and CASH. The large absolute reduction in the risk of death in MUSTT-I (31%) translates into an NNT of 5 over 36 months. Drug therapy was not associated with a survival advantage over best medical therapy.

The prognostic significance of inducible arrhythmias during invasive electrophysiologic testing was evaluated in MUSTT-I.[102] During 5 years of follow-up, patients with an inducible sustained ventricular arrhythmia had a significantly higher risk of cardiac arrest or death due to arrhythmia (32%) than patients in whom a sustained arrhythmia was not inducible (24%; $P < .001$). Overall mortality was also statistically higher in patients in whom a sustained arrhythmia was inducible (48% vs. 44%; $P = .005$). However, the absolute difference in mortality (4% over 5 years) was small and of questionable clinical significance. On the basis of these and other data, the MUSTT-II trial will evaluate the efficacy of ICD therapy in patients in whom no arrhythmia is inducible (see later discussion of ongoing trials).

Patients with Heart Failure or Left Ventricular Dysfunction Alone

The details of the six studies that involved patients with heart failure or LV dysfunction alone can be found in Tables 11-3 and 11-4. Table 11-3 summarizes the inclusion criteria, primary endpoint(s), and main results for each of the six studies. Details of the study populations,

TABLE 11-3. Clinical Trials of ICD Therapy for Heart Failure or Left Ventricular Dysfunction Alone: Inclusion Criteria, Comparison Groups, and Main Results

Trial (Year)	Inclusion Criteria	Comparison	Primary Endpoint	Main Findings
Second Multicenter Automatic Defibrillator Implantation Trial (MADIT-II) (2002)	NYHA I-III, EF ≤ 0.30, remote MI (>1 mo)	ICD vs. best medical therapy	All-cause mortality	31% relative reduction in primary endpoint ($P = .02$) with ICD
Amiodarone Versus Implantable Cardioverter-Defibrillator Trial (AMIOVIRT) (2003)	NYHA I-IV, EF ≤ 0.35, dilated cardiomyopathy, NSVT	ICD vs. best medical therapy	All-cause mortality	No significant alteration ($P = .8$) with ICD
Cardiomyopathy Trial (CAT) (2002)	NYHA II-III, EF ≤ 0.30, dilated cardiomyopathy, recent-onset heart failure (≤9 mos)	ICD vs. best medical therapy	All-cause mortality	No significant alteration ($P = .6$) with ICD
Comparison of Medical Therapy, Pacing, and Defibrillation in Heart Failure (COMPANION) (2004)	NYHA III-IV, EF ≤ 0.35, nonrecent MI or CABG (≥60 days), QRS ≥ 120 msec, PR ≥ 150 msec, recent heart failure hospitalization (≤12 mos), and nonrecent onset of heart failure (>6 mos)	Resynchronization ICD vs. best medical therapy	All-cause death or hospitalization	20% relative reduction in primary endpoint ($P = .01$) with resynchronization ICD
Sudden Cardiac Death Heart Failure Trial (SCD-HeFT) (2005)	NYHA II-III, EF ≤ 0.35, nonrecent MI or revascularization (>30 days), nonrecent heart failure onset (>3 mos)	ICD vs. placebo	All-cause mortality	23% relative reduction in primary endpoint ($P < .01$) with ICD
Defibrillators in Non-Ischemic Cardiomyopathy Treatment Evaluation (DEFINITE) (2005)	NYHA I-III, EF ≤ 0.35, dilated cardiomyopathy, NSVT, or ≥10 PVCs/hr	ICD vs. best medical therapy	All-cause mortality	35% relative reduction in primary endpoint ($P = .08$) with ICD

CABG, coronary artery bypass graft surgery; EF, ejection fraction; ICD, implantable cardioverter-defibrillator; MI, myocardial infarction; NSVT, nonsustained ventricular tachycardia; NYHA, New York Heart Association functional class; PVC, premature ventricular complex.

TABLE 11-4. Clinical Trials of ICD Therapy for Heart Failure or Left Ventricular Dysfunction Alone: Population Details and Mortality Results

							Mortality Results: ICD vs. Other (%)			
Trial	N	Age (yrs)	Women (%)	NYHA > II (%)	Mean Ejection Fraction	Mean Follow-up (mos)	Annual Rate in Controls	Relative Risk Reduction	Absolute Risk Reduction	Number Needed to Treat (36 mos)
Second Multicenter Automatic Defibrillator Implantation Trial (MADIT-II)	1232	64	16	29	0.23	20	10	31	5.4	10
Amiodarone Versus Implantable Cardioverter-Defibrillator Trial (AMIOVIRT)	103	52	30	20	0.23	24	4	13	1.7	39
Cardiomyopathy Trial (CAT)	104	52	20	35	0.24	23	4	17	5.4	12
Comparison of Medical Therapy, Pacing, and Defibrillation in Heart Failure (COMPANION)*	903	67	32	100	0.22	15	19	36	7.3	5
Sudden Cardiac Death Heart Failure Trial (SCD-HeFT)*	1676	60	23	30	0.25	46	7	23	6.8	23
Defibrillators in Non-Ischemic Cardiomyopathy Treatment Evaluation (DEFINITE)	458	58	29	21	0.21	29	7	35	5.2	24

*Patient numbers reflect assignment to an ICD or medical therapy (COMPANION)/placebo (SCD-HeFT).
ICD, implantable cardioverter-defibrillator; NYHA, New York Heart Association functional class.

the risk of the population untreated (annual control group mortality), and the relative and absolute alterations in mortality with ICD therapy are provided in Table 11-4. These trials are often dichotomized on the basis of the underlying etiology of LV dysfunction (ischemic versus nonischemic). Three of the six trials (CAT, AMIOVIRT, DEFINITE; see later) included only patients with a nonischemic etiology for LV dysfunction, two (COMPANION study, SCD-HeFT; see later) included patients with both ischemic and nonischemic etiologies, and one (MADIT-II) was limited to patients with an ischemic etiology for LV dysfunction. It is important to recognize that the numbers of patients, the duration of follow-up, and the resultant statistical power of these six trials differ markedly. The COMPANION study was also different from the other trials in that all patients had a QRS complex duration longer than 120 msec as well as symptoms of advanced heart failure. The COMPANION study also assessed the combined use of CRT plus an ICD, whereas the other trials evaluated standard, nonresynchronization ICD therapy. The two larger and long-term trials that used nonresynchronization ICD therapy—SCD-HeFT and MADIT-II—provide the most reliable information on the efficacy of ICD therapy in patients with heart failure or LV dysfunction alone.

Second Multicenter Automatic Defibrillator Implantation Trial

Although MADIT-I showed a large benefit from ICD therapy, its study population represented a highly select group of patients (see Figs. 11-2 and 11-3). MADIT-II evaluated ICD therapy in a lower-risk group that accounts for a larger proportion of patients who will experience sudden death. MADIT-II enrolled 1232 patients from 71 centers in the United States and 5 centers in Europe from July 1997 to January 2002.[103] ICD therapy was compared with usual care in patients with severe ischemic LV dysfunction (ejection fraction ≤0.30). Patients who had experienced a recent MI (≥1 month before evaluation) or revascularization procedure (≤3 months) were not eligible. Patients who underwent invasive electrophysiologic testing and had inducible sustained arrhythmias, fulfilling the criteria for MADIT-I, were ineligible. Angiotensin-converting enzyme (ACE) inhibitors, β-blockers, and lipid-lowering therapies were prescribed to 70%, 70%, and 66% of participants, respectively, on the basis of data from the last follow-up visit. These rates are higher than those in the trials evaluating ICD efficacy in patients with spontaneous or inducible ventricular arrhythmias that were conducted prior to the wider recognition of the importance of these medications.

Patients were followed up for an average of 20 months. ICD therapy was associated with a 31% relative reduction in mortality (95% CI = 7% to 49%; $P < .02$). Over the 20 months, 19.8% of patients in the conventional therapy group died compared with 14.2% in the ICD group (5.4% absolute reduction). This translates into an NNT for ICDs of approximately 10 over 36 months. These risk reductions are large but not as great as those observed in patients with similar characteristics in whom inducible sustained ventricular arrhythmias were provoked. The NNT for ICDS in MADIT-II patients is more than three times larger than the NNT in MADIT-I patients. The investigators have not published cost-effectiveness data, but an analysis by Blue Cross estimated the cost-effectiveness of ICD therapy in MADIT-II to be $51,000 to $58,100 (U.S.) per quality-adjusted life-year, based on a 5- to 7-year lifespan of the ICD system, making it marginally attractive from an economic perspective.[50] This estimate has led some authorities to call for improved risk assessment in order to better identify MADIT-II patients who truly require ICDs.[61,104]

The MADIT-II researchers noted that the effect of ICD therapy was similar in subgroup analyses stratified by age, gender, ejection fraction, NYHA class, and QRS duration. However, patients with higher QRS values (>120 msec) had larger absolute and relative risk reductions that trended toward statistical significance. Some considered this finding to indicate that patients with QRS values higher than 120 msec benefit from ICD therapy and that patients with lower QRS values do not. It has long been recognized that patients with higher QRS values are at higher risk of death than those with relatively low QRS values.[105] Longer QRS complex has also been shown to predict a higher risk of death among patients receiving contemporary medical therapy.[106-108] It has been suggested that patients with higher QRS values may derive greater benefit from ICD therapy,[109,110] but this suggestion is controversial.[111] Some data indicate that QRS duration alone is not a reliable means of identifying patients more likely to benefit from an ICD.[112] Other noninvasive risk assessment tools, such as T-wave alternans assessment or heart rate turbulence, may better identify patients likely to benefit from an ICD,[69,113-115] but their usefulness is currently unknown (see discussion of ongoing trials).

The predictive ability of electrophysiologic testing to predict mortality and ICD efficacy was also assessed in MADIT-II.[116] An electrophysiologic inducibility study was performed on 593 patients randomly assigned to ICD therapy. A sustained ventricular arrhythmia was inducible in 36% of patients, and these patients were more likely to demonstrate spontaneous VT in follow-up. In contrast, patients who did not have a sustained inducible ventricular arrhythmia were more likely to experience spontaneous VT. Overall, patients in MADIT-II had a 20% rate of appropriate ICD therapies for VT or VT over 4 years of follow-up. The likelihood of development of VT or VT was similar for patients with and without inducible arrhythmias at baseline. Like the findings in MUSTT-I, the data from MADIT-II indicate that electrophysiologic testing is not useful in identifying which patients will benefit from an ICD.

Another post hoc analysis of MADIT-II evaluated the impact on ICD therapy based on the time from MI to enrollment.[117] An inclusion criterion in MADIT-II was that patients have experienced their MI at least 1 month before enrollment. The average time from MI to enrollment in MADIT-II was markedly longer (81 months). Patients were subdivided into quartiles of time after MI: less than 18 months (n = 300), 18 to 59 months (n = 283), 60 to 119 months (n = 284), and more than 120 months (n = 292). A survival benefit from ICD therapy was apparent in all three of the longer-after-MI groups (relative risk reductions of 38% to 50% with ICD therapy compared with medical care), but no benefit from ICD therapy was evident among patients whose MIs had occurred less than 18 months before enrollment (2% reduction). These data, along with those of DINAMIT (see later), suggest that ICD therapy may not be effective early after MI. The explanation may relate to alterations in coagulation, the mechanisms of death early after MI, the possibility that ventricular arrhythmias in these patients are simply a marker for progressive heart failure, or other factors. Other studies assessing the efficacy of ICD therapy early after MI are ongoing (see discussion of ongoing trials).

Amiodarone versus Implantable Cardioverter-Defibrillator Trial

The Amiodarone versus Implantable Cardioverter-Defibrillator Trial (AMIOVIRT) compared ICD therapy with amiodarone in patients with nonischemic LV dysfunction and asymptomatic NSVT at 10 centers in the United States between 1996 and 2000.[118] Patients were required to have a nonrecent (>6 months) diagnosis of LV dysfunction. The primary endpoint was total mortality. A total of 103 patients were enrolled, and the average follow-up was 2 years. A total of 13 deaths, 6 in the ICD group versus 7 in the amiodarone group, were observed ($P = .8$). AMIOVIRT was terminated early owing to futility. The trial was powered to detect a 50% relative (10% absolute) reduction in mortality with an ICD compared with amiodarone therapy. The observed mortality rate in amiodarone-treated patients was 12% at 3 years. AMIOVIRT neither supports nor refutes the value of ICD therapy in patients with nonischemic LV dysfunction and NSVT.

Cardiomyopathy Trial

The Cardiomyopathy Trial (CAT), conducted in 15 German centers from 1991 to 1997, compared ICD therapy with standard medical therapy in 104 patients with nonischemic LV dysfunction.[119] Unlike in the other five trials of ICD therapy in patients with heart failure or LV dysfunction alone, the patients in CAT were required to have recently diagnosed heart failure (<9 months before enrollment). The primary endpoint of CAT was all-cause mortality. Only 30 deaths were observed over a mean follow-up of 5.5 years. Of these, 13 occurred in the ICD group and 17 in the control group (P = .6). CAT was terminated owing to futility. The observed mortality rate in patients randomly assigned to no ICD at 1 year was 3.7%; this value was markedly lower than the anticipated mortality rate, 30%. The trial has been interpreted as not providing evidence in favor of prophylactic ICD implantation in patients with dilated cardiomyopathy of recent onset and impaired LV systolic function. Like AMIOVIRT, CAT was grossly underpowered, so no conclusions may be drawn from it regarding ICD efficacy in patients with nonischemic LV dysfunction.

Comparison of Medical Therapy, Pacing, and Defibrillation in Heart Failure Study

The Comparison of Medical Therapy, Pacing, and Defibrillation in Heart Failure (COMPANION) study evaluated the efficacy of CRT plus ICD (n = 595) versus that of medical therapy (n =308) and CRT plus pacemaker (n = 617) versus medical therapy in patients with advanced heart failure (NYHA III or IV) and QRS duration longer than 120 msec.[24] The 1520 patients were enrolled at 128 sites in the United States between January 2000 and December 2002. Patients with ischemic (55%) and nonischemic (45%) etiologies for LV dysfunction were included. Patients with a recent (<2 months before consideration) MI or revascularization were not eligible. The primary endpoint was a composite of death or hospitalization from any cause. Secondary endpoints were mortality and cardiac morbidity. Median follow-up was 12 months in the medical therapy group and 16 months in the pacemaker and ICD groups. An ACE inhibitor or angiotensin receptor antagonist, a β-blocker, and spironolactone were prescribed to 90%, 68%, and 54% of participants at baseline, respectively. Use of medication during follow-up was not reported. This review focuses on the 903 patients randomly assigned to medical therapy or CRT plus ICD.

The 12-month rate of death or hospitalization from any cause (primary endpoint) was 68% in the medical therapy group versus 56% in the CRT plus ICD group. This represents a 21% relative reduction (95% CI = 4% to 31%; P = .014). The 12% absolute reduction indicates that fewer than 8 patients need to be treated with CRT plus ICD in order to prevent one death or hospitalization from any cause over 12 months. If one assumes a linear effect, fewer than 3 patients would need to be treated with CRT plus ICD over 36 months in order to prevent one death or hospitalization from any cause. This is a very large effect size and reflects the risk of the population as well as the impact of the combined outcome of death or hospitalization from any cause.

There were 77 deaths (25%) in the medical therapy group and 105 deaths (18%) in the CRT plus ICD group. These values reflect a 36% relative risk reduction (95% CI = 14% to 52%; P = .003). The 7% absolute risk reduction indicates that slightly more than 14 patients need to be treated with CRT plus ICD in order to prevent one death over 12 months. The effects of CRT plus ICD and medical therapy on mortality were compared in a range of patient subgroups. Consistent benefit was evident when data were stratified by age, gender, QRS duration, etiology of LV dysfunction, severity of LV dysfunction, blood pressure, and medication use. If one assumes a linear effect, fewer than 5 patients would need to be treated with CRT plus ICD over 36 months in order to prevent one death. This is a very large mortality reduction, similar to that observed in patients with spontaneous or inducible ventricular arrhythmias (see Table 11-2). The reason for the reduction is unknown but may relate to the combined effect of CRT plus an ICD. Large reductions in mortality have been demonstrated with CRT plus a pacemaker in the COMPANION study (4% absolute mortality reduction over 12 months) and the CARE-HF trial (10% absolute mortality reduction over 29 months).[25]

It is important to note that although most of the baseline characteristics of patients in the COMPANION study are similar to those of participants in the other trials of ICD in heart failure or LV dysfunction alone (see Table 11-4), the annual control group mortality rate in the COMPANION study is two to five times greater than that of the other trials. Whether this reflects the fact that all patients in the COMPANION study had advanced heart failure symptoms, that these patients all had QRS values higher than 120 msec, or other factors is not known. The 1-year mortality rate among patients assigned to medical therapy in the CARE-HF trial, another CRT trial involving similar patients, was approximately 13%.[25] Thus, the brief duration of follow-up in the COMPANION study or other factors appear to be more likely explanations for the high mortality rate in the medical care group.

A number of potential limitations are related to the COMPANION study. Concern has been raised regarding the unequal randomization used in favor of ICD or pacemaker therapy. However, this strategy has been used in other randomized trials, including MADIT-II. A more significant problem relates to the fact that 26% of the patients assigned to medical therapy withdrew prematurely from the study. This problem was addressed in part through censoring the data of lost participants on the date of last contact. Another concern is that the definition of *all-cause hospitalization* was changed after the trial was under way, potentially influencing the primary endpoint. Specifically, *the treatment of decompensated heart failure with vasoactive drugs for more than 4 hours in an urgent care setting* was included as a hospitalization.

Unlike the other five trials discussed in this section, which used only low ejection fraction and heart failure symptoms as the main inclusion criteria, the COMPANION study limited participation to patients with advanced heart failure and a wide QRS complex. The study also compared CRT plus ICD with medical therapy, not an ICD alone. This difference likely influenced treatment efficacy for reasons that have been discussed. The relative efficacy of an ICD alone versus an ICD plus CRT is currently being evaluated (see discussion of ongoing trials).

Sudden Cardiac Death–Heart Failure Trial

The Sudden Cardiac Death–Heart Failure Trial (SCD-HeFT) compared the efficacies of an ICD (n = 829), amiodarone (n = 845), and placebo (n = 847) in patients with heart failure (NYHA II or III).[120] The 2521 patients were enrolled at 148 sites in the United States, Canada, and New Zealand from September 1997 through July 2001.[120] Randomization was stratified according to etiology of LV dysfunction and NYHA class. Similar proportions of patients with ischemic (52%) and nonischemic (48%) etiologies of LV dysfunction were enrolled. The majority of patients (70%) had NYHA II functional status limitation at baseline. Patients with a recent (<1 month before consideration) MI or revascularization procedure were not eligible.

The primary endpoint was all-cause mortality. Secondary endpoints consisted of arrhythmic cardiac mortality, nonarrhythmic cardiac mortality, morbidity, cost-effectiveness, and QOL. Patients were required to be treated with a vasodilator for at least 3 months prior to enrollment, and the use of β-blockers and spironolactone was strongly encouraged. An ACE inhibitor or angiotensin receptor antagonist was prescribed to 96% of patients at baseline, 87% of whom continued to receive these agents at last follow-up. β-Blockers and spironolactone were prescribed to 69% and 19% of participants at baseline, respectively, and to 78% and 31% of patients at last follow-up, respectively. Rates of heart failure medication use in SCD-HeFT were higher than the rates in MADIT-II and the COMPANION study. This fact needs to be taken into consideration when outcomes and ICD efficacy results for these trials are compared.

Median follow-up in SCD-HeFT was 45.5 months. The vital status for every patient was available for last scheduled follow-up. During 60 months of follow-up, 36.1% of patients randomly assigned to placebo died. Patients randomly assigned to amiodarone therapy had a similar risk of death (34.0%) over this time. Patients randomly assigned to an ICD had a significantly lower risk of death (28.9%) over the 60 months. This difference translates into a 23% relative reduction in mortality with ICD therapy versus placebo (95% CI = 4% to 38%; P = .007). The relative benefit of ICD therapy was similar in patients with nonischemic (27%) and ischemic (21%) etiologies of LV dysfunction. The absolute reduction in mortality of 7.2% over 60 months indicates that almost 14 patients would need to be treated with an ICD to prevent one death during that time. The absolute mortality reductions with ICD therapy over 60 months were also similar in patients with nonischemic (6.5%) and ischemic (7.3%) etiologies for LV dysfunction. To allow comparison with the other trials, one can calculate the absolute mortality reduction in SCD-HeFT over 36 months to be about 4.3%, which translates into needing to treat 23 patients over this time to prevent one death. As noted previously, QRS duration was not a reliable predictor of benefit from an ICD in SCD-HeFT.[112]

Preliminary cost-effectiveness data from SCD-HeFT has been presented.[121] Five-year cumulative costs were $49,443 (U.S.) for amiodarone, $43,078 for placebo, and $61,968 for an ICD. If one assumes a generator longevity of 5 years, the cost-effectiveness for an ICD versus amiodarone was $33,192 (U.S.) per life-year added. Similar cost-effectiveness was found for patients with ischemic ($33,603) and nonischemic ($32,170) etiologies for LV dysfunction. Despite the relatively small absolute reduction in mortality with ICD therapy in SCD-HeFT, these data indicate that the use of an ICD in this population is economically attractive. It is important to recognize that the substantially longer average follow-up in SCD-HeFT provides a more reliable and realistic estimate of cost-effectiveness, for reasons previously discussed.

Defibrillators in Non-Ischemic Cardiomyopathy Treatment Evaluation

The Defibrillators in Non-Ischemic Cardiomyopathy Treatment Evaluation (DEFINITE) compared the efficacy of ICD therapy with that of no ICD therapy in 488 patients with nonischemic LV dysfunction.[122] Patients were enrolled from participating sites in the United States from 1998 to 2003. In addition to a low ejection fraction, patients were required to have ambient arrhythmias (frequent premature ventricular beats or NSVT). Unlike in the CAT, the duration of heart failure was neither an inclusion nor an exclusion criterion for the DEFINITE. The primary endpoint was death from any cause. The secondary endpoint was sudden death. Mean follow-up was 29 months. ACE inhibitors (86%), angiotensin receptor blockers (11%), and β-blockers (85%) were prescribed to the majority of patients. As shown in Table 11-4, the mean ejection fraction in DEFINITE was somewhat lower (0.21) than the average values for patients in CAT (mean ejection fraction 0.24) and SCD-HeFT (mean ejection fraction 0.25). More than one half (57%) of the patients in DEFINITE had NYHA class II symptoms.

During the 29 months of follow-up, there were 28 deaths in the ICD group and 40 in the medical therapy group. This difference represents a 35% relative reduction in mortality with an ICD versus no ICD (95% CI = 6% increase to 60% decrease; P = .08). The absolute reduction in mortality at 2 years was 6.2%, so 24 patients would need to be treated with an ICD over 36 months in order to prevent one death. A significant reduction in sudden death (80%; 95% CI = 29% to 94%; P = .006) was also observed.

Preliminary data regarding QOL in DEFINITE have been presented.[37] These data suggest that ICD therapy may improve QOL. Interestingly, patients with the greatest functional status impairment at baseline (NYHA class III) had the greatest improvement in QOL over time. As with other studies assessing QOL, patients in DEFINITE had markedly impaired self-perceived QOL at baseline; also, for reasons that are unclear, patients randomly assigned to medical therapy appeared to have lower QOL at baseline than those assigned to ICD therapy. Whether this difference reflects the timing of these assessments (before versus after randomization) or other factors is unknown. These results are also limited by the fact that QOL data were incomplete for two thirds of the patients.

Given the lack of benefit from ICD therapy in CAT, a trial wherein patients were randomly assigned to therapy within 9 months of the onset of heart failure, a post hoc analysis of data from DEFINITE was undertaken to assess the impact of time from heart failure diagnosis on survival and ICD efficacy.[123] No statistically significant difference in survival between patients diagnosed with heart failure within 9 months of randomization (11%) versus those diagnosed more than 9 months before (17%) was apparent over 2.5 years of follow-up (P = .2). The relative risk reduction for ICD therapy for patients in whom duration of symptoms was 9 months or less (52%; 95% CI = 1% increase to 78%) was similar to or perhaps greater than that of the overall trial, indicating that the duration of heart failure symptoms does not appear to explain the lack of efficacy with ICD therapy found in CAT.

Pooled Analysis of Trials in Patients with Heart Failure or Left Ventricular Dysfunction Alone

A systematic review found a 26% relative reduction in mortality with ICD therapy when the results of the MADIT-II, AMIOVIRT, CAT, COMPANION, SCD-HeFT, and DEFINITE trials were combined with the MADIT-I results (95% CI = 17% to 33%).[29] With the MADIT-I data removed, a smaller but statistically significant relative risk reduction in mortality, 21%, was observed (95% CI = 6% to 34%; P = .009). The absolute mortality reduction in those patients with heart failure or LV dysfunction alone was 5.8% to 7.9%, depending on which trials are included in the analysis. This translates into an NNT of 13 to 17 for ICDs over about 34 months. The absolute mortality reduction afforded by ICDs in these trials should be compared with a 6.1% absolute risk reduction seen with ACE inhibitors and a 4.4% absolute risk reduction seen with β-blockers. The mortality reduction with ICDs is in addition to that provided by β-blockers and ACE inhibitors.

Patients with Left Ventricular Dysfunction in Specific Circumstances

The details of the individual studies that included patients with LV dysfunction in specific circumstances can be found in Tables 11-5 and 11-6. Table 11-5 summarizes the inclusion criteria, primary endpoint, and main results for the three studies. Details of the study populations, the risk of the population untreated (annual control group mortality), and the relative and absolute alterations in mortality with ICD therapy are provided in Table 11-6. These trials are considered separately because the other studies invariably excluded patients with recent coronary artery bypass surgery or a recent MI, the specific populations in which ICD therapy was evaluated in the three studies discussed here.

Coronary Artery Bypass Graft Patch Trial

The Coronary Artery Bypass Graft Patch (CABG Patch) trial was conducted at 35 centers in the United States and 2 centers in Germany from 1990 to 1997. Prophylactic ICD therapy was compared with usual care in 900

TABLE 11-5. Clinical Trials of ICD Therapy for Left Ventricular Dysfunction in Specific Circumstances: Inclusion Criteria, Comparison Groups, and Main Result

Trial (Year)	Inclusion Criteria	Comparison	Primary Endpoint	Main Finding
CABG-Patch Trial (1996)	EF ≤ 0.35, undergoing CABG, abnormal signal-averaged ECG	ICD vs. best medical therapy	All-cause mortality	No significant alteration (P = .6) with ICD
Defibrillators in Acute Myocardial Infarction Trial (DINAMIT) (2005)	NYHA I-III, EF ≤ 0.35, recent MI (6–40 days), depressed heart rate variability or elevated average 24-hr heart rate	ICD vs. best medical therapy	All-cause mortality	No significant alteration (P = .7) with ICD
BEta-blocker STrategy plus ICD (BEST-ICD) (2005)	EF ≤ 0.3 *and* one or more of the following: ≥10 PVCs/hr, reduced heart rate variability, abnormal signal-averaged ECG Recent MI (<1 mo)	Invasive strategy (ICD if inducible VT, otherwise medical therapy) vs. conservative strategy (medical therapy)	All-cause mortality	No significant alteration (P = .4) with an invasive strategy vs. a conservative strategy

CABG, coronary artery bypass graft surgery; EF, ejection fraction; ICD, implantable cardioverter-defibrillator; MI, myocardial infarction; NYHA, New York Heart Association functional class; PVC, premature ventricular complex; VT, ventricular tachycardia.

TABLE 11-6. Clinical Trials of ICD Therapy for Left Ventricular Dysfunction in Specific Circumstances: Population Details and Mortality Results

Trial	N	Age (yrs)	Women (%)	NYHA > II (%)	Mean Ejection Fraction	Mean Follow-up (months)	Mortality Results: ICD vs. Other (%)		
							Annual Rate in Control Group	Relative Risk Alteration	Absolute Risk Alteration
Coronary Artery Bypass Graft Patch (CABG Patch)	900	64	16	—	0.27	32	8	7 (increase)	1.7 (increase)
Defibrillators in Acute Myocardial Infarction Trial (DINAMIT)	674	62	24	13	0.28	30	7	8 (increase)	1.7 (increase)
BEta-blocker STrategy plus ICD (BEST-ICD)	148	66	29	—	0.31	17	14	13 (increase)	2.4 (increase)

ICD, implantable cardioverter-defibrillator; NYHA, New York Heart Association functional class.

patients with ejection fraction values of 0.35 or less and abnormal signal-averaged electrocardiogram (ECG) recordings who were undergoing coronary artery bypass graft (CABG) surgery.[80] No significant reduction in mortality was observed with ICD therapy (relative increased risk 7%; $P = .6$) over an average follow-up of 32 months. A secondary analysis found that the ICD significantly reduced the risk of sudden death compared with medical therapy.[124] Despite the attempt to identify a group of patients at high risk for sudden death, most of the deaths in the CABG Patch trial (71%) were nonarrhythmic.[124] Thus, the lack of benefit from ICD therapy appears to be related to a low risk of sudden death.

The reasons for the divergent results in the CABG Patch trial will likely never be fully understood. Characteristics of the patients in the trial (see Table 11-6) were similar to those of patients with ischemic LV dysfunction and no history of sustained or inducible ventricular arrhythmias who were enrolled in MADIT-II and the other ICD trials, apart from higher mean ejection fraction values (see Table 11-6). Whether this finding relates to the use of a signal-averaged electrocardiogram to select patients, the effect of revascularization, or statistical chance is not known. Early studies suggested that the presence of late potentials on signal-averaged electrocardiogram analysis were very predictive of death and serious arrhythmias.[125] Later data suggest, however, that the findings do not provide useful prognostic information in patients who have undergone revascularization.[126] One analysis that evaluated the impact of CABG on outcome in patients with LV dysfunction demonstrated that revascularization is associated with a 25% reduction in risk of death and a 46% reduction in risk of sudden death independent of ejection fraction and severity of heart failure symptoms.[127] As baseline ejection fraction declined, absolute reduction in risk of sudden death with prior CABG rose. When these data were applied to a group of patients with LV dysfunction who had not undergone prior surgery (Coronary Artery Surgery Study Registry), the predicted annual rates of death (8.2%) and sudden death (2.4%) were similar to those observed in the CABG Patch trial (7.9% and 2.3%, respectively).[127] Regardless of the reasons why ICD therapy did not alter mortality in the CABG Patch trial, this result highlights the need for restraint in the use of ICD therapy for the prevention of sudden death in patient groups in whom data on ICD efficacy are lacking.

QOL was also assessed in the CABG Patch trial. Six months after surgery, 490 of the 900 enrolled patients completed QOL assessments.[36] Compared with the ICD group, control patients were more likely to feel that their health status had improved over the preceding year and had both higher emotional role functioning and greater psychological well-being. The ICD and control groups were similar on the other measures of QOL. These results are somewhat at odds with those of the AVID trial and CIDS, in which QOL was similar for the ICD and amiodarone. The results are also the opposite of what was reported in DEFINITE. Whether these differences in QOL with ICD therapy relate to the populations assessed, the use of thoracotomy versus nonthoracotomy ICD systems, rates of incomplete data, or other factors is unknown. Additional data on the effect of ICD therapy in populations without a history of spontaneous or inducible ventricular arrhythmias are required.

Defibrillators in Acute Myocardial Infarction Trial

The Defibrillators in Acute Myocardial Infarction Trial (DINAMIT) tested the hypothesis that an ICD will reduce mortality in patients with a recent MI who are at high risk of arrhythmic death because of LV dysfunction and impaired autonomic tone, which manifests as low heart rate variability or a high resting heart rate.[81] A total of 674 patients were enrolled at 73 sites in 12 countries from April 1998 to September 2002. Unlike patients in all of the other published ICD trials, patients in DINAMIT were enrolled very soon (6-40 days) after experiencing MI. Patients who had NYHA class IV symptoms or in whom CABG surgery or three-vessel coronary angioplasty had been performed or was planned were excluded. The primary outcome was death from any cause. Arrhythmic death was a secondary outcome. Mean follow-up was 30 months. Most of the characteristics of patients in DINAMIT (see Table 11-6) were similar to those of patients with ischemic LV dysfunction and no history of sustained or inducible ventricular arrhythmias enrolled in MADIT-II and the other ICD trials involving patients without a history of sustained or inducible ventricular arrhythmias, apart from higher mean ejection fraction values (see Table 11-6). Interestingly, the mean ejection fraction values in the CABG Patch trial and DINAMIT were similar.

There were 62 deaths in the ICD group compared with 58 deaths in the conventional therapy group, translating into a statistically nonsignificant 8% higher (95% CI = 24% lower to 55% higher) risk of death with ICD therapy. In terms of the secondary endpoint, there were 12 arrhythmic deaths in the ICD group compared with 29 in the conventional therapy group, translating into a significant 38% (95% CI = 17% to 78%) lower risk with an ICD than with medical care ($P = .009$).

An important analysis related to the development of arrhythmias requiring appropriate ICD therapies and subsequent mortality in DINAMIT patients has been presented.[128] Over the 2.5 years of follow-up, 18% of patients randomly assigned to receive an ICD had appropriate ICD therapies. On average, these patients had baseline ejection fractions and degrees of autonomic tone impairment similar to those of patients who did not have appropriate ICD therapies, but were more likely to have NSVT. A minority of patients (7%) experienced one ICD therapy. Most (29%) experienced multiple therapies. The mortality rate in those who experienced appropriate ICD therapies (36%) was significantly greater than that in patients who experienced no therapies (15%) or were randomly assigned to not receive an ICD (17%). Most (75%) of the deaths in patients experiencing appropriate ICD therapies were categorized as nonarrhythmic. As in the AVID trial,[38] a very high risk of death from progressive heart failure was observed in the first 6 months after appropriate ICD therapies in DINAMIT.

As for the CABG Patch trial, the reasons why no benefit from ICD therapy was evident in DINAMIT will likely never be known. The inclusion of patients whose MIs had occurred very recently may in part explain the lack of benefit. A significant amount of LV remodeling occurs in the initial weeks after an MI,[129] and thus, the substrate for ventricular arrhythmias is evolving. In this situation, some patients believed to be at high risk very early after MI may not actually be so, whereas others initially considered to be at low risk actually have a higher risk of sudden death. The choice of impaired heart rate variability as an inclusion criterion may have selected a group of patients at high risk for death but, necessarily, death related to ventricular arrhythmias. Although impaired heart rate variability does identify patients at high risk of presumed arrhythmic death early after MI,[60] it is also a potent predictor of death from progressive pump failure in patients with LV dysfunction.[130] Whether alterations in heart rate variability early versus later after MI provide similar prognostic information is unknown. It is known that other risk assessment tools that provide reliable information late after MI do not provide useful prognostic information if measured earlier.[131] As already discussed, no benefit from ICD therapy was evident among patients within 18 months of an MI in MADIT-II.[117] Whether this lack of early benefit after MI is explained by inflammation or alterations in coagulation factors with ICD placement is unknown. The high risk of nonarrhythmic death after appropriate ICD therapies in DINAMIT also raises the possibility that ventricular arrhythmias in these patients may simply be a marker for progressive heart failure and that ICD therapy is unlikely to improve survival. Other studies assessing the efficacy of ICD therapy early after MI are ongoing (see discussion of ongoing trials).

BEta-blocker STrategy plus Implantable Cardioverter-Defibrillator Study

The BEta-blocker STrategy plus ICD (BEST-ICD study) evaluated the usefulness of an electrophysiologic study–guided ICD strategy in patients at high risk of sudden death early (<1 month) after MI.[132] Patients were enrolled from July 1998 to February 2003. The overall study design was complex. Patients were required to have LV dysfunction, to be able to tolerate therapy with a β-blocker, and to have at least one of the following abnormal findings on noninvasive tests: 10 or more premature ventricular complexes per hour (PVCs/hr), depressed heart rate variability, and an abnormal signal-averaged electrocardiogram. Eligible patients who agreed to participation were then randomly assigned (with a ratio of 3:2) to usual medical care (conventional therapy) or to an invasive electrophysiology study (invasive strategy). Patients in the invasive strategy group in whom a sustained ventricular arrhythmia was induced received an ICD, whereas those in whom no sustained arrhythmia was induced were crossed over to receive usual medical care (conventional therapy). On the basis of this algorithm, a total of 59 patients were randomly assigned to conventional therapy and 79 to invasive strategy. A sustained ventricular arrhythmia was induced in 24 of the 79 patients in the invasive strategy group; these 24 patients received an ICD. The remaining 114 patients received usual medical care. All participants received metoprolol, with an average dose of 68 mg/day at baseline. The majority of patients were prescribed an ACE inhibitor (81% at discharge and 78% at last follow-up) and aspirin (81% at baseline and 82% at last follow-up). The rate of statin use was low (22% at baseline and 25% at last follow-up). Few patients received amiodarone (7% at baseline and 12% at follow-up). Like patients in the CABG Patch study and DINAMIT, patients in the BEST-ICD study had a lesser degree of LV dysfunction (see Table 11-6) than those in MADIT-II or the other trials of patients with heart failure or LV dysfunction alone.

During a mean follow-up of 17 months, 26 of the BEST-ICD study patients (19%) died. Only nine deaths (7%) were categorized as sudden. Overall, 22% of the patients randomly assigned to conventional therapy died compared with 16% of patients of those randomly assigned to an invasive strategy ($P = .4$). The mortality rates were similar among patients who received an ICD because of an inducible arrhythmia (21%), those randomly assigned to the invasive strategy who did not have an inducible arrhythmia (15%), and those randomly assigned to conventional therapy (22%).

A major limitation of the BEST-ICD study is the small number of patients (n = 138), which prevents any conclusion related to the efficacy or lack of efficacy of ICD therapy in patients with recent MI. Another limitation is that the population was highly select. More than 15,000 patients were screened. Of these, 8% had an ejection fraction of 0.35 or lower. The majority (92%) of these patients had at least one abnormal noninvasive test result. A very large number of patients were excluded for other reasons. The major reasons listed were lack of informed consent (40%), intolerance of β-blocker (18%), early revascularization (16%), and NSVT (7%). These data call into question the external validity of the BEST-ICD results.

Both the CABG Patch trial and DINAMIT illustrate that the ICD is not effective in all patients with LV dysfunction and that clinicians should not infer that an ICD will be effective in populations having only some of the characteristics of the participants in trials in which the ICD has been proved to reduce mortality. These trials also highlight the potential pitfalls related to using outcomes other than total mortality in evaluating the efficacy of ICD therapy. The BEST-ICD study results also fail to show any benefit from ICD therapy early after MI but do not provide the same level of evidence as DINAMIT. It is also clear from all three of these studies that prospective evaluation of risk assessment tools is required to determine whether their use can identify patients likely to benefit from an ICD. Finally, these trials emphasize the need for continued research into the efficacy of ICD therapy in patients with special circumstances, particularly those with a recent MI. Some of these issues are being addressed in ongoing studies.

Guidelines for Implantable Cardioverter-Defibrillator Therapy

Standard definitions of levels of evidence and categorization of that evidence have been proposed by the American College of Cardiology (ACC) and the American Heart Association (AHA) to guide ICD therapy.[133,134] They are listed in Table 11-7. The latest published ACC, AHA, and Heart Rhythm Society (HRS) guidelines for the use of ICD therapy are from 2002.[134] The conditions in which ICD therapy is useful or may be useful (classes 1 and II) in those recommendations are summarized in Table 11-8. The conditions for which there is evidence or general agreement that ICD therapy is not useful or may be harmful (class III) in those recommendations are summarized in Table 11-9.

Several important randomized trials have been published since the latest ACC/AHA/HRS guidelines were released: MADIT-II, COMPANION, SCD-HeFT, DEFINITE, and DINAMIT. On the basis of the results of these trials, alterations in guidelines for ICD therapy have been proposed (Table 11-10). The Canadian Cardiovascular Society has published guidelines for the

TABLE 11-7. Standard Definitions: Classification of Recommendations and Level of Evidence

Classification	Details
I	Conditions for which there is evidence and/or general agreement that a given procedure or treatment is beneficial, useful, and effective.
II	Conditions for which there is conflicting evidence and/or divergence of opinion about the usefulness/efficacy of a procedure or treatment.
IIa	Weight of evidence/opinion is in favor of usefulness/efficacy.
IIb	Usefulness/efficacy is less well established by evidence/opinion.
III	Conditions for which there is evidence and/or general agreement that a procedure/treatment is not useful/effective and in some cases may be harmful.
Level of Evidence	**Definition**
A	Data derived from multiple randomized clinical trials or meta-analyses.
B	Data derived from a single randomized trial or nonrandomized studies.
C	Only consensus opinion of experts, case studies, or standard of care.

TABLE 11-8. Indications for ICD Therapy

Recommendation	Level of Evidence
Class I (general agreement of benefit with ICD therapy):	
1. Cardiac arrest due to ventricular fibrillation (VF) or ventricular tachycardia (VT) not due to a transient or reversible cause.	A
2. Spontaneous sustained VT in association with structural heart disease.	B
3. Syncope of undetermined origin with relevant, hemodynamically significant VT or VF induced when drug therapy is not tolerated or not preferred	A
4. NSVT in patients with coronary disease, prior myocardial infarction (MI), left ventricular (LV) dysfunction, and inducible VF or sustained VT at electrophysiologic study that is not suppressible by a Class I antiarrhythmic drug.	C
5. Spontaneous sustained VT in patients who do not have structural heart disease that is not amenable to other treatments.	C
Class IIa (weight of evidence is in favor of usefulness of ICD therapy):	B
1. Patients with an ejection fraction $\leq$0.30–0.35; $\geq$1 month post-MI and 3 months post coronary artery revascularization surgery, and/or non recent heart failure onset.	C
Class IIb (efficacy of the ICD is less well established):	
1. Cardiac arrest presumed to be due to VF when electrophysiologic testing is precluded by other medical conditions.	C
2. Severe symptoms (e.g., syncope) attributable to ventricular tachyarrhythmias in patients awaiting cardiac transplantation.	C
3. Familial or inherited conditions with a high risk for life-threatening ventricular tachyarrhythmias such as long-QT syndrome or hypertrophic cardiomyopathy.	B
4. NSVT with coronary artery disease, prior MI, LV dysfunction, and inducible sustained VT or VF at electrophysiologic study.	B
5. Recurrent syncope of undetermined etiology in the presence of ventricular dysfunction and inducible ventricular arrhythmias at electrophysiologic study when other causes of syncope have been excluded.	C
6. Syncope of unexplained etiology or family history of unexplained sudden cardiac death in association with typical or atypical right bundle branch block and ST-segment elevations (Brugada syndrome).	C
7. Syncope in patients with advanced structural heart disease in which thorough invasive and noninvasive investigation has failed to define a cause.	C

ICD, implantable cardioverter-defibrillator; MI, myocardial infarction; NSVT, nonsustained ventricular tachycardia; VF, ventricular fibrillation; VT, ventricular tachycardia.

TABLE 11-9. Circumstances in which ICD Therapy is Not Indicated

Recommendation	Level of Evidence
Class III (general agreement that an ICD is not effective and may be harmful):	
1. Syncope of undetermined cause in a patient without inducible VT or VF and without structural heart disease.	C
2. VF or VT resulting from arrhythmias amenable to surgical or catheter ablation (e.g., atrial arrhythmias associated with the Wolff-Parkinson-White syndrome, right ventricular outflow tract VT, idiopathic left ventricular tachycardia, or fascicular VT).	C
3. Ventricular tachyarrhythmias due to a transient or reversible disorder (e.g., acute MI, electrolyte imbalance, drugs, or trauma) when correction of the disorder is considered feasible and likely to substantially reduce the risk of recurrent arrhythmia.	B
4. Significant psychiatric illnesses that may be aggravated by device implantation or may preclude systematic follow-up.	C
5. Terminal illnesses with projected life expectancy of less than six months.	C
6. Patients with coronary artery disease with LV dysfunction and prolonged QRS duration in the absence of spontaneous or inducible sustained or nonsustained VT who are undergoing coronary bypass surgery.	B
7. NYHA IV drug-refractory congestive heart failure in patients who are not candidates for cardiac transplantation.	C

ICD, implantable cardioverter-defibrillator; LV, left ventricular; MI, myocardial infarction NYHA, New York Heart Association functional class; VF, ventricular fibrillation; VT, ventricular tachycardia.

TABLE 11-10. **Updated Guidelines for ICD Therapy**

Class	Details
Ia	ICD therapy is recommended to reduce total mortality by a reduction in sudden death in patients who have ischemic heart disease and whose MI was ≥40 days ago, with EF ≤ 0.30, NYHA II or III symptoms with optimal medical therapy, and a reasonable expectation of survival with a good functional status for more than 1 year (level of evidence: A).
Ib	ICD therapy is recommended to reduce total mortality by a reduction in sudden death in patients with dilated nonischemic cardiomyopathy, EF ≤ 0.30, NYHA II or III symptoms with optimal medical therapy, and a reasonable expectation of survival with a good functional status for more than 1 year (level of evidence: B).
IIa	Placement of an ICD is reasonable in patients who have dilated ischemic cardiomyopathy and whose MI was ≥40 days ago, with EF ≤ 0.30, NYHA I symptoms with optimal medical therapy, and with a reasonable expectation of survival with good functional status of more than 1 year (level of evidence: B).
IIb	Placement of an ICD might be considered in patients who have dilated nonischemic cardiomyopathy, with EF ≤ 0.30, NYHA I symptoms with optimal medical therapy, and no comorbidities that would otherwise limit survival (level of evidence: C).

EF, ejection fraction; ICD, implantable cardioverter-defibrillator; MI, myocardial infarction; NYHA, New York Heart Association functional class.

use of ICD therapy[135] that are similar to those proposed by the ACC/AHA/HRS. These changes reflect the common belief that patients with both ischemic and nonischemic LV dysfunction derive benefit from ICD therapy. Whether all patients with these characteristics should receive ICDs is controversial. Many researchers in arrhythmia believe that additional risk assessment is required to identify those patients with heart failure or LV dysfunction alone who require an ICD (see later discussion of risk assessment).

Ongoing Trials

Several ongoing trials are assessing the efficacy of ICD therapy early after MI, evaluating the usefulness of risk stratification tools, and comparing ICD therapy alone with ICD therapy and CRT. Details of the individual studies are provided in Table 11-11.

Implantable Cardioverter-Defibrillator Therapy Early after Myocardial Infarction

Immediate Risk-Stratification Improves Survival Study

The Immediate Risk-Stratification Improves Survival (IRIS) study is comparing ICD therapy with no ICD therapy in select high-risk patients early after MI.[136] Emphasis is placed on optimal acute and long-term medical therapy, including the use of β-blockers. This and other trials of ICD therapy early after MI are required to better define the role of ICD therapy in this period.

Southern European DEfibrillator Trial

The Southern European DEfibrillator Trial (SEDET) is evaluating the efficacy of ICD therapy in patients with recent MI who have not received reperfusion therapies. With the advent of aggressive revascularization after MI in many North American and European centers, the applicability of the SEDET results may be limited. Further data on the role or limitations of ICD therapy soon after MI are needed to determine appropriate care for these patients.

Evaluation of Risk Assessment Tools

Alternans Before Cardioverter-Defibrillator Study

The Alternans Before Cardioverter-Defibrillator (ABCD) study compares the rate of appropriate ICD therapies and NSVT in patients receiving an ICD for a positive T-wave alternans (TWA) test result or because of inducible sustained ventricular arrhythmias with invasive electrophysiologic testing. The rates of arrhythmias will be compared in the following groups: (1) positive TWA result and inducible arrhythmias, (2) inducible arrhythmias alone, (3) positive TWA test alone, and (4) no inducible arrhythmias and negative TWA test result. Given the uncertainty about the usefulness of appropriate ICD therapies as a surrogate for death, it is unclear what effect the results of the ABCD study will have. It may provide the foundation for additional research aimed at identifying patients most likely to benefit from an ICD.

Second Multicenter Unsustained Tachycardia Trial

The MUSTT-II trial is not yet under way but is included here for completeness. The working hypotheses of MUSTT-II are that an ICD can improve survival in MUSTT-MADIT patients, even if there is no inducible monomorphic VT, that spontaneous NSVT is irrelevant, and that invasive electrophysiologic testing performed soon (72 hours to 1 month) after an acute MI is a valid tool for risk stratification. The final design will require patients to undergo an invasive electrophysiology study. Those with sustained inducible ventricular arrhythmias will receive an ICD, and those without an inducible arrhythmia will be randomly assigned to ICD or medical care alone.

TABLE 11-11. **Ongoing ICD Trials: Population, Details, Comparison Groups, and Outcomes**

Trial	Population	Comparison	Details	Primary Endpoint(s)
Immediate Risk-Stratification Improves Survival (IRIS)	Recent MI (5–31 days), EF ≤ 0.40, heart rate ≥ 100, NSVT	ICD vs. no ICD	Planned n = 700 Randomized (1:1) to ICD vs. no ICD Ongoing	All-cause mortality
Southern European DEfibrillator Trial (SEDET)	Recent MI (1–3 weeks), no reperfusion treatment, EF 0.15 to 0.40, NSVT or ≥10 PVCs/hr	ICD vs. no ICD	Planned n = 650 Randomized (1:1), ICD vs no ICD Ongoing	All-cause mortality
Alternans Before Cardioverter Defibrillator (ABCD)	CAD, ≥1 month since MI or revascularization, EF ≤ 0.40, NSVT	Outcomes in patients receiving an ICD for inducible VT vs. positive T-wave alternans test	Planned n = 618 ICD therapy guided by TWA and EP study results. Enrollment completed in 2005	Ventricular tachyarrhythmias
Resynchronization/ Defibrillation for Advanced Heart Failure Trial (RAFT)	Heart failure (NYHA II), EF ≤ 0.30, intrinsic QRS ≥ 120 msec or paced QRS ≥ 200 msec	ICD vs. resynchronization ICD	Planned n = 2000 Randomized (1:1) to ICD vs. resynchronization ICD	All-cause mortality or hospitalization for heart failure
Multicenter Automatic Defibrillator Implantation Trial (MADIT-CRT)	Heart failure (NYHA I-II), CAD, EF ≤ 0.30, QRS ≥ 130 msec	ICD vs. resynchronization ICD	Planned n = 1820 Randomized (2:3) to ICD vs. resynchronization ICD	All-cause mortality or heart failure events

CAD, coronary artery disease; EF, ejection fraction; EP, electrophysiologic; ICD, implantable cardioverter-defibrillator; MI, myocardial infarction; NYHA, New York Heart Association functional class; TWA, T-wave alternans; VT, ventricular tachycardia.

Implantable Cardioverter-Defibrillator Alone versus Implantable Cardioverter-Defibrillator plus Cardiac Resynchronization Therapy

Resynchronization/Defibrillation for Advanced Heart Failure Trial (RAFT)

The Resynchronization/Defibrillation for Advanced Heart Failure Trial (RAFT) is evaluating the capacity of ICD therapy plus CRT to reduce the combined endpoint of all-cause mortality or heart failure hospitalizations in comparison with ICD therapy without CRT. Patients with LV dysfunction from an ischemic or nonischemic etiology were initially eligible if they had NYHA class II or III symptoms and an intrinsic QRS duration of 120 msec or longer or a paced QRS duration of 200 msec or longer. Based on the results of the CARE-HF trial,[25] only patients with NYHA class II symptoms are now being enrolled and the sample size has been increased to 2000 patients. Mortality and cardiac mortality are secondary outcomes. RAFT will provide essential information with respect to the effect of CRT beyond that of an ICD alone in patients with heart failure.

Multicenter Automatic Defibrillator Implantation Trial-Cardiac Resynchronization Therapy

MADIT-CRT is evaluating the capacity of ICD therapy plus CRT to reduce the combined endpoint of all-cause mortality or heart failure events compared with ICD therapy alone. Unlike RAFT, MADIT-CRT will involve only patients with coronary artery disease and uses an intrinsic QRS duration cutoff of 130 msec. The composite outcome in MADIT-CRT is not restricted to hospitalization for heart failure. MADIT-CRT will also add to our knowledge base related to CRT by evaluating patients with few, if any, symptoms related to heart failure.

Other Issues

Cost-Effective, Not Inexpensive

Regardless of one's philosophy related to costly interventions, a fundamental principle is that the choice to implant an ICD must be based on the principle of a *reasonable probability of success*. This notion must be considered in terms of a broad perspective (mortality,

QOL, potential complications, cost). Although we label therapies as "cost-effective" if they are similar in cost to other interventions (e.g., renal dialysis), this label does not mean that they are inexpensive. This issue is of particular relevance when we concurrently use multiple interventions in a single patient (e.g., renal dialysis, CABG, ICD). Ultimately, because of the evolving face of health care delivery, issues of cost influence the practice of medicine. It is also paramount to appreciate that estimates of cost efficacy derived from clinical trials may not mirror costs in the real world.

Are Implantable Cardioverter-Defibrillators Shocks a Reasonable Surrogate for Mortality Reductions?

Given the desire to reduce sample size and improve statistical power or to evaluate ICD therapy in populations in whom the number of potential recipients is modest, some studies have used a composite outcome of death or appropriate ICD therapy.[137,138] These studies have demonstrated that patients experience frequent ICD therapies in follow-up and that this finding justifies insertion of an ICD in patients with similar characteristics. A major concern with this approach is that the frequency of appropriate ICD therapies does not appear to be a reliable surrogate for ICD efficacy in terms of reducing mortality. For example, two studies of patients with nonischemic LV dysfunction found high rates (36% to 51%) of appropriate ICD therapies over 36 months of follow-up.[138,139] Randomized trials of patients with nonischemic LV dysfunction (see Table 11-3), however, have demonstrated that the mortality rate in these patients would be anticipated to be only 12% to 21% over this period.[118,119,122] Other analyses have also demonstrated poor correlation between mortality and appropriate ICD therapies.[140] Data from DEFINITE[141] indicate that the use of appropriate ICD shocks overestimates the risk of an otherwise fatal event in ICD recipients by a factor of 2. Thus, future trials of ICD therapy will likely continue to use total mortality or cardiac mortality as the primary outcome measure.

Is There a Need for Additional Risk Assessment?

There is controversy regarding the use of ICD therapy in all patients with ejection fraction values of 0.35 or less.[61,62] Although widespread use of ICD therapy for prevention of arrhythmic death is understandable, this approach is not without risk in terms of complications related to the initial implantation and subsequent revisions, alterations in QOL, and cost. Although extrapolation of the findings of past studies is reasonable and often necessary, it is prudent to consider a *reasonable probability of success*, including assessment of sudden death risk versus the risk of competing modes of death.

In an attempt to include a greater proportion of patients at risk for sudden death (see Fig. 11-2), marked LV dysfunction has been the only major inclusion criterion for study participation (see Table 11-3). Many of these lower-risk patients do not experience life-threatening arrhythmias in the near term. Studies indicate that the incidence of appropriate ICD therapies ranges from to 28% to 68% over the initial 2 to 5 years after ICD implantation, depending on the population studied and the duration of follow-up.[138,140,142] Most data indicate that patients receiving an ICD on the basis of heart failure or LV dysfunction alone have a two- to threefold lower risk for development of life-threatening arrhythmias in the initial 2 to 5 years of follow-up than patients who have a history of spontaneous sustained ventricular arrhythmias[143-145] and patients with inducible sustained ventricular arrhythmias.[146]

Although the relative efficacy values for an ICD are similar in *most* of the ICD trials (see Fig. 11-4), the absolute impacts of an ICD differ substantially. Among sudden death survivors[82-84] and patients with ischemic LV dysfunction and inducible arrhythmias,[85,86] the average absolute risk reduction is approximately 12%. Therefore, NNT for ICDs in this group is approximately 8. In contrast, among patients with only marked LV dysfunction,[103,120,122] the average absolute benefit is about 6%, translating into an NNT of 16 for ICDs. These data have been used to support the need for methods to better identify patients in whom ICD therapy leads to a greater absolute risk reduction and a lower NNT. Given the grave consequences of sudden death, it is imperative that a balance between identifying a population with a large absolute mortality reduction with ICD therapy (specificity) and identifying a greater proportion of patients at risk for sudden death (sensitivity) be achieved (see Fig. 11-3).

Real-World Effectiveness

The sites participating in the reviewed trials are typically high-volume, academically oriented centers. The success rates and complication rates achieved in these trials may not reflect the results in other centers. Little is known about the real-world success rates and complications of ICD placement. This issue is particularly relevant when the results of more complex ICD systems that include CRT are applied to less experienced centers, given the steep learning curve associated with implantation of LV leads.[147]

Large registries have been proposed to assess real-world effectiveness of ICD therapy in patients with heart failure or LV dysfunction alone and to better identify patients more or less likely to benefit from an ICD. The proposed minimal requirements for participation in these registries are that hospitals and providers be certified as competent in ICD implantation, report data on all patients undergoing ICD implantation for primary prevention, and be removed from the system if they do not comply with the data collection requirements. The proposed data elements are (1) baseline patient characteristics, (2) device type and characteristics, (3) facility and provider characteristics, (4) measures of the extent of disease progression, (5) periodic device interrogation for firing data, and (6) data related to long-term patient outcomes. Given the aforementioned problems related to using appropriate ICD therapies as a surrogate for mortality and a lack of standard methods of risk assessment, some authorities have questioned the usefulness of these registries.

Summary

With advances in ICD technology, the populations that may benefit from this therapy continue to expand. A large number of important trials have evaluated the efficacy of the ICD in a variety of settings. These studies have convincingly demonstrated that the ICD is superior to antiarrhythmic drug therapy in patients with spontaneous or inducible ventricular arrhythmias. Several randomized trials have now extended our knowledge, proving that ICD therapy improves the survival of patients with heart failure or LV dysfunction due to ischemic heart disease or dilated cardiomyopathy. However, patients with LV dysfunction in specific circumstances, notably those undergoing CABG surgery and those with recent MI, do not appear to benefit from ICD therapy. Ongoing and future studies will address the role of the ICD early after MI as well as issues of which patients benefit to the greatest extent from ICD therapy. Ongoing and future studies will assess the effect of ICD therapy combined with CRT in altering outcomes of patients with heart failure and those with largely asymptomatic LV dysfunction. Issues of reliability, cost, QOL, and real-world effectiveness will also feature prominently in future ICD studies.

A tremendous gratitude is owed to the thousands of patients who have helped us learn so much about the usefulness and limitations of ICD therapy over the past 20 years. Without the time and effort of these individuals, we would know far less, and our capacity to reduce the burden of sudden death and improve the lives of so many individuals would be greatly diminished.

REFERENCES

1. Fox CS, Evans JC, Larson MG, et al: Temporal trends in coronary heart disease mortality and sudden cardiac death from 1950 to 1999: The Framingham Heart Study. Circulation 110:522-527, 2004.
2. Bunch TJ, White RD, Friedman PA, et al: Trends in treated ventricular fibrillation out-of-hospital cardiac arrest: A 17-year population-based study. Heart Rhythm 1:255-259, 2004.
3. Kuller LH, Traven ND, Rutan GH, et al: Marked decline of coronary heart disease mortality in 35-44-year-old white men in Allegheny County, Pennsylvania. Circulation 80:261-266, 1989.
4. Josephson M, Wellens HJ: Implantable defibrillators and sudden cardiac death. Circulation 109:2685-2691, 2004.
5. Bayes de Luna A, Coumel P, Leclercq JF: Ambulatory sudden cardiac death: Mechanisms of production of fatal arrhythmia on the basis of data from 157 cases. Am Heart J 117:151-159, 1989.
6. Luu M, Stevenson WG, Stevenson LW, et al: Diverse mechanisms of unexpected cardiac arrest in advanced heart failure. Circulation 80:1675-1680, 1989.
7. Goraya TY, Jacobsen SJ, Belau PG, et al: Validation of death certificate diagnosis of out-of-hospital coronary heart disease deaths in Olmsted County, Minnesota. Mayo Clin Proc 75:681-687, 2000.
8. Goldman S, Johnson G, Cohn JN, et al: Mechanism of death in heart failure: The Vasodilator-Heart Failure Trials. The V-HeFT VA Cooperative Studies Group. Circulation 87:VI24-VI31, 1993.
9. Marcus FI, Cobb LA, Edwards JE, et al: Mechanism of death and prevalence of myocardial ischemic symptoms in the terminal event after acute myocardial infarction. Am J Cardiol 61:8-15, 1988.
10. Hinkle LE Jr, Thaler HT: Clinical classification of cardiac deaths. Circulation 65:457-464, 1982.
11. Narang R, Cleland JG, Erhardt L, et al: Mode of death in chronic heart failure: A request and proposition for more accurate classification. Eur Heart J 17:1390-1403, 1996.
12. Uretsky BF, Thygesen K, Armstrong PW, et al: Acute coronary findings at autopsy in heart failure patients with sudden death: Results from the Assessment of Treatment with Lisinopril and Survival (ATLAS) trial. Circulation 102:611–616, 2000.
13. Gottlieb SS: Dead is dead—artificial definitions are no substitute. Lancet 349:662-663, 1997.
14. Greenberg H, Case RB, Moss AJ, et al: Analysis of mortality events in the Multicenter Automatic Defibrillator Implantation Trial (MADIT-II). J Am Coll Cardiol 43:1459-1465, 2004.
15. Mirowski M, Mower MM, Langer A, et al: A chronically implanted system for automatic defibrillation in active conscious dogs: Experimental model for treatment of sudden death from ventricular fibrillation. Circulation 58:90-94, 1978.
16. Exner DV, Klein GJ, Prystowsky EN: Primary prevention of sudden death with implantable defibrillator therapy in patients with cardiac disease: Can we afford to do it? (Can we afford not to?) Circulation 104:1564-1570, 2001.
17. Schoels W, Swerdlow CD, Jung W, et al: Worldwide clinical experience with a new dual-chamber implantable cardioverter defibrillator system. J Cardiovasc Electrophysiol 12:521-528, 2001.
18. Wathen MS, DeGroot PJ, Sweeney MO, et al: Prospective randomized multicenter trial of empirical antitachycardia pacing versus shocks for spontaneous rapid ventricular tachycardia in patients with implantable cardioverter-defibrillators: Pacing Fast Ventricular Tachycardia Reduces Shock Therapies (PainFREE Rx II) trial results. Circulation 110:2591-2596, 2004.
19. Friedman PA, Dijkman B, Warman EN, et al: Atrial therapies reduce atrial arrhythmia burden in defibrillator patients. Circulation 104:1023-1028, 2001.
20. Adler SW 2nd, Wolpert C, Warman EN, et al: Efficacy of pacing therapies for treating atrial tachyarrhythmias in patients with ventricular arrhythmias receiving a dual-chamber implantable cardioverter defibrillator. Circulation 104:887-892, 2001.
21. Steinhaus D, Reynolds DW, Gadler F, et al: Implant experience with an implantable hemodynamic monitor for the management of symptomatic heart failure. Pacing Clin Electrophysiol 28:747-753, 2005.
22. Yu CM, Wang L, Chau E, et al: Intrathoracic impedance monitoring in patients with heart failure: Correlation with fluid status and feasibility of early warning preceding hospitalization. Circulation 112:841-848, 2005.
23. St John Sutton MG, Plappert T, Abraham WT, et al: Effect of cardiac resynchronization therapy on left ventricular size and function in chronic heart failure. Circulation 107:1985-1990, 2003.
24. Bristow MR, Saxon LA, Boehmer J, et al: Cardiac-resynchronization therapy with or without an implantable defibrillator in advanced chronic heart failure. N Engl J Med 350:2140-2150, 2004.
25. Cleland JG, Daubert JC, Erdmann E, et al: Cardiac Resynchronization-Heart Failure (CARE-HF) Study Investigators: The effect of cardiac resynchronization on morbidity and mortality in heart failure. N Engl J Med 352:1539-1549, 2005.
26. Kim SG, Pathapati R, Fisher JD, et al: Comparison of long-term outcomes of patients treated with nonthoracotomy and thoracotomy implantable defibrillators. Am J Cardiol 78:1109-1112, 1996.
27. Kleman JM, Castle LW, Kidwell GA, et al: Nonthoracotomy-versus thoracotomy-implantable defibrillators: Intention-to-treat

comparison of clinical outcomes. Circulation 90:2833-2842, 1994.

28. Connolly SJ, Hallstrom AP, Cappato R, et al: Meta-analysis of the implantable cardioverter defibrillator secondary prevention trials. AVID, CASH and CIDS studies. Antiarrhythmics vs Implantable Defibrillator study. Cardiac Arrest Study Hamburg. Canadian Implantable Defibrillator Study. Eur Heart J 21:2071-2078, 2000.
29. Nanthakumar K, Epstein AE, Kay GN, et al: Prophylactic implantable cardioverter-defibrillator therapy in patients with left ventricular systolic dysfunction: A pooled analysis of 10 primary prevention trials. J Am Coll Cardiol 44:2166-2172, 2004.
30. Al-Khatib SM, Sanders GD, Mark DB, et al: Implantable cardioverter defibrillators and cardiac resynchronization therapy in patients with left ventricular dysfunction: Randomized trial evidence through 2004. Am Heart J 149:1020-1034, 2005.
31. Steinbrook R: The controversy over Guidant's implantable defibrillators. N Engl J Med 353:221-224, 2005.
32. McCready MJ, Exner DV: Quality of life and psychological impact of implantable cardioverter defibrillators: Focus on randomized controlled trial data. Card Electrophysiol Rev 7:63-70, 2003.
33. McAlister FA, Ezekowitz JA, Wiebe N, et al: Systematic review: Cardiac resynchronization in patients with symptomatic heart failure. Ann Intern Med 141:381-390, 2004.
34. Schron EB, Exner DV, Yao Q, et al: Quality of life in the antiarrhythmics versus implantable defibrillators trial: Impact of therapy and influence of adverse symptoms and defibrillator shocks. Circulation 105:589-594, 2002.
35. Irvine J, Dorian P, Baker B, et al: Quality of life in the Canadian Implantable Defibrillator Study (CIDS). Am Heart J 144: 282-289, 2002.
36. Namerow PB, Firth BR, Heywood GM, et al: Quality-of-life six months after CABG surgery in patients randomized to ICD versus no ICD therapy: Findings from the CABG Patch Trial. Pacing Clin Electrophysiol 22:1305-1313, 1999.
37. Passman R, Anderson K, Subacius H, et al: Superior quality of life in patients with non-ischemic dilated cardiomyopathy and implantable cardioverter defibrillators: Results from the DEFINITE study. Circulation 110:II-625, 2004.
38. Exner DV, Pinski SL, Wyse DG, et al: Electrical storm presages nonsudden death: The Antiarrhythmics Versus Implantable Defibrillators (AVID) Trial. Circulation 103:2066-2071, 2001.
39. Hurst TM, Hinrichs M, Breidenbach C, et al: Detection of myocardial injury during transvenous implantation of automatic cardioverter-defibrillators. J Am Coll Cardiol 34:402-408, 1999.
40. Epstein AE, Kay GN, Plumb VJ, et al: Gross and microscopic pathological changes associated with nonthoracotomy implantable defibrillator leads. Circulation 98:1517-1524, 1998.
41. Trayanova N, Eason J: Shock-induced arrhythmogenesis in the myocardium. Chaos 12:962-972, 2002.
42. Pires LA, Hull ML, Nino CL, et al: Sudden death in recipients of transvenous implantable cardioverter defibrillator systems: Terminal events, predictors, and potential mechanisms. J Cardiovasc Electrophysiol 10:1049-1056, 1999.
43. Mitchell LB, Pineda EA, Titus JL, et al: Sudden death in patients with implantable cardioverter defibrillators: The importance of post-shock electromechanical dissociation. J Am Coll Cardiol 39:1323-1328, 2002.
44. Pacifico A, Hohnloser SH, Williams JH, et al: Prevention of implantable-defibrillator shocks by treatment with sotalol: d,l-Sotalol Implantable Cardioverter-Defibrillator Study Group. N Engl J Med 340:1855-1862, 1999.
45. Dorian P, Borggrefe M, Al-Khalidi HR, et al: Placebo-controlled, randomized clinical trial of azimilide for prevention of ventricular tachyarrhythmias in patients with an implantable cardioverter defibrillator. Circulation 110:3646-3654, 2004.
46. Sweeney MO, Wathen MS, Volosin K, et al: Appropriate and inappropriate ventricular therapies, quality of life, and mortality among primary and secondary prevention implantable cardioverter defibrillator patients: Results from the Pacing Fast VT REduces Shock ThErapies (PainFREE Rx II) trial. Circulation 111:2898-2905, 2005.
47. Mehta D, Nayak HM, Singson M, et al: Late complications in patients with pectoral defibrillator implants with transvenous defibrillator lead systems: High incidence of insulation breakdown. Pacing Clin Electrophysiol 21:1893-1900, 1998.
48. Zipes DP: Implantable cardioverter-defibrillator: A Volkswagen or a Rolls Royce: How much will we pay to save a life? Circulation 103:1372-1374, 2001.
49. Disclosure and performance: Expecting more, and better. CMAJ 173:457-459, 2005.
50. Hauser RG: The growing mismatch between patient longevity and the service life of implantable cardioverter-defibrillators. J Am Coll Cardiol 45:2022-2025, 2005.
51. Alter P, Waldhans S, Plachta E, et al: Complications of implantable cardioverter defibrillator therapy in 440 consecutive patients. Pacing Clin Electrophysiol 28:926-932, 2005.
52. Nichol G, Kaul P, Huszti E, Bridges JF: Cost-effectiveness of cardiac resynchronization therapy in patients with symptomatic heart failure. Ann Intern Med 141:343-351, 2004.
53. Simpson CS, Klein GJ, Hoffmaster B: Expensive medical technologies and "indication extrapolation:" The case of implantable cardioverter-defibrillators. Am Heart J 140:419-422, 2000.
54. Salukhe TV, Dimopoulos K, Sutton R, et al: Life-years gained from defibrillator implantation: Markedly nonlinear increase during 3 years of follow-up and its implications. Circulation 109:1848-1853, 2004.
55. Cannom DS, Prystowsky EN: Management of ventricular arrhythmias: Detection, drugs, and devices. JAMA 281:172-179, 1999.
56. Zipes DP, Wellens HJ: Sudden cardiac death. Circulation 98:2334-2351, 1998.
57. Myerburg RJ, Mitrani R, Interian A Jr, Castellanos A: Interpretation of outcomes of antiarrhythmic clinical trials: Design features and population impact. Circulation 97:1514-1521, 1998.
58. Rea TD, Pearce RM, Raghunathan TE, et al: Incidence of out-of-hospital cardiac arrest. Am J Cardiol 93:1455-1460, 2004.
59. Gorgels AP, Gijsbers C, de Vreede-Swagemakers J, et al: Out-of-hospital cardiac arrest—the relevance of heart failure. The Maastricht Circulatory Arrest Registry. Eur Heart J 24:1204-1209, 2003.
60. La Rovere MT, Bigger JT Jr, Marcus FI, et al: Baroreflex sensitivity and heart-rate variability in prediction of total cardiac mortality after myocardial infarction. ATRAMI (Autonomic Tone and Reflexes After Myocardial Infarction) Investigators. Lancet 351:478-484, 1998.
61. Buxton AE. Should everyone with an ejection fraction less than or equal to 30% receive an implantable cardioverter-defibrillator? Not everyone with an ejection fraction < or = 30% should receive an implantable cardioverter-defibrillator. Circulation 111:2537-2549, 2005; discussion, 2537-2549.
62. Moss AJ: Should everyone with an ejection fraction less than or equal to 30% receive an implantable cardioverter-defibrillator? Everyone with an ejection fraction < or = 30% should receive an implantable cardioverter-defibrillator. Circulation 111:2537-2549, 2005; discussion 2537-2549.
63. Traven ND, Kuller LH, Ives DG, et al: Coronary heart disease mortality and sudden death: Trends and patterns in 35- to 44-year-old white males, 1970-1990. Am J Epidemiol 142:45-52, 1995.
64. Northcote RJ, Flannigan C, Ballantyne D: Sudden death and vigorous exercise—a study of 60 deaths associated with squash. Br Heart J 55:198-203, 1986.
65. Domanski MJ, Exner DV, Borkowf CB, et al: Effect of angiotensin converting enzyme inhibition on sudden cardiac

death in patients following acute myocardial infarction: A meta-analysis of randomized clinical trials. J Am Coll Cardiol 33:598-604, 1999.
66. Dietary supplementation with n-3 polyunsaturated fatty acids and vitamin E after myocardial infarction: Results of the GISSI-Prevenzione trial. Gruppo Italiano per lo Studio della Sopravvivenza nell'Infarto miocardico. Lancet 354:447-455, 1999.
67. Mitchell LB, Powell JL, Gillis AM, et al: Are lipid-lowering drugs also antiarrhythmic drugs? An analysis of the Antiarrhythmics versus Implantable Defibrillators (AVID) trial. J Am Coll Cardiol 42:81-87, 2003.
68. Hallstrom AP, Ornato JP, Weisfeldt M, et al: Public-access defibrillation and survival after out-of-hospital cardiac arrest. N Engl J Med 351:637-646, 2004.
69. Bloomfield DM, Steinman RC, Namerow PB, et al: Microvolt T-wave alternans distinguishes between patients likely and patients not likely to benefit from implanted cardiac defibrillator therapy: A solution to the Multicenter Automatic Defibrillator Implantation Trial (MADIT) II conundrum. Circulation 110:1885-1889, 2004.
70. Hohnloser SH, Klingenheben T, Bloomfield D, et al: Usefulness of microvolt T-wave alternans for prediction of ventricular tachyarrhythmic events in patients with dilated cardiomyopathy: Results from a prospective observational study. J Am Coll Cardiol 41:2220-2224, 2003.
71. Schmidt G, Malik M, Barthel P, et al: Heart-rate turbulence after ventricular premature beats as a predictor of mortality after acute myocardial infarction. Lancet 353:1390-1396, 1999.
72. Barthel P, Schneider R, Bauer A, et al: Risk stratification after acute myocardial infarction by heart rate turbulence. Circulation 108:1221-1226, 2003.
73. Huikuri HV, Makikallio T, Airaksinen KE, et al: Measurement of heart rate variability: A clinical tool or a research toy? J Am Coll Cardiol 34:1878-1883, 1999.
74. Huikuri HV, Tapanainen JM, Lindgren K, et al: Prediction of sudden cardiac death after myocardial infarction in the beta-blocking era. J Am Coll Cardiol 42:652-658, 2003.
75. Makikallio TH, Barthel P, Schneider R, et al: Prediction of sudden cardiac death after acute myocardial infarction: Role of Holter monitoring in the modern treatment era. Eur Heart J 26:762-769, 2005.
76. O'Leary DH, Polak JF, Kronmal RA, et al: Carotid-artery intima and media thickness as a risk factor for myocardial infarction and stroke in older adults. Cardiovascular Health Study Collaborative Research Group. N Engl J Med 340:14-22, 1999.
77. van der Burg AE, Bax JJ, Boersma E, et al: Impact of viability, ischemia, scar tissue, and revascularization on outcome after aborted sudden death. Circulation 108:1954-1959, 2003.
78. Tan HL, Hofman N, van Langen IM, et al: Sudden unexplained death: Heritability and diagnostic yield of cardiological and genetic examination in surviving relatives. Circulation 112:207-213, 2005.
79. Wever EF, Hauer RN, Schrijvers G, et al: Cost-effectiveness of implantable defibrillator as first-choice therapy versus electrophysiologically guided, tiered strategy in postinfarct sudden death survivors. A randomized study [see comments]. Circulation 93:489-496, 1996.
80. Bigger JT Jr: Prophylactic use of implanted cardiac defibrillators in patients at high risk for ventricular arrhythmias after coronary-artery bypass graft surgery. Coronary Artery Bypass Graft (CABG) Patch Trial Investigators. N Engl J Med 337:1569-1575, 1997.
81. Hohnloser SH, Kuck KH, Dorian P, et al: Prophylactic use of an implantable cardioverter-defibrillator after acute myocardial infarction. N Engl J Med 351:2481-2488, 2004.
82. A comparison of antiarrhythmic-drug therapy with implantable defibrillators in patients resuscitated from near-fatal ventricular arrhythmias. The Antiarrhythmics versus Implantable Defibrillators (AVID) Investigators [see comments]. N Engl J Med 337:1576-1583, 1997.
83. Connolly SJ, Gent M, Roberts RS, et al: Canadian Implantable Defibrillator Study (CIDS): A randomized trial of the implantable cardioverter defibrillator against amiodarone. Circulation 101:1297-1302, 2000.
84. Kuck KH, Cappato R, Siebels J, Ruppel R: Randomized comparison of antiarrhythmic drug therapy with implantable defibrillators in patients resuscitated from cardiac arrest: The Cardiac Arrest Study Hamburg (CASH). Circulation 102:748-754, 2000.
85. Buxton AE, Lee KL, Fisher JD, et al: A randomized study of the prevention of sudden death in patients with coronary artery disease. Multicenter Unsustained Tachycardia Trial Investigators. N Engl J Med 341:1882-1890, 1999.
86. Moss AJ, Hall WJ, Cannom DS, et al: Improved survival with an implanted defibrillator in patients with coronary disease at high risk for ventricular arrhythmia. Multicenter Automatic Defibrillator Implantation Trial Investigators [see comments]. N Engl J Med 335:1933-1940, 1996.
87. Larsen G, Hallstrom A, McAnulty J, et al: Cost-effectiveness of the implantable cardioverter-defibrillator versus antiarrhythmic drugs in survivors of serious ventricular tachyarrhythmias: Results of the Antiarrhythmics Versus Implantable Defibrillators (AVID) economic analysis substudy. Circulation 105:2049-2057, 2002.
88. DeMets DL, Hardy R, Friedman LM, Lan KK: Statistical aspects of early termination in the beta-blocker heart attack trial. Control Clin Trials 5:362-372, 1984.
89. Stanton MS, Bell GK: Economic outcomes of implantable cardioverter-defibrillators. Circulation 101:1067-1074, 2000.
90. Domanski MJ, Sakseena S, Epstein AE, et al: Relative effectiveness of the implantable cardioverter-defibrillator and antiarrhythmic drugs in patients with varying degrees of left ventricular dysfunction who have survived malignant ventricular arrhythmias. AVID Investigators. Antiarrhythmics Versus Implantable Defibrillators. J Am Coll Cardiol 34:1090-1095, 1999.
91. Assmann SF, Pocock SJ, Enos LE, Kasten LE: Subgroup analysis and other (mis)uses of baseline data in clinical trials [see comments]. Lancet 355:1064-1069, 2000.
92. Exner DV, Reiffel JA, Epstein AE, et al: Beta-blocker use and survival in patients with ventricular fibrillation or symptomatic ventricular tachycardia: The Antiarrhythmics Versus Implantable Defibrillators (AVID) trial. J Am Coll Cardiol 34:325-333, 1999.
93. Wyse DG, Friedman PL, Brodsky MA, et al: Life-threatening ventricular arrhythmias due to transient or correctable causes: High risk for death in follow-up. J Am Coll Cardiol 38:1718-1724, 2001.
94. Raitt MH, Renfroe EG, Epstein AE, et al: "Stable" ventricular tachycardia is not a benign rhythm: Insights from the Antiarrhythmics Versus Implantable Defibrillators (AVID) registry. Circulation 103:244-252, 2001.
95. O'Brien BJ, Connolly SJ, Goeree R, et al: Cost-effectiveness of the implantable cardioverter-defibrillator: Results from the Canadian Implantable Defibrillator Study (CIDS). Circulation 103:1416-1421, 2001.
96. Sheldon R, Connolly S, Krahn A, et al: Identification of patients most likely to benefit from implantable cardioverter-defibrillator therapy: The Canadian Implantable Defibrillator Study. Circulation 101:1660-1664, 2000.
97. Sheldon R, O'Brien BJ, Blackhouse G, et al: Effect of clinical risk stratification on cost-effectiveness of the implantable cardioverter-defibrillator: The Canadian Implantable Defibrillator Study. Circulation 104:1622-1626, 2001.
98. Exner DV, Sheldon RS, Pinski SL, et al: Do baseline characteristics accurately discriminate between patients likely versus

unlikely to benefit from implantable defibrillator therapy? Evaluation of the Canadian Implantable Defibrillator Study Implantable Cardioverter Defibrillator efficacy score in the Antiarrhythmics Versus Implantable Defibrillators trial. Am Heart J 141:99-104, 2001.

99. Exner DV: Quality of life in patients with life-threatening arrhythmias: Does choice of therapy make a difference? Am Heart J 144:208-211, 2002.
100. Mushlin AI, Hall WJ, Zwanziger J, et al: The cost-effectiveness of automatic implantable cardiac defibrillators: Results from MADIT. Multicenter Automatic Defibrillator Implantation Trial. Circulation 97:2129-2135, 1998.
101. Andresen D, Steinbeck G, Bruggemann T, et al: Can the MADIT results be applied to myocardial infarction patients at hospital discharge? J Am Coll Cardiol 31:308A, 1998.
102. Buxton AE, Lee KL, DiCarlo L, et al: Electrophysiologic testing to identify patients with coronary artery disease who are at risk for sudden death. Multicenter Unsustained Tachycardia Trial Investigators. N Engl J Med 342:1937-1945, 2000.
103. Moss AJ, Zareba W, Hall WJ, et al: Prophylactic implantation of a defibrillator in patients with myocardial infarction and reduced ejection fraction. N Engl J Med 346:877-883, 2002.
104. Gehi A, Haas D, Fuster V: Primary prophylaxis with the implantable cardioverter-defibrillator: The need for improved risk stratification. JAMA 294:958-960, 2005.
105. Greco R, Siciliano S, D'Alterio D, et al: 10-year follow-up of patients with intraventricular conduction defects associated with myocardial infarction: The meaning of QRS duration. G Ital Cardiol 15:1147-1154, 1985.
106. Iuliano S, Fisher SG, Karasik PE, et al: QRS duration and mortality in patients with congestive heart failure. Am Heart J 143:1085-1091, 2002.
107. Baldasseroni S, Opasich C, Gorini M, et al: Left bundle-branch block is associated with increased 1-year sudden and total mortality rate in 5517 outpatients with congestive heart failure: A report from the Italian network on congestive heart failure. Am Heart J 143:398-405, 2002.
108. Kalahasti V, Nambi V, Martin DO, et al: QRS duration and prediction of mortality in patients undergoing risk stratification for ventricular arrhythmias. Am J Cardiol 92:798-803, 2003.
109. Horwich T, Lee SJ, Saxon L: Usefulness of QRS prolongation in predicting risk of inducible monomorphic ventricular tachycardia in patients referred for electrophysiologic studies. Am J Cardiol 92:804-809, 2003.
110. Bode-Schnurbus L, Bocker D, Block M, et al: QRS duration: A simple marker for predicting cardiac mortality in ICD patients with heart failure. Heart 89:1157-1162, 2003.
111. Buxton AE, Sweeney MO, Wathen MS, et al: QRS duration does not predict occurrence of ventricular tachyarrhythmias in patients with implanted cardioverter-defibrillators. J Am Coll Cardiol 46:310-316, 2005.
112. Poole J, Anderson J, Johnson G, et al: Baseline ECG data and outcome in the Sudden Cardiac Death-Heart Failure Trial. In Program and Abstracts from the Heart Rhythm 25th Annual Scientific Sessions, 2004.
113. Cohen RJ: Enhancing specificity without sacrificing sensitivity: Potential benefits of using microvolt T-wave alternans testing to risk stratify the MADIT-II population. Card Electrophysiol Rev 7:438-442, 2003.
114. Malik M, Hnatkova K, Batchvarov VN: Post infarction risk stratification using the 3-D angle between QRS complex and T-wave vectors. J Electrocardiol 37(Suppl):201-208, 2004.
115. Wichterle D, Camm AJ, Malik M: Turbulence slope after atrial premature complexes is an independent predictor of mortality in survivors of acute myocardial infarction. J Cardiovasc Electrophysiol 15:1350-1356, 2004.
116. Moss AJ: Correcting misconceptions. Ann Noninvasive Electrocardiol 8:177-178, 2003.
117. Wilber DJ, Zareba W, Hall WJ, et al: Time dependence of mortality risk and defibrillator benefit after myocardial infarction. Circulation 109:1082-1084, 2004.
118. Strickberger SA, Hummel JD, Bartlett TG, et al: Amiodarone versus implantable cardioverter-defibrillator: Randomized trial in patients with nonischemic dilated cardiomyopathy and asymptomatic nonsustained ventricular tachycardia-AMIOVIRT. J Am Coll Cardiol 41:1707-1712, 2003.
119. Bansch D, Antz M, Boczor S, et al: Primary prevention of sudden cardiac death in idiopathic dilated cardiomyopathy: The Cardiomyopathy Trial (CAT). Circulation 105:1453-1458, 2002.
120. Bardy GH, Lee KL, Mark DB, et al: Amiodarone or an implantable cardioverter-defibrillator for congestive heart failure. N Engl J Med 352:225-237, 2005.
121. Mark DB, Nelson CL, Anstrom KJ, et al: Cost-effectiveness of ICD therapy in the sudden cardiac death in heart failure trial (SCD-HeFT). Circulation 111:1727-1727, 2005.
122. Kadish A, Dyer A, Daubert JP, et al: Prophylactic defibrillator implantation in patients with nonischemic dilated cardiomyopathy. N Engl J Med 350:2151-2158, 2004.
123. Kadish A, Schaechter A, Subacius H, et al: Patients with recently diagnosed non-ischemic cardiomyopathy benefit from ICD implantation. In: Heart Rhythm Society: Program and abstracts from the Heart Rhythm 2005 26th Annual Scientific Sessions, May 4-7, 2005, New Orleans.
124. Bigger JT Jr, Whang W, Rottman JN, et al: Mechanisms of death in the CABG patch trial: A randomized trial of implantable cardiac defibrillator prophylaxis in patients at high risk of death after coronary artery bypass graft surgery. Circulation 99:1416-1421, 1999.
125. Bailey JJ, Berson AS, Handelsman H, Hodges M: Utility of current risk stratification tests for predicting major arrhythmic events after myocardial infarction. J Am Coll Cardiol 38:1902-1911, 2001.
126. Bauer A, Guzik P, Barthel P, et al: Reduced prognostic power of ventricular late potentials in post-infarction patients of the reperfusion era. Eur Heart J 26:755-761, 2005.
127. Veenhuyzen GD, Singh SN, McAreavey D, et al: Prior coronary artery bypass surgery and risk of death among patients with ischemic left ventricular dysfunction. Circulation 104:1489-1493, 2001.
128. Dorian P, Connolly S, Hohnloser SH: Why don't ICDs decrease all-cause mortality after MI? Insights from the DINAMIT study. Circulation 110:502-502, 2004.
129. St John Sutton M, Lee D, Rouleau JL, et al: Left ventricular remodeling and ventricular arrhythmias after myocardial infarction. Circulation 107:2577-2582, 2003.
130. Nolan J, Batin PD, Andrews R, et al: Prospective study of heart rate variability and mortality in chronic heart failure: Results of the United Kingdom heart failure evaluation and assessment of risk trial (UK-heart). Circulation 98:1510-1516, 1998.
131. Tapanainen JM, Still AM, Airaksinen KE, Huikuri HV: Prognostic significance of risk stratifiers of mortality, including T wave alternans, after acute myocardial infarction: Results of a prospective follow-up study. J Cardiovasc Electrophysiol 12:645-652, 2001.
132. Raviele A, Bongiorni MG, Brignole M, et al: Early EPS/ICD strategy in survivors of acute myocardial infarction with severe left ventricular dysfunction on optimal beta-blocker treatment. The BEta-blocker STrategy plus ICD trial. Europace 7:327-337, 2005.
133. Gregoratos G, Cheitlin MD, Conill A, et al: ACC/AHA Guidelines for implantation of cardiac pacemakers and antiarrhythmia devices: Executive Summary—a report of the American College of Cardiology/American Heart Association Task Force on Practice Guidelines (Committee on Pacemaker Implantation). Circulation 97:1325-1335, 1998.
134. Gregoratos G, Abrams J, Epstein AE, et al: ACC/AHA/NASPE 2002 guideline update for implantation of cardiac pacemakers

and antiarrhythmia devices: Summary article—a report of the American College of Cardiology/American Heart Association Task Force on Practice Guidelines (ACC/AHA/NASPE Committee to Update the 1998 Pacemaker Guidelines). Circulation 106:2145-2161, 2002.

135. Tang AS, Ross H, Simpson CS, et al: Canadian Cardiovascular Society/Canadian Heart Rhythm Society position paper on implantable cardioverter defibrillator use in Canada. Can J Cardiol 21(Suppl A):11–18, 2005,

136. Steinbeck G, Andresen D, Senges J, et al: Immediate Risk-Stratification Improves Survival (IRIS): Study protocol. Europace 6:392-399, 2004.

137. Maron BJ, Shen WK, Link MS, et al: Efficacy of implantable cardioverter-defibrillators for the prevention of sudden death in patients with hypertrophic cardiomyopathy [see comments]. N Engl J Med 342:365-373, 2000.

138. Grimm W, Hoffmann JJ, Muller HH, Maisch B: Implantable defibrillator event rates in patients with idiopathic dilated cardiomyopathy, nonsustained ventricular tachycardia on Holter and a left ventricular ejection fraction below 30%. J Am Coll Cardiol 39:780-787, 2002.

139. Grimm W, Flores BT, Marchlinski FE: Shock occurrence and survival in 241 patients with implantable cardioverter-defibrillator therapy. Circulation 87:1880-1888, 1993.

140. Klein RC, Raitt MH, Wilkoff BL, et al: Analysis of implantable cardioverter defibrillator therapy in the Antiarrhythmics Versus Implantable Defibrillators (AVID) Trial. J Cardiovasc Electrophysiol 14:940-948, 2003.

141. Ellenbogen KA, Levine JH, Berger RD, et al: Are implantable cardioverter defibrillator shocks a surrogate for sudden cardiac death in patients with nonischemic cardiomyopathy? Circulation 113:776-782, 2006.

142. Theuns DA, Klootwijk AP, Simoons ML, Jordaens LJ: Clinical variables predicting inappropriate use of implantable cardioverter-defibrillator in patients with coronary heart disease or nonischemic dilated cardiomyopathy. Am J Cardiol 95:271-274, 2005.

143. Theuns DA, Thornton AS, Klootwijk AP, et al: Outcome in patients with an ICD incorporating cardiac resynchronisation therapy: Differences between primary and secondary prophylaxis. Eur J Heart Fail 7:1027-1032, 2005.

144. Wilkoff BL, Hess M, Young J, Abraham WT: Differences in tachyarrhythmia detection and implantable cardioverter defibrillator therapy by primary or secondary prevention indication in cardiac resynchronization therapy patients. J Cardiovasc Electrophysiol 15:1002-1009, 2004.

145. Capoferri M, Schwick N, Tanner H, et al: Incidence of arrhythmic events in patients with implantable cardioverter-defibrillator for primary and secondary prevention of sudden cardiac death. Swiss Med Wkly 134:154-158, 2004.

146. Backenkohler U, Erdogan A, Steen-Mueller MK, et al: Long-term incidence of malignant ventricular arrhythmia and shock therapy in patients with primary defibrillator implantation does not differ from event rates in patients treated for survived cardiac arrest. J Cardiovasc Electrophysiol 16:478-482, 2005.

147. Kautzner J, Riedlbauchova L, Cihak R, et al: Technical aspects of implantation of LV lead for cardiac resynchronization therapy in chronic heart failure. Pacing Clin Electrophysiol 27:783-790, 2004.

148. Bokhari F, Newman D, Greene M, et al: Long-term comparison of the implantable cardioverter defibrillator versus amiodarone. Eleven-year follow-up of a subset of patients in the Canadian Implantable Defibrillator Study (CIDS). Circulation 110:112-116, 2004.

Chapter 12

Clinical Trials of Cardiac Resynchronization Therapy: Pacemakers and Defibrillators

LESLIE A. SAXON • TERESA DE MARCO • KENNETH A. ELLENBOGEN

The major acute and chronic clinical trials of cardiac resynchronization therapy (CRT) alone and CRT with a defibrillator (CRT-D), performed worldwide, are reviewed in this chapter. The positive results of these studies herald a new era in the treatment of advanced heart failure due to systolic dysfunction. Building on impressive improvements in symptom status and mortality achieved with medical therapies for heart failure that modulate the effects of neurohormonal activation that accompanies heart failure, large-scale randomized clinical trials of CRT have further improved symptoms and longevity in the population with advanced heart failure and QRS delay.[1-10]

Resynchronization devices now represent roughly one third of all implantable cardioverter-defibrillators (ICDs) implanted in the United States.[11] This proportion is expected to grow as the clinical trials in progress, aiming to expand the population pool of patients eligible for CRT to include those with less severe functional status, patients with an indication for a bradycardia device, and patients with systolic dysfunction and mechanical dyssynchrony but no QRS delay, are completed.[12-15]

Another, often overlooked factor that will serve as an additional driver for CRT implants in the future is that a sizable proportion of patients with indications for a primary prevention ICD under the broad umbrella of New York Heart Association functional class (NYHA class) II symptoms and left ventricular ejection fraction (LVEF) of less than 35% also have indications for a CRT device.[16,17] Review of clinical trial data shows that at least one third of the patients for whom ICDs are indicated would qualify for a CRT-D device. Although the implant procedure for a CRT-D is technically more challenging than that for an ICD, CRT has the added advantage of making patients feel better, causing reverse ventricular remodeling, and reducing heart failure hospitalizations—three important goals for anyone offering device therapy to a population with heart failure.[2,9,18-20]

Future advances in technology and device features for delivering CRT itself or as accompaniments to CRT, such as remote device follow-up and other CRT–heart failure hybrid device therapies, are reviewed in this chapter.[21-25]

Treatment of the heart failure disease substrate with a device-based therapy such as CRT has allowed for the expansion of our thinking about the potential uses of a heart failure device—that is, the development of a device that not only treats heart failure but also possesses features and technologies that diagnose and prevent heart failure exacerbations and that assist in the overall management and tracking of the status of the heart failure patient.

Heart Failure and QRS Delay: Scope of the Problem

The single largest expense for the Medicare Trust Fund in the United States is incurred in the treatment of heart failure.[26-29] The majority of this expense is in the acute management of heart failure hospitalizations, which often require intensive care unit management.[29] There are not only nearly one million heart failure hospitalizations yearly but also 300,000 heart failure deaths yearly. These deaths are primarily due to progressive pump dysfunction and sudden cardiac death, both of which can be addressed with CRT or CRT-D.[8,9,30] As heart failure severity increases, characterized by both mechanical and electrical remodeling, the primary cause of cardiovascular death typically is pump failure, although the absolute number of sudden deaths in the setting of advanced heart failure and QRS prolongation is significant, accounting for roughly one third of all deaths.[31,32]

When it accompanies heart failure due to systolic dysfunction, QRS delay itself adds significant morbidity and mortality.[33-38] Affecting 30% to 50% of patients with NYHA class III to IV heart failure, QRS delay, which is predominantly left bundle branch block (LBBB), adversely affects cardiac function by introducing intraventricular dyssynchrony. Conduction delay also worsens atrioventricular (AV) and interventricular dyssynchrony, but intraventricular dyssynchrony results in worsening LV function as measured by dP/dT and filling times.[39-41] Interestingly, even in those patients with right BBB (RBBB) or intraventricular conduction delay, significant electrical delay to the LV is observed on detailed activation mapping, suggesting that RBBB in this setting often represents "concealed" LBBB.[42,43]

Studies of Cardiac Resynchronization Therapy in the Acute Setting: How Does It Work?

Cardiac resynchronization therapy, defined as the stimulation of the left ventricle or simultaneous stimulation of both the right and left ventricles after atrially sensed or paced events or in atrial fibrillation (AF) demonstrates that CRT works by partially or wholly correcting AV, interventricular, and, most importantly, intraventricular dyssynchronies.[40,44-50] The predominant effects are on measures of systolic function. These beneficial effects are summarized in Table 12-1 and discussed in detail in Chapter 14.

In the first closed-chest study of CRT, in 27 subjects with heart failure and QRS delay, Blanc and associates[44] demonstrated improvements in systolic blood pressure, pulmonary capillary wedge pressure, and V-wave

TABLE 12-1. Mechanisms of Acute Improvements in Cardiac Function with Cardiac Resynchronization Therapy (CRT)

Effect of CRT	Mechanism(s)/Measure(s)
Atrioventricular resynchronization	Diminished mitral regurgitation Lengthened diastolic filling time Optimization of filling pattern
Inter/intraventricular resynchronization	Increases in left ventricular efficiency/systolic blood pressure, dP/dt, pulse pressure, stroke volume, and stroke work Decrease in left ventricular end-systolic volume

amplitude with LV or biventricular (BiV) stimulation in comparison with baseline or right ventricular (RV) pacing. Kass and colleagues[40] and Aurrichio and coworkers[45] subsequently demonstrated that the effects of CRT could be further optimized by AV delay timing to achieve immediate increases in dP/dt and pulse pressure of 12% to 25% with LV or BiV stimulation in studies performed in a total of 45 patients.[40,45] Figure 12-1 demonstrates the effects of pacing site on pressure-volume loops obtained in a patient with heart failure and LBBB. Neither RV pacing site alters the abnormal loop. Both LV free wall (LVFW) and BiV stimulation result in reductions in end-systolic volume, stroke volume, and stroke work (increased loop width and area). These changes correlated with improvements in pulse pressure. Interestingly, in the setting of AF and heart block, greater immediate improvements in LV function are achieved with BiV or LV-RV offset stimulation than with single-site LV stimulation, presumably owing to avoidance of interventricular dyssynchrony induced by LV-only stimulation in the setting of heart block.[49]

Acute predictors of a beneficial hemodynamic response to CRT were identified to be baseline extent of QRS delay (but not subsequent shortening with pacing) and mechanical dyssynchrony.[47,50] LVFW rather than true anterior LV stimulation sites appear to elicit a more robust acute hemodynamic response.[48] Acute myocardial energetics improve with CRT because of greater contractile efficiency.[51]

Controlled Trials of Cardiac Resynchronization Therapy Devices

The design, inclusion criteria, and results of the controlled clinical trials of CRT and CRT-D devices are summarized in Table 12-2. In general, inclusion criteria were similar: symptomatic NYHA class III to IV heart failure, LVEF of less than 0.35, prolonged QRS duration (>120, >130, or >150 msec), and stability of proved medical therapies for heart failure prior to enrollment.[3,5,7-10,52-55]

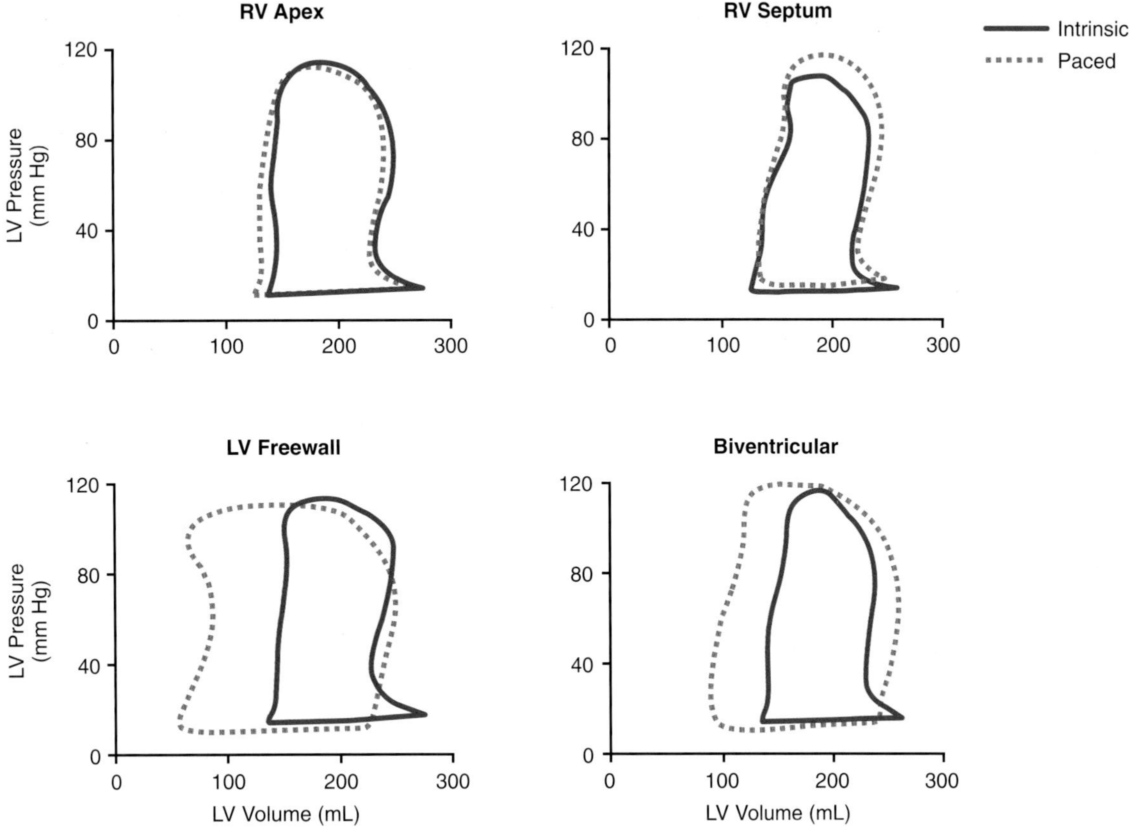

Figure 12-1. Pressure-volume graphs from a patient with baseline left bundle branch block as a function of varying pacing sites. Data are shown for optimal atrioventricular interval at each site. Solid line *indicates NSR control, and* dashed line, *VDD pacing. There was a negligible difference between right ventricular apex and septum pacing. However, left ventricular pacing produced loops with greater area (stroke work) and width (stroke volume) and a reduced systolic volume. The last finding is consistent with increased contractile function and thus with elevation of dP/dt_{max}. These results were similar in a subset of patients in whom data were measurable. (From Kass DA, Chen CH, Curry C, et al: Improved left ventricular mechanics from acute VDD pacing in patients with dilated cardiomyopathy and ventricular conduction delay. Circulation 30;99:1567-1573, 1999.)*

Only two early trials used epicardial LV leads, placed via limited thoracotomy for LV stimulation.[4,52] The Multisite Stimulation in Cardiomyopathy Sinus Rhythm (MUSTIC) trial used a stylet-driven coronary sinus lead, and the remaining trials used over-the-wire leads to achieve LV stimulation via a coronary sinus branch vein.[3,7-10,52-55] The earliest U.S. CRT study using an epicardial LV lead, the VIGOR-CHF trial was not completed owing to insufficient patient enrollment for the primary functional endpoint of peak $\dot{V}O_2$. Also, the emergence of the coronary sinus branch vein lead resulted in reluctance on the parts of patients and physicians to continue to use a more invasive procedure for LV stimulation. The results of the echocardiographic substudy were published, however, and, like data from the first European Pacing Therapies in Congestive Heart Failure (PATH I) study, demonstrated a level of improvement in several measures of response to CRT comparable with those seen in studies using transvenous LV stimulation for CRT.[19,41,52] The VIGOR-CHF trial demonstrated a decrease in LV and left atrial volumes as well as improvements in LV outflow tract, aortic velocity, and myocardial performance index with just 12 weeks of CRT. The severity or grade of mitral regurgitation as well as mitral deceleration, a measure of improvement of diastolic LV function, also improved.

In the two early U.S. trials that were the basis for attaining the initial approvals from the U.S. Food and Drug Administration (FDA) for CRT-D—CONTAK CD and MIRACLE ICD (see later)—patients with NYHA class II were included, but FDA labeling was not requested for this patient subset and was granted only for patients with NYHA classes III and IV.[7,8,14] Exclusion criteria included the presence of an implanted device and requirement for bradycardia pacing support or permanent AF. The early U.S. trials used parallel design; devices were implanted in all patients, who were then randomly assigned to "CRT on" or "CRT off" status for a period of 6 months. Two principal investigators at each enrolling center were designated in most trials, so that the physician managing the medical therapies (heart failure) was blinded as to the treatment assignment and the implanting physician (electrophysiologist) followed the device performance.

The study endpoints in CRT trials evolved over time. Although all trials have included safety and efficacy

TABLE 12-2. **Published Controlled Trials of Cardiac Resynchronization Therapy Alone or with an Implantable Cardioverter-Defibrillator (ICD)**

Study (Location)	Type and Duration of Trial	Enrollment (Publication) Dates	Inclusion Criteria	Endpoints	N*	Results
Multisite Stimulation in Cardiomyopathy Sinus Rhythm (MUSTIC SR) (Europe)	Prospective, randomized, single-blind crossover study of HF 3 mos	1998-1999 (2001)	NYHA class III, LVEF < 0.35, LVEDD > 60 mm, QRS ≥ 200 msec, 6MWD < 450 m	6MWD, peak Vo_2, QOL, NYHA class† Hospitalization, patient treatment preference, all-cause mortality, echocardiographic indices	67	Improvements in 6MWD, peak Vo_2, QOL, and NYHA class; reduced hospitalizations; patients preferred CRT
Multisite Stimulation in Cardiomyopathy Atrial Fibrillation (MUSTIC AF) (Europe)	Prospective, randomized, single-blind crossover VVIR-BiV study of HF 2-3 mos	1998-1999 (2002)	NYHA class > III, LVEF < 0.35, LVEDD > 60 mm, paced QRS ≥ 200 msec during ventricular pacing, 6MWD < 450 m	6MWD, peak Vo_2, QOL, NYHA class† Hospitalization, patient treatment preference, all-cause mortality, echocardiographic indices	59	Improvements in 6MWD, peak Vo_2, QOL, and NYHA class; reduced hospitalizations; patients preferred CRT
Pacing Therapies in Congestive Heart Failure (PATH-CHF) (Europe)	Longitudinal study of CRT with second placebo control phase; first and third periods are crossovers between LV and BiV 3 mos	1995-1998 (2002)	NYHA class III or IV, QRS > 120 msec, sinus rate ≥ 55 bpm, PR ≥ 150 msec	Peak Vo_2, 6MWD, NYHA class, QOL†	41	Improvements in exercise capacity, functional status, and QOL
PATH-CHF II (Europe)	Crossover randomized trial of no CRT vs. CRT in LV only; 2 patient groups: QRS 120-150 msec and QRS > 150 msec 3 mos	1998 (2003)	NYHA class II-IV, LVEF ≤ 0.30, QRS ≥ 120 msec, optimal therapy for HF; patients with ICDs may be included	Peak Vo_2, peak Vo_2 AT, 6MWD, QOL, NYHA class† Hospitalization	86	In group with QRS 120–150 msec, no improvement In group with QRS >150 msec, improvements in Vo_2, AT, 6MWD, and QOL
Multicenter InSync Randomized Clinical Evaluation (MIRACLE) (U.S.)	Prospective, randomized, double-blind, parallel, controlled trial 6 mos	1998-2000 (2002)	NYHA class III-IV, LVEF ≤ 0.35, LVEDD ≥ 55 mm, QRS ≥ 130 msec; patients with pacing indication not admitted; stable optimal medical therapy	NYHA class, 6MWD, QOL† Echocardiography indices, peak Vo_2, mortality, hospitalization, QRS duration, neurohormone levels	453	Improvements in NYHA class, 6MWD, QOL, LVEF, ventricular volumes, mitral regurgitation, peak Vo_2; reduced hospitalizations
Multicenter InSync ICD Randomized Clinical Evaluation—(MIRACLE-ICD) (U.S.)	Prospective, randomized, double-blind, parallel, controlled trial evaluating safety and efficacy of CRT in patients with HF and indication for ICD 6 mos	1999-2001 (2003)	NYHA class III-IV, LVEF ≤ 0.35, LVEDD ≥ 55 mm, QRS ≥ 130 msec, ICD indication	QOL, NYHA class, 6MWD† Peak Vo_2, exercise duration, HF composite (death, HF hospitalization, NYHA class, and patient global self assessment), safety of CRT-D	369	Improvements in QOL, NYHA class, and clinical composite endpoints; CRT-D safe to use
CONTAK CD (U.S.) Bi-Ventricular Pacing Study	Started as a 3-mo crossover between BiV CRT and no CRT; modified to 6-mo parallel, double-blind trial between CRT and no CRT, starting 1 mo after implantation 6 mos	1998-2001 (2003)	NYHA class II-IV, LVEF ≤ 0.35, QRS ≥ 120 msec; ICD indication; stable optimal medical therapy	Composite index: all-cause mortality, HF-related hospitalization, or VT/VF resulting in device therapy† Peak Vo_2, QOL, 6MWD, NYHA class, echocardiographic parameters, neurohormone levels	490	Primary endpoint not met; lead and system effectiveness and safety endpoints met; improvements in peak VO_2, 6MWD, QOL, and functional class in NYHA class III-IV patients

TABLE 12-2. **Published Controlled Trials of Cardiac Resynchronization Therapy Alone or with an Implantable Cardioverter-Defibrillator (ICD)—cont'd**

Study (Location)	Type and Duration of Trial	Enrollment (Publication) Dates	Inclusion Criteria	Endpoints	N*	Results
Comparison of Medical Therapy Pacing and Defibrillation in Heart Failure (COMPANION) (U.S.)	Randomized (1:2:2), open-label, 3-arm study to determine whether optimal drug therapy + CRT or drug therapy + CRT-D is superior to drug therapy alone	2000-2002 (2004)	NYHA class III or IV, LVEF ≤ 0.35, QRS ≥ 120 msec, PR > 150 msec, no indication for pacemaker or ICD HF hospitalization in the past year	Combined all-cause mortality and all-cause hospitalization† QOL, functional capacity, peak exercise performance, cardiac morbidity	1520	Stopped early owing to reduced all-cause mortality and hospitalization with CRT; reduced all-cause mortality with CRT-D
Cardiac Resynchronization in Heart Failure (CARE-HF) (Europe)	Open-label, randomized, controlled trial of CRT + optimal medical therapy vs. optimal medical therapy alone	2001-2003 (2004)	NYHA class III or IV, LVEF ≤ 0.35, LVEDD ≥ 30 mm/m (height), QRS > 50 msec or QRS ≥ 120 msec + echocardiographic criteria of dyssynchrony; stable optimal medical therapy	All-cause mortality or unplanned cardiovascular hospitalization† All-cause mortality, all-cause mortality or hospitalization for HF, NYHA class, QOL, echocardiographic LV function, neurohormone levels, economic impact	800	Improvements in morbidity and mortality/ cardiovascular hospitalization

*Accrual or accrual goals.

†Primary endpoint.

6MWD, 6-minute walk distance; AT, anaerobic threshold; AV, atrioventricular; BiV, biventricular; CRT, cardiac resynchronization therapy; CRT-D, CRT with defibrillator; ICD, implantable cardioverter-defibrillator; HF, heart failure; ICD, implantable cardioverter-defibrillator; LV, left ventricle; LVEDD, left ventricular end-diastolic diameter; NYHA class, New York Heart Association functional class; QOL, quality of life; RV, right ventricle; Vo_2, oxygen uptake; VF, ventricular fibrillation; VT, ventricular tachycardia.

Adapted from Saxon LA, De Marco T, Prystowsky EN, et al: Executive Summary: Resynchronization Therapy for Heart Failure. Executive Consensus Conference, May 8, 2002. Available online at http://www.hrsonline.org/positionDocs/CRT_12_3.pdf/

endpoints, the initial trials assessed only measures of heart failure functional status, LV systolic function (LVEF), and LV remodeling (LV end-systolic and diastolic dimensions). The later, larger studies targeted mortality and hospitalization endpoints (Table 12-3). The use of these multiple endpoint measures is standard for heart failure trials evaluating medical therapies and has created an interesting issue with regard to defining benefit from CRT.[1,6] One can define *response* as consisting only of symptom improvement or can require that all three of the measures of heart failure show benefit, as outlined in Table 12-3. To further complicate the issue, there does not appear to be a 1:1 correlation between these measures of response. As already described, the CONTAK CD and MIRACLE ICD studies enrolled patients with NYHA class II in addition to those with NYHA classes III and IV status. In the NYHA II group, significant improvements in measures of functional status were not uniformly observed, yet some of these patients experienced a positive reverse remodeling response.[7,14] Clearly, the therapy has a positive effect on decreasing LV size, but it does not affect symptom status that was not severely compromised at baseline. In spite of this improvement, the less symptomatic NYHA II subset of patients has not been well studied and is currently not included in FDA-labeled indications for CRT devices.[56]

TABLE 12-3. **Study Endpoints Evaluation in Trials of Cardiac Resynchronization Therapy Devices**

Measures of functional status	Quality of life 6-minute walk distance Cardiopulmonary exercise test
Measures of heart failure progression	Left ventricular ejection fraction, ventricular volume, dimension Mitral regurgitation Serum catecholamines, brain natriuretic protein, heart rate variability
Measures of heart failure outcome	Hospitalization Mortality

The Multisite Stimulation in Cardiomyopathy Studies

Published in 2001 and 2002, the MUSTIC European studies provided the first long-term controlled trial data on the efficacy of CRT, delivered as BiV stimulation, for 3-month intervals, in comparison with normal sinus rhythm or continuous RV-based pacing in AF.[3,54]

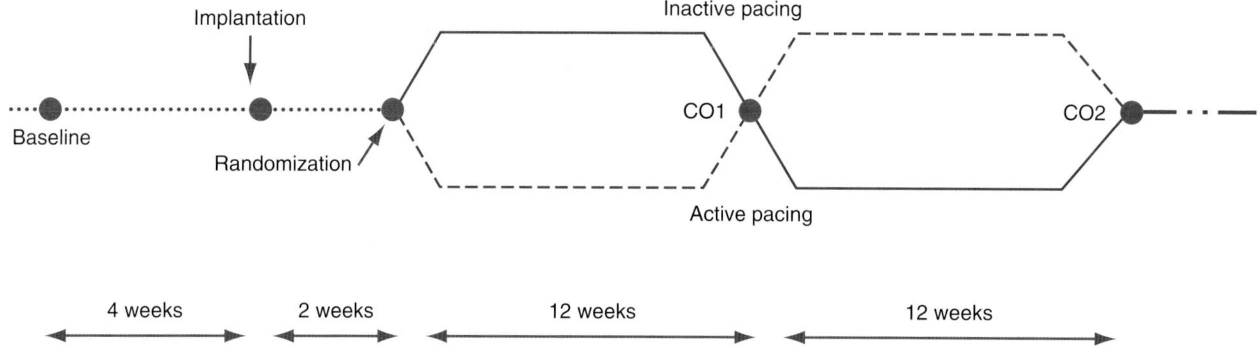

Figure 12-2. Patients were randomly assigned to 3 months each of inactive pacing (ventricular, inhibited at a basic rate of 40 beats per minute [bpm]) and active pacing (atriobiventricular). CO1 denotes the end of crossover period 1, and CO2 the end of crossover period 2. (From Cazeau S, Leclercq C, Lavergne T, et al: Multisite Stimulation in Cardiomyopathies (MUSTIC) Study Investigators: Effects of multisite biventricular pacing in patients with heart failure and intraventricular conduction delay. N Engl J Med Mar 22;344:873-880, 2001.)

Figure 12-2 illustrates the crossover study design of the MUSTIC and MUSTIC AF studies. Although only 48 patients completed the two 3-month crossover study periods, all leads placed in the trial were transvenous and there were no significant safety issues. Eligibility for patient enrollment included NYHA class III with a QRS duration longer than 150 msec. In those patients with normal sinus rhythm, quality of life (QOL) score improved by 32%, 6-minute walk distance (6MWD) improved by 23% and peak Vo_2 improved by 8%. Although the study was not statistically powered to determine a reduction in rate of hospitalization, hospitalizations after CRT initiation decreased by two thirds.[3] At the end of the crossover phase, patients (who were blinded to treatment) were asked to choose which 3-month period they preferred; 85% chose the pacing period during which they had been assigned to VDD, 10% had no preference, and 4% chose ODO (no pacing). Four patients had severe episodes of congestive heart failure exacerbation during the ODO pacing period.

In the patients with permanent AF and continuous RV pacing, 37 of 59 who underwent CRT implantation completed both 3-month crossover phases and had documentation of 97% to 100% CRT delivery. Because of the significant number of dropouts (42%), the intention-to-treat analysis did not show a significant improvement with CRT. In the 37 patients with a complete data set and documentation of CRT, QOL measure did not improve, but 6MWD and peak Vo_2 increased significantly by 9% ($P = .05$) and 13% ($P = .04$), respectively.[54] When the entire 6-month crossover phase is considered, 10 of 44 patients were hospitalized for heart failure decompensation during RV pacing, whereas only 3 patients were hospitalized for heart failure during the CRT period. Eighty-five percent of patients preferred the CRT period. There was a trend toward a better QOL among patients with CRT (11% improvement; $P = .09$). Subsequent uncontrolled trials in patients with permanent AF and continuous RV pacing have shown a more robust improvement in these measures as well as demonstrating a reverse remodeling response with CRT compared with RV pacing alone.[57,58] The PAVE trial (see later) also showed improvement with CRT but did not target patients with heart failure per se for enrollment.[55]

Pacing Therapies in Congestive Heart Failure

The two Pacing Therapies in Congestive Heart Failure (PATH I and II) European studies were groundbreaking in that chronic device programming was based on acute hemodynamic measures of cardiac performance. In addition, these same measures were used to optimize AV delay programming.[52,53] These trials were begun in 1995 and completed in 1998. They were performed in Europe and enrolled patients with NYHA III or IV congestive heart failure, sinus rate higher than 55 beats per minute (bpm), and QRS duration longer than 120 msec.

In PATH I, patients were crossed over between LV and BiV stimulation with a 1-month interval of no stimulation. A second study phase lasted 9 months and used the CRT mode that achieved what the follow-up physician determined was the most optimal mode. There were no differences in the acute or chronic response whether patients were programmed to LV or BiV CRT. Statistically significant improvements in peak Vo_2 anaerobic threshold (24% improvement; $P < =.001$), 6MWD (25% improvement; $P < .001$) and QOL (59% improvement; $P < .001$) were observed at 3 months and 12 months during follow-up. Twenty-one of 29 patients followed up to 12 months improved from NYHA class III or IV to class I or II. Heart failure hospitalizations were decreased from 76% in the year prior to implantation to 31% during the year after implantation. It should be noted that LBBB was the type of conduction delay in more than 87% of patients; most CRT trials enroll up to 30% of patients with either interventricular condition delay (IVCD) or RBBB.[4-6,9] This difference may account for the fact that LV stimulation in PATH I resulted only in an equivalent response to BiV stimulation to achieve CRT, although the study was not statistically powered to demonstrate a difference between the two modalities and the long-term data were pooled from both modes. The best that one can say is that in small numbers of patients who undergo hemodynamic optimization programming during implantation that shows equivalence between LV and BiV stimulation to achieve CRT, long-term symptom responses appear to be equivalent.

Extending the observations from PATH I, PATH II evaluated LV-only CRT compared with no CRT in a 3-month crossover design.[53] In all patients with LBBB (88% of subjects), LV pacing was identified as the optimal single-chamber pacing mode (compared with RV only) on the basis of immediate hemodynamic response, and AV delay timing was optimized in all patients. Patients were further divided by QRS duration according to whether the QRS was more than 120 msec but less than 150 msec ("short QRS") or more than 150 msec ("long QRS"). Unfortunately, only 35 patients, slightly less than one half of all patients enrolled, completed both 3-month crossover intervals. Nonetheless, the study did demonstrate improvements in peak Vo_2, anaerobic threshold, 6MWD, and QOL score in the patients with long QRS duration. For example, 71% of patients in the long QRS group and 38% of patients in the short QRS group had an increase in the peak oxygen uptake of more than 1 mL/kg/min with active pacing. The short QRS group did not have an improvement in peak oxygen uptake or any other endpoint measure. This was the first study to demonstrate that QRS duration predicts the magnitude of symptom response to CRT delivered as LV-only stimulation. Subgroup analysis of all but one of the larger U.S. long-term studies of BiV CRT has also suggested that the magnitude of benefit may be greater in patients with longer QRS duration at baseline.[5,7,8-10]

Multicenter InSync Randomized Clinical Evaluation

The Multicenter InSync Randomized Clinical Evaluation (MIRACLE) study was the only U.S. trial of CRT for heart failure that used a CRT device only.[5] The numbers of patients randomly allocated in U.S. clinical trials was much greater those in the European trials until the CARE-HF trial (see later). All 453 patients enrolled in the MIRACLE study underwent implantation of the CRT device and were then randomly assigned to "CRT on" or "CRT off" status for a period of 6 months. Figure 12-3 illustrates the study design of the MIRACLE, MIRACLE ICD, and CONTAK CD U.S. trials. Unlike the COMPANION trial (see later), in which patients were randomly assigned after consent was obtained and before device implantation, these earlier U.S. trials randomly assigned patients only after a successful CRT implant. The U.S. trials also employed strict protocol-mandated criteria relative to appropriate and stable heart failure medical regimen requirements prior to consent and device implantation.

The primary endpoints, including 6MWD, QOL score, and NYHA class, were all favorably influenced by CRT, and the effects of CRT were apparent as early as 1 month after therapy initiation. Patients who underwent CRT showed 13% improvement in 6MWD, 13% improvement in QOL, a roughly 1 mL/kg/min improvement in exercise capacity, and an increase in total exercise time of approximately 60 seconds. Unlike in the

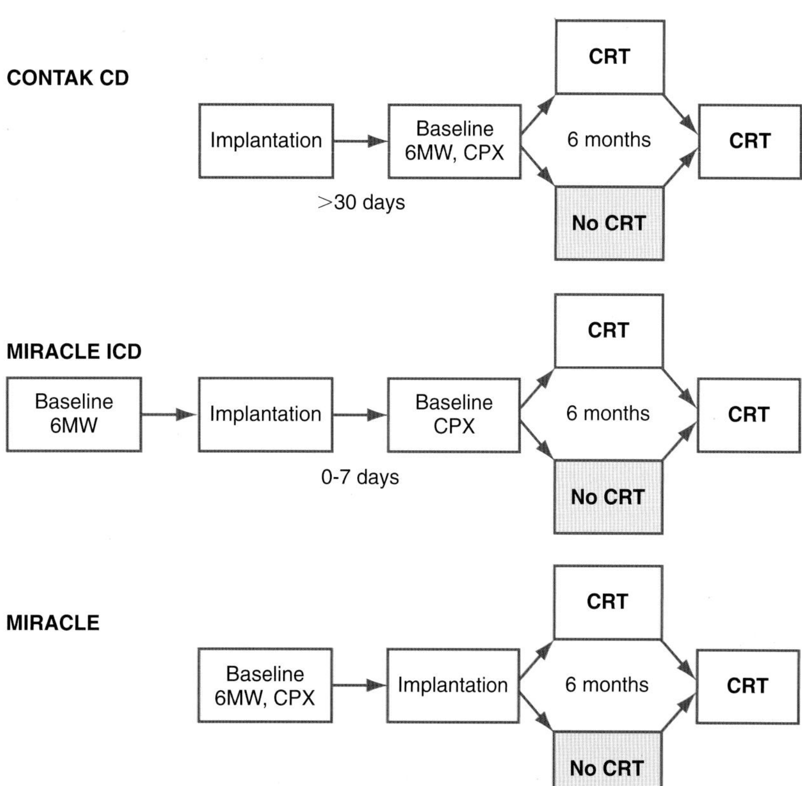

Figure 12-3. Study design of three U.S. trials: CONTAK CD Biventricular Pacing Study (CONTAK CD), Multicenter InSync ICD [implantable cardioverter-defibrillator] Randomized Clinical Evaluation (MIRACLE ICD), and Multicenter InSync Randomized Clinical Evaluation (MIRACLE). 6MW, 6-mile walk distance; CPX, cardiopulmonary exercise test; CRT, cardiac resynchronization therapy.

European and acute hemodynamic studies, neither baseline QRS duration nor type of bundle branch block influenced response to CRT in the MIRACLE study. The secondary endpoints, of Vo_2 and LVEF, also improved with CRT, as did episodes of heart failure worsening, including heart failure hospitalizations. At 6 months, CRT was associated with a reduction in LV end-diastolic and end-systolic volumes, reduced LV mass, increased ejection fraction (+3.6%), reduction in mitral regurgitation jet area (−2.5 cm^2), and improvement in the myocardial index. Improvements in LV end-diastolic volume and ejection fraction were twofold greater in patients with nonischemic cardiomyopathy.

CONTAK CD and Multicenter InSync ICD Randomized Clinical Evaluation

Concurrent with the MIRACLE trial enrollment, two large-scale trials of CRT-D for patients with heart failure and either primary or secondary indications for an ICD were also enrolling subjects. These were the Multicenter InSync ICD Randomized Clinical Evaluation (MIRACLE ICD) and the CONTAK CD Biventricular Pacing Study. Unlike in the MIRACLE study, the 950 patients randomly assigned to different therapies in the CRT-D studies had primarily ischemic cardiomyopathy (61% to 75%,[7,8]) and roughly one half of the patients had a secondary indication for the ICD. In patients with NYHA class III to IV status, both studies demonstrated improvements in functional measures of heart failure status. In the CONTAK CD study, patients with NYHA class II status did not experience benefit in all measures of functional status. Neither study showed a difference in the incidence of treated episodes of VT/VF with CRT on or off, indicating a neutral effect of CRT on the arrhythmia substrate early after device implantation. A subsequent analysis of the MIRACLE ICD study data indicated that patients with secondary ICD indications experienced more ICD therapies for VT, whereas those with primary ICD indications had more therapy for VF.[60] The incidence of ICD therapy was, as expected, higher in those with secondary prevention indications. In CONTAK CD, the incidence of ICD therapy over the 6-month follow-up interval was 16% for both VT and VF.

Improvements in LVEF and ventricular size and dimension and degree of mitral regurgitation were noted in the VIGOR-CHF, MIRACLE, MIRACLE ICD, and CONTAK CD studies, all of which had central core echocardiographic laboratories performing echocardiographic analysis with excellent intraobserver and interobserver variability.[19,41] As mentioned earlier, even the patients with NYHA class II benefited from CRT in terms of an echocardiographic response of reverse remodeling.[7,14] These CRT-related effects were independent of the use of β-blocker therapy.[19] This finding suggests that CRT can exert beneficial effects on the remodeling process across a spectrum of heart failure severity, much like that observed with angiotensin-converting enzyme (ACE) inhibitor therapy.[1] Subsequent study of the effects of CRT on ventricular function, volume, and dimension have shown that the beneficial effects occur as early as 4 weeks and are sustained for a time even after CRT is suspended, indicating that CRT affects cardiac structure.[61]

Another measure of heart failure progression, level of plasma neurohormones, did not improve or worsen with CRT in the MIRACLE ICD or MIRACLE study. This neutral effect may be due to the fact that medical therapy with neurohormonal antagonists was optimized before device implantation or the possibility that the duration of follow-up may have been inadequate.[7]

Comparison of Medical Therapy, Pacing, and Defibrillation on Heart Failure Study

The Comparison of Medical Therapy, Pacing, and Defibrillation on Heart Failure (COMPANION) study was the first and only U.S. trial statistically powered to assess the impact of CRT on hospitalization and mortality endpoints.[9,62] At the time of the COMPANION study design, it was unclear whether ICD therapy in addition to CRT would reduce mortality in advanced heart failure in comparison with medical therapy. Therefore, the study randomly assigned patients to optimal medical therapy for heart failure (OPT), a CRT device alone, or a CRT with an ICD (CRT-D). The patients were assigned in a 1:2:2 ratio, respectively, to maximize the number of patients receiving devices. There was not sufficient statistical power to directly compare CRT with CDT-D (both were compared with OPT), but the highest-order secondary endpoint was mortality. In order to enrich the anticipated event rate in the trial, patients were additionally required to have been hospitalized for heart failure in the year prior to enrollment but to be receiving stable medical therapy at enrollment and to have no history of hospitalization in the month preceding enrollment. Unlike the prior trials of CRT, patients were assigned for therapy and data were analyzed after they had provided informed consent, not after they had undergone a successful implantation. The design of the COMPANION study is provided in Figure 12-4. The clinical characteristics of COMPANION patients are listed in Table 12-4. Like MIRACLE study patients, and unlike the patients in the CRT-D studies, an equal proportion of patients in the COMPANION study had both ischemic and nonischemic etiologies for LV dysfunction. This was the first trial to enroll patients with advanced heart failure who were medically treated with “triple therapy,” consisting of angiotensin-converting enzyme inhibitors, β-receptor blockers, and aldosterone antagonists.

The primary study endpoint was a composite of all-cause hospitalization and mortality. The primary secondary endpoint was mortality. A total of 1520 patients were enrolled. Figure 12-5 shows the event-free survival curves for the primary and secondary endpoints and demonstrates the 20% 12-month reductions in death or hospitalization from any cause observed with both CRT and CRT-D devices compared with OPT. It is also noteworthy that the risk of one of these events was 68% in OPT patients, attesting to the severity of heart failure in this population. The CRT device did reduce mortality by 24%, but this reduction was not statistically significant

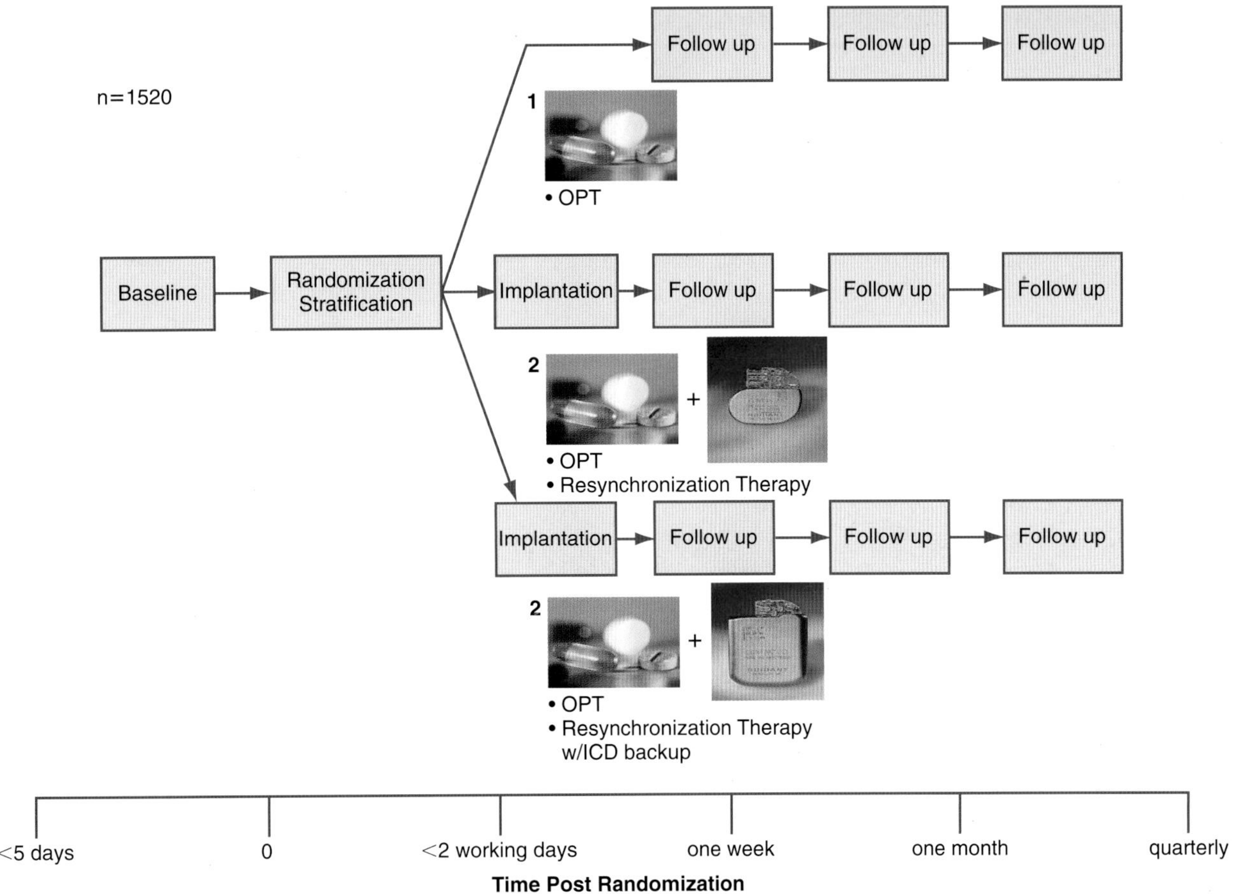

Figure 12-4. Study design of the Comparison of Medical Therapy, Pacing, and Defibrillation on Heart Failure (COMPANION) study. ICD, implantable cardioverter-defibrillator; OPT, optimal medical therapy.

($P = .06$). The CRT-D device alone reduced mortality by 36% ($P = .003$) compared with OPT. Close inspection of the mortality curves shows that CRT survival parallels OPT survival until 6 months, when CRT shows benefit. In contrast, the CRT-D and OPT curves separate immediately. These observations may be interpreted as follows: The ICD portion of the CRT-D has an immediate effect to prevent sudden arrhythmic deaths, whereas the reductions in sudden death with CRT alone may be mediated through stabilization of heart failure status, which may be time dependent. Subsequent analysis showed that the reduction in mortality with CRT-D was due to a reduction in sudden cardiac death as adjudicated by an events committee.[62]

Subgroup analyses were remarkably consistent in demonstrating CRT benefit in all patient subgroups. There appeared to be equal benefit in women and men, in either ischemic or nonischemic etiologies of heart failure, regardless of LVEF greater or less than 20% (0.20) and LV size greater or less than 67 mm. Those patients with longer QRS duration did appear to experience greater benefit with CRT, as did those with LBBB rather than RBBB or IVCD. Figure 12-6 provides the subgroup analysis from the COMPANION study, comparing CRT and CRT-D with OPT therapy for the primary and secondary endpoints.

The COMPANION data expand the role of CRT to achieve the three primary therapeutic goals in treating patients with heart failure—to improve symptoms, to retard disease progression, and to reduce rates of hospitalization and mortality. There are two primary reasons for selecting a CRT-D over CRT alone. The COMPANION data support early sudden death protection with CRT-D, and the majority of patients with CRT indications also have ICD indications in single-chamber primary prevention ICD trials.[16,17] In an abstract presentation of the ICD discharge rate in COMPANION, the 12-month appropriate ICD therapy rate was reported to be 15%, suggesting that the risk of development of a potentially fatal, ventricular arrhythmia is significant in the first year after CRT.[63]

Cardiac Resynchronization–Heart Failure Study

The Cardiac Resynchronization–Heart Failure (CARE-HF) study, enrolling 813 patients at 82 European centers, compared CRT only with optimal medical therapy.[10] Over a mean follow-up of 29 months, CRT resulted in significant reductions in the primary composite endpoint of death or cardiovascular hospitalization. Additionally, reductions in the secondary

TABLE 12-4. **Clinical Characteristics of the 1520 COMPANION Study Patients***

Characteristic	Optimal Pharmacologic Therapy (N = 308)	Cardiac Resynchronization Therapy	
		Pacemaker (N = 617)	Pacemaker-Defibrillator (N = 595)
Age (yrs)	68	67	66
Male sex (%)	69	67	67
NYHA class III (%)	82	87	86
Duration of heart failure (yrs)	3.6	3.7	3.5
LV ejection fraction	0.22	0.20	0.22
LV end-diastolic dimension (mm)	67	68	67
Heart rate (bpm)	72	72	72
Blood pressure (mm Hg):			
Systolic	112	110	112
Diastolic	64	68	68
Distance walked in 6 min (m)	244	274	258
QRS interval (msec)	158	160	160
Ischemic cardiomyopathy (%)	59	54	55
Diabetes (%)	45	39	41
Bundle branch block (%):			
Left	70	69	73
Right	9	12	10
Pharmacologic therapy (%):			
ACE inhibitor†	69	70	69
ACE inhibitor or angiotensin-receptor blocker†	89	89	90
β-blocker	66	68	68
Loop diuretic	94	94	97
Spironolactone	55	53	55

*Median values are given for continuous measures. There were no significant differences among the groups.
†Patients who could not tolerate an ACE inhibitor received an angiotensin-receptor blocker.
ACE, angiotensin-converting enzyme; COMPANION, Comparison of Medical Therapy, Pacing, and Defibrillation in Heart Failure trial; LV, left ventricular; NYHA class, New York Heart Association functional class.
Adapted from Bristow MR, Saxon LA, Boehmer J, et al: Comparison of Medical Therapy, Pacing, and Defibrillation in Heart Failure (COMPANION) Investigators: Cardiac-resynchronization therapy with or without an implantable defibrillator in advanced chronic heart failure. N Engl J Med 350:2140-2150, 2004.

endpoint of mortality were achieved. Figure 12-7 illustrates the Kaplan-Meier curves for these endpoints.

Comparing CARE-HF with COMPANION, we observe that the COMPANION patients appear to have been a somewhat sicker group, perhaps owing to the requirement for a heart failure hospitalization in the year prior to enrollment.[9] The 12-month mortality rate in the medical therapy group in CARE-HF was 12.6%, versus 19% in COMPANION. Only 38% of the patients in CARE-HF had coronary artery disease, compared with 56% in COMPANION; the mean LV ejection fraction was 25% in CARE-HF, compared with 21% in COMPANION; and a higher percentage of patients in COMPANION had NYHA class IV status (16% vs. 6.5% in CARE-HF). Another issue is the positive effect of CRT on mortality in CARE-HF. The relative risk reduction with CRT in CARE-HF patients was equivalent to that of the COMPANION CRT-D patients (36%). The CRT group in the COMPANION study did show a 24% reduction in mortality, but this was not statistically significant ($P = .06$). These differences may be due to the shorter duration of follow-up in the COMPANION study, meaning that if follow-up had been longer in COMPANION, the value would have reached significance. Another important question is the risk of sudden death in the CARE-HF patients given CRT. Although only 7% of deaths in CRT patients in CARE-HF were adjudicated as sudden, these accounted for 37% of all deaths, and COMPANION data indicate such deaths may have been prevented with a CRT-D device.[62]

Several other important issues were answered by CARE-HF. The advantages of CRT over best medical management appear to increase over time, at least to 18 months. Before this trial, follow-up past 12 months was

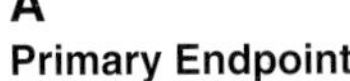

A
Primary Endpoint

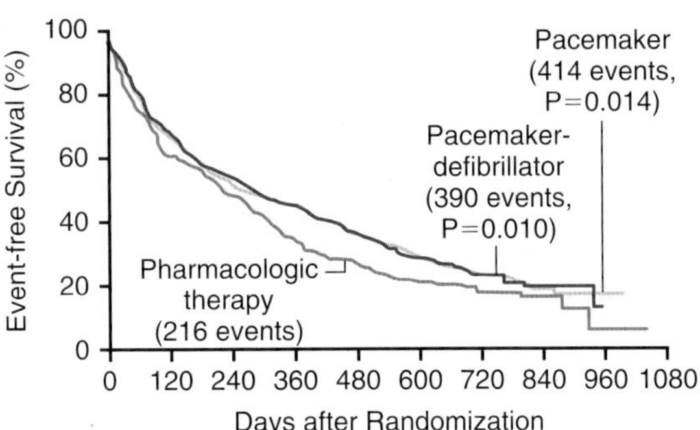

No. at Risk

Pharmacologic therapy	308	176	115	72	46	24	16	6	1
Pacemaker	617	384	294	228	146	73	36	14	3
Pacemaker-defibrillator	595	385	283	217	128	61	25	8	0

B
Secondary Endpoint

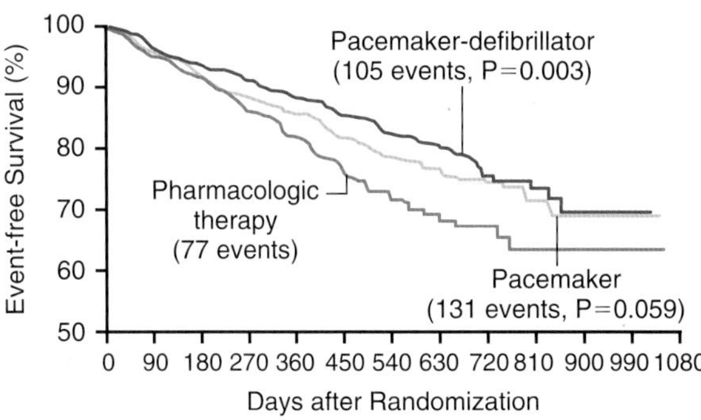

No. at Risk

Pharmacologic therapy	308	284	255	217	186	141	94	57	45	25	4	2
Pacemaker	617	579	520	488	439	355	251	164	104	60	25	5
Pacemaker-defibrillator	595	555	517	470	420	331	219	148	95	47	21	1

C
Death from or Hospitalization for Cardiovascular Causes

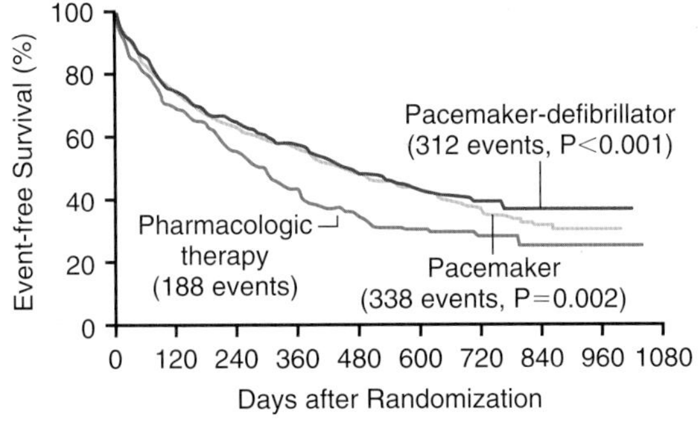

No. at Risk

Pharmacologic therapy	308	199	134	91	56	29	20	8	2
Pacemaker	617	431	349	282	194	102	51	22	5
Pacemaker-defibrillator	595	425	341	274	167	89	45	20	3

D
Death from or Hospitalization for Heart Failure

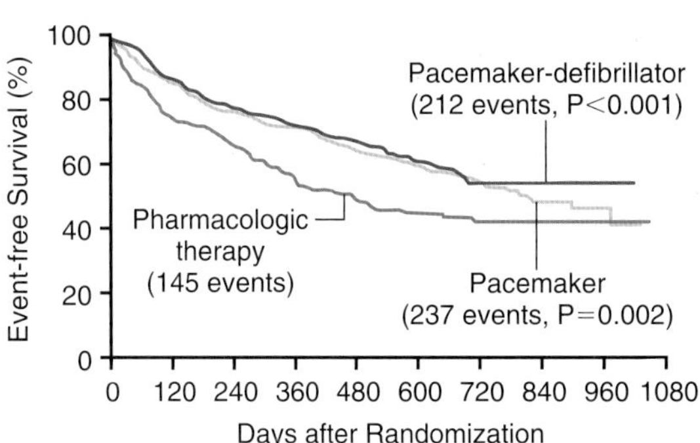

No. at Risk

Pharmacologic therapy	308	216	161	118	76	39	28	11	2
Pacemaker	617	498	422	355	258	142	75	35	9
Pacemaker-defibrillator	595	497	411	343	228	131	71	27	5

*Figure 12-5. Kaplan-Meier estimates of the time to the primary endpoint of death from or hospitalization for any cause (**A**), the time to the secondary endpoint of death from any cause (**B**), the time to death from or hospitalization for cardiovascular causes (**C**), and the time to death from or hospitalization for heart failure (**D**) in the Comparison of Medical Therapy, Pacing, and Defibrillation in Heart Failure (COMPANION) study. In **A**, The 12-month rates of death from or hospitalization for any cause—the primary endpoint—were 68% in the pharmacologic therapy group, 56% in the group that received a pacemaker as part of cardiac resynchronization therapy, and 56% in the group that received a pacemaker-defibrillator as part of cardiac resynchronization therapy. In **B**, the 12-month rates of death from any cause—the secondary endpoint—were 19% in the pharmacologic therapy group, 15% in the pacemaker group, and 12% in the pacemaker-defibrillator group. In Panel **C**, the 12-month rates of death from or hospitalization for cardiovascular causes were 60% in the pharmacologic therapy group, 45% in the pacemaker group, and 44% in the pacemaker-defibrillator group. In Panel **D**, the 12-month rates of death from or hospitalization for heart failure were 45% in the pharmacologic therapy group, 31% in the pacemaker group, and 29% in the pacemaker-defibrillator group. In the pharmacologic therapy group, death from heart failure made up 24% of the events, hospitalization for heart failure 72% of events, and the intravenous administration of inotropes or vasoactive drugs for more than 4 hours 4% of events. P values are for comparison with optimal pharmacologic therapy. (From Bristow MR, Saxon LA, Boehmer J, et al: Comparison of Medical Therapy, Pacing, and Defibrillation in Heart Failure (COMPANION) Investigators: Cardiac-resynchronization therapy with or without an implantable defibrillator in advanced chronic heart failure. N Engl J Med 20;350:2140-2150, 2004.)*

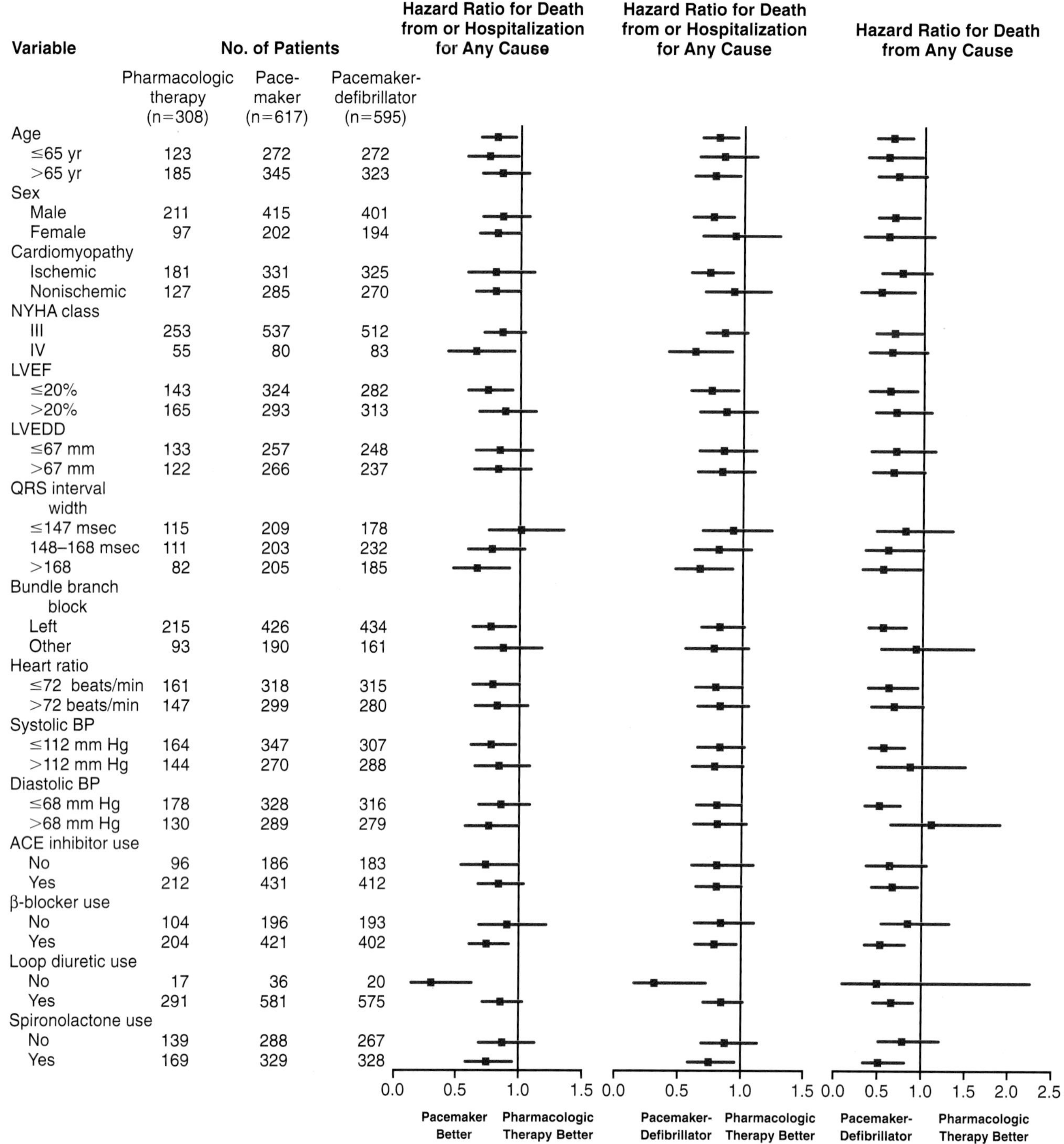

Figure 12-6. Hazard ratios and 95% confidence intervals for the primary endpoint, death from or hospitalization for any cause, and the secondary endpoint, death from any cause, according to the baseline characteristics of the patients in the Comparison of Medical Therapy, Pacing, and Defibrillation in Heart Failure (COMPANION) study. Echocardiographically determined values for left ventricular end-diastolic dimension (LVEDD) were not available for all patients. ACE, angiotensin-converting enzyme; BP, blood pressure; LVEF, left ventricular ejection fraction; NYHA, New York Heart Association functional class. (From Bristow MR, Saxon LA, Boehmer J, et al: Comparison of Medical Therapy, Pacing, and Defibrillation in Heart Failure (COMPANION) Investigators: Cardiac-resynchronization therapy with or without an implantable defibrillator in advanced chronic heart failure. N Engl J Med 350:2140-2150, 2004.)

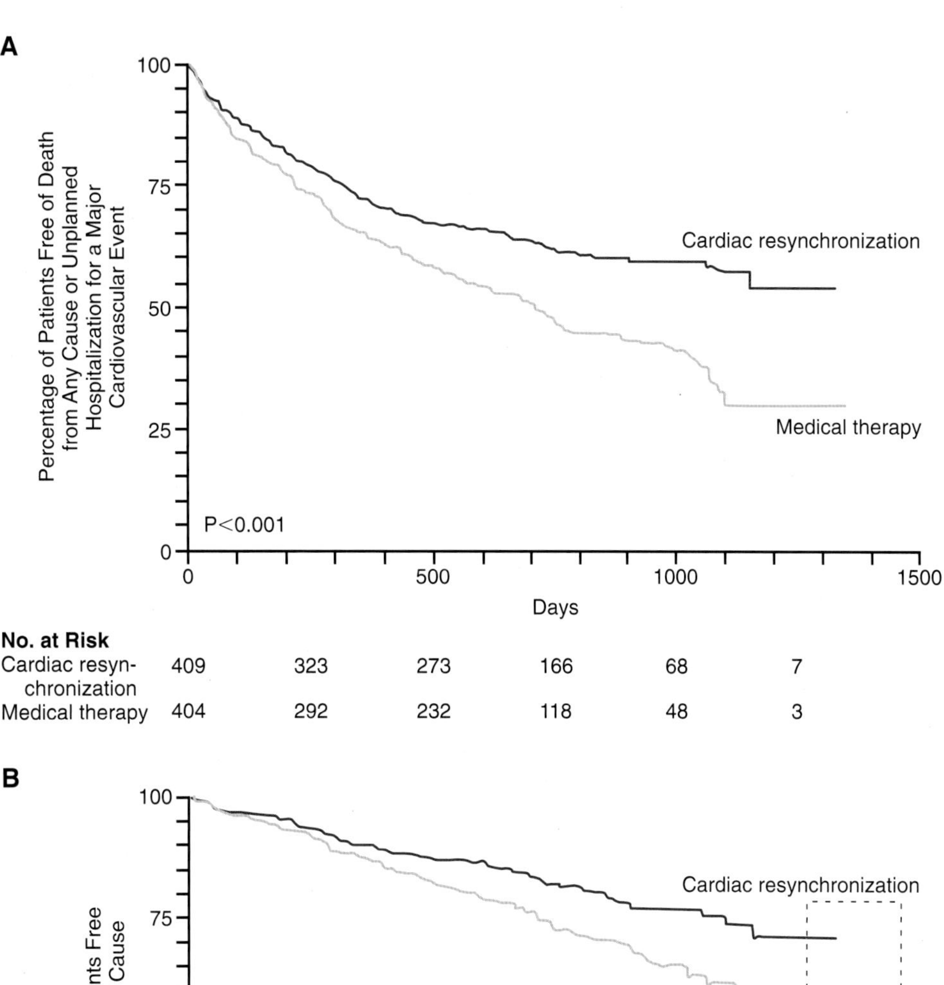

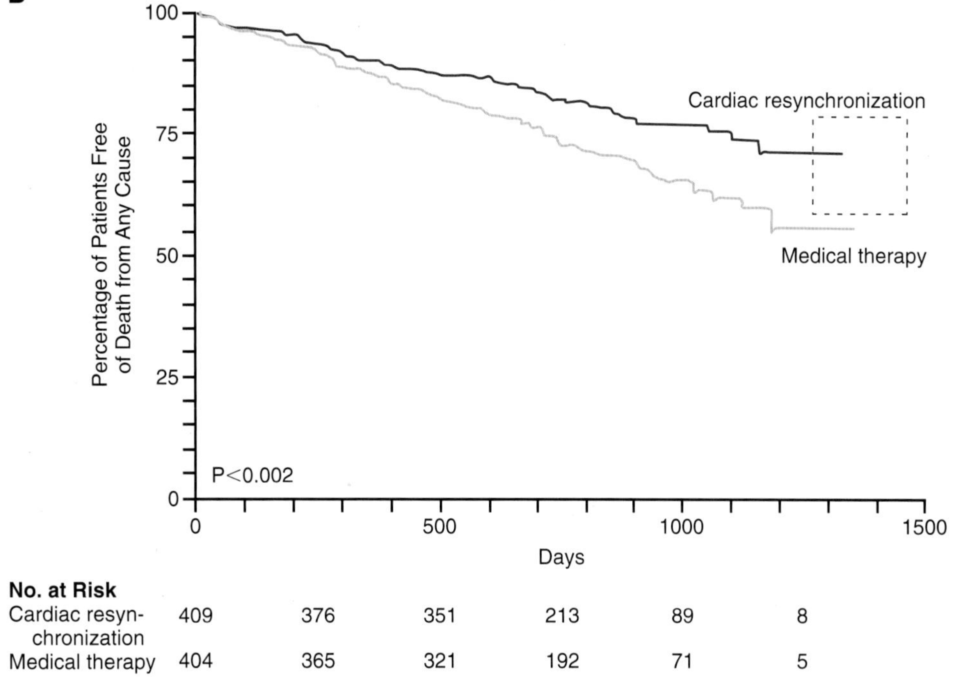

*Figure 12-7. Kaplan-Meier estimates of the time to the primary endpoint (**A**) and the principal secondary outcome (**B**) in the Cardiac Resynchronization–Heart Failure (CARE-HF) study. The primary outcome was death from any cause or an unplanned hospitalization for a major cardiovascular event. The principal secondary outcome was death from any cause. (From Cleland JG, Daubert JC, Erdmann E, et al: Cardiac Resynchronization-Heart Failure [CARE-HF] Study Investigators: The effect of cardiac resynchronization on morbidity and mortality in heart failure. N Engl J Med 352:1539-1549, 2005.)*

available for too few patients undergoing CRT. This is the first large trial to demonstrate benefit with respect to biomarker measurements as a surrogate of congestive heart failure severity with CRT. A nonsignificant decrease in *N*-terminal pro-brain natriuretic peptide (NT-BNP) was noted at 3 months, but by 18 months, there was a dramatic decrease of more than 1100 pg/mL (P = .0016). Finally, CARE-HF was the first large clinical trial to select patients on the basis of either a wide QRS >149 msec or a wide QRS >120 msec and the presence of additional dyssynchrony markers. It is likely that the selection of patients for CRT using measures of dyssynchrony served to better identify candidates for CRT and improve the response rate and outcome for patients in this trial.

Procedural Safety and LV lead Performance

In all of the clinical trials subsequent to the PATH I study and in patients enrolled early in the CONTAK CD study,

LV lead placement was performed through a coronary sinus branch vein with an over-the-wire unipolar lead. In general, lateral LV wall sites were chosen on the basis of results of trials of short-term implants demonstrating that the most robust hemodynamic response is located at this site in patients with LBBB.[48]

Figures 12-8 and 12-9 illustrate radiographs of CRT systems implanted long-term using two over-the-wire LV leads from two different manufacturers with a CRT and a CRT-D device. In both, the LV lead is in a lateral branch vein. In Figure 12-9, two RV defibrillating leads are shown because there was an insulation break in the long-term RV lead and a new one was placed at the time of CRT implantation.

Despite initial concerns about the additional risk of LV branch vein lead placement, particularly given the additional skills required for the procedure and extensive anatomic remodeling that occurs in the setting of advanced heart failure, which renders access to the coronary sinus and its branch veins more challenging, the procedural safety and LV lead performance have been very good. Table 12-5 lists the procedural safety and LV lead performance data observed in the long-term CRT studies. A learning curve does appear to be involved in CRT implantation, and the CONTAK CD study found the threshold for attaining a higher than 95% rate of successful LV implantation was 15 cases.[64]

The most common complication of LV lead placement is coronary sinus trauma, which occurs at a rate of 2% to 4%; and the incidence of true perforation resulting in cardiac tamponade is less than 1%. LV lead dislodgement requiring repositioning occurs in 1% to 3% of implants. Diaphragmatic stimulation requiring reoperation for lead repositioning occurs in 1% to 4% of cases, but this risk has been lowered with the introduction of bipolar LV leads.

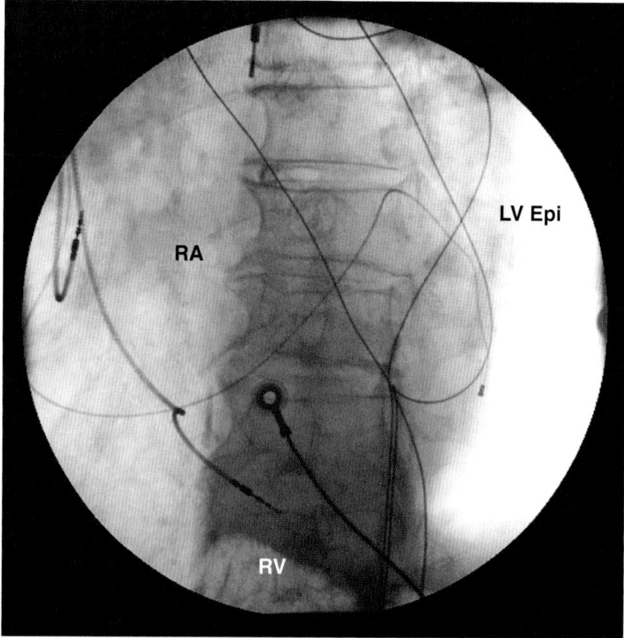

LAO

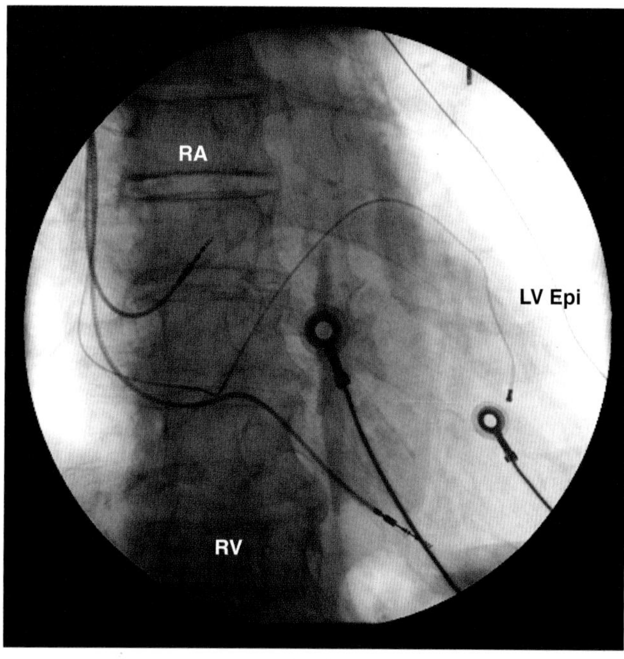

RAO

Figure 12-8. Left anterior oblique (LAO) and right anterior oblique (RAO) radiographs of a cardiac resynchronization therapy system implanted for long-term treatment. LV Epi, left ventricular epicardial lead; RA, right atrial lead; RV, right ventricular lead.

Trials of Long-Term Cardiac Resynchronization Therapy in Special Populations

The Post AV Nodal Ablation Evaluation Study

The Post AV Nodal Ablation Evaluation (PAVE) study compared CRT with RV pacing in patients with permanent AF who were undergoing AV nodal ablation.[55] Entry criteria for the study did not require patients to have symptomatic heart failure or systolic dysfunction. However, patients were required to have exercise limitation, defined as the inability to walk farther than 450 meters during a 6MWD test, which was also the primary study endpoint. Peak Vo_2 and QOL were assessed as secondary endpoints.

A total of 252 patients were randomly assigned to either CRT or RV pacing; 205 patients (mean age 69 years, 64% male, 51% NYHA class II, 32% NYHA class III, 46% with LVEF <0.45) completed 6 months of follow-up. Forty-seven patients (19%) were withdrawn before completing the 6-month follow-up, mostly owing to unsuccessful LV lead implantation (n = 21) or death (n = 16). Compared with RV pacing, which also produced improvements in the study endpoints, CRT resulted in greater 6MWD improvement (25.5 m), Vo_2 increase (2 mL/kg/min), and QOL improvements. Improvements in LVEF were observed with CRT but not with RV pacing (P = .03). In patients with LVEF values

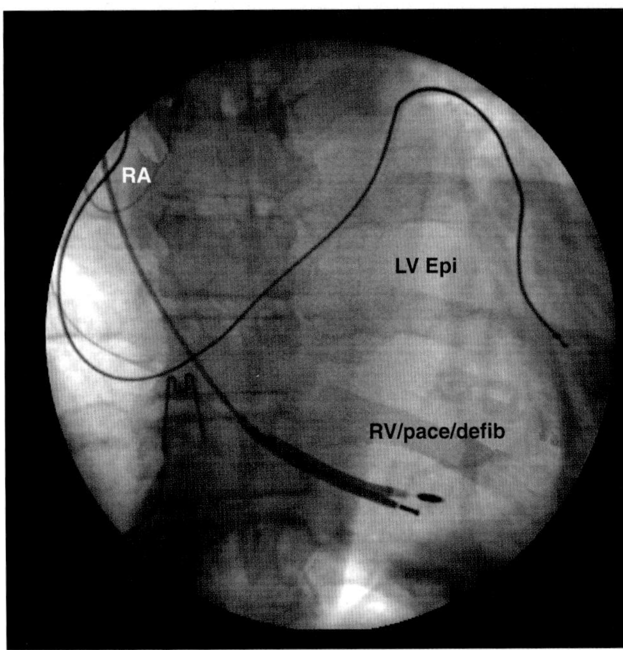

Figure 12-9. Radiograph of a cardiac resynchronization therapy system implanted for long-term treatment. LV Epi, left ventricular epicardial lead; RA, right atrial lead; RV/pace/defib, right ventricle defibrillating lead.

of 0.45 or less, the improvement in 6MWD in the CRT group was statistically significantly higher, by 41.0 m, than that in the RV pacing group (P = .04), and QOL measurements were higher as well. The magnitude of improvement was also more marked in patients with NYHA class II or III in 6MWD. In all cases, symptoms and walk distance improved immediately after CRT and continued to improve throughout the 6-month follow-up. In patients with LVEF values greater than 0.45 or NYHA class I status, CRT had no advantage over RV pacing in QOL improvements. More subjects in the RV pacing group died, but the difference was not statistically significant (P = .16).

We can conclude from this trial that CRT does provide greater improvement than RV pacing in the functional status of patients undergoing AV nodal ablation if they have significant baseline limitation of exercise capacity.

Trials Evaluating Device Features and Programming

A number of ongoing or completed clinical trials have evaluated the use of CRT device features or programming options. Some features, such as atrial antitachycardia pacing and defibrillation, are available in an FDA-approved RV ICD and have been tested for safety and efficacy in a CRT device.[23] In other cases, such as studies evaluating the usefulness of RV/LV offset programming for CRT, the feature is specific to a CRT device and intended to maximize response to therapy.[65-69]

In the Multicenter RENEWAL 3 AVT Clinical Study of Cardiac Resynchronization Defibrillator Therapy in Patients with Atrial Fibrillation (RENEWAL AVT study), the safety and efficacy of a CRT-D device capable of advanced atrial therapies and diagnostics, including atrial defibrillation, was tested in a CRT device.[23] In this single-arm study, enrolling 138 patients with a history of paroxysmal or persistent AF in the year prior to enrollment, the delivery of atrial and ventricular antitachycardia therapies was not compromised by the delivery of CRT. Conversely, CRT did not adversely affect the delivery of tachycardia therapies. Figure 12-10 shows an instance of AF occurring in the presence of ventricular fibrillation. In this instance, both atrial and ventricular diagnostics and therapies were programmed "on." The device correctly sensed both the atrial and ventricular fibrillation and prioritized treatment of ventricular fibrillation with a 17-J shock, which converted the rhythm to atrially paced CRT.

The Device Evaluation of CONTAK RENEWAL 2 and EASYTRAK 2: Assessment of Safety and Effectiveness in Heart Failure (DECREASE-HF) and the Rhythm ICD V-V Optimization Phase (Rhythm ICD) studies were designed to assess the effects of LV only or V-V offset against simultaneous BiV stimulation to achieve CRT.[65-67] The study endpoints are measures of functional status. In each study, an echocardiographic assessment is performed to determine the effects of the method of CRT delivery on cardiac function. Presented but not published, the results of the Rhythm ICD study suggest that greater long-term benefit in functional endpoint measures can be achieved with individualized short-term, echocardiographic assessment of best CRT method and that in most instances this method is not simultaneous BiV CRT but, rather, RV/LV offset pacing.[69] However, this study enrolled a relatively small number of patients (72) and was statistically powered to show only equivalence of alternative CRT delivery to BiV stimulation and not to detect differences between the groups. Currently, V-V timing offset is offered in two FDA-approved CRT devices. The data in support of this method of CRT delivery come from a substudy of the MIRACLE ICD study.[56]

The issue of long-term AV delay programming has not been systematically evaluated in clinical trials of long-term CRT, uncontrolled data on short- and long-term therapies based largely on echocardiographic assessment of LV filling profile and forward output have shown that for most subjects, AV delay programming during atrial sensing is optimal at 100 to 130 msec, although there are some exceptions.[20,45] One report demonstrated that altering programming in implanted CRT devices from atrially sensed VDD stimulation to DDD stimulation actually worsened intraventricular LV synchrony and curtailed LV filling and worsened the myocardial performance index, a measure of systolic and diastolic function.[67,68] These effects are most likely due to delay in intra-atrial conduction times. Compared to atrial sensing, pacing from a long-term implanted right atrial lead results in delayed left atrial to LV contraction. This is a very important observation, in that it suggests that

TABLE 12-5. Procedure Safety and LV Lead Performance in Clinical Trials of Cardiac Resynchronization Therapy

			Trial			
Parameter	**MUSTIC**	**MIRACLE**	**CONTAK CD**	**MIRACLE ICD**	**COMPANION**†	**CARE-HF**
No subjects	64	528*	289	421	1212	409
Rate of successful implantation (%):						
At first attempt	90	NA	87	NA	NA	86
Total	92	NA*	NA	88	89	95
Procedure Length (hrs)		2.7*			2.7	
Implantation problems (%):						
Failure	8	NA	13	12	11	5
Coronary	NA	NA	2	4	3	2.4
Sinus trauma						
Deaths	0	0.7	0	0	0.08	—
Other	4.5	—	15.2	38	—	1.5
Late complications (%):						
LV lead dislodgement /replacement	13.6	6*	6.8	8.6	4	6
Extracardiac stimulation	12		1.6	3	1.5	—
Pocket infection	3.4	1.3*	0	0	3.1	2.6
Loss of capture	0	—	0	0	0.2	—
Death	0	0.1	0	0	0.6	0.2
Other	3.4	—	1.8	1.3	—	—
Pacing thresholds (volts @ 0.5 msec ± SD):						
At implantation	1.36 ± 0.96	NA	NA	1.5-1.7 (Model 4189) 1.7-2.3 (Models 218 7/8)	2.1 ± 1.0	—
Long-term	2.4 (3 mos)	NA	1.8 ± 1.2 (13 mos)	NA	2.4 ± 1.8	—

*Patients followed up only after successful implantation.
†Cardiac resynchronization therapy with and without defibrillator treatment.
CARE-HF, Cardiac Resynchronization in Heart Failure; COMPANION, Comparison of Medical Therapy, Pacing, and Defibrillation in Heart Failure; CONTAK CD, CONTAK CD Biventricular Pacing Study; LV, left ventricular; MIRACLE, Multicenter InSync Randomized Clinical Evaluation; MIRACLE ICD, Multicenter InSync ICD [implantable cardioverter-defibrillator] Randomized Clinical Evaluation; MUSTIC, Multisite Stimulation in Cardiomyopathy; NA = not available.

echocardiographic evaluation and repeated AV delay optimization may be indicated in patients with CRT devices requiring atrial rate support to ensure that CRT efficacy is not compromised.

Enhancing Response to Cardiac Resynchronization Therapy

Depending on how response is defined, the major clinical trials of CRT indicate that the magnitude of response to CRT is clinically significant for a variety of endpoints but that a symptomatic improvement in functional endpoints in not seen in all CRT recipients. Table 12-6 summarizes the data from randomized clinical trial. Taken together, the data indicate that depending on the endpoint measure, up to 30% of patients may not receive at least one of the potential benefits of CRT. In addition, because the clinical trials could not consistently identify baseline predictors of response to CRT, such as QRS duration or QRS delay type, investigators have more recently focused on measures of mechanical dyssynchrony to improve the rate of response to therapy.[69-75]

Echocardiography, because it is noninvasive, is the most widely used method for short- and long-term assessments of both baseline mechanical dyssynchrony and response to therapy. Also, the advent of tissue Doppler ultrasound methods has led to a host of measures that assess regional and particularly intraventricular dyssynchrony.[69,70] One of the many interesting observations arising from this work is that up to 50% of patients without QRS delay who have depressed LVEF and symptomatic heart failure also have mechanical dyssynchrony.[74,75] Further, uncontrolled trials indi-

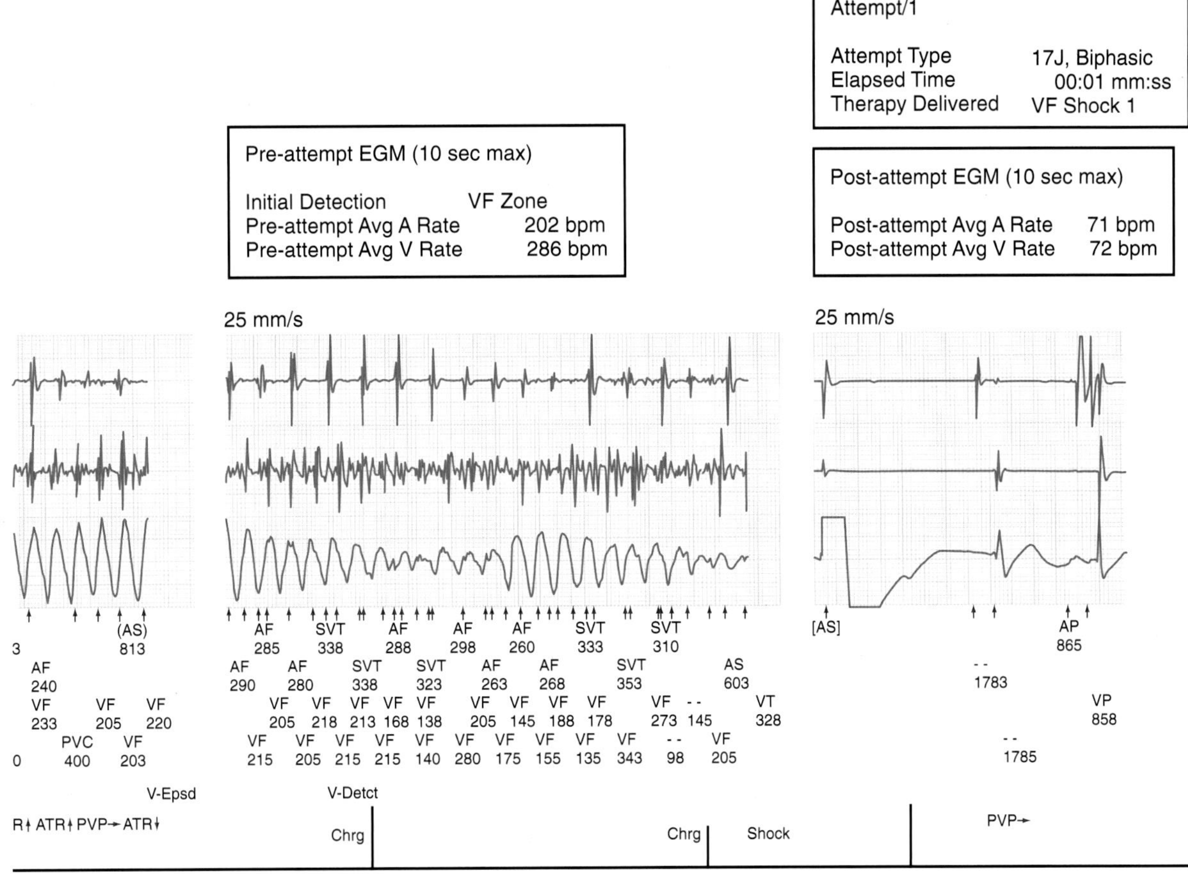

Figure 12-10. Concomitant conversion. (1) Atrial features and therapies were programmed "on"; (2) atrial fibrillation (AF) was induced and the device was allowed to detect AF; (3) ventricular fibrillation (VF) was induced; (4) the RENEWAL 3 AVT device (Guidant, Boston Scientific, Natick, Mass.) was allowed to detect the arrhythmia and deliver therapy; (5) VF was detected and therapy delivered during AF (ventricular detection takes precedence over atrial detection); (6) VF and AF were converted with a 17-J shock.

TABLE 12-6. **Summary of the Magnitude of Response to Cardiac Resynchronization Therapy in Randomized Controlled Trials***

Outline Measure	Magnitude Summary
Functional measures:	
Functional class improvement (% improving one NYHA class)	62 to 85
Quality-of-life score improvement	−18 to −24
6-minute walk distance improvement (m)	25 to 46
Peak VO_2 improvement (mL/kg/min)	0.8 to 2
Measures of heart failure progression:	
LV ejection fraction	0.03 to 0.07
LV end-systolic volume index (mL/m^2)	−3 to −7
LV end-diastolic dimension index (mm/m^2)	−3 to −6
Measures of heart failure outcome:	
Relative risk reduction in heart failure hospitalization/mortality (%)	40 to 52
Relative risk reduction in cardiovascular hospitalization/mortality (%)	36

*Data from references 2-10; 3-month to 3-year follow-up.
LV, left ventricular; NYHA class, New York Heart Association functional class.

cate that these patients demonstrate response to CRT and that this response is similar in magnitude to that in patients with wide QRS delay.[73,74] Because the tissue Doppler characterization is relatively new, there are no published acquisition standards. Additionally, the new tissue Doppler–derived criteria used for patient selection for CRT have not been prospectively tested in a randomized clinical trial against the standard selection criteria. It is also not clear whether or not patients with QRS delay but without echocardiographic evidence of mechanical dyssynchrony show response to CRT. Nonetheless, these various echocardiographic measures provide an elegant method for assessing mechanical dyssynchrony and resynchronization and offer important ancillary information. They can also be extremely valuable in attempts to optimize LV lead placement, if several candidate branch veins are present, as well as in programming of short- and long-term devices.[69-75]

The Predictors of Response to CRT (PROSPECT) Trial is a prospective study evaluating the role of echocardiographic measures to predict a positive response to CRT. Enrollment commenced in 2004, and the study intends to enroll 300 patients in European, U.S., and

Asian centers with a composite endpoint of clinical response and a measure of remodeling consisting of LV end-systolic volume.[15,76] Entry criteria are the same as those used in the major clinical trials of CRT.

Future Populations for Cardiac Resynchronization Therapy

In general, the new randomized clinical trials of CRT are attempting to build on observations made in previous studies to identify additional patients with heart failure who may stand to benefit from CRT. These studies are targeting two groups of patients, those with less symptomatic heart failure who may benefit from CRT through reverse remodeling and those who are scheduled to undergo device implantation or already have an implanted device because of heart failure and have RV pacing–induced LBBB.[77]

The Multi-Center Automatic Defibrillator Implantation Trial–Cardiac Resynchronization Therapy (MADIT-CRT) study, a randomized controlled trial, is comparing the use of CRT-D devices with RV-based ICDs in patients with QRS delay and depressed LVEF (<0.30) and NYHA class II symptoms. A composite endpoint, reduction in all-cause mortality and heart failure events, is the primary study endpoint, and LV volumes will be assessed. The study has initiated enrollment, with 196 patients enrolled at the time of this writing. The expected enrollment is 1800 patients.[12]

Two similar studies performed in smaller numbers of patients, the MIRACLE ICD II study and the Resynchronization Reverses Remodeling in Systolic Left Ventricular Dysfunction (REVERSE) trial, will also evaluate the effect of CRT in limiting the clinical progression of heart failure.[13,14] The REVERSE trial is enrolling patients with NYHA class I (previously symptomatic) or II symptoms, QRS duration of 120 msec or longer, LVEF 0.40 or less, and LV end-diastolic dimension 55 mm or more, without bradycardia, and with or without an ICD indication who are undergoing optimal medical therapy; they will be randomly assigned to "CRT off" or "CRT on" for 12 months. The primary endpoint is a clinical composite index (as in the MIRACLE study) and the secondary endpoint is the LV end-systolic volume index. The REVERSE trial will enroll 683 patients from 115 centers in the United States, Europe, and Canada.

Because of the potential for worsening of heart failure due to RV pacing–induced dyssynchrony as well as the findings of uncontrolled studies that "upgrading" RV devices to CRT devices in patients with heart failure improves symptoms and ventricular function, upgrading of RV devices is a common practice in experienced CRT implantation centers but falls outside FDA labeling.[57,58,77] There is currently no randomized trial evaluating CRT in this setting.

There is another group of patients, however, in whom a pacemaker is indicated and who have depressed ventricular function in whom a CRT device to prevent pacing-induced dyssynchrony may have a role. The Biventricular Versus Right Ventricular Pacing in Heart Failure Patients with Atrioventricular Block (BLOCK HF) study is evaluating the role of CRT in patients with depressed LVEF (≤0.45) and AV block in whom a pacemaker is indicated. The study will assess whether CRT limits the clinical progression of heart failure in comparison with DDD RV–based pacing. The primary composite endpoint consists of mortality, morbidity, and cardiac function. Enrollment was initiated in 2004.[13]

Managing Heart Failure with Implanted Devices: Additional Device Features

A number of device features offer potential assistance in the management of a patient with advanced heart failure who is receiving a CRT device. Assessment of the heart failure clinical status before an acute exacerbation of heart failure is very attractive, and a number of features that may predict heart failure worsening, such as the heart rate variability assessment, are already present in some CRT devices.[78] Some studies have shown that CRT induced a reduction in minimum heart rate and an increase in the standard deviation of the R-R interval. Event-free survival was better in patients with higher measures of heart rate variability. Another available feature is thoracic impedance monitoring, which measures thoracic impedance between the RV lead and the device pulse generator in devices implanted for the long term. Although the data to date are sparse, a decrease in impedance may reflect increased fluid volume and may be an early indicator of a heart failure exacerbation.[79]

Currently a stand-alone device, but one that may be incorporated into a CRT system, the implantable hemodynamic monitor measures pulmonary artery pressures and provides a reliable surrogate for pulmonary artery diastolic pressure both at rest and with activity.[20] The Chronicle Offers Management to Patients with Advanced Signs and Symptoms of Heart Failure (COMPASS) trial enrolled 274 patients from 40 centers in the United States with NYHA class III/IV status and at least one heart failure hospitalization within 6 months while undergoing optimal medical therapy. The primary endpoint was the rate of combined heart failure hospitalizations, emergency department visits, and urgent visits. The trial showed that access to these measurements may aid in the long-term management of patients with heart failure.[22]

The concept of adding CRT or defibrillator capability to a cardiac restraint or support device is also intriguing.[21]

Other techniques employing electrical impulses delivered to the heart for treatment of heart failure are under development. One such approach delivers high-current impulses from a pacemaker-like implantable pulse generator to the heart during the absolute refractory period and therefore does not elicit a new action potential; accordingly, the impulses are considered nonexcitatory signals. In isolated muscle preparations and intact hearts of animals and humans, these signals can modulate cardiac contractility. They have therefore been termed *cardiac contractility modulating* (CCM) signals.

The initial clinical study of CCM signals involved short-term (10-30 min) application of CCM signals through temporarily placed electrodes in patients with heart failure who had a clinical indication for an electrophysiology procedure (such as a CRT and/or ICD implantation or a study for evaluation of ventricular or supraventricular arrhythmias). The findings showed the feasibility of delivering CCM treatment in humans and demonstrated that contractile performance could be enhanced. The signals were applied to patients with normal and prolonged QRS complexes, and similar immediate effects were identified in both groups. In a subgroup of the patients with long QRS, CCM signals were also applied simultaneously with BiV pacing; the effects of CRT and CCM on acute contractile performance, as quantified by dP/dt_{max}, were shown to be additive in most patients.[3]

The initial experiences with long-term CCM signal applications were obtained in patients with NYHA class III symptoms and QRS duration of 120 msec or less.[79,80] This feasibility study was designed mainly to test the functionality of an implanted device that automatically delivers CCM signals, called the OPTIMIZER System (Impulse Dynamics USA, New York, NY), and to assess basic safety issues. The device operated as intended, no change in ambient ectopy was observed between baseline and 8 weeks of treatment, and no overt safety concerns were revealed. Additionally, improvements were reported in patient symptoms (assessed by NYHA class), QOL (assessed by the Minnesota Living with Heart Failure Questionnaire [MLWHFQ]) and ejection fraction. Notably, the extent of improvement in ejection fraction reported in this study after 8 weeks of treatment was comparable to that reported in response to CRT in patients with prolonged QRS duration.[1]

To date, however, completed studies of CCM are nonrandomized, are nonblinded (therefore subject to placebo effect), and have small sample sizes. Two multicenter, randomized, controlled studies of CCM are currently under way (one in Europe and one in the United States being performed under an investigational device exemption from the FDA) to definitively test the safety and efficacy of CCM as a treatment for heart failure. If these studies show CCM treatment in patients with normal QRS duration to be as safe and effective as CRT in patients with prolonged QRS, a new, easily deployable treatment will be made available to patients with otherwise untreatable symptoms. Future studies could also evaluate whether CCM is effective in patients with wide QRS nonresponsive to CRT or whether combining CRT with CCM is more effective than CRT alone. Testing of these hypotheses would be facilitated by development of a single device that incorporates pacing, antitachycardia therapies, and CCM.

Incorporation of microelectromechanical systems (MEMS) technology into LV leads themselves is another area of interest. Development of short- and long-term leads with this technology would provide for the opportunity to assess acute hemodynamic and regional cardiac performance.[81]

Another important offering to facilitate the management of patients with CRT devices is the introduction of remote monitoring capabilities.[24,82] Such systems, using telephone or RF communication, which allow device function to be monitored by the physician with the patient remaining at home, provide secure access to the information on the Internet so that device data can be frequently reviewed with ease. The opportunity for better patient management with "virtual," frequent patient encounters is available and is being investigated.[83] In addition, other aspects of the patient's condition, such as weight and blood pressure, can be added to the remote transmission to provide a broader view of the patient's clinical status.

Summary

In less than 10 years of clinical study, CRT devices have gained an established role in the treatment of patients with advanced heart failure due to systolic dysfunction in association with QRS delay. Patients not only feel better and can do more with CRT, they also live longer and are hospitalized less.

Extending the benefit of CRT to patients at earlier stages of heart failure and those with or about to receive RV pacing devices is being studied.

Other lead-based technologies capable of diagnosing or treating heart failure may also be incorporated into CRT devices in the future.

Expanding the flexibility and usefulness of information obtained from the device can also advance the treatment of heart failure in CRT recipients, and we are just beginning to appreciate the potential of the CRT device to provide immediate and ancillary data about the status of heart failure disease in a particular patient.

REFERENCES

1. Heart Failure Society of America (HFSA) practice guidelines: HFSA guidelines for management of patients with heart failure caused by left ventricular systolic dysfunction—pharmacological approaches. J Card Fail 5:357-382, 1999.
2. Hunt SA, Baker DW, Chin MH, et al: American College of Cardiology/American Heart Association Task Force on Practice Guidelines (Committee to Revise the 1995 Guidelines for the Evaluation and Management of Heart Failure); International Society for Heart and Lung Transplantation; Heart Failure Society of America: ACC/AHA Guidelines for the Evaluation and Management of Chronic Heart Failure in the Adult: Executive Summary—A Report of the American College of Cardiology/American Heart Association Task Force on Practice Guidelines (Committee to Revise the 1995 Guidelines for the Evaluation and Management of Heart Failure). Developed in Collaboration With the International Society for Heart and Lung Transplantation; Endorsed by the Heart Failure Society of America. Circulation 104:2996-3007, 2001.
3. Cazeau S, Leclercq C, Lavergne T, et al: Multisite Stimulation in Cardiomyopathies (MUSTIC) Study Investigators: Effects of multisite biventricular pacing in patients with heart failure and intraventricular conduction delay. N Engl J Med 344:873-880, 2001.

4. Saxon LA, Boehmer JP, Hummel J, et al: Biventricular pacing in patients with congestive heart failure: Two prospective randomized trials. The VIGOR CHF and VENTAK CHF Investigators. Am J Cardiol 83:120D-123D, 1999.
5. Abraham WT, Fisher WG, Smith AL, et al: for the MIRACLE Study Group: Cardiac resynchronization in chronic heart failure. N Engl J Med 346:1845-1853, 2002.
6. Saxon LA, Ellenbogen KA: Resynchronization therapy for the treatment of heart failure. Circulation 108:1044-1048, 2003.
7. Higgins SL, Hummel JD, Niazi IK, et al: Cardiac resynchronization therapy for the treatment of heart failure in patients with intraventricular conduction delay and malignant ventricular tachyarrhythmias. J Am Coll Cardiol 42:1454-1459, 2003.
8. Young JB, Abraham WT, Smith AL, et al: Multicenter InSync ICD Randomized Clinical Evaluation (MIRACLE ICD) Trial Investigators: Combined cardiac resynchronization and implantable cardioversion defibrillation in advanced chronic heart failure: The MIRACLE ICD Trial. JAMA 289:2685-2694, 2003.
9. Bristow MR, Saxon LA, Boehmer J, et al: Comparison of Medical Therapy, Pacing, and Defibrillation in Heart Failure (COMPANION) Investigators: Cardiac-resynchronization therapy with or without an implantable defibrillator in advanced chronic heart failure. N Engl J Med May 350:2140-2150, 2004.
10. Cleland JG, Daubert JC, Erdmann E, et al: Cardiac Resynchronization-Heart Failure (CARE-HF) Study Investigators: The effect of cardiac resynchronization on morbidity and mortality in heart failure. N Engl J Med 352:1539-1549, 2005.
11. Morgan Stanley: Equity Research—North America—Industry: Hospital Supplies and Medical Technology. September 2004.
12. University of Rochester Leads Worldwide Heart Research Project. University of Rochester Medical Center News Archives, November 23, 2004. Available online at http://www.urmc.rochester.edu/pr/news/story.cfm?id=695/
13. Medtronic, Inc: Medtronic Begins Clinical Trial To Evaluate Possible Expansion Of Cardiac Resynchronization Therapy In Heart Failure Patients With Mild Or No Symptoms: "REVERSE" study investigates if CRT can help limit the downward spiral of heart failure. News Release, July 6, 2004. Available online at http://wwwp.medtronic.com/Newsroom/NewsReleaseDetails.do?itemId=1097076282648&lang=en_US/
14. Abraham WT, Young JB, Leon AR, et al: Effects of cardiac resynchronization on disease progression in patients with left ventricular systolic dysfunction, an indication for an implantable cardioverter-defibrillator, and mildly symptomatic heart failure. Circulation 110:2864-2868, 2004.
15. Yu C-M, Abraham WT, Bax J, et al: Predictors of response to cardiac resynchronization therapy (PROSPECT)—study design. Am Heart J 149:600-605, 2005.
16. Bardy GH, Lee KL, Mark DB, et al: Sudden Cardiac Death in Heart Failure Trial (SCD-HeFT) Investigators: Amiodarone or an implantable cardioverter-defibrillator for congestive heart failure. N Engl J Med 352:225-237, 2005.
17. Moss AJ, Zareba W, Hall WJ, et al: the Multicenter Automatic Defibrillator Implantation Trial II Investigators: Prophylactic implantation of a defibrillator in patients with myocardial infarction and reduced ejection fraction. N Engl J Med 346:877-883, 2002.
18. De Marco T, Foster E, Chatterjee K, et al: Cardiac resynchronization therapy: Will ancillary atrial rate support promote greater utilization of β-blockers in heart failure. J Card Fail 6-3S: 40, 2000.
19. St. John Sutton MG, Plappert T, Abraham WT, et al: for the Multicenter InSync Randomized Clinical Evaluation (MIRACLE) Study Group: Effect of cardiac resynchronization therapy in left ventricular size and function in chronic heart failure. Circulation 107:1985-1990, 2003.
20. Saxon LA, De Marco T, Prystowsky EN, et al: Executive Summary: Resynchronization Therapy for Heart Failure. Executive Consensus Conference, May 8, 2002. Available online at http://www.hrsonline.org/positionDocs/CRT_12_3.pdf/
21. Mann DL: Results of a multicenter randomized clinical trial for the assessment of a cardiac support device (CSD) in patients with heart failure. Presented at the American Heart Association Scientific Sessions, New Orleans, November 7-10, 2004.
22. Bourge R, for the COMPASS Investigators: The Chronicle Offers Management to Patients with Advanced Signs and Symptoms of Heart Failure (COMPASS-HF) study. Presented at ACC 54th Annual Meeting, March 6-9, 2005; Orlando, Fla. J Am Coll Cardiol 45(Suppl B):30B-32B, 2005.
23. Saxon LA, Crandall BG, Nydegger CC, et al: Results of the Multicenter CONTAK RENEWAL 3 AVT clinical study of cardiac resynchronization defibrillator therapy in patients with atrial fibrillation (abstract AB9-6). Presented at Heart Rhythm 2005. Abstracts of the 26th Annual Meeting of the Heart Rhythm Society. May 4-7, 2005, New Orleans. Heart Rhythm 2(Suppl): S18, 2005.
24. Medtronic, Inc: Medtronic CareLink Network. Available online at http://www.medtronic.com/carelink/
25. Guidant Corporation: LATITUDE Patient Management. Available online at https://www.latitude.guidant.com/
26. Cleland JGF, Khand A, Clark AL: The heart failure epidemic: Exactly how big is it? Eur J Heart Fail 22:623-626, 2001.
27. Haldeman GA, Croft JB, Giles WH, et al: Hospitalization of patients with heart failure: National Hospital Discharge Survey, 1985-1995. Am Heart J 137:352-360, 1999.
28. Havranek EP, Abraham WT: The healthcare economics of heart failure. Heart Fail 14:10-18, 1998.
29. O'Connel JB: The economic burden of heart failure. Clin Cardiol 23(Suppl 3):III6-III10, 2000.
30. Beta-Blocker Evaluation of Survival Trial Investigators: A trial of the beta-blocker bucindolol in patients with advanced chronic heart failure. N Engl J Med 344:1659-1667, 2001.
31. Cohn JN, Goldstein SO, Greenberg BH, et al: A dose-dependent increase in mortality with vesnarinone among patients with severe heart failure. Vesnarinone Trial Investigators. N Engl J Med 339:1810-1816, 1998.
32. Pitt B, Zannad F, Remme WJ, et al: The effect of spironolactone on morbidity and mortality in patients with severe heart failure. Randomized Aldactone Evaluation Study Investigators. N Engl J Med 341:709-717, 1999.
33. Shenkman HJ, McKinnon JE, Khandelwal AK, et al: Determinants of QRS prolongation in a generalized heart failure population: Findings from the Conquest Study. Circulation 102(Suppl II):1, 2000.
34. Aaronson KD, Schwartz JS, Chen TM, et al: Development and prospective validation of a clinical index to predict survival in ambulatory patients referred for cardiac transplant evaluation. Circulation 95:2660-2667, 1997.
35. Farwell D, Patel NR, Hall A, et al: How many people with heart failure are appropriate for biventricular resynchronization? Eur Heart J 21:1247-1250, 2000.
36. Shamim W, Francis DP, Yousufuddin M, et al: Intraventricular conduction delay: A prognostic marker in chronic heart failure. Int J Cardiol 70:171-178, 1999.
37. Baldasseroni S, Opasich C, Gorini M, et al: Left bundle-branch block is associated with increased 1-year sudden and total mortality rate in 5517 outpatients with congestive heart failure: A report from the Italian Network on Congestive Heart Failure. Am Heart J 143:398-405, 2002.
38. Gottipaty VK, Krelis SP, Fei L, et al: for the VEST Investigators: The resting electrocardiogram provides a sensitive and inexpensive marker of prognosis in patients with chronic heart failure [abstract 847-4]. J Am Coll Cardiol 33:145A, 1999.
39. Xiao HB, Brecker S, Gibson DG: Effects of abnormal activation on the time course of left ventricular pressure in dilated cardiomyopathy. Br Heart J 68:403-407, 1992.

40. Kass DA, Chen CH, Curry C, et al: Improved left ventricular mechanics from acute VDD pacing in patients with dilated cardiomyopathy and ventricular conduction delay. Circulation 99:1567-1573, 1999.
41. Saxon LA, De Marco T, Schafer J, et al: for the VIGOR-CHF Investigators: Effects of chronic biventricular stimulation for resynchronization on echocardiographic measures of remodeling. Circulation 105:1304-1310, 2002.
42. Fantoni C, Kawabata M, Massaro R, et al: Right and left ventricular activation sequence in patients with heart failure and right bundle branch block: A detailed analysis using three-dimensional non-fluoroscopic electroanatomic mapping system. J Cardiovasc Electrophysiol 16:112-119, 2005.
43. Saxon LA: If only rights were really lefts. J Cardiovasc Electrophysiol 16:120-121, 2005.
44. Blanc JJ, Etienne Y, Gilard M, et al: Evaluation of different ventricular pacing sites in patients with severe heart failure: Results of an acute hemodynamic study. Circulation 96:3273-3277, 1997.
45. Auricchio A, Stellbrink C, Block M, et al: Effect of pacing chamber and atrioventricular delay on acute systolic function of paced patients with congestive heart failure. The Pacing Therapies for Congestive Heart Failure Study Group. The Guidant Congestive Heart Failure Research Group. Circulation 99:2993-3001, 1999.
46. Nelson GS, Berger RD, Fetics BJ, et al: Left ventricular or biventricular pacing improves cardiac function at diminished energy cost in patients with dilated cardiomyopathy and left bundle-branch block. Circulation 102:3053-3059, 2000.
47. Nelson GS, Curry CW, Wyman BT, et al: Predictors of systolic augmentation from left ventricular preexcitation in patients with dilated cardiomyopathy and intraventricular conduction delay. Circulation 101:2703-2709, 2000.
48. Butter C, Auricchio A, Stellbrink C, et al: Pacing Therapy for Chronic Heart Failure II Study Group: Effect of resynchronization therapy stimulation site on the systolic function of heart failure patients. Circulation 104:3026-3029, 2001.
49. Hay I, Melenovsky V, Fetics BJ, et al: Short-term effects of right-left heart sequential cardiac resynchronization in patients with heart failure, chronic atrial fibrillation, and atrioventricular nodal block. Circulation 110:3404-3410, 2004.
50. Leclercq C, Faris O, Tunin R, et al: Systolic improvement and mechanical resynchronization does not require electrical synchrony in the dilated failing heart with left bundle-branch block. Circulation 106:1760-1763, 2002.
51. Nelson GS, Curry CW, Wyman BT, et al: Predictors of systolic augmentation from left ventricular preexcitation in patients with dilated cardiomyopathy and intraventricular conduction delay. Circulation 101:2703-2709, 2000.
52. Auricchio A, Stellbrink C, Sack S, et al: Pacing Therapies in Congestive Heart Failure (PATH-CHF) Study Group: Long-term clinical effect of hemodynamically optimized cardiac resynchronization therapy in patients with heart failure and ventricular conduction delay. J Am Coll Cardiol 39:2026-2033, 2002.
53. Auricchio A, Stellbrink C, Butter C, et al: Pacing Therapies in Congestive Heart Failure II Study Group; Guidant Heart Failure Research Group: Clinical efficacy of cardiac resynchronization therapy using left ventricular pacing in heart failure patients stratified by severity of ventricular conduction delay. J Am Coll Cardiol 42:2109-2116, 2003.
54. Linde C, Braunschweig F, Gadler F, et al: Long-term improvements in quality of life by biventricular pacing in patients with chronic heart failure: Results from the Multisite Stimulation in Cardiomyopathy study (MUSTIC). Am J Cardiol 91:1090-1095, 2003.
55. Doshi R, Daoud E, Fellows C, Turk et al: The PAVE trial: The first prospective, randomized study evaluating bv pacing after ablate and pace therapy. Presented at the American College of Cardiology Annual Scientific Session 2004 Late-Breaking Clinical Trials, March 8, 2004. Abstract available online at http://www.sjm.com/resources/pave.aspx/
56. U.S. Food and Drug Administration, Center for Devices and Radiological Health: Premarket Approval (PMA) Database. Available online at http://www.accessdata.fda.gov/scripts/cdrh/cfdocs/cfPMA/pma.cfm.
57. Baker CM, Christopher TJ, Smith PF, et al: Addition of a left ventricular lead to conventional pacing systems in patients with congestive heart failure: Feasibility, safety, and early results in 60 consecutive patients. Pacing Clin Electrophysiol 25:1166-1171, 2002.
58. Horwich T, Foster E, De Marco T, et al: Effects of resynchronization therapy on cardiac function in pacemaker patients "upgraded" to biventricular devices. J Cardiovasc Electrophysiol 15:1284-1289, 2004.
59. Touiza A, Etienne Y, Gilard M, et al: Long-term left ventricular pacing: Assessment and comparison with biventricular pacing in patients with severe congestive heart failure. J Am Coll Cardiol 38:1966-1970, 2001.
60. Wilkoff BL, Hess M, Young J, Abraham WT: Differences in tachyarrhythmia detection and implantable cardioverter defibrillator therapy by primary or secondary prevention indication in cardiac resynchronization therapy patients. J Cardiovasc Electrophysiol 15:1002-1009, 2004.
61. Yu CM, Chau E, Sanderson JE, et al: Tissue Doppler echocardiographic evidence of reverse remodeling and improved synchronicity by simultaneously delaying regional contraction after biventricular pacing therapy in heart failure. Circulation 105:438-445, 2002.
62. Carson P, Anand I, O'Connor C, et al: Relation of cardiac device therapy to mode of death in advanced heart failure—COMPANION Trial. Circulation 108:IV628-IV629, 2003.
63. Saxon LA, Bristow MR, DeMarco T, Krueger SK: Procedural outcomes and device performance in the COMPANION trial of resynchronization therapy for heart failure. Circulation 110:III-443, 2004.
64. Higgins S, Giudici M, Hummel J, et al: Procedure time and success rates for the placement of a coronary venous lead designed for left ventricular pacing [abstract]. J Am Coll Cardiol 39:77A, 2002.
65. De Lurgio DB, Foster E, Higginbotham MB, et al: A comparison of cardiac resynchronization by sequential biventricular pacing and left ventricular pacing to simultaneous biventricular pacing: Rationale and design of the DECREASE-HF clinical trial. J Card Fail 11:233-239, 2005.
66. Baker J, Turk K, Pires LA, et al, and the Rhythm ICD V-V Optimization Phase Investigators: Optimization of interventricular timing delay in biventricular pacing: Results from the Rhythm ICD V-V Optimization Phase Study [abstract P3-96]. Presented at Heart Rhythm 2005. Abstracts of the 26th Annual Meeting of the Heart Rhythm Society. May 4-7, 2005, New Orleans. Heart Rhythm 2(Suppl):S205, 2005.
67. Bernheim A, Ammann P, Sticherling C, et al: Right atrial pacing impairs cardiac function during resynchronization therapy: Acute effects of DDD pacing compared to VDD pacing. J Am Coll Cardiol 45:1482-1487, 2005.
68. Tei C, Ling LH, Hodge DO, et al: New index of combined systolic and diastolic myocardial performance: A simple and reproducible measure of cardiac function—a study in normals and dilated cardiomyopathy. J Cardiol 26:357-366, 1995.
69. Bax JJ, Ansalone G, Breithardt OA, et al: Echocardiographic evaluation of cardiac resynchronization therapy: Ready for routine clinical use? A critical appraisal. J Am Coll Cardiol 44:1-9, 2004.
70. Ansalone G, Giannantoni P, Ricci R, et al: Doppler myocardial imaging in patients with heart failure receiving biventricular pacing treatment. Am Heart J 142:881-896, 2001.
71. Sogaard P, Egeblad H, Pedersen AK, et al: Sequential versus simultaneous biventricular resynchronization for severe heart failure: Evaluation by tissue Doppler imaging. Circulation 106:2078-2084, 2002.

72. Sogaard P, Egeblad H, Kim WY, et al: Tissue Doppler imaging predicts improved systolic performance and reversed left ventricular remodeling during long-term cardiac resynchronization therapy. J Am Coll Cardiol 40:723-730, 2002.
73. Gasparini M, Mantica M, Galimberti P, et al: Beneficial effects of biventricular pacing in patients with a "narrow" QRS. Pacing Clin Electrophysiol 26:169-174, 2003.
74. Achilli A, Sassara M, Ficili S, et al: Long-term effectiveness of cardiac resynchronization therapy in patients with refractory heart failure and "narrow" QRS. J Am Coll Cardiol 42:2117-2124, 2003.
75. Yu CM, Lin H, Zhang Q, Sanderson JE: High prevalence of left ventricular systolic and diastolic asynchrony in patients with congestive heart failure and normal QRS duration. Heart 89:54-60, 2003.
76. Packer M: Proposal for a new clinical end point to evaluate the efficacy of drugs and devices in the treatment of chronic heart failure. J Card Fail 7:176-182, 2001.
77. Wilkoff BL, Cook JR, Epstein AE, et al: Dual Chamber and VVI Implantable Defibrillator Trial Investigators: Dual-chamber pacing or ventricular backup pacing in patients with an implantable defibrillator: The Dual Chamber and VVI Implantable Defibrillator (DAVID) Trial. JAMA 288:3115-3123, 2002.
78. Medtronic, Inc: InSync Sentry CRT-D Device. Available online at http://www.medtronic.com/physician/hf/insync_sentry.html
79. Pappone C, Rosanio S, Burkhoff D, et al: Cardiac contractility modulation by electric currents applied during the refractory period in patients with heart failure secondary to ischemic or idiopathic dilated cardiomyopathy. Am J Cardiol 90:1307-1313, 2002.
80. Pappone C, Augello G, Rosanio S, et al: First human chronic experience with cardiac contractility modulation by nonexcitatory electrical currents for treating systolic heart failure: Mid-term safety and efficacy results from a multicenter study. J Cardiovasc Electrophysiol 15:418-427, 2004.
81. MEMS and Nanotechnology Clearinghouse: What is MEMS Technology? Available online at http://www.memsnet.org/mems/what-is.html
82. Guidant Corporation: LATITUDE Patient Management System Fact Sheet. Available online at http://www.guidant.com/webapp/emarketing/newsroom/newspg.jsp?dir=latitude&file=fact
83. Schricker A, Shinbane J, Contrafatto I, et al: Remote device follow-up: New technologies for patient management in an era of increasing device use for heart failure. J Card Fail 11(6):S148, 2005.

Chapter 13

Pacing for Sinus Node Disease: Indications, Techniques, and Clinical Trials

ANNE M. GILLIS*

Sinus node disease (SND) is the most common indication for a cardiac pacing system in North America.[1] SND is characterized by electrophysiologic abnormalities of the sinus node and atria. These electrophysiologic abnormalities include disturbances of impulse generation and exit from the sinus node to atrial tissue, impaired impulse transmission within the atria and/or specialized cardiac conduction system, failure of subsidiary pacemaker activity, and paroxysmal or chronic atrial tachycardias, including atrial fibrillation (AF).[2,3] The electrocardiographic manifestations of SND are (1) sinus bradycardia, (2) sinus pauses or sinus arrest, (3) sinoatrial exit block, (4) atrial tachycardia (AT), (5) AF, which is initially paroxysmal in nature, and (6) sinus node chronotropic incompetence.[2,3] Brady-arrhythmias alternating with paroxysmal atrial flutter or fibrillation are common in SND. The natural history of SND can be recurrent syncope, heart failure, stroke, and/or AF.

*Supported by the Canadian Institutes for Health Research and the Heart and Stroke Foundation of Alberta. Dr. Gillis is a Medical Scientist of the Alberta Heritage Foundation for Medical Research.

Pathophysiology of Sinus Node Disease

Cellular Electrophysiology

The sinoatrial node is a heterogenous tissue with multiple cell types and a complex structure.[4,5] It is crescent-like in shape and is typically at least partially subepicardial with irregular margins and multiple nodal radiations. Approximately 1% of the sinoatrial node acts as the leading pacemaker site.[5] This site is usually in the center of the sinoatrial node. From the center of the node to the periphery there is a gradient in ionic current densities, connexin expression, myofilament density, cell size, and action potential characteristics. A variety of ionic currents contribute to normal sinus node automaticity. The sinus node generates phase 4 depolarization by activating a hyperpolarization-activated inward current, I_f. Other inward currents, including the L- and T-type calcium currents—$I_{Ca(L)}$, $I_{Ca(T)}$—and the tetrodotoxin-sensitive sodium current, contribute to the pacemaker potential. Outward currents that govern sinus node automaticity include the sodium-potassium (Na^+-K^+) pump, the delayed rectifier current, and the potassium channel activated by the muscarinic receptor I_{KACh}. The sodium-calcium exchanger also plays an important role in sinus node automaticity. Abnormalities of one or more of these ionic currents may contribute to sinus node dysfunction. In addition, connexin 43 disappears from the sinus node during aging, possibly contributing to abnormalities of conduction within the sinus node.[5,6]

Mutations of the hyperpolarization-activated cyclic nucleotide-gated channel 4 gene, *HCN4*, have been reported to be associated with reduced membrane expression and with decreased I_f currents in conjunction with abnormalities of sinus node dysfunction.[7-9] In an experimental model of heart failure, drops in the intrinsic sinus rate have been observed in association with significant decreases in I_f.[10] Mutations of the α-subunit of the sodium channel that cause one form of the long QT syndrome have also been associated with SND.[11] Such mutations may lead to the presence of a persistent inward current and a negative shift in voltage dependence of inactivation that either separately or in combination may cause a reduction in the sinus rate. Congenital SND that is characterized by bradycardia progressing to atrial inexcitability has also been reported to be associated with mutations of the α-subunit of the sodium channel that cause loss of function or significant impairments in channel gating (inactivation) resulting in reduced myocardial excitability.[12]

Knockout of *ERG1 B*, the gene that encodes I_{Kr}, in mice has also been reported to be associated with episodic sinus bradycardia.[13] Mutations of the *KCNQ1* gene that encodes the KvLQT1 potassium channel are also associated with SND.[14] Thus, decrease or loss of I_{Kr} or I_{Ks} in the long QT syndrome may contribute to SND in that setting. Maternal antibodies may contribute to sinus node dysfunction in the setting of congenital complete heart block by inhibition of I_{CaL} and I_{CaT}.[15] Knockout of I_{CaL} in transgenic mice has been reported to be associated with SND.[16,17] Some experimental models of ventricular hypertrophy have been reported to be associated with sinus node dysfunction and/or AF.[18-20] Thus, the causes of SND are likely multifactorial. Abnormalities of one or more ionic channels, transporters, or receptors that are inherited or that develop under pathophysiologic states, including aging, likely contribute to the substrate for SND.

Clinical Electrophysiology

Electroanatomic mapping in patients with SND has demonstrated significant increases in atrial refractory periods at all right atrial sites, increased atrial conduction times along the lateral right atrium and coronary sinus, and greater number and duration of double potentials along the crista terminalis.[21] The sinus node complex has also been noted to be more often unicentric and localized to the low crista terminalis (Fig. 13-1). Significant regional conduction slowing with double potentials and fractionation associated with areas of low voltage and electrical silence has also been observed in the right atrium. Impairment of sinus node function and increases in atrial refractory periods have been reported in association with aging.[22]

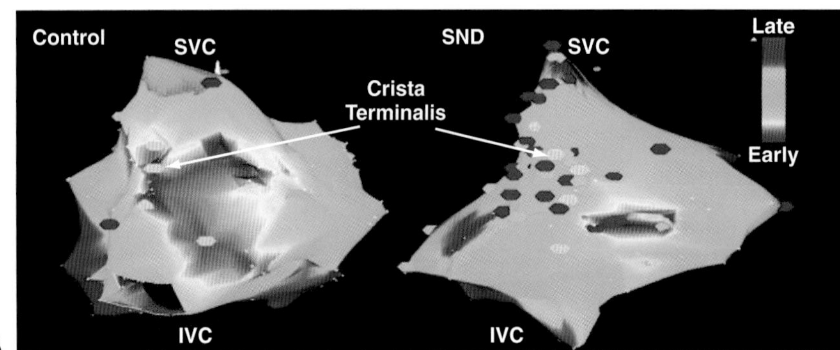

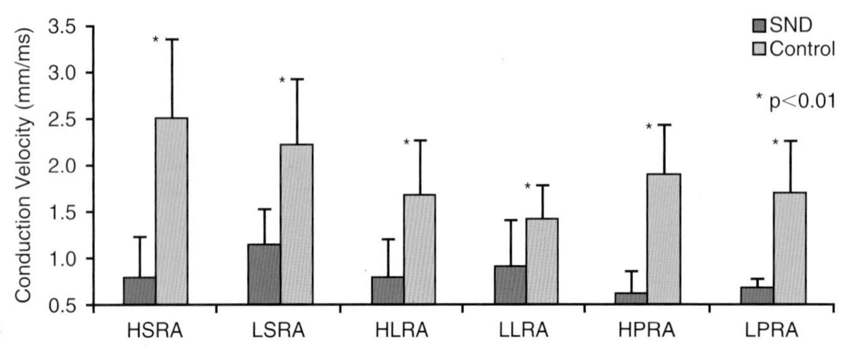

Figure 13-1. ***A,*** *Activation mapping in sinus rhythm in a patient with sinus node disease (SND)* (right) *and an age-matched control* (left). *Both atria are oriented such that posterior right atrium (crista terminalis, shown in* yellow dots*) is en face to demonstrate sinus node complex. Patient with SND demonstrates significantly greater number of points with double potentials* (blue dots) *and fractioned electrograms* (brown dots) *and earlier activity (sinus node complex) over a greater extent of the crista terminalis.* ***B,*** *Regional conduction velocity. IVC, inferior vena cava. (From Sanders P, Morton JB, Kistler PM, et al: Electrophysiological and electroanatomic characterization of the atria in sinus node disease: Evidence of diffuse atrial remodeling. Circulation 109:1514-1522, 2004.)*

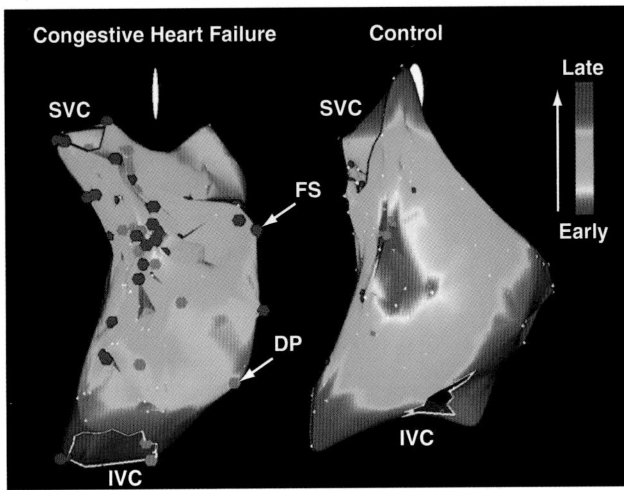

Figure 13-2. *Activation mapping to demonstrate the sinus node complex in a patient with congestive heart failure (CHF)* (left) *and an age-matched control subject* (right). *Both atria are oriented so that the crista terminalis is en face. Note the localized region of early sinus activation* (red) *in the patient with CHF and points demonstrating double potentials (DP;* blue dots*) and fractionated electrograms (FS;* brown dots*) along this structure. IVC, inferior vena cava; SVC, superior vena cava. (From Sanders P, Morton JB, Kistler PM, et al: Electrophysiological and electroanatomic characterization of the atria in sinus node disease: Evidence of diffuse atrial remodeling. Circulation 109:1514-1522, 2004.)*

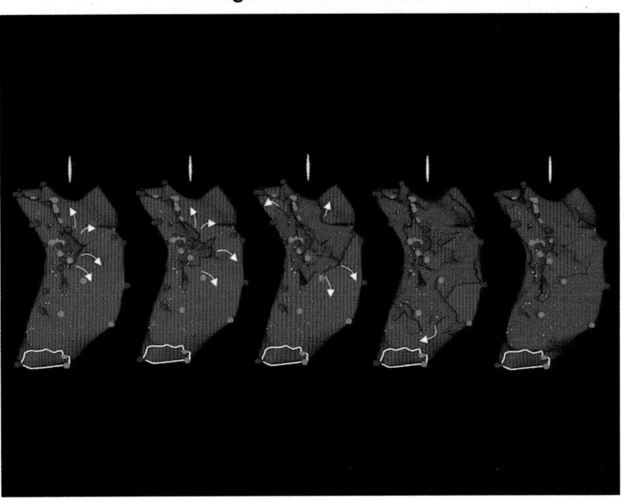

Figure 13-3. *Propagation map of the sinus impulse in a patient with congestive heart failure. Atria are oriented so that the crista terminalis is en face. Sinus activity exits to atria from anteroinferior margin of the crista terminalis. With delayed activation across the crista terminalis, activation fronts were observed to break cranially, caudally, and through gaps along this anatomic structure.* Blue dots *indicate points with double potentials, and* brown dots, *those with fractionated electrograms.* Arrows *indicate the direction of activation. (From Sanders P, Morton JB, Kistler PM, et al: Electrophysiological and electroanatomic characterization of the atria in sinus node disease: Evidence of diffuse atrial remodeling. Circulation 109:1514-1522, 2004.)*

Patients with congestive heart failure (CHF) have significant sinus node remodeling, characterized by anatomic and structural changes along the crista terminalis and a reduction in functional sinus node reserve (Fig. 13-2).[23,24] Compared with age-matched controls, patients with CHF have greater prolongation of the intrinsic sinus cycle length, greater prolongation of sinus node recovery times, caudal origin of sinus activity, prolongation of sinoatrial conduction time, greater number and duration of fractionated electrograms or double potentials along the crista terminalis, loss of voltage amplitude along the crista terminalis, and abnormal and circuitous propagation of the sinus impulse (Fig. 13-3). In addition, atrial refractoriness and regional conduction times are prolonged, and these changes may contribute to the propensity to AF in this setting.[24]

Experimental and clinical data suggest that AF causes reverse remodeling of the sinus node.[25-31] Prolonged sinus pauses after paroxysms of AF may result from depression of sinus node function that is eliminated by curative ablation of AF.[30] Sinus node recovery times are prolonged immediately after successful cardioversion and shorten over time.[31] The long-term loss of atrioventricular (AV) synchrony induced by VVI pacing is also associated with atrial electrical remodeling that is characterized by nonuniform prolongation of atrial refractoriness as well as prolongation of both atrial conduction time and sinus node recovery times.[25] These electrophysiologic changes are reversible after restoration of AV synchrony with DDD pacing. Together, the changes in atrial and sinus node electrophysiology may contribute to the higher incidence of AF that has been observed in patients treated with VVI pacing than in those treated with AV sequential pacing. The cellular mechanisms resulting in the association between sinus node dysfunction and atrial tachyarrhythmias remain unknown.

Clinical Presentation

The most common symptoms for which patients with SND seek medical attention are presyncope, syncope, palpitations, decreased exercise tolerance, and fatigue (Table 13-1).[2,3] Symptoms are usually intermittent and may be of variable duration. Many patients with electrocardiographic evidence of SND may be asymptomatic. Symptoms secondary to systemic thromboembolism may also be observed. Syncope may be

TABLE 13-1. Symptoms of Sinus Node Disease

Major symptoms	Syncope Presyncope
Less specific symptoms	Fatigue Decreased exercise tolerance Palpitations Confusion Memory loss

TABLE 13-2. Diagnostic Evaluation of Sinus Node Function

Electrocardiography (ECG): 12-lead ECG, including carotid sinus massage Ambulatory ECG monitoring Event recorders (patient activated, memory storage capability) Implantable loop recorder
Exercise treadmill testing
Autonomic testing: Tilt table testing Pharmacologic interventions
Invasive electrophysiologic assessment: Sinus node recover time (SNRT) Sinoatrial conduction time (SACT) Sinus node effective refractory period (SNERP) Direct recording of sinoatrial electrogram Effect of autonomic blockade on SNRT, SACT, SNERP

secondary to bradycardia, asystole, or atrial tachycardias. Syncope may occur without warning or may be heralded by dizziness or palpitations. The physical findings are frequently unremarkable, although sinus bradycardia or AF should raise suspicion of this disorder. However, sinus bradycardia is frequently observed in normal healthy individuals in all age ranges. Clinical correlation with symptoms is important.

Diagnosis

The diagnostic tools currently available for diagnosing SND are summarized in Table 13-2. Owing to the intermittent nature of this syndrome, the diagnosis is often time consuming and frustrating. The usefulness of both noninvasive tests and invasive electrophysiologic studies to identify SND as a potential cause of syncope are low (4% to 16%).[2] Implantable loop recorders have been reported to improve the likelihood of diagnosing bradycardia as the cause of syncope in patients with SND, and this approach has been shown in select patients to be more cost-effective than a strategy of serial noninvasive studies followed by invasive studies.[32-34]

Natural History

The course of SND is unpredictable; periods of symptomatic sinus node dysfunction may be separated by long periods of normal sinus node function.[2] SND is believed to evolve over 10 to 15 years, commencing with an asymptomatic phase and ultimately progressing to complete failure of sinus node activity and the emergence of subsidiary pacemaker escape rhythms or the development of chronic AF. Menozzi and colleagues[35] performed a prospective study in 35 untreated patients with SND. These subjects had a mean sinus rate at rest of ≤50 beats per minute (bpm) and/or intermittent sinoatrial block as well as symptoms attributable to SND. The patients were monitored for up to 4 years (mean 17 ± 15 months). During follow-up, the majority of patients (57%) experienced at least one cardiovascular event that required treatment. Syncope occurred in 23%, symptomatic heart failure in 17%, permanent AF in 11%, and symptomatic paroxysmal atrial tachyarrhythmias in 6%. The actuarial rates of occurrence of all cardiovascular events were 35%, 49%, and 63% after 1, 2, and 4 years, respectively. Older age, left ventricular end-diastolic diameter, and associated left ventricular dysfunction were independent predictors of cardiovascular events. The rates of occurrence of syncope were 16%, 31%, and 31% after 1, 2, and 4 years, respectively. Although a favorable outcome was observed in 43% of patients, the cohort studied was small, and duration of follow-up was relatively short.

In a cohort of 213 patients with symptomatic SND who were treated with atrial pacing, the incidence of permanent AF during follow-up has been reported to be 1.4% per year.[36] The risk of development of AF rose substantially with age 70 years or more at the time of pacemaker implantation. The risk of high-grade AV block was 1.8% per year, and this risk was much greater in patients with complete bundle branch block or bifascicular block (35%) than in patients without such conduction disturbances (6%). Survival rates in this population were similar to those of a matched general population (97% at 1 year, 89% at 5 years, and 72% at 10 years). Retrospective data also support the conclusion that survival in patients with SND treated with pacemaker therapy is similar to that of patients in a general matched population.[37]

Clinical Outcomes

Potential Detrimental Effects of Ventricular Pacing in Sinus Node Disease

A conceptual model illustrating the potential detrimental effects of ventricular pacing is shown in Figure 13-4. Ventricular dyssynchrony arising from right ventricular (RV) pacing and the loss of the contribution of atrial contraction to cardiac filling may alter cardiac hemodynamics and contribute to the development of cardiac dysfunction over time. Ventricular pacing is proarrhythmic. Ventricular pacing is associated with increased valvular regurgitation. This and contraction of the atrium when the AV valves are closed may cause adverse electrical remodeling of the atria and sinus node that create a substrate for AF.[22-31] Persistent AF may further contribute to the development of left ventricular dysfunction and ultimately the development of CHF.[28-31] Whether this is due to altered myocardial mechanics or to inadequate rate control, which leads to the development of tachycardia-induced myopathy, is unclear.

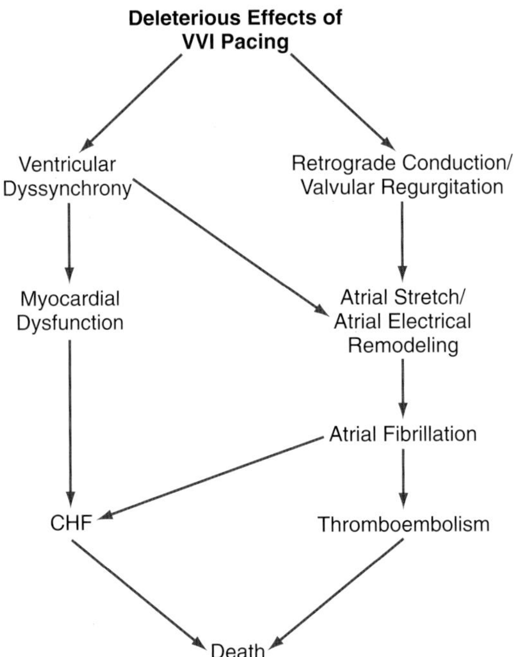

Figure 13-4. Potential deleterious effects of ventricular pacing. CHF, congestive heart failure.

Pacing and Survival

A number of retrospective studies[38] and one prospective study[39] have reported that atrial pacing is associated with better survival than ventricular pacing in patients with symptomatic bradycardia secondary to SND. Andersen and coworkers[39] randomly allocated 225 patients (mean age of 76 years) with sinus-node dysfunction, normal AV conduction, and a normal QRS complex to AAI or VVI pacing.[39] Over a mean of 5.5 years of follow-up, fewer cardiac deaths occurred in the atrial pacing group (19%) than in the ventricular pacing group (34%; $P = .0065$). The annual mortality rate was 3.0% in the atrial pacing group compared with 6.4% in the ventricular pacing group.

However, these results have not been confirmed in three larger clinical trials. The Pacemaker Selection in the Elderly (PASE) trial randomly assigned 407 patients 65 years or older to receive a dual-chamber pacemaker programmed to either DDDR mode or VVIR mode.[40] Overall mortality rates were similar in the two pacing groups. Of the 175 patients with SND as the primary indication for pacing in this study, overall mortality was slightly higher in the VVIR group (8.8% per yr) than in the DDDR group (5.2% per yr; $P = .09$).

The Canadian Trial of Physiologic Pacing (CTOPP) investigators randomly allocated 2568 patients from a general pacemaker population, but without permanent AF, to receive either a ventricular (n = 1474) or atrial (n = 1094) pacemaker.[41] Forty-two percent of the study population had SND as an indication for pacing. Over a mean follow-up period of 3.1 years, overall mortality rates were similar in both groups (6.3% per yr in the physiologic pacing group compared with 6.6% per yr in the ventricular pacing group; $P = .92$). Because the effects of atrial pacing for prevention of AF were delayed in the CTOPP population and similar observations were reported by Andersen and colleagues (in the Danish study),[39] the follow-up in CTOPP was extended. Over a follow-up of 6.4 years, the primary composite outcome of cardiovascular death or stroke occurred at a rate of 6.1% per year in patients assigned to ventricular pacing and at a rate of 5.5% per year in patients assigned to physiologic pacing.[42] The relative risk reduction was 8.1% with physiologic pacing (95% confidence interval [CI] −6.5 to 20.7; $P = .26$).

The MOde Selection Trial (MOST) investigators randomly assigned 2010 patients with SND to rate-modulated ventricular or dual-chamber pacing.[43] Over a mean follow-up period of 2.76 years, annual mortality rates were similar in the two groups (7.1% per yr in the physiologic pacing group compared with 7.4% per yr in the ventricular pacing group; $P = .65$) (Fig. 13-5).

Subgroup analysis in CTOPP suggested that patients in the ventricular pacing group who were pacemaker dependent experienced higher mortality than patients in the atrial pacing group, although this effect did not persist over the long term.[44] Subgroup analysis in the MOST population suggested that a high proportion of ventricular pacing despite maintenance of AV synchrony was associated with a higher risk of hospitalization for heart failure and an increased risk for development of AF.[45] These results, in conjunction with the results of the Dual-Chamber and VVI Implantable Defibrillator (DAVID) Trial,[46] have raised concerns that unnecessary RV pacing imposed by programming relatively short AV delays may have adversely influenced clinical outcomes in CTOPP and MOST. At present, a number of clinical trials are under way exploring the potential clinical benefits of reducing ventricular pacing in patients with intrinsic AV conduction.[47]

Pacing and Stroke

Thromboembolism secondary to AF occurs in SND. In the Danish study, thromboembolic events were significantly less likely to occur in the atrial pacing group (12%, 2.1% per yr) than in the ventricular pacing group (23%, 4.3% per yr; $P = .023$).[39] In the Danish study, the use of anticoagulation therapy was very low. However, the larger clinical trials failed to show a benefit of atrial pacing for prevention of stroke. In CTOPP, the annual incidences of stroke were similar for the atrial pacing group (1.0% per yr) and ventricular pacing group (1.1% per yr).[40,41] In MOST, the annual incidences of stroke were similar for the dual-chamber pacing (1.5%) and ventricular-pacing (1.8%) groups.[42,48]

The failure to show a benefit of reducing stroke by preventing AF in these larger trials may be due to other factors. The etiology of stroke in an elderly pacemaker population is multifactorial, not merely secondary to emboli originating in the left atrium as a consequence of AF.[47] Furthermore, the impact of randomized clinical trials of anticoagulation for the prevention of stroke may have led to greater use of antithrombotic therapy in patients with pacemakers and AF.[49] In MOST, 72% of patients were taking antiplatelet therapy or warfarin.

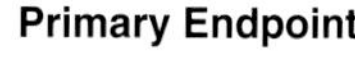

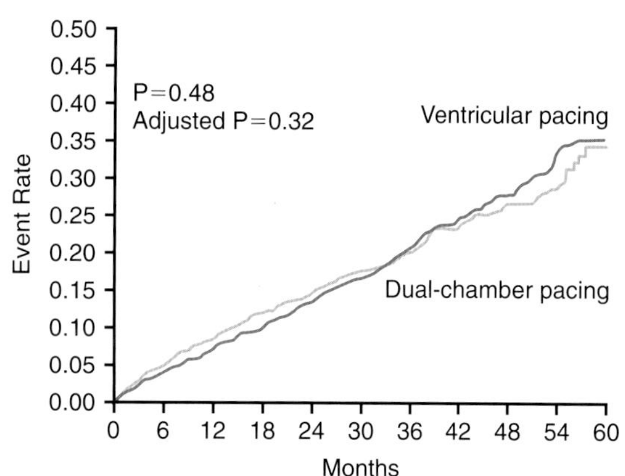

No. at Risk											
Ventricular pacing	996	934	897	813	678	557	431	320	218	125	39
Dual-chamber pacing	1014	963	930	833	693	555	431	328	214	120	28

Hospitalization for Heart Failure, Stroke, or Death

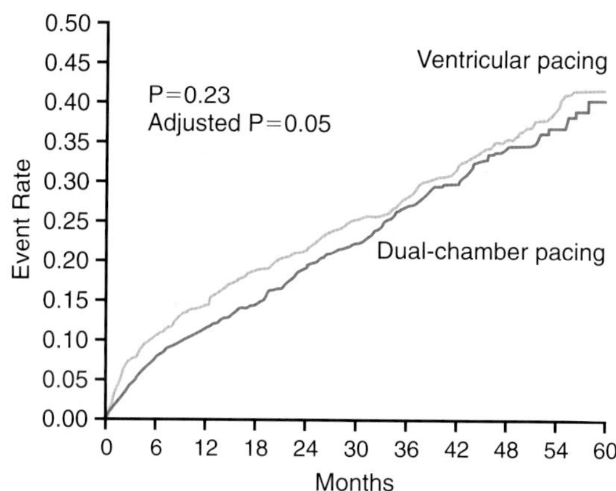

No. at Risk											
Ventricular pacing	996	880	839	752	624	504	388	287	193	110	35
Dual-chamber pacing	1014	926	889	793	649	518	394	297	188	105	26

Hospitalization for Heart Failure

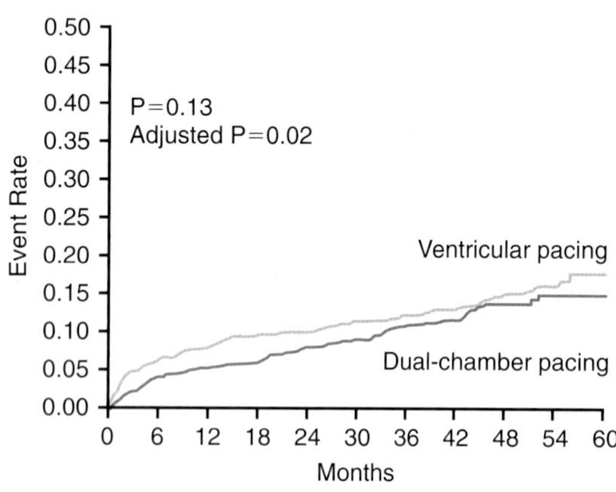

No. at Risk											
Ventricular pacing	996	890	855	766	637	516	402	300	200	116	36
Dual-chamber pacing	1014	932	894	801	658	528	406	307	191	106	27

Atrial Fibrillation

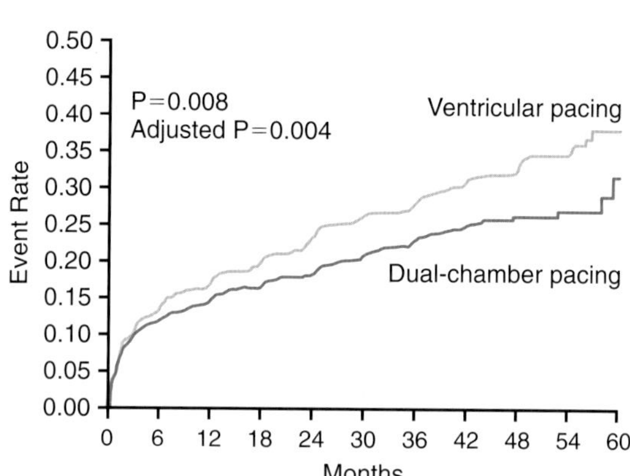

No. at Risk											
Ventricular pacing	996	815	761	668	542	432	333	242	162	92	27
Dual-chamber pacing	1014	852	795	700	572	444	341	248	148	77	20

Figure 13-5. Rates of clinical events according to the mode of pacing in the MOde Selection Trial. (From Lamas GA, Lee KL, Sweeney MO, et al: MOde Selection Trial in Sinus-Node Dysfunction: Ventricular pacing or dual-chamber pacing for sinus-node dysfunction. N Engl J Med 346:1854-1862, 2002.)

A pooled analysis of the five largest randomized trials comparing atrial pacing with ventricular pacing did demonstrate a significant reduction in stroke with atrial pacing (hazard ratio = 0.81, 0.67-0.99; $P = .038$) which was similar among patients with SND and AV block.[50]

Pacing and Atrial Fibrillation

Paroxysmal AF, atrial flutter, and AT occur commonly in SND.[51] Atrial tachyarrhythmia detection and data storage features are now present in many dual-chamber pacemakers that facilitate the diagnosis and treatment of AF.[51-54] Newer devices also have special algorithms developed specifically for the prevention and treatment of atrial tachyarrhythmias.[52,54,56]

Atrial Fibrillation Detection in Pacemakers

Accurate detection of atrial tachyarrhythmias, including atrial flutter and AF, by implantable devices with advanced atrial tachyarrhythmia management features is important for a number of reasons. Accurate detection ensures the appropriateness of automatic mode switching, which is a limitation of many current devices. Accurate arrhythmia detection ensures the appropriateness of device therapies for atrial tachyarrhythmias, including atrial antitachycardia pacing (ATP) and atrial cardioversion shocks. Many implantable devices provide a wide range of diagnostic data, including the frequency of atrial tachyarrhythmias, duration of atrial tachyarrhythmia episodes, the quantity of atrial tachyarrhythmia (burden), ventricular rate control during AF, and symptomatic AT/AF events (Fig. 13-6).[52,54,57,58] Such information may be valuable for managing antiarrhythmic and anticoagulation drug therapy.[59] In addition, many later clinical device trials have used device-based indices of arrhythmia recurrence, frequency, and burden as surrogates for clinical endpoints.[52]

Some investigators have reported comparatively low values for appropriate atrial tachyarrhythmia episode detection using traditional pacemaker mode-switching and detection algorithms.[60-62] It is important that pacemakers be programmed to optimize detection of atrial tachyarrhythmias with careful attention to the atrial sensitivity and postventricular atrial blanking period. Atrial lead position is an important factor for appropriate atrial tachyarrhythmia detection, because some sites (e.g., near the coronary sinus os) are associated with a high incidence of far-field R wave oversensing that may be inappropriately classified as AF. Interelectrode lead spacing (e.g., 5-mm interelectrode distance) may also minimize far-field R wave sensing. Attention to these issues permits high sensitivity and specificity of atrial tachyarrhythmia detection.[62] In the experience of the Atrial Pacing Periablation for Paroxysmal Atrial Fibrillation (PA^3) study investigators in applying these parameters, the sensitivity of atrial tachyarrhythmia detection was 97% for sustained episodes 5 minutes or more in duration.[63] Some devices have incorporated newer detection algorithms that include pattern recognition to facilitate detection of atrial tachyarrhythmias and minimize inappropriate detections due to far-field oversensing.[62,64] Such algorithms have been reported to have high sensitivity (>95%) and specificity for atrial tachyarrhythmia detection.[62,64,65]

Atrial Pacing for Prevention of Atrial Fibrillation

Several prospective randomized clinical trials have reported that atrial or dual-chamber pacing prevents paroxysmal and permanent AF in patients with symptomatic bradycardia as the primary indication for cardiac pacing (Table 13-3; see Fig. 13-5). The Danish investigators reported a 46% relative risk reduction for the development of AF in the atrial pacing group (P = .012).[39] The CTOPP investigators reported an 18% risk reduction in the development of AF (P = .05) in patients

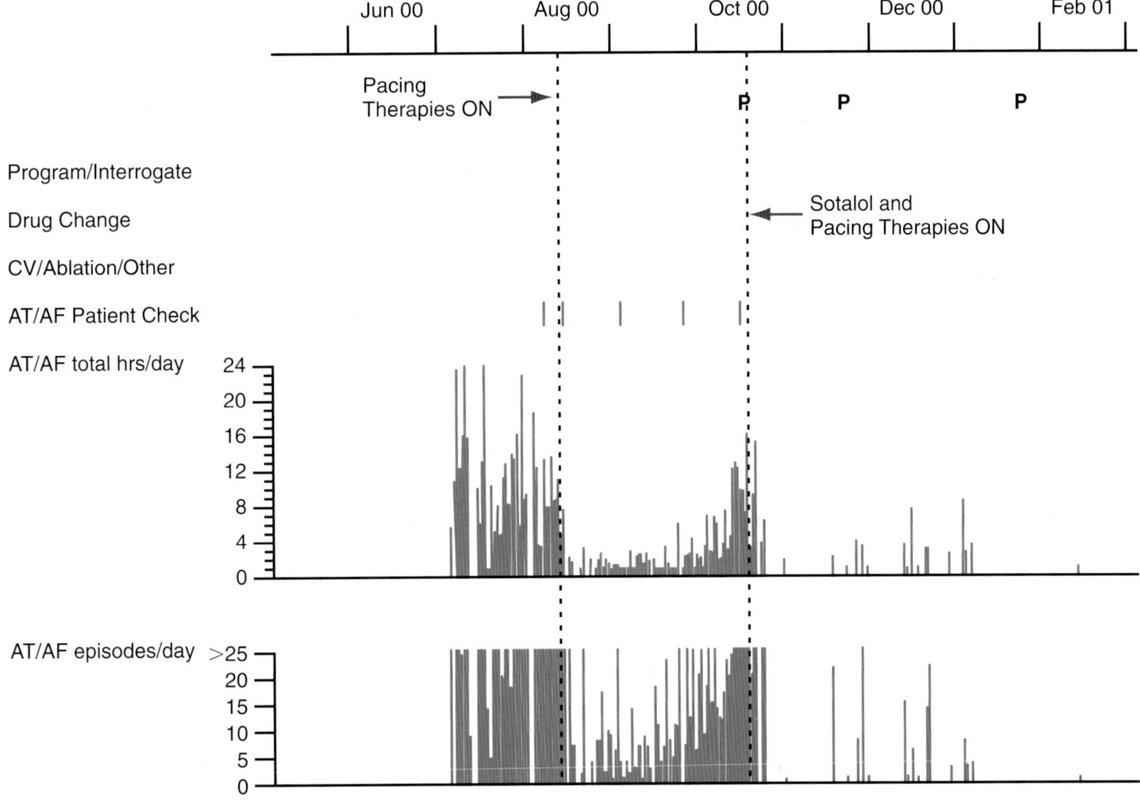

Figure 13-6. Data on atrial tachyarrhythmia burden (hr/day) and AT/AF frequency (episodes/day) over time, retrieved from a patient with a Medtronic AT 501 (Medtronic, Inc, Minneapolis, Minn). Atrial antitachycardia pacing (ATP) and AF pace prevention therapies were programmed "on" 1 month after device implantation. AT/AF burden decreased from 46% to 16% over the next 3 months, whereas AT/AF frequency was unchanged. With the addition of sotalol 4 months after pacemaker implantation, further reductions in atrial tachyarrhythmia burden and frequency were maintained over long-term follow-up. (Courtesy of A. M. Gillis.)

TABLE 13-3. **Randomized Trials of Physiologic Pacing and Impact on AF**

	Andersen et al[39]	Connolly et al[41]	Kerr et al[42]	Lamas et al[43]	Nielsen et al[68]
Trial or mode	AAI vs. VVI	CTOPP	Extended CTOPP	MOST	AAI vs. DDD
Number	225	2568	2568	2050	177
Age (yrs)	71 ± 17	73 ± 10	73 ± 10	74 (67–80)	74 ± 9
Pacing indication	SND-AAI	All pacemaker patients	All pacemaker patients	SND	SND-AAI
Follow-up (yr)	5.5	3.1	6.4	2.7	2.9
Pacing modes	AAI vs. VVI	Physiologic vs. VVIR	Physiologic vs. VVIR	DDDR vs. VVIR	AAI vs. DDDR-s vs. DDDR-l
AF risk (%/yr)	4.1 vs. 6.6	5.3 vs. 6.3	4.5 vs. 5.7	7.9 vs. 10	2.4 vs. 8.3 vs. 6.2
Relative risk reduction (%)	46	18	20	21	73
P value	0.012	0.05	0.009	0.008	0.02

AF, atrial fibrillation; DDDR-l, long atrioventricular delay; DDDR-s, short atrioventricular delay; RR, relative risk; SND, sinus node disease.

randomly allocated to atrial-based pacing compared with those given ventricular pacing[40,66]; this effect was sustained over long-term follow-up (20% risk reduction at 6 years; $P = .009$).[42] Patients with structurally normal hearts were most likely to derive benefit from atrial pacing.[66] Although a retrospective subgroup analysis in CTOPP suggested that pacemaker-dependent patients were most likely to enjoy the benefit of physiologic pacing for prevention of AF, this effect was not confirmed over long-term follow-up.[42,44] The PASE researchers reported a 32% reduction in AF in patients with SND as the primary indication for pacing who were randomly assigned to dual-chamber pacing mode compared with those assigned to ventricular pacing mode ($P = .06$).[40] The MOST investigators reported a 21% relative risk reduction in the development of AF ($P = .008$) and a 56% relative risk reduction in the development of permanent AF ($P < .001$) in patients randomly allocated to dual-chamber pacing compared with those given ventricular pacing.[42] The results of these clinical trials are summarized in Table 13-3. In contrast, the United Kingdom Pacing and Cardiovascular Events (UKPACE) Trial investigators, who randomly allocated 2021 patients 70 years or older with high-grade AV block to dual-chamber or ventricular pacing did not observe a benefit for dual-chamber pacing in prevention of AF.[67] These data suggest that the primary benefit of atrial pacing for prevention of AF is observed in patients with SND.

The MOST investigators reported that ventricular pacing adversely influenced the development of AF independent of AV synchrony.[45] Patients with pacemakers programmed to DDDR mode were more likely to be paced in the ventricle (90%) than patients with pacemakers programmed to VVIR mode (58%; $P = .001$). AF was more likely to develop in patients who were more frequently paced in the ventricle. The risk for development of AF rose approximately 1% for each 1% increase in ventricular pacing. Nielsen and associates[68,69] also reported adverse effects of AV sequential pacing compared with atrial pacing on the development of AF. They randomly assigned 177 patients with sick sinus syndrome to AAIR pacing, DDDR pacing with a short (≤150 msec) AV interval (DDDR-short) or DDDR pacing with a long (300 msec) AV interval (DDDR-long). AF during follow-up was significantly less common in the AAIR group (7.4%) than in the DDDR-short group (23.3%) or the DDDR-long group (17.5%; $P = .03$). Together, these data suggest that RV pacing creates ventricular dyssynchrony even when AV synchrony is preserved, leading to adverse atrial electrical remodeling and thereby raising the risk for AF (see Fig. 13-4).

The results of these studies have generated much debate about alternate ventricular pacing sites.[70-74] It is important to remember, however, that many patients with SND have intrinsic AV conduction and do not require ventricular pacing most of the time. Consequently, considering strategies that minimize ventricular pacing (e.g., AAIR pacing) when clinically indicated[75,76] and programming long AV delays to minimize ventricular pacing, including use of AV delay hysteresis algorithms or even backup ventricular pacing at a low rate, may be sufficient for the majority of patients with SND.[72] Some newer pacemakers have introduced algorithms that switch from AAIR to DDD/R mode when AV conduction fails. Such algorithms have been reported to substantially reduce the amount of ventricular pacing from 90% to 1% in select patient populations, including those with SND.[77,78] Whether such algorithms will prevent the development of AF in patients with SND requires further study.

In the CTOPP population, the number of patients needed to treat (NNT) to prevent any AF over the course of 10 years (the ideal longevity of a dual-chamber pacemaker) was 9.[54,55] In the MOST popula-

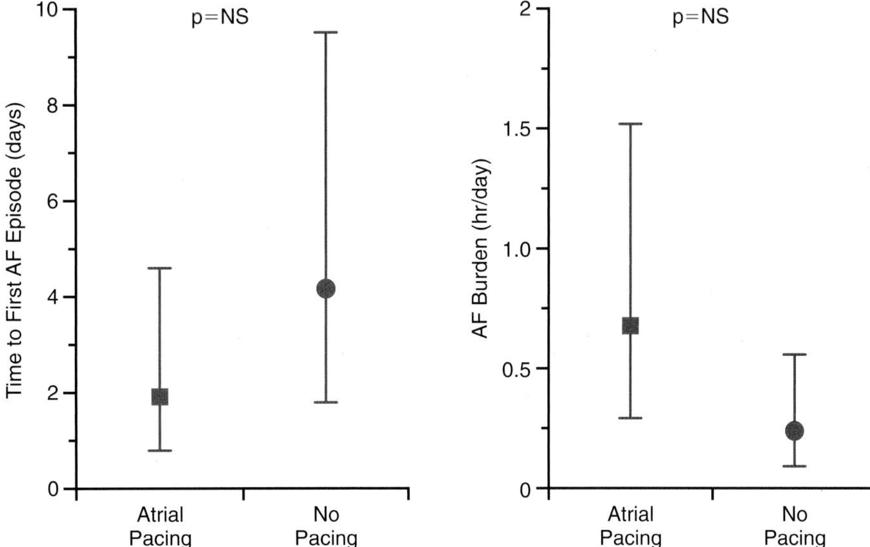

Figure 13-7. Time to first recurrence of sustained atrial fibrillation (AF) (left) *and AF burden measured during the 3-month follow-up period from the diagnostic counters in the pacemaker* (right) *in patients randomly allocated to atrial pacing and patients allocated to no atrial pacing in the Atrial Pacing Periablation for Paroxysmal Atrial Fibrillation (PA³) trial. Data are geometric mean data with 95% confidence intervals. (Data from Gillis AM, Wyse, DG, Connolly SJ, et al: Atrial pacing peri-ablation for prevention of paroxysmal atrial fibrillation. Circulation 99:2553-2558, 1999.)*

tion, the NNT to prevent permanent AF in patients with SND over 3 years was 9. The additional cost of atrial pacing compared with ventricular pacing in CTOPP was $2500.[79] The additional cost of atrial pacing is approximately $1 per day. In patients with pacemakers, AF commonly goes unrecognized, anticoagulation is often underutilized, and classes I through III antiarrhythmic drug therapy for prevention of AF may be proarrhythmic. Accordingly, atrial pacing may be a cost-effective therapy for the prevention of a condition that causes substantial morbidity.[79,80] However, to date, no study has shown that prevention of AF in this patient population translates into a substantial clinical benefit, such as better quality of life (QOL), improved functional capacity, or reduction in rates of hospitalization or health care utilization.

Atrial Pacing for Prevention of Atrial Fibrillation in Patients without Symptomatic Bradycardia

The potential mechanisms of atrial pacing for prevention of AF are (1) prevention of bradycardia-induced dispersion of atrial repolarization—a substrate for AF,[52-54,81] (2) suppression of frequent supraventricular premature beats (SVPBs), which are triggers for AF,[52-54,81] by atrial overdrive pacing, and (3) prevention of adverse atrial electrical remodeling that predisposes to AF by preservation of AV synchrony.[52-54,81] It has been hypothesized that atrial pacing may prevent paroxysmal AF in patients without symptomatic bradycardia as an indication for pacing. To test this hypothesis, the PA³ Study randomly allocated 97 patients with frequent paroxysmal AF who were being considered for AV junction ablation either to a trial of atrial pacing or to no pacing therapy.[81] The time to first recurrence of AF and total AF burden documented over a 3-month follow-up period were similar in the two groups (Fig. 13-7).[82] In phase II, the PA³ trial tested the hypothesis that atrial pacing would prevent AF more effectively than AV synchrony.[81] After AV junction ablation, 76 patients were randomly allocated to either DDDR or VDD pacing. The time to first recurrence of sustained AF and the total AF burden over time were similar in the two groups. Furthermore, AF burden increased progressively over time, and permanent AF had developed in 42% of the study population within 1 year of ablation. Patients who underwent constant antiarrhythmic drug therapy throughout the PA³ study experienced significant increases in AF burden and were more likely to have permanent AF very early after AV junction ablation compared with patients in whom ablation was deferred.[83]

Together, the trials of atrial pacing for prevention of AF in patients with and without bradycardia indications for pacing suggest that atrial pacing is not antiarrhythmic but that ventricular pacing is proarrhythmic, as summarized in Figure 13-4.

Site-Specific Atrial Pacing for Prevention of Atrial Fibrillation

Clinical and experimental studies have demonstrated that septal pacing, dual-site right atrial pacing, and biatrial pacing reduce total atrial conduction times and dispersion of atrial refractoriness.[84-86] A number of randomized trials conducted in the cardiac surgery population have reported that right atrial, dual-site right atrial, and biatrial pacing prevent postoperative AF.[87] In patients with symptomatic bradycardia, the efficacy of selective atrial pacing sites for the prevention of AF has been evaluated in a number of clinical trials. Patients randomly allocated to pacing at Bachmann's bundle were less likely to have permanent AF (47%) than patients assigned to pacing in the right atrial appendage (75%; $P < .05$).[88] In a small series of patients, Padeletti and colleagues[89] reported a significant reduction in AF frequency and AF burden in patients randomly assigned to pacing near the triangle of Koch compared with those receiving pacing in the right atrial appendage.

Other studies have not confirmed these benefits, however.[90,91] In the largest randomized trial conducted to

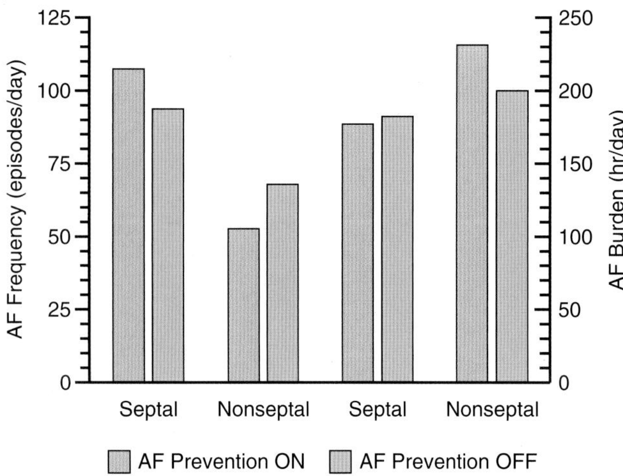

Figure 13-8. AF frequency (left, blue bars) *and AF burden* (right, yellow bars) *in 298 patients randomly allocated to either septal pacing or nonseptal pacing and crossover to trials of three atrial pacing algorithms for prevention of AF (AF Prevention Rx). AF frequency and burden were similar at the two pacing sites. The pacing prevention therapies did not reduce AF frequency or burden. Data are median* (lines) *and 25th and 75th percentiles (*lower and upper borders of boxes, *respectively). (Data from Padeletti L, Purerfellner H, Adler SW, et al: Worldwide ASPECT Investigators: Combined efficacy of atrial septal lead placement and atrial pacing algorithms for prevention of paroxysmal atrial tachyarrhythmia. J Cardiovasc Electrophysiol 14:1189-1195, 2003.)*

date comparing right atrial appendage pacing with atrial septal pacing, a significant reduction in AF frequency or AF burden was not observed between the two sites over short-term follow-up (Fig. 13-8).[90] Dual-site right atrial, right atrial appendage, and coronary sinus os lead locations have been reported to confer a modest benefit for the prevention of AF in comparison with the right atrial appendage.[92] The benefit of dual-site right atrial pacing was greatest in patients treated with antiarrhythmic drug therapy. Biatrial pacing has been reported to prevent paroxysmal AF and the development of permanent AF in patients with marked intra-atrial conduction delays.[93] This finding may in part be secondary to atrial hemodynamic benefits associated with biatrial pacing.[94] At present, the role of selective atrial lead site for prevention of AF in the pacemaker population remains uncertain.[95] A hybrid approach, consisting of aggressive antiarrhythmic therapy combined with dual-site right atrial pacing and right atrial linear ablation, has been reported to provide effective AF rhythm control in select patients.[96] Nevertheless, a single-site atrial lead location would be preferable, given the higher expense and complexity of additional leads.

Pacing Algorithms for Prevention of Atrial Fibrillation

Specific pacing algorithms have been developed for the purpose of AF prevention.[52-56] These algorithms are summarized in Table 13-4. The mechanism(s) by which these algorithms might work are as follows:

1. Prevention of a pause after an atrial premature beat may increase dispersion of atrial repolarization—a substrate for AF.[54,55,81]
2. Atrial overdrive suppresses atrial premature beats—reducing triggers for AF.[52-56,90,97]
3. Continuous atrial pacing at select sites may reduce total atrial activation time, thus preventing intra-atrial reentry when an atrial premature beat occurs.[52-56,90,97]

The Dynamic Atrial Overdrive pacing algorithm was evaluated in the Atrial Dynamic Overdrive Pacing Trial (ADOPT).[97] The investigators randomly allocated 399 patients with SND and paroxysmal AF to a trial of either DDDR pacing or DDDR pacing plus the overdrive atrial pacing algorithm. Patients were assessed at 1, 3, and 6

TABLE 13-4. Pacing Algorithms for Prevention of AF

			Manufacturer*			
Mechanism	**Biotronik**	**ELA**	**Guidant**	**Medtronic**	**St. Jude**	**Vitatron**
Continuous atrial pacing	DDD +	Sinus rhythm overdrive	Atrial preference pacing	Atrial pacing preference	Dynamic atrial overdrive	Pace conditioning
Overdrive pacing after PAC		Acceleration on PAC			Pro-Act	PAC suppression
Prevent pause after PAC		Post-extrasystolic pause suppression		Atrial rate stabilization		Post-PAC response
Overdrive pacing after AF			Post-atrial therapy pacing	Post-mode switch overdrive pacing		Recurrence prevention

*Biotronik GMbH & Co., Berlin, Germany; ELA Medical, Sorin Group, Milan; Guidant, Boston Scientific, Natick, Mass.; Medtronic, Inc., Minneapolis, Minn.; St. Jude Medical, St. Paul, Minn.; Vitatron B.V., Arnheim, The Netherlands.

AF, atrial fibrillation; PAC, premature atrial contraction.

months after pacemaker insertion. The primary study outcome was symptomatic AF burden, defined as percentage of days in symptomatic AF. Both groups experienced a substantial reduction in symptomatic AF over time. In addition, the ADOPT investigators reported a modest but statistically significant reduction in symptomatic AF associated with the atrial overdrive algorithm during follow-up (Fig. 13-9, *upper panel*). However, the absolute risk reduction diminished over time, from 1.25% at 1 month to 0.36% at 6 months. Moreover, overall AF burdens, calculated from the mode-switch device diagnostics in the device, were similar in the two groups and indeed increased over time, suggesting that the overdrive pacing algorithm had no effect on total AF burden over time (Fig. 13-9, *lower panel*).

Other studies have not demonstrated a significant impact of overdrive atrial pacing for prevention of AF. The Atrial Septal Pacing Clinical Efficacy Trial (ASPECT) researchers randomly assigned 298 patients with paroxysmal AF and associated symptomatic bradycardia to conventional DDDR pacing or to DDDR pacing plus three additional atrial pacing algorithms specifically designed for prevention of AF at atrial septal or right atrial appendage pacing sites.[90] After a 3-month treatment period, patients were crossed over to the other pacing strategy and monitored for 3 months longer. AF burden, determined from the diagnostic counters in the pacemaker and measured as percentage of time in AF, was the primary study outcome. The three AF prevention algorithms (Atrial Pacing Preference, Atrial Rate Stabilization, and Post Mode Switch Overdrive Pacing) did *not* reduce AF burden or AF frequency despite suppression of atrial premature beat frequency (see Fig. 13-8).

The Pacing in Prevention of AF (PIPAF) study investigators randomly allocated 192 patients with bradycardia and AF to a trial of three atrial pacing AF prevention algorithms.[98] The primary outcomes, total mode-switch duration, were similar when the AF prevention algorithms were programmed "on" (11.9 ± 27.7 days) and "off" (11.6 ± 26.5 days; P = NS). The investigators reported that these AF prevention algorithms reduced AF burden in the group that was infrequently paced in the ventricle. Blanc and colleagues[99] reported similar results in a smaller series of patients.

To date, the published studies evaluating the effect of AF pace prevention algorithms have demonstrated modest to minimal incremental benefit compared with atrial pacing for the prevention of AF. Further studies are required to determine whether subgroups can be identified who are more likely to benefit from these therapies and to establish the long-term (>6 months) efficacy of the algorithms. Future studies also need to demonstrate that any incremental reductions in AF burden are associated with a clinically relevant outcome, such as better QOL, improved functional capacity, or reduction in health care utilization.

Pacing Algorithms for Termination of Atrial Fibrillation

Episodes of atrial tachycardia (AT) and atrial flutter occur commonly in patients with AF, and AT or atrial flutter frequently transition between episodes of AF.[57,63,98-100] Figure 13-10 shows an example of AF that organizes into atrial flutter and is then effectively terminated by atrial ATP. Atrial ATP therapy has been incorporated into some pacemakers and implantable

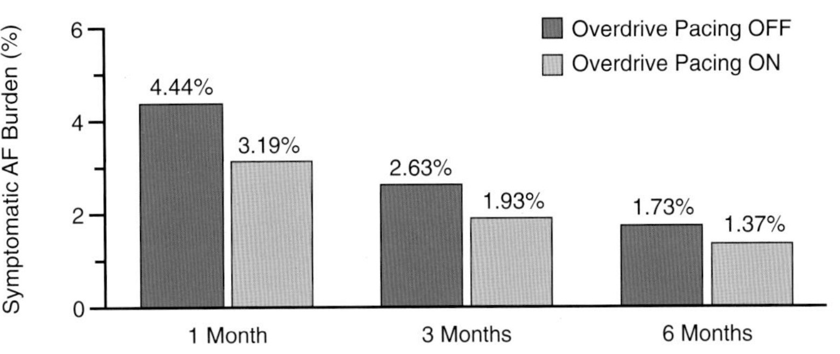

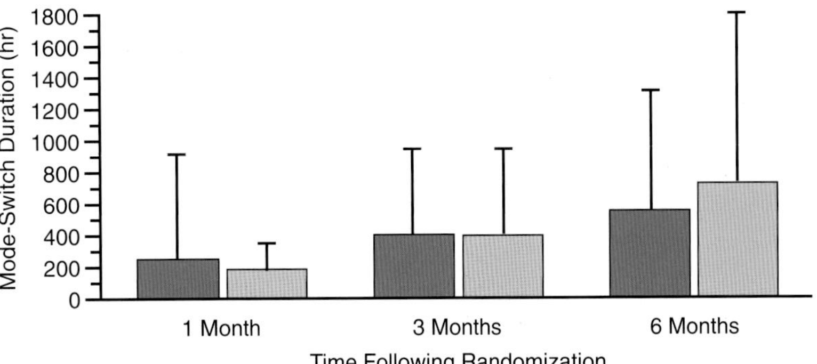

Figure 13-9. Time spent in symptomatic atrial fibrillation (AF) (top) and AF burden estimated from the mode-switch duration counters retrieved by pacemaker interrogation (bottom) *at 1-, 3-, and 6-month follow-ups in 399 patients randomly allocated to DDDR pacing with dynamic atrial overdrive (DAO) programmed "on"* (yellow) *or "off"* (blue). *(Data from Carlson MD, Ip J, Messenger J, et al: Atrial Dynamic Overdrive Pacing Trial [ADOPT] Investigators: A new pacemaker algorithm for the treatment of atrial fibrillation: Results of the Atrial Dynamic Overdrive Pacing Trial [ADOPT]. J Am Coll Cardiol 42:627-633, 2003.)*

defibrillators. A number of clinical studies have reported the efficacy of atrial ATP for termination of atrial tachycardia and atrial flutter to range from 30% to 54%.[100-105] In select individuals, atrial ATP therapy has been reported to reduce atrial tachyarrhythmia burden over time.[57,103,106] The hypothesis that successful pace termination of atrial tachycardia or atrial flutter would prevent the development of AF over time was tested in the Atrial Therapy Efficacy and Safety Trial (ATTEST).[102] In a parallel study design, 370 patients received a Medtronic AT 500 (Medtronic, Inc., Minneapolis, Minn.) and were randomly assigned to either DDDR pacing or DDDR pacing with atrial ATP therapies and atrial pace prevention therapies programmed "on." Over a 3-month follow-up period, 15,000 episodes of an atrial tachyarrhythmia were treated by atrial ATP therapies, and the device-classified efficacy was 41%. However, AF frequency and AF burden (Fig. 13-11) were not reduced by the delivery of prevention therapies or atrial ATP therapies.

Friedman and coworkers[107] randomly allocated 405 patients with a history of AF who had received an implantable cardioverter-defibrillator for standard indications to atrial prevention and termination therapies "on" (n = 199) or "off" (n = 206). Patients were monitored for 7 months. The mean AT/AF burden was 4.3 ± 20.0 hr/month in patients with AT/AF prevention and termination therapies programmed "on," compared with 9.0 ± 50.0 hr/month in the group with these therapies programmed "off" ($P = .11$).

The discrepancy between the reported high atrial ATP efficacy for termination of AT and the failure to demonstrate a significant reduction in AT/AF burden may be due to several factors.[53] Device-classified efficacy may be exaggerated because of spontaneous termination of many episodes of AT.[64] Indeed, in ATTEST[102] and in a trial reported by Gillis and colleagues,[64] which evaluated the GEM III AT (Medtronic, Inc.), approximately one half of the episodes that the pacemakers classified as atrial tachyarrhythmias were less than 10 minutes in duration. By design, these devices define ATP efficacy if sinus or atrial paced rhythm occurs before redetection of atrial tachyarrhythmia.[64] Although the redetection time is usually less than 1 minute, these devices may allow up to 3 minutes from the last-delivered ATP therapy for rede-

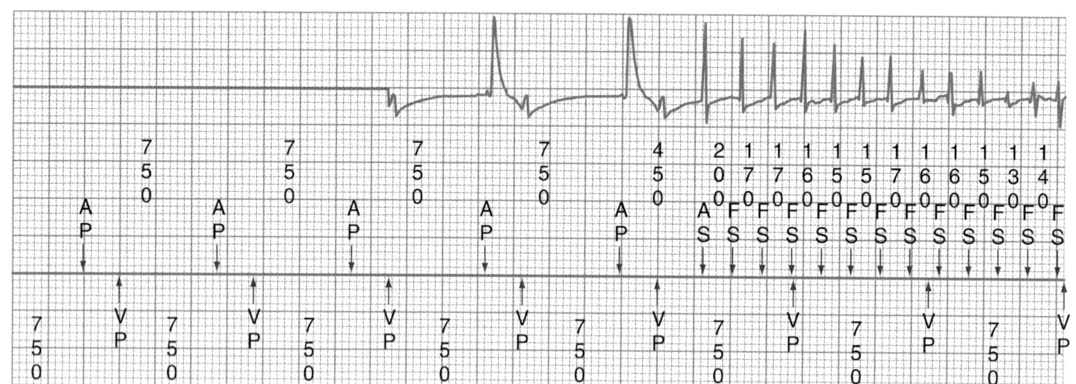

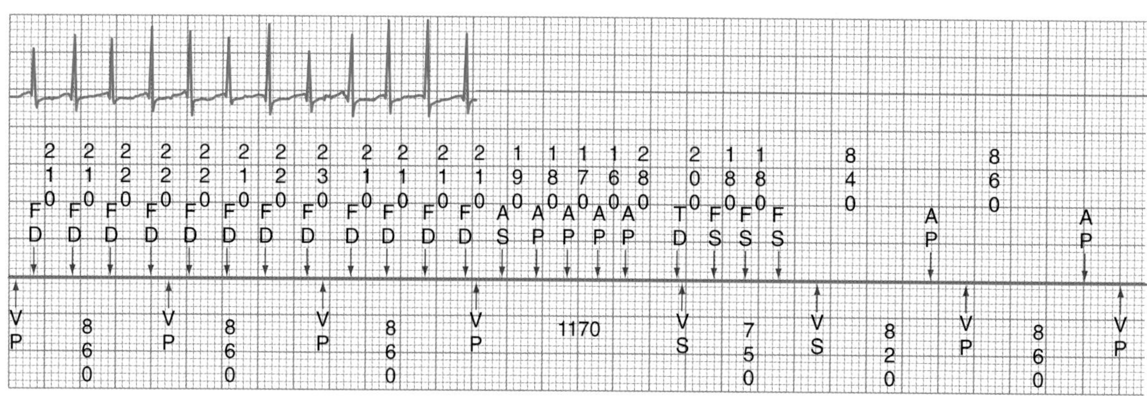

Figure 13-10. An example of atrial fibrillation (AF) organizing into atrial flutter. The atrial electrogram (EGM) and the annotated markers indicating how the pacemaker classifies each atrial and ventricular event as well as the cycle length (in msec) of each interval are displayed in each panel. The initial rhythm is AF (upper panel), *which subsequently organizes into atrial flutter (cycle length 210 msec). The atrial flutter is terminated by a ramp atrial antitachycardia pacing (ATP) therapy that restores atrial paced rhythm. The marker channel notations indicate how the device classifies each beat. Interbeat intervals are also shown (in msec). AP, atrial paced event; VP ventricular paced event; AR, atrial event sensed in atrial refractory period; FS, AF sensed event; TD, tachycardia detected; TS, tachycardia sensed event; Rx, pharmaceutical therapy.*

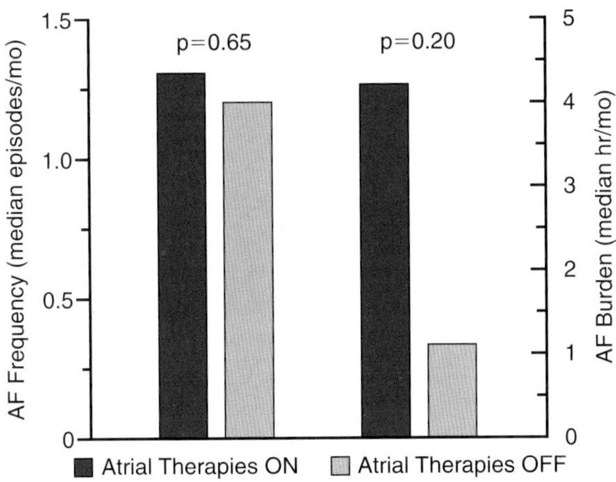

Figure 13-11. Left, *Atrial fibrillation (AF) frequency in patients randomly allocated to atrial antitachycardia pacing (ATP) therapy and three AF pace prevention therapies "on" or "off" in the Atrial Therapy Efficacy and Safety Trial (ATTEST). Patients were followed for 3 months.* Right, *AF burden over 3 months of follow-up in the two treatment groups. Median data are shown. (Data from Lee MA, Weachter R, Pollak S, et al: ATTEST Investigators: The effect of atrial pacing therapies on atrial tachyarrhythmia burden and frequency: Results of a randomized trial in patients with bradycardia and atrial tachyarrhythmias. J Am Coll Cardiol 41:1926-1932, 2003.)*

tection to occur. Gillis and colleagues[64] showed that if a more conservative definition of efficacy—termination of AT or AF within 20 seconds of delivery of atrial ATP therapy—is used, atrial ATP efficacy is lower than previously reported; these researchers found that atrial ATP terminated only 26% of all atrial tachyarrhythmias and 32% of AT episodes. Furthermore, the incorporation of 500-Hz burst pacing algorithms into atrial defibrillators has not been shown to terminate AF.[64]

In the studies evaluating atrial ATP efficacy for prevention of AF, not all patients received maintenance class I/III antiarrhythmic drug therapy, which may be important in facilitating ATP therapy and preventing early recurrence of atrial tachyarrhythmia.[108,109] Some episodes of AT are not reentrant in mechanism, and some episodes classified as AT may have been AF, which cannot be pace terminated.[110] Certain patients do benefit from atrial ATP therapy for prevention of AF (see Fig. 13-8).[57,106] Patients with high atrial ATP efficacy for termination of AT (>60% of all treated episodes effectively terminated) experience a significant reduction in AF burden.[111,112] As many as 30% of patients with SND and paroxysmal AF may benefit from atrial ATP therapy. Also, more aggressive programming of atrial ATP therapy, rather than use of the nominal values in these devices, may improve the efficacy of therapy.[113]

Pacing and Pacemaker Syndrome in Sinus Node Disease

The *pacemaker syndrome* consists of a constellation of signs and symptoms that occur due to the loss of AV synchrony during ventricular pacing (Table 13-5).[2,47] The definition and diagnostic criteria of pacemaker syndrome have varied, but symptoms include fatigue, dyspnea on

TABLE 13-5. Symptoms of Pacemaker Syndrome

Severe	Syncope Presyncope
Moderate	Dizziness Dyspnea Chest pain Jaw pain Confusion
Mild	Venous pulsation in neck Fatigue Weakness Palpitations Fullness in chest

exertion, paroxysmal nocturnal dyspnea, orthopnea, orthostatic hypotension, and syncope. In MOST, pacemaker syndrome was prospectively defined as either (1) new or worsened dyspnea, orthopnea, elevated jugular venous pressure, rales, and edema with ventriculoatrial conduction during ventricular pacing or (2) symptoms of dizziness, weakness, presyncope or syncope, and a reduction in systolic blood pressure of more than 20 mm Hg during VVIR pacing in comparison with atrial pacing or sinus rhythm.[43,114] The incidence of pacemaker syndrome was 13.8% at 6 months, 16.0% at 1 year, 17.7% at 2 years, 19.0% at 3 years, and 19.7% at 4 years. Univariate predictors of pacemaker syndrome were a higher percentage of ventricular paced beats, a higher programmed lower pacemaker rate, and a slower underlying sinus heart rate. However, only a higher percentage of ventricular pacing was an independent predictor of developing pacemaker syndrome. QOL, measured with a variety of metrics, diminished in association with the diagnosis of pacemaker syndrome and improved after the pacemaker was reprogrammed to a physiologic mode.[114] Of the 204 patients randomly allocated to VVIR pacing mode in the PASE trial, 26% crossed over to DDDR mode because of intolerance to ventricular pacing.[40] The incidence of pacemaker syndrome was reported to be 2% in the Danish study[39] and 2.7% at 3 years in CTOPP.[41] The incidence of pacemaker syndrome was likely underestimated in these last two trials, because treatment would have required a surgical intervention. It is possible that pacemaker syndrome was overestimated in MOST and the PASE trial, because it was easy to cross patients over to the DDDR pacing mode.[47]

Pacing and Congestive Heart Failure in Sinus Node Disease

In the Danish study, New York Heart Association functional class and diuretic use were significantly higher during follow-up in the ventricular pacing group than in the atrial pacing group.[39] In CTOPP, the annual incidences of hospitalization for CHF were similar in the ventricular pacing group (3.5%) and the atrial pacing group (3.1% relative risk reduction 7.9%; 95% CI, −18.5% to 28.3%; $P = .52$).[41] In MOST, the annual incidences of hospitalization for heart failure were similar in patients receiving dual-chamber pacing (3.7%) and those receiving ventricular pacing (4.4%; hazard ratio, 0.82; 95% CI, 0.63 to 1.06; $P = .13$).[43] During follow-up, patients receiving dual-chamber pacing had a lower heart failure score than those receiving ventricular pacing (average points per visit during follow-up: ventricular pacing, 1.75; dual-chamber pacing, 1.49; $P < .001$).

Pacing and Quality of Life in Sinus Node Disease

Dual-chamber pacing has been reported to be associated with better physiologic parameters, including cardiac output, exercise capacity, and exercise oxygen consumption, than ventricular pacing.[47] However, none of the large clinical trials conducted to date has demonstrated substantial improvements in QOL measures associated with atrial and ventricular pacing.[115,116] The PASE trial investigators did not show higher values for measures of QOL in patients treated with dual-chamber pacing than in those treated with ventricular pacing, although they did report a modest improvement in some scales of the Medical Outcomes Study 36-Item Short Form Health Survey (SF-36) at 3 months of follow-up in the subgroup with SND.[40] In MOST, dual-chamber pacing resulted in a small but measurably higher QOL than ventricular pacing.[43] In CTOPP, QOL improved after pacemaker implantation in both atrial pacing and ventricular pacing groups, but no significant health-related QOL difference was observed between the two groups.[115] Thus, atrial pacing appears to confer some improvements in QOL in patients with SND, particularly the group at risk for pacemaker syndrome.[114]

Treatment of Sinus Node Disease

Pacing Modalities in Sinus Node Disease

The indications for pacing in the setting of SND are shown in Table 13-6. Although none of the large randomized clinical trials has shown a survival benefit of atrial pacing, dual-chamber pacemakers are commonly implanted in North America.[1] Atrial pacing should be considered in the setting of SND for prevention of AF and pacemaker syndrome.[47,116,117] There is some controversy about the American College of Cardiology/American Heart Association/North American Society for Pacing and Electrophysiology (ACC/AHA/NASPE) classification of these recommendations. Some experts have assigned a class I indication to the selection of dual-chamber pacing over ventricular pacing for prevention of AF in patients with SND (level of evidence A).[47] In contrast, this recommendation was assigned a class IIa recommendation by a Canadian Cardiovascular Society–sponsored Consensus Conference on Atrial Fibrillation.[117] This lower class was assigned on the basis of the absence of data showing that prevention of AF in this population is associated with significant clinical benefit, such as reduction in rates of stroke or mortality.[118] Certainly, on the basis of all the available data from multiple clinical studies, an AAIR system should be considered if the patient has intact AV conduction.[39,75,76] A cost-effectiveness analysis performed in the MOST population has reported that during the first 4 years of the trial, dual-chamber pacemakers increased quality-adjusted life expectancy by 0.013 year per subject at an incremental cost-effectiveness ratio of $53,000 per quality-adjusted year of life gained.[80] This cost could be further reduced by increasing the use of AAIR pacing over that of DDDR pacing in select patients.

AAIR Pacing

As many as 20% of patients with symptomatic SND are potential candidates for AAIR pacing systems.[1,39,54] Because of the high incidence of chronotropic incompetence in patients with SND, a rate-adaptive pulse generator should be considered.[47] Although the most economical approach to providing atrial pacing in this population, this modality is used for less than 1% of implants in North America.[1] Concerns about progression of AV block and the development of chronic AF

TABLE 13-6. Indications for Pacing in Sinus Node Disease

Class I	General consensus that pacing is indicated	Sinus node dysfunction with documented symptomatic bradycardia Symptomatic chronotropic incompetence
Class II: IIa IIb	Divergence of opinion on need for pacing	Sinus node dysfunction with heart rate <40 bpm without a clear association between symptoms and documented bradycardia Minimally symptomatic with heart rate <30 bpm while patients are awake
Class III	General consensus that pacing is not indicated	Sinus node dysfunction in asymptomatic patients Sinus node dysfunction in patients with symptoms suggestive of bradycardia documented not to be associated with bradycardia Sinus node dysfunction secondary to nonessential drug therapy

Data from Gregoratos G, Abrams J, Epstein AE, et al: American College of Cardiology/American Heart Association Task Force on Practice Guidelines/North American Society for Pacing and Electrophysiology Committee: ACC/AHA/NASPE 2002 guideline update for implantation of cardiac pacemakers and antiarrhythmia devices: Summary article: A report of the American College of Cardiology/American Heart Association Task Force on Practice Guidelines (ACC/AHA/NASPE Committee to Update the 1998 Pacemaker Guidelines). Circulation 106:2145-2161, 2002.

likely explain the low use of the AAIR modality in SND. However, these concerns appear to be unfounded if the patient is carefully selected for such treatment.[36,75,76] The risk of progression to AV block is less than 1% per year if the patient has normal AV conduction and no intraventricular conduction delays on the surface electrocardiogram (ECG) at the time of implant. The likelihood of development of permanent AF is small (<1.5% per yr) if the patient is younger than 70 years at the time of implant, has no history of paroxysmal AF prior to implantation,[75,76,119] and shows no evidence of marked intra-atrial conduction delays.[120] Given the concerns that dual-chamber pacing may result in unnecessary ventricular pacing that promotes the development of AF and CHF,[45,46,68-72] higher use of AAIR pacing should be considered in patients with SND. The contraindications to AAIR pacing are shown in Table 13-7. The Danish Multicenter Randomized Study on Atrial Inhibited versus Dual-Chamber Pacing in Sick Sinus Syndrome (DANPACE) is comparing AAI pacing with DDD pacing programmed to have a short AV delay in patients eligible for AAI pacing.[47] The impact of AV hysteresis algorithms or newer pacing algorithms that switch mode from AAI to DDD and thus minimize the amount of unnecessary ventricular pacing are also undergoing clinical investigation to determine whether such modalities are associated with reduced adverse cardiovascular outcomes.

Automatic Mode Switching in Dual-Chamber Pacing

Automatic mode-switching algorithms permit switching from the DDD/R mode to a nontracking mode (DDI/R or VDI/R) for the duration of an episode of atrial tachyarrhythmia, thus preventing atrial tracking at inappropriately high rates (Fig. 13-12). Upon arrhythmia termination, the pacemaker reverts back to the DDD/R mode. Some mode-switching algorithms impose restrictions on maximum programmable AV delays in order to provide adequate windows for AT/AF detection. Shorter AV delays may increase the proportion of unnecessary ventricular pacing.[45] Automatic mode-switching algorithms have been shown to reduce the need for pacemaker reprogramming due to symptomatic rapid ventricular pacing during AT/AF. However, in a large pacemaker population, this feature has not been shown to improve QOL or to reduce overall cardiovascular symptoms.[121]

TABLE 13-7. Contraindications to AAI/AAIR Pacing

Absolute contraindications	AV block documented except during sleep AV block during carotid sinus massage PR interval > 220 msec IVCD on electrocardiogram
Relative contraindications	Age > 70 yr Wenckebach block during atrial pacing <120 bpm HV interval >75 msec Infra-Hisian block during atrial pacing

AV, atrioventricular; IVCD, intraventricular conduction delay; HV, His-ventricular interval.

Rate-Adaptive Pacing in Sinus Node Disease

Chronotropic incompetence is common in SND, and rate-adaptive pacing is beneficial in select patients. Some investigators have reported that rate-adaptive pacing was beneficial in preventing AF in patients with chronotropic incompetence.[122] However, Duff and colleagues have not demonstrated any improvement in QOL in patients after AV junction ablation when they compared fixed-rate VVI at 80 bpm with rate-adaptive VVIR pacing. Furthermore, rate-adaptive VVIR pacing after AV junction ablation has been associated with more dispersion of ventricular repolarization than fixed-rate VVI pacing in this population.[123]

Alternative Ventricular Pacing Sites in SND

There has been some debate about the optimal ventricular pacing site for minimizing the risk of heart failure or AF in patients receiving dual-chamber pacemakers.[72] There have even been calls to consider biventricular pacing for the prevention of heart failure in this patient population.[71] It is important to remember, however, that the vast majority of patients with SND have intrinsic AV conduction the vast majority of the time. Accordingly, strategies of minimizing ventricular pacing whenever possible should be pursued, including the judicious use of AAI pacing when suitable, the optimal use of AV search hysteresis algorithms, and the use of newer algorithms that switch mode from AAI to DDD pacing when atrial conduction fails (Fig. 13-13). These algorithms include the MVP (Managed Ventricular Pacing, Medtronic, Inc.) and the AAIsafeR, (ELA Medical, Sorin Group, Milan). These algorithms promote intrinsic AV conduction and normal ventricular activation while avoiding iterative reprogramming of the AV interval. The MVP algorithm, for example, avoids interlocks that limit upper rate programming or AV interval programming. Clinical studies have demonstrated that the amount of ventricular pacing can be substantially reduced with these newer pacing algorithms, even in patients in whom AV block is the primary indication for pacing.[77,78] Large controlled trials are under way evaluating the impact of these algorithms on heart failure, incidence of AF, and cardiac mortality, including the use of the MVP algorithm in patients undergoing implantation of DDD implantable cardioverter-defibrillators (ICDs), AV search hysteresis in patients with DDD ICDs, and AAIsafeR in patients undergoing implantation of DDD pacemakers. There are no data to date to suggest that biventricular pacing prevents heart failure in patients without significant systolic dysfunction.[74] RV outflow tract and high RV septal pacing sites may be associated with less ventricular dyssynchrony than RV apical pacing.[73] However, no large clinical trials demonstrating that any of these pacing sites are superior to the

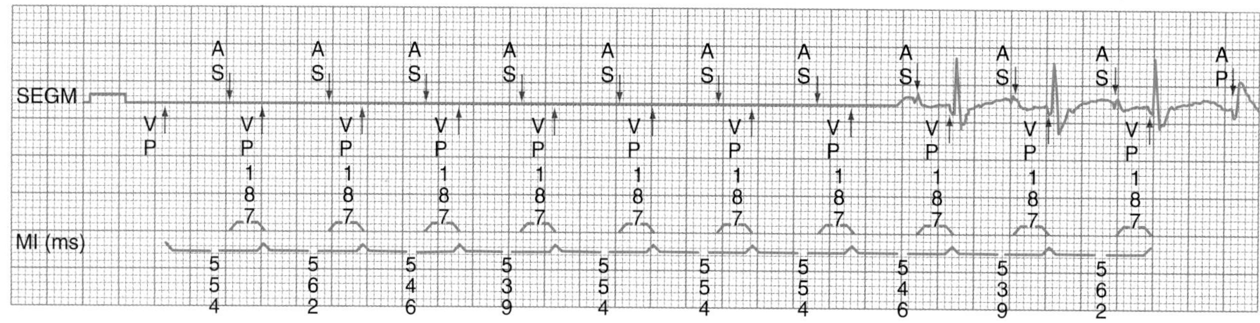

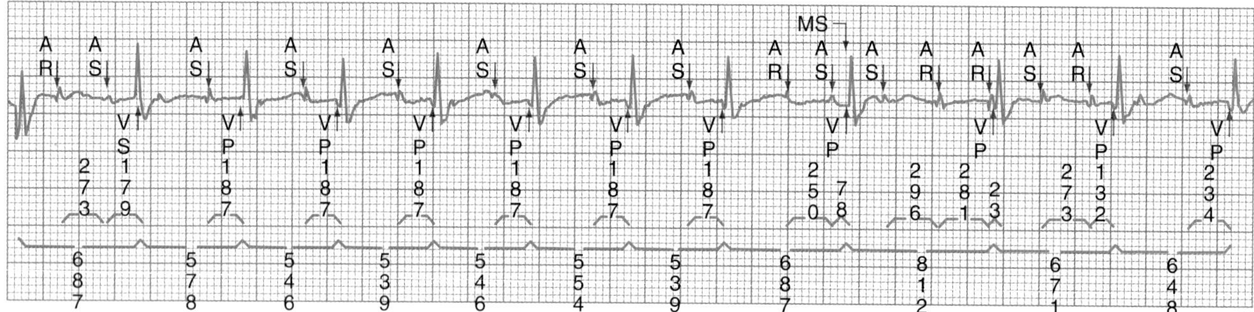

Figure 13-12. Example of atrial flutter onset followed by automatic switching from DDDR to DDIR mode. The upper trace illustrates atrial and ventricular electrograms as well as Marker Channel annotations. The numbers represent interatrial or interventricular cycle lengths (in msec). Note the slowing of the ventricular pacing rate after the mode-switch (MS) event. AS, atrial sensed event; VP, ventricular paced event; AR, atrial event sensed in the atrial refractory period.

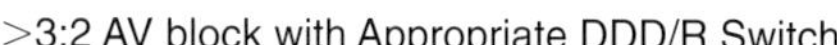

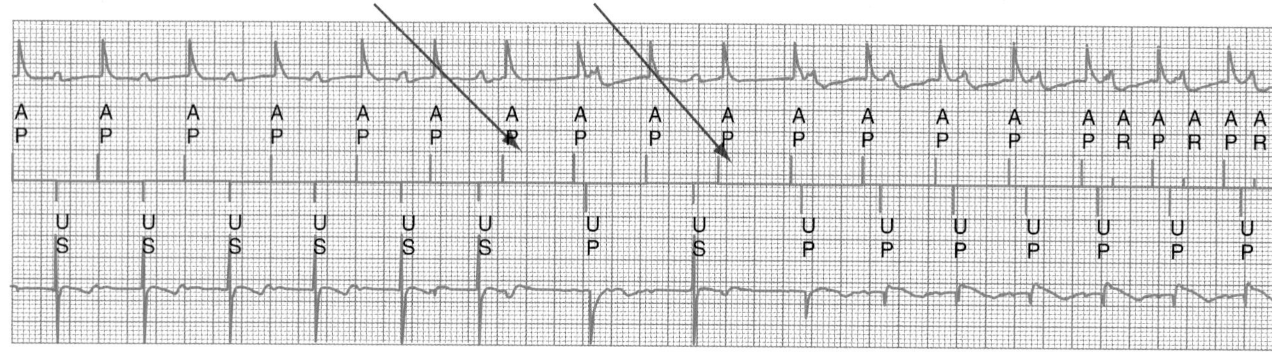

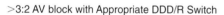

Figure 13-13. Example of MVP (Minimal Ventricular Pacing, Medtronic, Inc.) algorithm showing switch from AAI pacing to DDDR with failure of AV conduction. The algorithm monitors AV conduction; if AV conduction fails, the mode returns to DDD(R). The backup ventricular pace occurs after any A-A interval in which there is no ventricular sensed event.

traditional RV apical pacing site have been reported to date.

Diagnostic Data for Atrial Fibrillation in Pacemakers

Most dual-chamber pacemakers now provide some data on frequency and duration of atrial tachyarrhythmias or information about the number and duration of mode switches. Some pacemakers and ICDs designed for the management of patients with AF have more sophisticated AF detection and data storage features (see Fig. 13-6). Such information may be of value in the management of AF. Response to antiarrhythmic drug therapy can be monitored over the long term.[57] Willems and associates[59] have reported that patients with AF associated with episodes of rapid ventricular rates are more likely to experience hospitalization for cardiovascular events (Fig. 13-14). Identification of such episodes led to changes in antiarrhythmic drug therapy. Clinical studies are under way to determine whether the availability of such diagnostic data has clinical value.

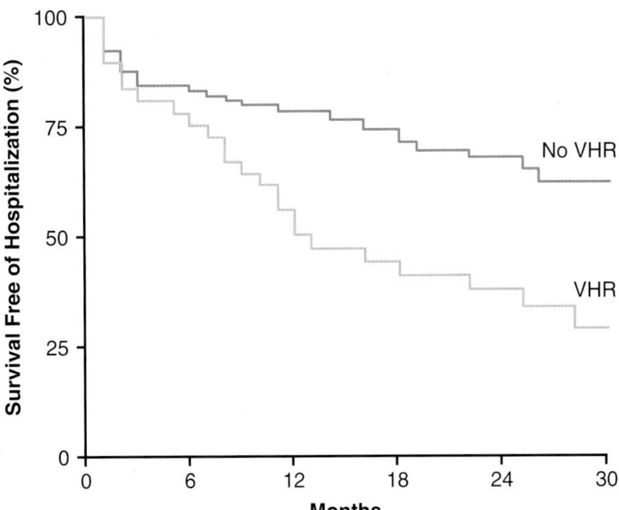

Figure 13-14. Survival free of hospitalization for cardiovascular symptoms. Patients who experienced ventricular high rate (VHR) episodes predominantly due to atrial fibrillation with a rapid ventricular response (yellow line) were more likely to be hospitalized than patients without VHR episodes (blue line; Log rank P =.001). (From Willems R, Morck ML, Exner DV, Gillis AM: Ventricular high rate episodes in pacemaker diagnostics identify a high-risk subgroup of patients with tachy-brady syndrome. Heart Rhythm 1:414-421, 2004.)

Implantable Atrial Cardioverter

Atrial pacing does not prevent all episodes of AF, nor do atrial ATP therapies terminate AF. The Metrix Atrioverter (Guidant, Boston Scientific, Natick, Mass.) was the first implantable device designed for detection and cardioversion of AF.[124] It consisted of two atrial defibrillation leads, one placed in the right atrium and one in the coronary sinus, as well as a ventricular lead, which was used to synchronize shocks to the ventricular electrogram. The initial efficacy of this device in terminating AF was 90%. Because the shocks are usually painful, sedation was usually required before device activation, and this approach significantly improved patient acceptability of atrial shock therapy.[125] No instances of ventricular proarrhythmia have been reported. During more than 40 months of follow-up in the initial cohort of 136 patients to receive the first implantable atrial cardioverter, only 39 patients were actively delivering therapy with the device.[126] This device lacked bradycardia pacing and ventricular defibrillation capabilities and is no longer manufactured.

Atrial tachyarrhythmias occur frequently in patients receiving ICDs.[127,128] Combined atrial and ventricular defibrillators have been approved by the U.S. Food and Drug Administration (FDA). Discrimination of AF from ventricular tachyarrhythmias has been reported to be high.[64,129,130] Shocks for AF can be activated by the patient or can be delivered automatically at a prespecified time, such as in the early morning while the patient is asleep. Shock efficacy for termination of AF has been reported to range from 85% to 93%.[129-131] Patients are more likely to accept an atrial cardioverter-defibrillator if they have less psychosocial distress and lower AF symptom burden.[132] Regular early use of the atrial defibrillator has been reported to increase the duration of sinus rhythm in a minority of patients during long-term follow-up.[133]

Ricci and associates[134] monitored 40 patients who received a dual defibrillator (Medtronic 7250, Medtronic, Inc.) with atrial ATP therapies and atrial cardioversion therapies for 15 ± 4 months.[134] Eighty-five percent of patients had recurrences of atrial tachyarrhythmias during follow-up. Among 1366 treated episodes, device-classified efficacy was 60.1% for atrial ATP therapy and 88.2% for atrial shock efficacy. These investigators reported a significant reduction in arrhythmia-related hospitalization within the first year after implant (hospitalization number decreased from 1.5 ± 2.0 to 0.4 ± 0.8; $P < .01$). Measures of QOL improved after device implantation. The patients assigned to early delivery of atrial shock after AF onset experienced a significant reduction of AF burden, a higher reduction in hospitalization numbers, and a greater improvement of QOL than the patients who did not accept atrial shock therapy.

A strategy of maintaining sinus rhythm over the long term with an atrial ICD is feasible in select patients. This approach has been reported to be associated with improvements in QOL.[135] However, patient selection is critical, and this therapy is ideal for only a small percentage of the population with AF.

Future Therapies

Overexpression of *HCN2* into a localized region of atrium has been reported to generate an I_f-based biologic pacemaker in dogs, offering a promising gene therapy for pacemaker disease. Much more experimental work is required before such an approach can be tested in humans.[136,137]

REFERENCES

1. Mond HG, Irwin M, Morillo C, Ector H: The world survey of cardiac pacing and cardioverter defibrillators: Calendar year 2001. Pacing Clin Electrophysiol 27:955-964, 2004.
2. Gillis AM: Sinus node disease. In Ellenbogen KA, Kay GN, Wilkoff BL (eds): Clinical Cardiac Pacing, 2nd ed. Philadelphia, WB Saunders, 2000, pp 405-425.
3. Brignole M: Sick sinus syndrome. Clin Geriatr Med 18:211-227, 2002.
4. Boyett MR, Honjo H, Kodama I: The sinoatrial node: A heterogeneous pacemaker structure. Cardiovasc Res 47:658-687, 2000.
5. Boyett MR, Dobrzynski H, Lancaster MK, et al: Sophisticated architecture is required for the sinoatrial node to perform its normal pacemaker function. J Cardiovasc Electrophysiol 14:104-106, 2003.
6. Jones SA, Lancaster MK, Boyett MR: Ageing-related changes of connexins and conduction within the sinoatrial node. J Physiol 560:429-437, 2004.
7. Schulze-Bahr E, Neu A, Friederich P, et al: Pacemaker channel dysfunction in a patient with sinus node disease. J Clin Invest 111:1537-1545, 2003.
8. Stieber J, Hofmann F, Ludwig A: Pacemaker channels and sinus node arrhythmia. Trends Cardiovasc Med 14:23-28, 2004.

9. Ueda K, Nakamura K, Hayashi T, et al: Functional characterization of a trafficking-defective HCN4 mutation, D553N, associated with cardiac arrhythmia. J Biol Chem 279:27194-27198, 2004.
10. Verkerk AO, Wilders R, Coronel R, et al: Ionic remodeling of sinoatrial node cells by heart failure. Circulation 108:760-766, 2003.
11. Veldkamp MW, Wilders R, Baartscheer A, et al: Contribution of sodium channel mutations to bradycardia and sinus node dysfunction in LQT3 families. Circ Res 92:976-983, 2003.
12. Benson DW, Wang DW, Dyment M, et al: Congenital sick sinus syndrome caused by recessive mutations in the cardiac sodium channel gene (SCN5A). J Clin Invest 112:1019-1028, 2003.
13. Lees-Miller JP, Guo J, Somers JR, et al: Selective knockout of mouse ERG1 B potassium channel eliminates I(Kr) in adult ventricular myocytes and elicits episodes of abrupt sinus bradycardia. Mol Cell Biol 23:1856-1862, 2003.
14. Demolombe S, Lande G, Charpentier F, et al: Transgenic mice overexpressing human KvLQT1 dominant-negative isoform. Part I: Phenotypic characterisation. Cardiovasc Res 50:314-327, 2001.
15. Hu K, Qu Y, Yue Y, Boutjdir M: Functional basis of sinus bradycardia in congenital heart block. Circ Res 94:e32-e38, 2004.
16. Platzer J, Engel J, Schrott-Fischer A, et al: Congenital deafness and sinoatrial node dysfunction in mice lacking class D L-type Ca2+ channels. Cell 102:89-97, 2000.
17. Zhang Z, Xu Y, Song H, et al: Functional Roles of Ca(v)1.3 (alpha(1D)) calcium channel in sinoatrial nodes: Insight gained using gene-targeted null mutant mice. Circ Res 90:981-987, 2002.
18. Gillis AM, Kavanagh KM, Mathison HJ, et al: Heart block in mice overexpressing calcineurin but not NF-AT3. Cardiovasc Res 64:488-495, 2004.
19. Opthof T, Coronel R, Rademaker HM, et al: Changes in sinus node function in a rabbit model of heart failure with ventricular arrhythmias and sudden death. Circulation 101:2975-2980, 2000.
20. Hong CS, Cho MC, Kwak YG, et al: Cardiac remodeling and atrial fibrillation in transgenic mice overexpressing junctin. FASEB J 16:1310-1312, 2002.
21. Sanders P, Morton JB, Kistler PM, et al: Electrophysiological and electroanatomic characterization of the atria in sinus node disease: Evidence of diffuse atrial remodeling. Circulation 109: 1514-1522, 2004.
22. Kistler PM, Sanders P, Fynn SP, et al: Electrophysiologic and electroanatomic changes in the human atrium associated with age. J Am Coll Cardiol 44:109-116, 2004.
23. Sanders P, Kistler PM, Morton JB, et al: Remodeling of sinus node function in patients with congestive heart failure: Reduction in sinus node reserve. Circulation 110:897-903, 2004.
24. Sanders P, Morton JB, Davidson NC, et al: Electrical remodeling of the atria in congestive heart failure: Electrophysiological and electroanatomic mapping in humans. Circulation 108:1461-1468, 2003.
25. Sparks PB, Mond HG, Vohra JK, et al: Electrical remodeling of the atria following loss of atrioventricular synchrony: A long-term study in humans. Circulation 100:1894-1900, 1999.
26. Sparks PB, Jayaprakash S, Vohra JK, Kalman JM: Electrical remodeling of the atria associated with paroxysmal and chronic atrial flutter. Circulation 102:1807-1813, 2000.
27. Kalman JM, Sparks PB: Electrical remodeling of the atria as a consequence of atrial stretch. J Cardiovasc Electrophysiol 12:51-55, 2001.
28. Manios EG, Kanoupakis EM, Mavrakis HE, et al: Sinus pacemaker function after cardioversion of chronic atrial fibrillation: Is sinus node remodeling related with recurrence? J Cardiovasc Electrophysiol 12:800-806, 2001.
29. Hadian D, Zipes DP, Olgin JE, Miller JM: Short-term rapid atrial pacing produces electrical remodeling of sinus node function in humans. J Cardiovasc Electrophysiol 13:584-586, 2002.
30. Hocini M, Sanders P, Deisenhofer I, et al: Reverse remodeling of sinus node function after catheter ablation of atrial fibrillation in patients with prolonged sinus pauses. Circulation 108:1172-1175, 2003.
31. Raitt MH, Kusumoto W, Giraud G, McAnulty JH: Reversal of electrical remodeling after cardioversion of persistent atrial fibrillation. J Cardiovasc Electrophysiol 15:507-512, 2004.
32. Krahn AD, Klein GJ, Yee R, Skanes AC: Randomized assessment of syncope trial: Conventional diagnostic testing versus a prolonged monitoring strategy. Circulation 104:46-51, 2001.
33. Krahn AD, Klein GJ, Yee R, et al: Cost implications of testing strategy in patients with syncope: Randomized assessment of syncope trial. J Am Coll Cardiol 42:495-501, 2003.
34. Solano A, Menozzi C, Maggi R, et al: Incidence, diagnostic yield and safety of the implantable loop-recorder to detect the mechanism of syncope in patients with and without structural heart disease. Eur Heart J 25:1116-1119, 2004.
35. Menozzi C, Brignole M, Alboni P, et al: The natural course of untreated sick sinus syndrome and identification of the variables predictive of unfavorable outcome. Am J Cardiol 82:1205-1209, 1998.
36. Brandt J, Anderson H, Fahraeus T, Schuller H: Natural history of sinus node disease treated with atrial pacing in 213 patients: Implications for selection of stimulation mode. J Am Coll Cardiol 20:633-639, 1992.
37. Jahangir A, Shen WK, Neubauer SA, et al: Relation between mode of pacing and long-term survival in the very elderly. J Am Coll Cardiol 33:1208-1216, 1999.
38. Connolly SJ, Kerr C, Gent M, Yusuf S: Dual-chamber versus ventricular pacing: Critical appraisal of current data. Circulation 94:578-583, 1996.
39. Andersen HR, Nielsen JC, Thomsen PEB, et al: Long-term follow-up of patients from a randomized trial of atrial versus ventricular pacing for sick-sinus syndrome. Lancet 350:1210-1216, 1997.
40. Lamas GA, Orav EJ, Stambler BS, et al: Quality of life and clinical outcomes in elderly patients treated with ventricular pacing as compared with dual-chamber pacing. Pacemaker Selection in the Elderly Investigators. N Engl J Med 338:1097-1104, 1998.
41. Connolly SJ, Kerr CR, Gent M, et al: Effects of physiologic pacing versus ventricular pacing on the risk of stroke and death due to cardiovascular causes. Canadian Trial of Physiologic Pacing Investigators. N Engl J Med 342:1385-1391, 2000.
42. Kerr CR, Connolly SJ, Abdollah H, et al: Canadian Trial of Physiological Pacing: Effects of physiological pacing during long-term follow-up. Circulation 109:357-362, 2004.
43. Lamas GA, Lee KL, Sweeney MO, et al: MOde Selection Trial in Sinus-Node Dysfunction: Ventricular pacing or dual-chamber pacing for sinus-node dysfunction. N Engl J Med 346:1854-1862, 2002.
44. Tang AS, Roberts RS, Kerr C, et al: Relationship between pacemaker dependency and the effect of pacing mode on cardiovascular outcomes. Circulation 103:3081-3085, 2001.
45. Sweeney MO, Hellkamp AS, Ellenbogen KA, et al; MOde Selection Trial Investigators: Adverse effect of ventricular pacing on heart failure and atrial fibrillation among patients with normal baseline QRS duration in a clinical trial of pacemaker therapy for sinus node dysfunction. Circulation 107:2932-2937, 2003.
46. Wilkoff BL, Cook JR, Epstein AE, et al; Dual Chamber and VVI Implantable Defibrillator Trial Investigators: Dual-chamber pacing or ventricular backup pacing in patients with an implantable defibrillator. The Dual Chamber and VVI Implantable Defibrillator (DAVID) Trial. JAMA 288:3115-3123, 2002.
47. Lamas GA, Ellenbogen KA: Evidence base for pacemaker mode selection: From physiology to randomized trials. Circulation 109:443-451, 2004.

48. Greenspon AJ, Hart RG, Dawson D, et al; MOST Study Investigators: Predictors of stroke in patients paced for sick sinus syndrome. J Am Coll Cardiol 43:1617-1622, 2004.
49. Kerr CR: Stroke and pacing mode: Is pacing mode important? J Am Coll Cardiol 43:1623-1624, 2004.
50. Healey JS, Toff WD, Lamas GA, et al: Prevention of stroke with atrial-based pacing: A meta-analysis of randomized trials using individual patient data. Can J Cardiol 21:Supple 173C, 2005.
51. Gillis AM, Morck M: Atrial fibrillation after DDDR pacemaker implantation. J Cardiovasc Electrophysiol 13:542-547, 2002.
52. Gillis AM: Rhythm control in atrial fibrillation: Endpoints for device-based trials. Can J Cardial 21:Supple 173C, 2005.
53. Gillis AM: Pacing to prevent atrial fibrillation. Cardiol Clin 18:25-36, 2000.
54. Gillis AM: Clinical trials of pacing for maintenance of sinus rhythm. J Interv Card Electrophysiol 10(Suppl 1):55-62, 2004.
55. Willems R, Gillis AM: New indications for pacing. Curr Cardiol Rep 5:369-374, 2003.
56. Cooper JM, Katcher MS, Orlov MV: Implantable devices for the treatment of atrial fibrillation. N Engl J Med 346:2062-2068, 2002.
57. Gillis AM, Morck M, Fitts S: Antitachycardia pacing therapies and arrhythmia monitoring diagnostics for the treatment of atrial fibrillation. Can J Cardiol 18:992-995, 2002.
58. Glotzer TV, Hellkamp AS, Zimmerman J, et al; MOST Investigators: Atrial high rate episodes detected by pacemaker diagnostics predict death and stroke: Report of the Atrial Diagnostics Ancillary Study of the MOde Selection Trial (MOST). Circulation 107:1614-1619, 2003.
59. Willems R, Morck ML, Exner DV, Gillis AM: Ventricular high rate episodes in pacemaker diagnostics identify a high-risk subgroup of patients with tachy-brady syndrome. Heart Rhythm 1:414-421, 2004.
60. Passman RS, Weinberg KM, Freher M, et al: Accuracy of mode switch algorithms for detection of atrial tachyarrhythmias. J Cardiovasc Electrophysiol 15:773-777, 2004.
61. Plummer CJ, McComb JM; STOP AF trial: Detection of atrial fibrillation by permanent pacemakers: Observations from the STOP AF trial. Card Electrophysiol Rev 7:333-340, 2003.
62. Purerfellner H, Gillis AM, Holbrook R, Hettrick DA: Accuracy of atrial tachyarrhythmia detection in implantable devices with arrhythmia therapies. Pacing Clin Electrophysiol 27:983-992, 2004.
63. Fitts SM, Hill MR, Mehra R, Gillis AM: High rate atrial tachyarrhythmia detections in implantable pulse generators: Low incidence of false-positive detections. The PA^3 Clinical Trial Investigators. Pacing Clin Electrophysiol 23:1080-1086, 2000.
64. Gillis AM, Unterberg-Buchwald C, Schmidinger H, et al; for the GEM III AT Worldwide Investigators: Safety and efficacy of advanced atrial pacing therapies for atrial tachyarrhythmias in patients with a new implantable dual chamber cardioverter-defibrillator. J Am Coll Cardiol 40:1653-1659, 2002.
65. Kouakam C, Kacet S, Hazard JR, Ferraci A, et al; Ventak AV Investigators: Performance of a dual-chamber implantable defibrillator algorithm for discrimination of ventricular from supraventricular tachycardia. Europace 6:32-42, 2004.
66. Skanes AC, Krahn AD, Yee R, et al: Canadian Trial of Physiologic Pacing: Progression to chronic atrial fibrillation after pacing: The Canadian Trial of Physiologic Pacing. CTOPP Investigators. J Am Coll Cardiol 38:167-172, 2001.
67. Toff WD: UK PACE trial. Presented at the American College of Cardiology Scientific Sessions, Chicago, March 30-April 2, 2003.
68. Nielsen JC, Kristensen L, Andersen HR, et al: A randomized comparison of atrial and dual-chamber pacing in 177 consecutive patients with sick sinus syndrome: Echocardiographic and clinical outcome. J Am Coll Cardiol 42:614-623, 2003.
69. Kristensen L, Nielsen JC, Mortensen PT, et al: Incidence of atrial fibrillation and thromboembolism in a randomised trial of atrial versus dual chamber pacing in 177 patients with sick sinus syndrome. Heart 90:661-666, 2004.
70. Kass DA: Pathophysiology of physiologic cardiac pacing: Advantages of leaving well enough alone. JAMA 288:3159-3161, 2003.
71. Barold SS: Adverse effects of ventricular desynchronization induced by long-term right ventricular pacing. J Am Coll Cardiol 42:614-623, 2003.
72. Gillis AM, Chung MK: Pacing the right ventricle: To pace or not to pace. Heart Rhythm 2:201-206, 2005.
73. Stambler BS, Ellenbogen K, Zhang X, et al; ROVA Investigators: Right ventricular outflow versus apical pacing in pacemaker patients with congestive heart failure and atrial fibrillation. J Cardiovasc Electrophysiol 14:1180-1186, 2003.
74. Daoud E, Doshi R, Fellows C, et al, and the investigators of the PAVE Study: Ablate and pace with cardiac resynchronization therapy for patients with reduced ejection fraction: Sub-analysis of PAVE study. Heart Rhythm 1:s59, 2004.
75. Kristensen L, Nielsen JC, Pedersen AK, et al: AV block and changes in pacing mode during long-term follow-up of 399 consecutive patients with sick sinus syndrome treated with an AAI/AAIR pacemaker. Pacing Clin Electrophysiol 24:358-365, 2001.
76. Andersen HR, Nielsen JC, Thomsen PE, et al: Atrioventricular conduction during long-term follow-up of patients with sick sinus syndrome. Circulation 98:1315-1321, 1998.
77. Gillis AM, Purerfellner H, Israel C, et al: Reduction of unnecessary right ventricular pacing with the managed ventricular pacing (MVP) mode in patients with symptomatic bradycardia: Benefit for both sinus node disease and AV block indications. PACE (in press).
78. Sweeney MO: Multicenter, prospective, randomized trial of a new atrial-based managed ventricular pacing mode (MVP) in dual chamber ICDs. Circulation 110:III-444, 2004.
79. Gillis AM, Kerr CR: Whither physiologic pacing? Implications of CTOPP. PACE 23:8:1193-1196, 2000.
80. Rinfret S, Cohen DJ, Lamas GA, et al: Cost-effectiveness of dual-chamber pacing compared with ventricular pacing for sinus node dysfunction. Circulation 2005 111:165-172, 2005.
81. Gillis AM, Connolly SJ, Lacombe P, et al; for the PA^3 Investigators: A randomized crossover comparison of DDDR versus VDD pacing post-AV node ablation for prevention of atrial fibrillation. Circulation 102:736-741, 2000.
82. Gillis AM, Wyse, DG, Connolly SJ, et al: Atrial pacing peri-ablation for prevention of paroxysmal atrial fibrillation. Circulation 99:2553-2558, 1999.
83. Willems R, Wyse DG, Gillis AM; for the Atrial Pacing Periablation for Paroxysmal Atrial Fibrillation (PA^3) Study Investigators: Total AV nodal ablation increases atrial fibrillation burden in patients with paroxysmal AF despite continuation of antiarrhythmic drug therapy. J Cardiovasc Electrophysiol 14:1296-1301, 2003.
84. Yu WC, Chen SA, Tai CT, et al: Effects of different atrial pacing modes on atrial electrophysiology: Implicating the mechanism of biatrial pacing in prevention of atrial fibrillation. Circulation 96:2992-2996, 1997.
85. Prakash A, Delfaut P, Krol RB, Saksena S: Regional right and left atrial activation patterns during single- and dual-site atrial pacing in patients with atrial fibrillation. Am J Cardiol 82:1197-1204, 1998.
86. Papageorgiou P, Anselme F, Kirchhof CJ, et al: Coronary sinus pacing prevents induction of atrial fibrillation. Circulation 96:1893-1898, 1997.
87. Crystal E, Connolly SJ, Sleik K, et al: Interventions on prevention of postoperative atrial fibrillation in patients undergoing heart surgery: A meta-analysis. Circulation 106:75-80, 2002.
88. Bailin SJ, Adler S, Giudici M: Prevention of chronic atrial fibrillation by pacing in the region of Bachmann's bundle: Results of a multicenter randomized trial. J Cardiovasc Electrophysiol 12:912-917, 2001.

89. Padeletti L, Porciani MC, Michelucci A, et al: Interatrial septum pacing: A new approach to prevent recurrent atrial fibrillation. J Interv Card Electrophysiol 3:35-43, 1999.
90. Padeletti L, Purerfellner H, Adler SW, et al; Worldwide ASPECT Investigators: Combined efficacy of atrial septal lead placement and atrial pacing algorithms for prevention of paroxysmal atrial tachyarrhythmia. J Cardiovasc Electrophysiol 14:1189-1195, 2003.
91. Hermida JS, Kubala M, Lescure FX, et al: Atrial septal pacing to prevent atrial fibrillation in patients with sinus node dysfunction: Results of a randomized controlled study. Am Heart J 148:312-317, 2004.
92. Saksena S, Prakash A, Ziegler P, et al: Improved suppression of recurrent atrial fibrillation with dual-site right atrial pacing and antiarrhythmic drug therapy. J Am Coll Cardiol 40:1140-1150, 2002.
93. D'Allonnes GR, Pavin D, Leclercq C, et al: Long-term effects of biatrial synchronous pacing to prevent drug-refractory atrial tachyarrhythmia: A nine-year experience. J Cardiovasc Electrophysiol 11:1081-1091, 2000.
94. Doi A, Takagi M, Toda I, et al: Acute haemodynamic benefits of biatrial atrioventricular sequential pacing: Comparison with single atrial atrioventricular sequential pacing. Heart 90:411-418, 2004.
95. Gammage MD, Marsh AM: Randomized trials for selective site pacing: Do we know where we are going? Pacing Clin Electrophysiol 27:878-882, 2004.
96. Madan N, Saksena S: Long-term rhythm control of drug-refractory atrial fibrillation with "hybrid therapy" incorporating dual-site right atrial pacing, antiarrhythmic drugs, and right atrial ablation. Am J Cardiol 93:569-575, 2004.
97. Carlson MD, Ip J, Messenger J, et al; Atrial Dynamic Overdrive Pacing Trial (ADOPT) Investigators: A new pacemaker algorithm for the treatment of atrial fibrillation: Results of the Atrial Dynamic Overdrive Pacing Trial (ADOPT). J Am Coll Cardiol 42:627-633, 2003.
98. Mabo P, Funck R, De Roy L, et al: Impact of ventricular pacing on atrial fibrillation prevention. PACE 24:II-621, 2002.
99. Blanc JJ, De Roy L, Mansourati J, et al; PIPAF Investigators: Atrial pacing for prevention of atrial fibrillation: Assessment of simultaneously implemented algorithms. Europace 6:371-379, 2004.
100. Israel CW, Hugl B, Unterberg C, et al: Pace-termination and pacing for prevention of atrial tachyarrhythmias: Results from a multicenter study with an implantable device for atrial therapy. J Cardiovasc Electrophysiol 12:1121-1128, 2001.
101. Israel CW, Ehrlich JR, Gronefeld G, et al: Prevalence, characteristics and clinical implications of regular atrial tachyarrhythmias in patients with atrial fibrillation: Insights from a study using a new implantable device. J Am Coll Cardiol 38:355-363, 2001.
102. Lee MA, Weachter R, Pollak S, et al; ATTEST Investigators: The effect of atrial pacing therapies on atrial tachyarrhythmia burden and frequency: Results of a randomized trial in patients with bradycardia and atrial tachyarrhythmias. J Am Coll Cardiol 41:1926-1932, 2003.
103. Friedman PA, Dijkman B, Warman EN, et al: Atrial therapies reduce atrial arrhythmia burden in defibrillator patients. Circulation 104:1023-1028, 2001.
104. Adler SW 2nd, Wolpert C, Warman EN, et al: Efficacy of pacing therapies for treating atrial tachyarrhythmias in patients with ventricular arrhythmias receiving a dual-chamber implantable cardioverter defibrillator. Circulation 104:887-892, 2001.
105. Stephenson EA, Casavant D, Tuzi J, et al; ATTEST Investigators: Efficacy of atrial antitachycardia pacing using the Medtronic AT500 pacemaker in patients with congenital heart disease. Am J Cardiol 92:871-876, 2003.
106. Israel CW, Gronefeld G, Li YG, Hohnloser SH: Usefulness of atrial pacing for prevention and termination of atrial tachyarrhythmias in a patient with persistent atrial fibrillation. Pacing Clin Electrophysiol 25:1527-1529, 2002.
107. Friedman PA, Ip JH, Jazayeri M, et al; RID-AF Investigators: The impact of atrial prevention and termination therapies on atrial tachyarrhythmia burden in patients receiving a dual-chamber defibrillator for ventricular arrhythmias. J Interv Card Electrophysiol 10:103-110, 2004.
108. Camm AJ, Savelieva I: Rationale and patient selection for "hybrid" drug and device therapy in atrial and ventricular arrhythmias. J Interv Card Electrophysiol 9:207-214, 2003.
109. Murgatroyd FD: "Pills and pulses:" Hybrid therapy for atrial fibrillation. J Cardiovasc Electrophysiol 13:S40-S46, 2002.
110. Konings KT, Kirchhof CJ, Smeets JR, et al: High-density mapping of electrically induced atrial fibrillation in humans. Circulation 89:1665-1680, 1994.
111. Gillis AM, Morck M, Willems R, et al: Atrial antitachycardia pacing therapy and reduction in atrial tachyarrhythmia burden. PACE 26:II-973, 2003.
112. Gillis AM, Koehler J, Mehra R, Hettrick DA: High atrial ATP therapy efficacy is associated with a reduction in atrial tachyarrhythmia burden. Heart Rhythm 1:S66, 2004.
113. Hugl B, Israel CW, Unterberg C, et al; AT500 Verification Study Investigators: Incremental programming of atrial anti-tachycardia pacing therapies in bradycardia-indicated patients: Effects on therapy efficacy and atrial tachyarrhythmia burden. Europace 5:403-409, 2003.
114. Link MS, Hellkamp AS, Estes NA 3rd, et al; MOST Study Investigators: High incidence of pacemaker syndrome in patients with sinus node dysfunction treated with ventricular-based pacing in the Mode Selection Trial (MOST). J Am Coll Cardiol 43:2066-2071, 2004.
115. Newman D, Lau C, Tang AS, et al; CTOPP Investigators: Effect of pacing mode on health-related quality of life in the Canadian Trial of Physiologic Pacing. Am Heart J 145:430-437, 2003.
116. Gregoratos G, Abrams J, Epstein AE, et al; American College of Cardiology/American Heart Association Task Force on Practice Guidelines/North American Society for Pacing and Electrophysiology Committee: ACC/AHA/NASPE 2002 guideline update for implantation of cardiac pacemakers and antiarrhythmia devices: Summary article: A report of the American College of Cardiology/American Heart Association Task Force on Practice Guidelines (ACC/AHA/NASPE Committee to Update the 1998 Pacemaker Guidelines). Circulation 106:2145-2161, 2002.
117. Gillis AM, Crystall E, Kerr CR: Atrial pacing for prevention of atrial fibrillation (Consensus Conference on Atrial Fibrillation). Can J Cardiol 21:Supple 41B-44B, 2005.
118. Wyse DG, Waldo AL, DiMarco JP, et al; Atrial Fibrillation Follow-up Investigation of Rhythm Management (AFFIRM) Investigators: A comparison of rate control and rhythm control in patients with atrial fibrillation. N Engl J Med 347:1825-1833, 2002.
119. De Sisti A, Attuel P, Manot S, et al: Electrophysiological determinants of atrial fibrillation in sinus node dysfunction despite atrial pacing. Europace 2:304-311, 2000.
120. De Sisti A, Leclercq JF, Stiubei M, et al: P wave duration and morphology predict atrial fibrillation recurrence in patients with sinus node dysfunction and atrial-based pacemaker. Pacing Clin Electrophysiol 25:1546-1554, 2002.
121. Sweeney MO, Hellkamp AS, Ellenbogen KA, et al; MOST Investigators: Prospective randomized study of mode switching in a clinical trial of pacemaker therapy for sinus node dysfunction. J Cardiovasc Electrophysiol 15:153-160, 2004.
122. Bellocci F, Spampinato A, Ricci R, et al: Antiarrhythmic benefits of dual chamber stimulation with rate-response in patients with paroxysmal atrial fibrillation and chronotropic incompetence: A prospective, multicentre study. Europace 1:220-225, 1999.

123. Duff HJ, Raj SR, Exner DV, et al: Randomized controlled trial of fixed rate versus rate responsive pacing after radiofrequency atrioventricular junction ablation: Quality of life, ventricular refractoriness, and paced QT dispersion. J Cardiovasc Electrophysiol 14:1163-1170, 2003.
124. Daoud EG, Timmermans C, Fellows C, et al: Initial clinical experience with ambulatory use of an implantable atrial defibrillator for conversion of atrial fibrillation. Metrix Investigators. Circulation 102:1407-1413, 2000.
125. Boodhoo L, Mitchell A, Ujhelyi M, Sulke N: Improving the acceptability of the atrial defibrillator: Patient-activated cardioversion versus automatic night cardioversion with and without sedation (ADSAS 2). Pacing Clin Electrophysiol 27:910-917, 2004.
126. Geller JC, Reek S, Timmermans C, et al: Treatment of atrial fibrillation with an implantable atrial defibrillator—long term results. Eur Heart J 24:2083-2089, 2003.
127. Wolpert C, Jung W, Spehl S, et al: Incidence and rate characteristics of atrial tachyarrhythmias in patients with a dual chamber defibrillator. Pacing Clin Electrophysiol 26:1691-1698, 2003.
128. Gillis AM, Wyse DG, Sheldon RS, et al: Prevalence and time course of atrial fibrillation development following implantation of an implantable cardioverter defibrillator. Heart Rhythm 1:S176, 2004.
129. Gold MR, Sulke N, Schwartzman DS, et al; Worldwide Jewel AF-Only Investigators: Clinical experience with a dual-chamber implantable cardioverter defibrillator to treat atrial tachyarrhythmias J Cardiovasc Electrophysiol 12:1247-1253, 2001.
130. Swerdlow CD, Schwartzman D, Hoyt R, et al; Worldwide Model 7250 AF-Only Investigators: Determinants of first-shock success for atrial implantable cardioverter defibrillators. J Cardiovasc Electrophysiol 13:347-354, 2002.
131. Boriani G, Biffi M, Camanini C, et al: Efficacy of internal cardioversion for chronic atrial fibrillation in patients with and without left ventricular dysfunction. Int J Cardiol 95:43-47, 2004.
132. Burns JL, Sears SF, Sotile R, et al: Do patients accept implantable atrial defibrillation therapy? Results from the Patient Atrial Shock Survey of Acceptance and Tolerance (PASSAT) Study. J Cardiovasc Electrophysiol 15:286-291, 2004.
133. Spurrell P, Mitchell A, Kamalvand K, et al: Does sinus rhythm beget sinus rhythm? Long-term follow-up of the patient activated atrial defibrillator. Pacing Clin Electrophysiol 27:175-181, 2004.
134. Ricci R, Quesada A, Pignalberi C, et al: Dual defibrillator improves quality of life and decreases hospitalizations in patients with drug refractory atrial fibrillation. J Interv Card Electrophysiol 10:85-92, 2004.
135. Newman DM, Dorian P, Paquette M, et al; Worldwide Jewel AF AF-Only Investigators: Effect of an implantable cardioverter defibrillator with atrial detection and shock therapies on patient-perceived, health-related quality of life. Am Heart J 145:841-846, 2003.
136. Qu J, Plotnikov AN, Danilo P Jr, et al: Expression and function of a biological pacemaker in canine heart. Circulation. 107:1106-1109, 2003.
137. Rosen MR, Brink PR, Cohen IS, Robinson RB: Genes, stem cells and biological pacemakers. Cardiovasc Res 64:12-23, 2004.

Chapter 14

Pacing for Atrioventricular Conduction System Disease

BRUCE S. STAMBLER • SHAHBUDIN H. RAHIMTOOLA • KENNETH A. ELLENBOGEN

Anatomy

The sinus node lies near the junction of the superior vena cava and the right atrium (RA). It is supplied by the sinus nodal artery, which originates from the proximal few centimeters of the right coronary artery (RCA) in about 55% of human subjects and from the proximal few centimeters of the left circumflex (LCX) artery in the remainder (Fig. 14-1).[1-4]

The atrioventricular (AV) node lies directly above the insertion of the septal leaflet of the tricuspid valve and just beneath the RA endocardium.[2-4] The AV junction is a structure encompassing the AV node with its posterior, septal, and left atrial (LA) approaches as well as the His bundle and its bifurcation. The AV node is a small subendocardial structure located within the interatrial septum at the distal convergence of the preferential internodal conduction pathways that course through the atria from the sinus node.[1] Like the sinus node, the AV node has extensive autonomic innervation and an abundant blood supply.

Three regions, the transitional cell zone, the compact node, and the penetrating bundle, compose the AV node and are distinguished by functional and histologic differences (Fig. 14-2). The transitional cell zone, which consists of cells constituting the atrial approaches to the compact AV node, has the highest rate of spontaneous diastolic depolarization. The compact node is composed of groups of cells that have extensions into the central fibrous body and the anulus of the mitral and tricuspid valves. These cells appear to be the site of most of the conduction delay through the AV node.[5-7] The penetrating bundle consists of cells that lead directly into the His bundle and its branching portion.

Only the proximal two thirds of the AV node are supplied by the AV nodal artery[4]; the distal segment of the AV node has a dual blood supply in 80% of human hearts from the same AV nodal artery and the left anterior descending (LAD) artery. In 90% of patients, the AV nodal artery originates from the RCA. During acute myocardial infarction (AMI), conduction disturbances in the AV node are usually the consequence of an occlusion proximal to the origin of the AV nodal artery. The conduction abnormalities, therefore, are usually associated with inferior MI. The AV nodal tissue merges with the His bundle, which runs through the inferior portion of the membranous interventricular septum and then, in most instances, continues along the left side of the crest of the muscular interventricular septum. The His bundle usually receives a dual blood supply from both the AV nodal artery and branches of the LAD artery.[6] Unlike the sinus and AV nodes, the bundle of His and Purkinje system have relatively little autonomic innervation.

The right bundle branch (RBB) originates from the His bundle. It is a narrow structure that crosses to the right side of the interventricular septum and extends along the right ventricular (RV) endocardial surface to the region of the anterolateral papillary muscle of the RV, where it divides to supply the papillary muscle, the parietal surface of the RV, and the lower part of the RV

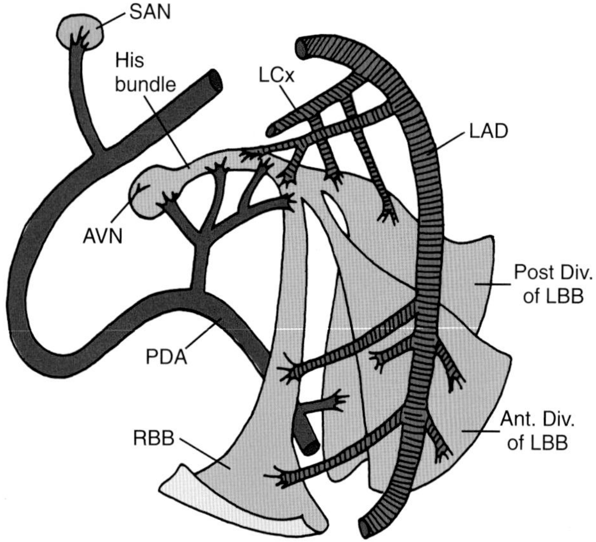

Figure 14-1. A diagrammatic representation of the conduction system and its blood supply. Ant, anterior; AVN, atrioventricular node; div, division; LAD, left anterior descending artery; LBB, left bundle branch; LCx, left circumflex artery; PDA, posterior descending artery; Post, posterior; RBB, right bundle branch; SAN, sinoatrial node. (From de Guzman M, Rahimtoola SH: What is the role of pacemakers in patients with coronary artery disease and conduction abnormalities? In Rahimtoola SH: Controversies in Coronary Artery Disease. Philadelphia, FA Davis, 1983.)

surface.[7] The proximal portion of the RBB is supplied by branches from the AV nodal artery or the LAD artery, whereas the more distal portion is supplied mainly by branches of the LAD artery.

The left bundle branch (LBB) is anatomically much less discrete than the RBB. It may divide immediately as it originates from the bundle of His or may continue for 1 to 2 cm as a broad band before dividing.[4,7] The LBB fibers spread out over the left ventricle (LV) in a fanlike manner, like a "cascading waterfall," with many subendocardial interconnections that resemble a syncytium rather than two anatomically discrete, distinct branches or fascicles.[7,8] As originally proposed by Rosenbaum, however, it is clinically useful to consider the LBB as dividing into an anterior branch or fascicle and a larger and broader posterior branch or fascicle, both of which radiate toward the anterior and posterior papillary muscles of the LV, respectively.[9] The LBB and its anterior fascicle have a blood supply similar to that of the proximal portion of the RBB; the left posterior fascicle is supplied by branches of the AV nodal artery, the posterior descending artery, and the circumflex coronary artery.

Diagnosis of Atrioventricular Conduction Disturbances

Electrocardiography

First-degree AV block usually is due to conduction delay within the AV node. Much less commonly, first-degree AV block is due to intra-atrial or infra-Hisian conduction delay.[10] Localization of the site of second-degree AV block to the AV node or His-Purkinje system can be obtained by His bundle recording during invasive electrophysiologic testing, but in most cases, careful analysis of the electrocardiogram (ECG) and the effect of various pharmacologic agents on the block will suffice.[11] Adherence to precise definitions of second-degree AV block, particularly in cases of 2:1 AV block and suspected type II AV block, is critical to avoiding diagnostic errors that could result in potentially unnecessary permanent pacemaker implantation.[12] Furthermore, type I and type II designations refer only to ECG patterns and not to the anatomic site of block.

Classic type I (Wenckebach) second-degree AV block has the following three characteristics: (1) progressive P-R interval prolongation before the nonconducted beat, (2) progressive decrease in the increment of P-R interval prolongation, and (3) progressive decrease in the R-R interval, parallel to the progressive decrease in the increment of change in the P-R interval.[13] All patterns of type I second-degree AV block not having this pattern are called "atypical" patterns, although in actuality, they may occur more commonly than the classic variety (Fig. 14-3).[14,15] As a general rule, type I second-degree AV block with a narrow QRS is almost always due to delay within the AV node. Delay within the His bundle (intra-Hisian block), however, is a rare cause of type I second-degree AV block with a narrow QRS and requires an electrophysiologic study for definitive diagnosis. Intra-Hisian block should be suspected in a patient with a narrow QRS if type I second-degree AV block is provoked by exercise. In contrast, type I AV nodal block at rest improves with exercise. When type I second-degree AV block is associated with concomitant bundle branch block (BBB), the site of delay or block is in the His-Purkinje system (infranodal) in up to 60% to 70% of cases.[13-15]

Type II second-degree AV block is defined as a single nonconducted sinus P wave associated with fixed P-R intervals before and after the blocked beat (Fig. 14-4). The sinus rate must be stable (i.e., constant P-P intervals), and there must be at least two consecutive conducted P waves to determine the P-R interval, which can be either normal or prolonged. Type II second-degree AV block should not be diagnosed in the case of a nonconducted atrial premature beat or if there is simultaneous sinus slowing and AV nodal block (e.g., hypervagotonia). Type I block with relatively long Wenckebach sequences and small increases in AV nodal conduction time may be confused with type II AV block but should not be classified as such (even though the site of block may be either AV nodal or infranodal in such cases). Type II second-degree AV block is most commonly encountered when the QRS is prolonged (in about 70% of cases) and is localized within the His-Purkinje system; in contrast, type II AV block with a narrow QRS is within the His bundle (i.e., intra-Hisian). Sudden AV block of more than one impulse with stable sinus rhythm and 1:1 AV conduction with constant P-R and P-P intervals before and after the block has been labeled "advanced AV block," "paroxysmal AV block," and

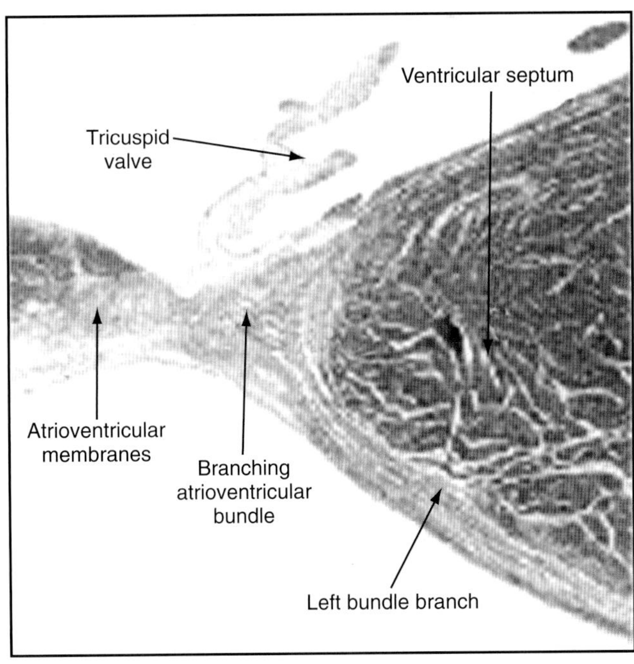

A

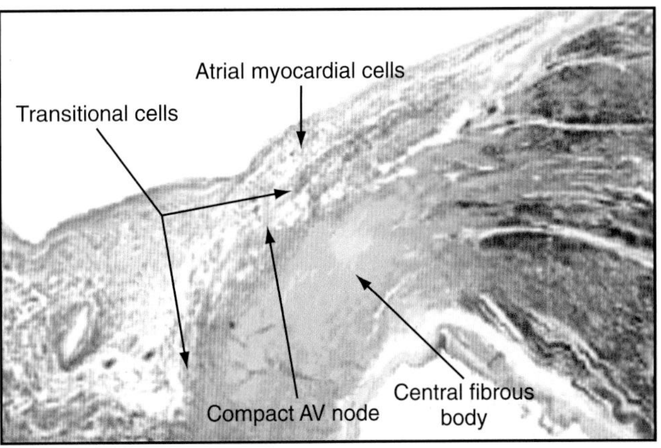

B

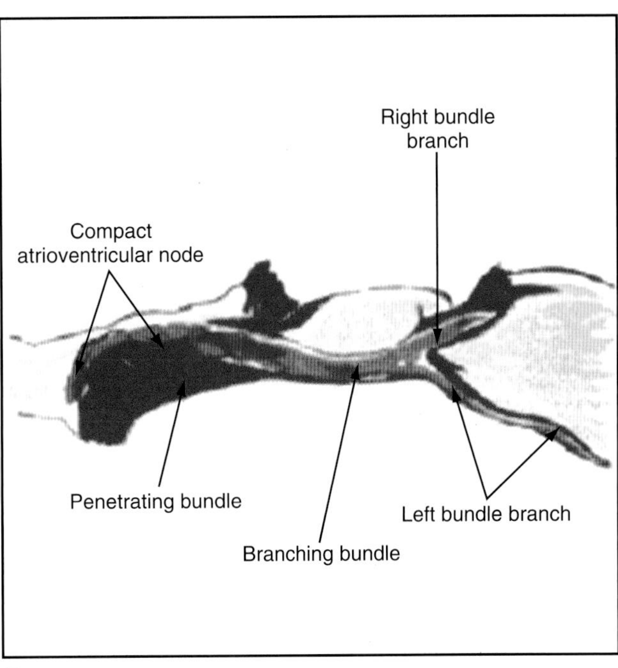

C

Figure 14-2. ***A,*** *Section through the crest of the muscular ventricular septum of the human heart, oriented in attitudinally correct fashion, shows the insulated nature of the branching atrioventricular bundle and the left bundle branch.* ***B,*** *Section (trichrome stain) from a human child's heart shows the region of the atrioventricular node. The cells of the compact node are joined to the atrial myocardial cells through short regions of transitional cells. The node itself is part of the atrial wall, with no fibrous sheath interposed between the histologically specialized tissues and the working atrial myocardium.* ***C,*** *Illustration scanned from Tawara's monograph of 1906, reoriented to attitudinally correct position and relabeled. It shows the axis of conduction tissue (orange), extending from the atrial myocardium (yellow), penetrating the insulating plane (red), and branching on the crest of the muscular ventricular septum, (also yellow). Compare with* ***A*** *and* ***B****. (From Anderson RH, Ho SY, Becker AE: Anatomy of the human atrioventricular junctions revisited. Anat Rec 260:81, 2000.)*

"type II AV block." Although this rhythm does not conform to the strict definition of type II block (i.e., a single block beat), it does suggest that the anatomic site of AV block is infranodal, and permanent pacing is indicated. On the other hand, Wenckebach periodicity before the development of high-grade AV block is suggestive of an AV nodal site of block.

Lange and colleagues[16] reported on their experience with a large number of patients with transient second-degree AV block and narrow QRS complexes detected on ambulatory Holter monitoring. The researchers emphasized the many ways in which second-degree AV block can be manifested. Classic type I AV block with progressive PR prolongation to more than 40 msec during at least three beats before the blocked P waves was seen in only 50% of patients. Another pattern observed was a more subtle Wenckebach periodicity with minor PR prolongation of 20 to 40 msec before a blocked P wave in 29% of patients. A third pattern, seen in 8% of patients and termed *pseudo–Mobitz type II AV block,* demonstrated nearly constant P-R intervals before the blocked P wave, followed by PR shortening on the subsequent conducted beat (see Fig. 14-3). Classic Mobitz type II second-degree AV block with constant P-R intervals for at least three beats before the blocked P wave followed by the same P-R interval after the blocked P wave was seen in 4% of patients (see Fig. 14-4). A mixed type I Wenckebach and pseudo–Mobitz type II AV block were seen in 6% of all patients. Of all patients showing periods of pseudo–Mobitz type II block, 44% also demonstrated classic Wenckebach conduction patterns at some time.[16] Slowing of the sinus cycle length often preceded the blocked P wave in both classic and pseudo–Mobitz type II AV blocks (Fig. 14-5).

Diagnosis of the site of AV block may be problematic with 2:1 AV block, which should not be classified as type I or type II block. The anatomic site of block in 2:1 AV block can be in the AV node or His-Purkinje system (Fig. 14-6). The most likely site of AV block can often be determined by noting the company that the 2:1 AV block keeps. When 2:1 AV block is associated with a wide QRS, the block is in the His-Purkinje system in 80% of cases and in the AV node in 20% (Fig. 14-7). A long P-R interval (>0.30 sec) on conducted beats during 2:1 AV block with a narrow QRS complex is suggestive of an AV nodal site of block, whereas a normal P-R interval favors intra-Hisian block.

In general, the response of the block, particularly 2:1 AV block, to pharmacologic agents may help to determine the site of the block. Atropine generally improves AV conduction in patients with AV nodal block; however, atropine is expected to worsen conduction in patients with block localized to the His-Purkinje system, owing to its effect on increasing sinus rates without improving His-Purkinje conduction (Fig. 14-8). Carotid sinus stimulation is expected to worsen block localized to the AV node, whereas it either has no effect or improves conduction in patients with His-Purkinje system disease by causing sinus node slowing. The effect of any given drug, however, may be difficult to predict because its effect on the sinus node may be greater than its effect on the AV node. For example, atropine may improve AV node conduction, but if

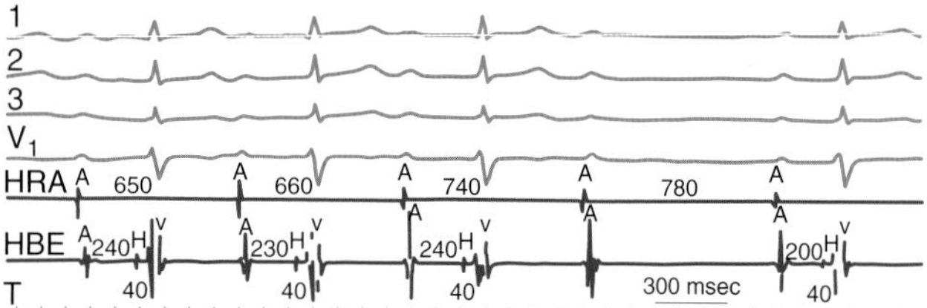

Figure 14-3. Example of atypical or uncommon type I second-degree atrioventricular (AV) block in the AV node. Surface leads I (1), II (2), III (3), and V1 are displayed with intracardiac electrograms recorded from the high right atrium (HRA), His bundle (HBE), and right ventricular apex (RV). There is little alteration in the A-H interval before the fourth atrial complex not conducting to the ventricle. The true nature of this arrhythmia is revealed by the first-conducted P wave (A, atrial electrogram) after the pause, which is associated with substantial shortening of the A-H interval from 230 to 240 msec to 200 msec. (From Josephson ME: Clinical Cardiac Electrophysiology: Techniques and Interpretations, 3rd ed. Philadelphia, Lippincott Williams & Wilkins, 2002, pp 92-109.)

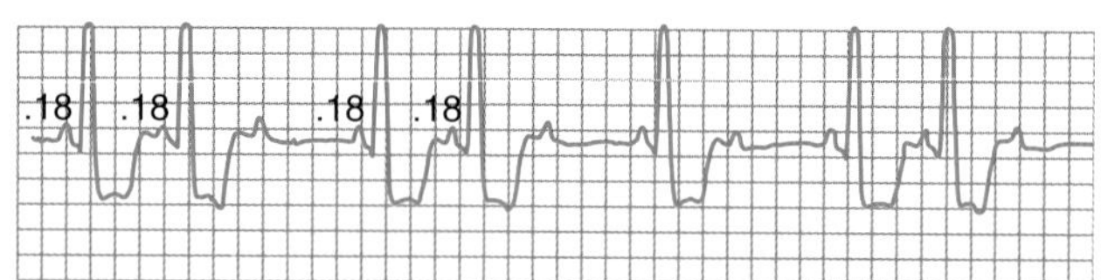

Figure 14-4. Example of type II second-degree atrioventricular (AV) block showing repeating episodes of block. Note that the P-R interval is constant both before and after the nonconducted P wave and that there is associated bundle branch block.

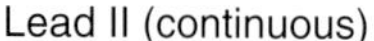

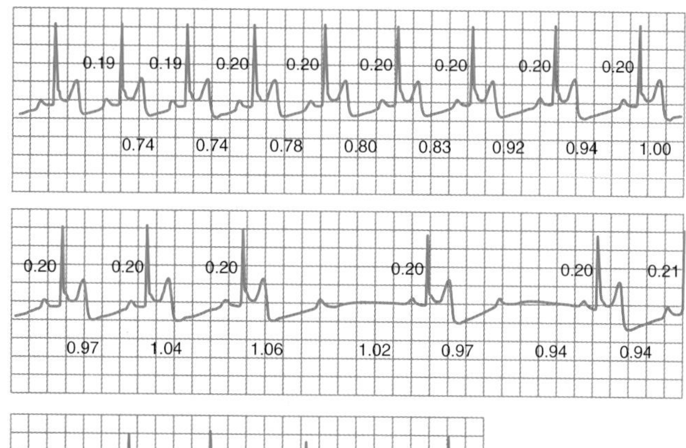

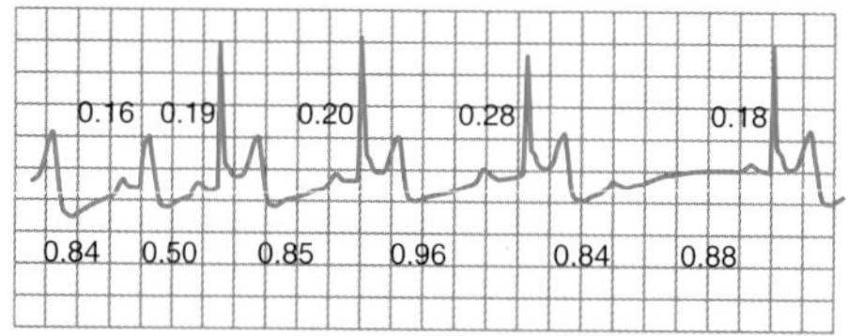

Figure 14-5. Rhythm strip demonstrating vagally mediated second-degree atrioventricular (AV) block. Note the progressive slowing of the heart rate before the first episode of block, although no change in P-R interval can be discerned. During the second episode of block, both sinus slowing and P-R interval prolongation occur, confirming the presence of type I second-degree AV block.

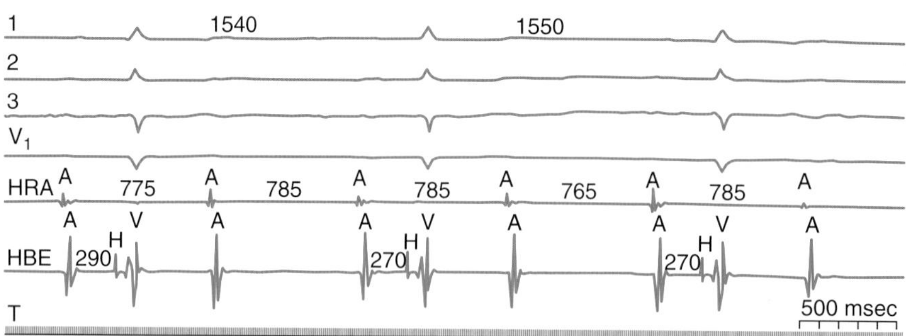

Figure 14-6. Spontaneous 2:1 (high-grade) atrioventricular (AV) block localized to the AV node. Surface leads I (1), II (2), III (3), and V1 are displayed with intracardiac electrograms recorded from the high right atrium (HRA), His bundle (HBE), and right ventricular apex (RV). Alternate atrial depolarizations (A) are not followed by either a His bundle or a ventricular depolarization. On the basis of a surface electrocardiogram, the finding of 2:1 AV block with a narrow QRS is compatible with a block at either the AV node or an infra-Hisian bundle site. The intracardiac recordings localize the site of block to the AV node. (From Josephson ME: Clinical Cardiac Electrophysiology: Techniques and Interpretations, 3rd ed. Philadelphia, Lippincott Williams & Wilkins, 2002, pp 92-109.)

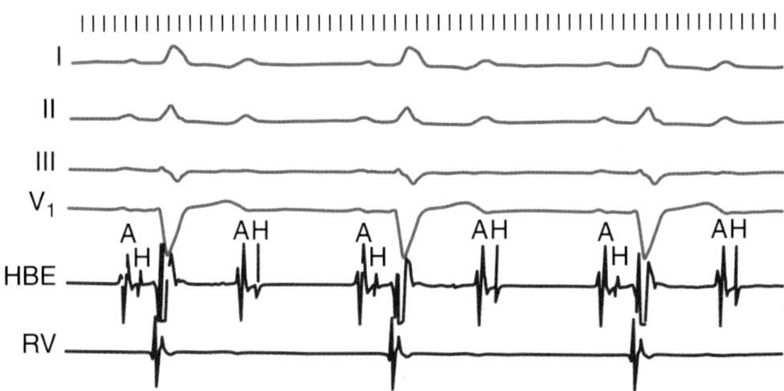

Figure 14-7. Intracardiac tracing of 2:1 second-degree atrioventricular (AV) block located in the His-Purkinje system. Sinus rhythm with left bundle branch block is present. Surface leads I, II, III, and V1 are displayed with intracardiac electrograms recorded from the high right atrium (HRA), His bundle (HBE), and right ventricular apex (RV). The A-H intervals are constant, but every other atrial complex fails to activate the ventricle even though each atrial depolarization is followed by a His bundle deflection. This finding shows that the site of AV block is within the His-Purkinje system. (From Josephson ME: Clinical Cardiac Electrophysiology: Techniques and Interpretations, 3rd ed. Philadelphia, Lippincott Williams & Wilkins, 2002, pp 92-109.)

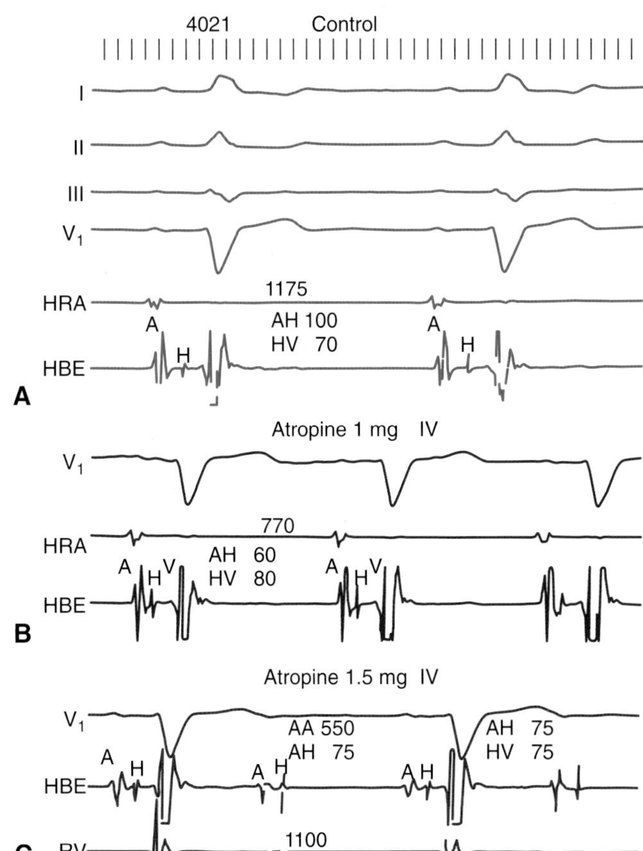

Figure 14-8. His-Purkinje atrioventricular block after an atropine-induced increase in sinus rate. Surface leads I, II, III, and V1 are displayed with intracardiac electrograms recorded from the high right atrium (HRA), His bundle (HBE), and right ventricular apex (RV). ***A,*** *Sinus rhythm at a cycle length of 1175 msec with 1:1 AV conduction. Left bundle branch block is present, and the H-V interval is slightly prolonged, to 70 msec.* ***B,*** *After injection of 1 mg of atropine, the sinus rate speeds up to 770 msec and the H-V interval increases to 80 msec, but 1:1 AV conduction is still present. The A-H interval shortens despite the faster sinus rate, because of the direct effect of atropine on AV nodal conduction.* ***C,*** *After injection of 1.5 mg of atropine, the sinus cycle length decreases further to 550 msec, and 2:1 AV block occurs below the His bundle. Atropine worsens AV conduction in this patient, not through a direct drug effect but because the improvement in AV nodal conduction caused by atropine stresses the already abnormal His-Purkinje system. (From Miles WM, Klein LS: Sinus nodal dysfunction and atrioventricular conduction disturbances. In Naccarelli GV: Cardiac Arrhythmias: A Practical Approach. Mt Kisco, NY, Futura, 1991, pp 243-282.)*

atropine causes excessive sinus node acceleration, AV conduction may improve marginally or not at all. The response to infusion of isoproterenol is less clear. Isoproterenol may improve conduction disorders localized in the AV node as well as occasionally in the His-Purkinje system.

The diagnosis of complete heart block (CHB) rests on demonstration of complete dissociation between atrial and ventricular activation. Care must be taken to distinguish transient AV dissociation due to competing atrial and junctional or ventricular rhythms with similar rates (so-called isorhythmic AV dissociation). If sufficiently long monitoring strips are available, intermittent conduction of appropriately timed atrial events is seen. Temporary atrial pacing can be performed to accelerate the atrial rate to overdrive the competing junctional or ventricular arrhythmia, demonstrating intact AV conduction. In the presence of atrial fibrillation (AF), CHB can be inferred when the ventricular rate becomes regular rather than the typical irregular ventricular response (Fig. 14-9). Digoxin toxicity may be the cause of heart block with AF, and this and other drug toxicity should be ruled out before one assumes that structural AV conduction disease is present. In patients with AF, regular R-R interval may on occasion be due to "concealed" sinus rhythm and not heart block.[17]

The escape rhythm in CHB may be generated by the AV junction, His bundle, bundle branches, or distal conduction system. Rarely, the underlying rhythm arises from the ventricular myocardium or, for all practical purposes, is absent. The site of AV block is important, in that it determines to a great extent the rate and reliability of the underlying escape rhythm. The site of origin of the escape rhythm in cases of advanced AV block is more important than the escape rate itself.[10,18] For example, in heart block associated with inferior AMI or congenital CHB, the escape rhythm is usually generated by the AV junction, and permanent pacing may not be required. Nevertheless, it is worth emphasizing that *symptomatic* AV block requires pacing regardless of the site, morphology, or rate of the escape rhythm.

Trifascicular block is present when bifascicular block is associated with HV prolongation. *Trifascicular block*, however, is often applied loosely to the electrocardiographic patterns of bifascicular block (RBB block [RBBB] plus left anterior hemiblock, RBBB plus left posterior hemiblock, or LBB block [LBBB]) plus first-degree AV block. The use of the term trifascicular block to describe these AV conduction disturbances on the ECG is misleading, because the site of block in such

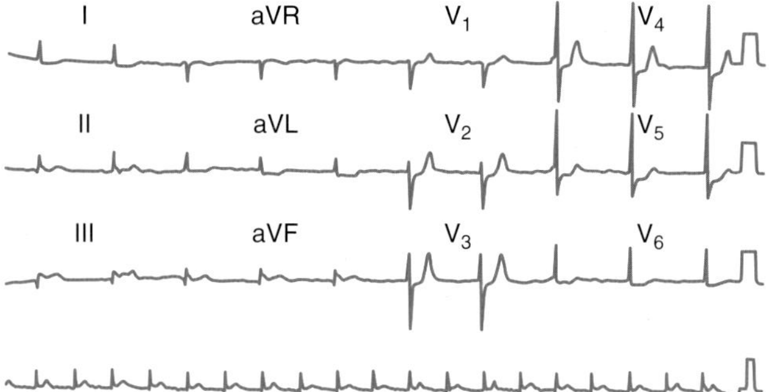

Figure 14-9. Twelve-lead electrocardiogram from a patient with recent aortic valve surgery and atrial fibrillation treated with digoxin. Surface leads I, II, III, and V1 are displayed with intracardiac electrograms recorded from the high right atrium (HRA), His bundle (HBE), and right ventricular apex (RV). The QRS complexes are narrow and occur at a regular rate of 56 bpm, illustrating complete heart block with a junctional escape rhythm in the setting of atrial fibrillation. Despite discontinuation of digoxin, complete heart block persisted in this patient.

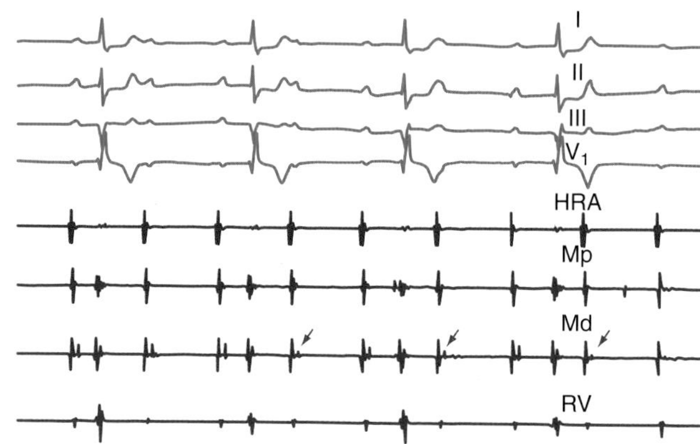

Figure 14-10. Surface leads I, II, III, and V1 reveal sinus rhythm with 2:1 AV conduction, marked P-R interval prolongation during conducted beats, and right bundle branch block. Intracardiac electrograms from the high right atrium (HRA), proximal and distal poles of the His bundle catheter (Mp and Md, respectively), and the right ventricle (RV) are shown. The distal pole of the His bundle catheter registers a His bundle potential, which can be seen as a discrete sharp potential between the atrial and the ventricular electrograms on that channel. During nonconducted atrial complexes, spontaneous infra-Hisian block is apparent because the His bundle potential (arrow) is not followed by a ventricular electrogram.

cases may be located in the AV node or His-Purkinje system.[12] The P-R interval does not identify those patients who have prolonged H-V intervals in such cases. Up to 50% of patients with bifascicular block and prolonged P-R intervals have prolongation of the A-H interval (i.e., AV nodal conduction time).[19] *Trifascicular block* should be used only to refer to alternating RBBB and LBBB, RBBB with a prolonged H-V interval (regardless of the presence or absence of left anterior or posterior fascicular block), and LBBB with a prolonged H-V interval. In addition, the term can be used in a patient with second- or third-degree AV block in the His-Purkinje system with permanent block in all three fascicles, permanent block in two fascicles with intermittent conduction in the third, permanent block in one fascicle with intermittent block in the other two fascicles, or intermittent block in all three fascicles. Thus, according to its strict definition, when one is interpreting an ECG in the absence of a His bundle recording, *trifascicular block* should be applied only to the patterns of alternating RBBB and LBBB or RBBB with intermittent left anterior and posterior hemiblocks. These situations are class I indications for permanent pacing even in asymptomatic individuals.

Electrophysiologic Study

Invasive electrophysiologic study (e.g., His bundle recording) is a useful means of evaluating AV conduction in patients who have symptoms and in whom the need for permanent pacing is not obvious (Fig. 14-10). Electrophysiologic studies (strictly for evaluation of the conduction system and site of block) are not required in patients with symptomatic high-grade or complete AV block recorded on surface ECG tracings, ambulatory Holter monitoring, or transtelephonic recordings. The need for permanent pacing has already been established in these patients (class I indication). However electrophysiologic studies may be indicated in patients with high-grade AV block if another arrhythmia is suspected or is a likely cause of symptoms. For example, even if high-grade AV block is documented on spontaneous recordings, ventricular tachycardia may still be the cause of syncope in patients who have suffered extensive MI. In patients with alternating BBB, electrophysiologic testing almost invariably demonstrates a high degree of His-Purkinje system disease. These patients typically have very long H-V intervals and are at very high risk of progression to CHB in a short time. Pacing in these patients is indicated on clinical grounds, and electrophysiologic testing may not be necessary.[10] Electrophysiologic studies are also not indicated in patients whose symptoms are shown to not be associated with a conduction abnormality or block. In addition, patients without symptoms who have intermittent AV block associated with sinus slowing, gradual PR prolongation before a nonconducted P wave, and a narrow QRS complex should not undergo electrophysiologic study, given the benign prognosis of these findings.

The incidence of progression of bifascicular block to CHB is variable, ranging from 2% to 6% per year. The method of patient selection affects this incidence, with patients who have asymptomatic bifascicular block progressing to CHB at a rate of 2% per year, and patients with symptoms (e.g., syncope or presyncope) progressing at a rate closer to 6% per year.[20-22] Many of these studies emphasize the high mortality associated with BBB and bifascicular block. It is worth emphasizing that the mortality associated with the presence of structural heart disease predominantly reflects death due to AMI, heart failure, or ventricular tachyarrhythmias rather than bradyarrhythmias.

Three large studies of patients with chronic BBB have been performed to assess the role of His bundle conduction (e.g., H-V interval) measurements in predicting progression to CHB. The measurement of the H-V interval represents the conduction time through the His bundle and bundle branches until ventricular activation begins. Because these studies included both asymptomatic and symptomatic patients, care must be taken to ensure that similar patient populations are compared for proper interpretation of these results. Dhingra and colleagues[20] prospectively followed 517 patients with BBB and measured the time required for progression to second- and third-degree block. In their study, only 13% of patients presented with syncope; the remainder did not have symptoms. The cumulative 7-year incidence of progression to AV block was 10% in the group with a normal H-V interval and 20% in the group with H-V interval prolongation. The cumulative mortality rate at 7 years was 48% in patients with a normal H-V interval and 66% in patients with a prolonged H-V interval.[20] This study emphasized that despite the high mortality associated with the presence of bifascicular block, there is only a low rate of progression to more advanced AV block.

McAnulty and associates[23] studied 554 patients with "high-risk" BBB, defined as LBBB, RBBB and left- or right-axis, RBBB with alternating left and right axis, or alternating RBBB and LBBB. The cumulative incidence of AV block, either type II second-degree or CHB, was 4.9%, or 1% per year, in patients with a prolonged H-V interval and 1.9% in patients with a normal H-V interval (difference not significant). H-V interval prolongation did not predict a higher risk of development of CHB. In this study, 8.5% of patients experienced syncope after entry into the study. The incidence of complete AV block was 17% in patients with syncope, compared with 2% in patients without a history of syncope.

Scheinman and colleagues[21] studied 401 patients with chronic BBB for about 30 months. This study, in contrast to the Dhingra[20] and McAnulty[23] studies, primarily included patients with symptoms referred for electrophysiologic study. About 40% of the patients in the Scheinman study had a history of syncope.[21] In patients with an H-V interval of more than 70 msec, the incidence of progression to spontaneous second- or third-degree AV block was 12%. The incidence of complete AV block was 25% for those with an H-V interval of 100 msec or greater. The yearly incidence of spontaneous AV block was 3% in those with a normal H-V interval and 3.5% in those with a prolonged H-V interval.

Thus, these findings suggest that there is a relationship between a prolonged H-V interval and the development of CHB during the ensuing years in patients with intraventricular conduction disturbances. It also seems that the risk varies directly with the extent of H-V prolongation. Symptomatic patients with syncope or presyncope are at much higher risk than asymptomatic patients. The overall risk of CHB in an unselected, symptom-free group of patients with chronic BBB is low (<6%/yr). Current recommendations are not to perform electrophysiologic studies in patients with asymptomatic BBB.[24]

A number of studies evaluated the clinical usefulness of electrophysiologic testing in patients with *BBB* and *syncope*.[25] These studies were performed prior to the current era of ICD implantation in patients with syncope and advanced structural heart disease. In one study, 112 patients with chronic BBB and syncope or near-syncope underwent electrophysiologic testing.[25] A normal result predicted a good long-term prognosis. About 25% of patients were found to have a significant conduction system disorder, underwent pacemaker implantation, and experienced recurrence of symptoms at a rate of only 6%. In the study reported by Morady and associates,[26] 28% of patients (7 of 32) had sustained induced monomorphic ventricular tachycardia, whereas about 20% had conduction disturbances at electrophysiologic study. Six of the 7 patients who received pacemakers had no recurrent symptoms.

Thus, electrophysiologic studies may be useful in patients with BBB or bifascicular block and syncope for several reasons. First, negative results of electrophysiologic studies may identify a group of patients at low risk for cardiac events, especially in the absence of advanced structural heart disease. Induction of sustained ventricular tachycardia during electrophysiologic testing identifies patients who are at risk for life-threatening ventricular arrhythmias and require ICDs. Programmed ventricular stimulation in patients with BBB and syncope may induce bundle branch reentrant ventricular tachycardia, which may be readily cured with radiofrequency catheter ablation. Finally, electrophysiologic testing also identifies those patients with advanced conduction system disease (e.g., prolonged H-V interval with BBB) who need pacemakers.

Later clinical trials, which established the role of the ICD for both primary and secondary prevention of sudden death, have significantly affected the management of patients with BBB and syncope. Current guidelines recommend ICD implantation in patients with syncope of undetermined etiology in the setting of advanced structural heart disease because these patients are likely to have an arrhythmic cause of syncope. Thus, if LV dysfunction is present (LV ejection fraction ≤35%-40%) in patients with BBB and syncope, ICD implantation is indicated, and many centers may choose not to perform electrophysiologic studies in these patients. Electrophysiologic studies may be still be considered in patients with syncope or near syncope and BBB with no, minimal, or mild structural heart disease (LV ejection fraction >40%).

Methods Used to Identify Patients at Risk for Atrioventricular Block

In patients with symptomatic BBB or bifascicular block, electrophysiologic testing with measurement of H-V intervals has been used for several decades. A markedly prolonged H-V interval (100 msec or longer) is predictive of development of symptomatic heart block. As noted earlier, Scheinman and colleagues[21] demonstrated that an H-V interval of 100 msec or longer identified a group of patients who had a 25% risk of development of heart block over a mean follow-up of 22 months. According to current guidelines published by the American College of Cardiology/American Heart Association

Task Force on Practice Guidelines/North American Society for Pacing and Electrophysiology (ACC/AHA/NASPE), an H-V interval of 100 msec or longer in an asymptomatic patient documented as an incidental finding on an electrophysiologic study is a class IIa indication for permanent implantation of a pacemaker. Although the finding of a markedly prolonged H-V interval is quite specific, it is very insensitive because H-V intervals of 100 msec or longer are very uncommon.

Atrial pacing to stress the His-Purkinje system may provide additional information to identify patients at risk of spontaneous AV block. Most healthy subjects do not experience second- or third-degree infra-Hisian block during atrial pacing when the atrial rate is gradually increased, as would occur spontaneously. Certain pacing protocols with abrupt onset of pacing at rapid rates are more likely to induce infra-Hisian block, even in healthy subjects, but this rarely occurs at pacing rates below 150 beats per minute (bpm). Because AV nodal dysfunction is frequently seen in patients with significant His-Purkinje system disease, AV nodal block may occur at lower pacing rates than those necessary to demonstrate infra-Hisian block. This "protective" effect of AV nodal dysfunction during resting states may lead to the incorrect conclusion that significant His-Purkinje disease is not present. A second trial of atrial pacing after administration of atropine or isoproterenol to facilitate AV nodal conduction, however, may demonstrate infra-Hisian block. Dhingra and colleagues[27] reported a 50% rate of progression to type II or complete AV block in patients in whom block develops distal to the His bundle at paced rates of less than 150 bpm. In a later study, Petrac and coworkers[28] evaluated 192 patients with chronic BBB and syncope, of whom 18 (9%) had incremental atrial pacing–induced infra-Hisian second-degree AV block at a paced rate of 150 bpm or less (mean pacing rate, 112 ± 10 bpm). During a mean follow-up of 68 ± 35 months, 14 of the 18 patients (78%) demonstrated spontaneous second- or third-degree AV block, confirming that this abnormal finding identifies a subgroup at a high risk for development of heart block. However, like an H-V interval of 100 msec or less, His-Purkinje block during incremental atrial pacing at physiologic rates is an uncommon finding in patients with BBB and syncope. According to current guidelines, if atrial pacing–induced infra-Hisian block that is "not physiologic" is demonstrated as an incidental finding on an electrophysiologic study, permanent pacing is recommended (class IIa indication).

Provocative drug tests have been suggested as another means of evaluating the distal conduction system (Fig. 14-11).[29] Pharmacologic stress testing is often considered in patients with BBB and syncope in whom the H-V interval at baseline is 70 msec or higher but less than 100 msec and infra-Hisian block is not demonstrated. There are only limited available data describing the experience with intravenous type Ia (procainamide, ajmaline, or disopyramide) or type Ic (flecainide) antiarrhythmic drugs.[20,30-32] Only intravenous procainamide is available in the United States. Administration of these agents may result in a marked increase in the H-V interval (>15-20 msec), an H-V interval greater than 100 msec, or precipitation of spontaneous type II second- or third-degree AV block, all of which may indicate a higher risk for development of CHB. Intravenous disopyramide has the potential benefit of facilitating AV nodal conduction by its anticholinergic properties while accentuating underlying infra-Hisian disease through its membrane-stabilizing effects.[31] Tonkin and associates[32] administered procainamide at a dose of up to 10 mg/kg to 42 patients with BBB and syncope and produced intermittent second- or third-degree His-Purkinje block or H-V prolongation to more than 15 msec during sinus rhythm in 11 patients (26%).[33] However only 2 of the 11 patients (18%) with a positive result had documented high-grade AV block during 38 months of follow-up, and 3 of 5 asymptomatic control patients with BBB (60%) had a positive procainamide challenge test result. Other studies of class I antiarrhythmic drug testing to stress the His-Purkinje system likewise suffer from limited patient numbers, lack adequate control groups or follow-up, and seem to indicate that this test has low predictive value. Current permanent pacing guidelines do not include a recommendation regarding the need for permanent pacing on the basis of results of pharmacologic stress testing of the His-Purkinje system.

Electrophysiologic testing has recognized limitations for identifying patients with significant AV nodal or His-Purkinje dysfunction.[34] Although finding an abnormality on an electrophysiologic study may be helpful, the sensitivity of electrophysiologic testing is low and cannot be used to entirely exclude a significant AV conduction disturbance. In a small study conducted by Fujimura and associates,[34] 13 patients with documented symptomatic transient second- or third-degree AV block referred for implantation of a permanent pacemaker underwent AV conduction testing at the time of pacemaker insertion. These tests included facilitation of AV nodal conduction with atropine and pharmacologic stress of His-Purkinje conduction with low doses of procainamide. Surprisingly, only 2 of the 13 patients showed significant abnormalities in the AV conduction system (inducible infra-Hisian block in both cases) during electrophysiologic testing, yielding a sensitivity of 15.4%. Two other patients had moderately prolonged H-V intervals, although they were much shorter than 100 msec. If these 2 patients are included in the diagnostic data, the sensitivity of electrophysiologic testing is increased to 46%. Thus, this study raised important questions about the sensitivity of electrophysiologic testing for identifying patients at risk for development of symptomatic AV block.

Classification, Epidemiology, and Natural History of Atrioventricular Conduction Disturbances

AV block can be classified clinically on the basis of electrocardiographic findings, anatomic site of block, onset,

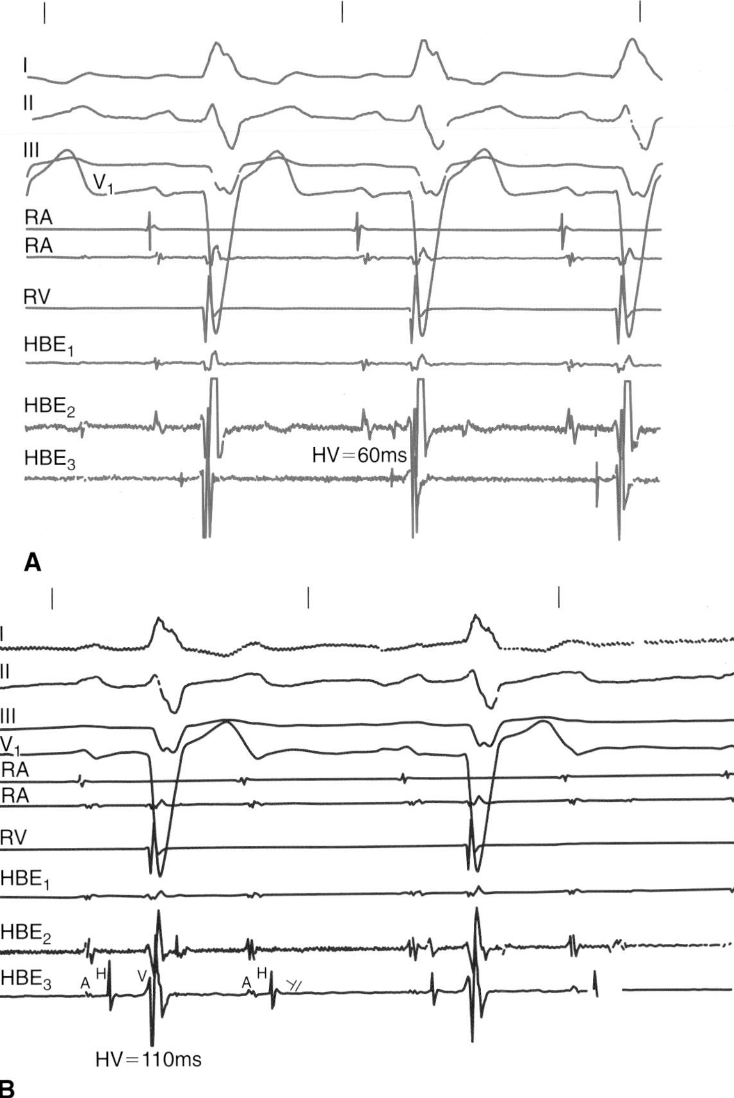

Figure 14-11. **A,** *Electrophysiologic testing in the baseline state in a patient with syncope reveals a left bundle branch block pattern during sinus rhythm. There is 1:1 atrioventricular (AV) conduction with an H-V interval of 60 msec.* **B,** *After a loading dose of procainamide, 2:1 AV conduction develops. The first and third atrial activations are conducted to the ventricles with an H-V interval of 110 msec. The third and fourth atrial activations conduct through the AV node to generate a His bundle potential without subsequent ventricular activation. Thus, this test illustrates spontaneous infra-Hisian block induced by procainamide. HBE1, HBE2, and HBE3 are proximal, middle, and distal His bundle catheter recordings, respectively; RA, right atrial recordings; RV, right ventricular recording.*

extent of severity, clinical presentation, underlying etiology, or associated conditions. Each of these classifications provides insight into the basis and management of these clinical disorders.

Patients who present with symptomatic first-, second-, or third-degree AV block usually have symptoms of syncope, dizziness, decreased energy, palpitations, or recurrent presyncope or dizziness. Other symptoms, which primarily reflect inadequate cardiac output or tissue perfusion, are fatigue, angina, and congestive heart failure. The most severe symptom is recurrent Stokes-Adams attacks or documented episodes of polymorphic ventricular tachycardia. Patients with long P-R intervals may have symptoms suggestive of pacemaker syndrome and may demonstrate resolution of symptoms with institution of dual-chamber pacing. It is important to emphasize that symptoms can be subtle or nonspecific in some patients or may be of sufficiently long duration that a high index of suspicion is warranted. Some clinicians recommend temporary pacing to document improvement of symptoms or reversal of long-standing problems, but the usefulness of this intervention has not been demonstrated in prospective studies.

First-Degree AV Block

The prognosis and natural history in patients with primary first-degree AV block and moderate PR prolongation are almost always benign.[35] Progression to CHB over time occurred in about 4% of patients in the study by Mymin and coworkers.[35] Most of the patients (66%) had only mild to moderate PR prolongation, to about 0.22 to 0.23 seconds. In the great majority of subjects, the P-R interval remained within a narrow range, changing by less than 0.04 seconds. Patients with markedly prolonged P-R interval may or may not be symptomatic at rest, but may demonstrate a pseudo-pacemaker syndrome due to AV dyssynchrony, particularly during exertion. They are more likely to become symptomatic during exercise, because the P-R interval may not shorten appropriately as the R-R interval decreases. Zornosa and colleagues[36] described occurrence of PR prolongation after radiofrequency ablation as a result of injury of the fast pathway in patients with AV nodal reentry who were undergoing ablation. Symptoms due to long P-R intervals resolved after DDD pacing was performed. Kim and associates[37] also described a patient with intermittent failure of fast pathway conduction who experienced light-headedness, weakness, and chest fullness when the P-R interval suddenly shifted from between 160 and 180 msec to 360 msec; this patient's condition improved after pacing.[36,37]

Implantation of permanent pacemakers is recommended in patients with first-degree AV block with symptoms similar to those of pacemaker syndrome (class IIa indication). Previous versions of the ACC/AHA/NASPE guidelines required documentation of alleviation of symptoms with temporary AV pacing prior to permanent pacing. However, this requirement was removed from the latest (2002) revision of the guidelines, in part because a temporary AV pacing study may not demonstrate symptomatic improvement at rest and is often impractical to perform during exercise. Thus, it is reasonable to institute permanent pacing in symptomatic patients with very long P-R intervals (≥0.30 sec) that do not shorten during exercise. Current guidelines also recommend permanent pacemaker implantation in patients with LV dysfunction, congestive heart failure, and marked first-degree AV block (>0.30 sec) in whom a shorter A-V interval results in hemodynamic improvement (class IIb indication). A study in patients with first-degree AV block suggested that systolic performance measured using a Doppler echocardiography–derived aortic flow time velocity integral improved after institution of DDD pacing at a rate of 70 bpm if the intrinsic AV conduction time (A-R interval) was longer than 0.27 seconds.[38] The optimal AV delay in this study was 159 ± 22 msec, which is consistent with that in most other studies, in that the optimal AV delay is around 150 msec at rest.

Second-Degree AV Block

Controversy exists regarding the prognosis and need for permanent pacing in patients with chronic type I second-degree AV block in the presence of a narrow QRS complex. Some consider this condition benign only in young people or athletes without organic heart disease. The natural history of 56 patients with chronic type I second-degree AV block, some of whom were younger than 35 years or were well-trained athletes, was described by Strasberg and colleagues in 1981.[39] They concluded that progression to CHB is relatively uncommon in this patient population and that this finding carries a benign prognosis in the absence of structural heart disease. A 1985 report by Shaw and coworkers[40] in 1985 suggested that patients with type I second-degree AV block have a worse prognosis than age- and sex-matched individuals unless the patients already had permanently implanted pacemakers. Their patient population consisted of 214 patients with chronic second-degree AV block with a mean age of 72 years who were monitored over a 14-year period; the patients were divided into three groups—those with type I block (77 patients), those with type II block (86 patients), and those with 2:1 or 3:1 block (51 patients). The 3- and 5-year survival times were similarly poor regardless of the type of AV block. Patients with type I block without BBB did not fare any better than those with type II block. Patients with type I second-degree AV block who received permanent pacemakers had a survival similar to that of an age- and sex-matched control population.

In 1991, a working group of the British Pacing and Electrophysiology Group (BPEG) suggested that pacing should be considered in adults in whom type I second-degree AV block occurs during much of the day or night irrespective of the presence or absence of symptoms.[41] In 2004, Shaw and associates[42] reported again on the prognosis of patients with type I second-degree AV block and once again concluded that type I second-degree AV block is not a benign condition in patients 45 years or older. The majority of their patients with type I second-degree AV block who were 45 years or older progressed to higher-degree AV block, experienced symptomatic bradycardia, or died prematurely if they did not receive pacemakers. These investigators recommended pacemaker implantation in patients with type I second-degree AV block even in the absence of symptoms or structural heart disease, except in those younger than 45 years. According to current ACC/AHA/NASPE guidelines however, permanent pacemaker implantation in asymptomatic type I second-degree AV block that is at the supra-His (AV node) level or is not known to be intra-Hisian or infra-Hisian is considered insupportable by current evidence (class III indication). It seems prudent, on the basis of available data, to at least monitor closely any elderly patient with asymptomatic type I AV block or 2:1 AV block with narrow QRS complexes, because these ECG abnormalities may be markers for progressive conduction system disease.

The natural history of asymptomatic type II second-degree AV block initially was addressed in a study from the University of Illinois reported in 1974.[43] Most patients monitored in this study were found to experience symptoms within a relatively short period. In the study by Shaw and colleagues[40] reported in 1985, 86 patients (mean age 74 years) seen and monitored between 1968 and 1982 with chronic Mobitz type II second-degree heart block had a 5-year survival rate of 61%. The five-year survival of those who underwent permanent pacemaker implantation was significantly better than those who did not. These observations form the basis for recommendations to institute permanent pacing in all patients with type II second-degree AV block regardless of symptoms (class IIa indication).

Complete Heart Block

The natural history of spontaneously developing asymptomatic CHB in adult life dates back to the days before pacemaker therapy was available.[44-46] Today, almost all adult patients with CHB eventually have symptoms and undergo pacemaker placement. Several studies published in the 1960s emphasized the poor prognosis of patients with CHB. The 1-year survival rate of patients who experienced Stokes-Adams attacks due to CHB and did not receive pacing was only 50% to 75%, significantly less than that of a sex- and age-matched control population.[45-47] The "best" prognosis was in patients with an idiopathic or unknown cause of CHB. At least 33% of deaths were related to CHB and Stokes-Adams attacks. These differences in survival persisted even after 15 years of follow-up and appear to be related to the considerably higher incidence of sudden death.[46] There is some debate about whether the presence of syncope is associated with a worse prognosis in patients with documented CHB. The prognosis for transient CHB was poor as well, with a 36% 1-year mortality rate reported in at least one study from the 1970s.[45] Whether this poor prognosis applies today to patients with transient CHB who have not received pacing is unknown.

Edhag and Swahn[45,46] reported in the 1960s and 1970s on the long-term prognosis of 248 patients with high-grade AV block, most of whom had complete heart AV block, with a mean 6.5 years of follow-up. The mean age at pacemaker implantation was 66 years, and the 1-year survival rate of patients who received pacemakers was 86%, slightly lower than the 95% 1-year survival rate of an age- and sex-matched group of Swedish patients. After the first year, survival in the patients with pacemakers was similar to that in the general population. Edhag[46] compared survival in different age groups, found no difference in survival between elderly patients with heart block who underwent permanent pacing and the age- and sex-matched general population. In contrast, younger patients with heart block had an increased mortality even after pacing than sex- and age-matched controls from the general population.[46] It is likely that this higher mortality is a reflection of the underlying structural heart disease that is responsible for high-grade AV block.

CHB can be described as acute or chronic depending on its onset. Acute AV block associated with myocardial ischemia is rare but may occur and result in transient AV block. High-grade AV block is strictly defined as 3:1, 4:1, or higher AV ratios in which AV synchrony is intermittently present. As in complete AV block, block may be localized anywhere in the conduction system (Fig. 14-12). In some patients, block may be present at multiple levels in the conduction system. Generically, the term *high-grade AV block* has been used to describe any form of AV block that suggests an increased risk for CHB or symptomatic bradycardia. This typically includes type II second-degree block, 2:1 AV block, strictly defined high-grade AV block, and CHB. The generic use of the term *high-grade AV block* may be best avoided because the multiple forms of AV block included have variable pathogeneses and prognoses that blur the clinical usefulness of the term.

Paroxysmal AV Block

Paroxysmal AV block is defined as the sudden occurrence, during a period of 1:1 AV conduction, of block of sequential atrial impulses resulting in a transient total interruption of AV conduction.[49,50] It is thus the onset of a paroxysm of high-grade AV block associated with a period of ventricular asystole before conduction returns or a subsidiary pacemaker escapes. Paroxysmal AV block may occur in a variety of clinical conditions but has been described most often in association with vagal reactions, such as during vomiting, coughing, or swallowing, after urination, or with abdominal pain, carotid sinus massage, coronary angiography, or head-up tilt table testing. Patients with neurally mediated syncopal syndromes may have transient heart block, typically with associated sinus slowing. It may occur in some patients with tachycardia-dependent AV block in the His-Purkinje system (phase 3 block), during or after exertion, with the abrupt onset of bradycardia (phase 4 block), and in type II second-degree AV block. One report described the clinical experience in 20 patients (mean age, 63 ± 14 years) with paroxysmal AV block seen at a single institution over a 12-year period.[51] Paroxysmal AV block in these patients was related to a vagal reaction, AV-blocking drugs, or distal conduction disease. The AV block in these patients lasted from 2.2 to 36 seconds. Fifteen patients experienced syncope, and one patient had bradycardia-induced polymorphic ventricular tachycardia that required electrical cardioversion. About one half the patients had structural heart disease and a wide QRS duration.

Complete AV block can be classified as congenital or acquired. In patients with *acquired complete AV block*, the site of block is localized distal to the His bundle in about 70% to 90% of patients, to the His bundle in 15% to 20%, and within the AV node in 16% to 25%.[10] In patients with congenital heart block, the escape rhythm is more often found in the proximal His bundle or AV node.

Bundle-Branch Block

Most patients with chronic BBB or bifascicular block have underlying structural heart disease, the prevalence of which ranges from 50% to 80%.[20,21,23,25] Historically, it was believed that progression from chronic bifascicular block to trifascicular block was common. Retrospective studies in patients with chronic bifascicular block suggested that the risk of progression to complete AV block was 5% to 10% per year. In the early 1980s, the results of several large prospective studies questioned assumptions about the incidence and clinical implications of the progression of conduction system disease in this patient population. Prospective studies of groups of symptom-free patients with bifascicular block who were found to have prolonged H-V intervals on electrophysiologic study showed that such patients are at increased risk for CHB but that the absolute risk remains very low, about 1% to 2% per year.[20,23] In the study by McAnulty and colleagues,[23] the risk for development of CHB was 5% in 5 years. A prolonged H-V interval was associated with higher values for both total cardiovascular mortality and sudden death. It is likely that a prolonged H-V interval is associated with more extensive structural heart disease. Furthermore, these studies demonstrated that in the absence of symptoms, routine His bundle recordings are of limited usefulness in patients with bifascicular block. Asymptomatic individuals with chronic BBB need no further evaluation than an occasional ECG.

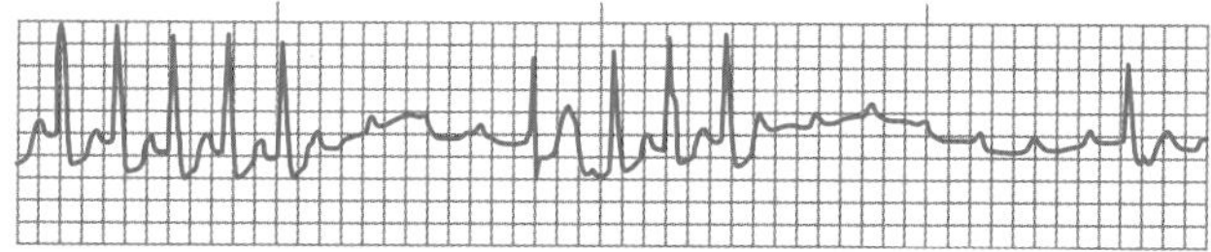

Figure 14-12. Rhythm strip of high-grade atrioventricular (AV) block. The baseline rhythm is sinus tachycardia, in which the P wave occurs simultaneously with the T wave. After the fifth QRS complex, there is an abrupt, or paroxysmal, onset of AV block with four consecutive P waves that do not conduct to the ventricles. The sixth QRS complex probably represents a junctional escape rhythm followed by three conducted complexes and then a longer episode of high-grade AV block. Before both episodes of high-grade AV block, there is no obvious P-R interval prolongation, nor is there slowing of the sinus rate to suggest hypervagotonia as a cause of this patient's block.

On the other hand, patients with *syncope* and *bifascicular block* represent a different clinical problem. If a thorough clinical evaluation, including a history, physical examination, and ECG, do not uncover a cause of syncope, an electrophysiologic study may be useful.[25,26] Linzer and associates[48] found that the presence of first-degree AV block or BBB increased the odds ratio of finding abnormalities suggesting risk of bradyarrhythmia (predominantly heart block) by three- to eightfold during electrophysiologic studies in patients with unexplained syncope (Table 14-1). Electrophysiologic studies may uncover other causes of syncope, such as sinus node dysfunction, rapid supraventricular tachycardias, and inducible monomorphic ventricular tachycardia. In some studies, monomorphic ventricular tachycardia was inducible in at least 30% of patients with BBB and syncope.[25,26] A minority of patients are found to have a markedly prolonged H-V interval, abnormal or fragmented His bundle electrogram, or block distal to the His bundle with atrial pacing, suggesting the need for permanent implantation of a pacemaker.

Congenital AV Block

Congenital CHB traditionally was diagnosed in the first month after birth in a child in whom a slow heart rate was detected and certain infectious etiologies rarely seen today, such as diphtheria, rheumatic fever, and congenital syphilis, were excluded.[52,53] Currently, with fetal echocardiography, many cases are diagnosed in utero and, if associated with structural heart disease, are associated with a high rate of fetal death. The incidence of congenital CHB is estimated to be 1 in 15,000 to 1 in 22,000 live births. More than one half of fetuses found to have congenital CHB have structural heart disease, including congenitally corrected transposition of the great arteries, and often have a poor prognosis in infancy. When congenital CHB is detected in utero in a child with a structurally normal heart, the condition is frequently associated with intrauterine exposure to maternal autoantibodies to Ro and La (i.e., neonatal lupus); this situation has a better prognosis than congenital heart disease. The development of AV block in a child with a structurally normal heart is uncommon but should not be confused with congenital CHB. Childhood-onset heart block often is presumed to be due to viral myocarditis.

TABLE 14-1. Odds Ratio for Abnormality on Electrophysiologic Testing in Patients with Syncope

Clinical Variable	Multivariable	95% Confidence Interval for Multivariable
Age	1.01	0.99-1.03
Duration (months)	1.00	0.98-1.02
Sex (male)	1.76	0.79-3.93
Organic heart disease	1.53	0.71-3.33
Sudden loss of consciousness	1.93	0.89-4.16
Left ventricular ejection fraction	0.99	0.93-1.06
ECG variables:		
Bundle branch block	2.97*	1.23-7.21
Sinus bradycardia	3.47*	1.12-10.71
First-degree heart block	7.89†	2.12-29.31
Premature ventricular contractions (PVSs)	1.47	0.37-5.82
Holter monitoring variables:		
Sinus bradycardia	0.68	0.21-2.23
Sinus pause	1.04	0.26-4.23
Mobitz I atrioventricular block	0.63	0.06-6.33
PVCs	0.87	0.35-2.13

*$P < .05$.
†$P < .001$.
Adapted from Linzer M, Prystowsky EN, Divine GW, et al: Predicting the outcomes of electrophysiologic studies of patients with unexplained syncope: Preliminary validation of a derived model. J Gen Intern Med 6:113, 1991.

In patients with congenital CHB, the mean resting heart rate is between 40 and 60 bpm but decreases with age. The indications for permanent pacemaker implantation are controversial in these young patients but may include symptomatic bradycardia manifested by long naps or nightmares, heart rate of less than 55 bpm in a neonate, an average heart rate of less than 50 bpm in a child, pauses in heart beat of more than 3 seconds while a child is awake or more than 5 seconds during sleep, associated congenital heart disease or ventricular dysfunction, exercise intolerance due to chronotropic incompetence, prolonged QTc, wide ventricular escape rhythm, and complex ventricular ectopy. A 2004 study demonstrated, however, that long-term transvenous RV apical pacing was associated with deleterious LV remodeling and reduced exercise capacity after 10 ± 3 years of follow-up in patients with congenital CHB.[54] Thus, alternative ventricular pacing sites, including RV septum and outflow tract and LV, have been proposed in patients with congenital CHB, who may require many decades of ventricular pacing.

Inherited causes of AV conduction disturbances have been recognized, representing an exciting new development in our understanding of the AV conduction system.[55] Insights have also been provided from genetic animal models in which molecular genetic causes of AV block are beginning to be identified. Many of the identified cases of inherited AV conduction disease were previously classified as idiopathic or having an unknown cause. Familial clustering in some cases has been seen with an autosomal dominant pattern of inheritance and associated congenital heart malformations and cardiomyopathy. For example, mutations of lamin A/C gene (LMNA), referred to as "laminopathy," cause dilated cardiomyopathy with AV conduction defects. A large Japanese family with 21 of 224 members affected by this genetic defect, which manifests clinically as progressive AV block, dilated cardiomyopathy, progressive heart failure, and sudden death, has been described.[56] Electrophysiologic studies in affected individuals demonstrated AV nodal dysfunction (marked prolongation of A-H interval) and normal H-V and QRS durations. Histologic evaluation of postmortem heart specimens from affected members showed preferential degeneration of the AV nodal region.

Acquired Causes of AV Block

Acquired AV block may be secondary to a number of causes of generalized myocardial scarring (Table 14-2). These causes include atherosclerosis, dilated cardiomyopathy, hypertension, infiltrative cardiomyopathies, inflammatory disorders, and infectious diseases. In most cases, the specific etiology is clinically unknown and, with few exceptions (e.g., Lyme disease, endocarditis, sarcoidosis), is relatively unimportant from a therapeutic point of view. The most common cause of chronic acquired AV block is related to aging of the cardiac cytoskeleton. An entity known as idiopathic bilateral bundle branch fibrosis, or *Lev's disease*, is characterized by slowly progressive replacement of specialized conduction tissue by fibrosis, resulting in progressive

TABLE 14-2. Causes of Acquired Atrioventricular (AV) Block

Idiopathic fibrodegenerative diseases	Lev's disease Lenègre's disease
Ischemic heart diseases	Myocardial infarction Ischemic cardiomyopathy
Nonischemic cardiomyopathies	Myocarditis Idiopathic dilated cardiomyopathies Hypertensive heart disease
Cardiac surgery	Coronary artery bypass Aortic, mitral, or tricuspid valve replacement/repair Ventricular septal defect repair Congenital heart disease repair Septal myomectomy
Ablation	His bundle ablation Ablation of septal accessory connections Ablation of slow or fast AV nodal pathway for AV nodal reentrant tachycardia Catheter-based septal ablation for hypertrophic cardiomyopathy
Trauma	Chest trauma
Infections	Endocarditis Chagas' disease Lyme disease Acute rheumatic fever Other: bacterial, viral, rickettsial, fungal
Neuromuscular diseases	Myotonic dystrophy Fascioscapulohumeral dystrophy Other muscular dystrophies Kearns-Sayre syndrome Friedreich's ataxia
Infiltrative diseases	Amyloidosis Sarcoidosis Hemochromatosis Carcinoid
Neoplastic diseases	Postradiation therapy Primary and metastatic tumors
Connective tissue diseases	Rheumatoid arthritis Systemic lupus erythematosus Systemic scleroderma Ankylosing spondylitis Others
Drugs	β-blockers Calcium channel antagonists Digoxin and other cardiac glycosides (e.g., oleandrin) Amiodarone Procainamide Flecainide Adenosine Chemotherapeutic agents (arsenic trioxide) Antimalarials (chloroquine) Tricyclic antidepressants Phenothioazines Donepezil
Miscellaneous causes	Exercise Vagal mediation (hypervagatonia, neurocardiac, vasovagal) Temporal lobe epilepsy Hyperkalemia

fascicular block and BBB.[57] Lev[57] proposed that damage to the proximal LBB and adjacent main bundle or main bundle alone is the result of an aging process exaggerated by hypertension and arteriosclerosis of the blood vessels supplying the conduction system. Another variant of idiopathic conduction system disorder is *Lenègre's disease*, which occurs in the younger population and is characterized by loss of conduction tissue, predominantly in the peripheral parts of the bundle branch.[58]

Patients with sick sinus syndrome are known to be at risk for concomitant symptomatic heart block.[59,60] The block may be due to progressive fibrodegenerative disease extending from the sinus node region to the AV conduction system. The relative frequency of this association varies between studies. Rosenqvist and Obel[61] pooled the data from 28 published studies and reported a mean incidence of development of second- or third-degree AV block to be 0.6% per year (range, 0%/yr to 4.5%/yr) in patients in whom permanent atrial pacemakers have been implanted for symptomatic sinus node dysfunction. The total prevalence of second- or third-degree AV block was 2.1% (range, 0% to 11%). In a retrospective review of 1395 patients with sick sinus syndrome who were monitored for a mean of 34 months, Sutton and Kenny[62] estimated that the development of conduction system diseases had an annual incidence of 3%; such conduction diseases included significant first-degree AV block, BBB, H-V prolongation, and a low Wenckebach heart rate. Thus, AV conduction system disease occurs relatively frequently in patients with sinus node dysfunction. Similarly, sinus node dysfunction, particularly chronotropic incompetence, may occur commonly in patients with acquired CHB.

Complete AV block may occur after cardiac surgical or interventional catheter-based procedures. CHB occurs more commonly (3%-6% incidence) after replacement of aortic, mitral, or tricuspid valves, given the proximity of their anuli to the AV junction, than after isolated coronary artery bypass graft surgery, in which the incidence is less than 1% to 2%.[63,64] CHB is seen commonly after surgical procedures to repair ventricular septal defects, tetralogy of Fallot, AV canal defects, or subvalvular aortic stenosis.[65,66] Heart block is also a potential complication of septal myomectomy and catheter-based septal ablation to relieve LV outflow tract obstruction in hypertrophic cardiomyopathy.[67,68] The incidence of heart block requiring permanent pacing after alcohol septal ablation is reported to vary from 10% to 33%.

The time course of conduction defects after bypass surgery was investigated in one study.[69] Operative technique consisted of cold, hyperkalemic cardioplegia, and conduction defects resolved partially or completely in 50% of patients. Patients with conduction defects generally had longer cardiopulmonary bypass times, longer aortic cross-clamp times, and more vessels requiring bypass. In three of the four patients with CHB, the heart block eventually resolved after discharge and implantation of a permanent pacemaker. Reasons for conduction abnormalities after cardiac surgery include ischemic injury to the conduction system, direct surgical manipulation or trauma to conduction tissue, traumatic disruption of the distal conduction system, edema, dissecting hematomas, and alterations in conduction caused by cardioplegia.

Surgery for correction of valvular heart disease commonly leads to conduction defects. After discontinuation of cardiopulmonary bypass, a variety of cardiac rhythm disturbances may be seen, including sinus arrest, junctional rhythm, BBB, AV block, and sinus bradycardia. Many of these rhythm disturbances are transient, resolving within 5 to 7 days. Transient BBB is quite common, occurring in 4% to 35% of patients and generally resolving within 12 to 24 hours.[63] In one study, newly acquired, persistent BBB developed in 15.6% of patients after aortic valve replacement and was associated with a higher adverse event rate.[70] The investigators recommended that prophylactic implantation of a pacemaker be considered soon after surgery in patients who demonstrate persistent BBB. Conduction disturbances are particularly common both in patients with aortic valve disease and after aortic valve replacement, with 5% to 30% of patients experiencing some conduction abnormality after valve replacement. Most of these abnormalities are transient; however, chronic CHB may occur. Postoperative AV block that is not expected to resolve after cardiac surgery is a class I indication for permanent pacing. The incidence of conduction disorders requiring permanent pacing in patients after aortic valve replacement is reported to be 3% to 6%.[71]

Intraoperative heart block does not predict the need for permanent pacing.[72] One study found that risk factors for irreversible AV block requiring permanent pacemaker implantation after aortic valve replacement were previous aortic regurgitation, MI, pulmonary hypertension, and postoperative electrolyte imbalance.[71] In another study, Koplan and associates[73] developed and validated a preoperative risk score to predict the need for permanent pacing after cardiac valve surgery, through the use of a large database from patients undergoing cardiac valve surgery at a single institution from 1992 to 2002.[73] Preoperative predictors of the need for permanent pacing after cardiac valve surgery were age more than 70 years, previous valve surgery, multiple valve surgery (especially involving the tricuspid valve), preoperative BBB (especially RBBB), and first-degree AV block. The incidence of permanent pacemaker implantation ranged from 25% in high-risk patients to 3.6% in low-risk patients, with risk based on preoperative variables. Glikson and colleagues[74] showed that postoperative complete AV block was the most important predictor of subsequent pacemaker dependency. They recommended earlier decisions on the timing of permanent pacemaker implantation, by the sixth postoperative day in patients with a wide QRS complex escape rhythm and by the ninth postoperative day in patients with a narrow QRS complex escape rhythm. In most institutions, permanent pacing would be instituted earlier, probably by the fourth to sixth postoperative day.

Persistent heart block occurs infrequently (0.5%-2% of patients) after radiofrequency catheter ablation of septal accessory pathways or the slow AV nodal pathway in patients with AV nodal reentrant tachycardia.[75] Transient, intraprocedural AV block during ablation performed in close proximity to the AV septum does not necessarily indicate that permanent pacemaker implantation is required. Ablation of the fast pathway in AV nodal reentrant tachycardia in the anterior septum is associated with a higher risk of transient AV block than ablation of the slow pathway in the posterior septum. In one large series of more than 500 patients, transient second- or third-degree AV block was seen in 20% of patients during fast pathway ablation, in 2.3% during slow pathway ablation, and in 42% during combined fast and slow pathway attempted ablation.[76] Within 7 days after the ablation procedure, however, persistent AV block was seen in 3.4%, 0.2% and 0% of patients in these groups, respectively.

Late occurrence of unexpected heart block after radiofrequency catheter ablation of AV nodal reentry (using a posterior approach) or posteroseptal accessory pathways is rare (<0.5% incidence) and often resolves after a few weeks.[77] In patients who experience this rare complication of radiofrequency catheter ablation, prolonged clinical observation and monitoring rather than immediate pacemaker implantation is a reasonable approach. The risk for development of heart block should decrease with the use of cryoablation for the treatment of AV nodal reentry and accessory pathways near the AV node. A higher incidence of heart block (1%-10% of patients) was observed when patients underwent surgical ablation for the Wolff-Parkinson-White syndrome, especially when the accessory pathway was in an anteroseptal, intermediate septal, or posteroseptal location, or after surgical modification of the AV node for treatment of AV nodal reentrant tachycardia.[78]

Radiofrequency catheter ablation is used to create permanent complete AV block in patients with paroxysmal and chronic atrial tachyarrhythmias (most commonly AF). This treatment option is reserved for the small group of patients in whom AV node–blocking drugs cannot control the heart rate or who are intolerant, unwilling, or unable to take drugs to maintain sinus rhythm or control the ventricular response during AF. In most studies, radiofrequency ablation of the AV junction can be accomplished in more than 90% of patients with a right-sided approach through placement of an ablation catheter across the tricuspid valve and recording of a His bundle potential or, less frequently, by placement of the catheter in the LV on the septum underneath the noncoronary cusp of the aortic valve to record a His bundle potential.[79]

Radiofrequency ablation of the AV junction should be performed only in patients with a previously implanted permanent pacemaker or at the time of permanent pacemaker implantation (class I indication for pacing). There are no studies to assess outcome without permanent pacing after catheter ablation of the AV junction. Radiofrequency current ablation of the AV junction usually results in a junctional escape rhythm that has a rate generally ranging from 40 to 50 bpm. In one study, about 65% of patients had an escape rhythm with an average rate of 39 bpm, with a new RBBB in 24%, a new LBBB in 6%, and an idioventricular rhythm in 19%.[80] Several studies have shown AV junction ablation with pacemaker therapy to be highly effective at controlling symptoms and to result in improved quality of life in patients with paroxysmal and chronic AF. In patients with depressed LV function, significant improvements in ventricular function are measured after ablation and pacing in 20% to 40% of patients in some series.[80,81] Currently, many patients with depressed LV function who undergo AV junction ablation receive devices with biventricular pacing capabilities.

AV nodal modification is a catheter ablation procedure designed to impair but not fully destroy AV nodal conduction in patients with rapid ventricular rates during AF.[82] Radiofrequency energy is delivered in and around the slow AV nodal pathway in the posterior septum in an attempt to leave conduction intact over the fast AV nodal pathway. At present, however, AV nodal modification has fallen out of favor and is performed infrequently in patients with AF. In some patients, AV nodal modification results in a slower ventricular response during AF and possibly avoids permanent pacemaker placement, but in other patients, there is an unpredictable decrease in the ventricular rate. Patients who undergo AV nodal modification may remain symptomatic because of recurrent rapid AV conduction or the irregularity of the ventricular response during AF and may subsequently require complete AV nodal ablation. A bimodal RR histogram during AF has been suggested as indicative of dual AV nodal physiology and may be a predictor of successful outcome after AV nodal modification.[83] The risk of sudden death or syncope due to unexpected late CHB is a significant concern with this procedure, however. The rate of inadvertent AV block during the procedure may be as high as 25%.[83] The incidence of long-term AV block is quite variable as well as controversial, with estimates for late development of CHB ranging from 0% to more than 20% in different series.[84]

In patients who have suffered blunt or penetrating chest trauma, a variety of conduction disturbances, including AV block, have been reported, but they appear to be rare complications of this type of injury.[85,86] The reported conduction abnormalities after chest trauma consist of BBB and varying degrees of AV block, including CHB. The most common abnormality is RBBB followed by first-degree AV block, and the least common is CHB. Most AV conduction defects after traumatic chest injury are transient and resolve early. A few cases of persistent heart block requiring permanent pacemaker implantation have been described. Delayed development of complete AV block—occurring 15 to 30 days after injury—has been seen, suggesting that patients suffering blunt chest trauma should be monitored for late complications. The severity of injury does not always correlate with the development of posttraumatic complications, including conduction disorders. The mechanism of conduction defects in this setting is believed to be related to ischemia and/or infarction of the conduction system.

CHB has been described in a large variety of infectious diseases. They include bacterial, viral, fungal, protozoan, and rickettsial infections. Heart block may occur with endocarditis and may be either transient or permanent. In most infectious diseases, heart block is transient and resolves with treatment of the underlying infection. In some cases, transient heart block may recur, and permanent pacing is required. This is particularly true in patients with entities such as endocarditis, in which a valve ring abscess may erode into the conduction system, and in patients with infections such as Chagas' disease.[87-90] AV block occurs in up to 25% of patients with endocarditis complicated by perivalvular abscess, the aortic valve being much more commonly involved than the mitral valve.

Lyme disease is the most common cause of reversible AV block in younger individuals. This systemic illness, first described in 1975, was characterized later as an infection caused by a spirochete, *Borrelia burgdorferi*, which is transmitted to humans by a tick bite. This illness is often characterized by a rash, erythema chronicum migrans, which is followed by cardiac and neurologic abnormalities and then, in some cases, by arthritis.[91] Cardiac involvement may occur in 8% to 10% of patients, is generally transient, and may consist of a myocarditis or a myopericarditis.[92] Varying degrees of AV block are a common manifestation of carditis, occurring in about 75% of patients. More than 50% of patients with AV block have symptomatic high-grade or complete AV block that requires temporary pacing. Most often, the site of block is localized to the AV node, although occasional cases have been reported in which the site of block is intra-Hisian or infra-Hisian.[93,94] Continuous cardiac monitoring is recommended in all patients with second-degree AV block and a prolonged P-R interval of more than 0.30 seconds because of the risk of development of complete AV block. Complete AV block generally resolves within 1 to 2 weeks. Recurrent AV block has not been reported. Rarely, some patients may have symptomatic AV block as the sole manifestation of Lyme disease.[95] Permanent pacing is rarely required except for persistent CHB, which is uncommon. Two important axioms worth repeating are that (1) heart block associated with infectious disease usually resolves with appropriate and prompt antibiotic treatment and (2) conduction disease is rarely the only manifesting feature of an infectious illness.

Heart block may occur rarely after radiation therapy or chemotherapy. Heart block may occur after radiation therapy if radiation is directed at the mediastinum, as may be the case for Hodgkin's and some non-Hodgkin's lymphomas.[96] Radiation therapy may induce fibrosis of the cardiac conduction system as well as the atrial and ventricular myocardium and may accelerate coronary atherosclerosis. Rarely, tumors, including mesothelioma of the AV node, cardiac lymphoma, and metastatic disease to the heart from breast, lung, or skin cancer, may involve the conduction system.[97] AV block has been reported as a rare complication of chemotherapeutic agents (e.g., arsenic trioxide treatment for leukemia). In general, however, it is unusual for toxicity to antineoplastic drugs, such as doxorubicin, to result in damage to the cardiac conduction system.

Certain neuromuscular diseases may give rise to progressive and insidiously developing cardiac conduction system disease. The disorders include Duchenne's muscular dystrophy, fascioscapulohumeral muscular dystrophy, X-linked muscular dystrophy, myasthenia gravis, myotonic dystrophy, and Friedreich's ataxia.[98] Abnormalities of conduction manifest as infranodal conduction disturbances resulting in fascicular block or CHB. This has been noted particularly in Kearns-Sayre syndrome (progressive external ophthalmoplegia with pigmentary retinopathy), Guillain-Barré syndrome, myotonic muscular dystrophy, slowly progressive X-linked Becker's muscular dystrophy, and fascioscapulohumeral muscular dystrophy. Myotonic muscular dystrophy and Kearns-Sayre syndrome are both associated with a high incidence of conduction system disease that frequently is rapidly progressive and cannot be predicted by the ECG or isolated His bundle recordings. His-Purkinje disease can culminate in fatal Stokes-Adams attacks unless anticipated by insertion of a pacemaker. In a study of 49 patients with myotonic dystrophy (46 ± 9 years old) and an H-V interval of 70 msec or more, high-grade paroxysmal AV block was recorded after pacemaker implantation in 47% of patients who had had no known bradycardia on entry into the study.[99] These findings led the researchers to conclude that prophylactic implantation of permanent pacing should be considered in patients with myotonic dystrophy in whom the H-V interval is 70 msec or more even without bradycardia-related symptoms. Waiting for the development of complete AV block in patients with neuromuscular diseases may expose them to significant risk of sudden death or syncope related to AV block. Permanent pacing should be considered early in the course of neuromuscular disease and should be offered to the asymptomatic patient once any conduction abnormality is noted.

Heart block may occur with amyloid and other infiltrative diseases, including hemochromatosis, porphyria, oxalosis, Refsum's disease, carcinoid, Hand-Schüller-Christian disease, and sarcoidosis.[100] Sarcoidosis should be considered in the differential diagnosis in a young patient presenting with CHB. Cardiac manifestations of sarcoidosis are uncommon but can include heart block, ventricular tachyarrhythmias, intracardiac masses, ventricular aneurysms, and dilated cardiomyopathy.[101] Clinical evidence of cardiac involvement is present in less than 5% of patients with sarcoidosis.[102] Virtually all patients with sarcoid heart disease have extracardiac involvement that manifests either clinically or on biopsy. Isolated cardiac involvement in sarcoidosis is extremely rare and usually precedes future systemic sarcoidosis. Newer imaging modalities such as magnetic resonance imaging may be helpful in the diagnosis of cardiac sarcoid, which can be difficult in some cases owing to the lack of definitive criteria. Cardiac involvement, unlike isolated pulmonary disease in sarcoidosis, implies a poor prognosis and an increased risk of sudden death. Heart block in patients with sarcoid heart disease generally warrants a permanent pacemaker. However, AV block may resolve after long-term treatment with corticosteroids alone or in combination with other immunosuppressive therapy.[103] An ICD should be considered strongly in patients with sarcoidosis undergoing device implantation for AV block,

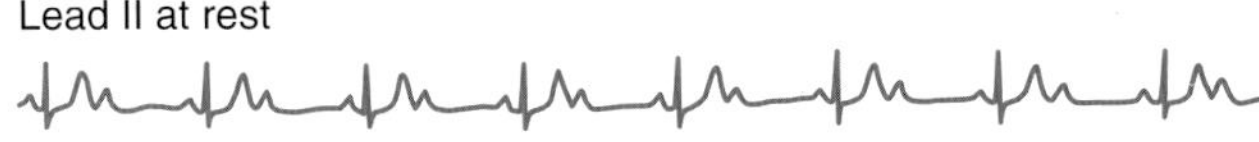

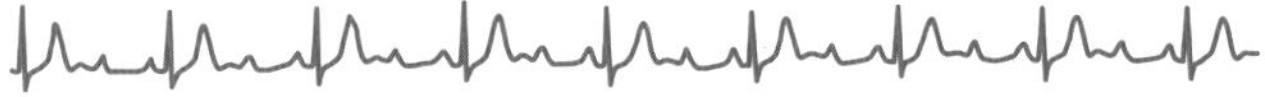

Figure 14-13. Upper panel, Lead II rhythm strip from a patient with syncope and frequent 2:1 atrioventricular (AV) block with an incomplete right bundle branch block and a sinus rate of 97 bpm. Periods of 3:2 AV conduction were not available to determine whether the patient's 2:1 AV conduction was due to type I or type II AV block. Lower panel, Rhythm strip obtained 2 minutes into treadmill testing shows 3:1 AV conduction with an increase in heart rate to 142 bpm. The development of high-grade AV block despite exercise-induced increases in sympathetic tone and decrease in parasympathetic tone suggests infra- or intra-Hisian block and the need for permanent pacing.

because of the risk of ventricular tachyarrhythmias and sudden death.

Connective tissue disorders giving rise to conduction system disease include periarteritis nodosa, rheumatoid arthritis, polymyositis, mixed connective tissue disorders, Reiter's syndrome, ulcerative colitis, scleroderma, Takayasu's arteritis, systemic lupus erythematosus, and ankylosing spondylitis.[104,105] In one study of 50 consecutive patients with scleroderma, electrophysiologic studies demonstrated conduction abnormalities in up to 50% of patients, suggesting that a much higher level of cardiac involvement may be present in patients than is readily apparent clinically. However, CHB is uncommon.[106] Most patients with AV conduction disorders have other clinical manifestations of the connective tissue disease. AV block has been reported as a rare complication of antimalarial therapy used to treat systemic autoimmune diseases (e.g., chloroquine for rheumatoid arthritis or systemic lupus erythematosus).

Exercise-induced transient AV block is a relatively rare condition that is usually due to a block in the His-Purkinje system (Fig. 14-13).[107,108] The incidence of exercise-induced AV block during treadmill exercise testing is between 0.1% and 0.5%.[109] Donzeau and colleagues[110] reported 14 symptomatic patients with exercise-induced AV block, in 9 of whom block was localized to an infranodal site. Other studies have confirmed that exercise-induced AV block is primarily infra-Hisian.[111,112] In these studies, about 25% to 75% of patients had underlying BBB. Several reports of patients with cardiac asystole after exertion have demonstrated postexercise sinus arrest with ventricular asystole.[113] Some researchers proposed that transient ischemia of the conduction system is a mechanism of exercise-induced AV block in patients with severe right coronary artery lesions and chronic infranodal conduction disturbances.[109] A case of pseudo–AV block during exercise due to His bundle parasystole has been reported.[114] Permanent pacing is recommended in patients with exercise-induced AV block, even in the asymptomatic state, because of the high incidence of development of symptomatic AV block.

Drug-induced bradycardia is a common and important clinical problem that remains poorly characterized and has not been well studied in clinical trials.[115] Many commonly prescribed drugs, including β-blockers, calcium channel antagonists, digoxin, antiarrhythmic drugs, tricyclic antidepressants, phenothiazines, and donepezil (a cholinesterase inhibitor used to treat Alzheimer's disease), can cause AV conduction disturbances. In patients presenting with drug-induced AV block, drug therapy can be stopped entirely, reduced in dosage, or continued if there is no acceptable alternative. In the last case, if drug-induced AV block results in symptomatic bradycardia, permanent pacemaker implantation is recommended (class I indication). On the other hand, if the offending agent causing drug-induced AV block can be stopped, pacemaker implantation is generally considered unnecessary according to current guidelines.

The 2002 ACC/AHA/NASPE practice guidelines state that permanent pacemaker implantation is not supported by current evidence as beneficial if AV block is a result of drug toxicity, expected to resolve, and unlikely to recur (class III indication). A provocative study by Zeltser and colleagues,[116] however, challenges this conventional clinical practice and suggests that in the majority of patients presenting with presumed drug-induced AV block, discontinuation of the offending medications does not obviate the need for pacemaker implantation. In this study, AV block persisted after drug discontinuation in most patients. Furthermore, even if AV block resolved when drugs were discontinued, patients remained at risk of recurrent AV block in the absence of offending drugs. Among a consecutive series of 169 mostly elderly patients with structural heart disease presenting with second- or third-degree AV block not related to AMI, vasovagal syncope, digitalis toxicity, or radiofrequency ablation, 92 patients (54%) had drug-induced AV block while receiving β-blockers and/or verapamil or diltiazem. Drug therapy was discontinued in 79 patients; in 32 of these patients (41%), AV block resolved within 48 hours. However, in 18 (56%) of the 32 patients with drug-induced AV block who experienced spontaneous resolution of AV block after drug discontinuation, AV block recurred. Ten of these patients had syncope during the subsequent 3 weeks of follow-up without drug therapy. On the basis of this experience, the researchers estimated that the medications caused only 8% of all cases of AV block and only 15% of occurrences of AV block in patients receiving medications. It must be recognized, however, that recommending permanent pacing in patients with drug-induced bradycardia exposes these patients to the potential harmful effects of ventricular desynchronization imposed by RV pacing. Thus, recommendations regarding the optimal management of patients with drug-induced bradycardia are not straightforward, especially with regard to the need for permanent pacing and the optimal pacing mode. Additional controlled clinical trials addressing this issue are warranted so that future updates to pace-

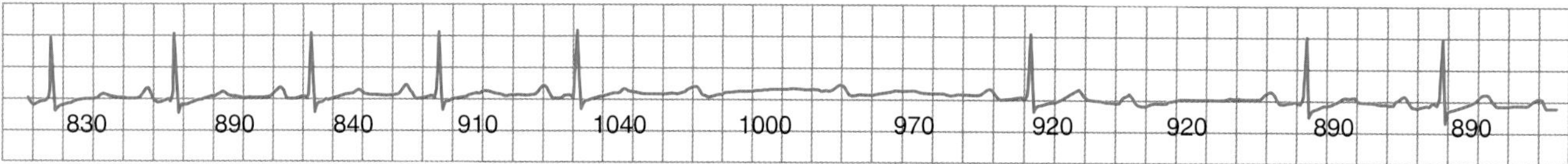

Figure 14-14. Rhythm strip from a 44-year-old man with asymptomatic paroxysmal high-grade atrioventricular (AV) block, but without structural heart disease. The rhythm strip shows sudden, transient total interruption of AV conduction with ventricular asystole. The AV block is preceded by 1:1 AV conduction with a narrow QRS complex and is associated with concomitant prolongation in the sinus cycle length (indicated by the numbers in msec). These findings are consistent with vagally induced AV block at the level of the AV node and usually do not require permanent pacing.

maker practice guidelines can be formulated from an evidence-based approach.

Vagally mediated AV block infrequently requires a permanent pacemaker, especially in the absence of recurrent syncope or profound asystole. AV block may occur in the setting of increased vagal tone in response to various stimuli, such as carotid sinus hypersensitivity, coughing, swallowing, and visceral distention.[117-119] Because vagally mediated AV block often occurs in young, otherwise healthy patients, especially during sleep, it must be differentiated from type II second-degree AV block because the latter patients require implantation of a permanent pacemaker.[120] In most cases, vagally induced AV block occurs at the level of the AV node and is associated with a narrow QRS complex.[121] As a general rule, vagally mediated AV nodal block shows obvious heart rate slowing, even if only slight, before the onset of block, owing to the concomitant effect of increased vagal tone on the sinus node (Fig. 14-14). Rarely, vagal stimulation may precipitate phase IV or bradycardia-mediated block in the His-Purkinje system.[49]

Indications for Permanent Pacing in Chronic Atrioventricular Block

Historically, chronic or acquired AV block with syncope was the first indication for cardiac pacing. Intermittent or chronic high-grade AV block still accounts for a large but varying number of permanent pacemaker implantations, depending on the series. The proportion of pacing related to AV block without AF, according to world and U.S. surveys, ranged from 21% to 54% of pacemakers in 1997.[122,123] Despite published guidelines, permanent pacemaker implantation continues to be underused in patients with CHB. During the period of 1996 to 2001, there were 165,541 admissions to U.S. hospitals with a primary diagnosis of CHB. Only 74% to 83% of patients with a primary diagnosis of CHB received permanent pacemakers before hospital discharge.[124] Furthermore, African-Americans and ethnic minorities were significantly less likely (68% and 60% implantation rates, respectively) than white patients (80% implantation rate) to receive pacemakers for CHB.

In 1984, a subcommittee of the ACC-AHA Task Force on Assessment of Cardiovascular Procedures formulated a set of guidelines for the indications for permanent pacing.[125] These guidelines were revised in 1991, 1998, and 2002.[47,126,127] Permanent pacing indications for acquired AV block and chronic bifascicular and trifascicular block in the 2002 ACC/AHA/NASPE revised guidelines are listed in Tables 14-3 and 14-4.[127]

Indications for pacemaker implantation are categorized into three classes as follows:

- *Class I:* Conditions for which there is evidence or general agreement that pacemaker implantation is beneficial, useful, and effective. There is general agreement among physicians that a permanent pacemaker should be implanted. This implies that the condition is chronic or recurrent but not due to drug toxicity, acute myocardial ischemia or infarction, or electrolyte imbalance.
- *Class II:* Conditions for which cardiac pacemakers are generally found acceptable or necessary, but there is some divergence of opinion. In a *class IIa* indication, the weight of evidence and opinion is in favor of the usefulness and efficacy of implantation. In a *class IIb* indication, the usefulness or efficacy is less well established by evidence and opinion.
- *Class III:* Conditions for which adequate benefit from permanent pacemakers is considered insupportable by current evidence and for which there is general agreement that a pacemaker is not indicated.

Recommendations supported by studies based on data derived from multiple randomized clinical trials with large numbers of patients are ranked at level of evidence A; those based on a limited number of trials involving smaller numbers of patients from well-designed data analyses of nonrandomized studies or observational data registries are ranked at level of evidence B; and those based on expert consensus and years of clinical experience are ranked at level of evidence C.

Acute Myocardial Infarction

Prior to the era of reperfusion therapy for AMI, AV block occurred in 12% to 25% of all patients with AMI; first-degree AV block occurred in 2% to 12%, second-degree block in 3% to 10%, and third-degree block in 3% to 7%.[128-130] It is unclear whether thrombolytic therapy has altered the overall incidence of AV conduction defects in patients with AMI.[131-133] In one study, use of a thrombolytic agent was associated with a higher rate of occurrence of complete AV block (odds

TABLE 14-3. Indications for Permanent Pacing for Acquired Atrioventricular (AV) Block in Adults

Class I	Third-degree and advanced second-degree AV blocks at any anatomic level, associated with any one of the following conditions: Bradycardia associated with symptoms presumed to be due to AV block, including syncope or presyncope, congestive heart failure, mental confusion improving with temporary pacing, symptomatic ventricular ectopy, nonsustained or sustained ventricular tachycardia, and ventricular fibrillation related to an inadequate or slow escape rhythm (level of evidence: C) Arrhythmias and other medical conditions requiring drugs that result in symptomatic bradycardia (level of evidence: C) Documented periods of asystole ≥3 seconds or any escape rhythm <40 bpm in awake, symptom-free patients (levels of evidence: B, C) After catheter ablation of the AV junction (levels of evidence: B, C) Postoperative AV block that is not expected to resolve after cardiac surgery (level of evidence: C) Neuromuscular diseases with AV block, such as myotonic muscular dystrophy, Kearns-Sayre syndrome, Erb's (limb-girdle) dystrophy, and peroneal muscular atrophy with or without symptoms, because there may be unpredictable progression of AV conduction disease (level of evidence: B) Second-degree AV block regardless of the type or the site of block with associated symptomatic bradycardia (level of evidence: B)
Class IIa	Asymptomatic third-degree AV block at any anatomic site with average, awake ventricular rates ≥to 40 bpm, especially if cardiomegaly or left ventricular dysfunction is present (levels of evidence: B, C) Asymptomatic type II second-degree AV block with a narrow QRS; when type II second-degree AV block occurs with a wide QRS, pacing becomes a class I recommendation (level of evidence: B) Asymptomatic type I second-degree AV block at intra-Hisian or infra-Hisian level found incidentally at electrophysiologic study performed for other indications (level of evidence: B) First- or second-degree AV block with symptoms similar to those of pacemaker syndrome (level of evidence: B)
Class IIb	Marked first-degree AV block >0.30 sec in duration in patients with left ventricular dysfunction and symptoms of congestive heart failure in whom a more physiologic A-V interval results in hemodynamic improvement, presumably by decreasing left atrial filling pressure (level of evidence: C) Neuromuscular diseases, such as myotonic muscular dystrophy, Kearns-Sayre syndrome, Erb's (limb-girdle) dystrophy, and peroneal muscular atrophy, with any degree of AV block (including first-degree AV block) with or without symptoms, because there may be unpredictable progression of AV conduction disease (level of evidence: B)
Class III	Asymptomatic first-degree AV block (level of evidence: B) Asymptomatic type I second-degree AV block at the supra-Hisian (AV node) level or not known to be intra- or infra-Hisian (levels of evidence: B, C) AV block that is expected to resolve and is unlikely to recur (e.g., drug toxicity, Lyme disease, and during hypoxia in sleep apnea syndrome in the absence of symptoms) (level of evidence: B)

TABLE 14-4. Indications for Permanent Pacing in Chronic Bifascicular and Trifascicular Blocks

Class I	Intermittent third-degree AV block (level of evidence: B) Type II second-degree AV block (level of evidence: B) Alternating bundle branch block (level of evidence: C)
Class IIa	Syncope not demonstrated to be due to AV block when other likely causes have been excluded, specifically ventricular tachycardia (level of evidence: B) Incidental finding at electrophysiologic study of markedly prolonged H-V interval (>100 msec) in a symptom-free patient (level of evidence: B) Incidental finding at electrophysiologic study of atrial pacing–induced infra-Hisian block that is not physiologic (level of evidence: B)
Class IIb	Neuromuscular diseases, such as myotonic muscular dystrophy, Kearns-Sayre syndrome, Erb's (limb-girdle) dystrophy, and peroneal muscular atrophy with any degree of fascicular block with or without symptoms, because there may be unpredictable progression of AV conduction disease (level of evidence: C).
Class III	Fascicular block without AV block or symptoms (level of evidence: B) Fascicular block with first-degree AV block without symptoms (level of evidence: B)

AV, atrioventricular; BBB, bundle branch block.

ratio = 1.44) but a tendency toward a lower rate of occurrence of BBB (odds ratio = 0.68).[132] Another study suggested that thrombolytic therapy was associated with a tendency toward a lower rate of third-degree AV block in anterior AMI but a higher rate in inferior AMI.[133] Among 6657 patients admitted with AMI between 1990 and 1992 and included in the TRAndolapril Cardiac Evaluation (TRACE) randomized trial in Denmark, 340 (5.1%) experienced third-degree AV block during their hospitalization.[133] The incidence of third-degree AV block was higher among patients with inferior AMI (193 of 2061 [9.4%]) than among those with anterior AMI (44 of 1747 [2.5%]).[133] Likewise, in pooled data from 75,993 patients with ST-segment elevation AMI treated with thrombolytic therapy, 5251 patients (6.9%) had second- or third-degree AV block. AV block occurred in 9.8% of those with inferior AMI and in 3.2% of those with anterior AMI.[134]

The onset of AV block usually occurs 2 to 3 days after the infarction but has a range of a few hours to 10 days. The mean duration is usually 2 to 3 days and the range of duration is 12 hours to 16 days. In one large study, third-degree AV block occurred within 48 hours of symptom onset in 81% of patients and a trend was observed toward later onset of third-degree AV block in anterior rather than in inferior AMI.[134]

Clinicopathologic studies indicate that there is a relationship between the anatomic location of an AMI and involvement of the conduction system.[8,135] The development of AV and intraventricular blocks during anterior AMI is related to the extent of the ischemic/infarcted area. AV block in patients with inferior AMI more often results from vagal reflexes or local metabolites occurring early within the AV node in a transient fashion.

Several mechanisms have been proposed for AV block in the presence of inferior AMI. These include Bezold-Jarisch reflex, reversible ischemia or injury of the conduction system, local accumulation of adenosine or its metabolites, and local AV nodal hyperkalemia.

Stimulation of the Bezold-Jarisch reflex causes an abnormally increased output of vagal nerve traffic; it is initiated by ischemia of the afferent nerves in the area of the inferoposterior LV. Reperfusion of the RCA with thrombolytic agents is a strong stimulus for the Bezold-Jarisch reflex.[136,137] Despite this, the second Thrombolysis in Myocardial Infarction (TIMI II) study did not show an increase in AV block in patients with inferior AMI who received thrombolytic therapy and had a patent infarct-related artery.[138]

In inferior or posterior AMI, obstruction of the RCA produces reversible ischemia of the AV node. In patients who experienced AV block after inferior AMI, pathologic studies demonstrated little or no necrosis, structural damage, or histologic degenerative changes in the conduction system in most cases.[8,135,139] Bilbao and colleagues,[140] however, identified a subgroup of patients with fatal inferior or posterior AMI and AV block who had necrosis of the prenodal atrial myocardial fibers. These necrotic fibers were absent in patients without AV block. Clinically, the transient nature of the AV block supports the concept that injury to the AV node is reversible.[141] The anatomic data reported by Bassan and associates[128] support the concept that the blood supply of the AV node is dual. In their prospective study, 11 of 51 patients who survived an inferior AMI had some degree of transient AV block, and about 90% of the patients with AV block had simultaneous obstruction of the RCA (or left coronary artery [LCA] when it was dominant) and the proximal segment of the LAD artery. Moreover, patients with inferior AMI and LAD artery obstruction had a sixfold higher risk for development of AV block than those without LAD artery obstruction. The TIMI II data do not support this finding, however; in study patients with inferior AMI and AV block, the incidence of disease in the LAD was low and was similar to that in patients with inferior AMI without AV block.[138] The Thrombolysis and Angioplasty in Acute Myocardial Infarction (TAMI) study group also showed no increase in incidence of LAD disease in patients with inferior AMI and complete AV block.[142]

Local accumulation of endogenous adenosine or its metabolites also has been suggested to play a mechanistic role in AV block occurring as an early complication of inferior AMI.[143] Patients with "early" AV block (occurring less than 24 hours into their hospital course) are less likely to show response to atropine.[144] Several case reports or small series have suggested that aminophylline, a competitive adenosine antagonist, reverses atropine-resistant AV block in patients with inferior AMI.[145] Current practice guidelines for management of ST-segment elevation AMI, however, recommend against giving aminophylline to treat bradyarrhythmias because it increases myocardial oxygen demand and is arrhythmogenic.[146]

A higher level of potassium was found in the lymph draining from the infarcted inferior and posterior cardiac walls of dogs after experimental RCA occlusion, suggesting that local AV nodal hyperkalemia may play a role in the development of AV block in the presence of inferior AMI.[147] Sugiura and colleagues[148] found that serum potassium value was an independent predictor of the occurrence of fascicular blocks in anteroseptal AMI.

Anterior or anteroseptal AMI results from obstruction of the LAD artery. Occurrence of AV block and BBB in patients with anterior AMI is usually the result of necrosis of the septum and the conduction system below the AV node and reflects more extensive and permanent myocardial damage with severe LV dysfunction.[139,149,150] Wilber and colleagues,[151] however, reported on two patients with anterior AMI and complete AV block in whom 1:1 conduction returned within minutes after late reperfusion (>40 hours) with angioplasty. Their experience suggests that reversible ischemia rather than necrosis of the conduction system occurs in some patients. Some experimental studies in dogs with anterior AMI suggest that extensive but reversible ischemia of the infranodal conduction tissue occurs, as evidenced by recovery from complete AV block. Several clinical studies also report that most patients with anterior AMI and high-grade AV block who are discharged from the hospital show late recovery of 1:1 AV conduction.[152-156]

Atrioventricular Block without Bundle Branch Block

Incidence

In a series of 684 consecutive patients with AMI admitted to the Los Angeles County–University of Southern California Medical Center (LAC-USCMC) Coronary Care Unit (CCU) between 1966 and 1970, 110 had AV block (16%); 79 of 110 patients (72%) with AV block did not have BBB.[157] The total percentages of patients who had

TABLE 14-5. **Atrioventricular (AV) Block in Acute Myocardial Infarction (AMI) without Bundle Branch Block***

Incidence (%):	12 (79/684 patients)
First-degree AV block	6 (44/684 patients)
Second-degree AV block	7 (50/684 patients)
Third-degree AV block	4 (29/684 patients)
Site of infarction (%):	
Inferior	79
Anterior	18
Combined	6
Progression (%):	
First-degree AV block to second- or third-degree AV block	59
Second-degree AV block to third-degree AV block	36
Outcome (%):	
Hospital mortality	29
Return to 1:1 conduction in survivors	95

*Data from 684 consecutive patients with AMI at Los Angeles County–University of Southern California Medical Center (LAC-USCMC), Los Angeles.

Adapted from de Guzman M, Rahimtoola SH: What is the role of pacemakers in patients with coronary artery disease and conduction abnormalities? In Rahimtoola SH (ed): Controversies in Coronary Artery Disease. Philadelphia, FA Davis, 1983, pp 191-207.

first-, second-, or third-degree AV block at some time were 6%, 7%, and 4%, respectively (Table 14-5).

Site of Infarction

AV block is more commonly associated with inferior infarction, and in those who experience second- and third-degree blocks, inferior AMI is present two to four times as often as anterior AMI. The site of block in inferior infarction is above the His bundle in about 90% of patients, whereas in anterior infarction, the conduction abnormality is usually localized below the His bundle in the distal conducting system.[158] In the LAC-USCMC series, of the 79 patients with AV block who did not have BBB, 60 (76%) had an inferior infarction, 14 (18%) an anterior infarction, and 5 (6%) a combined infarction (Table 14-6).

Progression of Atrioventricular Block

In patients with inferior AMI, progression of AV block commonly occurs in stages, whereas in those with anterior AMI, it may occur in stages, or third-degree AV block or ventricular asystole may develop suddenly (Fig. 14-15).[141]

Outcome

AV block complicating AMI is associated with a high mortality rate (24% to 48%), two to three times that for AMI without AV block (9% to 16%). Even with the use of thrombolytic therapy and primary percutaneous coronary interventions, if AV block occurs in the setting of AMI, mortality remains high, especially in anterior MI.[138,142,159,160] This poor prognosis generally reflects the larger ischemic/infarcted region associated with devel-

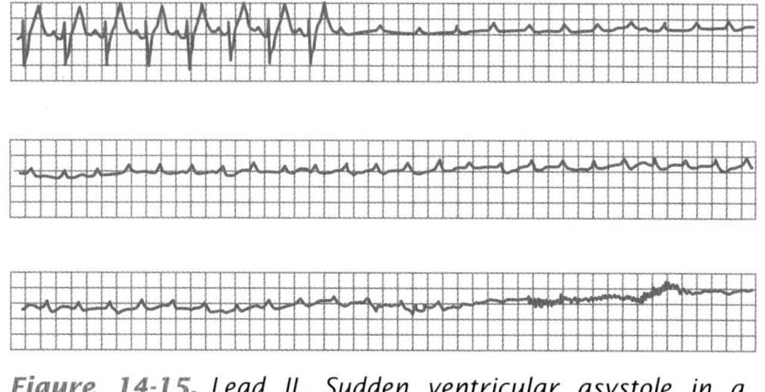

Figure 14-15. Lead II. Sudden ventricular asystole in a patient with acute myocardial infarction complicated by right bundle branch block and left axis deviation. (From de Guzman M, Rahimtoola SH: What is the role of pacemakers in patients with coronary artery disease and conduction abnormalities? In Rahimtoola SH: Controversies in Coronary Artery Disease. Philadelphia, FA Davis, 1983.)

TABLE 14-6. **Atrioventricular (AV) Block in Anterior and Inferior-Posterior Acute Myocardial Infarction (AMI)**

Feature	Anterior AMI	Inferior-Posterior AMI
Pathophysiology	Extensive necrosis of septum	Reversible ischemia, injury of conduction system
Site of block	Infranodal	Intranodal
Frequency	Less frequent	Two to four times more frequent
Progression to complete AV block	Sudden	Gradual
Intraventricular conduction defect	Common	Rare
Escape focus	Ventricular	Junctional
Escape rate (per minute)	20-40	40-60
Prognosis	High mortality	Lower mortality

opment of AV block in the setting of AMI. Although AV block that occurs during inferior AMI predicts a higher risk of in-hospital death, it may be less predictive of long-term mortality in patients who survive to hospital discharge.[138,142] Before the reperfusion era, Tans and coworkers[130] reported that in patients with inferior AMI, those with high-grade AV block and no severe pump failure had a higher in-hospital mortality rate (17%) than those without high-grade AV block (9%).[130] The major cause of death in patients who have AV block in the setting of AMI is pump failure.[161] In the LAC-USCMC series, the hospital mortality rate was 29% (32 of 110 patients); 29 of the 32 deaths (91%) were due to pump failure. Survival, therefore, is greatly influenced by the severity of the hemodynamic disturbance and is less dependent on the degree of heart block. Death is related primarily to extensive myocardial damage, but in an important minority of patients, it can be attributed to sudden ventricular asystole or severe bradycardia.

Atrioventricular Block with Bundle Branch Block

Prior to the widespread use of thrombolytic therapy, BBB was present during hospitalization in 8% to 18% of patients with AMI.[162-167] The presence of a persistent intraventricular conduction defect during the hospitalization increases the risk of high-grade AV block as well as other complications and is associated with poor survival in patients with AMI. In patients receiving thrombolytic therapy, the incidence of persistent intraventricular conduction defects appearing during the hospitalization is reduced to about 4% to 9%.[131-133,168] However, the adverse risk associated with intraventricular conduction defects (except for isolated left anterior hemiblock) has persisted even in the modern era of AMI reperfusion therapy.

In an older series of 2779 patients with AMI admitted from 1966 to 1977 to the LAC-USCMC coronary care unit, 257 (9%) had BBB (Table 14-7).[157] Of the 257 patients, 83 (32%) had LBBB, 80 (31%) had RBBB, 72 (28%) had RBBB plus left-axis deviation, 21 (9%) had RBBB plus right-axis deviation, and one had alternating BBB. The conduction abnormality was "new" in 60%—that is, the BBB developed during the infarction and was documented by serial ECGs or was present on admission and was not seen on previous ECGs or reverted to normal conduction later as documented by serial ECGs. When the site of infarction was not obscured by the BBB in the LAC-USCMC series, the block was associated with anterior AMI about three times as often as with inferior AMI.

TABLE 14-7. Bundle Branch Block in Acute Myocardial Infarction

Incidence (%):	9 (257/2779 patients)*
LBBB	32 (83/257 patients)
RBBB	31 (80/257 patients)
RBBB + LAD obstruction	28 (72/257 patients)
RBBB + RAD obstruction	9 (21/257 patients)
Onset of BBB (%):	
New	60
Old	40
Site of infarction (%):	
Inferior	21
Anterior	52
Combined	4
Indeterminate	18
Nontransmural	5
Incidence of AV block (%):	29 (75/257 patients)
First-degree	10 (25/257 patients)
Second-degree	5 (13/257 patients)
Third-degree	14 (37/257 patients)
Progression of AV block (%):	
First-degree AV block to second- or third-degree AV block	32
Second-degree AV block to third-degree AV block	46
Progression to high-grade AV block	18 (46/257 patients)
Bilateral BBB + first-degree AV block	50
New *bilateral* BBB + first-degree AV block	43
First-degree AV block	30
New BBB + first-degree AV block	29
Bilateral BBB	18
New BBB	16
New bilateral BBB	15
Outcome (%):	
Hospital mortality	20
Return to 1:1 conduction in survivors	89

AMI, acute myocardial infarction; AV, atrioventricular; BBB, bundle branch block; L, left; LAD, left anterior descending (artery); R, right; RAD, right anterior descending (artery).

*Data from 2779 AMI patients seen from October 1966 to March 1977 at Los Angeles County–University of Southern California Medical Center (LAC-USCMC), Los Angeles.

Adapted from de Guzman M, Rahimtoola SH: What is the role of pacemakers in patients with coronary artery disease and conduction abnormalities? In Rahimtoola SH (ed): Controversies in Coronary Artery Disease. Philadelphia, FA Davis, 1983, pp 191-207.

Progression of Atrioventricular Block

In the LAC-USCMC series conducted before the thrombolytic era, progression of AV block occurred in 75 of the 257 patients (29%) with AMI and BBB (see Table 14-7).

Of the 28 patients with AV block and BBB who initially had a normal P-R interval, 13 (46%) experienced first-degree AV block. Nine of the 13 (69%) remained in first-degree block, 2 (15%) progressed to second-degree block type II only, 1 (8%) had type II second-degree block that progressed to third-degree AV block, and 1 had third-degree block without first having second-degree block. Six patients had type II second-degree block without initially having first-degree AV block; 4 of the 6 (67%) went on to have third-degree AV block.

Of the total 41 patients who had first-degree AV block and BBB, 13 (32%) progressed to high-grade block. Twenty-eight (68%) were admitted in first-degree AV block. Sixteen of the 28 (57%) remained in first-degree block; 3 (11%) progressed to type II second-degree AV block, 1 of whom went on to third-degree block; 5 (18%) progressed to type I second-degree block, 2 of whom went on to third-degree block; and 4 (14%) patients had third-degree block without initially having second-degree AV block.

Of the total 24 patients who had second-degree AV block and BBB, 11 (46%) progressed to third-degree block. Six had second-degree AV block on admission; of these, type II block occurred in 4, 1 of whom progressed to third-degree block, and type I occurred in 2, 1 of whom progressed to third-degree block.

There were 37 patients with third-degree AV block and BBB, 13 (35%) of whom were admitted in third-degree block. Of the 24 who progressed to third-degree block, 11 (46%) had demonstrated second-degree block; 7 of the 11 had type II second-degree block. Consistent with the LAC-USCMC series, AV block occurred in other studies in about one third of patients with AMI and BBB.[157,169-172]

Two large, older studies from the 1970s and 1980s developed a data bank on patients with BBB in association with MI. One was a large collaborative multicenter study involving five centers,[156] and the other was a study conducted at LAC-USCMC.[157] Both studies have limitations because (1) the data were obtained retrospectively and (2) at the time, no guidelines existed pertaining to pacemaker insertion, which was performed at the physician's discretion in all cases. Thus, although these studies are unable to provide definitive answers about the natural history of BBB in association with AMI, they nevertheless do offer valuable clinical information.

In the multicenter study reported by Hindman and coworkers,[156] high-grade AV block (third- or second-degree block with a type II pattern) occurred in 55 of 432 patients (22%). To determine which patients were at considerable risk for development of high-grade AV block while hospitalized with AMI, several variables were analyzed. Combinations of the three following ECG findings identified high-risk patients: (1) first-degree AV block, (2) bilateral BBB (if both bundle branches were involved [e.g., RBBB plus left- or right-axis deviation] or alternating RBBB and LBBB), and (3) "new" BBB. The absence of all variables or the presence of only one of the three defined variables was associated with a lower risk (10% to 13%) for development of high-grade AV block during hospitalization. The risk was moderate for patients with first-degree AV block with either new BBB or bilateral BBB (19% to 20%), and highest (31% to 38%) for new bilateral BBB regardless of the P-R interval (Fig. 14-16).

In the LAC-USCMC study, high-grade AV block occurred in 46 of 257 patients (18%). The absence of all three variables (first-degree AV block, bilateral BBB, and new BBB) or the presence of either bilateral BBB or new BBB or new bilateral BBB was associated with the lowest risk (10% to 18%) for development of high-grade AV block during hospitalization with AMI.[157] The risk was moderate for first-degree AV block with or without new BBB (29% to 30%) and highest (50%) for bilateral BBB plus first-degree AV block, regardless of whether the BBB was old or new (Fig. 14-17).

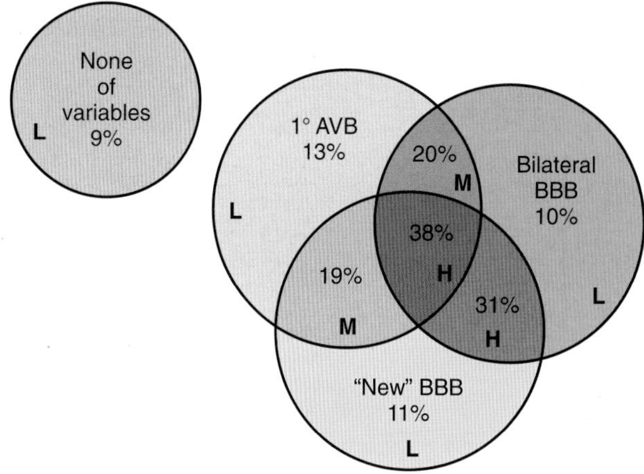

Figure 14-16. Venn diagram for 432 patients in the multicenter study, depicting the risk for high-grade atrioventricular block (AVB) in patients with acute myocardial infarction (AMI) and bundle branch block (BBB). (From Hindman MC, Wagner GS, JaRo M, et al: The clinical significance of bundle branch block complicating acute myocardial infarction. 2: Indications for temporary and permanent pacemakers. Circulation 58:689, 1978. Copyright 1978, American Heart Association.)

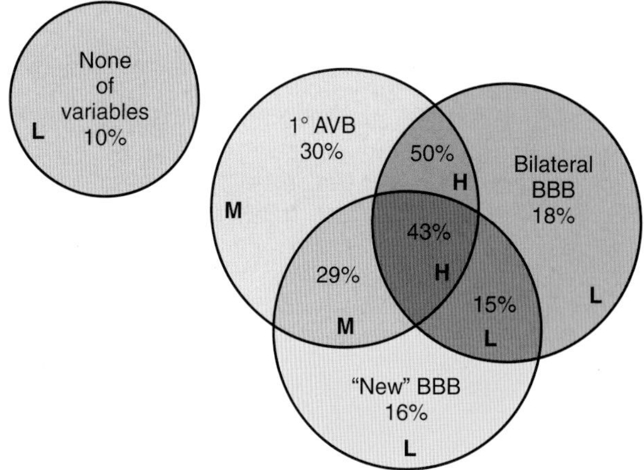

Figure 14-17. Venn diagram for 257 patients in the Los Angeles County–University of Southern California Medical Center (LAC-USCMC) study, depicting the risk for high-grade atrioventricular block (AVB) in patients with acute myocardial infarction (AMI) and bundle branch block (BBB). (From de Guzman M, Rahimtoola SH: What is the role of pacemakers in patients with coronary artery disease and conduction abnormalities? In Rahimtoola SH: Controversies in Coronary Artery Disease. Philadelphia, FA Davis, 1983.)

Despite some differences in the findings between the two studies, both studies found that the following subgroups of patients were at highest risk for high-grade AV block: (1) those with new bilateral BBB plus first-degree AV block (risks, 38% in the Hindman[156] study and 43% in the LAC-USCMC[157] study), (2) those with bilateral BBB plus first-degree AV block (risks, 20% and 50%, respectively), and (3) new BBB plus first-degree AV block (risks, 19% and 29%, respectively). Subgroups in whom the findings of the two studies show different risks can be considered to be at moderate risk for high-grade AV

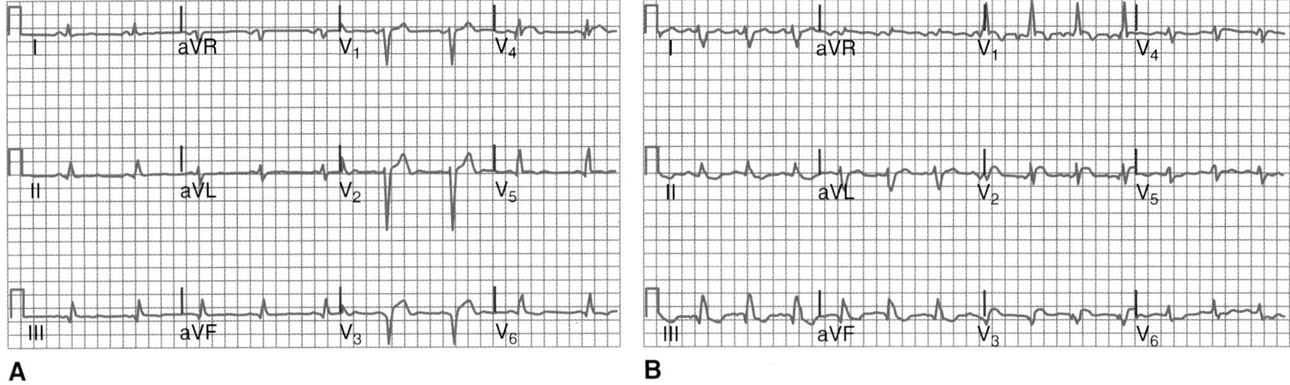

Figure 14-18. ***A** and **B**, Electrocardiograms of a patient with anterior acute myocardial infarction (AMI) and development of "new" bilateral bundle branch block (BBB)—left BBB and right BBB with right-axis deviation. This patient had sudden ventricular asystole.*

block. These subgroups include patients with (1) new bilateral BBB (risks, 31% and 15%, respectively) (Fig. 14-18), (2) first-degree AV block (risks, 13% and 30%, respectively), and (3) bilateral BBB (risks, 10% and 18%, respectively). The remaining subgroups of patients with AMI and BBB can be considered to be at lowest risk (≤10%) for development of high-grade AV block.

The database assembled by the Multicenter Investigation of the Limitation of Infarct Size (MILIS) was used to develop a simplified method of predicting the occurrence of CHB. Data from 698 patients with proved MI were analyzed, and the presence or absence of ECG abnormalities of AV or intraventricular conduction was determined for each patient. Risk factors for development of CHB were as follows: first-degree AV block, Mobitz type I AV block, Mobitz type II AV block, left anterior hemiblock, left posterior hemiblock, RBBB, and LBBB. A risk score for the development of CHB was devised that consisted of the sum of each patient's individual risk factors. Incidences of CHB of 1.2%, 7.8%, 25%, and 36% were associated with risk scores of 0, 1, 2, and 3 or more, respectively (Fig. 14-19). The risk score was subsequently tested on the published results of six studies for a combined total of 2151 patients.[173] The limitations of this scoring system include the lack of differentiation between newly appearing and old BBB, a factor that has been shown to be of predictive value. It is likely that consideration of such factors would further improve the accuracy of the scoring system, but it would also add to its complexity. Another criticism of the scoring system is that it would assign a risk score of only 1 to a patient with isolated Mobitz type II AV block, a disorder usually believed to be highly predictive of progression to CHB. Isolated Mobitz type II AV block is, however, relatively rare.

It must be recognized that the algorithms and clinical databases used to estimate the risk for occurrence of CHB in the setting of AMI were developed in the prethrombolytic era and, thus, must be interpreted cautiously when applied to the modern post-AMI patient population. The availability of transcutaneous pacing and early primary percutaneous coronary interventions has had an important effect on the clinical management of these patients in the setting of AMI in the current era. The actual clinical decision whether to institute prophylactic temporary pacing should be individualized according to the patient-related risk factors and the available personnel and equipment at each institution.

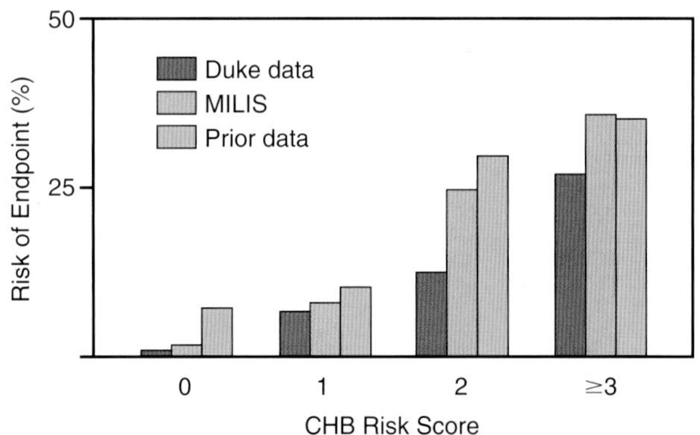

Figure 14-19. Comparison of the incidence of complete heart block (CHB) predicted by the CHB risk score method (blue bars), the observed incidence of CHB in the Duke University myocardial infarction database (orange bars), and the observed incidence of CHB or CHB and Mobitz II atrioventricular (AV) block in six reported studies (yellow bars). MILIS, Multicenter Investigation of the Limitation of Infarct Size. (From Lamas GA, Muller JE, Turi AG, et al: A simplified method to predict occurrence of complete heart block during acute myocardial infarction. Am J Cardiol 57:1213, 1986.)

Outcome

The short- and long-term mortality and sudden death rates are higher in patients with AMI and BBB (25% to 50%) than in those without BBB (15%).[130,162-166,174] The one exception is the isolated finding of left anterior fascicular block in patients with AMI, which appears not to carry an unfavorable prognosis. When the infarction is extensive and produces diffuse conduction system abnormalities progressing to high-grade AV block, it is also extensive enough to damage a large amount of myocardial muscle. Therefore, affected patients often die from pump failure and from ventricular tachyarrhythmias, and the adverse prognosis is not necessarily due to development of high-grade AV block. Nevertheless, some of these patients do *not* die from heart failure or ventricular arrhythmias, and in these patients, the conduction abnormality may be contributory and can be the major cause of death if prophylactic pacing is not undertaken. In some patients, sudden third-degree AV block or asystole is abrupt and fatal if untreated. It is interesting that in the LAC-USCMC study, 75% of patients with BBB and AMI had either no heart failure or, at worst, mild heart failure.[157] These results as well as those of Hindman and coworkers[156] showed that high-grade AV block influenced hospital mortality independently of pump failure.

Impact of Thrombolytic Therapy

Several prospective trials involving thrombolytic therapy of AMI provide data pertaining to the effect of such therapy on the development of high-grade (second- or third-degree) AV block and BBB.[138,142]

The study by Clemmensen and associates[142] was designed to examine the effect of thrombolytic therapy and adjunctive angioplasty as a treatment strategy for AMI (TAMI trial) after inferior AMI.[142] In all patients, treatment was initiated with thrombolytic agents within 6 hours of symptom onset. There were 373 patients with an inferior AMI, of whom 50 (13%) had complete AV block; 54% of these patients had complete AV block on admission. In all but 2 patients, the block was manifest within 72 hours of onset of symptoms. The duration of block was less than 1 hour in 25% and less than 12 hours in 15%; the median duration of block was 2.5 hours. There was no difference in the rate of infarct vessel patency between those with and those without AV block (90% and 91%, respectively). A precipitating clinical event—vessel reperfusion, performance of percutaneous transluminal coronary angioplasty (PTCA)—or vessel reocclusion was identifiable in 38% of instances of complete AV block. At the predischarge angiogram, the vessel patency rate was 11% lower in the group with AV block than in the group without it (71% vs. 82%, respectively). Those in whom AV block developed showed a decrease in ejection fraction between the early post-thrombolytic angiogram and the predischarge angiogram. Also, those who experienced AV block had a higher in-hospital mortality, 10 of 50 (20%) versus 12 of 323 (4%; $P < .001$). When age, LV ejection fraction in the acute phase, number of diseased vessels, and grade of blood flow through the culprit lesion were entered into a multivariate model, the development of complete AV block still contributed significantly to the risk for in-hospital death. After a median follow-up period of 22 months, mortality rates for patients with and without AV block were equivalent (2%). These data suggest that, compared with the prethrombolytic era, use of thrombolytics and angioplasty has not altered either the incidence of complete AV block nor the associated greater ventricular dysfunction or in-hospital mortality of inferior MI.

In another study of 1786 patients with inferior AMI who received recombinant tissue-type plasminogen activator (rt-PA) within 4 hours of symptom onset, high-grade (second- or third-degree) AV block developed in 214 (12%) (TIMI II trial).[138] Of the group who had AV block, 113 (6.3% of the total, or 52% of those who ever had AV block) had this finding on admission. The remaining 101 patients (5.7%) experienced heart block during the 24 hours after treatment with thrombolytics. Patients who already had high-grade AV block before receiving thrombolytic therapy tended to be older and had a higher prevalence of cardiogenic shock than those without heart block. Nevertheless, the presence of heart block did not carry a higher 21-day mortality rate independent of other variables such as shock, and the 1-year mortality rate was similar to that in the group without heart block. Patients in this study were randomly assigned to coronary arteriography 18 to 48 hours after admission. Among those who had heart block after admission, the infarct-related artery was less frequently patent than in those without heart block (28 of 39 [72%] vs. 611 of 723 [84.5%]; $P = .04$]). The RCA was the infarct-related artery more often in patients who had heart block than in those who did not (36 of 69 [92.3%] vs. 542 of 723 [75.1%], respectively; $P = .04$). Among patients without heart block at the time of hospital admission, death occurred within 48 hours in 4 of 9 patients (44%) with new heart block and in 8 of 68 (12%) without new heart block at 24 hours. The 21-day mortality rate was higher in the group with AV block than in the group without block (10 of 101 [9.9%] versus 35 of 1572 [2.2%], respectively; $P < .001$), as was the 1-year mortality rate (15 of 101 [14.9%] versus 65 of 1572 [4.2%], respectively; $P = .001$). A temporary pacemaker was inserted in about one third of patients who had heart block on admission and in almost 30% of patients who experienced heart block after institution of thrombolytic therapy, whereas only 6.5% of patients without heart block received temporary pacemakers. None of the patients who had heart block on admission or who experienced heart block later received permanent pacemakers, but 4 patients without heart block at 24 hours went on to receive permanent pacemakers. Heart block was not listed as a primary or contributing cause of death in any patient.

The data from these two studies of thrombolytic therapy suggest that aggressive treatment with thrombolytic agents or thrombolytic therapy plus angioplasty is not associated with a lower incidence of high-grade or complete AV block in patients with inferior AMI than was seen in the prethrombolytic era; the incidence remains about 10% to 13%, with about one half of cases appearing as new AV block during hospitalization. The infarct-related vessel is more often the RCA, and there is a lower vessel patency rate after thrombolysis among patients in whom AV block complicates inferior AMI. In-hospital and early posthospitalization mortality rates are higher in patients with than in those without AV block among patients treated with thrombolytics, with or without angioplasty. It has not been clear, however, that patients with acute AV block continue to be at greater risk of death over the long term if they survive the initial hospitalization. A study that pooled data

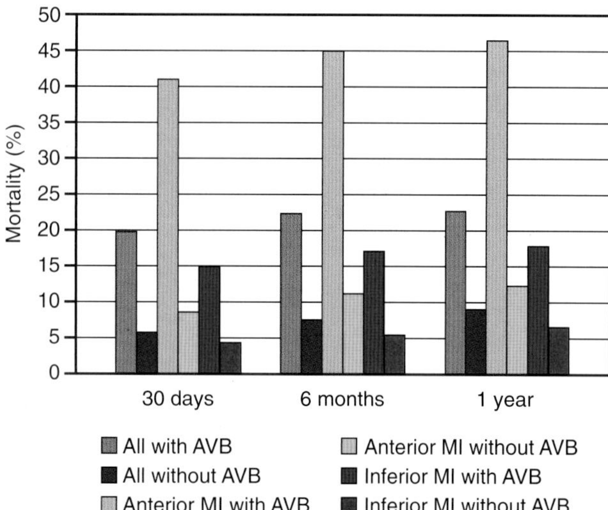

Figure 14-20. Unadjusted mortality rates in patients with and without atrioventricular block (AVB). MI, myocardial infarction. (From Meine TJ, Al-Khatib SM, Alexander JH, et al: Incidence, predictors, and outcomes of high-degree atrioventricular block complicating acute myocardial infarction treated with thrombolytic therapy. Am Heart J 149:670, 2005.)

from four large randomized clinical trials involving 70,000 patients with AMI treated with thrombolytic therapy evaluated the short- and long-term mortality rates associated with second- and third-degree AV blocks.[134] Compared with patients with AMI and no AV block, patients with AMI and AV block were more than three times more likely to die within 30 days and 1.5 times more likely to die during 1 year of follow-up. The higher short- and long-term mortality rates were observed in the setting of inferior as well as anterior AMI (Fig. 14-20). The presumption remains, as before the era of thrombolytic therapy, that the presence or development of AV block is associated with a higher mortality because it tends to indicate the presence of more extensive infarction or injury.

In trials conducted with thrombolytic therapy in AMI, BBB is reported present on admission in up to 2% to 4% of patients.[173] In the first Global Utilization of Streptokinase and tissue-type plasminogen activator for Occluded Coronary Arteries (GUSTO-I) trial, among 26,003 North American patients, 420 (1.6%) had left (n = 131) or right (n = 289) BBB on admission ECG.[175] Interestingly, reversion of BBB occurred in 24% of patients during hospitalization and was associated with a 50% relative risk reduction in 30-day mortality, from 20% to 10%. Prognosis for patients who recovered normal intraventricular conduction (i.e., transient BBB) was similar to that for patients who never had BBB. Another study examined the significance of RBBB in AMI in the prethrombolytic era and compared it with the incidence and prognostic significance of new RBBB in the thrombolytic era.[176] In a multicenter prospective study of 1238 patients with 1-year follow-up, a higher rate of new and transient RBBB and lower rate of bifascicular block were found in patients receiving thrombolytic therapy. The overall prognostic implications of RBBB, however, were unchanged and included a higher rate of heart failure, greater chance of needing a permanent pacemaker, and a higher 1-year mortality rate.[176]

Bundle Branch Block after Recovery from Acute Myocardial Infarction

The subset of patients with persistent BBB and transient high-grade AV block during AMI are at increased risk of late mortality.[156,177,178] It is now recognized that most of these deaths are sudden and result from ventricular tachyarrhythmias. In a previous era, however, whether these patients were at high risk for sudden death from a bradyarrhythmia was debated and controversial.[154,172,179-181] A number of investigators suggested that patients with persistent BBB plus transient AV block during the acute infarction had a higher risk of dying suddenly as a result of CHB. These investigators attempted to identify the subset of patients at highest risk of late sudden death due to AV block in order to maximize the therapeutic benefit of permanently implanting a pacemaker.

The multicenter study by Hindman and coworkers[156] supported the previous reports by Atkins and colleagues[177] and Ritter and associates,[178] who found that the subset of patients with chronic BBB and transient high-grade AV block during AMI were at increased risk of late sudden death. These data showed that patients who did not receive pacing had a higher incidence of sudden death or recurrent high-grade AV block during follow-up (65%) than those who were given permanent pacing (10%), suggesting that implantation of a permanent pacemaker protected against sudden death in these patients. Waugh and coworkers[182] likewise recommended permanent pacemaker therapy to prevent syncope or sudden death in another group of high-risk patients, those with bilateral BBB plus transient high-grade AV block (type II progression).

Other studies from the same era, however, questioned whether these patients are at high risk for sudden death from a bradyarrhythmia.[154,174,179-181] For example, in the study by Nimetz and associates,[172] late sudden death occurred in 4 of 13 (31%) survivors with BBB and second- or third-degree AV block and in 14 of 41 (34%) survivors without AV block. In a study by Ginks and coworkers,[154] of patients with anterior MI complicated by CHB with return to normal sinus rhythm but with persistent BBB, 4 of 14 hospital survivors (29%) with anterior MI, persistent BBB, and transient AV block died, and 2 of 4 (50%) with permanent pacemakers died during a follow-up period averaging 49 months. In a study by Murphy and associates[180] of patients surviving AMI complicated by BBB, none of the deaths resulted from heart block, even in patients with transient AV block during the AMI. Lie and colleagues[181] reported on a group of 47 patients who had survived anterior infarction complicated by BBB and who were kept for 6 weeks in the monitoring area; 17 of the 47 patients (36%) sustained late ventricular fibrillations. Likewise, the Birmingham Trial of permanent pacing in patients with persistent intraventricular defects after AMI showed no significant difference in survival between patients with and without heart block during up to 5 years of follow-up.[183] Finally, in a prospective long-term study by Talwar and colleagues,[184] 18 patients with anterior AMI, intraventricular defects, and transient complete AV block were monitored for a mean of 2 years; pacemakers were permanently implanted in 8 patients. There was only one death, in the unpaced group, and it was due to a cerebrovascular accident. Clearly, these older studies were limited by the small number of patients with AMI enrolled and monitored and may not be applicable to the current era of post-AMI management. Despite the controversy regarding whether late sudden death in patients with BBB is caused by heart block, permanent ventricular pacing is indicated for transient advanced second- or third-degree infranodal AV block and associated BBB after AMI, according to current practice guidelines (class I indication).[127]

Role of Electrophysiologic Studies in Atrioventricular Block and Bundle Branch Block in Acute Myocardial Infarction

Electrophysiologic studies with recording of the His bundle electrogram (HBE) are not performed routinely today for risk stratification of patients with AV block after AMI. HBE studies after AMI were used primarily in the 1970s and 1980s to identify the sites of AV conduction disturbances, which were shown to be either in the AV node (proximal block) or in the distal conduction system (distal block). The presence of distal block identifies patients at high risk for development of high-grade AV block. In individual cases in which the diagnosis is uncertain (e.g., type I second-degree AV block in patients with BBB) or infranodal or multilevel block is suspected, an electrophysiologic study is helpful in identifying the sites of AV block (Fig. 14-21).

In patients with inferior AMI, the site of AV block is usually proximal. Harper and colleagues[185] showed that 30 of 32 patients (94%) with inferior AMI and third-degree AV block had AV nodal block during HBE; the remaining two patients were in normal sinus rhythm during the study and had a normal P-R interval and normal A-H and H-V intervals. Thus, in this group of patients, HBE offered no advantage over conventional ECG criteria in localizing the site of block.

In anterior AMI, the block is frequently in the distal conduction system. In the study by Harper and colleagues,[185] 50% of patients (9 of 18) with BBB and a normal P-R interval on ECG had a prolonged H-V interval.[185] Of the 22 patients who experienced AV block and BBB, 5 had proximal block, 14 had distal block, and 3 had both proximal and distal blocks. Thus, in both groups of patients, HBE was the only means of localizing the block in the proximal or distal portion of the conduction system. Distal block indicates disease in either the His bundle or the remaining bundle branches; clinically, this finding is a common antecedent to sudden asystole and a poorer prognosis. Despite the fact that a prolonged H-V interval could identify a group of patients who may be at high risk for high-grade AV block, several studies have shown that it does not help in assessing the short- or long-term prognosis of patients after AMI.[185,186]

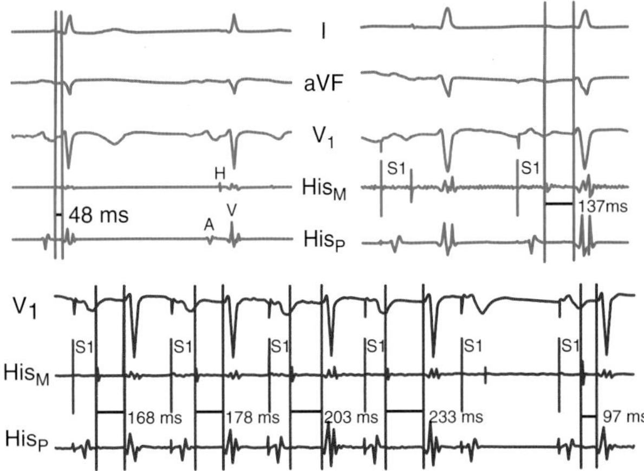

Figure 14-21. Simultaneous surface electrocardiogram (leads I, aVF, and V1) and intracardiac recordings from the His bundle region (His_M and His_P) in a 65-year-old patient with ischemic cardiac disease and a history of syncope. Left upper panel shows sinus rhythm with normal baseline H-V interval (48 msec) and a narrow QRS complex with a left anterior fascicle block pattern. Right upper panel shows prolonged H-V interval (137 msec) during atrial overdrive pacing (S1S2 = 650 msec). Lower panel shows H-V Wenckebach conduction during atrial overdrive pacing (S1S1 = 600 msec). This case and figure show that serious infranodal conduction disease may be localized to within the His bundle and may be "masked" by a normal QRS as well as a normal P-R interval during sinus rhythm. (Courtesy of Drs. Yanfei Yang and Melvin Scheinman, University of California San Francisco/Cardiac Electrophysiology, San Francisco.)

Intracardiac electrophysiologic studies have been evaluated as a means of attempting to predict which patients with MI and BBB are most likely to die. Harper and associates[179] reported on 72 patients with AMI complicated by AV block, BBB, or both who underwent His bundle recording or electrophysiologic (HBE) studies during their coronary care unit stay. Thirty of 32 patients (94%) with AV block and narrow QRS complexes had a proximal block. Hospital mortality was low (13%), and HBE studies provided no information additional to that obtained from the surface ECG. Of 18 patients with BBB and a normal P-R interval, 9 had distal block, but there were no hospital deaths in this group of patients. Of 22 patients with BBB and AV block, 5 had proximal block, 14 distal block, and 3 proximal and distal blocks. Hospital mortality in these patients, who progressed to second- or third-degree AV block, was higher (9 of 12 patients, 75%) than in those who remained in first-degree AV block (2 of 10 patients, 20%). Lichstein and colleagues[187] and Lie and associates[155] also concluded that patients with BBB and AMI who had HBE evidence of a distal block had higher hospital mortality (73% and 81%, respectively) than those with normal H-V intervals (25% and 47%, respectively). On the other hand, in the study by Gould and coworkers,[188] the presence or absence of a prolonged H-V interval did not affect mortality.

Indications for Pacing after Acute Myocardial Infarction

Temporary Pacing in Acute Myocardial Infarction

The use of temporary transvenous pacing in the post-AMI period has diminished in recent years with the greater and more widespread reliance on transcutaneous pacing. Situations in which temporary transvenous pacing is recommended or should be considered according to practice guidelines are listed in Table 14-8.[146] Current practice guidelines and recommendations for temporary pacing in the setting of AMI, however, are based primarily on clinical experience rather than well-controlled clinical trials. Essentially no trials have evaluated the risks versus the benefits of temporary pacing during the current era of AMI treatment. Furthermore, RV pacing (VVI) may have potential deleterious hemodynamic effects even when compared with spontaneous intrinsic bradycardic rhythms in the absence of BBB (e.g., sinus node dysfunction or heart block with junctional escape rhythms). In addition, there is little scientific evidence of an advantage of temporary RV pacing over intrinsic rhythm in patients with bradycardia after AMI. Thus, temporary ventricular pacing should not be used for hemodynamic support but should be used primarily as "backup pacing" for prophylactic indications to prevent catastrophic bradycardia or to treat sudden CHB without an adequate ventricular escape mechanism.

TABLE 14-8. Recommendations for Temporary Pacing in Patients with Acute Myocardial Infarction

Symptomatic AV block	Marked bradycardia (ventricular rate <40 bpm) Hypotension Heart failure or reduced cardiac output Cardiogenic shock Altered mental status Pause-dependent polymorphic ventricular tachycardia
Asymptomatic AV block without BBB	Third-degree AV block Second-degree AV block, type II: Patients with anterior AMI Patients with inferior AMI and narrow QRS complex if block recurs or persists despite atropine administration
Asymptomatic AV block with BBB	Third-degree AV block Second-degree AV block: Type I Type II Prophylactic pacing for those at high risk for high-grade AV block: Bilateral BBB: Alternating LBBB and RBBB RBBB with alternating LAHB and LPHB New BBB with first-degree AV block Indeterminate-age RBBB with LAHB or LPHB and first-degree AV block

AMI, acute myocardial infarction; AV, atrioventricular; BBB, bundle branch block; LAHB, left anterior hemiblock; LBBB, left bundle branch block; LPHB, left posterior hemiblock; RBBB, right bundle branch block.

After temporary pacing is instituted, the temporary pacing generator should be programmed to minimize RV pacing (i.e., prolonging the AV delay). Atrial or dual-chamber pacing (AV synchronous) leads to better cardiac output than temporary ventricular pacing.[189-191] Thus, when hemodynamic support is required in patients with AMI who need temporary pacing, physiologic pacing should be considered. In general, however, because of the risks of infection, limitation in venous access, and difficulties in maintaining stability of atrial pacing during temporary pacing for prolonged periods, and unless there are contraindications, patients who need permanent pacing after AMI (see later) should undergo permanent rather temporary pacemaker implantation as soon as is feasible. The requirement for temporary pacing in AMI does not by itself mandate an indication for permanent pacing.

Administration of thrombolytic therapy is a priority in AMI and should not be delayed by the need to insert a temporary pacing wire. If necessary in the bradycardic patient, temporary transcutaneous pacing can be instituted while thrombolytic therapy is being given. Pharmacologic therapies (with isoproterenol, aminophylline) to treat bradycardia are not recommended in AMI because of their arrhythmogenic effects and adverse effects on myocardial oxygen demand.[146] Atropine is generally well tolerated in inferior AMI, but in some cases of inferior AMI, AV block does not respond to atropine. When infranodal conduction disturbances are present, especially in anterior infarction, atropine raises the sinus rate and may worsen AV conduction and decrease the ventricular rate. When temporary pacing is required because of continued hemodynamically significant bradycardia or profound asystole after thrombolytic therapy or in fully anticoagulated patients, the temporary pacing wire should be inserted by an experienced operator. It also is best to avoid the left subclavian approach for temporary pacemaker insertion because this is the most popular site for permanent pacemaker implantation.

Regardless of the site of infarction, a temporary pacemaker should be placed whenever AV block is associated with marked symptomatic bradycardia (<40 bpm), asystole, hypotension, reduced cardiac output, heart failure, altered mental status, shock, or ventricular irritability (such as pause-dependent polymorphic ventricular tachycardia).

In almost all cases, patients with a normal QRS complex or old or new fascicular block (left anterior fascicular block [LAFB] or left anterior hemiblock [LAHB]) and first-degree AV block or type I second-degree AV block with normal hemodynamics and patients with inferior AMI and block above the His bundle (i.e., normal QRS width) do not require insertion of a temporary pacemaker. These patients are not at risk for sudden asystole. It must be appreciated that a small number of patients with type I second-degree AV block and narrow QRS complexes have block in the His bundle and not in the AV node. Nevertheless, some clinicians believe that the relatively uncommon clinical manifestation of intra-Hisian block in inferior AMI is almost always reversible and rarely requires pacing.[192]

Insertion of a temporary transvenous pacemaker is recommended in patients with an anterior AMI complicated by any of the following conditions: (1) type I second-degree AV block with a wide QRS complex in which the block is presumed to be below the His bundle (class IIa or IIb indication, depending on whether the BBB is new or old), (2) type II second-degree AV block with a normal (class IIa indication) or wide QRS complex (class I or IIa indication, depending on whether BBB is new or old), or (3) complete or advanced AV block (class I indication).[146] These patients are at risk for sudden asystole in the setting of anterior AMI.

In the setting of a nonanterior wall AMI, temporary transvenous pacing likewise is recommended in patients with (1) type I second-degree AV block with a wide QRS complex in whom the block is presumed to be below the His bundle (class IIa or IIb indication, depending on whether the BBB is new or old), (2) type II second-degree AV block with a normal (class IIa indication) or wide QRS complex (class I or IIa indication, depending on whether the BBB is new or old), and (3) complete or advanced AV block (class I indication).[146] As noted previously, however, in most cases of AV block complicating inferior MI, AV block is almost always located in the AV node, is reversible, is associated with a junctional (narrow complex) escape rhythm, and does not predict the development of sudden asystole. Thus, temporary pacing can almost always be avoided in these patients.

Prophylactic temporary transvenous pacing in the early post-infarction period also is indicated for patients considered at high risk for development of sudden high-grade AV block.[146] Such patients are identified by (1) new or indeterminate-age bilateral BBB (alternating LBBB and RBBB or RBBB with alternating left anterior hemiblock/left posterior hemiblock) with or without first-degree AV block (class I indication), (2) new BBB with first-degree AV block (class IIa indication), or (3) indeterminate-age RBBB with fascicular and first-degree AV blocks (class IIa indication). Because of the risk of sudden asystole, these subgroups of patients probably should receive temporary pacemakers or be considered for early implantation of permanent pacemakers. Even in these high-risk patients, however, it must be recognized that prophylactic temporary ventricular pacing has not gained widespread acceptance because it does not improve in-hospital survival and may be associated with serious complications. Thus, the use of standby transcutaneous pacing may be a preferred alternative.

Other patient subgroups at moderate risk for development of high-grade AV block who may have to be considered for temporary prophylactic transvenous pacing are those with (1) new BBB without first-degree AV block (class IIb indication), (2) old BBB with first-degree AV block (class IIb indication), or (3) indeterminate-age RBBB with fascicular block but without first-degree AV block (class IIb indication). However, placement of external pacing pads with the ability to provide prophylactic transcutaneous pacing as standby with close telemetry monitoring may be preferred in these patient subgroups during the acute phase of AMI.[146] Furthermore, in the absence of higher-grade AV block, patients with persistent first-degree AV block in the presence of old or indeterminate-age BBB do not require permanent ventricular pacing after AMI.

Permanent Pacing in Patients Recovering from the Acute Phase of Myocardial Infarction

The ACC/AHA/NASPE current guidelines for permanent pacemaker implantation after AMI are listed in Table 14-9.[127] All patients who have an indication for permanent pacing after AMI should also be evaluated for ICD and cardiac resynchronization therapy indications.

Patients with AV conduction disturbances after AMI in whom documented, symptomatic bradyarrhythmias develop should receive permanent pacemakers. In

TABLE 14-9. Indications for Permanent Pacing after the Acute Phase of Myocardial Infarction

Class I	Persistent second-degree AV block in the His-Purkinje system with bilateral BBB or third-degree AV block within or below the His-Purkinje system after acute myocardial infarction (level of evidence: B) Transient advanced (second- or third-degree) infranodal AV block and associated BBB; if the state of block is uncertain, an electrophysiologic study may be indicated (level of evidence: B) Persistent and symptomatic second or third-degree AV block (level of evidence: C)
Class IIa	None
Class IIb	Persistent second- or third-degree AV block at the AV node level (level of evidence: B)
Class III	Transient AV block in the absence of intraventricular conduction defects (level of evidence: B) Transient AV block in the presence of isolated left anterior fascicular block (level of evidence: B) Acquired left anterior fascicular block in the absence of AV block (level of evidence: B) Persistent first-degree AV block in the presence of BBB that is old or of indeterminate age (level of evidence: B)

AV, atrioventricular; BBB, bundle branch block.

Adapted from Gregoratos G, Abrams J, Epstein AE, et al; American College of Cardiology/American Heart Association Task Force on Practice Guidelines/North American Society for Pacing and Electrophysiology Committee: ACC/AHA/NASPE 2002 guideline update for implantation of cardiac pacemakers and antiarrhythmia devices: Summary article: A report of the American College of Cardiology/American Heart Association Task Force on Practice Guidelines (ACC/AHA/NASPE Committee to Update the 1998 Pacemaker Guidelines). Circulation 106:2145, 2002.

patients with persistent and symptomatic second- or third-degree AV block, permanent ventricular pacing has a class I indication. Of patients who have second- or third-degree block in the hospital, regardless of infarction or block location, return to 1:1 conduction is seen in 95% of those without BBB and in 89% of those with BBB who survive the infarction and are discharged eventually from the hospital.[157] Thus, in patients recovering from AMI who demonstrate AV block, the major determinant of the need for prophylactic permanent pacing beyond symptomatic bradycardia is the presence of intraventricular conduction defects. Patients with persistent second-degree AV block in the His-Purkinje system with bilateral BBB and those with persistent third-degree AV block located within the His-Purkinje system after AMI should receive permanent pacemakers (class I indication).

Patients with persistent second- or third-degree AV block at the AV nodal level without BBB may also be considered for permanent pacing (class IIb indication). However, permanent pacing is rarely needed in patients with an inferior wall AMI and narrow QRS. It may take up to 16 days for AV conduction to return. Some conservative clinicians recommend pacemaker implantation only when second- or third-degree AV block is present for more than 3 weeks after inferior wall MI.[193] On the basis of their review of prior literature, Barold and Hayes[194] asserted that patients who reportedly had type II AV block with a narrow QRS in the setting of inferior AMI were misclassified according to incorrect criteria for the diagnosis of type II second-degree AV block.[194] Thus, transient or persistent second-degree AV block with inferior AMI is virtually always AV nodal in origin and not an indication for permanent pacing. Development of complete AV block during inferior AMI is associated with a higher in-hospital mortality, which is not altered by temporary or permanent pacing, but a favorable long-term prognosis in those who survive to hospital discharge.[142]

When transient advanced second- or third-degree infranodal AV block is associated with persistent BBB, permanent ventricular pacing is indicated (class I indication).[127,142] An electrophysiologic study may be helpful if the site of block is uncertain. Development of a new intraventricular conduction delay in the setting of an anterior or inferior infarction reflects extensive myocardial damage. Patients with AMI who demonstrate BBB have an unfavorable prognosis and a higher risk of sudden death. Although these patients may be at risk for serious bradyarrhythmias in the posthospitalization period, their adverse prognosis is not necessarily related to the development of high-grade AV block. These patients are at high risk for other post-MI complications, including pump failure and ventricular tachyarrhythmias. In the past, the decision to implant a permanent pacemaker in a survivor of AMI complicated by transient complete or second-degree AV block and persistent BBB during the hospitalization was not always straightforward. In the previous edition of this textbook, it was suggested that there were at least three possible ways of managing these patients, as follows: (1) all should receive permanent pacemakers, (2) only those with documented bradyarrhythmias should receive permanent pacemakers, or (3) patients should undergo a diagnostic evaluation, including measurement of LV ejection fraction, ambulatory 24-hour ECG monitoring, and possibly His bundle studies, and then the need for permanent pacemaker implantation may be considered in some of the patients.

In the current era, however, the decision to implant a permanent pacemaker to provide bradycardia support in these patients is less of an issue. Most patients with AMI with AV block and BBB have LV dysfunction and thus are eligible for implantation of an ICD for primary prevention of sudden death and/or a biventricular pacing system to provide cardiac resynchronization therapy. However, the timing of ICD implantation may complicate management of such patients, because Medicare reimbursement guidelines for ICD implantation established in 2005 indicate that patients must not have had an AMI within the past 40 days.[195] Furthermore, an important consideration in selection of the mode of pacing and the need for an ICD is the recognition that the extent of myocardial dysfunction in patients with ischemic heart disease may not be a permanent condition. Stunning and hibernation of the myocardium, leading to apparent dysfunction, may resolve as the ischemia resolves and after adequate time has passed for recovery.[196,197]

Permanent pacing is not recommended for patients with AMI and transient AV block in the absence of intraventricular conduction defects or in the presence of isolated left anterior fascicular block. Patients with persistent first-degree AV block in the presence of BBB after AMI do not require permanent pacing for bradycardia indications; if advanced LV dysfunction is present, however, such patients should be evaluated for ICD and cardiac resynchronization therapy indications.

Selection of Pacing Mode in Atrioventricular Block

Several important factors that should be considered in the choice of appropriate pacing mode in patients with AV block are the status and activity level of the patient, the importance of AV synchrony, the presence of chronotropic incompetence, the underlying cardiac substrate, and the estimated likelihood of the frequency and duration of pacing. The importance of each of these factors varies from patient to patient.

The selection of pacing mode for patients with acute AV block usually takes into account many of the same considerations used for mode selection for chronic AV block. In the setting of acute AV block, however, it should be appreciated that if the patient was in sinus rhythm, loss of chronotropic competence will have been recent and abrupt and that loss of AV synchrony is usually associated with varying degrees of ventricular dysfunction, which may be severe. For temporary pacing of patients with acute AV block, single-chamber RV VVI pacing usually provides adequate rate correction of the bradyarrhythmia. If there is no or minimal hemodynamic compromise of cardiac function, this mode of pacing may be sufficient to tide the patient over what is usually a transient period of high-grade or complete AV block. If the underlying rhythm before acute AV block was AF, single-chamber ventricular pacing should provide a satisfactory rate, with no compromise of hemodynamic status because there was no preexisting AV synchrony. In the presence of sinus rhythm or of sinus bradycardia with or without chronotropic competence, restoration of AV synchrony even in the acute situation of temporary pacing may be a desirable therapeutic goal in patients with acute AV block. Dual-chamber pacing with sensing of the native atrial complex and synchronous pacing of the ventricle restores both chronotropic response to activity (provided that sinus node activity is normal) and AV synchrony. Restoration of AV synchrony may result in substantial hemodynamic improvement in a patient in whom correction of bradyarrhythmia by ventricular pacing alone fails to increase cardiac output in the presence of acute RV infarction.[189] Similar benefit has been shown for AV sequential pacing in the presence of acute anterior infarction.[190,191] It is apparent, however, that optimization of the AV delay is also crucial, because an excessively long A-V interval may result in deterioration with complete loss of the advantages of AV sequential pacing over ventricular pacing alone.[198,199]

According to world pacing surveys, about 50% of patients with AV block receive permanent dual-chamber pacing devices.[122,123,200] In patients with complete persistent AV block and underlying intact sinus node function, dual-chamber pacing maintains or restores AV synchrony at rest and also allows the rate to rise with activity. If sinus node function is impaired and chronotropic incompetence is present, the DDDR mode restores both AV synchrony and rate response to activity, albeit with substitution of a physiologic parameter other than the P wave. To simulate the physiologic behavior of the P-R interval during exercise, DDD and DDDR units are able to shorten the AV delay during activity-induced increases in heart rate.[199]

If the indication for permanent pacing is transient advanced AV block and the patient is expected to be predominantly in sinus rhythm with normal AV conduction, a simple single-chamber VVI system may be adequate as a backup to provide a reasonable minimum heart rate. Restoration of chronotropic adaptation to activity may be achieved through VVIR and DDDR pacing, in which sensor detection of changes in various physiologic stimuli are used to adjust the pacing rate. The selection of a VVIR unit in preference to a VVI unit may be appropriate for patients with more frequent dependence on the pacemaker and a higher projected activity level, in the anticipation that increased cardiac output with activity is a desirable and reasonable therapeutic goal. If, for example, the patient has other comorbid conditions, such as a major stroke, and has minimal chance of regaining even modest levels of activity, little would be gained through the use of the more expensive rate-adaptive VVIR mode. On the other hand, although rate-adaptive VVIR pacing can achieve increases in work performance and cardiac output, the maintenance of AV synchrony is desirable, particularly at slower heart rates and in patients with impaired ventricular function. Therefore, it has become accepted that in such patients, dual-chamber pacing is advantageous,[201] and the VVIR mode would appear to be appropriate only for patients with no preexisting AV synchrony, such as those with permanent AF, those with atrial standstill (i.e., inability to pace the atrium), and those in whom the rate and hemodynamic demands on the pacemaker system are minimal even at rest.

Another consideration that might influence the choice of pacing mode is the presence of concomitant paroxysmal supraventricular tachyarrhythmias. DDD(R) pacing units have mode-switch algorithms designed to detect and automatically change the pacing mode during atrial tachyarrhythmia episodes. These algorithms automatically switch the device from atrial tracking (DDD) to nontracking modes (DDI or VVI) during atrial tachyarrhythmias to prevent upper rate tracking. The benefits of AV synchrony are maintained during sinus rhythm because the tachyarrhythmia is monitored and the unit automatically switches back to DDD(R) pacing when the arrhythmia terminates.

For permanent pacing, the benefit of restoring the patient's ability to increase heart rate with activity (chronotropic competence) should be considered. This may be accomplished through the use of VVIR/DDDR modes in patients with chronotropic incompetence or VDD/DDD modes in patients with normal sinus node function.[202] In the absence of an ability to raise heart rate with activity, the only remaining mechanism for increasing cardiac output is to increase stroke volume. The magnitude of increase in cardiac output (<25%) achieved by this mechanism, however, is relatively small compared with what can be achieved by an increase in heart rate.[203] Additionally, in the presence of myocardial dysfunction, the contribution of change in stroke volume to the adaptive response to activity is even more limited. Therefore, if chronotropic competence is impaired in patients with AV block, rate-responsive pacing is considered the preferred mode for improving cardiac output and work capacity during activity in patients with AV block. Furthermore, chronotropic incompetence may develop in subsequent years after the pacemaker has been implanted either as an acquired condition or as the result of medications, such as β-blockers and antiarrhythmic drugs.[204] More than 95% of all pacemaker generators implanted in the United States have rate modulation as a programmable option. Despite this common clinical practice, however, preliminary results from two randomized controlled trials—Rate Modulated Pacing and Quality of Life (RAMP) and Advanced Elements of Pacing Trial (ADEPT), which included patients with AV block and chronotropic incompetence—evaluation of the effects of rate responsive pacing failed to demonstrate a benefit of this mode of pacing on quality of life.[205] It certainly is possible that the adverse effects of ventricular dyssynchrony imposed by RV pacing may negate the potential benefits of rate responsiveness.

The long-term outcome of patients with AV block who require permanent pacing is most strongly affected by the extent of myocardial dysfunction or the severity of the underlying coronary disease and ischemia. In a 2-year follow-up study of 2021 patients with permanent pacing, the leading causes of the 249 recorded deaths were stroke (30%) and sudden cardiac death (22%).[206] The presence of BBB, which was seen predominantly in patients with AV block and MI, was a predictor of sudden cardiac death because 28% of all patients with BBB and 35% of patients with bifascicular or trifascicular block died suddenly. In comparison, the prevalence of sudden death in the remaining 138 patients without such block was 18%.

Alpert and colleagues[207] compared the prognoses of 132 patients with high-grade AV block and VVI pacemakers and of 48 patients with DDD pacemakers for high-grade AV block during a 1- to 5-year follow-up period. Permanent dual-chamber pacing enhanced survival to a greater extent than permanent VVI pacing in a subgroup of patients with preexisting congestive heart failure. However because this was a nonrandomized trial, selection bias may have affected the results. The causes of congestive heart failure were variable; about 50% of patients had underlying ischemic heart disease, and the rest had hypertension, valvular heart disease, or idiopathic dilated cardiomyopathy. Most deaths in the patient group with VVI pacemakers were due to AMI or congestive heart failure.

An important clinical trial evaluating pacing mode selection in patients with chronic AV block was the United Kingdom Pacing and Cardiovascular Events (UKPACE) trial.[208] UKPACE was designed to compare the long-term clinical impact and cost effectiveness of DDD vs. VVI or VVIR pacing in patients 70 years or older with high-grade AV block undergoing their first pacemaker implantation. Between 1995 and 1999, 2021 patients (mean age, 80 years) were enrolled at 46 centers. One half the patients were randomly assigned by pacing system hardware to single-chamber pacing (25% VVI and 25% VVIR) and one half to dual-chamber pacing. Patients were followed up for a median of 4.6 years, and clinical events were censored at last follow-up for up to 3 years. There was no significant difference after 5 years of follow-up in the primary endpoint, all-cause mortality, between the single-chamber and dual-chamber groups. Likewise, there were no significant differences in the rates of atrial fibrillation, heart failure, or thromboembolism between the group with single-chamber pacing and that with dual-chamber pacing. Thus, in elderly patients with AV block, dual-chamber pacing does not influence all-cause mortality or cardiovascular outcomes within the first 5 years after pacemaker implantation.

VDD(R) Pacing

Despite its availability for more than 20 years, VDD pacing is used in less than 1% of patients receiving pacemakers in the United States and in only 4% in Canada, according to the world survey of cardiac pacing for the calendar year 2001.[200] VDD pacing is used more widely in other areas of the world, but its use from country to country is highly variable, ranging from 0% to 24% in South America, Europe, and the Asian-Pacific and Middle East regions.

A VDD pacing system uses a single-pass lead with far-field, floating atrial sensing bipoles as well as ventricular electrodes for pacing and sensing. The single VDD lead offers a simpler approach to provide AV synchronous pacing that avoids implantation of two separate pacing leads, thus limiting implanted hardware. VDD or VAT pacing allows preservation of normal AV synchrony and rate responsiveness and is an appropriate pacing mode for patients with high-grade block or CHB and normal sinus node function.[202,209] Furthermore, VDD pacemaker implantation can be performed at lower cost and with shorter implantation time than other dual-chamber systems.[210-212] Therefore, VDD pacing is a viable alternative to DDD pacing for treatment of patients with high-grade AV block, normal sinus node function, and no need for atrial pacing.[127,210-214]

The implantation procedure for a VDD system consists of fixing the ventricular tip to allow the atrial electrodes to lie as close as possible to a high-middle location of the lateral RA wall (Fig. 14-22). Care must be taken to ensure an adequate safety margin and amplitude of the atrial signal (>2.0 mV) at implantation to avoid significant atrial undersensing. An atrial signal should be measured at rest, during deep breathing, and during coughing as well as during arm and shoulder movements. The lowest acceptable atrial electrogram signal during any maneuver should be at least 0.5 to 1.0 mV during deep inspiration.[202,209] In one study, the mean maximum and minimum values of atrial

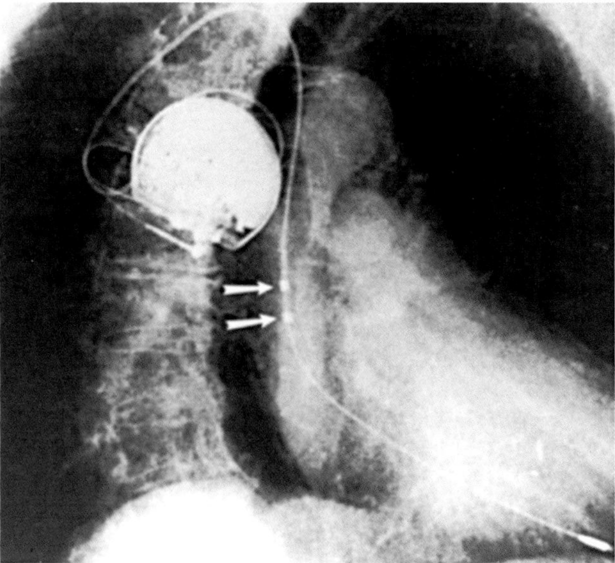

Figure 14-22. Lateral chest radiograph showing single atrioventricular (AV) lead with narrow-spaced AV ring electrodes connected to a LEM Biomedica/Cardiac Control Systems VDD pacemaker. Arrows indicate atrial electrodes. (From Antonioli EG, Ansani L, Barbieri D, et al: Single-lead VDD pacing. In Barold SS, Mugica J: New Perspectives in Cardiac Pacing 3. Mt. Kisco, NY, Futura, 1993, pp 359-381.)

electrogram characteristics within a whole respiratory cycle were 2.64 ± 1.05 mV and 1.65 ± 0.38 mV amplitude (maximum) and 0.31 ± 0.12 mV and 0.18 ± 0.09 mV (minimum).[209,213-215] In general, there is considerable variability between patients and within individuals from moment to moment with respect to atrial electrogram amplitude. For example, the atrial electrogram amplitude can decrease markedly during exercise. Single-lead VDD pacing is best avoided if the atrial chamber diameter of the RA is greater than 3 × 3 cm and if the LA is larger than 4 × 3 cm in the echocardiographic apical four-chamber view. Patients with paroxysmal supraventricular tachyarrhythmias probably should not receive VDD pacemakers.

Various electrode configurations for VDD leads have been studied, including bipolar leads with narrow and wide spacing and orthogonal and diagonal atrial electrodes. The optimal spacing of two poles of the floating bipolar lead was found to range between 0.5 and 1 cm. Factors influencing atrial electrogram detection include electrode spacing, distance from the atrial wall, orientation of electrodes relative to atrial tissue, and electrode size. Lau and associates[216] compared the clinical performance of two systems with different electrode configurations, one using a diagonally arranged bipole and one using closely spaced bipolar ring electrodes. The clinical performance of atrial sensing was similar despite different electrode configurations.

Concerns have been expressed about the long-term reliability of VDD pacing systems with regard to atrial sensing performance of floating VDD leads. Studies with early models of VDD leads reported a high incidence of atrial lead dislodgment as well as deterioration of atrial pacing and sensing characteristics over time. In one early study, Ramsdale and Charles[217] reported difficulty in obtaining an adequate P wave amplitude at implantation, resulting in prolonged implantation times. In their series, almost 60% of patients showed intermittent failure of P wave sensing. Marked fluctuations in the paced ventricular rate were noted especially during exercise, when intermittent failure to sense P waves occurred. In other older series, however, atrial pacing and sensing were maintained for 5 years in almost 90% of patients.[218]

In a 2003 study, Huang and colleagues[219] compared the long-term reliability and complication rates of VDD pacing in 112 consecutive patients with symptomatic AV block and intact sinus node function who received a single-pass bipolar VDD system and in 80 patients who received DDD pacing for the same indication.[219] Implantation times were shorter for VDD systems than for DDD systems (63 ± 20 vs. 97 ± 36 minutes; $P <$ .0001). P wave amplitude at implantation was lower in the VDD patients but remained stable during long-term follow-up, such that AV synchrony was maintained in 94% to 99% of beats in the VDD group and only 2 patients in the VDD group required reprogramming to VVIR mode during the follow-up period (18 ± 10 months). Thus, clinical trials of VDD pacing systems have shown overall good clinical performance.[220]

Linde-Edelstam and associates[221] performed a case-controlled study comparing consecutive patients who received VDD pacemakers with the first-available VVI patients who fulfilled certain "predetermined characteristics." The two groups were similar with respect to other concomitant diseases and severity of congestive heart failure. The investigators compared survival in 74 patients treated with VVI pacemakers and in 74 patients with VDD pacemakers over a mean follow-up period of 5.4 years. The overall survival was better in patients with the VDD pacing mode than in the age- and sex-matched general Swedish population. Survival was no different between patients paced in the VVI and VDD modes if congestive heart failure was absent.

Pacemaker programming of VDD systems should take into account atrial sensitivity as well as programming of the postventricular atrial refractory period (PVARP), AV delay, and lower rate. Some degree of atrial undersensing (≈5% of beats) is often seen during ambulatory ECG monitoring and exercise testing of VDD systems, but rarely is this a clinically significant problem when the pacemaker is programmed at high atrial sensitivity (≤0.3 mV). P wave amplitude should be tested during maneuvers that simulate daily activities, such as coughing, hyperventilation, arm swinging, isometric exercises, and respiration. Some generators allow programming of the bandwidth of the atrial amplifier. This may attenuate interference and oversensing from myopotentials as well as retrograde P waves in patients with ventricular ectopy.[215] VDDR generators with programmable atrial amplifier bandwidths allow the implanter to minimize the sensing of myopotentials and retrograde P waves, thus avoiding the need for programming long postventricular atrial refractory periods. This period should be programmed to contain retrograde P waves.

The AV delay must take into account the delay in detecting atrial depolarization. The lower rate should be programmed to a value below the minimum sinus rate noted during a 24-hour Holter recording. Patients with retrograde VA conduction may experience symptoms if their sinus rate frequently falls below the lower programmed rate, leading to VVI pacing at the lower rate. One can avoid this problem by obtaining a 24-hour Holter monitor recording and then programming the lower rate to a rate below the slowest recorded sinus rate. Atrial oversensing from the floating dipole during upper-body isometric exercises involving the pectoral muscles is an uncommon clinical problem. Use of the VDDR pacing mode allows the option of employing the sensor to differentiate sinus tachycardia from the tracking of myopotentials. The implanted sensor can be used to judge the appropriateness of the atrial rate. In addition, the rate-adaptive sensor allows for rate smoothing of upper rate behavior. However, ventricular pacing and loss of AV synchrony can arise during exercise if the sensor rate exceeds the sinus rate or when the atrial rate is slower than the programmed lower rate.

Enthusiasm for the VDD pacing mode in North America likely will remain very limited, because implantation of atrial pacing leads is routine and highly reliable with a very low complication rate. In the practices of most implanters, the additional risk and work of positioning an atrial lead do not outweigh the disadvantage of not having atrial pacing. On the other hand, if a patient experiences sinus node dysfunction and a need for atrial pacing arises, upgrading to a DDDR pacing system can be easily performed.[222]

Optimal Atrioventricular Interval Programming

Hemodynamics during dual-chamber pacing is influenced by the A-V interval. During dual-chamber pacing in patients with high-grade AV block, an appropriate electrical A-V interval must be programmed to maintain mechanical synchronization of cardiac chambers (i.e., mechanical AV synchrony). Programming excessively short A-V intervals may result in cannon A waves (i.e., atrial contraction against a closed mitral valve), whereas diastolic mitral regurgitation may occur with excessively long programmed A-V intervals. The A-V interval is considered optimal if it results in maximum cardiac output. A-V interval optimization provides the best timing of LA filling and LA systole. Appropriately timed atrial systole improves LV performance, reduces mean atrial pressure, and maximizes LV end-diastolic pressure by coordinating AV valve closure, facilitating venous return, and increasing preload. Optimal AV synchrony not only maximizes cardiac output by increasing ventricular preload, thus lowering mean atrial pressure, but also minimizes diastolic mitral regurgitation.

Under most circumstances in patients with normal LV function at rest, the optimal A-V interval lies between 100 and 200 msec.[223,224] However, shorter A-V intervals have been proposed as a means of achieving higher cardiac output in patients with AV block and dilated cardiomyopathy. Hochleitner and coworkers[225] generated interest when they reported functional improvement in patients with dilated cardiomyopathy who were treated with AV pacing using a short AV delay of 100 msec. Unfortunately, results of this original uncontrolled study could not be reproduced by others. Subsequent studies suggested that the benefit of such an approach with a very short AV delay may be confined to patients with long PR intervals and significant diastolic mitral regurgitation.[226,227] On the other hand, very long A-V intervals may be required to provide effective LA systole in occasional patients with high-grade interatrial conduction delay in the presence of atrial disease and either sick sinus syndrome or heart block. The usual nominally programmed A-V intervals, 125 to 175 msec, may not provide optimal AV synchrony in these patients, and sometimes, AV delays as long as 250 to 350 msec are required.[223] Such very long A-V intervals have the disadvantage, however, of resulting in long total atrial refractory periods and limiting the upper rate possible during exercise. An alternative approach is to shorten intra-atrial conduction time in these patients with RA septal or biatrial pacing.[224]

Some investigators suggest that when the AV delay is selected empirically, it is incorrectly programmed in approximately two thirds of patients and the potential contribution of a correctly timed AV delay to cardiac output varies from 13% to 40%.[228,229] The optimal A-V interval can vary considerably from patient to patient and is difficult to predict beforehand. Furthermore, AV optimization may be a difficult task to achieve in any particular patient, and although the interval is generally measured while the patient is supine and at rest, the value may not be applicable while the patient is upright and active.

Although many factors are important in the attempt to define the optimal A-V interval—the atrial pacing site, intra-atrial conduction time, atrial size, ventricular function, heart rate, body position, autonomic tone, catecholamine levels, whether the atrial event is paced or sensed—and their interrelationships are variable and complex, a major determinant of the optimal AV delay in an individual patient is the interatrial conduction time. The duration of the optimal A-V interval varies among individuals, substantially as a result of differences in interatrial conduction. The interatrial conduction time determines when the LA depolarization begins and therefore directly determines the LA-LV timing interval. Programming differential A-V intervals for sensing and pacing may give rise to small but significant increases in cardiac output in patients with LV dysfunction, owing to differences in paced versus sensed atrial conduction times.[223,224]

A variety of techniques have been used to determine the optimal A-V interval by comparing the calculated stroke volume at different A-V intervals as measured by continuous-wave cardiac Doppler echocardiography of the aortic valve, right heart catheterization, radionuclide ventriculography, myocardial thallium scintigraphy, or transthoracic impedance cardiography.[230] Ritter's method of A-V interval optimization, which uses Doppler echocardiography of the mitral valve inflow profile, is the most widely applied technique (Fig. 14-23).[231] This technique is based on the assumption that the AV delay that maximizes cardiac output is the one that provides the longest LV filling time without interruption of the A wave (atrial contraction wave) and allows ventricular systole to begin immediately subsequent to maximum diastolic ventricular filling, thus avoiding cannon A waves and diastolic mitral regurgitation. The technique has been validated in patients with both normal and depressed LV function. However there are limitations to the Ritter method; it is time-consuming, is subject to significant variability between consecutive measurements, cannot be reliably performed during exercise, and is not readily available in routine pacemaker follow-up clinics. An alternative simplified approach has been proposed that uses the surface ECG alone and defines the optimal AV delay on the basis of a delay of 100 msec from the end of the surface P wave to the peak/nadir of the paced ventricular complex (Fig. 14-24).[232]

Rate-adaptive A-V interval shortening or automatic rate-adaptive AV delay is a programmable feature on many DDD pacemaker generators designed to mimic the normal physiologic response of the P-R interval to rising heart rates.[233] A-V intervals may be shortened

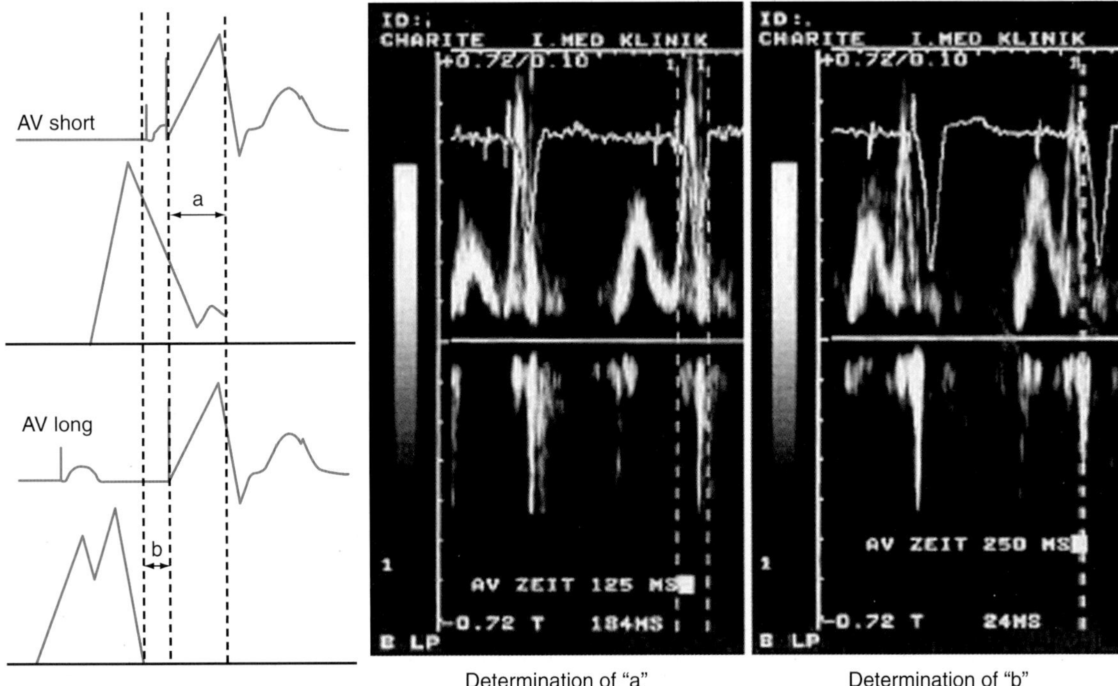

Figure 14-23. Ritter's method for determination of the optimal atrioventricular (AV) interval using the following formula: $AV_{opt} = AV_{long} - (a - b)$. The first step is determination of a for a nonphysiologically short A-V interval (e.g., 125 msec), followed by determination of b for a nonphysiologically long A-V interval (e.g., 250 msec). The value a, the temporal interval between the ventricular contraction spike and the end of the A wave, designates the electromechanical delay between right ventricular stimulation and the beginning of the left ventricular systole (i.e., closure of the mitral valve). The value b is the temporal interval between the ventricular contraction spike and the end of the A wave. (From Melzer C, Borges A, Knebel F, et al: Echocardiographic AV-interval optimization in patients with reduced left ventricular function. Cardiovasc Ultrasound 2:30, 2004.)

further during atrial tracking; when the patient exercises and the heart rate increases, the sensed P wave to ventricular pacing stimulus can be shortened. This can be accomplished as one-step shortening or multistep shortening in discrete, nonprogrammable, or linear steps as the atrial rate increases. Compared with fixed A-V interval without rate adaptation, rate-adaptive A-V interval shortening improves exercise tolerance by improving stroke volume and prolonging systolic ejection time.[234,235] The assumption behind the shortening of the P-V or A-V interval is that it maintains the proper timing of the atrial contraction and thereby optimizes stroke volume (Fig. 14-25).

With the shortened P-V (or A-V) intervals, however, there may be a greater proportion of ventricular pacing in patients with intermittent or catecholamine-sensitive AV conduction. If this results in fewer intrinsic beats and more RV pacing, there may be no improvement in hemodynamics and potentially even a worsening of hemodynamics in some patients. The minimum value below which the AV delay is not shortened is calculated on the basis of the programmed pacing rate and the upper ventricular rate limit. In the DDDR mode, the paced AV delay shortens as the pacing rate increases in response to the sensor. The sensed AV delay can also be adapted to the atrial rate on a beat-by-beat basis, with linear shortening occurring between maximal and minimal values, the net result being a shortening of the total atrial refractory period, thereby allowing higher 1:1 tracking rates.

Site-Specific Ventricular Pacing in Atrioventricular Block

The RV apex (RVA) has been accepted as the traditional ventricular pacing site for decades. The RVA site allows easy placement of endocardial leads while providing stable and reliable long-term pacing parameters. RVA pacing imposes ventricular desynchronization, however, and leads to a myriad of adverse effects on LV systolic and diastolic function, hemodynamics, coronary perfusion, and myocardial structure.[236-248] The harmful effects of RVA pacing, manifested clinically as an increased risk of heart failure hospitalization or death associated with an increased frequency of cumulative RV pacing in the Dual Chamber and VVI Implantable Defibrillator (DAVID) study, the MOde Selection Trial (MOST), and the second Multicenter Automatic Defibrillator Implantation Trial (MADIT-II).[249-251] In none of these trials, however, was AV block the indication for permanent pacing. In the Post AV Nodal Ablation Evaluation (PAVE) trial, patients with chronic AF refractory to pharmacologic therapy underwent radiofrequency catheter ablation of the AV

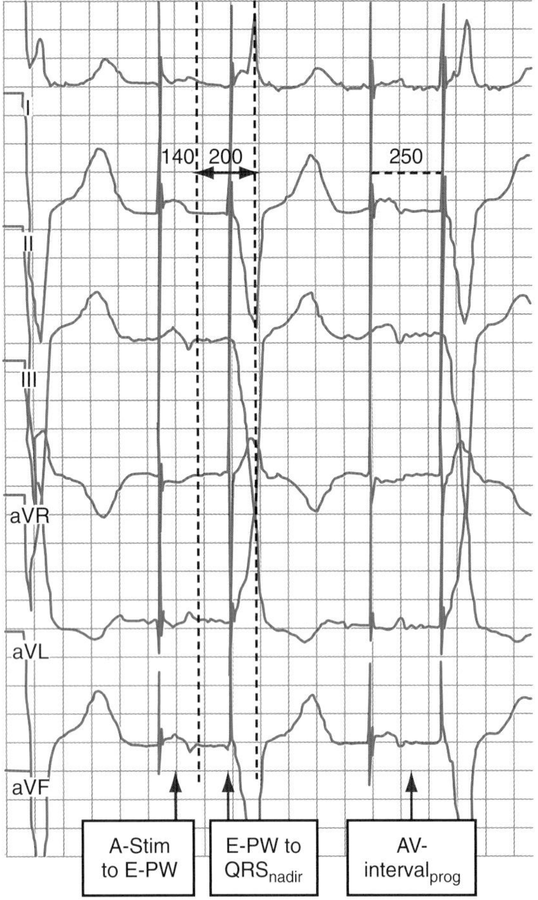

Figure 14-24. *Determination of optimal paced atrioventricular (AV) delay (AVD_{opt}) by surface electrocardiogram. First, a long AV delay of 250 msec was programmed (AVD_{prog}, programmed interval from atrial to ventricular stimulus). The interval from the end of the P wave to the peak/nadir of the paced ventricular complex (T) was 200 msec. The interval atrial stimulus to the end of P wave (= global atrial conduction time) was 140 msec. According to the algorithm $AVD_{opt} = AVD_{prog} + 100 - T$, the optimized AV delay was 150 msec. A-Stim to E-PW, interval between the pacing stimulus and the end of P wave deflection; E-PW to QRS_{nadir}, end of P wave (E-PW) to peak/nadir of paced QRS; AV-$interval_{prog}$, long AV delay programmed for testing. (From Strohmer B, Pichler M, Froemmel M, et al; ELVIS Study Group: Evaluation of atrial conduction time at various sites of right atrial pacing and influence on atrioventricular delay optimization by surface electrocardiography. Pacing Clin Electrophysiol 27:468, 2004).*

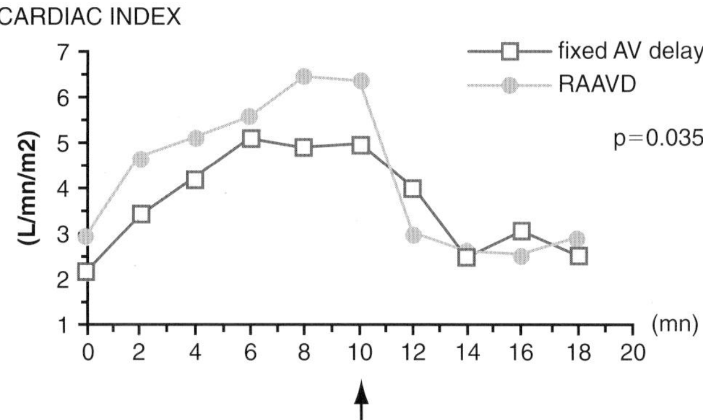

Figure 14-25. *Comparison of an automatic rate-responsive atrioventricular delay (RAAVD) and a fixed but individually optimized (by Doppler echocardiography) AV delay in a patient with a DDD pacemaker implanted over the long term for complete AV block. At each exercise level, and especially at peak exercise (arrow), rate-responsive AV delay produced a significantly higher cardiac index (CI) than the fixed value. (From Daubert C, Ritter P, Mabo P, et al: AV delay optimization in DDD and DDDR pacing. In Barold SS, Mugica J: New Perspectives in Cardiac Pacing 3. Mt Kisco, NY, Futura, 1993, pp 259-287.)*

junction, which was followed in a randomized manner by either RVA or biventricular pacing.[252] LV ejection fraction in the RVA pacing group declined from 44.9% prior to implantation time to 40.7% at 6 months. In contrast, the LV ejection fraction in the biventricular pacing group remained stable over the follow-up period (45.6% vs. 46.0%, respectively) and the ejection fraction was significantly lower in the RVA group than in the biventricular group after 6 months (46.0% vs. 40.7%; $P = .03$). The deleterious long-term effects of RVA pacing were also demonstrated in a study of 23 young adult patients (24 ± 3 years) with congenital complete AV block who underwent at least 5 years of RVA pacing.[54] After 10 ± 3 years of RVA pacing, these patients exhibited abnormal indices of LV intraventricular dyssynchrony, asymmetrical hypertrophy, and dilatation and lower exercise capacity compared with values in the patients before pacemaker implantation and with values found in matched healthy control subjects. Thus, RVA pacing may lead to deterioration of LV function and congestive heart failure due to LV desynchronization.

Growing recognition of the long-term adverse effects of RVA pacing has stimulated interest in strategies to promote physiologic pacing and to minimize or eliminate the deleterious effects of RVA pacing. There is controversy, however, regarding the optimal ventricular pacing sites and approach in patients undergoing permanent pacemaker implantation for AV block in whom ventricular pacing cannot be avoided.[253] Some investigators advocate LV or biventricular pacing, whereas others suggest that there is a role for selective-site RV pacing. Alternative RV pacing sites (i.e., non-RVA), including the His bundle, RV septum, RV outflow tract (RVOT), and dual-site RV, have been investigated, but the benefits of alternative site pacing remain unresolved.[253-265] The mixed results in studies of alternative site RV pacing in general are difficult to interpret because of small numbers of patients, wide ranges of LV function and underlying heart disease, lack of standardization of alternative RV pacing sites, differing endpoints, and short durations of follow-up.

The His bundle is an ideal RV stimulation site from a hemodynamic standpoint. However, the technical challenge of long-term implementation of permanent His bundle pacing using current lead technology is the major obstacle to its reliable application in routine clinical practice. In a report that demonstrated the feasibility of this approach in a small number of patients after AV junction ablation, excessively high pacing thresholds, unreliable sensing, and failure to achieve consistent pacing were found in a subset of patients.[254] Furthermore, the complexity of achieving selective His bundle pacing and the potential for unpredictable distal

His-Purkinje conduction make it unlikely to become an accepted alternative RV pacing site in the future. Other studies evaluating long-term stimulation of the interventricular septum from the RV as a potential alternative site demonstrate encouraging preliminary results in a small number of patients.[264,265]

A review of randomized studies published prior to 2003 concluded that pacing from the RVOT results in a modest but significant benefit in terms of acute hemodynamic function, particularly in patients with impaired ventricular function.[262] However, in the RV Outflow Versus Apical pacing (ROVA) trial, RVOT and dual-site RV pacing (from the RVOT and RVA sequentially) shortened paced QRS duration but did not consistently result in better quality of life, functional class, exercise capacity, or ejection fraction than RVA pacing after 3 months.[261] The ROVA trial enrolled patients with chronic AF, New York Heart Association (NYHA) functional class II or III heart failure, and LV systolic dysfunction (ejection fraction ≤0.40) who were undergoing permanent VVIR pacing for bradycardia indications, which included AV junction ablation in 64% and chronic AV block in the remaining patients. Likewise, at least two other studies that limited follow-up to 3 to 6 months failed to demonstrate a benefit of RVOT pacing.[257,263] Only one published study evaluated long-term RVOT pacing. Tse and associates[260] investigated the effects of ventricular pacing site on myocardial perfusion and LV function in 24 patients with high-grade AV block who were randomly assigned to receive RVA or RVOT pacing leads. At 6 months, the incidences of myocardial perfusion defects, regional wall motion abnormalities, and ejection fraction were similar during RVA and RVOT pacing; at 18 months, however, patients with RVOT pacing had fewer myocardial perfusion defects, fewer regional wall motion abnormalities, and higher ejection fractions than those with RVA pacing.

In view of the lack of sufficient long-term data, it seems premature to entirely abandon the traditional RVA pacing site in hopes of preserving ventricular function in patients who require ventricular pacing for AV block. Large, long-term, randomized, multicenter studies are needed to determine the impact of nonapical RV pacing sites on major clinical outcomes, including heart failure hospitalization and death, before a definitive recommendation can be made that selective site RV pacing prevents the deleterious effects of RVA pacing. Furthermore, in patients with significant LV dysfunction (ejection fraction ≤0.35), biventricular pacing seems to be a more attractive approach than RVOT or RV septal pacing. The Biventricular versus RV Pacing in Heart Failure Patients with Atrioventricular Block (BLOCK HF) study is an ongoing, prospective randomized trial comparing RV with biventricular pacing in patients with mild to moderate heart failure (NYHA functional class I, II, or III), LV dysfunction (LV ejection fraction ≤0.50), and AV block. This study is designed to determine whether biventricular pacing will slow progression of heart failure. As of 2006, enrollment and follow-up in Block HF is ongoing. This study's findings may further enlarge the population of patients in whom biventricular pacing is indicated.

Summary

AV conduction system disease is relatively common in the general population, and its prevalence rises with advancing age. Most diagnoses of AV conduction disturbances can be made through careful analysis of the surface ECG. The traditional electrocardiographic classification of AV and intraventricular blocks provides insight into the prognosis and natural history of these disorders and remains clinically useful. Thorough noninvasive and, if necessary, invasive screening for structural heart disease should be performed when AV conduction disturbances are identified on electrocardiogram. Electrophysiologic testing has limitations but in select cases remains a useful diagnostic tool, especially when the anatomic site of AV block is not certain.

Many causes of AV block and conduction system disease are recognized, but in most instances it is difficult to ascribe a specific cause in an individual case. Reversible causes of AV block frequently have a benign prognosis and should be excluded. Structural heart disease is commonly associated with AV conduction system disorders and has a major effect on prognosis. When AV conduction disorders occur in the setting of structural heart disease, other rhythm disturbances, including atrial and ventricular tachyarrhythmias, are common and increase morbidity and mortality. The development of AV conduction disturbances during AMI is related to the extent of the ischemic/infarcted myocardial region. When AV block is associated with intraventricular conduction disturbances in the setting of MI, the risks of mortality and sudden death remain high even in the reperfusion era. In the future, new insights into the molecular genetic basis of AV conduction disturbances undoubtedly will have a major effect on the evaluation and management of these disorders in children and adults.

In a patient with an AV conduction disturbance, the decision to institute permanent pacing is based on a correlation of symptoms with an abnormal ECG rhythm and recognition of the likelihood of progression to high-grade AV block. Chronic or intermittent AV block is a major indication for cardiac pacing that is likely to remain so during the next decade. In patients who have experienced AMI, however, there has been greater reliance on transcutaneous rather than transvenous temporary pacing. The decision to institute permanent pacing for AV block in the setting of AMI is based in large measure on the presence of intraventricular conduction defects, which appear to be less common in the thrombolytic era. Thus, permanent pacing for AV block is not commonly required after MI. Furthermore, expanded indications for ICD and cardiac resynchronization in the current era have largely eliminated the prior debate regarding the need for and benefit of permanent pacing after MI.

Clinical trials have not demonstrated clear superiority of dual-chamber over single-chamber ventricular pacing. However, it is likely that dual-chamber pacing with separate atrial and ventricular leads will remain the major pacing modality for most patients with heart block. Pacing from the RVA has been used traditionally during both dual-chamber and single-chamber ventricular pacing for AV block. Growing recognition of the potential for deleterious effects of RVA pacing has stimulated interest in ventricular pacing from alternative RV, dual-site RV, LV, or biventricular pacing sites in patients in whom ventricular pacing cannot be avoided. Large, long-term, multicenter studies demonstrating that non-RVA or biventricular pacing prevents the deleterious effects of RVA pacing are needed before a definitive recommendation can be made to entirely abandon the traditional RVA pacing site. In the decades to come, development of biologic pacemakers using gene therapy or stem cells may supplement or replace electronic implantable pacemakers in the treatment of AV conduction system disease.

REFERENCES

1. James TN: Anatomy of the coronary arteries and veins: Anatomy of the conduction system of the heart. In Hurst JW (ed): The Heart. New York, McGraw-Hill, 1978, pp 33-56.
2. James TN: Anatomy of the coronary arteries in health and disease. Circulation 32:1020, 1965.
3. Lev M, Bharati S: Anatomic basis for impulse generation and atrioventricular transmission. In Narula OS (ed): His Bundle Electrocardiography and Clinical Electrophysiology. Philadelphia, FA Davis, 1975, p 1.
4. Van der Hauwaert LG, Stroobandt R, Verhaeghe L: Arterial blood supply of the atrioventricular node and main bundle. Br Heart J 34:1045, 1972.
5. Frink RJ, James TN: Normal blood supply to the human His bundle and proximal bundle branches. Circulation 47:8, 1973.
6. Massing GK, James TN: Anatomical configuration of the His bundle and bundle branches in the human heart. Circulation 53:609, 1976.
7. Pruitt RD, Essex HE, Burchell BH: Studies on the spread of excitation through the ventricular myocardium. Circulation 3:418, 1951.
8. Hunt D, Lie JT, Vohra J, et al: Histopathology of heart block complicating acute myocardial infarction: Correlation with the His bundle electrogram. Circulation 48:1252, 1973.
9. Rosenbaum MB: Types of left bundle branch block and their clinical significance. J Electrocardiol 2:197, 1969.
10. Josephson ME: Clinical Cardiac Electrophysiology: Techniques and Interpretations, 3rd ed. Philadelphia, Lippincott Williams & Wilkins, 2002, pp 92-109.
11. Zipes DP: Second-degree atrioventricular block. Circulation 60: 465, 1979.
12. Barold SS: ACC/AHA guidelines for implantation of cardiac pacemakers: How accurate are the definitions of atrioventricular and intraventricular conduction blocks? PACE 16:1221, 1993.
13. Cabeen WR, Roberts NK, Child JS: Recognition of the Wenckebach phenomenon. West J Med 129:521, 1978.
14. Denes P, Levy L, Pick A, Rosen KM: The incidence of typical and atypical A-V Wenckebach periodicity. Am Heart J 89:26, 1975.
15. Ursell S, Habbab MA, El-Sherif N: Atrioventricular and intraventricular conduction disorders: Clinical aspects. In El-Sherif N, Samet P (eds): Cardiac Pacing and Electrophysiology, 3rd ed. Philadelphia, WB Saunders, 1991, pp 140-169.
16. Lange HW, Ameisen O, Mack R, et al: Prevalence and clinical correlates on non-Wenckebach narrow complete second-degree atrioventricular block detected by ambulatory ECG. Am Heart J 115:114, 1988.
17. DeMotss H, Brodeur MTH, Rahimtoola SH: Concealed sinus rhythm: A cause of misdiagnosis of digitalis intoxication. Circulation 50:632, 1974.
18. Puech P, Grolleau R, Guimond C: Incidence of different types of A-V block and their localization by His bundle recordings. In Wellens HJJ, Lie KI, Janse MJ (eds): The Conduction System of the Heart: Structure, Function, and Clinical Implications. Leiden, HE Stenfert Kroese BV, 1976, pp 467-484.
19. Denes P, Dhingra RC, Wu D, et al: H-V interval in patients with bifascicular block (right bundle branch block and left anterior hemiblock): Clinical, electrocardiographic, and electrophysiologic correlations. Am J Cardiol 35:23, 1975.
20. Dhingra RC, Palileo E, Strasberg B, et al: Significance of the H-V interval in 517 patients with chronic bifascicular block. Circulation 64:1265, 1981.
21. Scheinman MM, Peters RW, Morady F, et al: Electrophysiologic studies in patients with bundle branch block. PACE 6:1157, 1983.
22. Bauernfeind RA, Welch WJ, Brownstein SL: Distal atrioventricular conduction system function. Cardiol Clin 4:417, 1986.
23. McAnulty JH, Rahimtoola SH, Murphy E, et al: Natural history of "high risk" bundle branch block: Final report of a prospective study. N Engl J Med 307:137, 1982.
24. Zipes DP, Gettes LS, Akhtar M, et al: Guidelines for clinical intracardiac electrophysiologic studies: A report of the American College of Cardiology/American Heart Association Task Force on Assessment of Diagnostic and Therapeutic Cardiovascular Procedures. J Am Coll Cardiol 14:1827, 1989.
25. Click RL, Gersh BJ, Sugrue DD, et al: Role of invasive electrophysiologic testing in patients with symptomatic bundle branch block. Am J Cardiol 59:817, 1987.
26. Morady F, Higgins J, Peters RW, et al: Electrophysiologic testing in bundle branch block and unexplained syncope. Am J Cardiol 54:587, 1984.
27. Dhingra RC, Wyndham C, Bauernfeind R, et al: Significance of block distal to the His bundle induced by atrial pacing in patients with chronic bifascicular block. Circulation 60:1455, 1979.
28. Petrac D, Radic B, Birtic K, Gjurovic J: Prospective evaluation of infrahisal second-degree AV block induced by atrial pacing in the presence of chronic bundle branch block and syncope. Pacing Clin Electrophysiol 19:784, 1996.
29. Englund A, Bergfeldt L, Rosenqvist M: Pharmacological stress testing of the His-Purkinje system in patients with bifascicular block. Pacing Clin Electrophysiol 21:1979, 1998.
30. Scheinman MM, Weiss AN, Shaffar A, et al: Electrophysiologic effects of procainamide in patients with interventricular conduction delay. Circulation 49:522, 1974.
31. Bergfeldt L, Rosenqvist M, Vallin H, et al: Disopyramide-induced second- and third-degree atrioventricular block in patients with bifascicular block: An acute stress test to predict atrioventricular block progression. Br Heart J 53:328, 1985.
32. Tonkin AM, Heddle WF, Tornos P: Intermittent atrioventricular block: Procainamide administration as a provocative test. Aust N Z J Med 8:594, 1978.
33. Twidale N, Heddle WF, Tonkin AM: Procainamide administration during electrophysiology study—utility as a provocative test for intermittent atrioventricular block. Pacing Clin Electrophysiol 11:1388, 1988.
34. Fujimura O, Yee R, Klein GJ, et al: The diagnostic sensitivity of electrophysiologic testing in patients with syncope caused by transient bradycardia. N Engl J Med 321:1703, 1989.
35. Mymin D, Mathewson FAL, Tate RB, et al: The natural history of first-degree atrioventricular heart block. N Engl J Med 315:1183, 1986.
36. Zornosa JP, Crossley GH, Haisty WK Jr, et al: Pseudopacemaker syndrome: A complication of radiofrequency ablation of the AV junction [abstract]. PACE 15:590, 1992.
37. Kim YH, O'Nunain S, Trouton T, et al: Pseudo-pacemaker syndrome following inadvertent fast pathway ablation for

atrioventicular nodal reentrant tachycardia. J Cardiovasc Electrophysiol 4:178, 1993.

38. Iliev II, Yamachika S, Muta K, et al: Preserving normal ventricular activation versus atrioventricular delay optimization during pacing: The role of intrinsic atrioventricular conduction and pacing rate. Pacing Clin Electrophysiol 23:74, 2000.
39. Strasberg B, Amat-Y-Leon F, Dhingra RC, et al: Natural history of second-degree atrioventricular nodal block. Circulation 63:1043, 1981.
40. Shaw DB, Kerwick CA, Veale D, et al: Survival in second-degree atrioventricular block. Br Heart J 53:587, 1985.
41. Clarke M, Sutton R, Ward D, et al: Recommendations for pacemaker prescription for symptomatic bradycardia: Report of a working party of the British Pacing and Electrophysiology Group. Br Heart J 66:185, 1991.
42. Shaw DB, Gowers JI, Kekwick CA, et al: Is Mobitz type I atrioventricular block benign in adults? Heart 90:169, 2004.
43. Dhingra RC, Denes P, Wu D, et al: The significance of second-degree atrioventricular block and bundle branch block: Observations regarding site and type of block. Circulation 49:638, 1974.
44. Johansson BW: Complete heart block: A clinical hemodynamic and pharmacological study in patients with and without an artificial pacemaker. Acta Med Scand 180(Suppl 451):1, 1966.
45. Edhag O, Swahn A: Prognosis of patients with complete heart block or arrhythmic syncope who were not treated with artificial pacemakers. Acta Med Scand 200:457, 1976.
46. Edhag O: Long-term cardiac pacing: Experience of fixed-rate pacing with an endocardial electrode in 260 patients. Acta Med Scand 502(Suppl):64, 1969.
47. Gregoratos G, Cheitlin MD, Conill A, et al: ACC/AHA guidelines for implantation of cardiac pacemakers and antiarrhythmia devices: A report of the American College of Cardiology/American Heart Association Task Force on Practice Guidelines. J Am Coll Cardiol 31:1175, 1998.
48. Linzer M, Prystowsky EN, Divine GW, et al: Predicting the outcomes of electrophysiologic studies of patients with unexplained syncope: Preliminary validation of a derived model. J Gen Intern Med 6:113, 1991.
49. Sherif N, Scherlag BJ, Lazzara R, et al: The pathophysiology of tachycardia-dependent paroxysmal atrioventricular block after myocardial ischemia: Experimental and clinical observations. Circulation 50:515, 1974.
50. Rosenbaum MB, Elizari MV, Levi RJ, et al: Paroxysmal atrioventricular block related to hyperpolarization and spontaneous diastolic depolarization. Chest 63:678, 1973.
51. Shohat-Zabarski R, Iakobishvili Z, et al: Paroxysmal atrioventricular block: Clinical experience with 20 patients. Int J Cardiol 97:399, 2004.
52. Rosenthal E: Fetal Heart Block. In Allan L, Hornberger L, Sharland G (eds): Textbook of Fetal Cardiology. London, Greenwich Medical Media, 2000, pp 438-451.
53. Friedman RA, Fenrich AL, Kertesz NJ: Congenital complete atrioventricular block. Pacing Clin Electrophysiol 24:1681, 2001.
54. Thambo JB, Bordachar P, Garrigue S, et al: Detrimental ventricular remodeling in patients with congenital complete heart block and chronic right ventricular apical pacing. Circulation 110:3766, 2004.
55. Benson DW: Genetics of atrioventricular conduction disease in humans. Anat Rec A Discov Mol Cell Evol Biol 280:934, 2004.
56. Otomo J, Kure S, Shiba T, et al: Electrophysiological and histopathological characteristics of progressive atrioventricular block accompanied by familial dilated cardiomyopathy caused by a novel mutation of lamin a/c gene. J Cardiovasc Electrophysiol 16:137, 2005.
57. Lev M: The pathology of complete AV block. Prog Cardiovasc Dis 6:317, 1964.
58. Lenegre J: Etiology and pathology of bilateral bundle branch fibrosis in relation to complete heart block. Prog Cardiovasc Dis 6:409, 1964.
59. Narula OS: Atrioventricular conduction defects in patients with sinus bradycardia. Circulation 44:1096, 1971.
60. Evans R, Shaw DB: Pathological studies in sino-atrial disorder (sick sinus syndrome). Br Heart J 39:778, 1977.
61. Rosenqvist M, Obel IWP: Atrial pacing and the risk for AV block: Is there a time for change in attitude? PACE 12:97, 1989.
62. Sutton R, Kenny RA: The natural history of sick sinus syndrome. PACE 9:1110, 1986.
63. Caspi J, Amar R, Elami A, et al: Frequency and significance of complete atrioventricular block after coronary artery bypass grafting. Am J Cardiol 63:526, 1989.
64. Keefe DL, Griffin JC, Harrison DC, et al: Atrioventricular conduction abnormalities in patients undergoing isolated aortic or mitral valve replacement. PACE 8:393, 1985.
65. Rosenbaum MB, Corrado G, Oliveri R, et al: Right bundle branch block with left anterior hemiblock in surgically induced tetralogy of Fallot. Am J Cardiol 26:12, 1970.
66. Van Lier TA, Harinck E, Hitchcock JF: Complete right bundle branch block after surgical closure of permembranous ventricular septal defect. Eur Heart J 6:959, 1985.
67. Maron BJ, Merrill WH, Freier PA, et al: Long-term clinical course and symptomatic status of patients after operation for hypertrophic subaortic stenosis. Circulation 57:1205, 1978.
68. Talreja DR, Nishimura RA, Edwards WD, et al: Alcohol septal ablation versus surgical septal myectomy: Comparison of effects on atrioventricular conduction tissue. J Am Coll Cardiol 44:2329, 2004.
69. Baerman JM, Kirsh MM, de Buitleir M, et al: Natural history and determinants of conduction defects following coronary artery bypass surgery. Ann Thorac Surg 44:150, 1987.
70. El-Khally Z, Thibault B, Staniloae C, et al: Prognostic significance of newly acquired bundle branch block after aortic valve replacement. Am J Cardiol 94:1008, 2004.
71. Limongelli G, Ducceschi V, D'Andrea A, et al: Risk factors for pacemaker implantation following aortic valve replacement: A single centre experience. Heart 89:901, 2003.
72. Chu A, Califf RM, Pryor DB, et al: Prognostic effect of bundle branch block related to coronary artery bypass grafting. Am J Cardiol 59:798, 1987.
73. Koplan BA, Stevenson WG, Epstein LM, et al: Development and validation of a simple preoperative risk score to predict the need for permanent pacing after cardiac valve surgery. J Am Coll Cardiol 41:795, 2003.
74. Glikson M, Dearani JA, Hyberger LK, et al: Indications, effectiveness, and long-term dependency in permanent pacing after cardiac surgery. Am J Cardiol 80:1309, 1997.
75. Scheinman M, Calkins H, Gillette P, et al: NASPE policy statement on catheter ablation: Personnel, policy, procedures, and therapeutic recommendations. Pacing Clin Electrophysiol 26:789, 2003.
76. Delise P, Sitta N, Zoppo F, et al: Radiofrequency ablation of atrioventricular nodal reentrant tachycardia: The risk of intraprocedural, late and long-term atrioventricular block. The Veneto Region multicenter experience. Ital Heart J 3:715, 2002.
77. Pelargonio G, Fogel RI, Knilans TK, Prystowsky EN: Late occurrence of heart block after radiofrequency catheter ablation of the septal region: Clinical follow-up and outcome. J Cardiovasc Electrophysiol 12:56, 2001.
78. Ferguson TB Jr, Cox JL: Surgical treatment for the Wolff-Parkinson-White syndrome: The endocardial approach. In Zipes DP, Jaliffe J (eds): Cardiac Electrophysiology: From Cell to Bedside. Philadelphia, WB Saunders, 1990, pp 897-906.
79. Jackman WM, Wang X, Friday KJ, et al: Catheter ablation of atrioventricular junction with radiofrequency current in 17

patients: Comparison of standard and large-tip catheter electrodes. Circulation 83:1562, 1991.
80. Kay GN, Ellenbogen KA, Guidici M, et al: The Ablate and Pace Trial: A prospective study of catheter ablation of the AV conduction system and permanent pacemaker implantation for treatment of atrial fibrillation. J Intervent Cardiac Electrophysiol 2:121, 1998.
81. Brignole M, Giafranchi L, Menozzi C, et al: Assessment of atrioventicular junction ablation and DDDR mode-switching pacemaker versus pharmacological treatment in patients with severely symptomatic paroxysmal atrial fibrillation: A randomized controlled study. Circulation 96:2617, 1977.
82. Williamson BD, Man KC, Daoud E, et al: Radiofrequency catheter modification of atrioventricular conduction to control the ventricular rate during atrial fibrillation. N Engl J Med 331:910, 1994.
83. Rokas S, Gaitanidou S, Chatzidou S, et al: Atrioventricular node modification in patients with chronic atrial fibrillation: Role of morphology of RR interval variation. Circulation 103:2942, 2001.
84. Garratt CJ, Skehan JD, Payne GE, Stafford PJ: Effect of sequential radiofrequency ablation lesions at fast and slow atrioventricular nodal pathway positions in patients with paroxysmal atrial fibrillation. Heart 75:502, 1996.
85. Benitez RM, Gold MR: Immediate and persistent complete heart block following a horse kick. PACE 22:816, 1999.
86. Lazaros GA, Ralli DG, Moundaki VS, Bonoris PE: Delayed development of complete heart block after a blunt chest trauma. Injury 35:1300, 2004.
87. Anderson DJ, Bulkley BH, Hutchins GM: A clinicopathologic study of prospective valve endocarditis in 22 patients: Morphologic basis for diagnosis and therapy. Am Heart J 94:325, 1977.
88. Maguire JH, Hoff R, Sherlock I, et al: Cardiac morbidity and mortality due to Chagas' disease: Prospective electrocardiographic study of a Brazilian community. Circulation 75:1140, 1987.
89. Hagar JM, Rahimtoola SH: Chagas' heart disease. Curr Probl Cardiol 20:825, 1995.
90. Hagar JM, Rahimtoola SH: Chagas' heart disease in the United States. N Engl J Med 325:763, 1991.
91. Steere AC: Lyme disease. N Engl J Med 321:586, 1989.
92. Steere AC, Batsford WP, Weinberg M, et al: Lyme carditis: Cardiac abnormalities of Lyme disease. Ann Intern Med 93:8, 1980.
93. Van der Linde MR, Crijns HJGM, De Koning J, et al: Range of atrioventricular conduction disturbances in Lyme borreliosis: A report of four cases and review of other published reports. Br Heart J 63:162, 1990.
94. McAlister HF, Klementowicz PT, Andrews C, et al: Lyme carditis: An important cause of reversible heart block. Ann Intern Med 110:339, 1989.
95. Kimball SA, Janson PA, LaRaia PJ: Complete heart block as the sole presentation of Lyme disease. Arch Intern Med 149:1897, 1989.
96. Cohen IS, Bharati S, Glass J, et al: Radiotherapy as a cause of complete atrioventricular block in Hodgkin's disease. Arch Intern Med 141:676, 1981.
97. Almange C, Lebrestec T, Louvet M, et al: Bloc auriculo-ventriculaire complet par métastase cardiaque: A propos d'une observation. Sem Hôp Pans 54:1419, 1978.
98. Perloff JK: The heart in neuromuscular disease. In O'Rourke RA (ed): Current Problems in Cardiology. Chicago, Yearbook, 1986, pp 513-557.
99. Lazarus A, Varin J, Babuty D, et al: Long-term follow-up of arrhythmias in patients with myotonic dystrophy treated by pacing: A multicenter diagnostic pacemaker study. J Am Coll Cardiol 40:1645, 2002.
100. Wynne J, Braunwald E: The cardiomyopathies and myocarditides. In Braunwald E (ed): Heart Disease: A Textbook of Cardiovascular Medicine, 4th ed. Philadelphia, WB Saunders, 1992, pp 1349-1450.
101. Bargout R, Kelly RF. Sarcoid heart disease: Clinical course and treatment. Int J Cardiol 97:173, 2004.
102. Silverman KJ, Hutchins GM, Bulkley BH: Cardiac sarcoid: A clinicopathologic study of 84 unselected patients with systemic sarcoidosis. Circulation 58:1204, 1978.
103. Kato Y, Morimoto S, Uemura A, et al: Efficacy of corticosteroids in sarcoidosis presenting with atrioventricular block. Sarcoidosis Vasc Diffuse Lung Dis 20:133, 2003.
104. Hurd ER: Extraarticular manifestations of rheumatoid arthritis. Semin Arthritis Rheum 8:151, 1979.
105. Owen DS: Connective tissue diseases and the cardiovascular system: A review. Virginia Med 110:426, 1983.
106. Janosik DL, Osborn TG, Moore TL, et al: Heart disease in systemic sclerosis. Semin Arthritis Rheum 19:191, 1989.
107. Rozanski JJ, Castellanos A, Sheps D, et al: Paroxysmal second-degree AV block induced by exercise. Heart Lung 9:887, 1980.
108. Egred M, Jafary F: Exercise induced atrio-ventricular (AV) block: Important but uncommon phenomenon. Int J Cardiol 97:559, 2004.
109. Finzi A, Bruno A, Perondi R: Exercise-induced paroxysmal atrioventricular block during nuclear perfusion stress testing: Evidence for transient ischemia of the conduction system. G Ital Cardiol 29:1313, 1999.
110. Donzeau JP, Dechandol AM, Bergeal A, et al: Blocs auriculo-ventriculaires survenant à l'effort: Considerations generales à propos de 14 cas. Coeur 15:513, 1985.
111. Woelfel AK, Simpson RJ, Gettes LS, et al: Exercise-induced distal atrioventricular block. J Am Coll Cardiol 2:578, 1983.
112. Petrac J, Gjuroivic J, Vukoskovic D, et al: Clinical significance and natural history of exercise-induced atrioventricular block. In Belhassen B, Feldman S, Copperman Y (eds): Cardiac Pacing and Electrophysiology: Proceedings of the VIII World Symposium on Cardiac Pacing and Electrophysiology. Jerusalem, R & L Creative Communications, 1987, p 265.
113. Huycke EC, Card HG, Sobol SM, et al: Postexertional cardiac systole in a young man without organic heart disease. Ann Intern Med 106:844, 1987.
114. Kasaoka Y, Ajiki K, Hayami N, Murakawa Y: His-bundle parasystole masquerading as exercise-induced 2:1 atrioventricular block. J Cardiovasc Electrophysiol 12:965, 2001.
115. Ovsyshcher IE, Barold SS: Drug induced bradycardia: To pace or not to pace? Pacing Clin Electrophysiol 27:1144, 2004.
116. Zeltser D, Justo D, Halkin A, et al: Drug-induced atrioventricular block: Prognosis after discontinuation of the culprit drug. J Am Coll Cardiol 44:105, 2004.
117. Jonas EA, Kosowsky BD, Ramaswamy K: Complete His-Purkinje block produced by carotid massage. Circulation 50:192, 1974.
118. Hart G, Oldershaw PJ, Cull RE, et al: Syncope caused by cough-induced complete atrioventricular block. PACE 5:564, 1982.
119. Wik B, Hillestad L: Deglutition syncope. Br Med J 3:747, 1975.
120. Strasberg B, Lam W, Swiryn S, et al: Symptomatic spontaneous paroxysmal AV nodal block due to localized hyperresponsiveness of the AV node to vagotonic reflexes. Am Heart J 103:795, 1982.
121. Zaman L, Moleiro F, Rozanski JJ, et al: Multiple electrophysiologic manifestations and clinical implications of vagally mediated AV block. Am Heart J 106:92, 1983.
122. Ector H, Rickards AF, Kappenberger L, et al: The World Survey of Cardiac Pacing and Implantable Cardioverter Defibrillators: Calendar year 1997-Europe. PACE 24:863, 2001.
123. Bernstein AD, Parsonnet V: Survey of cardiac pacing and implanted defibrillator practice patterns in the United States in 1997. PACE 24:842, 2001.

124. Hreybe H, Saba S: Effects of race and health insurance on the rates of pacemaker implantation for complete heart block in the United States. Am J Cardiol 94:227, 2004.
125. Frye RL, Collins JJ, DeSanctis RW, et al: Guidelines for permanent cardiac pacemaker implantation, May 1984: A report of the Joint American College of Cardiology/American Heart Association Task Force on Assessment of Cardiovascular Procedures (Subcommittee on Pacemaker Implantation). Circulation 70:331A, 1984.
126. Dreifus LS, Fisch C, Griffin JC, et al: Guidelines for implantation of cardiac pacemakers and antiarrhythmia devices: A Report of the American College of Cardiology/American Heart Association Task Force on Assessment of Diagnostic and Therapeutic Cardiovascular Procedures (Subcommittee on Pacemaker Implantation). J Am Coll Cardiol 18:1, 1991.
127. Gregoratos G, Abrams J, Epstein AE, et al; American College of Cardiology/American Heart Association Task Force on Practice Guidelines/North American Society for Pacing and Electrophysiology Committee: ACC/AHA/NASPE 2002 guideline update for implantation of cardiac pacemakers and antiarrhythmia devices: Summary article: A report of the American College of Cardiology/American Heart Association Task Force on Practice Guidelines (ACC/AHA/NASPE Committee to Update the 1998 Pacemaker Guidelines). Circulation 106:2145, 2002.
128. Bassan R, Maia IG, Bozza A, et al: Atrioventricular block in acute inferior wall myocardial infarction: Harbinger of associated obstruction of the left anterior descending coronary artery. J Am Coll Cardiol 8:773, 1986.
129. Forsberg SA, Juul-Moller S: Myocardial infarction complicated by heart block: Treatment and long-term prognosis. Acta Med Scand 206:483, 1979.
130. Tans AC, Lie KI, Durrer D: Clinical setting and prognostic significance of high degree atrioventricular block in acute inferior myocardial infarction: A study of 144 patients. Am Heart J 99:4, 1980.
131. Archbold RA, Sayer JW, Ray S, et al: Frequency and prognostic implications of conduction defects in acute myocardial infarction since the introduction of thrombolytic therapy. Eur Heart J 19:893, 1998.
132. Escosteguy CC, Carvalho Mde A, Medronho Rde A, et al: Bundle branch and atrioventricular block as complications of acute myocardial infarction in the thrombolytic era. Arq Bras Cardiol 76:291, 2001.
133. Aplin M, Engstrom T, Vejlstrup NG, et al; TRACE Study Group: Prognostic importance of complete atrioventricular block complicating acute myocardial infarction. Am J Cardiol 92:853, 2003.
134. Meine TJ, Al-Khatib SM, Alexander JH, et al: Incidence, predictors, and outcomes of high-degree atrioventricular block complicating acute myocardial infarction treated with thrombolytic therapy. Am Heart J 149:670, 2005.
135. Sutton R, Davies M: The conduction system in acute myocardial infarction complicated by heart block. Circulation 38:987, 1968.
136. Wei JY, Markis JE, Malagold M, et al: Cardiovascular reflexes stimulated by reperfusion of ischemic myocardium in acute myocardial infarction. Circulation 67:796, 1983.
137. Koren G, Weiss AT, Ben-David Y, et al: Bradycardia and hypotension following reperfusion with streptokinase (Bezold-Jarisch reflex): A sign of coronary thrombolysis and myocardial salvage. Am Heart J 112:468, 1986.
138. Berger PB, Ruocco NA, Ryan TJ, et al, and the TIMI II Investigators: Incidence and prognostic implications of heart block complicating inferior myocardial infarction treated with thrombolytic therapy: Results from TIMI II. J Am Coll Cardiol 20:533, 1992.
139. Blondeau M, Maurice P, Reverdy, et al: Troubles du rythme et de la conduction auriculo-ventriculaire dans l'infartus du myocarde récent: Considérations anatomiques. Arch Mal Coeur 60:1733, 1967.
140. Bilbao FJ, Zabalza IE, Vilanova JR, et al: Atrioventricular block in posterior acute myocardial infarction: A clinicopathologic correlation. Circulation 75:733, 1987.
141. Rosen KM, Ehrsani A, Rahimtoola SH: Myocardial infarction complicated by conduction defect. Med Clin North Am 57:155, 1973.
142. Clemmensen P, Bates ER, Califf RM, et al, and the TAMI Study Group: Complete atrioventricular block complicating inferior wall acute myocardial infarction treated with reperfusion therapy. Am J Cardiol 67:225, 1991.
143. Wesley RC Jr, Lerman BB, DiMarco JP, et al: Mechanism of atropine-resistant atrioventricular block during inferior myocardial infarction: possible role of adenosine. J Am Coll Cardiol 8:1232, 1986.
144. Shah PK, Nalos P, Peter T: Atropine resistant post infarction complete AV block: Possible role of adenosine and improvement with aminophylline. Am Heart J 113:194, 1986.
145. Bertolet BD, McMurtrie EB, Hill JA, Belardinelli L: Theophylline for the treatment of atrioventricular block after myocardial infarction. Ann Intern Med 123:509, 1995.
146. Antman EM, Anbe DT, Armstrong PW, et al; American College of Cardiology; American Heart Association; Canadian Cardiovascular Society: ACC/AHA guidelines for the management of patients with ST-elevation myocardial infarction—executive summary: A report of the American College of Cardiology/American Heart Association Task Force on Practice Guidelines (Writing Committee to revise the 1999 guidelines for the management of patients with acute myocardial infarction). J Am Coll Cardiol 44:671, 2004.
147. Cohen HC, Gozo EG Jr, Pick A: The nature and type of arrhythmias in acute experimental hyperkalemia in the intact dog. Am Heart J 82:777, 1971.
148. Sugiura T, Iwasaka T, Takayama Y, et al: The factors associated with fascicular block in acute anteroseptal infarction. Arch Intern Med 148:529, 1988.
149. Rotman M, Wagner GS, Wallace AG: Bradyarrhythmias in acute myocardial infarction. Circulation 45:703, 1972.
150. Hunt D, Lie JY, Vohra J, et al: Histopathology of heart block complicating acute myocardial infarction. Circulation 48:1252, 1973.
151. Wilber D, Walton J, O'Neill W, et al: Effects of reperfusion on complete heart block complicating anterior myocardial infarction. J Am Coll Cardiol 4:1315, 1984.
152. Norris RM: Heart block in posterior and anterior myocardial infarction. Br Heart J 31:352, 1969.
153. Brown RW, Hunt D, Sloman JG: The natural history of atrioventricular conduction defects in acute myocardial infarction. Am Heart J 78:460, 1969.
154. Ginks WR, Sutton R, Winston DH, et al: Long-term prognosis after acute myocardial infarction with atrioventricular block. Br Heart J 39:186, 1977.
155. Lie KI, Wellens HJ, Schuilenburg RM, et al: Factors influencing prognosis of bundle branch block complicating acute anteroseptal infarction. Circulation 50:935, 1974.
156. Hindman MC, Wagner GS, JaRo H, et al: The clinical significance of bundle branch block complicating acute myocardial infarction. 2: Indications for temporary and permanent pacemakers. Circulation 58:689, 1978.
157. de Guzman M, Rahimtoola SH: What is the role of pacemakers in patients with coronary artery disease and conduction abnormalities? In Rahimtoola SH (ed): Controversies in Coronary Artery Disease. Philadelphia, FA Davis, 1983, pp 191-207.
158. Rosen KM, Loeb HS, Chiquimia R, et al: Site of heart block in acute inferior myocardial infarction. Circulation 42:925, 1970.
159. Goldberg RJ, Zevallos JC, Yarzebski J, et al: Prognosis of acute myocardial infarction complicated by complete heart block

(the Worcester Heart Attack Study). Am J Cardiol 69:1135, 1992.
160. Behar S, Zissman E, Zion M, et al, for the SPRINT Study Group: Prognostic significance of second-degree atrioventricular block in inferior wall acute myocardial infarction. Am J Cardiol 72:831, 1993.
161. Kostuk WJ, Beanlands DS: Complete heart block with acute myocardial infarction. Am J Cardiol 26:380, 1970.
162. Bigger JT, Dresdale RJ, Heissenbuttal RH, et al: Ventricular arrhythmias in ischemic heart disease: Mechanism, prevalence, significance, and management. Prog Cardiovasc Dis 19:255, 1977.
163. Mullins CB, Atkins JM: Prognoses and management of ventricular conduction blocks in acute myocardial infarction. Mod Concepts Cardiovasc Dis 45:129, 1976.
164. Hindman MC, Wagner GS, JaRo H, et al: The clinical significance of bundle branch block complicating acute myocardial infarction. 1: Clinical characteristics, hospital mortality, and one-year follow-up. Circulation 58:679, 1978.
165. Norris RM, Croxson MS: Bundle branch block in acute myocardial infarction. Am Heart J 79:728, 1970.
166. Scheinman M, Brenman B: Clinical and anatomic implication of intraventricular conduction blocks in acute myocardial infarction. Circulation 46:753, 1972.
167. Lie KI, Wellens HJ, Schuilenburg RM: Bundle branch block and acute myocardial infarction. In Wellens HJ, Lie KI, Janse MI (eds): The Conduction System of the Heart: Structure, Function, and Clinical Implications. Philadelphia, Lea & Febiger, 1976, pp 662-672.
168. Newby KH, Pisano E, Krucoff MW, et al: Incidence and clinical relevance of the occurrence of bundle-branch block in patients treated with thrombolytic therapy. Circulation 94:2424, 1996.
169. Godman MJ, Lassers BW, Julian DG: Complete bundle branch block complicating acute myocardial infarction. N Engl J Med 282:237, 1970.
170. Scanlon PJ, Pryor R, Blount G: Right bundle branch block associated with left superior or inferior intraventricular block. Circulation 42:1135, 1970.
171. Godman MJ, Alpert BA, Julian DG: Bilateral bundle branch block complicating acute myocardial infarction. Lancet 2:345, 1971.
172. Nimetz AA, Shubrooks SJ, Hutter AM, et al: The significance of bundle branch block during acute myocardial infarction. Am Heart J 90:439, 1975.
173. Lamas GA, Muller JE, Turi AG, et al: A simplified method to predict occurrence of complete heart block during acute myocardial infarction. Am J Cardiol 57:1213, 1986.
174. Roos C, Dunning AJ: Right bundle branch block and left axis deviation in acute myocardial infarction. Br Heart J 32:847, 1970.
175. Sgarbossa EB, Pinski SL, Topol EJ, et al: Acute myocardial infarction and complete bundle branch block at hospital admission: clinical characteristics and outcome in the thrombolytic era. GUSTO-I Investigators. Global Utilization of Streptokinase and t-PA [tissue-type plasminogen activator] for Occluded Coronary Arteries. J Am Coll Cardiol 31:105, 1998.
176. Melgarejo-Moreno A, Galcera-Tomas J, Garcia-Alberola A, et al: Incidence, clinical characteristics, and prognostic significance of right bundle-branch block in acute myocardial infarction: A study in the thrombolytic area. Circulation 196:1139, 1997.
177. Atkins J, Leshin S, Blomqvist CG, et al: Ventricular conduction blocks and sudden death in acute myocardial infarction. N Engl J Med 288:281, 1973.
178. Ritter WS, Atkins J, Blomqvist G, et al: Permanent pacing in patients with transient trifascicular block during acute myocardial infarction. Am J Cardiol 38:205, 1976.
179. Harper R, Hunt D, Vohra J, et al: His bundle electrogram in patients with acute myocardial infarction complicated by atrioventricular or intraventricular conduction disturbances. Br Heart J 37:705, 1975.
180. Murphy E, DeMots H, McAnulty J, et al: Prophylactic permanent pacemakers for transient heart block during myocardial infarction? Results of a prospective study. Am J Cardiol 49:952, 1982.
181. Lie K, Liem KL, Schuilenberg RM, et al: Early identification of patients developing late in-hospital ventricular fibrillation after discharge from the coronary care unit: A $5^1/_2$-year retrospective and prospective study of 1,897 patients. Am J Cardiol 41:674, 1978.
182. Waugh RA, Wagner GS, Haney TL, et al: Immediate and remote prognostic significance of fascicular block during acute myocardial infarction. Circulation 47:765, 1973.
183. Watson RDS, Glover DR, Page AJF, et al: The Birmingham Trial of permanent pacing in patients with intraventricular conduction disorders after acute myocardial infarction. Am Heart J 108:496, 1984.
184. Talwar KK, Kalra GS, Dogra B, et al: Prophylactic permanent pacemaker implantation in patients with anterior wall myocardial infarction complicated by bundle branch block and transient complete atrioventricular block: A prospective long-term study. Indian Heart J 39:22, 1987.
185. Harper R, Hunt D, Vohra J, et al: His bundle electrogram in patients with acute myocardial infarction complicated by atrioventricular or intraventricular conduction disturbances. Br Heart J 37:705, 1975.
186. Gould L, Reddy CVR, Kim SG, et al: His bundle electrogram in patients with acute myocardial infarction. PACE 2:428, 1979.
187. Lichstein E, Gupta P, Liu MM, et al: Findings of prognostic value in patients with incomplete bilateral bundle branch block complicating acute myocardial infarction. Am J Cardiol 32:913, 1973.
188. Gould L, Reddy CV, Kim SG, et al: His bundle electrogram in patients with acute myocardial infarction. PACE 2:428, 1979.
189. Topol EJ, Goldschlager N, Ports TA, et al: Hemodynamic benefit of atrial pacing in right ventricular myocardial infarction. Ann Intern Med 96:594, 1982.
190. Chamberlain DA, Leinbach RC, Vassaux CE, et al: Sequential atrioventricular pacing in heart block complicating acute myocardial infarction. N Engl J Med 282:577, 1970.
191. Murphy P, Morton P, Murtagh JG, et al: Hemodynamic effects of different temporary pacing modes for the management of bradycardias complicating acute myocardial infarction. Pacing Clin Electrophysiol 15:391, 1992.
192. Barold SS, Herweg B, Gallardo I: Acquired atrioventricular block: The 2002 ACC/AHA/NASPE guidelines for pacemaker implantation should be revised. Pacing Clin Electrophysiol 26:531, 2003.
193. Barold SS: American College of Cardiology/American Heart Association guideline for pacemaker implantation after acute myocardial infarction: What is persistent advanced block at the atrioventricular node? Am J Cardiol 80:770, 1997.
194. Barold SS, Hayes DL: Second-degree atrioventricular block: A reappraisal. Mayo Clin Proc 76:44, 2001.
195. McClellan MB, Tunis SR: Medicare coverage of ICDs. N Engl J Med 352:222, 2005.
196. Rahimtoola SH: The hibernating myocardium. Am Heart J 117: 211, 1989.
197. Braunwald E, Rutherford JD: Reversible ischemic left ventricular dysfunction: Evidence for the "hibernating myocardium." J Am Coll Cardiol 8:1467, 1986.
198. Nordlander R, Hedman A, Pehrsson SK: Rate-responsive pacing and exercise capacity: A comment. PACE 12:749, 1989.
199. Luceri RM, Brownstein SL, Vardeman L, et al: PR interval behavior during exercise: Implications for physiological pacemakers. PACE 13:1719, 1990.

200. Mond HG, Irwin M, Morillo C, Ector H: The world survey of cardiac pacing and cardioverter defibrillators: Calendar year 2001. Pacing Clin Electrophysiol 27:955, 2004.
201. Dreifus LS, Fisch C, Griffin JC, et al: Guidelines for implantation of cardiac pacemaker and antiarrhythmia devices: A report of the American College of Cardiology/American Heart Association Task Force on Assessment of Diagnostic and Therapeutic Cardiovascular Procedures (Committee on Pacemaker Implantation). Circulation 84:455, 1991.
202. Lau CP: Rate-Adaptive Cardiac Pacing: Simple and Dual Chamber. Mt Kisco, NY, Futura, 1993, pp 249-264.
203. Benditt DG, Milstein S, Buetikofer J, et al: Sensor-triggered rate-variable cardiac pacing. Ann Intern Med 107:714, 1987.
204. Gwinn N, Lemen R, Kratz J, et al: Chronotopic incompetence: A common and progressive finding in pacemaker patients. Am Heart J 123:1216, 1992.
205. Lamas GA, Ellenbogen KA: Evidence base for pacemaker mode selection: From physiology to randomized trials. Circulation 109:443, 2004.
206. Zehender M, Buchner C, Meinertz T, et al: Prevalence, circumstances, mechanisms, and risk stratification of sudden cardiac death in unipolar single-chamber ventricular pacing. Circulation 85:596, 1992.
207. Alpert MA, Curtis JJ, Sanfelippo JF, et al: Comparative survival after permanent ventricular and dual-chamber pacing for patients with chronic high-degree atrioventricular block with and without preexistent congestive heart failure. J Am Coll Cardiol 7:925, 1986.
208. Toff WD, Camm AJ, Skehan JD, et al: Single-chamber versus dual-chamber pacing for high-grade atrioventricular block. N Engl J Med 353:145, 2005.
209. Antonioli GE, Anscani L, Barbieri D, et al: Single-lead VDD pacing. In Barold SS, Mugica J (eds): New Perspectives in Cardiac Pacing 3. Mt Kisco, NY, Futura, 1993, pp 359-381.
210. Wiegand UK, Potratz J, Bode F, et al: Cost-effectiveness of dual chamber pacemaker therapy: Does single lead VDD pacing reduce treatment costs of atrioventricular block? Eur Heart J 22:174, 2001.
211. Ovsyshcher IE, Crystal E: Permanent and temporary single-lead VDD and DDD pacemakers: State of the art. In Barold SS, Mugica J (eds): The Fifth Decade of Cardiac Pacing. New York, Blackwell Scientific, 2003.
212. Ovsyshcher IE, Crystal E: VDD pacing: Under evaluated, undervalued, and underused. Pacing Clin Electrophysiol 27:1335, 2004.
213. Lau CP, Tai YT, Li JPS, et al: Initial clinical experience with a single pass VDDR pacing system. PACE 15:1894, 1992.
214. Antonioli GE, Ansani L, Barbieri D, et al: Italian multicenter study on a single-lead VDD pacing system using a narrow atrial dipole spacing. PACE 15:1890, 1992.
215. Sermasi S, Marconi M: VDD single pass lead pacing: Sustained pacemaker-mediated tachycardias unrelated to retrograde atrial activation. PACE 15:1902, 1992.
216. Lau CP, Leung S-K, Lee IS-F: Comparative evaluation of acute and long-term clinical performance of two single lead atrial synchronous ventricular (VDD) pacemakers. PACE 19:1574, 1996.
217. Ramsdale DR, Charles RG: Rate-responsive ventricular pacing: Clinical experience with the RS4-SRT pacing system. PACE 8:378, 1985.
218. Gross JN, Moser S, Benedek ZM, et al: DDD pacing mode survival in patients with a dual-chamber pacemaker. J Am Coll Cardiol 19:1536, 1992.
219. Huang M, Krahn AD, Yee R, et al: Optimal pacing for symptomatic AV block: A comparison of VDD and DDD pacing. PACE 26:2230, 2003.
220. Wiegand UK, Bode F, Schneider R, et al: Atrial sensing and AV synchrony in single lead VDD pacemakers: A prospective comparison to DDD devices with bipolar atrial leads. J Cardiovasc Electrophysiol 10:513, 1999.
221. Linde-Edelstam C, Gulberg B, Norlander R, et al: Longevity in patients with high-degree atrioventricular block paced in the atrial synchronous mode or the fixed-rate ventricular inhibited mode. PACE 15:304, 1992.
222. Nakata Y, Ogura S, Tokano T, et al: VDD pacing with a previously implanted single-lead system. PACE 15:1425, 1992.
223. Wish M, Fletcher RD, Gottdiener JS, et al: Importance of left atrial timing in the programming of dual-chamber pacemakers. Am J Cardiol 60:566, 1987.
224. Daubert C, Ritter P, Mabo P, et al: AV delay optimization in DDD and DDDR pacing. In Barold SS, Mugica J (eds): New Perspectives in Cardiac Pacing 3. Mt Kisco, NY, Futura, 1993, pp 259-287.
225. Hochleitner M, Hortnagl H, Ng CK, et al: Usefulness of physiologic dual-chamber pacing in drug-resistant idiopathic dilated cardiomyopathy. Am J Cardiol 66:198, 1990.
226. Nishimura RA, Hayes DL, Holmes DR Jr, Tajik AJ: Mechanism of hemodynamic improvement by dual-chamber pacing for severe left ventricular dysfunction: An acute Doppler and catheterization hemodynamic study. J Am Coll Cardiol 25:281, 1995.
227. Brecker SJ, Xiao HB, Sparrow J, Gibson DG: Effects of dual-chamber pacing with short atrioventricular delay in dilated cardiomyopathy. Lancet 340:1308, 1992.
228. Crystal E, Ovsyshcher IE: Cardiac output-based versus empirically programmed AV interval—how different are they? Europace 1:121, 1999.
229. Ovsyshcher IE: Toward physiological pacing: Optimization of cardiac hemodynamics by AV delay adjustment. PACE 20:861, 1997.
230. Ovsyshcher I, Zimlicheman R, Katz A, et al: Measurement of cardiac output by impedance cardiography in pacemaker patients at rest: Effects of various atrioventricular delays. J Am Coll Cardiol 21:761, 1993.
231. Ritter P, Dib JC, Lelievre T: Quick determination of the optimal AV delay at rest in patients paced in DDD mode for complete AV block [abstract]. Eur J CPE 4:A163, 1994.
232. Strohmer B, Pichler M, Froemmel M, et al; ELVIS Study Group: Evaluation of atrial conduction time at various sites of right atrial pacing and influence on atrioventricular delay optimization by surface electrocardiography. Pacing Clin Electrophysiol 27:468, 2004.
233. Haskell RJ, French WJ: Physiological importance of different atrioventricular intervals to improved exercise performance in patients with dual-chamber pacemakers. Br Heart J 61:46, 1989.
234. Khairy P, Talajic M, Dominguez M, et al: Atrioventricular interval optimization and exercise tolerance. Pacing Clin Electrophysiol 24:1534, 2001.
235. Sheppard RC, Ren JF, Ross J, et al: Doppler echocardiographic assessment of the hemodynamic benefits of rate adaptive AV delay during exercise in paced patients with complete heart block. Pacing Clin Electrophysiol 16:2157, 1993.
236. Wiggers CJ: The muscle reactions of the mammalian ventricles to artificial surface stimuli. Am J Physiol 73:346, 1925.
237. Barold SS: Adverse effects of ventricular desynchronization induced by long-term right ventricular pacing. J Am Coll Cardiol 42:624, 2003.
238. Burkhoff D, Oikawa RY, Sagawa K: Influence of pacing site on canine left ventricular contraction. Am J Physiol 251:J428, 1986.
239. Rosenqvist M, Bergfeldt L, Haga Y, et al: The effect of ventricular activation sequence on cardiac performance during pacing. Pacing Clin Electrophysiol 19:1279, 1996.
240. Tantengco MV, Thomas RL, Karpawich PP: Left ventricular dysfunction after long-term right ventricular apical pacing in the young. J Am Coll Cardiol 37:2093, 2001.

241. Betocchi S, Piscione F, Villari B, et al: Effects of induced asynchrony on left ventricular diastolic function in patients with coronary artery disease. J Am Coll Cardiol 22:1124, 1993.
242. Lee MA, Dae MW, Langberg JJ, et al: Effects of long term ventricular apical pacing on left ventricular perfusion, innervation, function and histology. J Am Coll Cardiol 24:225, 1994.
243. Tse HF, Lau CP: Long-term effect of right ventricular pacing on myocardial perfusion and function. J Am Coll Cardiol 29:744, 1997.
244. Prinzen FW, Augustijn CH, Arts T, et al: Redistribution of myocardial fiber strain and blood flow by asynchronous activation. Am J Physiol 259:330, 1990.
245. Van Oosterhout MFM, Prinzen FW, Arts T, et al: Asynchronous electrical activation induces inhomogeneous hypertrophy of the left ventricular wall. Circulation 98:588, 1998.
246. Prinzen FW, Cheriex EM, Delhaas T, et al: Asymmetric thickness of the left ventricular wall resulting from asynchronous electrical activation: A study in patients with left bundle branch block and in dogs with ventricular pacing. Am Heart J 130:1045, 1986.
247. Adomian GE, Beazell J: Myofibrillar disarray produced in normal hearts by chronic electrical pacing. Am Heart J 112:79, 1986.
248. Karpawich PP, Rabah R, Haas JE: Altered cardiac histology following apical right ventricular pacing in patients with congenital atrioventricular block. Pacing Clin Electrophysiol 22:1372, 1999.
249. Wilkoff BL, Cook JR, Epstein AE, et al: Dual-chamber pacing or ventricular backup pacing in patients with an implantable defibrillator: The Dual Chamber and VVI Implantable Defibrillator (DAVID) Trial. JAMA 288:3115, 2002.
250. Sweeney MO, Hellkamp AS, Ellenbogen KA, et al, for the MOST Investigators: Adverse effect of ventricular pacing on heart failure and atrial fibrillation among patients with normal baseline QRS duration in a clinical trial of pacemaker therapy for sinus node dysfunction. Circulation 107:2932, 2003.
251. Steinberg JS, Maniar P, Zareba W, et al, for the MADIT-II Investigators: The relationship between right ventricular pacing and outcomes in MADIT-II patients. Presented at the North American Society of Pacing and Electrophysiology Annual Scientific Sessions, Washington, DC, May 14-17, 2003.
252. Doshi R, Daoud E, Fellows C, et al: Left ventricular-based cardiac stimulation post AV nodal ablation evaluation (the PAVE study). J Cardiovasc Electrophysiol 16:1160, 2005.
253. Gammage MD, Marsh AM: Randomized trials for selective site pacing: Do we know where we are going? PACE 27:878, 2004.
254. Deshmukh P, Casavant DA, Romanyshyn M, Anderson K: Permanent, direct His-bundle pacing: A novel approach to cardiac pacing in patients with normal His-Purkinje activation. Circulation 101:869, 2000.
255. Giudici MC, Thornburg GA, et al: Comparison of right ventricular outflow tract and apical permanent pacing on cardiac output. Am J Cardiol 79:209, 1997.
256. Buckingham TA, Candinas R, Attenhofer C, et al: Systolic and diastolic function with alternate and combined site pacing in the right ventricle. Pacing Clin Electrophysiol 21:1077, 1998.
257. Victor F, Leclercq C, Mabo P, et al: Optimal right ventricular pacing site in chronically implanted patients: A prospective randomized crossover comparison of apical and outflow tract pacing. J Am Coll Cardiol 33:311, 1999.
258. Schwaab B, Frohlig G, Alexander C, et al: Influence of right ventricular stimulation site on left ventricular function in atrial synchronous ventricular pacing. J Am Coll Cardiol 33:317, 1999.
259. Mera F, DeLurgio DB, Patterson RE, et al: A comparison of ventricular function during high right ventricular septal and apical pacing after His-bundle ablation for refractory atrial fibrillation. Pacing Clin Electrophysiol 22:1234, 1999.
260. Tse HF, Yu C, Wong KK, et al: Functional abnormalities in patients with permanent right ventricular pacing: The effect of sites of electrical stimulation. J Am Coll Cardiol 40:1451, 2002.
261. Stambler BS, Ellenbogen K, Zhang X, et al; ROVA Investigators: Right ventricular outflow versus apical pacing in pacemaker patients with congestive heart failure and atrial fibrillation. J Cardiovasc Electrophysiol 14:1180, 2003.
262. de Cock CC, Giudici MC, Twisk JW: Comparison of the haemodynamic effects of right ventricular outflow-tract pacing with right ventricular apex pacing: A quantitative review. Europace 5:275, 2003.
263. Bourke JP, Hawkins T, Keavey P, et al: Evolution of ventricular function during permanent pacing from either right ventricular apex or outflow tract following AV junctional ablation for atrial fibrillation. Europace 4:219, 2002.
264. Victor F, Mansour H, Pavin D, et al: Optimal right ventricular pacing site in classical pacemaker indications: A randomized crossover comparison of apical and septal pacing [abstract]. Heart Rhythm 1:S70, 2004.
265. Peschar M, Marsh AM, Verbeek XAAM, et al: Site of right ventricular pacing in patients with atrioventricular block. Heart Rhythm 1:S245, 2004.

Chapter 15

Evolving Indications for Pacing: Hypertrophic Cardiomyopathy, Sleep Apnea, Long QT Syndromes, and Neurally Mediated Syncope Syndromes*

ROBERT S. SHELDON • AHMAD HERSI

Given the tremendous progress in pacemaker technology and our growing insight into the physiology of various cardiovascular disorders, pacing therapy has been explored for several new conditions. In this chapter, we review the recent progress in determining whether pacemakers are useful in the management of hypertrophic cardiomyopathy, long QT syndrome, sleep apnea, and the neurally mediated syncope syndromes.

*This study was supported in part by grant 73-1976 from the Canadian Institute for Health Research (CIHR).

Hypertrophic Cardiomyopathy

Clinical Perspective

The World Health Organization defines *hypertrophic cardiomyopathy* (HCM) as a unique process of primary muscle hypertrophy that may exist with or without a dynamic left ventricular (LV) outflow tract (LVOT) gradient. Hypertrophic cardiomyopathy is the most common heritable cardiovascular disease, with a reported prevalence of 0.1% to 0.2% in the general population. It is defined by the finding of LV hypertrophy in the absence of an identifiable cause. Although the diagnosis can be suspected on the basis of abnormal physical findings or electrocardiogram results, the primary diagnostic test is two-dimensional echocardiography.

Hypertrophic cardiomyopathy is the most common cause of sudden death in the young.[1] However, this risk is not homogeneous in the young. Early reports suggested that high mortality rates were based on data from tertiary referral centers with extraordinarily adverse patient selection. Subsequent population-based studies revealed the relatively common prevalence (1:500) and annual mortality rates, which range from 1% to as high as 5% in a subset of high-risk patients. There are, however, families with multiple early sudden deaths. Identifying the few patients who belong in this latter group remains one of the more difficult challenges in the management of HCM. Death can be sudden and unexpected and is most common in young adults; a substantial proportion of patients die during or just after vigorous physical activity. Hypertrophic cardiomyopathy is the most common cause of sudden death among young competitive athletes and thus represents a medical exclusion from participation in competitive athletics.

The mechanism of sudden death has been inferred from patients experiencing discharges from implantable defibrillators.[2-4] Ventricular tachycardia and fibrillation appear to be the primary mechanism; however, other arrhythmias may also play a role, including asystole, rapid atrial fibrillation, and pulseless electrical activity. Many patients eventually demonstrate progressive myocardial wall thinning, a reduction in systolic performance, and an increase in LV dimension. Progressive wall thinning may be especially common in patients with initially severe hypertrophy. In one series of 106 patients with initial wall thickness of 30 mm or more, more than 5 mm of wall thinning was seen in 41 (58%); the duration of follow-up was a significant predictor of thinning. In patients with HCM, obstruction of the LVOT results in shortness of breath, syncope, presyncope, fatigue, angina, and cardiac arrest.

Rationale for Pacing

The rationale for dual-chamber pacing in obstructive HCM is based on the ability of right ventricular (RV) pacing to increase LVOT diameter (Fig. 15-1). With RV pacing, the paced activation sequence of the septum leads to a larger LVOT diameter, a diminished LVOT gradient, and less systolic anterior motion of the mitral valve during systole.[5-7] These changes, which are due to alterations in ventricular activation sequence, were

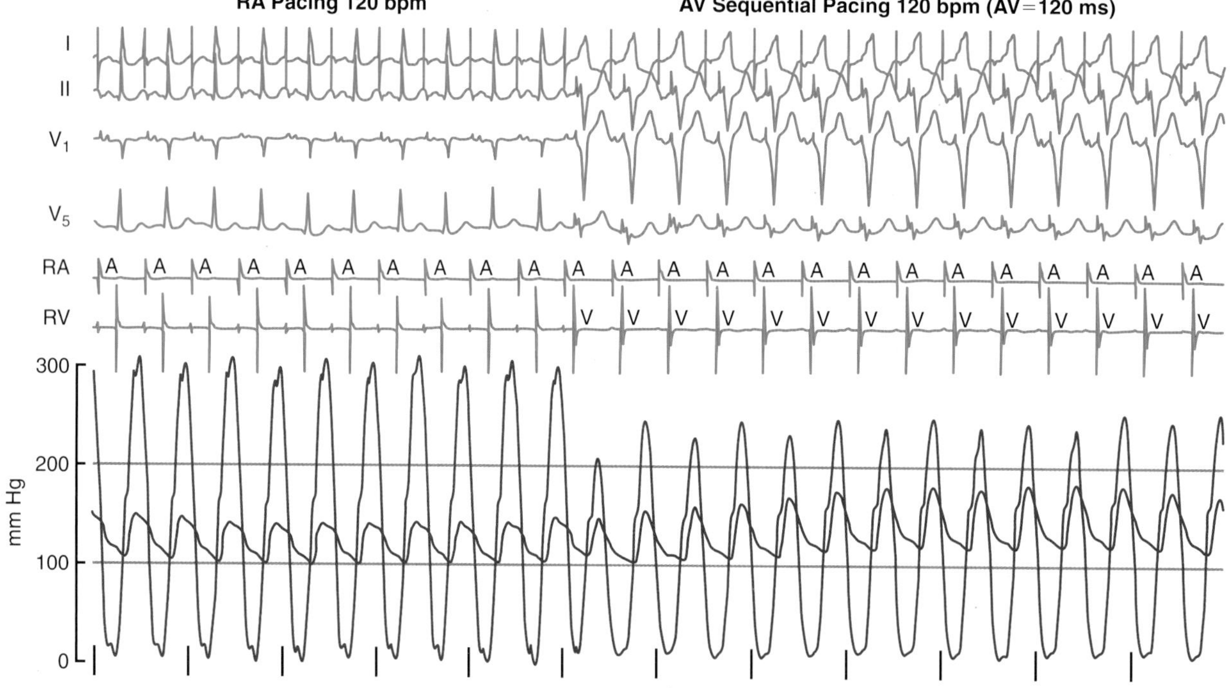

Figure 15-1. Tracing showing the impact of atrioventricular (AV) sequential pacing on left ventricular and femoral arterial pressure in an individual patient. On the left, during right atrial (RA) pacing at 120 bpm, the maximum left ventricular pressure is 330 mm Hg and the left ventricular outflow gradient is 170 mm Hg. On the right, an acute change in AV sequential pacing at the same rate is made with an AV interval of 120 msec to pre-excite the ventricular septum. The left ventricular systolic pressure is reduced to 250 mm Hg, and a left ventricular outflow tract gradient to 70 mm Hg is shown. These changes were accompanied by an improvement of the femoral arterial systolic and pulse pressures. Shown, from top *to* bottom, *are surface electrocardiogram leads I, II, III, V1, and V5; RA, right atrial intracardiac recording; A and V, atrial and ventricular intracardiac electrograms. (From Fananapazir L, Cannon RO III, Tripodi D, et al: Impact of dual chamber permanent pacing in patients with obstructive hypertrophic cardiomyopathy and symptoms refractory to verapamil and β-adrenergic blocker therapy. Circulation 85: 2149, 1992. Copyright 1992 by the American Heart Association.)*

believed to be the basis of relieving severe symptoms refractory to drug therapy.[8] These benefits from dual-chamber pacing may also extend to a small subset of patients with HCM who do not have LVOT obstruction at rest but have a severe gradient provoked by either the Valsalva maneuver or an isoproterenol infusion.[9,10] This mechanism, however, cannot explain all of the benefit due to pacing. It does not account for the ability of dual-chamber pacing to reduce LV obstruction in patients with preexisting left bundle branch block. An alternative explanation is that the asynchrony due to pacing results in a depression in contractility, manifested as a rightward shift of the end-systolic pressure-volume curve, which reduces apical cavity compression and cardiac work.[11] Finally, the change in LVOT gradient with pacing does not correlate with the presence or absence of clinical improvement.

Evidence of Clinical Benefit

Observational Studies

Several early observational studies suggested that dual-chamber pacing with a short atrioventricular (AV) delay has clinical benefit in HCM.[6,10,12] The benefit can consist of short- and medium-term decreases in symptoms and improvement in exercise capacity associated with reductions of LVOT gradient in the region of 60%. Fananapazir and colleagues[13] reported that 89% of patients with HCM undergoing DDD pacing with a short AV delay were either asymptomatic or had a dramatic improvement in symptoms after 2.3 years of follow-up. This finding was associated with regional regression of LV hypertrophy, suggesting that pacing may be associated with LV remodeling. However, these results were all from open-label, nonrandomized observational studies, with the possibility of a placebo effect. Accordingly, three randomized clinical trials were performed.

Randomized Studies

All three randomized trials enrolled patients with obstructive HCM and drug-refractory symptoms. They were all randomized, double-blind, crossover trials in which all patients received pacemakers. The patients were randomly allocated to either 3 months of DDD pacing or 3 months of minimum-rate backup pacing (either AAI or VVI at 30 beats per minute [bpm]), then crossed over to the alternative pacing mode. A study performed at the Mayo Clinic enrolled 21 patients with a mean age of 58 years who had severe, drug-refractory symptoms.[14] The LVOT gradient decreased from 76 ± 61 mm Hg at baseline to 55 ± 38 mm Hg during DDD pacing but was unchanged (83 ± 59 mm Hg) during the AAI phase. Quality of life score and exercise duration during DDD pacing were significantly better than baseline values but not significantly different from improvements noted during AAI pacing. Overall, 63% of patients had subjective improvement in dyspnea during DDD pacing, although 42% also improved while programmed to AAI (30 bpm), the placebo arm of "no pacing." There were no significant differences in the average New York Heart Association (NYHA) functional classes between baseline and either of the two pacing modes. The improvement in symptoms with AAI pacing suggests that there is an important placebo effect, underscoring the importance of randomized double-blind trials in assessing pacemaker therapy.

The European Pacing in Cardiomyopathy (PIC) study was the largest trial, enrolling 83 patients who had symptoms refractory to conventional drug treatment or who did not tolerate the drugs.[7] An important inclusion criterion was that patients were required to have experienced a reduction in the peak pressure gradient of more than 30 mm Hg as demonstrated by angiography and/or echocardiography during a hemodynamic study of dual-chamber pacing. These were therefore patients whom screening identified as likely to have a significant clinical response to DDD pacing. In 64 patients (77%), pacing induced an acute peak gradient reduction of more than 30% (from a mean of 78.5 mm Hg to 32.4 mm Hg) during short-term testing; those patients were classified as group A. In 18 patients (22%), the gradient reduction was less than 30% (from a mean of 85.3 mm Hg to 70.2 mm Hg); these patients were classified as group B. Both groups were randomly assigned to either an inactive mode (AAI) or an active mode (DDD) of pacing. After 12 weeks, the group A patients were assessed and were then crossed over to the other pacing mode. The mean LVOT gradient decreased from 53 mm Hg at baseline to a 26 mm Hg during DDD pacing ($P <$ .0001). In Group B, the mean gradient decreased from 69 mm Hg to 54 mm Hg ($P =$ .004). Exercise duration was not significantly increased, except in a subgroup of patients with more severely limited exercise tolerance (<10 minutes of the Bruce protocol).

In both groups in the PIC study, the walking times of these highly symptomatic patients improved significantly, by 21% ($P <$ .008), with active pacing. Dyspnea, angina, and functional class were better during active pacing than in the inactive phase ($P =$ .001), and 95% of patients preferred pacing. A placebo effect was once again seen, with significant improvement in symptoms compared with baseline even during the inactive AAI backup phase. Interestingly, when DDD pacing was activated after crossover, there was a significant improvement in symptoms and quality of life scores. Conversely, when patients were crossed over from DDD to AAI pacing, they showed significant deterioration in peak LVOT pressure gradient from 33 mm Hg to 59 mm Hg ($P <$ .0001). After the crossover phase, patients remained in their preferred pacing mode for 6 months and were re-evaluated 1 year after the baseline assessment. Seventy-six of 83 patients opted for active pacing. The observed gradient reduction was sustained for up to 1 year, with further improvement in symptoms and quality of life. In this study, both hemodynamic and symptomatic improvement occurred in patients with active DDD pacing.

The Multicenter Study of Pacing Therapy for Hypertrophic Cardiomyopathy (M-PATHY)[15] randomly allocated 44 patients with a mean age of 53 ± 17 years who had severe refractory symptoms to 3 months each of active (DDD) and inactive (AAI backup at 30 bpm) pacing in a double-blind crossover study design. After 6 months, all patients were offered an additional 6 months of open-label active pacing. There were no significant differences in subjective or objective measures of symptoms or exercise capacity, including NYHA functional class, quality of life, treadmill exercise time, and peak oxygen consumption, between active and inactive pacing. Importantly, however, many patients reported symptomatic improvement after pacemaker implantation, suggesting a potent placebo effect. After 6 months of open-label, nonrandomized pacing, both functional class and quality of life were improved over baseline ($P < .01$), but peak oxygen consumption was unchanged. The LVOT gradient decreased with active pacing from a mean of 82 ± 33 mm Hg after 3 months of pacing to 48 ± 32 mm Hg ($P < .001$) after 12 months, but there was marked interindividual variability in responses. In contrast to earlier nonrandomized studies, M-PATHY showed no evidence of remodeling, as assessed by change in LV wall thickness at 12 months. There also were no differences in LV diastolic and systolic functional parameters between DDD and AAI modes. Therefore active DDD pacing may have a hemodynamic benefit, but the benefit does not appear to translate into a symptomatic improvement. The symptomatic improvement that does occur with pacing seems more likely to be due to a placebo effect.

How do pacing and myectomy compare? Ommen and associates[16] compared outcome in a concurrent cohort study of 19 patients treated with dual-chamber pacing and 20 patients who underwent surgical myectomy. Symptomatic improvement was seen more frequently in those undergoing surgery (90% vs. 47%). There was a greater reduction in the LVOT gradient with surgery (mean: 76 mm to 9 mm) than after pacing (mean: 77 mm to 55 mm; $P = 0.02$ for comparison with myectomy). Similarly, exercise duration increased significantly after myectomy but *not* with pacing. Maximal oxygen consumption increased after myectomy but not in the paced group. Therefore, patients have better hemodynamic and clinical improvement with myectomy than with pacing.

Patient Selection

The randomized trials provide, at best, inconsistent evidence of clinical benefit of dual-chamber pacing in HCM. Pacemaker implantation appears to have a strong placebo effect. There are no data to support the contention that pacing alters the clinical course of the disease or improves survival or quality of life. These trials led the American College of Cardiology/American Heart Association Task Force on Practice Guidelines/North American Society for Pacing and Electrophysiology (ACC/AHA/NASPE) consensus conference to classify permanent DDD pacing as a class IIb indication for patients with significant gradients (>30 mm Hg at rest or >50 mm Hg provoked gradient; Table 15-1).[17] The evidence does not rule out the possibility of some benefit in the most significantly symptomatic patients, and it might be reasonable to try pacing in patients in whom a myectomy is contraindicated or unlikely to help.

TABLE 15-1. Pacing and Hypertrophic Cardiomyopathy

Goal	Reduce left ventricular outflow track obstruction Reduce heart failure symptoms
Level of evidence for success	Randomized short-term controlled trials Modest evidence of benefit
Consensus recommendations	Class IIb for patients with gradients >30 mm Hg at rest or >50 mm Hg provoked
Patient selection	Medically refractory heart failure with significant gradient at rest or provoked Consider the benefit of myectomy
Programming considerations	Use echocardiography to optimize atrioventricular (AV) delay Shortest AV delay that is associated with the greatest gradient reduction Pace/sense offset feature and rate-responsive AV delay

Programming

The pacemaker should have the following features: (1) flexible programming to permit the AV delay to be short, (2) a pace/sense offset feature, and (3) a rate-responsive AV delay feature. The programming of the AV delay should be individualized. The AV delay should be the longest interval that results in full apical preexcitation both at rest and during exercise.[8,12] The AV delay should be 40 to 80 msec shorter than the PR interval. The AV delay should also be greater than or equal to the P wave duration to prevent interference with left atrial emptying, and thus to avoid a decrease in stroke volume with short AV delay pacing. The use of echocardiography may help select the shortest AV delay that is associated with the greatest gradient reduction and that also does not adversely affect left atrial emptying. In some cases, normal AV conduction is very rapid, possibly leading to failure to capture the ventricle. This in turn may cause an incomplete response to pacing. The problem might be overcome through the use of AV nodal ablation. Gadler and colleagues[18] reported that in a series of 6 patients, AV nodal modification could be used to permanently prolong the native AV interval sufficiently to facilitate full apical pre-excitation without using prohibitively short AV delays.

The positioning of the ventricular lead is crucial. The hemodynamic outcome is better when pacing is performed from the RV apex than from the RV mid-septum or outflow tract.[19,20] Gadler and colleagues[20] showed that RV apical pacing is important for gradient reduction and does not reduce cardiac output. During follow-up visits, pacemaker programming should be optimized to achieve the best possible hemodynamic results. The AV delay may require adjustment with time, especially with a change in medication that slows AV conduction. Finally, in all the pacing trials, optimal medical therapy was established for all patients prior to device implantation.

Long QT Syndrome

Clinical Perspective

Patients with congenital long QT syndrome (LQTS) have a diverse group of myocardial repolarization disorders that makes their diagnosis, risk stratification, and therapy interesting and challenging. The prevalence of congenital LQTSs in the United States is about 1 in 7000 to 10,000.[21] The syndromes are usually caused by autosomal dominant genetic mutations. Long QT types LQT1, LQT2, and LQT3 account for more than 90% of cases of congenital LQTS, with LQT1 and LQT2 more common than LQT3.[22,23] Seven causal genes have been identified; five are associated with potassium channels, one with ankyrin B, and one with the sodium channel. These patients are at high risk of syncope and sudden death, usually due to a polymorphic ventricular tachycardia called torsades de pointes. This tachycardia is typically preceded by pauses or bradycardia.

Rationale for Pacing

Pacing is used in LQTS with the intent of preventing potentially arrhythmogenic pauses and bradycardia. Interestingly, there is an association between the specific genotypes and different situational triggers of this arrhythmia.[23] Exercise, emotion, and noise are more likely to trigger ventricular tachycardia in LQT1 and LQT2 than in LQT3 (85% and 67% vs. 33%, respectively). Sensitivity of patients with LQT1 to exercise may be due to prolongation of the QT interval during exercise.

Patients with LQT3 are at highest risk of event at rest or sleep.[23] Arrhythmias that occur during sleep are more often pause-dependent torsades de pointes.[24] Schwartz and colleagues[23] reported that patients with LQT3 may have fewer events with exercise or stress because they significantly shorten their action potentials during faster rates and therefore become less susceptible to catecholamine-induced arrhythmia. These findings are consistent with the clinical observation that these patients derive no benefit from therapy with β-blockers.[25] Although these findings suggest that patients with LQT3 might derive particular benefit from pacing therapy not available to patients with LQT1 and LQT2 mutations, there is no published evidence for this. The pause dependence of torsades de pointes does suggest, however, that permanent pacing might prevent it in many patients.

Evidence of Clinical Benefit

Observational Studies

There is strong evidence that in acquired LQTS, transvenous pacing is a life-saving procedure.[26,27] Similarly, observational studies[28-30] and the International Long QT Syndrome Registry[31] suggest that cardiac pacing, with concomitant β-blocker therapy, may reduce the rates of recurrent syncope and sudden death. The registry reported that in 124 patients who underwent pacing for long QT syndrome, there was an approximately 50% reduction in the incidence of cardiac events. Many of the patients received concomitant β-blocker therapy, making interpretation of results difficult. There were 30 patients, however, who received a pacemaker after failure of β-blockers without a subsequent increase in drug dose. These patients experienced a significant reduction in the incidence of syncope. However, pacing should not be implemented without concomitant β-blocker therapy and β-blocker therapy should not be stopped after a pacemaker is implanted. Of the 10 patients in whom β-blockers were withdrawn after pacemaker implantation, 3 died suddenly during the 2 years of follow-up. The benefit of pacing in such patients may be due to the prevention of bradycardia and pauses together with rate-related shortening of the QT interval.

Randomized Studies

There are no randomized controlled trials of pacing in LQTS.

Patient Selection

There is no evidence that pacing is more useful in patients with specific genotypes of LQTS or that patients with specific repolarization abnormalities or family histories respond better than others (Table 15-2). Pacing should not be used in patients who have had sustained ventricular tachyarrhythmias, who prob-

TABLE 15-2. Pacing and Long QT Syndrome

Goal	Prevent bradycardia-related QT prolongation, torsades de pointes VT, and sudden death
Level of evidence for success	Observational only
Consensus recommendations	None
Patient selection	Definite congenital long QT syndromes Patients with pause-related or bradycardia-dependent QT prolongation Syncope due to torsades de pointes Exclude cardiac arrest survivors, who should receive a defibrillator
Programming considerations	Dual-chamber pacemaker Bradycardia support rate >70 bpm Disable features that might result in transient pauses or bradycardias Avoid oversensing Consider post-extrasystole rate-smoothing algorithms

ably would do better with an implanted defibrillator. Finally, many clinicians choose a DDD defibrillator rather than a DDD pacemaker for patients with LQTS because of the unpredictable risk of sudden death.

Programming

Insertion of a dual-chamber pacemaker (rather than a single-chamber device) is the norm for patients with LQTS. Although sinus bradycardia is very common in such patients,[32] there have been several reports of functional AV block immediately before the onset of torsades de pointes ventricular tachycardia.[33,34] Careful attention to pacemaker programming is essential.[35] More rapid pacing both shortens the QT interval and reduces dispersion of repolarization. Hence high lower rates—higher than 80 bpm[36]—may be required, with the attendant disadvantages of reduced battery life and the potential risk of tachycardia-induced cardiomyopathy.[37] Patients with a lower rate limit—lower than 70 bpm—have a higher chance of recurrence of symptoms, suggesting that pacing rates lower than 70 bpm may not confer optimal protection.[29] Hysteresis and sleep function, which permit slowing of the heart rate below a safe lower rate limit, should be turned off. Meticulous programming is essential to prevent failure to capture or oversensing.

Other features that require attention are rate search hysteresis and algorithms that extend the postventricular atrial refractory period, because both can cause pauses. Rate-smoothing algorithms may prevent pause-dependent ventricular tachycardia.[38] When rate smoothing is programmed on, extrasystoles trigger pacing at a relatively fast rate for a few beats, followed by a gradual slowing until the lower rate limit is reached. This arrangement prevents post-extrasystolic pauses and relative bradycardias.

Sleep Apnea

Clinical Perspective

The *obstructive sleep apnea syndrome* is usually defined by daytime sleepiness and other sequelae attributable to frequent obstructive apneas or hypopneas during sleep. It occurs in 9% of adults, most of whom have obstructive rather than central sleep apnea. Patients with this condition are at increased risk of systemic hypertension, cardiovascular disease, including bradyarrhythmias and atrial fibrillation, and exacerbation of congestive heart failure. Several studies report improvement in sleep-disordered breathing after pacemaker implantation in patients with sinus node dysfunction and AV block.

Rationale for Pacing

The mechanism underlying the apparent improvement with pacing in sleep apnea is unclear. It might be that greater sympathetic activity during pacing might counteract sustained increases in vagal tone or that there is a central mechanism affecting both respiratory rhythm and pharyngeal motor neuron activity.[39] The studies reported results with patients who had conventional reasons for pacing, and it is unknown whether patients with sleep apnea who do not have a conventional indication for pacing would have a similar benefit.

Evidence of Clinical Benefit

Observational Studies

Permanent pacing may improve sleep apnea in patients with sinus node dysfunction and AV block.[40,41] Mizutani and coworkers[40] examined the relationship of pacing mode and sleep in a total of 16 patients (8 men and 8 women; mean age 72 years) with DDD pacemakers. Of these patients, 8 had complete AV block and 8 had sick sinus syndrome. The recording was done twice in VVI and DDD modes. Between VVI mode and DDD mode, sleep latency time, frequency of temporary waking, the number of episodes of apnea, the apnea-hypopnea index, and efficacy of sleep were all significantly lower when the patients received dual-chamber pacing. There was no significant difference in total sleep time or in total duration of temporary waking between the two groups. This study showed a significant reduction in sleep disturbance when dual-chamber pacing rather than single-chamber ventricular pacing was used.

Randomized Studies

Atrial overdrive pacing has been assessed in a randomized crossover trial.[42] The trial involved 15 patients with sleep apnea confirmed by polysomnography who had a bradycardia indication for pacing. Patients underwent sleep studies on three consecutive nights. The first night provided baseline evaluation; during the second and third nights, the patients were randomly assigned to either atrial overdrive pacing or backup ventricular pacing in a crossover design (Figs. 15-2 and 15-3). The hypopnea index was 9 ± 4 during spontaneous rhythm and 3 ± 3 during atrial overdrive pacing ($P < .001$). The combined apnea and hypopnea index was 28 ± 22 during spontaneous rhythm and 11 ± 14 ($P < .001$) during atrial overdrive pacing.

Two groups have performed randomized studies of atrially based dual-chamber pacing in patients with sleep apnea. Preliminary results of these two randomized trials do not show any benefit from pacing on indices of sleep disturbance, hypopnea/apnea episodes, or heart failure in patients in whom pacemakers were implanted for the treatment of bradycardia. Although there were differences in the patient populations studied in all these trials, the evidence that pacing improves sleep apnea is at best controversial.

Cardiac resynchronization therapy may also reduce central sleep apnea (in patients with heart failure and sleep-related breathing disorders). In a 2004 study, cardiac resynchronization therapy improved sleep apnea and sleep quality in patients with central sleep

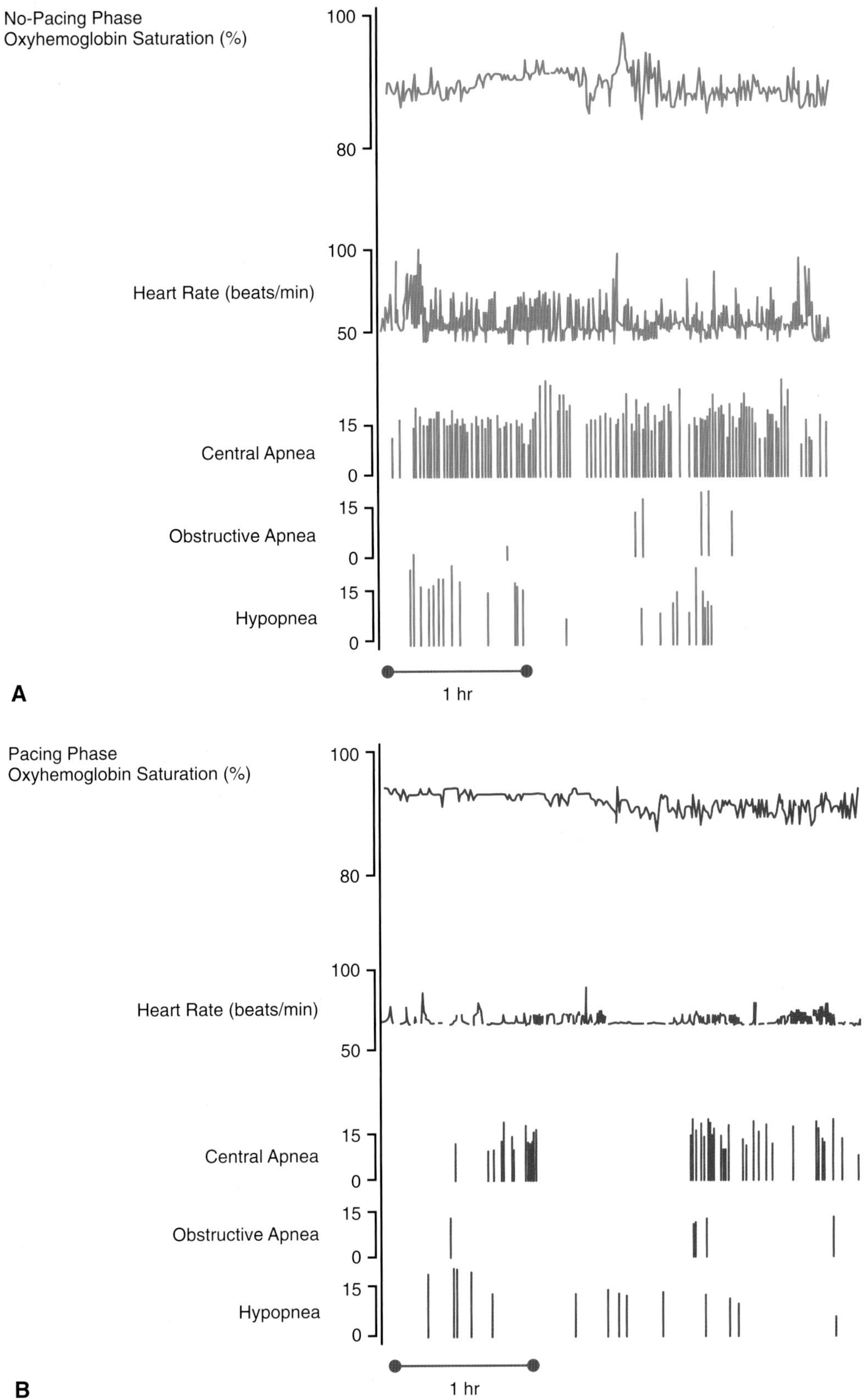

*Figure 15-2. Polysomnographic recordings in a patient with predominantly central apnea obtained with the pacemaker programmed to a fixed basic rate of 40 beats per minute (bpm) (no-pacing phase) (**A**) and with atrial overdrive pacing at 72 bpm (pacing phase) (**B**).The patient presented with very frequent episodes of central sleep apnea. Each episode of apnea or hypopnea is represented by a* vertical line; *the height of the line indicates the duration of the episode in seconds. (From Garrigue S, Bordier P, Jais PM, et al: Benefit of atrial pacing in sleep apnea syndrome. N Engl J Med 346:404, 2002.).*

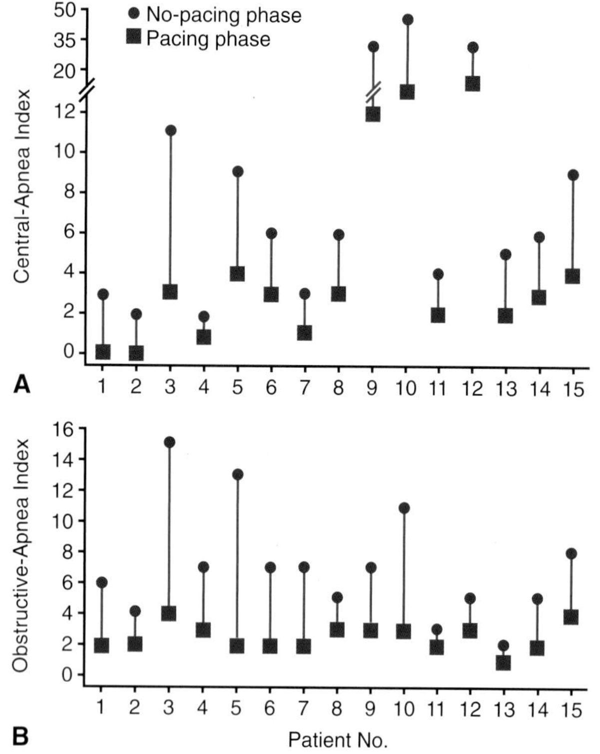

*Figure 15-3. Effect in 15 patients of atrial overdrive pacing on central sleep apnea (**A**) and on episodes of obstructive sleep apnea (**B**). The central-apnea and obstructive-apnea indexes were calculated as the number of episodes divided by the number of hours of sleep. (From Garrigue S, Bordier P, Jais PM, et al: Benefit of atrial pacing in sleep apnea syndrome. N Engl J Med. 346:404, 2002.)*

apnea, but not in patients without central sleep apnea.[43] This finding is best explained as simply an improvement in congestive heart failure.

Patient Selection

There is no published evidence that pacing improves sleep apnea in the absence of another indication for pacemaker therapy (Table 15-3).

Programming

The evidence published to date has centered on dual-chamber pacing in patients with sleep apnea.

TABLE 15-3. Pacing and Sleep Apnea

Goal	Reduce apneic episodes and their sequelae
Level of evidence for success	Early randomized studies of pacemaker patients
Consensus recommendations	None
Patient selection	Patients with sleep apnea and another indication for pacing Evidence better for central sleep apnea
Programming considerations	Use atrially based pacing (usually dual-chamber)

Neurally Mediated Syncope Syndromes

Syncope is the transient loss of consciousness with subsequent complete resolution and without focal neurologic deficits, resulting from cerebral hypoperfusion, and not requiring specific resuscitative measures. The neurally mediated syncope syndromes are a collection of clinical disorders of heart rate and blood pressure regulation caused by autonomic reflexes.[44,45] These often include bradycardia, which has led to attempts to use cardiac pacing as a therapy for carotid sinus syncope (CSS), and vasovagal syncope, the most common form of the neurally mediated syncopes.

Vasovagal syncope generally begins at a much younger age, usually occurs in the absence of any underlying structural heart disease, and can have a long and sporadic course lasting decades. Terminology is still variable, and diagnostic synonyms include ventricular syncope, empty heart syndrome, neurally mediated syncope, cardioneurogenic syncope, neurocardiogenic syncope, and neurally mediated hypotension bradycardia. We prefer the term *vasovagal syncope*, partly for historical deference, partly because of its descriptive accuracy, and partly in the absence of a compelling reason to adopt another term. In contrast to vasovagal syncope, CSS occurs in the elderly and is often associated with hypertension, peripheral vascular disease, or coronary artery disease. There are now several expert consensus conferences and position papers on these syndromes.[46,47]

Carotid Sinus Syncope

Clinical Perspective

Carotid sinus syncope is a syndrome of syncope associated with a consistent clinical history, carotid sinus hypersensitivity, and the absence of other potential causes of syncope. Historical features that suggest the diagnosis are syncope or presyncope occurring with carotid sinus stimulation that reproduces clinical symptoms, and fortuitous Holter monitoring or other documentation of asystole during syncope after maneuvers that could presumably stimulate the carotid sinus.[48-52] The incidence of CSS is low, being perhaps 35 per million cases per year.[53] CSS occurs in older patients, mainly in men. It tends to occur abruptly, with little prodrome, and only one half of patients may recognize a precipitating event. Such events most typically are wearing tight collars, shaving, head turning (as in looking to back up a car), coughing, heavy lifting, and looking up.

Symptoms of CSS range from mild presyncope to profound loss of consciousness, occasionally with significant injuries. Some patients may not recall losing consciousness, instead presenting with unexplained falls. In Britain, fits, faints, and falls are often investigated in an integrated setting with a comprehensive clinical pathway. Elderly patients with unexplained falls may have positive responses to carotid sinus massage (CSM), suggesting that CSS is responsible for many unexplained or recurrent falls.[54,55] However, physiologic carotid sinus hypersensitivity is far more common than CSS, and care should be taken in the interpretation of these results.

Natural History

Little is known about the natural history of CSS. Even though it may have a substantial effect on quality of life, it has not been shown to significantly affect mortality, and patients with CSS who receive therapy do not appear to have worse prognoses than the general population. Even in the absence of pacing, only 25% of patients may have a syncope recurrence.[56,57]

Rationale for Pacing: Physiology

The carotid sinus reflex is an integral component of the homeostatic mechanisms of blood pressure regulation.[58] Increases in intrasinus pressure stimulate mechanoreceptors, which participate in an afferent arc terminating in the brainstem. The efferent arc travels to peripheral end organs through vagal efferents, which augment cardiac vagal input and slow heart rate, and through the spinal cord to inhibit peripheral sympathetic activity in skeletal vasculature, resulting in peripheral vasodilation. This reflex maintains blood pressure within a narrow range.

An abnormal carotid sinus reflex can cause exaggerated responses of heart rate and blood pressure. There is some evidence that the major defect in carotid sinus hypersensitivity does not reside in the carotid sinus, in its neural efferents,[60] or in the brainstem. Rather, the neuromuscular structures surrounding the carotid sinus may be involved in CSS. Blanc and colleagues[61] found similar results in 30 patients without known carotid sinus hypersensitivity or syncope. Abnormal sternocleidomastoid electromyogram findings were associated with abnormal responses to CSM. It may be that because the denervated sternocleidomastoid muscle cannot provide or contribute information to the central nervous system baroreflex centers, any output from the carotid sinus is inappropriately interpreted as heightened blood pressure.

Other Therapies

When CSS is the likely cause of syncopal episodes, the initial treatment recommendation should be simple elimination of any recognized maneuvers that may precipitate an event. Discontinuation of the wearing of tight collars and ties and shaving more carefully may help. Hypovolemia should be corrected. The addition of high salt intake, of volume expanders such as fludrocortisone (Florinef),[62] or of oral vasopressors such as midodrine hydrochloride (ProAmatine) may be helpful, but such measures are frequently limited in older patients by comorbidities such as hypertension and heart failure.

In the pre-pacemaker era, recalcitrant cases of CSS were treated with carotid sinus denervation by surgical technique.[63] Surgical sinus denervation is currently reserved for cases that are secondary to head or neck tumors or lymphadenopathy, or is performed in conjunction with carotid endarterectomy or in patients with severe refractory CSS of the pure vasodepressor variety.

Evidence of Clinical Benefit

Observational Studies. Although permanent pacing is almost universally accepted for the treatment of CSS, there are no randomized, placebo-controlled trials of pacemaker therapy, patient selection, or pacemaker mode. A comprehensive summary of studies of pacing for CSS is shown in Table 15-4.[56,64-68] Earlier studies tended to be retrospective reports of pacing practices for CSS and therefore were inherently biased toward patients with a clear diagnosis of CSS who would truly benefit from pacing.

Randomized Studies. Later prospective, randomized trials examined outcomes on the basis of presence of pacing and mode. A prospective randomized trial from Reggio, Italy, reaffirmed the important role of permanent pacing for CSS.[57] Sixty patients with CSS were randomly allocated either to pacing (32 patients) or to no pacing (28 patients). During a follow-up of about 3 years, syncope recurred in 16 patients in the nonpacing group (51%) and in 3 (9%) of the pacing group (P = .002). This observation to some extent confirms the usefulness of pacing for the prevention of CSS, although a significant placebo effect cannot be excluded (see later). Finally, Kenny and associates[58a] reported the SAFE PACE trial, in which older patients (mean age: 73 ± 10 years, 60% women) with unexplained falls and cardioinhibitory response to carotid sinus massage were randomly assigned to receive either a dual-chamber pacemaker with rate-drop responsiveness or no placebo. This was an open-label trial involving 187 subjects. The investigators found that patients who received a pacemaker had a highly significant (58%) reduction in falls and a 40% reduction in syncope. Injurious events were reduced by 70% (202 in the control group, compared with 61 in the pacing group). Although these results suggest that many unexplained falls in the elderly are due to CSS and that they can be prevented with pacing, one must remember that this was an open-label trial. Trials of similar design involving patients with vasovagal syncope have been fraught with large placebo effects (see later). Finally, Kenny has also suggested that amnesia for loss of consciousness is the most likely reason why elderly patients with CSS and syncope present with falls rather than syncope.[68a]

TABLE 15-4. **Clinical Studies of Pacing for Carotid Sinus Syncope***

Study and Treatment	Study Type	Follow-Up (mos)	Patients (n)	Syncope-Free (%)
Sugrue et al:[65]	OBS			
No pacing		39	11	73
Pacing		23	23	91
Huang et al:[56]	OBS			
No pacing		42	8	88
VVI		42	9	100
DDD		42	4	100
Morley et al:[66]	OBS			
VVI		18	54	89
DVI		18	13	92
DDD		18	3	66
Brignole et al:[68]	RCT			
No pacing		8.4	19	53
Pacing		7.2	16	100
VVI		7.2	11	100
DDD		7.2	5	100
Brignole et al:[67]	Crossover			
VVI		2	26	92
DDD		2	26	100

*No differences were statistically significant. The most striking feature is how well patients appear to do regardless of attempted therapy.
OBS, observation; RCT, randomized controlled trial.

Patient Selection

Careful patient selection may help provide effective and efficient therapy for CSS (Table 15-5). Permanent pacemaker therapy is indicated for patients with recurrent, frequent, or severe CSS, and in particular for predominantly cardioinhibitory syncope.[69,70] Predictors of success with permanent pacing include multiple episodes before implantation, episodes that occur while the patient is upright or sitting, and episodes that are preceded by a recognized stimulus.[71] When syncope recurs after implantation of a permanent pacemaker, it may be due to a major persistent vasodepressor component.

TABLE 15-5. **Pacing and Carotid Sinus Syncope**

Goal	Prevent reflex bradycardia and compensate for reflex hypotension Prevent syncope
Level of evidence for success	Observational and open-label randomized controlled studies No double-blind studies
Consensus recommendations	Class I: Recurrent syncope, with syncope induced by carotid sinus massage Class IIa: Recurrent syncope, with profound bradycardia induced by carotid sinus massage
Patient selection	Syncope and positive carotid sinus massage
Programming considerations	Atrioventricular sequential pacing

Physical Diagnosis with Carotid Sinus Massage

The carotid sinus is located high in the neck below the angle of the mandible. Carotid sinus massage (CSM) is contraindicated in the presence of bruits or a history of cerebral vascular disease, transient ischemic attacks, or carotid endarterectomies. Sequential applications of carotid sinus massage to the left and right carotid arteries should be performed with at least 10 to 20 seconds between applications. The duration of CSM should be 5 to 10 seconds, and the massage should be terminated with the onset of characteristic asystole or severe presyncope. In most series, the predominant responses to carotid massage are obtained on the right side.[48] CSM should be performed while the patient is both supine and upright—either sitting or while secured safely on a tilt table. It may be difficult to document transient hypotension with standard sphygmomanometric methods, and noninvasive continuous digital plethysmography is often used.

Physiologic Responses. Carotid sinus massage (CSM) elicits both cardioinhibitory and vasodepressor responses (Fig. 15-4). A cardioinhibitory response to CSM is defined as 3 seconds or longer of ventricular standstill or asystole. Ventricular asystole usually occurs as a consequence of a sinus pause due to sinus node exit block[72] but can be due to AV block as well. A vasodepressor response to CSM, defined as a drop in systolic blood pressure of 50 mm Hg or more during

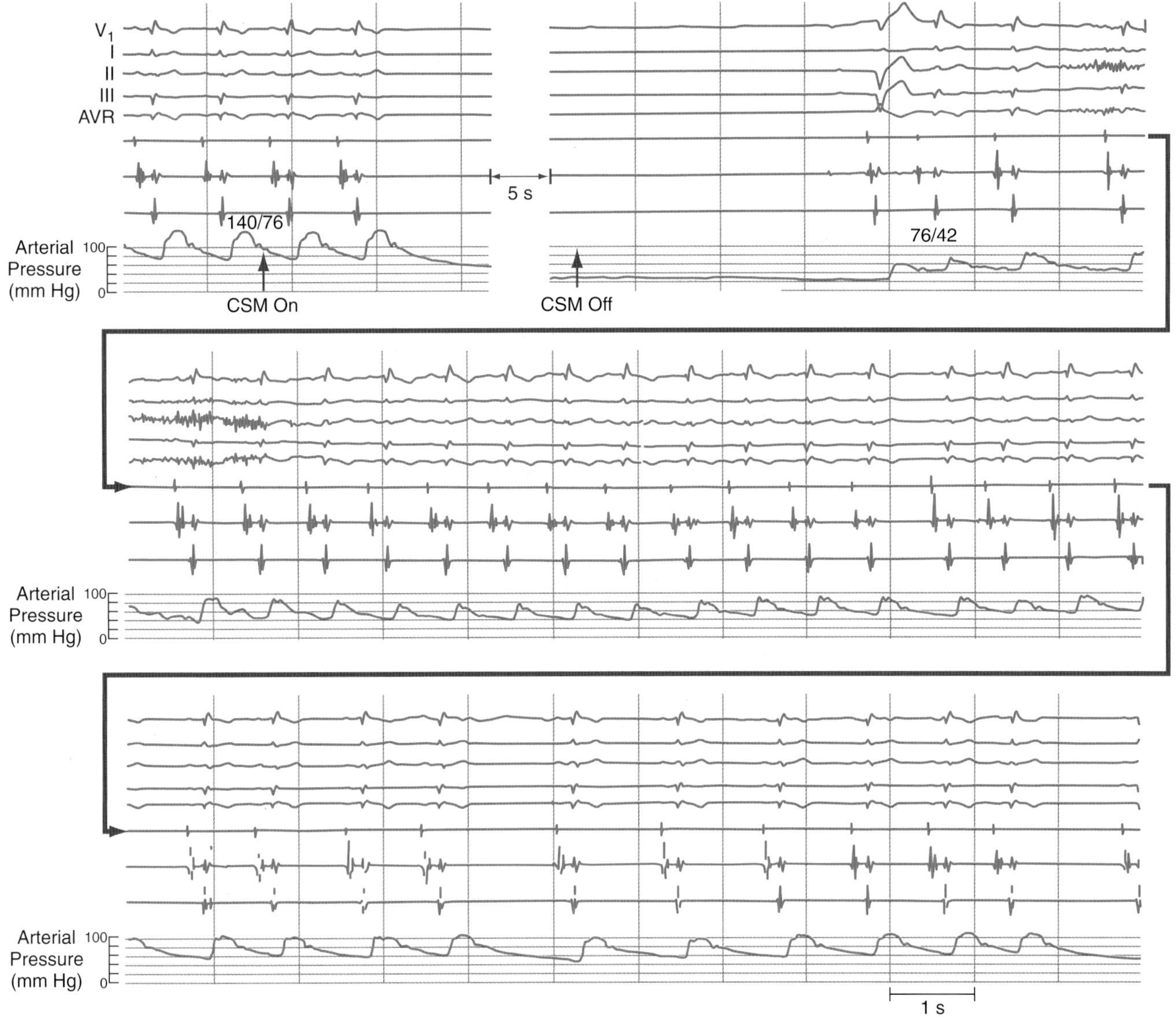

Figure 15-4. Combined cardioinhibitory and vasodepressor response to carotid sinus massage (CSM). Note the slow return of blood pressure despite the resolution of asystole. (From Almquist A, Gornick C, Benson W, et al: Carotid sinus hypersensitivity: Evaluation of the vasodepressor component. Circulation 71:927, 1985. Copyright 1985 American Heart Association.)

massage; this response may be difficult to demonstrate in patients who have a significant cardioinhibitory component. In contrast to the induced cardioinhibitory component of carotid sinus hypersensitivity, the vasodepressor response may have a more insidious, slower onset and a more prolonged resolution.

Carotid Sinus Hypersensitivity and Carotid Sinus Syncope. *Carotid sinus hypersensitivity* denotes the abnormal physiologic responses, either cardioinhibitory or vasodepressor or both, to CSM. The presence of asymptomatic carotid sinus hypersensitivity is quite common in populations of older adults. For example, a positive cardioinhibitory response to CSM was noted in 32% of patients undergoing coronary angiography.[73] CSS is the syndrome of syncope in association with carotid sinus hypersensitivity and in the absence of other apparent causes of syncope.

Complications. CSM is quite safe if done carefully. It is contraindicated in patients with a history of cerebrovascular disease or carotid bruits, in whom it can cause cerebrovascular accidents. In a review of 3100 episodes of CSM performed on 1600 patients, there were seven complications (0.14%), all of which were neurologic and transient.[74] Rare arrhythmic complications include asystole and ventricular fibrillation.[75]

Programming

AAI pacing is contraindicated in CSS because many patients may eventually demonstrate associated reflex AV block.[76] In general, patients appear to benefit most from AV sequential pacing, even when a significant component of vasodepressor CSS is present. VVI pacing should not be used in patients with intact VA conduction,[77] because of possible pacemaker syndrome. Lack of VA conduction at a given point in time, however, does not ensure against its future development. Therefore, we recommend dual-chamber pacemakers for patients with CSS and normal sinus rhythm.

Few studies have examined the role of rate-responsive pacing in CSS. Patients are generally older and therefore may have bradycardia comorbidities such as sick sinus syndrome and chronotropic incompetence, either intrinsic or due to medications. Therefore, rate-responsive pacing might be beneficial. Similarly, few studies have prospectively examined pacing with rate-drop or hysteresis capabilities, which has the theoretical advantage of providing rapid, higher-rate, AV sequential pacing to counteract the vasodepressor component during attacks of CSS.[78]

Vasovagal Syncope

Clinical Perspective

Vasovagal syncope is the most common of the neurally mediated syncopal syndromes (Table 15-6). Most people who faint probably do not seek medical attention for isolated events. Prolonged standing, sight of blood, pain, and fear are common precipitating stimuli for this, the common faint. Patients experience nausea, diaphoresis, pallor, and loss of consciousness as a result of hypotension with or without significant bradycardia. Return to consciousness after seconds to 1 or 2 minutes is the norm. Those with adequate warning may be able to use physical counterpressure maneuvers, or simply sit or lie down, to prevent a full faint. For some patients, however, there is little or no prodrome or recognized precipitating stimulus and no marked bradycardia accompanies the faint.[79-83] These patients have sparked interest in the use of permanent pacing as a therapy.

TABLE 15-6. Principles of Management of Vasovagal Syncope

Diagnosis and prognosis	Confirm diagnosis with history, tilt-table tests, loop recorder Assess likelihood of syncope recurrence (>2 spells or recent worsening)
Assess patient needs	Insight into diagnosis Cause of syncope Probability of syncope recurrences Treatment options
Conservative advice	Limit salt and fluid intake Physical counterpressure maneuvers Driving and reporting to authorities Avoidance and management of triggers
Medical options	Fludrocortisone (weak evidence) Midrodine HCl (good evidence) Serotonin reuptake inhibitors (weak evidence) β-Blockers in patients >42 years old (modest evidence)
Permanent pacing	Weak evidence

Although we prefer the term *vasovagal syncope* to signify reflex fainting due to bradycardia and/or hypotension, there are numerous synonyms—emotional faint, reflex syncope, empty heart syndrome, neurally mediated syncope, situational syncope, vasomotor syncope, ventricular syncope, neurocardiogenic syncope, hypotension-bradycardia syndrome, and autonomic syncope. In addition, the terms *convulsive syncope* and *venipuncture fits* have been used to describe those patients with vasovagal syncope who experience generalized muscle movements that may resemble epilepsy.[84,85]

Epidemiology of Vasovagal Syncope. About 40% of people faint at least once in their lives, and at least 20% of adults faint more than once.[86,87] Fainters usually present first in their teens and twenties and may faint sporadically for decades. This long, usually benign, and sporadic history can make for difficult decisions about therapy. Syncope is responsible for 1% to 6% of emergency room visits and 1% to 3% of hospital admissions.[88-90] Tilt table tests are commonly used as a diagnostic tool, although they are limited by difficulties with sensitivity, specificity, reproducibility, and little evidence-based agreement on methodologic details and outcome criteria. Positive tilt table test results (Fig. 15-5) are characterized by presyncope, syncope, bradycardia, and hypotension, and a reproduction of the patient's pre-syncope symptoms.[91,92] Although many patients of all ages simply have vasovagal syncope, clinicians must remain vigilant and look for other causes, including valvular and structural heart disease, sick sinus syndrome, CSS, and orthostatic hypotension.

Symptom Burden and Quality of Life. The vasovagal syncope syndrome has an extremely wide range of symptom burden, from a single syncopal spell in a lifetime to daily faints. Some patients have very sporadic presentations, with periods of intense symptoms interspersed with long periods of quiescence. Several observational studies and randomized clinical trials reported that patients have a median of 5 to 15 syncopal spells

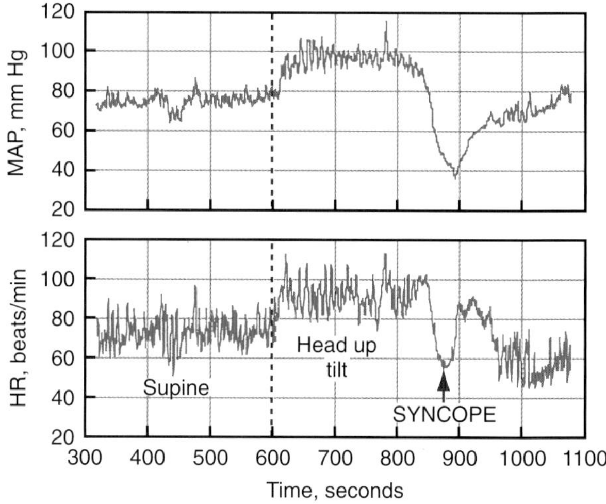

Figure 15-5. Hypotension and bradycardia induced during a positive drug-free passive tilt table test response.

and a duration of fainting of 2 to 60 years.[93-96] Patients with recurrent syncope are impaired much like those with severe rheumatoid arthritis or chronic low back pain or like psychiatric inpatients.[93] The quality of life decreases as the frequency of syncopal spells rises.[94]

After clinical assessment, many patients continue to do poorly. After 1, 2, and 3 years, 28%, 38%, and 49% of patients, respectively, faint again.[97] Interestingly, several studies reported a 90% reduction in the total number of faints in the population after a tilt table test. The cause for this apparently great reduction in syncope frequency after assessment is unknown, but it does leave a large number of patients who request further treatment. Therefore, when assessing syncope patients, clinicians must be alert to the surprising impairment of quality of life that many patients endure, must provide a perspective that lasts decades, and must remember that the clinical state of such a patient will probably fluctuate.

Rationale for Pacing

Physiology of Vasovagal Syncope. Syncope is a transient loss of neurologic function due to a global reduction of cerebral blood flow. Sudden cessation of cerebral blood flow results in loss of consciousness within 4 to 10 seconds.[98] Lesser reductions in blood flow may result in presyncope. Almost all vasovagal syncope occurs while the patient is in an upright position and is usually associated with heightened physiologic or psychological stress, such as prolonged orthostatic stress, arising quickly and walking, pain, fear, or other strong emotion, seeing blood or medical procedures, or heavy exercise.

There is no unified hypothesis that explains all the aspects of the pathophysiology of vasovagal syncope. The classic explanation, advanced by Sharpey-Shafer, is based on animal models suggesting that LV mechanoreceptors located primarily in the inferoposterolateral LV can trigger vagally mediated bradycardia and decrease sympathetic output to the peripheral arteriolar vasculature, resulting in vasodilation and hypotension. This model is based on the Bezold-Jarisch reflex: Orthostatic stress increases sympathetic tone, and the resultant increase in β-adrenoreceptor stimulation causes either increased contractility or increased gain in the LV baroreceptors. Thus, a relatively hypovolemic, vigorously contracting ventricle is the presumed trigger of the reflex.

There are three main concerns with this model. The first is the uncertainty that the particular animal models and measurements appropriately illuminate the human condition. Second, vasovagal syncope can be provoked in patients with heart transplants, which are centrally denervated for at least one year after transplantation.[99,100] Third, there is relatively little evidence from echocardiographic studies of loss of LV volume preceding the onset of the vasovagal reaction on tilt table tests. Other important factors may include reduced plasma volume and salt sensitivity,[101] blunting of vagal and sympathetic baroreflex response to orthostatic stress,[102,103] altered peripheral vascular and endothelial reflex responses,[104] and impaired cerebral autoregulation.[105,106]

Transient hypotension is the most common hemodynamic manifestation of vasovagal syncope. Many patients have inappropriate peripheral sympathetic responses to physiologic and psychological stressors. Under conditions in which the normal response may be vasoconstriction, patients with syncope usually fail to demonstrate it. Abnormalities have been documented in arteriolar vasoconstriction, splenic venoconstriction, and venous capacitance. The ultimate cause of hypotension is an abrupt cessation of vascular sympathetic traffic, causing withdrawal of α-adrenergic tone.

Evidence for Bradycardia in Vasovagal Syncope. Permanent pacemaker therapy could be effective if bradycardia is a common and symptomatically important feature of vasovagal syncope. The evidence for clinically important bradycardia comes from studies that have used tilt table tests, pacemaker memory, and implantable loop recorders to record heart rate during syncopal spells.

Tilt Table Tests. Bradycardia frequently occurs during vasovagal syncope induced by tilt table testing.[107,108] The mean heart rate during syncope induced by passive head-up tilt table tests is 30 bpm, and asystole longer than 3 seconds is often documented. However, there is uncertainty about the relationship between hemodynamics observed on tilt table testing and clinical vasovagal syncope. For example, the investigators in the International Study on Syncope of Uncertain Etiology (ISSUE; see later) found no relationship between the heart rate during syncope on tilt table testing and the heart rate during syncope occurring spontaneously in the community.[109] Patients with tilt table test–induced bradycardia frequently do not have bradycardia during clinical syncope.[102,103] Therefore, although bradycardia is the rule rather than the exception during a positive tilt table test response, the bradycardia evoked on a tilt table test may not resemble the hemodynamics during syncope in that patient during day-to-day living.

Pacemaker Memory. Is asystole in patients in the community commonly associated with syncope? Evaluation of frequent fainters with pacemakers programmed to act as event recorders demonstrated that although transient asystole is common during documented syncope, many other asymptomatic asystolic episodes also occurred. Only 0.7% of asystolic events lasting 3 to 6 seconds and 43% of events lasting more than 6 seconds resulted in symptoms of presyncope or syncope.[110] Therefore, even asystole of several seconds' duration does not necessarily cause syncope.

Implantable Recorders. The implantable loop recorder (ILR) permits prolonged electrocardiographic monitoring, and its use is a reasonable approach to the diagnosis of patients with infrequent syncope. Current ILRs weigh only 17 grams and have battery lives of 14 months. The electrocardiographic signal is stored in a buffer that can be frozen with a manual activator. The ILR has programmable automatic rate detection parameters for high and low rates as well as pause detection. In a Canadian study of 206 patients with syncope, symptoms recurred in 69% of patients; bradycardia was detected more frequently than tachycardia (17% vs. 6%).[111,112]

The ISSUE investigators studied 111 patients with syncope who had previously undergone tilt table testing. Not all tilt table test responses were positive.[113] In both patient groups, those with positive and those with negative tilt table test results, clinical events occurred in 34% of patients group over a follow-up of 3 to 15 months. Marked sinus bradycardia or asystole was detected during syncope (46% and 62%, respectively). Therefore, quite a wide range of bradycardic episodes is reported during syncope: Between 17% and 62% of patients with vasovagal syncope had significant bradycardia during syncope in the ILR studies.[111-113] The heart rate response during tilt table testing did not predict spontaneous heart rate response, asystole being observed more frequently than expected on the basis of the tilt table test response. Thus, many patients with positive tilt table test results may have some degree of bradycardia at the time of presyncope or syncope, and pacing may be a plausible treatment.

Conservative Therapy

Pacing should be tried only in patients with vasovagal syncope who have not shown responses to other treatments or are not candidates for them. Currently, most clinicians first teach the patients about the causes of syncope, encourage fluid and salt intake, and coach physical counterpressure maneuvers. If this initial approach is unsuccessful, attempts at pharmacologic therapy with drugs such as fludrocortisone, midodrine, β-blockers, and serotonin reuptake inhibitors are made. Only after these options have been explored should permanent pacing be considered.

Reassurance and Education. Most patients with vasovagal syncope simply require reassurance and education. Many of the patients with more frequent syncope also benefit from these conservative measures. Patients have four broad areas of learning needs—etiology, management, natural history, and prognosis.[114] These areas should be covered in efforts to provide patients with reassurance and education. In particular, patients should be taught to recognize their prodromal symptoms and to sit or lie down as quickly as possible to minimize injury during recurrences and lessen the severity of attacks.

Salt and Fluids. Blood volume is an important factor in the pathophysiology of vasovagal syncope. Syncope almost always occurs in the upright position, and many patients faint solely from orthostatic stress in situations such as attendance at religious services, cadet parades, outdoor band practices, and showering. Prolonged drug-free head-up tilt provokes syncope in a large number of patients with syncope, depending on the duration and angle of the head-up tilt.[115] Finally, many patients report avoiding dietary salt and have a low daily urinary sodium excretion.[101]

Two studies reported that acute volume loading prevented syncope on tilt table testing in adolescents with vasovagal syncope and a previously positive tilt table test response. A combined 53 of 62 patients had a subsequent negative response after receiving 10 to 15 mL/kg of saline intravenously.[116,117] El-Syed and Hainsworth[101] reported a small, placebo-controlled study of salt supplements in patients with vasovagal syncope. Eight weeks of salt supplements increased plasma volume and urinary sodium excretion and also increased time to presyncope during a combination of head-up tilt and lower-body negative pressure. Similarly, Claydon and Hainsworth[118] showed that orthostatic cerebral and vascular control improved after the administration of 100 mmol/day of slow-release sodium for 2 months. Thus, orthostatic stress causes vasovagal syncope, and salt supplements and acute volume loading help prevent it. Unless contraindicated, patients should drink at least 2 liters of water per day and should consume high-salt meals. Salt tablet administration can be useful in patients with a urinary sodium excretion of less than 170 mmol per day. Salt supplementation should be avoided in patients with a history of hypertension or heart failure.

Physical Counterpressure Maneuvers. Physical counterpressure maneuvers may be quite helpful, although no blinded, controlled studies confirming their usefulness have been reported. Patients must have a prodrome long enough that they can react by isometrically tightening muscles using maneuvers such as squatting, leg crossing, and fist clenching. Brignole and associates[119] showed that vigorous isometric arm tensing around a small ball raised blood pressure 30% to 40% and prevented 80% to 90% of presyncope and syncope responses on tilt table testing. Similarly, leg crossing raises blood pressure 50% to 60% and eliminates symptoms on tilt table testing.[120] There are two remaining problems with counterpressure techniques. Patients must have enough warning to act on them, and symptoms, including syncope, often recur when the muscles are relaxed. Whether these techniques will help during daily life is unknown. A randomized clinical trial, the Physical Counterpressure Trial, has finished and is under review.

Medical Therapy

There are no therapies that have been proved in large randomized clinical trials to prevent vasovagal syncope. Few have been subjected to rigorous clinical trials, and when interpreting results of open-label studies, one should remember that most patients appear to improve after assessment. There is an estimated 90% reduction in syncope in the population after tilt table testing.[121] The four major drug classes that are used are α_1-adrenergic agonists, β-adrenergic blockers, serotonin-specific reuptake inhibitors, and salt-retaining mineralocorticoids.

Vasopressors. There is reasonable evidence for the effectiveness of the α_1-adrenergic agonist midodrine. A pro-drug, midodrine was shown to reduce symptoms of syncope and presyncope in three small, randomized clinical trials. Ward and associates[122] reported that compared with placebo, midodrine significantly increased the number of symptom-free days in 16 highly symptomatic patients. Subsequently, Perez-Lugones and colleagues[123] reported an open-label randomized study of 61 patients showing that patients who received midodrine had significantly fewer syncopal spells than patients who did not.[123] This study was not blinded, and thus, a placebo effect cannot be excluded. Finally, Kaufmann and associates[124] reported that midodrine reduced the likelihood of a positive tilt table test result to 17%, compared with a 67% likelihood in patients receiving placebo. The major limitations of midodrine are the need for frequent dosing and its tendency to raise supine blood pressure. The latter side effect is usually seen at higher doses (>30 mg/day). Midodrine should not be used in patients with hypertension. It also causes piloerection and crawling paresthesias in the scalp.

Serotonin-Specific Reuptake Inhibitors. Numerous small open-label studies of serotonin-specific reuptake inhibitors in the early 1990s reported that serotonin-specific reuptake inhibitors prevented the induction of syncope on tilt table tests and reduced symptoms in patients in the community. Paroxetine, a selective serotonin reuptake inhibitor, was found to be effective in preventing syncope in one randomized placebo-controlled study[125] and numerous case report series. In contrast, Takata and associates[126] reported that paroxetine did not block the vasovagal reaction elicited by lower-body negative pressure. These drugs do not appear to be used widely for the prevention of syncope.

β-Blockers. The evidence for the effectiveness of β-blocker therapy is mixed. It has a strong physiologic rationale, as well as positive results in two and negative results in one open-label study involving 42 to 153 patients.[127-129] Five randomized clinical trials have evaluated the efficacy or effectiveness of β-adrenergic blockers for the prevention of syncope.[130-134] Although the results are not completely consistent, they do suggest strongly that β-blocker therapy does not prevent vasovagal syncope. Mahanonda and coworkers,[130] studying 42 patients with an unspecified mix of historical presyncope and syncope and positive tilt table test results, reported that after 1 month, 71% of patients receiving atenolol and only 29% of patients receiving placebo reported feeling better and had fewer combined presyncopal and syncopal spells.

Madrid and associates[131] randomly assigned 50 patients with vasovagal syncope to either treatment with atenolol 50 mg daily, or placebo.[131] Patients were monitored for up to 1 year, during which a nonsignificantly higher number of patients in the group taking atenolol had recurrent syncope than those taking placebo. Flevari and colleagues[132] performed a prospective, randomized crossover study of nadolol, propranolol, and placebo in 30 patients with recurrent vasovagal syncope and positive tilt table test responses. These investigators found a remarkable 80% to 90% reduction in all measures of presyncope and syncope in all three treatment arms, with no significant difference among the three arms. Ventura and coworkers[133] randomly allocated 56 patients with recurrent syncope either to treatment with β-blockers or to no treatment. In a 1-year follow-up, syncope recurred in 71% of untreated patients and only 29% of patients who received β-blockers. The strength of the conclusions of this study is weakened by its lack of placebo control and blinding.

Sheldon and colleagues[134] performed the Prevention of Syncope Trial, whose design has been described elsewhere. It was a randomized, placebo-controlled, double-blind trial designed to assess the effects of metoprolol in vasovagal syncope over a 1-year treatment period. Nearly 40% of the subjects had at least one recurrence of syncope during the 1-year observation period, as predicted in the initial power calculations. Metoprolol was no more effective than placebo in preventing vasovagal syncope in the study population as a whole. Taken together with the results of the previous four smaller studies, these data indicate that metoprolol and atenolol, and possibly β-adrenergic receptor blockade in general, are ineffective in preventing vasovagal syncope in the broad patient population. A substudy showed a possible benefit in middle-aged and elderly patients.

Fludrocortisone Acetate. Fludrocortisone acetate has mineralocorticoid activity without appreciable glucocorticoid effect at doses up to 0.2 mg, which are the commonly used clinical doses for various disorders.[135] The immediate actions of fludrocortisone acetate are sodium and water retention at the expense of urinary potassium excretion. Two open-label trials examined fludrocortisone in neurocardiogenic syncope. Both demonstrated clinical improvement but neither was placebo controlled.[136,137] Salim and Di Sessa[138] reported a small, placebo-controlled, randomized clinical trial of fludrocortisone acetate (Florinef) in children with vasovagal syncope. Patients taking the drug did significantly worse ($P < .04$) than those taking placebo. Other drugs have been studied, but not in adequately powered, placebo-controlled, randomized clinical trials.

Evidence of Clinical Benefit of Pacing in Vasovagal Syncope

Four groups assessed the effect of pacing in preventing syncope induced by tilt table testing (Table 15-7). Forty-one patients with a positive initial tilt table test result and a marked bradycardia underwent a second tilt table test with temporary pacing at rates around 85 to 100 bpm.[107,108,110,138-143] Taken together, the studies showed that temporary dual-chamber pacing prevented the development of syncope in 24 of 41 subjects (57%).[139-141] However almost all the conscious patients experienced the vasovagal reaction and had significant presyncope. Temporary pacing may be partly effective in preventing vasovagal syncope but does not prevent presyncope.

Rate Drop–Responsive Pacemakers. The strategy that emerged in the early 1990s was to attempt to use cardiac pacing not only to overcome transient brady-

TABLE 15-7. **Clinical Studies of Rate Drop–Responsive Pacing in Vasovagal Syncope**

Study	Type	Patients (n)	Treatment Tested	Results
Petersen et al[144]	2-period	31	Rate hysteresis	62% stopped fainting
Benditt et al[78]	2-period	28	Rate drop	78% stopped fainting
Sheldon et al[145]	2-period	12	Rate smoothing	50% stopped fainting
First North American Vasovagal Pacemaker Study (VPS I)[146]	Unblinded RCT	54	Rate drop	Hazard ratio down 85% 78% stopped fainting
Vasovagal Syncope International Study (VASIS)[147]	Unblinded RCT	42	Rate hysteresis	Hazard ratio down 80% 95% stopped fainting
Syncope Diagnosis and Treatment (SYDAT) Study[148]	Unblinded RCT	93	Rate drop vs. atenolol	Hazard ratio down 87% 95% stopped fainting
Ammirati et al[149]	Unblinded RCT	20	Rate drop vs. rate hysteresis	Rate drop better than rate hysteresis
VPS II[154]	Blinded RCT	100	DDD-rate drop vs. ODO	No significant difference
McLeod et al[153]	Blinded RCT	12	No pacing vs. VVI–rate hysteresis vs. DDD–rate drop	Pacing better than not; pacing modes equivalent
Vasovagal Syncope and Pacing Trial (SYNPACE)[155]	Blinded RCT	29	DDD–rate drop vs. ODD	No difference

RCT, randomized controlled trial.

cardia during syncope but also to provide enough heart rate support to compensate for the transient hypotension that is part of the vasovagal reflex. The major issues in the development of pacing strategies are the detection of the onset of syncope and whether pacing is effective at all during the episode. Given the modest efficacy of simple bradycardia support in preventing syncope induced by tilt table tests, investigators soon turned to more flexible and more sophisticated modes of sensing and pacing.

Sensors of Transient Heart Rate Drops. Three combined sensing and pacing options have been assessed clinically in some detail: rate hysteresis, rate smoothing, and rate-drop sensing. Rate hysteresis is the oldest. With this approach, pacing at a relatively high rate is triggered by a drop in heart rate below a low detect rate. An example of settings might be a sensing rate of 40 bpm and a pacing response rate of 90 bpm. Typically the high rate pacing might be interrupted periodically to permit the pacemaker to detect an underlying rate, and might cease pacing if the rate is high enough.

Rate smoothing is used to avoid abrupt and sustained changes in heart rate. An abrupt drop in heart rate over only one to three beats elicits a pacing response at a slightly lower rate, and this pacing rate gradually slows until it is below the accelerating intrinsic heart rate. Rate drop–responsive pacing is a more sensitive and sophisticated variant of rate hysteresis. An abrupt drop in heart rate of a programmable magnitude over a programmable duration elicits a burst of high rate pacing for 1 to 2 minutes. The drop in heart rate need only be on the order of 10 bpm, over a few seconds, and the high rate might be around 90 to 110 bpm.

Observational Studies. Three groups reported studies on the usefulness of long-term pacing in the prevention of vasovagal syncope. Petersen and colleagues[144] reported the first clinical study of dual-chamber pacing with rate hysteresis in 37 patients with syncope. The patients had experienced a median of six syncopal spells, and a positive tilt table test response with bradycardia. Of the 37 patients, 31 received pacemakers with rate hysteresis. Over a mean follow-up of 50 months 62% of the patients remained free of syncope, and the number of syncopal spells in the total population fell from an expected number of 136 to only 11. Benditt and associates[78] reported equally encouraging results in a study of 36 patients with predominantly vasovagal syncope. The patients were very symptomatic, with a median of 10 syncopal spells over about 2 years, or about 5 spells yearly. All patients received a pacemaker with rate drop responsiveness. The patients were monitored for a mean of 6 months. During this time, syncope recurred in only 6 patients, compared with expected recurrences in about 30 patients. Therefore, in this relatively short-term study, pacing may have benefited about 80% of patients.

Sheldon and associates[145] studied 12 extremely symptomatic patients who had had a median syncope frequency of three spells per month.[145] All had a positive tilt table test response and recurrent syncope while receiving medical therapy. All received a pacemaker with a rate-smoothing feature but without a high rate response. After implantation of the pacemaker, the actuarial syncope-free survival increased 20-fold, the syncope frequency dropped by 93%, and the improvement in quality of life was highly significant. These were all sequential design studies, with no control for time-dependent effects or for the placebo effect of pacemaker implantation.

Open-Label Randomized Studies of Rate-Drop Responsiveness. The first North American Vasovagal Pacemaker Study (VPS I) tested whether permanent pacing with rate-drop responsiveness would reduce the likelihood of syncope in patients with frequent vasovagal syncope.[146] Patients were eligible if (1) they had fainted six or more times before tilt table testing or they had fainted within the first year after a positive tilt table test result and (2) they had a predefined degree of bradycardia. Patients were randomly allocated either to receive a pacemaker with automatic rate-drop responsiveness or to receive the best medical therapy according to their treating physicians. The 54 patients were randomly allocated evenly to pacemaker or no pacemaker. There was a lower rate of syncope recurrence in the pacemaker patients (6/27) than in the medically treated patients (19/27). The hazard ratio for a recurrence of syncope in the pacing group compared with the medically treated group was 0.087 (P = .000016). The likelihood of a first syncope recurrence among patients randomly assigned to receive a pacemaker (or not) in VPS I is shown in Figure 15-6.

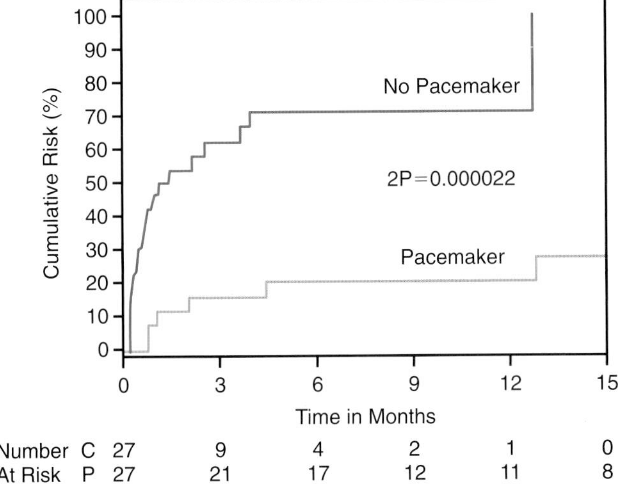

Figure 15-6. *Cumulative likelihood of a recurrence of syncope in patients randomly assigned to receive or not to receive a pacemaker in the North American Vasovagal Pacemaker Study. C, control; P, pacemaker. (From Connolly SJ, Sheldon RS, Roberts RS, Gent M: The North American Vasovagal Pacemaker Study: A randomized trial of permanent cardiac pacing for the prevention of vasovagal syncope. J Am Coll Cardiol 33:16, 1999.)*

Although VPS I was the first randomized trial to show benefit from pacing, it appeared to have a number of limitations. First, it was an open-label study. The investigators believed that there was insufficient evidence of pacemaker effectiveness to enable them to implant a device in all subjects and therefore selected an open-label design. Second, the patients were highly select: They had all fainted frequently, had positive tilt table test responses with the development of bradycardia, and agreed to participate in a study with only a 50% chance of receiving new therapy—that is, a pacemaker. The pacemaker could have benefited these patients through either conventional bradycardia support or by the sophisticated rate-drop responsiveness algorithm. Finally, medical therapy was not standardized.

Ammirati and colleagues[148] performed a small, randomized clinical trial comparing rate hysteresis and rate drop responsiveness. Twenty patients with moderately frequent syncope received a pacemaker with either rate hysteresis or rate-drop responsiveness. Three patients with rate hysteresis fainted during follow-up, whereas no patients with rate-drop responsiveness did so ($P < .05$). This small study suggested that rate-drop responsiveness is superior to rate hysteresis in preventing syncope, and therefore that not all of the pacemaker effect was due to placebo.

In the Vasovagal Syncope International Study (VASIS), 19 patients were randomly assigned to receive a dual-chamber pacemaker with rate hysteresis, and 23 patients to no pacemaker implant.[147] The patients all had experienced three or more syncopal spells over the preceding 2 years, with a median of 6 spells, and a cardioinhibitory response to tilt table testing. The VASIS subjects had a lower syncope burden than the subjects in VPS I. During a mean follow-up of 3.7 ± 2.2 years there was a lower likelihood of a syncope recurrence in the pacemaker group than in the no pacemaker group (5% vs. 61%; P = .0006). The intention-to-treat results are shown in Figure 15-7. Similar to VPS I, VASIS was an open-label study that involved highly select patients and could not eliminate a placebo effect.

The Syncope Diagnosis and Treatment (SYDAT) trial tested whether pacemakers or atenolol better prevented vasovagal syncope.[148] Ninety-three patients were randomly assigned to receive a DDD pacemaker with rate-drop responsiveness (n = 46) or to atenolol therapy (n = 47). All patients were older than 35 years, had had more than 3 syncopal spells in the preceding 2 years, and had a positive tilt table test response with a trough heart rate lower than 60 bpm. There was at least one syncope recurrence in 4.3% of the pacing group, compared with 26% of the atenolol group (Odds Ratio 0.13; P = .004). This was another open-label study of pacing in vasovagal syncope using a highly select population. One confounding issue is a possible deleterious effect of the atenolol rather than a beneficial effect of pacemaker implantation. This possibility seems unlikely, given the overall neutral effect of β-blockers in the randomized clinical trials summarized in the preceding section.

In summary, observational reports[78,144,145] and four randomized, open-label, controlled studies[146,147,149] sug-

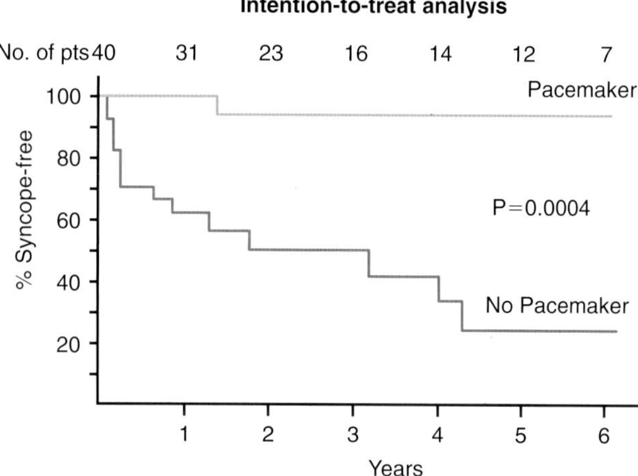

Figure 15-7. Cumulative likelihood of a recurrence of syncope in patients randomly assigned to receive or not to receive a pacemaker in the Vasovagal Syncope International Study. (From Sutton R, Brignole M, Menozzi C, et al: Dual-chamber pacing in the treatment of neurally mediated tilt-positive cardioinhibitory syncope: Pacemaker versus no therapy: A multicenter randomized study. The Vasovagal Syncope International Study (VASIS) Investigators. Circulation 102:294, 2000.)

gested strongly that patients have less syncope after they receive a permanent pacemaker. But is this effect real? All of these studies were unblinded for both patients and physicians. Syncope is an outcome that can be difficult to verify objectively. Surgical procedures can have a placebo effect.[150-152] Patients receiving a pacemaker may have benefited from the psychological effects of receiving a surgical procedure from enthusiastic health professionals. Given these uncertainties, the invasiveness and cost of pacing mandated placebo-controlled or blinded trials to determine the true beneficial effect of pacing in vasovagal syncope.

Blinded Randomized Studies of Rate-Drop Responsiveness. Three blinded studies have compared the benefit of rate-drop responsive pacemakers with what was anticipated to be lesser therapy. McLeod and associates[153] reported the efficacy of rate drop–responsive, dual-chamber pacing in the prevention of vasovagal syncope in 12 highly symptomatic young children who had frequent syncope associated with asystolic pauses longer than 4 seconds. This was a three-way, double-blind, randomized crossover study in which the pacemakers were programmed to no active pacing, ventricular pacing with rate hysteresis, or dual-chamber pacing with rate-drop responsiveness. The two pacing modes were equivalently more effective than no pacing in preventing syncope, and dual-chamber pacing was superior to ventricular pacing in preventing presyncope. This small study concluded that rate drop–responsive pacing was more efficacious than no pacing in preventing vasovagal syncope in children.

To ascertain the true therapeutic effect size of permanent pacing in vasovagal syncope, Connolly and associates[154] performed the second North American Vasovagal Pacemaker Study (VPS II), a larger double-blind trial.[154] The investigators expected that the risk of syncope in the control group would be reduced to some extent by the placebo effect of device implantation, so they increased the study sample size accordingly. VPS II was a multicenter, double-blind, placebo-controlled randomized clinical trial. Patients were eligible if they had recurrent vasovagal syncope with at least six lifetime syncope spells, or at least three spells in the 2 years prior to enrollment, and a positive response on a tilt table test performed according to the protocol in use in each center. A requirement for a specific degree of bradycardia during tilt table testing was not included because trough heart rate during tilt table testing did not correlate in patients with heart rate during clinical syncope,[115] and because trough heart rate during tilt table testing did not appear to predict response to pacing.[5,24]

After receiving dual-chamber pacemakers, all patients were randomly assigned either to dual-chamber pacing with rate-drop responsiveness or to sensing without pacing. The patients' health care providers remained blinded to treatment allocation, except for an unblinded nurse or physician who did all the programming but disclosed no details. The study was designed to have 80% power to detect a 50% relative reduction in the risk of recurrent syncope from a rate of 60% in the control group to 30% in the treatment group. There were 100 patients in the study, who were evenly divided into active pacing and sensing only groups. A total of 38 patients had syncope during the 6-month follow-up period. Twenty-two of 52 patients randomly assigned to sensing-only mode had recurrent syncope within 6 months, compared with 16 of 48 in the active pacing group. The cumulative risk of syncope at 6 months was 40% (95% confidence interval [CI] = 25% to 52%) for the sensing-only group and 31% (95% CI = 17% to 43%) for the rate drop–responsive group (Fig. 15-8). The relative risk reduction in time to syncope with active pacing was 30% (95% CI = −33% to 63%; one-sided $P = .14$). A retrospective analysis did not identify any variable that predicted benefit from pacing except in patients who received isoproterenol during the tilt table test.

Most importantly, VPS II found no statistically significant benefit in favor of pacemaker therapy for the prevention of syncope. The most important difference between the results of VPS I and VPS II is the observed risk of syncope in the nonpacing group. In VPS I, almost 80% of control patients fainted within 6 months, whereas in VPS II, only 41% of control patients fainted within 6 months. In contrast, the 6-month likelihoods of syncope in the patients receiving active pacing therapy were similar in the two studies: 20% in VPS I and 31% in VPS II.

The Vasovagal Syncope and Pacing (SYNPACE) trial involved 29 patients who had had a median of 12 lifetime syncopal spells, a positive tilt table test response, and bradycardia during the syncope induced by the tilt table test.[155] They received a dual-chamber rate drop–responsive pacemaker and were randomly allocated to either active pacing or no pacing modes. The trial was stopped early, after the VPS II results were released. Thirteen patients had at least one syncope recurrence,

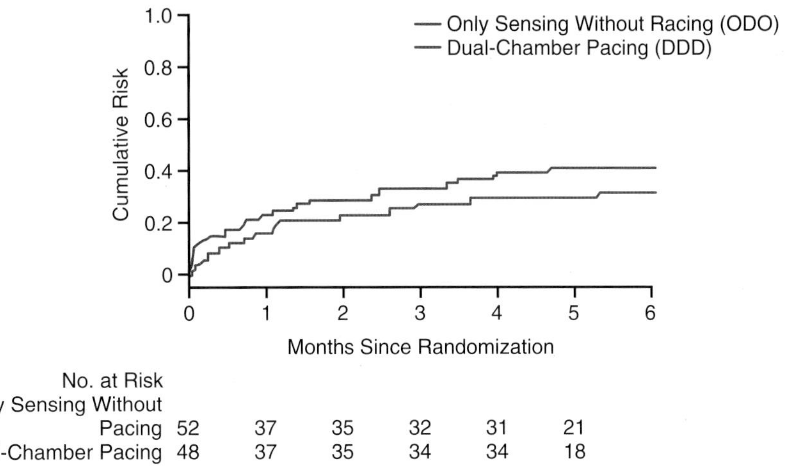

Figure 15-8. Kaplan-Meier plots of the time to the first recurrence of syncope among 48 patients randomly assigned to receive active dual-chamber pacing and 52 patients randomly assigned to receive a pacemaker in the sense-only mode, by intention-to-treat analysis in the second Vasovagal Syncope Pacemaker Study (VPS 2). (From Connolly SJ, Sheldon R, Thorpe KE, et al; on behalf of the VPS II Investigators: The Second Vasovagal Pacemaker Study [VPS II]: A double-blind randomized controlled trial of pacemaker therapy for the prevention of syncope in patients with recurrent severe vasovagal syncope. JAMA 289:2224, 2003.)

and there was no benefit from active pacing with rate-drop responsiveness. Although extremely underpowered, the SYNPACE trial did not provide any support for the usefulness of pacing in the prevention of vasovagal syncope.

Why Did VPS II and SYNPACE Not Show Benefit for Pacing? Both VPS II and the SYNPACE trial did not demonstrate a statistically significant benefit of pacemaker therapy for the prevention of vasovagal syncope. Although the SYNPACE trial was underpowered because of early termination, VPS II was the largest randomized trial of pacemaker therapy for vasovagal syncope, whether open label or double blinded. The researchers made a considerable effort to maintain blindedness, and there were no known protocol violations. This strict adherence sets the standard for randomized trials of treatments for vasovagal syncope. The possible reasons for the negative outcomes are (1) a simple play of chance, (2) early termination of previous studies, (3) the lack of bradycardia on tilt table testing as an inclusion criterion, (4) insufficiently accurate patient selection, (5) inadequate sensing with the rate drop criterion, (6) a placebo effect in open-label studies, and (7) inability to overcome vasodepression with high rate pacing.

Play of Chance. VPS II was designed to detect a relative risk reduction of 50% due to pacing. The observed relative risk reduction was 30% with a wide 95% confidence interval. Nevertheless, the very large relative risk reductions in the four unblinded randomized trials are well outside the 95% confidence interval of the relative risk reduction seen in VPS II. This trial did have reasonable power to detect a relative risk reduction of 50%, which may be the minimum effect size that would justify permanent pacing.

Early Termination of Open-Label Studies. An important difference between VPS II and the four open-label trials was that three of the four previous trials were stopped prematurely. Early termination of a trial for unexpected efficacy tends to overestimate the treatment effect.

Lack of Demonstrated Bradycardia at Baseline. A common speculation about the interpretation of the results of VPS II is that the lack of a requirement for a prespecified bradycardia provoked by tilt table testing may have contributed to selecting a population less amenable to the benefits of pacing. This seems unlikely for several reasons.

Patients in the VASIS and the SYDAT studies had more pronounced bradycardia and documented asystole.[147] This raises the possibility that the patient selection was insufficiently accurate and that a prespecified bradycardia during syncope on tilt table testing might identify patients more likely to have a response. However the tilt table–induced bradycardia noted during syncope on the baseline test was similar in VPS I, and heart rate changes during tilt table testing neither correlate with heart rate changes during clinical syncope nor predict responses to pacing. As well, tilt table test bradycardias during VPS I and VPS II were quite similar. For example, in VPS I, 12 of 54 patients enrolled (22%) had a rate lower than 40 bpm during tilt, compared with 19 of 100 patients (19%) in VPS II. Therefore, numbers of patients with extreme bradycardia at the time of positive tilt table test response in the two studies were similar, and this minor difference in study design is probably not the reason for the different results of the two studies.

Furthermore, the SYNPACE trial, which required a prespecified bradycardia during syncope on tilt table testing, also had a negative result. Indeed, the predictive ability of bradycardia on tilt table testing may not be useful. For example, trough heart rate during tilt table testing does not predict improvement after pacemaker insertion. Petersen and colleagues[144] found that the extent of cardioinhibition did not correlate with the level of benefit from permanent pacing. The ISSUE investigators also reported that asystole during tilt table testing did not predict asystole during follow-up[143]; indeed, some patients with tilt table–induced asystole had syncope without bradycardia (vasodepressor syncope). An asystolic response during recurrent syncope was found even if the patient had a vasodepressor response during the tilt table test. Taken together, these data suggest that the hemodynamic response during tilt table testing (including trough heart rate) does not predict the hemodynamic responses during spontaneous syncope and does not predict the response to permanent pacemaker insertion.

Strictly speaking, VPS II and the SYNPACE trial simply failed to demonstrate a significant benefit, and it remains possible that there is a small benefit, either in each patient or in a fraction of the population. We recently examined the long-term benefit from pacemaker insertion for vasovagal syncope. This open-labeled, observational study evaluated 40 patients with severe syncope. Thirty-five patients had positive tilt table testing. Pacemakers were programmed to rate drop-responsiveness or rate-smoothing algorithms in equal numbers. Rate-drop responsive pacemakers were implanted in 20 patients, and 20 patients received rate-smoothing pacemakers.

Raj and associates[156] found an overall 87% decrease in the median frequency of syncope over an approximate 5-year follow-up period (0.46 vs. 0.06 spells/month; $P = .04$). However, only 32.5% of their subjects continued to be syncope-free at 60 months. Patients were labeled "responders" to pacing therapy if they experienced reduction of syncopal episodes by more than 75% after implantation. With use of this definition, 55% of patients were long-term "responders." There was no difference in response according to pacing algorithm, as was previously expected. Patient characteristics of "responders" and "nonresponders" were similar, thus making predictions about which patients might benefit from pacing unlikely. Of particular relevance to this discussion, trough heart rate during tilt table testing was found *not* to predict long-term response to cardiac pacing. The findings of this study were entirely consistent with the overall negative results of VPS II and the SYNPACE trial.

Vasodepression Cannot Be Paced. Prevention of bradycardia is the main physiologic mechanism by which a pacemaker can prevent attacks of syncope. During positive tilt table test responses, however, reductions in blood pressure begin earlier than the development of bradycardia.[140,141] Pacing therapy might not help patients with hypotension due to vasodepression even if bradycardia or asystole also occurs at the time of syncope. The results of VPS II and the SYNPACE trial suggest that most episodes of vasovagal syncope may be associated with profound vasodepression as the cause of syncope, rather than simply bradycardia. In this light, pacing per se may simply be ineffective in the setting of profound vasodepression, and future progress in device therapy might best target implantable drug delivery systems.

Placebo Effect in Open-Label Studies. The history of attempts to treat patients with implanted devices has other examples of an initial promise of therapeutic success followed by subsequent well-controlled studies with negative results. For example, open-label studies suggested that dual-chamber pacing causes a marked improvement in the hemodynamics and functional status of patients with HCM. Later randomized, controlled, blinded studies revealed evidence of a much smaller effect size. Similarly, preliminary open-label studies suggested that atrially based pacing might prevent atrial fibrillation, but well-controlled, randomized, crossover trials showed much less benefit from conventional atrially based pacing for the prevention of atrial fibrillation.[157,158] Finally, large, open-label studies provided strong evidence for the ability of atrially based pacing to reduce stroke and death in patients with pacemakers. A large, randomized, blinded, controlled study showed that patients with atrially based pacemakers derived no benefit with respect to death, stroke, quality of life, or exercise tolerance for several years after implantation in comparison with patients with single-lead ventricular pacemakers.[159] From this experience, it appears that care should be taken in the assessment of results of open-label or nonrandomized pacemaker studies. The placebo effect can be substantial.

There are several reasons why pacemaker therapy may be associated with an initial spurious benefit. First, patients receiving expensive or invasive therapy may be loath to admit the possibility that such a therapy might be ineffective. Particularly with surgical procedures, the placebo effect can be pronounced.[150-152] Second, many patients with vasovagal syncope appear to improve spontaneously after tilt table testing.[90,95,96] This effect may account for up to 90% of the apparent benefit. The mechanism is unknown but may involve the counseling received at the time of the clinic visit, a regression to the mean, and the sporadic nature of the timing of manifestations of vasovagal syncope. This effect is similar in magnitude to the beneficial effect of pacing in sequential design trials. It is possible, in the unblinded studies, that some patients, hoping to have received a pacemaker and disappointed by being randomly allocated not to receive one, may have been more prone to report syncope. Conversely, patients receiving a pacemaker may have benefited from the psychological effects of receiving a surgical procedure from enthusiastic health care professionals. The double-blind trial design, to a considerable extent, removes this type of potential bias.

Patient Selection

Patients should have a definite history of vasovagal syncope based on a positive tilt table test response, suggestive loop recorder findings, or scrupulous history (Table 15-8). Given the weakness of the evidence supporting the efficacy of pacing, it is reasonable to institute pacing only in patients with documented profound bradycardia or asystole during syncope. Only patients at high risk of syncope recurrences should undergo pacing. The frequency and number of syncopal spells preceding positive tilt table test responses are independent risk factors that predict an early recurrence of syncope after the test. Criteria such as having more than six syncopal spells over any duration of time, or at least two syncopal spells in the preceding year, or any recurrence of syncope within a year of tilt table testing, generally select patients who have a more than 50% risk of at least one syncopal spell in the next 2 years. Otherwise, similar patients with syncope and either negative or positive tilt table test responses have similar likelihoods of syncope after assessment.[160,161]

TABLE 15-8. Pacing and Vasovagal Syncope

Goal	Prevent reflex bradycardia and compensate for reflex hypotension Prevent syncope
Level of evidence for success	Limited evidence for benefit based on double-blind randomized controlled trials May be a subset of patients with proved bradycardia who benefit
Consensus recommendations	Class IIa. Recurrent vasovagal syncope with clinically documented bradycardia, or bradycardia induced on tilt test
Patient selection	Medically refractory, frequent, disabling vasovagal syncope Documented pauses during syncope Tilt test results not helpful
Programming considerations	Dual-chamber pacemaker Benefit from specific sensor to drive rate response or pacing algorithm (rate-drop response, ventricular impedance) not proved

The result of the tilt table test (negative versus positive) does not predict subsequent clinical outcome. Similarly, the lowest heart rate (including asystole) during tilt table testing does not predict the eventual likelihood of syncope in clinical follow-up.[115,144]

Programming

There is an inexorable trade-off between sensitivity and specificity in programming rate-responsive pacemakers to detect the early stages of syncope. The main detection features are the range over which heart rate must fall, the time interval during which the drop must take place, and the number of confirmation beats below the minimum detection heart rate. Decreasing the specified heart rate range or number of confirmation beats improves the sensitivity, as does lengthening the time during which the heart rate fall must occur. Generally, the pacemakers greatly overdetect, with therapies delivered many times daily. This arrangement is usually well tolerated, particularly if the patient perceives a benefit in syncope prevention, but in some patients, the palpitations are intolerable. This can be particularly true at night, when respiratory sinus arrhythmia is larger and the patient is quieter. Although there is an understandable tendency to program the rate-drop feature "off" at night, doing so affords the patient no potential protection at night should he or she arise. This can be a problem, because patients have usually not had any fluids for hours and can have syncope provoked by either orthostatic changes or micturition.

Pacing therapy is usually a relative high rate burst. The pacemaker should be programmed to deliver atrially based pacing at rates of 90 to 110 bpm for 1 to 2 minutes. There is no evidence of greater benefit from any particular rate or duration.

Evolving Paradigms and Technology

Contractility Sensors. The search continues for alternative sensing strategies, such as QT interval, respiratory volume or frequency, RV pressure transduction (dP/dt), and indices of contractility. These are intended to sense either early hypovolemia or early rises in sympathetic activity that may precede frank syncope. There is some evidence that contractility can be estimated with measures of endocardial acceleration, with use of a microaccelerometer in the pacemaker lead to estimate RV myocardial contractility,[162,163] or with intracardiac impedance measurements.[164,165] The theory behind contractility sensors is that vasovagal syncope might be preceded by small but significant increases in contractility due to a sympathetic surge. These devices increase pacing rates in response to increases in apparent contractility, and then slowly decrease their rates after contractility subsides toward baseline. Discouragingly, Brignole and colleagues[162] found that endocardial acceleration did not predict the occurrence of tilt table–induced syncope.

The use of closed-loop stimulation (CLS) was evaluated in a preliminary study in 2002.[165] CLS pacemaker technology reacts to a change in the RV intracardiac impedance, which is believed to be a surrogate measure of contractility and, therefore, sympathetic tone. This study of 22 patients demonstrated that syncope is predicted by impedance changes and could be prevented on tilt table testing of patients with cardioinhibitory syncope. A subsequent study used CLS prospectively in 34 patients with recurrent vasovagal syncope.[166] Over 12 to 50 months of follow-up, 30 of 34 patients had not experienced a recurrent syncopal event. On the basis of this pilot study, a larger, multicenter randomized trial, the Inotropy Controlled Pacing in Vasovagal Syncope (INVASY) study, was planned and partially carried out.[167] Twenty-six patients with recurrent vasovagal syncope and a positive tilt table test response with induced bradycardia received dual-chamber pacemakers with CLS. Asymmetric randomization assigned patients to simple DDI pacing (9 of 26) and/or to dual-chamber pacing with CLS. This was an open-label trial. It was stopped early, after a preliminary analysis (Fig. 15-9) at a mean of 19 months showed that 7 of the 9 patients in the DDI group and none of the 17 patients in the CLS group had syncope recurrences ($P < .0001$). These positive results suggest three possible conclusions: (1) pacing can be useful in patients with vasovagal syncope, (2) CLS based on RV impedance changes is effective sensing for syncope, and (3) this may be the placebo effect once again. A larger and properly blinded study is being planned.

Automatic Drug Delivery Systems. Current pacemaker therapies focus only on heart rate support. This might not be as useful in patients with a predominantly vasodepressor response. Giada and coworkers[168] described a study assessing a novel implantable system that delivers phenylephrine when activated at the onset of syncope (prodrome with a drop in blood pressure). When treated with the phenylephrine, 15 of 16 patients had an immediate rise in blood pressure and a termination

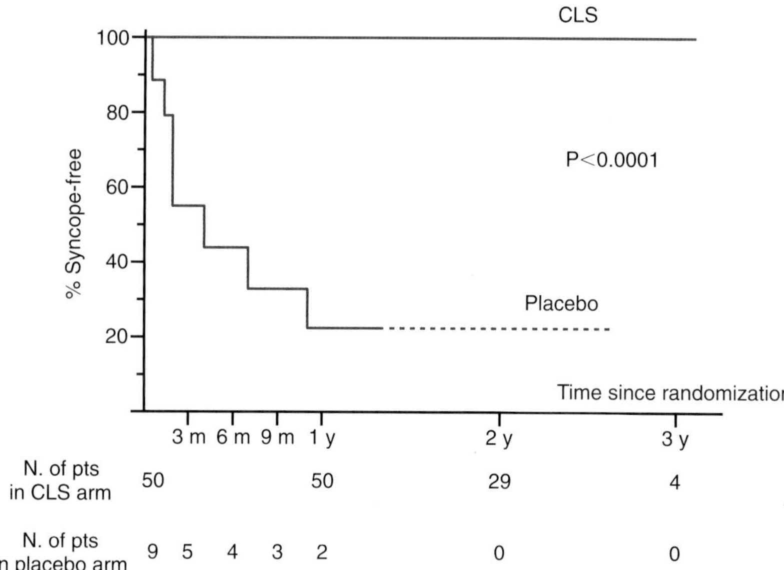

Figure 15-9. Probability of remaining free of syncopal recurrences according to Kaplan-Meier estimation in 41 patients in the closed-loop stimulation arm and 9 patients in the control group in the Inotropy Controlled Pacing in Vasovagal Syncope (INVASY) study. (From Occhetta E, Bortnik M, Audoglio R, Vassanelli C; INVASY Study Investigators: Closed loop stimulation in prevention of vasovagal syncope. Inotropy Controlled Pacing in Vasovagal Syncope (INVASY): A multicentre randomized, single blind, controlled study. Europace 6:538, 2004.)

of their tilt table–induced syncope, despite ongoing tilt table testing. In contrast, none of the patients was able to abort the episodes when a placebo infusion was delivered. The one patient who fainted despite the phenylephrine experienced a severe cardioinhibitory response to the tilt table test. This small study suggests the promise of a combined approach using pacing for the cardioinhibitory component and immediate pharmacologic support for the vasodepressor component of syncope.

Implications for Future Trials

Several lessons can be learned from this discussion. First, clinical trials of vasovagal syncope must be placebo-controlled and double-blinded to mitigate the sizable potential for the placebo effect. Second, the potential for the placebo effect must be considered when population sample is calculated. Third, initial efforts might be directed toward understanding whether there are physiologic differences between patients who faint during pacing and those who do not. Fourth, accurate patient selection may be important.

Guidelines for Pacing in Vasovagal Syncope

At the least, pacing should not be used early in patients with vasovagal syncope. First, it should be reserved for patients with frequent, highly symptomatic vasovagal syncope whose quality of life is markedly diminished and whose syncope has not responded to lifestyle and dietary changes, education, reassurance, the use of counterpressure maneuvers,[46,47] and at least three medication attempts. Second, pacing might be more effectively used in patients with documented asystole at the time of syncope. Third, all patients should have frank and detailed education about the limited (at best) evidence of its efficacy. In light of this, a revision of the ACC/AHA/NASPE pacing guidelines issued in 2002 should be reconsidered,[17] because they recommended permanent pacemaker implantation for patients with symptomatic and recurrent neurocardiogenic syncope associated with bradycardia documented spontaneously or at the time of tilt table testing.

REFERENCES

1. Maron BJ: Hypertrophic cardiomyopathy. Lancet 350:127, 1997.
2. Maron BJ, Shen WK, Link, MS, et al: Efficacy of implantable cardioverter defibrillation for the prevention of sudden death with hypertrophic cardiomyopathy. N Engl J Med 342:365, 2000.
3. Elliott PM, Sharma S, Varnava, A, et al: Survival after cardiac arrest or sustained ventricular tachycardia in patients with hypertrophic cardiomyopathy. J Am Coll Cardiol 33:1596, 1999.
4. Silka MJ, Kron J, Dunnigan A, Dick M 2nd: Sudden cardiac death and the use of implantable cardioverter defibrillator in pediatric patients: The Pediatric Electrophysiology Society. Circulation 87:800, 1993.
5. McDonald KM, Maurer B: Permanent pacing as treatment for hypertrophic cardiomyopathy. Am J Cardiol 68:108, 1991.
6. McDonald K, McWilliams E, O`Keeffe B, et al: Functional assessment of patients treated with permanent dual chamber pacing as a primary treatment for hypertrophic cardiomyopathy. Ann Thorac Surg 47:236, 1988.
7. Kappenberger L, Linde C, Daubert C, et al: Pacing in hypertrophic obstructive cardiomyopathy: A randomized crossover study. Eur Heart J 18:1249, 1997.
8. Fananapazir L, Cannon RO, Tripodi D, et al: Impact of dual chamber permanent pacing in patients with obstructive hypertrophic cardiomyopathy with symptoms refractory to verapamil and beta-blocker therapy. Circulation 85:2149, 1992.
9. Slade AKB, Sadoul N, Shapiro L, et al: DDD pacing in hypertrophic cardiomyopathy, a multicenter clinical experience. Heart 75:44, 1996.
10. Gadler F, Linde C, Juhli-Dannfeldt A, et al: Long-term effects of dual chamber pacing in patients with hypertrophic cardiomyopathy without outflow tract obstruction at rest. Eur Heart J 18:636, 1997.
11. Pak PH, Maughan WL, Baughman KL, et al: Mechanism of acute mechanical benefit from VDD pacing in hypertrophied heart: Similarity of responses in hypertrophic cardiomyopathy and hypertensive heart disease. Circulation 98:242, 1998.

12. Jeanrenaud X, Goy J, Kappenberger L, et al: Effects of dual-chamber pacing in hypertrophic obstructive cardiomyopathy. Lancet 339:1318, 1992.
13. Fananapazir L, Epstein ND, Curiel RV, et al: Long-term results of dual-chamber (DDD) pacing in obstructive hypertrophic cardiomyopathy: Evidence for progressive symptomatic and hemodynamic improvement and reduction of left ventricular hypertrophy. Circulation 90:2731, 1994.
14. Nishimura RA Trusty JM, Hayes DL, et al: Dual-chamber pacing for hypertrophic obstructive cardiomyopathy: A randomized, double-blind crossover trial. J Am Coll Cardiol 29:435, 1997.
15. Maron BJ, Nishimura RA, McKenna WJ, et al: Assessment of permanent dual-chamber pacing as a treatment for drug-refractory symptomatic patients with obstructive hypertrophic cardiomyopathy: A randomized, double-blind, crossover study (M-PATHY). Circulation 99:2927, 1999.
16. Ommen SR, Nishimura RA, Squires RW, et al: Comparison of dual-chamber pacing versus septal myectomy for treatment of patients with hypertrophic obstructive cardiomyopathy: A comparison of objective hemodynamic and exercise end points. J Am Coll Cardiol 34:191, 1999.
17. Gregoratos G, Abrams J, Epstein AE, et al; American College of Cardiology/American Heart Association Task Force on Practice Guidelines/North American Society for Pacing and Electrophysiology Committee: ACC/AHA/NASPE 2002 guideline update for implantation of cardiac pacemakers and antiarrhythmia devices: Summary article: A report of the American College of Cardiology/American Heart Association Task Force on Practice Guidelines (ACC/AHA/NASPE Committee to Update the 1998 Pacemaker Guidelines). Circulation 106:2145, 2002.
18. Gadler F, Linde C, Darpo B: Modification of atrioventricular conduction as adjunct therapy for pacemaker-treated patients with hypertrophic obstructive cardiomyopathy. Eur Heart J 19:132, 1998.
19. Chang AC, Atiga WL, McArevey D, et al: Relief of left ventricular outflow tract obstruction following inadvertent left ventricular apical pacing in a patient with hypertrophic cardiomyopathy. Pacing Clin Electrophysiol 18:1450, 1995.
20. Gadler F, Linde C, Juhli-Dannfeldt A, et al: Influence of right ventricular pacing site on left ventricular outflow tract obstruction in patients with hypertrophic obstructive cardiomyopathy. J Am Coll Cardiol 27:1219, 1996.
21. Schwartz PJ: The long QT syndrome. Curr Probl Cardiol 22:297, 1997.
22. Splawski I, Shen J, Timothy KW, et al: Spectrum of mutations in long-QT syndrome genes: KVLQT1, HERG, SCN5A, KCNE1, and KCNE2. Circulation 102:1178, 2000.
23. Schwartz PJ, Prior SG, Spazzolini C, et al: Genotype-phenotype correlation in long-QT syndrome: Gene-specific triggers for life-threatening arrhythmia. Circulation 103:89, 2000.
24. Benhorin J, Medina A: Congenital long QT syndrome. N Engl J Med 336:1568, 1997.
25. Moss AJ, Zareba W, Hall WJ, et al: Effectiveness and limitations of beta-blocker therapy in congenital long-QT syndrome. Circulation 101:616, 2000.
26. Sclarovsky S, Strsberg B, Lewin R, et al: Polymorphous ventricular tachycardia: Clinical features and treatment. Am J Cardiol 44:339, 1979.
27. DiSegni E, Klein HO, David D, et al: Overdrive pacing in quinidine syncope and other long QT-interval syndromes. Arch Intern Med 140:1036, 1980.
28. Elder M, Griffin JG, Hare V, et al: Combined use of beta adrenergic blocking agents and long-term cardiac pacing for patients with long QT syndrome. J Am Coll Cardiol 20:830, 1992.
29. Moss AJ, Liu JE, Gottlieb S, et al: Efficacy of permanent pacing in the long QT syndrome. Circulation 84:1524, 1991.
30. Eldar M, Griffin JG, Abbott JA, et al: Permanent cardiac pacing in patients with the long QT syndrome. J Am Coll Cardiol 10:600, 1987.
31. Zareba W, Priori SG, et al: Permanent pacing in the long QT syndrome patients. Pacing Clin Electrophysiol 20:1097, 1997.
32. Schwartz PJ, Periti M, Malliani A: The long QT syndrome. Am Heart J 89:378, 1975.
33. Van Hare GF, Franz MR, Roge C, et al: Persistent functional atrioventricular block in two patients with prolonged QT interval: Elucidation of the mechanism of block. Pacing Clin Electrophysiol 13:608, 1990.
34. Scott W, Dick M: Two to one atrioventricular block in infants with congenital long QT syndrome. Am J Cardiol 60:1409, 1987.
35. Viskin S: Cardiac pacing in the long QT syndrome: Review of available data and practical recommendation. J Cardiovasc Electrophysiol 11:593, 1999.
36. Viskin S, Alla SR, Baron HV, et al: Mode of onset of torsades de points in congenital long QT. J Am Coll Cardiol 28:1262, 1996.
37. Klein H, Levi A, Kaplinsky E, et al: Congenital long QT syndrome: Deleterious effect of long-term high rate ventricular pacing and definitive treatment by cardiac transplantation. Am Heart J 132:1079, 1996.
38. Viskin S, Fish R, Roth A, Copperman Y: Prevention of torsades de points in the congenital long QT syndrome: Use of a pause prevention pacing algorithm. Heart 79:417, 1998.
39. Gottlieb DJ: Cardiac pacing—a novel therapy for sleep apnea? N Engl J Med 346:444, 2002.
40. Mizutani N, Waseda K, Asai K, et al: Effect of pacing mode on sleep disturbance. J Artif Organs 6:106, 2003.
41. Kato I, Shiomi T, Sasanabe R, et al: Effect of physiological cardiac pacing on sleep-disordered breathing in patients with chronic bradydysrhythmias. Psychiatry Clin Neurosci 55:257, 2001.
42. Garrigue S, Bordier P, Jais O, et al: Benefit of atrial pacing in sleep apnea syndrome. N Engl J Med 346:404, 2002.
43. Sinha AM, Skobel EC, Breithardt OA, et al: Cardiac resynchronization therapy improves central sleep apnea and Cheyne-Stoke respiration in patients with chronic heart failure. J Am Coll Cardiol 44:68, 2004.
44. Benditt DG, Remole S, Milstein S, et al: Causes, clinical evaluation and current therapy. Ann Rev Med 43:283, 1992.
45. Brignole M, Alboni P, Benditt DG, et al: Guidelines on management (diagnosis and treatment) of syncope: Update 2004: Executive Summary. Eur Heart J 25:2054, 2004.
46. Brignole M, Alboni P, Benditt DG, et al; Task Force on Syncope, European Society of Cardiology: Guidelines on management (diagnosis and treatment) of syncope: Executive Summary. Eur Heart J 22:1256, 2001.
47. Gregoratos G, Cheitlin MD, Conill A, et al: ACC/AHA/ Guidelines for Implantation of Cardiac Pacemakers and Antiarrhythmic Devices: Executive Summary—a report of the American College of Cardiology/American Heart Association Task Force on Practice Guidelines (Committee on Pacemaker Implantation). Circulation 97:1325, 1998.
48. Thomas JE: Hyperactive carotid sinus reflex and CSS. Mayo Clin Proc 13:2065, 1969.
49. Volkmann H, Schnerch B, Kuhnert B: Diagnosis value of carotid sinus hypersensitivity. Pacing Clin Electrophysiol 13:2065, 1990.
50. Hartzler GO, Maloney JD: Cardioinhibitory carotid sinus hypersensitivity. Arch Intern Med 137:727, 1977.
51. Weiss S, Baker JP: The carotid sinus reflex in health and disease: Its role in the causation of fainting and convulsions. Medicine 12:297, 1933.
52. Zee-Cheng CS, Gibbs HR: Pure vasodepressor carotid sinus hypersensitivity. Am J Med 81:1095, 1986.
53. Morley CA, Sutton R: Carotid sinus syncope. Int J Cardiol 6:287, 1984.
54. Kenny RA, Traynor G: Carotid sinus syndrome: Clinical characteristics in elderly patients. Age Ageing 20:499, 1991.

55. Richardson DA, Bexton RS, Shaw FE, Kenny RA: Prevalence of cardioinhibitory carotid sinus hypersensitivity in patients 50 years or over presenting to the accident and emergency department with "unexplained" or "recurrent" falls. Pacing Clin Electrophysiol 15:820, 1997.
56. Huang SKS, Ezi MD, Hauser RG: Carotid sinus hypersensitivity in patients with unexplained syncope: Clinical, electrophysiological, and long term follow-up observations. Am Heart J 116:989, 1988.
57. Brignole M, Menossi C, Lolli G: Long-term outcome of paced and non-paced patients with severe carotid sinus syndrome. Am J Cardiol 69:1039, 1992.
58. Lown B, Levine SA: The carotid sinus: Clinical value of its stimulation. Circulation 23:766, 1961.
58a. Kenny RA, Richardson DA, Steen N, et al: Carotid sinus syndrome: A modifiable risk factor for nonaccidental falls in older adults (SAFE PACE). J Am Coll Cardiol 38:1491, 2001.
59. Baig MW, Kaye GC, Perrins EJ: Can central neuropeptides be implicated in carotid sinus reflex hypersensitivity? Med Hypotheses 28:255, 1989.
60. Strasburg B, Sagie A, Erdman S: Carotid sinus hypersensitivity and carotid sinus syndrome. Prog Cardiovasc Dis 31:376, 1989.
61. Blanc JJ, L`Heveder G, Mansourati J: Assessment of a newly recognized association, carotid sinus hypersensitivity and denervation of sternocleidomastoid muscles. Circulation 95:2548, 1997.
62. DaCosta D, McIntoch S, Kenny RA: Benefits of fludrocortisone in the treatment of symptomatic vasodepressor carotid sinus syndrome. Br Heart J 69:308, 1993.
63. Trout HH, Brown LL, Thompson JE: Carotid sinus syndrome: Treatment by carotid sinus denervation. Ann Surg 189:575, 1979.
64. Katritsis D, Ward DE, Camm AJ: Can we treat carotid sinus syndrome? Pacing Clin Electrophysiol 14:1367, 1991.
65. Sugrue DD, Gersh BJ, Holmes DR: Symptomatic "isolated" carotid sinus hypersensitivity: Natural history and results of treatment with anticholinergic drugs or pacemaker. J Am Coll Cardiol 158:1986, 1986.
66. Morley CA, Perrins EJ, Grant P: Carotid sinus syncope treated by pacing. Br Heart J 47:411, 1982.
67. Brignole M, Menozzi C, Lolli G: Validation of a method for choice of pacing mode in carotid sinus syndrome with or without sinus bradycardia. Pacing Clin Electrophysiol 14:196, 1991.
68. Brignole M, Menossi C, Lolli G: Natural and unnatural history of patients with severe carotid sinus hypersensitivity: A preliminary study. Pacing Clin Electrophysiol 11:1678, 1988.
68a. Parry SW, Steen IN, Bapfist M, Kenny RA: Amnesia for loss of consciousness in carotid sinus syncope: Implications for presentation with falls. J Am Coll Cardiol 45:1840, 2005.
69. Madigan NP, Flaker GC, Curtis JJ: Carotid sinus hypersensitivity: Beneficial effects of dual-chamber pacing. Am J Cardiol 53:1034, 1984.
70. Stryjer D, Friedensohn A, Schlesinger Z: Ventricular pacing as the preferable mode for long-term pacing in patients with carotid sinus syncope of the cardio inhibitory type. Pacing Clin Electrophysiol 9:705, 1986.
71. Walter F, Crawley IS, Dorney ER: Carotid sinus hypersensitivity and syncope. Am J Cardiol 42:396, 1978.
72. Gang ES, Oseran DS, Mandel WJ: Sinus node electrogram in patients with the hypersensitivity carotid syndrome. J Am Coll Cardiol 5:1484, 1985.
73. Brown KA, Maloney JD, Smith HC: Carotid sinus reflex in patients undergoing coronary angiography: Relationship of degree and location of coronary artery disease to response to carotid sinus massage. Circulation 62:697, 1980.
74. Munro NC, McLintoch S, Lawson J: Incidence of complications after carotid sinus massage in older patients with syncope. J Am Geriatr Soc 42:1248, 1994.
75. Alexander S, Ding WC: Fatal ventricular fibrillation during carotid sinus stimulation. Am J Cardiol 18:289, 1966.
76. Probst P, Muhlberger V, Lederbauer M, et al: Electrophysiologic findings in carotid sinus massage. Pacing Clin Electrophysiol 6:689, 1983.
77. Alicandri C, Fouad FM, Tarazi RC: Three cases of hypotension and syncope with ventricular pacing. Am J Cardiol 42:137, 1978.
78. Benditt DG, Sutton R, Gammage MD, et al: Clinical experience with Thera DR rate-drop response pacing algorithm in carotid sinus syndrome and vasovagal syncope. Pacing Clin Electrophysiol 20:832, 1997.
79. Maloney JD, Jaeger FJ, Fouad-Tarazi FM: Malignant vasovagal syncope: Prolonged asystole provoked by head-up tilt. Case report and review of diagnosis, pathophysiology and therapy. Cleve Clin J Med 55:543, 1988.
80. Sutton R: Vasovagal syncope: Could it be malignant? Eur Heart J 2:89, 1992.
81. Fitzpatrick AP, Ahmed R, Williams S: A randomized trial of medical therapy in "malignant vasovagal syndrome" or " neurally-mediated bradycardia/hypotension syndrome." Eur J Cardiac Pacing Electrophysiol 2:99, 1991.
82. Fitzpatrick AP, Sutton R: Tilting toward a diagnosis in recurrent unexplained syncope. Lancet 1(8639):658, 1989.
83. Grubb BP, Temesy-Armos P, Moore J: Head-upright tilt-table testing in the evaluation and management of the malignant vasovagal syndrome. Am J Cardiol 69:904, 1990.
84. Jaeger FJ, Schneider L, Maloney JD: Vasovagal syncope: Diagnostic role of head-up tilt test in patients with positive ocular compression test. Pacing Clin Electrophysiol 13:1416, 1990.
85. Grubb BP, Gerard JG, Roush K: Differentiation of convulsive syncope and epilepsy with head-up tilt testing. Ann Intern Med 115:871, 1991.
86. Ganzeboom KS, Colman N, Reitsma JB, et al: Prevalence and triggers of syncope in medical students. Am J Cardiol 91:1006, 2003.
87. Sheldon R, Sheldon A, Connolly SJ, et al; for the Investigators of the Syncope Symptom Study and the Prevention of Syncope Trial: Age of first faint in patients with vasovagal syncope. J Cardiovasc Electrophysiol 17:49, 2006.
88. Day SC, Cook EF, Funkenstein H, Goldman L: Evaluation and outcome of emergency room patients with transient loss of consciousness. Am J Med 73:15, 1982.
89. Savage DD, Corwin L, McGee DL, et al: Epidemiologic feature of isolated syncope: The Framingham Study. Stroke 16:626, 1985.
90. Dermkasian G, Lamb LE: Syncope in a population of healthy young adults. JAMA 168:1200, 1958.
91. Benditt DG, Ferguson DW, Grubb BP, et al: Tilt table testing for assessing syncope. J Am Coll Cardiol 28:263, 1996.
92. Mosqueda-Garcia R, Furlan R, Tank J, Femandez-Violante R: The elusive pathophysiology of neurally mediated syncope. Circulation 102:2898, 2000.
93. Linzer M, Pontinen M, Gold DT, et al: Impairment of physical and psychosocial function in recurrent syncope. J Clin Epidemiol 44:1037, 1991.
94. Rose MS, Koshman ML, Spreng S, Sheldon RS: The relationship between health related quality of life and frequency of spells in patients with syncope. J Clin Epidemiol 53:1209, 2000.
95. Lamb L, Green HC, Combs JJ, et al: Incidence of loss of consciousness in 1980 Air Force personnel. Aerospace Med 12:973, 1960.
96. Murdoch BD: Loss of consciousness in healthy South African men: Incidence, causes and relationship to EEG abnormality. South African Med J 57:771, 1980.
97. Sheldon R, Flanagan P, Koshman ML, Killam S: Risk factors for syncope recurrence after a positive tilt-table test in patients with syncope. Circulation 93:973, 1996.
98. Rossen R, Kabat H, Anderson JP: Acute arrest of cerebral circulation in man. Arch Neurol Psych 50:510, 1943.

99. Giannattasio C, Grassi C, Mancia G: Vasovagal syncope with bradycardia during lower body negative pressure in a heart transplant recipient. Blood Press 2:309, 1993.
100. Scherrer, Vissing S, Morgan BJ, et al: Vasovagal syncope after infusion of a vasodilator in a heart-transplant recipient. N Engl J Med 322:602, 1990.
101. El-Syed H, Hainsworth R: Salt supplement increases plasma volume and orthostatic tolerance in patients with unexplained syncope. Heart 75:134, 1996.
102. Thomson HL, Atherton JJ, Khafagi FA, Frenneaux MP: Failure of reflex venoconstriction during exercise in patients with vasovagal syncope. Circulation 93:953, 1996.
103. Thomson HL, Wright K, Frenneaux MP: Baroreflex sensitivity in patients with vasovagal syncope. Circulation 95:395, 1997.
104. Manyari DE, Rose S, Tyberg JV, Sheldon RS: Abnormal reflex venous function in patients with neuromediated syncope. J Am Coll Cardiol 27:1730, 1996.
105. Bechir M, Binggeli C, Corti R: Dysfunctional baroreflex regulation of sympathetic nerve activity in patients with vasovagal syncope. Circulation 107:1620, 2003.
106. Dietz NM, Halliwill JR, Speilman JM: Sympathetic withdrawal and forearm vasodilation during vasovagal syncope in humans. J Appl Physiol 82:1785, 1997.
107. Morillo CA, Eckberg DL, Ellenbogen KA, et al: Vagal and sympathetic mechanisms in patients with orthostatic vasovagal syncope. Circulation 96:2509, 1997.
108. Mosqueda-Garcia R, Furlan R, Tank J, et al: Sympathetic and baroreceptor reflex function in neurally mediated syncope evoked by tilt. J Clin Invest 11:2736, 1997.
109. Moya A, Brignole M, Menozzi C, et al; International Study on Syncope of Uncertain Etiology (ISSUE) Investigators: Mechanism of syncope in patients with isolated syncope and in patients with tilt-positive syncope. Circulation 104:1261, 2001.
110. Menozzi C, Brignole M, Lolli G, et al: Follow-up of asystolic episodes in patients with cardioinhibitory, neurally mediated syncope and VVI pacemaker. Am J Cardiol 72:1152, 1993.
111. Krahn AD, Klein GJ, Fitzpatrick A, et al: Predicting the outcome of patients with unexplained syncope undergoing prolonged monitoring. Pacing Clin Electrophysiol 25:37, 2002.
112. Krahn AD, Klein GJ, Yee R: Randomized assessment of syncope trial: Conventional diagnostic testing versus a prolonged monitoring strategy. Circulation 104:46, 2001.
113. Krahn AD, Klein GJ, Yee R, et al: Cost implication of testing in patients with syncope: Randomized assessment of syncope trial. J Am Coll Cardiol 42:495, 2003.
114. White WD, Sheldon RS, Ritchie DA: Learning needs in patients with vasovagal syncope. Can J Cardiovasc Nurs 13:26, 2003.
115. Sheldon R: Tilt testing for syncope: A reappraisal. Curr Opin Cardiol 1:38, 2005.
116. Burklow TR, Moak JP, Bailley JJ, Makhlouf FT: Neurally mediated cardiac syncope: Autonomic modulation after normal saline infusion. J Am Coll Cardiol 33:2059, 1999.
117. Mangru NN, Young ML, Mas MS, et al: Usefulness of tilt table test with normal saline infusion in management of neurocardiogenic syncope in children. Am Heart J 131:953, 1996.
118. Claydon VE, Hainsworth R: Salt supplementation improves orthostatic cerebral peripheral vascular control in patients with syncope. Hypertension 43:809, 2004.
119. Brignole M, Menozzi C, Solano A, et al: Isometric arm counterpressure maneuvers to abort impending vasovagal syncope. J Am Coll Cardiol 40:2053, 2002.
120. Krediet CT, van Dijk N, Linzer M, et al: Management of vasovagal syncope: Controlling or aborting faints by leg crossing and muscle-tensing. Circulation 106:1684, 2002.
121. Sheldon RS, Rose S, Flanagan P, et al: Risk factors for syncope recurrence after a positive tilt-table test in patients with syncope. Circulation 93:973, 1996.
122. Ward CR, Gray JC, Gilroy JJ, Kenny RA: Midodrine: A role in the management of neurocardiogenic syncope. Heart 79:45, 1998.
123. Perez-Lugones A, Schweikert R, Pavia S, et al: Usefulness of midodrine in patients with severely symptomatic neurocardiogenic syncope: A randomized control study. J Cardiovasc Electrophysiol 12:935, 2001.
124. Kaufmann H, Saadia D, Voustianiouk A: Midodrine in neurally mediated syncope double-blind, randomized, crossover study. Ann Neurol 52:342, 2002.
125. Di Girolamo E, Di Lorio C, Sabatini P, et al: Effects of paroxetine hydrochloride, a selective serotonin reuptake inhibitor, on refractory vasovagal syncope: A randomized, double-blind, placebo-controlled study. J Am Coll Cardiol 33:1227, 1999.
126. Takata TS, Wasmund SL: Serotonin reuptake inhibitor (Paxil) does not prevent vasovagal reaction association with carotid sinus massage and/or lower body negative pressure in healthy volunteers. Circulation 106:1500, 2002.
127. Sheldon R, Rose S, Flanagan P, et al: Effect of beta blockers on the time to first syncope recurrence in patients after a positive isoproterenol tilt table test. Am J Cardiol 78:536, 1996.
128. Cox MM, Perlman BA, Mayor MR, et al: Acute and long term beta-adrenergic blockade for patients with neurocardiogenic syncope. J Am Coll Cardiol 26:1293, 1995.
129. Alegria JR, Gersh BJ, Scott CG, et al: Comparison of frequency of recurrent syncope after beta-blocker therapy versus conservative management for patients with vasovagal syncope. Am J Cardiol 92:82, 2003.
130. Mahanonda N, Bhuripanyo K, Kangkagate C: Randomized, double-blind, placebo-controlled trial of oral atenolol in patients with unexplained syncope and positive upright tilt table test results. Am Heart J 130:1250, 1995.
131. Madrid AH, Ortega J, Rebollo JG, et al: Lack of efficacy of atenolol for the prevention of neurally mediated syncope in a highly symptomatic population: A prospective, double-blind, randomized and placebo controlled study. J Am Coll Cardiol 37:5554, 2001.
132. Flevari P, Livanis EG, Theodorakis GN, et al: Vasovagal syncope: A prospective, randomized, crossover, evaluation of the effect of propranolol, nadolol and placebo on syncope recurrence and patients' well being. J Am Coll Cardiol 40:499, 2002.
133. Ventura R, Maas R, Zeidler D: A randomized and controlled pilot trial of beta-blockers for the treatment of recurrent syncope in patients with a positive or negative response to head-up tilt test. Pacing Clin Electrophysiol 25:816, 2002.
134. Sheldon RS, Connolly S, Rose S, et al: The Prevention of Syncope Trial (POST): A randomized, placebo-controlled study of metoprolol in the prevention of vasovagal syncope. Circulation 113:1164-1170, 2006.
135. Schimmer BP, Parker KL: Adrenocorticotropic hormone: Adrenocortical steroids and their synthetic analogue; inhibitors of the synthesis and actions of adrenocortical hormones. In Hardman JG, Limbird LE, Gilman AG (eds): Goodman & Gilman's The Pharmacological Basis of Therapeutics, 10th ed. New York, McGraw-Hill, 2001, pp 1649-1677.
136. Balaji S, Oslizlok PC, Allen MC, et al: Neurocardiogenic syncope in children with a normal heart. J Am Coll Cardiol 23:779, 1994.
137. Scott WA, Pongiglione G, Bromberg BI, et al: Randomized comparison of atenolol and fludrocortisone acetate in the treatment of pediatric neurally mediated syncope. Am J Cardiol 76:400, 1995.
138. Salim MA, Disessa TG: Effectiveness of fludrocortisone and salt in preventing syncope recurrence in children. J Am Coll Cardiol 45:484, 2005.
139. el-Bedawi KM, Wahba MA, Hainsworth R: Cardiac pacing does not improve orthostatic tolerance in patients with vasovagal syncope. Clin Auton Res 4:233, 1994.

140. Fitzpatrick AP, Theodorakis G, Ahmed R, et al: Dual chamber pacing aborts vasovagal syncope induced by head-up 60 degrees tilt. Pacing Clin Electrophysiol 14:13, 1991.
141. Samoil D, Grubb BP, Brewster P, et al: Comparison of single and dual chamber pacing techniques in prevention of upright tilt induced vasovagal syncope. Eur J Cardiac Pacing Electrophysiol 1:36, 1991.
142. Sra JS, Jazayeri MR, Avitall B: Comparison of cardiac pacing with drug therapy in the treatment of neurocardiogenic (vasovagal) syncope with bradycardia or asystole. N Engl J Med 328:1085, 1993.
143. Moya A, Brignole M, Menozzi C, et al; International Study on Syncope of Uncertain Etiology (ISSUE) Investigators: Mechanism of syncope in patients with isolated syncope and in patients with tilt-positive syncope. Circulation 104:1261, 2001.
144. Petersen ME, Chamberlain-Webber R, Fitzpatrick AP, et al: Permanent pacing for cardioinhibitory malignant vasovagal syndrome. Br Heart J 71:274, 1994.
145. Sheldon R, Koshman ML, Wilson W, et al: Effect of dual-chamber pacing automatic rate-drop sensing on recurrent neurally mediated syncope. Am J Cardiol 81:158, 1998.
146. Connolly SJ, Sheldon RS, Roberts RS, Gent M: The North American Vasovagal Pacemaker Study. J Am Coll Cardiol 33:16, 1999.
147. Sutton R, Brignole M, Menozzi C, et al: Dual-chamber pacing in the treatment of neurally mediated tilt-positive cardioinhibitory syncope: Pacemaker versus no therapy: A multicenter randomized study. The Vasovagal Syncope International Study (VASIS). Circulation 102:294, 2000.
148. Ammirati F, Colivicchi F, Santini M: Permanent cardiac pacing versus medical treatment for the prevention of recurrent vasovagal syncope: A multicenter randomized, controlled trial. Circulation 104:52, 2001.
149. Ammirati F, Colivicchi F, Toscano S: DDD pacing with rate drop response function versus DDI with rate hysteresis pacing for cardioinhibitory vasovagal syncope. Pacing Clin Electrophysiol 21:2178, 1998.
150. Beecher HK: Surgery as placebo. JAMA 176:1102, 1961.
151. Moerman DE, Jonas WB: Deconstructing the placebo effect and finding the meaning response. Ann Intern Med 136:471, 2002.
152. Redelmeier DA, Tu JV, Schull MJ, et al: Problems for clinical judgement. 2: Obtaining a reliable past medical history. Can Med Assoc J 164:809, 2001.
153. McLeod KA, Wilson N, Hewitt J: Cardiac pacing for severe childhood neurally mediated syncope with reflex anoxic seizures. Heart 82:721, 1999.
154. Connolly SJ, Sheldon R, Thorpe KE, et al; VPS II Investigators: Pacemaker therapy for prevention of syncope in patients with recurrent severe vasovagal syncope. Second Vasovagal Pacemaker Study (VPS II): A randomized trial. JAMA 289:2224, 2003.
155. Raviele A, Giada F, Menpzzi C, et al: A randomized, double-blind, placebo-controlled study of permanent cardiac pacing for the treatment of recurrent tilt-induced vasovagal syncope: The vasovagal syncope and pacing trial (SYNPACE). Eur Heart J 25:1741, 2004.
156. Raj SR, Koshman ML, Sheldon R: Outcomes of patients with dual-chamber pacemakers implanted for the prevention of neurally mediated syncope. Am J Cardiol 91:565, 2003.
157. Gillis AM, Connolly SJ, Lacombe P, et al: Randomized crossover comparison of DDDR versus VDD pacing after atrioventricular junction ablation for prevention of atrial fibrillation. The Atrial Pacing Peri-Ablation for Paroxysmal Atrial Fibrillation Study investigators. Circulation 102:736, 2000.
158. Gillis AM, Connolly SJ, Lacombe P, et al: Atrial pacing periablation for prevention of paroxysmal atrial fibrillation. Circulation 99:2553, 1999.
159. Connolly SJ, Kerr CR, Gent M, et al: Effects of physiological pacing versus ventricular pacing on the risk of stroke and death due to cardiovascular causes. Canadian Trial of Physiologic Pacing Investigators. N Engl J Med 342:1385, 2000.
160. Sheldon R, Rose S, Koshman ML: Comparison of patients with syncope of unknown cause having negative or positive tilt-table tests. Am J Cardiol 80:581, 1997.
161. Grimm W, Degenhardt M, Hoffman J, et al: Syncope recurrence can better be predicted by history than by head-up tilt testing in untreated patients with suspected neurally mediated syncope. Pacing Clin Electrophysiol 18:1465, 1997.
162. Brignole M, Menozzi C, Corbucci G: Detecting incipient vasovagal syncope: Intraventricular acceleration. Pacing Clin Electrophysiol 20:801, 1997.
163. Osswald S, Cron T, Gradel C: Closed-loop stimulation using intracardiac impedance as a sensor principle: Correlation of right ventricular dp/dt_{max} and intracardiac impedance during dobutamine stress test. Pacing Clin Electrophysiol 23:1502, 2000.
164. Binggeli C, Duru F, Corti R: Autonomic nervous system-controlled cardiac pacing: A comparison between intracardiac impedance signal and muscle sympathetic nerve activity. Pacing Clin Electrophysiol 23:1632, 2000.
165. Griesbach L, Huber T, Knote B, et al: Closed loop stimulation: Therapy for malignant neurocardiogenic syncope. Prog Biomed Res 7:242, 2002.
166. Occhetta E, Bortnik M, Vassanelli C: The DDDR closed loop stimulation for the prevention of vasovagal syncope: Results from the INVASY prospective feasibility registry. Europace 5:153, 2003.
167. Ochetta E, Bortnik M, Audoglio R, Vassanelli C; for the INVASY Study Investigators: Closed loop stimulation in prevention of vasovagal syncope. Inotropy Controlled Pacing in Vasovagal Syncope (INVASY): A multicentre randomized, single blind, controlled study. Europace 6:538, 2004.
168. Giada F, Raviele A, Gasparini G: Efficacy of a patient-activity drug delivery system using phenylephrine as active drug in aborting tilt-induced syncope [abstract]. Pacing Clin Electrophysiol 24:573, 2001.

Chapter 16

Sensor-Driven Pacing: Device Specifics

CHU-PAK LAU • HUNG-FAT TSE • G. NEAL KAY

The ideal characteristics of an implantable sensor for rate adaptation have been addressed in Chapter 5. In clinical practice, many of the special lead sensors, such as the oxygen saturation sensor, have not been used for rate-adaptive pacing. Clinicians remained concerned about the stability and reliability of special leads and the future implications of their replacement. Thus the majority of clinically used rate-adaptive devices employ standard pacing leads. These include body movement sensing, minute ventilation sensing, QT interval sensing, and their combinations. The sensing of peak endocardial acceleration (PEA) and regional impedance changes at the pacemaker lead, used by the so-called closed-loop stimulation (CLS) sensors, are the more recently available methods of rate adaptation.

Activity-Sensing and Accelerometer-Based Pacemakers

Activity sensing has achieved wide clinical acceptance as a rate-controlling parameter for implantable cardiac pacemakers. The rate-adaptive pacemaker incorporating sensors that monitor body activity was the first to be implanted and is the standard used for rate-adaptive pacemakers in all companies.[1,2] Activity sensing is also the sensor method that is combined with other sensors. Because activity-based pacemakers are operationally simple and do not require a special sensor outside the pulse generator casing, they work with any type of pacing lead, have excellent long-term stability, and are highly reliable. Implantation of activity-guided pacemakers is no different from that of conventional pacemakers. Although they may not be excellent proportional sensors, activity sensors react promptly to the start and end of physical exercise. The first activity sensors were piezoelectric crystals that responded mostly to the frequency of vibrations that were transmitted to the pulse generator.

The specific use of an activity sensor for pacemaker rate augmentation was described first by Dahl[3] in 1979 (an accelerometer configuration) and then by Anderson and colleagues[4] in 1983 (a pressure-vibration configuration).

In 1987, the possibility of using accelerometer-based activity sensing for pacing rate control was reported for the first time.[5,6] Activity sensing has potential application for detecting daily activity, as in monitoring for heart failure, to detect the posture of the patient, and to adjust the lower pacing rate by defining the resting state.

Physical Principle of Activity Sensing

Body movements, especially walking, result in vibrations that are transmitted to the upper chest or generate acceleration forces in the body. In the pacemaker scenario, acceleration forces acting on the body during exercise are best detected by a device inside the pacemaker box. With triaxially mounted accelerometers placed on the surface of an externally attached pacemaker, acceleration signals during a variety of exercises have been measured, permitting the study of the acceleration forces during these exercises.[5] The axes used are referred to as "anteroposterior" (x-axis), "lateral" (y-axis), and "vertical" (z-axis). Because of the sloping of the chest and the swaying of the body (and hence the pacemaker) during walking, these axes are not the same as true horizontal (x or y) or true vertical (z) axes. The acceleration signals are transformed by fast Fourier method with respect to the frequency. The root mean square value of acceleration is used to quantify the acceleration force. The following findings have been reported:[5]

- *Axes most relevant to detect walking:* A recording of acceleration signals in a typical subject during walking is shown in Figure 16-1. It is apparent that either the x-axis or z-axis is useful to detect the acceleration forces during walking. On the other hand, the y-axis is useful only to detect body swinging. In the construction of an activity sensor in an implanted pacemaker, the anteroposterior (x) axis would be more practical than the z-axis because the "top" of the pacemaker can vary according to how the pacemaker is implanted and is likely to be influenced by subsequent pacemaker rotation in the pocket, whereas the anteroposterior axis remains relatively fixed over time.
- *Effects of walking speed and gradient on the acceleration signals:* Acceleration forces are represented by the integrated root mean square value of accelerations. Walking at a higher speed will induce significant increase in acceleration signal (Fig. 16-2). Although walking upslope also increases the acceleration forces, the increase is less than that induced by walking faster. Thus, activity sensors as a whole are less sensitive to this form of exercise.
- *Frequency range of acceleration forces during walking:* During normal walking, the fast Fourier transformed acceleration shows that the majority of the signal is less than 4 Hz (see Fig. 16-1). Relatively little signal is lost by low-pass filtering at 4 Hz, and filtering may also improve the proportionality of the acceleration force to the level of workload (Fig. 16-3).

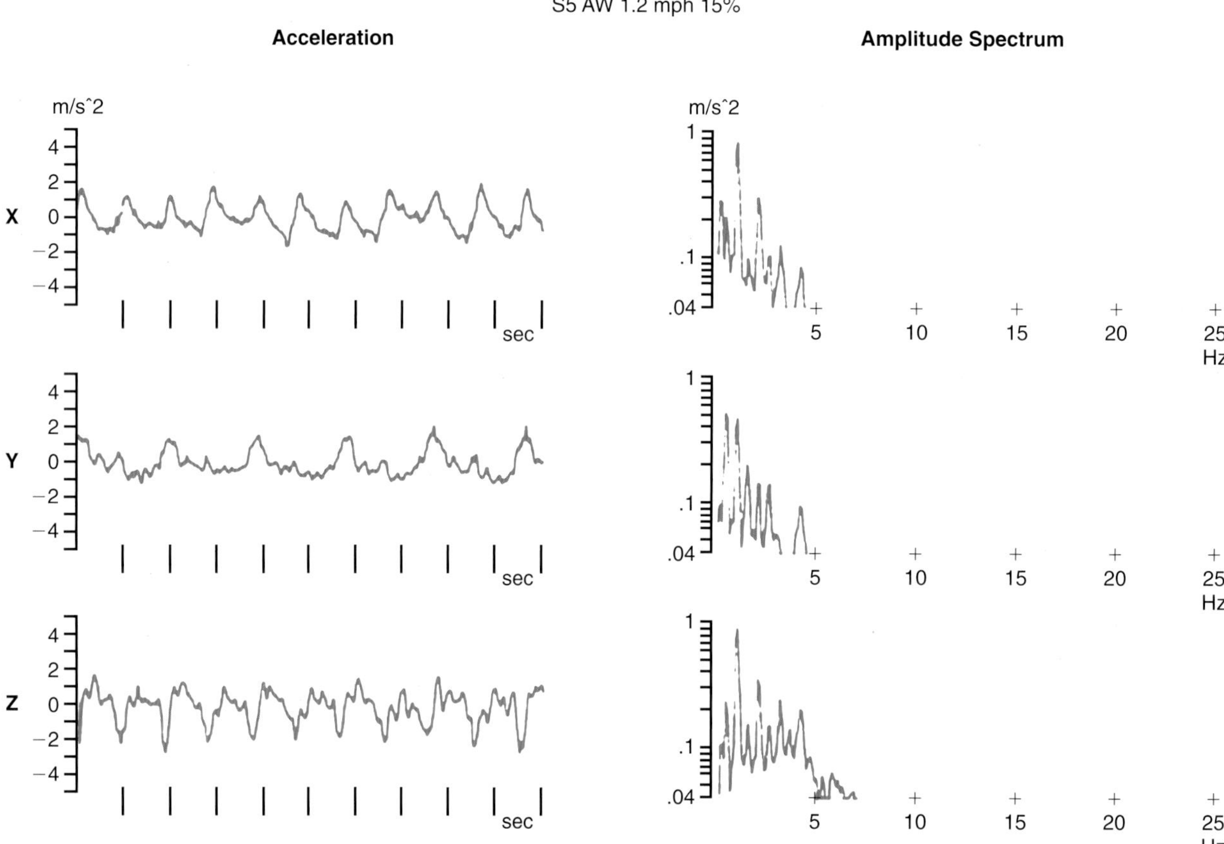

Figure 16-1. Representative acceleration signals recorded in a typical subject during walking at 1.2 mph at a 15% gradient on a treadmill. Each strip represents 10 seconds' duration on the treadmill, and each peak of the curves in the x- and z-axes on the left side represents one step on the treadmill. Left, *The number of peaks in the lateral (y-) axis is one half of either that of the x- or z-axis. This represents the swaying of the shoulder, which occurs once per complete walking cycle, which this axis principally detects.* Right, *Fourier-transformed acceleration amplitudes at different frequencies are shown graphically. Most of the acceleration forces are less than 4 Hz. (From Lau CP, Stott JR, Toff WD, et al: Selective vibration sensing: New design of activity-sensing rate-responsive pacing. PACE 11:1299, 1988.)*

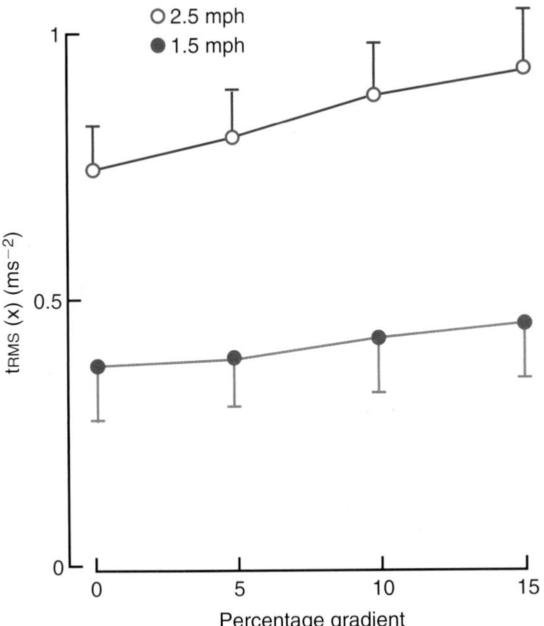

Figure 16-2. Total root mean square acceleration (tRMS) in the x-axis during walking at different speeds and gradients. tRMS increases as a function of both speeds and gradients ($P < .001$). Each error bar represents 1 SEM. (From Lau CP, Stott JR, Toff WD, et al: Selective vibration sensing: New design of activity-sensing rate-responsive pacing. PACE 11:1299, 1988.)

- *Other forms of exercise*: Appropriate increase in acceleration force occurs during running (Fig. 16-4). However, because the acceleration force encountered during arm exercise is small in the pectoral area, particularly if the x-axis is used, the forces measured during cycling and weightlifting would be lower than would be expected from the amount of workload. Although accelerations during arm movements are better detected in the horizontal axis, this direction is difficult to use in a pacemaker, which is liable to change its position inside the pocket after implantation.

Sensors

The three different types of clinically used activity sensors are a piezoelectric sensor and an accelerometer using either piezoelectric or piezoresistive materials (Fig. 16-5). The piezoelectric crystal is attached to the inside of the pacemaker casing, and pressure waves initiated in the skeleton and soft body tissues by physical activity result in a physical deformation of the piezoelectric element (see Fig. 16-5A).[4,7] Because deformation of the piezoelectric sensor induces a voltage that is proportional to the amount of structural disturbance, measurement of these induced voltages permits estimation of the level of physical activity. Because the piezoelectric element is usually attached to the posterior surface of the pulse generator can during manufacturing, it is typically positioned directly against the pectoralis major muscle to ensure good physical contact with the skeletal muscles. The pacemaker can be implanted with the sensor facing away from the muscle activity if the activity threshold or the rate response can be programmed to compensate for the reduced signal amplitude with this orientation. Generally, the piezoelectric element produces potentials in the range of 5 to 50 mV during rest and as much as 200 mV during vigorous activity. The range of frequencies to which these systems are most sensitive is generally about 10 Hz, close to the typical resonant frequency of the human body.[5,6] Given these signal characteristics, activity-based pacemakers that use a piezoelectric element bonded to the inside of the pacemaker case appear to offer good correlation with upright physical movement involving walking or running.

An accelerometer is a sensor designed to measure *acceleration*, defined as the rate of change in velocity. Accelerometers can be made of piezoelectric crystal, mounted on a cantilever mounted on the circuit board (see Fig. 16-5B), or as an integrated circuit using silicon wafers sandwiching a suspended mass, the so-called piezoresistive accelerometer (see Fig. 16-5C). Physiologic studies have shown that rhythmic body motions, such as walking and riding a bicycle, fall within a narrow

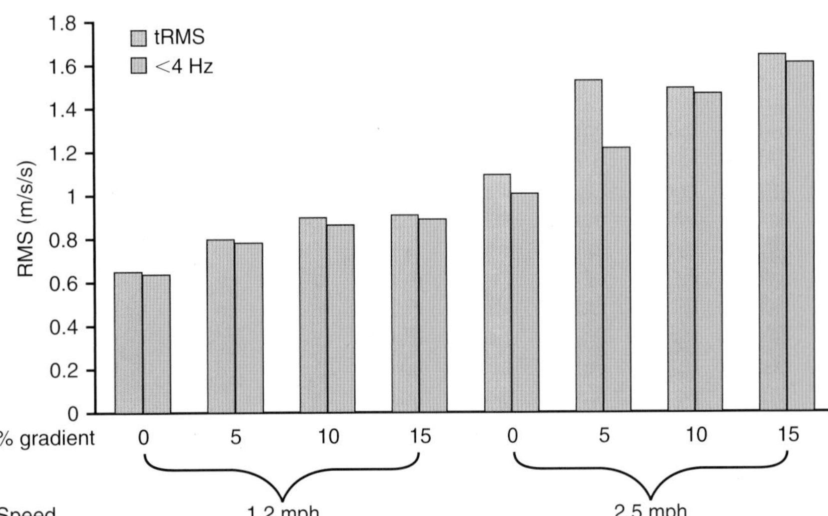

Figure 16-3. Total root mean square acceleration (tRMS) and low-pass RMS (<4 Hz) in a typical subject during treadmill exercise at different speeds and gradients. (From Lau CP, Stott JR, Toff WD, et al: Selective vibration sensing: New design of activity-sensing rate-responsive pacing. PACE 11:1299, 1988.)

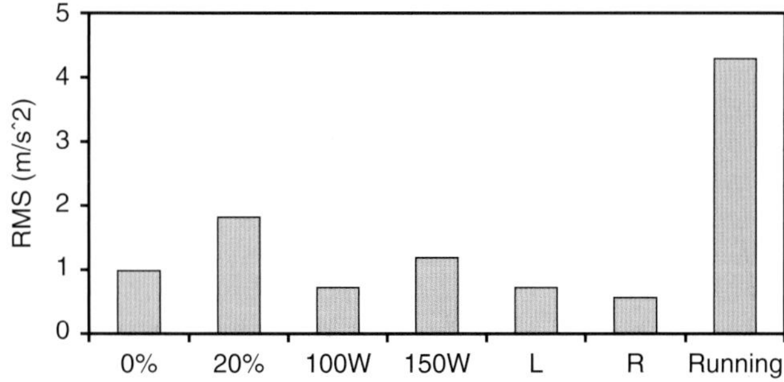

Figure 16-4. Acceleration level (filtered root mean square [RMS]) during different exercises. "Arm exercise" refers to the lifting of a 1-kg mass by 1 meter up from the ground and back down. (From Lau CP, Stott JR, Toff WD, et al: Selective vibration sensing: New design of activity-sensing rate-responsive pacing. PACE 11:1299, 1988.)

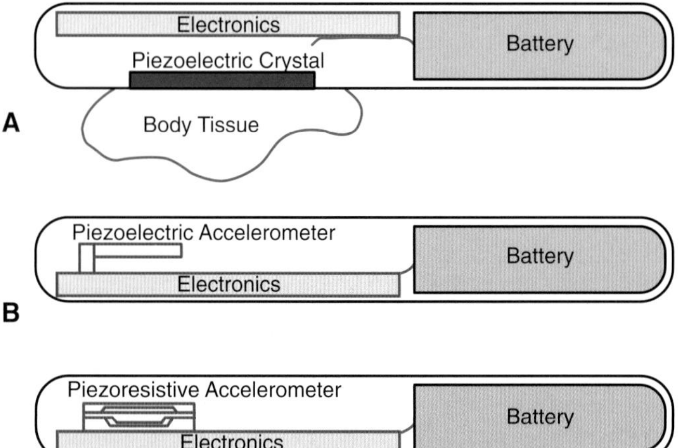

Figure 16-5. Three different types of activity sensors. ***A,*** *The piezoelectric sensor is bound to the inside surface of the pacemaker case. Vibration is sensed through tissue contact. The mechanical forces are transmitted by the surrounding connective tissue, fatty tissue, and muscles. The extent of contact and the coupling mass of the mechanical forces can vary considerably.* ***B*** *and* ***C,*** *The accelerometer is mounted on the pacemaker's hybrid circuitry. The seismic mass of the accelerometer is fixed. Therefore, measured accelerations are independent of surrounding tissue and patient physical properties.*

frequency range, typically 1 to 4 Hz,[5,6] in which accelerometers are most sensitive. When an accelerometer device is implanted, no special orientation of the pulse generator is needed. It may be flipped over or rotated in the pocket, and excess lead may be coiled beneath it.

The main difference between an accelerometer and a piezoelectric crystal sensor that measures vibration is in the actual mass that, on activity, deforms the piezoelectric or piezoresistive material; this is referred to as the *coupling mass*. In the case of the vibration-measuring device, the crystal is bonded to the inside of the pulse generator casing (see Fig. 16-5A). The coupling mass is the body tissue in close proximity to the sensor, which actually exerts a force on the pulse generator casing during activity. This mass, consisting of the connective tissue and muscles surrounding the pacemaker, may vary considerably among patients. Therefore, variation in rate response from patient to patient for the same level of activity can be expected from the vibrational piezoelectric crystal sensor.

In accelerometers, the coupling mass is a small seismic mass, typically weighing less than 100 mg, suspended on one or more levers. The structure is mechanically insulated from the pulse generator can. On acceleration, this mass deflects the lever by an amount that is proportional to the change in velocity and the direction of acceleration. In accelerometers, this deflection can be translated into an electric signal by piezoelectric or piezoresistive material applied to the suspension levers. Because the pulse generator moves with the patient, the accelerometer detects acceleration or deceleration associated with body motion. The main advantage can be found in the fact that the seismic mass of the accelerometer is constant. Equal acceleration forces induce equal sensor signals independent of the tissue mass surrounding the pacemaker and the physical characteristics of the patient, such as weight and height—allowing a more predictable rate response.

The characteristic properties of the piezoelectric crystal, the piezoelectric accelerometer, and the piezoresistive accelerometer are summarized in Table 16-1. The ability of the accelerometers to detect physiologic vibrations rather than noise significantly improves the specificity of these devices (Fig. 16-6).

Algorithms

Peak Count Systems

The first version of activity-sensing pacemakers to incorporate a piezoelectric sensor, the Medtronic Activitrax (Medtronic, Inc., Minneapolis, Minn.), used the peak counting method.[4-7] After filtering and amplification of the raw signal, the signal was passed through a threshold discriminator. Three thresholds and 10 programmable slopes were available. An algorithm that monitors the number of piezoelectric signals that exceed a programmable threshold (activity threshold) characterizes the peak counting method. As the intensity of physical activity increases, further increase in the amplitude of the piezoelectric signal does not affect the rate response if the peak has already crossed the threshold (Fig. 16-7). This results in a sensor that characteristically responds to exercise in a relatively "on" or "off" manner.[8,9] In clinical studies with this sensor, treadmill exercise testing with increased speed (increasing step frequency) resulted in an incremental rise in the pacing rate. On the other hand, tests of patients on a treadmill at a constant speed with a changing incline from 0% to 15% did not result in further rise in pacing rate despite the increase in workload. Therefore, this processing method involves a weaker correlation between changes in pacing rate and changes in metabolic workload (r = 0.2) than that with the integration method (Fig. 16-8).[5] Obviously, mental stress and non-exercise-related rate response will not be detected. There is also underdetection of upper limb movements. Postexercise rate recovery has to follow an arbitrary

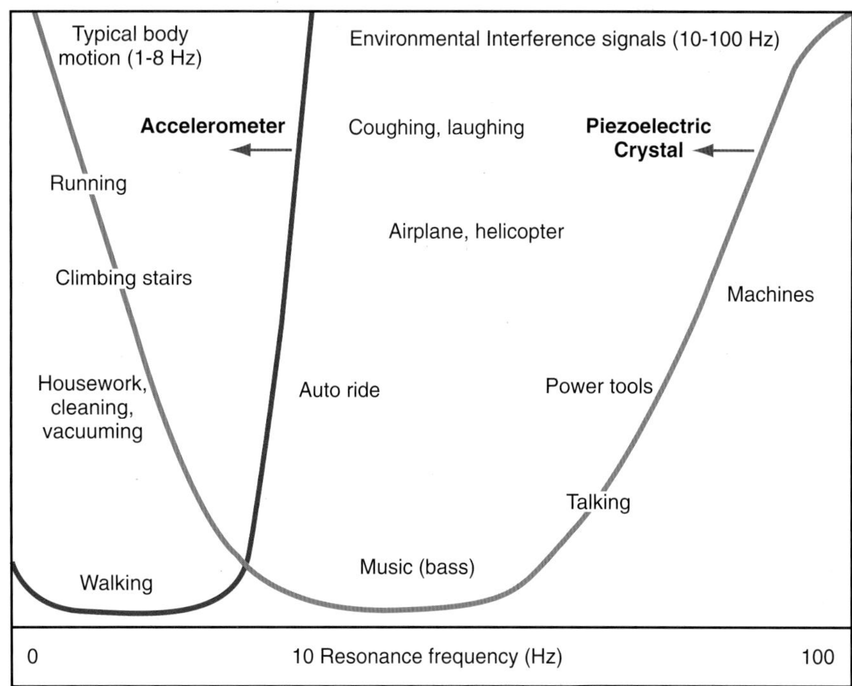

Figure 16-6. The low-filter bandpass accelerometer technology detects mechanical resonance frequencies associated with typical body motion in the low-frequency range. Environmental signals larger than 8 Hz, which can distort rate response, are undetected.

TABLE 16-1. Characteristics of Three Types of Activity Sensors Used for Adaptive-Rate Pacing

Characteristic	Piezoelectric	Piezoelectric Accelerometer	Piezoresistive Accelerometer
Activity sensor	Crystal bonded to can	Accelerometer	Accelerometer
Indicator	Vibration	Body motion	Body motion
Mechanics	Bonded to pacemaker	Mounted on hybrid	Integrated chip
Coupling mass	Body tissue	85-mg seismic mass	12-mg seismic mass
Sensitivity	10-15 Hz	1-4 Hz	1-8 Hz
Current drain	0.0 mA	0.0 mA	3-4 mA
Signal analysis	Frequency dominant	Frequency and amplitude	Frequency and amplitude
Approximate size	About 4 × 20 mm	4.6 × 3.8 × 1.5 mm	6.0 × 6.0 mm × 1.5 mm

decay as activity counts cease at the end of exercise, which may not be entirely physiologic.

Despite these limitations, the most useful and clinically most important characteristic of an activity-based, adaptive-rate pacemaker is its ability to provide a prompt pacing response at the onset of physical activity, which is achieved with a piezoelectric crystal. Improvement in cardiopulmonary exercise testing and clinical response have been documented from this simple system.[10-13] The peak counting method can be made sensitive to workload through dynamic variation in threshold, as detailed later.

Signal Integration Algorithms

A better correlation of workload with pacing rate can be achieved with signal integration (Fig. 16-9). Signals from either the piezoelectric sensor or the accelerometer are rectified and integrated to determine the pacing rate through a number of algorithms. The Siemens Sensolog (Siemens-Elema AB, Solna, Sweden) was a piezoelectric sensor that attempted to use a signal integration algorithm to determine the pacing rate. It was more effective than the Activitrax in detecting upper limb movements.[9,14,15] On the other hand, because of the limitation of a can-bonded piezoelectric crystal in its specificity, the device needed frequent adjustment of the programming setting over time, and its response depended on the patient's footwear.[14,16]

Accelerometers are ideal for signal integration algorithm, because the signal frequency is limited to the physiologic range, making them less susceptible to interference. The first version of accelerometer device was the Intermedics Dash/Relay rate-adaptive system.[17,18]

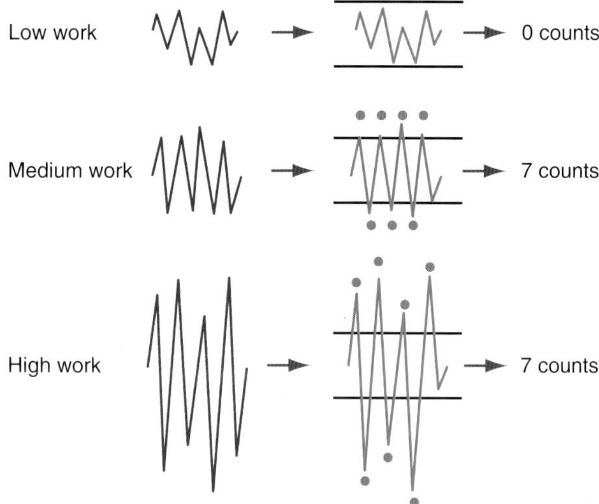

Figure 16-7. Peak counting method of signal processing. Note that at low levels of exertion, the amplitude of the sensor signals does not exceed the threshold amplitude, producing a sensor count of 0. At medium and high workloads, the amplitude of the sensor signals rises. Because this processing method counts only the number of threshold crossings, identical sensor counts are produced by medium and high workloads.

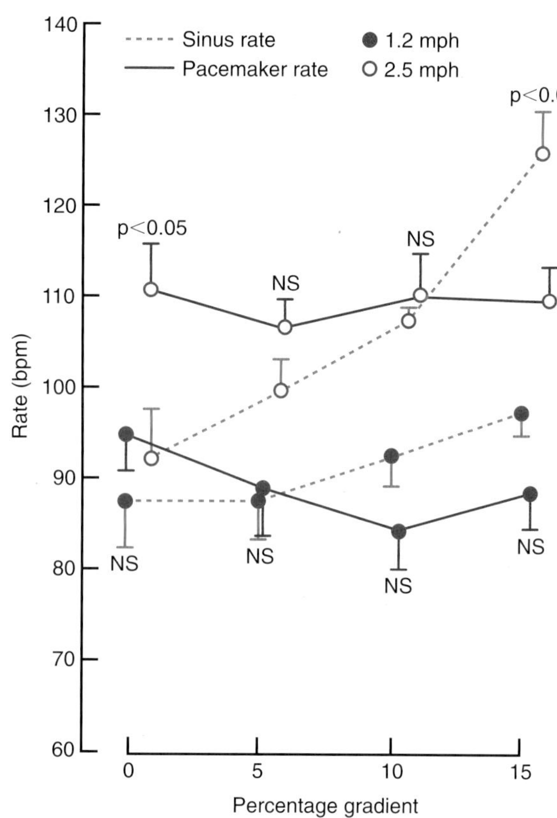

Figure 16-8. Pacing rates of six subjects with externally attached Activitrax pacemakers during treadmill exercises at different speeds and gradients. Each point represents a 3-minute exercise on the treadmill at a combination of two speeds (1.2 and 2.5 mph) and four gradients (0%-15%). Although there was an increase in pacing rate as the patients walked at a faster speed, there was no increase in rate as the subjects walked at higher gradients. The sinus rate, however, shows a rise in rate as the subjects walked at higher gradients and at faster speeds. (From Lau CP, Stott JR, Toff WD, et al: Selective vibration sensing: New design of activity-sensing rate-responsive pacing. PACE 11:1299, 1988.)

The device introduced a "triphasic" rate-responsive curve, so that the activity of daily living rate was linked to a range of acceleration signals to enhance rate stability. Approach to upper rate was allowed at the higher workload (Fig. 16-10). Both the accelerometer sensor and the implanted clock were used to determine a circadian rate. Current devices using accelerometers have since incorporated more sophisticated algorithms.

Currently Available Activity-Sensing Devices

The currently available activity-sensing devices are described here by manufacturer.

Medtronic, Inc.: Thera, Kappa 700, 900, and 400, Enpulse, and EnRhythm

The Thera devices are the traditional activity-sensing system, based on the Activitrax predecessor. A piezoelectric crystal is bonded to the inside of the pacemaker casing. Activity levels that exceed a programmable threshold are counted, and the number of counts that exceed a programmable threshold is used to determine the rate response. The physician adjusts the overall rate response by programming the activity threshold and the rate-response slope. Typically, this instrumentation allows a good response from the lower rate to about 100 beats per minute (bpm) during daily activities. The response to the upper rate is more difficult, and depends on the patient and the programming setting.

In the Kappa (700 and 900), EnPulse, and EnRhythm series, both the hardware and the software of the activity-sensing system have been changed. Instead of a

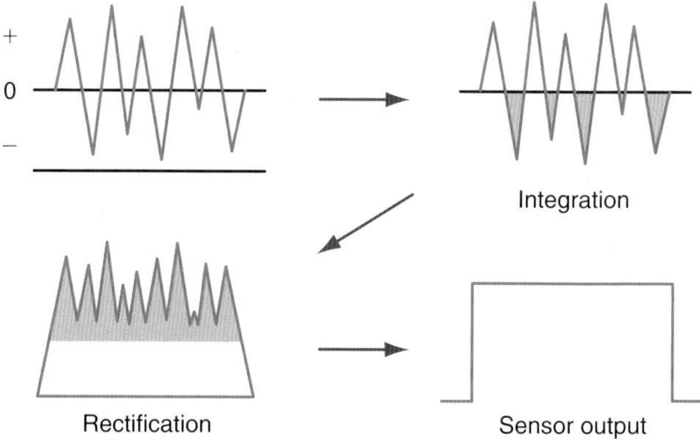

Figure 16-9. Integration method of signal processing. The raw activity signal (upper left) *is processed by integration of the area under the curve inscribed by the sensor* (upper right). *The integrated area is then rectified so that a uniform polarity is generated* (lower left). *The rectified sensor signal is then converted into a square wave that is directly related in duration to the area under the curve* (lower right).

Figure 16-10. Pacing rate profile in a patient with an activity-sensing rate-adaptive pacemaker (Relay, Intermedics, Inc., Angleton, Tex.) using accelerometry during treadmill and walking exercise at a slope of "5." The projected pacing rate at a slope of "10" can be estimated graphically without requiring the patient to repeat the exercise. Note that with the use of a more sensitive slope, the maximum rate during treadmill exercise can be reached without affecting the rate during walking because the latter falls within the flat intermediate portion of the rate-adaptive curve.

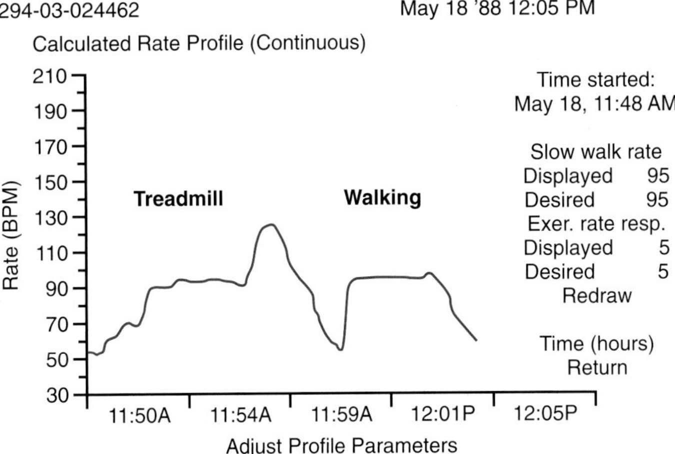

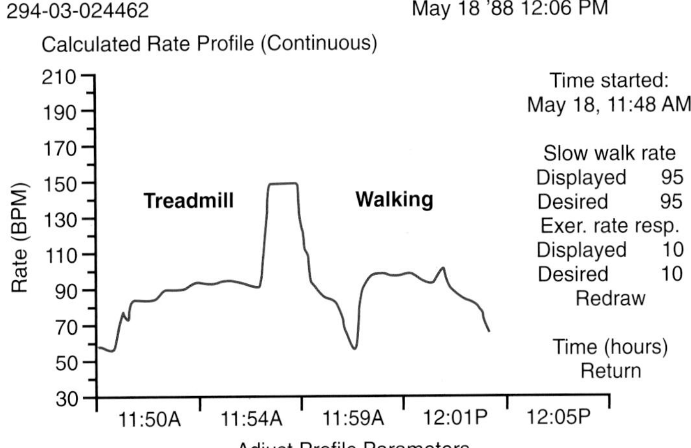

piezoelectric crystal, a "beam accelerometer" is attached to the circuit board to detect movement in the anteroposterior plane. Instead of a fixed threshold, a "rolling threshold" is used to provide a count of activity that depends not only on the frequency of counts that cross the threshold but also on the strength of these counts. The rolling threshold uses a 2-second window, the threshold is increased to 2x and 4x on the next two 2-second time frame, and the number of counts that occur in the last 6 seconds is averaged to give the rolling average of counts for every 2 seconds (Fig. 16-11). This rolling threshold, in effect, minimizes the detection of low-intensity but high-frequency accelerations, such as those occurring during a car ride, but allow detection of high-intensity signals during physical activities. The weighted sensor counts are used to derive a target rate, and the pacing rate matches the target rate within a time constant to smooth the rate response.

The response of the sensor can be further adjusted by the use of "Activity of Daily Living" (ADL) and "Exertion Response" (ER) programming (Fig. 16-12). The physician decides on the lower rate limit (LRL),

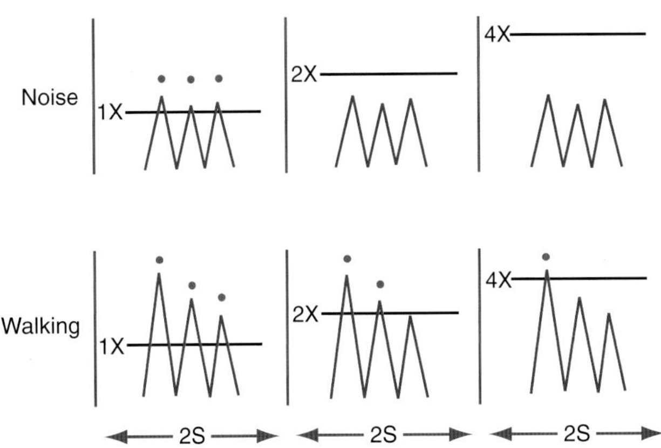

Figure 16-11. The "rolling threshold" of the Medtronic activity sensing pacemakers. As the threshold increases, the number of accelerations above the threshold that will be integrated will be filtered off. On the other hand, because an exercise such as walking results in higher acceleration levels, these signals will be taken in even when the threshold increases. See text for details.

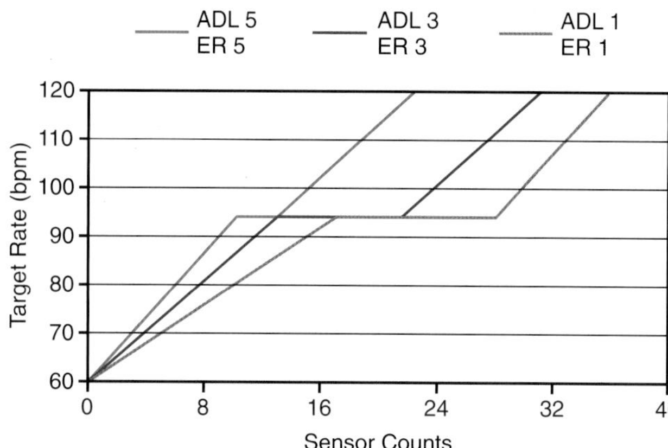

Figure 16-12. Triphasic rate-responsive curve of the Medtronic Kappa 600, 700, 900, Enrhythm, and Enpulse accelerometer activity-sensing pacemakers. ADL, activity of daily living response; ER, exertion response.

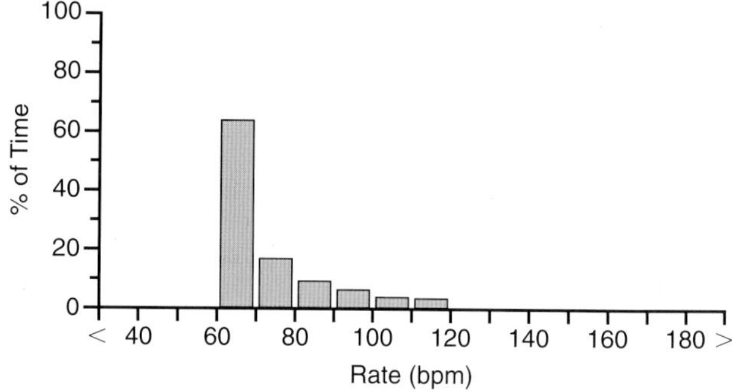

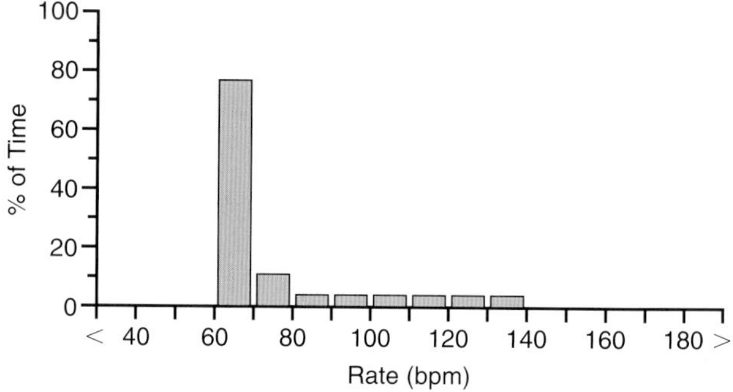

Figure 16-13. Sensor profiles of two patients with Medtronic Enpulse pacemakers at the following identical settings: activity of daily living (ADL) = 3; exertion response (ER) = 3; lower rate limit (LRL) = 60 bpm; sensor-driven upper rate limit (SURL) = 130 bpm. Patient A was a sedentary worker. Patient B was an active person, in whom larger rate ranges were encountered.

the ADL rate, and the sensor-driven upper rate limit (SURL) (see Fig. 16-12). In the nominal setting of ADL response of 3 (out of 5), counts that exceed 12 will achieve the ADL rate. Counts between 12 and 20 will also give the ADL rate, so that the rate response is stable. When counts exceed 20, ER will occur to the maximum programmed SURL. The flat portion of the response curve corresponds to 25% of the total counts. Adjustment of the ADL and ER to a more sensitive setting (e.g., 5 in both cases) decreases the number of counts to reach between ADL rate and SURL, and shortens the ADL rate portion of the response curve.

The actual number of counts to effect a rate response is not fixed but differs with the patient. Rather, an ADL response of 3 implies that the patient spends up to 30 minutes a day at a sensor rate at or above the ADL. This is achieved by adjusting the rate/count relationship to achieve this percentage of rate response. Similarly, an ER value of 3 means that the patient spends about 20 minutes per week at the higher rates, for example between 105 and 120 bpm. Thus, in effect, the physician is adjusting the target rate profile for a patient by adjusting the ADL and ER, on the basis of the medical condition of the patient and his or her activities. This is termed "rate profile optimization." It is interesting to note that although the percentage of time spent at or above ADL and ER may be the same at the same setting in two individuals, the actual time spent at each rate will be different, depending on the specific patient and the programmed threshold setting (Fig. 16-13).

The Kappa 400 is a combined activity and minute ventilation sensing device. The general hardware and software implementation is similar to that for the Kappa 700/600 series. However, the actual amount of time spent in the ADL and ER is greater in the Kappa 400, because a more aggressive rate response is allowed by the higher specificity of the dual-sensor system.

St. Jude Medical: Affinity, Integrity, Identity

The activity-sensing devices manufactured by St. Jude Medical (Sylmar, Calif.) use an "Omnisense" accelerometer bonded to the circuit board, which is sensitive to accelerations that occur in the anteroposterior axis. Activity counts above a programmable threshold (1 = most sensitive, 7 = least sensitive) will be integrated and translated to a rate response using a rate-response slope (1 = least sensitive, 16 = most sensitive) (Fig. 16-14A).

The threshold level can be adjusted manually or automatically ("AUTO"). In the "AUTO" setting, the device measures the sensor activity level over the preceding 18 hours to determine the threshold parameter. The physician can further raise or lower this threshold using "AUTO" threshold offset. Similarly, the slope level can be adjusted manually or automatically. In the slope AUTO adjustment, the device records the activity variance over the last 7 days, and the slope is adjusted to achieve a rate response such that almost 1% heart rate occurs beyond 23% of heart rate reserve (see Fig. 16-14B). Typically the slope adjusts by a factor of 2 each week. In the event that the patient is immobile for the last week, as indicated by the small activity variance, the slope setting will be held constant. Again, the physician can apply an AUTO offset to raise or lower the rate response. Alternatively, the patient can be instructed to perform an exercise at a prescribed slope. The "Prediction Model" in these devices attempts to suggest an alternative slope based on the detected rate response. In addition, the onset and recovery kinetics are separately programmable.

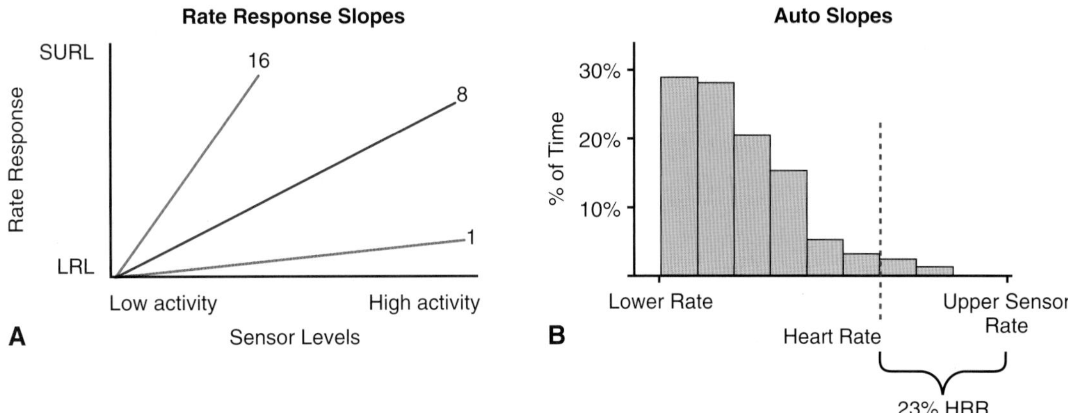

Figure 16-14. ***A,*** *Rate-response curves from St. Jude Medical activity sensors.* ***B,*** *Autoslope ensures that about 1% of the pacing rate will reach >23% of the heart rate reserve (HRR) over time. Note that the sensor-driven upper rate limit (SURL) may not be reached at a low slope setting. LRL, lower rate limit.*

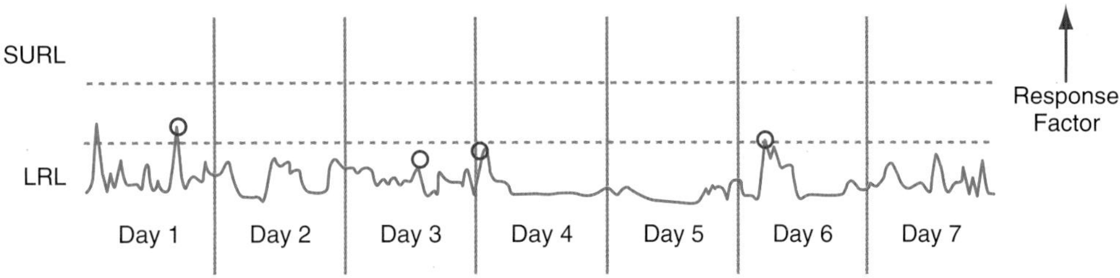

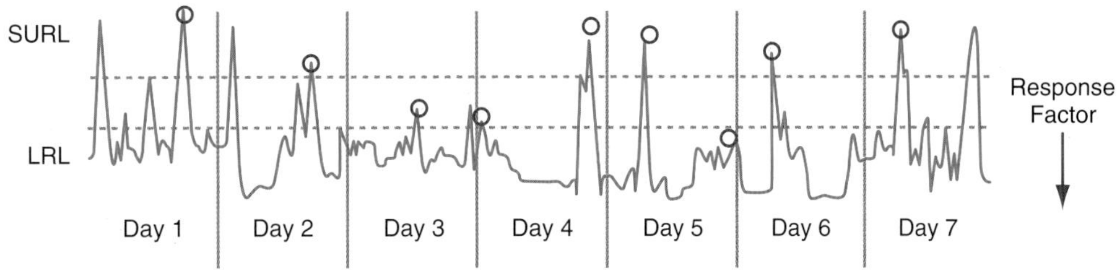

Figure 16-15. Automatic evaluation of rate response in the Guidant Insignia pacemaker. The "Response Factor" will be scaled upward or downward according to the average peak daily rates and compared with the programmed "Sensor Rate Target" accelerations above a moving average. LRL, lower rate limit; SURL, sensor-driven upper rate limit.

Guidant: Insignia, Pulsar Max

In the devices manufactured by Guidant (Boston Scientific, Natick, Mass.), an accelerometer mounted in the circuit board is used to detect anteroposterior acceleration. Four parameters are used to determine the rate response: response factor (1 = least sensitive, 16 = most sensitive), activity threshold (very low, low, medium-low, medium-high, high, and very high), reaction time, and recovery time. Programming can be effected either manually or automatically with the "Automatic Response Factor." In this method, the physician uses the "Expert Ease" feature in the programmer to decide the LRL, SURL, and the so-called Sensor Rate Target, on the basis of the patient's age, gender, exercise frequency, and target heart rate during exercise from a population average. After these parameters are input, an initial nominal slope, such as 8 (1 through 16 are available), is programmed. The "Automatic Response Factor" will track the maximum sensor rate each day for a week, and the average of this maximum will be compared with the "Sensor Rate Target." The response factor will then be scaled to effect either a more aggressive or a more conservative response, depending on whether the average rate falls below or exceeds the "Sensor Rate Target" by 5 bpm (Fig. 16-15).

Other Manufacturers

Sorin Biomedica CRM (Sorin Group, Milan) has introduced a gravitational sensor that is used either alone (Swing) or in combination with a PEA sensor (MiniLiving).

The gravitational sensor uses the vibrations from a mercury ball to measure body activity.

ELA Medical (Sorin Group, Milan) has an accelerometer activity sensor (Opus G) that uses a half-bridge variable-capacitance accelerometer. The accelerometer detects anteroposterior axis at a frequency range of 0.6 to 6 Hz, and samples acceleration signals every 1.56 seconds. The device can be programmed manually or automatically using the "Autocalibration." The level of acceleration at rest is reset daily according to the lowest mean acceleration of 64 consecutive measurements. The maximum mean acceleration of 8 consecutive accelerations is used to match the programmed upper sensor rate. In 43 patients with Opus G rate-adaptive pacing, the rate-response was reported to be proportional to workload on walking and descending stairs in comparison with normal and vibration sensors, but the rate-response on stair climbing remained inadequate.[18]

Clinical Results

Clinical studies have convincingly demonstrated that activity-based pacing systems offer the potential for greater exercise capacity and fewer exertionally related symptoms than do fixed-rate (VVI) pacemakers. In an early clinical study of a piezoelectric vibration-based, adaptive-rate pacemaker, Benditt and colleagues[12] used cardiopulmonary treadmill exercise tests to compare exercise tolerance during fixed-rate VVI pacing with that during VVIR pacing. Adaptive-rate pacing prolonged exercise duration by 35% and led to similar improvements in peak oxygen consumption and oxygen consumption at anaerobic threshold. Adaptive-rate pacing also reduced the patient's perception of exertion at comparable exercise levels,[12] and the benefit was sustained when exercise testing was repeated after an average of 5 months of follow-up. Furthermore, at the time of follow-up exercise testing, reversion of the pacing system to a fixed rate (VVI) mode resulted in prompt deterioration of both observed oxygen consumption and exercise duration. Thus, the ability of a single-chamber piezoelectric vibration-based pacing system to provide immediate and long-term improvements in exercise tolerance was clearly demonstrated.

Other investigators have also reported better exercise capacity with adaptive-rate pacemakers based on activity sensors, although the results from studies using bicycle exercise have been less dramatic than those observed with treadmill exercise.[19,20] The effect of ventricular function on exercise responses of 16 patients with piezoelectric vibration-based, adaptive-rate pacemakers in the VVI and the VVIR modes has been reported.[21] The findings indicate that the provision of appropriate heart rate responsiveness by this technique resulted in a substantial increase in cardiac index that was independent of baseline ejection fraction. Another study using mainly activity-sensing devices found that the potential hemodynamic benefits of adaptive-rate pacing in 22 patients was proportional to the extent of systolic dysfunction, with a greater benefit in those with poorer ventricular function.[22]

Activity-based VVIR pacing has also been compared with atrial-tracking, dual-chamber pacing modes (VDD, DDD),[23] which showed similar exercise tolerance in the two modes (VVIR, 68 ± 15 W/min vs. DDD, 70 ± 18 W/min), but more patients preferred the DDD mode, suggesting the importance of AV synchrony. On the other hand, other studies found no significant differences between the DDD and VVIR modes with respect to symptom scores, maximal exercise performance (treadmill), or plasma concentrations of epinephrine, norepinephrine, and atrial natriuretic peptide.[24,25] Surprisingly, venous epinephrine and norepinephrine levels were not higher during exercise in the VVIR mode, as might have been expected given comparable exercise levels. These data suggest that the role of atrial contribution is less in patients with heart block.

Several studies comparing the behavior of accelerometer-based devices with that of piezoelectric crystal devices reported that the accelerometer devices showed a better response to walking, jogging, and standing.[9,17,26] It was observed that the subject's footwear had no significant effect on the results seen with the accelerometer, as opposed to the results obtained with piezoelectric vibrational devices. Increasing grade of the treadmill had a significant effect on pacing rate with the accelerometer device, whereas there was no change in pacing rate with the piezoelectric vibrational sensors. The investigators concluded that, compared with the vibrational device, the accelerometer sensor-controlled devices showed a better rate-response and were less susceptible to direct pressure or to tapping on the pulse generator, unlike what was observed with the piezoelectric crystal.[26,27]

Using a strapped-on accelerometer, Charles and colleagues[27] found that the response of an accelerometer-based device (CPI Excel; CPI is now part of Guidant, St. Paul, Minn.) to graded treadmill testing was more strongly correlated with the patient's intrinsic heart rate (r = 0.80) than that of a vibrational adaptive-rate device (r = 0.27). The accelerometer responded appropriately when subjects walked up stairs (103 bpm) and walked down stairs (98 bpm). The response of the vibrational devices was paradoxical, giving a slower pacing rate when subjects walked up stairs (83 bpm) than when they walked down stairs (89 bpm). This multicenter study on the Excel has documented good response during daily activities.[27]

Schuster and associates[28] evaluated the efficacy of automatic "Rate Profile Optimization" over time. Eleven patients with Kappa 700 pacemakers performed treadmill testing at 1 month, 1 year, and 2 years after implantation. On the basis of the sinus profile at follow-up, the investigators found that the use of a more aggressive slope was needed to match the sinus rate profile. This required the change of ADL response from 3 to 4 and of ER from 3 to 4 at 1 year, and the change of activity threshold from medium/low to low at 2 years. These adjustments enabled better approximation of pacing rate to sinus rate during treadmill exercise. Exercise capacity was maintained during the 2 years.

In another study, activity level variation ("Activity Variance"), as detected by an accelerometer, was used to determine sleeping time in devices manufactured by St. Jude Medical.[29] The results showed good agreement with an actigraph that recorded patient movement externally. However, minor movement of the subject during sleep would reactivate the device, so that long periods of sleep rate pacing were not possible with the current algorithm.[29]

Raj and coworkers[30] examined the ability of the activity sensor to simulate heart rate variability, an important measure in heart failure.[30] They found that activity response contributed to long-term measures of heart rate variability through heart rate changes during exercise but had no effect during short-term measures, which depend on autonomic changes unrelated to exercise. This study suggested that rate modulation by activity sensors during exercise is an important element of heart rate variability.

Limitations

Activity sensing may give inappropriate heart rate-responses when subjected to environmental vibrations, such as those induced by the movement of a motor vehicle over rough terrain or those resulting from air travel or the use of appliances or machinery. The piezoelectric vibrational sensor also responds to the application of static pressure on the pulse generator, which may be important when the patient is prone. This false-positive response to pressure is less of a problem with pacemakers that incorporate an accelerometer.[31]

Matula and colleagues[32] assessed the effects of various means of locomotion on pacing rate for different activity-based pacemakers. Three different activity-based pacing systems (peak counting algorithm, integration type, and accelerometers) were strapped to the chests of volunteers. Bicycling on the street resulted in higher pacing rates than stationary bicycling for each type of pacemaker, although none of the pacemakers reached the heart rate achieved by the normal sinus node. During driving, the pacemakers raised the pacing rate, although the intrinsic sinus rate continued to be higher. In passively riding passengers, the pacemakers tended to produce a higher pacing rate than that of the normal sinus node. Of interest, the accelerometer-based system responded mainly to acceleration and curves, whereas vibration sensors responded primarily to vibrations and rough roads. Independent of the sensor, activity-initiated rate-response depends on the manner in which activity is being carried out rather than on the exercise workload, and proportionality is generally limited. Activity sensors may manifest paradoxically slower heart rates during walking uphill than during walking downhill. Non–exercise-related stresses such as emotional changes are not detected, limiting the sensor's sensitivity.

Minute Ventilation Sensing

Of all impedance-based sensors, the sensing of minute ventilation (MV) is the most commonly used technique and has been the concept for a physiologic system since 1966.[33,34] Although a respiratory rate–sensing pacemaker had been in use as early as 1983, it was limited by the need of an auxiliary subcutaneous electrode and easy interference by arm movement because of unipolar impedance sensing. All subsequent generations of respiratory sensors detect MV for rate adaptation.

Physiologic Principle

Relationship Between Heart Rate and Respiratory Parameters during Exercise

Changes in heart rate during exercise are closely related to changes in oxygen uptake (Vo_2) at all levels of exertion. At metabolic workloads of less than anaerobic threshold, Vo_2 and heart rate are also directly proportional to MV, with correlation coefficients greater than 0.9 in most studies.[35-39] On the other hand, the correlation between respiratory rate and oxygen uptake during submaximal exercise is less than 0.54.[35-37] The reason is that the ventilatory response at the onset of exercise is predominantly due to a change in tidal volume rather than in respiratory rate.[38,39] In a number of studies, it was noted that the tidal volume increased to a plateau within 2 minutes after the onset of exercise. The relative speed of changes in respiratory rate and MV (the product of tidal volume and respiratory rate) during exertion is shown in Figure 16-16.[39] The respiratory rate not only rises slowly during exercise but also declines faster than tidal volume at the cessation of exercise.

Anaerobic Threshold

With more strenuous exercise, the heart is unable to meet the increased oxygen demand of the working muscles completely, and anaerobic metabolism is initiated, resulting in greater production of lactic acid. Lactic acid dissociates into lactate and H^+, which is buffered by bicarbonate, resulting in an abrupt rise in carbon dioxide production. Because MV is largely controlled by carbon dioxide production and blood pH rather than Vo_2, the higher rate of carbon dioxide production induces a rise in MV that is out of proportion to the increase in Vo_2. Vo_2 is linearly related to the normal sinus rate throughout exercise, so at workloads above anaerobic threshold, MV will increase disproportionately relative to Vo_2 and the sinus rate. This has important implications in an MV-controlled pacemaker, which needs special rate-adaptive curves to avoid overpacing above the anaerobic threshold.

Effect of Pulmonary Disease and Congestive Heart Failure on Minute Ventilation Sensing

In patients with chronic obstructive pulmonary and restrictive lung diseases, it is the pulmonary system that usually limits exercise, not the cardiovascular system. In a healthy patient at peak exercise, MV is about 50% of the maximum voluntary ventilation. In a patient with pulmonary disease, this reserve is smaller and, in many

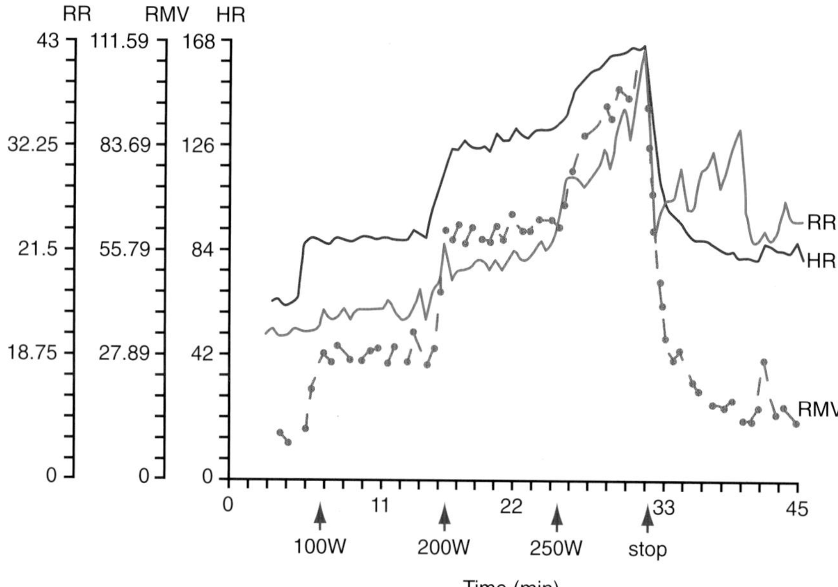

Figure 16-16. Changes in respiratory variables during progressive exercise. Minute ventilation (RMV, in L/min) closely parallels the change in heart rate (HR, in bpm), whereas there is little change in respiratory rate (RR, in breaths/min) at the beginning of exercise. (From Alt E, Heinz M, Hirgestetter C, et al: Control of pacemaker rate by impedance-based respiratory minute ventilation. Chest 92:247, 1987.)

cases, disappears before the anaerobic threshold, indicating that the patient will not reach this condition. The transthoracic estimate of MV is often higher for the same Vo_2 in patients with pulmonary disease, providing a strong signal for the implantable device to control heart rate, although the pacing rate change has to be limited. To date, only a limited number of case reports have suggested the safety and feasibility of using MV sensors in lung disease.[40]

In the era of biventricular pacing for heart failure, the use of MV rate-adaptive sensors during exercise and for monitoring heart failure is of interest. Like the resting heart rate, MV is higher at rest but achieves a lower maximum level in patients with congestive heart failure.[41] It has been suggested that the ratio of peak MV to resting MV in healthy patients is close to twice that in patients with congestive heart failure, thus providing a natural limit to the extent of rate adaptation. When patients with congestive heart failure undergo a regimen of exercise training, their peak MV increases, as does their maximum heart rate. On the cardiovascular side, patients with heart failure often have associated chronotropic incompetence, but the range of heart rate changes is small given the higher resting heart rate. Because of the lesser importance of atrial contribution during exercise in patients with heart failure, rate adaptation assumes a greater significance.[22] Patients with biventricular pacing may still derive benefit from rate-adaptive pacing if their maximum predicted heart rate during exercise is below 70% of the age-predicted maximum.[42]

Cheyne-Stokes respiration is a waxing and waning of tidal volume and respiratory rate with a periodicity of about 0.02 Hz. More than 60% of the patients with congestive heart failure show overt Cheyne-Stokes respiration or some form of pulsed breathing during sleep,[43] owing to prolonged transit time of blood flow to the brain. Manifestation of Cheyne-Stokes respiration during exercise[44] and activities of daily living[45] tends to carry a poor prognosis. Sleep apnea and Cheyne-Stokes respiration can be effective indices of congestive heart failure that a pacemaker, measuring MV, could monitor to guide therapy.

Despite these interesting data, MV sensing is best avoided in patients with significant lung disease. The usefulness of MV sensors in patients with heart failure and cardiac resynchronization therapy remains to be tested. No MV sensor–driven biventricular device has yet been introduced.

Sensors

The measurement of impedance in biomedical applications is commonly referred to as *plethysmography* and has its basis in Ohm's law. This law states that the ratio of the applied voltage (V) to the current (I) flowing is as follows:

$$R = V/I$$

where R is the impedance. If the current (I) is kept constant, then the voltage (V) that is measured will reflect changes in resistance. The value of R is related to the resistivity (ρ) of the medium (blood and tissue, etc.), by the length of the path (L), and inversely by the cross-sectional area ($A + \Delta A$) of the conducting medium, as indicated by the following equation:

$$R = \rho(L/A + \Delta A)$$

Note that the cross-sectional area is displayed as having two components, a constant component (A) and a dynamic component (ΔA) that changes with respiration (and other factors).

Placing any two electrodes subcutaneously across the human torso results in the impedances shown in Figure 16-17. A measurement of this type is termed a *bipolar* measurement. The resistances, R_1 and R_2, and the capacitances, C_1 and C_2, are due to the effects of polarization at the electrode-electrolyte interface (polar-

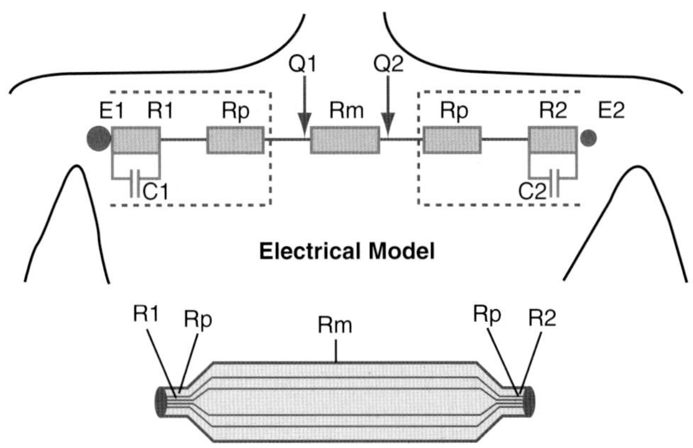

Figure 16-17. Constituents of impedance measurement across the human torso. When voltage is applied between electrodes E1 and E2, separate measurement points Q1 and Q2 give respiration changes independent of contact resistances. R1, C1, R2, and C2 are polarization elements; RP, contact resistance; RM, torso resistance containing respiration signal.

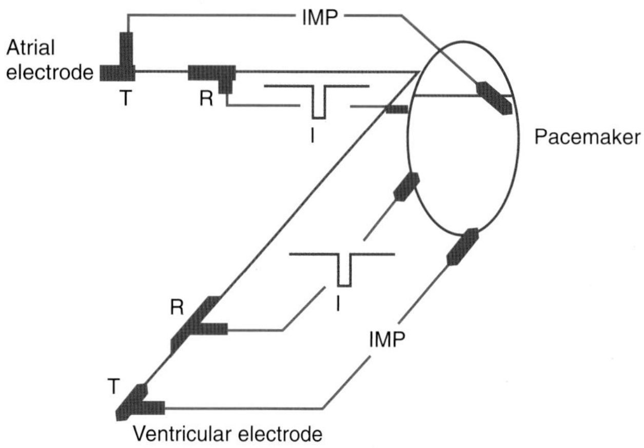

Figure 16-18. Measurements explored for conventional pacing electrode configurations for minute volume (MV) measurement. Measurements in both chambers of the heart are shown. I, constant-current pulse; IMP, impedance measured; R, ring; T, tip.

ization effects). The values of these parameters depend on the frequency of the measurement current. At frequencies above a few thousand hertz, their contribution becomes negligible. For this reason, as well as for the purposes of minimizing battery drain and maintaining patient safety, the measurements in implantable devices are performed with high frequencies or very narrow pulse widths. As an example, a current pulse used in one early MV pacing system is 0.015 msec wide, roughly equivalent to a frequency of 33 kHz (Meta MA, Telectronics Pacing Systems, Sylmar, Calif.). This frequency eliminates all polarization effects.

A fluid-flow analogy can be used to understand the bipolar impedance measurement. With this model, the impedance can be conceptualized to comprise three "conduits" that impede the flow of electric current. The narrow conduits (R_p) are related to contact resistance at the electrode-tissue interfaces and have a considerably larger impedance than the wider conduit R_m, which is related to resistance across the torso (the two R_p values are shown as equal for convenience). The impedance R_m contains the respiration signal that we want to measure to control the pacing rate of a rate-adaptive pacemaker. As a rule, the values of R_p are greater than those of R_m, especially for electrodes with a small surface area. This makes the regions around the electrodes prone to artifacts related to movement of the skin and underlying tissues. To eliminate this source of inaccuracy, normally either a four-electrode (quadripolar) system, as shown by the measurement points Q1 and Q2 in Figure 16-17, is used, or the electrodes are made large, thereby minimizing this funneling. The usual tip electrode-tissue impedance of a pacing lead is on the order of 400 ohms, and that around a pacemaker case is usually less than 20 ohms. The impedance across the torso is on the order of 50 ohms. The change in R_m that is related to respiration (the value that we want to measure) is in the vicinity of 1 ohm. To detect small changes in minute ventilation, a resolution of 0.06 ohms is required. This example gives some indication of how sensitive the measurement system has to be.

Rossi and colleagues[34] used an auxiliary lead tunneled across the chest as one pole of a bipolar system. This arrangement was successful in detecting respiratory rate, but the auxiliary lead is prone to erosion and movement artifacts from the chest cage.

With these disadvantages in mind, Nappholz, in collaboration with Maloney and Simmons of the Cleveland Clinic, carried out a series of studies to explore the use of transvenous electrodes to measure MV in exercising patients.[46,47] The impedance measurements were made using a quadripolar system in the superior vena cava at first in dogs and subsequently in patients. The correlation of changes in impedance with actual changes in MV was excellent ($r > 0.9$). In human studies, a cutaneous defibrillation pad was placed over the prepectoral region (the site of the pacemaker case), and the measurement current was generated between the right ventricle and the cutaneous pad. The results confirmed that the use of a common electrode for both generating the current pulses and measuring the impedance was appropriate and that the impedance of a cutaneous pad was about the same as that for a pulse generator case (<20 ohms). At the same time, with this approach and with all subsequent approaches, the highest impedance was through the thoracic cavity, which dominated the measurement.

In subsequent implanted systems, the current pulse was generated between the pulse generator case and the ring electrode (atrial or ventricular electrodes), with the measurement taken between the tip electrode and the case (Fig. 16-18). These measurements validated the application of this sensor for either atrial or ventricular pacemakers.

In later work, Pioger and associates[48] used implanted Chorus RM 7034 and Opus RM 4534 pacemakers (both from ELA Medical) to evaluate the effect of injecting current in the atrial or ventricular tip on the accuracy of MV measurement. In each of these cases, MV was

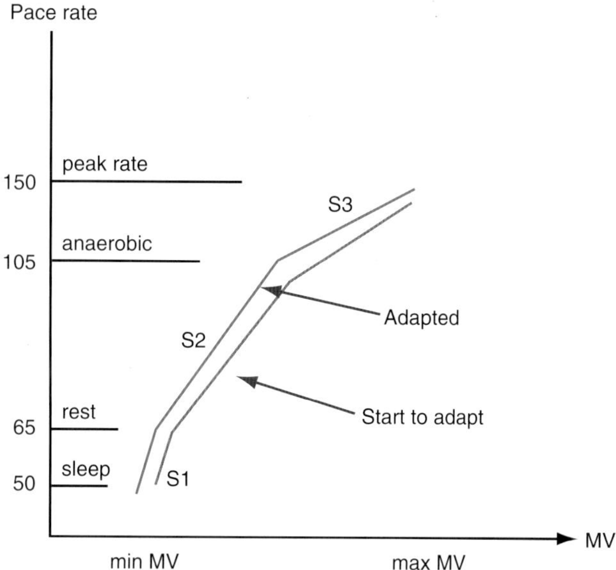

Figure 16-19. The comprehensive relationship between minute volume (MV) and heart rate in an automatic rate-adaptive pacemaker. MV issued to determine a sleep rate and a daytime rest rate (50 and 65 bpm, respectively; S1 portion of curve), and exercise MV–heart rate will follow either S2 or S3 (gentler curves), depending on the anaerobic threshold. The relationship adapts in time, as indicated, according to empirically derived rate profiles.

measured off the corresponding atrial and ventricular ring, except in the case of a single-pass lead, in which the MV was measured off the atrial sensing ring. In every case, the correlation with Vo_2 was better than 0.8.

Algorithm: The Ideal Response Curve

The relationship between MV and heart rate is shown in Figure 16-19, in which the curve is segmented into three regions. S1 is the segment controlling rate changes from sleep to daytime rest rates, S2 determines the relationship for light exercise, and S3 sets the relationship for anaerobic activity. The anaerobic threshold is set to about 75% of the maximum heart rate,[48] which corresponds to about 40% of maximum MV. This basic type of MV–pacing rate curve is used in current devices.

Clinical Experience

MV is an indirect but reliable marker of metabolic demands, and in the first generation of MV pacers (Meta MV, Telectronics Pacing Systems), the rate-response was proportional to the level of exertion and correlated with the sinus response.[49,50] It was superior to the respiratory rate–based rate-adaptive system.[51] When respiratory gas exchange was measured, the pacing rate was shown to be significantly correlated with Vo_2, MV, respiratory quotient, tidal volume, and respiratory rate.[52,53] Compared with VVI pacing, minute ventilation–driven VVIR pacing increased exercise capacity by 33%,[54] and maximal Vo_2 and cardiac output are significantly better. In one study on 10 patients with the first version of MV driven–VVIR pacing, pacing rate was highly correlated with measured MV (r = 0.89), respiratory quotient (r = 0.89), Vco_2 (r = 0.87), tidal volume (r = 0.87), Vo_2 (r = 0.84) and respiratory rate (r = 0.84). Maximum Vo_2 increased from 13.4 ± 3.4 to 16.3 ± 4.1 mL/kg/min (P = .0004).

Improvements in symptoms were also documented in the VVIR mode.[54] Minute ventilation has good long-term stability, programming of the sensor is relatively simple, and the rate-response was appropriate during daily activities. Figure 16-20 shows the rate response of the MV sensor in relation to ideal rate behavior based on the workload.[56] Compared with activity pacing, MV is significantly better in achieving a near-normal pacing rate–workload relationship, whereas activity sensing tends to overpace at low levels of exercise and to underpace at the peak exercise and in the recovery period. As expected with all impedance systems, the MV sensor is liable to interference by electromagnetic interference, arm swinging, coughing, and hyperventilation.[49] Artificial ventilation induces an unphysiologic rate so that MV sensor needs to be disabled in this setting.

Current Minute Ventilation–Sensing Devices

Medtronic Kappa 400

The Medtronic MV pacer is marketed as a dual-sensor device. The MV component requires a bipolar lead. Subthreshold 30-μg biphasic pulses at 1 msec are injected between the electrode (either atrial or ventricle) and pacemaker case at 16 Hz, and the resulting impedance is measured between the lead tip and the case. Changes in MV are measured as MV counts over a 32-second short-term moving average to avoid transient events like coughing. The short-term average is compared over an 18-hour long-term average to effect a change.

The Medtronic Kappa 400 has been evaluated with the use of symptom-limited treadmill exercise testing.[57] All patients underwent cardiopulmonary gaseous analysis in conjunction with simultaneous recording of MV-induced impedance changes. The calibrations between them during resting, supine, and sitting and the type of exercise (bicycle or treadmill) were made. The impedance-derived MV was smaller for sitting than for the supine position, for shallow than for slow breathing, and for bicycle than for treadmill exercise. The investigators concluded that this difference may be attributed to static or dynamic geometry of the intrathoracic viscera. Correlation coefficients of the best-fit line for measured and device-based MV values were high (>0.9 in first-, second-, and third-order polynomial equations; Fig. 16-21).[58] Furthermore, the calibration between measured MV and impedance MV changed over time (between 1 week and 1 month).[59] However, the changes were not correlative. This finding has implications for the need for continual automatic adaptation and the potential use of the sensor for MV monitoring.

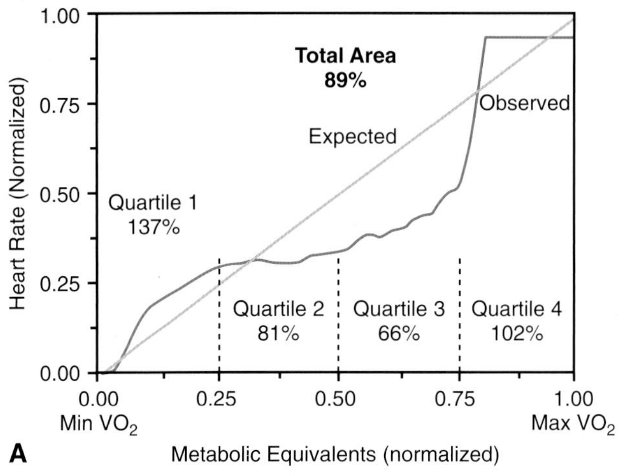

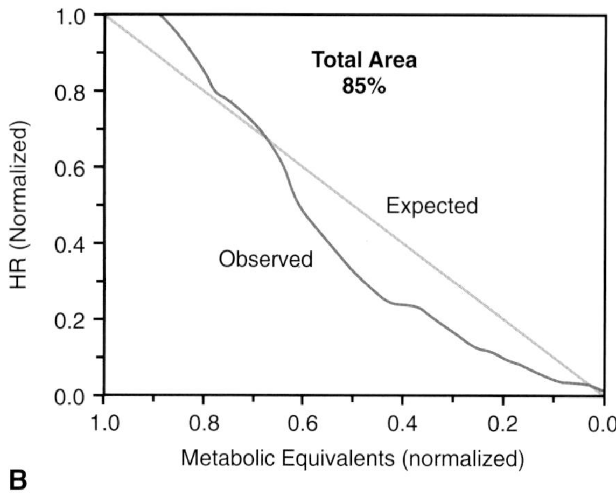

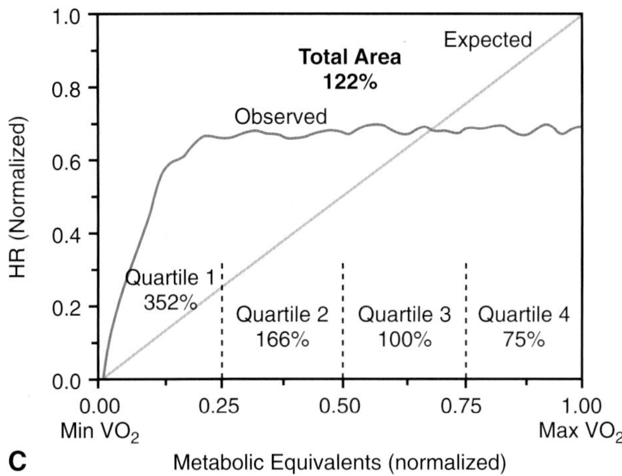

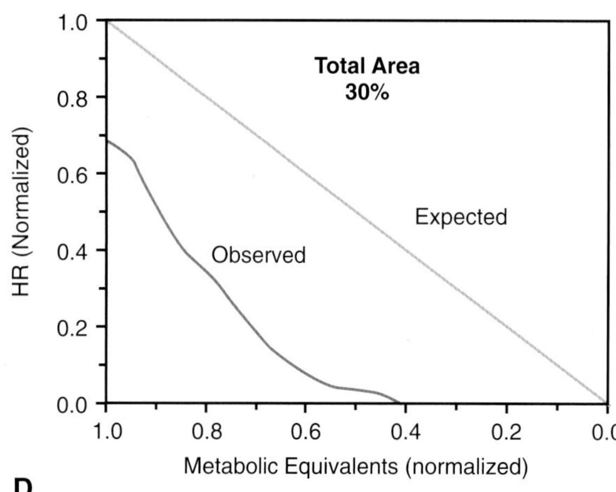

Figure 16-20. Quartification of pacing percentage of minute volume (MV) and activity pacer during graded treadmill exercise. ***A*** *shows the results of the normalized heart rate and workload in one patient. There is overpacing in quartile 1 (137%), underpacing in quartiles 2 and 3 (81% and 66%, respectively), and near-ideal pacing in quartile 4.* ***B*** *shows the near-ideal rate recovery of the MV sensor.* ***C*** *and* ***D*** *show the exercise response of an activity sensor with overpacing during most of the time, but inadequate rate recovery. (From Kay GN: Quartification of chronotropic response: Comparison of methods for rate-modulated permanent pacemakers. J Am Coll Cardiol 20:1533, 1992.)*

Guidant Devices

In the minute ventilation–sensing devices manufactured by Guidant, the Pulsar Max, and the Insignia, MV is available in conjunction with an accelerometer sensor, although the rate-adaptive function can be used either alone or blended with the accelerometer. MV collected by either the atrial or ventricular lead (programmable) over 24 hours is used as an average against which future changes in MV are compared for a rate response. The minimum time for achieving a baseline is 4 minutes (thus 4 → On). A linear response curve is used, and a total of 16 response factors can be chosen below the judged pacing rate for anaerobic threshold. This rate is also programmable. In between the pacing rate for anaerobic threshold and the maximum predicted heart rate, a gentler “High Rate Response” can be programmed. The adaptation can be made faster by activating the 4-minute walk within 30-minute option, in which the subject is instructed to exercise to achieve the maximal MV change.

Telemetered MV impedance signals from a Guidant MV device have been compared with measured MV in 20 patients.[60] Respiratory rate was accurately measured by the device during hyperventilation, with a difference of less than 0.2 breaths/minute. During 10-minute cycle ergometry at 50 W, the correlation between MV measured directly and that measured by the device was 0.99. There are large individual variations between the measured and impedance MV slopes, requiring specific rate-response curves for particular patients.

Sorin Group–ELA Medical Minute Ventilation–Sensing Devices

The MV devices manufactured by ELA Medical and its parent company, Sorin Group, are the Chorus, Talent,

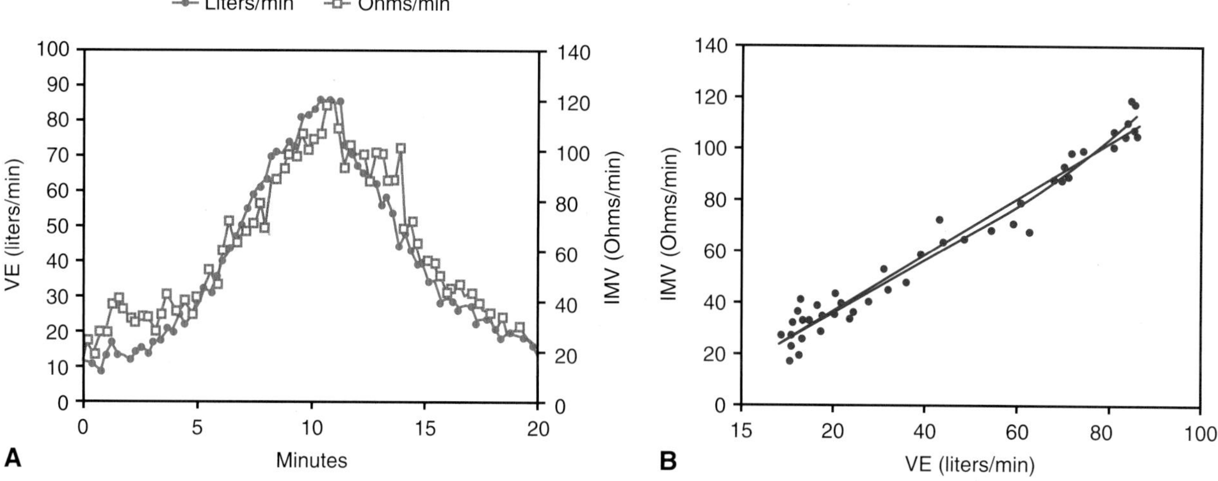

Figure 16-21. ***A,*** *Transthoracic impedance minute ventilation (IMV) and measured minute ventilation (VE) by duration of the exercise test and recovery for an individual subject. The two parameters show good correlation.* ***B,*** *Regression analysis for the same subject showing first-, second-, and third-order regression lines, which are practically superimposed. (From Cole CR, Jensen DN, Cho Y, et al: Correlation of impedance minute ventilation with measured minute ventilation in a rate responsive pacemaker. PACE 24:989, 2001.)*

Opus, Synphony, and Rhapsody. The automatic slope algorithm in the Chorus determines the resting and maximum MV values on a daily basis. The device calculates the exercise MV signal by looking for the maximal MV signal and recalculates this value every eighth cycle during which a change has occurred. The exercise MV value is increased or decreased in 6% intervals. The mean resting and exercise MV values are used to adjust the rate-response slope automatically over the range of values from 1 to 15 in steps of 0.1. By automatically adjusting the rate-response slope in this manner, the Chorus may be able to provide rate-response that is individualized for each patient and can vary it as physiologic conditions evolve. The algorithm used by the Chorus has now been tested extensively and found to be effective.[61,62] Furthermore, the use of different impedance-sensing electrode configurations has been evaluated—atrial bipolar, ventricular bipolar, double unipolar, and "floating" configurations in a unipolar lead.[63] The mean correlations for these four configurations between impedance-based MV values and MV values measured during exercise were 0.89 ± 0.08, 0.95 ± 0.05, 0.87 ± 0.14, and 0.88 ± 0.05, respectively, suggesting the possibility of using the MV sensor in a wide range of populations.

In addition, if the MV value over 128 cycles remains below the 24-hour mean MV, the lower rate decreases to the rest rate, which is set below the lower rate limit. In a Holter monitoring study of 46 patients with the Chorus RM pacemaker,[64] the MV successfully decreased the base rate during the sleep period, with the diurnal pacing rate at 68 ± 5 bpm and a nocturnal rate of 60 ± 4 bpm. Similarly, at the upper rate, if MV continues to increase, the device automatically decreases the linear rate-response slope to reach the higher MV on a subsequent exercise. In another study, the response of the Talent DR (ELA Medical) during exercise was compared in 81 patients. The correlation coefficient between the sinus rate and the programmer-derived sensor rate was 0.983 ± 0.005, and a linear relationship was observed between heart rate reserve and MV reserve.[61]

Limitations

The use of MV devices in patients with lung disease and heart failure remains controversial. Because of filtering of the cardiac component, the MV sensor does not accurately reflect rate adaptation at high respiratory rates, which occur commonly in children. A 1998 study found good correlation in 5 of 11 children between sinus rate and MV-driven rates.[65] In a later study, Cabrera and associates[66] measured MV in 38 healthy children and used computer simulation of the Kappa MV algorithm to define the intrinsic heart rate. They found good correlation between predicted heart rate within 80% of heart rate reserve. However, particularly in small children with body surface areas of less than 1.1 m^2, inadequate rate response occurred (26 ± 16 bpm lower than expected) because the respiratory rate at 65 breaths/minute exceeds the pacemaker MV processing capability, which is set at 48 breaths/minute. Thus, in children, MV is a feasible alternative with appropriate selection of subjects. In conjunction with an activity sensor, MV sensing may enhance metabolic response of patients with pacemakers, a capability that is particularly relevant in active children.

The speed of rate response of the earlier-generation MV sensing pacemakers was slow and had a delay of 30 to 45 seconds compared with an activity-sensing pacemaker. This slowness was due partly to the MV-averaging algorithm used and the curvilinear rate-adaptive curve, which resulted in a slow increase of rate at the onset but reached the maximal rate earlier during exercise compared with the sinus rate. The pacing rate may also remain high after exercise for 1 to 2 minutes before returning gradually to the baseline. This limitation is addressed with the use of more complex curves in modern MV devices. A bipolar atrial/ventricular lead is needed for MV sensing. The battery current for MV sensing may take up to about 2% of the total current of a dual-chamber pacemaker.

It is possible for some sense amplifiers to sense the small impedance pulses unless some preventive steps are taken. In some products, a blanking period of about 1 msec is applied to the amplifiers to "blind" them to these pulses. In other cases, special balancing of the pulse is carried out, achieving the same objective.

Sensing of the impedance pulses by a surface electrocardiogram monitor is always a possibility and depends on the sensitivity of the electrocardiogram machine. The pulse width and the balancing of the impedance pulse influence this possibility.

The impedance is measured only for the duration of the narrow, microsecond pulses. As long as the electric signal does not change during this short interval, interference from underlying electric signals is rejected. Sixty hertz takes about 7000 msec to change from its minimum to its maximum value. In the 15 msec required to make the impedance measurement, an intracardiac signal, obviously, changes very little. Hence, the effect of an intracardiac electrogram on the impedance pulse is negligible.

Frequencies above a few kilohertz, such as those generated by electrocautery and electrosurgery, are detected by the rate-response circuitry and could drive a pacemaker to its maximum rate, so it is recommended that the rate-response function of a pacemaker be turned off whenever a patient is to undergo electrosurgery. Respiration is also potentially influenced by phonation and coughing, which have no relevance to cardiac output.

Evoked QT Interval–Based Pacemakers

In 1920, Bazett[67] showed that changes in heart rate induced by exercise result in a progressive shortening of the QT interval on the surface electrocardiogram. The normal QT interval was found to be longer at relatively slow heart rates than at faster rates, and a nonlinear formula to correct the QT interval for changes in heart rate was proposed. In 1981, Rickards and Norman[68,69] found that QT interval shortening during exercise consisted of two components, an effect induced by exercise alone and an effect of an increased heart rate. They measured QT intervals during exercise in patients with normal sinus rhythm (in whom the QT interval was influenced by both factors), during atrial pacing at different rates with the patients at rest (a pure heart rate influence), and during exercise in patients with VVI pacemakers (a pure exercise influence). These observations led to the design of a cardiac pacemaker that uses the QT interval to modulate the pacing rate.[70]

The first QT interval–driven, rate-responsive pacemaker, the TX1(Vitatron Medical, Dieren, The Netherlands), was implanted in 1982. Experience gained with this and later models have proved the clinical applicability of this concept and have led to a series of pacemakers characterized by progressive improvement in rate-modulating behavior (Table 16-2).

Physical Principle

With exercise or psychological stress, the metabolism of the myocardium and the heart rate (sinus node) rise, mainly as a result of adrenergic stimulation. Available data indicate a relatively strong linear correlation between atrial rate and cardiac sympathetic activation. The ionic currents responsible for cardiac depolarization and repolarization periods parallel these changes. At low levels of exercise, the catecholamine release is relatively low, and the cardiac rate increase is primarily due to vagal withdrawal. This implies that as a biosensor, the QT interval (catecholamine influence) may be slow to respond at the start of exercise, although its major dependence on the sympathetic nervous system should result in its being a specific sensor. Indeed, a correlation between the QT driven pacing rate and the level of circulating adrenaline of more than 0.9 was found in a group of 9 patients in one study.[71]

To study the influence of various factors (e.g., drugs, autonomic influence, heart rate) on cardiac repolarization, investigators have looked for formulas to describe

TABLE 16-2. **Evolutions of Different Generations of QT Interval–Driven Rate-Responsive Pacemakers**

Year	Model*	Improvement	Technology
1985	Quintech TX	T-wave detection T-wave detection	Fast-recharge pulse Dual fast-recharge pulse
1988	Rhythmyx	Slope programming Onset of rate response	QT interval combined with activity
1992 Current device	Topaz Diamond, Selection	Sensor specificity	Sensor cross-checking

*All manufactured by Vitatron (a subsidiary of Medtronic, Inc., Minneapolis, Minn.).

the QT interval–heart rate relationship under these different circumstances. Several studies have shown that Bazett's formula is relatively accurate at heart rates between 60 and 100 bpm but is not correct in describing the relationship between the QT interval and heart rate over a wider range of rates because of the adrenergic influence on the QT interval.[72-74] Figure 16-22 shows electrocardiographic data obtained with the atrium paced at a constant rate of 130 bpm, and the QT interval measured before and after the administration of isoproterenol. The QT interval clearly shortens, independent of the heart rate, after the administration of the drug. A different QT interval–heart rate relationship was observed after administration of propranolol, a β-adrenergic blocker.[74] There are also large interindividual differences in the QT interval–heart rate relationship. A later study reported a curvilinear relationship between QT interval and heart rate, with a small QT interval change at low heart rates and a larger QT change at high heart rates.[75]

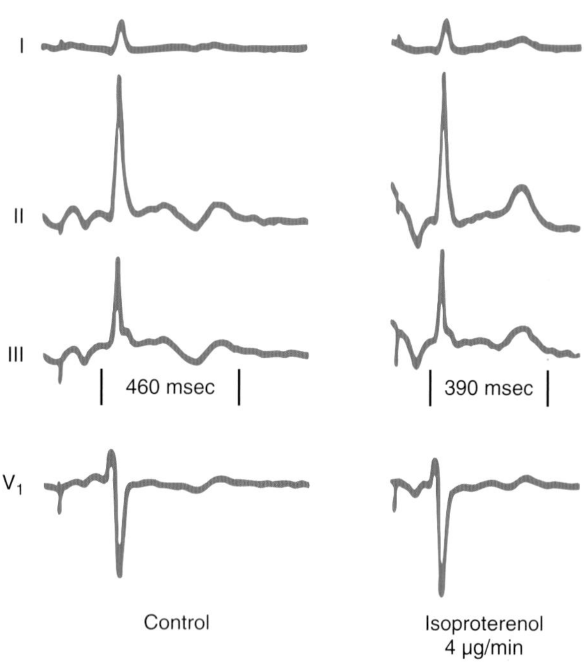

Figure 16-22. Fixed-rate atrial pacing at a pacing cycle length (PCL) of 450 msec and the influence of a catecholamine-mimicking drug, isoprenaline, on the length of the QT interval. (From Browne KF, Prystowsky E, Heger JJ, Zipes DP: Modulation of the Q-T interval by the automatic nervous system. PACE 6:1050, 1983.)

Sensor

The QT interval in rate-adaptive pacemakers is defined as the interval between the pacing stimulus and the evoked endocardial T wave. Detection of the evoked T wave should occur by means of the same electrode that is used for pacing. After a conventional pacing stimulus, a slowly decaying voltage can be observed with an amplitude of several hundred millivolts that gradually dissipates over a period of more than 300 msec, interfering with normal assessment of the T wave. These polarization after-potentials can be minimized by using a fast recharge. After a blanking period of 200 msec to avoid detection of an evoked R wave, the first negative derivative of the endocardial signal allows the pacemaker to sense the downslope of the evoked T wave (Fig. 16-23).[68,69,76] Boute and colleagues[77] used this method to evaluate the reliability of evoked T-wave sensing. T-wave sensing was possible in 99.5% of patients (n = 368). Mean evoked T-wave amplitude was 3.0 ± 1.3 mV at implantation and 2.2 ± 0.9 mV 3 months later, thus allowing for reliable sensing with a maximum T-wave sensitivity of 0.5 mV. Older, long-term leads tend to show slightly smaller T-wave amplitudes (1.6 ± 0.6 mV, vs. 2.3 ± 0.9 mV with newly implanted leads), mainly as a result of their electrode characteristics, such as larger surface area and nonporous surface structure.[77]

The QT Interval Rate-Adaptive Algorithm

In 1987, Baig and associates,[75,78-80] conducting a reappraisal of the relationship between the evoked QT interval and ventricular pacing rate, found a nonlinear relationship between pacing and evoked QT intervals in individual patients. They found that the extent of QT interval shortening is least at low heart rates. This finding resulted in the development of a new rate-adaptive algorithm that featured a rate-dependent slope—

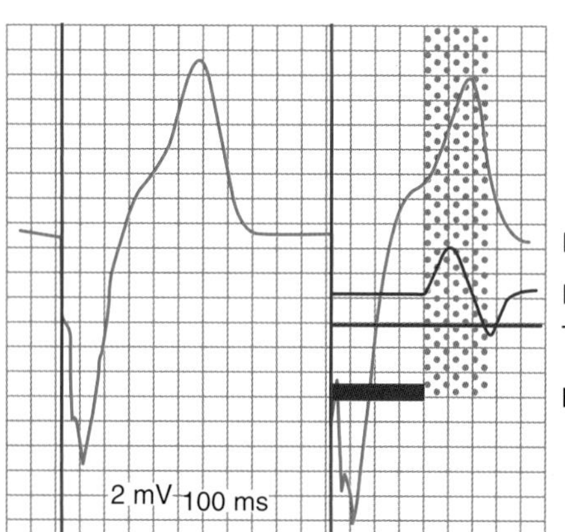

Figure 16-23. Recording of the paced evoked response from the pacing electrode using a dual-fast-recharge technique to eliminate polarization afterpotentials. The first derivative of the evoked T wave is compared with the programmed T-wave sensitivity.

that is, the slope is highest at low heart rates and decreases gradually as the heart rate increases.[78] The slope setting for low rates is adjusted automatically every night by measuring the QT interval at two different rates near the lower rate limit (daily learning). At the upper rate, the slope is adjusted in such a way that pacing at the upper rate occurs at the patient's shortest QT interval. Further shortening of the QT interval during pacing at the upper rate, an indication that the patient reached the upper rate at submaximal exercise levels, causes the slope at high rates to decrease (see Fig. 5-17).

Evaluation of the effectiveness of this new algorithm showed a faster initial acceleration of the pacing rate at the onset of exercise (a 10-bpm rate increase was obtained after 126 seconds, versus 255 seconds with the linear algorithm; n = 11; $P = .02$) and fewer instances of rate instability.[79,80] Baig and associates[81] also evaluated the long-term stability of the automatic slope adjustments. Slope settings were found to change considerably in the first 2 weeks, from relatively low settings initially to steeper values 2 weeks after implantation (n = 17; pacing cycle length–QT interval slope at lower rate limit changing from 3.7 msec/ msec at implantation to 5.8 msec/ msec after 2 weeks; $P < .001$). During the 1-year follow-up period, only minor slope adjustments were found, resulting in satisfactory and reproducible rate modulation.

Vitatron Combined QT Interval–Activity Devices: Topaz, Diamond, Selection

The main limitation of the QT sensor is its slow rate to initiate a rate-response. Despite algorithmic improvement, the QT sensor is still limited by the relatively slow onset of rate response. In one study, rate response was observed in the recovery phase of a short exercise.[82] On the other hand, an activity sensor gives an immediate rate response but is not proportional to the workload. Thus, it is logical to combine these two sensors to give a proportional and rapid response kinetics. In the currently available QT devices, the QT sensor is used with a piezoelectric activity sensor. In addition to improving the pattern of rate adaptation, the overall sensor specificity can be improved by continuous cross-checking of the information from the two sensors. If the two sensors provide consistent information, either exercise or recovery is confirmed, and the pacing rate increases or decreases, respectively. If false-positive activity signals are received (rises in the activity counts without a change in the QT interval), the pacemaker initially increases the pacing rate. If the QT interval still does not indicate an exercise condition after about 1 minute, a function called "sensor cross checking" is activated. This slowly decreases the pacing rate toward the QT interval–indicated rate. In case of false-positive activity sensing, the pacing rate gradually returns to the lower rate limit. Conversely, when the QT interval shortens while no activity is detected, mental stress or isometric exercise is most probable. Under these circumstances, the pacemaker is designed to increase the pacing rate, although its magnitude is limited.

The Topaz (Vitatron Medical) is the first dual-sensor VVIR device; QT and activity can be blended as follows: QT < Activity (ACT), QT = ACT, or ACT > QT.[82] In one study, 45 patients exercised according to a modified chronotropic assessment exercise protocol (CAEP) (stage 1 was made identical to stage 2) (Fig. 16-24).[83] In 30 patients, the rate adaptation was judged to be appropriate; that is, heart rate increased after 1 minute of exercise between 25% and 50% of the rate range and after 2 minutes between 50% and 75% of the rate range. In 12 patients, the initial response was too slow, and their pacemakers were reprogrammed to a blending pattern of QT < ACT; in three other patients, however, the initial response was judged to be too aggressive; these patients underwent reprogramming to QT > ACT.

Sharp and coworkers[84] evaluated heart rate and oxygen uptake at rest and at low exercise levels in

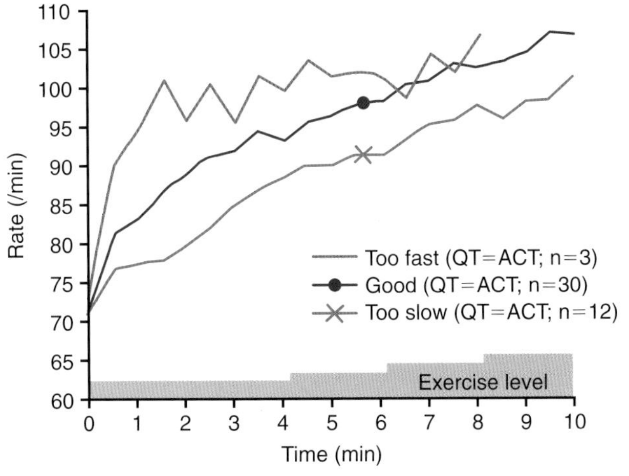

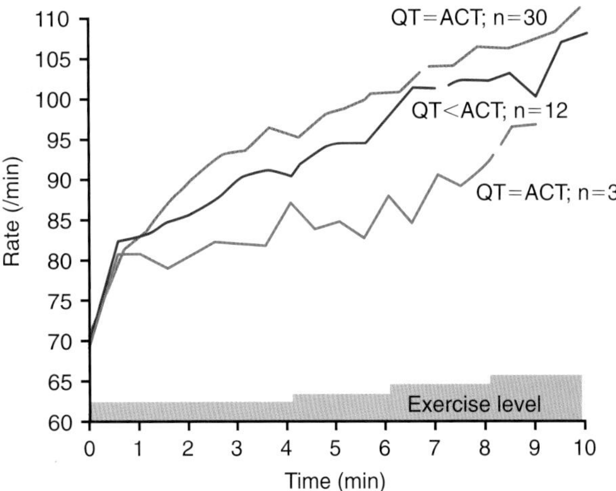

Figure 16-24. Effect of reprogramming "Sensor Blending" on the rate-response pattern. Initially, all patients exercised in the QT = ACT (activity) setting (left). *Two subgroups underwent pacemaker reprogramming because of a suboptimal rate response. A second exercise test* (right) *confirmed that the desired effect was actually obtained.*

patients with left ventricular dysfunction in the fixed-rate VVI mode and compared them with VVIR pacing based on the activity sensor only, the QT sensor only, and blending of both sensors. The dual-sensor chronotropic response reproduced the theoretical linear relationship among metabolic workload, heart rate, and oxygen uptake, suggesting the usefulness of this sensor in patients with stable left ventricular dysfunction.

The effectiveness of "sensor cross checking" was tested during continuous levels of false-positive activity: gentle and vigorous tapping on the pacemaker case and applying massage equipment over the pacemaker, which created excessive activity signals.[82] In all cases, "sensor cross checking" prevented unphysiologic rate accelerations. The time taken for the pacing rate to decrease from its peak (85 ± 8 bpm) to about the lower rate limit was 2.7 ± 1.7 minutes with gentle tapping and 8.3 ± 2.4 minutes with the massage equipment.

The ability of the combined sensor to simulate the normal sinus activity on a daily basis was studied in patients with the DDDR Diamond pacemaker.[85] A special software contained an additional diagnostic feature that continuously stored the difference between the sensor and the sinus rate during a 1-month ambulatory period. Sinus and dual-sensor rates were significantly correlated ($P < .001$; correlation coefficients > 0.90; mean difference throughout exercise and recovery 2.8 ± 6.1 bpm). During the ambulatory period, sensor and sinus rate differences were classified according to three activity levels (see Fig. 5-13). Nearly 90% of the sensor-driven beats were within 8 bpm of the sinus rate at medium and low levels of exercise. However, the difference was larger at higher levels of exercise.

Other Applications of the Evoked QT Interval Sensor

The evoked QT interval sensor is one of the few clinically available sensors that reflect cardiac metabolism. Several investigators have indicated other applications for the evoked QT interval sensor, as described here.

Dynamic Pace Refractory Period

Because the T wave marks the end of cardiac refractoriness, it can be used to match the pacemaker's paced ventricular refractory period, automatically and dynamically, to cardiac refractoriness.[86] This behavior is implemented in the current pacemaker models and provides optimized detection of early premature ventricular contractions, especially during exercise. Under exercise conditions, the ventricular pace refractory period automatically shortens with the measured QT interval, thus allowing earlier ventricular sensing.

Optimal Atrioventricular Interval

In patients at rest and during pacing in the atrium at a fixed rate, a positive correlation was observed between the longest QT interval, the highest cardiac output or cardiac index, and the programmed atrioventricular (AV) delay.[87] In the implanted Diamond pacemaker, the evoked QT interval value, derived from a downloadable software, was found to be longest at the optimal AV delay as assessed by the maximum Doppler mitral valve inflow.[88] Furthermore, QT interval–determined AV interval also minimized mitral regurgitation. It is of interest to see whether the optimal AV interval in cardiac resynchronization therapy can be similarly determined.

Recognition of Ventricular Fusion Beats

Boute and associates[89] demonstrated in dogs that the amplitude of the evoked T wave significantly decreases during fusion. Recognition of ventricular fusion is important for reliable and effective operations such as automatic capture detection as well as to avoid unnecessary fusion pacing, which may influence the ventricular contraction pattern and battery current wastage. On detection of fusion, a dual-chamber pacemaker could automatically extend its AV interval to allow the conducted R waves to prevail. Finally, in patients with hypertrophic obstructive cardiomyopathy, one would like to maintain ventricular pacing to obtain consistent septal preexcitation. In these patients, detection of ventricular fusion may shorten its AV interval, thereby providing an effective therapy through full ventricular capture.

Other Applications

A circadian variation in the QT interval has been reported.[90] The difference in the QT interval at 60 bpm between being awake and being asleep was 19 ± 7 msec,[91] reflecting greater vagal tone or sympathetic withdrawal. This difference could be used to automatically decrease the LRL during those hours of the day that the patient is asleep.

The evoked T-wave amplitude after cardiac transplantation has been tested in 13 patients during the immediate post-transplantation period. In 11 patients, the initial biopsy that proved rejection was associated with a significant decrease in the evoked T-wave amplitude from 1.3 to 0.6 mV ($P < .005$), which began 1 to 4 days before the biopsy. The paced evoked response can be used to evaluate drug-induced changes in myocardial repolarization.[93] Furthermore, Donaldson and coworkers[94] showed that subendocardial ischemia can be detected with the paced evoked response.

Unipolar Ventricular Impedance (Closed-Loop Stimulation Sensor)

Physiologic Principle

Cardiac contractility of the ventricle increases during catecholamine stimulation, as occurs during exercise and emotional stresses. In the absence of an adequate rate response, exercise induces a higher contractility, which decreases when rate response is adequate, thus establishing a negative feedback loop and a new steady-contractility state. On the other hand, rises in pacing rate per se can increase contractility, the so-called Treppe effect, although this effect has not been important in clinical practice.

Sensor and Algorithm

The CLS sensor is based on unipolar impedance at the tip of a pacing lead.[95] Subthreshold pulses of automatically selected outputs (ranging from 100 to 400 μA), with a biphasic duration of 46 msec, are emitted 50 to 300 msec after a sensed (Vs) or paced (Vp) ventricular event. Because two pulses are required for an impedance measurement, eight samples are taken per cardiac cycle (Fig. 16-25A). During diastole (immediately after a Vp or Vs), there is significant amount of blood around the electrode tip, and the impedance is low. On the other hand, as contraction occurs, the walls surrounding the electrode tip get closer, and impedance rises. A baseline waveform occurs, which depends on the conduction state of the heart: AsVs, AsVp, ApVs, ApVp, where As and Ap refer to atrial sensing and pacing, respectively. In addition, the impedence waveform changes with the heart rate and the time of the cardiac cycle. Because the field strength falls off rapidly with distance from the lead tip, approximately 90% of impedance is reflected in a diameter of 1 cm from the tip. Thus, the effect of respiration is limited. Baseline CLS waveforms are acquired only when the associated accelerometer indicates no activity, and a waveform is discarded within 48 hours if not referenced. An average template of the baseline CLS waveform will take 2 to 3 days to optimize.

As contractility increases during exercise, unipolar impedance changes (Fig. 16-26A). The time-integrated difference between the exercise and baseline impedance waveforms is converted to a pacing rate using an "Auto Response Factor, " until SURL is reached for the first time. This "Auto Response Factor" is continually adaptive and is patient specific. Thereafter, the response is determined by a programmable "Exertion Threshold Rate" (ETR) [very low, low, medium, high, and very high]. The ETR, acting through the "Auto Response Factor," determines that 80% of the heart rate will occur below the ETR and 20% above the ETR (see Fig. 16-26B). A young and active individual will probably require a higher ETR than an inactive sedentary elderly person. Again, the type of rate profile attained will be determined by the cardiac condition, the patient's physical state, and the patient-specific "Auto Response Factor," even though the ETR is programmed similarly. The maximum ETR is limited to less than 80 bpm above the LRL.

Although this is strictly not a dual-sensor pacemaker, the incorporated accelerometer performs an "on-off" function to decide on the acquisition of baseline CLS waveform and the CLS-driven response. Full CLS driven-rate according to the programmed ETR will be allowed only if the accelerometer registers exercise; otherwise only 20 bpm above the LRL is allowed to enable a nonexercise increase rate. In case of neurocardiogenic syncope, this rate-limiting algorithm can be inactivated for full overdrive response, as occurs during a syncopal episode.

Biotronik Closed-Loop Stimulation Pacemakers: Inos, Protos

Schaldach and Hutten[95] took immediate measurements of the CLS parameter (previously known as ventricular

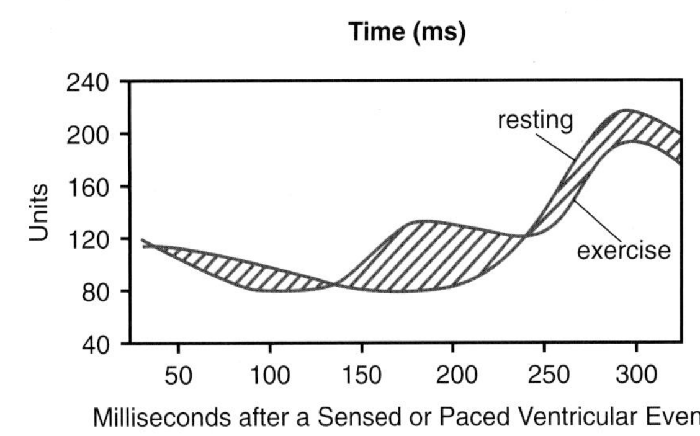

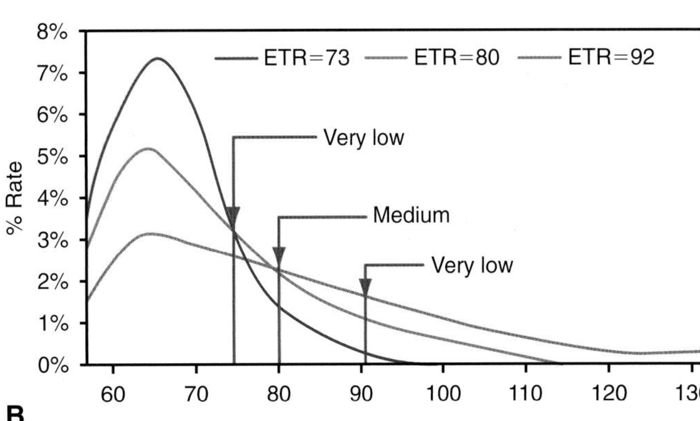

Figure 16-25. ***A,*** *Changes in closed-loop stimulation (CLS) parameter during exercise. The hatched area represents the difference between baseline and exercise CLS waveforms, and is converted to a rate using the "Exertion Transfer Rate" (ETR).* ***B,*** *The impact of ETR on the rate response of CLS. "Medium" ETR corresponds to a rate of 80 bpm (20 bpm above the lower rate limit). Programming this rate will ensure a rate response of 80% less than this rate and 20% above this rate. A higher or lower ETR will result in different rate responses.*

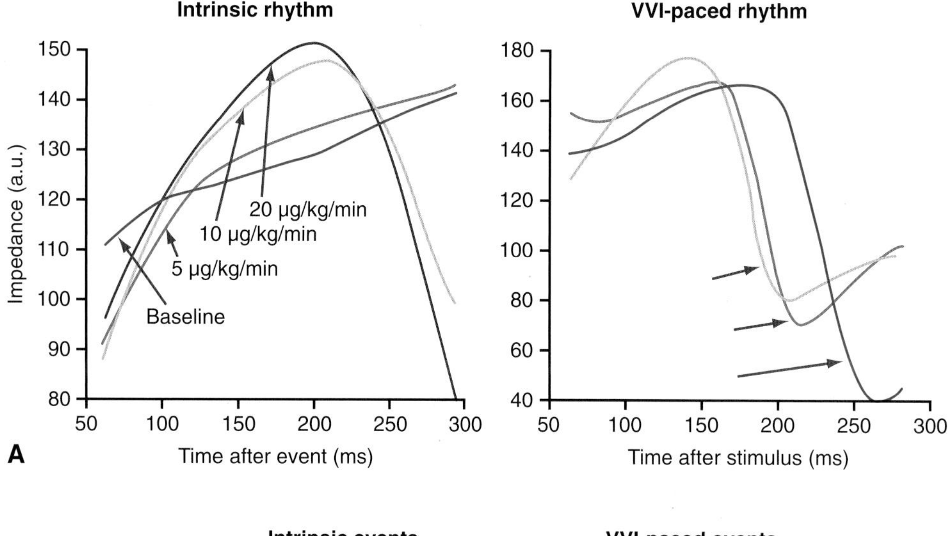

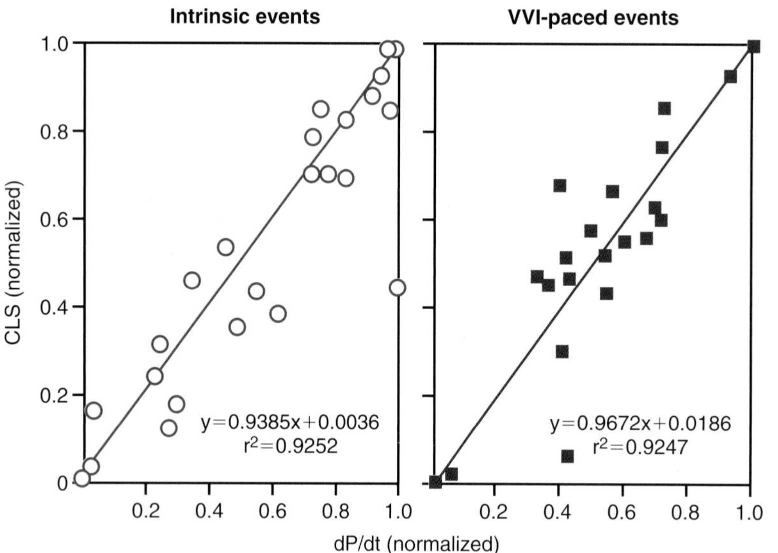

Figure 16-26. ***A,*** *The curves on the left show typical impedance curves at different dobutamine doses in the same patient during intrinsic rhythm, which in this case was sinus rhythm with a narrow QRS complex. Note that the shapes of these impedance curves were substantially different from those during ventricular paced rhythm (right) in the same patient. However, in both situations, a region of interest could be defined that provided an optimal curve separation. For intrinsic and VVI-paced rhythm, the difference in slope (measured slope – baseline slope of the corresponding curve pattern) was used to calculate a rhythm-specific sensor signal for each inotropic state of the heart. a.u. = arbitrary units.* ***B,*** *These graphs show the correlation between CLS and dP/dt_{max} separated for intrinsic (left) and VVI-paced rhythm (right). There was a comparably strong correlation between the CLS signal and right ventricular dP/dt_{max} for both types of rhythm. (From Osswald S, Cron T, Gradel P, et al: Closed-loop stimulation using intracardiac impedance as a sensor principle: Correlation of right ventricular dP/dt_{max} and intracardiac impedance during dobutamine stress test. PACE 23:1502, 2000.)*

inotropic index) in 82 patients with long-term implanted unipolar ventricular leads at the time of pulse generator replacement. A wide fluctuation of baseline impedance was observed (500 Ω to 1500 Ω), although CLS fluctuated by about 4 Ω to 25 Ω, with a good correlation between CLS and the baseline impedance. Using an investigational VVIR pacemaker with telemetry (Biotronik Neos-PEP, Biotronik, Lake Oswego, Oregon) in 158 patients, these investigators[95] demonstrated that rate adaptation can be achieved with this sensor. In individual patients, it was reported that rate adaptation close to that of the sinus node was observed with this sensor during exercise, although it was necessary to individually adjust the CLS detection algorithm (Fig. 16-27). A delay in the onset of an increase in pacing rate was observed, compared with onset in the normal sinus rhythm in some patients, possibly because the normal sinus rate at the onset of exercise is due to parasympathetic withdrawal rather than sympathetic increase.

A clinical study involving 205 patients was performed to evaluate the CLS pacemaker.[96] A significant proportion of these patients were young subjects with complete AV block due to Chagas' disease. Satisfactory rate modulation was reported in 93% of the patients. In the remaining 7% of patients, rate adaptation could not be achieved because of such factors as poor exercise tolerance, severe myocardial dysfunction, and intermittent AV conduction. In a multicenter study that involved 178 VVIR (Biotronik Neos-PEP) and 84 DDDR pacemakers (Biotronik Diplos-PEP and Inos²DR), physiologic rate adaptation was possible in 93% and 96% of patients with these devices, respectively.[97] Apart from exercise rate response, this study also involved mental stress testing using color-word matching and the infusion of inotropic agents. A moderate level of rate response was documented in some patients with CLS pacemakers during these nonexercise stresses. During stress echocardiography, the increase in CLS-driven pacing rate was similar to the changes observed with sinus rhythm.[98]

In some patients with the CLS pacemaker undergoing angioplasty, balloon inflation in the artery supplying the myocardium around the pacing electrode led to

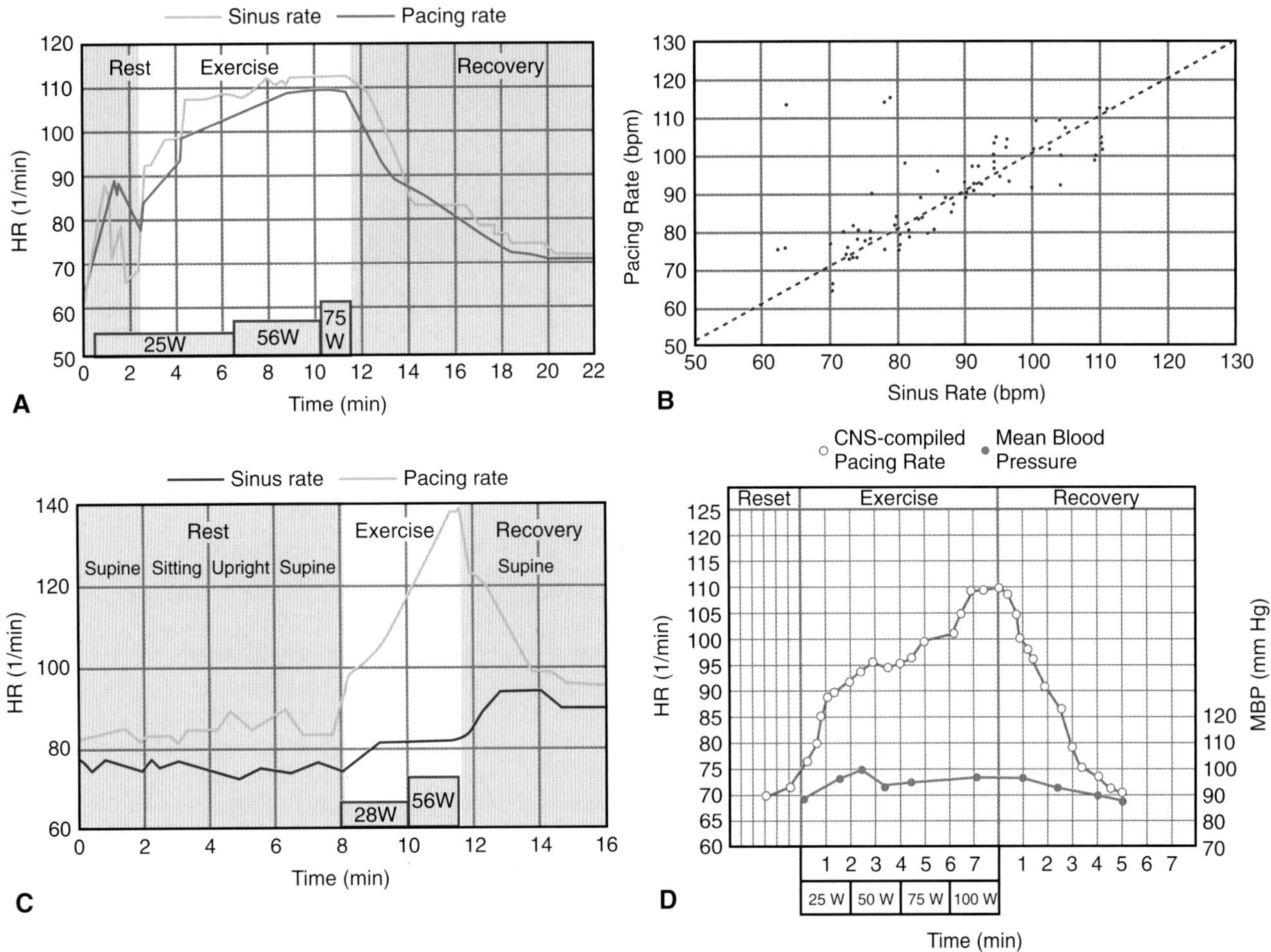

Figure 16-27. *Simultaneous recording of the sinus-derived and closed-loop stimulation (CLS)–derived pacing rates in a patient with atrioventricular block with a Neos-VVIR pacemaker (Biotronik GmbH & Co., Berlin).* ***A,*** *Appropriate rate response during graded cycle ergometry.* ***B,*** *Good correlation of sinus rate and CLS-driven pacing rate.* ***C,*** *Inappropriately adjusted CLS detection with failure of rate response.* ***D,*** *Maintenance of constant mean arterial pressure during exercise with appropriate rate response. HR, heart rate; MBP, mean blood pressure. (From Schaldach M, Hutten H: Intracardiac impedance to determine sympathetic activity in rate responsive pacing. PACE 15:1778, 1992.)*

a decrease in CLS, suggesting that CLS reflected a change in local contractility of the myocardium. Within an increase in pacing rate from 70 to 90 bpm at rest, there was no observable change in CLS. This finding suggests that within the rate range studied, there is no potential positive-feedback loop.

Osswald and associates[99] reported that the intrinsic and ventricular paced QRS has substantial influence on the rate response. In their study, infusion of dobutamine increased both intrinsic and paced CLS parameters in a dose-dependent manner, and the changes in CLS parameter in either case were proportional to the measured dP/dt. This finding suggests that rate adaptation is possible for both intrinsic and paced QRS complexes, provided that a correct reference waveform is used. However, the rate-adaptive behaviors of intrinsic and paced acquired CLS conditions have not been formally compared. During cardiopulmonary testing with the older version of a CLS device that has an activity sensor (Inos), Cook and coworkers[100] found excellent correlation between the pacing rate with the measured Vo_2 and cardiac output ($P < .01$ in both instances). The rate responses during daily activities have also reported to be appropriate in a multicenter study,[101] with rate responses of 104 ± 18 bpm, 95 ± 15 bpm, and 88 ± 11 bpm during ascending stairs, descending stairs, and walking, respectively. The CLS level is also correlated with skeletal muscle sympathetic nerve activity.[102] Furthermore, rate-adaptive pacing using the CLS sensor has been reported to simulate the rate response during phases II and IV of the Valsalva maneuver.[103] On the other hand, a delayed increase of heart rate was observed after nitroglycerine infusion.[103] These data indicate that the CLS sensor responds, at least in part, to the changes in autonomic tone.

There is interest in the possible use of this sensor to detect posture. Passive upright tilt, which depletes intravascular volume, increases the inotropic state of the heart.[104] This may cause a false-positive rate increase. This is now prevented by using an associated accelerometer to detect exercise.

In a multicenter study entitled INotropy Controlled pacing in Vasovagal SYncope (INVASY), [105] 50 patients with severe vasovagal syncope and positive head-up tilt test response were randomly assigned to DDD-CLS or DDI mode at 40 bpm.[105] Seven of the 9 patients in the DDI arm experienced syncope within 1 year, whereas only 4 of 41 patients in the DDD-CLS arm had presyncope. The investigators recommended the efficacy of this approach, although a placebo effect of pacing was suspected to have occurred in 22% of patients. Of special interest is the use of CLS sensor rate-adaptive pacing in patients who had bradycardia and heart failure. From a preliminary study,[106] in which the pacing rate was "titrated" according to the cardiac contractility, Bailey and Hull[106] suggested that CLS pacing may avoid (or even prevent) worsening of heart failure, preserving ejection fraction, and improving functioned class. This possibility has to be confirmed in further studies. The use of CLS in the left ventricle, as in a cardiac resynchronization therapy device, would be of interest.

Advantages and Limitations

The CLS sensor appears to be an interesting sensor to measure contractility of the heart, and CLS can be achieved using a conventional ventricular pacing electrode. The demands on pacing energy are acceptable. As a contractility sensor, it is sensitive not only to exercise but also to nonexercise requirements, and it may therefore be used for monitoring cardiac contractility for non-rate augmentation purposes. Like the QT sensor, the CLS sensor can be used only in a pacing mode that incorporates a ventricular lead. The effects of pacing rate on CLS have not been completely studied, and the difference in changes in preload and the CLS during pacing and intrinsic conduction may affect the resultant rate response. It is likely that CLS is affected by right ventricular ischemia or cardioactive medications. These factors may influence rate adaptation with the CLS sensor, although automatic adjustment may permit long-term function. CLS sensors are not suitable for a small proportion of patients because of severely impaired right ventricular function, although it may be possible to identify such patients preoperatively.

Peak Endocardial Acceleration Sensing

Sensor and Algorithm

The contractile state of the heart can be identified from the maximal velocity of shortening of unloaded myocardial contractile elements, which can be measured with a catheter-tip accelerometer attached to the ventricular wall. The PEA represents the endocardial vibration measured by the accelerometer in the right ventricle during the isovolumetric contraction phase of the ventricles. This signal is in close relationship to the intensity of the first heart sound. The sensor, developed by Sorin Biomedica Cardio, S.p.A., is termed the BEST (Biomechanical Endocardial Sorin Transducer) sensor. The microaccelerometer consists of an acceleration sensor built into an indeformable capsule located on the tip of a standard unipolar ventricular pacing lead. The lead is placed against the right ventricular wall so as to be sensitive to its acceleration and insensitive to the pressure of blood and myocardium (Fig. 16-28). This system has a frequency response of up to 1 kHz and a sensitivity of 5 mV/G (1 G = 9.8 m/sec/sec).

In preliminary experience in animals, and using an external system and an implantable radiotelemetry system, Occhetta and colleagues[107] found that the PEA was not affected by heart rate but was significantly raised by emotional stress, exercise stress testing, and inotropic stimulation. The PEA signal changes in parallel to the maximal left ventricular dP/dt and appears to measure the global left ventricular contractile performance rather than the regional mechanical function.[108,109] The PEA signal occurs at 150 msec after the R wave and corresponds to the isovolumetric contraction phase of the left ventricle (Fig. 16-29). This is also called the PEA-1, is the signal for cardiac contractility, and is proportional to the positive dP/dt during inotropic stimulation (r = 0.83).[110] A smaller signal also occurs in the 100-msec period after the T wave, the so-called PEA-2, which corresponds to the isovolumetric left ventricular relaxation. PEA-2 is related to peak

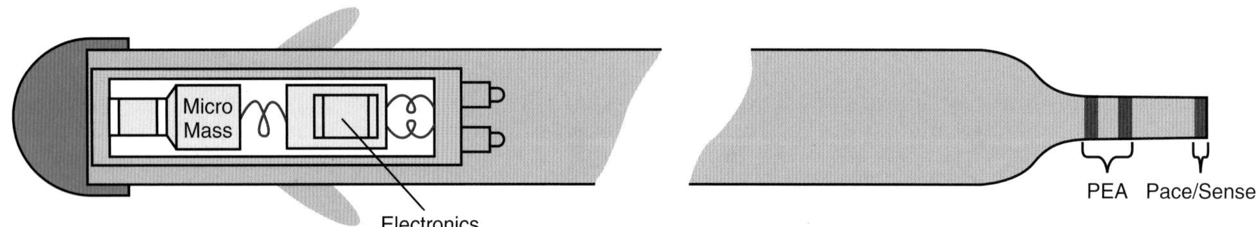

Figure 16-28. The Biomechanical Endocardial Sorin Transducer (BEST) sensor (Sorin Biomedica Cardio, S.p.A., Sorin Group, Milan) consists of a microaccelerometer located inside a rigid capsule at the tip of a standard ventricular pacing lead. This is connected to a triple header of the device. PEA, peak endocardial acceleration.

negative dP/dt ($r = 0.92$) and aortic diastolic pressure ($r = 0.91$).[110]

The BEST Sensor Rate-Adaptive Pacemakers: MiniLiving D and MiniLiving S

Sorin manufactures the MiniLiving D and MiniLiving S pacemakers, which use a dedicated unipolar ventricular pace/sense lead, that is IS1 compatible. Together with the two electrodes for PEA signals, a tripolar connector is necessary. These devices also incorporate an activity sensor using the vibration from a mercury ball (gravitational sensor). Vibrations during exercise result in greater excursion frequency and magnitude of the mercury ball, leading to an increase in output from the vibration sensor.

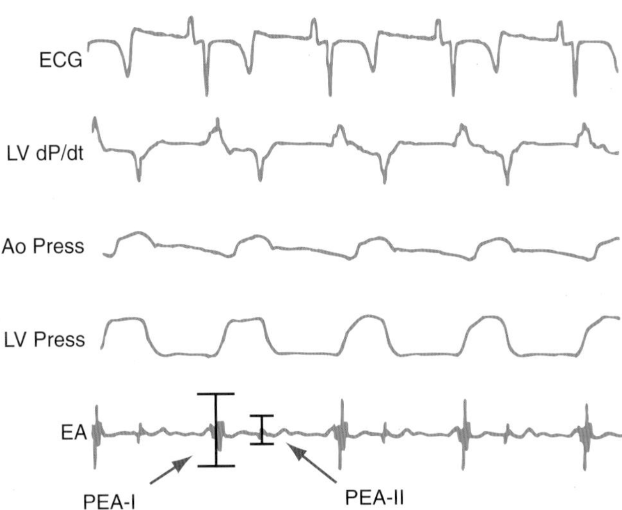

Figure 16-29. Electrocardiographic (ECG), left ventricular dP/dt (LV dP/dt), aortic pressure (Ao press), and E: accelerometer tracing (EA) recordings in a sheep with the Biomechanical Endocardial Sorin Transducer (BEST) sensor. The peak of the accelerometer tracing during the isovolumic diastole (PEA-II) occurs in a 100-msec period after the T wave on ECG. (From Plicchi G, Mercelli E, Parlapiano M, et al: PEA I and PEA II based implantable haemodynamic monitor: Preclinical studies in sheep. Europace 4:49, 2002.)

The MiniLiving pacemakers can be programmed in either the single-sensor or dual-sensor mode. In single-sensor, PEA mode, continuous PEA signal collected over time is used as a reference, with which the change in PEA is compared. A linear pacing rate to PEA signal rate-adaptive curve is used to control the rate response. Six different rate-response curves are available. If the maximum level of PEA occurring over time is below the maximum PEA signal change permitted by the curve, a more aggressive slope is advised. On the other hand, if the PEA exceeds the maximum change in the curve, a gentler slope will need to be programmed. Optimal PEA programming occurs when the maximum PEA change equals the maximum PEA level allowed for that rate-response slope (Fig. 16-30A).

In dual-sensor mode, the combined output from the two sensors is used to drive the rate to a middle rate level; further rate increase will be effected with output from the PEA sensor alone (see Fig. 16-30B). The rise time and recovery times are separately programmable. In addition, prolonged absence (about 45 minutes) of signals from both the gravitational and PEA sensors allows the basic rate to drop to the programmable rest rate. On the other hand, once the sensors are active, approach to rate response will be rapid.

The device also incorporates short-term (20 minutes) and long-term (3, 6, 12, and 24 hours) trends of both the PEA and heart rate signals to assess rate adaptation. In addition, the automatic AV search function

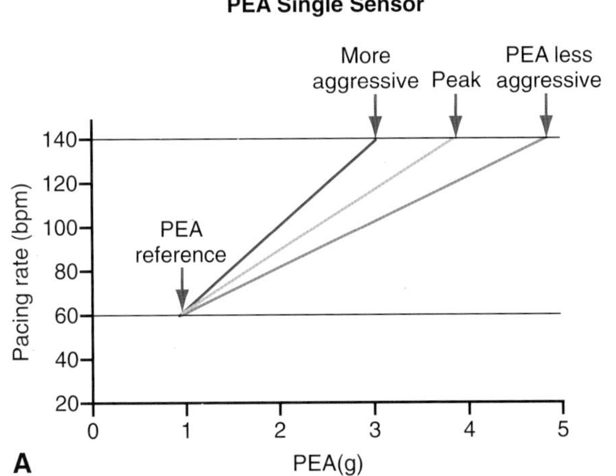

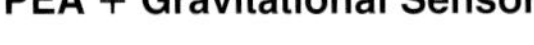

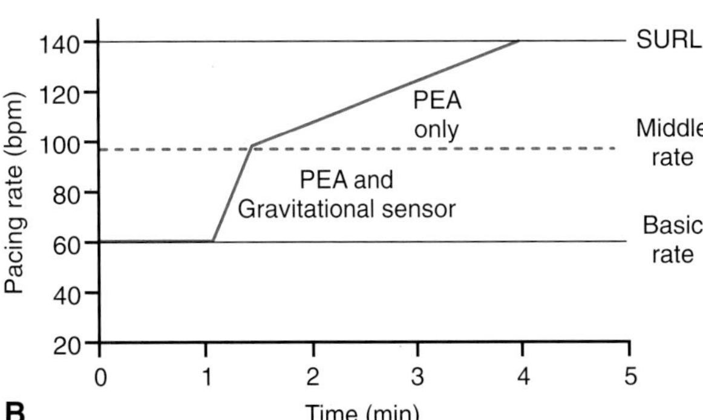

Figure 16-30. **A,** *Rate-adaptive algorithm of the MiniLiving (Sorin Biomedica CRM) at nominal settings. The ΔPEA (change in peak endocardial acceleration) allowed is 3 g to reach the sensor-driven upper rate limit (SURL) of 140 bpm at about 4 g. A more aggressive slope allows the SURL to be reached at a ΔPEA of 3 g, whereas a gentler curve may require a ΔPEA of 5g to reach the SURL.* **B,** *In a combined-sensor mode, initial exercise to a middle rate is contributed by the combined sensors, whereas the approach to the upper rate is contributed by the PEA sensor alone.*

allows the AV interval that corresponds to the minimum level of PEA to be derived automatically.

Clinical Results

Preliminary studies of pacemakers using the PEA sensor have shown a good correlation between the sinus rate and PEA sensor–indicated rate during daily life activities and submaximal stress test.[111,112] Similar results were obtained in patients being tested during electrophysiologic studies through the use of an external system; the changes in PEA were found to be linearly related to the right ventricular dP/dt during dobutamine infusion.[107,113] PEA is not affected by ischemia of the area in which the senor is attached. The performance of the PEA sensor with exercise-related and non–exercise-related stress was studied in 17 patients. The PEA sensor showed a quick response to exercise, and it also responded to both hand grip and the Valsalva maneuver.[114] During maximal treadmill exercise testing in 15 patients, the rise in PEA was found to have a good correlation with the increase in exercise workload (change in PEA to Mets, $r = 0.97$).[115] The correlation was best at the higher stages of exercise; the PEA changes at lower levels of exercise are less discriminative.[114,115]

PEA signals have been used to monitor hemodynamic function and for programming the AV interval. In 13 patients with end-stage heart failure in whom DDD-PEA devices with custom lead arrangements were implanted,[116] PEA level during right ventricular, left ventricular, and biventricular pacing were compared. Both left ventricular and biventricular pacing resulted in higher stroke volume than right ventricular pacing (+21 and +37%, respectively), and mean PEA changes over a 15-minute duration were also higher (+43 and +38%, respectively). In addition, there appears to be a minimum PEA level at the optimal AV interval, and this finding has shown some promise for automatic detection of the optimum AV interval in a dual-chamber device.[117] An increase in PEA during head-up tilting has been observed, and the use of PEA-driven overdrive pacing in patients with vasovagal syncope has been reported.[118] Patients randomly assigned to DDDR pacing have a lower frequency of syncope than those assigned to DDI pacing. These data suggest the potential use of PEA sensor for hemodynamic monitoring. The role of PEA-2 in assessing diastolic function and aortic pressure remains to be investigated.[110]

Advantages and Limitations

The PEA sensor is a proportional sensor that shows good correlation to workload, especially at the higher ranges. During daily activities in one study, the rate response was correlated with sinus rate, but the actual rates achieved were significantly lower.[119] Apart from using a higher baseline rate, the combination with the gravitational sensor may be advantageous for lower levels of exercise loads. There are many preliminary communications on the ability of the PEA sensor to monitor hemodynamics. Although these reports are interesting and potentially important, they must be validated by larger trials. The PEA sensor is limited by the need for a specialized lead, as well as by concern about its longer-term stability and the use of this lead at the time of a pacemaker replacement in which a different sensor is used.

Current Combined-Sensor Devices

Experience with sensors has suggested that fast-responding sensors such as activity sensors are not proportional at higher levels of workload, whereas a proportional sensor is usually slow in response. Furthermore, single sensors may be limited by insensitivity to non-exercise stress and are liable to be interfered with by nonphysical causes. Thus, it is logical to enhance the rate-response profiles of the various sensors by combining two or more sensors in a single pacemaker.

There are two principles of sensor combination, sensor blending and sensor cross-checking (see Chapter 5). *Sensor blending* involves combining the sensor-driven rates from individual sensors in a certain ratio. This can be the "faster win" method in which the higher rate is chosen as the dual-sensor rate, or ratios of the individual rates are added together to compile the ultimate rate response. *Sensor cross-checking* enhances the specificity of each sensor. If a more specific sensor registers no exercise or physiologic stresses, changes in the other, less specific sensor are ignored or its response is attenuated. In some situations, sensor blending and cross-checking may not be clear-cut but occur in combination to derive the rate adaptation. The instrumentation of current dual-sensor devices is summarized in Table 16-3. Details of the combinations of QT, activity, CLS, and PEA sensors have already been presented.

Kappa 400

In Medtronic's Kappa 400 pacemaker, a piezoelectric sensor is used for activity sensing, and MV is sensed from a bipolar ventricular lead. Differential sensor blending is used. Up to the ADL rate, activity input predominates, whereas MV-driven pacing will predominate at the SURL (see Fig. 5-15). Activity and MV sensors are checked against each other. In the absence of piezoelectric sensor indications of exercise, MV pacing will only reach the ADL rate, and vice versa. Only when both the MV and activity sensors signify exercise will pacing above the ADL rate occur.

The activity sensor can be programmed with the use of the conventional threshold and slope. In the dual-sensor mode, rate adaptation is achieved automatically using the "Rate Profile Optimization." This requires the input of the ADL and ER rates, together with the percentage of time spent in each rate (range 1 to 5), similar to the programming of the Kappa accelerometer devices.

Clinical Performance

The dual-sensor rate response has been reported to be reliable for both maximal and submaximal activities,

TABLE 16-3. **Types of Dual-Sensor Pacemakers in Current Use**

Sensors	Manufacturer	Models	Sensors	Algorithms	Cross-checking	Automaticity
ACT + MV	Medtronic, Inc.	Kappa 400	ACT = piezoelectric MV = impedance	Blending: ≤ADL range: ACT + MV; ADL-ER range: mainly ACT	ACT(0) and MV(+): up to ADL rate; ACT (+) and MV(0): up to ADL rate	"Rate Profile Optimization"
	Guidant	Pulsar Max Insignia	ACT = accelerometer MV = impedance	Blending: Low heart rate: ACT 80%, MV 20%; High heart rate: ACT 40%, MV 60%	ACT(0) and MV(+): MV rate; ACT(+) and MV(0): limited rate	"AutoLife style"
	ELA Medical	Chorus Talent Symphony Rhapsody	ACT = accelerometer MV = impedance	No Blending: MV-determined rate response if ACT indicates exercise	ACT(+) and MV(0): initial limited rate response; ACT(0) and MV(+): rate recovery	Automatic matching MV sensor to LRL and SURL
ACT + QT	Vitatron	Topaz Diamond Selection	ACT = accelerometer QT = unipolar evoked QT	Blending: ACT > QT ACT = QT ACT < QT	ACT(0) and QT(+): limited rate ACT(+) and QT(0): decrease to LRL	Automatic matching QT sensor to LRL and SURL
CLS + ACT	Biotronik GmBH	Inos Protos	CLS = unipolar ventricular impedance ACT = accelerometer	No blending: No ACT rate contribution Rate response determined by CLS only	ACT(0) and CLS(+): limited rate response; ACT(+) and CLS(0): no rate response	"Auto Response Factor" adjusts CLS data to reach rate distribution determined by the programmed "Exertion Threshold Rate"
PEA + ACT	Sorin Biomedica CRM	MiniLiving	PEA = accelerometer at ventricular lead tip ACT = gravitational sensor	Blending: Up to Middle rate: PEA + ACT > Middle rate: PEA only	Nil	Manual adjustment to match peak PEA from trend data to the desired SURL

ACT, activity sensor; CLS, closed-loop stimulation sensor; LRL, lower rate limit; MV, minute ventilation sensor; PEA, peak endocardial acceleration sensor; QT, QT interval–driven sensor; SURL, sensor-driven upper rate limit.

and resistant to non-physiologic interference.[120] Compared with MV sensor alone, dual sensor mode reduces oxygen deficit acquired during exercise by enhancing the initial rate response.[121] "Rate Profile Optimization" was found to be a useful method for rate-adaptive programming, and comparable with manual programming.[122] On the other hand, in a series of 11 patients followed up for 3 years with the accelerometer programmed by "Rate Profile Optimisation,"[28] repeated programming was still necessary to optimize the response of the activity sensor to treadmill exercise.

Insignia and Pulsar Max

An accelerometer activity sensor is integrated with the MV sensor in Guidant's Insignia and Pulsar Max pacemakers. A differential sensor blending is used. At low heart rate, approximately 80% of the blended sensor rate is contributed by the accelerometer, and 20% by MV sensor. These proportions change to 40% and 60%, respectively, near the SURL. In addition, if the MV-indicated rate is higher than the accelerometer rate, the dual-sensor rate follows the MV level.

Cross-checking occurs only against the activity sensor, because MV is considered to be more specific. An interim rate is allowed only in the event that the activity sensor alone indicates exercise and the MV sensor is inactive.

The programming of the dual sensor involves either a manual adjustment or use of the automatic sensor adjustment. In brief, after a "Sensor Rate Target" is chosen on the basis of the "Expert Ease" system, the combined sensor is adjusted according to the average of the maximum combined sensor activities and its difference from the "Sensor Rate Target" (see Fig. 16-15). Individual adjustments can be made with the use of trend data during a structured exercise test.

In the Insignia Ultra pacemaker, automatic adjustment of the dual sensor (or the MV only) is available. The "MV Response Factor" (10 nonprogrammable slopes) is adjusted on a weekly basis, on the basis of the detected "MV Max Long-term" value. The latter is derived from the maximum impedance–derived MV that has been confirmed by the accelerometer. The accelerometer further identifies this MV as occurring during mild, moderate, or vigorous exercise before "deciding" whether the MV is the maximum that occurs during vigorous exertion. The "MV Max Long-term" value is updated by 10% if it exceeds the value from last week, or decreased by 15% if it is above. Note that the "MV Max Long-term" value is linked to the age-predicted heart rate and is independent of the programmed SURL. In the MV mode, the accelerometer contributes only to the "MV Max Long-term" measurements. In the dual-sensor mode, the accelerator's input is differentially blended as previously described (Fig. 16-31).

Clinical Results

A preliminary study has addressed the use of automatic sensor adjustment in the Pulsar Max. The sensitivity of the MV sensor was changed in 36% of patients, whereas the accelerometer reactivity was increased in almost all patients. In another study, Pieragnoli and colleagues[124] randomly assigned 120 patients with Insignia pacemakers to accelerometer single-sensor mode, MV single-sensor mode, or dual-sensor mode, each for a 3-month period. Using the implanted "Activity Log" to determine the mean percentage and intensity of activity, these investigators assessed quality of life and New York Heart Association (NYHA) functional classes at the end of each period. Overall, either single-sensor DDDR mode led to better "Activity Log," quality of life, and NYHA scores than DDD pacing, but there was no difference between the two sensors. Dual-sensor mode did not provide additional benefit. Results of this study, which may have been limited by the prolonged triple-crossover design, nevertheless suggest that rate-adaptive pacing is more beneficial than DDD mode, but the clinical differences between sensors and their combinations in effecting a better adaptation are likely to be small.

Chorus, Talent, Symphony, Rhapsody

An accelerometer and a MV sensor are combined in the ELA Medical's dual-sensor pacemakers. Sensor blending and cross-checking are both operative to effect rate adaptation during exercise. When the accelerometer is active but MV has not increased, as may occur at the beginning of exercise, rate response occurs according to a fixed activity response curve to a limited rate (Fig. 16-32A). When MV increases, rate response follows the MV sensor–driven rate. Persistent absence of accelerometer signal is regarded as cessation of exercise and this drives the pacing rate in a recovery curve to the LRL even though MV remains higher than baseline. An "Autocalibration" function enables automatic matching of the MV sensor data to the upper and lower rate limits (see Fig. 16-32B). If the SURL is reached but the sensor level is still rising, the rate response is reduced in steps so that the SURL is reached later. Lower rate is considered when the MV value over 128 respiratory cycles is below the mean MV over the last 24 hours. In addition, persistent absence of either sensor signal forces the rate response to return to the LRL.

Clinical Results

Results of a multicenter study of 81 patients with the Talent pacemaker have been reported.[61] In patients who underwent exercise stress testing at 1 month of follow up, sensor-driven rate was found to be well correlated with the sinus rate ($r = 0.92 \pm 0.07$; $P < .001$), with the slope of linearity of 1.0 ± 0.2. With metabolic reserve used to relate to heart rate reserve, a slope of 1.1 ± 0.2 was obtained, suggesting a close relationship between the dual-sensor rate and the metabolic workload.

Conclusions

Current rate-adaptive devices have evolved to incorporate newer sensor technologies and increasingly sophisticated algorithms to enhance rate adaptation. Because single-sensor rate response may be limited by the speed of response, lack of proportionality, sensitivity, and specificity, sensors have been combined to enhance the overall rate-adaptive behavior. Almost all single- and

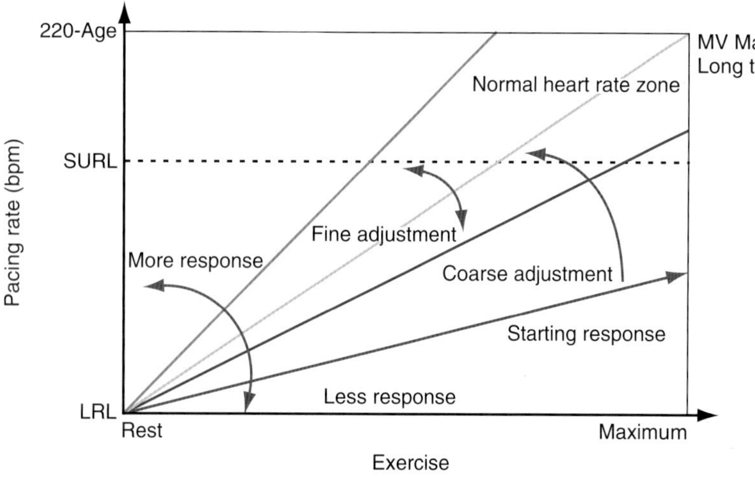

Figure 16-31. "AutoLife style" sensor adjustment of the Insignia Ultra Maximum MV (Guidant) will be updated on a weekly basis and confirmed by the accelerometer, indicating vigorous exercise. Note that the sensor-driven upper rate limit (SURL) is independent of the "MV Max Long-term." LRL, lower rate limit; MV, minute ventilation. See text for further discussion.

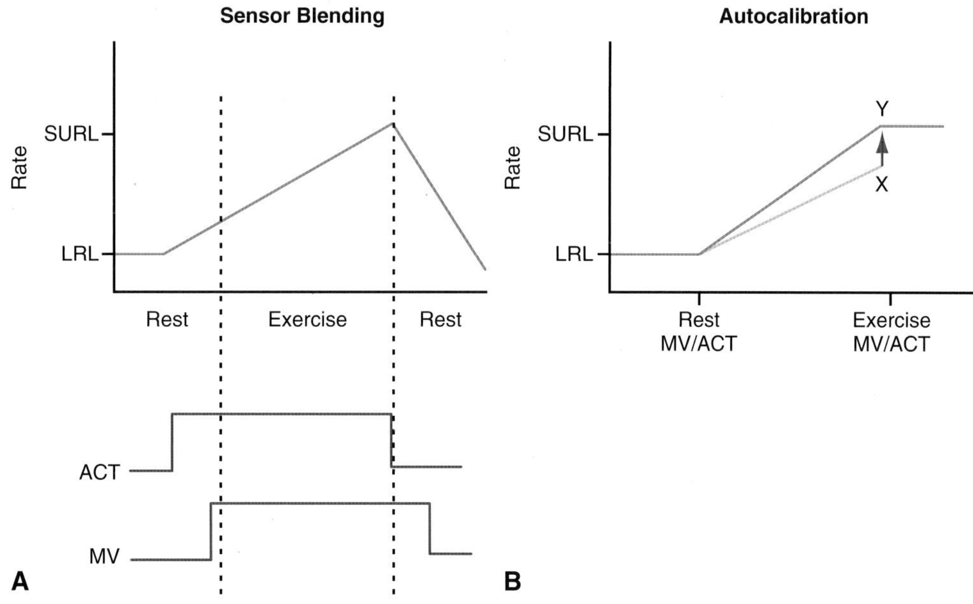

*Figure 16-32. Dual-sensor algorithm of the Symphony (ELA Medical, Sorin Group). **A,** A combination of activity (ACT) and minute ventilation (MV) inputs during exercise. **B,** "Autocalibration" of the sensor. If the maximum sensor level is reached before the sensor-driven upper rate limit (SURL; indicate by X), then the slope is adjusted in steps to Y to match the SURL to the maximum sensor level. LRL, lower rate limit.*

dual-sensor devices are now self-programmable, and physician input can be kept to a minimum. On the other hand, understanding of the interplay between sensors and their algorithms will be needed to fine-tune rate response in some patients. Apart from avoiding false rate acceleration, the clinical role of dual-sensors over single-sensor pacing remains to be addressed.

REFERENCES

1. Richards AF, Donaldson RM: Rate-responsive pacing. Clin Prog Pacing Electrophysiol 1:12, 1983.
2. Benditt DG, Milstein S, Buetikofer J, et al: Sensor-triggered, rate-variable cardiac pacing: Current technologies and clinical implications. Ann Intern Med 107:714, 1987.
3. Dahl JD, inventor: Variable rate timer for a cardiac pacemaker. US patent 4 140, 32. February 20, 1979.
4. Anderson K, Humen D, Klein GJ, et al: A rate variable pacemaker which automatically adjusts for physical activity. PACE 6:12, 1983.
5. Lau CP, Stott JR, Toff WD, et al: Selective vibration sensing: New design of activity-sensing rate-responsive pacing. PACE 11:1299, 1988.
6. Alt E, Matula M, Theres H, et al: The basis for activity controlled rate variable cardiac pacemakers: An analysis of mechanical forces on the human body induced by exercise and environment. PACE 12:1667, 1989.
7. Humen DP, Kostuk WJ, Klein GJ: Activity-sensing, rate-responsive pacing: Improvement in myocardial performance with exercise. PACE 8:52, 1985.
8. Lau CP, Mehta D, Toff W, et al: Limitations of rate response of activity-sensing rate-responsive pacing to different forms of activity. PACE 11:141, 1988.
9. Stangl K, Wirtzfeld A, Lochschmidt O, et al: Physical movement-sensitive pacing: Comparison of two "activity"-triggered pacing systems. PACE 12:102, 1989.
10. Lipkin DP, Buller N, Frenneaux M, et al: Randomized crossover trial of rate response Activittrax and conventional fixed rate ventricular pacing. Br Heart 58:613, 1987.
11. Lindemans FW, Rankin IR, Murtaugh R, et al: Clinical experience with an activity-sensing pacemaker. PACE 9:978, 1986.
12. Benditt DG, Mianulli M, Fetter J, et al: Single-chamber cardiac pacing with activity-initiated chronotropic response: Evaluation by cardiopulmonary exercise testing. Circulation 75:184, 1987.
13. Perrins EJ, Morley CA, Chan SL, et al: Randomized controlled trial of physiological and ventricular pacing. Br Heart J 50:112, 1983.
14. Kubisch K, Peters W, Chiladakis I, et al: Clinical experience with the rate-responsive pacemaker Sensolog 703. PACE 11:1829, 1988.
15. Lau CP, Tse WS, Camm AJ: Clinical experience with Sensolog 703: A new activity-sensing rate-responsive pacemaker. PACE 11: 1444, 1988.
16. Ahern T, Nydegger C, Mc Cormick DJ, et al: Incidence and timing of activity parameter changes in activity response pacing system. PACE 15:762, 1992.
17. Lau CP, Tai YT, Fong PC, et al: Clinical experience with an accelerometer based activity sensing dual chamber rate adaptive pacemaker. PACE 15:334, 1992.
18. Garrigue S, Gentilini C, Hofgartner F, et al: Performance of a rate responsive accelerometer-based pacemaker with autocalibratoin during standardized exercise and recovery. PACE 25:883, 2002.
19. Smedgard P, Kristensson BE, Kruse I, et al: Rate-responsive pacing by means of activity sensing versus single rate ventricular pacing: A double-blind cross-over study. PACE 10: 902, 1987.
20. Lau CP, Wong C-K, Leung W-H, et al: Superior cardiac hemodynamics of atrioventricular synchrony over rate-responsive pacing at submaximal exercise: Observations in activity-sensing DDDR pacemakers. PACE 13:1832, 1990.
21. Buckingham TA, Wodruf RC, Pennington G, et al: Effect of ventricular function on the exercise hemodynamics of variable rate pacing. J Am Coll Cardiol 11:1269, 1988.

22. Lau CP, Camm AJ: Role of left ventricular function and Doppler derived variables in predicting hemodynamic benefits of rate-responsive pacing. Am J Cardiol 62:906, 1988.
23. Menozzi C, Brignole M, Moracchini PV, et al: Intrapatient comparison between chronic VVIR and DDD pacing in patients affected by high-degree AV block without heart failure. PACE 13:1816, 1990.
24. Oldroyd KG, Rae AP, Carter R, et al: Double-blind crossover comparison of the effects of dual-chamber pacing (DDD) and ventricular rate-adaptive (VVIR) pacing on neuroendocrine variables, exercise performance, and symptoms in complete heart block. Br Heart J 65:188, 1991.
25. Linde-Edelstam C, Hjemdahl P, Pehrsson SK, et al: Is DDD pacing superior to VVIR? A study on cardiac sympathetic nerve activity and myocardial oxygen consumption at rest and during exercise. PACE 15:425, 1992.
26. Millerhagen J, Bacharach D, Street G, et al: A comparison study of two activity pacemakers: An accelerometer versus piezoelectric crystal device. PACE 14:665, 1991.
27. Charles RG, Heemels JP, Westrum BL, et al: Accelerometer-based pacing: A multi-center study. PACE 16:418, 1993.
28. Schuster P, Faerestrand S, Ohm OJ et al: Proportionality of rate response to metabolic workload provided by a rate adaptive pacemaker with automatic rate profile optimization. Europace 7:54, 2005.
29. Duru F, Block KE, Weilenmann D, et al: Clinical evaluation of a pacemaker algorithm that adjusts the pacing rate during sleep using activity variance. PACE 23:1509, 2000.
30. Raj SR, Boach DE, Koshmen ML, et al: Activity-responsive pacing products long-term heart rate variability. J Cardiovasc Electrophysiol 15:179, 2004.
31. Wilkoff BL, Shimokochi DD, Schaal SF: Pacing rate increase due to application of steady external pressure on an activity-sensing pacemaker. PACE 10:423, 1987.
32. Matula M, Alt E, Fotuhi P, et al: Rate adaptation of activity pacemakers under various types of means of locomotion. Eur J Cardiac Pacing Electrophysiol 2:49, 1992.
33. Krasner JL, Voukydis PC, Nardella PC: A physiologically controlled cardiac pacemaker. J Assoc Adv Med Instrum 1:14, 1966.
34. Rossi P, Rognoni G, Occhetta E, et al. Respiration-dependent ventricular pacing compared with ventricular and atrial-ventricular synchronous pacing: Aerobic and hemodynamic variables. J Am Coll Cardiol 6:646, 1985.
35. Weber KT, Kinasewitz GT, Janicki JS, Fishmann AP: Oxygen utilization and ventilation during exercise in patients with chronic cardiac failure. Circulation 65:1213, 1982.
36. McElroy P, Weber KT, Nappholz TA: Heart rate, ventilation, mixed venous temperature, pH, and oxygen saturation during incremental upright exercise. Presented at Third Asian Pacific Symposium on Cardiac Pacing and Electrophysiology, Melbourne, Australia, October 1985.
37. Vai F, Bonnet JL, Ritter PH, Pioger G: Relationship between heart rate and minute ventilation, tidal volume and respiratory rate during brief and low level exercise. PACE 11:1860, 1988.
38. Beaver WL, Wassermann K: Tidal volume and respiratory rate change at start and end of exercise. J Appl Physiol 29:872, 1970.
39. Alt E, Heinz M, Hirgestetter C, et al: Control of pacemaker rate by impedance-based respiratory minute ventilation. Chest 92: 247, 1987.
40. Kay GN, Bubien SR, Epsten AE, Plumb VJ: Rate-modulated pacing based on transthoracic impedance measurements of minute ventilation: Correlation with exercise gas exchange. J Am Coll Cardiol 15:1283, 1989.
41. Sullivan MJ, Higginbotham MB, Cobb FR: The anaerobic threshold in chronic heart failure. Circulation 81(Suppl II):II-47, 1990.
42. Tse HF, Siu CW, Lee KLF, et al: The incremental benefit of rate-adaptive pacing on exercise performance during cardiac resynchronization therapy. J Am Coll Cardiol 46:2292, 2005.
43. Mortara A, Sleight P, Pinna GD, et al: Abnormal awake respiratory patterns are common in chronic heart failure and may prevent evaluation of automatic tone by measures of heart rate variability. Circulation 96:246, 1997.
44. Ben-Dov I, Sietsema KE, Casaburi R, Wasserman K: Evidence that circulatory oscillations accompany ventilatory oscillations during exercise in patients with heart failure. Am Rev Respir Dis 145:776, 1992.
45. Andreas S, Hagenah G, Möller C, et al: Cheyne-Stokes respiration and prognosis in congestive heart failure. Am J Cardiol 78:1260, 1996.
46. Nppholz TA, Valenta H, Maloney J, Simmons A: Electrode configurations for a respiratory impedance measurement suitable for rate-responsive pacing. PACE 9:960, 1986.
47. Simmons A, Maloney, Abi-Samra F, et al: Exercise-responsive intravascular impedance changes as a rate controller for cardiac pacing. PACE 9:285, 1986.
48. Pioger G, et al: Comparison of different electrode configurations in minute ventilation measurement. Eur J Cardiol Pacing 6(1): 1996.
49. Lau CP, Antoniou A, Ward DE, Camm AJ: Reliability of minute ventilation as a parameter for rate-responsive pacing. PACE 12:321, 1989.
50. Mond HG, Kertes PJ: Rate responsive pacing using a minute ventilation sensor. PACE 11:1866, 1988.
51. Lau CP, Ward DE, Camm AJ: Single-chamber cardiac pacing with two forms of respiration-controlled rate-responsive pacemaker. Chest 95:352, 1989.
52. Kay GN, Bubien RS, Epstein AE, et al: Rate-modulated cardiac pacing based on transthoracic impedance measurements of minute ventilation: Correlation with exercise gas exchange. J Am Coll Cardiol 14:1283, 1999.
53. Lau CP, Butrous GS, Ward DE, et al: Comparison of exercise performance of six rate-adaptive right ventricular cardiac pacemakers. Am J Cardiol 63:833, 1989.
54. Lau CP, Antoniou A, Ward DE, et al: Initial clinical experience with a minute ventilation sensing rate modulated pacemaker: Improvements in exercise capacity and symptomatology. PACE 11:1815, 1998.
55. Candinas R, Eugster W, MacCarter D, et al: Does rate modulation with a minute ventilation pacemaker simulate the intrinsic heart rate response observed during representative patient daily activities? Eur J Cardiac Pacing Electrophysiol 2:89, 1995
56. Kay GN: Quantitation of chronotropic response. Comparison of methods for rate-modulated permanent pacemakers. Am Coll Cardiol 20:1533, 1992.
57. Duru F, Radicke D, Wilkoff BL, et al: Influence of posture, breathing pattern, and type of exercise on minute ventilation estimation by a pacemaker transthoracic impedance sensor. PACE 23:1767, 2000.
58. Cole CR, Jensen DN, Cho Y, et al: Correlation of impedance minute ventilation with measured minute ventilation in a rate responsive pacemaker. PACE 24:989, 2001.
59. Duru F, Cho Y, Wilkoff BL, et al: Rate responsive pacing using transthoracic impedance minute ventilation sensors: A multicenter study on calibration stability. PACE 25:1679, 2002.
60. Simon R, Ni Q, Willems R, et al: Comparison of impedance minute ventilation and direct measured minute ventilation in a rate adaptive pacemaker. PACE 26:2127, 2003.
61. Bonnet JL, Geroux L, Cazeau S; on behalf of the French Talent DR Pacemaker Investigators: Evaluation of a dual sensor rate responsive pacing system based on a new concept. PACE 25:2198, 1998.
62. Le Helloco A, et al: Optimal rate modulation slope provided by an automatic function in a DDDR pacemaker. Eur J Cardiac Pacing Electrophysiol 6:172, 1996.
63. Bonnet JL, Ritter P, Pioger G: Measurement of minute ventilation with different DDDR pacemaker electrode configurations.

Investigators of a Multicenter Study Evaluating the Chorus RM and Opus RM Pacemakers. PACE 21:4, 1998.
64. Defaye P, Pepin JL, Poezevara Y, et al: Automatic recognition of abnormal resporatory events during sleep by a pacemaker transthoracic impedance sensor. J Cardiovasc Electrophysiol 15:1034, 2004.
65. Celiker A, Ceviz N, Alehan D, et al: Comparison of normal sinus rhythm and pacing rate in children with minute ventilation single chamber rate adaptive permanent pacemakers. PACE 21:2100, 1998.
66. Cebrera ME, Portzline G, Aach S, et al: Can current minute ventilation rate adaptive pacemakers provide appropriate chronotropic response in pediatric patients? PACE 25:907, 2002.
67. Bazett HC: An analysis of time relations of electrocardiograms. Heart 7:353, 1920.
68. Rickards AF, Norman J: Relation between QT interval and heart rate: New design of a physiologically adaptive cardiac pacemaker. Br Heart J 45:56, 1981.
69. Rickards AF, Norman J: The use of stimulus-T interval to determine cardiac pacing rate. Am J Cardiol 47:435, 1981.
70. Donaldson RM, Rickards AF: Initial experience with a physiological, rate responsive pacemaker. Br Med J 286:667, 1983.
71. Jordaens L, Backers J, Moerman E, Clement D: Catecholamine levels and pacing behavior of QT-driven pacemakers during exercise. PACE 13:603, 1990.
72. Milne JR, Ward DE, Spurrel RAJ, Camm AJ: The ventricular paced QT interval: The effects of rate and exercise. PACE 5:352, 1982.
73. Browne KF, Prystowsky E, Heger JJ, Zipes DP: Modulation of the Q-T interval by the autonomic nervous system. PACE 6:1050, 1983.
74. Sarma JSM, Venkataraman K, Samant DR, Gadgil UG: Effect of propranolol on the QT intervals of normal individuals during exercise: A new method for studying interventions. Br Heart J 60:434, 1988.
75. Baig MW, Boute W, Begemann M, Perrins EJ: Nonlinear relationship between pacing and evoked QT intervals. PACE 11:753, 1988.
76. Brouwer J, Nagelkerke D, De Jongste MJL, et al: Analysis of the morphology of the unipolar endocardial paced evoked response. PACE 13:302, 1990.
77. Boute W, Derrien Y, Wittkampf FHM: Reliability of evoked endocardial T-wave sensing in 1, 500 pacemaker patients. PACE 9:948, 1986.
78. Boute W, Gebhardt U, Begemann MJS: Introduction of an automatic QT interval driven rate responsive pacemaker. PACE 11:1804, 1988.
79. Baig MW, Wilson J, Boute W, et al: Improved pattern of rate responsiveness with dynamic slope setting for the QT sensing pacemaker. PACE 12:311, 1989.
80. Baig MW, Green A, Wade G, et al: A randomized double-blind, cross-over study of the linear and nonlinear algorithms for the QT sensing rate adaptive pacemaker. PACE 13:1802, 1990.
81. Baig MW, Boute W, Begemann M, Perrins EJ: One-year follow-up of automatic adaptation of the rate response algorithm of the QT sensing, rate adaptive pacemaker. PACE 14:1598, 1991.
82. Landman MA, Senden PJ, van Rooijen H, van Hemel NM: Initial experience with rate adaptive cardiac pacing using two sensors simultaneously. PACE 13:1615, 1990.
83. Connelly DT and the Topaz Study Group: Initial experience with a new single chamber, dual sensor rate responsive pacemaker. PACE 16:1833, 1993.
84. Sharp C, Busse E, Burgess J, Haennel R: Non-linearity of the oxygen uptake: Heart rate relationship in pacemaker patients with left ventricular dysfunction. In Vardas PE (ed): Proceedings of Europace 97. Athens, Monduzzi Editore, 1997, p 517.
85. Lau CP, Leung SK, Guerola M, Crijns HJGM: Comparison of continuously recorded sensor and sinus rates during daily life activities and standard exercise testing: Efficacy of automatically optimized rate adaptive dual sensor pacing to simulate sinus rhythm. PACE 19:1672, 1996.
86. Begemann MJS, Boute W: Automatic refractory period. PACE 11:1684, 1988.
87. Sugano T, Ishikawa T, Ogawa H, et al: Relationship between atrioventricular delay and QT interval or cardiac function in patients with implanted DDD pacemakers. PACE 20:1544, 1997.
88. Ishikawa T, Sugeno T, Sumitas et al: Optimal atrioventricular delay setting determined by QT sensor of implanted DDDR pacemaker. PACE 35:195, 2002.
89. Boute W, Cals GLM, den Heijer P, Wittkampf FHM: Morphology of endocardial T-waves of fusion beats. PACE 11:1693, 1988.
90. Djordjevic M, Kocovic D, Pavlovic S, et al: Circadian variations of heart rate and stim-T interval: Adaptation of nighttime pacing. PACE 12:1757, 1989.
91. Browne KF, Prystowsky E, Heger JJ, et al: Prolongation of the Q-T interval in man during sleep. Am J Cardiol 52:55, 1983.
92. Grace AA, Newell SA, Cary NRB, et al: Diagnosis of early cardiac transplant rejection by fall in evoked T wave amplitude measured using an externalized QT driven rate responsive pacemaker. PACE 14:1024, 1991.
93. Donaldson RM, Rickards AF: Evaluation of drug-induced changes in myocardial repolarization using the paced evoked response. Br Heart J 48:381, 1982.
94. Donaldson RM, Taggart P, Swanton H, et al: Intracardiac electrode detection of early ischaemia in man. Br Heart J 50:213, 1983.
95. Schaldach M, Hutten H: Intracardiac impedance to determine sympathetic activity in rate responsive pacing. PACE 15:1778, 1992.
96. Pichlmaier AM, Braile D, Ebner E, et al: Autonomic nervous system controlled closed loop cardiac pacing. PACE 15:1787, 1992.
97. Witte J, Reibis R, Pichlmaier AM, et al: ANS-controlled rate-adaptive pacing: Clinical evaluation. Eur J Cardiac Pacing Electrophysiol 6:53, 1996.
98. Christ T, Shier M, Brattstrom A, et al: Rate-adaptive pacing using intracardiac impedance shows no evidence of positive feeback duing dobutanine stress rest. Europace 4:311, 2002.
99. Osswald S, Cron T, Gradel P, et al: Closed-loop stimulation using intracardiac impedance as a sensor principle: Correlation of right ventricular dP/dt_{max} and intracardiac impedance during dobutamine stress test. PACE 23:1502, 2000.
100. Cook L, Hamilton D, Busse E, et al: Impact of adaptive rate pacing controlled by a right ventricular impedance sensor on cardiac output response to exercise. PACE 26:244, 2003.
101. Griesbach L, Gestrich B, Wojciechowski D, et al: Clinical performance of automatic closed-loop stimulation systems. PACE 26:1432, 2003.
102. Bingelli C, Duru F, Corti R, et al: Autonomic nervous system-controlled cardiac pacing: A comparison between intracardiac impedance signal and much sympathetic nerve activity. PACE 23:1632, 2000.
103. Filho MM, Nishioke SAD, Lopes M, et al: Neurohumoral behaviour in recipients of cardiac pacemakers controlled by closed-loop autonomic nervous system-driven sensor. PACE 23:1778, 2003.
104. Cron TZ, Hilti P, Schächiger H, et al: Rate response of a closed-loop stimulation pacing system to changing preload and after-load conditions. PACE 26:1504, 2003.
105. Occhetta E, Bortnik M, Audoglio R, et al: Closed loop stimulation in prevention of vasovagal syncope. Inotropy Controlled Pacing in Vasovagal Syncope (INVASY): A multicenter randomised, single blind, controlled study. Europace 6:538, 2004.
106. Bailey WM, Hull D: Closed loop stimulation improves ejection fraction and NYHA class in patients with congestive heart failure and/or ejection fraction ≤40%. Heart Rhythm 2:S285, 2005.

107. Occhetta E, Perucca A, Rognoni G, et al: Experience with a new myocardial acceleration sensor during dobutamine infusion and exercise test. Eur J Cardiac Pacing Electrophysiol 5:204, 1995.
108. Bongiorni MG, Soldati E, Arena G, et al: Is local myocardial contractility related to endocardial acceleration signals detected by a transvenous pacing lead? PACE 19:1682, 1996.
109. Wood JC, Festen MP, Lim MJ, et al: Regional effects of myocardial ischemia on epicardially recorded canine first heart sounds. J Appl Physiol 76:291, 1994.
110. Plicchi G, Mercelli E, Parlapiano M, et al: PEA I and PEA II based implantable haemodynamic monitor: Preclinical studies in sheep. Europace 4:49, 2002.
111. Clementy J: Dual chamber rate responsive pacing system driven by contractility: Final assessment after 1-year follow-up. The European PEA Clinical Investigation Group. PACE 21:2192, 1998.
112. Langenfeld H, Krein A, Kirstein M, et al: Peak endocardial acceleration-based clinical testing of the "BEST" DDDR pacemaker. European PEA Clinical Investigation Group. PACE 21:2187, 1998.
113. Rickards AF, Bombardini T, Corbucci G, et al: An implantable intracardiac accelerometer for monitoring myocardial contractility. The Multicenter PEA Study Group. PACE 19:2066, 1996
114. Leung SK, Lau CP, Lam C, et al: Performance of a sensor measuring intracardiac cardiac acceleration signals during submaximal exercise. Pacing Electrophysiol 22:A106, 1999.
115. Greo EM, Ferrario M, Romano S: Clinical evaluation of peak endocardial acceleration as a sensor for rate response pacing. PACE 26:812, 2003.
116. Bordachar P, Garrigue S, Reuter S, et al: Hemodynamic assessment of right, left and biventricular pacing by peak endocardial acceleration and echocardiography in patients with end-stage heart failure. PACE 23:1726, 2000.
117. Leung SK, Lau CP, Lau CT: Automatic optimization of resting a peak endocardial acceleration sensor: Validation with Doppler echocardiography and direct cardiac output measurements. PACE 23:1762, 2000.
118. Deharo JC, Brunetto A, et al: DDDR pacing driven by contractility versus DDI pacing in vasovagal syncope: A multicenter, randomized study. PACE 26:447, 2003.
119. Clementy J, Kobeissi A, Gamigue S, et al: Validation by serial standardization testiny of a new rate-responsive pacemaker sensor based on variations in myocardial contractility. Europace 3:124, 2001.
120. Leung SK, Lau CP, Tang MO, et al: New integrated sensor pacemaker: Comparison of the rate responses between an integrated minute ventilation and activity sensor and single sensor modes during exercise and daily activities and non-physiological interference. PACE 19:1664, 1996.
121. Leung SK, Lau CP, Tang MO: Cardiac output is a sensitive indicator of difference in exercise performance between single and dual sensor pacemakers. PACE 21:35, 1998.
122. Leung SK, Lau CP, Tang MO, et al: An integrated dual sensor system automaticity optimized by target rate histogram. PACE 21:1559, 1998.
123. Boland J, Scherer M, Hartnung W: Clinical evaluation of an automatic sensor response algorithm in patients with DR pacemakers: A multicenter study. PACE 22:A102, 1999.
124. Pieragnoli P, Colella A, Moro E, et al: Blended dual sensor does not give additional benefits to single sensor in DDDR PM patients: Results from the DUSISLOG study. Heart Rhythm 2:S40, 2005.

Chapter 17

Testing and Programming of Implantable Defibrillator Functions at Implantation

MARK W. KROLL • PATRICK J. TCHOU

Since the inception of clinical implantation of automatic defibrillators in the early 1980s, testing of the device function at implantation has been an integral part of the surgical procedure. Implantable defibrillators serve to terminate life-threatening cardiac arrhythmias, so it is imperative that such a device sense a tachyarrhythmia appropriately and terminate it successfully. Verification of these functions at implantation involves measurement of the detected ventricular and—more recently—atrial electrograms, both during the normal rhythm and during ventricular fibrillation (VF) and ventricular tachycardia (VT). Testing of sensing and detection is especially important during VF, in which the amplitudes of the recorded ventricular complexes can vary greatly from beat to beat. Such variation can cause failure of arrhythmia detection as a result of automatic adjustment of sensitivity in the recording amplifiers or detection thresholds. Dropout of electrograms during detection may result in prolonged delays in tachycardia detection and termination of VF.

A measurement of defibrillation threshold (DFT) is important to ensuring that the implanted device has the shock strength to terminate VF in a reliable manner. Although biphasic shocks and newer electrode systems are more reliable in defibrillation, one occasionally still encounters a patient in whom the DFT is high. An implanting physician must be familiar with an approach to such a patient.

Antitachycardia pacing (ATP) plays a critical role in the treatment of VT by terminating VT without a shock. Thus, ATP therapy may be tested at implantation.

Strength, Duration, and Probabilistic Nature of the Shock Response

The most important function of the implantable cardioverter-defibrillator (ICD) is its ability to reliably terminate a life-threatening ventricular tachyarrhythmia. Thus, testing of this function is an important aspect of implanting an ICD. The process of terminating VF can best be described in a three-dimensional relationship of shock strength (voltage or current), shock duration (milliseconds; msec) and the probability of success of the shock. Conceptually, a defibrillation shock has certain similarities to a pacing impulse. The strength-duration relationship of pacing has been well defined.

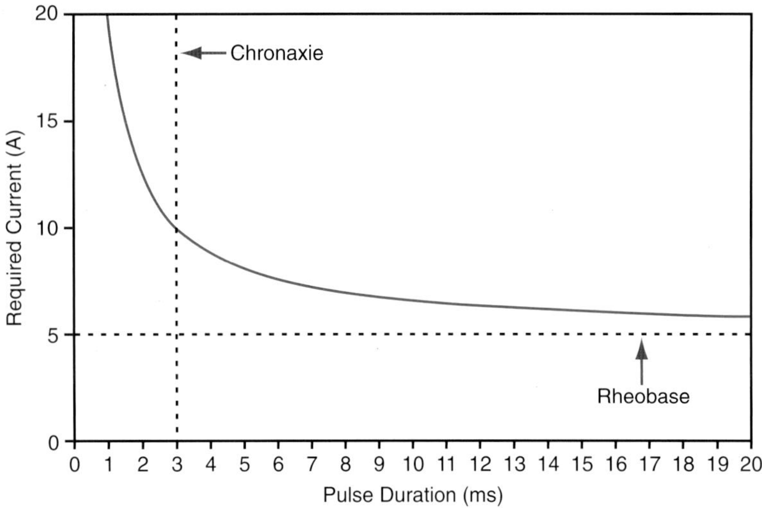

Figure 17-1. A generalized strength duration curve for defibrillation. The rheobase current in the human heart is generally in the range of 2-6 A, whereas the chronaxie is typically 2-4 msec. Optical mapping measurements of the transmembrane response to a shock show that the membrane time constant is in the same approximate range as the chronaxie.

Similarly, there is a strength-duration relationship for defibrillation shocks.[1-7] This relationship, shown in Figure 17-1, applies to monophasic shocks and the first phase of biphasic shocks. If one considers a rectangular monophasic shock waveform, there exists a rheobase voltage/current below which pulses will not defibrillate regardless of pulse duration. As one shortens the pulse width, the voltage/current required to defibrillate the heart increases. This relationship of pulse width to voltage and current has been well established in experimental models. The slope of this curve rises as the pulse width shortens, such that the voltage/current rises asymptotically when the pulse width approaches zero.

For pacing, such a strength-duration curve gives a good description of myocardial capture, because the threshold of myocardial capture is essentially an all-or-none phenomenon—that is, the probability of capture rises very steeply as the parameters of a pacing impulse (strength and duration) traverse the strength-duration curve. One essentially finds 100% capture on one side of the curve and no capture on the other side of the curve except for the well-known hysteresis effect.

Such is not the case for defibrillation. The probabilistic nature of defibrillation cannot be adequately described with a single strength-duration curve. The strength-duration relationship of defibrillation is best described as a family of curves in which each curve has a particular probability of successful defibrillation. Thus, another manner of looking at the defibrillation phenomenon is described by the defibrillation success curve.

This sigmoidal dose-response curve has been commonly described as a logistic regression curve.[8] In fact, this would suggest that at very low levels one could occasionally "get lucky" and defibrillate the heart. However, a more appropriate curve is one that rises steeply from a 0% probability and then asymptotically approaches 100%, as shown in Figure 17-2.[9,10] The use of extremely high energies can also reduce the efficacy of a defibrillation shock because of the deleterious effects of high energies, as discussed later. This problem is relatively rare at the voltages used with current ICDs, especially with anodal biphasic shocks.

The postulated mechanisms by which a shock terminates VF have undergone modifications over the years. These have been reviewed elsewhere, and a thorough discussion is beyond the scope of this chapter.[11,12] Although the defibrillation phenomenon and its probabilistic nature are still incompletely understood, several factors contribute to the difference between a pacing threshold and a defibrillation threshold. A pacing impulse is delivered at a time when the myocardium is in a relatively homogenous state—diastole. Furthermore, pacing capture occurs within a small volume of myocardium in the immediate vicinity of the pacing electrode. Thus, the electrical state of the myocardium within this small volume at the time of impulse delivery is highly homogenous. In contrast, defibrillation involves the influence of an electrical shock across the entire myocardium. Reproducibly

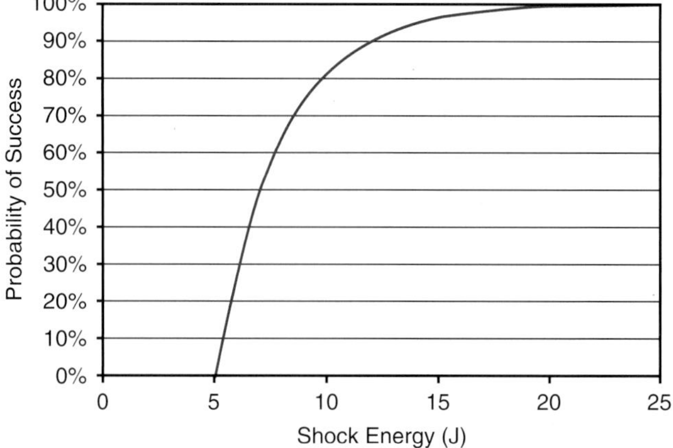

Figure 17-2. A typical defibrillation success curve showing the probability of successful defibrillation according to the amount of energy used. This type of success curve can just as easily be described for the average current or voltage of the shock. More effective waveforms would shift this curve to the left and generate a steeper slope.

successful defibrillation shocks must achieve minimum voltage gradients of about 5 V/cm at nearly all myocardial sites.[13] The defibrillation shock is delivered at a time when the myocardium is in a highly nonhomogenous state of activation.

There may be several reasons why defibrillation behaves in a probabilistic fashion. The number and size of wavelets or rotors existing at any time in the myocardium during VF can vary. The distance of any dominant wavefronts from the shocking electrode can vary. Furthermore, this nonhomogenous state is changing rapidly over time. Thus, the timing of the shock is not synchronized to dominant wavelets or rotors. Experiments in which the defibrillating shock was synchronized to a large-amplitude wave on a surface electrocardiogram (ECG) during VF, presumably a time when there is a large dominant wave, have demonstrated lowered DFTs.[14] Thus, spatial and temporal heterogeneity of ventricular myocardium is a likely explanation for the probabilistic nature of defibrillation.

Why Perform Defibrillation Threshold Testing?

With proper implantation of the ICD leads, today's biphasic waveforms in implantable defibrillators can achieve reliable defibrillation in a large percentage of patients. However, some form of testing to verify that an implanted device is capable of accomplishing the task of defibrillation reliably is needed at the time of implantation. This testing allows one to ensure that the device can deliver a shock waveform of sufficient amplitude to accomplish reliable defibrillation and provides an opportunity to make changes in the device to improve the defibrillation efficacy, if needed. Because defibrillation is a probabilistic phenomenon, a single success at a shock strength near the maximum output of the device is not adequate assurance that the device will work well in clinical circumstances when defibrillation is needed. Furthermore, clinical circumstances may be complicated by additional variables that may alter defibrillation energy requirements. The variability of serum electrolyte levels, changes in sympathetic tone, the rise and fall of serum antiarrhythmic drug levels, and the diastolic filling pressures of the heart are factors that may influence defibrillation energy requirements.

When testing demonstrates that defibrillation is reproducibly successful at relatively low shock strengths, one can program the device to deliver the first shock at a lower shock strength. This lower-energy output would require a shorter capacitor charge time and shorten the time from the initiation of ventricular tachyarrhythmia to the delivery of the first shock. Such a shortened device response time can mean the difference between maintenance and loss of consciousness. Sudden and unexpected loss of consciousness is usually an undesirable occurrence because it can increase patient morbidity and even cause death. Although awareness of the psychological stresses that may complicate sensed shocks, especially multiple sequential shocks, is growing, one must balance the potential generation of anxiety and depression against the real possibility of injuries to the patient and others brought on by loss of consciousness.[15]

The lower shock strengths that can be programmed after defibrillation testing may also have the advantage of decreasing the probability of myocardial damage, especially if the patient experiences circumstances that produce multiple shocks over a short period, because of either a "storm" of ventricular arrhythmias or inappropriate device discharges in response to atrial fibrillation with rapid ventricular response or device malfunction. The use of a lower shock strength can also accelerate post-shock hemodynamic recovery. One study showed that shocks stronger than 10 joules (J) tend to depress hemodynamic recovery by about 20% for as long as 4 minutes.[16] Lower shock strengths can also lengthen longevity of the device battery. Another advantage of determining the actual DFT is that the parameter can be monitored for increases during follow-up, providing an indication of changes in the lead position or myocardial substrate.

However, a thorough understanding of the DFT would require multiple fibrillation/shock sequences during implantation testing. The value of an accurate DFT measurement is further diminished by the knowledge that this threshold can vary from day to day in response to clinical changes in a patient's physiologic status and medication levels. Patients who receive defibrillator implants frequently have markedly depressed ventricular function as a reflection of the underlying substrate that puts them at risk for ventricular tachyarrhythmias. In such patients, multiple shocks for determining the DFT may cause deterioration of ventricular function during the implantation and thus may raise the risk of the procedure.[17] During clinical implantation of a defibrillator, therefore, one needs to strike a balance among the safety of the patient, the adequate performance of the implanted device, and a sufficient understanding of the DFT to enable one to program the first shock strength appropriately.

The most common definition of *defibrillation threshold* is the shock amplitude that provides a 50% chance of success. This is the definition we use as the default. When there is danger of confusion, we use DFT_{50} to refer to this parameter. Other useful DFTs are DFT_{70}, DFT_{80}, and DFT_{90} (see Fig. 17-2).

Alternatively, one can simply verify that the device, at its maximum output, has an adequate safety margin to defibrillate the heart reliably. The role of *verification* is to merely "verify" that the DFT is below a certain level and that the device can thus be safely implanted.[10,18] The advantage of a verification approach is that one minimizes the number of shocks during the implantation and shortens the duration of the procedure. If the device to be implanted is capable of a maximum energy shock of 30 J and if a single shock at 15 J or two successive shocks at 20 J are successful in converting VF, one can have some confidence that 30 J will be sufficient. The advantages of this approach are simplicity and brevity. In patients in whom one wishes to minimize the number of VF inductions and shocks, this approach would allow the implantation of a device with a minimal amount of testing. The drawbacks of using a verification approach are that the first shock energy may be set unnecessarily high and that there is no baseline DFT for tracking changes. There will also be no DFT data for scientific comparison. Thus, this approach is inadequate for comparative evaluation of different waveforms or shock electrode positions.

The main method for determining the DFT during ICD implantation or for postimplantation testing is to induce VF in the patient, wait approximately 10 seconds, and deliver a shock of a given energy. If this shock is successful, VF is induced again, and a lower-energy shock is tried. If the shock was unsuccessful, a rescue shock at a higher energy or an external shock is delivered. Next, a shock of energy intermediate between those of the last successful shock and the failed shock can be tried. Various protocols, discussed later, are used to determine the sequence of shocks and the number of shocks as well as to calculate the DFT. In experimental studies, a longer sequence of shocks may be necessary to provide an estimate of the DFT_{50} that is accurate enough for comparison purposes. However, during standard clinical implantation of an ICD, a step-down or step-up approach, starting at 15 J output with increments of 5 J, usually provides an adequate endpoint.

Animal studies have shown that prolonged DFT testing with multiple inductions of VF can lead to hemodynamic compromise and diminished cardiac function.[19] Human results are mixed, however, and there is no clear consensus. One study showed no decrease in the mean ejection fraction (EF) but reported one patient whose EF fell from 0.20 to 0.11.[20] Two studies found the only hemodynamic damage from VF testing to be a significant impairment in diastolic filling.[21,22] Another study found that, in the first hour after VF, there is no hemodynamic deterioration and, in fact, diastolic filling is *enhanced*.[23] Other studies have suggested that there is no morbidity from VF inductions for patients with left ventricular EF (LVEF) values in excess of 0.30.[17] Patients with lower EFs can have a serious reduction in cardiac index, however, with one report of prolonged inotropic support being necessary. Another human study, which looked specifically at patients with an LVEF of 0.35 or less, found no deterioration even with an average of nine inductions each.[24] In the Medtronic PCD trials, physicians were encouraged to find a combination of leads that would allow the implantation of the monophasic sequential shock device. Many of these patients received more than 50 shocks with no reported trends in mortality and morbidity.

Thus, there is considerable variation in the tolerance of repeated VF induction and defibrillations even in patients with reduced EFs. However, most implanting physicians have encountered the occasional patient—usually with very poor LV function—who showed marked hemodynamic deterioration mostly of limited duration following several VF inductions and shock sequences. It is important to use clinical judgment at the time of implantation to assess the safety of repeated VF inductions. Patients with EFs of less than 0.3 may need closer hemodynamic monitoring during and immediately after the implantation procedure, but the vast majority of patients undergo DFT testing with no problem at all. When defibrillation is followed by a prolonged episode of hypotension or marked bradycardia, it would be prudent to limit DFT testing to a verification protocol.

Initial electroencephalogram (EEG) data suggested that exceeding six inductions can cause transient cerebral dysfunction (defined as an increase in delta-wave power longer than 2.5 minutes).[25] Later studies have shown that the duration of EEG changes are correlated with VF duration.[26,27] These changes occur within 8 to 12 seconds of induction and last about 1 minute on average.[26] A study of 36 patients with 286 inductions of VF found that although EEG recovery time was correlated with VF duration, it was negatively correlated with the *number* of inductions.[28] Thus, there was no indication that any cumulative effect on the EEG occurred with repeated induction of VF. Defibrillation testing involves delivery of high-voltage shocks through the ICD leads. Thus, patients should be well sedated during the process to avoid undue stress.

Methods of Determining Defibrillation Threshold

Induction Methods

Before one can directly test a defibrillation shock, one must induce fibrillation. The four common methods for inducing VF are: (1) stimulating at extremely high rates, (2) delivering a shock on the T-wave, (3) applying direct current (DC) across the defibrillation electrodes, and (4) applying alternating current (AC). The classic approaches to inducing VF were to perform high-rate pacing and to deliver alternating current through an external testing device.

One method used today is extremely high-rate stimulation on the order of power-line frequencies. Pulses at a rate of 50 Hz (ICDs manufactured by Medtronic, Inc., Minneapolis, Minn.) or of 20 or 33 Hz (ICDs manufactured by Guidant [Boston Scientific, Natick, Mass.]), or programmable rates from 10 to 50 Hz (ICDs manufactured by St. Jude Medical, St. Paul, Minn.) are delivered until VF is induced. Direct delivery of the pulses through the ICD pacing leads has the advantage of being painless. However, the efficacy of inducing VF may be limited.

A popular method now used is to deliver a shock on the peak of the T-wave. This can be performed during sinus rhythm or ventricular pacing. It has the advantage of more reliably inducing VF. This approach is based on the principle of the "zone of vulnerability" surrounding the T-wave, where a range of shock strengths will initiate VF.[29] The upper limit of this zone of shock strength correlates well with reliable defibrillation. T-wave shocking is available with all current ICDs. In clinical practice, VF is generally initiated through delivery of a low-level shock, around 1 J, timed to the peak of the T-wave during a paced ventricular rhythm. A commonly used approach is to pace the ventricle at 400 msec for eight beats, followed by a 1-J shock at around 300 msec after the last paced impulse. The coupling interval of the shock can be adjusted if VF is not reliably induced. At times, several adjustments of the timing and, occasionally, the energy may be needed to achieve induction of VF. In general, shocks delivered before the peak of the T-wave are most reliable for inducing VF. This approach is available with all current ICD models. A subtlety of this approach is that fibrillation is induced most reliably with a cathodal right ventricular (RV) shock, yet defibrillation is most reliable with anodal RV polarity.[30]

The third method is to apply a low DC voltage, around 5 to 12 V, across the defibrillation electrodes. This was classically done with an external source of DC, such as a 9-volt battery, connected to the implanted epicardial leads. Current implantation techniques generally do not allow the use of an external source of DC. Thus, one uses the internal power of the ICD generator to deliver this current. One advantage of this approach is the high success rate for induction without the need for alignment to a T-wave. The method also appears to out-perform the T-wave shock in reliably inducing VF.[31] This DC fibrillation feature is currently available in St. Jude Medical devices.

The final method for induction is the use of low-voltage AC coupled directly to the defibrillation leads. Either 50- or 60-Hz AC (depending on the continent) has proved to be extremely effective in this role.[32] Transformer reduction to a 3-V level provides sufficient current to induce VF within 2 to 4 seconds in almost any subject. This method is now seldom used in ICD implantation, however, because it is not available for delivery through the devices. It may still be used occasionally when an ICD is implanted in a patient undergoing open-chest surgery for some other reason.

Defining the Defibrillation Threshold

It is important to understand the DFT both for historical and clinical reasons. The DFT must not exceed the capability of the device. In addition, even when the DFT is not evaluated explicitly, it must be evaluated implicitly through assessment of an upper bound so as to verify that the device has a shock of sufficient magnitude to defibrillate the heart reliably. This is what Singer and Lang[18] refer to as a "verification approach." Finally, an explicit DFT must often be calculated for research purposes to demonstrate that a certain waveform or lead system has advantages over others.

The definition of *defibrillation threshold* is deceptively simple: It is the electrical dosage required to defibrillate the heart. This definition, however, is complicated by two major subtleties. The first one is the choice of units for the dosage. This issue is dealt with later in the chapter; see "The Energy Crisis." Historically, energy has been chosen to compare efficiency in comparisons of the DFT values obtained in two different defibrillation systems. Although the use of energy is an acceptable means of comparing DFTs, one must be aware that just raising the amount of "delivered" energy does not necessarily translate to a better safety margin for defibrillation. For example, increasing the delivered energy by delaying the truncation to prolong the duration of a truncated exponential waveform may actually lower the defibrillation efficacy. Because of the ease with which the shock energy is measured and the historical precedent of reporting defibrillation success as shock energy, however, it has become accepted practice to use energy to describe DFTs and to discuss safety margins in units of energy. Fortunately, in current devices, increases in energy are tied to increases in voltage and current and not just to prolongation of pulse duration. Thus, the discussion of DFT in this chapter is focused on joules or energy for defibrillation. However, it is crucial to understand that DFT is most closely correlated to the current delivered through the leads.

The second subtlety in the definition of the DFT is the apparently probabilistic nature of the dose-response curve for defibrillation.[33] The probabilistic character of defibrillation efficacy inherent in this curve may be due to random variation in the size of the myocardial mass,[34] to conductive properties of myocardial cells,[35] or to systematic alteration of cellular or tissue electrophysiologic characteristics involved in the initiation and perpetuation of VF.[36] The "Progressive Depolarization" hypothesis offered by Dillon and Kwaku[11] holds that progressively stronger shocks depolarize progressively more refractory myocardium, to progressively prevent postshock wavefronts, and prolong and synchronize postshock repolarization, in a progressively larger volume of the ventricle, to progressively decrease the probability of fibrillation after the shock. These multiple functions, requiring different current densities acting on different phases of cellular activation potentials, which are distributed differently with wavefront positions, generate multiple degrees of freedom that help explain the apparent probabilistic nature of defibrillation. One might say "apparently" probabilistic because no one has been able to establish that the dose-response relationship is truly probabilistic on a level comparable with that of, say, electron position in quantum mechanics. In fact, evidence suggests that a large portion of the "probabilistic" nature of the shock response is actually due to our inability to better time the shock.[37-39]

Defibrillation Threshold Testing Protocols

The simplest protocol for determining the DFT and the one most commonly used in clinical practice is to reduce the shock amplitude until a shock fails to defibrillate the heart; this is known as a *step-down* protocol. The lowest successful shock level is then called the DFT. This approach gives, on average, a DFT estimate that approximates the 70% success (DFT_{70}) level.[40-42] However, given the probabilistic nature of a shock's success in converting VF, such a determination of DFT may have (occasionally) as low an overall success rate as 25%. Thus, one would need a device that has a maximum output of around twice the energy of the DFT to be confident that it would defibrillate reliably.

For example, a DFT of 15 J would require that the device have a maximum output of 30 J. When the DFT measured in this manner is 20 J, one does not have the confidence that this device would convert VF at all times. One means of reducing the need for such a large safety margin is to require two consecutive successful shocks at the lowest successful energy level. This DFT has been referred to as a *DFT+*, indicating the extra success of shocks at this energy level.[17] With a DFT+ determination, there is a greater likelihood that this DFT is near the upper end of the DFT curve. Thus, one can reduce the required safety margin. For a patient with a DFT+ of 20 J, one might implant a 35-J device. Similarly, with three consecutive successful shocks at 25 J (DFT++), one might consider implanting a device with a 35-J maximum output, or a device with a maximum output 10 J higher than the DFT++.

To arrive at a more accurate estimate of DFT, in experimental protocols, for example, one could average a step-down value and a step-up value.[43] The most popular method for determining a DFT has been the classic step-up/step-down method first popularized by Purdue University researchers. With this protocol, the attempted shock strength begins at a high level. It is then reduced at fixed steps until failure occurs. Typical fixed steps are 2 J or 100 V. After failure to defibrillate occurs, the direction of changes is reversed, and the shock strengths are raised by finer steps, such as 1 J or 50 V. This protocol is simple to perform, and the DFT is defined as the lowest amplitude at which a shock is successful. The disadvantage of this protocol is that it can require many shocks and is not very accurate; the mean estimate tends to overestimate the DFT_{50} with a fairly wide error band.

A variant on the step-up/step-down approach is the *three-reversal* approach.[44] With this approach, the step sizes are kept fixed. After stepping the shock strength down to defibrillation failure, the direction of change is reversed, and the strength is raised in same fixed steps until defibrillation is successful. At this point, the shock strength is changed again, and stepped down until defibrillation failure occurs. At this point, the third reversal is assumed "on paper"—that is, one more step-up would result in success. All of the shock energies from the lowest successful shock energy in the first step-down to the final "paper" shock are then averaged. This approach has the advantage of giving a more accurate estimate of the DFT and has proved very useful in research studies comparing the relative benefits of different waveforms.[45] The disadvantage of this reversal approach is that it requires numerous shocks.

An example of the three-reversal approach is as follows. Shock energies are reduced by 1 J at a time, with the lowest successful shock being 8 J. A reduction of shock strength to 7 J finds failure. The first reversal is then performed, and the shock strength is increased up to 8 J (another failure) and then to 9 J before defibrillation occurs. The second reversal is then performed, the shock being reduced to 8 J, which fails to terminate VT. The final reversal then is the "paper shock," which assumes that a 9-J shock would be successful. The DFT estimate then is the average of the shocks (in order) of 8, 7, 8, 9, 8, and 9 J, which is 8.2 J. The inclusion of the higher "paper shock" value balances the downward bias from inclusion of the failure shocks and results in an accurate, unbiased estimation of DFT_{50}.

During clinical ICD implantation, it is typical to use a step-down method with very coarse steps such as 5 J. This allows the determination of an approximate DFT while exposing the patient to a minimum number of shocks. In an attempt to achieve a high-resolution DFT estimate while staying with a lower number of shocks, the *binary search* technique was suggested. With this approach, the range of possible values for the DFT is continually cut in half to rapidly focus in on the DFT. This approach is best explained with an example: For a 32-J device, the first attempt at a shock is 16 J. If that shock is successful, the energy range is bifurcated, at 8 J. Assuming that the 8 J shock is a failure, the next energy attempted is halfway between 8 and 16 J, or 12 J. If the 12 J shock is a failure, the energy range is cut in half again, and 14 J is tried. The procedure is continued until the desired resolution is obtained. The advantage of a binary search is that it gives high resolution with very few shocks. The disadvantage is that the high resolution may be misleading in that it is not necessarily associated with high accuracy.

Malkin has derived a unique approach, which would appear to combine the best features of all of the DFT protocol techniques in his Bayesian technique.[46] This approach has also proved useful in scientific studies.[47] Depending on the number of shocks one is willing to use, Malkin and colleagues supply tables and formulas to give the exact sequence of shocks. Then, depending on the success and failure of each of the shocks, there is an optimal Bayesian estimate of the actual DFT. One version combines this with the upper limit of vulnerability (ULV; see later) approach.[48]

Another approach possible with Guidant ICDs is the *step-up*. A series of five, increasing energy shocks are programmed in for a therapy regimen. VF is induced, and then the shocks of increasing energy are given until defibrillation occurs. This approach allows for a reasonably accurate DFT determination without multiple inductions. The drawbacks are the length of the individual fibrillation episode and the possible influence of VF duration on the DFT.

Upper Limit of Vulnerability Approach to Determining the Defibrillation Threshold

There is a time interval near the peak of the T-wave (within 40 msec) known as the *vulnerable period,* during which a shock of sufficient but not too great magnitude induces VF (Fig. 17-3). According to the ULV theory of defibrillation, when such a shock generates an electrical field with its voltage gradient not parallel to a repolarizing wavefront, it initiates a spiraling wavefront around a critical point that can initiate VF. As one raises the shock strength, there is a limit above which VF can no longer be induced. This *upper limit of vulnerability* to VF has been demonstrated to correlate well with the DFT; that is, shocks with energies above the ULV should defibrillate the heart as well.[49] This concept can also

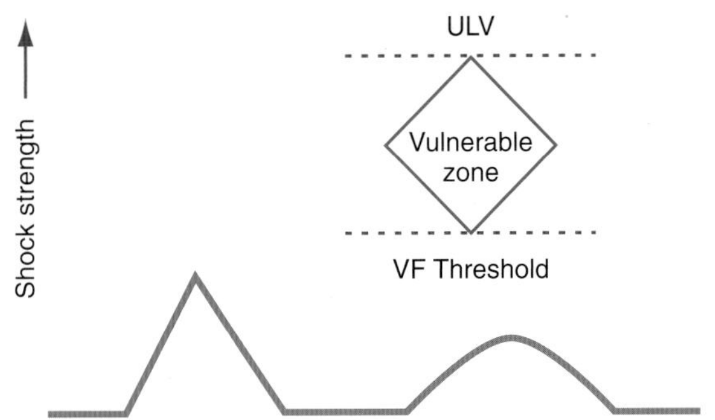

Figure 17-3. The vulnerable zone is a region of shock amplitude and time in which shocks will usually produce VF. The time period is within the T-wave and the shock strength lies between the VF threshold and the upper limit of vulnerability.

explain the probabilistic nature of defibrillation. In the myocardial regions of relative low voltage gradients, the exact orientation of a repolarizing wavefront with the local voltage gradient generated by a shock is a random phenomenon. Thus, the vulnerable zone of shock strengths for initiating (or reinitiating) VF in that region should follow a probabilistic distribution. It should be noted, however, that other theories also account for the clinical ULV phenomenon that do not rely on the ULV theory of defibrillation.[11]

The clinical attraction of the ULV approach is that one could perform implantation testing of DFT with the use of only one actual VF induction. Shocks are delivered synchronized with the T-wave (in sinus or paced rhythm) at a high energy and decreased in a stepwise fashion with successive shocks. If the 20-J shock fails to induce VF, that level must be higher than the ULV and hence higher than the DFT. Note that the patient has not been put into fibrillation with that shock. The shock strength then is reduced successively until either a sufficiently weak shock does not induce VF (which means that there was no induction of VF) or the first episode of VF occurs, which in turn has significance similar to that of a failed defibrillation shock. The timing of the shock within the T-wave is critical. The peak ULV within the vulnerable zone is not necessarily at the peak of the T-wave and can vary from patient to patient. In isolated rabbit hearts, accuracy with monophasic shocks appears to be optimized with a shock delivery during the T-wave upslope, whereas shocks at or after the peak may be better for biphasic waveforms.[50] Accuracy and repeatability are improved with multiple shock positions within the T-wave. For example, the shock can be delivered at the peak of the T-wave and 20 msec before.[51] One can add a third shock positioned 40 msec before the T-wave peak.[52,53] To use this method as a reliable approach to predict successful defibrillation, one should apply this approach at varying intervals before the peak of the T-wave, for example, 0, 20, and 40 msec.

Although there are occasional significant differences between the ULV and DFT,[54] the two values correlate well regardless of the pacing site,[55] the presence of ischemia,[56] whether testing is acute or chronic,[57] electrode polarity,[58] and waveform durations.[58] The disadvantage of the ULV approach is the number of shocks to be delivered for a reliable determination of defibrillation efficacy. The advantage is that one can minimize the number of inductions of VF. The ULV and DFT are both predictors of a shock strength that defibrillates the heart with a given probability of success. The prediction of defibrillation efficacy is actually more important than the precise correlation between ULV and DFT.

Verification

With the verification approach, one ensures that the maximum output of the ICD is well above the DFT without actually determining a DFT. Singer and Lang[18] have provided a classification of various approaches to verification. With their one-shock verification protocol, one low-energy shock was given which was successful in defibrillating the heart. This protocol assumes that this shock was so low in strength that even though it was tested only once, there was a large margin between that low-energy shock and the much higher output of the device. For example, if the low-energy shock of 10 J terminated VF, then one can have reasonable confidence that a device output of 27 J will defibrillate reliably. Similarly, one could use a two-shock protocol, in which two shocks of identical energy are used to defibrillate the heart. With this "2S" protocol, one can reduce the margin between the successful shock energy and the ICD output. A more detailed discussion of this topic can be found in the literature.[17, 59]

Equipment for Defibrillation Threshold Testing

Classically, external implant support devices were used to induce VF and provide defibrillation shocks. With the advent of the pectoral implantation approach, however, external device–based testing is rarely used today.[60,61]

The advantages of device-based testing rather than external support device testing are numerous, as follows: (1) one can be sure that there is a perfect match between the waveform for the testing and the waveform that will be used for therapy; (2) one can be certain that the measurements of shock amplitude and impedance are identical; (3) the lead connections are all being tested with each delivered shock; (4) the same sensing circuit and algorithms are tested; and (5) storage and maintenance of the external device are avoided. Major disadvantages of the external devices are that they are not updated as frequently as the actual ICDs and that the sensing amplifiers, filters, and sensing algorithms are rarely identical to those found in the ICD being currently implanted. Thus, in many cases, sensing performance is not adequately tested with the external system. Also, the waveforms have been, in some cases, significantly different with external device–based testing.

The advantages of using the external device are as follows: (1) the ICD longevity is enhanced because it is not used to deliver any shocks during testing; (2) one has the capability of higher-energy rescue shocks, should "bailout" be necessary; and (3) the use of the external support device for defibrillation testing gives the physician the flexibility of choosing a lower-energy ICD (presumably much smaller) for the final implant. This last procedure can be performed without breaking the sterility of the smaller device, which may be a risk if it is unable to perform the defibrillation.

Regardless of the device used for testing DFT, backup defibrillation is essential. The most common approach is to use a biphasic external defibrillator with flexible adhesive patches attached to the patient's chest. Two defibrillators with a biphasic waveform should be available during DFT testing. It is important to verify proper placement of the patches, especially in larger patients in whom the required defibrillation energy may be near the maximal output of the defibrillator. The adhesive patch electrodes are relatively radiolucent and generally do not obstruct the fluoroscopic view during the implantation procedure. A typical anterior-posterior placement of these electrodes keeps them out of the operating field. Optimal anterior placement is over the apex of the heart, and optimal posterior placement is over the spine at the upper border of the heart shadow in the AP view with fluoroscopy.

It is important to verify the proper placement of the internal defibrillation leads as well as the absence of a pneumothorax prior to initiation of VF for DFT testing. Occasionally, with a pneumothorax, even the external device does not successfully defibrillate the heart.[62] Pneumothorax defibrillation failure is very rare now with external biphasic defibrillators, but when external defibrillation is unsuccessful, one may consider—in addition to poor external electrode positions and pneumothorax—whether intramyocardial current is being shunted in some manner. Such shunting can occur, for example, if a posterior electrode such as a subcutaneous coil, a coronary sinus electrode, or an azygous shocking coil is connected to the superior vena cava (SVC) electrode port of the ICD header. Although this shunting is usually not of concern, it may make the difference between success and failure of defibrillation in a patient with high transthoracic impedance and high external DFT. Disconnecting the ICD electrode from the ICD header under those circumstances would solve the problem. In desperate circumstances, one can consider using the external biphasic defibrillator by connecting the apical patch electrode to the RV ICD electrode and use the posterior patch to deliver larger energy shocks in the 50- to 100-J range. Finally, should all external defibrillating attempts fail, extracorporeal cardiopulmonary bypass using peripheral vessel access can be tried if such equipment is readily available.

How Much Shock Energy Is Enough?

There are two main issues regarding the adequacy of energy output, as follows:

1. Does the device have an adequate safety margin with respect to its output above the DFT to ensure reliable therapy for the patient?
2. At what energy output should the first (and maybe second) shock amplitude be set?

Although there is some overlap in the consideration of these two questions, they really are quite different.

For the first question, let us presume that the DFT or an upper bound for the DFT has been determined through a verification protocol. How much additional energy must the device have in order to give an adequate safety margin for implant? Early systems occasionally had DFT shifts greater than 10 J, and patient deaths resulted or electrode revisions were required.[63,64] The classic rule of thumb was that a 10-J safety margin was sufficient, and this rule has achieved the status of accepted medical practice. Others have championed a safety margin equal to the DFT.[88] In other words, the device's maximal shock capability must be equal to *twice* the DFT for successful implantation. Originally this was a significantly more conservative approach than the 10-J safety margin. However, with thresholds now typically in the single digits, this rule is actually more liberal than the 10-J safety margin.[65] In one study, with a DFT of less than 6 J, a shock at twice the DFT gave a 95% success rate, whereas a classic DFT plus 10 J rule yielded a 99.5% rate for successful defibrillation.[65] When the DFT is very low, such as 4 J or less, using twice the DFT energy may yield only a 67% successful first shock rate.[66] Thus, when the DFT is less than 5 J, it would be more reliable to set the first shock energy with a safety margin of at least 7 J to achieve a first shock defibrillation success rate of 96%.

Finally, one should not take excessive comfort from a low DFT, because such numbers may have less stability (or confidence) associated with them. In another study, the shock of twice the energy yielded a success rate of 98% for patients with a DFT higher than 4 J but of only 67% for those with a DFT of less than 4 J.[67] The Malkin Bayesian approach may be used to calculate the shock strength required to achieve a conversion rate of 95%.[68,69]

The safety margin is needed to cover two basic problems. First, because of the probabilistic nature of the defibrillation dose-response curve, a shock must have higher energy than the DFT to give a reasonable confidence of defibrillation success (i.e., the shock strength should be the value that would suggest a near 100% probability of success). Second, it is difficult to estimate the required level of "insurance" against long-term drift in the DFT. Long-term rises in DFT have been reported by some investigators with the early monophasic devices,[70-73] but others found no increase in DFTs with these devices.[74] It is not clear that this drift is a problem with modern biphasic transvenous devices.[75-77] One study has reported a long-term rise in biphasic thresholds,[78] but the typical result is a rise over the first month or two, followed by a gradual return to the implant values. Although an early study in an animal model using epicardial patches suggested that rapid pacing–induced cardiomyopathy would elevate DFT,[79] a later animal study of transvenous endocardial defibrillation has shown that progressive heart failure does not increase the DFT.[80] The mean values of DFT in these studies using transvenous lead systems do not seem to show marked increases. However, there clearly are individual cases in which significant rises in DFTs do occur. In fact, one study found a DFT rise of 10 J or greater at 1- or 2-year follow-up testing in 15% of patients.[81] The reasons for long-term changes in DFT are not well understood. One can imagine that fibrosis might tend to increase resistance, and it often does. However, these increases in resistance have not been correlated with the rises in DFT that one might expect. Lead microdislodgement can significantly affect the DFT, although confirmed cases of a long-term DFT being affected by a change in lead position (short of a macro-dislodgment) are relatively rare. There are also circadian changes in the DFT, with a somewhat higher value in the morning than in the afternoon corresponding to the peak incidence of failed first shocks in response to clinical tachycardias.[82] The need for antiarrhythmic drug therapy could arise in patients who have ICDs either for the treatment of atrial arrhythmias or for suppression of frequent ventricular arrhythmias. These can also affect the DFT, as discussed later. A pneumothorax can lead to an increase in the DFT.[62,83,84] Thus, multiple factors can lead to changes in DFT after implantation that would make an adequate safety margin of the shock energy important.

The Low Energy Safety Study (LESS) is often miscited in support of the use of small safety margins such as 5 J.[85,86] This study excluded 10% of the enrolled patients—largely for high DFTs. Thus, by design, the study clearly did not address the patient with a high DFT. In this study, the DFT was defined as the DFT++. Because this definition required three consecutive successful shocks at the DFT, it was essentially a DFT_{88} ($0.88 = 1 - 2^{-3}$, which is the probability of failing to throw three out of three "heads" in a coin toss.). For a typical patient, as shown in Figure 17-2, the DFT++ is about 6 J above the DFT_{50}; thus, adding 5 J for the first two shock energies in LESS actually resulted in a setting about 11 J above the DFT_{50}. In spite of that, 4% of the patients required one to three maximal-energy rescue shocks for their spontaneous VF episodes.

Table 17-1, which shows the predicted performances of various verification techniques for defibrillator implantation testing, gives a sobering view and very well explains why a small number of patients who pass standard defibrillation testing may require multiple shocks at maximum output to terminate spontaneous VF. Using a large database of successful and unsuccessful defibrillation shocks, Smits and DeGroot[87] evaluated the popular ICD implantation defibrillation testing techniques for performance. Table 17-1 reflects the results of their computer simulation. They assumed a device with a 35-J maximum output. Patients with high DFTs would have a less than 90% chance of defibrillation with a single shock of 35 J. Those having a greater than 90% chance would be regarded as having low DFTs. The "Criterion"(column 2 of Table 17-1) is the lowest successful energy output for the testing protocol used. This is best explained by example. The row with protocol S1 and a criterion of 15 J means that a single shock verification at 15 J will be successful (Pass) in 91% of patients. The sensitivity value 94% means that this test will detect 94% of the patients with low DFTs. However, the specificity of 52% means that defibrillation with a 35-J shock failed in only 52% of patients with high DFTs; therefore, the test will miss 48% of patients with high DFTs. Approximately 3.4% of the patients who "pass" this test nevertheless belong in the high-DFT group.

Setting the First Shock Energy

Traditionally, it was believed that the shock energies for VF should all be set to the maximum output of the device. This was reflected by the philosophy that one "just could not take a chance." However, now with typical thresholds below 10 J, this practice has come into question. There are several problems with using excessive shock energy. The first is that the charge time is (at least) increasing proportionally with the shock energy. Thus, the charge time for a 10-J shock will be less than one third of that for a 30-J shock. This delayed therapy can potentially increase DFTs, exacerbate postshock dysfunction, and significantly raise the chance of syncope and accompanying sequelae.

In addition, the idea that a maximum-energy shock has a better chance of success than a low-energy shock is not universally accurate. The dose-response curve for defibrillation is not monotonic—especially for monophasic shocks. With shock energy above a certain level, the success rate may begin to go down from near 100%. The output of clinical biphasic devices does not typically generate this phenomenon, but it may still be seen clinically from time to time.[88] A report comparing the setting of the first shock to twice the DFT with the device maximum of 34 J demonstrated no significant

TABLE 17-1. **Predicted Performance of Various Verification Techniques**

Protocol	Criterion (J)	Pass (%)	Sensitivity (%)	Specificity (%)
S2	24	93	96	53
S1	15 12	91 87	94 90	52 61
Step-down	≤24 ≤18	96 87	98 91	32 74
Binary	≤24 ≤12	99 87	100 90	11 61

Data from Smits KF, DeGroot P: A Bayesian approach to reduced implant testing of a ventricular defibrillator: A computer simulation. Europace 6(Suppl):97, 2004.

difference in incidences of first biphasic shock conversion of spontaneous ventricular tachyarrhythmia. The lower setting actually trended toward a *higher* first shock conversion rate (98.5% vs. 92%).[88]

The third problem with the use of maximum-energy shocks is that higher-energy shocks can temporarily cause depressed ventricular function. Although seen only occasionally, this stunning may last for multiple seconds, delaying the hemodynamic recovery from VF.[16] Thus, if the goal is to have the patient regain good cardiac output and consciousness as soon as possible, the use of a maximum-energy shock could actually be counterproductive.

Factors that Affect the Defibrillation Threshold

Lead Systems

The current generation of defibrillation leads typically has either a single shocking electrode located in the right RV or two shocking electrodes, the second of which is located on the proximal portion of the lead, positioning it in the SVC. The advantage of the two-coil lead is its ease of use. It has the pace/sense electrodes and both shocking electrodes on one lead, allowing implantation with a single insertion (the single-pass lead). However, separate leads for the two shocking electrodes may allow better positioning of the proximal electrode. Occasionally, better results are reported for placement of the proximal electrode in the innominate vein[89,90] or the subclavian vein.[91] In general, placement in the left brachiocephalic vein does not appear to offer better DFTs.[92] In various patients, DFTs are lowest with this proximal lead in different locations.[93] When the proximal electrode is positioned too close to the RV, in the right atrium, for example, there may be energy shunting that could reduce defibrillation efficacy. Thus, locating this lead in the SVC or higher would optimize the position. In larger patients, leads that provide various positionings of the SVC electrode may be of help in ensuring that the proximal electrode is properly positioned.

Pectoral implantation of the ICD generator has become standard. Inclusion of the housing electrode has reduced DFTs by about 30% in comparison with previous, purely transvenous lead systems.[94,95] In fact, these so-called unipolar systems now offer thresholds that are comparable with those seen with monophasic shocks using epicardial patches. In most patients, using the RV shocking electrode in conjunction with the can electrode provides an adequate DFT for implantation of a device without the need for another electrode. This configuration can allow use of a thinner transvenous lead. Furthermore, such a unipolar lead may be more reliable because no high-voltage differences would exist within the lead body itself.

Adding a patch, subaxillary array, or a subcutaneous coil can result in lower DFTs than with the use of a simple transvenous system.[96,97] A subcutaneous patch may actually be as effective as an epicardial patch.[98] Because of crinkling problems, such patches are almost never used today. The addition of an array may be helpful in reducing DFT through two primary mechanisms. The first and most direct mechanism is that the overall system impedance decreases, and therefore, for a given maximum voltage from the ICD, the current increases. For a tilt-based waveform, the resistance lowering of the array will reduce the shock time constant, diminish the pulse widths, and possibly improve the efficiency of the waveform. Second, with a more posterior placement of the coils, the current from the RV coil may be more posteriorly directed, improving voltage gradients in the posterior LV portion of the myocardium. Thus, a subcutaneous coil must be inserted as posterior as possible at a level near the base of the ventricular shadow. This position may, however, increase the chance of back pain.

The most important electrode in transvenous defibrillation systems is the one placed in the RV, although it obviously cannot function in isolation. Although this coil is typically placed in the RV apex, there is some evidence that even better DFTs can be obtained with placement of the coil in the septum, near the outflow tract.[99,100]Assuming an RV coil and a can electrode in the left pectoral region, a natural question arises, "To what extent will the addition of an SVC lead reduce DFTs?" One study suggested that it probably makes no difference for most patients.[101] Practically, that may be the case. Later studies have demonstrated that inclusion of an SVC electrode can lower energy and voltage DFTs.[102,103] However, these studies were performed with fixed-tilt waveforms, so the automatic reductions in the pulse durations may have exerted a dominating influence by bringing the waveform closer to optimal durations. One report demonstrated that the addition of an SVC electrode lowers DFT energy but *increases* the current at DFT.[103] Because an increased current is associated with higher tissue voltage gradients, the lower DFT energy was actually associated with a higher DFT tissue gradient, implying a less efficient distribution of voltage gradients. DFTs using the RV coil–pectoral can defibrillation pathway typically are 10 J or less, so it is unclear whether using a "single-pass, two-electrode" lead has any significant advantage over using a lead with only one RV shocking electrode. However, in patients with higher DFTs, use of an SVC coil may improve DFTs enough to provide an adequate safety margin.

In certain clinical circumstances, the left pectoral region is not available for implantation of an ICD generator. Infection, a preexisting pacemaker, or other anatomic problems (e.g., ipsilateral breast cancer) may prevent implantation in that region. Although a left-sided approach gives the best DFTs for the endocardial-can electrode systems,[104] data from animal[105] and clinical[106-108] studies suggest that placement of the generator on the right side or even over the abdomen[105,109] allows achievement of reasonable DFTs. With the abdominal implantation site, the use of an SVC lead appears to offer significant advantage and should probably be used routinely even with a "hot" can.[110] With the continued down-sizing of the generator that has occurred since the early 1990s, one may question whether reduction of the can electrode size may influence DFT. However, the can size, at least within the anticipated range of potential reductions, does not appear to significantly influence the DFT.[111,112] Interestingly, the radius of the RV electrode[113] and the surface area of the RV electrode,[114] within reasonable bounds, have little effect on the DFT. One study found a small benefit in using an 11F rather than a 7F SVC electrode.[115] The polarization of the RV electrode during shock delivery may contribute to greater impedance and may also affect DFT.

Shock Waveforms

Because of the clearly demonstrated benefits of biphasic waveforms for converting VF, all ICDs today have biphasic waveforms.[116] However, several factors affect the efficiency of biphasic waveforms. Nevertheless, one must note that there is no evidence of the superiority of biphasic waveforms for converting VT.

A Primer on Defibrillation

Defibrillation involves more questions than answers. However, the knowledge of the basic principles of defibrillation has advanced to the point that waveforms may be optimized with the use of simple first-order theories. The recitation and use of these theories to optimize defibrillation are by no means meant to give the impression that these simple models represent the state of knowledge of defibrillation.

The monophasic shock acts as a super pacing pulse that synchronizes the fibrillating heart. (This is also true of the first phase of the biphasic shock.) During fibrillation, most cells are in phase 2 or 3; thus, the shock typically interacts with the membrane passive response, as seen in Figure 17-4. The membrane is charged up until the new activation potential begins. Numerous optical and electrode mapping studies have demonstrated this membrane response. Indirect human data have shown that the typical time constant for human myocardial cells is about 3.5 msec. In the situation represented by Figure 17-4, the capacitor is charged to 400 V and then delivers its charge to the heart. The cell membrane is charged up as the capacitor is discharged. Note that the membrane response peaks at 4 msec, yet the shock is prolonged to "deliver more energy" or "achieve a certain tilt." However, the membrane response clearly shows that the energy delivered after 4 msec is wasted. Actually, it is worse than wasted—it is actually counterproductive because it is reducing the final membrane response. This simple analysis shows why shock truncation can have such a dramatic effect on DFTs.

Figure 17-5 shows a low-capacitance waveform and a high-capacitance waveform. The 22-J low-capacitance waveform has the same delivered charge (area under the curve) in the critical first 4 msec as the 27-J high-capacitance waveform. The high capacitance (160-μF) system has a maximum voltage of around 600 V. Because of this low voltage, it requires a great deal more time to deliver its energy. Also, the durations are not programmable but are fixed with a 60% phase 1 tilt and a 50% phase 2 tilt. For a patient with a resistance of 50 Ω, durations would be 7.3 and 4.9 msec, respectively. These durations are about twice optimal. In fact, the first phase is almost as long as the entire duration of the low-capacitance waveform. During the "golden" 4 msec, however, the high-capacitance shock delivers about 22 J. Thus, about 3 of the 5 J of the

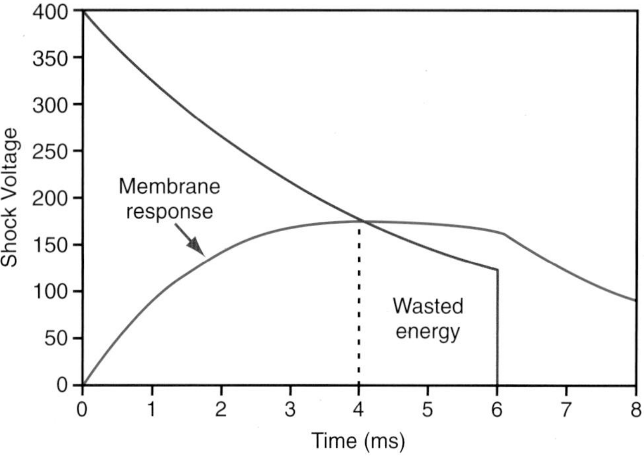

Figure 17-4. A 400-volt capacitive discharge shock waveform is shown as the purple *line. A typical passive cardiac membrane response is identified by the* arrow *and the* red *line. Note that the energy delivered does not help charge the cardiac membrane and is actually counterproductive. This applies to a monophasic shock as well as to the first phase of a biphasic shock.*

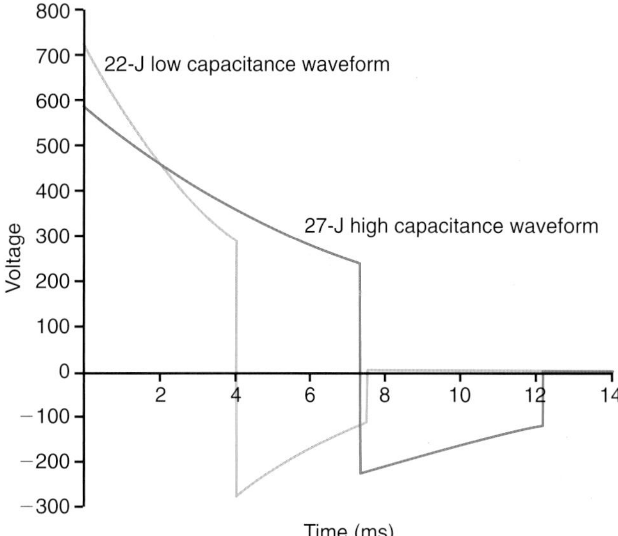

Figure 17-5. The waveforms from the highest and lowest capacitance ICDs available clinically. Note that the 22-J low capacitance waveform (yellow) *has the same delivered charge (area under the curve) in the critical first 4 msec as does the 27-J high capacitance waveform* (blue). *About 3 of the 5 J delivered by the high capacitance waveform between 4 and 7.3 msec is wasted. Hence the low capacitance waveform has at least a 3 J DFT advantage over the high capacitance waveform.*

shock is wasted. The excessively long second phase further reduces efficacy. This is the simple reason why the high-capacitance, lower-voltage shock is less efficient and has higher-energy DFTs.

Effect of Capacitance

One now has a choice of defibrillation capacitance values over a range of 85 to 160 μF. Theoretical models of defibrillation all show that the optimal capacitance is inversely related to the inter-electrode resistance.[117-119] To be precise, the product of the resistance and the capacitance should be about 80% of the chronaxie value.[117] Thus, for a patient with a chronaxie of 5 msec[120] and a resistance of 50 Ω, the optimal capacitance is 80 μF. Numerous animal and clinical studies have shown the benefits of reductions in the capacitance value from the conventional values of 140 to 150 μF.[45,121-124]

The benefit of the reduced capacitance values is, of course, more dramatic in patients with higher resistance.[125] The converse is also true. With extremely-low-resistance pathways, there is little to no benefit. For example, one study with an average resistance of 32 Ω found no difference between a 125-μF and 450-μF capacitor—although the tilts and durations were not held constant.[126]

The benefits of the smaller capacitance values probably accrue from the shortening of the first phase so that its duration is closer to the defibrillation chronaxie. In addition, the second phase is closer to the passive membrane time constant required for optimum membrane discharge, as described by the "burping theory."[127] A simple example explains why this is so critical for the patient with a high resistance. Imagine a device with a capacitance of 140 μF and a patient with an impedance of 70 Ω who underwent implantation of an ICD with a 65% tilt for both phases. The first phase duration is 10 msec and a second phase duration is also about 10 msec. These durations are significantly longer than the chronaxie (3-5 msec) and passive membrane time constant (2-4 msec), respectively. If, in the same situation, the output capacitance were 70 μF, these durations would be halved and much closer to optimal.

For the average patient, the best capacitance value is probably about 90 μF.[128] One concern about using lower capacitance values is that—even though they lower energy DFTs—they store less energy for a given fixed voltage level. With the limits of capacitor voltages under current technology, the maximum stored energy would be reduced in proportion to the capacitance. Thus, the resulting safety margin may not, in fact, be improved. However, if future technology would permit higher voltages in capacitors, smaller capacitors, in the range of 50 to 60 μF, may be optimal. In addition, for patients with DFTs below 10 J, a maximum energy of 18 to 20 J can provide appropriate safety margins. With current and improving lead systems, a majority of patients may belong in this category. Thus, for these patients, a smaller capacitance would allow the use of a smaller device. Last, the use of a smaller capacitance tends to improve the DFT in patients with high shock electrode impedance at implantation. Because the impedance stays relatively constant with implanted lead systems, smaller capacitance values may be most helpful in these patients.[117,128,129]

For a given stored energy, the capacitance is inversely related to the voltage. Hence the data supporting the small capacitance waveforms also directly support the use of a higher-voltage shock. Current ICDs use shock voltages ranging from 600 to 830 V. If the shock voltage is not given on the labeling or the programmer, the implanting physician should insist on obtaining the voltage value (and by implication, the capacitance value) from the manufacturer's representative before attempting an implantation in a patient with a potentially high DFT.

Effect of Pulse Durations

Let us assume that the ICD already has the optimum capacitance for defibrillation. It is now well understood that a major function of the first phase is to act as a monophasic shock designed to synchronize the vast majority of the myocytes by extending their refractory periods.[127,130] Thus, the first phase should be set at between 3 and 5 msec, the typical range for the human chronaxie.[120,128] However, if one has a large capacitance value (i.e., >120 μF), a compromise is in order. A duration roughly equal to the average of the chronaxie and the shock time constant is required, so as to achieve a balance between the chronaxie and the need to deliver a charge from the capacitor. Consider a patient with a resistance of 50 Ω and a 140-μF capacitor. This time constant is simply the product of these two variables, or 7 msec. If one chooses a 4-msec chronaxie, the optimal first phase duration should then be the average of 4 msec and 7 msec, or about 5.5 msec.

The second phase is far simpler. Regardless of the shock time constant or the impedance, the second phase duration should be set at slightly less than the passive membrane time constant in order to actively "burp" the cell membrane.[47,127,131] The burping theory of the biphasic shock holds that the function of the first phase is to extinguish as many wavefronts as possible by "capturing" a majority of the cells in the broad sense. The function of the second phase is to counter the three side effects of the first phase—marginal stimulation, electroporation, and cathodal launching of new wavefronts. The term burping came from the analogy of the removal of excess gas from a baby. This duration should be in the order of 2.5 to 3 msec for optimal performance.

The burping model is illustrated in Figure 17-6. The first phase charges up the membrane of each cell. If the cell is captured, there is an extended activation potential, and everything is wonderful. There is nothing for phase two to do. If the cell is only marginally charged up, the second phase will remove the charge, and the cell will go back to normal.

If the cell is electroporated, the second phase, by quickly removing the excess charge sitting on the membrane, immediately will heal the cell. Finally, the

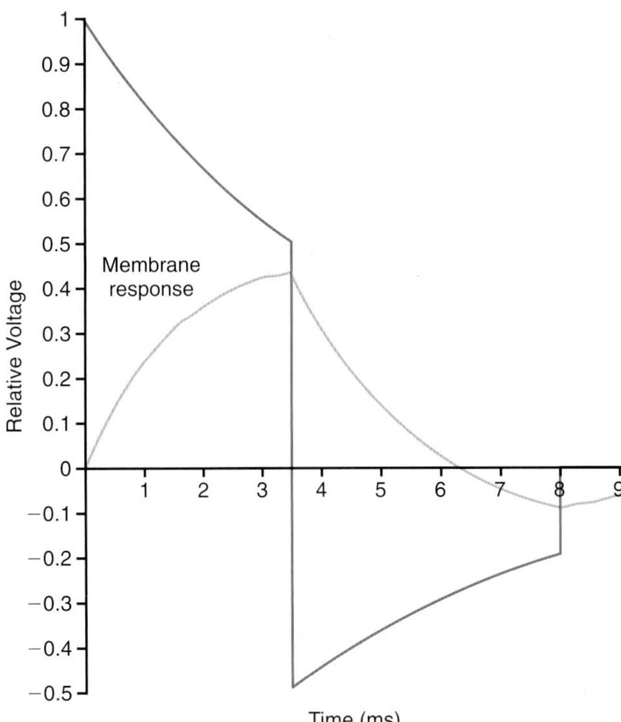

Figure 17-6. The biphasic shock voltage is shown in blue. *The typical membrane response is shown in* yellow. *The burping theory of the biphasic shock holds that the function of the first phase is to maximally charge the membrane, and the function of the second phase is to discharge the membranes of the uncaptured cells back to zero. In this example, the second phase is too long as the membrane is pulled past zero.*

second phase will tend to discharge virtual electrodes and reduce the launching of new wavefronts.[132] In the example shown in Figure 17-6, we can see that the second phase, at 3.5 msec, is too long and the membrane is actually discharged and taken slightly negative; this result is suboptimal. But a 2.5-msec duration would have been optimal. This is how one can calculate the optimal durations for the second phase.

All predictions of the burping theory have been verified in animal or clinical studies.[133-136] Nevertheless, an unwritten myth persists, in some circles, that the second phase somehow captures cells that were missed by the first phase. That spoken myth may have impeded proper programming of the second phase. Simply reducing the second (and first) phase duration from "standard" settings tends to lower DFTs in clinical studies.[134,137-139] The effect of optimizing the first and second phase durations is sometimes quite dramatic, as can be seen in studies using devices in which these durations are programmable.[140]

Some devices have their phases determined only in terms of the classic tilt instead of fixed durations in milliseconds. This approach arose from the invention of the truncated capacitive waveform by Schuder and colleagues.[141] They used a single time constant for truncation (which one would now refer to as a 63% tilt). This gave a duration for the *monophasic* shock close to optimum for the low-resistance epicardial patches then in use. Unfortunately, this one lucky datum led to the false belief that tilt-based waveforms were somehow optimal. It is commonly believed that the dependence of the tilt-based durations on resistance is helpful because it was hoped that the duration changes are a possibly correct adjustment. However, the first phase significantly over-adjusts to resistance changes, and the second phase is actually adjusted in the wrong direction.[127]

Imagine the case of a patient's impedance rising to 100 Ω with a 140-μF capacitor and 65% tilt. This would result in a first phase duration of 14 msec, at least *triple* the chronaxie. For the second phase, use of the tilt-based duration is highly nonoptimal according to current understanding of the operation of the biphasic waveform. The tilt approach would tend to make the second phase increase in proportion to impedance, whereas the burping theory suggests that the second phase duration should actually *decrease* slightly with increases in resistance.[127,131]

More complex waveforms currently under study may lower thresholds even further than those achieved with the use of a lower capacitance. These so-called parallel-series waveforms achieve a more ascending first phase while leaving enough charge for a fully functioning second phase to operate. Such a waveform operates by running multiple capacitors in parallel for a few milliseconds and then, after they have discharged sufficiently, switching them to series, which brings the upper voltage back up to near the initial voltage.[142,143]

The use of fixed pulse durations dramatically reduces the DFT with the use of tilt. Denman reported on a series of 56 patients in whom DFTs were determined both for tilt and msec pulse durations.[140] The mean DFT was reduced by 20% and the DFT for those starting over 15 J was reduced by 30%. Impressively, the population peak DFT was reduced by 40%. Keane[144] studied a series of 17 patients with DFTs of 30 J or higher who would have had an insufficient safety margin without an array—with tilt-based waveforms. By using msec pulse durations instead of tilt, Keane was able to reduce the DFT to 25 J or less in all 17 cases and thereby remove the need for an array. Thus, in patients with high DFTs, especially those with higher shock impedance, it is advantageous to use ICDs with independently adjustable first and second phase pulse durations (or tilts). Doing so allows optimization of the first and second phases separately rather than locking the two phases to the same pulse width. This concept is illustrated by the following case study.

An 18-year-old man with a nonischemic cardiomyopathy underwent implantation of a single-chamber ICD (Contour, St. Jude Medical) with a 150-μF capacitance and 750-V maximum voltage shock. The impedance was 38 Ω. A classic 65% tilt-equivalent waveform was attempted. This gave phase durations of 6 msec for both phases. A maximum energy (38 J delivered) shock succeeded once but then failed. Application of the burping theory suggested 5 and 3 msec as optimal phase durations. The implanter was reluctant to shorten the waveform so drastically, because it would "deliver less energy." So only the second phase was shortened to 3 msec for the first iteration. There were two successful defibrillations at 27 J, followed by two more successes at 22 J. No further waveform adjustments were made.

Shock Polarity

The defibrillating shock polarity can influence the DFT, especially with suboptimal biphasic and monophasic shocks. Unfortunately, the polarity is typically set incorrectly in most implants. Because most ventricular pacing is done with the tip as a cathode, this polarity was naturally assumed to be appropriate for defibrillation. However, it is clear that with monophasic waveforms, the use of "anodal" defibrillation leads to significantly lower thresholds than those found with cathodal defibrillation.[145,146] The same changes have been found, although not as dramatic or as consistent, for biphasic waveforms. A listing of reports on the influence of the first phase polarity of biphasic shocks on DFT is shown in Table 17-2. These reports involved 110 patients and showed an average reduction in DFTs of 16% when the RV electrode started the shock as an anode. This was the best polarity for 46% of patients, whereas 42% had equal DFTs with either polarity.

Animal studies with more "optimal" biphasic waveforms, those using shorter phase 1 and phase 2 durations closer to optimal "burping," have shown no superiority of either polarity.[147] It appears that polarity makes little difference in "optimal" biphasic waveforms as the anodal polarity tends to prevent the main first phase side effect, which is treated by the second phase—namely, cathodal waveform launching.

Observations by Efimov and associates[148] of cells surrounding the RV shock electrode provide some support for this hypothesis. The passive membrane response to a shock is the opposite of the electrode polarity (e.g., it is negative for cells nearer the anode and positive for cells nearer the cathode). The cells act as if they are either near the anode or near the cathode, with essentially no graded response; this is referred to as the *virtual electrode* effect. During fibrillation, most cells are in their plateau phase. The transmembrane potential of such cells in the virtual anode tends to be reduced from near zero to, say, −80 mV. Thus, they are, at least temporarily, masquerading as repolarized cells and very amenable to capture. On the other hand, cathodal shocks generate positive transmembrane potentials, which tend to "pace" the cells in the virtual anode. Hence, the virtual cathode launches new wavefronts into the virtual anode.[132] If the RV coil is an anode, these wavefronts merely go toward the coil and are usually extinguished. If the RV coil is cathodal, however, the wavefronts are launched into the rest of the ventricle and are proarrhythmic.

Biphasic shocks, through the "burping" function, appear to counteract the persistence of the virtual electrode effect. If this were to be the primary mechanism by which biphasic shocks are superior to monophasic ones, optimized biphasic shocks would not demonstrate a polarity preference in defibrillation because they would eliminate or minimize the virtual electrode effect. In fact, Mowry and colleagues[132] have demonstrated a second phase burping of the virtual electrode potential back to near zero.

A common clinical practice, especially in a patient with a high DFT, of programming five or six cathodal shocks and then finally making the polarity anodal has no scientific support. A common practice at the Cleveland Clinic is to program the ICD to anodal shock configuration before it is tested. Given that one cannot truly determine whether a particular biphasic waveform is optimized for a given patient, it would make sense to test DFT in the anodal configuration. It is important to appreciate the different polarities of the various ICD models. St. Jude devices are shipped anodal and thus require no polarity "reversal." Guidant devices are always cathodal and thus should be reversed before usage. Older Medtronic models require reversal, but the Intrinsic (and presumably later models) are already anodal polarity.

Timing of the Shock

Timing of the shock during VF may be important. At present, a shock is synchronized to ventricular activation at the sensing electrode, usually located at the RV

TABLE 17-2. **Influence of Right Ventricular Electrode Polarity on Defibrillation Threshold**

Study	N	RV+ (J)	RV− (J)	Reduction in Mean (%)	Lower RV+	Equal DFT	Lower RV+
Schauerte et al[252]	27	11.1	13.3	17	10	14	3
Shorofsky & Gold[253]	26	11.1	12.2	9			
Natale et al[254]	20	16.3	21.5	24	12	6	2
Strickberger et al[255]	15	9.9	9.5	−4	3	9	3
Keelan et al[256]	10 12	6.6 12	10.8 16.3	39 26	7 7	3 3	0 2
Total or merged *% of patients*	110			16	39 46	35 42	10 12

DFT, defibrillation threshold.

apex or sometimes in the RV outflow or mid-septum. However, in the future, this timing may change. VF may have periods of greater organization or susceptibility to shock termination. For example, timing the shock to large amplitude points on the ECG may reduce DFT.[149,150] The absence of such timing in shock delivery during DFT determination and in current ICDs may be a factor contributing to the probabilistic nature of defibrillation.[38,39,150,151] Greater coherence of myocardial activation suggests fewer random wavefronts. Shocks delivered during periods of fibrillation with greater coherence of ventricular activation appear to have a better chance of success, that is, lower DFT, than shocks delivered during other periods.[152]

The influence of VF duration on DFT is somewhat controversial. Many studies have shown that the DFT rises steadily over time for monophasic shocks.[153,154] This can be shown for shocks delivered anywhere from 2 seconds to 9 minutes after induction of VF and has been attributed to rises in adenosine levels.[155,156] However, the situation for biphasic shocks is much more controversial. Although early animal studies suggested that the DFT for biphasic shocks also rises with time, later papers have challenged this concept and suggested that the threshold may actually dip to a minimum at about 20 seconds after VF initiation.[157] In the interval between onset of VF and delivery of first or even second shock from an ICD, however, it is unlikely that VF duration would affect defibrillation efficacy. Finally, the time of day affects the DFT; DFTs are higher in the morning,[81] which is unfortunately when the incidence of tachyarrhythmias also peaks.[158]

TABLE 17-3. Antiarrhythmic Drugs: Effects on Defibrillation Threshold (DFT)*

Drugs that increase DFT	Ajmaline[257] Amiodarone[167,168,170,172,173,174,177] Atropine[214] Bidisomide[166] Diltiazem[257] Encainide[160] ODE[160] Recainam[165] Verapamil[179] Carvedilol[180]
Drugs that cause no change in DFT	Atenolol[216] Disopyramide[258,191] MODE[160] Phenylephrine[216] Phentolamine[216] Procainamide[182,184,193] Propafenone[194] Azimilide[212]
Drugs for which reports on effect on DFT are conflicting	Amiodarone[161,167,171,259,260] Bretylium[179,181,197,198] Flecainide[159,161-164,205,191] Isoproterenol[214-216] Lidocaine[184,187,193,195,257,261] Moricizine[190-192] Mexiletine[187-189] Quinidine[180,185,186]
Drugs that decrease DFT	Clofilium[262] E-403[205,206] Ibutilide[203,204] LY-190147[263] MS-551[207,264] Sotalol[209-211] Tedisamil[208] Dofetilide[199]

*Superscript numbers indicate chapter references.

Effects of Drugs on the Defibrillation Threshold

Most antiarrhythmic and anesthetic drugs can affect the DFT. However, reports on these influences are mixed and results may depend on whether a monophasic or a biphasic waveform was used in the study. The discrepancies are, at least in part, related to the lack of standardized testing from one report to another. Details of the studies are listed in Table 17-3. Pharmacologic therapy is often used in patients with ICDs to minimize the frequency of therapy delivery by the device. Because some antiarrhythmic drugs also affect DFT, the effects of antiarrhythmic therapy on DFT must be considered when safety margins are being established during ICD implantation and/or testing and when the pharmacologic therapy is modified.

Drugs that Raise the Defibrillation Threshold

Class Ic drugs, such as encainide, can increase DFT.[159] Fain and colleagues[160] reported on intravenous encainide and the two metabolites, O-dimethyl encainide (ODE) and 3-methoxy-ODE (MODE). Intravenous encainide and ODE increased the average DFT in dogs by 129% and 76%, respectively, from control values. The DFT returned to normal after drug washout. No significant drop in DFT was reported with MODE. For another class Ic drug, flecainide, widely divergent effects on DFT were reported in different animal species. In dogs, this agent markedly raised DFTs so that defibrillation was nearly impossible with the existing equipment.[161] Another study, however, reported flecainide to have no effect on DFT in pigs.[162,163] Flecainide has also been found to reduce the atrial DFT in humans.[164] The investigational class Ic drug recainam has been shown to elevate DFT.[165] Bidisomide (SC-40230), an investigational class Ia/Ib agent, raises the DFT in dogs.[166]

Amiodarone, a multiple-class drug, tends to elevate DFTs. Short-term administration of amiodarone has been reported to both lower the DFT[167] and to raise it.[168] Long-term oral administration of amiodarone tends to raise DFT.[169-171]

Guarnieri and associates found larger increases in the DFT in patients receiving amiodarone who were undergoing generator change.[172] DFTs rose from 10.9 ± 4.3 J to 20 ± 4.7 J. The mean DFT decreased for patients taking no antiarrhythmics or only class Ia agents. Pelosi and colleagues found a 60% DFT increase in patients after an average of 73 days of amiodarone therapy, a finding that showed a does-response relationship (r^2 = 0.36).[173] Epstein and associates[174] found that 52% of patients with high DFTs (>25 J) at implantation were taking amiodarone. However, such elevated

DFTs may reflect preselection of patients with poor prognosis rather than an intrinsic effect of amiodarone on the DFT. For example, one clinical study found no difference with long-term amiodarone use.[171] These differences may be caused by a metabolite and the total body load of amiodarone.[175] Amiodarone and its metabolite, desethylamiodarone, are stored in cardiac tissue, delaying the drug's action on the myocardium; such storage can explain the increase in DFTs in patients taking the drug long term.[176] Zhou and coworkers[177] found levels of desethylamiodarone to have a larger impact on the DFT than amiodarone itself.

The selective potassium blocker barium lowers the DFT.[178] Ajmaline and calcium channel blockers tend to increase the DFT.[179]

The combined β_1, β_2, and α receptor blocker carvedilol is widely used for the treatment of heart failure and does not appear to affect the mean DFT in most patients, although there are case reports of significant DFT increases in individual patients.[180]

Drugs with Minimal Effects or with Conflicting Reports of Effect

Class Ia drugs have minimal effects on DFT. Dorian and associates[181] found no changes in DFT with quinidine infusion. In dogs and pigs, intravenous infusion of procainamide (15 mg/kg) had no significant influence on DFT.[182,183] Procainamide generally has no effect on DFT in humans at the usual therapeutic doses.[184] Guarnieri and associates reported that DFTs were actually lower in patients taking class Ia agents at the time of generator replacement than at the time of device implantation.[172] Rises in DFT were reported by Woolfolk and colleagues[185] and Babbs and coworkers[186] with the use of very high doses of quinidine in animal studies.

The class Ib drug mexiletine increased DFTs in a case report.[187] Animal studies, however, have shown little or no increase in the DFT with its use.[188,189] Moricizine does not affect DFTs in pigs[190] but increases DFTs in dogs,[191] especially in the presence of lidocaine.[192] One clinical report found a decrease in DFT, whereas another found an increase.[190,193] Oral propafenone does not affect human DFT.[194] Lidocaine raises the DFT in dogs,[193,195] especially with monophasic waveforms.[196] One study in dogs found that lidocaine did not increase DFT with the use of chloralose for anesthesia but a large increase with the use of pentobarbital.[193]

Bretylium did not affect DFT in two animal studies.[181,197] Interestingly, in another study in dogs, the DFT was reported to be lowered 15 to 90 minutes after intravenous injection of bretylium tosylate (10 mg/kg IV).[198] A pig study also showed a reduction in DFTs.[179]

Drugs that Decrease DFT

Pure class III agents tend to decrease DFT.[193,199,200] This effect is most likely due to lengthening of the refractory period.[201] Clofilium blocks outward potassium current and can directly defibrillate the heart. Tacker and colleagues[198] found that clofilium lowers the DFT in dogs,[198] possibly owing to its ability to lengthen the refractory period extension associated with a defibrillating shock.[202]

Ibutilide significantly lowers DFTs and occasionally causes spontaneous defibrillation.[203,204] The research class III drug E-4031 cut DFTs in *half* in a dog study,[205] even in the presence of isoproterenol.[206] The experimental class III agent LY-190147 also lowers the DFT,[201] as does MS-551 (nifekelant hydrochloride). Murakawa and associates[207] found that although MS-551 lowered the DFT_{50}, it had minimal effect on the DFT_{90}. Tedisimal increases the electrogram coherence and reduces the DFT.[208] D-Sotalol and DL-sotalol decrease the DFT in humans.[209-211] Azimilide appears to reduce the DFT by increasing spatial organization.[212]

What is the effect of β-adrenergic modulation? A dog study showed that isoproterenol reduced the DFT, which returned to baseline value after β-blockade.[213] However, others have reported a rise in DFT with isoproterenol in dogs[214,215] but no change of DFT in pigs.[216] Aminophylline has been reported to lower DFTs.[217]

Anesthetic Agents

Fentanyl can increase the DFT in humans by 41% compared with nitrogen dioxide.[218] However, fentanyl reduced the DFT in animals, unlike pentobarbital and enflurane.[219] The common inhalation agents and barbiturates, however, do not appear to have significant effects on measured DFTs in dog studies,[220] with the possible exception that pentobarbital may interact with lidocaine to increase DFT as noted previously.

Noncardiac Drugs

A 2005 study found that 100 mg IV of sildenafil citrate in 20- to 30-kg swine raised the mean DFT from 12 to 19 J.[221] Although the applied dosage was rather large (typical adult human dosage is 50-100 mg), patients with low shock safety margins should be counseled regarding the use of sildenafil. The risk of VF induction by sexual activity does suggest that the probability of an interaction leading to a failure to defibrillate is real.

The Energy Crisis

Energy is used as the primary defibrillation dosage unit for unfortunate historical and nonscientific reasons. Although it is the dosage unit of common medical practice, energy simply does not defibrillate. Defibrillation requires the generation of an adequate voltage gradient across the myocardium. A myocardial voltage gradient, given a stable myocardial impedance, will generate a current. Thus, current is a good reflection of defibrillation efficacy for a constant set of electrode positions. For relatively stable electrode impedances, voltage correlates with current and can also be a good reflection of defibrillation efficacy. Consideration of shock energy may be useful in considering battery longevity, but it does not necessarily correlate to defibrillation efficacy.

A simple gedanken (thought) experiment shows why that is the case. Imagine that one could merely turn on a pacemaker battery output of 6 V for 120 seconds. Assuming an impedance of 100 Ω, total energy delivered would be 21.6 J. This would eliminate the need for the bulky capacitors and inverter that determine the size of the present ICD. This is energy delivered directly to the heart, yet no one would ever imagine that it would defibrillate the heart.[222] In fact, delivery of energy at a constant low voltage is an excellent way to induce fibrillation.[223]

The confusion of energy with defibrillation has led to some accepted practices that are not justified. Scientifically, for example, the idea that energy defibrillates the heart led to the corollary that the capacitance probably did not matter. As long as the capacitor stored enough energy, it did not matter whether it was a small-value capacitance or a large-value capacitance. This assumption delayed the arrival of the smaller-capacitance, higher-efficiency waveforms.

As unfortunate as the concept of energy for defibrillation is for understanding and optimization, the concept of "delivered" energy is even more damaging. This concept held that the more energy delivered to the heart, the better. A related theme held that some systems are not subject to the vagaries of electrode impedance changes because they are able to "guarantee" a certain energy delivery.

Simple reflection demonstrates that the concept of delivered energy has no scientific basis. It was demonstrated more than 20 years ago that truncating the shock (consider the monophasic waveform momentarily) significantly decreases the DFT—in fact by up to 50%.[141] More recently, shortening of the exponential shock waveform by truncation did not demonstrate any deterioration in the DFTs of delivered energy until the pulse width was shortened to the range of 5 to 6 msec. Truncation of the shock, however, means less energy is delivered, violating the philosophy that *delivered energy* is the critical parameter for defibrillation.[117] Transthoracic modeling studies have shown that current is far superior to an energy-based dosage parameter.[224] This finding is confirmed in actual clinical studies.[225] Current, of course, has a direct relationship with tissue voltage gradient. That is, for a fixed electrode configuration, a higher current is associated with a higher tissue voltage gradient. In some situations, an increase in delivered energy may actually have a negative relationship with the average current of the pulse.

A more pernicious and damaging effect of the concept that more delivered energy would defibrillate better and provide greater safety margin is the idea of increasing delivered energy by lengthening the waveform. This approach, which has been blamed for patient deaths, can actually generate negative safety margins. In an older investigational device, high-energy shocks of 21, 24, 28, and 33 J were available. Although the voltage rose very slightly between the lowest and the highest of these four high-energy shocks, the pulse widths increased dramatically from 4 to 12 msec. However, the 33-J shock did in fact "deliver" the most energy, but its average current was as low as or lower than any of the other shocks. Thus, patients whose DFT was found to be equal to one of the lower applied shocks (i.e., 21 J) could actually have a zero or negative safety margin when the device was set at the 33 J.

A further harmful effect comes from the attempt to apply the delivered energy concept to biphasic waveforms. By confusing the role of the second phase as just another means of delivering additional energy, some devices extend the second phase out proportionally to the resistance (by maintaining the same tilt) in order to guarantee the "delivered energy" of the whole waveform. This results in second-phase durations that are significantly suboptimal, especially for patients with high resistance.

In spite of the significant problems in the use of energy as the defibrillation dosage measurement, it is supported by a wealth of published literature and is given by every manufacturer. It has become accepted practice to measure thresholds in terms of joules. It is acceptable to use energy as a dosage measurement so long as the model of device, the lead resistance, the capacitance value, and the pulse duration are not changing.[226] (If the model changes, then one might assume that the capacitance values and durations are also changing.) If any of those four items is changing and one needs to make a DFT comparison, the average current should be calculated. Average current is very easy to calculate, as follows:

$$\text{Average current} = \frac{\text{Capacitance} \times \text{Peak voltage} \times \text{Tilt}}{\text{Pulse (msec)}}$$

This calculation applies to the first phase.

Dosage calculations for the second phase are irrelevant and misleading. As recent literature would support, the small amount of charge delivered in a second phase merely functions as a counterbalance (albeit a very important one) for the deleterious actions of the first phase,[47,127,131] including the virtual electrode effects.[148]

A capacitor is best viewed as a tank holding a "gas of electrons." One can store a gas in a large tank at low pressure or in a small tank at high pressure. The advantage is with the low capacitance, because it delivers its charge in a time much closer to the optimal timing of the cardiac cells. For the same delivered energy, the shock from a high-capacitance, low-voltage shock is less efficacious. For example, for a 30-J device, a shock from a 600-V, 160-μF capacitor will tend to have DFTs that are higher than those from an 830-V, 85-μF capacitor (see Fig. 17-5). Use of such low-voltage ICDs resulted in significant increases in the number of patients with high DFTs in the Multi-Center Inductionless Defibrillator Implant Study (MIDIS).[227]

Approach to the Patient with a High Defibrillation Threshold

Although certain clinical characteristics may be associated with high DFTs, the predictive value of these characteristics are generally not very accurate because of the wide variation of patients. A number of studies have attempted to predict the DFT from clinical data available before implantation. The results are mixed. Several studies have found no clinical predictors of high DFT, possibly owing to limited sample size.[228-230] Other studies have found statistically significant predictors of a high DFT.[231-236] The most common predictors are large cardiac size, large body size, wide QRS, high New York Heart Association (NYHA) functional class, VF as the manifesting arrhythmia, and low EF. These characteristics are helpful in alerting the implanting physician to the potential for a higher DFT, but their predictive value in an individual is not good enough to be reliable. Thus, a large patient with an enlarged heart may not necessarily have a high DFT. Another and perhaps more reliable item to consider is the obvious one of the previously determined threshold. If the DFTs at prior implantations in a patient were high, assuming that the electrodes were positioned in appropriate locations, one should expect a high DFT at a device change-out or when implanting a new system in that patient.

In a typical pectoral implantation of a "hot can" system (in which the device housing is a defibrillation electrode), one occasionally encounters a patient with high DFTs. Several approaches can be used to lower the DFT. The first is to check that the RV electrode is in a reasonable position. Attempts can be made to reposition the RV electrode as far into the apex as possible. This may increase the voltage gradients in the area of low voltage gradient located at the apical region of the LV free wall. An alternative is to position the tip of the electrode in the high mid-septum/RV outflow tract region and the proximal end of the electrode toward the apex. This configuration may also improve the DFT by bringing the main body of the electrode closer to the septum.

The addition of a right atrial/SVC lead can sometimes improve the DFT.[103,237] The mechanism of such lowering consists primarily of lowering the shock impedance, increasing the current of the shock delivered through the RV coil and reducing pulse width. However, this benefit has not been established for millisecond waveforms. Although pectoral implantation of an ICD is clearly the standard, clinical circumstances occasionally prevent pectoral implantation. Implantation in the abdominal area may still be necessary in a few patients. In the past, such implantation used a long "single-pass" lead containing both the RV electrode and an SVC electrode. Incorporating the device canister into the shocking configuration by connecting the SVC and the abdominal can, so as to have the same polarity can significantly improve DFT.[105] When an independent SVC electrode is available, one can consider positioning that electrode higher into the left innominate vein[85] or into the azygos vein[238] to attempt to improve the DFT.[90] However, withdrawing the SVC electrode too far into the brachiocephalic region may reduce any benefit of such an electrode because of higher impedance in this location.[92]

Similarly, use of the subcutaneous array tends to lower the DFT. The use of a long subcutaneous electrode such as the model made by Medtronic or Guidant may help lower DFT through more than one mechanism. This electrode is designed to be inserted at the lateral edge of the pectoral pocket and tracked subcutaneously along the back to a position near the spine. The tip of the electrode should be near the base of the ventricular shadow on an AP fluoroscopic view. This large surface electrode will reduce impedance of the shock as well as potentially redirect current posteriorly. Two other locations of an additional coil could be of help, the high lateral coronary sinus and the azygos vein. It may be more difficult to anchor the electrode in the coronary sinus. However, a coronary sinus lead would provide an excellent vector in combination with a RV apical electrode. The azygos vein, however, can provide an excellent position for a shock vector from the RV as well as a stable location. The azygos vein enters the SVC near the right atrial junction posteriorly. The ostium can be searched with a curved sheath or even a curved stylet inserted into the lead.

Another potential placement for an SVC lead to improve DFTs can be exploited in patients with persistent left-sided SVC. Insertion of the ICD lead through the left-sided SVC, across the coronary sinus, and into the RV usually paces the proximal "SVC" coil in the coronary sinus. This would provide an excellent vector for defibrillating the heart. Alternatively, a separate SVC coil can be placed in the lower part of the left-sided SVC, positioning it near the lateral portion of the coronary sinus. Lastly, the hemi-azygos vein, when present in adequate size, can serve as the location of a proximal coil. Because of the more posterior nature of these veins, positioning a proximal coil in any of them would provide an excellent shock vector for improving DFTs.

The presence of epicardial patches from a prior ICD implantation may affect DFT. Animal studies have suggested that locating an inactive epicardial patch in low-voltage-gradient areas of the apical LV free wall, a not unusual area for such a patch, can markedly increase the DFT.[239,240] However, a clinical study in patients in whom pectoral "hot can" systems were used did not demonstrate an unusually high DFT.[241]

For every trick to lower the patient's DFT, there is a cost and a benefit. There is certainly a cost in terms of physician time, but there are also going to be material costs. Probably more significantly, there are patient costs with each trial at threshold lowering, resulting from additional time in VF and delivery of possibly unwanted additional shocks. Longer procedure time may also be associated with higher infection risks. Thus, one should try to follow an optimal path toward obtaining an acceptable DFT. Additional leads bring additional potential complications.[242] Table 17-4 summarizes the various approaches to lowering DFT, listing them in order from least costly to most costly.[242a]

In our experience, these maneuvers seldom fail to achieve an adequate DFT in patients demonstrating high DFTs when implanted with a standard transvenous ICD. However, if all of these maneuvers fail to provide an adequate safety margin for defibrillation, one can still consider implanting the device if defibrillation can be achieved with the highest output of the

TABLE 17-4. **Approaches to Reducing Defibrillation Threshold in Patients Undergoing Implantation of a Pectoral Device***

Approach	Benefit(s)	Drawback(s)	Note(s)
Verify RV coil polarity is positive (anodal)	Lower or equal DFT in 88% of patients	Must be changed in some models	No "downside"
Add SVC coil	—	Dangerous to remove in presence of infection	May not help with programmable outputs
Use high-voltage device	DFT reduction ≤25%	Some devices are not labeled for voltage	Refers to benefit of going from 600 to 800 V
Program output durations to theoretical optimal	DFT reduction ≤40%	—	Only in devices with programmable pulse widths
Add subcutaneous coils	Reduces durations for nonprogrammable devices	Infection risk, back pain Difficult to implant	—
Add lead in coronary sinus or azygos or hemi-azygos vein	Good current vector	Possibly difficult to implant	—

DFT, defibrillation threshold; RV, right ventricular; SVC, superior vena cava.
*Listed in order from least costly to most costly.

device. Clinical evidence would suggest that such patients nevertheless benefit from such an implant.[243] The alternative at present is to proceed to an epicardial or pericardial implantation.

Evaluation of Sensing

A most critical function of the ICD, of course, is to sense VF. Inappropriate shocks quickly destroy the patient's quality of life. Unlike ventricular electrograms during sinus rhythm, electrograms during VF can vary widely in amplitude. ICD manufacturers have different engineering approaches to accommodate this variability. Thus, the best approach to assessment of VF detection is to actually induce VF and assess this function of the implanted device. The availability of annotation on the stored or telemetered electrogram indicating detection of ventricular beats is helpful in analyzing the reliability of detection. Owing to the variability of VF amplitude, some dropout of detection from a beat-to-beat basis may be present in all devices. However, one must be assured that such dropout will not be long enough to divert the device from progressing to delivery of therapy.

A second sensing function that must be tested is interference from electrical pulses delivered from another device, typically a pacemaker. Although this problem may become less important as dual-chamber ICDs become more commonly used, such testing must ensure that the pacemaker will not interfere with the ICD's detection of VF. For implantation of an ICD lead into the RV where a previous pacemaker lead is already present, it is ideal to implant the ICD lead remote from the pacemaker lead and to have its sensing electrode oriented more or less perpendicular to the pacer electrodes.[244] With bipolar pacemaker electrodes, one can generally reduce the pacing artifact to a small enough amplitude to minimize cross-sensing. An additional improvement can be obtained by using ICD leads with dedicated bipolar sensing rather than "integrated bipolar" sensing, which incorporates the RV shocking electrode into the sensing circuit.[245,246] The dedicated bipolar sensing leads use two closely spaced electrodes at the lead tip for sensing, thus minimizing any far-field sensing. The disadvantage of such a lead is that the RV shocking electrode is moved further away from the tip of the lead to accommodate the sensing electrodes, possibly reducing its efficacy somewhat. In most circumstances, however, when one wants to use such a lead, there is a pacemaker lead in the RV apex, and the ICD lead should be place higher on the septum. With such placement, the position of the shocking coil near the tip of the lead may not be important.

A further advantage of such a dedicated bipolar lead is that it may be possible to implant it even with a unipolar pacemaker, a circumstance generally considered a contraindication to ICD implantation. Because of the dedicated bipolar sensing of such a lead, even unipolar pacing artifacts may be small enough to not interfere with VF sensing. Such a system, of course, should be thoroughly tested at implantation to ensure lack of interference by programming the pacemaker to its maximal output in the VOO or DOO mode during VF induction. One must not forget about the potential sensing interference that the atrial lead may generate when a dual-chamber pacemaker is present. The output of the leads from both chambers should be maximized during VF testing to ensure that they will not interfere with ICD sensing of VF.

With the advent of dual-chamber defibrillators, sensing in the atrium may also play a role in detection of tachycardia and delivery of therapy. Because automatic gain controls may amplify the atrial signals considerably, it is important to locate the atrial lead in an area where minimal or no ventricular electrogram is detectable even with high gain. This would avoid potential confounding of the detection enhancements available with such devices, which incorporate atrial sensing as part of a detection algorithm. Such optimal placement would also be important in functions such as atrial tachycardia detection and mode switching.

Testing and Programming of Antitachycardia Pacing

ATP is an important therapeutic modality of the ICD. Shocks from the ICD even at very low energy outputs, such as 2 to 5 J, are usually perceived as painful. Most clinical shocks from the device are received in the conscious state, sometimes causing marked anxiety in the patient, so the ability to terminate tachycardia with pacing offers a relatively pain-free approach that is sometime imperceptible to the patient. The role of ATP can vary considerably from patient to patient. Testing of ATP may be important in those patients in whom empirically programmed approaches were clinically unsuccessful in terminating tachycardia. In patients with frequently occurring clinical VT, testing of ATP may also be useful in establishing the most effective means of terminating the tachycardia without promoting acceleration. However, testing in the electrophysiology laboratory with the patient sedated may not be the same as clinical tachycardia occurring during daily life, in which there may be varying degrees of sympathetic tone. Even for faster tachycardia, empirically programmed ATP can be quite useful in terminating a majority of clinical events.

Several reports have indicated the usefulness of activating the ATP feature of the ICD even in the patient who has not yet experienced an episode of clinical sustained ventricular tachyarrhythmia. Retrospective analyses of stored electrogram data in the ICDs of patients with recurrent episodes of VT showed that about 90% of tachycardia can be terminated with ATP.[247,248] It had been assumed that faster VTs were less likely to respond to ATP, having a higher chance of accelerating with the pacing. Thus, in general, ATP has not been commonly used for tachycardia faster than rates of 180 to 200 bpm. However, two clinical trials have demonstrated the efficacy of ATP in tachycardia with rates up to 250 bpm. The PAcing Fast VT REduces Shock ThErapies (PainFREE Rx) clinical trial enrolled 220 patients with coronary artery disease who underwent ICD implantation for standard clinical indications.[249] A fast VT zone was programmed in all patients to allow ATP for tachycardia with a CL shorter than 320 msec but longer than 240 msec. Two bursts of ATP, 8 beats each, were programmed for this zone. The first burst was programmed at 88% of tachycardia CL, whereas the CL of the second burst was shortened by 10 msec. Over a mean follow-up of 6.9 months, 52 patients experienced 446 episodes of fast VT. Eighty-five percent of the VT episodes were terminated with the trial prescribed ATP therapy in this zone. Approximately three fourths of the patients who experienced fast VT experienced successful termination of their fast VT episodes and did not receive a shock. Several patients did experience syncope. However, owing to the nonrandomized nature of this pilot study, it was unclear whether shock therapy could have prevented syncope.

The PainFREE Rx II trial was a randomized study in which patients were assigned to either initial ATP therapy for fast VT or to immediate shock therapy.[250] The ATP therapy was programmed as a single ATP sequence, 8 beats, at 88% of the tachycardia CL. The results indicated that more than 70% of tachycardia episodes with rates in the range of 188 to 250 bpm could be terminated by one burst of ATP. The incidence of syncope was no higher in patients programmed to receive this empiric ATP therapy than in those who were programmed to receive immediate shocks. In this trial, median numbers of VT episodes were similar for the patients undergoing primary prevention (248 of the 582 patients) and those undergoing secondary prevention.[251] Thus, patients receiving ICDs for primary prevention of ventricular arrhythmia–related deaths, in whom the first episode of tachycardia could reasonably be expected to have a faster rate, can nevertheless benefit from empiric programming of a tachycardia zone where ATP is used. Avoidance of shocks reduces the morbidity of ICD therapy in this patient population. Quality-of-life assessment of patients in the PainFREE Rx II trial demonstrated better physical and mental outlooks in those receiving the ATP therapy than in those receiving shocks.

Clinical programming of an empiric tachycardia zone should take into account several factors, including the expected heart rates during exercise, any known history of atrial fibrillation, the use of β-blockers, and any prior documented sustained VT. In a young patient (<20 years), for example, one should expect that sinus rates of 180 bpm can be easily achieved during exercise. Treatment with β-blockers may reduce this rate if the patient is compliant with the medication. Ventricular rates during atrial fibrillation may vary considerably among patients. Lastly, the safety of the patient should be the primary concern. Multiple attempts at pace termination of VT with relatively rapid rates should be avoided, because syncope may result prior to VT termination.

REFERENCES

1. Koning G, Schneider H, Hoelen AJ, et al: Amplitude-duration relation for direct ventricular defibrillation with rectangular current pulses. Med Biol Eng 13:388-395, 1975.
2. Gold JH, Schuder JC, Stoeckle H, et al: Transthoracic ventricular defibrillation in the 100 Kg calf with unidirectional rectangular pulses. Circulation 56:745-750, 1977.
3. Bourland JD, Tacker WA, Geddes LA: Strength duration curves for trapezoidal waveforms of various tilts for transchest defibrillation in animals. Med Instrum 12:38-41, 1978.

4. Geddes LA, Bourland JD, Tacker WA: Energy and current requirements for ventricular defibrillation using trapezoidal waves. Am J Physiol 238:H231-H236, 1980.
5. Niebauer MJ, Babbs CF, Geddes LA, et al: Efficacy and safety of defibrillation with rectangular waves of 2 to 20-milliseconds duration. Crit Care Med 11:95-98, 1983.
6. Geddes LA, Niebauer MJ, Babbs CF, et al: Fundamental criteria underlying the efficacy and safety of defibrillating current waveforms. Med Biol Eng Comp 23:122-130, 1985.
7. Wessale JL, Bourland JD, Tacker WA, Geddes LA: Bipolar catheter defibrillation in dogs using trapezoidal waveforms of various tilts. J Electrocardiol 1:359-65, 1980.
8. Davy JM, Fain ES, Dorian P, Winkle RA: The relationship between successful defibrillation and delivered energy in open-chest dogs: Reappraisal of the "defibrillation threshold" concept. Am Heart J 113:77-84, 1987.
9. Malkin RA, Souza JJ, Ideker RE: The ventricular defibrillation and upper limit of vulnerability dose-response curves. J Cardiovasc Electrophysiol 8:895-903, 1997.
10. Degroot PJ, Church TR, Mehra R, et al: Derivation of a defibrillator implant criterion based on probability of successful defibrillation. PACE 20:1924-1935, 1997.
11. Dillon SM, Kwaku KF: Progressive depolarization: A unified hypothesis for defibrillation and fibrillation induction by shocks. J Cardiovasc Electrophysiol 9:529-552, 1998.
12. Chen PS, Swerdlow CD, Hwang C, Karacueuzian HS: Current concepts of ventricular defibrillation. J Cardiovasc Electrophysiol 9:552-62, 1998.
13. Zhou X, Daubert JP, Wolf PD, et al: Epicardial mapping of ventricular defibrillation with monophasic and biphasic shocks in dogs. Circ Res 72:145-160, 1993.
14. Hsu W, Lin Y, Lang DJ, Jones JL: Improved internal defibrillation success with shocks timed to the morphology electrogram. Circulation 98:808-812, 1998.
15. Hegel MT, Griegel LE, Black C, et al: Anxiety and depression in patients receiving implanted cardioverter-defibrillators: A longitudinal investigation. Int J Psychiatry Med 27:57-69, 1997.
16. Tokano T, Bach D, Chang J, et al: Effect of ventricular shock strength on cardiac hemodynamics. J Cardiovasc Electrophysiol 9:791-797, 1998.
17. Steinbeck G, Dorwarth U, Mattke S, et al: Hemodynamic deterioration during ICD implant: Predictors of high-risk patients. Am Heart J 127:1064-1067, 1994.
18. Singer I, Lang D: The defibrillation threshold. In Kroll M, Lehmann M (eds): Implantable Cardioverter Defibrillator Therapy: The Engineering Clinical Interface. Boston, Kluwer Academic, 1996.
19. Spotnitz HM: Does ventricular fibrillation cause myocardial stunning during defibrillator implantation? J Card Surg 8(Suppl):249-256, 1993.
20. Antunes ML, Spotnitz HM, Livelli FD Jr, et al: Effect of electrophysiological testing on ejection fraction during cardioverter/defibrillator implantation. Ann Thorac Surg 45: 315-318, 1988.
21. Poelaert J, Jordaens L, Visser CA, et al: Transoesophageal echocardiographic evaluation of ventricular function during transvenous defibrillator implantation. Acta Anaesth Scand 40:913-918, 1996.
22. Runsio M, Bergfeldt L, Brodin LA, et al: Left ventricular function after repeated episodes of ventricular fibrillation and defibrillation assessed by transoesophageal echocardiography. Eur Heart J 18:124-131, 1997.
23. Stoddard MF, Redd RR, Buckingham TA, et al: Effects of electrophysiologic testing of the automatic implantable cardioverter-defibrillator on left ventricular systolic function and diastolic filling. Am Heart J 122:714-719, 1991.
24. Meyer J, Mollhoff T, Seifert T, et al: Cardiac output is not affected during intraoperative testing of the automatic implantable cardioverter defibrillator. J Cardiovasc Electrophysiol 7:211-216, 1996.
25. Singer I, van der Laken J, Edmonds HL Jr, et al: Is defibrillation testing safe? PACE 14:1899-1904, 1991.
26. Behrens S, Spies C, Neumann U, et al: Cerebral ischemia during implantation of automatic defibrillators. Z Kardiol 84:798-807, 1995.
27. de Vries JW, Visser GH, Bakker PF J: Neuromonitoring in defibrillation threshold testing: A comparison between EEG, near-infrared spectroscopy and jugular bulb oximetry. Clin Monit 13:303-307, 1997.
28. Vriens EM, Bakker PF, Vries JW, et al: The impact of repeated short episodes of circulatory arrest on cerebral function: Reassuring electroencephalographic (EEG) findings during defibrillation threshold testing at defibrillator implantation. Electroencephalogr Clin Neurophysiol 98:236-242, 1996.
29. Swerdlow CD, Martin DJ, Kass RM, et al: The zone of vulnerability to T wave shocks in humans. J Cardiovasc Electrophysiol 8:145-154, 1997.
30. Yamanouchi Y, Cheng Y, Tchou PJ, Efimov IR: The mechanisms of the vulnerable window: The role of virtual electrodes and shock polarity. Can J Physiol Pharmacol 79:25-33, 2001.
31. Sharma AD, Fain E, O'Neill PG, et al: Shock on T versus direct current voltage for induction of ventricular fibrillation: A randomized prospective comparison. PACE 27:89-94, 2004.
32. Cua M, Veltri EP: A comparison of ventricular arrhythmias induced with programmed stimulation versus alternating current. PACE 16:382-386, 1993.
33. Rattes MF, Jones DL, Sharma AD, Klein GJ: Defibrillation threshold: A simple and quantitative estimate of the ability to defibrillate. PACE 10:70-77, 1987.
34. Zipes DP, Fisher J. King RM, et al: Termination of ventricular fibrillation in dogs by depolarizing a critical amount of myocardium. Am J Cardiol 36:37-44, 1975.
35. Jones JL, Jones RE: Improved defibrillator waveform safety factor with biphasic waveforms. Am J Physiol 245:H60-H65, 1983.
36. Mower MM, Mirowski M, Spear JF, et al: Patterns of ventricular activity during catheter defibrillation. Circulation 49:858-861, 1974.
37. Deale OC, Wesley RC Jr, Morgan D, Lerman BB: Nature of defibrillation: Determinism versus probabilism. Am J Physiol 259:H1544-H1550, 1990.
38. Province RA, Fishler MG, Thakor NV: Effects of defibrillation shock energy and timing on 3-D computer model of heart. Ann Biomed Eng 21:19-31, 1993.
39. Hsia PW, Mahmud R: Genesis of sigmoidal dose-response curve during defibrillation by random shock: A theoretical model based on experimental evidence for a vulnerable window during ventricular fibrillation. PACE 13:1326-1342, 1990.
40. McDaniel WC, Schuder JC: The cardiac ventricular defibrillation threshold: Inherent limitations in its application and interpretation. Med Instrum 21:170-176, 1987.
41. Rattes MF, Jones DL, Sharma AD, et al: Defibrillation threshold: A simple and quantitative estimate of the ability to defibrillate. PACE 10:70-77, 1987.
42. Davy JM, Fain ES, Dorian P, et al: The relationship between successful defibrillation and delivered energy in open-chest dogs: Reappraisal of the "defibrillation threshold" concept. Am Heart J 113:77-84, 1987.
43. Church T, Martinson M, Kallok M, Watson W: A model to evaluate alternative methods of defibrillation threshold determination. PACE 11:2002-2007, 1988.
44. Gill RM, Sweeney RJ, Reid PR: The defibrillation threshold: A comparison of anesthetics and measurement methods. PACE 16:708-714, 1993.
45. Leonelli FM, Kroll MW, Brewer JE: Defibrillation thresholds are lower with smaller storage capacitors. PACE 18:1661-1665, 1995.

46. Malkin RA, Burdick DS, Johnson EE, et al: Estimating the 95% effective defibrillation dose. IEEE Trans Biomed Eng 40:256-265, 1993.
47. Swerdlow CD, Fan W, Brewer JE: Charge-burping theory correctly predicts optimal ratios of phase duration for biphasic defibrillation waveforms. Circulation 94:2278-2284, 1996.
48. Malkin RA, Pilkington TC, Ideker RE: Estimating defibrillation efficacy using combined upper limit of vulnerability and defibrillation testing. IEEE Trans Biomed Eng 43:69-78, 1996.
49. Chen PS, Feld GK, Kriett JM, et al: Relation between upper limit of vulnerability and defibrillation threshold in humans. Circulation 88:186-192, 1993.
50. Behrens S, Li C, Franz MR: Timing of the upper limit of vulnerability is different for monophasic and biphasic shocks: Implications for the determination of the defibrillation threshold. PACE 20:2179-2187, 1997.
51. Hwang C, Swerdlow CD, Kass RM, et al: Upper limit of vulnerability reliably predicts the defibrillation threshold in humans. Circulation 90:2308-2314, 1994.
52. Swerdlow CD, Ahern T, Kass RM, et al: Upper limit of vulnerability is a good estimator of shock strength associated with 90% probability of successful defibrillation in humans with transvenous implantable cardioverter-defibrillators. J Am Coll Cardiol 27:1112-1118, 1996.
53. Swerdlow CD, Davie S, Ahern T, Chen PS: Comparative reproducibility of defibrillation threshold and upper limit of vulnerability. PACE 19:2103-2111, 1996.
54. Souza JJ, Malkin RA, Ideker RE: Comparison of upper limit of vulnerability and defibrillation probability of success curves using a nonthoracotomy lead system. Circulation 91:1247-1252, 1995.
55. Fan W, Gotoh M, Chen PS: Effects of the pacing site, procainamide, and lead configuration on the relationship between the upper limit of vulnerability and the defibrillation threshold. PACE 18:1279-1284, 1995.
56. Behrens S, Li C, Franz MR: Effects of myocardial ischemia on ventricular fibrillation inducibility and defibrillation efficacy. J Am Coll Cardiol 29:817-824, 1997.
57. Martin DJ, Chen PS, Hwang C, et al: Upper limit of vulnerability predicts chronic defibrillation threshold for transvenous implantable defibrillators. J Cardiovasc Electrophysiol 8:241-248, 1997.
58. Huang J, KenKnight BH, Walcott GP, et al: Effects of transvenous electrode polarity and waveform duration on the relationship between defibrillation threshold and upper limit of vulnerability. Circulation 96:1351-1359, 1997.
59. Singer I, Lang D: Defibrillation threshold: Clinical utility and therapeutic implications. PACE 15:932-949, 1992.
60. Grimm W, Timmann U, Menz V, et al: Simplified Implantation of single lead pectoral cardioverter defibrillators using device based testing. Am J Cardiol 81:503-505, 1998.
61. Rugge FP, Savalle LH, Schalij MJ: Subcutaneous single-incision implantation of cardioverter defibrillators under local anesthesia by electrophysiologists in the electrophysiology laboratory. Am J Cardiol 81:302-305, 1998.
62. Schuchert A, Hoffman M, Steffgen F, Meinertz T: Several unsuccessful internal and external defibrillations during active can ICD implantation in a patient with pneumothorax. PACE 21:471-473, 1998.
63. Marchlinski FE, Flores B, Miller JM, et al: Relation of the intraoperative defibrillation threshold to successful postoperative defibrillation with an automatic implantable cardioverter defibrillator. Am J Cardiol 62:393-398, 1988.
64. Daoud EG, Man KC, Morady F, Strickberger SA: Rise in chronic defibrillation energy requirements necessitating implantable defibrillator lead system revision. PACE 20:714-719, 1997.
65. Neuzner J: Safety margins: Lessons from the Low Energy ENDOTAK Trial (LEET). Am J Cardiol 78:26-32, 1996.
66. Strickberger SA, Man KC, Souza J, et al: Prospective evaluation of two defibrillation safety margin techniques in patients with low defibrillation energy requirements. J Cardiovasc Electrophysiol 9:41-46, 1998.
67. Strickberger SA, Daoud EG, Davidson T, et al: Probability of successful defibrillation at multiples of the defibrillation energy requirement in patients with an implantable defibrillator. Circulation 96:1217-1223, 1997.
68. Compos AT, Malkin RA, Ideker RE: An up-down Bayesian, defibrillation efficacy estimator. PACE 20:1292-1300, 1997.
69. Malkin RA, Burdick DS, Johnson EE, et al: Estimating the 95% effective defibrillation dose. IEEE Trans Biomed Eng 40:256-265, 1993.
70. Poole JE, Bardy GH, Dolack GL, et al: Serial defibrillation threshold measures in man: A prospective controlled study. J Cardiovasc Electrophysiol 6:19-25, 1995.
71. Higgins SL, Rich DH, Haygood JR, et al: ICD restudy: Results and potential benefit from routine predischarge and 2-month evaluation. PACE 410-417, 1998.
72. Tummala RV, Riggio DR, Peters RW, et al: Chronic rise in defibrillation threshold with a hybrid lead system. Am J Cardiol 78:309-312, 1996.
73. Venditti FJ Jr, Martin DT, Vassolas G, Bowen S: Rise in chronic defibrillation thresholds in nonthoracotomy implantable defibrillator. Circulation 89:216-223, 1994.
74. Hsia HH, Mitra RL, Flores BT, Marchlinski FE: Early postoperative increase in defibrillation threshold with nonthoracotomy system in humans. PACE 17:1166-1173, 1994.
75. Neuzner J, Pitschner HF, Stohring R, et al: Implantable cardioverter/defibrillators with endocardial electrode systems: Long-term stability of the defibrillator's effectiveness. Z Kardiol 84:44-50, 1995.
76. Schwartzman D, Callans DJ, Gottlieb CD, et al: Early postoperative rise in defibrillation threshold in patients with nonthoracotomy defibrillation lead systems: Attenuation with biphasic shock waveforms. J Cardiovasc Electrophysiol 7:483-493, 1996.
77. Newman D, Barr A, Greene M, et al:. A population-based method for the estimation of defibrillation energy requirements in humans: Assessment of time-dependent effects with a transvenous defibrillation system. Circulation 96:267-273, 1997.
78. Martin DT, John R, Venditti FJ Jr: Increase in defibrillation threshold in non-thoracotomy implantable defibrillators using a biphasic waveform. Am J Cardiol 76:263-266, 1995.
79. Lucy SD, Jones DL, Klein GJ: Pronounced increase in defibrillation threshold associated with pacing-induced cardiomyopathy in the dog. Am Heart J 127:366-376, 1994.
80. Friedman, PA, Foley DA, Christian TF, Stanton MS: Stability of the defibrillation probability curve with the development of ventricular dysfunction in the canine rapid paced model. PACE 21:339-351, 1998.
81. Tokano T, Pelosi F, Flemming M, et al: Long-term evaluation of the ventricular defibrillation energy requirement. J Cardiovasc Electrophysiol 9:916-920, 1998.
82. Venditti FJ Jr, John RM, Hull M, et al: Circadian variation in defibrillation energy requirements. Circulation 94:1607-1612, 1996.
83. Luria D, Stanton MS, Eldar M, Glikson M: Pneumothorax: An unusual cause of ICD defibrillation failure. PACE 21:474-475, 1998.
84. Cohen TJ, Lowenkron DD: The effects of pneumothorax on defibrillation thresholds during pectoral implantation of an active can implantable cardioverter defibrillator. PACE 21:468-470, 1998.
85. Mann DE, Klein RC, Higgins SL, et al; LESS Investigators: The Low Energy Safety Study (LESS): Rationale, design, patient characteristics, and device utilization. Am Heart J 143:199-204, 2002.
86. Gold MR, Higgins S, Klein R, et al; Efficacy and temporal stability of reduced safety margins for ventricular defibrillation: Primary results from the Low Energy Safety Study (LESS). Circulation 105:2043-2048, 2002.

87. Smits KF, DeGroot P: A Bayesian approach to reduced implant testing of a ventricular defibrillator: A computer simulation. Europace 6(Suppl):97, 2004.
88. Winters SL, Casale AS, Inglesby TV, Curwin JH: Setting of relatively low energy outputs may permit implantation of a nonthoracotomy automatic cardioverter defibrillator system when high energy outputs prove ineffective. PACE 19:1516-1518, 1996.
89. Nitta J, Khoury DS: Role of proximal electrode position in transvenous ventricular defibrillation. Ann Biomed Eng 24:418-423, 1996.
90. Stajduhar KC, Ott GY, Kron J, et al: Optimal electrode position for transvenous defibrillation: A prospective randomized study. J Am Coll Cardiol 27:90-94, 1996.
91. Markewitz A, Kaulbach H, Mattke S, et al: Influence of anodal electrode position on transvenous defibrillation efficacy in humans: A prospective randomized comparison. PACE 20:2193-2199, 1997.
92. Block M, Hammel D, Bocker D, et al: Bipolar transvenous defibrillation: Efficacy of two different positions of the anode. PACE 18:1995-2000, 1995.
93. Trappe HJ, Pfitzner P, Fain E, et al: Transvenous defibrillation leads: Is there an ideal position of the defibrillation anode? PACE 20:880-892, 1997.
94. Gold MR, Shorofsky SR: Transvenous defibrillation lead systems. J Cardiovasc Electrophysiol 7:570-580, 1996.
95. Bardy GH, Johnson G, Poole JE, et al: A simplified, single-lead unipolar transvenous cardioversion-defibrillation system. Circulation 88:543-547, 1993.
96. Kall JG, Kopp D, Lonchyna V, et al: Implantation of a subcutaneous lead array in combination with a transvenous defibrillation electrode via a single infraclavicular incision. PACE 18:482-485, 1995.
97. Kuhlkamp V, Khalighi K, Dornberger V, Ziemer G: Single-incision and single-element array electrode to lower the defibrillation threshold. Ann Thorac Surg 64:1177-1179, 1997.
98. Obadia JF, Janier M, Chevalier P, et al: Defibrillation threshold and electrode configurations: An experimental study testing three configurations in twelve pigs. J Cardiovasc Surg (Torino) 38:495-499, 1997.
99. Tang AS, Hendry P, Goldstein W, et al: Nonthoracotomy implantation of cardioverter defibrillators: Preliminary experience with a defibrillation lead placed at the right ventricular outflow tract. PACE 19:960-964, 1996.
100. Singer I, Goldsmith J, Maldonado C: Transseptal defibrillation is superior for transvenous defibrillation. PACE 18: 229-232, 1995.
101. Bardy GH, Dolack GL, Kudenchuk PJ, et al: Prospective, randomized comparison in humans of a unipolar defibrillation system with that using an additional superior vena cava electrode. Circulation 89:1090-1093, 1994.
102. Gold MR, Foster AH, Shorofsky SR: Effects of an active pectoral-pulse generator shell on defibrillation efficacy with a transvenous lead system. Am J Cardiol 78:540-543, 1996.
103. Gold MR, Foster AH, Shorofsky SR: Lead system optimization for transvenous defibrillation. Am J Cardiol 80:1163-1167, 1997.
104. Epstein AE, Kay GN, Plumb VJ, et al: Elevated defibrillation threshold when right-sided venous access is used for nonthoracotomy implantable defibrillator lead implantation. The ENDOTAK Investigators. J Cardiovasc Electrophysiol 6:979-986, 1995.
105. Yamanouchi Y, Mowrey KA, Niebauer MJ, et al: Additional lead improves defibrillation efficacy with an abdominal 'hot can' electrode system. Circulation 96:4400-4407, 1997.
106. Natale A, Sra J, Geiger MJ, et al: Right side implant of the unipolar single lead defibrillation system. PACE 20:1910-1912, 1997.
107. Jensen SM, Pietersen A, Chen X: Implantation of active can implantable defibrillators in the right pectoral region. PACE 21:476-477, 1998.
108. Flaker GC, Tummala R, Wilson J, et al: Comparison of right- and left-sided pectoral implantation parameters with the Jewel active can cardiodefibrillator. PACE 21:447-451, 1998.
109. Neuzner J, Schwarz T, Strasser R, et al: Effect of the addition of an abdominal hot can cardioverter/defibrillator pulse generator on the defibrillation energy requirements in a single-lead endocardial defibrillation system. Eur Heart J 18:1655-1658, 1997.
110. Yamanouchi Y. Mowrey KA, Niebauer MJ, et al: Additional lead improves defibrillation efficacy with an abdominal 'hot can' electrode system. Circulation 96:4400-4407, 1997.
111. Jones GK, Poole JE, Kudenchuk PJ, et al: A prospective randomized evaluation of implantable cardioverter-defibrillator size on unipolar defibrillation system efficacy. Circulation 92:2940-2943, 1995.
112. Newby KH, Moredock L, Rembert J, et al: Impact of defibrillator-can size on defibrillation success with a single-lead unipolar system. Am Heart J 131:261-265, 1996.
113. Leonelli FM, Wright H, Latterell ST, et al: A long thin electrode is equivalent to a short thick electrode for defibrillation in the right ventricle. PACE 18:221-224, 1995.
114. Tomassoni G, Pendekanti R, Dixon-Tulloch E, et al: Importance of electrode conductive surface area and edge effects on ventricular defibrillation efficacy. J Cardiovasc Electrophysiol 8:1246-1254, 1997.
115. Halperin BD, Reynolds B, Fain ES, et al: The effect of electrode size on transvenous defibrillation energy requirements: A prospective evaluation. PACE 20:893-898, 1997.
116. Kroll MW, Anderson KM, Supino CG, Adams TP: Decline in defibrillation thresholds. PACE 16:213-217, 1993.
117. Kroll MW: A minimal model of the monophasic defibrillation pulse. PACE 16:769-777, 1993.
118. Irnich W: Optimal truncation of defibrillation pulses. PACE 18:673-688, 1995.
119. Cleland BG: A conceptual basis for defibrillation waveforms. PACE 19:1186-1195, 1996.
120. Gold MR, Shorofsky SR: Strength-duration relationship for human transvenous defibrillation. Circulation 96:3517-3520, 1997.
121. Rist K, Tchou PJ, Mowrey K, et al: Smaller capacitors improve the biphasic waveform. J Cardiovasc Electrophysiol 5:771-776, 1994.
122. Bardy GH, Poole JE, Kudenchuk PJ, et al: A prospective randomized comparison in humans of biphasic waveform 60-microF and 120-microF capacitance pulses using a unipolar defibrillation system. Circulation 91:91-95, 1995.
123. Poole JE, Kudenchuk PJ, Dolack GL, et al: A prospective randomized comparison in humans of 90-mu F and 120-mu F biphasic pulse defibrillation using a unipolar defibrillation system. J Cardiovasc Electrophysiol 6:1097-1100, 1995.
124. Swerdlow CD, Kass RM, Davie S, et al: Short biphasic pulses from 90 microfarad capacitors lower defibrillation threshold. PACE 19:1053-1060, 1996.
125. Swerdlow CD, Kass RM, Chen PS, et al: Effect of capacitor size and pathway resistance on defibrillation threshold for implantable defibrillators. Circulation 90:1840-1846, 1994.
126. Block M, Hammel D, Bocker D, et al: Biphasic defibrillation using a single capacitor with large capacitance: Reduction of peak voltages and ICD device size. PACE 19:207-214, 1996.
127. Kroll MW: A minimal model of the single capacitor biphasic defibrillation waveform. PACE 17:1782-1792, 1994.
128. Swerdlow CD, Brewer JE, Kass RM, Kroll MW: Application of models of defibrillation to human defibrillation data: Implications for optimizing implantable defibrillator capacitance. Circulation 96:2813-2822, 1997.
129. Kroll MW, Lehmann MH, Tchou PJ: Defining the defibrillation dosage. In Kroll M, Lehmann (eds): Implantable Cardioverter Defibrillator: The Engineering-Clinical Interface. Boston, Kluwer Academic, 1996.

130. Dillon SM: Synchronized repolarization after defibrillation shocks: A possible component of the defibrillation process demonstrated by optical recordings in rabbit heart. Circulation 85:1865-1878, 1992.
131. Walcott GP, Walker RG, Cates AW, et al: Choosing the optimal monophasic and biphasic waveforms for ventricular defibrillation. J Cardiovasc Electrophysiol 6:737-750, 1995.
132. Mowrey KA, Cheng Y, Tchou PJ, Efimov R: Kinetics of defibrillation shock-induced response: Design implications for the optimal defibrillation waveform. Europace 4:27-39, 2002.
133. White JB, Walcott GP, Wayland JL Jr, et al: Predicting the relative efficacy of shock waveforms for transthoracic defibrillation in dogs. Ann Emerg Med 34:309-320, 1999.
134. Schauerte P, Schondube FA, Grossmann M, et al: Influence of phase duration of biphasic waveforms on defibrillation energy requirements with a 70 μF capacitance. Circulation 97:2073-2078, 1998.
135. Schauerte PN, Zeigert K, Waldmann M, et al: Effect of biphasic shock duration on defibrillation threshold with different electrode configurations and phase 2 capacitances. Circulation 99:1516-1522, 1999.
136. Mouchawar G, Kroll M, Val-Mejias JE, et al: ICD waveform optimization: A randomized, prospective, pair-sampled multicenter study. PACE 23:1992-1995, 2000.
137. Swartz JF, Fletcher RD, Karasik PE: Optimization of biphasic waveforms for human nonthoracotomy defibrillation. Circulation 88:2646-2654, 1993.
138. Natale A, Sra J, Krum D, et al: Relative efficacy of different tilts with biphasic defibrillation in humans. PACE 19:197-206, 1996.
139. Sweeney MO, Natale A, Volosin KJ, et al: Prospective randomized comparison of 50%/50% versus 65%/65% tilt biphasic waveform on defibrillation in humans. PACE 24:60-65, 2001.
140. Denman RA, Umesan C, Martin PT, et al: Benefit of millisecond waveform durations for patients with high defibrillation thresholds. Heart Rhythm 3:536-541, 2006.
141. Schuder JC, Stoeckle H, West JA, Keskar PY: Transthoracic ventricular defibrillation in the dog with truncated and untruncated exponential stimuli. IEEE Trans Biomedical Eng 13:410-415, 1971.
142. Yamanouchi Y, Brewer JE, Mowrey KA, et al: Sawtooth first phase biphasic defibrillation waveform: A comparison with standard waveform in clinical devices. J Cardiovasc Electrophysiol 8:517-528, 1997.
143. Yamanouchi Y, Mowrey KA, Nadzam GR, et al: Large change in voltage at phase reversal improves biphasic defibrillation thresholds: Parallel-series mode switching. Circulation 94:1768-1773, 1996.
144. Keane DTJ, Sheahan RG, Cripps T, et al: Use of millisecond biphasic waveforms in lieu of subcutaneous arrays. PACE 2007, under review.
145. Strickberger SA, Hummel JD, Horwood LE, et al: Effect of shock polarity on ventricular defibrillation threshold using a transvenous lead system. J Am Coll Cardiol 24:1069-1072, 1994.
146. Thakur RK, Souza JJ, Chapman PD, et al: Electrode polarity is an important determinant of defibrillation efficacy using a nonthoracotomy system. PACE 17:919-923, 1994.
147. Yamanouchi Y, Mowrey KA, Nadzam GR, et al: Effects of polarity on defibrillation thresholds using a biphasic waveform in a hot can electrode system. PACE 20:2911-2916, 1997.
148. Efimov IR, Cheng YN, Biermann M, et al: Transmembrane voltage changes produced by real and virtual electrodes during monophasic defibrillation shock delivered by an implantable electrode. J Cardiovasc Electrophysiol 8:1031-1045, 1997.
149. Clayton RH, Murray A, Campbell RWF: Evidence for electrical organization during ventricular fibrillation in the human heart. J Cardiovasc Electrophys 6:616-624, 1995.
150. Hsia PW, Frerk S, Allen CA, et al: A critical period of ventricular fibrillation more susceptible to defibrillation: Real-time waveform analysis using a single ECG lead. PACE 19:418-430, 1996.
151. Murakawa Y, Yamashita T, Ajiki K, et al: Electrophysiological background of individual variability in electrical defibrillation efficacy. Am J Physiol 271:H1094-H1098, 1996.
152. Hsia PW, Fendelander L, Harrington G, Damiano RJ: Defibrillation success is associated with myocardial organization: Spatial coherence as a new method of quantifying the electrical organization of the heart. J Electrocardiol 29(Suppl):189-197, 1996.
153. Yakaitis RW, Ewy GA, Otto CW, et al: Influence of time and therapy on ventricular defibrillation in dogs. Crit Care Med 8:157-163, 1980.
154. Winkle RA, Mead RH, Ruder MA, et al: Effect of duration of ventricular fibrillation on defibrillation efficacy in humans. Circulation 81:1477-1481, 1990.
155. Lerman BB, Engelstein ED: Increased defibrillation threshold due to ventricular fibrillation duration: Potential mechanisms. J Electrocardiol 28(Suppl):21-24, 1995.
156. Lerman BB, Engelstein ED: Metabolic determinants of defibrillation: Role of adenosine. Circulation 91:838-844, 1995.
157. Windecker S, Kay GN, KenKnight BH, et al: The effects of ventricular fibrillation duration and a preceding unsuccessful shock on the probability of defibrillation success using biphasic waveforms in pigs. J Cardiovasc Electrophysiol 8:1386-1395, 1997.
158. Tofller GH, Gebara OCE, Mittleman MA, et al: Morning peak in ventricular tachyarrhythmias detected by time of implantable cardioverter defibrillator therapy. Circulation 92:1203-1208, 1995.
159. Reiffel JA, Coromilas J, Zimmerman JM, et al: Drug-device interactions: Clinical considerations. PACE 8:369-373, 1985.
160. Fain ES, Dorian P, Davy JM, et al: Effects of encainide and its metabolites on energy requirements for defibrillation. Circulation 73:1334-1341, 1986.
161. Hernandez R, Mann DE, Breckinridge S, et al: Effects of flecainide on defibrillation thresholds in the anesthetized dog. J Am Coll Cardiol 14:777-781, 1989.
162. Szabo TS, Jones DL, McQuinn RL, Klein GJ: Flecainide acetate does not alter the energy requirements for direct ventricular defibrillation using sequential pulse defibrillation in pigs. J Cardiovasc Pharmacol 12:377-383, 1988.
163. Natale A, Jones DL, Kleinstiver PW, et al: Effects of flecainide on defibrillation threshold in pigs. J Cardiovasc Pharmacol 21:573-577, 1993.
164. Boriani G, Biffi M, Capucci A, et al: Favorable effects of flecainide in transvenous internal cardioversion of atrial fibrillation. J Am Coll Cardiol 33:333-341, 1999.
165. Frame LH, Sheldon JH: Effect of recainam on the energy required for ventricular defibrillation in dogs as assessed with implanted electrodes. J Am Coll Cardiol 12:746-752, 1988.
166. Hackett AM, Gardiner P, Garthwaite SM: The effect of bidisomide (SC-40230), a new class Ia/Ib antiarrhythmic agent, on defibrillation energy requirements in dogs with healed myocardial infarctions. PACE 16:317-326, 1993.
167. Fain ES, Lee JT, Winkle RA: Effects of acute intravenous and chronic oral amiodarone on defibrillation energy requirements. Am Heart J 114:8-17, 1987.
168. Nielsen TD, Hamdan MH, Kowal RC, et al: Effect of acute amiodarone loading on energy requirements for biphasic ventricular defibrillation. Am J Cardiol 88:446-448, 2001.
169. Fogoros RN: Amiodarone-induced refractoriness to cardioversion. Ann Intern Med 100:699-700, 1984.
170. Jung W, Manz M, Pizzulli L, et al: Effects of chronic amiodarone therapy on defibrillation threshold. Am J Cardiol 70:1023-1027, 1992.
171. Huang SK, Tan de Guzman WL, Chenarides JG, et al: Effects of long-term amiodarone therapy on the defibrillation threshold and the rate of shocks of the implantable cardioverter-defibrillator. Am Heart J 122:720-727, 1991.

172. Guarnieri T, Levine JH, Veltri EP: Success of chronic defibrillation and the role of antiarrhythmic drugs with the automatic implantable cardioverter/defibrillator. Am J Cardiol 60:1061-1064, 1987.
173. Pelosi F Jr, Oral H, Kim MH, et al: Effect of chronic amiodarone therapy on defibrillation energy requirements in humans. J Cardiovasc Electrophysiol 11:736-740, 2000.
174. Epstein AE, Ellenbogen KA, Kirk K, et al: Clinical characteristics and outcome of patients with high defibrillation thresholds: A multicenter study. Circulation 86:1206-1216, 1992.
175. Holt DW, Tucker GT, Jackson PR, et al: Amiodarone pharmacokinetics. Am Heart J 106:840-847, 1983.
176. Barbieri E, Conti F, Zampieri P, et al: Amiodarone and desethylamiodarone distribution in the atrium and adipose tissue of patients undergoing short and long-term treatment with amiodarone. J Am Coll Cardiol 8:210-213, 1986.
177. Zhou L, Chen BP, Kluger J, et al: Effects of amiodarone and its active metabolite desethylamiodarone on the ventricular defibrillation threshold. J Am Coll Cardiol 31:1672-1678, 1998.
178. Dorian P, Witkowski FX, Penkoske PA, Feder-Elituv RS: Barium decreases defibrillation energy requirements. J Cardiovasc Pharmacol 23:107-112, 1994.
179. Jones DL, Kim YH, Natale A, et al: Bretylium decreases and verapamil increases defibrillation threshold in pigs. PACE 17:1380-1390, 1994.
180. Melichercik J, Goepfrich M, Breidenbach T, Von Hodenberg E: Rise of defibrillation energy requirement under carvedilol therapy. PACE 24:1417-1419, 2001.
181. Dorian P, Fain ES, Davy JM, et al: Effect of quinidine and bretylium on defibrillation energy requirements. Am Heart J 112:19-25, 1986.
182. Echt DS, Black JN, Barbey JT, et al: Evaluation of antiarrhythmic drugs on defibrillation energy requirements in dogs: Sodium channel block and action potential prolongation. Circulation 79:1106-1117, 1989.
183. Deeb GM, Hardesty RL, Griffith BP, et al: The effects of cardiovascular drugs on the defibrillation threshold and the pathological effects on the heart using an automatic implantable defibrillator. Ann Thorac Surg 4:361-366, 1983.
184. Echt DS, Gremillion ST, Lee JT, et al: Effects of procainamide and lidocaine on defibrillation energy requirements in patients receiving implantable cardioverter defibrillator devices. J Cardiovasc Electrophysiol 5:752-760, 1994.
185. Woolfolk DI, Chaffee WR, Cohen W, et al: The effect of quinidine on electrical energy required for ventricular defibrillation. Am Heart J 72:659, 1966.
186. Babbs CF, Yim GKW, Whistler SJ, et al: Elevation of ventricular defibrillation energy requirements. Am Heart J 112:19, 1986.
187. Marinchak RA, Friehling TD, Line RA, et al: Effect of antiarrhythmic drugs on defibrillation threshold: Case report of an adverse effect of mexiletine and review of the literature. PACE 11:7-12, 1988.
188. Sato S, Tsuji MH, Naito H: Mexiletine has no effect on defibrillation energy requirements in dogs. PACE 17:2279-2284, 1994.
189. Murakawa Y, Inoue H, Kuo TT, et al: Prolongation of intraventricular conduction time associated with fatal [correction of fetal] impairment of defibrillation efficiency during treatment with class I antiarrhythmic agents. J Cardiovasc Pharmacol 25:194-199, 1995.
190. Pharand C, Goldman R, Fan C, et al: Effect of chronic oral moricizine and intravenous epinephrine on ventricular fibrillation and defibrillation thresholds. PACE 19:82-89, 1996.
191. Avitall B, Hare J, Zander G, et al: Cardioversion, defibrillation, and overdrive pacing of ventricular arrhythmias: The effect of moricizine in dogs with sustained monomorphic ventricular tachycardia. PACE 16:2092-2097, 1993.
192. Ujhelyi MR, O'Rangers EA, Kluger J, et al: Defibrillation energy requirements during moricizine and moricizine-lidocaine therapy. J Cardiovasc Pharmacol 20:932-939, 1992.
193. Echt DS, Black JN, Barbey JT, et al: Evaluation of antiarrhythmic drugs on defibrillation energy requirements in dogs: Sodium channel block and action potential prolongation. Circulation 79:1106-1117, 1989.
194. Stevens SK, Haffajee CI, Naccarelli GV, et al: Effects of oral propafenone on defibrillation and pacing thresholds in patients receiving implantable cardioverter-defibrillators. Propafenone Defibrillation Threshold Investigators. J Am Coll Cardiol 28:418-422, 1996.
195. Dorian P, Fain ES, Davy JM, et al: Lidocaine causes a reversible, concentration-dependent increase in defibrillation energy requirements. J Am Coll Cardiol 8:327-332, 1986.
196. Ujhelyi MR, Schur M, Frede T, et al: Differential effects of lidocaine on defibrillation threshold with monophasic versus biphasic shock waveforms. Circulation 92:1644-1650, 1995.
197. Kerber RE, Pandian NG, Jensen SR, et al: Effect of lidocaine and bretylium on energy requirements for transthoracic defibrillation: Experimental studies. J Am Coll Cardiol 7:397-405, 1986.
198. Tacker WA, Niebauer MJ, Babbs CF, et al: The effect of newer antiarrhythmic drugs on defibrillation threshold. Crit Care Med 8:177-180, 1980.
199. Davis DR, Beatch GN, Dickenson DR, Tang AS: Dofetilide enhances shock-induced extension of refractoriness and lowers defibrillation threshold. Can J Cardiol 15:193-200, 1999.
200. Qi X, Dorian P: Antiarrhythmic drugs and ventricular defibrillation energy requirements. Chin Med J (Engl) 112:1147-1152, 1999.
201. Beatch GN, Dickenson DR, Tang AS: Effects of optical enantiomers CK-4000(S) and CK-4001(R) on defibrillation and enhancement of shock-induced extension of action potential duration. J Cardiovasc Electrophysiol 6:716-728, 1995.
202. Sweeney RJ, Gill RM, Steinberg MI, Reid PR: Effects of flecainide, encainide, and clofilium on ventricular refractory period extension by transcardiac shocks. PACE 19:50-60, 1996.
203. Wesley RC Jr, Farkhani F, Morgan D, Zimmerman D: Ibutilide: Enhanced defibrillation via plateau sodium current activation. Am J Physiol 264:H1269-H1274, 1993.
204. Labhasetwar V, Underwood T, Heil RW Jr, et al: Epicardial administration of ibutilide from polyurethane matrices: Effects on defibrillation threshold and electrophysiologic parameters. J Cardiovasc Pharmacol 24:826-840, 1994.
205. Murakawa Y, Sezaki K, Inoue H, et al: Shock-induced refractory period extension and pharmacologic modulation of defibrillation threshold. J Cardiovasc Pharmacol 23:822-825, 1994.
206. Sezaki K, Murakawa Y, Inoue H, et al: Effect of isoproterenol on facilitation of electrical defibrillation by E-4031. J Cardiovasc Pharmacol 25:393-396, 1995.
207. Murakawa Y, Yamashita T, Kanese Y, Omata M: Effect of a class III antiarrhythmic drug on the configuration of dose response curve for defibrillation. PACE 22:479-486, 1999.
208. Dorian P, Newman D: Tedisamil increases coherence during ventricular fibrillation and decreases defibrillation energy requirements. Cardiovasc Res 33:485-494, 1997.
209. Wang M, Dorian P: DL and D sotalol decrease defibrillation energy requirements. PACE 12:1522-1529, 1989.
210. Dorian P, Newman D: Effect of sotalol on ventricular fibrillation and defibrillation in humans. Am J Cardiol 72:72A-79A, 1993.
211. Dorian P, Newman D, Sheahan R, et al: d-Sotalol decreases defibrillation energy requirements in humans: A novel indication for drug therapy. J Cardiovasc Electrophysiol 7:952-961, 1996.
212. Qi XQ, Newman D, Dorian P: Azimilide decreases defibrillation voltage requirements and increases spatial organization during ventricular fibrillation. J Interv Card Electrophysiol 3:61-67, 1999.
213. Ruffy R, Schechtman K, Monje E, et al: Beta-adrenergic modulation of direct defibrillation energy in anesthetized dog heart. Am J Physiol 248:H674-677, 1985.

214. Wang M, Dorian P, Ogilvie RI: Isoproterenol increases defibrillation energy requirements in dogs. J Cardiovasc Pharmacol 19:201-208, 1992.
215. Wang M, Dorian P, Ogilvie RI: Isoproterenol increases defibrillation energy requirements in dogs. J Cardiovasc Pharmacol 19:201-208, 1992.
216. Rattes MF, Sharma AD, Klein GJ, et al: Adrenergic effects on internal cardiac defibrillation threshold. Am J Physiol 253:H500-H506, 1987.
217. Ruffy R, Monje E, Schechtman K: Facilitation of cardiac defibrillation by aminophylline in the conscious, closed-chest dog (abstract). J Electrophysiol 2:450, 1988.
218. Weinbroum AA, Glick A, Copperman Y, et al: Halothane, isoflurane, and fentanyl increase the minimally effective defibrillation threshold of an ICD: First report in humans. Anesth Analg 95:1147-1153, 2002.
219. Wang M, Dorian P: Defibrillation energy requirements differ between anesthetic agents. J Electrophysiol 3/2:86-94, 1989.
220. Gill RM, Sweeney RJ, Reid PR: The defibrillation threshold: A comparison of anesthetics and measurement methods. PACE 16:708-714, 1993.
221. Shinlapawittayatorn K, Sangoon R, Chattipakorn S, Chattipakorn N: Effects of sildenafil citrate on defibrillation efficacy. J Cardiovasc Electrophysiol 17:292-295, 2006.
222. Valentinuzzi ME: Defibrillation, either in clinical practice or in basic and applied research, uses mainly energy (expressed by and large in joules) as the reference parameter to dose the discharge or to describe thresholds. PACE 18:1465-1466, 1995.
223. Sharma AD, Fain E, O'Neill PG, Skadsen A, et al: Shock on T versus direct current voltage for induction of ventricular fibrillation: A randomized prospective comparison. PACE 27:89-94, 2004.
224. Lehr JL, Ramirez IF, Karlon WJ, Eisenberg SR: Test of four defibrillation dosing strategies using a two-dimensional finite-element model. Med Biol Eng Comput 30:621-628, 1992.
225. Lerman BB, DiMarco JP, Haines DE: Current-based versus energy-based ventricular defibrillation: A prospective study. J Am Coll Cardiol 12:1259-1264, 1988.
226. Wesley RC Jr, Farkhani F, Porzio D, et al: Transepicardial defibrillation dose response: Current versus energy. PACE 16:193-197, 1993.
227. Day JD, Freedman RA, Zubair I, et al: Feasibility of inductionless ICD implants: Correlation of upper limit of vulnerability testing to defibrillation threshold testing at ICD implantation (abstract). PACE 26:1010, 2003.
228. Neuzner J, Bahawar H, Berkowitsch A, et al: Clinical predictors of defibrillation energy requirements. Am J Cardiol 79:205-206, 1997.
229. Schwartzman D, Concato J, Ren JF, et al: Factors associated with successful implantation of nonthoracotomy defibrillation lead systems. Am Heart J 131:1127-1136, 1996.
230. Raitt MH, Johnson G, Dolack GL, et al: Clinical predictors of the defibrillation threshold with the unipolar implantable defibrillation system. J Am Coll Cardiol 25:1576-1583, 1995.
231. Brooks R, Garan H, Torchiana D, et al: Determinants of successful nonthoracotomy cardioverter-defibrillator implantation: Experience in 101 patients using two different lead systems. J Am Coll Cardiol 22:1835-1842, 1993.
232. Leitch JW, Yee R: Predictors of defibrillation efficacy in patients undergoing epicardial defibrillator implantation. The Multicenter Pacemaker-Cardioverter-Defibrillator (PCD) Investigators Group. J Am Coll Cardiol 21:1632-1637, 1993.
233. Strickberger SA, Brownstein SL, Wilkoff BL, Zinner AJ: Clinical predictors of defibrillation energy requirements in patients treated with a nonthoracotomy defibrillator system. The ResQ Investigators. Am Heart J 131:257-260, 1996.
234. Gold MR, Khalighi K, Kavesh NG, et al: Clinical predictors of transvenous biphasic defibrillation thresholds. Am J Cardiol 79:1623-1627, 1997.
235. Khalighi K, Daly B, Leino EV, et al: Clinical predictors of transvenous defibrillation energy requirements. Am J Cardiol 79:150-153, 1997.
236. Horton RP, Canby RC, Roman CA, et al: Determinants of nonthoracotomy biphasic defibrillation. PACE 20:60-64, 1997.
237. Gold MR, Olsovsky MR, Pelini MA, et al: Comparison of single- and dual-coil active pectoral defibrillation lead systems. J Am Coll Cardiol 31:1391-1394, 1998.
238. Cesario D, Bhargava M, Valderrabano M, et al: Azygos vein lead implantation: A novel adjunctive technique for implantable cardioverter defibrillator placement. J Cardiovasc Electrophysiol 15:780-783, 2004.
239. Callihan RL, Idriss SF, Dahl RW, et al: Comparison of defibrillation probability of success curves for an endocardial lead configuration with and without an inactive epicardial patch. J Am Coll Cardiol 25:1373-1379, 1995.
240. Fotuhi PC, Ideker RE, Idriss SF, et al: Influence of epicardial patches on defibrillation threshold with nonthoracotomy lead configurations. Circulation 92:3082-3088, 1995.
241. Nasir N Jr, Cedillo-Salazar FR, Doyle TK, et al: Effect of preexisting epicardial patch electrodes on defibrillation thresholds of unipolar defibrillators. Am J Cardiol 79:1408-1409, 1997.
242. Schwartzman D, Nallamothu N, Callans DJ, et al: Postoperative lead-related complications in patients with nonthoracotomy defibrillation lead systems. J Am Coll Cardiol 26:776-786, 1995.
242a. Mainigi SK, Callans DJ: How to manage the patient with a high defibrillation threshold. Heart Rhythm 3:492-495, 2006.
243. Epstein AE, Ellenbogen KA, Kirk KA, et al: Clinical characteristics and outcome of patients with high defibrillation thresholds: A multicenter study. Circulation 86:1206-1216, 1992.
244. Spotnitz HM, Ott GY, Bigger JT, et al: Methods of implantable cardioverter-defibrillator pacemaker insertion to avoid interactions. Ann Thor Surg 53:253-257, 1992.
245. Haffajee C, Casavant D, Desai P, et al: Combined third generation implantable cardioverter-defibrillator with dual-chamber pacemakers: Preliminary observations. PACE 19:136-142, 1996.
246. Brooks R, Garan H, McGovern BA, et al: Implantation of transvenous nonthoracotomy cardioverter-defibrillator systems in patients with permanent endocardial pacemakers. Am Heart J 129:45-53, 1995.
247. Mont L, Valentino M, Sambola A, et al: Arrhythmia recurrence in patients with a healed myocardial infarction who received an implantable defibrillator: Analysis according to the clinical presentation. J Am Coll Cardiol 34:351-357, 1999.
248. Grosse-Meininghaus D, Siebels J, Wolpert C, et al; German Ventritex MD-Investigators: Efficacy of antitachycardia pacing confirmed by stored electrograms: A retrospective analysis of 613 stored electrograms in implantable defibrillators. Z Kardiol 91:396-403, 2002.
249. Wathen MS, Sweeney MO, DeGroot PJ, et al; for the PainFREE Investigators: Shock reduction using antitachycardia pacing for spontaneous rapid ventricular tachycardia in patients with coronary artery disease. Circulation 104:796-801, 2001.
250. Wathen MS, DeGroot PJ, Sweeney MO, et al; for the PainFREE Rx II Investigators: Prospective randomized multicenter trial of empirical antitachycardia pacing versus shocks for spontaneous rapid ventricular tachycardia in patients with implantable cardioverter-defibrillators-pacing fast ventricular tachycardia reduces shock therapies (PainFREE Rx II) trial results. Circulation 110:2591-2596, 2004.
251. Sweeney MO, Wathen MS, Volosin K, et al: Appropriate and inappropriate ventricular therapies, quality of life, and mortality among primary and secondary prevention implantable cardioverter defibrillator patients: Results from the Pacing Fast VT Reduces Shock ThErapies (PainFree Rx II) trial. Circulation 111:2898-2905, 2005.

252. Schauerte P, Stellbrink C, Schondube FA, et al: Polarity reversal improves defibrillation efficacy in patients undergoing transvenous cardioverter defibrillator implantation with biphasic shocks. PACE 20:301-306, 1997.
253. Shorofsky SR, Gold MR: Effects of waveform and polarity on defibrillation thresholds in humans using a transvenous lead system. Am J Cardiol 78:313-316, 1996.
254. Natale A, Sra J, Dhala A, et al: Effects of initial polarity on defibrillation threshold with biphasic pulses. PACE 18:1889-1893, 1995.
254. Strickberger SA, Man KC, Daoud E, et al: Effect of first-phase polarity of biphasic shocks on defibrillation threshold with a single transvenous lead system. J Am Coll Cardiol 25:1605-1608, 1995.
256. Keelan ET, Sra JS, Axtell K, Maglio C, et al: The effect of polarity of the initial phase of a biphasic shock waveform on the defibrillation threshold of pectorally implanted defibrillators. PACE 20:337-342, 1997.
257. Anvari A, Mast F, Schmidinger H, et al: Effects of lidocaine, ajmaline, and diltiazem on ventricular defibrillation energy requirements in isolated rabbit heart. J Cardiovasc Pharmacol 29:429-435, 1997.
258. Murakawa Y, Sezaki K, Inoue H, et al: Shock-induced refractory period extension and pharmacologic modulation of defibrillation threshold. J Cardiovasc Pharmacol 23:822-825, 1994.
259. Behrens S, Li C, Franz MR: Effects of long-term amiodarone treatment on ventricular-fibrillation vulnerability and defibrillation efficacy in response to monophasic and biphasic shocks. J Cardiovasc Pharmacol 30:412-418, 1997.
260. Frame LH: The effect of chronic oral and acute intravenous amiodarone administration on ventricular defibrillation threshold using implanted electrodes in dogs. PACE 12:339-346, 1989.
261. Lake CL, Kron IL, Mentzer RM, Crampton RS: Lidocaine enhances intraoperative ventricular defibrillation. Anesth Analg 65:337-340, 1986.
262. Dorian P, Wang M, David I, et al: Oral clofilium produces sustained lowering of defibrillation energy requirements in a canine model. Circulation 83:614-621, 1991.
263. Beatch GN, Dickenson DR, Wood RH, Tang AS: Class III antiarrhythmic effects of LY-190147 on defibrillation threshold. J Cardiovasc Pharmacol 27:218-225, 1996.
264. Murakawa Y, Yamashita T, Kanese Y, Omata M: Can a class III antiarrhythmic drug improve electrical defibrillation efficacy during ventricular fibrillation? J Am Coll Cardiol 29:688-692, 1997.

Section Three

Implantation Techniques

Chapter 18

Permanent Pacemaker and Implantable Cardioverter-Defibrillator Implantation

PETER H. BELOTT • DWIGHT W. REYNOLDS

The approach to cardiac pacemaker implantation has evolved during the past half century.[1] From the initial epicardial implants of Senning[2] and transvenous implantation by Furman and Schwedel,[3] cardiac pacemaker implantation has undergone radical changes not only in the implanted hardware but also in the preoperative planning, anatomic approach, personnel, and implantation facilities. The early trend from the epicardial approach to the simpler transvenous cutdown led the way to the percutaneous technique developed by Littleford and Spector.[4] Preoperative planning and, in particular, device selection, which once were simple, have become complex. The pacemaker system, both device and electrodes, must be individualized to the patient's particular clinical and anatomic situation. The implantation procedure, previously the exclusive domain of the cardiovascular surgeon, has also become the purview of the invasive cardiologist. Similarly, the procedure has undergone a transition from the operating room to the cardiac catheterization laboratory or special procedures room. Except in special instances, the luxury of an anesthesiologist has disappeared, with the implanting physician assuming additional responsibilities. Finally, because of concerns about cost containment, the usual in-hospital postoperative observation period has been dramatically reduced or replaced by an ambulatory approach to pacemaker implantation.

Similarly, since Mirowski and colleagues[5] implanted the first implantable cardioverter-defibrillator (ICD) in 1980, its evolution has been comparable with that of the cardiac pacemaker. The initial epicardial ICD placement with an abdominal pocket has given way to a transvenous approach and a pectoral pocket. The surgery initially performed in the operating room exclusively by a cardiovascular surgeon is now carried out by nonsurgeons in the catheterization or electrophysiology laboratory. Also, protracted hospital stays have been replaced by much shorter hospital stays, even outpatient situations. The once simple ICD device is now much more complex, offering total arrhythmia control as well as backup dual-chamber rate-adaptive pacing.

The advent of cardiac resynchronization therapy (CRT) has added a new level of complexity to pacemaker and defibrillator implantation. Not only is a third lead required but also reliable left ventricle (LV) stimulation is essential for positive clinical results. CRT has brought new challenges to device implantation with respect to venous access, coronary sinus cannulation, lead positioning, effective stimulation, and new complications. And finally, the new popularity of selective or alternative site pacing for optimal hemodynamics and arrhythmia management has challenged the traditional sites of lead placement. All of these changes have not been without a price: New techniques have brought new challenges as well as problems and concerns. This chapter attempts to explore all aspects of modern pacemaker and ICD implantations from a practical point of view. It also addresses these new challenges, problems, and concerns.

Pacemaker Implantation

Personnel

Implanting Physician or Surgeon

Traditionally, pacemaker implantation procedures were performed exclusively by a thoracic or cardiac surgeon. The skills were acquired during a residency or fellowship. Early pacemaker implantations involved more extensive surgery and, at times, an open-chest procedure for placement of epicardial electrodes. The pulse generator and electrodes were large, requiring considerable dissection and surgical skill. Since 1980, diminishing pacemaker size has limited the more extensive surgery previously required. Today, the knowledge and skills required for dual-chamber pacing are well suited for the physician trained in cardiac catheterization.

It has become generally well accepted that the pacemaker-implanting physician may be either a thoracic surgeon or an invasive cardiologist.[6] At times, the two may even act as a team, with the surgeon isolating the vein and the cardiologist positioning the electrodes. With the current reimbursement structure and the changing economic environment, however, this team approach is rapidly becoming burdensome; in any event, it is frequently unnecessary. Today, the credentialing for pacemaker implantation procedures poses a dilemma. The trainee in thoracic surgery has ever-diminishing exposure to pacemaker implantation as the procedure becomes more the responsibility of the cardiologist. At the same time, the cardiologist has little or no exposure to proper surgical technique, the use of surgical instruments, and preoperative and postoperative care.

Considerable controversy exists about what constitutes an appropriate implantation experience and how long that experience should extend. *One thing that appears certain is that physicians with limited training and ongoing experience have unacceptable complication rates.*[7] It has been suggested that to remain proficient, one must perform a minimum of 12 procedures per year.

There is a definite need for formal training programs specifically designed to teach cardiac pacing.[8-10] Such programs should be offered to both cardiologists and surgeons interested in cardiac pacing. The ideal program should be comprehensive and integrated, involving not only all implantations but also follow-up and troubleshooting. To be an effective implanter, one must understand the problems of follow-up and troubleshooting. Formal didactic experience and hands-on exposure are necessary. Although a formal, year-long, comprehensive, integrated training program is ideal, consideration of physicians who are out of formal training programs requires, at times, combining more intensive didactic programs with extended, supervised hands-on experience. Training is important for the implantation and non-implantation aspects of pacing. It has been our frequent experience that there is substantially less enthusiasm for the pre- and post-surgical aspects of pacing. We ardently believe such mastery is crucial to becoming an effective implanter.

Regardless of how one has become trained to implant pacemakers, careful review (by those responsible for credentialing in a given institution) of the training and experience of individuals in pacing will help prevent inadequately trained individuals from performing independent, unsupervised pacemaker implantation. Criteria for adequate training and experience should involve a minimum number of pacemaker procedures, including single-chamber and dual-chamber implantations, lead replacements, pulse generator replacements, and upgrades to dual-chamber from single-chamber systems. Also, some documentable experience in an active pacemaker service clinic should be required.[11]

Support Personnel

Support personnel are crucial to the success and safety of any pacemaker procedure. Historically, whether in a large medical center or a small community hospital, the procedure was performed in the operating room. This had its drawbacks because each case could be a first-time experience for the operating room staff. Pacemaker procedures were commonly added at the end of a busy operating room schedule and were assigned to the first available room with support personnel, who changed from procedure to procedure. Personnel not familiar with the procedure can interrupt the flow of the case. Even with the transition to the cardiac catheterization laboratory for pacing procedures, the same problems can apply. Conversely, depending on the volume of procedures in the operating room and the cardiac catheterization laboratories, there may be a greater opportunity for consistent, recurrent availability of cardiovascular technicians, nurses, and radiography personnel in the latter. These more focused staff members tend to have a certain appreciation for the procedure and are better equipped to deal with the unique problems that may be encountered during pacemaker implantation.

Whether implantation takes place in the operating room or catheterization laboratory, the minimal personnel required are the same:

- A scrub nurse or technician familiar with each operator's surgical preferences
- A circulating nurse to support the personnel who have scrubbed; this support generally involves delivery of supplies and equipment to the sterile field as needed and patient monitoring and med-

ication administration, although this latter function is somewhat limited in the operating room when an anesthesiologist is present

- An individual responsible for the performance of electrical testing

It is also useful to have access to an experienced cardiovascular radiology technician, which generally is more easily accomplished in the cardiac catheterization laboratory than in the operating room.

The presence of an anesthesiologist or nurse anesthetist is becoming something of a luxury. Initially an essential member of the implantation team, an anesthesiologist in many centers is now involved only in special situations requiring airway support in an unstable or otherwise problematic patient. Anesthesiology staff should always be available for emergency situations and consulted if problems are anticipated.

The participation of the pacemaker manufacturer's representative as support personnel has always been a subject of debate. This person's role varies from center to center.[12] At one extreme, the representative merely delivers the pacemaker and leads to the hospital. At the other extreme, he or she is a vital member of the support team, retrieving threshold data, filling out registration forms, and at times, offering technical advice. The latter extreme is particularly true in smaller institutions with less pacemaker activity. A well-trained, experienced pacemaker representative can be an important member of the support team. An experienced representative dedicated to cardiac pacing commonly has broad experience and a knowledge base in problems especially unique to his or her company's products. Although such a representative of industry can be helpful, such a person, no matter how experienced or knowledgeable, should not be considered an acceptable alternative to a knowledgeable, skilled, and experienced physician implanter. If an industrial representative is to be used during implantations for support, hospital approval is advisable.

When the support personnel requirements of the operating room and the catheterization laboratory are compared, there are the previously noted general advantages to the latter. There is one other important concern, relating to sterile technique. The regular operating room personnel tend to be more keenly aware of sterile technique and are scrupulous in this regard. In contrast, the cardiac catheterization laboratory personnel are not routinely trained in operating room and sterile techniques, and if these procedures are not strongly reinforced, they can be disastrously neglected.

Implantation Facility and Equipment

The cardiac catheterization laboratory and special procedures room appear well suited for permanent pacemaker procedures.[13,14] Early concerns about safety and sterility have been shown to be unfounded when these issues are appropriately addressed prospectively. The unique capabilities from a radiologic point of view are invaluable. High-resolution images, unlimited projections, and angiographic capabilities can be extremely helpful in venous access and electrode placement as well as in variable image magnification, digital image acquisition, and image imposition techniques and storage. In addition, these facilities tend to be equipped for ready access with all of the catheters, guidewires, sheaths, and angiographic materials that might be required for special situations. The implantation facility is also typically the location of the most sophisticated physiologic monitoring and recording equipment (Fig. 18-1), offering continuous surface and endocardial electric recordings as well as extensive hemodynamic monitoring capabilities. The importance of staffing with qualified cardiovascular nurses and technicians has already been mentioned.

Concerns about the potential for infection must be addressed. These facilities are designated as intermediate-sterile areas. The sterile precautions tend to be less rigid than in the operating room. The cardiac catheterization laboratory also tends to be a high-traffic area. A rigid protocol for sterile technique must be established, and the room sealed from traffic after it has been cleaned for the surgical procedure. Everyone entering this area must wear scrub clothing, a hat, and a mask. The ventilation system should also meet the standards for an intermediate-sterile area.

The cardiac catheterization laboratory and special procedures room generally have another drawback. Most do not allow the patient to be placed in the Trendelenburg position, which can be important in the percutaneous approach to pacemaker implantation. This problem can be obviated, however, by the use of a wedge under the legs early in the procedure.

Of course, the ideal is a room or suite dedicated to pacemaker procedures and containing all of the capabilities previously noted as well as skilled staffing as previously described. The ability to maintain sterility, as well as dedicated equipment and staff, in such a room is attractive, although it is clearly the exception at present. As growth occurs in the number of transvenously implantable defibrillators, the establishment of rooms dedicated to pacemaker and defibrillator implantation will likely also increase.

The strongest arguments for implanting a pacemaker in the operating room are sterility and patient control. The operating room is typically the area of best sterility and sterile technique. A pacemaker represents a foreign body; therefore, one prime concern is infection. A procedure in the operating room generally offers the maximum in protection from infection. In addition, patient control is better because most operating rooms, as a matter of policy, require that an anesthesiologist be available for any procedure. Presence of the anesthesiologist allows for more effective airway control and ventilation in the unstable or uncooperative patient. The anesthesiologist is available to intubate the patient, and even to administer general anesthesia, if necessary. Another small advantage of an operating room is the seemingly endless availability of surgical instruments and supplies. It can also be argued that if a catastrophe should occur requiring more extensive surgery, such as an open-chest procedure, the patient is already in the operating room. Conversely,

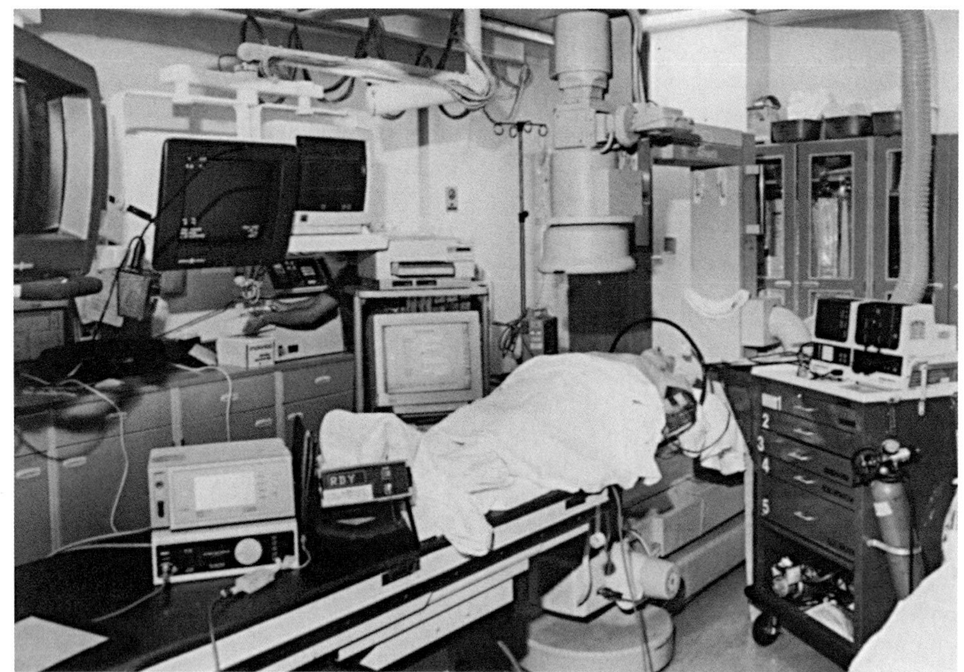

Figure 18-1. Cardiac catheterization laboratory. The patient is surrounded by sophisticated monitoring equipment, including a pulse oximeter, a physiologic recorder, an external defibrillator, an automatic blood pressure cuff, and an emergency "crash" cart.

in our independent experience, this advantage is only theoretical.

The biggest pitfall of the operating room is the fluoroscopy equipment. It is usually of lesser quality and of limited capability compared with that available in the catheterization laboratory. In addition, the operating room equipment is frequently shared with other services, such as orthopedics. Conflicts can occur when more than one service is trying to use it at the same time. The lack of immediate access to angiographic materials and catheterization equipment is another drawback to using the operating room for pacemaker procedures. Unless pacemaker implantation is given special consideration and is performed in a specific operating room with equipment and supplies under the control of a pacemaker physician and staff, there is a tendency for lack of technical preparation. This lack disrupts the flow of the procedure and can adversely affect the outcome. This same caveat holds, however, for a busy catheterization laboratory.

The monitoring equipment used for a pacemaker procedure is variable. A multichannel electrocardiogram (ECG) recording system is frequently recommended; such systems are able to monitor and record a minimum of three surface and one intracardiac ECGs.[15] From a more practical point of view, all that is absolutely required is continuous ECG monitoring on an oscilloscope. The ECG pattern need only be clear. Selection of ECG leads should demonstrate adequate atrial and ventricular morphology for defining underlying rhythm, arrhythmias, and atrial and ventricular capture.

Threshold information can be obtained from the combined use of a pacing system analyzer (PSA) (see later) and an oscilloscope. Sensing data can be obtained from a reliable PSA alone. Multichannel recorders provide more thorough evaluation and documentation and occasionally are extremely valuable in discerning arrhythmias, capture, capture morphology, timing, and so on. The multichannel recorder also allows retrieval of intracardiac signals, precise waveform analysis, and assessment of ventriculoatrial conduction. High-quality hard copy for analysis is also generally available with these more sophisticated recording devices, which tend to be ubiquitous in the catheterization laboratory but uncommon in the operating room.

Patient monitoring should also include reliable means for blood pressure and arterial oxygen saturation determinations. This can usually be accomplished adequately with the use of an automatic noninvasive blood pressure cuff and a transcutaneous oxygen saturation monitor (some institutions place indwelling arterial lines for blood pressure monitoring, although this practice is generally not necessary and has some associated morbidity). These devices are of particular value when an anesthesiologist is not in attendance. Continuous oxygen saturation monitoring can detect hypoventilation from sedation, pneumothorax, and air embolization. A direct current (DC) defibrillator and complete emergency cart should be in the room where the pacemaker procedure is performed. The cart must include an Ambu bag and intubation equipment.

The surgical instruments for a pacemaker procedure usually call for something akin to a "minor surgical" setup (Fig. 18-2). Depending on the institution, the contents of a minor surgical setup can be rather overwhelming, particularly for the nonsurgeon implanting physician. The rows of unnamed clamps and retractors

TABLE 18-1. Pacemaker Surgical Instrument Tray

2 Adson forceps with teeth
1 mouth-tooth forceps
1 smooth forceps
1 medium blunt Weitlaner retractor
1 small Weitlaner retractor
2 Senn retractors
1 Army-Navy retractor
4 baby towel clips
5 curved mosquito clamps
1 Peers clamp
2 curved Kelly clamps
1 small Metzenbaum scissors
1 curved Mayo scissors
1 No. 3 knife handle
2 small needle holders
1 Goulet retractor
1 Bozeman uterine dressing forceps
1 pkg 1-0 silk 18-inch suture material
1 pkg 2-0 polyglactin mesh nonabsorbable suture material
1 pkg of 4-0 polyglactin mesh nonabsorbable suture material
1 No. 3 or 4 French eye needle
1 No. 10 scalpel blade

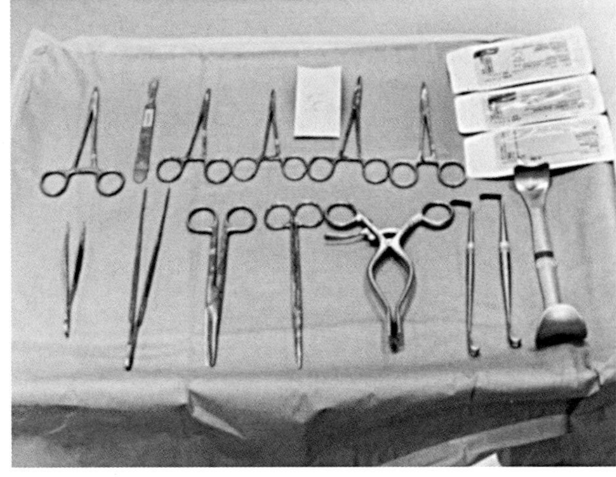

Figure 18-2. Minor surgical tray displaying the minimum required surgical instruments and supplies. From the top left and clockwise*: needle holder, scalpel, four sizes of curved hemostats and clamps, Goulet retractor, two Senn retractors, Weitlaner self-retaining retractor, Metzenbaum scissors, suture scissors, nontoothed forceps, and toothed forceps. The four packages are one of "free needles" and three of resorbable and nonresorbable sutures.*

would suggest that some major body cavity might have to be entered. Actually, a pacemaker procedure can be performed efficiently with only a few, well-selected instruments,[16] and there are many acceptable variations and personal preferences. Problems can occur, however, with the nonsurgeon implanting physician who is unfamiliar with the instruments and their appropriate uses.

Table 18-1 lists the contents of an acceptable basic surgical tray for pacemaker implantations. There are several valuable retractors worthy of individual comment. The Gelpi and/or Weitlaner retractors can be used throughout the procedure for improved visual exposure (see Fig. 18-2). The Senn retractor is used for more delicate retraction (see Fig. 18-2). One end is shaped in an L and the other has tiny claws. This instrument allows the more delicate lifting of tissue edges. Another useful retractor is the Goulet retractor (see Fig. 18-2), which can be replaced with a Richardson retractor. It is extremely helpful in retraction when one is creating the pacemaker pocket. Unlike other large retractors, the smooth, scalloped ends of these retractors are gentle to the tissues while affording a generous area of exposure. Army-Navy retractors can also be helpful for this purpose. Other instruments, such as forceps (with or without "teeth"), hemostats, scissors (tissue and other), needle holders, and clamps, are necessary, but their use does not require explanation here. It is important to add that proper use and care of the instruments are crucial, and replacement of worn-out instruments is mandatory for avoiding frustration, delays, and suboptimal work.

Pacemaker procedures performed in the operating room typically benefit from excellent lighting. Multiple high-intensity lamps light the surgical field. This is not the case for pacemaker procedures performed in the catheterization laboratory or special procedures room, where lighting is frequently marginal at best. One solution to this problem is the use of a high-intensity headlamp (Fig. 18-3). A headlamp is extremely useful when one is creating the pocket and inspecting for bleeders, particularly when one's head blocks out other light. The use of the headlamp can initially be frustrating and requires practice. Once one is facile with its use, it will become the major light source for creating the pocket. Even in the operating room, despite all the lighting, the headlamp can be very helpful.

The final piece of equipment to be discussed is the electrocautery device. This device can be useful, and some experienced implanters consider it essential to any pacemaker procedure. Its use, however, has been the subject of controversy.[17-19] Historically, the use of electrocautery equipment for cutting or coagulation during a pacemaker procedure was considered taboo. Concerns have been raised with respect to its causing burns at the myocardium-electrode interface, destruction of the pulse generator, and damage to the pacemaker leads. There is a growing consensus that the use of an appropriately grounded electrocautery device is

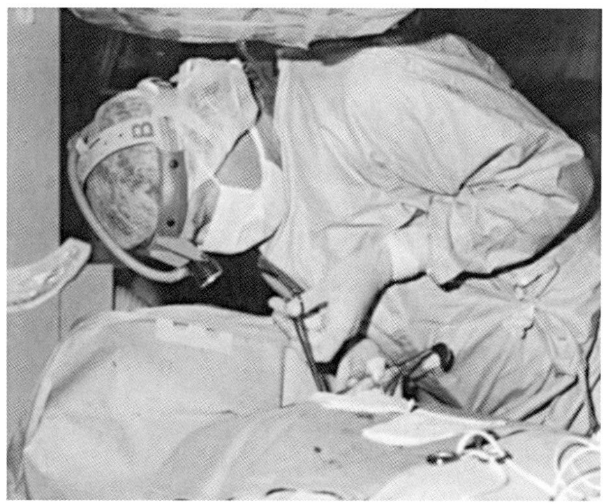

Figure 18-3. High-intensity headlamps optimize visualization in situations of limited lighting experienced frequently in the catheterization laboratory and sometimes in the operating room.

safe when the following precautions are taken. First, active cautery should never touch the exposed proximal pin of the electrode. Second, the use of all electrocautery should cease when the pulse generator is in the surgical field.

During pulse generator changes, electrocautery can be extremely useful. Cutting with electrocautery expedites the freeing up of the pulse generator and, at the same time, avoids the misfortune of cutting the lead. At times, even in the most experienced hands, a tedious dissection ends with the scalpel or scissors nicking or cutting the electrode insulation. Use of rapid strokes with cautery avoids the buildup of heat, preventing injury to leads.

Experience leads us to believe that there are no important untoward effects on the myocardium if the cautery touches the pulse generator. There is, however, a risk of causing a permanent no-output situation by destroying the pulse generator. This appears to be particularly true in certain pulse generators. The risk to the patient of a sudden lack of output can be prevented by placing a temporary pacemaker in patients who are pacemaker dependent; this consideration is fundamental to all pacemaker procedures whether or not electrocautery is used.

The PSA is extremely valuable during pacemaker procedures. Even when stimulators and recorders are available, a PSA, the circuitry (especially sensing) of which mimics that of the planned pulse generator, will more accurately predict the performance of the pulse generator. In some institutions, the PSA is provided by the pacemaker manufacturer. The early PSAs were simple and were designed to measure the pacing and sensing thresholds for single-chamber ventricular pacing. They were unable to perform (or were cumbersome when performing) the tasks required for atrial and dual-chamber pacing.[20] Today's PSA should be able to perform all of the measurements required for any pacemaker procedure for both the pulse generator and the pacing electrode. At the same time, it should offer backup pacing support during parameter measurements. The modern PSA should be able to function in any mode and should measure from either chamber, offering a clear digital display as well as extensive programmability. It should have emergency capabilities of high output and high rate. The capacity to generate a hard copy for analysis and record keeping is also desirable. An example of a PSA is the Medtronic model 2090 (Medtronic, Inc., Minneapolis, Minn.; Fig. 18-4); Table 18-2 summarizes its desirable features. Some of the pacemakers driven by sensors, for example, temperature and oxygen sensors, require special additional sensor analysis by a specialized PSA tool. Whether supplied by the institution or the manufacturer, a good PSA is a must.

There never seem to be enough spare parts during a pacemaker procedure. It is certainly common that just when you need it, the key spare part is unavailable. Most manufacturers offer service kits containing splice kits, stylets, lead adapters, wrenches, lubricant, lead caps, wire cutters, and so on (Table 18-3). It is advisable to set up a pacemaker cart stocked with all the supplies you are likely to need. This cart should hold (1) a temporary pacemaker tray that contains the materials for venous insertion as well as the temporary pulse generator and leads, (2) an assortment of sheath sets, dilators, and guidewires, (3) the service kits from the manufacturers of the most commonly used pacemakers, (4) the equipment for lead retrieval, and (5) if they are used, a supply of polyester (Parsonnet) pouches (C. R. Bard, Inc., Billerica, Mass.; Fig. 18-5). Someone should be designated to make sure supplies are reordered and up to date.

Other, rarely used supplies can be obtained from the operating room or central supply facility. Examples are a Jackson-Pratt drain (Fig. 18-6) for managing hematomas and various sizes of Penrose drains that may be used for tunneling.

Preoperative Planning

The planning that goes into a pacemaker procedure is important if the case is to proceed smoothly. It starts with the evaluation of the patient. A history elucidating patient symptoms, medications the patient is taking, and associated conditions is essential. The physical examination may demonstrate the effects of bradycardia, including altered vital signs, evidence of cardiac decompensation, and neurologic deficits. Anatomic issues potentially affecting the implant can also be uncovered. One of the most important preoperative considerations is the documentation of the bradyarrhythmia. This can be accomplished with the 12-lead ECG, Holter monitor, event recordings, or in-hospital critical care unit or telemetry unit monitoring. Supporting laboratory data, such as digitalis levels, thyroid parameters, and blood chemical analysis, provide documentation that the bradycardia is not secondary to another condition. The evaluation of the patient should substantiate the indications outlined by the American College of Cardiology/American Heart Association/North American Society of Pacing and

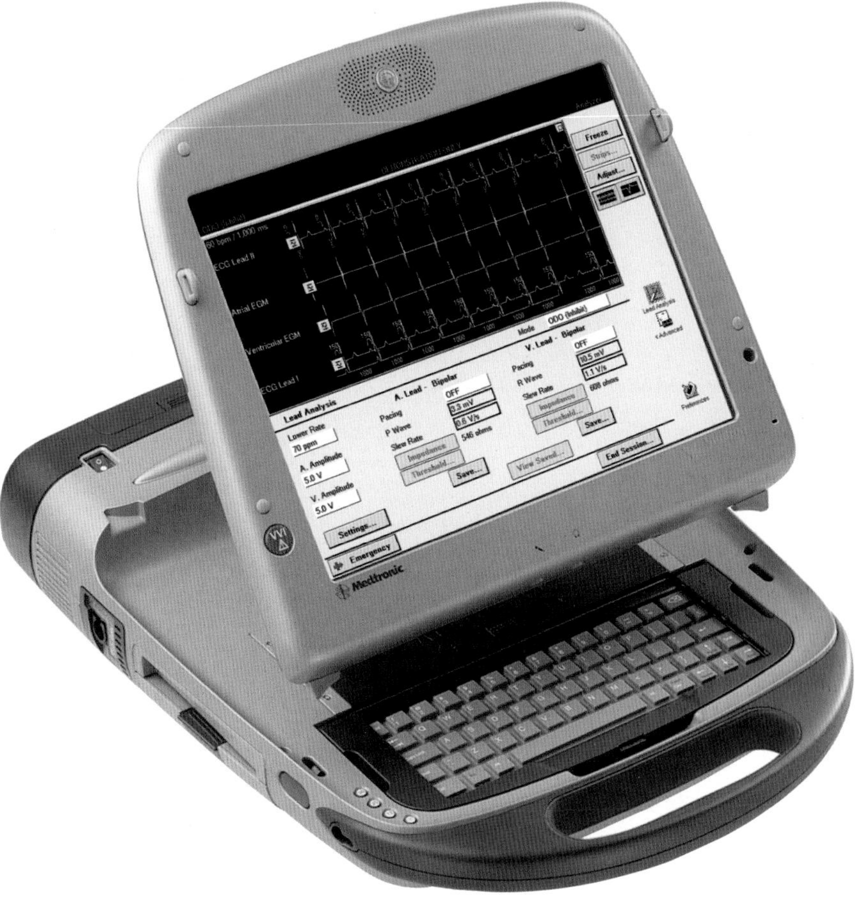

Figure 18-4. The multifunction Medtronic 2090 (Medtronic, Inc., Minneapolis, Minn.) pacemaker system analyzer. This device determines the pacing and sensing functions of the electrode and the pulse generator as well as the electrical integrity of the electrode. (From Barold SS: Modern Cardiac Pacing. Armonk, NY, Futura, 1985, p 444.)

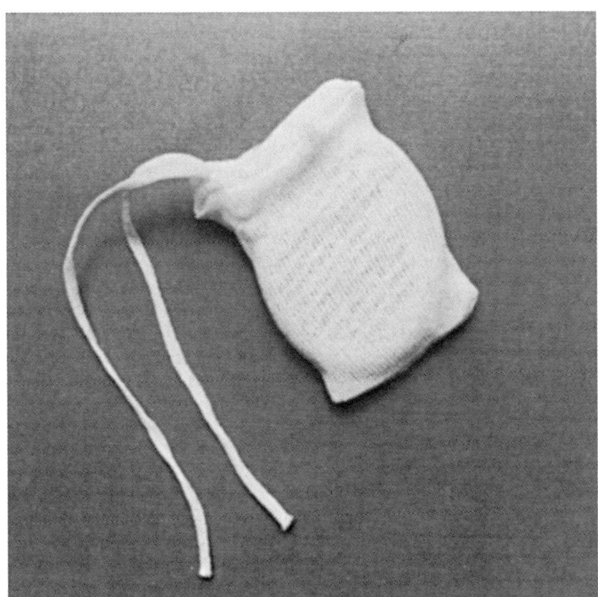

Figure 18-5. The polyester (Dacron) Parsonnet pouch (C.R. Bard, Inc., Billerica, Mass.) is useful in patients with little subcutaneous tissue. The pouch is usually soaked in povidone-iodine (Betadine) before the pacemaker is inserted into the pouch, which is then inserted into the pacemaker pocket.

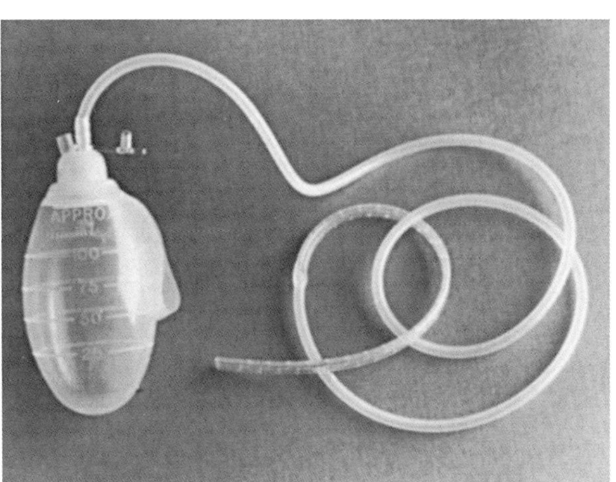

Figure 18-6. The Jackson-Pratt drainage system allows for sterile closed-wound drainage. The negative-pressure squeeze bulb has a one-way valve that prevents drainage from returning to the wound.

TABLE 18-2. Operating Features of the Medtronic CareLink Programmer 2090 Pacing System Analyzer

Parameter	Range
Models	VOO, VVI, AOO, AAI, DOO, DDD, VDD, ODO
Lower rate:	
AOO, AAI, VOO, VVI, DOO	30-220
DDD, VDD	30-110
Upper rate	80-220
Amplitudes (A and V)	0.1-10.0 V
Pulse width (A and V)	0.02-1.5 msec
AV interval:	
Sensed	20-350 msec
Paced	20-350 msec
Rapid atrial stimulation	200-800 min. (ppm)
Atrial refractory	200-500 msec
Ventricular refractory	250 msec
Atrial sensitivity	0.25-20 mV
Ventricular sensitivity	0.5-20 mV
Polarity (A and V)	Unipolar/bipolar
Atrial blanking:	
After atrial pace	160-300 msec
After atrial sense	160-300 msec
After ventricular pace:	
VVI/VOO	150-350 msec
DDD/VDD	200-220 msec
After ventricular sense	150 msec
Ventricular blanking:	
After atrial pace	40 msec
After ventricular sense	125 msec
After ventricular pace	200 msec
Measurement parameters:	
P-wave amplitude	0.3-30 mV
R-wave amplitude	0.6-30 mV
Impedance (A and V)	200-2499
	2500-4000
Slew rate	0.1-4.0 V/s
Pacing current	0.1-25 Max
Special features:	
Rapid stimulation	AOO, VOO, DOO modes
Rates	180-800 ppm
Emergency pacing	VVI rate at 70 at 10 V and 1.5 msec

A, atrium/atrial; AV, atrioventricular; V, ventricle/ventricular.
*Medtronic, Inc., Minneapolis, Minn.

Electrophysiology (ACA/AAH/NAPSE) joint task force.[21] The documentation should be readily available and is usually affixed to the patient's chart.

Inpatient versus Outpatient Procedure

With all of the documentation obtained and indications met, the next step is the scheduling of the pacemaker procedure. Pacemaker surgery can be performed on either an inpatient or an outpatient basis. Traditionally, pacemaker procedures have been performed on an inpatient basis, which involves formal admission of the patient to the hospital for the procedure. The preoperative evaluation (in most cases), the pacemaker procedure, and early postoperative care are carried out in the hospital. Generally, the patient has already been admitted to the hospital because of symptoms (e.g., syncope), and the diagnosis of a bradyarrhythmia subsequently established. The pacemaker procedure is then scheduled. Alternatively, some or most of the evaluation is completed before admission; after the need for a pacemaker is determined, the patient is admitted for the pacemaker procedure and postoperative care. In some cases, this inpatient approach is inefficient and not cost-effective.

The early pacing systems were large, had brief longevity, and were prone to catastrophic complications, such as lead dislodgment, perforation, and wound infection. Postoperatively, patients were managed with extreme caution because of these concerns, and an abbreviated hospital stay seemed radical, whereas the concept of an ambulatory procedure was unthinkable. Today, complications are rare, the pacemakers are small, venous access is easy and quick with the introducer technique, and the procedure is relatively minor. Refinements of the electrode systems with active and passive fixation have reduced the dislodgment rate to near zero. In addition, the indications have been expanded to include more patients who are less pacemaker dependent. Finally, and perhaps most directly, there is a growing mandate for cost containment. The very technology that has made cardiac pacing physiologic, reliable, and safe has resulted in higher cost. For all these reasons, it seems logical that an ambulatory approach for pacemaker procedures could be at once safe and effective as well as less expensive.

TABLE 18-3. Supplies and Spare Parts for Pacemakers

Lead stylets: Varying lengths; Varying stiffness
Straight and variable J-shaped retention wire curve
Silicone oil
Helical coil adaptor with 5-mm pin
Sterile medical adhesive
Wire crimper-cutter
Lead connector caps: 3.2, VS-1, and 5-mm sizes
Step-up and step-down adapters
Adapter sleeves
Screwdriver kit and torque wrenches
One set of connecting cable introducer sets, 11F and 12F

There is a trend toward performing pacemaker procedures on an ambulatory basis. The experiences at several centers, in both Europe and the United States, have clearly supported the safety and efficacy of this approach.[22,23] Concerns about potential complications continue to be expressed.[24-26] Questions about lead selection, the timing of discharge, and the intensity of follow-up are frequently raised. In addition, the economic impact has yet to be fully appreciated. We believe that more pacemaker procedures are being performed on an ambulatory basis, but this impression has not been reflected in the pacing literature. Since the original reports of Zegelman and colleagues[22] and Belott,[23] Haywood and associates[27] have reported a randomized, controlled study of the feasibility and safety of ambulatory pacemaker procedures. Although the study group was small (50 patients), the results were similar to those of one of the authors (PHB). There was good patient acceptance, no evidence of a higher complication rate, and cost savings of £540 (at that time, about $810 U.S.).

Since the initial report of 181 new pacemaker implants in 1987, our own ambulatory experience continues to be gratifying. During a 13-year span reported in 1996, that experience comprised 1474 pacemaker procedures, 1043 (69%) of which were performed on an ambulatory basis.[28] The experience also included pulse generator changes, all of which we have performed on an outpatient basis since 1987. On the basis of this experience, it appears that between 60% and 75% of new pacemaker implantations can be successfully performed as ambulatory procedures (Table 18-4). There have been no additional ambulatory failures, pacemaker-related emergencies, or deaths in the ambulatory procedures. (An *ambulatory failure* is an implantation that is initiated as an ambulatory procedure but for which the hospital stay is extended to admitting the patient because of a complication.) The complications encountered in ambulatory cases included one hemothorax detected 2 weeks after discharge. This was successfully managed by hospitalization and chest tube drainage. Three hematomas were managed on an ambulatory basis with reoperation, control of bleeding, and drain placement. Two small pneumothoraces that did not require chest tubes occurred fortuitously in hospitalized patients in whom an ambulatory procedure had not been planned.

These experiences underscore the safety of the ambulatory approach. At present, one of the authors (PHB) approaches all elective pacemaker procedures (new implantations, electrode repositioning, upgrade procedures, electrode extractions, and pulse generator changes) on an ambulatory basis. A simple protocol is used, and the patients often go home 1 to 2 hours after the procedure. They are seen the following day in the pacemaker clinic. A simple outpatient protocol is outlined in Table 18-5.

In most institutions, patients can remain in the hospital overnight and still be considered outpatients. This practice conforms to the present U.S. Health Care Financing Administration's definition of *ambulatory surgery* for reimbursement in the United States, as

TABLE 18-4. Analysis of Ambulatory Pacemaker Procedures, 1983-1995

Year	Total No. Patients	No. Patients Ambulatory	No. Patients Discharged on Day of Procedure	No. Patients Discharged <24 Hrs after Procedure*	Percentage of Ambulatory Procedures
1983	99	34	8	26	34
1984	102	34	16	18	34
1985	112	56	44	12	50
1986	110	60	56	4	60
1987	112	78	78	0	69
1988	123	87	86	1	70
1989	100	70	68	2	70
1990	107	87	83	4	77
1991	135	124	124	0	91
1992	119	94	90	4	78
1993	145	128	125	3	88
1994	113	104	102	2	92
1995	97	87	87	0	88
Total	1474	1043	967	76	69

*Patients were hospitalized overnight.

TABLE 18-5. Outpatient Protocol

- Surgery scheduled as an outpatient procedure with outpatient number assigned
- Preoperative blood analyses, electrocardiogram, and chest x-ray study performed on an outpatient basis within 24 hours before admission
- Patient instructed to fast after midnight of the evening before the procedure
- Patient instructed to report to the outpatient department on the morning of the day of procedure
- Postoperative electrocardiogram and chest x-ray study performed
- Patient discharged when fully awake and vital signs stable
- Patient instructed to report to the pacemaker center the next morning

follows: "When a patient with a known diagnosis enters a hospital for a specific minor surgical procedure or treatment that is expected to keep him or her in a hospital for only a few hours (less than 24) and this expectation is realized, he or she will be considered an outpatient regardless of the hour of admission, whether or not he or she occupied a bed, and whether or not he or she remained in the hospital past midnight."[23a] An important caveat of ambulatory pacemaker procedures is that if there is any doubt or concern about the patient's well-being, the hospital stay can be extended.

For ambulatory procedures to become more widely practiced, reasonable and equitable reimbursement schedules will have to be instituted. As of this writing, such schedules are lacking, and this fact may be contributing to a slower than optimal transition toward the performance of more ambulatory procedures.[29]

Preoperative Patient Assessment

The preoperative patient assessment consists of the synthesis of all patient information, including history, physical findings, old records, cardiac rhythm strips, and laboratory data. With this information, appropriate decisions can be made about the pacemaker mode, leads, and general approach.

The first such decision is whether the patient requires a single-chamber or dual-chamber pacemaker. With the expansion of options in devices, we need to also consider whether the patient's condition would be better served with an ICD or a cardiac resynchronization device. As a rule, if the patient has intact atrial function, every effort is made to preserve atrial and ventricular relationships. Single-chamber ventricular pacing is usually reserved for the patient with chronic atrial fibrillation or atrial paralysis. A device is selected with acceptable size, longevity, and programmability. If the heart is chronotropically incompetent, a device that offers some form of rate adaptation is considered.

Just as important is the lead selection, which is more completely addressed in Chapter 4. One necessary decision is whether to use passive-fixation or active-fixation leads. Generally, an active-fixation electrode is selected when problems of dislodgment are expected, such as in the patient with a dilated right ventricle (RV) or amputated atrial appendage. Active-fixation leads are one of several factors that enhance removability of the lead, if it is necessary in the future. Also important is the pacing configuration (unipolar vs. bipolar). This decision relates to both electrodes and the pulse generator. Although the use of bipolar pacing and sensing has definite advantages, bipolar leads have historically been more complicated and prone to more problems. Bipolar leads are also larger in diameter. The compatibility of electrodes and the pulse generator is extremely important, particularly when one is using an older existing electrode with a modern pulse generator. If they are incompatible, an appropriate adapter must be obtained. Directly related to the device selection process is whether an ICD or cardiac resynchronization system should be placed. These decisions also affect the type of device selected and the lead systems employed.

If an ambulatory approach is being considered, the patient is assessed with respect to the risk of this approach. An unstable patient should always be admitted to the hospital. If the patient is critically ill, pacemaker dependent, or unstable, a temporary pacemaker is considered. It is commonly better to take the few extra minutes and place a temporary pacemaker. Doing so can avoid moments of "terror" during the procedure if asystole occurs. This statement is particularly true in patients with complete atrioventricular (AV) block, in whom an apparently stable escape rhythm can suddenly disappear, a common situation after initial pacing has been established.

The timing of the procedure usually relates to the stability of the patient. In the critically ill patient in whom there are concerns about the stability of the cardiac rhythm or temporary pacemaker, an early permanent procedure is in order. Conversely, in a patient whose survival is in doubt, one may appropriately decide to wait for stabilization. At times, the procedure is delayed because of systemic infection or sepsis. A permanent pacemaker implantation performed in a septic patient may lead to the seeding of bacteria on the pacemaker or electrode. It has been our approach that if there is active infection, the procedure is deferred until the patient is afebrile and no longer septic, to reduce the risk for pacemaker system infection.

Decisions with regard to the implantation site are not as important currently as they were when only large pulse generators were available. The currently available devices, weighing less than 30 g, make the site, in most situations, moot. They tend to be tolerated well in almost any location. There are, however, special circumstances that deserve mention. These are hobbies, recreational and occupational activities, cosmetic issues, and previous medical conditions. In the patient who hunts, for instance, the pacemaker should be placed on the side opposite from the side where the patient places the rifle butt. Similar considerations are appropriate for the tennis enthusiast or golfer (although our experience with the golfer indicates that whether placing the pacemaker on the backswing or follow-through side varies). In a young person, placement of the pacemaker under the breast (women) or in the axilla may be more desirable from a cosmetic point of view. Medical conditions, such as previous surgery, radiation therapy, and skeletal or other anatomic abnormalities, should also be considered. In the patient who is small with little subcutaneous tissue, a subpectoralis muscle (subpectoral) implantation may be required. This calls for the use of a bipolar system to avoid stimulation of skeletal muscles.

Preoperative Orders

The preoperative orders for pacemaker implantation are generally simple. The patient fasts for at least 6 hours before the procedure. If the implantation is being performed on an ambulatory basis, the patient is instructed to report to the hospital on the day of the procedure, with enough time to obtain the necessary preoperative testing; generally, 2 hours are adequate. The preoperative procedures consists of posteroanterior and lateral chest radiographs, an ECG, a complete blood count, prothrombin time, partial thromboplastin time, and measurements of serum electrolytes, blood urea nitrogen, and serum creatinine. Because the patient is fasting, adequate hydration is maintained with a stable intravenous (IV) line. Hydration is extremely important for subsequent venous access and prevention of air embolization during the procedure. It can be frustrating and dangerous to try to gain venous access in a patient who is dehydrated after prolonged fasting without IV hydration. We generally request that the IV line be started on the side of the planned procedure, so as to facilitate venography during attempts at venous access if this becomes a problem.

The management of pacemaker surgery in the patient taking anticoagulants is controversial. There is a paucity of information throughout the literature with respect to the handling of a patient who requires anticoagulation. One thing is clear: The patient receiving anticoagulants, including heparin and platelet antagonists, is at risk for hematoma formation. It is commonly held that in patients who require oral anticoagulants, the prothrombin time should be brought to normal before implantation. Anticoagulant therapy can be resumed between 24 and 48 hours after pacemaker implantation. Reducing the prothrombin time to normal in a patient requiring anticoagulants, such as a patient with an artificial heart valve, puts the patient at grave risk for thromboembolic complications. To address this issue, many operators choose to admit the patient to the hospital and start intravenous heparin while the warfarin is withheld and the prothrombin time brought to normal values. This process often takes several days. When the prothrombin time has reached the control value, the patient is scheduled for surgery. On the day of surgery, the heparin is stopped, and in some situations, the anticoagulation reversed and the procedure carried out. Several hours after operation, the heparin is resumed. Then, after 24 to 48 hours with no evidence of significant hematoma, the warfarin is resumed; when therapeutic levels are reached, the heparin is stopped, and the patient is discharged with oral warfarin therapy.

In this day of cost control and managed care, the proceeding process is problematic. In addition, despite vigorous attempts at hemostasis, significant hematomas have resulted from the use of heparin. This problem is anecdotal, but in our general experience, the greatest risks for bleeding complications, hemorrhage, and hematoma occur with the use of heparin or platelet antagonists such as aspirin. Having encountered a patient in whom a devastating thromboembolic complication from withdrawal of warfarin, as well as multiple large hematomas from the use of heparin, one of us (PHB) has chosen to perform pacemaker and ICD procedures with the patient still undergoing anticoagulation with oral warfarin. This policy has been in effect for at least 15 years. As a rule, patients taking oral anticoagulants have their INR reduced to about 2. There have been no devastating hematomas or thromboembolic events. It is our opinion that pacemaker and ICD procedures can be performed safely with the patient anticoagulated in this way. This approach has been supported by a 4-year experience reported by Goldstein and colleagues.[30] These investigators found no difference in incidental bleeding complications between patients receiving warfarin and those without anticoagulation. There were no wound hematomas, blood transfusions, or clinically significant bleeding in any patients receiving warfarin. In a later, large series of patients, Giudici and associates[31] further substantiated the safety and efficacy of implanting devices without reversing warfarin therapy.[31]

The medicolegal risks of interrupting continuous anticoagulant therapy and a resultant thromboembolic event are not insignificant. Although there is a risk for hemorrhage during and after pacemaker procedures in patients with therapeutic levels of anticoagulation, the risk appears to be minimal. The bleeding can generally be treated with local measures, such as the placement of drains or reoperation. The risk of bleeding is greatly outweighed by the risk of thromboembolism after withdrawal of anticoagulant therapy. The issue of pacemaker and ICD surgery in the patient undergoing anticoagulant therapy is becoming more prevalent as more patients are prescribed these therapies for atrial fibrillation.

The patient is instructed to continue maintenance oral medications, which may be taken with small sips of water. Patients taking a hypoglycemic agent are instructed to reduce the preoperative dose by 50%. The administration of prophylactic antibiotics is controversial. Our individual preferences call for a broad-spectrum cephalosporin, such as cefazolin, to be given intraoperatively. Many others use vancomycin, which covers all the gram-positive, potentially pathogenic organisms. We also have the patient scrub the chest, neck, shoulders, and supraclavicular fossae with a povidone-iodine (Betadine) sponge the evening and the morning before the procedure. In most instances, shaving of the surgical area is carried out in the procedure room. Finally, we ask the patient to empty the bladder before coming to the procedure room.

Pacemaker Implantation: General Information

On arrival at the procedure room, the patient is transferred to a radiography table. In the catheterization laboratory or special procedures area, the table's radiolucent properties are expected. In the operating room, prior arrangements are made for a special radiolucent operating table. In this latter situation, it is advisable to test the fluoroscopy equipment's ability to penetrate the table. It is also helpful to establish proper x-ray tube orientation. Attention to these details can avoid considerable hassle later, when it is discovered that the patient is on the wrong table, the radiographic equipment is inoperative, or the image is upside down, backward, or both. Almost immediately, the patient is connected to physiologic monitoring (ECG, pulse oximetry, and automatic blood pressure cuff). If it has not already been accomplished, a reliable venous line is established, preferably on the side of the operative site. The circulating nurse must have easy access to the IV line for drug administration and introduction of radiographic materials. Oxygen can be administered by nasal cannula or mask. If a temporary pacemaker is to be placed, the appropriate site is shaved and prepared, and the temporary pacemaker is placed with use of the Seldinger technique. It is important to secure the lead and sheath adequately to maintain accessibility, so that they can be easily removed at the end of the procedure.

Site Preparation and Draping

When effective patient support has been established, focus turns to the operative site. If not already accomplished, shaving and skin cleansing are carried out, which should be generous in scope and include the neck, supraventricular fossae, shoulders, and chest. The operative site, shaved and cleansed, is now formally prepared and draped. There are several ways to accomplish this. One can use a povidone-iodine scrub, followed by alcohol, followed by povidone-iodine solution, with skin drying before the final povidone-iodine solution is applied. This older, more time-consuming, although effective, scrub can be replaced by the use of povidone-iodine solution gel, which is a gelatinous preparation of povidone-iodine. It is spread liberally over the operative site. Within 30 seconds, an optimal bactericidal effect is achieved. With this approach, scrubbing the area is not required. In the case of patients who are allergic to povidone-iodine, a chlorhexidine (Hibiclens) or hexachlorophene (pHisoHex) scrub can be used.

The draping process is a matter of personal preference. One of the authors (DWR) applies a sterile, see-through plastic adhesive drape (impregnated with an iodoform solution) over the entire operative area. The other (PHB) uses one or more sterile plastic drapes with adhesive along one side (Fig. 18-7); the adhesive surface is applied from shoulder to shoulder at the level of the clavicle, which serves to create a sterile barrier from the shoulder level down. Depending on the situation, other barriers can be created. In both cases, the use of the plastic drape is to optimize sterility.

After some form of sterile barrier is established, the operative site is draped with sterile towels, and one or

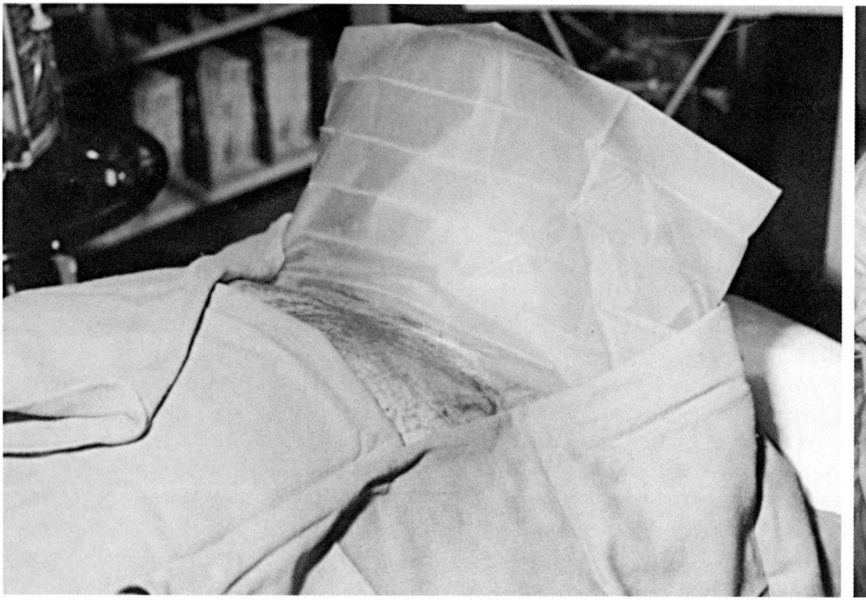

A

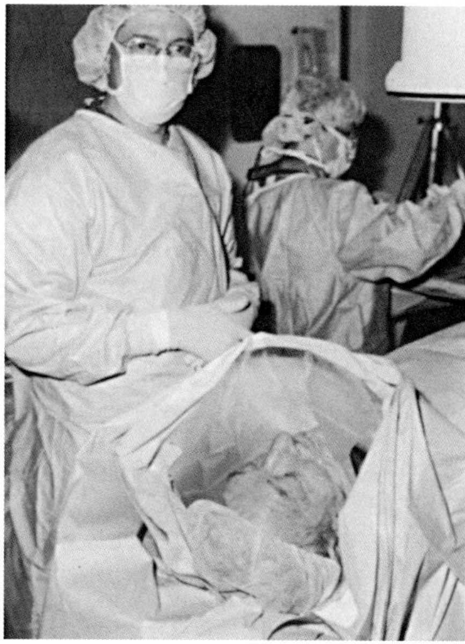

B

Figure 18-7. ***A,*** *Application of a 3M (Minneapolis, Minn.) 10/10 drape to create a sterile barrier.* ***B,*** *The drape folds over the support of common house (Romex) wire, creating an effective sterile barrier and preventing patient claustrophobia.*

more large sterile surgical sheets are applied. Care is taken to avoid smothering the patient and causing claustrophobia, best achieved by keeping the drapes off the patient's face and maintaining the cephalic aspect of the main drape perpendicular to the patient's neck. This arrangement allows unrestricted access to the patient's head and neck. The main drape is clipped to some form of support on both sides of the patient. The support can consist of IV poles placed on each side of the patient.

Such an arrangement may not be possible in laboratories, where it interferes with radiographic equipment. Alternatively, the drape may be fixed to the C-arm or image intensifier. This solution is less than optimal, because the drapes pull away every time the C-arm or radiographic table is repositioned, increasing the risks of contamination and breaks in sterile technique. A simple, cost-effective solution to this problem has now been developed. A length of common house wire (8/3-gauge Romex) is shaped into an arc over the patient's neck. The ends of the wire are bent at right angles to the arc and tucked under the x-ray table padding at the level of the patient's shoulders (Fig. 18-8). The weight of the patient's shoulders supports the wire arc. The wire can be shaped to fit any patient. The wire positioned under the shoulder is checked with fluoroscopy to avoid interference with the radiographic field of view. The house wire is strong enough to keep its shape under the weight of the surgical drape, offering optimal patient comfort and a reliable sterile barrier. There is no interference with the C-arm, and claustrophobia is avoided. The traditional use of a Mayo stand over the patient's face is problematic, in that it can cause claustrophobia, makes access to the patient's airway difficult in an emergency, and may interfere with the x-ray equipment.

From the moment the catheterization laboratory or special studies room is cleaned, it must be treated as a surgical suite. All personnel must wear surgical clothing, hats, and masks. There should be an attempt to seal the room, limiting traffic and restricting access to personnel participating in the procedure.

Anesthesia, Sedation, and Pain Relief

Most pacemaker procedures are performed with local anesthesia and the addition of some form of sedation and pain reliever.[32] Local anesthesia alone is inadequate for optimal patient comfort. Even in the best of circumstances, the effect of local anesthesia does not avoid the discomfort associated with the creation of the pacemaker pocket. For this reason, the additional combination of a narcotic and sedative is recommended. The use of sedation alone is frequently inadequate. The challenge to the physician in charge is to achieve patient comfort without risking oversedation or respiratory depression. If an anesthesiologist or nurse anesthetist is part of the implantation team, patient comfort is usually achieved easily and safely. In this situation, if respiratory depression occurs, the patient can easily be ventilated. In the circumstance in which the implanting physician orders the sedation and narcotics, the patient must be carefully monitored by the circulating nurse. It is recommended that the medications be administered slowly.

The selection of local anesthetic and the dose delivered are also important considerations. The use of a local agent in therapeutic concentration that provides rapid onset of action and sustained duration is desirable. Local agents can be used in combination to achieve the desired effect. An example is the use of lidocaine for its rapid onset and bupivacaine for its sustained action. There is also an upper limit of total local anesthetic dose that should not be exceeded. Toxic blood levels of commonly used local anesthetics can result in profound neurologic abnormalities, including obtundation and seizures. Table 18-6 lists the pharmacologic properties of commonly used local anesthetic agents.

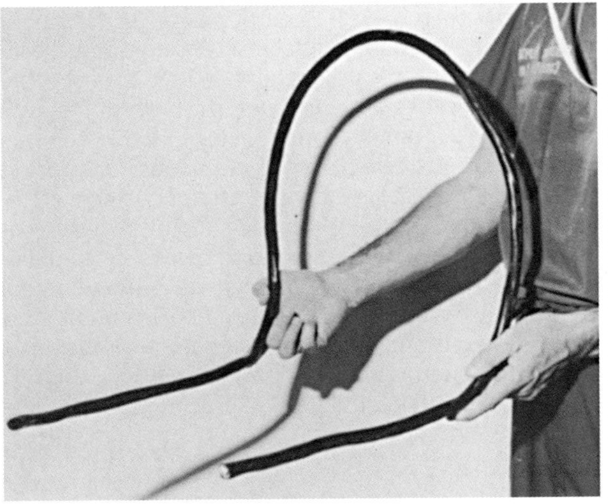

A

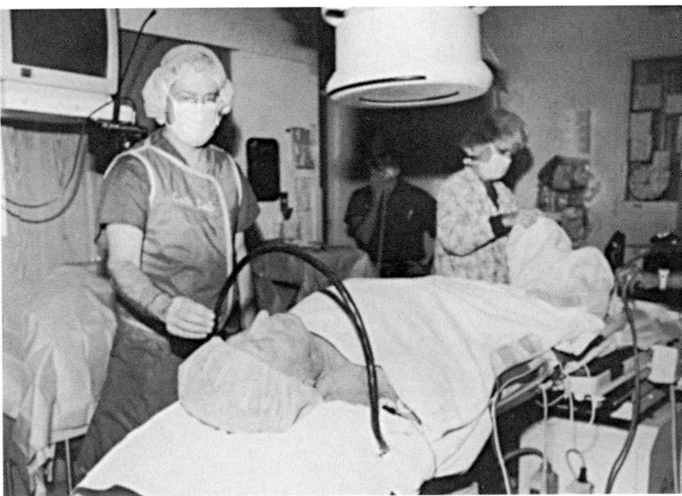

B

Figure 18-8. ***A*** *and* ***B,*** *House (Romex) wire shaped to form an arch over the patient's head is positioned under the patient's mattress and bent to accommodate differences in patients and circumstances.*

TABLE 18-6. Pharmacologic Properties of Commonly Used Local Anesthetic Agents

Agent	Onset (min)	Duration (hr)	Protein Binding (%)	Maximum Adult Dose
Esters:				
Chloroprocaine (Nesacaine)	Slow (5-10)	Short (0.5-1.5)	5	800 mg (11 μg/kg)
Procaine (Novocain)	Fast (5-15)	Short (0.5-1.5)	—	800 mg (11 μg/kg)
Tetracaine	Slow (20-30)	Long (3-5)	85	200 mg
Amides:				
Bupivacaine (Marcaine)	Moderate (10-20)	Long (3-5)	82-96	100 mg
Lidocaine (Xylocaine)	Fast (5-15)	Moderate (1-3)	55-65	300 mg (4 μg/kg)

TABLE 18-7. Drug Protocols for Conscious Sedation

Drug Name	Route of Administration	Dosage	Maximum	Comments
Meperidine	IM or IV	25-100 mg	100 mg	Long-acting
Morphine	IM or IV	1.5-15 mg	20 mg	Long-acting
Fentanyl	IM or IV	50-100 μg	100 mg	Very short-acting
Valium	IV	2-10 mg	10 mg	—
Droperidol	IV	8-17 mg/kg	17 mg/kg	—
Midazolam	IV	1-2.5 mg	5 mg	—
Nitrous oxide	Inhalation	30%-50%	50%	—
Thiopental	IV	1-4 mg/kg	—	Temporary LOC
Ketamine	IV	0.5 mg/kg	0.5 mg/kg	Temporary LOC

IM, intramuscular; IV, intravenous; LOC, loss of consciousness.

The selection of sedative and narcotic depends on personal preference. We use midazolam and fentanyl. The operator should become familiar with one or more sedative agents as well as an analgesic, preferably a narcotic. Many newer agents are available. The selection of a benzodiazepine in combination with a semi-synthetic narcotic can achieve ideal sedation, amnesia, and analgesia. A cooperative, relaxed, and pain-free patient is fundamental to the success of the procedure and the avoidance of complications. Pentothal and nitrous oxide have been used to effect brief periods of complete sedation at times of anticipated maximum discomfort, but the use of these drugs requires the expertise of an anesthetist because temporary respiratory support is frequently needed.

In the United States, the Joint Commission on Accreditation of Hospitals mandates that institutions establish a policy and protocol for patients receiving intravenous sedation. Pacemaker procedures would be included in such a protocol. In essence, the protocol requires formal patient assessment before sedation. Resuscitation equipment must be present at all times in the sedation and recovery areas, and patients undergoing intravenous sedation must be monitored with pulse oximetry, continuous ECG rhythm monitoring, and automatic blood pressure recordings. Monitoring of the patient should continue for at least 30 minutes after the last intravenous sedative drug administration and for at least 90 minutes after intramuscular sedative drug administration. There are also strict discharge criteria. Common intravenous sedation drug protocols are shown in Table 18-7.

On May 3, 1995, a National Association of Pacing and Electrophysiology (NASPE; now renamed Heart Rhythm Society) Policy Conference on IV sedation was held in Boston. An NASPE Expert Consensus document on the use of IV sedation/analgesia by non-anesthesia personnel in patients undergoing arrhythmia-specific diagnostic, therapeutic, and surgical procedures was generated.[33] The policy conference (1) reviewed the current state of the art with respect to conscious (intravenous) sedation, (2) reviewed current position statements developed by other relevant health professional groups, (3) reviewed the legal and licensing applications of IV sedation, (4) developed recommendations for the use of IV sedation, (5) specified the minimum training requirements for professionals administering IV sedation for arrhythmia-specific procedures, and (6) reviewed the cost-effectiveness and economic implications of IV sedation.

Antibiotic Prophylaxis and Wound Irrigation

The use of prophylactic antibiotics to reduce the incidence of postoperative wound infection in a pacemaker procedure is controversial.[34] It is important to point out that antibiotics are not a substitute for good infection control practices, an adequate surgical environment, and good surgical technique. The use of antibiotics in a pacemaker procedure follows the principle of prophylaxis, in which the risk for infection is low but the monetary penalty or morbidity is high.[35-37] The selection of antibiotics is based on site-specific flora for wound infection and the spectrum, kinetics, and toxicity of the antimicrobial agent. The risk factors for infection have been well defined. The National Research Council for Wound Classification places the risk for infection from an elective procedure with primary closure at less than 2%. One important factor to be considered is the higher risk for infection in operations lasting longer than 2 hours.

Although not formally studied, the use of prophylactic antibiotics in the low-risk, high-morbidity group, such as patients receiving pacemakers, appears justified. There are no specific references in the literature to antibiotic prophylaxis for pacemaker procedures, only for prosthetic devices. The spectrum of the antibiotic prophylaxis need only cover the gram-positive skin flora, primarily *Staphylococcus epidermidis* and *Staphylococcus aureus*. In the case of pacemakers and cardiac procedures, the cephalosporins appear ideal (i.e., 1 to 2 g of cefazolin IV, pre-anesthesia). Because many institutions have a high incidence of methicillin-resistant *S. aureus* or *S. epidermidis*, vancomycin should be considered (i.e., 1 g of vancomycin IV given slowly preoperatively). Postoperative doses are left to clinical judgment. Generally, 1 g of either drug may be given intravenously up to 8 hours postoperatively. Occasionally, the postoperative doses of cephalosporin are given orally for several days. These drug guidelines are also reflected in the January 1992 issue of *Medical Letter*[38]; it is interesting to note that this issue specifically does not recommend antibiotic prophylaxis for pacemaker procedures.

An additional strategy in the prevention of infection is topical antibiotic prophylaxis or antibiotic wound irrigation.[39] Controlled trials evaluating the benefit of antibiotic irrigations are lacking. The concept of irrigation is to provide a high concentration of antibiotic at the site of potential infection at the time of contamination. The technique has proved most efficient in the absence of established infection. It calls for the use of nonabsorbable antibiotics. Historically, aminoglycosides and bacitracin combinations have been used, but there are many regimens varying in number, type, concentration, and duration of antibiotic use. Systemic toxicity with antibiotic irrigation is a major concern. When large volumes of irrigating solutions are used in combination with systemic antibiotics, the therapeutic range can be greatly exceeded. The superiority of irrigation over systemic antibiotic administration has never been proved, and given the potential toxicity, caution in its use is recommended. Some popular antibiotic irrigation protocols are listed in Table 18-8.

Despite the controversial nature of prophylactic systemic antibiotics and topical irrigation, the experience of one of the authors (PHB) at the Pacemaker and Arrhythmia Center, El Cajon, California, has been very gratifying. A protocol of intravenous antibiotics and wound irrigation has been followed at this facility since 1978. In each case, 1 g of cefazolin was given intraoperatively, followed by cefadroxil monohydrate, 500 mg, twice daily for 4 days. A sponge soaked in povidone-iodine is placed in the pacemaker pocket just after pocket formation and is removed at the time of wound closure. In more than 1500 pacemaker procedures, there have been two wound infections. A similar low incidence of infection has occurred at the other author's (DWR) institution, University of Oklahoma College of Medicine, Oklahoma City, Oklahoma; since 1980, this institution's regimen has consisted of a preoperative dose of cefazolin, 1 g IV, followed by 1 g IV for one to five more doses every 8 hours (depending on length of stay), as well as pocket irrigation with a solution of bacitracin, gentamicin, and polymyxin. Although the issue is admittedly controversial, all the implanting physician needs to experience is one pacemaker infection with all of its problems to become convinced that infection should be avoided at all cost.

TABLE 18-8. Common Antimicrobial Irrigation Protocols

Agent	Concentration
Bacitracin	50,000 units in 200 mL of saline
Cephalothin	1 g/L of saline
Cefazolin	1 g/L of saline
Cefuroxime	750 mg/L of saline
Vancomycin	200-500 mg/L of saline
Povidone-iodine	Concentrated or diluted in aliquots of saline

Anatomic Approaches for Implantation

There are two basic anatomic approaches to the implantation of a permanent pacemaker.[40,41] From a historical perspective, the first is the epicardial approach, and the second the transvenous approach. The epicardial approach calls for direct application of pacemaker electrodes on the heart. This requires general anesthesia and surgical access to the epicardial surface of the heart. The transvenous approach is usually performed with local anesthesia and IV sedation. Each approach can be accomplished by several unique techniques. Today, 95% of all pacemaker implantations are performed transvenously.

The epicardial approach is generally reserved for patients who cannot undergo safe or effective pacemaker implantation by the transvenous route. The major epicardial techniques involve either applying the electrode(s) directly to a completely exposed heart or performing a limited thoracotomy through a subxiphoid incision (Fig. 18-9). A third technique places the leads via mediastinoscopy. There is even a fourth technique, which combines epicardial and endocardial lead placement.

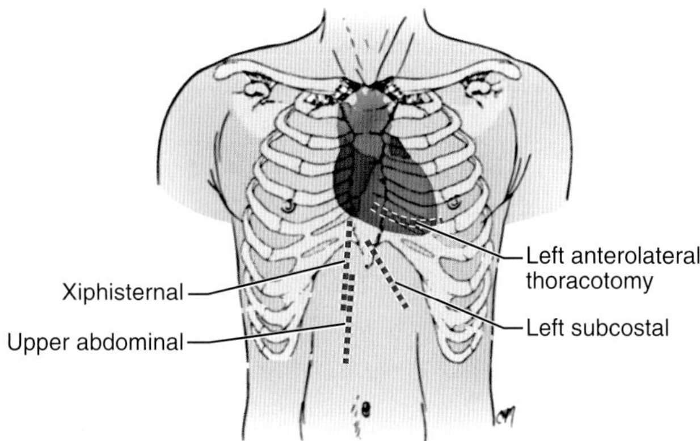

Figure 18-9. Location of surgical incisions for the placement of epimyocardial systems.

Several techniques are used for the transvenous approach. All involve a venous surgical cutdown, percutaneous venous access, or a combination of both (Table 18-9). The pros and cons of the various approaches and techniques are reviewed here.

A thorough knowledge of the anatomic structures of the neck, upper extremities, and thorax is essential for cardiac pacing (Fig. 18-10). The precise location and orientation of the internal jugular, innominate, subclavian, and cephalic veins are important for safe venous access.[42,43] Their anatomic relations to other structures is crucial to avoiding complications.

The venous anatomy of interest, from a cardiac pacing point of view, starts peripherally with the axillary vein.[43] This vessel is a large venous structure that represents the continuation of the basilic vein. It starts at the lower border of the teres major tendon and latissimus dorsi muscle. The axillary vein terminates immediately beneath the clavicle at the outer border of the first rib, where it becomes the subclavian vein. The axillary vein is covered anteriorly by the pectoralis minor and pectoralis major muscles and the costocoracoid membrane. It is anterior and medial to the axillary artery, which it partially overlaps. At the level of the coracoid process, the axillary vein is covered only by the clavicular head of the pectoralis major muscle (Fig. 18-11). At this juncture, the axillary vein receives

TABLE 18-9. Techniques for Axillary Venous Access

Techniques
Blind percutaneous puncture using surface landmarks
Blind puncture through the pectoralis major muscle using deep landmarks
Direct cutdown on the axillary vein
Fluoroscopy: Needle the first rib for reference
Contrast venography
Doppler guidance
Ultrasound guidance

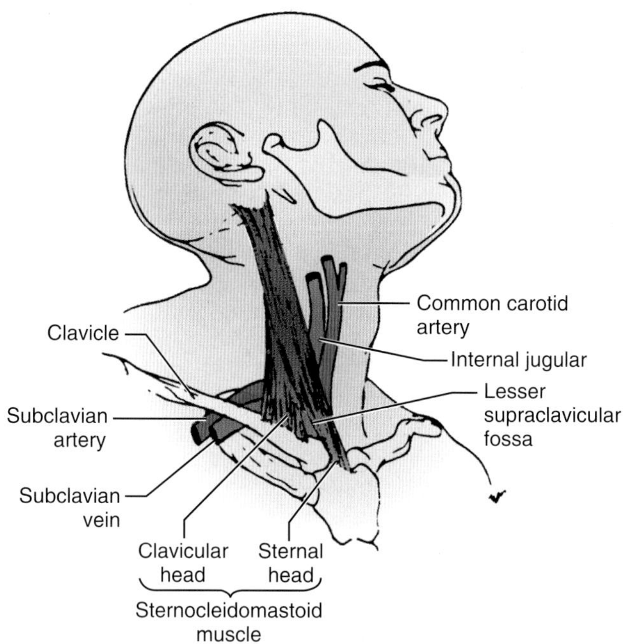

Figure 18-10. Anatomic relationship of the vascular structures in the neck and superior mediastinum.

the more superficial cephalic vein. The cephalic vein terminates in the deeper axillary vein at the level of the coracoid process beneath the pectoralis major muscle. The cephalic vein commonly used for pacemaker venous access is classified as a superficial vein of the upper extremity. This vein, which actually commences near the antecubital fossa, travels along the outer border of the biceps muscle and enters the deltopectoral groove. The deltopectoral groove is an anatomic structure formed by the deltoid muscle and clavicular head of the pectoralis major. The cephalic vein traverses the deltopectoral groove and superiorly pierces the costocoracoid membrane, crossing the axillary artery and terminating in the axillary vein just below the clavicle at the level of the coracoid process.

The subclavian vein is a continuation of the axillary vein. The subclavian vein extends from the outer border of the first rib to the inner end of the clavicle, where it joins with the internal jugular vein to form the brachiocephalic trunk or innominate vein. The subclavian vein is just inferior to the clavicle and subclavius muscle. The subclavian artery is located posterior and superior to the vein. These two structures are separated internally by the scalenus anticus muscle and phrenic nerve. Inferiorly, the subclavian vein is associated with a depression in the first rib and on the pleura. The brachiocephalic trunks or innominate veins are two large venous trunks located on each side of the base of the neck. The right innominate vein is relatively short. It starts at the inner end of the clavicle and passes vertically downward to join with the left innominate vein just below the cartilage of the first rib to form the superior vena cava (SVC). The left innominate vein is larger and longer than the right, passing from left to right for approximately 2.5 inches, where it joins with the right

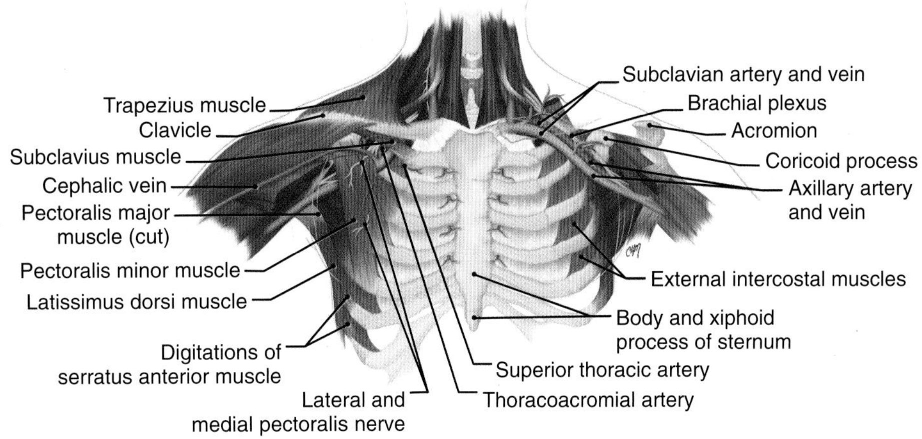

Figure 18-11. Detailed anatomy of the anterolateral chest demonstrating the axillary vein with the pectoralis major and pectoralis minor muscles removed.

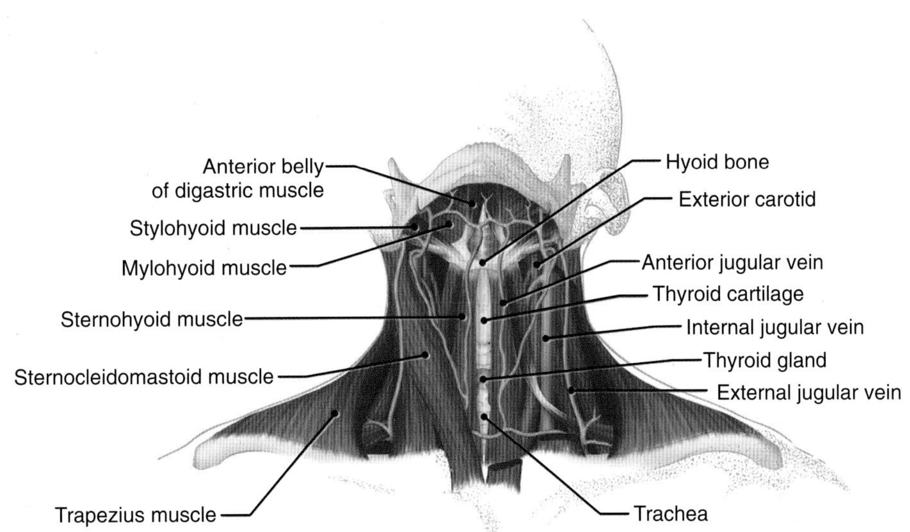

Figure 18-12. Detailed anatomy of the neck demonstrating the relationship of venous anatomy to the superficial and deep structures.

innominate vein to form the SVC. The left innominate vein is in the anterior and superior mediastinum.

The internal and external jugular veins have also been used for pacemaker venous access. The external jugular vein is a superficial vein of the neck that receives blood from the exterior cranium and face. This vein starts in the substance of the parotid gland, at the angle of the jaw, and runs perpendicular down the neck to the middle of the clavicle. In this course, it crosses the sternocleidomastoid muscle and runs parallel to its posterior border. At the attachment of the sternocleidomastoid muscle to the clavicle, this vein perforates the deep fascia and terminates in the subclavian vein just anterior to the scalenus anticus muscle. The external jugular vein is separated from the sternocleidomastoid muscle by a layer of deep cervical fascia. Superficially, it is covered by the platysma muscle, superficial fascia, and skin. The external jugular vein can vary in size and may even be duplicated. Because of its superficial orientation, the external jugular vein is less commonly used for cardiac pacing venous access (Fig. 18-12).

The internal jugular vein is an unusual site for pacemaker venous access. Because of its larger size and deeper and more protected orientation, however, the internal jugular vein is used more frequently than the external jugular vein,. The internal jugular vein starts just external to the jugular foramen at the base of the skull. It drains blood from the interior of the cranium as well as superficial parts of the head and neck. This vein is oriented vertically as it runs down the side of the neck. Superiorly, it is lateral to the internal carotid and inferolateral to the common carotid. At the base of the neck, the internal jugular vein joins the subclavian vein to form the innominate vein. The internal jugular vein is large and lies in the cervical triangle defined by the lateral border of the omohyoid muscle, the inferior border of the digastric muscle, and the medial border of the sternocleidomastoid muscle. The superficial cervical fascia and platysma muscle cover the vein, which is easily identified just lateral to the easily palpable external carotid artery.

From a venous access perspective, the location of the subclavian vein may vary from a normal lateral course to an extremely anterior or posterior orientation in elderly patients. Byrd[44] has described the subclavian venous anatomy of two distinct deformities, both of

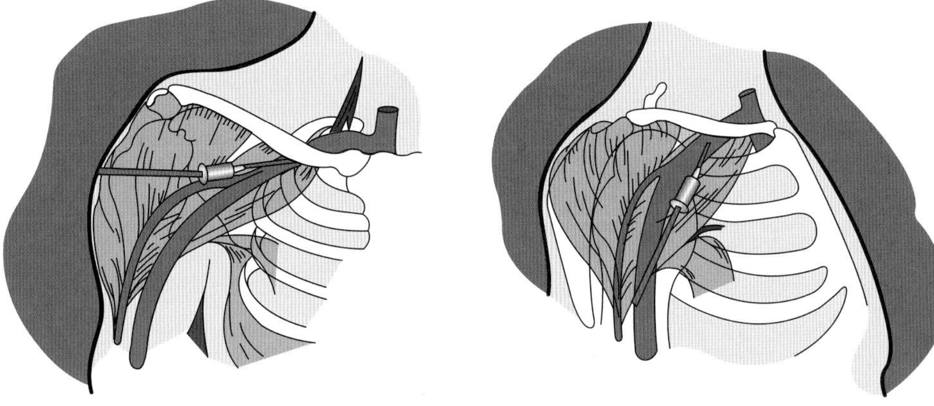

Figure 18-13. Posterior displacement of the clavicle, signified by a horizontal rather than oblique position of the deltopectoral groove. (From Byrd CL: Current clinical applications of dual-chamber pacing. In Zipes DP [ed]: Proceedings of a Symposium. Minneapolis: Medtronic, Inc, 1981, p 71.)

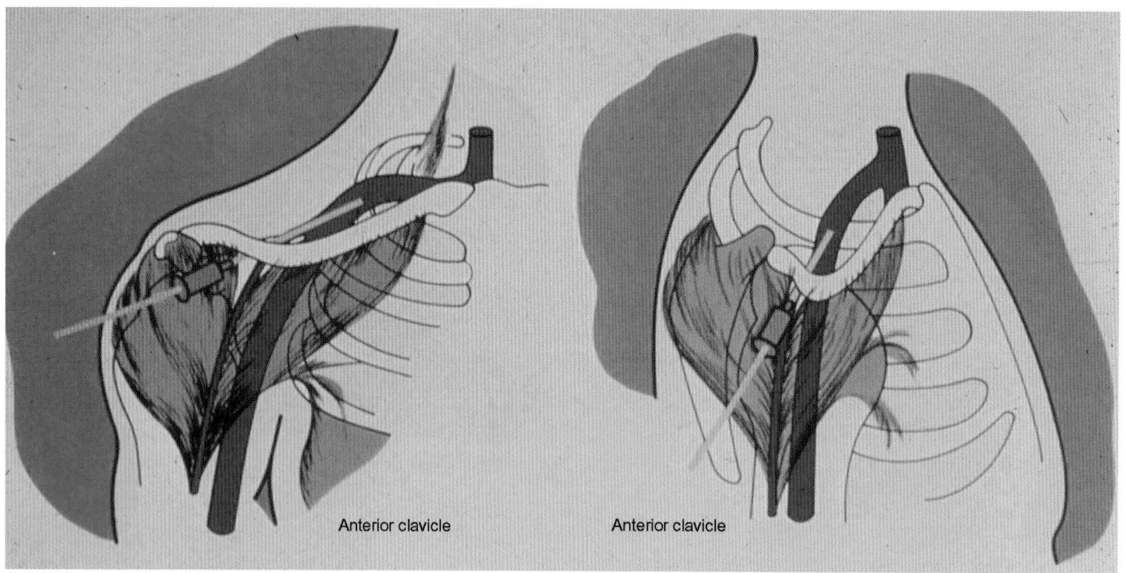

Figure 18-14. Anterior displacement of the clavicle. The deltopectoral groove is nearly vertical. (From Byrd CL: Current clinical applications of dual-chamber pacing. In Zipes DP [ed]: Proceedings of a Symposium. Minneapolis: Medtronic, Inc, 1981, p 71.)

which make venous access more difficult and hazardous. The first deformity involves a posteriorly displaced clavicle (Fig. 18-13). This is commonly seen in patients with chronic lung disease and anteroposterior chest enlargement. Such patients can be identified from the presence of a horizontal deltopectoral groove and the posteriorly displaced clavicle. The second deformity is an anteriorly displaced clavicle (Fig. 18-14), which is found occasionally, especially in elderly women. In this situation, the clavicle is anteriorly bowed or actually displaced anteriorly. It is important that the implanting physician recognize such variations so as to avoid complications such as pneumothorax and hemopneumothorax when using the percutaneous approach.

It is assumed that the implanting physician is also completely familiar with the anatomy of the heart and great vessels.[45] However, their spatial orientation is at times confusing, particularly with respect to the right atrium (RA) and RV. In the frontal plane, the border of the right side of the heart is formed by the RA. The border of the left side of the heart is composed of the LV. Importantly, the RV is located anteriorly (Fig. 18-15) and is triangular. The apex of the RV is the generally accepted initial "target" for ventricular lead placement. Unfortunately, the location of the apex of the RV can vary. Its normal location, distinctly to the left of midline, depends on the rotation of the heart, which is affected by various pathologic and anatomic conditions. At times, it may be located directly anterior to or even to the right of midline. A lack of appreciation of these variations can lead to considerable difficulty in electrode placement.

The choice of site for pacemaker implantation is also occasionally important anatomically. This decision is typically made most appropriately on the basis of the patient's dominant hand, occupation, recreational activities, and medical conditions. The decision should

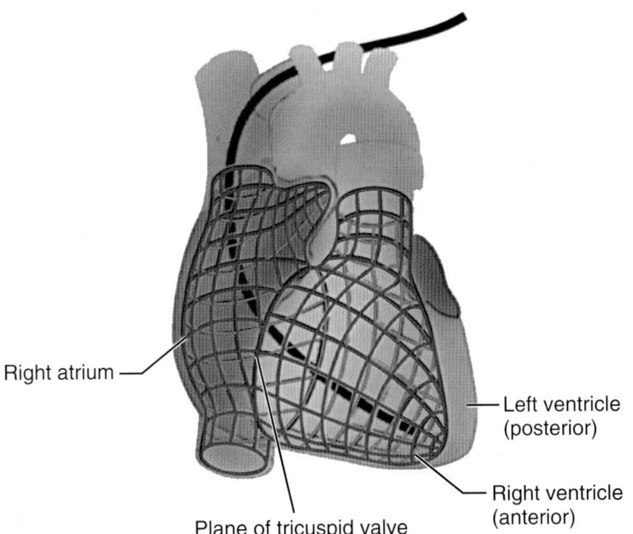

Figure 18-15. The spatial orientation of the right ventricle as an anterior structure in relationship to the left or posterior ventricle or coronary sinus, which is also posterior.

not be made according to the dominant hand of the implanting physician. There are, however, some fundamental differences between the anatomy of the right side and that of the left side. These differences can result in frustration when one is passing a pacemaker electrode. It seems to be easier for many right-handed implanters to work on the right side of the patient (and vice versa), but from a surgical point of view, catheter manipulation from the right can be a frustrating experience. When entering the central venous circulation from the left upper limb, the pacemaker electrode tracks along a smooth arc to the RV. There are generally no sharp angles or bends (Fig. 18-16A). Conversely, when approaching from the right, the electrode is forced to negotiate a sharp angle or bend at the junction of the right subclavian and internal jugular veins, where the innominate vein is formed (see Fig. 18-16B). This acute angulation can make the manipulation of the pacemaker electrode difficult when a curved stylet

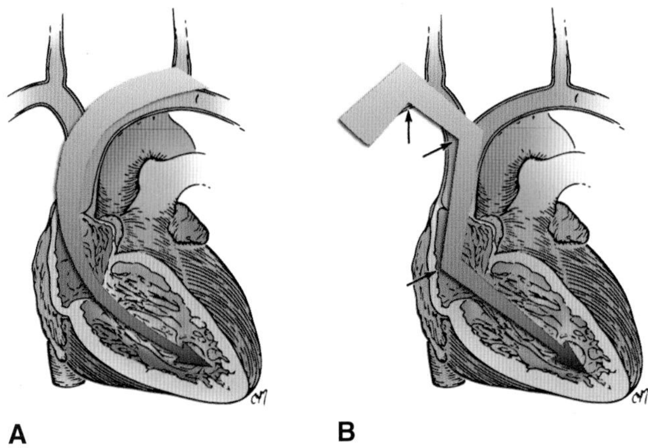

*Figure 18-16. **A,** Smooth course of an electrode entering from the left side. **B,** Acute angulation of the catheter course when the lead enters the venous system from the right.*

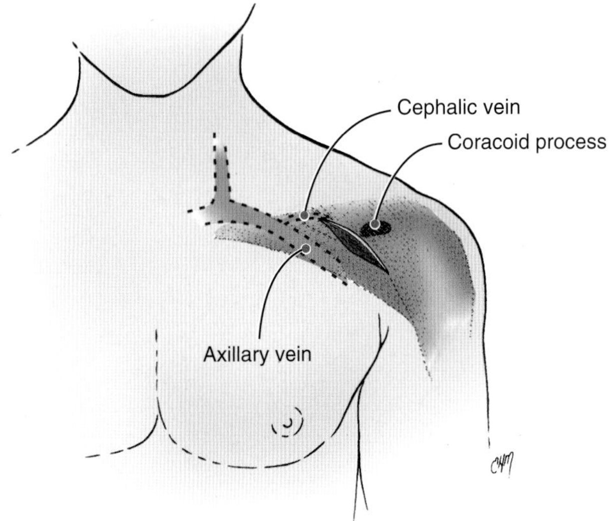

Figure 18-17. Anatomy of the deltopectoral groove.

is fully inserted. Another anatomic pitfall occurs when there is a persistent left SVC, making passage to the heart from the left more difficult and, if there is no right SVC, makes passage from the right impossible. These situations are considered later, in the discussion of ventricular electrode placement.

Transvenous Pacemaker Placement

Cephalic Venous Access

The right or left cephalic vein is the most common vascular entry site for insertion of pacemaker electrodes by the cutdown technique.[46] The cephalic vein is located in the deltopectoral groove (Fig. 18-17), which is formed by the reflections of the medial head of the deltoid and the lateral border of the greater pectoral muscles. The groove can be precisely located by palpating the coracoid process of the scapula. The dermis along the deltopectoral groove is infiltrated with local anesthetic, encompassing the anticipated length of the incision. A vertical incision is made adjacent to and at the level of the coracoid process. It is extended for about 2 to 5 cm. Care is taken to keep the scalpel blade perpendicular to the surface of the skin. One can create smooth skin edges by making an initial single stroke that carries through the dermis to each corner of the wound. The subcutaneous tissue is infiltrated with local anesthetic along the edges of the incision. The Weitlaner retractor is applied to the edges of the wound, and the subcutaneous tissue is placed under tension. The tension is released by light strokes of the scalpel from corner to corner of the wound in the midline. As the subcutaneous tissue falls away, tension is restored by reapplication of the Weitlaner retractor. This process is continued down to the surface of the pectoral fascia. The fascia is left intact. At this level, the borders of the pectoral and deltoid muscles forming the deltopectoral groove are identified. A Metzenbaum scissors is used to dissect along the groove by separating the muscles' fibrous attachments. The Weitlaner

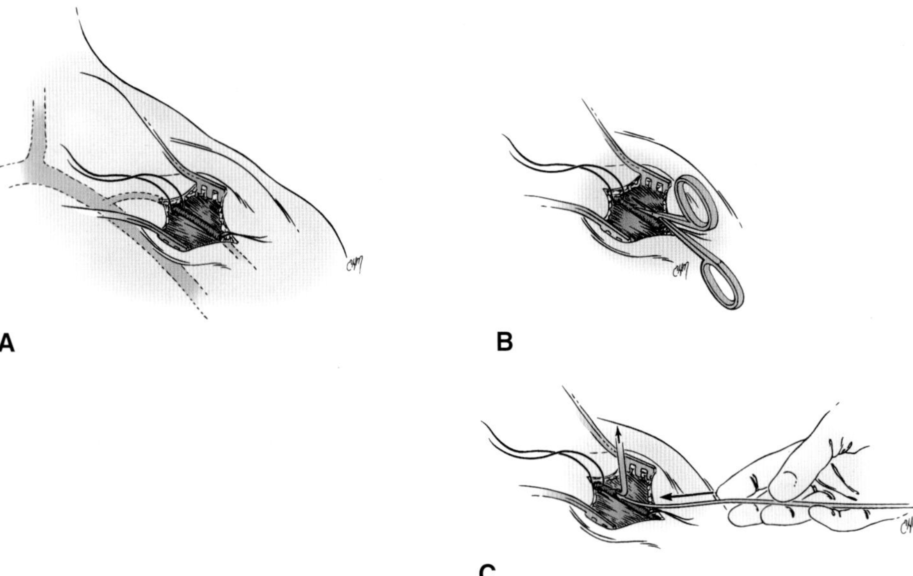

Figure 18-18. ***A,*** *Introduction of a lead into the cephalic vein, which is isolated and tied off distally.* ***B,*** *Venotomy performed with iris scissors.* ***C,*** *Lead inserted while venotomy is held open with a vein pick.*

retractor is reapplied more deeply to retract the muscle. Gradual release of the fascial tissue between the two muscle bodies will expose the cephalic vein.

At times, the cephalic vein is diminutive or atretic and unable to accommodate a pacemaker lead. In this case, the cephalic vein can be dissected, centrally, to the axillary vein, and this larger vein catheterized. Once the vein to be catheterized is localized, it is freed of all fibrous attachments. Ligatures are applied proximally and distally (Fig. 18-18A). The distal ligature is tied and held by a small clamp. The proximal ligature is not tied but is kept under tension with another clamp. An arbitrary entry site is chosen between the two ligatures. The anterior one half of the vein at this site is grasped with a smooth forceps, and the vein is gently lifted. A small horizontal venotomy is made with iris scissors (see Fig. 18-18B) or a No. 11 scalpel blade. The vein is continuously supported by the forceps. The venotomy is held open by any of several means: a mosquito clamp, forceps, or vein pick. Gentle traction is applied on the distal ligature while tension is released on the proximal ligature. With the venotomy held widely open, the electrode or electrodes are inserted and advanced into the central venous circulation (see Fig. 18-18C).

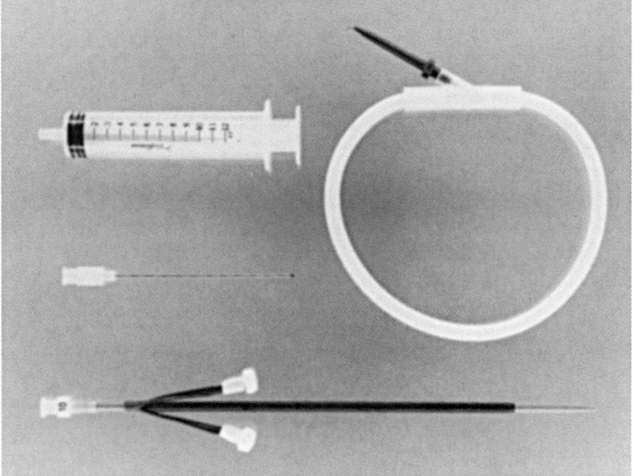

Figure 18-19. Prepackaged introducer set with 18-gauge needle, guidewire, and sheath with rubber dilator.

Subclavian Venous Access

For many years, vascular access has been achieved for many purposes through the use of the Seldinger technique. This simple approach calls for the percutaneous puncture of the vessel with a relatively long, large-bore needle; passage of a wire through the needle into the vessel; removal of the needle; and passage of a catheter or sheath over the wire into the vessel with removal of the wire. An 18-gauge, thin-walled needle 5 cm in length is commonly used, although smaller needles are available. These needles come prepackaged with most introducer sets (Fig. 18-19), but an extra supply should be available. The historical problem limiting the use of this technique in cardiac pacing was the inability to remove the sheath from the pacemaker lead. The development of a peel-away sheath by Littleford solved this problem.[47-50]

Use of the percutaneous approach requires a thorough knowledge of both normal and abnormal anatomy to avoid complications. The subclavian vein is generally the intended venous structure used for percutaneous venous access in cardiac pacing. Given the previously discussed anatomic variations, the subclavian vein puncture is typically made near the apex of the angle formed by the first rib and clavicle.[51] This defines the "subclavian window" (Fig. 18-20). At this puncture site (and after both skin infiltration with local anesthetic and a 1-cm incision at the site, which generally is 1 to 2 cm inferolateral to the point where the clavicle and first rib actually cross), the needle is aimed in a medial and cephalic direction. It is important to make the puncture with the patient in a "normal"

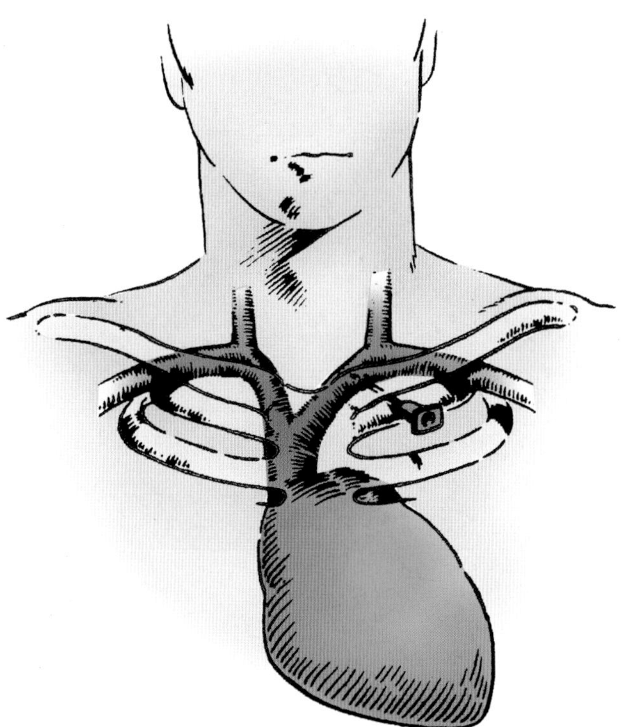

Figure 18-20. The subclavian window. (From Barold SS, Mugica J: New Perspectives in Cardiac Pacing. Armonk, NY, Futura, 1988, p 257.)

anatomic position. The infraclavicular space or costoclavicular angle should not be artificially opened by maneuvers such as extending the arm or placing a towel roll between the scapulae. These maneuvers can open a normally closed or tight space and lead to undesirable puncture of the costoclavicular ligament or subclavius muscle, which in turn can result in lead entrapment and crush. With the patient in the normal anatomic position, access to the subclavian window is medial yet usually avoids the costoclavicular ligament. The more medial puncture and needle trajectory of this approach vastly improves the success rate and dramatically reduces the risks of pneumothorax and vascular injury compared with a more lateral approach. With this medial position, the vein is a much larger target and the apex of the lung is more lateral. This safer approach is a departure from the conventional subclavian venous puncture, which calls for introduction of the needle in the middle third of the clavicle.

There are legitimate concerns that this medial approach, although safer, results later in higher rates of complications and of failure from conductor fracture and insulation damage.[51] It is postulated that the extreme medial position results in a tight fit, subjecting the lead to compressive forces and causing binding between the first rib and the clavicle. Occasionally, this binding can even crush the lead and today is called the *subclavian crush phenomenon*. This phenomenon is more common in larger, complex leads of the in-line bipolar, coaxial design. Fortunately, the incidence of this complication is low. Fyke[53,54] first reported insulation failure of two leads placed side by side with use of the percutaneous approach through the subclavian vein, where there was a tight costoclavicular space. This issue has now been addressed thoroughly by two independent groups. Jacobs and associates[55] analyzed a series of failed leads for the mechanism of failure. They used autopsy studies to correlate the anatomic relationship of lead position to compressive forces (Fig. 18-21). These autopsy data demonstrated generation of significantly higher pressure when leads were inserted in the costoclavicular angle than with a more lateral puncture. They concluded that the tight costoclavicular angle should be avoided. Magney and colleagues[56] derived similar data from cadaveric studies and suggested that lead damage is caused by soft tissue entrapment by the subclavius muscle rather than bony contact. This soft tissue entrapment causes a static load on the lead at that point, and repeated flexure around the point of entrapment may be responsible for the damage.

Concern about this problem has also been communicated by pacemaker manufacturers in company literature.[57,58] Reduction in lead diameter and, perhaps, modification of lead technology may be required to eliminate this problem. In the meantime, technique modification appears to be effective at reducing the occurrence of this problem. In our experience, if a pacemaker lead feels tight in the costoclavicular space, it is more susceptible to being crushed; it has become our practice at the University of Oklahoma (DWR) to remove the lead from the vein in this situation and repuncture the vein in a slightly different location with reintroduction of the lead. We believe that this practice has reduced the incidence of crush, although more substantial modifications in technique, described later, may be indicated.

Addressing this issue, along with other introducer- or percutaneous-related complications, Byrd[59] has described a "safe introducer technique." This technique consists of a "safety zone" associated with precise conditions ensuring a safe puncture. Byrd also describes a new technique for cannulating the axillary vein if this safety zone cannot be entered. Byrd's safety zone is defined as a region of venous access between the first rib and the clavicle, extending laterally from the sternum in an arc (Fig. 18-22A). As a condition for puncture, the site of access must be adequate for ease of insertion to avoid friction and puncture of bone, cartilage, or tendon. With this technique, subclavian vein puncture should never be made outside the safety zone or in violation of the preceding conditions. If the safety zone is inaccessible, or the preceding conditions are not met, an axillary vein puncture is recommended. As previously mentioned, the axillary vein is actually a continuation of the subclavian vein after it exits the superior mediastinum and crosses the first rib. The axillary vein is also frequently referred to as the *extrathoracic portion* of the subclavian vein (Fig. 18-23).

Axillary Venous Access

The axillary vein approach is actually not new. In 1987, on the basis of cadaveric studies that established reli-

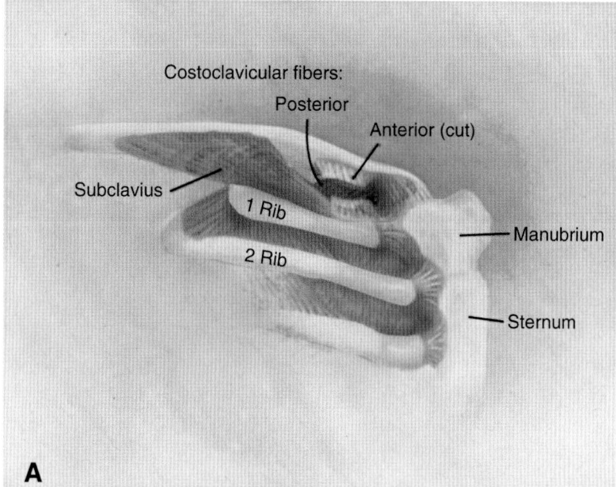

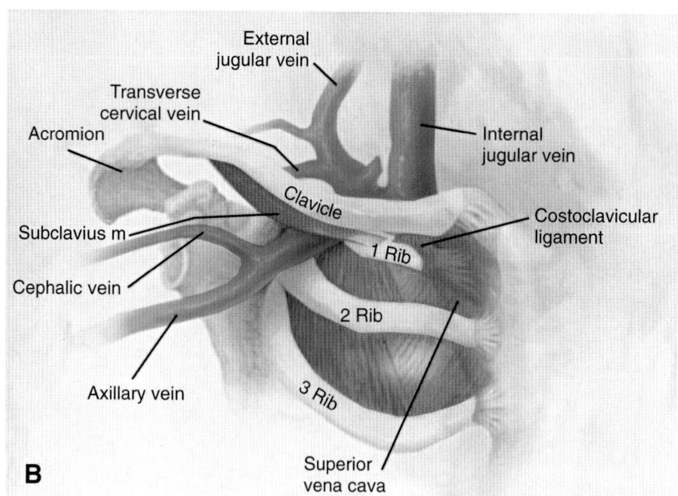

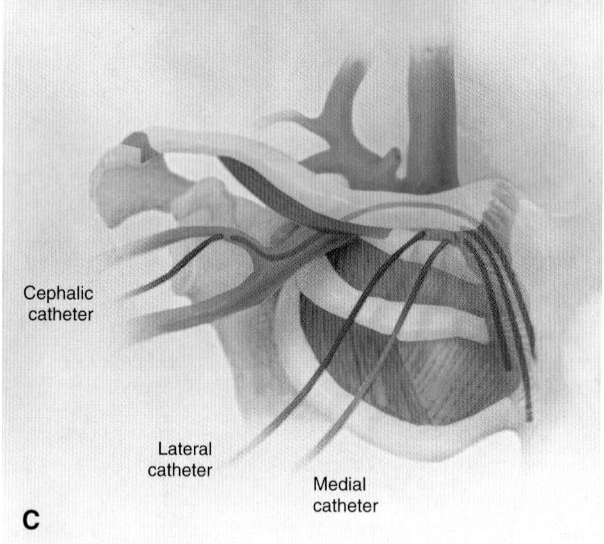

Figure 18-21. ***A,*** *Musculoskeletal anatomy of the infraclavicular space.* ***B,*** *The relationship of the venous structures to clavicle, first rib, and costoclavicular ligaments.* ***C,*** *Course of leads through the venous structures demonstrating how the pacemaker electrode can become entrapped. (From Jacobs DM, Fink AS, Miller RP, et al: Anatomical and morphological evaluation of pacemaker lead compression. PACE 16:434, 1993.)*

able surface landmarks, Nichalls[60] and Taylor and Yellowlees[61] reported this approach as an alternative safe route of venous access for large central lines. The axillary vein has a completely infraclavicular course. The needle path must always be anterior to the thoracic cavity, avoiding risks of pneumothorax and hemothorax. The suggested landmarks for this infraclavicular course of the axillary vein are as follows (Fig. 18-24).

The axillary vein starts medially at a point below the aspect of the clavicle where the space between the first rib and the clavicle becomes palpable. The vein extends laterally to a point about three fingerbreadths below the inferior aspect of the coracoid process. The skin is punctured along the medial border of the smaller pectoralis muscle at a point above the vein as it is defined by the surface landmarks. One punctures the axillary vein by passing the needle anterior to the first rib, maneuvering posteriorly and medially corresponding to the lateral to medial course of the axillary vein. The needle never passes between the first rib and the clavicle, but stays lateral to this juncture. Some implanters have found it useful to abduct the arm 45 degrees when using this approach.

In the technique described by Byrd, the axillary vein puncture is performed as a modification of the standard subclavian vein procedure without repositioning of the patient (Fig. 18-25; see Fig. 18-20B). The introducer needle is guided by fluoroscopy directly to the medial portion of the first rib. The needle is held perpendicular to, and touches, the first rib. The needle, held perpendicular to the rib, is "walked" laterally and posteriorly, touching the rib with each change of position. Once the vein is punctured, as indicated by aspiration of venous blood into the syringe, the guidewire and the introducer are inserted with use of standard technique. This approach essentially guarantees a successful and safe venipuncture without compromising the leads if the conditions for entering the safety zone are adhered to and if the first rib is touched to maintain orientation. The only complication not prevented by this approach is inadvertent puncture of the axillary artery.

Byrd[62] has reported success in a series of 213 consecutive cases in which the extrathoracic portion of the subclavian vein (axillary vein) was successfully cannulated as a primary approach. Magney and associates[63] subsequently reported a new approach to per-

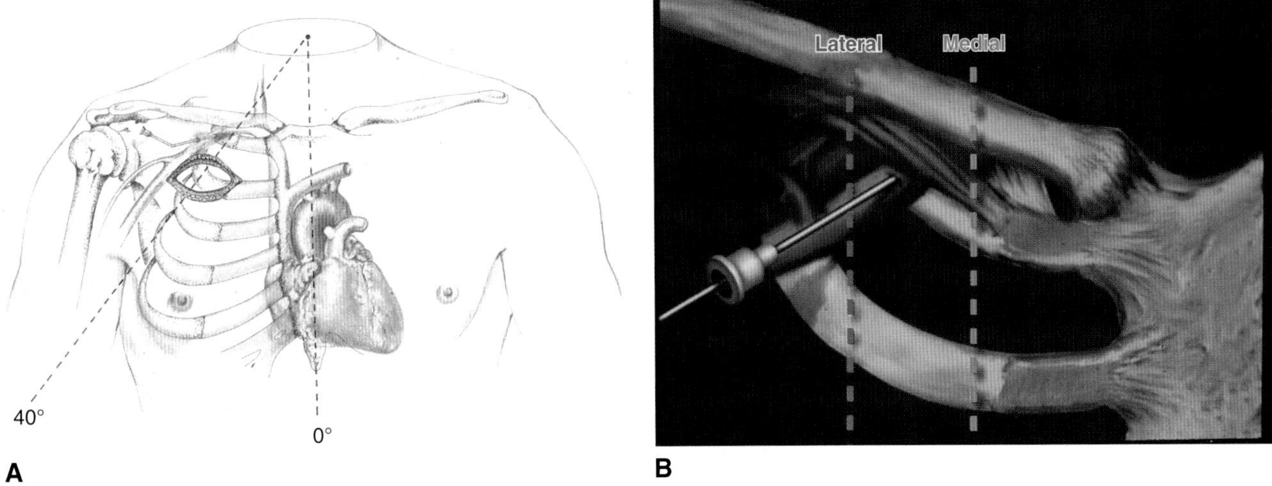

Figure 18-22. ***A,*** *Anatomic orientation of the "safety zone" for intrathoracic subclavian vein puncture.* ***B,*** *Safe access to the extrathoracic portion of the subclavian vein as described by Byrd. (**A** from Barold SS, Mugica J: New Perspectives in Cardiac Pacing 2. Armonk, NY, Futura, 1991, p 108; **B** from Byrd CL: Recent developments in pacemaker implantation and lead retrieval. PACE 16:1781, 1993.)*

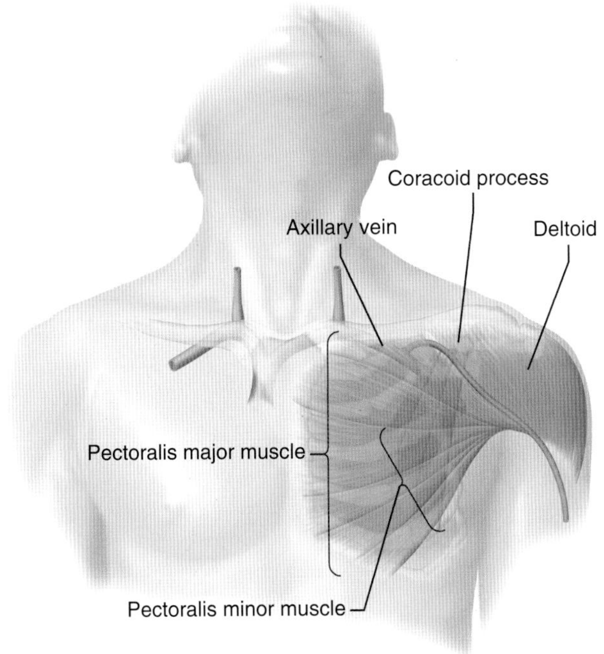

Figure 18-23. Anatomic relation of the axillary vein to the pectoralis minor muscle. The pectoralis major muscle has been removed. Note the cephalic vein draining directly into the axillary vein at approximately the first intercostal space. (From Belott PH, et al: Unusual access sites for permanent cardiac pacing. In Barold SS, Mugica J [eds]: Recent Advances in Pacing for the 21st Century. Armonk, NY, Futura, 1998, p 139.)

cutaneous subclavian venipuncture to avoid lead fracture. This technique is very similar to Byrd's and uses extensive surface landmarks for venipuncture (Fig. 18-26). It involves puncture of the extrathoracic portion of the subclavian vein. Magney and associates[63] define the location of the axillary vein as the intersection with a line drawn between the middle of the sternal angle and the tip of the coracoid process. This is generally near the lateral border of the first rib.

Belott[64] described blind axillary venous access using a modification of the Byrd and Magney recommendations. In this technique, the deltopectoral groove and coracoid process are primary landmarks. The deltopectoral groove and coracoid process are palpated, and the curvature of the chest wall is noted (Fig. 18-27). An incision is made at the level of the coracoid process. It is carried medially for about 2.5 inches and is perpendicular to the deltopectoral groove (Fig. 18-28). The incision is carried to the surface of the pectoralis major muscle. The deltopectoral groove is visualized on the surface of the muscle. The needle is inserted at an angle 45 degrees to the surface of the pectoralis muscle and parallel to the deltopectoral groove and 1 to 2 cm medial (Fig. 18-29). If the vein is not entered, fluoroscopy is then used to define the first rib (Fig. 18-30), which is an extremely reliable landmark for axillary venous access. With fluoroscopy guidance, the needle is advanced to touch the first rib. Caution should be used so as to avoid passing the needle into the interspace between the first and second ribs, which would cause a pneumothorax. The needle tip should be placed over the rib with fluoroscopic guidance; the needle angle should be gradually increased while being advanced until the rib is touched. Then one can "walk" the needle along the rib medially and laterally until the vein is entered.

At present, the blind venous access approach has been abandoned (PHB) for this first rib approach, because it reduces the risk of pneumothorax to zero. Critical to its success is the ability to identify the first or second rib on a radiograph. In addition, if the first rib is poorly visualized or set too far under the clavicle, one can always use the second rib in a similar fashion. Sequential needle punctures are "walked" laterally and posteriorly until the vein is entered (Fig. 18-31). Occasionally, in a thin patient, the axillary artery can

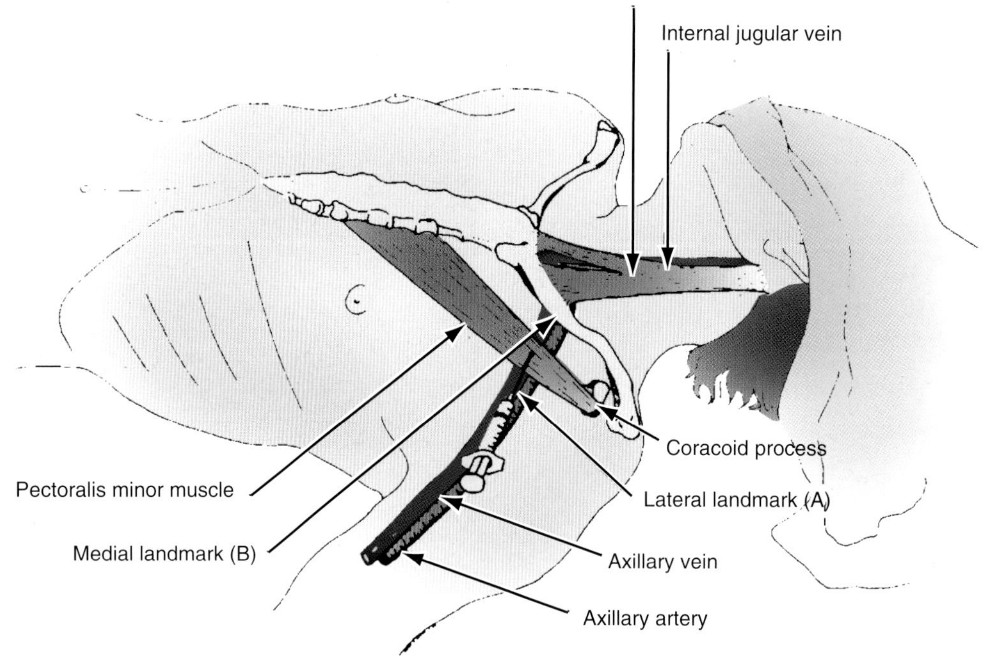

Figure 18-24. Nichalls' landmarks for axillary venipuncture. (From Belott PH, Byrd CL: Recent developments in pacemaker implantation and lead retrieval. In Barold SS, Mugica J [eds]: New Perspectives in Cardiac Pacing. Armonk, NY, Futura, 1991.)

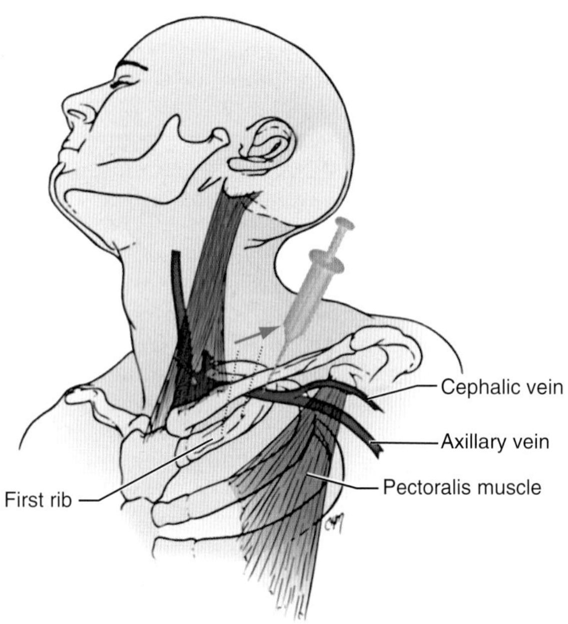

Figure 18-25. Byrd's technique for access to the extrathoracic portion of the subclavian vein. Sequential needle punctures are walked posterolateral along the first rib. (From Belott PH, Byrd CL: Recent developments in pacemaker implantation and lead retrieval. In Barold SS, Mugica J [eds]: New Perspectives in Cardiac Pacing. Armonk, NY, Futura, 1991.)

be easily palpated. This makes the axillary vein stick easy, because the percutaneous puncture can be made just medial and inferior to the palpable axillary pulse. Because one cannot always palpate the axillary pulse, it is not a reliable landmark. The axillary artery and brachial plexus are usually much deeper and more posterior structures. This simple technique, which uses basic anatomic landmarks of the deltopectoral groove and a blind venous stick, has been used successfully in 168 consecutive pacemaker and ICD procedures. There have only been three failures requiring an alternative approach. With a thorough knowledge of the regional anatomy, one can safely use the axillary vein as a primary site for venous access.

Access to the axillary vein may also be achieved by direct cutdown. With Metzenbaum scissors, fibers of the pectoralis major muscle are separated adjacent to the deltopectoral groove at the level of the coracoid process. This is just above the level of the superior border of the pectoralis minor. If the pectoralis major muscle is split in this area and the fibers are gently teased apart in an axis parallel to the muscle bundle, the axillary vein can be found directly beneath the pectoralis major muscle. A purse-string stitch is applied to the axillary vein, which can then be cannulated by a direct puncture or cutdown technique. The purse-string stitch will serve for hemostasis and ultimately assists in anchoring the electrodes after positioning.

A number of techniques can facilitate access to the axillary vein. Varnagy and coworkers[65] described a technique for isolating the cephalic and axillary veins by introduction of a radiopaque J-tipped polytetrafluoroethylene guidewire through a vein in the antecubital fossa under fluoroscopic control (Fig. 18-32). The metal guidewire is then palpated in the deltopectoral groove or identified with fluoroscopy. This guides the subsequent cutdown or puncture of the vessel with fluoroscopy. A cutdown can be performed on a vein, and the intravascular guidewire pulled out of the venotomy

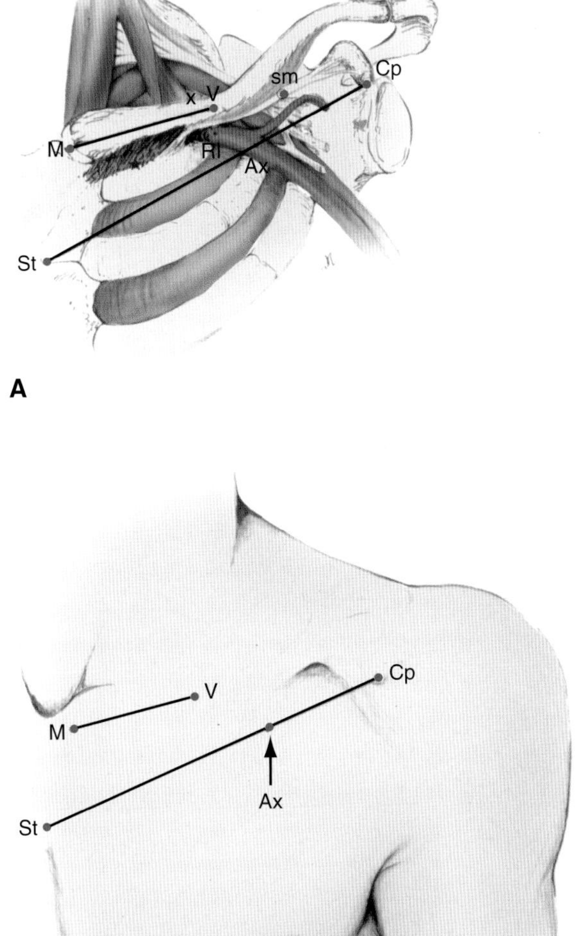

*Figure 18-26. Deep (**A**) and superficial (**B**) anatomic relationships of the Magney approach to subclavian venipuncture. Point M indicates the medial end of the clavicle. X defines a point on the clavicle directly above the lateral edges of the clavicular/subclavius muscle (tendon complex) (R1). The* arrow *indicates the center of the subclavian vein as it crosses the first rib. Ax, axillary vein; Cp, coracoid process; sm, subclavius muscle; St, center of the sternal angle.* Arrow *points to Magney's ideal point for venous entry. (From Magney JE, Staplin DH, Flynn DM, et al: A new approach to percutaneous subclavian needle puncture to avoid lead fracture or central venous catheter occlusion. PACE 16:2133, 1993.)*

to allow the application of an introducer. If a percutaneous approach is used, the puncture can always be extrathoracic, with fluoroscopy used to guide the needle to the guidewire. This technique offers the benefit of rapid venous access while avoiding the risk of pneumothorax associated with the percutaneous approach.

Contrast venography, described subsequently, can also be used for axillary venous access. The venous anatomy can be observed with contrast fluoroscopy in the pectoral area and, if possible, recorded for repeat viewing. The needle trajectory and venipuncture are guided by the contrast material in the axillary vein. Laboratories with sophisticated imaging capabilities can create an image "mask" (see later). Spencer and colleagues[66,67] reported the use of contrast material for localizing the axillary vein in 22 consecutive patients. Similarly, Ramza and associates[68] demonstrated the safety and efficacy of using the axillary vein for placement of pacemaker and defibrillator leads when guided with contrast venography. They successfully accomplished lead placement in 49 of 50 patients using this technique.

Access to the axillary vein can also be guided by Doppler flow detection and ultrasound techniques. Fyke[69] has described use of an extrathoracic introducer insertion technique in 59 consecutive patients (total of 100 leads) with a simple Doppler flow detector. A sterile Doppler flow detector is moved along the clavicle. Once the vein is defined, the location and angulation of probe are noted, and the venipuncture is carried out (Fig. 18-33). Care is taken to avoid directing the Doppler beam beneath the clavicle. Gayle and coworkers[70,71] have developed an ultrasound technique that directly visualizes the needle puncture of the axillary vein. A portable ultrasound device with sterile sleeve and needle holder are used. The ultrasound head is placed over the skin surface in the vicinity of the axillary vein. Once the vein is visualized, the puncture technique can be used. This technique has been used with considerable success for both pacing and defibrillator electrodes. There have been no reports of pneumothoraces. This technique can be carried out transcutaneously or through the incision on the surface of the pectoralis muscle (Figs. 18-34 and 18-35).

In summary, the axillary vein is becoming a common venous access site for pacemaker and defibrillator implantations, because of concerns about subclavian crush and the requirement for insertion of multiple electrodes for dual-chamber pacing and at least one large complex electrode for transvenous defibrillation. A number of reliable techniques are available for axillary venous access (see Table 18-9). Given the recent interest in the axillary vein, it is recommended that the implanting physician become thoroughly familiar with the relevant anatomy. The interested physician must visit the anatomic laboratory to refresh and review the regional anatomy and surface landmarks.

For a more conventional subclavian vein approach, Lamas and colleagues[72] have even recommended fluoroscopic observation of the needle trajectory for achieving a successful and safe subclavian vein puncture. They initially identify the clavicle on the side of the puncture, noting its course and landmarks. The skin is entered about 2 cm inferior to the junction of the medial and lateral halves of the clavicle, aiming with fluoroscopic guidance for the caudal half of the clavicular head.

The various techniques of transvenous pacemaker lead placement—the subclavian window, the safety zone, the axillary vein puncture, or fluoroscopic guidance—have some common features. Needle orientation is always medial and cephalad, almost tangential to the chest wall. All needle probing should use a forward motion. Lateral needle probing should be avoided

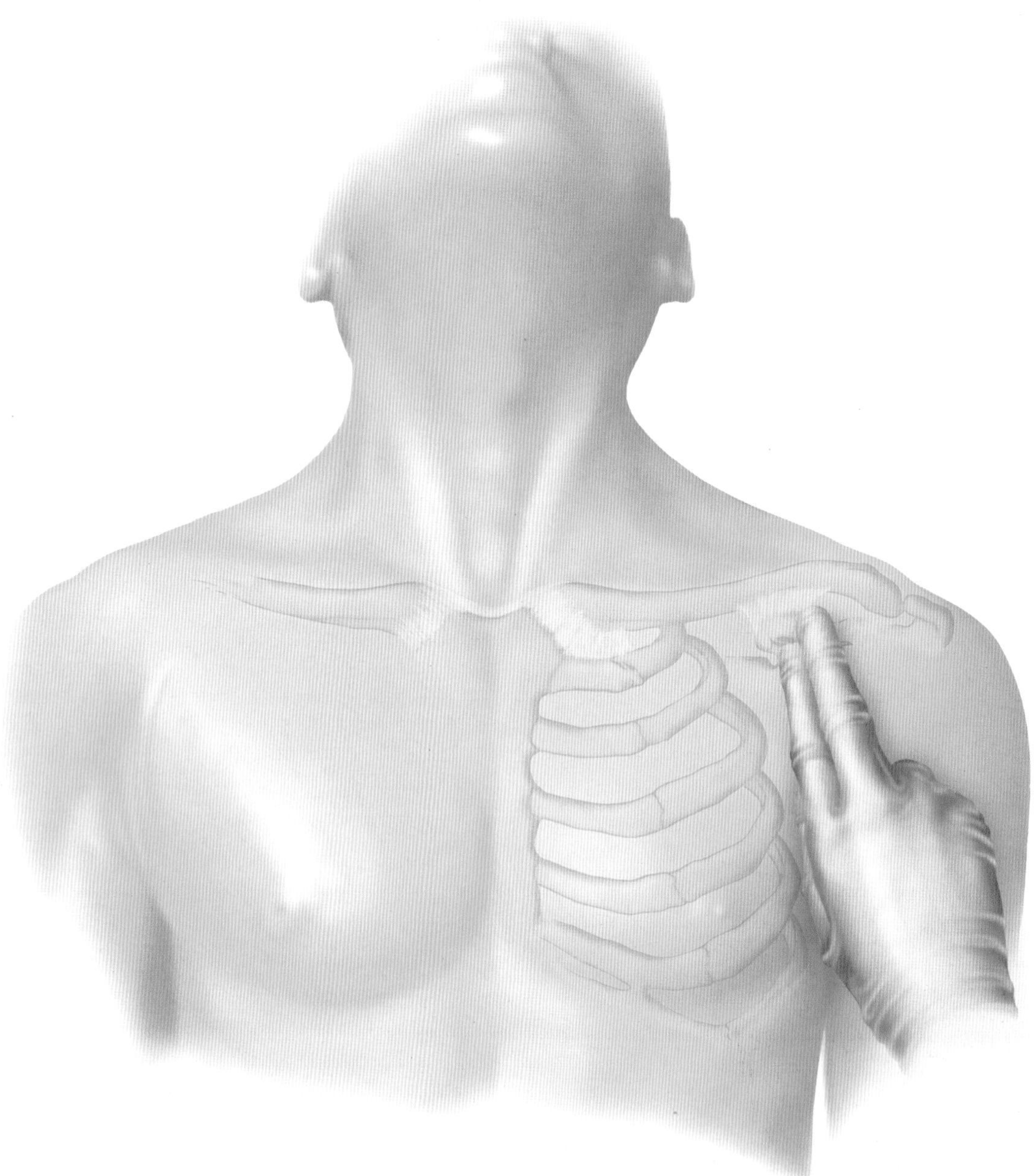

Figure 18-27. Superficial landmarks of the deltopectoral groove. Palpation of the deltopectoral groove and coracoid process.

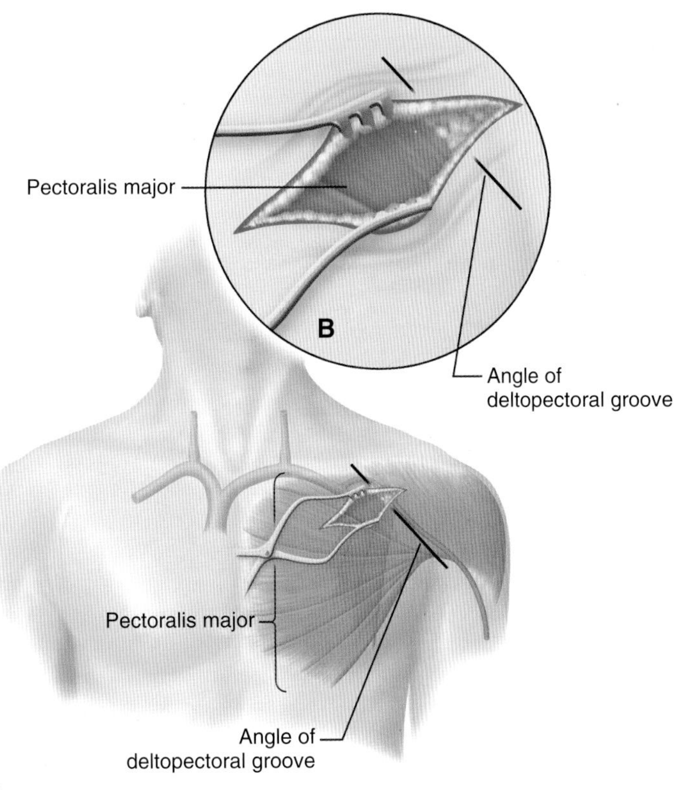

Figure 18-28. ***A,*** *Incision perpendicular to the deltopectoral groove at the level of the coracoid process.* ***B,*** *Close-up view of incision demonstrating the plane of the deltopectoral angle and the plane of the deltopectoral groove and pectoralis muscle.*

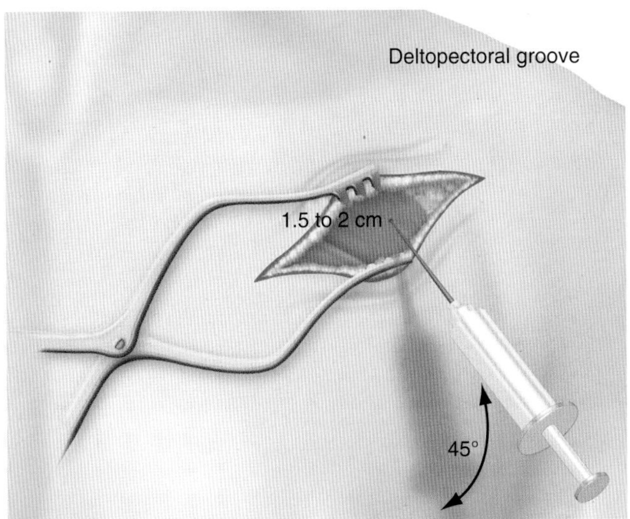

Figure 18-29. Needle and syringe trajectory and angle with respect to the deltopectoral groove and chest wall.

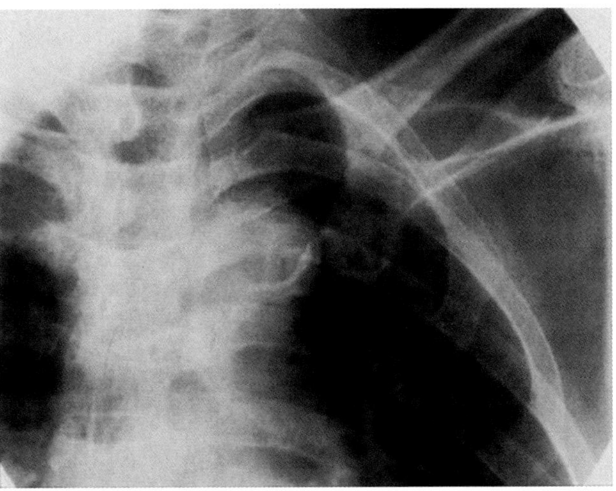

Figure 18-30. Radiograph demonstrating the location of the first rib.

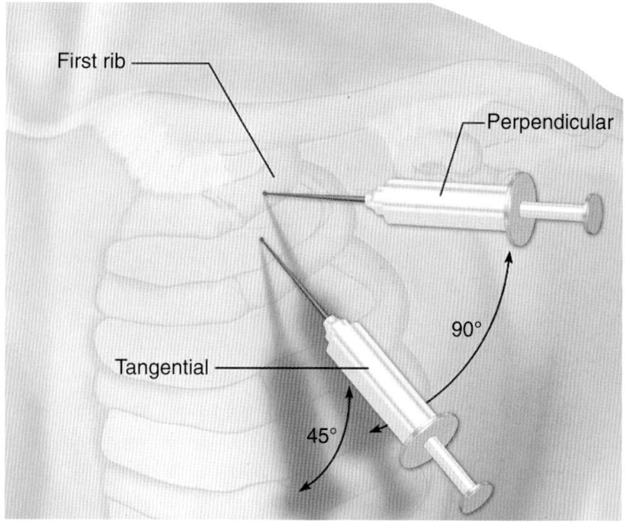

Figure 18-31. Needle trajectory in relationship to the first rib for axillary vein puncture. Note that when the needle is held tangential, there is little risk of pneumothorax or of entering the intercostal space.

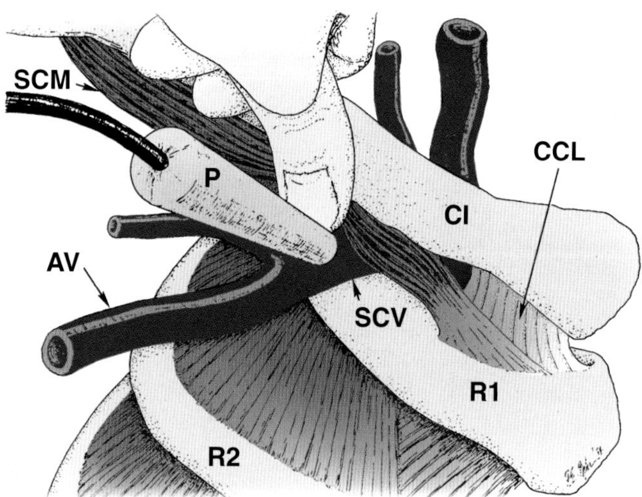

Figure 18-33. Doppler ultrasound location of the axillary vein crossing the first rib. AV, axillary vein; CCL, costoclavicular ligament; Cl, clavicle; P, Doppler probe; R1, first rib; R2, second rib; SCM, subclavius muscle; SCV, subclavian vein.

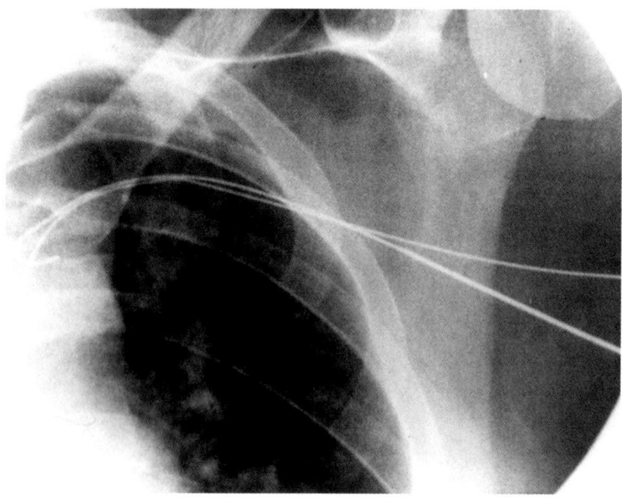

Figure 18-32. Percutaneous access to the axillary vein using a J wire introduced by means of the antecubital vein for reference.

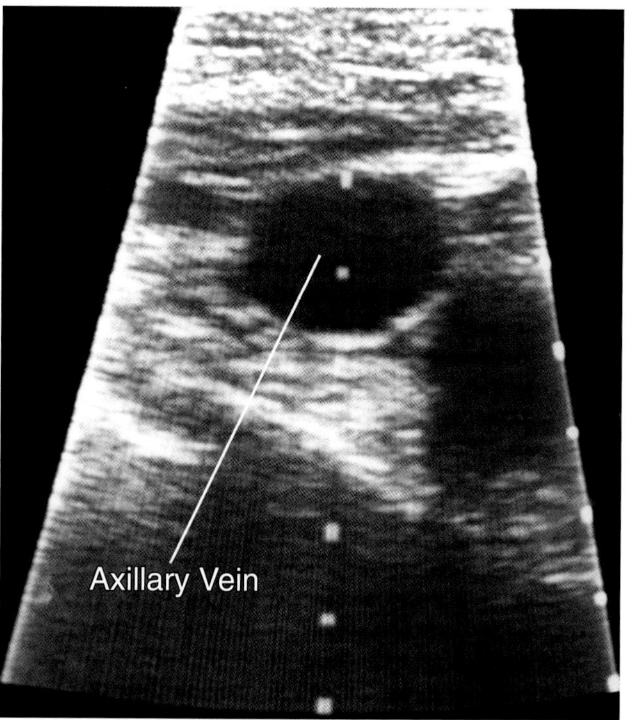

Figure 18-34. Ultrasonic image of the axillary vein.

because it could lacerate important structures. Anatomic landmarks are defined, and the puncture is made, with rare exception, with the patient in the anatomic position. The costoclavicular angle is not artificially opened by maneuvers. Although the essence of the nonaxillary approaches is medial placement to avoid the lung, the undesirable puncture of the costoclavicular ligament should be avoided. In the obese patient, the tendency is to orient the needle more perpendicular to the chest wall in an attempt to pass between the clavicle and first rib. This perpendicular angle is to be avoided with the medial approaches because it is associated with a higher incidence of pneumothorax. In this circumstance, a more inferior skin puncture is recommended, allowing the needle to slip between the first rib and clavicle. The needle is, therefore, kept almost tangential to the chest wall, avoiding the lung. Some implanters bend the needle in an attempt to slip under the clavicle. We do not recommend this maneuver because it is associated with a higher incidence of pneumothorax and vascular trauma. We instead recommend that in the morbidly obese patient, the subclavian puncture be carried out after direct visualization of the pectoral muscle. This can be done only by making an initial skin incision and carrying it down to the pectoral muscle. Once the

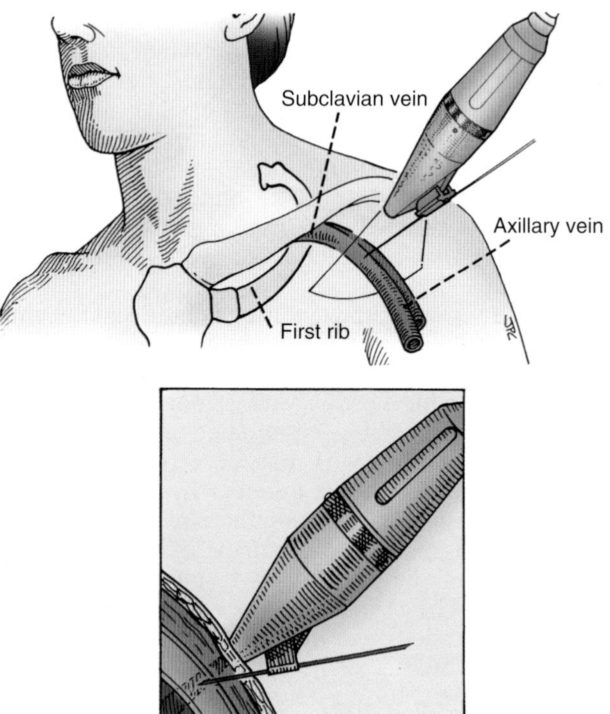

Figure 18-35. Ultrasound-guided puncture of the axillary vein with use of the Site-Rite device (Site Rite Ultrasound System, Salt Lake City, Utah).

anatomic landmarks are defined, the needle is slipped between the first rib and the clavicle with a trajectory that is nearly tangential to the chest wall and directed cephalad and medial.

This last recommendation raises the question whether the skin incision should routinely be made first, with percutaneous venous access carried out through the incision, or whether an initial percutaneous venous puncture should be performed, followed by the incision. It is, arguably, better for one not to commit oneself with an initial pocket-length incision and subsequent venipuncture. Doing so avoids the embarrassment of having to explain matching incisions if venous access could not be achieved through the initial incision and one is forced to move to the patient's other side. It is difficult enough explaining multiple unsuccessful skin punctures. As an acceptable alternative, and one that has been in regular use for some time at the University of Oklahoma, a 1 cm–long stab wound can be made initially, through which the venipunctures can be accomplished. This approach allows easy incorporation of the puncture sites (especially if two separate punctures are used for a dual-chamber pacing system) into a single incision that is extended after successful venipuncture. A full incision is made to the greater pectoral fascia before one gains access to the vein.

As with axillary vein access techniques, the subclavian puncture can be facilitated by the use of contrast venography.[73] It is helpful in patients in whom venous access can be anticipated to be a problem. It should be considered before any puncture in which venous patency is in doubt or abnormal anatomy is suspected.

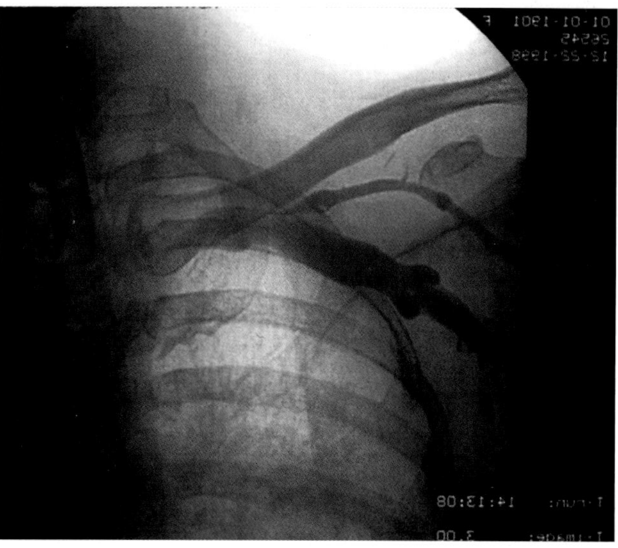

Figure 18-36. Contrast venography–guided venipuncture. With contrast material, the needle is guided under fluoroscopic guidance directly to the vein.

The technique has been described by Higano and colleagues.[73] A venous line is established in the arm on the side of planned pacemaker venous access. The line should be reliable and 20-gauge or larger. One must ensure that the patient does not have an allergy to radiographic contrast material. The contrast material injection is performed by a nonsterile assistant. From 10 to 50 mL of contrast material (non-ionic or ionic) is injected rapidly into the IV line in the forearm, followed by a saline bolus flush. The contrast medium moves slowly in the peripheral venous system and can be moved along by massage of the arm through or under the sterile drapes. The venous anatomy is observed with fluoroscopy in the pectoral area and, if possible, recorded for repeated viewing (Fig. 18-36). The needle trajectory and venipuncture are guided by the contrast material in the subclavian vein. In more sophisticated radiologic laboratories, a mask or map can be made for guidance after the contrast medium has dissipated. The process can be repeated as necessary.

The actual percutaneous puncture is carried out with a syringe attached to the 18-gauge needle. A common practice is to fill the syringe partially with saline. The theory behind this practice is that if a pneumothorax occurs, it will be detected by air bubbles aspirated through the saline. In addition, the saline can be used to flush out tissue plugs that may obstruct the needle and prevent aspiration. We avoid this practice because we believe that one does not need air bubbles to detect an inadvertent pneumothorax. More important, the syringe even partially filled with saline makes it difficult to differentiate between arterial and venous blood, because when blood (arterial or venous) mixes with the saline, it takes on the color of oxygenated blood. If saline is not used, which vascular structure has been entered is more readily apparent.

When proceeding with a percutaneous venipuncture, one should hold the syringe in the palm of the hand with the dorsal aspect of the hand resting on the patient.

This gives support and control as the needle is advanced. With the needle held this way, tactile sensation is enhanced, and one can frequently feel the needle enter the vein. Once the vessel is entered, the guidewire is inserted, and the tip advanced to a position in the vicinity of the RA (Fig. 18-37). We prefer to use J-shaped or curved-tip guidewires for safety reasons. If resistance is encountered, the wire is withdrawn slightly and advanced again. If the resistance persists, the wire position is checked with fluoroscopy. If the wire just outside the tip of the needle appears coiled, it is probably extravascular. In this case, the wire and needle are removed, and a new venous puncture is carried out. Extremely rarely, one may not be able to re-enter the vein. This may be due to collapse of the vein by a resultant hematoma caused by a small tear in the vein from the misdirected guidewire. In this case, one should probably proceed to an alternative approach or site of venous access, to avoid an unnecessary waste of time and a higher risk of pneumothorax with multiple subsequent unsuccessful percutaneous punctures.

Occasionally the guidewire tracks up the internal jugular vein. Changing the angle of the needle slightly to a more medial and inferior direction while the guidewire is still in the internal jugular vein, withdrawing the guidewire back into the needle, and then advancing again usually results in passage of the guidewire through the innominate vein and SVC into the RA. This maneuver may have to be repeated several times with varying needle angulations. Care must be exercised to avoid tearing the vein. The application of a 5F or 6F dilator can sometimes help steer the guidewire in the right direction. In rare instances, the guidewire and needle must be removed, and a new puncture site selected. The key point is that once venous access has been achieved, every effort is made to retain it.

When air is withdrawn through the needle during attempted venipunctures, suggesting lung puncture and raising the possibility of a pneumothorax, our practice is to withdraw the needle, wait a moment or two to make certain that a rapid-onset, large, markedly symptomatic pneumothorax is not occurring, and then proceed (obviously with a different needle trajectory) with further attempts at venipuncture. In our experience, most lung punctures occurring with forward (not lateral!) needle motion do not result in a clinically apparent (on chest radiography) pneumothorax. If a pneumothorax does develop, it may do so in this setting over a matter of hours and may not even be apparent radiographically at the end of the procedure. If a lung puncture has occurred, obtaining another upright chest radiograph 6 hours after completion of the procedure is advisable. If a pneumothorax has

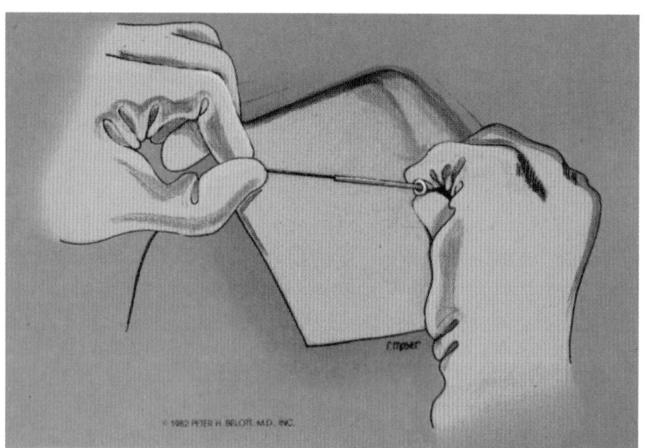

A

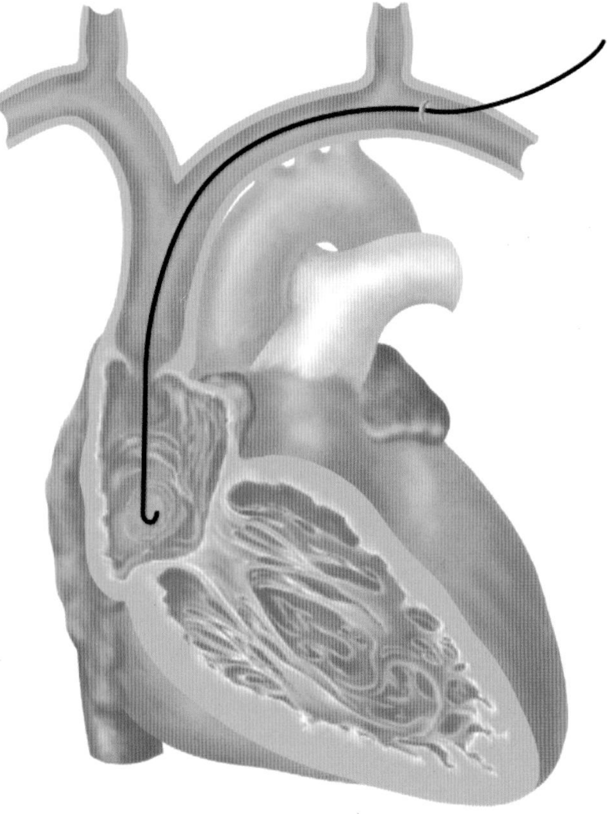

B

Figure 18-37. ***A,*** *Once venous access is achieved, the needle is supported with one hand and the guidewire with tip occluder is advanced with the other hand.* ***B,*** *Guidewire tip advanced to the middle right atrium. (**A** from Belott PH: Retained guide wire introducer technique, for unlimited access to the central circulation. Clin Prog Pacing Electrophysiol 1:59, 1983.)*

developed, a chest tube or catheter evacuation procedure may be necessary, although frequently, a small to moderate pneumothorax that is not expanding can be managed conservatively without evacuation.

Similarly, if an arterial puncture occurs inadvertently, our approach has consisted of removal of the needle, compression at the site of the puncture for 5 minutes or so, followed by repeated venipuncture attempts with a different needle path. It is rare for such arterial punctures to result in a hemothorax, provided that no tearing of the artery has occurred (avoidance of lateral needle motion is crucial here also). Follow-up chest radiographs taken 6 to 18 hours after the procedure are advisable, and postoperative hemoglobin and hematocrit measurements are suggested. The most important problem to avoid if the artery has been punctured is nonrecognition and placement of a sheath into the artery. If there is any doubt about whether the artery has been punctured, a blood sample withdrawn through the needle and subjected to oximetric analysis should clarify the situation.

Once the wire is successfully positioned in the vein, some implanters place a purse-string suture in the tissue around the point of entry of the wire into the tissue. Alternatively, a figure-of-eight stitch can be applied (Fig. 18-38). This step can be helpful later for hemostasis.[74] Such sutures require that an incision be made beginning at the needle and extending inferiorly to the depth of the pectoral fascia.

Once the guidewires are in the subclavian vein, it is usually a simple procedure to advance the appropriate-sized dilator and peel-away sheath over the wire into the venous circulation. Occasionally, there is substantial resistance to dilator-sheath advancement, and repetitive dilation with progressively larger dilators is necessary. Alternatively, a 15- to 20-degree bending of the tip of the full-sized introducer may facilitate advancement over the wire. If difficulty with advancement occurs, we generally remove the sheath from the dilator and use only the dilator initially to dilate the track into the vein. This protects the rather delicate sheaths from damage. After successful advance of the dilator alone over the wire, the dilator can be withdrawn, the sheath added, and both then advanced over the wire. We have found that gentle back-pressure on the guidewire while the dilator-sheath is advanced also facilitates advancement in difficult or tortuous vessels.

After the sheath has been successfully passed over the guidewire to the vicinity of the SVC, the dilator and guidewire can be removed, and the lead advanced through the sheath. Problems can be encountered when the lead is passed through the sheath. Occasionally, in the process of introduction, the sheath buckles at a point in the venous system where there is a bend (Fig. 18-39).[75] This usually occurs after the removal of the dilator. It can also occur if the sheath is advanced against the lateral wall of the SVC; if a buckle occurs, the lead will not pass this point. Forcing the lead can result in damage to the cathode and insulation. This kink can usually be observed on fluoroscopy. There are several solutions to this problem. If the guidewire and dilator have both been removed, both can be replaced down the sheath. The dilator with wire inside is now functioning not only as a way to stiffen the sheath but also as a tip occluder, and both can be passed back down the sheath. The tapered tip of the dilator will straighten the buckle. One can change the position of the buckle point by either slightly advancing or retracting the sheath. The dilator is removed but the guidewire can be retained. It is hoped that the retained guidewire will act as a stent, preventing the buckle

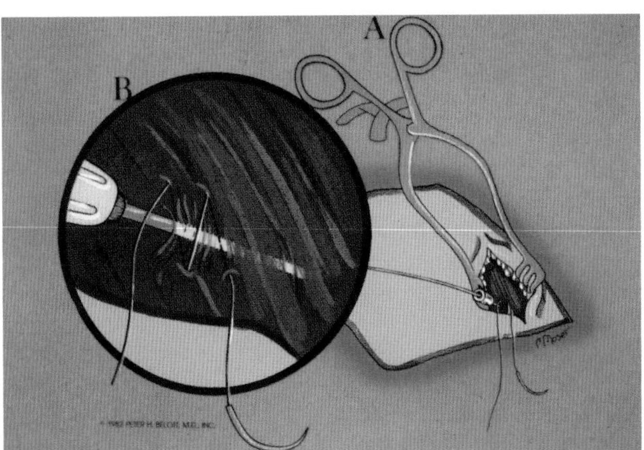

Figure 18-38. Placement of the figure-of-eight stitch to enhance hemostasis. (From Belott PH: Retained guide wire introducer technique, for unlimited access to the central circulation. Clin Prog Pacing Electrophysiol 1:59, 1983.)

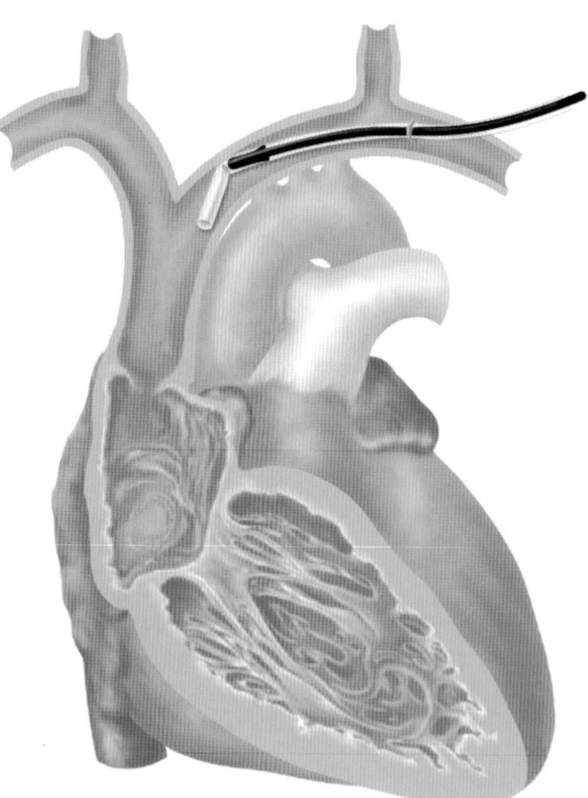

Figure 18-39. Buckling of the introducer sheath prevents the passage of the electrode.

from recurring and thus allowing the electrode to pass completely down the sheath. Another option when buckling of sheath occurs is to advance the lead to within a couple of centimeters of the buckle and then slowly withdraw the sheath, holding the lead position stationary. The sheath, including the buckle point, may occasionally be easily withdrawn over the tip of the lead, and the lead can be cautiously advanced. In this situation, it is sometimes necessary to withdraw the stylet from the tip of the lead to allow easy advancement of the lead beyond the buckle point. Inexperienced implanters should be cautious with this latter technique, however, because it may damage the distal electrodes.

If these maneuvers fail, the guidewire and dilator are reinserted and the sheath and dilator are removed, leaving the guidewire in the vein. Tissue compression or traction is applied to the purse-string suture for hemostasis. The sheath is inspected for buckling. At this point, the implanter should consider advancing a sheath of the next larger size over the retained guidewire, because application of the same-sized sheath usually results in recurrence of the same problem. The important point is that despite this frustrating experience, one must be reluctant to relinquish the vein once it has been catheterized. Generally, the larger sheath is less likely to buckle, especially if the guidewire is retained to act as a stent. With successful electrode introduction, the sheath is briskly pulled back out of the circulation, and skin compression or traction is applied to the purse-string or figure-of-eight suture for hemostasis.

The risk of air embolization is substantial with the percutaneous approach. This issue has been addressed by the recommendation that the Trendelenburg patient position be used. With the shift of the pacemaker procedure to the cardiac catheterization laboratory or special procedures room, however, it is commonly impossible to place the patient in the Trendelenburg position. Consequently, the patient is at greater risk for air embolization if the percutaneous approach is used. It is most important that the implanting physician be aware of the danger and take steps necessary to avoid this potential catastrophe (Table 18-10). The physician must be aware that removal of the sheath dilator in a patient who is fasting and somewhat volume depleted can rapidly cause aspiration of large quantities of air. Because the luxury of the Trendelenburg position is unlikely to be available in the catheterization laboratory, other steps must be taken. Contrary to some practices, the patient about to undergo pacemaker implantation should be kept in a euvolemic or even a relatively volume-overloaded state if there is no contraindication. Instead of administration of intravenous fluids at a restricted rate, adequate hydration should be maintained. We routinely place a large wedge sponge under the patient's legs to enhance blood return and increase central venous pressure.

An assessment of the state of hydration can be carried out during the procedure. With the sheath in the central venous circulation, careful withdrawal of the dilator from the sheath can allow the state of hydration and venous pressure to be observed: After the dilator is withdrawn in the hydrated patient with adequate venous pressure, there is continuous blood flow out of the sheath despite the cycle of respiration. In the dehydrated patient, withdrawal of the dilator results in little or no flow of blood. The blood meniscus is barely visible. More important, on inspiration, the blood meniscus is observed to move substantially inward. If this is observed, the dilator can be rapidly advanced back into the sheath; alternatively, the sheath can be pinched and additional precautions taken to avoid air embolization. If a wedge has not been placed under the patient's legs, this can be done now and is frequently helpful. Also, at this point, it is most important to have the cooperation of the patient. If the patient is sleeping, he or she should be aroused. The patient should be coached to reduce the depth of respirations and avoid the sudden large inspiration that can result in the aspiration of a lethal volume of air into the vein. At the same time, administration of intravenous fluids is increased to enhance hydration. Having the patient hold the breath after maximal inspiration offers the greatest latitude in time, because the patient will have to exhale before inhaling, thereby causing negative intrathoracic pressure and aspiration of air into the vein. This gives the implanter time to insert the lead. Pinching of the sheath with the lead going through it to avoid air embolization is ineffective and gives a false sense of security. A peel-away sheath with a hemostasis valve would be useful. In the patient who is substantially sedated or uncooperative, adequate hydration and elevation of the lower extremities are the only solutions. Careful planning of the lead insertion procedure also helps. Expeditious lead insertion is important. For example, positioning the electrodes with the sheath in

TABLE 18-10. Prevention of Air Embolism during Permanent Pacemaker Procedures

In the normal patient	Remember that air embolism is possible Ensure that the patient is well hydrated, avoiding long periods of prohibiting oral intake Be aware of increased risk (i.e., with open sheath in vein) Assess hydration by observing central venous pressure
In the high-risk patient	Increase hydration (i.e., with wide-open IV lines) Ensure that patient is awake and cooperative Elevate patient's lower extremities and place wedge under legs Use Trendelenburg position (if available) Plan for expeditious lead placement and sheath removal Check for introduction of air Monitor patient continuously (vital signs, oxygen saturation, blood pressure)
In an extremely high-risk, uncooperative patient	Intubation and sedation causing temporary loss of consciousness may be required

situ is unwise, because it may result in air embolism or unnecessary blood loss.

Once the lead has been inserted, the introducer should be rapidly withdrawn. The practice of peeling away the sheath while part of it is in an intravascular location should be avoided; doing so is a waste of time and increases the risk for air embolization and blood loss. In this regard, the actual peeling away of the sheath is not even a necessity at this point so long as it is completely extravascular. It can be peeled away later at one's convenience. In fact, the tabs of the unpeeled sheath can be used to pin the lead to the drapes during threshold testing, preventing inadvertent dislodgment of the lead onto the floor. With the sheath withdrawn completely from the circulation, hemostasis is achieved by applying tension to the purse-string or figure-of-eight suture or by applying skin compression over the entry site.

A variation of the introducer technique involves retaining the guidewire. Instead of being removed together with the dilator, the guidewire is left in place, so that the lead is passed through the sheath alongside it. The sheath is subsequently removed and peeled away (Fig. 18-40). Occasionally, the size of the electrode and the sheath precludes the passage of the lead alongside the guidewire. In this case, the guidewire is removed, the lead is passed down the sheath, and the guidewire is reinserted behind the electrode. The reason this maneuver can work is that, in most cases, it is the electrode that will not pass alongside the guidewire, whereas the lead body is thinner and leaves enough room in the sheath to accommodate the guidewire. Certain leads (especially those with bipolar electrodes) and sheath combinations are too tight to allow passage of both the electrode and guidewire. In this case, a larger sheath can be used.

When the guidewire is reintroduced, the tip occluder is not used because it can wind up in the central circulation fairly easily. Reusing the dilator as a tip occluder during reinsertion of the guidewire works well. The retained guidewire may provide unlimited venous access and the ability to exchange or introduce additional electrodes by simply applying another sheath set to the guidewire. The retained guidewire should be held to the drape with a clamp to avoid inadvertent dislodgment. The retained guidewire can serve as a ground for unipolar threshold analysis instead of a grounding plate. It can also be used as an intracardiac lead for recording of the atrial electrogram (to confirm atrial capture) or as an electrode for emergency pacing. We routinely retain an intravascular guidewire in both single-chamber and dual-chamber procedures until a satisfactory lead position is obtained.

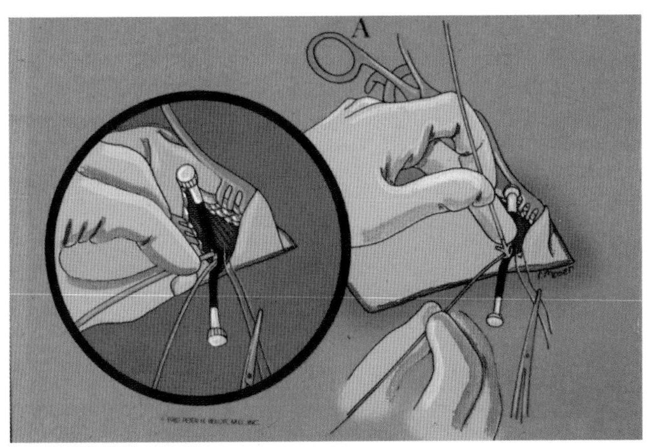

A

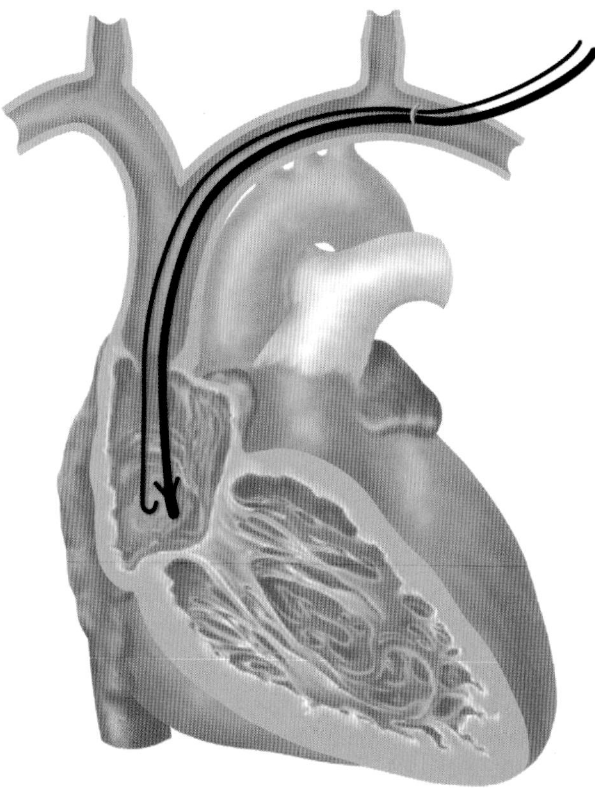

B

Figure 18-40. ***A,*** *The guidewire with dilator removed remains in the sheath. The lead has been inserted and advanced (inset) alongside the guidewire.* ***B,*** *Both the guidewire and the lead are advanced to the vicinity of the middle right atrium. Additional introducers can be advanced over this retained guidewire to place additional leads. (**A** from Belott PH: Retained guide wire introducer technique, for unlimited access to the central circulation. Clin Prog Pacing Electrophysiol 1:59, 1983.)*

TABLE 18-11. Options for Venous Access for Single- and Dual-Chamber Pacing

Venous cutdown	Isolation of one or two veins With cephalic vein guidewire (Ong-Barold technique)
Percutaneous	Two separate sticks and sheath applications Two electrodes down one large sheath Retained guidewire (Belott's technique) Access to the extrathoracic portion of the subclavian vein (Byrd's technique)

Methods of Dual-Chamber Venous Access

The percutaneous approach is particularly useful in dual-chamber pacing and has eliminated the earlier dilemma of having to introduce two leads into a vein exposed by cutdown that may barely accommodate a single lead and the resultant need for a second venous access site. The options for dual-chamber venous access are shown in Table 18-11. For dual-chamber pacing, at least four methods that involve the percutaneous approach are described here. The first three can be used with any of the previously described percutaneous approaches.

Two Separate Percutaneous Sticks and the Use of Two Sheath Sets. Parsonnet and colleagues[76] have described the insertion of two sets of permanent electrodes, with a third set for a cardiac venous lead. Two separate punctures raise the risk of complications related to the venipuncture process, and there is also the possibility of not finding the vessel the second time. The advantage of this method is that even relatively large bipolar leads can be easily and independently manipulated after introduction, with little risk of unwanted and frustrating movement of the other lead.

One Percutaneous Puncture and Use of a Large Sheath with the Passage of Both Electrodes. The passage of two electrodes down one sheath reduces the risk of making two separate punctures.[77,78] However, the large sheath may increase the risk of substantial air embolism and blood loss. In our experience, there is also frequent frustration from lead interaction, entanglement, and dislodgment.

The Retained Guidewire Technique. The retained guidewire technique can be used alone as a method for the introduction of two leads or can be incorporated into any of the other techniques for the introduction of two leads.[79,80] One of the authors (PHB) uses this technique alone, preferentially for dual-lead introductions, and the other (DWR) uses it as backup in combination with the two separate puncture techniques described previously. This approach is most desirable because it provides unlimited access to the central circulation. The implanter using this technique can easily add and exchange leads, an important advantage in dual-chamber pacing, in which the initially chosen atrial lead is occasionally unacceptable for a given anatomic situation. Less commonly, it is also helpful to be able to exchange ventricular leads. When using the retained guidewire technique for dual-chamber implantation, one usually positions the ventricular electrode first, a practical and safe step. The ventricular electrode can be more easily stabilized and is less susceptible to dislodgment from positioning of the second electrode. One can then stabilize the ventricular electrode by leaving the stylet pulled back in the lead in the vicinity of the lower RA (Fig. 18-41). A stitch should be placed proximally around the lead and suture sleeve and secured about 1 to 2 cm from the puncture site in the subcutaneous tissue on the surface of the pectoral muscle.

After ventricular electrode stabilization, a second sheath can be advanced over the retained guidewire. The atrial electrode is introduced, positioned, tested, and secured. Alternatively, the retained guidewire technique can be employed to introduce both leads into the SVC, RA, or inferior vena cava areas before positioning of either of the electrodes. This procedure may eliminate some of the risk of dislodgment of the initially positioned electrode incurred by introduction of the second sheath. Regardless of variation, the guidewire is removed only after all leads have been placed and tied down (Fig. 18-42). A purse-string or figure-of-eight suture can be tied loosely to achieve hemostasis around the puncture site.

The Sheath Set Technique in Conjunction with the Cutdown Approach. Ong and associates[81] described a modified cephalic vein guidewire technique for the introduction of one or more electrodes. The Ong-Barold technique appears to be a safe and reasonable alternative to the percutaneous subclavian vein introducer technique.[82] It is particularly recommended for the inexperienced implanter. It is also recommended for use in patients at high risk of complications with the percutaneous approach and in situations in which one can anticipate the percutaneous approach to be difficult if not impossible.

This technique requires an initial cutdown to the cephalic vein as previously described. For a single-lead introduction, the size of the vein is irrelevant. All that is necessary is the introduction of the guidewire, which is accomplished with needle puncture under direct visualization. The cephalic vein is sacrificed because it seems to invaginate into the subclavian vein with advancement of the sheath set over the guidewire (Fig. 18-43). Hemostasis is achieved with pressure or the application of a figure-of-eight stitch. Despite sacrifice of the cephalic vein, there have been no reported venous complications. When two leads are required, the retained guidewire technique and sheath set technique can be used in this approach.

Complications of Percutaneous Venous Access and Blind Subclavian Puncture

There is ongoing debate with respect to the safety and efficacy of the blind subclavian puncture. Although the blind subclavian puncture technique has proved very

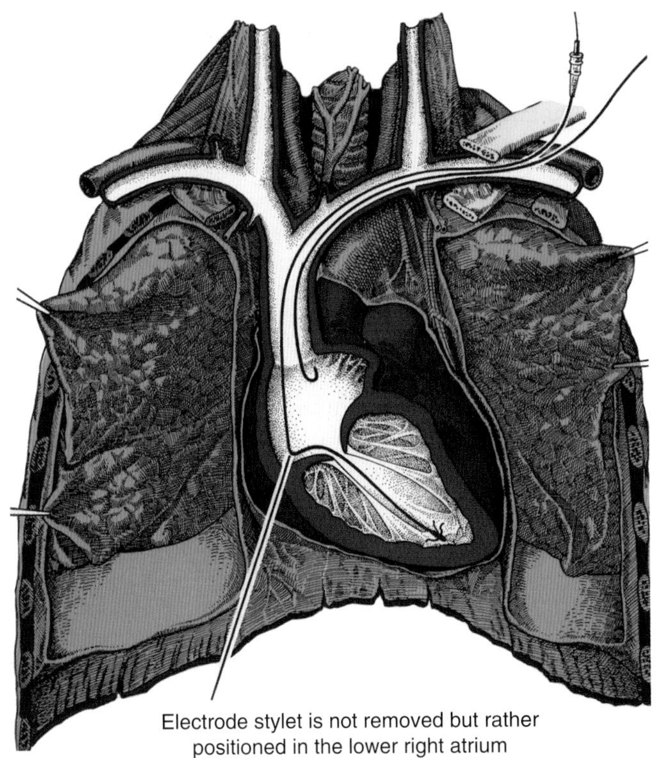

Figure 18-41. The ventricular lead has been placed first. The guidewire has been retained, and the lead stylet is positioned in the lower right atrium for stability.

useful, it has generated considerable controversy with respect to the incidence of serious complications and even death (Table 18-12). Parsonnet and Bernstein[83] reported a 0.4% incidence of serious complications in a survey of 11 implanting physicians in a review of 2500 cases. Furman[84] has demonstrated the remarkable efficiency of the cutdown approach for single-chamber and dual-chamber pacing, particularly with unipolar leads. The cutdown technique, however, was less useful for the introduction of bipolar leads via a single cephalic vein. Furman[85] reported no vascular or pleural complications in a large series of 3500 cases in which the cutdown approach was used for single-chamber and dual-chamber pacemaker implantations. Parsonnet and colleagues[86] analyzed the pacemaker implantation complication rates with respect to contributing factors. They reviewed 632 consecutive implantations over a 5-year period performed by 29 implanting physicians at a single institution. There were 37 perioperative complications. Complications were analyzed with respect to experience of the implanting physician. Percutaneous venous access was associated with the highest complication rate and contributed significantly to a 5.7% overall complication rate. When the complications related to the percutaneous approach were excluded, the complication rate dropped to a more acceptable 3.5%. The highest complication rate was among physicians implanting fewer than 12 pacemakers a year and with the least pacing experience.

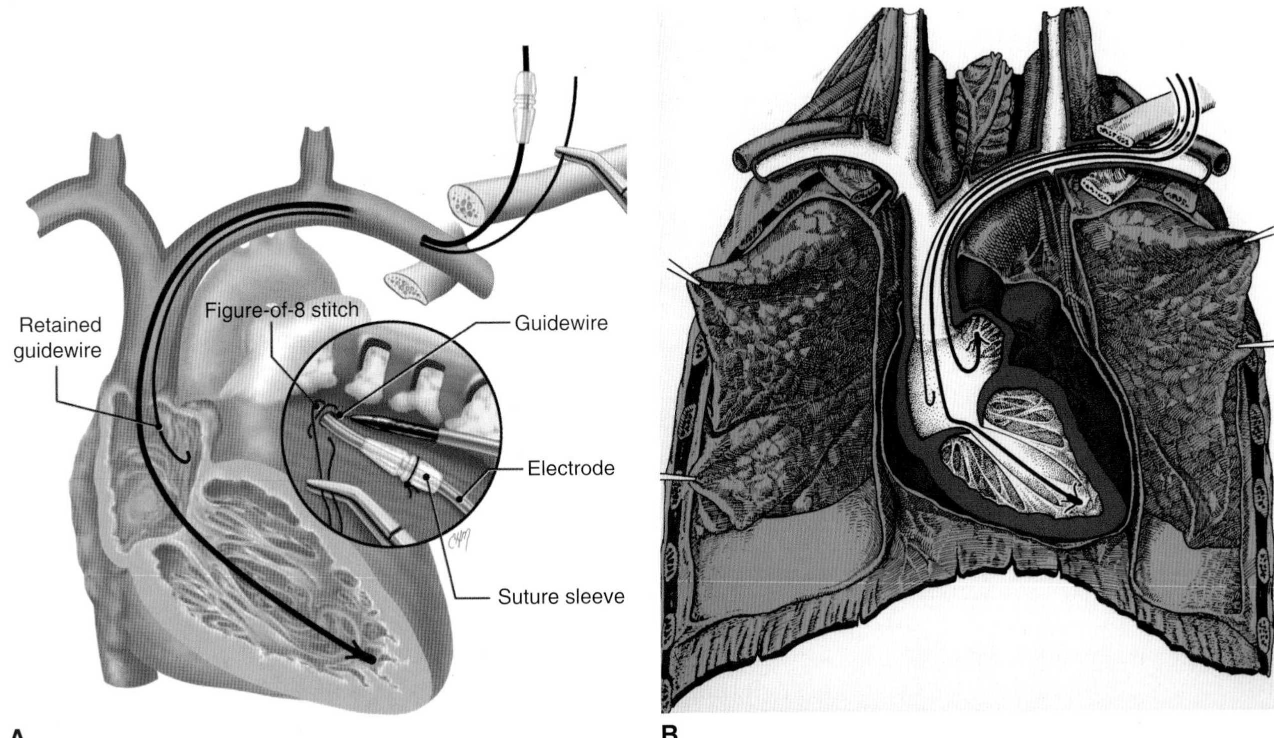

*Figure 18-42. **A,** The ventricular electrode and retained guidewire are demonstrated in the main drawing. The inset demonstrates the ventricular lead anchored by suture around its suture sleeve and the second sheath advancing over the retained guidewire. A hemostat on the figure-of-eight suture maintains hemostasis. **B,** The atrial and ventricular electrodes have been positioned, yet the guidewire is still retained. (**A** from Barold SS, Mugica J: New Perspectives in Cardiac Pacing 2. Armonk, NY, Futura, 1991, p 110.)*

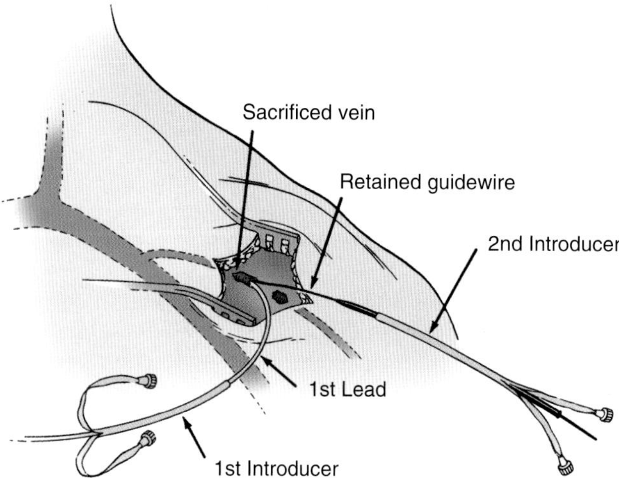

Figure 18-43. Cephalic vein guidewire technique uses the guidewire as access to the vein for one or more electrodes. The distal connection of the cephalic vein is sacrificed (Ong-Barold technique). (From Barold SS, Mugica J: New Perspectives in Cardiac Pacing 2. Armonk, NY, Futura, 1991, p 112.)

TABLE 18-12. Complications of Percutaneous Venous Access and Blind Subclavian Puncture

Pneumothorax
Hemothorax
Hemopneumothorax
Laceration of subclavian artery
Arteriovenous fistula
Nerve injury
Thoracic duct injury
Chylothorax
Lymphatic fistula

Sutton and Bourgeois,[87] in reviewing complications of pacemaker insertion, noted an overall 1% incidence of subclavian vein puncture leading to pneumothorax. Arterial puncture occurred more commonly, at a rate of about 3%, but generally was not associated with any morbidity. Similarly, in their analysis of thrombotic complications, axillary vein thrombosis was rare, occurring in 0.5% to 1% of cases. Interestingly, partial venous obstruction in the great veins was almost the rule and occurred to some degree in up to 100% of cases. Clinical pulmonary embolism, however, was extremely rare. As a rule, partial or silent inconsequential thrombosis is considered extremely common but generally of no clinical significance.[88]

Placement of the Ventricular Electrode

Many techniques for placing the ventricular electrode are described throughout the published pacing literature,[88] essentially reflecting the approach with which any particular clinician has facility. There is no one correct technique. Ventricular electrode placement is largely independent of the route of venous access. The implanting physician must draw on experience to deal with the variety of situations that will be encountered in any given patient. In time, one develops one's own technique. The following fundamental principles and maneuvers are common to all: (1) simultaneous manipulation of lead and stylet, (2) documentation of passage into the right side of the heart, and (3) manipulation of the electrode into the apex or other desired location in the RV.

One must grasp the concept that pacemaker placement involves a "symphony" of lead and stylet movements. Without the two working together, proper electrode positioning is impossible. The lead without stylet is somewhat like a limp piece of spaghetti. During positioning of the ventricular electrode, the lead must negotiate a course through the chambers of the right side of the heart and, ultimately, to the apex of the RV. This is typically accomplished through preforming of the lead stylet. Preforming enables easier manipulation of the lead and is probably the best way to position a pacemaker electrode effectively. A curve is applied to the distal aspect of the stylet. The size or tightness of the curve and how it is created are personal preferences. As a rule, a curve that is too gentle will fail to negotiate the tricuspid valve, making passage into the pulmonary artery difficult. Conversely, a curve that is too tight may fail to negotiate the venous structures in the superior mediastinum, such as the innominate vein and SVC. At times, however, unusual circumstances call for extremes of wire curvature for effective positioning of the electrode. In every case, the ideal curve for the stylet is slightly different.

There are several ways to form the curve on the stylet. Some implanters choose to use a blunt instrument, such as the tip of a clamp or scissors. The stylet is pulled between the thumb and the blunt instrument with a rotary motion of the wrist, forming the curve. Another method is to form the curve by pulling the guidewire between the thumb and index finger, gently shaping the curve. Whatever method is used, the curve should be a bend that is not sharp, because a sharp bend in a stylet generally precludes its passage through the lead. The aim of the curve is to enable the curved stylet to direct the electrode to the appropriate position.

Unlike diagnostic catheters, the pacemaker lead cannot be steered or torqued into position. Positioning of a pacemaker electrode solely depends, therefore, on the manipulation of lead and stylet together. The basic technique of lead positioning involves advancing the electrode, with curved stylet in place, through the chambers of the right side of the heart. A more sophisticated variation of this technique involves simultaneously advancing the electrode while retracting and readvancing the stylet. The retraction of the stylet renders the lead tip floppy. With the use of a slightly retracted although curved stylet and pointing the electrode body in the proper direction, the lead, with 1 to 2 cm of its floppy tip, in most instances, can make for more precise and expeditious electrode placement.

An alternative, related technique, and one that can expedite ventricular lead implantation—although it is clearly more difficult to master—involves the use of a straight stylet. The stylet is retracted to allow the floppy lead tip to "catch" on a structure in the RA, with subsequent advancement of the lead. The lead body then prolapses through the tricuspid valve into the RV. The stylet can then be cautiously advanced to stiffen the lead body and, generally, free the tip from the catch. It is possible, even likely, that these techniques involving prolapse of the leads across the tricuspid valve present less likelihood of damaging the valve or entangling subvalvular structures than techniques involving direct advancement of stiff-tipped leads.

The fluoroscope should be used for the entire lead positioning process and can be used initially in the posteroanterior (PA) projection or in the right anterior oblique (RAO) projection. The latter helps delineate the apex of the RV to the left of the spine and toward the left lateral chest wall. The RAO projection creates the illusion that the "mind's eye" expects, with respect to the location of the apex of the RV, specifically, that the RV apex is near the apex of the cardiac silhouette. In many patients, however, the RV apex tends to be more anterior than leftward. Much time can be wasted trying to position a ventricular electrode to the left of the spine toward the apex of the cardiac silhouette (in the PA projection) when, in reality, the RV apex is directly anterior to the spine. This anterior position results in an electrode position that is over the spine or nearly so and appears in the PA projection to be erroneously placed in the RA or in the less desirable proximal aspect of the RV. Rotating the image intensifier unit into the RAO projection in this situation superimposes the RV apex over the apex of the cardiac silhouette in the left side of the chest, confirming the appropriate position (Fig. 18-44). Whether or not the initial choice of projection is the RAO, it should be used freely to facilitate ventricular lead placement.

We recommend that the electrode be passed initially across the tricuspid valve and then out into the pulmonary artery (Fig. 18-45A to C). This maneuver confirms passage into the right side of the heart and precludes erroneous placement in the coronary sinus.

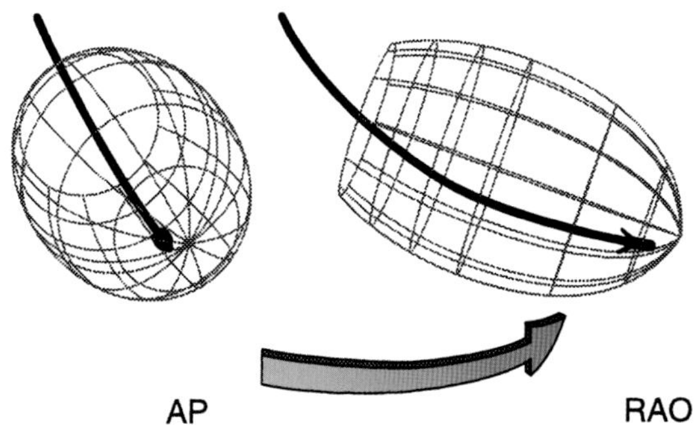

Figure 18-44. Wire frame demonstrating the orientation of the lead in the right ventricular apex in the anteroposterior (AP) and right anterior oblique (RAO) projections. Note that in the AP projection, the electrode appears to be vertical, whereas in the RAO, the lead is horizontal from right to left.

The RAO projection is also helpful in making certain the lead is not in the coronary sinus. If the lead is appropriately placed in the apex of the RV, there will be no posterior component of the course of the lead on the RAO projection. If the lead is in the coronary sinus, it will have a posterior course on this projection. If it courses down the middle cardiac vein, the lead will have a posterior course as it traverses the coronary sinus and then an anterior course as it traverses this branch.

There are several techniques for the actual placement of the electrode into the RV apex. They involve the combined manipulation of the lead stylet and electrode body. If one chooses to pass the electrode to the pulmonary artery as an indicator of being across the tricuspid valve, the next maneuver is to advance the stylet to the tip of the electrode. With the stylet advanced to the electrode tip and the electrode tip in the pulmonary artery, the electrode is slowly withdrawn from the pulmonary artery, dragging the tip down along the interventricular septum. This may result in premature ventricular contractions or runs of nonsustained ventricular tachycardia. When the electrode tip has reached the lower third of the septum, the stylet may be retracted about 2 to 3 cm, making the tip floppy; this can be done with a curved or straight stylet (see Fig. 18-45D). The lead tip can be observed to move up and down with the flow of blood, the motion of the tricuspid valve, and the contractions of the RV. As it does so, it will intermittently point toward the apex of the RV. If one coordinates the advancing of the lead body (with or without the stylet fully inserted, although generally only straight stylets should be fully inserted at this point) with the appropriate lead trajectory, one can gently seat the tip in the RV apex. This maneuver can be repeated by withdrawal and readvance of the electrode until the desired fluoroscopic location is achieved for threshold testing.

After satisfactory electrode tip placement, the curved stylet is withdrawn and replaced with a straight stylet if a curved stylet was initially used and if it was not already replaced (some implanters replace the curved stylet with a straight one while the lead tip is still in the pulmonary artery). The straight stylet is advanced to the electrode tip, and the electrode with stylet in place is gently advanced toward the RV apex until it is fully inserted and resistance is encountered. Care should be taken not to dislodge the electrode tip with the straight stylet. Dislodgment is a common occurrence, especially in patients with an enlarged RA. In the process of being advanced to the electrode tip, the straight stylet can force the electrode body inferiorly to the lower RA and inferior vena cava, consequently dragging the tip of the electrode out of the RV apex back into the RA. This phenomenon can obviously be extremely frustrating. Ways to avoid this problem include using a more flexible stylet that will be guided more easily by the electrode coil than will the stiff stylet. Also, before advancing the stylet, one can straighten the lead body as it crosses the tricuspid valve by gently pulling back on the lead; this usually avoids the looping of the lead in the lower RA.

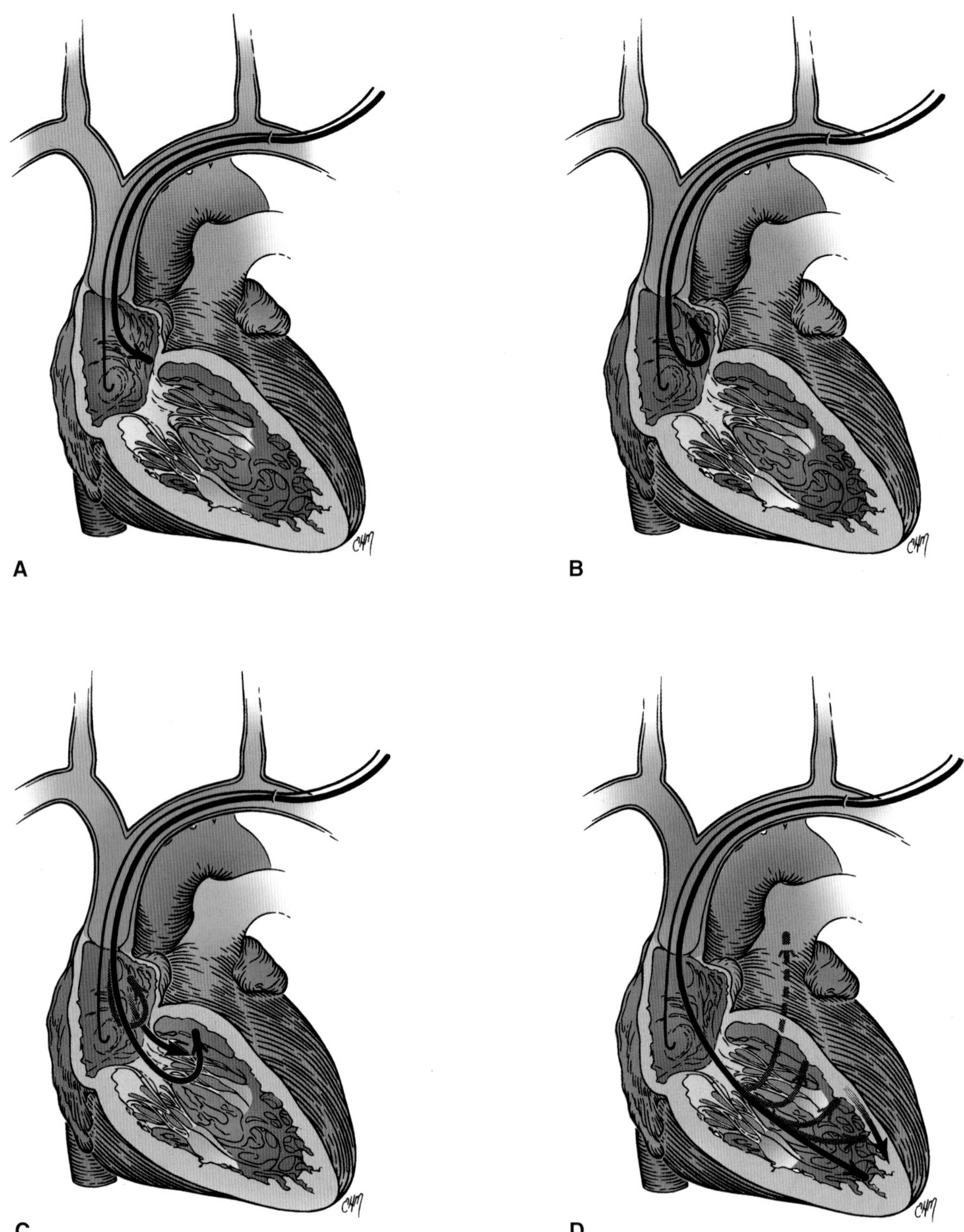

Figure 18-45. ***A,*** *Lead with curved stylet approaching the tricuspid valve.* ***B,*** *Lead being pushed against the tricuspid valve.* ***C,*** *Lead snapping across the tricuspid valve into the right ventricle.* ***D,*** *Lead passed to the pulmonary artery, then withdrawn to the right ventricular apex.*

Lead fixation in the RV can be validated with a gentle pull on the electrode until resistance, both tactile and visual, is encountered. This is a good method for ensuring reliable fixation if a tined or other passive-fixation lead is being used. In the case of an active-fixation lead, the best method for determining that reliable fixation is accomplished is a subject of debate. Some believe that threshold measurements, and not retraction of the lead tip to the point of resistance, is a better way of validating fixation. It is argued that the strength of fixation in the tissue with a screw-in electrode is impossible to gauge from the sensation of resistance on retraction and that, all too often, the bond is disrupted when one pulls back on the screw-in electrode to the point of resistance. Conversely, others argue that the same gentle lead retraction, coupled with achievement of acceptable thresholds, is more appropriate validation for achievement of active fixation. The argument here is that acceptable thresholds may be achieved without adequate fixation and that adequate fixation easily prevents the disruption of an acceptable bond by gentle retraction.

If the initial stylet choice was straight, or after the electrode with the curved stylet has been passed to the pulmonary artery and is replaced with a stiff, straight stylet, the tip of the straight stylet can be positioned just across the tricuspid valve. It usually points to the RV apex. Simultaneous advancement of the stylet and retraction of the electrode drags the electrode tip down the interventricular septum to the end of the stylet, which is tracking toward the RV apex. Once the electrode tip has snapped into a straight position, now in line with the trajectory of the stylet, both are advanced to the RV apex. In both cases, when one is seating the electrode in the RV apex, one can more easily avoid perforations by simultaneously advancing the electrode body while retracting the stylet. Thus, the stylet is not acting as a battering ram but is merely pointing the way. In all cases, if there is any doubt about the location of the electrode in the RV apex, the fluoroscope is merely rotated into the steep RAO or lateral projection. As previously noted, a correctly placed electrode is observed to curve anteriorly, with the electrode tip appearing to almost touch the sternum. If the electrode curves posteriorly toward the spine, it is likely in the coronary sinus.

Although the means of venous access has little bearing on electrode placement, there is some difference between the left and right sides. Placement of the ventricular electrode after venous access has been achieved from the left side generally appears to be more expeditious. The ventricular lead with a curved stylet in place will track in a gentle curve from the point of venous entry through to the SVC, RA, RV, and pulmonary outflow tract (see Fig. 18-16A). Typically, little or no difficulty is encountered. There are generally no acute bends or angles. The only occasional impediment is the tricuspid valve, which can be negotiated with one of several techniques. One may be able to advance the tip across the valve without hang-up. If the lead tends to hang up on the valve, retracting the stylet and using the floppy tip technique already described frequently solves this impasse. There is also the possibility of using a technique in which the curved tip of the electrode is pushed across the valve through the building of a loop. Whatever technique is used, because of the anatomic configuration, passage from the left typically presents little difficulty. One exception is in the elderly patient with an extremely tortuous left subclavian-innominate venous system. In such a patient, the venous structure may have one or more sharp angles or bends in the superior mediastinum before entry into the RA. It would be a truly extreme case for such tortuosity to preclude passage of the electrode from the left.

Passage and placement of the ventricular electrode after right venous access may be much more challenging. Intrinsic to this approach is one acute angle or bend in the venous system (see Fig. 18-16B). This bend occurs at the junction of the right subclavian vein and internal jugular vein, where the innominate vein is formed. More important is the fact that this bend is clockwise. Because of this fact, when a lead with a curved stylet is placed in the vein from the right, the electrode is typically directed clockwise or to the lateral RA wall (Fig. 18-46A). In this situation, routing the tip across the tricuspid valve, which is in the other direction, may call on all of one's skill, ingenuity, and luck. One method involves building a loop in the RA in an attempt to prolapse the lead and to back the electrode across the valve, with the tip ultimately flipping into the RV (see Fig. 18-46B). If the lead has tines, they may get caught on the tricuspid valve and prevent transit to the RV. Another method of crossing the tricuspid valve that is somewhat more successful is the floppy-tip technique. If the curved stylet is withdrawn to the high RA, with the lead tip in the lower RA, the lead will no longer point to the lateral atrial wall. Its trajectory may now be medial, toward the tricuspid valve. Advancing the body of the lead, even though the tip is floppy, allows the lead tip to cross the tricuspid valve into the RV. With this approach, it is important to avoid extreme stylet curves, which serve to increase the tendency for the lead tip to move toward the lateral RA wall. It is hoped that future lead designs will incorporate some steering mechanism in either the stylet or the lead.

A benefit of modern lead design is the various fixation mechanisms that have resulted in a near 0% dislodgment rate. One should become familiar with the lead handling characteristics of the various active-fixation and passive-fixation designs. It is important to become familiar with the passive-fixation mechanism of tines. Learning to recognize when tines are stuck on an endocardial structure and to not be intimidated by the resistance encountered when traction is applied is a must. There has yet to be a reported case of endocardial trauma from a tined electrode, even though one may occasionally get the impression that the tines have permanently attached themselves to an endocardial structure during attempts at lead placement. It is this same feeling of resistance that ensures us that the electrode will not dislodge once an ideal location is found. When the tip of a tined lead becomes caught on a structure in an undesirable position, it is usually impossible to advance the lead. The lead must be pulled free and usually withdrawn to the RA, no matter what force must be applied. Sometimes, it may take multiple electrode advances and withdrawals with the tines hanging up and preventing placement in the RV apex. Subtle adjustments in the stylet manipulation, as well as persistence, will ultimately overcome this problem.

The active-fixation leads offer a new set of problems. There are some unique problems in placement directly related to design. There are basically two types of active-fixation leads in use, both involving a helix or "screw" as the fixation mechanism. First, there is the fixation tip design with an exposed or fixed screw. Because the screw is continually exposed, its tip may catch onto any endocardial structure. As one would

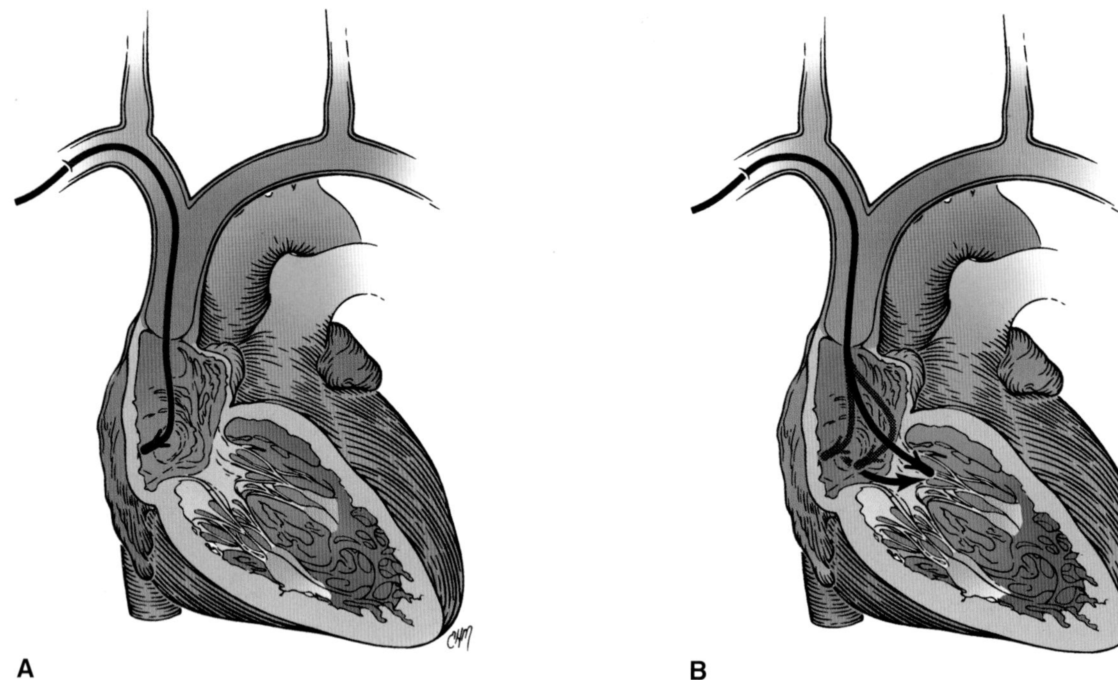

Figure 18-46. ***A,*** *Acute bends encountered with right venous access orient the lead to the lateral wall of the right atrium when a stylet with a modest curve is inserted into the electrode.* ***B,*** *The lead must be backed into the right ventricle, across the tricuspid valve when a right-sided approach is used. Rotation or partial withdrawal of the stylet is sometimes helpful in moving the electrode across the valve.*

expect, this type of helix has a high propensity for getting caught, particularly on the chordae of the tricuspid valve. Unlike tines, the screw, when caught, cannot be pulled free without some fear of damaging endocardial structures. It can usually be freed easily with counterclockwise rotation of the lead body, which results in unscrewing of the tip (the available screws are made with a clockwise helix). Some manufacturers have attempted to resolve this problem by coating the exposed screw with a sugar compound that ultimately dissolves, exposing the screw. This can work well, provided that one is consistently able to place the lead in an optimal position quickly. Doing so requires significant skill and experience, among other things, including luck. Once the coating has dissolved, the screw can hook endocardial structures if there is a difficult positioning or a need to reposition or withdraw to the RA. The exposed screw does, however, offer a reliable fixation mechanism. The second type of active-fixation lead employs an extendable-retractable screw that is mechanically extended from its "resting" retracted position. This lead is generally easier to work with because the problem of helix hang-up is avoided. In fact, the extendable-retractable screw-in type leads may be the easiest of all leads to position. Placement of both types of fixation mechanisms uses the stylet techniques previously described.

When the implanting physician is satisfied with electrode placement, the stylet may be withdrawn to the vicinity of the lower RA (Fig. 18-47)[89] or, alternatively, completely removed. Threshold testing is then carried out. If thresholds are acceptable, the ventricular elec-

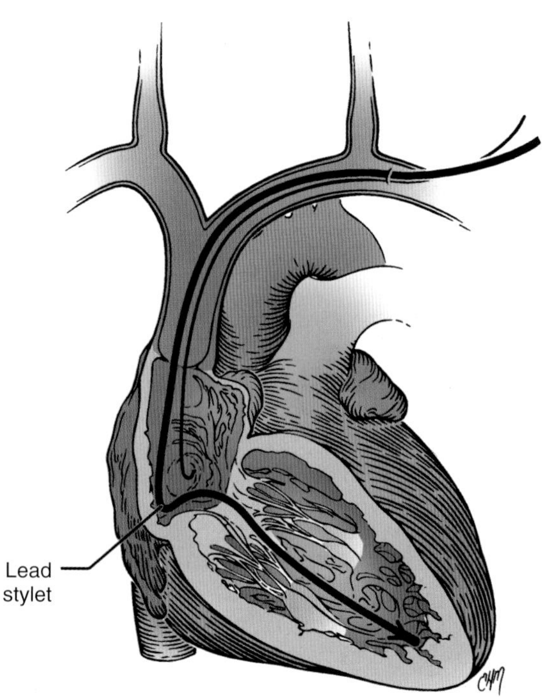

Figure 18-47. The stylet of the ventricular electrode is left in the lead but is withdrawn to the lower right atrium to permit threshold testing and assessment of the appropriate amount of lead redundancy.

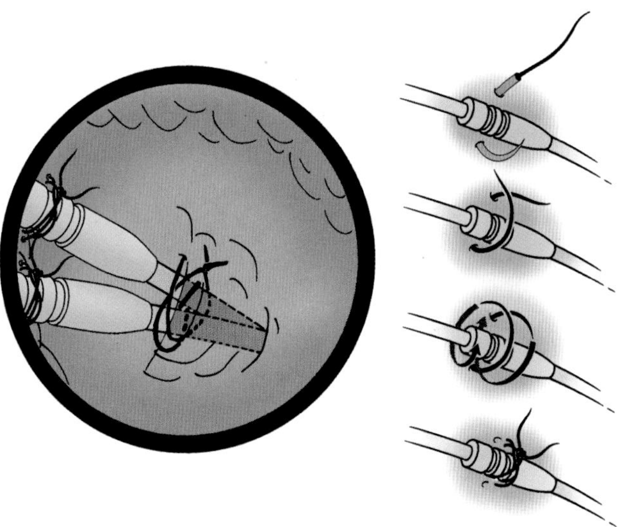

Figure 18-48. Using the suture sleeve to secure the ventricular electrode to the pectoral muscle.

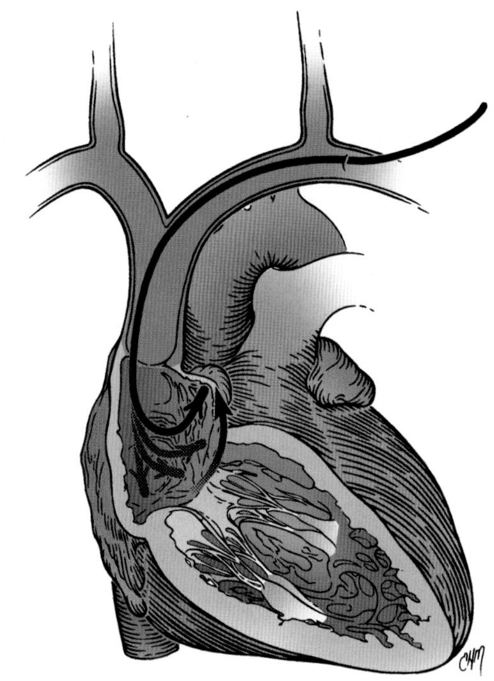

Figure 18-49. Positioning a preformed atrial J electrode by partial withdrawal of the lead stylet.

trode may be secured. Some implanters leave the stylet in the lead with the tip in the lower RA and secure the lead with the anchoring sleeve. This practice reduces the risk for ventricular lead dislodgment during placement and positioning of the atrial lead. Other implanters remove the stylet completely for testing and securing the lead but not for atrial lead placement and positioning, because there is general agreement that the stylet helps stabilize the ventricular lead during atrial lead manipulation, which otherwise can frequently dislodge the ventricular lead.

The suture sleeve is advanced down the shaft of the lead body to the vicinity of venous entry. One to three ligatures are applied around the suture sleeve and lead, incorporating a generous amount of pectoral muscle (Fig. 18-48). It has been our experience that multiple ligatures that are not excessively tight make lead slippage as well as lead damage less likely than a single, tightly applied ligature. Securing the ventricular electrode immediately after satisfactory positioning is important. Early securing helps prevent inadvertent dislodgment whether or not an atrial electrode is to be placed. The ventricular electrode should be oriented somewhat horizontally in a plane roughly parallel to the clavicle. This orientation avoids excessive bending of the lead at the point where it exits the vein.

Placement of Atrial Electrodes

Atrial electrode placement can be extremely easy but has been the nemesis of many implanting physicians. It has even been responsible for the resistance of many implanters to the dual-chamber approach to cardiac pacing. This, we believe, is largely because the clinician has not been exposed to proper placement technique. Once again, it must be appreciated that the proper placement of any pacemaker electrode is a symphony of lead and stylet. The lead, by itself, cannot be steered or twisted into place.

Two fundamental techniques relate directly to lead design. The first is placement of an electrode with a preformed curve or atrial J electrode.[90] This electrode can have either active-fixation or passive-fixation mechanisms. More commonly, a lead with passive-fixation tines is used. After insertion into the venous system, the lead tip is positioned with a straight stylet fully inserted in the middle to lower RA. The preformed J has been straightened with the straight stylet. Fluoroscopy can be applied in either the PA or the RAO projection. Under fluoroscopic observation, the straight stylet is withdrawn several centimeters. The atrial lead tip can be observed to begin assuming its J configuration, with the tip beginning to point upward. The lead body is then slowly advanced at the venous entry site (Fig. 18-49). On fluoroscopy, the lead tip is observed to continue its upward motion, eventually seating in the atrial appendage. If the lead tip is too low in the RA, it may catch on or cross the tricuspid valve as the stylet is withdrawn. In this case, the lead is simply withdrawn a bit and the maneuver repeated slightly higher in the RA. If the lead tip is too high in the RA or is in the SVC, the tip will not move upward adequately. In this case, the electrode is repositioned more inferiorly. As one gains comfort with this maneuver, it can be repeated over and over. With experience, the act of retracting the stylet slightly can be performed briskly. This brisk move "snaps" the lead tip into the atrial appendage, at times resulting in better electrode-endocardium contact. Frustration and failure may occur if one attempts atrial placement by briskly removing the entire stylet and expecting the electrode to jump into the atrial appendage. This maneuver usually results in the electrode's coiling on itself in the

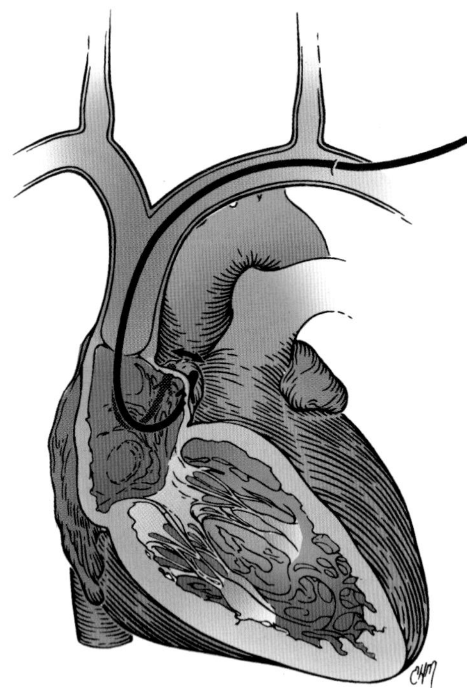

Figure 18-50. The to-and-fro, medial-to-lateral motion of a well-placed atrial lead in the atrial appendage when viewed in the posteroanterior projection.

SVC or RA. With the stylet coiled in this fashion, further attempts at positioning are impossible until it has been reinserted and the process begun again.

Good atrial positioning consists of a generous J loop, with the tip moving from medial to lateral in a to-and-fro fashion in the PA radiographic projection (Fig. 18-50).[91,92] In the lateral projection, the tip should be anterior and observed to "bob" up and down. With the firmly seated tip in the atrial appendage, the lead body should be twisted or torqued to the left and right to establish a position of neutral torque. Sometimes, in the process of positioning, torque can build up. If it is not released, electrode dislodgment could result. This same maneuver of twisting can also result in better electrode-myocardium contact. With experience, one gets a sense of the proper J or loop size, which can be a source of frustration. Too much or too little loop can result in dislodgment, depending somewhat on the lead model. Another frustrating event can occur in relation to conformational changes in the vasculature with postural movement. With the patient supine, just the right loop appears to have been created, but as soon as the patient becomes upright, the conformational change occurs, and it appears as though the mediastinal vasculature shifts inferiorly, pulling up on the lead, and obliterating the loop. Unfortunately, this situation may not be discovered until the postimplantation chest radiograph is reviewed. Attempts at gauging the loop size by having the patient take deep inspirations are frequently unrewarding. As a general rule, it is better to create a more generous loop.

Positioning the preformed J lead with an active-fixation screw-in mechanism uses the same basic technique described earlier. After positioning in the atrial appendage, however, the active-fixation mechanism must be activated. This step usually involves the extension of a screw or helix. The exposed or fixed screw described previously is not available in a preformed atrial J configuration.

The second fundamental technique of atrial electrode placement involves the use of a straight or non-preformed lead. This lead is positioned in the atrium with the use of a stylet that is preformed into a J shape and can be modified into other configurations. The stylets typically come with the lead already preformed into the J shape, or if desired, a straight stylet can be shaped into the J or other configurations via the same technique described for curving the ventricular lead stylet. The stylet can then be positioned in the atrium, frequently in the atrial appendage, although it has become increasingly evident that other locations in the atrium, especially the anterior and lateral free walls, can be easily and safely targeted.[93] Manipulation of the stylet is required to gain access to the various atrial locations. Not uncommonly, modification of the preformed stylet shape is required. At the University of Oklahoma (DWR), the modification of the J stylet into a shape similar to that of an Amplatz coronary artery catheter (several varieties) has been helpful in gaining access to a number of positions in the RA. The principal advantage of the non-preformed leads (which use stylets of various shapes) with active-fixation mechanisms is that one is not restricted to the atrial appendage; this issue is discussed in more detail later. With a straight or non-preformed active-fixation lead, either a fixed screw or an extendable-retractable screw can be used.

Reports have been made of successful placement of a straight, tined lead in the atrial appendage without dislodgment. Because of the risk for dislodgment and the high success rate of both the active-fixation and preformed atrial J leads, however, this is not recommended, especially early in one's experience. The use of an active-fixation lead in the atrium is ideal in patients who have undergone open heart surgery during which the atrial appendage was amputated.

There are several other advantages to using an active-fixation lead in the atrium. The first, as already noted, is the ability to choose the placement site and/or map the atrium for optimal electrical threshold. By extending and retracting an extendable-retractable screw or attaching and detaching a fixed screw, one can analyze multiple positions. The straight active-fixation lead can be placed essentially anywhere in the atrium. On the other hand, the preformed atrial J lead can typically and easily be placed only in the atrial appendage. The second advantage of the active-fixation lead is its ease of retrievability. The ability to remove a lead implanted for long-term function, if removal becomes necessary in the future, is probably more easily accomplished if it is an active-fixation lead.

Proper or adequate placement of active-fixation leads is reflected by good electrical threshold measurements. Adequate active lead fixation has been shown to relate to a current of injury. The development of a current of injury indicates that within 10 minutes of fixation, pacing thresholds return to acceptable limits and indicate good fixation.[94] As discussed in the section on ventricular electrode placement, there are differences of opinion about whether, in addition to the achievement of optimal electrical parameters, a gentle tug on the lead after fixation is helpful in determining whether good mechanical fixation is achieved. Although some implanters use a floppy-tip technique for unusual or precise lead placement, some types of active-fixation leads (especially of the extendable-retractable variety) require full insertion of the stylet to activate the screw-in mechanism. The floppy-tip approach is not effective in this situation. This problem is not encountered with the fixed screw and some of the extendable-retractable screws.

Occasionally, one encounters difficulty while attempting to place leads in the atrial appendage with the preformed atrial J stylet. In certain situations, the lead with J stylet in place does not assume an adequate J shape to enter the atrial appendage or make contact with atrial muscle. The reason may be that the stylet is too limp or does not have enough curve or that the atrium is large. In this situation, one may have to use a stiffer stylet and preform it with an exaggerated curve or J. One can also have difficulty when trying to maneuver stiffer stylets down through the electrode as well as during negotiation of the venous system in the superior mediastinum. A trial-and-error approach using multiple stylet configurations is almost always ultimately rewarded by success.

The side of venous access has little effect on trial electrode placement. Whether placement is from the right or the left, the preformed J electrode or the straight electrode with preformed J stylet can generally provide easy access to the atrial appendage. Venous access may affect placement of the electrode in unusual atrial positions. Precise placement through the use of stylet and electrode manipulation may be more difficult from the right side. As discussed for ventricular lead placement, the electrode, depending on the shape of the stylet curve, may seek a right lateral orientation.

Securing the atrial lead is similar to securing the ventricular lead. When being secured after percutaneous venous access and placement, the atrial lead, like the ventricular lead, should be oriented in a generally horizontal plane, roughly parallel to the clavicle. If the pocket has not already been made, the infraclavicular space is opened by means of dissection with Metzenbaum scissors. Dissection is carried to the surface of the greater pectoral muscle near its attachment point under the clavicle. The fibers of the platysma muscles are severed. A 1-0 silk suture is placed in a generous "bite" of the pectoral muscle under the anticipated site of attachment. The suture sleeve is advanced down the lead to the vicinity of the suture. Care should be taken not to dislodge or change the atrial lead position in the process.

Occasionally, the suture sleeve binds to the electrode, making it difficult to position. One can best manage this difficulty by lubricating the lead with sterile saline or other fluid and using smooth forceps to then slide the sleeve into position. Once the suture sleeve is in position, the suture is secured around it. Many implanters first put a knot in the suture on the surface of the muscle. The two ends of the suture are then wrapped around the suture sleeve and tied. This second tie is directly around the lead and is designed to prevent lead slippage. Some implanters use multiple sutures rather than a single one, as discussed for ventricular electrode placement. Care must be taken to make the tie snug and yet avoid injury to the lead. It is important to orient the electrode horizontally. As with ventricular leads, doing so orients the lead in a plane similar to that of the axillary vein, reduces the bend of the lead, and may decrease the likelihood of the crush phenomenon or other stress-related lead damage.

If venous access and electrode placement have been achieved with venous cutdown, there is essentially no risk of the classic crush injury. Generally, the suture sleeve and lead are anchored to the pectoral muscle parallel to the vein. Similar precautions concerning lead injury should be observed. The securing process is the same, and one should avoid acute angulation of the lead and the creation of points of lead stress.

Upgrading Techniques

An upgrading procedure is necessary in patients with the pacemaker syndrome. With the growing acceptance of dual-chamber pacing, all patients who have been implanted with VVI systems and who have intact atrial function are now being considered for a pacemaker system upgrade with the addition of an atrial lead. In addition, some patients with an existing pacemaker system need an upgrade to an automatic ICD or a biventricular system for resynchronization. Such patients also need a pacing and shocking electrode and/or an LV lead. Generally, this change is deferred until the time of pulse generator power depletion, but greater awareness of the pacemaker syndrome or the need for an ICD or resynchronization has resulted in earlier pacemaker system upgrades.

The upgrade procedure requires new venous access for the introduction of one or more new leads. It may also involve the introduction of a new ventricular lead because of problems with the existing lead. Most pacemaker system upgrades require the replacement of the pulse generator, although occasionally, the existing pulse generator used in the ventricle can be used for atrial pacing. Most of the time, upgrade procedures involve a conventional approach using one of the previously described percutaneous techniques or a venous cutdown. If the first ventricular lead was placed through the cephalic vein, the percutaneous approach is almost mandatory for the upgrade. Conversely, in patients treated with an initial percutaneous subclavian approach, the new lead can be introduced either by cutdown of the cephalic vein or through percutaneous venous access. In the case of an initial percutaneous approach, the ventricular electrode can serve as a map. Using fluoroscopy, one can use the existing ventricular lead as a target to guide the percutaneous needle. Care should be taken not to touch or damage the first lead with the needle. The lead should be used as a reference landmark for the expected location of the subclavian vein. Bognolo and associates[95,96] have described a technique to reestablish venous access using the old ventricular lead. The patency of the venous structures can be assessed as previously described with the injection of radiographic contrast material.[73]

If access to the subclavian vein cannot be obtained by following the axioms of the safe introducer technique previously described by Byrd,[59] an extrathoracic puncture of the axillary vein can be carried out. The puncture of the vein can be expedited with a simple technique: A guidewire or catheter is passed to the vicinity of the subclavian vein through a vein in the arm. The guidewire or catheter can be palpated or viewed fluoroscopically, thus serving as a reference for venous access. In the case of a cutdown on a previously unused cephalic vein, the Ong-Barold percutaneous sheath set technique can be used.[81]

Lead compatibility is important when one is considering a pacemaker system upgrade. To avoid embarrassment, one must be aware of the new pulse generator's compatibility with the chronic lead system.

Occasionally, ipsilateral venous access is impossible. Either the vessel is thrombosed or there is some form of obstruction that precludes the placement of a second (atrial) lead from the same side. In this case, contralateral venous access can be achieved, and the lead tunneled back to the original pocket (Fig. 18-51). Early injection of radiographic contrast material may expedite the decision to use this approach. The use of the contralateral subclavian (rather than cephalic) vein is recommended for this approach.[97] The distance to the original pocket is less, and the new lead is not as susceptible to dislodgment. The same percutaneous techniques and precautions are used as previously described for the percutaneous approach. The only difference is the size of the skin incision, which is limited to about 1 to 1.5 cm. The incision need only be large enough to allow anchoring of the lead and securing of the suture sleeve. As in an initial implantation, the incision should be carried down to the pectoral fascia. Once the lead has been positioned and secured, it can be tunneled to the original pocket.

The maneuver of passing an electrode or catheter through tissue from one location to another is referred to as *tunneling*. It always involves the passage of a catheter from one wound through tissue to a second wound remote from the first. An example is the placement of a pacemaker lead through the internal jugular vein. The lead is passed from the jugular incision through the tissue over (or under) the clavicle to the pacemaker pocket in the pectoral area. With the development of implantable defibrillator lead and patch systems that do not require thoracotomy, tunneling has become popular and necessary.

A number of techniques are available for tunneling. They differ in level of trauma to the tissue and lead. As a rule, the least traumatic technique is desirable. A popular technique is to place the proximal end of the lead or leads to be tunneled in a 14-inch Penrose drain (Fig. 18-52A). A gentle, nonconstricting tie is applied around the drain just distal to the lead connector (see

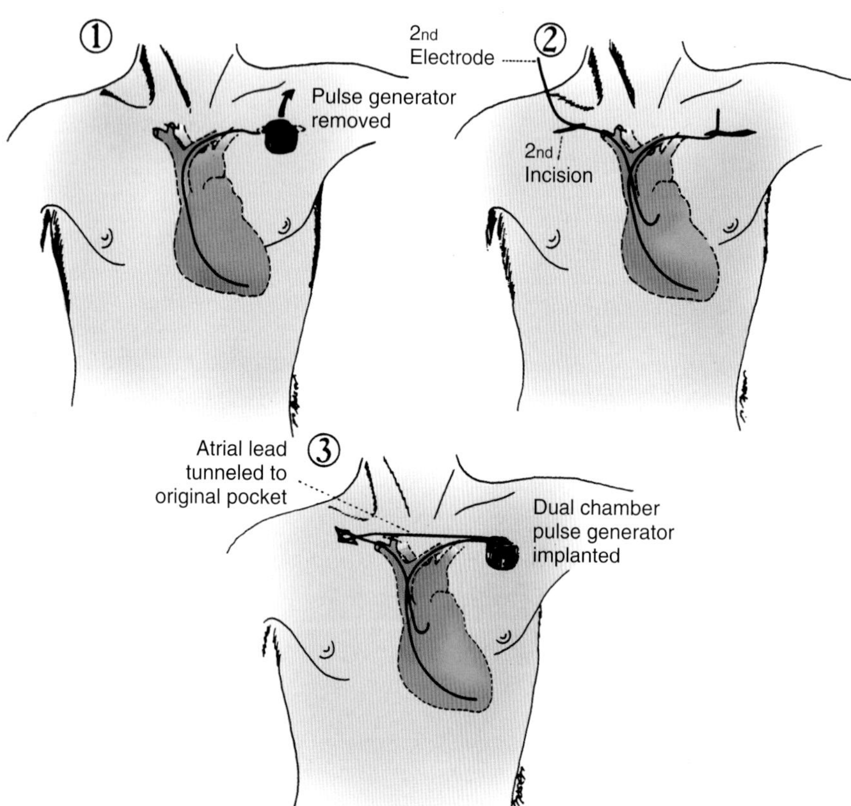

Figure 18-51. Pacemaker upgrade using the contralateral subclavian vein: (1) the pacemaker pocket is opened, and the old pulse generator and lead are dissected free, externalized, and disconnected; (2) the second lead is inserted by means of the contralateral subclavian vein; and (3) the second lead is tunneled back to the initial pocket. (From Belott PH: Use of the contralateral subclavian vein for placement of atrial electrodes in chronically VVI paced patients. PACE 6:781, 1983.)

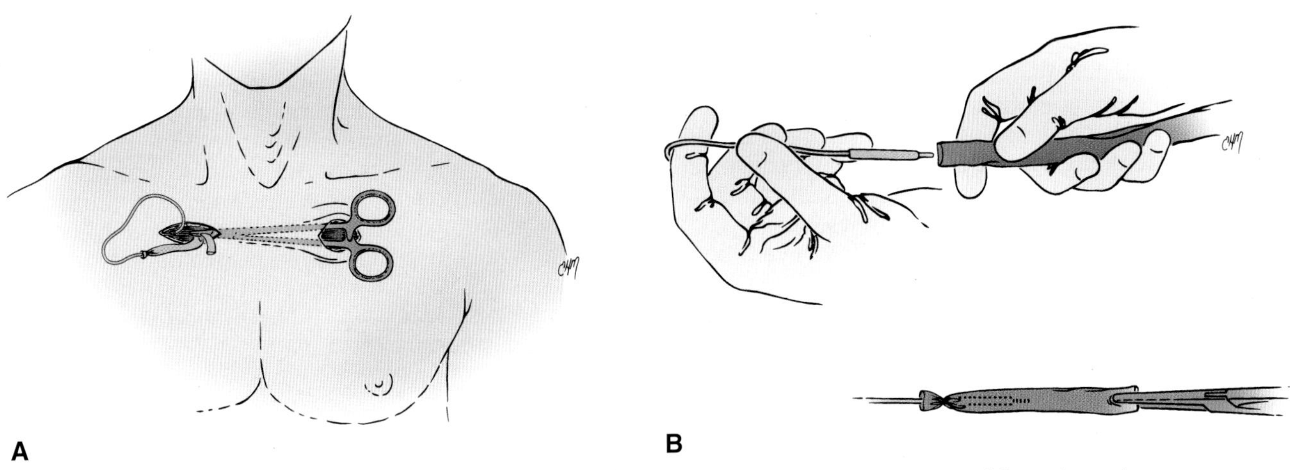

Figure 18-52. ***A,*** *Penrose drain and lead grabbed by a clamp that has been passed from the recipient wound to the donor site. The Penrose drain and lead(s) are pulled back to the recipient wound.* ***B,*** *Tunneling from one wound to another by placing the electrode(s) in a Penrose drain. The lead(s) are placed in a 14-inch Penrose drain and tied. The Penrose drain is then grabbed with a long clamp.*

Fig. 18-52B). The track of the tunnel, from the satellite wound to the pocket, is infiltrated with local anesthesia by means of an 18-gauge spinal needle. The free end of the Penrose drain is then brought to the receiving wound from the satellite wound in the subcutaneous tissue. This can be accomplished with several techniques. The first technique involves the use of a Kelly clamp or uterine packing forceps. The tip of the clamp is pushed bluntly in the subcutaneous tissue from the receiving wound directly to the satellite wound. Care is taken to keep the tunnel as deep as possible, usually on the surface of the muscle. The free end of the Penrose drain is grasped and pulled back from the satellite wound to the receiving wound. The remainder of the Penrose drain containing the electrode connector pin is pulled through the track to the receiving wound. The tie is released, and the Penrose drain is removed.

A second technique delivers the Penrose drain to the receiving wound by use of a "passer," usually a knitting needle or dilator. In this technique, the free end of the Penrose drain is fixed to the back end of the passer with a tie. The pointed tip of the passer is inserted into the satellite wound and pushed to the receiving wound. The tip of the passer is grasped and pulled into the receiving wound with the Penrose drain attached. The remainder of the Penrose drain with the lead is then pulled into the receiving wound.

A variation of this technique uses the percutaneous technique to establish the tunnel. After the track of the tunnel is infiltrated with an 18-gauge spinal needle, the needle is passed from the wound of origin to the receiving wound. A guidewire is passed through the needle into the receiving wound. A standard peel-away introducer is then passed over the guidewire from the satellite incision to the receiving wound. The sheath can then be used to pass the lead, and the sheath is eventually removed and peeled.

Another variation uses the dilator of the sheath set to tunnel and the guidewire to pull the Penrose drain from wound to wound. After the dilator is used to create the tunnel from one wound to the other, the guidewire is passed through the dilator. The dilator is removed, and the guidewire is attached to the loose end of the Penrose drain. The implanter then brings the Penrose drain to the receiving wound by pulling the guidewire.

A technique that is similar in principle to the use of the Penrose drain, but that may be more traumatic, involves the use of a small chest tube and a Pean clamp. The size of the chest tube is determined by the size and number of leads to be tunneled at one time. The length is determined by the distance from the initial wound to the receiving wound. The tube may be cut to size and the end beveled to a point. The leads at the wound of origin are placed in the back end of the chest tube. The Pean clamp is bluntly passed from the receiving wound to the wound containing the leads. The pointed end of the chest tube is grasped by the Pean clamp and is pulled into and through the receiving wound. Although more traumatic to tissue, this technique is protective of the electrodes.

Another related technique involving the use of a chest tube requires blunt passage of the chest tube, with the trocar in place, through the subcutaneous tissue from the site of origin to the receiving wound with the lead or leads placed in the "back end" of the tube after removal of the trocar. The tube can then be pulled through into the receiving wound.

Finally, new tunneling tools have been developed for use with implantable defibrillators. These tools may be used for pacemaker lead tunneling also.

The preceding techniques and principles are used whenever tunneling is required. Tunneling with a clamp and directly grasping the lead should always be avoided because of the risk of damage to the lead.

Placement of Epicardial Electrodes

Epicardial pacemaker implantation was the earliest, and once the most common, implantation technique, but it has limited use and usefulness today, largely because of the unparalleled success of transvenous implantation. Today, epicardial implantation is reserved mainly for patients undergoing cardiac surgery. In fact, in many centers, even in patients needing permanent pacing who are undergoing cardiac surgery, temporary epicardial electrodes are applied, with subsequent implantation of permanent transvenous pacing systems. Modern transvenous leads have largely eliminated the problems of exit block and dislodgment. These leads have proved more reliable than epicardial leads. In addition, the abdominal pacemaker location of epicardial systems may cause more discomfort than a prepectoral location. Today, only unusual circumstances dictate an epicardial implantation; they are (1) patients undergoing cardiac surgery for another indication (with the preceding caveat), (2) patients with recurrent dislodgments of transvenous systems, (3) patients with prosthetic tricuspid valves or congenital anomalies, such as tricuspid atresia, and (4) more recently, patients undergoing CRT in whom coronary sinus lead placement has been unsuccessful. There are multiple reasons for unsuccessful coronary sinus lead placement, including unsuccessful coronary sinus cannulation, poor branch anatomy location, poor lead stability, unacceptable capture thresholds, and diaphragmatic or phrenic nerve stimulation.

This chapter has dealt extensively with transvenous electrode placement, but epicardial placement is treated more superficially.

There are several surgical approaches for epicardial lead placement. The most common is probably the median sternotomy performed as a secondary procedure at the time of other, related cardiac surgery. In this case, both the atria and ventricles are mapped for optimal pacing thresholds and other electrophysiologic parameters. The electrodes are attached directly to the epicardium. The electrode is tunneled via the chest tube technique to a subcutaneous pocket in the upper abdomen.

For epicardial electrode placement performed as a primary procedure, there are three distinct approaches: the subxiphoid approach, the left subcostal approach, and the left anterolateral thoracotomy. The first two avoid a "formal" thoracotomy. The pericardium is entered through an abdominal incision that is supradiaphragmatic. The subxiphoid approach exposes the diaphragmatic surface of the heart and mainly the RV. The RV can be thin, and care should be taken to avoid laceration, which can require urgent thoracotomy and, possibly, cardiopulmonary bypass. The left subcostal approach exposes more of the LV. The left lateral thoracotomy favors LV electrode placement. With this approach, an incision is made in the fifth intercostal space. The incision extends from the left parasternal border to the left anterior axillary line. Care must be taken to avoid the phrenic nerve.

All of the epicardial pacemaker implantation techniques require general anesthesia. The median sternotomy and left lateral implantation procedures generally require chest tube placement. The epicardial procedures are performed in an operating room by a thoracic surgeon trained specifically in epicardial pacemaker implantation.

Epicardial lead placement has also been accomplished by additional, minimally invasive techniques, such as the same small-incision techniques used for coronary or valve surgery. In addition, thoracoscopic and robotic surgical techniques are now more frequently attempted for LV lead placement. Finally, like the techniques used for ablation, techniques for percutaneous access to the pericardium are under development. These leads will probably be placed without general anesthesia.

Securing Leads, Creating Pockets, and Closure

When all electrodes are in position, it is time to establish permanent venous stasis and secure the leads. These maneuvers pertain to the transvenous approach only. In the epicardial procedures, the electrodes have already been secured directly to the heart, and no vascular structure has been entered that requires comparable attainment of venous stasis. In the case of the transvenous approach, one or more leads must be secured and the venous port of entry must be permanently sealed. If the cutdown approach has been used, the proximal and distal ligatures must be tied. One should take care not to injure or cut the lead when securing the ligature around the vein containing the lead. The venous ties are merely to effect hemostasis, not to secure the lead. These ties should be gentle and as nonconstricting as possible. The securing process using the anchoring sleeves has already been described. We reiterate here that the leads should be secured and oriented in a plane that is roughly parallel to the subclavian or axillary vein to reduce the risk for subclavian crush injury. As with the ligatures around the leads, the suture sleeves should be secured snugly but not overtightened (Fig. 18-53).

If the figure-of-eight or purse-string suture has been used in conjunction with the percutaneous approach, it can be tied after all leads are in position and no

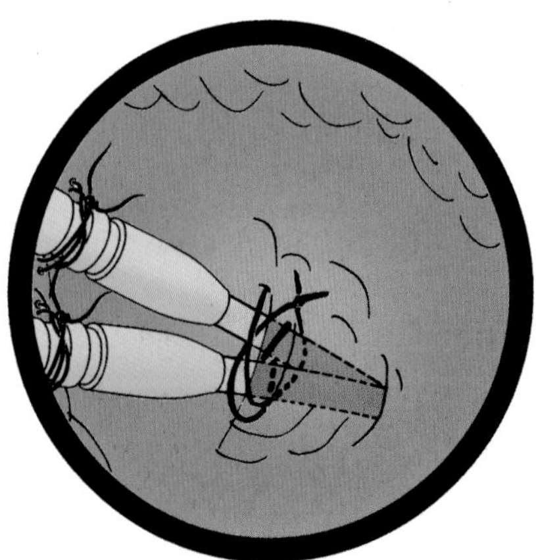

Figure 18-53. Secured atrial and ventricular electrodes with the suture sleeves. Hemostasis is effected at the puncture site, when necessary, with a loose nonconstricting tie.

further venous entry is desired. Also at this time, the retained guidewire can be removed, although it is not essential to do so. The retained guidewire can be removed later, just before wound closure; in this case, if the figure-of-eight or purse-string suture has been tied properly, there will be no back-bleeding. The guidewire should, in any case, be retained until the last moment, when no further venous access is required. It should be removed only after the implanter is completely satisfied with electrode placement and there is no need for replacement or exchange. Like the venous ligatures used in the cutdown technique, the figure-of-eight or purse-string suture requires only enough tension to collapse the vein or the tissue surrounding the leads near their point of entry into the vein. It is not intended to anchor the leads. If tied too tightly, it may injure the lead or leads. As mentioned before, the retained guidewire need not be removed before the figure-of-eight stitch is tied. The retained guidewire can be removed much later, just before wound closure.

Once the leads have been secured, it is time to create the pacemaker pocket if this step has not already been accomplished. Traditionally, the step is performed at the end of the procedure. The actual timing of the pocket creation, however, is at the discretion of the implanting physician. Some implanters prefer to create the pocket early in the procedure, even as the initial step in a pacemaker implantation. In this case, a rudimentary pocket is created and packed with gauze, allowing time for natural hemostasis. Toward the end of the procedure, the packing is removed, and the pocket is reinspected for hemostasis and surgically modified as necessary. The alternative approach involves creation of the pacemaker pocket after the leads have been secured. There are arguments for both approaches. Proponents of early pocket creation argue that bleeding is more easily controlled and the risk for damage to leads is lower. Proponents of late pocket creation argue that to make the pocket early is "putting the cart before the horse" and that the highest priority is to establish pacing early to protect the patient. Creation of the pacemaker pocket is of lower priority. In addition, early creation of the pocket may result in embarrassment if the pocket is not used because venous access was unsuccessful.

A reasonable modification of the early pocket approach avoids the risk of embarrassment if the vein on that side is not used for access. It involves percutaneous venous access with placement and maintenance of an intravenous guidewire before pocket creation, which, in turn, precedes placement of the leads using the guidewire. This approach ensures venous access before formation of the pocket and achieves the advantages of early pocket formation noted previously.

Before the pacemaker pocket is created, the area is generously infiltrated with a local anesthetic agent, assuming that local anesthesia is used. If an earlier incision has been made to facilitate lead placement and securing, anesthesia is best achieved through infiltration along the edge of the incision directly into the subcutaneous tissue. The incision is carried down to the anterior surface of the pectoral fascia. The pacemaker pocket is best formed predominantly inferior and medial to the incision, although many implanters also form a small portion of the pocket superior and lateral to an incision directed from the venipuncture site in an inferolateral vector. The advantage of this approach is that the pulse generator, with leads coiled deep, can then be placed directly under the incision, making subsequent pacing procedures, such as pulse generator replacement, both easy and safe with an incision at the same site.

A plane of dissection is created at the junction of the subcutaneous tissue and pectoral fascia. This is best achieved by putting the subcutaneous tissue under slight tension with some form of retraction, to better define the plane of dissection. The Senn retractor can be used initially and then is replaced by the Goulet retractor. The plane of dissection can be started with either the Metzenbaum scissors or the cutting function of electrocautery. After a plane of dissection has been established, the remainder of the pocket can be created with blunt dissection. Some argue that blunt dissection is less traumatic to the tissues. The problems with blunt dissection are the lack of adequate visualization and the lack of control with respect to tissue depth. Optimally, the pacemaker pocket should be as deep as possible right on top of the fascia of the pectoral muscle. This arrangement offers the optimal subcutaneous tissue thickness necessary to avoid erosion. Unfortunately, with blunt dissection, this ideal plane can be lost, creating inconsistent pocket thickness with greater risk of erosion. Today's pacemaker is small, limiting the amount of dissection required and the pocket size needed. The pocket can easily be created with direct visualization instead of blindly. As previously noted, the subcutaneous tissue is held under gentle tension, defining the plane of dissection. Sharp dissection with Metzenbaum scissors, the cutting function of electrocautery, or both is then used to form the pocket. This technique is less traumatic than blunt dissection. The pocket created by precise dissection over the pectoral muscle provides optimal tissue thickness. Thus, the pocket is created under direct vision, and the plane of dissection is well controlled. The headlamp as a light source can be helpful here. There is less risk for hematoma because all bleeding is directly visualized and managed with electrocautery.

Occasionally, the patient has little or no subcutaneous tissue. In this situation, a subpectoralis subpectoral implantation should be considered. Fortunately, with the dramatically reduced size of today's pacemakers and the availability of the Parsonnet pouch (see Fig. 18-5), this approach is rarely necessary.[98] If required, placement of the pacemaker under the pectoral muscle represents only a slight departure from the techniques already described. The one major concern with using this approach is the increased chance of bleeding and hematoma formation. But if one understands the anatomy and performs the procedure correctly, little or no bleeding is encountered when the subpectoral space is entered. However, typically an increased risk for hematoma formation is observed. In subpectoral implantation, the incision has already been carried down to the surface of the pectoral muscle, and the leads secured. The pectoralis major muscle is inspected for a separation or seam between parallel muscle fibers. Metzenbaum scissors are used to open the fascia over the seam. Using the blunt ends of two Senn retractors, one can gently separate the muscle bellies and lift the pectoralis major muscle lifted off the chest wall. The chest wall is usually identified from its yellow fatty tissue.

Once the space is entered, one can insert an index finger gently, lifting the pectoralis major muscle bluntly creating a space under the pectoralis major muscle and on top of the pectoralis minor muscle. Occasionally a vascular pedicle is seen, which can be moved to one side. If this pedicle is inadvertently torn, hemostasis is easily achieved with vascular staples. If one is careful to avoid tearing of the muscle and tissue, little or no bleeding is encountered. If bleeding is encountered, it is most effectively managed with electrocautery. Incisions should be made through the muscle parallel to the muscle fibers. The muscle is separated, and a plane of dissection is established on the chest wall. This pocket is best created with blunt dissection. As already described, considerable bleeding can be encountered with subpectoral implantations. This bleeding is best controlled with electrocautery. Careful visual inspection using a Goulet retractor and good lighting is important. All bleeding sources should be identified and either sutured, stapled or electrocoagulated. Pocket drainage is rarely required.

Use of electrocautery has been a traditional taboo in cardiac pacing. It can cause fibrillation or burns at the myocardium-electrode interface and can reprogram or even irreparably damage the pulse generator. However, electrocautery can be extremely useful in a pacemaker procedure in both coagulation and cutting modes. It is the surest and most expeditious way to control bleeding and create the pacemaker pocket. It can be used safely, provided that one is aware of the dangers and takes a few precautions. Today's electrocautery systems are extremely safe from an electrical hazard point of view. Built-in mechanisms protect against improper grounding. A few simple rules should be followed that are specific to the use of electrocautery systems in pacemaker implantation procedures. First, the use of electrocautery should be avoided when the pulse generator is in the surgical field. Second, the cautery must never touch the exposed pin of the pacemaker lead. Finally, the cautery must never touch the retained guidewire if the wire is in the heart.

Wound drainage is required in patients who manifest excessive bleeding. The term *wet pocket* has been used to describe this condition. This situation is being encountered more frequently with the growing use of anticoagulants. In patients taking aspirin, warfarin, or heparin, a wet pocket often occurs, and medical indications often preclude cessation of such drugs. If a patient is taking warfarin, a prothrombin time that is 1 to 1.5 times the control level is less likely to cause a problem than a value greater than 1.5 times the control level. In the latter situation, the procedure should be postponed until the prothrombin time reaches a more reasonable level. Heparin and platelet antagonists appear to cause the greatest problem. Despite diligent efforts to establish hemostasis, the pockets may continue to ooze diffusely. In this circumstance, some implanters have resorted to the topical application of thrombin.

The patient who is taking anticoagulants and whose pacemaker pocket appears wet should be considered for some form of drainage. As a general rule, if reasonable hemostasis cannot be achieved, the pacemaker pocket should be drained (although drainage should not be considered an alternative to adequate attempts to attain hemostasis). This is accomplished by placing a Jackson-Pratt drain or Blake drain. A trocar connected to the drainage tubing is passed from the inferior aspect of the pacemaker pocket to a satellite exit wound remote from the pacemaker pocket. The distal end of the tubing in the pacemaker pocket is specially designed of soft rubber with multiple drainage ports. This end can be cut to the desired size to avoid excessive tubing in the pocket. After the pacemaker pocket is closed, the proximal end of the drainage tubing is connected to a closed-suction system. The Jackson-Pratt system is preferred because it has a one-way valve that allows emptying yet prevents inadvertent flushing of old drained fluids back into the pocket. It is small and of little encumbrance to the patient. To avoid infection, the drainage system is removed within 24 hours. If drainage is copious, a longer period may be required. In the case of persistent bloody drainage, the wound should be reexplored and the culprit bleeding vessel ligated or cauterized.

Wound irrigation is largely a matter of personal preference, with no clearly established mandate by investigations to perform it. Drainage options range from simple saline lavage to concentrated solutions of multiple antibiotics. It is likely that such antibiotic solutions are unnecessary, especially if systemic antibiotics are used. This issue has been previously addressed. In addition to irrigation of the wound, some implanters place antibiotic-soaked gauze pads in the pocket early to achieve not only antibiosis but also hemostasis through compression with the pads.

Closure of the pacemaker pocket consists of initial approximation of the subcutaneous tissues and subsequent skin closure. The subcutaneous tissue can be approximated by single or multiple layers of interrupted or running sutures. The number of layers is a function of the thickness of the subcutaneous tissue. The suture material used by most implanters for subcutaneous closure is an absorbable semisynthetic product that is fairly strong, usually 2-0 or 3-0. There are several techniques of skin closure. The choice of technique relates to the desired cosmetic effect and time spent. An ideal cosmetic effect can be achieved with the subcuticular suture. This is best accomplished with 4-0 semisynthetic absorbable suture material, which does not require removal. The use of interrupted sutures has the least pleasing cosmetic result, and the sutures must be removed. The resulting scar may have visible cross-hatches. Many skin closures are performed with surgical staples or clips, which are cosmetically appealing and extremely fast. The only drawback to the use of staples is that they require removal in 7 to 10 days. After closure of the skin, the wound is coated with an antiseptic ointment, and a dry sterile dressing is applied. Because a pocket has been created that can fill with blood, some form of pressure dressing may be used, although it is often not easy to maintain the pressure in an ambulatory or otherwise active patient.

Immediate Postoperative Care

The intensity of monitoring after implantation varies considerably from center to center, although there is general agreement that postoperative intensive care monitoring is not usually required. Patients who were in the intensive care unit before implantation may be transferred to a bed on a nursing unit for continuous cardiac rhythm monitoring, unless, of course, there is another reason for the patient to be in an intensive care setting. Other patients electively admitted to the hospital specifically for pacemaker implantation are also returned to a cardiac monitoring area. Basic rhythm monitoring would appear to be all that is necessary. The activity level allowed the patient in the immediate postoperative period is subject to the implanter's personal preference and philosophy. In the early days of pacing, the patient was kept on strict bed rest with restricted activity for many days. Today's lead systems with both active-fixation and passive-fixation mechanisms offer a new dimension of security. The historic dislodgment rates of nearly 20% have been dramatically reduced.

In most centers, the current philosophy is to have the patient active immediately or shortly after arriving in the monitoring area. The intention is early identification of patients with potential pacemaker system malfunctions. The patient with a precariously placed electrode who is kept on strict bed rest may not demonstrate malfunction, giving a false sense of security at the time of discharge. The active patient gives a better indication whether reliable pacemaker sensing and capture are occurring. This approach is important in the patient being managed on an ambulatory basis. The practice of placing the patient's arm on the side of implantation in a sling should be avoided. This only gives one a false sense of security and can result in a frozen shoulder. If the pacemaker or defibrillator leads had been placed so poorly that simple motion of the extremity on the side of the implant results in dislodgment and pacemaker system failure, the operator would want to be aware of this problem immediately. Hiding this potential problem with a sling is counterproductive. If the patient will be staying in the hospital postoperatively, noninvasive pacemaker evaluation and programming may be carried out. They might include re-evaluation of sensing and pacing thresholds as well as initial activation and setup of the rate-adaptive system. If the patient is to be managed as an outpatient, these functions can be carried out at the time of the initial postoperative visit to the pacemaker clinic.

The documentation of the pacemaker procedure is crucial from both a clinical and a medicolegal point of view. It is essential to have a surgical report that identifies indications; pacemaker and lead manufacturer, make, and model; details of the implantation procedure; and pacemaker-programmed settings. A clear description of the procedure, including problems encountered as well as electrical testing data, is important. Copies of the surgical report should be sent to the pacemaker clinic as well as to the referring and follow-up physicians. Further documentation includes the manufacturer's registration forms for all pacemaker, ICD, and biventricular systems. In addition, on January 27, 2005, the U.S. Center for Medicare and Medicaid Services mandated a national registration of all primary prevention ICDs in the United States for all covered patients. It is extremely important to have multiple resources for retrieving pacemaker implantation information. Many manufacturers supply convenient stickers containing pulse generator and lead data for the patient's chart.

A postoperative chest radiograph is extremely important for documentation of the lead position immediately after surgery. It can be used for comparison if subsequent dislodgment is suspected. In the case of a percutaneous procedure, the chest radiograph is essential to rule out a pneumothorax. Generally, it is useful to obtain both PA and lateral films for documentation of lead position. The postoperative radiograph should be overpenetrated.

Similarly, a 12-lead ECG with and without magnet application is essential to document initial appropriate pacemaker sensing and capture. The chest radiograph and ECG also have medicolegal value if a question arises subsequently.

The timing of patient discharge is controversial, with considerable variability among institutions. Today, there is a trend toward a more abbreviated hospital stay. For example, at the University of Oklahoma, patients are now discharged routinely the day after implantation unless there is a specific reason for prolonging the hospital stay. During the short stay, the patient ambulates within 2 hours of completion of the procedure, a chest radiography study and ECG are performed, and preliminary interrogation, threshold testing, and programming are accomplished. Even markedly pacemaker-dependent patients are approached this way. No complications or morbidity after discharge that would have been averted by longer hospitalization have been observed. Some centers use the first and second postoperative days for more extensive testing of the pacemaker system and the patient-pacemaker system interface. Such testing might include Holter monitoring, extensive reprogramming with particular attention to pacing and sensing thresholds, and exercise testing to adjust rate-adaptive parameters. In some centers, the pacemaker-dependent patient may be hospitalized longer.

At the other end of the spectrum is a completely ambulatory approach. Patients are discharged on the same day, immediately after the pacemaker procedure, regardless of whether or not they are pacemaker dependent. This has been the approach at the El Cajon Pacemaker Center. This experience in the United States, in addition to a large series of ambulatory procedures in Europe, has been very encouraging. The El Cajon experience is now longer than 20 years and includes more than 1000 ambulatory pacemaker procedures. There have been no postoperative pacemaker deaths or pacemaker emergencies. The El Cajon experience suggests that between 70% and 75% of pacemaker procedures can be safely conducted on an ambulatory basis. It is likely that patients referred for a pacemaker procedure on an ambulatory basis are at no greater risk from the bradyarrhythmia than they were before they entered the hospital, in the unlikely event the entire system were to fail postoperatively. If there are specific concerns about the pacemaker-dependent patient, the hospital stay can always be extended. As previously noted, it is important to have patients who undergo ambulatory procedures active during the monitored postoperative period so that potential problems can be detected. This philosophy also applies to any patient who is considered to be at higher risk for a problem or complication.

The timing of initial follow-up varies according to the timing of discharge and which physician will perform follow-up of the pacing system. If the implanting physician is to discharge the patient and perform the follow-up, there should be excellent continuity of care. Parenthetically, we have a strong bias that implanting physicians must be involved substantially in both short- and long-term follow-ups of the pacemaker recipient, to enable them to understand and appreciate many important aspects of the process as they relate to implantation.

Even if the discharging physician did not perform the procedure but is responsible for the follow-up, there may again be good continuity of care. Of concern is the situation in which the implanting physician discharges the patient to someone else for follow-up. In this case, there is the possibility that ideal pacemaker follow-up will not take place. This situation is common when a patient is discharged to a nursing home. In this case, the implanting or discharging physician must arrange some form of reliable follow-up. It is important that patients whose procedure has been performed on an ambulatory basis be seen the following day for an initial follow-up visit. At the other extreme are patients who have been hospitalized and evaluated intensively for days postoperatively with Holter monitoring and extensive reprogramming; these patients may not need to be seen for a week or even a month.

Special Considerations and Situations

Use of the Jugular Vein

If initial venous access is unsuccessful, jugular vein placement may be considered.[77] This is less desirable than subclavian, axillary, or cephalic vein placement because of the greater risk for lead fracture and the potential for erosion. An acute bend must be created in the lead after it exits the venous structure and is brought down to the pacemaker pocket under or over the clavicle. In addition, some form of tunneling is

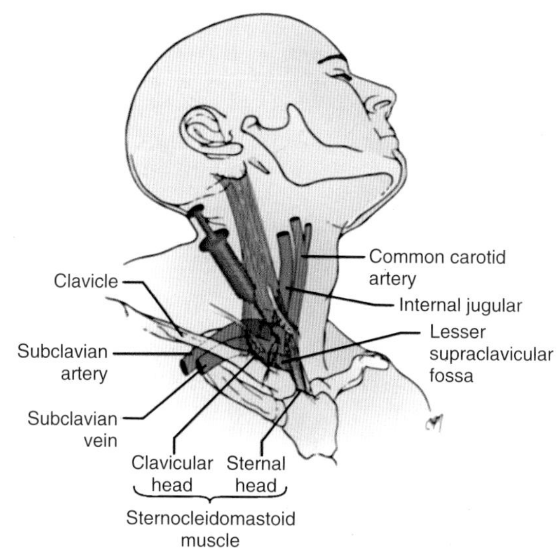

Figure 18-54. Venous anatomy for the right internal jugular approach.

required to bring the lead to the pacemaker pocket. If one tunnels under the clavicle, there is increased risk of vascular injury. If the lead is tunneled over the clavicle, the tissue is typically thin, and there is a greater chance of erosion.

Both the internal and external jugular veins have been used. Generally, the right jugular approach is preferred (Fig. 18-54). For a jugular venous approach, two separate incisions are required, one above and one below the clavicle. Many detailed descriptions have been published of anatomic dissection involving both the internal and external jugular veins. In these, particular attention is paid to precise anatomic landmarks. An alternative percutaneous technique is proposed that is simple, requiring little attention to anatomic landmarks or dissection. Additionally, an initial supraclavicular incision is not required. This approach involves the percutaneous access of the right internal jugular vein.

Once the decision is made to place the electrodes through the jugular vein, the neck must be prepared and draped accordingly in sterile fashion. To save time, this step may be performed in the initial preparation. If done in such a manner, the sterile field can be moved directly to the right supraclavicular area. If not, an effective sterile barrier can be created with the use of an iodoform-impregnated, see-through plastic drape. Access to the internal jugular vein is best obtained with the patient in the normal anatomic position, with the head facing anteriorly. Turning the head to the left should be avoided because doing so may distort the anatomy. The carotid artery is palpated in the lower third of the neck. The internal jugular vein is lateral to the common carotid artery. The two structures are parallel and lie side by side. Standing on the right side of the patient (for a right jugular vein approach), the implanting surgeon places the left middle finger along the course of the common carotid artery. The course of the internal jugular vein is under the implanter's index finger. In fact, the index and middle fingers are, side by side, generally analogous in size and orientation on the surface of the skin to the internal jugular vein and common carotid artery as they run side by side underneath the skin. A puncture anywhere along this course should enter the internal jugular vein. The higher the puncture is in the neck, the less the risk of pneumothorax. Some prefer to make the needle puncture roughly perpendicular to the plane of the neck rather than angled; this maneuver also helps avoid a pneumothorax.

Once the vein is entered, the needle and syringe can be gently angled inferiorly for passage of the guidewire. If the carotid artery is inadvertently punctured, the needle is removed, pressure over the puncture site is maintained briefly, and a second attempt at venipuncture is made a little lateral to the initial stick. The remainder of the lead placement technique is essentially identical to the previously described percutaneous technique. A small incision is carried laterally down the shaft of the needle to the surface of the muscle (sternocleidomastoid). If more tissue depth is required, the muscle can be split, and the incision carried down to the vein. A small Weitlaner retractor is used for retraction. A figure-of-eight or purse-string suture can be applied for hemostasis. Two leads for dual-chamber pacing can be placed via the retained guidewire technique. After the leads have been placed, the hemostasis suture is tied, and the leads are anchored to the muscle with the anchoring sleeve. A second incision for pocket formation is made infraclavicularly. A pacemaker pocket is created with conventional techniques. The leads are then tunneled to the pocket with the techniques previously described.

The tunneling technique described by Roelke and colleagues[99] for submammary implantation of a pacemaker may also be used for transclavicular tunneling. A long 18-gauge spinal needle can be passed from the infraclavicular incision to the supraclavicular incision. The guidewire is passed, and the sheath set is applied and tunneled to the supraclavicular incision. The rubber dilator is removed. The lead to be used is inserted in the distal end of the sheath and tied down. Once the lead is secured, the lead and sheath are pulled through the infraclavicular incision (Fig. 18-55). The external jugular vein is less commonly used for venous access because it is more inferiorly located and there is a high risk of pneumothorax and vascular complications. Its location, as previously stated, is less precise, and successful cannulation may be frustrating. If the electrodes are tunneled under the clavicle, care must be taken to avoid vascular trauma. Conversely, when tunneling over the clavicle, the implanter should make every effort to ensure optimal tissue thickness.

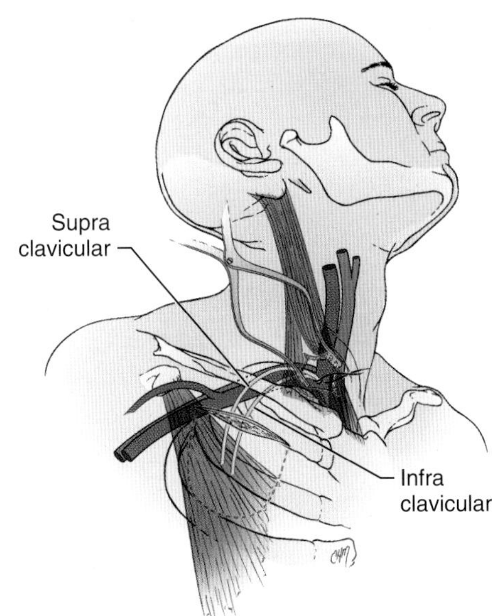

Figure 18-55. Lead(s) tunneled over and under the clavicle to the infraclavicular pocket. (From Belott PH: Pacemaker implantation: The old and new. In Singer L, Barold SS, Camm AJ: Nonpharmaceutical Therapy of Arrhythmias for the 21st Century. Armonk, NY, Futura, 1998, p 726.)

Use of the Iliac Vein

Ellestad and French[100,101] reported a 90-patient experience using the iliac vein as an alternative source of venous access for both single-chamber and dual-chamber pacemaker implantations (Fig. 18-56). The vein can be used for transvenous lead placement when an abdominal pocket is desired, such as when patients have little pectoral tissue, in patients who have just undergone bilateral radical mastectomy, in patients with extensive pectoral radiation damage, and for a variety of cosmetic reasons. A small incision is made just above the inguinal ligament over the vein (just medial to the palpable artery) and carried down to the fascia above the vein. The vein is punctured through the use of the sheath set technique with the guidewire retained for dual-chamber implantations. A figure-of-eight or purse-string suture is placed for hemostasis through the fascia around the lead as it enters the vein. Long (85-cm) leads are positioned in a conventional manner and secured to the fascia with a tie around the suture sleeve and lead. A second horizontal incision is made lateral to the umbilicus and is carried to the surface of the rectus abdominis sheath. A pacemaker pocket is created with blunt dissection. Preparations are made to tunnel the leads from the initial incision to the pacemaker pocket through use of one of the previously described techniques.

Active-fixation leads are recommended for both atrial and ventricular lead placement. Lead dislodgment is the major weakness of this approach, with 9 of 42 (21%) of the atrial and 5 of 67 (7%) of the ventricular leads in the Ellestad and French[100] experience requiring repositioning. Lead fracture and venous thrombosis do not appear to be problems, although the published experience with this approach is relatively small and the latter especially could be difficult to discern. The complication of pneumothorax essentially does not exist with this approach. Extraction of these leads can be challenging because many of the conventional tools used for extraction of leads placed in the axillary subclavian and cephalic veins are not long

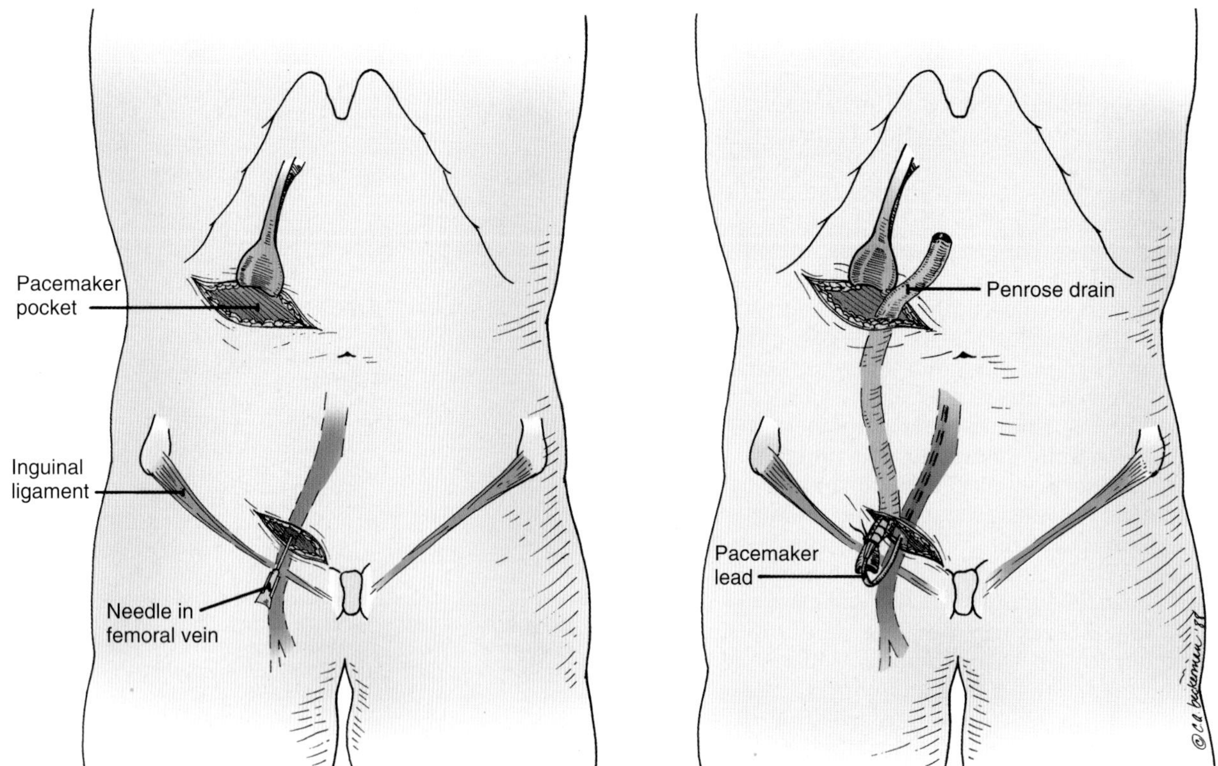

Figure 18-56. Use of the right iliac vein for placement of pacemaker lead(s). Percutaneous capture of the iliac vein is performed, and the lead is tunneled up to an upper-quadrant pacemaker pocket with the use of a Penrose drain. (From Ellestad MH, French J: Iliac vein approach to permanent pacemaker implantation. PACE 12:1030, 1989.)

enough to handle these significantly longer systems. Iliac vein implantation is particularly useful when both the left and right subclavian approaches are unavailable because of venous occlusion or after extraction of an infected system. This approach has been also used for ICD implantation.

Alternative (Cosmetic) Locations for the Pacemaker Pocket

If the patient is greatly concerned about the negative cosmetic effects of standard pacemaker pocket location, at least two alternative techniques may be considered.[102] Both can be performed with local anesthesia, but they may best be performed with general or modified general anesthesia for patient comfort because they involve more extensive surgery. Both procedures lend themselves well to the percutaneous approach for both single-chamber and dual-chamber pacing. In both procedures, after the subclavian vein is accessed, a limited (1.5-cm) initial skin incision is made. The incision is carried to the surface of the pectoral muscle, allowing only enough room to secure the lead or leads. A second incision is then made. For one of the alternative pocket locations, an incision is made under the breast along the breast fold or reflection. A standard pacemaker pocket is created under the breast, with care taken to keep the incision line on the pectoral fascia (Fig. 18-57). The pocket is carefully inspected for

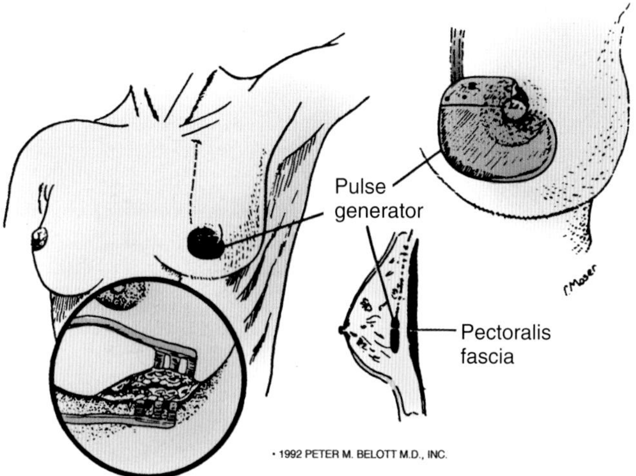

Figure 18-57. Inframammary placement of a pulse generator after percutaneous lead placement for optimal cosmetic effect. A small incision is made near the clavicle, and the pocket incision is made in the hidden fold under the breast. The lead is tunneled deep to the breast, between the incisions. (From Belott PH, Bucko D: Inframammary pulse generator placement for maximizing optimal cosmetic effect. PACE 6:1241, 1983.)

hemostasis. Similarly, as another alternative pocket location, a second incision can be made in the axilla with the patient's arm abducted 60 degrees. This incision can be carried to a depth that exposes the muscle fascia, where a pocket can be formed with appropriate attention to hemostasis. With either of these approaches, tunneling of leads can be carried out with the previously described techniques.

As previously noted, Roelke and colleagues[103] have described a submammary pacemaker implantation technique that uses unique tunneling. In this technique, a 1-cm horizontal incision is made over the deltopectoral groove 1 cm inferior to the clavicle. A direct subclavian-axillary puncture or cephalic cutdown for venous access is carried out. The electrodes are positioned and anchored. A 2- to 3-cm horizontal incision is made in the medial third of the inframammary crease. The incision is carried down to the level of the pectoralis fascia, and blunt dissection is used to create a pocket superficial to the pectoralis fascia behind the breast. A 20-cm, 18-gauge pericardiocentesis needle is directed from the inframammary pocket to the infraclavicular incision. A 145-cm J wire is then passed from the submammary pocket through the needle and to the infraclavicular incision. The needle is removed and, with use of the retained guidewire technique, two appropriate-sized introducer dilators are passed consecutively over the guidewire. The free ends of the atrial and ventricular electrodes from the infraclavicular incision are placed in the sheaths and secured with a suture (Fig. 18-58). The sheath sets are then withdrawn to the infraclavicular pocket. This innovative tunneling technique has been extremely successful and well tolerated.

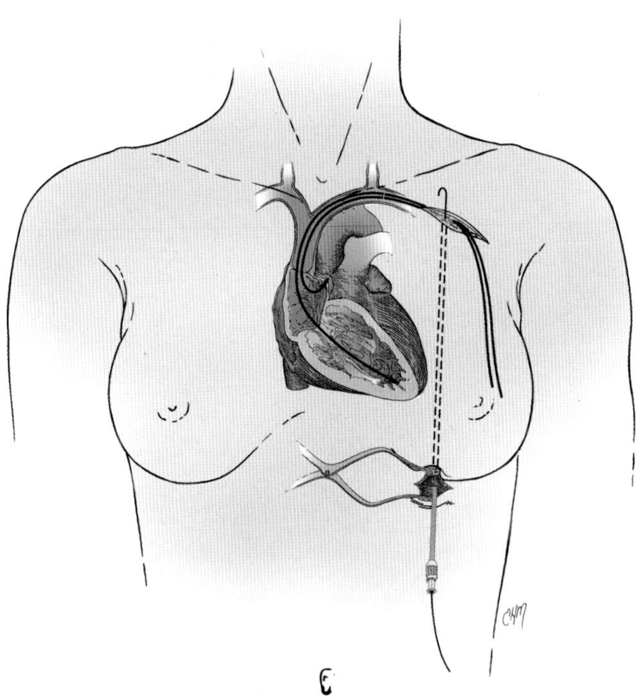

Figure 18-58. Subcutaneous tunneling with guidewire and sheath. (Redrawn from Roelke M, Jackson G, Hawthorne JW: Submammary pacemaker implantation: A unique tunneling technique. PACE 17:1793, 1994.)

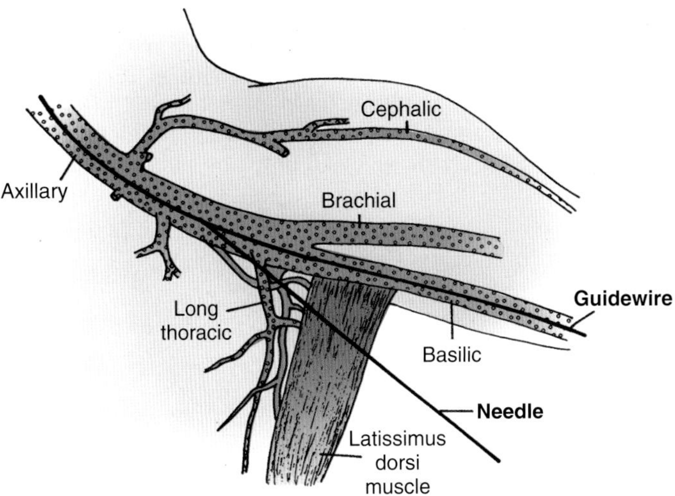

Figure 18-59. Stylized illustration of axillary venipuncture using the guidewire as a landmark.

Shefer and associates[104] have described a retropectoral transaxillary percutaneous technique for optimal cosmetic effect. This technique is performed with local anesthesia and intravenous sedation. Venography is used to confirm the relationship of the axillary vein to the surface anatomy. A marker is then placed in the axillary vein through the antecubital fossa (Fig. 18-59). This marker usually consists of a temporary transvenous pacing wire or an 0.03-inch guidewire. The skin in the ipsilateral axilla is then prepared and draped. With local anesthesia and under fluoroscopic control, a 16-gauge, thin-walled needle is inserted and guided medially in a cranial and anterior direction to meet and cross the temporary pacing wire marker in the axillary vein (Fig. 18-60). The axillary vein is punctured when

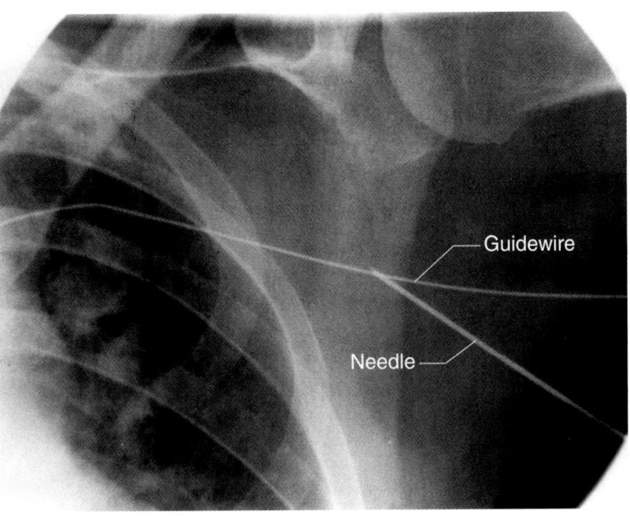

Figure 18-60. Radiograph of needle accessing the axillary vein using the guidewire as a landmark. (From Shefer A, Lewis SB, Gang ES: The rectopectoral transaxillary permanent pacemaker: Description of a technique for percutaneous implantation of an invisible device. PACE 16:1646, 1996.)

the tip of the needle touches and moves the marker wire. Venipuncture is confirmed by aspiration of venous blood. A 0.038-inch guidewire is then introduced, and the needle discarded. A longitudinal incision is made along the posterior border of the pectoralis muscle in the axilla (Fig. 18-61). The pectoralis fascia is then exposed with blunt dissection, and the retropectoral space opened. One or two pacing electrodes can then be placed via conventional techniques. The electrodes are secured by their suture sleeve to the pectoralis fascia. The leads are then connected to the pacemaker and inserted in the retropectoral pocket. At the completion of the operation, the temporary pacing lead and guidewire marker are removed. This technique offers excellent cosmetic results, and results in no restriction in physical activity or movement of the shoulder joint (Fig. 18-62).

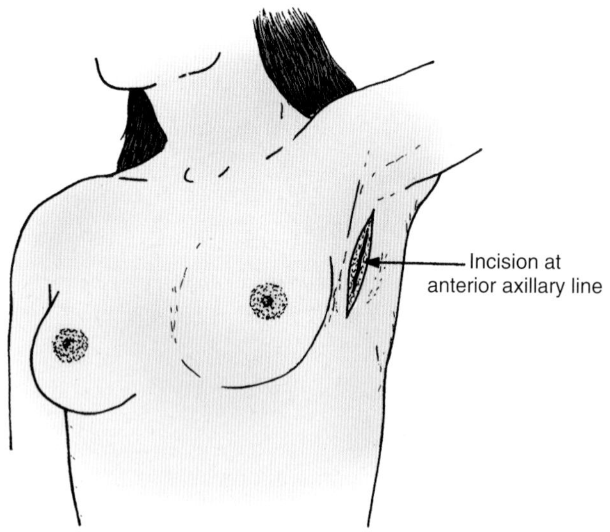

Figure 18-61. Incision in the anterior axillary line for optimal cosmetics. (From Shefer A, Lewis SB, Gang ES: The rectropectoral transaxillary permanent pacemaker: Description of a technique for percutaneous implantation of an invisible device. PACE 16:1646, 1996.)

With any of these techniques, the pulse generator and leads are connected, and the incisions closed. A polyester (Dacron) Parsonnet pouch (see Fig. 18-5) can be used to prevent rotation of the pulse generator and leads in the tissue. To avoid the problems of diaphragmatic stimulation, a bipolar system should be used, especially with the inframammary pocket.

Transvenous Lead Placement in Infants and Children

Historically, the predominance of epicardial pacing has persisted substantially longer in children than it has in adolescents and adults. Explanations for this fact are manifold. Much of the need for pacemaker implantation during infancy and childhood has occurred as a comorbidity of cardiac surgery for congenital heart disease.[105] In this context, epicardial implantation at the time of surgery has been typical. Additionally, certain forms of congenital heart disease (e.g., tricuspid

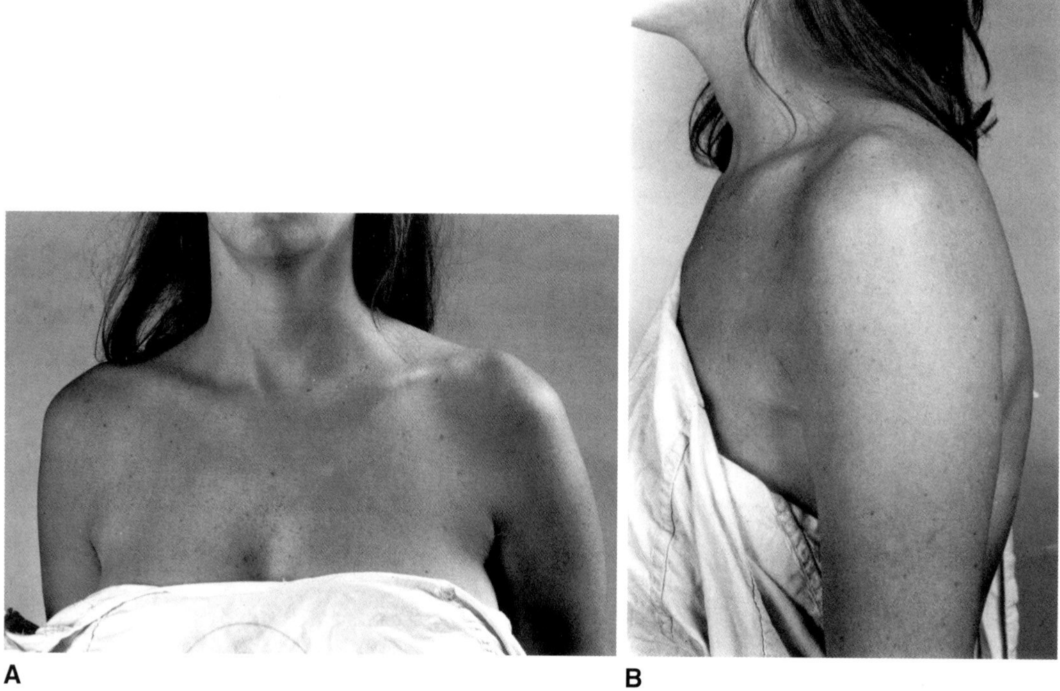

*Figure 18-62. Frontal (**A**) and lateral (**B**) views of patient after transaxillary retropectoral pacemaker implantation. There are no visible scars. (From Shefer A, Lewis SB, Gang ES: The rectropectoral transaxillary permanent pacemaker: Description of a technique for percutaneous implantation of an invisible device. PACE 16:1646, 1996.)*

atresia) make transvenous pacing difficult if not impossible. Expertise in transvenous pacing in children has also been difficult to acquire because of the relatively smaller number of patients in this age group who need pacemaker therapy.[106] Also, there has been a perception that the relatively rapid growth in body size that occurs in childhood makes transvenous pacing problematic with respect to the intravascular length of leads. Also, parents and physicians have been reluctant about placement of pacemakers in the traditional prepectoral area in children, with, instead preferring abdominal implantation of pulse generators. Finally, the lead diameters for transvenous pacemaker system implantation and pulse generator sizes have been believed to be too large for conventional techniques of transvenous implantation in children.

Conversely, as problems with epicardial pacemaker implantation have been more clearly elucidated, especially the problems of epicardial lead fracture and epicardial exit block, transvenous approaches have been appropriately reconsidered.[105] Encouraging in this reconsideration is the evolution of transvenous pacemaker implantation expertise by pediatric cardiologists or in concert with pacemaker implantation experts and pediatric cardiologists. More sophisticated lead placement techniques, coupled with smaller-diameter leads and smaller pulse generators, have also encouraged this relatively recent trend toward transvenous implantation in this age group.[108] New technologies in electrodes that help prevent the exit block problem have also been a motivator for the trend toward transvenous systems. Finally, the clear capacity to implant transvenous pacing systems successfully in patients in a variety of pediatric age groups with a range of congenital cardiac problems has been a crucial factor. With all of these considerations, especially with anticipated future developments in pacing technology, there is little question that transvenous pacing will become progressively dominant in children as it has in adolescents and adults.

As noted previously, the relative infrequency of pediatric pacemaker implantation, compared with the frequency in the adult population, makes acquisition of expertise in implantation in children difficult. It is, perhaps, ideal when one can use individuals specifically expert in pediatric implantation, although the level of regionalization necessary to do so might be unrealistic. A team approach is a reasonable alternative, pairing an expert in pacemaker implantation (adult cardiologist or cardiac surgeon) with an invasive pediatric cardiologist or pediatric electrophysiologist. Although this type of redundancy in physician services is generally inefficient and is not often well compensated by third-party payers, it may be the most attractive of a variety of options.

Pediatric pacemaker implantation can be carried out with local anesthesia and relatively substantial intravenous sedation and pain control without the services of an anesthesiologist. Conversely, although uncommon in children, excessive sedation must be monitored closely by someone experienced in doing so. It is appropriate to consider general anesthesia for pediatric pacemaker implantation, and in many cases, general anesthesia is the safest approach to use.[109]

For transvenous pacemaker implantation in children, the techniques of venous access are precisely those described for adults. Smaller venipuncture needles and guidewires are available, although they typically are not necessary except, perhaps, in infants. An important consideration in children is blood loss. Generally speaking, the younger and smaller the patient, the more crucial any blood loss. Special attention to this matter is warranted in young patients, unlike in their older counterparts.

The choice of pacemaker leads for pediatric implantation is also worthy of brief discussion. The five most important considerations in this regard are the choice of bipolar or unipolar leads, the lead diameters, the fixation mechanisms (active versus passive), the higher incidence of exit block in children, and lead length. Bipolar leads and the resulting bipolar (and optional unipolar) pacing systems have distinct advantages, but in small infants or in certain situations in which maximal lead flexibility is necessary, unipolar leads and pacing systems may be appropriately chosen. Most children beyond infancy tolerate not only the thicker bipolar systems but also dual-chamber bipolar systems. As lead (and pulse generator) technology moves toward smaller diameters, bipolar dual-chamber systems may be more comfortably used in even smaller patients. The fixation mechanism is another important consideration. The advantages of the types of fixation are not categorically different from those previously discussed. The flexibility for placement of leads in a variety of locations using active-fixation leads is attractive. It is also an unproved hypothesis that active-fixation leads may be less likely to become dislodged than their passive counterparts in a population of patients not able to understand the importance of temporary immobilization of the shoulder and arm after implantation.

In contrast, electrode technologies such as that of steroid elution have proved useful in reducing the problem of exit block, which occurs in substantially greater frequency in children. This steroid elution technology has been married more effectively with passive-fixation leads. Finally, and possibly most importantly, lead length is a crucial issue in children. Excessive lead that must be coiled in the pacemaker pocket beneath the pulse generator creates formidable bulk in these small patients. Leads of various lengths should be available, and the choices for a specific patient carefully made. In this regard, one should remember that these patients will grow significantly, so an adequate extra length of lead to accommodate this growth is desirable. One of the advantages in unipolar lead technology is that leads can be shortened or lengthened with splicing techniques, although they are certainly an imperfect solution to this vexing problem.

Once the leads have been positioned, the implanter may secure them (if such a procedure is desired) in the manner previously described using the anchoring sleeve. Alternatively, one may use an absorbable suture material for securing the leads with the anchoring sleeve. This latter approach has the advantage of good security of the lead while the electrode-myocardium interface is unstable and dislodgment is most likely; it also provides for eventual elimination of the fixation to the pectoral fascia and muscle by dissolution of the suture material, facilitating movement of the lead through the anchoring sleeve and into the vein as growth occurs. Another alternative is to use active-fixation leads and avoid the anchoring sleeve completely.

The formation of the pacemaker pocket follows the same guidelines outlined previously for adults. There has been greater enthusiasm for subpectoral implantation of pacemakers in children, although as pulse generators decrease in size, this trend may wane.

There are certain unusual situations, especially those that relate to congenital anomalies and their surgical correction, that mitigate creativity. One example involves the need to pace the LV, left atrium, or both in patients who have undergone a Mustard-type baffle procedure for transposition of the great arteries. Another example is successful transvenous pacing in patients with tricuspid atresia. This can be accomplished with passage of a transvenous lead through the RA into the coronary sinus and, respectively, into one of the posterior ventricular veins, such as the middle cardiac vein. A caveat here relates to the higher risk of diaphragmatic pacing, especially if a unipolar system is employed. In children with congenital heart disease, intracardiac shunting creates the need for special concern about the risks of systemic embolization related to placement of endocardial pacing systems. Normally, placement of endocardial systems should not be the procedure of choice in these patients before the shunts are surgically corrected.

Although a question often arises about the minimum age or size that would be considered acceptable for transvenous pacing, the answer is not easily provided. At the University of Oklahoma (and in many other medical centers), transvenous implantation is considered appropriate for infants weighing 10 pounds or more, although it is likely that as leads and pulse generators are progressively diminished, this minimum size will also decrease.

Alternatives to Radiography during Implantation

The use of radiography may be problematic in certain situations, such as during pregnancy. The prospect of implanting a pacemaker in a pregnant patient becomes particularly challenging. Guldal and colleagues[109] have described an implantation technique for single-chamber (ventricular) pacemakers using two-dimensional echocardiography and intracardiac ECG. The technique involves subcostal visualization of the structures of the right side of the heart and the lead with two-dimensional echocardiography. The electrode position is verified by recording an intracardiac electrogram, and adequate capture is ensured by intermittent pacing. More recently, Lau and Wong[110] used ultrasound to position an electrode in a patient with severe pulmonary tuberculosis. In this patient, collapse of the right side of the chest caused deviation of the heart to the right, making fluoroscopic visualization impossible. A passive-fixation lead was introduced by means of a left cephalic cutdown and was passed with fluoroscopic visualization to an ill-defined cardiopulmonary shadow in the right side of the chest. The lead could then apparently no longer be visualized adequately on fluoroscopy. Two-dimensional echocardiography identified the lead in relation to the anatomy and assisted in its final placement. Lead placement was verified by the intracardiac electrogram.

Repositioning of Electrodes

Repositioning of a malpositioned or dislodged permanent pacemaker electrode traditionally requires a surgical procedure—the pacemaker pocket must be surgically reopened, and the pacemaker and leads freed of adhesions and disconnected. A nonsurgical approach has been described by Morris and associates.[111] The technique uses principles similar to those of lead extraction through the femoral vein. The malpositioned lead is hooked and pulled into the inferior vena cava with the use of a 3-mm J-shaped deflecting wire passed through a catheter placed in the femoral vein. This is accomplished by forming a closed loop in the deflecting wire and "capturing" the lead tip with the loop. The lead tip in the inferior vena cava is snared by a loop formed with a 300-cm 0.021-inch exchange wire. The loop is passed through an 8F catheter with a 2-cm radius curve steamed into its tip. The snared lead tip is then repositioned in the apex of the RV. Iatrogenic repeated dislodgment is avoided by release of the snare, which is accomplished by advancing one end of the 0.0210-inch guidewire, forming a large loop, while retracting the other end of the wire from the catheter.

Alternatives to Transvenous Lead Placement

Transvenous endocardial lead placement is occasionally contraindicated, impractical, or impossible. Westerman and Van Devanter[112] have described a transthoracic technique requiring general anesthesia and a limited thoracotomy for electrode placement. The electrodes are passed and positioned transatrially through the sixth intercostal space (Fig. 18-63). The RA is identified, and the electrode is passed transatrially through an incision or by using a sheath set. Hemostasis is effected with a purse-string suture around the entry site. Fluoroscopy can be used for the ventricular placement of a tined or screw-in electrode. All of the electrodes are secured to the endocardial surface. A tined electrode can be directly secured to the atrial endocardium. Double-ended sutures are tied around the leads under the tines of the electrode. Before introduction of the lead, the needles are driven through the atriotomy into the atrial cavity and then out of the atrial muscle at the point of desired endocardial atrial fixation. The electrode is then pulled through the incision into the atrium and "snugged" to the endocardium by retraction and tying of the double-ended suture. In many situations, this approach may have more merit than the epicardial approach, because better long-term

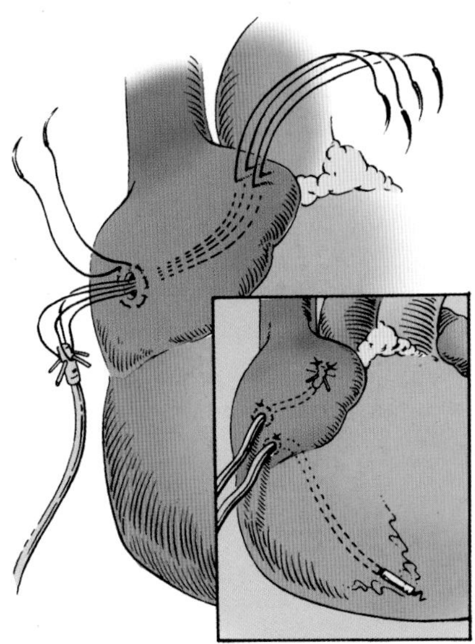

Figure 18-63. Transatrial endocardial lead placement during thoracotomy allows low-threshold transvenous leads to be implanted at the time of thoracic surgery. (From Barold SS, Mugica J: New Perspectives in Cardiac Pacing. Mt Kisco, NY, Futura, 1988, p 271.)

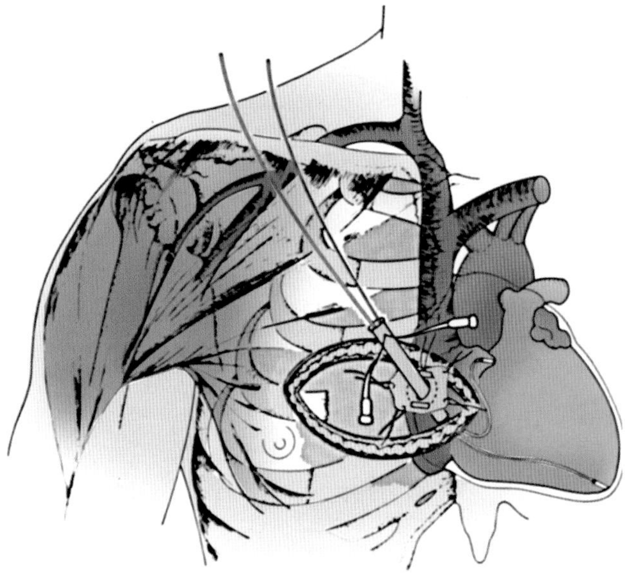

Figure 18-65. Endocardial lead placement by means of limited thoracotomy with removal of only the third and fourth costal cartilages. Standard fluoroscopy and peel-away introducer techniques are used with transatrial access. (From Byrd CL, Schwartz SJ, Siviona M, et al: Technique for the surgical extraction of permanent pacing leads and electrodes. J Thorac Cardiovasc Surg 89:142, 1985.)

electric thresholds are typically achieved. This technique may be useful for some pediatric implantations.

Hayes and colleagues[113] described a similar technique of endocardial atrial electrode placement at the time of corrective cardiac surgery (Fig. 18-64), avoiding atrial epicardial pacing because of poor pacing and sensing thresholds. In their patient, who had severe tricuspid regurgitation and had been implanted with a dual-chamber pacemaker and long-term endocardial electrodes, all four previously implanted endocardial leads and placement of a prosthetic tricuspid valve were required. New epicardial electrodes were placed on the ventricle. Stable atrial pacing and sensing were achieved with a transatrial endocardial placement in the RA appendage. In this case, the lead was secured by purse-string ligatures around the incision.

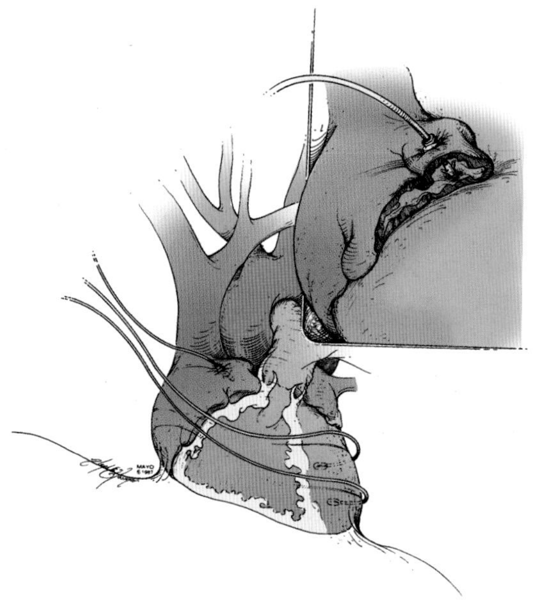

Figure 18-64. Transatrial endocardial atrial pacing in congenital heart disease. The ventricular leads were epicardial because the patient also needed a prosthetic tricuspid valve. (From Hayes DL, Vliestra RE, Puga FJ, et al: A novel approach to atrial endocardial pacing. PACE 12:125, 1989.)

Byrd and Schwartz[114] described another epicardial approach based on experience in five patients. The technique also allows conventional transvenous leads to be implanted in patients requiring an epicardial approach, including those with SVC syndrome or anomalous venous drainage as well as young patients with one innominate vein occluded by thrombosis. The technique uses a limited surgical approach with general anesthesia. The RA appendage is exposed through a 4- to 5-cm incision. The third and fourth costal cartilages are excised. A sheath set is placed inside an atrial purse-string suture and secured in a vertical position. The atrial and ventricular leads are passed down the sheath into the atrium (Fig. 18-65). The electrodes are positioned with the use of standard techniques, including fluoroscopy. Once the electrodes are positioned, the sheath is removed, and the purse-string suture around the atriotomy is secured. The pacemaker is placed in a pocket created at the incision on the anterior chest wall.

The advantage of this technique for patients in whom conventional transvenous systems are contraindicated or impossible is that it provides for implantation of a more conventional transvenous pacing system with minimal morbidity compared with a standard epicardial implantation. The chest is not entered (except for the atrium), and the time required is similar

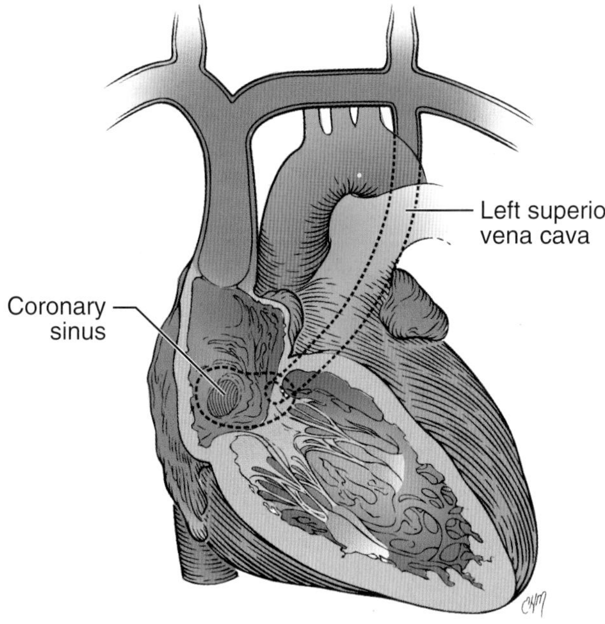

Figure 18-66. Persistent left superior vena cava.

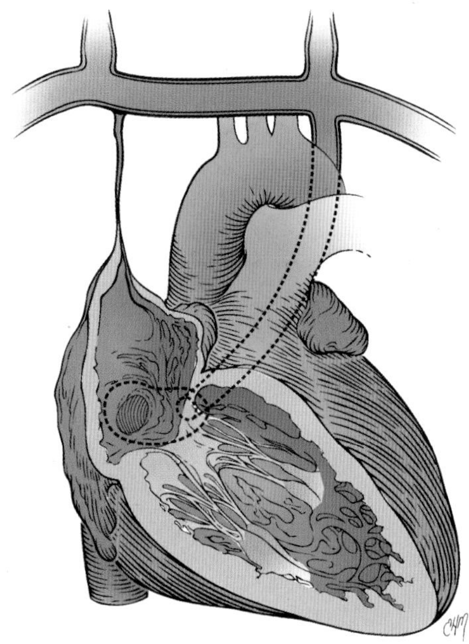

Figure 18-67. Persistent left superior vena cava with absence of the right superior vena cava.

to that for transvenous implantation. The disadvantages (although not necessarily in relation to other nonstandard transvenous techniques) include the requirement for general anesthesia, violation of the pericardia and epicardia, and the necessity of a right-sided approach (which may not be possible because of prior infection, mastectomy, and so on).

Occasionally, one encounters an anomalous venous structure, such as a persistent left SVC. Embryologically, the normal left SVC becomes atretic. There is, however, a 0.5% incidence of structural persistence of patency connected with the coronary sinus. Persistence of the left SVC usually represents failure in the development of the left innominate vein. This vein normally forms from communication of the right and left anterior cardinal veins. In this situation, the left anterior cardinal vein persists and continues to drain to the brachiocephalic veins and sinus venosus. It ultimately develops into a left SVC, which empties directly into the coronary sinus (Fig. 18-66). Normally, the left innominate vein develops as an anastomosis between the left and right anterior cardinal veins. Occasionally, with persistent left SVC, there is an associated atresia and incomplete absence of the right SVC system (Fig. 18-67). In 10% to 15% of patients, one encounters total absence of the right SVC. In this situation, venous access for pacing from the right is virtually impossible. Despite the fact that there are reported classic physical and radiographic findings for absence of the right SVC, the diagnosis is typically discovered unexpectedly at the time of pacemaker or ICD implantation.

Placement of electrodes through a persistent left SVC can prove challenging, if not impossible.[115-120] A knowledge of anatomy and radiographic orientation is essential. If one proceeds from the left and is confronted with a persistent left SVC, one must realize that the lead or leads actually are passed through the coronary sinus and out its ostium into the RA. For RV apex lead positions to be achieved, the lead must then be manipulated at an acute angle to cross the tricuspid valve. One can best accomplish this by having the lead form a loop on itself, using the lateral RA wall for support (Fig. 18-68). This maneuver can prove extremely challenging. Occasionally, depending on anatomy, such efforts prove unsuccessful, and one must consider changing

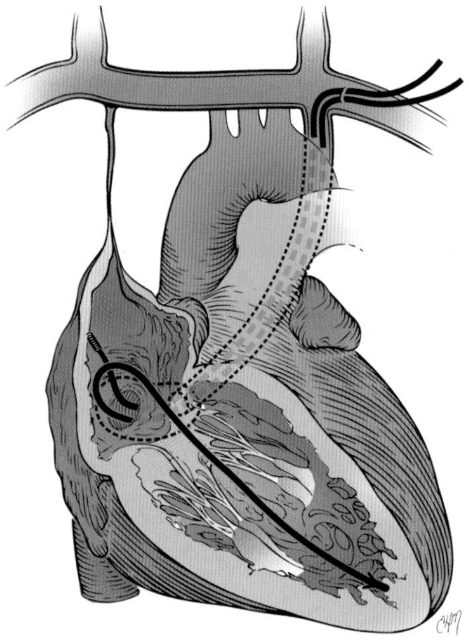

Figure 18-68. Placement of atrial and ventricular electrodes through persistent left superior vena cava in a patient with absence of the right superior vena cava. (From Belott PH: Unusual access sites for permanent cardiac pacing. In Barold SS, Mugica J: Recent Advances in Cardiac Pacing for the 21st Century. Armonk, NY, Futura, 1998.)

the site of venous access. At this point, it is prudent to assess the patency of the right venous system with contrast administration and angiographic techniques.[119] This can be carried out by advancing a standard end-hole catheter from the left SVC to the vicinity of the right SVC. Occasionally, such communication does not exist. If the right SVC is absent, the iliac vein approach, as previously described by Ellestad and French,[100] or one of the epicardial approaches is recommended.

In the case of persistent left SVC in which an atrial electrode is required, a positive-fixation screw-in electrode is recommended.[122,123] The use of a preformed atrial J wire will prove difficult if not impossible. Dislodgment of the preformed J is also a concern. When using a positive-fixation electrode, one should take care to avoid pacing of the right phrenic nerve. This can be accomplished by high-output pacing after fixation. As a rule, the anterior RA position is preferred.

Discovery of absence of the right SVC during a right-sided approach may also require changing approach sites. In this case, if an attempt is to be made from the right, the expected venous tortuosity of the persistent left SVC should alert one to request longer electrodes. At times, an 85-cm lead is required. Again, it is advisable to use positive-fixation leads in anticipation of dislodgment problems.

Permanent pacemakers have also been implanted through the inferior vena cava via a retroperitoneal approach. West and associates[124] reported the case of a 48-year-old man with congenital heart disease. The patient had undergone multiple procedures to correct transposition of the great vessels with a functional single ventricle and subvalvular pulmonic stenosis. The patient had undergone multiple operations, including a palliative Blalock shunt and Glenn procedures. At 47 years of age, the patient demonstrated a complete AV block. Given the complex congenital anomalies and subsequent corrective procedures, venous access to the RA and ventricle was complicated by loss of continuity between the RA and SVC, precluding a standard transvenous access. An epicardial approach was also less desirable because of the multiple surgical procedures already performed. West and associates[124] selected a retroperitoneal approach through a transvenous right flank incision. The inferior vena cava was infiltrated and cannulated retroperitoneally (Fig. 18-69). Bipolar active-fixation screw-in electrodes were used in both the atrium and the ventricle. The venous insertion site was secured and hemostasis effected by purse-string sutures. The pulse generator was implanted in a subcutaneous pocket formed in the anterior abdominal wall.

In a similar fashion, pacemaker leads have been placed through transhepatic cannulation. Fischberger and colleagues[125] have described percutaneous transhepatic cannulation using fluoroscopic guidance (Fig. 18-70). Once venous access has been achieved percutaneously with the guidewire inserted transhepatically, a sheath set is applied, affording the subsequent introduction of a permanent pacemaker electrode. This procedure, which has been reserved for use in complex congenital anomalies that preclude venous access through a superior vein, avoids a thoracotomy.

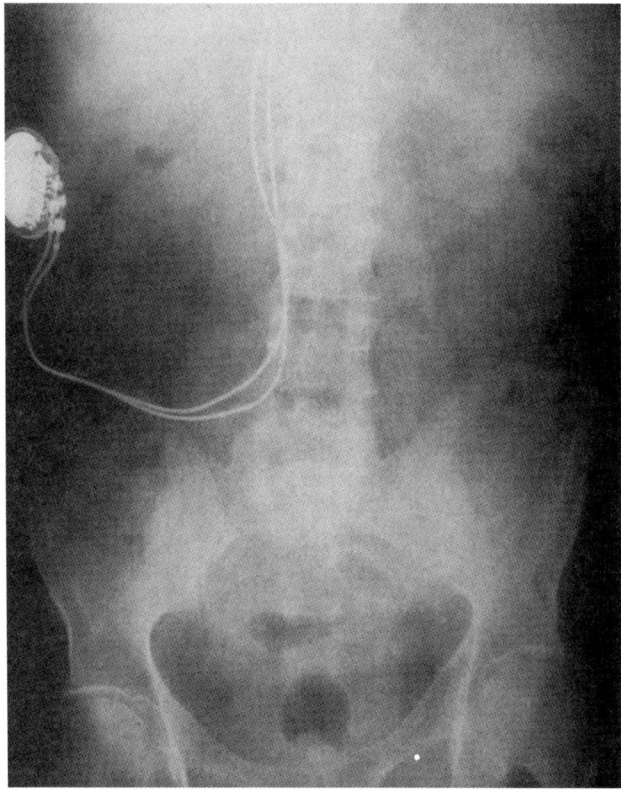

Figure 18-69. *Posteroanterior abdominal radiograph showing the position of the pacemaker and generator lead inserted into the inferior vena cava. (From West JNW, Shearmann CP, Gammange MD: Permanent pacemaker positioning via the inferior vena cava in a case of a single ventricle with loss of right atrial to vena cava continuity. PACE 16:1753, 1993.)*

The coronary sinus has been used for pacing both by design and by accident (Fig. 18-71). Today the evolution of CRT, which is discussed in Chapter 19, has placed the coronary sinus center stage. In the past, the coronary sinus per se has been unreliable for ventricular pacing and has generally been avoided, although posterior and lateral cardiac veins and sometimes the middle cardiac vein are used more commonly now to achieve LV pacing. The main coronary sinus can be an acceptable location for atrial pacing.[126,127] The problems with coronary sinus atrial pacing have been access and lead stability. Before the development of reliable atrial electrodes, the coronary sinus was a popular site of lead placement for atrial pacing. The best place for atrial pacing is the proximal coronary sinus. It is also the least stable location. Special coronary sinus leads have been developed to enhance position stability. These leads have a flexible, elongated tip that reaches deep into the coronary sinus, wedging in the great cardiac vein for stability. Gaining access to the coronary sinus requires experience (unless one is trying to avoid it, in which case it seems to be routinely entered). With the growing number of implanting electrophysiologists who use the coronary sinus routinely for diagnostic studies, this experience becomes a moot point. In addition, as more implantations are performed in the catheterization laboratory, which is equipped

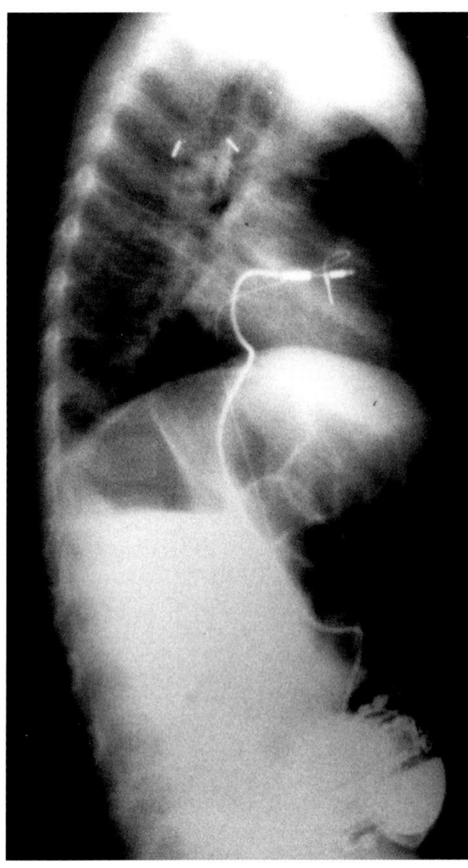

Figure 18-70. Lateral view demonstrating transhepatic lead implantation.

with sophisticated radiographic equipment including biplane fluoroscopy, the required beneficial fluoroscopic projections for placement are easily achieved.[128]

Placement of a coronary sinus lead is generally easier from the left side. A generous curve is required on the lead stylet. Coronary sinus placement is confirmed by visualization of a posterior lead position on lateral fluoroscopy. In addition, lead placement is not associated with ventricular ectopy.

Although it was once a popular approach to atrial pacing, use of the coronary sinus is uncommon today. This change is largely the result of the development of extremely reliable atrial leads equipped with fixation devices and tips that preclude dislodgment and ensure effective capture.

Misplacement of Lead in Left Ventricle

A final cautionary note on lead placement involves the risk of inadvertently placing a permanent ventricular pacing lead in the left rather than right ventricle (Fig. 18-72A). This can occur if the lead is passed from the RA through a patent foramen ovale into the left atrium (LA) and then advanced into the LV across the mitral valve. The radiographic appearance can be deceptive in an anteroposterior projection. A lateral radiographic projection (see Fig. 18-72B) and an ECG showing an RBBB QRS pattern during ventricular pacing (see Fig. 18-72C) can usually clarify this occurrence. Computed tomography scans can also identify the mislocation of the lead on the left side of the heart (see Fig. 18-72D).

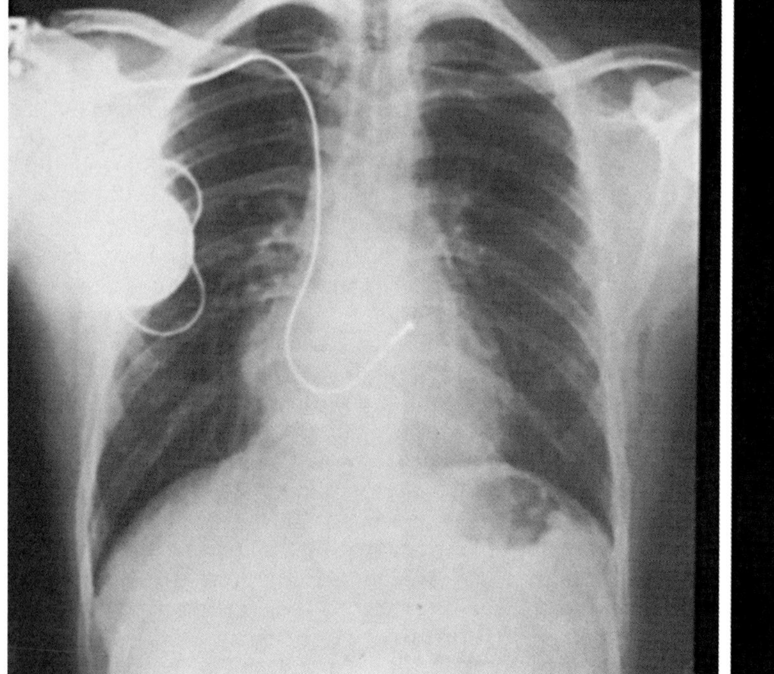

A

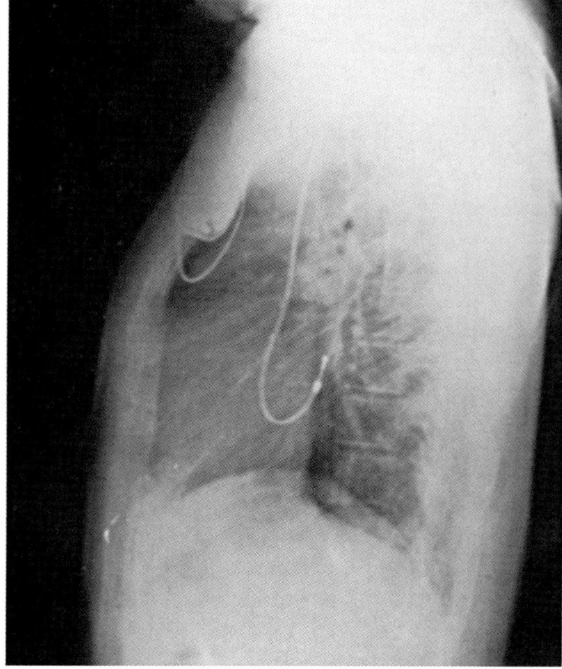

B

*Figure 18-71. **A,** Posteroanterior radiograph of a patient with a coronary sinus permanent pacemaker electrode. The lead tip is superior and to the left side across the midline. **B,** Lateral film showing that the coronary sinus and the lead curve posteriorly and superiorly, precluding right ventricular placement.*

If the mislocation is promptly detected, repositioning within 24 hours is the reasonable course of action. If the detection delay is longer, long-term anticoagulation without repositioning of the lead is advisable.

Implantation of Implantable Cardioverter-Defibrillators

A variety of ICD implantation techniques have been developed employing both epicardial and transvenous approaches. Initially, all ICD systems were placed via an epicardial approach for placement of rate-sensing and pacing leads as well as defibrillation patch electrodes. The mere size of the ICD pulse generator required an abdominal pocket. With the development of the transvenous pacing and defibrillating electrodes and active can defibrillator systems, there has been a shift to a nonthoracotomy approach. The radical reduction in the size of ICD devices has allowed their placement in pectoral pockets. Today, the overwhelming majority of ICD systems are placed via a nonthoracotomy transvenous approach and in a subcutaneous or subpectoral pocket.[129-132] The epicardial approach is reserved for unique and extenuating circumstances. Many more ICD procedures are now performed in the electrophysiology or catheterization laboratory with intravenous sedation.[133,134] The various ICD epicardial and nonthoracotomy implantation techniques are reviewed here, along with the equipment, personnel, and preparation for safe and expeditious ICD implantation.

Personnel and Equipment

The personnel required for insertion of an ICD are similar to those needed for pacemaker implantation. The primary surgeon may be an electrophysiologist, a cardiologist, or a cardiothoracic surgeon. Of course, if an epicardial approach is employed, the cardiothoracic

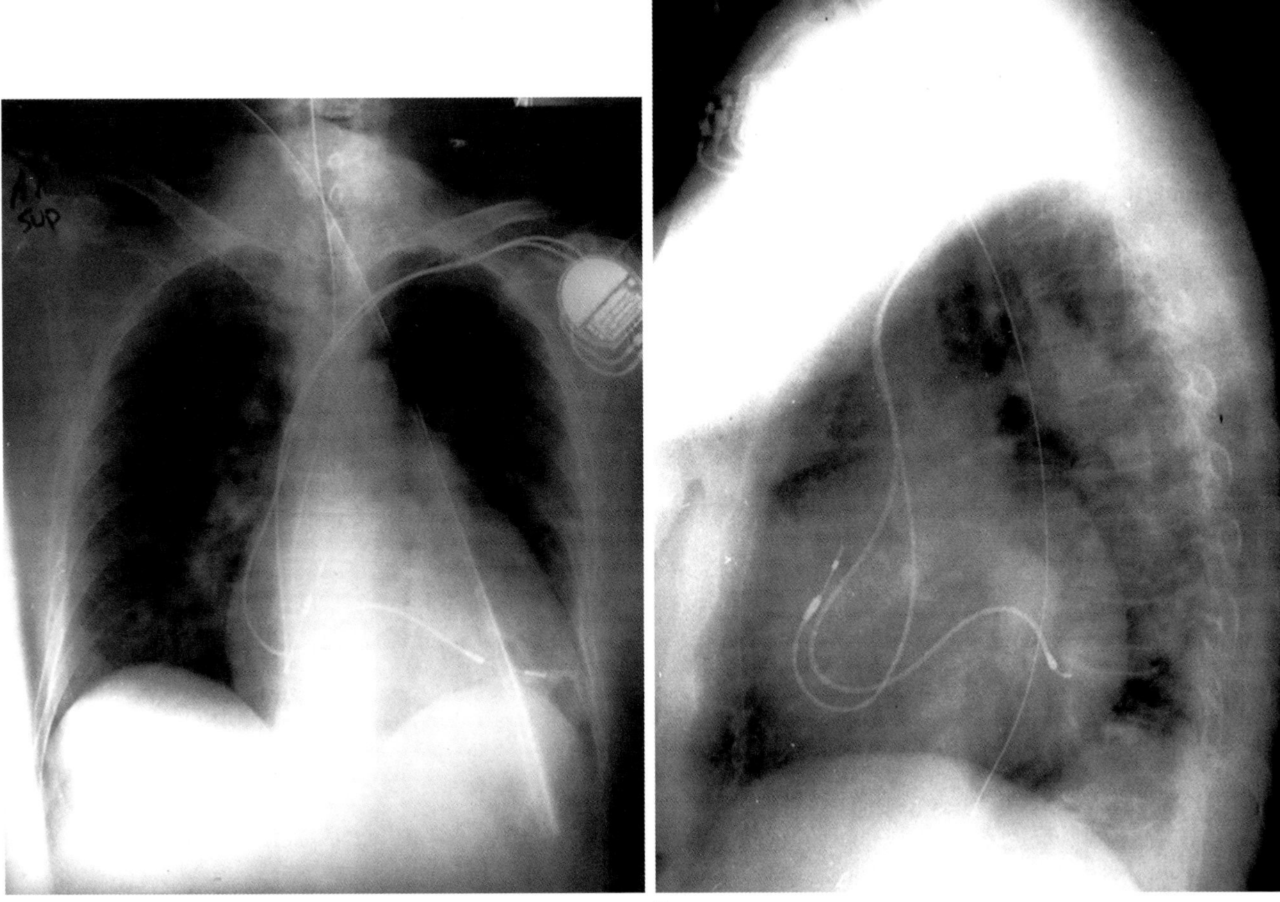

Figure 18-72. ***A,*** *Anteroposterior chest radiograph with the ventricular electrode placed in the lateral wall of the left ventricle. This view can be very deceiving. At first glance, the electrode appears to be appropriately placed in the apex of the right ventricle. The high takeoff across the tricuspid valve is a clue that the lead is in reality crossing a patent foramen ovale.* ***B,*** *Lateral radiographic projection of the same patient clearly demonstrates the posterior placement of the ventricular electrode.* *Continued*

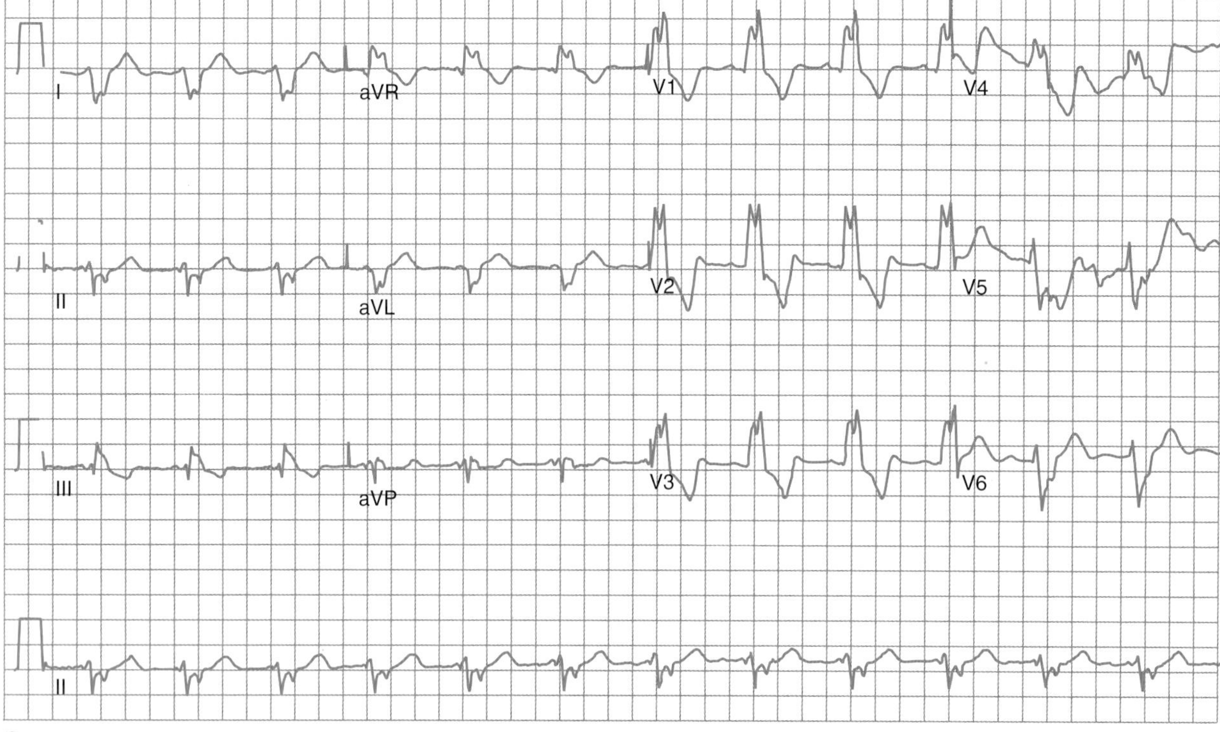

RV
RA
LV

D

Figure 18-72, cont'd. ***C,*** *Twelve-lead electrocardiogram of the same patient. Note the prominent right bundle branch block pattern in the precordial leads.* ***D,*** *Computed tomography (CT) scan of the same patient. LV, left ventricle; RA, right atrium; RV, right ventricle.*

surgeon is mandatory, but the skills usually obtained during an electrophysiology fellowship are needed to evaluate defibrillation efficacy and choose the programmed parameters.[135,136] Although the practice is controversial, the ICD manufacturer's representative can be an important member of the implantation team and can prove to be invaluable for providing leads, defibrillators, and support equipment. The earlier ICD implantations that were limited to epicardial placement required a minimum of two trained physicians, an electrophysiologist and a cardiothoracic surgeon. With the transition to the nonthoracotomy approach, a device specialist (electrophysiologist, cardiologist, or cardiothoracic surgeon) working with the ICD manufacturer's representative may be all that is required. If general anesthesia is to be used, a nurse anesthetist or anesthesiologist is also needed.[137] The ideal constitution of an ICD implantation team is listed in Table 18-13.[138]

Each member of the ICD implantation team should be completely familiar with the unique requirements of an ICD implantation, including a protocol for patient rescue. The circulating nurse should be responsible for operating the external defibrillator for rescue as directed by an electrophysiologist or implanting

TABLE 18-13. Personnel Required for Implantation and Testing of Implantable Cardioverter-Defibrillators

Implanting physician (cardiothoracic surgeon, electrophysiologist)
Anesthesiologist
Electrophysiologist
Technical support personnel: Engineer Technician Electrophysiology nurse Device manufacturer's representative

physician. Similarly, the manufacturer's representative should be responsible not only for equipment and supplies but also for threshold testing, programming, arrhythmia induction, and even rescue; this person functions under the guidance of the implanting physician or electrophysiologist.

As the ICD implantation procedure becomes less electrophysiologically complex, there is a growing desire on the part of non-electrophysiologists to implant ICDs. The technique for ICD implantation, now almost exclusively transvenous, has become very similar to that for a permanent pacemaker implantation. The Heart Rhythm Society has published formal guidelines for documenting skills and obtaining privileges for the insertion of implantable defibrillators and cardiac resynchronization devices.[139] These guidelines, published as a clinical competency statement and endorsed by the American College of Cardiology, set forth an alternative pathway for physicians not trained during an electrophysiology fellowship to document their ICD and CRT implantation skills. The stringent curriculum requirements are (1) documentation of current pacemaker implantation experience, (2) proctored ICD implantation experience, (3) completion of a formal didactic course, and (4) passing a formal examination such as the NASP exam. Monitoring of patient outcomes and complications as well as maintenance of competence are also recommended.

One must remember that there are two parts to ICD implantation: first, the implantation of a lead and device, and second, the intraoperative electrophysiologic measurements, which comprise not only pace and sense threshold determinations but also arrhythmia induction, defibrillation threshold determination, patient rescue, and, finally, defibrillator programming. The second part of an ICD implantation can best be performed by a trained electrophysiologist; in any case, one should be immediately available.

Although the initial ICD implantations took place solely in the operating room with the patient under general anesthesia, ICD implantation now may be performed either in the cardiac catheterization laboratory or the operating room. The choice of the implantation facility is subject to operator preference, hospital policy, and economics. The safety and efficacy of ICD implantation in the cardiac catheterization laboratory have been well established.[140-144] In many institutions, the ICD implantation may take place in either venue and with IV sedation. The concerns about infection appear to be unfounded even with complex tunneling and abdominal ICD placement. As previously stated, it is well accepted that the operating room offers a strict sterile environment and unlimited surgical supplies as well as ease of emergency thoracotomy, but these advantages do not preclude performance of the procedure in the cardiac catheterization laboratory, where imaging and support equipment is optimal. It would also appear that the catheterization laboratory offers a less expensive procedure with lower hospital charges.[145,146] The basic required equipment for nonthoracotomy ICD insertion is identical to that for permanent pacemaker insertion. Additional considerations are arterial blood pressure monitoring as well as the equipment and supplies unique to the ICD, such as high-voltage cables, programmable stimulator, external defibrillator with sterile external and internal paddles, alternating current (AC) fibrillator, sterile programming wand for ICD communication, an external programmer, and the tunneling tools unique to ICD implantation (Table 18-14).[147,148]

As for the pacemaker implantation procedure, one cannot have too many supplies and spare parts for ICD implantation.

TABLE 18-14. Equipment and Supplies Recommended for Implantation of Cardioverter-Defibrillators

Alternating current (AC) fibrillator box
Lead adapter sleeves and caps
External defibrillator
Large Parsonnet (Dacron) pouches (1.5 × 6 inches)
Guidewires
Imaging contrast material
Introducers (long and short lengths, 9F-12F and 14F)
Jackson-Pratt drainage system
Multiple stylets
Multiple torque wrenches
Tunneling tool with multiple lead adapters
Transvenous rate sensing lead
Subcutaneous patches
Y-Adapters
Subcutaneous array
Extra transvenous rate-sensing leads
Lead extensions
Lead repair kit

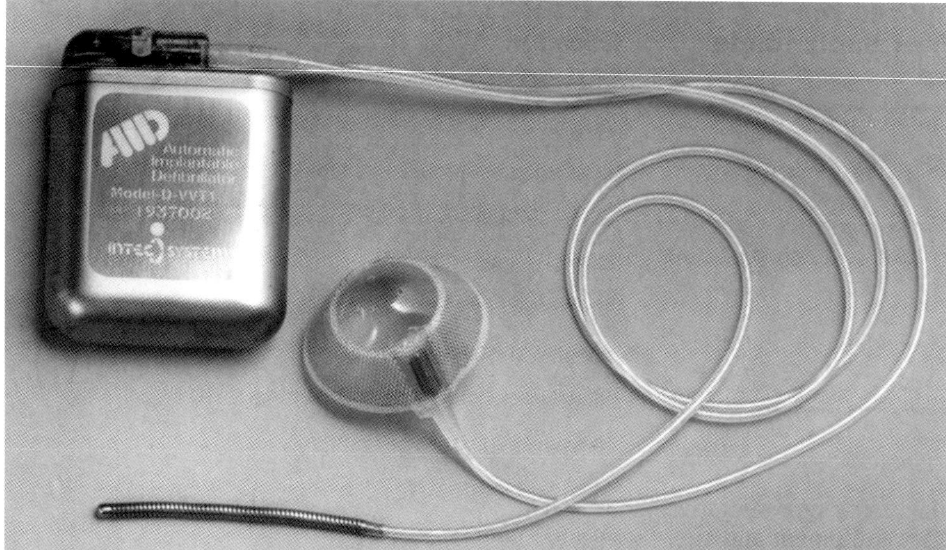

Figure 18-73. Epicardial cup and helical spring electrodes.

General Considerations

By and large, the general considerations are identical to those of a permanent pacemaker implantation. There are some subtle additional differences. Although not mandatory, many centers require intra-arterial blood pressure monitoring for ICD insertion. In addition, appropriate device selection and choice of anesthesia must be determined. Because of the drastically reduced ICD size and required surgery, as well as protocols for more expeditious device testing, the procedures are now even performed on an outpatient basis.

The choice of anesthesia is related to operator preference or, in some cases, hospital protocol.[149-151] As previously mentioned, the procedure may be performed with either general anesthesia or intravenous sedation. In a patient in whom multiple defibrillation threshold determinations as well as subpectoral dissection are required, general anesthesia might be a better selection.[152] General anesthesia offers optimal patient comfort and airway control. At many centers where subcutaneous prepectoral muscle ICD implantation is performed, IV sedation with local anesthesia for periods of ventricular fibrillation arrhythmia induction is used, and the patient receives brief periods of deeper sedation with a short-acting medication such as midazolam, methohexital, propofol, or fentanyl.[153-155]

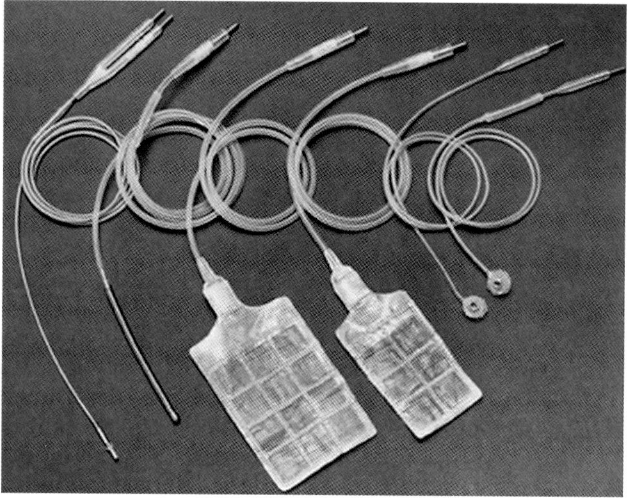

Figure 18-74. Assortment of electrodes available for the automatic implantable cardioverter-defibrillator. From left to right: *Endocardial bipolar rate-sensing lead, superior vena cava shocking coil, large epicardial patch lead, small epicardial patch lead, and epicardial screw-in rate-sensing electrodes. (Courtesy of Guidant, Boston Scientific, Natick, Mass.)*

Approaches to Implantation

Epicardial Approach

The epicardial approaches that were used for cardiac pacing have been employed for ICD implantation. In addition to those approaches previously mentioned, the median sternotomy[146-158] has become the approach of choice for combination of open heart surgery and ICD implantation.[159,160] The common approaches for epicardial ICD implantation are the subxiphoid approach, subcostal approach, left lateral thoracotomy, and sternotomy. The goal of the epicardial approach is to configure the fibrillation patches around the heart for optimal defibrillation thresholds.

Historically, the first clinical implants used an epicardial cup electrode on the ventricular apex in conjunction with a helical spring electrode in the SVC (Fig. 18-73).[161] High defibrillation thresholds from this system ultimately led to the preference of two epicardial patch electrodes.[162] The epicardial patches may even be placed on the external surface of the pericardium. This modification reduces epicardial adhesions. The epicardial patches come in a variety of sizes and shapes and vary among manufacturers (Fig. 18-74). The basic principle is for each patch to cover as large a surface of myocardium as possible. To avoid short-circuiting, the patches must not touch each other.

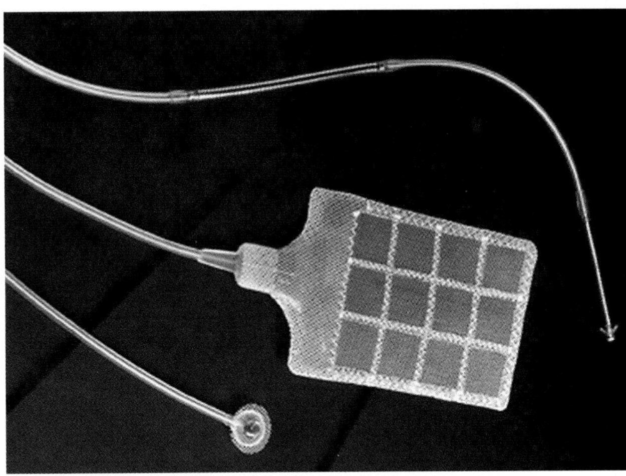

Figure 18-75. Leads and electrodes for an implantable cardioverter-defibrillator. Left, *Epicardial screw-in, rate-sensing electrode. Center, Rectangular epicardial patch electrode.* Right, *Transvenous rate-sensing electrode. (Courtesy of Guidant, Boston Scientific, Natick, Mass.)*

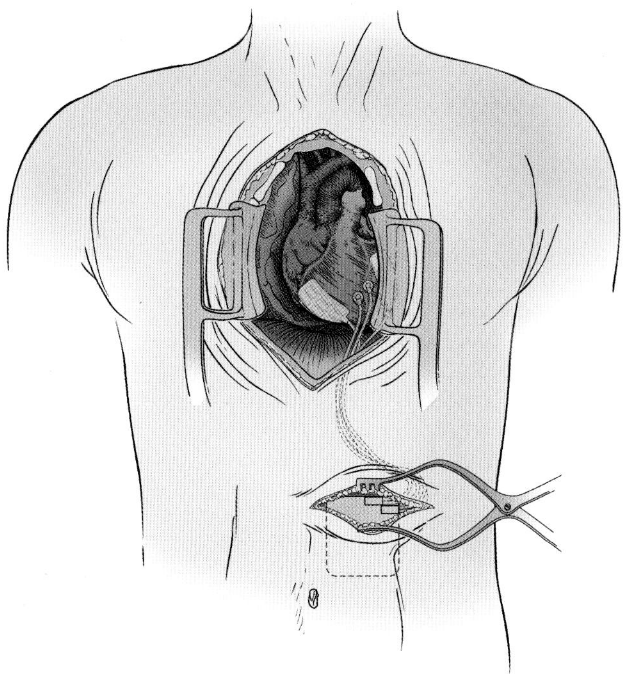

Figure 18-76. Median sternotomy with epicardial rate-sensing and patch electrodes tunneled to an implantable cardioverter-defibrillator pocket in the left upper quadrant.

In addition to the patches, rate-sensing leads must be applied. Usually, this involves the placement of two sutureless screw-in electrodes side by side (Fig. 18-75). These electrodes serve both pacing and sensing functions. Because epicardial pacing and sensing electrodes have less optimal long-term performance characteristics, the rate-sensing and pacing electrodes may be placed transvenously using standard techniques. These leads are then tunneled to the device pocket via the standard tunneling technique previously outlined. Epicardial lead and patch placement has historically involved an abdominal pocket because of the larger sizes of the devices. Abdominal pockets could be achieved by creation of a subcutaneous pocket or, if optimal comfort and cosmetics are desired, placement under the rectus abdominis muscle.

Median Sternotomy Approach. The median sternotomy is preferred by most cardiothoracic surgeons because it provides optimal exposure and access to the entire heart. It is generally used in patients undergoing an open heart procedure who also require ICD implantation. A median sternotomy incision is not necessary for satisfactory placement of defibrillator leads. This approach is usually well tolerated and associated with much less patient discomfort. The median sternotomy usually allows for the placement of two large patches in an extrapericardial location (Fig. 18-76). Because this approach is usually performed during cardiopulmonary bypass, the lungs can be deflated, and excellent exposure achieved. The phrenic nerves and coronary artery bypass graft should be identified to avoid their injury. The rate-sensing electrodes are directly screwed into the surface of the heart. These can be placed on either ventricle. One patch is typically placed on the surface of the RV. Because of the smaller RV surface area, smaller patch sizes are frequently required. The patches are then sutured to the pericardium (or, in the case of an intrapericardial implant, directly on the surfaces of the ventricles). The median sternotomy approach for ICD placement is the procedure of choice of most cardiothoracic surgeons. This is true even for isolated ICD implantation, because the median sternotomy results in less pain and optimal exposure.[163]

Left Anterolateral Thoracotomy Approach. The left thoracotomy approach, like the median sternotomy, is attractive because it allows for excellent exposure of the heart and, more specifically, the LV. The heart is exposed through an incision created in the fifth intercostal space (Fig. 18-77). The skin incision is made

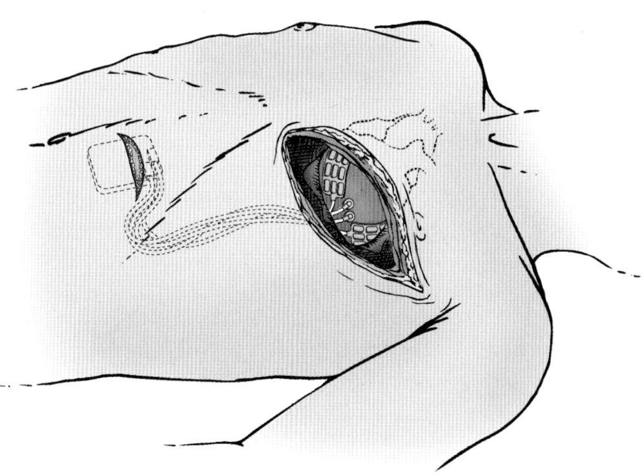

Figure 18-77. Left lateral thoracotomy with epicardial rate-sensing and patch electrodes tunneled to subcutaneous pocket in the left upper quadrant.

along the inframammary fold. This approach is ideal for the extrapericardial placement of a large patch electrode over the posterior surface of the LV as well as a smaller patch anteriorly between the sternum and pericardium. Occasionally, a small right minithoracotomy is required for additional exposure and placement of a patch electrode on the right side of the heart. The left lateral thoracotomy is ideal for epicardial placement of a LV lead for cardiac CRT. This is generally reserved for cases in which coronary sinus lead placement has failed or is unacceptable. In some centers it has been used as a primary approach to CRT. The left lateral thoracotomy exposes the posterolateral aspect of the LV and, as such, is ideal for resynchronization.

The anterior thoracotomy is associated with considerable postoperative pain—its major detraction. This pain can also result in atelectasis and transient pleural effusions. One can reduce the postoperative wound pain by working through a more lateral incision. An additional disadvantage of the left thoracotomy is seen in patients who have had prior cardiac surgery. The common postoperative adhesions usually preclude the anterior placement of an extrapericardial patch and also raise the hazard of damaging coronary bypass grafts. A more lateral approach has been adapted that eliminates pain associated with division of the latissimus dorsi muscle. The more lateral incision offers an excellent exposure of the LV and avoids injury to the costal cartilages as well as division of thoracic musculature. The leads are tunneled to the abdominal pocket through the use of a small chest tube and hemostat. An LV lead being placed for resynchronization can be directly connected to the previously placed biventricular pulse generator in the left pectoral area, with little or no tunneling.

Subxiphoid Approach. The subxiphoid approach was developed for patients undergoing an isolated ICD implantation. This approach offers decreased morbidity and discomfort compared with the median sternotomy and thoracotomy,[164] even though it is associated with a slight increase in defibrillation thresholds.[165] This approach requires the least surgical dissection.

A midline incision is made just above the xiphosternal junction and is carried inferiorly for about 6 cm. The xiphoid process is usually excised. With traction, the sternum is elevated and the pericardium identified. The pericardium is incised with an anterior or transverse incision. Patches are placed over the right anterior and diaphragmatic surfaces of the heart (Fig. 18-78). One then merely extends the subxiphoid incision and creates a subcutaneous or subfascial pocket. The pocket can also be created by means of a separate incision in the left upper quadrant with the leads tunneled to the pocket. The major disadvantages of this approach are limited surgical exposure and the requirement for intrapericardially placed patches. Occasionally, because of unacceptable defibrillation thresholds, an additional transvenous coil must be placed. This requires substantial subcutaneous tunneling from the subclavian vein to the abdominal pocket. Also, because of limited exposure, the subxiphoid approach is generally not used in patients with prior cardiac surgery.[166]

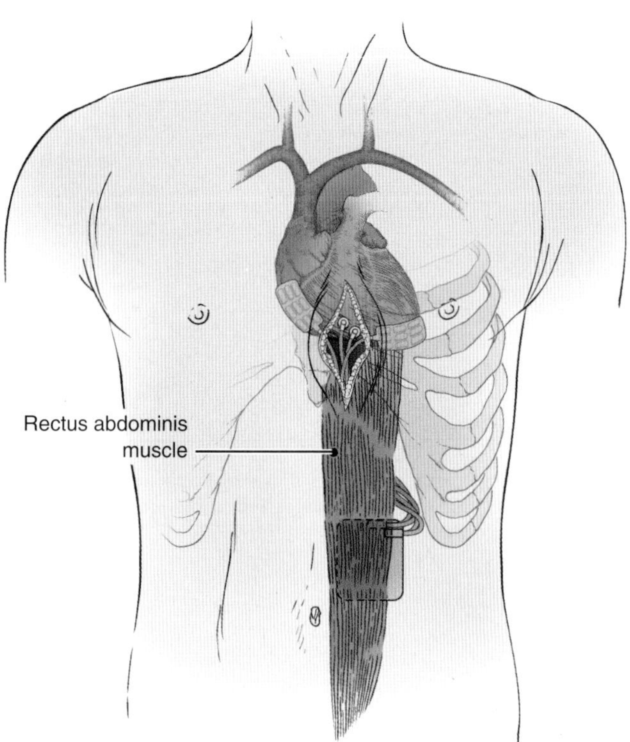

Figure 18-78. Subxiphoid epicardial approach with rate-sensing and patch electrodes tunneled to a subrectus abdominis muscle pocket in the left upper quadrant.

Left Subcostal Approach. The left subcostal approach was originally developed for placement of epicardial pacing and sensing electrodes.[167] A technique has been developed that expands this approach for the placement of ICD patches. Like the subxiphoid approach, the left subcostal approach is associated with minimal morbidity.[168,169] Surgical exposure is somewhat better than with the subxiphoid approach. The left subcostal approach is carried out with an incision in the left subcostal area (Fig. 18-79). This incision is carried down to the rectus abdominis muscle, which is divided. The posterior rectus sheath is identified. With blunt dissection under the costal margin, the pericardium is exposed. Retraction of the costal margin enhances exposure. With proper dissection, patches may be placed extrapericardially. This approach can be used in patients who have had prior cardiac surgery.[170,171] Because the posterior rectus sheath has been left intact, a subrectus pocket may be created for placement of a pulse generator.

The advantages of the subcostal approach are similar to those of the subxiphoid approach. Because the left subcostal approach is extrathoracic, it avoids the complications of a thoracotomy. As previously mentioned, the exposure in the subcostal approach is somewhat better than that in the subxiphoid technique. Because the subcostal approach requires division of the left rectus muscle, there is greater postoperative discomfort. In essence, the subcostal approach improves

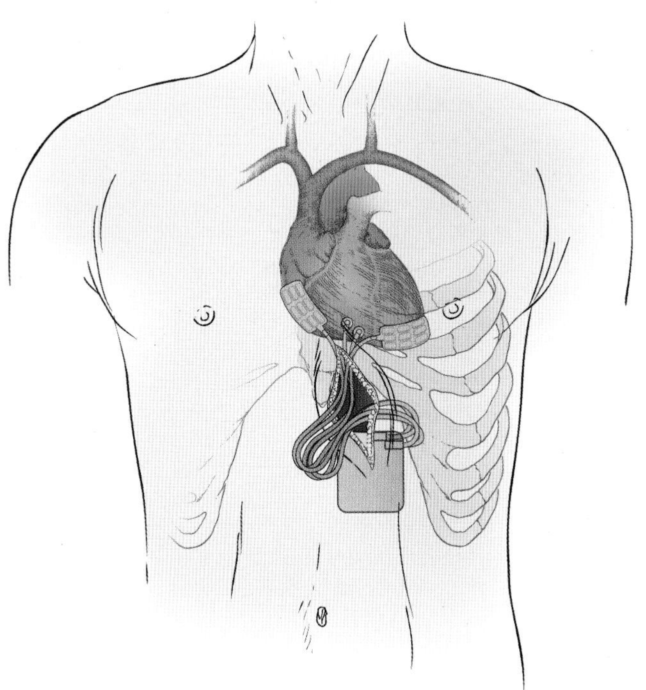

Figure 18-79. Left subcostal epicardial approach with rate-sensing and patch electrodes tunneled to subcutaneous pocket in the left infracostal space.

exposure over the subxiphoid approach while at the same time minimizing pulmonary complications and problems. It also allows one to insert the defibrillator through the same incision.

A transdiaphragmatic approach has been described that offers the same advantages and disadvantages as the subcostal approach.[172,173] It uses a longitudinal epigastric extraperitoneal incision for access to the heart. An initial skin incision is carried to the surface of the peritoneum. The diaphragm is identified, and an incision is made through its central tendon. Possibly because of potential violation of the abdominal cavity, the transdiaphragmatic approach has not gained popularity.

Thoracoscopic Approach. ICD patches can be placed by means of a thoracoscope.[174,175] A small incision is made on the left anterior chest, and the defibrillator patches are introduced into the left pleural space (Fig. 18-80). The thoracoscope is then used to grab the patches, guide them, and subsequently attach them to the surface of the pericardium. This is a relative new approach, and its safety and efficacy have not been fully defined. Because this approach avoids thoracotomy and sternotomy, it carries the lowest morbidity of all the epicardial approaches.[176] Robotic techniques are also being developed for epicardial lead placement.[177]

Endocardial Approach

The endocardial, or nonthoracotomy, approach was initially described in 1987 when the ENDOTAK (Guidant, Boston Scientific, Natick, Mass.) was introduced (Fig.

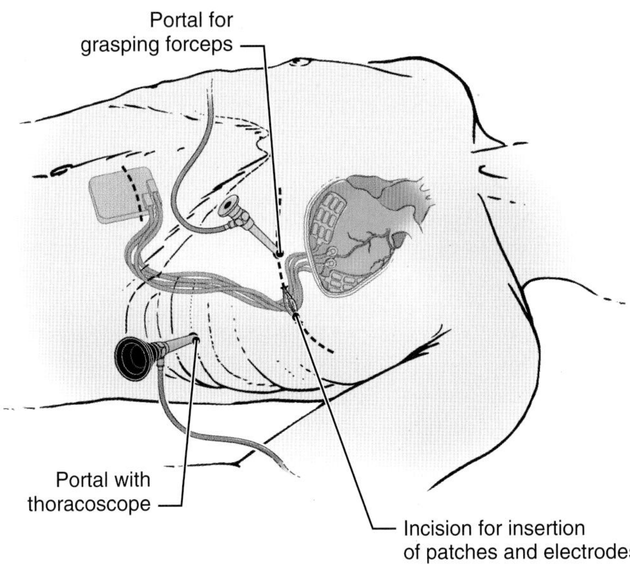

Figure 18-80. Thoracoscopic epicardial rate-sensing and patch electrode placement. Electrodes tunneled subcutaneously to implantable cardioverter-defibrillator pocket in the left upper quadrant.

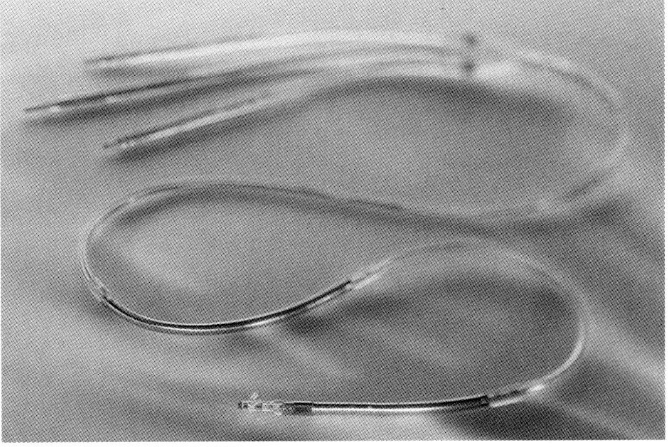

Figure 18-81. ENDOTAK transvenous endocardial pace and shock electrode. (Courtesy of Guidant, Boston Scientific, Natick, Mass.)

18-81).[178,179] Unfortunately, the early experience was associated with a high incidence of lead fractures, which slowed its initial acceptance.[180] Today, most manufacturers offer an endocardial pacing and shocking electrode, and the endocardial approach has become the technique of choice. Initially, the endocardial and transvenous electrode system required a subcutaneous patch to achieve effective acceptable defibrillation thresholds.[181,182] With the development of new electrical defibrillation waveforms and lead configurations, electrically active can systems, and efficient energy delivery systems, the transvenous approach is now the main technique for ICD implantation.[183]

The transvenous lead systems vary in configuration from manufacturer to manufacturer, but venous access is identical, and lead positioning nearly identical, to the techniques previously described for the ventricular pacing electrode. Because of concerns about the subclavian crush syndrome, cephalic cutdown or percutaneous access to the axillary vein is recommended.[184,185] If more than one electrode is to be inserted, a simple venous puncture is made with use of the retained guidewire technique or two separate punctures can be used. Left-sided venous access is preferred. As with pacemaker systems, the left-sided venous access offers a more direct and facile approach to the RV apex. If a two-coil system is used, the proximal coil is more easily and effectively positioned against the lateral RA wall or in the left innominate or subclavian vein from the left subclavian venous approach. Finally, defibrillation thresholds appear to be higher for an active ("hot") can when a right-sided approach is used.[186-188]

The techniques for endocardial placement of defibrillator electrodes are identical to those for pacing. An RV apex position is desired. This position can frequently be facilitated with a right anterior oblique fluoroscopic projection. Once positioned, the leads are secured to the pectoralis muscle with the suture sleeve. Because the early nonthoracotomy lead systems were frequently tunneled to an abdominal pocket, the tie-down sleeves were often used to reduce strain by being fashioned into an S shape just proximal to the venous entry site. This provided slack to prevent dislodgment during manipulation of the pulse generator. A complete loop should be avoided because this tends to form pressure points that may lead to erosion. The need for a strain-reducing S configuration has been lessened by the use of pectoral pockets and smaller generators.

Pocket Creation

Initially, ICD pockets were created almost exclusively in the left upper quadrant of the abdomen. The reasons were the predominance of the epicardial approach and the rather generous size of the device. With the advent of the nonthoracotomy approach, the ICD pocket is almost exclusively placed in the left pectoral area. Most abdominal pockets are subcutaneous, but if excellent cosmetics and comfort are desired, an intra–rectus abdominis sheath or even a submuscular approach can be used. In the pectoral area, because of device size, many centers initially used a submuscular approach. With the radical reduction in device size, the subcutaneous pocket is becoming much more common. The concern associated with a subcutaneous pocket, whether abdominal or pectoral, is the higher risk of erosion (Table 18-15).

Abdominal Pocket

If an abdominal pocket is to be created, the implanting surgeon must be completely familiar with the anatomy of the anterior abdominal wall, including the multiple muscular and fascial layers (Fig. 18-82). One must be able to identify the anterior rectus abdominis sheath, rectus muscle, posterior rectus sheath, linea alba, and peritoneum. Failure to understand the anatomy of the abdominal wall may result in inadvertent access of the peritoneal cavity. An abdominal pocket is created with an initial 3- to 4-inch transverse incision high in the left upper quadrant. This incision is carried through the subcutaneous tissue and fat to the surface of the anterior rectus sheath. The incision can be held apart with one or two Weitlaner retractors. A Goelet or Richardson retractor may then be applied to retract the subcutaneous tissue; then, with the electrocautery unit in cutting function, an inferior pocket is created just on top of the anterior rectus sheath. A plane is created directly on top of the anterior rectus sheath, and an attempt is made not to violate this structure. The subcutaneous tissue is separated from the anterior rectus sheath, creating a pocket large enough to accommodate the particular pulse generator. The pocket is carefully inspected for hemostasis and lavaged with antibacterial solution. The pocket should be low enough to avoid the costal margin and yet above the belt line. The pocket receives the leads by means of standard tunneling techniques (see later). When epicardial approaches are used, most leads are tunneled with a small chest tube and Kelly clamp for guidance. When transvenous leads are tunneled to an abdominal pocket, a special tunneling tool may be used (Fig. 18-83). Whether a tunneling tool or elongated clamps is used, care should be taken to achieve optimal depth of the tunneling track so as to avoid future lead erosion.

A modification of the subcutaneous approach calls for the creation of a submuscular abdominal pocket. This pocket allows placement of the ICD in a space created between the posterior rectus sheath and the rectus muscle. This space may be approached via a vertical incision through the anterior rectus sheath at either its medial or lateral margin. The muscle can then be easily retracted off the posterior rectus sheath.

TABLE 18-15. Subcutaneous versus Submuscular Pocket for Implantable Cardioverter-Defibrillators

Site	Advantages	Disadvantages
Subcutaneous	Limited surgery Better control of bleeding Better analgesia Easier pulse generator change	Less cosmetic Greater risk of erosion Higher risk of dislodgment due to twiddler's syndrome
Submuscular	Optimal cosmetics Less risk of dislodgment due to twiddling Greater patient acceptance	Increased problems with hemostasis Greater postoperative pain Potential lateral migration to the axilla

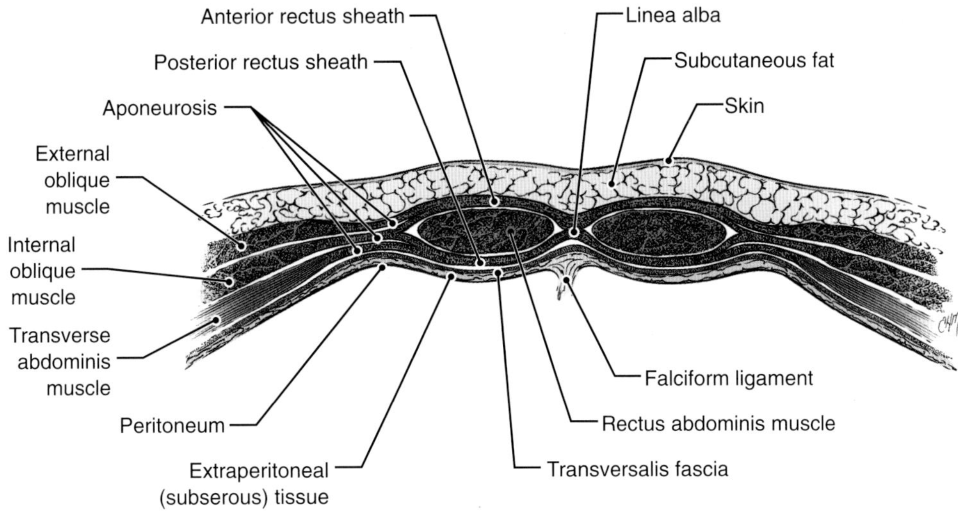

Figure 18-82. Cross-sectional anatomy of the rectus sheath above the arcuate line.

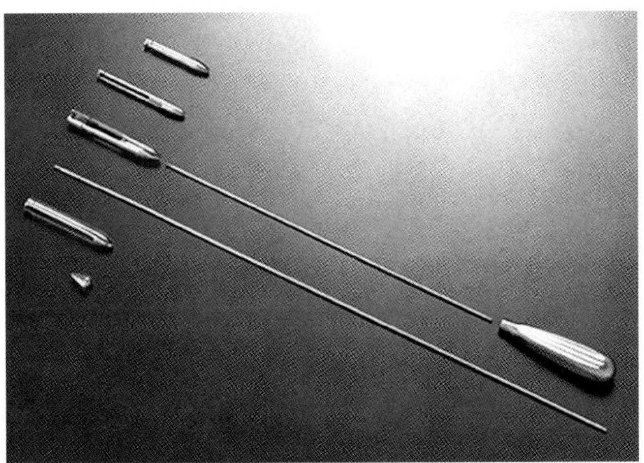

Figure 18-83. Subcutaneous tunneling tool with interchangeable handle, tunneling rod, and tunneling bullet. (Courtesy of Guidant, Boston Scientific, Natick, Mass.)

Occasionally, vascular pedicles are encountered; these should be clipped with vascular staples. Once this submuscular compartment has been carefully inspected for hemostasis, the ICD may be inserted. A redundant lead can be placed in a separate subcutaneous space.

The aponeuroses and subcutaneous tissue are then reapproximated with standard closure techniques. Once again, the deeper submuscular approach is associated with potential violation of the peritoneal cavity as well as postoperative erosion into the peritoneal cavity (Fig. 18-84). As a general rule, the abdominal pocket should not be located or placed over previous abdominal surgery, including previous abdominal incisions and drain sites. Such scar tissue raises the risk of direct communication between the ICD pocket and the peritoneal cavity. Similarly, one should avoid placing an abdominal pocket in the vicinity of abdominal hernias, which have the propensity to extend into an ICD pocket. Finally, if one is aware of potential future abdominal surgical requirements, an alternate abdominal location or pectoral approach should be considered.

Tunneling Techniques

The initial epicardial ICD systems required tunneling of leads from the epicardium to an abdominal pocket. This step was usually carried out with a large chest tube. The proximal ends of the electrodes were stuffed into the back end of a chest tube for protection, and the chest tube was guided by a large clamp subcutaneously to the abdominal pocket. The tip of the chest tube was grasped with a large, curved Kelly clamp, and with use of an index finger for palpation, the clamp guided the chest tube through the tissue to the abdominal pocket. The distance from the epicardium to the abdominal pocket was relatively short, and this tunneling technique proved simple and expeditious.

This is not the case when one is tunneling from a transvenous insertion site in the upper chest to an abdominal pocket. To assist in long stretches of tunneling, CPI (now CPI/Guidant) developed a tunneling tool to resolve this problem. The tunneling tool had multiple components and basically consisted of a rod with a handle at one end and a distal bullet that could be replaced with a lead adapter (see Fig. 18-83).

Tunneling should never be carried out until acceptable lead position and defibrillation thresholds have been achieved. Even with the tunneling tool, tunneling over large areas can prove to be extremely challenging. It is important to maintain optimal depth of the tunneled track. Care should be taken to avoid intrathoracic entry as well as superficial cutaneous exit. The tunneling device may be introduced either through the abdominal pocket or via a venous access incision. Care should be taken to avoid an intramuscular track to prevent hematoma formation (see Fig. 18-84).

Once the tunneling track has been established, the bullet is exchanged for the lead adapter. With the leads placed in the adapter, a suture is sometimes required

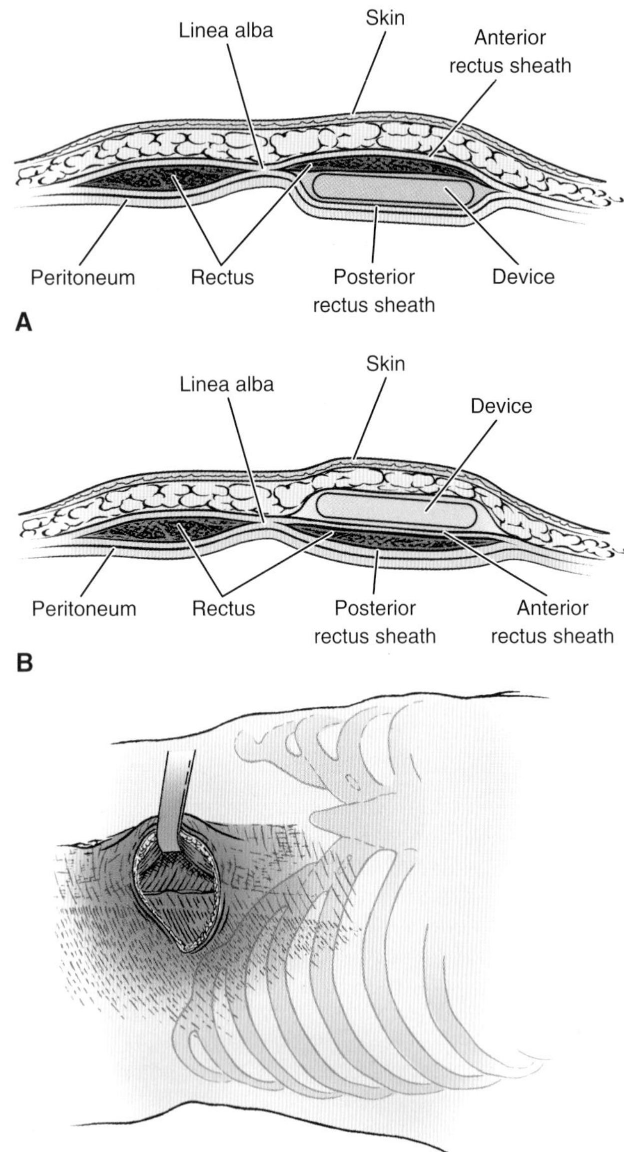

Figure 18-84. Cross-sectional anatomy of the rectus sheath above the arcuate line with implantable cardioverter-defibrillator placement. ***A,*** *Implantable cardioverter-defibrillator (ICD) placed on top of the posterior rectus sheath beneath the rectus muscle.* ***B,*** *ICD placed anterior to the anterior rectus sheath in a subcutaneous pocket above the rectus muscle.* ***C,*** *Smooth retractor exposing the posterior rectus sheath with gentle retraction of the rectus abdominis muscle positioned anteriorly.*

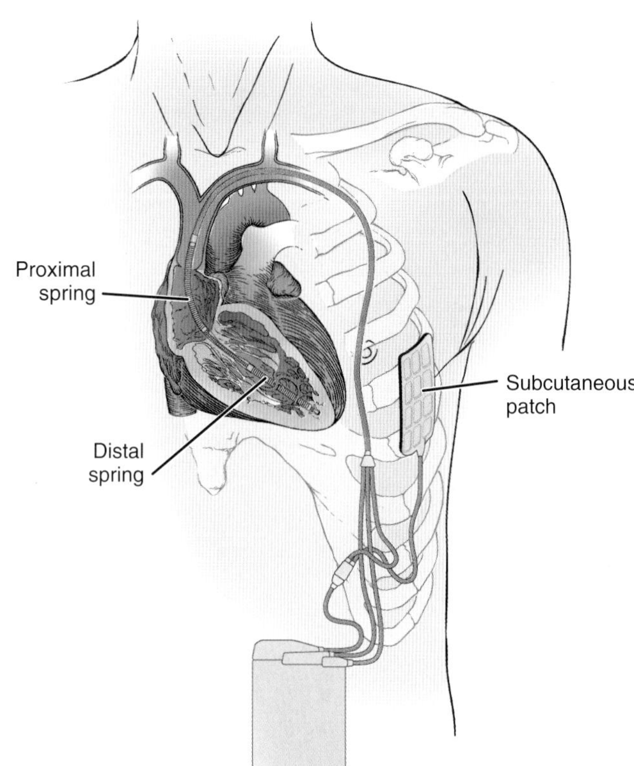

Figure 18-85. Endocardial pacing and shocking electrode positioned in the apex of the right ventricle. The electrode has been tunneled to the implantable cardioverter-defibrillator (ICD) in the right upper quadrant; the subcutaneous patch has been placed and similarly tunneled to the ICD.

to secure them in place. After the leads are secured to the adapter, the tunneling tool is retracted back to the abdominal pocket, and the leads are released from the adapter. If the tunneling tool was initially passed from the venous entry incision, the handle and bullet must be exchanged. The tunneling tool comes with two rod sizes: The shorter 12-inch rod is used for tunneling over short distances, and the longer 20-inch rod is used for pectoral-to-abdominal communication. The short rod is reserved for tunneling of subcutaneous array, for pocket-to-pocket communication, and for venous entry site-to-pectoral pocket communication. After tunneling, pacing and defibrillation parameters should be reconfirmed.

Subcutaneous Patch and Array

Occasionally, the endocardial lead system alone fails to provide an adequate defibrillation threshold. In this case, a small electrode patch may be added through a small left anterior chest incision (Fig. 18-85).[189] This incision is usually placed along the left inframammary skin fold. A subcutaneous pocket is developed in the vicinity of the anterior axillary line. The patch is sutured to the chest wall, and the proximal lead tunneled to the ICD pocket. A variation on this system is the subcutaneous array developed by Guidant (Fig. 18-86).[190] The array consists of three flexible defibrillator leads that are joined at a common connector. The leads are designed to be placed subcutaneously along the contour of the left chest wall. The leads fuse as a common electrode that connects to the ICD. The array is placed through a small incision to the left lateral inframammary skin fold. The incision is created down to the muscular fascia. Three subcutaneous tracks are created with a blunt-tipped malleable stylet. The stylet is then loaded with a sheath, which is advanced down each of the tracts. The stylet is removed, and the limbs

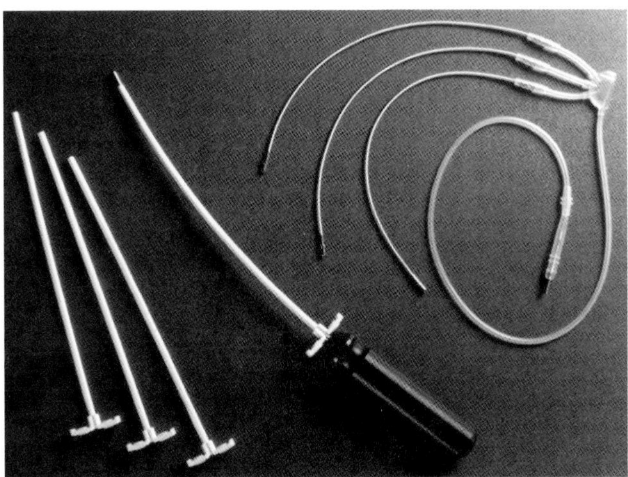

Figure 18-86. Subcutaneous array system. Left, *sheaths;* middle, *tunneling tool loaded with sheath;* right, *subcutaneous array. (Courtesy of Guidant, Boston Scientific, Natick, Mass.)*

of the array are passed down each sheath. The sheaths are split and retracted, leaving the array limb in position (Figs. 18-87 and 18-88). The proximal end of the array lead is connected to the ICD, and additional ICD defibrillation thresholds are obtained. The hub of the array is fixed to the chest wall to prevent dislodgment. Once acceptable defibrillation thresholds have been achieved, the proximal end of the lead is tunneled to the device pocket.

Similarly, Medtronic manufactures a single subcutaneous coil that is implanted through a single slittable sheath. The sheath is first loaded onto a blunt-tipped, malleable stylet that is hand-molded to slide subcutaneously from the prepectoral pocket around the lateral chest wall to the middle of the posterior chest wall at the level of the mid-LV and medial, 1 to 2 cm from the spine. The lead is inserted into the sheath after removal of the stylet, and then the sheath is slit for removal. The subcutaneous patch, the array, or the coil can be connected directly into the header or often is Y-connected with the SVC coil into the header with an adapter.

Pectoral Pocket

The creation of a pectoral pocket is generally reserved for ICDs inserted via the endocardial approach. The success and acceptance of the pectoral pocket are largely due to the considerable reduction of the ICD pulse generator. The ICD has now reached the size of the permanent transvenous pacemakers that were routinely placed in pectoral pockets in the early 1970s. Occasionally, because of the smaller ICD pulse generator, epicardial leads have been tunneled to a pectoral pocket. With the ICDs of 40 to 50 cm^3 and a thickness of 1.5 cm, pectoral pockets can easily be achieved. The pocket can be created in either the right or left pectoral area, although the left is preferred because of lower achievable defibrillation thresholds with an active can device.[188]

The pocket created can be either subcutaneous or submuscular. If the subcutaneous approach is used, it is identical to that described for a permanent transvenous pacemaker. The benefit of a subcutaneous pocket is its simplicity and avoidance of deep dissection. Creation of the pocket is also the same as that described for the permanent transvenous pacemaker. We cannot overemphasize that maximum subcutaneous depth should be achieved, with the pocket created directly on top of the pectoralis muscle to avoid potential erosion. The disadvantage of the subcutaneous approach is the concern about erosion. If the pocket is not created deep enough, the corners of the ICD can create pressure points and potential erosion. If the pocket is not made large enough and the pocket is under tension, there is a great risk for erosion. The final disadvantage of the subcutaneous pocket with the ICD at its current size is cosmetic. The subcutaneous approach results in a visible bulge that does not occur with a deeper, submuscular approach. The less attractive cosmetic result of a subcutaneous placement of an ICD has been a concern for some patients.

For the patient in whom twiddler's syndrome is a possibility, a Parsonnet pouch can be used.[191] The Parsonnet pouch is also of benefit in the asthenic patient with little subcutaneous tissue in the hope of precluding potential erosion. During creation of a subcutaneous pocket, some attention should be directed toward appropriate incision length as well as pocket size to avoid skin tension along the suture line, which can result in erosion. The management of pocket hematomas is the same in an ICD pocket as in a permanent pacemaker pocket. When recognized, the hematoma should be evacuated early, and a Jackson-Pratt drain placed. This drain is removed within 24 hours. Antibiotic lavage of the pocket is also identical to that for a permanent pacemaker pocket. One cannot excessively underscore the necessity for strict adherence to antiseptic technique.

Submuscular Pectoral Pocket

The submuscular pectoral pocket remains a popular practice for ICD implantation, because of its optimal cosmetics and virtual freedom from erosion. Vital to the submuscular pectoral approach is a complete understanding of the regional anatomy.[192] The superficial landmarks of the clavicle, deltoid muscle, pectoralis muscle, and deltopectoral groove should be clearly identified (Fig. 18-89). The pectoralis major muscle is superior to the pectoralis minor. The pectoralis major muscle has two major subdivisions. The clavicular head of the muscle attaches to the clavicle and the sternal head attaches to the lateral border of the sternum. Both heads ultimately fuse and attach to the humerus. The fascial plane that separates these two heads represents an attractive plane of dissection for access to the subpectoral space for creation of a pocket. The much smaller pectoralis minor muscle has two connections. Its superior head is attached to the coracoid process. The muscle then fans out inferiorly, attaching to the anterior ribs.

The thoracoacromial neurovascular bundle can be easily identified on the outer surface of the pectoralis

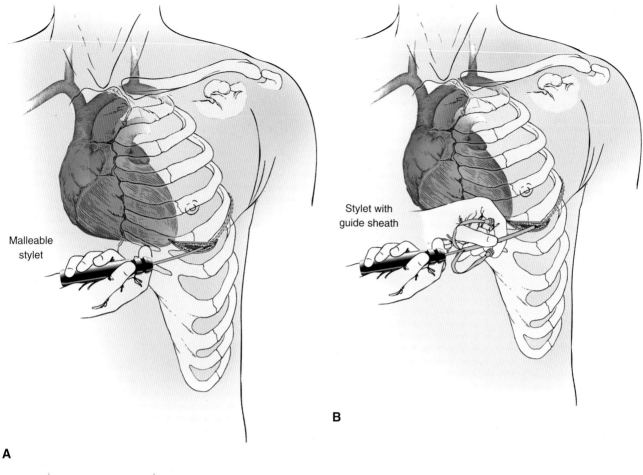

Malleable stylet

A

Stylet with guide sheath

B

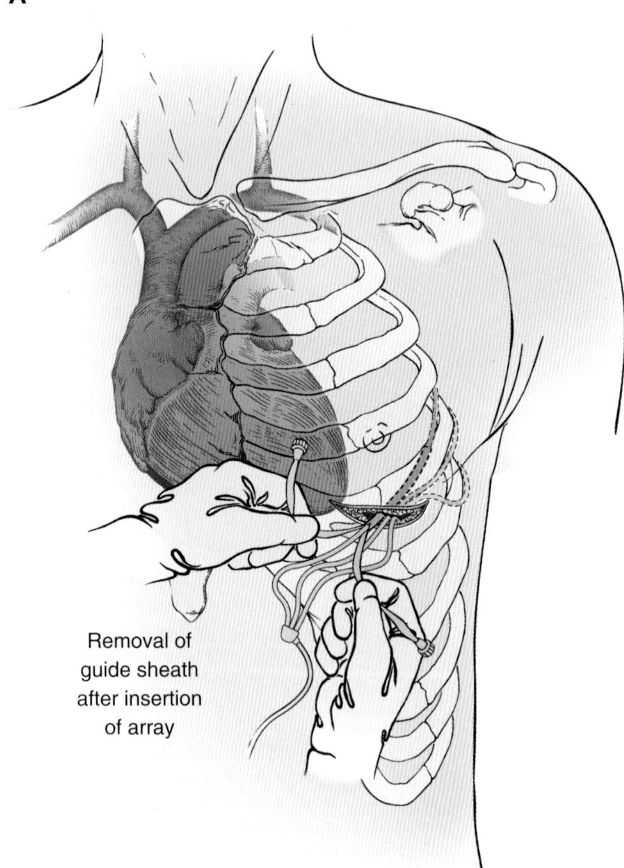

Figure 18-87. ***A,*** *Malleable tunneling stylet passed laterally, creating a tract in the subcutaneous tissue of the intercostal space.* ***B,*** *Malleable tunneling stylet loaded with sheath passed along previously created track in the subcutaneous tissue of the intercostal space.* ***C,*** *Arms of the subcutaneous array passed down previously placed sheaths. Sheaths are then peeled away, and the array is fixed to the chest wall.*

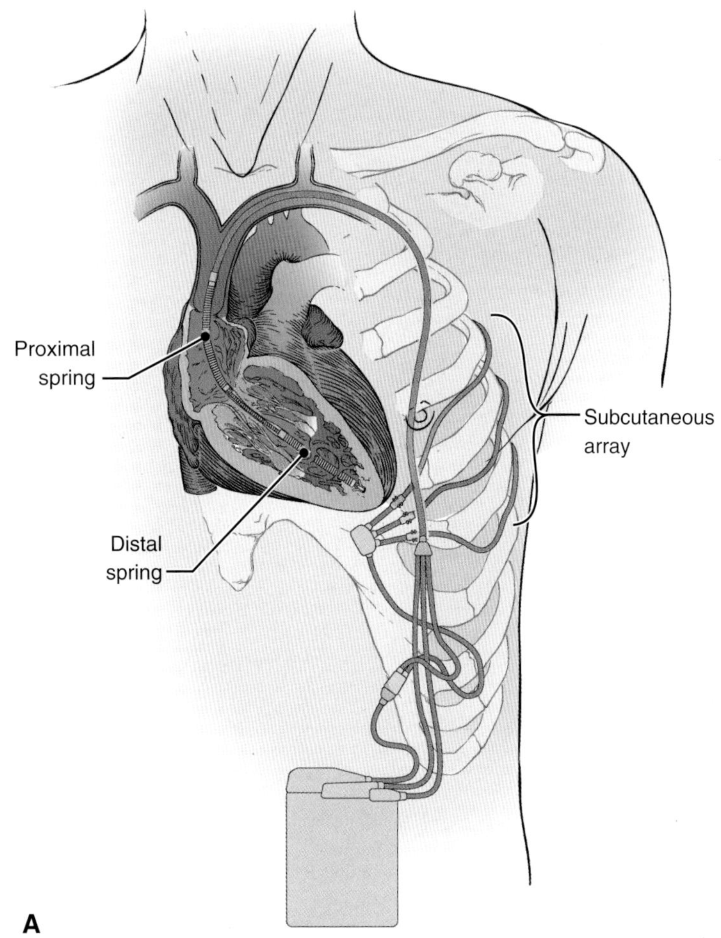

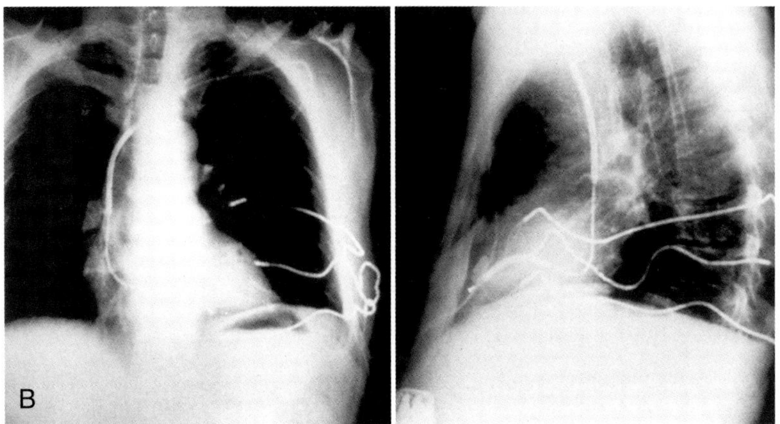

Figure 18-88. ***A,*** *Endocardial pacing and shocking electrode tunneled to the pocket in the left upper quadrant. Subcutaneous array similarly positioned and fixed to the left anterior chest wall and tunneled to the device.* ***B,*** *Anteroposterior and lateral radiographic views of the ENDOTAK subcutaneous array system.*

minor muscle (Fig. 18-90). With creation of a submuscular pectoral pocket, this bundle should always be identified and avoided, because it is a potential source of complication. Tearing the artery or vein may result in pocket hematoma, and interruption of the nerve may result in pectoral muscle dysfunction. The deltopectoral groove is defined by the lateral border of the clavicular head of the pectoralis major muscle. The anterior axillary fold is defined by the inferolateral border of the sternal pectoralis major muscle head. Today, with the active can and in combination with the dual-coil lead system, the submuscular pectoral approach may be performed from either the right or left pectoral area. The left pectoral approach, however, results in lower defibrillation thresholds.[193] Occasionally, if the right submuscular pectoral approach is used, a patch or array system may be required.

There are three distinct submuscular pectoral approaches. The first is the anterior subpectoral approach, created between the clavicular and sternal

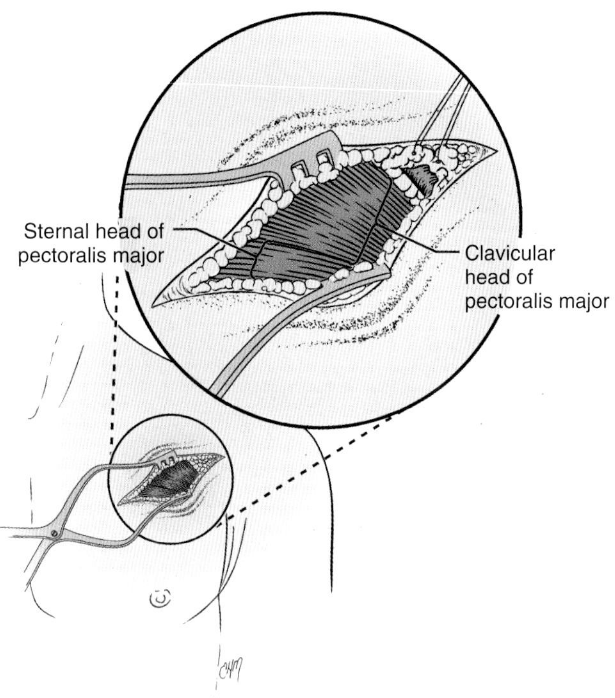

Figure 18-89. Initial incision for subpectoralis muscle placement of implantable cardioverter-defibrillator. Inset, *The deltopectoral groove and the clavicular and sternal heads of the pectoralis major muscle.*

heads of the pectoralis major (Fig. 18-91). The second submuscular pectoral approach is through a lateral reflection of the clavicular head of the pectoralis major (Fig. 18-92), and the third is a lateral submuscular pectoral approach or anterior axillary approach through the inferolateral border of the pectoralis major muscle (Fig. 18-93). Each approach has its benefits and potential complications. The anterior approach is similar to that for a subcutaneous pacemaker pocket creation. It requires the creation of a dissection plane between the sternal and clavicular portions of the pectoralis muscle. The resultant pocket is anterior and does not interfere with the axilla. The lateral approach requires dissection of the pectoralis major muscle along the deltopectoral groove. Because this approach is more lateral, there is a tendency for the ICD to drift into the axilla. Similarly, the axillary approach requires dissection and establishment of a plane at the anterior axillary fold, and there is a tendency for the device to drift into the axilla and cause discomfort. Surgical techniques to help prevent this device drift from occurring have been described. With both the lateral and axillary approaches, there is also the risk of interrupting the long thoracic nerve, leading to "wing" scapula.

The skin incision for the anterior approach is similar to that used for a permanent pacemaker pocket. One palpates the coracoid process and notes the angle of the deltopectoral groove. The incision is initiated just medial to the coracoid process and is carried from the level of the coracoid process inferomedially and per-

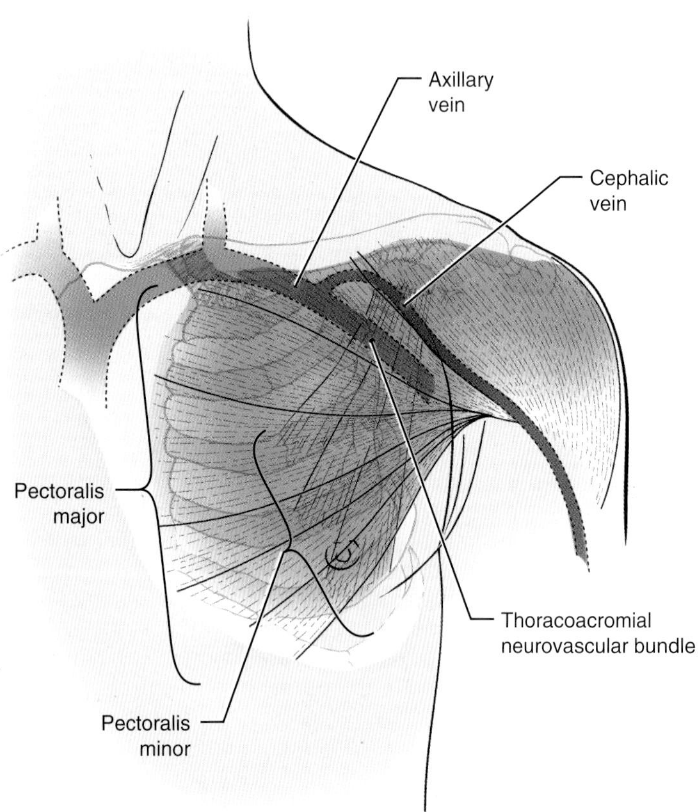

Figure 18-90. Superficial and deep anatomy of the deltopectoral area, demonstrating the relationship of the superficial pectoralis major and deep pectoralis minor muscles, axillary and cephalic veins, and thoracoacromial neurovascular bundle.

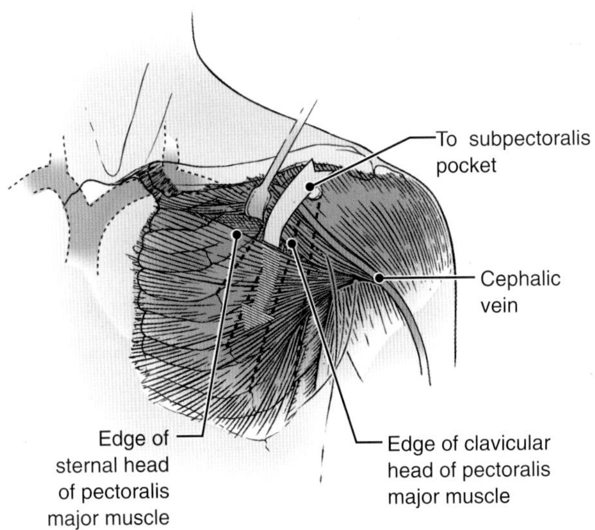

Figure 18-91. Anterior subpectoralis muscle approach. The clavicular and sternal heads of the pectoralis major muscle are gently retracted, and a plane of dissection is established postpectorally.

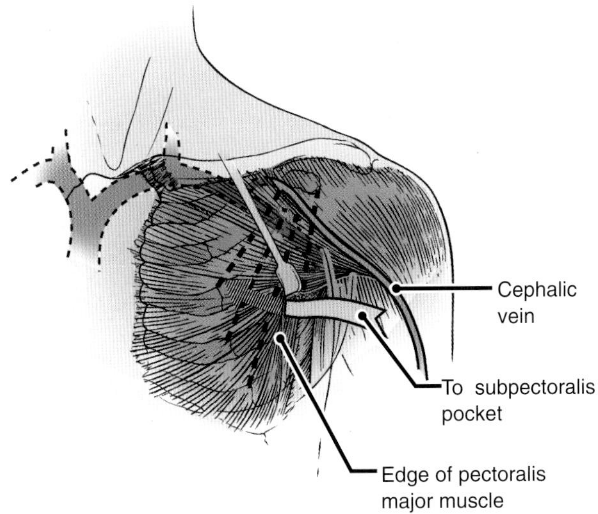

Figure 18-93. Anterior axillary fold, subpectoralis muscle approach. The lateral border of the pectoralis major sternal head at the anterior axillary fold is gently retracted, and a plane of dissection is established retropectorally.

pendicular to the deltopectoral groove for about 3 inches. With a Weitlaner retractor for retraction and electrocautery, the incision is carried down to the surface of the pectoralis fascia. With this approach, one may access the cephalic vein, the axillary vein, or the subclavian vein. After venous access is achieved and the leads are positioned, the leads are anchored to the pectoralis muscle with the suture sleeve. One creates the submuscular pectoral pocket by first identifying the border between the clavicular and sternal heads of the pectoralis muscle—usually as a line of fat. Using the smooth end of two Senn retractors, one establishes a plane of dissection between the two heads of muscle, which are gently peeled back until the surface of the chest wall is visualized as a clear plane of fatty tissue

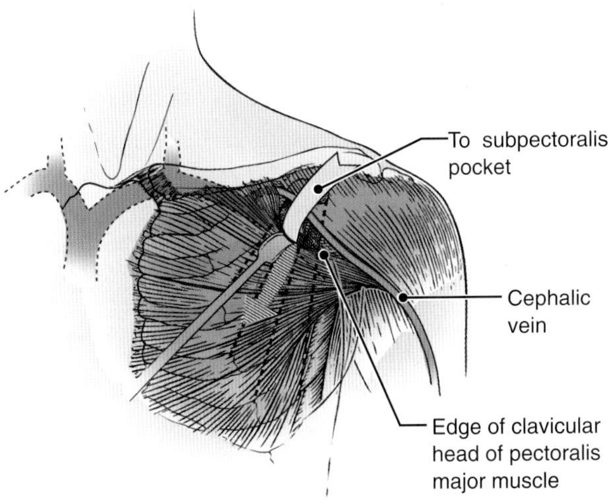

Figure 18-92. Deltopectoral groove, subpectoral approach. The lateral border of the pectoralis major muscle's clavicular head is gently retracted, and a plane of dissection is established medially, behind the pectoralis muscle.

(Fig. 18-94). One can then insert a finger and continue the dissection bluntly. Underneath the pectoralis major muscle, one can palpate superiorly the leads entering the axillary vein and identify the fibers of the pectoralis minor as well as the thoracoacromial neurovascular bundle. Occasionally, this bundle may be torn, and electrocautery or vascular clamps may be applied to effect hemostasis. Care should be taken to avoid interrupting the nerve.

Once the subpectoral pocket has been established, a Goulet clamp may be inserted, and the pocket visually inspected for any unusual bleeding. The leads are connected to the ICD, which is inserted into the submuscular pectoral pocket. It is recommended that longer lead lengths be used for this anterior pocket. Particularly in a dual-chamber ICD system, the atrial electrodes should be a minimum of 52 cm long. After successful, thorough testing, the device may be rendered inactive and removed from the pocket. The pocket is carefully inspected for hemostasis as well as lavaged with antiseptic solution. The device is then reinserted into the pocket, and a multilayer closure is completed. Closure usually involves the placement of several interrupted sutures to approximate the clavicular and sternal portions of pectoralis muscle and then standard subcutaneous skin closure.

If the lateral submuscular approach through reflection of the lateral clavicular head is to be used, an initial vertical incision along the deltopectoral groove is recommended. Dissection is carried down to the surface of the pectoralis fascia. After venous access and lead placement are achieved through the cephalic, axillary, or subclavian vein, the lateral border of the clavicular head of the pectoralis major is retracted medially, and a plane of dissection on top of the pectoralis is established. Care should be taken to extend the pocket sufficiently medially to avoid interference with the abductor motion of the lateral humeral head. After

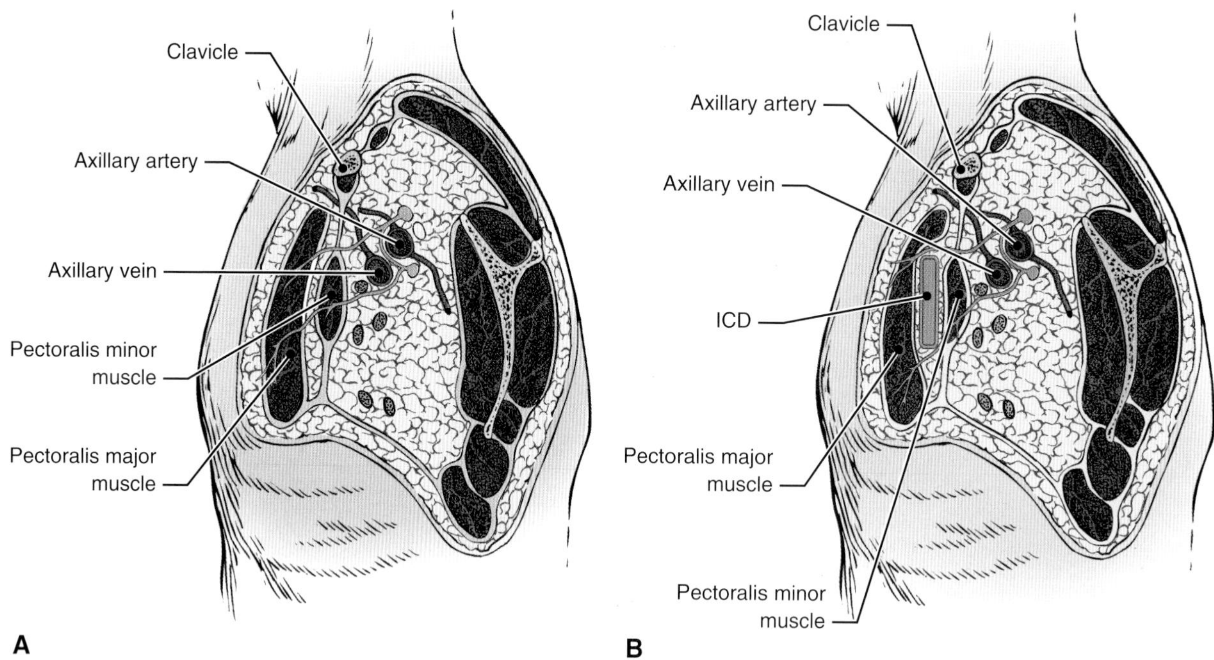

Figure 18-94. ***A,*** *Sagittal section of the shoulder girdle demonstrating the superficial and deep anatomy.* ***B,*** *Sagittal section of the shoulder girdle demonstrating superficial and deep anatomy with placement of automatic implantable cardioverter-defibrillator under the pectoralis major muscle.*

through device testing and careful pocket inspection for hemostasis, a multilayer closure is effected as described for the anterior approach.

The lateral anterior axillary submuscular pectoral approach calls for creation of a dissection plane in the anterior axillary fold.[194] If this approach is to be used, careful sterile skin preparation of the entire axilla should be carried out. Some operators prefer this approach because it is less traumatic. A dissection plane is easily established in the separation of planes created between the pectoralis major and pectoralis minor muscles. This approach is usually carried out with the patient's left arm in abduction. A skin incision is created inferiorly along the anterolateral axillary fold. The incision is carried down to the surface of the pectoralis major muscle, the pectoralis major and minor muscles are identified and separated, and a plane of dissection is created between them. This approach usually requires a separate incision for venous access and tunneling to the axillary fold incision. One has the option of cephalic, axillary, or subclavian venous access. Some operators also create a small subcutaneous pocket for placement of the strain-relief loop and excess lead. The inferolateral margin of the pectoralis major muscle is easily separated from the adjacent subcutaneous tissue for establishing a large plane of dissection. The plane of blunt dissection is created on top of the pectoralis minor muscle.

After the pocket is created, the electrodes and ICD are united, and thorough device testing is carried out. The ICD should be placed as medially as possible, with the leads lateral to the generator to avoid the risk of can abrasion. With the ICD in the pocket, a multilayer closure is used. The lateral margin of the anterior axillary soft tissue and pectoralis major muscle are approximated. Care should be taken to avoid suturing the pectoralis major and pectoralis minor muscles together because doing so would limit motion of the upper extremity. The leads are anchored to the pectoralis muscle through the separate incision for venous access. As mentioned previously, with this approach as well as the lateral approach, care should be taken to avoid interrupting the long thoracic nerve.

All three approaches call for a multilayer closure. The submuscular layer is closed by gentle approximation of the muscular heads. Care is taken to avoid tight ties that may damage the muscular tissue. The subcutaneous tissue and skin are approximated as previously discussed.

Selective Site Pacing

The preceding traditional implantation techniques describe positioning the transvenous leads in the RV apex or RA appendage. Historically these techniques have been unproved and unscientific, their evolution largely driven by available techniques and technology. A clear example is the transition from the epicardial to the endocardial approach and RV apex. This is because the RV apex is readily available, reliable, and proved to be stable over time. In addition, it is easily achieved. More recently, the conventional sites for placement of RA and ventricular leads have been challenged as inadequate and nonphysiologic.[195,196] RV apex pacing has been demonstrated to cause LV dysfunction. The resultant contraction from RV apex pacing has been shown to produce abnormalities in regional systolic fiber shortening, mechanical work, blood flow, and oxygen consumption.[197]

RV apex pacing has also been shown to result in a higher incidence of atrial fibrillation,[198] which has been underscored by the recent experience with CRT. Atrial pacing has been shown to have a beneficial effect with respect to preventing atrial fibrillation.[199-202] It is believed that the prolonged times of signal conduction from high to low atrium that can occur with pacing from the atrial appendage may play an important role in the induction of atrial fibrillation. Low atrial selective and multisite atrial pacings have been shown to reduce the incidence of atrial fibrillation.[203-208]

As a result, the conventional approach to cardiac pacing has been challenged. The term "alternative sites" has entered the cardiac pacing literature. In an attempt to optimize cardiac function, RV leads are no longer simply placed in the RV apex but are being positioned along the intraventricular septum and outflow tract.[209] The atrial leads are no longer simply placed in the high RA or atrial appendage but are now being positioned in one or more sites in the RA and sometimes LA in an attempt to suppress atrial fibrillation.[208] These concepts have resulted in the term "selective site pacing" as the preferred means of cardiac stimulation in any given patient.

Selective site pacing has resulted in new challenges for implantation, from venous access to final lead position. A thorough knowledge of cardiac anatomy and, more specifically, radiographic cardiac anatomy is essential. In addition, the tools and techniques for achieving a selective site are evolving. There are also many problems to be solved and questions to be answered if selective site pacing is to become the standard of care. First, the scientific community must define the best sites to pace in the heart. At present, the suggested selective sites include the interatrial septum, RV septum and outflow tract, the His bundle, and the coronary sinus ostium. Precise lead placement requires identification of locations that will have optimal clinical benefit. The following discussion reviews the current state of the art of selective site pacing with respect to lead location, implantation techniques, and tools. LV pacing implantation techniques are reviewed in Chapter 19.

General Considerations

For the most part, the general considerations are identical to those for permanent pacemaker implantation. There are, however, several important issues. The recommended location for the procedure is the cardiac catheterization or electrophysiology laboratory, because selective site pacing requires high-quality imaging equipment and the ability to easily achieve multiple radiographic projections. In addition, a physiologic recorder capable of obtaining high-quality electrograms for mapping is essential. The choice of anesthesia is related to operator preference. Most procedures can be conducted with intravenous sedation and on an outpatient basis.

Venous access for selective site pacing is essentially the same as previously discussed for conventional pacing techniques. The challenges involve the addition of multiple electrodes, which is best achieved with the retained-guidewire technique.[89] Simply retaining the guidewire enables one to introduce multiple additional pacing leads into the central circulation. This ability becomes important with multiple-site atrial pacing and biventricular pacing, in which three or more leads are introduced into the venous system. If one anticipates the addition of multiple electrodes after venous access is achieved, a 6F sheath set can be placed over the guidewire, and additional guidewires, corresponding to the number of required leads, can be passed down the sheath and retained. The extra guidewires are then pinned to the drape for future use.

If multisite atrial pacing is to be performed, lead Y adapters are usually needed to connect the atrial leads to the pacemaker. An assortment of adapters for any given situation should be kept on hand at all times.

Selective site pacing requires the use of active-fixation leads, either extendable, retractable, or with a fixed extended helix. Positioning the lead for the selected site can be quite challenging. At times, a selected site is almost inaccessible with conventional leads, particularly in the atrial septum or for direct His bundle pacing. Special J-shaped stylets are often required. Two types of delivery systems are now available for such difficult clinical situations. The first is a steerable stylet (Fig. 18-95). In its current design, the curves achieved by the stylet preclude access to some selective sites. A steerable stylet is connected to a handle with a slide bar. This activates and adjusts the curve. The stylet is actually inside a 0.0016-mm tube that is attached to the slide bar on the handle. The tube is passed down the pacing lead to be inserted. The lead is slipped over the tube and attached to the handle, and the desired curve is made with the lead in the heart. The handle is also used to turn the lead around its axis, maneuvering the curve clockwise or counterclockwise. The stylet can also be manually curved to achieve desired secondary curves, which can help achieve stability of the lead in the SVC. The stylet curves the distal 4 cm of the pacing lead. This system was used successfully by De Voogt and colleagues[210] in 100 patients to position leads in the low RA septum.

The second system builds on the concept of a catheter delivery system. Unlike in the catheter delivery systems for CRT that had fixed curves, a family of steerable catheters (Selectsite, models 10634-39 and 10635-49, Medtronic, Inc.) has been developed to guide pacing leads to selective sites (Fig. 18-96). In these products, the 4F active-fixation lead is passed down the steerable catheter to the desired position for fixation. This lead is a simple cable and has no guiding stylet, being delivered by a guide catheter.

Anatomic Considerations

A complete understanding of the gross and radiographic cardiac anatomy is essential for successful selective site pacing. An appreciation of the RA

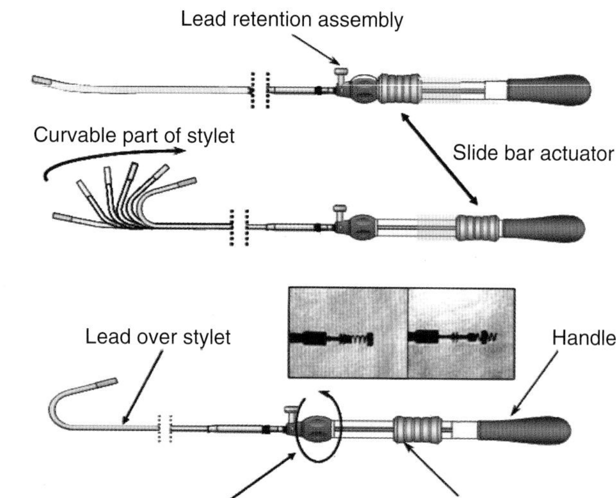

Figure 18-95. *Steerable stylet (locator, St. Jude Medical model 4036, St. Jude Medical, St. Paul, Minn.).* Top, *The slide lies next to the clamp and the tip of the stylet is straight.* Middle, *The slide is moved from the clamp toward the handle resulting in the tip of the stylet being curved.* Bottom, *The lead retention assembly is rotated to activate the screw active fixation mechanism. (From De Voogt WG, Van Mechelen R, Van Den Bos A, et al: A technique of lead insertion for low atrial septal pacing. PACE 28:639, 2005.)*

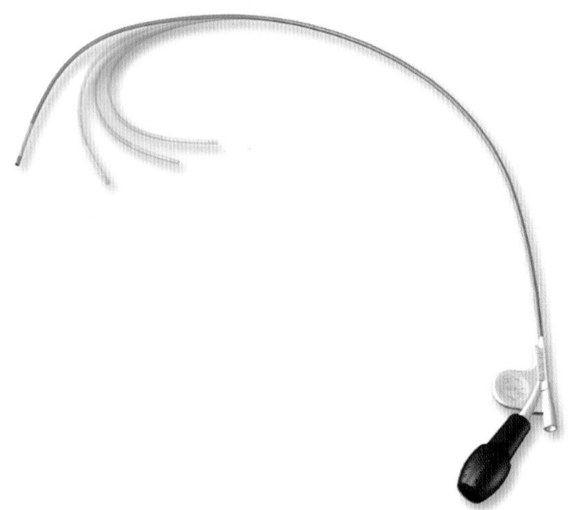

Figure 18-96. Top, *The Selectsite steerable catheter (model 10634-39, Medtronic, Inc., Minneapolis, Minn.). (From Mond HG, Grenz D: Implantable transvenous pacing leads: The shape of things to come. PACE 27:892, 2004.)*

anatomy is necessary for targeting of the low atrial septum and cannulation of the coronary sinus. As previously mentioned, appreciation of the RV spatial orientation is important for direct His bundle, RV septal, and outflow tract pacing.

Right Atrium. In the frontal plane, the RA cavity is located to the right and anteriorly. The LA is located to the left and mainly posterior to the interatrial septum; when viewed in the transverse plane, it runs obliquely from a left anterior position to a right posterior position. The RA is somewhat larger than the left, but its walls are thinner. Traditionally, the RA is considered to consist of two parts, a posterior smooth-walled part into which the superior and inferior vena cava enter and a very thin-walled trabeculated part located anterolaterally.[211]

The two parts of the RA are separated by a muscular ridge called the crista terminalis. The ridge consists of muscle that is more prominent superiorly, tapering toward its inferolateral end. Externally, the crista terminalis corresponds to a seam known as the sulcus terminalis, the pectinate muscles travel laterally in a parallel fashion from the crista terminalis along the RA's free wall. The atrial wall between the pectinate muscle bundles is almost paper thin and translucent. The RA appendage is the triangular superior portion of the RA. It is filled with pectinate muscles. The eustachian valve is a fold of tissue that guards the anterior border of the inferior vena caval ostium. In humans it demonstrates considerable variability and may even be absent. Occasionally, the eustachian valve is perforated and even fenestrated, forming a lacelike network known as the network of Chiari. Anterior and medial to the eustachian valve, the coronary sinus enters the RA. The thebesian valve is a valvelike fold of tissue that guards the orifice of the coronary sinus. The interatrial septum forms the posterior or medial wall of the RA. The central ovoid portion, which is thin and fibrous, forms a shallow depression known as the fossa ovalis. The remainder of the septum is muscular, forming a ridge known as the limbus fossa ovalis (Fig. 18-97).

Developments in interventional electrophysiology, CRT, and selective site pacing have mandated a better understanding of atrial anatomy. Contemporary anatomists Ho and Anderson have led the way to a better understanding of the RA anatomy as it relates to the cardiac electrophysiologic interventions.[212,213] Ho considers the RA to consist of three components, the appendage, a venous part, and the vestibule (Fig. 18-98). The interatrial septum, a fourth component, is shared by the RA and LA. When viewed from the epicardium, the atrial appendage is a triangular structure located anteriorly and laterally. The sulcus terminalis corresponding to the crista terminalis can be seen running along the lateral wall as a fat-filled groove. Epicardially, the sinus node is located in this groove adjacent to the SVC-RA junction. The RA musculature extends from the SVC externally and terminates at the

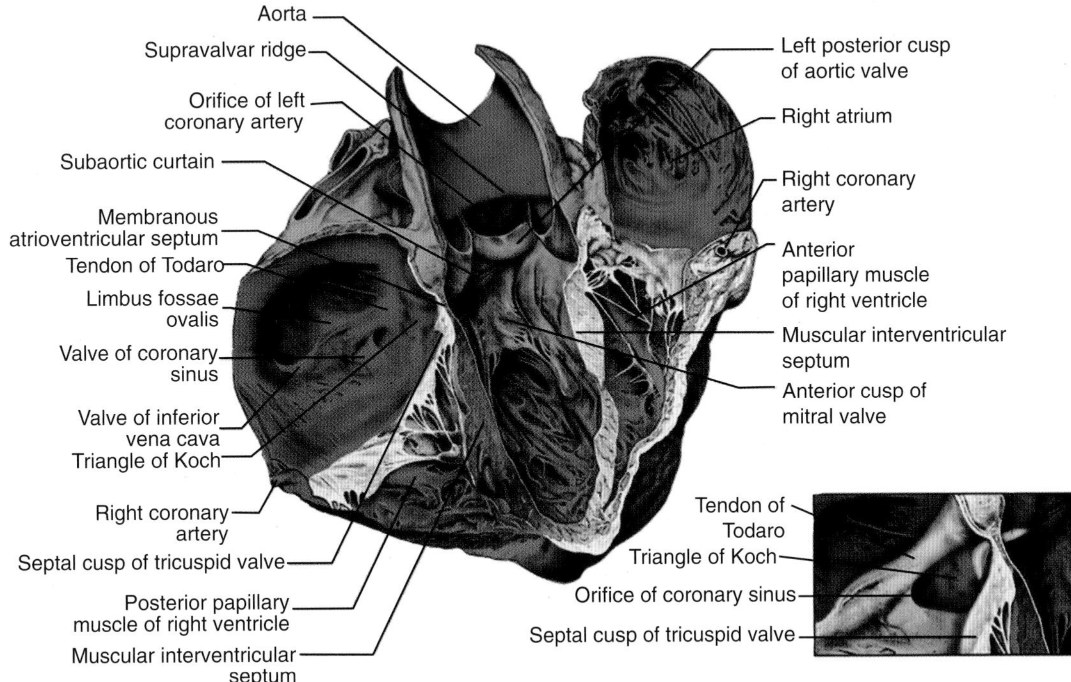

Figure 18-97. The interior of the heart, which one can reveal by incising it along its right and lower surfaces and excising the pulmonary trunk and infundibulum. The rest of the heart has been turned over to the left. (From David Johnson: Heart and great vessels. In Standring S: Gray's Anatomy: The Anatomical Basis of Clinical Practice. Philadelphia, Elsevier, 2005, p 1002.)

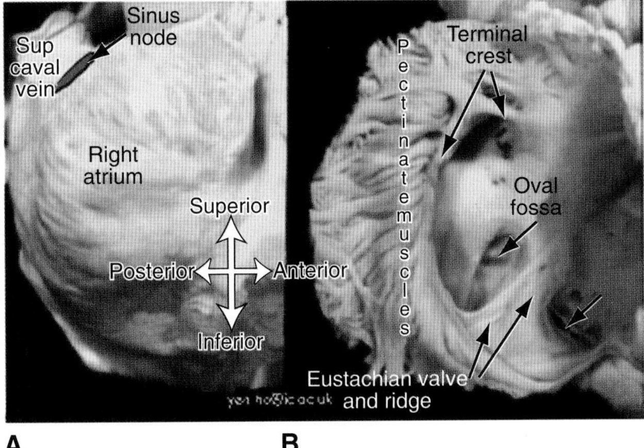

*Figure 18-98. **A,** Right anterior view of the right atrium (RA) from outside showing the relationship of the superior vena cava and atrial appendage. The RA is thin walled with a rough texture. The sinus node is shown. **B,** Interior of the RA as seen from the right anterior oblique view. The RA free wall is retracted posteriorly. The septal aspect and the venous components are visible. The pectinate muscles arise from the terminal arch of the crista terminalis. The eustachian ridge and valve as well as a fenestrated thebesian valve are seen. (From Ho S: Understanding atrial anatomy: Implications for atrial fibrillation ablation. In Cardiology International for a Global Perspective on Cardiac Care. London, Greycoat Publishing, 2002, pp S17-S20.)*

entrance of the inferior vena cava. When viewed externally, the pectinate muscles, as previously noted, can be seen radiating from the terminal crest. The pectinate muscles spread throughout the entire wall of the atrial appendage, extending to the lateral and inferior walls of the atrium. The pectinate muscles never reach the orifice of the tricuspid valve.

The vestibule is a smooth muscular rim that surrounds the tricuspid valve orifice (Fig. 18-99). The posterior smooth wall of the atrium constitutes the venous component. The terminal crest marks the division between the venous smooth and trabeculated parts of the atrium. The terminal crest is a muscular bundle that begins on the superior aspect of the medial wall and passes anteriorly and laterally to the orifice of the SVC. It then descends obliquely along the lateral atrial wall. Its terminal portion consists of a number of smaller muscle bundles extending to the vestibule and orifice of the inferior vena cava. The eustachian valve, a triangle or flap of fibromuscular tissue, guards the entrance of the inferior vena cava. This valve inserts medially and forms the eustachian ridge or sinus septum, which is the border between the fossa ovalis and the coronary sinus. The eustachian valve may be quite large, fenestrated, perforated, or delicate. The free border of the eustachian valve extends as a tendon that runs into the musculature of the sinus septum. Called the tendon of Todaro, it forms the posterolateral border of Koch's triangle.

The anterior border is marked by a hinge of the septal leaflet of the tricuspid valve. The vestibular portion of the RA that surrounds the valvular orifice is the common location for slow-pathway ablations of AV node reentrant tachycardia. The thebesian valve is a small, flat, crescentic flap of fibrous tissue that guards the orifice of the coronary sinus. It varies considerably in size and thickness and is occasionally fenestrated.

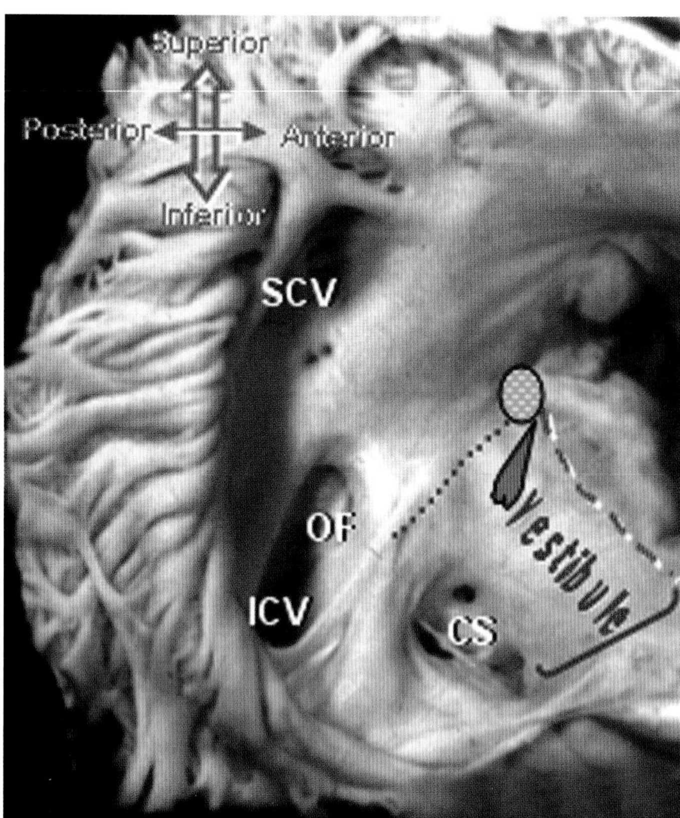

Figure 18-99. The landmarks of the triangle of Koch are superimposed on the exposed right atrial cavity. The relationship of the structural landmarks to the coronary sinus (CS) is seen. ICV, inferior vena cava: OF, flap valve: SCV, superior caval vein. (From Ho S: Understanding atrial anatomy: Implications for atrial fibrillation ablation. In Cardiology Interatrial for a Global Perspective on Cardiac Care. London, Greycoat Publishing, 2002, pp S17-S20.)

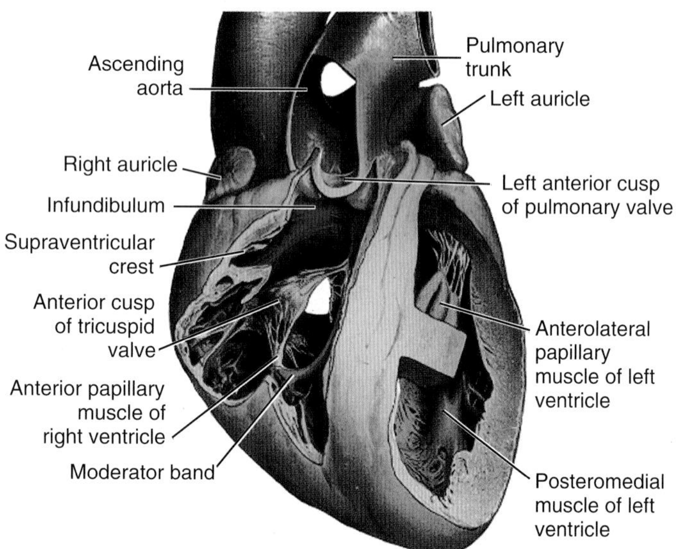

Figure 18-100. Dissection opening the ventricles, viewed from the front. (From David Johnson: Heart and great vessels. In Standring S: Gray's Anatomy: The Anatomical Basis of Clinical Practice. Philadelphia, Elsevier, 2005, p 1002.)

The atrial wall inferior to the coronary sinus os often forms a pouch known as the subeustachian sinus. The coronary sinus, the terminal portion of the great cardiac vein, is located posteriorly in the left AV groove. It is frequently covered by muscular fibers of the LA. The coronary sinus receives the veins draining the LV, including the great cardiac vein, posterior cardiac vein, left cardiac vein, and anterior cardiac veins. The coronary sinus terminates in the inferoposterior aspect of the RA and forms the inferior border of Koch's triangle.

Right Ventricle. As previously stated, the RV is an anterior mediastinal structure, extending from the RA ventricular orifice to the cardiac apex (Fig. 18-100). It ascends leftward to become the infundibulum or conus arteriosus, reaching the pulmonic valve. The RV consists of an inlet component supporting the tricuspid valve, and an apical component, a coarsely trabeculated and muscular infundibulum or outlet that attaches to the pulmonic valve. The anterior surface of the RV is convex and constitutes the majority of the heart under the anterior thoracic wall. Its inferior aspect is flat, resting on the diaphragm. The RV left and posterior walls constitute the ventricular septum. This structure is slightly curved and bulges into the ventricular chamber.

The RV inlet and outlet components that support the tricuspid and pulmonic valves are separated and covered by the roof of the RV. These are separated in the roof of the RV by a prominent supraventricular crest called the crista supraventricularis. This is a thick muscular structure that extends obliquely forward and to the right from a septal extension on the interventricular septal wall to a mural or parietal extension on the anterolateral RV wall. The inlet and outlet regions extend apically into the ventricle. The inlet component is trabeculated, whereas the outlet is predominantly smooth walled. It is the myriad of irregular muscular ridges and protrusions that are responsible for the trabeculated appearance. The protrusions and grooves result in great variation in wall thickness. The papillary muscles are prominent protrusions from the ventricular wall. The septal marginal trabecula or septal band is a prominent protrusion in the RV chamber. It supports the septal surface at its base and divides into limbs that embrace the supraventricular crest. The apex of the septal band supports the anterior papillary muscle. At this point it crosses to the parietal wall of the ventricle and is called the moderator band. The infundibulum or outflow tract is smooth walled and extends leftward below the arch of the supraventricular crest to the pulmonary orifice.

Radiographic Anatomy. In addition to understanding the gross anatomy of the RA, coronary sinus and RV, one must have a thorough knowledge of the radiologic and angiographic anatomy in order to succeed in selective site pacing and CRT. Previously, few studies were devoted to the angiographic anatomy of the right heart, but with the popularity of CRT, the coronary sinus angiographic anatomy has now been extensively described.

Farré and colleagues[214] have elegantly described the gross and fluoroscopic cardiac anatomy for interventional electrophysiology. They recommend the use of the visible human slice and surface server developed by Hersch for understanding and correlating the cardiac anatomy to the fluoroscopic projections. It is important to understand the fluoroscopic anatomy in the frontal and oblique projections when one is implanting leads. The frontal view is generally used for introduction and positioning of leads in the RV apex and high RA. For selective site pacing, it is difficult to locate with certainty the position of the lead by means of a single fluoroscopic projection. This is when oblique views are very important to help position the pacemaker lead within the three dimensions of the heart. The RAO and left anterior oblique (LAO) projections define what is anterior, posterior, inferior, and superior in cardiac planes that are parallel to the input of the image intensifier (Fig. 18-101).

In the frontal plane, the RV occupies most of the cardiac silhouette as an anterior structure. The upper half of the right heart border is formed by the SVC, and the lower portion is formed by the lateral wall of the RA. The plane of the lateral valve is sandwiched between the anterior RV and posterior LV. It can be conceptualized as an oval ring tipped somewhat to the left. The coronary sinus is located at the inferior aspect of the cardiac silhouette at the level of the diaphragms, approximately in the midline. The RAO projection rolls the RV to the left. In this view, the superior and inferior vena cavae and RA become an anterior structure. The plane of the tricuspid and mitral valves becomes more vertical and perpendicular to the anteroposterior plane (Fig. 18-102). The RV is pushed to the left. In the LAO projection, the plane of the tricuspid and mitral valves becomes frontal, with the coronary sinus tipped in a horizontal position and crossing over the spine as it courses to the left, crossing over the spine from right to left and turning superiorly along the left heart border (Fig. 18-103).

For placement of a pacemaker lead in the RA appendage, the frontal projection is preferred. The tip of the RA appendage is superior and anterior. When the lead tip is placed in the apex of the atrial appendage, it moves from right to left. In the RAO projection, the tip points to the right, and in the LAO projection, it points to the left. The triangle of Koch is in

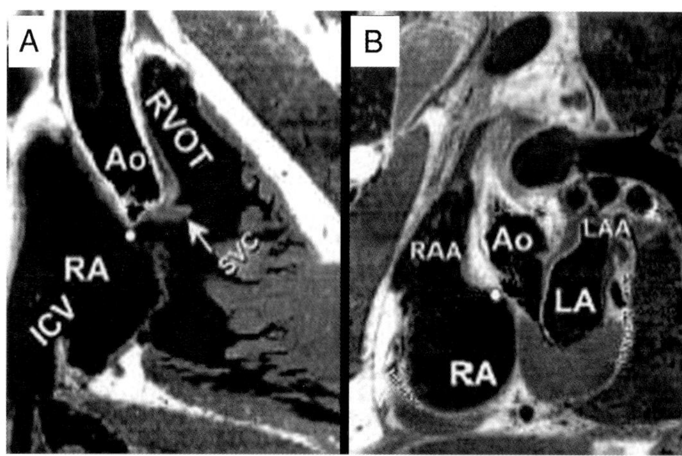

Figure 18-101. ***A,*** *Right anterior oblique projection;* ***B,*** *left anterior oblique (LAO) projection. Sections of the male heart (obtained from the Ecole Polytechnique Fédérale de Lausanne: Visible Human Surface Server. Online at visiblehuman.epfl.ch).* ***A*** *shows the inferior caval vein (ICV), the supraventricular crest (SVC), the aorta (Ao), and right ventricular outflow tract (RVOT). The* white dot *identifies the site corresponding to the membranous septum or the area the maximal His bundle potential is usually recorded. In the LAO projection, the right atrial appendage (RAA) and the right and left atria (RA and LA, respectively) at the level of the atrioventricular junctions are depicted. As in A, white* dot *signals the area where the His bundle potential is recorded. The left atrial appendage (LAA) is superior. (From Farré J, Anderson RH, Cabrera JA, et al: Fluoroscopic cardiac anatomy for catheter ablation of tachycardia. PACE 25:88, 2002.)*

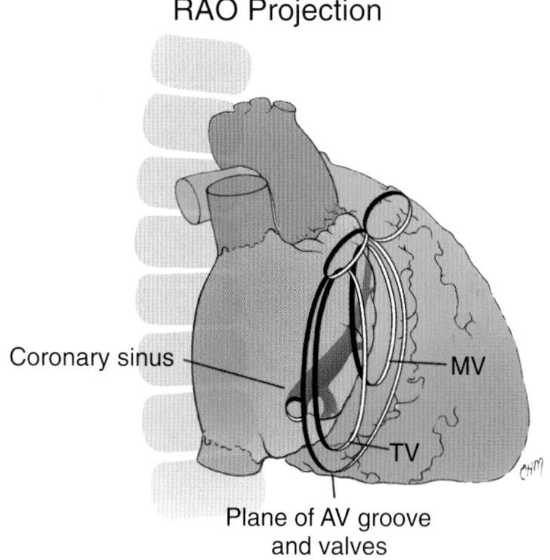

Figure 18-102. Heart rotated in the right anterior oblique (RAO) view showing the relationship of the atrioventricular (AV) groove and spine. (From Belott PH: Implantation techniques for cardiac resynchronization therapy. In Barold SS, Mugica J: The fifth decade of cardiac pacing. Armonk, NY, Futura, 2004, p 6.)

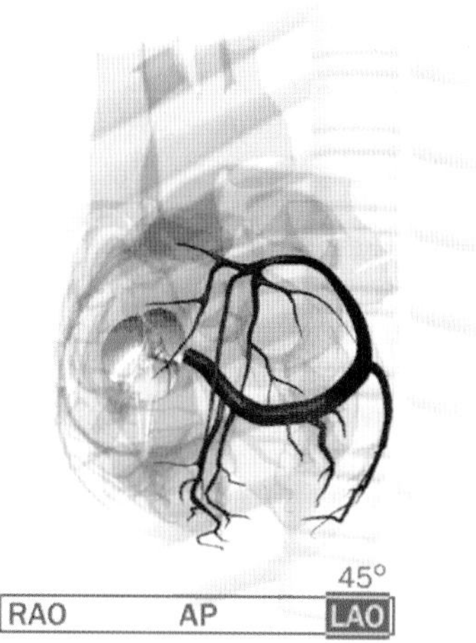

Figure 18-104. Coronary sinus (CS) in the left anterior oblique (LAO) projection. The plane of the sinus is more horizontal and posterior. The posterior and lateral branches are directed inferiorly and to the left, whereas the anterior branches are directed superiorly to the right. (From Belott PH: Implantation techniques for cardiac resynchronization therapy. In Barold SS, Mugica J: The fifth decade of cardiac pacing. Armonk, NY, Futura, 2004, plate 1.4.)

the inferior paraseptal RA region. This region is important for RA septal and His-bundle selective site pacing. In the RAO projection, the plane of Koch's triangle is parallel to the image intensifier. The LAO projection helps differentiate paraseptal lead positions. The region of the His bundle is located superiorly, and the coronary sinus os inferiorly. In the RAO and LAO projections, the os of the coronary sinus can be found at the inferior aspect of the cardiac silhouette at the level of the diaphragms just to the right of the spine.

Rotating from the RAO to the LAO projection and back becomes important in attempts to cannulate the coronary sinus os. As a simple example, the frontal projection makes the catheter appear to be in the vicinity of the coronary sinus os with the trajectory pointing inferiorly and to the left; when the image is rotated to the LAO projection, however, the catheter is seen to be actually 180 degrees away from the coronary sinus os, pointing anteriorly and to the right. After the catheter is adjusted to a posterior and leftward position, the RAO projection may show the catheter pointing laterally to the right, away from the coronary sinus os. This simple example points to the importance of multiple views in achieving a selected site.

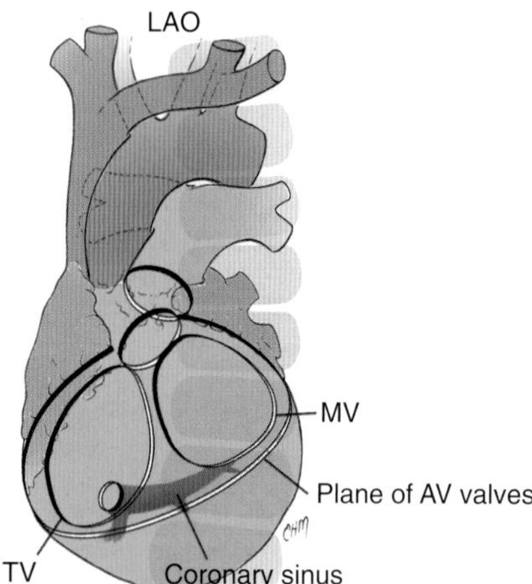

Figure 18-103. Heart rotated in the left anterior oblique (LAO) view in which the atrioventricular groove is tipped horizontally. AV, atrioventricular; MV, mitral valve; TV, tricuspid valve. (From Belott PH: Implantation techniques for cardiac resynchronization therapy. In Barold SS, Mugica J: The fifth decade of cardiac pacing. Armonk, NY, Futura, 2004, p 6.)

With respect to the coronary sinus, the LAO projection is extremely important in distinguishing anterior and posterior tributaries of this sinus (Fig. 18-104). In the frontal and RAO projections, tributaries of the coronary sinus appear to run perpendicular to the coronary sinus, obliquely from a superior to an inferior direction (Fig. 18-105). The branches appear to be parallel, making differentiation of anteroseptal, lateral, and posterolateral branches almost impossible.

Atrial Septal Pacing

Atrial fibrillation, the most common sustained tachycardia arrhythmia in clinical practice, is associated with considerable morbidity and mortality. It is believed that atrial pacing might help prevent the onset of atrial fibrillation through a variety of mechanisms. Atrial pacing should prevent relative bradycardia, which is often a trigger for atrial fibrillation. In addition, atrial pacing should suppress bradycardia-induced dispersion of refractoriness in the atrium as well as escape atrial ectopy, which are potential causes of atrial fibrillation.

In 1907, Bachmann described a distinct band of muscle tissue extending from the base of the LA appendage, called the anterior interatrial band.[215] Bachmann's bundle was later defined as a band of fibers traversing the LA, curving posteriorly within the interatrial septum and reaching the crest of the AV node.[216] RA activation mapping, when the heart is being paced from the LA and coronary sinus, has demonstrated preferential sites of the transseptal conduction (Figs. 18-106 and 18-107). The earliest RA activation has been found to be near the insertion of Bachmann's bundle.[217-220] Electroanatomic mapping has confirmed the role of Bachmann's bundle in intra-atrial propagation. Bachmann's bundle may therefore be an ideal selective site for prevention of atrial fibrillation.[217]

The selective sites for RA pacing include the high RA septum and the low RA septum in the vicinity of the coronary sinus os. The area of the high RA septum involves the crista terminalis, and Bachmann's bundle is particularly difficult to pace with conventional tools. The selective site for low RA septum is the mouth or os of the coronary sinus. The usual target for lead attachment is just superior to the coronary sinus os. Atrial septal pacing from this position will result in negative P waves in leads II, III, and aVF.

For atrial septal pacing, a permanent pacing lead is placed in the posterior RA septal wall. To achieve a selective site, an active fixation lead is mandatory. The triangle of Koch is situated in the lower aspect of the interatrial septum. It is confined by the borders of the tricuspid valve anulus and the eustachian ridge superiorly. The base of the triangle, as mentioned previously, is formed by the coronary sinus. The posterior aspect of the triangle is the muscular part of the interatrial septum. The 45-degree LAO fluoroscopic projection is used to guide the pacing lead at a right angle into the intra-atrial septum. The interatrial septum is oriented at about 45 degrees from right posterior to left anterior. The 45-degree LAO projection helps confirm lead fixation to the triangle of Koch (Fig. 18-108).

Selective site atrial septal lead placement is next to impossible with the frontal or RAO projection. These views can be used only for secondary confirmation of

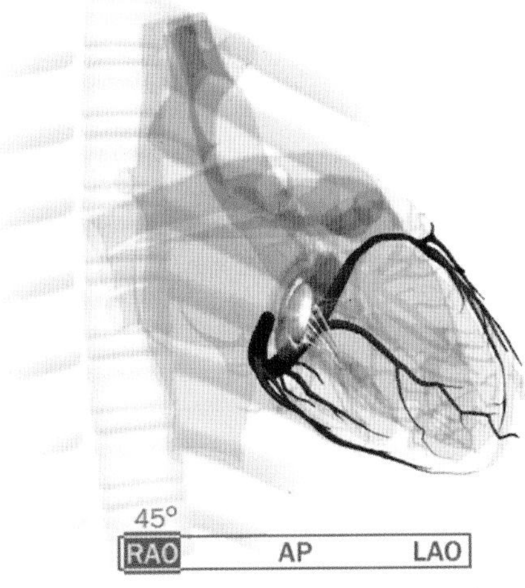

Figure 18-105. Coronary sinus (CS) seen in the right anterior oblique projection. The plane of the sinus is vertical with the branch tributaries at a right angle. In this view all the branches come into coronary sinus at nearly a right angle and are directed slightly inferiorly into the left. (From Belott PH: Implantation techniques for cardiac resynchronization therapy. In Barold SS, Mugica J: The fifth decade of cardiac pacing. Armonk, NY, Futura, 2004, plate 1.3.)

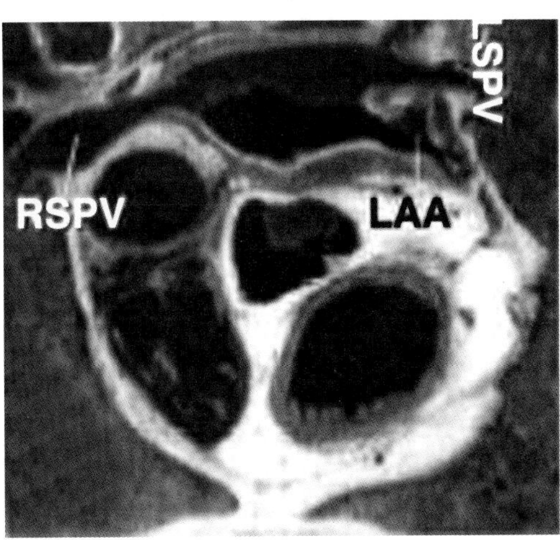

Figure 18-106. Axial section of the heart (obtained from the Ecole Polytechnique Fédérale de Lausanne: Visible Human Surface Server. Online at visiblehuman.epfl.ch). LAA, left atrial appendage; LSPV, left superior pulmonary vein; RSPV, right superior pulmonary vein. (From Farré J, Anderson RH, Cabrera JA, et al: Fluoroscopic cardiac anatomy for catheter ablation of tachycardia. PACE 25:88, 2002.)

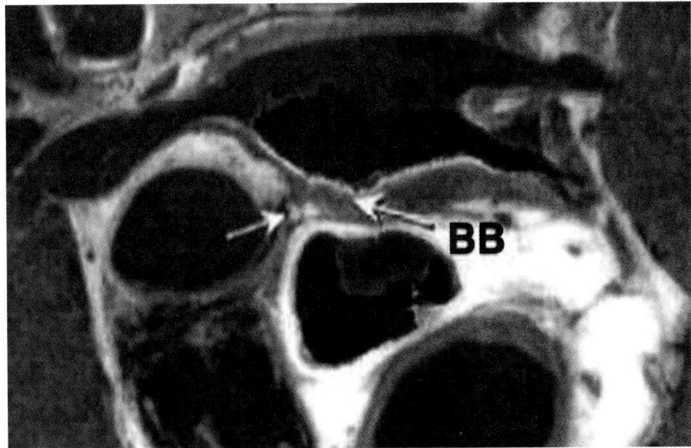

Figure 18-107. Axial section of the heart and magnification of Figure 18-106 (obtained from the Ecole Polytechnique Fédérale de Lausanne: Visible Human Surface Server. Online at visiblehuman.epfl.ch.), depicting the area of Bachmann's bundle (BB, arrow*). (From Farré J, Anderson RH, Cabrera JA, et al: Fluoroscopic cardiac anatomy for catheter ablation of tachycardia. PACE 25:88, 2002.)*

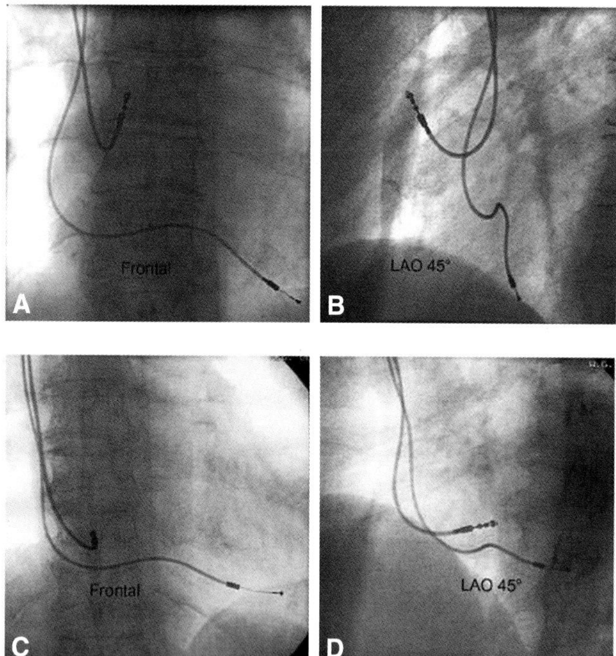

Figure 18-108. ***A*** *and* ***B,*** *Fluoroscopic images of the position of the right atrial appendage (RAA) lead. The frontal view is shown in* ***A*** *and a left anterior oblique 45-degree angulation in* ***B,*** *where the RAA lead is directed superior and anterior.* ***C*** *and* ***D,*** *Fluoroscopic images of the position of the low atrial septum (LAS) lead. The frontal view in* ***C*** *and a left anterior oblique 45-degree angulation* ***D,*** *where the LAS lead is directed at 90-degree angles at the interatrial septum. (From de Voogt WG, van Mechelen R, van den Bos AA, et al: Electrical characteristics of low atrial septum pacing compared with right atrial appendage pacing. Europace 7:62, 2005.)*

appropriate lead position. In the frontal plane, the lead appears in the neutral position or somewhat directed to the left, depending on the contraction phase of the atrium. Unlike the fluoroscopic movement of the lead tip in the RA appendage—that is, to and fro—the RA septal lead tip moves up and down. If the ventricular lead has been implanted before the atrial lead, its undulation over the tricuspid valve marks the position of the structure. The ventricular lead marks the inferior part of the tricuspid ostium. The coronary sinus ostium has also been used to locate the interatrial septum with active fixation leads placed just superior to the coronary sinus os. This site is recommended for dual-site RA pacing.[221] The second lead is usually placed in the atrial appendage. Achieving the desired location is directly related to stylet management and the skill of the operator.

Local electrogram and stimulation analysis, which is important for the recognition of far-field R-wave detection, can cause inappropriate mode switching. The height of any far-field R-wave recorded on the atrial channel must be measured. During an implantation, far-field R-wave analysis in sinus rhythm and normal AV conduction can be masked by the current of injury caused by the active fixation of the atrial septal lead. Far-field R-wave signals become superimposed on the current of injury. To avoid this problem, far-field R waves can be measured during VVI pacing, in which the far-field R wave can be seen to precede the atrial complex when VA conduction is present or can be seen between beats during VA dissociation. Far-field R-wave voltages should be less than the P-wave voltage. If high far-field R-wave voltages are found, lead repositioning should be considered. In addition, high far-field R waves may also mean that the screw-in mechanism of the atrial lead is protruding into the ventricular myocardium. This possibility can be evaluated with high-output pacing from the atrium, which produces simultaneous atrial and ventricular stimulation if the lead is in the ventricular myocardium. Malpositioning of an atrial septal lead can be deleterious, possibly causing pacemaker syndrome or, if high-rate atrial tachyarrhythmia therapy pacing is used, resulting in inappropriate, dangerously high ventricular rates.

Right Ventricular Selective Site Pacing

The search for an alternative RV pacing site has gone on for many years. The results of a 2003 quantitative review suggest that the RV outflow tract (RVOT) is the ideal site.[222] Yet the variability of anatomic, electrocardiographic, and functional criteria used to describe specific locations of the RV pacing lead in many studies is huge and conflicting.[223] The heterogenicity of selective site RV pacing studies does not allow the definition of a single beneficial site. It may be that the single hemodynamically best site in any given patient must be individually sought. Some studies have suggested that the width of the paced QRS complex could indicate the most favorable site, but this concept has been questioned.

At present, the best selected site for RV pacing is in the RVOT. In a 2004 review, Lieberman and associates[224] defined the RVOT as a broad area of the RV that is poorly defined and encompasses all areas except the apex. In the frontal projection, the lower border of the RVOT is a line extending from the apex of the tricuspid valve to the border of the RV (Fig. 18-109). The RVOT's superior limit is the pulmonic valve. Fluoroscopic images and associated ECG patterns are used to define the RVOT. The lower border can be defined by extending an electrophysiologic catheter parallel to the RV inferior border from the tricuspid valve apex to the lateral RV border in the frontal RAO projection (Fig. 18-110). The superior border of the RVOT is determined by positioning the catheter across the pulmonic valve. Monitoring electrograms allows identification of the junction between the RVOT and the pulmonic valve.

Once the RVOT boundaries have been defined, the selective site needs to be identified. One does so by dividing the RVOT into four quadrants. The RVOT is divided horizontally by a line midway between the pulmonic valve and the lower border, defining an upper and lower half. These halves are divided vertically by a line that connects the pulmonic valve to the RVOT lower border, dividing the RVOT into a septal wall and a free wall. Thus, the RVOT can be divided into four quadrants, high infundibular and low (outflow) septal RVOT, and high infundibular and low (outflow) free wall RVOT. The RAO fluoroscopic projection is used to determine high and low positions. The 40-degree LAO

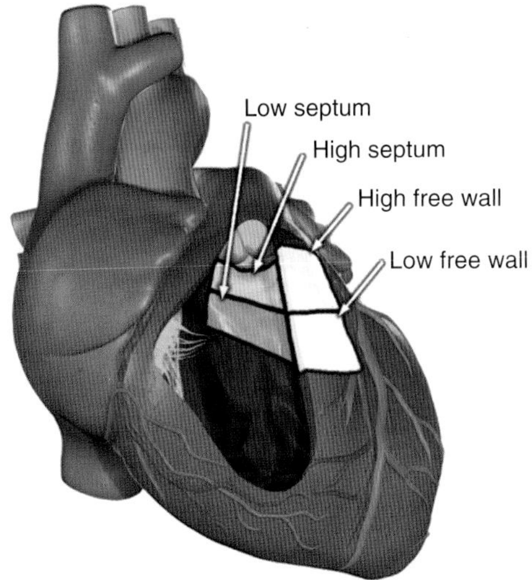

Figure 18-109. Anteroposterior view of the right ventricle. The right ventricular outflow tract has been divided into four segments, two on the septum and two on the free wall. (From Lieberman R, Grenz D, Mond HG, et al: Selective site pacing: Defining and reaching the selected site. PACE 27:883, 2004.)

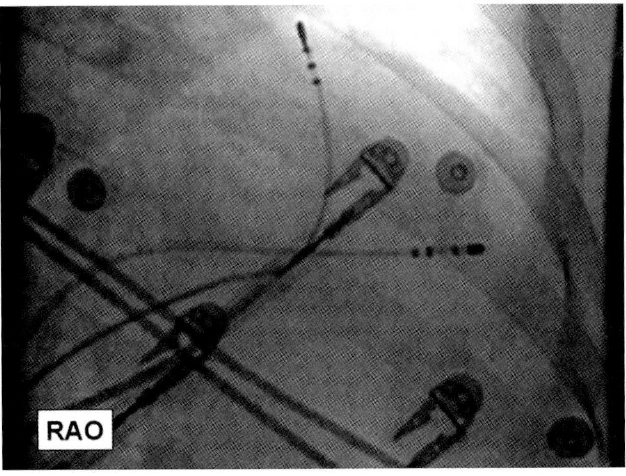

Figure 18-110. Right anterior oblique (RAO) fluoroscopic image of the heart with two catheters in the right ventricle to define the upper and lower limits of the right ventricular outflow tract. (From Lieberman R, Grenz D, Mond HG, et al: Selective site pacing: Defining and reaching the selected site. PACE 27:883, 2004.)

projection is used to differentiate RVOT, septal, and free wall positions (Fig. 18-111).

The ECG is used to confirm pacing from the RV septum. In this position, the QRS in lead I is negative. When the RV free wall is paced, the QRS in lead I is positive. Lead aVF may be used to differentiate high and low positions. Ventricular pacing in the high position results in an upright QRS in lead aVF; lower positions result in a less positive QRS.

Direct His Bundle Pacing

The normal His-Purkinje activation of the myocardium results in a rapid sequential depolarization of myocardial cells and efficient ventricular contraction. Therefore, it is believed that the His bundle would be an ideal target for selective site pacing. This site should prevent ventricular dyssynchrony and maintain normal ventricular activation sequence. There is very little human clinical experience with direct His bundle pacing. In 1992, Karpawich and associates[225] described a permanent approach to His bundle pacing in open chests of dogs. They used a specifically designed screw-in lead passed through a mapping introducer. The introducer was delivered through a right atriotomy. When an entirely transvenous approach was used, considerable difficulty was encountered directing the lead tip into the desired target.

In 2004, Deshmukh and coworkers[226] reported on attempts to perform direct His-bundle pacing in 54 patients.[225] All patients had a narrow QRS complex (<120 msec), persistent atrial fibrillation requiring AV node ablation, and a dilated cardiomyopathy. A hexapolar catheter introduced via the femoral vein was used to map and localize the His bundle with use of the RAO projection. Once localized, the His bundle was paced. Criteria for His bundle capture included (1) His-Purkinje–mediated cardiac activation and repolarization, as evidenced by ECG concordance of the QRS and T-wave complexes, (2) the paced ventricular interval identical to the His ventricular interval, and (3) His bundle capture in an all-or-none fashion, meaning that the QRS did not widen at a lower pacing output. This last criterion was critical in differentiating para-Hisian pacing or indirect capture of the His bundle from direct His bundle pacing. Once the His bundle was localized, an active fixation pacing lead was advanced into the septum. Conventional lead placement was difficult and required a specially modified, J-shaped stylet with a secondary distal curve orthogonal to the J plane, which allowed the lead to be positioned medially toward the AV septum. An attempt was made to position the lead near the mapping catheter. Once the lead was in position, an electrophysiologic study was carried out,

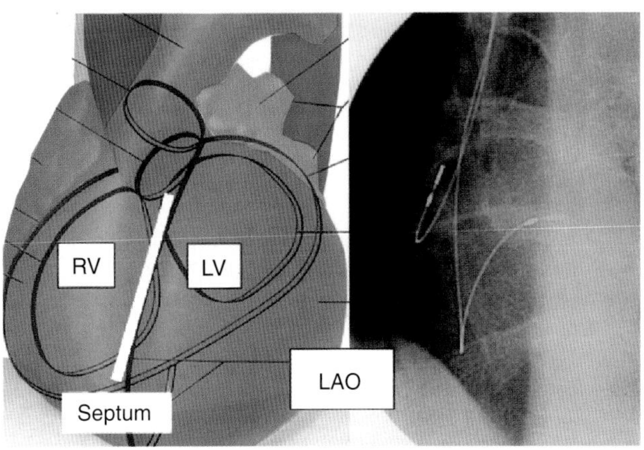

Figure 18-111. Left anterior oblique (LAO) views of the heart. Left, *Anatomic diagram to show the position of the right ventricle and septum.* Right, *Fluoroscopic image to show the pacing lead in the low septum. (From Lieberman R, Grenz D, Mond HG, et al: Selective site pacing: Defining and reaching the selected site. PACE 27:883, 2004.)*

measuring His ventricular and paced ventricular intervals. Occasionally, because of rapid ventricular rates, radiofrequency ablation was performed. These investigators reported successful direct His bundle pacing in 39 patients. It is clear from their experience that direct His bundle pacing is feasible. Electrophysiologic mapping is critical to the procedure. Precise placement of a permanent pacing lead is extremely difficult, requiring special stylets for lead manipulation. Some form of catheter delivery system needs to be developed for this selective site.

The Future of Selective Site Pacing

It is clear that selective site pacing in the atria and ventricles is evolving There are many studies supporting this approach in either chamber. Unfortunately, most of these studies have been small and reflect conflicting and confusing data. The long-term harmful effects of RV apex pacing have been well cataloged and accepted. Unfortunately there is a paucity of long-term data from carefully designed long-term studies. It is clear that patients with compromised LV function are at the greatest risk from RV apex pacing. The incidence of harm from RV apex pacing in patients with normal LV function is unknown, however, because no large, carefully designed studies have been performed. The large landmark trials, such as the Dual Chamber and VVI Implantable Defibrillator (DAVID) study, instruct us to minimize RV apex pacing and use atrium-based modes that promote AV conduction.

But what about the patient who requires ventricular pacing? The results of pacing from alternative sites have been disappointing. There is no sound basis to do so from any site other than the RV apex. There are problems defining the ideal alternate selective site as well as accurate, reliable, and stable lead placement. The RVOT is a poorly defined, broad area that needs definition of boundaries, both fluoroscopic and electrocardiographic. The scientific community must identify the best site to pace the heart, determine the location that provides optimal hemodynamic benefit, and create the tools to meet the challenge. There are also issues of training necessary for the implanting physician, who must let go of the old techniques and embrace new ones. If selective site pacing proves to be better, safe, user-friendly, and cost effective tools that require a minimum of advanced training must be developed.

With the preceding considerations, there is a need for long-term, randomized studies that involve a well-defined patient population and use multiple well-defined pacing sites to evaluate functional hemodynamics, lead stability, extractability, and complication data. Until results of such studies become available, pacing at the RA appendage and RV apex, which has proved reliability, stability, and simplicity, should not be abandoned.

REFERENCES

1. Schecter DC: Modern era of artificial cardiac pacemakers. In Schecter DC: Electrical Cardiac Stimulation. Minneapolis, Medtronic, 1983, pp 110-134.
2. Senning A: Discussion of a paper by Stephenson SE Jr, Edwards WH, Jolly PC, Scott HW: Physiologic P-wave stimulator. J Thorac Cardiovasc Surg 38:639, 1959.
3. Furman S, Schwedel JB: An intracardiac pacemaker for Stokes-Adams seizures. N Engl J Med 261:948, 1959.
4. Littleford PO, Spector SD: Device for the rapid insertion of permanent endocardial pacing electrode through the subclavian vein: Preliminary report. Ann Thorac Surg 27:265, 1979.
5. Mirowski M, Reid PR, Mower MM, et al: Termination of malignant ventricular arrhythmias with an implantable automatic defibrillator in human beings. N Engl J Med 303:322, 1980.
6. Parsonnet V, Furman S, Smyth NP, Bilitch M: Optimal resources for implantable cardiac pacemakers. Pacemaker Study Group. Circulation 68:226A, 1983.
7. Parsonnet V, Bernstein AD, Lindsay B: Pacemaker implantation complication rates: An analysis of some contributing factors. J Am Coll Cardiol 13:917, 1989.
8. Harthorne JW, Parsonnet V: Seventeenth Bethesda Conference: Adult cardiac training. Task Force VI: Training in cardiac pacing. J Am Coll Cardiol 7:1213, 1986.
9. Parsonnet V, Bernstein AD: Pacing in perspective: Concepts and controversies. Circulation 73:1087, 1986.
10. Parsonnet V, Bernstein AD, Galasso D: Cardiac pacing practices in the United States in 1985. Am J Cardiol 62:71, 1988.
11. Hayes DL, Naccarelli GV, Furman S, et al: Training requirements for permanent pacemaker selection, implantation, and follow-up. PACE 17:6, 1994.
12. Bernstein AD, Parsonnet V: Survey of cardiac pacing in the United States in 1989. Am J Cardiol 69:331, 1992.
13. Stamato NJ, O'Toole MF, Enger EL: Permanent pacemaker implantation in the cardiac catheterization laboratory versus the operating room: An analysis of hospital charges and complications. PACE 15:2236, 1992.
14. Hess DS, Gertz EW, Morady F, et al: Permanent pacemaker implantation in the cardiac catheterization laboratory: The subclavian approach. Cathet Cardiovasc Diagn 8:453, 1982.
15. Andersen FH, Crossland S, Alexander MB: Use of a three-channel electrocardiographic recorder for limited intracardiac electrocardiography during single- and double-chamber pacemaker implantation. Ann Thorac Surg 39:485, 1985.
16. Sutton R, Bourgeois I: Techniques of implantation. In Sutton R, Bourgeois I (eds): The Foundations of Cardiac Pacing: An Illustrated Practical Guide to Basic Pacing, Vol I, Part 1. Mt Kisco, NY, Futura, 1991.
17. Levine PA, Balady GJ, Lazar HL, et al: Electrocautery and pacemakers: Management of the paced patient subject to electrocautery. Ann Thorac Surg 41:313, 1986.
18. Belott PH, Sands S, Warren J: Resetting of DDD pacemakers due to EMI. PACE 7:169, 1984.
19. Chauvin M, Crenner F, Brechenmacher C: Interaction between permanent cardiac pacing and electrocautery: The significance of electrode position. PACE 15:2028, 1992.
20. Hauser RG, Edwards LM, Guiffe VW: Limitation of pacemaker system analyzers for evaluation of implantable pulse generators. PACE 4:650, 1981.
21. Gregoratos G, Abrams J, Epstein AE, et al: ACC/AHA/NASPE 2002 Guideline Update for Implantation of Cardiac Pacemakers in Arrhythmia Devices—summary article: A report of the American College of Cardiology/American Heart Association Task Force on Practice Guidelines (ACC/AHA/NASPE Committee to Update the 1998 Pacemaker Guidelines). J Am Coll Cardiol 40:1703, 2002.
22. Zegelman M, Kreyzer J, Wagner R: Ambulatory pacemaker surgery: Medical and economical advantages. PACE 9:1299, 1986.
23. Belott PH: Outpatient pacemaker procedures. Int J Cardiol 17:169, 1987.

23a. Health Care Financing Administration: Hospital Manual, publication 10, section 210A.

24. Dalvi B: Insertion of permanent pacemakers as a day case procedure. Br Med J 300:119, 1990.
25. Hayes DL, Vliestra RE, Trusty JM, et al: Can pacemaker implantation be done as an outpatient? J Am Coll Cardiol 7:199, 1986.
26. Hayes DL, Vliestra RE, Trusty JM, et al: A shorter hospital stay after cardiac pacemaker implantation. Mayo Clin Proc 63:236, 1988.
27. Haywood GA, Jones SM, Camm AJ, et al: Day case permanent pacing. PACE 14:773, 1991.
28. Belott PH: Ambulatory pacemaker procedures: A 13-year experience. PACE 19:69, 1996.
29. Belott PH: Ambulatory pacemaker procedures. Mayo Clin Proc 63:301, 1988.
30. Goldstein DJ, Losquadro W, Spotnitz HM: Outpatient pacemaker procedures in orally anticoagulated patients. PACE 21:1730, 1998.
31. Giudici MC, Barold SS, Paul DL: Pacemaker and implantable cardioverter defibrillator implantation without reversal of warfarin therapy. PACE 27:358, 2004.
32. Philip BK, Corvino BG: Local and regional anesthesia. In Wetchler BV (ed): Anesthesia for Ambulatory Surgery, 2nd ed. Philadelphia, JB Lippincott, 1991, pp 309-334.
33. Bubien RS, Fisher JD, Gentzel JA, et al: NASPE expert consensus document: Use of IV (conscious) sedation/analgesia by nonanesthesia personnel in patients undergoing arrhythmia-specific diagnostic, therapeutic, and surgical procedures. PACE 21:375, 1998.
34. Page CP, Bohen JMA, Fletcher R, et al: Antimicrobial prophylaxis for surgical wounds: Guidelines for clinical care. Arch Surg 128:79, 1993.
35. Muers MF, Arnold AG, Sleight P: Prophylactic antibiotics for cardiac pacemaker implantation: A prospective trial. Br Heart J 46:539, 1981.
36. Ramsdale DR, Charles RG, Rowlands DB: Antibiotic prophylaxis for pacemaker implantation: A prospective randomized trial. PACE 7:844, 1984.
37. Bluhm G, Jacobson B, Ransjo U: Antibiotic prophylaxis in pacemaker surgery: A prospective trial with local and systemic administration of antibiotics at pulse generator replacement. PACE 8:661, 1985.
38. Antimicrobial prophylaxis in surgery. Med Lett Drugs Ther 34:5-8, 1992.
39. Golightly LK, Branigan T: Surgical antibiotic irrigations. Hosp Pharm 24:116, 1989.
40. Smyth NPD: Techniques of implantation: Atrial and ventricular, thoracotomy and transvenous. Prog Cardiovasc Dis 23:435, 1981.
41. Smyth NPD: Pacemaker implantation: Surgical techniques. Cardiovasc Clin 14:31, 1983.
42. Netter FH: Atlas of Human Anatomy, 5th printing. West Caldwell, NJ, Ciba Geigy Medical Education, 1992.
43. Gray H, Pick TP, Howden RE: Anatomy, Descriptive and Surgical, 1901 ed. Philadelphia, Running Press, 1974, p 60.
44. Byrd C: Current clinical applications of dual-chamber pacing. In Zipes DP (ed): Proceedings of a Symposium. Minneapolis, Medtronics, 1981, p 71.
45. Netter FH: The Ciba Collection of Medical Illustrations, Vol 5: Heart. Summit, NJ, Ciba Medical Education Division, 1981, pp 22-26.
46. Furman S: Venous cutdown for pacemaker implantation. Ann Thorac Surg 41:438, 1986.
47. Feiesen A, Kelin GJ, Kostuck WJ, et al: Percutaneous insertion of a permanent transvenous pacemaker electrode through the subclavian vein. Can J Surg 10:131, 1977.
48. Littleford PO, Spector SD: Device for the rapid insertion of permanent endocardial pacing electrodes through the subclavian vein: Preliminary report. Ann Thorac Surg 27:265, 1979.
49. Littleford PO, Parsonnet V, Spector SD: Method for rapid and atraumatic insertion of permanent endocardial electrodes through the subclavian vein. Am J Cardiol 43:980, 1979.
50. Miller FA Jr, Homes DR Jr, Gersh BJ, Maloney JD: Permanent transvenous pacemaker implantation via the subclavian vein. Mayo Clinic Proc 55:309, 1980.
51. Belott PH, Byrd CL: Recent developments in pacemaker implantation and lead retrieval. In Barold SS, Mugica J (eds): New Perspectives in Cardiac Pacing 2. Mt Kisco, NY, Futura, 1991, pp 105-131.
52. Stokes K, Staffeson D, Lessar J, et al: A possible new complication of the subclavian stick: Conductor fracture. PACE 10:748, 1987.
53. Fyke FE III: Simultaneous insulation deterioration associated with side by side subclavian placement of two polyurethane leads. PACE 11:1571, 1988.
54. Fyke FE III: Infraclavicular lead failure: Tarnish on a golden route. PACE 16:445, 1993.
55. Jacobs DM, Fink AS, Miller RP, et al: Anatomical and morphological evaluation of pacemaker lead compression. PACE 16:373, 1993.
56. Magney JE, Flynn DM, Parsons JA, et al: Anatomical mechanisms explaining damage to pacemaker leads, defibrillator leads, and failure of central venous catheters adjacent to the sternoclavicular joint. PACE 16:445, 1993.
57. Subclavian venipuncture reconsidered as a means of implanting endocardial pacing leads. Angleton, TX, Issues Intermedics, December 1987, pp 1-2.
58. Subclavian puncture may result in lead conductor fracture. Medtronic News, 16:27, 1986-1987.
59. Byrd CL: Safe introducer technique for pacemaker lead implantation. PACE 15:262, 1992.
60. Nichalls RWD: A new percutaneous infraclavicular approach to the axillary vein. Anesthesia 42:151, 1987.
61. Taylor BL, Yellowlees I: Central venous cannulation using the infraclavicular axillary vein. Anesthesiology 72:55, 1990.
62. Byrd CL: Clinical experience with the extrathoracic introducer insertion technique. PACE 16:1781, 1993.
63. Magney JE, Staplin DH, Flynn DM, et al: A new approach to percutaneous subclavian needle puncture to avoid lead fracture or central venous catheter occlusion. PACE 16:2133, 1993.
64. Belott PH: Blind percutaneous axillary venous access. PACE 22:1085, 1999.
65. Varnagy G, Velasquez R, Navarro D: New technique for cephalic vein approach in pacemaker implants. PACE 18:1807a, 1995.
66. Spencer W III, Kirkpatrick C, Zhu DWX: The value of venogram-guided percutaneous extrathoracic subclavian venipuncture for lead implantation. PACE 19:700, 1996.
67. Spencer W III, Zhu DWX, Kirkpatrick C, et al: Subclavian venogram as a guide to lead implantation. PACE 21:499, 1998.
68. Ramza BM, Rosenthal L, Hui R, et al: Safety and effectiveness of placement of pacemaker and defibrillator leads in the axillary vein guided by contrast venography. Am J Cardiol 80:892, 1997.
69. Fyke FE III: Doppler-guided extrathoracic introducer insertion. PACE 18:1017, 1995.
70. Gayle DD, Bailery JR, Haistey WK, et al: A novel ultrasound-guided approach to the puncture of the extrathoracic subclavian vein for surgical lead placement. PACE 19:700, 1996.
71. Nash A, Burrell CJ, Ring NJ, Marshall AJ: Evaluation of an ultrasonically guided venipuncture technique for the placement of permanent pacing electrodes. PACE 21:452, 1998.
72. Lamas GA, Fish DR, Braunwald NS: Fluoroscopic technique of subclavian venous puncture for permanent pacing: A safer and easier approach. PACE 11:1398, 1987.
73. Higano ST, Hayes DL, Spittell PC: Facilitation of the subclavian-introducer technique with contrast venography. PACE 15:731, 1992.

74. Belott PH: Implantation techniques: New developments. In Barold SS, Mugica J (eds): New Perspectives in Cardiac Pacing. Mt Kisco, NY, Futura, 1988, pp 258-259.
75. Bognolo DA: Recent advances in permanent pacemaker implantation techniques. In Barold SS (ed): Modern Cardiac Pacing. Mt Kisco, NY, Futura, 1985, pp 206-207.
76. Parsonnet V, Werres R, Atherly T, et al: Transvenous insertion of double sets of permanent electrodes. JAMA 243:62, 1980.
77. Bognolo PA, Vijayanagar RR, Eckstein PR, et al: Two leads in one introducer technique for A-V sequential implantation. PACE 5:217, 1982.
78. Vander Salm TJ, Haffajee CI, Okike ON: Transvenous insertion of double sets of permanent electrodes through a single introducer: Clinical application. Ann Thorac Surg 32:307, 1981.
79. Belott PH: A variation on the introducer technique for unlimited access to the subclavian vein. PACE 4:43, 1981.
80. Gessman LJ, Gallagher JD, MacMillan RM, et al: Emergency guidewire pacing: New methods for rapid conversion of a cardiac catheter into a pacemaker. PACE 7:917, 1984.
81. Ong LS, Barold SS, Lederman M, et al: Cephalic vein guidewire technique for implantation of permanent pacemakers. Am Heart J 114:753, 1987.
82. August DA, Elefteriades JA: Technique to facilitate open placement of permanent pacing leads through the cephalic vein. Ann Thorac Surg 42:112, 1986.
83. Parsonnet V, Bernstein AD: Cardiac pacing in the 1980's: Treatment and techniques in transition. J Am Coll Cardiol 1:399, 1983.
84. Furman S: Venous cutdown for pacemaker implantation. Ann Thorac Surg 41:438, 1986.
85. Furman S: Subclavian puncture for pacemaker lead placement. PACE 9:467 1986.
86. Parsonnet V, Bernstein AD, Lindsay B: Pacemaker-implantation complication rates: An analysis of some contributing factors. J Am Coll Cardiol 13:917, 1989.
87. Sutton R, Bourgeois I: The Foundations of Cardiac Pacing. I: An Illustrated Practical Guide to Basic Pacing. Mt Kisco, NY, Futura, 1991, pp 235-243.
88. Barrold SS, Mugica J: Recent Advances in Cardiac Pacing: Goals for the 21st Century, Vol 19. Mt Kisco, NY, Futura, 1998, pp 213-231.
89. Belott PH: Retained guidewire introducer technique, for unlimited access to the central circulation: A review. Clin Prog Electrophysiol Pacing 1:59, 1981.
90. Bognolo DA, Vijayanagar R, Ekstein PF, et al: Anatomical suitability of the right atrial appendage for atrial J lead electrodes. In Proceedings of the Second European Pacing Symposium, Florence, Italy: Cardiac Pacing. Padova, Italy, Piccin Medical, 1982, p 639.
91. Bognolo DA, Vigayanagar R, Ekstein PF, et al: Implantation of permanent atrial J lead using lateral fluoroscopy. Ann Thorac Surg 316:574, 1981.
92. Thurer RJ: Technique of insertion of transvenous atrial pacing leads: The value of lateral fluoroscopy. PACE 4:525, 1981.
93. Jamidar H, Goli V, Reynolds DW: The right atrial free wall: An alternative pacing site. PACE 16:959, 1993.
94. Saxonhouse SJ, Conti JB, Curtis AB: Current of injury predicts adequate active lead fixation in permanent pacemaker/defibrillation leads. J Am Coll Cardiol 45:412, 2005.
95. Bognolo DA, Vijaranagar RR, Eckstein PF, Janss B: Method for reintroduction of permanent endocardial pacing electrodes. PACE 5:546, 1982.
96. Bognolo DA, Vijay R, Eckstein P, Jeffrey D: Technical aspects of pacemaker system upgrading procedures. Clin Prog Pacing Electrophysiol 1:269, 1983.
97. Belott PH: Use of the contralateral subclavian vein for placement of atrial electrodes in chronically VVI paced patients. PACE 6:781, 1983.
98. Parsonnet V: A stretch fabric pouch for implanted pacemakers. Arch Surg 105:654, 1972.
99. Roelke M, Jackson G, Hawthorne JW: Submammary pacemaker implantation: A unique tunneling technique. PACE 17:1793, 1994.
100. Ellestad MH, French J: Iliac vein approach to permanent pacemaker implantation. PACE 12:1030, 1989.
101. Antonelli D, Freedberg NA, Rosenfeld T: Transiliac vein approach to a rate-responsive permanent pacemaker implantation. PACE 16:1637, 1993.
102. Belott PH, Bucko D: Inframammary pulse generator placement for maximizing optimal cosmetic effect. PACE 6:1241, 1983.
103. Roelke M, Jackson G, Hawthorne JW: Submammary pacemaker implantation: A unique tunneling technique. PACE 17:1793, 1994.
104. Shefer A, Lewis SB, Gang ES: The retropectoral transaxillary permanent pacemaker: Description of a technique for percutaneous implantation of an invisible device. PACE 16:1646, 1996.
105. Young D: Permanent pacemaker implantation in children: Current status and future considerations. PACE 4:61, 1981.
106. Smith RT Jr: Pacemakers for children. In Gillette PC, Garson A Jr (eds): Pediatric Arrhythmias: Electrophysiology and Pacing. New York, Grune & Stratton, 1990, pp 532-558.
107. Smith RT Jr, Armstrong K, Moak JP, et al: Actuarial analysis of pacing system survival in young patients. Circulation 74(Suppl II):120, 1986.
108. Gillette PC, Zeigler VL, Winslow AT, Kratz JM: Cardiac pacing in neonates, infants, and preschool children. PACE 15:2046, 1992.
109. Guldal M, Kervancioglu C, Oral D, et al: Permanent pacemaker implantation in a pregnant woman with guidance of ECG and two-dimensional echocardiography. PACE 10:543, 1987.
110. Lau CP, Wong CK, Leung WH, et al: Ultrasonic assisted permanent pacing in a patient with severe pulmonary tuberculosis. PACE 12:1131, 1989.
111. Morris DC, Scott IR, Jamesson WR: Pacemaker electrode repositioning using the loop snare technique. PACE 12:996, 1989.
112. Westerman GR, Van Devanter SH: Transthoracic transatrial endocardial lead placement for permanent pacing. Ann Thorac Surg 43:445, 1987.
113. Hayes DL, Vliestra RE, Puga FJ, et al: A novel approach to atrial endocardial pacing. PACE 12:125, 1989.
114. Byrd CL, Schwartz SJ: Transatrial implantation of transvenous pacing leads as an alternative to implantation of epicardial leads. PACE 13:1856, 1990.
115. Dosios T, Gorgogiannis D, Sakorafas G, et al: Persistent left superior vena cava: A problem in transvenous pacing of the heart. PACE 14:389, 1991.
116. Hussaine SA, Chalcravarty S, Chaikhouni A: Congenital absence of superior vena cava: Unusual anomaly of superior systemic veins complicating pacemaker placement. PACE 4:328, 1981.
117. Ronnevik PK, Abrahamsen AM, Tollefsen J: Transvenous pacemaker implantation via a unilateral left superior vena cava. PACE 5:808, 1982.
118. Cha EM, Khoury GH: Persistent left superior vena cava. Radiology 103:375, 1972.
119. Colman AL: Diagnosis of left superior vena cava by clinical inspection: A new physical sign. Am Heart J 73:115, 1967.
120. Dirix LY, Kersscochot IE, Fiernen SH, et al: Implantation of a dual-chambered pacemaker in a patient with persistent left superior vena cava. PACE 11:343, 1988.
121. Giovanni QV, Piepoli N, Pietro Q, et al: Cardiac pacing in unilateral left superior vena cava: Evaluation by digital angiography. PACE 14:1567, 1991.
122. Robbens EJ, Ruiter JH: Atrial pacing by unilateral persistent left superior vena cava. PACE 9:594, 1986.
123. Hellestrand KJ, Ward DE, Bexton RS, et al: The use of active fixation electrodes for permanent endocardial pacing via a persistent left superior vena cava. PACE 5:180, 1982.

124. West JNW, Shearmann CP, Gammange MD: Permanent pacemaker positioning via the inferior vena cava in a case of single ventricle with loss of right atrial to vena caval continuity. PACE 16:1753, 1993.
125. Fishberger SB, Cammanas J, Rodriguez-Fernandez H, et al: Permanent pacemaker lead implantation via the transhepatic route. PACE 19:1124, 1996.
126. Moss AJ, Rivers RJ Jr: Atrial pacing from the coronary vein: Ten-year experience in 50 patients with implanted pervenous pacemakers. Circulation 57:103, 1978.
127. Greenberg P, Castellanet M, Messenger J, Ellestad MH: Coronary sinus pacing. Circulation 57:98, 1978.
128. Hewitt MJ, Chen JTT, Ravin CE, Gallagher JJ: Coronary sinus atrial pacing: Radiographic considerations. Am J Radiol 136: 323, 1981.
129. Trappe H, Pfitzner P, Heintze J, et al: Cardioverter-defibrillator implantation in the catheterization laboratory: Initial experiences in 46 patients. Am Heart J 129:259-264, 1995.
130. Koukal C, Hemmer W, Oertel F, et al: ENDOTAK lead alone configuration, a new standard when using biphasic shocks [abstract]? PACE 18:1189, 1995.
131. Bardy GH, Johnson G, Poole JE, et al: A simplified, single-lead unipolar transvenous cardioversion-defibrillation system. Circulation 88:543, 1993.
132. Raitt MH, Bardy GH: Advances in implantable cardioverter-defibrillator therapy. Curr Opin Cardiol 9:23, 1994.
133. Parsonnet V, Bernstein AD, Lindsay B: Pacemaker-implantation complication rates: An analysis of some contributing factors. J Am Coll Cardiol 13:917, 1989.
134. Bernstein AD, Parsonnet V: Survey of cardiac pacing in the United States in 1989. Am J Cardiol 69:331, 1992.
135. Flowers NC, Abildskov JA, Armstrong WF, et al: ACC Policy Statement: Recommended guidelines for training in adult clinical cardiac electrophysiology. J Am Coll Cardiol 18:637, 1991.
136. Scheinman M, Akhtar M, Brugada P, et al: Teaching objectives for fellowship programs in clinical electrophysiology. Report for the Ad Hoc Committee of the North American Society of Pacing and Electrophysiology. J Am Coll Cardiol 12:255, 1988.
137. Natale A, Kearney MM, Brandon MJ, et al: Safety of nurse-administered deep sedation for defibrillator implantation in the electrophysiology laboratory. J Cardiovasc Electrophysiol 7:301, 1996.
138. Lehmann MH, Saksena S: Implantable cardioverter defibrillators in cardiovascular practice: Report of the Policy Conference of the North American Society of Pacing and Electrophysiology. PACE 14:969, 1991.
139. Curtis AB, Ellenbogen KA, Hammill SC, et al: Clinical competency statement: Training pathways for implantation of cardioverter defibrillators in cardiac resynchronization devices. Heart Rhythm 1:371, 2004.
140. Fitzpatrick AP, Lesh MD, Epstein LM, et al: Electrophysiological laboratory, electrophysiologist-implanted, nonthoracotomy-implantable cardioverter defibrillators. Circulation 89:2503, 1994.
141. Strickberger SA, Hummel JD, Daoud E, et al: Implantation by electrophysiologist of 100 consecutive cardioverter-defibrillators with nonthoracotomy lead systems. Circulation 90:868, 1994.
142. Strickberger SA, Niebauer M, Ching Man K, et al: Comparison of implantation of nonthoracotomy defibrillators in the operating room versus the electrophysiology laboratory. Am Heart J 75:255, 1995.
143. Bardy GH, Hofer B, Johnson G, et al: Implantable cardioverter-defibrillators. Circulation 87:1152, 1993.
144. Brooks R, Garan H, Torchiana D, et al: Determinants of successful nonthoracotomy cardioverter-defibrillator implantation: Experience in 101 patients using two different lead systems. J Am Coll Cardiol 22:1835, 1993.
145. Luceri RM, Zilo P, Habal SM, David IB: Cost and length of hospital stay: Comparisons between nonthoracotomy and epicardial techniques in patients receiving implantable cardioverter defibrillators. PACE 18:168, 1995.
146. Stanton MS, Hayes DL, Munger TM, et al: Consistent subcutaneous prepectoral implantation of a new implantable cardioverter defibrillator. Mayo Clin Proc 69:309, 1994.
147. Mower M, Mirowski M, Pitt B, et al: Ventricular defibrillation with a single intravascular catheter system having distal electrode in left pulmonary artery and proximal electrode in right ventricle or right atrium [abstract]. Clin Res 20:389, 1972.
148. Schuder JC, Stoeckle H, West JA, et al: Ventricular defibrillation with catheter having distal electrode in right ventricle and proximal electrode in superior vena cava [abstract]. Circulation 43/44:99, 1971.
149. Tung RT, Bajaj AK: Safety of implantation of a cardioverter-defibrillator without general anesthesia in an electrophysiology laboratory. Am J Cardiol 75:908, 1995.
150. Lipscomb KJ, Linker NJ, Fitzpatrick AP: Subpectoral implantation of a cardioverter defibrillator under local anesthesia. Heart 79:253, 1998.
151. Pacifico A, Cedillo-Salazar FR, Nasir N Jr, et al: Conscious sedation with combined hypnotic agents for implantation of implantable cardioverter-defibrillators. J Am Coll Cardiol 30:679, 1997.
152. Moerman A, Herregods L, Foubert L, et al: Awareness during anaesthesia for implantable cardioverter defibrillator implantation: Recall of defibrillation shocks. Anaesthesia 50:733, 1995.
153. Hunt GB, Ross DL: Comparison of effects of three anesthetic agents on induction of ventricular tachycardia in a canine model of myocardial infarction. Circulation 78:221, 1988.
154. Natale A, Jones DL, Kim Y-H, et al: Effects of lidocaine on defibrillation threshold in the pig: Evidence of anesthesia related increase. PACE 14:1239, 1991.
155. Gill RM, Sweeney RJ, Reid PR: The defibrillation threshold: A comparison of anesthetics and measurements methods. PACE 16:708, 1993.
156. Shepard RB, Goldin MD, Lawrie GM, et al: Automatic implantable cardioverter defibrillator: Surgical approaches for implantation. J Card Surg 7:208, 1992.
157. Watkins L Jr, Taylor E Jr: The surgical aspects of automatic implantable cardioverter-defibrillator implantation. PACE 14:953, 1991.
158. Watkins L Jr, Guarnieri T, Griffith LS, et al: Implantation of the automatic implantable cardioverter defibrillator. J Card Surg 3:1, 1998.
159. Daoud EG, Strickberger SA, Man KC, et al: Comparison of early and late complications in patients undergoing coronary artery bypass graft surgery with and without concomitant placement of an implantable cardioverter defibrillator. Am Heart J 130:780, 1995.
160. Trappe HJ, Klein H, Wahlers T, et al: Risk and benefit of additional aortocoronary bypass grafting in patients undergoing cardioverter-defibrillator implantation. Am Heart J 127:75, 1994.
161. Watkins L Jr, Mirowski M, Mower MM, et al: Automatic defibrillation in man: The initial surgical experience. J Thorac Cardiovasc Surg 82:492, 1981.
162. Troup PJ, Chapman PD, Olinger GN, et al: The implanted defibrillator: Relation of defibrillating lead configuration and clinical variable to defibrillation threshold. J Am Coll Cardiol 6:1315, 1985.
163. Shepard RB, Goldin MD, Lawrie GM, et al: Automatic implantable cardioverter defibrillator: Surgical approaches for implantation. J Cardiac Surg 7:208, 1992.
164. Watkins L Jr, Mirowski M, Mower MM, et al: Implantation of the automatic defibrillator: The subxiphoid approach. Ann Thorac Surg 35:515, 1982.
165. Flaker G, Boley T, Walls J, et al: Comparison of subxiphoid and traditional approaches for ICD implantation. PACE 15:1531, 1992.

166. Beckman DJ, Crevey BJ, Foster PR, et al: Subxiphoid approach for implantable cardioverter defibrillator in patients with previous coronary bypass surgery. PACE 15:1637, 1992.
167. Lawrie GM, Griffin JC, Wyndham CRC: Epicardial implantation of the automatic implantable defibrillator by the left subcostal thoracotomy. PACE 7:1370, 1984.
168. Shahian DM, Williamson WA, Streitz JM Jr, Venditti FJ: Subfascial implantation of implantable cardioverter defibrillator generator. Ann Thorac Surg 54:173, 1992.
169. O'Neill PG, Lawrie GM, Kaushik RR, et al: Late results of the left subcostal approach for automatic implantable cardioverter. Am J Cardiol 67:387, 1991.
170. Lawrie GM, Kaushik RR, Pacifico A: Right mini-thoracotomy: An adjunct to left subcostal automatic implantable cardioverter defibrillator implantation. Ann Thorac Surg 47:780, 1989.
171. Damiano RJ Jr, Foster AH, Ellenbogen KA, et al: Implantation of cardioverter defibrillators in the post-sternotomy patient. Ann Thorac Surg 53:978, 1992.
172. Obadia JF, Claudel JP, Rescigno G, et al: Subdiaphragmatic implantation of implantable cardioverter defibrillator generator. Ann Thorac Surg 59:239, 1995.
173. Shapira N, Cohen AI, Wish M, et al: Transdiaphragmatic implantation of the automatic implantable cardioverter defibrillator. Ann Thorac Surg 48:371, 1989.
174. Frumin H, Goodman GR, Pleatman M: ICD implantation via thoracoscopy without the need for sternotomy or thoracotomy. PACE 16:257, 1993.
175. Krasna MJ, Buser GA, Flowers JL, et al: Thoracoscopic versus laparoscopic placement of defibrillator patches. Surg Laparosc Endosc 6:91, 1996.
176. Tobin M, Ching E, Firstenberg M, et al: Thoracoscopy ICD implantation compared to a subxyphoid approach [abstract]. Eur J Cardiac Pacing Electrophysiol 4:118, 1994.
177. Jansens JL, Jottrand M, Treumont N, et al: Robotic-enhanced biventricular resynchronization: An alternative to endovenous cardiac resynchronization therapy in chronic heart failure. Ann Thorac Surg 76:413, 2003.
178. Saksena S, Parsonnet V: Implantation of a cardioverter/defibrillator without thoracotomy using a triple electrode system. JAMA 259:69, 1988.
179. Saksena S, Tullo NG, Krol RB, Mauro AM: Initial clinical experience with endocardial defibrillation using an implantable cardioverter/defibrillator with a triple-electrode system. Arch Intern Med 149:2333, 1989.
180. Tullo NG, Saksena S, Krol RB, et al: Management of complications associated with a first-generation endocardial defibrillation lead system for implantable cardioverter-defibrillators. Am J Cardiol 66:411, 1990.
181. McCowan R, Maloney J, Wilkoff B, et al: Automatic implantable cardioverter-defibrillator implantation without thoracotomy using an endocardial and submuscular patch system. J Am Coll Cardiol 17:415, 1991.
182. Trappe H, Klein H, Fieguth H, et al: Initial experience with a new transvenous defibrillation system. PACE 16:134, 1993.
183. Bhandari AK, Isber N, Estioko M, et al: Efficacy of low-energy T wave shocks for induction of ventricular fibrillation in patients with implantable cardioverter defibrillators. J Electrocardiol 31:31, 1998.
184. Roelke M, O'Nunain SS, Osswald S, et al: Subclavian crush syndrome complicating transvenous cardioverter defibrillator systems. PACE 18:1968, 1995.
185. Lawton JS, Wood MA, Gilligan DM, et al: Implantable transvenous cardioverter-defibrillator leads: The dark side. PACE 19:1273, 1996.
186. Kirchhoffer JB, Cook JR, Kabell GG, et al; the Jewel Investigators: Right-sided implantation of defibrillators using nonthoracotomy lead system is feasible. PACE 18:874, 1995.
187. Epstein AE, Kay GN, Plumb VJ, et al: Elevated defibrillation threshold when right-sided venous access is used for nonthoracotomy implantable defibrillator lead implantation. The ENDOTAK Investigators. J Cardiovasc Electrophysiol 6:979, 1995.
188. Bardy GH, Yee R, Jung W: Multicenter experience with a pectoral unipolar transvenous cardioversion-defibrillation. Active Can Investigators. J Am Coll Cardiol 28:400, 1996.
189. Saksena S, DeGroot P, Krol RB, et al: Low-energy endocardial defibrillation using an axillary or a pectoral thoracic electrode location. Circulation 88:2655, 1993.
190. Jordaens L, Vertongen P, van Bellegham Y: A subcutaneous lead array for implantable cardioverter defibrillators. PACE 16:1429, 1993.
191. Crossley GH, Gayle DD, Bailey JR, et al: Defibrillator twiddler's syndrome causing device failure in a subpectoral transvenous system. Pacing Clin Electrophysiol 19:376-377, 1996.
192. Eastman DP, Selle JG, Reames MK Sr: Technique for subpectoral implantation of cardioverter defibrillators. J Am Coll Surg 181:475, 1995.
193. Bardy GH, Yee R; the International Active Can Investigators: World wide experience with the Jewel 7219C unipolar, single lead active can implantable pacer-cardioverter/defibrillator. PACE 18:806, 1995.
194. Foster AH: Technique for implantation of cardioverter defibrillators in the subpectoral position. Ann Thorac Surg 59:764, 1995.
195. Wilkoff BL, Cook JR, Epstein AE, et al; DAVID Trial Investigators: Dual chamber pacing or ventricular backup pacing in patients with an implantable defibrillator. The Dual Chamber and VVI Implantable Defibrillator (DAVID) trial. JAMA 288: 3115, 2002.
196. Nielson JC, Kristensen L, Anderson HR, et al: A randomized comparison of atrial and dual-chambered pacing in 177 consecutive patients with sick sinus syndrome. J Am Coll Cardiol 42:614, 2003.
197. Prinzen FW, Peschar M: Relationship between the pacing-induced sequence of activation and left ventricular pump function in animals. PACE 25:484, 2002.
198. Rosenqvist M, Isaaz K, Botvinick EH, et al: Relative importance of activation sequence compared to atrial ventricular synchrony in left ventricular function. Am J Cardiol 67:148, 1991.
199. Rosenqvist M, Brandt J, Schuller H: Long-term pacing in sinus node disease: Effects of stimulation mode on cardiovascular morbidity and mortality. Am Heart J 116:16, 1988.
200. Stangl K, Seitz K, Wirtzfeld A, et al: Differences between atrial single-chamber pacing (AAI) and ventricular single-chamber pacing (VVI) with respect to prognosis and antiarrhythmic effect in patients with sick sinus syndrome. PACE 13:2080, 1990.
201. Brandt J, Anderson H, Fahraeus T, et al: Natural history of sinus node disease treated with atrial pacing in 213 patients: Implications for selection of stimulation mode. J Am Coll Cardiol 20:633, 1992.
202. Anderson HR, Thuesen L, Bagger JP, et al: Prospective randomized trial of atrial versus ventricular pacing in sick sinus syndrome. Lancet 344:1523, 1994.
203. Daubert C, Gras D, Berder V, et al:[Permanent atrial resynchronization by synchronous bi-atrial pacing in the preventive treatment of atrial flutter associated with high degree interatrial block]. Arch Mal Coeur Vaiss 87:1535, 1994.
204. Saksena S, Prakash A, Hill M, et al: Prevention of recurrent atrial fibrillation with chronic dual-site right atrial pacing. J Am Coll Cardiol 28:687, 1996.
205. Levy T, Walker S, Rochelle J, Ball V: Evaluation of biatrial pacing, right atrial pacing, and no pacing in patients with drug-refractory atrial fibrillation. Am J Cardiol 84:426, 1999.
206. Levy T, Walker S, Rex S, et al: No incremental benefit of multisite atrial pacing compared to right atrial pacing in patients with drug-refractory atrial fibrillation. Heart 85:48, 2001.
207. Leclercq JF, DeSisti A, Fiorello P, et al: Is dual site better than single site atrial pacing in the prevention of atrial fibrillation? PACE 23:2101, 2000.

208. Padeletti L, Porciani MC, Michelucci A, et al: Intraatrial septum pacing: A new approach to prevent recurrent atrial fibrillation. J Intervent Cardiac Electrophysiol 3:35, 1999.
209. Frohlig G, Schwaab B, Kindermann M: Selective site pacing: The right ventricular approach. PACE 27:855, 2004.
210. De Voogt WG, Van Mechelen R, Van Den Bos A, et al: A technique of lead insertion for low atrial septal pacing. PACE 28:639, 2005.
211. Netter FH: Atria and ventricles, right atrium. In Yonkman FF (ed): CIBA Collection of Medical Illustrations, Vol 5: Heart. Newark, NJ, CIBA-GEIGY, 1969, p A.
212. Yen Ho S, Anderson RH, Sanchez-Quintana D: Gross structure of the atriums: More than an anatomical curiosity. PACE 25:842, 2002.
213. Ho S: Understanding atrial anatomy: Implications for atrial fibrillation ablation. In Cardiology International for a Global Perspective on Cardiac Care. London, Greycoat Publishing Ltd., 2002, S17 through S20.
214. Farré J, Anderson RH, Cabrera JA, et al: Fluoroscopic cardiac anatomy for catheter ablation of tachycardia. PACE 25:76, 2002.
215. Bachmann G: The interauricular time interval. Am J Physiol 1:1, 1907.
216. James TN, Sherf L: Specialized tissues and preferential conduction in the atria of the heart. Am J Cardiol 28:414, 1971.
217. Roithinger FX, Cheng J, Sippens A, et al: Use of electroanatomical mapping to delineate transseptal atrial conduction in humans. Circulation 100:1791, 1999.
218. Anderson RH, Ho SY: The architecture of the sinus node, the atrioventricular conduction axis in the intranodal atrial myocardium. J Cardiovasc Electrophysiol 9:1233, 1998.
219. Chauvin M, Shah DC, Hauissaguerre M, et al: The anatomic basis of connections between the coronary sinus musculature and the left atrium in humans. Circulation 101:647, 2000.
220. DePonti R, Ho SY, Salerno-Uriarte JA, et al: Electroanatomical analysis of sinus impulse propagation in normal human atria. J Cardiovasc Electrophysiol 13:1, 2002.
221. Saksena S, Prakash A, Hill M, et al: Prevention of recurrent atrial fibrillation with chronic dual-site right atrial pacing. J Am Coll Cardiol 28:687, 1996.
222. de Cock CC, Giudici MC, Twisk JW: Comparison of the hemodynamic effects of right ventricular outflow tract pacing with right ventricular apex pacing: A quantitative review. Europace 5:275, 2003.
223. Stambler BS, Ellenbogen KA, Zhang X, et al: Right ventricular outflow versus apical pacing in pacemaker patients with congestive heart failure and atrial fibrillation. J Cardiovasc Electrophysiol 14:1180, 2003.
224. Lieberman R, Grenz D, Mond HG, et al: Selective site pacing: Defining and reaching the selected site. PACE 27:883, 2004.
225. Karpawich P, Gates J, Stokes K: Septal His-Purkinje ventricular pacing in canines: A new endocardial electrode approach. PACE 15:2011, 1992.
226. Deshmukh PM, Romanyshyn M: Direct His-bundle pacing, present and future. PACE 27:862, 2004.

Chapter 19

Left Ventricular Lead Implantation

SETH WORLEY

Each step in the implantation must prepare for the most difficult conceivable anatomy.

—*The golden rule of CRT implantation*

The approach described in this chapter is intended for the physician who is determined to achieve an uncompromising left ventricular (LV) lead position for his/her patient without surgery. It is intended for the physician who will analyze a failed initial attempt to determine what needs to be done to be successful for the patient and avoid surgery. Unless the physician is motivated to learn new tools and techniques, this chapter has little to offer. The approach presented here is for the implanter who will learn to do whatever it takes to be successful for the patient. The reader is taken from patient preparation through room setup to initial venous access for the LV lead to the final adjustment of lead slack before the lead is tied down. The implantation tools and techniques used for each step are designed to ensure that the operator is prepared to deal with the potential problems that might be encountered in subsequent steps. For example, if a stenotic area in the subclavian vein is not completely relieved, each subsequent step will be impeded; to ensure that the subsequent steps are unencumbered, venoplasty is required. If the implanter is unwilling to learn venoplasty of the subclavian vein on behalf of the patient, the likelihood of achieving a successful implantation is substantially reduced, either because "catheter" manipulation is restricted or the implanter must use the contralateral side.

What about setting a time limit on the transvenous LV implantation, and then, if this attempt is unsuccessful, referring the patient for surgery, as suggested by several writers?[1] This mindset is certainly practical and appropriate if the implanter is using the same approach over and over without effect. However, there is a tremendous advantage, to both the patient and the implanting physician, to seeking counsel with interventional colleagues or other implanting physicians to develop another approach based on the experience gained with the first attempt. Rather than a dead end, the implanting physician should regard an initially failed attempt as an opportunity to enlarge his/her armamentarium. For instance, it might represent an opportunity to learn the use of the third-generation guiding systems or venoplasty on a second attempt. The new techniques learned with a second attempt can then be applied early in subsequent cases in which the same issue arises. The implanting physician might even design a tool for general use to solve the same problem for other patients and physicians. Interestingly, some physicians who have advocated surgical referral also describe bringing patients back for another implantation attempt that is ultimately successful.

The chapter is divided into the following sections:

- Room setup
- Venous access
- Cannulation of the coronary sinus (CS)
- Cardiac venous anatomy

Unless otherwise credited, all illustrations are copyright © Seth J. Worley.

- Delivery systems and tools for lead placement
- Matching the LV lead to the venous anatomy
- Coronary vein venoplasty
- Removing the guide, sheath, and stylet

Background

With the undeniable demonstration that cardiac resynchronization therapy (CRT) reduces the chance of hospitalization, improves quality of life, and lowers mortality from congestive heat failure (CHF),[2-5] transvenous placement of LV pacing leads in specific locations became important.[6-9] As with most new therapeutic procedures, the recognition of what needs to be accomplished precedes development of the required tools and techniques. The ability to initially demonstrate the therapeutic concept and to then safely and cost-effectively implement the advance into clinical practice depends on the development of tools and techniques.[10] The pioneering physician and early adopter initially develops his/her own technique, employing a combination of the limited tools specifically designed for the procedure and existing tools that proved useful through improvisation, reflecting his/her particular talents. Because the early tools are not well adapted to the procedure, each approach has its strengths and weaknesses. Each approach works to some extent for some physicians, usually those with similar talent and experience. In this case, "tips and tricks" often apply only to those with talents similar to those of the trickster. As a result of experience-based innovation, improved tools and techniques specifically designed for the procedure are introduced. The procedure evolves. The new tools and techniques that are successful dominate, and the less successful become of historical interest. Since CRT began, there has been a convergence of the multiple approaches initially used for LV lead placement. If the tools and techniques presented in this chapter had been available at the advent of CRT, there would now be a greater convergence of implantation techniques. It is likely that over the next several years the remaining strategies will merge and, with refinements, approximate the approach presented in this chapter.

Despite the convergence brought on by improved tools, skilled pioneering physicians—commonly in academic medical centers—who have mastered the procedure despite limited tools often rightfully see no need to change their approach. On occasion they take considerable pains to denigrate a new approach, extolling the virtues of the method they invested so much to master. This behavior is typical in the evolution of new tools and techniques. For an example, let us regard cardiac catheterization as analogous to CS cannulation for LV lead placement. Dr. Mason Sones, pioneered the classic brachial artery technique for cardiac catheterization, whereby arterial access was obtained through exposure of the brachial artery and insertion of the catheters under direct visualization. Coronary angiography was performed using a Sones catheter; either the catheter tip had to be deflected off the aortic valve cusps or the catheter was shaped during the procedure with the use of boiling water or an alcohol lamp. After the procedure, the arteriotomy and then the skin were sutured closed. The Sones approach has a steep learning curve and multiple areas for potential complications. Dr. Melvin Judkins developed new tools and techniques for performing coronary angiography via the femoral artery that require separate preformed catheters for the right and left coronary arteries and a pigtail catheter for the left ventriculogram. Although the physician must learn a new approach to arterial access and several new catheters, the Judkins technique is safer and easier and has a shorter learning curve for the starting physician than the Sones method. Nevertheless, skilled physicians who invested the time and effort to master the Sones method were slow to adopt the Judkins technique, particularly in academic centers. With the development of the Judkins technique, it made little sense to teach diagnostic cardiac catheterization via the Sones method. However, the masters of the Sones method often continued to teach it and extol its virtues. Continuing to cannulate the CS with use of an electrophysiology (EP) catheter for LV lead placement is still advocated,[11] but in my mind such advocacy is analogous to continuing to use the Sones method for cardiac catheterization.

Let us continue the analogy, this time as it relates to the statement often made by those teaching LV lead implantation that "you should stick with what you know." Consider the physician who is learning to perform percutaneous transluminal coronary angioplasty (PTCA) after mastering Sones cardiac catheterization. If the physician continues to use the Sones method rather than learning the Judkins technique, learning PTCA will be more comfortable and have a shorter learning curve. However, the operator who sticks with the Sones method will quickly be limited by multiple issues, including lack of guide support for the angioplasty balloon and stent. Similarly, the implanting physician who sticks with the familiar EP approach to CS cannulation will be quickly limited by multiple issues, including lack of guide support—in this case for the venoplasty balloon and pacing lead. Despite an initially short and comfortable learning curve, the "stick with what you know" approach will ultimately limit the physician's rate of success in LV lead implantation. Further, some of the "successes" will likely entail compromised lead positions from the desire to avoid surgery. It is most important to insist that lead position is not compromised in order to "complete" the procedure with transvenous techniques. Implanters who do not want to step outside their comfort zones and learn the new tools and techniques for their patients should refer the patient either for transvenous lead placement by an operator experienced in the interventional approach or for surgical positioning of the LV lead. Surgical epicardial placement can and should be used to achieve functional and hemodynamically advantageous lead positions. A variety of approaches to surgical epicardial LV lead placement

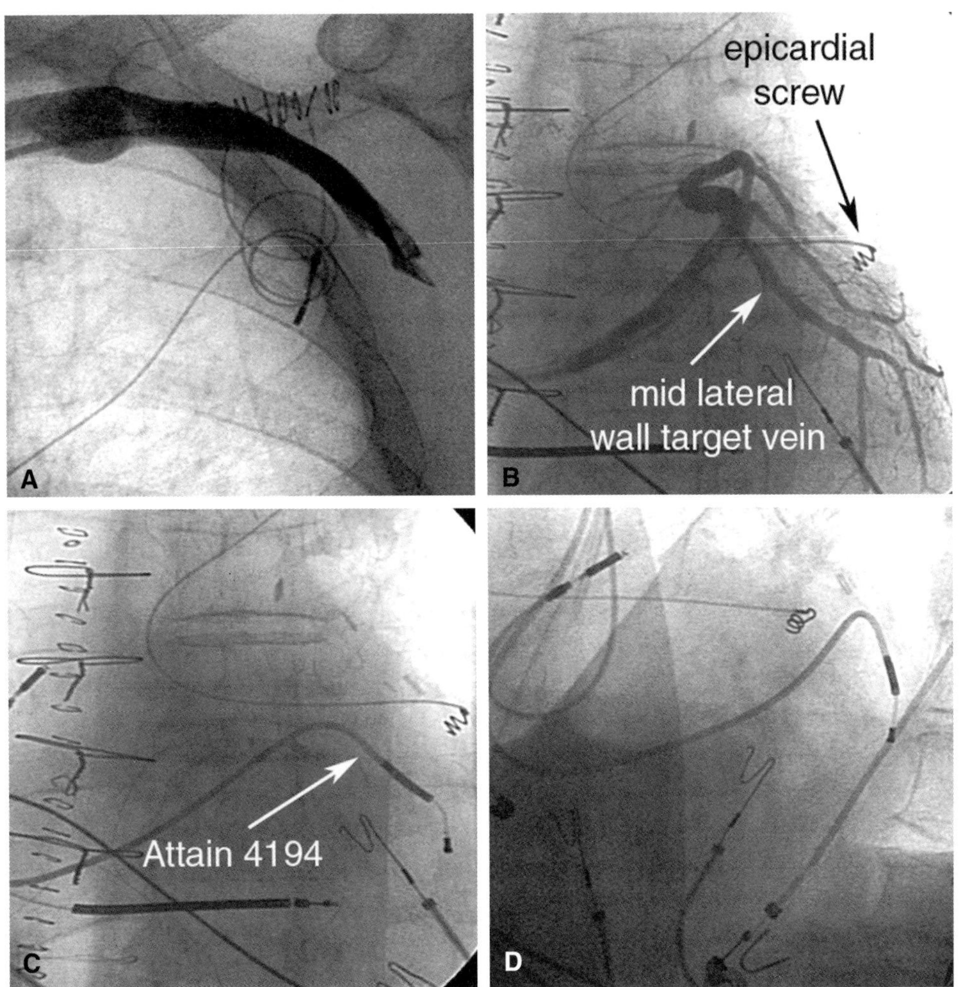

Figure 19-1. Epicardial versus transvenous lead placement for biventricular pacing. ***A,*** *The IS-1 connector end of the epicardial lead is shown in relation to the axillary vein.* ***B,*** *The epicardial screw-in lead and the occlusive coronary sinus (CS) venogram are shown.* ***C,*** *Anteroposterior view of the Attain 4194 lead (Medtronic, Inc., Minneapolis, Minn.) and the epicardial lead.* ***D,*** *Left anterior oblique view of the Attain 4194 and epicardial lead. The transvenous lead is in an ideal anatomic position on the midlateral wall according to the CS venogram. The epicardial lead is not in the ideal anatomic position.*

have been described,[12] including a robotically assisted approach.[13] However, surgically placed LV pacing leads do not always reach the midlateral free wall. Figure 19-1 shows a patient who underwent lead placement via an epicardial approach, showed no response, and then experienced improvement with a transvenously placed lead. It is equally important to insist that the surgically placed and transvenously placed leads are located on the midlateral free wall.

Although surgical lead placement is effective and always appropriate when other surgical intervention is planned, how often is it required for LV stimulation? In the experience of the author and his colleagues with 300 patients undergoing lead implantation between March 2003 and November 2004 in our Lancaster, Penn., practice, successful transvenous implantation was achieved with the first attempt in 293 (97.7%). Second, successful attempts were made in 3 of the 7 patients with initial failures. The average time to CS access was 72 seconds, and the average time to a tied-down LV lead was 59.3 minutes. To accomplish these times, 44 cardiac vein venoplasties (14.7%) were performed. The frequency of surgical intervention can approach zero, but only when all of the tools and techniques presented in this chapter are enthusiastically embraced by the implanting physician. In cases in which the CS drains into the left atrium (LA), a modified transseptal approach can be employed.[14] Thus, a 99% rate of uncompromised success is available to the implanter who is willing to step outside his/her comfort zone and embrace the tools and techniques presented in this chapter.

On the basis of experience garnered from more than 1400 CRT implantations, I have come to the conclusion that if one is intent on a successful LV lead implantation for each patient with no compromise in lead position, then *each step in the implant must prepare for the most difficult conceivable anatomy.* I have adopted this approach as the "golden rule" of CRT implantation. To follow this rule, one must know the techniques and have the tools on hand at the start of the procedure and must possess the self-discipline to follow the steps in order. Tip and tricks were in vogue when the procedure was new and many tools were improvised. As the procedure matured, better tools evolved. Now the best tip is that there are no tricks, only better tools and techniques. Anyone who wants to learn how to implant without compromise must enthusiastically adopt new tools and methods. The reward is a paradoxically reduced learning curve, shorter implantation times, and greater overall success. In the long run, it is more efficient to learn a new method designed for the procedure than to try to force a familiar but intrinsically flawed technique to fit. Once the tools and techniques are mastered, the implanting physician is in a position to follow the golden rule of CRT implantation.

When a biventricular (BiV) implantation is begun, there is no way to predict what lies ahead. A CRT implantation ultimately fails as a result of patient anatomy for which the implanter is not prepared. In effect, the implanting physician and the patient are "victimized" by the patient's anatomy. To succeed, the implanter must be prepared to deal with whatever anatomy is encountered, starting with venous access and ending with the final removal of the stylet. For example, it may be difficult to find the vein, the subclavian vein may be stenotic or occluded, the CS os may be difficult to locate, and the main CS may be tortuous. The CS venogram may reveal a range of target veins from very easy to extremely difficult (Fig. 19-2). Once the lead is in the target vein, the implanter must be prepared to deal with phrenic pacing or high pacing thresholds. Once the lead is in a satisfactory location, the implanter must anticipate and prevent the lead from being displaced either spontaneously or as the final catheter or stylet is removed. The tools and techniques presented in this chapter have been used to safely implant the LV lead without compromising location in more than 98% of patients. Disciplined, systematic use of the tools and techniques described here may not change the implantation time in a patient with favorable anatomy. However, the time saved when the method eliminates just one obstacle makes it worthwhile.

The approach presented in this chapter is based on tools and techniques developed to specifically address the technical challenges that arise during the course of an agressive approach to CRT implantation. This chapter takes the position that although there are many approaches to "successful" CRT implantation, the strategies presented here are for those who refuse to accept a suboptimal lead position and are willing to do what it takes to (safely) avoid surgery. Specifically, the implanting physician must be willing to accept and use contrast material to locate and cannulate the CS, to cannulate the target vein, when needed, with a preformed catheter large enough to deliver the pacing lead directly, and to learn venoplasty of the subclavian/brachiocephalic and cardiac veins (Tables 19-1 to 19-3).

Use of Contrast Material

The use of contrast agents in patients with CHF often causes concern among noninterventional cardiologists. However, interventional cardiologists routinely perform procedures on patients with CHF that require the use

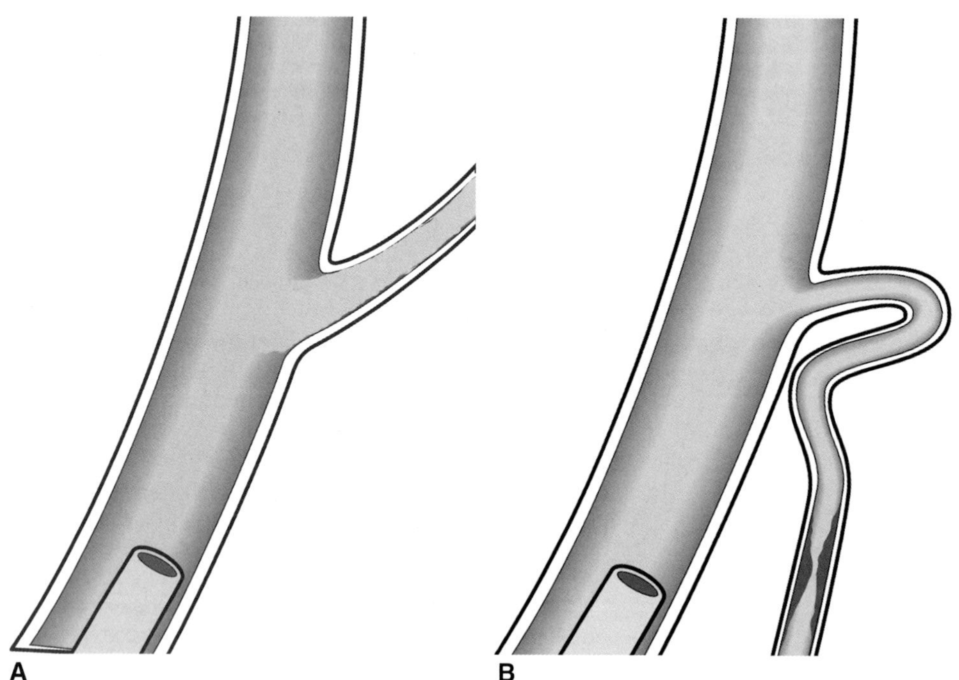

Figure 19-2. Range of venous anatomy encountered at the time of venography. ***A,*** *The target vein is easily accessible from the main coronary sinus. The left ventricular (LV) lead is easily placed.* ***B,*** *The target vein is acutely angulated, tortuous, and stenotic. Without proper tools, placement of an LV lead in this vein is physically impossible. With a third-generation telescoping delivery system and venoplasty, placement of a lead in this vein is easily accomplished.*

TABLE 19-1. **Definition of Terms**

Catheter	When used, indicates that the tubing may be braided or unbraided with or without a hemostatic hub that may or may not be removable or sliceable. For example, a catheter in the coronary sinus may be braided or peel-away.
Guiding catheter	A catheter with metal braid in the walls that provides torque control and with a lumen large enough to accept the pacing lead to be delivered. The *French size* refers to the outside diameter. The inner diameter of the guiding catheter is approximately 2 French sizes smaller than the outer diameter. For example a 9F guiding catheter has a 7F lumen and can deliver a 7F or smaller pacing lead.
Directional catheter	A catheter with braid in the walls that provides torque control and with a lumen only sufficient to accept a guidewire and inject contrast material. It is intended to identify veins and direct a wire into a vein for subsequent lead placement. A directional catheter must be withdrawn over the wire before the pacing lead can be advanced over the wire. Examples are any diagnostic catheter from cardiology or radiology as well as the IC 90 (Guidant, Boston Scientific, Natick, Mass.) and the Attain Select (Medtronic, Inc., Minneapolis, Minn.). The French size refers to the outer diameter.
Sheath	A catheter that is used to obtain venous access and through which a directional catheter, guiding catheter, or pacing lead is inserted. The proximal end may be open, hemostatic and removable, or hemostatic and fixed. Sheaths do not have metal braid in their walls and thus do not have torque control but may be peel-away. The French size of a sheath refers to the inner diameter. The outer diameter is typically 2 French sizes larger than the internal diameter. For example, the lumen of a 9F sheath is large enough to accept a 9F or smaller directional or guiding catheter or a 9F or smaller pacing lead.
Introducer	Traditionally thought of as a removable (by cutting or peeling) nonbraided catheter that is being used to obtain venous access and through which a pacing lead is placed. In the current context, *introducer* and *sheath* are used interchangeably.
Lateral vein introducer (LVI)	A group of guiding catheters (metal braid in the walls) whose shape is designed to selectively cannulate a specific vein configuration in the coronary sinus, analogous to the variously shaped Judkins catheter designed to selectively cannulate the coronary arteries. The French size refers to the outer diameter. For example, the lumen of a 9F LVI is approximately 7F.
French size of guide vs. introducer/sheath	The French size of a directional catheter and guide refers to *outer* diameter. The French size of a sheath refers to the *inner* diameter. Thus, for example, a 9F guide fits inside a 9F sheath.

TABLE 19-2. **Steps to Left Ventricular (LV) Lead Placement via the Cardiac Venous System**

1. Gain unrestricted venous access with a sheath that is:
   a. Long enough to extend from the pocket into the mid–coronary sinus (mid-CS)
   b. Large enough to accept a third-generation preshaped guide for direct lead delivery
   c. Anatomically shaped to prevent kinking and avoid lead-dislodging "spring-back" when removed from the CS
   d. Designed to have sufficient torque control to readily manipulate the tip of the sheath within the right heart
2. Locate the CS os using contrast material and a properly shaped guide, as follows:
   a. Set up a contrast injection system that facilitates catheter manipulation, contrast injection, and guidewire insertion.
   b. Use CS area anatomy to facilitate location of the CS.
3. Establish a stable platform in the CS by advancing the long sheath from the os into the CS using:
   a. The telescoping feature of a sheath with an extendable braided-core introducer
   b. Wire insertion into the CS with tracking of the braided-core introducer followed by the sheath
4. Fully define the coronary venous anatomy with three-view occlusive CS venography.
5. Select a mid–lateral LV free wall location for LV lead placement, and devise a plan to "get there" using the available venous structures as well as collateral vessels to the area from large veins not on the lateral midwall.
6. Select the largest LV pacing lead possible, on the basis of the size of the vein(s) or collateral vessels, that facilitates access to the desired location.
7. Select a third-generation telescopic guide on the basis of:
   a. Size of the vein
   b. Origin of the vein from the CS (proximal, mid-, distal)
   c. Initial angle of takeoff of the vein from the CS
   d. Course of the vein after its origin from the CS
8. Place the LV pacing lead on the midlateral wall of the LV. In addition to a telescopic guide, this step may require:
   a. Advanced guidewire techniques (buddy wire)
   b. Venoplasty of small or stenotic coronary veins
   c. Venoplasty to enter the target area in a retrograde fashion using collateral vessels from large veins outside the target area
9. Test the LV pacing lead to ensure adequate pacing thresholds (<3 V @ 0.5 msec) and lack of phrenic pacing.
10. Remove the directional guide (if used) and the CS platform without disrupting the LV lead position.
11. Remove the stylet without disrupting the LV lead position.

TABLE 19-3. Anatomic Pitfalls to a Successful Implantation and Their Solutions

Occlusion of axillary/subclavian vein	Learn venoplasty and/or lead extraction
Difficult catheter manipulation at the shoulder:	
Binding at the clavicle	Axillary vein approach
Binding in a stenotic vein	Learn venoplasty
Coronary sinus (CS) os difficult to locate	Prepare for and use contrast material Understand how torque affects a catheter in the CS area and how an extendable braided-core torque device can change the shape of the cannulating assembly
CS difficult to cannulate owing to shape, size, position, stenosis, or a valve	Prepare for and use contrast material Understand and employ the progressive support rail approach Understand how a telescoping sheath system can be used to change the shape and trajectory of the catheter Learn venoplasty Understand the effect of changing from a standard-curve to a large-curve sheath
No target vein to the midlateral wall	Always perform a three-view occlusive CS venogram Consider double-inflating the occlusive balloon if the CS is very large Try to selectively cannulate the veins with a telescoping system Be familiar with the use of third-generation guides for direct lead delivery Understand how to use collateral vessels and venoplasty to reach areas without direct venous access
Target vein difficult to cannulate owing to shape, size, position, or stenosis	Be familiar with and use third-generation guides to cannulate the target vein Use first-generation directional catheters inside third-generation guides to facilitate insertion of the larger guide Learn venoplasty to facilitate insertion of third-generation guides into the target vein
LV lead cannot be advanced despite cannulation of the target vessel with a third-generation guide	Venoplasty and the buddy-wire technique
Absence of anatomic support or backing out of guide/sheath from CS as lead is advanced	Use a long peel-away sheath you can use for coronary sinus access instead of the subclavian vein Keep track of sheath location and use a sheath with an extra-large proximal curve
High pacing thresholds	Understand the "personalities" of the available LV leads Use collaterals Learn venoplasty
Phrenic stimulation before or after the guide is removed	Understand the "personalities" of the available LV leads Learn venoplasty Use collateral vessels
Lead dislodgment as/after the guide/sheath is removed	Learn and follow implantation etiquette Examine the course of the LV lead in the left anterior oblique projection to determine the amount of slack required Be systematic in approach, keeping track of tools, wires, and cables

of contrast material. What is the real risk of contrast material-induced nephrotoxicity? On the basis of experience in an unselected patient population of 220 patients who received 122 ± 90 mL of contrast material (75% received a high-osmolarity agent), Solomon and colleagues[15] reported, "There is little risk of clinically important nephrotoxicity attributable to contrast material for patients with diabetes and normal renal function or for nondiabetic patients with preexisting renal insufficiency. The risk for those with both diabetes and preexisting renal insufficiency is about 9% which is lower than previously reported."[15] None of their patients required dialysis. Despite this report, noninterventional physicians contend that patients with CHF who need cardiac resynchronization are unique and at higher risk than other patients. However, Meisel and associates[16] used 169 ± 105 mL of contrast material in 129 patients with ventricular tachycardia and CHF to locate and investigate the CS anatomy. They reported, "Transient renal failure occurred . . . in 1 of 129 patients. Several unsuccessful attempts to enter the coronary sinus . . . resulted in the use of 420 mL of contrast agent. Serum creatinine level increased from 1.5 mg/100 mL before the procedure to 2.64 mg/100 mL after the procedure. The patient recovered completely (without dialysis)."[16] Thus, the objective data do not support the fear of using contrast material in patients with CHF. Nevertheless, proper respect must be paid to the potential for nephrotoxic effects in such patients with CHF because of the day-to-day variability in their serum creatinine levels.

The three varieties of iodinated contrast agents are (1) standard ionic, (2) low-osmolar nonionic, and (3) iso-osmolar nonionic. Prospective evaluation of data comparing standard with low-osmolar nonionic contrast agents found no difference in the incidence of nephrotoxicity.[17,18] However, another study comparing iodixanol (iso-osmolar, nonionic, dimeric contrast medium) with iohexol (low-osmolar, nonionic, monomeric contrast medium) found that nephropathy is less likely to develop in high-risk patients when iodixanol is used. Thus, the iso-osmolar nonionic contrast medium iodixanol is the preferred agent.[19]

Gadolinium-based contrast agents are more expensive and less radiopaque than iodinated contrast agents. However, gadolinium-based agents are less nephrotoxic, with the iso-osmolar variety possibly less nephrotoxic than the standard gadolinium agent. Figure 19-3 shows an occlusive venogram produced with gadolinium. Balloon occlusion improves the visibility.

Patient Preparation to Prevent Renal Insufficiency

Several precautions have been demonstrated to reduce the renal insufficiency associated with administration of iodinated contrast material, as reviewed here:

- *Hydration:* The most important step in reducing contrast nephrotoxicity in patients with renal insufficiency is hydration. Patients should be pretreated with 0.45% saline 1 mL/kg/hour 12 hours before and 12 hours after the procedure. The volume infused is intended to compensate for insensible losses while the patient is on NPO ("nothing by mouth") status and rarely results in an exacerbation of CHF.
- *Acetylcysteine:* The prophylactic oral administration of the antioxidant acetylcysteine (Mucomyst) along with hydration has been reported to prevent the reduction in renal function induced by iodinated contrast agents in patients with chronic renal insufficiency.[20,21]
- *Ascorbic acid:* In a double-blind, randomized, placebo-controlled trial, ascorbic acid—administered as 3 gm 2 or more hours before, 2 gm the night after, and 2 gm the morning after angiography or intervention—was demonstrated to reduce the risk of contrast agent–mediated renal dysfunction.[22]
- *Bicarbonate:* In one study, hydration with sodium bicarbonate was found to be more effective in reducing renal insufficiency after administration of iodinated contrast material in 119 patients.[23] A particular advantage of bicarbonate hydration is that it can be started shortly before the procedure.

A reasonable approach, which we have successfully adopted, is as follows: Because the serum creatinine levels of patients with class III or IV CHF vary from day to day, we regard all patients undergoing CRT as having renal insufficiency and use the iso-osmolar nonionic contrast agent iodixanol. Recognizing that diabetic patients with elevated creatinine concentrations are at highest risk, we use a gadolinium-based contrast agent in all such patients. In addition, all patients are pretreated with acetylcysteine and hydration. Specifically, we hydrate all hospitalized patients with 0.45% saline,

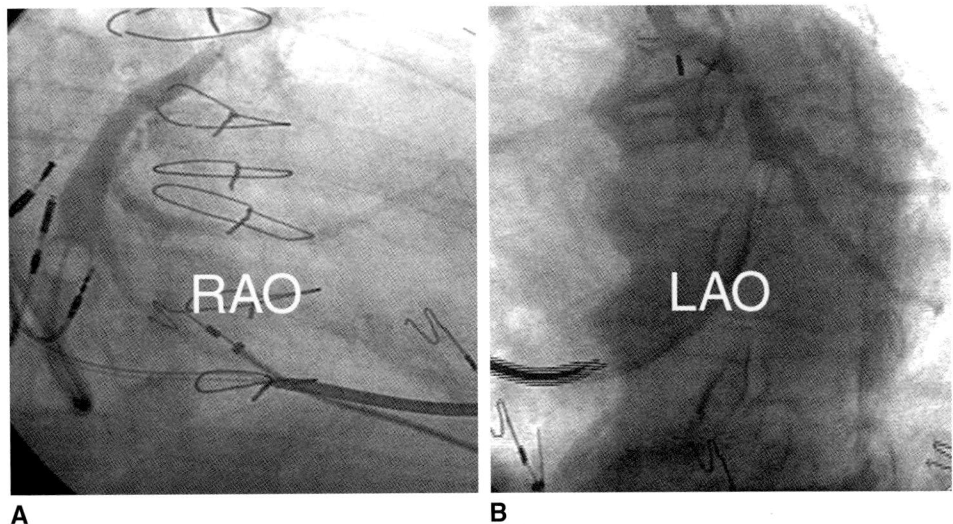

Figure 19-3. Gadolinium-based occlusive venogram. ***A,*** *Right anterior oblique (RAO) projection;* ***B,*** *left anterior oblique (LAO) projection. In both projections, the venous anatomy is well enough seen to visualize the takeoff and size of the target vein.*

1 mL/kg/hour starting 12 hours before the procedure and continuing during the procedure (while the patient's status is NPO) and for 12 hours after the procedure. For day surgery patients and hospitalized patients, for whom overnight hydration is not possible, we recommend hydration with sodium bicarbonate. Considering the possibility of converting chronic CHF to acute CHF via hydration, it is important to remember that the patients are taking nothing in by mouth and continue to receive diuretics. We also pretreat all patients with the antioxidant acetylcysteine (600 mg every 12 hours the day before, the day of, and the day after the procedure), which is inexpensive and nontoxic.

Low-osmolar nonionic contrast agents do not lessen the risk of renal insufficiency, but iso-osmolar nonionic contrast agents do.[19] Thus, iodixanol is currently the preferred contrast agent. Not all nonionic contrast agents are the same. It is important to specify iodixanol. Judicious use of contrast agent (iodixanol or a gadolinium-based agent) in the properly prepared (hydrated and premedicated) patient improves the efficiency and safety of CRT.

Electrophysiology Catheter–Based versus Contrast Agent–Based Implantation

A contrast material–based LV lead implantation approach has several advantages over the EP catheter–based approach. Use of contrast material is essential to an understanding of the individual patient's CS and coronary venous anatomy, to facilitating localization of, and advancing into, the CS, and to reaching the target area of the LV. Use of contrast material identifies the "catheter" location at all times, limiting unintentional trauma. When open-lumen catheters and contrast agents are used, staining quickly identifies a misstep. The same misstep with an EP catheter commonly goes unrecognized until occlusive CS venography is performed or pain or hypotension announces its presence. Thus, the potential for staining with a contrast agent is what makes it safe.

Contrast staining can occur at the time of CS venography but is not of hemodynamic significance. Staining can result from one of three mechanisms:

- *Unmasking of CS trauma inflicted by the EP catheter used to cannulate the CS:* Physicians commonly used a (deflectable) EP catheter to cannulate the CS and to serve as a wire over which to advance a guide (guidewire). The EP catheter is not designed to prevent vascular trauma. It does not have a soft tip (like an open-lumen catheter) nor does it have a J-shaped tip (like a guidewire) to prevent vascular trauma; thus, unrecognized trauma to the CS is likely with such a catheter but becomes apparent only when contrast material is injected under pressure in the CS. Occlusive CS venography does not cause the staining but unmasks the unrecognized trauma inflicted by the sharp, stiff EP catheter (Fig. 19-4).
- *Local extravasation of contrast material at the tip of the balloon:* If the tip of the balloon becomes lodged in a small venous branch during injection of contrast material, the vein is disrupted, and contrast material is extravasated into the interstitial space, causing a stain.
- *Balloon-induced trauma due to overinflation of a noncompliant balloon:* Balloon trauma is limited by careful inflation of the balloon in the CS under fluoroscopic guidance while contrast material is being injected. Inflation is stopped when the balloon occludes the CS, preventing reflux of contrast material. When overinflation occurs, a non-

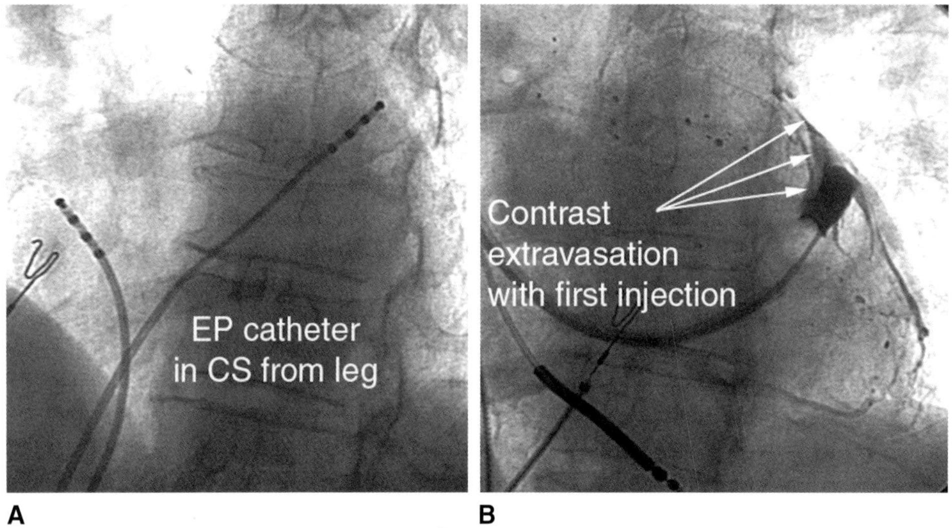

Figure 19-4. Extravasation of contrast material from electrophysiology (EP) catheter–induced coronary sinus (CS) trauma. ***A,*** *The EP catheter is used to find the CS from the leg.* ***B,*** *Contrast material extravasates freely into the pericardial space through the perforation caused by the EP catheter.*

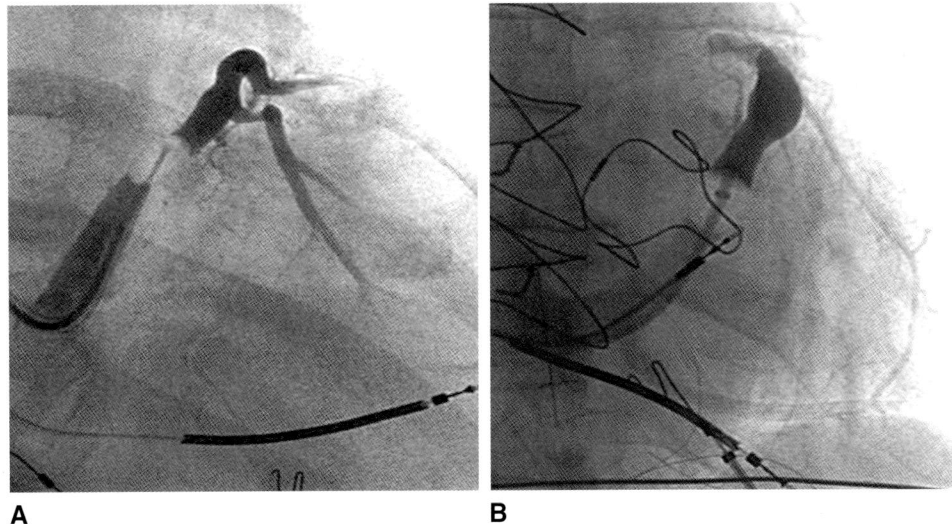

*Figure 19-5. Compliant versus noncompliant balloons for occlusive coronary sinus venography. **A,** The compliant balloon deforms to fit in the coronary sinus. **B,** The noncompliant balloon maintains its shape independent of the patient anatomy.*

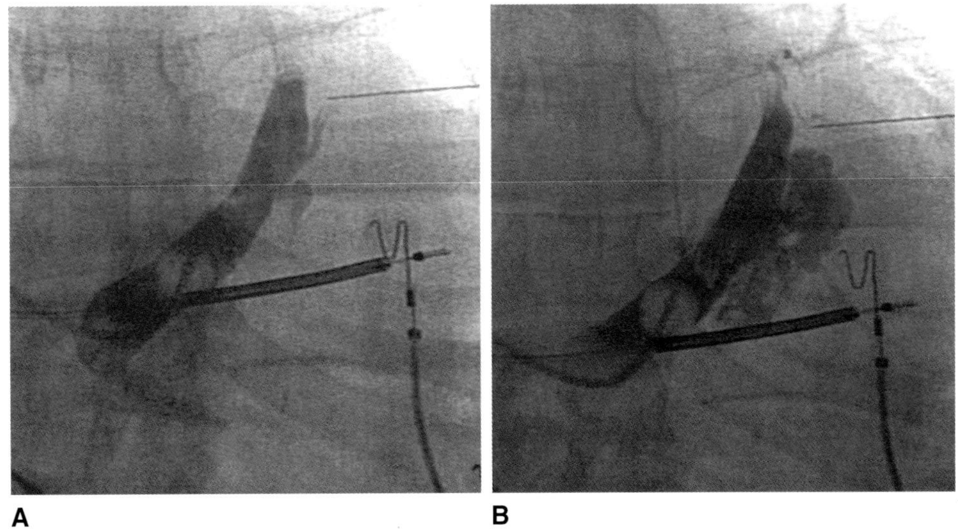

*Figure 19-6. Contrast staining at the time of occlusive coronary sinus venography. **A,** The balloon is inflated and contrast material fills the coronary sinus in retrograde fashion. **B,** The tip of the balloon catheter engages a small venous branch, and contrast material extravasates into the interstitial tissue. Despite their ominous appearance, contrast stains rarely result in hemodynamic complications. At their worst they obscure the venous anatomy for 10 to 15 minutes.*

compliant (nondeformable) balloon is more likely to inflict CS trauma than a compliant balloon. When a compliant balloon is overinflated for the size of the CS, it becomes distorted and conforms to the CS (Fig. 19-5). When a noncompliant balloon is overinflated, it enlarges without conforming to the CS, possibly resulting in local trauma (Fig. 19-6).

When Is Occlusive Coronary Sinus Venography Potentially Dangerous?

If a compliant occlusive balloon is used and the tip of the balloon is watched during injection, CS venography rarely produces a stain, let alone hemodynamic consequence. There are two exceptions to this rule. Both arise when occlusive venography is performed after initial CS trauma is inflicted; they are as follows:

- When the EP catheter used to identify the CS from the leg and/or to deliver the sheath/guide to the CS inflicts unrecognized trauma.
- When the *occlusive* CS venogram is repeated during the same procedure after venous trauma is recognized.

The balloon occlusion increases venous pressure distally, forcing blood into the traumatized area. When contrast material is injected with the balloon inflated,

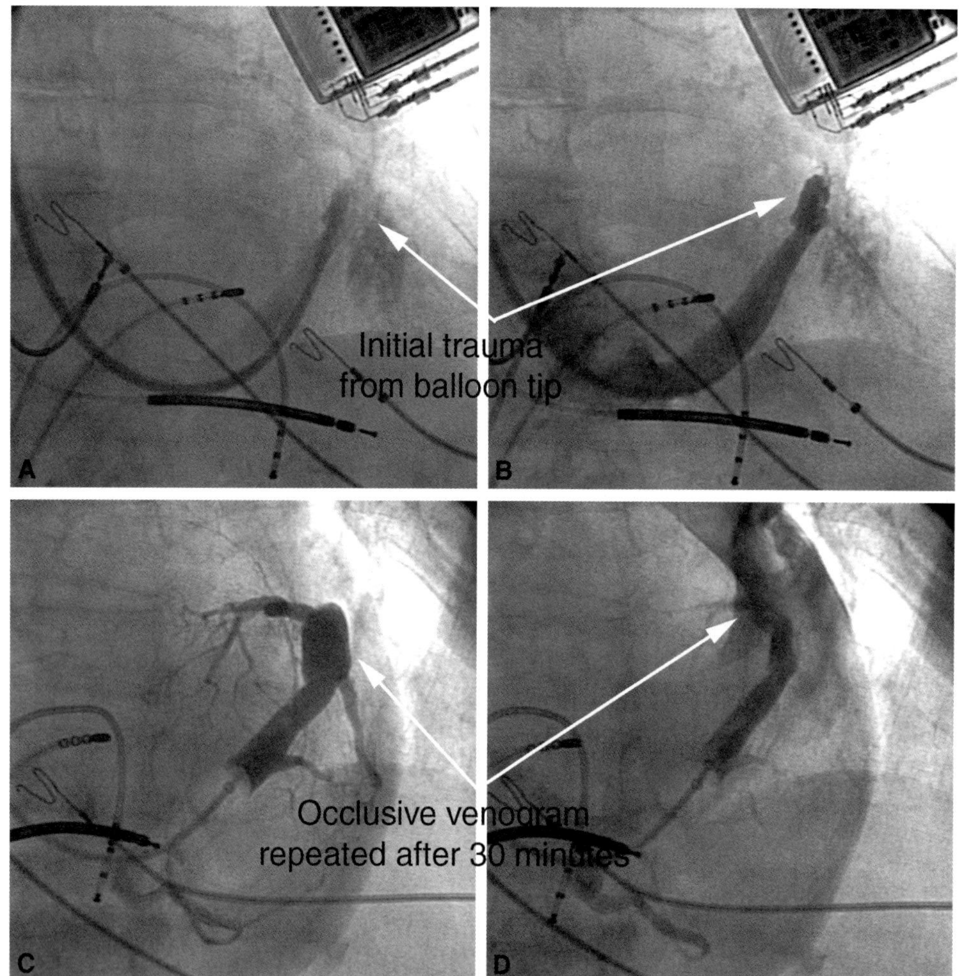

Figure 19-7. Coronary sinus (CS) aneurysm formation and rupture with second occlusive CS venogram. ***A*** *and* ***B****, The tip of the balloon produces trauma and staining of the CS.* ***C,*** *An aneurysmal dilatation of the CS expands as the balloon is inflated, and contrast material is injected 30 minutes after the initial CS trauma.* ***D,*** *With balloon occlusion and contrast injection, the aneurysmal area bursts, forcing blood and contrast material into the pericardial space.*

the distal pressure increases, further forcing blood and contrast material into and through the venous disruption. Enough blood and contrast material can be forced into the pericardial space to result in hemodynamic compromise, as illustrated in Figure 19-7.

Manipulation of Open-Lumen "Catheters" in and around the Coronary Sinus

EP physicians are often not comfortable (owing to a lack of experience) with the manipulation of open-lumen catheters in the heart, yet they feel safe with fixed-curve or deflectable EP catheters. Objective comparison of a soft-tip, open-lumen catheter with an EP catheter shows that the EP catheter is much stiffer and more prone to inflict vascular trauma. Further, there is concern that manipulation of catheters in and around the coronary venous structures is intrinsically more "dangerous" than in and around the arteries because veins are "thin-walled structures." Nothing is further from the truth. Consider the three possible effects of trauma to the coronary veins and compare the same events in a coronary artery, as follows:

- *Dissection:* It is useful to compare the effect of an intimal disruption in a coronary artery with that in a coronary vein. In an artery, the blood is under high pressure and will get under the flap and extend the dissection. In a vein, the blood is flowing in the opposite direction from the flap and is under low pressure, so the dissection is not extended (Fig. 19-8).
- *Occlusion:* If catheter trauma results in coronary artery closure, the consequences are abrupt and profound, leading to an acute myocardial infarction. However, the effect of catheter-induced trauma resulting in closure of a venous structure is of no acute or long-term significance other than the lack of venous access. Figure 19-9 demonstrates occlusion of a lateral wall target vein.
- *Perforation:* When "catheter"-induced trauma results in coronary artery perforation, the situation is

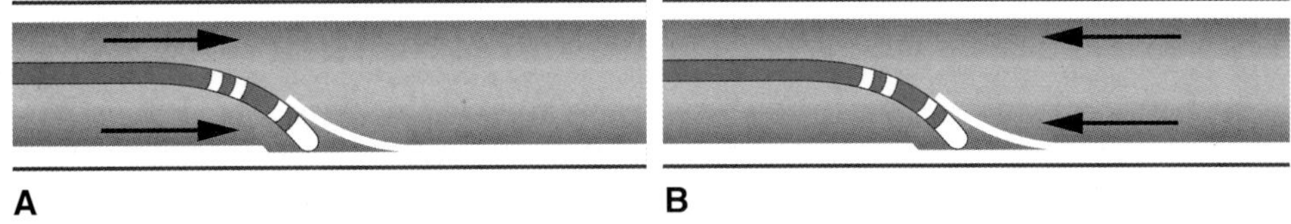

Figure 19-8. Comparison of the effect of an intimal flap in an artery and a vein. ***A,*** *Catheter trauma created an intimal flap in an artery. High pressure and the direction of blood flow in the artery* (arrows) *will lift the flap and extend the dissection.* ***B,*** *Catheter trauma created an intimal flap in a vein. The direction of blood flow in the vein* (arrows) *will close and seal the flap.*

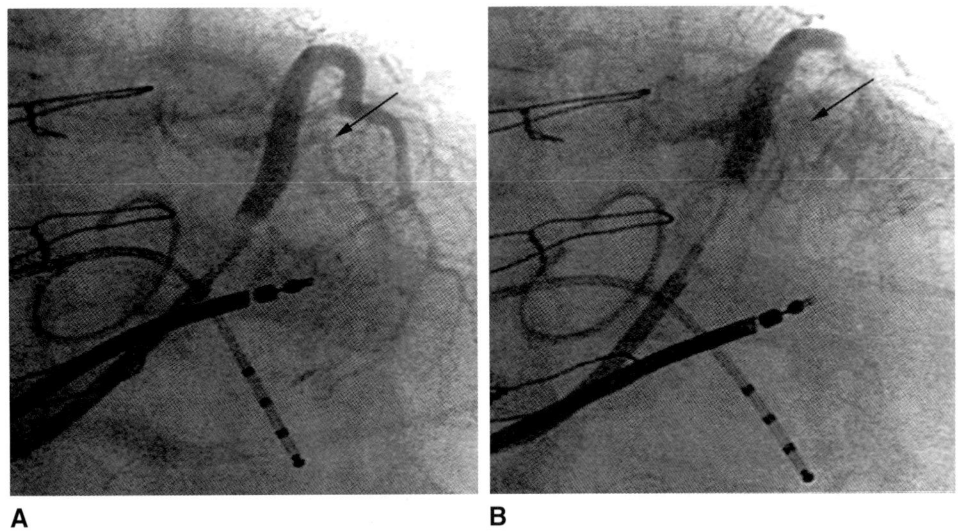

Figure 19-9. Occlusion of a lateral wall target vein. ***A,*** *A small lateral wall target vein* (arrow) *can be seen during the initial occlusive coronary sinus venography.* ***B,*** *The target vein is no longer visible on a second venogram performed after an unsuccessful venoplasty. The patient suffered no ill effects. An alternative lateral wall target vein was used for placement of a left ventricular lead.*

difficult because the pressure gradient forces blood into the pericardial space, rapidly leading to cardiac tamponade. With perforation of a coronary vein, on the other hand, the pressure gradient is in the opposite direction. After a venous perforation, blood within the vein follows the pressure gradient into the CS and to the right atrium (RA). The exception is if occlusive CS venography is performed after the perforation (see Fig. 19-7).

Lead Perforation

It appears to be far more likely for stylet-driven pacing leads to perforate the coronary veins than catheters, guides, or sheaths. Stylet-driven pacing leads, like EP catheters, have solid metal tips with wire-reinforced shafts. A considerable amount of tip force can be delivered, as evidenced by the ability of such catheters to perforate the right ventricle (RV). However, unlike RV perforation, coronary venous perforation rarely if ever causes tamponade, because the pressure in the RV is much higher than that in the pericardial space, causing a pressure gradient favoring tamponade. The pressure in a vein is much lower than that in the RV, and a pressure gradient exists from distal to proximal in the vein. Thus, the pressure gradient favors the flow of blood into the more proximal vein rather than out into the pericardial space (Figs. 19-10 and 19-11).

"Responders" versus "Nonresponders" and Left Ventricular Lead Position

Chest Radiograph versus Fluoroscopy to Document Lead Position

The left anterior oblique (LAO) view on fluoroscopy at the time of implantation should define the LV lead position. However, if the fluoroscopy is not performed in a standard fashion, it can be deceptive. Kistler and associates[24] describe a case in which it became apparent, from analysis of the electrocardiogram (ECG), that a lead that was fluoroscopically demonstrated to be in the LV at the time of implantation was actually in the RV. Another example of fluoroscopic error is shown in Figures 19-12 and 19-13. The LAO fluoroscopic image in Figure 19-12A appeared to document a lateral position. However, the lateral chest radiograph (see Fig. 19-12B) demonstrated the anterior location. In Figure 19-13A, the steeper LAO projection reveals the anterior nature of the first ("nonresponder") LV lead position. It is important for the implanting physician to take personal responsibility for reviewing the final

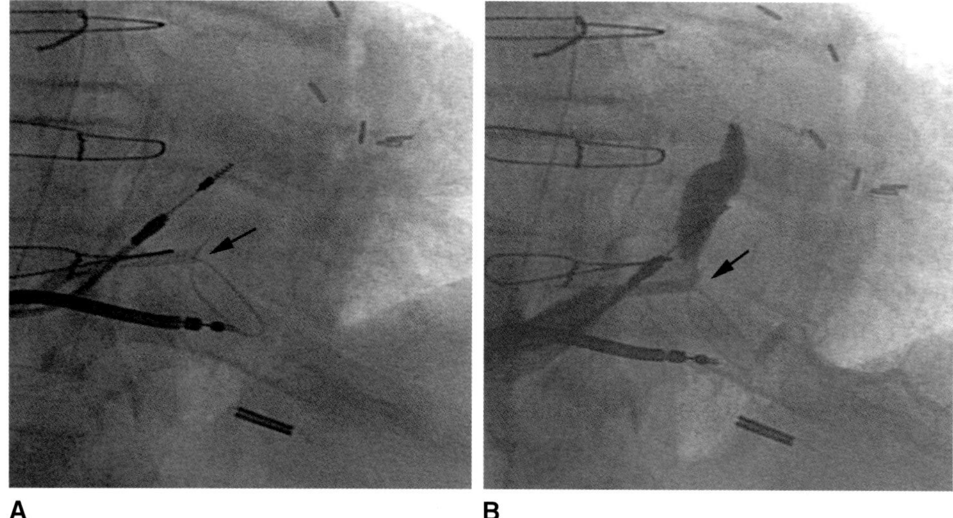

Figure 19-10. *Contrast staining from a Medtronic, Inc. (Minneapolis, Minn.), Attain 6218 guide.* ***A,*** *The guide is advanced over a wire and small catheter (second-generation telescoping system) into the lateral wall target vein.* ***B,*** *Two milliliters of contrast material are injected to confirm that the guide is coaxial in the target vein before the Attain 2187 LV pacing lead (Medtronic, Inc.) is advanced. The tip of the guide is not coaxial with the lumen of the vein, and 1 mL of contrast material is extravasated into the tissues around the vein. On the basis of this appearance, the position of the guide was adjusted, and the lead was advanced without incident. Vein perforation rather than staining is likely if the pacing lead is advanced without injection of contrast material.*

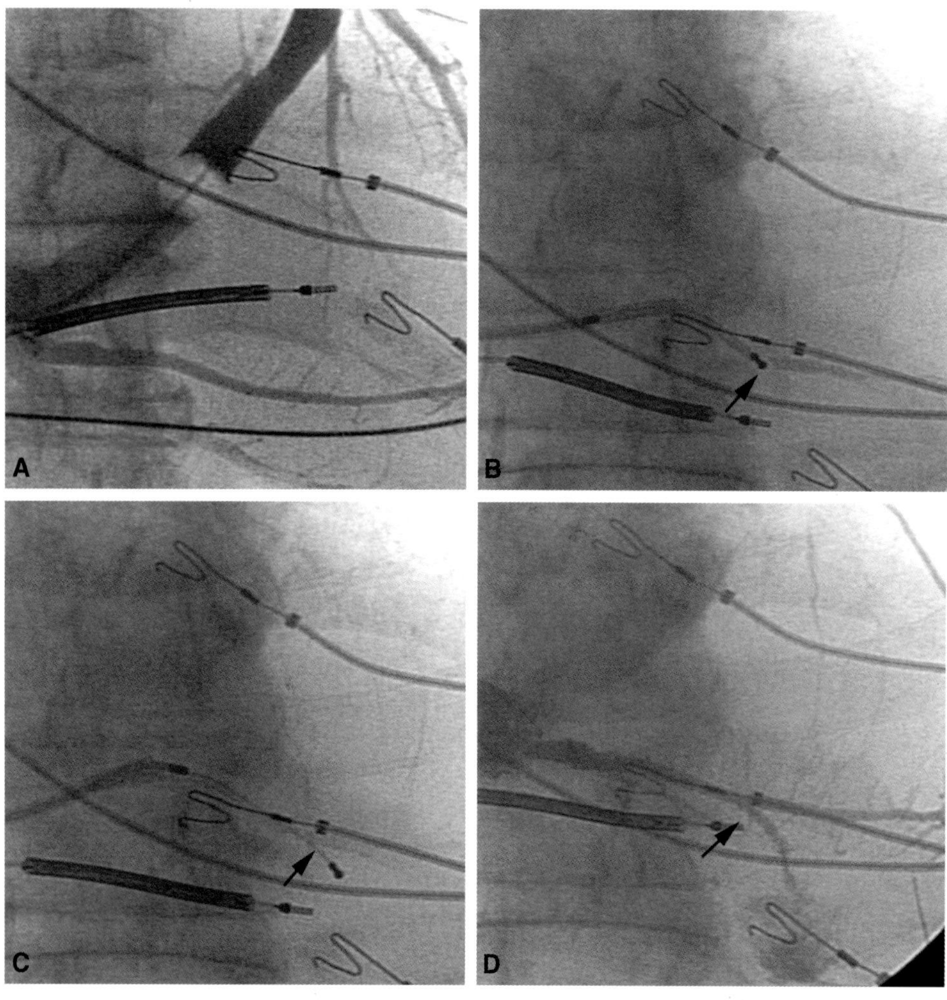

Figure 19-11. *Pacing lead–induced vein perforation with free flow of contrast material into the pericardial space.* ***A,*** *The posterior lateral target vein is demonstrated with occlusive coronary sinus venography.* ***B,*** *The Attain 2187 LV pacing lead* (arrow) *(Medtronic, Inc., Minneapolis, Minn.) is advanced into the vein.* ***C,*** *The tip of the lead* (arrow) *advances beyond the limits of the vein.* ***D,*** *The lead is removed, and contrast material is injected into the posterior lateral vein. Contrast material under pressure from the injection (3 mL) exits the vein freely* (tip of arrow) *into the pericardial space. Despite this ominous appearance, no pericardial effusion was found on echocardiography and there were no hemodynamic consequences. The lead was successfully placed in an anterior lateral vein during the same procedure.*

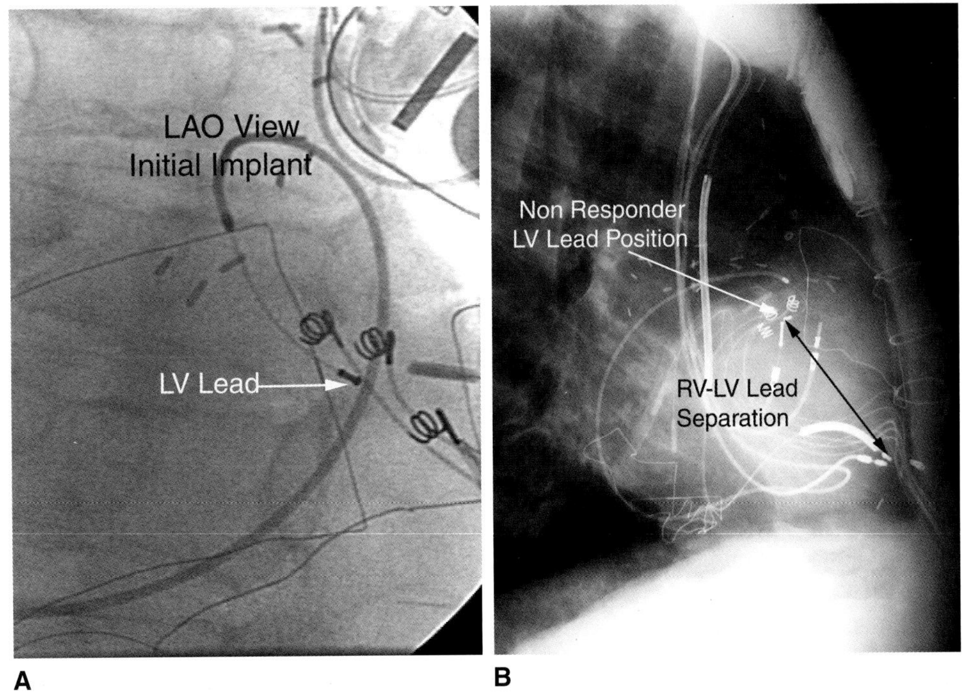

Figure 19-12. Left anterior oblique (LAO) fluoroscopy and lateral chest radiography at initial implantation of a left ventricular (LV) lead. ***A,*** *The LAO view demonstrates the LV lead in what appears to be a lateral position next to the epicardial screw-in leads from a prior implantable cardioverter-defibrillator (ICD).* ***B,*** *The lateral chest radiograph shows that the LV lead (labeled Non Responder LV Lead Position) is actually anterior.* Black arrow *indicates the separation between the right ventricular and LV leads.*

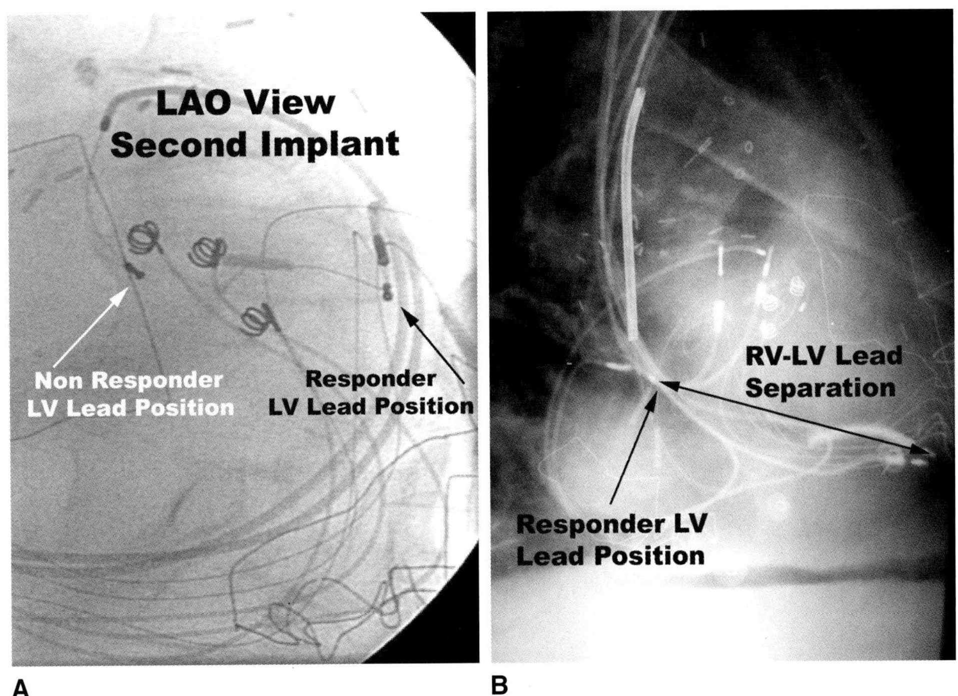

Figure 19-13. Left anterior oblique (LAO) fluoroscopy and lateral chest radiograph from the second implantation. ***A,*** *The steep LAO view reveals the original left ventricular (LV) lead position (labeled Non Responder LV Lead Position) to be anterior. The new LV lead position (labeled Responder LV Lead Position) is midlateral.* ***B,*** *The lateral chest radiograph taken after the second LV lead was implanted confirms the posterior lateral lead position.*

location of the LV lead, to ensure that the patient has received the best possible lead position. In addition, one of the most important pieces of data in the evaluation of a CRT "nonresponder" is the final location of the LV lead on a chest radiograph.

Heist and colleagues[25] documented that the acute hemodynamic effect of CRT is predicted by the LV-RV interlead distance as measured on the lateral chest radiograph taken after the procedure. In follow-up of patients after implantation, I have found the LV-RV lead separation on the lateral chest radiograph essential in evaluating "nonresponders" in whom LV lead placement has been "successful."[26] The appropriate placement of the LV lead on the lateral wall of the LV is critical to successful CRT. Placement of the LV lead on the anterior surface of the LV is at best suboptimal and may worsen LV function. Unless convincing, specific information to the contrary is available, the midlateral free wall of the LV is the optimal position for the LV lead. When the LV lead is on the midlateral wall, its position on a lateral chest radiograph is directly posterior. Figure 19-14 shows the typical post-implantation chest radiographs of a "responder" in whom the LV lead is located on the midlateral wall of the LV. Note that the LV and RV leads are maximally separated on the lateral chest radiograph.

Figure 19-15 shows the lateral chest radiographs of two patients who did not show response to CRT. Figure 19-15A is the lateral chest radiograph of a "nonresponder" in whom the lead was placed in the anterior interventricular vein; patients with a lead in this location are not expected to show response. Figure 19-15B, however, is the lateral chest radiograph of a patient who showed no response even though the LV lead had been placed in the vein to the midlateral free wall. What happened? The LV lead is advanced distally in the midlateral vein, which wraps around anteriorly toward the septum. Although the lead was started in the vein to the midlateral free wall, it ended up anterior, close to the RV lead. Note that in Figure 19-15A and B, the tip of the LV pacing lead is closer to the RV pacing lead than the ideal position seen in Figure 19-14B.

The clinical question raised is whether repositioning the LV lead of the patient in Figure 19-15B to a more proximal position in the same vein, thus increasing the RV-LV separation, would change a "nonresponder" to a "responder." Figure 19-16 illustrates the original and new, more proximal positions in the same vein of a patient in whom such repositioning was performed. The RV-LV lead separation was increased, and the patient demonstrated a marked symptomatic improvement, objectified by reductions in both serum creatinine level and dose of diuretics.

Figure 19-17A is the lateral chest radiograph of a patient in whom the original implanting physician was not prepared to perform coronary vein venoplasty. The vein to the midlateral wall was distal to a stenosis in the main body of the CS. Although the implantation was regarded as "successful," the pacing lead was not placed on the midlateral wall of the LV. The patient did not improve after the procedure, was regarded as a CRT "nonresponder," and was listed for heart transplantation. He was evaluated at our facility, where the lead position on the lateral chest radiograph was discovered. He subsequently underwent venoplasty of the main body of the CS, and the lead was placed on the lateral wall of the LV; dramatic resolution of symptoms eliminated the need for a heart transplant. Both the acute hemodynamic effect and the subsequent clinical response to CRT are predicted by the RV-LV lead separation on the lateral chest radiograph. On the basis of the work of Heist and colleagues,[25] the RV-LV separation in the horizontal plane is more important than the total RV-LV separation, and the RV-LV separation in the vertical plane is not predictive.

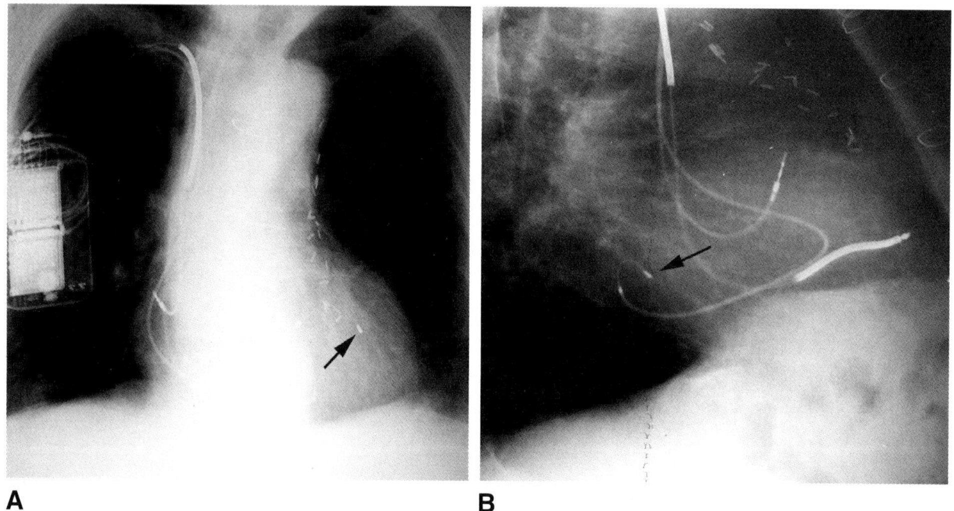

*Figure 19-14. The posteroanterior and lateral chest radiographs of a patient showing response to cardiac resynchronization therapy. **A,** Anteroposterior view; **B,** lateral view. Arrow indicates the tip of the Attain 2187 left ventricular (LV) pacing lead (Medtronic, Inc., Minneapolis, Minn.) On the lateral chest radiograph, the LV lead is located directly posterior the maximal distance from the right ventricular lead. This is the lateral chest radiograph of an LV lead on the midlateral wall.*

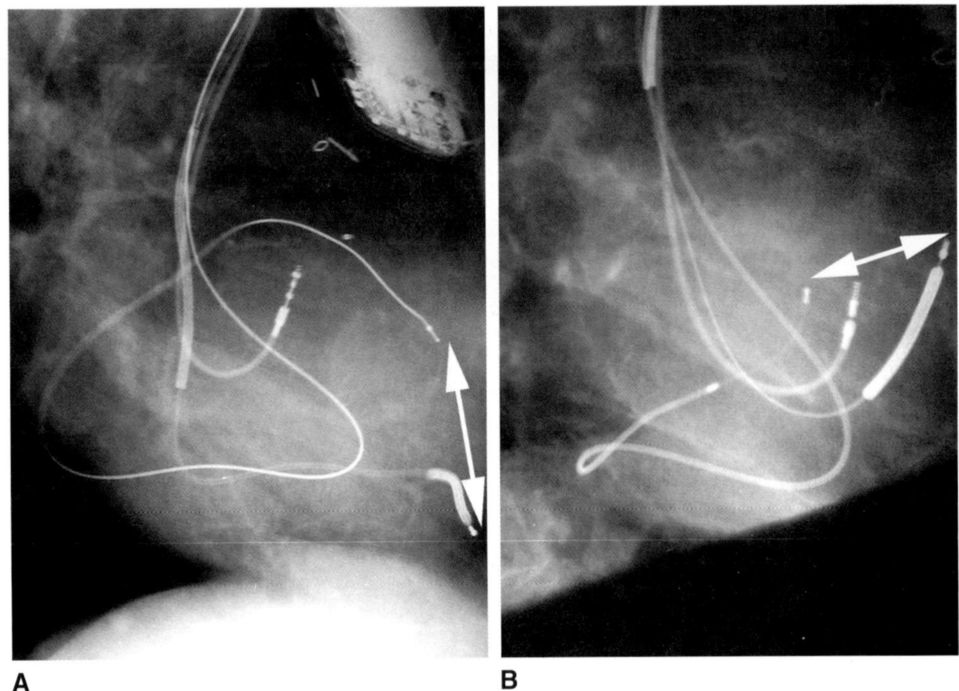

Figure 19-15. *Chest radiographs of two "nonresponders" with an anterior left ventricular (LV) leads placed via different veins.* ***A,*** *The LV lead is in the anterior vein.* ***B,*** *The lead starts in the lateral wall target vein but is well beyond the ideal location. In both* **A** *and* ***B,*** *the physical separation between the right ventricular (RV) and LV leads* (white arrows) *is suboptimal. In both patients, new leads were placed in positions similar to those shown in Figure 19-4, with marked improvement in symptoms.*

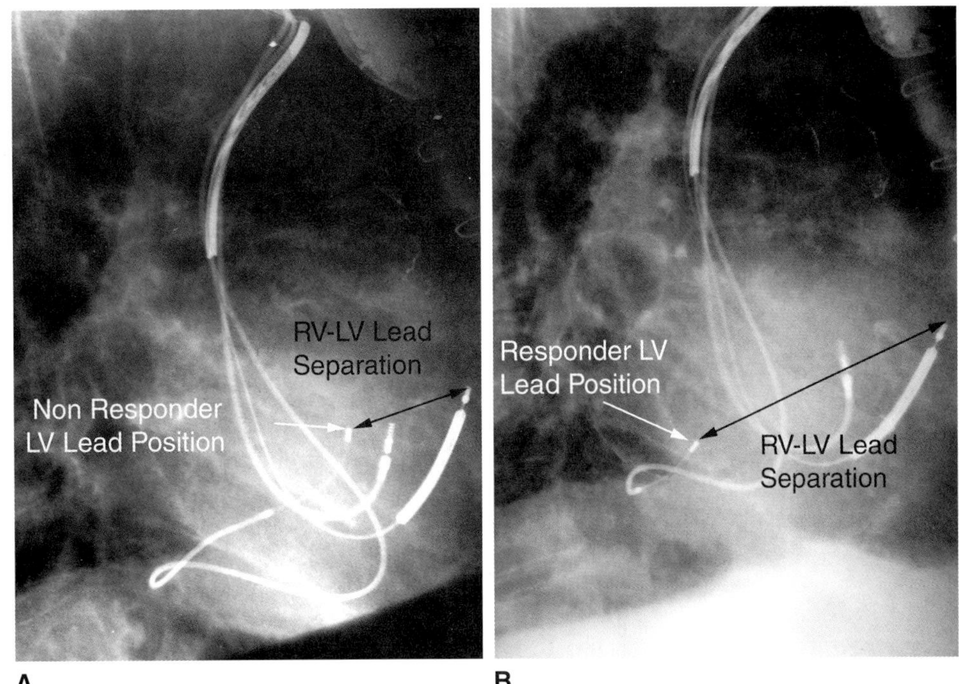

Figure 19-16. *Lateral chest radiographs before and after repositioning.* ***A,*** *The left ventricular (LV) lead is anterior near the right ventricular (RV) lead. There is little RV-LV lead separation* (black arrow). ***B,*** *The LV lead is lateral. The RV-LV lead separation* (black arrow) *is larger. Although the LV lead was placed in a mid-lateral wall vein, it was advanced distally, resulting in a more anterior position and lack of symptom response. When the lead was withdrawn more proximally in the same vein, the RV-LV lead separation increased, and the patient's symptoms improved.*

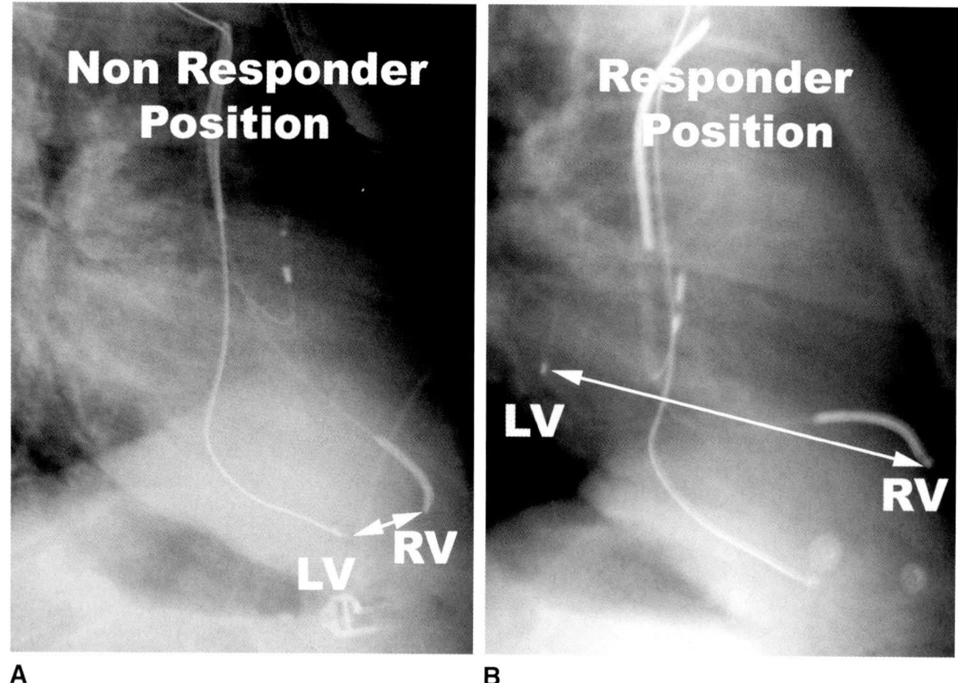

Figure 19-17. *Lateral chest radiographs of a "nonresponder" before and after coronary sinus (CS) venoplasty and repositioning of the left ventricular (LV) lead.* ***A,*** *The LV lead is anterior, near the right ventricular (RV) lead, on the lateral chest radiograph. Because of a stenosis in the main CS, the LV lead was placed in a posterolateral vein. To ensure stability and low pacing thresholds, it is advanced distally. There is little RV-LV lead separation.* ***B,*** *Venoplasty of the main CS was performed to provide access to the vein to the midlateral wall of the LV. The LV lead is directly posterior on the lateral chest radiograph. The RV-LV lead separation is markedly increased. With venoplasty of the main CS and placement of the LV lead on the lateral wall, the clinical response was dramatic and the patient's name was removed from the heart transplant list.*

It is important to remember that surgical placement of LV pacing leads does not ensure their placement on the midlateral free wall, as shown in Figure 19-1.

Equipping and Setting Up the Room to Be Able to Follow the "Golden Rule"

Four of the most important and most easily overlooked parts of BiV pacing lead implantation are mechanical issues that can be easily resolved before the procedure starts. Careful attention to these issues can make the difference between an agonizing unsuccessful attempt and a 15-minute LV lead placement. Actions to avoid these issues are discussed here.

Collect Available Biventricular Implantation Equipment and Review Its Use

Possibly the worst mistake that can be made is to assume that the equipment required for a successful efficient LV lead implantation either is in the room or has been provided by the manufacturer. Some of the equipment is readily available in the hospital but is not part of the usual repertoire of many implanting physicians. Knowledge of the equipment used in interventional radiology and interventional cardiology can be extremely useful during an LV lead implantation (Table 19-4). The technical staff and physicians from interventional cardiology and radiology commonly have helpful ideas for solving the mechanical problems posed by an LV lead implantation, and equipment specifically tailored to LV lead placement is slowly making its way into the world of electrophysiology. Access to these new tools can make the difference between an easy success and a painful, demoralizing failure.

Organize the Equipment to be Readily Available in the Room

It is important to remember that the equipment one needs is not commonly available in a room that is used for either pacer implantation or an electrophysiology study. To avoid spending more time looking around in the interventional cardiology and radiology laboratories than actually working on the patient, one should make certain of having the most basic equipment in the room. These tools are additional to the device company equipment and sheaths used for pacemaker implantation. To be certain we have the proper tools regardless of the room, our staff created a "BiV Cart." This cart

TABLE 19-4. **Essential Biventricular Implantation Equipment***

Product and Description	Length (cm)	Diameter	Manufacturer	Order No.
Coronary sinus access and telescoping system platform:				
9F SafeSheath-CSG Worley STD with braided core	40	11F OD, 9F ID	Pressure Products, Inc., San Pedro, Calif.	CSG/Worley/BCor-1-09-STD
9F SafeSheath-CSG Worley Jumbo with braided core	49	11F OD, 9F ID	Pressure Products, Inc.	CSG/Worley/BCor-1-09-LRG
SafeSheath-Worley telescoping braided guides for direct lead delivery to target vein:†				
Renal Shape Worley Braided Telescopic Guide	60	9F OD, 7F ID	Pressure Products, Inc.	LVI/Tele/B-60-07-RE
Hockey Stick Worley Braided Telescopic Guide	60	9F OD, 7F ID	Pressure Products, Inc.	LVI/Tele/B-60-07-HS
Multipurpose Worley Braided Telescopic Guide	60	9F OD, 7F ID	Pressure Products, Inc.	LVI/Tele/B-60-07-MP
Balloon for occlusive coronary sinus venography	—	—	Pressure Products, Inc.	BVCS6180
Angioplasty guidewires for over-the-wire LV pacing lead:‡				
Medium-support guidewire (e.g., Luge)	180	0.014 in.	Boston Scientific Corp., Natick, Mass.	12130-01/12100-01
Low-support or "floppy" wire (Choice PT Floppy)	180	0.014 in.	Boston Scientific Corp.	12160-01/12154-01
Extra-support wire (Choice PT Extra Support)	180	0.014 in.	Boston Scientific Corp.	12161-01/12155-01
Super-support wire (e.g., Platinum Plus or Iron Man)	300	0.014 in.	Boston Scientific Corp.	1752
Torque device (steering handle) for the angioplasty wire				
Introducer for the angioplasty wire				
Guidewires for sheaths and telescopic braided guides:§				
Terumo Angled Glidewire	150	0.035 in.	Terumo Medical Corp., Somerset, N.J.	GR 3506
Torque device (steering handled) for Angled Glidewire				
Emerald Guidewire	180	0.032 in.	Cordis, Miami, Fla. (a division of Telectronics, St. Jude Medical, Sylmar, Calif.)	502-454
Tetrafluroethylene-coated curve (J-tip) Amplatz Extra-Stiff Wire	180	0.032 in.	Cook Vascular, Inc., Leechburg, Penna.	121649
Simplified contrast agent injection system:¶				
10-mL contrast injection control syringe				
Three-way stopcock				
30-mL syringe (to serve as contrast reservoir)				
12 to 18 inches of tubing with male and female ends				
Y-adapter with luer lock				

*In addition to either Medtronic, Inc. (Minneapolis, Minn.), or Guidant (Boston Scientific, Natick, Mass.) implantation equipment, at least two of each of these items must be in the implantation room for each case.

†For difficult veins, these guides are inserted through the SafeSheath/CSG (Coronary Sinus Guide) Worley (Thomas Medical Products Inc, Malvern, Penna.) (9F guide fits through a 9F sheath) directly into the target vein. Both Medtronic Attain (2187 and 4193) and Guidant leads fit through these 9F OD/7F ID guides. The 9F Worley telescopic braided guides will also accept a 0.014-inch angioplasty wire with the Attain leads (buddy wire) if needed. Pressure Products, Inc., released this line of braided guides with hemostatic valves in the fall of 2003.

‡The brand of wire is not critical. Most companies make a floppy, a medium-support, and an extra-support wire.

§Here the brand and description of the wire are important.

¶The components of the contrast injection system must be on the procedure table and assembled before the procedure starts.

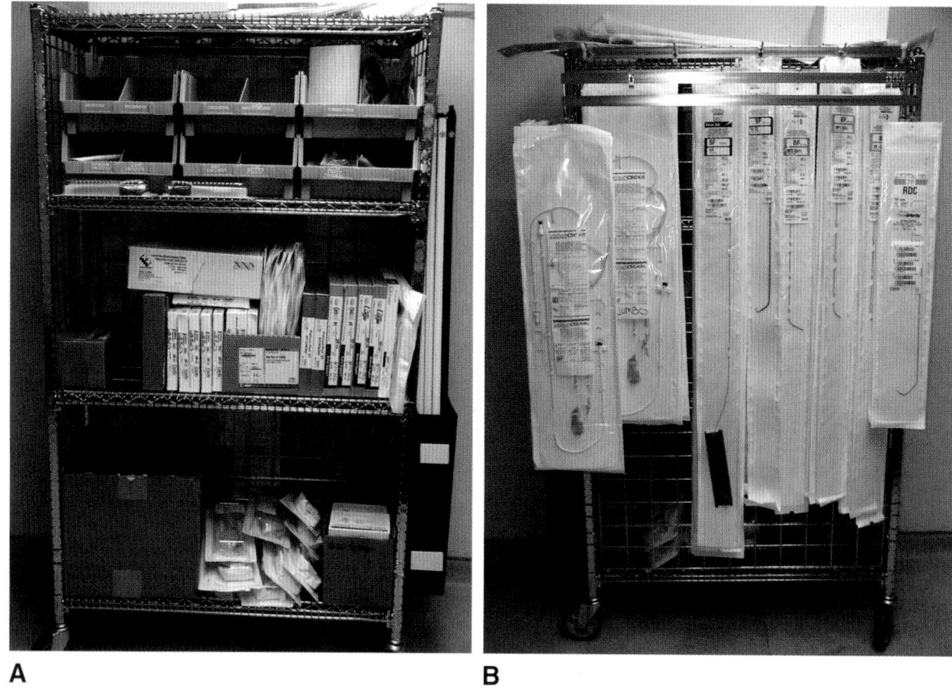

Figure 19-18. Biventricular (BiV) cart for keeping equipment readily available in any implantation room when needed. ***A,*** *Front view;* ***B,*** *back view.*

also contains equipment for performing subclavian and coronary vein venoplasties (Fig. 19-18A and B).

Assemble the "Always Used" Equipment on the Table before Starting

Having a routine and setting the table with equipment needed for the procedure give the operator the freedom to concentrate on the procedure and help avoid "rethinking" the tools for each implantation (Fig. 19-19).

Pay Careful Attention to the Orientation of the Instrument Table during Various Stages of the Procedure

It is truly remarkable how important the position of the instrument table can be to a successful implantation. It is even more remarkable how frequently even an experienced implanter forgets to change to a table position appropriate to the stage of the procedure until either the support staff provides a gentle reminder or something that should be easy feels difficult. Figure 19-20A demonstrates the usual "backfield" position of the instrument table. We keep the table in this position until we start CS access, at which point the table is turned perpendicular to the patient (see Fig. 19-20B). Once the LV lead is in place and it is time to start removing the guide and/or sheath, the table is returned to the "backfield" position so the assistant can support the sheath and lead during sheath and guide removal.

The perpendicular position of the table from the start of CS cannulation until removal of the guide and or sheath can be cumbersome with standard tables, for the following reasons:

- The legs of the table closer to the patient interfere with the position of the operator's feet and the fluoroscopy pedals.
- The legs of the table interfere with rotation of the fluoroscopy unit, particularly in the right anterior oblique (RAO) position.
- The height of the standard instrument table is lower than the height of the patient, as shown in Figure 19-20B. As a result, wires and catheters do not make a smooth transition from the patient to the table.

The custom-built table shown in Figure 19-21A addresses all three issues. The legs are recessed to provide room for the fluoroscopy unit, the operator's feet, and fluoroscopy pedals. The height is adjustable so that the top of the table can be raised to reduce the vertical stepoff between the patient and the table. Testing the LV and RV simultaneously for pacing thresholds can be very difficult with standard testing cables. Simply attaching an additional alligator eliminates this problem (see Fig. 19-21B).

Venous Access

At first, venous access may seem like a minor issue, but one must keep in mind the cascade of events that follows a difficult venous access. If compression between the clavicle and first rib, friction between the

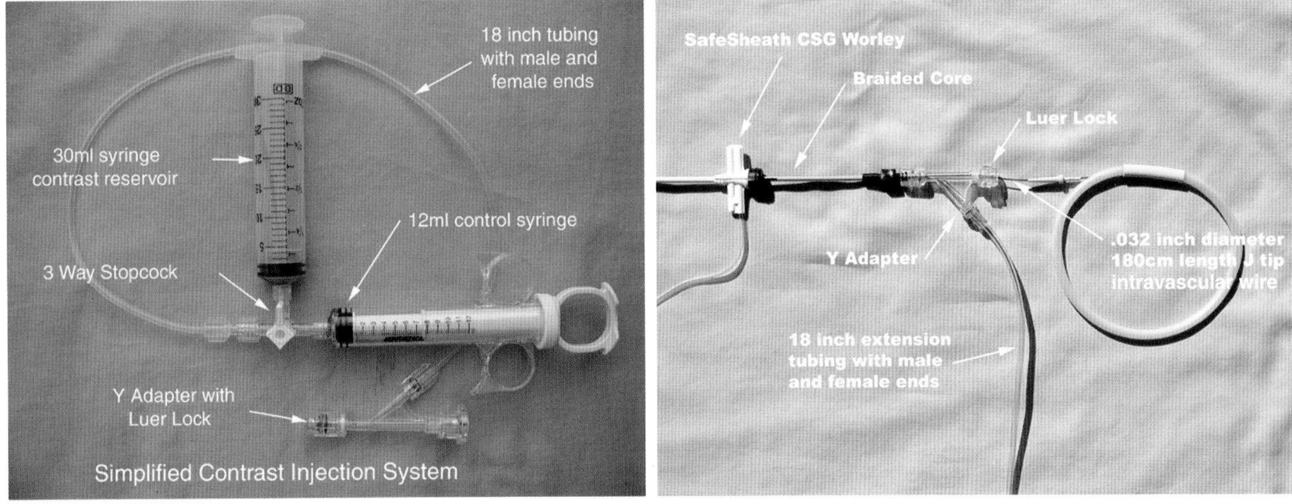

Figure 19-19. ***A,*** *Simplified contrast injection system. Placement of a pacing lead on the lateral wall of the left ventricle (LV) almost always requires the injection of contrast material to find the coronary sinus (CS) os and define the CS anatomy. The simplified system shown here can be constructed from equipment readily available in most laboratories. The scrub technician should have the pieces on the table and assembled before notifying the implanting physician to scrub for surgery.* ***B,*** *The simplified contrast injection system attached to the hub of the braided core of the SafeSheath-CSG Worley sheath (Pressure Products, Inc., San Pedro, Calif.). An intravascular J-tip guidewire is inserted into the braided core through the luer lock of the Y adapter. The same contrast injection system can be attached to the balloon for occlusive CS venography and to the Worley telescoping braided guides for target veins.*

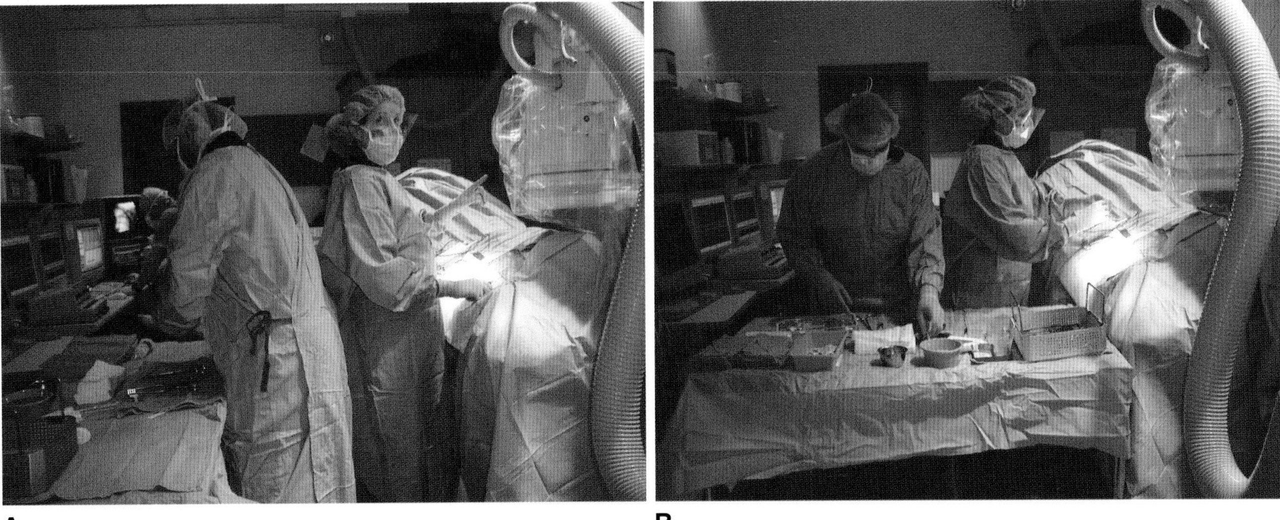

Figure 19-20. Positioning the instrument table during various stages of the implantation procedure. ***A,*** *The instrument table is in the traditional "backfield" position. With the table in this position, the assistant has access to the field when standing beside the operator. Procedures such as retraction for pocket formation and trimming suture are best accomplished with the table in this position. However, the long wires, sheaths, and guide either must be folded along the side of the patient; or if allowed to remain straight, they will project out perpendicular to the long axis of the patient and fall to the floor unless they are supported.* ***B,*** *The instrument table is perpendicular to the patient. As soon as the operator begins to obtain venous access for the left ventricular (LV) pacing lead, the instrument table is moved into a position perpendicular to the patient. The long wires, sheaths, and guides may thus be kept straight as they exit the body. The assistant works at the table beside the operator where he/she can assist with contrast injection, control the long guidewires, sheaths, and torque devices, and insert the pacing lead onto the wire as the procedure progresses. Ideally, the table would be at the same height as the patient's chest. Some centers use a Mayo stand for this purpose, but my colleagues and I value the additional table length over the ideal height. If the table is not turned perpendicular, the guides and sheaths kink near the hub as they are manipulated by the operator parallel to the patient's body. In addition, if wires, guides, and sheaths are draped along the patient's body, there is the constant risk that they will dislodge, fall to the side, and become contaminated. However, the perpendicular table position blocks the assistant's access to the field. The table must be returned to the standard "backfield" position when it is time to slice the guide and/or peel the sheath.*

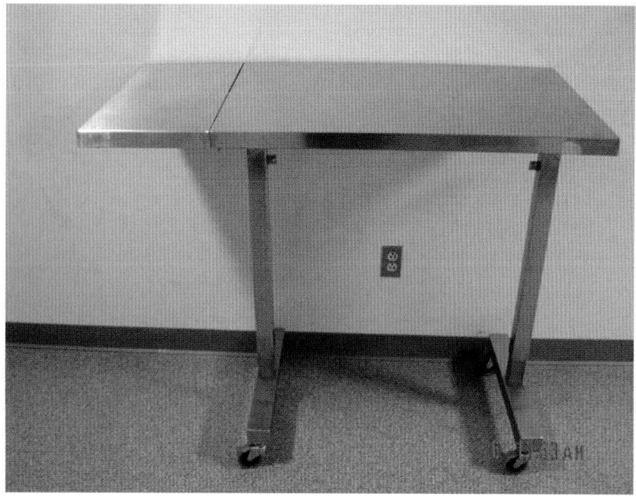

A

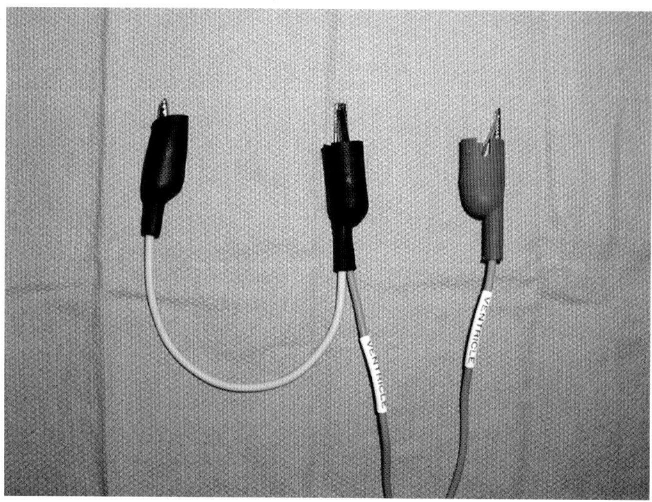

B

Figure 19-21. Custom-made equipment to facilitate implantation of the left ventricular (LV) pacing lead. ***A****, Custom-designed biventricular (BiV) implantation table. The importance my colleagues and I place on the perpendicular position of the table is exemplified by the time and energy we devoted to optimizing the table for the LV lead implantation phase of the procedure; we (1) moved the supporting legs of the table back 18 inches from one end and (2) added height adjustment to the table. When placed perpendicular to the patient, the legs of a standard table interfere with the position of the foot pedal for fluoroscopy as well as the operator's feet. In addition, the legs interfere with the table position when the radiograph tube is rotated for a right anterior oblique projection. Moving the supporting legs of the table back 18 inches from one end allows the table edge to approximate the patient without interfering with either radiography or the operator's feet. The height of the table is adjustable to ensure a smooth transition of catheters and wires from the patient to the table while the operator is working perpendicular to the patient (BiV position).* ***B****, Biventricular pacing cables. When determining LV and right ventricular (RV) pacing thresholds to a single cathode, it is time consuming and tedious to attach both anodes of the pacing leads to a single alligator clip. Something as simple as having a second anode alligator clip makes a tremendous difference to this phase of the procedure.*

leads, or subclavian stenosis restricts manipulation of the leads or sheath, the operator is handicapped for every subsequent step. The operator is not prepared for difficult anatomy in subsequent steps if the result of the first step is limiting. Further, if the initial basic venous access for the LV lead does not extend to the CS, the operator's options are immediately limited, and the risk of LV lead displacement at the end may be increased. The impact of initial venous access extends from start to finish of lead placement. The outcome of a poorly considered initial venous access is a good example of what can happen if one does not follow the "golden rule" of CRT implantation.

Preventing Restricted Catheter/Lead Movement

Separate Access for Each Lead

It is valuable to have separate access sites for each lead to reduce the interaction among the three leads. If it is possible to obtain only two access sites, the RV and RA leads should be placed through the same access site to minimize the potential for movement of either lead to displace the LV lead. When leads share the same access, friction between the two may result in the stable lead's being withdrawn by manipulation of the other lead. To help prevent the lead from being withdrawn, one should keep the stylet of the stable lead at the junction between the inferior vena (IVC) cava and superior vena cava (SVC) until manipulation of both leads is complete, even after the stable lead is tied down. Without a stylet, the stable lead can withdraw, even when tied to the muscle, by forming an S configuration within the subclavian distal to the tie-down, as shown in Figure 19-22.

Axillary versus Subclavian Access

With subclavian vein access, compression between the first rib and clavicle can restrict lead manipulation. In a non-BiV or an easy BiV implantation, restricted manipulation of the leads may be only a mild annoyance. However, precise manipulation is required, and the friction may make it impossible to place the LV lead. Axillary vein access ensures that lead manipulation will be unrestricted by compression between the clavicle and first rib. Axillary vein access also minimizes the risk of lead fractures and/or pneumothorax (Fig. 19-23).

Response to a Stenosis between the Axillary Vein and the Right Atrium

In patients with previously implanted leads, one or more stenotic areas may develop between the site of

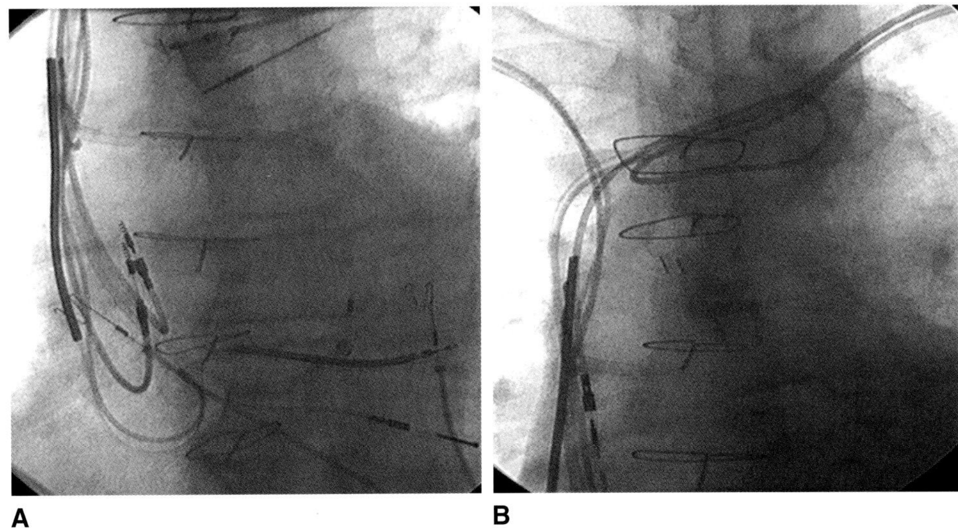

Figure 19-22. Friction between lead and guide pulls the lead back even though it is sewn down. ***A,*** The atrial lead is in place and secured to the muscle. ***B,*** The atrial lead is pulled back, creating a loop in the subclavian vein created by friction during manipulation of the other pacing leads, sheaths, and guides that share the same vein. After a lead is positioned and sewn down, it is prudent to reinsert a stylet into the superior vena cava–right atrium junction until manipulation of other sheaths, guides, and leads is complete.

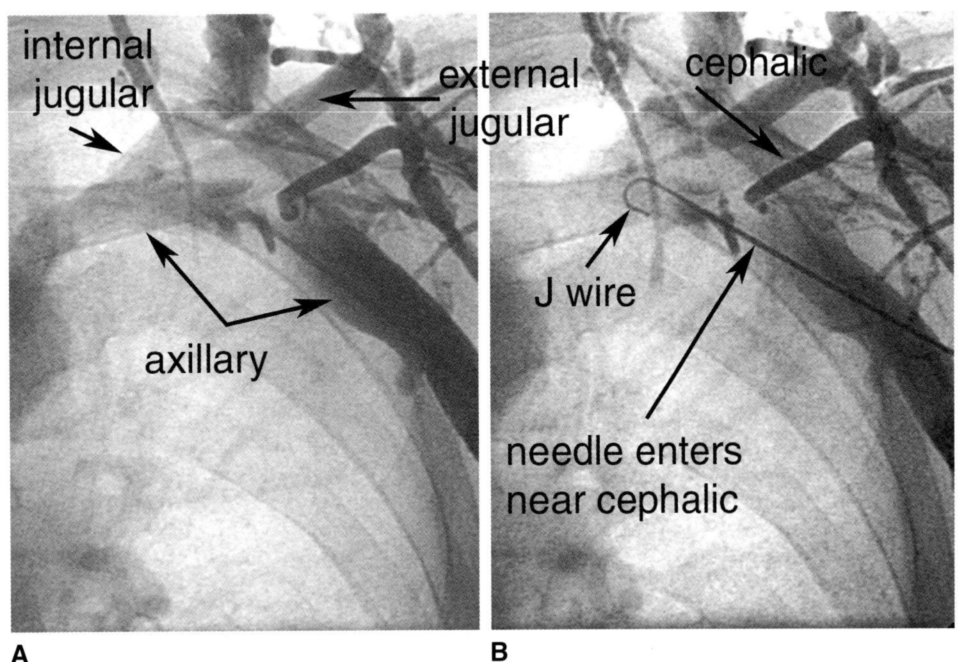

Figure 19-23. Axillary vein venogram before and after insertion of the 0.035-inch J-shaped retention wire. ***A,*** The anatomy of the venous system proximal to the brachiocephalic vein is well outlined with contrast material. ***B,*** The needle enters the axillary vein near the junction of the cephalic and axillary veins. The 0.035-inch J-wire is advanced from the axillary vein into the subclavian vein.

venous insertion and the RA (Fig. 19-24). Prior to the advent of LV lead placement, the response of the implanting physician to a subclavian stenosis was to advance progressively larger dilators until the introducer could be advanced. Dilator opening of a stenotic area, if possible, is always incomplete. The stenotic area continues to restrict manipulation. Furthermore, distal stenotic areas are not addressed. Venoplasty solves the problem (Fig. 19-25).

In patients with previously implanted leads, venoplasty may be required anywhere between the RA and the axillary vein. The lumen of the balloon must be large enough to accommodate the wire across the stenotic area (usually a 0.035-inch angled Glidewire

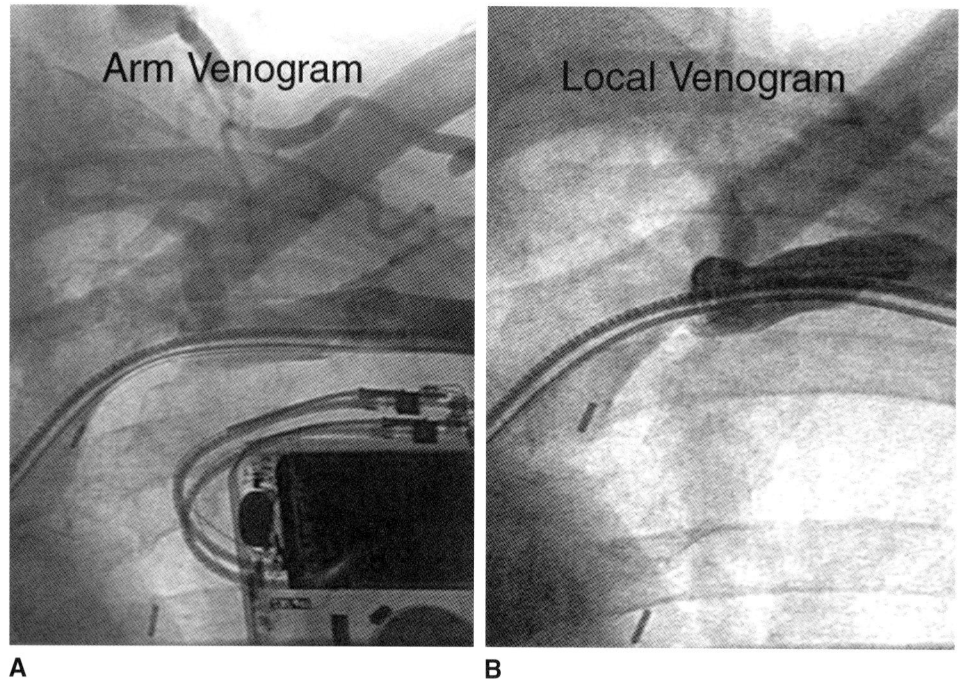

Figure 19-24. Arm and local venograms of a typical high-grade stenosis at the axillary vein–subclavian vein junction. ***A,*** *Fifteen to 20 mL of contrast material is injected into a vein in the distal left arm, revealing a stenosis at the junction of the axillary and subclavian veins.* ***B,*** *The contrast material is injected through a 5F sheath inserted in the axillary vein proximal to the stenosis. To create a flexible stable platform from which to approach the occlusion, one obtains venous access and inserts a 5F sheath percutaneously in the axillary vein as distal to the stenosis as possible. If venous access is too close to the occlusion, it will also be difficult to direct the wire to different potential routes through the stenosis.*

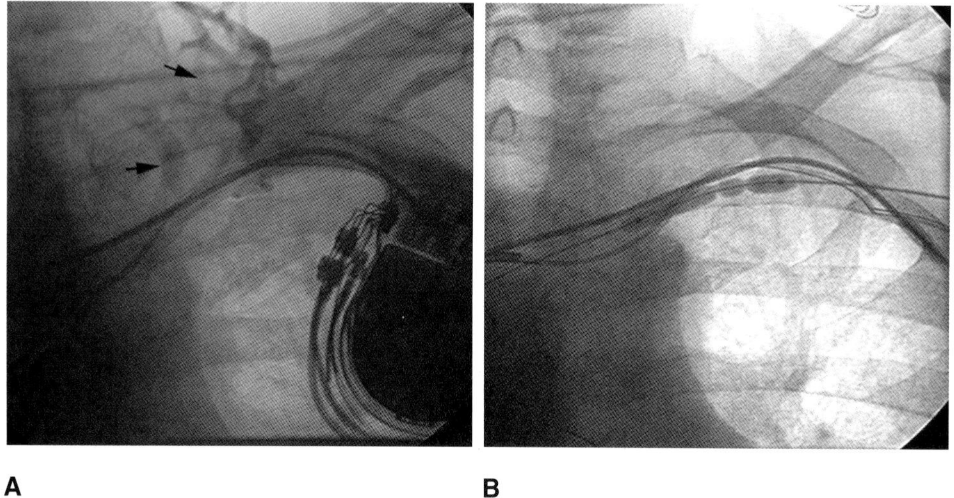

Figure 19-25. Dilation of a proximal subclavian vein occlusion. ***A,*** *Collateral vessels are seen* (arrows) *around the subclavian vein occlusion that developed in association with the leads of a previous implantable cardioverter-defibrillator (ICD).* ***B,*** *Despite what appeared to be a total occlusion, a 0.035-inch angled Glidewire (Terumo Medical Corporation, Somerset, NJ) crossed the occlusion and advanced through the heart into the pulmonary artery. A 6-mm-diameter, 4-cm-long balloon with a 0.038-inch wire lumen is across the occlusion and inflated to 15 atm, where two residual waists are seen. With inflation to 20 atm, both waists were eliminated.*

[Terumo Medical Corporation, Somerset, NJ]). In addition, the inflated diameter of the balloon must be large enough for the 9F sheath (9F ID/11F OD) to pass freely after dilation (6 mm). Finally, the balloon must be long enough to dilate from the RA to the axillary vein with three to five inflations (4 cm). Initially, the balloon is inflated to the "nominal pressure" (listed on the package). At the nominal pressure, the balloon reaches the labeled diameter. The pressure is then increased until the "waist" (the indentation in the balloon created by the obstruction) opens or the balloon bursts. A balloon typically used by interventional radiologists is the PowerFlex P3, which is 6 mm × 4 cm with a 0.038-inch lumen (Cordis, Miami, Fla. [a division of Telectronics, St. Jude Medical, Sylmar, Calif.]). If the stenosis does not submit to the initial balloon, an ultra-noncompliant (aramid fiber [Kevlar]), high-pressure balloon (Conquest PTA Dilatation Catheter [Bard Peripheral Vascular, Inc., Tempe, Ariz.] or equivalent) may be used. Once the proximal stenosis is dilated, the balloon is advanced to the RA-SVC junction and inflated to nominal pressures from the RA back to the axillary vein in an overlapping manner. In this way, any occult distal stenotic areas are revealed and opened (Fig. 19-26).

Which Balloons Are Used for Subclavian Vein Venoplasty?

Why not use coronary balloons for subclavian vein venoplasty? We switched from coronary balloons to interventional radiology balloons for several reasons, including the diameter of the access wire and the diameter and length of the balloons available. Surprisingly, the diameter of the tracking wire is a major consideration. Interventional radiology balloons track over wires 0.038 inch or less in diameter, whereas coronary balloons track over wires 0.018 inch or less. In the process of dealing with stenotic veins in one patient, we found that we had a Glidewire across the lesion. To use a coronary balloon, we were faced with downsizing to a 0.014-inch angioplasty wire. In addition, it is common to find an area of narrowing that is longer than most coronary balloons. The lengths of balloons available for interventional radiology are much more suitable as well. We have had experience in 40 cases using a 6 mm × 4 cm balloon inflated to 15 atm (Fig. 19-27).

A coronary balloon may be necessary when the only wire to cross the occlusion is 0.014-inch or 0.018-inch angioplasty wire. The HI-TORQUE CROSS-IT 300XT (Guidant, Boston Scientific, Natick, Mass.) and the 0.014-inch Crosswire (Terumo Medical) are specifically designed to cross total coronary occlusions. They may be used to cross a subclavian occlusion when the 0.035-inch wire will not advance. When the only wire that will cross the lesion is a 0.014-inch, we start with a 2- to 3-mm coronary balloon. Once the stenosis is dilated with the coronary balloon, the peripheral balloon may track over the 0.014-inch wire or it may be necessary to advance a 4F dilator or a Micro Guide Catheter (LuMend, Inc., Redwood City, Calif.) across the residual stenosis and exchange it for a 0.035-inch Amplatz Extra Stiff Wire Guide (Cook Vascular, Inc., Leechburg, Penna.). The 6 mm × 4 cm interventional balloon is then tracked over the 0.035-inch wire.

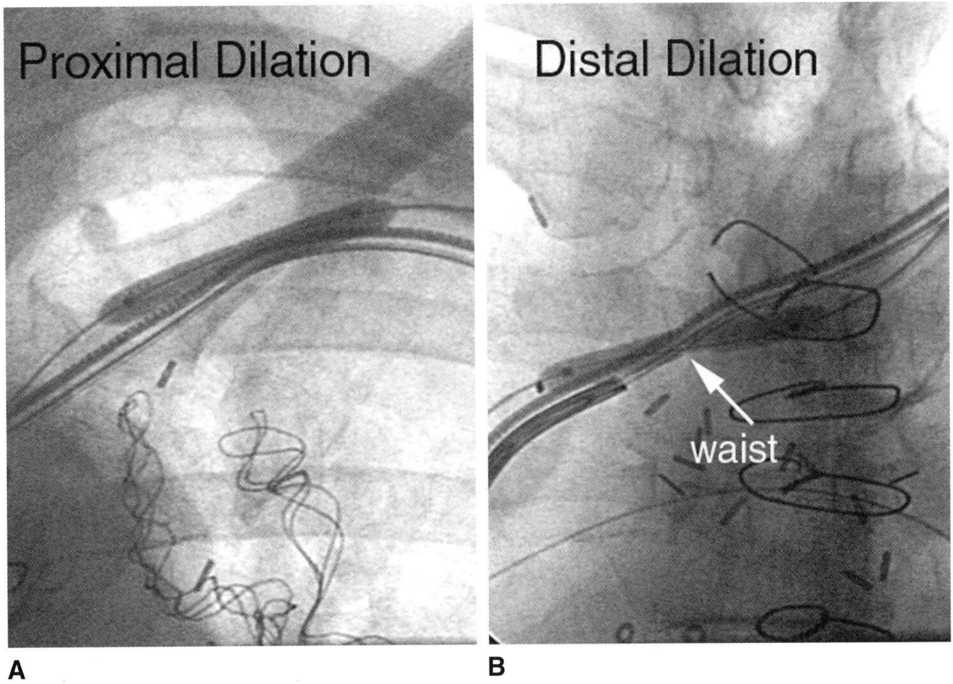

Figure 19-26. Dilation of both proximal and distal subtotal venous occlusions encountered in the same patient. ***A,*** *The balloon is inflated at the site of the proximal occlusion to 15 atm with elimination of the waist and proximal stenosis.* ***B,*** *The balloon is advanced to the junction of the superior vena cava and the brachiocephalic vein and inflated, demonstrating a waist in the balloon in the second stenotic location.*

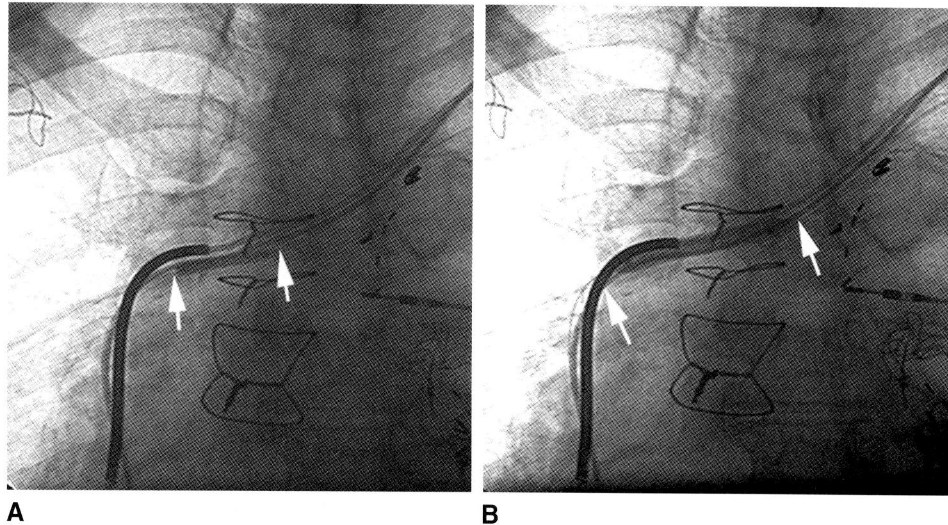

Figure 19-27. Comparison of a "long" coronary balloon to a "peripheral" balloon for dilation of an occlusion at the junction of the brachiocephalic vein and the superior vena cava. ***A,*** *The proximal vein is open, but the distal vein near the right atrium (RA) appears to be totally occluded.* ***B,*** *A wire designed to cross total occlusions is advanced into the RA. A short balloon is inflated at the site of occlusion.*

In summary, coronary balloons are too short, their diameters too small, and their lumens too narrow for the typical 0.035-inch access wire (see Fig. 19-26). Coronary balloons are used only when a 0.014- or 0.018-inch wire is the only one that will cross the occlusion. As soon as the stenosis is partially dilated, the 0.014- or 0.018-inch wire is replaced with a 0.035-inch wire (Fig. 19-28).

Short Balloons for Distal Stenosis at the Superior Vena Cava–Brachiocephalic Vein Junction

As previously noted, many patients with a proximal stenosis also have a second distal stenosis, as shown in Figure 19-26. Progressive sheath dilation of the proximal occlusion leaves the distal stenosis untouched, further restricting lead manipulation. In some patients, only a distal occlusion is encountered. Short balloons (<20 mm) are usually chosen for an occlusion on a sharp bend. Figure 19-29 shows a distal-only occlusion on a sharp bend dilated with a short balloon at multiple sites.

Kevlar Balloons for Resistant Stenosis

In some patients, the stenosis is particularly resistant to dilation, requiring special balloons. An example is illustrated in Figure 19-30. The patient experienced worsening CHF after receiving a dual-chamber defibrillator and needed ventricular pacing support. The wire for the sheath would not advance from the site of axillary access. The venogram (see Fig. 19-26) revealed a high-grade stenosis in the subclavian vein. A polytetrafluoroethylene (Teflon)–coated, 0.035-inch angled Glidewire was manipulated across the stenosis, but the sheath would not advance. The stenosis was dilated with a 6 mm × 4 cm balloon delivered over the Glidewire. Figure 19-30A demonstrates the balloon dilated at 16 atm; at 20 atm, the balloon ruptured without eliminating the stenosis. A Kevlar balloon (Conquest) was then advanced across the occlusion. Once the second balloon was inflated to 22 atm, the stenosis was relieved, and the 9F sheath (9F ID/11F OD) passed easily.

"Complications" of Subclavian–Brachiocephalic Venoplasty

Despite our initial concerns, we find balloon dilation of venous structures remarkably safe. In the case of dilating at the site of stenosis associated with existing leads, concern with safety is understandable. Because the stenosis and leads are surrounded by fibrous tissue, it is fibrous tissue, not a vein, that is being dilated. In addition, one must consider the relative trauma inflicted by extraction of a lead with a 14F to 16F laser sheath that cuts through the tissue surrounding the lead. By comparison, balloon venoplasty in the same area is much less traumatic. We have seen contrast staining related to our attempts to manipulate a wire through the stenosis, but our patients have experienced no clinically significant complications (Fig. 19-31). When contrast staining occurs, we continue the procedure and perform venoplasty as long as we can get the wire across the stenosis.

Total Occlusion (No Wire Will Cross the Occlusion)

McCotter and coworkers[27] reported successfully crossing chronic total occlusions of the subclavian vein with a guidewire followed by venoplasty or dilation. In some patients, however, the total occlusion cannot be crossed with a 0.035-inch Glidewire or even with a 0.014-inch

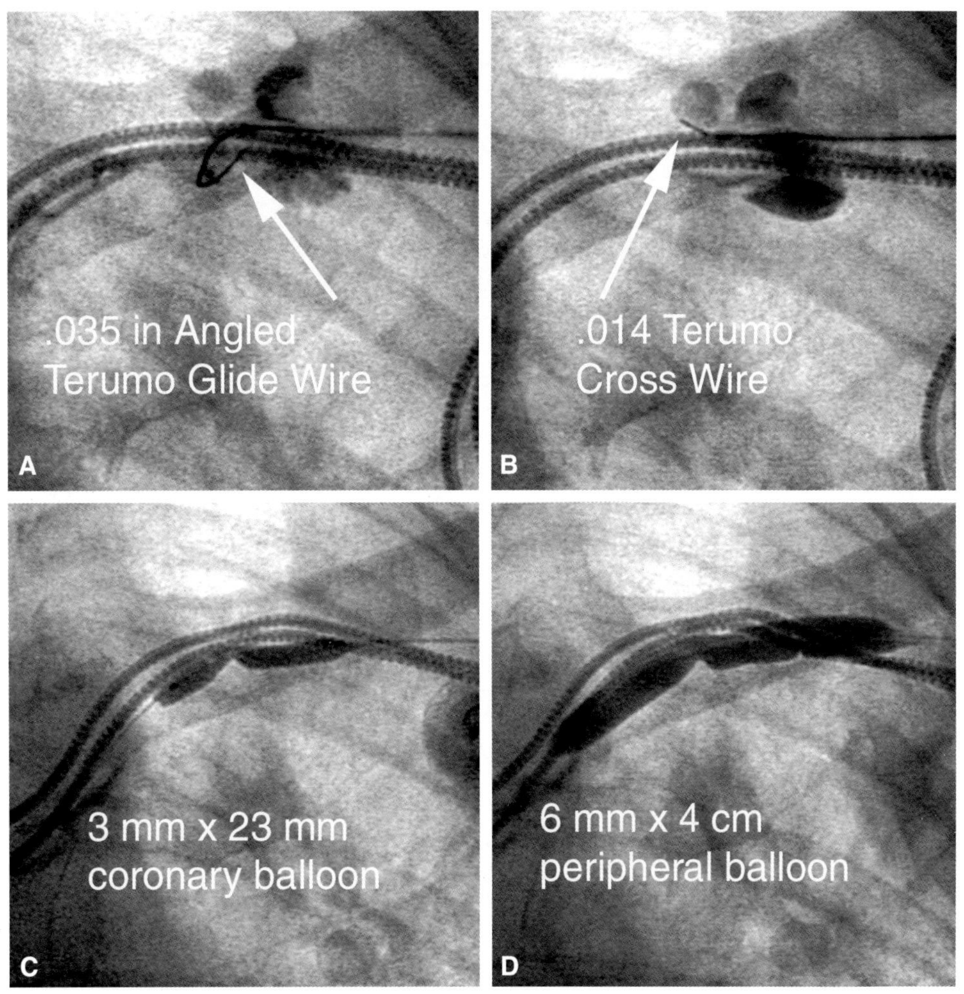

*Figure 19-28. Opening of a totally occluded subclavian vein with a 0.014-inch Terumo Crosswire (Terumo Medical Corporation, Somerset, NJ). **A,** The 0.035-inch angled Glidewire (Terumo Medical) will not cross the total occlusion. **B,** The 0.014-inch Crosswire is used to cross the total occlusion. **C,** A coronary balloon is inflated at the site of occlusion. **D,** The 6-mm-diameter, 4-cm-long peripheral balloon with an 0.038-inch lumen is advanced over the 0.014-inch Crosswire and inflated.*

wire specifically designed to cross total occlusions (e.g., Crosswire, CROSS-IT 300XT). In these cases, the options are (1) lead extraction with preservation of the lumen, (2) abandonment of the site and transfer to the other side, and (3) opening of the total occlusion. Several devices for crossing total occlusions are available. The Frontrunner CTO Catheter (LuMend) is a device designed for microdissection through total occlusions in interventional radiology (Fig. 19-32). For short total venous occlusions, the Frontrunner is very successful in crossing the occlusion (Fig. 19-33).[28] However, long total occlusions can require an extensive procedure. In several of our cases, the catheter has been beyond the total occlusion in the fibrous tissue surrounding the lead, and we have not been able to redirect the catheter back into the lumen even with the addition of the Outback Re-Entry Catheter (LuMend) (Figs. 19-33 through 19-35).

The inability to reenter the true lumen is addressed with the OutBack Re-Entry Catheter (Fig. 19-36). The OutBack is an open-lumen catheter with a curved, extendable, retractable 21-gauge needle on the distal end. The Outback with needle retracted is advanced through the channel created by the Frontrunner catheter, until the tip is in the fibrous tissue outside the distal true lumen. The needle is advanced with the tip angled toward the true lumen. A 0.014-inch guidewire is then advanced into the distal true lumen, the OutBack catheter is withdrawn over the wire, and venoplasty is performed.

Venous Access for the Left Ventricular Lead

Typically, short peel-away sheaths are used to access the venous circulation for insertion of leads in the RA and RV. However, starting with a short peel-away sheath to access the venous circulation for insertion of the LV lead severely limits the options available to the operator if difficult anatomy is encountered. That is, if the tip of the 9F peel-away sheath ends in the CS, a 9F

Text continued on p. 683

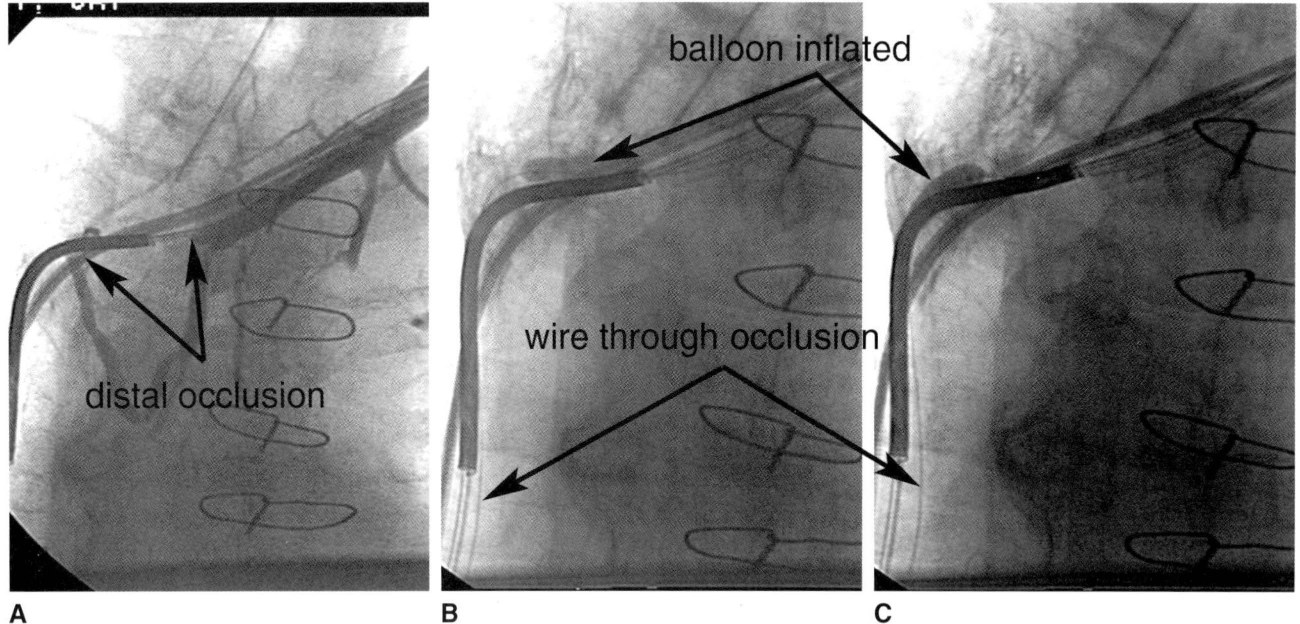

Figure 19-29. *Dilation of a total occlusion on a bend with short balloons.* ***A,*** *The proximal subclavian vein is open, but the distal vein at the junction with the superior vena cava (SVC) is totally occluded. Collateral vessels have developed around the occlusion.* ***B,*** *Despite what appears to be chronic total occlusion, an angioplasty wire designed to cross total arterial occlusions is successfully advanced into the right atrium. A short (23-mm) balloon is inflated at the site of occlusion.* ***C,*** *The short balloon is again inflated, this time more distally. The short balloon is chosen because the occlusion occurs on a bend. Contrast material used to facilitate crossing of the total occlusion can be seen staining the tissues at the site of previous occlusion. No adverse clinical event occurred despite the contrast stain.*

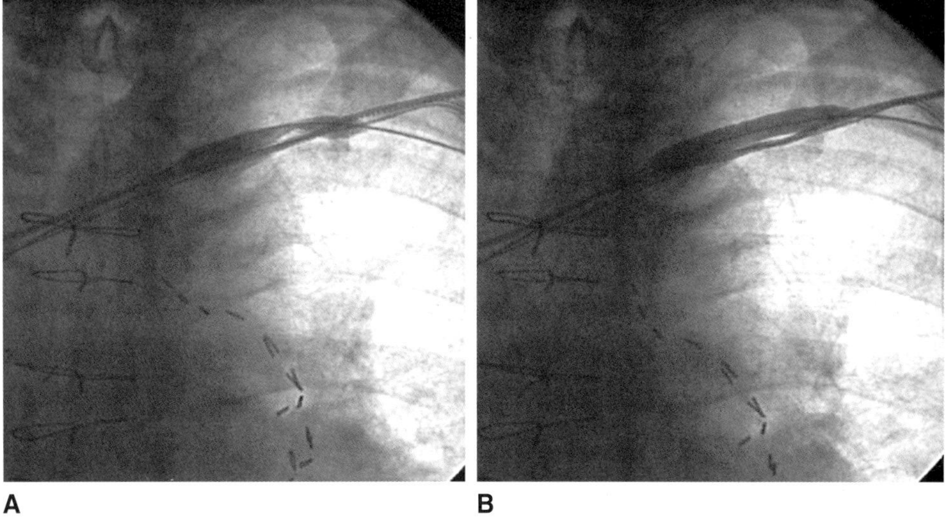

Figure 19-30. *Venoplasty of a stenotic subclavian vein that required an aramid fiber (Kevlar) balloon to eliminate the waist.* ***A,*** *The subclavian vein stenosis can be seen at the site of the patient's previously implanted defibrillator leads. Collateral filling can be seen distal to the stenosis (arrows).* ***B,*** *A The 6-mm-diameter, 4-cm-long peripheral balloon is inflated at the site of stenosis. Despite the stenosis seen in* ***A,*** *it was possible to pass a 0.0350-inch angled Glidewire (Terumo Medical Corporation, Somerset, NJ) across the stenosis. The balloon was then advanced over the Glidewire and inflated to 16 atm, relieving the stenosis and allowing for easy passage of a 9F sheath (9F ID/11F OD). Subsequent manipulation of pacing leads in the coronary sinus was not hindered by the stenosis.*

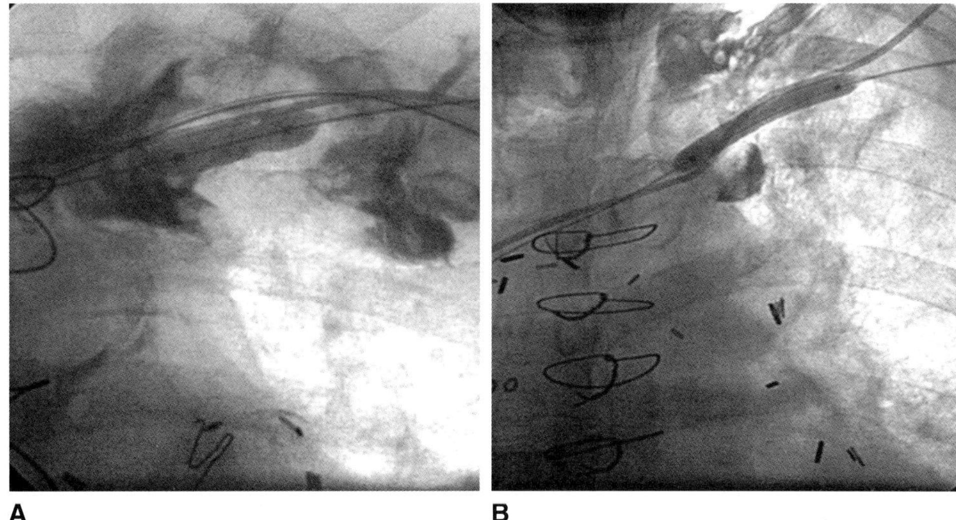

Figure 19-31. Extensive "stains" created with injection of contrast material during manipulation of wires to cross total occlusions seen at the time of subclavian venoplasty. ***A,*** *An extensive contrast stain can be seen in the tissue surrounding the subclavian occlusion. The stain developed as contrast material was injected to facilitate advancing the wire across the occlusion.* ***B,*** *A similar extensive contrast stain can be seen in the tissue surrounding the subclavian occlusion. Like that shown in* ***A,*** *The stain in* ***B*** *developed as contrast material was injected to facilitate advancing the wire across the occlusion. In neither case did the contrast stain have any clinical effect.*

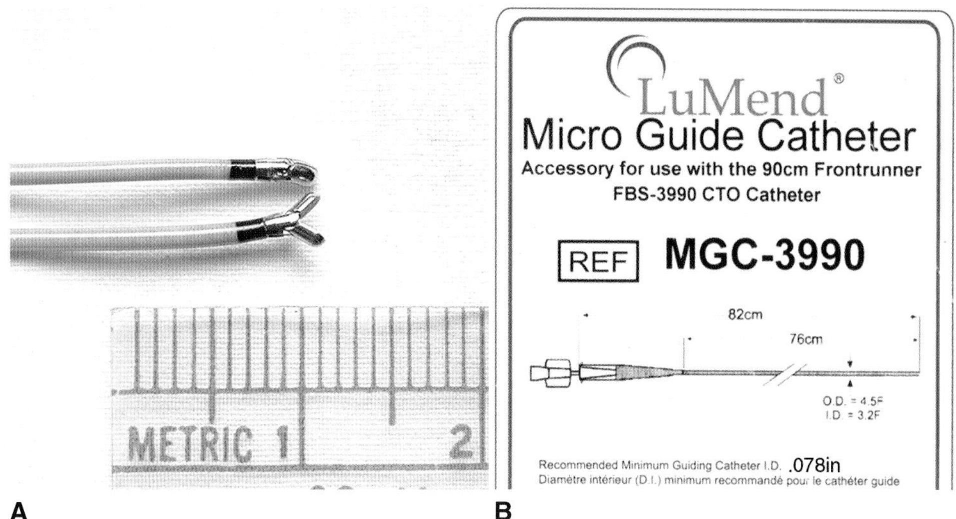

Figure 19-32. Frontrunner CTO Catheter, a blunt microdissection system (LuMend, Inc., Redwood City, Calif.). ***A,*** *The Frontrunner with jaws closed (top) and open (bottom). The ruler provides a reference for the size of the device.* ***B,*** *The Micro Guide Catheter through which the Frontrunner is passed. The lumen of the Micro Guide easily tracks over a 0.014-inch guidewire, but the lumen is large enough to accommodate two 0.014-inch guidewires. The Micro Guide is also very useful alone in other phases of the left ventricular (LV) lead implantation procedure. For example, when a single 0.014-inch guidewire passes through an occlusion or a tortuous segment, the wire may be bent or one may need to pass a second wire through the occlusion. The Micro Guide is advanced over the wire until the radiopaque tip can be seen beyond the stenotic or tortuous segment. Once the tip of the Micro Guide is beyond the difficult section, the damaged wire can be easily exchanged for a new wire and/or a second wire added without having to cross through the stenotic or tortuous segment. The second wire advanced distally into the target vein can serve either as a "buddy wire" (see Figs. 19-202 and 19-203) or as a "side-wire" to facilitate elimination of a resistant stenosis (see Fig. 19-216).*

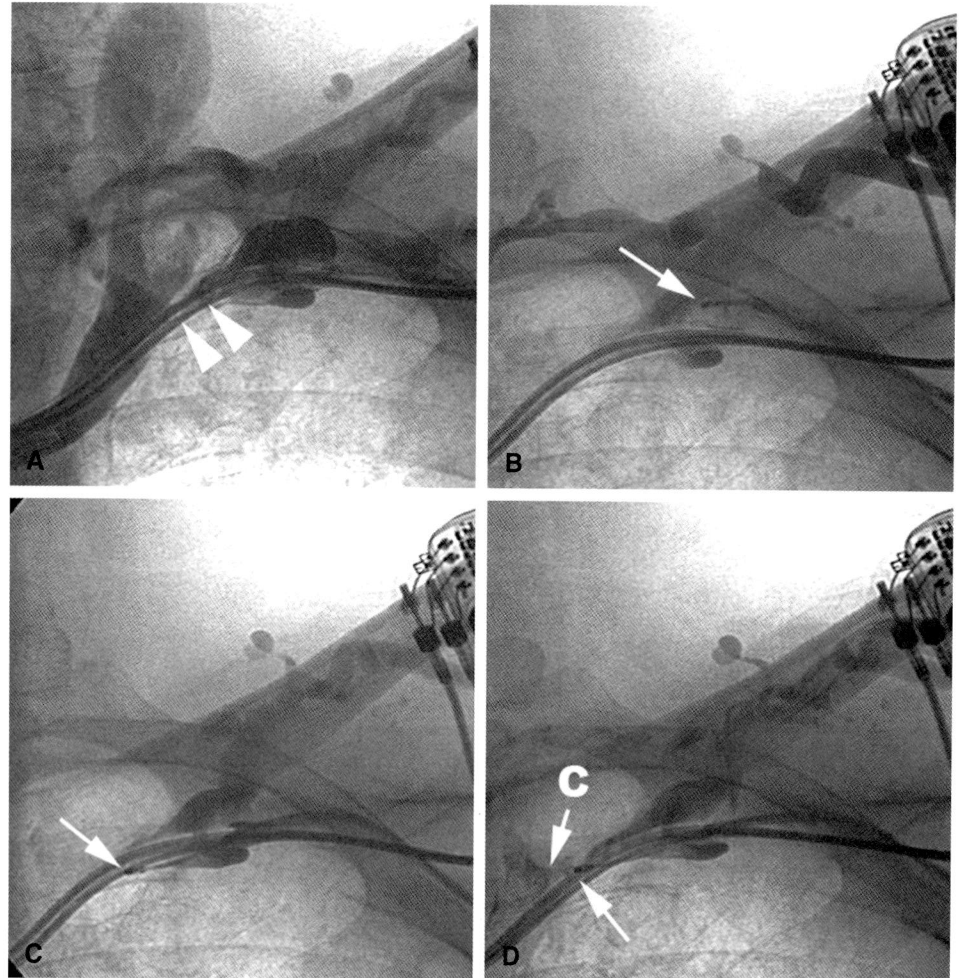

Figure 19-33. Frontrunner CTO Catheter, a blunt microdissection system (LuMend, Inc., Redwood City, Calif.), successfully crosses a total occlusion. ***A,*** *The length of the total occlusion (between the two arrowheads) is short (3 to 5 mm).* ***B,*** *When the Frontrunner is advanced through the 6F sheath in the proximal axillary vein, it tends to be directed superior to the interface between the pacing leads and the occlusion.* ***C,*** *A short (65-cm) 6F multipurpose guide is advanced through the 6F sheath to direct the Frontrunner to the occlusion adjacent to the pacing leads.* ***D,*** *The Frontrunner (arrow) is across the lesion in the vein which is filled with contrast (C-arrow). The Micro Guide catheter (LuMend) is then advanced over the Frontrunner into the venous lumen, the Frontrunner is removed, a wire is advanced through the Frontrunner into the vein, and the Micro Guide is removed. Venoplasty is then performed.*

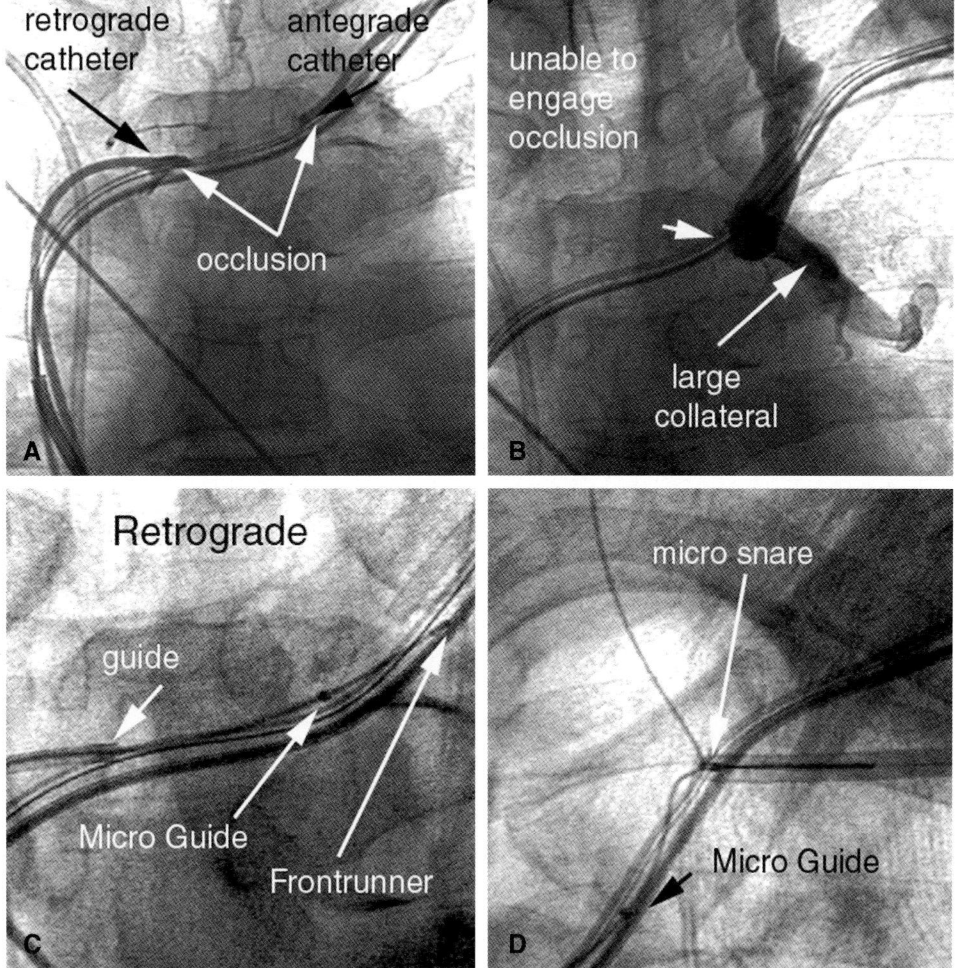

*Figure 19-34. Retrograde microdissection of a long total occlusion. **A,** Both retrograde and antegrade catheters define the occlusion, which extends from the subclavian vein to the superior vena cava. **B,** Attempts to engage the occlusion are unsuccessful. Despite the use of various guide shapes, the Frontrunner CTO Catheter (LuMend, Inc., Redwood City, Calif.) repeatedly went into the collateral vein. **C,** Microdissection is successful in reaching the level of the open vein. However, on the first attempt, the Frontrunner will not reenter the lumen. On the second try, starting at the inferior vena cava, the lumen of the vein is entered. The Micro Guide catheter through which the Frontrunner passes is advanced into the true lumen proximally. **D,** A microsnare is advanced through the sheath in the proximal vein. The wire originating in the femoral vein is snared into the sheath, providing access to the heart for lead placement.*

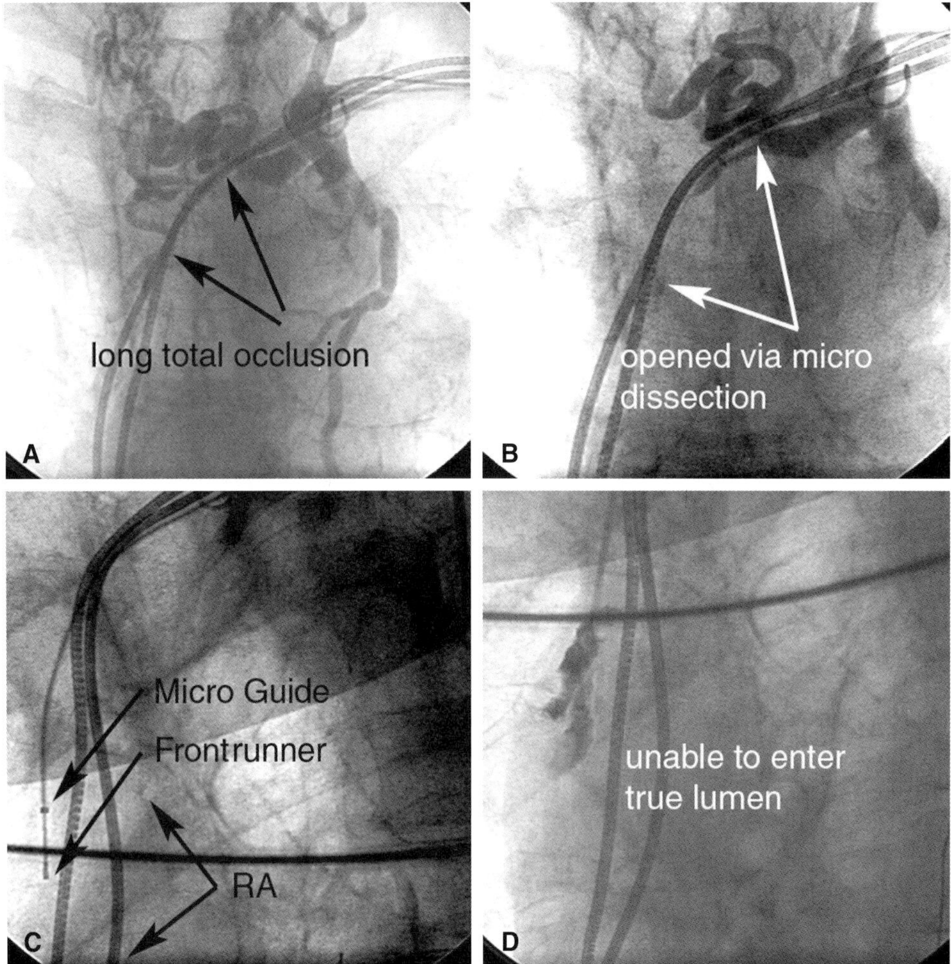

Figure 19-35. *Frontrunner CTO Catheter, a blunt microdissection system (LuMend, Inc., Redwood, Calif.), fails to reenter the true lumen despite successful microdissection beyond the occlusion.* ***A,*** *The long total occlusion from the brachiocephalic vein to the superior vena cava (SVC) with extensive collateral vessels is shown.* ***B,*** *The long total occlusion is successfully crossed via antegrade microdissection along the inner curve of the leads. However, the Frontrunner does not cross into the true lumen, but remains in the fibrous tissue surrounding the pacing leads.* ***C,*** *The Frontrunner and Micro Guide (LuMend) catheters are again advanced beyond the total occlusion, this time along the outer curve of the lead, but remain in the fibrous tissue surrounding the pacing leads.* ***D****, Contrast material injected into the Micro Guide catheter shows that it is in the tissues outside the SVC. Attempts to direct the Frontrunner into the true lumen of the SVC are unsuccessful. The contrast staining had no clinical impact.*

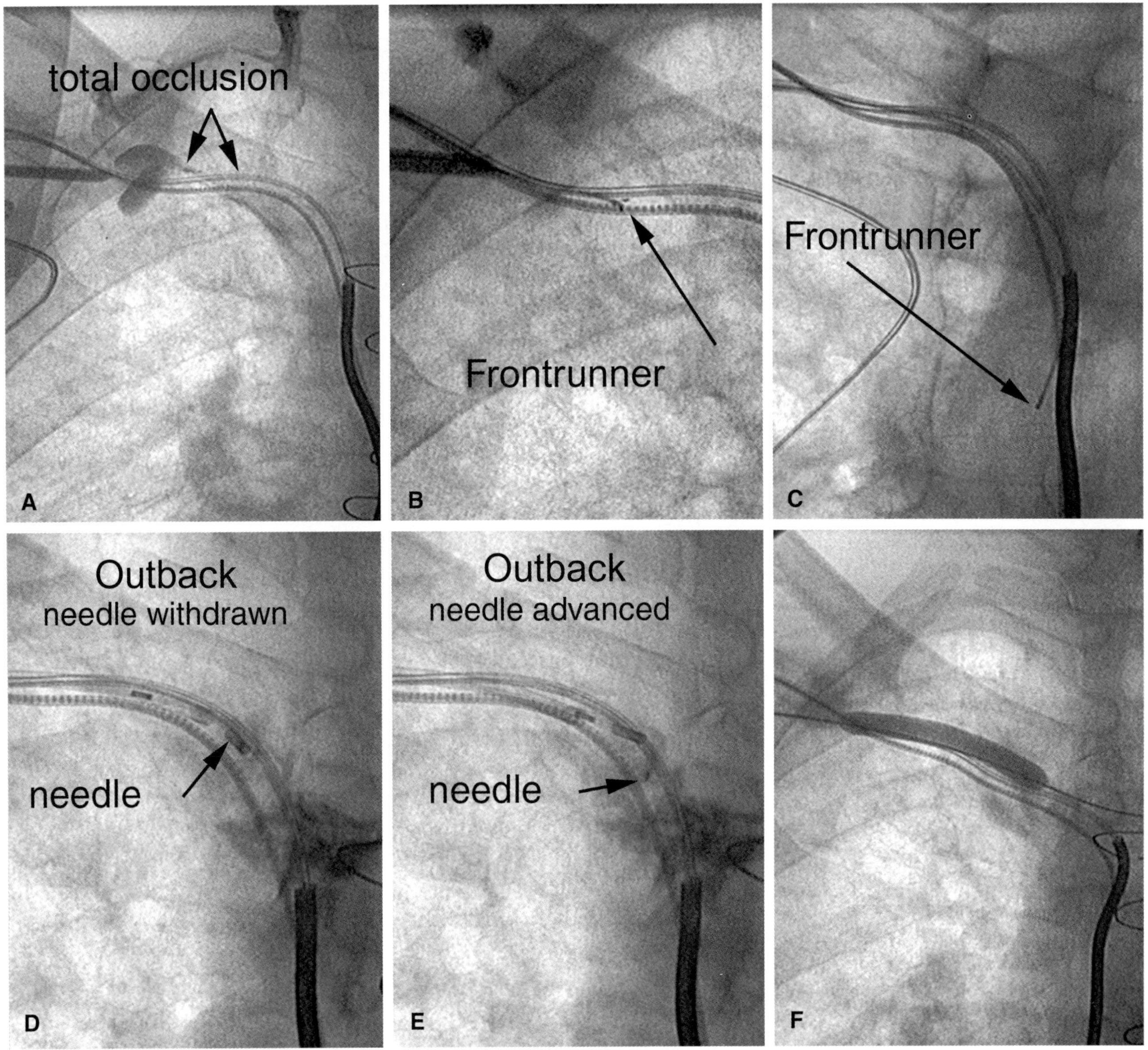

Figure 19-36. Outback Re-Entry Catheter (LuMend, Inc., Redwood City, Calif.) used to reenter the distal true lumen. ***A,*** *The short total occlusion with proximal and distal true lumen* (arrows). ***B,*** *The jaws of the Frontrunner CTO Catheter are open in the proximal portion of the occlusion.* ***C,*** *The Frontrunner and Micro Guide (LuMend) catheters will not reenter the true lumen from track created in the fibrous tissue created by microdissection well beyond the distal true lumen.* ***D,*** *The Outback Re-Entry catheter with needle retracted is advanced to the proximal portion of the distal true lumen.* ***E,*** *The curved hollow needle is advanced into the true lumen, and a 0.014-inch guidewire into the distal true lumen.* ***F,*** *Final venoplasty is performed with an interventional radiology 6-mm-diameter, 4-cm-long balloon over a 0.035-inch Amplatz wire; predilation was performed with a 3-mm-diameter, 23-mm-long coronary balloon over the 0.014-inch guidewire, which was then changed for the 0.035-inch wire using the Micro Guide catheter.*

introducer with a 7F lumen specifically shaped to cannulate target veins can be inserted directly into the CS. However, if the same 9F sheath ends in the subclavian vein, the 8F or 9F introducer must be shaped to cannulate the CS, which is usually not suitable to directly cannulate the target vein. Further, as discussed later, peeling away a long sheath is more familiar and less likely to displace the LV lead than cutting away a guide as the last step. Long peel-away sheaths are shown in Figures 19-37 through 19-39.

The long sheath offers the advantage of greater support during LV lead placement (see Fig. 19-39). When a guide is placed through the long sheath, the sheath supports the LV lead during cutting. In addition, CS access is maintained after the guide is removed, in case the lead is unstable or paces the phrenic nerve and must be replaced or repositioned.

The operator must remain aware that peel-away sheaths kink at sharp turns unless they are preshaped to fit the anatomy.

Cutting versus Peeling

Peeling is a familiar, easy procedure that can be performed in a stable, controlled manner. With a long sheath in place in the CS, the last step of lead placement is to peel the sheath away once the lead is positioned.

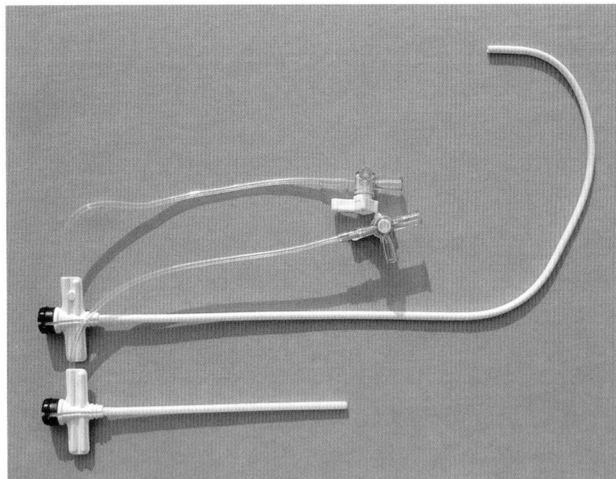

Figure 19-37. Straight short (bottom) *and anatomically shaped long* (top) *9F sheaths. The straight short sheath is the sheath usually used for access to the venous circulation to place leads in the right heart. When in place, the tip of the sheath is in the proximal brachiocephalic vein, severely limiting the options open to the operator when used for left ventricular (LV) lead venous access. The anatomically shaped, long, 9F peel-away sheath is designed for venous access for the LV lead, coronary sinus cannulation (when used with the braided core), a conduit for preshaped guides (lateral vein introducers [LVIs]) designed for target vein cannulation and delivery of the LV pacing lead to the target vein.*

When a short sheath is used for LV lead venous access, the last step of lead placement is to remove the CS guide after the lead is positioned. The steel mesh in the wall of the guide must be cut to allow removal of the guide. Cutting is unfamiliar to most implanting physicians, who find it clumsy and difficult. Many physicians have displaced leads while cutting. If one does not *start* with a long preformed peel-away sheath as the venous access for the LV lead, the risk of lead displacement at the *end* is increased. This issue is covered in detail in the section on removing the guide sheath.

Long peel-away sheaths are not routinely used for initial LV lead venous access for the following two reasons:

1. Peel-away sheaths do not have the torque control required for reliable CS cannulation. Metal braid added to the walls of catheters provides the necessary torque control but cannot be peeled. The solution is to place a braided catheter inside a long peel-away sheath to provide the torque control for CS cannulation. Once the peel-away

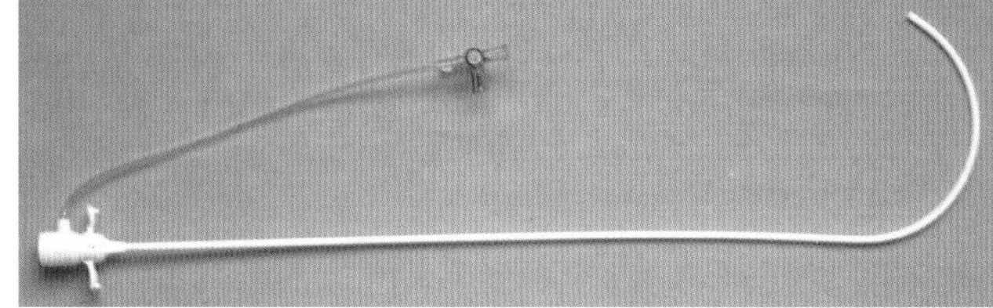

Figure 19-38. An 8F long sheath designed for venous access for the left ventricular (LV) lead, coronary sinus cannulation, and delivery of the LV pacing lead to the target vein.

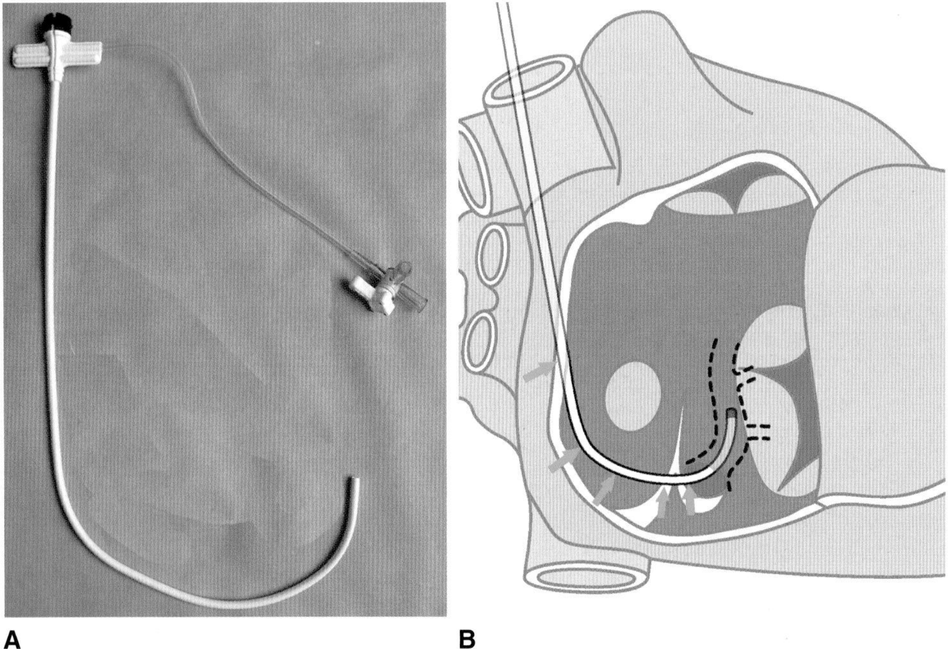

Figure 19-39. The properly curved sheath in the coronary sinus provides support by resting on the eustachian ridge, floor of the right atrium (RA), and superior vena cava (SVC). ***A,*** *The 9F sheath designed for left ventricular (LV) lead venous access.* ***B,*** *The properly curved sheath in the coronary sinus provides support by resting on the eustachian ridge, floor of the RA, and SVC* (arrows).

sheath is in the CS, the braided catheter is removed, leaving the peel-away sheath in place. This issue is covered in more detail in the section on CS cannulation.

2. Straight peel-away sheaths kink at sharp bends. Stainless steel braid in the walls of the catheter reduces kinking but renders it nonpeelable. The problem of kinking is resolved by bending the sheath at the time of manufacture in anticipation of sharp turns in the anatomy—such sheaths are called anatomically shaped.

Cannulation of the Coronary Sinus

Al-Khadra[29] points out that failure to cannulate the CS continues to contribute significantly to failure of LV lead implantation. Multiple approaches to aid in CS cannulation have been reported.[30] However, even with *successful* cannulation of the CS, using an ill-considered catheter contributes significantly to failure of LV lead implantation because it (1) lacks support, (2) displaces the lead as it is removed, and (3) is too small to deliver anything but the pacing lead. The catheter to be used for CS cannulation should be chosen before venous access is begun. One should keep in mind that the catheter chosen not only must be capable of cannulating the CS but, once in the CS, also must allow one to be prepared for the most difficult possible anatomy in subsequent steps. For example, there is little benefit cannulating the CS with a catheter that is too small to deliver a pacing lead. If the catheter cannulating the CS is only large enough to accommodate the pacing lead, one's options are limited. To be optimally prepared, venous access for the LV lead must extend to the CS rather than ending in the brachiocephalic vein. A 9F sheath connecting the pocket to the mid-CS rather than ending in the subclavian vein provides the most options for dealing with difficult anatomy. If the 9F sheath ends before the mid-CS, one loses (1) the convenience of direct access to the CS, (2) the safety of peeling rather than cutting as the last step in the procedure, (3) the added support provided by the sheath, and (4) the option of using a third-generation telescoping catheter capable of direct delivery of larger, more stable pacing leads.

Although placing a catheter in the CS is usually easy in patients with supraventricular tachycardia (SVT), it can be quite difficult in patients with CHF who present for CRT. Use of contrast material greatly reduces the mean time to CS cannulation. When contrast material is used, cannulation of the CS becomes a two-step process, (1) locating the CS os and (2) advancing the sheath or guide into the CS.

Find the Coronary Sinus Os

Whether or not contrast material is used, it is important to understand the anatomy surrounding the CS and the effect of torque on a catheter in the area of the CS os.

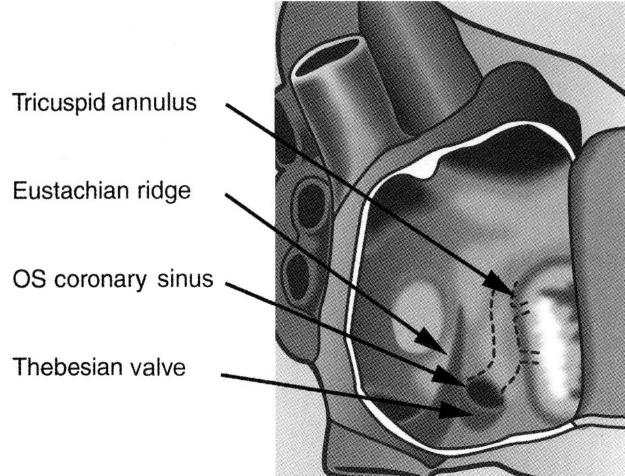

Figure 19-40. Anatomy of the structures surrounding the coronary sinus os. The eustachian ridge protrudes into the right atrium from the posterior wall of the atrium. The ridge is most prominent inferiorly near the inferior vena cava. As the coronary sinus is approached from the right atrium, the os is located behind the eustachian ridge The thebesian valve protrudes from the posterior wall of the right atrium and forms the inferior boundary of the os. The posterior inferior tricuspid annulus forms the boundary of the os on the right.

Anatomy of the Coronary Sinus Os

Successful location of the CS os is facilitated by a complete understanding of the anatomy. In Figure 19-40, the structures that affect locating the os are demonstrated. The key to easy, rapid location of the CS os is using the eustachian ridge and thebesian valve to direct the catheter toward (not away from) the os. In Figure 19-41A, it is clear that a catheter approaching the CS os along the posterior wall of the right atrium (RA) will be deflected away from the os by the eustachian ridge. When one approaches the CS from below (see Fig. 19-41B), catheter entrance is blocked by the thebesian valve.

An examination of the anatomy explains why some physicians find femoral CS cannulation easier. When one is cannulating the CS from below, the catheter approaches the os as illustrated in Figure 19-42A. The curve of the catheter reaches over the eustachian ridge, approaching the os from above. When done properly, femoral CS cannulation uses the eustachian ridge and thebesian valve to direct the tip into the os.

Similarly, if one approaches the CS os from the posterior superior tricuspid annulus (see Fig. 19-42B), the eustachian ridge and thebesian valve direct the catheter tip into the os. A properly shaped catheter can be made to approach the CS os from the posterior superior tricuspid annulus inferiorly toward the RA to use the eustachian ridge and thebesian valve to guide the tip of the catheter toward the os.

Directing a Catheter into the Coronary Sinus from Above

As shown in Figure 19-42, it is easier to enter the CS os from the posterior superior tricuspid annulus with use

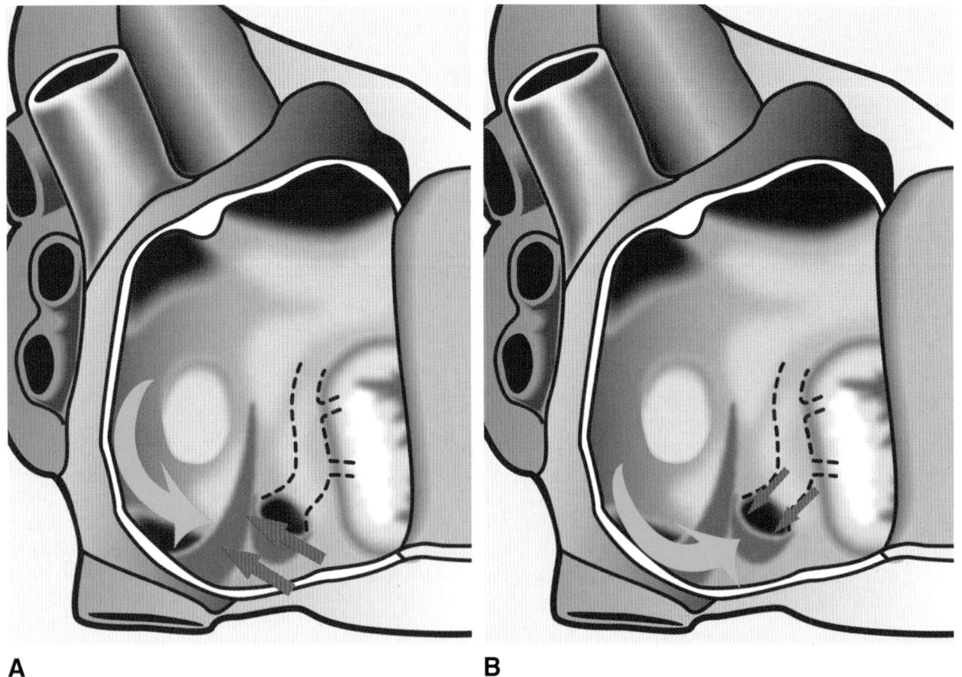

Figure 19-41. Eustachian ridge and thebesian valve inhibit coronary sinus (CS) cannulation. ***A,*** *The eustachian ridge* (small arrows) *blocks entrance to the CS os as it is approached from the atrium along the posterior wall* (large arrow). ***B,*** *The thebesian valve* (small arrows) *blocks the entrance to the CS os as it is approached from below* (large arrow).

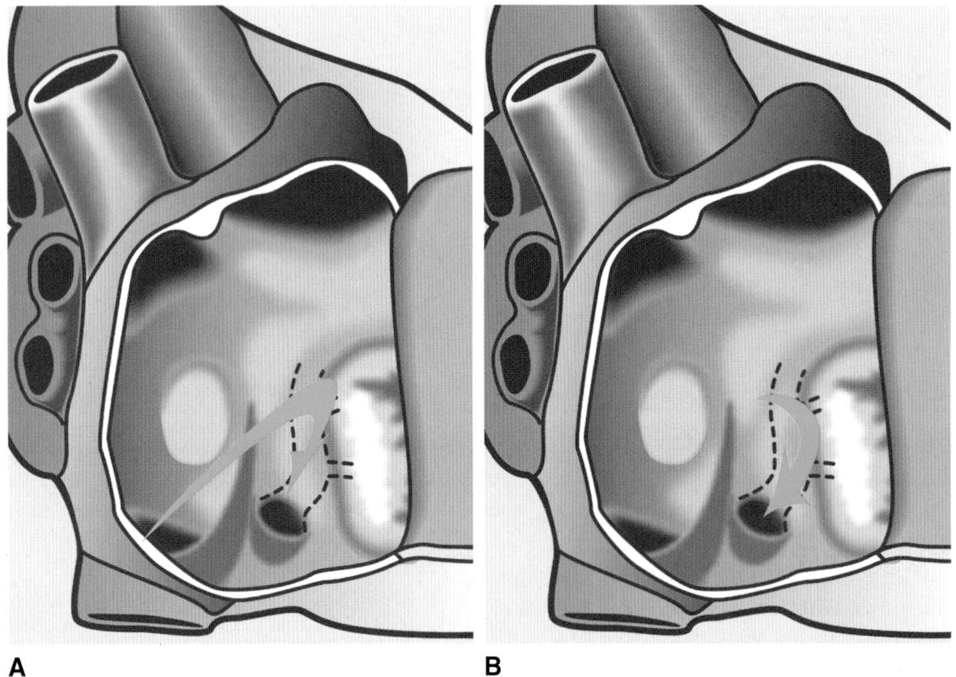

Figure 19-42. Thebesian valve and eustachian ridge assist coronary sinus (CS) cannulation. ***A,*** *The femoral approach to the CS uses the eustachian ridge and thebesian valve to advantage by approaching the CS from above as the catheter is deflected.* ***B,*** *Both the eustachian ridge and thebesian valve direct the tip of the guide into the CS os as the os is approached from the posterior superior tricuspid annulus.*

of the eustachian ridge and thebesian valve to direct the catheter into the os. Thus, it is not surprising that some physicians find it easier to cannulate the CS through the femoral approach. The trajectory of a femoral catheter is demonstrated in Figure 19-42A. With the femoral approach, the tip of the catheter approaches the CS from above. Thus, the eustachian ridge and thebesian valve form a pocket to catch the tip of the catheter and direct it into the CS. Because physicians who approach the CS as shown in Figure 19-41 continue to have difficulty locating and cannulating the CS, Al-Khadra[29] advocates first using the femoral approach to locate the CS, plan the implantation on the basis of venography, and facilitate CS cannulation from above. However, if the correctly shaped sheath and proper technique are used from the subclavian vein, the CS is approached from above as illustrated in Figure 19-42B.

Figure 19-43 demonstrates the effect of counterclockwise torque on the tip of a catheter with torque control to direct the catheter path. When counterclockwise torque is applied, the tip is directed posteriorly until it contacts the heart. As more torque is applied, the heart limits the posterior direction of the tip. Additional torque directs the tip inferiorly and toward the RA. The shape and position of the catheter with torque control are adjusted through the application of counterclockwise torque.

Interestingly, some clinicians caution that approaching the CS from above is prone to causing dissection.[1] In our experience this is not the case. Further, physicians who cannulate the CS using the femoral approach also approach the CS from above (see Fig. 19-42A) without reports of dissection or CS trauma. In addition, the shape of the well-received and popular Guidant Rapido Advance extended hook is designed to enter the CS from above. To my knowledge, there are no reports either formal or informal of dissection or CS trauma with the use of this "new" shape. Finally, the latest CS cannulating Attain guide shape from Medtronic, Inc. (Minneapolis, Minn.), (see Fig. 19-122A, far right), with the proximal curve and long vertical tip section, is also designed to approach the CS from above.

For counterclockwise torque to be effective in location of the os, the starting position of the catheter tip must be superior to and on the RV side of the os. If the tip starts above the CS on the tricuspid annulus, application of torque directs the tip posteriorly and inferiorly toward the RA into the CS. If the guide starts at or below the CS os, however, torque moves the tip inferiorly away from the os. As an aside: Clockwise torque will direct the tip of the guide anteriorly away from the os into the RA.

Ideal Catheter Shape for Cannulation of the Coronary Sinus in Patients Undergoing Cardiac Resynchronization Therapy

Using the eustachian ridge and thebesian valve to direct the guide into the os from above requires the initial

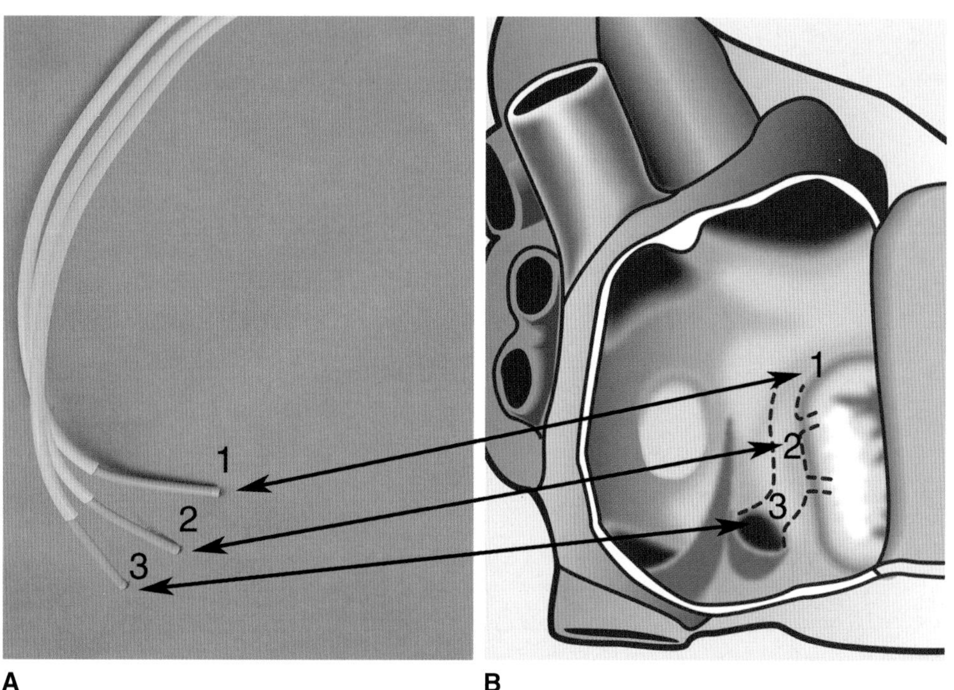

Figure 19-43. Effect of counterclockwise torque on a catheter with torque control when the tip of the catheter starts above the coronary sinus. ***A,*** *Three positions of a catheter with progressive application of torque are superimposed: 1, Initial counterclockwise torque at the hub of the guide directs the tip of the guide back. 2, With additional counterclockwise torque, the guide tip can no longer move back. Torque directs the tip of the guide down and to the left. 3, As more counterclockwise torque is added, the tip of the guide continues to move down and to the left. At positions 2 and 3, the proximal section of the catheter lifts off the surface (out of the plane of the illustration).* ***B,*** *1 is the initial position on the posterior superior tricuspid annulus; additional counterclockwise torque moves the tip to positions 2 and 3.*

catheter position to be above the CS on the tricuspid annulus. In patients with CHF, the natural rest position of many available catheter shapes places the tip of the guide at or below the CS in the RA (Fig. 19-44). Counterclockwise torque directs the guide posteriorly and inferiorly away from the os.

The addition of a "proximal curve" to the catheter (Fig. 19-45) places the tip above the CS on the tricuspid annulus or in the RV rather than in the RA. Counterclockwise torque directs the guide with the "proximal curve" inferiorly, posteriorly, and toward the RA into the os.

Catheters with a "Proximal Curve"

A catheter with a "proximal curve" can be purchased or created in a variety of ways, as illustrated in Figures 19-45 and 19-46. In Figure 19-46, a proximal curve is added to an 8F multipurpose guide.

The "proximal curve" shape is available or can be created in a variety of ways (Fig. 19-47). The combination of an 8F multipurpose guide and deflectable EP catheter, a 6F multipurpose catheter within a standard 9F multipurpose guide, the Guidant version of the "proximal curve" guide (CS-W), and the Pressure Products, Inc. (San Pedro, Calif.) peel-away sheath with the "proximal curve" all have a proximal curve to carry the tip of the guide across the RA to the tricuspid annulus above the CS. However, the peel-away sheath does not have torque control. Application of torque to the peel-away sheath does not result in the tip movement required to cannulate the CS. Figure 19-47B shows a modified peel-away sheath in which torque control is provided and shape retained by the addition of a preshaped 8F multipurpose 2 Cyber guide.

As mentioned previously, the implanting physician is in the best position to respond to difficult anatomy if the peel-away sheath used for venous access ends in the CS and not in the brachiocephalic vein. Also, removing a peel-away sheath from the CS as the final step rather than cutting a guide may reduce the risk of lead dislodgment. However, torque control is required for the tip of the catheter to be directed posteriorly, inferiorly, and toward the RA when counterclockwise torque is applied to the hub.

Peel-away sheaths lack torque control, making them difficult to manipulate into the CS, but the addition of a braided catheter inside a peel-away sheath gives it the torque control needed to cannulate the CS. The braided catheter provided by St. Jude Medical (St. Paul, Minn.) to insert their peel-away sheaths is the LiveWire Cannulator, a deflectable EP catheter (see Fig. 19-129). Biotronik GmbH & Co. (Berlin) also provides long peel-away sheaths but does not specify how their sheaths

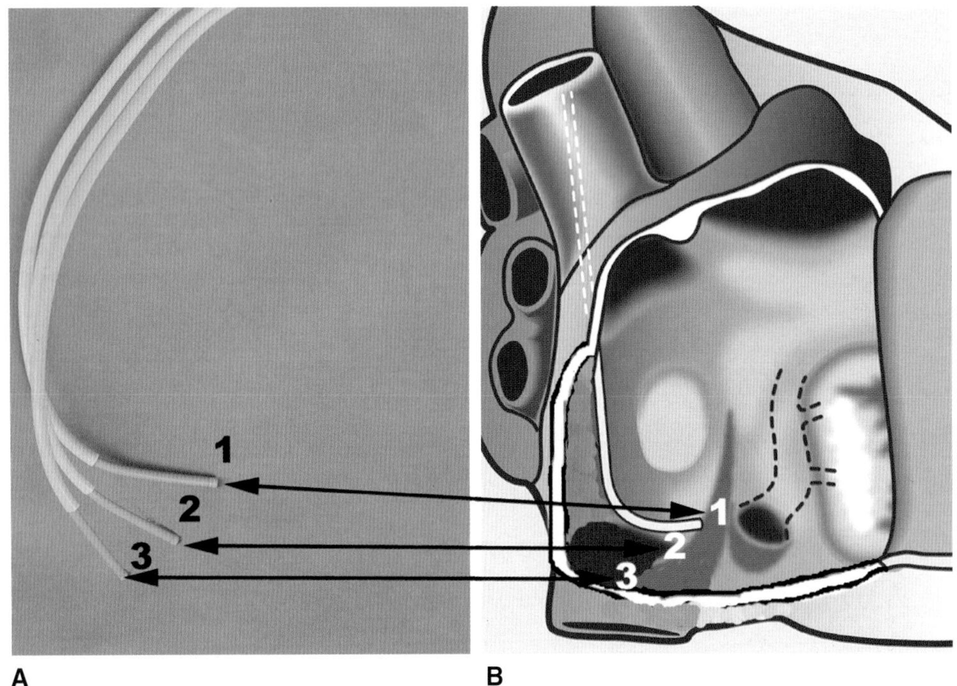

*Figure 19-44. Effect of counterclockwise torque on a catheter with torque control when the tip of the catheter starts below the coronary sinus (CS). **A,** Three positions of a catheter with progressive application of torque are superimposed: 1, Initial counterclockwise torque at the hub of the guide directs the tip of the guide back. 2, With additional counterclockwise torque, the guide tip can no longer move back. Torque directs the tip of the guide down and to the left. 3, As more counterclockwise torque is added, the tip of the guide continues to move down and to the left. At positions 2 and 3, the proximal section of the catheter lifts off the surface (out of the plane of the illustration). **B,** 1 is the initial position on the eustachian ridge below the CS. Additional counterclockwise torque moves the tip to positions 2 and 3, down and away from the CS os.*

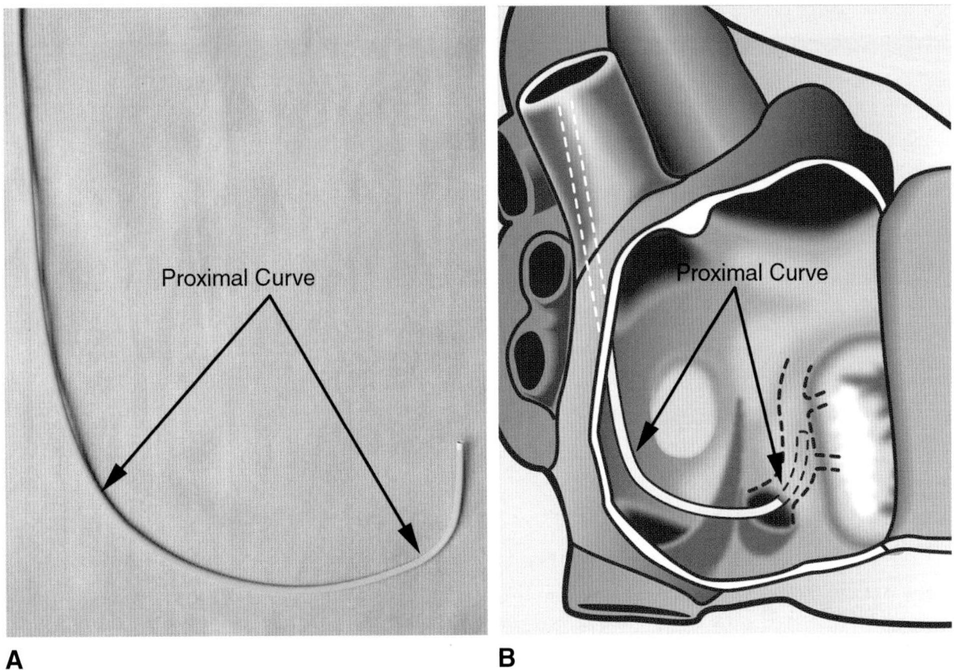

*Figure 19-45. Starting position of a catheter with a "proximal curve." **A,** The guide shape with a "proximal curve." **B,** The position of the guide (*black dotted lines*) in the heart. Note that the proximal curve carries the tip of the catheter across the right atrium and lifts the tip above the os of the coronary sinus. When counterclockwise torque is applied, the tip will be directed posterior and inferior toward the os. The eustachian ridge and thebesian valve direct the tip into the os.*

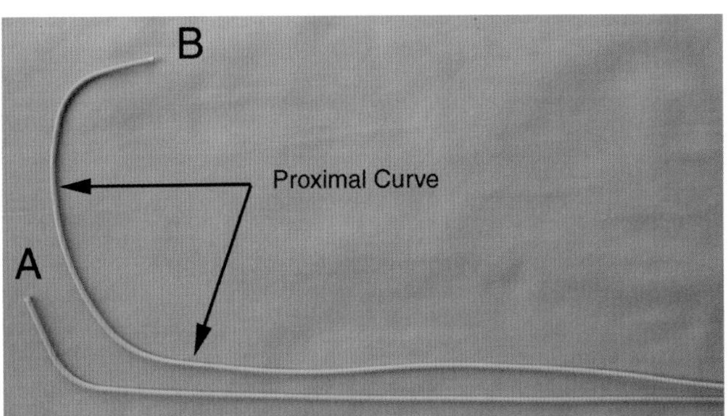

*Figure 19-46. "Proximal curve" added to a Multipurpose 2 Cyber Guide catheter (Boston Scientific, Natick, Mass.). A proximal curve is introduced by running the MP2 between the thumb and forefinger from proximal to distal starting 5 to 7 inches from the tip of the catheter, much like shaping a pacing stylet. The tip length on an MP2 is longer than that on an MP1 Cyber Guide. If a proximal curve is added to an MP1, the tip is too short to reliably reach above the coronary sinus os. The Cyber Guide catheter material responds well to shape changes applied by hand. Attempts to add a proximal curve to other guides frequently results in collapse of the lumen. **A,** The guide prior to shaping. **B,** The guide after shaping for the proximal curve.*

are to be inserted (see Fig. 19-115). Pressure Products provides a braided guiding catheter referred to as the "braided core" (Figs. 19-48 and 19-49).

Once the peel-away sheath is in the CS and the LiveWire Cannulator or braided core is removed, the peel-away sheath extends from the pocket to the mid-CS. The combination of a long peel-away sheath and a longer braided catheter has the added advantage of enabling the implanter to change trajectory and shape by holding the sheath in position and advancing the braided catheter or moving the two together as a unit (see Fig. 19-48C and Fig. 19-49B).

When torque is applied to the braided catheter (see Fig. 19-49A), it directs the tip of the long peel-away sheath posteriorly, inferiorly, and toward the RA. When the braided catheter is extended out the tip of the peel-away sheath, a variety of shapes may be created. If the sheath is held in position as the braided core is advanced, the trajectory of the tip cannot be matched by advancing a catheter alone.

Whether to Use Contrast Material in Cannulating the Coronary Sinus

The noncontrast material method of CS cannulation is familiar to many operators, who typically use the combination of a deflectable EP catheter inside a multipurpose guide (see Fig. 19-47) or a long peel-away sheath (see Fig. 19-112). Electrograms may or may not be recorded. As noted previously, however, finding the os and placing a catheter in the CS can be quite difficult in patients with CHF who present for CRT. The limitations of both the contrast and noncontrast methods are discussed here.

Limitations of the Noncontrast Method.

The Catheter Must Advance into the Coronary Sinus to Confirm Location. In many cases the problem is not finding the CS os but advancing the catheter beyond it.

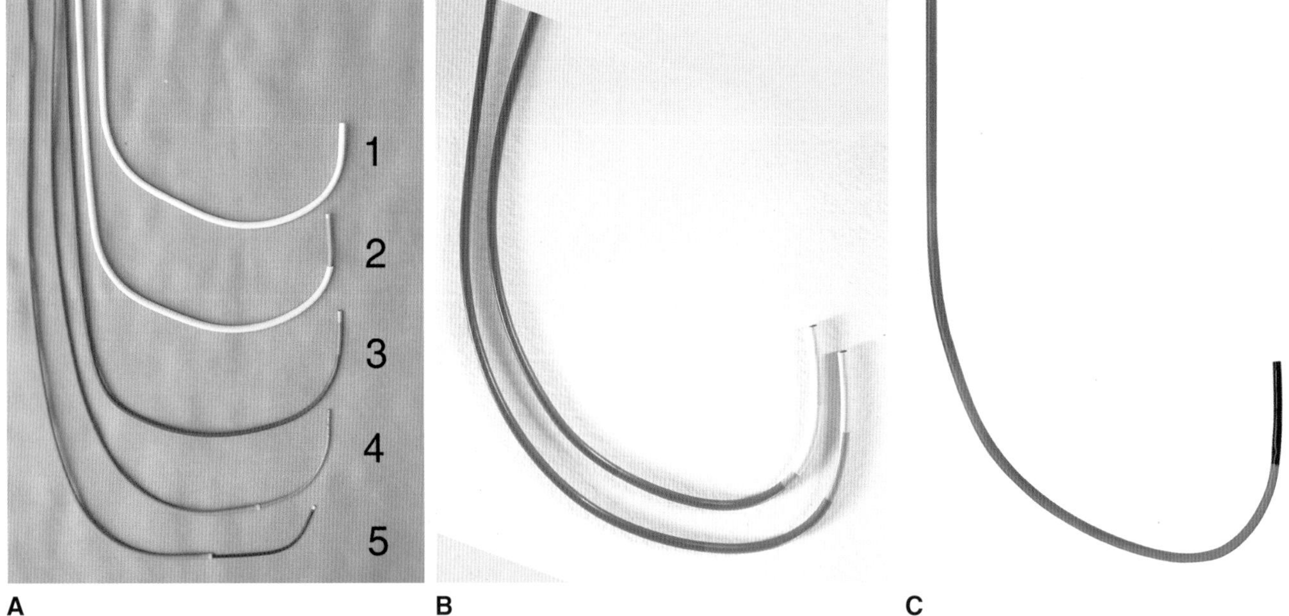

Figure 19-47. *Multiple catheter configurations with a "proximal curve."* ***A,*** *Peel-away sheath with a proximal curve (1); peel-away sheath with an 8F Cyber multipurpose 2 guide (Boston Scientific, Natick, Mass.) inserted for torque control (2); Guidant (Boston Scientific, Natick, Mass.) coronary sinus–W shape (3); Medtronic, Inc. (Minneapolis, Minn.) 6216 guide with deflectable catheter (4); Medtronic 6216 guide with 5F multipurpose catheter (5). To the right are B Guidant's and C Medtronic's latest fixed-curve shapes, which use the proximal curve concept.* ***B,*** *Guidant Rapido Coronary Sinus Extended Hook.* ***C,*** *Medtronic Attain Extended Hook Guide.*

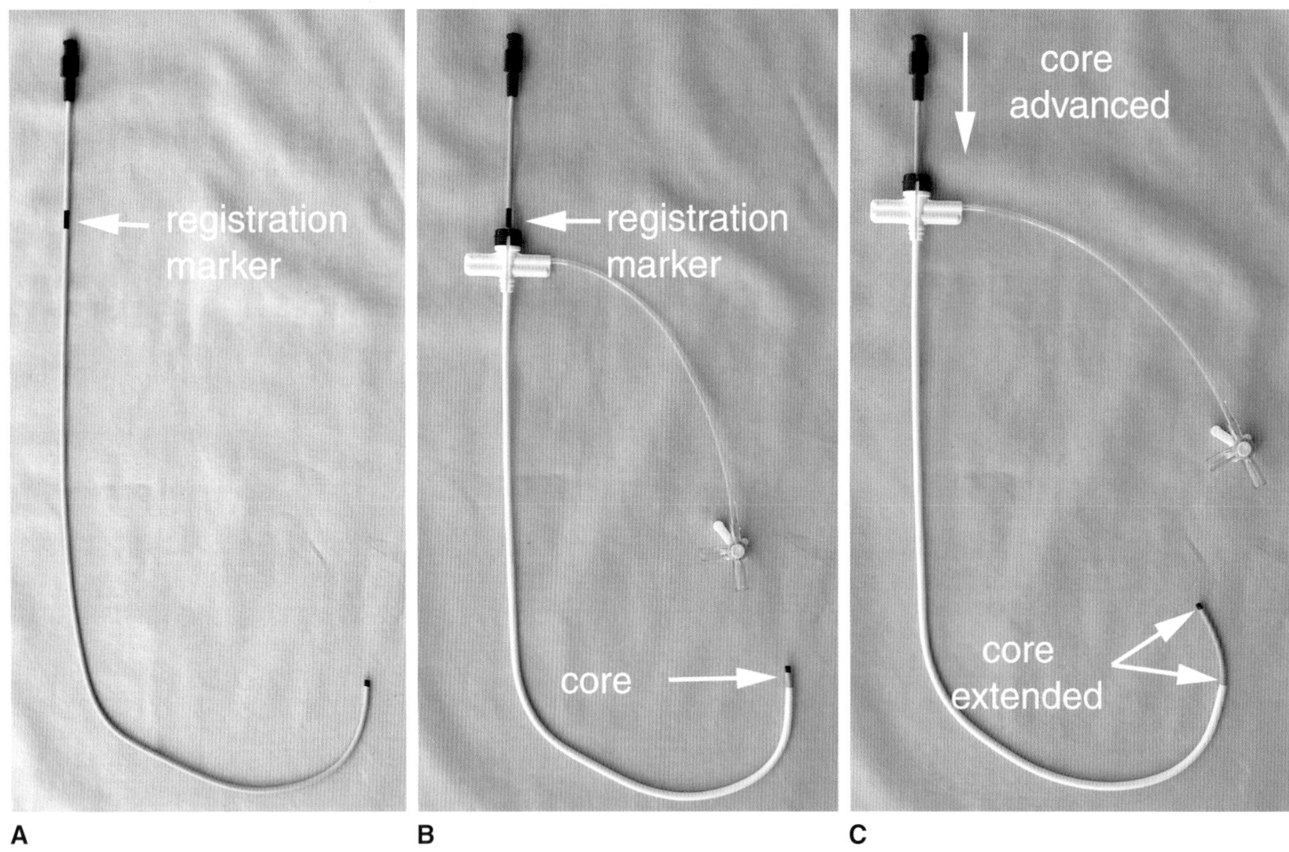

Figure 19-48. *Braided guide (core) for torque control and shape modification.* ***A,*** *The braided guide (core) has torque control. A black band (registration marker) identifies the length to be inserted into the sheath.* ***B,*** *The braided guide (core) is inserted into the peel-away sheath, giving it torque control. The braided core is 5 cm longer than the peel-away sheath. When the registration marker is at the hemostatic hub, the tip of the core extends 3 mm out of the sheath.* ***C,*** *The core is advanced beyond the registration marker, extending the core out the tip of the sheath and creating a new shape. In addition to creating new shapes, advancing the core while holding the sheath stable creates tip trajectories not possible with a single catheter.*

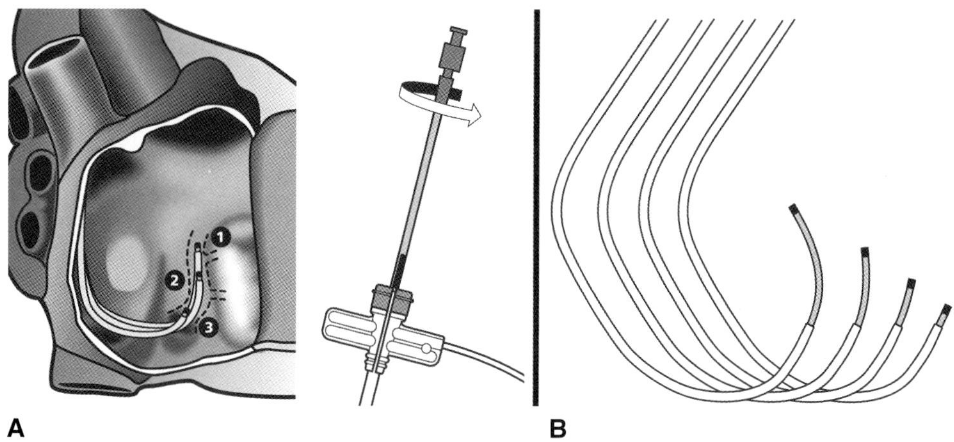

Figure 19-49. Demonstration of torque control and change in shape and trajectory. ***A,*** *The effect of applying counterclockwise torque to the braided core. The core gives the peel-away sheath torque control to facilitate finding the coronary sinus. As more and more torque is applied, the tip of the sheath/core combination moves posteroinferior to and toward the right atrium (RA) (1, 2, and 3).* ***B,*** *The effect of advancing the core while holding the sheath constant creates a variety of tip trajectories and catheter shapes not possible with a single catheter.*

The noncontrast method assumes (incorrectly) that if the tip of the catheter can be placed in the os, it will advance easily into the CS. Without using a contrast agent, the operator recognizes that the tip of the catheter was in the os only when the catheter advances into the CS. Recognition that the catheter has advanced into the CS is best appreciated in the LAO projection. Working in the LAO projection to cannulate the CS is uncomfortable and increases radiation exposure. However, even if working in the LAO projection and monitoring electrograms, the operator may have no idea that the catheter is or was in the os if it does not advance beyond the os into the CS. Figure 19-50 demonstrates two cases in which it was easy to find the os with a contrast agent but difficult to advance the catheter beyond the os. In these two cases the operator did not recognize that the tip of the catheter was in the os and spent hours continuing to look for the CS. A simple puff of contrast agent reveals that the tip of the catheter is in the CS os but will not advance.

The Catheter Does Not Provide Anatomic Landmarks to Assist in Locating the Os. With the noncontrast method, the catheter does not provide the anatomic landmarks provided by contrast injection to help guide the operator toward the CS os. For example, the operator may spend hours looking for the CS, not recognizing that the tip of the catheter is only a few

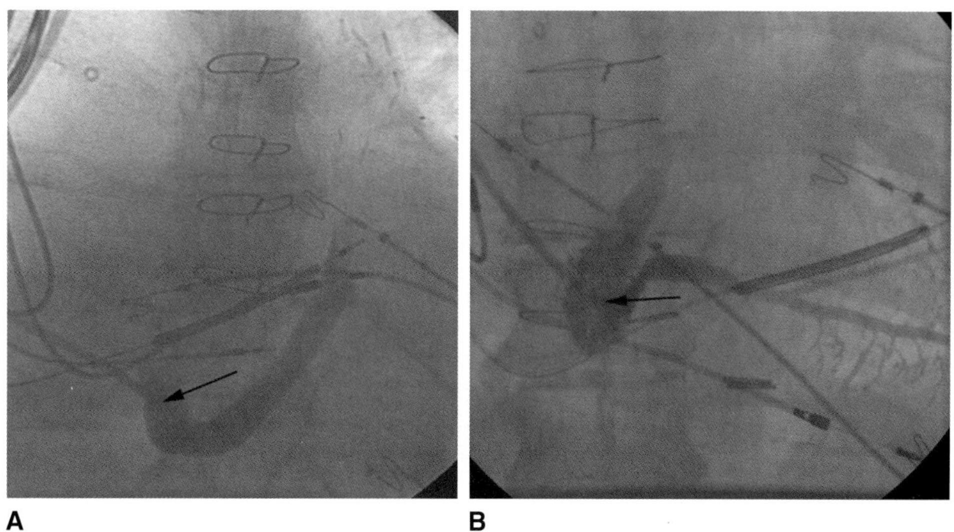

Figure 19-50. Difficulty advancing the guide beyond the os; sigmoid coronary sinus and large proximal vein. ***A,*** *The hook shape of the proximal coronary sinus (CS) makes it difficult to advance the guide* (arrow)*.* ***B,*** *A large posterior vein catches the tip of the guide* (arrow)*, preventing it from advancing into the vertically oriented CS. In both cases, without use of contrast material, the operator would be unaware that the tip of the guide was at or beyond the CS os. Contrast material not only confirms location but also defines why it is difficult to advance the catheter.*

millimeters from the os. In this situation, a 2-mL puff of contrast agent will reveal the location of the os and allow the operator to adjust the trajectory of the catheter accordingly. Recording electrograms does not provide the same type of information (Fig. 19-50).

Limitation of the Contrast Method. Transient renal insufficiency may result from administration of contrast agents, but this risk can be minimized as discussed previously.

How to Locate the Os of the Coronary Sinus with a Guide and Contrast Injection System

A simplified contrast injection system is pictured in Figure 19-51. The injection syringe is attached to a three-way stopcock. The reservoir syringe is also connected to the stopcock. A short (8- to 12-inch) piece of extension tubing is connected from the stopcock to a Y-adapter with a Touhy-Borst valve. The extension tubing allows the operator to manipulate the guide while the assistant injects contrast material. The braided guide is connected to the Y-adapter. The reservoir syringe is filled from a small bowl of contrast agent (not shown). One can fill the injection syringe several times from the reservoir syringe by rotating the stopcock open to the reservoir syringe. A Terumo Glidewire can be inserted through the Touhy-Borst valve on the Y-adapter if needed. Note that the entire system is contained on the table to help preserve sterility.

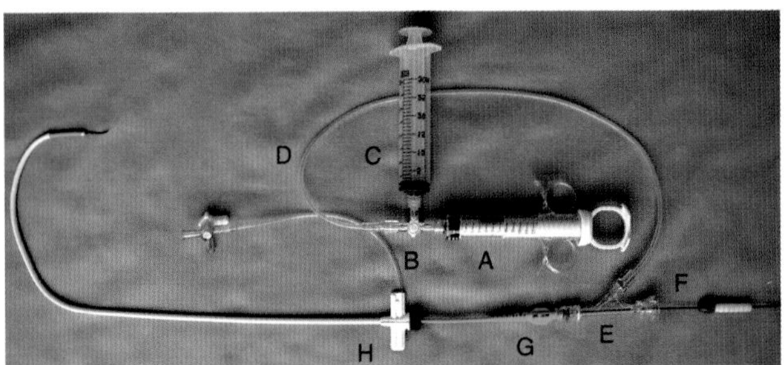

Figure 19-51. Simplified contrast material injection system. A, Injection syringe; B, three-way stopcock; C, reservoir syringe; D, 8-inch extension tubing; E, Touhy-Borst Y-adapter with hemostatic valve; F, Angled tip 0.035-inch Glidewire with steering handle (Terumo Medical Corporation, Somerset, NJ); G, Boston Scientific Corporation (Natick, Mass.) Cyber 8F 55-cm multipurpose 2 guide (proximal curve shaped by hand); H, Pressure Products, Inc. (San Pedro, Calif.), SafeSheath-CSG Worley STD.

Coronary Sinus Cannulation: A Two-Step Process with Contrast Injection

Step 1: Locating the Os of the Coronary Sinus

The variable location of the CS os in patients with CHF explains why it can be difficult to find even with contrast injection (Figs. 19-52 and 19-53). The location of the os varies owing to the combination of cardiac rotation, cardiac dilatation, and distortion from previous open-heart surgery (OHS). When viewed on the fluoroscopy screen in the AP view, the os can be to the right or left of the spine, as seen in Figure 19-52. Note that in both cases shown, the os of the CS is at the proximal end of the distal coil.

In addition, the os may be high or low relative to the floor of the tricuspid annulus, as seen in Figure 19-53. Systematic use of contrast injection with an understanding of the anatomy (Figs. 19-54 to 19-60) allows the operator to quickly recognize where the catheter tip is in relation to the CS os. The direction of the catheter can then be adjusted.

Anatomy Surrounding the Coronary Sinus Os as Defined by Contrast Injection. The RV, tricuspid annulus, eustachian ridge (valve of the inferior vena

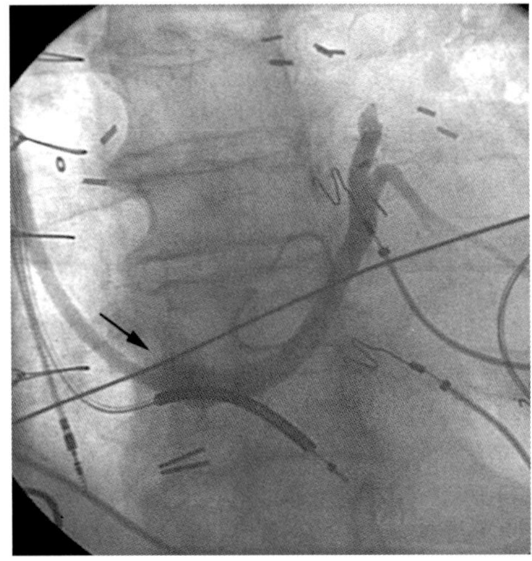

A

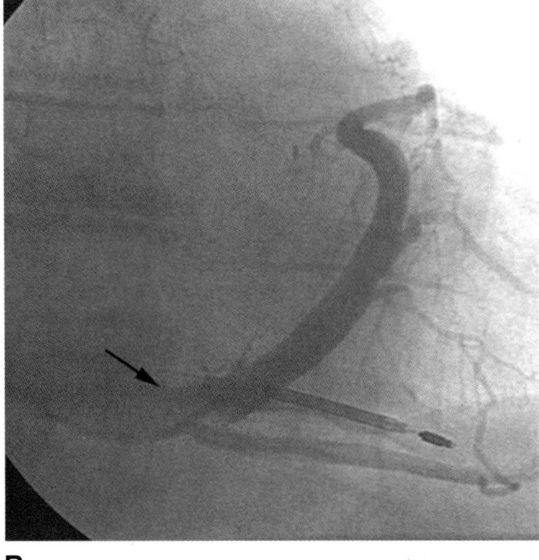

B

*Figure 19-52. Variability of the coronary sinus (CS) os seen on the anteroposterior projection. **A,** The os of the CS* (arrow) *is on the left border of the spine. **B,** The os of the CS* (arrow) *is to the right of the spine. "Right" and "left" are as viewed on the fluoroscopy screen in the AP view. Note that in both cases, the os of the CS is at the proximal end of the distal coil.*

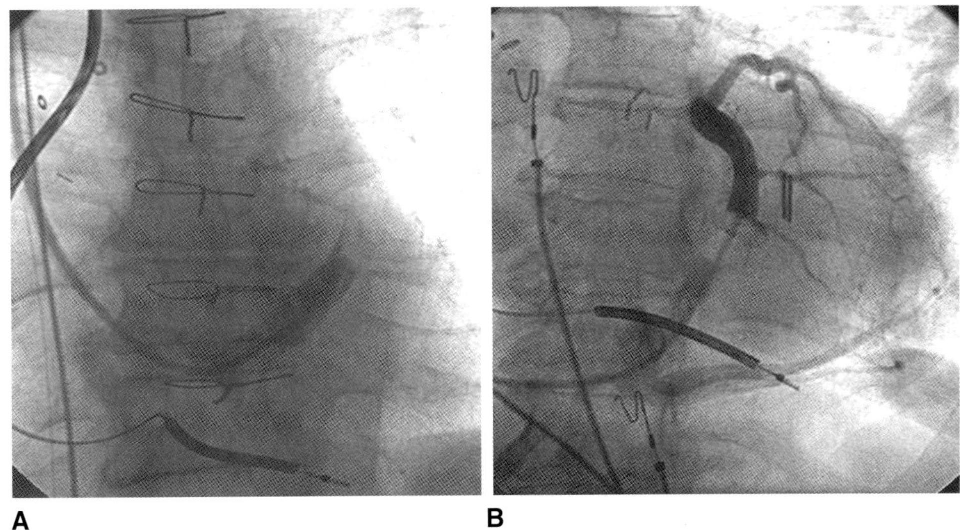

Figure 19-53. High-to-low variability of the coronary sinus (CS) os. ***A,*** *The os is high relative to the floor of the tricuspid valve.* ***B,*** *The os is low. In both views, the floor of the tricuspid valve is defined by the pacing lead.*

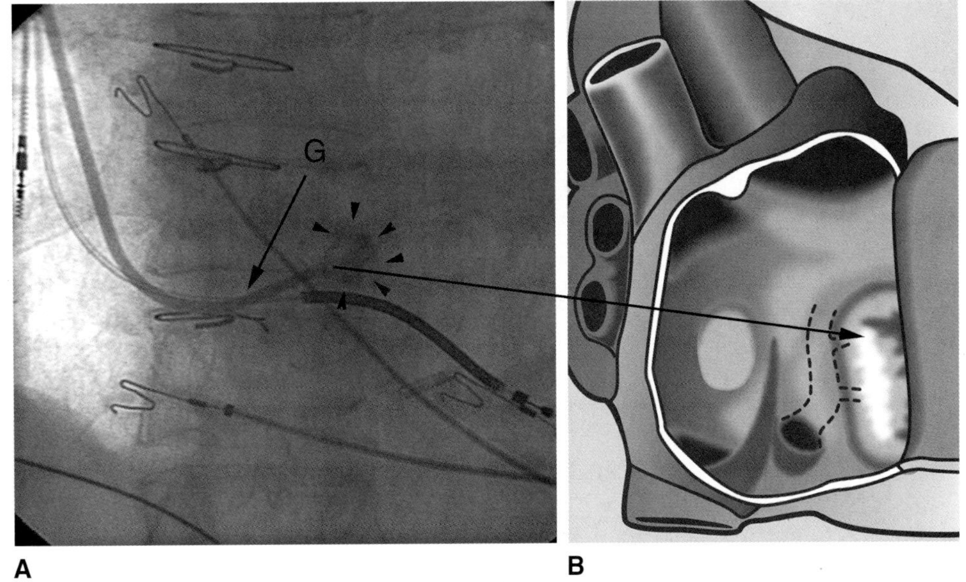

Figure 19-54. Composite illustration with the guide high in the right ventricle. ***A,*** *Anteroposterior projection with the guide (G) rotated 20 to 30 degrees counterclockwise, placing the tip of the guide posterior and superior to the pacing lead. A 2-mL puff of contrast material outlines the trabeculae (arrowheads), confirming that the tip of the guide is in the right ventricle.* ***B,*** *Drawing of the heart corresponding to* ***A,*** *showing the location of the tip of the guide (long arrow).*

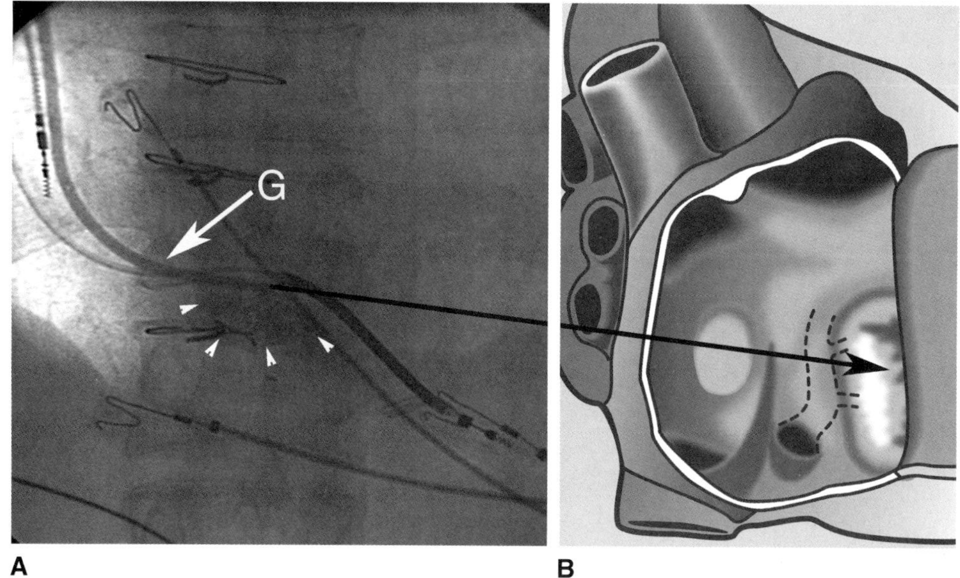

Figure 19-55. *Composite illustration with the guide in the right ventricle.* ***A,*** *Anteroposterior projection with the guide (G) rotated 20 to 30 degrees further counterclockwise than in Figure 19-54. The additional counterclockwise torque directs the tip down toward the coronary sinus os. A 2-mL puff of contrast material outlines the trabeculae* (arrowheads), *confirming that the tip of the guide is in the right ventricle. The guide is inferior to the position of the guide in Figure 19-54.* ***B,*** *Drawing of the heart corresponding to* ***A,*** *showing the location of the tip of the guide (*long arrow*).*

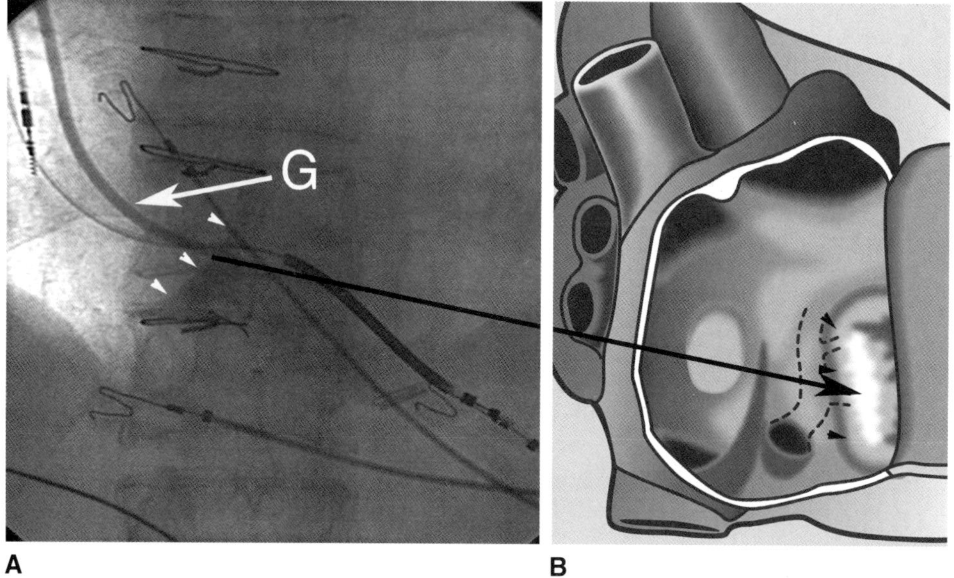

Figure 19-56. *Composite illustration with the guide at the tricuspid annulus.* ***A****, Anteroposterior projection of the guide (G) in the right ventricle just under the tricuspid valve. Contrast material fills the space between the right ventricle and the tricuspid valve, outlining the tricuspid annulus* (arrowheads) *from the ventricular side.* ***B,*** *Drawing of the heart corresponding to* ***A,*** *showing the location of the tip of the guide (*long arrow*).*

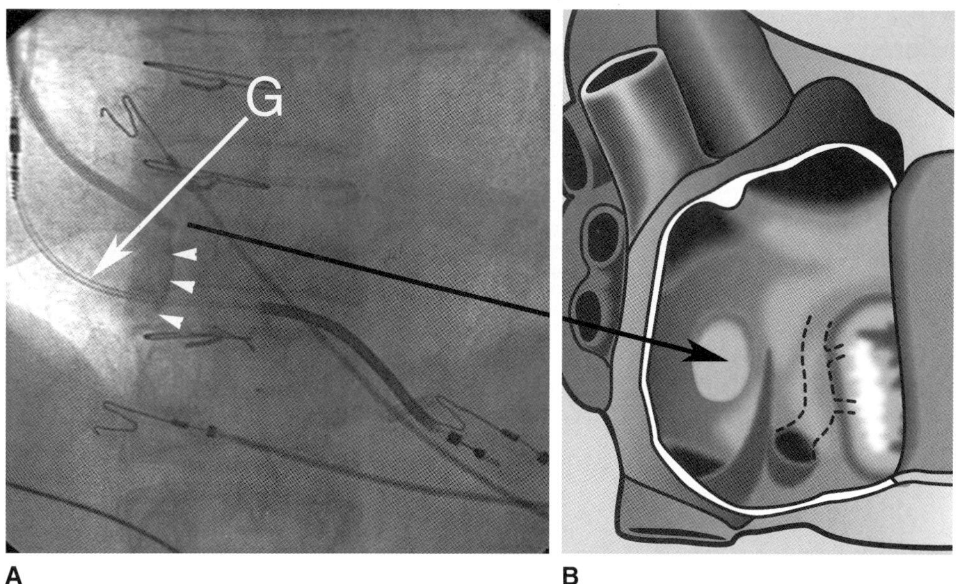

Figure 19-57. Composite illustration of the guide in the right atrium. ***A,*** *Anteroposterior projection with a linear stream of contrast material without trabeculae* (arrowheads) *formed with a 2-mL injection of contrast material. The position of the pacing lead and the lack of trabeculae confirm the position of the guide in the right atrium.* ***B,*** *Drawing of the heart corresponding to* ***A,*** *showing the location of the tip of the guide* (long arrow).

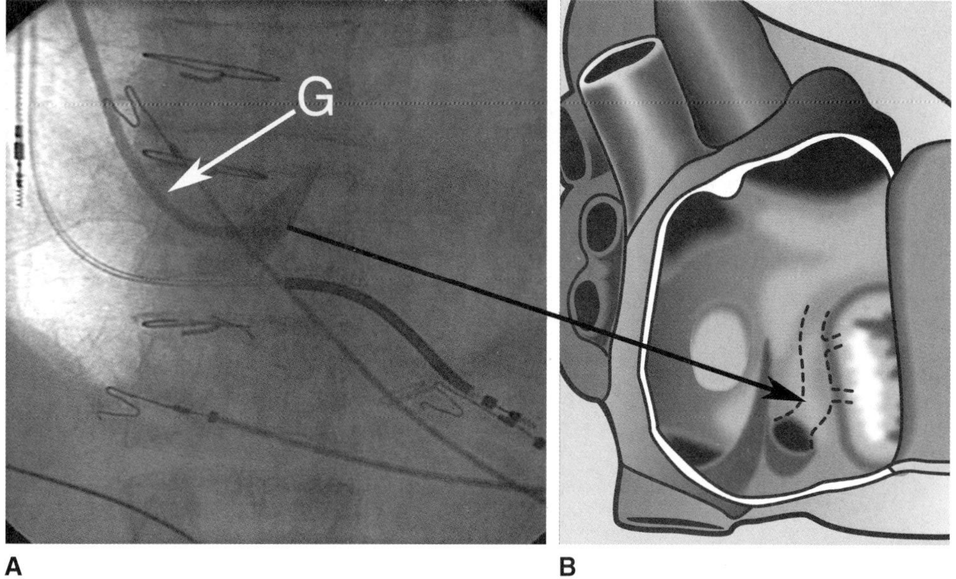

Figure 19-58. Composite illustration with the guide in the coronary sinus. ***A,*** *Anteroposterior projection with the guide (G) is in the CS.* ***B,*** *Drawing of the heart corresponding to* ***A,*** *showing the location of the tip of the guide* (long arrow).

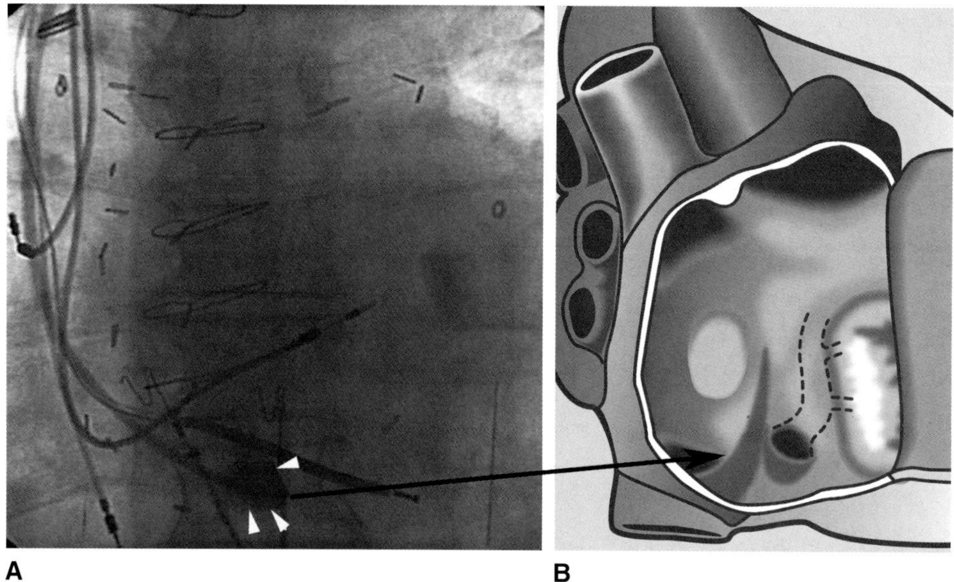

Figure 19-59. Composite illustration of a catheter in the subeustachian space. ***A,*** *Anteroposterior projection of the guide tip (G) is in the subeustachian space* (arrowheads) *below and on the atrial side of the coronary sinus os. Contrast material outlines the subeustachian space.* ***B,*** *Drawing of the heart corresponding to* ***A,*** *showing the subeustachian valve* (arrowheads) *as well as the tip of the guide* (long arrow).

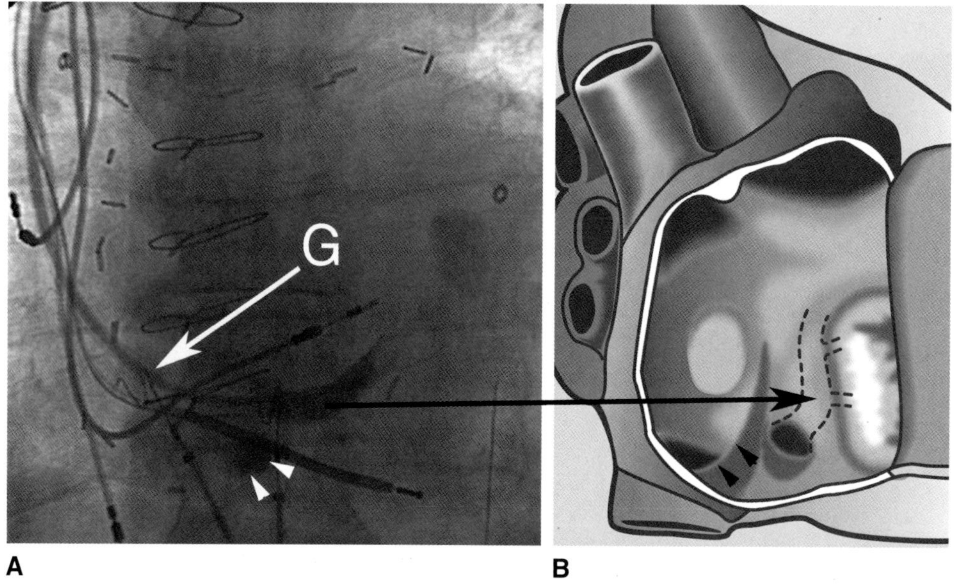

Figure 19-60. Composite illustration of the catheter in the coronary sinus. ***A,*** *Anteroposterior projection of the tip of the guide (G) in the os of the CS. Residual contrast pooling can be seen in the subeustachian space* (arrowheads). ***B,*** *Drawing of the heart corresponding to* ***A,*** *showing the eustachian valve* (arrowheads) *as well as the location of the tip of the guide* (long arrow).

cava), thebesian valve (valve of the CS), os of the CS, and subeustachian space are all important structures in the search for the CS os. These landmarks are readily identified with contrast injection. In Figure 19-54, the tip of the guide is across the tricuspid annulus and directed posteriorly with 20 to 30 degrees of counterclockwise torque. A 2-mL puff of contrast agent outlines the trabeculae and confirms the location of the guide in the RV. In Figure 19-55, additional counterclockwise torque directs the tip inferiorly and toward the RA. Trabeculae confirm that the guide is still in the RV. In Figure 19-56, contrast agent is trapped between the tricuspid valve and posterior wall of the RV, outlining the tricuspid annulus. In Figure 19-57, the tip of the guide is in the RA near the fossa ovalis. In Figure 19-58, the tip of the guide enters the CS os. Figures 19-59 and 19-60 demonstrate the subeustachian space, another important landmark defined by contrast injection. One must recognize that when the guide is in the subeustachian space, it is too low and on the atrial side of the CS os. The tip of the guide must be directed superiorly and advanced across the tricuspid valve into the RV. This can be accomplished by withdrawing the guide 1 cm, applying 20 degrees of clockwise torque to orient the tip toward the tricuspid valve, and then advancing the guide into the RV. If the tip of the guide remains in the RA, a wire may be advanced through the Touhy-Borst valve and through the tip of the guide into the RV, as illustrated in Figure 19-61. Once the wire is in the RV, the guide is advanced over the wire into the RV (Fig. 19-62).

Summary. The procedure for quickly finding the CS os with use of a contrast agent is to start with a catheter that has both torque control and a "proximal curve" that takes the tip across the RA to a position on the tricuspid annulus above the os and then to proceed as follows:

1. Apply 20 degrees of counterclockwise torque to the hub of the guide, directing the tip to the posterior superior tricuspid annulus.
2. Confirm location with a 2-mL contrast injection.
3. Apply an additional 20 to 40 degrees of counterclockwise torque, watching the tip of the guide for inferior deflection.
4. As the tip of the guide "walks" inferiorly and toward the RA in response to the torque, inject 2-mL puffs of contrast agent to visualize the structures demonstrated in Figures 19-54 through 19-60.
5. On the basis of the anatomy demonstrated by the contrast agent, the guide can be either advanced or withdrawn and either more or less torque can be applied to direct the tip into to the os.

Anatomic Variants May Make It Difficult to Find the Coronary Sinus Os. The anatomic variants that make

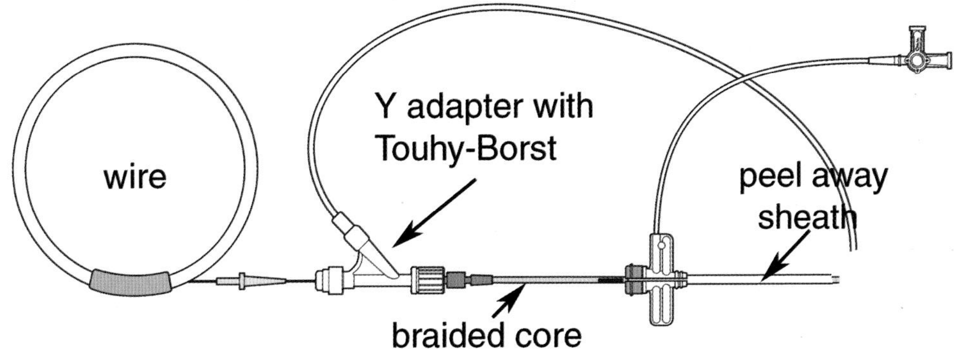

Figure 19-61. Insert a wire into the Touhy-Borst valve.

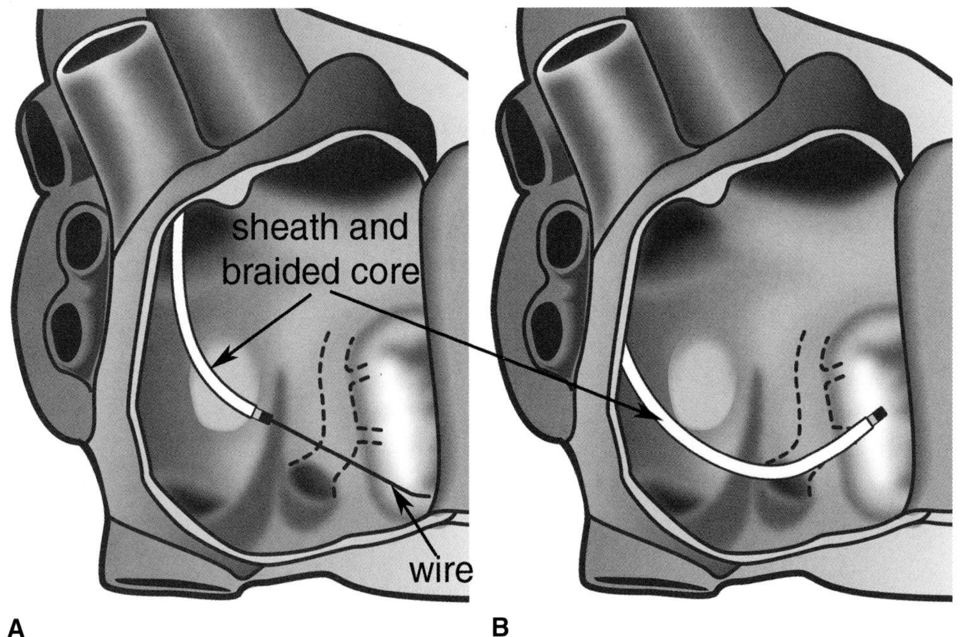

*Figure 19-62. Advance the catheter over the wire into the right ventricle (RV). **A,** The wire inserted through the Touhy-Borst valve extends out the catheter into the RV. **B,** The wire is held taut and used as a rail to advance the catheter across the tricuspid valve into the RV.*

it difficult to locate the CS os include the high CS, tricuspid ring, huge RA, and a CS that empties into the LA.

The High Coronary Sinus Os. The os location most difficult to find can be in the high CS. The CS os in Figure 19-63 is well above the usual location. Using a catheter with a proximal curve places the tip high on the tricuspid annulus. Adding counterclockwise torque with the tip of the catheter high makes it more likely to find the high CS. Counterclockwise torque only directs the tip of the guide posteriorly and inferiorly. The curve on many catheters places the tip too low. Counterclockwise torque will direct the tip of the catheter posteriorly and inferiorly, away from the CS os.

Tricuspid Valve Ring. Patients with severe CHF often have tricuspid regurgitation requiring a tricuspid valve repair at the time of left side valve repair/replacement or coronary artery bypass grafting (CABG). The tricuspid repair/ring may distort the anatomy, making it difficult to find the os. In Figure 19-64, the CS os is easily found in one case (A) and difficult to find in another case (B).

The Giant Right Atrium. The RA may be extremely large owing to permanent atrial fibrillation (AF) or a massively dilated right heart. In this situation, even when a guide/sheath with a large proximal curve is used, the catheter tip usually ends in the RA below the tricuspid valve. Unless the shape of the catheter is

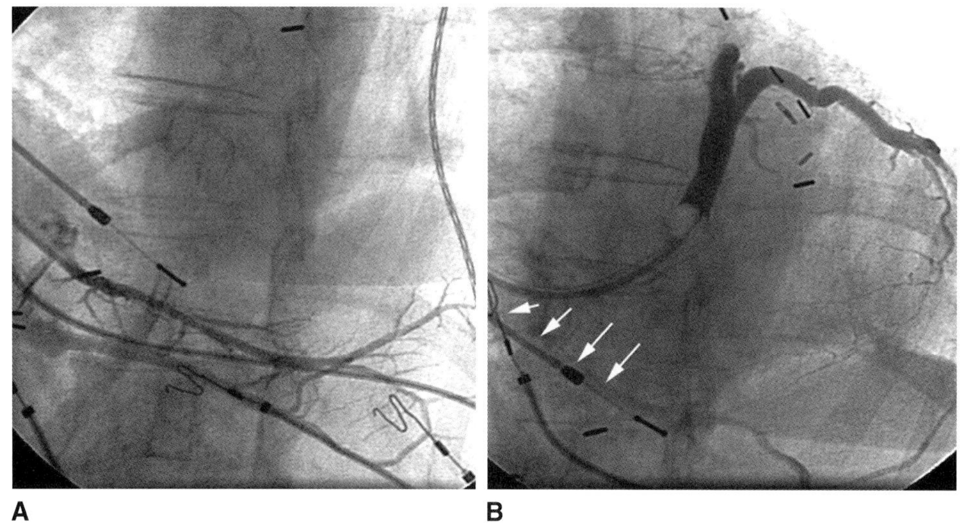

Figure 19-63. The high coronary sinus (CS) os is hard to locate. ***A,*** *The only vein found on the initial attempt by a previous operator is low.* ***B,*** *The high CS os is easily cannulated with use of the approach described in Figure 19-62. Retrograde filling of the previously injected vein can be seen (arrows).*

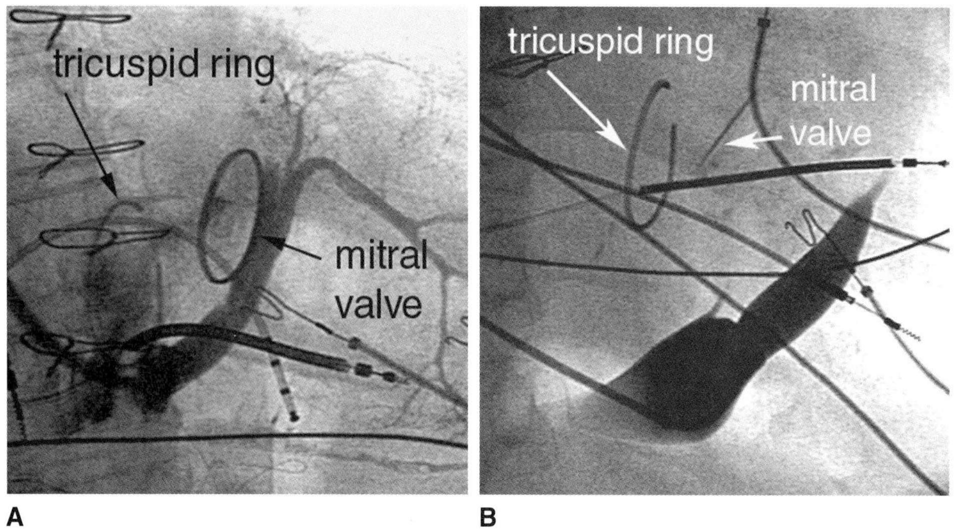

Figure 19-64. Variable location of the coronary sinus (CS) os in two patients with tricuspid rings. ***A,*** *The CS os is located just below the tricuspid ring.* ***B,*** *The CS os is located well below the tricuspid ring.*

changed significantly, the tip will flail about aimlessly in the RA. A 2-mL injection of contrast agent will confirm that the tip is in the RA, not the RV, because of the lack of trabeculae. A guidewire inserted through the Touhy-Borst valve of the Y-adapter and advanced out the tip of the guide/sheath into the RV can help to get the tip of the guide into the RV. Alternatively, a sheath/guide with an extended proximal curve specifically designed for the massive RA may be selected (Fig. 19-65).

The Coronary Sinus Empties into the Left Atrium. In rare cases, the CS empties into the LA, as illustrated in Figure 19-66. Injection of contrast material into a coronary artery with imaging of the venous phase demonstrates the location of the CS os. In addition, a small vein leading to the CS is cannulated. The only way to reach the CS is via the transseptal approach.

Step 2: Advancing a Sheath or Guide into the Coronary Sinus

As mentioned previously, cannulation of the CS is a two-step process. Once the os of the CS is located, it may be easy or difficult to advance the sheath or guide into the CS because of the following anatomic features:

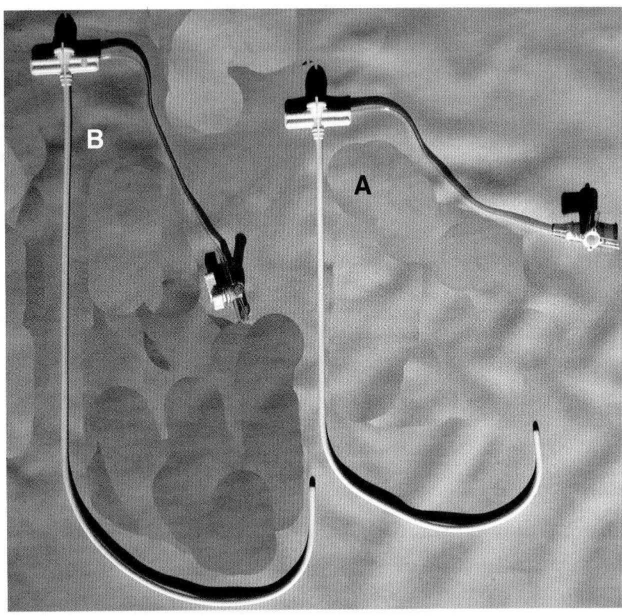

*Figure 19-65. Standard **(A)** and jumbo **(B)** versions of the proximal curve. The larger version was specifically designed for massively dilated hearts with huge right atria. The reach of the curve is sufficient for the tip to reach across the tricuspid valve.*

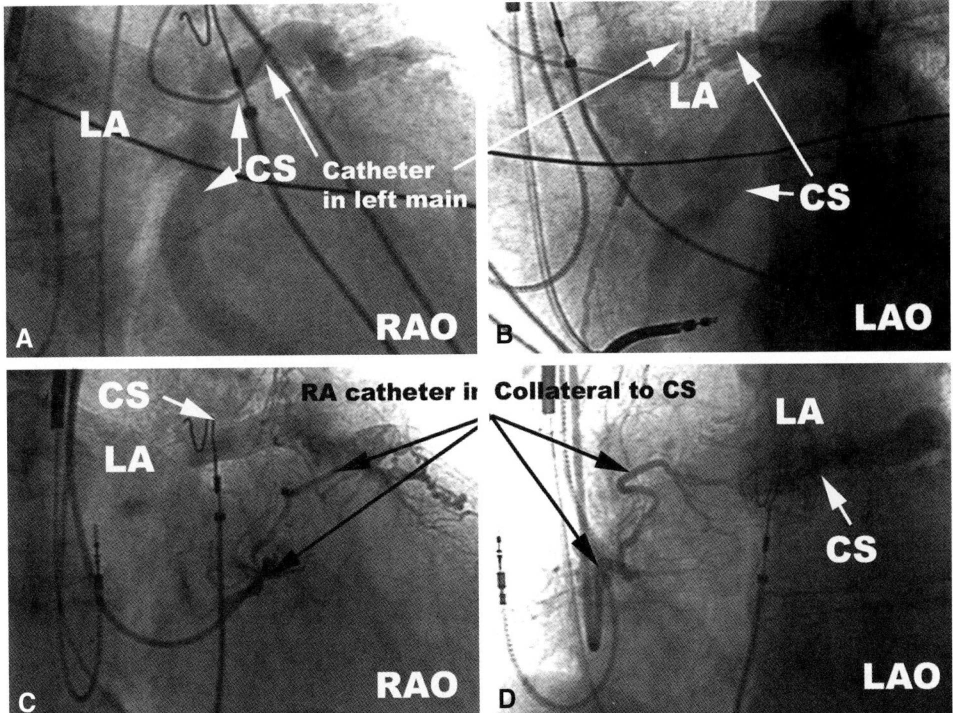

*Figure 19-66. The coronary sinus (CS) drains into the left atrium (LA). **A,** Contrast material is injected into the left main artery in the right anterior oblique (RAO) projection with delayed imaging to demonstrate the venous return. The CS drains into the LA. **B,** The venous return of the left main artery injection draining into the LA is shown in the left anterior oblique (LAO) projection. The contrast material stays to the right. **C,** RAO projection of the CS filling from an injection of a collateral vessel found in the RA. **D,** LAO projection of the CS filling from an injection of a collateral vessel in the RA. The course of the collateral vessel helps define the limits of the RA and LA.*

- A proximal vein branch that catches and misdirects the tip of the guide
- The initial angle of approach from the RA to the CS os
- The thebesian valve
- A vertical CS
- A sigmoid CS
- CS stenosis from previous surgery
- A mid-CS valve
- A double-os CS

If the Sheath/Guide is Difficult to Advance. If the sheath/guide is difficult to advance, it is important to first establish why. Inject 1 to 2 mL of contrast agent into the os while observing the LAO and RAO projections to establish the nature of the problem and to suggest a solution. For example, the tip of the guide may be caught in a large proximal venous branch. Simply withdrawing the guide a few millimeters and applying additional torque may free the tip and allow the guide to advance. Other reasons for difficulty advancing the sheath/guide are as follows:

- The large proximal branch (Fig. 19-67)
- The tortuous CS (Fig. 19-68)
- The sigmoid CS (Fig. 19-69)

Creating a Rail to Advance a Catheter through a Difficult Area. The ability to track a catheter or sheath over a wire into the CS depends on the course of the CS and the flexibility of the catheter as well as the wire. In cases in which the CS is very tortuous and neither a stiff guidewire (Amplatz 0.035-inch Extra Support) nor a Glidewire will advance, only a floppy angioplasty wire will advance fully. Thin floppy wires are easier to

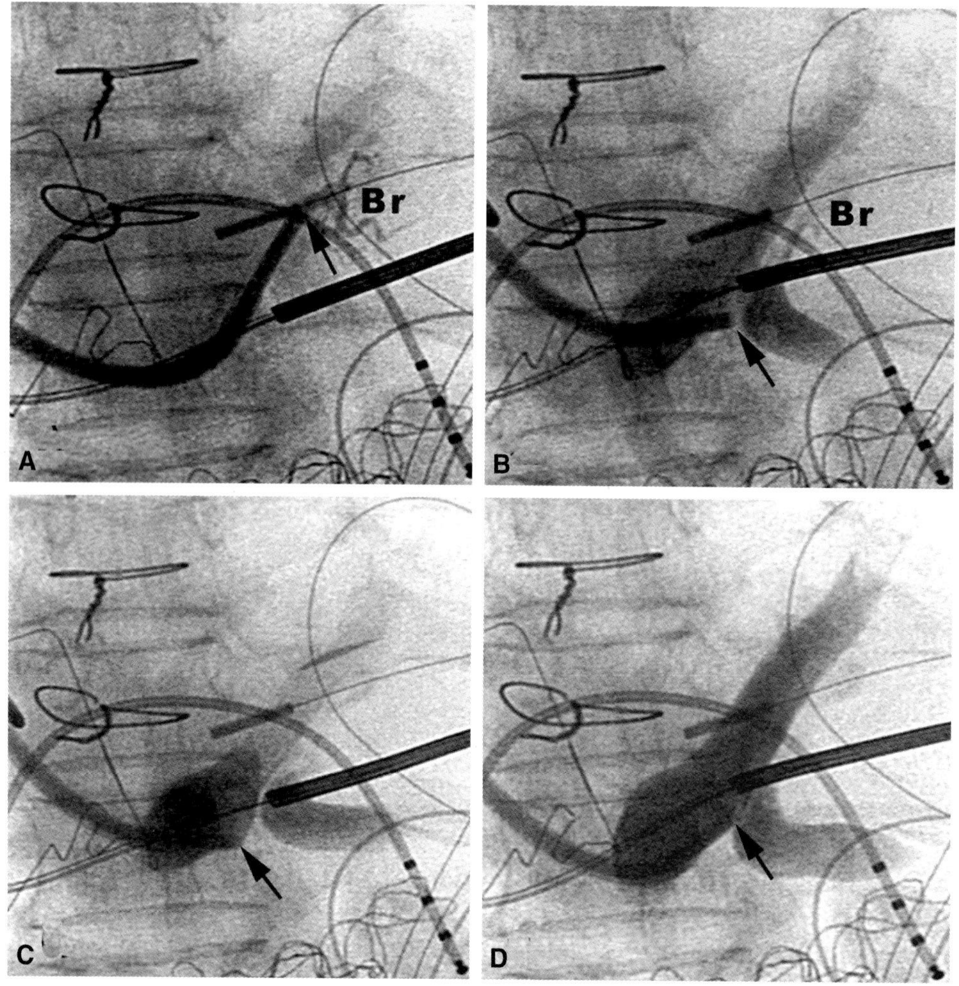

*Figure 19-67. Counterclockwise torque to redirect the guide out of the large posterior lateral vein into the coronary sinus. **A,** The tip of the guide* (arrow) *is in a venous branch (Br) of the posterior lateral vein. **B,** The tip of the guide* (arrow) *is withdrawn back into the posterior lateral vein with counterclockwise torque. The branch (Br) is still visible. **C,** The tip of the guide* (arrow) *is back in the coronary sinus. Additional counterclockwise torque is added. **D,** The tip of the guide* (arrow) *is advanced beyond the ostium of the posterior lateral vein into the coronary sinus. With limited experience, the entire procedure is accomplished in a single motion with 3 to 5 mL of contrast material.*

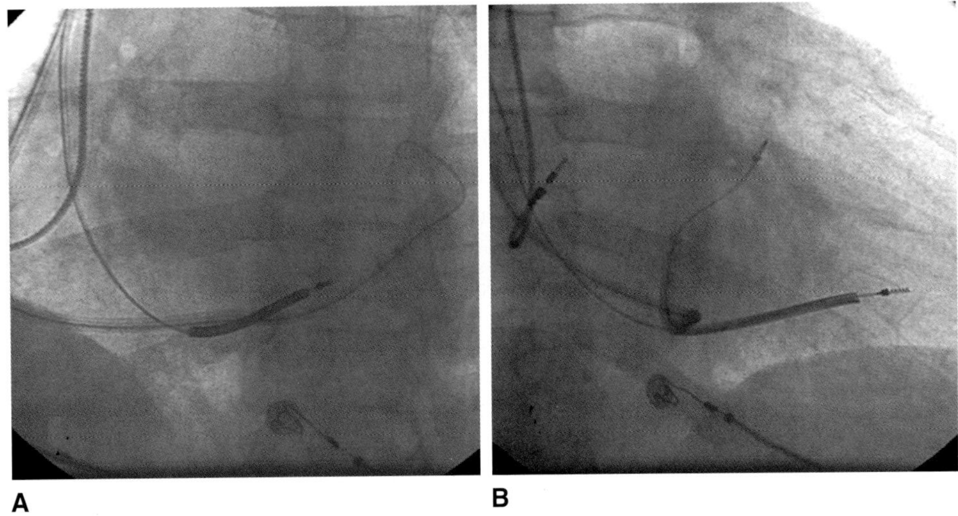

Figure 19-68. The coronary sinus (CS) in this patient is difficult to cannulate because of a tortuous initial segment. ***A****, Anteroposterior projection showing the result of attempts to advance the guide into the CS: The guide is laid out on the floor of the right atrium (RA).* ***B****, The right anterior oblique projection demonstrates that the forces are directed from left to right initially, rather than up into the CS. Application of torque to the catheter to provide a straight approach can resolve the problem. Reviewing the line of the guiding catheter into the CS in various projections is important to understanding how to adjust the torque to keep the catheter as straight as possible as it is advanced.*

advance, but a stiff wire provides more support once in place.

A rail is created to increase the support provided by a wire. Starting with the most supportive wire that will fully advance into the CS, the operator adds progressively more support as follows: With the wire held taut, a catheter is advanced over the wire. The size and flexibility of the catheter depend on the wire. If only an angioplasty wire will advance, a small flexible catheter should be next. Once in place, the wire and first catheter are held taut, and the next larger catheter is advanced over the wire and first catheter. For example, a Glidewire followed by a 5F or 6F multipurpose guide followed by an 8F guide followed by a 9F sheath may work in some cases. Such cases make the importance of establishing a stable CS platform from which to work abundantly clear.

Using the Inflated Coronary Sinus Venogram Balloon to "Pull" the Sheath into the Sinus. In some cases, the only wire that will advance into the CS is a 0.014-inch guidewire. Attempts to advance a catheter over the angioplasty wire results in wire displacement. In this case a trackable compliant balloon is advanced deep into the CS over the wire and inflated to create an anchor. The sheath is then pulled over the shaft of the balloon catheter into the CS, as illustrated in Figure 19-70. Two critically important issues must be addressed for this maneuver to be completed successfully:

1. The balloon must be compliant—that is, it must deform to fit into the CS rather than maintain its shape, or else it will traumatize the CS (see Fig. 19-5).
2. The compliant balloon must be trackable—that is, the catheter on which the balloon is mounted must advance readily over the 0.014-inch angioplasty wire.

Coronary angioplasty balloons are highly trackable, but the balloons are typically noncompliant. Many balloons used for occlusive CS venography neither are trackable nor have compliant balloons. The balloons supplied by Pressure Products and others are reasonably trackable and compliant.

Coronary Sinus with a Valve, Stenosis, or Downward Sigmoid Shape. Sometimes advancing a catheter alone results in the following problems:

- Valve located near the os of the CS (Fig. 19-71)
- Stenotic CS (Fig. 19-72)
- Downward sigmoid CS (Figs. 19-73 and 19-74)

In such cases, the telescoping approach can be used to direct the forces differently. If the sheath is placed on the lip of the CS and held in position, and the guide is advanced out the sheath, the sheath will help support the guide and resist the downward trajectory, allowing the guide (core) to advance into the CS rather than dropping down into the RA. This concept is shown diagrammatically in Figure 19-75 and in a patient in Figure 19-76.

Coronary Sinus Venous Anatomy

Compared with the coronary arterial system, the coronary venous system receives little attention. With CRT for heart failure, the coronary venous system is used to access target areas and implant the LV pacing lead.[13] In the early days of CRT, implanters were forced to use a "take what's

Text continued on p. 706

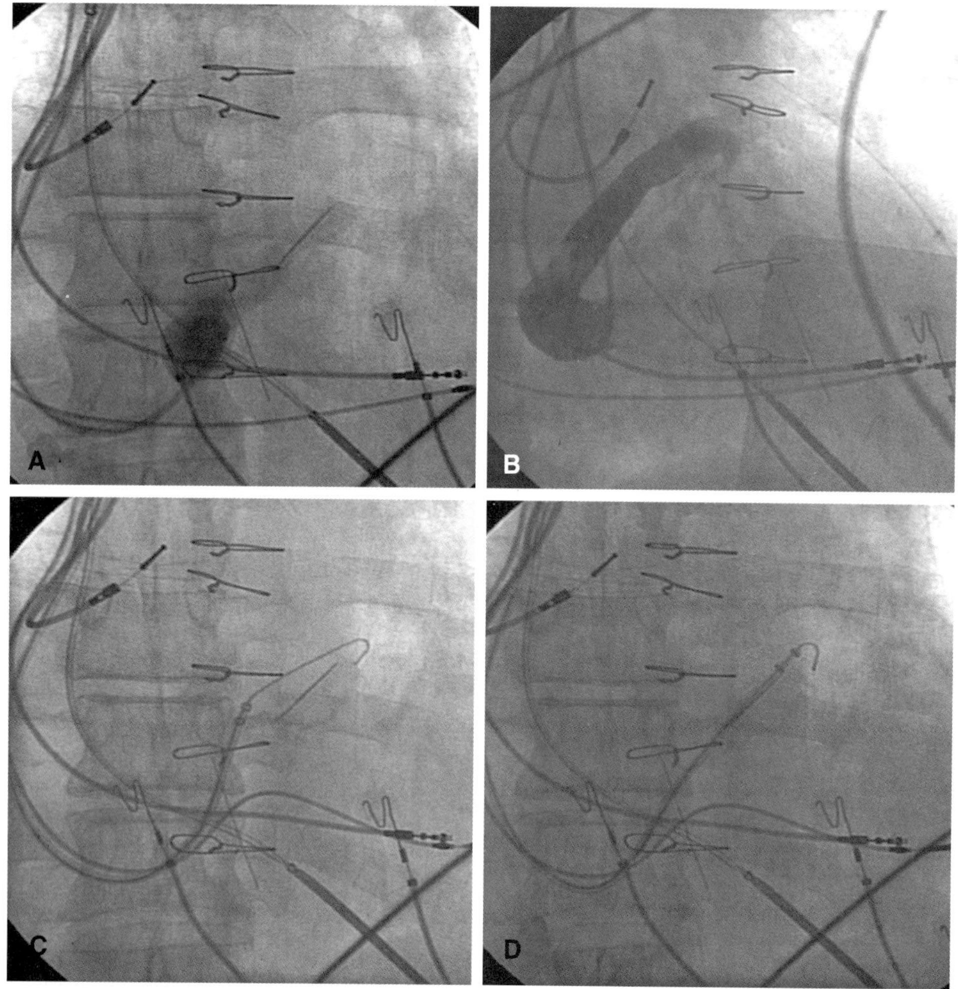

Figure 19-69. *Sigmoid coronary sinus in a patient with previous mitral valve repair.* ***A,*** *The tip of the guide rests at the os but will not advance into the coronary sinus (CS).* ***B,*** *After injection of contrast material, right anterior oblique projection reveals the sigmoid shape of the proximal CS.* ***C,*** *A J-tip guidewire is advanced out the tip of the guide deep into the CS.* ***D,*** *The guidewire is held taut, and the guide is advanced over the guidewire deep into the CS. Several important points are demonstrated in sequence. First, without the use of contrast material, the operator would not be aware that advancing into the CS rather than finding the CS was the problem. Contrast material also demonstrated the nature of the anatomic variant, which provided a potential solution (use of a guidewire). Advancing the guidewire through the sigmoid section of the CS is possible because the guide provides support for the wire as it is advanced. The wire, once in place deep in the CS, supports a track by which to advance the wire. It is important to hold the wire taut to create a rail as the guide is advanced over the wire.*

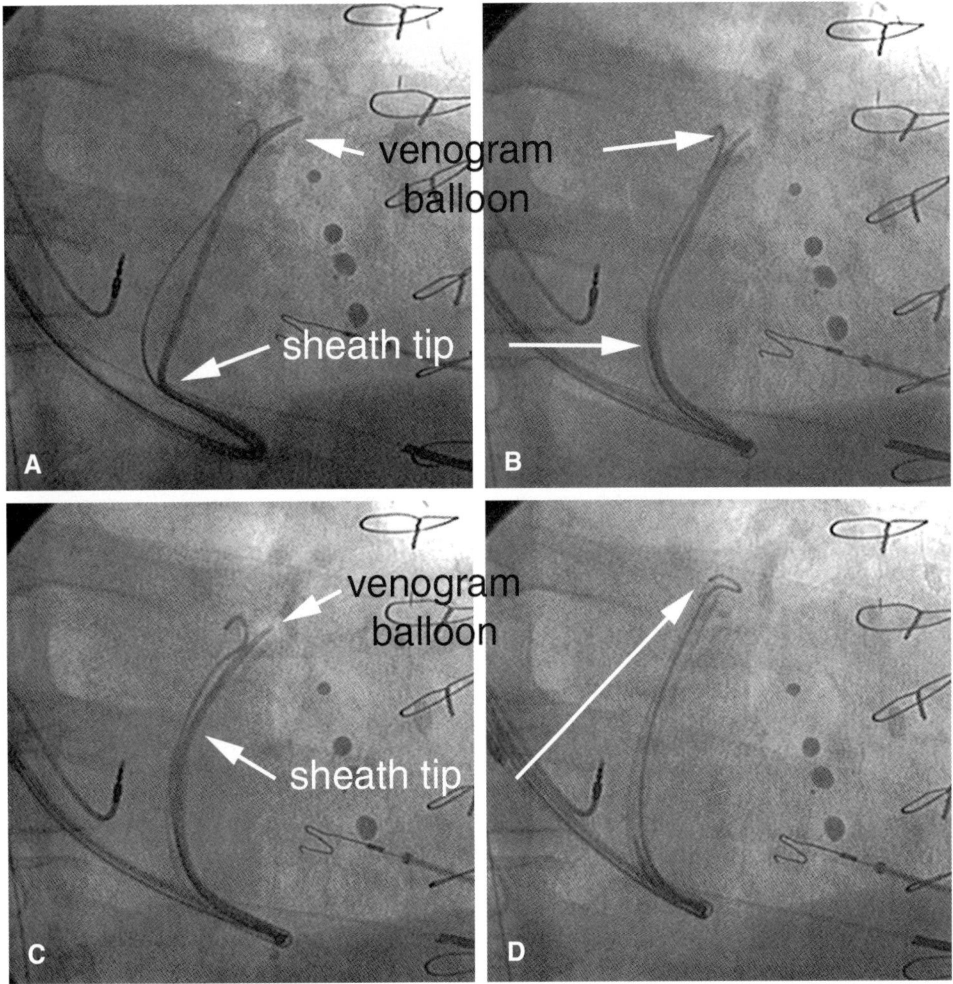

Figure 19-70. Compliant trackable balloon catheter used as an anchor to "pull" the sheath into the coronary sinus (CS). ***A,*** *The tip of the sheath is at the os of the backward sigmoid coronary sinus. The compliant trackable balloon is advanced into the distal CS over the 0.014-inch guidewire and inflated with 2 mL of air. With the additional support provided by the anchoring balloon, an Amplatz stiff wire (J-tip wire) is advanced into the CS to add support.* ***B*** *and* ***C,*** *The sheath is "pulled" over the balloon catheter and Amplatz wire deep into the CS.* ***D,*** *The balloon catheter is removed.*

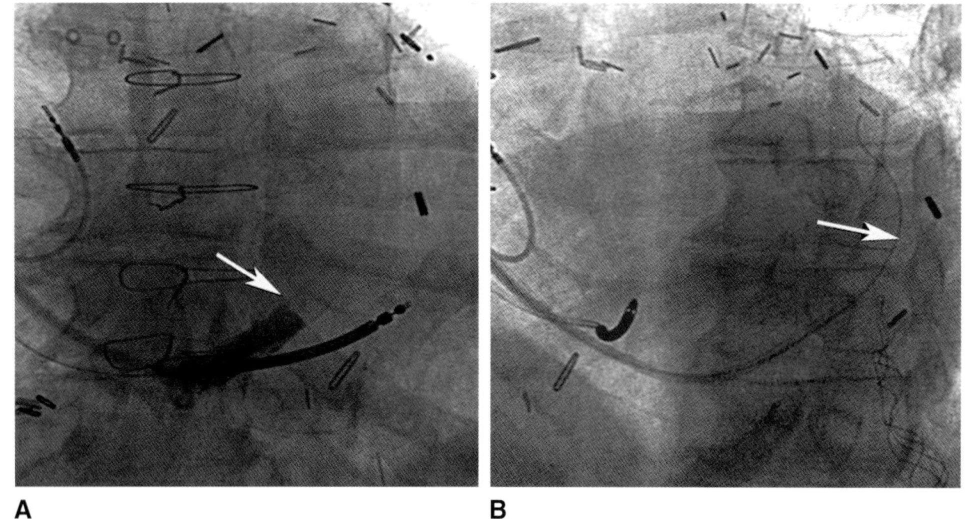

Figure 19-71. Valve near the os of the coronary sinus (CS) prevents guide from advancing. ***A,*** *Anteroposterior projection demonstrating the valve* (arrow). ***B,*** *Left anteroposterior projection with the Glidewire (Terumo Medical Corporation, Somerset, NJ) beyond the valve. The guide would not advance despite normal takeoff of the CS. Manipulation of the catheter did not succeed in advancing the guide beyond the valve. A 0.035-inch angled Glidewire was advanced through the hemostatic valve in the Y-adapter and out the tip of the guide. With manipulation, the Glidewire advanced beyond the valve. The wire was held taut, and the catheter is advanced over the wire beyond the valve.*

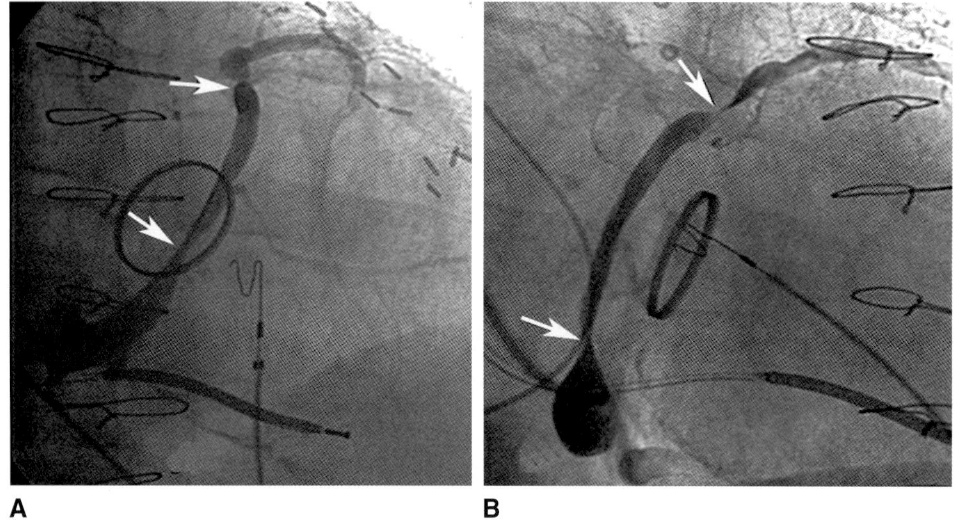

Figure 19-72. Coronary sinus stenosis preventing advancement of the guide. ***A,*** *Anteroposterior projection reveals the proximal stenosis* (arrows). ***B,*** *Right anterior oblique projection shows the proximal stenosis as well as the distal stenosis* (arrows) *in the body of the coronary sinus. Without venoplasty (covered later), this case would require surgical implantation of epicardial leads.*

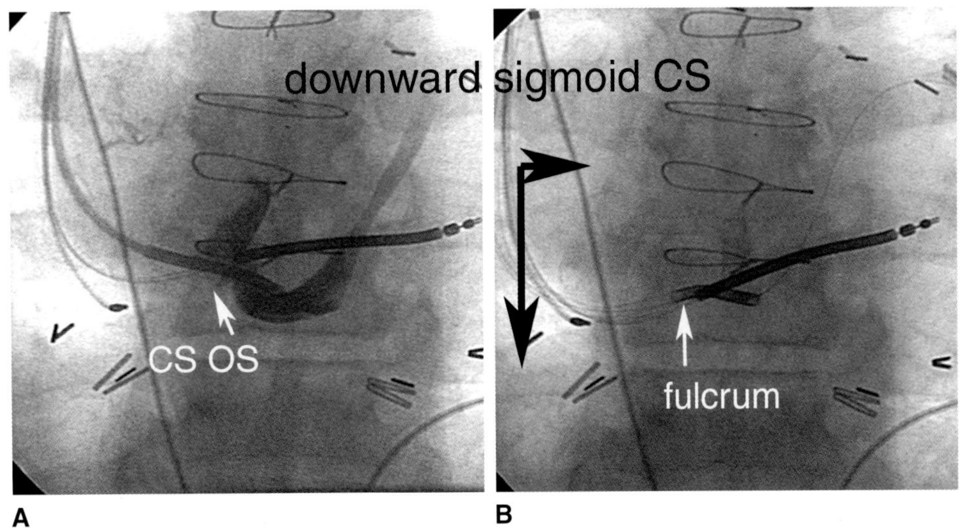

Figure 19-73. The downward sigmoid coronary sinus (CS). **A,** The os of the CS is not difficult to find but it is hard to advance the guide beyond the os. **B,** The effect of trying to advance the guide is a downward trajectory. The majority of the force is directed inferiorly, with little force to advance the catheter into the CS.

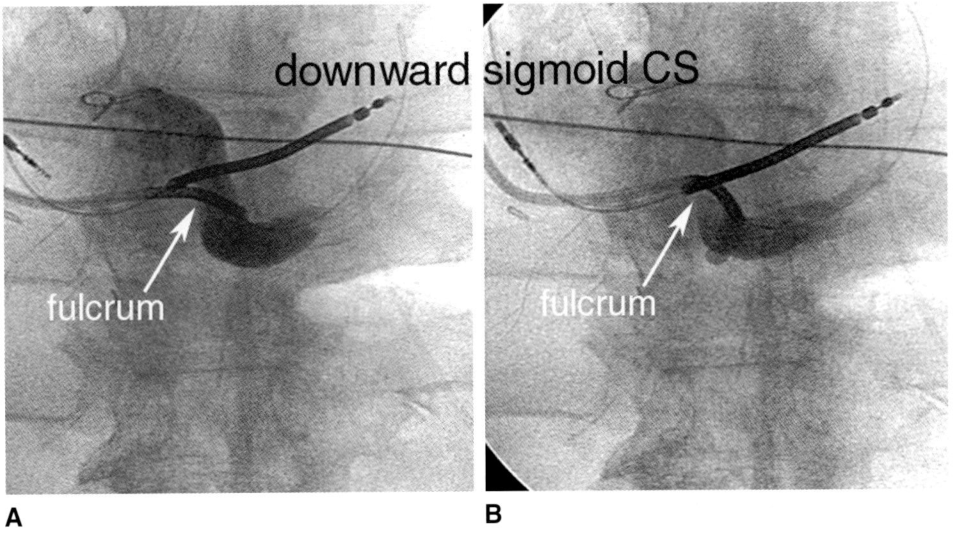

Figure 19-74. Second example of the downward sigmoid coronary sinus (CS). **A,** The tip of the guide is in the CS, and a wire is advanced into the CS. **B,** During attempts to advance the guide, the lip of the CS acts as a fulcrum. The forces are directed down toward the inferior vena cava.

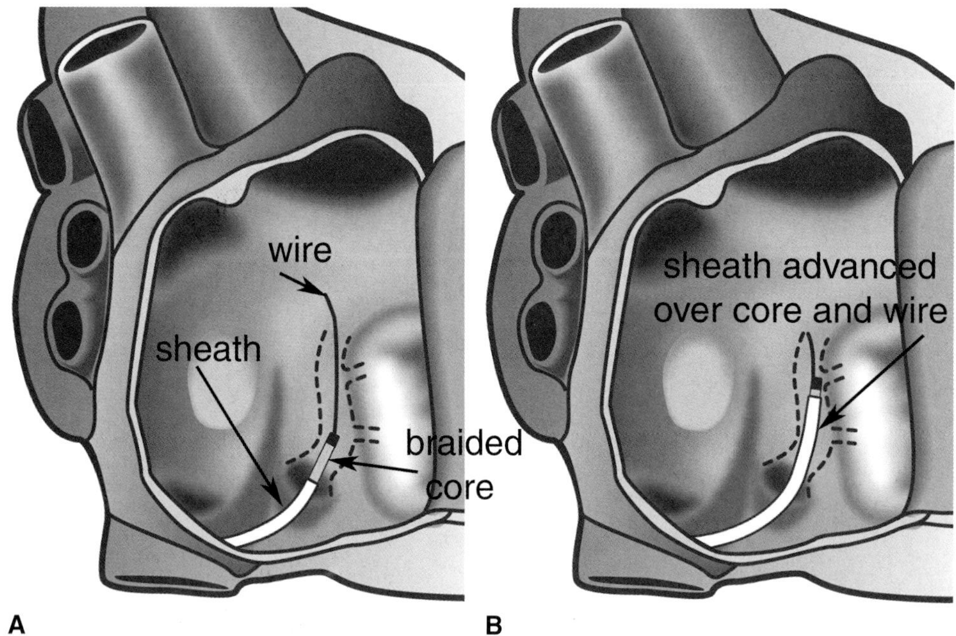

*Figure 19-75. Core is advanced into coronary sinus (CS) over a wire, followed by the sheath. **A,** The wire is advanced into the CS and held taut. The sheath is held fixed at the CS os while the braided core is advanced into the CS. The trajectory cannot be achieved by advance of a catheter alone. **B,** The wire and braided core are held taut to form a rail over which the sheath is advanced.*

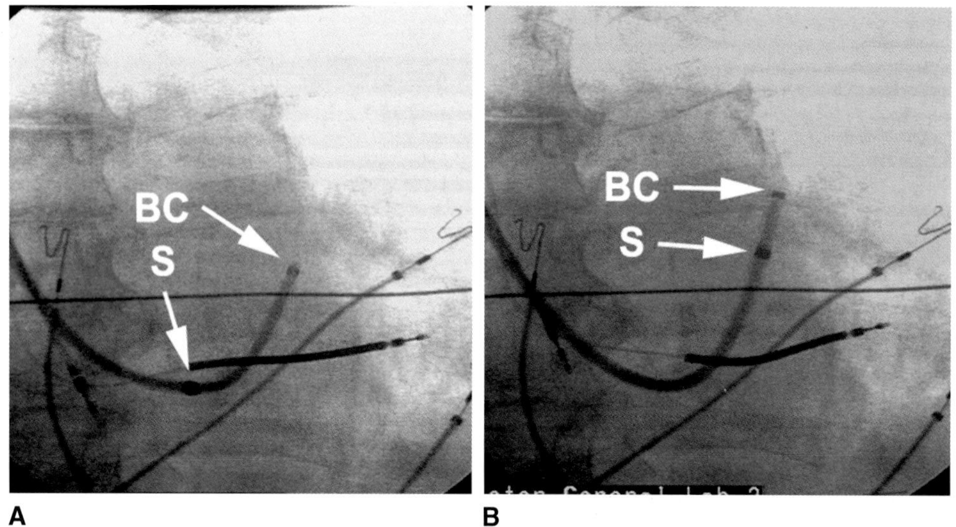

*Figure 19-76. Using the telescopic features of the braided core–sheath combination to cannulate the coronary sinus (CS). **A,** The sheath (S) is held at the os of the CS while the braided core (BC) is advanced into the CS. **B,** The braided core is held in place as the sheath is advanced over the core into the CS. The core is then removed.*

available" approach to LV lead implantation. As experience grows and the implantation tools mature, physicians are increasingly inclined to place the lead in a specific location. As a result, the implanting physician will need to study the patient's coronary venous circulation to determine the best way to get the LV lead to the desired location. Under these circumstances, a complete set of well-performed cine-venograms is important.

In the absence of knowledge to the contrary (such as tissue Doppler ultrasonography information), the midlateral wall of the LV is the location of choice. When tissue Doppler ultrasonography (or another method) defines a specific area for LV lead placement, the operator studies the coronary veins to decide how to use the available anatomy to reach the chosen destination.

Half-Strength versus Full-Strength Contrast Agent

Some favor the use of half-strength contrast agent for occlusive CS venography to reduce the load. However, half-strength contrast agent does not fully define the coronary venous anatomy: Collateral vessels are not well seen, retrograde filling of proximal veins is difficult to appreciate, and a potential venous approach to the target area may be missed. Even when any lateral vein is acceptable, subsequent contrast injections are often required because of difficult anatomy (stenotic areas, phrenic pacing, or high pacing thresholds). Because of incomplete visualization on the initial half-strength venogram, the total contrast load may be ultimately greater than if full-strength contrast agent had been used in the first place. Using full-strength contrast agent for the occlusive CS venogram is following the "golden rule" of implantation.

Figure 19-77 is an example of the limited visualization obtained with occlusive CS venography using half-strength contrast agent. Full-strength contrast agent provides much better visualization of the venous system, both antegrade and retrograde filling (Fig. 19-78). Full-strength contrast agent also visualizes venous collateral vessels that may be used for retrograde placement of the LV lead if the antegrade approach is problematic (Fig. 19-79). Full-strength contrast agent also visualizes venous anomalies that may be important to lead placement (Fig. 19-80).

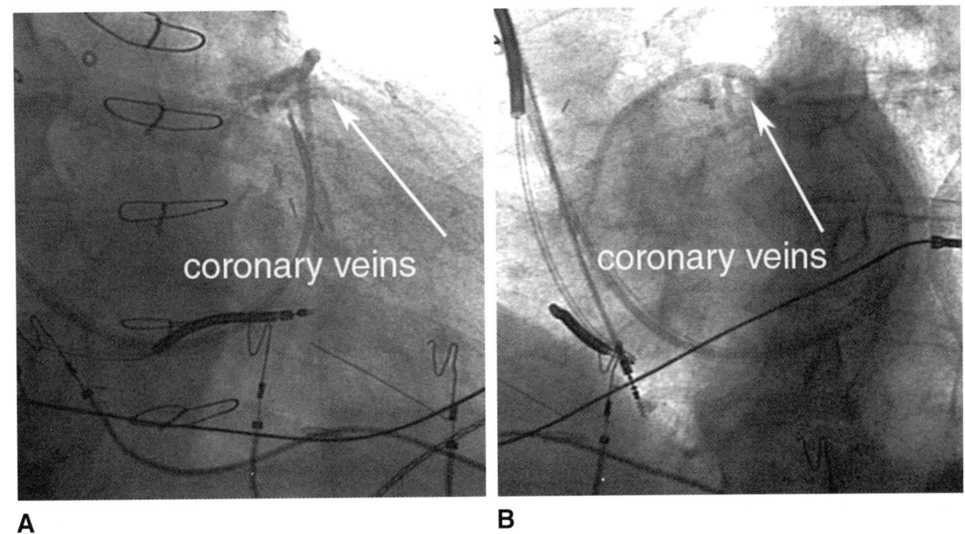

Figure 19-77. Occlusive coronary sinus (CS) venogram performed with half-strength contrast material. ***A,*** *On the right anterior projection, the venous anatomy is difficult to define.* ***B,*** *Left anterior oblique projection of the CS venogram with half-strength contrast material. As with* ***A,*** *it is difficult to appreciate the lateral wall target veins.*

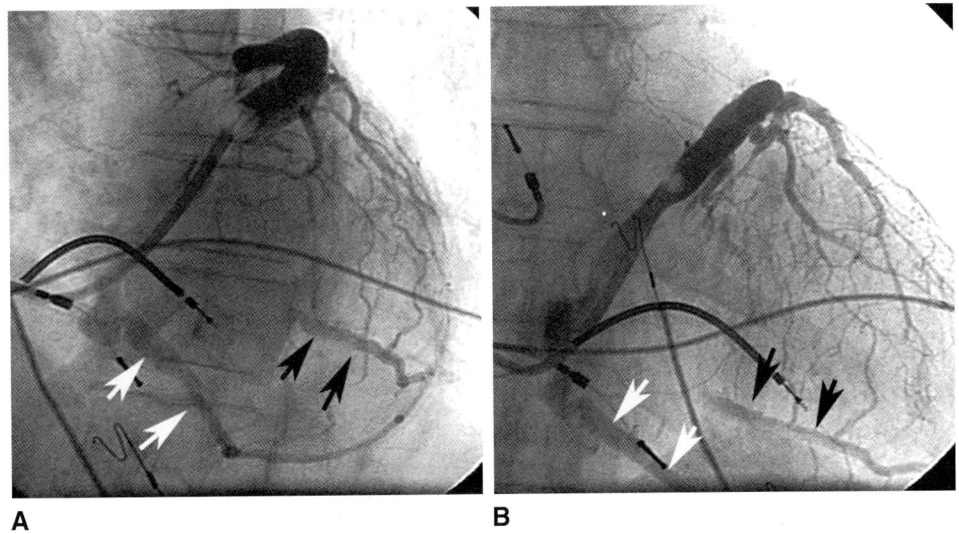

Figure 19-78. ***A*** *and* ***B,*** *Occlusive coronary sinus venogram performed with full-strength contrast material. The veins can be well seen beyond the balloon occlusion. Retrograde filling clearly identifies the middle cardiac vein* (white arrows) *and the posterior lateral cardiac vein (*black arrows*).*

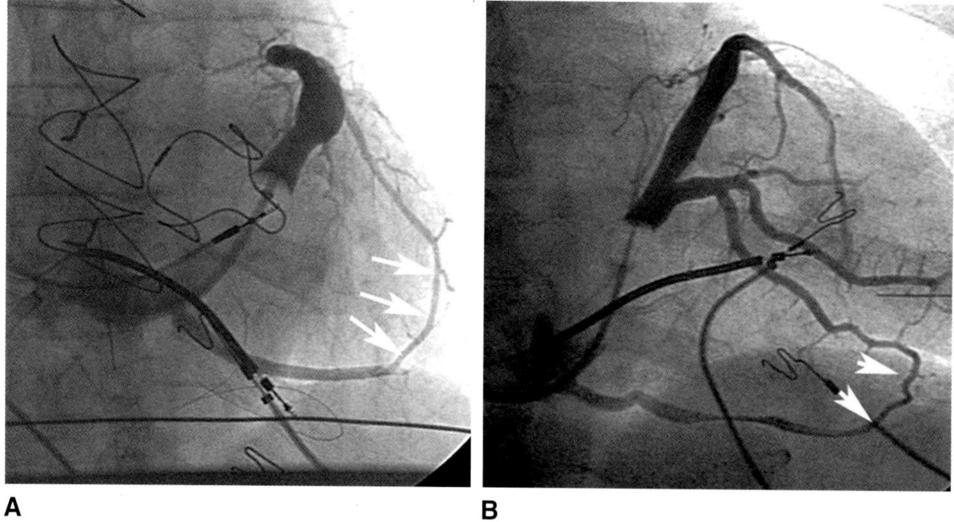

Figure 19-79. ***A*** *and* ***B,*** *Two examples of occlusive coronary sinus venogram with full-strength contrast material, demonstrating collateral vessels. Large collateral vessels that can be used to place the left ventricular lead retrograde are well shown. The patient in* ***A*** *had undergone prior open heart surgery, but the patient in* ***B*** *had not. The arrows point to venous collateral.*

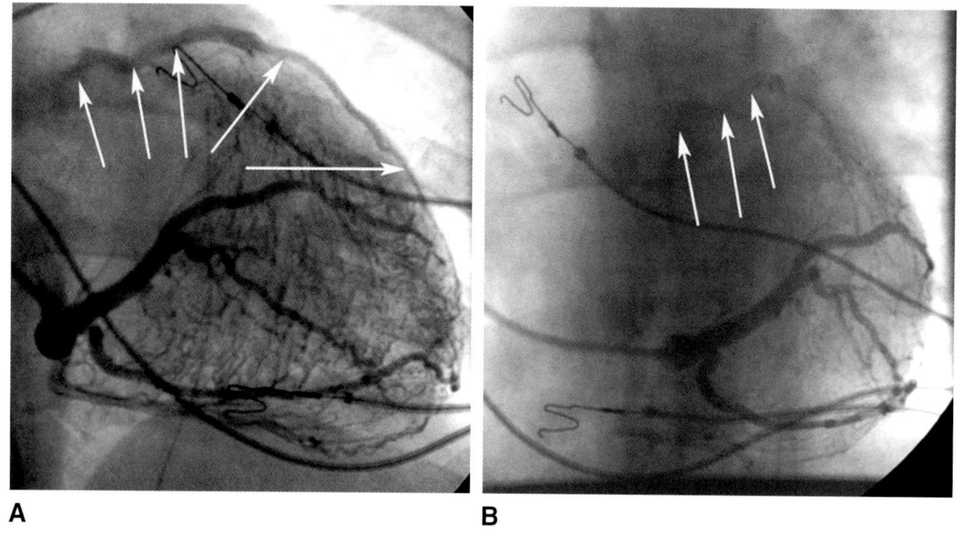

Figure 19-80. ***A*** *and* ***B,*** *Occlusive coronary sinus (CS) venogram with full-strength contrast material demonstrating anomalous venous return. The veins that drain the anterior wall of the left ventricle* (arrows) *form a second CS that empties into the left atrium with a separate CS os.*

Occlusive Coronary Sinus Venography

When imaging the coronary venous system, one must remember the "golden rule" of implantation. It might be tempting to "jump ahead" after the first injection of contrast agent, but when the goal is to place the LV lead in a specific location, a single injection will not fully define the veins to the target area for lead placement.

For efficient, effective lead placement in *every* case, it is essential to obtain all three views of the occlusive CS venogram. Unless all three views are obtained, the coronary venous anatomy is not fully visualized. In many cases, the critical anatomic information required to simply get the lead in the vein is apparent in only one view. Even when the goal of the implanter is to simply find a vein (any vein) to place the lead, a single view often leads to a blind alley. Without the additional views, the implanter may work for hours on the basis of a false assumption about the venous anatomy.

In the case illustrated in Figure 19-81, both the AP (not shown) and LAO venogram views make it appear that the patient's venous anatomy is straightforward with no further contrast agent required. After more than one hour of unsuccessful lead manipulation, the RAO CS venogram showed the proximal takeoff and parallel course of the target vein. With the venous anatomy understood, the lead was quickly placed. The time wasted because of the lack of knowledge about the venous anatomy in one case easily justifies

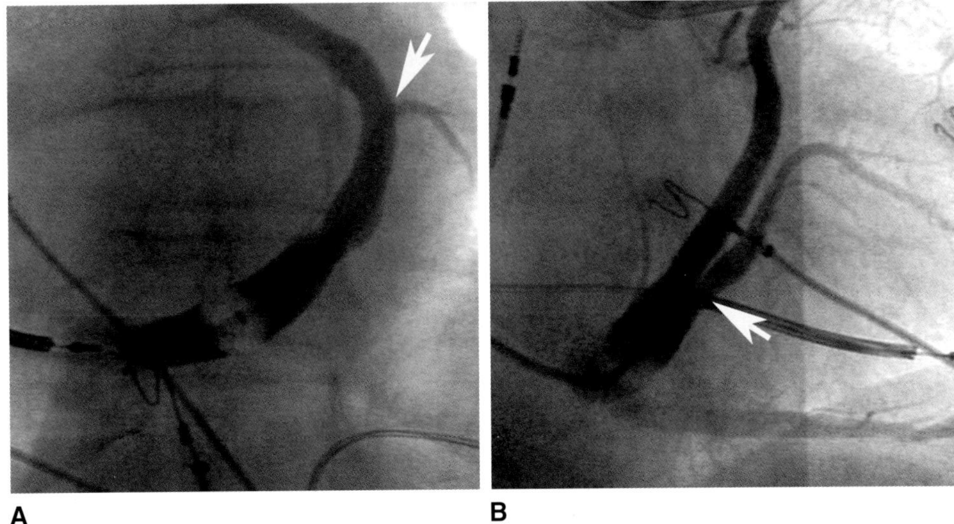

*Figure 19-81. Proximal origin of the lateral wall vein can be seen only on the right anterior oblique (RAO) venogram. The origin of the lateral wall target vein appeared to be in the midcoronary sinus (CS) in both the anteroposterior projection (not shown) and the left anterior oblique projection (**A,** arrow). **B,** The RAO view shows that the origin of the vein is close to the CS os (arrow). Hours were lost trying to advance the left ventricular pacing lead into the vein from the mid-CS in this patient, until the RAO venogram (originally omitted) revealed the proximal origin of the vein.*

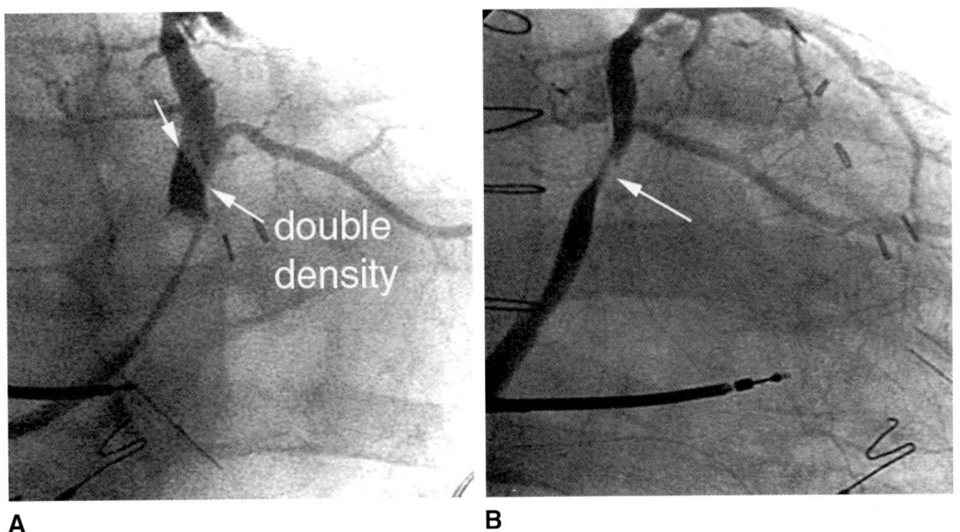

*Figure 19-82. Stenotic coronary sinus (CS) proximal to the lateral wall vein can be seen only on the right anterior oblique (RAO) venogram. **A,** The initial CS venogram indicates simple venous anatomy. Closer inspection, once additional projections are obtained, shows a double density (arrows) near the os of the lateral wall vein. **B,** The RAO venogram reveals the stenotic segment of the main CS proximal to the target vein. Without knowledge of the CS stenosis, the operator could have spent hours trying to advance a lead into the vein.*

multiple additional occlusive venogram projections. Figure 19-82 is another example of the importance of multiple views. In retrospect, careful inspection of the first view suggests more complex venous anatomy than is initially appreciated. Figure 19-83 is another example of the importance of multiple views. In retrospect, the dilated segment of the main CS on the first view could have indicated more complex venous anatomy.

Even with a three-view occlusive CS venogram, however, CS anatomy can be deceiving. Any suspicious areas should be investigated with additional views to make sure the anatomy is completely understood before the lead and method of delivery are chosen. Each step in the implantation procedure must prepare for the most difficult conceivable anatomy.

Figure 19-84 illustrates a case in which all three initial projections of the occlusive venogram suggest a simple takeoff of a large mid–lateral wall vein. However, the density in the LAO projection raises the possibility of an unusual origin of the vein. A steeper LAO projection reveals the complex origin. As shown

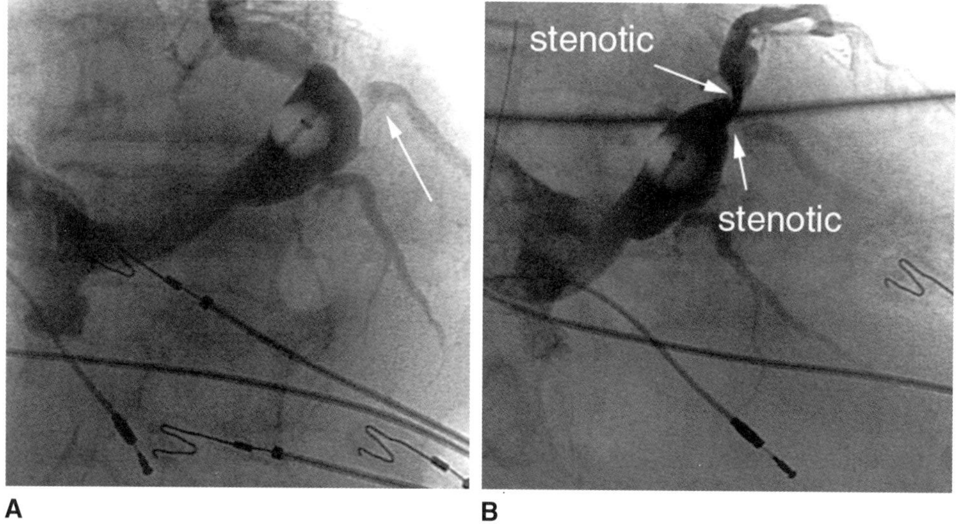

Figure 19-83. *Stenotic coronary sinus (CS) and lateral wall vein seen only in the right anterior oblique (RAO) projection.* ***A,*** *On the anteroposterior (AP) occlusive CS venogram, the lateral wall vein* (arrow) *appears easily accessible.* ***B,*** *RAO view shows, however, that the main CS and target vein are stenotic. What initially appeared to be an easy case on the basis of appearance on the AP and left anterior oblique (not shown) projections is revealed to be difficult only in the RAO projection. Recognition of the stenotic areas affects the approach to the midlateral wall, the choice of left ventricular lead, and the choice of delivery system.*

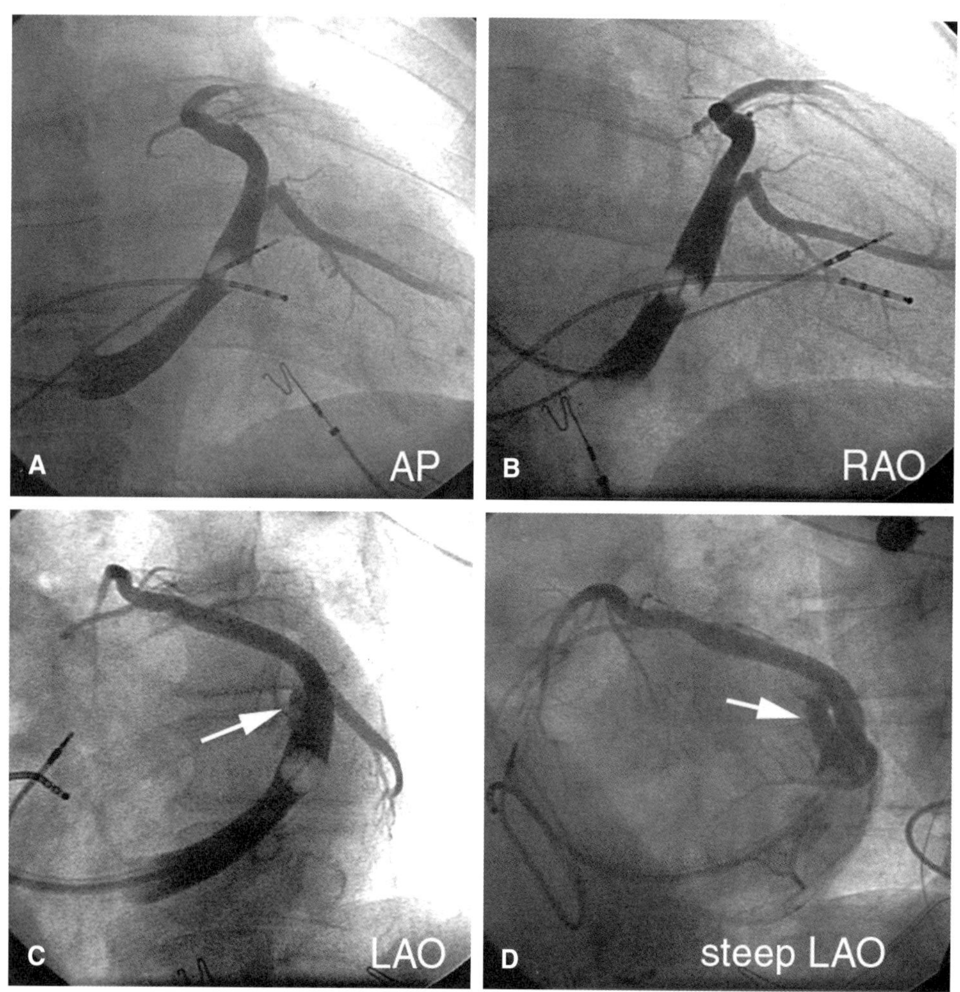

Figure 19-84. *Complex origin of the lateral wall vein only seen in a steep left anterior oblique (LAO) projection.* ***A,*** *Anteroposterior projection;* ***B,*** *right anterior oblique (RAO) projection;* ***C,*** *LAO projection. The density along the medial wall of the coronary sinus raises the possibility of a complex takeoff.* ***D,*** *Steep LAO projection taken to clarify the origin of the target vein. The origin of the vein from the coronary sinus is medial, rather than lateral as suggested by the initial images. If such a situation is unrecognized, the implanter will spend time in the fruitless attempt to direct the wire/lead laterally.*

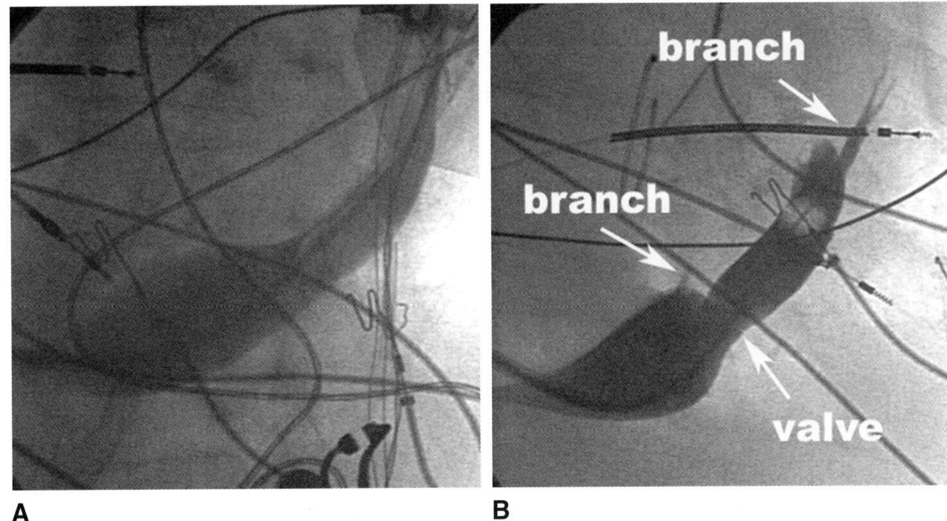

*Figure 19-85. In the left anterior oblique (LAO) projection (**A**), the coronary sinus appears to be dissected. The contrast material appears to be in the pericardial space. **B,** The venous branches of the coronary sinus are evident in the anteroposterior (AP) coronary sinus venogram. Without the AP images, it is difficult to be certain that what can be seen in **A** is not a dissection.*

in Figure 19-85, additional projections of the occlusive venogram may demonstrate that things are not as bad as they seem on the initial venogram. In some cases, the multiview occlusive venogram shows the unexpected. In Figure 19-86 a lateral wall target vein is not appreciated in the initial occlusive venograms. After additional projections, it becomes clear that the defibrillator lead is in the lateral wall vein.

Measures to Overcome Failure to Visualize the Coronary Venous Anatomy

Failure to visualize the coronary venous anatomy with the occlusive CS venogram usually results from incomplete occlusion of the CS. The four options for visualizing the veins that must be draining into the CS are distal occlusion with retrograde filling, double inflation of the balloon, selective vein injection, and coronary artery injection with venous-phase images.

Distal Occlusion with Retrograde Filling

The occlusive balloon is advanced further into a narrow portion of the CS and inflated. Full-strength contrast agent will provide visualization of the vessels proximal to the occlusion as they fill retrograde from the contrast agent injected into the distal veins. In some cases, when the balloon is inflated distally, it slides back proximally and will not occlude the vessel or produce an adequate venogram.

Double Inflation of the Balloon

When the occlusive balloon is too small to occlude the mid-CS, it may be double inflated. Specifically, a full syringe of air is injected into the balloon and the valve is closed. The syringe is detached and filled with air and is connected to the valve. Then the valve is opened, and additional air injected into the balloon.

Selective Vein Injection

Because veins must drain into the CS, a preformed catheter is manipulated within the CS with puffs of contrast agent until a target vein is found. Selective occlusive injection of one target vein will demonstrate the other veins through retrograde filling (Fig. 19-87).

Coronary Artery Injection with Venous-Phase Images

If no veins draining the lateral wall of the LV can be visualized with the first three approaches, injection of the coronary artery with delayed images for venous return can be effective (Figs. 19-88 and 19-89).

Basic Patterns of the Coronary Venous Anatomy

The variability of the venous anatomy may at first seem infinite, but there are basic patterns. Recognition of the venous pattern is important in selecting an approach to the target area and the type of lead. The venous anatomy can be classified according to the size of the vein that drains a particular area and characterized from the angle the vein takes as it comes off the CS.

Size Distribution

The four patterns in the proximal to distal caliber of veins draining into the CS are as follows:

1. Midlateral dominant (Fig. 19-90A).
2. Posterior lateral dominant (see Fig. 19-90B).
3. Balanced (Fig. 19-91A).
4. Anterior lateral dominant (see Fig. 19-91B).

Text continued on p. 716

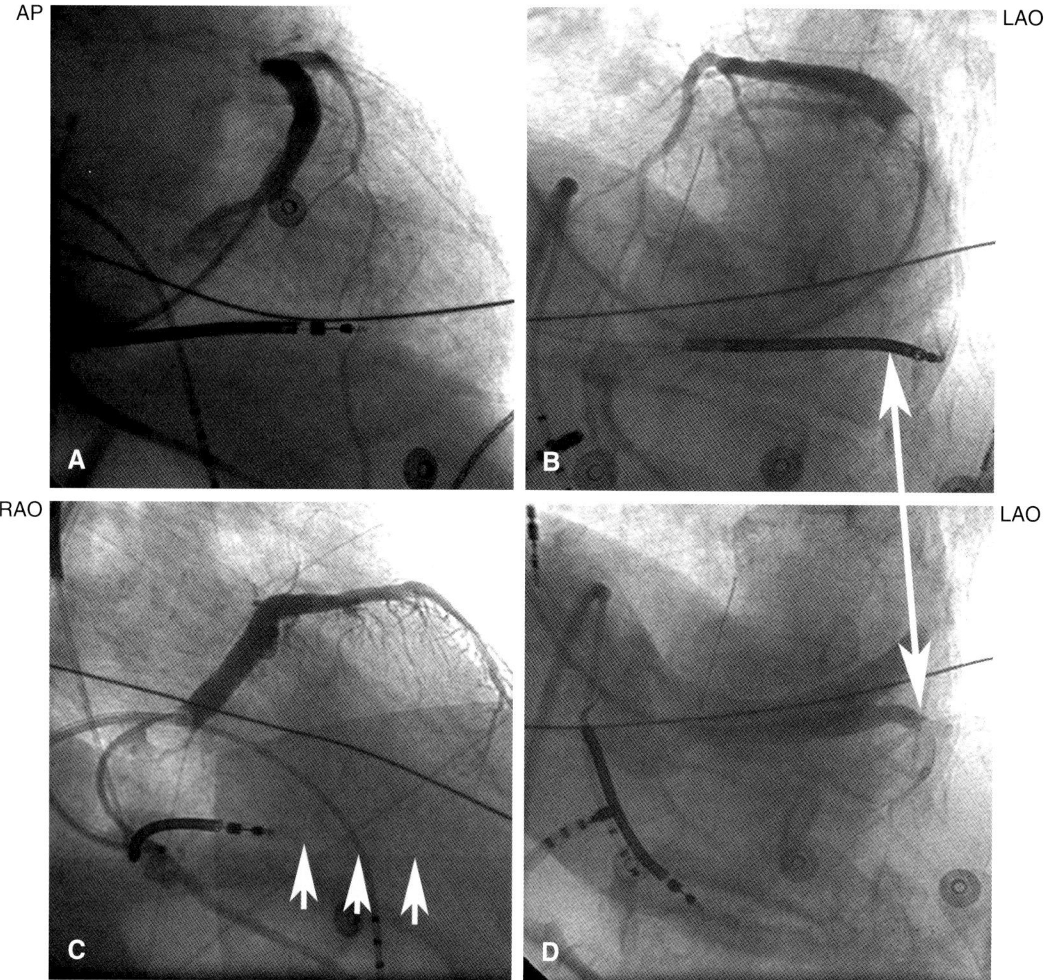

Figure 19-86. The defibrillator lead in the large posterior large lateral vein. ***A,*** *No lateral wall target vein is identified in the anteroposterior projection. The defibrillation lead appears to be placed in the mid–right ventricular (RV) septum.* ***B,*** *No lateral wall target veins are identified on this left anterior oblique (LAO) projection. However, the location of the defibrillator lead is unusual for the midseptum.* ***C,*** *The right anterior oblique projection reveals that the defibrillator lead is in the large posterior lateral wall vein, not the RV septum as was originally thought.* Arrows *mark subtle retrograde filling of the vein.* ***D,*** *The defibrillator lead is removed from the posterior lateral wall vein. The LAO projection now shows the vein previously obscured by the lead. In* ***B, C,*** *and* ***D*** *the* arrows *indicate the location of the posterior lateral wall vein.*

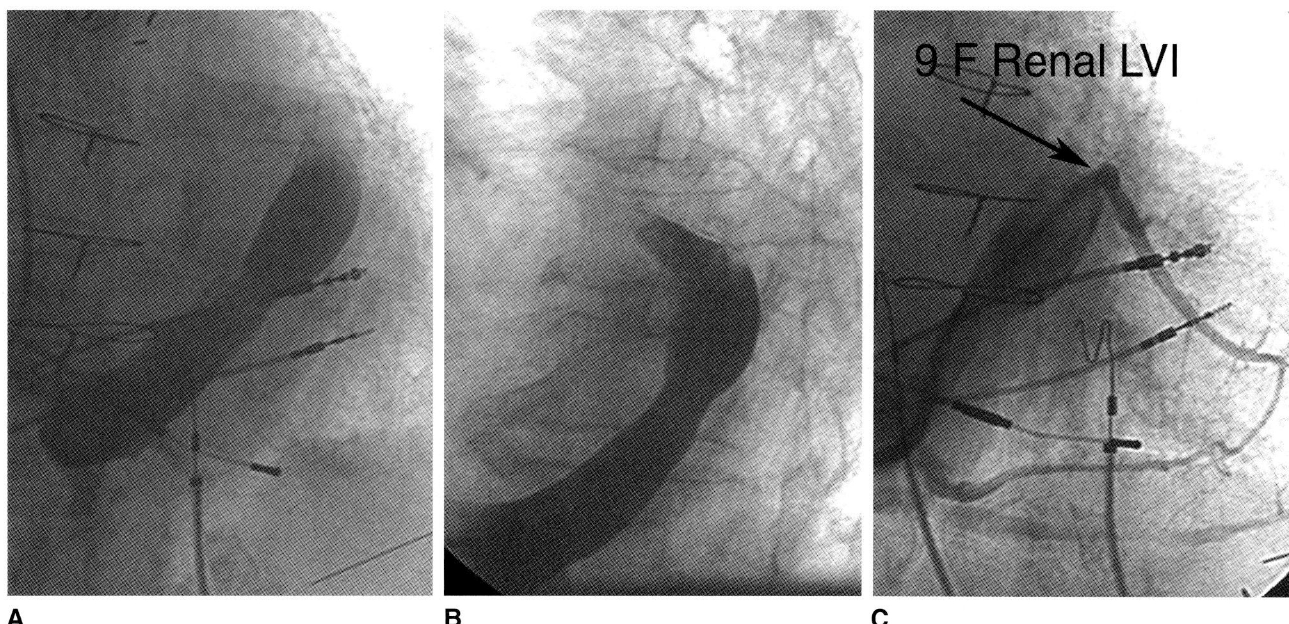

Figure 19-87. Lateral wall veins identified with selective injection of contrast material. ***A,*** *No lateral wall vein is identified despite double inflation of the balloon and injection of full-strength contrast material.* ***B,*** *No lateral wall veins are identified.* ***C,*** *a 9F OD/7F ID guide with a renal shape (renal lateral vein introducer) is advanced through a 9F sheath located in the coronary sinus to selectively engage a target vein. Injection of contrast material in the anterior lateral vein also fills the posterior lateral vein retrograde.*

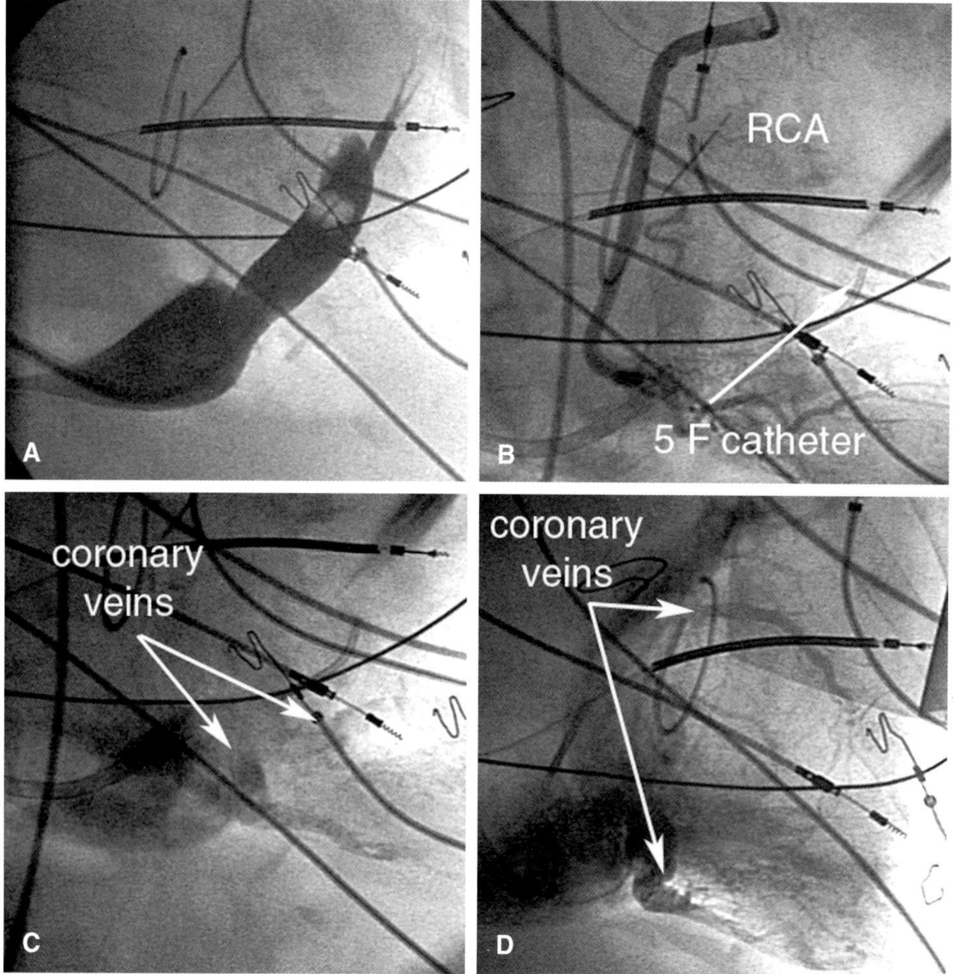

Figure 19-88. The coronary veins are identified only on delayed images after injection of contrast material into the coronary artery. ***A,*** *The coronary sinus (CS) is identified. Despite multiple attempts, including double balloon inflation and injection of full-strength contrast material, the veins draining the lateral wall are not visualized.* ***B,*** *Attempts are made to selectively cannulate and inject veins to the lateral wall with a 5F catheter. After the veins have not been identified by either occlusive venography or selective retrograde injection, arterial access is obtained, and selective injection of the right coronary artery (RCA) is performed. The RCA is shown with imaging during the initial contrast injection.* ***C,*** *The left anterior oblique projection of delayed imaging after RCA injection shows the coronary veins draining into the CS.* ***D,*** *The right anterior oblique projection of delayed imaging after RCA injection reveals the coronary veins draining into the CS.*

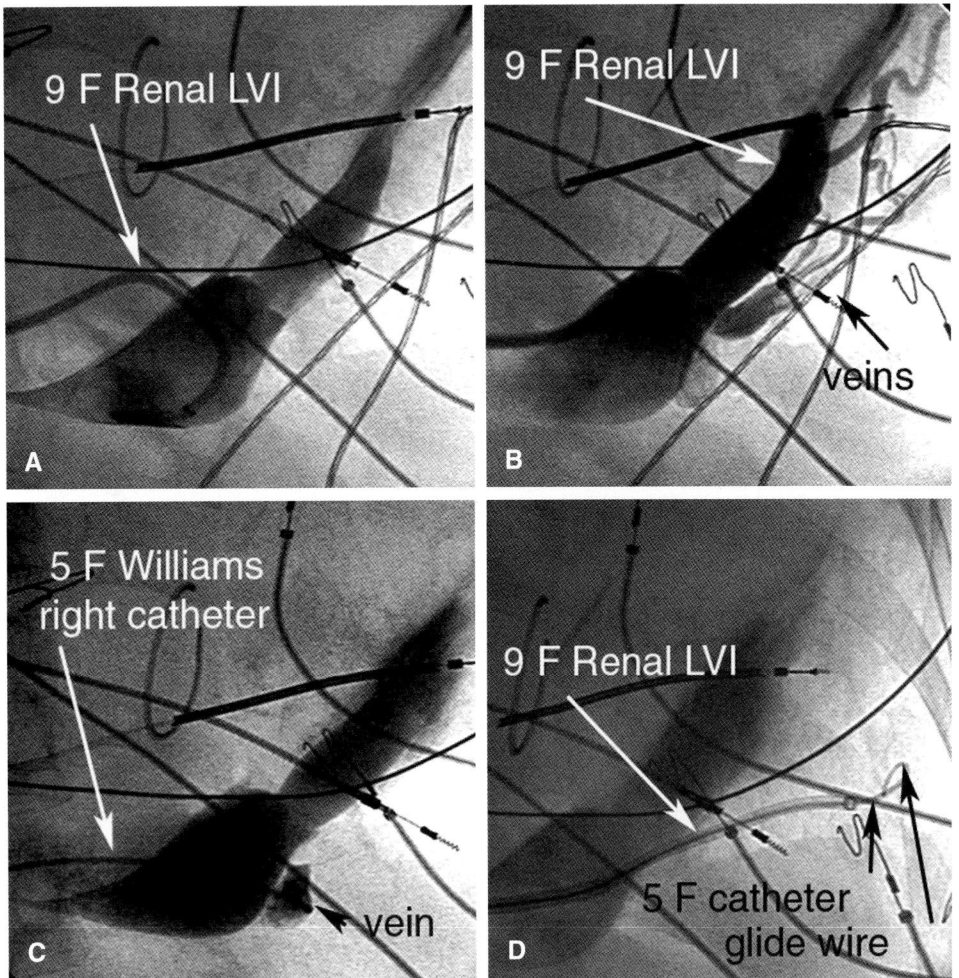

Figure 19-89. *Selective cannulation of the coronary veins identified on delayed images after arterial injection.* ***A,*** *Manipulation of a 9F OD/7F ID renal-shaped guide (renal lateral vein introducer [renal LVI]) in the coronary sinus is unable to locate and cannulate the target vein identified in the venous phase after injection of the right coronary artery.* ***B,*** *After selective injection of the anterior coronary vein, the lateral coronary veins are seen to fill retrograde.* ***C,*** *A 5F Williams right catheter is inserted into the 9F renal LVI. The combination is used to successfully cannulate the lateral wall vein.* ***D,*** *The renal LVI is advanced into the vein using the combined support of a Terumo Glidewire (Terumo Medical Corporation, Somerset, NJ) and the 5F Williams catheter.*

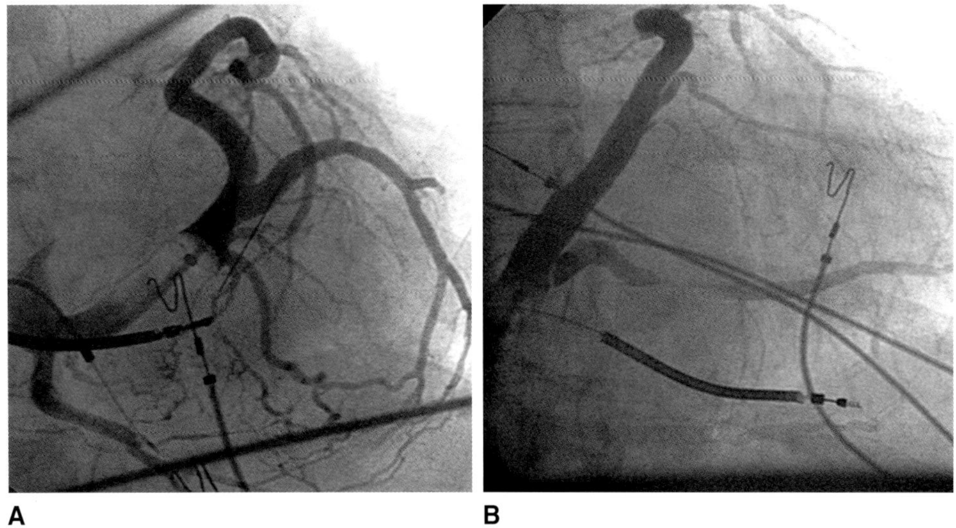

Figure 19-90. Midlateral and posterior-lateral dominant patterns of coronary veins. ***A,*** *The largest coronary vein drains into the midportion of the coronary sinus (CS) and is thus midlateral dominant.* ***B,*** *The largest coronary vein drains into the posterior CS and is thus posterior-lateral dominant.*

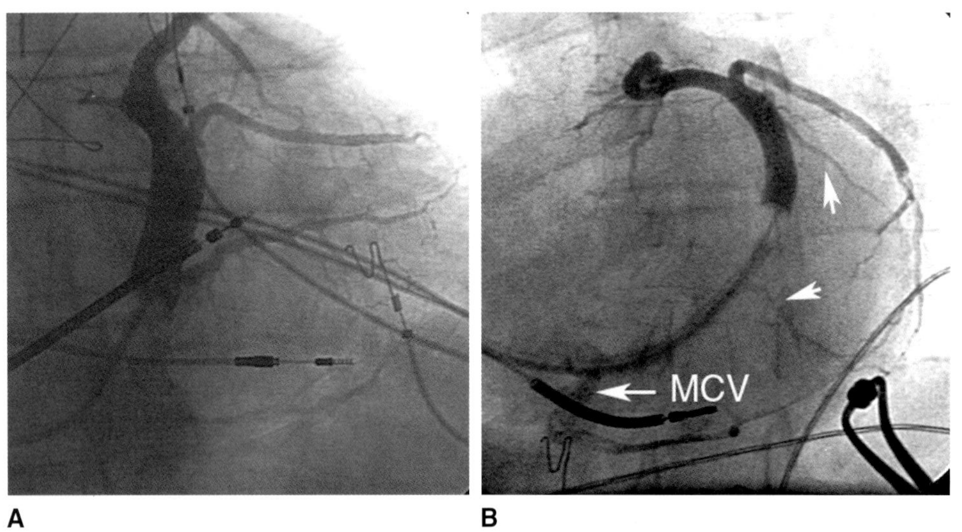

Figure 19-91. Balanced and anterior lateral dominant patterns of coronary veins. ***A,*** *The lateral wall target veins are of approximately equal size.* ***B,*** *The midlateral wall veins are small* (upper two arrows). *The anterior lateral vein is large and thus dominant. The lower* arrow *points to the middle cardiac vein (MCV).*

Angle of the Vein as It Empties into the Coronary Sinus

The angle that a vein forms as it empties into the CS further defines the coronary venous anatomy. Although some angles are easy to place wires through (Fig. 19-92), others are more difficult (see Fig. 19-97).

Effect of Prior Cardiac Surgery on the Venous Circulation

The greatest challenges arise in the patient with prior mitral valve repair or replacement, presumably owing to the distortion of the CS and associated venous structures during repair or replacement of the valve. Figure 19-93 demonstrates the tortuous vein segments frequently seen in such patients.

Delivery Systems/Tools for Site-Specific Implantation of Left Ventricular Pacing Leads: Evolution to Third-Generation Telescoping and Beyond

Delivery Systems versus Improved Pacing Leads

At first, transvenous lateral wall LV pacing was performed with modified stylet-driven leads inserted into a coronary vein from a catheter in the CS. In many patients, it was impossible to advance the stylet-driven lead into a coronary vein with a stylet from the CS. Initially, physicians and device companies focused almost

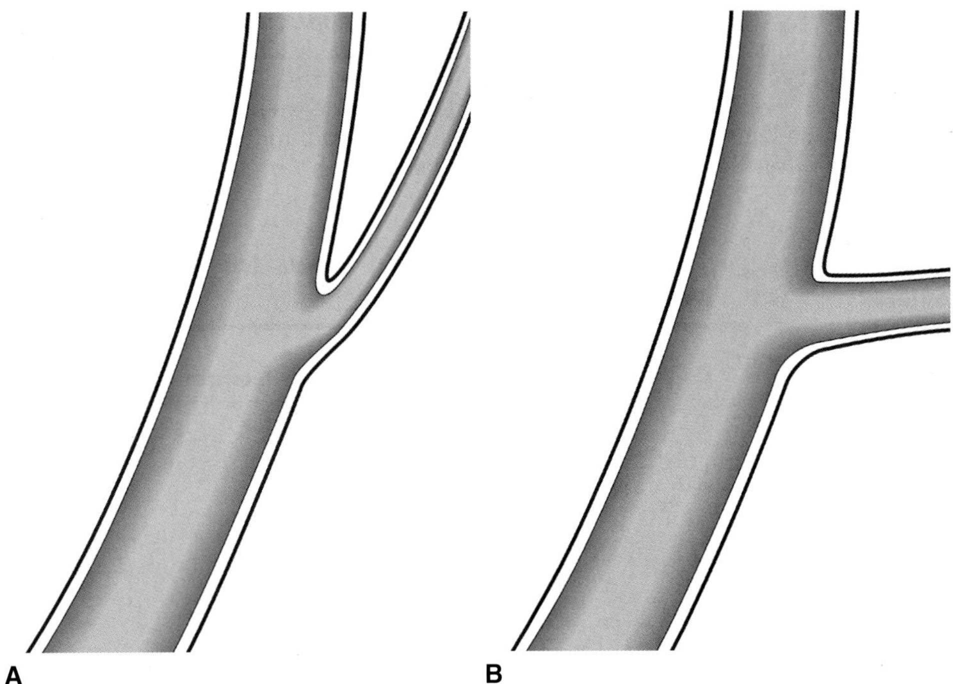

Figure 19-92. Illustrations of coronary veins that are easy to cannulate from the main coronary sinus. ***A,*** *The vein enters the coronary sinus (CS) on an angle that is very easy to cannulate.* ***B,*** *The vein enters the CS on an angle that is easy to cannulate.*

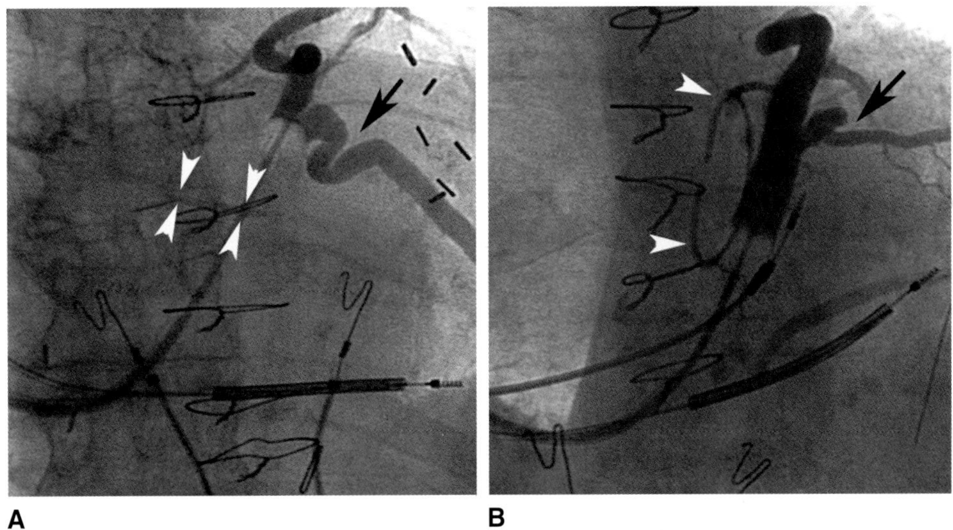

Figure 19-93. Two patients with highly tortuous proximal coronary veins after mitral valve replacement/repair. ***A,*** *This patient has a St. Jude Medical (St. Paul, Minn.) mitral valve (*arrowheads*). Note the tortuous lateral wall vein (*black arrow*).* ***B,*** *This patient underwent placement of a mitral ring (*arrowheads*). The lateral wall vein is highly tortuous (*black arrow*). In both cases, initial attempts at left ventricular (LV) lead placement were unsuccessful. With the use of a third-generation delivery system, LV lead placement on the lateral wall was successful. Highly tortuous proximal coronary veins are commonly seen after mitral valve replacement/repair, presumably because of distortion of the mitral annulus.*

exclusively on improvements in the LV pacing lead as the means to successful implantation. On occasion, an angioplasty guidewire inserted beside the lead into the vein ahead of the pacing lead made it possible to advance the stylet-driven lead into the vein. This maneuver, referred to as the *buddy wire technique*, is depicted in Figure 19-202. On the basis of this approach and the relative ease of directing a guidewire into a vein, it was reasoned that over-the-wire was a superior design for LV pacing leads. LV pacing leads deliverable over the angioplasty wire became available in the United States in 1998. With these leads, the guidewire is directed into the coronary vein from a catheter in the CS. The pacing lead is then tracked over the wire into the vein. Initially, over-the-wire leads were believed to be all that was necessary for successful LV lead placement in most patients. With experience, however, the limitations of over-the-wire pacing leads became apparent.[31] In addition, the importance of precise LV lead placement to the success of CRT was recognized. It became clear that the successful LV lead placement required a better means of delivering the lead to coronary vein, "a delivery system" (Table 19-5).

TABLE 19-5. Tools Available for Placement of LV Pacing Leads for Cardiac Resynchronization Therapy*

	Biotronik	Cook	ELA	Guidant	Medtronic	Pressure Products	St. Jude
Long peel-away sheath	Yes	Yes	No	No	No	Yes	Yes
Anatomically shaped long peel-away sheath	No	No	No	No	No	Yes	No
Braided guide to access the CS	Yes	No	Yes	Yes	Yes	Yes (in peel-away)	No
Shape 1	Standard multipurpose		Standard multipurpose	Rapido Advance	Straight (1)	Standard	
Shape 2	Large multipurpose		Hook	Large multipurpose	Large multipurpose	Jumbo	
Shape 3	Standard hook			CS-Wide	Extended multipurpose	Mini	
Shape 4	Large hook			Large hook	Amplatz		
Shape 5	Amplatz			Amplatz	Extended hook		
Braided deflectable open-lumen catheter	No	No	No	No	Yes	No	No
Deflectable EP catheter for CS cannulation	No	No	No	No	Mariner	No	LiveWire
First-generation telescoping:	No	No	No	Yes	Attain Select	No	No
Shape 1				IC-50	Straight		
Shape 2				IC-90	90-degree		
Shape 3					Hook		
Deflectable catheter for wire placement	No	No	No	No	Yes—Attain Prevail	No	No
Second-generation telescoping				Yes (1)	Yes (1)	No	
Third-generation telescoping	No	No	No	No	No	Yes	No
Shape 1						Renal	
Shape 2						Hockey-stick	
Shape 3						Multipurpose	
Shape 4						Hook	

CS, coronary sinus; EP, electrophysiology; LV, left ventricular.

*Biotronik GmBh & Co., Berlin; Cook Vascular, Inc., Leechburg, Penna.; ELA Medical, Sorin Group, Milan; Guidant, Boston Scientific, Natick, Mass.; Medtronic, Inc., Minneapolis, Minn.; Pressure Products, Inc., San Pedro, Calif.; St. Jude Medical, St. Paul, Minn.

Analysis of a Delivery System for Left Ventricular Lead Placement

All LV pacing lead delivery systems divide the process into two independent but interrelated steps, (1) CS cannulation and (2) advancement of the guidewire/lead into the target vein. Dividing the process into two steps allows equipment design to be more specific to the requirement of the step. In order to fully describe an LV lead delivery system, we must first define the following: sheath, introducer, catheter, and guide.

For the purposes of this discussion, *sheath* and *introducer* are used synonymously. In most cases introducers/sheaths do not have braided-wire walls. The absence of braid means that introducers/sheaths are prone to kinking, do not have torque control, but can be peeled away. The French (F) size of introducers/sheaths reflects the inner diameter (ID). For example, a 9F introducer/sheath has an ID of 9F and an outer diameter (OD) of 11F. Sheaths/introducers are typically used to obtain arterial or venous access through which to insert a pacing lead or another catheter.

The terms *catheter* and *guide* have similar but not identical meanings. In the context of a delivery system for LV pacing leads, the word *catheter* refers to an open-lumen catheter unless otherwise specified. A catheter is usually thought of as being used to inject a fluid or advance a wire. A *guide* is usually thought of as not only capable of being used to inject a fluid or advance a wire but also large enough to serve as a conduit for a pacing lead or another device, such as a balloon catheter. Within the context of this discussion, catheters and guides have braided-wire walls. The presence of braid means that the catheter/guide is less prone to kinking, does have torque control, but cannot be peeled away. Guides and catheters are typically placed in the body through a sheath introducer of the same or larger French size. The French size of a catheter/guide refers to the outer diameter, whereas the French size of introducers/sheaths, as already mentioned, refers to the ID.

Finally, a generic term is needed to refer to any long open-lumen tubing of unspecified size, structure, and function. For this purpose I will use catheter. Thus, *catheter* can mean catheter, guide, sheath, or introducer.

Overview of Left Ventricular Pacing Lead Delivery Systems

At times the catheter used to cannulate the CS inadvertently advances into a coronary vein. Once the vein is selectively cannulated, it is "easy" to advance a stylet-driven lead, an over-the-wire lead, or an angioplasty wire into the vein, depending on the relative sizes of the catheter in the vein and the pacing lead. An important step in the development of modern delivery systems is the recognition that selective cannulation of the coronary veins is safe. With the recognition of the safety and ease of implantation after selective cannulation, telescoping delivery systems began to be developed.

A *telescoping LV lead delivery system* is defined by the selective cannulation of a coronary vein with a second catheter that is advanced (telescoped) through the catheter used for access to the CS. Under these circumstances, the catheter in the CS through which the second catheter is advanced is designated as the *platform* for the telescoping system. The characteristics (size, shape, and composition) of the catheter that serves as the platform of a telescoping system have a major impact on the ultimate success of the LV lead placement. The catheter in the CS serving as the CS platform is discussed separately, after the evolution of telescoping system is described.

Initially there were no commercially available telescoping delivery systems designed for BiV pacing. Many successful implanters created their own by adapting sheaths, guides, and catheters from interventional cardiology and radiology. Over the last several years, telescoping systems have evolved from the first to the third generation. Each step in the evolutionary process of the LV lead delivery systems was stimulated by the limitations of the preceding system. Third-generation telescoping delivery systems offer the greatest procedural flexibility. They are able to function as nontelescoping or with first-, second-, and/or third-generation capacity, depending on the requirements of the anatomy.

Figure 19-94 illustrates the limitations encountered by an over-the-wire lead with each of the first three delivery systems, starting with the nontelescoping delivery system. Stylet-driven leads encounter similar limitations with less difficult venous anatomy. Second-generation telescoping systems use the smaller catheter to deliver the wire and then attempt to deform the tip of the catheter used to cannulate the CS to fit into the target vein. When the smaller catheter is removed, the pacing lead is delivered directly through the deformed guide without the need for wire exchange. The third-generation telescoping delivery system is distinguished from previous systems by having the catheter pre-shaped to fit the anatomy large enough to deliver the lead directly to the target vein. Of note is the difference in the venous access between third-generation and the other three forms of delivery systems, assuming that all use a 9F sheath. With the third-generation delivery system, the 9F sheath used for venous access extends from the pocket into the CS. With the other three systems, the 9F catheter for venous access ends in the subclavian vein. The 8F or 9F guide that is inserted through the short 9F venous access must be designed to locate and cannulate the CS. When the 9F sheath extends into the CS, the 8F or 9F guide that is inserted into the sheath can be designed for selective vein cannulation.

Evolution of the Left Ventricular Pacing Lead Delivery System

Step 1: The Nontelescoping Delivery System

The initial step in the evolution of an LV pacing lead delivery system is the ability to reliably establish a nontelescoping system via CS access. Figure 19-95 illustrates a case in which the pacing lead easily advances

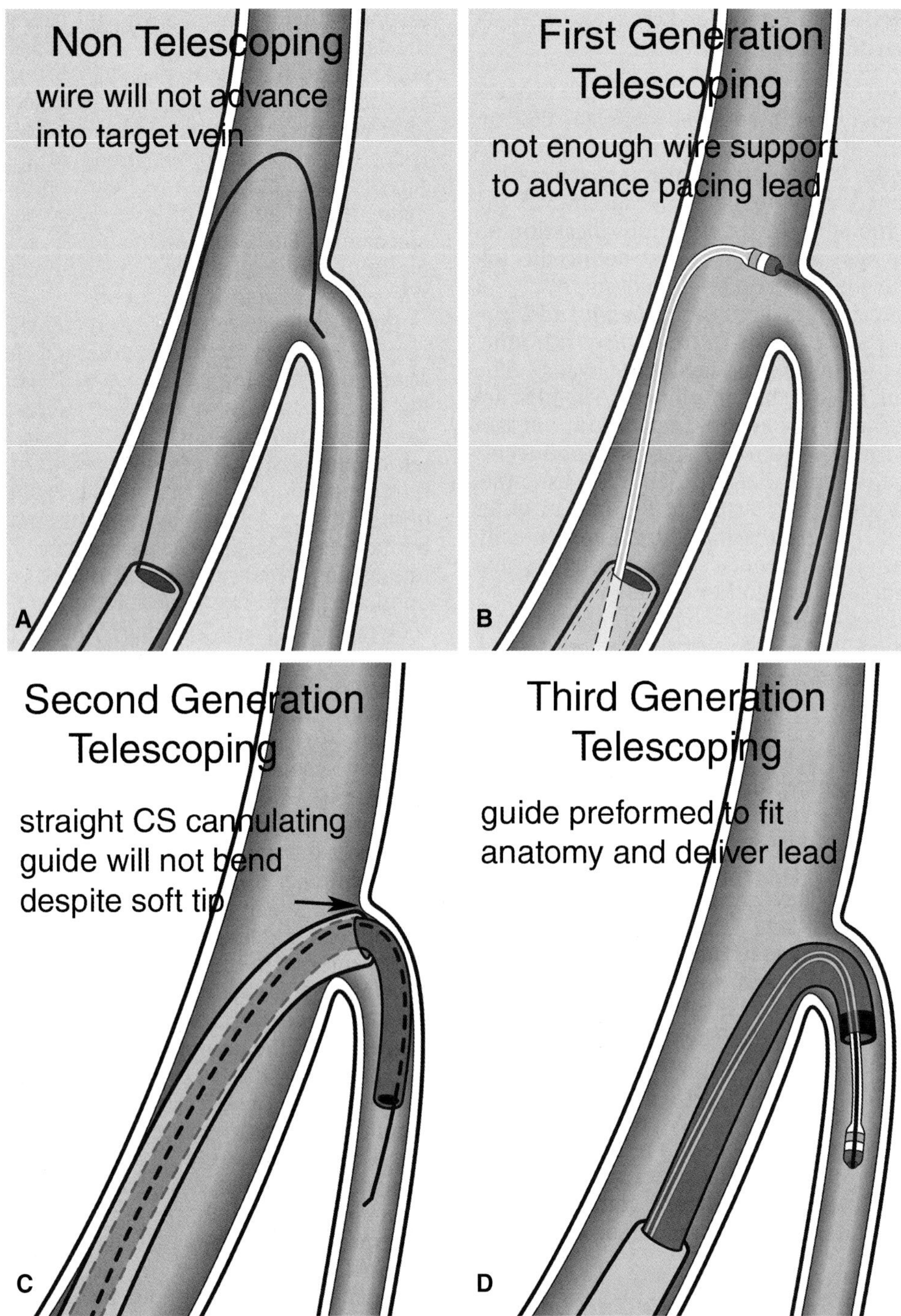

*Figure 19-94. Nontelescoping through third-generation telescoping left ventricular (LV) lead delivery systems. **A,** The nontelescoping approach is illustrated. The guide/sheath is placed in the coronary sinus (CS). It is physically impossible to direct a pacing lead or angioplasty wire into the target vein. **B,** A first-generation telescoping delivery system is used. A small preformed or deflectable catheter delivers the angioplasty wire, but there is not enough wire support to advance the LV lead into the target vein. **C,** A second-generation telescoping delivery system is used. The angioplasty wire and smaller catheter are advanced into the target vein. The straight tip of the same guide used to cannulate the CS will not track over the wire into the target vein. **D,** A third-generation telescoping delivery system is used. A preformed guide large enough to deliver the angioplasty wire and pacing lead is used. The tip configuration of the preformed guide matches the target vein. It does not need to be deformed to fit the anatomy and easily advances into the vein over the wire for LV lead delivery. The sheath in the CS serves only for CS cannulation and as the conduit for the preformed guide. The CS cannulation catheter is not intended to be deformed by smaller catheters to fit into the target vein. Its sole purpose is to provide a conduit for the pacing lead or preformed catheter used to deliver the lead.*

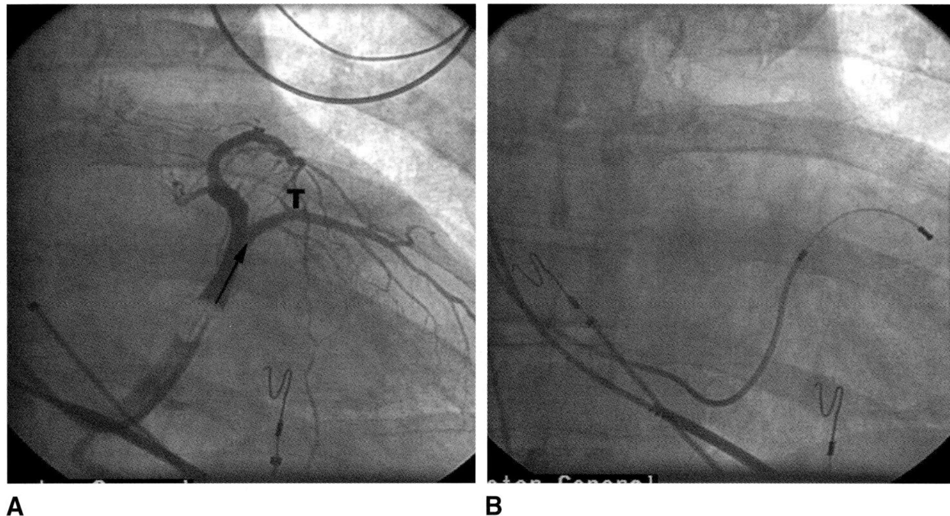

Figure 19-95. Placement of a left ventricular (LV) pacing lead on the lateral wall through ideal venous anatomy. ***A,*** *Anteroposterior (AP) projection of the coronary sinus venogram.* ***B,*** *AP projection of the Medtronic, Inc. (Minneapolis, Minn.), Attain 2187 LV pacing lead in place. The stylet-driven lead easily advances into the lateral wall target vein. The takeoff of the target vein lines up with the sheath. The forward vector of the lead is not degraded by the need to change direction to enter the target vein. In addition no twists, turns or stenotic segments limit access to the vein.*

from the CS onto the epicardial surface of the LV through the lateral wall target vein once CS access is obtained. In patients with CHF, establishing the most basic LV delivery system—that is, CS access—is not a given, but better physician training for CS was believed to be all that was necessary. As a result of the combined expectation that over-the-wire pacing leads would eliminate problems with LV lead placement and that training and experience would eliminate problems with CS cannulation, there was little focus on improving the delivery system. However, even with training and experience, CS cannulation using the catheters provided with the pacing leads was unreliable regardless of the method employed—contrast injection or EP catheter. As discussed in detail in the section on CS cannulation, rapid reliable access to the CS is facilitated by an anatomically shaped catheter, an understanding of the anatomy surrounding the CS, torque control, and use of contrast material. Thus, the first step in the evolution of an LV pacing lead delivery system was the development of a catheter shape suitable for CS cannulation in patients with CHF.

In many cases, however, even with the availability of catheter shapes to rapidly cannulate the CS and the availability of over-the-wire pacing leads, the angioplasty wire/LV lead does not advance because of a difficult takeoff or small, tortuous, or stenotic target vein, as illustrated in Figure 19-96. The operator successfully implants the LV lead in an alternative, less desirable position. In some cases, as a result of unfavorable anatomy, the pacing lead may be placed in the anterior or middle cardiac vein, a location that may actually worsen LV function. The actual rate of success using a nontelescoping system, defined as placement in the most anatomically desirable position, is unknown but in my estimate is only 50%.

Limitations of Nontelescoping Delivery Systems. The wire/lead in a nontelescoping delivery system has an initial forward vector imparted by the operator at the shoulder as the wire is advanced. The force of the final forward vector is defined as the force at the tip of the wire that allows it to advance. For a wire/lead to advance, the force of the forward vector applied at the shoulder must overcome the resistive forces along the length of the wire/lead without buckling it. In the venous system, turns, vessel size, and the presence of a focal stenosis result in resistance to forward progress through friction along the length of the wire/lead, axial stability factors, and change in wire/lead direction.

Friction. The initial forward vector is degraded by friction acting along the length of the wire. The initial and final forward vectors are similar in magnitude as long as the wire is in a low-friction environment along a straight line, such as in support tubing. However, as soon as the wire exits the tubing, the initial forward vector is degraded by the high-friction environment of the veins. When the wire changes direction from the original course, additional frictional forces are applied. These are discussed in more detail in the section on change in direction.

Axial Stability. The intrinsic axial stability of the wire is defined as its ability to resist buckling from distal forces. When the wire is in the guide, its axial stability is enhanced. The stability produced by the combination of the wire and sheath is the total axial stability. Once the wire exits into the CS, it is no longer supported. The further the wire extends from the support tubing, the lower the total axial stability.

Change in Direction. As the wire is advanced from the shoulder to the CS, the guide/sheath provides a low-

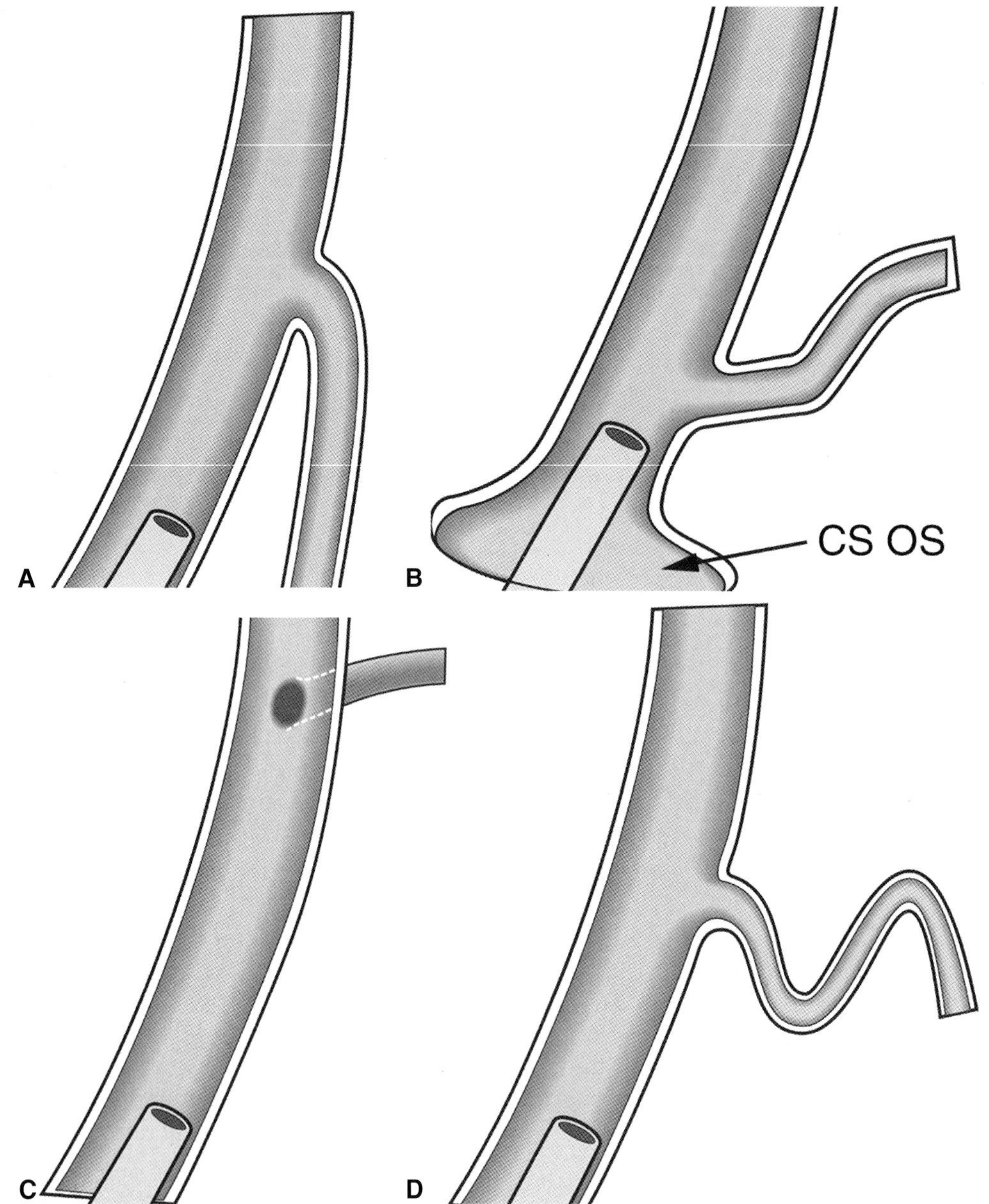

*Figure 19-96. Difficult target vein anatomy. **A,** An acutely angulated target vein. **B,** A vein with a proximal takeoff. **C,** A target vein with a posterior takeoff. **D,** A tortuous target vein. In all four views, the guide/sheath for coronary sinus (CS) access is located just inside the CS os.*

friction environment for it. The wire easily negotiates twists and turns between the shoulder and the CS within the support tubing without significant loss of the forward force or control. The direction of the wire outside the guide/sheath is controlled by the venous anatomy.

When a wire changes direction outside the support tubing, the forward vector is broken down into the displacement vector and the residual forward vector. The residual forward vector is the component of the initial forward vector that advances the wire/lead in the desired direction. The displacement vector is the component of the initial forward vector that follows the original direction of the wire as it exits the sheath. When the displacement vector exceeds the residual forward vector, the wire is displaced rather than advanced by additional force. Each time the direction of the wire is changed within a vein, the forward vector is degraded by the displacement vector. The number of times the wire changes direction and the magnitude of the change in direction of each turn determine the residual forward vector.

Whether a wire continues to move outside the support tubing depends on how much of the initial forward vector is lost to the displacement vector at each turn. Figure 19-97 illustrates the minimal degradation found when the takeoff of the target vein is along the same line as the sheath. Little if any of the initial forward vector is lost as the lead enters the target vein, and the lead passes easily. Figure 19-98 shows the mod-

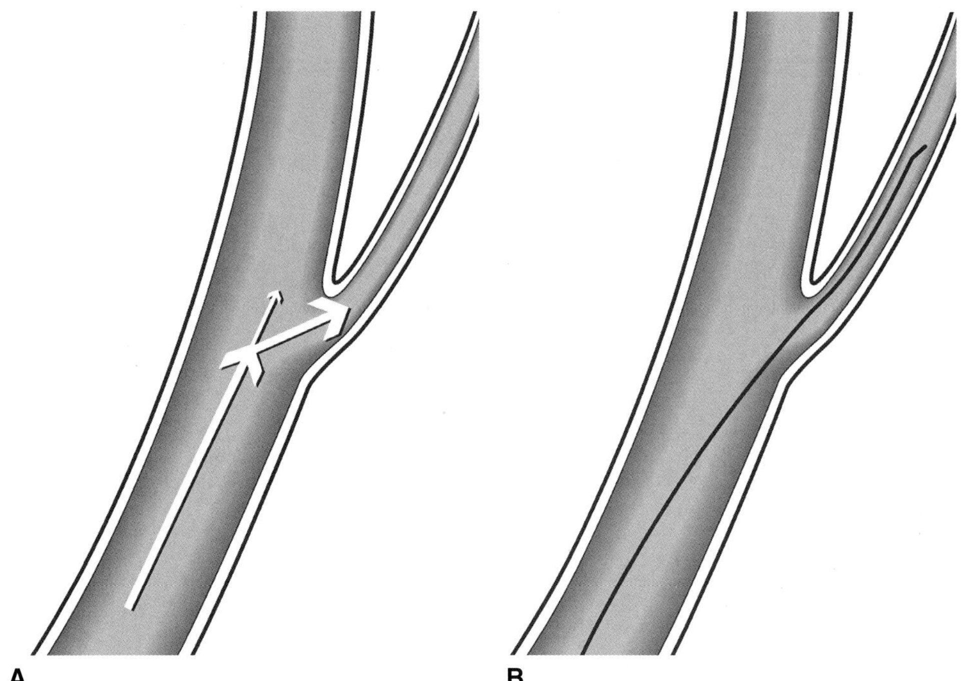

*Figure 19-97. Minimal degradation of forward vector (<45 degrees). **A,** The wire requires little change in direction to enter the target vein. The initial forward vector* (arrow before branch) *before the turn and the residual forward vector* (arrow into branch) *after the turn are almost equal. The wire is minimally displaced from the original direction. **B,** The wire is in the target vein. The wall of the vein redirects the wire. The friction between the wire and the wall of the vein reduces the forward vector and impedes movement of the tip when torque is applied at the shoulder. Because the direction of the wire was only minimally changed, there is minimal friction between the wire and vein to degrade the forward vector or reduce torque control.*

erate degradation of the forward vector as the direction change needed to enter the target vein is changed considerably from the direction of the sheath in the CS. Figure 19-99 shows the severe degradation of the forward vector as the wire essentially reverses direction. The displacement vector is larger than the forward vector. It becomes physically impossible to direct the wire down into the target vein.

Physical Properties of a Directional Device. The directional device is the key to all telescoping delivery systems. The pacing lead or guidewire/lead is contained within the directional device after it exits the catheter in the CS. As a result, the directional device:

- Preserves the initial forward vector and the ability to manipulate the wire tip
- Provides wire direction, axial stability, and back support
- Straightens tortuous veins
- Provides support to the lead (when the directional device is large enough to deliver the lead directly)

In order to take optimal advantage of directional devices, the operator must understand how they work.

Preservation of the Initial Forward Vector and Tip Control. Consider the effect of the support tubing of the directional device on preservation of the forward vector and the operator's ability to manipulate and direct the tip of a wire. As long as the wire remains in the unkinked support tubing (of the directional device), the tip of the wire is easily directed by application of torque at the shoulder. However, once the wire is outside the tubing, the frictional force from changes in wire direction or a small and/or stenotic vein segment not only degrade the initial forward vector but also impede manipulation of the tip of the wire.

When the operator applies torque at the shoulder to redirect the tip of the wire, the rotational movement is resisted at all the sites of friction along the length of the wire. The ability of the operator to direct the tip of the wire is severely degraded. If the wire remains in the low-friction support tubing without kinks (sheath/guide/catheter), neither the forward vector nor torque control is lost. Figure 19-100 demonstrates how a tortuous vein segment affects a wire without and with the support tubing of a directional device. The support tubing restores not only the forward vector but also the ability to manipulate the tip of the wire.

Axial Stability and Back-Support. When the operator initially advances the wire at the shoulder, the forward vector moves the wire ahead through the sheath into the CS. Resistance encountered at the tip of the wire tends to cause the wire to bend or buckle. As more forward force is applied at the shoulder, there is a greater tendency to buckle. Two factors determine how much force can be applied before a wire will buckle, the axial stability (stiffness) of the wire itself and the support

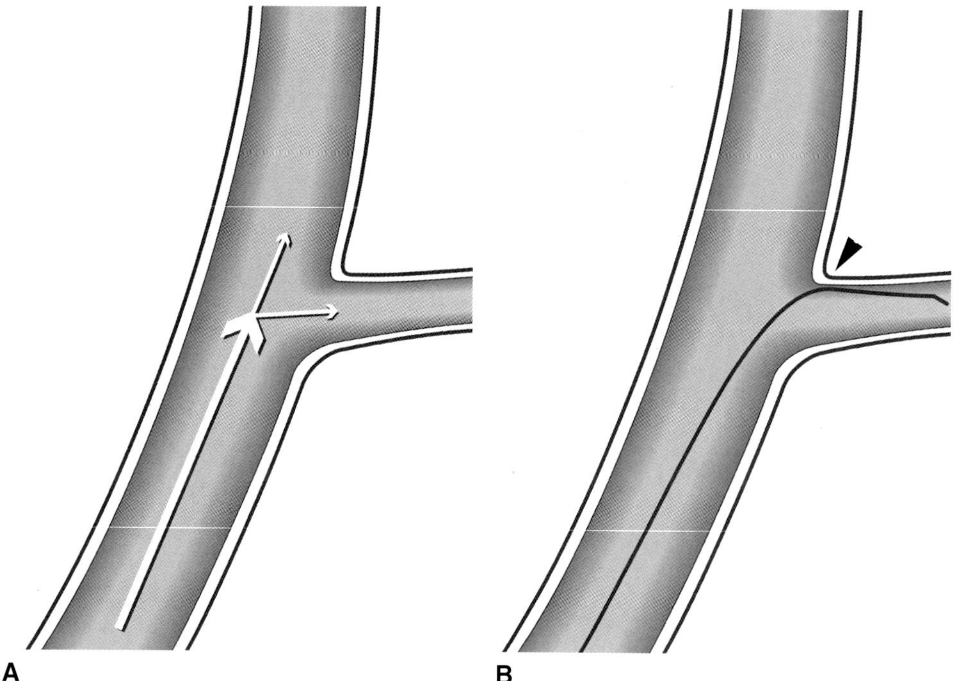

Figure 19-98. Moderate degradation of forward vector (45 to 90 degrees). ***A,*** *The wire must change direction considerably to enter the target vein. The initial forward vector* (large arrow before branch) *is divided into equal residual forward* (arrow into branch) *and displacement vectors* (arrow after branch). ***B,*** *The wire is in the target vein. The wall of the vein redirects the wire. The friction between the wire and the wall of the vein* (arrowhead) *reduces the forward vector and impedes movement of the tip when torque is applied at the shoulder. Because the direction of the wire is changed considerably, there is more friction between the vein and the wire to degrade the forward vector and reduce torque control.*

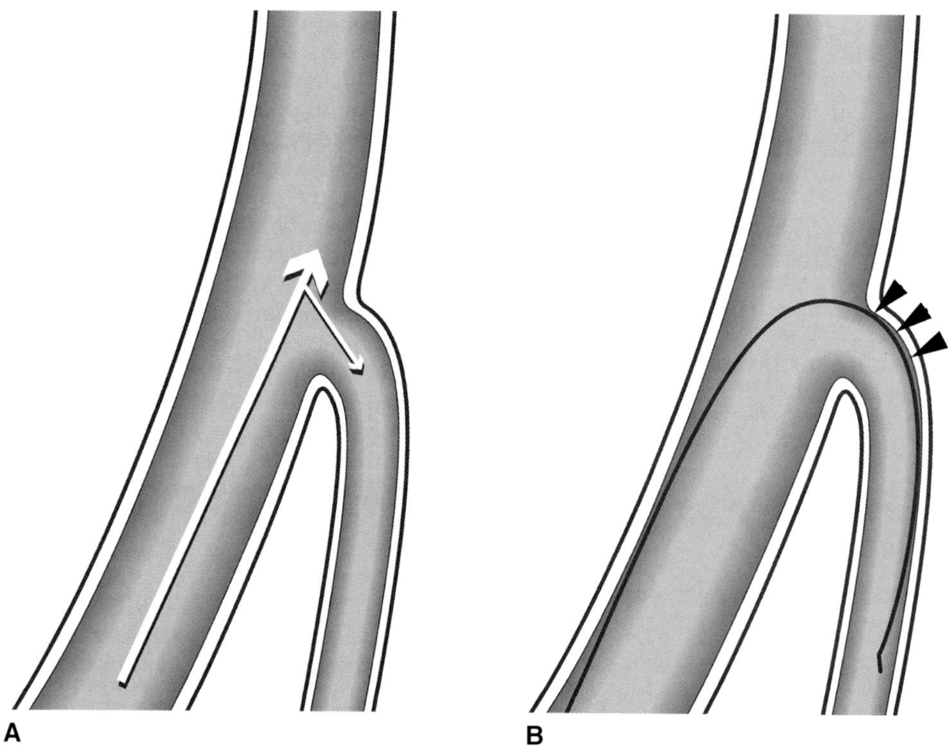

Figure 19-99. Severe degradation of forward vector (>90 degrees). ***A,*** *The wire must reverse the initial direction to enter the target vein. The initial forward vector* (large arrow before branch) *is divided into a small residual forward* (arrow into branch) *and a large displacement* (arrow after branch) *vector.* ***B,*** *The wall of the vein redirects the wire. The friction between the wire and the wall of the vein* (arrowheads) *degrades the forward vector and impedes movement of the tip when torque is applied at the shoulder. Because the direction of the wire is changed markedly, there is more friction between the vein and the wire. The greater the change in wire direction, the more force applied at the shoulder is lost to friction redirecting the tip of the wire/lead into the target vein. The residual forward vector is far less than the original forward vector. In this case, the residual forward vector may be too small to advance the wire.*

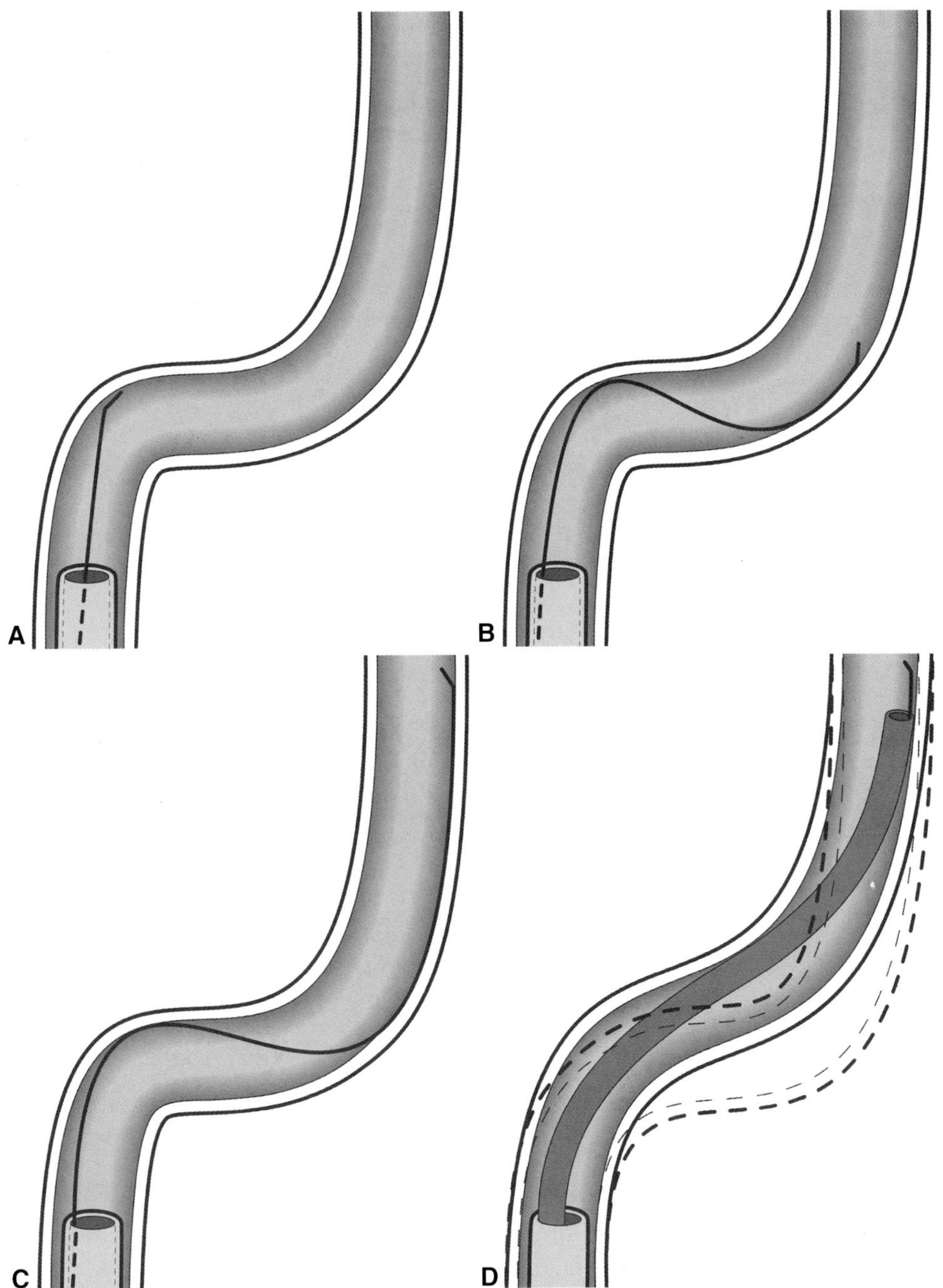

Figure 19-100. Support tubing in a tortuous vein improves wire movement. ***A,*** *The wire encounters a turn in the vein after it exits the sheath.* ***B,*** *The first bend in the vein redirects the tip of the wire perpendicular to the original direction. As the wire is advanced, there is friction between the wire and the vein with loss of forward force. Some of the forward force applied at the shoulder is lost to friction at the first turn. A degree of torque control is also lost.* ***C,*** *The wire is advanced beyond the second bend in the vein. There is further loss of forward force and torque control owing to friction between the vein and the wire.* ***D,*** *A directional device* (dark grey) *is advanced beyond the curved vein segment. The directional device straightens the vein* (dotted lines *indicate the original position of the vein) as well as providing a low friction environment for the wire. In this example, the directional device provides the following four of the six functions of a directional device: (1) preservation of the initial forward vector (straightens the vein and provides a low friction environment); (2) preservation of the ability to manipulate the tip of the wire (less friction in the two areas where the wire changes direction); (3) axial stability; and (4) wire direction.*

around the wire. For example, an angioplasty wire may have little if any axial stability on its own. If the wire is contained within the support tubing of a directional device, the axial stability of the wire is amplified by that of the support tubing. As long as the wire is within the walls of the tubing it will not buckle. Figure 19-101 demonstrates how the limited axial stability of a wire is enhanced by the support tubing of the directional catheter. The angioplasty wire buckles and the tip retracts out of the target vein when it encounters the

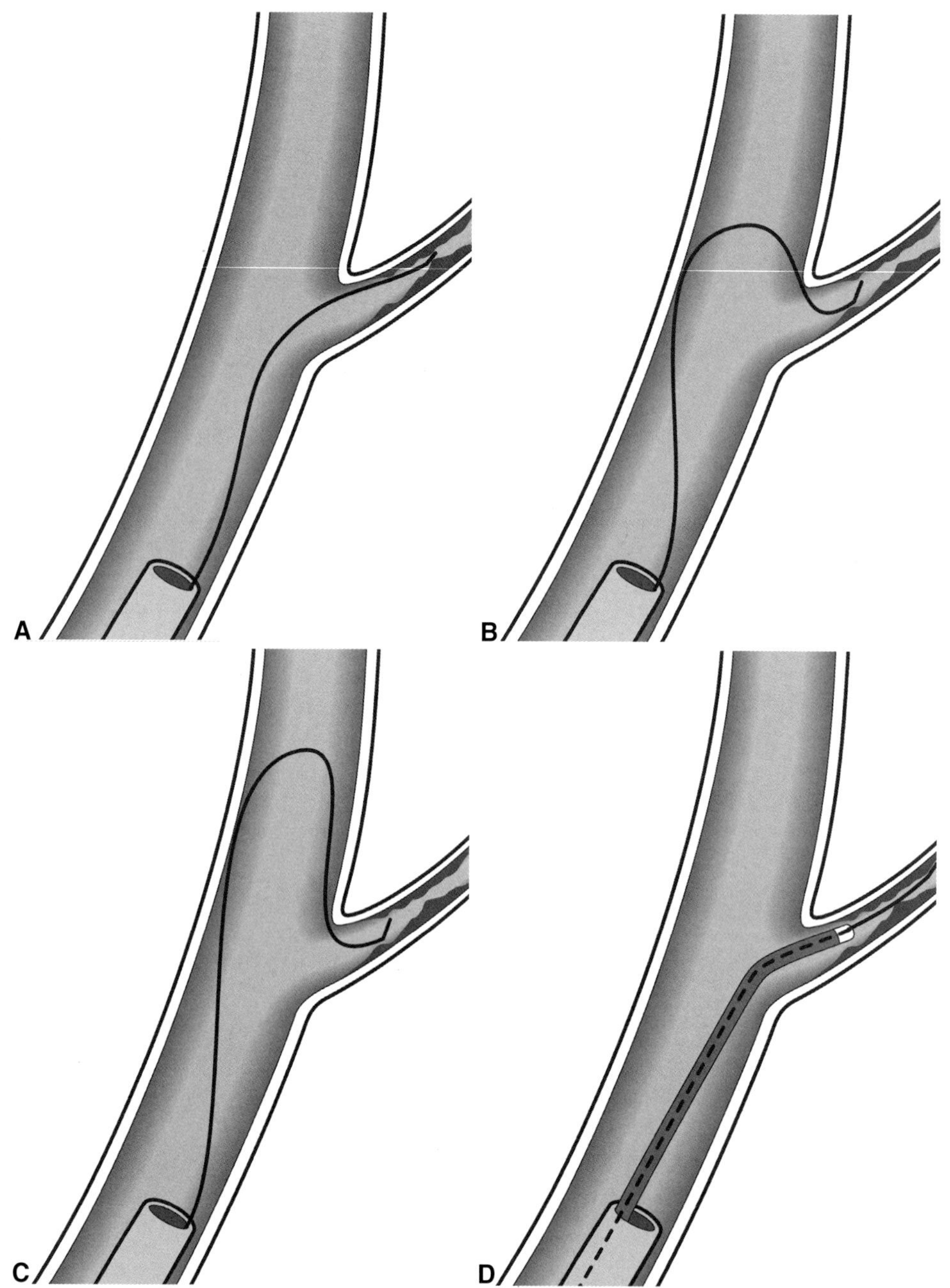

Figure 19-101. *Directional catheter increases axial stability of a wire.* ***A,*** *The wire is easily directed into the target vein without loss of the initial forward vector; however, the wire encounters the resistance of a stenotic vein segment and stops moving forward.* ***B,*** *Additional force is applied at the shoulder in an attempt to cross the stenotic segment. The wire does not have sufficient axial stability (stiffness) to transmit the added force to the tip and starts to buckle.* ***C,*** *As more forward force is applied at the shoulder, the wire buckles further and the tip pulls out of the vein.* ***D,*** *The wire is supported within the directional catheter, which is inserted into the target vein. The axial support provided by the catheter allows the additional forward force applied at the shoulder to be transmitted directly to the stenosis without buckling the wire. As long as the guide is not displaced, the forward force applied at the shoulder is directed at the stenosis. If the catheter is displaced, there is insufficient back-support. The size, stiffness, and shape of the directional device determine the amount of back-support it provides. A directional catheter with a curve that rests on the wall of the coronary sinus is less likely to be displaced than the catheter in* ***D.***

stenosis. A directional catheter adds axial support. As the wire is advanced, the catheter may be displaced rather than the wire advancing. The ability of the catheter to resist being displaced is the *back-support*. If the catheter is not displaced, the wire will not buckle.

The stiffness of the lead also adds to or subtracts from axial stability of the lead and the back-support of the guide catheter. This is best demonstrated by a comparison of the stiffer polyurethane of the lead body of the St. Jude leads with the softer silicone rubber lead body of the Guidant leads. The stiffness of the leads offered by Medtronic, Inc. is intermediate between the leads of the other two manufacturers. The physical characteristics of LV pacing leads are discussed in detail in the section on pacing leads.

Step 2: The First-Generation Telescoping Delivery System

Addition of a Directional Catheter to the Catheter Cannulating the Coronary Sinus. The ID of the directional device and the size of the pacing lead determine whether the directional device functions as a directional catheter or directional guide. When the ID of the directional device is large enough to deliver only the angioplasty wire, the device is referred to as a *directional catheter.* It provides direction, support, and a low-friction environment only for an angioplasty wire. In first-generation telescoping systems, catheters are used to place the wire into the target vein, as depicted in Figure 19-102. This figure demonstrates the use of a directional catheter to insert a wire into a target vein that is in the opposite direction to the wire as it enters the CS. Prior to the commercial availability of these devices, some implanters successfully used catheters designed for interventional cardiology and radiology.

Both Guidant and Medtronic offer directional catheters as part of their current delivery systems (see Figs. 19-118 and 19-121), but the shapes available are limited. The directional catheters offered by these companies provide little in addition to what is already available from other specialties and are significantly more expensive. We continue to use small catheters from interventional radiology to create a first-generation delivery system. Figure 19-103 is a photograph of several diagnostic and interventional radiology catheters with preformed fixed shapes that we have found useful as directional catheters to "aim" the angioplasty wire into the target vein. We keep several of each shape in the room. On the basis of the requirements of the patient's venous anatomy, we select one of the shapes and create a first-generation telescoping system if the anatomy is appropriate. All major catheter companies produce similar shapes. Some but not all of these shapes are also available in the cardiac catheterization laboratory as well. However, the catheter length used in interventional radiology (55 to 65 cm) is easier to work with at the shoulder than the length used in cardiology (90 to 100 cm).

Limitations of the First-Generation Systems. Despite the tremendous improvements seen with first-generation delivery systems, they have several important limitations. First, the ID of the directional device determines whether the lead can be advanced directly through the device into the vein (directional guide as seen in third-generation telescoping systems) or whether it must be removed first (directional catheter). Recall that the French size of a catheter refers to its OD. The ID 4F of all 6F OD and smaller catheters is too small to accept the available pacing leads. Thus 6F and smaller catheters can deliver only the angioplasty wire. The option of using a directional catheter to place an angioplasty wire is not relevant to stylet-driven leads. In addition, removing the directional catheter without displacing the wire from the vein can be difficult, and occasionally, the position of the wire in the target vein is lost in the process.

Figure 19-104 depicts the pitfalls of removing a directional catheter while retaining the angioplasty wire in place. Note that if too much or two little wire is advanced as the catheter is withdrawn, the wire will be dislodged from the target vein. This process is particularly cumbersome when a standard 100-cm diagnostic cardiology catheter is used as the directional catheter, because an exchange-length (300-cm) angioplasty guidewire is required. When a 65-cm catheter from interventional radiology is chosen, the exchange process can be accomplished using a standard-length (192-cm) angioplasty guidewire.

A second disadvantage of removing the directional catheter after the wire is in place in the vein is that there is nothing to support the lead as it tracks over the wire. The wire alone may not provide enough support to redirect the over-the-wire lead when there is a sharp curve or small stenotic vessel. Figure 19-105 depicts what happens when the operator tries to advance over-the-wire pacing lead into an acutely angulated target vein. The angioplasty wire is first placed with a directional catheter and then removed, leaving the wire in place. As the pacing lead starts to turn into the target vessel, the friction between the vein and the combined lead and wire causes the pacing lead to become dislodged.

Figure 19-106 is an example of the same situation in a patient. The vein is acutely angulated. Attempts to advance a wire without a directional catheter were futile. The maximum forward vector (F) (forward into the target vein) was far exceeded by the displacement vector (D). A 5F Soft-Vu Hook(1) from AngioDynamics, Inc. (Queensbury, NY; shown in Fig. 19-103, extreme *bottom right*), was advanced into the vein, a wire was delivered, and the catheter was removed. The wire did not provide enough support, however, and as the pacing lead approached the hook curve, it pulled the wire out.

A similar situation is demonstrated in Figure 19-107 in a patient with a posterior lateral dominant circulation. In Figure 19-107A, the acutely angulated target vein is indicated with an *arrow*. A less suitable but easier to access large posterior lateral vein is labeled as a "bail out" vessel to indicate that it is not optimal in location. The target vein is selectively engaged with a 5F Williams right diagnostic catheter. An angioplasty wire is advanced down the vein. The wire is displaced

Text continued on p. 732

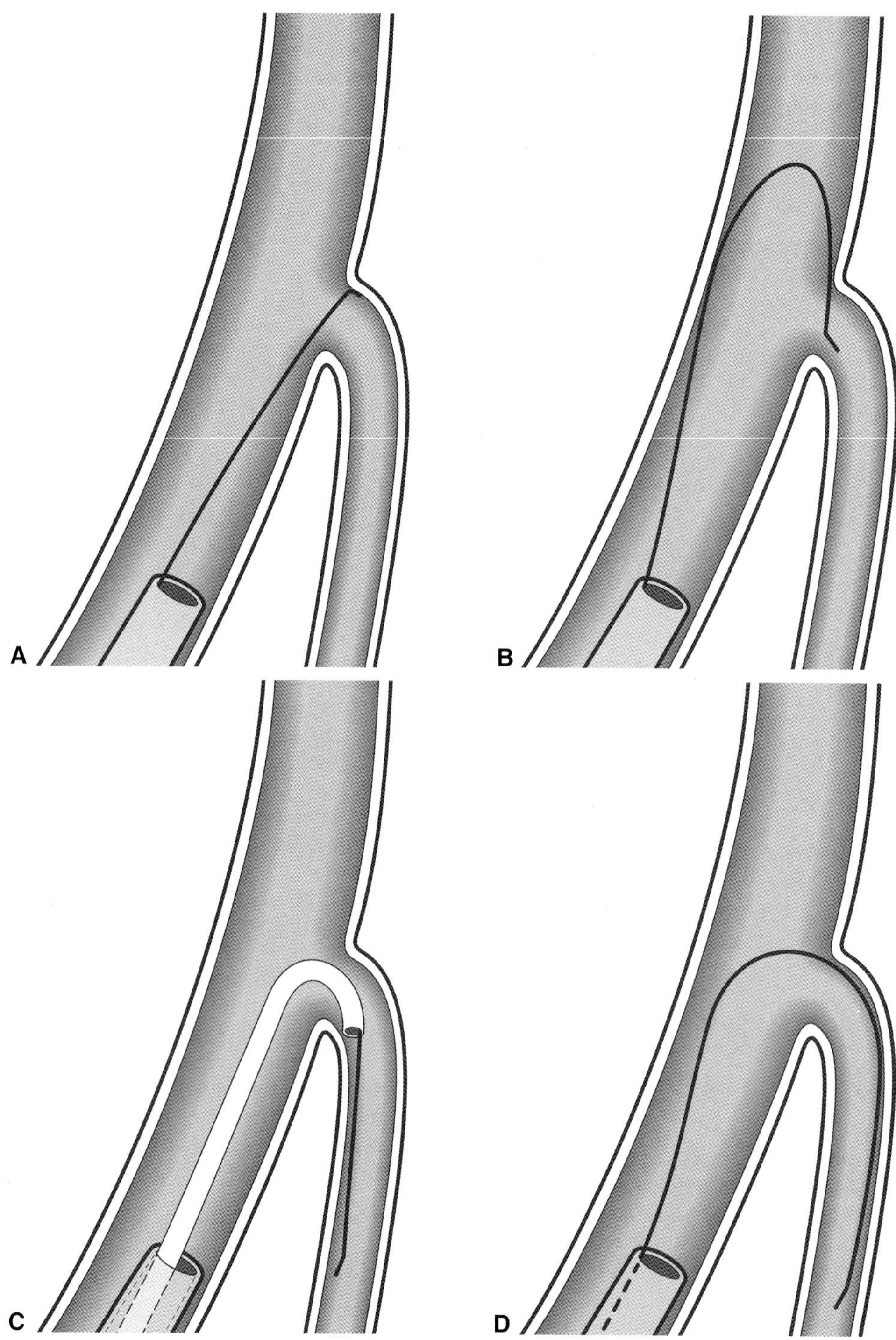

Figure 19-102. *Directional catheter for acutely angulated target vein.* ***A,*** *The angioplasty wire approaches an acutely angulated target vein.* ***B,*** *The wire buckles into the coronary sinus (CS) as it is advanced.* ***C,*** *The wire is directed into the target vein with a directional catheter.* ***D,*** *The directional catheter is removed, leaving the wire in place. The direction of the target vein is in the opposite direction of the wire as it exits the CS platform into the CS. It is physically impossible to redirect the wire down the target vein without an additional piece of equipment—the directional device. With a properly shaped directional device in the target vein, the wire is easily redirected into the target vein. The directional catheter is only large enough for the angioplasty wire and must be withdrawn off the back of the wire before the left ventricular lead can be placed.*

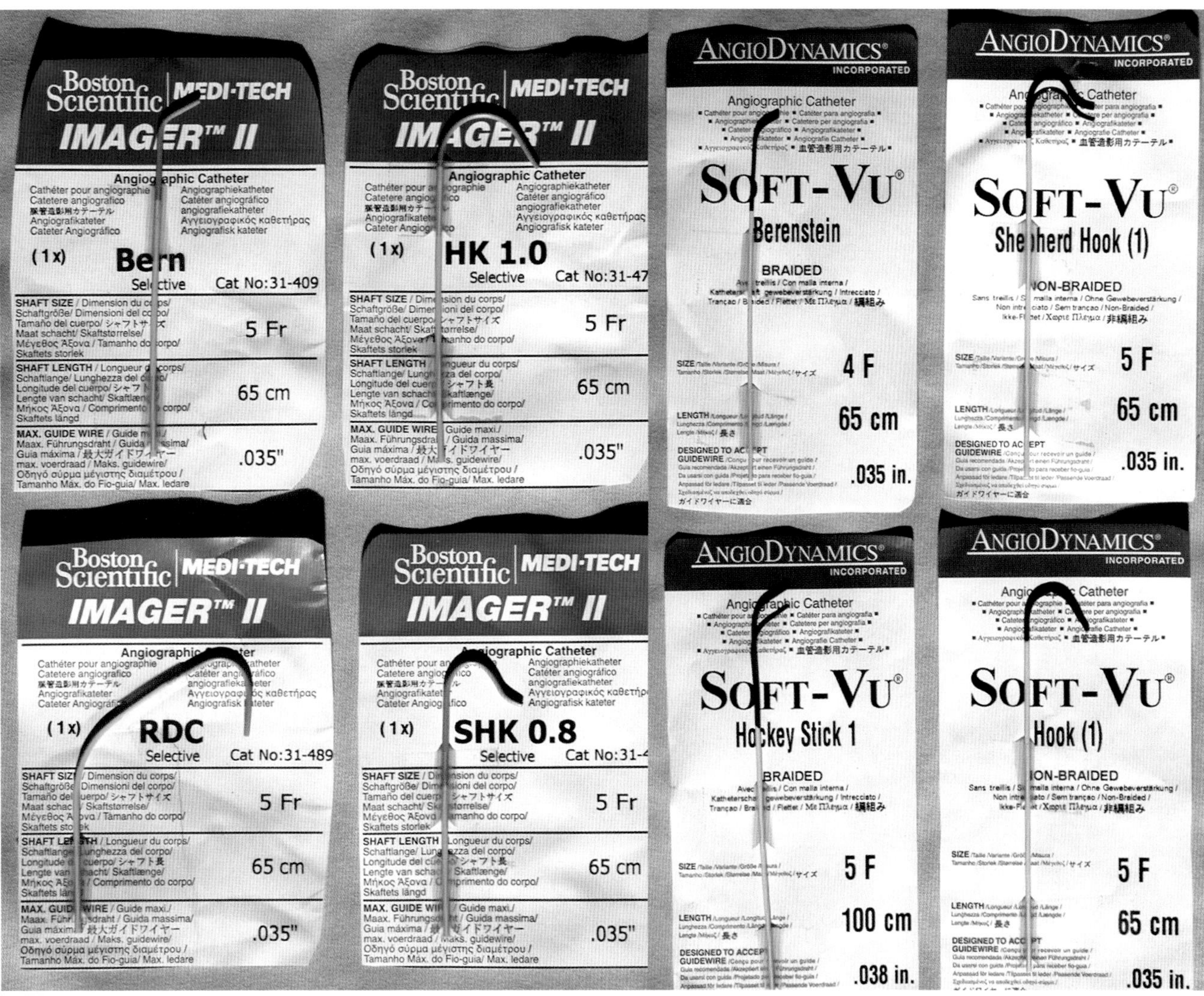

Figure 19-103. Directional catheters available from various companies. A variety of shapes are available from the interventional radiology divisions of large catheter companies. The shapes demonstrated here are more useful than most cardiac shapes. In addition, the 65-cm length used in radiology is more appropriate for use in lead implantation. The shorter length is easier to manipulate and does not require an exchange-length angioplasty wire. The directional catheters available from the device companies are essentially identical but are more expensive and available in only a few shapes. These catheters are used as parts of second- and third-generation delivery systems as well. (Boston Scientific/Medi-Tech catheters, Boston Scientific Corporation, Natick, Mass.; AngioDynamics, Inc., Queensbury, NY.)

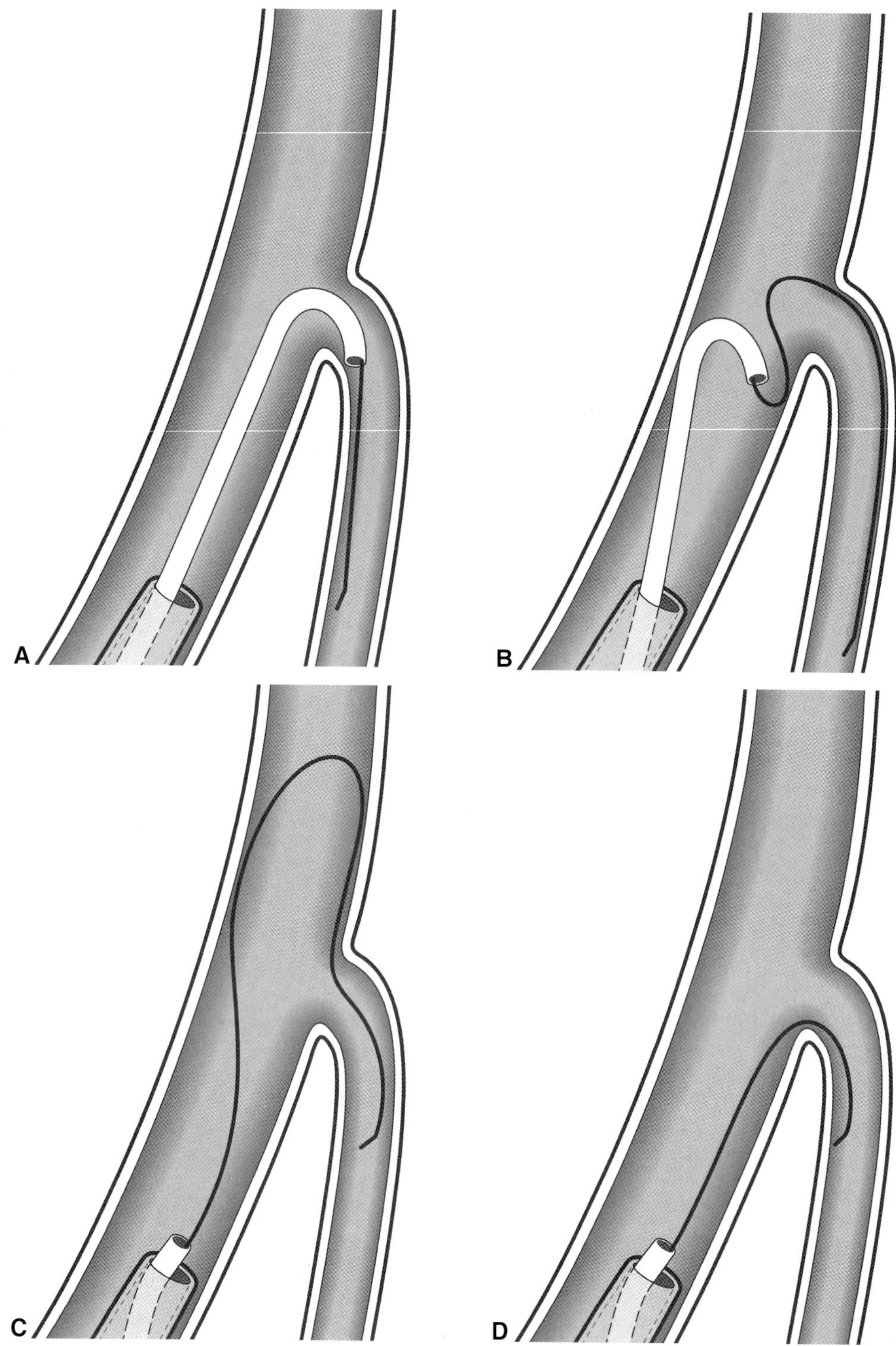

Figure 19-104. *Removal of directional catheter from target vein.* ***A,*** *The guidewire is inserted into the target vessel by means of a preshaped 4F to 6F OD directional catheter.* ***B,*** *The wire is advanced and the catheter is withdrawn out of the target vein into the coronary sinus (CS).* ***C,*** *Too much wire is advanced, and a loop of wire forms in the CS distal to the target vein. Advancing the wire further would create a larger loop in the CS and pull the wire further out of the target vein.* ***D,*** *Not enough wire is advanced as the catheter is removed. The tip of the wire is pulled back proximally in the target vein, and the wire is taut. From this diagram, it is clear that great care must be taken to advance just enough but not too much wire as the catheter is removed.*

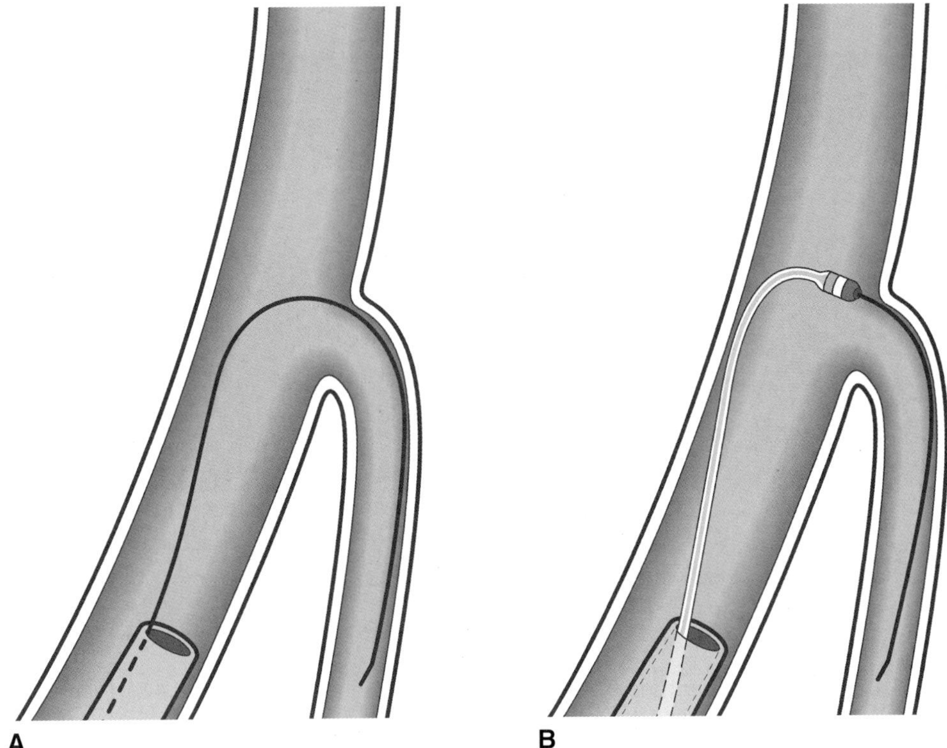

Figure 19-105. Despite wire placement, the pacing lead does not track into the target vein. ***A,*** The wire is advanced into the target vein by means of a directional catheter. ***B,*** The angioplasty wire does not provide adequate support for the acute angle. The angioplasty wire and lead pull out of the vein.

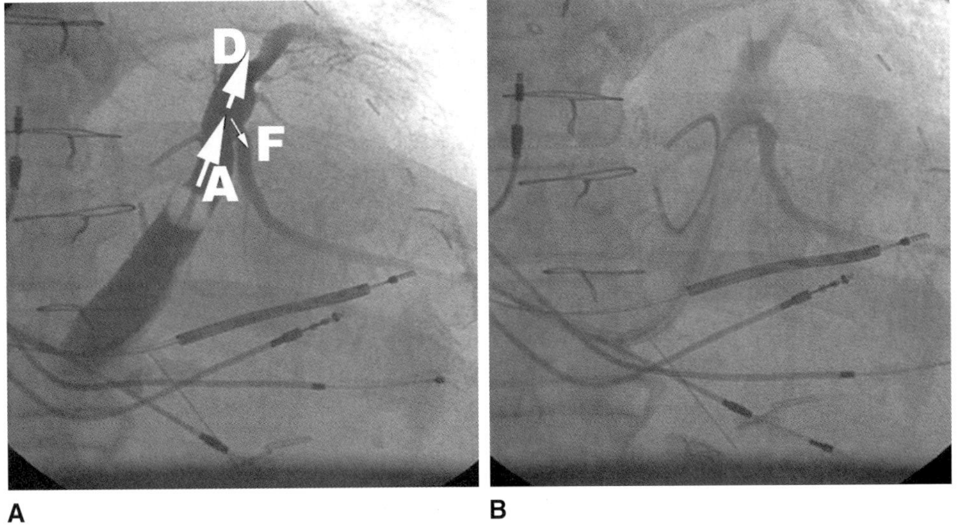

Figure 19-106. Example of failure of a first-generation telescoping system. ***A,*** The acutely angulated target vein can be seen on the anteroposterior coronary sinus (CS) venogram. The axial vector (arrow *A*) of the lead/wire as it exits the sheath is in the opposite direction from the required forward vector (arrow *F*). The displacement vector (arrow *D*) is the dominant force. ***B,*** A 5F hook catheter (shown in Fig. 19-103) is in the target vein and points the wire into the vein. However, the wire alone does not provide sufficient support to counteract the displacement vector. Attempts to advance the Attain 4193 (Medtronic, Inc., Minneapolis, Minn.) into the target vein dislodges the wire as the lead turns into the target vein.

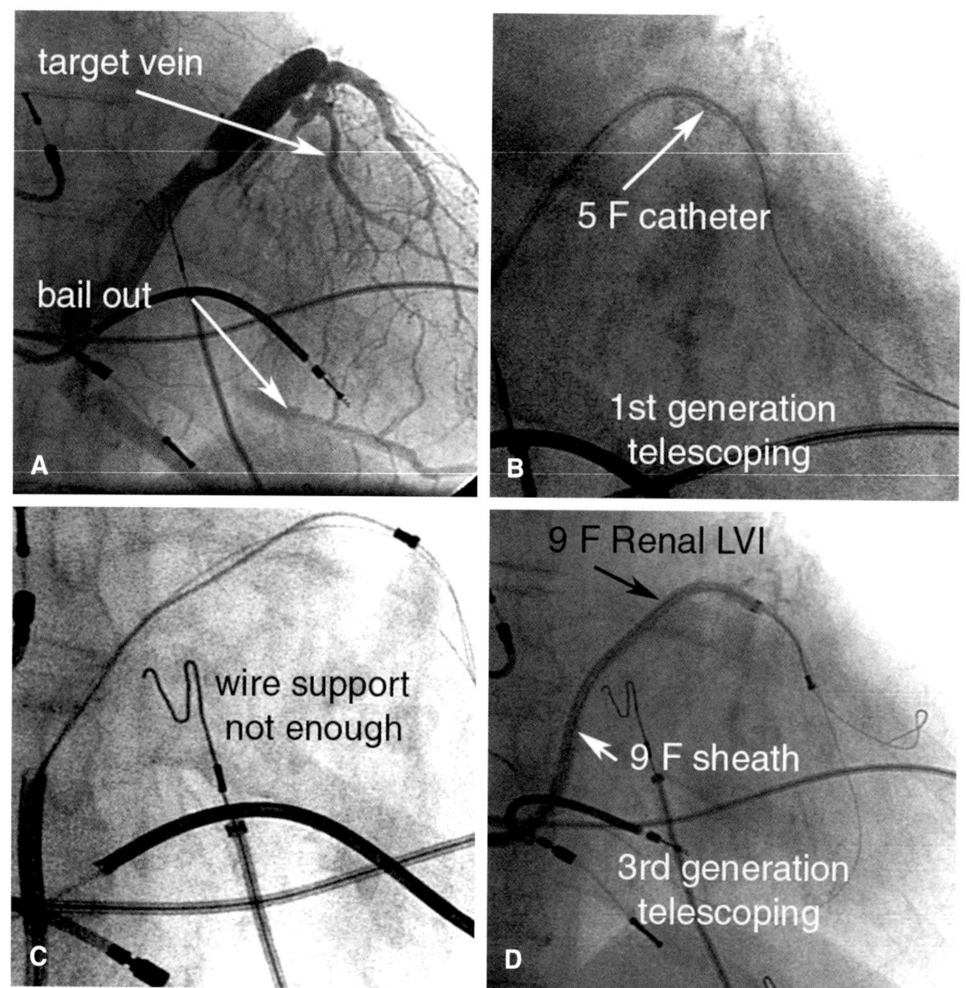

Figure 19-107. ***A*** *through* ***D,*** *First-generation telescoping system fails but third-generation system succeeds.*

as the pacing lead enters the vein. A "stiff" buddy wire and "floppy" tracking wire are advanced into the vein when it is recannulated with the 5F catheter, as explained in the section on venoplasty techniques (two 0.014-inch wires fit into the lumen of a 5F catheter). Despite straightening of the vein with the aid of the second wire, the pacing lead still will not advance into the target vein. This example represents the failure of a first-generation system despite the addition of the buddy wire. In Figure 19-107D, a preshaped catheter with a lumen large enough to directly deliver the lead cannulates the vein. The support provided by the catheter (9F OD, 7F ID renal shape lateral vein introducer [LVI]) was sufficient to advance the lead directly into the vein. Cases such as these instigated the development of second- and third-generation telescoping pacing lead delivery systems.

Step 3: The Second-Generation Telescoping Delivery System

In a second-generation telescoping system, the directional catheter is used to advance both the angioplasty wire and the CS cannulating guide into the target vein. The LV lead is then advanced directly into the target vein through the guide. The guide that cannulates the CS is also the platform for the telescoping system and the guide to selectively cannulate the target vein for direct lead delivery. Although Guidant and Medtronic systems can be used in this manner, using directional catheters to bend the straight tip of the CS cannulation catheter can be difficult (or impossible), depending on the angle of the vein (Fig. 19-108A). Forcing the CS cannulation catheter into the target vein can cause perforation (see Fig. 19-108B).

Figure 19-109 illustrates our attempt to deflect the straight tip of a 9F CS cannulation guide into a target vein in a patient (see Fig. 19-109C). In the process of forcing the straight guide into the target vein (see Fig. 19-109D), the tip perforated the vein, resulting in the contrast stain (see Fig. 19-109E). More importantly, the pacing lead would not advance into the vein. When a 9F guide preshaped to fit into the target vein was introduced into the CS through a 9F sheath, it readily advanced into the target vein and delivered the lead (see Fig. 19-109F). In this case, the second-generation telescoping system failed, but the third-generation system was able to deliver the lead.

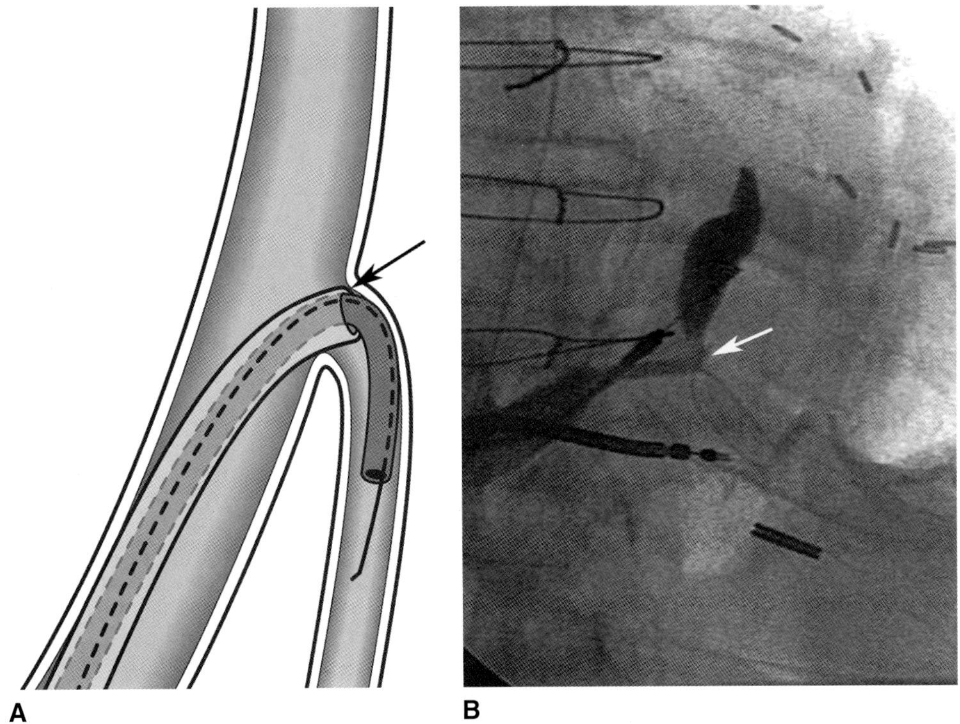

Figure 19-108. The straight tip of a second-generation telescoping guide perforates the vein as it is advanced around the curve. ***A,*** *Illustration of the limitations of the second-generation telescoping approach. The wire and directional catheter are in the target vein. Attempts to bend the straight tip of the coronary sinus (CS) cannulating guide into the target vein are not successful. The tip of the guide digs into the vein, causing a perforation.* ***B,*** *Real-life example of the diagram. A contrast stain can be seen at the tip of the guide where it would not "turn the corner" into the target vein.*

Step 4: The Third-Generation Telescoping Delivery System

As already suggested, third-generation telescoping systems use an 8F or 9F OD preshaped directional guiding catheter.[32] The lumen of the 8F or 9F guiding catheter is large enough (6F or 7F) to deliver the LV lead directly into the target vein. The 8F or 9F OD preshaped directional guiding catheter used to selectively cannulate the target vein is not suitable for cannulating the CS. The catheter used to cannulate the CS must have an ID sufficient to accept an 8F or 9F guiding catheter (i.e., 9F sheath). With the third-generation telescoping system, the 9F sheath (9F ID/8F OD) used for venous access is long, is shaped to cannulate the CS, and extends from the pocket into the CS. As stated previously, the 9F sheath (9F ID/8F OD) used for venous access in the other three approaches to LV lead placement is the same diameter as that in the third-generation system sheath but does not reach the CS, ending instead in the subclavian vein. Therefore the 8F or 9F guide that is inserted through the short 9F venous access must be designed to locate and cannulate the CS, not shaped to cannulate a coronary vein. Again, when the 9F sheath extends into the CS, the 8F or 9F guide that is inserted into the sheath can be designed for selective vein cannulation.

In the third-generation telescoping system, the shape of the directional guide used depends on the venous anatomy. Once the directional guide is coaxially seated in the target vein, the lead is inserted and the hub is removed. With the lead tested in the target vein, the guide is cut away. Until recently, the operator was forced to shape existing interventional guides to create a third-generation telescoping system, (Fig. 19-110). Directional guides are now available commercially in four shapes specifically designed for LV lead placement. Although we continue to use diagnostic catheters for wire placement (first-generation telescoping system), we no longer use interventional guides for direct lead delivery because they must be reshaped, the hub must be cut off before the lead is advanced, and the guide can be difficult to cut. Figure 19-111 illustrates the creation of a third-generation telescoping system with use of an interventional guide and a long sheath with a proximal curve. Figures 19-107 and 19-109 show cases in which the first-generation (Fig. 19-107) and second-generation (Fig. 19-109) telescoping systems failed to deliver the lead to the initial vein of interest. In these cases, a third-generation telescoping system (preshaped 9F guiding catheter inserted through a 9F sheath in the CS) successfully implanted the LV lead in the vein of choice (see Figs. 19-107D and 19-109F).

In the rare event that a third-generation telescoping system must still be created from a long sheath and interventional guide, the following information is useful:

- An interventional guide with an ID of 0.078 inches (2.0 mm) or greater is large enough to deliver a

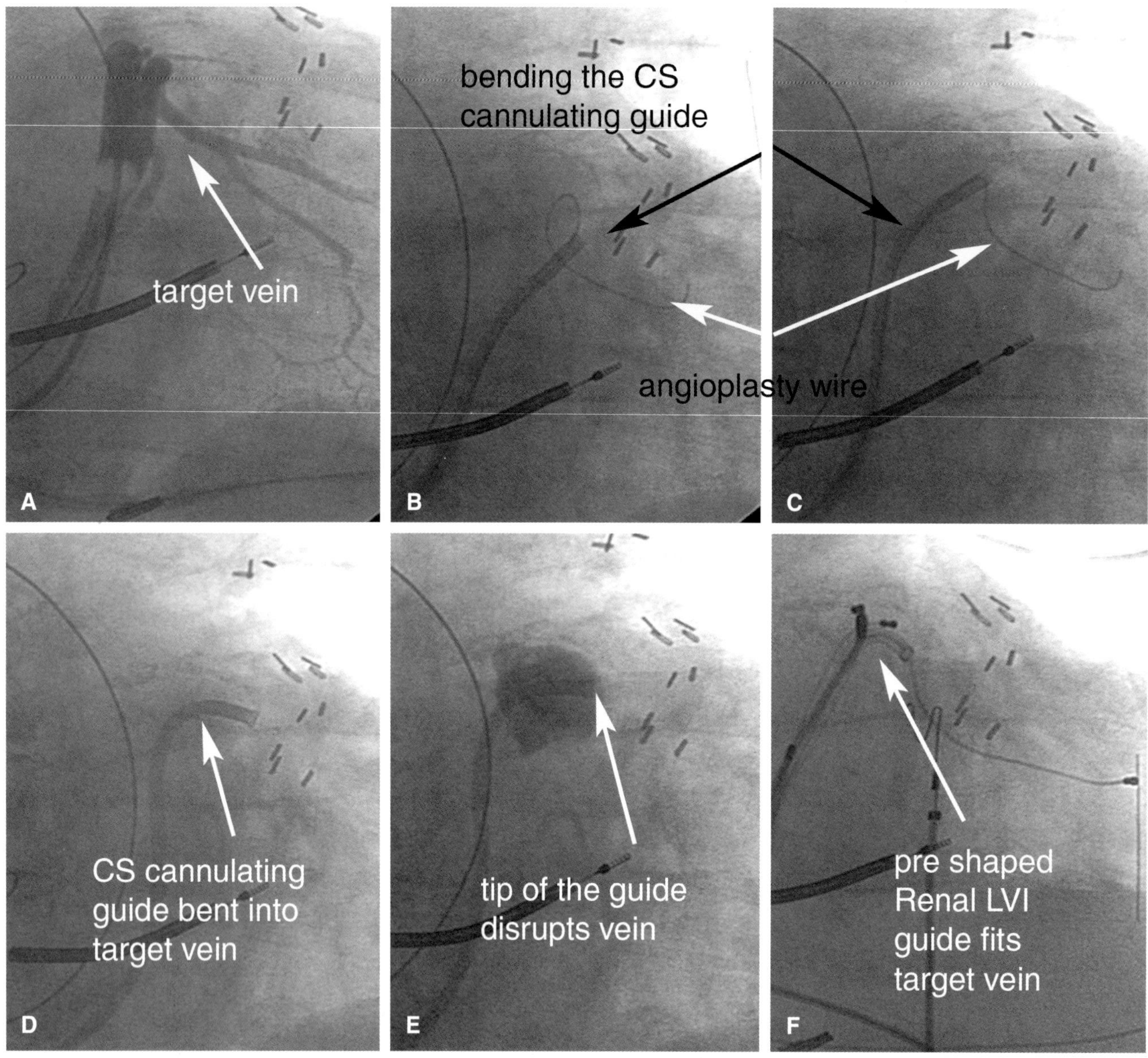

Figure 19-109. *The third-generation preshaped guide succeeds where the second-generation guide fails.* ***A,*** *The tortuous, acutely angled takeoff of the target vein is shown.* ***B,*** *The angioplasty wire is advanced and the straight tip of the coronary sinus (CS) cannulating guide is advanced to the proximal segment of the target vein.* ***C,*** *The straight guide is advanced further into the target vein over a wire and directional catheter (second-generation telescoping system).* ***D,*** *The straight tip guide is successfully advanced well in the target vein. However the tip of the guide digs into the vein. The lead will not advance.* ***E,*** *Injection of contrast material reveals that the tip of the straight guide disrupted the vein as it was forced around the acute angle of the vein. The second-generation approach to delivery was not successful.* ***F,*** *The straight tip guide is replaced with a preformed renal lateral vein introducer whose intrinsic shape matches the shape of the vein. Its preformed shape is designed to fit coaxially into the vein without being forced, reducing the likelihood of trauma to the vein.*

Medtronic Attain 4193 lead directly into the target vein.

- All 8F OD interventional guides have sufficient ID to accommodate the Attain 4193 LV lead.
- The Attain 2187 lead requires a guide with an ID of 0.088 inches (2.2 mm) or greater.
- Some 8F OD interventional guiding catheters (e.g., Vistabritetip RDC[1] interventional guide, Cordis) and all 9F OD interventional guiding catheters have an adequate ID for the Guidant EASYTRAK family of LV pacing leads as well as the St. Jude QuickSite LV pacing lead. (Recall that a guide's French size refers to its OD; a 9F directional guide [9F OD/7F ID] is large enough to accept all commercially available LV pacing leads.)

The Platform for a Telescoping Left Ventricular Pacing Lead Delivery System. As mentioned earlier,

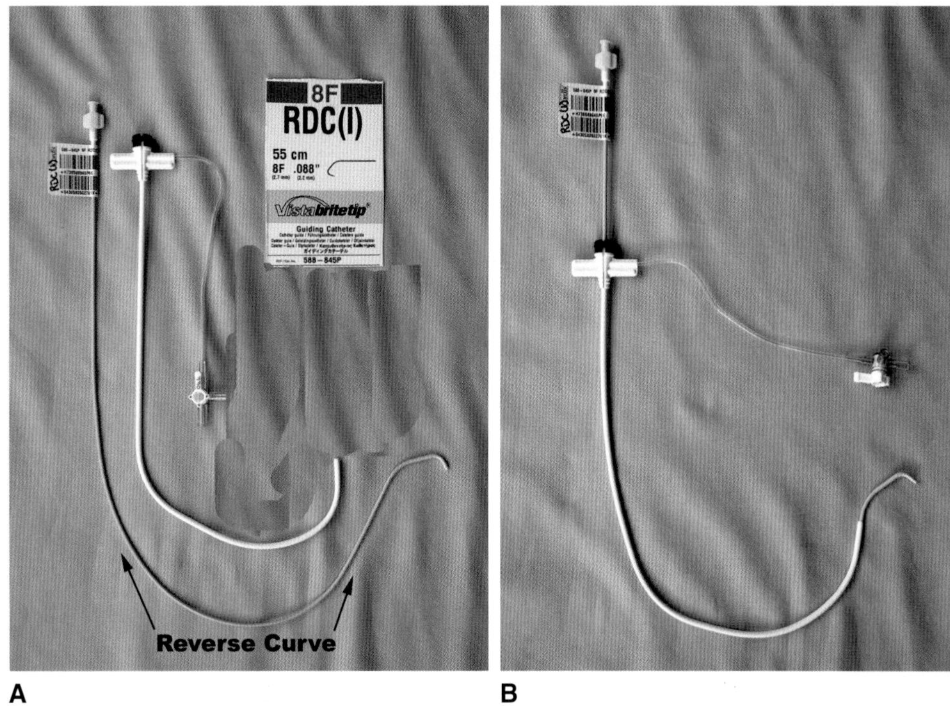

Figure 19-110. Improvised third-generation telescoping system, composed of a long 9F sheath with a proximal curve to serve as the coronary sinus (CS) Platform and a modified renal shape interventional guide to serve as the directional guide. ***A,*** *The 8F Vistabritetip RDC(1) interventional guide (Cordis, Miami, Fla.) is modified by placing a curve in the direction opposite to the tip curve, a "reverse curve." The interventional guide with reverse curve and the 9F sheath with proximal curve are shown side by side.* ***B,*** *The improvised directional guide is inserted into the CS sheath. Note that the curve placed on the body of the guide is in the opposite direction to the curve at the tip. When inserted into the sheath, the tip curve points outward toward the target veins, reducing the amount of torque required in the CS. The internal diameter of the 8F Vistabritetip guide is large enough to deliver any of the following pacing leads: Attain OTW 4193, Attain 2187, and CapSure SP 4023 (all from Medtronic, Inc., Minneapolis, Minn.). The hub of the guide must be cut off before the lead is inserted into the guide. Once the lead is in place and pacing thresholds have been confirmed, the guide is cut away with a cutter (Medtronic or Guidant [Boston Scientific, Natick, Mass.]).*

the characteristics (size, shape, and composition) of the catheter that serves as the platform of a telescoping system has a major impact on the ultimate success of LV lead placement. The ID of the catheter in the CS serving as the platform should be large enough to accept a directional guide capable of direct delivery of the chosen pacing lead. For example, if the pacing lead is 6F, the ID of the directional guide/introducer must be ≥6F. A ≥6F ID translates to an ≥8F outside diameter. The CS ID of the CS platform therefore must be ≥8F, which is the same as saying that the sheath in the CS serving as the platform must be ≥8F. An ≥8F guide in the CS will not do. The ID of an 8F guide is only 6F and will not accept a directional introducer with a 6F ID.

In addition, the optimal platform for a telescoping LV lead delivery system must be capable of rapid CS access, stability in the CS, and ease of removal without displacing the LV lead. Either a sheath (no braid) or guide (with braid) or a combination may be used to cannulate the CS and serve as a platform. In first-generation telescoping systems, the guide or sheath used to cannulate the CS for the nontelescoping approach is used both as the platform for the directional catheter and for delivery of the lead to the vein from the CS. In second-generation telescoping systems, the guide or sheath used to cannulate the CS for the nontelescoping approach is used as the platform for the directional catheter as well as to cannulate the vein and deliver the lead.

Details of the Coronary Sinus Platform for a Telescoping System. The first step in deploying a telescoping system is to establish a stable platform in the CS from which to work that maintains CS access throughout the procedure. The CS platform must have the following features:

Easy to place in the CS: The details of CS cannulation have been discussed previously. Peel-away catheters (which lack metal braid in the walls) do not have torque control, making it difficult to manipulate them into the CS even if the shapes are designed for rapid CS cannulation. Many of the available shapes are difficult to get into the CS because they lack a proximal curve

Stable within the CS: The shape should follow the anatomy in patients with CHF and should fit within the RA with the tip in the CS. In many cases, this requires

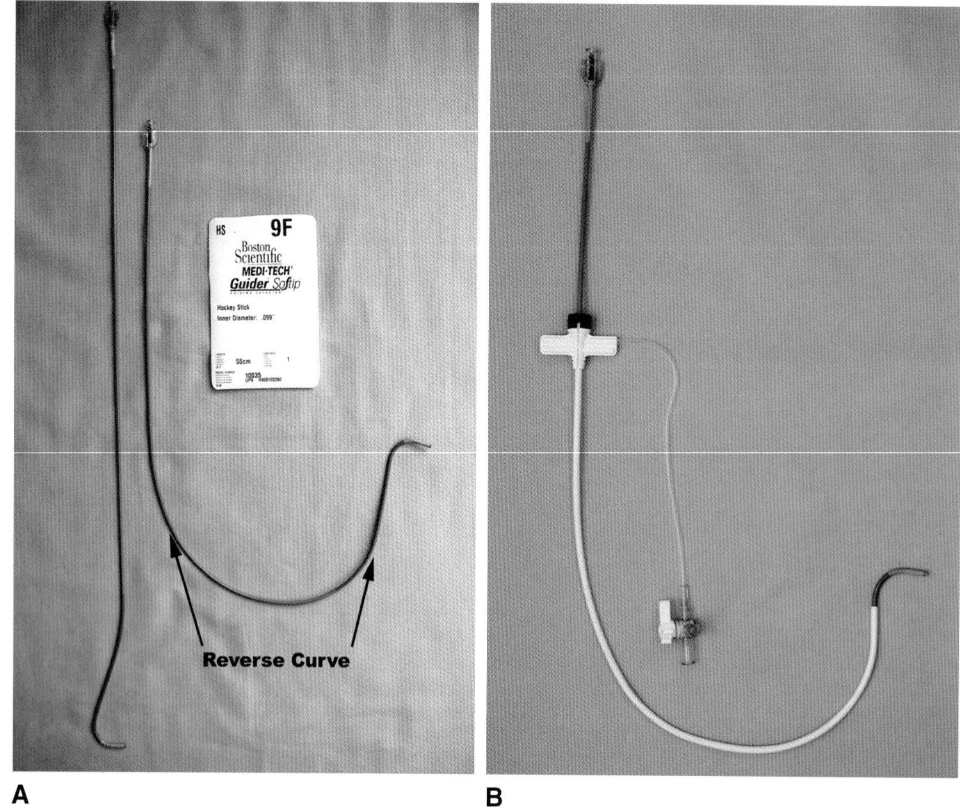

*Figure 19-111. Modified hockey stick guide for use in improvised third-generation telescoping system. **A,** A 9F hockey stick guide (Boston Scientific/Medi-Tech Guider Softip, from Boston Scientific Corporation, Natick, Mass.) is shown before (left) and after (right) the shape of the guide is changed to include the reverse curve. **B,** The hockey stick guide with reverse curve is inserted into the long 9F sheath with proximal curve. Within the sheath, the reverse curve of the guide directs the tip of the guide toward the target veins as it emerges from the sheath. The snout of the hockey stick is long enough to cross the tortuous segment.*

a wide radius of curvature with both a proximal curve and a distal curve. The distal curve lifts the tip up into the CS os. The straight midsegment rests on the eustachian ridge or floor of the RA. The proximal curve directs the sheath up into the SVC.

Highly resistant to kinking: Kinking is defined as the collapse of the lumen of a catheter. Catheters tend to kink under the following stresses or combination of stresses:

- Acute bends
- Application of torque to one end of the catheter with resistance to torque along or at the distal end of the catheter (longer catheters tend to kink with the application of torque than shorter catheters)
- Compressive forces

The combination of any of the three forces tends to be synergistic in lumen collapse. Resistance to kinking from all three forces is achieved by incorporation of wire braid in the walls of the catheter, which prevents the catheter from being peeled. To resist lumen collapse from torque and/or compressive forces without wire braid, the walls of the catheter are made thicker and stiffer. Thick stiff walls can increase the tendency for lumen collapse when a catheter is bent acutely by the demands of the anatomy. There is no tendency for the lumen to collapse if the sheath (catheter without wire braid) is preshaped (usually at the time of manufacture) to accommodate the anatomically required bend. Figure 19-112 is a photograph of two peel-away sheaths of somewhat different shapes that lack proximal bends. Figure 19-112A shows the original Pressure Products 9F SafeSheathCSG. Figure 19-112B is one of the four sheath curves of the St. Jude Apeel CS Catheter delivery system. Biotronik provides peel-away sheaths of similar shape as part of their Scout CS Utility Tools (see Fig. 19-115B).

Figure 19-113A shows a catheter approaching the CS that is not preshaped to fit the anatomy between the body surface on the left and the CS (without a proximal curve). Note that for the sheath to enter the CS, it must be deformed or bent to fit the anatomy Even if the walls of the catheter are thick and stiff, they will collapse unless supported by a wire braid. However, if the sheath is precurved in anticipation of the anatomic demands (see Fig. 19-113B), kinking will not occur. Figure 19-114 shows a case example. In Figure 19-114A, a long Pressure Products sheath (the original SafeSheath CSG) without a proximal curve was introduced into the CS

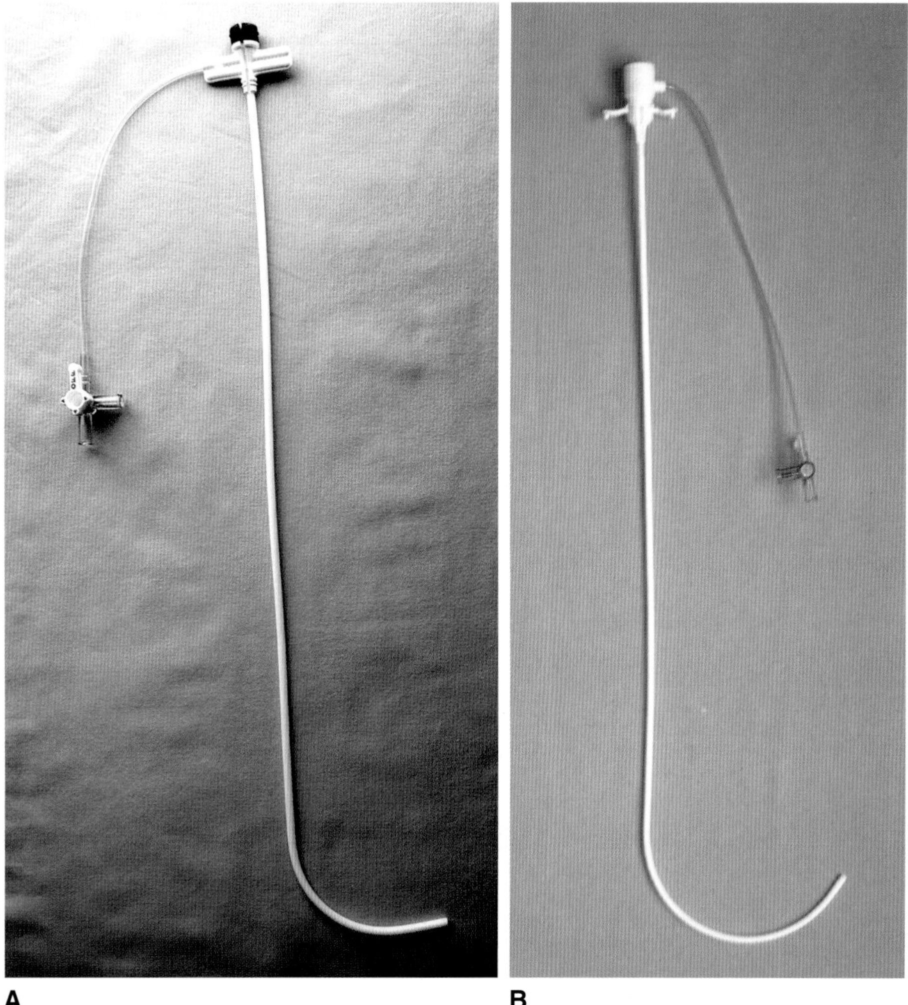

A **B**

Figure 19-112. Long peel-away sheaths that lack a proximal bend. ***A,*** *The original 9F SafeSheathCSG (Pressure Products, Inc., San Pedro, Calif.).* ***B,*** *Apeel CS Catheter (St. Jude Medical, St. Paul, Minn.). Without the proximal curve that anticipates the anatomic curves between the body surface and the coronary sinus, such sheaths are prone to kink. To provide torque control, an electrophysiology (EP) catheter or a braided guide must be inserted into the sheath.*

using a preshaped braided angioplasty guide. When the guide was removed, the lumen of the sheath collapsed. In Figure 19-114B, a Pressure Products sheath with a proximal curve (SafeSheath CSG–Worley) was introduced into the CS. The proximal curve molded into the sheath in anticipation of the anatomic demands eliminated the need for the catheter to be "bent acutely" to enter the CS. The sheath is said to be anatomically shaped.

Dislodgment of the LV pacing lead as it is removed: As discussed, many guides and sheaths must be deformed from their original shapes by the operator to fit the cardiac anatomy; thus, to maintain the shape while it is in the CS, such a sheath/guide is under tension. As the sheath/guide is withdrawn from the CS, it loses support and suddenly resumes the original shape, directing its tip to the floor of the RA, a movement that may pull the lead out of the target vein. By comparison, an anatomically shaped guide/sheath is not under tension as it rests in the CS. When removed, the tip of such a guide rises above the CS. This concept is covered in a later section (see Figs. 19-226 to 19-228).

Commercially Available Delivery Systems

Each of the CRT device manufacturers offers an LV lead delivery system, ranging in sophistication from nontelescoping to second-generation telescoping. Other companies manufacture sheaths and/or guides designed for use in the CS. Finally, suitable catheters designed for other cardiac and noncardiac applications may be used for placement of LV pacing leads. More advanced delivery systems are created by combining sheaths and guides from various sources.[33] The following discussion describes the sheaths/guides designed for use in the CS, in alphabetical order by company name.

Most of the tools that have been provided by all sources have been designed for a left-sided approach, but the ability to implant from both sides is crucial.

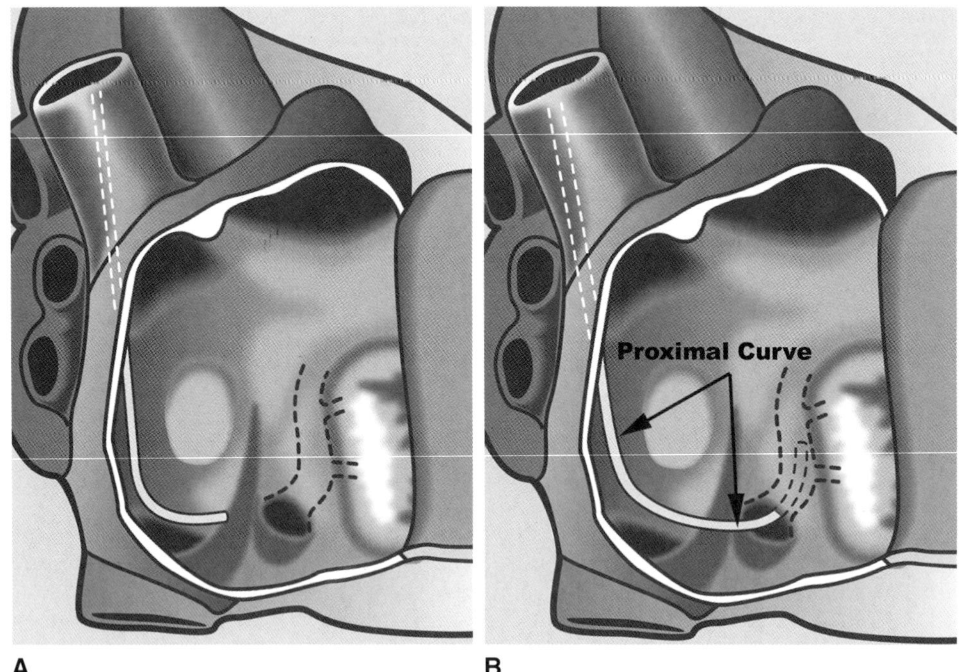

*Figure 19-113. Position of "catheters" inside the right heart of a patient with congestive heart failure. **A,** The shape without a proximal curve is shown with the tip at the level of the coronary sinus (CS). To place the sheath in the CS, the shape must be reformed using another catheter or the endocardial surface of the heart. A catheter without braided walls will likely kink as it is bent to fit into the CS. A catheter with wire mesh walls is less likely to kink but will spring back to its original shape when the support provided by the CS is removed. **B,** A sheath or guide with a proximal curve is shown with the tip in the CS. Because of the proximal curve, the tip rests in the CS without being reformed. A catheter without wire mesh walls will not kink because the curves are preformed. The proximal curve is supported by the eustachian ridge. As force is applied within the CS to deliver the left ventricular lead, the proximal curve provides the required counter force.*

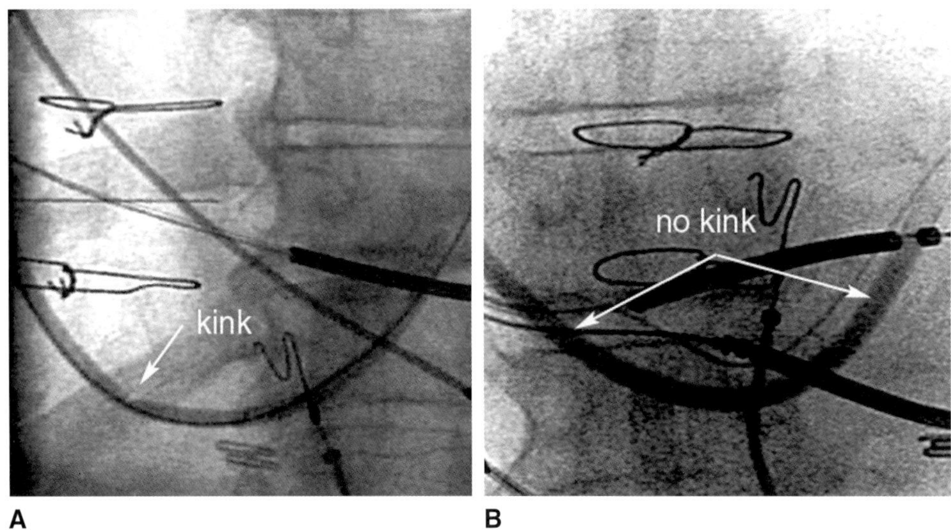

*Figure 19-114. Kinking of a nonpreformed sheath (**A**) and no kinking in the preformed sheath (**B**).*

Right-sided implantation tools are an area prime for further development.[34]

Biotronik GmbH & Co.

The delivery system designed for implanting Biotronik LV pacing leads has the following components:

- Scout CS Utility Tools
- The ScoutPro Introducer System
- Scout Tracing Tool

The Scout CS Utility Tools consists of two 8F introducers, a dilatator, a hemostatic valve, and a balloon catheter

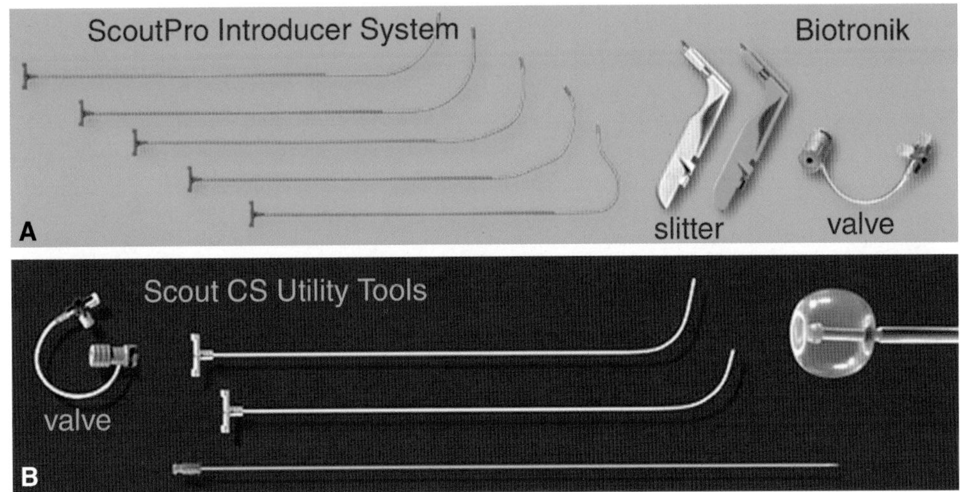

*Figure 19-115. Delivery system for left ventricular (LV) pacing leads from Biotronik GmbH & Co. (Berlin, Germany). **A,** The ScoutPro Introducer System for placement of LV pacing leads. The walls of the introducer catheters have wire mesh walls for kink resistance and distal radiographic markers. There are five different curve shapes. The introducer system also contains a hemostatic valve and slitter tool. **B,** The Biotronik Scout Coronary Sinus Utility Tools: two 8F peel-away introducers, a dilator, a hemostatic valve, and a venogram balloon catheter for performing an occlusive coronary sinus (CS) venogram. Neither the introducers with wire mesh walls nor the peel-away sheaths are anatomically shaped. If the introducer can be deformed to fit into the CS, it is prone to springing back and displacing the lead when removed. If the peel-away sheath can be deformed to fit into the CS, it is likely to kink.*

for performing an occlusive angiography of the coronary venous system (Fig. 19-115B). The ScoutPro Introducer System consists of a selection of five catheter curves with an integrated wire mesh for kink resistance and a distal radiograph marker. The introducer system also contains a hemostatic valve and slitter tool (see Fig. 19-115A). The Scout Tracing Tool (*not shown*) is for mechanical and/or electrical tracing of the ostium of the CS.

Cook Vascular, Inc.

Cook Vascular produces a 9F ID/11F OD sheath that is long enough to cannulate the CS. The shape of the sheath does not include a proximal curve, nor does it have torque control; thus the sheath can be difficult to get into the CS. Usually, the dilator is removed and a catheter with torque control is employed to direct the catheter into the CS. Depending on the demands of the anatomy, kinking can be a problem when the dilator or braided catheter is removed. In addition, it does not have a hemostatic hub. The absence of a hemostatic hub is not a major issue when the sheath is removed as soon as the pacing lead is the venous circulation. However, when the sheath is used as a nontelescoping delivery system, there is a continued tendency for air emboli and/or blood loss around the pacing lead throughout LV lead manipulation, which can be prolonged. If the 9F polytetrafluoroethylene sheath is used in conjunction with sheaths or guides from other manufacturers (for example, the straight Medtronic 6218 or the Guidant IC 50, IC 90, or Rapido Advance), bleed-back and air emboli around the guide/sheath remain problems that limit the applicability of this sheath as an LV lead implantation tool.

ELA Medical

The delivery system for LV pacing leads offered by ELA Medical (Sorin Group, Milan) is the ELA Situs LVAS Kit, an LV introducer kit for the Situs OTW. Components are the guiding catheter (two shapes available), dilator, guidewire, lead extender for guide catheter removal without slitting, and stylet for guide catheter removal (Fig. 19-116).

Guidant

Over the years, Guidant has introduced several fixed-curve shapes for CS access and LV lead delivery (Fig. 19-117). The latest offering has primary and secondary curves designed to take advantage of the RA anatomy. The curves are designed to use the high right lateral wall of the RA and low right lateral wall of the SVC as a fulcrum to probe the fossa between the tricuspid valve, the thebesian valve, and the eustachian ridge. One version, the Rapido Advance, has a straight but flexible tip that can be advanced into side branches. This design, because it is not preformed to fit into the side branches, is a second-generation system. In addition, once the sheath is advanced into the side branch, the support provided by the primary curve is no longer in position to provide the support for lead advancement (Fig. 19-118). The inner directional catheters (Fig. 19-119) can be used to advance the guidewires into the side branches but also can aid in the advancement of the flexible tip into the side branch. In addition, using the higher structures for the fulcrum has allowed the development of CS cannulation guides for right-sided implantation (Fig. 19 120).[34]

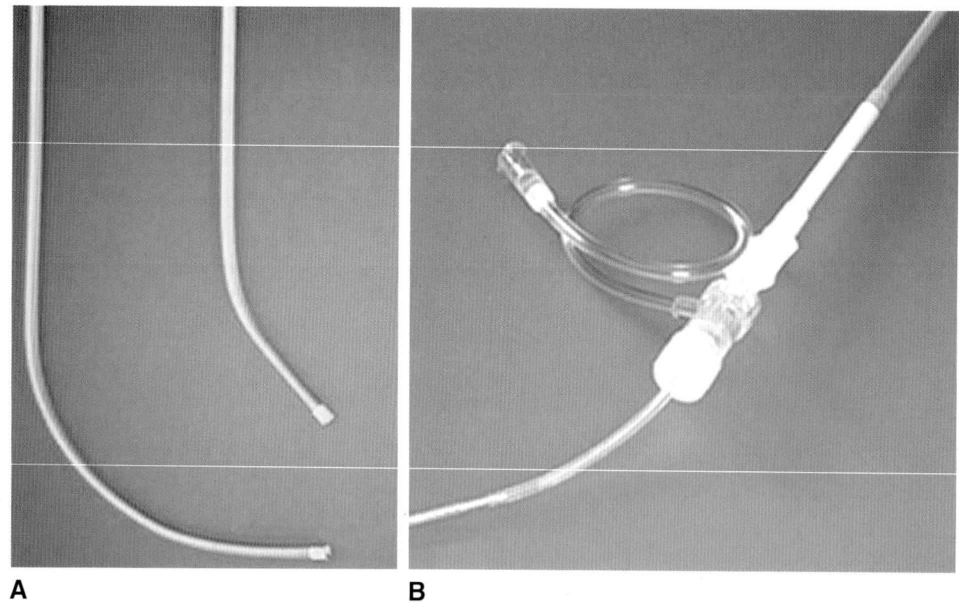

Figure 19-116. *Delivery system for left ventricular (LV) pacing leads from ELA Medical (Sorin Group, Milan).* ***A,*** *The two available guiding catheter shapes with wire mesh walls.* ***B,*** *The hemostatic valve is attached to the hub of the guiding catheter. The lead extender for removal of the guide without slitting is shown attached to the distal end of the pacing lead. Both of the guiding catheter shapes lack a proximal curve and thus must be deformed to cannulate the coronary sinus (CS). They are prone to springing back and displacing the pacing lead as they are removed from the CS.*

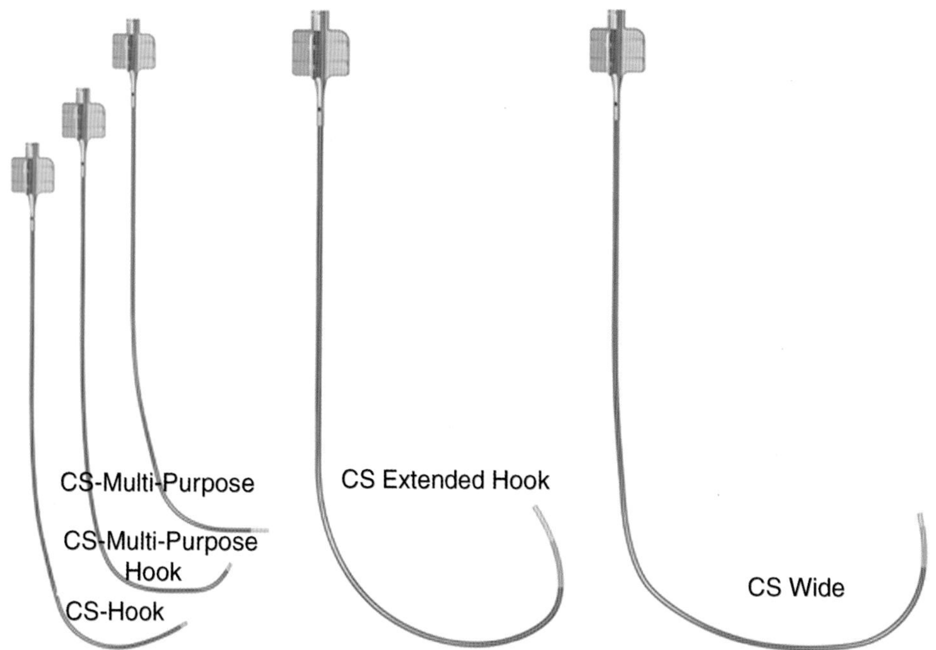

Figure 19-117. *The range of guiding catheter shapes that have been introduced by Guidant (Boston Scientific, Natick, Mass.) over the last 5 years. The extended-hook Rapido Advance is the most widely used and successful of this manufacturer's shapes, presumably because it is designed to approach the coronary sinus from above.*

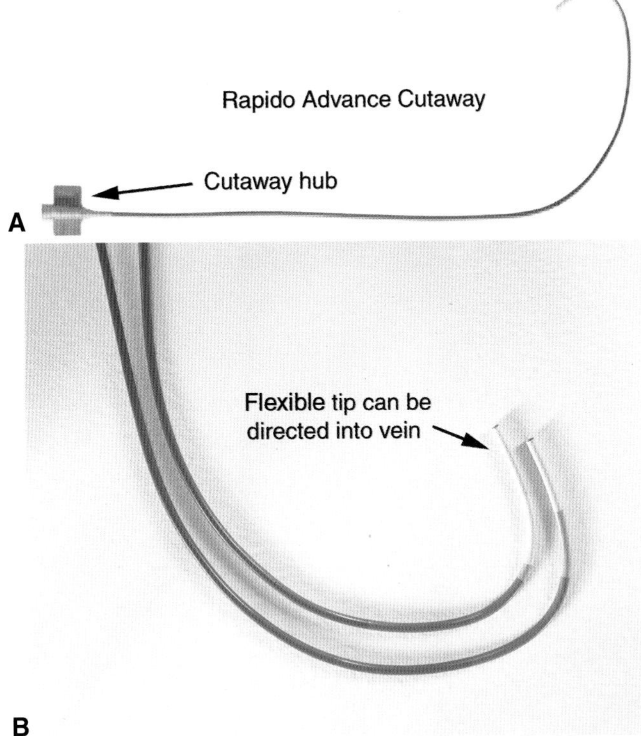

Figure 19-118. The Rapido Advance Cutaway Guide Catheter system (Guidant, Boston Scientific, Natick, Mass). ***A,*** *The extended-hook shape of the Rapido Advance with cutaway hub is shown. The wall of the catheter contains wire mesh for kink resistance and torque control. The shape includes a proximal curve, which facilitates coronary sinus (CS) cannulation and reduces "springback" as it is removed.* ***B,*** *The distal portion of the Rapido Advance CS cannulating guide is shown in detail. The flexible tip of the guide can be directed into the target vein for direct lead delivery using the Guidant coronary sinus inner catheter CS-IC 50 or CS-IC 90 (see Fig. 19-119). The combination of the Rapido Advance system and the IC 50/IC 90 directional catheter represents a second-generation telescoping system: The guide shape used to cannulate the CS (Rapido Advance) is deformed to selectively cannulate the coronary vein with a removable directional catheter.*

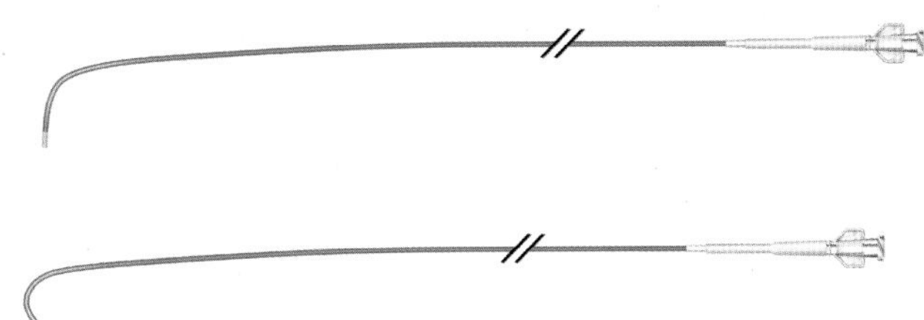

Figure 19-119. Rapido Coronary Sinus Inner Catheters 90 (CS-IC 90, top) and 50 (CS-IC 50, bottom) (Guidant, Boston Scientific, Natick, Mass.). The Guidant GuideCaths are used in a telescoping fashion through the Rapido Advance guiding catheter to facilitate coronary sinus (CS) cannulation. Once in the CS, the catheters may be used to selectively cannulate coronary veins for guidewire placement. Once the guidewire and the GuideCath are in the vein, the Rapido Advance Cutaway Guide Catheter system can be advanced into the vein. With the Rapido Advance securely in the vein, the GuideCath is removed and the pacing lead is delivered. The combination of the Rapido Advance and the IC 50/IC 90 directional catheters represents a second-generation telescoping system: The guide shape used to cannulate the CS (Rapido Advance) is deformed to selectively cannulate the coronary vein with a removable directional catheter.

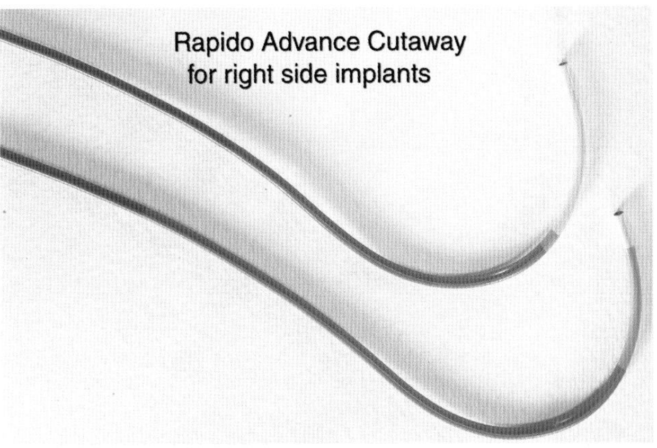

Figure 19-120. Coronary sinus cannulation guides for right-side implantation (Rapido Advance Cutaway Guide Catheters from Guidant, Boston Scientific, Natick, Mass.).

Medtronic, Inc.

Several fixed guide shapes and a deflectable guide intended for both CS access and LV lead delivery are available from Medtronic. None of them is peel-away. The guides are designed to be inserted into the venous circulation through a peel-away 9F sheath. Because the ends of the straight guides are flexible, they can also be advanced into the target side branch. This is particularly useful if the peel-away sheath used for venous access is long enough to cannulate the CS and does not kink. Medtronic also provides a line of three small fixed-curve catheters and one deflectable-curve catheter for selection of target veins off the main CS (Fig. 19-121). All the smaller catheters are too small for direct lead delivery. Once the angioplasty wire is delivered to the target vein, the catheter must be removed over the wire before the lead is placed. As discussed previously, the availability of the smaller catheter to deliver the wire to the target vein represents a step forward but is limited by the inability to deliver the lead directly except when the larger guide is advanced over the smaller catheter into the side branch. However, even if this is accomplished, the CS access guide must be cut away once the lead is in place and tested, raising the risk of lead dislodgment (Fig. 19-122).

Pressure Products, Inc.

Pressure Products offers the first third-generation telescoping system. It is capable of delivering all of the available LV pacing leads. It is composed of a peel-away sheath that acts as the platform and preformed braided guides to cannulate the target veins and deliver the lead. There are three peel-away sheaths designed for cannulating the CS, as discussed in the section on CS cannulation. Because they are anatomically shaped, the

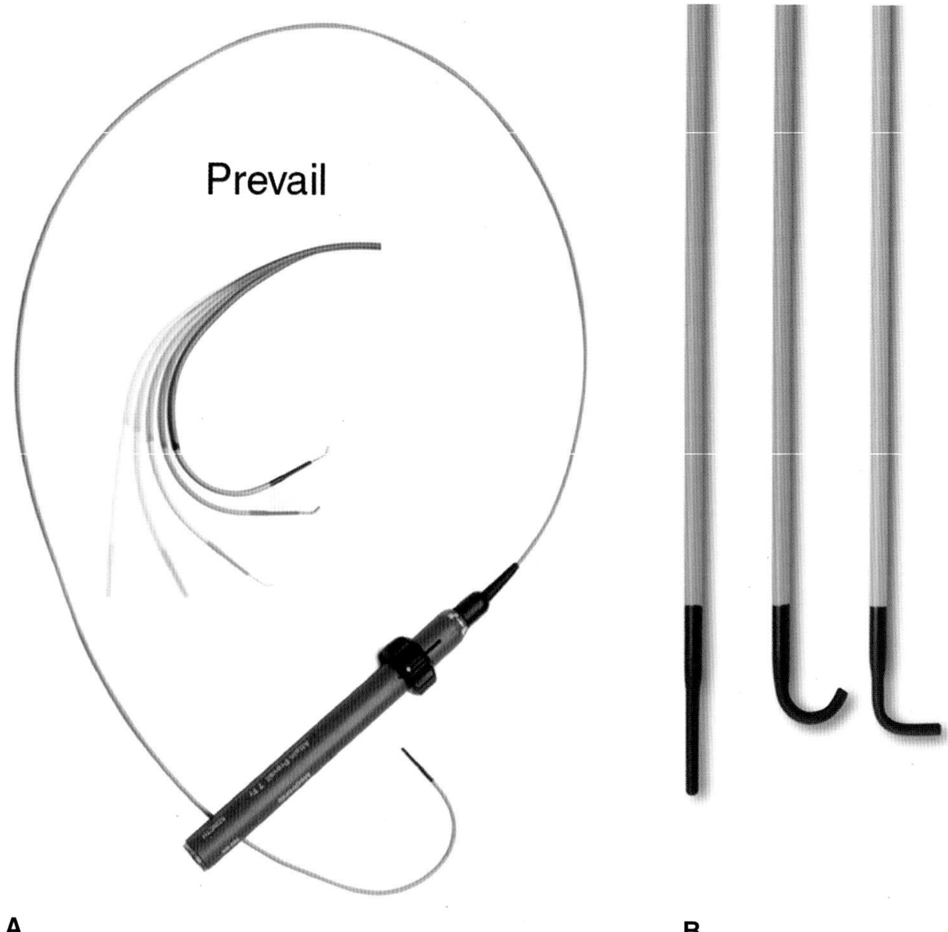

Figure 19-121. "Small" open-lumen catheters to facilitate coronary sinus (CS) and coronary vein cannulation from Medtronic, Inc. (Minneapolis, Minn.). **A,** The Prevail deflectable open-lumen catheter is shown alone and inside an Attain fixed-curve CS cannulation catheter. The Prevail–fixed-curve combination is a first-generation telescoping system when the angioplasty wire is directed into the target vein with the Prevail catheter. When the Prevail catheter directs the tip of the CS cannulation catheter into the target vein, it becomes a second-generation telescoping system. **B,** The Attain Select fixed-curve directional catheters. These catheters are used in conjunction with an Attain fixed-curve CS cannulation catheter to create either a first-generation (wire down target vein) or second-generation (Attain guide into the target vein) telescoping system.

risk of kinking is low. Torque control for CS cannulation is provided by the removable "braided core." The tips of both the peel-away sheath and the braided core are radiopaque. Figure 19-123A is a photograph of the standard size peel-away CS sheath. Figure 19-123B is a photograph of the four 9F OD/7F ID preformed braided guides available to cannulate specific target veins and deliver the lead. They are referred to as lateral vein introducers (LVIs). Figures 19-124 through 19-127 illustrate the veins for which the LVI shapes are designed. The LVI has a breakaway hemostatic valve; the larger side remains attached to the LVI and serves as a handle to assist in slicing (Fig. 19-128).

Details on how to use the Pressure Products third-generation telescoping system and examples of its use in patients are presented later (see Figs. 19-138 through 19-159). The discussion deals with guide support, coaxial placement of the LVI, and use of wires, small catheters, and balloons to advance the tip of the LVI into the target vein.

St. Jude Medical

St. Jude Medical provides the Apeel CS Catheter Delivery System (Figs. 19-129 and 19-130), including the LiveWire Cannulator, which is designed for LV placement of the QuickSite lead. This system is composed of a peel-away sheath with a hemostasis valve (Apeel Valve) attached to the proximal end. The distal end of the sheath is equipped with a radiopaque marker. The LiveWire steerable/deflectable catheter provides torque control of the peel-away sheath for placement into the CS, after which the catheter is removed. Once the lead is in place, the valve is removed over the back of a standard IS-1 lead. The sheath is then peeled away. The advantages of a peel-away sheath were listed earlier. The disadvantage of the Apeel CS Catheter Delivery System is the lack of a means to deliver contrast agent to assist in cannulating the CS. In addition, some of the Apeel peel-away sheaths are not anatomically shaped to avoid kinking.

Text continued on p. 748

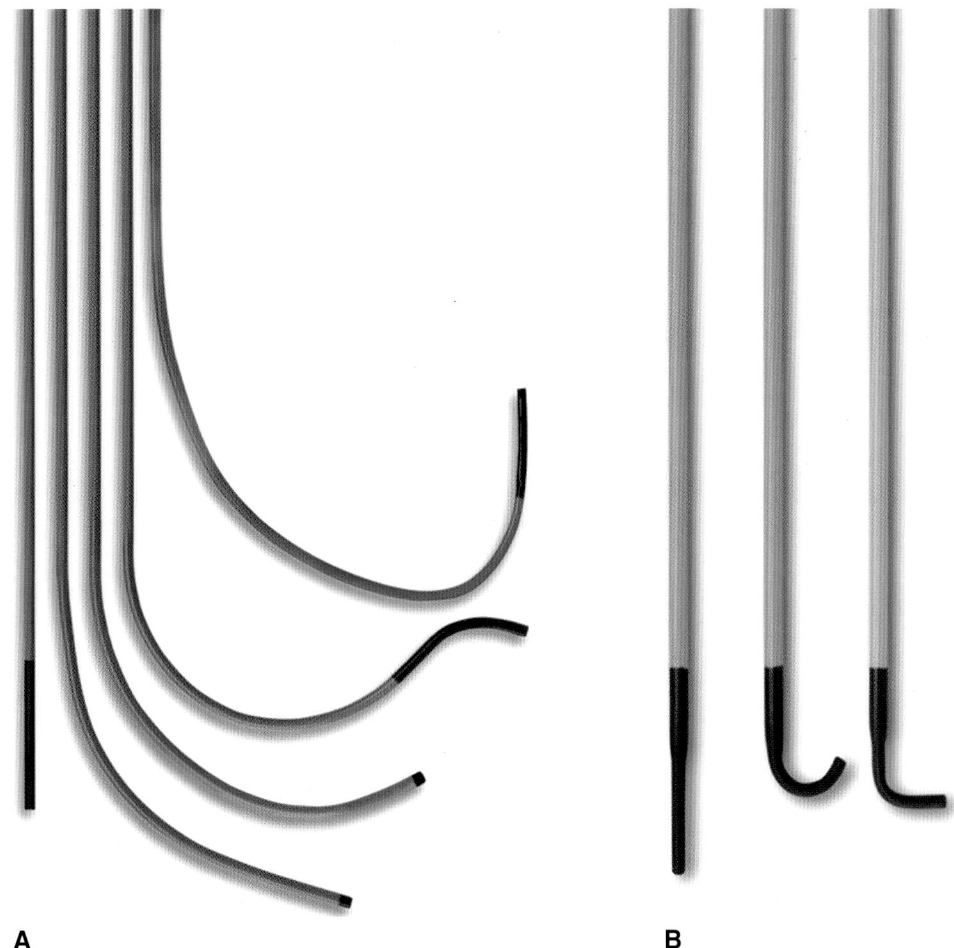

*Figure 19-122. Fixed-curve (Attain) and inner (Attain Select), guides from Medtronic, Inc. (Minneapolis, Minn.). **A,** The fixed-curve coronary sinus cannulation guide shapes currently available from Medtronic. The wall of the catheter contains wire mesh for kink resistance and torque control. The fifth shape (most medial) has a proximal curve to facilitate coronary sinus cannulation and reduce spring-back. **B,** The inner guides fit through the fixed-curve coronary sinus cannulation guide and facilitate the cannulation of side branches with a guidewire for over-the-wire access of the lead.*

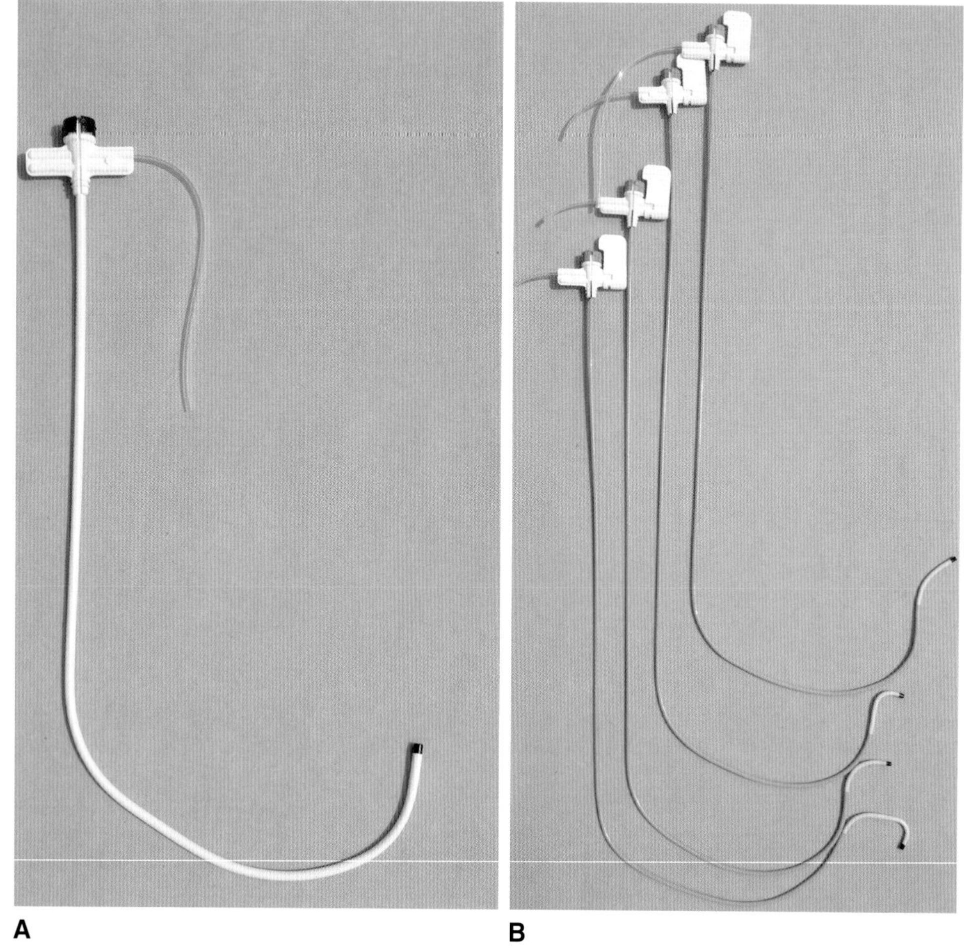

Figure 19-123. *Components of the third-generation telescoping system from Pressure Products, Inc. (San Pedro, Calif.).* ***A,*** *The standard size peel-away coronary sinus (CS) sheath.* ***B,*** *The four 9F OD/7F ID preformed braided guides designed to cannulate specific target veins and deliver the lead. They are referred to as lateral vein introducers (LVIs).*

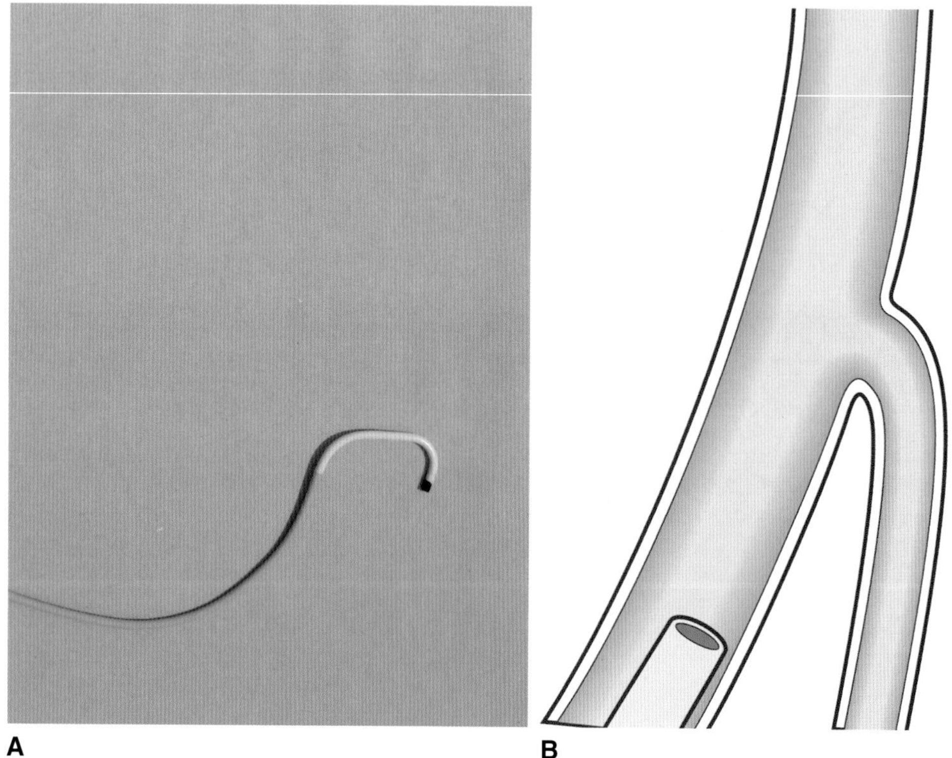

Figure 19-124. *Renal lateral vein introducer (Pressure Products, Inc., San Pedro, Calif.) (**A**) with a diagram of the intended anatomy (**B**).*

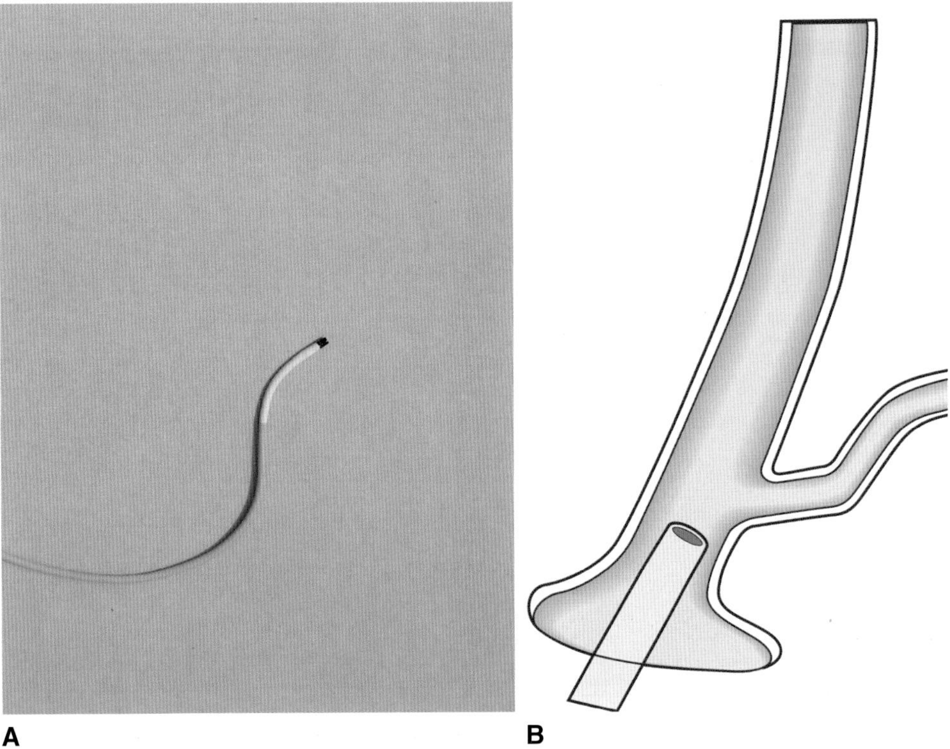

Figure 19-125. *Multipurpose lateral vein introducer (Pressure Products, San Pedro, Calif.) (**A**) with a diagram of the intended anatomy (**B**).*

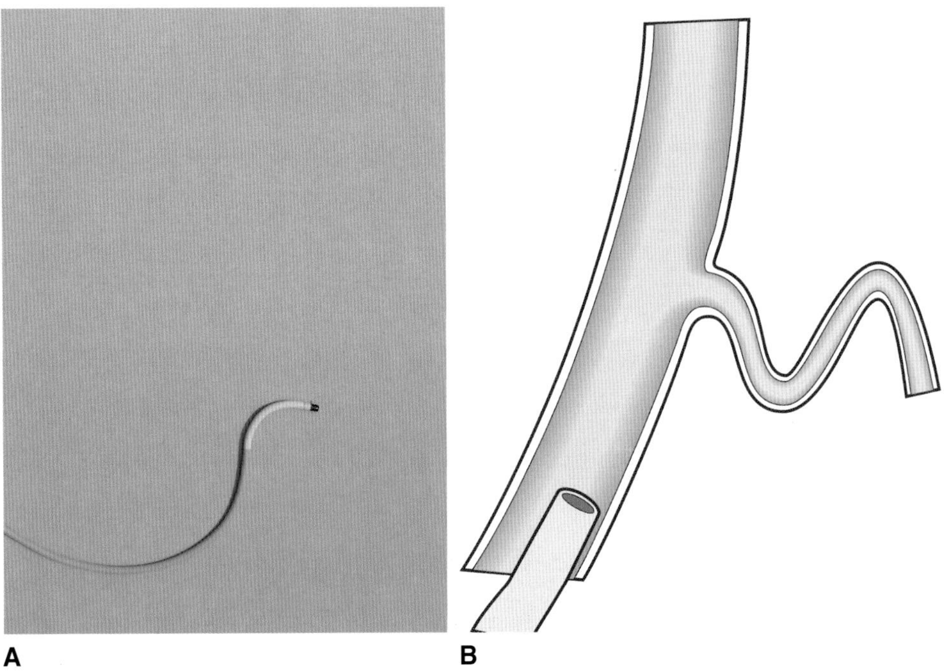

Figure 19-126. *Hockey stick lateral vein introducer (Pressure Products, San Pedro, Calif.) (**A**) with a diagram of the intended anatomy (**B**).*

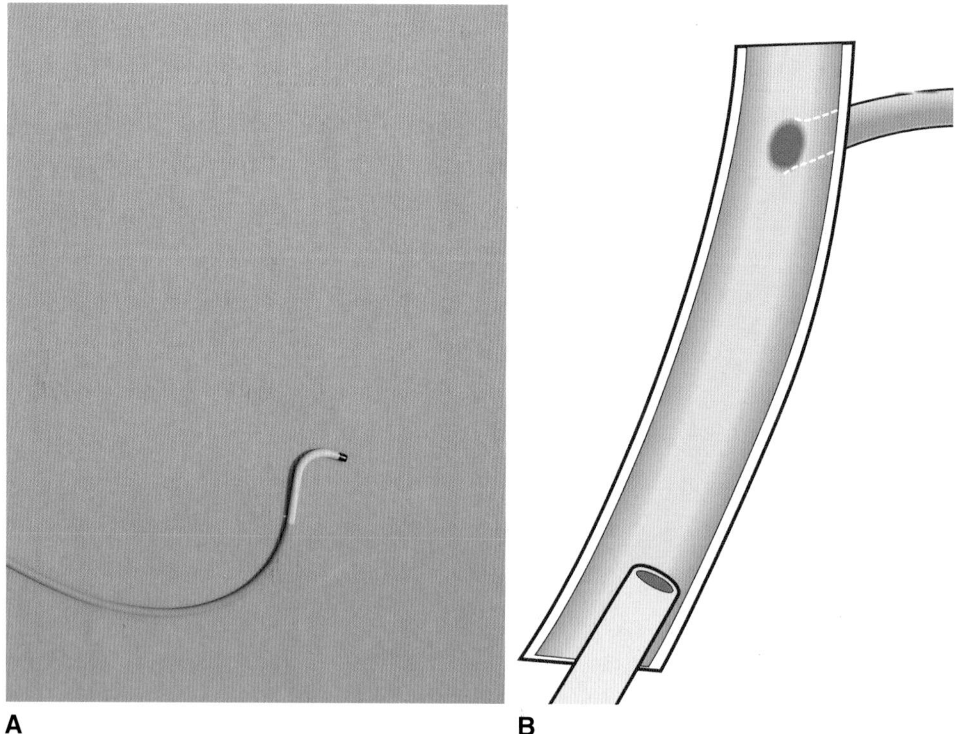

*Figure 19-127. Hook lateral vein introducer (Pressure Products, San Pedro, Calif.) (**A**) with a diagram of the intended anatomy (**B**).*

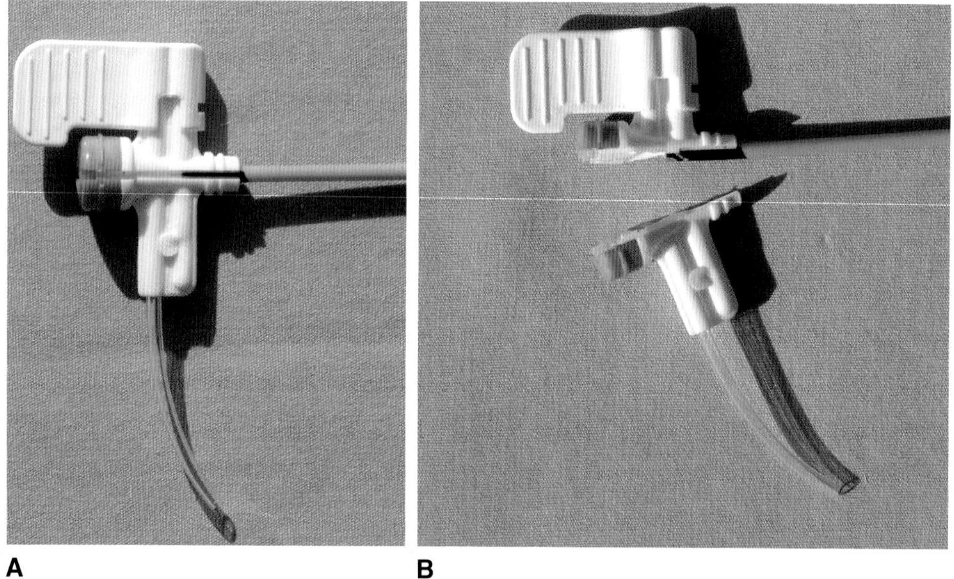

*Figure 19-128. Break-away hemostatic valve. **A,** The hemostatic valve is intact and attached to the proximal end of a lateral vein introducer. One of the flanges is larger than the other. **B,** The valve is cracked open. The larger wing of the hemostatic valve remains attached to the braided guide and will serve as a handle for the slicing process.*

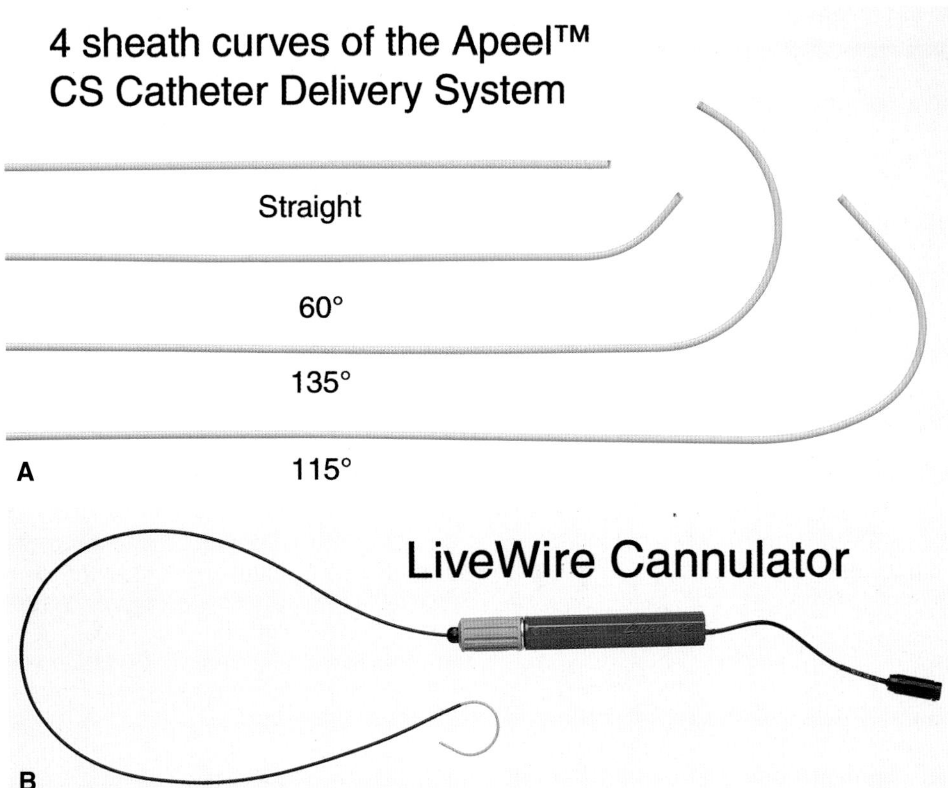

*Figure 19-129. The Apeel CS Catheter Delivery System and LiveWire Cannulator from St. Jude Medical (St. Paul, Minn.). **A,** The four shapes of the Apeel (peel-away) system sheaths are illustrated. **B,** The LiveWire Cannulator, a steerable/deflectable bipolar electrophysiology (EP) catheter, is designed to enhance access of the 8F Apeel peel-away sheath to the coronary sinus (CS). The cannulator is inserted through the peel-away sheath into the CS. Then the sheath is advanced over the cannulator into the CS, and the cannulator is removed.*

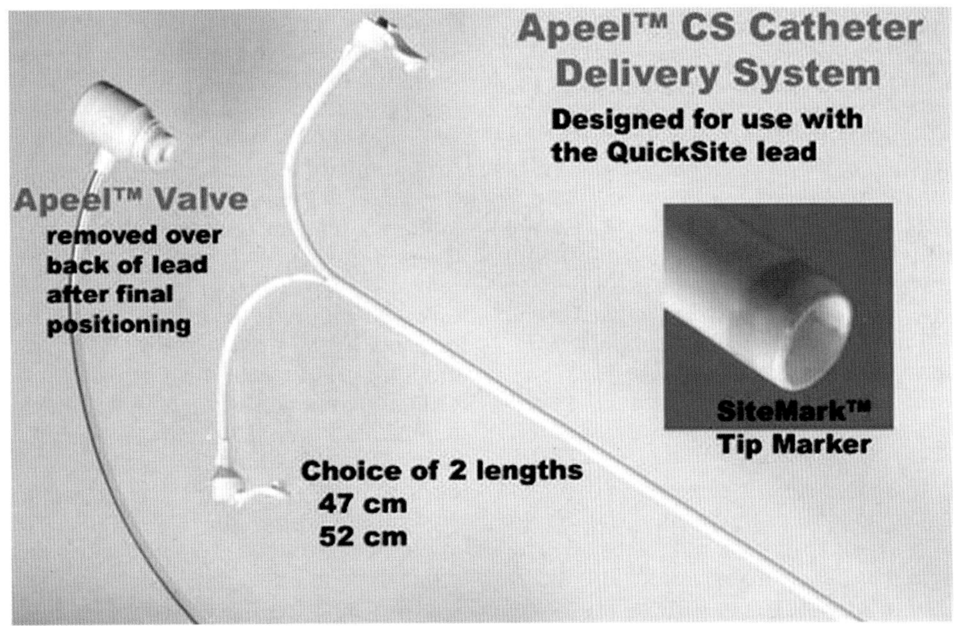

Figure 19-130. The Apeel CS Catheter Delivery System, including the Apeel Valve, from St. Jude Medical (St. Paul, Minn.). The peel-away sheath is an 8F ID, and the tip is radiopaque. It is available in two lengths, 47 cm and 52 cm. The lumen of the Apeel Valve is large enough to slide over an IS-1 connector of the pacing lead.

St. Jude Medical has not provided a line of smaller catheters with which to create a first-generation telescoping system from the Apeel CS Catheter delivery system. Adopting diagnostic or interventional radiology directional catheters easily solves this problem. The peel-away sheath of the St. Jude system does not have a flexible tip and thus is not easily distorted into the target vein, so it cannot be adapted into a second-generation delivery system.

How to Use the Guides of a Third-Generation Telescoping System

When using third-generation guides for direct LV lead delivery, the implanter must advance the guide into the CS over a wire. It is also important to understand coaxial placement and guide support. In addition, the guide size and shape must match the target vein. Finally, care must be taken that the CS is not stenotic at or before the target vein.

Advance the Guide over a Small Catheter and Wire

To upgrade to a third-generation telescoping system, a sheath large enough to accept the guide is placed in the CS at the start of the procedure. The transition from first- and second-generation to third-generation telescoping system is easier if the small catheter (Rapido, Attain Select, etc.) is inserted inside the telescoping guide. The small catheter is advanced over a wire into the CS to cannulate the target vein. The LVI/guide is advanced out of the sheath over the catheter and wire into the target vein. The small catheter is then removed (Fig. 19-131).

Advance the Guide with a Wire into the Coronary Sinus

As the operator becomes familiar with the feel of the third-generation telescoping guides, he/she may no longer need to cannulate the target vein first with the small catheter. In some patients with large target veins and a large CS, there may be a temptation to advance the third-generation telescoping guide directly into the vein without first advancing it above the vein over the wire. However, when directional guides are used for direct LV lead delivery, it is prudent to advance the guide over a wire to reduce the risk of contrast staining and CS perforation (Figs. 19-132 and 19-133).

Guide Support

With third-generation telescoping systems, the guides are specifically designed for the target veins. The shapes are not limited by the need to also cannulate the CS. The shape of the guide can be tailored to provide optimal guide support. *Guide support* refers to how much the guide resists being pushed back out of the target vein by attempts to advance the LV lead. The greater the support, the more the guide resists being pushed out of the target vein as the lead is advanced. Lead advancement may be resisted by a small, tortuous, or stenotic vein segment. When the operator attempts to advance against resistance, the lead may advance or, if the resistance is excessive, the guide may be displaced.

Whether or not the guide is displaced depends on the shape, composition, wall thickness, and French size of the guide. A 9F guide provides more guide support than an 8F guide with the same shape and composition. In addition, the shape that the guide takes in the CS can have a major impact on guide support. If the shape of the guide places the back of the curve against the wall of the CS, it will provide far more support than the same guide with a different shape (Figs. 19-134 and 19-135).

Coaxial Guide Placement

When the tip of the guide is in the target vein, the lumen of the guide should be aligned with the lumen of the vein. In Figure 19-136A, the 5F hook catheter is coaxial with the vein. In Figure 19-136B, the 8F guide is not coaxial with the vein. Ideally, before the LV lead is advanced, the lumen of the guide is coaxial with the vein. A guide with more bend in the tip, similar to the 5F hook, is desirable.

Directional Guides Available for Left Ventricular Lead Placement

Until recently, using a third-generation telescoping system required significant operator improvisation. The reverse curve had to be added, the hub had to be cut off before the lead was placed, and the interventional guides were hard to cut. Now, third-generation guides that address these issues are commercially available. The 9F guides are designed to be used with a 9F sheath that has a prominent proximal curve. The guides have a reverse curve proximally to ensure that the tip points laterally toward the target veins. The importance of the proximal curve is illustrated in Figure 19-137. Without the reverse curve in the guide, the tip of the guide points medially, away from the target vein. Substantial torque must be exerted to turn the tip laterally toward the target veins. If torque is released at any time, the guide will flip back medially out of the target vein. With the proximal curve in the guide, the tip exits the sheath laterally and often requires little if any torque. In addition, with a guide with the reverse curve, there is less pressure at the tip to tear the vein than with a straight guide that has been twisted laterally.

Every commercially available guide has a removable hemostatic hub attached to its proximal end that reduces the blood loss and risk of air embolization that occurred with the improvised systems when the hub was cut off to place the lead. With the removable hemostatic hub, contrast material can be injected and the guide repositioned if it becomes dislodged from the vein or there is phrenic pacing or high pacing thresholds. Once the lead is in place and pacing thresholds and phrenic pacing have been evaluated, the hub is cracked. The hub section containing the tubing falls

Text continued on p. 753

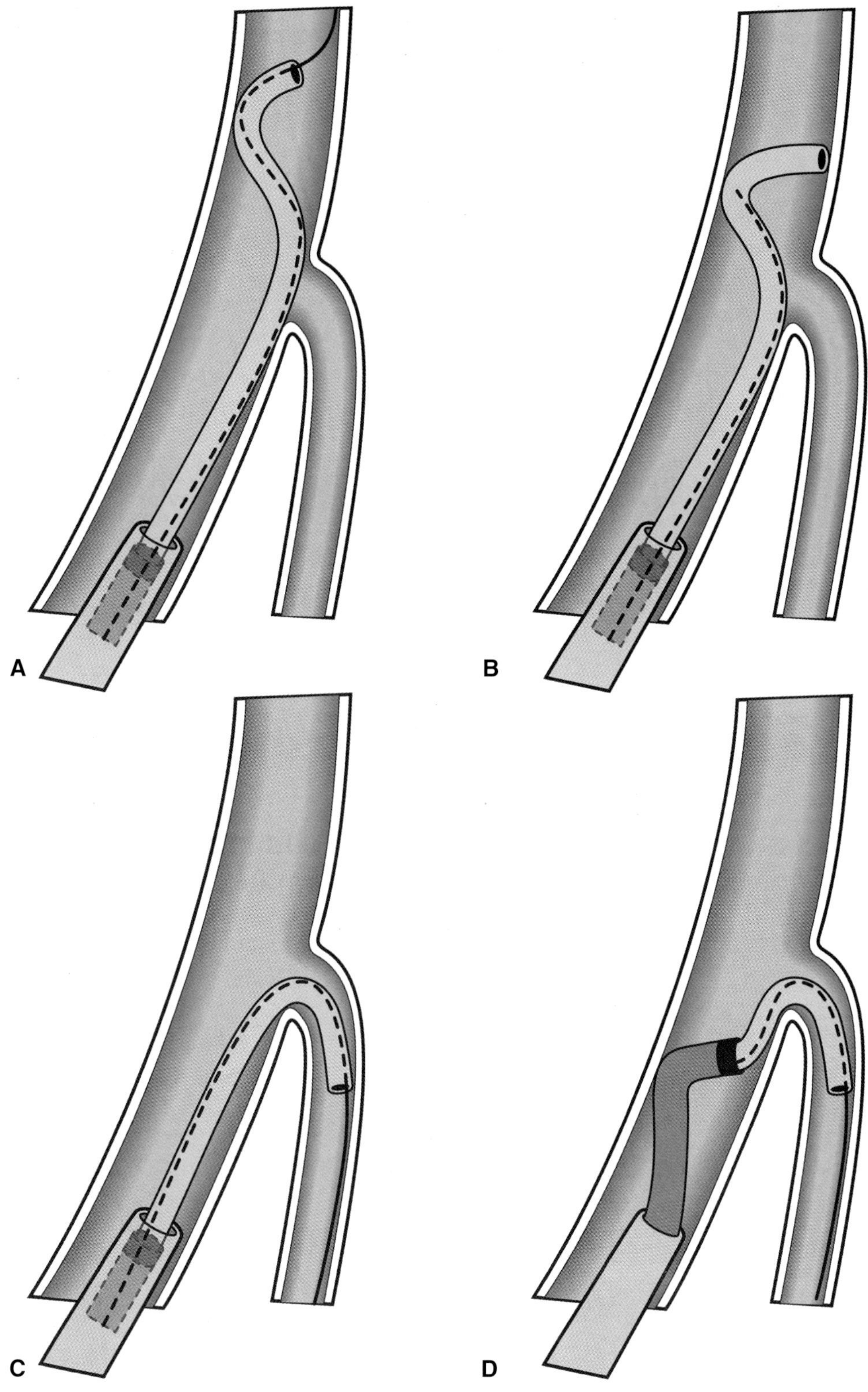

Figure 19-131. *Use of a small catheter to assist the placement of a third-generation telescoping guide.* ***A,*** *The directional catheter is through the third-generation telescoping guide into the main coronary sinus (CS) over a wire to a position above the target vein. The third-generation telescoping guide (renal lateral vein introducer [renal LVI]) remains in the sheath. The peel-away sheath is at mid-CS level.* ***B,*** *The wire is withdrawn into the small directional catheter. Small catheter manipulation with puffs of contrast material identifies and cannulates the target vein. The peel-away sheath and renal LVI remain in position.* ***C,*** *The small catheter is seated in the target vein, and the wire is advanced deep into the target vein. The peel-away sheath and renal LVI remain in position.* ***D,*** *The third-generation telescoping guide is advanced out of the peel-away sheath over the small catheter and wire into the target vein. The wire and small catheter are held taut to create a rail supporting and directing the delivery catheter as it is advanced into the target vein. The small catheter is removed from the target vein, leaving the wire and guide in the vein for lead delivery.*

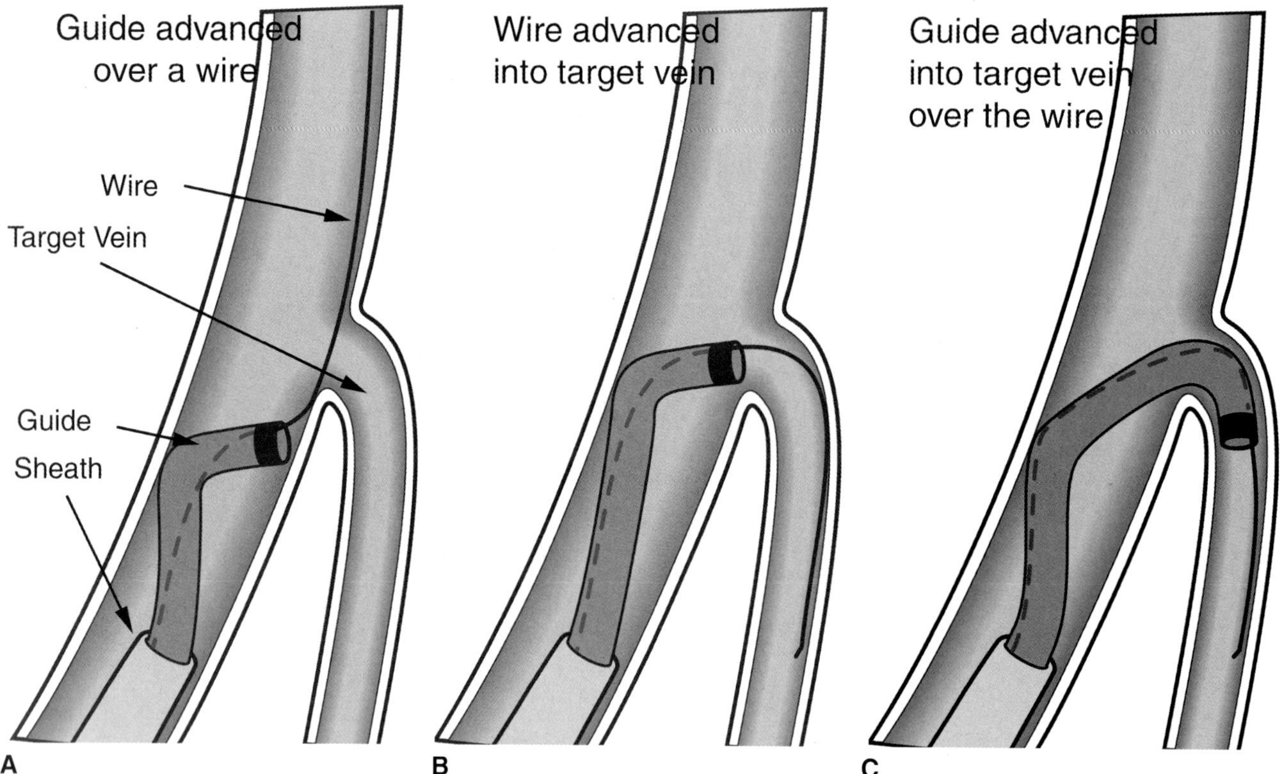

Figure 19-132. Wire used to facilitate placement of the guide into the target vein. ***A,*** *The guide is advanced out of the sheath into the coronary sinus (CS) over a wire.* ***B,*** *After the guide is advanced over the wire above the target vein, the wire is withdrawn into the guide. The guide is withdrawn, followed by puffs of contrast material until the vein is identified. The wire is then advanced down the target vein.* ***C,*** *The guide is advanced over the wire into the target vein.*

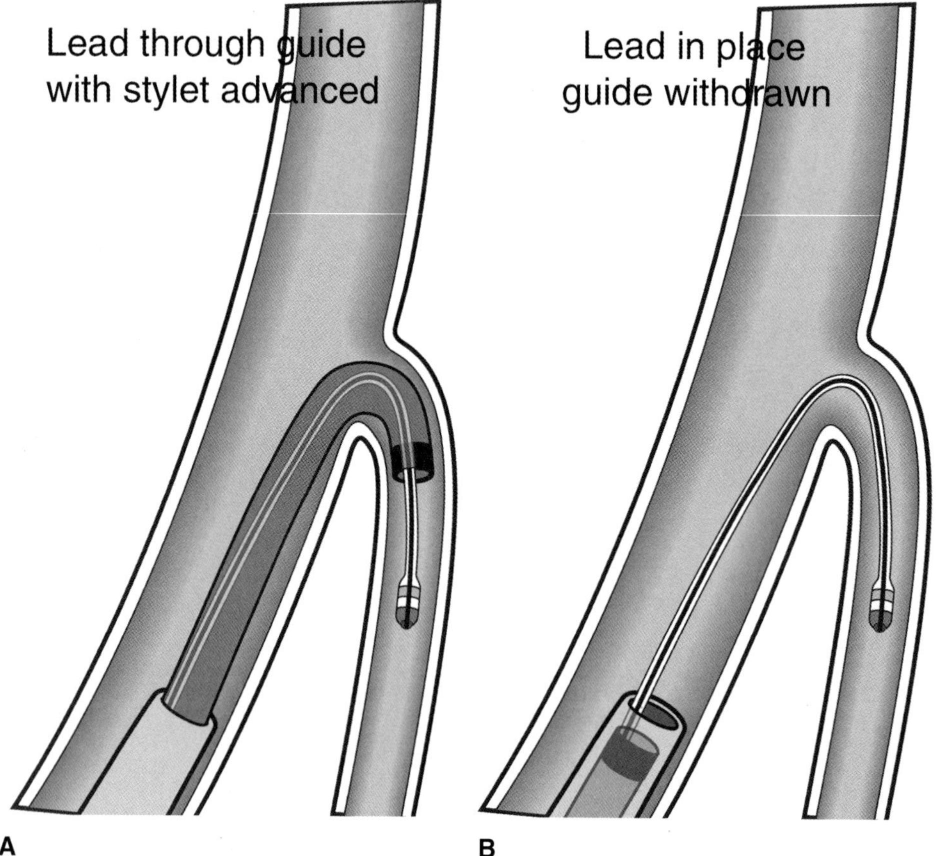

Figure 19-133. Final lead placement with a third-generation telescoping system. ***A,*** *The guide supports the lead in the vein while the angioplasty wire is removed and the stylet is advanced to the tip of the lead.* ***B,*** *The guide withdraws into the sheath as it is cut away. The sheath supports the lead and straightens the guide as it is cut away.*

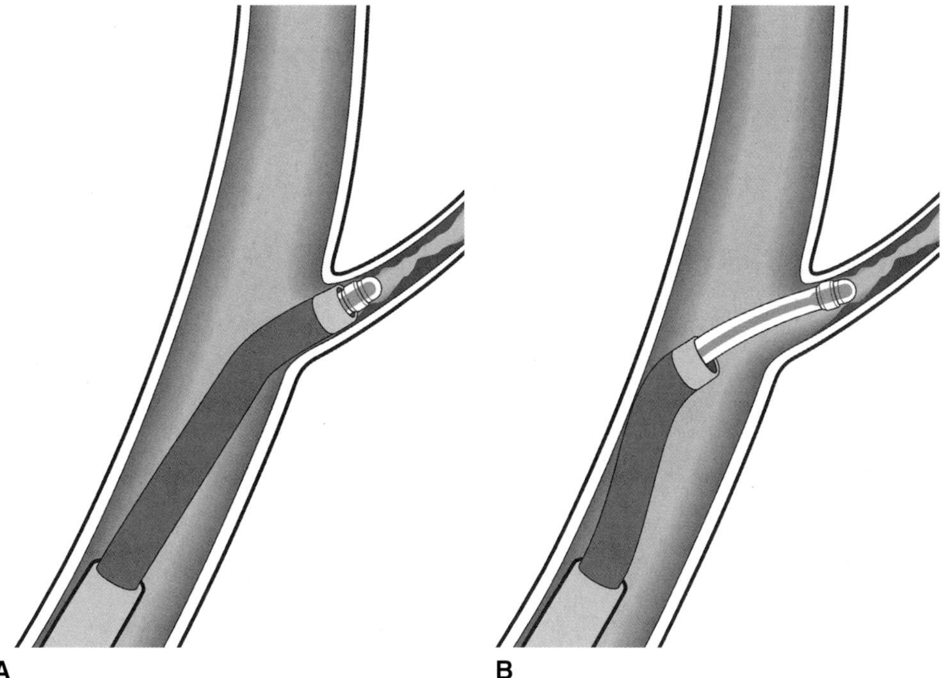

*Figure 19-134. The shape of the guide provides little support. **A,** The shape of the guide directs the pacing lead into the target vein. **B,** The guide is displaced as the operator attempts to advance the pacing lead against the stenosis. The support provided by the guide is not sufficient. The guide is displaced. As the guide backs out, the pacing lead loses the axial support provided by the guide and starts to buckle.*

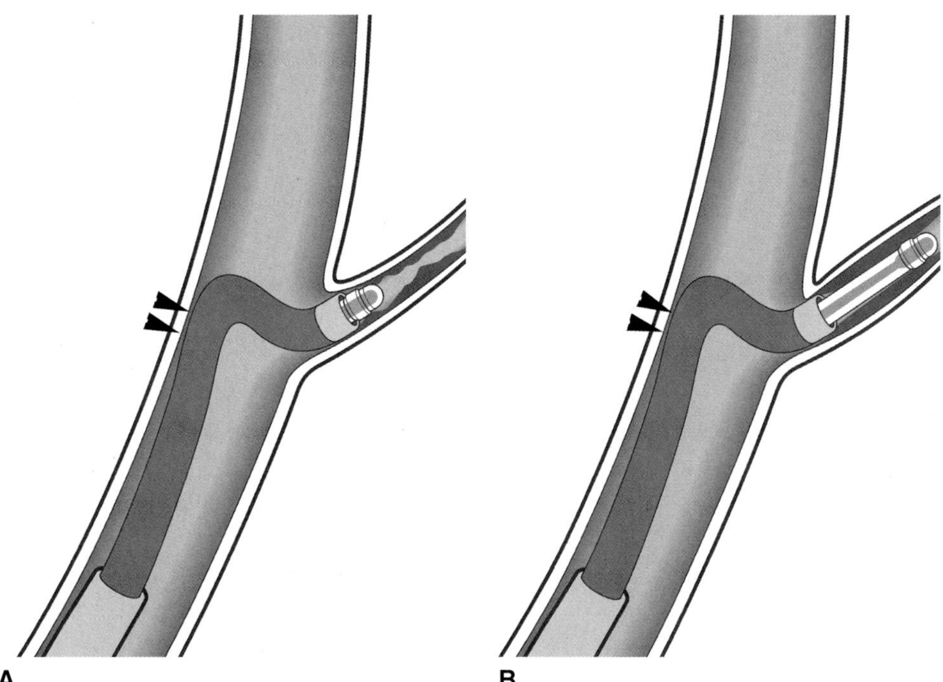

*Figure 19-135. The shape of the guide provides good support. **A,** The shape of the guide places the proximal curve against the wall of the coronary sinus (CS) when the tip is in the target vein. **B,** The pacing lead is advanced through the stenotic lesion. As the lead is advanced, the proximal curve resting against the back of the CS resists displacement of the guide. The axial support provided by the guide is maintained at the site of stenosis as the pacing lead exits the guide, and the lead does not buckle.*

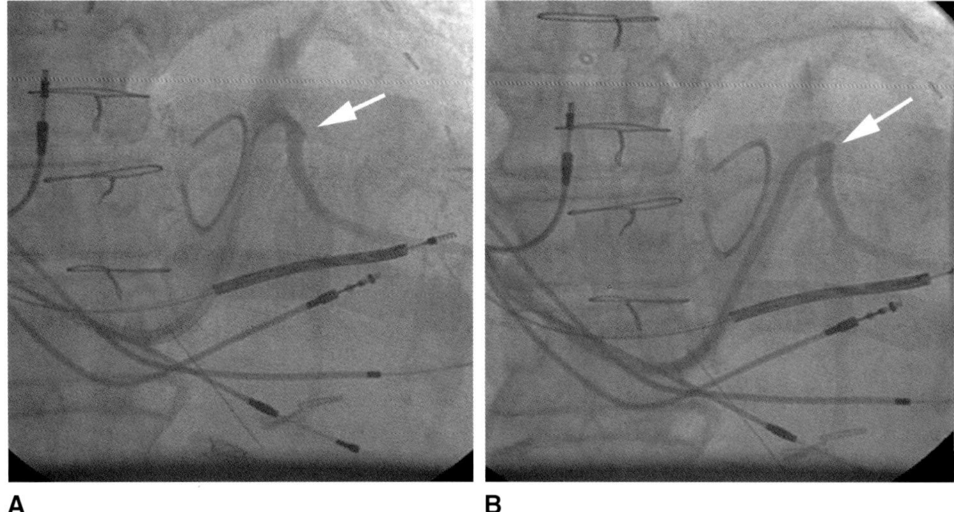

Figure 19-136. Coaxial versus noncoaxial placement of catheters and guides in target veins. ***A,*** *The catheter is coaxial. The lumen of the catheter and lumen of the vein are in line* (arrow). *When the catheter/guide is coaxial, the wire/lead is directed into the lumen of the vein.* ***B,*** *The tip of the guide in the preformed improvised third-generation telescoping delivery system is not coaxial. The lumen of the guide points toward the wall of the vein* (arrow). *When the catheter/guide is not coaxial, the wire/lead is directed at the wall of the vein, either perforating the vein or increasing resistance to passage of the wire/lead. The tip curve on the tip of the guide needs more inferior cant. In some cases, one can make the guide coaxial by advancing a wire into the vein and then advancing the guide over the wire. Before inserting the lead into the guide, one should attempt to improve the position of the guide tip in the vein. There is no risk of perforation during advancement of an over the wire lead if the wire is deep in the vein.*

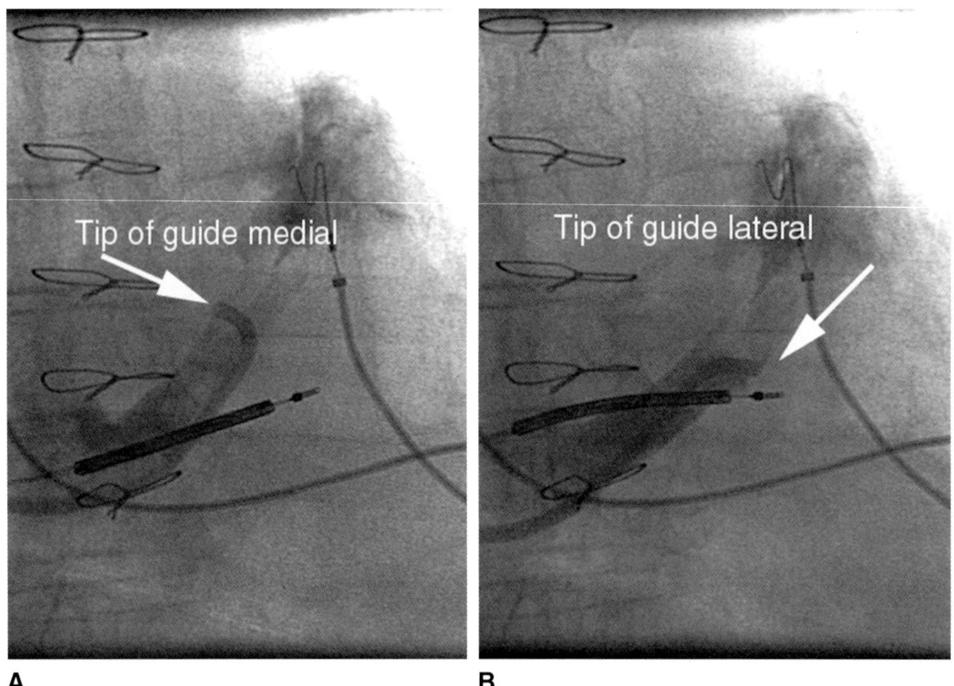

Figure 19-137. Braided directional guide in the coronary sinus (CS) without "back curve." ***A,*** *The renal shaped 9F guide without back curve is advanced into the CS, and the wire is removed. In the neutral state (no torque added), the tip of the guide points medially, away from the origin of the target veins.* ***B,*** *Counterclockwise torque is applied at the hub of the guide, turning the tip laterally toward the target veins. If the torque is released, the guide snaps back to the medial position even if the tip of the guide is in the target vein.*

away, and the other half remains attached to the guide as a handle for slicing. With the sheath in the CS to provide support, the guide is cut away.

Using the Third-Generation Telescoping System to Deal with Difficult Venous Anatomy

The most common venous variants that make LV lead placement difficult or impossible are as follows:

- Acute-angle vein
- Tortuous vein
- Proximal vein
- Partially obstructed vein
- Posterior vein

The current third-generation telescoping system provides four guide shapes to specifically deal with these vein anatomies (Fig. 19-138). The four guide shapes are based on the shapes found to be successful with an improvised third-generation telescoping system.

For the beginner as well as experienced operator facing a small tortuous vein, we recommend first cannulating the target vein with a small directional catheter and then sliding the third-generation guide into the target vein over the small catheter (see Fig. 19-131). In all cases, to avoid venous trauma, the guide should always be advanced over a wire to a site above the os of the target vein (Figs. 19-132 and 19-139). In addition, the operator must be certain the CS is not stenotic at or before the target vein. Finally, the vein and guide size and shape must be matched appropriately. Attempts to cannulate a vein that is too small for the guide or that does not match the guide shape can result in venous trauma (Figs. 19-140 and 19-141).

Acute-Angle Vein

Although the renal LVI is the appropriate shape for a large percentage of difficult target veins, it has a short distal segment that does not fit deep into the target vein. As a result, it will not extend beyond tortuous vein segments (Fig. 19-142).

Tortuous Veins

Third-generation telescoping delivery systems are also used to straighten tortuous vein segments. Second-generation telescoping systems can be used but are far less likely to succeed.

To straighten a vein, the operator advances a wire through the vein segment. The third-generation guide is then advanced over the wire. The ease with which the operator can advance the guide over the wire depends on the support provided by the wire, among other factors. With wire support, the thicker and stiffer the wire, the greater the support. Thus, a "floppy" 0.014-inch angioplasty wire provides little support,

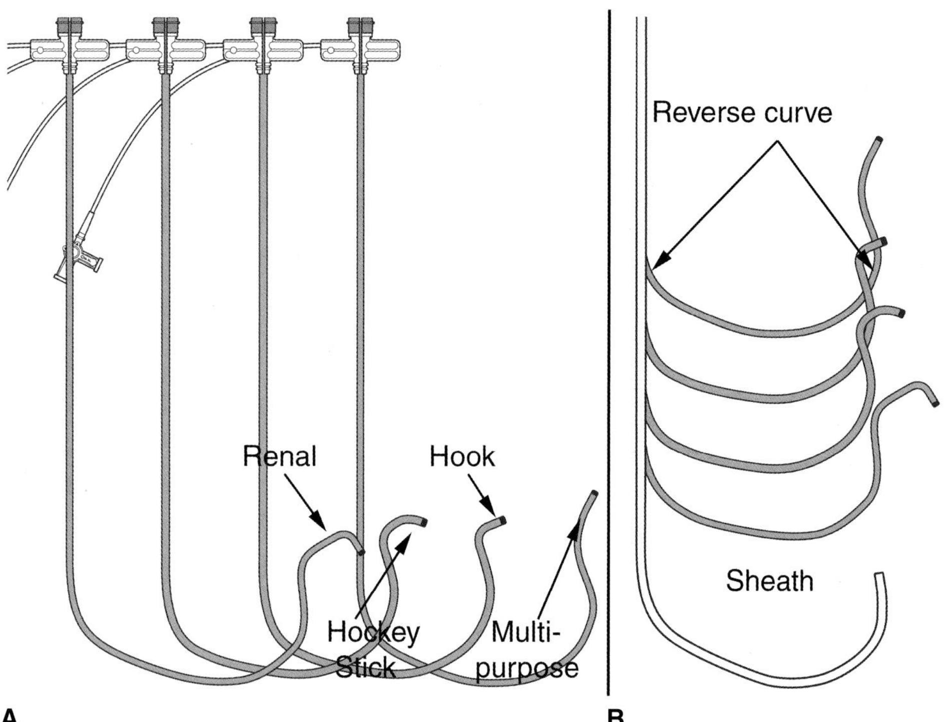

Figure 19-138. The four preformed guide shapes of the third-generation telescoping system. ***A,*** *The four guide shapes are shown: renal, hockey stick, hook, and multipurpose. The hemostatic break-away hub is on the proximal end of each.* ***B,*** *The four shapes are superimposed on and aligned with the matching sheath. All four shapes have the same curve proximal to the tip "back curve" that ensures that the tip of the guide points laterally.*

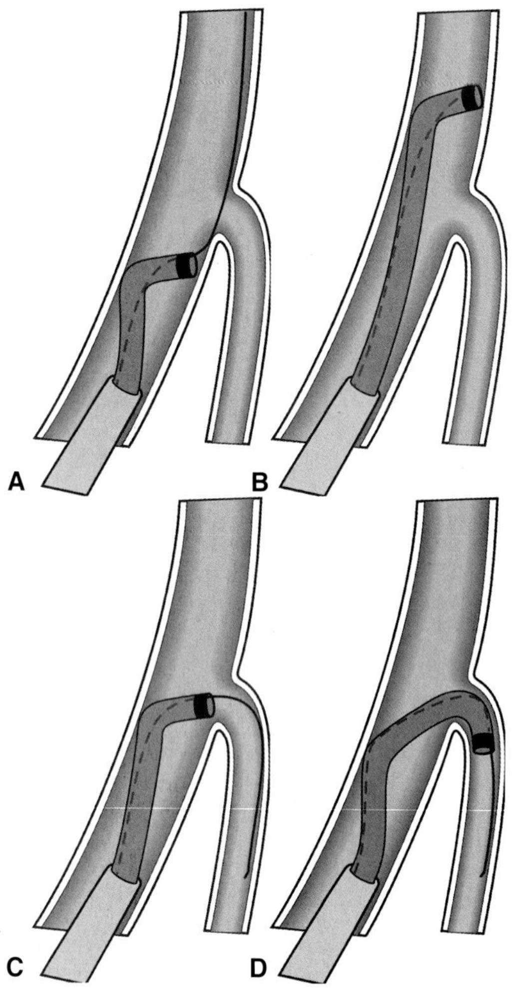

Figure 19-139. Insertion of a third-generation guide (lateral vein introducer) over a guidewire and into a coronary vein. **A,** Guidewire is advanced to straighten the guide and permit advancement beyond the side branch. **B,** The guidewire is pulled back and the guide is slowly withdrawn until it cannulates the side branch. **C,** The guidewire is advanced down the side branch so that the guide follows coaxial to the branch. **D,** The guide is advanced over the guide into the side branch.

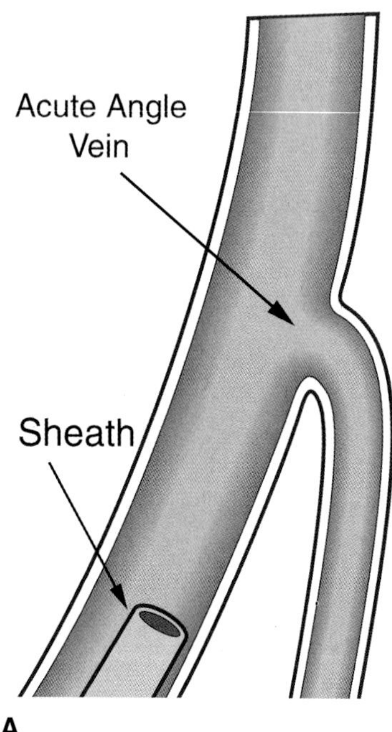

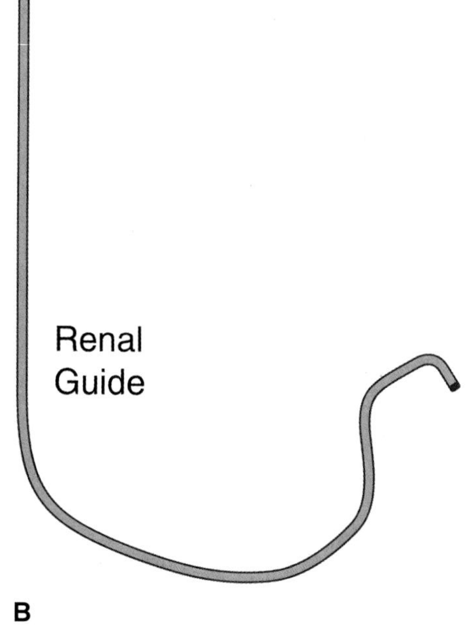

Figure 19-140. Acutely angled vein and third-generation renal telescoping system. **A,** An acutely angled target vein is depicted with the sheath at midcoronary sinus level. It would be difficult to direct a wire/pacing lead into the target vein from the position of the sheath. **B,** The third-generation renal guide designed for this anatomy is selected. The angle on the tip of the guide ensures that it will be coaxial with the lumen of the vein. The pacing lead is inserted directly into the vein through the guide.

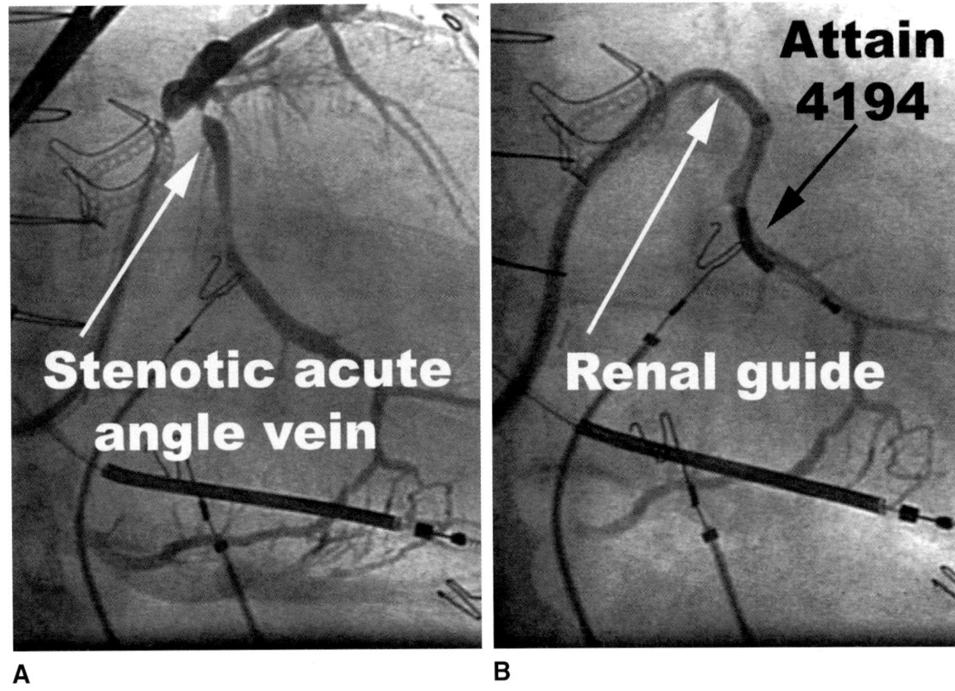

*Figure 19-141. Third-generation renal telescoping guide in a stenotic, acutely angled vein. **A,** The occlusive coronary sinus (CS) venogram identifies the midlateral wall target vein with a stenosis near the os. **B,** The telescoping renal guide is advanced over a glidewire (Terumo Medical Corp., Somerset, NJ.) without venoplasty into the target vein. The lumen of the guide and vein are coaxial. The Attain 4194 lead (Medtronic, Inc., Minneapolis, Minn.) advances into the vein.*

whereas a 0.035-inch Amplatz Extra Support wire will provide much greater support. A stiff wire is more difficult to advance through a tortuous vein segment. The 0.035-inch Terumo Radiofocus Glidewire is a good choice in most cases. Once the wire is through the tortuous vein segment, the guide is advanced over it. The tip shape of the guide (in addition to size and stiffness) has a major impact on whether it will advance into the target vein. If the angle of the tip of the third-generation guide matches the takeoff angle of the target vein, the guide is likely to advance against the friction of the tortuous vein segment. In contrast, if a second-generation telescoping system is employed, the CS cannulating guide must overcome the friction of being bent to the shape of the takeoff as well as the friction of the tortuous segment.

In some cases, even with a properly shaped third-generation telescoping system, it can be difficult to advance the guide. Advancing a series of progressively larger catheters over the wire can be effective. For example, if the goal is to advance a 9F guide through a tortuous vein segment, it may be necessary to first advance a 5F directional catheter through the 9F Guide, over-the-wire. Once the 5F catheter is across the area, the 9F guide may follow the over-the-wire/5F catheter combination. In some cases, even more support will be required, such as a 5F-7F-9F sequence. Initially the 5F catheter is inserted into the 7F catheter. The 7F catheter is advanced into the 9F catheter. At the tortuous area, first the 5F catheter is advanced over the wire, and then the 7F is advanced over the 5F catheter. Finally, with the wire and 5F and 7F catheters held in place, the 9F catheter is advanced over the combination. The guidewire/5F/7F combination is shown in Fig. 19-143. The combination of the sequential upsizing of the guidewires and sheaths and the hockey stick–shaped LVI (guide) leads can be advanced through tortuous venous target veins to the distal position, as demonstrated in Figures 19-144 and 19-145.

As noted previously, the deformation of the mitral annulus produced by mitral valve repair/replacement distorts the veins of the CS, particularly near their origins. Figure 19-146 shows a large extremely tortuous target vein being negotiated in a patient with mitral valve repair.

Proximal Vein

The target vein with its origin near the CS os is often difficult to cannulate. As the guide is withdrawn, the tip tends to disengage from the CS and fall to the floor of the RA. In response to this problem, a guide with a laterally directed tip is useful (Figs. 19-147 and 19-148).

Examples of the use of the multipurpose shape are presented here. In the first example (Figs. 19-149 and 19-150), attempts were made to advance the same guide used for CS cannulation into the target vein to deliver the lead (second-generation telescoping system). Although the tip of the guide advanced into the vein, it would not advance far enough to deliver the over-the-wire lead. When the guide was exchanged for a

Text continued on p. 761

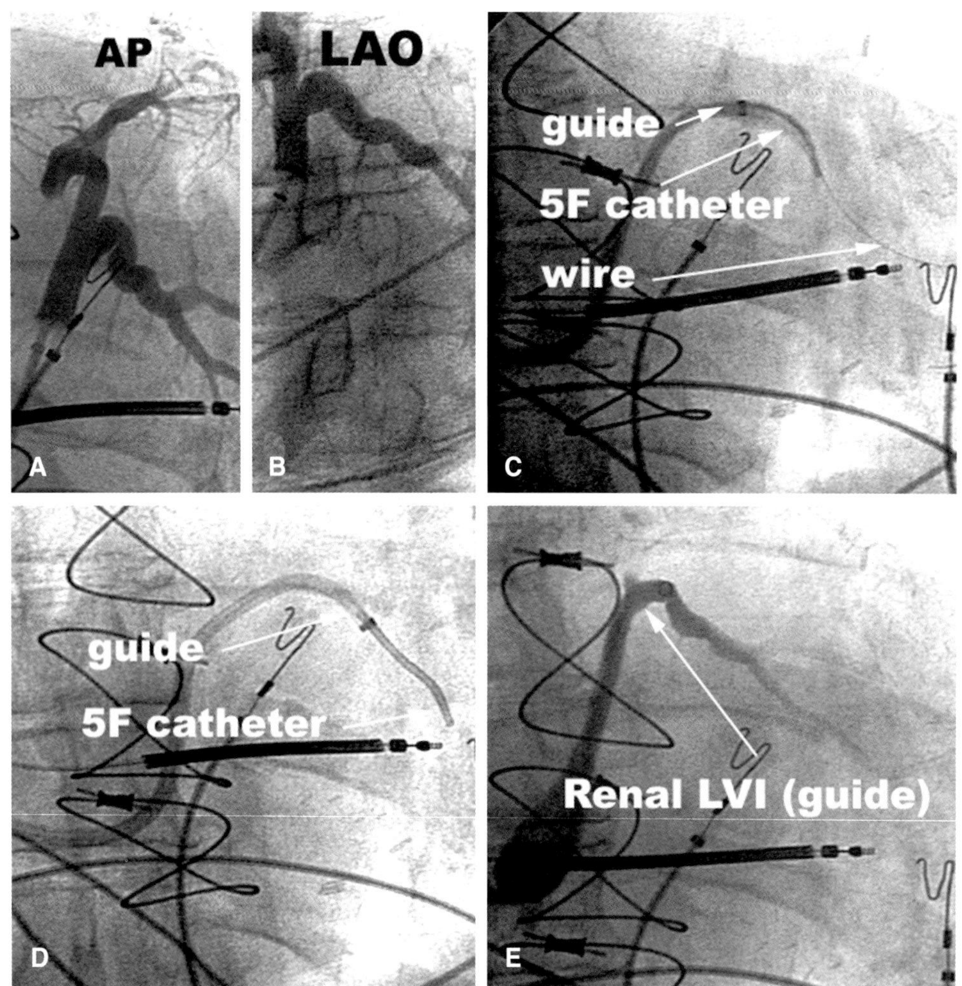

Figure 19-142. *Tip of a renal lateral vein introducer (renal LVI; guide) is too short; a hockey stick LVI is a better choice. The tortuous vein segment is shown in anteroposterior (**A**) and left anterior oblique (**B**) views. **C,** The 9F OD/7F ID renal LVI is advanced through the 9F ID/11F OD peel-away sheath into the os of the target vein over a 6F Attain Select catheter (Medtronic, Inc., Minneapolis, Minn.) and an angioplasty wire. **D,** The renal LVI is advanced over the 5F catheter beyond the tortuous segment. **E,** When the 5F catheter is removed, the tip of the guide retracts proximal to the tortuous vein segment.*

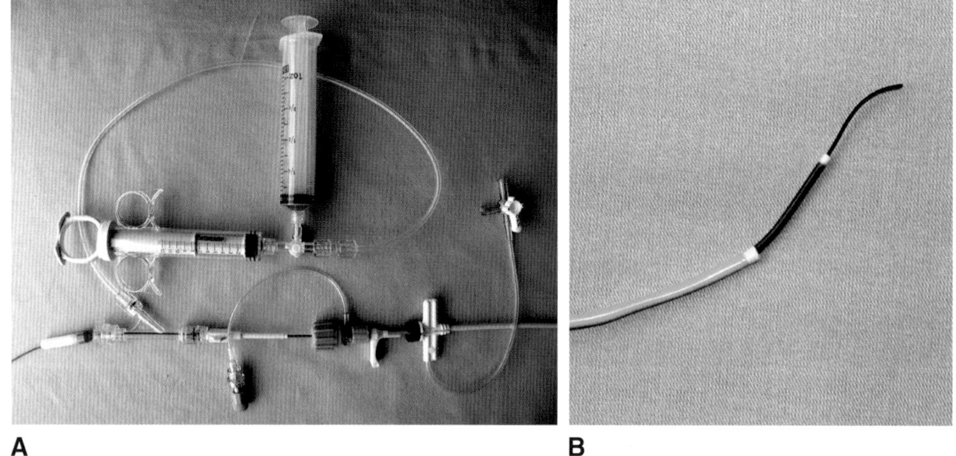

Figure 19-143. *Sequential combination of wire and guide to straighten tortuous vein. The glidewire is advanced into the tortuous vein, followed by the 5F catheter with the 7F guide advanced over it. Ultimately, the third-generation guide long enough to deliver the lead is advanced over the combination. **A,** Hub end of the assembly. **B,** Tips of the guides and guidewire of the assembly.*

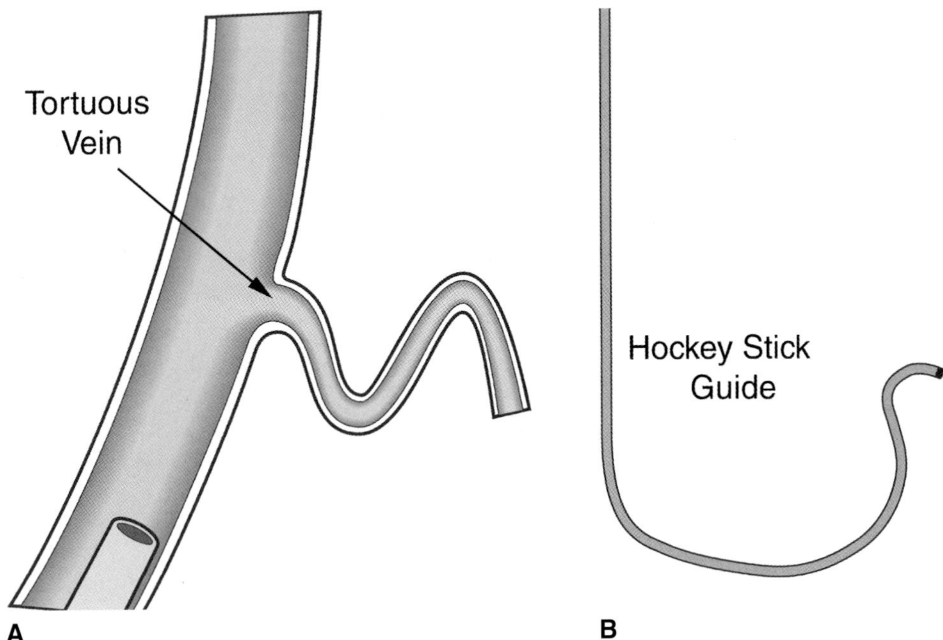

Figure 19-144. *The hockey stick–shaped guide of a third-generation system for a tortuous lateral wall target vein.* ***A,*** *The tortuous lateral wall target vein is depicted with the sheath at midcoronary sinus (CS) level. It will be difficult to advance the lead into the target vein and through the tortuous segment without buckling of the lead or displacement of the sheath out of the CS as attempts are made to advance the lead from this level.* ***B,*** *The hockey stick–shaped directional guide. When inserted into the sheath, the tip of such a guide extends laterally and advances through the tortuous segment. The guide then provides support and a smooth low-friction conduit for the lead from the sheath to beyond the tortuous vein segment.*

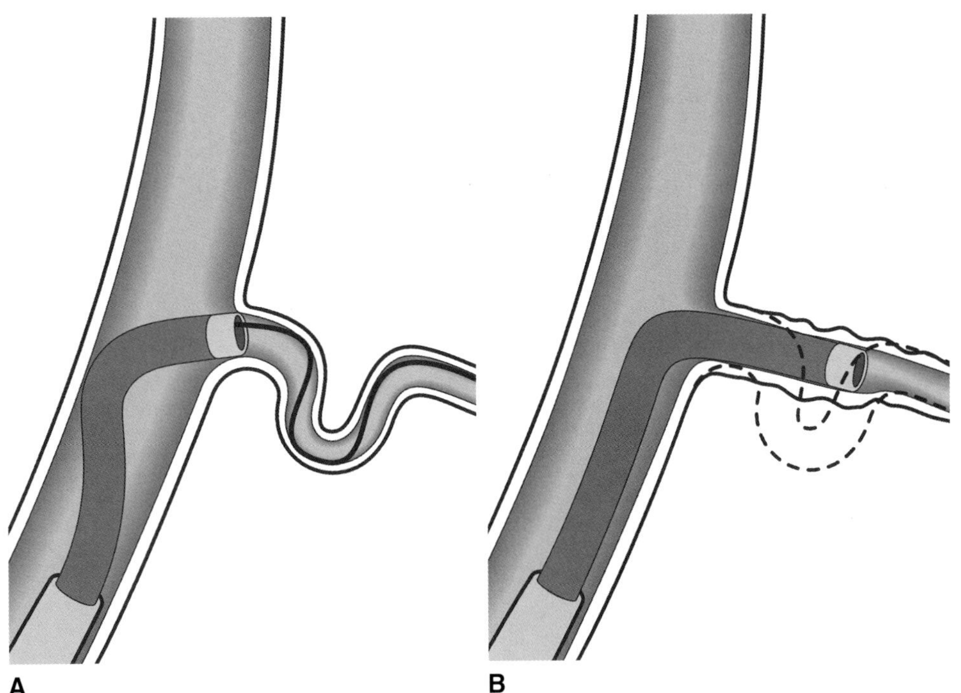

Figure 19-145. *A third-generation telescoping hockey stick guide passing through a tortuous segment.* ***A,*** *The tip of the guide is at the mouth of the target vein. The angle of takeoff of the vein and the angle of the guide match.* ***B,*** *The guide is advanced over the wire through the tortuous vein segment until the tip of the guide is beyond the tortuous segment. The pacing lead now has a smooth low-friction environment to traverse between the skin and the tip of the sheath.*

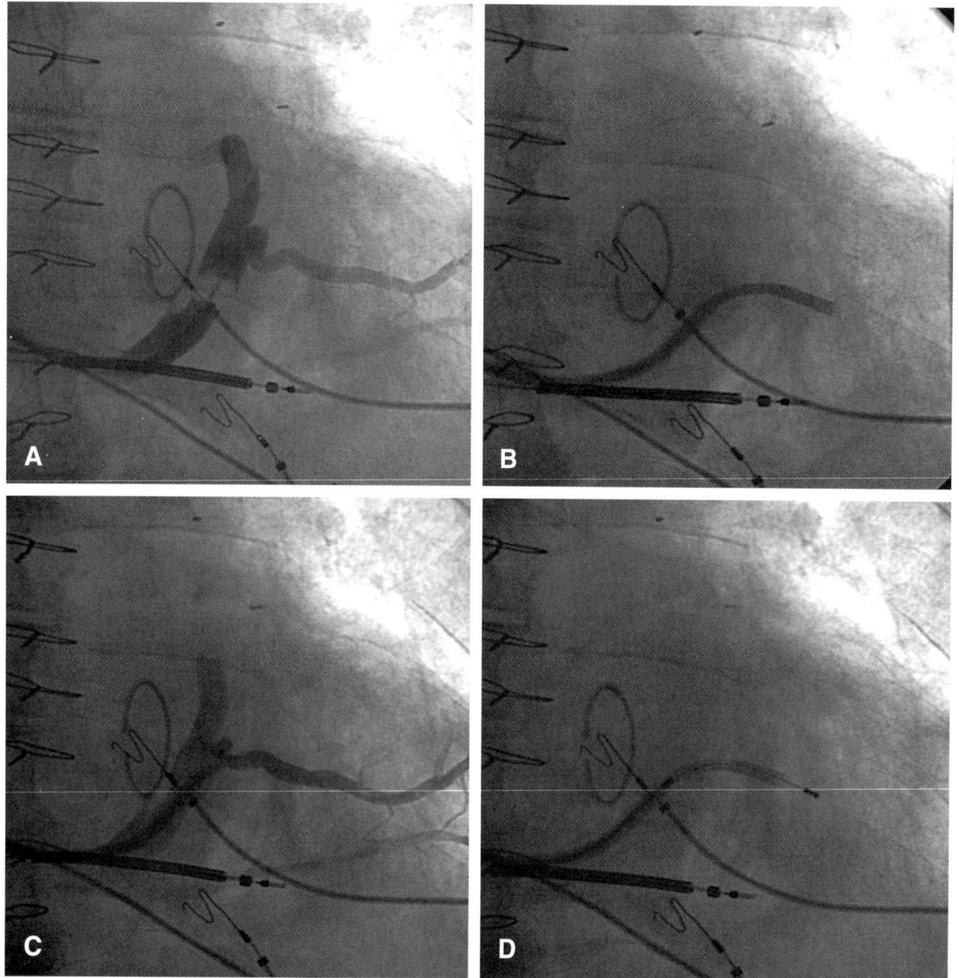

Figure 19-146. Improvised third-generation telescoping hockey stick guide passing through a tortuous vein segment. ***A,*** *The tortuous vein segment in a patient with prior mitral valve surgery.* ***B,*** *The 9F hockey stick guide is inserted through the 9F sheath with proximal curve into the tortuous vein.* ***C,*** *Contrast material is injected to confirm that the guide is coaxial and the tip is beyond the tortuous segment of the vein.* ***D,*** *The Attain 2187 left ventricular pacing lead (Medtronic, Inc., Minneapolis, Minn.) is advanced through the guide into the target vein. Before the 2187 lead was inserted into the guide, the hub was cut off after satisfactory pacing thresholds are confirmed.*

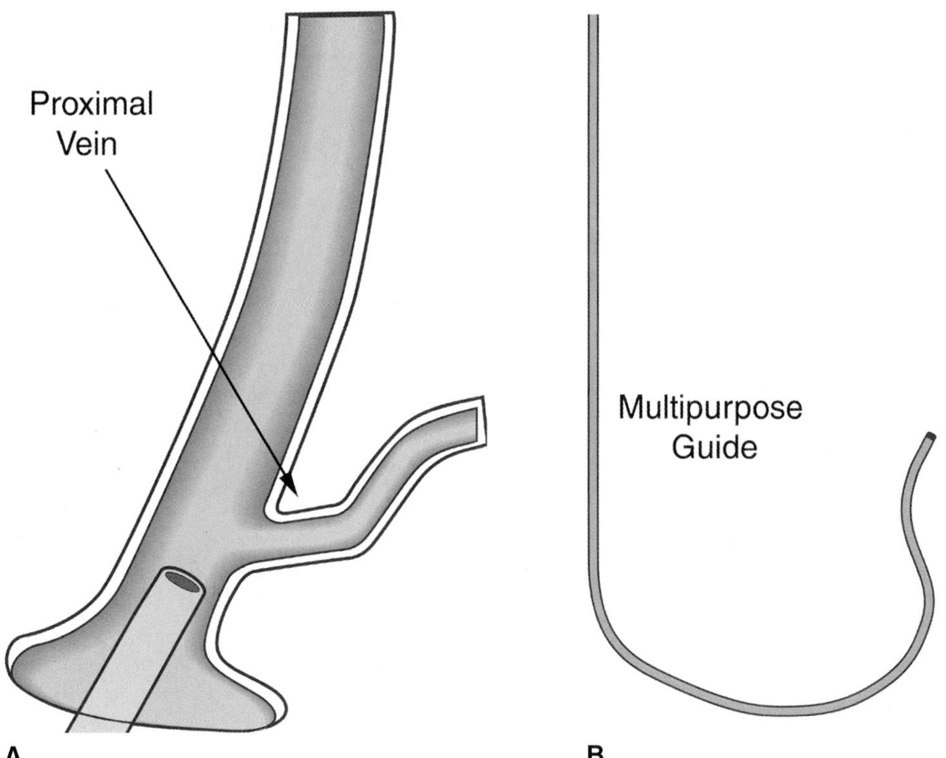

Figure 19-147. Proximal vein and third-generation multipurpose telescoping system, with a multipurpose shape guide for the proximal takeoff of the target vein. ***A,*** *The target vein has a proximal takeoff. It can be difficult to advance a lead into the vein without having it fall out of the coronary sinus.* ***B,*** *The multipurpose shape guide points laterally.*

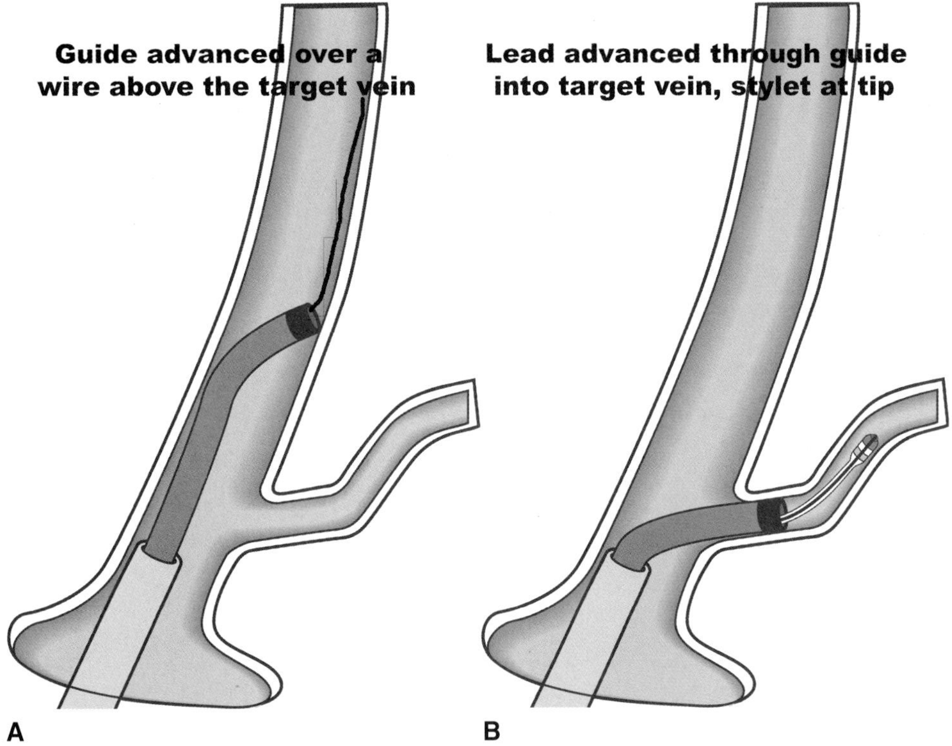

Figure 19-148. Cannulating a vein with a proximal takeoff using a third-generation multipurpose telescoping system. ***A,*** *The multipurpose guide is advanced above the target vein over a wire. The angioplasty wire is withdrawn into the guide. The guide is withdrawn toward the coronary sinus os until the multipurpose guide enters the side branch.* ***B,*** *The lead is advanced to the final position in the side branch through the multipurpose guide.*

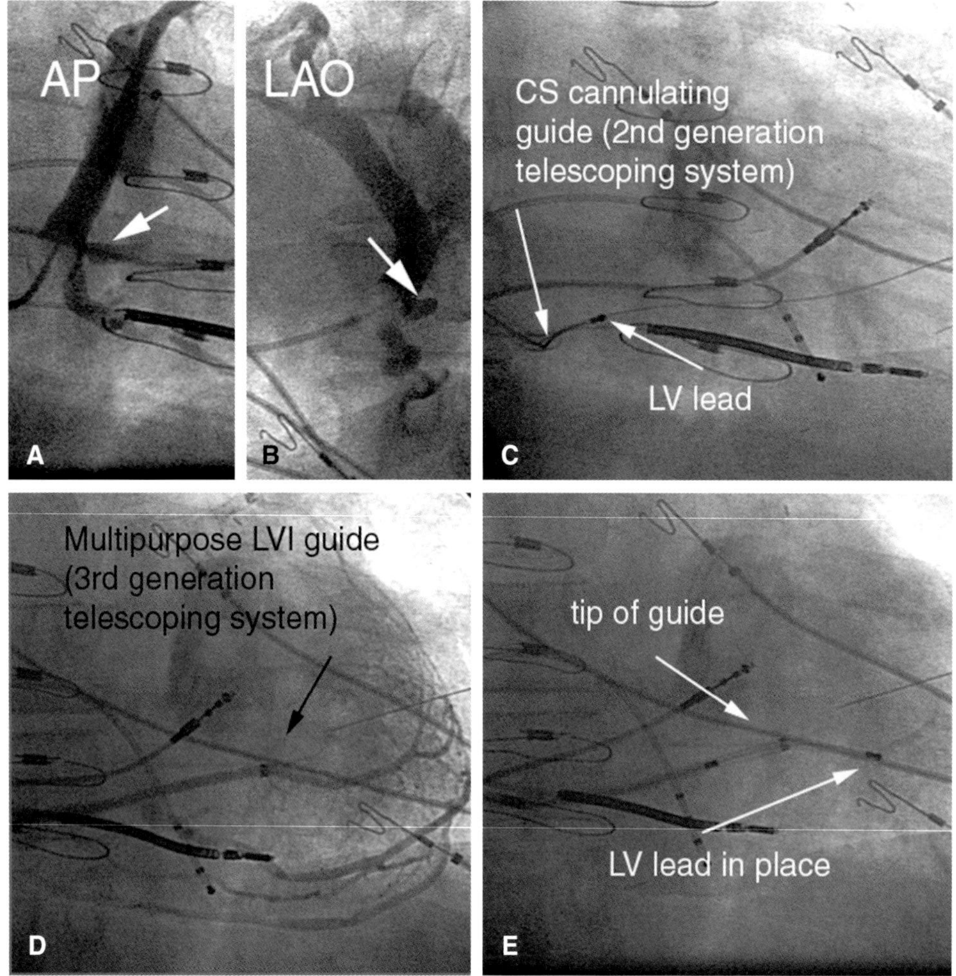

Figure 19-149. *Second-generation telescoping guide fails, but third-generation multipurpose lateral vein introducer (LVI) succeeds. Anteroposterior (**A**) and left anterior oblique (**B**) views of the target* (arrows)*.* ***C,*** *The angioplasty wire is in the target vein with the coronary sinus (CS) cannulation guide (second-generation telescoping system) advanced as far as possible (just inside the os of the target vein). The left ventricular (LV) lead will not advance further.* ***D,*** *The second-generation system is replaced with a third-generation telescoping system (CS cannulation guide exchanged for 9F ID/11F OD peel-away sheath). A multipurpose LVI guide is advanced through the peel-away sheath over the angioplasty wire into the target vein. A selective target vein venogram is made with the wire removed.* ***E,*** *A stylet-driven Attain 2187 pacing lead (Medtronic, Inc., Minneapolis, Minn.) is advanced into the target vein.*

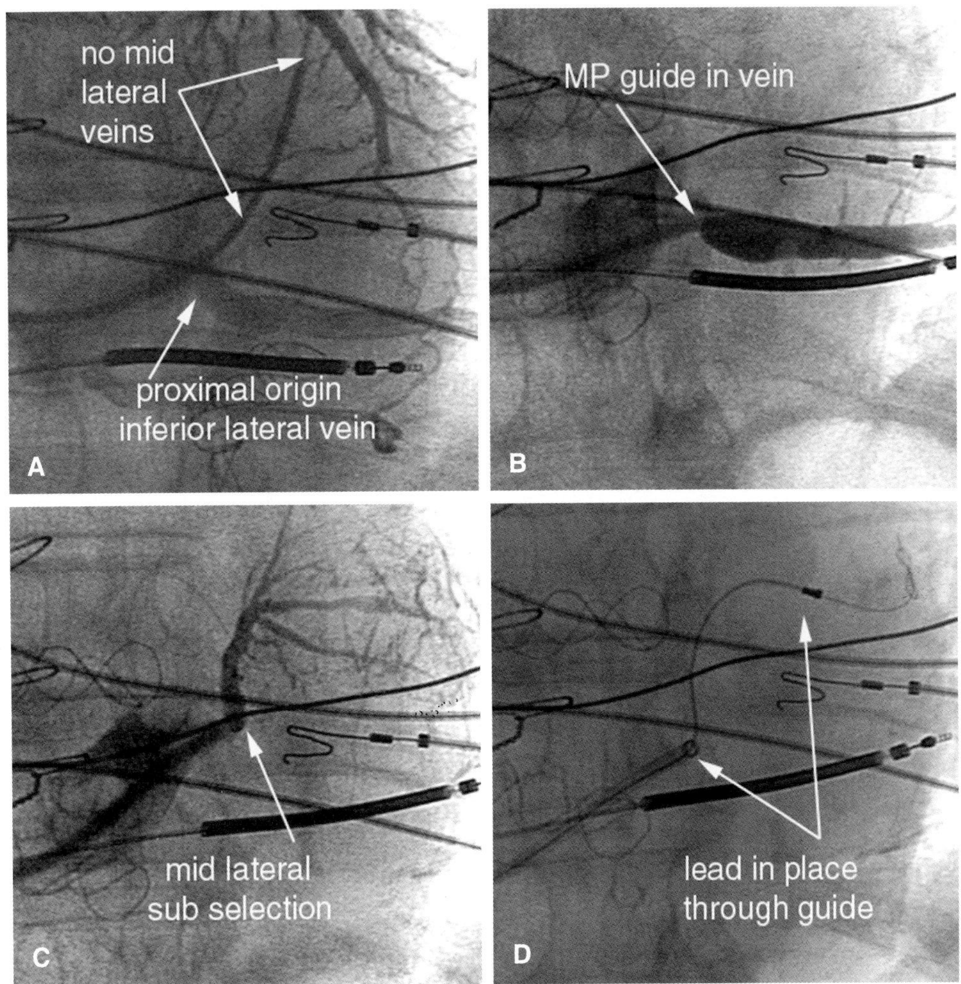

Figure 19-150. Multipurpose lateral vein introducer (LVI) (9F preshaped guide) for midlateral wall left ventricular (LV) lead placement in a vein with a proximal origin. ***A,*** *No identifiable midlateral wall veins can be seen. A large inferior lateral vein with origin near the coronary sinus (CS) os is visible.* ***B,*** *The multipurpose guide is advanced into the vein by means of selective venography.* ***C,*** *A branch of the inferior vein to the mid–lateral wall vein is subselected. Venography demonstrates lateral wall distribution.* ***D,*** *The left ventricular lead is advanced into the lateral wall branch using support from the guide.*

peel-away sheath and a preshaped guide suitable to the target vein was inserted into the target vein (third-generation telescoping system), the guide advanced further into the vein. With the guide deep in the vein, any 7F or smaller lead can be delivered.

The multipurpose LVI also works to provide support for a partially obstructed target vein (Figs. 19-151 and 19-152), and for lead placement in small lateral veins (Fig. 19-153).

As with the renal and hockey stick LVIs, the multipurpose shape guide may be initially selected but may turn out to be the incorrect shape for the vein. If the wrong shape guide is selected for the target vein, lead delivery may not be successful until the guide is replaced with the correct shape guide (Fig. 19-154).

When the target vein has a posterior origin, neither the renal, the multipurpose, nor the hockey stick LVI may fit the anatomy. For this situation the hook LVI is available (Figs. 19-155 and 19-156).

As physicians become more facile with the larger lead-delivering guides, they may skip using the 5F and 6F guides through the lead delivery guide. Sometimes, it is difficult to cannulate the target vein with the guide or even to advance a wire into the vein with the lead delivery guide. In these cases it is important to remember to use the small directional catheters through the larger lead delivery catheter. As mentioned earlier, it may be essential to insert a small catheter through the lead delivery guide (LVI) to cannulate the vein and assist placement of the lead delivery guide. Figure 19-157 demonstrates the use of a Rapido catheter to assist placement of a renal LVI telescoping guide. Figure 19-158 is a case example of the use of the Rapido inside the renal LVI to facilitate the placement of the guide into the os of the vein.

The shapes of small assist catheters available from both Guidant and Medtronic are limited. In some cases a different shape may be needed. In the case illustrated

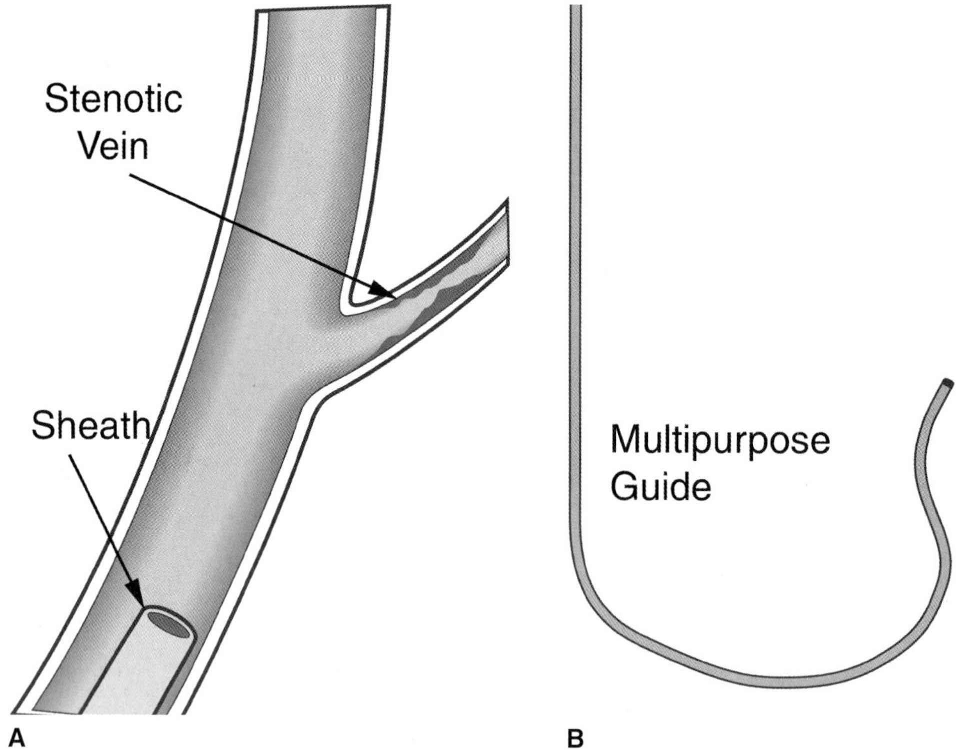

Figure 19-151. Multipurpose lateral vein introducer (9F preshaped guide) for partially obstructed vein. ***A,*** *The sheath is shown resting in the midcoronary sinus. The angle of the lateral wall target vein is not acute, but there is an obstruction in the vein that will inhibit lead placement. The wire/lead may buckle between the sheath and the obstruction.* ***B,*** *The multipurpose shape guide is shown. When this guide is inserted into the sheath, the tip of the guide will rest in the mouth of the target vein. Because the pacing lead is supported by both the sheath and the guide up to the point of obstruction, it will be less likely to buckle. The third-generation multipurpose guide can also be used to selectively cannulate lateral wall target veins with origins near the os of the coronary sinus, as shown in Figures 19-147 and 19-148.*

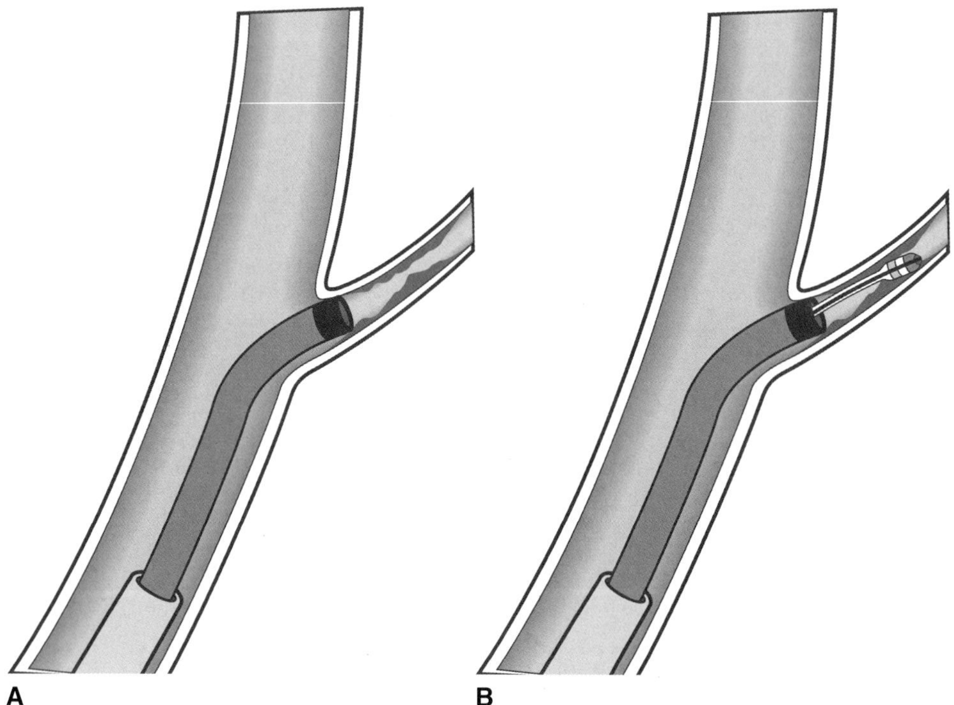

Figure 19-152. Multipurpose lateral vein introducer in a stenotic vein to deliver the left ventricular pacing lead. ***A,*** *The guide is advanced into the stenotic vein from the sheath in the coronary sinus (CS).* ***B,*** *The pacing lead is advanced directly into the vein from the guide in the vein.*

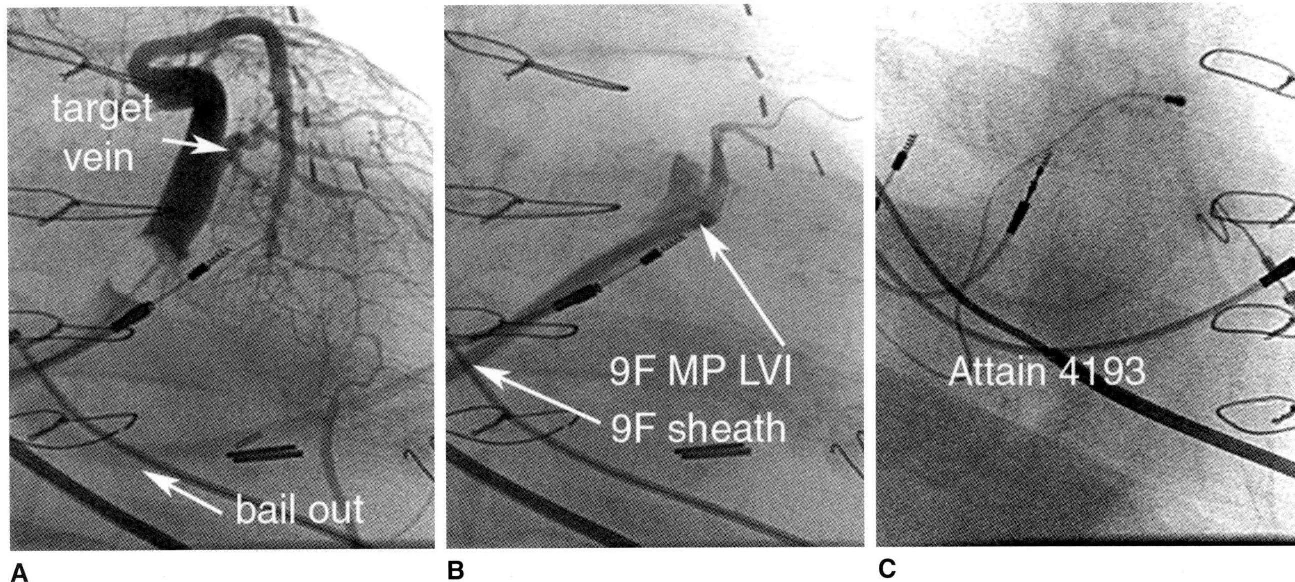

Figure 19-153. Multipurpose lateral vein introducer (LVI) (9F preshaped guide) for lead placement in a small vein. ***A,*** *The midlateral wall target vein is small. A less desirable vein on the low lateral wall is also seen ("bailout" vein).* ***B,*** *The multipurpose LVI is advanced through the 9F peel-away sheath over a wire into the vein.* ***C,*** *The Attain 4193 pacing lead (Medtronic, Inc., Minneapolis, Minn.) is advanced into the small vein with the guide support provided by the third-generation guide.*

in Figure 19-159, the standard shapes were not successful in cannulating the target vein. Several of the additional shaped catheters shown in Figure 19-138 were tried until the 5F hook successfully engaged the target vein. The wire and hook catheter were held taut to form a rail over which the 9F renal LVI (guide) was advanced into the target vein.

Delivery System Is Key to Placement of Lead on Lateral Wall

Reliably placing the LV lead in the *desired* position on the lateral wall is determined more by the delivery system than the type of angioplasty wire, the LV lead, or even experience of the operator. A system capable of placing larger, less flexible leads is essential when pacing thresholds are high or the lead is unstable or paces the phrenic nerve distally. Delivery systems have changed significantly since the advent of CRT. However, they have not finished evolving. Use of a third-generation telescoping delivery system coupled with new LV pacing leads and venoplasty techniques will generally reduce the LV lead implantation time to 15 minutes in most cases. More importantly, the location of the lead placement can be uncompromising. Even patients with persistent left-sided SVC can be successfully implanted with preformed catheters.[35] Currently, the major device manufacturers provide proprietary LV lead delivery systems. The properties of the delivery system reflect the expertise available within each manufacturing organization. Independent manufacturers have developed delivery systems to address the perceived deficiencies of current equipment. The operator must be aware of all the available delivery systems, because although none is perfect, each possesses qualities the operator may need for a particular case.

Matching the Left Ventricular Lead to the Venous Anatomy

Choice of Leads

Pacing the LV via the coronary venous system is safe, and thresholds remain stable.[9,36] However, before a selection of leads became available, fruitless hours were spent and a variety of approaches were employed in attempts to make a lead of the wrong size and shape work in the target vein.[37] With only one lead available, high pacing thresholds, phrenic pacing, and/or an unstable lead position frequently resulted in the use of a less desirable target vein or even implantation failure. If one matches the LV lead to the target vein without regard to manufacturer, the time required for successful LV lead implantation is dramatically reduced. With today's selection of leads, a patient in whom implantation previously failed or resulted in a compromised lead position can undergo successful lead implantation through selection of the lead appropriate for the vein.[38] Variables that effect how an LV lead behaves in a given vein are as follows:

- Lead size
- Location of the pacing electrode (tip versus ring)
- Presence or absence of tines
- Preformed lead shape (straight or curved)

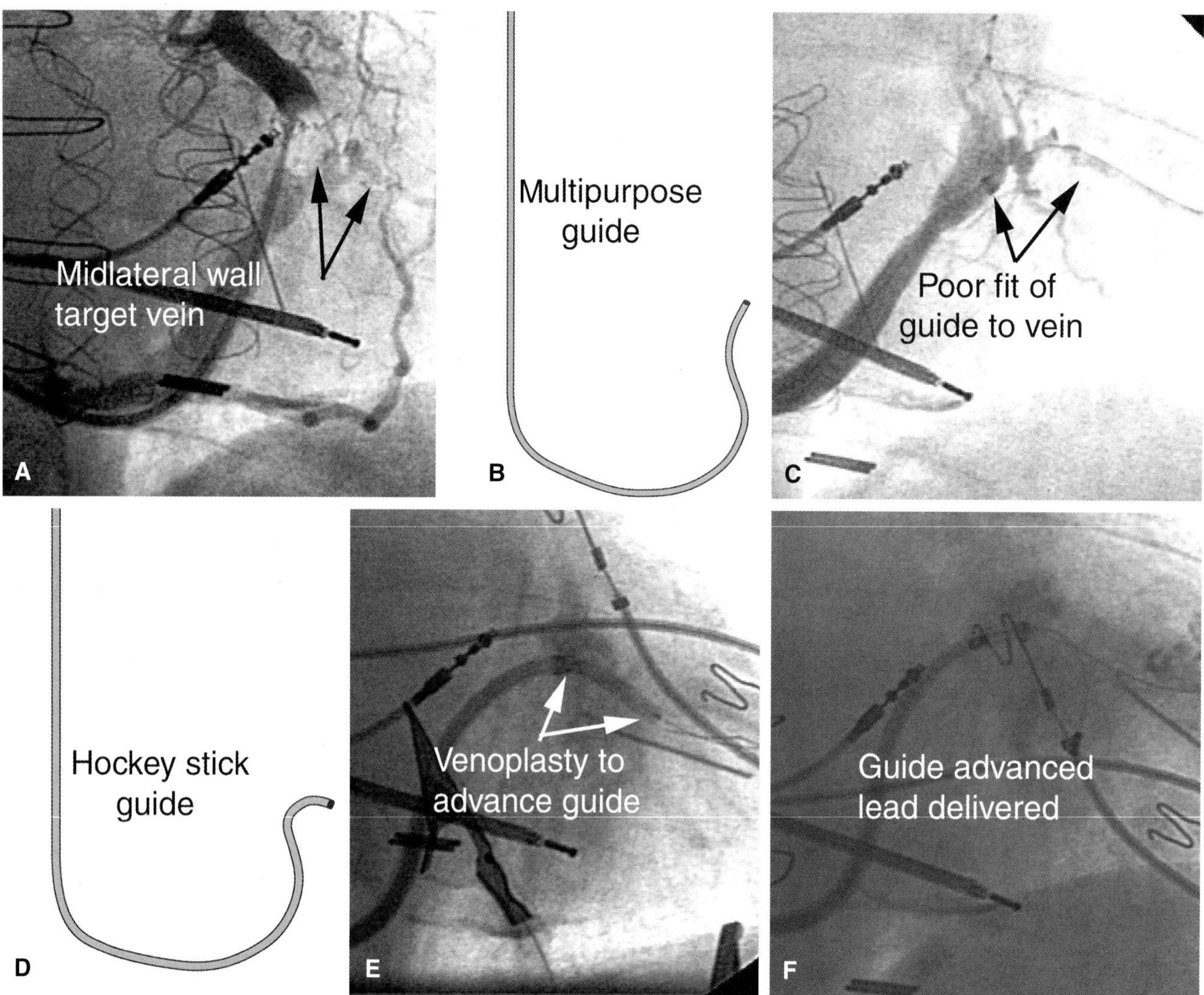

Figure 19-154. Proper match of guide and vein shape is critical to successful lead placement in the target vein. ***A,*** *The midlateral wall vein is identified as the target. The vein is tortuous at the origin and possibly stenotic.* ***B,*** *A third-generation multipurpose telescoping guide is selected for lead delivery.* ***C,*** *The angles of the guide and vein are poorly matched. Despite venoplasty, the left ventricular (LV) lead will not advance. The tip of the guide will not advance into the target vein.* ***D,*** *A third-generation hockey stick guide is selected as a better match to the vein.* ***E,*** *The hockey stick guide is advanced to the os of the target vein. A 30-mm balloon is inflated just distal to the tip of the guide. The guide is advanced into the vein as the balloon is deflated. Contrast stains from the failed attempt with the multipurpose guide are evident above the hockey stick guide.* ***F,*** *The hockey stick guide is advanced into the vein, and the LV pacing lead is delivered.*

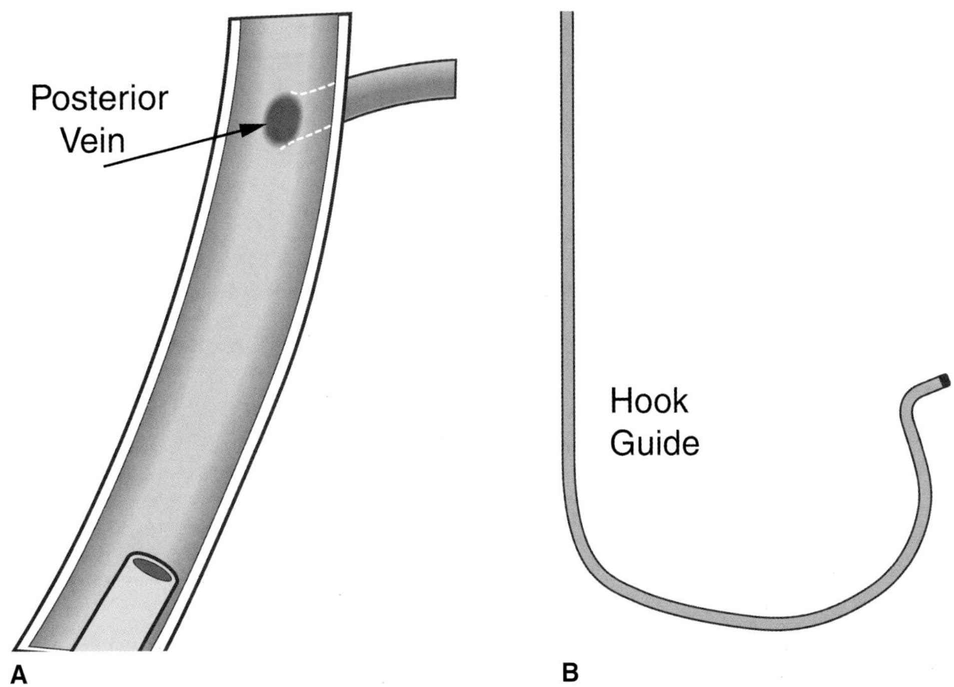

*Figure 19-155. Hook-shape guide of a third-generation telescoping system for veins with posterior takeoff. **A,** The posterior target vein is depicted with the sheath at midcoronary sinus level. It would be difficult to advance the angioplasty wire/lead into the target vein. **B,** A hook-shape directional guide, which is braided, will direct wire/lead into the vein. Once in place, the guide provides direction, support, and a low-friction conduit for the angioplasty wire/lead from the sheath into the vein.*

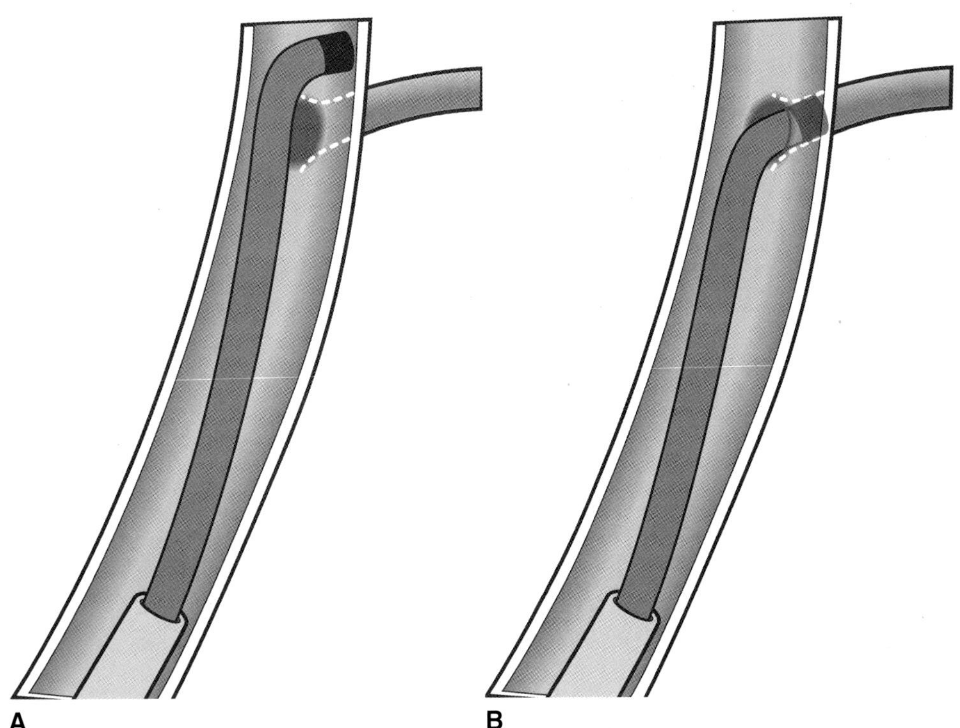

*Figure 19-156. Cannulation of posterior vein with a third-generation hook-shape braided guide. **A,** The guide is advanced over the wire to a position above the vein. The wire is withdrawn into the guide. After a puff of contrast material identifies the origin of the vein, the guide is manipulated toward the os of the vein. **B,** The wire is advanced into the vein. The guide is then advanced over the wire into the vein. The pacing lead is then advanced through the guide into the vein.*

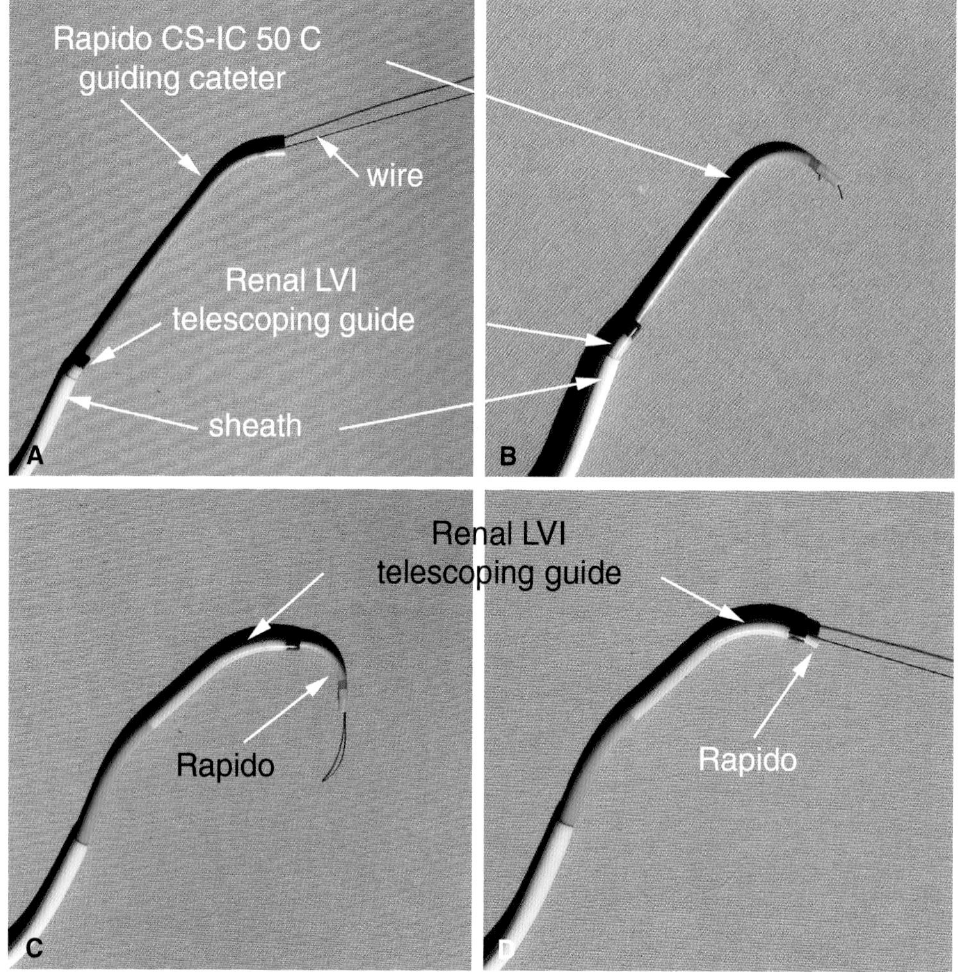

Figure 19-157. *Technique for using the Rapido CS-IC 50 catheter (Guidant, Boston Scientific, Natick, Mass.) to assist placement of a renal lateral vein introducer (renal LVI) telescoping guide in vitro.* ***A,*** *The renal LVI remains just outside the peel-away sheath. The CS-IC 50 catheter is inserted through the renal LVI over an angioplasty wire above the target vein.* ***B,*** *The wire is withdrawn into the Rapido catheter. The renal LVI remains just outside the sheath. Puffs of contrast material are used to identify the target vein as the catheter is withdrawn toward the level of the target vein.* ***C,*** *The Rapido catheter and wire are in the target vein. The renal LVI is advanced out of the sheath over the wire and catheter toward the target vein. The catheter and wire are held taut to form a rail over which the renal LVI is advanced.* ***D,*** *The wire is advanced into the target vein. The Rapido catheter is withdrawn over the wire, leaving the renal LVI in the target vein. The lead is then advanced over the wire through the renal LVI into the target vein.*

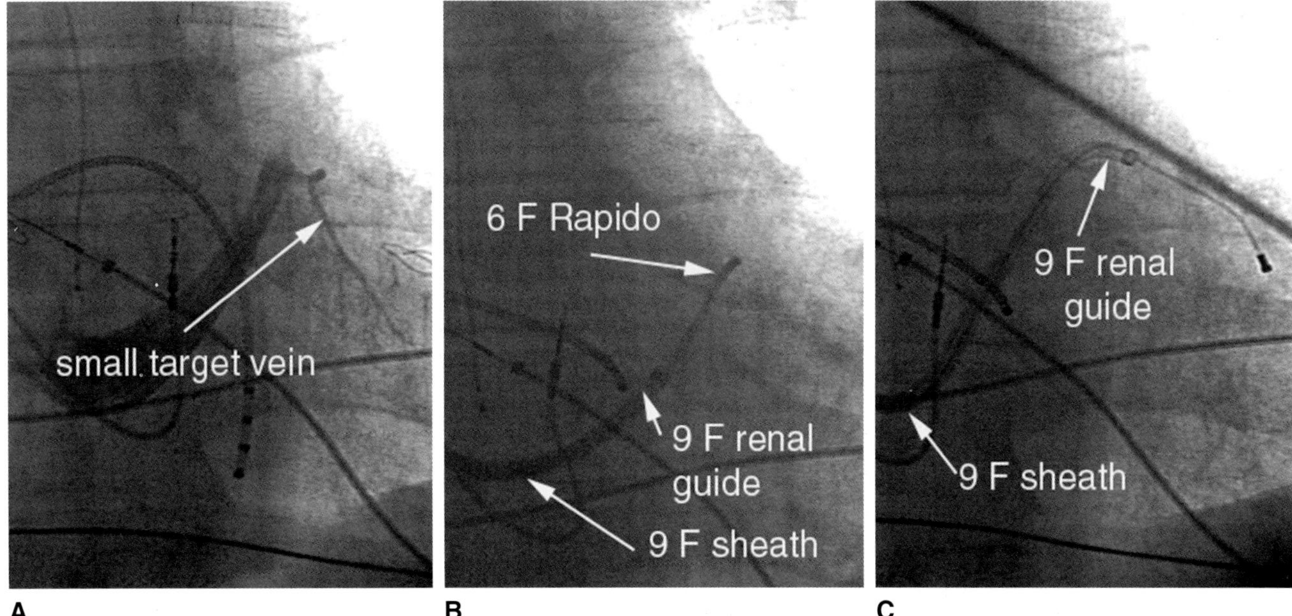

*Figure 19-158. Placement of a renal lateral vein introducer (renal LVI telescoping guide) into a small target vein with the assistance of a Rapido IC90 (Guidant, Boston Scientific, Natick, Mass.). **A,** The ideal target vein is identified. It is small with a tortuous takeoff. **B,** The Rapido is inserted through the renal LVI into the target vein with position confirmed via contrast material. The LVI remains in the sheath. **C,** The renal LVI is advanced over the Rapido into the target vein. The Rapido is removed over the wire. The pacing lead is advanced over the wire through the guide into the target vein. The wire is removed, and the curved soft stylet is advanced to the tip of the lead.*

- Over-the-wire or stylet-driven design
- Bipolar or unipolar design
- Steroid-eluting or bare metal construction

Lead Size

For this discussion on lead size, the reader must remember that a guide is designed to be placed in the human body through a sheath; thus, a 7F guide fits through a 7F sheath. The French size refers to the OD. By comparison, *sheath sizes* refer to the ID. Matching the size of the lead to the target vein is the most important first step. It is obvious that if the LV lead is too large for the target vein, it will not advance into the vein. However, a too small lead in a large target vein will be unstable and have high thresholds. The Medtronic 2188 Bipolar Coronary Sinus Lead is the largest lead; it will pass through a 9F ID sheath (which has the same ID as an 11F guide). The Medtronic Attain OTW 4193 LV Pacing Lead is the smallest lead; it will pass through a 5F sheath (or a 7F guide).

Electrode Location

An LV lead with the pacing electrode at the tip will behave differently from a lead with a ring set back from the tip. The Guidant EASYTRAK LV pacing leads are the only ones with the distal electrode composed of a ring set back from the tip. In order for the electrode on the EASYTRAK lead to make contact with the myocardium, the lead must be wedged into the target vein. By comparison, when the pacing electrode is at the tip, and depending on the shape, the electrode may contact the myocardium without being wedged.

Presence or Absence of Tines

Tines are added to the tip of the pacing lead to help ensure stability. In the RA and RV, the tines catch in the trabeculae. The mechanism by which tines promote stability in a venous branch of the CS is less clear. The tines are intended to wedge in the vein as it is advanced distally. The Guidant EASYTRAK 1 and 2 LV pacing leads are the only leads specifically designed for LV pacing that have tines. When the Medtronic CapSure SP 4023 lead is adapted for LV pacing, two of the four tines are usually removed.

Preformed Lead Shape

The Medtronic Attain LV 2187 and 2188 and Attain OTW 4193 and 4194 LV pacing leads, the Guidant EASYTRAK 3, the St. Jude Medical QuickSite OTW, and the Aescula stylet-driven LV leads (St. Jude Medical) are designed with unique preformed distal shapes intended to promote stability and orient the tip electrodes toward the myocardium.[38] Although the body of the lead is straight, the tip of the Medtronic 2188 Bipolar Coronary Sinus Lead is canted. When the CapSure SP 4023 lead is adapted for LV pacing, the tip of the lead may be canted by hand to resemble the 2188 lead. Although intended to promote stability, the preformed shapes of the 2187, 4193, and 4194 leads may

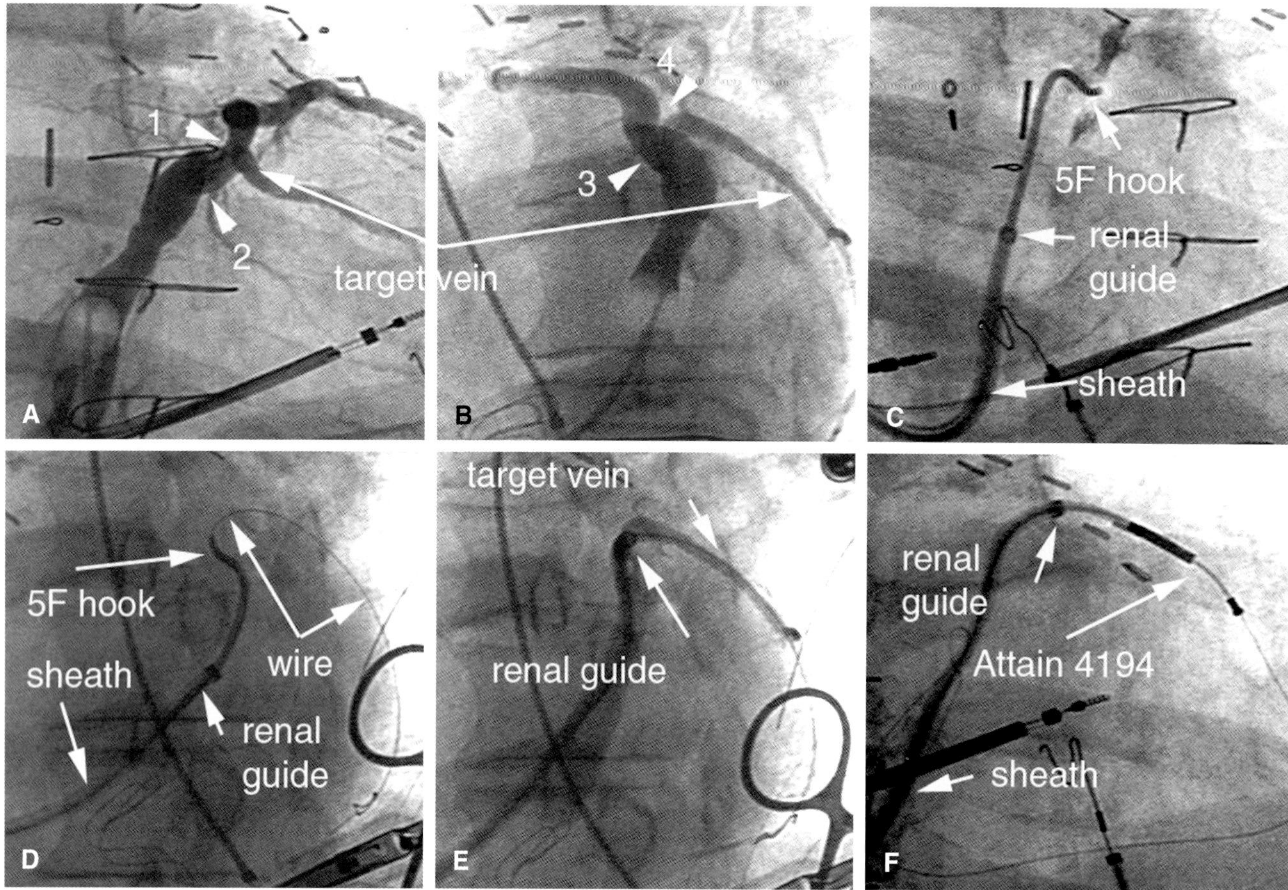

Figure 19-159. *Attain 4194 lead (Medtronic, Inc., Minneapolis, Minn.) placed via a 5F hook catheter and a third-generation renal LVI (lateral vein introducer) (guide).* ***A,*** *The target vein is identified in the right anterior oblique view. At the os of the vein, the coronary sinus (CS) is irregular* (arrow *1), and double density of the contrast material* (arrow *2) indicates that the veins are superimposed.* ***B,*** *The target vein is identified in the left anterior oblique (LAO) view. The double density of contrast material* (arrow *3) indicates overlapping, superimposed veins. Despite several angulated views, a clear origin of the vein from the CS is not identified* (arrow *4).* ***C,*** *When a wire will not find the vein, a 5F hook catheter (see Fig. 19-127) is advanced through the renal guide. The target vein is selectively engaged with the hook catheter by means of manipulation and injection of contrast material.* ***D,*** *With use of the LAO view, the wire is advanced into the target vein. The 5F hook is advanced into the vein, providing additional support for the 9F renal guide. The 9F guide is advanced over the 5F hook into the vein. The sheath remains in the CS for support.* ***E,*** *The renal guide is in the vein. Contrast material is injected to demonstrate the target vein.* ***F,*** *The Attain 4194 lead is advanced into the vein through the guide over the wire. The tip of the 9F sheath is in the CS, providing support.*

actually induce lead dislodgment or less desirable pacing thresholds in some cases. Once the stylet or wire is removed, the lead attempts to return to its original (preformed) shape within the confines of the coronary vein. The tip may migrate forward or back (usually back) a few millimeters to a stable position within the particular vein. On occasion, the physical characteristics of the CS vein and the preformed lead shape result in "walking back" of the lead to a very proximal location or out of the vein entirely.

Over-the-Wire or Stylet-Driven Design

LV leads come in two basic types according to the method of delivery, traditional stylet-driven and newer over-the-wire. The Guidant EASYTRAK family of leads, the Medtronic Attain OTW 4193 and 4194, the St. Jude Medical QuickSite, and the ELA Situs OTW Coronary Sinus Lead are over-the-wire LV pacing leads. The 4193 and 4194 leads may also be used with the included stylet.

Stylet-driven leads without the over-the-wire options are:

- Medtronic's 2187, 2188, and 4193 leads
- ELA Medical's stylet-driven pacing leads
- Biotronik's Corox + LVH-UP CS Lead (75 and 85 cm, unipolar, stylet-driven helical fixation); Corox LA-H CS Lead (bipolar, stylet driven); Corox LV-H CS Lead, Corox LV-S CS Lead, and Corox OTW-UP Steroid (unipolar, over-the-wire, 75- and 85-cm lengths)

The option to use a lead either over the wire or via a stylet offers greater procedural flexibility.[39] Stylet-driven leads, as a rule, are more difficult to advance to the lateral wall than over-the-wire leads, particularly without a third-generation telescoping delivery system. However, when the tip of a directional guide is placed in the target vein, stylet-driven leads are easily placed and may work in a target vein in which an over-the-wire lead failed. One inserts over-the-wire leads by first advancing a conventional angioplasty wire into the target vein, then advancing the pacing lead over the wire. The characteristics of the angioplasty wire (floppy, standard, or extra support) influence not only the ability of the wire to advance into the target vein but also the ability of the pacing lead to be advanced over the wire. Stiff angioplasty wires (e.g., Platinum Plus or Choice PT Extra Support [Boston Scientific Corporation, Natick Mass.]) are more difficult to advance into the target vein but tend to provide more support for the lead once in place. Conversely, softer wires may pass easily into the target vein but may not provide enough support for the lead. Generally, a middle-weight angioplasty wire (Luge [Pressure Products] or the equivalent) is the best choice. More details on the selection of angioplasty wires are given in the venoplasty discussion. Lead characteristics can dramatically alter the wedged distal position (Fig. 19-160).

Type, Size, and Personality of Left Ventricular Pacing Lead

Each lead has a size, shape, and electrode configuration that produces a "personality" that will have advantages and disadvantages when the lead is used in different veins of differing anatomies (Table 19-6).

Medtronic Attain LV 2187 Pacing Lead

The Attain LV 2187, a transvenous, unipolar LV cardiac vein pacing lead, is a stylet-driven lead with the electrode at the tip. The electrode is not steroid eluting. The lead can be difficult to deliver without a telescoping system. However, once in place in a large target vein, the Attain 2187 provides the best position on the lateral LV free wall with the lowest pacing thresholds. Once in place with the stylet and guide/sheath removed, the Attain 2187 lead will not advance further into a target vein even if additional slack is deployed. When a lot of slack is added, the 2187 has enough body to displace itself from the target vein.

The Attain 2187 will pass through any 7F sheath. When a second- or third-generation telescoping system is used, the Attain 2187 fits in any guide with an ID greater than 0.088 inch (2.2 mm). For improvising a third-generation telescoping delivery system, it is worth knowing that some 8F guides and all 9F or greater guides have an ID of 0.088 inch or greater. The Cordis Vistabritetip is an 8F interventional guide with an ID of 0.088 inch, whereas the Boston Scientific/Medi-Tech Guider Softip (Boston Scientific) must be 9F to have sufficient ID for direct lead delivery. The Attain 2187 lead passes through the Pressure Products series of LVIs (Figs. 19-161 and 19-162).

Medtronic Attain OTW 4193 LV Pacing Lead

The Attain OTW 4193 LV pacing lead is a steroid-eluting, transvenous, unipolar, LV, over-the-wire, cardiac vein pacing lead with the electrode at the tip (Fig. 19-163A). It assumes a preformed box shape when the stylet or wire is removed. The box shape is designed to direct the tip toward the myocardium and stabilize the lead in the target vein. It is delivered over a 0.014-inch or 0.018-inch angioplasty wire or with a stylet. Because the Attain 4193 is smaller and can be delivered over an angioplasty wire, it is easier to place than the Attain 2187. Like the 2187, it does not tend to migrate more distally in the target vein. However, it will migrate proximally if the target vein is large or the proximal bend is not within the target vein. As a result, the

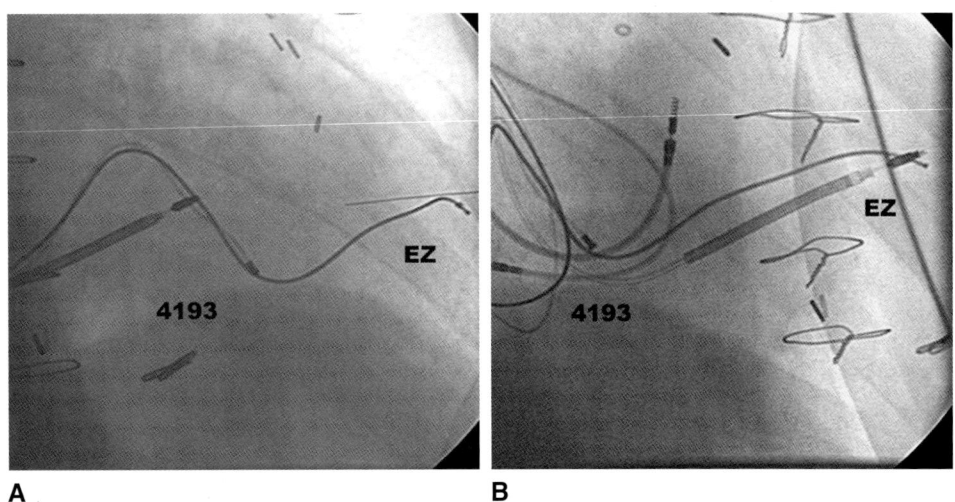

*Figure 19-160. EASYTRAK 1 (Guidant, Boston Scientific, Natick, Mass.) lead (EZ) advances several centimeters further into the vein than the Attain model 4193 (4193) lead (Medtronic, Minneapolis, Minn.) producing a more posterior position and improved capture thresholds. **A,** Left anterior oblique projection. **B,** Right anterior oblique projection.*

TABLE 19-6. **Available LV Pacing Leads for Cardiac Resynchronization Therapy***

	Biotronik	ELA	Guidant	Medtronic	St. Jude
Lead option #1:					
Name	Corox + LVH-UP CS	Situs OTW	EASYTRAK 1	Attain LV 2187	QuickSite Unipolar
Method of fixation	Helical shape	Silicone screw	Tines	Single curve	Undulations
No. of poles	Unipolar	Unipolar	Unipolar	Unipolar	Unipolar
Stylet or OTW or both	Stylet	OTW	OTW	Stylet	Both
Steroid tip	No	No	Yes	No	Yes
Lead option #2:					
Name	Corox + LVH-H CS	Situs LV UL28D	EASYTRAK 2	Attain 4193	QuickSite Bipolar
Method of fixation	Helical shape	Dual curve	Tines	Double curve	Undulations
No. of poles	Unipolar	Bipolar	Bipolar	Unipolar	Bipolar
Stylet or OTW or both	Stylet	Stylet	OTW	Both	Both
Steroid tip	No	No	Yes	Yes	Yes
Lead option #3:					
Name	Corox LV-S CS Lead	Situs LV UL28C	EASYTRAK 3	Attain 4194	
Method of fixation	None	Dual curve	Helical shape	Double curve	
No. of poles	Unipolar	Bipolar	Bipolar	Bipolar	
Stylet or OTW or both	Stylet	Stylet	OTW	Both	
Steroid tip	None	No	Yes	Yes	
Lead option #4:					
Name	Corox OTW-UP			Attain CS 2188	
Method of fixation	Double curve			Canted tip	
No. of poles	Unipolar			Bipolar	
Stylet or OTW	OTW			Stylet	
Steroid tip	Yes			No	
Lead option #5:					
Name	Corox LA-H CS			CapSure SP 4023	
Method of fixation	Single curve			Tines	
No. of poles	Bipolar			Unipolar	
Stylet or OTW	Stylet			Stylet	
Steroid tip	No			Yes	

CS, coronary sinus; LV, left ventricular; OTW, over-the-wire.
*Biotronik GmBh & Co., Berlin; ELA Medical, Sorin Group, Milan; Guidant, Boston Scientific, Natick, Mass.; Medtronic, Inc., Minneapolis, Minn.; St. Jude Medical, St. Paul, Minn.

operator tendency at the time of implantation is to advance the 4193 more distally than is desirable for optimal resynchronization. Distal locations are also more prone to phrenic stimulation. In situations in which the 4193 lead has high pacing thresholds (large target vein) or diaphragmatic/phrenic stimulation, replacing it with the Attain 4194 or 2187 frequently solves the problem.

The Attain OTW 4193 lead can be delivered through a directional guide with an ID of 0.076 inch (1.93 mm) or greater. The ID of most 7F guides is more than 0.076 inch. The 4193 will pass through any 5F introducer/sheath. The size of the 4193 makes it suitable for placement in small lateral wall veins directly, either antegrade after balloon dilation or retrograde after dilation of the collateral vessels (Figs. 19-164 through 19-166).

Medtronic Attain OTW 4194 LV Pacing Lead

The Attain OTW 4194 LV pacing lead is a steroid-eluting, transvenous, bipolar, LV over-the-wire (or stylet-driven) cardiac vein pacing lead with the distal electrode at the tip (Fig. 19-167A). The tip-to-anode spacing is 11 mm. The 5.4-mm-diameter tip electrode is platinum alloy that contains 1.0 mg of dexamethasone. The anode is a platinum/iridium coil 5.4 mm in diameter with a surface area of 38 mm^2. The lead body is 2 mm with outer polyurethane insulation and inner silicone insulation. The lead's preformed shape is straightened with either the 0.018-inch stylet or an angioplasty wire (0.014 or 0.018 inch). The preformed box shape is designed to direct the tip toward the myocardium and stabilize the lead in the target vein. It is delivered over a 0.014-inch or 0.018-inch angioplasty wire or with a stylet.

The pacing threshold of the 4194 is usually lower than that of an Attain 4193 in the same vein. Because the Attain 4194 is deliverable over an angioplasty wire, it is easier to place than the Attain 2187. Like the 2187, the 4193 does not tend to migrate more distally in the target vein *after* initial stabilization. However, it will migrate proximally if the target vein is large or the proximal bend is not within the target vein. As a result, the operator tendency at the time of implantation is to advance the 4194 more distally than is desirable for optimal resynchronization. Distal locations are also more prone to phrenic stimulation. The recommended

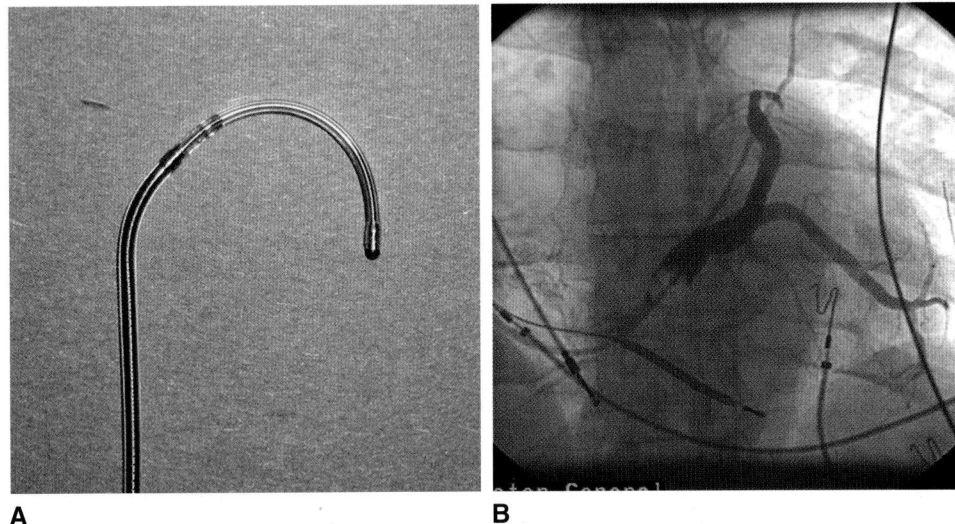

Figure 19-161. *The Attain 2187 left ventricular (LF) pacing lead (Medtronic, Inc., Minneapolis, Minn.) and a suitable target vein in a patient with a midlateral dominant coronary venous pattern.* ***A,*** *The 2187 lead is shown with the stylet removed.* ***B,*** *A target vein suitable for a 2187 lead is demonstrated. If an Attain 4193 (Medtronic), EASYTRAK 1 or 2 (Guidant, Boston Scientific, Natick, Mass.), or QuickSite (St. Jude Medical, St. Paul, Minn.) pacing lead is placed in this vein, the pacing thresholds are likely to be high and the leads unstable unless the tip is wedged into a distal branch, a location that is more likely to result in phrenic pacing. Leads placed distally in a target vein are usually anterior, a location at which there may be no response. The EASYTRAK 3 and the Attain 4194 or 2188 are all well suited to this vein as well.*

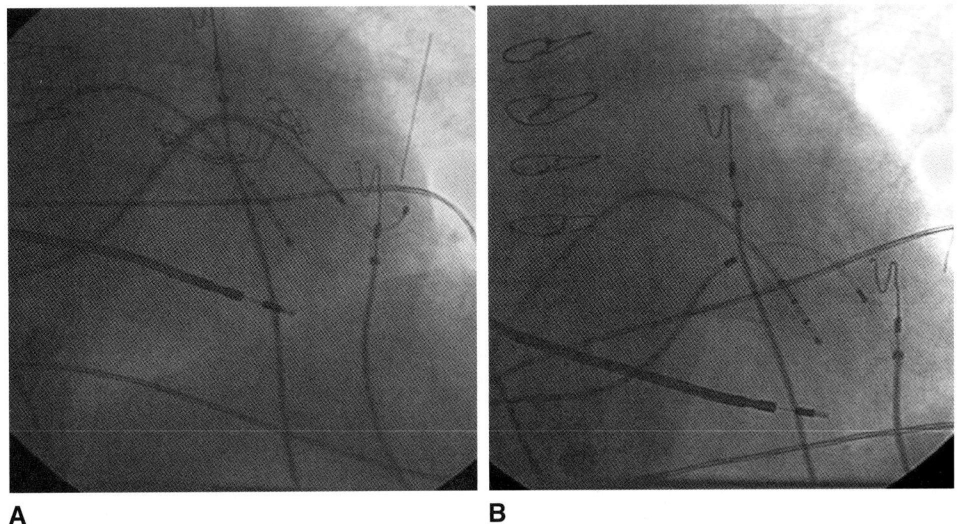

Figure 19-162. *The Attain LV 2187 pacing lead (Medtronic, Inc., Minneapolis, Minn.) spontaneously retracts from its original distal position.* ***A,*** *The lead is located distally in the lateral wall target vein.* ***B,*** *The lead has spontaneously migrated back to a more proximal position despite being tied down. This type of spontaneous retraction occurs within 3 to 5 minutes of lead placement. Spontaneous retraction reoccurs if the lead is replaced in the same position.*

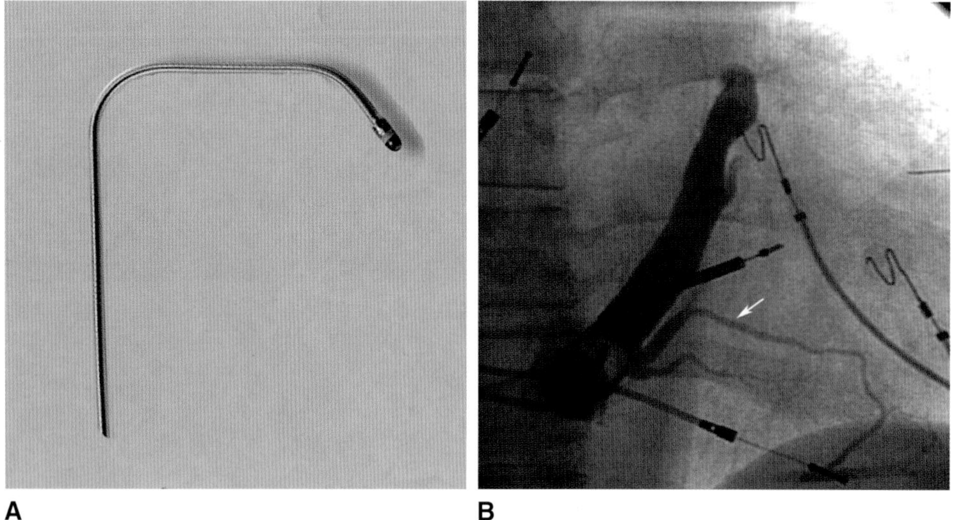

Figure 19-163. ***A,*** *The Attain OTW 4193, a steroid-eluting, transvenous, unipolar, left-ventricular over-the-wire pacing lead (Medtronic, Inc,. Minneapolis, Minn.). The preformed shape of the lead and tip electrode can be seen.* ***B,*** *Target vein* (arrow) *of suitable size for this lead.*

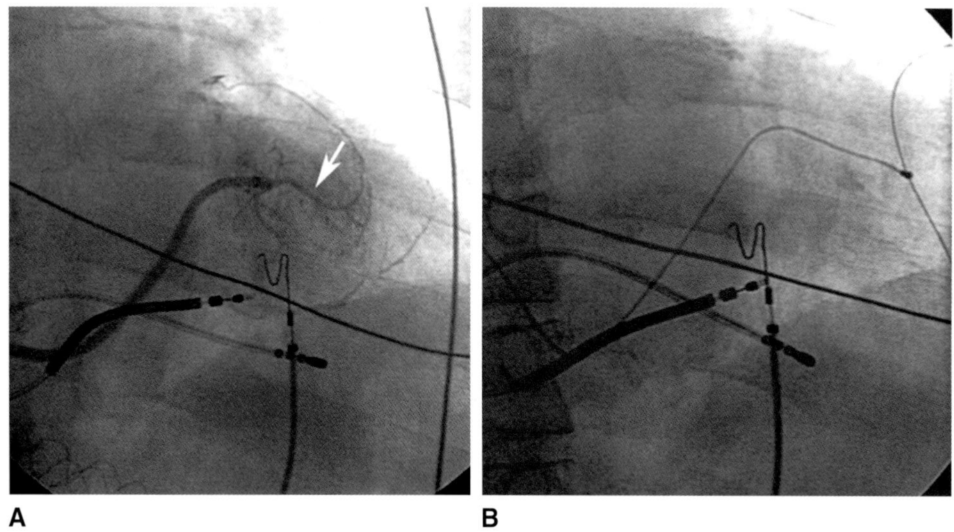

Figure 19-164. The Attain OTW 4193 pacing lead (Medtronic, Inc., Minneapolis, Minn.) is placed in a small vein using a third-generation telescoping system (Renal Shape Worley Braided Telescopic Guide, Pressure Products, Inc., San Pedro, Calif. [Renal LVI]) and venoplasty. ***A,*** *The small vein to the midlateral wall* (arrow) *is cannulated with the Renal LVI.* ***B,*** *The lead is in place after venoplasty of the small vein with direct delivery of the lead into the target vein.*

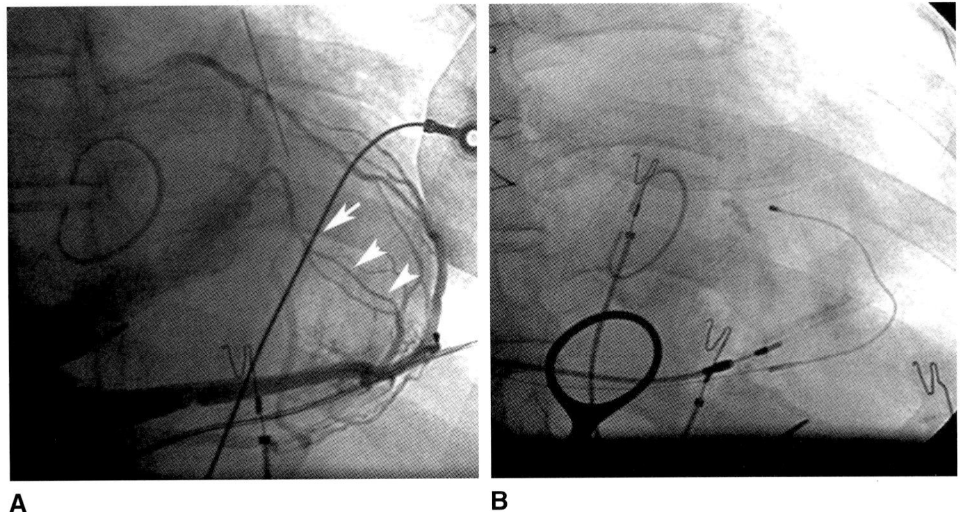

Figure 19-165. *Attain OTW 4193 pacing lead (Medtronic, Inc., Minneapolis, Minn.) placed in a midlateral wall target vein via a retrograde approach after venoplasty of the collateral vessels; the antegrade approach was unsuccessful.* ***A,*** *The midlateral wall vein* (arrow) *is filled retrograde via collaterals* (arrowheads) *from the large posterior lateral vein.* ***B,*** *After venoplasty the Attain 4193 lead is in the midlateral wall vein.*

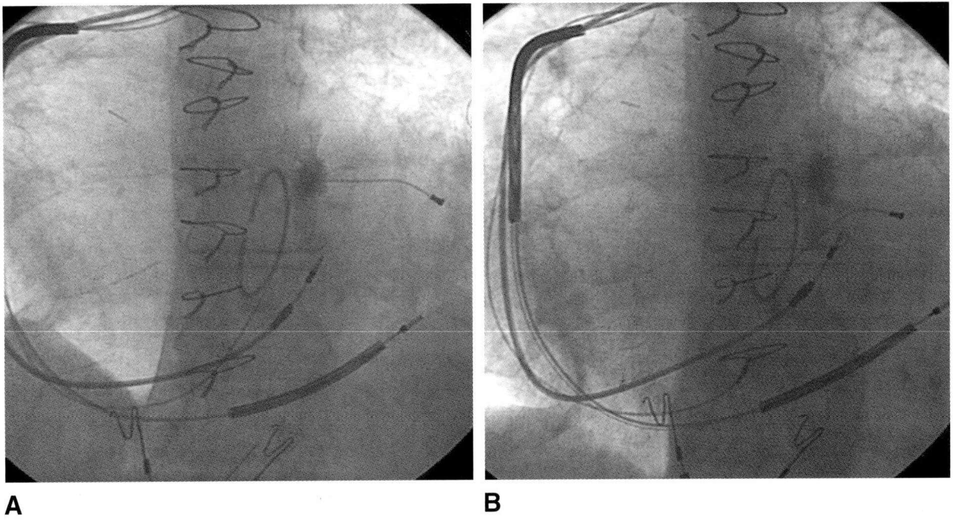

Figure 19-166. *Attain OTW 4193 (Medtronic, Minneapolis, Minn.) pacing lead dislodging from a lateral wall target vein.* ***A,*** *The tip of the lead is in the target vein, but its proximal curve is in the coronary sinus (CS).* ***B,*** *The lead works its way back into the CS. In general, unless the proximal curve of the lead is in the target vein, the lead tends to dislodge out of the vein.*

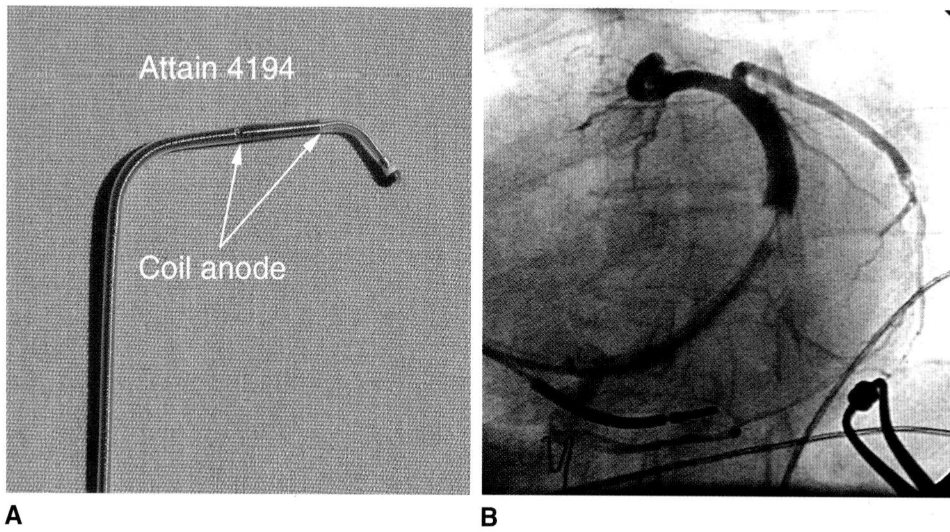

Figure 19-167. Attain Bipolar OTW 4194 pacing lead (Medtronic, Inc., Minneapolis, Minn.) and a suitable coronary vein. ***A,*** *The anode of the 4194 is a coil rather than a typical ring. The greater surface area reduces pacing thresholds, but the coil section of the lead is less flexible, reducing ease of implantation.* ***B,*** *A large anterior lateral vein suitable for the 4194. The coronary veins suitable for the Attain 2187 (Medtronic) and 4194 leads are similar. The difference in shape is important when spontaneous migration of a lead to attain stability results in phrenic pacing or high pacing thresholds.*

ID of the sheath/guide for delivery of the 4194 is 2.3 mm (7F sheath/9F guide) (Figs. 19-167 and 19-168).

Even with favorable venous anatomy, it is at times difficult to advance the Attain 4194 far enough to achieve stability. The proximal curve of the lead must be within the target vein to be stable. If the tip or anode coil meets resistance, the lead may not advance far enough to be stable. In the example shown in Figure 19-169, the venous anatomy appeared well suited to the Attain 4194. After several attempts with different wires, however, the lead retracted after the wire was removed. An attempt to advance the lead with a stylet was also unsuccessful. Only with the support of a preshaped guide was the lead advanced to a stable position, thus underscoring the importance of a guide capable of direct lead delivery.

Even when the Attain 4193 is in a stable position in a medium to large vein, the pacing threshold of the Attain 4194 would usually be lower (Fig. 19-170).

After insertion of the lead and removal of the stylet (or angioplasty wire), the proximal and distal bends of the Attain 4194 migrate to their most stable position. Such migration of the bends may cause the 4194 to move either proximally or distally in the vein. The early migration caused by the bends is usually complete within 1 to 2 minutes but may on rare occasions extend to 5 minutes immediately after the lead is placed. Similar early migration is seen with the Attain 2187 and Attain 4193 leads (Figs. 19-171 and 19-172).

The distance from the tip of the lead to the proximal bend is occasionally too long for the target vein. As a result, the proximal bend develops in the CS, pulling the tip of the lead back out of the vein (Fig. 19-173). A shorter tip-to–proximal bend distance would allow the distal part of the proximal curve to fit within the target vein, producing stability.

St. Jude Medical Leads

The QuickSite Unipolar and QuickSite Bipolar (1056T) are the LV pacing leads available from St. Jude. Both leads can be placed over the wire or with a stylet. The undulations in the distal segment provide some stability in veins larger than the lead diameter (Figs. 19-174 through 19-177). The relatively diminutive undulations in the QuickSite leads may be problematic for lead stability in the proximal portion of large veins (see Fig. 19-177).

Guidant EASYTRAK LV Family of Leads

The Guidant EASYTRAK LV family of pacing leads is shown in Figure 19-178. The last two digits of the model number define the length of the lead. For example, models 4510, 4511, 4512, and 4513 are 65, 72, 80, and 90 cm, respectively. Initially, EASYTRAK leads had a unique connector (LV-1) that was smaller than the standard IS-1 connector (Fig. 19-179C). The LV-1 connector made the lead isodiametric, so the guide could be withdrawn over the lead. With the introduction of the Guidant Rapido Advance Cutaway delivery system, the leads became available with either IS-1 or LV-1 connectors. Oscor, Inc. (Palm Harbor, Fla.) manufactures adapters to convert an LV-1 connector to IS-1 connector, and vice versa, if needed. The distal pacing electrode is a ring that is located 2 mm from the tip on the EASYTAK 1 and 2 leads (see Fig. 19-179B) and 5 mm from the tip of the EASYTRAK 3. The proximal electrode on the EASYTRAK 2 and 3 leads is a ring similar to the distal electrode separated by 11 mm. A steroid collar is contiguous with the ring electrode (white band). The EASYTRAK family of leads is delivered over a 0.014-inch angioplasty wire.

Text continued on p. 781

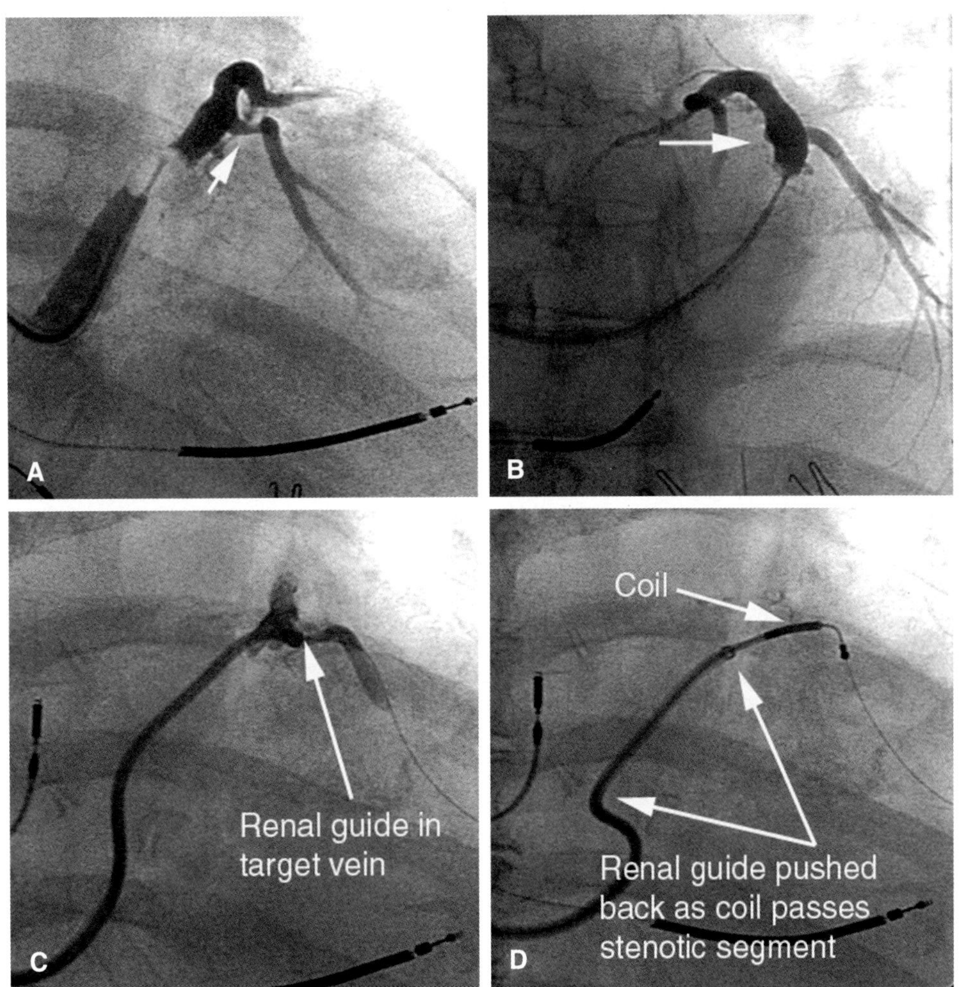

Figure 19-168. *The coil anode of the Attain OTW 4194 pacing lead (Medtronic, Inc., Minneapolis, Minn.) reduces lead flexibility, necessitating guide support to advance through a narrow tortuous area.* ***A,*** *The target vein can be seen in the anteroposterior view. The origin of the vein is narrowed (arrow).* ***B,*** *The left anterior oblique view reveals the complex origin of the vein from the coronary sinus (CS). Rather than having a direct lateral takeoff, the vein loops under the CS and proceeds medially and then laterally.* ***C,*** *The tip of a third-generation renal telescoping guide is advanced over a wire into the proximal segment of the vein. The narrow area is apparent on the selective venogram.* ***D,*** *The lead is advanced into the vein. The distal portion of the lead advances easily. When the coil anode reaches the narrow area, attempts to advance the lead push the guide out of the vein. The guide abuts the back wall of the CS, providing additional support for advancing the lead. Without the support of the guide, the lead would not advance into the vein.*

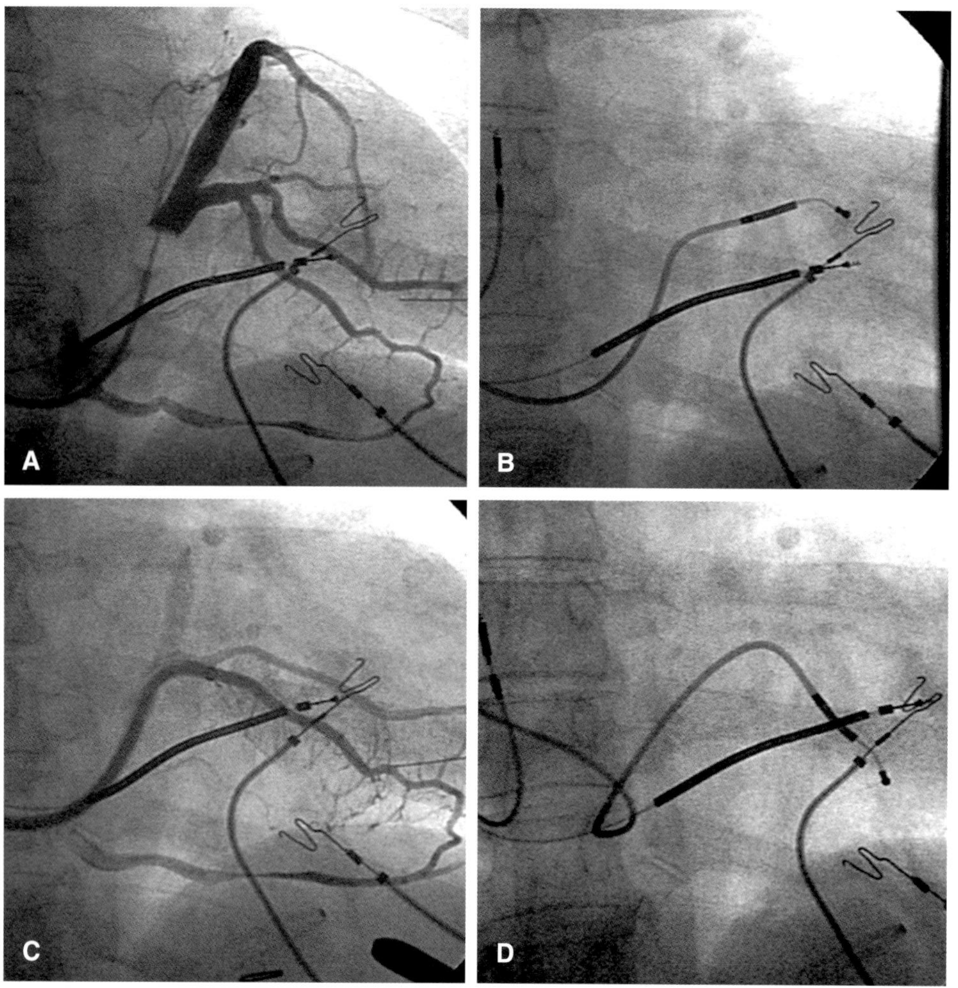

Figure 19-169. The Attain 4194 pacing lead (Medtronic, Inc., Minneapolis, Minn.) requires a third-generation guide despite favorable anatomy. ***A,*** *The target vein appears readily accessible without the need for a guide.* ***B,*** *The 4194 is placed in the vein directly through the 9F ID/11FOD peel-away sheath in the main coronary sinus (CS). It will not advance any further even when the angioplasty wire is replaced with a stylet. The proximal curve remains in the main CS, and the lead is not stable.* ***C,*** *A third-generation 9F OD/7F ID renal lateral vein introducer (renal LVI; renal-shape telescoping guide) is advanced through the 9F ID/11F OD peel-away sheath (already in the main CS) into the target vein. Because the operator started with the 9F ID/11F OD sheath that ended in the CS rather than in the subclavian vein, conversion from a nontelescoping system to a third-generation telescoping system required only adding the 9F OD/7F ID directional guide. The 9F renal LVI (guide) is large enough to deliver any of the left ventricular (LV) pacing leads directly.* ***D,*** *With the support provided by the long 9F sheath (with a proximal curve) and the 9F renal LVI (guide), the 4194 lead is advanced into the vein until its proximal curve is within the vein. The lead is now stable.*

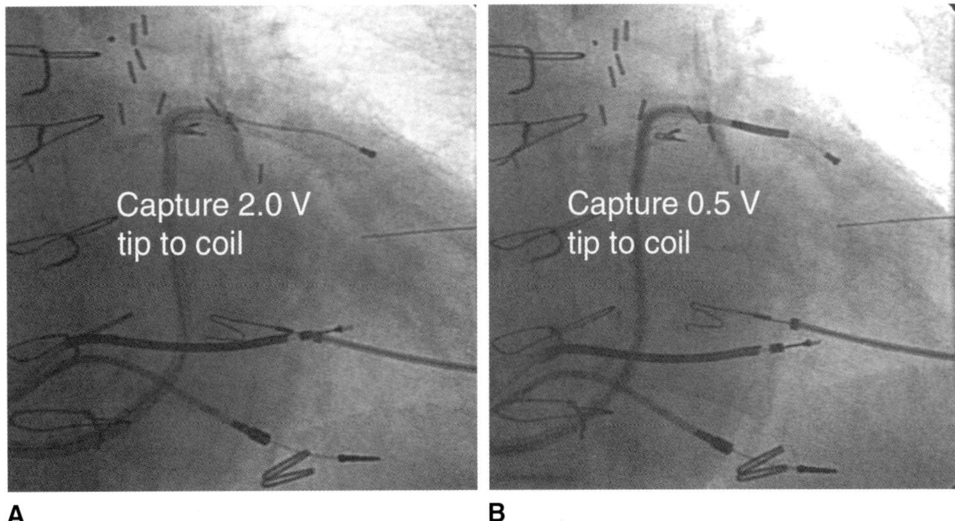

Figure 19-170. The pacing threshold of the Attain 4194 lead is lower than that of the Attain 4193 pacing lead (both from Medtronic, Inc., Minneapolis, Minn.) in most cases. ***A,*** *The threshold of the 4193 is 2.0 volts.* ***B,*** *The threshold of the 4194 is 0.5 volts. The two leads are in the same patient at the same location and were placed through a third-generation renal telescoping delivery system.*

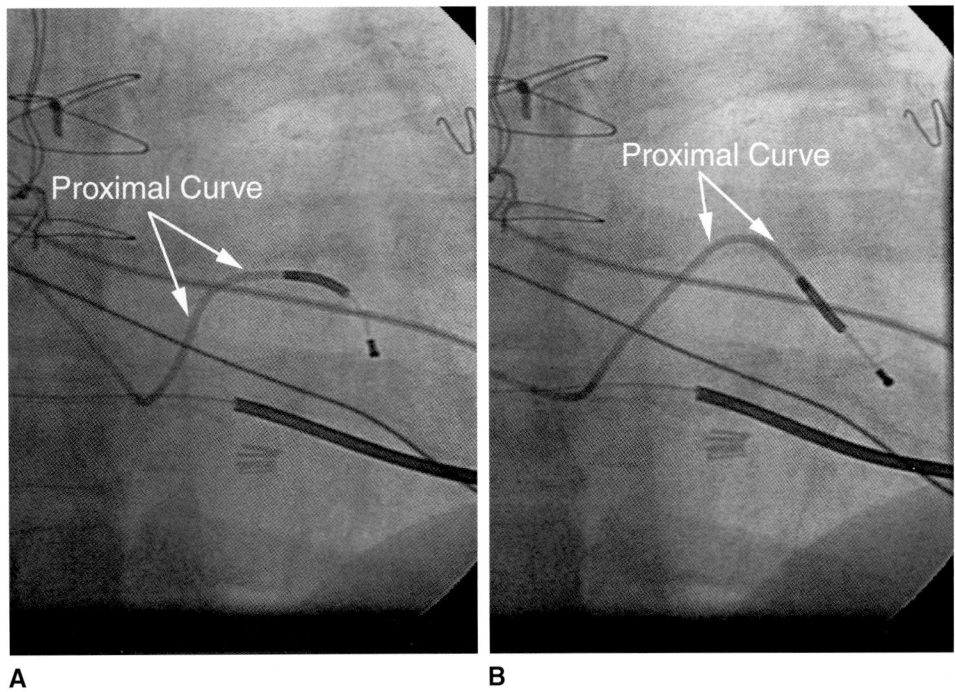

Figure 19-171. When the proximal curve on the Attain 4194 pacing lead (Medtronic, Inc., Minneapolis, Minn.) aligns with the vein's anatomy it advances distally to pace the phrenic nerve. ***A,*** *The lead is withdrawn to prevent phrenic pacing. The proximal curve of the lead is just inside the os of the vein. In this position, the lead does not pace the phrenic nerve. However, the curve of the vein and the curve of the lead are not aligned. The lead is not stable in this position.* ***B,*** *The lead advances spontaneously so that its proximal curve aligns with the venous anatomy. In this position, the proximal curve of the lead and vein match. The lead is stable, but phrenic pacing occurs with the tip in this position. The only way to prevent the lead from advancing in this vein is to change the location of its proximal curve.*

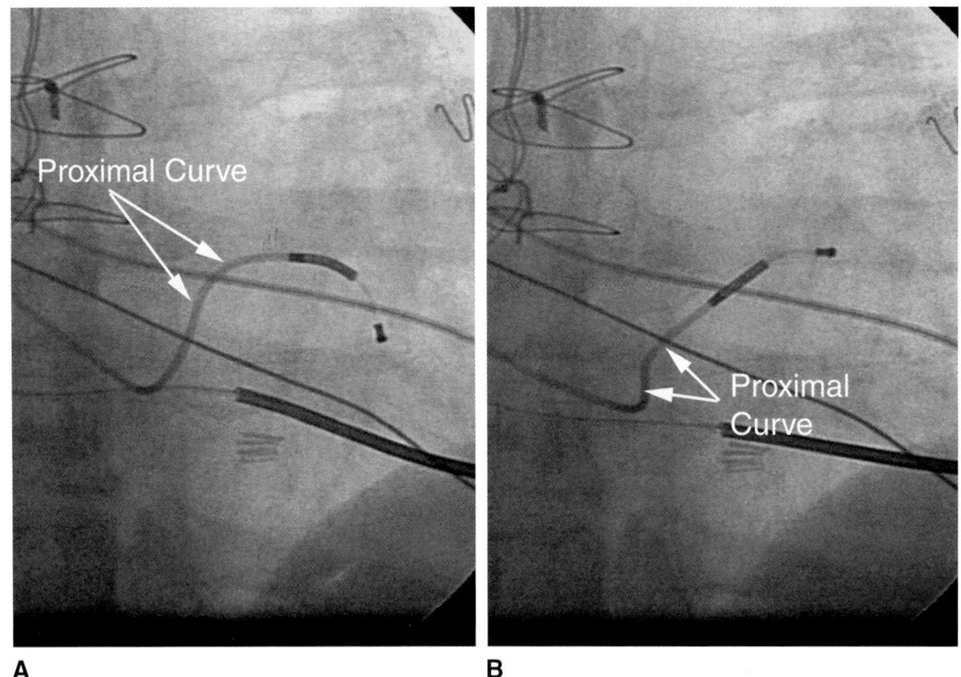

Figure 19-172. When the proximal curve on the Attain 4194 pacing lead (Medtronic, Inc., Minneapolis, Minn.) is in a stable position, it aligns with the curve in the vein, withdrawing the lead out of the target vein. ***A,*** *The proximal curve of the lead is positioned at the os of the target vein. In this position, phrenic pacing is not present at 10V. With the proximal curve slightly deeper in the vein, the lead spontaneously advances, with resumption of phrenic pacing.* ***B,*** *The 4194 lead spontaneously withdraws from the target vein as the proximal curve aligns with the venous anatomy.*

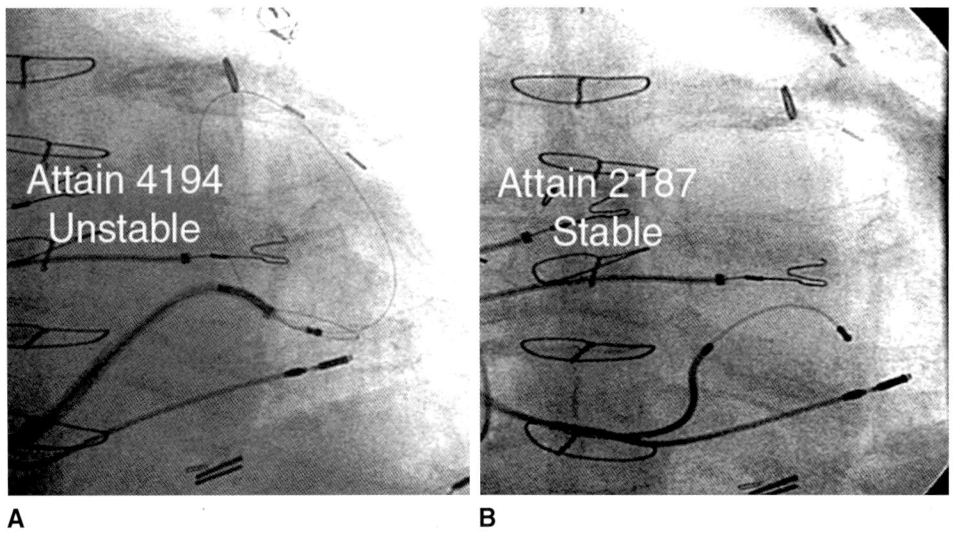

Figure 19-173. The unstable Attain 4194 pacing lead is replaced with an Attain 2187 pacing lead (both from Medtronic, Inc., Minneapolis, Minn.). ***A,*** *The proximal bend of the 4194 is too proximal for the target vein. As the proximal bend stabilizes, the lead retracts into the coronary sinus, pulling the tip back.* ***B,*** *The curve on the Attain 2187 lead is stable in the vein.*

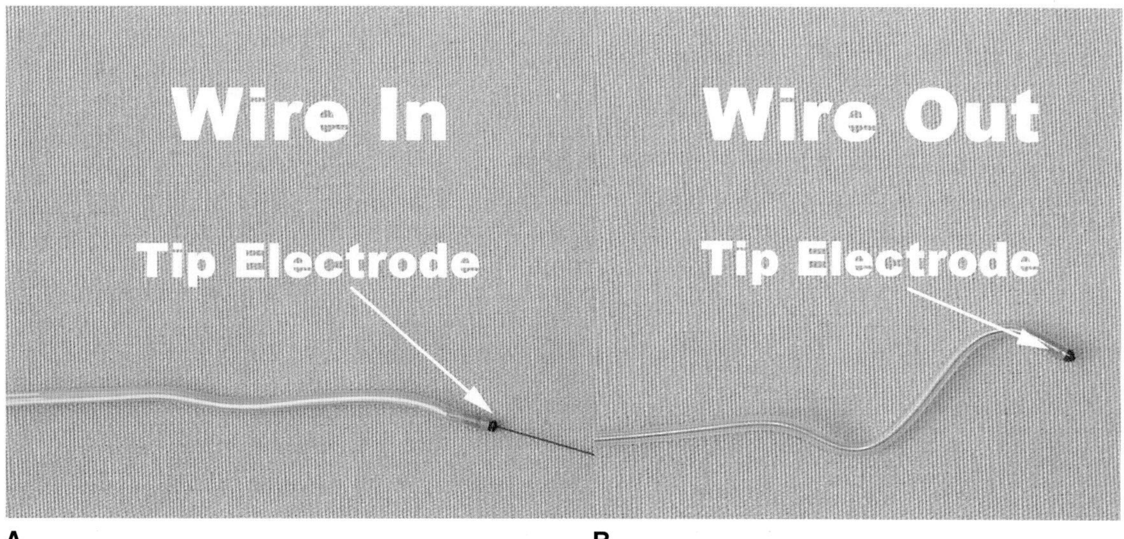

Figure 19-174. *QuickSite Unipolar over-the-wire LV (left ventricular) pacing lead (St. Jude Medical, St. Paul, Minn.).* ***A,*** *The angioplasty wire is in place, and the lead is straightened.* ***B,*** *The angioplasty wire is withdrawn and assumes its preformed shape. The preformed shape is intended to stabilize the lead within the vein and direct the tip toward the myocardium.*

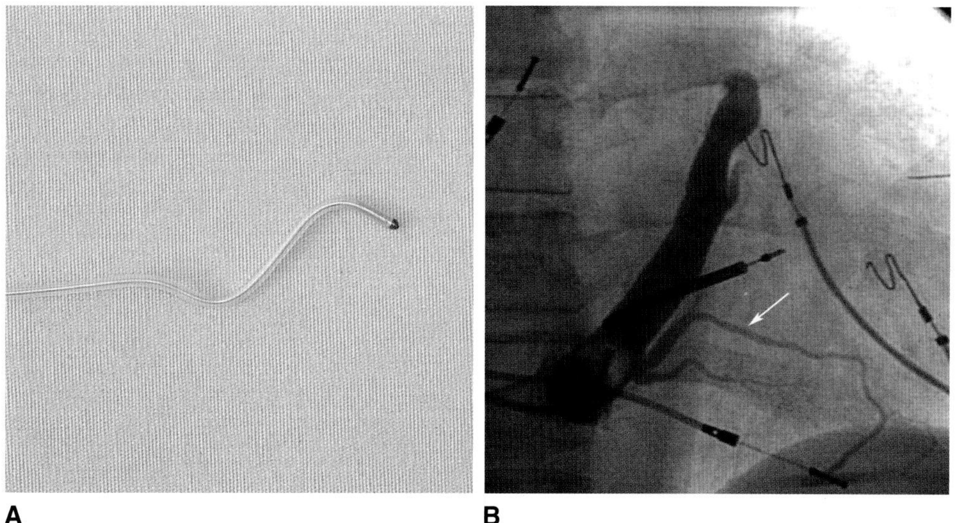

Figure 19-175. *QuickSite Unipolar over-the-wire LV (left ventricular) pacing lead (St. Jude Medical, St. Paul, Minn.) (**A**) and a suitable coronary vein (**B,*** arrow*).*

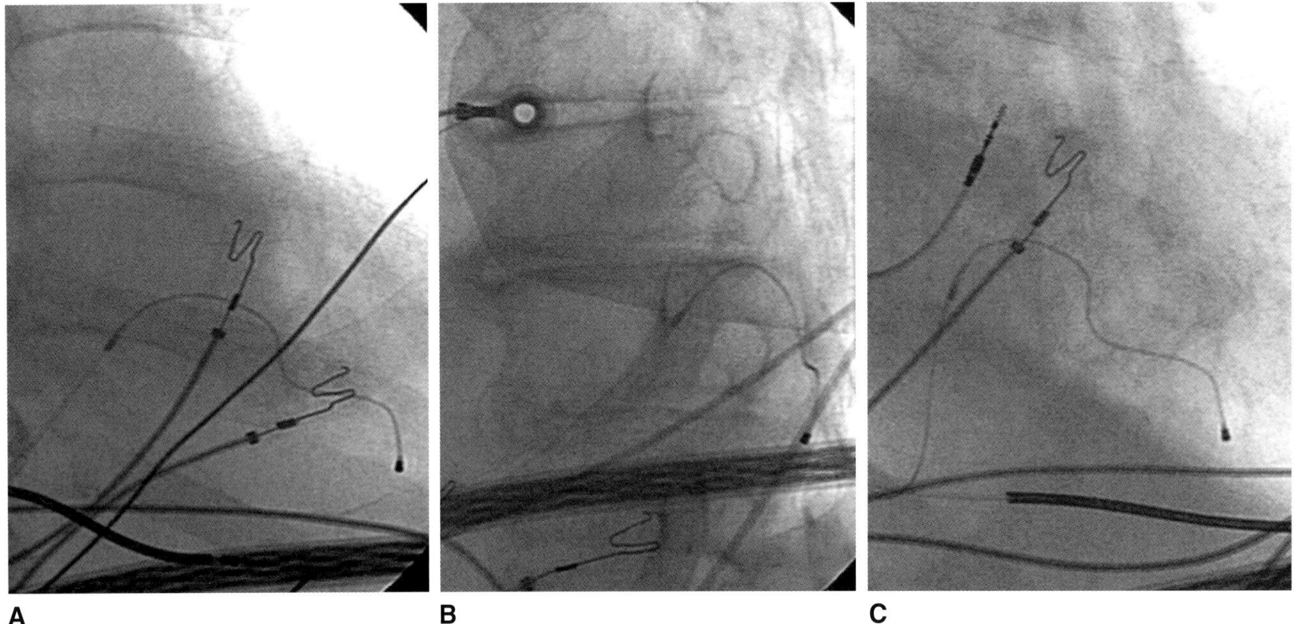

*Figure 19-176. QuickSite LV (left ventricular) pacing lead (St. Jude Medical, St. Paul, Minn.) in a target vein in anteroposterior (**A**), left anterior oblique (**B**), and right anterior oblique (**C**) projections.*

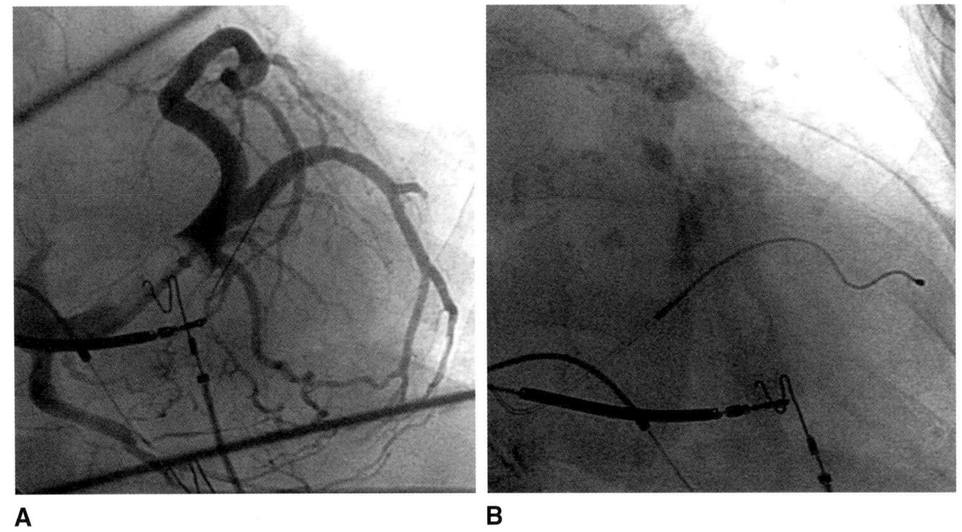

*Figure 19-177. Large target vein with the QuickSite LV (left ventricular) pacing lead (St. Jude Medical, St. Paul, Minn.) in place distally. **A,** The target vein is large with an easy takeoff from the coronary sinus. **B,** The lead is advanced distally, placing it anteriorly near the septum.*

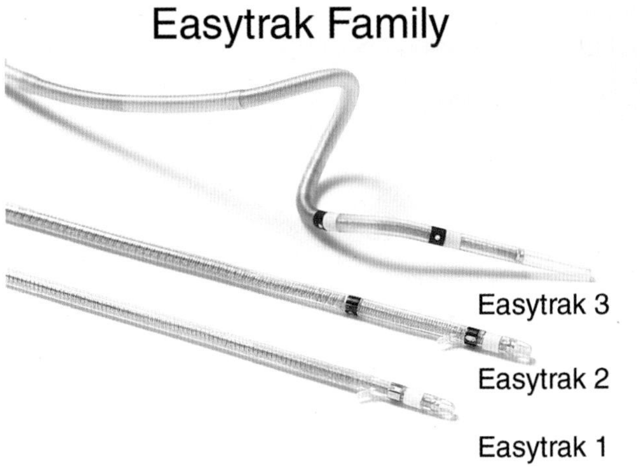

Easytrak Family

Easytrak 3

Easytrak 2

Easytrak 1

Figure 19-178. *EASYTRAK "family" of left ventricular pacing leads (Guidant, Boston Scientific, Natick, Mass.).*

EASYTRAK 1 and 2 Leads. The EASYTRAK 1 and 2 leads are similar, except that the EASYTRAK 2 is bipolar. Both have tines at the tip and tend to migrate either proximally or distally unless wedged in a small branch of the target vein. Also, because the pacing electrodes of the EASYTRAK 1 and 2 leads are not at the tip, the leads must be wedged in a small branch to achieve optimal thresholds. With these leads, it is often difficult or even impossible to find a suitable location in a large target vein because of diaphragmatic/phrenic stimulation distally with high pacing thresholds and lead instability proximally. In our experience with 38 sequential procedures in which an EASYTRAK 1 lead was placed in the ideal target vein, 11 were unsuccessful owing to high pacing thresholds or diaphragmatic/phrenic stimulation, but the leads were successfully replaced with Attain 2187 or 4193 leads in the same vein.

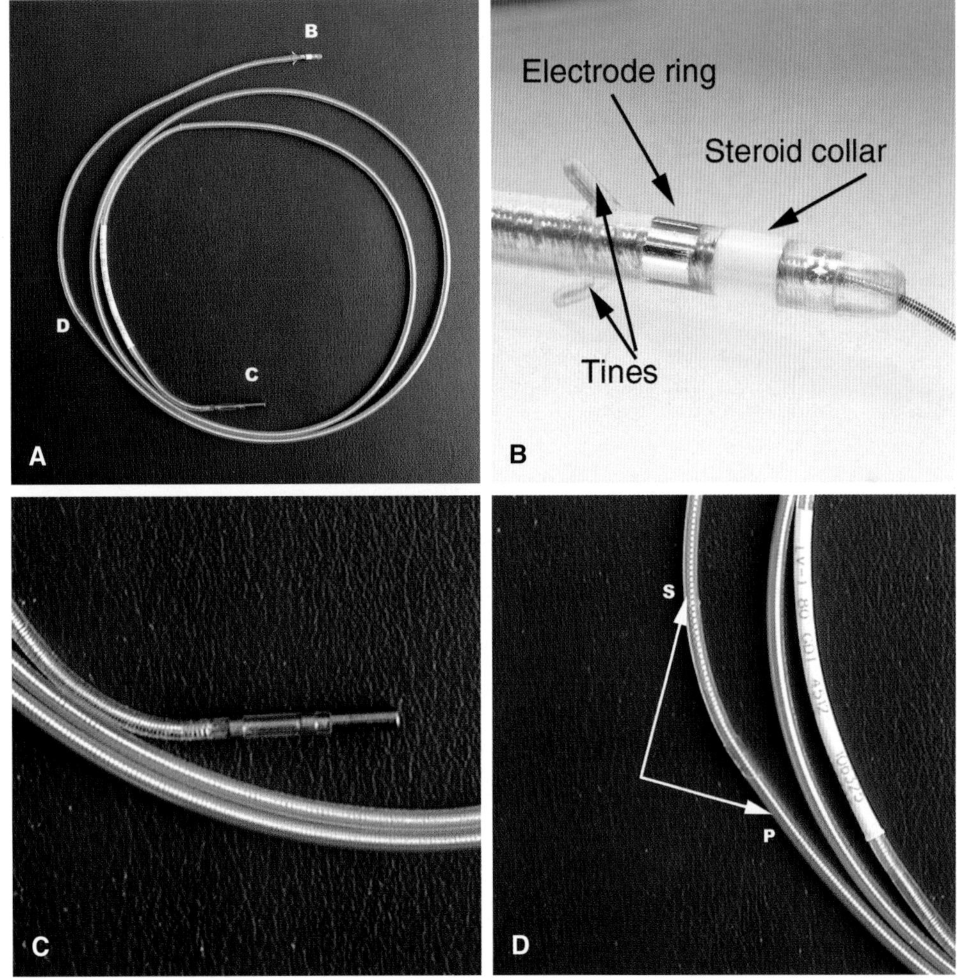

Figure 19-179. *EASYTRAK 1 left ventricular pacing lead (Guidant, Boston Scientific, Natick, Mass.). **A,** The entire lead. **B,** Close-up of the tip of the lead. Note that there are two tines at 180 degrees proximal to the pacing ring electrode. The white band is the steroid-eluting collar. The ring pacing electrode is 2 mm proximal to the tip of the electrode. Unless the lead is wedged in a small target vein (or a branch of a large target vein), the ring electrode does not make good contact with the myocardium, and pacing thresholds are high. **C,** Close-up of the LV-1 connector. It does not fit in a standard IS-1 connector. **D,** The transition from polyurethane sheath over silicone (P) to silicone alone (S). The lead is insulated with silicone but also has an abrasion-resistant polyurethane coating that extends from the connector to a point 5 cm from the tip of the lead. The polyurethane coating increases the stiffness of the lead. Unless the lead is deep enough in the target vein that the polyurethane-coated body is within the target vein, the lead tends to become dislodged.*

In addition, failure of clinical response to resynchronization occurred in five of our patients with a distally placed EASYTRAK lead, who experienced improvement after a lead was placed proximally in the same vein (Fig. 19-180). On the other hand, the EASYTRAK lead wedges well in much smaller veins without dislodgment (Fig. 19-181). The EASYTRAK 3 lead has solved the problem of lead position in large as well as medium veins.

The handling characteristics of the EASYTRAK 2 lead are quite similar to those of the EASYTRAK 1. The advantage of the EASYTRAK 2 is the ability to selectively pace the proximal ring if the distal ring is too distal and/or paces the phrenic nerve.

EASYTRAK 3 Lead. The EASYTRAK 3 lead is an important addition to our "quiver" of LV pacing leads (Fig. 19-182). The helical shape is straightened with an angioplasty wire for delivery into the target vein (Fig. 19-183). Once at the desired location, the wire is removed and the lead resumes a helical shape, securing it in place. Because of the helical design, a larger surface area of lead is in contact with the vessel wall (Fig. 19-184). My experience is that with the EASYTRAK 3 in a large vein, the pacing thresholds are not as low as those with a large lead with the electrode at the tip. However, the EASYTRAK 3 lead may be more stable. Most important, the location of the lead can be controlled more precisely than those of other leads (Fig. 19-185). If high pacing thresholds or phrenic pacing is encountered at a specific site, the lead can be straightened out and moved proximally or distally. When the wire is removed, the lead will remain at that location. Straight leads and preformed leads may move back to the original site (Figs. 19-186 and 19-187). In some cases, it is important that the proximal marker of the EASYTRAK 3 be in the target vein (Fig. 19-188). In this case, the Attain 4194 is the best lead choice.

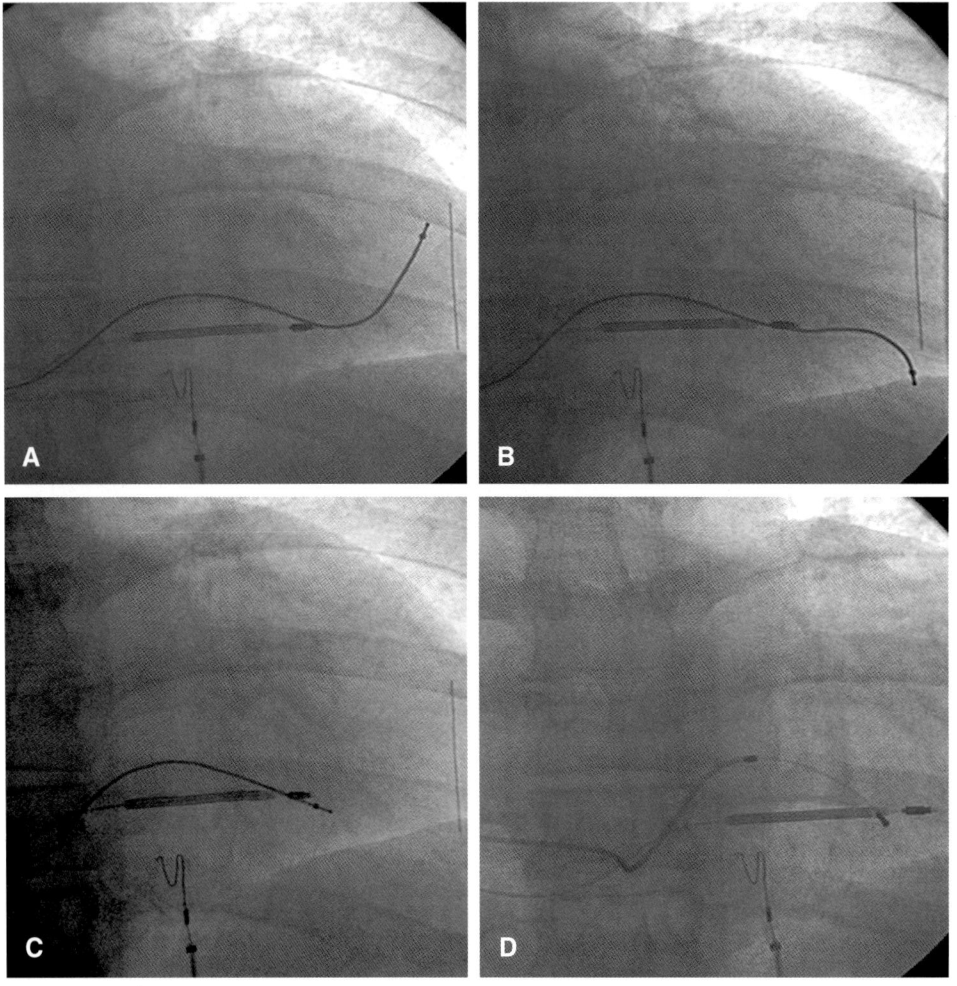

Figure 19-180. Failure of an EASYTRAK 1 LV (left ventricular) pacing lead (Guidant, Boston Scientific, Natick, Mass.) in a large target vein. ***A*** *and* ***B,*** *The distal location of the lead resulted in phrenic pacing.* ***C,*** *The proximal location of the lead resulted in pacing thresholds over 5 V.* ***D,*** *An Attain 2187 lead (Medtronic, Inc., Minneapolis, Minn.) paced at 0.7 V. Without the option of an alternative lead, the target vein would have to be abandoned. This figure demonstrates the problem of placing an EASYTRAK 1 lead in a large target vein.*

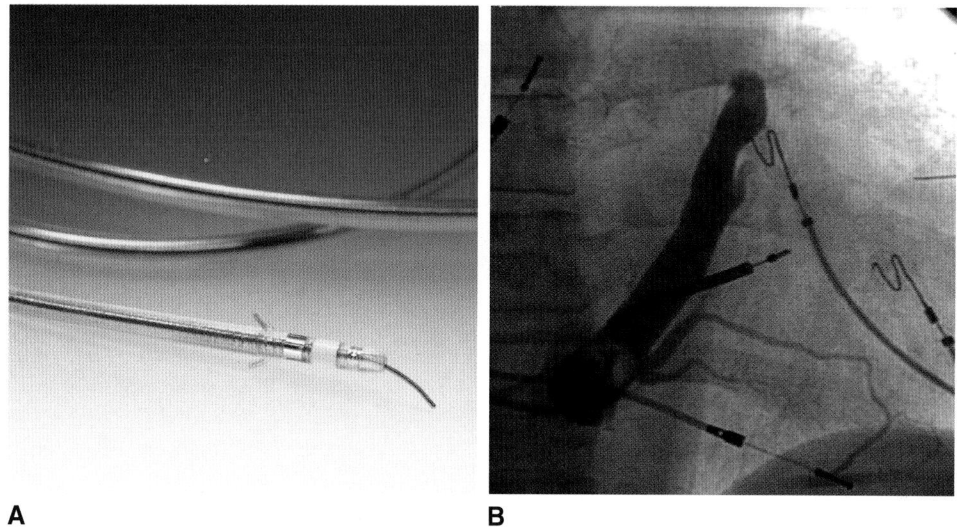

Figure 19-181. *EASYTRAK 1 unipolar LV (left ventricular) pacing lead (Guidant, Boston Scientific, Natick, Mass.) (**A**) and a suitable coronary vein (**B**).*

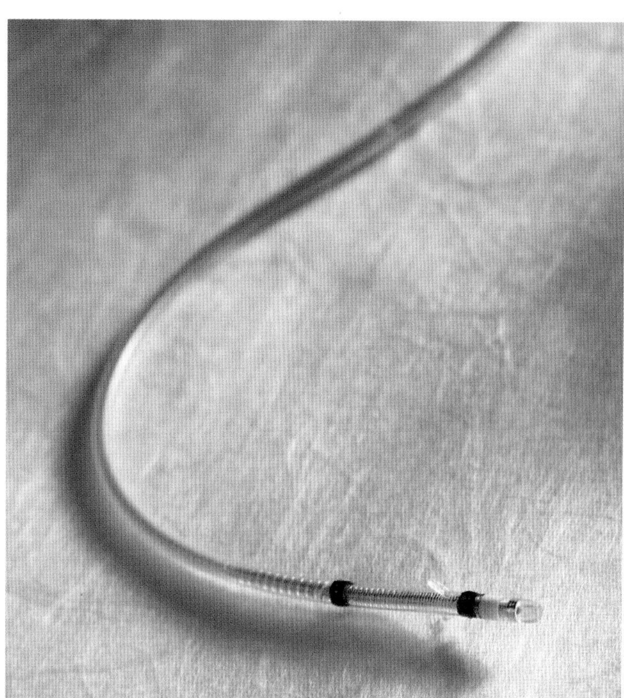

Figure 19-182. *EASYTRAK 2 bipolar steroid-eluting LV (left ventricular) pacing lead (Guidant, Boston Scientific, Natick, Mass.).*

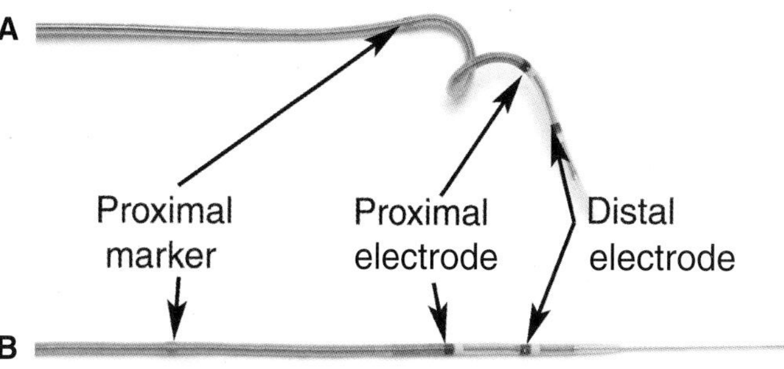

Figure 19-183. *EASYTRAK 3 LV (left ventricular) pacing lead (Guidant, Boston Scientific, Natick, Mass.) with and without guidewire. **A,** With the guidewire removed, the lead assumes its intrinsic shape. **B,** The wire is inserted, straightening the lead for placement into the vein. When the lead is placed, the proximal marker should be within the target vein. The distal electrode is back from the tip. Steroid collars (white bands) are just distal to both ring electrodes.*

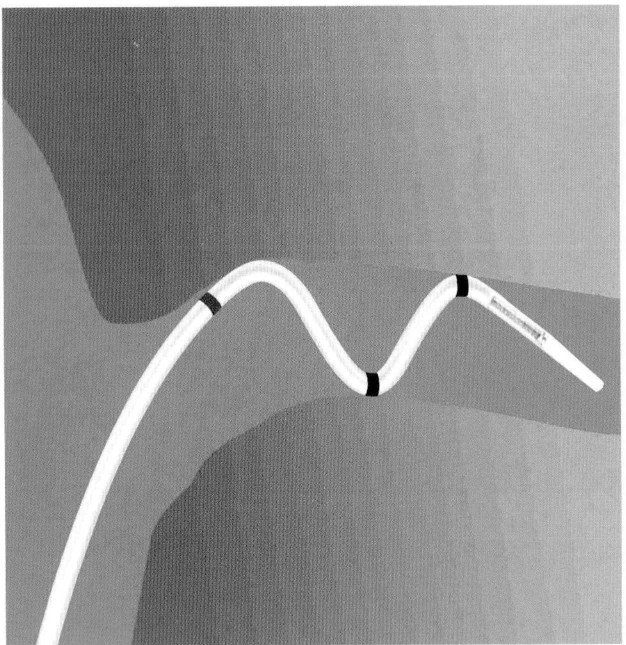

Figure 19-184. The EASYTRAK lead (Guidant, Boston Scientific, Natick, Mass.) is deployed in a large vein. Note that the proximal marker is within the vein. The two ring electrodes are in contact with the walls of the vein. Importantly, the lead is in contact with the walls of the vein not only at the areas shown but also along the entire length of the vein.

Medtronic 2188 Bipolar Coronary Sinus Lead

The Medtronic 2188 Bipolar Coronary Sinus Lead is a bipolar lead originally designed to pace the atrium from the ostium of the CS (Fig. 19-189A). In an occasional case it may be placed in an extremely large target vein. The 2188 lead has a canted tip, which may provide lead stability not possible with other leads. The 2188 fits through the 9F or 11F guide.

Medtronic CapSure SP 4023 Lead

The Medtronic CapSure SP 4023 pacing lead is a steroid-eluting, unipolar, implantable, tined ventricular transvenous lead. It is insulated with polyurethane and is available in 65- and 85-cm lengths. The 4023 is not specifically designed for use in LV pacing but is essential for an occasional case. Other unipolar or bipolar leads could be used but are not available off the shelf in lengths exceeding 58 cm. A 58-cm lead is usually not long enough to reach a lateral wall target vein in a patient with heart failure and a dilated heart. The recommended introducer/sheath size is 7F. The 4023 lead fits through most 8F or larger guides.

The 4023 lead is usually modified for LV pacing: Two tines at 180 degrees are removed. The tip of the lead may be bent 30 degrees to improve contact and allow the lead tip to negotiate tight curves. Figure 19-190 illustrates a patient with a single lateral wall target

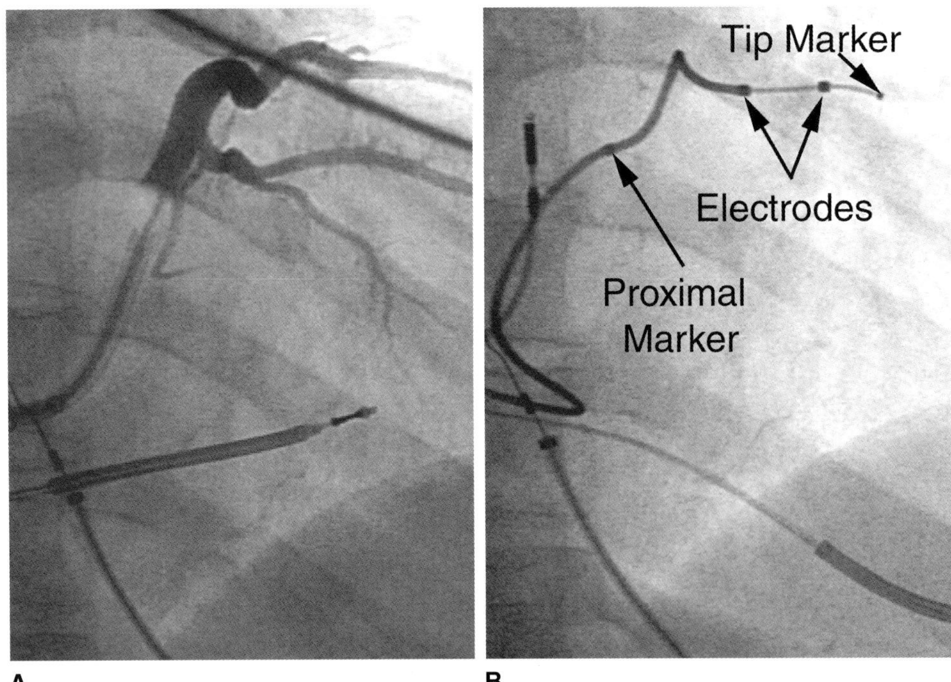

*Figure 19-185. Lateral wall target vein before and after placement of the EASYTRAK 3 pacing lead (Guidant, Boston Scientific, Natick, Mass.). **A,** The vein is shown. Initially an EASYTRAK 2 lead was placed, but satisfactory pacing thresholds were achieved only when it was advanced distally. **B**, The EASYTRAK 3 lead is placed in the same vessel. The angioplasty wire is withdrawn when the tip electrode is in the desired location. Even though the proximal marker is not within the target vein, the lead is stable, and the pacing threshold is 1.5 V.*

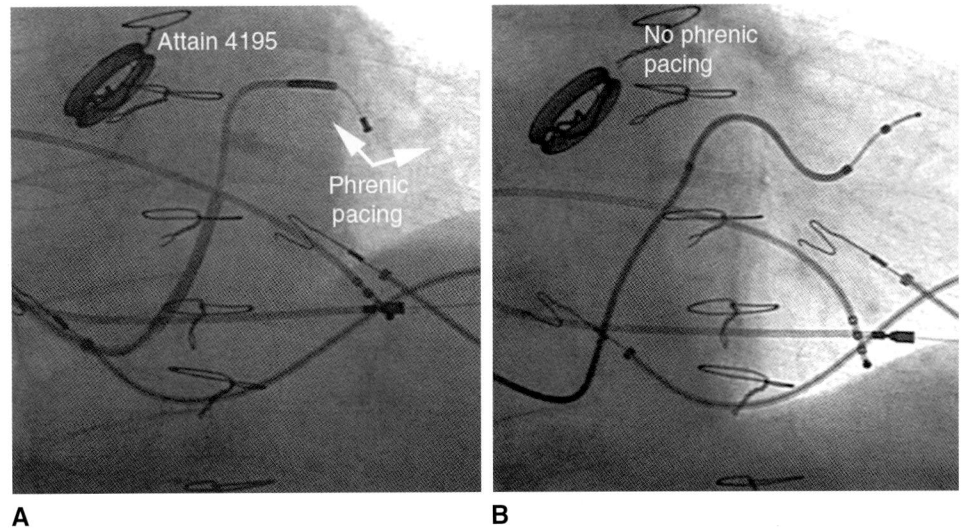

Figure 19-186. *Phrenic pacing with an Attain 4195 lead but not with an EASYTRAK 3 lead.* ***A,*** *The shape of the Attain 4195 lead (Medtronic, Inc., Minneapolis, Minn.) directs the tip inferior. Phrenic pacing is found along the inferior portion of the vein.* ***B,*** *The shape of the EASYTRAK 3 lead (Guidant, Boston Scientific, Natick, Mass.) in the same vein directs the electrodes superiorly, where phrenic pacing is not encountered.*

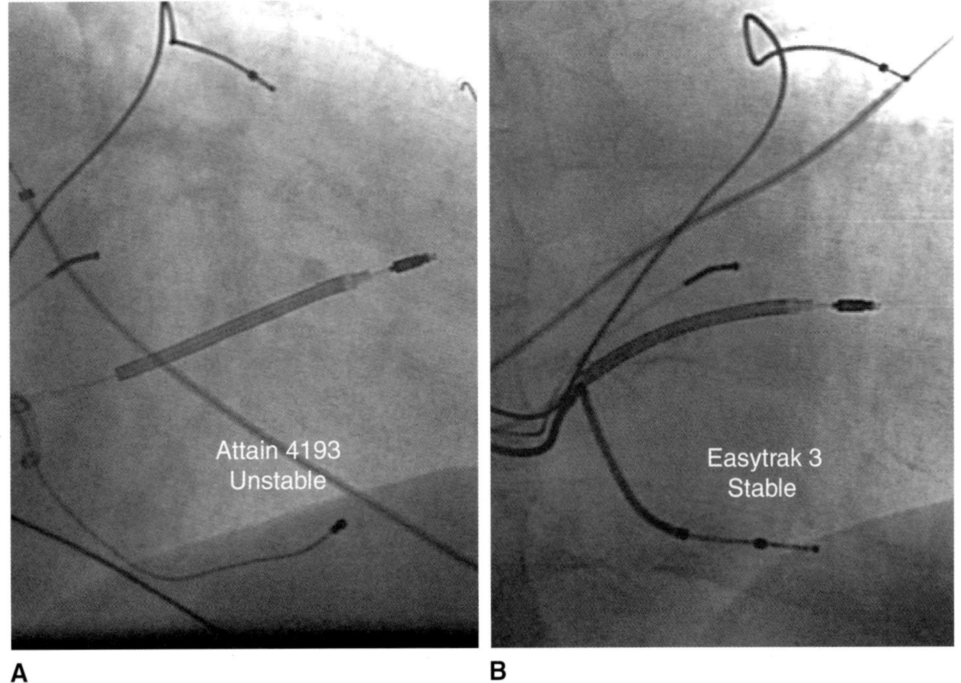

Figure 19-187. *An Attain 4193 lead is unstable in the vein and is successfully replaced with an EASYTRAK 3 lead.* ***A,*** *The Attain 4193 pacing lead (Medtronic, Inc., Minneapolis, Minn.) repeatedly became dislodged from the vein after the stylet was removed.* ***B,*** *The EASYTRAK 3 lead (Guidant, Boston Scientific, Natick, Mass.) is stable with pacing thresholds of 1.2 V in the same position.*

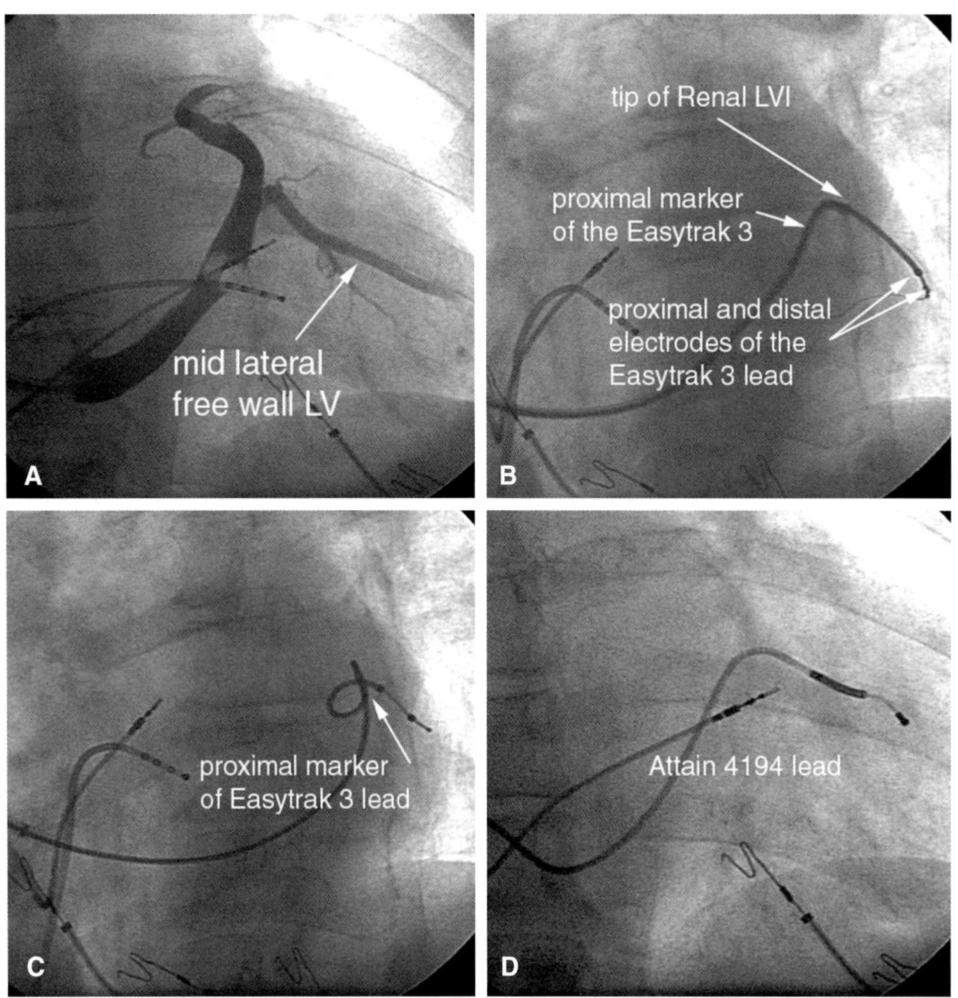

Figure 19-188. The EASYTRAK 3 lead is unstable with the proximal marker in the coronary sinus (CS); the Attain 4194 lead is a better choice. ***A,*** *Anteroposterior projection of the CS venous anatomy. The ideal location of the tip of the left ventricular (LV) pacing lead is pointed out.* ***B,*** *An EASYTRAK 3 lead is placed in the vessel with a renal lateral vein introducer (renal LVI). To place the distal electrode on the midlateral wall, the proximal marker is not in the target vein.* ***C,*** *The EASYTRAK 3 lead has withdrawn into the CS.* ***D,*** *An Attain 4194 pacing lead (Medtronic, Inc., Minneapolis, Ind.) is in a stable position with the proximal bend in the target vessel and the tip on the midlateral wall of the left ventricle.*

vessel in whom both the Attain 2187 and 4193 leads caused phrenic pacing. However, the 4023 lead delivered to the same vessel was placed in a different position that did not cause phrenic pacing.

ELA Left Ventricular Pacing Leads

ELA Medical manufactures two transvenous LV cardiac venous leads. The Situs OTW (Fig. 19-191) is a polyurethane-coated lead that is isodiametric with a lead body silicone insulation and an IS-1 sleeve that screws onto the lead body. The Situs LV (Fig. 19-192), which is a dual-curve passive-fixation lead, is stylet-driven with a 2-mm half-ring electrode.

Biotronik Left Ventricular Leads

The Biotronik leads are shown in Figure 19-193. The Corox + LVH-UP CS lead comes in 75- and 85-cm lengths. The lead is unipolar and stylet-driven with helical fixation. The Corox OTW-UP Steroid Lead is also unipolar and comes in the same lengths, but is delivered over the wire. The Corox LV-H CS Lead, LV-S CS Lead, and LA-H CS Lead are bipolar and stylet-driven.

Epicardial Left Ventricular Pacing Leads

On occasion, transvenous LV lead placement is not possible with the tools and techniques the implanting physician has chosen to learn and use. In our experience, using a third-generation telescoping delivery system and venoplasty for the last 400 patients, epicardial LV lead placement was considered in only 1 patient in whom the CS emptied into the LA. Transseptal LV lead placement is an alternative to epicardial LV lead placement in patients in whom aggressive use of venoplasty, modern leads, and a third-generation telescoping delivery system are unsuccessful.

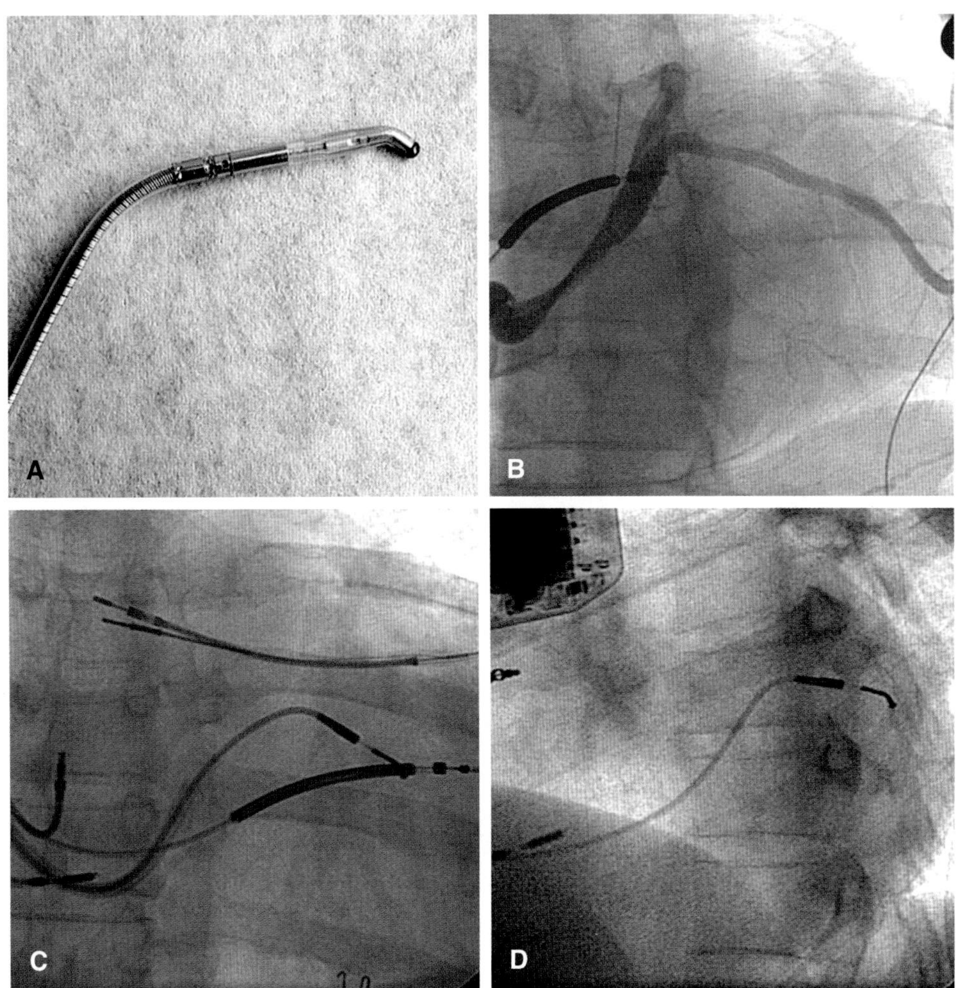

Figure 19-189. *Attain CS 2188 pacing lead (Medtronic, Inc., Minneapolis, Minn.). **A,** Note the canting of the lead tip. **B,** Venogram demonstrating the vein into which the 2188 lead was placed. The lead is shown in place in the anteroposterior (**C**) and left anterior oblique (**D**) projections.*

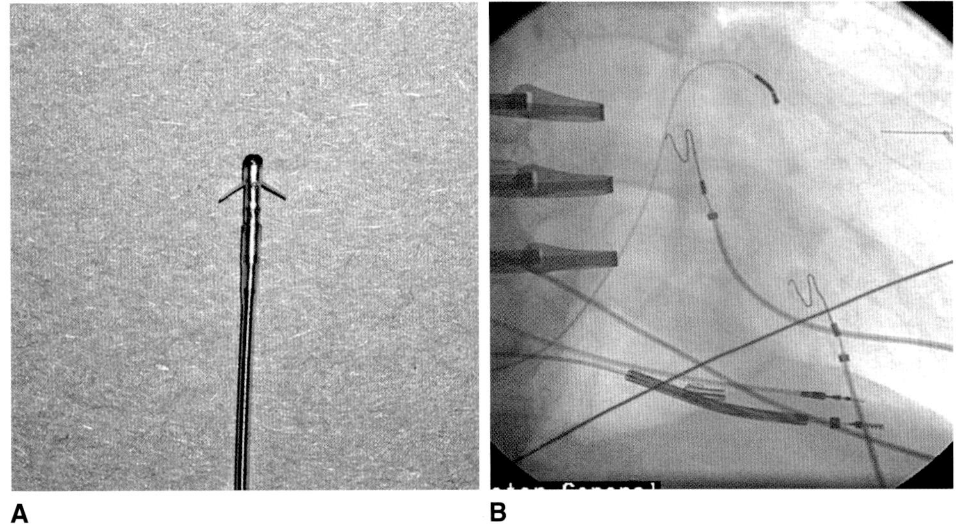

Figure 19-190. *CapSure SP 4023 pacing lead (Medtronic, Inc., Minneapolis, Minn.). **A,** The lead with two tines removed. **B,** The lead in place on the lateral wall of the left ventricle in a location where both the Attain 2187 and Attain 4193 pacing leads (Medtronic) caused phrenic pacing. No other suitable target veins were available. The tip of the 4023 lead was bent to allow the lead to turn the corner into the vein. Bending the tip also seems to improve contact and lower pacing thresholds.*

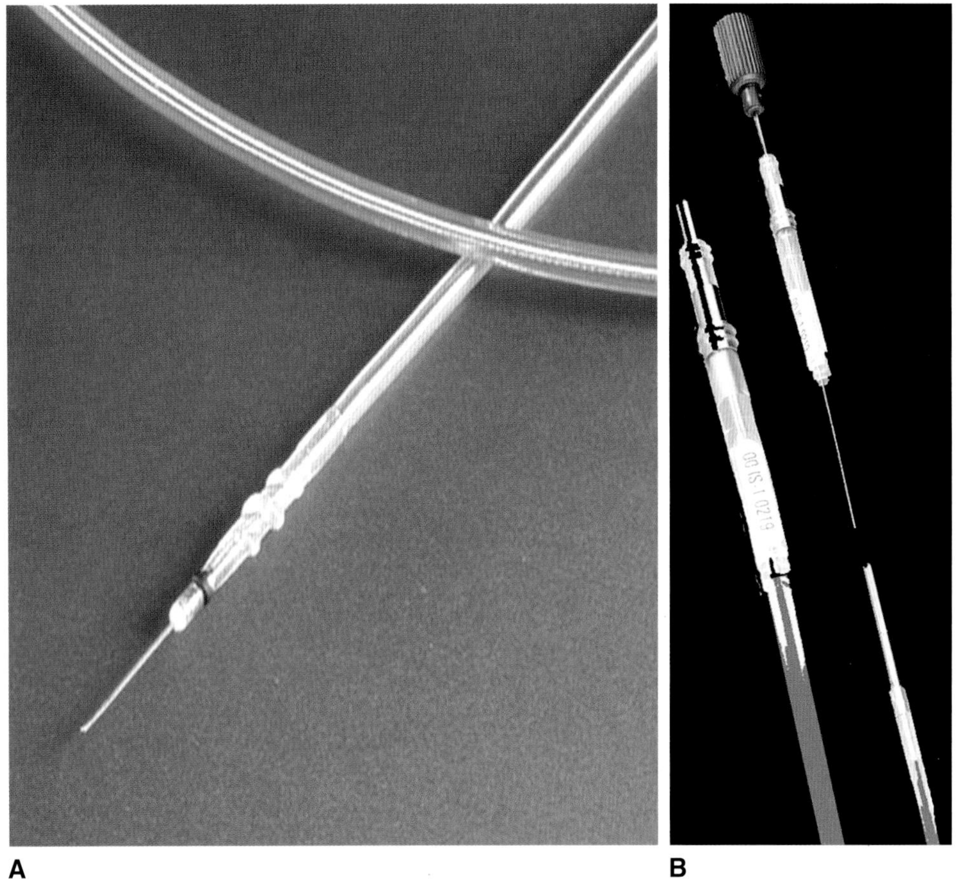

*Figure 19-191. Situs OTW Coronary Sinus Lead (ELA Medical, Sorin Group, Milan) (**A**) and IS-1 sleeve (**B**).*

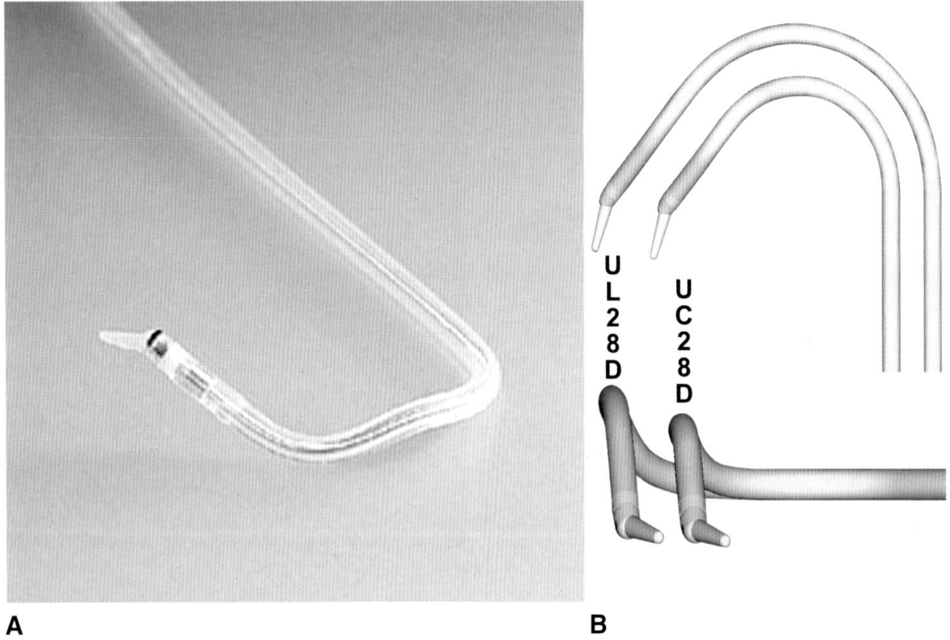

*Figure 19-192. **A,** Stylet-driven pacing leads available from ELA Medical (Sorin Group, Milan). **B,** Same leads inserted into implantation sheaths.*

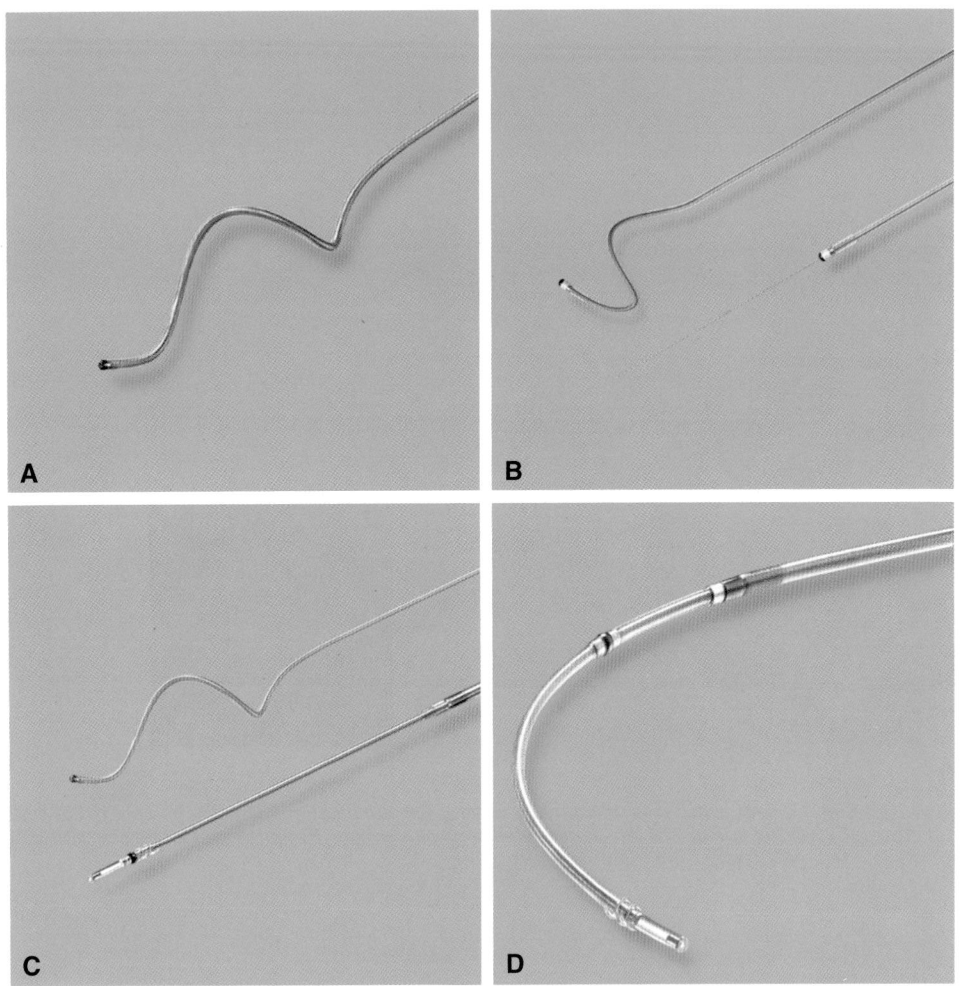

Figure 19-193. *Left ventricular pacing leads available from Biotronik GmbH & Co. (Berlin, Germany). See text and Table 19-6 for details.* ***A,*** *Corox + LVH-UP CS.* ***B,*** *Corox OTW-UP Steroid.* ***C,*** *Corox LVH CS* (top); *Corox LV-S CS* (bottom). ***D,*** *Corox LA-H CS.*

The tools designed for epicardial lead placement have only recently advanced from the technology of the 1970s, when epicardial lead placement was more commonly performed. Tools are available for placement of leads on the posterior and lateral walls, usually in the segment of the myocardium near the base just lateral to the circumflex artery (Fig. 19-194). The same tools can be used through mini-thoracotomies or through small ports during thoracoscopic implantation (Fig. 19-195). Although sew-on steroid electrodes often have better long-term electrical performance, their placement is reasonable only during a sternotomy or thoracotomy because of otherwise limited access. Consequently, the lead offerings from Guidant (Fig. 19-196) and St. Jude Medical (Fig. 19-197) are screw-in electrodes and are now available as bipolar leads. The implantation tool from Enpath Medical, Inc. (Plymouth, Minn.; Fig. 19-197), demonstrates the value of using tools from multiple sources during lead implantation.

Biotronik offers unipolar and bipolar leads for epicardial pacing. The bipolar lead has a sewing patch, whereas the unipolar lead is a screw-in lead (Fig. 19-198; see Table 19-6).

With epicardial pacing leads, the location of the LV pacing leads relative to the midlateral LV free wall is not always clear. Figure 19-199 illustrates a patient with both epicardial leads and transvenous leads for comparison. It is clear that surgically placed leads are located in segments that are distinct from those achieved with transvenous leads, but the clinical responses are similar as long as the LV free wall is the target (Fig. 19-200).

Test for Viability and Phrenic Pacing before Lead Placement

Before one makes the effort to insert a pacing lead into the target vein, it is useful to know where phrenic pacing will be found and to obtain a rough estimate of myocardial viability. This goal can be accomplished by using an angioplasty wire as a test pace system. Any angioplasty wire with an uncoated tip—the Luge but not the Choice PT—can be used as a unipolar test system. However, because the length of the exposed tip is 3 to 5 cm, pacing is not very specific unless the tip is covered up to the last 5 mm with insulation. The Cordis 3F Transit Infusion

Text continued on p. 793

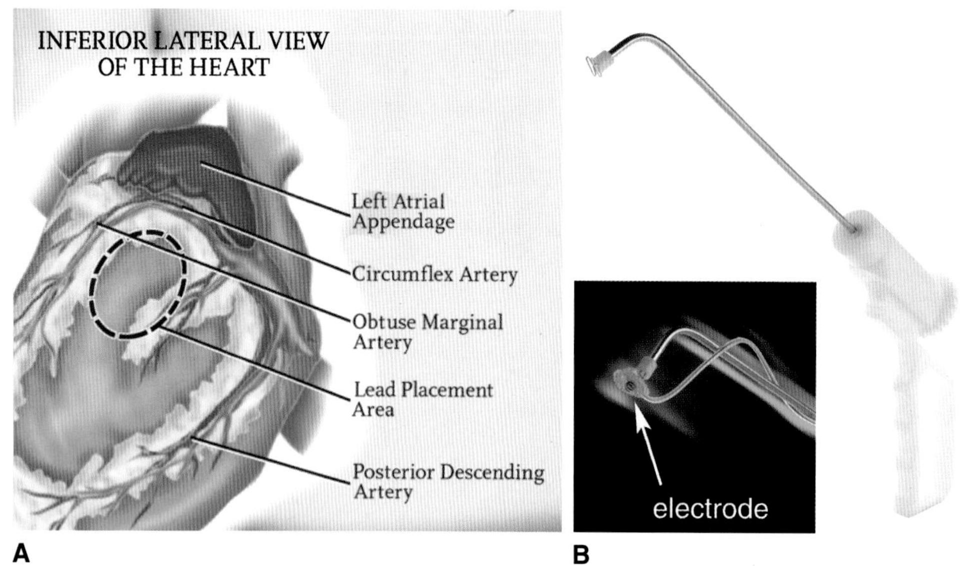

Figure 19-194. Target zone and placement device for surgical placement of epicardial leads. ***A,*** *The target zone for epicardial left ventricular lead placement.* ***B,*** *Epicardial electrode and placement device from Medtronic, Inc. (Minneapolis, Minn.).*

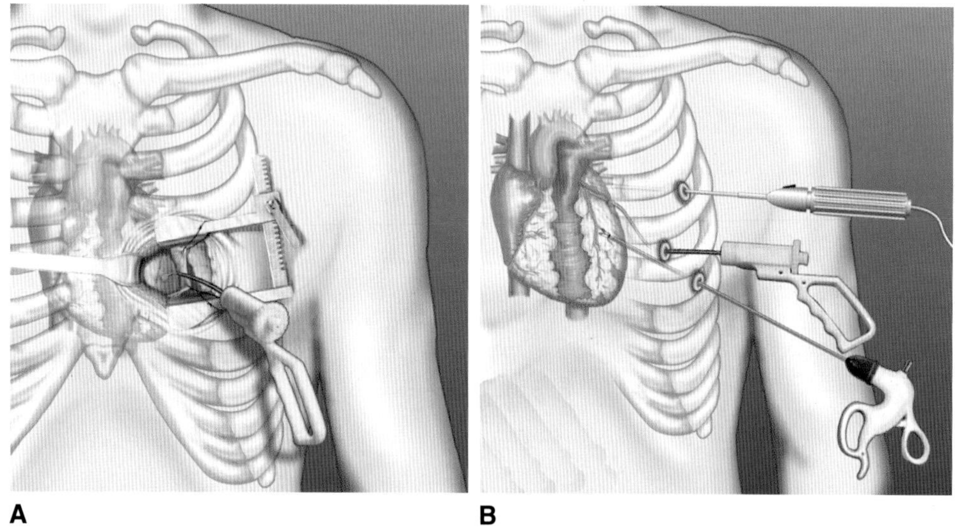

Figure 19-195. Mini-thoracotomy and thorascopic approach to left ventricular lead placement. ***A,*** *The mini-thoracotomy approach with lead placement device.* ***B,*** *The thorascopic approach using the Medtronic, Inc. (Minneapolis, Minn.) placement device.*

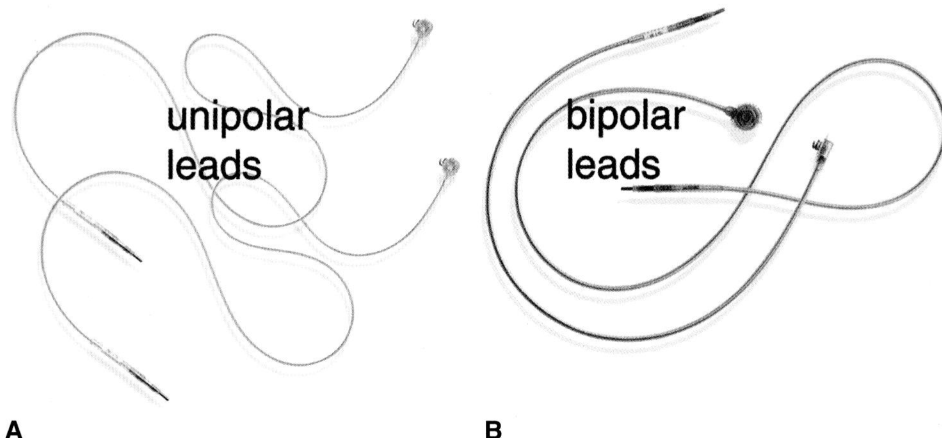

Figure 19-196. Unipolar and bipolar epicardial leads available through Guidant (Boston Scientific, Natick, Mass.).

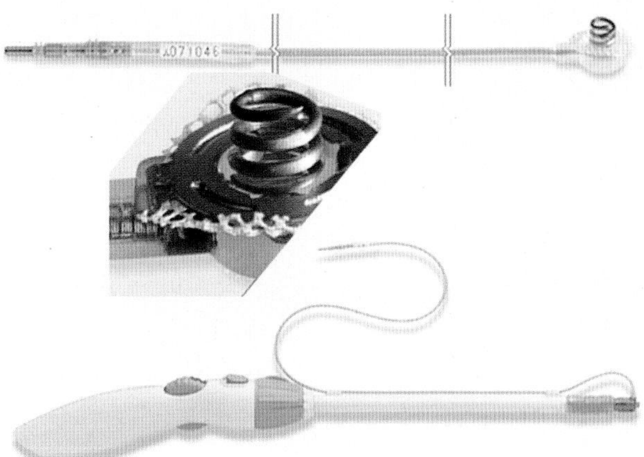

Figure 19-197. Top, *MyoPore Sutureless Bipolar Epicardial Pacing Lead.* Middle, *Close-up of the electrode portion of the lead.* Bottom, *FasTac Flex Epicardial Lead Implant Tool with a pacing lead attached. (Devices made by Enpath Medical, Inc., Plymouth, Minn., and marketed by St. Jude Medical, St. Paul, Minn.).*

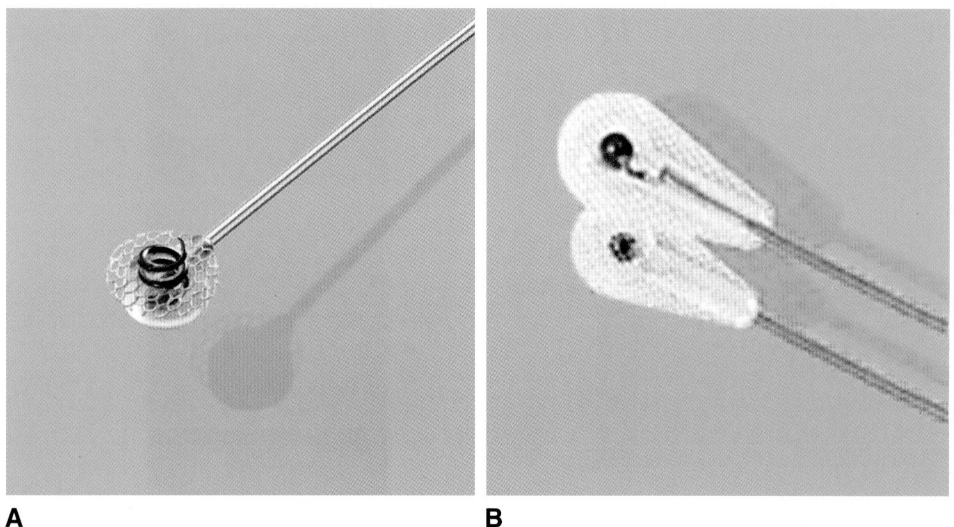

*Figure 19-198. Screw in **(A)** and sew on **(B)** epicardial leads from Biotronik GmbH & Co. (Berlin, Germany).*

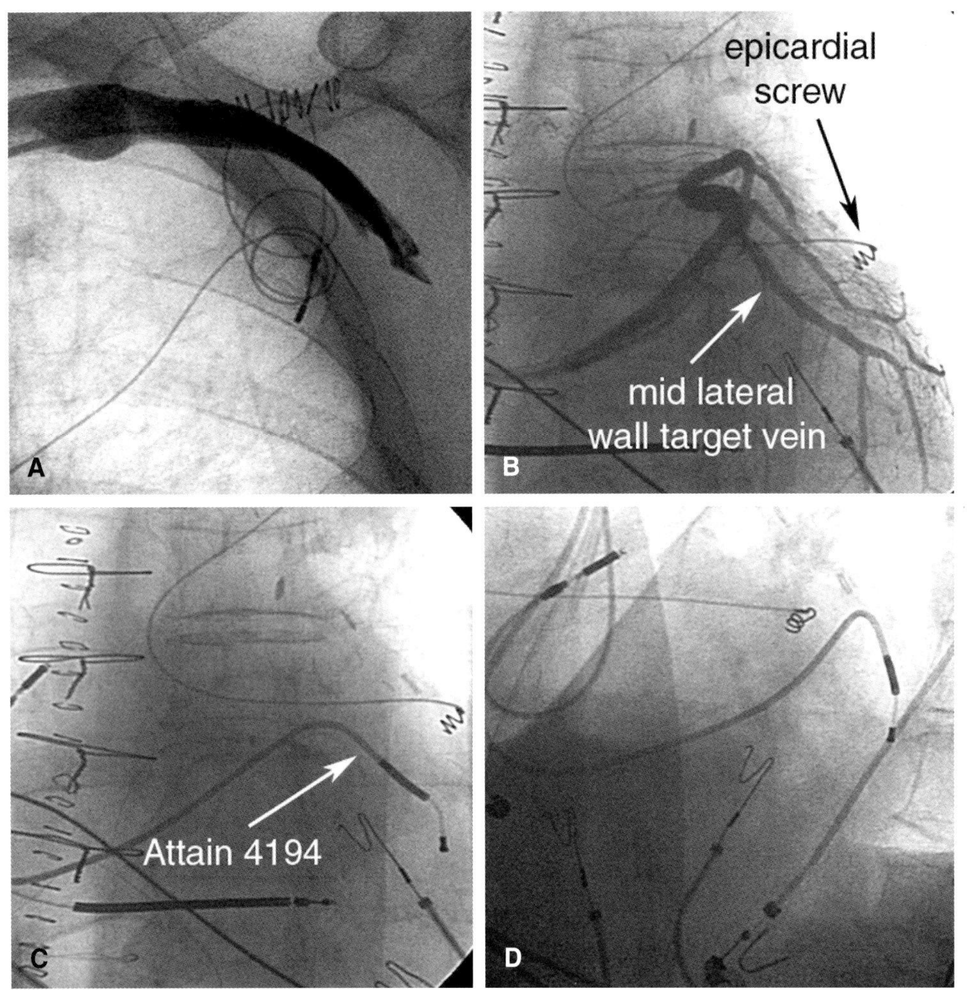

Figure 19-199. *Epicardial versus transvenous lead placement for biventricular pacing.* ***A,*** *The IS-1 connector end of the epicardial lead is shown in relation to the axillary vein.* ***B,*** *The epicardial screw-in lead and the occlusive coronary sinus venogram are shown.* ***C,*** *The anteroposterior view of the Attain 4194 transvenous lead (Medtronic, Inc., Minneapolis, Minn.) and epicardial lead are shown.* ***D,*** *The left anterior oblique view of the Attain 4194 and epicardial lead are shown. On the basis of the coronary sinus venogram, the transvenous lead is in the ideal anatomic position on the midlateral wall. The epicardial lead is not in the ideal anatomic position.*

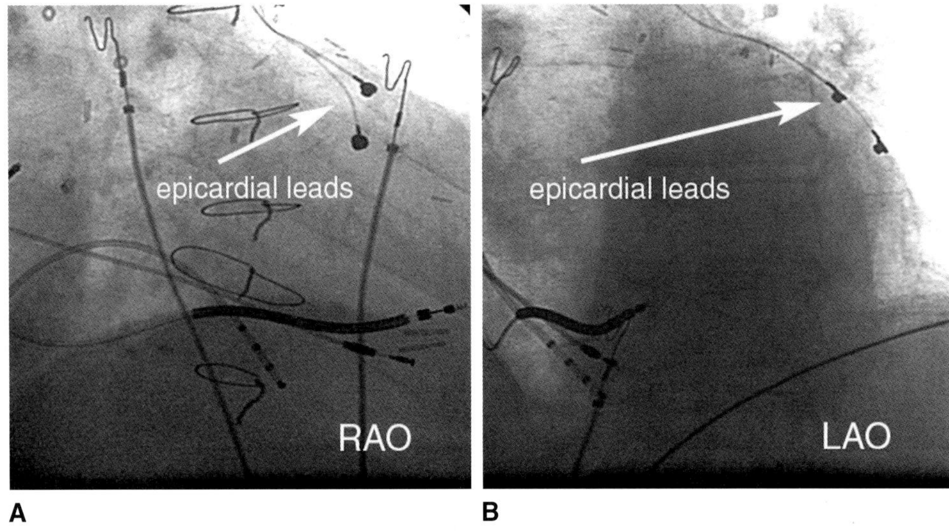

Figure 19-200. *Right anterior oblique (RAO) (**A**) and left anterior oblique (LAO) (**B**) views of epicardial leads placed at the time of open heart surgery for biventricular pacing.*

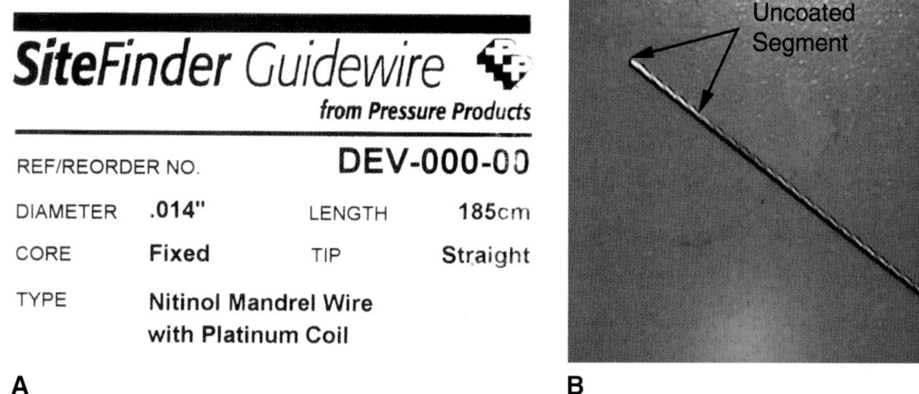

Figure 19-201. Pacing angioplasty wire to test for viability and phrenic pacing before lead placement. ***A,*** *Label for the SiteFinder Guidewire (Pressure Products, Inc., San Pedro, Calif.).* ***B,*** *A photomicrograph of the tip of the SiteFinder showing the uncoated distal 5 mm of the tip of the wire. The resistance between the tip and proximal end is 45 Ω.*

catheter can be used as insulation to cover the wire except at the tip. Alternatively, the SiteFinder Guidewire (Pressure Products, Inc.; Fig. 19-201) can be used. The SiteFinder is insulated with a lubricious coating except at the proximal and distal 5 mm.

Extraction of a Transvenous Left Ventricular Pacing Lead

A section on LV pacing leads is not complete without a comment on lead extraction. Limited data are available on LV lead extraction.[40,41] To date there have been no reported complications, presumably because of the age of the patient at the time of implantation and the duration of the implant. Given a fixed set of clinical criteria (patient age at the time of implantation and implant duration), ease of extraction can be predicted on the basis of the presence or absence of tines, coils, or an expanded tip. Each of these physical characteristics makes it more difficult to withdraw a lead through a thick fibrous capsule surrounding it. If the lead is isodiametric or tapers at the tip, there will be less resistance to removal. For example, the Attain 2187 lead, which tapers slightly from its tip, and the QuickSite and EASYTRAK 3 leads, which are isodiametric, would be easier to remove than an Attain 4193 (expanded tip), Attain 4194 (coil and expanded tip), or EASYTRAK 1 or 2 lead (tines).

Venoplasty Techniques for Cardiac Resynchronization

The Buddy Wire Technique

The buddy wire technique is used to advance a pacing lead beyond a tortuous area without the need for venoplasty. With the buddy wire technique, a stiff angioplasty wire (the buddy wire) is used to straighten a tortuous or looped vascular segment, allowing the LV lead to pass more easily.[31,42] The ability to advance the stiff part of the wire through the tortuous vein segment requires a stable CS platform; otherwise, the sheath will be displaced and the wire will not advance. After the vein is straightened, the stiff wire is left in place, and the lead is delivered over a second, softer wire (tracking wire) or with a stylet. The straightening wire should be an extra-support wire (e.g., Choice PT Extra Support or Platinum Plus ST), whereas the tracking wire should be a floppy wire (e.g., Choice PT Floppy). Figure 19-202 is a diagrammatic representation of the method; Figure 19-203 illustrates a patient in whom the lead would not pass beyond the tortuous area despite support from the sheath in the CS and an LVI in the target vein. With a stiff wire straightening the vein, however, the pacing lead encountered less resistance and was advanced over the soft wire.

Coronary Sinus and Percutaneous Coronary Venoplasty

The ability to confidently perform coronary vein venoplasty revolutionizes the operator's approach to LV lead placement. With venoplasty, leads are placed transvenously in areas that were previously accessible only via surgery. With venoplasty, the operator is far less dependent on the venous anatomy. Venoplasty of the main CS, stenotic target veins, and/or collateral vessels between two veins virtually eliminates failed implantations and the need to accept a suboptimal LV lead position. With coronary vein venoplasty, the operator is empowered to place LV leads in a target area rather than being constrained by the venous anatomy.[43,44] Despite the advantages of venoplasty, however, the technique is not yet widely used.[1]

To perform coronary vein venoplasty successfully, the operator must establish a stable platform in the CS from which to work. First, a long sheath is placed in the CS that is large enough to accept a preshaped LVI (guide), which is in turn large enough for the pacing lead to fit through. Currently, this requires a 9F sheath (9F ID/11F OD) and an 8F or 9F LVI (guide; 8F OD/6F ID or 9F OD/7F ID). After occlusive CS venography, a preshaped guiding catheter suitable for the anatomy is selected. The preshaped guide is advanced through the CS sheath

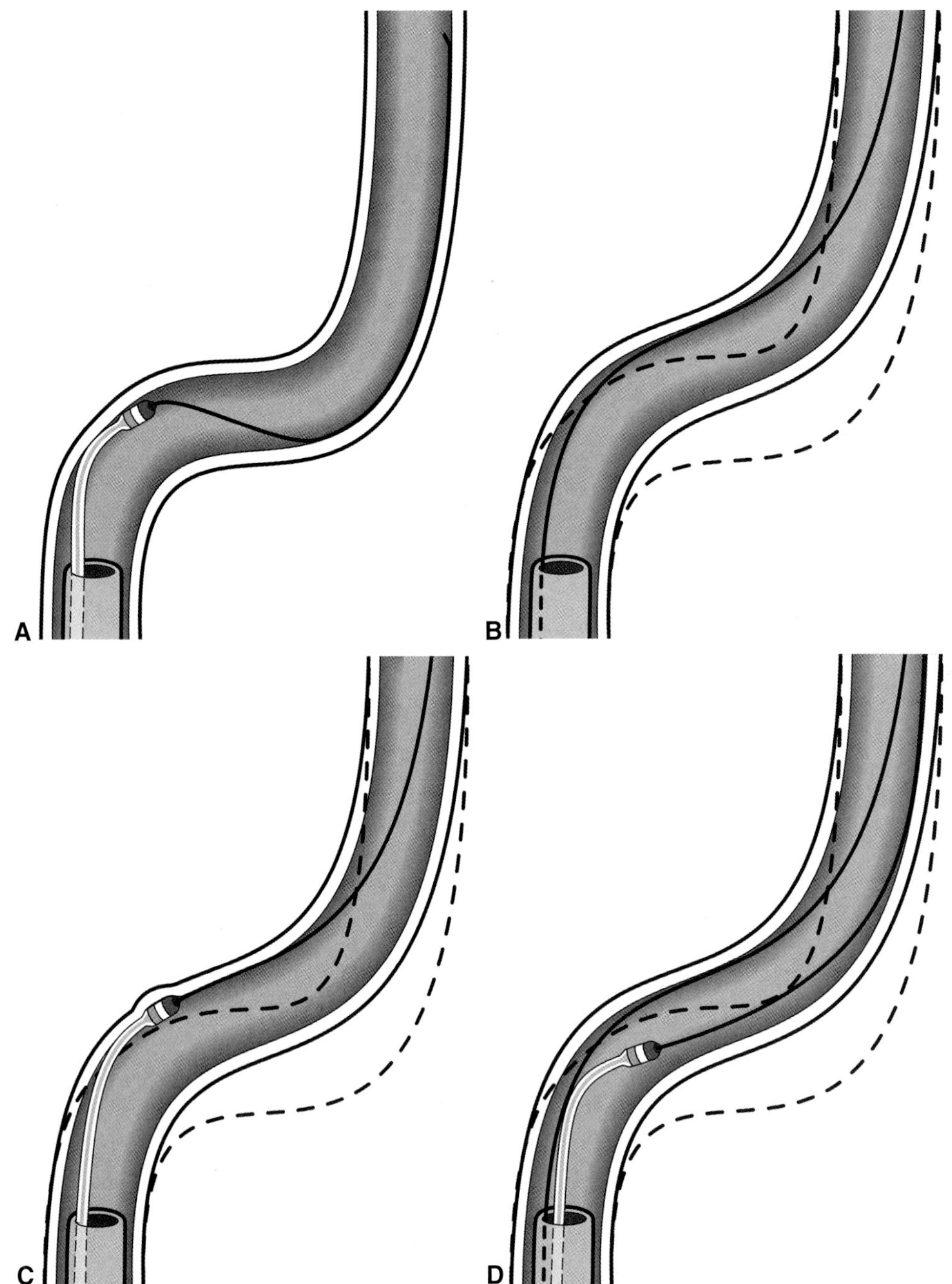

Figure 19-202. Buddy wire used to straighten a tortuous vein segment. ***A,*** *The vein segment is too tortuous to allow the lead to advance over the wire.* ***B,*** *A "stiff" angioplasty wire is advanced beyond the tortuous segment, straightening the vein.* Dotted lines *indicate the course of the vein before it was straightened by the stiff wire.* ***C,*** *The pacing lead is advanced over the stiff wire but gets stuck as the lead is forced into the roof of the vein.* ***D,*** *The stiff wire is left in place to straighten the vein, becoming the* buddy wire. *The pacing lead is delivered over a second, softer wire, the* tracking wire. *To keep the tracking wire and lead centered, one must keep as much tension on the wire as possible without pulling it out of the vein.*

to the target vein (third-generation telescoping system). Although some angioplasty techniques can be accomplished with only a first- or second-generation telescoping system, the absence of the direction and support provided by a third-generation telescoping system increases the difficulty and reduces success (see later).

A stenotic lesion in the main body of the CS or the lateral wall target vein often prevents placement of the LV pacing lead in the ideal location on the lateral wall of the LV. In other cases the target vein may be too small or even occluded, preventing access to the desired area on the LV free wall. Percutaneous coronary venoplasty (PCV) is a safe and effective alternative to either implantation failure or accepting a less desirable lead position.

We have performed PCV in 158 of 1400 patients since our first CRT case in 1999. Initially, we used PCV

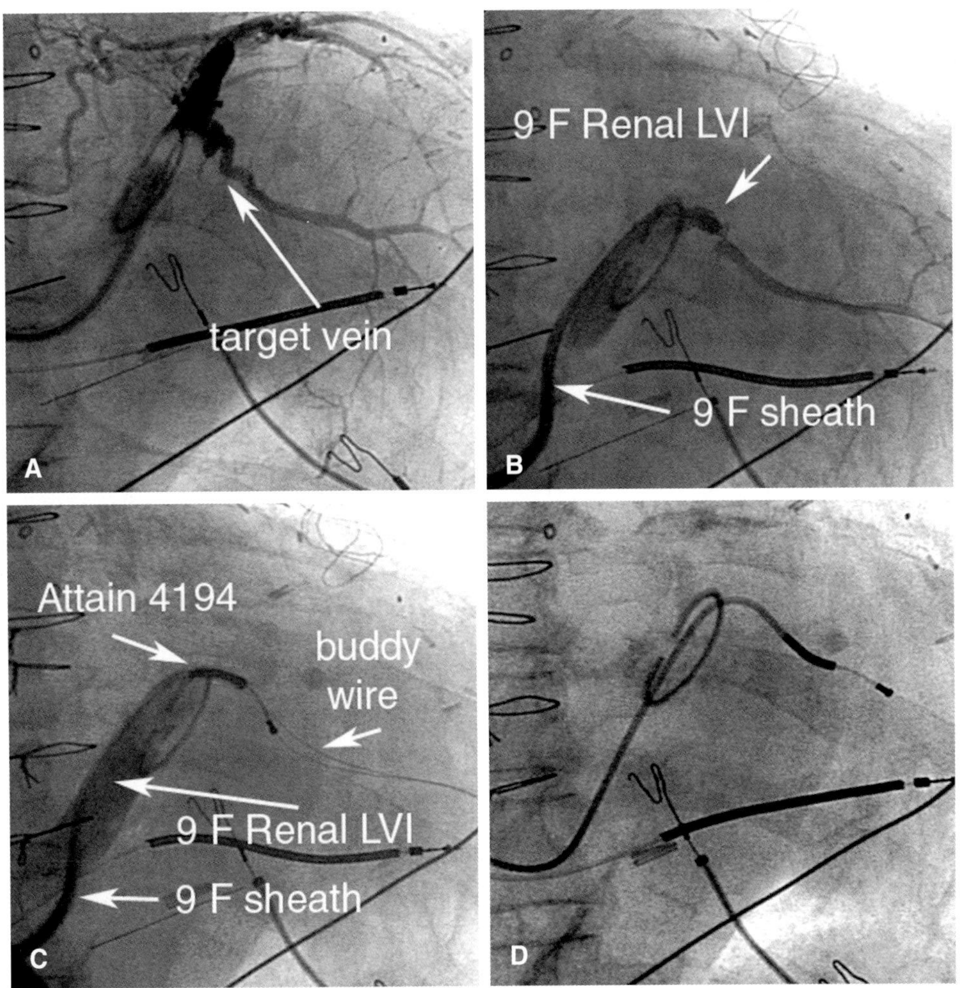

Figure 19-203. Buddy wire used to straighten vein for left ventricular (LV) lead placement. ***A****, The midlateral wall target vein is demonstrated to be tortuous.* ***B,*** *A 9F OD/7F ID renal lateral vein introducer (LVI) is inserted into the target vein through a 9F sheath in the main coronary sinus (CS). A tortuous (or stenotic) segment remains beyond the tip of the guide, preventing the lead from advancing.* ***C,*** *A stiff buddy wire is advanced into and straightens the target vein. The pacing lead is tracked over a floppy angioplasty wire. Both wires are introduced directly into the target vein through the renal LVI. The combined effect of the buddy wire and the support provided by the LVI is enough to advance the lead beyond the tortuous area into a stable position.*

as a last resort. As we became comfortable with the safety and efficacy of the procedure, we used it more often. The importance of a specific LV location further increased use. The rate of first-attempt success in our last 300 patients with first-time implantations was 98%. Venoplasty is credited with success or ideal placement in 15%. Our first-attempt success rate in the last 50 patients with a previously failed attempt was 98%. Venoplasty is credited with successful/ideal lead placement in 40%. The majority of our patients undergoing coronary vein venoplasty (79%) had prior OHS. The overall success rate for coronary vein venoplasty (defined as the ability to pass the lead beyond the stenosis) was 75%. Cine-review of our first 100 cases showed that venoplasty failed when a straight guide was used, whereas failure was rare with a preshaped guide directed into the os of the target vein. Recognition of the importance of directing the preshaped guide into the target vein improved our success rate to 95% in the last 50 cases. Venoplasty can fail from lack of guide support (Fig. 19-204).

If a preshaped guide is used, lateral pressure will direct the tip of the guide into the vein beyond the stenosis as the balloon is deflated. In some cases, venoplasty will fail owing to the use of a straight guide (Fig. 19-205). To ensure success, a guide preformed to fit into the takeoff of the vein is advanced over the balloon into the vein as the balloon is deflated. With the tip of the guide beyond the stenosis, the lead will advance.

Venoplasty of the Main Coronary Sinus

On occasion, a fixed stenosis in the main CS completely prevents advancement of the pacing lead. Balloon venoplasty is used to relieve the stenosis and permit lead placement. To get the wire past the stenosis, we occasionally use a multipurpose catheter (4F to 6F) passed through the CS platform to provide additional

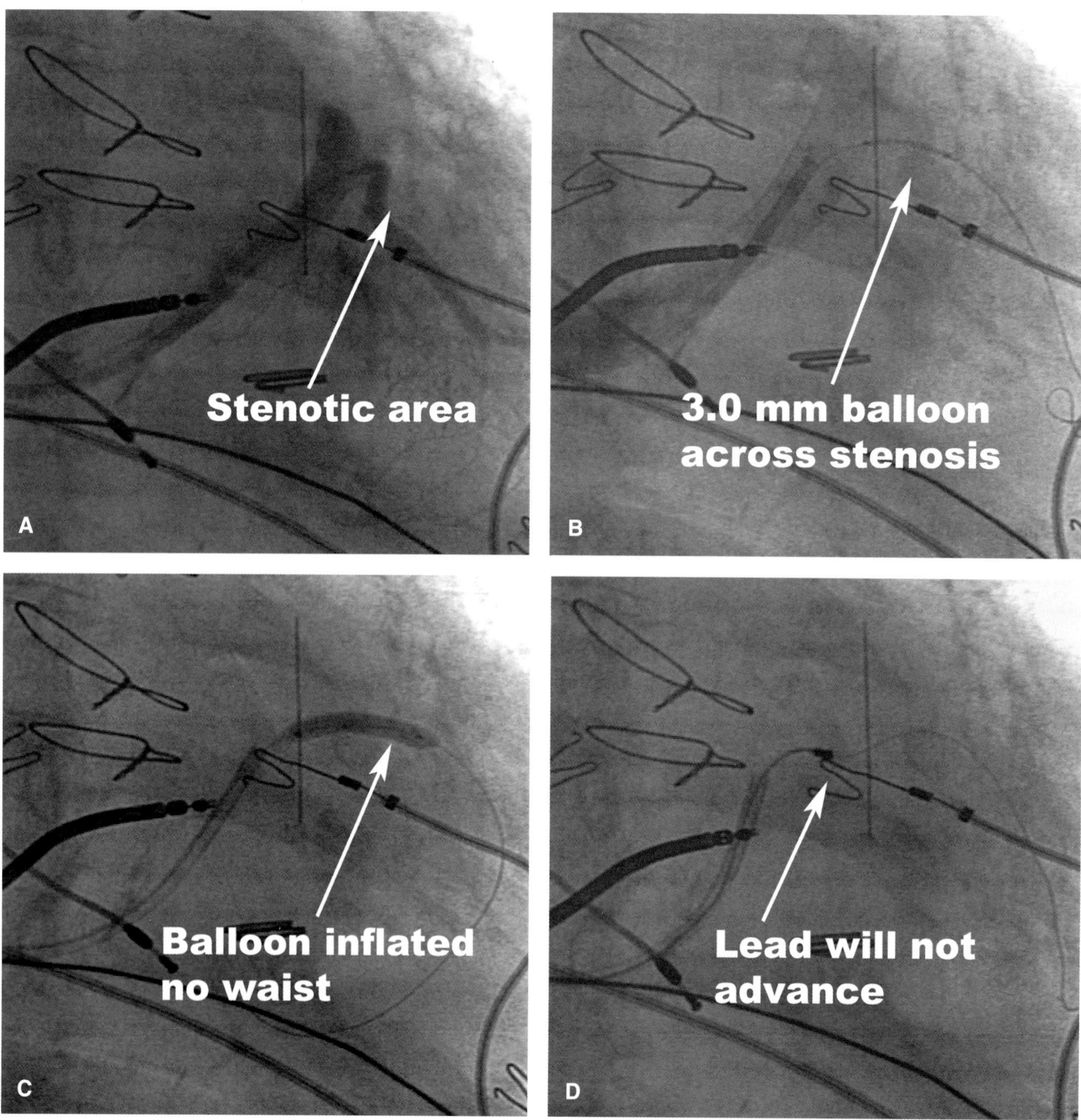

Figure 19-204. Venoplasty fails owing to lack of guide support. ***A,*** *The stenotic area of the vein is identified as a first-generation telescoping system delivers the wire.* ***B,*** *After the pacing lead fails to advance, a 3-mm balloon is placed across the narrowing.* ***C,*** *The balloon is inflated to 15 atm with elimination of the waist, indicating that the stenosis is eliminated.* ***D,*** *Despite successful balloon dilation, the pacing lead does not advance. Venoplasty has failed because of the lack of guide support. This situation required a preformed directional guide (third-generation telescoping system).*

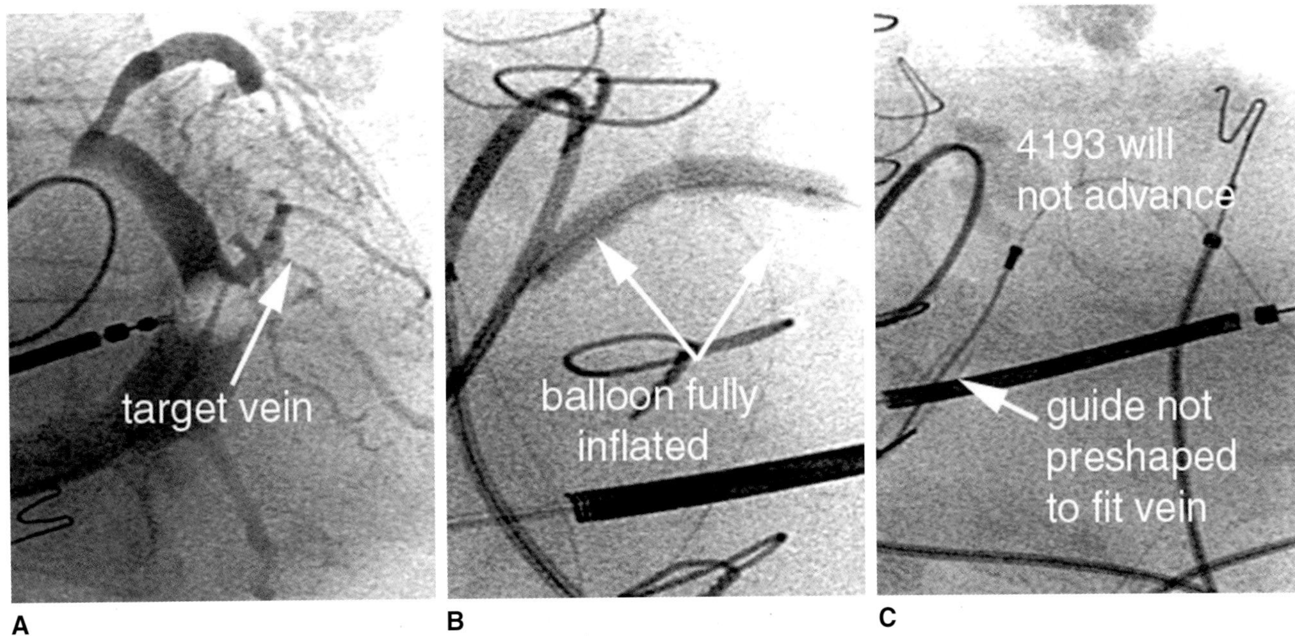

Figure 19-205. Venoplasty using a straight guide fails. ***A,*** *The target vein is shown.* ***B,*** *There is no residual stenosis when the 3-mm balloon is inflated to 16 atm.* ***C,*** *The left ventricular lead (Attain 4193 pacing lead, Medtronic, Inc., Minneapolis, Minn.) will not advance from the straight guide over the wire into the target vein.*

wire support and direction. With the small catheter beyond the stenosis, contrast material is injected to confirm wire position before balloon dilation. Figure 19-204 is an example of a high-grade stenosis preventing the pacing lead from reaching the target vein. After dilation, the lead is delivered through a preshaped guide advanced through the sheath into the vein (Fig. 19-206).

Venoplasty of Small or Stenotic Target Veins

When the tip of the third-generation guide is in the os of the target vein, the fine points of guidewire manipulation are less critical because the guide supports the balloon. To ensure that the balloon is advanced only over the firm segment of the wire (not the soft tip), the operator should advance the angioplasty wire beyond the stenosis as far as possible before attempting to advance the balloon. To keep the wire straight as the balloon is advanced, the operator applies gentle traction to the wire. When the wire is advanced distally into the collateral vessels, more traction can be placed on the wire to keep it straight without causing it to retract. If the wire does retract somewhat as the balloon is advanced, sufficient wire is left within the target vein to continue advancing the balloon over the firm section of the wire. When a preshaped telescoping guide fits securely in the os of a large vein, the angioplasty wire can be advanced distally against the resistance of the stenosis and the venous structures beyond without buckling. Thus, it is easier to perform venoplasty in a large vein with a discrete stenosis than in a small vein, because the tip of the guide is outside the os of a small vein.

Figure 19-207 depicts the use of PCV to enlarge a diffusely small and stenotic vessel. Occlusive CS venography showed extremely limited options for target veins. A preshaped guide was placed at the os of the target vein. The lead would not follow despite the use of a buddy wire. A 3-mm balloon was advanced and inflated to 20 atm. The "bone" indicating residual stenosis was eliminated. Contrast injection showed that the target vein was large enough to accept the lead, which was easily placed and yielded a pacing threshold of 0.8 V at 0.5 msec without phrenic pacing. Preformed guides specific to the anatomy of the side branch can be the key to venoplasty and lead implantation (Fig, 19-208). When there is no suitable preformed guide for the anatomy, the balloon may be used to "pull" the guide into the target vein (Fig. 19-209).

Angioplasty of Venous Collateral Vessels

Placement of the LV lead on the lateral wall may be foiled by phrenic pacing, high pacing thresholds, or veins that are extremely small or totally occluded. When the veins to the midlateral LV free wall are too small or stenotic to accept the LV lead, an alternative or "bailout vein" is used. Although such a procedure is a technical success, the lead has not been placed where the implanter believes is optimal. When there is no bailout vessel, the implantation fails. Venoplasty of venous collateral vessels is used to avoid failure and suboptimal lead position.

The angioplasty wire frequently passes from one vein to another through a collateral vessel and reenters

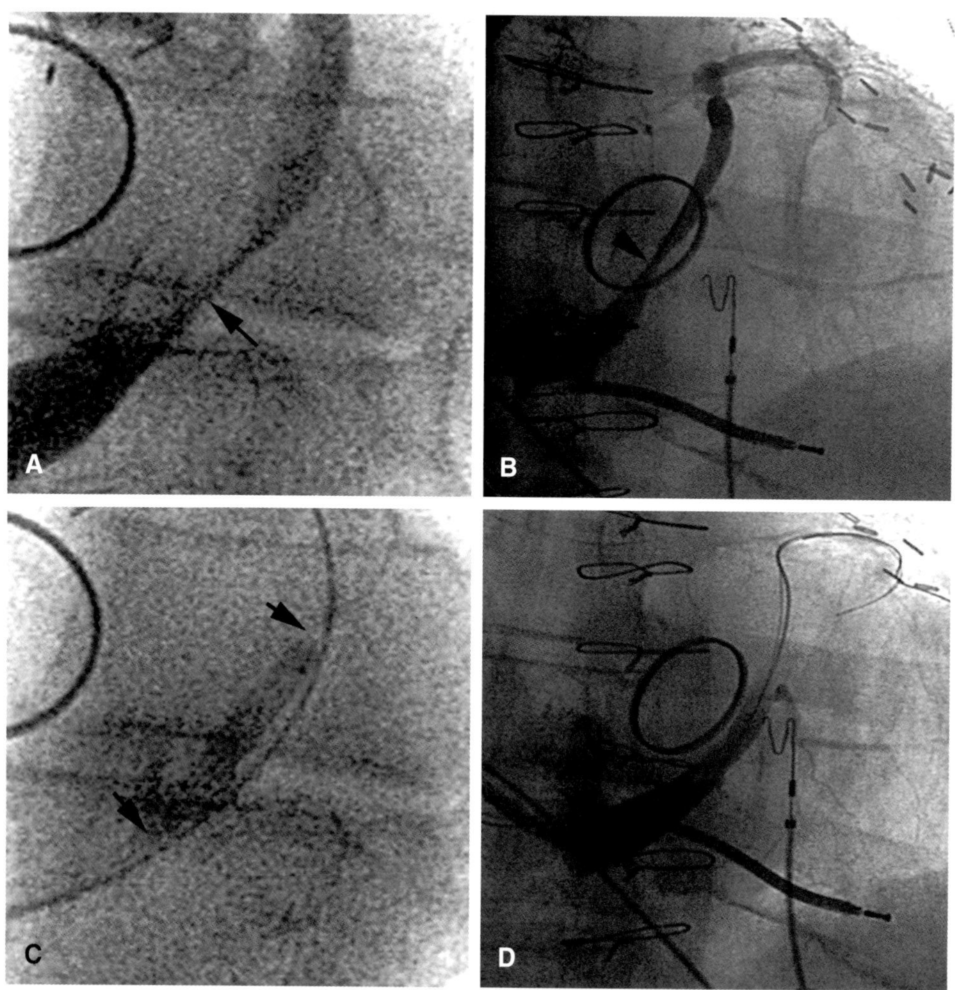

Figure 19-206. Balloon venoplasty of the main coronary sinus. ***A,*** *The stenosis* (arrow) *can be seen on the left anterior oblique projection.* ***B,*** *On the anteroposterior projection, the lateral wall target vein is at the 2-o'clock position on the mitral valve ring* (arrow). ***C,*** *A 40-mm balloon is inflated at the site of the stenosis. The proximal and distal ends of the balloon are indicated by* arrows. ***D,*** *The site of stenosis after balloon angioplasty.*

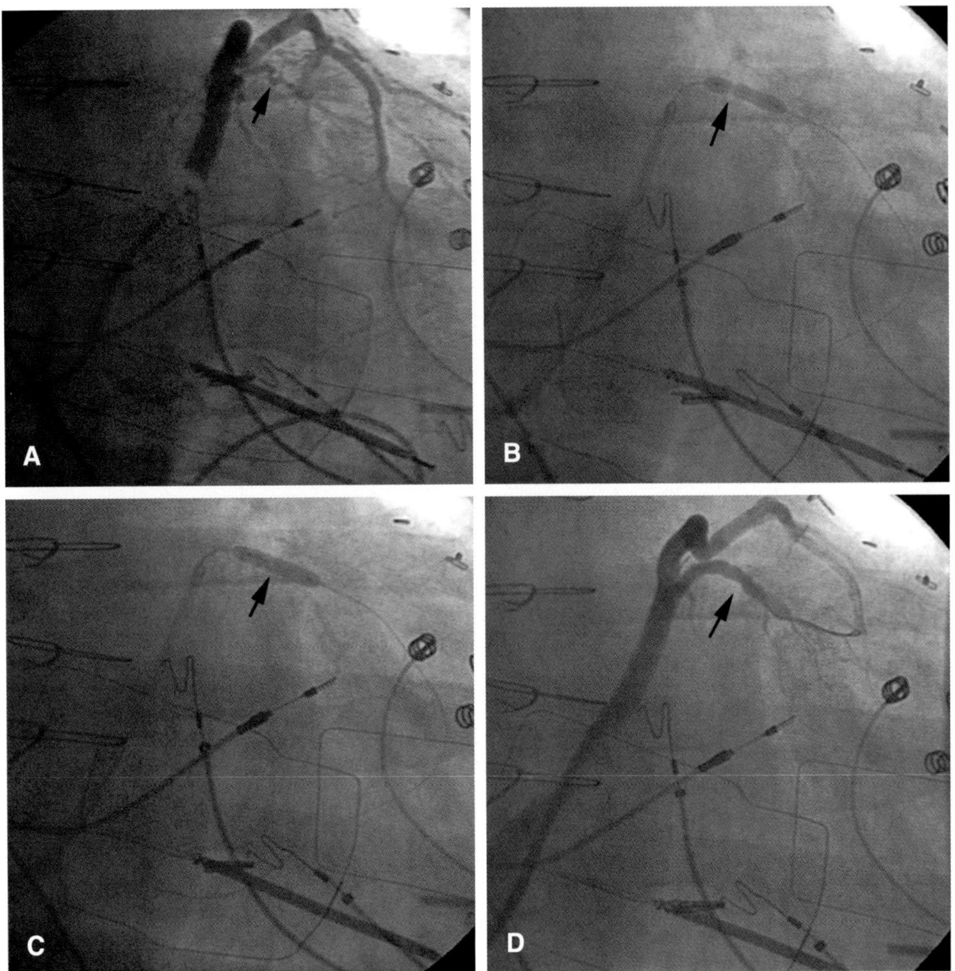

Figure 19-207. Diffusely small and stenotic vein enlarged with venoplasty. ***A,*** *The only lateral wall target vein* (arrow) *is too small to permit placement of a left ventricular (LV) pacing lead.* ***B,*** *A 3.5 mm × 18 mm, noncompliant balloon is inflated in the target vein. A stenotic segment is signified by the indentation in the balloon* (arrow) *at 15 atm.* ***C,*** *The balloon is inflated to 20 atm, and the stenosis is eliminated* (arrow)*.* ***D,*** *The enlarged target vein is filled with contrast material from the guiding catheter in the vein.*

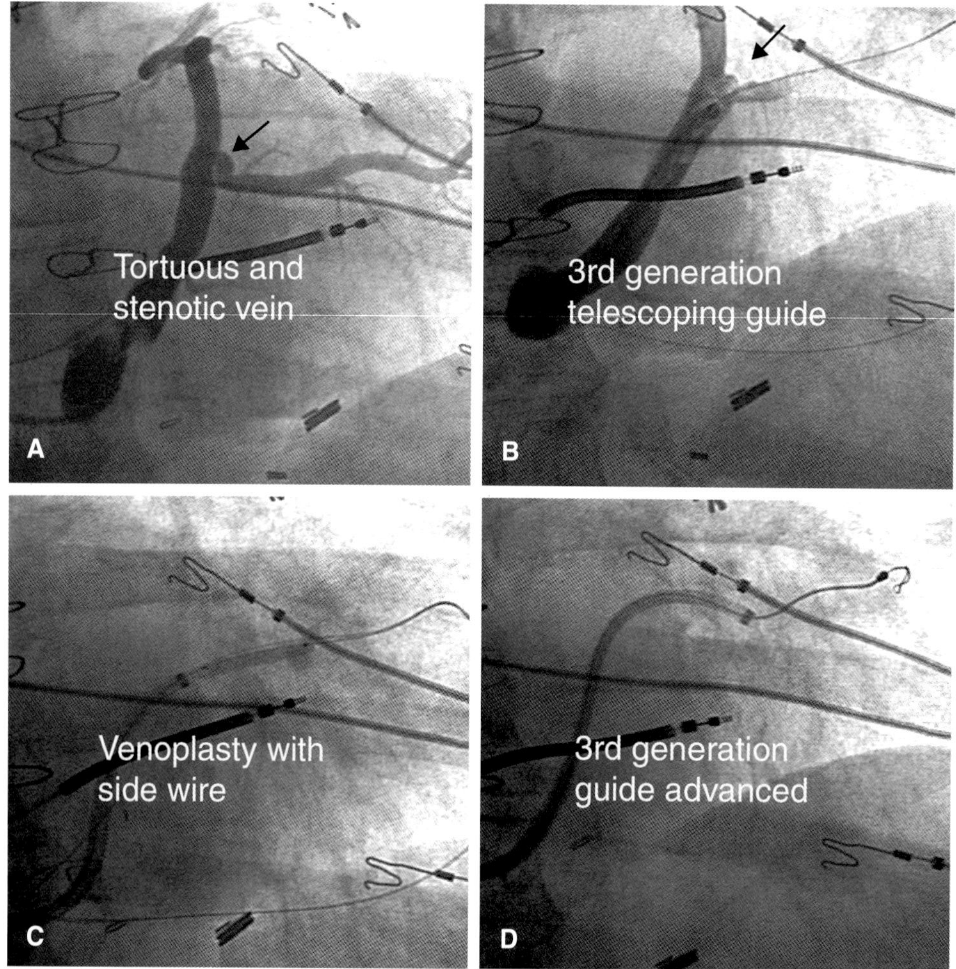

Figure 19-208. Successful venoplasty of a tortuous stenotic vein with a third-generation preformed guide (hockey stick lateral vein introducer [LVI]). ***A,*** *The origin of the vein is tortuous, as indicated by the double density of the coronary sinus (CS) near the origin of the vein* (arrow) *and the course of the vein beyond the CS.* ***B,*** *A third-generation preformed guide, selected to place the tip beyond the tortuous segment, is advanced over a wire into the CS above the vein. As the guide is withdrawn and contrast material is puffed in, the vein is identified. The wire is advanced from the guide into the vein. Neither the guide nor the left ventricular (LV) lead advances into the vein. A stenosis is identified at the origin of the vein* (arrow). ***C,*** *A stiff second wire is added to straighten the vein (buddy wire). The lead still will not advance. A 30-mm balloon is centered at the os and inflated. As the balloon deflates, the preshaped guide advances into the vein.* ***D,*** *The tip of the guide is beyond the tortuous and stenotic segment. The LV lead is easily placed.*

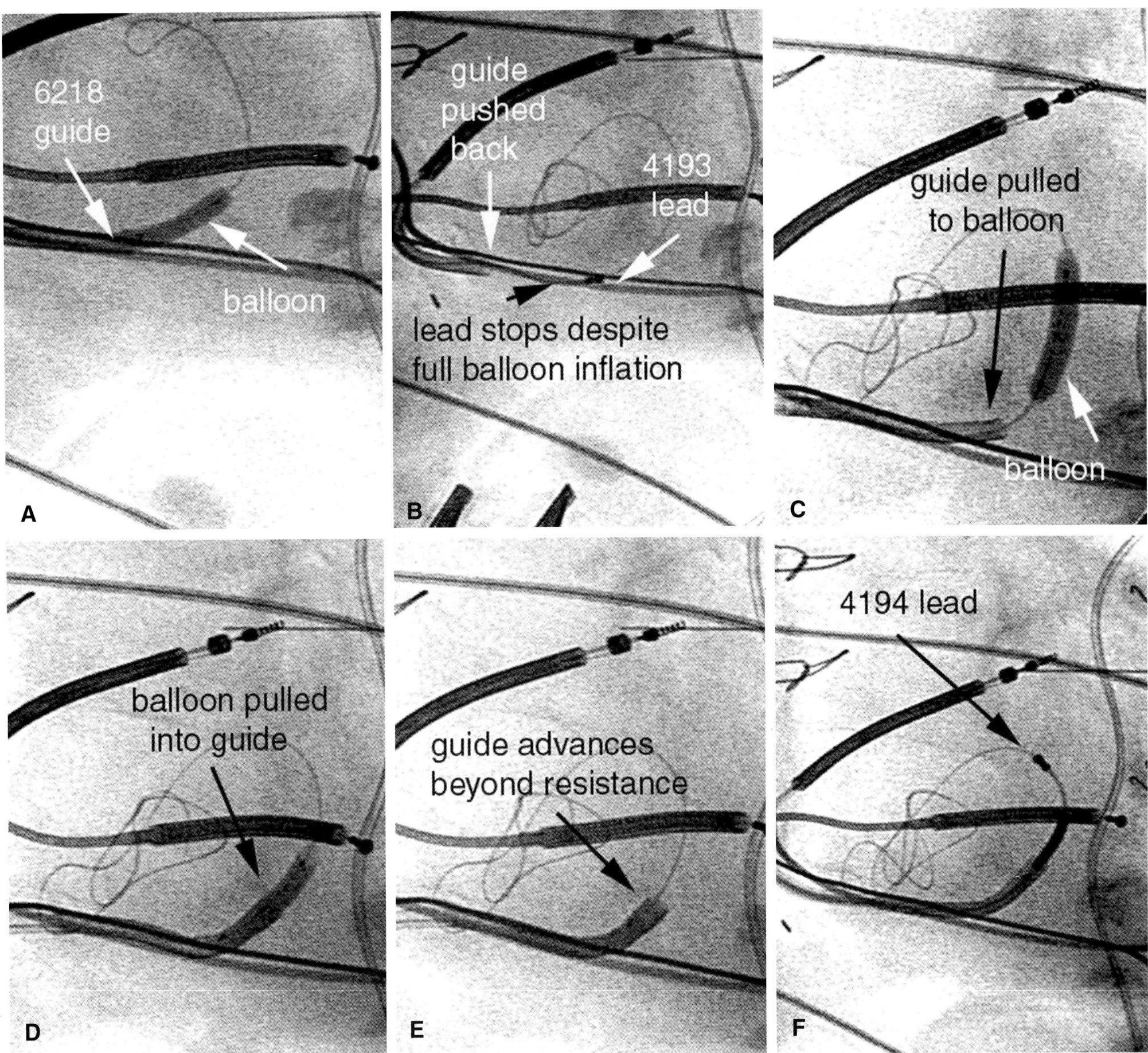

*Figure 19-209. Straight guide pulled into a small branch with angioplasty balloon. **A,** The 3-mm balloon is inflated in a small branch to the lateral wall off the large posterior branch, with an Attain 6218 guide (Medtronic, Inc., Minneapolis, Minn.). **B,** Despite full balloon inflation in the small branch, the Attain 4193 pacing lead (Medtronic, Inc.) will not track over the wire. Attempts to advance the lead caused the guide to back out. **C,** The 3.5-mm balloon is inflated in the small branch and used as an anchor. The guide is pulled toward the balloon. **D,** The guide is pulled over the balloon into the dilated branch. **E,** The balloon is deflated and removed. The tip of the guide is turned up into the vein. **F,** With the tip of the guide beyond the area of difficulty, the larger lead (Attain 4194, Medtronic, Inc.) will advance.*

the CS through the second vein (Fig. 19-210). In patients with previous OHS, these collaterals are freely used to reach the target area. Figure 19-210 demonstrates the dilation of the venous collateral between the posterior lateral and midlateral coronary veins. Previous attempts to place an LV lead on the lateral wall in the patient had failed because of phrenic pacing, high pacing thresholds, and limited access.

Although we primarily dilate collateral vessels in patients with previous heart surgery, there are situations in which the collaterals are large enough to be dilated in patients without prior cardiac surgery (Fig. 19-211).

With preshaped guiding catheters and the venoplasty techniques described here, successful placement of the LV lead on the lateral wall is possible in virtually every patient. Examples of multiple anatomic pitfalls overcome with guide support and venoplasty are shown in Figures 19-212 and 19-213.

Usually, percutaneous venous angioplasty (PCVA) is required in patients with a prior heart surgery, presumably owing to scar tissue or clips. Occasionally,

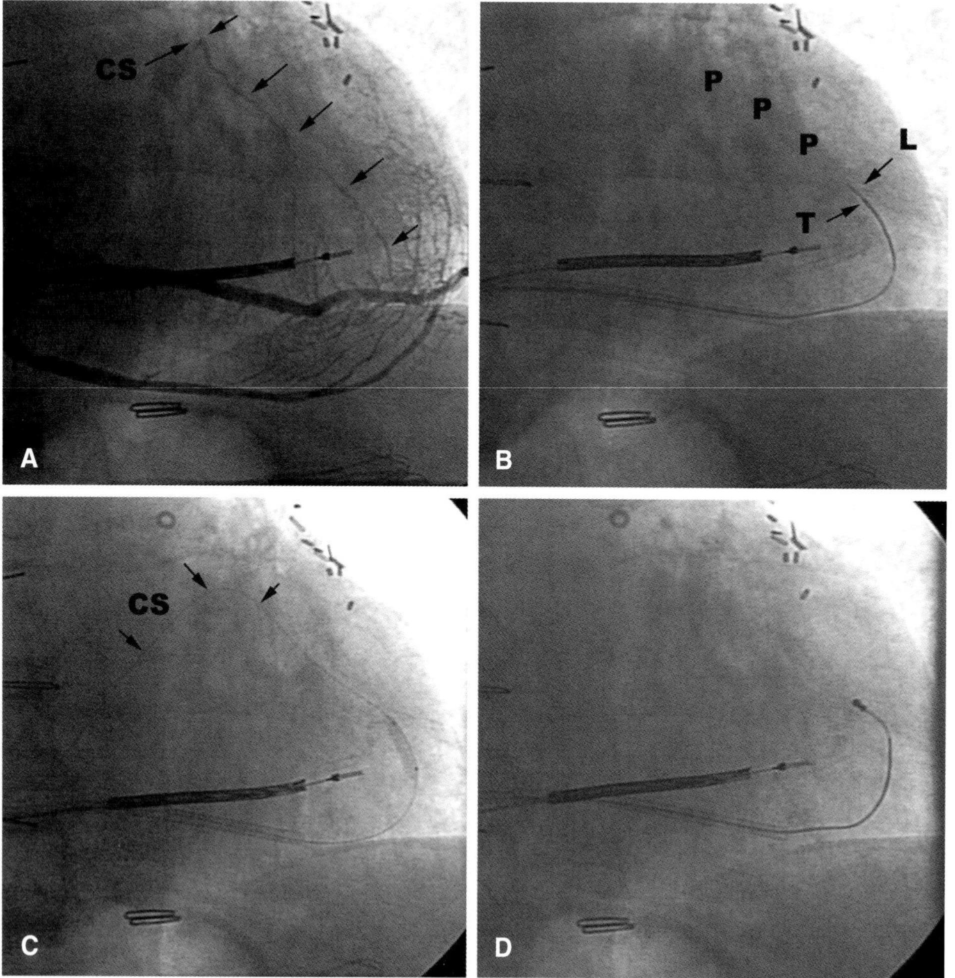

Figure 19-210. *Angioplasty of collateral vein in a patient with previous open heart surgery.* ***A,*** *Selective injection reveals the collateral vein connecting the posterior lateral coronary vein to the lateral vein* (arrows)*. Contrast material injected into the posterior lateral vein can be seen entering the coronary sinus (CS) through the lateral vein as a blush at the* upper arrow. *The lateral wall target vein could not be entered from the CS. Prior to proceeding with angioplasty of the collateral vein, the operator test-paced the target area with a Luge angioplasty wire insulated except at the tip (Pressure Products, Inc., San Pedro, Calif.) and a Cordis Transit infusion catheter (Cordis, Miami, Fla.).* ***B,*** *The Luge angioplasty wire (L) covered with the Transit catheter (T) is directed into the collateral vein to confirm pacing without phrenic stimulation before balloon dilation. The distal marker of the Transit catheter is indicated by an* arrow *from T. The exposed electrically active segment of the Luge is indicated by the* arrow *from L. Pacing with this device establishes where phrenic pacing is a problem (indicated by P). The Transit catheter was then removed, leaving the angioplasty wire in place.* ***C,*** *The angioplasty wire* (arrows) *that starts in the posterior lateral vein returns to the CS through the lateral vein via collateral vessels. A 3.5-mm balloon is advanced into the collateral vein and inflated to 18 atm to create a channel for the pacing lead. The area of phrenic pacing, marked with a P, was not dilated.* ***D,*** *The left ventricular pacing lead is advanced into position, capturing at 0.5 V without phrenic pacing at 10 V.*

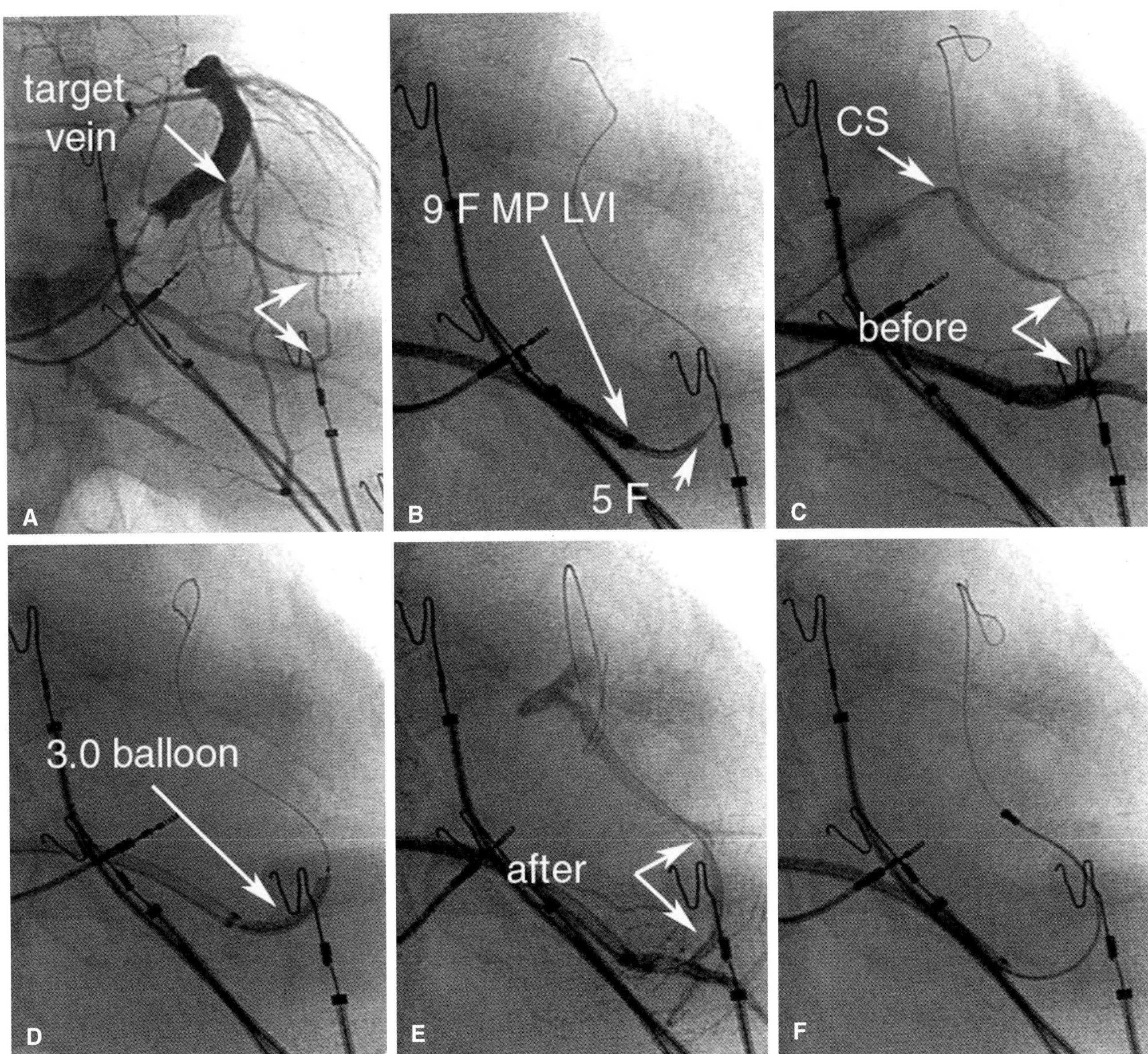

Figure 19-211. *Angioplasty of collateral vein in a patient without previous open heart surgery.* ***A,*** *A collateral venous structure connects the posterior lateral wall coronary vein to the midlateral vein (arrows).* ***B,*** *The angioplasty wire is placed in the collateral vein with use of a 5F Bernstein catheter inserted through a 7F ID/9F OD multipurpose lateral vein introducer (MP LVI).* ***C,*** *The 5F catheter is removed over the wire, leaving the LVI in place. Contrast material injected into the posterior lateral vein enters the coronary sinus (CS) retrograde through the lateral vein (the blush at the upper arrow labeled CS).* ***D,*** *A 3.0 mm × 15 mm noncompliant balloon (PowerSail, Guidant, Boston Scientific, Natick, Mass.) is advanced into the collateral vein and inflated to 12 atm to create a channel for the pacing lead.* ***E,*** *Injection of contrast material shows that the collateral vessel has been enlarged.* ***F,*** *An Attain OTW 4193 LV pacing lead (Medtronic, Inc., Minneapolis, Minn.) is advanced into position. The lead captured at 0.5 V without phrenic pacing at 10 V.*

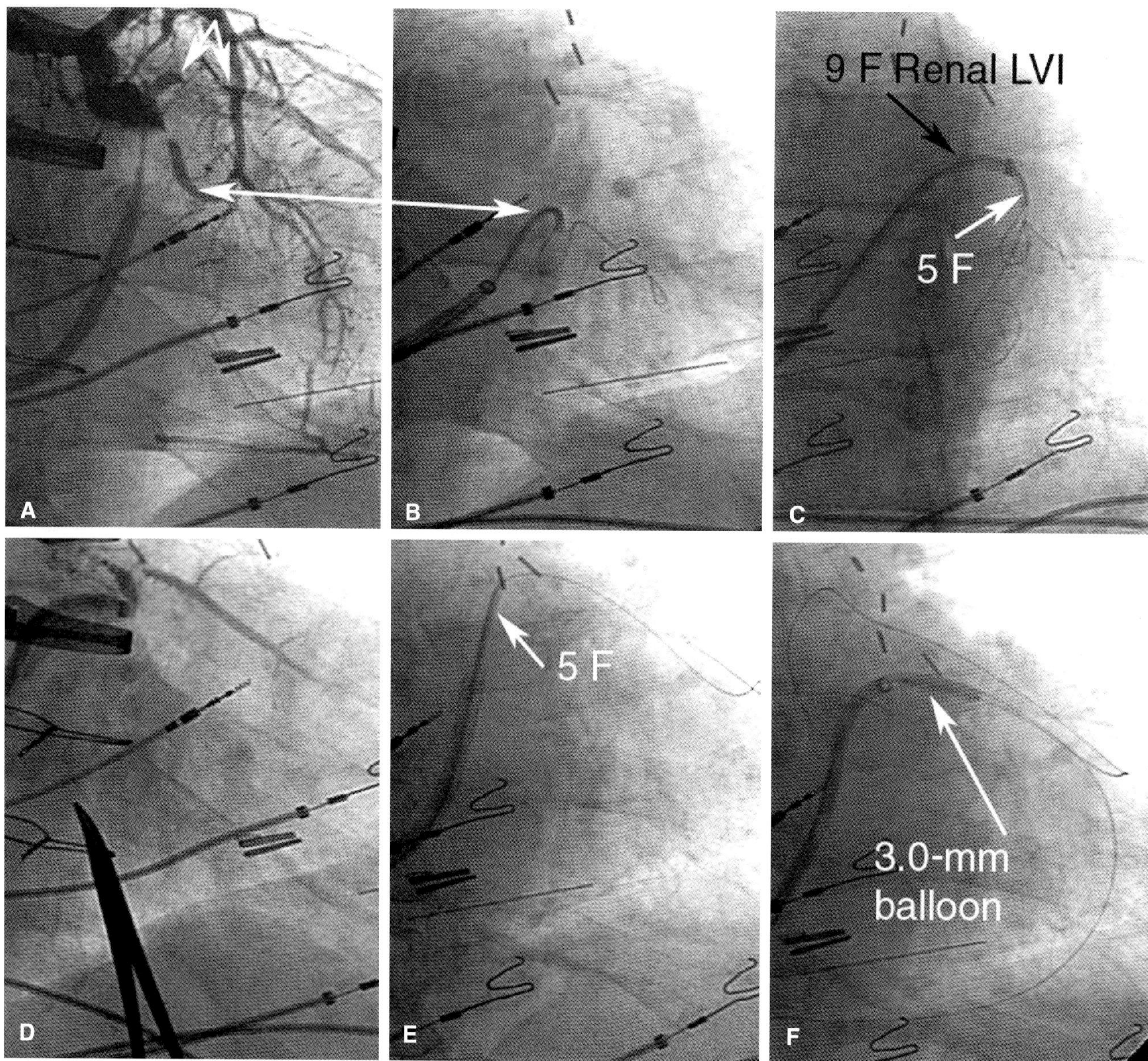

*Figure 19-212. Placement of a left ventricular lead despite the virtual absence of target veins and the presence of phrenic pacing, part 1. **A,** The occlusive coronary sinus (CS) venogram shows only two lateral wall target veins. The lower of the two (long arrow to **B**) is small with an acute takeoff. There is a subtotal occlusion in the higher lateral wall branch. **B,** The lower branch is cannulated with a 5F internal mammary artery (IMA) catheter catheter inside the 9F renal lateral vein introducer (LVI) (guide). **C,** The 9F renal LVI is advanced into the vein by means of the wire and used as a rail. The lead is placed, but pacing thresholds are higher than 5 V. **D,** The renal LVI is advanced to the mouth of the higher target vein. Injection of contrast material confirms the tortuous course of the vein and the subtotal occlusion. **E,** A 5F Bernstein catheter is inserted through the 9F guide into the vein, and an angioplasty wire is advanced deep into the vein beyond the stenosis. The wire and 5F IMA catheter are used as a rail to advance the renal LVI to the mouth of the target vein. **F,** The preformed shape of the guide directs the tip laterally into the target vein but is stopped by the stenosis. A 3-mm balloon is advanced across the occlusion and inflated.*

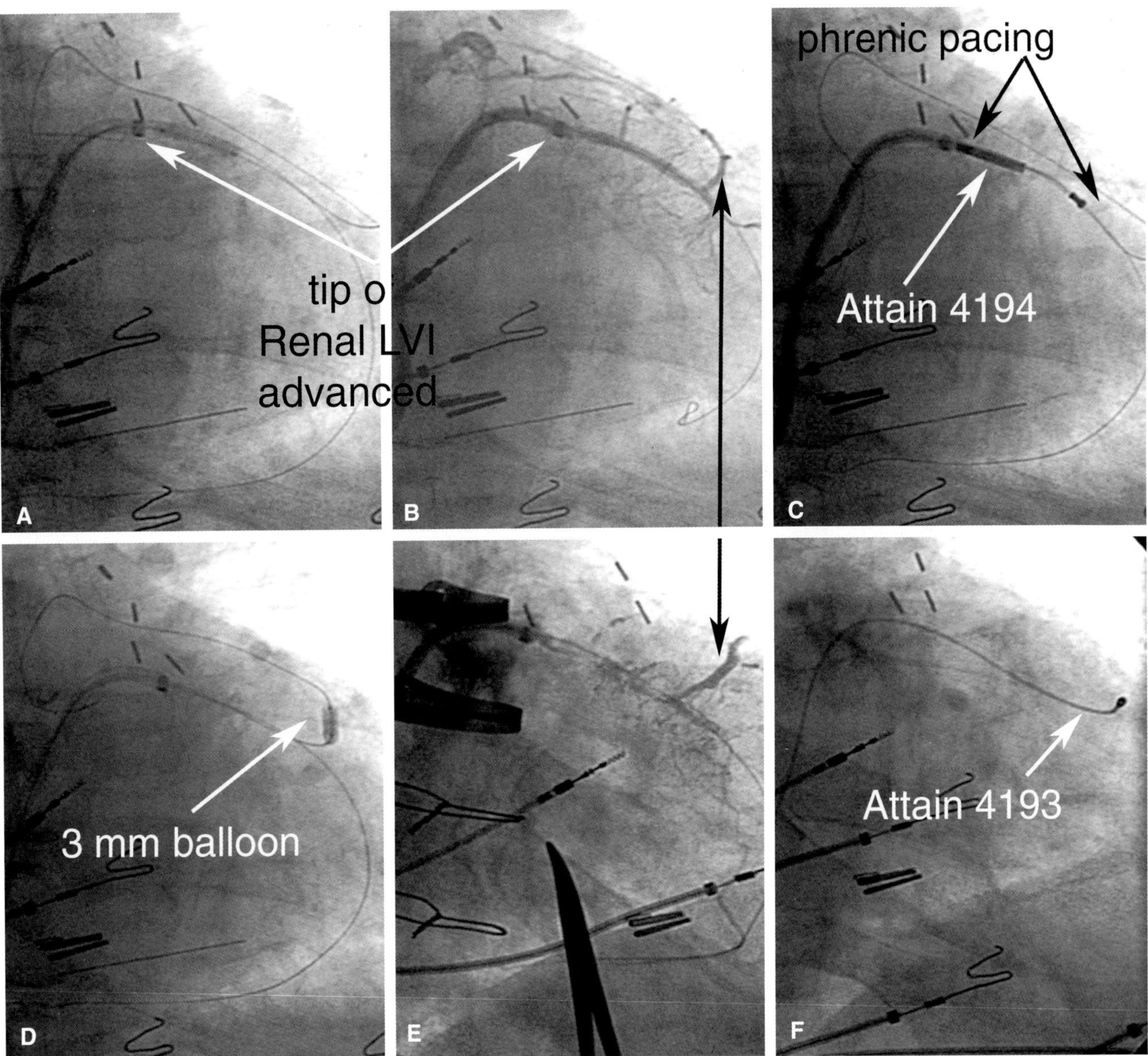

Figure 19-213. Placement of a left ventricular (LV) lead despite the virtual absence of target veins and the presence of phrenic pacing, part 2. ***A,*** *The balloon is inflated in the proximal stenosis with the tip of the renal lateral vein introducer (LVI) (guide) directed into the os of the target vein. Because of the shape of the guide, there is lateral pressure at the tip of the guide directing it into the vein. The guide will not advance because of the stenosis.* ***B,*** *Lateral pressure at the tip of the guide (resulting from its preformed shape) advances it into the target vein as the balloon deflates. Injection of contrast material confirms that the tip of the guide is beyond the stenotic segment.* ***C,*** *The Attain 4194 pacing lead (Medtronic, Inc., Minneapolis, Minn.) is advanced through the guide into the target vein. Phrenic pacing at outputs of less than 2 V is found in the vein.* ***D,*** *A 3-mm balloon is inflated in the small branch seen in* ***B*** *(black arrow).* ***E,*** *Injection of contrast material confirms that the small branch seen in* ***B*** *is enlarged (black arrow).* ***F,*** *The LV pacing lead, an Attain 4193 lead (Medtronic, Inc.) is placed in the dilated branch vein, where phrenic pacing is not encountered.*

however, a venous branch is stenotic in a patient without prior heart surgery (Fig. 19-214). We usually use a 3.0-mm balloon and limit the inflation pressure to 18 atm in patients without prior cardiac surgery. Figure 19-214 shows a patient without prior thoracotomy in whom the stenotic segment did not respond to application of 18 atm of pressure for more than 2 minutes. This represents one of our PCV failures.

What happens if the balloon bursts during the attempt to relieve a stenosis? Figure 19-215 demonstrates a patient with previously failed implantation who was denied surgical LV lead placement. The only target vein is cannulated with a preshaped guide large enough to place the lead directly.

In some cases even an ultra-noncompliant balloon (Boston Scientific NC Monorail or equivalent) taken to

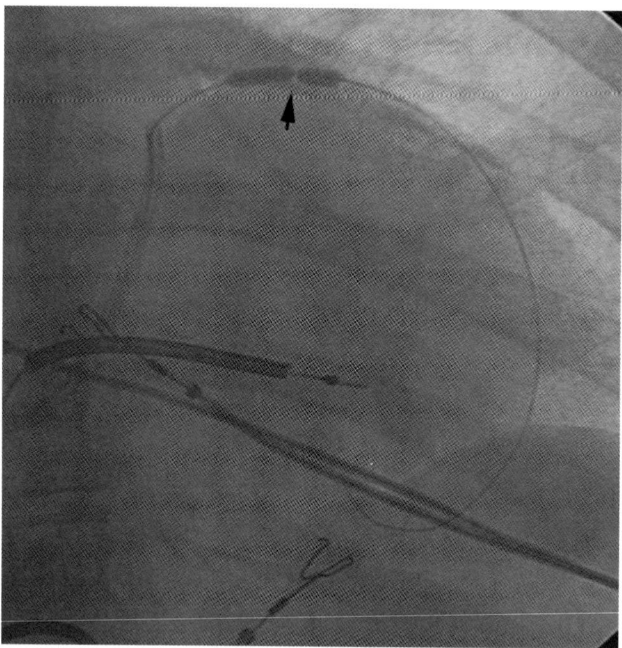

Figure 19-214. Persistent stenosis in a patient without prior open heart surgery. The 30-mm × 18-mm PowerSail balloon (Guidant, Boston Scientific, Natick, Mass.) is inflated to 18 atm. The stenosis is not eliminated, as indicated by the residual indentation (arrow) *in the balloon.*

the maximum pressure of the inflation device (25 atm) will not eliminate the stenosis. In this case, either the side-wire technique (Fig. 19-216) or a cutting balloon (Fig. 19-217) is used, usually in patients with prior cardiac surgery. The patient whose procedure is shown in Figure 19-216 had not had prior OHS.

Venoplasty with Stent Placement

A tortuous vein segment can usually be overcome with a third-generation telescoping system with or without the buddy wire technique. However, in some cases, the vein may be folded back on itself because of prior surgery, particularly mitral valve ring, repair, or replacement. In these cases, a stent may be required to straighten the vein long enough to allow the pacing lead to pass.[45] Figure 19-218 demonstrates a case in which the target vein was folded back on itself and required a stent to place the lead.

One of the questions frequently asked is, "What happens to the vein after venoplasty?" In the patient shown in Figure 19-219, initial placement of the LV lead required PCV with a 3.0-mm balloon. The LV lead became dislodged. Six days later, a second occlusive CS venogram demonstrated a widely patent vein. With use of a third-generation renal telescoping LVI, a larger, more stable LV lead was placed.

Choice of Angioplasty Balloon and Inflation Pressure for Venoplasty

Choice of angioplasty balloon is influenced by several interacting variables, as follows.

Composition of the Balloon

The composition of balloons may be compliant, noncompliant, or ultra-noncompliant. Ultra-noncompliant balloons are composed of thicker, less flexible material that makes them more difficult to advance across a stenosis. When inflated, they are more likely to eliminate the waist but reduce overexpansion of the proximal and distal sides of the waist. For coronary venoplasty, a "noncompliant balloon" (midrange in the compliance scale) is a good place to start. Such balloons track easily and relieve most stenotic areas. If the balloon will not advance across the stenosis, the first step is to reevaluate the guide support. After a guide with a size and shape suitable for the target vein is in place, the operator should consider downsizing the balloon, using one of the same composition (e.g. 3-mm to 2-mm) and/or changing to a more compliant balloon. Once the smaller or less compliant balloon is inflated across the lesion, the 3.0-mm balloon should be reinserted and inflated. If there is a residual waist after full inflation of a noncompliant balloon, an ultra-noncompliant balloon (e.g., NC Monorail) should be tried. The addition of a second (stiff) angioplasty wire beside the balloon before inflation will focus the force of the balloon on the narrowing.

Diameter of the Balloon

With PTCA, the size of the balloon an operator should start with is based on the estimated size of the normal coronary artery proximal and distal to the stenosis. However, with PCVA, the size of the pacing lead determines the size of the balloon. A 3.0-mm balloon inflated to at least nominal pressure or until the waist is eliminated is satisfactory for most situations. In patients with prior heart surgery, a 3.5-mm balloon may be required, and a 4.0-mm balloon for the distal main CS and a 5.0-mm balloon for the proximal main CS.

Length of the Balloon

The length of noncompliant balloon suitable for coronary venoplasty is 15 to 21 mm. For enlargement of a straight, diffusely narrow vein segment, a longer balloon may be chosen. Longer balloons tend to be more difficult to advance because of their greater surface area of resistance in the stenotic vein segment. If a very tight discrete stenosis is encountered, a shorter balloon with less resistance may be a better choice. However, longer balloons tend to be a bit more stable in the vein as well. The composition of the balloon material also influences the length. When an ultra-noncompliant or a cutting balloon is required, 9 to 10 mm is usually the best starting length The material required to construct the ultra-noncompliant balloon is relatively thick and stiff and thus is difficult to track through any curved vein segments, particularly if the balloon is long.

Inflation Pressure

Reviewing the packing material included with the balloon gives the best indicator of the appropriate pressure, with the following definitions kept in mind:

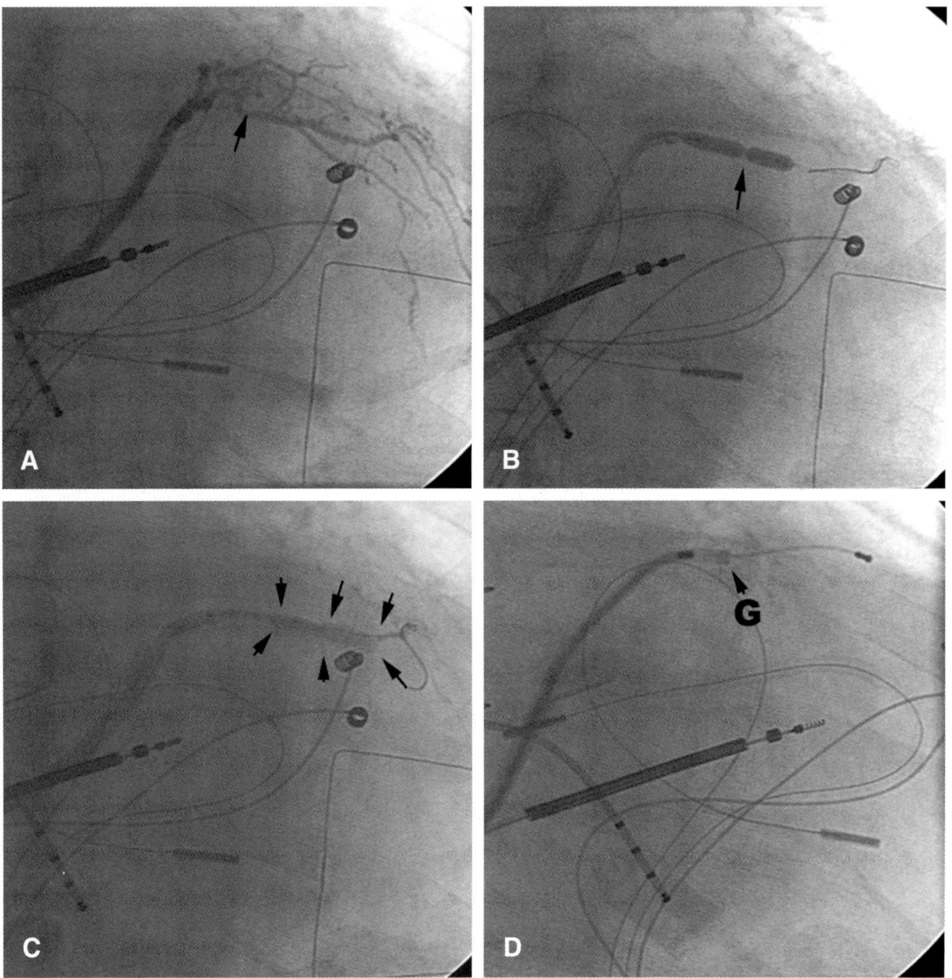

Figure 19-215. Angioplasty balloon bursts at 24 atm. ***A,*** *The only viable target vein* (arrow) *is identified. An improvised third-generation renal telescoping guide (8F, 55-cm Vistabritetip RDC-1, Cordis, Miami, Fla.) cannulates the vein. Neither a 4193 nor an Attain 2187 lead (Medtronic, Minneapolis, Minn.) could be advanced into the target vein.* ***B,*** *A 3.5 mm × 18 mm, noncompliant PowerSail balloon (Guidant, Boston Scientific, Natick, Mass.) is inflated to 24 atm without relief of the stenosis* (arrow). ***C,*** *The balloon ruptures from overinflation. Contrast material* (arrows) *can be seen in the pericardial space, limited by adhesions from prior open heart surgery.* ***D,*** *After inflation of an NC Monorail Balloon (ultra-noncompliant) (Boston Scientific Corporation, Natick, Mass.) to atm, the tip of the guide (G) advances further into the target vein. An Attain 4193 lead was initially placed, but it was removed because of high pacing thresholds. With the tip of the guide in the vein, an Attain 2187 lead (Medtronic, Inc., Minneapolis, Minn.) is advanced, yielding a pacing threshold lower than 2 V.*

- *Nominal pressure*—the pressure required for that balloon to achieve the rated size in an open system. If the balloon is not inflated to the nominal pressure, it will not reach the rated size. For example, the nominal pressure for a Cordis 3.5-mm RaptoRail is 6 atm, but that for a Boston Scientific 3.5-mm Quantum Maverick balloon is 12 atm. In other words, the RaptoRail will reach 3.5 mm at 6 atm and the Quantum Maverick will reach 3.5 mm at 12 atm.
- *Over-inflated*—the size of the balloon if the nominal pressure is exceeded. Whereas the 3.5-mm RaptoRail goes to 3.7 mm at 12 atm (6 atm above nominal), the 3.5-mm Quantum Maverick goes to 3.62 mm at 18 atm (6 atm above nominal). The size of the balloon at pressures that exceed nominal is printed on the packaging along with the nominal pressure.
- *Rated burst pressure*—the pressure above which the balloon will burst (usually). For example, burst pressure for the RaptoRail is 16 atm, and that for the Quantum Maverick is 22 atm.
- *Effective pressure*—the pressure required to relieve the obstruction. The effective pressure varies according to the nature of the stenosis. In patients with prior OHS, significant fibrosis or even suture material may be contributing to the obstruction. The effective pressure is judged from observation of the balloon. The pressure is effective when the balloon achieves a uniform size and the waist is eliminated.

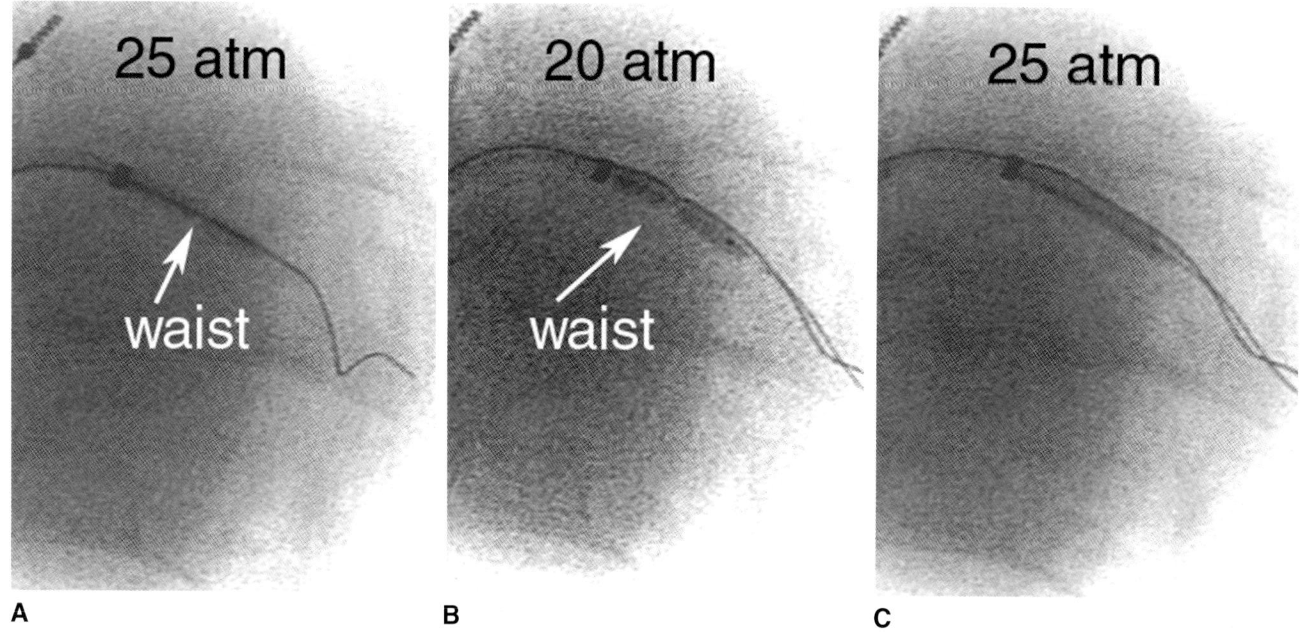

Figure 19-216. Persistent waist eliminated by means of a side wire and ultra-noncompliant balloon. ***A,*** *Waist remains despite inflation of, first, a noncompliant balloon (PowerSail, Guidant, Indianapolis, Ind.) to 20 atm and, then, an ultra-noncompliant balloon (NC Monorail Balloon, Boston Scientific Corporation, Natick, Mass.) to 25 atm.* ***B,*** *A stiff second wire is advanced beyond the stenosis using a Micro Guide (LuMend, Inc., Redwood City, Calif.). The NC Monorail is inflated on the softer wire with the stiff angioplasty wire balloon beside the balloon. The side wire augments the effect of the balloon on the waist.* ***C,*** *The waist is eliminated at 25 atm.*

Removing the Guide, Sheath, and Stylet without Displacing the Left Ventricular Lead

Once the LV pacing lead is in place with satisfactory pacing thresholds and no phrenic or diaphragmatic pacing, the guide, sheath, and stylet must be removed without dislodging the lead. The type of delivery system (nontelescoping, first-, second-, or third-generation telescoping) used to place the lead influences the risk of lead dislodgment. Third-generation systems allow larger, more stable leads to be placed and ensure that the stylet is advanced to the tip of the lead; the last step with such systems is peeling, not cutting.

When over-the-wire pacing leads are used, it is critical to remove the angioplasty wire and replace it with a soft stylet or fixing wire to stabilize the lead before guide/sheath removal. If the guide/sheath is removed with the angioplasty wire in place, friction between the guide/sheath and the pacing lead slides the lead back over the wire (Fig. 19-220). Figure 19-221 illustrates one of the advantages of using a telescopic guiding system large enough to deliver the lead directly to the vein. The telescoping guide supports the lead in the target vein while the angioplasty wire is removed and the stylet is advanced.

Before the stabilizing stylet is inserted, the distal 8 to 10 cm of the stylet should be gently curved (Fig. 19-222). The importance of using a soft curved stylet becomes apparent once guides and sheaths are removed.

The stylet should always be advanced to the tip of the pacing lead. If the stylet is not at the tip of the lead, friction between the guide/sheath and pacing lead will slide the lead back over the stylet (Fig. 19-223). If the stylet is at the tip, the lead position will remain constant as long as the position of the stylet is fixed (Fig. 19-224).

The stylet should never be left at the mid-CS level, but should be advanced all the way to the tip of the lead. The telescoping guide supports the lead so the stylet can be advanced to the tip of the lead without fear of displacing the lead out of the target vein (Fig. 19-225). Once the stabilizing stylet is in place, the preformed telescoping guide of a third-generation system is cut away.

Before the telescoping guide is removed, the operator should ensure that the long sheath is secured at the mid-CS level. The hemostatic hub is removed, and a cutter is used to remove the third-generation braided telescoping guide. As the telescoping guide is sliced away, the long sheath maintains CS access and helps support the lead.

The next step is removal of the braided guide or the long peel-away sheath (depending on the initial decision for venous access). If the sheath or guide initially used to cannulate the CS is not anatomically shaped, two interrelated issues tend to result in lead displacement. First, the shape of the nonanatomic guide or sheath in the CS is maintained by contact between the

Text continued on p. 814

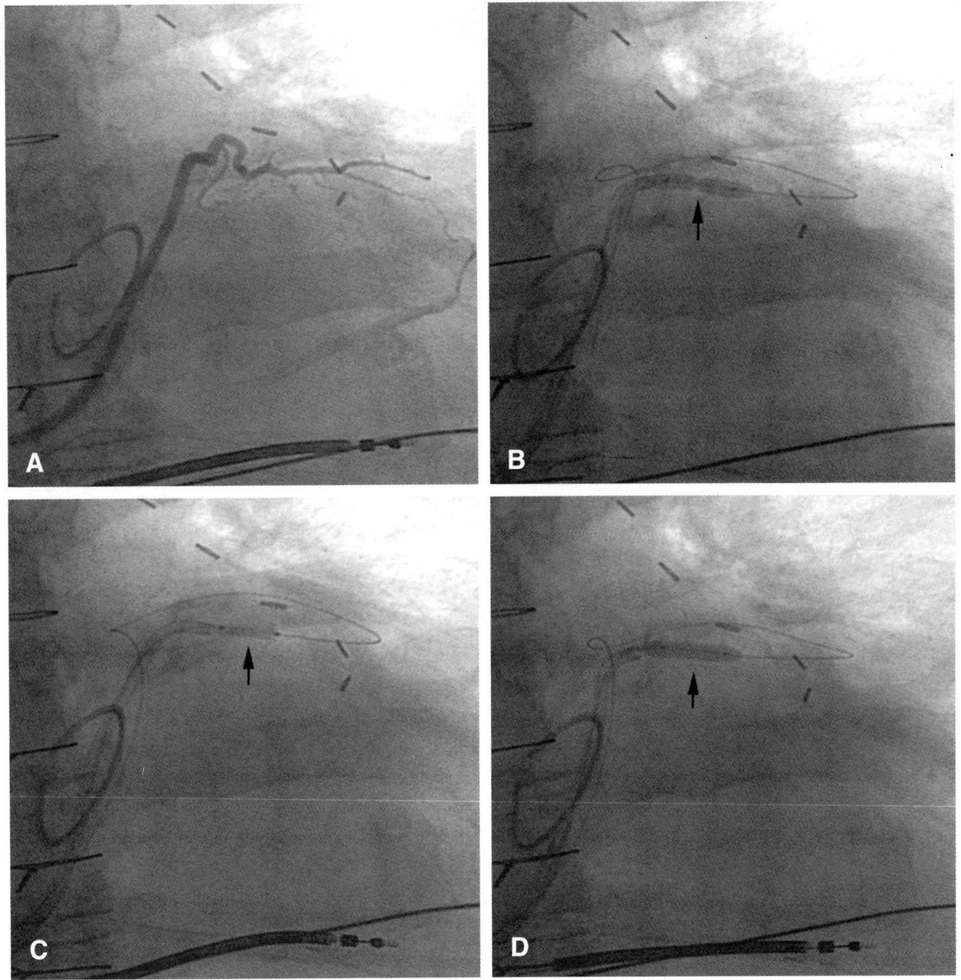

Figure 19-217. *Cutting balloon used to open stenotic target vein.* ***A,*** *The only lateral wall target vein is selectively engaged with an improvised third-generation renal telescoping system (8F Vistabritetip RDC-1, Cordis, Miami, Fla.). Contrast material is injected to confirm the location and proper position of the guide.* ***B,*** *The 3.5 mm × 23 mm PowerSail balloon (Guidant, Indianapolis, Ind.) is inflated to 20 atm without relief of the stenosis* (arrow). ***C,*** *A 2.5 mm × 10 mm cutting balloon (Boston Scientific Corporation, Natick, Mass.) is inflated to 8 atm at the site of stenosis* (arrow). ***D,*** *With the PowerSail balloon inflated to 18 atm, the stenosis is no longer seen* (arrow).

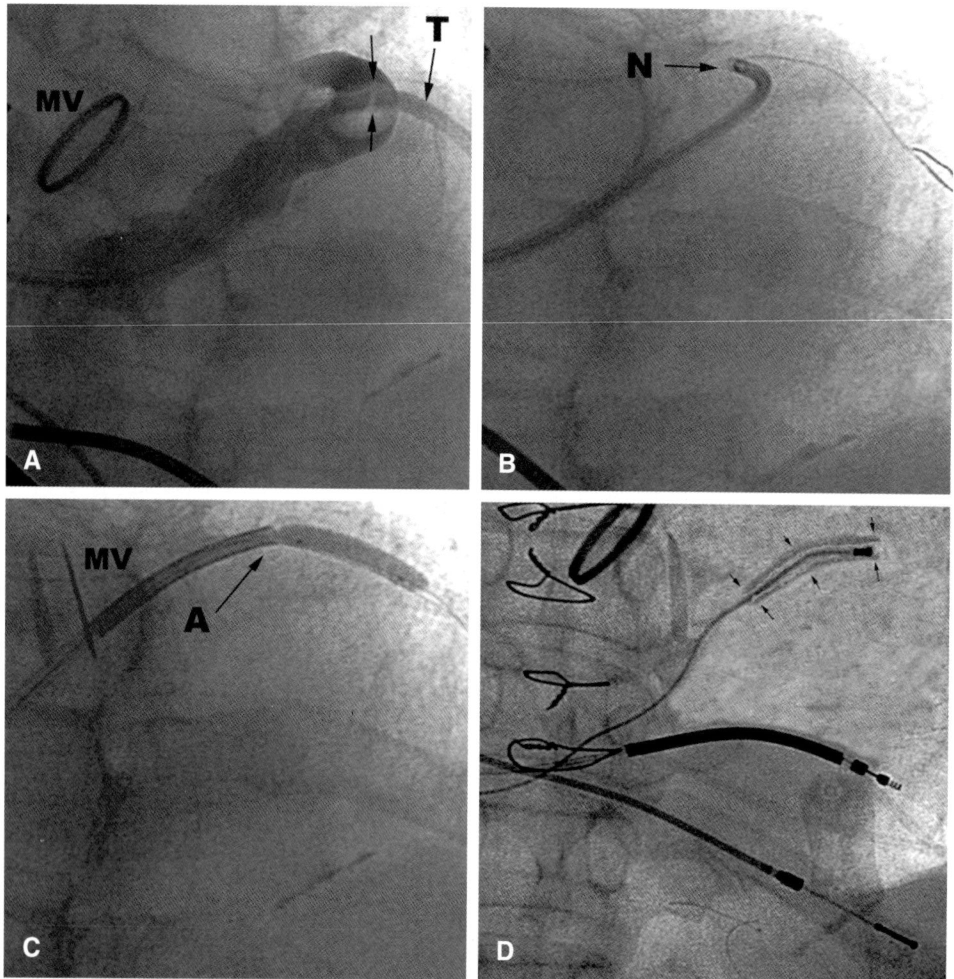

Figure 19-218. *Stent to straighten folded cardiac vein.* ***A,*** *The target vein (T) can be seen folded back on itself* (arrow)*; MV, ring of mitral valve. Nothing will advance beyond the fold in the vein.* ***B,*** *An 8F NAVIPORT deflectable-tip guiding catheter (Cardima, Inc., Fremont, Calif.) (N) is in place at the ostium of the lateral wall target vein. An angioplasty wire is in place in the vein.* ***C,*** *The Naviport is replaced with the Attain guide (Medtronic, Inc., Minneapolis, Minn.) (A). A 3.5 mm × 18 mm PowerSail balloon (Guidant, Boston Scientific, Natick, Mass.) is shown inflated in the target vein. Note that there is no waist in the balloon but the lead still will not advance. After the balloon deflates, the vein is folds back on itself, preventing the lead from being advanced. To keep the vein from folding back, stents are deployed.* ***D,*** *An Attain 4193 pacing lead (Medtronic, Inc.) is in place just inside the two 3.5-mm Multi-Link Zeta stents Guidant* (arrows)*.*

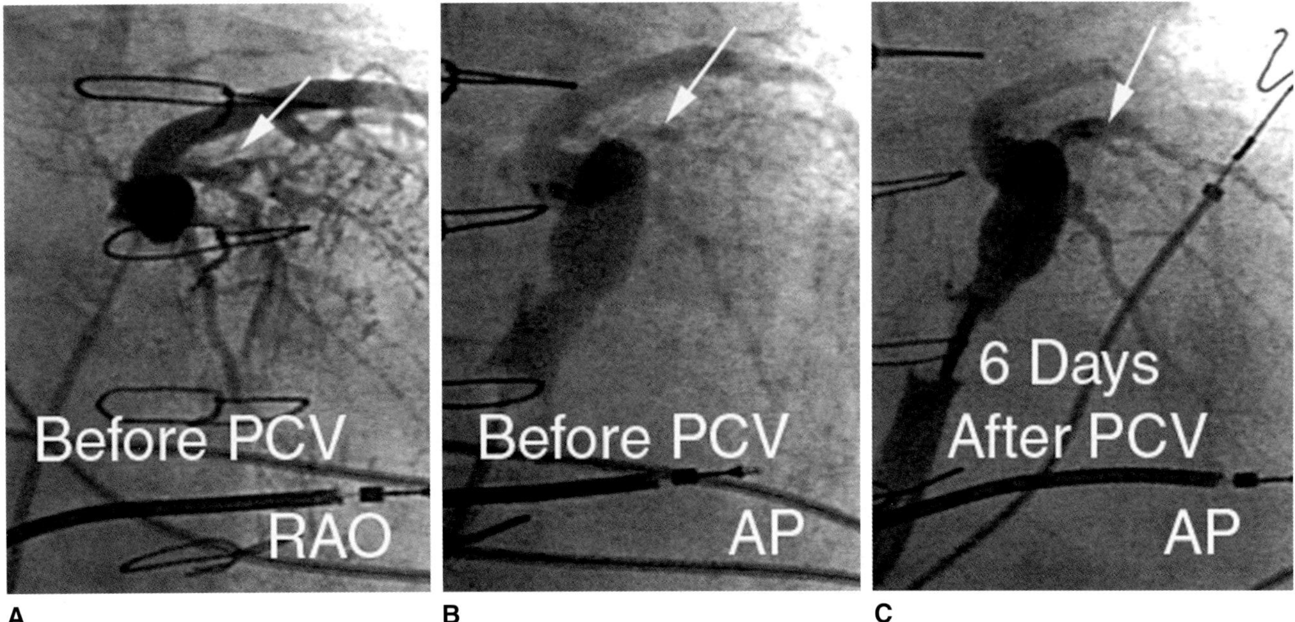

Figure 19-219. *Coronary vein before and 6 days after venoplasty. Right anterior oblique (**A**) and anteroposterior (AP) (**B**) occlusive venograms showing small stenotic vein* (arrow). ***C,*** *AP occlusive venogram taken 6 days after venoplasty, showing the same vein.*

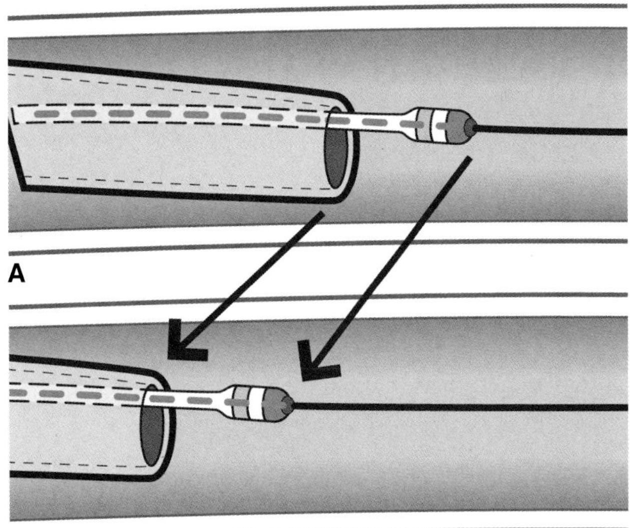

Figure 19-220. *The pacing lead slides back on the angioplasty wire.* ***A,*** *The pacing lead is free to slide on the angioplasty guidewire.* ***B,*** *As the sheath is withdrawn, friction between the guide/sheath and the pacing lead slides the pacing lead back along the angioplasty wire.*

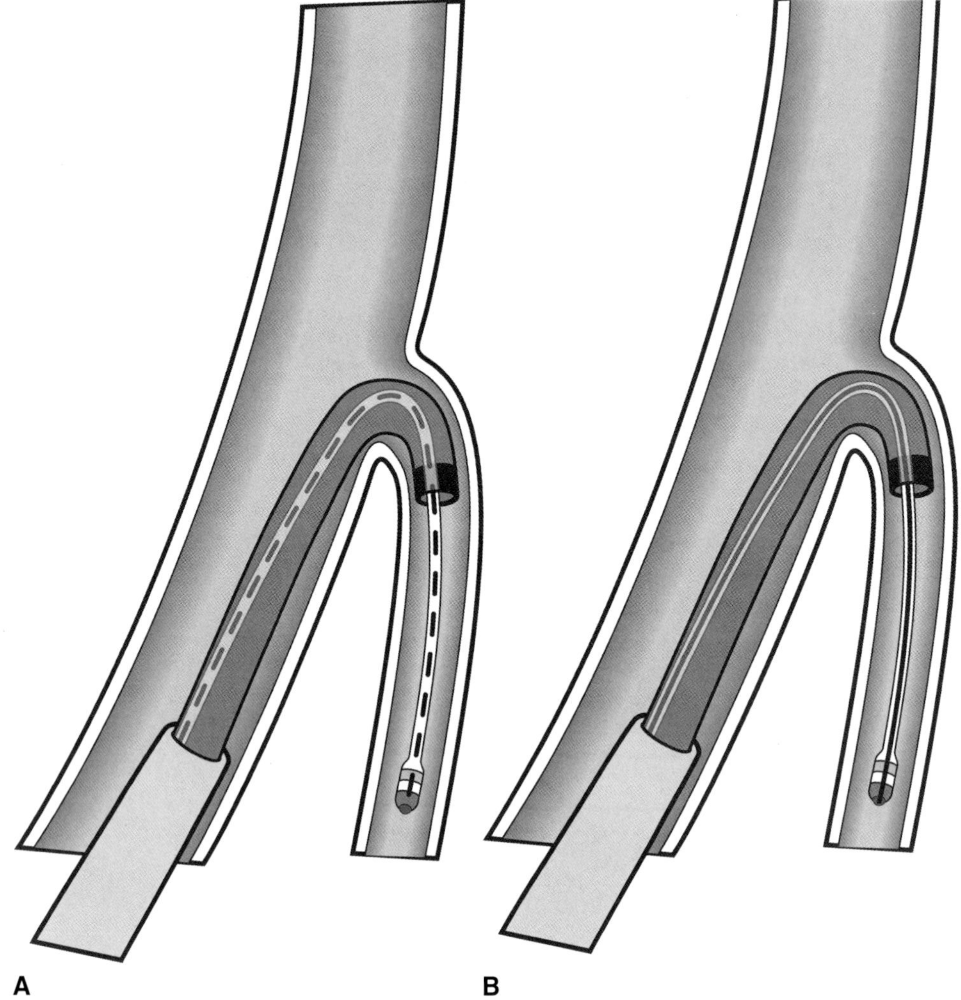

Figure 19-221. The third-generation guide supports the lead as the stylet is advanced to the tip. ***A,*** *The angioplasty wire is removed. The telescoping guide holds the lead in place.* ***B,*** *The stylet is advanced to the tip of the left ventricular (LV) pacing lead. The third-generation telescoping guide ensures that the stylet can be advanced to the tip without displacing the lead. With the stylet at the tip, the lead is less likely to become dislodged during the removal process.*

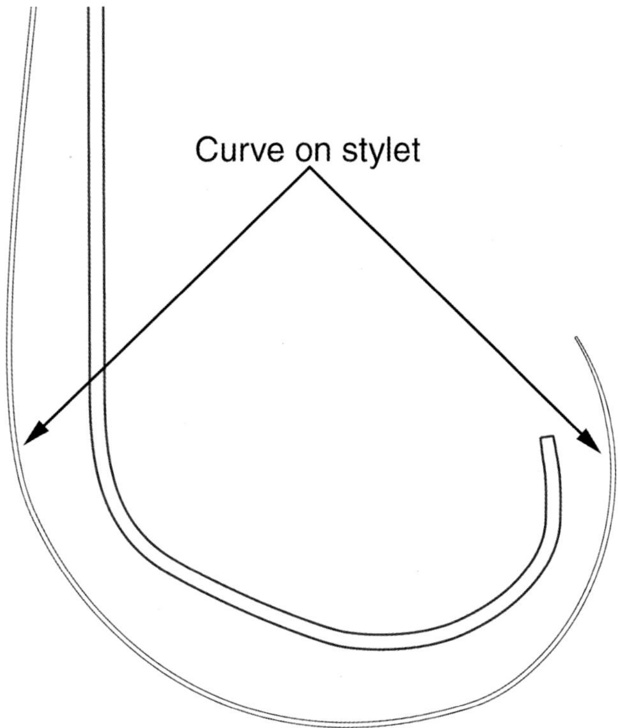

Figure 19-222. Gently curved, soft stabilization stylet. A stabilization stylet is formed by curving the distal 10 cm of a soft stylet to the shape of a peel-away sheath with a proximal curve.

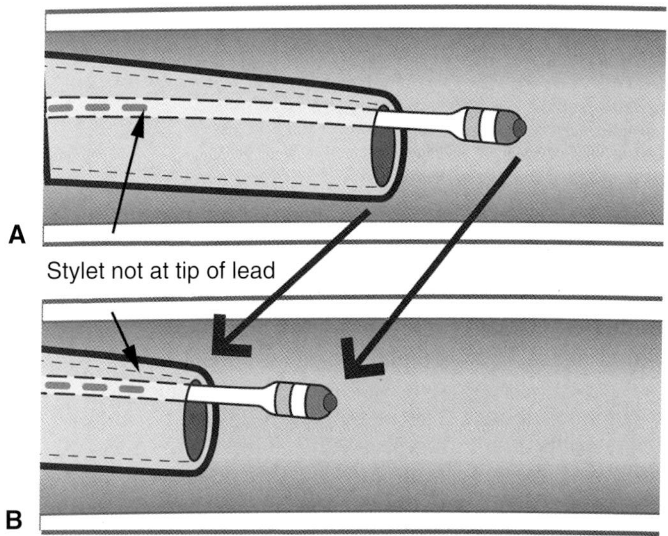

Figure 19-223. When the stylet is not at the tip, the pacing lead can slide back. ***A,*** *The stylet is not at the tip of the pacing lead. The pacing lead can slide back on the stylet until the tip of the stylet is at the tip of the lead.* ***B,*** *Even when the position of the stylet is fixed, friction between the guide/sheath and pacing lead can slide the lead back until the tip of the stylet reaches the tip of the lead.*

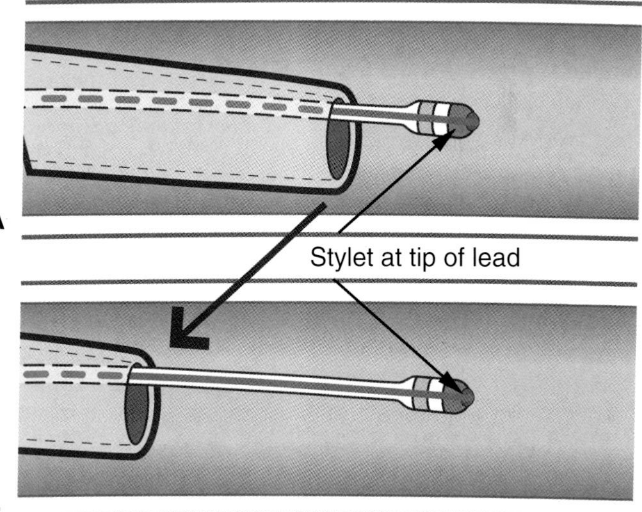

Figure 19-224. When the stylet is advanced to the tip, the pacing lead cannot slide back further on the stylet. ***A,*** *The stylet at the tip the pacing lead. The pacing lead cannot be moved more proximally.* ***B,*** *The guide/sheath is withdrawn. Despite friction between the guide/sheath and lead, the lead will not slide back over the stylet as the sheath is withdrawn, as long as the position of the stylet is fixed.*

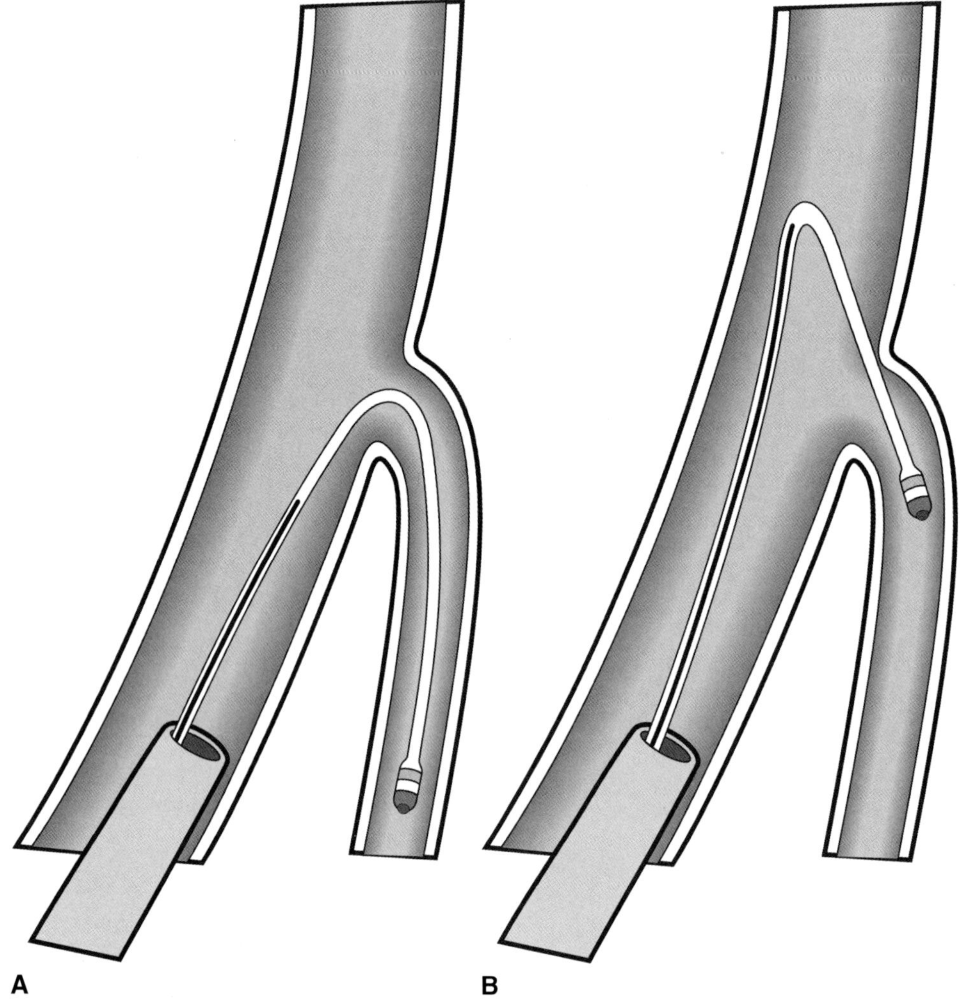

Figure 19-225. Effect of unintentionally advancing the lead/stylet when the stylet is advanced to midcoronary sinus (CS) level prior to guide/sheath removal. ***A,*** *The stabilization stylet is not advanced to the tip of the left ventricular (LV) pacing lead before the telescopic sheath is removed.* ***B,*** *The lead/stylet is inadvertently advanced in the process of removing the guide/sheath. The tip of the lead is displaced from the target vein. If the stylet is advanced to the tip of the lead before removal of the guide/sheath, unintentionally advancing the lead/stylet forces the lead further into the vein.*

sheath and the CS. When the tip of sheath/guide clears the CS os, it loses CS support and resumes its intrinsic shape, falling into the RA and potentially displacing the lead (Fig. 19-226). If the guide is anatomically shaped, it does not require CS support to maintain its shape. When it clears the CS, it does not fall into the RA (Fig. 19-227). Figure 19-228 illustrates withdrawal of an anatomically shaped sheath from the CS.

Second, additional lead length will be required once a nonanatomic guide/sheath is removed (Fig. 19-229). With the guide in place, the length of lead required to reach the CS is determined by the guide's length between the body surface and the CS. Sheaths or guides that are not anatomically shaped take a more direct course from the SVC across the RA to the CS than anatomically shaped sheaths. As a result, if the guide/sheath is removed without advancement of additional lead into the body, the lead length will be inadequate. The lead will be stretched due to tension and may be displaced between the time the guide is removed and the time the operator can advance additional lead. Lead displacement should be less of a problem if the stylet is at the tip of the lead.

Independent of whether the guide/sheath is anatomically shaped, the operator will have to take one of the following steps to remove the catheter, depending on the pacing lead and delivery system employed at the start of the procedure:

- Slide the guide back off the lead (LV-1 connector leads)
- Cut the guide
- Peel a long sheath

When the pacing lead has an LV-1 connector, the guide/sheath is withdrawn over the connector with use of a finishing wire to control the lead while the entire lead is in the guide. With the Cook Vascular, St. Jude,

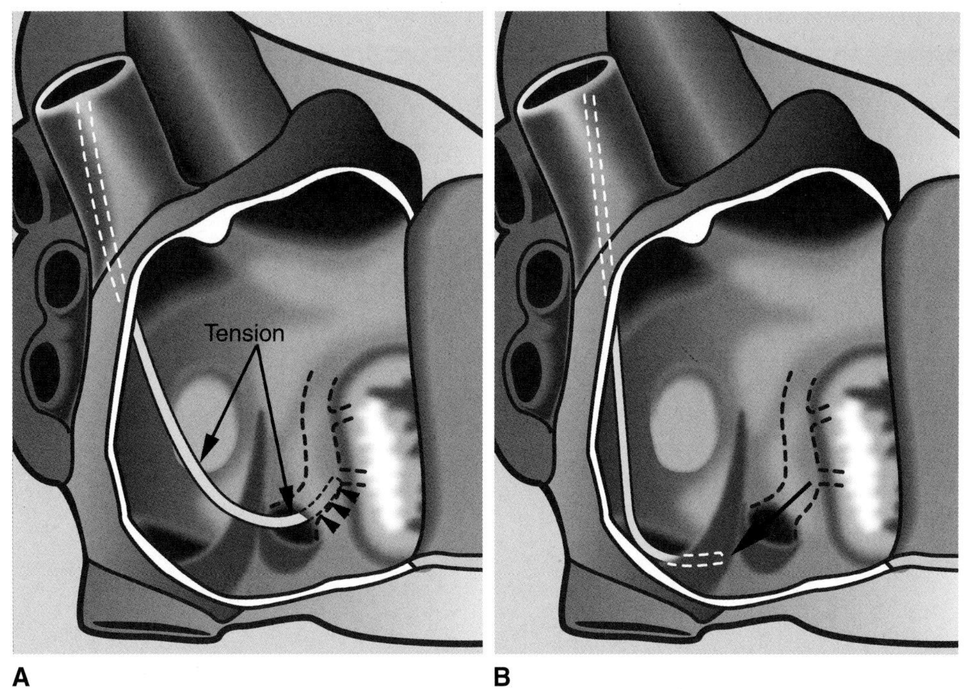

*Figure 19-226. Removal of a guide/sheath without a proximal curve from the coronary sinus (CS). **A,** The native shape of a guide/sheath without a proximal curve is deformed to fit into the CS. The shape of the guide/sheath is the result of the bending forces exerted on the guide as it was inserted. The shape is maintained by pressure on the distal section of the sheath* (arrows) *as it rests in the CS. **B,** The tip of the guide is withdrawn from the CS. The distorted shape is no longer supported by the CS. The guide resumes its native resting shape and falls to the floor of the right atrium* (arrow), *an event that can dislodge the left ventricular (LV) lead.*

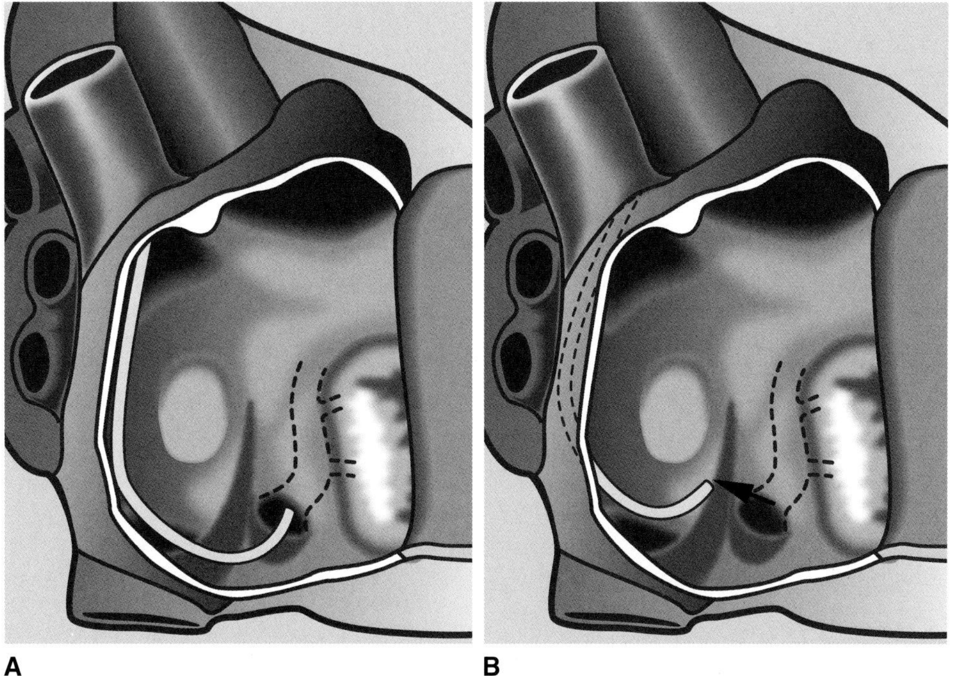

*Figure 19-227. Removal of an anatomically shaped guide/sheath. **A,** The sheath is withdrawn to the os of the coronary sinus (CS). Because the proximal curve is preformed, the tip is not under tension. **B,** The sheath is withdrawn from the CS. Because it is not under tension, it does not uncoil and fall to the floor of the right atrium (RA) as the tip clears the os. The tip of the sheath lifts upward* (arrow) *into the RA as it is withdrawn.*

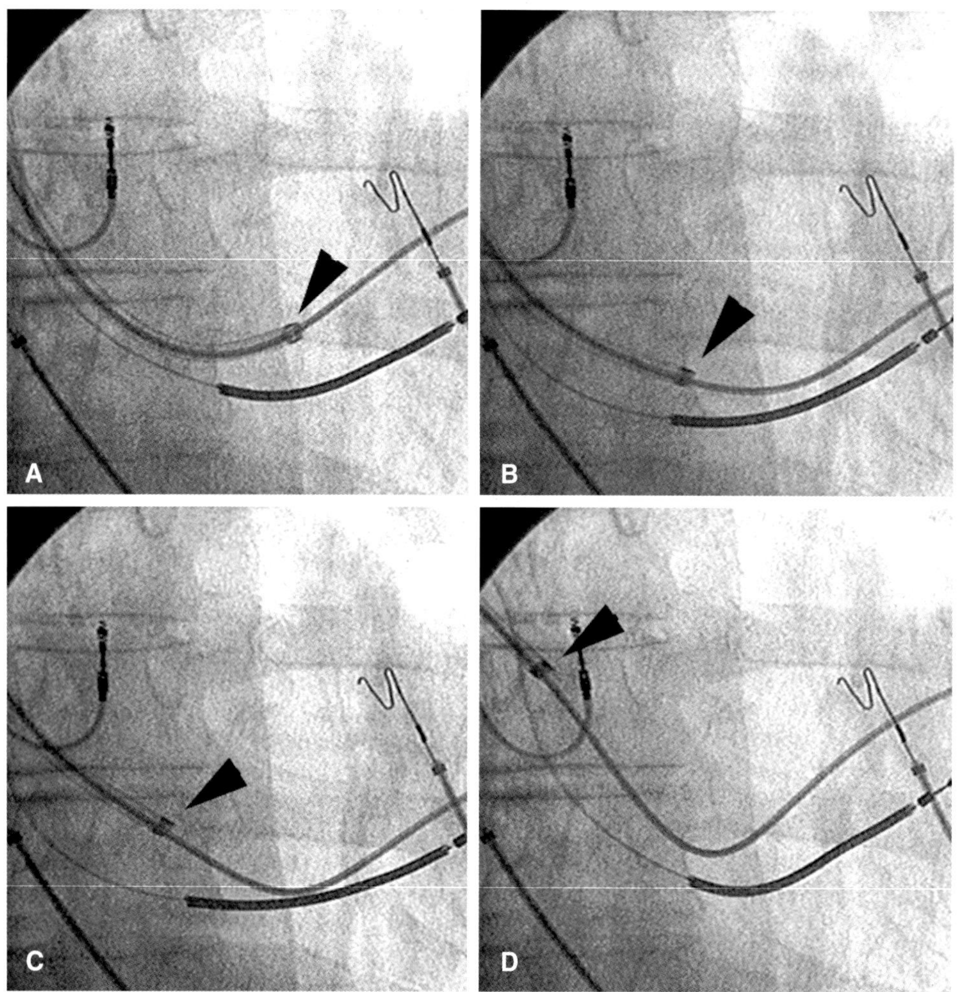

Figure 19-228. Removing an anatomically shaped sheath from the coronary sinus (CS). ***A,*** *The sheath is in the CS with the tip* (arrowhead) *just inside the os.* ***B,*** *The tip of the sheath* (arrowhead) *is withdrawn to just beyond the CS os. Note that the tip of the sheath is at the level of the CS os.* ***C,*** *The sheath is withdrawn further. Note that the tip of the sheath* (arrowhead) *is now well above the CS.* ***D,*** *The sheath is withdrawn still further. The tip of the sheath* (arrowhead) *distorts the shape of the lead slightly. Note that the left ventricular (LV) lead remains in place in the target vein. Because of the proximal curve, it is not under tension and does not drop to the floor of the right atrium as it clears the CS.*

and Pressure Products delivery systems, the long peel-away sheath is last to be removed from the CS. With the other delivery systems, the braided guide is the last to be removed (by cutting). The method of final CS sheath/guide removal influences the risk of lead displacement.

Methods of Guide/Sheath Removal

Intact Guide

When the connector on the LV pacing lead is an LV-1, the guide may be withdrawn over the lead. This method is cumbersome and has been largely replaced by one of the other two methods.

Cutting or Peeling

When the connector on the LV pacing lead is IS-1, the guide/sheath must be cut or peeled. Catheters with metal braid (guides) must be sliced along their length to be removed. Cutting a guide requires either removal of the hub before the lead is placed or presence of a hub that can be cut (Figs. 19-230 and 19-231). The Pressure Products break-away hub exposes one half the circumference of the proximal end of the guide (Fig. 19-232; see also Fig. 19-128). With this action, the guide is sliced from the lead without the need to cut through the hub. Cutting through the hub is one of the five issues that can result in pacing lead displacement as the guide is sliced away.

Cutting the guide will displace the lead if the directions are not carefully followed to the letter. The five troublesome issues with cutting are as follows:

1. Fixing the lead to the cutter/cutting hand and pulling the guide over the cutter.
2. Stabilizing the cutting hand as the guide is pulled over the cutter.

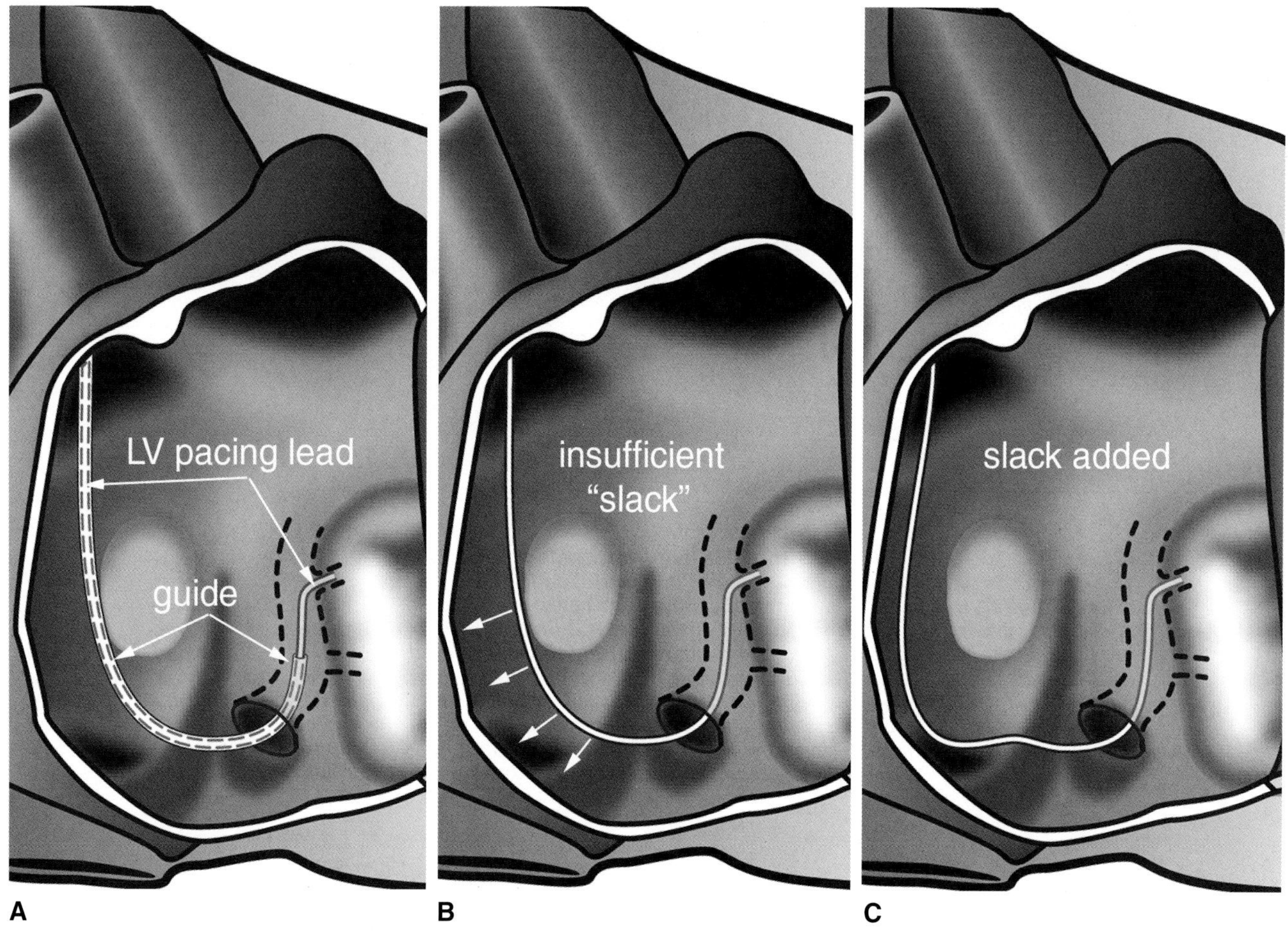

Figure 19-229. More lead length is required when the final guide/sheath is removed. ***A,*** *The left ventricular (LV) pacing lead is in place in the target vein. The lead is supported within the guide/sheath between the skin and the proximal coronary sinus. The sheath determines the length of the lead in the body, particularly in the right atrium (RA).* ***B,*** *The guide/sheath is removed without advance of additional lead. Without the support of the guide/sheath, the length of the lead in the RA is insufficient. Because the lead is on stretch, it may displace the tip of the lead from the target vein.* ***C,*** *Additional slack is added to ensure that the tip of the lead is not dislodged when the patient breathes or stands up. After guide/sheath removal, the length of additional lead required is determined from the shape of the guide/sheath. There is more pacing lead in the heart when an anatomically shaped sheath is removed because of the lead in the long curved section in the RA. With a straight or nonanatomic shape, the course of the guide/sheath through the RA is more direct, resulting in less lead in the body when the guide/sheath is removed.*

3. Cutting through the hub-to-guide transition (see later for details).
4. Keeping the split hub/guide from grabbing and displacing the lead (Fig. 19-233).
5. The need for additional slack once the final guide/sheath is removed and the LV pacing lead is no longer supported in the RA (see Fig. 19-226). The need for additional slack is more pronounced if the guide/sheath is not anatomically shaped. If the lead and cutting hand are fixed as the guide is cut away, the additional slack must await the complete slicing of the guide and removal of the slicing tool from the lead. During this time, the lead will be on stretch, possibly resulting in lead displacement.

Cutting through the hub-to-guide transition occurs as the tip of the guide loses support of the CS and is prone to fall into the RA. It is extremely difficult to both draw the guide over the cutting hand and advance the lead at the same time, raising the risk of dislodgment. In addition, the resistance to cutting changes abruptly as the blade passes through the heavy plastic hub into the guide. The sudden change in resistance can cause the cutting hand to jump at the same time as the guide is prone to fall into the RA. Together, these factors tend to displace the lead in a synergistic fashion.

Keeping the Split Hub/Guide from Grabbing and Displacing the Lead

After it is cut, the thick plastic of the hub of the guide can close around the lead. Unless the lead is carefully removed from the grip of the cut hub, the lead and guide will be jerked abruptly when the hub reaches the IS-1 connector (Fig. 19-234).

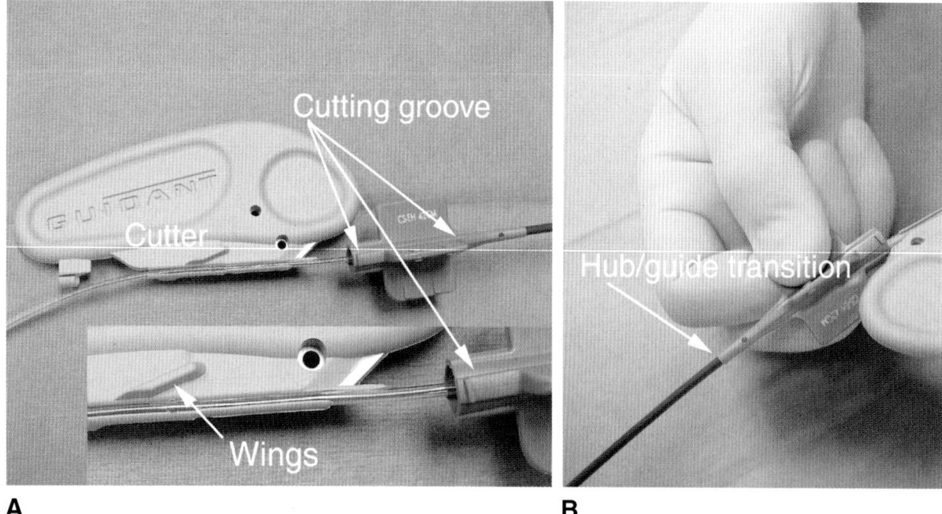

Figure 19-230. Cutting tool and sliceable hub from Guidant (Boston Scientific, Natick, Mass.) ***A,*** *The cutter is attached to the left ventricular (LV) lead. The lead is attached to the cutter where it exits the hub of the guide. The hemostatic valve is removed from the hub over the IS-1 connector of the lead. Between each of the four fins of the hub is a line of thin plastic that extends from the proximal end to the body of the guide to facilitate cutting the hub (the cutting groove).* ***B,*** *The blade of the guide is engaged in the cutting groove of the hub. The operator holds the cutter fixed in position with the nondominant hand. The hub is grasped by one of the wings opposite the cutting groove. The guide is pulled back, first cutting the hub then the guide. At the hub-guide transition, resistance to cutting changes abruptly, which can cause the cutting hand to leap forward and displace the lead. Fins on the cutter spread the plastic of the hub to prevent the hub from catching the lead.*

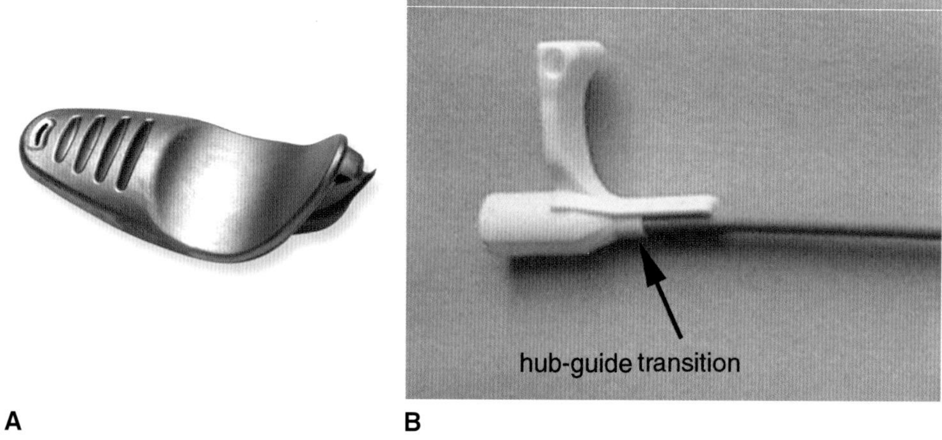

Figure 19-231. Universal Slitter and guide hub from Medtronic, Inc. (Minneapolis, Minn.). ***A,*** *The Universal Slitter is used with all size leads. The operator's thumb secures the lead to the bottom of the slitter, preventing the cut hub from grabbing and dislodging the lead.* ***B,*** *The plastic hub of the guide with hub-guide transition is shown. At the hub-guide transition, resistance to cutting changes abruptly, which can cause the cutting hand to leap forward and displace the lead.*

A valuable technique to avoid the five troublesome issues of cutting that occur just as the catheter clears the CS is to withdraw the braided guide over the lead as far as the lead length will permit, often moving the tip above the RA before cutting. This technique can also be used with peel-away sheaths. It permits easier adjustment of the lead length in the RA as the tip clears the CS os. Separating the step of removing the sheath/guide from the CS from the step of cutting or peeling is a valuable technique that permits advancement of the lead if it demonstrates its location to be unstable. However, cutting a guide that has been withdrawn to the IS-1 connector can be problematic. There is no way to stabilize the lead and no place to support the cutting hand. Peeling, by comparison, is better suited to this approach, as described later.

This concept is demonstrated in Figure 19-235, which shows that lead stability and hemostasis are facilitated if the operator does not remove the hemostatic valve and withdraw the sheath over the pacing lead to the IS-1 connector. As the sheath is withdrawn, both the portion in the atrium and tip of the LV lead

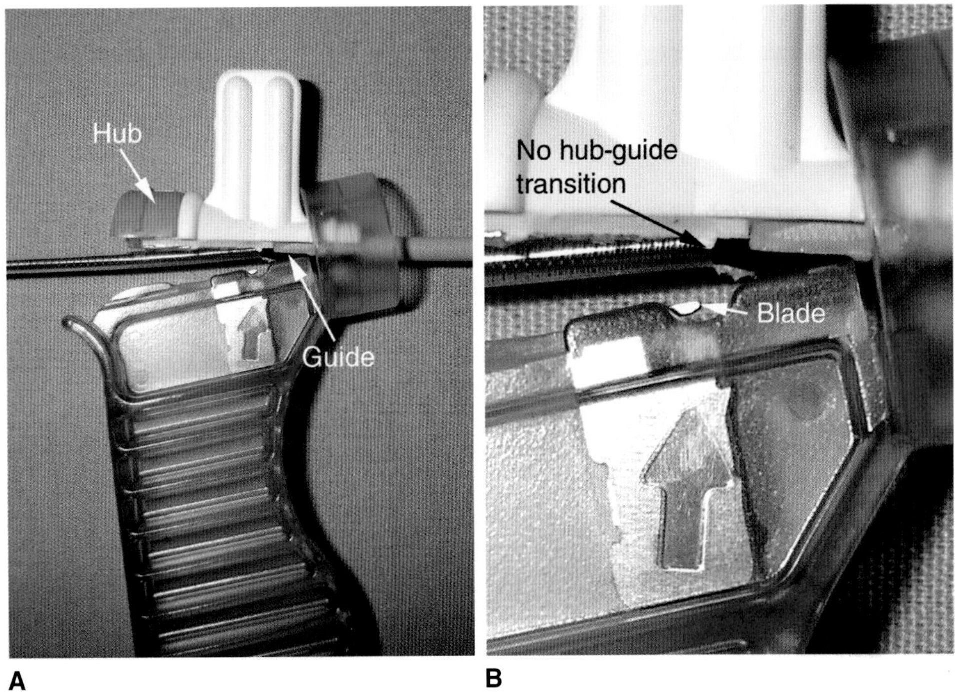

Figure 19-232. *Cutter and telescoping hub guide from Pressure Products, Inc. (San Pedro, Calif.).* ***A,*** *The cutter is used with leads of all sizes. The operator's thumb secures the lead to the back of the slitter, preventing the cut hub from grabbing and dislodging the lead.* ***B,*** *After the hemostatic hub is cracked, one half of the hub detaches from the guide. The blade of the cutter engages the guide directly (not the hub). There is no transition in resistance to cutting to cause the cutting hand to leap forward.*

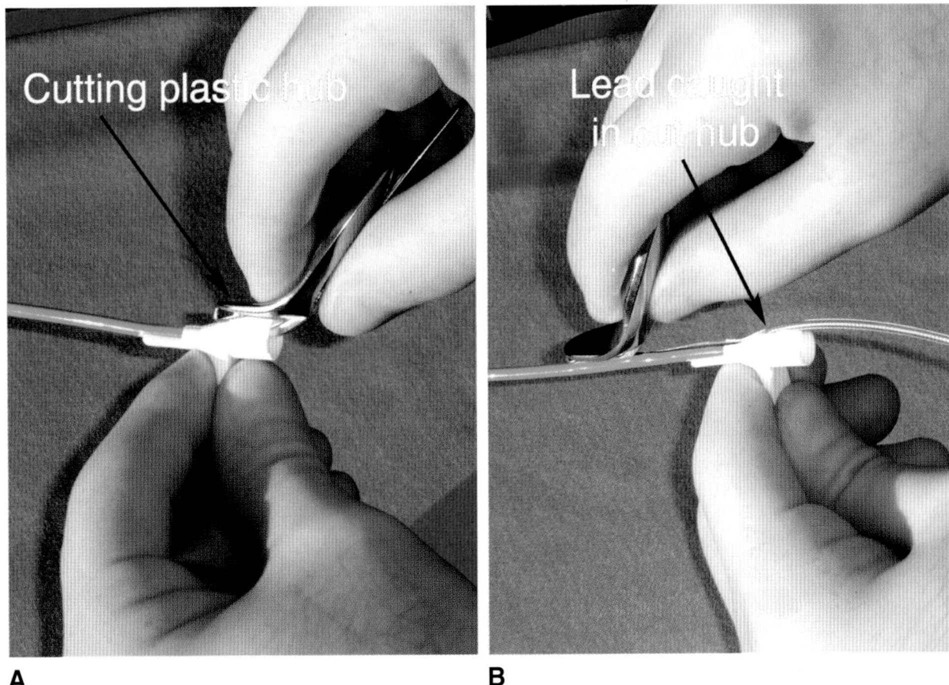

Figure 19-233. *The pacing lead caught in the cut plastic hub as the guide is sliced.* ***A,*** *The Universal Slitter (Medtronic, Inc., Minneapolis, Minn.) cuts the plastic hub of the guide. The lead is fixed to the back of the cutter with the thumb. As the hub is split, the lead pulls clear of the plastic.* ***B,*** *The lead is not fixed to the cutter with the thumb. The split hub closes around the lead. As the guide is pulled back, it pulls the lead back.*

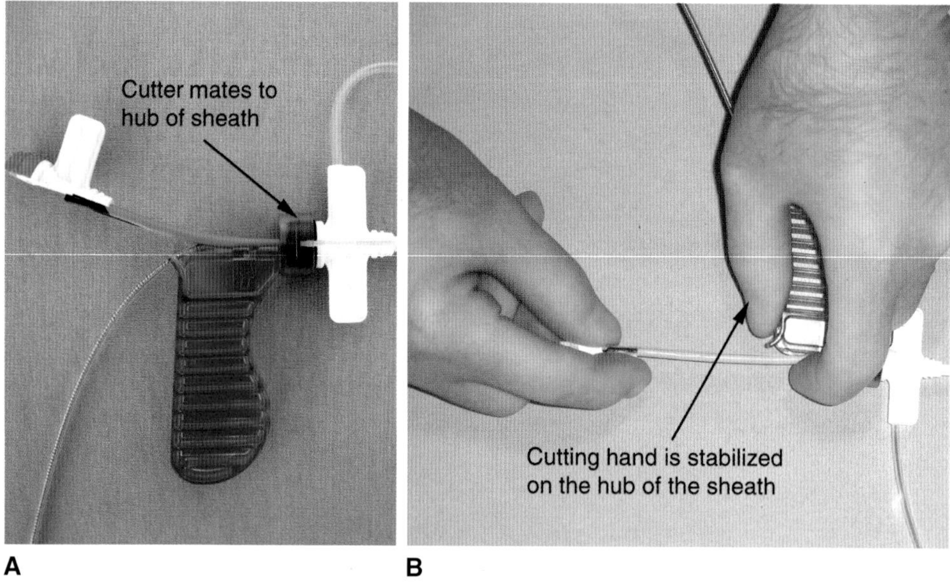

Figure 19-234. The hand holding the Pressure Products, Inc. (San Pedro, Calif.), cutter is stabilized on the hub of the sheath. ***A,*** *The lead is NOT attached to the cutter. Without moving the lead, the operator cuts the third-generation guide down to the hub of the safe sheath. The curved front of the cutter is mated to the hub of the sheath. The operator removes the lead from the cut guide and secures it to the cutter by placing the lead in the notch of the cutter under the thumb.*

should be in the fluoroscopic field so that the operator can judge the length of lead required as the supporting sheath is removed. This approach minimizes blood loss and the risk of air embolization because the hemostatic valve is not removed until it is withdrawn to the IS-1 connector. Pinching the lead between the walls of the sheath reduces the bleeding and risk of air embolization once the valve is removed. A guide with wire mesh walls is more difficult to collapse than a plastic peel-away sheath, so pinching a guide with wire mesh walls to stabilize the lead distally may not be effective.

After the assistant releases the sheath/lead, the rest of the sheath is drawn back over the lead under fluoroscopic observation. As the tip of the sheath exits the body and the pacing lead becomes visible, the assistant secures the lead position with fingers in the pocket.

Stylet Removal

The final step is to remove the stylet. Care is needed. Many successful implantations have been lost during this step. The two issues of importance are the physical characteristics of the stylet and how the stylet is withdrawn.

Stylet Characteristics. When the stylet is in the lead within the CS, the shape of the lead/stylet combination is determined by the course of the CS. Once outside the CS, the stylet is no longer supported. When the shape of the stylet and course of the LV pacing lead do not match, the stylet determines the ultimate shape of the lead/stylet combination, often by withdrawing the tip from the target vein. The stiffer the stylet, the greater the displacing force applied to the lead. Placing a gentle curve on the stylet that approximates the final course of the lead through the RA reduces the tendency for the stylet to displace the lead because of a shape mismatch. A softer stylet exerts less displacing force when the shape of the stylet and course of the lead do not match despite the curve. Earlier I advised that a soft, gently curved stylet be advanced to the tip of the lead (see Fig. 19-222). Figure 19-236 illustrates what can happen if a stiff straight stylet is used.

How the Stylet Is Withdrawn. As already discussed, when the shape of the stylet and course of the LV pacing lead do not match, the stiffer stylet will prevail, often by displacing the lead. The longer the stylet remains in a position prone to displacing the lead, the more likely the lead will be displaced. To prevent the stylet from displacing the pacing lead when the course of the lead and the shape of the stylet do not match, the stylet is removed quickly (like pulling the cord on a lawn mower). This maneuver gives the stylet less time to displace the lead. Prior to insertion into the LV pacing lead, the stylet should be curved as shown in Figure 19-222.

Final Slack on the Lead

The final step in LV lead placement is to be certain that the lead has adequate slack. Appearance on AP and RAO projections can be deceptive about this issue. The LAO projection is best for judging the amount of slack in the lead. In the LAO projection, the RV and LV leads should appear to touch low in the RA and continue parallel in close proximity as they leave the RA into the SVC. Figure 19-237 is an example of dislodgment of the lead because of insufficient slack. Note the trajectory in the LAO projection with insufficient slack

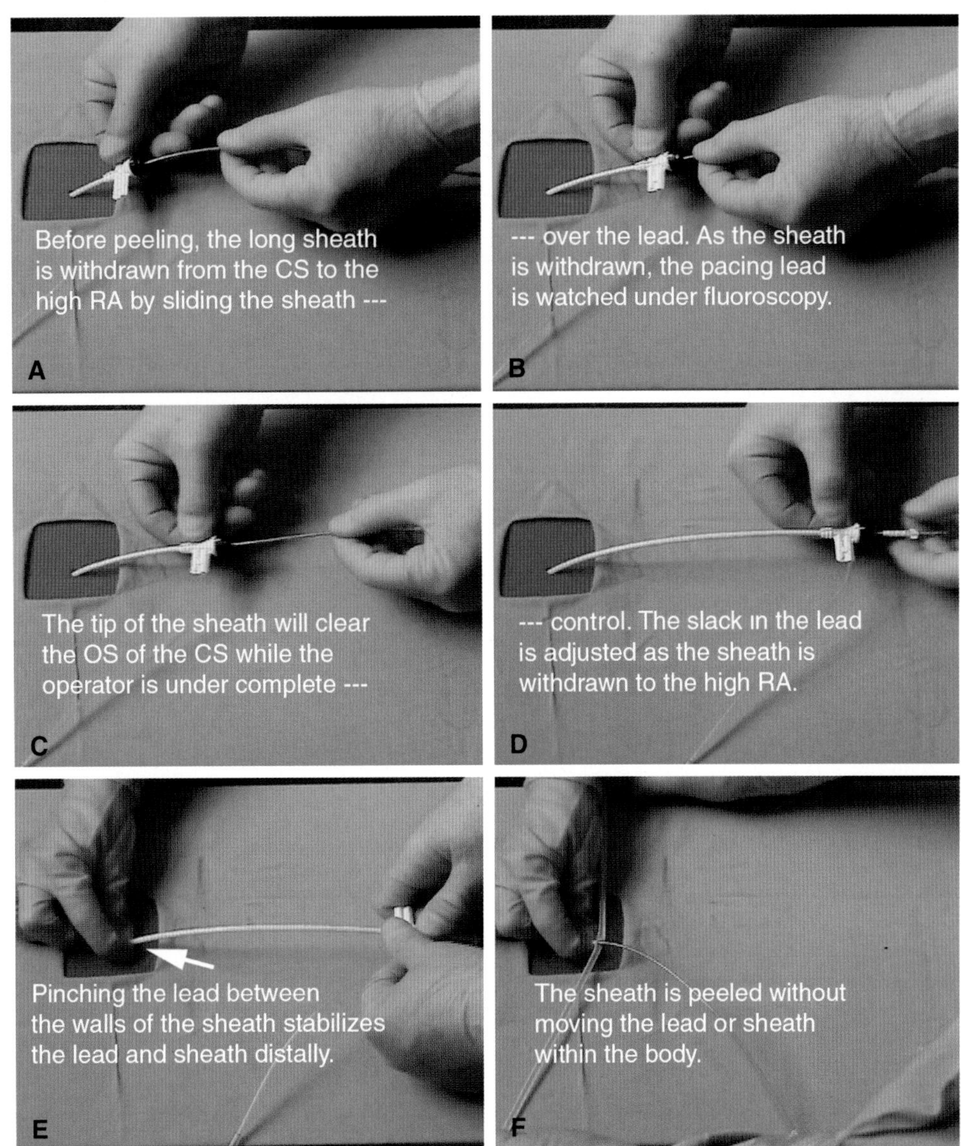

Before peeling, the long sheath
is withdrawn from the CS to the
high RA by sliding the sheath ---
A
--- over the lead. As the sheath
is withdrawn, the pacing lead
is watched under fluoroscopy.
B
The tip of the sheath will clear
the OS of the CS while the
operator is under complete ---
C
--- control. The slack in the lead
is adjusted as the sheath is
withdrawn to the high RA.
D
Pinching the lead between
the walls of the sheath stabilizes
the lead and sheath distally.
E
The sheath is peeled without
moving the lead or sheath
within the body.
F

Figure 19-235. Removing the long peel-away sheath from the coronary sinus (CS) without displacing the left ventricular (LV) lead. ***A,*** *The left hand holds the lead (with stylet advanced to the tip) fixed in place 5 cm from the hemostatic valve. The right hand holds the peel-away sheath and is ready to withdraw the sheath back to the left hand.* ***B,*** *The right hand withdraws the sheath to the left hand holding the lead. The operator performs this step in a careful and controlled manner, watching the lead with fluoroscopy as the tip of the sheath transitions from the CS to the right atrium (RA). Frequently, additional slack is required as the sheath is withdrawn. Adding slack is easily accomplished by advancing the lead with the right hand as the left hand withdraws the sheath.* ***C,*** *The lead is again fixed 5 cm from the hemostatic valve with the left hand. The right hand grasps the hub of the sheath and is ready to withdraw the sheath toward the left hand.* ***D,*** *The sheath is withdrawn to the IS-1 connector. The tip of sheath is now in the superior vena cava (SVC), where inadvertent motion is not likely to cause displacement of the LV lead.* ***E,*** *An assistant pinches the pacing lead firmly between the walls of the sheath where it exits the body in the pacemaker pocket. With the assistant stabilizing the LV lead and sheath, the operator prepares to remove the hemostatic valve.* ***F,*** *With the lead and sheath both stabilized by the assistant, the operator removes the hemostatic valve and rapidly peels the sheath down to the fingers of the assistant, who continues to pinch the lead between the walls of the sheath. Pinching the lead between the walls of the sheath not only stabilizes the sheath and LV lead but also reduces bleeding and the risk of air embolization. In this figure, a long SafeSheath (Pressure Products, Inc., San Pedro, Calif.) is shown. The technique applies for any long peel-away sheath. As the sheath is withdrawn, the slack on the lead can be adjusted.*

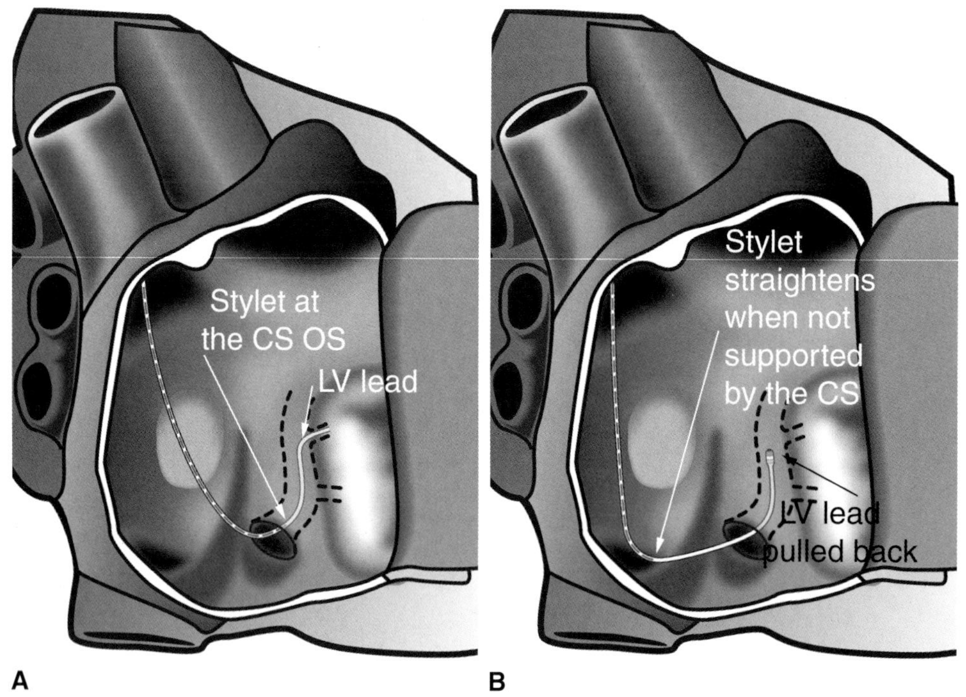

Figure 19-236. Straight stiff stylet dislodges the left ventricular (LV) pacing lead as it is slowly withdrawn from the coronary sinus (CS). ***A,*** *The straight stiff stylet is withdrawn from the tip of the pacing lead to the CS os. The curve on the stylet is maintained through contact of the lead with the wall of the CS.* ***B,*** *The stylet is withdrawn from the CS. The stylet springs back to its native straight shape, pulling the LV lead out of the vein. The stiffer the stylet, the more displacement force is exerted as it springs back to its native straight shape. To avoid loss of lead position at the time of stylet removal, one should use an anatomically shaped, soft stylet. In addition, rapid removal of the stylet reduces the duration of the displacement force acting to withdraw the lead from the vein.*

(see Fig. 19-237B) compared with adequate slack (see Fig. 19-237D). To ensure adequate slack on the LV pacing lead, the operator should inspect the steep LAO projection to confirm that the LV and RV leads appear to touch in the low RA.

Conclusion

To optimize success and minimize implant time: *Each step in the implant procedure must anticipate the most difficult conceivable anatomy.*

Tip and tricks were in vogue when the LV implantation procedure was new and many tools needed to be improvised. As the procedure matured, better tools evolved. Now the best tip is "There are no tricks, only better tools and techniques." An implanting physician who wants to learn how to implant without compromise must embrace new tools and methods. The reward consists of a paradoxically reduced learning curve, shorter implantation times, and greater overall success. In the long run, it is more efficient to learn a new method designed for the procedure than to try to force a familiar but intrinsically flawed technique. Once the tools and techniques are mastered, the implanting physician is in a position to follow the golden rule of CRT implantation.

When a BiV implantation is begun, there is no way to predict what lies ahead. A CRT implantation ultimately fails as a result of patient anatomy for which the implanter is not prepared. In effect, the implanting physician and the patient are "victimized" by the patient's anatomy. To succeed, the implanter must be prepared to deal with whatever anatomy is encountered, starting with venous access and ending with the final removal of the stylet. This chapter takes the position that although there are many approaches to "successful" CRT implantation, the strategies presented here are more likely to consistently succeed. The approach is predicated on the use of tools and techniques specifically developed to overcome the obstacles that prevent success with the other methods. For example, finding the vein may be difficult, followed by discovery of a stenotic or occluded subclavian vein, followed by difficulty locating the CS os, followed by a tortuous main CS. At that point, the CS venogram may show a range of target veins from very easy to extremely difficult. Once the pacing lead is in the vein, phrenic pacing or high pacing thresholds may be encountered. A pacing lead of different size or shape may solve the problem. Once the lead is in a satisfactory location, it can be displaced as the final guide/sheath is removed because (1) the deformed guide/sheath springs back into the RA as the tip disengages from the CS and its native shape is restored,

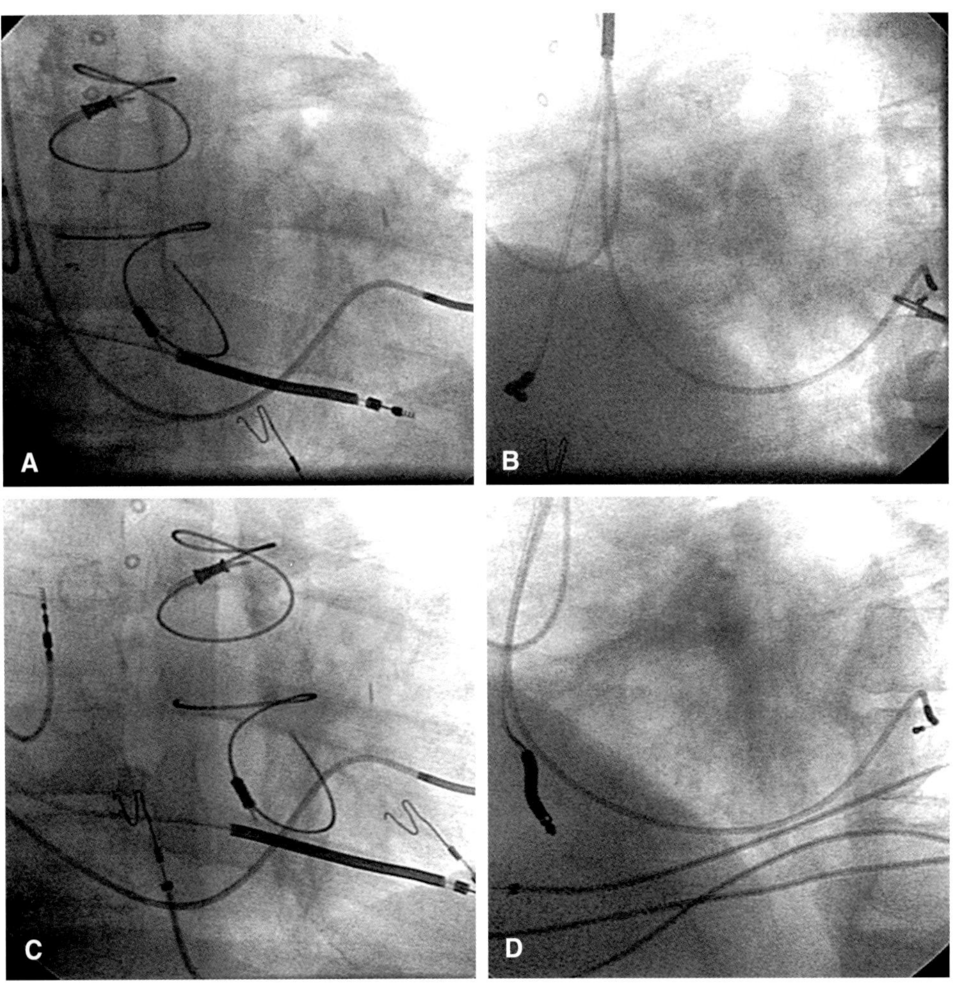

*Figure 19-237. Insufficient slack in the left ventricular (LV) pacing lead results in displacement. **A,** On the anteroposterior (AP) projection of the final LV pacing lead position, the amount of slack seems adequate. **B,** On the left anterior oblique (LAO) projection, there is not enough slack. Note distance from right ventricular (RV) lead in the atrium. **C,** The AP projection after advancing the lead. **D,** The LAO projection with appropriate slack. Note the course of the LV lead next to the RV lead on the right atrium.*

(2) the lead/stylet is unintentionally advanced with the stylet at mid-CS level, or (3) lead length is not added as the sheath is removed. Withdrawing the stylet can dislodge the lead if it is straight or stiff or is removed slowly. Finally, inadequate slack in the lead after tie-down will result in late lead displacement.

The tools and techniques presented in this chapter take these issues into consideration and have been used to safely implant LV leads without compromising location in more than 98% of my patients. In addition, most if not all patients in whom either implantation is initially unsuccessful or clinical response has not occurred because of an unsatisfactory lead location can undergo successful implantation via a second transvenous attempt that employs the methods presented here. Disciplined, systematic use of these tools and techniques will not shorten the implantation time in a patient with favorable anatomy. However, the time saved when the method eliminates just one obstacle makes it worthwhile.

Much of what is presented in this chapter may be new to the reader. When one is learning a new technique or the use of a new piece of equipment, it is critical not to try it in a fit of desperation when all else has failed. The "last gasp" approach is doomed to failure and is certain to confirm the operator's initial feeling that the new tool or approach is no good and that he/she should go back to using the old way. If a new technique or tool is to be learned, it must be performed or used repeatedly when the operator is not exhausted, harried, and frustrated but fresh and relaxed. Only after one tries the new tool in this way is it accurate to say that the new tool has been "tried." It must be assumed that trying a new tool or technique only as a last resort is an indication that the operator is not really interested in learning to use it.

CS cannulation using contrast material and a properly shaped catheter is a good example. No matter how facile a physician is with cannulating the CS using an EP catheter, he or she will cannulate safer and faster if he/she is willing to give up a familiar technique and spend the time to learn the new method. The time required to achieve successful CS access in the first 50 patients is shorter with the unfamiliar contrast method than with the "familiar" EP method, even when the time spent learning the contrast method is added to the total time. The experience gained with the technique used in less challenging cases will then be available when the more challenging cases arise. If an operator is truly interested in deciding whether a new approach is valuable, he/she must evaluate it under the same set of conditions as the old, familiar approach.

Setting a time limit on the transvenous LV implantation attempt and then, if the attempt is unsuccessful, referring the patient directly to the surgeon is practical and appropriate if the implanter is using the same approach over and over without effect and is not interested in learning new techniques on behalf of the patient. However, there is a tremendous advantage to both the patient and the implanting physician to seeking counsel with interventional colleagues or other implanting physicians to develop another approach based on the experience gained with the first attempt. Rather than a frustrating dead end, an initially failed attempt should be regarded as an opportunity to enlarge the implanting physician's armamentarium. For instance, it might represent the opportunity to learn the use of the third-generation guiding systems or venoplasty on a second attempt. The new techniques learned with a second attempt can then be applied early in subsequent cases in which the same issue arises. The implanting physician might even design a tool for general use to solve the same problem for other patients and physicians. The physician who sends a patient in whom lead implantation has failed for surgical lead placement without first seeking counsel from his/her interventional colleagues and or other implanting physicians assumes a great deal. Interestingly, the same physicians who advocate surgical referral also describe bringing patients back to the implantation room for another attempt that turns out to be successful.

REFERENCES

1. Leon AR, Delurgio DB, Mera F: Practical approach to implanting left ventricular pacing leads for cardiac resynchronization. J Cardiovasc Electrophysiol 16:100, 2005.
2. Abraham WT, Fisher WG, Smith AL, et al: Cardiac resynchronization in chronic heart failure. N Engl J Med 346:1845, 2002.
3. Abraham WT, Young JB, Leon AR, et al: Effects of cardiac resynchronization on disease progression in patients with left ventricular systolic dysfunction, an indication for an implantable cardioverter-defibrillator, and mildly symptomatic chronic heart failure. Circulation 110:2864, 2004.
4. Bristow MR, Saxon LA, Boehmer J, et al: Cardiac-resynchronization therapy with or without an implantable defibrillator in advanced chronic heart failure. N Engl J Med 350:2140, 2004.
5. Cleland JGF, Daubert J-C, Erdmann E, et al: The effect of cardiac resynchronization on morbidity and mortality in heart failure. N Engl J Med 352:1539, 2005.
6. Auricchio A, Stellbrink C, Block M, et al: Effect of pacing chamber and atrioventricular delay on acute systolic function of paced patients with congestive heart failure. Circulation 99:2993, 1999.
7. Butter C, Auricchio A, Stellbrink C, et al: Effect of resynchronization therapy stimulation site on the systolic function of heart failure patients. Circulation 104:3026, 2001.
8. Cazeau S, Leclercq C, Lavergne T, et al: Effects of multisite biventricular pacing in patients with heart failure and intraventricular conduction delay. N Engl J Med 344:873, 2001.
9. Albertsen AE, Nielsen JC, Pedersen AK, et al: Left ventricular lead performance in cardiac resynchronization therapy: Impact of lead localization and complications. PACE 28:483, 2005.
10. Auricchio A, Abraham WT: Cardiac resynchronization therapy: Current state of the art: Cost versus benefit. Circulation 109:300, 2004.
11. Kautzner J, Riedlbauchova L, Cihak R, et al: Technical aspects of implantation of LV lead for cardiac resynchronization therapy in chronic heart failure. PACE 27:783, 2004.
12. Fisher JD, Garcia J, Kim SG, et al: Easy surgical approach for completion of biventricular pacing. J Cardiovasc Electrophysiol 15:1462, 2004.
13. DeRose JJ Jr, Ashton RC Jr, Belsley S, et al: Robotically assisted left ventricular epicardial lead implantation for biventricular pacing. J Am Coll Cardiol 41:1414, 2003.
14. Ji S, Cesario DA, Swerdlow CD, Shivkumar K: Left ventricular endocardial lead placement using a modified transseptal approach. J Cardiovasc Electrophysiol 15:234, 2004.
15. Solomon R, Werner C, Mann D, et al: Effects of saline, mannitol, and furosemide on acute decreases in renal function induced by radiocontrast agents. N Engl J Med 331:1416, 1994.
16. Meisel E, Pfeiffer D, Engelmann L, et al: Investigation of coronary venous anatomy by retrograde venography in patients with malignant ventricular tachycardia. Circulation 104:442, 2001.
17. Schwab S, Hlatky M, Pieper K, et al: Contrast nephrotoxicity: A randomized controlled trial of a nonionic and an ionic radiographic contrast agent. N Engl J Med 320:149, 1989.
18. Parfrey P, Griffiths S, Barrett B, et al: Contrast material-induced renal failure in patients with diabetes mellitus, renal insufficiency, or both: A prospective controlled study. N Engl J Med 320:143, 1989.
19. Aspelin P, Aubry P, Fransson S-G, et al: Nephrotoxic effects in high-risk patients undergoing angiography. N Engl J Med 348: 491, 2003.
20. Shyu K-Gi, Cheng J-J, Kuan P: Acetylcysteine protects against acute renal damage in patients with abnormal renal function undergoing a coronary procedure. J Am Coll Cardiol 40:1383, 2002.
21. Tepel M, van der Giet M, Schwarzfeld C, et al: Prevention of radiographic-contrast-agent-induced reductions in renal function by acetylcysteine. N Engl J Med 343:180, 2000.
22. Spargias K, Alexopoulos E, Kyrzopoulos S, et al: Ascorbic acid prevents contrast-mediated nephropathy in patients with renal dysfunction undergoing coronary angiography or intervention. Circulation 110:2837, 2004.
23. Merten GJB, Burgess W, Gray LV, et al: Nephropathy with sodium bicarbonate: A randomized controlled trial. JAMA 291:2328, 2004.
24. Kistler PM, Mond HG, Corcoran SJM: Biventricular pacing: It isn't always as it seems. PACE 26:2185, 2003.
25. Heist EK, Fan D, Mela T, et al: Radiographic left ventricular-right ventricular interlead distance predicts the acute hemodynamic response to cardiac resynchronization therapy. The Am J Cardiol 96:685, 2005.
26. Worley SJ: Cardiac resynchronization failures: The lateral chest radiograph identifies patients who benefit from a new LV lead position. Presented at the 8th Annual Scientific Meeting of the Heart Failure Society of America, Toronto, September 9-14, 2004.
27. Mccotter CJ, Angle JF, Prudente LA, et al: Placement of transvenous pacemaker and ICD leads across total chronic occlusions. PACE 28:921, 2005.
28. Worley SJ, Gohn DC, Smith TL: Micro-dissection to open totally occluded subclavian veins. EP Lab Digest, September, 2003.
29. Al-Khadra A: Use of preshaped sheath to plan and facilitate cannulation of the coronary sinus for the implantation of cardiac resynchronization therapy devices: Preshaped sheath for implantation of biventricular devices. PACE 28:489, 2005.
30. Bashir JG, Frank G, Tyers O, et al: Combined use of transesophageal ECHO and fluoroscopy for the placement of left

ventricular pacing leads via the coronary sinus. PACE 26:1951, 2003.

31. Debruyne P, Geelen P, Janssens L, Brugada P: Useful tip to improve electrode positioning in markedly angulated coronary sinus tributaries. J Cardiovasc Electrophysiol 14:415, 2003.
32. Worley SJ, Gohn D, Smith TL: Telescoping delivery system for unsuccessful biventricular implants. Presented at Cardiostim 2002, Nice, France, June 19-22, 2002.
33. Leon AR: New tools for the effective delivery of cardiac resynchronization therapy. J Cardiovasc Electrophysiol 16:S42, 2005.
34. Romeyer-Bouchard C, Da Costa A, Abdellaoui L, et al: Simplified cardiac resynchronization implantation technique involving right access and a triple-guide/single introducer approach. Heart Rhythm 2:714, 2005.
35. Lane RE, Chow AWC, Mayet J, Davies DW: Biventricular pacing exclusively via a persistent left-sided superior vena cava: Case report. PACE 26:640, 2003.
36. Daoud EG, Kalbfleisch SJ, Hummel JD, et al: Implantation techniques and chronic lead parameters of biventricular pacing dual-chamber defibrillators. J Cardiovasc Electrophysiol 13:964, 2002.
37. De Cock CC, Jessurun ER, Allaart CA, Visser CA: Repetitive intraoperative dislocation during transvenous left ventricular lead implantation: Usefulness of the retained guidewire technique. PACE 27:1589, 2004.
38. Schuchert A, Seidl K, Pfeiffer D, et al: Two-year performance of a preshaped lead for left ventricular stimulation. PACE 27:1610, 2004.
39. Ellery S, Paul V, Prenner G, et al: A new endocardial "over-the-wire" or stylet-driven left ventricular lead: First clinical experience. PACE 28:S31, 2005.
40. Frank G, Tyers O, Clark J, et al: Coronary sinus lead extraction. PACE 26:524, 2003.
41. Burke MC, Morton J, Lin AC, et al: Implications and outcome of permanent coronary sinus lead extraction and reimplantation. J Cardiovasc Electrophysiol 16:830, 2005.
42. Chierchia G-B, Geelen P, Rivero-Ayerza M, Brugada P: Double wire technique to catheterize sharply angulated coronary sinus branches in cardiac resynchronization therapy. PACE 28:168, 2005.
43. Worley SJ, Gohn DC, Smith TL, et al: Percutaneous coronary venous angioplasty for left ventricular lead placement in cardiac resynchronization therapy: Analysis of 35 cases. J Am Coll Cardiol 41:115A, 2003.
44. Worley SJ, Gohn DC: Coronary venoplasty reduces mortality in resynchronization therapy. Heart Rhythm 1:S55, 2004.
45. Van Gelder BM, Meijer A, Basting P, et al: Successful implantation of a coronary sinus lead after stenting of a coronary vein stenosis. PACE 26:1904, 2003.

Chapter 20

Approach to Generator Change

STEVEN P. KUTALEK • BHARAT K. KANTHARIA • J. MARCH MAQUILAN

At some time in the life of any patient who has a pacemaker or defibrillator, replacement of the device's pulse generator may be required. Although this need is most often the result of the finite life span of the battery, replacement of the device may be precipitated by such diverse causes as infection,[1-9] erosion,[10] trauma,[11-13] device malfunction or migration,[14-20] and the need for system upgrade (Table 20-1).[21,22] Lead replacement or revision may also result secondarily in generator change,[23-28] especially if the generator is already near the end of its service. Lead malfunction, in particular low lead impedance, may secondarily require premature battery replacement owing to high current drain.

Although device or lead replacement includes surgery, the success of the procedure depends on an accurate preoperative evaluation as well as on good surgical technique. This chapter addresses the preoperative evaluation of the patient and the pacing or defibrillation system as well as the surgical process of device replacement and revision.

Because of the variety of indications for replacement of pacemaker or defibrillator generators, considerations regarding the approach to be used for generator change or lead revision begin at the initial implantation of the system. Meticulous technique in the positioning of endocardial leads to minimize pacing thresholds and maximize sensing capabilities allows optimal programming of the pacing function of the pulse generator to reduce long-term battery drain, thereby prolonging the life of the generator.[29] Careful lead positioning also reduces the likelihood of lead dislodgement that would require reoperation.[26,27,30,31] Caution in venous entry, lead fixation, lead-generator connection, pocket location, and handling of components enhances long-term pacing and sensing function. Ensuring that leads in the generator pocket are placed posterior to the pulse generator improves the likelihood of expeditious pulse generator replacement without damage to the lead. Bulkier defibrillator leads or lead headers may be placed in the same surgical plane next to the device. Ensuring that the pocket is of adequate size to accommodate the pulse generator and lead coils without undue tension diminishes the likelihood of damage to the leads in the pocket due to excessive bending. Thus, the primary implanting physician prepares the stage for successful reoperation (Table 20-2).

Special Considerations for Implantable Cardioverter-Defibrillators

Since the first surgical placement of an implantable cardioverter-defibrillator (ICD) in 1980,[32] the role of ICDs in the management of patients with life-threatening ventricular tachyarrhythmias has become well established. Advances in engineering technology and implantation methods—particularly the nonthoracotomy approach—have enabled widespread use of ICDs in clinical practice. Furthermore, the indications for ICD implantation have been expanding. Many patients outlive the life span of the first ICD generator. Like

TABLE 20-1. Indications for Replacement of Pacemaker or Implantable Cardioverter-Defibrillator (ICD) Generator

Primary indications	Generator end of service: Elective replacement indication Complete failure due to end of service Loss of output Sensing malfunction Generator upgrade: Unipolar to bipolar (pacemaker) Single- to dual-chamber Need for high-energy ICD Pocket twitch: Due to generator insulation break Due to lead insulation break Due to unipolar system Unanticipated generator failure Device recall
Secondary indications*	Pocket issues: Generator migration Persistent pain Pronounced pocket effusion or hematoma Erosion Infection of pacing system Trauma Lead issues: Need for lead revision High thresholds (pacing or sensing) High defibrillation threshold Lead conductor fracture Lead insulation break Loose lead-generator connection Myopotential sensing Diaphragmatic pacing or sensing Twiddler's syndrome Change bifurcated bipolar to unipolar due to malfunction of one conductor (rare)

*These are due to factors other than the pulse generator itself. They require reoperation but may or may not require generator replacement.

pacemakers, ICDs are prone to complications such as infection and malfunction, necessitating replacement or revision of the generator or leads. Although the approach to ICD generator change, lead evaluation, and reoperation can be extrapolated from the approach to pacemaker revision, certain aspects of ICD generator change and revision deserve special consideration. They are indications for replacement or revision, the need to upgrade to more complex lead systems or pacing modes (including cardiac resynchronization), lead malfunction, inadequate defibrillation thresholds, change of implantation site, and interchangeability of older devices and leads from various manufacturers. Each of these issues is addressed in the chapter in relation to special considerations for ICD devices.

Patient Evaluation

Noninvasive Evaluation

Before performing a surgical procedure for pacemaker or defibrillator revision or generator replacement, one must document the need for intervention. Specific indications are approached with a well-defined plan of evaluation.

TABLE 20-2. Technical Factors of Device Implantation that May Reduce the Need for Reoperation

Appropriate connections of leads in the generator header
Gentle treatment of tissues
Hemostasis
Secure closure of subcutaneous tissues and skin
Pocket large enough for generator and leads, without tension
Generator set-screws secure
Appropriate pocket location, intruding on neither clavicle nor axilla Lead issues: Meticulous care in positioning for pacing, sensing, or defibrillation thresholds Fixation Lead selection appropriate for patient Integrity of lead insulation maintained Gentle handling of stylets Anchoring sleeve secured with nonabsorbable suture Placement posterior to, or beside, pulse generator Appropriate connections: A or V to generator Proximal and distal high-energy coils, array, patch Leads fully advanced into generator head Adapters secure and not kinked Set-screws sealed

TABLE 20-3. Indicators of Pacemaker Battery Depletion

Primary indicators	Abrupt decrease in magnet-paced rate Gradual decrease in magnet-paced rate Mode switch (especially DDD to VVI or DOO to VOO magnet mode) Abrupt loss of pacing or sensing capability Interrogated marker of battery depletion
Secondary indicators	Rise in internal battery impedance Drop in battery voltage Pulse width stretch Battery depletion curve

Documentation of Pacemaker Pulse Generator Battery Depletion

Most bradycardia pacemaker pulse generators provide direct or indirect indicators of battery depletion, documenting the need for enhanced follow-up, elective generator replacement, or incipient battery failure. Additionally, certain nonspecific indicators may alert the physician to early signs of battery wear (Table 20-3). Because most pacemaker patients are followed by transtelephonic monitoring systems more frequently

TABLE 20-4. **General Magnet Responses of Pulse Generators**

Pacemaker	Battery depletion indicators: Mode switch (DOO to VOO) Rate change—gradual or abrupt Noise reversion modes: DOO—usual asynchronous operation in dual-chamber system AAT, VVT—usual asynchronous operation in single-chamber system P, R synchronous pacing OOO Magnet rate: Fixed Variable First few complexes faster Last few complexes faster Output: Fixed Variable Voltage or pulse width decremented in first or last few complexes for threshold margin test, or pulse width reduced after magnet withdrawal Duration: Continuous as long as magnet is applied Fixed number of paced complexes
Defibrillator	Inhibition of sensing—especially useful to avoid initiation of tachyarrhythmia with magnet application Reset of tachyarrhythmia sensing Activation/inactivation of device

than by full evaluation in the physician's office, it is not surprising that battery depletion for permanent pacemaker patients is most often detected through transtelephonic recording.[33-36] Methods for transtelephonic evaluation of defibrillator systems are also being developed to allow interrogation after arrhythmic events and to assess battery capacity.[37]

A change in magnet-activated paced rate remains the most common indicator of reduced battery output voltage for pacemakers (Table 20-4). Some pacemaker pulse generator models respond to declining voltages through a gradual reduction in magnet-activated pacing rate; reduced rates indicate the need for enhanced follow-up, with still slower rates indicating elective or obligatory replacement. Other models demonstrate an abrupt shift in the magnet-activated paced rate at the enhanced follow-up period or at the time of elective replacement. A demand mode switch from DDD to VVI (DOO to VOO in magnet mode) may occur at the elective replacement time or as an obligate replacement indicator for dual-chamber systems before complete battery failure (Table 20-5). Inability to reprogram the device, inaccurate measurement of lead impedances, and loss of data collection may also occur as the generator approaches obligate replacement time.

In the office, other secondary parameters suggest gradual battery depletion. The usual battery impedance in a new pulse generator is less than 1000 Ω. As lithium iodide batteries are depleted, internal battery impedance increases, providing a secondary indicator (Fig. 20-1). With high internal battery impedance, some devices compensate for reduced current output by increasing the pulse width to maintain adequate energy delivery to the lead tip. The extent of pulse width stretching is measurable and may be precipitated by high-output pacing; it serves as another secondary indicator of battery depletion. Replacement is not required, however, until more definitive indicators appear, such as a change in magnet-activated pacing rate or mode switch.

Telemetered battery depletion curves (Fig. 20-2) or internal calculations of anticipated device longevity at current programmed settings, as well as a general knowledge of the expected performance of various generators, assist in anticipating and documenting a pacemaker generator's end of service. Ultimately, loss of sensing and pacing capabilities occurs with battery exhaustion. The rate of battery depletion may accelerate as the device reaches end of service, making timely replacement in dependent patients very important.

Indicators for Replacement of Implantable Cardioverter-Defibrillator Generators

Because the rate of defibrillator generator depletion depends on both the frequency of bradycardia pacing and the delivery of high-energy shocks to terminate tachyarrhythmias, the precise longevity of ICD battery systems is more difficult to predict. Nevertheless, documentation of ICD battery drain remains crucial to evaluation of the safe function of the defibrillator system. Various manufacturers have developed relatively straightforward methods to document impending ICD battery depletion. These methods fall into the following three major categories: (1) a measurable reduction in battery voltage that can be acquired through telemetry, (2) an increase in measured charge times to levels that indicate elective replacement time, and (3) various device-specific markers that indicate a particular degree of generator depletion (Table 20-6). Measurement of charge time to a maximal voltage on the device capacitors is the oldest method for estimating the remaining longevity of an ICD. Most early systems included such markers. This method of determining elective replacement time, however, requires fully charging the capacitors and usually necessitates an office visit. Charge times can also be obtained if the device spontaneously charges and delivers therapy at maximum output, but this process does not always occur opportunely between office visits.

Recording a reduced battery voltage provides a readily useful method of determining generator depletion; the value can be obtained telemetrically. This method is now the most common for marking elective replacement time and end of service for ICDs. Specifically, telemetered voltage can be obtained on initial interrogation of the device. It is now remotely retrievable in some devices.

Some specific ICD models use battery voltage to produce labels that indicate the beginning, middle, or end of service for pulse generators. These labels can be obtained directly through interrogation of the device in the office. End of service is clearly indicated (see Table 20-6).

TABLE 20-5. **Examples of Specific Pacemaker Magnet Responses**

Manufacturer	Model	BOL Mode	ERI Mode	EOL Mode	BOL Rate (ppm)	ERI Rate (ppm)	EOL Rate (ppm)	Output (<ERI)	Duration Magnet Response
Biotronik GmbH & Co., Berlin	178	DOO	VDD	VOO	PR	PR − 11% (AD)	PR − 11%	PO	C
Cardiac Control Systems, Inc., Palm Coast, Fla.	505	DOO	DOO	VOO	80*	80-70 (AD)	50 (alt cycles)	PO	C
Cook Vascular, Inc., Leechburg, Penna.	500	VOO	VOO	NSI	100	90 (AD)	NSI	PO	C
Cordis, Miami, Fla. (now a division of Telectronics, St. Jude Medical, Sylmar, Calif.)	233 GL	DOO	DOO	VOO	70	62.5 (AD)	52.5†	PO	C
Guidant, Boston Scientific, Natick, Mass.	1230	DOO	DOO	DOO	100	90 (AD)	85	PO	C
ELA Medical, Sorin Group, Milan	2550	DOO	DOO	DOO	96	80 (GD)	69.8	PO‡	C
Intermedics, Inc., Angleton, Tex.	294-09	DOO	VOO	VOO	5C 90, to PR	4C 90, to 80	80	PW 50% 5th cycle	64 Cx + 5 Cx @ 90
Medtronic, Inc., Minneapolis, Minn.	E2DR01	DOO	VOO	NSI	3C 100, to 85	65 (AD)	NSI	PW 25% 3rd cycle	C
St. Jude Medical, St. Paul, Minn.	5376	DOO	DOO	NSI	PR	PRI + 100 msec (AD)	NSI	PO	C
Telectronics Pacing Systems, Englewood, Col. (now Pacesetter, part of St. Jude Medical, Sylmar, Calif.)	1256	DOO	DOO	DOO	100	82.5 (GD)	At EOL, rate response suspends and the device goes to VVI at 63 ppm, nonprogrammable	PO	C

*80 ppm × 16 C, then PR for 16 C, then 80 ppm.
†62.5 ppm for serial numbers ≥4000.
‡Output is increased to 5.0 V and 0.49 ms (if programmed for less than these values) during magnet application, then is reduced to PO for 6 complexes at the magnet rate after magnet removal with shortening of the AV interval.
AD, abrupt decrease; BOL, beginning of life; C, continuous; Cx, complexes; EOL, end of life; ERI, elective replacement indication; Fx, fixed; GD, gradual decrease—indicated rate defines ERI or EOL; PO, programmed output; NSI, no specific additional EOL indicator before battery failure; ppm, pulses per minute; PR, programmed rate; PRI, programmed rate interval; PW, pulse width.

Regardless of the method used by the device to document an approach to the end of its service, the clinician has the responsibility to increase the frequency of follow-up visits as the unit nears elective replacement time to ensure continued safe function of the system and protection of the patient from tachyarrhythmias. In the event that the patient receives frequent shocks just before the need for device replacement, one must keep in mind that the elective replacement time may occur earlier than was originally anticipated.

Documentation of Lead Malfunction

A variety of causes of lead malfunction require reoperation,[29,38] owing to primary lead dysfunction or secondarily to premature battery depletion as a result of

Pacing rate		60	ppm
Pacing interval		1003	ms
Cell voltage		2.61	volts
Cell impedance		6.75	KOhms
Cell current		20.9	UA
	ATRIAL	VENTRICULAR (UNI)	
Sensitivity	1.6	1.5	mV
Lead impedance	613	504	ohms
Pulse amplitude	2.49	4.97	volts
Pulse width	0.50	0.50	ms
Output current	3.8	9.3	mA
Energy delivered	4.4	20.8	UJ
Charge delivered	1.94	4.66	UC

Figure 20-1. Acquired telemetry data from an Intermedics, Inc. (Angleton, Tex.), Cosmos II 284-05 dual-chamber (DDD) pacemaker programmed to the unipolar mode. Cell impedance has increased to 6750 Ω, a secondary indicator of battery depletion. Pulse amplitude and pulse width are maintained. Lead impedance in both chambers is acceptable.

excessive current drain (see Table 20-1). Primary lead malfunction may be due to outer insulation break,[39-45] inner insulation break in a bipolar coaxial lead,[46,47] lead conductor fracture,[11,13,48] or lead dislodgement.[26,27,30,31,49] Current drain may be increased by (1) high pacing thresholds[23,25,50] through a need to increase output voltage, (2) failure to optimize generator output for long-term pacing after lead maturation (about 3 months after implantation), or (3) inner insulation break with a resultant low pacing impedance. All of these scenarios can result in premature battery depletion. Before reoperation for lead malfunction is performed, consideration should be given to upgrading or replacing the pulse generator, especially if the battery is old.

Lead malfunction can usually be documented by noninvasive telemetric evaluation.[21,51] A measured bipolar pacing lead impedance less than 200 Ω suggests an inner insulation break between the two coaxial pacing coils. An outer insulation break may be the result of lead wear or may have been inadvertently caused during surgery; an inner insulation break between the two coils of a bipolar system occurs most commonly at the subclavian insertion site as the result of crush injury to the lead, especially with leads inserted into the subclavian vein and tied securely in a far medial position in patients with a tight clavicle–first rib space. Telemetry for lead diagnostics may demonstrate markedly low impedance in bipolar pacing in patients with an inner insulation break. The impedance may vary with manipulation of the pacemaker, which causes intermittent shorting of the two lead conductors (Fig. 20-3).

High pacing lead impedance (>1200 Ω) may be the result of lead conductor fracture or an incomplete circuit caused by a loose lead–pulse generator connection. The introduction of high-impedance leads makes it essential to compare the impedance at implantation with follow-up impedance measurements and acceptable impedance ranges for each lead. Depending on the point of discontinuity, lead impedance may vary with manipulation of the pulse generator or with respiration. Lead conductor fractures may be evident on chest radiographs or fluoroscopy; however, absence of visual

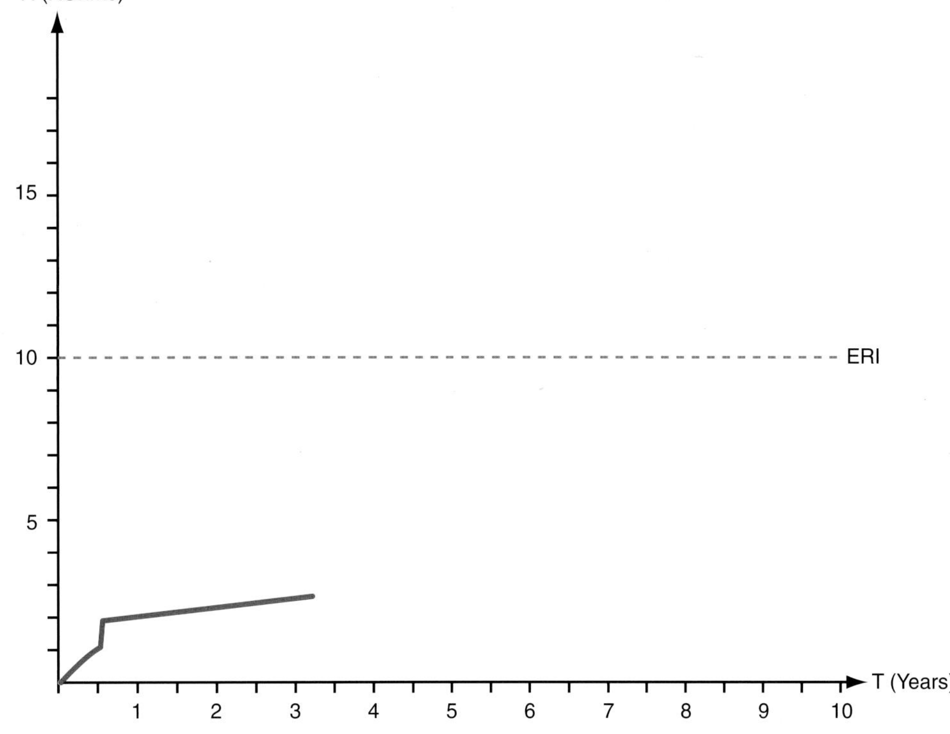

Figure 20-2. Example of a battery depletion curve from an ELA Medical (Sorin Group, Milan) Chorus RM 7034 dual-sensor DDDR pacemaker. The curve graphically presents the true increase in internal battery impedance (R) over time, with an indication of the anticipated impedance at elective replacement time (ERI). Changes in programming that affect battery current drain alter the slope of the battery depletion curve. In this example, the battery impedance has reached about 2.5 kΩ after 3.5 years of use.

TABLE 20-6. **Indicators for Elective Replacement of Commonly Used Implantable Cardioverter-Defibrillators (ICDs)**

Manufacturer	ICD Model	Indicator for Elective Replacement
ELA Medical, Sorin Group, Milan	Defender II 9201 Alto DR 614	BV < 4.90 V BV < 4.90 V
Guidant, Boston Scientific, Natick, Mass.	Ventak Mini, Mini 1740, 1745, 1746 Ventak Mini II, 1742, 1753, 1762, 1763 Ventak Prizm 2 DR 1851 Contak CD 1823 Contak Renewal series	BV < 2.45 V or 2nd CT > 18 sec BV < 2.45 V or 2nd CT > 18 sec BV < 2.45 V or 2nd CT > 20 sec BV > 4.90 V Programmer indicated
Intermedics, Inc., Angleton, Tex.	Res-Q, 101-01, 101-01R Res-Q Micron, 101-05, 101-09	BV < 4.75 V or CT > 30 sec* BV < 4.75 V or 2nd CT > 18 sec
Medtronic, Inc., Minneapolis, Minn.	MicroJewel 7221B, Cx, E, 7223Cx Marquis DR 7274	BV < 4.91 V or 2nd CT > 60 sec BV < 2.62 V or CT > 7.5 sec
St. Jude Medical, St. Paul, Minn.	Profile MD V-186 Atlas + DR V-243 Epic HF V-337	BV < 2.55 V BV < 2.45 V BV < 2.45 V
Telectronics Pacing Systems, Englewood, Col. (now Pacesetter, part of St. Jude Medical, Sylmar, Calif.)	Guardian ATP, 4210 Guardian ATPII, ATPIII, 4211, 4215	Remaining battery life <5% Remaining cell capacity <20%
Ventritex, Sylmar, Calif. (now part of St. Jude Medical, Sunnyvale, Calif.)	Contour, V-135AC, D, V-145AC, D	BV, 2.55 Volts

*After capacitor reform.
BOL, beginning of life; BV, battery voltage; CT, charge time;

evidence does not exclude lead fracture. A break in the connection of the lead to the generator, or within the lead itself, can produce intermittent loss of energy delivery to the heart, which in turn results in absence of pacemaker spikes. Undersensing, or oversensing due to chatter, may also occur with lead conductor fracture.

Lead dislodgement produces intermittent noncapture or failure to sense that may be related to respiration. Pacing thresholds needed to achieve consistent capture may rise significantly. Lead impedance increases or remains unchanged. Fluoroscopy may demonstrate a loose or displaced lead tip but is not always diagnostic.

Special Issues Regarding Implantable Cardioverter-Defibrillator Leads

Evaluation of the ICD generator and its lead system poses a special problem in patients who remain free of arrhythmic events after ICD implantation. The ICD lead remains the weak link in the ICD system for the patient. Oversensing due to diaphragmatic impulses or extraneous signals may inhibit pacing therapy or lead to inappropriate delivery of "treatment" for presumed ventricular tachyarrhythmias that actually represent noise sensing (Figs. 20-4 and 20-5).[52] Further, although fracture and degradation of transvenous leads have become less common with transvenous, as opposed to epicardial, ICD lead systems, they can nevertheless occur with some frequency, necessitating reprogramming or reoperation.[53]

Depleted battery status is readily evident on routine ICD follow-up (as described previously and in Table 20-6), and integrity of the ICD shocking conductors can be evaluated easily in most current devices. High shocking electrode impedance measurements may indicate lead discontinuity due to conductor fracture or a lead-generator interface problem.

Measuring high-energy electrode impedance traditionally required delivery of a shock, either for a clinical tachyarrhythmia or as part of a noninvasive testing protocol. In the absence of consensus or guidelines for performing noninvasive programmed stimulation routinely during follow-up (during which shock electrode integrity may be documented),[54] it was not uncommon in patients with early ICD devices and infrequent shocks for the first documentation of high-energy conductor fracture to occur when they presented for generator replacement. About 10% of patients undergoing ICD generator replacement due to battery depletion were found to have a previously undetected sensing or defibrillation system failure.[55] The operator therefore should test the lead system carefully during the replacement procedure and should be prepared to deal with malfunctioning leads at the time of generator change.

Pacing rate	68	ppm
Pacing interval	873	ms
Average cell voltage	2.63	volts
Cell impedance	<1.00	KOhms
Sensitivity	8	mV
Lead impedance	41	ohms
Pulse amplitude	7.42	volts
Pulse width	0.45	ms
Output current	96.5	mA
Energy delivered	173.2	UJ
Charge delivered	42.85	UC
Tachycardia detected	No	

Figure 20-3. Acquired telemetry data from an Intermedics, Inc. (Angleton, Tex.), Intertach 262-14 VVICP antitachycardia pacemaker connected through a bipolar coaxial lead to the right ventricular apex. Battery voltage and cell impedance are normal. Measured lead impedance of 41 Ω is, however, extremely low. In this patient, measured lead impedance was normal in the supine position but decreased with sitting or when the device was pulled inferiorly. This behavior indicates a break in the inner insulator between the coaxial conductor strands in the area of the clavicle. With movement, the conductors contact each other, resulting in low impedance and preventing delivery of electric current to the heart. Because output voltage is fixed, the low lead impedance results in a high delivered current (96.5 mA) and energy.

Newer systems automatically measure high-energy lead impedance at device interrogation in a manner similar to that used for standard pacing and sensing electrodes. The lower-energy impulses delivered by these devices may be more sensitive to the detection of microfractures than would higher-energy shocks.

Determination of Pulse Generator–Lead Interface Malfunction

Pulse generator–lead interface problems may be grouped into the following three categories: (1) loose, incomplete, or uninsulated connections, (2) reversal of atrial and ventricular leads in the pulse generator connector block (for ICDs, reversal of shocking electrode polarity may also occur), and (3) pulse generator–lead mismatch.

A loose pace/sense lead connection should become apparent with noninvasive testing. The device may fail to deliver pacing spikes when appropriate, it may intermittently fail to sense, and/or it may oversense as a result of chatter due to intermittent contact with the

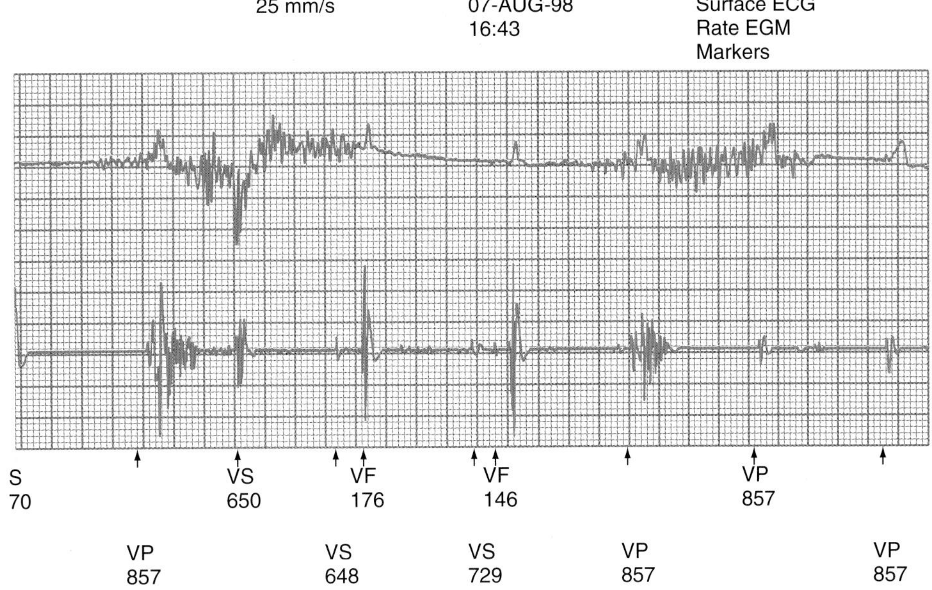

Figure 20-4. Sensing of diaphragmatic myopotential during periods of deep inspiration can lead to inappropriate triggering of the antitachycardia functions of an implantable cardioverter-defibrillator (ICD) (Endotak, CPI, St. Paul, Minn). These electrograms are recorded from an ICD placed with a passive-fixation endocardial lead that incorporates integrated bipolar sensing and high-energy shocking coils in the right ventricular apex and the superior vena cava. Surface electrocardiogram (ECG), rate-sensing electrograms (EGMs), and marker channels all record spurious signals that represent inappropriate sensing of extracardiac electrical potentials. The frequency of these signals is high, and they occur after paced events as well as after sensed events. Pacing increases the gain of the device to avoid undersensing of low-amplitude signals of ventricular fibrillation. An underlying paced rhythm exists at a cycle length of 857 msec, but even this is altered by oversensing. The first paced complex (VP 857) is followed by two inappropriately sensed events (VS 650 and VS 648) that inhibit ventricular pacing output. Because the next native QRS complex occurs close to an inappropriately sensed signal, it is interpreted by the device to represent sensing in the ventricular fibrillation zone (VF 176). After that, another myopotential is inappropriately sensed (VS 729), and the native QRS is again sensed in the VF zone (VF 146). Finally, three sequential paced events occur at intervals of 857 msec, despite the presence of spurious electrical signals, which are not of sufficient amplitude to trigger sensing. Repetitive events such as these could lead to inappropriate antitachycardia therapies or prolonged periods of inhibition of pacing. This lead was extracted and replaced with an active-fixation endocardial defibrillation lead positioned distally on the lower region of the interventricular septum. (Photography by Todd Forkin, Hahnemann University Hospital, Philadelphia.)

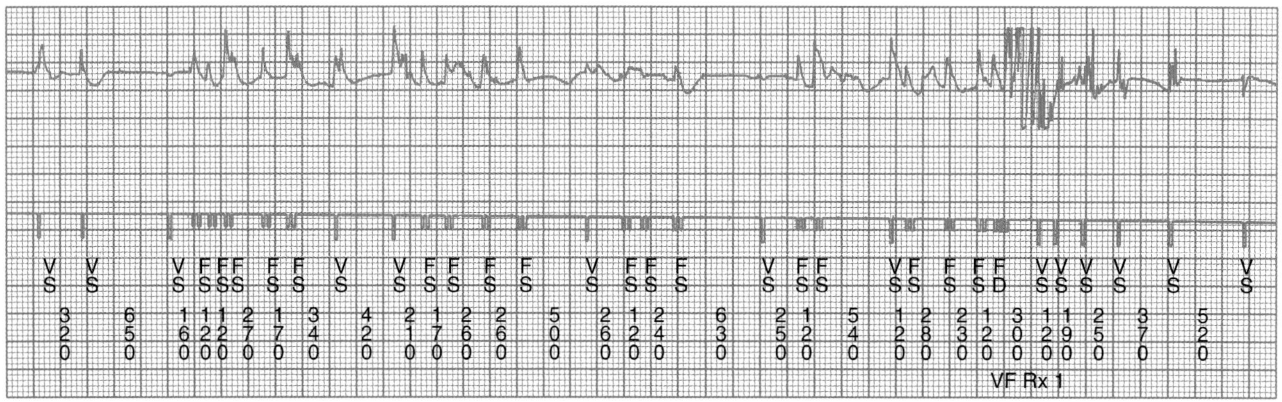

Figure 20-5. Conductor fracture with intermittent contact of the broken ends of the lead wire may result in inappropriate sensing of noise chatter, as demonstrated in this example. Underlying native QRS complexes are difficult to discern. Noise sense intervals vary from 120 to 650 msec. The high degree of variability of sensed intervals, as well as frequent nonphysiologic intervals shorter than 200 msec, lead to the diagnosis of noise sensing. In this example, the number of sensed intervals in the ventricular fibrillation zone is great enough to trigger the VF detection algorithm of the device; this is recorded by the marker channel (FD). Ventricular fibrillation therapy was inappropriately delivered (VF Rx 1). Lead replacement, or placement of a new rate-sensing lead, is indicated. The top tracing is a ventricular electrogram, and the bottom tracing is an interpretation channel with interval measurements. (Photography by Todd Forkin, Hahnemann University Hospital, Philadelphia.)

setscrew. Oversensing can result in inappropriately high tracking rates or inhibition of ventricular output. Capture or sensing problems may be exacerbated by manipulation of the device. An uninsulated connection most commonly produces current leakage (an electrical short circuit in the system) that inhibits pacing or sensing. Leakage can occur if a setscrew is not properly insulated or tightened or if sealing rings on the lead header do not prevent body fluid from oozing into the pulse generator connector block around a loosely fitting lead. Leakage around lead header sealing rings may result from a loose lead connection or lead–pulse generator mismatch. Lead impedance in pulse generator–lead interface problems varies, depending on the specific situation. A loose, unconnected lead that remains in the pulse generator connector block, so that lead header sealing rings prevent fluid from entering, causes a break in the electric circuit and a very high impedance. If fluid enters the pulse generator connector block around a loose lead or at the level of a setscrew and maintains contact with body fluids, however, the resultant electric short circuit can produce very low measured impedance. As with lead fractures, impedance can vary with manipulation of the device.

Reversed lead connections (i.e., atrial lead in the ventricular port, and vice versa) should be evident before the patient leaves the implantation laboratory, allowing immediate correction. Some atrial and ventricular leads are marked to enable easy identification; however, it is not uncommon to place "generic" leads into both chambers, especially straight screw-in leads, which may not be marked. Likewise, atrial and possibly the left and right ventricular lead pace/sense headers for insertion into ICD ports are both of the International Standard IS-1, so the implanter must exercise care in placing these leads properly into the appropriate locations in the ICD generator connector block. It is also possible, in patients in whom a pacemaker or ICD remains inhibited because of native electrical activity, to see no pacing spikes initially after implantation. To be certain that the pulse generator–lead system functions appropriately immediately after implantation, the device should be programmed to an atrioventricular (AV) delay shorter than the intrinsic PR interval, the device should be checked with a programmer or (for a pacemaker) one should place a magnet over the device after the leads are attached to document appropriate function before the pocket is closed. Caution exercised at implantation should avoid reversed leads; for example, we always connect the ventricular lead first to ensure pacing in the proper chamber.

Beyond ensuring the presence of adequate and appropriate lead connections to the pulse generator, the battery connector block and leads must be compatible (see later).[56-58] This issue is especially important with older lead models for device upgrades or generator replacements. Incompatibility can result in fluid leakage or loose connections, with resultant loss of pace/sense or shocking capabilities, requiring reoperation.

Detection of Need for Reoperation for Other Reasons

Other indications for pacemaker or ICD generator replacement or lead revision (see Table 20-1) generally become apparent through careful patient evaluation. Abrupt pulse generator failure with no antecedent sign of battery depletion is rare but can occur, producing symptoms in pacemaker-dependent patients. In others, abnormal pacing output or rate, lack of pacing output, or inappropriate sensing due to generator malfunction may be detected by remote interrogation at home or in the physician's office.[17] Of particular importance to patients with ICDs are the possibilities of no output when required to terminate tachyarrhythmias, inappropriate shocks due to oversensing of diaphragmatic or lead chatter artifact (see Figs. 20-4 and 20-5), and oversensing of extraneous electromagnetic signals, such as surveillance systems or high-voltage generators, that can be sensed as ventricular fibrillation or can inhibit ventricular pacing output. Cellular telephones rarely present substantial interference due to variations in signal frequency.[59,60]

Development of pacemaker syndrome in patients with implanted ventricular demand (VVI), ventricular rate-responsive (VVIR), or atrial rate-responsive (AAIR)[22] pacemakers presents another indication for device revision. This need should be apparent from history and physical examination, although confirmatory blood pressure or cardiac output measurements may be required. Documentation of hemodynamic improvement with dual-chamber synchronization may require placement of a temporary atrial lead before reoperation for upgrading to a dual-chamber system. Pacemaker syndrome occurring with an implanted functioning dual-chamber pacemaker must be managed by reprogramming.[61,62]

Interchangeability of Products from Different Manufacturers

Unlike pacemaker leads, most early ICD leads from different manufacturers were compatible only with ICD pulse generators from the same manufacturer. For later models, manufacturers have adhered to standard header designs for ICDs, including IS-1 ports for the pace/sense lead heads from both atrial and ventricular leads. Defibrillation ports now also follow a standard for defibrillation lead headers, DF-1, a 3.2-mm unipolar lead head with sealing rings. The newest agreed-on IS-4 standard, which provides four electrical connections combining the functions of a bipolar pace/sense connection with up to two high-voltage connections, should reduce some of the confusion. However, there are two IS-4 connections, one for devices with and one for devices without high-voltage (defibrillation) capacity. In the end, this situation should simplify connections except when extra leads for defibrillation are adapted into the lead system.

For procedures involving old, nonstandard ICD connector blocks, however, the operator must be familiar with the existing system of leads and generator in the patient before surgery, and technical support from the manufacturer may be required at the time of the operation. A full range of adapters, or various header designs, to mate a replacement generator to the existing leads must be available. Ensuring tight and proper connections between the generator and the lead, and any adapters and lead extenders, avoids malfunction and current leak. Although older adapters used an uncured medical adhesive to seal set-screws in the connector block of the device, some newer adapters use set-screw seals similar to those found in pacemaker pulse generators.

Special Indications for Replacement of Implantable Cardioverter-Defibrillator Generators

In addition to the indications outlined in Table 20-1, the ICD generator may need to be replaced for the reasons discussed here.

Malfunction of the Generator with or without Lead Malfunction. Hardware or software errors in the ICD generator—or, more commonly, malfunctioning ICD leads—may result in the need to revise the ICD system. The overall reported incidence of lead-related complications has ranged from 2% to 28%.[63,64] These complications commonly manifest as inappropriate shocks resulting from oversensing of noise (see Fig. 20-5) or as ineffective shocks from the shunting of defibrillation energy due to an inner insulator breach.

Upgrading the Device to Incorporate Tiered Therapy and Multiple Zones of Therapy. Older devices incorporated monophasic shock energy for defibrillation, which was more likely to achieve an inadequate defibrillation threshold (DFT) than biphasic lead systems. The success of current ICD generators is attributed primarily to the use of biphasic shocking waveforms[65-68] and tiered therapy, incorporating antitachycardia pacing. Certain older ICD systems and "stripped-down" shock-only rescue units were designed to deliver only shock therapy. In the rare instance that a shock-only ICD is still in place and requires replacement by an ICD that offers more sophisticated therapies, including tiered therapies for different arrhythmia zones, reoperation is required.

Upgrading to a Higher-Energy Device or Addition of Hardware for an Inadequate Defibrillation Threshold. Occasionally, through invasive or noninvasive testing, the physician determines that the best function of the device may be achieved through a change in its hardware configuration. This may involve reoperation to place a generator capable of delivering higher defibrillation energy to respond to an elevated DFT, repositioning the right ventricular apical (RVA) shocking electrode, or the addition of various other lead systems, including superior vena cava coils and subcutaneous coils, arrays, or patches. Clearly, location of the RVA lead as close to the cardiac apex as possible affords the lowest DFT. Similarly, addition of various other leads to better distribute current around the heart can also reduce the DFT,[69,70] often concomitantly lowering shocking electrode impedance for higher current delivery. Finally, if these invasive adjustments fail to reduce the DFT, waveform adjustments[65] or replacement of the pulse generator with a higher-energy system may be warranted.

Many patients with ICDs continue to require treatment with antiarrhythmic medications, which can affect the appropriate functioning of ICDs. The most common antiarrhythmic medication–ICD interaction observed is that of an elevated DFT. This is particularly evident with potent sodium channel–blocking drugs and with amiodarone.[71,72] In this regard, reoperation may be required for antiarrhythmic drug changes that lead to substantial alterations in the DFT, although elimination of the offending medication provides a more straightforward solution. When that is not possible, the physician may consider use of a device that delivers higher energy for defibrillation. Addition of a superior vena cava (SVC) coil or subcutaneous array may be indicated.

Upgrading to Incorporate Dual-Chamber Pacing Capability. With an established role for β-blockers in the treatment of congestive heart failure and coronary artery disease, as well as a baseline frequency of developing sinus node dysfunction or AV conduction disorders, substantial numbers of patients with implanted defibrillators require dual-chamber bradycardia pacing backup. This problem is easily resolved in the new implant but can require considerable deliberation when substantial hardware is already in place. Several scenarios may be encountered, each with unique potential solutions. Some of these situations, with possible approaches, are described here.

The patient may have a previously implanted abdominal single-chamber ICD with a fully functional epicardial lead system. In this situation, the operator has three primary options, as follows: (1) to place an endocardial atrial pacing lead through the subclavian system and tunnel the lead subcutaneously to the abdominal pocket, while upgrading the device to a dual-chamber ICD, (2) to abandon the abdominal ICD and place an entirely new AV sequential ICD system in the pectoral area, and (3) to place a totally separate dual-chamber permanent pacemaker system with atrial and ventricular leads and perform device interaction testing to ensure that neither of the two devices inhibits the other.

There are various advantages and disadvantages to each of these techniques. For the first option, the advantage of long-term stability of thresholds for endocardial pace and sense leads speaks for the approach of adding an endocardial atrial lead and tunneling it to the abdomen, but it also requires that the lead be long enough to tunnel to the abdominal site. This makes manipulation and positioning of the lead in the atrium more challenging. Alternatively, a lead extender may be attached to a shorter lead, but this arrangement adds another weak link in the system in the form of an adapter. Finally, this approach requires opening both the abdominal pocket and the subclavian site simultaneously, which could raise the risk for cross-infection of the abdominal site. Accordingly, we prefer not to have two pockets open at the same time, especially when one involves an epicardial lead system, where infection could be disastrous.

Abandoning the abdominal site altogether, the second option, may be the preferred technique because it eliminates the need to open two pockets simultaneously; it also eliminates the need to depend on *any* epicardial leads, which have a higher failure rate than endocardial leads. The new pulse generator and lead system are placed in the standard manner in the pectoral area, and DFT testing is performed at implantation; the previous abdominal pocket remains closed during this operation, eliminating the possibility of cross-infection between sites. Electrical shielding afforded by the epicardial patches may affect the endocardial DFT. This problem may well be offset, however, by the improved long-term reliability of the endocardial lead system. The abdominal generator may be turned off and left in place, or it can be removed after implantation of the new system, preferably during a separate procedure. This approach is particularly useful in patients in whom a new high-energy ventricular coil is needed, which can be placed endocardially.

The third option, placement of a totally endocardial dual-chamber pacemaker system with atrial and ventricular bradycardia pacing leads, also eliminates the need to open the two pockets simultaneously. It also affords the advantages of prolonging ICD battery life (through a separate pacemaker battery) and provides consistent and separate bradycardia pacing backup through a device designed primarily for bradycardia support. Implantation of a separate pacemaker and an ICD may, however, lead to various device-device interactions, including undersensing of ventricular fibrillation.[72] The availability of combined dual-chamber pacemaker and ICD systems should reduce the physician's concern about device interaction. This option is our least-favored approach.

Upgrade to a Biventricular, Cardiac Resynchronization System. Upgrade to a biventricular (BiV), cardiac resynchronization system has become one of the most common indications for ICD reoperation, either as a de novo device upgrade or at the time of generator replacement.[73] Upgrade to a biventricular system requires device generator replacement and insertion of a new coronary sinus/LV electrode. We perform venography to ensure patency of the vasculature for the new lead if any difficulty is encountered in accessing the axillary vein. Implantation of the new lead and device often requires a pocket revision to accommodate the larger generator.

Change of Implantation Site. Older ICD generators, because of their bulky nature, were routinely implanted in the abdominal wall. With the availability of active can electrodes and ICD generators of smaller size, consideration should be given to changing the implantation site to the pectoral area when leads need to be revised. This issue was addressed previously with respect to placement of atrial leads; it should also be considered when ventricular lead malfunction necessitates reoperation, especially with a long nonthoracotomy ICD lead tunneled from the subclavian area to the abdominal wall. Another example is malfunction of epicardial ventricular sensing electrodes due to conductor fracture, high pacing threshold, or oversensing. Options for such a situation are placing a ventricular endocardial sensing electrode and tunneling it to the abdominal pocket or abandoning the abdominal pocket to place an entirely new completely endocardial ICD system in a pectoral location. We prefer the latter approach, again because it eliminates the need to open the two pockets simultaneously in a patient with epicardial leads and patches, in whom infection could be devastating, and because it eliminates the danger of fracture of the epicardial leads due to wear.

The implantation site may also need to be changed in the event of incipient erosion, or outright infection, of the device site. Clearly, a staged approach is most useful here. If the site is infected with a malignant organism such as *Staphylococcus aureus*, the pulse generator and leads should be removed, with use of appropriate antibiotic coverage; a separate surgical procedure will be needed for implantation of a pectoral, contralateral ICD system. The two pockets should not be opened at the same operation. Most commonly, removal of the entire system is required for cure of the infection.

Tunneling a lead from a location in the abdomen to one in the pectoral area can damage the tunneled lead, especially the header. There is no definitive way to avoid this risk, although gentleness with respect to lead manipulation and use of a standard dilator or tunneling tool reduces the tendency to damage. The lead needs first to be positioned in the ventricle through manipulation at the shoulder, because a long lead would be difficult to maneuver from an abdominal location through a tunnel. Only after it is carefully positioned can it be tunneled; therefore, the connector head of the lead will be tunneled from the shoulder to the abdominal pocket. Such tunneling can place significant stress on the lead connector, which could damage it. When preexisting tunneled leads must be replaced, the tract can be dilated with extraction sheaths, although this procedure is time-consuming and complex. As noted previously, whenever possible, adapters should be avoided because they merely add another weak link in the chain of possibilities for lead malfunction.

Complications of Pacemaker or Implantable Cardioverter-Defibrillator Implantation that Require Reoperation. Reoperation may be required for complications resulting from the initial implantation procedure.[10,15,16,74-80] Decisions about surgery in patients with large pocket hematomas or effusions, cardiac chamber perforation by a lead, or a need to reposition the pulse generator must be made on an individual basis. Most small to moderate hematomas resolve; the risk of secondarily introducing infection through reoperation or aspiration can thus be avoided. Large hematomas or effusions that do not resolve and that compromise the blood supply through pressure on the overlying skin of the pacemaker or ICD pocket require evacuation followed by primary closure, because the pocket cannot be left open with a device in place. Bolus dosing of heparin, use of enoxaparin, and large loading doses of warfarin should be avoided whenever possible to reduce hematoma risk.

Pocket twitch (due to lead insulation break, loose lead-generator connection, exposed set-screw, battery insulation break, inverted unipolar insulated pacemaker pulse generator, or the need for high-output pacing in a unipolar system), diaphragmatic pacing, or skeletal muscle stimulation or myopotential inhibition[81] (Fig. 20-6) may require surgical intervention if such problems cannot be solved by reprogramming.

Identification of Pulse Generator Make and Model

The most straightforward means of identifying a pulse generator showing signs of malfunction or operating in a mode that suggests end of service is to obtain information directly from the patient (Table 20-7). An identification card is provided by the manufacturer for each pacemaker and patient with an ICD, specifying the type of device, model and serial number, implantation date, name of implanting or monitoring physician, and, often, lead model and serial numbers. This information may also be obtained from records kept by the manufacturer, the implanting physician, the monitoring physician, the transtelephonic service that monitors the patient, or the institution at which the device was placed. If none of these sources of information is helpful, alternative methods must be used to identify the pulse generator. Identification of the make and model of the existing pulse generator is crucial to determining its true functional status and, with older leads, to have the necessary information to select a compatible replacement or upgraded device. In the rare instance in which a pulse generator cannot be identified before surgery, the implanting physician must have a full array of leads, generators, and adapters available at the time of reoperation.

Magnet Response. The response of a bradycardia pacemaker pulse generator to placement of a magnet can assist in the identification of its manufacturer (Fig. 20-7; see Table 20-5). Most pacemaker pulse generators

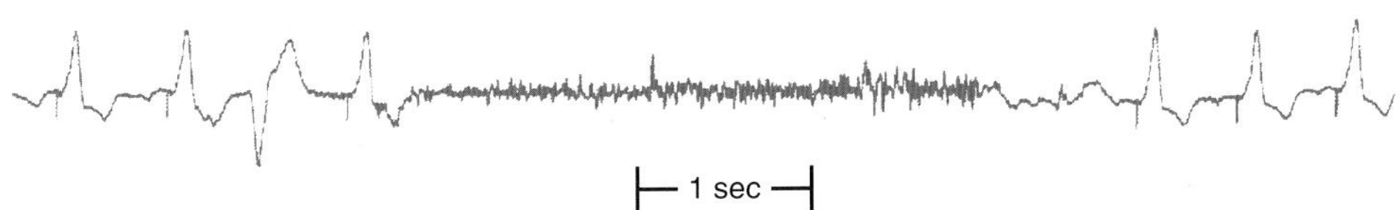

Figure 20-6. Myopotential inhibition in a unipolar dual-chamber pacing system induced by pectoral muscle contraction in a patient who noted recurrent lightheadedness with activity. Atrial sensitivity is programmed to 0.5 mV, and ventricular sensitivity to 2.5 mV. Two atrially tracked complexes are followed by a ventricular premature depolarization. The fourth QRS complex occurs early as a result of atrial myopotential tracking. Thereafter, ventricular pacing output is inhibited by myopotentials for nearly 6 seconds, after which normal DDD function resumes. Intrinsic QRS complexes occurring during the period of inhibition may be obscured by myopotential activity. Programming the ventricular sensitivity to 5 mV avoided myopotential inhibition and the need for lead revision. Although atrial sensitivity could not be adjusted because of the low intrinsic P wave amplitude, atrial myopotential tracking remained asymptomatic.

TABLE 20-7. Identification of the Pulse Generator

Manufacturer code and serial number code
Implantation data
Identification card
Transtelephonic monitoring records
Manufacturer's implantation records
Monitoring physician's records
Noninvasive testing
Size, shape, thickness
Magnet response (pacemakers)
Interrogation (if manufacturer identified)
Fluoroscopy: Size, shape Connector block Unipolar or bipolar (pacing) Single- or dual-chamber Number of ports for implantable cardioverter-defibrillator leads Identifying markings/codes
Lead: Unipolar or bipolar (pacing) Active or passive fixation Number of high-energy coils
Invasive testing: Direct identification of pulse generator Lead—manufacturer code and serial number code Type of connector Size of lead header

respond to magnet application by entering a fixed-rate single-chamber or dual-chamber pacing mode corresponding to the type of generator and the programmed mode. Magnet rates vary among manufacturers and may provide a clue to the origin of the device. To undergo a magnet-activated test, the patient must be connected to an electrocardiographic recorder before the magnet is applied and must remain connected until after the magnet is removed. The first few paced complexes after magnet application may occur at a rate or output other than that seen later in the recording, providing identification data as well as information regarding the integrity of the pulse generator and lead system (e.g., the delivered pulse width may be reduced during the first few paced complexes to ensure that capture still occurs with an adequate safety margin). Furthermore, with constant magnet application over the pacemaker, some devices continue to pace at a fixed rate, whereas others cease pacing after a programmed number of intervals. Devices temporarily reprogrammed to a backup mode by electrical interference (e.g., electrocautery during surgery) may exhibit magnet responses that vary from the standard for such.

Radiographic or Fluoroscopic Identification of the Pulse Generator. Most pulse generators—both pacemakers and ICDs—can be identified from their appearance under radiography. This is the most helpful method of identifying unknown devices. The shape and size of the generator may characterize a particular manufacturer (e.g., square, oval, elongated ellipsoid, round). Pulse generator shape can vary significantly from one device model to another, however, even when produced by the same manufacturer. Considering that the life span of some pacemaker devices may exceed 10 or 12 years, various shapes and sizes may be encountered.

More specific to identification of the pulse generator are radiopaque markings placed near the connector block that code for manufacturer and device model. These markings appear most clearly under magnified fluoroscopic or radiographic examination when the device is positioned perpendicular to the x-ray beam (Fig. 20-8).

The shape and orientation of internal components, which can often be identified radiographically, provide further clues to the device type, manufacturer, and model. Comparison of these radiographic features (size and shape, identification markings, internal components) with compiled x-ray photographs available from manufacturers facilitates identification of the pulse generator.

Finally, an attempt to interrogate a pulse generator with an "army" of different programmers may identify the pulse generator, unless the battery is so depleted that telemetry communication is not possible.

Radiographic or Fluoroscopic Identification of Leads. Radiographic examination of leads serves two purposes.[82] First, it allows the physician to ascertain the presence of unipolar versus bipolar distal electrodes and, frequently, the fixation mechanism. Distal active-fixation screws may often be seen directly on radiography, whereas passive-fixation leads often have a bulbous tip. Second, radiographic examination identifies lead conductor fractures in which the conductor has clearly separated, leaving a gap; this identification may require magnified views. Lead information of this sort is important for programming (bipolar vs. unipolar), for selecting an appropriately compatible generator, and for identifying leads for extraction. Fluoroscopy also gives some indication of the degree of fibrosis evident through the real-time motion of the lead, information that could be useful if extraction is required.

Radiography of leads involves an examination of the insertion site (e.g., subclavian, axillary, cephalic, jugular, or epicardial), acute bends or fractures in the lead, the location of lead coils beneath the pulse generator in the event that they need to be freed for lead repositioning or extraction, the position of the pulse generator connector block, and a general preview of the character of the connector block–lead interface (see Fig. 20-8). The lead should be examined fluoroscopically throughout its course for kinking, fracture, or excessive tension as well as for fixation at the distal tip. A thorough radiographic examination of lead integrity and pulse generator–lead interface before reoperation

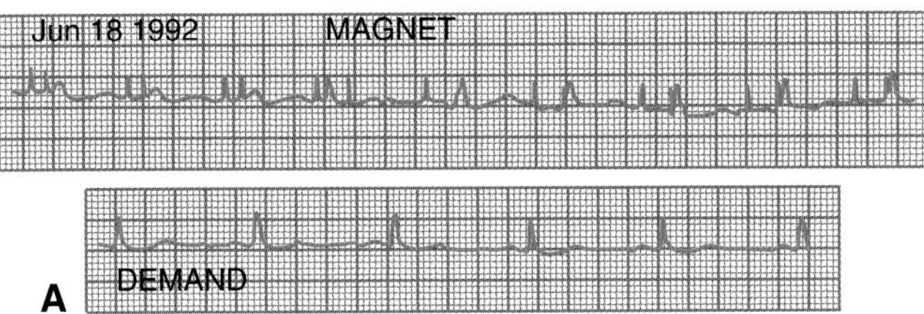

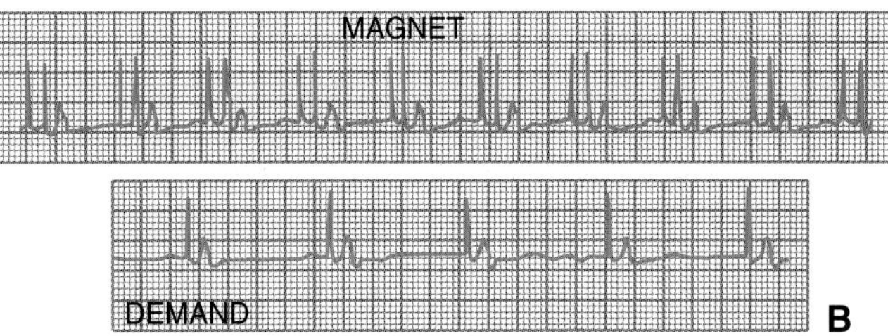

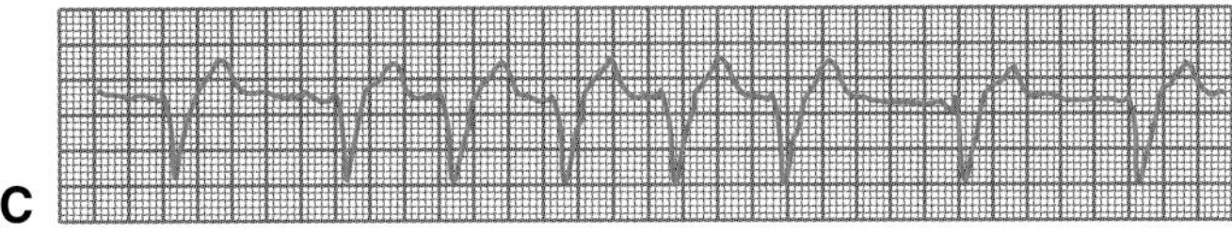

*Figure 20-7. Examples of normal pacemaker generator magnet response. Tracings **A** and **B** were recorded transtelephonically during routine follow-up. Upper tracings in both **A** and **B** show magnet response (DOO), and lower tracings show demand mode with the magnet off. Tracing **C** was recorded by real-time surface electrocardiography at follow-up in the office. **A,** Representative tracings from Medtronic, Inc. (Minneapolis, Minn.), dual-chamber pacing systems, here from a model 7070 Synergyst II device programmed DDD. The first three atrioventricular (AV) sequentially paced complexes are delivered at a rate 10% higher than the magnet rate; the AV interval is shortened to ensure both atrial and ventricular capture. The first two AV complexes are delivered at programmed atrial and ventricular outputs, whereas the delivered pulse width of the third complex is reduced by 25% ("threshold margin test"). Thereafter, the device delivers AV sequentially paced complexes at a fixed rate of approximately 85 bpm at programmed output. The device in this example remains entirely inhibited in the demand mode. **B,** Representative tracings from ELA Medical (Sorin Group, Milan) dual-chamber pacing systems, here from a model 6034 Chorus device programmed DDD. Magnet application results in fixed-rate DOO pacing at a rate of 96 bpm at the programmed AV interval. The AV interval in this example is short owing to activation of the rate-adaptive AV delay. Output during magnet application may be increased but reverts to programmed levels for six complexes after magnet withdrawal (see Table 20-5). The pacemaker appropriately tracks in the demand mode. **C,** Representative electrocardiographic recording from Intermedics, Inc. (Angleton, Tex.), dual-chamber pacing systems, here from a model 294-03 Relay device programmed DDD. The first four complexes are delivered at 90 bpm with a shortened AV delay. Programmed pulse width for the fourth complex is reduced by 50%. Thereafter, the device delivers AV sequentially paced complexes in a fixed mode (DOO) at the programmed rate, while the magnet remains in place for a total of 60 AV complexes in the DOO mode.*

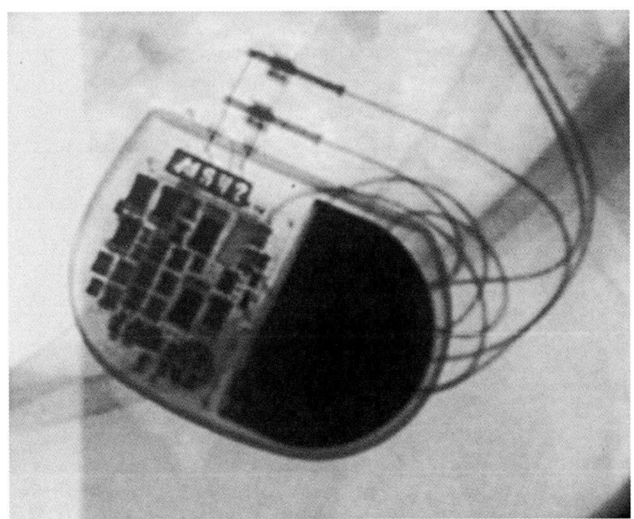

Figure 20-8. Radiographic identification of a pulse generator. The unit is clearly connected to two leads, and each lead has only a single electrically active pole (i.e., unipolar). Although the shape and arrangement of electronic components assist in identification, the specific radiopaque code block inside the pulse generator provides the primary means of identifying the device. Here, a Medtronic logo, followed by S W 2, indicates that the pulse generator is a Medtronic, Inc. (Minneapolis, Minn.), Synergyst II model 7071 DDDR unit with a connector block that will accept two (atrial and ventricular) 5-mm or 6-mm unipolar leads.

in pacemaker and ICD patients saves much distress when the pocket is opened.

Invasive Evaluation

After as much information as possible has been gathered noninvasively about the hardware of the pacing system and the functional status of all its components, further invasive evaluation may proceed at the time of reoperation. Invasive evaluation does not supplant noninvasive analysis but adds to it. Invasive evaluation involves (1) measuring the functional capacity of implanted leads, (2) examining the structural integrity of leads and the lead-generator interface, and (3) venography.

Measuring the Functional Capacity of Implanted Leads

By far one of the most crucial parts of invasive analysis during reoperation involves measurement of pacing and sensing capabilities in existing long-term leads. Vigorous noninvasive evaluation should provide the operator with a significant amount of information regarding lead viability and functional status as well as a determination of pulse generator end of life.[28,29,35,43,51] Verification of lead integrity and precise DFT determination must, however, be performed at reoperation. If surgery is undertaken for pulse generator replacement, demonstrating viability of existing leads is vital to the appropriate long-term performance of the new battery. Surgery for lead repair or revision itself involves extensive testing of long-term leads to confirm the lead as the source of malfunction, ensure normal operation of other leads, and evaluate new leads for optimal positioning inside the heart.

After the pacemaker or ICD pocket is opened, the pulse generator is disconnected from the leads to enable testing of lead sensing and pacing functional capacity.[83] The lead must be disconnected from the pulse generator cautiously in pacemaker-dependent patients; to avoid prolonged ventricular asystole, the operator must be prepared to connect the lead immediately to a cable attached to a functioning external pacing system. The external device should be activated and should be delivering pacing impulses before the ventricular lead is disconnected from the pulse generator in a pacemaker-dependent patient. Alternatively, although it is not usually necessary, a temporary pacing wire may be placed before lead disconnection in a pacemaker-dependent patient; such additional instrumentation, however, may raise the risk of infection. Of course, the operator must exercise care in the removal of the pulse generator and dissection of the lead to maintain lead integrity.

Invasive Testing of the Sensing and Pacing Capabilities of Leads that Have Been Implanted for a Long Time

One of the most important aspects of invasive testing involves measurement of pacing and sensing thresholds in long-term pacemaker and ICD leads. Pace and sense lead thresholds rarely remain as low as those at initial lead implantation. Most leads show some deterioration in pacing and sensing thresholds during the first 4 to 8 weeks after implantation, then reach a relatively stable level for the long term.[23,50] It is possible, however, for thresholds to continue to increase over time, a change that may not be recognized by transtelephonic monitoring alone. The change in threshold from baseline appears greatest with active-fixation, non–steroid-eluting leads; threshold increases are reduced with passive-fixation and steroid-eluting leads, even if the steroid is applied to active-fixation systems. Noninvasive testing should give the operator some clues to the usefulness of long-term leads, but invasive testing confirms their functional utility.

Both atrial and ventricular leads must be tested. If bipolar, they should be evaluated in both unipolar and bipolar configurations. The external pacing analyzer is connected to the lead; pacing and sensing thresholds and lead impedance are determined. The voltage pacing threshold at a fixed pulse width is recorded as the threshold that produces reliable capture. Delivered current can then be measured. Pacing lead impedance is best determined at an increased output voltage (e.g., 5 V) to ensure accuracy.

Low-voltage pacing thresholds are desirable for long-term leads. This allows programming of the pulse generator output to a reduced level, enhancing battery longevity. For leads that have been in place for several years, the operator may decide to accept a pacing threshold (at 0.5-msec pulse width) of up to 2.5 V because this provides a two-times pacing safety margin for most pulse generators and because long-term leads generally show little additional increase in threshold over time. However, a pacing threshold of 2.5 V that occurs early after implantation (e.g., within 6 months) may not be acceptable. This situation suggests excessive early fibrosis around the lead tip and the possibility that exit block and noncapture will develop in the future if the pacing threshold continues to increase. Care at initial implantation helps ensure lower long-term pacing thresholds and improved sensing capabilities.

Thresholds for sensing likewise tend to increase after lead implantation. Acceptable measurable intracardiac electrogram amplitudes depend on the maximum programmable sensitivity of the new pulse generator. For most systems, a P wave amplitude of 1 mV or more and R wave amplitude of 3 mV or more constitute minimally acceptable long-term values. Such low amplitudes, however, leave little room for further deterioration in lead function. Values of 1.5 mV or more and of 4 mV or more for P and R sensing, respectively, provide an additional safety margin. If atrial or ventricular ectopy is present, the operator should determine electrogram amplitude of ectopic complexes to ensure appropriate sensing by the pacemaker. In patients with paroxysmal atrial fibrillation, excellent atrial sensing may be required to detect atrial fibrillation reliably when it occurs, without signal dropout. Higher-amplitude electrograms are required for unipolar (versus bipolar) leads to allow programming of lower sensitivities to avoid myopotential sensing interference.

Inadequate sensing or pacing thresholds at the time of generator replacement are indications for placement of a new lead in the affected chamber. This may entail either capping an old lead and leaving it in place or removing it. The new lead can usually be placed through the same subclavian or axillary vein, although it is preferable to avoid having too many leads (especially more than three) pass through the same vessel, to reduce the chance of venous occlusion and thrombosis. A single new lead may also be placed through the internal jugular vein, external jugular vein, or contralateral subclavian or axillary vein. The proximal tip can be tunneled to the original pocket to meet a second, functional long-term lead for a dual-chamber pacemaker system if required. Alternatively, an entirely new generator or lead system may be placed on the contralateral side.[84]

Invasive Testing of the Defibrillation Capacity of High-Energy Leads that Have Been Implanted for a Long Time

DFT testing of ICD leads can be performed after evaluation of the pace and sense functions of the multifunctional lead and proceeds according to standard DFT testing techniques. Stability of the intracardiac electrogram recording should be ensured, and visual inspection should demonstrate no significant abnormalities in lead appearance, consistent with lead structural integrity.

Examining the Structural Integrity of Leads and the Lead-Generator Interface

Visual inspection at surgery provides clues to lead integrity. Fluid inside the lead body suggests an outer insulation break but, especially in low-voltage leads, does not mandate lead replacement. Undue tension on the lead near the fixation site may cause kinking, conductor uncoiling, conductor fracture, or thinning of the electric insulator. A hazy appearance of the insulator surrounding an area of tension or repeated stress is common in older leads. This appearance represents surface erosion of the lead insulator and does not itself imply lead malfunction. The finding should, however, alert the operator to the possibility of lead damage in areas of stress to the insulation. An examination of the suture location ensures that the ligature remains around the suture sleeve, and gentle tension on the lead body ensures its fixation at the venous entry site. Visual inspection of the specific course of a coiled lead in the pocket may be hampered by a significant thickness of overlying capsule scar; fluoroscopy can assist in this regard.[39-42]

Direct examination of the lead connector can assist in the identification of the lead model if not previously known.[56-58] This issue is particularly important for lead models that have been found to have excessive premature failure rates; such leads in the ventricular position should be replaced in pacemaker-dependent patients.

Venography

Venography is becoming more commonly required as part of the device replacement procedure. It plays an important role when insertion of replacement leads into the subclavian vein is rendered difficult, because the evaluation can ensure patency of the subclavian and SVC systems, demonstrate the point of venous occlusion, or show the course of the axillary venous system for direct access.

Venography is indicated when the subclavian, axillary, or cephalic veins cannot be accessed (to demonstrate their locations) and when the veins are accessed but a guidewire cannot be passed into the SVC. Inability to access the subclavian vein that carries a previously implanted lead suggests either an incorrect needle insertion angle or an occluded subclavian or brachiocephalic venous system.[85-89] Finding an appropriate location to insert the access needle can be facilitated by advancing the needle fluoroscopically in the direction of the chronic electrode under the clavicle, with care taken not to damage the implanted lead. The vein should be approached with the bevel of the needle facing the implanted lead. If access is not possible, venography may provide better delineation of the course of the axillary or subclavian vein. In this situation, radiopaque dye must be injected distal to the veins to be visualized, that is, into the basilic or median cubital vein.

Occasionally, access to the axillary or subclavian vein is possible, but the guidewire will not pass freely to the SVC. If needle placement in the vessel is adequate, failure to pass suggests proximal venous occlusion.[90-94] Venography demonstrates whether occlusion is indeed present and, if so, its site. Chronic venous occlusion may occur asymptomatically in conjunction with the development of collateral venous circulation around the shoulder. Delineation of the location and length of occlusion indicates to the operator an appropriate needle insertion site for placement of a new lead. It also ensures patency of the SVC. Dye is injected directly into the subclavian vein. Occlusion of the subclavian system proximal to the junction of the internal jugular vein excludes the ipsilateral jugular system as an alternative site for a new lead. Alternatively, if the subclavian vein is occluded and the internal jugular vein remains patent, a new lead may still be placed using the jugular approach. Occlusion of the SVC precludes the use of any new endocardial lead placed from a superior site unless the vessel is dilated after lead extraction.[95] Although venoplasty is acceptable, stents should never be placed into veins without removal of the leads, so as to avoid trapping of the leads between a stent and the vein wall.

Anomalies of the left SVC (which usually drain into the coronary sinus) make placement of right ventricular endocardial leads difficult or impossible.[96,97] Venography defines the anatomy of the venous system in such a situation, which may be suggested by an unusual intravascular guidewire course. Finally, leakage of venography dye into perivascular tissues or into the pericardial space suggests vessel or cardiac chamber perforation, respectively.

The technique is performed by injection of 10 to 20 mL of radiopaque dye (a 50% dilution generally suffices) into a vein peripheral to the occlusion site. The dye may be injected directly into the subclavian vein or, if subclavian access is not possible, into the antecubital or brachial vein. Fluoroscopy with permanent storage of cine images is necessary to evaluate flow.

Generator Lead Adaptability

Lead Connectors

Replacing a pulse generator onto one or more long-term leads requires that the pulse generator connector block be compatible with the proximal lead tip.[56-58] Through years of development by multiple manufacturers, pacemaker leads have evolved to an IS-1 proximal lead connector configuration, which consists of (1) a 3.2-mm lead connector with a short pin that is electrically connected to the distal electrode tip, (2) a lead connector ring wired to the proximal pacing pole (the ring is electrically active in a bipolar lead), and (3) sealing rings. The proximal lead connector configuration is the same

TABLE 20-8. **Common Configurations for Endocardial Lead Connectors**

Designation	Unipolar (U) or Bipolar (B)?	Linear (L) or Bifurcated (B)?	Pin L/S	Connector Diameter (mm)	Sealing Rings? (Y/N)	Fixation (A/P)	Atrial J Available? (Y/N)
IS-1	U or B	L	S	3.2	Y	A or P	Y
DF-1	U	—	S	3.2	Y	—	N
VS-1	U or B	L	S or L	3.2	Y	A or P	Y
3.2-mm low-profile	U or B	L	L	3.2	Y or N	A or P	Y
5-mm	U	—	L	5.4	Y	A or P	Y
5-mm	B	B	L	5.4	Y	A or P	Y
6-mm	U or B	L or B	S or L	6.4	Y	A or P	Y

A/P, active or passive; DF-1, Standard for high-energy defibrillator lead connectors; IS-1, International Standard for pacemaker lead connectors; L/S, long or short; VS-1, Voluntary Standard for pacemaker lead connectors; Y/N, yes or no.

for unipolar and bipolar leads, except that the ring is inactive in unipolar leads. Modern pulse generators have connector block specifications that conform to IS-1 leads and that also fit the prior Voluntary Standard (VS-1) lead type. Thus, generator replacement onto implanted leads of either of these two types poses no difficulty because of the wide array of compatible pulse generators from multiple manufacturers.

In a similar manner, ICD leads have evolved to incorporate IS-1 pace/sense connectors with concomitant IS-1 atrial and ventricular ports in the generator connector block to attach these leads. Early-generation ICDs, however, used a wide variety of lead port sizes and configurations, requiring the operator to have available generators with various header port sizes, adapters, and upsizing sleeves for reoperation of old ICD generators implanted before the adoption of a uniform standard. Even coronary sinus lead ports have evolved from an LV-1 configuration without sealing rings to the IS-1 configuration.

As discussed previously, high-energy defibrillation lead headers have also evolved into a standard configuration, DF-1, which consists of (1) a lead pin that is electrically connected to the corresponding high-energy coil or patch, (2) sealing rings, and (3) a single lead head for each coil of an endocardial lead to allow various hardwire configurations. A single DF-1 connector attaches to all three coils of a subcutaneous array or to a single patch. As with pace/sense leads, defibrillator lead heads had a variety of different end configurations before the adoption of the DF-1 standard, resulting in greater complexity at the time of generator or lead replacement.

Because a variety of other lead connector configurations had previously been developed (Table 20-8; Fig. 20-9) and because implanted leads may remain useful for many years, a number of these older lead connector configurations remain in use. If sensing and pacing thresholds are adequate, old leads with such configurations may be used, but a pacemaker or ICD pulse generator with a compatible connector block should be selected. Like pacemakers, ICD generator connector blocks from some manufacturers are available in a variety of configurations and port sizes to attach directly to existing implanted leads (Fig. 20-10). An alternative (but less desirable) approach involves using an adapter to fit odd-sized lead connectors into available ports on an ICD header block. Most old pacemaker leads are unipolar; upgrading to a bipolar system should be considered but is not always necessary.

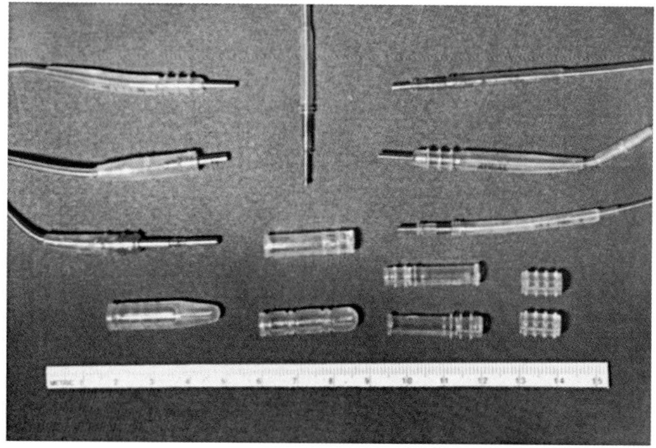

Figure 20-9. A variety of pacemaker lead connectors (top), nonconducting adapters (bottom right five), and lead caps (bottom left two). The lead connectors shown are (clockwise from bottom left) Intermedics, Inc. (Angleton, Tex.), 6-mm linear bipolar; Intermedics 6-mm unipolar; Medtronic, Inc. (Minneapolis, Minn.), 5-mm unipolar; Cordis (Miami) 3.2-mm linear bipolar, Pacesetter IS-1; Medtronic atrial 5-mm unipolar; and Medtronic IS-1. Lead caps are 5-mm cap (bottom left) and 3.2-mm low-profile or IS-1/VS-1 (bottom left, center). Upsizing sleeves are 5-mm to 6-mm (top left, center), 3.2-mm to 5-mm (top right, center), and 3.2-mm to 6-mm (bottom right, center). Unipolarizing sleeves for 6-mm bipolar leads are shown on bottom right. (Photography by Andrew C. Floyd, Hahnemann University Hospital, Philadelphia.)

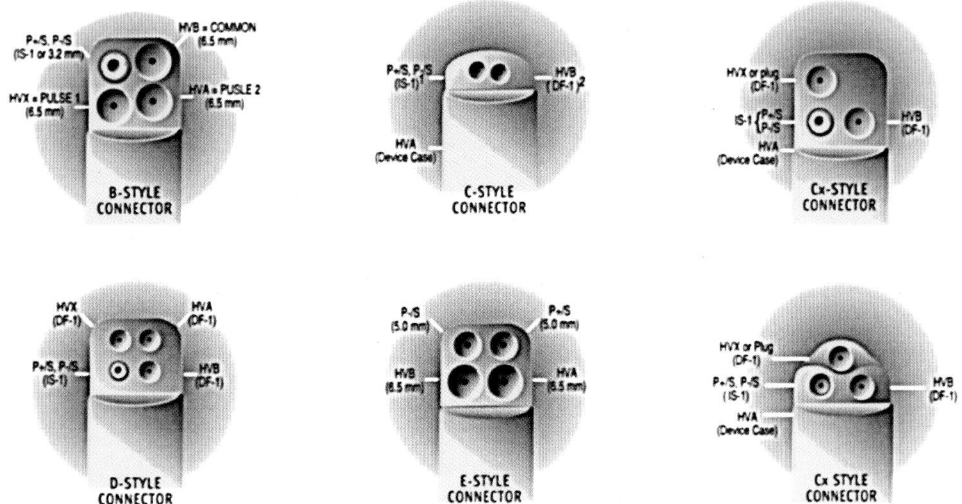

Figure 20-10. Examples of a variety of implantable cardioverter-defibrillator (ICD) header connector block configurations. These various styles of header configurations are designed to connect directly to different types of implanted rate-sensing and pacing leads (pace and sense, P/S) and to high-voltage lead connectors (HVA, HVB, HVX). All rate/sense lead ports are of the IS-1 configuration. This means that any rate/sense leads that are of different connector configurations must be adapted to fit into these ports. Likewise, high-energy lead ports are of the DF-1 or 3.2-mm configuration. Adapters may be required here as well to provide a direct connection into the ICD header. Many forms of adapters are available for pace and sense leads (see Fig. 20-14). A variety of adapters for high-energy leads are also available (see Fig. 20-15). (From ICD Replacement Guide. Minneapolis, Minn., Medtronic, Inc., 1997.)

Before the availability of IS-1 and VS-1 lead connector configurations,[56,57] the most commonly used pacemaker leads were 3.2-mm low-profile leads (unipolar or linear bipolar), 5-mm or 6-mm unipolar and linear bipolar leads, and bifurcated bipolar systems. Pacemaker pulse generators available from some manufacturers remain compatible with each of these lead models, especially 3.2-mm and 5- or 6-mm linear bipolar and unipolar leads. Precise compatibility, however, is essential to ensure that no fluid leaks into the pulse generator connector block and that electrical continuity to proximal and distal poles remains intact. The physician must be particularly cautious to ensure that sealing rings are located either on the lead connector or in the pulse generator connector block, because not all older lead models had sealing rings placed on the lead connector itself.

Review of manufacturers' specifications of devices should provide the necessary details regarding lead and pulse generator compatibility. Because the lead model may not always be known before reoperation and because it may not be determined even with visual inspection, careful evaluation of the lead connector configuration may be required in the laboratory after the old pulse generator has been removed. Although the lead and pulse generator should have been compatible at the initial implantation, the physician cannot make this assumption without visual inspection of the type of lead connector at reoperation. Lead-generator incompatibility may be the cause of presumed lead malfunction or premature generator depletion.

Bifurcated bipolar leads were implanted primarily with ventricular demand pacing systems with 5- to 6-mm lead connectors that plugged side by side into the pulse generator connector block. Some of these leads continue to function because they are so heavily insulated. Replacement of the pulse generator entails selection of a new battery with a compatible connector block to maintain bipolar capability, use of an adapter to convert the bifurcated bipolar lead to a linear bipolar system, or conversion to unipolar through the use of only one pole of the bifurcated lead, with the other capped. The last option is particularly useful in the event that only one pole of a bifurcated bipolar lead functions well. Either of the last two options allows conversion to a dual-chamber pacing system, if desired, by placement of a new IS-1 atrial bipolar lead and adaptation of the functional pole of the old lead in a unipolar configuration to an IS-1 connector. If the bifurcated bipolar lead is adapted to linear bipolar, placement of a linear bipolar atrial lead can convert the system to bipolar DDD.

Defibrillator (high voltage) and pacemaker (low voltage) standards continue to progress with the proposal of a quadripolar 3.2-mm standard. Likely this will be introduced as DF-4 for combined pacing and shocking applications and IS-4 for dedicated low-voltage applications (Figs. 20-11 and 20-12). The terminal pin and first ring will carry low-voltage impulses in both applications and for all four poles in the low-voltage application. The most anticipated application, DF-4 replaces the trifurcated ICD lead combining the function of one IS-1 and up to two DF-1 connectors (Fig. 20-13). However, the introduction of this connector creates new problems with needs for new adapters and need for care during intraoperative testing with correct placement of the alligator clips.

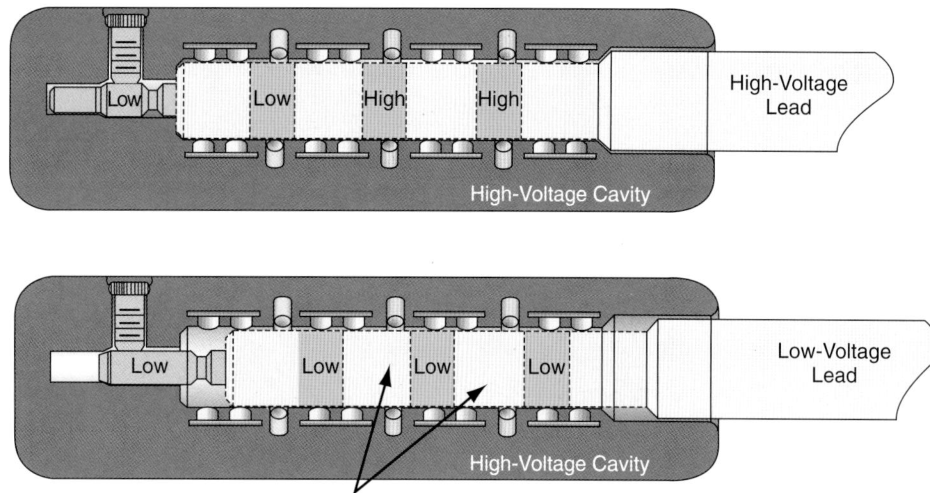

Figure 20-11. Drawing of the proposed quadripolar low- and high-voltage lead pin configuration and header configuration. The specifications for the pins and the header are extremely precise, permitting the interchange of leads between models and manufacturers. Although both configurations are quadripolar, the low-voltage leads will not fit into the cavity of the high-voltage cavity. Although both leads are 3.2 mm in diameter, the diameter of the distal pin is larger for the low-voltage leads. (From Proposed IS-4 Standard. American Association of Medical Instrumentation presentation at Cardiostim, Nice, France, June 2004.)

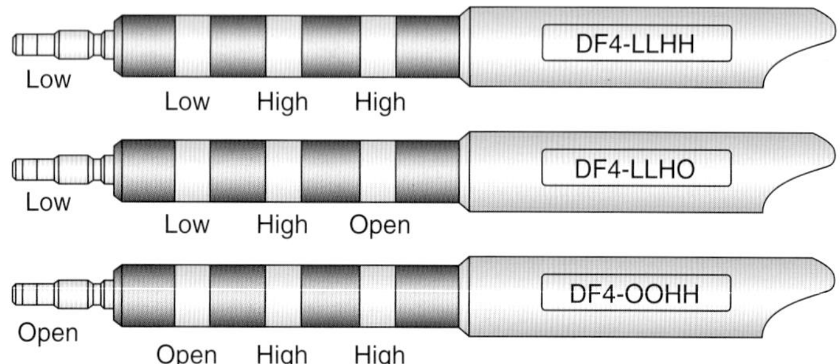

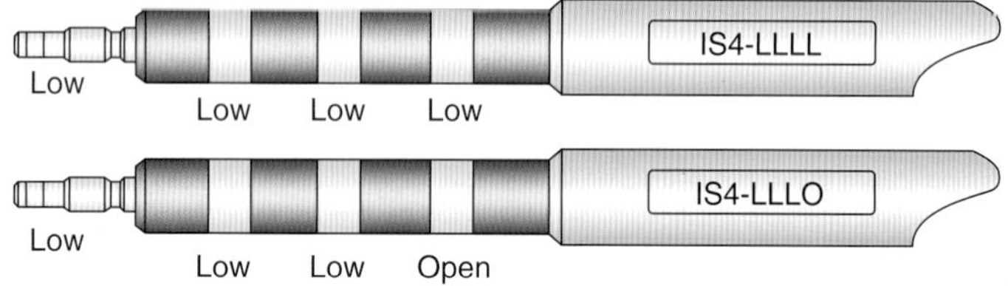

Figure 20-12. Drawing of three high-voltage and two low-voltage lead configurations as proposed by the American Association of Medical Instrumentation. In all configurations, the connections flow from the distal extent of the lead proximally and connect at the pin, most distal to most proximal, and so forth. In all configurations, the pin and next electrode are reserved for low-voltage functions. Each pole is labeled either L or H, depending on its function. (From Proposed IS-4 Standard. American Association of Medical Instrumentation presentation at Cardiostim, Nice, France, June 2004.)

Adapters

The following two general categories of adapters are available: (1) electrically conducting units that change the size or configuration of lead connectors to fit specific pulse generators and (2) upsizing sleeves that allow IS-1 or 3.2-mm, low-profile leads to fit into 5- or 6-mm pulse generator connector blocks while maintaining a fluid seal (Table 20-9 and Fig. 20-14).

Electrically conducting adapters necessarily contain wires attached on one end to a lead pin to enter the new pulse generator and a socket on the other to accept the old lead as well as a mechanism to connect the old lead, generally a set-screw. Produced by most manufacturers, adapters are available in an array of types (see Table 20-9). The most common pacemaker adapters downsize 5- or 6-mm leads to IS-1 unipolar or bipolar configurations or adapt 3.2-mm low-profile connectors to the IS-1 variety. Adapters are also available to convert bifurcated bipolar leads to the linear IS-1 bipolar configuration; they may be particularly useful in a patient who requires upgrading from VVI to DDD pacing when maintenance of bipolar pacing is important, as occurs when a permanent pacemaker is placed in conjunction with an implanted defibrillator (rarely done now, as it would be better to place an entirely new ICD system), or to avoid myopotential sensing.

Adapters for ICD leads may be used either for the rate-sensing (pace/sense) leads or for the high-energy leads, patches, or arrays (Fig. 20-15). These small units are most helpful for adapting epicardial lead connectors found in an abdominal pocket to newer-generation

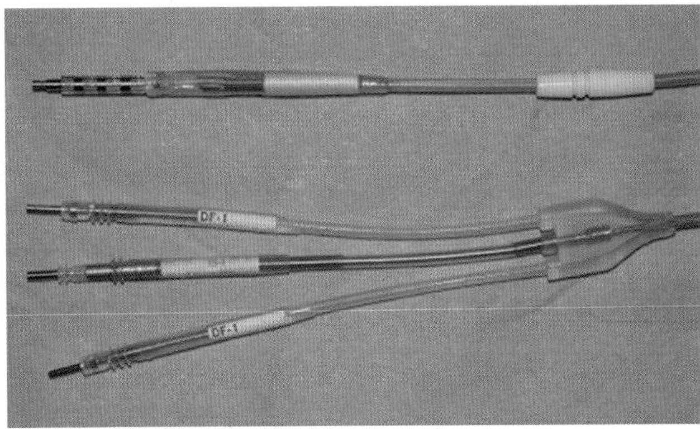

Figure 20-13. Pictures of the proximal portions of leads intended for a dual-coil implantable cardioverter-defibrillator lead. The traditional connection with a yolk dividing into two DF-1 connectors and one IS-1 connector is replaced with a single-connection, 3.2-mm in diameter, permitting all four electrical connections and a simplified lead configuration proposed to be labeled DF4. (From Proposed IS-4 Standard. American Association of Medical Instrumentation presentation at Cardiostim, Nice, France, June 2004.)

TABLE 20-9. **Common Configurations for Pacemaker Adapters***

From (Lead)	To (Generator)
Conducting adapters:	
6-mm UNI	5-mm UNI
6-mm BIF	3.2-mm LP BI
6-mm BI	3.2-mm LP BI
5-mm BIF	3.2-mm LP BI
5-mm BIF	*IS-1 BI*
5-mm UNI	*IS-1 UNI*
3.2-mm LP BI	5-mm BIF
3.2-mm LP	*IS-1 BI*
Nonconducting upsizing sleeve adapters:	
3.2-mm LP BI	5-mm or 6-mm UNI (± pin extender)
IS-1 UNI or BI	5-mm or 6-mm UNI
5-mm UNI	6-mm UNI
LV-1	*IS-1*

*Adapters shown in *italics* are those most commonly used.
BI, linear bipolar; BIF, bifurcated bipolar; LP, low profile; UNI, unipolar.

ICD batteries, that is, attaching nonstandard lead connectors to IS-1 pacing and DF-1 shocking ports in an ICD header block. The adapters may also be used when older transvenous leads must be attached to newer, standard-connect ICD pulse generators.

One additional special use for ICD lead adapters involves connecting high-energy leads in parallel to enable them to function as a single unit with the same polarity. For example, a subcutaneous patch or array may have to be added to a system because of a high DFT. This additional hardware can be connected in parallel with a proximal high-energy coil located in the SVC. Lead connectors from both the subcutaneous lead and the proximal coil are inserted side by side into an adapter, which then attaches to a *single* port in the ICD header. This lead system thereby functions as a single electrically connected unit with the same polarity.

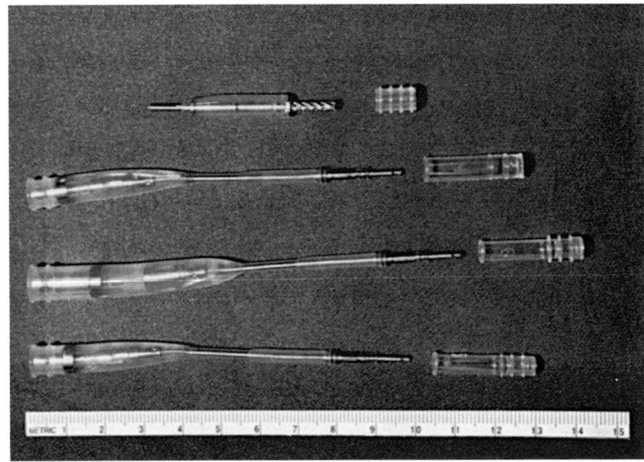

Figure 20-14. Eight pacing lead adapters: four conducting (left) and four nonconducting (right). Conducting adapters shown are (top to bottom) 6-mm lead pin replacement; 3.2-mm low-profile linear bipolar (to accept a lead connector without sealing rings) to VS-1 linear bipolar; 6-mm linear bipolar to 3.2-mm linear bipolar; and 3.2-mm low-profile linear bipolar to VS-1 linear bipolar. Nonconducting adapters shown are (top to bottom): unipolarizing sleeve for 6-mm bipolar lead; upsizing from 5 to 6 mm; upsizing unipolarizing sleeve from 3.2 to 6 mm; upsizing unipolarizing sleeve from 3.2 to 5 mm. (Photography by Andrew C. Floyd, Hahnemann University Hospital, Philadelphia.)

Despite the available variety of electrically conducting adapters, these units prove bulky in the pacemaker or ICD pocket. Furthermore, they provide another weak link, that is, one additional set of connections in the pacing circuit for delivery of current to the patient and for sensing, increasing the chance of malfunction, compared with direct attachment of a lead into a pulse generator connector block. Some adapter set-screws must be sealed with medical adhesive after being fastened to the lead; a poor seal can result in a short circuit in the system. Because of internal connections, not all adapters have the reliability inherent in most pacemaker or ICD leads directly connected to the generator.

Tools

Several specially designed tools assist the operator in replacing pacemaker and ICD pulse generators and repairing leads (Table 20-10 and Fig. 20-16). Most important are wrenches to loosen set-screws in the pulse generator connector block to allow the old lead to be withdrawn. Most set-screw sizes are now standardized, but if the old generator manufacturer and model are known, a specific wrench may be required. If these are not known, it is best to have available an array of small Allen wrenches to remove the hexagonal set-screw. Some pulse generators must be removed from the lead with a small flat screwdriver. Some pulse generators are connected to the lead without set-screws through pressing of an attachment unit into place; to loosen this unit requires that a small probe be inserted into the side of the connector block to push open the locking mechanism. It is unusual to lose set-screws

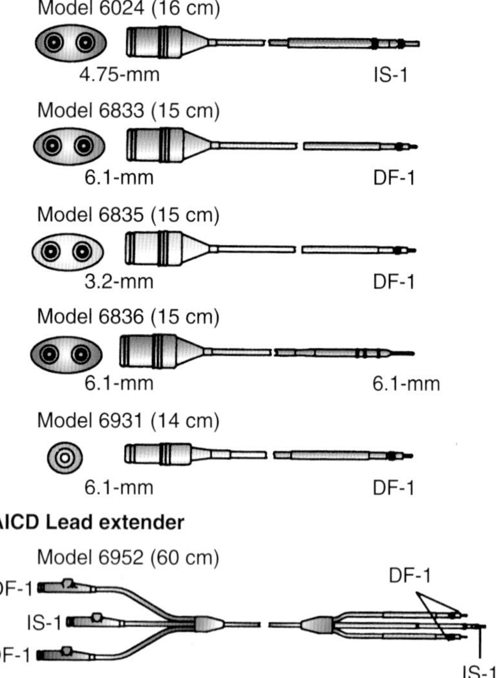

Figure 20-15. A variety of implantable cardioverter-defibrillator (ICD) lead adapters. As indicated, several different sizes of lead connectors can be inserted side by side to be adapted to the appropriate size to fit directly into the ICD header port. Additionally, linear adapters used merely to change the size of a lead connector may also be required, as indicated. Lead extenders are used to attach rate-sensing and high-energy leads placed through the subclavian system to an ICD pulse generator inserted in the abdomen. As the size and weight of ICDs have been reduced, however, the need to place the ICD pulse generator in the anterior abdominal wall has diminished markedly. (From Multiple Options for Customized Therapy. Guidant Corporation, Cardiac Pacemakers [CPI], St. Paul, Minn., 1996.)

because they are generally held in place by a seal. It is advisable, however, to have additional set-screws available in a busy pacing laboratory.

Occasionally, repair can salvage an old lead, as long as the conductor fracture or insulation break is accessible at least several centimeters from the point at which the lead enters the vascular system. Lead insulation breaks can be repaired by gluing on a polymeric silicone (Silastic) sleeve with medical adhesive. The operator can repair a conductor fracture by (1) severing the lead, (2) placing the two cut conductor ends into an electrically conducting sleeve, which is crimped down onto both ends of the lead conductor, and (3) gluing a silicone sleeve over the insulator with medical adhesive. This procedure is recommended only for a lead on which the patient is not dependent, because recurrent conductor fracture may occur. It is also not recommended for repair of high-energy defibrillation lead conductors. Repair of polyurethane leads can prove functionally inadequate because adhesive may not bond properly with the lead insulator, as it does with silicone. A more viable approach in any of these situations may be to extract or cap the culprit lead and replace it entirely.

TABLE 20-10. Commonly Used Tools for Generator Replacement, Lead Replacement, Lead Revision, or Lead Repair

Probes (to unlock lead connector block in some devices)
Allen wrenches*: 0.035-inch (No. 2) 0.050-inch (No. 4) 0.062-inch (No. 6) 0.093-inch (No. 10)
Screwdrivers: 0.100-inch 0.200-inch
Set-screws
Anchoring sleeves
Lead repair kit: Conductor with crimp ends Crimping tool Insulating sleeve Medical adhesive
Lead end-caps: 6.5-mm 5-mm 3.2-mm LP IS-1

*Specific torque wrenches may be available from some manufacturers; these are especially important for tightening set-screws with appropriate force. Wrench numbers are standardized for ease of identification.

Surgical Considerations

Device replacement or revision in a tertiary care institution with an active electrophysiology service and long-term follow-up may account for more than one quarter of all pacemaker or ICD procedures (Table 20-11). The timing of intervention depends on the specific indication. Most patients require reoperation for elective battery replacement or battery or lead revision, whereas 1% to 6% of patients return to the laboratory for other problems, such as pocket hematoma, pocket twitch, diaphragmatic pacing, and pocket relocation (Table 20-12).

Elective Device Replacement or Revision

Most reimplantation procedures are either elective or performed for repair or replacement of prior devices. Preoperative blood analysis is performed. In our laboratory, aspirin and clopidogrel are not stopped prior to the procedure. Warfarin should generally be discontinued for 3 to 5 days for procedures in which the major vessels will be instrumented, although not all laboratories follow this approach. Because the risk of hematoma development is much higher with heparin

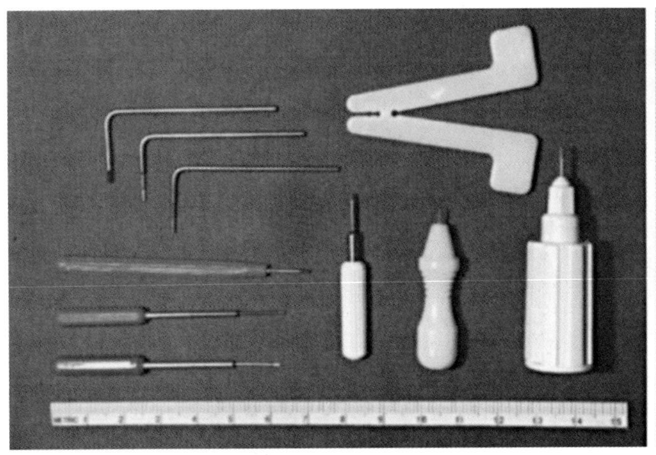

A

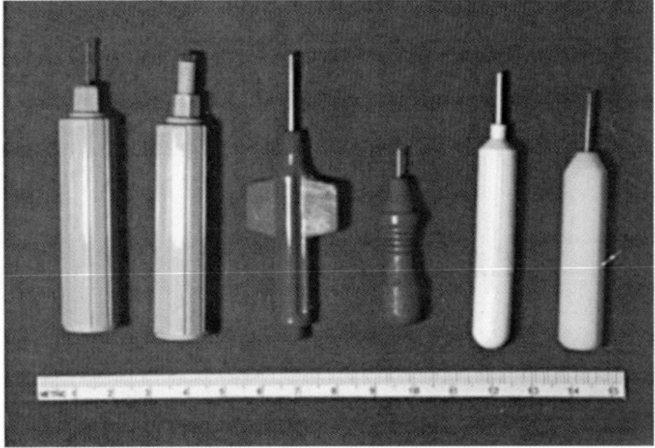

B

Figure 20-16. Tools commonly required for reoperation. ***A,*** *Three nondeformable Allen wrenches (top left) of various sizes; a pinch-on tool (Medtronic, Inc., Minneapolis, Minn.) (top right) to extend and retract the distal screw of an active-fixation lead; three wrenches (bottom left); two torque wrenches (Medtronic and CPI/Guidant, St. Paul, Minn.) (bottom right) on either side of a probe (Intermedics, Inc., Angleton, Tex.) used to unlock a pacemaker connector block. Some wrenches are deformable to avoid placing excess torque on the set-screw, whereas others are not; caution is required in use of the various systems (see text).* ***B*** *(left to right), Intermedics ratchet torque wrench; Intermedics flat-bladed ratchet torque screwdriver; Cordis (Miami) No. 6 Allen wrench; unlocking probe; two Allen wrenches with handles (not deformable). (Photography by Andrew C. Floyd, Hahnemann University Hospital, Philadelphia.)*

TABLE 20-11. **Rates of Pacemaker Pulse Generator Implantations, Revisions, and Replacements***

Procedure	Rate (%)
DDD implantation	51
VVI implantation	23
Revision or replacement	26

*The frequency of dual-chamber (DDD-R) and single-chamber (VVI-R) pulse generator implantations and battery or lead revisions or replacements over a $5^1/_2$-year period at Hahnemann University Hospital, Philadelphia.

and enoxaparin than with warfarin, we may elect to perform simple device replacements in patients with full warfarin anticoagulation.

The patient fasts from midnight and receives preoperative antibiotics, most commonly being admitted on the day of the procedure. Elevated coagulation times may be corrected with fresh-frozen plasma if absolutely necessary. Procedures are routinely performed with local or regional anesthesia, supplemented by intravenous conscious sedation. For ICDs, the patient is given general anesthesia for ventricular fibrillation induction and testing of shock therapies. Most institutions use a combination of a short-acting, amnestic benzodiazepine such as midazolam together with an intravenous narcotic for analgesia. Continuous electrocardiographic monitoring, pulse oximetry, and sterile preparation and draping are standard procedures. Preoperative antibiotics are administered intravenously.

TABLE 20-12. **Pacemaker Reoperations: Frequency of Various Indications**

Indications	Frequency (%)
Generator indications:	
Battery end of service	53
Battery insulation break	1.1
DDD to VVIR conversion	1.1
Lead indications:	
Lead revision (exit block or lead injury)	17
Diaphragmatic pacing	2.2
Lead fracture	1.1
Lead insulation break	1.1
Battery or lead indications:	
Battery end of service and lead replacement	6.8
VVI to DDD conversion	4.4
Unipolar DDD to bipolar DDD	1.1
Pocket twitch	1.1
Surgical indications:	
Pocket relocation	5.6
Pocket effusion	2.2

The frequency of indications for pacemaker reoperation over a $5^1/_2$-year period at Hahnemann University Hospital, Philadelphia.

General Guidelines and Techniques

There is no substitute for careful surgical planning in approaching the established pacemaker pocket and gentle handling of the tissues. Perfect hemostasis, avoidance of a tight-fitting pacemaker or ICD pocket, and multilayered incision closure are the basic principles that help prevent future difficulties. These principles are similar to those required at initial implantation (see Table 20-2). To avoid induction of ventricular fibrillation, development of fibrosis at the lead tip, and damage to the generator itself, electrocautery must not be used directly over an implanted pulse generator with unipolar leads. This issue has become much less of a problem with bipolar leads. Electrocautery also must not be used during battery changes with the generator disconnected when pacemaker leads are grounded to the patient for testing, because current may be shunted directly to the heart. Hemostasis at reoperation can usually be secured with electrocautery or direct ligature. Use of surgical absorbable cellulose or topical thrombin assists in treating persistently oozy pockets. Clinical judgment should be used in the application of various technical approaches (Fig. 20-17).

Specific Techniques

Local anesthesia is administered most commonly as 1% lidocaine (Xylocaine) infiltrated into the scar line from the previous procedure; additional lidocaine may be given under direct vision once the capsule of the pocket has been defined.

The surgical incision is placed directly over the previous incision. The skin and subcutaneous tissues are opened with sharp dissection, which is required to penetrate the tough scar tissue and dermal layer. Deeper dissection with Metzenbaum scissors is carried out to delineate the pacemaker capsule. Once the pocket is reached, the fibrous capsule is sharply incised with a blade to make a small opening, which is then extended with scissors under direct visualization of the implanted pulse generator and leads (Fig. 20-18). Alternatively, electrocautery may be used to open the pacemaker capsule.

The capsule must be opened far enough to allow extraction of the pulse generator and lead connector assembly without undue force. The posterior capsule may have to be carefully dissected away from the leads to allow mobility. Access to leads and generator may be facilitated through the use of self-retaining retractors. Extreme care is required throughout the procedure to preserve the integrity of the leads and lead connectors; they must not be punctured with anesthetic needles or cut with blades or scissors. If electrocautery is used to remove tissue from the leads in dissecting them from scar tissue in the posterior capsule, the probe must keep moving over the lead so as to not overheat the lead insulation and thereby damage it. Leads with very thin insulation, including most coronary sinus electrodes used with biventricular systems, are more prone to heat damage from electrocautery.

Once the generator is delivered out of the pocket, the leads are disconnected and analyzed, as described earlier. Leads from pacemaker-dependent patients need to be expeditiously reconnected to an external pacemaker (Fig. 20-19). Unipolar pacemaker leads require direct grounding to subcutaneous tissue; the active part of the unipolar generator must remain in contact with the patient before the lead is disconnected. Grounding can best be accomplished through a large surface area ground electrode placed directly into the open pocket. Making contact with this electrode onto the active surface of a unipolar pulse generator allows the generator to be removed safely from the pocket before the lead is disconnected, even in a pacemaker-dependent patient.

After being secured to temporary pacing cables, leads can be completely freed of adhesions up to their entry point into the subclavian vein, if necessary, to examine lead integrity or for extraction. We use low-energy electrocautery sparingly to dissect the leads free of adhesions because the scar tissue could be especially tough and adherent to lead structures. If lead replacement or repair is not necessary, and if the function of previously implanted leads is adequate, dissection of the complete course of each lead may not be necessary.

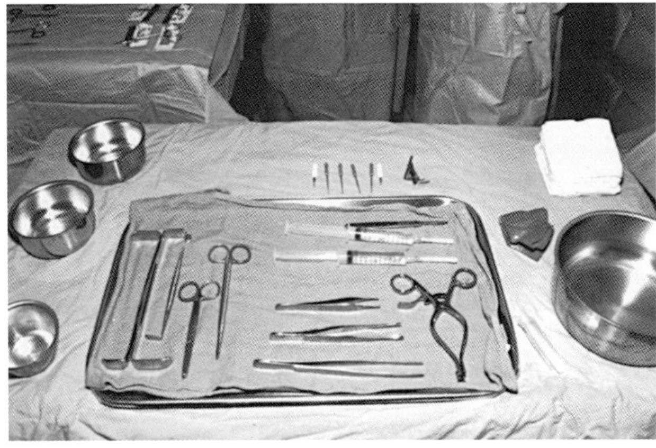

Figure 20-17. Preparation for surgery. A typical array of instruments required for reoperation. Foreground, Retractors, scissors, forceps, scalpel, syringes filled with lidocaine anesthetic, sterile saline solution, sponges, and a variety of wrenches. Background, Hemostats and absorbable and nonabsorbable sutures. (Photography by Andrew C. Floyd, Hahnemann University Hospital, Philadelphia.)

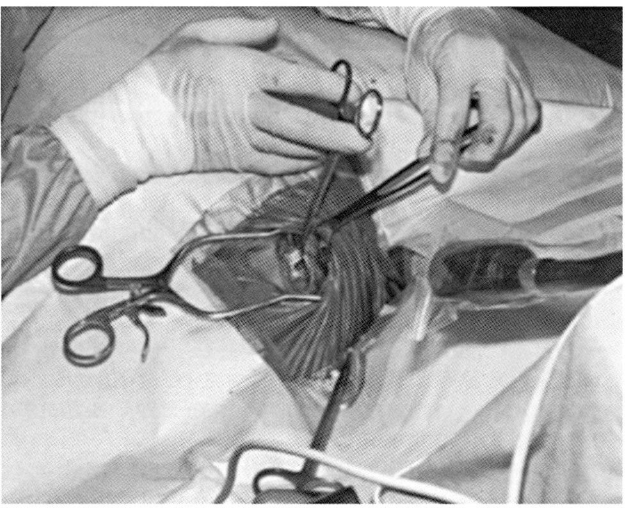

Figure 20-18. Opening the capsule of the long-term generator pocket to expose the pulse generator. (Photography by Andrew C. Floyd, Hahnemann University Hospital, Philadelphia.)

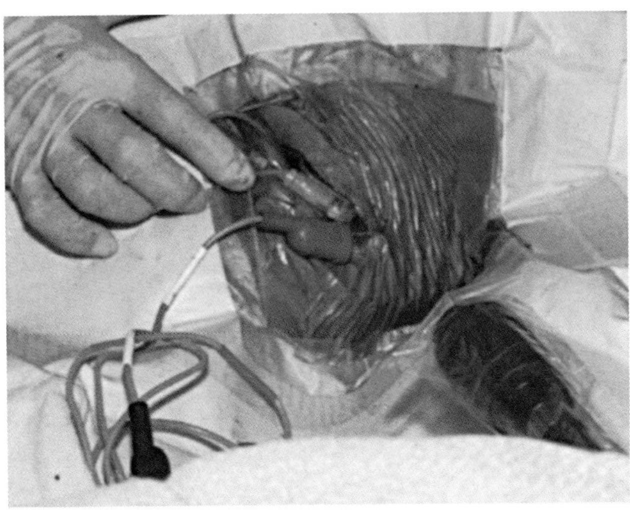

Figure 20-19. *Disconnecting the previously implanted lead. The active surface of the unipolar pacemaker pulse generator remains in contact with the open pocket to maintain pacing output until the lead is withdrawn from the connector block. The surgeon has adequately mobilized the proximal portion of the 5-mm lead to allow rapid connection to an external pacing cable, one end of which has already been securely grounded to the patient. A ligature previously placed around the lead connector block entry post has been removed. After the external pacemaker has been activated, the surgeon will loosen the set-screw (here covered by a seal on the top right side of the connector block) and withdraw the lead from the pulse generator, immediately connecting it to the negative pole of the external pacing cable. (Photography by Andrew C. Floyd, Hahnemann University Hospital, Philadelphia.)*

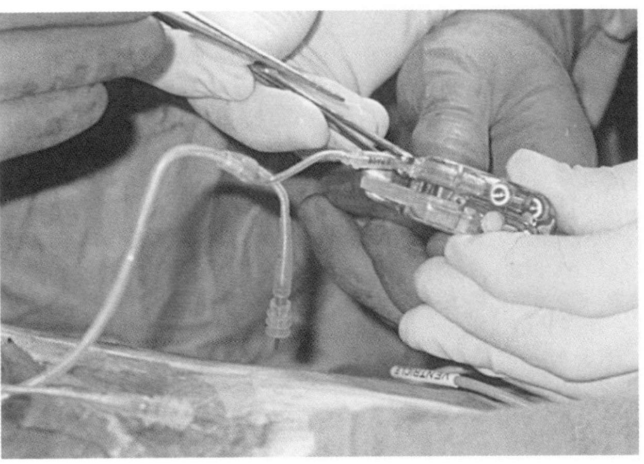

Figure 20-20. *Adapting and inserting rate-sensing and high-voltage defibrillator leads into the implantable cardioverter-defibrillator (ICD) connector block. The incision is made in the left upper quadrant of the abdomen over the scar line from the previous device implant. The old ICD generator has been removed, and the leads have been freed up by gentle electrocautery to allow them to be easily manipulated and to be placed into the header of the new pulse generator without undue tension or bending. Basic pacing and sensing thresholds have been tested; this testing also includes delivery of low-energy (5-V) pacing impulses through the high-energy leads to measure lead impedance and thus ensure structural integrity of the high-voltage conductors. The new ICD device to be implanted has been placed on the surgical field, and its connection to the lead system has begun. A plug is first inserted into the upper right port because the port will not be used. The set-screw has already been tightened onto this plug, and a required cap has been placed over the set-screw. The surgeon is inserting a unipolar lead connector from the rate-sensing portion of the defibrillator lead into the ICD connector block. This lead head is connected to the distal tip of a right ventricular endocardial integrated lead system (497-05 lead, Intermedics, Inc., Angleton, Tex.); it is inserted into the appropriate sensing port of the ICD. Sealing O-rings are evident on the ICD header and are used in this device to prevent fluid leakage around a cap placed over the set-screw. Also evident just within the forceps is a thickened area of the lead that represents a sleeve glued in place with medical adhesive to cover a minor break in the outer insulator of the lead (i.e., an insulator repair). A plug has been inserted into an unused port of the ICD connector block; the sealing cap has already been placed over the set-screw for this plug. The dangling high-voltage lead connector has been inserted through an upsizing sleeve before being placed in the ICD connector block. The original lead connector is a 4-mm configuration; the sleeve passes over the insulator on the head to increase its diameter to fit into a 6-mm high-voltage port in the ICD connector block. The remaining lead connector evident on the patient attaches to a subcutaneous high-voltage patch used in the defibrillation circuit. The tip of this lead is also adapted through the use of a similar sleeve to fit a 6-mm port. (Photography courtesy of Todd Forkin, Hahnemann University Hospital, Philadelphia.)*

The physician, however, must ascertain whether the lead connector mobility is sufficient to attach it to a new pulse generator without tension.

Inadequate implanted lead pacing or sensing thresholds may require placement of one or two new leads. Upgrade from a single-chamber to a DDD pacemaker system or to a biventricular system may require placement of an additional lead. If a previously implanted lead is extracted through a dilating sheath, a guidewire can usually be inserted into the vascular system through the extraction sheath to maintain a conduit for replacement. In other cases, repeated axillary or subclavian vein puncture, brachiocephalic cutdown, or an internal jugular approach provides an alternative means of inserting a new lead. If new leads are placed through the same subclavian system by direct puncture, the operator must be careful to avoid lead damage.

After the old pulse generator has been detached from leads and the lead integrity and functional status have been ascertained, a new pulse generator can be attached. The principles of generator-lead compatibility must be maintained (Fig. 20-20). Redundant lead coils are placed posterior to the pulse generator, and the pocket is closed with three layers of absorbable suture—two subcutaneous and one subcuticular. ICD leads may be tested for defibrillation threshold before, or concomitant with, final pocket closure. We also open the capsule inside the device pocket, usually in a medial and inferior direction, for two reasons. First, a new device, even if an identical model to the one removed, will never fit perfectly in the original pocket, and second, doing so allows for absorption of fluid and fresh blood flow, which are not possible if the relatively avascular capsule is left intact.

For generator replacement, the previous pacemaker or ICD pocket location is used most commonly, usually opposite the patient's dominant side. Because most pacemakers and most ICDs are placed inferior to the clavicle in a subcutaneous location anterior to the pectoralis fascia, the location of replacement devices is similar. Various modifications suit individual patient needs. In very thin patients, subpectoral or axillary locations may be required. One can access the subpectoral plane by locating the junction between the sternal and clavicular heads of the pectoralis major muscle and making entry at that point, taking care to avoid damage to penetrating neurovascular bundles. Alternatively, the muscle fibers of the pectoralis major can be teased apart longitudinally to allow entry to the subpectoral plane, which can also be accessed through the deltopectoral groove. Axillary subcutaneous placement of a pacing device is generally avoided because of the possibility of lateral migration of the device, which can be uncomfortable for the patient and can, especially with larger ICDs, lead to erosion. When required, however, the axillary location can be entered through direct extension from a subclavian pocket or through a separate axillary incision. The device may be placed in a subpectoral location at that site for more stability. The abdominal wall, subcostal, and intrathoracic positions represent other alternatives for a replacement pulse generator. Nevertheless, a subcutaneous prepectoral approach is appropriate in most patients for both pacemaker and ICD reimplantations.

For replacement of an abdominal ICD, dissection can be difficult if the device is located behind the rectus abdominis muscle. We usually begin over the area where the device is most easily palpated, carefully spreading the muscle apart in the area of prior scarring. The scar tissue is carefully divided to expose the pulse generator, which is then handled in the usual manner. The physician must be cautious not to exert undue force to remove the generator in order to avoid rupture into the peritoneal cavity. Electrocautery is avoided over the muscle if the patient is not under general anesthesia.

Approach to the Eroding Device

Although relatively uncommon, chronic erosion through the skin by the pulse generator or lead can occur.[1,10,77] Incipient erosion manifests as localized erythema in an area of thinned skin that is adherent to the underlying device. The area gradually becomes necrotic and may drain serosanguineous fluid. Outright erosion and drainage necessarily imply that the pacemaker pocket is no longer sterile[1,98]; in such instances, the system (generator and leads) should be removed if possible.[5,8] Occasionally, the pocket heals with removal of the pulse generator alone, but only when skin integrity has not been breached. After removal of the pulse generator and leads, eroded pockets are packed for secondary closure or they can be fully débrided and closed primarily, leaving a drain in place for 2 to 3 days. Administration of intravenous antibiotics proceeds for 1 to 6 weeks (the longer duration if bacteremia has occurred).

A new device should be implanted on the contralateral side only after all signs of infection have resolved at the old pacemaker site, if the patient has not experienced recurrent fever, and if there is no elevation of the white blood cell count. Five to 7 days of intravenous antibiotic administration appear sufficient before device replacement, as long as bacteremia has resolved and there are no large intracardiac vegetations. Replacement of the pulse generator on the original side is not recommended but may be possible if complete erosion did not occur, the pocket could be closed after primary removal of the generator, and there are no signs of active infection after antibiotics have been discontinued. Alternative approaches are discussed in Chapter 21.

Antibiotic Prophylaxis

Compared with pacemaker generator change, the overall procedure time for ICD generator change may be lengthier because of the larger size of the device and greater extent of dissection, the frequent need for upgrade, and the added time for DFT testing during the procedure. The surgical wound may, therefore, be open for a longer time, although closure may be started before all testing is complete. Furthermore, the generator change could involve a larger incision in an abdominal site. We recommend routine use of broad-spectrum antibiotics for antimicrobial prophylaxis during all procedures involving generator or lead revision, especially because these procedures use combinations of previously implanted hardware with new equipment. Whether and how long to use postoperative antibiotic prophylaxis has been debated.[98]

Intervention for Acute Problems

Indications for acute intervention include primary complications of pacemaker or ICD implantation (e.g., pocket hematoma, infection,[1-3] or cardiac perforation[73-77]) as well as other, less crucial indications, such as iatrogenic lead damage and lead dislodgement.

Pocket hematomas occur most commonly in patients receiving anticoagulants, especially heparin and enoxaparin, and in patients with platelet dysfunction, which is common in those undergoing long-term hemodialysis. The range in hematoma size varies from a contained, small amount of fluctuance and ecchymosis to a large hematoma that may drain through the skin. A minor hematoma requires only observation, whereas a breach of skin integrity after operation may require evacuation of the hematoma or, if it has become secondarily infected, complete removal of the generator and lead system. If the patient remains pacemaker dependent, a temporary wire must be placed when the original system is removed; after an appropriate course of intravenous antibiotic therapy, a new pacemaker can be placed on the contralateral side. Prolonged antibiotic therapy may be required in some cases. Antibiotic therapy alone and conservative surgical approaches other than complete removal of an eroded or infected generator and leads prove unsatisfactory.[5-8]

Immediate reoperation may also be required for cardiac perforation.[73-77,79] Perforation is suggested by curvature of the lead beyond the confines of the right ventricular apex, an abrupt rise in pacing threshold or deterioration of sensing, precordial pain that increases with inspiration, hypotension, and hemodynamic collapse. Although most perforations close spontaneously, development of a large pericardial bleed or tamponade requires immediate intervention.[79] Pericardiocentesis usually suffices, but occasionally, a subxiphoid approach to pericardial drainage is necessary. Proper lead selection to match the patient's anatomy and gentle technique are vital to avoiding acute perforation. Subcostal placement of epicardial screw-in leads has been associated with a high incidence of serious or fatal ventricular perforations; chronic perforation by endocardial leads is distinctly rare.[24]

Early surgical exploration is indicated to confirm the diagnosis of iatrogenic lead insulation damage. This is an uncommon complication that manifests early in the form of pocket twitch,[81] failure to capture, or failure to sense, with associated low measured lead impedance.[51] Chronic lead damage has been associated with excessively tight anchoring sutures, especially if they are placed around the lead and not the anchoring sleeve. The damaged lead, whether passive or active fixation, should be removed and replaced, if possible; alternatively, it may be repaired, although repair is difficult if damage has occurred near the venous insertion site.

Lead dislodgement occurs most commonly during the first 24 to 48 hours after system implantation.[26,27] It can occur later, however, as a result of a loose anchoring sleeve, incomplete fixation of the distal lead tip, excessive diaphragmatic motion, or patient manipulation of the device (i.e., twiddler's syndrome).[49] Before the development of leads with active fixation or a fin-like mechanism at the distal tip, the incidence of lead dislodgement ranged as high as 5% to 18%. With careful technique and selection among a variety of active-fixation and passive-fixation leads, the incidence should range no higher than 1% to 2%.[30,31,99] Most spontaneous dislodgements occur with atrial passive-fixation leads. The diagnosis may be facilitated by chest radiography or fluoroscopy; pacing analysis reveals an increased pacing threshold with, usually, normal lead impedance. The operator has the option of repositioning or replacing the lead. If a distinct cause cannot be identified, placement of an active-fixation lead may avoid a second dislodgement. To prevent recurrent lead dislodgement in twiddler's syndrome, leads must be sutured to prepectoral fascia or firm pacemaker pocket fibrous tissue with nonabsorbable sutures around anchoring sleeves at more than two points; the pacemaker connector block may also be anchored to the pectoralis fascia. A polyester (Dacron) pouch has been used in the past to improve device stability in this syndrome and in patients with very loose subcutaneous tissue,[100] but it is rarely required today.

Interval or Unscheduled Intervention

In the course of pacemaker or ICD follow-up and before the patient requires elective replacement, interval intervention may be needed to correct other complications. These include pulse generator migration,[15] lead dislodgement,[16,23,26,27,31,49] high pacing thresholds,[23,50] pocket twitch or diaphragmatic pacing,[24,81] lead insulation break or lead fracture,[11,13,26] premature generator failure (which could be due to intrinsic component failure or the result of externally induced failure, such as that caused by electrocautery, irradiation, or cardioversion),[19,20] and the need for upgrade of the system.[73] The pacemaker clinic may prove particularly useful in recognizing early surgical or functional problems.[37] Evaluation and technique follow the principles described earlier.

Summary

Successful pacemaker or ICD replacement is the result of accurate preoperative evaluation and careful surgical intervention. The preoperative status of the pulse generator battery and lead pacing and sensing function as well as the appropriateness of both to future pacing or defibrillating systems need to be determined to enable surgical planning. There should be no surgical surprises, and all the tools, adapters, leads, and generators should be ready for the intervention. The goal should be to avoid reoperation for as long as possible with careful initial implantation and programming. When properly planned, surgery is likely to proceed smoothly.

REFERENCES

1. Bonchek LI: New methods in the management of extruded and infected cardiac pacemakers. Ann Surg 176:686, 1972.
2. Corman LC, Levison ME: Sustained bacteremia and transvenous cardiac pacemakers. JAMA 233:264, 1975.
3. Morgan G, Ginks W, Siddons H, Leatham A: Septicemia in patients with an endocardial pacemaker. Am J Cardiol 44:221, 1979.
4. Wohl B, Peters RW, Carliner N, et al: Late unheralded pacemaker pocket infection due to *Staphylococcus epidermidis*: A new clinical entity. PACE 5:190, 1982.
5. Prager PI, Kay RH, Somberg E, et al: Pacemaker remnants-another source of infections. PACE 7:763, 1984.
6. Mansour KA, Kauten JR, Hatcher CR Jr: Management of the infected pacemaker: Explantation, sterilization, and reimplantation. Ann Thorac Surg 40:617, 1985.
7. Buch J, Mortensen SA: Late infections of pacemaker units due to silicone rubber insulation boots. PACE 8:494, 1985.
8. Ruiter JH, Degener JE, Van Mechelen R, Bos R: Late purulent pacemaker pocket infection caused by *Staphylococcus epidermidis*: Serious complications of in situ management. PACE 8:903, 1985.
9. Vilacosta I, Zamorano J, Camino A, et al: Infected transvenous permanent pacemakers: Role of transesophageal echocardiography. Am Heart J 125:904, 1993.
10. Garcia-Rinaldi R, Revuelta JM, Bonnington L, Soltero-Harrington L: The exposed cardiac pacemaker: Treatment by subfacial pocket relocation. J Thorac Cardiovasc Surg 89:136, 1985.
11. Kronzon I, Mehta SS: Broken pacemaker wire in multiple trauma: A case report. J Trauma 14:82, 1974.
12. Tegtmeyer CJ, Bezirdjian DR, Irani FA, Landis JD: Cardiac pacemaker failure: A complication of trauma. South Med J 74:378, 1981.
13. Grieco JG, Scanlon PJ, Pifarre R: Pacing lead fracture after a deceleration injury. Ann Thorac Surg 47:453, 1989.

14. Wallace WA, Abelmann WH, Norman JC: Runaway demand pacemaker: Report, in vitro reproduction, and review. Ann Thorac Surg 9:209, 1970.
15. Bello A, Yepez CG, Barcelo JE: Retroperitoneal migration of a pacemaker generator: An unusual complication. J Cardiovasc Surg 15:256, 1974.
16. Kim GE, Haveson S, Imparato AM: Late displacement of cardiac pacemaker electrode due to heavyweight pulse generator. JAMA 228:74, 1974.
17. Austin SM, Kim CS, Solis A: Electrical alternans of pacemaker spike amplitude: An unusual manifestation of permanent pacemaker generator malfunction. PACE 4:313, 1981.
18. Campo A, Nowak R, Magilligan D, Tomlanovich M: Runaway pacemaker. Ann Emerg Med 12:32, 1983.
19. Venselaar JL, Van Kerkeorle HL, Vet AJ: Radiation damage to pacemakers from radiotherapy. PACE 19:538, 1987.
20. Lewinn AA, Serago CF, Schwade JG, et al: Radiation-induced failures of complementary metal oxide semiconductor containing pacemakers: A potentially lethal complication. Int J Radiol Oncol Biol Phys 19:1967, 1984.
21. Halperin JL, Camunas JL, Stern EH, et al: Myopotential interference with DDD pacemakers: Endocardial electrographic telemetry in the diagnosis of pacemaker-related arrhythmias. Am J Cardiol 54:97, 1984.
22. den Dulk K, Lindemans FW, Brugada P, et al: Pacemaker syndrome with AAI rate-variable pacing: Importance of atrioventricular conduction properties, medication, and pacemaker programmability. PACE 11:1226, 1988.
23. Aris A, Shebairo RA, Lepley D Jr: Increasing myocardial thresholds to pacing after cardiac surgery. Surg Forum 24:167, 1973.
24. Gaidula JJ, Barold SS: Elimination of diaphragmatic contractions from chronic pacing catheter perforation of the heart by conversion to a unipolar system. Chest 66:86, 1974.
25. Contini C, Papi L, Pesola A, et al: Tissue reaction to intracavitary electrodes: Effect on duration and efficiency of unipolar pacing in patients with A-V block. J Cardiovasc Surg 14:282, 1973.
26. Holmes DR Jr, Nissen RG, Maloney JD, et al: Transvenous tined electrode systems: An approach to acute dislodgement. May Clin Proc 54:219, 1979.
27. Snow N: Elimination of lead dislodgment by the use of tined transvenous electrodes. PACE 5:571, 1982.
28. Alt E, Volker R, Blomer H: Lead fracture in pacemaker patients. Thorac Cardiovasc Surg 35:101, 1987.
29. Woscoboinik JR, Maloney JD, Helguera ME, et al: Pacing lead survival: Performance of different models. PACE 15:1991, 1992.
30. Morse D, Yankaskas M, Johnson B, et al: Transvenous pacemaker insertion with a zero dislodgment rate. PACE 6:283, 1983.
31. Hakki AH, Horowitz LN, Reiser J, Mundth ED: Improved pacemaker fixation and performance using a modified finned porous surfaced tip lead. Int Surg 69:291, 1984.
32. Mirowski M, Reid PR, Mower MM, et al: Termination of malignant ventricular arrhythmias with an implanted automatic defibrillator in human beings. N Engl J Med 303:322, 1980.
33. Mond H, Twentyman R, Smith D, Sloman G: The pacemaker clinic. Cardiology 57:262, 1972.
34. Starr A, Dobbs J, Dabolt J, Pierie W: Ventricular tracking pacemaker and teletransmitter follow-up system. Am J Cardiol 32:956, 1973.
35. Janosik DL, Redd RM, Buckingham TA, et al: Utility of ambulatory electrocardiography in detecting pacemaker dysfunction in the early postimplantation period. Am J Cardiol 60:1030, 1987.
36. Mugica J, Henry L, Rollet M, et al: The clinical utility of pacemaker follow-up visits. PACE 9:1249, 1986.
37. Joseph GK, Wilkoff BL, Dresing T, et al: Remote interrogation and monitoring of implantable cardioverter defibrillators. J Interv Card Electrophysiol 11:161, 2004.
38. Kertes P, Mond H, Sloman G, et al: Comparison of lead complications with polyurethane tined, silicone rubber tined, and wedge tip leads: Clinical experience with 822 ventricular endocardial leads. PACE 6:957, 1983.
39. van Gelder LM, El Gamal MI: False inhibition of an atrial demand pacemaker caused by an insulation defect in a polyurethane lead. PACE 6:834, 1983.
40. Sanford CF: Self-inhibition of an AV sequential demand (DVI) pulse generator due to polyurethane lead insulation disruption. PACE 6:840, 1983.
41. Timmis GC, Westveer DC, Martin R, Gordon S: The significance of surface changes on explanted polyurethane pacemaker leads. PACE 6:845, 1983.
42. Chawla AS, Blais P, Hinberg I, Johnson D: Degradation of explanted polyurethane cardiac pacing leads and of polyurethane. Biomater Artif Cells Artif Organs 16:785, 1988.
43. Van Beek GJ, den Dulk K, Lindemans FW, Wellens HJ: Detection of insulation failure by gradual reduction in noninvasively measured electrogram amplitudes. PACE 9:772, 1986.
44. Stokes KB, Church T: Ten-year experience with implanted polyurethane lead insulation. PACE 9:1160, 1986.
45. Phillips R, Frey M, Martin RO: Long-term performance of polyurethane pacing leads: Mechanisms of design-related failures. PACE 9:1166, 1986.
46. Barold SS, Gaidula JJ: Demand pacemaker arrhythmias from intermittent internal short circuit in bipolar electrode. Chest 63:165, 1973.
47. Adler SC, Foster AJ, Sanders RS, Wuu E: Thin bipolar leads: A solution to problems with coaxial bipolar designs. PACE 15:1986, 1992.
48. Barold SS, Scovil J, Ong LS, Heinle RA: Periodic pacemaker spike attenuation with preservation of capture: An unusual electrocardiographic manifestation of partial pacing electrode fracture. PACE 1:375, 1978.
49. Bayliss, CE, Beanlands DS, Baird RJ: The pacemaker-twiddler's syndrome: A new complication of implantable transvenous pacemakers. Can Med Assoc J 99:371, 1968.
50. Starr DS, Lawrie GM, Morris GC Jr: Acute and chronic stimulation thresholds of intramyocardial screw-in pacemaker electrodes. Ann Thorac Surg 31:334, 1981.
51. Ferek B, Pasini M, Pustisek S, et al: Noninvasive detection of insulation break. PACE 7:1063, 1984.
52. Sandler MJ, Kutalek SP: Inappropriate discharge by an implantable cardioverter defibrillator: Recognition of myopotential sensing using telemetered intracardiac electrograms. PACE 17:665, 1994.
53. Korte T, Jung W, Spehl S, et al: Incidence of ICD lead related complications during long-term follow-up: Comparison of epicardial and endocardial electrode systems. PACE 18:2053, 1995.
54. Schwartzman D, Callans DJ, Gottlieb CD, et al: Early postoperative rise in defibrillation threshold in patients with nonthoracotodefibrillation lead systems: Attenuation with biphasic shock waveforms. J Cardiovasc Electrophysiol 7:483, 1996.
55. Goyal R, Harvey M, Horwood L, et al: Incidence of lead system malfunction detected during implantable defibrillator generator replacement. PACE 19:1143, 1996.
56. Calfee RV, Saulson SH: A voluntary standard for 3.2-mm unipolar and bipolar pacemaker leads and connectors. PACE 9:1181, 1986.
57. Doring J, Flink R: The impact of pending technologies on a universal connector standard. PACE 9:1186, 1986.
58. Tyers GF, Sanders R, Mills P, Clark J: Analysis of setscrew and sidelock connector reliability. PACE 15:2000, 1992.
59. Hayes DL, Wang PJ, Reynolds DW, et al: Interference with cardiac pacemakers by cellular telephones. N Engl J Med 336:1473, 1997.
60. Fetter JG, Ivans V, Benditt DG, Collins J: Digital cellular telephone interaction with implantable cardioverter-defibrillators. J Am Coll Cardiol 31:623, 1998.

61. Torresani J, Ebagosti A, Allard-Latour G: Pacemaker syndrome with DDD pacing. PACE 7:1183, 1984.
62. Cunningham TM: Pacemaker syndrome due to retrograde conduction in DDI pacemaker. Am Heart J 115:478, 1988.
63. Schwartzman D, Nallamothu N, Callans DJ, et al: Postoperative lead-related complications in patients with nonthoracotomy defibrillation lead system. J Am Coll Cardiol 26:776, 1995.
64. Lawton JS, Wood MA, Gilligan DM, et al: Implantable cardioverter defibrillator leads: The dark side. PACE 19:1273, 1996.
65. Swartz JF, Fletcher RD, Karasik PE: Optimization of biphasic waveforms for human nonthoracotomy defibrillation. Circulation 88:2646, 1993.
66. Neuzner J, Pitschner HF, Huth C, et al: Effect of biphasic waveform pulse on endocardial defibrillation efficacy in humans. PACE 17:207, 1994.
67. Natale S, Sra J, Axtell K, et al: Preliminary experience with a hybrid nonthoracotomy defibrillating system that includes a biphasic device: Comparison with a standard monophasic device using the same lead system. J Am Coll Cardiol 24:406, 1994.
68. Block M, Hammel D, Bocker D, et al: A prospective randomized cross-over comparison of mono- and biphasic defibrillation using nonthoracotomy lead configuration in humans. J Cardiovasc Electrophysiol 5:581, 1994.
69. Gold MR, Foster AH, Shorofsky SR: Lead system optimization for transvenous defibrillation. Am J Cardiol 80:1163, 1997.
70. Bardy GH, Dolack GL, Kudenchuck PJ, et al: Prospective comparison in humans of a unipolar defibrillation system with that using an additional superior vena cava electrode. Circulation 89:1090, 1994.
71. Almassi GH, Olinger GN, Wetherbee JN, et al: Long-term complications of implantable cardioverter defibrillator lead system. Ann Thorac Surg 55:888, 1993.
72. Brode SE, Schwartzman D, Callans DJ, et al: ICD-antiarrhythmic drug and ICD-pacemaker interactions. J Cardiovasc Electrophysiol 8:830, 1997.
73. Baker CM, Christopher TJ, Smith PF, et al: Addition of a left ventricular lead to conventional pacing systems in patients with congestive heart failure: Feasibility, safety, and early results in 60 consecutive patients. PACE 25:166, 2002.
74. Peters RW, Scheinman MM, Raskin S, Thomas AN: Unusual complications of epicardial pacemaker: Recurrent pericarditis, cardiac tamponade and pericardial constriction. Am J Cardiol 45:1088, 1980.
75. Phibbs B, Marriott HJ: Complications of permanent transvenous pacing. N Engl J Med 312:1428, 1985.
76. Villaneuva FS, Heinsiner JA, Burkman MH, et al: Echocardiographic detection of perforation of the cardiac ventricular septum by a permanent pacemaker lead. Am J Cardiol 59:370, 1987.
77. Hill PE: Complications of permanent transvenous cardiac pacing: A 14-year review of all transvenous pacemakers inserted at one community hospital. PACE 10:564, 1987.
78. Pizzarelli G, Dernevik L: Inadvertent transarterial pacemaker insertion: An unusual complication. PACE 10:951, 1987.
79. Sandler MA, Wertheimer JH, Kotler MN: Pericardial tamponade associated with pacemaker catheter manipulation. PACE 12: 1085, 1989.
80. Mueller X, Sadeghi H, Kappenberger L: Complications after single- versus dual-chamber pacemaker implantation. PACE 13:711, 1990.
81. Ekbom K, Nilsson BY, Edhag O, Olin C: Rhythmic shoulder girdle muscle contractions as a complication in pacemaker treatment. Chest 66:599, 1974.
82. Chun PK: Characteristics of commonly utilized permanent endocardial and epicardial pacemaker electrode systems: Method of radiologic identification. Am Heart J 102:404, 1981.
83. Angello DA: Principles of electrical testing for analysis of ventricular endocardial pacing leads. Prog Cardiovasc Dis 27:57, 1984.
84. Kemler RL: A simple method for exposing the external jugular vein for placement of a permanent transvenous pacing catheter electrode. Ann Thorac Surg 26:266, 1978.
85. Sethi GK, Bhayana JN, Scott SM: Innominate venous thrombosis: A rare complication of transvenous pacemaker electrodes. Am Heart J 87:770, 1974.
86. Fritz T, Richeson JF, Fitzpatrick P, Wilson G: Venous obstruction: A potential complication of transvenous pacemaker electrodes. Chest 83:534, 1983.
87. Sharma S, Kaul U, Rajani M: Digital subtraction venography for assessment of deep venous thrombosis in the arms following pacemaker implantation. Int J Cardiol 23:135, 1989.
88. Antonelli D, Turgeman Y, Kaveh Z, et al: Short-term thrombosis after transvenous permanent pacemaker insertion. PACE 12:280, 1989.
89. Spittell PC, Vlietstra RE, Hayes DL, Higano ST: Venous obstruction due to permanent transvenous pacemaker electrodes: Treatment with percutaneous transluminal balloon venoplasty. PACE 13:271, 1990.
90. Wertheimer M, Hughes RK, Castle CH: Superior vena cava syndrome: Complication of permanent transvenous endocardial cardiac pacing. JAMA 224:1172, 1973.
91. Toumbouras M, Spanos P, Konstantaras C, Lazarides DP: Inferior vena cava thrombosis due to migration of retained functionless pacemaker electrode. Chest 82:785, 1982.
92. Blackburn T, Dunn M: Pacemaker-induced superior vena cava syndrome: Consideration of management. Am Heart J 116:893, 1988.
93. Goudevenos JA, Reid PG, Adams PC, et al: Pacemaker-induced superior vena cava syndrome: Report of four cases and review of the literature. PACE 12:1890, 1989.
94. Mazzetti H, Dussaut A, Tentori C, et al: Superior vena cava occlusion and/or syndrome related to pacemaker leads. Am Heart J 125:831, 1993.
95. Pace JN, Maquilan M, Hessen SE, et al: Extraction and replacement of permanent pacemaker leads through occluded vessels: Use of extraction sheaths as conduits-balloon venoplasty as an adjunct. J Interv Cardiol Electrophysiol 1:271, 1997.
96. Chaithiraphan S, Goldberg E, Wolff W, et al: Massive thrombosis of the coronary sinus as an unusual complication of transvenous pacemaker insertion in a patient with persistent left, and no right superior vena cava. J Am Geriatr Soc 22:79, 1974.
97. Kennelly BM: Permanent pacemaker implantation in the absence of a right superior vena cava: A case report. S Afr Med J 55:1043, 1979.
98. Wade JS, Cobbs CG: Infections in cardiac pacemakers. Curr Clin Topics Infect Dis 9:44, 1988.
99. Boake WC, Kroncke GM: Pacemaker Complications: Cardiac Pacing. Philadelphia, Lea & Febiger, 1979.
100. Parsonnet V: A stretch fabric pouch for implanted pacemakers. Arch Surg 105:654, 1972.

Chapter 21

Managing Device-Related Complications and Transvenous Lead Extraction

CHARLES L. BYRD

Management of device-related complications is an established and essential branch of electrophysiology. The prerequisites include proficiency in device implantation; knowledge of the etiology, pathophysiology, and treatment of each type of complication; and acquisition of the procedural skills necessary to administer the treatment. In this chapter, emphasis is placed on both procedure-related technical skills and management of individual complications. A divergence is made from the classic historical description of topics in order to emphasize the current clinical relevance of the various types of complications.

The two essential skills are lead extraction and lead implantation. In the past, extraction procedures were on the leading edge of technical development, evolving rapidly, and potentially dangerous; patient management revolved around the lead extraction procedure. Today, lead extraction plays the same essential role in managing device-related complications as does lead implantation for insertion of a device. Mastery of extraction and implantation skills is a necessary prerequisite to managing device-related complications.

Complications

A device-related complication is a potential or actual morbid process or event associated with an implanted device. This definition of a device-related complication mirrors the definition for any medical complication, except for the identification of a "potential process or event." Potential is used because, in some situations, the probability of occurrence of a morbid process or event elevates it to the level of a complication. A morbid process pertains to a disease or clinical event. By this definition, a device-related event (DRE) may not be a complication. For example, a device component failure does not qualify as a complication unless it causes a potential or actual clinical event.

Classifications of Device-Related Complications

A uniform classification of device-related complications does not exist. Device-related complications encompass a diverse collection of DREs, clinically ranging from trivial to life-threatening, and some may not require therapeutic intervention. DREs involve the device itself, the biophysical interface between the device and tissue, and communication between the device and the heart and blood vessels. For a complication to exist, the DRE must cause a local clinical event involving heart rhythm, mechanically induced hemodynamic events, and/or electric field effects. The local clinical event may cause systemic clinical events, which involve organ perfusion and compensatory mechanics. The name given to a complication should reflect the associated DRE, the local clinical event, and the systemic clinical event. The challenge is to construct a logical classification system that meets this objective.

It is not surprising that current practices label a device-related complication with a superficial descriptive name associated with an event, such as loss of capture, loss of sensing, venous occlusion, phrenic nerve stimulation, or infection. Although some of these labels are unique, relate to symptoms, reflect the magnitude of the clinical sequelae, and define the cause, most do not. For example, the descriptive device-related complication name "loss of pacing" signifies that there is no evidence the device is pacing the heart. It does not indicate whether pacing spikes are present or why the loss of capture occurred (e.g., conductor coil fracture, battery failure, component failure in the pulse generator, exit block, low output voltage, oversensing). The label is obviously not unique.

"Loss of capture" implies that a pacing spike was present and narrows the list to conductor coil fracture, exit block, and low output voltage. To further define the problem, additional test data, such as impedance and stimulation threshold data, are needed, along with more descriptive labels to reflect the testing. In addition, more labels are required to describe the magnitude of the problem: signs and symptoms related to the heart, central nervous system (CNS), pulmonary system, renal system, and so on. Assume all of these labels qualify as a complication. Which label is to be listed as the complication? This is not a logical or uniform classification system.

A pictorial classification is descriptive and complete, and its meaning is intuitively obvious. Pictures can easily demonstrate any complicated scenario. Unfortunately, unless the picture can be standardized, incorporated into a classification scheme, or communicated in a simple fashion, its integration into a logical uniform classification system is too complicated. An abstract classification tries to integrate the complexities depicted in a picture into a simple, uniform, and logical classification using words and/or symbols. The reverse is also true: an abstract description can also be presented as a picture. A classification of a device-related complication must include all of the DREs (Fig. 21-1).

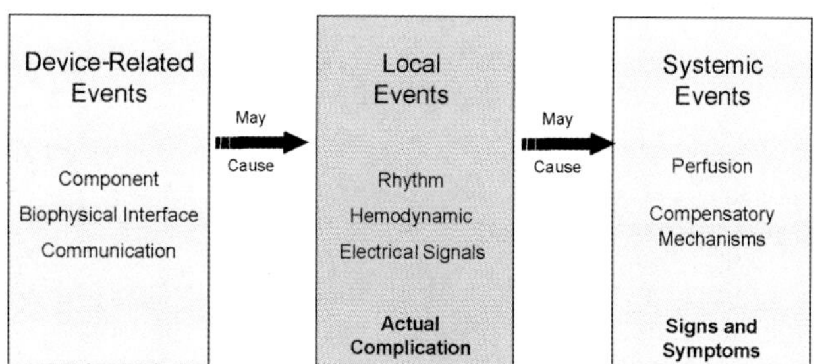

Figure 21-1. Device-related complications. Device-related complications are separated into device-related events (DREs), local events, and systemic events. DREs include all events and may or may not cause a clinical complication. DREs are separated into component failures, biophysical interface issues, and problems of communication between the pulse generator and the heart. A local event is a complication caused by a DRE and is an actual complication. Local events manifest as abnormal rhythms, hemodynamic parameters, and electrical signals. A systemic event is the systemic manifestation of a local complication. Systemic events are the signs, symptoms, and organ failures caused by perfusion or compensatory mechanisms.

Device-Related Events

DREs are separated into problems with the physical device components (e.g., pulse generator, leads, adaptors), interaction of the device with the biophysical interface, and communication of the device with tissues (cardiac, muscular, neural, and vascular). An abstract classification based on components, biophysical interface, and communication physically defines all DREs, and these events can be presented as pictures. All complications are DREs, but not all DREs are complications. A DRE must have actual or potential clinical sequelae to qualify as a complication. DREs must be an integral part of any classification system. Component events are issues associated with the device hardware. Examples of component events are pulse generator failures (battery and pulse generator circuit) and lead failures (insulation and conductor coil). Biophysical interface events are stress related. Physical, metabolic, and chemical stresses injure the tissue, causing inflammatory tissue reactions (encapsulating fibrous tissue, exit block, venous occlusion, and vegetation on leads) and mechanical tissue disruption (resulting in lead dislodgment, perforation, and mechanical stimulation of heart). Physical stress refers to mechanical stresses (traction, shearing, and compression forces) that injure the surrounding tissue. Chemical stress relates primarily to toxins associated with bacterial infections.

Communication events involve the electrical signals delivered to and received from the cardiac, muscular, and neural tissues. It also involves the logic of the commands sent to the heart and how they interact. Examples include programming variables (voltage output, sensing levels, and refractory period), appropriateness of device logic interactions (conduction system and pathologic rhythms), interaction with skeletal muscle (stimulation and oversensing), and nerve stimulation (phrenic nerve stimulation).

Clearly, an abstract separation into components, biophysical interface, and communication events is all-inclusive with respect to DREs. Despite the fact that this abstract presentation defines DREs and reflects the pictorial information, clinical information is needed for an event to qualify as a device-related complication.

Local Clinical Events

Local clinical events (see Fig. 21-1) include the rhythm, hemodynamic, and electric field effects caused by DREs. A rhythm event is the resultant rhythm caused by a DRE. A rhythm event can be described using the same classic terminology used for all rhythms. Sinus bradycardia, Mobitz II atrioventricular block, and pacemaker-mediated tachycardia are all acceptable descriptions for a rhythm event. Hemodynamic clinical events are the hemodynamic sequelae of a DRE. Examples are swelling from venous occlusion, shunting from pulmonary emboli, ascites from tricuspid valve insufficiency, and cardiac tamponade from disruption of the superior vena cava (SVC).

An electric field effect is a DRE caused by a remote action of the electric field. Examples are crosstalk between the atrial and ventricular electrodes, stimulation of the phrenic nerve, stimulation of the pectoral muscle, and sensing of myopotentials. The local clinical events (rhythm, hemodynamic, and electric field effects) include all of the DREs that qualify as a complication. For a complication name (label) to be descriptive, both the local clinical event and the DRE must be combined in some fashion. Although the combined label is a satisfactory description of a device-related complication, system-related events and the clinical magnitude of an event are not known.

Systemic Clinical Events

Systemic clinical events are caused by local clinical events superimposed on the system's underlying pathophysiology. Acute effects are related to perfusion and chronic effects to compensation. Perfusion issues are controlled by blood flow and pressure gradients. Tissue perfusion is intuitively obvious. A low cardiac output can result in decreased blood pressure and/or elevated venous pressure, both of which can result in poor tissue perfusion. Examples of poor perfusion to the brain are dizziness, syncope, and coma; to the kidneys, prerenal failure; and to the skeletal muscle, fatigue. Examples of elevated venous pressure are stiff lungs and pulmonary edema.

"Compensatory mechanism" is a name given for the cardiovascular system's attempt to correct a perfusion problem. Compensatory mechanisms all represent pathologic states, even though they may restore satisfactory tissue perfusion. For example, a dilated cardiomyopathy is the heart's compensatory mechanism for low output (bradycardia, tachycardia, decreased muscle power, and/or valvular stenosis and insufficiency) and for conduction abnormalities altering the filling of the left ventricle (right ventricular apical pacing and left bundle branch block). Formation of collateral veins or arteries is the compensatory mechanism for venous or arterial occlusion.

The labeling for a systemic clinical event should reflect the magnitude of the insult and/or its potential risk. This includes both the heart and the vascular system. Performing this task for each organ system is not practical. Use of accepted integrated clinical labels such as signs and symptoms will suffice. In describing an acute poor perfusion state, statements such as cardiovascular collapse, low-output syndrome, weakness and fatigue, syncope, dizziness, and asymptomatic are all acceptable. If multiple signs and symptoms apply, the one reflecting a worst-case scenario should be used. For compensatory states, the situation is less clear. The patient may be asymptomatic even though the pathologic state caused by the local clinical event is significant. In these cases, the label should include the compensatory mechanism modified by symptoms (e.g., symptomatic dilated cardiomyopathy, heart failure with dilated cardiomyopathy). Compensatory states are usually reversible with correction of the local clinical event. For example, a dilated cardiomyopathy with failure symptoms secondary to a chronic heart rate of 30 beats per minute will reverse itself once the heart rate is returned to normal.

Summary of Abstract Classification

The abstract classification presented here defines a device-related complication. The word presentation of events (device-related, local, systemic) gives a complete picture that is intuitively obvious; examples include conductor coil fracture, loss of pacing and sensing, asymptomatic or exit block, loss of capture, and asymptomatic dilated cardiomyopathy. Although these labels are easy to understand when read, their formulation is complicated. Facility with this type of classification forces one to develop a clear understanding and organization of device-related complications. Once understood, the uniformity of the classification and the completeness of the definitions are rewards for the effort. The author has no delusions that this is the only way or even the best way to construct a uniform classification system. The usefulness of such a classification will be apparent as the chapter progresses.

Device-Related Events

DREs constitute the basis for all complications. Understanding a DRE is necessary for both diagnosis and management of a device-related complication. DREs are separated into events related to device components, device interaction at the biophysical interface, and communication between the device and the tissue. The first two types of DREs will be discussed here. The third type is the subject of the chapters on stimulation, sensing, and arrhythmia detection (Chapters 1 and 3).

Component-Related Problems

Battery Failure and Pulse Generator Circuit Failure

A battery and/or pulse generator circuit failure is an industry-related misadventure. The physician can neither cause nor prevent these types of complications. Pulse generator reimplantation is the only definitive treatment for these failures. Reimplantation is simple and direct and relieves the problem. The company should be notified and the pulse generator returned. Even if this was a known random failure mode, it is best to be safe and notify the company. No further action is needed. If the mode of failure is unknown or new, it may require some form of advisory or recall action. In both circumstances, the pulse generator should be returned to the manufacturer.

A company's advisory or recall notice usually states that reimplantation should be performed immediately should a failure occur, if there is a high probability of failure occurring, or if there is a chance that failure may be life-threatening. Reimplantation for generator failure or high probability of failure is obvious. The language "chance of a life-threatening failure" leaves the decision to replace the pulse generator in the hands of the physician. Two variables are implied in this subjective language: the incidence of failure and the patient's intrinsic conduction. If the incidence of failure is low and/or the patient is not "pacemaker dependent," continued close follow-up is recommended, as well as notification and counseling of the patient. In those situations where the manufacturer can be precise and recommend a logical plan of action, most physicians will follow those recommendations. If the recommendations are not precise and the physician has to make the reimplantation decision, confusion and insecurity often ensue, and the pulse generator is replaced. Although replacement resolves the pulse generator problem, the probability of a complication associated with replacement, such as infection, lead damage requiring a corrective action, or physiologic decompensation or death, may be greater than the risk of continued close patient monitoring.

A brief discussion of pulse generator failure is in order. It will be separated into battery failure and failure of other circuit components. Battery failure seems to be a trivial event, because all batteries fail with normal depletion of their energy stores. This is not a component failure as long as the battery depletes with time as designed. A true battery failure is rare, but when it does occur, it causes global pulse generator failure. The most common forms of battery failure are caused by some form of short circuit in the system. For example, a short circuit caused by a circuit component failure may manifest as a battery failure. If the system is short circuited and the battery overheats, the temperature change is felt by the patient. There are examples in the past of overheated batteries rupturing their containers, but tissue damage has not been reported. Examples of circuit failure are shunting of the high-energy circuit to a low-energy circuit, reed switch failure, grommet failure, and other random individual component failures. Stress-related issues usually occur over time. Examples of time-dependent stress-related failures are battery failure in the Marquis family implantable cardioverter-defibrillator (ICD) and cardiac resynchronization therapy defibrillator (CRT-D) (Medtronic, Minneapolis, Minn.), which was caused by a manufacturing error,[1] and shunting of energy from the high-energy circuit to the low-energy circuit in the PRIZM 2 ICD (Guidant, Boston Scientific, Natick, Mass.), with destruction of the low-energy circuit.[2]

A brief discussion and recognition of causes of past failures are informative and may be useful if similar mechanisms occur in the future. A circuit failure mode that plagued all manufacturers in the past was the presence of dendritic growth of conductive crystals causing a short circuit. This unique failure mode was prevented by hermetically sealing the circuit. Another form of battery failure was caused by failure of the artificial baffles placed between the chemical components within the battery. This is not an issue with the lithium/iodine battery currently in use in pacemakers. The baffle is formed by the reaction of the two components, lithium and iodine. This reaction generates the charge and forms the baffle at the same time. Rechargeable batteries failed not because of battery issues, but because they failed to gain patient acceptance due to the necessity of frequently recharging the battery. The most odious battery technology was the nuclear battery. A nuclear cell generated heat, which was converted into electricity. This battery was cloaked in red tape by the nuclear regulatory agency and was expensive. Red tape, expense, and the frequent advances in pulse generator performance negated the advantages of a long-acting battery, dooming it to failure.

Lead Failure

Lead failure is a common complication. A pacemaker lead failure is defined as failure of 1% per year for 5 years (i.e., 95% lead survival at 5 years).[1] ICD leads are more complicated and fail at a higher rate, and their failure rate has not been well defined. Despite their complexity, both pacemaker and ICD leads should be judged by the same standards. Lead failures include conductor coil fractures and loss of integrity of the inner and/or outer insulation. The mechanisms of failure are well defined for both types of leads.

The mechanisms for lead failure relating to the conductor coil include binding and excessive torque. The mechanisms for conductor coil failure are mechanical and are best illustrated by clinical examples. Failures relating to the insulation include environmental stress cracking (ESC), metal ion–induced oxidation (MIO), compression erosion or abrasion, cold flow, and tears. Insulation failures have general mechanical and chemical properties common to all polymers. Clinical examples specific to polyurethane and silicone rubber are discussed in more detail later. Two types of polyurethane are still used today: Pellethane 80A and Pellethane 55D. The difference between these two polymers is the percentage of short-chain polyurethane. Pellethane 80A has 70% short chain and is soft and supple, making it ideal for bipolar leads. Because of its insulation properties, bipolar leads could be made small for the first time. Pellethane 55D has 30% short chain and is harder and less supple. These leads were too stiff for bipolar configuration but were ideal for unipolar leads.

Conductor Coil Fracture

Conductor coil fracture is a break of one or more of the wires going from the pulse generator to the electrode (Fig. 21-2). A mental picture of a lead failure with the two ends separated or, at best, making intermittent contact is valid immediately after the break. The space between the broken ends acts as a perfect insulator with an infinite impedance (i.e., no pacing or sensing).

Chronic fractures are different. The space at the fracture site is filled with an electrolytic fluid within a short time period. It then behaves like two electrodes in an electrolytic medium (leaking capacitor), allowing some current to flow and generating a voltage at the pacing electrode. If the voltage is high enough, it can continue to pace the heart. The impedance is high, in the range of 1000 to 2000 ohms. Intermittent contact can cause a transmitted current spike, resulting in a voltage sufficient to pace or generate an electrical signal (a form of make-break signal) which, if seen by the sense ampli-

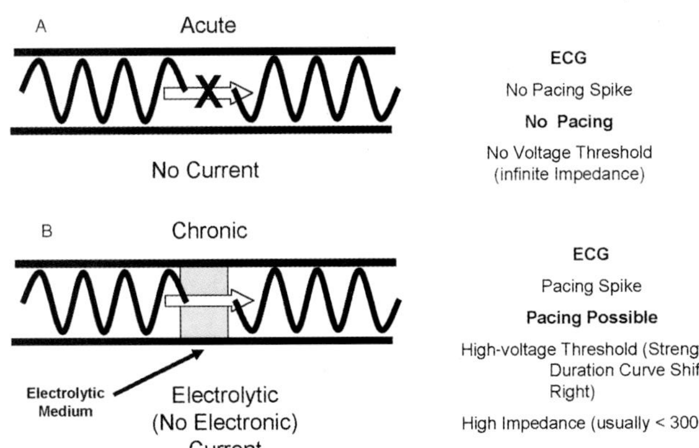

Figure 21-2. Conductor coil fracture. Conductor coil fractures can have an acute or a chronic presentation. ***A,*** *An acute fracture and separation of the conductor coil result in no current flow to the electrode and an infinite impedance. The result is no pacing spike on electrocardiogram (ECG) and loss of pacing.* ***B,*** *A chronic fracture has accumulated electrolytic fluid in the fracture space. The ends of the fractured wire behave as electrodes, and current can flow between the two ends of conductor coils at a high impedance. In many cases, the charge density on the electrodes is sufficient to pace, and a pacing spike is present on ECG.*

fier, will be acted on, causing a sensing abnormality. In some situations, both the inner and outer coils break, along with the insulation, leaving the entire lead in two separate pieces.

In regard to mechanisms of failure, the first example involves the medial placement of leads between the clavicle and the first rib in the thoracic inlet. This complication is related to lead binding. Passing the introducer needle through the subclavius muscle or the costoclavicular ligament can result in calcification of those structures. Lead binding occurs when the lead body becomes entrapped in the encapsulating calcifying fibrous tissue. If a lead with a helical conductor coil is rigidly bound, the helix cannot bend to relieve deformation stresses when the conductor coil is flexed on either side of the binding site. This situation is similar to a wire being bent back and forth in a narrow site. The stress at the flex site causes heat and, finally, breakage (fracture) of the wire. This same wire, configured as a helix, will bend back and forth without causing stress at the flex site. The helix is flexed, preventing deformation of the wire itself. Binding of the helix prevents it from flexing, causing the wire to be deformed at the junction between the bound and unbound helix, resulting in conductor coil fracture.

Another mechanism of failure involves the crimp and weld joints. These types of conductor coil fractures are caused by the torque and motion stresses applied to the joints by extension and retraction of the helix on an active fixation lead. Turning the inner conductor coil is a common mechanism used to extend and retract an active fixation helix. Excessive torque can break a crimp and weld joint between the conductor coil and the terminal pin or the helix (or both), resulting in a loss of integrity of the wire and mimicking a conductor coil fracture. The excessive torque at the terminal pin is usually caused by the conductor coil's binding against the stylet along a circuitous route. Similarly, excessive torque can be applied to the distal crimp and weld joint at the helix when the helix is bound inside the housing. Breakage at the terminal pin is more common and is associated with a circuitous path, whereas breakage at the helix is related to a manufacturing defect or to blood and tissue ingress that wedges the helix in the housing.

Insulation Failure

Lead insulation failure (Fig. 21-3A) became a significant clinical issue in the late 1970s with the use of polyurethane (Pellethane 80A).[3-6] Failure of the polyurethane insulation in unipolar leads was shown to be caused by ESC. Once the residual strains were relieved by changing the manufacturing practices, this problem was resolved. Normal stresses applied at the biophysical interface will cause some minor ESC. A far more sinister problem, MIO, also arose and is still with us today. MIO is the breakage of the short-chain ether linkages in Pellethane 80A by metal ions diffusing from the conductor coil into the insulation. MIO causes dissolution of the insulation at the molecular level. Current state-of-the-art leads have minimized, but not eliminated, the problem. Pellethane 55D is primarily long-chain polyurethane and is more resistant to MIO than Pellethane 80A.

Cold flow is a property of plastics caused by compression. The polymer flows away from the compression site, thinning the insulation. Cold flow can cause a loss of the insulation's integrity. This is a problem for both polyurethane and silicone. It is seen at sites of compression, such as suture tie sites on the suture sleeve, points where two leads press against one another, between the clavicle and first rib, and at points where the pulse generator is pinning the lead against the bone in a submuscular pocket. Formulations of silicone designed to withstand compression are more resistant to cold flow than silicones designed to stretch.

The effects of loss of insulation integrity depend on the arrangement of the conductor coils. Each conductor coil needs an insulator. A unipolar lead with one insulated conductor coil has only one configuration. Most bipolar leads with two helical conductor coils are coaxial, with the insulation around the inner and outer coils. Failure modes for the unipolar and coaxial bipolar leads are well known. Clinical experience with ICD leads that have multiple individually insulated conductor coils or individually insulated high-voltage coils has been good. There are few insulation failures. Although the failure modes for new leads with more sophisticated arrangements are unknown, failures caused by known mechanisms should still be apparent.

An outer insulation covers both unipolar and bipolar leads. Unipolar leads have one conductor coil connecting the pulse generator to the electrode (see Fig. 21-3B). A loss of insulation integrity creates an alternative current pathway between the lead and the pulse generator. These defects behave the same as another

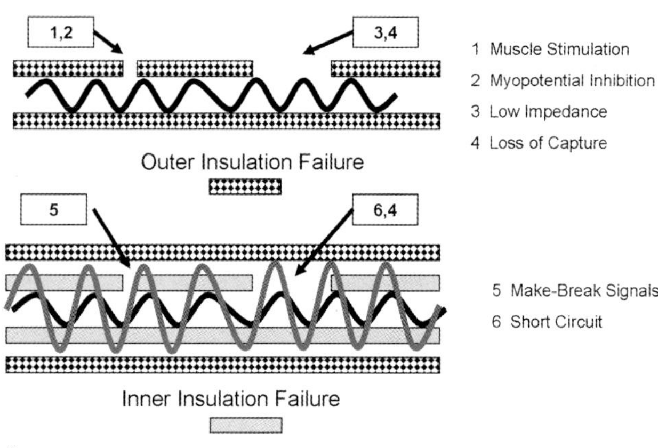

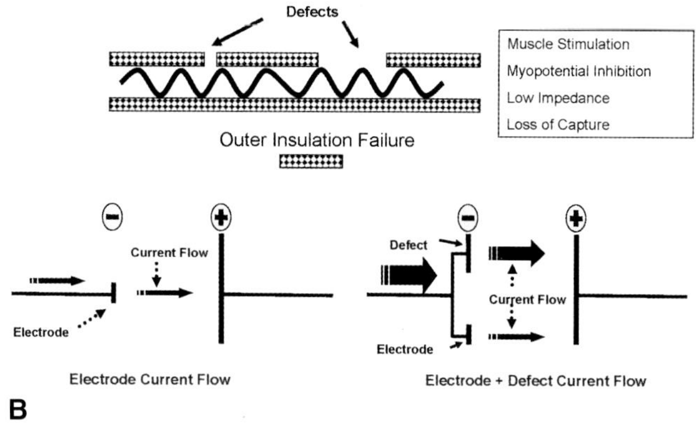

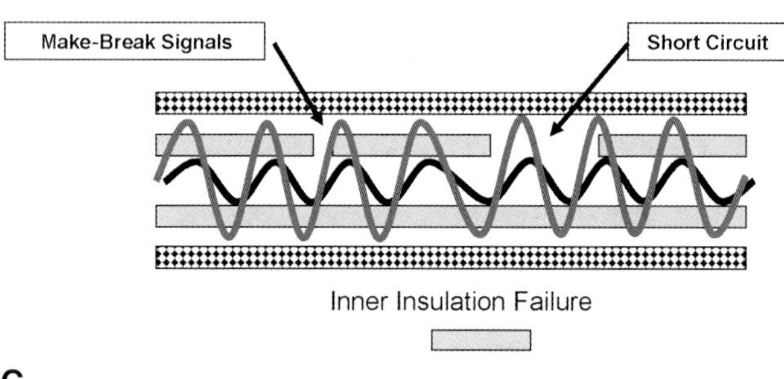

*Figure 21-3. Lead insulation failure. **A,** Outer insulation failure exposes the conductor coil to the surrounding tissue. Inner insulation failure allows the two conductor coils to communicate. **B,** Unipolar configuration has only one conductor coil and an outer insulation. Defects in the insulation act as electrodes, with the potential of simulating tissue (muscle and nerve stimulation) and/or sensing electrical activity (myopotential inhibition). The stimulation circuit is parallel to the pacing circuit, resulting in a decrease in impedance. Current flow may exceed the maximum discharge current from the capacitor, causing a decrease in voltage to the pacing electrode (loss of capture). **C,** Both outer and inner insulation failure can occur in bipolar configuration. Outer insulation failure in the bipolar configuration differs from that in the unipolar configuration. Sensing abnormalities can still occur, because electrical activity can be seen by the sensing circuit. Stimulation pathways similar to the unipolar configuration do not exist. Inner insulation failure has the potential to create make-break signals and to short-circuit the pacing circuit. Small defects in the inner insulation act as a small capacitor between the inner and outer coils, charging and discharging. These discharge signals can be seen by the sense amplifier, causing inhibition. A large defect causing shunting of current between the inner and outer coil lowers the impedance and potentially causes loss of capture (exceeding the output current of the capacitor).*

negative electrode capable of stimulating muscle and/or nerve tissue and sensing myopotential signals. The electric circuit created by the defect is in parallel with the pacing circuit. The resultant circuit obeys the laws governing a parallel circuit. The impedance across the parallel circuit decreases as the size of the defect gets larger and the current flow increases. Because the pulse generator's output current from the discharge of the capacitor is limited (approximately 17 mA), at some point the current to the pacing electrode will be insufficient to generate a threshold voltage, causing failure to pace. Also, the increased current drainage depletes the battery, shortening its life. If the electrode at the site of the defect is near skeletal muscle, myopotential signals can be detected by the sense amplifier, causing inhibition of pacing (same as a bipolar lead). Multiple defects in the insulation create multiple electrodes and multiple parallel circuits. Except for differences in location, multiple defects behave like one large alternative site electrode in parallel with the pacing electrode.

Bipolar leads have both outer and inner insulation. A loss of integrity of the outer insulation in a bipolar lead exposes the outer conductor coil to the tissue in the same manner as for a unipolar lead. This might lower the impedance slightly, but it does not change the pacing threshold. A conductor coil exposed to skeletal muscle acts as a sensing electrode and sends myopotential signals to the sense amplifier, causing oversensing and inhibition of pacing. The voltage is usually too low on the outer conductor coil to stimulate muscle or nerve tissue. Inner insulation failure has meaning only for bipolar leads (see Fig. 21-3C). Loss of integrity of the inner insulation creates a pathway to the outer conductor coil (electrical short-circuit). The size of the defect determines the current flow through the defect and its influence on the pacing electrode's voltage. In addition, a small defect behaves like a capacitor with the two wires separated by a dielectric. As the voltage builds across the defect, the dielectric breaks down, shunting current from the inner to the outer coil. The sense amplifier may see this make-break signal. Sensing abnormalities caused by make-break signals are an early sign of inner insulation failure. As the defects become larger, they no longer act as a capacitor, and current is shunted from the inner to the outer coils. This defect creates low-impedance parallel circuits. The increased current decreases battery longevity. Once the pulse generator's current output from its capacitor is maxed out, voltage on the pacing electrode will decrease, just as for a unipolar lead.

The first example of this mechanism of failure is related to the lead's being pinched (crush injury) between the clavicle and the first rib. This type of compression injury damages the lead body insulation. The loss of integrity of the polymers caused by compression injury results in inner insulation failure, resulting in make-break signals and short-circuiting between the inner and outer coils. Outer insulation failure is of consequence only if the exposed wire senses electrical signals and causes oversensing.

Silicone rubber and polyurethane are the two common polymers used for lead body insulation. Silicone deforms, cracks, and breaks when subjected to physical stress. Deformation by cold flow is the most common type of silicone compression, resulting in a flow (cold flow) of the polymer away from the compression stress. Once the stress is relieved, the flow stops. Continued stress will result in thinning to the point of loss of integrity. Excessive shearing and traction stresses result in cracking (breaking of molecular bonds) along stress lines, which can lead to loss of polymer and/or loss of lead integrity. Polyurethane deforms, cracks, and breaks when subjected to physical stress in a fashion similar to silicone. However, it seems to be more sensitive to stress. Compression easily causes cold flow, and excessive stress (shearing, traction, and compression) causes cracking (breaking of ether bonds) along stress lines ESC. ESC occurs at sites of applied stresses to the lead. The initial failure mechanism for Pellethane 80A was massive ESC caused by residual manufacturing stress left in the insulation from a solvent expansion-contraction technique used to place the insulation over the conductor coil. In the early 1980s, a new failure mechanism was found. Metal ions that diffused into the Pellethane 80A polymer broke the ether linkages in the polyurethane polymer, causing dissolution (crumbling) of the insulation. This was called MIO of the polymer, and it caused a non–stress-related failure with loss of polymer integrity. The insulation seemed to just melt away.

Historically, a potentially dangerous type of lead failure occurred due to protrusion of a retention wire through the insulation and into the surrounding tissue. This type of failure was the first example of a destructive lead failure. It had the potential to be destructive (i.e., to penetrate or tear tissue locally or remotely after migration), but it did not cause a problem with the electrical performance of the leads. The Telectronics 330-801 and 330-854 leads (St. Jude Medical, Sylmar, Calif.) had a component called a retention wire that was designed to hold a J configuration in the atrium. This wire had the potential of breaking (fracture) and eroding through the insulation without a loss of its electrical integrity; pacing and sensing characteristics were unchanged. The eroded retention wire could penetrate the superior veins, atrium, or aorta, causing a cardiovascular emergency.

This failure mechanism had a particularly important historical impact on the development of lead extraction expertise in the physician community. Because of the potential for fatal bleeding, hundreds of physicians were motivated to use these techniques. However, not everyone who extracted these leads was experienced or well trained, and the disadvantage of extraction became immediately apparent as the risk of extraction in the hands of some operators greatly exceeded the risk of fatal intrathoracic bleeding from penetration of the aorta by the J wire.[7-10] Although the specific techniques required for the removal of these leads are of historical interest (almost all were removed or the patients have died of old age), the risk-benefit analysis done for this situation is core to the decisions patients and physicians make every day for lead extraction or even for device change in the event of a device notification (recall).[11] The bottom line is that lead extraction training is essential, and tailoring extraction techniques to the specific lead construction and failure mechanism is crucial.

Biophysical Interface

The biophysical interface is the boundary between an implanted device and the body's tissue. If the device injures the tissue, there is an interaction between device and tissue called the inflammatory reaction.[12] The author's modeling of the interactions between implanted devices and surrounding tissue is based on general knowledge and experiences. Depending on the magnitude of the inflammatory reaction, it is considered a normal event, in the same sense as wound healing (primary intention) by an inflammatory reaction is considered normal. For example, the electrode is the perfect example of a critical device component whose function is dependent on a normal inflammatory reaction at the biophysical interface.

Device-related tissue injury is caused by applied stresses, including mechanical stresses (pressure and traction), traumatic disruptions (penetration, tears, and ruptures), metabolic insults (supply of oxygen and other nutrients), and chemical toxins (infections). Applied stresses are separated naturally into physical, metabolic, and chemical stresses (Fig. 21-4). Allergic reactions to device components have been postulated, speculated, and alleged but never proved to exist. The applied stresses cause an inflammatory reaction ranging from minor tissue injury to tissue disruption. To help avoid confusion, discussion of injury-related events at the biophysical interface are separated into inflammatory reactions and applied stresses.

Inflammatory Reactions

The inflammatory reaction is the body's physiologic response to tissue injury or death caused by any form of stress applied to the tissue. This includes the organization of blood clots in the bloodstream into fibrous tissue. Inflammatory reaction is hypothesized to be the same for all tissue, but there are various tissue-related presentations. In the vascular space, clot plays a predominant role. The following is a pictorial discussion modeling an inflammatory reaction (Fig. 21-5).

If one assumes an event happening in extravascular tissue (e.g., soft tissue), the initiation of an inflamma-

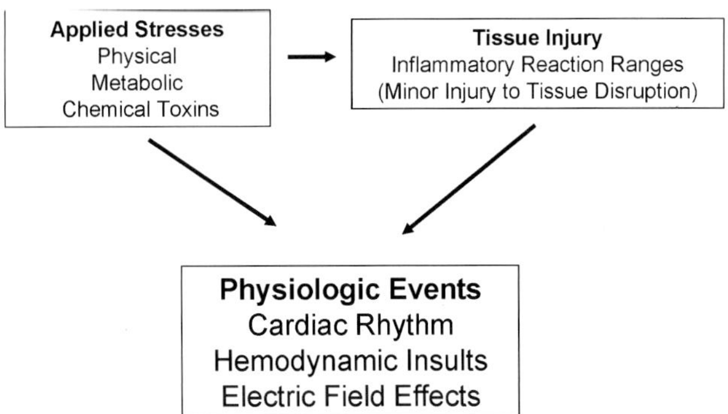

Figure 21-4. Biophysical interface. Applied stresses at the biophysical interface are caused by physical stresses (mechanical forces), metabolic issues, and chemical toxins (bacterial toxins). Applied stresses injure tissue, initiating an inflammatory reaction. Both the applied stresses and the inflammatory reaction cause physiologic events such as cardiac rhythm disorders, hemodynamic insults, and electric field complications (phrenic nerve stimulation).

tory reaction begins with emigration of cellular elements in the blood into the extravascular space. In normal laminar blood flow, cellular elements, such as red and white blood cells, are located in the center cellular zone, and the smaller blood components, such as proteins, are in the peripheral plasmatic zone (see Fig. 21-5A). Normally, there are no cellular elements in the plasmatic zone near the vessel walls. Imagine this arrangement as a natural consequence of blood flowing above a certain velocity.

The known sequence of events after injury to a mass of tissue in which the blood vessels remain structurally intact includes multiple steps. The first event is the dilation and subsequent increase in flow of small blood vessels in and near the injured tissue. The initial cause of this dilation is not clear. At this point, except for dilated vessels and increased flow, the physiology at the capillary level is still normal: the arterial pressure (hydrostatic pressure) forces electrolytic fluid out of the first part of the capillaries and into the extravascular space. This increases the concentration of the proteins, increasing the intravascular oncotic pressure and viscosity. The blood flow slows, and fluid is pulled back into the capillaries on the venous side (see Fig. 21-5B). Ideally, equal volumes are forced out and pulled back in.

The next event is a swelling of the endothelial cells that line the vessels in the capillary bed. This allows a fluid exudate containing both electrolytic fluids and protein material to move into the extravascular space, resulting in edema and dilution. The protein loss decreases the oncotic pressure and the intravascular volume, causing further slowing of blood flow. With this loss of fluid exudate and slowing of blood flow, the blood cells migrate from the center of the bloodstream into the plasmatic zone and to the wall (see Fig. 21-5C). The vessels then become more porous, resulting in neutrophil emigration and forcing out of red blood cells by hydrostatic pressure. The presence of fluid exudate and neutrophils marks the beginning of the full

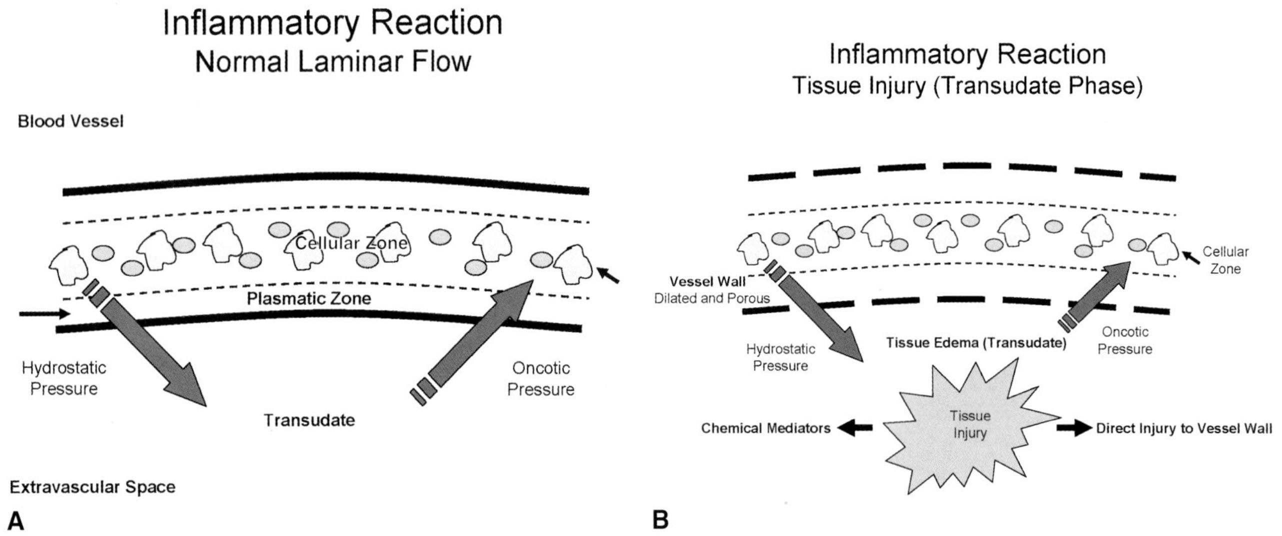

Figure 21-5. Inflammatory reaction (normal physiology). Inflammatory reaction is the body's response to tissue injury. The extravascular inflammatory reaction represents the microbiologic and macrobiologic physiologies of an inflammatory reaction. ***A,*** *Normal physiology at a microbiologic level involves the flow of blood through small blood vessels and capillaries supplying the metabolic needs of uninjured tissue and removing metabolic waste. Blood flow through these vessels is laminar, with blood cells flowing in the central cellular zone and proteinaceous material flowing in the peripheral plasmatic zone. Hydrostatic pressure forces transudate out of the blood vessels with the nutrients, and oncotic pressure draws the transudate back into the blood vessels with the metabolic waste.* ***B,*** *Tissue injury starts the transudate phase. Chemical mediators and direct injury to the vessel walls cause the vessels to become more porous. The hydrostatic pressure forces more fluid out than the oncotic pressure draws back in, resulting in tissue edema.*

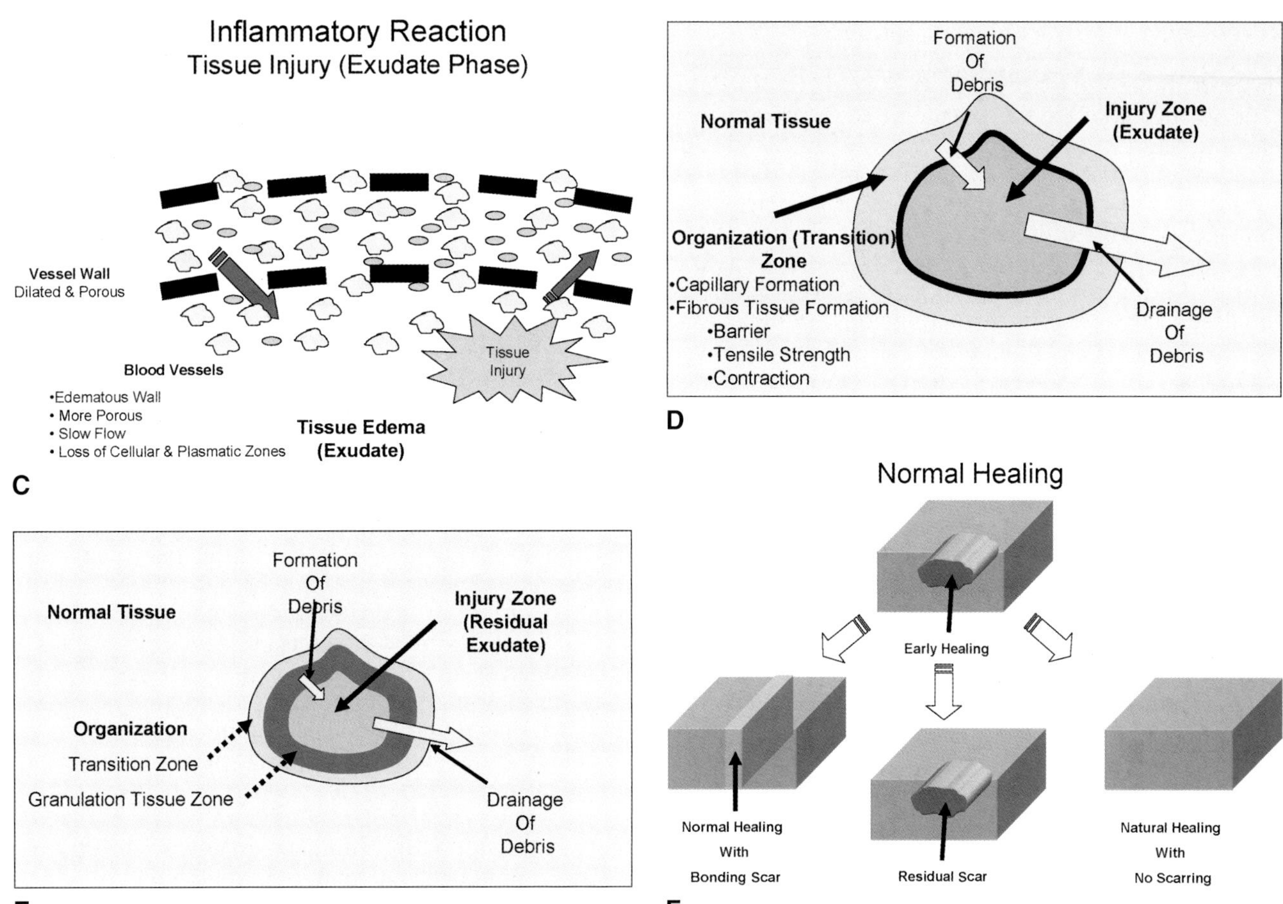

Figure 21-5, cont'd. ***C,*** *The exudative phase occurs when cellular elements pass through the blood vessel wall and into the injured tissue. As the injury persists, the vessel walls become more porous, and cellular elements migrate to the walls. Emigration of neutrophils and the hydrostatic pressure force red blood cells out of the blood vessels and into the edematous tissue exudate. This marks the beginning of the full inflammatory reaction. The intensity of the inflammatory reaction depends on the magnitude of the tissue injury.* ***D,*** *The organizational phase is a dynamic event, with formation and drainage of exudate and debris. In the early organization phase, an exudative effusion occurs as the result of poor drainage. A transition zone between the injury zone and normal tissue has capillary and fibrous tissue formation. The transition zone creates a barrier between the injury zone and normal tissue. Barrier formation consists of contraction and cross-linkage of the fibrous tissue, which increases the tensile strength. Contraction also decreases the vascularity in the transition zone as the tissue injury subsides. Continued tissue injury decreases the contraction, increasing the vascularization and formation of fibrous tissue. This dynamic reaction persists until the barrier is protective. This reaction is most intense at the interface between the transition zone and the injury zone.* ***E,*** *The late organization phase is characterized by maturation of the interface between the transition zone and injury zone into a granulation tissue zone. Granulation tissue is the vascular fibrous tissue barrier that separates the injury zone from normal tissue. As the barrier becomes more effective, the transition zone decreases.* ***F,*** *In the normal early healing stage, scar tissue is still present and is continuously remodeling. Natural healing is complete resolution of scar tissue, leaving normal tissue. Natural healing occurs when the scar tissue mass is not large and tissue stresses are not present. Bonding scar (healed incision) occurs when the tensile strength of the normal tissue is insufficient to hold it together without stress and strain, injuring normal tissue. A permanent bonding scar supplies the tensile strength necessary to remove stress from normal tissue. A residual scar exists when the mass of scar tissue is so large and dense that it stresses the surrounding tissue, causing a low-grade tissue injury that perpetuates the scar. This scar mass usually resolves over time.*

inflammatory reaction, with plasma factors such as fibrinogen and chemical mediators being released from the cells. The continued evolution of the inflammatory reaction depends on the tissue involved and the magnitude of the injury.

Now picture a lead located in the middle of the bloodstream, with the cellular elements and blood components flowing past at some velocity, and assume that a clot forms on the lead. (The terms "clot" and "thrombus" are the same and are used interchangeably; thrombus is used clinically to describe events associated with clot.) Clot can lyse in two ways. It can lyse completely without an inflammatory reaction, or it can lyse as a part of an inflammatory reaction. For an inflammatory reaction to take place, the clot and lead must first contact the vessel wall, injuring the tissue. The inflammatory reaction in the vessel wall is the same as an extravascular reaction. The inflammatory reaction extends into the clot, with lysis of the clot or organization of the clot to form a mural thrombus (organized clot attached to the vessel wall). Except for drainage, most of the other factors are similar. If the cleaning phase is incomplete (i.e., lysis of clot and fibrin), the remaining tissue organizes. This granulation tissue acts as a barrier, isolating the thrombus from the bloodstream. The granulation tissue transforms the thrombus into the encapsulating fibrous tissue surrounding the lead or becomes a mural thrombus.

Now picture the lead touching the wall, applying enough pressure to injure the tissue. The injured tissue initiates the inflammatory reaction. Clot forms on the injured tissue and around the lead as a result of chemical mediators associated with the inflammatory reaction and other factors, such as negative surface charge, turbulence, and stasis. It does not matter whether free clot is contiguous with the vessel wall or the lead touches and injures the wall—the end result is the same. The clot is completely dissolved, or it is organized into encapsulating fibrous tissue and/or a mural thrombus.

The properties of an inflammatory reaction are dependent on the tissue type and magnitude of the injury. From a macrobiologic point of view, the inflammatory reaction cleans and drains the area, organizes fibrous tissue to wall off the cause of injury, bonds tissue together, and promotes cellular regeneration where applicable. To clean the injury site, phagocytosis kills bacteria and degrades necrotic cellular debris, and enzymes lyse fibrin and clot to facilitate lymphatic drainage. Organization is the formation of granulation tissue at the edges of the damaged tissue (see Fig. 21-5D). Granulation tissue is composed of endothelial cells forming capillaries and fibroblasts laying down a fibrous tissue network. The granulation tissue protects normal tissue from injury by constructing a fibrous tissue barrier at the biophysical interface (see Fig. 21-5E). It uses its tensile strength to bind tissue and its contractile properties to obliterate dead spaces. An example of regeneration is new skin covering the injury site. Soft tissue and cardiovascular tissues do not regenerate.

Applied Stresses

Physical Stresses. To avoid confusion, physical stresses are separated into extravascular and intravascular stresses. There are significant differences in the initiation and presentation of an intravascular inflammatory reaction. Intravascular inflammatory reaction is complicated by the clotting mechanism, blood flow, and the circulating cellular and protein components in the bloodstream. The physiologic effects of physical stresses are common to both extravascular and intravascular inflammatory tissue reactions.

Implantation of a pulse generator, leads, adaptors, arrays, and so on, in the soft tissue causes an inflammatory reaction. The physical stresses create a tissue injury zone by tissue disruption (surgically forming the pocket) and by pressure (compression) on surrounding tissue at the biophysical interface. The pressure is caused by the exudative fluid in the pocket (hemorrhagic fluid) and by the implanted devices themselves. The tissue disruption far exceeds the criteria set in the microbiologic view for initiating an inflammatory reaction. The tissue is disrupted by both sharp and blunt dissection, leaving a surface of exposed tissue with exposed ends of blood vessels and lymph channels, drainage of extracellular fluid, exposed injured and dying cells, and an injury zone extending from the pocket edge. The tissue injury and exudative fluid media mark the beginning of the inflammatory reaction. Excessive bleeding into the cavity with clotting creates a biodegradable foreign body which, along with the cellular and proteinaceous debris, must be dissolved and drained. The inflammatory reaction in the injury zone is caused by pressure applied to the tissues by the implanted device, the diffusion of chemical mediators released from injured and dying cells after tissue disruption, and the fluid exudate.

Surgical closure of the incision leaves in progress an inflammatory reaction associated with tissue-to-tissue healing by primary intention and an inflammatory reaction associated with a cavity containing an exudate and a foreign body, hopefully healing by secondary intention. The inflammatory reaction associated with closure of a wound by primary intention is called wound healing. Lymphatic drainage removes the cellular debris, proteinaceous material, and blood products. Organization by a thin layer of granulation tissue between the two layers vascularizes the tissue and bonds the two sides with fibrous tissue. As the fibrous tissue matures, its tensile strength increases, by way of collagen cross-linkage, and becomes greater than that of the native tissue. The skin regenerates on the thin scar. The cavity contains a device, exudate, and a cavity wall of injured tissue. Drainage is the same as for wound healing. The difference is in the amount of material to be drained, the time it takes to prepare the material for drainage, and the capacity of the lymphatics. Organization takes place along the cavity wall. Granulation tissue forms on the edge and functions as a barrier, relieving stress to the tissue by forming a fibrous tissue interface (pocket or biophysical interface).

The biophysical interface is, in effect, a protective barrier of encapsulating fibrous tissue that separates and protects the normal tissue from device-related physical stresses. Because the goal of the barrier is to eliminate the physical stress to the tissue, the thickness of the biophysical interface is determined by the physical stress. Without this stimulus, new granulation tissue is not formed and the fibrous tissue contracts, constricting blood vessels. The resultant devascularized fibrous tissue is called scar tissue when it is acting primarily as a bonding agent, as in wound healing. When it acts as a protective barrier, as in a device pocket, it is called encapsulating fibrous tissue. If the inflammatory reaction is minimal, tissue bonding and a protective barrier are not required. Fibrous tissue is absorbed, leaving normal tissue. This is called natural healing (see Fig. 21-5F).

Scar tissue and encapsulating fibrous tissue are continuously remodeled along stress lines. A simple explanation for this is that a dynamic equilibrium exists at the biophysical interface between the device and the surrounding tissue. The inflammatory reaction caused by tissue injury results in organization, reinforcing fibrous tissue, and the absence of injury results in dissolution of the fibrous tissue. This dynamic process continuously remodels the fibrous tissue along lines of stress.

Intravascular leads implanted in a vein and in the right side of the heart demonstrate different inflammatory reaction properties than those in soft tissue. In the bloodstream, lead-related injury to the endothelial cells lining the vein and heart wall may be a dominant factor contributing to the encapsulating fibrous tissue and to mural thrombus formation (defined as a thrombus attached to the vein or heart wall). However, blood flow factors (stasis and turbulence) and surface properties of the lead also contribute to encapsulating fibrous tissue and thrombus formation. Inflammatory reaction is also involved with incorporation of the lead into the vein wall and, in some cases, exclusion of a segment of the lead from the vein.

Assume that a small area of vein wall is traumatically injured, with damage to the endothelial cells. Because the wall of the vein does not contain a vascular component, the normal sequence for injury, small vessel dilatation, and fluid exudation cannot take place. However, the injured cells do swell, change polarity to positive, and liberate clotting factors. Platelets drawn to the wall by opposite charge or by random migration into the plasmatic zone adhere to the injured site. Once a small mound of platelets forms, the local turbulence and stasis cause more platelets to migrate into the plasmatic zone and adhere to the mounded platelets, releasing more clotting factors. Once red blood cells migrate to the area and fibrinogen is converted into fibrin by the clotting factors, a clot is formed. This clot is called a mural thrombus. Depending on the magnitude of the injury, blood flow, and the effectiveness of clot lysis, the thrombus will grow, remain stable, or dissolve (Fig. 21-6). A persistent mural thrombus will eventually attract other cells, including fibroblasts. Organization of the thrombus by an inflammatory reaction will replace the clot with fibrous tissue. Unless further clot forms on the fibrous tissue mass, it will remodel along stress lines with time, leaving a contracted scar at the injury site. Continuous clot formation will result, with continuous organization in a large pedunculated fibrous tissue mass.

Now assume that a small area is injured by an implanted lead that is applying pressure to the wall. A mural thrombus can form, as described, from the injury to the wall. In addition, the presence of the lead can cause turbulent flow, accelerating the migration of platelets and red blood cells to the wall. Also, stasis of flow can occur between the vein wall and segments of the lead. This further aids in the migration of platelets, red blood cells, and fibroblasts to the wall. The influence of continued pressure causes injury to the wall; turbulence and stasis practically guarantee mural thrombus formation, and that is exactly what happens clinically. The organization of the thrombus into encapsulating fibrous tissue surrounding the lead and involving the vein wall can persist in some form for the duration of the implant (dynamic modeling). If clot formation persists because of turbulence, stasis, and/or surface issues, organization can result in exuberant encapsulating fibrous tissue (Fig. 21-7). Also, if the exuberant fibrous tissue mass causes tissue injury, a recursive reaction can be started. The mass of fibrous tissue injures the vein wall, generating more fibrous tissue, which causes further clotting, perpetuating the process. In time, fibrous tissue increases in tensile strength, and at some sites it mineralizes (primarily calcium deposits), creating a bonelike structure. In children and young adults, mineralization occurs after 4 to 5 years, and in the elderly after 8 to 10 years.[13]

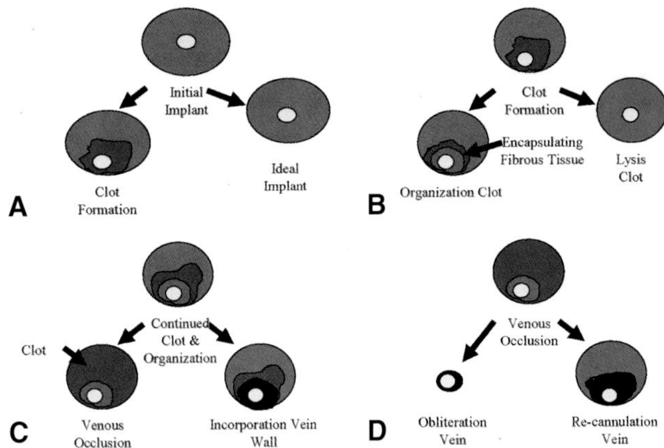

Figure 21-6. Intravascular inflammatory reactions. Intravascular inflammatory reactions involve clot and differ from extravascular reactions. Clot can form without causing an inflammatory reaction, or the clot (clot and lead) can injure the vein wall and cause an inflammatory reaction. ***A,*** *Clot forms when leads injure the vascular wall, cause stasis and turbulence of flow, and/or have thrombogenic surface texture properties.* ***B,*** *Clot can lyse, removing all clot from the lead surface, or it can become involved in an inflammatory reaction at the vessel wall, forming a mural thrombus, which can organize into encapsulating fibrous tissue.* ***C,*** *Secondary clot formation on the organizing thrombus occludes veins and causes thrombi in the atrium. Lead pressure on the wall causes inclusion of the lead into vessel or heart wall.* ***D,*** *Thrombosed veins can recanalize into patent veins or be obliterated by the inflammatory reaction into scar tissue surrounding the lead.*

A lead in the bloodstream may be free of encapsulating fibrous tissue, leaving the blood as the biophysical interface. However, other leads in this same situation can be covered with a thin layer of encapsulating fibrous tissue. Chemical structure and the texture of the lead's surface can stimulate fibrous tissue formation on the surface of the lead, even if these leads are in a high flow area in the center of the blood stream.[14] The cellular elements are also in the center of flow, and the surface properties can attract platelets and other cell elements. Microturbulence can increase their contact with the lead's surface. For example, the old rough silicone surfaces were usually covered with a thin layer of encapsulated fibrous tissue, whereas the smooth polyurethane surfaces were free (Fig. 21-8).[9] Also, the interstices of the conductor coils on ICD leads

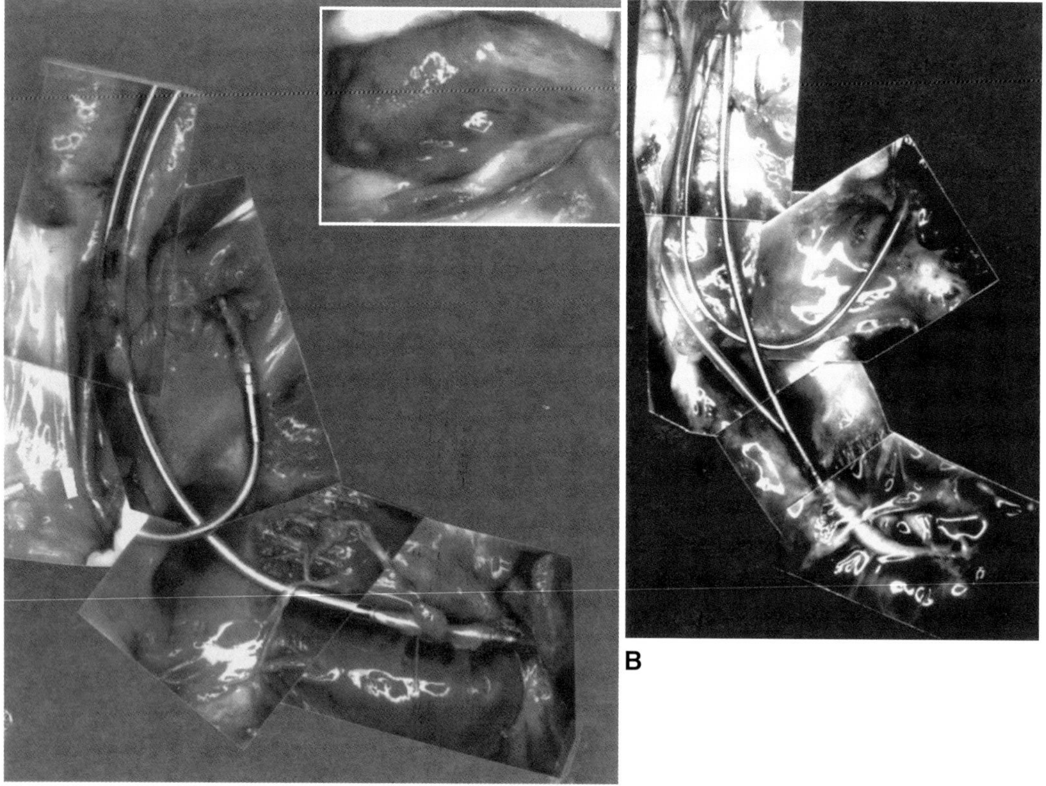

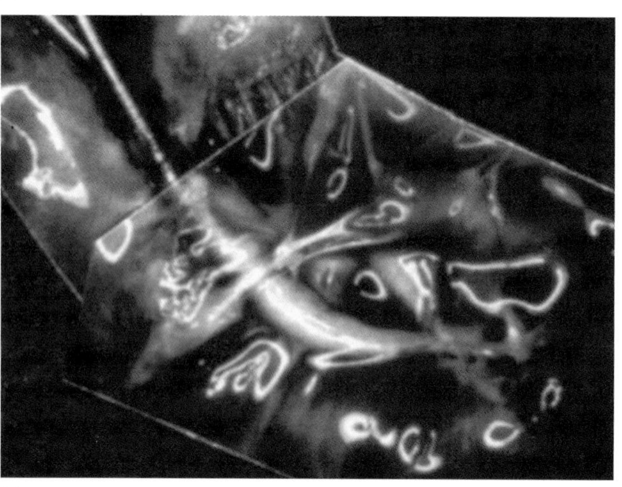

Figure 21-7. Thrombus formation. ***A,*** *Acute thrombus formation 1 week after implantation in a dog. Thrombus has formed at each site where the lead touches the wall and in some regions where there was stasis or eddying of blood flow. Most of this early thrombus lyses. It persists and organizes at sites of continued pressure on the wall and in areas with stagnant blood flow. Inset demonstrates a close-up of thrombus.* ***B,*** *Organized fibrous tissue encapsulating the lead forms chronically at sites of pressure. It progresses from fibrous tissue to cartilaginous tissue and, finally, to bone.* ***C,*** *Magnified view of chronic encapsulation shows the magnitude of the fibrous tissue to be ablated in extracting the lead.*

are ideal for fibrous tissue ingrowth. Conditioning the surface to make it smooth or changing its chemical properties is becoming a priority with industry. Covering conductor coils with a conductive material such as ePTFE (expanded polytetrafluoroethylene), known as Gore-Tex (Guidant), and back filling with silicone (Medtronic) are two current examples.

Multiple leads increase the vein wall injury sites, and the lead configuration can increase turbulence and create areas of stasis. Mural thrombus formation occurs at the contact points along the walls.

Metabolic Stresses. Metabolic stresses clinically refer to those situations that cause oxygen deprivation to cells. Local ischemia is caused by entrapment of the arterial blood vessels in encapsulating scar tissue, which obstructs blood flow. Acute oxygen deprivation injures or kills cells, liberating chemical mediators and initiating an inflammatory reaction. Complications such as migration, erosion, and tissue gangrene are caused by metabolic stresses.

Chemical Toxins (Infection). Bacteria can liberate chemical toxins (exotoxins and endotoxins) that injure and kill tissue, initiating an inflammatory reaction. Exotoxins are classified as neurotoxins (nerve), enterotoxins (intestine), and cytotoxins (all tissue). Cytotoxins are of primary interest with device-related complica-

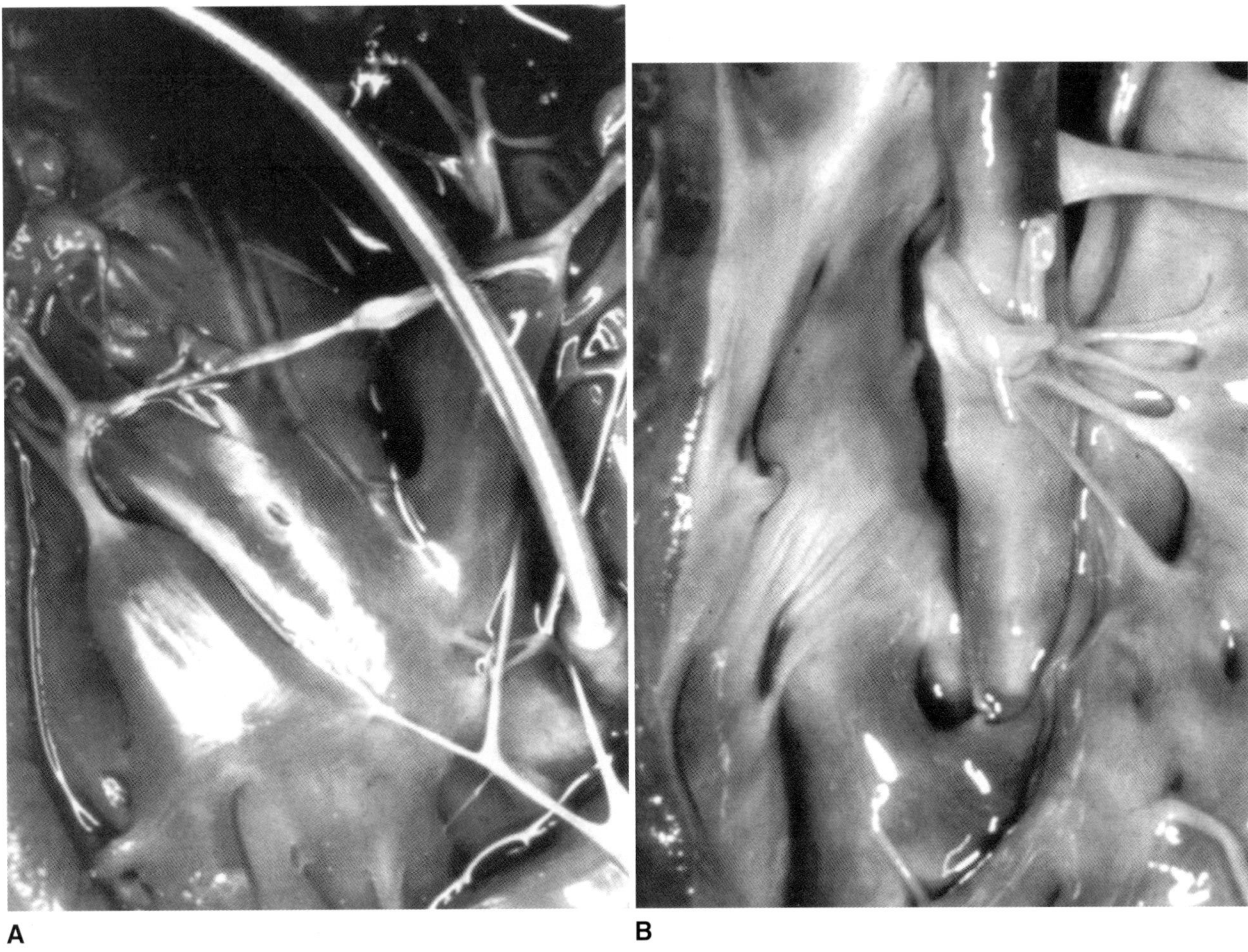

*Figure 21-8. Lead surface reaction canine model. Reaction to polyurethane **(A)** and silicone rubber **(B)** in leads implanted for 12 weeks. **A,** The polyurethane lead has minimal encapsulation, whereas the silicone rubber lead is completely encapsulated. **B,** A surface thrombogenicity phenomenon not related to the mechanical properties of the lead. The magnitude of the surface encapsulation is probably responsible in part for the greater difficulty of extraction of silicone leads in the first 2 to 3 years after implantation, compared with polyurethane.*

tions, although *Staphylococcus aureus* can produce all three toxins, causing a lethal infection if left untreated. Endotoxins are released by gram-negative bacteria and are not a common problem with device-related infections. Endotoxins usually activate the Hageman factor (factor XII), which can activate the coagulation, fibrinolytic, complement, and/or kininogen systems.

By definition, an infection is just the presence and multiplication of bacteria or any other organism. If a symbiont bacterium causes harm or lives at the expense of the host, it is classified as parasitic. A parasitic bacterium that causes harm is called a pathogen, and the infection becomes an infectious disease. All bacteria associated with an implanted device are parasitic, and, in this chapter, infection refers to an infectious disease caused by pathogenic parasitic bacteria, whether the infection is active or dormant (latent or clinically occult).

Pathogenic bacteria have properties such as virulence (intensity), invasiveness (ability to spread, grow, or reproduce), and infectivity (ability to establish a focal point). These properties and the organism's pathogenic potential (morbidity caused by its toxigenicity) determine the magnitude of the infection and its clinical sequelae. However, toxigenicity is usually not a major issue in device-related infections.

Other properties, such as adhesins, may be just as important as pathogenicity. Examples of adhesin properties are slime layer, capsule, and S layer, which facilitate the adherence of bacteria to smooth surfaces, especially implant devices. Slime production may be the primary criterion for the pathogenicity of *S. aureus*. It is a factor in both the initiation and the persistence of a device-related infection. For example, the inability to cure a device-related infection with antibiotics may be related to presence of adhesins.

Clinical Concepts

Requisite Skills

Prerequisites for managing device-related complications include a general knowledge base, patient preparation, anesthesia, procedure room issues, soft tissue surgical skills, lead extraction skills, and lead implantation skills. Most physicians practicing electrophysiology accept lead extraction as a skill to be learned. However, they may not recognize the need to expand and perfect their soft tissue surgical and implantation skills to perform at the advanced level necessary to manage device-related complications.

Patient Information and Preparation

All patients presenting for a procedure must have a standard history and physical examination with a detailed description of all DREs, including the company and the model of the pulse generator and all leads. The procedure notes should be carefully reviewed for any problems observed during the implantation, such as difficult access. Also, if infection is present, detailed information reflecting the time line, organism, susceptibilities, and antibiotic therapy is needed. Basic laboratory work including white blood cell count, hematocrit and hemoglobin, platelet count, blood urea nitrogen, creatinine, potassium, sodium, liver profile, and prothrombin time is generally indicated. The patient's blood should have been typed and cross-matched for a possible blood transfusion. A current chest X-ray and electrocardiogram (ECG) are mandatory. An echocardiogram is mandatory for two groups of patients before the procedure, even if transesophageal echocardiography (TEE) is routinely available in the procedure room: those with infection, to rule out vegetation in the right atrium; and those with heart failure, to define cardiac function.

The patients are given antibiotics before the procedure. Antibiotic coverage ranges from a cephalosporin to combinations such as vancomycin and gentamicin, covering both gram-positive and gram-negative organisms. The author uses vancomycin and gentamicin in an attempt to cover most of the common organisms infecting implantable devices. If the infecting organism and susceptibilities are known, an antibiotic specific to the known organism is administered. Although some question the need for prophylactic antibiotics, most physicians believe they are beneficial. Da Costa and colleagues[15] performed a meta-analysis that demonstrated a favorable effect of antibiotic prophylaxis in pacemaker implantation. There were seven available randomized trials for new implants or replacement pacemaker procedures. The incidence of endpoint events in the control groups ranged from 0% to 12%. The meta-analysis suggested a consistent protective effect of antibiotic pretreatment ($P = .0046$). Overall, the surgical literature emphasizes the importance of having the antibiotics administered so that good levels are present at the moment that the incision is made. This has become the standard of care.

The patient is continuously monitored via ECG, an arterial pressure line, oxygen saturation, and Foley catheter. A reliable intravenous line should be placed. The author prefers a triple-lumen catheter placed in a femoral vein (or internal jugular vein) for all extraction procedures. In addition, a femoral arterial line is used for patients needing continuous vasopressor support and for those being sent to an intensive care unit. Patients are prepared from chin to midthigh for all transvenous and cardiac surgical approaches, including an emergency cardiac surgical procedure, if needed.

Anesthesia

The types of anesthesia available include local anesthesia, conscious sedation, managed anesthesia care (MAC), laryngeal mask anesthesia (LMA), and general endotracheal anesthesia. The rationale for using a specific type of anesthesia is based on factors such as the type of procedure, physician comfort level with general anesthesia, perceived risk of a given type of anesthesia, and availability of general anesthesia.

General Endotracheal Anesthesia

General endotracheal anesthesia is the only type of anesthesia that is suitable for all procedures, and it is essential for some. General anesthesia consists of an "anesthesia package:" anesthesiologist, compliance with preoperative anesthesia protocols, anesthesia and monitoring machines, and general anesthetic agents and gases. It requires procedure room space, scheduling, and an anesthesia recovery room. In addition, the electrophysiologist (EP) and anesthesiologist must work as a team to manage the patient. Most surgeons acquire this teamwork skill early in their training; a medical EP may have to learn it.

The merits of placing a patient at any desired level of anesthesia and providing a satisfactory environment to perform any type of surgical procedure are obvious and are accepted by all when presented in this abstract fashion. However, the practical demands of the anesthesia package and the fundamental questions relating to the safety of general anesthesia limit its use. The perceived risk of anesthesia causes insecurity and a lack of confidence. The potential risks associated with general anesthesia range from small to negligible. If the risk of anesthesia is combined with the risk of performing a more complicated implantation, a lead extraction, or a cardiac surgical procedure, the risk is not trivial. The procedure risks should remain separate from the actual technical risks associated with anesthesia. The procedure risk is associated with the EP procedure and patient management, including coordination between the anesthesiologist and the EP.

The anesthesiologist is a trained professional in possession of certain technical skills. Giving anesthesia for EP procedures is complicated and stressful and frequently involves patients with significant compromise to their cardiovascular system. This type of procedure is not for everyone, just as cardiac surgical procedures are not for everyone. Consequently, choosing an anesthesiologist is an important decision, one that can potentially affect the outcome of the procedure.

The anesthesiologist's goal is to provide an optimal anesthetic for both the patient and the surgeon. These professionals are presented with patients whose physical status ranges from American Society of Anesthesiologists (ASA) class I through V for the full spectrum of surgical procedures, and they often have the feeling that keeping the patient alive is their sole responsibility. In many cases, this feeling is justified. They do what is necessary to manage the patient, and give the surgeon only the information they think he or she needs to know. Even in cardiac surgical procedures, the anesthesiologist manages the renal, respiratory, and metabolic status in most situations and shares cardiovascular management issues with the cardiac surgeon and pump technician. In EP procedures, management is generally more challenging: there is no specific EP training for these procedures, the rhythm and filling pressures are changing continuously, and metabolic insults caused by low cardiac output are rapidly precipitated. To safely manage these events, the EP and anesthesiologist must communicate and share the management responsibilities. The EP cannot delegate this responsibility.

The author's experience with general anesthesia is positive and is presented here to highlight important issues. All procedures, including pacemaker implantation, are performed under some form of general anesthesia. The risk of anesthesia is negligible, if it exists at all. This statement requires a detailed explanation, because it is based on rigid guidelines for giving anesthesia, a patient management philosophy, and a defining of the responsibilities of the anesthesiologist and EP. There is no dispute regarding performance by the EP or anesthesiologist of technical procedures related to their specialty. However, protocols or guidelines for adjusting anesthesia for EP procedures are in order. The author strongly believes that use of central venous lines and continuous arterial pressure monitoring are warranted, and, once the patient is intubated, paralytic agents are discontinued. Also, fundamental decisions must be made with respect to patient management responsibilities. The need for central venous and arterial lines is intuitively obvious. Views on paralytic agents and management responsibilities require some explanation.

Most anesthesiologists feel uncomfortable operating without paralytic agents. The indications for paralytic agents are intubation and relaxation of skeletal muscle. Fortunately, when the chest is opened, breathing can be suppressed with other agents. In some situations, the combination of paralytic and amnestic agents allows the anesthesiologist to decrease the level of inhalation agents, making it easier to manage a hemodynamically compromised patient. This approach results in less than optimal anesthesia, potentially masking serious hemodynamic issues that could cause cardiovascular collapse or other hemodynamic sequelae later in the case. For example, if a patient requires norepinephrine (Levophed) and/or high-dose dopamine while paralyzed and receives only an amnestic agent, marked vasoconstriction may develop, causing a low cardiac output, poor tissue perfusion, and acidosis resulting in cardiovascular collapse. Also, nerve stimulation from electrosurgery or pacing stimuli is masked by paralytic agents, increasing the risk for destruction or inadvertent chronic stimulation of the phrenic nerve. Both of these complications can be prevented by avoiding paralytic agents.

To give anesthesia without paralytic agents requires a change in philosophy and reliance on inhalation agents, narcotics, and short-term agents such as propofol (Diprivan). Separating anesthesia management from cardiovascular management is essential. The same level of anesthesia should be given despite the presence of cardiovascular issues. These issues are treated separately. For example, suppression of the myocardium and vascular dilatation are considered the "cost of giving anesthesia" and not a reason to modify the anesthetic regimen. It is not a complication to give an appropriate vasopressor by injection or infusion as needed to compensate for these expected events.

It is the EP's responsibility to manage the cardiovascular system. The EP's actions during the procedure are continuously influencing the rhythm and filling pressures; the sequelae of these actions, superimposed on the intrinsic cardiac function, are best managed primarily by the EP. Many of the maneuvers performed during a lead extraction can reduce filling pressure. Traction on an atrial lead may block the SVC and reduce blood flow to the heart. Traction on a ventricular lead reduces the compliance of the chamber wall during diastole or, if strong enough, can pull the wall to the tricuspid valve, reducing blood flow. Immediate injections of a short-term α-adrenergic stimulant such phenylephrine (Neo-Synephrine) or Levophed constrict the cardiovascular system, causing an increase in both filling pressure and systemic blood pressure. This is frequently required throughout the case to compensate for these transient iatrogenic insults. Their use in no way reflects on the safety and efficacy of general anesthesia. In conclusion, the risk of anesthesia is related to the procedure and not the general anesthesia.

Laryngeal Mask Anesthesia

Laryngeal mask anesthesia is general anesthesia without the use of an endotracheal tube or paralytic agents. For less complicated procedures in which patients are allowed to breathe spontaneously, LMA is an excellent form of general anesthesia. Inhalant anesthesia is uniform, eliminating problems encountered with MAC or conscious sedation. For procedures such as pacemaker or ICD implantation, it is ideal. Contraindications are airway obstruction, history of esophageal regurgitation, peptic ulcer disease, and the need for TEE. At the end of the procedure, the inhalation agents are turned off and the patient wakes up.

Managed Anesthesia Care and Conscious Sedation

MAC is essentially conscious sedation managed by an anesthesiologist. Conscious sedation is anesthesia managed by the physician who is performing the procedure. The rationale for use of this type of anesthetic includes the following points: it is effective for most procedures, it removes the general "anesthesia package" from the procedure room, and the option of general anesthesia is available. MAC and conscious sedation are satisfactory for less extensive procedures and for those procedures that seem less likely to involve a procedure-related complication. Short-acting drugs such as midazolam (Versed) and Diprivan, given intravenously, provide sedation and cause amnesia. Combined with a local anesthesia, they are effective for most procedures. The issue with this type of anesthesia is the maintenance of a uniform level of sedation. When patients become too "light," they may behave like a "bad drunk," becoming impossible to control and possibly making the procedure dangerous.

When patients get too deeply sedated, they begin to have difficulties with ventilation and/or snoring. A potentially lethal volume of air may be sucked into the heart during snoring or deep breathing. If an air lock develops in the right ventricle, blood flow will be compromised. The cardiovascular system must be supported, and rolling the patient onto the left side may facilitate the passage of air out into the lung field. Compromise of cardiac output, perfusion to the alveoli, and air exchange in the lungs may be marked, requiring time to resolve. The most effective treatment is to pass a catheter into the right side of the heart and out into the pulmonary artery, sucking out the air as you go. In less severe cases, although it takes time to clear, support of blood pressure and high-pressure hyperventilation will help. The author has not had to take additional steps to resolve this problem.

Local Anesthesia

Performing device-related complication procedures using only a local anesthetic is a rare occurrence today. Once an intravenous sedative of any kind is given, it becomes conscious sedation. With the anesthetic agents available today, it is difficult to find an indication for using only local anesthesia. It is effective for local pain control in a normal tissue environment. The vascular environment associated with an acute inflammatory reaction diminishes the effectiveness, and the large doses needed increase the potential for an overdose complication. For example, high doses of lidocaine can cause a catatonic CNS reaction, incapacitating the patient and usually terminating the procedure.

Procedure Room

EP procedures are currently performed in general operating room suites, device implantation procedure rooms, EP procedure rooms, catheterization laboratories, and fully equipped cardiovascular operating rooms. The room must be large enough to support the procedure. Small procedure rooms are sufficient for a device implantation but not large enough for a complicated lead extraction procedure. There should also be space to accommodate emergency procedures and/or a more extensive surgical EP procedure. Procedures should not be performed in smaller rooms without a contingency plan for an emergency.

The author's vision of a complete procedure room suitable for handling the most complicated procedure is described. Scaling down for lesser procedures should be intuitively obvious. The ideal procedure room should meet most of the requirements for an operating room, especially those requirements related to room cleaning, patient draping, gown and gloving, and instrument sterility. It should have the full "anesthesia package" including continuous monitoring of ECG, arterial pressures, and oxygen saturation. Specialty equipment such as fluoroscopy, TEE, pacemaker system analyzer, and other external EP devices to ensure pacing and defibrillation; electrosurgery; and an excimer laser and/or dedicated electrosurgical unit for lead extraction are essential. In addition, for minimally invasive cardiac surgical procedures, lighted retractors, access to thoracoscopy equipment, and an emergency tray to open the chest should be available. Additional safety devices to help protect physicians and nurses include lead drapes for radiation protection, smoke evacuators, and chairs for sitting when appropriate during the procedure. Physicians wearing lead aprons, thyroid collars, or a lead face shield have less musculoskeletal issues if they can sit during long procedures.

Pocket Surgery

Pocket surgery is a requisite skill that is essential for both implantation and explantation procedures. It is soft tissue surgery and centers on the creation, debridement, and abandonment of a pocket. Some pocket procedures, such as extensive debridement or revision, can be challenging for experienced surgeons. In extreme tissue debridement and reconstruction situations, it is the EP's responsibility to provide an experienced surgeon and to ensure that the procedure is performed in a proper fashion. These procedures can be performed in any procedure room, with the patient prepared and draped in a sterile fashion. Instruments needed include basic surgical instruments, suction, sutures, ties and staples (optional), an electrosurgical unit, and an assortment of retractors. Also needed is an antibiotic irrigation solution. Two additional pieces of equipment that are useful for these extensive procedures are a lighted retractor to see clearly under subcutaneous tissue and muscle flaps, and a smoke evacuator (same as for laser and orthopedic surgery) to remove the airborne debris. In the author's opinion, a smoke evacuator is helpful for extensive debridement of noninfected pockets and for all infected pockets.

Pocket Location

A pulse generator can, in theory, be implanted almost anywhere, limited only by anatomic and device-related constraints. Proved and popular locations are on the left or right anterior surface of the chest wall and in the upper quadrants of the anterior abdominal wall. Other locations are not used routinely because they are uncomfortable, are inconvenient, require special equipment such as longer leads, and/or have poor durability.

Anterior Chest Wall. Implantation on the anterior chest wall is a natural location. It is close to the vein entry site and is not influenced by body movement. For example, shoulder motion does not influence the pocket or the lead tunneled to the vein entry site. Because of the variations in chest wall anatomy, it is not always intuitively obvious where to place the pocket on the anterior chest wall. There are two general approaches. One approach is to make an incision convenient to the vein entry site and intended pocket location. The second approach is to uncouple the vein entry and pocket procedures. If the vein entry procedure cannot be performed from within the pocket incision, a separate vein entry incision is made. The author uses the second approach, placing the pocket in a predetermined location (Fig. 21-9). The medial aspect of the incision is made at the intersection of two landmarks. Imagine a horizontal line crossing at a point 5 cm below the sternal notch and a vertical line drawn inferior from the middle of the clavicle. Placement of the medial margin of the incision near this site compensates for variations in the chest wall and provides uniformity in pocket location. Also, for most chest wall configurations, the vein can be cannulated from within the incision using a percutaneous introducer approach.

There are no rigid rules, but several principles should be followed. Do not place the pocket near the deltopectoral groove. Frequent contact between the head of the humerus and the pulse generator causes pain. Do not place the pocket immediately below the clavicle, because the pulse generator's contact with the clavicle causes pain. A minor consideration is a location remote from the vein entry site. If the leads are long enough and the tunnel is deep, a remote site is not a problem. Caution should be used in placing the

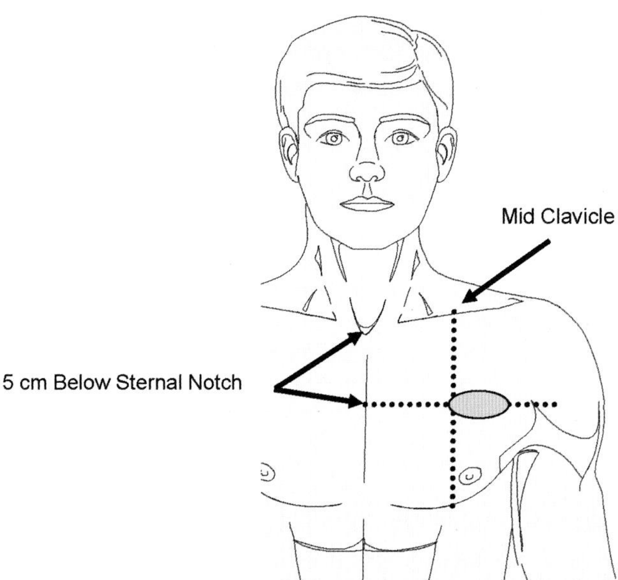

Figure 21-9. Skin incision site. Placing the skin incision in a uniform location on the chest wall is difficult because of the variations in the chest wall. The sternal notch and the clavicle are two relatively constant landmarks that can be used for reference. Placing the medial aspect of the skin incision at the intersection of a horizontal line approximately 5 cm below the sternal notch and a vertical line extending down from the clavicle is one technique to achieve uniformity.

pocket beneath the breast in a female or beneath the nipple in a male patient. The anatomic considerations for this location are a potential issue. Part of the pocket will be below the origin of the pectoralis muscle on the chest wall, and in males the subcutaneous tissue may be of insufficient thickness. This is not an issue for females, and many young women request that the generator be placed in the tissue space beneath the breast for cosmetic reasons. Regardless of gender, the pulse generator must be carefully anchored, especially in women, to prevent migration and erosion through the skin below the breast.

Subcutaneous Tissue Pocket. Historically, the classic location is in normal tissue on the anterior superior portion of the chest wall, in the relatively avascular fascial plane between the subcutaneous tissue and the surface of the pectoralis major muscle. The pocket is made with sharp and blunt dissection, and/or by electrocautery. If the fascia is cut or torn, the muscle frequently separates in the direction of its fibers, exposing the intramural portion of the muscle. Torn muscle should be sutured back together using an absorbable suture. Separation of the muscle fibers is the most common cause of bleeding into the pocket, and it is caused by the small arteries that run in the direction of the muscle fibers on or just beneath the surface. For safety, all arterial bleeding sites in the subcutaneous tissue should be suture-ligated. The pocket can migrate within the fascial plane. A suture securing the generator to the muscle prevents migration within the plane. It usually takes a traumatic or vascular event for it to break out of the plane and migrate to the surface.

Submuscular Pocket. Construction of a pocket in the tissue plane posterior to the pectoralis major and anterior to pectoralis minor is another natural location. Historically, submuscular pockets were used as an alternative location. Indications were related to the size of the generator, the condition of an old pocket, erosion of an old pocket, and cosmetic considerations. Today, the indications are essentially the same. If the thickness of the subcutaneous tissue is considered inadequate for the size of the pulse generator, the physician's concern for migration, erosion, or ischemic injury may motivate the change to a submuscular pocket.

During reimplantation of a pulse generator, issues may be discovered with the old pocket, such as exuberant fibrous tissue, granulation tissue, calcification, or a gelatinous material from an old clot. If the pocket is not suitable for reimplantation after debridement, a submuscular pocket is used.

Erosion with secondary infection is one of the most common complications. Once the infection is treated and the old pocket abandoned, the new pocket is frequently placed beneath the muscle at a remote site as protection against erosion at the new site. Today, pulse generators are smaller, but many patients do not want the device showing on their chest wall. A submuscular pocket may still show a bulge, but the outline cannot be seen. Cosmetic concerns are becoming more common.

Four approaches are described to construct a submuscular pocket; these are the clavicular, second intercostal, third intercostal, and axillary approaches. The author uses the second and third intercostal approaches. The standard pocket incision is over the second intercostal space and is the preferred approach. An incision over the third intercostal space is used for pocket creation and epicardial lead implantation. An incision below the clavicle, near the vein entry site, is at a natural separation between the clavicular and sternocostal origins of the pectoralis major muscle. The lateral approach is a plastic surgical approach. An incision is made in the axilla, and the pocket is created by a lateral dissection onto the chest wall.

For the clavicular, second intercostal, and third intercostal approaches, the pectoralis muscle is split in the direction of its fibers, using blunt dissection. The pocket is constructed in the avascular plane beneath the pectoralis major muscle and anterior to the pectoralis minor. The pectoralis minor helps to prevent the projection of the pocket into the axilla when the arm is raised. In the clavicular approach, the muscle is separated between the clavicular and sternocostal portion of the pectoralis major muscle, exposing the same avascular plane beneath the pectoralis major and minor. This is a satisfactory approach if the pocket is placed inferior enough to prevent the pulse generator from being pushed superiorly against the clavicle and laterally into the deltopectoral groove. The pulse generator must be secured to full-thickness muscle to prevent migration. The axillary approach is a surgical variation using a lateral dissection into the same fascial plane. Short-term cosmetic issues need to be convincing for the author to use this approach.

Abdominal Pockets. Abdominal pockets are still used today. In the past, large pulse generators were routinely placed into abdominal pockets. Once their size was reduced, they met the subjective criteria for a pectoral pocket near to the vein entry site. However, there are still indications for an abdominal pocket: infection, mastectomy, injury, pain, convenience, and patient preference. The pockets for short-term epicardial implants in patients being treated for vegetative endocarditis are usually placed in the abdomen. Pockets for femoral vein implants are also placed in the abdomen. Leads are tunneled from the implant site to the abdominal pocket. Tunneling should be deep in the subcutaneous or submuscular tissues whenever possible. Tunneling substernal, within the chest and/or pericardium, is also acceptable, especially for cardiac surgical procedures. For example, transatrial and epicardial leads can be tunneled to any convenient location through the pericardium and/or chest.

The same rules apply to subcutaneous tissue implants in the abdomen as in the pectoral region. If the subcutaneous tissue is adequate for the pulse generator, the pocket is best placed in the fascial plane between the subcutaneous tissue and muscle. The pocket is usually placed in the left or right upper quadrant. The pocket must be placed inferior to the costal margins and away from the belt line. This is relatively easy to do, because body motion and position are predictable in the upper quadrant. Placement in a lower quadrant is necessary for femoral implants. Lower quadrant pockets need to be selected with care. Body motion, especially positions such as bending and sitting, influence these pockets. Placement away from the iliac crest prevents painful contacts. In some cases, pockets cannot be placed out of harm's way in the lower abdomen because of the extreme ranges of pocket motion. Complications seen by the author with lower quadrant pockets include pain and erosion of the pocket into the abdomen. If a lower quadrant implant is necessary (e.g., femoral vein implant), awareness and avoidance of these issues are essential.

A submuscular pocket in the abdomen can safely be made under the rectus abdominus muscle. A device under the muscle in any other location can erode into the abdomen. It is safe to place the pocket within the rectus sheath, under the rectus abdominus muscle in the upper quadrant. The sheath is strong enough to prevent erosion into the abdomen. This is not true for the lower quadrants. The plane between the muscle and the posterior sheath in the upper quadrant is traversed by large neurovascular bundles, passing from the abdomen to the muscle. To prevent a hematoma, these bundles should be suture ligated. An arterial bleed causes a dramatic hematoma. If it is not corrected immediately, the pressurized pocket enlarges by dissection within the rectus sheath or decompresses by rupturing through the incision. Also, do not open the posterior rectus sheath; it could result in herniation of the omental apron or bowel into the pocket. Tears or cuts must be closed with suture material.

Reimplantation or re-exploration in an abdominal pocket is a potentially dangerous operation. The inflammatory reaction involving the posterior sheath frequently causes exuberant fibrous tissue reactions, especially in large pulse generator pockets. Attempts to modify and/or debride this suboptimal pocket is technically challenging. Misadventures resulting in loss of integrity of the posterior wall can damage the colon and small bowel contiguous to this site. Loss of integrity of the colon or small bowel wall requires an extensive emergency surgical procedure such as a colostomy. All device hardware must be removed from this site and temporary devices implanted at a remote site. Loss of integrity of the colon or small bowel that is not recognized during the procedure can cause a lethal infection. All defects in the wall must be repaired to avoid herniation. Consequently, it is recommended that only surgical EPs, qualified surgeons, or medical EPs with extensive experience perform these procedures.

The pocket is closed with the use of conventional surgical techniques. First, the pocket is irrigated extensively with an antibiotic solution. If a submuscular pocket was used, the pocket is closed with *permanent* suture material. The subcutaneous and subcuticular tissues are then closed with suture material that dissolves by hydrolysis (e.g., Dexon, Vicryl). Skin closures are made according to the physician's preference, and almost anything works. Subcuticular closures have plastic surgery appeal. They work well as long as there is no reaction to the suture or infection associated with the suture. In those cases, the suture line becomes red, swollen, warm and may or may not become suppurative. Sutures are placed perpendicular to the incision and are, in effect, a sinus tract through the subcutaneous tissue that can cause a pressure injury to the surface of the skin. Staples are an alternative and are used by the author. Staples are fast and can be applied to any incision regardless of the condition of the tissue. An occlusive dressing should be applied until the suture line seals (about 24 hours). Liquid skin adhesives are used by some; the author does not believe they are acceptable for closure when there has been a pocket complication.

Pocket Complications

Pocket complications, summarized in Table 21-1, include pocket hematoma, wound dehiscence, migration, erosion, pain, and infection. Hematoma formation and wound dehiscence are acute events and are usually related to implantation technique. A pocket hematoma may form late in anticoagulated patients, especially those treated with heparin or enoxaparin (Lovenox), or if the pocket is subjected to trauma. Migration, erosion, and pain are related to device–tissue interaction. Infection is caused by contamination of the pocket and is associated with implantation technique and tissue made susceptible by an abnormal device–tissue interaction.

Pocket Hematoma. A hematoma that develops immediately after an implantation procedure is one of the most common complications associated with a device implant. Although this is a technique-related complication, experienced implanters occasionally have difficulty obtaining hemostasis. Three conditions predispose to hematoma formation: a tear outside the fascial plane, arterial bleeding, and extrusion of venous blood back along the leads and into the pocket. Tears outside the fascial plane were discussed in the section on pocket construction.

Arterial bleeding within the pocket causes the most dramatic hematoma and should be considered an urgent or emergent situation, depending on how fast the hematoma is expanding. A hematoma develops rapidly; if not corrected immediately, the pressurized pocket enlarges by dissection into the tissue planes or decompresses by rupturing through the incision. The arterial pressure can cause extensive tissue dissection, enlarging the pocket area multiple times. If a larger artery is torn, the expanding hematoma can contain more than 500 mL of clot and blood. If it is left unchecked for a period of time, the tissue pressure and resultant ischemia can cause tissue necrosis and/or disruption of a recent incision. A small artery running in the direction of the pectoralis muscle fibers, on or just beneath the surface, and the small artery running parallel to the cephalic vein in the deltopectoral groove are the two most common causes of arterial bleeding. External forces applied to the pulse generator can cause a traumatic rupture of the pectoralis muscle, causing

TABLE 21-1. **Pocket Complications**

Complication	Predisposing Factors or Causes	Treatment
Pocket hematoma	Tear outside fascial plane Arterial bleeding Extrusion of venous blood along leads	If it is large enough to be palpated: Remove clot and debris Obtain hemostasis Reduce pocket size if necessary Use closed drainage system if hemostasis is difficult to achieve *Avoid repeated needle aspirations*
Wound dehiscence	Excessive stress on suture line by hematoma, hemorrhagic effusion, or trauma Error in surgical technique	Immediate: attempt to salvage site Delayed: treat as infected pocket
Migration	Unknown	No treatment unless another complication exists
Erosion	Device implanted outside correct plane Sustained insult forcing device out of correct plane (compromised blood supply, trauma, sequestered effusion)	Before pocket sticks to skin: debride and relocate pocket After pocket sticks to skin or skin is broken: treat as infected (abandon site)
Pain	Unknown	Relocate pocket if necessary
Infection	Perioperative contamination Chronic site may have poorer defenses against infection Metastatic (seeding from remote infection or procedure such as teeth cleaning) Chronic occult infection becomes acute Note: pocket infection may manifest as respiratory distress if infection decompresses into venous system	Most infections: Antibiotic treatment and abandon site (removing device and leads) If no septicemia, no inflammatory buildup around leads near insertion site, and >2.5 cm from pocket to suture sleeve, antibiotic treatment and abandonment of pocket may be sufficient

rupture of an artery when a sedated patient changes position in bed or uses the ipsilateral arm to lift a heavy object.

Blood forced retrograde out of the implant vein along the leads and into the pocket causes a hematoma. Although the pocket may be dry, an elevated venous pressure from heart failure, Valsalva maneuver, or coughing can extrude blood along the leads, filling the pocket with venous blood. With an introducer approach, extrusion of blood is prevented by placing a suture around the leads at the muscle entry site. If the cephalic vein is used, a suture around the vein and lead (or leads) at the entry site will suffice. The suture also prevents debris collected within the pocket from being forced back into the venous circulation.

Once clot forms in the pocket, it is subjected to both lysis and organization. Lysis creates particulate debris, increases the osmotic pressure, and pulls fluid into the pocket, thereby creating a hemorrhagic effusion. As the hemorrhagic effusion increases, the resultant tension on the pocket wall continues to enlarge the pocket by dissection or ruptures a recent incision. Both of these complications require immediate surgical intervention for correction.

Excessive granulation tissue, formed during the organization of a large clot, may be present years later. In addition, only the surface of a massive clot may organize, leaving a residual gelatinous portion of partially organized clot debris. These pockets are not healthy, behave similar to pockets with exuberant fibrous tissue, and should be debrided.

A pocket hematoma that is large enough to be palpated should be treated. The only successful treatment is immediate pocket exploration. Prolonged observation and procrastination must be avoided. This is especially true if the pocket wall is tense. Wound dehiscence with spontaneous evacuation of the hematoma can occur if the pressure generated by the effusion is great enough. Other complications of an untreated hematoma include chronic wound dehiscence, migration or erosion, and infection. The goal is to remove all clot and tissue debris and obtain hemostasis. The pocket must be opened and the hemorrhagic effusion, clot, and tissue debris removed. Needle aspiration is ineffectual and dangerous, because clot cannot be aspirated through a needle, and percutaneous needle puncture is a potential source for introduction of bacteria. If the pocket has been enlarged, the dissected region should be excluded with suture material, leaving only an appropriate-sized pocket. If adequate hemostasis is difficult to achieve, a closed drainage system (e.g., Jackson-Pratt) is placed in the excluded pocket to prevent the hematoma from reoccurring. In the author's experience, the immediate surgical correction of a hematoma and placement of a closed drainage system do not adversely affect the healing of the pocket.

Wound Dehiscence. Wound dehiscence is a rare event. It occurs within the first few days or weeks after implantation (Fig. 21-10). During the acute wound healing phase, suture material is required to reapproximate and reinforce the tissue. Most wound dehiscences are caused by excessive stress placed on the suture line by a hematoma, effusion, or trauma. Traumatic disruption is rare. Dehiscence, without a predisposing cause, is caused by an error in surgical technique. Treatment consists of salvaging the site by intervening immediately (within hours) after a dehiscence, similar to treating a hematoma. It is usually successful and, considering the consequences, worth the attempt. A delayed intervention allows gross contamination, and an infection is likely to develop. If intervention is delayed, the case is treated as an infected pocket, with the removal and discard of expensive leads and pulse generator, debridement of the pocket, insertion of a closed drainage system, and abandonment of the pocket.

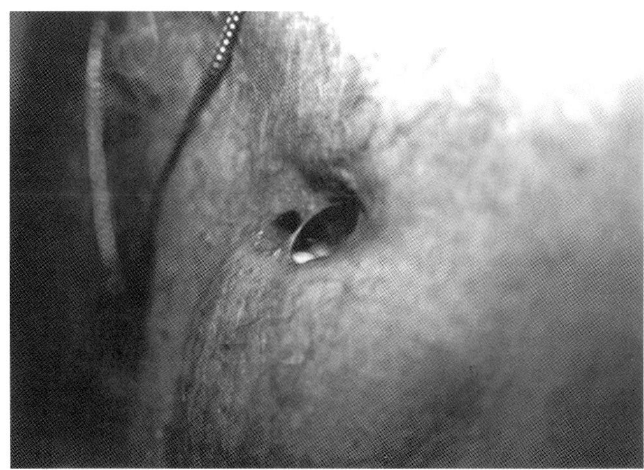

Figure 21-10. Wound dehiscence. A wound dehiscence left unattended for more than a week. The pacemaker pocket developed a hematoma that evacuated spontaneously, rupturing the incision. At this point, the pocket is considered infected and is treated as such.

Migration. Migration is the movement of a device through the surrounding tissue. In the past, migration was more common due to the large size and pointed shape of some devices, even when contained within a Dacron (Parsonnet) pouch. Most migrations are slow, occurring over a period of years; most move in an inferior-lateral direction and do not cause a complication. The author does not know the exact mechanism for migration, but size and weight of the pulse generator are factors. One possible scenario relates to the motion between the device and the musculoskeletal system, which creates directed forces (pressures) that compress and/or stretch the fibrous capsule and surrounding tissues. This would cause a low-grade inflammatory reaction, initiating a cycle of fibrous tissue lysis and formation (organization), with remodeling of the tissue to relieve the stress on the wall. This could result in migration of the pocket through the tissue. A migrated device is not usually treated unless the potential for an actual complication exists.

Erosion. Erosion is the exteriorization of the device after loss of skin wall integrity. Infection is the most common cause of erosion and is discussed later. For all other erosions, the pacemaker pocket sticks to the skin before erosion occurs (pre-erosion). Before the pocket becomes adherent to the skin, it moves freely. At this point, if infection is not present, debridement and relocation of the pocket are usually successful. However, once an inflammatory reaction begins, the skin sticks to the pocket, skin integrity is lost, and bacteria cross the skin, contaminating the pocket. Pockets treated after the skin sticks or after frank erosion are treated as infected pockets.

Implant Fascial Plane. Flat devices, such as pulse generators, do well when implanted in a natural tissue plane (fascial plane) between two tissue types (subcutaneous tissue and pectoralis muscle or pectoralis muscle and chest wall). Minimal pressures are exerted by the flat surfaces against the two tissue types. The device's curved surfaces apply the greatest pressures. It may migrate in the plane, but it will not erode. For an erosion to occur, the pulse generator would have to be implanted with a portion of a curved surface extending out of the fascial plane, or it would have to sustain an insult forcing it out of the plane. Such insults include compromise of the blood supply with loss of tissue, trauma with tissue disruption, and a sequestered effusion applying pressure to the pocket wall. In these situations, erosions occurring within the first few months after an initial implantation are not uncommon.

A current trend is to place the pocket within the subcutaneous tissue. This pocket must be perfect and without applied stress to prevent migration and erosion. Anchoring the pulse generator to the soft tissue is not sufficient to prevent free migration when the device is subjected to an applied force. Another factor is significant weight loss. Loss of the subcutaneous tissue barrier between the pulse generator and the skin can result in erosion, especially if the pocket is subjected to some form of trauma. Most of the eroding pockets seen by the author were placed in the subcutaneous fatty tissue away from the tissue planes.

Pacemaker pulse generators placed under the pectoralis major muscle sometimes protrude into the axilla when the muscle is flexed. The resulting migration into the axilla can cause pain or erosion. This complication is avoided by placing the device more medially under the pectoralis major, over the pectoralis minor, and anchoring the device by placing a suture through the full thickness of the muscle.

Compromise of the blood supply causes tissue loss. Blood supply is compromised by mechanical factors and by exuberant fibrous tissue, which causes pressure and/or constricts the entrapped vessels. If the blood supply to a region of subcutaneous tissue and skin is compromised, the resultant dissolution of the subcutaneous tissue (pre-erosion) is caused by lack of nutrition (Fig. 21-11A). If this is severe enough, tissue necrosis develops, leaving only ischemic or gangrenous skin (see Fig. 21-11B).

Trauma and sequestered effusion may rupture the fibrous capsule barrier around the device. A traumatic rupture is intuitively obvious, resulting in device migration through the rupture site. A sequestered effusion or a hematoma can generate sufficient pressure to erode through the subcutaneous tissue and skin, draining to the outside like a decompressing abscess. Other con-

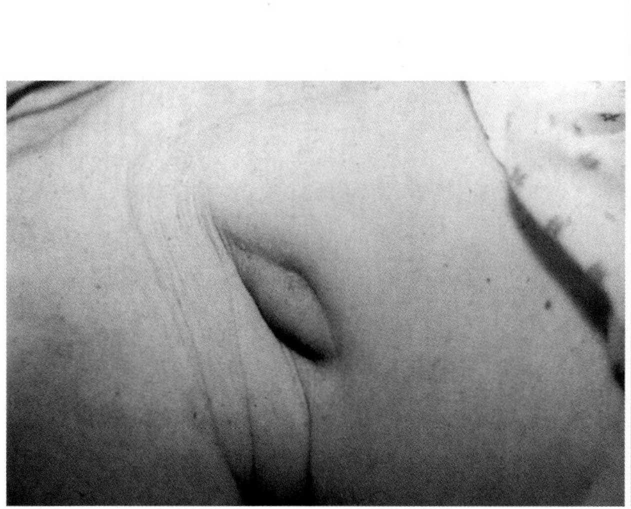

A

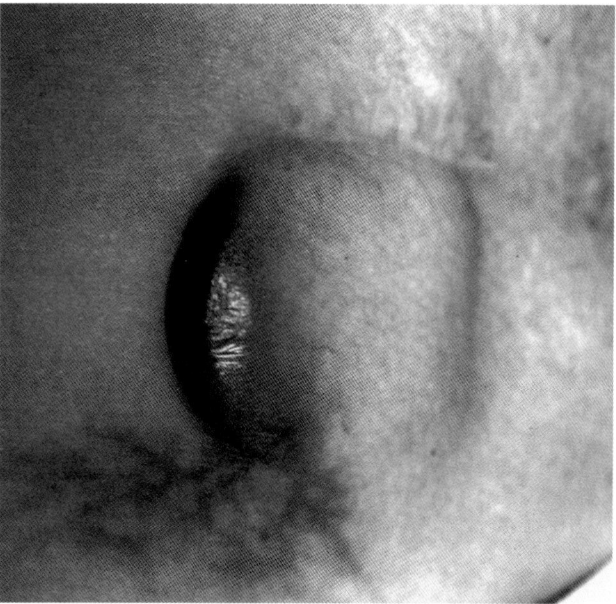

B

Figure 21-11. Compromised blood supply. Compromise of the blood supply to the subcutaneous tissue and skin causes a decrease in the supply of nutrients to the cells. ***A,*** *In the early stages (pre-erosion), the fatty tissue begins to lose mass. During the latter pre-erosion stages, the tissue becomes ischemic, and skin changes occur. The last stage before erosion is adhesion of the skin to the fibrous tissue pocket.* ***B,*** *Complete loss of blood supply to the skin results in gangrene of the skin before erosion.*

tributing mechanisms include tissue ischemia and an intense inflammatory reaction.

Pain. Occasionally, patients complain of pain in or near the pocket. History and physical examination are the only diagnostic tools available. Pain is a complication regardless of the cause. Pain is a difficult complication to manage. Acutely, some patients heal without any complaints of pain. Others have severe pain. The cause of pain may be nerve entrapment, inflammation of the scar tissue, migration, or injury to the musculoskeletal system. Pain associated with no physical signs may be related to nerve entrapment. Because nerves cannot be seen, a diagnostic exploration of the pocket is not an option. The best chance for a successful treatment is to remove the generator and leads, abandon the site, and reimplant on the opposite side.

A worst-case scenario for a normal healing process is a patient involved in strenuous physical activity. This type of patient should be given more time for postimplantation pain to subside. If the pain is caused by such activities, it will subside when the body adjusts to the applied stresses causing the pain. The author believes that patients are going to subject themselves to these activities at some point and encourages them to continue their activities. If a normal activity causes pain, the patient is treated with pain medication and the activity is allowed to continue. If the pain does not subside, the pocket is relocated; a subcutaneous tissue pocket is changed to a submuscular pocket, or vice versa. The pocket area must eventually be made pain free, regardless of the patient's activity. Limitation of activity is not an option.

Chronic pain is not normal, and complaints of pain should be taken seriously. An implanted device is like a watch: the patient should be aware of its existence only when something draws attention to it. Pain on the chest wall can cause other symptoms. For example, chronic chest wall pain can cause muscle spasm.

Inflammation of the scar tissue is usually obvious. The scar is exuberant, red, and painful to the touch. It has the appearance of a red keloid. Injection with steroid reduces the inflammation and will eventually alleviate the symptoms.

Pain associated with injury to the musculoskeletal system can be related to the initial placement of the pocket, migration, or trauma. Pain is usually caused, not by the migration per se, but by some traumatic event associated with the new anatomic position. Trauma to a rib or at the costochondral junctions is the most common pain complaint. This pain can be similar to a broken rib: intense and even debilitating. Injury to the pectoralis major muscle from sutures, tears, or erosions into the muscle can also cause pain. In most cases, the pain is typical of muscle spasm and the insertion site on the humerus is tender (bursitis). Spasm of the neck muscle is not uncommon in this situation. This pain usually goes away when the muscle injury heals.

Placement of the pocket near the deltopectoral groove can injure the head of the humerus, mimicking bursitis. A similar, but less specific cause of pain is trauma to the tissue beneath the clavicle. Pocket relocation to another subcutaneous area or placement beneath the pectoralis major muscle may be effective.

Tissue Debridement

Tissue debridement is the surgical removal of all inflammatory and damaged native tissues, leaving only normal native tissue behind (Fig. 21-12). The need for tissue debridement in normal pockets seen on routine reimplantation is minimal. On opening an old pocket, the debridement goal is to remove any exuberant inflammatory tissue (fibrous tissue), leaving only thin healthy fibrous tissue (biophysical interface) or normal native tissue behind. The fibrous tissue present is involved in the chronic remodeling inflammatory reaction; rarely is an acute inflammatory reaction present. This is important, because exuberant fibrous tissue masses, which are the result of an inflammatory reaction, can injure adjacent tissue, continuing the inflammatory reaction (recursive reaction). Also, if this tissue is contaminated by bacteria, it becomes a nidus for infection (bacteria stick to the smooth surface of the exuberant encapsulating tissue, and the body's immunodefense mechanisms cannot reach the bacteria). Leads entrapped in the encapsulating fibrous tissue may be under undue stress if the pulse generator is not placed back in the same position. Tissue debridement and freeing of the leads rectify this situation.

Initially, tissue debridement was performed using a scalpel. This was tedious, bloody, and time-consuming, deterring all but the most dedicated. Fortunately, modern electrosurgical units provide the frequency options and control of power needed to cut and coagulate in an efficient, tissue-friendly manner. Tissue debridement with a modern electrosurgical unit is recommended.

Tissue debridement, even in infected cases, is rarely extensive and can be treated as described earlier. However, there is occasionally a situation, usually involving an infection, in which the pocket must be extensively debrided and then abandoned. If an acute inflammatory reaction is extensive, debridement is tedious because of the presence of acute and chronic inflammatory material and/or proximity of large blood vessels and important nerves. Knowledge of local anatomy is mandatory in this situation. In some cases, the inflammatory tissue can be more than 2.5 cm thick, extending above and below the pectoralis major muscle with fingers to the clavicle, and damaging a large amount of skin. In these cases, skin loss is significant, and reapproximation of skin edges is challenging. Once the debridement is complete, hemostasis is difficult to achieve, especially on the muscles. Whenever possible, muscle fascia should be reapproximated.

Tissue Closure

Healing by primary intention is the closing of an open wound by reapproximation of tissue (muscle, subcutaneous tissue, and skin) using suture material. The suture material holds the tissue in place until the tensile

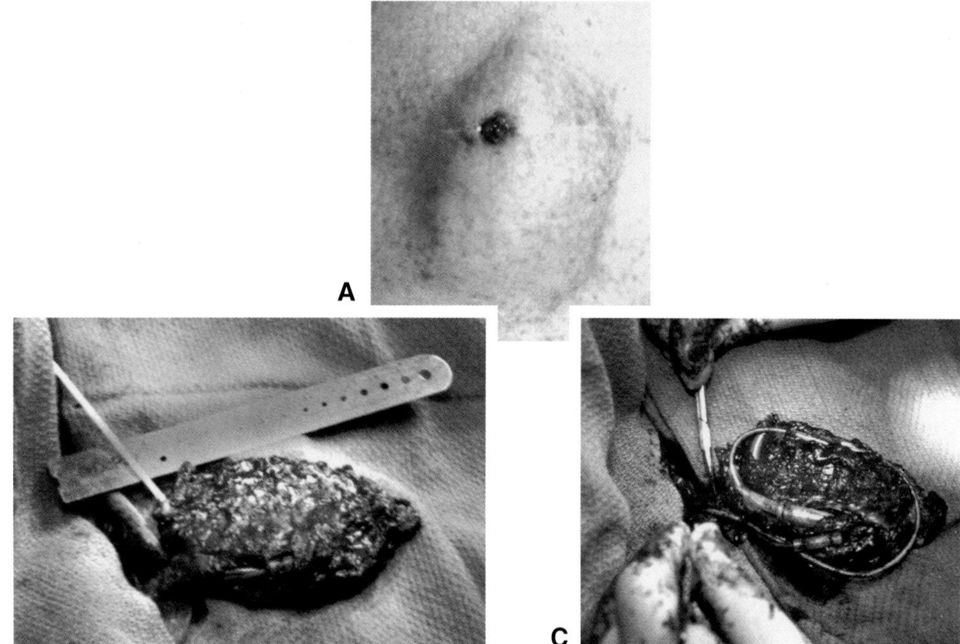

Figure 21-12. Debridement of a chronically infected pocket. ***A,*** *Chronic draining sinus tracking to an infected pocket lined with granulation tissue.* ***B,*** *Surgical debridement. To close the pocket, with healing by primary intention, the pocket must be completely debrided of all inflammatory material, including the tissue encapsulating the lead near the vein entry site. The excised mass includes a thin layer of normal tissue, organizing inflammatory tissue protecting the normal tissue, and the inner surface of granulation tissue. The swab stick marks the location of the sinus track.* ***C,*** *Extravascular encapsulating fibrous tissue. Leads are dissected free, demonstrating the tissue surrounding the leads.*

strength of the bonding fibrous tissue produced by the inflammatory reaction is sufficient to permanently keep the tissue together. All initial and reimplanted pockets are closed in a conventional fashion by reapproximation of the tissue with suture material and allowed to heal by primary intention. Chronic pockets are debrided of all exuberant inflammatory material before closure.

The author also closes those pockets that are not suitable for reimplantation, because of inadequate tissue or infection, before abandoning the pocket. These pockets are debrided and closed using a closed drainage system (Jackson-Pratt) placed in the debrided pocket, applying suction to prevent the development of effusions or clot, and keeping normal tissue contiguous with normal tissue. This is the author's method for closure of all complicated pockets and has been successful. The author has not left a pocket or any other type of soft tissue wound open since the early 1970s. A large defect, resulting from loss of tissue during debridement, is sometimes a challenge to close. In extreme cases, a major defect requires an experienced surgeon or a plastic surgeon, especially if a flap is needed. Skin grafts are not used, because the areas of tissue loss are made permanent, creating cosmetic issues.

Another philosophy is that pockets that have debridement defects or are infected should be left open. Once the device (foreign body) is removed, the infection will heal, so why not let it heal by secondary intention? This rationale shortens the procedure and is an accepted method of healing. Infection is not an issue, and it avoids the need for acquiring surgical debridement and closure skills. Also, a qualified surgeon may be hard to find on short notice. Concerns such as morbidity, extensive healing time, long-term antibiotic therapy, the requirement for constant professional care of the wound, and the possible need for some form of surgical intervention, including skin grafting, are considered the natural cost of healing the wound. Healing by primary intention, on the other hand, does not have these issues. Healing by secondary intention was used a long time ago as the only way to heal an open wound. The healing stages were well documented: suppuration, granulation, closure of defect, and, finally, skin closure. This was the recommended method of treating contaminated wounds by surgeons up and until the 1980s. Since the 1970s, however, primary closure of debrided infected pockets has been successfully and almost exclusively used to manage device-related infections.

Lead Extraction Skills

Lead extraction is a fundamental skill that is required to manage device-related complications. Lead extraction, like lead implantation, is a requisite skill with predictable and expected results. This was not always the case. From its inception in the early 1980s until the late 1990s, the procedures evolved rapidly. The management of a device-related complication centered on the lead extraction procedure, overshadowing all other aspects of management. This was because unexpected tears in the SVC and heart wall sometimes occurred without warning, despite the rigid protocols followed. The technology and those rigid protocols have evolved into today's procedures. The procedures are less stressful and have predictable results. Predictability allows an extractor to recognize an approach that has a potential for a bad result and change to an approach with a predictably good outcome.

Lead extraction is discussed in its entirety in this chapter, including indications, extraction techniques, and medical/surgical EP approaches. A goal is to show that once lead extraction is mastered, it becomes a requisite skill and, like lead implantation, a routine component of the procedure. Indications range from the author's simplistic list to a more extensive list with conditional and subjective statements. An attempt is made to add perspective to this controversy. Extraction techniques are much simpler today and are explained in detail. Unfortunately, some of the old, more complicated techniques are also needed to manage an occasional rare situation. Consequently, some of these techniques are presented in the same detail as the more modern techniques. Presentation of the extraction techniques and approaches from the medical and surgical EP's point of view has been challenging. The common ground is that most of the extractions involve transvenous leads. These are extracted using the techniques and approaches common to both groups. The alternative approaches are sometimes different for surgical and medical EPs. For example, in addition to the transvenous approaches, surgeons have the option of a transatrial or epicardial approach. Although these surgical approaches are not mainstream, they are essential to the management of certain complications. Though medical EPs cannot perform these procedures, they must be able to direct a non-EP surgeon enlisted to perform the procedure.

Indications for Extraction

There is considerable divergence of opinion in regard to the indications for lead extraction. In addition, there has been significant evolution of the tools, techniques, and number of experienced physicians since the lead extraction policy conference was convened in May of 1997.[16] The author's indications for lead extraction are the presence of a device-related infection, creation of a conduit, and superfluous leads. For the indications to be accepted, the risk of not extracting a lead in a *specific patient* must be greater than the risk of extracting (risk-benefit ratio). The author's earlier classification of indications into mandatory, necessary, and discretionary indications reflected the magnitude of the risk (Fig. 21-13).[17] The author's current descriptive classification of indications into infection, creation of a conduit, and superfluous leads does not reflect actual or potential risk. The relation between the two is straightforward. Infection is a mandatory indication, and creation of a conduit is a necessary indication. Superfluous leads, based on the earlier discussion, become a discretionary indication. The change from a risk-based to a descriptive indication evolved over the

Magnitude of Risk (Initial Classification)	Descriptive (Current Classification)
Mandatory (Class I)	Infection
Necessary (Class II)	Creation of Conduit
Discretionary (Class III)	Superfluous Leads
A	B

Figure 21-13. Indications for lead extraction. Indications are difficult to describe because of the complexities associated with device-related complications and the procedure-related risk. ***A,*** *Magnitude of risk. The author's first attempt was to classify indications based on the magnitude of the perceived risk. This approach presents a classification based on risk of the complication relative to the perceived risk of the procedure.* ***B,*** *Descriptive. The author's second attempt is a descriptive classification based on three clinical situations. The rationale for these indications is clinical and is not based on procedure risk. The author assumes that the risks are negligible for an experienced physician trained in the management of device-related complications.*

years as the risk and morbidity associated with lead extraction have become less dominant factors. In other words, the concept of "arm twisting" to justify the risk of extracting leads has changed to the concept of "managing an actual or potential complication." The potential dangers associated with the procedure have not changed. However, today, a large number of procedures have been performed, and an individual extractor's experience is known. The risk of extraction decreases to an acceptable level with training and experience. Consequently, the focus has shifted from risk to management of the potential or actual complication.

Infection. Infection is an intuitively obvious indication for lead extraction. Most physicians accept the hypothesis that antibiotic therapy, pocket debridement, and local relocation are palliative and that all device components, including leads, must be removed to cure the infection. Also, the morbidity associated with a local pocket infection, the lethal sequelae of septicemia, and the potential risk of infected thrombus formation in the heart are well known. Because leaving an infected lead in the body is potentially lethal, the risk of the procedure is clearly less than the risk of lead extraction (i.e., the risk of not extracting far exceeds the risk of extracting). The risk of *S. aureus* device infection without extraction was supported by a series of 33 patients from the Duke Medical Center, in which 10 (47.6%) of 21 patients died without lead extraction, and 2 (16.7%) of 12 died despite lead extraction, and none from lead extraction.[18] The safety and efficacy of complete lead extraction, with debridement and delayed reimplantation at a remote anatomic site, were demonstrated in 123 patients at the Cleveland Clinic Foundation with device infection. Despite infections with a wide range of bacterial organisms, mostly coagulase-negative staphylococci and *S. aureus*, extraction was associated with no major complications. Infection reoccurred only in those four patients who had incomplete extraction or reimplantation concurrent with the extraction.[19]

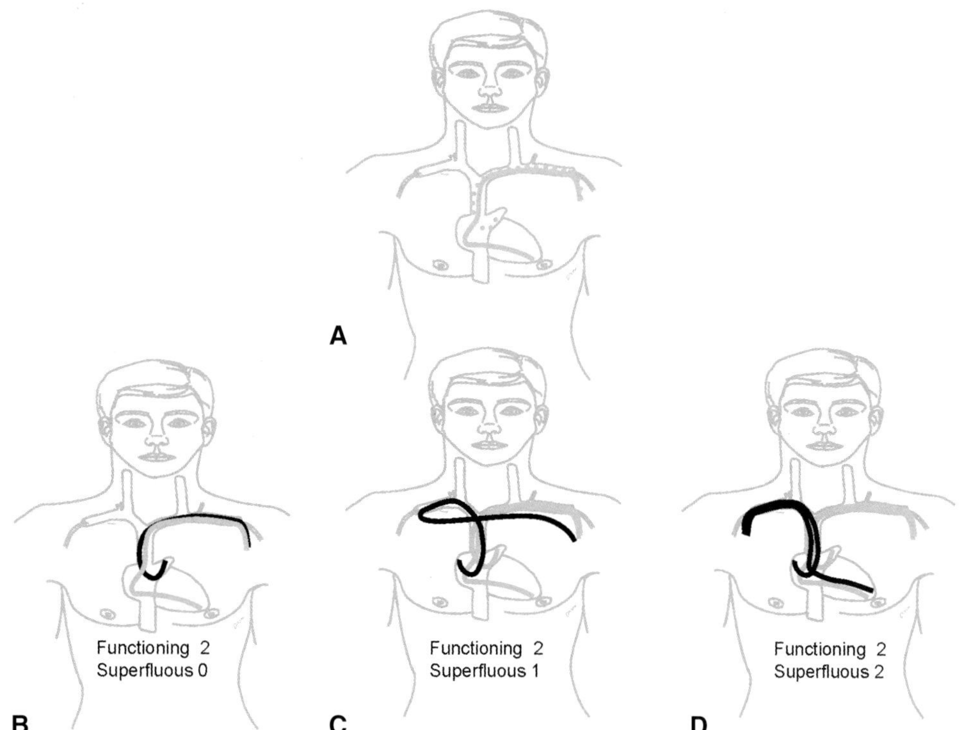

Figure 21-14. Creation of a conduit. ***A,*** *Atrial lead failure caused by a conductor coil fracture and an occluded ipsilateral subclavian-brachiocephalic vein.* ***B,*** *Extraction of the old atrial lead and implantation of a new lead through the extraction site (two functioning leads).* ***C,*** *Insertion of a new lead through the contralateral subclavian vein, tunneled to the old pocket (two functioning leads and one superfluous lead).* ***D,*** *Insertion of an atrial lead, a ventricular lead, and a new pocket on the contralateral side (two functioning leads and two superfluous leads).*

Creation of a Conduit. Creation of a conduit is a more subtle indication for lead extraction. The rationale for this indication is applicable to component failures. An example is the best way to define this problem. Consider a patient with a dual-chamber pacemaker and an atrial lead conductor coil fracture. This patient has a normal ventricular lead, an occlusion of the brachiocephalic vein, and the need to implant a new atrial lead. The only way to insert the new lead through the same vein entry site is to extract one of the old leads and reinsert two new leads through the extraction conduit (Fig. 21-14A and B). This same logic would apply to other situations, such as the addition of a new lead (Fig. 21-15A and B). For example, a patient with a dual-chamber ICD needs a cardiac vein implant for biventricular pacing. The alternatives are doing nothing, implanting the new lead through a contralateral vein or a transfemoral vein, and using a cardiac surgical approach.

Sometimes, when there is severe stenosis with or without symptoms from the obstruction of flow, physicians have initiated balloon venoplasty and stenting without extraction of the leads. This produces a particularly difficult scenario if either infection or reocclusion occurs, because extraction now becomes impossible without extensive open surgery. A more appropriate approach includes extraction, venoplasty, stenting, and reimplantation through the stent, as reported by Chan and associates[20] in a subclavian occlusion that progressed to an SVC occlusion.

Doing nothing is an option in some cases, such as with patients who rarely use their device, who have chronic atrial fibrillation or flutter, who have complete heart block, or who have high filling pressures where the atrial contraction has negligible effect. In these patients, loss of an atrial lead will go unnoticed, cause occasional palpitations, or result in an unnoticed chronic compromise in hemodynamic function. If the example had been loss of the ventricular pacing lead in a patient with frequent ventricular pacing, doing nothing would not be an option.

Implantation through a contralateral vein seems logical, especially if it is the implanter's only skill level option. The simplest alternative is to abandon the two old leads on the ipsilateral side and implant the new leads on the contralateral side. In the example of a conductor coil fracture, the patient has the risk of having two functioning and two superfluous leads in the heart and the risk of instrumentation of the superior veins on the opposite side (see Fig. 21-14D). In the example of adding a biventricular pacing lead, the patient has the risk of having three functioning leads and two superfluous leads in the heart and the risk of instrumentation of the superior veins on the opposite side (see Fig. 21-15D). These risks are weighed against the risk of extracting the one atrial lead. The resultant risk of having a complication is the sum of the individual risk factors.

For these two examples, another approach would be to implant the new atrial lead or biventricular lead

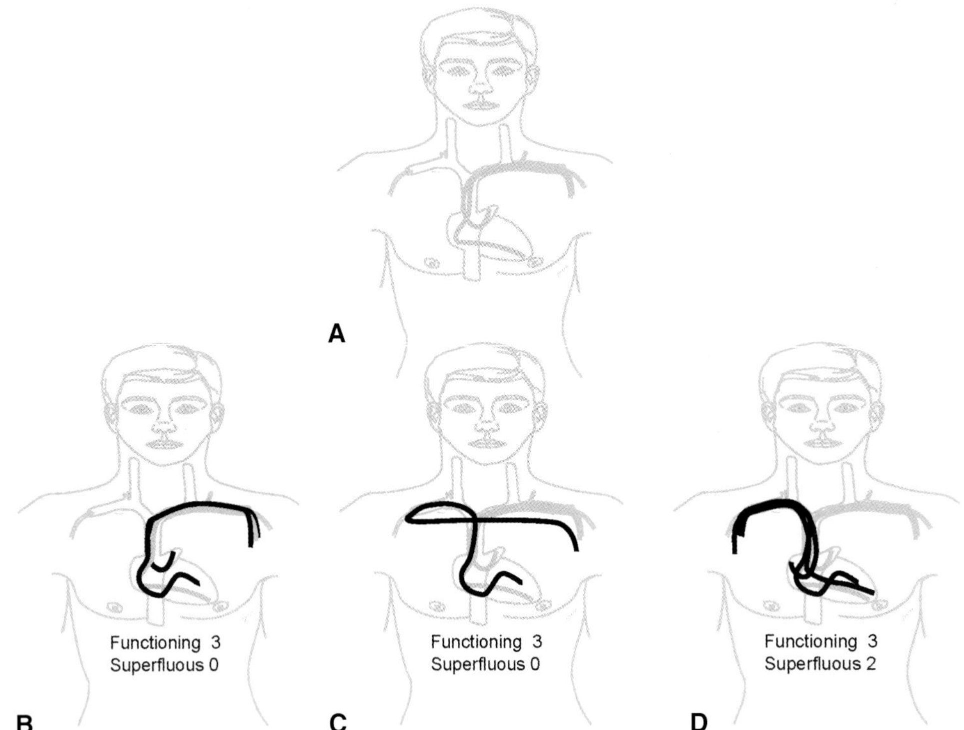

Figure 21-15. Creation of a conduit. ***A,*** *Addition of a cardiac vein lead in a patient with an implantable cardioverter-defibrillator (ICD), an occluded subclavian-brachiocephalic vein, and heart failure.* ***B,*** *Extraction of the atrial lead and implantation of a new atrial and cardiac vein lead (three functioning leads).* ***C,*** *Insertion of the new lead through the contralateral subclavian vein, tunneled to the old pocket (two functioning leads and one superfluous lead).* ***D,*** *Insertion of a new atrial lead, ICD lead, cardiac vein lead, and new pocket on the contralateral side (three functioning leads and two superfluous leads).*

on the contralateral side and tunnel it across to the pulse generator and ventricular lead. In addition to the risk of instrumentation of the superior veins and tunneling, the patient with conductor coil fracture will have two functioning leads and one superfluous lead in the heart (see Fig. 21-14C), and the patient with the biventricular lead will have three functioning leads in the heart (see Fig. 21-15C). In the *author's opinion*, the combined risks associated with not extracting often exceed the risk of extracting in both these cases, but clearly the risks will vary in individual patients.

Total bilateral occlusion of the superior veins further complicates the problem. The transfemoral approach is the only approach available to the medical EP. The surgical EP has the options of a transatrial or epicardial approach. The risks associated with these choices make the decision to extract the atrial lead easier. However, without extraction skills, the medical and surgical EPs may choose these alternatives.

The risk/benefit ratio is crucial to the rationale for extracting these leads. For example, the life-threatening risk associated with infection in effect forces an EP to extract the lead and abandon the pocket. The risk of not creating a conduit to insert new leads is a potential risk for a future complication related to bilateral implants, superfluous leads, multiple implanted leads, and/or tunneling. This risk is obviously less than the life-threatening risk of infection. In the situation of lead failure, the alternatives presented provide an acceptable short-term solution and can be performed by implanters without lead extraction skills. Potential risks are not as compelling a reason for action as the immediate risks associated with lead extraction. However, physicians with experience in lead extraction may not be happy with the scenario of abandoning two leads (i.e., creating two superfluous leads) and leaving a total of four or five leads implanted. Many would probably accept the tunneling of a lead from the opposite side, leaving only three leads in the heart. Although three leads may be acceptable to many, there is still a stigma associated with four leads. The discussion comparing the risk of not extracting with the risk of extracting may be helpful in resolving these issues.

Superfluous Leads. A rationale for extraction of superfluous leads is not easy to construct. This situation differs from creation of a conduit. For example, if the ipsilateral vein is patent, insertion of a new biventricular lead should be uneventful. However, the addition of a new atrial lead and abandonment of the old atrial lead create a superfluous lead. The disposition of superfluous leads causes controversy, confusion, and, at times, an emotional debate. Many questions need to be answered. Why should a lead be removed, if the lead itself is not causing a problem such as penetration or perforation, is not dislodged, or is not broken?[21] A discussion of the risks of lead extraction ensues.

Risk of Extracting Versus Risk of Not Extracting

The risks associated with lead extraction are tamponade (tearing of the SVC and/or heart), hemothorax (tearing into the thorax), arteriovenous fistula and/or dissecting hematoma (tear of the aortic arch), and failure to extract the lead (attempted lead extraction). The latter is usually not considered a risk; however, a failed lead extraction may lead to additional procedures or may be a precursor for dangerous situations in the future.

There are two situations in which the risk of tearing the SVC and/or heart is negligible to nonexistent. The first situation is those patients who have previously undergone an open heart surgical procedure. The pericardial space has been obliterated, and fibrous tissue reinforces the SVC and heart wall. The author has not had a cardiac tamponade in a patient with an obliterated pericardial space. The second situation is an implant of short duration: less than 2 years for pacemaker leads, or less than 1 year for ICD leads. The forces involved in freeing these leads *usually* are not sufficient to tear the SVC or heart.

Extraction centers from the continental United States and Hawaii voluntarily submitted data for a national registry between December 1988 and December 1999.[22,23] The most recent published report, from 1996, included data from 226 centers, 2338 patients and 3540 leads and demonstrated major complications in 1.4% of the cases (<1% for centers with >300 extraction procedures).[24] The total U.S. data, including 7823 extraction procedures and 12,833 leads, were presented at Cardiostim in June of 2000. Multivariate analysis of the data from 1994 through 1999 demonstrated four predictors of major complications (1.6%): (1) implant duration of oldest lead, (2) female gender, (3) ICD lead removal, and (4) use of laser extraction technique. Major complications were (1) death, 0.3%; (2) nonfatal hemopericardium or tamponade, 0.7%; (3) nonfatal hemothorax, 0.2%; (4) transfusion for bleeding/hypotension, 0.1%; (5) pneumothorax requiring a chest tube, 0.1%; and (6) other nonfatal events, 0.2% (including 4 arteriovenous fistulae, 2 pulmonary embolisms, 2 thoracotomies for defibrillator leads trapped in sheaths, 2 respiratory arrests, 2 strokes, 2 cases of renal failure, 1 anoxic encephalopathy, and 1 open surgical retrieval of a device fragment).

It is otherwise clear that the risk of lead extraction is dependent on the extractor's experience, duration of implant, age of patient, and condition of patient. There is no ongoing national database or registry, and the risks depend on the individual, the assembled team, and the institution. For example, the experiences and opinions of this author, a cardiac surgeon, must be judged accordingly. If a complication occurs, it is managed by the author. The most reliable indicator of risk is the individual extractor's personal statistics. It is important that each institution and individual keep track of complications and effectiveness.

Risks are caused by maturation of the encapsulating fibrous tissue, which is related to the duration of the implant and the patient's age. With time, the tensile strength of the encapsulating fibrous tissue increases; it may calcify in 3 to 4 years in children and in 8 to 10 years in older adults. Sedentary patients increase their tensile strength more slowly, and the tissue takes longer to mineralize. In sedentary elderly patients, the tensile strength seems to decrease with time. The influences of duration and age are apparent in the extremes. Also, patients with calcium metabolism abnormalities can calcify at any age in a short duration. Although the properties of encapsulated fibrous tissue are known, it is difficult to apply general principles to a specific patient and assign a risk.

Condition refers to the patient's physical status and mental state. It is a dominant factor in assessing the risk of the procedure for a given patient. Condition relates to the capability of a patient to survive a worst-case complication, such as a tear of the SVC or heart, or management of a difficult medical condition, such as refractory heart failure. Patients who have an ejection fraction of less than 10% or who have ascites and renal failure caused by cardiac cirrhosis are considered end-stage. The risk of a procedure in such an individual is extremely high. The risk is related to the postoperative management of these patients and not to the procedure itself. In the author's experience, except for the two high-risk examples, patients survive. Condition also influences procedure decisions in patients who have an altered mental state or function, especially those confined to an extended care facility. Decisions in regard to these philosophical and social issues, although influenced by the physician, are usually based on family preference, medical ethics, and legal factors.

Potentially lethal complications requiring extensive surgical procedures include tear of the vein and heart wall causing tamponade, arterial tears causing arterial-venous fistulae and/or dissecting hematoma, and tears into the thoracic cavity causing a hemothorax (Fig. 21-16). The procedure-related complications are discussed in detail later. Time and the surgeon's experience are the two factors related to survival. The influence of time is obvious: low blood pressure and poor tissue perfusion are time-dependent events. Being prepared for a cardiovascular emergency is the only way to meet time constraints. This includes having a cardiovascular surgeon available, along with the proper instrumentation and experienced support personnel. A cardiovascular surgeon has the technical skill to manage these complications but may need direction from the extractor on the proper approach. Once a complication resulting in poor or no perfusion is recognized, the repair should begin immediately. The fear of needlessly subjecting the patient to extensive surgery and morbidity pales in comparison to that of applying the therapy late because of confusion or procrastination. Failure to recognize the complication in a timely fashion or the lack of access to qualified personnel, not patient condition, is the cause of a lethal outcome.

In regard to the risk of not extracting, a decision to abandon a lead creates a superfluous lead—one of the

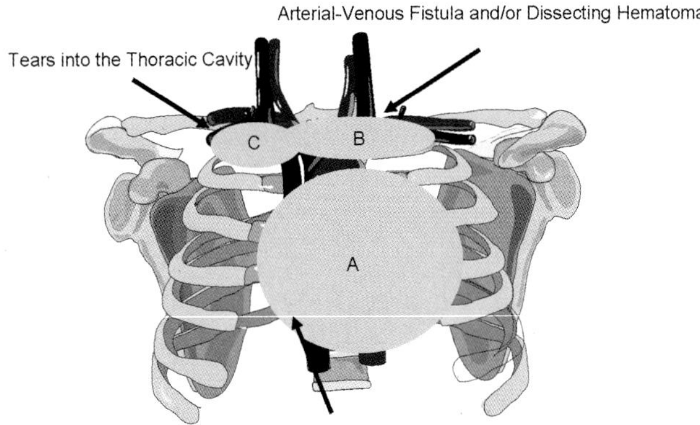

Figure 21-16. Potentially lethal complications. These potentially lethal complications all result from vascular tissue disruption during lead extraction. Disruptions are caused by tears, cutting, perforations, or avulsions of a vascular wall. Tearing or cutting of the superior vena cava (SVC) or atrial wall (A) is the most common complication resulting in cardiac tamponade. Leads that are contiguous with or embedded in the subclavian artery, innominate artery, or aorta can tear these vessels during lead extraction (B). Acutely, a dissecting hematoma develops, having the potential of rupture into the thorax or, chronically, of developing an arteriovenous fistula. Disruption of the right brachiocephalic vein into the right thoracic cavity (C) is insidious; it occurs during a difficult lead extraction when the vein and pleura are adherent or when a dissecting hematoma ruptures the pleura.

author's indications for lead extraction. It must be stated that the author's indication classification is not accepted by all. In fact, a superfluous lead is considered a class II or III indication for lead extraction in the guidelines published by the North American Society of Pacing and Electrophysiology in 2000.[16] Using the logic applied in the previous section to justify extraction of these leads, the risk of not extracting has to be greater than the risk of extracting. The risk of extracting is not known, except as it pertains to the skill and experience of the individual extractor, and data do not exist on the risk of not extracting. Acquiring some knowledge of the risk of not extracting a lead is totally different from the knowledge base for extracting a lead. Each physician performing lead extraction must draw on his or her own experience. Although individual statistics are the most important for a given lead extraction, statistics relative to the population of lead extractors are not known. In contrast, if you make a decision *not* to extract a lead, creating a superfluous lead, it is unlikely that the outcome of that decision will be known in the short term, if at all. Lack of detailed outcome data and issues with logic make it difficult to establish the presence of a superfluous lead as an indication for lead extraction. Despite this dilemma, an attempt will be made. The only tools available are logical discussions based on the author's experiences and the consequences to the biophysical interface of a chronic lead implant.

Complications related to superfluous leads are the same as for a functioning lead. To justify the prophylactic removal of a superfluous lead, a potential biophysical interface problem relating to the presence of multiple leads and the duration of the implant must exist. Arguments not related to the biophysical interface involving lead component and communication failures do not apply to superfluous leads. Questions such as, "What is the evidence that a biophysical interface issue will develop over time?" and "If three functioning leads are acceptable, why are two functioning leads and one superfluous lead not acceptable?" must be answered. Statements such as, "It is intuitively obvious," "The X-ray looks better," and "What would you have done?" cannot be used. Also not to be used are arguments suggesting that the superfluous lead may interfere with the electrical performance of the new lead (e.g., electrical noise created by contact between two ICD leads). Biophysical interface issues are known to occur with multiple leads over time. They include thrombus formation in the SVC and right atrium, damage to the tricuspid valve, and lead removal issues at lead–lead binding sites caused by an organized thrombus. These events have the same potential of forming regardless of the number of leads, functional or superfluous. For example, outcome with three functioning leads is the same as with combinations of functional and superfluous leads, such as one functioning and two superfluous leads or two functioning and one superfluous lead. The only difference is that the functioning leads provide a benefit justifying the potential risk. Based on this line of reasoning, there is no need to remove superfluous leads.

The author's view is based on experiences gained in dealing with the complications associated with multiple leads. Insight into how multiple leads increase the potential for a complication to occur and the added difficulty of managing those complications, including lead removal, are discussed. To avoid confusion, complications known to occur at the biophysical interface are presented for each vein and cardiac region in both single and multiple leads. The complications known to occur include clot formation, thrombus formation, encapsulating fibrous tissue, vascular occlusion and obliteration, embedding of the lead into the vascular wall, lead exclusion from a vein, tricuspid valve insufficiency, and, rarely, tricuspid valve stenosis.

For a lead or leads passing through the ipsilateral axillary-subclavian-brachiocephalic veins, all of the complications listed have occurred, regardless of the number of implanted leads. The incidence of a complication with a single lead is not known, and it is only *assumed* that the probability of a complication increases with multiple leads. The clinical sequelae of these complications are rarely significant and are the same regardless of the number of leads involved. Consequently, the complications associated with multiple leads (used or superfluous) in these ipsilateral veins cannot be used as an argument. The same is not true of an occlusion or obliteration of both the ipsilateral and contralateral brachiocephalic veins. The occlusion of the brachiocephalic vein also occludes the internal jugular and collateral veins draining into the brachiocephalic vein. Bilateral occlusion of the brachiocephalic veins is equivalent to occlusion of the proximal SVC. A proximal SVC occlusion causes an SVC syndrome, which is incapacitating in an active patient. Contralateral vein implants should be avoided whenever possible. This is especially true if the removal of superfluous leads prevents a contralateral vein implant from being used.

The interaction in the SVC of a lead with the vein wall, resulting in thrombus formation, maturation of the thrombus into encapsulating fibrous tissue, and embedding in or exclusion from the vein wall, have been discussed for both single and multiple leads. It is hard to make an argument that extracting a superfluous lead will prevent a future embedding and exclusion complication, because the potential for this to occur is unknown. More importantly, embedding and exclusion have not caused a known complication. The presence of embedding or exclusion is not apparent unless a complication occurs in extracting these leads.

Lead–lead interactions cause complications such as thrombus formation that can result in stenosis or occlusion of both the proximal and distal SVC. The author *believes* that the presence of more leads increases the probability of such an event. This is especially true over time. Changes in flow and lead binding cause stasis and turbulence. It can be argued that increasing the number of leads passing through the SVC increases the potential for a complication. The distal SVC, at the junction between the SVC and atrium, has the same potential for a complication as the proximal SVC. Multiple lead interactions in this narrowed area cause stenosis or occlusion resulting in SVC syndrome. The potential for this complication increases with the presence of multiple leads.

Thrombus formation in the atrium is common. Progression of thrombus to occlusion of the atrium has been seen by the author only in association with severe infection. The reason for an increased incidence of thrombus formation in the atrium is probably related to its larger size and lower flow. The potential for this complication increases with the presence of multiple leads. A lead passing through the tricuspid valve damages the valve by interaction with the valve leaflets. Thrombus formation between multiple leads makes the situation worse. The clinical sequela of tricuspid valvular insufficiency caused by leaflet damage is hemodynamic dysfunction. Stenosis of the tricuspid valve is a rare complication seen only once by the author. This is caused by organization of a lead–lead thrombus. As the scar tissue contracts, the stenosis worsens. It is logical to assume that the potential for this complication increases with the presence of multiple leads.

Multiple lead implants in the right ventricle cause a change in compliance of the ventricular wall. Multiple stiff leads can decrease the compliance of the ventricular wall without lead–lead thrombus interactions. The sequelae of thrombus formation and organization with scarring only make the situation worse. To compensate for the resultant decrease in chamber volume and wall compliance, the filling pressure increases. The potential for this complication increases with the presence of multiple leads.

Multiple lead implants have the potential for obstructing venous return with or without lead interactions and thrombus formation. Examples of initial compensatory mechanisms are formation of collateral venous drainage and elevated venous pressure. Successful compensation for these insults may leave the patient asymptomatic, especially if the insults occur over an extended period. The gradual decrease in activity may go unnoticed or misdiagnosed. Although the number of patients with venous occlusions is unknown, the author's experiences suggest that it is a significant chronic implant problem.

Lead Extraction Techniques

Segments of chronically implanted leads are encased in encapsulating fibrous tissue and bound to the vein and/or heart wall, bound to another lead, or both. Lead extraction is the removal of chronically implanted leads from these binding sites. Because the tensile strength of encapsulating fibrous tissue is greater than that of the surrounding tissue, leads cannot easily be removed without risking a tear or avulsion of the vein or heart wall. The word *ablation* best describes the removal, separation, and freeing of leads from encapsulating fibrous tissue. Ablation techniques include traction, countertraction, counterpressure, and tissue disruption cutting locally with an instrument, laser, or electrosurgery unit. Lead extraction techniques are designed to free the lead from the encapsulating fibrous tissue (countertraction) or to free the encapsulating fibrous tissue (counterpressure) from the vein or heart wall.[25] Telescoping sheaths are used to remotely apply countertraction and counterpressure at the selected binding sites. Lead extraction procedures are those procedures used to apply the sheaths and remove the lead in a safe and efficacious manner.

Traction, Countertraction, and Counterpressure. In the 1960s and early 1970s, transvenous leads were large, bipolar, and without fixation devices. These leads were usually isodiametric, implanted for 1 to 2 years, and removed by traction. With the introduction of tines and pulse generators lasting 4 to 6 years, leads were entrapped in encapsulating fibrous tissue with significant tensile strength. These leads could not be safely removed by traction alone.

Traction is the force exerted on the lead by pulling. Applying traction to the lead pulls directly on the binding site. Once the encapsulating tissue has a greater tensile strength than the venous or cardiac tissue, the tissue will tear or avulse. Disruption of the vein or heart wall can be lethal. Because the relative tensile strengths are not known, traction should be used with caution. This being said, traction is an acceptable extraction technique if it is applied in a judicious manner. The force applied when pulling on a lead is related to lead size, lead tensile strength, how the lead is grasped, use of locking stylets, and, most importantly, the extracting physician's catecholamine level. The catecholamine level is an important factor in determining the actual traction force. When the extractor is

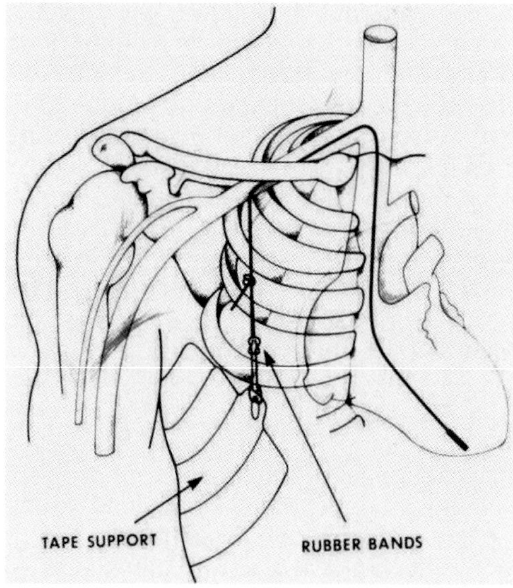

Figure 21-17. Direct traction. Direct traction is being applied by pulling on the proximal portion of the lead. Rubber bands are used in this case. Variations include using free weights and applying weights via an orthopedic traction apparatus. If a locking stylet is inserted, the traction point is moved distal to the locking site, usually near the electrode.

relaxed and calm, the perceived force may be realistic. When he or she is upset, agitated, or mad, the force is much greater than perceived. Consequently, "giving it a little tug" is not wise.

Direct Traction. All current lead extraction procedures use some form of traction, or pulling force (Fig. 21-17).[26] Pulling on leads was a successful method of extracting leads during the early years of pacing, when leads lacked efficient fixation devices and were implanted for short periods of time. Traction was applied manually for minutes or applied using various weights or elastic bands for days. Traction proved unsafe and had a high incidence of failure when applied to leads with efficient fixation devices and leads implanted for longer periods of time. The amount of traction required increases and becomes more dangerous as the duration of the implant and the tensile strength of the fibrous tissue increase. Leads with efficient passive fixation devices may be difficult to remove 4 to 6 months after implantation. A failed previous attempt to extract a lead frequently damaged the lead, making future extraction attempts more difficult.

Traction must be applied judiciously to minimize the risk to the patient. The pulling force applied to the proximal portion of the lead is distributed to sites where fibrous tissue binds the lead or electrode and makes contact with the vein or heart wall. Multiple leads may be bound to the vein or heart wall and to each other. Because the pulling force is not focused, the distribution of force to the binding sites is unknown. It is possible to inadvertently tear a vein or the heart wall.

Traction, in some form, is integral to lead extraction. The physician must consciously limit the pulling force and apply a continuous, steady traction. Never jerk the lead, because impulse forces tear. Accidents are not predictable and frequently happen without warning, in part because it is impossible to accurately judge the level of force applied to the lead. In an attempt to gauge the applied force, most direct traction techniques try applying sufficient force to feel the rhythmic tugging of the heart without producing arrhythmias, hypotension, or chest pain. These are crude and unreliable end points and are not reflective of the tensile strength of the lead or the tissue. Breaking the lead, tearing a vein, or avulsing or tearing the heart wall all represent complications. Although applying "just a little tug" to see if the lead will come out may not be safe, following basic principles and guidelines acquired from practical experience will help minimize the risk.

It is important to understand the difference between pulling from above and pulling from below. The mediastinal structures are not bound from below. If you pull upward on the heart, it will move, along with the lungs, diaphragm, and rest of the mediastinal contents, in that direction. If you pull downward, the superior veins and surrounding structures are bound to the musculoskeletal system and do not move downward. Assume that traction is applied from above to a lead implanted in the right ventricle. With continuous traction, the right ventricle starts to evaginate, decreasing the compliance of the wall and finally obstructing the flow of blood through the tricuspid valve. At the same time, the heart is pulled into the superior portion of the mediastinum. This maneuver is safe as long as the hemodynamic status is monitored and the process is reversible. Reversibility means that traction-induced deterioration in hemodynamic function is corrected on cessation of the traction, and the right ventricle, along with remainder of the mediastinal structures, returns to its normal position. Most of the time, the structures do return to normal. The danger is slippage of the lead body through a binding site. On release of the traction, the mediastinal forces pulling downward are insufficient to pull the lead back through the binding site. The forces required to elevate the mediastinum to this position are still applied to the heart. Any hemodynamic compromise such as decreased blood flow through the right ventricle persists, creating a cardiovascular emergency. If the lead body cannot be released by manipulation, including use of a stiff stylet to help push it through the binding site, an emergency median sternotomy is required to manually retract the heart.

Once a lead is freed from a distal binding site, the lead and associated fibrous material can then become wedged in a more proximal binding site. For example, a lead removed from the right ventricle can become wedged at a binding site in the atrium, SVC, or axillary-subclavian-brachiocephalic veins. With direct traction, the lead is freed from the binding sites, distal to proximal. The strongest binding site determines the outcome of an extraction attempt, regardless of its proximal or distal location.

Indirect Traction. Elevation of the mediastinum with traction is the main reason why traction from above is not as effective at pulling a lead through a binding site as is pulling from below. When traction is applied from below, the mediastinum is not pulled down (inferior), because the superior veins and surrounding tissues are bound to the musculoskeletal system. Traction forces applied to the binding sites are directed at freeing the lead, and not at moving structures. The limit to the force applied to the axillary-subclavian-brachiocephalic veins is determined by the tensile strength of the lead. If the lead binding in these veins is extensive enough to require that kind of force, the veins are probably occluded, atretic, or encapsulating sheaths. Disruption of these veins by tearing and/or avulsion is of no consequence. Binding sites in the SVC, however, must be treated in the same manner as in the heart. Disruption of the wall of the SVC has the same consequences as disruption of the heart wall.

The safety and efficacy (higher success rate) of applying indirect traction from below should be apparent from these comments. Indirect traction is traction applied by an instrument, such as a snare passed into the heart, usually through a femoral vein. The lead is entrapped in the snare, and traction is applied by pulling or pushing. The difficulty is in grasping the lead in a fashion that allows sufficient traction to be applied. Only a few snares, such as the Dotter basket snare (Cook), have sufficient strength to support extraction forces. The lead must first be freed from the superior veins and then from the heart. The lead is pulled out of the superior veins and into the atrium or inferior vena cava (IVC). It can be regrasped, if necessary, and traction can be applied to the heart. The techniques for applying indirect traction are the same as for grasping and manipulating the leads in other approaches, such as applying countertraction sheaths, and are described later. The risks eliminated by indirect traction are tearing of superior veins, wedging of the lead in the atrium or in a superior vein, and creating a low cardiac output caused by failure of the lead to return to its original position after traction. Indirect traction has the same potential for breaking the lead or tearing the heart wall as direct traction, if their tensile strengths are exceeded.

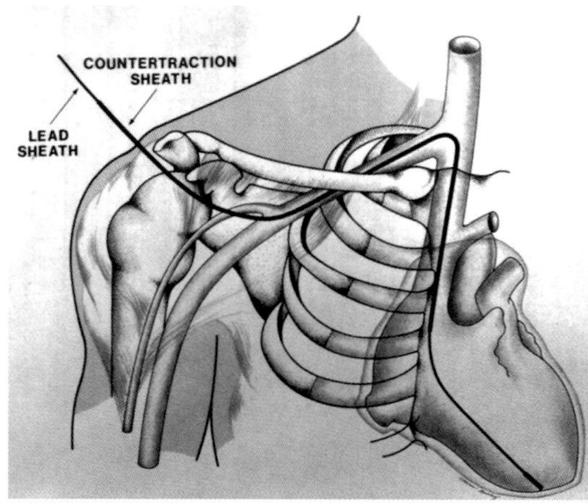

Figure 21-18. Countertraction. Telescoping sheaths are passed over the lead and maneuvered from binding site to binding site, breaking through each one primarily by countertraction. When necessary, the application of counterpressure peels the encapsulating fibrous tissue from the wall. At the electrode myocardial interface, countertraction is the only safe method that can be used to remove the lead.

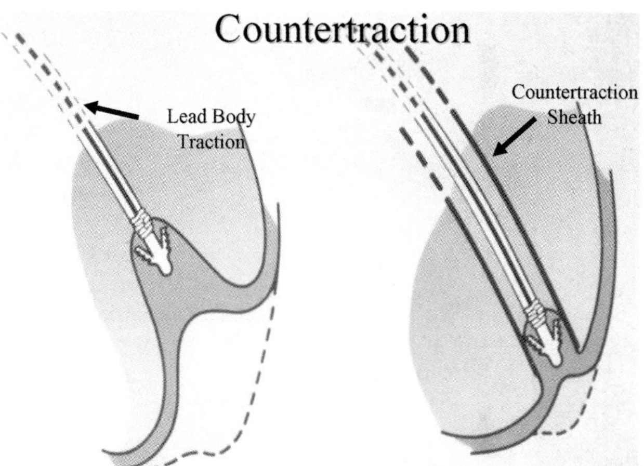

Figure 21-19. Countertraction. Countertraction is a safe method extirpating a lead or electrode from a vein or heart wall. Traction on the lead body with evagination of the right ventricular wall (left) *decreases the compliance on the wall and pulls it toward the tricuspid valve. Complications include decreased flow through the right ventricle and disruption of the ventricular wall instead of the scar tissue, with tearing of the wall and/or avulsion of tissue. Placing a sheath near the heart wall applying traction* (right) *causes the traction force to be countered by the sheath. The limit on the traction force applied is the tensile strength of the lead. The lead is extirpated from the scar tissue, and the heart returns to its normal position.*

Countertraction. Countertraction is the technique used to free the lead from compliant encapsulated fibrous tissue. Countertraction was first used to remove a lead from an implantation site in the right ventricle or atrium. Although the technique for extracting leads from the heart wall is discussed first, this is the last step in a normal lead extraction procedure, using any type of sheath. Extraction sheaths free leads from binding sites, proximal to distal (Fig. 21-18). Once the sheath is passed over the lead and down to the implantation site, traction on the lead pulls the site to the sheath (Fig. 21-19). The traction force is countered by the circumference of the sheath. The countertraction sheath focuses the traction force at the tip of the sheath, limiting the excursion of the heart wall. This prevents compliance changes and blockage of the tricuspid valve with possible perforation, tearing, and avulsion of the heart wall. The countertraction forces are limited by the tensile strength of the lead. At some point, the electrode is freed from the encapsulating fibrous tissue, allowing the heart wall to fall away and the electrode to be pulled out of the sheath.

The way countertraction actually frees the lead is postulated but not known. It is imagined that the traction force wedges the lead against the countertraction sheath. The pulling force on the electrode tries to evaginate the encapsulating fibrous tissue. The electrode is then imagined to be freed either by a plastic deformation of the tissue that allows it to slide out of the encapsulating tissue as the countertraction sheath peels the tissue off the electrode or by an actual disruption or bursting of the encapsulating tissue that frees the electrode, or both. For a passive electrode, the tines are removed intact with the electrode; for an active fixation electrode, the fixation mechanism is ideally retracted or unscrewed before countertraction is applied. In some cases, continued "unscrewing" of an active fixation lead results in complete lead removal without the need for countertraction because of the absence of significant binding at other sites along the lead.[27] If the helix will not retract, the electrode and fixation mechanism are removed together. The same scenario is envisioned for removal of electrodes from the atrial wall.

Countertraction is also used to free the lead from the encapsulating fibrous tissue at binding sites along the vein and heart wall (see Fig. 21-19). This is possible only if the encapsulating fibrous tissue still has plastic qualities (compliant). The tissue at the binding site is pulled against or into the sheath and is removed by evagination, peeling, or tissue rupture. Countertraction can be performed with either the inner or the outer sheath.

Counterpressure. Counterpressure was the name given to the removal technique used for noncompliant encapsulating fibrous tissue (mineralized tissue). A sheath larger than the solid encapsulating tissue is used, and the tissue is pulled into the sheath. The encapsulating fibrous tissue is usually attached to the vein, tricuspid valve, or heart wall. The sheath counters the traction force applied to the tissue mass by converting this force into a pressure concentrated locally between the edge of the sheath and the vein wall (counterpressure sheath). This local action peels the calcified mass off the vein or heart wall. The encapsulating tissue is included with the lead inside the sheath (inclusion). The force applied is limited by the tensile strength of the lead and/or the wall. Because the magnitude of the counterpressure force actually focused on the wall is unknown, application of force is subjective. Counterpressure is potentially dangerous and should be approached with caution. It is believed by some that mineralization of tissue may lead to a higher risk associated with lead extraction. The inability to safely pass a binding site using counterpressure is the primary reason for abandoning this approach and changing to a transfemoral or transatrial approach. These approaches allow the lead to be pulled out of the superior veins from below, through the binding site.

It is unknown whether the lead is being removed by countertraction or counterpressure (Fig. 21-20). In the past, counterpressure was used to describe the removal of tissue from all sites other than the electrode implantation site. In most cases, removal is still credited to counterpressure; compliant tissue is removed primarily by countertraction, and noncompliant tissue by counterpressure. Not discussed are leads bound to one another by the calcified encapsulating tissue. Separation of the two leads is safe, and the traction force is limited only by the tensile strength of the lead.

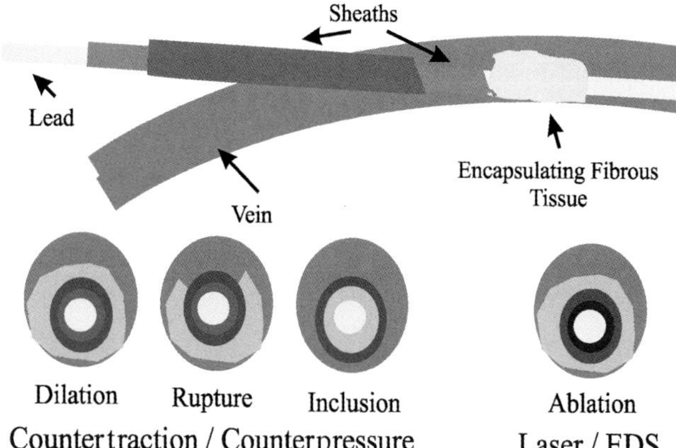

Figure 21-20. Mechanical and powered sheaths. Telescoping sheaths are inserted transvenously and passed to the first binding site. Countertraction, counterpressure, and/or power ablation is applied to extirpate the lead. Countertraction dilates and/or ruptures the binding site, liberating the lead. The laser and electrosurgical dissection sheath (EDS) is a powered sheath that vaporizes the tissue. Counterpressure is used to pass the sheath over the entire calcified encapsulating fibrous tissue mass (inclusion). Counterpressure is the actual manipulation of the telescoping sheaths to peel the encapsulating tissue off the vein or heart wall.

Extraction Instruments. Lead extraction instruments are separated into mechanical sheaths, powered mechanical sheaths, and snares.

Mechanical Sheaths. Mechanical sheaths are telescoping sheaths made of Teflon, polypropylene, or stainless steel (Fig. 21-21). These telescoping sheaths are designed to pass over the lead, which acts as a rail guiding the sheaths through the veins and down to the heart wall. Countertraction and counterpressure are applied as the sheaths move down the lead from one binding site to another. The outer sheath also acts as a workstation. As a workstation, it facilitates the free movement of the inner sheath and lead by eliminating binding, and it protects the surrounding vascular structures. The leading edges of the sheaths are beveled. The rotation of the beveled tips facilitates maneuvering past obstructions and through the narrow channels along the tortuous paths surrounding the lead body. This is especially true in the superior veins. For the sheaths to pass down the lead in a true fashion, the lead must be stiff enough to act as a guide rail. The lead is stiffened by pulling it taut. The lead must be stiff enough to resist bending or kinking as the sheaths are passed over it (lead stiffness > sheath stiffness). The telescoping action of the sheaths allows the more supple inner sheath to track over the lead. The larger outer sheath is then advanced using the combination of taut lead and inner sheath as the guide rail. The lead is made taut by traction (pulling on it). A locking stylet is inserted, and a suture is usually tied to the lead, acting as both an extender and a traction handle.

As described earlier, experience and judgment are required to avoid tearing and avulsing vein and heart wall tissues. Also, if the traction force exceeds the lead's tensile strength, it can cause lead disruption

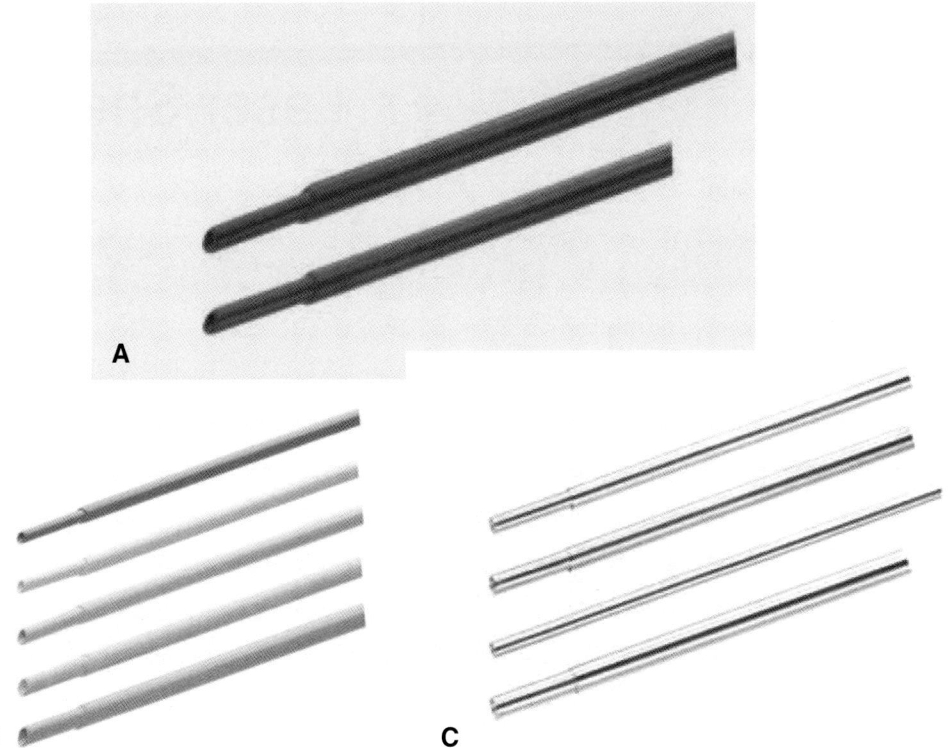

Figure 21-21. Mechanical sheaths. Mechanical telescoping sheaths have a beveled tip and come in various sizes. ***A,*** *Teflon sheaths are softer and more supple; they were the original sheaths.* ***B,*** *Polypropylene sheaths are stiffer and allow more force to be applied at the binding site.* ***C,*** *Stainless steel sheaths are rigid and are used to bore through bone or calcified tissue at the vein entry site. The stainless steal sheaths should not be passed into the brachiocephalic vein.*

and/or breakage. Insertion of a locking stylet adds some stiffness to the lead and focuses the traction force to a locking site near the electrode. Except for simple cases, in which leads have been implanted for a short duration, a locking stylet should be inserted. Despite these efforts, as the tensile strength increases it becomes more difficult and more time-consuming to free the lead from its binding site. The forces involved frequently exceed the tensile strength of the lead, resulting in lead disruption and breakage.

Powered Mechanical Sheaths. Powered cutting tips positioned at the leading edge of the mechanical sheath have changed the nature of lead extraction. The ability to free the leads by cutting tissue significantly decreases the countertraction forces. Reduction in the applied force has made lead breakage and separation of the lead body from the distal electrode rare events. The expectation is that any lead should be completely extracted regardless of its tensile strength. Before the advent of powered sheaths, a lead breakage rate of 15% to 20% was common for leads with satisfactory tensile strengths. The first powered sheath was the excimer laser sheath (Spectranetics, Colorado Springs, Colo.) developed in the mid-1990s. The second was the electrosurgical dissection sheath (EDS; Cook) in the early 2000s. Both of these sheaths are used successfully today.

Excimer Laser Sheath. The development of the excimer laser was a milestone for lead extraction (Fig. 21-22). The excimer laser generated a high-energy 308-nm laser beam known to disrupt tissue (both cells and hydrated proteins) by an explosive vaporization of intracellular water. The rapid vaporization helped to cool the site. These were appealing properties for lead extraction. Unfortunately, the laser did not ablate mineralized tissue. If the laser could not be maneuvered through this tissue in grinding fashion, counterpressure techniques had to be used.

The development of the excimer laser sheath was a technical achievement. It required expertise in polymer chemistry and optic fibers to develop a small-diameter, flexible sheath capable of withstanding the excessive forces applied during a lead extraction. At the time, optic fibers were bundled in a circumferential fashion inside a cylindrical metal housing. The metal housing protected the optic fibers from the applied forces generated while maneuvering the tip through the encapsulating tissue. Initially, the only sheath meeting all the clinical requirements was a 12F sheath that was interchangeable with the 12/16F mechanical Teflon sheaths. In time, larger 14F and 16F sheaths were perfected. These sizes were sufficient to manage all sizes of pacing leads up to the largest ICD leads. The last iteration of the laser sheath was to place a 15-degree bevel at the tip. It is the largest angle permitted by the circular configuration of the optic fibers at the electrode. The laser is controlled by a foot switch. By design, the laser is on for 10 seconds and off for 5 seconds. The

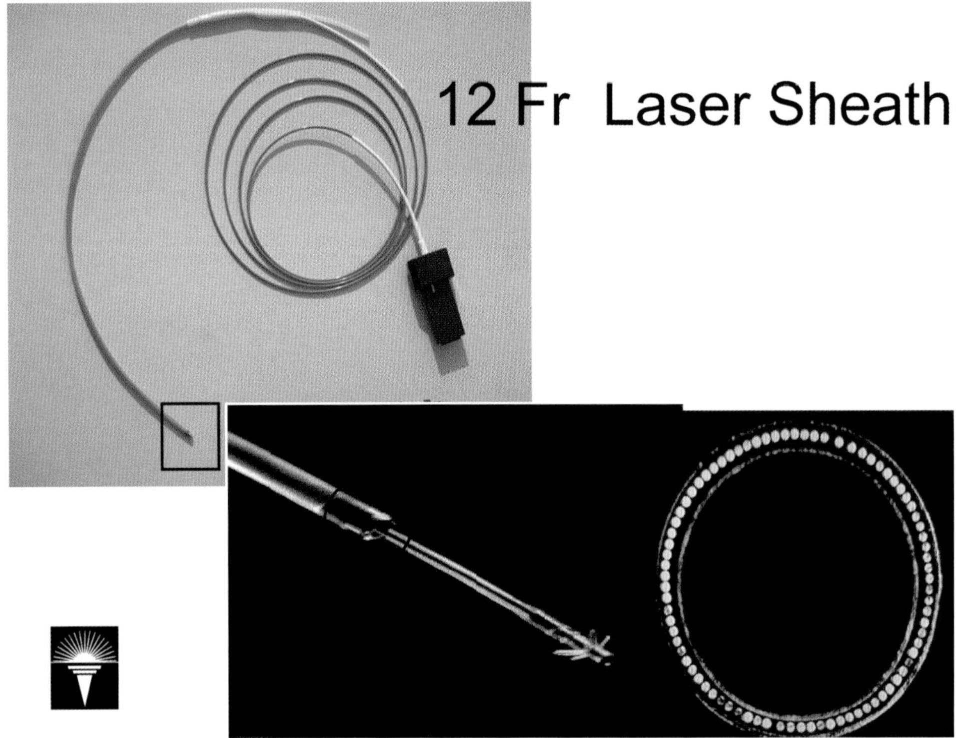

Figure 21-22. *Excimer laser sheath. The laser sheath plugs into the CVX-300 excimer laser system with a black connector at the proximal end. A blue fiberoptic cable conducts the pulsed ultraviolet light to the working section, which is tubular in shape. The inset gives an idea of how the laser sheath is designed to slide over the lead body as it threads its way through the veins to the heart. A micrograph of the tip shows how the 83 fibers are arranged in a single circumferential row at the tip. When the laser light comes out of these fibers, it cuts the fibrotic tissue that binds the lead to the vein walls.*

sound caused by the rapid pulsing of the laser furnishes a unique sound indicating the laser is on. The laser beam is a light cone that ablates tissue up to a distance of 1 mm. The water vapor generates bubbles that are clearly visible on echocardiography. Although the bubbles and other particulate debris are filtered out in the lungs, there are no apparent clinical sequelae. The cutting action of the laser can disrupt the SVC or the atrial wall if the lead is embedded in the wall. Because there is no way to know when a lead is embedded in the wall, the same emergency precautions apply to the laser as to the mechanical sheaths.

The laser sheath technique was evaluated prospectively in two clinical trials. The first, the Pacing Lead Extraction with the Excimer Sheath (PLEXES) trial, included only the initial version of the 12F sheath. Although there have been substantial subsequent improvements in the 12F sheath, including an outer sheath, better mechanical properties to prevent crushing of the optical fibers, lubrication, a flexible distal and a more still proximal segment, and certainly better understanding of how to use the tool, the PLEXES trial was a dramatic success. This was a randomized clinical trial comparing mechanical extraction tools with laser-assisted lead extraction, and it was used to support the clinical release of this technology. The complete lead removal rate was 94% in the laser group and 64% in the nonlaser group ($P = .001$). Failed nonlaser extraction was completed with the laser tools 88% of the time. The mean time to achieve a successful lead extraction was significantly reduced for patients randomized to the laser tools: 10.1 ± 11.5 minutes compared with 12.9 ± 19.2 minutes for the nonlaser techniques ($P < .04$). There was only one death, but it was in the laser group; and there were two other potentially life-threatening bleeding episodes in the laser group.[28]

After the trial with the 12F sheaths, a second, nonrandomized cohort trial was done with 14F and 16F sheaths. This was particularly important, because implantable defibrillator leads required the 16F sheaths, and many of the bipolar leads (almost all) were better approached with the 14F sheath. In contrast to other, nonlaser sheaths, upsizing of the laser sheath to pass over (include) the fibrosis or calcification is frequently a very effective maneuver. In this study, 863 patients underwent extraction of 1285 leads. Expanding the number of research sites from fewer than 10 to 52 gave a broader view of this tool in general practice. The patients treated with the 14F device tended to have older leads than patients in the 12F population; the 16F population, composed mostly of defibrillator patients, were younger, had younger leads, and were more often male than the 12F population. Clinical success (extraction of the entire lead or of the lead body minus the distal electrode) was observed in 91% to 92% of cases for all device sizes. The overall complication rate was 3.6%, with a 0.8% perioperative mortality rate. The incidence of complications was independent of laser sheath size.[29]

Ultimately, a cohort comparison trial of defibrillator and pacemaker leads extracted with laser assistance was done at the Cleveland Clinic Foundation. ICD extraction results were compared with the results for a matched cohort of patients undergoing extraction of ventricular pacemaker leads from a national registry and with the experience with pacemaker lead extraction at the Cleveland Clinic Foundation. Successful complete extraction of ventricular nonthoracotomy implantable defibrillator leads, in the absence of major complications, was achieved in 96.9% of attempts to extract leads from 161 patients. Clinical success was achieved in 98.1% of patients. There were three major complications, including one death. ICD lead extraction was done at an experienced center with equal risk and no significant difference in procedure or fluoroscopy time.[30]

The total investigational experience with laser sheaths was also reported, encompassing the period from October 1995 to December 1999, including 2561 pacing and defibrillator leads in 1684 patients at 89 sites in the United States. Of these leads, 90% were completely removed, 3% were partially removed, and 7% were failures. Major perioperative complications (tamponade, hemothorax, pulmonary embolism, lead migration, and death) were observed in 1.9% of patients, with in-hospital deaths in 13 (0.8%). Minor complications were seen in an additional 1.4% of patients. Multivariate analysis showed that implant duration was the only preoperative independent predictor of failure, and female sex was the only multivariate predictor of complications. Success and complications were not dependent on laser sheath size. At follow-up, various extraction-related complications were observed in 2% of patients. The learning curve showed a trend toward fewer complications with experience.[31] A similar experience was observed in Europe.[32]

Electrosurgical Dissection Sheaths. The EDS has two bipolar electrodes positioned at the tip of the bevel (Fig. 21-23). The sheath is connected to an interface plate inserted on a conventional electrosurgery unit (Valley Lab Force V; PEMED, Denver, Colo.), placed in a bipolar cutting configuration, and activated with a foot switch. The interface plate is attached to the front panel of the electrosurgery unit to ensure that the EDS is connected in a bipolar configuration. The interface also has an attachment to pulse the electrosurgery unit 80 times per minute. A plasma arc is generated between the electrodes. The plasma arc extends out from the electrodes and vaporizes the tissue to a depth of about 1 mm. On continuous discharge, desiccated tissue debris shunts the arc between the electrodes, preventing it from cutting. Also, on continuous discharge, if one of the electrodes touches a conductor coil, a parallel alternate current (AC) circuit is created consisting of the EDS electrode in contact with the conductor coil, the conductor coil down to an electrode in the heart, and back to the other EDS electrode. An AC current applied to the heart in a unipolar configuration can fibrillate the heart. To ensure cutting and avoid fibrillating the heart, the EDS is operated in a pulsed mode at 80 pulses/min. In the pulsed mode, if a conductor coil is touched, it paces the heart.

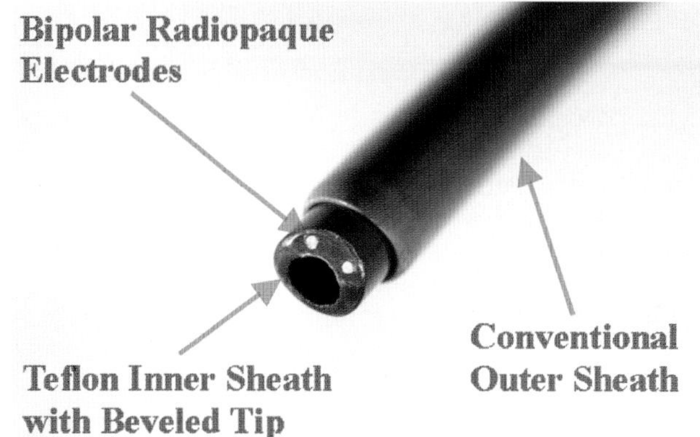

Figure 21-23. Electrosurgical dissection sheath (EDS). The EDS is a telescoping, Teflon, beveled sheath set with two electrodes in a bipolar configuration at the tip of the inner sheath. Encapsulating tissue is ablated with the use of radiofrequency energy delivered as needed in a pulsed fashion at 80 Hz. The electrodes are radiopaque, allowing precise placement.

The EDS is a conventional Teflon mechanical sheath with two tungsten electrodes embedded in the polymer. Placement of the EDS electrodes in a bipolar configuration at the tip of the inner telescoping sheath endows the EDS sheath with properties of mechanical sheaths: it can maneuver through tortuous veins, and it can be used to apply countertraction and counterpressure. These sheaths are currently available in sizes 7F, 9F, 11F, and 13F (circumference of the inner sheath).

The electrodes and sheath are radiopaque, allowing visualization during fluoroscopy. The electrodes' positions are continuously adjusted by rotation of the sheath. For example, around a curve, the electrodes are placed on the inner curvature passing down the lead. Also, the electrodes are rotated away from skeletal muscle and nerves to avoid stimulation. Stimulation of skeletal muscle and/or the phrenic nerve does not harm the patient and is not an issue for patients under general anesthesia. However, skeletal muscle and diaphragmatic contractions can be discomforting and even frightening if the patient is awake. At present, this is the only clinical issue associated with the EDS. The same emergency precautions applicable to mechanical and laser sheaths also apply to the EDS.

Clinical evaluation of the EDS has been formally published only in an observational study from five centers, involving 265 patients with extraction of 459 leads.[33] During the investigation, only the 9F and 11F sheaths were used, excluding almost all ICD leads from consideration for extraction. As in all extraction series, some of the leads came out easily and others were more difficult to remove, and the techniques consisted more of an approach than of universal use of one tool to remove all leads. In this case, 542 leads were potentially presented for extraction, but about 15% were removed with direct traction, yielding 459 for which the EDS was employed. The laser tool was used in fewer than 3% of the leads. The average implant duration of the patient's oldest lead was 8.4 ± 5.0 years; 31% of patients had leads implanted for longer than 10 years. Major complications occurred in 2.6% of patients, including cardiac tamponade in 4 patients (1 surgical repair, 1 after switching to a femoral approach), 1 hemothorax, 1 arteriovenous fistula (surgical repair), and 1 death that was associated with the mechanical removal of an oversized SVC lead for which the EDS was not used. For the 459 leads with attempted removal by the EDS, 99.4% were removed (95.9% completely, 3.5% subtotally with ≤4 cm of lead remaining), and only 0.6% were not removed. Overall, the experience with the EDS has been good. The application of 7F and 13F sheaths with intermittent pulsing of the electrosurgical energy has been useful in removing smaller and larger leads and in making the sheath more powerful in cutting through the fibrosis.

EVOLUTION Mechanical Dilation Sheath. Cook Vascular has recently introduced a new mechanically powered lead extraction sheath set, the EVOLUTION Mechanical Dilation Sheath. A rotating inner sheath with a threaded barrel metal tip was designed to function as a dilating drill. This bores through the encapsulating fibrous tissue as it advances down the lead through the binding sites. The outer sheath is a conventional beveled plastic sheath. The rotation of the inner sheath is powered by a pistol grip handle squeezed by the operator (mechanical power). Multiple inner diameter sizes (7, 9, 11 and 13 French) are available. In the author's initial clinical experience with 19 patients (leads implanted from 1 to 17 years), the leads were successfully removed. In the absence of calcified encapsulating tissue, the device moves at an impressive rate along the lead. Although this tool has not been tested by multiple operators, it appears to be useful and an advance in the technology of lead extraction.

Locking Stylets. Locking stylets were developed after the mechanical sheaths. From the beginning, the major pacing companies (Medtronic, Cordis [St. Jude Medical], and Pacesetter [Guidant]) all attempted to make a universal locking stylet (one size stylet to fit all). These initial attempts were unsuccessful because of breakage of the locking mechanism. The tensile strength was inadequate to withstand the traction forces. Cook Pacemaker, Inc., (now Cook Vascular Inc., Vandergrift, Penna.) took another approach; they abandoned the concept of a universal stylet. Their first-generation locking stylet came in various sizes to fit a variety of conductor coil diameters (Fig. 21-24). The conductor coil had to be measured before selecting the locking stylet. This locking mechanism was a small wire welded to the tip of the stylet and wrapped around the lead. Once the lead was passed down the conductor coil to the electrode, it was rotated counterclockwise, bundling the free wire and causing it to bind against the conductor coil. The greater the traction, the greater the binding force. The locking stylet bound to the inner conductor coil, ideally at the distal electrode, functioned as a lead extender for applying traction and focused the traction force at the binding site. Focusing the traction force helped maintain the integrity of the lead but did not prevent lead disruption if excessive force was applied or if the lead had poor tensile strength. Also, the locking stylet was conductive, and the heart could be paced during parts of the lead extraction procedure if needed. This was the first effective locking stylet.

Cook's second-generation locking stylet (Wilkoff Locking Stylet) had a different locking mechanism (Fig. 21-25). These stylets had a small flange at the tip that was designed to stay flat against the stylet until the

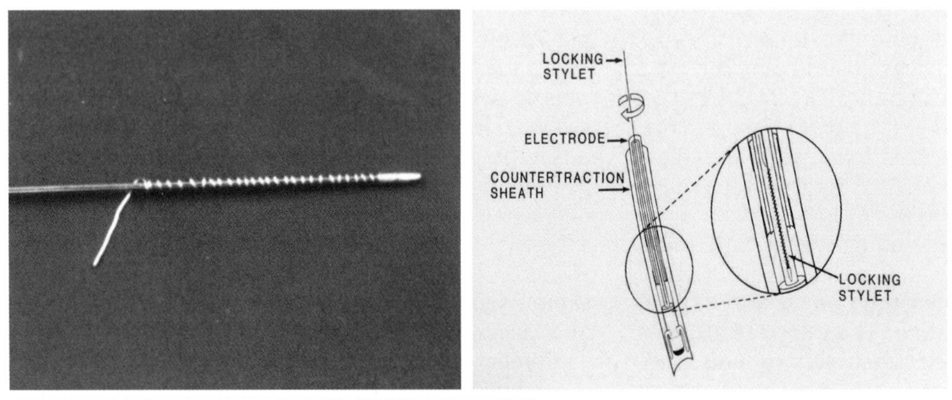

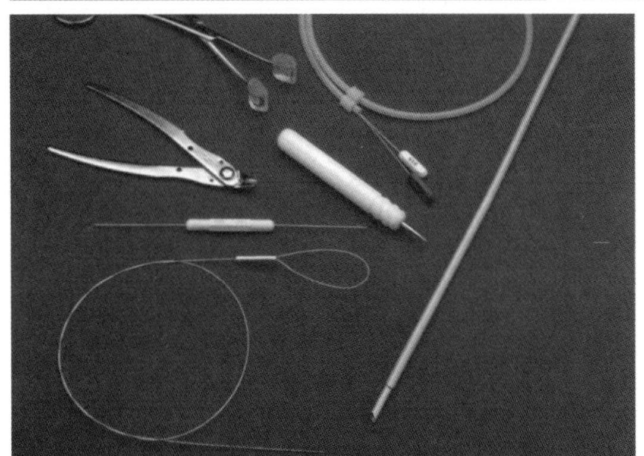

Figure 21-24. ***A,*** *Cook first-generation locking stylet. Ideally, the locking stylet is passed to the electrode and secured. The locking mechanism is a wire that is secured to the tip and wrapped around the stylet.* ***B,*** *When the stylet is turned counterclockwise, the wire bundles together, binding the stylet to the conductor coil. The locking stylet acts primarily as a lead extender to apply traction and secondarily to keep the lead intact during the extraction. When the stylet is positioned at the electrode, the lead has its best chance of remaining intact. If the stylet is positioned near the proximal end, the fragile leads will be pulled apart when traction is applied.* ***C,*** *Clockwise from lower left: locking stylet, sizing pin, lead cutter, corical coil expander, soft grip hemostat, standard stylets, and polypropylene telescoping sheaths.*

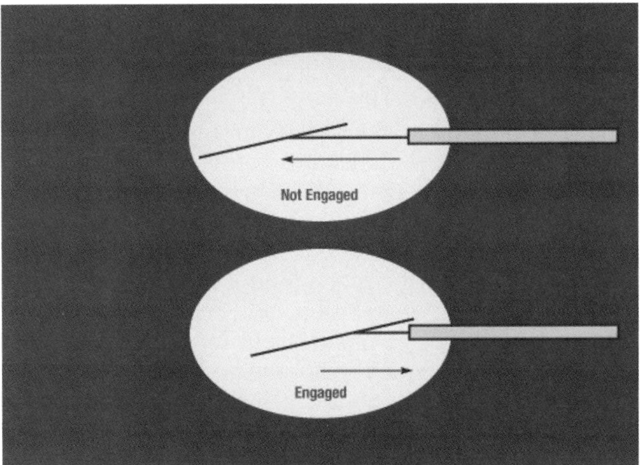

Figure 21-25. Cook second-generation locking stylet (Wilkoff Locking Stylet). The Wilkoff Locking Stylet employs a different mechanism for applying traction to the lead conductor at the tip of the lead. It also functions as a lead extender to lengthen the lead so that the sheaths can be advanced to the endocardial surface. The locking mechanism does not require precise measurement of the internal diameter of the conductor coil, and each size of the Wilkoff stylet bridges three sizes of the original locking stylet. The mechanism is activated by advancement of the thin cylinder, which nudges the hook to the side, engaging it between the coils of the conductor. This mechanism can be reversed and relocked but does not tolerate rotation. The response to rotation can be an advantage if the stylet needs to be removed.

preloaded thin cylinder was advanced; the cylinder deflected the flange to lock into the conductor coil. This was an efficient locking stylet that was easy to implant and could be removed by rotating the stylet, breaking the flange. However, it could not be used if the conductor coil diameter was 0.016 inches or less, and it could not be used with extendable/retractable screw-in leads. Spectranetics made the first near-universal locking stylet (Lead Locking Devices 1, 2, and 3), with three sizes to fit all leads. It used a long wire mesh that bundled and bound the stylet to the conductor coil. This type of locking stylet was efficient and functioned well. Cook's most resent locking stylet (Liberator Locking Stylet) is a true universal locking stylet (one size fits all). It uses a wire coil, which is compressed by a reloaded cylinder, expanding the wire coil and binding it against the conductor coil (Fig. 21-26). This is the only universal stylet on the market, and it has excellent performance.[34]

As mentioned earlier, the goals for inserting the locking stylet were to provide a lead extender and to focus the traction force at the tip to help maintain lead integrity. Although these goals were met, the insulation still has to be secured with a suture. Without traction to the insulation, it can "snow plow" and tear more easily, making passage of the extraction sheaths difficult, and in some cases preventing their passage. Therefore, traction should be applied to both the suture

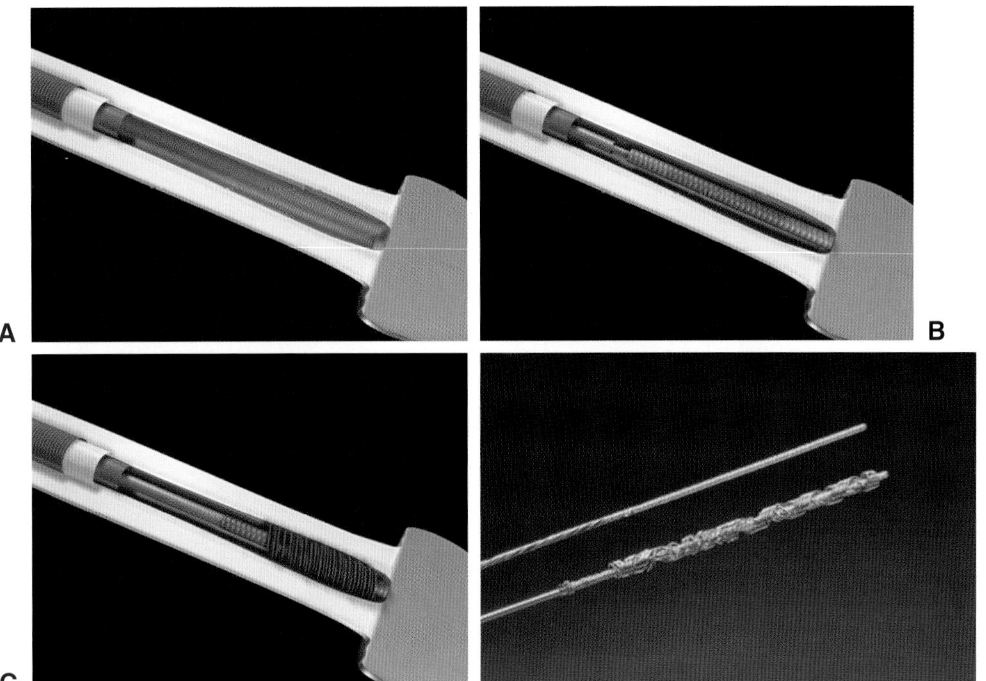

*Figure 21-26. Cook third-generation locking stylet (universal locking stylet). The universal locking stylet works by binding the locking stylet to the conductor coil. A wire coil is ideally positioned at the tip of the lead, near the distal electrode. The coil is expanded, binding the stylet to the lead's inner conductor coil. Traction increases the binding force. A universal locking stylet is possible today because of advances in technology. It is now possible to manufacture a stylet to fit the smallest conductor coil and still have sufficient tensile strength to support a wire coil large enough to bind to the largest diameter conductor coil. **A,** Lead conductor without the locking stylet. **B,** The liberator locket stylet has been advanced to the tip of the lead. **C,** The cylinder is pushed to crush the wire coil at the tip of the lead, locking to the conductor. **D,** Comparison of the inner wire with and without the wire coil at the tip of the universal or liberator locking stylet.*

(insulation) and the locking stylet (conductor coil) to be most effective.

Snares. Snares are used to grasp leads and to remove tissue in the bloodstream from the vein or transatrial entry site. The vein entry sites commonly used are the subclavian, internal jugular, and femoral veins. Only a few snares are safe to maneuver in the cardiovascular system or have the tensile strength to support the forces involved in a lead extraction procedure. The Dotter snare, Needle's Eye Snare (Cook), and Amplatz Goose Neck snare (ev3/Vasocare, Seoul, Korea) are discussed as examples of the types of snares available. The Dotter snare, together with a deflection catheter, is prepackaged in the femoral workstation. Before the availability of powered sheaths, lead breakage and the need to use a femoral approach were common. The only substitute for a snare is a cardiac surgical procedure. Consequently, facility with snares still is a requisite skill. Also, there are still extractors who do not use powered sheaths, relying only on the mechanical sheath extraction, and snares are integral to these procedures.

Reversible Loop. With the Dotter snare, a reversible loop is created around the lead body to pull the proximal end of the lead out of the superior veins into the IVC, without placing traction on the electrode myocardial interface (Fig. 21-27). A loop must be created and bound to the lead body. It is mandatory that the binding of the loop be reversible. Irreversibly binding the lead, or inability to remove the loop from around the lead, may result in dangerous traction maneuvers being performed in desperation while trying to extract the lead and snare. Failure to extract the lead subjects the patient to more invasive procedures to remove both the lead and snare.

Creating a reversible loop using two snares is a complicated maneuver requiring practice to perfect. One technique is to use a Cook deflecting wire guide and a Dotter basket snare. The Cook deflecting wire guide is wrapped more than 360 degrees around the lead body. Next, the tip of the deflection catheter is passed into the Dotter basket snare. When the basket snare is pulled into the workstation, the basket closes, grasping the deflection catheter and completing the loop. The loop is pulled into the workstation, tightly binding the lead body to the workstation, and traction is applied. If needed, the loop is relaxed and repositioned on the lead body. This sequence is repeated until the lead is pulled out of the superior veins, through the right atrium, and into the IVC. The reversible loop is then released, and the deflection catheter is removed.

The Needle's Eye Snare is a more efficient method of grasping the lead in a reversible fashion (Fig. 21-28). This snare has a wire loop that is passed over the lead body. A small wire loop tongue is then passed over the opposite side of the lead and into the larger wire loop tongue. Pulling this apparatus into the workstation binds the lead in a reversible manner for safe indirect traction. Also, the binding forces are more diffuse, resulting in fewer lead breakages.

The Goose Neck Snare is a radiopaque noose that is slipped over the free proximal end of a lead (Fig. 21-29). In situations in which the proximal end is floating in the SVC, heart, or a pulmonary vein, the free end can be lassoed and extracted.

Extraction Procedure Approaches

Extraction procedure approaches involve transvenous and cardiac surgical extraction techniques. Transve-

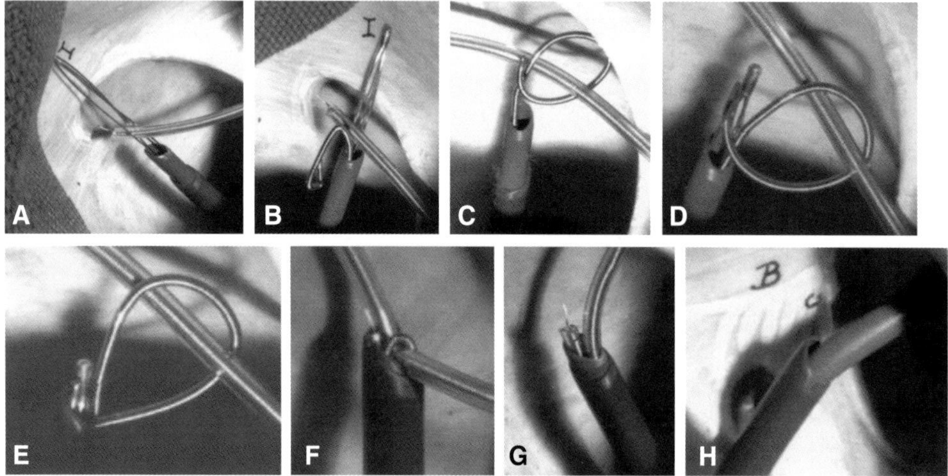

Figure 21-27. Cook femoral workstation (Byrd WorkStation). The workstation's two snares (Dotter basket and Cook deflection) were the first found by the author to have the versatility and tensile strength suitable for lead extraction. ***A,*** *Telescoping Teflon sheaths and Dotter snare advanced to the right atrium with lead body entangled in the snare. Pulling the lead into the sheaths for lead extraction is possible but not recommended because it is not reversible.* ***B,*** *Dotter snare and deflection catheter in atrium.* ***C,*** *Looping the lead body with the deflection catheter.* ***D,*** *Entangling the tip of the deflection catheter in the Dotter snare.* ***E*** *to* ***G,*** *Tightening the loop and pulling it into the Teflon sheaths.* ***H,*** *Sliding the telescoping sheaths to the electrode for removal using countertraction. At any time, the process can be reversed, freeing the lead.*

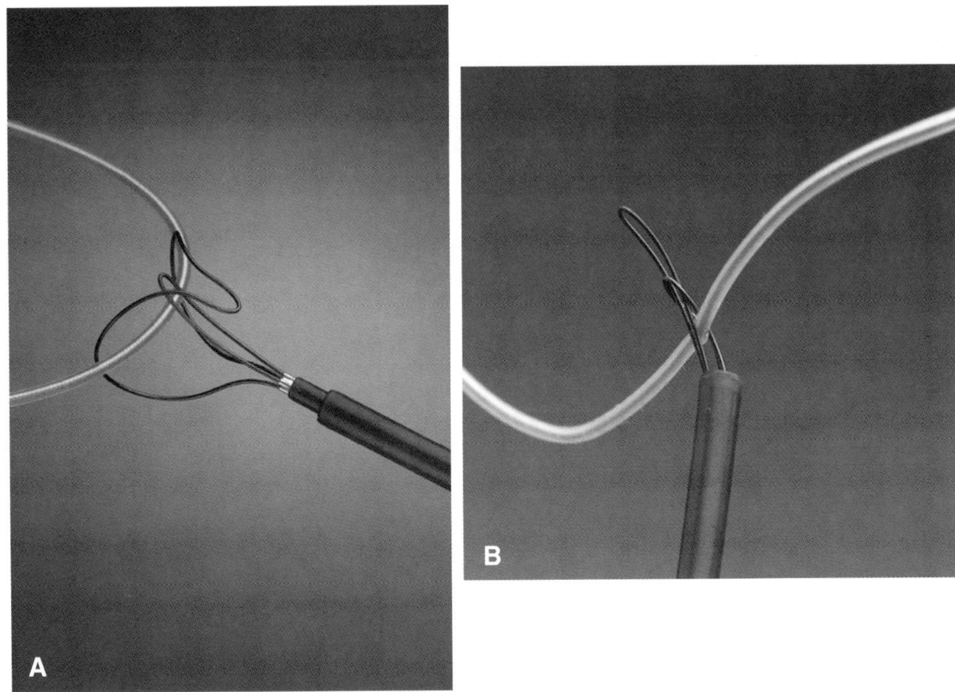

Figure 21-28. *Needle's Eye Snare. Cook's Needle's Eye Snare is the only reversible snare designed specifically for removing leads.* ***A,*** *The lead body is hooked, usually in the atrium, and the tongue is extended, forming a reversible loop.* ***B,*** *The lead body is pulled into the telescoping sheaths for lead removal.*

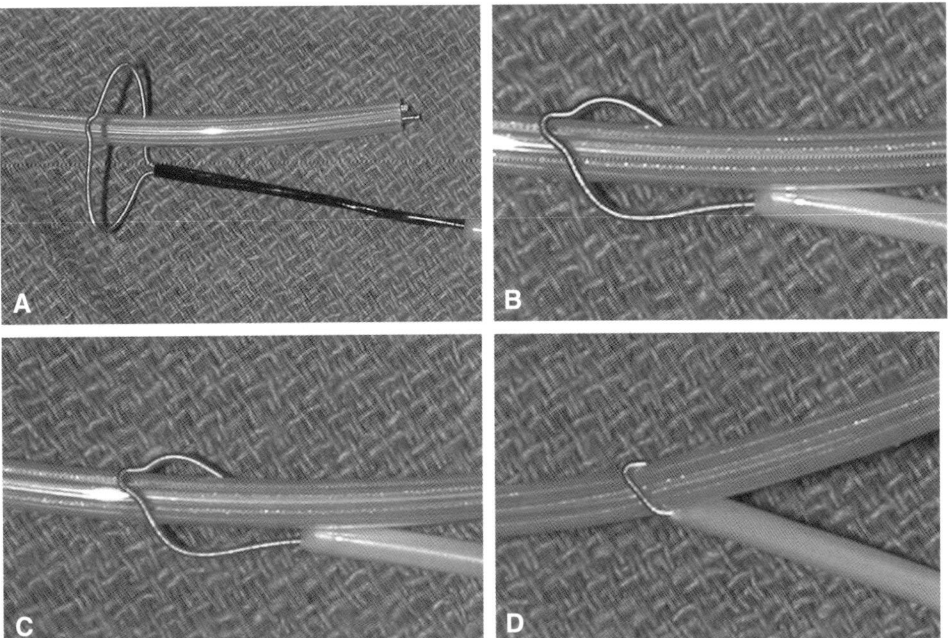

Figure 21-29. *Amplatz Goose Neck snare.* ***A*** *to* ***D,*** *The Goose Neck snare places a noose around the end of a lead and is pulled taut. The Goose Neck assembly is then pulled into telescoping sheaths for lead removal. This snare is reversible unless the assembly binds in the telescoping sheaths. In the author's experience, this snare is most effective for removal of small lead segments (e.g., electrodes, lead body segment) from small vessels such as hepatic veins, pulmonary arteries, azygos veins, and pelvic veins.*

nous approaches are usually performed through the lead implant site, but any other vein suitable for the extraction instruments may be used. Suitable veins include the axillary-subclavian-brachiocephalic, external jugular, internal jugular, and femoral-iliac. Cardiac surgical approaches to intravascular leads are transatrial, right ventriculotomy, and open heart surgery. All epicardial lead extractions are cardiac surgical procedures.

In the past, procedure approaches were separated into SVC and IVC approaches. An SVC approach is defined as the passage of lead extraction instruments through the vein entry site and down the SVC to the heart. The IVC approach was defined as a transfemoral approach using remote extraction instruments inserted in a femoral vein and passed through the IVC into the heart. This classification was based on the two types of extraction tools available at that time. Today, a more descriptive classification is to separate the approaches into transvenous and cardiac surgical procedures. Transvenous procedures are further divided into procedures through the vein entry site and those through a remote vein. Cardiac surgical procedures are separated into the individual cardiac surgical approaches: transatrial, ventriculotomy, and open heart.

The approach selected depends on the experience, extraction skills, and extraction instruments available to the physician; the reason for the lead extraction; and situations that arise during lead extraction. For example, a transvenous lead implanted in the right ventricle with a conductor coil fracture is ideally extracted from the vein entry site, using a powered sheath. A change in approach must be considered if this same lead is found to be attached to the lateral wall in the distal half of the SVC by a calcified mass of encapsulating tissue. A determination to continue the approach or a decision to choose a new one depends on experience and extraction skills. Two safe approaches are through the femoral vein using snares and via a transatrial cardiac surgical approach. If this same lead is found to have large solid thrombi measuring 4 × 8 cm, it is best extracted through a transatrial or an open heart procedure.

Extracting leads is dangerous if it is not properly performed. Procedures with these inherent dangers can be made safe only by knowledge of the pathology, pathophysiology, extraction skills, and available approaches. An example illustrating a potentially dangerous situation made safe by knowledge, training, and experience is flying. Flying an airplane has inherent, potentially life-threatening risks, but with proper training, experience, and "flying by the numbers," it is safe. A lead extraction performed in an organized step-by-step fashion, following known principles and proved guidelines, is equivalent to "flying by the numbers." The antithesis is "flying by the seat of your pants" or extracting a lead in a reckless, cavalier fashion, hoping for the best. While reading this section, remember that life-threatening complications are rare. During the evolution of lead extraction, the author and many others helped define the procedures, techniques, and approaches to minimize and hopefully eliminate complications of all types. The material presented represents more than 25 years of experiences that form the basis for current lead extraction procedures.

Transvenous Approaches

Lead Vein Entry Site. A transvenous approach through the lead vein entry site is a natural approach. After the pocket debridement procedure, which includes freeing the leads to near the vein entry site, it is natural to continue and remove the lead from this site. In some situations, the lead is broken or cut and retracted into the axillary-subclavian-brachiocephalic veins. If this lead can be grasped by an instrument passed into the vein and exteriorized, it is then considered to be a lead passing through the vein entry site for the purposes of this discussion. The lead can be extracted by direct traction, if applicable, or by a mechanical or powered telescopic sheath. This natural approach is used by most extractors today. Working through the vein entry site is efficient and subjects the patient and physician to the least amount of radiation. Efficiency includes the least number of maneuvers and the least amount of time required. Radiation exposure is related to the amount of fluoroscopy time. Also, once the lead is removed, a new lead may be readily inserted through the conduit created during the extraction.

Direct traction is the term used when traction is applied by pulling directly on the lead manually, with a suture or locking stylet or both. This is in contrast to *indirect traction,* which refers to grasping the lead with a snare and applying traction by the snare. Some leads are easily removed by direct traction.

The vein entry site is not always easily accessed. In some situations, the lead is entrapped in calcified encapsulating tissue and cannot be entered using the nonmetal extraction sheaths, with or without power. The cause of the calcified encapsulating tissue at the vein site is usually related to introducer technique. If the introducer needle scores the clavicle or first rib, elevating the periosteum, the periosteum will reform about the lead, entrapping it in a bone sheath. If the introducer needle passes through the costoclavicular ligament, this damaged tissue will mineralize and entrap the lead. It can also be postulated that natural maturation of a thrombus into fibrous tissue, which mineralizes with time, also leads to this problem. Although this can occur, the problem usually is associated with the periosteum and/or costoclavicular ligament. In this situation, metal sheaths are used.

Telescoping stainless steel metal sheaths look dangerous but are safe and effective if properly used (Fig. 21-30). The principle is simple: keep the sheaths tracking true over the lead, and apply the force needed to destroy this tissue. A combination of pushing and rotation of the beveled tip is most effective. Once the metal sheaths break into the vein, they are removed and replaced by plastic extraction sheaths. Tracking true is a principle used for all sheath maneuvers. All sheath maneuvering must be performed under fluoroscopy. This is to ensure that the sheaths are tracking over the lead. Any kinking or other deviation of the vein course

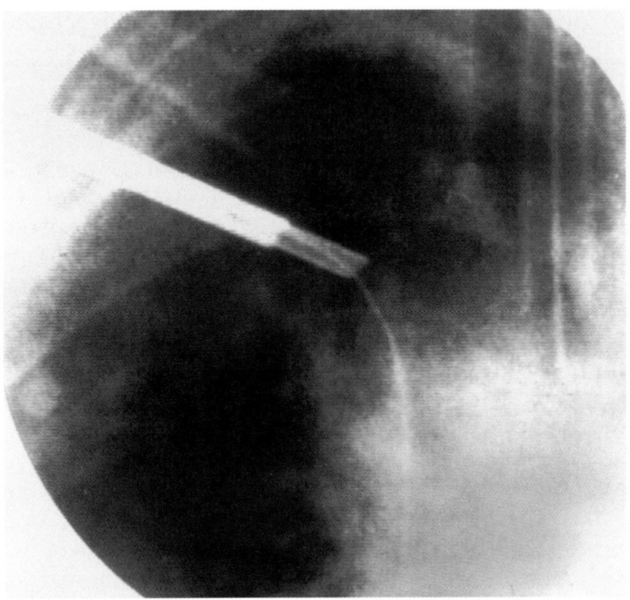

Figure 21-30. Stainless steel sheaths. Stainless steel sheaths are invaluable for freeing leads at the vein entry site that are entrapped in calcified tissue or bone (clavicle). They are remarkably safe when fluoroscopy is used to monitor all maneuvers and the sheath is not inserted past the end of the subclavian vein.

is dangerous. It creates a false passage that may be extravascular and may damage nearby structures.

Complications. Telescoping sheaths use a combination of countertraction, counterpressure, and tissue ablation (powered sheaths) to maneuver past the intravenous and intracardiac binding sites to the heart wall. These techniques, used with various types of sheaths, have already been described in detail. The maneuvering of these sheaths over the lead and down to the heart is separated into the three anatomic regions: axillary-subclavian-brachiocephalic veins, SVC, and intracardiac. This is the most dangerous portion of the procedure, and a detailed understanding of the issues unique to these three regions is essential for a safe and successful lead extraction. Complications associated with lead extraction involving loss of vein or heart wall integrity are tearing (including bone spicules), avulsion, rupturing, penetration, embedding of lead into the wall, and exclusion of the lead from the vascular space. The sequelae of these events are related to the anatomy of the region. The presence of fibrous tissue must be borne in mind when considering the anatomy of the region. Inflammatory reaction and the resultant fibrous tissue formation increase the tensile strength of the tissue. For example, a dissecting arterial hematoma or pericardial effusion is rarely seen in patients with previous open heart surgery, because scar tissue has the positive effect of reinforcing the tensile strength of the surrounding tissue. The forces required to tear aorta, subclavian, or innominate arteries or heart wall reinforced with scar tissue exceed those normally applied during lead extraction.

The axillary veins are surrounded by soft tissue on both sides, and the loss of vein wall integrity causes a low-pressure extravasation of blood, which is usually of no consequence. The subclavian-brachiocephalic veins are surrounded by structures which, if damaged, could lead to life-threatening consequences. On the left side, the vein is contiguous with the subclavian artery and aorta. During an inflammatory reaction, if the lead becomes embedded in the vein wall and involves the wall of the subclavian artery, innominate artery, or aorta, passage of extraction sheaths over the lead could tear these contiguous vessels, causing an arteriovenous fistula or a dissecting hematoma or both. The arteriovenous fistula could cause high-output heart failure, and the dissecting hematoma could cause major blood loss. If the hematoma ruptures into the left thoracic cavity, the resultant hemorrhage could be lethal. Immediate surgical intervention is required for a dissecting hematoma. An emergency median sternotomy provides satisfactory surgical exposure. If time permits, a minimally invasive approach may be preferable, especially for correction of a small arteriovenous fistula.

Also on the left side, it is common to maneuver in and out of the subclavian-brachiocephalic veins, causing low-pressure extravasation. After vein occlusion and organization, frequently all that is left is an atretic encapsulating fibrous tissue sheath (sometimes mineralized). For a single lead, the telescoping sheaths are, at times, larger than the circumference of this fibrous tissue sheath, and the entire capsule may be included along with the lead in the telescoping sheaths. If two or more leads are present, the circumference of the telescoping sheaths will remove at least one wall of the encapsulating sheath entirely or in segments. The resulting extravasation is not clinically significant with reasonable venous pressures. In those exceptional cases in which the venous pressure reaches a systemic level of 70 to 90 mm Hg, a dissecting hematoma would ensue, causing the same clinical scenario as described earlier.

The right-sided vein is contiguous with the right pleura. If the encapsulating fibrous tissue and embedded lead constitute the inferior vein wall, a tear in the pleura will result in hemorrhage into the right thoracic cavity. This can be lethal without immediate surgical intervention. The area is hard to reach through a median sternotomy or an anterior thoracotomy. Because of the time constraints, a median sternotomy with elevation of the clavicle and right anterior chest wall is radical but provides adequate exposure. In less urgent situations, the patient may be repositioned for a less extensive approach. Venous bleeding into the right chest, if not massive, can be insidious and may not be recognized until the onset of cardiovascular collapse. It is not painful, and the signs and symptoms associated with blood volume depletion can be masked by anesthesia or by increased catecholamines compensating for the low filling pressures. With sufficient blood loss, compensation is no longer possible, blood pressure falls, metabolic acidosis develops, and cardiovascular collapse ensues.

The SVC passes from the brachiocephalic veins to the right atrium. Along the upper half of the SVC, the lateral surface is contiguous with the right pleura, and the lower half is within the pericardium. Loss of integrity of the upper half results in blood loss into the right thoracic cavity; in the lower half, it causes cardiac tamponade. The sequelae of blood loss into the right chest are identical to those described for the right subclavian-brachiocephalic veins. In an emergency, a median sternotomy provides adequate exposure to either the upper or lower half of the SVC.

Cardiac Tamponade. Bleeding into the pericardial space causes a cardiac tamponade (pathologic cardiac compression). Small amounts of blood (approximately 200 mL), accumulating rapidly in the pericardium, will cause symptoms. Rapid accumulation increases ventricular wall compliance, decreasing filling of the ventricles and the resultant stroke volume. Rapidly accumulating blood in the pericardial space clots, whereas a slow accumulation does not. Clot formation can localize the compression, and some parts of the heart are more sensitive to compression than others. A 1-cm tear causes immediate tamponade with instantaneous decrease in systolic pressure. A precipitous drop of systolic blood pressure with failure to recover within 2 to 3 minutes is an emergency requiring immediate surgical intervention. The author uses this short time to confirm that the drop in pressure is real and not secondary to a technical issue by viewing the TEE and checking the pressure lines. The patient and operating field are then prepared for a median sternotomy. The TEE is usually definite, but if it is not, and no other cause is apparent, a tamponade must be considered the cause. The time constraints force a decision to be made within 2 to 3 minutes to prevent irreversible brain damage. A median sternotomy is used to decompress the pericardium, manually remove the clot, and surgically repair the tear. Needle aspiration and tube drainage are ineffectual for removing clot.

A tear in the lower half of the SVC measuring 2 mm is an example of a slow-onset pericardial effusion. A slow onset of tamponade, while maintaining a blood pressure, allows more time to confirm the tamponade and to make the decision of whether to use a less invasive pericardial drainage procedure. Pericardial drainage tubes inserted into a pericardial effusion are therapeutic in relieving the compression, with immediate restoration of blood pressure. It provides a drainage system for monitoring bleeding and in some cases for blood replacement, cell saver, or direct reinfusion, and it buys time to set up for a corrective surgical procedure. A rushed insertion of a percutaneous pericardial tube without an effusion being present can be a disaster. This is especially true in an enlarged heart if the diaphragm is penetrated and torn during insertion of the tube, creating the need for surgical correction. The only safe way to insert a pericardial tube without clear confirmation of the effusion is under direct vision. The safest approach is through a small subxyphoid incision that opens the pericardium under direct vision. Although the incision is slightly larger than for a percutaneous approach, it is safe.

Other conditions mimicking a tamponade are mechanical occlusion of the SVC, lead traction applied to the right ventricular wall decreasing compliance and filling, tachyarrhythmia, and metabolic acidosis from poor perfusion. Reflex therapeutic actions for a drop in blood pressure during lead removal include pausing lead extraction maneuvers (including lead traction), immediate intravenous administration of a vasopressor (Neo-Synephrine or Levophed), cardioversion of arrhythmias, and administration of sodium bicarbonate in low cardiac output situations. These reflex actions are used throughout any procedure, at any time, to compensate for transient decreases in filling pressure from the causes mentioned. They should be considered routine maintenance and not emergency treatment.

The right atrium and ventricle are also contained within the pericardium, and loss of wall integrity from a penetration, tear, or tissue avulsion can cause cardiac tamponade as described earlier. The treatment is the same. There are four mechanisms for tearing the wall not previously discussed: bone spicule laceration of the right atrium, chronic penetration of the right ventricle, fibrous tissue between the electrode and the heart wall, and size disparity between the electrode and the sheath.

The first mechanism involves a variation of the encapsulating tissue seen only in some extreme cases of mineralization. An example is a large silicone lead (>10F) that was in place for more than 20 years and making contact with the inferior-lateral atrial wall. The encapsulating tissue was completely mineralized, with "bonelike spicules" embedded within the wall. With any traction on the encapsulating sheath, the "bonelike spicules" acts as a knife blade, causing a surgical incision in the wall. This scenario is rare, but the author has seen it on two occasions. It has not been seen with any of the silicone leads manufactured since the late 1970s. To be safe, a lead bound to the lateral wall of the atrium should be removed with caution.

A second mechanism involves the application of countertraction in removing a lead from the ventricular wall. For example, an ICD lead implanted for 12 years is attached to the thin anterior wall of the right ventricle. The tissue at the electrode removed during the extraction contains epicardial fat, indicating a defect in the ventricular wall and suggesting that the electrode had penetrated the wall, most likely during implantation. Unless the lead has perforated and is positioned within the pericardial space, it is undetectable. Fortunately, this is a rare occurrence. This mechanism for tearing the heart has been observed twice by the author.

A third mechanism that could potentially tear the heart wall has not been seen by the author. It involves a band of tissue attached to the extracted electrode which is still connected to the heart wall. Continued traction on the freed lead could avulse the tissue or tear the heart wall. When this is seen, the sheath (preferably powered) is maneuvered until the band is cut. With mechanical sheaths, care must be taken with the force used to break the band. This mechanism is readily on fluoroscopy, and once it is recognized, care is taken.

A fourth mechanism is caused by a large size disparity between the extraction sheath and the lead.

Although this mechanism has been reported, it has not been seen by the author. If an attempt is made to apply countertraction with a sheath larger than the lead, the electrode and the ventricular wall will both be pulled into the sheath, potentially tearing the wall. Once the ventricular wall tissue is pulled into the sheath, it becomes a form of direct traction and not countertraction. For this to happen, the size difference between the lead and the sheath must be sufficient to accommodate the electrode-tissue mass. The cardiac tissue being pulled into the sheath cannot be seen. The only protection is avoiding large size differences between the lead and the sheath. Unfortunately, this is not always possible. For example, the smallest laser sheath is 12F with a 16F outer sheath, so extracting a 4F lead involves a sizable mismatch, and care must be taken. Also, a 9F sheath may have to be changed to an 11F sheath to include calcified encapsulating tissue, resulting in a size mismatch during countertraction.

Today, the vast majority of leads are successfully removed through the vein entry site. The current procedures and extraction tools provide a safe, reliable, and effective method of removing these leads from most of the pathologic environments created at the biophysical interface. Recognizing the limits of an extraction approach (i.e., a dangerous situation) and changing to a more appropriate, safe approach is the key to eliminating complications. A national lead extraction database no longer exists, and extraction data are now kept by individual practitioners. Individual data are considered anecdotal, and the data from one individual cannot be extrapolated to another. Consequently, it is impossible to quote meaningful lead extraction statistics, and the author's experiences must be placed in this context. These comments apply to most of the lead extraction discussions.

Remote Vein Sites. A remote vein site is a vein other than the lead vein entry site. A remote vein site requires a remote instrument, such as some type of snare, to manipulate the lead. The femoral vein was the first remote vein site used. During the early evolution of lead extraction, removing leads with mechanical sheaths from the superior veins via the vein entry site was frequently a failure and potentially dangerous. A more difficult approach through a femoral or other remote vein site was more effective and safer. The problems were related to maneuvering the long telescoping mechanical sheaths from the femoral vein to the heart wall and the complexities associated with grasping the lead body. With the advent of powered sheaths, the safety and efficacy of removing leads from the vein entry site improved dramatically. Although most of the leads can be removed from the vein entry site, there are still dangerous situations and lead breakages. In these cases, a remote vein or a transatrial cardiac surgical procedure are the only options. In many cases, the femoral vein approach is still the best remote vein approach. However, other remote veins (contralateral external jugular, internal jugular, or axillary-subclavian-brachiocephalic) may be more suitable and easier to use. Some physicians have developed combination approaches, applying mechanical sheaths from both the vein entry site and a remote vein site. This combination constitutes a safe and efficacious approach that is still used by some extractors today. For cases such as lead breakage, use of a snare to grasp the lead and the subsequent removal of the lead using direct traction or a powered sheath is advantageous. Powered sheaths are usually not long enough for a femoral approach. Consequently, these approaches are confined to the superior veins, via both remote and vein entry sites.

The techniques used involve manipulation of snares to grasp the lead body. Although these techniques are simple in principle, they can be difficult to achieve in a timely fashion. Initially, there were no snares designed for lead removal, so a suitable off-the-shelf ("off-label") snare designed for other purposes had to be found. The author's criteria for such a snare included the tensile strength to withstand the forces applied during lead extraction, safety of the surrounding tissue when maneuvering the snare, and reversibility of the grasping mechanism. The Dotter snare was the first snare to meet the tensile strength requirements. When the Dotter snare was combined with the Cook deflection snare, the safety and reversibility requirements were met. Later, two snares were manufactured meeting these requirements: Cook developed the Needle's Eye snare and the Amplatz Goose Neck snare, which are still in use today.

A classification of remote vein approaches deviates from the historic use of the IVC (femoral vein) approach. A natural classification is to employ the removed vein (e.g., femoral approach, internal jugular approach). A detailed discussion of remote vein site usage will be made based on this natural classification. The goal is the same as for the vein entry discussion: to define the approach, procedure techniques, and expected results in relation to the pathology and pathophysiology associated with the implanted lead.

Femoral Approach. Before the advent of powered sheaths, the femoral approach was used extensively. The indications for its use were failure to extract leads from the superior veins by any technique, lead breakage, and avoidance of the application of excessive force with the mechanical sheaths. The techniques used have not evolved significantly over the past 15 years. The transvenous approach through a femoral vein requires a special sheath set (Byrd WorkStation) that functions as an introducer, as a workstation for manipulation of snares, and as countertraction sheaths (Fig. 21-31). The set consists of an introducer needle, a guidewire, a 16F workstation, an 11F tapered dilator, an 11F telescoping sheath, a Cook deflection snare, and a Dotter basket snare. The workstation serves many functions. Initially, it acts as a protective sheath. The outer sheath prevents the insertion, withdrawal, and manipulation of the inner sheath and snares from damaging the veins or heart. To prevent clot formation, the workstation has a valve (Check-Flo) to continuously irrigate the sheath. The workstation and snares form a reversible loop to pull the proximal portion of the lead out of the superior veins; the workstation also acts as the outer

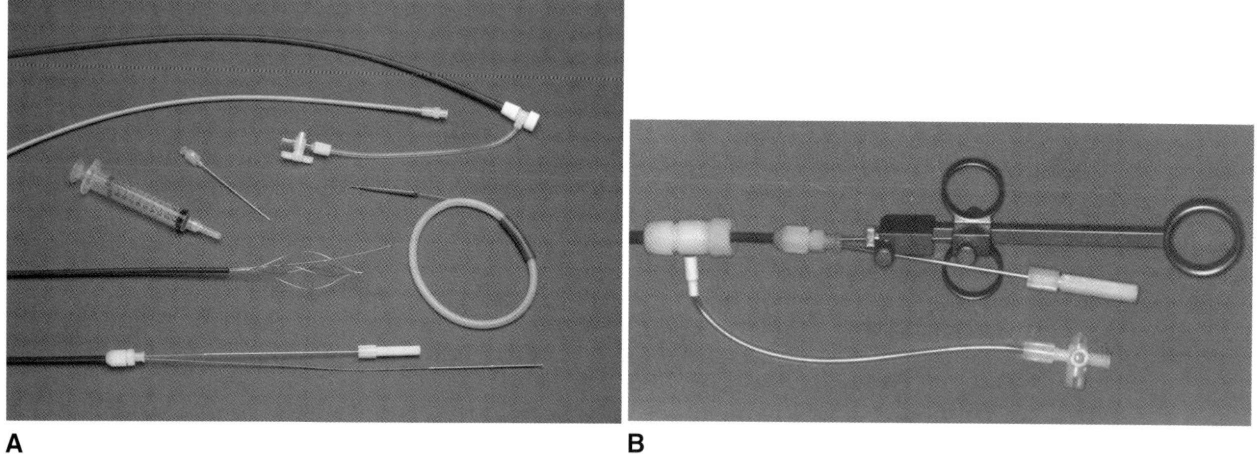

A B

Figure 21-31. *Byrd Femoral WorkStation. Telescoping sheaths are passed to the heart. The outer sheath functions as a workstation protecting the vein and heart wall during maneuvering of the inner sheath. Once the lead is secured by the reversible loop, the sheaths are advanced to the electrode to apply countertraction.* ***A,*** *The workstation is packaged with telescoping sheaths, guidewire, and dilator to be inserted like an introducer. The dilator is removed and the snares inserted.* ***B,*** *Check-Flo valve with the Dotter snare and deflection catheter. The deflection catheter requires a special, nondisposable handle to manipulate the tip of the deflection catheter, forming a reversible loop. The Dotter snare can be maneuvered using a plastic knob or a surgical clamp.*

telescoping countertraction sheath. The safe insertion and removal of the workstation is a prerequisite for an extraction procedure through a femoral vein. The workstation is 16F and must be inserted with care. Fluoroscopic monitoring is mandatory. Once the guidewire is passed into the heart, the workstation with its tapered dilator must be maneuvered through the iliac vein and IVC and into the right atrium. The route can be circuitous, especially from the left side. In rare cases, the curvature may be too sharp for the stiff dilator to follow the guidewire. Forcing the dilator in this situation is unsafe, and the approach should be abandoned. A torn retroperitoneal iliac vein or IVC is a serious complication. Once the workstation is inserted, irrigation fluids are run continuously through the Check-Flo valve to prevent clotting.

Pulling leads down and out of the superior veins has been remarkably successful. Many leads freed from the heart cannot be pulled up through these same veins. The lead binding forces caused by the circumferential bands of fibrous tissue are the same in both directions. The author's hypothesis for this difference is the free upward mobility of the mediastinal structures and the inability to pull the superior veins downward. The mediastinum is easily pulled upward, compressing the veins. This compression of the fibrous tissue bands around the lead as they bunch together is postulated to increase the binding strength. The superior veins cannot be pulled downward, and irreversible lead slippage through the binding sites is not an issue. Cardiac function is not influenced by pulling leads downward out of the superior veins. Failures to extract the proximal lead from the superior veins using this technique are rare and are usually caused by other complicating factors. Examples of complicating factors are thrombosis of the superior veins and excessive fibrosis around the lead caused by a previous extraction attempt that left the conductor coil exposed or pulled the lead taut against the heart and vein wall. Such leads are removed using approaches such as the transatrial approach, which are reserved for more complicated extractions.

To apply countertraction through the workstation, the proximal end of the lead must be entangled in the basket snare. This is accomplished by placing the basket snare in close proximity to the lead and rotating it slowly. The lead will flip into the basket. The basket closes when the 11F sheath is advanced over the snare. For most leads, the snare and lead are pulled into the 11F sheath. The workstation and 11F sheaths are then worked in a telescoping fashion to a point near the electrode. At this point, countertraction is applied to extract the electrode, as previously described. Removal of the workstation must be carefully performed. Once the lead is extracted, clot and debris may be attached to the end of the tubing. If this material dislodges in the femoral vein entry site, it can act as a nidus, forming a thrombus or initiating thrombophlebitis and its sequelae. To prevent this complication, blood is aspirated during the withdrawal of the workstation. If the entry site does not bleed freely after withdrawal of the workstation, a surgical exploration of the vein is recommended. Bleeding is controlled by applying pressure over the vein entry site after withdrawal of the sheath and during Valsalva maneuvers induced by the anesthesiologist. A suture or staple is required to close the skin. A potential complication is thrombophlebitis and pulmonary embolus. Fear of this complication was the incentive for the workstation. Postoperatively, anti-emboli stockings (pneumatic, if possible) and subcutaneous heparin (5000 units twice a day) are the only precautions taken.

The technique for grasping the lead in a reversible loop using a Cook deflection catheter and a Dotter snare is more complicated. Once mastered, it is an effective method of performing precision extraction. For example, a patient may have six leads in the heart. Two new leads are connected to a pacemaker and are to be saved. Four leads are abandoned and are to be extracted. The abandoned atrial and ventricular leads can be extracted, leaving the newly implanted leads intact. The IVC approach allows this level of precision.

Superior Vein Approaches. The other transvenous approaches include the external, internal jugular, and axillary-subclavian-brachiocephalic veins, usually on the contralateral side. The telescoping sheaths used with the femoral approach are mechanical (powered sheaths are not available). The creation of a conduit by the powered sheaths from the vein entry site encourages the use of snares passed through these sheaths to remove leads (e.g., broken free floating leads). A snare is used to grasp the lead, and, if needed, sheaths are passed over the snare to the lead. The difference is in the extraction tools available. For example, the femoral workstation is too long and is not applicable for the superior vein approaches. Using standard introducer techniques, a guidewire is inserted and telescoping mechanical sheaths are passed into the SVC or heart. These sheaths then act as a workstation for passage and manipulation of a snare. The same snares used for the femoral approach are usable with the superior vein approaches. The Needle's Eye Snare has a shorter, easier to use version for the superior veins. Once snared, the lead can be removed using indirect traction, mechanical sheaths, or powered sheaths. The noose snares are also effective from the superior approaches. All of the principles and guidelines for lead extraction apply to these approaches.

Combined Vein Entry and Remote Entry Approaches. To some degree, most remote approaches are a combination of a vein entry site and a femoral vein approach. An extensive effort may have been used to free the lead from the superior veins; this was always in preparation for the intended use of the remote approach. From its inception, some physicians championed the use of a combined approach. Initially, the vein entry approach and femoral vein approach were combined, sometimes with two teams working, one for each approach. The goal was to free the lead by applying the extraction techniques from both approaches and removing the lead in an opportunistic fashion (the resultant easiest approach). It was not uncommon to have the EP working from the vein entry site and a radiologist from the femoral vein site. Although this approach was successful, it was overkill for most lead extractions. This was especially true once powered sheaths became available.

A combination of the vein entry site approach and a right internal jugular approach is used by some physicians as their primary approach to lead extraction. They use snares and/or a grasping instrument passed through the internal jugular vein into the SVC to pull the lead out of the axillary-subclavian-brachiocephalic veins and, if necessary, to pull the lead into the atrium. Mechanical sheaths are then applied to complete the extraction (to date, powered sheaths are not used).[35]

The techniques used with remote approaches can be applied through the vein entry site. A lead may have broken or been cut, retracting into the axillary-subclavian-brachiocephalic veins, floating in the SVC or heart, or migrating into the pulmonary veins. If the lead can be reached and grasped inside the axillary-subclavian-brachiocephalic veins by a surgical instrument, it can be pulled out of the vein entry site and secured with a suture or a locking stylet, or both. The lead can then be extracted using the vein entry approach. If the lead cannot be grasped by an instrument but a snare can be passed into the SVC from the vein entry site or a contralateral vein, the lead is grasped and removed using mechanical and/or powered sheaths. Before powered sheaths became available, the femoral approach was commonly used by the author, but today it is rarely used. Surgical EPs have the transatrial approach as a viable alternative. Regardless of the frequency of use today, the transfemoral approach is a requisite procedure required for managing device-related complications.

Surgical Approaches

The surgical approach to lead extraction is a cardiac surgical procedure. There are three procedures used for transvenous endocardial implants: the transatrial approach, right ventriculotomy, and an open heart procedure using cardiopulmonary bypass (CPB). In the author's opinion, these procedures should be performed only by experienced cardiac surgeons. The technical and patient management skills possessed by an experienced cardiac surgeon negate the normal risk associated with the increased magnitude and complexity of the surgical procedure.

The transatrial procedure is a general procedure that can be used for both extraction and implantation of leads. It can be used instead of the transvenous remote approach for lead extraction. It has the added advantage of being an implantation site that bypasses the SVC and IVC. The right ventriculotomy is a technique for removing leads from the right ventricle in special situations. Today, an open heart procedure is reserved for removing thrombotic material (usually infected) from the right atrium and ventricle and for removing leads implanted in the left ventricle.

Transatrial Approach. The transatrial approach was first described by the author in 1985.[36] This surgical EP procedure is suitable for intracardiac EP implantation, explantation, and ablation procedures. The only disadvantages are the morbidity associated with surgical thoracic pain and the fact that a medical EP must work with a cardiac surgeon to perform this procedure. It is a primary approach for noninfected patients who are candidates for a transatrial lead implantation. Younger patients with occlusion of one brachiocephalic vein or with an SVC syndrome have the old leads extracted through a transatrial approach, followed by implantation of new leads. The advantage of the transatrial approach is the ability to remove leads that are not accessible or removable by the SVC or IVC approach.

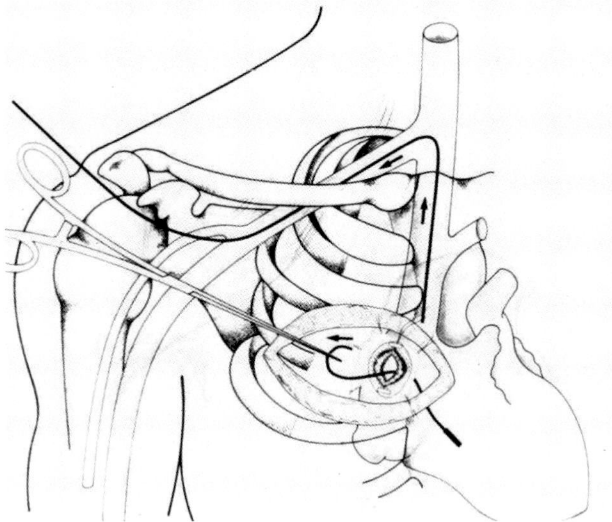

Figure 21-32. Transatrial approach. This is a minimally invasive cardiac surgical approach. The third or fourth cartilage is removed, and a pursestring suture is placed in the right atrium. A pituitary rongeur is inserted through the atriotomy incision and used to grasp the lead. The proximal portion of the lead body is removed from the superior veins by direct traction, and the distal lead is removed by mechanical and/or powered sheaths and countertraction.

Most of the transatrial extractions are failures of the IVC approach. Rarely, failure of a SVC approach will lead directly to a transatrial approach (e.g., when the workstation cannot be passed via the femoral veins into the heart). Infected patients who are candidates for transatrial lead implants will have the leads extracted by an SVC or IVC approach and the transatrial implantation performed after the infection is properly treated.

The transatrial approach is performed as originally described, through a limited surgical incision on the right anterior chest wall (Fig. 21-32). The right atrium is exposed by removal of the third or fourth right costal cartilage (determined by fluoroscopy). The pericardium is opened and suspended, and a pledgeted pursestring suture placed in the right atrium. If the pericardium has been obliterated from a previous procedure or disease process, a small region of the lateral wall of the right atrium is dissected free. Using fluoroscopy, a pituitary biopsy instrument is inserted through the purse string. The lead body is grasped in the atrium and pulled out. The lead is then cut, extracting the proximal and distal segments separately. The proximal portion of the lead can usually be pulled out by direct traction. The only limitation to the force employed is the tensile strength of the lead. On those occasions where the tensile strength is insufficient, telescoping powered sheaths may be required. The distal segment is extracted by inserting a locking stylet, advancing telescoping powered sheaths to the wall, and removing the electrode from the wall using countertraction. This procedure is repeated for each lead to be extracted. On completion of the lead extraction, the atriotomy site is used to insert new leads, or to perform another EP procedure, or the pursestring is tightened, tied, and abandoned.

After transatrial extraction, patient management is more involved than for the transvenous extraction techniques. The pericardium must be drained, in most cases by a closed drainage system such as a chest tube, if the pleural space is free; by a mediastinal tube, if the pleural space is obliterated; or by a Jackson-Pratt closed drainage system, if both the pleural and pericardial spaces are obliterated. The thoracic cavity is occasionally entered and a chest tube inserted to drain both the pericardium and pleura. These drainage tubes are removed in 2 to 3 days. The procedure-related morbidity increases the hospital stay by 1 or 2 days, compared with a transvenous procedure. Patients must be managed in an intensive care setting until the thoracic pain sequelae are controlled.

Right Ventriculotomy. A right ventriculotomy is a cardiovascular surgical procedure. This approach is rare for the author to use, and its frequency of use by others is unknown. Because this procedure is virtually unknown, a cursory discussion of indications for use is in order. Initially, it was reserved for infected broken leads retained in the right ventricle that were not reachable by the other approaches. These are fragile leads that break near the ventricular wall or within a fibrous tissue tunnel along the ventricular wall and are impossible to grasp using transvenous or transatrial techniques. It is also used in conjunction with lead penetration requiring lead removal and a repair of the heart wall, and possibly for an emergency tear in the ventricular wall caused by an attempt to remove a lead. In the latter, the defect is turned into a ventriculotomy site for lead extraction.

The first ventriculotomy procedures were performed by the author in the late 1980s. The heart is exposed through a median sternotomy incision. The heart is then elevated on a pad, exposing the right ventricle. The tip of the electrode is localized by fluoroscopy and by using needles for triangulation of the electrode. A pursestring suture is placed around the electrode, and a ventriculotomy incision is made to the electrode. The electrode is grasped with a clamp and pulled out of the heart. Because the lead segment is being pulled in the direction of the tines, the tines slip out of the embedding scar without resistance. Today, the procedure is performed through a minimally invasive incision on the anterior surface of the left chest through the fifth intercostal space. The pursestring and extraction techniques are the same. The author performs no more than one or two of these procedures a year. This is a stressful procedure, and it is not known how many procedures need to be done to acquire some comfort level. As long as there is a need for the procedure, continuing attempts will be made to perfect it.

Open Heart Procedure. The concept of using CPB to perform an open heart procedure is intuitively obvious. It is a standard cardiac surgical procedure involving a median sternotomy incision. Because of its familiarity, the issues associated with this approach need no further discussion. Right-sided leads were initially

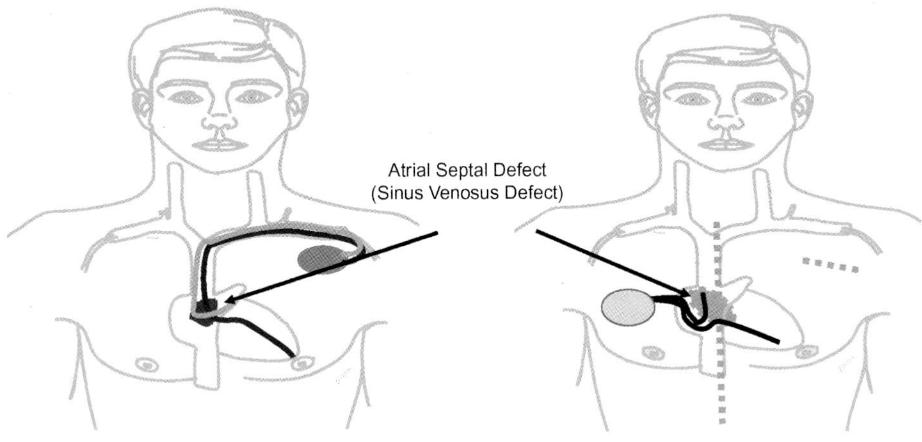

Figure 21-33. Left-sided implantation. Transvenous implantation in the left atrium and/or ventricle or a transarterial implantation through the aortic valve into the left ventricle is rare. A transvenous implantation through an atrial septal defect (ASD) such as a sinus venosus defect is the most common (left). *The anatomy guides the leads into the left atrium. Extraction of these leads is dangerous because of the potential for an arterial embolization of debris. The author performs these procedures with the use of cardiopulmonary bypass, repairing the congenital defect after lead extraction* (right). *After extraction, the left ventricle is monitored by transesophageal echocardiography, and all debris is removed through an incision in the aorta before bypass support is removed. The new pacemaker or ICD is implanted transatrially to avoid passing the lead through the junction of the superior vena cava and atrium.*

removed by direct traction and under direct vision during open heart surgery. Transvenous and transatrial lead extraction techniques evolved to eliminate the need for an open heart surgical procedure.

Implantation of leads in the left atrium and ventricle is a notable exception (Fig. 21-33). Leads are implanted into the left ventricle in two ways: through a congenital atrial or ventricular septal defect, or retrograde through the aortic valve. The author is amazed at the diversity of opinions expressed concerning the management of these leads. All consider the presence of left-sided leads and embolic symptoms an urgent indication for lead removal. Most consider their presence, with the potential for a complication, to be an urgent indication for lead extraction. A few physicians believe that, in the absence of complications (cerebrovascular accident, coronary artery occlusion, infarction of another other organ, or the sequelae of a peripheral embolus), leaving the leads intact is an acceptable option. The rationale is that the extraction procedure is more dangerous than the presence of left-sided leads. In contrast, the author believes that the presence of these leads in the left atrium and/or ventricle is an indication for urgent lead removal. The views on lead removal are just as varied. Some believe the leads should be removed; the chambers debrided of vegetation; and congenital defects, if present, repaired with the use of CPB. Others think it is safe to extract the leads using the established right-sided techniques and protecting the brain from emboli by compressing the carotid arteries when necessary. The author believes the leads should be removed using total bypass with the aorta cross-clamped, and congenital defects should be repaired. If the second approach has any merit, it would be in removing newly implanted leads. If the newly implanted leads are proved to be free of vegetation and the procedure is monitored using TEE, it is probably safe to extract using direct traction. Specific data are not available on the numbers of physicians using these opinions.

The author's experience is based on the management of 10 consecutive patients, most of whom had chronic leads and were symptomatic. Symptoms included transient ischemic attack and/or cerebrovascular accident, and vegetation was apparent in symptomatic patients. All but one patient had leads passing from right to left through an atrial septal defect. One patient had a lead that was implanted through the subclavian artery and passed retrograde through the aortic valve into the left ventricle. The procedure included establishing CPB, using cardioplegia to stop ventricular contraction, cross-clamping the aorta as needed, extracting the leads using conventional tools, debriding the chambers, repairing the septal defects, continuously observing the left atrium and ventricle by TEE, and carefully restarting the heart with protection from inadvertent ejection of embolic material. A new transatrial right-sided implantation was performed off bypass with the use of fluoroscopy and the conventional approach. With this technique, the leads were all removed, the congenital defects were repaired, and the new devices were implanted without sequelae. From the encapsulating fibrous tissue and vegetation present, the author cannot envision a less complex procedure that would be safe. To develop a safe technique not employing an open heart procedure is difficult to imagine.

Special Situations

The most interesting development in lead extraction has been the interest in placing leads into the coronary sinus and cardiac veins. Left atrial leads for sensing and stimulation and defibrillator leads to improve defibrillation thresholds are nothing new, but they were not frequently used in the past. Cardiac resynchronization therapy has made this a frequent and evolving issue. The experience of extracting these leads has so far not been very interesting. Partially this is true because of the short implantation durations and partially it is related to the simple and extraction-friendly designs of the leads. Smooth, thin, single-diameter unipolar leads with good tensile properties are all characteristics that enhance the safe and quick removal of the leads. However, because physicians and manufacturers have been concerned with the stability of these leads in the cardiac veins, they have been developed into more complicated shapes, multipolar, and with fixation mechanisms. These leads are not likely to be so easily removed.

As an evaluation of extraction tools and a novel lead design technique to reduce the barriers to extraction of complicated leads, the author participated in a study that used a sheep model with atrial defibrillator leads placed into the coronary sinus to the great cardiac vein. The leads, originally designed for atrial defibrillation in the METRIX atrial defibrillator (InControl, Redmond, Wash.), were modified but kept their pigtail configuration for lead stability. Three configurations—one without modification of the defibrillation coil, one with medical adhesive backfill under the defibrillation coil, and one covered with ePTFE—were implanted in sheep and were subjected to extraction at either 6 or 14 months. The model proved to be an excellent one for developing profound fibrosis, and the unmodified leads were almost impossible to remove without hemopericardium. The medical adhesive backfill was much better, and there was almost no trouble removing the ePTFE-covered leads. The study also demonstrated that laser sheaths were dangerous in the coronary sinus, because the sheath approximated the size of the vein, and that a special 7F electrosurgical extraction sheath was relatively much safer to use. During the procedures, the electrosurgical sheath was rotated away from the pericardial and toward the myocardial surface.[37]

Overall, coronary sinus lead extraction has not become a clinical issue, but it will, and when it does, hopefully the implanters will have made sound decisions that promote the extraction of these leads. From the sheep experience, it appears clear that implanters should at all costs avoid construction that allows for tissue ingrowth.

Lead Implantation Skills

Implantation skills are possessed by all who practice device implantation. The implantation skills required to manage device-related complications are, at times, more demanding. In some situations, conventional implantation techniques are not suitable, and a more exotic approach is required, such as a transvenous femoral approach or a cardiac surgical transatrial or epicardial approach. Device implantation is covered in a rigorous manner in other chapters of this book. Only those principles and guidelines believed to be essential to managing device-related complications are reviewed here. Because the goal is to reimplant without creating another acute or chronic complication, emphasis is placed on the situations that cause complications and the techniques used to prevent them. To avoid confusion, implantation techniques are separated into components: reimplant location and lead insertion techniques, endocardial implantation techniques, and epicardial lead implantation techniques. Focusing on each of these components provides a natural order for discussion.

Reimplant Location and Lead Insertion Techniques

Reimplant location and implantation techniques are the primary determinants of implant longevity relative to a specific lead. For implanted leads to survive without a complication for 30 to more than 60 years requires a remarkable combination of events. Implantation decisions are believed to be one of the key factors influencing the duration of an implant.

Reimplantation locations include those sites that are accessible by transvenous approaches and cardiac approaches. Picking the appropriate site should be based on reason and not expedience. For example, questions such as, "Can a temporary lead be implanted after debridement at an infected vein entry site?" "Is the extraction site suitable for lead reimplantation?" "Which remote vein is useable?" "Do I have the knowledge and skill level to reimplant in this situation?" and "What are the long-term consequences of using a particular implant approach?" must all be answered in a satisfactory manner. The answers to these types of questions help prevent acute or chronic reimplantation complications. The only way to answer these questions is to have thorough understanding of the potential complications associated with various reimplantation locations and techniques. Most complications are related to anatomic considerations, and a presentation based on the anatomy is beneficial. Knowledge of complications based on anatomic considerations allows natural and rational reimplantation decisions.

To reimplant a lead at the lead extraction site, if appropriate, is natural and convenient. The goal is to use the old, damaged implant site for as long as possible. The most versatile technique is to insert a guide wire through the extraction sheath after removal of the old lead. The extraction sheath is then removed, leaving the guidewire in place. A conduit now exists for reimplantation using a long introducer set. A useful guideline is to keep a guidewire in place throughout the procedure for conduit security. Although some veins are patent, many are not, and the conduit created by the extraction sheath is a natural channel for reimplantation. To avoid losing this conduit, always insert a guidewire before removal of the extraction sheaths, and use an introducer that is long enough to reach the right atrium. The long introducer ensures lead passage through obstructions in the brachiocephalic vein and proximal SVC. Loss of the conduit requires the use of an alternative reimplantation approach.

An alternative technique is to leave the extraction sheath in place and insert the new lead and guidewire through the extraction sheath. Then, to remove the sheath, it has to be split (destroyed). Split-sheath technique cannot be used with powered sheaths. Powered sheaths can be used to remove more than one lead and cannot be destroyed. Mechanical sheaths are usually damaged and not reused, encouraging the split-sheath technique to avoid the use of a long introducer.

Permanent lead reimplantation through the vein entry site into the axillary-subclavian-brachiocephalic veins is contraindicated in the presence of a device-related infection, vein occlusion with poor collateral drainage, damage to arterial structures from improper implantation, or lead exclusion from the vein. These four contraindications are intuitively obvious. A lead placed back through a carefully debrided infected site will probably get infected. The one exception is the implantation of a temporary lead. Once the area is debrided, this is safe for at least 1 week. The remaining three conditions are contraindications for all types of leads due to the potential for propagation of vein thrombosis toward the arm, arterial bleeding from arteries damaged during the old lead implantation (healed or small arteriovenous fistulae), and the erosion of old leads into an artery. The rationale for not implanting a lead in the presence of arterial damage is clear, but venous occlusion with poor collateral flow needs further discussion. Venous occlusion is a common occurrence at the vein entry site due to tissue injury and initial clot formation (Fig. 21-34A). Venous occlusion in this area is rarely a complication, because the collateral venous drainage is usually adequate to support all activity levels. Unfortunately, the exact incidence is unknown. Occasionally, a patient will have poor collaterals and be symptomatic with pain and swelling usually in the arm. Placing a lead in this low-flow environment constitutes an ideal condition for continued vein thrombosis with retrograde propagation. Symptomatic patients are candidates for a venous stent (see Fig. 21-34B). In the past, placing a lead through a stent was considered unwise, but it has been done successfully with no reports of adverse consequences.[20] Placement of leads first, followed by a stent, leaves the lead pinned against the vein wall and difficult to extract. Treatment of adult patients with transposition of the great arteries after childhood surgical atrial baffle construction has yielded SVC stenosis in many, often after pacemaker or ICD placement. Because trapping of the leads is a far worse choice, extraction and reimplantation after stenting of the stenosis has been become the treatment of choice. However in the author's opinion, the presence of an occlusion with poor collateral drainage is a contraindication to lead implantation.

The presence of a contraindication related to the biophysical interface or loss of the conduit after lead

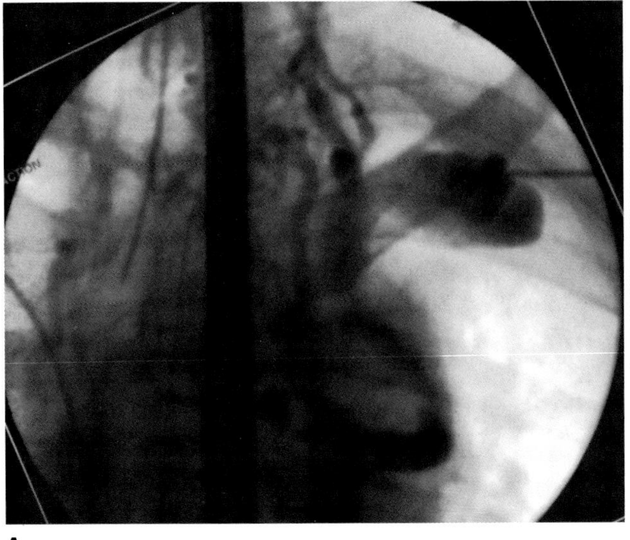

A

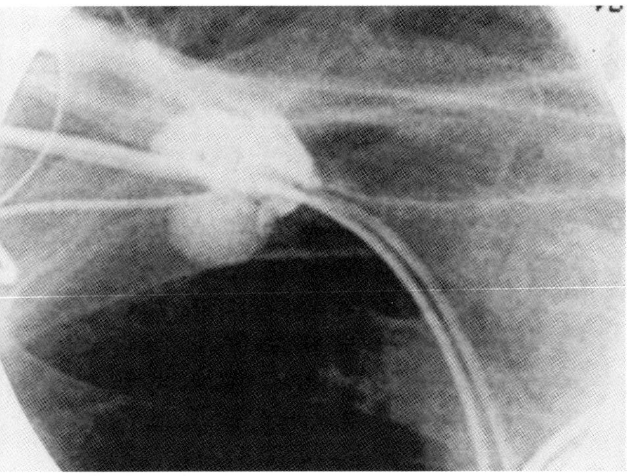

B

Figure 21-34. Occlusion of subclavian-brachiocephalic veins. Occlusion of the subclavian-brachiocephalic veins is common and is rarely symptomatic. Acute occlusion may cause transient signs and symptoms; chronic occlusions are usually asymptomatic. Collateral flow is rich in this area and quickly compensates. ***A,*** *Partial occlusion of the subclavian vein and total occlusion of the brachiocephalic with sufficient collateral flow. Implantation through a conduit created by lead extraction is not contraindicated.* ***B,*** *Occlusion of the subclavian vein with little collateral flow. An occluded subclavian vein must have adequate collateral vein formation and blood flow. The subclavian vein is the most commonly occluded superior vein. The presence of adequate collateral vein flow is a criterion for reimplantation through the conduit created during the lead extraction. If the patient is symptomatic, a stent may be effective, but implantation of a permanent lead through a created conduit could cause retrograde vein thrombosis.*

extraction necessitates reimplantation through a transvenous, transatrial, or epicardial approach. Use of the external jugular and internal jugular tributaries to the axillary-subclavian-brachiocephalic veins is included in the ipsilateral contraindications. Options for location and implantation technique depend on the status of the biophysical interface and the patient's age. Most patients have a contralateral vein in good condition, and it seems natural on an abstract level to use this vein. The technique for insertion of a new lead into the contralateral vein is the same as for inserting a new lead for a primary implantation. Unless the physician is experienced in managing device-related complications, an implantation technique based on preconceived beliefs acquired from training and other experiences may not meet the desired goal of having the highest probability of achieving a long-term, complication-free implant. The following discussion of implant technique, based on the anatomy of the axillary-subclavian-brachiocephalic veins and surrounding musculoskeletal system, is derived from the author's opinion and interpretation. Although the discussions are generally applicable to either the right or left side, exceptions will be noted.

Transvenous Approaches

Contralateral Veins. The contralateral veins include the cephalic, subclavian, brachiocephalic, internal jugular, and external jugular. The internal and external jugulars are of interest only if the proximal subclavian vein is occluded. The author has one relative and two absolute contraindications to contralateral vein implantation. These contraindications are based on the author's experiences and the availability of surgical procedures. Medical EPs should be familiar with the logic and, whenever possible, should work with a cardiac surgeon. Sending the patient to a cardiac surgeon without EP experience is usually unsatisfactory.

The relative contraindication involves young patients who have an occluded ipsilateral subclavian-brachiocephalic vein (Fig. 21-35A). These patients' internal and external jugular veins do not drain into the subclavian-brachiocephalic veins. Consequently, all the venous drainage is by collateral flow. Although the collateral flow may be adequate, it is a dynamic pathologic condition that can change with time. For example, the initial collateralization is usually through neck veins. With time, this can shift to the veins on the chest wall. If the transition is not smooth, the patient becomes symptomatic. Implantation in the contralateral vein could result in an occlusion of the contralateral subclavian-brachiocephalic veins, causing the equivalent of an SVC syndrome (poor drainage of the head and upper extremities). This potential complication should be prevented whenever possible, especially in younger patients. It is easier to prevent than to correct.

Partial occlusion of the SVC is an absolute contraindication to venous reimplantation (see Fig. 21-35B). Reimplantation from either side through the partial occlusion has a high probability of completely occluding the SVC. An occlusion occurring over a short

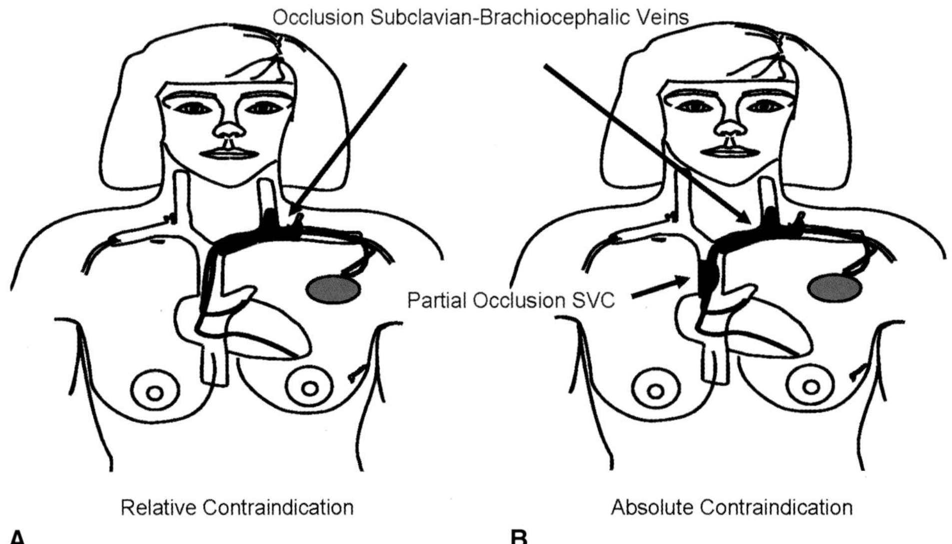

Figure 21-35. Contraindication to contralateral implantation. Occlusion of the ipsilateral subclavian-brachiocephalic veins is frequently an indication for a contralateral implantation. ***A,*** *A relative contraindication to contralateral implantation is a young patient at risk for a similar situation on the contralateral side, creating the equivalent of a superior vena cava (SVC) occlusion.* ***B,*** *Ipsilateral occlusion in conjunction with a partial occlusion of the proximal SVC is an absolute contraindication, because of its potential to completely occlude the SVC. The author uses the transatrial implantation approach to avoid the superior veins in these situations.*

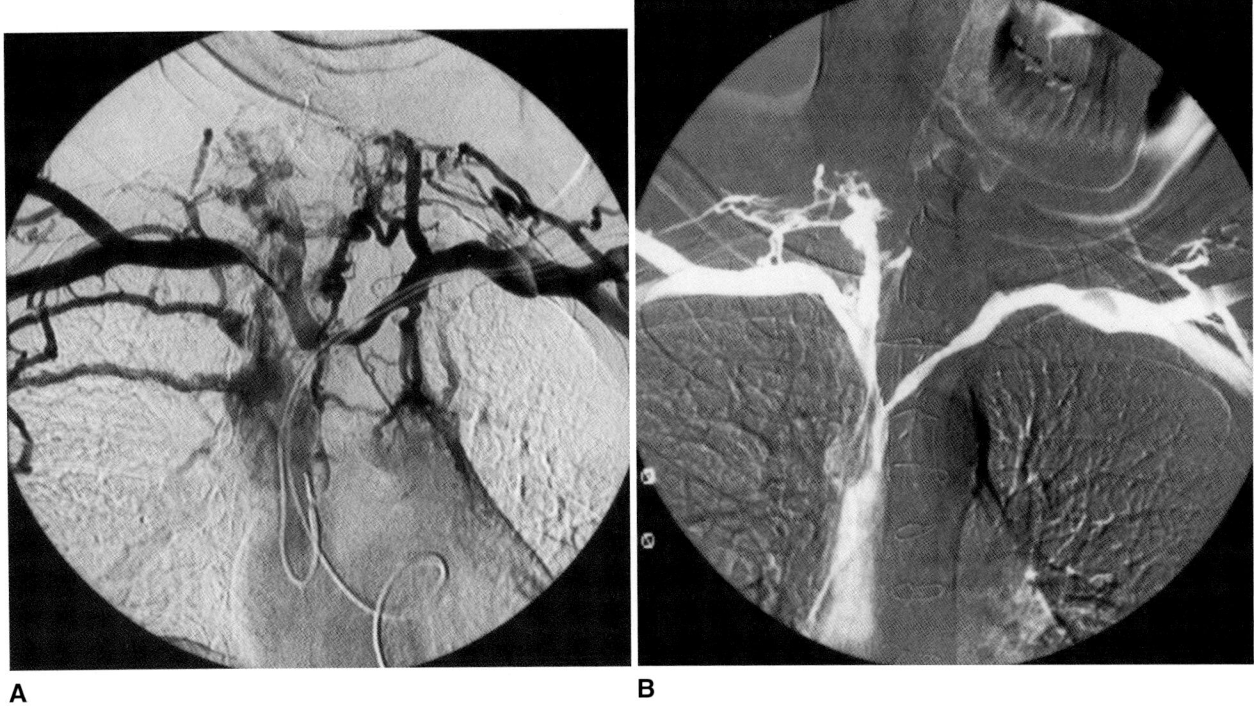

Figure 21-36. Occlusion of the superior vena cava (SVC). This 8-year-old occlusion of the SVC has inadequate collateral vein formation for an active young patient. ***A,*** *A venogram demonstrating occlusion of the SVC, collateral veins, and implanted atrial and ventricular leads.* ***B,*** *The brachiocephalic vein and SVC are shown to be patent 6 months after surgical correction. The veins are repaired by debridement of the organized intravenous inflammatory tissue and a vein patch angioplasty. The patient is symptom free and has a marked reduction of the collateral venous drainage.*

period of time will cause an SVC syndrome; if it occurs over a long period of time, the symptoms will depend on the adequacy of the collateral drainage and the activity level of the patient. Total occlusion of the SVC is an intuitively obvious contraindication (Fig. 21-36A). These patients are candidates only for a transatrial, epicardial, or femoral approach. Only the transatrial approach can duplicate a transvenous venous superior vein approach. The author repairs SVC occlusions in all physically active patients (see Fig. 21-36B). Initially, these procedures were performed through a median sternotomy incision. Today, they are performed using a right parasternal approach similar to the transatrial approach. These repairs are done without CPB through a minimally invasive procedure and have been successful. Despite the repair of the SVC, the pacemaker or ICD must be implanted using an alternative approach (e.g., transatrial).

The other absolute contraindication is the presence of anomalous venous drainage (Fig. 21-37). For example, abandonment of a right ipsilateral implantation and substitution of a contralateral implantation through a persistent left vena cava draining the left contralateral veins into the coronary sinus is not acceptable. The implantation of a lead through this congenital abnormality is possible, but difficult. Thrombosis and subsequent occlusion of the persistent vena cava are equivalent to occlusion of the brachiocephalic vein, and extraction of these leads is difficult and dangerous.

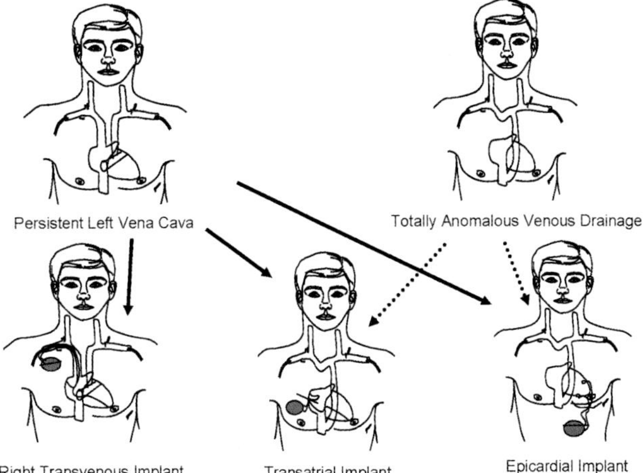

Figure 21-37. Anomalous drainage of the superior vena cava. Anomalous drainage of the superior veins is in many cases a contraindication to superior vein implantation, although it is technically possible. Implantation in a persistent left vena cava is contraindicated in the presence of an occlusion of the right subclavian-brachiocephalic vein. Implantation in any superior vein is contraindicated in the presence of totally anomalous drainage of the superior veins. The rationale for these statements is the perceived greater risk of occlusion of anomalous veins after lead implantation.

Because of these two potential problems, the author elevates this type implantation to an absolute contraindication. The same logic applies to initial implantation or reimplantation into a totally anomalous venous drainage, usually into the IVC. The difference is that a subsequent occlusion of the totally anomalous vein is equivalent to a SVC occlusion.

Axillary and Cephalic Veins. The axillary vein is the large vein that carries most of the venous drainage from an upper extremity. It begins at the confluence of the brachial and basilic veins near the teres major and subscapularis muscles. The axillary vein changes its name to subclavian vein as it crosses the outer border of the first rib. The cephalic vein drains into the middle to distal portion of the axillary vein. The distal axillary vein and cephalic veins are considered safe insertion sites.

An occlusion of the axillary vein at the confluence of the arm veins is a devastating complication. It is almost impossible to acquire acute collateral circulation sufficient to support the blood flow from the arm. The resultant venous distention causes a swollen, painful extremity. Any increase in cardiac output to the extremity from activity and/or anxiety makes the situation worse. In some cases, collateral circulation capable of supporting resting blood flow develops after many years. There is no known treatment for this complication. Anticoagulation helps prevent further thrombus formation and worsening of the situation. To help prevent this complication, the proximal portion of the axillary vein should never be used as an implantation site.

Cephalic vein implantation is argued by many to be the gold standard. It is a surgical cutdown on the vein within the deltopectoral groove. Insertion of the lead at this site is safe (i.e., no chance for a pneumothorax or hemothorax), and the lead passes over the first rib in the subclavian groove. A diminutive vein that is not suitable for a lead insertion can always be instrumented with a guidewire. This statement needs to be qualified: "always" is correct in the author's experience. However, it can be a technically challenging procedure requiring a variety of guidewires, fluoroscopy, and a venogram to be successful. Fortunately, the introducer approach offers an alternative to this approach. A small artery runs parallel to the cephalic vein. If it bleeds and is not controlled, a high-pressure hematoma can develop, applying pressure to the proximal portion of the axillary vein. External pressure can occlude the vein and cause vein thrombosis. This complication can be prevented by suture-ligation of the artery if it appears damaged or bleeds.

It should be mentioned that safe insertion into the distal axillary vein is relative. Occlusion near the vein entry site is common and would not affect the drainage from the arm. However, retrograde extension of clot from a thrombosed cephalic or subclavian vein into the confluence of the arm veins can result in an irreversible complication. This is rare. Usually, the collateral flow from the axillary vein is significant, and the fast venous flow prevents further retrograde propagation of a clot.

As the subclavian vein passes from the lateral to the medial border of the first rib, it is still outside the thoracic cavity (extrathoracic). Starting at the medial aspect of the first rib, it lies within the thoracic inlet and is intrathoracic. The thoracic inlet is the apex of the thorax, which is separated from the thoracic cavity by the pleura. The subclavian vein passes over the extrathoracic portion of the first rib in the subclavian vein groove and anterior to the attachment of the anterior scalene muscle. The distal portion of the axillary vein and the proximal portion of the subclavian vein on the first rib are usually free from implantation complications.

The intrathoracic approach was the initial introducer procedure. The goal was to cannulate the subclavian vein within the thoracic inlet. The technique is to pass the introducer needle under the clavicle and over the first rib and puncture the anterior surface of the subclavian vein. In an idealized approach, the introducer needle can be passed from within the pocket, cannulate the subclavian vein without entering the pleura, and avoid binding the lead between the clavicle and first rib. Despite the plethora of literature on this subject, experience and judgment are the only predictors of success.

Two extreme techniques introduced to help prevent complications were the "medial" and "lateral" approaches (Fig. 21-38). The medial technique was to pass the needle between the clavicle and first rib as medial as possible, through the costoclavicular ligament. This technique placed the needle into the anterior portion of the thoracic inlet, away from the pleura, helping prevent a pneumothorax. The disadvantage of

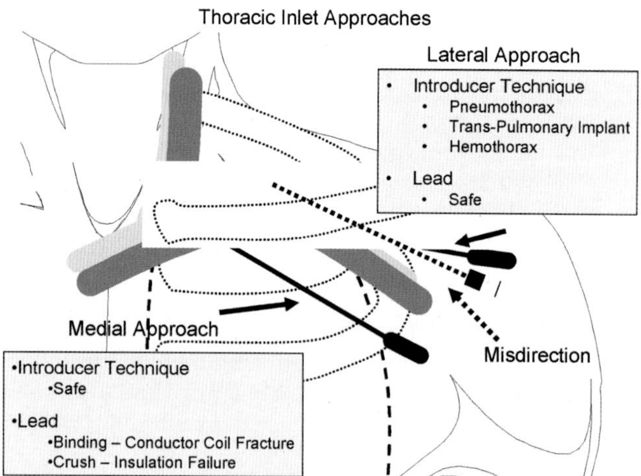

Figure 21-38. Intrathoracic (thoracic inlet) introducer approaches. Two introducer approaches, medial and lateral, demonstrate the issues associated with inserting introducers in the intrathoracic portion of the subclavian vein. The medial approach is safe, but the leads are subjected to crush (insulation failure) and binding (conductor coil fracture). The lateral approach is free from lead crush and binding, and it is safe when the needle is properly directed. Because of variation in chest wall anatomy, extensive experience is needed to avoid misdirection with the introducer needle and potentially lethal complications such as pneumothorax, hemothorax, or a transpulmonary-vein implantation.

this approach is the binding and compression to which the lead is subjected, which increases the probability of insulation and/or conductor coil failure. The lateral approach was designed to place the introducer needle in the anterior portion of the thoracic inlet, free from the binding and compression forces present in a more medial approach. Although this lateral approach was successful, it was more complicated. A lateral safe zone was defined by the author using fluoroscopy and based primarily on the presence of adequate spacing (>1 cm) between the clavicle and first rib.[38] This spacing was an attempt to ensure lead passage in the subclavian groove. An anatomic variable determined the location of the safe zone, but training, judgment, and experience were still factors in its application. The extrathoracic approach was published along with the lateral safe zone technique. It was presented as an alternative technique suitable for all situations. At the time it was presented, it was considered a more radical approach.

Misadventures with an introducer needle within the thoracic inlet can cause pneumothorax (needle puncture of the lung) and/or hemothorax (needle tear of the pleura and subclavian artery and/or vein). Also, insertion of a lead into the right brachiocephalic-SVC vein from the right side is difficult to do without passing through the apex of the right lung, causing both a pneumothorax and a hemothorax. Removal of an introducer or lead accidentally inserted within the subclavian artery can cause bleeding into the thoracic inlet, with the potential for a lethal rupture into the thoracic cavity. All of these complications are potentially life-threatening if not recognized and treated in a timely fashion. Treatment may include major thoracic and cardiovascular procedures. Because of the variations in anatomy, the only way to guarantee these complications can be avoided is to stay out of the thoracic inlet.

Two complications are associated with leads placed medially between the clavicle and first rib into the thoracic inlet. The first complication is related to lead binding. Passage of the introducer needle through the subclavius muscle or the costoclavicular ligament can result in calcification of those structures. Lead binding occurs when the lead body becomes entrapped in the encapsulating calcified tissue. If a lead with coaxial cabling is rigidly bound, the helix cannot bend to relieve stress, and the conductor coil at each end of the binding site becomes deformed. If the wire is configured as a helix, bending the helix back and forth does not affect the wire because the coils of the helix flex, preventing deformation of the wire itself. Binding of the helix prevents it from flexing, and the wire will be deformed at the junction between the bound and unbound helix. The second complication is related to pinching (crush injury) of the lead between the clavicle and first rib. This type of compression injury damages the lead body insulation. The loss of integrity of the polymers caused by compression injury results in inner insulation failure, resulting in make-break signals and short-circuiting between the inner and outer coils. Outer insulation failure is of consequence only if the exposed wire senses electrical signals, interfering with communication between the pulse generator and the heart.

The intrathoracic approach has been reallocated to a support role or an alternative approach for most physicians managing device-related complications. Although the extrathoracic approach is favored by most, there is still a place for the intrathoracic approach. For example, this approach combined with venography is useful for passing localized occlusions in the axillary and proximal subclavian veins. The distal subclavian and proximal brachiocephalic veins can be instrumented in some situations. However, to eliminate both the acute and the chronic complications associated with the thoracic inlet, an extrathoracic approach is recommended by the author. There are two extrathoracic approaches: introducer and cutdown. The author believes that the extrathoracic introducer approach is the safest, most efficient, and most versatile approach available. The lead is inserted into the subclavian vein as it passes over the first rib in the subclavian vein groove. This routing eliminates crush injury, pneumothorax, and intrathoracic arterial or venous bleeding associated with the thoracic inlet. This is a fluoroscopic technique; it should not be done without direct visualization of the first rib and the introducer needle in an anterior-posterior view. For orientation, the needle is passed from the pocket area to the clavicle. The needle is then passed posterior to the first rib. Without visualization, directing the needle posteriorly and missing the first rib would result in puncturing the lung and a pneumothorax. To maintain orientation, contact should actually be made with the first rib, followed by aspiration on withdrawal. The needle is marched anteriorly or posteriorly along the first rib until the vein is located. The subclavian artery marks the posterior boundary of the posterior march. The subclavian vein is always anterior to the artery. A direct puncture of the artery over the first rib is of no consequence because it is easy to apply pressure, if necessary, for a few minutes to prevent hematoma formation. Once the vein is located, a guidewire is passed to the heart, and a long curved introducer is inserted into the right atrium.

The location of the subclavian vein on the first rib is based on fluoroscopic landmarks. In an anterior-posterior view, the clavicle appears to cross over the first rib. The subclavian vein is in the region where the outer border of the clavicle crosses the rib (Fig. 21-39). To visualize the anatomy, the first rib is divided into three equal segments, starting anteriorly at the sternum. The clavicle most commonly crosses the first rib in the second segment, indicating that the subclavian vein most commonly crosses in the second segment. However, a few are located in the third segment or, rarely, in the first segment. This coincides with the three general chest wall types distinguished by the position of the shoulder.[39] A descriptive name such as an anterior rotation, normal rotation, and posterior rotation is sufficient to describe the visual appearance of the chest wall types. These terms correspond to passage of the subclavian vein over the first, second, and third segments of the first rib, respectively. Because

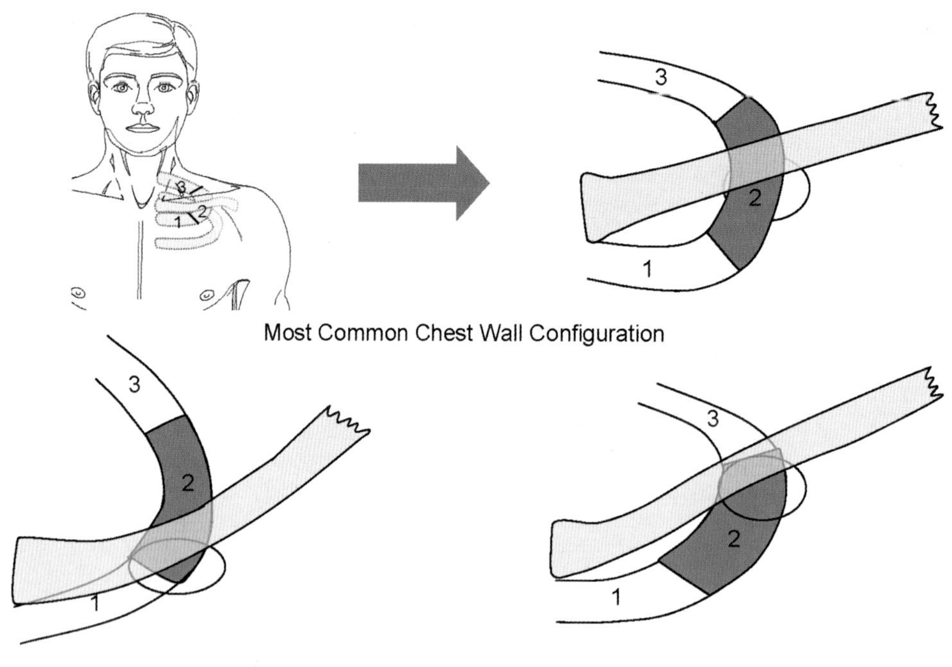

Figure 21-39. Extrathoracic introducer technique. The technique is to puncture the subclavian vein outside the thoracic cavity, in the subclavian groove as it passes over the first rib. This approach is safe and is free from lead-related issues, and the technique is the same for all chest wall configurations. The puncture site is the point at which the subclavian vein passes over the first rib beneath the anterior edge of the clavicle, as seen in an anterior-posterior fluoroscopic view. Three chest wall configurations are defined by where the clavicle crosses the first rib, which is divided visually into three equal segments (anterior to posterior). The most common crossing site is in the midportion of the second segment. Less frequent are anterior first segment crossings and posterior crossings near or on the third segment.

shoulder rotation and location of the subclavian vein are related, recognition of the type shoulder rotation may be helpful, but a fluoroscopic view showing the crossing of the clavicle and first rib is definitive. A subclavian vein passing over the first or second segment of the first rib can usually be instrumented from a conventional pocket incision. This is not usually possible with a posterior rotation of the shoulder, which positions the vein over the third segment. A needle puncture from within the pocket causes the angle between the long axis of the needle and the vein to approach 90 degrees. This is not satisfactory, and a separate small incision superior to the pocket incision is necessary to obtain an angle of 45 degrees or less. Otherwise, the lead-vein entry angle will cause problems maneuvering the lead, biophysical interface issues such as pain, and/or stress-related lead integrity issues such as insulation failure or conductor coil fracture.

A second extrathoracic approach is a cutdown to the cephalic vein. The cephalic vein travels through the deltopectoral groove and enters the distal portion of the axillary vein. This approach has always been touted as the gold standard. Because this vein is extrathoracic and pneumothorax-hemothorax is not an issue, comparing an introducer with this approach was like arguing against "motherhood and apple pie." In truth, a large, patent cephalic vein is easy to cannulate, and two leads can usually be inserted. Even a small vein can be dilated to accommodate multiple leads by using a guidewire and inserting an introducer. However, there are two disadvantages to a cutdown approach: small vein size and lead removal. The surgical dissection to locate a small cephalic vein (<1 mm diameter) with a circuitous route to the axillary vein can be challenging; skill and experience are required to cannulate and maneuver into the axillary vein. In these cases, even if the vein can be instrumented, passing a guidewire through the circuitous route requires fluoroscopy, venography, and an improvised technique to direct the guidewire. The most difficult anatomic variations are caused by a posterior rotation of the shoulder and third segment subclavian vein location. This anatomic variation makes the introducer technique more difficult. Lead extraction from the cephalic vein is often more difficult and is associated with more difficult hemostasis.

Both of these extrathoracic approaches achieve the same goals of lead passage in the subclavian groove over the first rib and elimination of the serious introducer-related complications. However, because of the efficiency of the introducer technique and the requirement of an introducer for a high percentage of cutdowns, only the inexperienced, masochistic, or "diehard cutdown enthusiast" can seriously argue for a primary cutdown approach.

Femoral-Iliac Vein. The transvenous femoral vein is the remaining alternative for medical EP implanters when the contralateral superior veins are occluded.[40]

The femoral-iliac veins are readily accessible and easy to implant but are limited in usefulness. The primary limitation is the lack of appropriate-length leads. In some patients, lead lengths of 80 to 100 cm may be required to travel from the implantation site in the heart, down to the vein entry site, and back onto the abdominal wall. Extenders may be used with pacemaker leads, but not with ICD leads. The clinical sequelae associated with instrumentation of the femoral-iliac veins are not known. The potential for an acute complication such as phlebitis and large clot formation caused by the leads damaging the vein walls is unknown. Pulmonary embolus is the major cause for concern, although this has not been a factor in the limited clinical experience. The question is not whether transfemoral implantation is technically feasible, but whether it is an acceptable long-term alternative. In general, any vein large enough to accept an introducer guidewire can be used as an implantation site. The author has used, in addition, the hepatic vein and the IVC near the junction with the atrium.

Transatrial Implantation

The other commonly used implantation approaches are the transatrial and epicardial cardiac surgical approaches. The transatrial approach combines surgical and endocardial implantation techniques and is the most efficacious alternative approach, in the author's opinion.

The transatrial cardiac surgical approach was described in detail in the section on lead extraction.[36] It is primarily an endocardial implantation procedure, using conventional state-of-the-art transvenous leads, and requires cardiac surgery only to access the atrium (Fig. 21-40). In the author's opinion, this is an ideal alternative to contralateral vein implantation. The procedure is safe and has demonstrated long-term results for both pacemaker and ICD implants. It is natural to combine the transatrial extraction and implantation procedures in a manner similar to transvenous implantations. Also, in the author's experience, for especially difficult or complicated cases, a transatrial lead extraction is safe and efficient, and, except for short broken leads in the right ventricle, all leads can be extracted using this approach. Again in the author's experience, transatrial extraction and/or implantation is considered a fail-safe procedure and a frequent alternative to the transvenous approach.

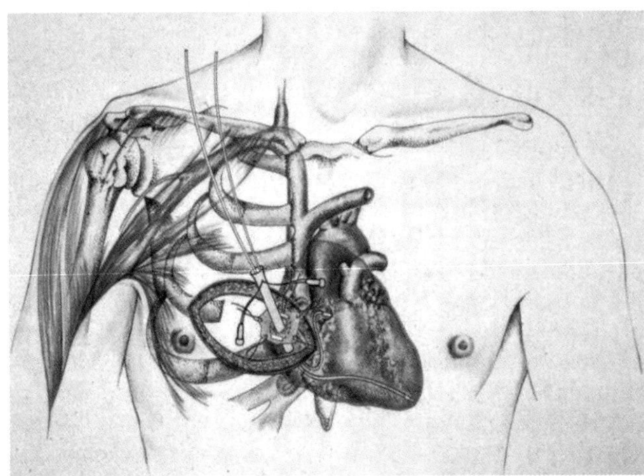

Figure 21-40. Transatrial implantation. This is a minimally invasive cardiac surgical approach to the right atrium through the bed of the third or fourth costal cartilage. State-of-the-art transvenous leads are implanted into the right atrium, coronary sinus, cardiac vein, and right ventricle. Epicardial leads can be implanted onto the right and left atria, including an epicardial implant into Bachman's bundle. Using the bed of the fifth costal cartilage, epicardial atrial and right ventricular leads can be implanted. In the author's opinion, any transvenous procedure can be performed using this versatile approach, sparing the superior veins.

Prevention of Complications. Phrenic nerve stimulation should be apparent when testing at 10 V. To eliminate the problem, move the lead to a site not causing the stimulation. To prevent masking of the phrenic nerve stimulation during electrical testing and to avoid cutting nerves using electrosurgery, it is imperative paralytic agents be used only in small doses for induction of general anesthesia.

Penetration is the burrowing of the electrode into the cardiac muscle in the right ventricle. Penetration does not occur in the atrium. The initial event causing penetration is not known, but, once started, the electrode can work its way out to the epicardium. Several conventional signs suggest penetration: exit block, poor sensing, low impedance, and phrenic nerve stimulation as the electrode nears the epicardial surface. The electrogram shows a continuous injury potential during penetration. Penetration is not a common event during the implantation procedure. The so-called high-impedance leads, with a small surface area electrode and large lead body, could generate enough pressure at the electrode-myocardial interface to initiate penetration at the time of implantation. Although this is not common during the implantation procedure, it can be a postimplantation complication, even weeks to months after implantation.[41] Lead configuration can increase the potential for penetration. If the lead body is lying in a straight configuration from the tricuspid valve to the implantation site, this is a setup for penetration. The straight (nonbending) configuration does not allow for absorption of the forces generated during cardiac contraction. Because the lead does not bend, the pressures generated at the electrode initiate penetration. To correct or prevent this situation from occurring, the lead should always be curved. Contraction forces will accentuate the bend in a curved lead, absorbing the forces without applying pressure at the electrode-myocardial interface and thus preventing penetration. Atrial leads are always curved and rarely penetrate in the atrial wall.

Perforation is puncture of the heart wall by a lead. Although knowledge of the mechanisms associated with puncture is helpful, it can be prevented only by proper training and judgment. It is caused by application of a force along the longitudinal axis of the lead with sufficient force to puncture the heart wall. Most commonly, the lead is in a straight configuration with a stylet inserted. Unlike a penetration, in which the electrode worms its way through the muscle fibers, perforation tears the tissue, leaving a defect in the wall. Perforation can result in hemorrhage into the pericardial space, which can lead to a tamponade. The hemorrhagic effusion must be drained, and, if bleeding persists, the pericardium must be explored and the puncture site surgically repaired. Once the sequelae of the perforation have been corrected, the implantation can proceed.

The final task is to adjust the curvature of the lead (allow for sufficient slack) to compensate for changes in orientation of the heart with diaphragmatic excursion. With inspiration, the diaphragm moves inferior and the heart follows. This causes the anterior surface of the heart to rotate inferiorly, and electrodes implanted near the atrial appendage and apex of the right ventricle will rotate along the maximal portion of the arc. The distance moved can exceed the redundant lead, or slack, and place traction on the electrode, elevating the threshold or dislodging the lead.

Epicardial Lead Implantation

An epicardial lead implantation is another cardiac surgical procedure. Currently, epicardial implantation is used to provide short-term pacing therapy (rarely ICD therapy) for patients with vegetative endocarditis, as a primary approach for pediatric patients, and as an alternative site for patients without useable veins. The rationale has expanded with the introduction of cardiac resynchronization therapy (CRT). Failure to achieve satisfactory lead placement in a cardiac vein for left ventricular pacing was the initial expanded indication. Techniques for epicardial lead implantation have evolved, and it is now used by the author as an alternative to the transvenous cardiac vein implantation procedure.

Epicardial implantation does involve certain issues: a cardiac surgeon should perform these procedures, the implantation options are limited, the long-term success of epicardial leads is in question, and pacing modality is usually limited to VVI because of difficulties implanting atrial leads in a location remote from the ventricular implantation site. In addition, an epicardial lead implantation is a minimally invasive thoracic surgical approach with associated morbidity, potential mortality, and patient management difficulties. In the author's recent experiences with more than 200 epicardial implantation procedures, the only concern was to keep the implanted electrode free from physical stress to prevent threshold elevation. The other issues were eliminated by the implantation approach, development of new implantation tools, and aggressive management protocols.

Surgical Approaches. The epicardial approaches described here are the conventional approaches. These approaches are specific to the chamber or chambers to be implanted. The chambers are exposed, freeing adhesions with sharp dissection as necessary. The electrode placement sites are remote from a rigid surface such as the sternum or ribs. Also, the lung is not a factor with these approaches and does not have to be retracted or decompressed (i.e., double-lumen endotracheal tubes are not required). Once the heart is exposed, electrical testing is required to find an optimal implantation site. The implanted lead should be secured to the pericardium or some other structure, leaving slack on the lead to avoid traction forces' being applied to the electrode. The leads are then tunneled to the pocket location.

The subxyphoid approach (epigastric approach) is used to provide access to the right ventricle and atrium; A midline epigastric incision is made from the xyphoid down approximately 8 to 10 cm. Large xyphoid bones are removed with a rongeur. The pericardium is opened, and adhesions, if present, are freed with sharp dissection. The basilar surface of the right ventricle and the inferior portion of the right atrium are accessible from this approach. There is a bare area on the basilar surface of the right ventricle that is suitable for implantation. Toward the apex, the muscle thickens as part of the confluence of the anterior, basilar, and septal walls. The inferior portion of the right atrium is more difficult to expose, but if the electrical signals are adequate, it is a satisfactory implantation site. Atrial and ventricular lead implantation allows atrioventricular sequential pacing to be performed. The lead or leads are usually tunneled to an abdominal pocket.

The anterior thoracotomy approach (to expose the right and left ventricles) is one of the original classic epicardial implantation incisions. A 6- to 10-cm incision through the fifth intercostal space exposes the anterior-lateral surface of the left ventricle near the apex. The apex can be retracted to access the basilar surface of the right ventricle. By enlarging the incision, the posterior-superior-lateral portion of the left ventricle and even the left atrium can be exposed. This is difficult to do and is not recommended as a standard approach. However, if necessary, dual-chamber (atrioventricular sequential) biventricular epicardial pacing can be performed by placing epicardial leads on the right ventricle, left ventricle, and left atrium. This is an efficient incision to be used for rapid access to the lateral wall of the right atrium or in those cases where the basilar surface of the right ventricle cannot be easily accessed through a subxyphoid approach due to previous surgery, obesity, or other reasons. The leads are tunneled to an abdominal or a left pectoral pocket.

The minimally invasive anterior thoracotomy through the third intercostal space is ideal for providing access to the posterior-superior-lateral surface of the left ventricle and to the left atrium. This is used primarily to implant a left ventricular lead for resynchronization of the left ventricle. The leads can be tunneled substernally to a right-sided pocket if necessary. Although this approach is to the superior portion of the left ventricle, pleural adhesions, pericardial adhesions, and the presence of coronary bypass grafts are not deterrents.

Other approaches, such as the lateral thoracotomy and thoracoscopy procedures, may be used, but they are not the most efficient way to access the heart and implant current leads. The lateral thoracotomy incision is not an efficient approach. Placing the patient in a lateral position takes away the option of using fluoroscopy and transvenous implantation in combination with the epicardial procedure. It limits it to an epicardial implantation procedure. In addition, it is remote from the usual implantation sites, and the lung frequently needs to be collapsed by means of a double-lumen endotracheal tube to obtain exposure. The thoracoscopy approaches are useful only in ideal situations, because enlarged hearts, pleural and pericardial adhesions, and the need to electrically map the surface of the heart cannot easily be done through this approach. In addition, the lung must be collapsed for visualization, and a large cannula must be inserted to implant current epicardial leads. Although this can be done, it is not a universal approach and is relegated to implanting in ideal situations.

Implantation Tools and Leads. Implantation tools have evolved, making both left and right ventricular implants and atrial implants possible. Epicardial leads that are implantable through small incisions were designed more than 35 years ago for a ventricular lead and 20 years ago for an atrial lead. For various reasons, these leads limit the usefulness and long-term survival of epicardial implants. Evolution of epicardial lead technology is one of the essential prerequisites to the evolution of epicardial implantation. The other is the development of percutaneous approaches designed to minimize the morbidity and potential mortality of these procedures. The implantation tool packaged with current epicardial leads is not satisfactory for implantation through a small incision around the curved surface of the heart. Medtronic was the first to make a usable implantation tool for their model 5071 lead.

There are various types of epicardial leads: helical (unipolar and bipolar), stab-on (unipolar), suture electrode (unipolar or bipolar), and two passive suture-on buttons (bipolar). These leads all have their advantages and disadvantages. A helical lead is the safest to implant through a small incision using the implantation tool. The helix, screwed into the epicardium, acts as the electrode and as an efficient fixation device. The disadvantage is its long-term performance. External stresses (traction or compression) injure the tissue and elevate the thresholds both acutely and chronically. Recursive reactions, such as mineralization of the external encapsulating tissue, prevent the electrode from moving freely with the heart, causing injury and threshold elevation.

Stab-on electrodes work well in the atrium. The electrode is stabbed through the atrial wall and secured with sutures remote from the electrode. The electrode works well acutely and chronically. It does not seem to be as sensitive as other types to external stresses. The disadvantages are its poor electrical performance in the ventricle and the dangers involved in implanting the lead in the thin atrial wall. Stabbing the lead into the ventricle works well acutely, but the electrode erodes to the surface with time, resulting in poor electrical performance. Stabbing the lead into the atrium is dangerous. It is easy to tear the atrial wall, causing significant bleeding. The only safe way to implant this electrode in the atrium is to secure the atrial tissue with a vascular clamp.

The suture electrode is an electrode configured as a suture. The electrode is sutured into the myocardial tissue. This electrode design has been used in cardiac surgical procedures as a temporary lead for many years. Its short-term performance is excellent. The long-term performance of permanent lead designs is unknown. Also, the safety of placing a suture into the left ventricle through a small incision, at a remote distance around a curved surface, is unknown.

Placing two small button electrodes on the heart and securing them with sutures has been effective in pediatric applications. The electrode performance has been satisfactory, and the application is safe through relatively large incisions. However, it is not feasible to implant these electrodes at a distance around a curved surface through a small incision. Securing the electrode with a suture and tying the suture are dangerous and difficult to do.

Patient Management. The magnitude of the management challenges associated with an epicardial surgical approach is much greater than for a transvenous implantation approach. Subjecting a patient to a thoracic surgical procedure under general endotracheal anesthesia requires aggressive management to ensure a successful outcome. In general, managing patients who have heart failure with or without comorbidity can be a challenging endeavor. Having a successful, low-morbidity procedure was a prerequisite to subjecting a patient to an epicardial procedure. A comprehensive management protocol must provide a uniform management scheme for cardiac, renal, and pulmonary support. The author devised such a protocol, which has been successful in eliminating the confusion and need to improvise in complex multisystem management scenarios. Its success has also eliminated surgical and postoperative management failures as a contraindication to epicardial pacing in patients with heart failure.

The goal of the protocol is to maintain an effective heart rhythm, a systolic blood pressure greater than 100 mm Hg, a urine output of 80 mL/hr, a physiologic respiratory function, and the metabolic status within a physiologic range. Transition to a chronic treatment program is made before discharge. Blood pressure is maintained with the use of pressors, if necessary. The most common cause of low blood pressure in patients with an ejection fraction greater than 25% is vasodilatation caused by pain medication. Renal management is designed to prevent prerenal failure. Immediately after the procedure, 100 mL/hr of normal saline is given intravenously, and the urine output is maintained at 80 mL/hr with diuretics as needed. Pulmonary management is routine. The metabolic status is checked with a blood gas analysis as needed to confirm the physiologic status. The cardiovascular system collapses when the pH falls to less than 7.15 regardless of the cause (respiratory or perfusion). The major morbidity occurs in patients with an ejection fraction between 10% and 20%, especially in the presence of comorbidities associated with a concomitant disease process. Except for pain-related morbidity, an epicardial procedure should be a successful, uneventful procedure in the absence of a concomitant disease process.

TABLE 21-2. **Database Population**

Period	No. Infected
1985-2000	1208
2000-May 2005	500
Total	1708

Device-Related Infections

Management of device infections is both complicated and technically challenging. It requires all the requisite skills, including knowledge of bacteria, soft tissue, lead extraction, and implantation, to manage these complications. In addition, the morbidity associated with infection superimposed on other concomitant disease processes adds to the management difficulties. The author has experience treating more than 1708 patients with a device-related infection since 1985, as shown in Table 21-2. Detailed information taken from the author's database is presented on 500 consecutive patients treated since 2000.

Device-related parasitic bacteria found at the site of infection are relatively few and are listed in Table 21-3. Two thirds of the cultures were positive, and one third were negative or unknown. The positive cultures are self-evident, but the negative and unknown cultures need some discussion. The exact cause for a negative culture is never known. There are five possibilities: extensive prior treatment with antibiotics, attempted culture of exudative effusion, slow-growing bacteria such as mycobacterium, material mishandled by the laboratory, and information lost from the referring physician. Negative cultures are seen most commonly in patients who have had extensive prior antibiotic therapy. Many of these patients were treated empirically for 1 week or longer before transfer to the author's care. However, tissue obviously related to an infection is debrided and cultured. It is postulated that the concentration of antibiotics in the tissue prevents bacterial growth on the culture media and/or the bacterial count is too low to culture. Culture of an exudative effusion is rarely successful, because bacteria are not in the effusion but against some smooth surface. A tissue biopsy is needed, especially with *Staphylococcus epidermidis.* A rare cause of a negative in-hospital culture is a slow-growing organism such as a mycobacterium that does not grow on common culture plates or discarding of the culture plates after a short hospital stay. In these cases, the patient has a recurrence and the bacteria are identified at that time. Another rare cause is a misadventure with the debrided tissue; if it is not cultured, the material is lost, or it arrives at the laboratory too late to be suitable for culture. In 21 patients, positive culture results from the referring physician were lost and the tissue cultures were negative. A recent study demonstrated that pocket tissue cultures are

TABLE 21-3. **Device-Related Pathogens**

Category	Organism	No. of Cases	Total
Staphylococcus			296 (59%)
	Coagulase-negative and *S. epidermidis*	176	
	S. aureus	103	
	Other (8)	17	
Gram-negative			28 (6%)
	Klebsiella pneumoniae	2	
	Alcaligenes xylosoxidans	1	
	Pseudomonas sp	11	
	Proteus mirabilis	6	
	Serratia marcescens	8	
Rare gram-positive	*Enterococcus faecalis*	4	
	Enterobacter cloacae	3	
	Mycobacterium fortuitum	1	
	Corynebacterium sp	1	
Contaminants			3 (1%)
	Nonpathogens	3	
No culture results			164 (32%)
	No growth	140	
	No information	24	
Total			500 (100%)

TABLE 21-4. **Positive Cultures (*N* = 336)**

Category	Frequency (%)
Staphylococcus	88
Gram-negative bacteria	9
Rare gram-positive bacteria	2
Contaminants	1

TABLE 21-5. **Staphylococcus Species**

Species	No. Cases	%
Coagulase-negative and *S. epidermidis*	175	60
S. aureus	103	35
S. haemolyticus	3	1
S. simulans	2	0.5
S. warneri	2	0.5
Other	4	1
Total	294	100

more effective than pocket swab cultures for isolation and identification of the pathogens in device infections.[42]

It is useful to assume that the incidence of bacteria found in the positive cultures mirrors that of the bacteria causing the infections with a negative culture. If the reasons for a negative culture are as postulated, this assumption is valid. Table 21-4 shows the frequency of bacteria identified in the positive cultures. The positive culture data are used for the remainder of this section. *S. epidermidis* and *S. aureus* are responsible for more than 83% of the infections with known cultures. Organisms such as *Pseudomonas, Klebsiella, Proteus,* and *Enterococcus* are seen less frequently (8%). Fungi and acid-fast mycobacteria are present on rare occasions. Some of these organisms may have caused the infection, and some may be secondary contaminants (e.g., yeast). Infections caused by a mycobacterium are rare, dangerous, and hard to treat. The unique features of staphylococci, gram-negative bacteria in general, and mycobacteria will be discussed in relation to device infection.

Staphylococci

Staphylococci cause most of the device-related infections (88%). Staphylococci are gram-positive bacteria, pyogenic, slime producers, and clinically separated into coagulase-positive and coagulase-negative types.[43] They are pyogenic (pus producers), demonstrating the effectiveness of their cytotoxins. Although some of these bacteria are capable of producing exotoxins, neurotoxins and endotoxins, they usually are not associated with device infections. Classification of staphylococci based on the presence or absence of a slime layer may have clinical significance. The pathogenic organisms may be the slime producers. Slime production definitely enhances their effectiveness as a pathogen in device infections. The ability to adhere to smooth surfaces, such as an implanted device and encapsulating fibrous tissue, is a major factor enhancing the infectivity of these bacteria. Slime helps protect the bacteria from the body's defense mechanisms and from antibiotics. Clinically, staphylococci are naturally separated in the identification phase into the pathogenic coagulase-positive species (e.g., *S. aureus*) and the relatively nonpathogenic coagulase-negative species (e.g., *S. epidermidis*). Table 21-5 shows the *Staphylococcus* species that were cultured.

Staphylococcus Epidermidis. Coagulase-negative staphylococci cause most device-related infections (52%). Most of the coagulase-negative staphylococci are eventually classified as *S. epidermidis.* In those cases where the final report is inconclusive, it is generally interpreted to be *S. epidermidis.* Coagulase-negative staphylococci are part of the normal flora found on the conjunctiva of the eye, on the skin, in the outer ear, in the nose, in the urethra, in the mouth, and in the oral pharynx. These symbiont bacteria are part of the normal host flora at these sites. These same bacteria within tissue become parasitic and are cytotoxic, injuring or killing tissues, causing an inflammatory reaction and an infectious disease. In the past, *S. epidermidis* was not taken as a serious cause of device infection, because of their presence throughout the body and their frequent labeling as a contaminant.

Coagulase-negative staphylococci are not very virulent or invasive and do not produce dangerous toxins. They are slime producers, adhering to smooth surfaces and injuring the tissue in some manner, causing an inflammatory reaction. The body reacts to tissue contamination with coagulase-negative staphylococci in one of three ways. The first example is bacterial contamination of normal tissue. The infectivity is low because of the absence of a smooth surface to which the bacteria can adhere. A small inoculum would be eradicated by the body's immunodefense mechanism. A postulated course would be that the bacteria and/or the method of inoculation injured or killed tissue, initiating an inflammatory reaction. A low-grade inflammatory reaction would be sufficient for the immunodefense system to eliminate the bacteria and clean the area without scar tissue formation. A large inoculum could increase the intensity of the infection (virulence) and cause an inflammatory reaction response sufficient to cause a small abscess. This abscess-forming infection could probably be managed by a healthy immunodefense system, leaving scar tissue. In a worst-case scenario, the body's defense would have to be supported with antibiotics.

In the second example, a small inoculum contaminates a device implantation site. With the production of slime, the presence of smooth surfaces on the device and in a chronic pocket, and exuberant encapsulating tissues, the adherence of bacteria to these surfaces is enhanced. The bacteria initiate a low-grade inflammatory reaction, and the body's defenses (with or without antibiotics) eliminate the bacteria in normal tissue and in injured tissue where the body's defenses have access to the bacteria. However, once the bacteria adhere to the smooth surfaces and the slime layer is sufficient to shield them from the body's defenses, antibiotics and natural defenses cannot eradicate the bacteria and cure the infection. The slime-protected bacteria continue to grow and invade the surrounding tissues, and a low-grade, subclinical inflammatory reaction persists (latent or occult infection). Unfortunately, this smoldering inflammatory reaction continues to organize, increasing the fibrous tissue barrier between the normal tissue and the bacteria-infested areas. This can continue for years, especially if clinical manifestations of the inflammatory reaction are suppressed with antibiotics. At some point, the encapsulating fibrous tissue barrier is sufficient to limit the effectiveness of the body's defenses and antibiotics. The resultant cavity is now an abscess. The effusion in the early stages of the abscess cavity is straw-colored and later becomes purulent. Culture of these effusions is rarely productive. To obtain a positive culture, tissue must be submitted. The effusion will continue to enlarge, creating pressure on the wall. The abscess will eventually erode through the wall, creating a draining sinus, or, in the worst case, it will decompress into the bloodstream. The clinical variations associated with this second example are related to the size of the inoculum, the status of a chronic pocket, and the status of the body's defenses. In a chronic pocket with a large inoculum, a marked amount of exuberant encapsulating fibrous tissue, and/or impairment of the body's defenses, the infection will accelerate, bypassing the latent stage, to abscess formation. Although the inflammatory reaction may be apparent within 1 or 2 weeks, it usually takes many weeks for the abscess to mature.

The first and second examples are realistic and mirror the thousands of typical coagulase-negative infections the author has treated. Together, they not only give a mental picture of this type of infection but also serve as a model to develop effective methods of prevention and treatment. An inoculum of bacteria cannot be prevented from coming in contact with an implant device. The author believes it is essential to eradicate these bacteria before they can establish their slime-producing colonies. In addition to the perfunctory surgical steps, such as sterility and minimizing tissue damage, intravenous antibiotics and antibiotic irrigation are necessary. Prophylactic antibiotic therapy is one of those things everybody does on a cursory level, but it probably should be administered in a more aggressive fashion. Copious irrigation of the pocket with an antibiotic solution is also important and should be routine. Debridement of the exuberant fibrous tissue from chronic pockets will remove those smooth, poorly vascularized surfaces. The author has not witnessed a postoperative infection using this treatment regimen. This suggests that proper surgical technique, mobilization of the body's defenses by the inflammatory reaction initiated by the surgical trauma, selective debridement, intravenous antibiotics, and antibiotic irrigation create a lethal environment for this type of bacterial inoculum.

The third example of the body's reaction to infection by coagulase-negative staphylococci involves an intravascular inoculum (bacteremia). This usually occurs once an infection has been established, causing septicemia. Bacteremia would be rare in the first example, and, if a low inoculum of these nonvirulent bacteria did occur, they would be filtered by the lungs or, rarely, by other organ tissues and eradicated. Adherence of coagulase-negative staphylococci to the heart wall, causing endocarditis, has not been seen by the author in this situation. In the second example, bacteremia could occur. It is easy to visualize conditions favorable for a bacteremia to evolve in the environment of a dynamic vascular inflammatory reaction. It is not uncommon for the occurrence of bacteremia causing septicemia to be the first symptom of an infection. In addition, the implanted device has leads entering the veins at a site near the pocket. The bacteria slimed to the device surface can become invasive by migrating along the lead to the vein entry site. On exploration, an encapsulating fibrous tissue sheath is commonly found around the lead at the vein entry site, confirming the presence of bacteria and the associated inflammatory reaction. The circulating bacteria can adhere to the lead body at intravenous sites of low blood flow and turbulence. These are the same sites favorable to clot formation. The bacteria can also be incorporated in clot formation. The slimed bacterial colonies also initiate clot formation. Regardless of which comes first, the combination of septicemia and clot or thrombus in the heart is labeled by the author as vegetative endocarditis. Endocarditis with vegetations is treated more vigorously, much the same as classic bacterial endocarditis. Septicemia without the presence of vegetation is not considered endocarditis by the author. Because septicemia is a clinical manifestation of bacteremia, which can occur without symptoms, the author has elected to not treat septicemia as endocarditis without evidence of intracardiac vegetation.

A brief discussion of bacteremia and septicemia is in order. Slime-producing bacteria can theoretically adhere to the lead body surface, creating slime colonies. In the thousands of cases treated by the author, not treating septicemia as endocarditis (i.e., with extraction of all leads and treatment for 6 to 8 weeks with an appropriate intravenous antibiotic), vegetative endocarditis occurs at some frequency on these leads. However, in the absence of vegetation, the author has not had a patient with septicemia develop endocarditis. The author's interpretation of these results is that either a clot forms first, followed by bacterial seeding, or that bacteria adhere to the lead body and a clot forms at the same time. Either of these interpretations would explain the data. Also, if the bacteria flow with the cellular elements in the central portion of the bloodstream and have sufficient velocity, adherence to the lead surface is prevented. Another clinical situation supporting this hypothesis is the liberation of a massive concentration of bacteria and other cellular and proteinaceous abscess cavity debris into the venous system. A clinical example is the presence of an abscess cavity at the vein entry site. This can also occur with a large channel along the leads, from a pocket abscess cavity into the implant vein. The effusion accumulates and decompresses almost in a rhythmic fashion. The decompression of this material is filtered in the lungs, causing clinical symptoms mimicking the flu. Symptoms include fever, shortness of breath, coughing, and, in some situations, desaturation. Radiographic studies shows interstitial edema throughout the lung fields. It is apparent that the decompressed effusion is trapped in the lung field, and the resultant inflammatory reaction causes interstitial edema. The lung seems to be well equipped to handle this insult and will recover within a few days. These patients are usually treated as having the flu. The bacteria in this situation do not adhere to the lead surface, supporting the working hypothesis. Clinical examples of specific infection presentations and treatment protocols are discussed later, as well as the requisite skills in patient management.

Staphylococcus Aureus. *S. aureus* is a coagulase-positive bacterium whose virulence, invasiveness, infectivity, and exotoxin production make it a potentially deadly pathogen. *S. aureus* is also a slime producer and pyogenic. Although *S. aureus* and *S. epidermidis* have many properties in common, the former is far more invasive and dangerous. Examining *S. aureus* infection in the three scenarios presented earlier indicates marked changes in the timing and intensity. The small inoculum in the first example could cause a significant purulent abscess requiring antibiotics and possibly incision and drainage. This could evolve over several days. The same inoculum in the second example will cause an abscess to form in the pocket within 1 week or less. With high-dose intravenous antibiotics, the infection may be suppressed with some resolution of the inflammatory reaction (cellulitis, effusion, and possibly fever). The infection should be suppressed for 1 or 2 weeks, allowing time to debride the pocket and remove the implanted device. Continued treatment with antibiotics results in failure, recurrence of the inflammatory reaction, and exacerbation of the symptoms. The infection is not as easy to control at this point. With each recurrence, the infection escalates, possibly stabilizing with spontaneous drainage of the effusion. Intravascular spread of the infection, as in the third example, is serious and can be lethal if not effectively treated in a timely fashion. The same treatment protocols are used as with the coagulase-negative infections; the only difference is that the inflammatory reactions and systemic sequelae are more intense.

Gram-Negative Bacteria

Pseudomonas, Klebsiella, Proteus, and *Serratia* are examples of gram-negative bacteria that occasionally cause a device-related infection (8%). Gram-negative infections behave differently from gram-positive ones. The incidence of these infections is low, so the clinical experience is not as great. Except for *Serratia,* these bacteria are part of the normal flora of the colon. *Serratia* grows in moist areas and in some solutions. It may be found growing in solutions, intravenous apparatus, transducers, and so on, and it is a potential cause of nosocomial infections. These gram-negative bacteria are opportunistic pathogens that cause device infections by metastatic spread (e.g., colon polyp removal) or by a loss of skin integrity and direct contamination. Acquisition of an inoculum of gram-negative bacteria found in the colon or a contaminated solution during a device procedure requires a major breach in sterility and/or surgical technique. A direct procedure-related complication is rare.

Gram-negative bacteria do not secrete a toxin as gram-positive bacteria do. Their endotoxins are part of the bacteria wall (lipopolysaccharide). Most are liberated during cell lysis, but some can be released during cell division (multiplication). These bacteria create a capsule-forming mucoid colony (*Klebsiella, Proteus,* and *Serratia*) or a slime layer (*Pseudomonas*). Like *Staphylococcus* infections, once established, they cannot be cured with antibiotics. Tissue debridement and device removal are the only ways to cure the infection.

Mycobacteria

The rare infection caused by a mycobacterium is extremely difficult to treat. Mycobacteria are found in soil and are occasionally present as part of the skin flora. Contaminations from the skin and a breach in sterility are two possible causes for this type infection. Mycobacterial infections are hard to identify and can take longer than 2 weeks to grow in culture media. The treatment protocol used for gram-positive and gram-negative bacteria does not apply and will fail. Consequently, an acid-fast infection will not be identified by routine culture during a normal hospital stay, and the presence of acid-fast mycobacteria is not known when the patient is discharged from the hospital. Slow growth and poor permeability of the cell wall to antibiotics are the two acid-fast properties responsible for conventional treatment failures.

The patient will return within a month with the previously closed debrided pocket now open and healing by secondary intention. The opened pocket will be covered with a perfect bed of granulation tissue. There is little, if any, cellular debris or purulent material. This is the characteristic appearance of these infections. The bacteria cause a low-grade, persistent inflammatory reaction that organizes with this perfect layer of granulation tissue. Except for the tissue beneath the granulating bed, the normal underlying tissues are effectively isolated from this persistent infection. It will not heal without antibiotics. Repair of the wound cannot be done until the infection has resolved, or at least until after sufficient coverage with antibiotics for 1 or 2 months.

Appropriate treatment for this granulating wound is possible only after an acid-fast culture identifies the type of mycobacterium and its antibiotic susceptibility. It can take months to treat a subcutaneous tissue infection, and infections at intrathoracic pacing leads and ICD patch sites can take much longer. The author has no solution to this problem. Culturing all tissue samples for acid-fast bacteria is not a solution. This would be expensive, and the damage would be done by the time the culture returned. Recognition of the characteristic appearance of the granulation tissue is currently the only solution.

Classification of Device-Related Infections

Patients with device infections present a variety of clinical problems that range from acute to chronic phases, from contaminated tissue to abscess formation, from extravascular to intravascular location, and from local morbidity to systemic, life-threatening sepsis. Without a classification system, dry pocket erosion with a positive culture would be placed in the same group as an acute pocket infection (i.e., *S. aureus* infection, cellulitis, a marked purulent effusion, and septicemia). However, dry pocket erosion may not represent an infection. It could have been caused by ischemic erosion with bacterial contamination but no cellulitis (inflammatory reaction), because the tissue is not invaded by bacteria or their toxins. Although the treatment for both these conditions is the same, the classification should be different. To avoid these ambiguities, the author has classified device infections into four groups (Table 21-6). This classification is based on the management of more than 2000 pacemaker and ICD infections. This classification scheme was designed to characterize the potential morbidity and mortality of infections and to serve as a basis for their management.

Infections frequently begin as a class III pocket infection. They either remain a class III; erode through the skin, changing into a relatively benign class IV; or convert to a potentially lethal class II by intravascular drainage. A class II infection may evolve into a class I-B. The author has never seen a class I-B or class II infection become a class III, either spontaneously or after maximal antibiotic therapy.

TABLE 21-6. Classification of Device-Related Infections

Class	Definition
I	Endocarditis
I-A	Infected cardiac tissue
I-B	Infected vegetation
I-C	Infected foreign body
II	Septicemia without endocarditis
III	Subcutaneous tissue infection
IV	Chronic stable exteriorized pocket
IV-A	Contaminated chronic pocket tissue
IV-B	Chronic granulation tissue barrier

Class I

Class I infections are a form of endocarditis. In the presence of a device implanted in the heart three types of infection are possible: classic viral or bacterial endocarditis, infected vegetative material associated with the implanted device, and a retained infected segment of an implanted device. The rationale for separating device-related endocarditis into two groups is based on the differences in the properties and treatment procedures.

Class I-A. The diagnosis of class I infections can be difficult because of their varied presentations. Consequently, class I infections contain three subgroups created to enhance the diagnosis. Class I-A is defined as a pure infection of cardiac tissue. Examples are an infected mitral, tricuspid, or aortic valve. One cannot make this diagnosis with device hardware in place; it is rare, a diagnosis of exclusion, and initially assumed not to exist. The author has seen only one such case, which involved a yeast infection of the tricuspid valve. Consequently, if a class I-A infection does exist, the patient will be inappropriately treated with short-term antibiotics and the reimplantation of endocardial leads. The tissue infection will persist and will probably infect the new device implant. Therefore, when a device is present, the diagnosis of a class I-A infection may become apparent only after recurrence of the infection.

Class I-B. A class I-B acute infection involves septicemia and vegetation in the right side of the heart but is not associated with infected cardiac tissue as in class I-A. A class I-B infection is a combination of septicemia and vegetation. The vegetation ranges from small, finger-like clots to massive thrombi. Because the infected status of vegetation cannot always be determined, some class II patients are overtreated as class I-B. The incidence of vegetation in patients with or without septicemia is unknown.

Class I-C. A partial lead extraction resulting from lead breakage with a retained segment and bacteria in the interstices of the insulation or within the lumen causes a class I-C endocarditis. The parts of the retained segment are embedded within the myocardium. Vegetation is not present at the site. The cause of these infections is (1) a failed lead extraction with breakage, leaving a lead segment behind, and (2) contamination of either the lumen or the interstices of a failed insulation with bacteria. For example, if the insulation has failed in the pocket and bacterial growth is in the lumen, contamination can extend the entire length of the lead. A small number of patients who have class II infection (<5%) with the electrode and insulation left in the heart have returned with a class I-C infection. In the past, lead breakage with retained segments in the myocardium was considered a potential outcome of lead extraction, with an incidence as high as 15% to

20% in some situations. Today, with powered sheaths, it is not an expected outcome. The incidence is dependent on the tensile strength of the lead.

Class II

Class II infections are not a form of endocarditis, despite the presence of septicemia. Septicemia alone is insufficient to make a diagnosis of endocarditis. Clinically, unless a vegetation is present, no relationship has been shown between septicemia and endocarditis. Otherwise, a class II infection is indistinguishable from a class I infection. Septicemia in class II infections is caused by drainage of bacteria and/or their toxins into the bloodstream through the vein entry site alongside the lead, through breaks in the lead insulation, through a venous tributary draining the pocket, or, hypothetically, through the lymphatics.

The motivation for a distinction between a class I and class II infection was based on the need to avoid treating all patients who have septicemia and/or positive blood cultures as if they had endocarditis. The selection of vegetation as the separation variable was arbitrary. As evidenced by the clinical results, it has proved to be a remarkably effective marker for selecting the group of patients who require more extensive antibiotics and temporary epicardial lead implants. Although there is a potential for overtreatment of an unknown number of class II infections and noninfected vegetations as class I-B, the clinical results show this number to be small. Also, to date, the author's experience suggests that class II and class I-B infections rarely coexist or evolve into class I-A.

Class III

Class I and class II infections include potentially lethal systemic sepsis and are generally associated with a pocket infection. An identical extravascular infection confined to the subcutaneous tissue pocket without septicemia is a class III infection. A class III infection is an abscess and will manifest the clinical properties associated with an abscess. A class III infection may or may not drain spontaneously through the skin.

As an abscess associated with an implanted device, clinically two factors determine its clinical presentation. The first is drainage (internal or external). If formation of the exudative debris exceeds the drainage, the effusion grows and pressure increases, worsening the signs and symptoms of the infection. Drainage of the effusion into the bloodstream is potentially lethal. Drainage to the exterior provides an immediate resolution of the signs and symptoms and offers the only chance for the inflammatory reaction to construct a protective barrier between the infection and normal tissue. The obvious conclusion from these comments is that it may be necessary to perform incision and drainage. The second factor is the presence of the implanted device. The infection cannot heal without removal of this material. In addition, it generally cannot heal by primary intention without removal of all inflammatory material.

Class IV

A chronic exteriorized class III infection organizes and develops a granulation tissue barrier that protects the normal subcutaneous tissue from the outside surface. This granulation tissue barrier is a self-perpetuating, chronic inflammatory reaction that prevents bacteria and their toxins from invading normal tissue. Although the surface of the granulation tissue is contaminated with bacteria and by definition infected, it is not an infectious disease. This is a class IV-B infection. A class IV infection is defined as a stable dynamic tissue barrier protecting normal tissue from the bacteria. When this tissue barrier is the encapsulating fibrous tissues, it is a class IV-A infection, and when it is granulation tissue, it is a class IV-B.

Class IV-A. Migration and erosion through the skin expose the pocket to bacteria. Contaminated pocket tissue without evidence of cellulitis is a class IV-A infection. In this situation, the chronic pocket tissue (encapsulating fibrous tissue) is the barrier protecting the normal subcutaneous tissue beneath. In the past, migration and erosion were more common and class IV-A infections occurred more frequently. In the author's experience, successful attempts to debride the pocket and reimplant the decontaminated devices were probably confined to class IV-A infections (see Salvage Procedures).

A class IV-A infection is not a permanent condition. An inflammatory reaction and cellulitis will eventually ensue, converting the encapsulating fibrous tissue into granulation tissue. Consequently, a class IV-A infection will evolve into a class IV-B.

Class IV-B. A class IV-B infection may manifest as an open granulating ulcer (proud flesh), or it may evolve into a chronic draining sinus. Once the granulation tissue barrier forms, it is usually protective as along as exudative debris freely drains to the surface. The most frequent complication associated with a class IV-B infection is blockage and accumulation of an effusion. The granulation tissue barrier fails, cellulitis returns, and the infection is again a class III.

Application of the Classification

This classification does not address the magnitude of infection. An extravascular infection with minimal cellulitis, no effusion, and occasional bacteremia (causing a low-grade fever) receives the same class II designation as a pocket abscess with marked cellulitis, a massive suppurative effusion, and debilitating septicemia.

The treatment is similar for all four classes of infections, except for the intensity of antibiotic therapy before and after surgical procedures. Curative therapy for all types consists of the surgical removal of all extravascular and intravascular inflammatory and foreign material, including intracardiac vegetation. All incisions are closed by first intention. A new transvenous device can then be implanted at a remote site, such as the opposite side, in classes II through IV infections, whereas an epicardial approach must be used for class I, because intravascular devices are contraindicated.

The relationship between bacteria and classification in the 500 patients analyzed is shown in Table 21-7. Using the same format as for the bacterial species, the number of patients and classifications are presented. Figure 21-41A shows the similarity in incidence between the positive and negative culture groups for each class. This suggests that the two groups are equivalent and that the data are representative of the combined patient population. The 24 patients with no

TABLE 21-7. Relationship between Bacteria and Classification

		Classification							
Category	**Organism**	**I-A**	**I-B**	**I-C**	**II**	**II**	**IV-A**	**IV-B**	**Total**
Staphylococcus									296
	Coagulase-negative and *S. epidermidis*	0	22	0	23	72	1	58	176
	S. aureus	0	11	0	44	22	0	26	103
	Other	0	3	0	4	6	0	4	17
Gram-negative									28
	Klebsiella pneumoniae	0	1	0	0	1	0	0	2
	Alcaligenes xylosoxidans	0	0	0	1	0	0	0	1
	Pseudomonas sp	0	0	0	2	6	0	3	11
	Proteus mirabilis	0	0	0	2	1	0	3	6
	Serratia marcescens	0	0	0	2	2	0	4	8
Rare gram-positive									9
	Enterococcus faecalis	0	2	0	2	0	0	0	4
	Enterobacter cloacae	0	1	0	0	0	0	2	3
	Mycobacterium fortuitum	0	0	0	0	1	0	0	1
	Corynebacterium sp	0	0	0	0	1	0	0	1
Contaminants									3
	Nonpathogens	0	0	0	1	2	0	0	3
(Subtotal)		0	41	0	80	114	1	100	336
No culture results									
	No growth	1	24	0	24	46	0	45	140
Total		1	65	0	104	160	1	146	476

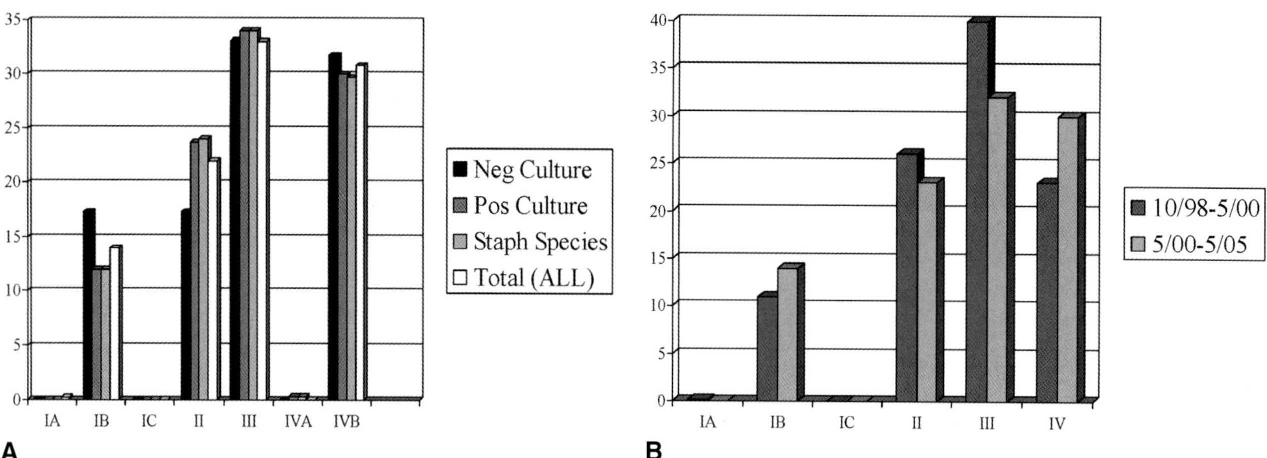

Figure 21-41. Culture results by classification: 68% of the 500 patients (May 2000 to May 2005) had positive cultures, and 59% of the total were a Staphylococcus *species. The culture results and classification data have been remarkably consistent over the years. See text for description of the classes of infection.* ***A,*** *Classifications of the infections in the cultured and noncultured groups show a similarity between the two groups. There is also a similarity between these groups and the presence of* Staphylococcus *species. This suggests to the author that the incidence of various bacterial species in the noncultured group is the same as for the cultured group.* ***B,*** *The results for the expanded group from 1998 show the same pattern.*

information were excluded, although from these data their statistics would be expected to be similar. The data on infection class from 1998 to 2000 is shown in Figure 21-41B. This is similar to the more recent data. The difference between the two groups is the greater incidence of class III and class IV infections in the earlier patients; the reason for this difference is unknown. The availability of powered sheaths minimizes breakage and accounts for the lack of patients in class I-C. Also, classification of class IV as class IV-A reflects the decrease in ischemic erosions. The reason may be related to the reduced size of the generator, but in the author's opinion, it is related to a delay in diagnosis. A class IV-A infection quickly evolves into class IV-B, and by the time the author receives the patient he or she is in class IV-B.

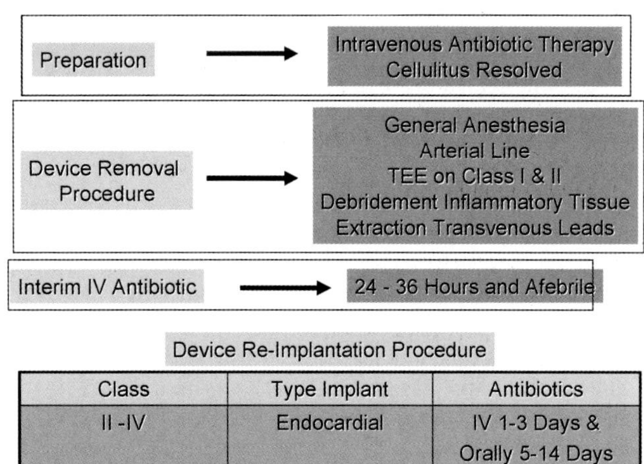

Class	Type Implant	Antibiotics
II -IV	Endocardial	IV 1-3 Days & Orally 5-14 Days
I	Epicardial	IV 6 – 8 Weeks

Figure 21-42. Device infection protocol. The device infection protocol includes patient preparation, the device removal procedure, interim intravenous (IV) antibiotic therapy, and the device reimplantation procedure including antibiotic therapy. The initial portions of the protocol are the same for all patients. However, the reimplantation and antibiotic management portions depend on the classification of the infection (see text). This protocol is conservative in requiring a minimum of 5 days in the hospital. Class-related antibiotic therapy is considered radical. TEE, transesophageal echocardiography.

Treatment of Device-Related Infections

Separation of device infections into classes was the first step toward the development of a treatment protocol. The need for an uncomplicated treatment protocol applicable to all patients is self-evident. For example, the treatment of a class I-B infection is accepted by all. The treatment consists of intravenous antibiotic therapy for 6 to 8 weeks, removal of implanted devices and vegetative material, debridement of all inflammatory tissue, abandonment of the pocket, and reimplantation using epicardial leads. Treatment recommendations for class II through class IV infections, with or without septicemia, based on the plethora of anecdotal information found in the literature, are confusing and frequently wrong or not applicable. Also, known principles, such as removal of foreign material, are often ignored because of perceived risk associated with lead extraction. To rectify this situation, the author developed a device infection treatment protocol that has been used to treat more than 2000 patients during the last 20 years.

Treatment Protocol

Mandatory. The devised treatment protocol is presented in Figure 21-42. This protocol includes antibiotic therapy, debridement of the pocket, removal of the implanted devices (pulse generator and leads), temporary pacing, approximately 36 hours of interim antibiotic therapy, and reimplantation of a device in a remote site. It is considered universal and applicable to all device infections, classes I through IV. The protocol is based on the hypothesis that antibiotic therapy, debridement of the pocket, removal of the implanted devices and any other foreign material, and reimplantation at a remote site are mandatory to ensure a successful result.

Necessary. The temporary pacemaker and the 36-hour time period between the destructive and reconstructive procedures are considered necessary by the author but are not mandatory. Before the reconstructive phase (reimplantation), the patient must be hemodynamically stable and afebrile. Although the author implants a temporary pacemaker, the need for a temporary pacemaker is a judgment decision a physician has to make. If a mistake is made, the patient can be paced externally and a temporary lead can be implanted at that time. Some believe that a 36-hour interval between phases is too short and use a longer interval, such as 72 hours to 2 weeks. This is to give the antibiotics sufficient time to treat the slowest-growing bacteria and rule out endocarditis. Others prefer to combine the destructive and reconstructive phases into one procedure. For example, at the end of the destructive phase, the disposable equipment can be removed and replaced with new equipment, the patient reprepared and draped, and new instruments obtained. The new pacemaker or ICD is then reimplanted at a remote site. The advantages of this approach are that it shortens the hospital stay by 2 hospital days and it eliminates the administration of a second general anesthetic. The author's choice of 36 hours (1 day on the floor) evolved over years in an attempt to compromise between the perceived need for long-term interim antibiotic coverage and the technical difficulties of preparing a contaminated procedure room for a sterile procedure. Initially, many physicians believed the interim time period should be longer. Today, many believe it should be eliminated. With experience, the author is convinced that an interim period is necessary to treat and/or correct problems associated with the initial procedure. These problems include septicemia, inadequate culture results, surgical complications associated with the initial procedure, and time to consider reimplantation options. A few patients develop septicemia after the initial procedure as a result of the pocket debridement, lead extraction, or inappropriate antibiotic coverage. Culture results from material obtained during the initial procedure can sometimes change the antibiotics needed and/or the infection class. A class II designation may change to class I-B, and vice versa. An initial procedure complication requiring surgery on the infected site is best performed before implantation with a new device. In some situations, reimplantation options are complicated; having time to consider those options is another advantage of the interim period. Mistakes (e.g., judgment error, wrong decisions) can cause morbidity and mortality, prolonged hospitalization, and significant device-related expense, especially if cross-contamination occurs.

The mandatory portion of the protocol should not be altered. Modifications of the mandatory procedure components will, in the author's opinion, affect the treatment outcome. For example, use of antibiotics alone, inadequate tissue debridement, failure to extract leads, pocket reuse, and so on, will result in treatment failures.

Antibiotics

Antibiotics are essential to the management of device infections. They are used in conjunction with the corrective surgical procedures. All device infections are treated with intravenous antibiotics before the corrective surgical procedures are performed. The morbidity, potential mortality, and economic considerations associated with device infections demand that they be treated in a timely fashion with administration of those antibiotics having the highest probability of success. Because the infecting bacterium and its susceptibilities usually are not known when therapy is instituted, 1 g of vancomycin and 60 mg of gentamicin are given to all patients before the surgical procedure. Antibiotics other than these are discontinued, unless culture susceptibilities show them to be effective. Vancomycin was chosen because most infections are caused by staphylococci, and almost all staphylococci are susceptible to vancomycin. In addition, allergic reactions to vancomycin are rare. Itching and flushed appearance caused by rapid infusion of the drug is not an allergy. Gentamicin was chosen for general gram-negative coverage, and a prophylactic dose is given. The choice of gentamicin was arbitrary and not based on the need to cover any specific organism. If a gram-negative infection is present, a therapeutic dose of gentamicin is given, unless the bacterium is known to be more susceptible to another antibiotic.

Ciprofloxacin (Cipro) and now levofloxacin (Levaquin) is the preferred oral antibiotic for treatment before and after discharge from the hospital. This was initially an arbitrary choice based on its broad-spectrum effectiveness against most offending organisms and patient acceptance. Over the years, most staphylococcal and many gram-negative infections have been shown to be susceptible to ciprofloxacin. Also, some strains of acid-fast mycobacteria are susceptible to this antibiotic. Antibiotic coverage is modified, as needed, depending on culture susceptibility data. Most bacteria not susceptible to ciprofloxacin have been found to be susceptible to doxycycline (Vibramycin).

The duration of antibiotic therapy before the procedure is determined by the magnitude of the infection. For example, an acute *S. aureus* class II infection with cellulitis, marked suppuration, and septicemia may require 1 week of antibiotic therapy, with or without an incision and drainage of the pocket, to resolve the cellulitis and render the patient afebrile. In contrast, a class IV infection with dry gangrenous erosion, without cellulitis, would need only the few hours required to reach an appropriate blood level of antibiotic. Regardless of the type of infection, two clinical conditions must be met before a surgical procedure is performed: (1) the cellulitis must be almost completely resolved, to allow a primary intention closure, and (2) the patient's temperature must be, at most, a low-grade fever, to avoid an anesthesia complication.

Antibiotic therapy is not curative and should not be tried alone as a curative approach. The negative historical experience was the rationale for combining antibiotics with the corrective surgical procedures. Antibiotics can cause a remission of the clinical signs and symptoms. The remission with virulent bacteria such as *S. aureus* is short term, and the signs and symptoms will reappear as soon as the antibiotic therapy is stopped. In contrast, the duration of remission with the less pathogenic *S. epidermidis* is unknown; most patients return within weeks or months. The length of the remission is usually related to the condition of the pocket. For example, in pockets subjected to latent (smoldering) infection, with a thick layer of encapsulating fibrous tissue, infection usually recurs within 1 or 2 weeks after the antibiotics are stopped. More normal pockets have longer remissions due to the ability of the body's biologic defense systems to engage the bacteria.

Another compelling reason for avoiding long-term treatment with antibiotics is the development of resistance to the drugs. For example, it is not uncommon for *S. epidermidis,* treated for months with ciprofloxacin, to be susceptible to only vancomycin and one or two orally administered antibiotics, such as tetracycline or clindamycin. The same is true for long-term vancomycin therapy. This nonabstract, real-world problem can be avoided if the treatment protocol is followed.

The relationship between device culture and antibiotics is shown in Table 21-8. The intravenous and oral antibiotics presented are used as described here (Fig. 21-43). The data confirm the clinical efficacy of using intravenous vancomycin and gentamicin preoperatively to cover the spectrum and levofloxacin as the primary oral agent. A large number of staphylococcus species (especially *S. epidermidis*) are susceptible to doxycycline and not levofloxacin. Fortunately, the susceptibilities are known before the intravenous antibiotics are stopped. Resistance to levofloxacin is seen commonly in *S. epidermidis* infections treated for long periods before transfer for definitive therapy.

Salvage Procedures

Salvaging an infected device is not possible, in the author's opinion. Salvage procedures have been a therapeutic goal from the beginning. The motivating factors were to eliminate the need for lead extraction and to

TABLE 21-8. **Antibiotic Therapy Given**

Category	Organism	No. of Cases	Vancomycin		Levaquin		Vibramycin		Clindamycin		Other Therapy		No Data	
			IV	PO	IV	PO	IV	PO	IV	PO	IV	PO	IV	PO
Staphylococcus		295												
	Coagulase-negative and *S. epidermidis*	176	143	0	10	85	8	38	7	9	6	15	2	29
	S. aureus	103	91	0	3	14	1	38	3	1	1	4	4	14
	Other	17	13	0	1	7	0	4	1	2	1	0	1	4
Gram-negative		29												
	Klebsiella pneumoniae	2	0	0	0	0	0	0	0	0	2	2	0	0
	Alcaligenes xylosoxidans	1	0	0	1	0	0	0	0	0	0	0	0	1
	Pseudomonas sp	11	0	0	7	0	0	0	0	0	4	4	0	7
	Proteus mirabilis	6	1	0	4	1	0	0	0	0	1	2	0	3
	Serratia marcescens	8	2	0	1	6	0	0	0	0	3	1	2	1
Rare gram-positive		9												
	Enterococcus faecalis	4	2	0	1	2	0	1	0	0	1	0	0	1
	Enterobacter cloacae	3	0	0	2	2	0	0	0	0	1	0	0	1
	Mycobacterium fortuitum	1	0	0	0	0	0	0	0	0	1	1	0	0
	Corynebacterium sp	1	1	0	0	0	0	0	0	0	0	0	0	1
Contaminants		3												
	Nonpathogens	3	1	0	1	1	0	0	0	0	1	1	0	1
Total		336												

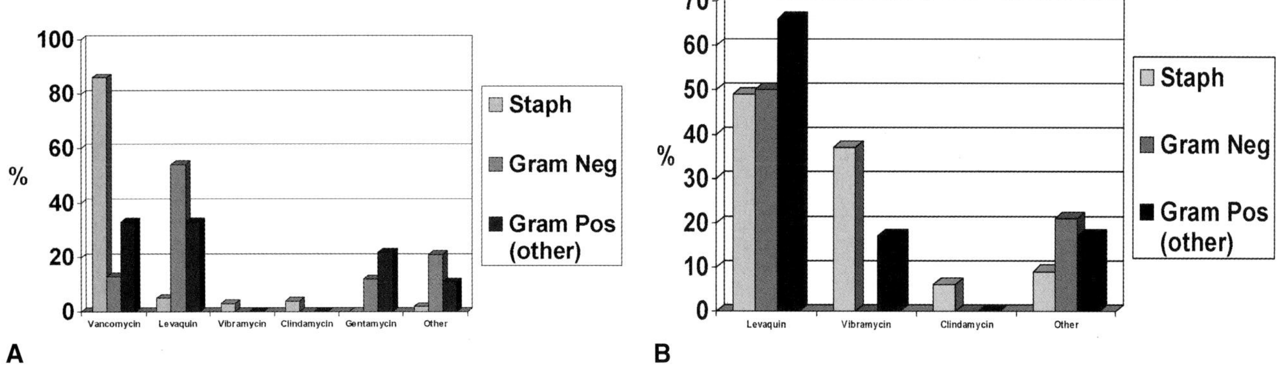

*Figure 21-43. Antibiotic therapy. Antibiotic coverage is instituted according to the protocol (see Table 21-8). The data justify the initial choice of both intravenous (**A**) and oral (**B**) antibiotics. Most patients present without culture results. This selection of antibiotics has the highest probability of the organism's being susceptible.*

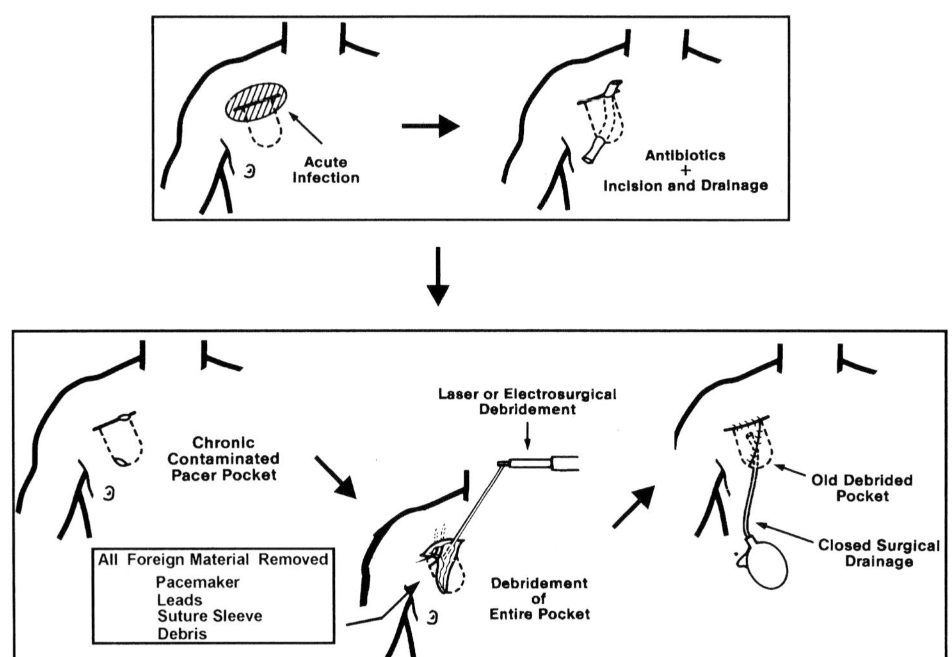

Figure 21-44. Abandoning the implantation site. Acute infections must first be converted into chronic, smoldering infections with a minimal amount of sequestered exudate. In some cases, an incision and drainage is performed, and the drain left in place. Chronic smoldering pockets are debrided of all inflammatory tissue with the use of a carbon dioxide laser. The pulse generator is decontaminated with Cidex, and the leads are cleaned with Betadine. The pulse generator is reimplanted in the debrided pocket, and the old portion of the debrided pocket is excluded. A closed drainage system (e.g., Jackson Pratt) is used in all cases.

avoid pocket abandonment and relocation. To cure a local device infection, it seemed logical to debride the pocket, chemically sterilize the leads to near the vein entry site, and treat with intravenous antibiotics for an extensive period. No bacteria were expected to survive this type of procedure. Some apparent successes did encourage the quest. Unfortunately, slime-producing bacteria, tissue invasion, inability to chemically sterilize implanted leads, and inadequate long-term follow-up doomed this quest to failure. Salvaging an implantation site is not a viable option because the failure rate is too high, the potential morbidity and mortality are too risky, and economic considerations are prohibitive. Since it is still being tried, a historical review may be beneficial. A pocket salvage procedure, at a minimum, includes debridement of all inflammatory tissue and debris, leaving only normal viable tissue. The old pulse generator must be chemically sterilized or a new device used. The old leads are chemically sterilized, and the pocket is closed with or without a closed drainage system (Fig. 21-44). An alternative lead salvage procedure would be to abandon the old debrided and drained pocket, tunnel the leads to a new location, and create a new pocket at the new location.

In the procedure for pocket salvage, the pocket is opened, the pulse generator removed, and the leads freed. All encapsulating and inflammatory tissue must be removed, including the fibrous sheaths tracking the lead (or leads) into the muscle to near the lead's vein entry site. Successful debridement of encapsulating and inflammatory tissue includes leaving a viable bed of normal tissue and obtaining meticulous hemostasis. All tissue dissections are currently performed using an electrosurgical unit, taking care to minimize the injury to normal tissue and to suture-ligate visible veins and all arteries. Skeletal muscle is reapproximated by direct surgical suturing techniques. Reconstitution of this tissue is necessary to achieve hemostasis. After the lead extractions, a closed drainage system (e.g., a flat Jackson-Pratt system) is inserted, and suction is applied to prevent the accumulation of an effusion, ensuring that normal tissue is contiguous to normal tissue. The pocket is then abandoned.

In the past, the pulse generator in infected cases was decontaminated with the use of glutaral (Cidex), and the leads were wiped clean with povidone-iodine (Betadine) and saline. Although Cidex had the potential to sterilize the pacemaker, it was applied for only a short time, and sterility was not assured. The efficacy of lead decontamination by cleaning the surface was dependent on the integrity of the insulation. Insulation with a rough surface and/or cracks, such as degraded polyurethane, could not be cleaned. Decontamination and reuse of a pulse generator is no longer an option. The warranty provided by the company is usually voided if an attempt is made to resterilize the pulse generator. Chemical resterilization may affect the polymers used to insulate the case, the header, and the grommets used to seal the set-screws. Sterilization using ethylene oxide also voids the warranty, due to the potential of heat-related damage. Therefore, if a device is to be reused after ethylene oxide resterilization, the patient must be made aware of the changes in the warranty and the potential of damage to the device.

Continuing the salvage procedure, the pacemaker was reimplanted in the pocket. Most pockets were enlarged after the extensive tissue debridement. If necessary, a portion of the debrided pocket was excluded using interrupted sutures, and the pacemaker was replaced in an appropriately sized space. A closed drainage system (e.g., a flat Jackson-Pratt drain) was routinely used to prevent fluid collection before the adherence of tissue flaps. An exudative or hemorrhagic effusion jeopardizes the success of the procedure by separating the tissues and acting as a culture medium. The closed drainage system was left in place until the drainage stopped and tissue flaps were stuck together (2 to 3 days). All incisions were closed primarily.

In the early 1980s, before the development of effective lead extraction, early salvage procedures were tried (Fig. 21-45). These procedures involved only class III or class IV infections. Class I-B, class I-C, and class II infections were never considered to be salvageable. Although a few were successfully treated, most failed with immediate recurrence of the infection. In addition, many early successes led to a recurrence of the infection 6 to 12 months after the procedure. A success was then defined by the author as no recurrence of infection for a least 1 year after the salvage procedure. Preselection exclusion criteria included septicemia, class I or II infection, gram-negative sepsis, thin subcutaneous tissue and ischemic skin, and a history of previous erosion at the site. These criteria excluded 25% of the patients. During the attempted salvage procedures, another 9% were excluded. In these cases, the debrided pocket was judged to be not suitable for a pacemaker reimplantation, or the inflammatory tissue could not be completely removed from the leads near the vein entry site. The exclusion criteria required judgment and experience in recognizing inflammatory tissue (subjective decisions). A total of 34% of the patients were excluded, and 33% of the procedures were considered failures. The success rate was 45%. During the early and mid-1980s, 45% salvage was an impressive cure rate. Unfortunately, it was impossible to accurately predict which patients would have a successful result. In addition, most of the successes were class IV-A infections with dry erosions. These were just contaminated pockets without tissue infection. Today, the success rate is 100% when following the author's protocol discussed earlier. Salvage procedures are never a viable option.

Exceptions to the Treatment Protocol

Abandonment of the Pocket without Removal of Leads. In one specific situation, the pocket can be abandoned, removing the proximal portion of the leads and leaving the distal portion intact. The infected chronic pocket must be remote (>2.5 cm from the lead insertion site) and free of any visible inflammatory response, and the lead lumen must be free of bacteria. Through a separate incision at the lead insertion site, the leads are inspected and, if found to be free of any inflammatory tissue, cut, clipped, and abandoned. Leads are secured and are not allowed to retract into the superior veins. Leads in the superior veins can migrate, causing another complication. This incision is closed. The infected pocket is then opened, the proximal portion of the leads are removed, all inflammatory tissue is debrided, and the pocket is closed primarily. In the author's opinion, experience is needed to determine whether a lead is free from infection at the vein entry site, and it is impossible to know whether the lumen is contaminated. The safest approach is to treat this situation according to the treatment protocol.

Surgical Creation of a Chronic Draining Sinus. Some patients with class III or class IV infection are not candidates for the treatment protocol. An alternative for these patients is to create a stable class IV-B infection. A class IV-B infection becomes class III when the draining sinus closes. The goal is to create a chronic draining sinus, which stays open and drains. This is accomplished by removing the pulse generator, debriding the pocket, cutting the leads long, and closing the pocket around the lead to create a chronic draining sinus. The leads should be anchored to the skin. As long as the leads protrude from the sinus tract, the

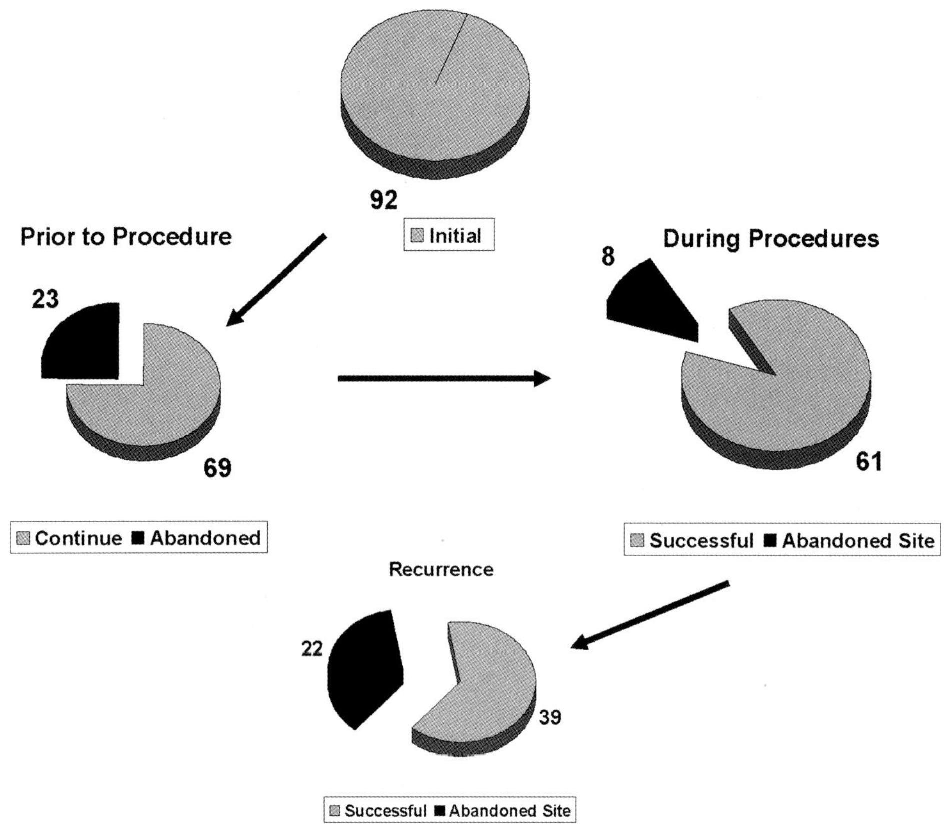

Figure 21-45. This series comprised 92 patients presenting with pocket infections. Only 42% of these patients were successfully treated by the salvage procedure. Of the 69 preselected patients, 8 patients were found to be unsuitable. Of the 61 salvage procedures performed, 22 had a recurrence of infection, leaving only 39 with a successful result. Most of the successful results were with class IV-A infections.

chronic draining sinus will persist. The only care required will be chronic dressing changes. Antibiotic therapy is necessary only for the 7 to 10 days required for the incision to heal. Although this procedure is palliative, it is effective in controlling class III and class IV infections.

These patients usually meet one of two criteria. One criterion is the presence of a concomitant disease process that precludes general anesthesia. General anesthesia may not be required for an uneventful lead removal, but it will be needed in a cardiovascular emergency. For example, a tear of the great veins or heart causing a hemothorax or pericardial tamponade must be corrected immediately via a thoracotomy or a median sternotomy. Although these accidents are rare (<0.5%), the patient must be a candidate for such a procedure to ensure survival. The other criterion is a short time to live, as in patients with a terminal illness and patients with dementia who are confined to a nursing home. In these two examples, it is hard to justify subjecting patients to the procedure in the lead extraction protocol. In such cases, antibiotic therapy is continued, and reimplantation is delayed for an interval of approximately 36 hours. Before reimplantation, two clinical conditions must be met: the patient must be hemodynamically stable and must have a near-normal temperature.

Management of Device-Related Infection Complications

Pocket Infection

Acute infections occurring after an initial implantation in normal tissue are rare and usually result from some breach in surgical technique that contaminates the pocket with a virulent bacterium. For example, inadvertent contamination of the pocket or devices with *S. aureus* will probably cause an acute infection. Most surgical sites are contaminated by mainly nonvirulent bacteria such as *S. epidermidis.* These sites do not become infected when patients are effectively treated with preoperative antibiotics and the pocket is irrigated with an antibiotic solution before closure. Combined with the body's defenses, a small inoculum of these bacteria can be eradicated. However, a large inoculation or the presence of a culture medium such as devitalized tissue or hematoma can negate these efforts, and an infection will ensue. An acute infection is characterized by cellulitis, a suppurative effusion within the pocket (abscess), and, in some cases, decompression into the blood, causing septicemia or discharge through the skin or both. If septicemia is present, the infection is life-threatening and demands immediate treatment. The magnitude of the cellulitis reflects the tissue reaction to the bacteria and their toxins.

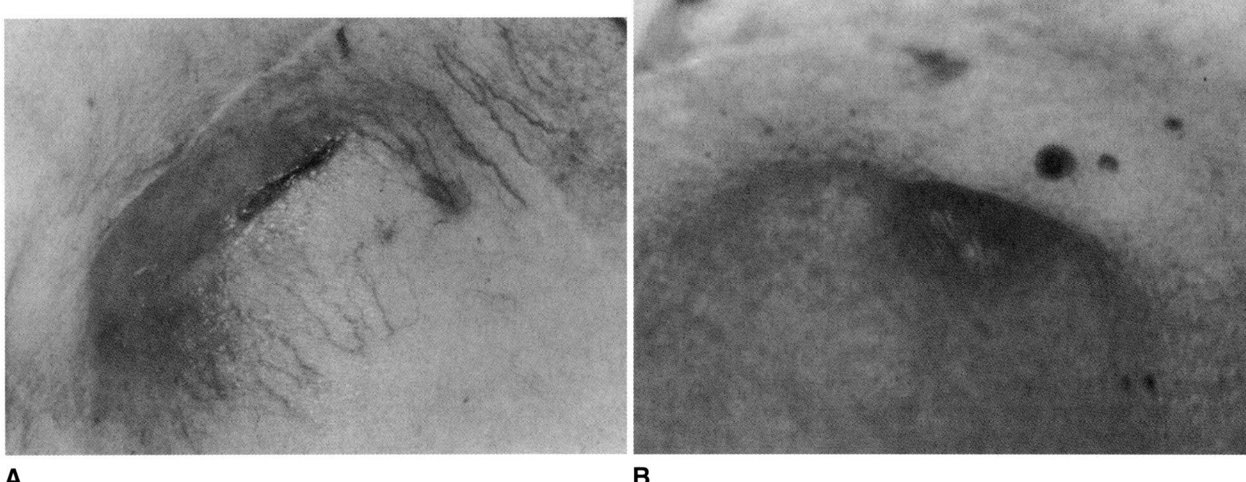

Figure 21-46. Acute infection. An acute infection occurring immediately after an implantation procedure is infrequent. This type of infection indicates a break in surgical technique or metastatic spread from a remote infection site. ***A,*** *The most common presentation is a pocket abscess. Rarely, the infectious debris drains intravenously, causing septicemia and a life-threatening systemic infection.* ***B,*** *An infrequent acute infection is a stitch abscess. This is usually remote from the pocket on the suture sleeve and represents a breach in surgical technique. This type of infection is classified as class III or class IV and treated accordingly.*

Class II, III, and IV-B infections involving old pockets are the most common types of device-related infections (Figs. 21-46A and B). These infections are caused by contamination at the time of pulse generator or lead reimplantation or by metastatic infections. Most of these pockets treated by the author became infected after a reimplantation procedure, usually after replacement of a new device back into the old pocket. Some chronic pacemaker pockets cannot tolerate minimal levels of contamination without developing an infection. For example, pockets with smooth surfaced, poorly vascularized, and exuberant fibrous tissue are ideally suited for an infection. There are two options for these pockets. One involves debridement of the exuberant fibrous tissue, which, in effect, reconditions the pocket. If this is not safe (e.g., hemostasis cannot be ensured), a subcutaneous tissue pocket can be abandoned and the device moved to a submuscular pocket, or vice versa. If other material is present in the pocket, such as granulation tissue or pannus of unorganized clot, the material should be debrided, drained with a closed system (e.g., Jackson-Pratt), excluded, and abandoned. A subcutaneous tissue pocket is moved submuscular, and a submuscular pocket is moved into the subcutaneous tissue in the same location. Rarely, a more remote pocket is necessary. It is the author's opinion that most physicians are not aware of the sequelae of implanting in pockets with exuberant inflammatory tissue. Consequently, they do not effectively debride the pocket, irrigate the pocket, and/or use adequate antibiotic coverage. To some, these maneuvers may seem aggressive for a simple reimplantation procedure, but they represent a practical solution to a potentially complicated, expensive, and even life-threatening problem for the patient.

Another cause of pocket infection is seeding of the pocket by bacteria from a remote infection or from a procedure such as teeth cleaning or colon polyp biopsy or resection. The question of coverage with prophylactic antibiotics in these situations is still unanswered in the literature. Soft tissue implants (pulse generators and leads in the pocket) and right-sided transvenous implants (leads) should be more susceptible to metastatic infections than left-sided arterial implants (prosthetic heart valves); low-flow, right-sided implants should be more susceptible than high-flow, left-sided implants. Although the consequences of acquiring an infection are not quite as serious for right-sided implants, the author believes that the antibiotic therapy used should be similar to that in the protocols published for patients with diseased or prosthetic heart valves.

The same logic used for prophylactic therapy in chronic implants also applies to acute implants. The same probability for metastatic spread exists for both these procedures. In addition, phlebitis and lymphadenitis caused by an infected intravenous fluid administration site has the potential of infecting a new device implant pocket and probably a chronic pocket. Therefore, intravenous fluids should not be administered on the same side as the implant.

Every attempt should be made to find out how an infection started. It is counterproductive to treat a device infection, implant a new device, and have it become reinfected because the infection was the result of metastatic spread from some remote infection (e.g., vertebral body abscess). Infections caused by a transient bacteremia due to teeth cleaning or by a biopsy or removal of a colon polyp may be prevented by use of prophylactic antibiotics.

Latent (Chronic Occult) Infection. In a latent (smoldering or occult) infection, some sort of balance has been reached between the bacteria and the body's defenses. Latent pocket infections are usually caused by *S. epidermidis.* On pocket exploration, exuberant fibrous tissue, with or without an exudative effusion, is found to be present. Granulation tissue may also be present. Bacteria are difficult to culture from effusions within these pockets; pocket tissue gives the best chance of obtaining a positive culture. A diagnosis can usually be made from the appearance of the pocket: exuberant fibrous tissue, yellow transudate-like effusion, and, in some cases, granulation tissue. Once the infection has reached a stage where it cannot be suppressed by the body's defenses, cellulitis and a suppurative effusion are present. On occasion, a chronic pocket is entered and a latent infection exposed. Once detected, it is treated as a class III pocket infection.

A chronic draining sinus is a stabilized chronic infection (see Fig. 21-12). Decompression of an acute infection through the skin and an erosion of a chronic pocket through the skin can both evolve into a chronic draining sinus. As the inflammatory response walls off the pocket from normal tissue and the pocket becomes lined with fibrous and granulation tissue, a steady state exists as long as the exudative debris is drained. If the sinus stops draining, the abscess cycle is repeated. For a chronic draining sinus to last, constant medical management is required. The sinus tract may have to be surgically enlarged from time to time, and if the sinus closes, a brief course of antibiotics may be necessary. In some cases, the entire pocket may not be infected. For example, an infected silk suture (stitch abscess) at the suture sleeve causes a localized abscess, which subsequently forms a draining sinus (see Fig. 21-46B). If a communication with the pocket cannot be found, the local infection can be successfully treated by excision of the sinus and abscess cavity. If a connection is found, or if the pocket infection occurs after treatment of the local abscess, it is treated as a class III or IV-B infection.

Pocket infections that decompress episodically into the venous system cause fever and pulmonary symptoms. The pulmonary symptoms result from an interstitial reaction caused by the filtering of bacteria and debris in the pulmonary capillary bed. An interstitial reaction is apparent on chest X-ray. Some patients develop significant respiratory distress when a large amount of material is decompressed or when the problem persists for an extensive period. Diagnosis is difficult, because in many cases there are no signs or symptoms of class III infection. Patients presenting initially with fever and a persistent cough are sometimes treated for a flulike illness. With antibiotics and time, the symptoms improve, but they recur after the next episode of bacteremia. In patients with these symptoms and an implanted device, a device infection should be suspected until proved otherwise.

Lead Infection

The sequelae of an infected permanent pacing lead range from subcutaneous tissue erosion resulting in a draining sinus (class IV) to a life-threatening systemic infection (classes I-B, I-C, and II). The author believes that most untreated intravascular lead infections are, in time, lethal. Also with time, with or without antibiotic therapy, infections progress in class. For example, class III infections advance to class II and then class I-B infections. It has been recommended that infected leads be removed because of their lethal potential, even in the elderly high-risk patient, using open heart surgery if necessary.

To make it clear how an infected lead is classified and treated, two examples are given. The first example is an infection involving only the extravascular portion of a lead. It is classified and treated as a class III or IV-B infection, regardless of the fact that the lead passes through the vein entry site and into the heart. The treatment consists of pocket debridement, removal of the pulse generator and leads, and reimplantation at a remote site. The second example is an infection that is localized to a segment of the lead in the axillary-subclavian-brachiocephalic veins. It can behave like an abscess and is called a suppurative phlebitis. Despite the fact the infection is confined to the veins, it must be treated the same as a class I-B infection (i.e., 4 to 6 weeks of intravenous antibiotic therapy, and transvenous leads cannot be implanted for 2 to 3 months). Epicardial leads are implanted as an interim solution for pacing. Patients with an ICD may be left unprotected, be monitored in the hospital, or wear an external ICD vest of some type.

Class I-B Infection. An acute class I-B infection involving a new lead implant is rare. These leads are free of encapsulating fibrous tissues, and the insulation is intact. There are two possible mechanisms for this type of infection: (1) clot formation secondarily infected by some source of bacteremia, and (2) a large inoculum of slime-forming bacteria colonizing the lead. Bacteria colonizing the lead would surely cause clot formation, making it difficult to know which came first.

In chronic (old) leads, the presence of encapsulating fibrous tissue, deteriorating insulation, and, in some cases, a mural thrombus offers a potential nidus for infection. Bacteria initially colonizing the encapsulating fibrous tissue causing infected clot formation, or a clot becomes secondarily infected; both mechanisms can cause the infected vegetation (clot or thrombus) necessary for a class I-B infection. Bacteria have been found within the interstices of a degraded insulation polymer and within the lumen, if a breach in the insulation is present. If the insulation has failed and bacteria growth is in the lumen, it can extend the entire length of the lead.

All leads associated with an infection are extracted. On extraction, if an infected clot lodges in the superior veins, a serious suppurative phlebitis will ensue. This is more common when the leads are removed by direct traction. The clot is usually included in an extraction sheath or sheared off the lead. A suppurative phlebitis is a dangerous infection causing septicemia, septic pulmonary emboli, and/or endocarditis. Although this infection can be successfully treated, the morbidity is great. The author has seen only one such case, and it was started by *S. aureus* contamination at the time of implantation from a known break in sterile technique. Fortunately, such breaks in sterile technique are extremely rare.

Class I-C Infection. Class I-C infection is a recurrent endocarditis caused by a retained infected lead segment. Broken leads and fragments abandoned during lead extraction are the sources of these infections. The current incidence of retained infected lead segments is not known exactly but is typically less than 10% The use of powered sheaths has dramatically reduced the incidence of lead breakage and increased the success rate for extraction of leads from the vein entry site. Lead breakage today is not expected and is considered an unsatisfactory outcome.

It is not always possible to extract Class I-B infected leads intact from the right atrium. A recurrent infection caused by a retained lead segment is called a class I-C infection. Different techniques are required for retained atrial and ventricular leads. In the atrium, lead segments with a sufficient portion of the lead body free in the bloodstream can usually be removed using a snare. If they cannot be removed with a snare, the author uses the transatrial approach. The incidence of retained atrial lead segments in patients with class I-B infection is low, and the incidence of recurrent class I-C infection is unknown (probably < 10%).

In the ventricle, embedded electrodes cannot be removed using a transatrial approach. They can be removed only through a right ventriculotomy or an open procedure using CPB. The incidence of recurrent class I-C infections was about 1%, or fewer than 10 patients in the author's database. The rationale for managing these patients was influenced by the perceived dangers associated with a right ventriculotomy. The danger is tearing the ventricle, creating a defect that can be repaired with the use of CPB. Tears on the anterior surface of the right ventricle are extremely difficult to repair, even with CPB. Scarring around the electrode seems to reinforce the tissue, providing sufficient tensile strength to withstand the forces involved in extracting the lead. In the patients with a class I-C infection, the distal and proximal electrode, with or without a short segment of lead body, or the distal electrode with a short segment of lead body insulation, were removed. Because of the potential danger, the author was initially reluctant to subject class I-B patients with a retained lead segment to a ventriculotomy. The electrodes were left in the right ventricle, and 6 to 8 weeks of intravenous antibiotic therapy was given. On completion of treatment, any recurrent infection was assumed to be caused by the retained lead segments. The author cannot find an example of a class I-C infection caused by a distal electrode without lead body insulation. Ventricular leads are now treated the same as atrial leads: all retained, potentially infected lead segments are removed.

Right Atrial Vegetation (Thrombus). Vegetation in the right atrium exists as clot or thrombus (mural or free) and after lead extraction as an encapsulating fibrous tissue. It can be noninfected or infected. From a clinical point of view, a clot is newly formed, soft, and has the potential to lyse; a thrombus is an organized, more solid mass. After lead extraction, ribbon-shaped segments of vegetation consist of encapsulating fibrous tissue peeled or stripped off the lead. This material was not present before lead extraction, and, although it is technically vegetation, it is iatrogenic in origin. Vegetation ranges in size from a few millimeters to a large pedunculated mass (4 to 10 cm). Also, some large masses are adherent to the atrial wall over a broad base, potentially occluding the right atrium. Vegetation is seen most commonly in infected patients and in patients with poor cardiac function. The presence of infected and/or large vegetation is an indication for lead extraction and removal of the vegetation. The connotation is that vegetation is "bad" and that, when it is present, both the vegetation and lead must be removed.

Vegetation, in relation to implanted leads, can be defined as a growth or excrescence, such as clot or thrombotic material. This broad definition appears satisfactory on first impression. However, on closer inspection, it has little clinical usefulness and is complicated and confusing to apply. By this definition, forms of vegetation include a small clot on the lead and the organizing encapsulating fibrous tissue. However, this type of vegetation is considered a naturally occurring pathologic event (oxymoron). This is a form of "good" vegetation, and it must be distinguished in some fashion from "bad" vegetation. To qualify, or place a condition in, the definition is a natural way to separate "good" vegetation from "bad." Separation must be done at a macrobiologic level using everyday tools, and it must be based on the known physical and clinical properties of vegetation. Vegetation is visible on echocardiography. Echocardiography has the same clinical usefulness for visualizing vegetation relative to the cardiac anatomy as fluoroscopy does for visualizing implanted leads. Modifying the definition to mean only those growths and excrescences that are visible echocardiographically satisfies both the physical and the clinical properties present at a macrobiologic level.

Vegetation begins as a clot forming on the lead, vascular wall, or most commonly on both. If a clot does not lyse, it will organize into encapsulating fibrous tissue and/or thrombus. A thrombus has the potential to grow by continued deposition of clot and organization. A clot is a supple, malleable, jelly-like mass that is easily deformable. In the bloodstream, it is subjected to the forces caused by flowing blood. Once the mass is of sufficient size, it begins to move, causing elongation (stretching). It then becomes visible echocardiographically and is called vegetation. Visibility on echocardiogram is the only way to know if vegetation exists. This separates vegetations based on size and the resolution of the echocardiographic technique. Small clots and noncalcified encapsulating fibrous tissue are not visible in a definitive fashion using current echocardiographic imaging. A discussion of class II and class I-B infections provides an excellent example of the clinical usefulness of this definition for vegetation.

Class II infections (septicemia with positive blood cultures) and the presence of vegetation on echocardiography are the criteria used for making a diagnosis of vegetative endocarditis (class I-B). The absence of vegetation keeps septicemia a class II infection, regardless of the magnitude of the signs and symptoms. This diagnosis is empirical and is based on clinical experience and the hypothesis that the presence of bacteria causes clot and/or causes a clot to grow into vegetation.

Classes II, III, and IV infections are all treated the same. This therapeutic modality is based on the hypothesis that if bacterial colonies on the lead and/or clot have not reached the size of vegetation, the surrounding tissues are not at risk of becoming infected. This hypothesis is based on the author's clinical observation that class I infections do not occur using this treatment protocol; there are no false-negative results. The confidence in the protocol treatment outcome is reinforced by the clinical behavior of class I infections. These malignant infections are lethal and do not go unnoticed. The success of the treatment protocol leads to two possible interpretations: an infected clot must reach vegetation size before it can infect other tissues (hypothesis), or treating class I-B infections with intravenous antibiotics for 4 to 6 weeks is unnecessary. The prevailing wisdom is that long-term intravenous antibiotic therapy is an essential part of the treatment protocol for class I-B infections. However, if the second interpretation is correct, the hypothesis would not have to be true; short-term oral antibiotics are effective enough to treat other infected tissues. A false-positive result cannot be determined clinically using the current treatment protocol. The incidence of a class II infection associated with noninfected vegetation is unknown. A research project designed to obtain a biopsy of the vegetation from a remote vein entry site would be necessary to attempt to determine the incidence. For the present, false-positive findings will be treated as class II infections.

A vegetation's actual status, clot or thrombus, is a histologic determination. However, making an educated guess based on the size, shape, and consistency is helpful in selecting a therapeutic modality. Size is apparent and easily measured by echocardiography. Size has clinical significance but is not a reliable method of separating clot from thrombus. Shape is important. A clot whipping around in the bloodstream is typically longer and more narrow than a thrombus (clot stretches more than thrombus). A thrombus is more globular and frequently has a defined stalk. The motion of the vegetation in the bloodstream (i.e., suppleness and ease of deformation) provides clues to its consistency. Clots are more supple and have a loose consistency. A thrombus is less supple and has a more rigid consistency. Combining shape and consistency is useful in clinically separating clot from thrombus.

Small vegetations (<2 cm) all appear the same: a finger-like mass of material whipping around in the bloodstream. A more detailed knowledge of small vegetations is not needed, because it would not change the clinical management. For class I-B infections, the leads and vegetation are removed. The vegetation frequently is not removed with the lead and must be removed separately. In the absence of infection, small vegetation is not always removed. Because the incidence and natural history of small vegetations is not known, treatment protocols have not been developed. Currently, treatment options include doing nothing, monitoring with echocardiography, embarking on a trial of heparin therapy, and making an attempt at transvenous removal by snare. The author's perspective is based on experience with a large number of patients with vegetation and is skewed, because most of the patients were referred for treatment of a complication. TEE was used in all procedures. The small vegetation status of all patients was recorded (infected and noninfected). The author was surprised at the number of noninfected patients who had small vegetations that would have gone undetected without TEE. The incidence is small for the general patient population, but it is higher among patients with multiple leads and those with low flow. Because most of the patients require lead removal and an attempt was made to remove the vegetation during the lead extraction, the natural history is unknown. In a few rare patients with multiple leads and low output not requiring lead extraction, the vegetation was left intact. The rationale for this decision was based on the premise that replacement of these leads with new leads did not preclude the recurrence of vegetation on the new leads. Also, there are areas in the atrium where vegetation cannot easily be reached with a snare.

The properties of large vegetations are determined with the use of TEE. If the vegetation is more clotlike, it appears suppler, thinner, and frequently has a parachute appearance. It sometimes billows out like a parachute; it waves around like a sheet in the wind. A solid pedunculated mass such as a thrombus is usually bulbous and will bounce around in the atrium but does not have wave motions or appear supple. Vegetations larger than 2 to 3 cm are considered "bad" and are removed. Large vegetations (>6 cm) must be considered dangerous. They can occlude the tricuspid valve or break free, causing pulmonary emboli. If one of these masses breaks free and wedges in the right ventricular outflow tract or main pulmonary artery, it can cause an immediate cessation of blood flow through the heart and cardiovascular collapse. Unless it is removed surgically or dislodged into a more distal left or right pulmonary artery, it is lethal. Occlusion of one of the large branches is tolerated for a period of time. There is time enough to initiate therapy such as intravenous infusion of thrombolytic agents and/or to perform a pulmonary embolectomy, with or without CPB. If the mass breaks up and the lungs are showered with small and large emboli bilaterally, the acute insult could be low cardiac output; right-sided heart failure caused by pulmonary artery hypertension ensues. The author has observed one such embolic event (mainly large fragments) partially occluding the pulmonary flow; it was successfully treated on an emergency basis by surgical embolectomy. In general, emergency aggressive therapy (embolectomy and/or thrombolytic agents) is required. It is obvious that removal of large vegetation should be approached with care, and a contingency plan should be available for emergencies.

The size, shape, and consistency of vegetation determine the removal approach. The type of mass, clot or thrombus, is at best an educated guess; it is frequently a mixture of both. It should be mentioned that removal of large vegetation from the right atrium is a work in progress, and removal procedures are evolving with experience. Experience is gained slowly, because the incidence of this type of vegetation is low. Fortunately, the clinical results are excellent as long as most of the vegetation is removed (extensive debulking procedure).

Transvenous snare removal is relegated to smaller clot removal (<4 cm). During lead extraction, the lead and vegetation are sometimes removed through the extraction sheath. If the vegetation is still present after extraction, the author attempts to remove it with a snare. A Dotter snare is passed through the sheath and into the atrium. It is easy to entangle the clot and ribbons of liberated encapsulating fibrous tissue in a Dotter snare and remove it. The snare is positioned and rotated, entangling the vegetation or shearing it off the atrial wall. The passage of small vegetation into the pulmonary vasculature is generally not a clinical problem. There are no apparent respiratory symptoms and no changes on chest radiography. By whatever mechanism, it seems to be handled in an expeditious fashion. Rarely, a larger solid thrombus passes into the periphery of the pulmonary vasculature, causing small wedge infarct and a painful local pleuritic reaction. This is usually an accident, because every attempt is made to remove a solid mass intact. Clot emboli detected in the pulmonary vasculature are treatable with thrombolytic agents. Clots larger than 4 cm are usually removed by the author using one of the transatrial techniques.

The author uses the transatrial approach as the primary approach for all large vegetation (>4 cm) and for bulbous pedunculated thrombi greater than 2 cm. The transatrial approach is the same as for lead implantation and extraction. Two techniques are used to remove the vegetation: grasping the vegetation with a pituitary rongeur and applying a suction apparatus. The lead is grasped proximal to the vegetation and pulled out of the atriotomy site. The vegetation, if adherent to the lead, is pulled to the atriotomy site and removed. If the vegetation is attached to the wall and not adherent to the lead, it is grasped with a pituitary rongeur. The instrument is guided to the vegetation by echocardiography; the rongeur replaces the snare, and the vegetation is removed through the atriotomy site. This technique has been successful in removing vegetations smaller than 4 cm. Large vegetations are more difficult to remove intact with the rongeur and are frequently removed piecemeal.

The author has developed a new technique using suction. A large suction catheter is inserted through the atriotomy site and guided to the vegetation by echocardiography. The suction apparatus is composed of the suction catheter, a trap, and connection to wall suction. Once the suction tip is placed against the vegetation, the clamp is released, applying maximum suction. Gelatinous material and friable thrombus along with blood are sucked into the trap. The contents in the trap are filtered, and the removed vegetation visually inspected. The trap can hold 100 mL of blood, and the blood loss is monitored. The process is repeated until all visible vegetation is removed. If a solid thrombus becomes firmly attached to the suction tip, it is pulled to the atriotomy site and teased out. This technique has been remarkably successful to date and is currently the procedure of choice. It is much faster and more efficient than the rongeur technique. Little or no material is lost to the lung field. This technique evolved from experiences removing clot with the atrium opened on CPB. Use of a large suction catheter was found to be one of the most efficient ways to clean the vegetation from the chamber. The more gelatinous vegetation was sucked out, and solid thrombus attached to the suction handle and was peeled off the atrial wall. The easiest way to remove vegetation is to place the patient on CPB and remove it under direct vision. Most cardiac surgeons do not have experience with the transatrial approach and feel insecure performing the procedure. Consequently, they use CPB instead of the transatrial approach as their primary procedure of choice. The presence of infection and the morbidity associated with the procedure usually discourage the initial use of this approach, positioning it as a procedure of last resort. No special techniques are required to remove vegetation under direct vision on CPB; it is a surgical dissection.

A large vegetative mass in the right atrium with both sessile and pedunculated components is primarily thrombus. This material is attached to the wall at all points of contact and, with time, becomes occlusive. The author has seen this complication only twice. With this limited experience, it is hard to generalize. Two statements are known to be true. First, because of the size of the mass and adherence to the wall, transvenous or transatrial debulking is not practical. Second, this material can be removed only under direct vision on CPB. It is not easy to use CPB with these patients. A total bypass with cannulation of the SVC and IVC is required. TEE is necessary to find a free channel and direct the cannula around the mass into the SVC and IVC. The thrombus must be peeled off the atrial wall, which is a tedious, time-consuming operation. Also, leads have to be removed. Although they can be removed under direct vision, the use of lead extraction tools in the right ventricle expedites this process.

Conclusion

The goal in managing device-related complications is to understand the mechanical, biologic, and technical factors responsible for their occurrence, in order to design biocompatible devices, develop complication-free implantation techniques, and develop safe, efficient procedures for treating complications.

The golden rule is to never send a patient treated for one complication home with another.

REFERENCES

1. Medtronic Product Performance Report, Marquis Family ICD and CRT-D Advisory Update, February 2005 and December 2005, http://www.medtronic.com/crm/performance/advisories/marquis-feb2005.html. Accessed July 23, 2006.
2. Ventak Prizm 2Dr Model 1861 Advisory Update, Guidant, May 9, 2006, update of June 17, 2005, physician advisory letter, http://www.guidant.com/physician_communications/prizm2_060509.pdf. Accessed July 23, 2006.
3. Stokes K, Urbanski P, Upton J: The in vivo auto-oxidation of polyether polyurethanes by metal ions. J Biomater Sci Polym Ed 1:207, 1990.
4. Stokes KB, Church T: Ten-year experience with implanted polyurethane lead insulation. PACE 9:1160, 1986.
5. Byrd CL, Schwartz SJ, Wettenstein E: Chronic analysis of polyurethane leads. PACE 8:A-83, 1985.
6. Byrd CL, McArthur W, Stokes K, et al: Implant experience with unipolar polyurethane pacing leads. PACE 6:868-882, 1983.
7. Kawanishi DT, Brinker JA, Reeves R, et al: Spontaneous versus extraction related injuries associated with Accufix J-wire atrial pacemaker lead: Tracking changes in patient management. PACE 21:2314-2317, 1998.
8. Kay GN, Brinker JA, Kawanishi DT, et al: Risks of spontaneous injury and extraction of an active fixation pacemaker lead: Report of the Accufix Multicenter Clinical Study and Worldwide Registry. Circulation 100:2344-2352, 1999.
9. Kawanishi DT, Brinker JA, Reeves R, et al: Cumulative hazard analysis of J-wire fracture in the Accufix series of atrial permanent pacemaker leads. PACE 21:2322-2326, 1998.
10. Kawanishi DT, Brinker JA, Reeves R, et al: Kaplan-Meier analysis of freedom from extraction or death in patients with an Accufix J retention wire atrial permanent pacemaker lead: A potential management tool. PACE 21:2318-2321, 1998.
11. Wilkoff BL: ICDs: Dealing with less than perfect. J Cardiovasc Electrophysiol 16:796-797, 2005.
12. Anderson JM: Inflammatory response to implants. ASAIO J 11:101-107, 1988.
13. Schoen FJ, Harasaki H, Kim KM, et al: Biomaterial-associated calcification: Pathology, mechanisms, and strategies for prevention. J Biomed Mater Res 22(A1):11-36, 1988.
14. Hecker JR, Scandrett LA: Roughness and thrombogenicity of the outer surfaces of intravascular catheters. J Biomed Mater Res 19:381-395, 1985.
15. Da Costa A, Kirkorian G, Cucherat M, et al: Antibiotic prophylaxis for permanent pacemaker implantation: A meta-analysis. Circulation 97:1796-1801, 1998.
16. Love CJ, Wilkoff BL, Byrd CL, et al: Recommendations for extraction of chronically implanted transvenous pacing and defibrillator leads: Indications, facilities, training. North American Society of Pacing and Electrophysiology Lead Extraction Conference Faculty. PACE 23:544-551, 2000.
17. Byrd CL, Schwartz SJ, Hedin N: Lead extraction: Indications and techniques. Cardiol Clin 10:735-748, 1992.
18. Chamis AL, Peterson GE, Cabell CH, et al: *Staphylococcus aureus* bacteremia in patients with permanent pacemakers or implantable cardioverter-defibrillators. Circulation 104:1029-1033, 2001.
19. Chua JD, Wilkoff BL, Lee I, et al: Diagnosis and management of infections involving implantable electrophysiologic cardiac devices. Ann Intern Med 133:604-608, 2000.
20. Chan AW, Bhatt DL, Wilkoff BL, et al: Percutaneous treatment for pacemaker-associated superior vena cava syndrome. PACE 25:1628-1633, 2002.
21. Suga C, Hayes DL, Hyberger LK, et al: Is there an adverse outcome from abandoned pacing leads? J Interv Card Electrophysiol 4:493-499, 2000.
22. Fearnot NE, Smith HJ, Goode LB, et al: Intravascular lead extraction using locking stylets, sheaths, and other techniques. PACE 13:1864-1870, 1990.
23. Smith HJ, Fearnot NE, Byrd CL, et al: Five-years experience with intravascular lead extraction. U.S. Lead Extraction Database. PACE 17:2016-2020, 1994.
24. Byrd CL, Wilkoff BL, Love CJ, et al: Intravascular extraction of problematic or infected permanent pacemaker leads: 1994-1996. U.S. Extraction Database, MED Institute. PACE 22:1348-1357, 1999.
25. Byrd CL, Schwartz SJ, Hedin N: Intravascular techniques for extraction of permanent pacemaker leads. J Thorac Cardiovasc Surg 101:989-997, 1991.
26. Bilgutay, AM, Jensen MK, Schmidt WR, et al: Incarceration of transvenous pacemaker electrode: Removal by traction. Am Heart J 77:377-379, 1969.
27. Karagoz T, Celiker A, Hallioglu O, Ozme S: Unusual extraction of an active fixation ventricular pacing lead with outer coil fracture in a child. Europace 5:185-187, 2003.
28. Wilkoff BL, Byrd CL, Love CJ, et al: Pacemaker lead extraction with the laser sheath: Results of the Pacing Lead Extraction with the Excimer Sheath (PLEXES) trial. J Am Coll Cardiol 33:1671-1676, 1999.
29. Epstein LM, Byrd CL, Wilkoff BL, et al: Initial experience with larger laser sheaths for the removal of transvenous pacemaker and implantable defibrillator leads. Circulation 100:516-525, 1999.
30. Saad EB, Saliba WI, Schweikert RA, et al: Nonthoracotomy implantable defibrillator lead extraction: Results and comparison with extraction of pacemaker leads. PACE 26:1944-1950, 2003.
31. Byrd CL, Wilkoff BL, Love CJ, et al: Clinical study of the laser sheath for lead extraction: The total experience in the United States. PACE 25:804-808, 2002.
32. Kennergren C: Excimer laser assisted extraction of permanent pacemaker and ICD leads: Present experiences of a European multi-centre study. Eur J Cardiothorac Surg 15:856-860, 1999.
33. Love C, Byrd C, Wilkoff BL, et al: Lead extraction using a bipolar electrosurgical dissection sheath: An interim report. Europace: 223-228, 2001.
34. Kennergren C, Schaerf RH, Sellers TD, et al: Cardiac lead extraction with a novel locking stylet. J Interv Card Electrophysiol 4:591-593, 2000.
35. Bongiorni MG, Giannola G, Arena G, et al: Pacing and implantable cardioverter-defibrillator transvenous lead extraction. Ital Heart J 6:261-266, 2005.
36. Byrd CL, Schwartz SJ: Transatrial implantation of transvenous pacing leads as an alternative to implantation of epicardial leads. PACE 13:1856-1859, 1990.
37. Wilkoff BL, Belott PH, Love CJ, et al: Improved extraction of ePTFE and medical adhesive modified defibrillation leads from the coronary sinus and great cardiac vein. PACE 28:205-211, 2005.
38. Byrd CL: Safe introducer technique for pacemaker lead implantation. PACE 15:262-267, 1992.
39. Byrd CL: Current clinical applications of dual-chamber pacing. In Zipes DP (ed): Proceedings of a Symposium. Minneapolis: Medtronic, Inc., 1981, p 71.
40. Erdogan O, Augostini R, Saliba W, et al: Transiliac permanent pacemaker implantation after extraction of infected pectoral pacemaker systems. Am J Cardiol 84:474-475, A9-A10, 1999.
41. Khan MN, Joseph G, Khaykin Y, et al: Delayed lead perforation: A disturbing trend. PACE 28:251-253, 2005.
42. Dy Chua J, Abdul-Karim A, Mawhorter S, et al: The role of swab and tissue culture in the diagnosis of implantable cardiac device infection. PACE 28:1276-1281, 2005.
43. Prescott LM, Harley JM, Klein DA (eds): Human diseases caused primarily by gram-positive and gram-negative bacteria. In Prescott LM, Harley JM, Klein DA (eds): Microbiology, 4th ed. Boston, WCB/McGraw-Hill, 1999, pp 766-796.

Chapter 22

Imaging in Pacing and Defibrillation

DHANUNJAYA R. LAKKIREDDY • ELIZABETH SAAREL • MINA K. CHUNG

Thoracic and, occasionally, abdominal imaging plays an important role in the implantation, maintenance, and removal of pacing and defibrillation systems. Many available contemporary modalities, including radiography, fluoroscopy, venography, echocardiography, computed tomography (CT) and magnetic resonance imaging (MRI), are frequently applied for the diagnosis and treatment of patients with pacemaker and implantable cardioverter-defibrillator (ICD) devices. Those most commonly used before, during, and after device implantation are radiography, fluoroscopy, and venography, critical tools for physicians who perform pacemaker and ICD surgery. In addition, echocardiography has widespread applications, ranging from confirmation of the acute procedural complication of cardiac rupture with cardiac tamponade to optimization of pacing in cardiac resynchronization therapy (CRT). CT imaging is primarily used in preoperative and postoperative settings to assess complex cardiac anatomy, especially in patients with corrected and uncorrected congenital heart conditions. In contrast, MRI may be used for preoperative assessment of cardiovascular anatomy but is more often employed for diagnosis of pathologic conditions outside the thoracic cavity. Its potential for electromagnetic interference with implanted pacemaker and ICD devices is discussed here.

Radiography

Radiographs provide essential information about the location, type, and integrity of the pulse generators and leads of both pacing and defibrillation systems. They also provide basic details of patient anatomy. Interpretation of a chest radiograph should be approached in a focused and systematic fashion, consisting of examination of the bony structures, cardiac silhouette, lung fields, trachea and aorta as well as the presence and location of all preexisting hardware, prosthetic valves, and valve rings or calcification (Fig. 22-1). Abdominal radiographs should be obtained when abdominal device implantation is anticipated.

Pre-Procedure Chest Radiography

Pre-procedure posteroanterior (PA) and lateral chest radiographs provide essential information about patient anatomy and help identify the location, type, and integrity of implanted lead and device hardware in patients with preexisting pacing and defibrillation systems.

Identification of Patient Anatomy

Chest wall deformities, such as scoliosis and kyphosis, can occasionally make the implantation of endovascular leads difficult because of distortion of venous and cardiac anatomy. Identification of massive cardiomegaly may influence the choice of lead length. Anomalies such as a right-sided aortic knob suggest the presence of congenital abnormalities. Congenital abnormalities are discussed later.

Identification of Pacing and Defibrillation Systems

It is important to identify the type and location of preexisting pacing or defibrillation systems, particularly in

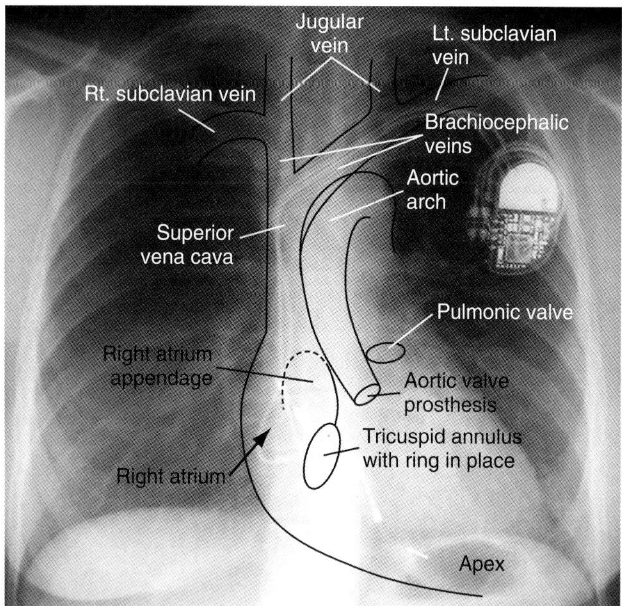

Figure 22-1. *Overlay of diagram on a posteroanterior chest radiograph demonstrating the typical location for the formation of the subclavian veins, brachiocephalic veins, the superior vena cava, and the right atrium along with their associated osseous landmarks. Lt, left; Rt, right. (From Castle LW, Cook S: Pacemaker radiography. In Ellenbogen KA, Kay GN, Wilkoff BL [eds]: Clinical Cardiac Pacing. Philadelphia, WB Saunders, 1995, p 538.)*

the significant and growing numbers of patients presenting for generator exchange, lead addition, lead extraction, or device upgrade. With expanding indications and longevity of patients, it is not uncommon for a patient to have multiple functional and abandoned leads or even separate pacemaker and ICD devices. The type and position of the generators as well as the type, position, and integrity of all leads should be examined. A thorough examination requires a PA as well as a lateral chest radiograph and, in the patient with an abdominally located device, an abdominal film.

Pacemaker and Implantable Cardioverter-Defibrillator Pulse Generators; Implantable Loop Recorders

For transvenous systems, the pulse generator is typically located in the subcutaneous, prepectoral region caudal to the clavicle, overlying the pectoralis major muscle. In some patients, the device is located in a subpectoral or submammary position (Fig. 22-2). In pediatric patients and patients with older, larger ICD pulse generators or epicardial ICD lead systems, devices may be located in the abdomen, typically in the left upper quadrant and occasionally in the right upper quadrant or epigastrium (Fig. 22-3).Although most pulse generators are implanted in the subcutaneous region in adult patients, many have been implanted below the rectus abdominis muscle in children and younger women. The pulse generator is also generally implanted abdominally in patients in whom a femoral vein approach is required (Fig. 22-4).

The generator manufacturer and type can be identified from radiography. Most pacemaker and ICD pulse generators have a radiopaque code or logo identifying the manufacturer and model of the device (Figs. 22-5 and 22-6). If the manufacturer can be determined, the proper programmer can be selected. Most current manufacturer programmers can auto-identify the specific devices of that manufacturer. Manufacturer technical support divisions may be able to aid in identification of lead systems and devices and can often access device data, such as leads implanted, pacing or shocking configurations, and implant thresholds. Some patients may have both pacing and ICD systems as well as leads or devices that originate from different manufacturers. Figure 22-7 shows the appearance of an implantable loop recorder.

The pacemaker or ICD connector block should be carefully examined radiographically. The connector pins should be advanced beyond the distal pin set-screw blocks (Fig. 22-8). It is usually difficult to determine radiographically whether set-screws are in contact with the electrodes. Clues to the polarity of pacing

Text continued on p. 938

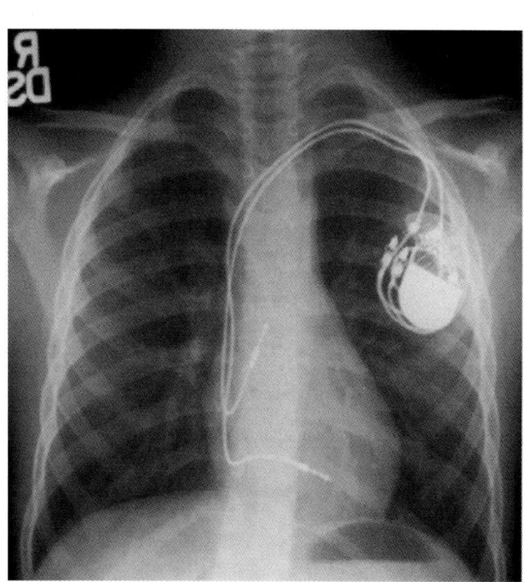

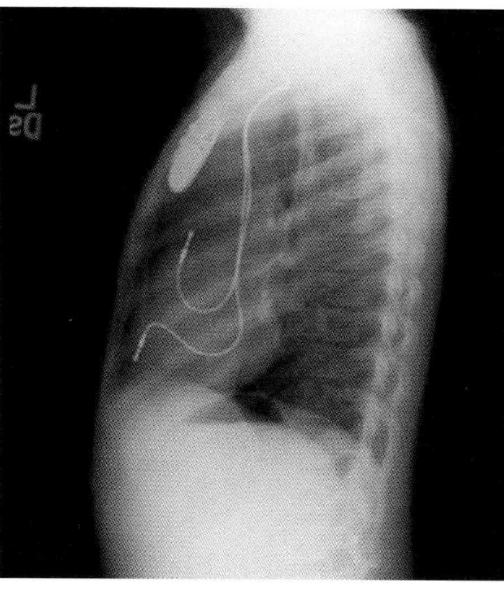

Figure 22-2. *Transvenous pacemaker system in subpectoral position. Posteroanterior and lateral chest radiographs in child with congenital complete heart block and dual-chamber pacemaker.*

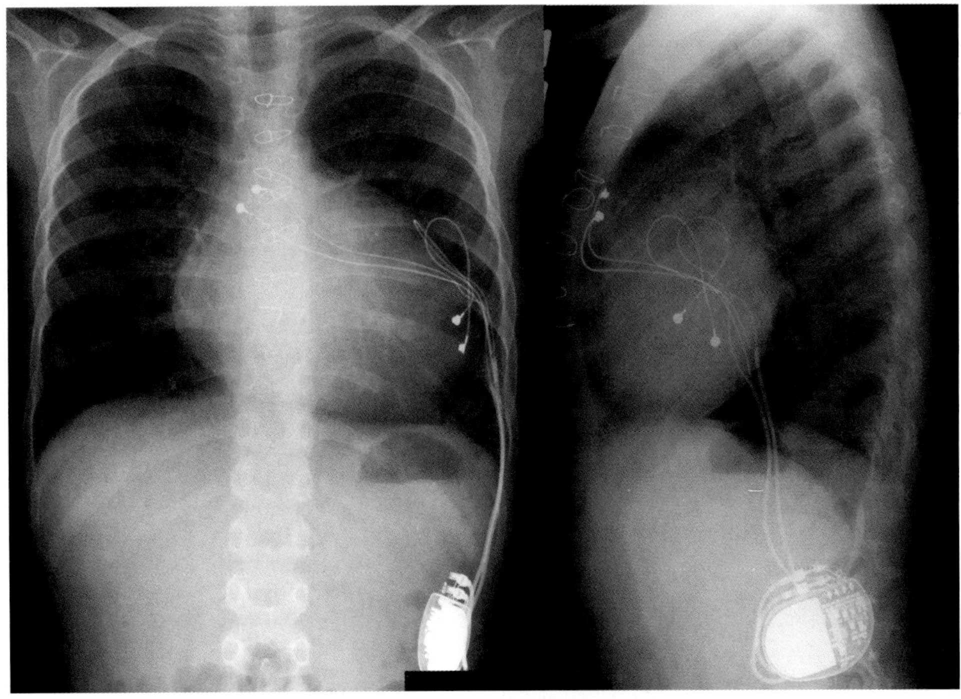

A

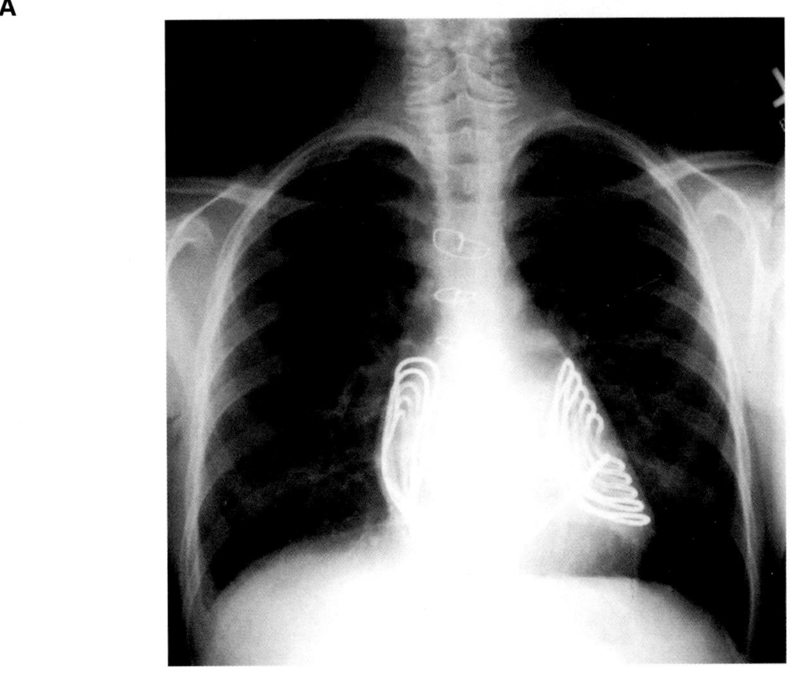

B

Figure 22-3. Abdominal pacemaker and implantable cardioverter-defibrillator (ICD) systems. ***A,*** *Posteroanterior and lateral chest radiographs of an abdominal pacemaker system with epicardial leads in a child with congenital heart disease.* ***B,*** *Abdominal ICD system with epicardial leads.*

Continued

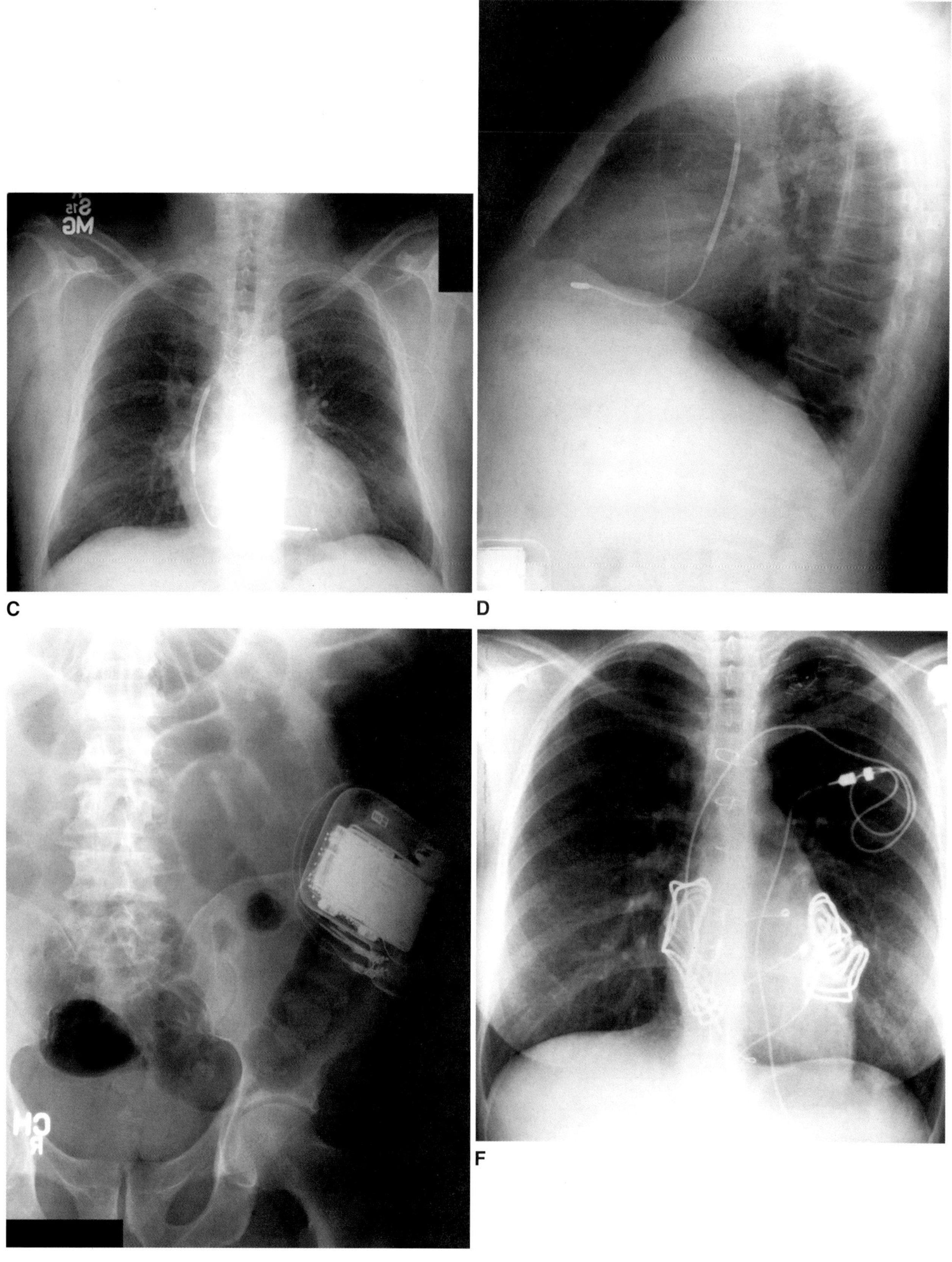

Figure 22-3, cont'd. ***C to E,*** *Abdominal ICD system with transvenous leads.* ***F,*** *Abdominal ICD lead system with an epicardial and a transvenous lead.*

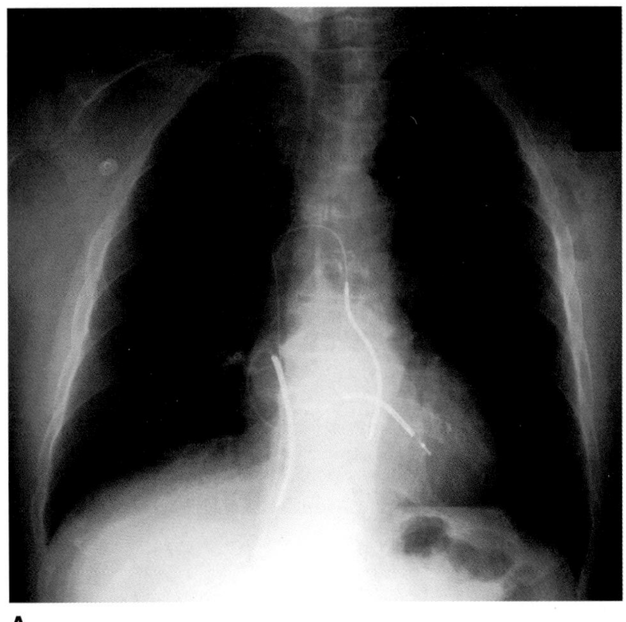

A

B

C

Figure 22-4. Implantable cardioverter-defibrillator (ICD) with defibrillation leads, including an azygos coil lead, inserted via a femoral vein approach. The leads are inserted via a right femoral vein approach. ***A,*** *Posteroanterior chest radiograph shows the coils of the dual-coil defibrillation–pace/sense lead are positioned in the right atrium and right ventricle. The second lead is placed in the azygos vein.* ***B,*** *Lateral chest radiograph demonstrates the posterior positioning of the azygos coil.* ***C,*** *Abdominal radiograph displays the leads are tunneled from the right femoral vein access site to the ICD device pocket in located in the left upper quadrant.*

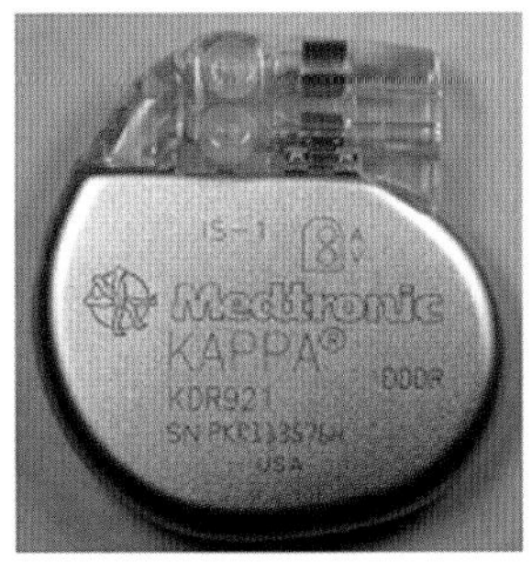

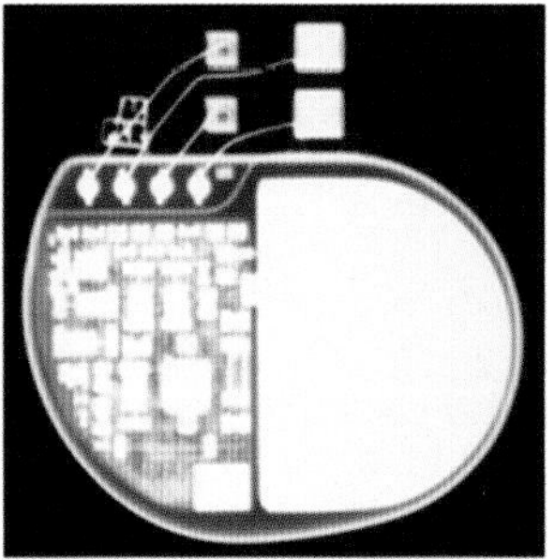
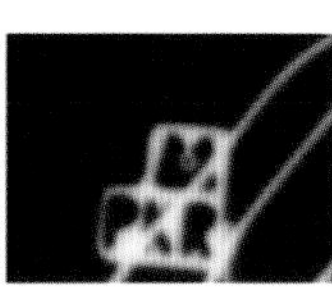

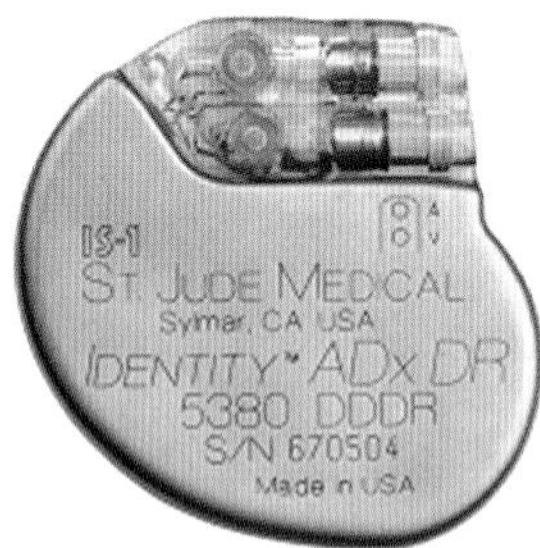

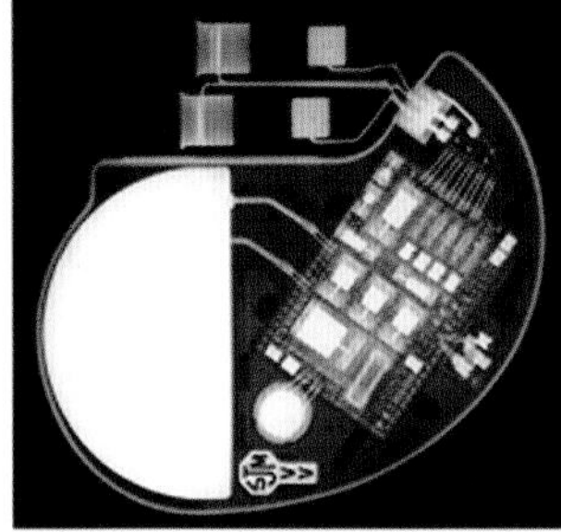
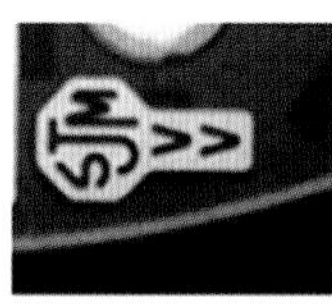

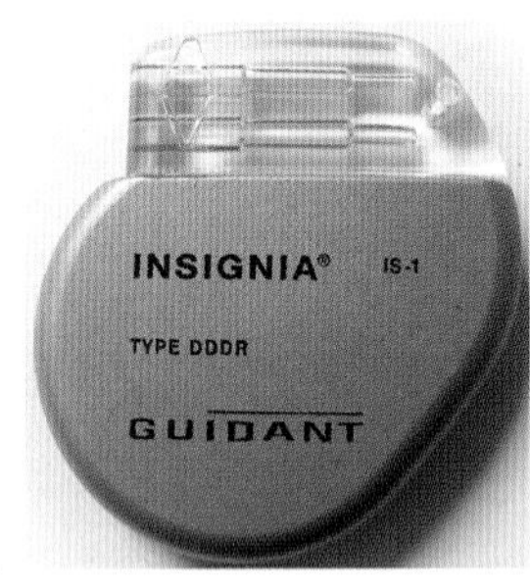

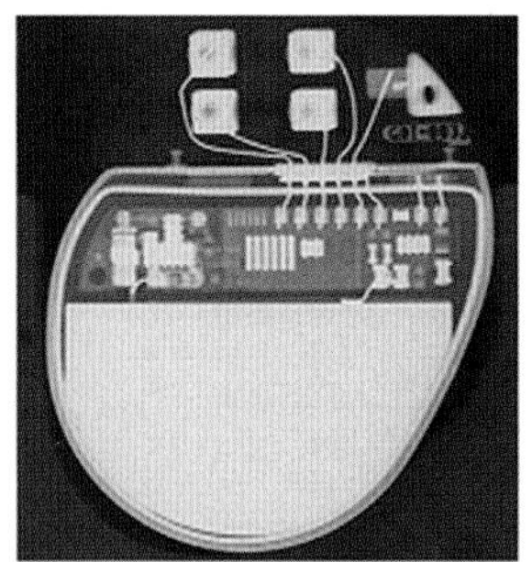
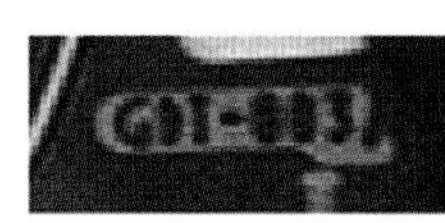

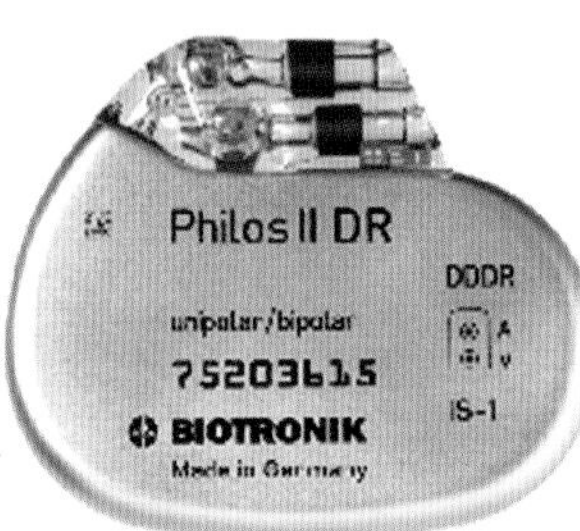

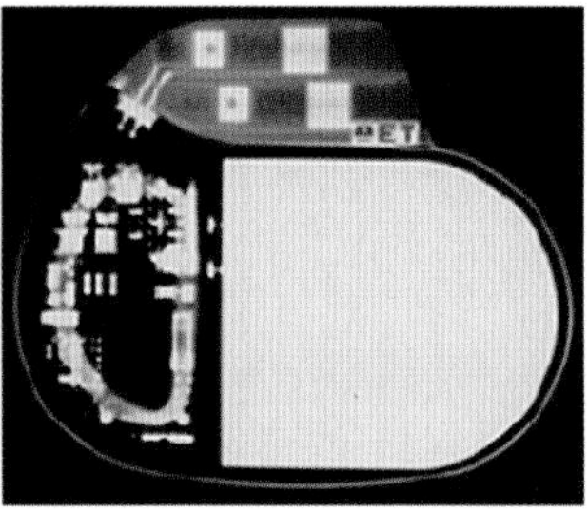
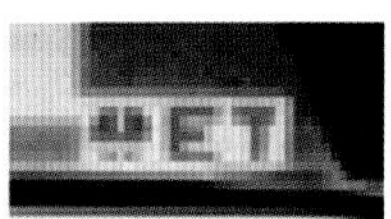

Figure 22-5. Radiographic appearance of various pacing pulse generators and their radiographic logos. (Courtesy of Medtronic, Inc., Minneapolis, Minn.; St. Jude Medical, St. Paul, Minn.; Guidant, Boston Scientific, Natick, Mass.; and Biotronik GmbH & Co., Berlin.)

Guidant Vitality

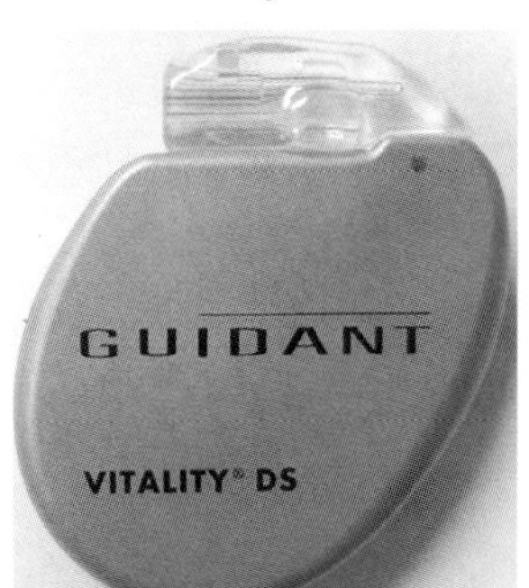

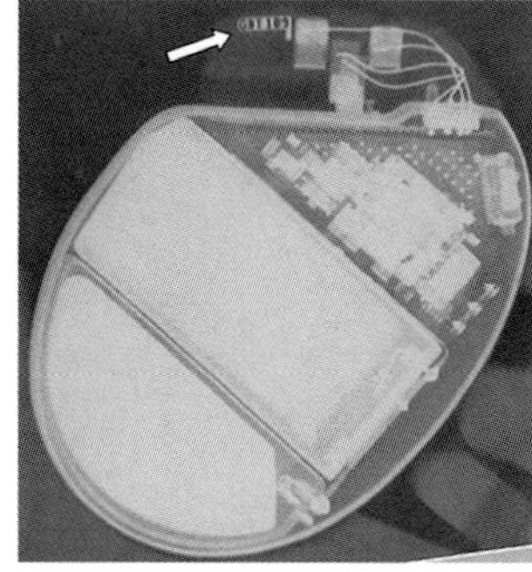

Guidant Renewal 3 HF

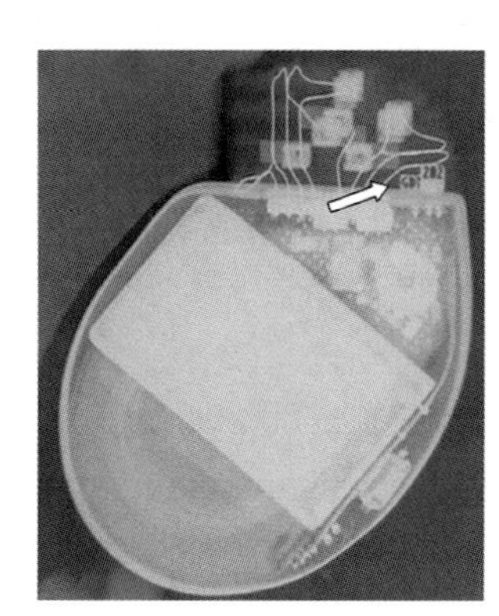

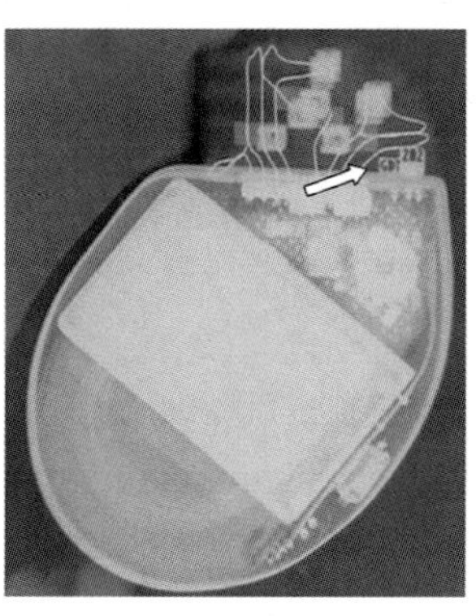

St. Jude Epic+ DR

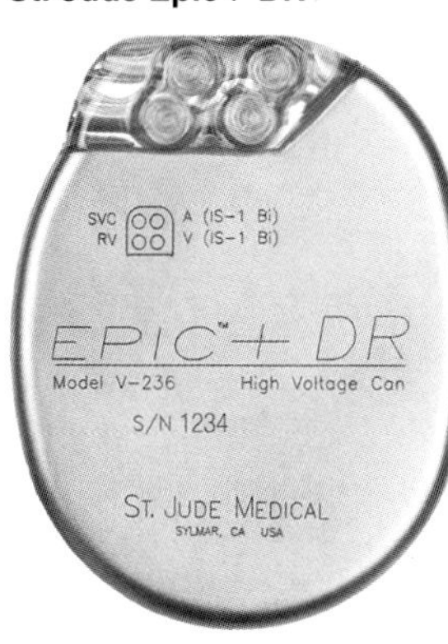

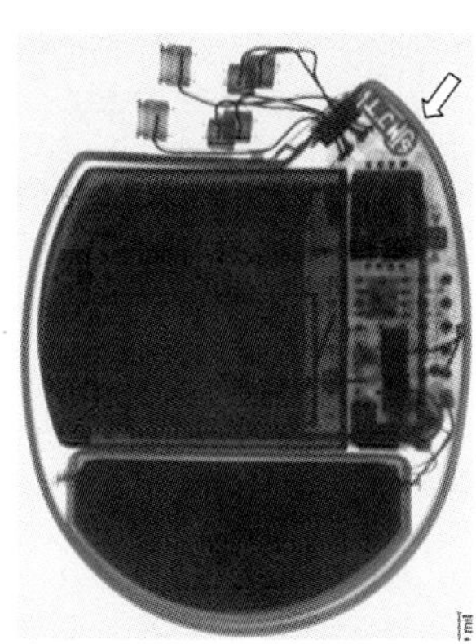

A

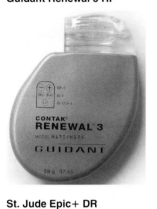

St. Jude Atlas + HF

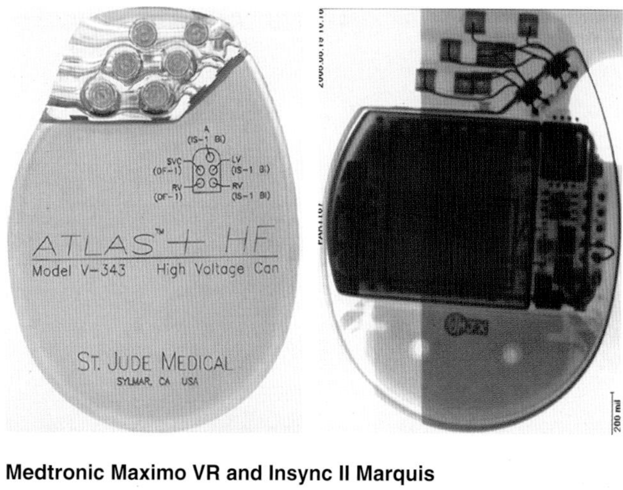

Medtronic Maximo VR and Insync II Marquis

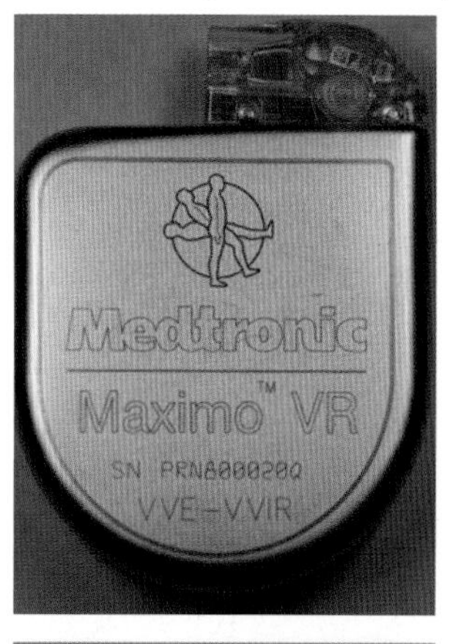

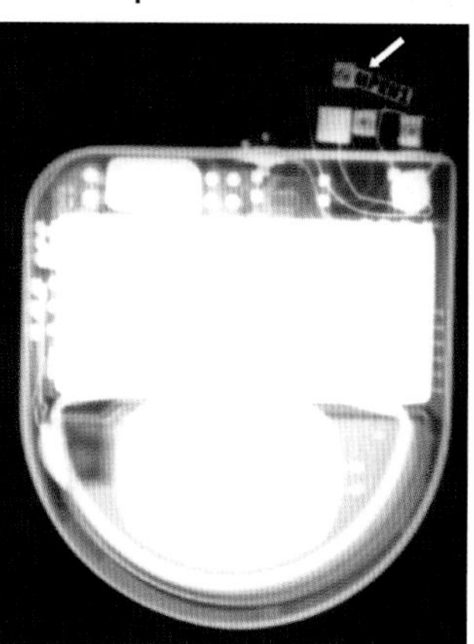

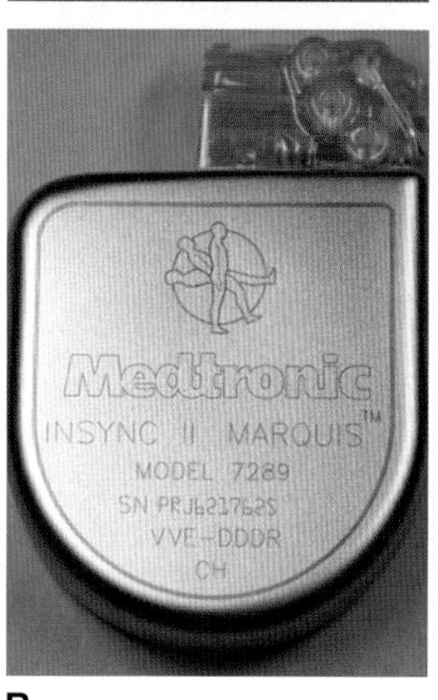

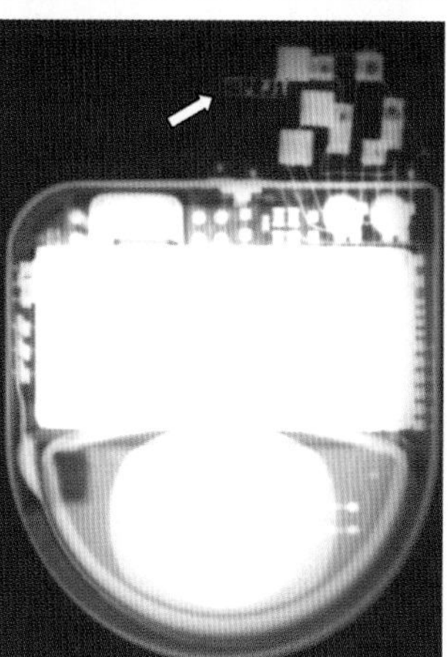

B

Figure 22-6. ***A to C,*** *Radiographic appearance of various ICD pulse generators. Arrows denote manufacturer's identification symbol. (Courtesy of Guidant, Boston Scientific, Natick, Mass.; St. Jude Medical, St. Paul, Minn.; Medtronic, Inc., Minneapolis, Minn.; Biotronik GmbH & Co., Berlin; and ELA Medical, Sorin Group, Milan.)*

Continued

Biotronik DR-T

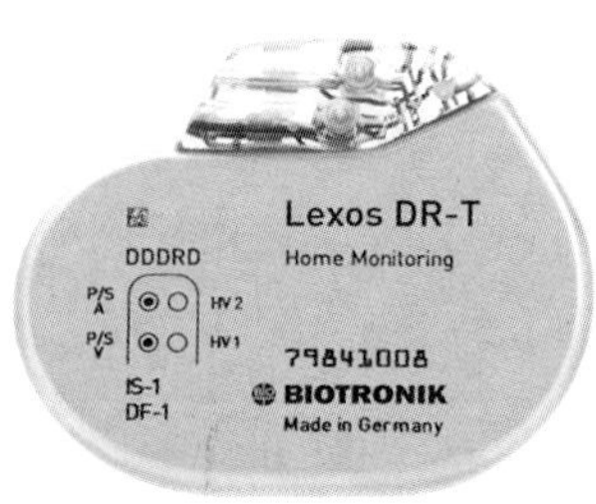

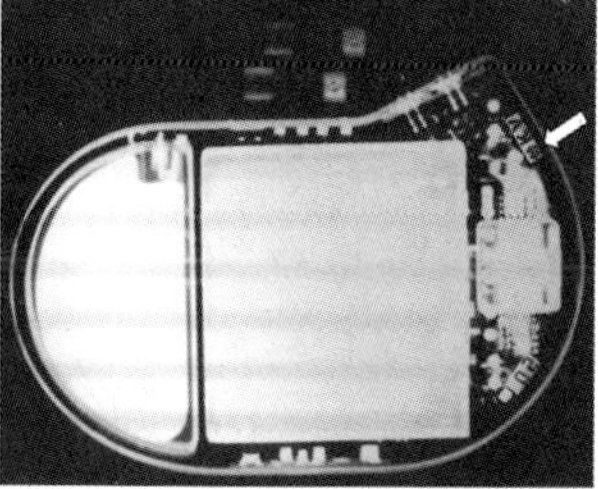

Ela Alto 2 DR

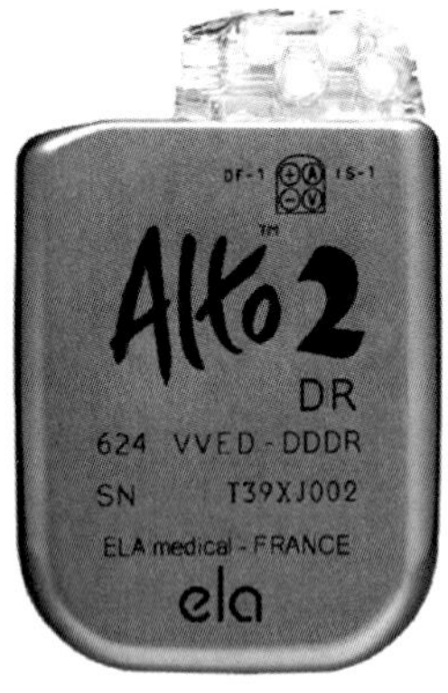

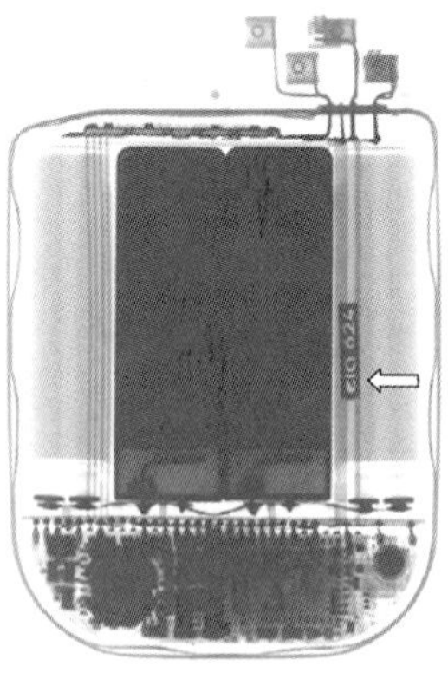

C

Figure 22-6, cont'd.

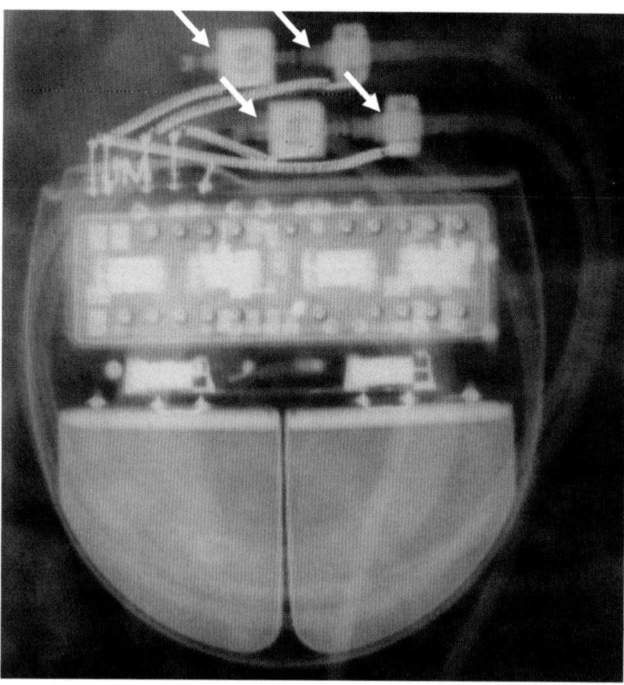

Figure 22-8. Examination of the device for lead connector pin insertion into the header. Pins can be visualized extending past the distal connector blocks (arrows).

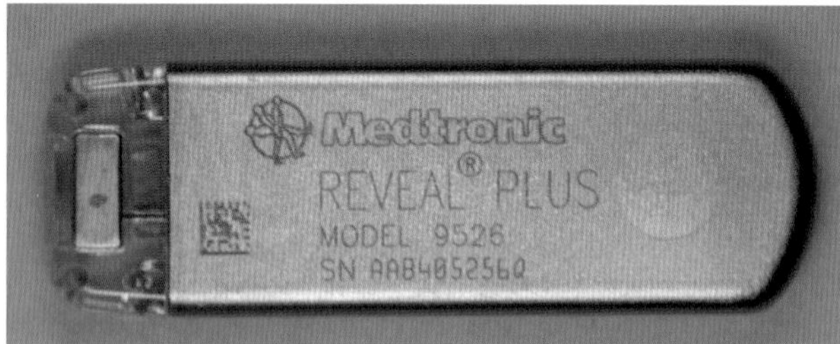

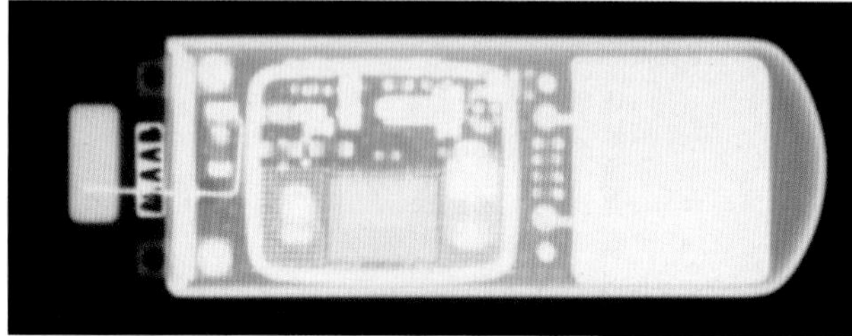

Figure 22-7. Implantable loop recorder. The Medtronic Reveal Plus implantable loop recorder and corresponding radiographic appearance. (Courtesy of Medtronic, Inc., Minneapolis, Minn.)

pulse generators include the number and type of connector pins. Determining the type of connector pins (International Standard 1 [IS-1], 3.2-mm Voluntary Standard [VS]-1, 5- or 6-mm) prior to device replacement is critical to avoiding an unfortunate intraoperative discovery that a compatible device is not readily available for the exchange. Radiographically, detection of connector pins that appear longer than the conventional IS-1 pins should prompt checking of lead connector type.

Migration of the pulse generator may be seen radiographically in older patients with loosened prepectoral fascia, patients who have lost significant amounts of weight, or with pulse generators implanted within larger areas of subcutaneous prepectoral fatty tissue.[1]

In patients who have symptoms associated with the current generator location, revision of the pocket or anchoring of the generator may be considered. The migration of the pulse generator may influence the sterile draping area prior to device replacements.

Pacing and Defibrillation Leads

When planning lead revision and/or extraction, one should assess the types, location, and integrity of all leads radiographically. Higher radiographic penetration may be required to more clearly demonstrate lead components. Dislodgement can be identified and is aided by comparison with old films. Leads generally do not have manufacturer-specific, characteristic radiopaque identifiers, but radiography may provide clues to the lead type (active or passive fixation; unipolar or bipolar) and integrity.[2]

Venous Anatomy for Localization of Lead Positions

Most pacemaker and ICD leads are inserted transvenously. The subclavian, axillary, and cephalic veins are most commonly employed for lead insertion, with the internal or external jugular or femoral veins being used rarely. The cephalic vein courses lateral to the biceps, continuing in a groove between the deltoid and pec-

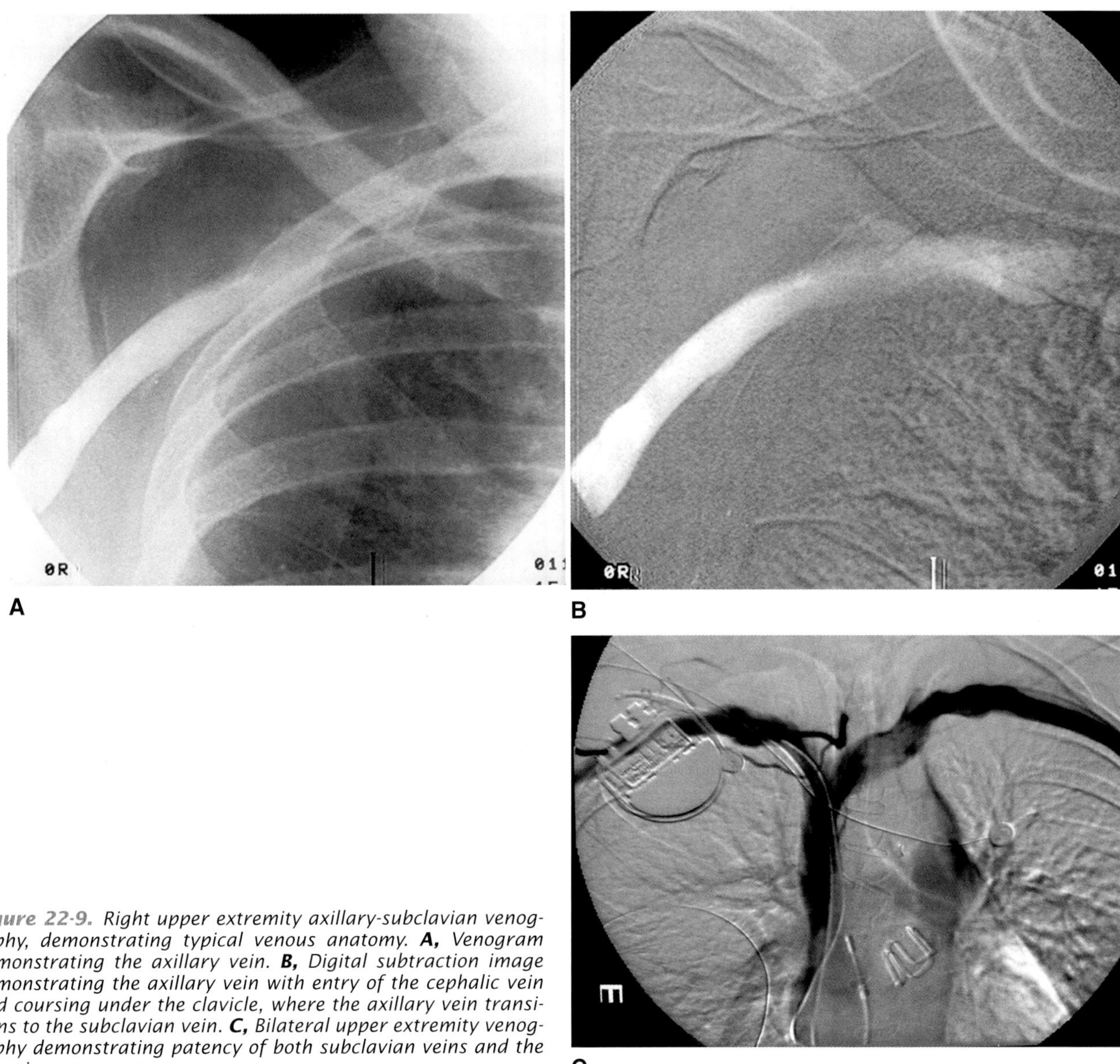

Figure 22-9. Right upper extremity axillary-subclavian venography, demonstrating typical venous anatomy. ***A,*** *Venogram demonstrating the axillary vein.* ***B,*** *Digital subtraction image demonstrating the axillary vein with entry of the cephalic vein and coursing under the clavicle, where the axillary vein transitions to the subclavian vein.* ***C,*** *Bilateral upper extremity venography demonstrating patency of both subclavian veins and the superior vena cava.*

toralis major muscles, then empties into the axillary vein (Fig. 22-9). The axillary vein drains the basilic and brachial veins, coursing medially over the lateral margin of the first rib to become the subclavian vein under the clavicle. This marks the usual site for insertion of pacemaker or defibrillator leads (see Fig. 22-1). A change in the directionality of the lead can sometimes indicate the location of the venous insertion site or suture tie-down sleeve. A more lateral insertion site suggests a cephalic or lateral axillary insertion site. Medial insertions into the subclavian vein should be inspected for evidence of lead crush injuries. Lateral axillary insertion sites should be examined for excessive angulation.

After entering the venous system, leads typically pass through the brachiocephalic veins, which are formed by the joining of the internal jugular and subclavian veins behind the head of the clavicle, to the superior vena cava (SVC), and then to the right atrium (RA) or right ventricle (RV). In a small percentage of patients, a persistent left SVC is present and drains into the coronary sinus (CS) (see later).[3]

On preparation for a procedure requiring insertion of a new lead, peripheral subclavian and SVC venography can be helpful in anticipating the need for lead extraction or preparation of a new site for venous access because of venous occlusion or severe stenoses (Fig. 22-10). Chronic venous occlusion is often marked by the presence of venous collaterals.

The CS, which enters the inferior septal region of the RA, just anterior and superior to the opening of the inferior vena cava, receives most of the venous drainage of the heart. The main CS traverses in the atrioventricular (AV) groove between the left atrium and left ventricle (LV). Tributaries include the middle cardiac vein, posterior ventricular branch, posterolateral, lateral,

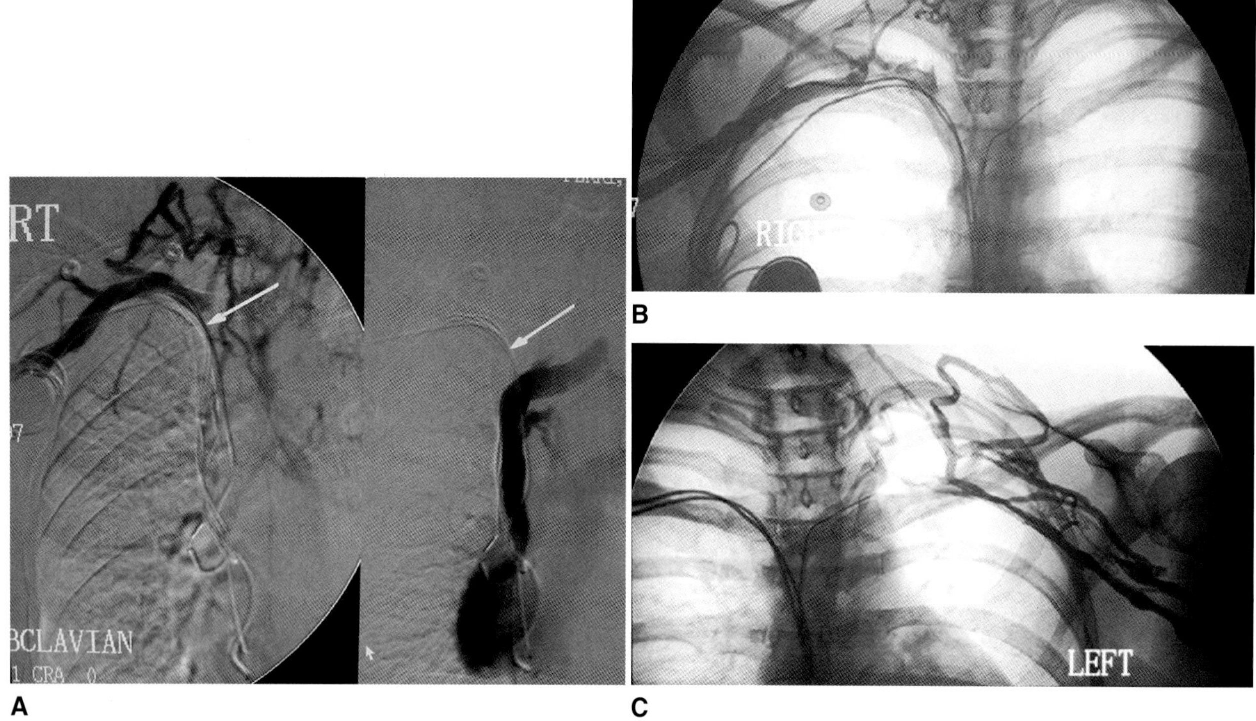

Figure 22-10. Peripheral venography demonstrating occlusion of the subclavian vein. ***A,*** Right panel *shows a peripheral right venogram demonstrating location of an occlusion* (arrows) *of the right subclavian vein with collateralization.* Left panel *shows patency of the left subclavian–brachiocephalic vein to the superior vena cava.* ***B,*** *Peripheral right venography exhibiting occlusion of the right subclavian vein.* ***C,*** *Peripheral left venography in the same patient as in* ***B,*** *demonstrating occlusion of the left subclavian vein with extensive collateralization.*

and anterolateral marginal branches, and the great cardiac vein overlying the RA. The posterior, posterolateral, and lateral branches of the CS are typical targets for LV or biventricular pacing in CRT devices (see Chapter 19). Chest radiography can be essential in determining whether absence of clinical response to CRT is due to inadequate lead position (e.g., lead placement in an anterior branch) or lead dislodgement.

The azygos vein, which enters the posterior wall of the SVC, is sometimes the target vessel for ICD coil lead implantation in patients with high defibrillation thresholds, as the vessel traverses posteriorly behind the heart, providing an additional favorable shock vector option (see Fig. 22-4; Fig. 22-11).[4]

Pacemaker Leads

Besides identification of the venous and cardiac insertion sites of pacing leads, chest radiographs can help determine polarity and fixation types. A unipolar lead has a single electrode at the tip of the lead; a bipolar lead has two electrodes separated by a space. Active-fixation leads have screws that extend from the tip of the lead (Fig. 22-12A). Passive-fixation leads have various types of tines that are radiolucent (cannot be visualized radiographically) (see Fig. 22-12B). Active-fixation leads may be fixed in the extended position or may have an extendable/retractable screw. Different manufacturers denote extension of the latter with various markers (Fig. 22-13).

Atrial Lead Positions. In patients who have not undergone cardiac surgery, most atrial leads are fixed to the RA appendage and will exhibit a J shape with an anteriorly directed curve on the lateral view.[5] Patients who have undergone cardiac surgery may not have suitable RA appendage remnants for fixation. Lead placement is generally guided by optimization of electrical characteristics, such as sensing and pacing thresholds and lead fixation stability. Leads may be implanted laterally, septally, caudally, or cranially in the RA, generally requiring active-fixation leads. Although most pacing systems use one atrial lead, pacing for atrial arrhythmia suppression may incorporate alternative-site or dual-site pacing.[6,7] Placements targeting Bachmann's bundle or the RA septum typically display lead tips directed near the high septum of the RA.[8,9] The CS or septum near the CS may also be targeted; leads placed in the CS generally exhibit a large, open posterior curve. Higher posterior crossings on lateral films may suggest passage of the lead via a patent foramen ovale or atrial septal defect to the left atrium or ventricle.[10]

Ventricular Lead Positions. Ventricular pacing leads have traditionally been targeted to the RV apex (RVA). The lead should display some slack, particularly as it

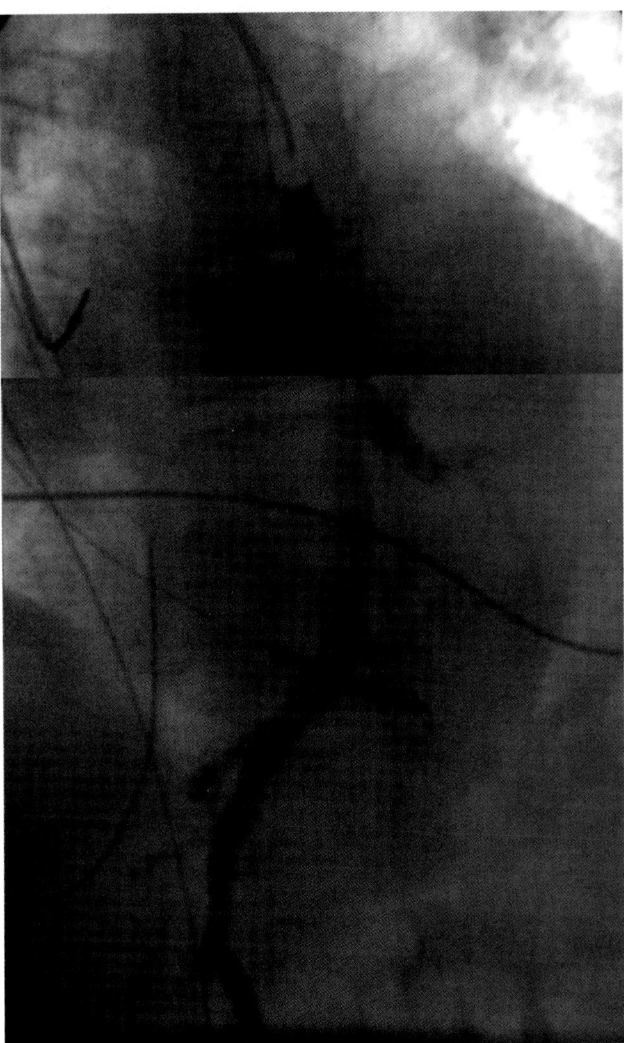

Figure 22-11. Azygos vein occlusive venography. A balloon catheter was inserted near the origin of the azygos vein to delineate the course of the vessel prior to the addition of a defibrillation coil, and was advanced to just above the diaphragm and behind the left ventricle. The atrial lead is in the upper left corner of the image, and the anterior or right ventricular defibrillation coil is in the lower portion. (Courtesy of Kalyanam Shivkumar, MD, PhD.)

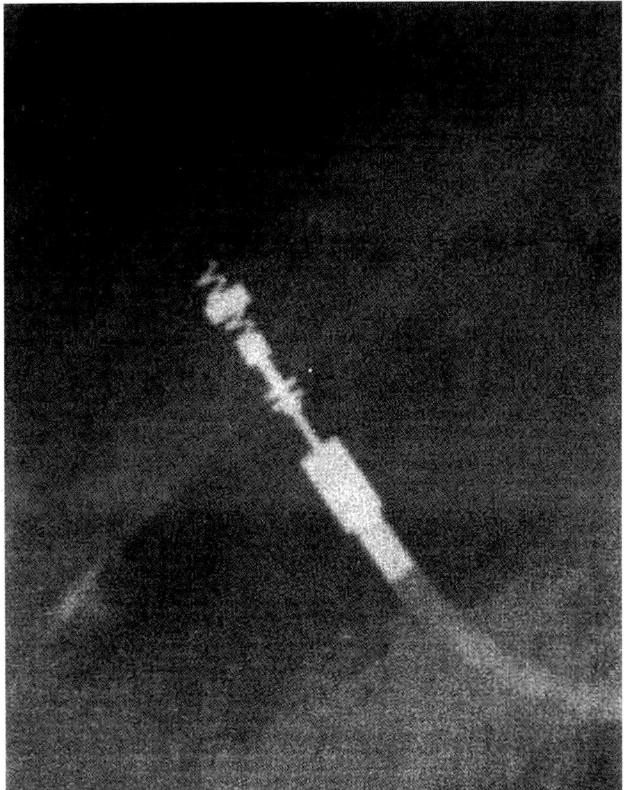

A

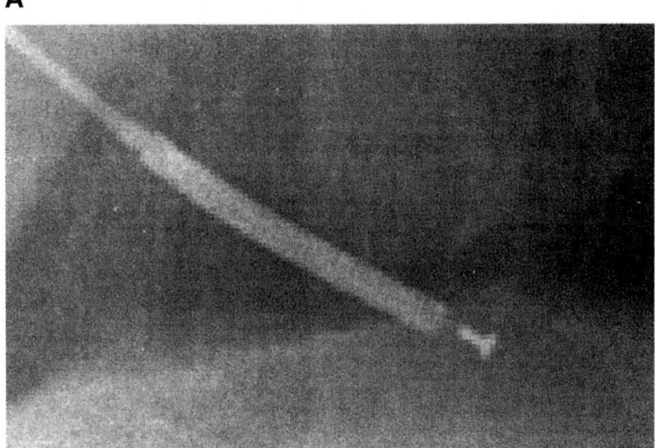

B

*Figure 22-12. Radiographic appearance of transvenous leads. **A,** Active-fixation, bipolar lead. **B,** Passive-fixation ICD lead.*

traverses and is lifted by the tricuspid valve. The RVA is generally located to the left of the spine on the PA view with a slight inferior direction. On the lateral view, the lead is usually directed anteriorly (Fig. 22-14), unless the septal aspect of the apex is targeted. A more posterior course suggests positioning in the CS or middle cardiac vein. A large posterior curve suggests possible passage through a patent foramen ovale or atrial or ventricular septal defect to the LV (Fig. 22-15).

Although the RVA has been the traditional site for ventricular pacing lead placement, awareness of the potential for LV dyssynchrony from RVA pacing has led to more frequent use of RV outflow tract (RVOT) or septal pacing (Fig. 22-16).[11] A position away from the RVA may also be sought when there are high pacing thresholds at the apex or if an ICD lead is present at the apex, to avoid device-device interactions (Fig. 22-17). His bundle pacing has been proposed as an alternative to RVA pacing in the absence of infra-Hisian conduction system disease.[12] An extra set of bipolar sensing electrodes present at the level of the RA on a ventricular lead body identifies a VDD single-lead pacing system, which is designed to sense in the atrium and allow atrial-synchronous ventricular pacing (Fig. 22-18).

Coronary Sinus Lead Positions. The branches of the CS are common targets for leads placed for LV or biventricular pacing for CRT.[13] Placement of the CS lead involves localization and cannulation of the CS, CS

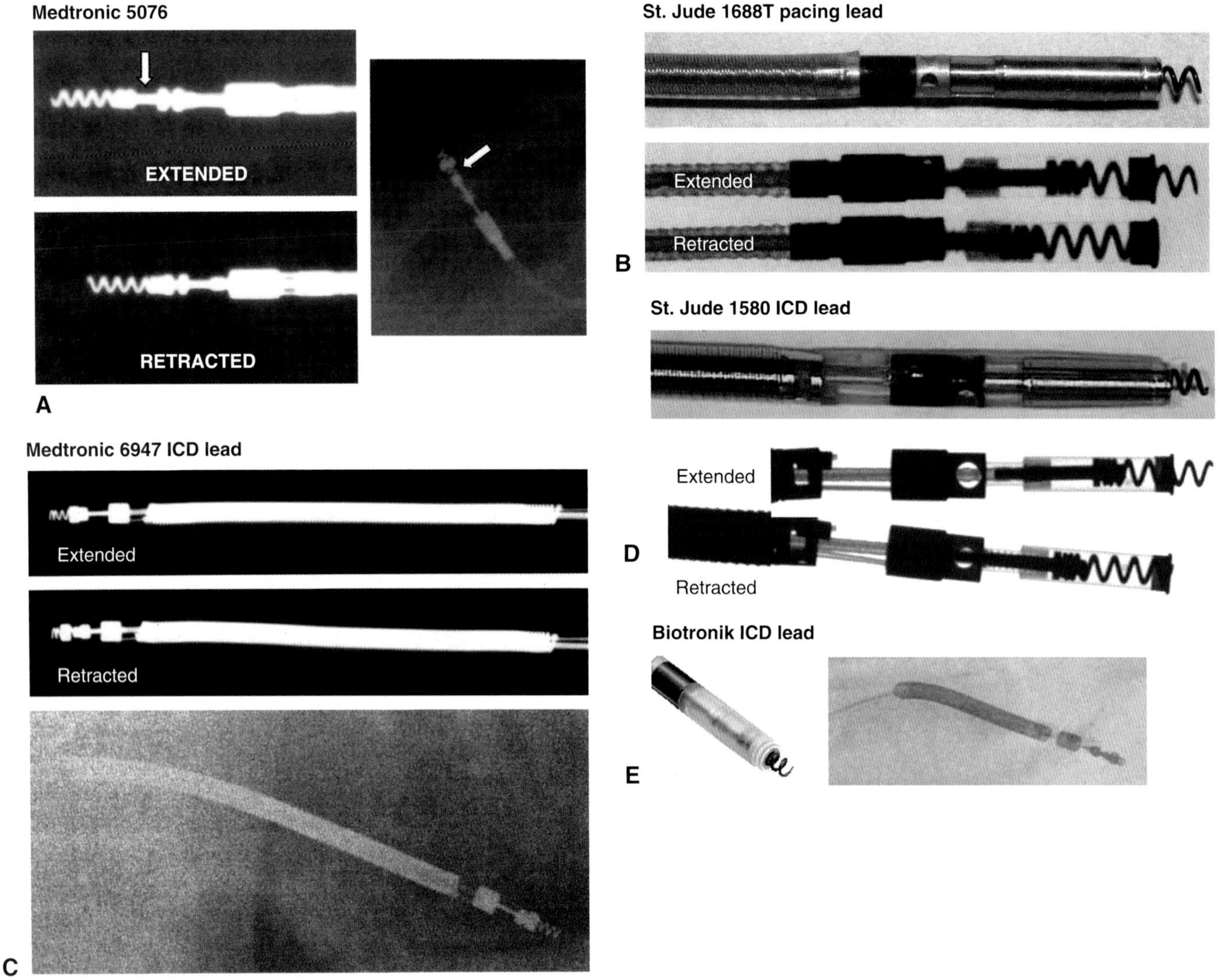

Medtronic 5076

EXTENDED

RETRACTED

A

St. Jude 1688T pacing lead

Extended

Retracted

B

St. Jude 1580 ICD lead

Extended

Retracted

D

Medtronic 6947 ICD lead

Extended

Retracted

C

Biotronik ICD lead

E

Figure 22-13. *Active-fixation screw positions.* ***A,*** *Medtronic 5076 bipolar pacing lead with extended and retracted screw positions. The fluoroscopy image shows the screw is extended with appearance of a space between the two distal radiopaque rings* (arrow). ***B,*** *St. Jude 1688T bipolar pacing lead with radiographs of extended and retracted screw positions. In the extended position, two helical turns of the screw are visible.* ***C,*** *Medtronic 6947 ICD lead with extended and retracted screw positions. The fluoroscopy image shows the screw is extended with* dis*appearance of the space between the two distal radiopaque rings.* ***D,*** *St. Jude 1580 ICD lead with radiographs of extended and retracted screw positions, showing two helical turns of the screw in the extended position.* ***E,*** *Biotronik ICD lead with screw extended. (Courtesy of Medtronic, Inc., Minneapolis, Minn.; St. Jude Medical, St. Paul, Minn.; and Biotronik GmbH & Co., Berlin.)*

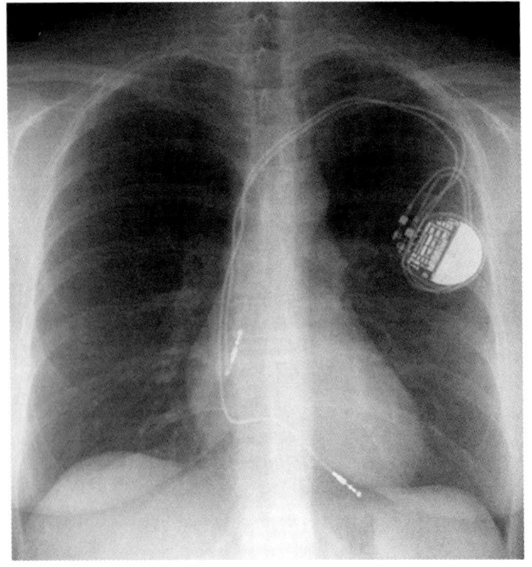

A

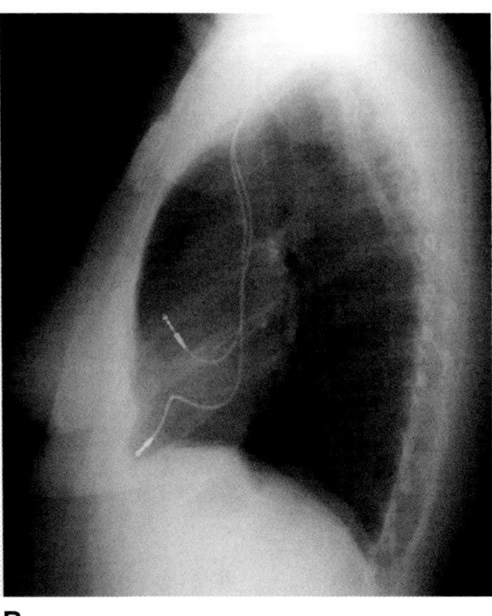

B

Figure 22-14. *Ventricular pacing lead position in the right ventricular apex and atrial lead in the right atrial appendage. Posteroanterior (**A**) and lateral (**B**) radiographs demonstrate the anterior course of the right atrial appendage lead and the apical anterior course of the right ventricular apex lead.*

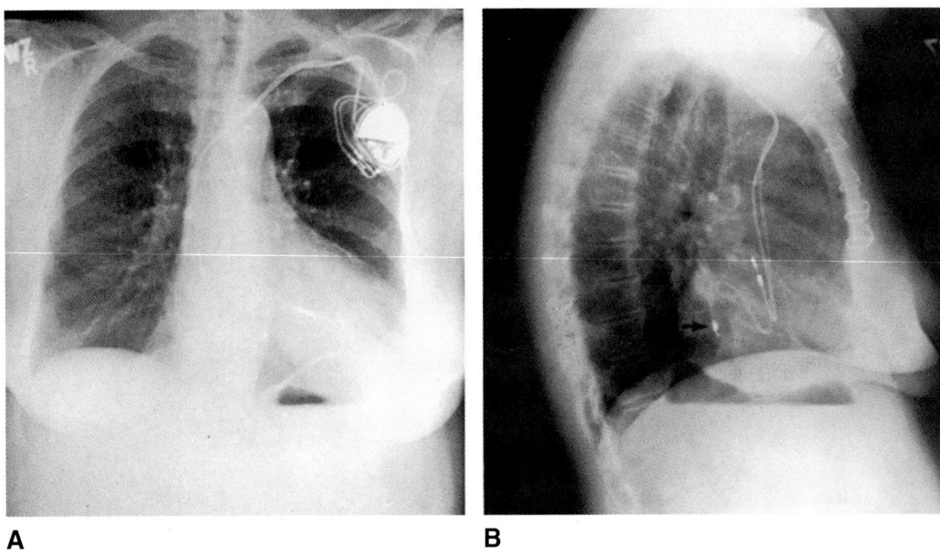

*Figure 22-15. Ventricular lead placement into the left ventricle. Posteroanterior (PA) (**A**) and left lateral (**B**) views demonstrating a dual-chamber pacing system. The ventricular wire has an unusual curve on the PA view; and on the lateral view, it can be seen to extend in a posterocranial direction, only then to curve back on itself with the tip of the wire in the wall of the left ventricle* (arrow). *This is an example of improper ventricular lead placement, with the wire traversing the foramen ovale and extending through the body of the left atrium, through the mitral valve, and into the left ventricle. (From Trohman RG, Wilkoff B, Byrne T, Cook S: Successful percutaneous extraction of a chronic left ventricular pacing lead. PACE 14:1448, 1991.)*

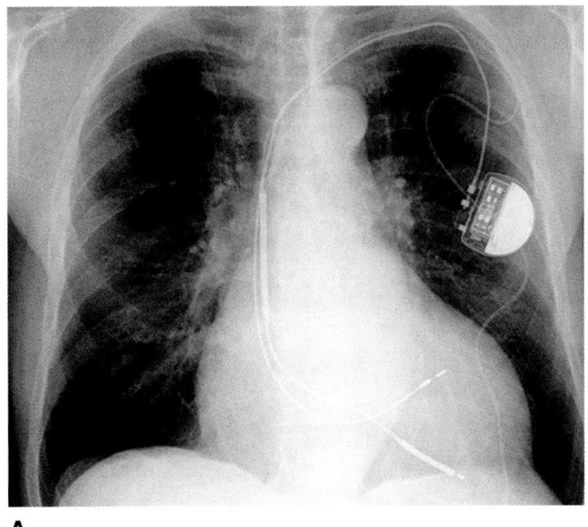

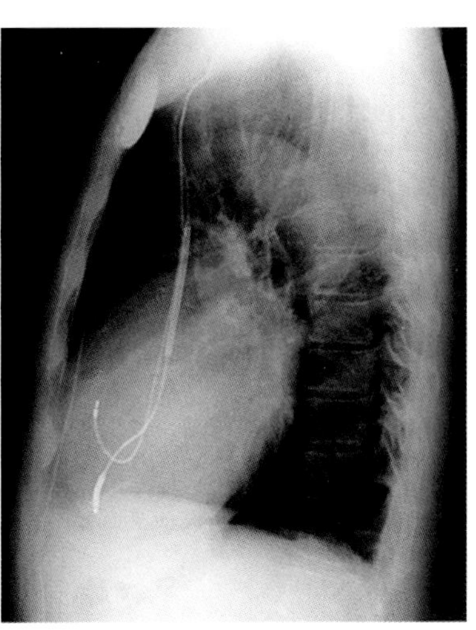

*Figure 22-16. Ventricular pacing lead position in the right ventricular outflow tract. Posteroanterior (**A**) and lateral (**B**) chest radiographs with a left-sided single-chamber pacemaker. The lead tip is in the anterior right ventricular outflow tract, and the abdominal transvenous ICD lead tip is placed in the right ventricular apex. (Courtesy of Walid Saliba, MD.)*

venography, and placement of the lead in the target branch. CS ostium cannulation is accomplished using an angiographic approach or electrophysiologic approach. Angiographic technique involves the use of a variety of guiding sheaths and diagnostic catheters (described in Chapter 19) with boluses of contrast agent for locating the CS ostium (os). The electrophysiologic technique involves the use of guiding sheaths with mapping catheters to help determine the presence of CS morphology on intracardiac electrograms.

Commonly, in patients with congestive heart failure, CS anatomy is extremely variable owing to cardiac dilatation as well as to rotation and alteration from prior cardiac operations, making localization of the ostium difficult. In addition, patients with atrial fibrillation may have markedly enlarged right atria for which larger-curve guiding sheaths or catheters may be helpful in cannulation of the ostium. A quick fluoroscopic visualization may show the extent of cardiomegaly or cardiac rotation, or anatomic markers, such as right coronary artery calcifications or the radiolucent fat pad in the AV groove. In the anteroposterior (AP) view, the CS ostium can be on either side of the spine and variable vertically, relative to the floor of the tricuspid valve. A thorough understanding of the RA anatomy with judicious use of contrast material helps the implanting physician assess the position of the catheter tip relative to the CS ostium.

After gaining access to the CS, one advances the outer guide sheath into the proximal portion of the CS

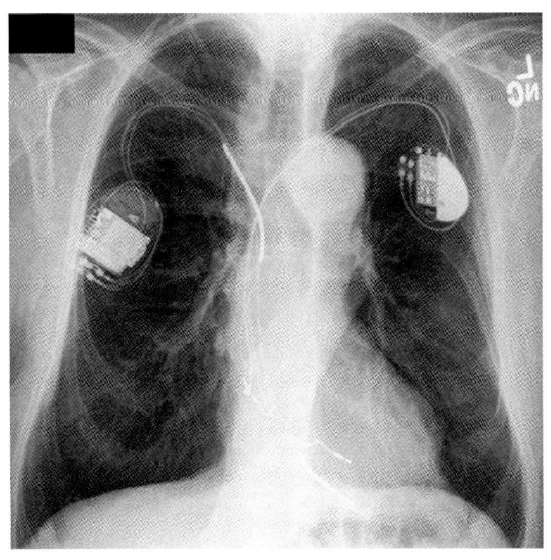
A

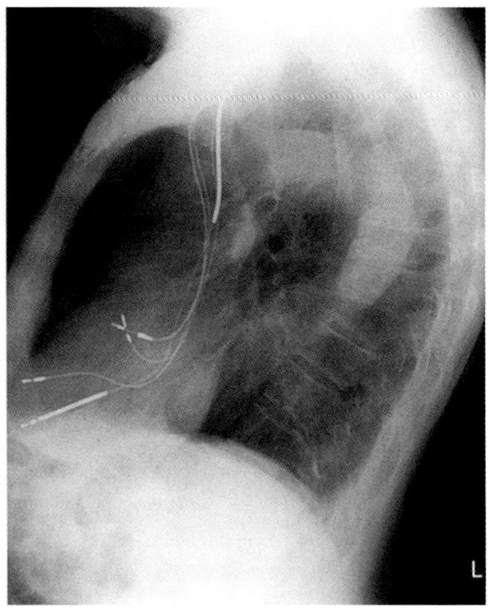
B

Figure 22-17. *Dual-chamber pacing system on the left with ventricular pacing lead placed higher on the right ventricular wall and a dual-chamber implantable cardioverter-defibrillator (ICD) system implanted on the right with the ventricular ICD lead at the apex. Posteroanterior (**A**) and lateral (**B**) chest radiographs. The ventricular pacing lead is implanted higher and away from the high-voltage ICD lead.*

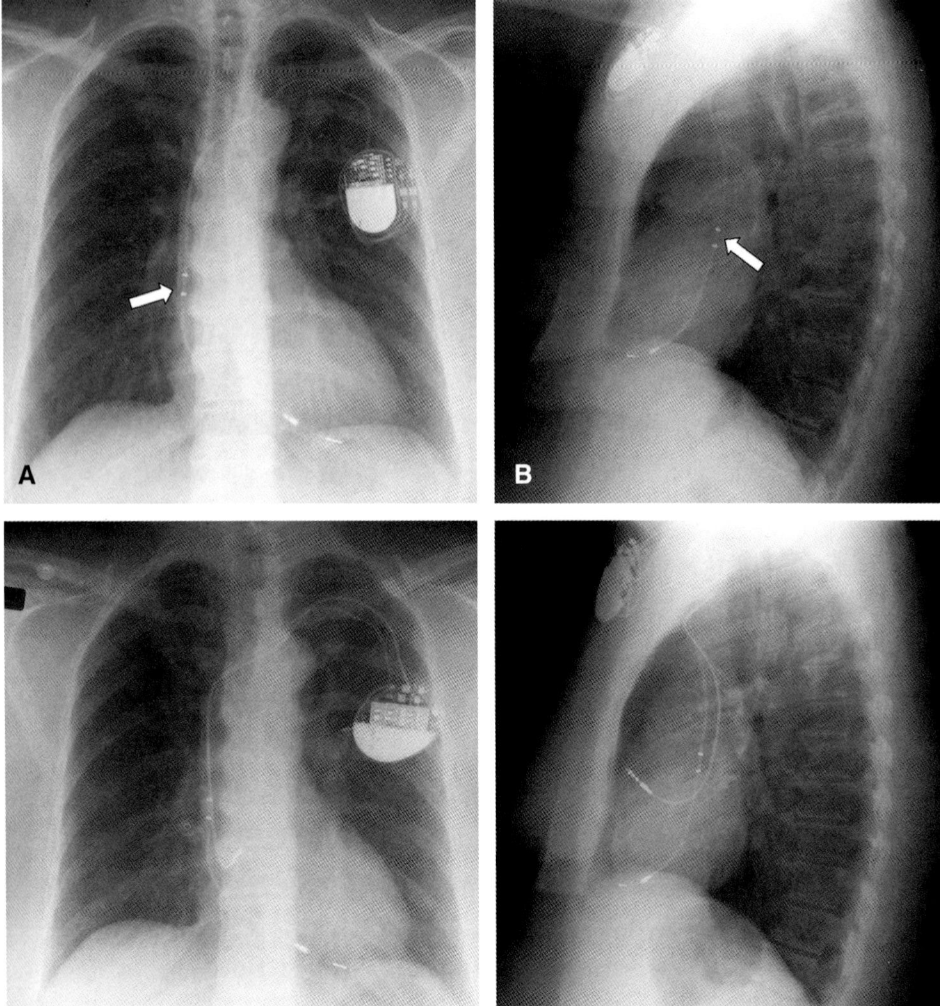

Figure 22-18. *Single-lead VDD pacing system with a bipolar atrial sensing electrode* (arrow) *and bipolar ventricular pace/sense electrodes. Posteroanterior (PA) (**A**) and lateral (**B**) views of the VDD pacing system. The system was subsequently upgraded with the addition of a new atrial bipolar lead, as shown on PA (**C**) and lateral (**D**) views, because of inadequate atrial sensing.*

at least 3 to 4 cm over a guidewire or a softer inner catheter to prevent mural dissection. Balloon occlusion CS contrast venography can then be performed to identify potential target tributaries, strictures, and collateral vessels to aid in selection of an optimal target vessel (Fig. 22-19). Balloon inflation must be performed with caution to avoid overinflation and dissection of the vein. After visualization of the distal vessels, the balloon is deflated to promote proximal runoff, thereby allowing visualization of tributaries proximal to the balloon tip. Continued acquisition of images for a few extra seconds after injection of contrast agent allows flow to tributaries through collaterals, which might highlight the posterior and posterolateral LV veins that could otherwise go unnoticed. Two radiographic planes are helpful for assessing the CS tributaries and ostia for optimal target vessel determination. The most common positions used are left anterior oblique (LAO) 25 to 45 degrees, AP, and right anterior oblique (RAO) 15 to 30 degrees.

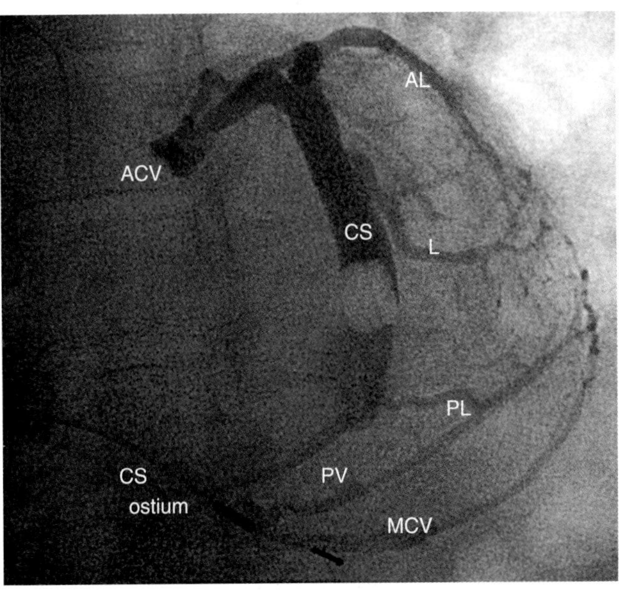

Figure 22-19. Coronary sinus balloon venography demonstrating branch anatomy in the left anterior oblique view. ACV, anterior cardiac vein; AL, anterolateral marginal vein; CS, coronary sinus; L, lateral marginal vein; MCV, middle cardiac vein; PL, posterolateral marginal vein; PV, posterior ventricular branch.

CS anatomy is variable, and no consensus has yet been reached regarding the nomenclature of CS branch anatomy; nevertheless, common nomenclature is depicted in Figure 22-19. From the CS ostium, the first branch is generally termed the middle cardiac vein. A posterior ventricular branch may enter near the middle cardiac vein. The distal CS becomes the great cardiac vein as it passes around the mitral annulus anteriorly and then becomes the anterior cardiac vein, which courses down the anterior interventricular groove. In between the middle cardiac and anterior cardiac veins, posterior, posterolateral, lateral, anterolateral, and/or anteroseptal branches may be present. Branches may be described by clock face positions as viewed in LAO projection. In this classification, the CS ostium generally is located at 7 o'clock, the middle cardial vein at about 6 o'clock, the posterior-lateral veins at 5 o'clock to 2 o'clock, and the great cardiac vein/anterior cardiac vein at 12 o'clock. If present, a persistent left SVC drains into the CS directly.[14] Typical lead tip positions are illustrated in Figure 22-20.

Epicardial Lead Positions. When placed for potential CRT, unipolar or bipolar leads are placed on the LV posterolateral free wall epicardium either after failure to place transvenous CS leads or at the time of concomitant valve or coronary bypass surgery (Fig. 22-21). Minimally invasive methods for implantation are available for patients not in need of concomitant cardiac surgery.[15-17] Epicardial leads may also be placed in

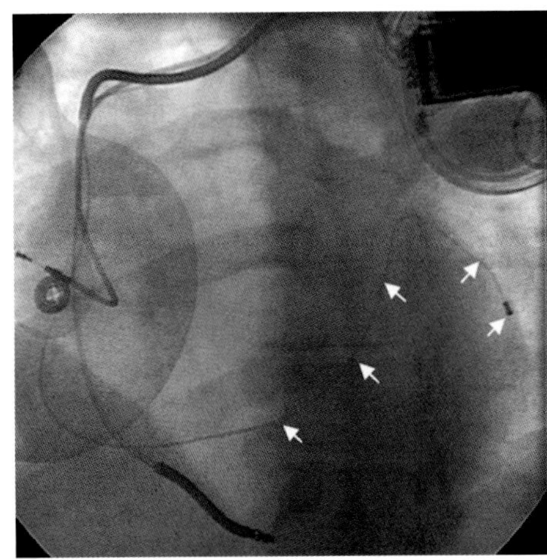
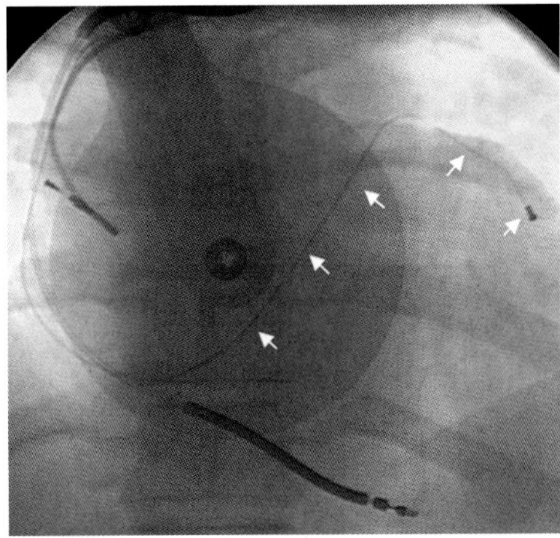

A

Figure 22-20. Coronary sinus (CS) lead positions in cardiac resynchronization therapy systems. **A,** *Left anterior oblique (LAO)* (left) *and posteroanterior (PA)* (right) *projections demonstrating positioning of a unipolar pacing lead in an anterolateral marginal branch of the coronary sinus.* Arrows *highlight the course of the CS leads.*

Continued

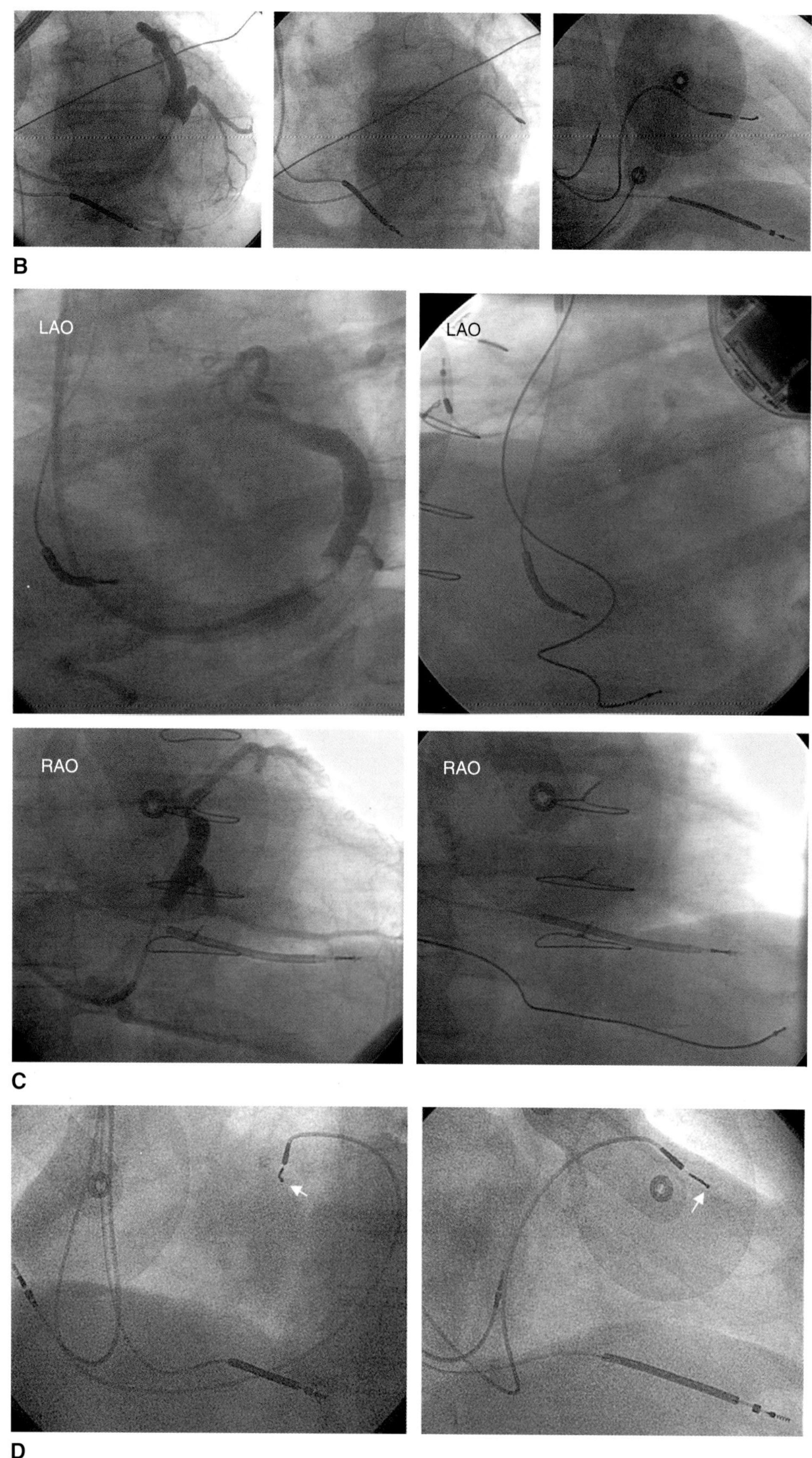

Figure 22-20, cont'd. ***B,*** *CS venography in the LAO projection demonstrating a large lateral branch of the CS* (left)*. LAO* (middle) *and RAO* (right) *projections after placement of a bipolar CS pacing lead show the tip to be in the middle to distal segment of the superior division of the lateral branch.* ***C,*** *LAO* (top) *and RAO* (bottom) *CS venograms* (left) *and projections demonstrating the CS lead tip positioned in the distal middle cardiac vein* (right)*. Positioning of the lead in the lateral branch resulted in unacceptable diaphragmatic stimulation.* ***D,*** *LAO* (left) *and RAO* (right) *projections showing the CS lead tip* (arrows) *in an anterior CS branch location.*

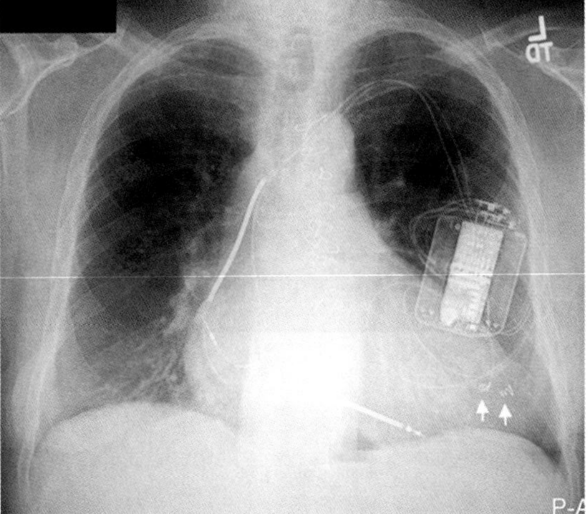

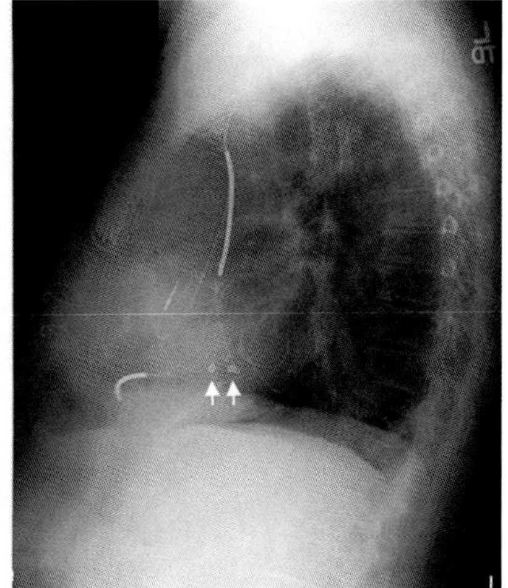

Figure 22-21. Left ventricular epicardial leads connected to a cardiac resynchronization therapy implantable cardioverter-defibrillator. Posteroanterior (left) *and lateral* (right) *chest radiographs show epicardial screw-tip leads placed on the left ventricular epicardium* (arrows).

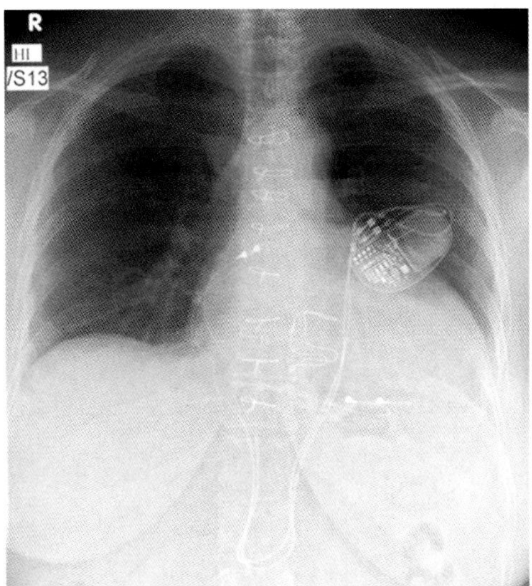

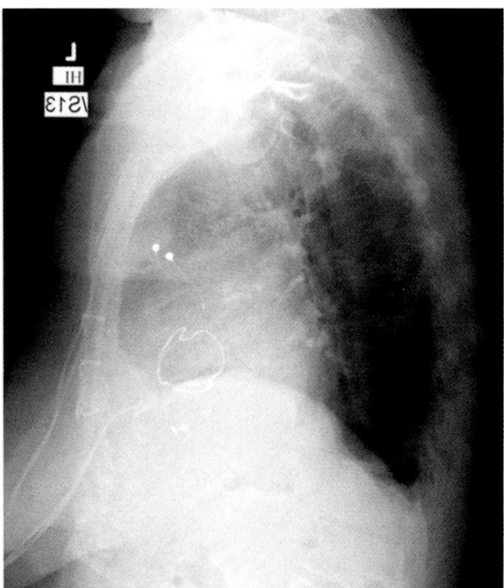

Figure 22-22. Epicardial atrial and ventricular pacing leads in a woman with a tricuspid valve prosthesis.

patients with congenital abnormalities or as part of cardiac surgical procedures with risk for or resulting in complete heart block (see Fig. 22-3), and in patients with prosthetic tricuspid valves (Fig. 22-22). In the past, epicardial leads had a higher incidence of malfunction than transvenous pacing leads, but newer lead designs may improve epicardial lead longevity. The leads are tunneled to the pulse generator pocket in either the pectoral or abdominal area. Evaluation may require chest and abdominal radiographs, depending on the location of the pacemaker or ICD device, to allow examination of integrity of a lead throughout its entire course.

Identification of Possible Pacemaker Lead Malfunction. The presence of abandoned leads usually indicates that the leads were malfunctioning or no longer needed. Examples of the latter situation are (1) permanent atrial fibrillation with change to a single-chamber from dual-chamber pacemaker at device replacement and (2) upgrade from a permanent pacemaker to an ICD with abandonment and capping of the ventricular pacing lead and implantation of an ICD lead. The proximal portion of the lead is usually capped, unattached to the generator, and free in the generator pocket. Some implanters cut the leads, but doing so risks retraction of a lead into the venous system, greatly increasing the difficulty of future extraction (Fig. 22-23). One should determine whether the abandoned lead is present in its entirety or whether its proximal portion has been severed or retracted into the vein (see Fig. 22-23B).

Active-fixation leads have a radiopaque screw that may be fixed (extended) or retractable-extendable. The chest radiograph should be examined to determine whether the screw is extended properly, although one must recognized that there may be alternative markers to screw extension besides apparent extension past the apparent tip electrode. Screw extension is marked in some cases by removal or creation of a space between radiopaque rings and in other cases by visualized extension of the screw past the tip (see Fig. 22-13A).

Particularly when troubleshooting device or lead malfunction prior to surgical exploration of a device

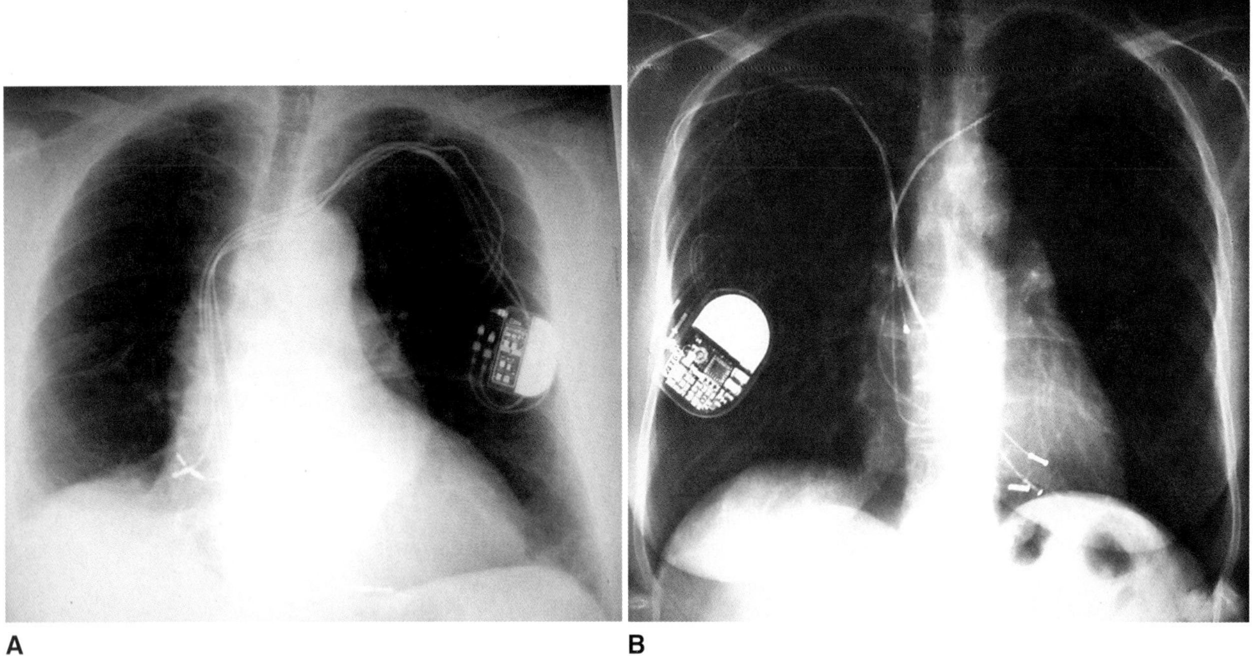

Figure 22-23. Abandoned leads. ***A,*** *Posteroanterior (PA) chest radiograph. Two of the pacing leads are connected to a left prepectoral dual-chamber pacemaker. Two leads have been cut with tips abandoned in the pocket.* ***B,*** *PA chest radiograph showing a right pacemaker system and abandoned leads, including a cut lead from the left stem that has retracted into the left subclavian vein.*

system, one must scrutinize the chest radiograph for lead integrity and connection to the device header. The header should be examined for any obvious disconnections. It is often possible to visualize the pin extending past the distal connector block (see Fig. 22-8). The lead coil should also be scrutinized for obvious discontinuity, abnormal angulation, and kinking, particularly between the pulse generator and the venous insertion site (Fig. 22-24). Medial venous insertion sites appear to be more prone to the subclavian clavicle–first rib crush syndrome, or subclavian crush syndrome (Fig. 22-25).[18,19] In addition, acute angulation of leads may lead to inner conductor fracture (Fig. 22-26). This situation may occur with insertions into the lateral axillary vein or with acute angulation out of the subclavian vein. Crimping of the lead insulation by tight ligatures around suture sleeves may cause the appearance of pseudofracture on a radiograph (Fig. 22-27).[20,21] Pacing characteristics may be unaffected by such crimping, but over time, lead insulation damage or coil fracture may result and should be monitored. Another type of pseudofracture describes a transition from a coaxial to a linear configuration, such as in ICD leads at the transition from the coil to the cable or where coils come together from a bifurcated (now obsolete) connector configuration.

Excessive unintentional or intentional coiling and knotting of the leads may occur because of a large generator pocket or loose, fatty subcutaneous tissue, allowing rotation or repeated flipping of the pulse generator with physical activity or from patient manipulation—the latter called twiddler's syndrome or reel syndrome (Fig. 22-28).[22,23] Chest radiography leads to diagnosis, and early identification of the problem with follow-up chest radiographs may help prevent its perpetuation. Such excessive coiling and knotting of the leads can lead to lead fracture, insulation breaks, or inappropriate defibrillator shocks.

A special situation in which radiographic imaging has been important has been for examination of the Telectronics Pacing Systems (Englewood, Colo.; now part of St. Jude Medical, Sylmar, Calif.) Accufix active-fixation and Encor passive-fixation atrial leads.[24,25] Designed to maintain a J shape, these leads have retention wires located within the insulation in the Accufix lead and inside the coil in the Encor lead. The retention wire may fracture, protrude, and migrate, leading to cardiovascular perforation. Open J shapes appear more prone to fracture than more closed shapes. Coned-in views with higher penetration and digital fluoroscopy have been used to assess the retention wire (Fig. 22-29). The Encor lead appears less prone to fracture complications, but fracture is more difficult to detect. It has been associated with angulation in the inter-electrode space. Chest radiographs and digital fluoroscopy with high magnification and multiple views should be used to optimize visualization of these retention wires.[26]

Implantable Cardioverter-Defibrillator Leads

The cornerstone of current ICD systems is a transvenous pace/sense-defibrillation lead placed into the RV and typically connected to an "active-can" ICD pulse

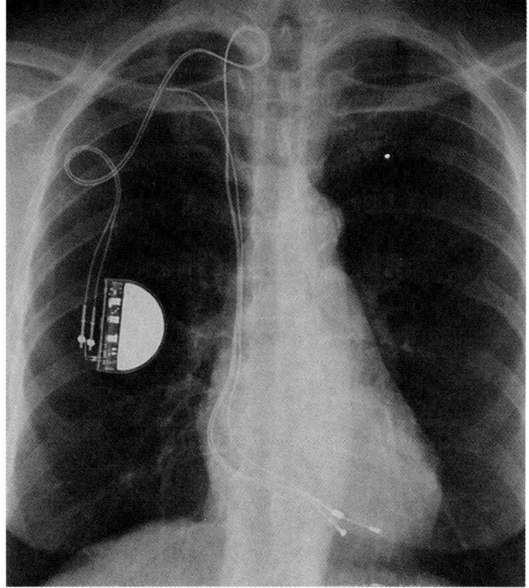
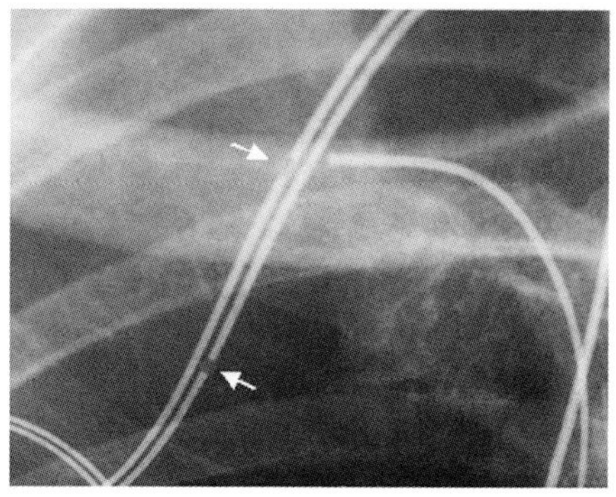

Figure 22-24. *Pacemaker lead conductor fracture. The right-sided dual-chamber pacemaker is connected to leads inserted via the right internal jugular vein* (left). *The expanded view* (right) *demonstrates that these leads contain conductor fractures* (arrows). *There is also an abandoned and cut right ventricular lead that has retracted into the right subclavian vein.*

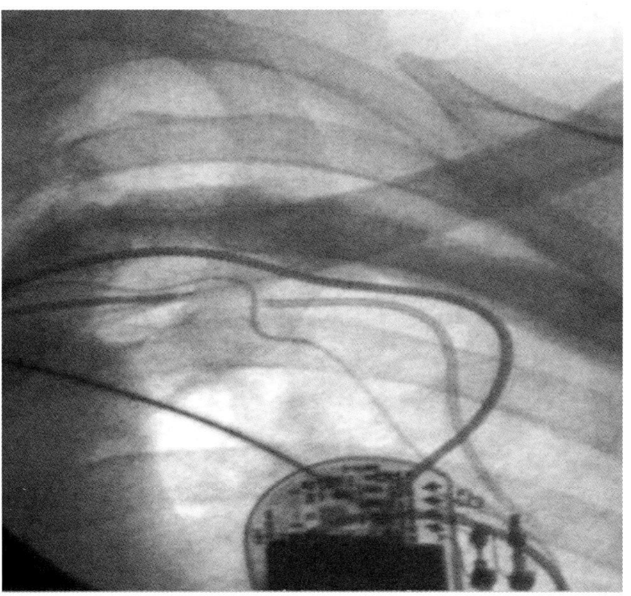

Figure 22-25. *Subclavian clavicle–first rib crush syndrome. There is a fracture with frank lead discontinuity at the clavicle–first rib. The venogram shows that the insertion of the leads into the subclavian vein was at a very medial site.*

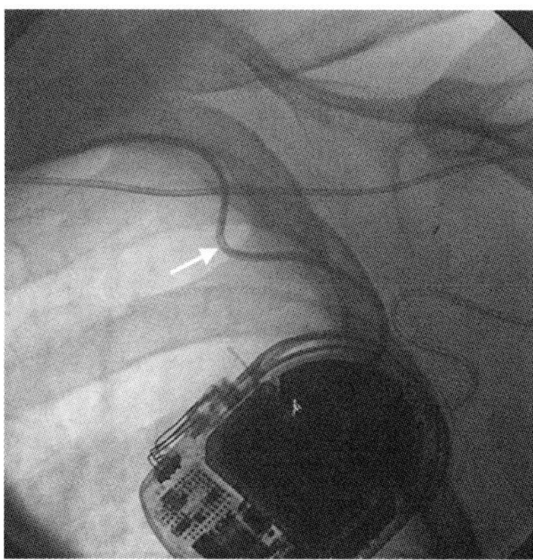
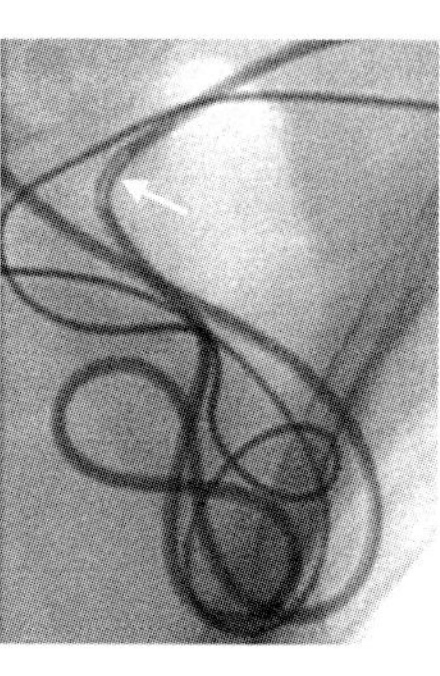

Figure 22-26. *Two examples of inner conductor fractures* (arrows) *due to acute angulation of pacing leads. (Courtesy of Ludwig Binner, MD, University of Ulm, Ulm, Germany.)*

generator located in the prepectoral region, most commonly on the left side.[27]

These leads may have a single high-voltage defibrillation coil, which should be situated in the RV, or two high-voltage coils, the distal coil being positioned in the RV, and the proximal coil positioned in the region of the SVC–high RA. The ventricular ICD lead tip is typically placed at the RV apex with enough lead slack to allow a lift at the tricuspid valve. ICD leads may also be placed in the RVOT (Fig. 22-30). In patients with high defibrillation thresholds, a separate SVC coil lead may also be placed in the SVC–brachiocephalic region, or a subcutaneous patch, coil, or array may be placed (Fig. 22-31). Subcutaneous electrodes are usually placed inferior and posterior to the axilla but may be placed in the left prepectoral region if the ICD is not an active-can device or if the ICD is located elsewhere (e.g., abdominal or right prepectoral region). Epicardial patch defibrillation leads (see Fig. 22-3B and F) were placed via sternotomy or lateral thoracotomy in early ICD systems but very rarely may still be required in patients who are not candidates for transvenous lead systems—because of absence of any venous vascular access, repeated infection with endocarditis, or tricuspid valve replacement, with some forms of congenital heart disease, and in small children.

CS defibrillation leads were used in an early atrial defibrillator device but are not in current standard ICD systems. The atrial defibrillator device (Metrix by InControl Inc., Redmond, Wash.) used an S-shaped lead to maintain stability in the CS (Fig. 22-32). However, this lead is not currently being marketed, and other straight leads may be at a higher risk for dislodgment. Moreover, placement of defibrillation coil leads in the

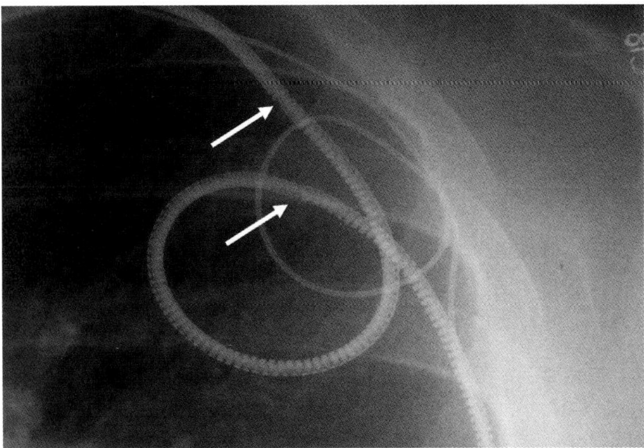

Figure 22-27. Implantable cardioverter-defibrillator (ICD) lead "pseudofracture." Two suture tie-down sleeves were positioned to produce a strain-relief loop on this ICD lead. The slight separation in the outer coil spacing (see arrows*) represents not disruption of the wire but merely too tight a placement of the ligature.*

main CS may preclude future access of this venous system for CRT leads.

The azygos vein may be cannulated for placement of ICD defibrillation leads (see Fig. 22-11; Fig. 22-33). This vein enters the SVC posteriorly, just below the confluence of the brachiocephalic veins, and can provide access to a position posterior to the heart for optimization of the defibrillation vector. Similarly, an additional defibrillation lead/array can be placed in the subcutaneous tissue along the posterolateral wall to change the defibrillation vector in patients who cannot achieve a safe defibrillation threshold through traditional dual-coil ICD leads.[28]

Identification of Lead Malfunction. Although defibrillation lead diameters have become smaller and some rival diameters of pacing leads, most ICD leads have a larger diameter relative to pacing leads. Thus, they may be more susceptible to subclavian crush syndrome. Chest radiographs should be inspected closely in the region near the venous insertion sites and the suture sleeve tie-down sites. Leads, patches, coils, and arrays should be inspected for fracture and excessive bending or kinking. This inspection may require abdominal films and customized views. "Phantom fracture" and pseudofracture are terms used to describe a pseudodiscontinuity of one manufacturer's ICD lead just distal to the proximal high-voltage coil (Fig. 22-34).[29] This appearance is a normal feature of this particular lead. A discontinuity of radiopaque markers on the perimeter of some epicardial patches is likewise no cause for concern, because these markers are not a part of the defibrillation electrode and do not indicate lead fracture (see Fig. 22-31E).

Special Considerations in Congenital Heart Disease

Congenital cardiovascular anomalies may result in unusual locations of pacing or ICD lead systems. An understanding of the native and corrected anatomy is essential for correct interpretation of radiographic imaging in patients with implanted devices. Epicardial pacing indications include residual intracardiac shunts, prosthetic pulmonary ventricular AV valves (usually tricuspid), severe RV endocardial fibroelastosis, lack of viable access to the heart through systemic veins, and prohibitively small stature (Fig. 22-35). Hence,

Text continued on p. 954

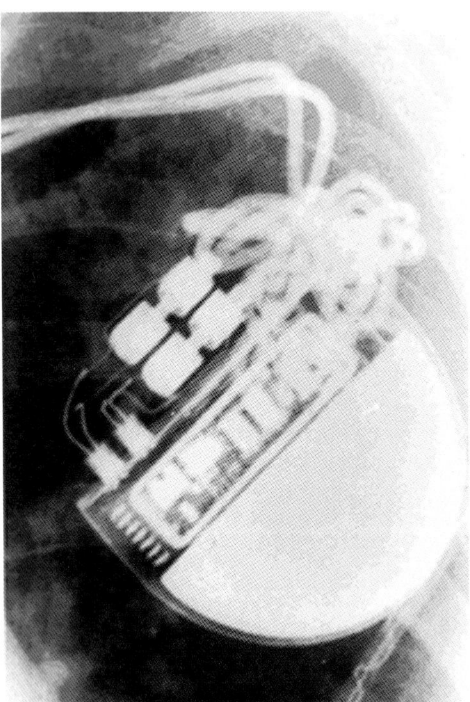

A

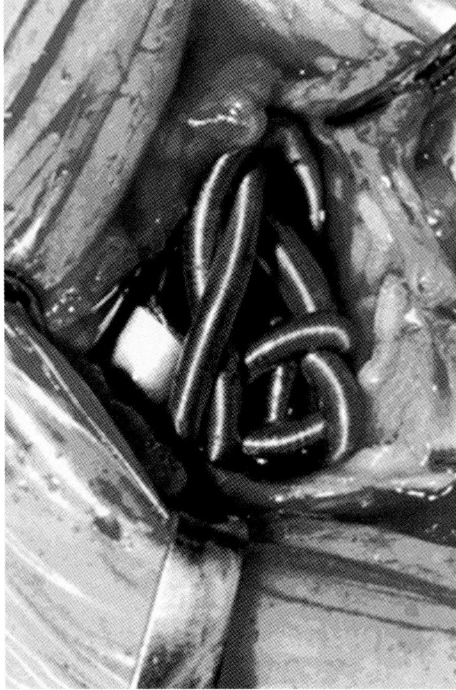

B

Figure 22-28. Twiddler's syndrome. ***A,*** *Magnified view of a radiograph of a patient with twiddler's syndrome.* ***B,*** *During surgical exploration, the pacer had to be twisted 18 revolutions to uncoil the leads. Note the wormlike characteristic of the multiple loops of the electrode wires, which are coiled on themselves. (From Castle LW, Cook S: Pacemaker radiography. In Ellenbogen KA, Kay GN, Wilkoff BL [eds]: Clinical Cardiac Pacing. Philadelphia, WB Saunders, 1995, p 560.)*

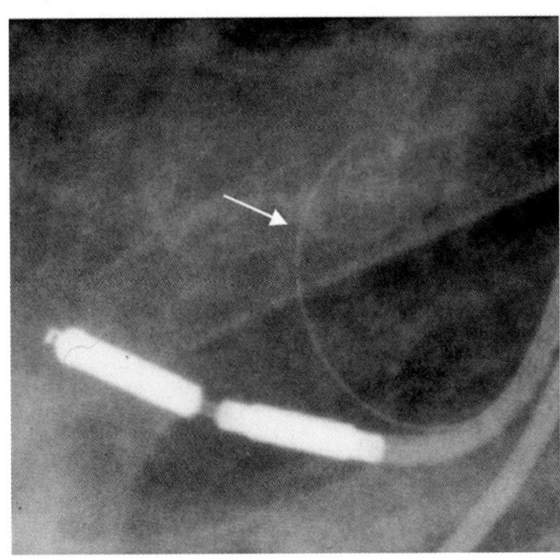

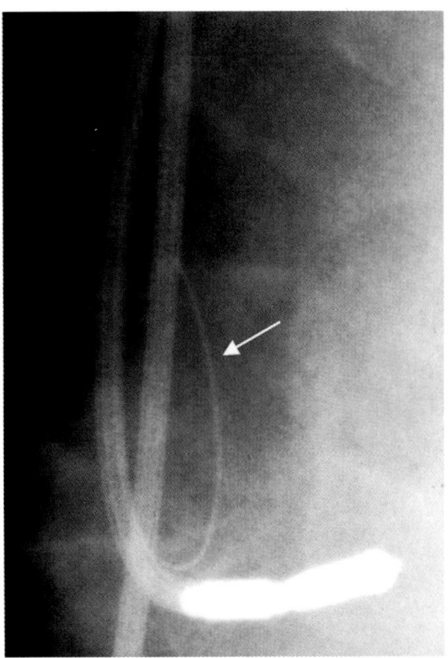

Figure 22-29. Telectronics (Englewood, Col.; now part of St. Jude Medical, Sylmar, Calif.) Accufix atrial lead with fracture and protrusion of the J retention wire (arrow) with migration into the right atrium. Detection of such protrusions is enhanced by the use of higher-penetration, coned-in views.

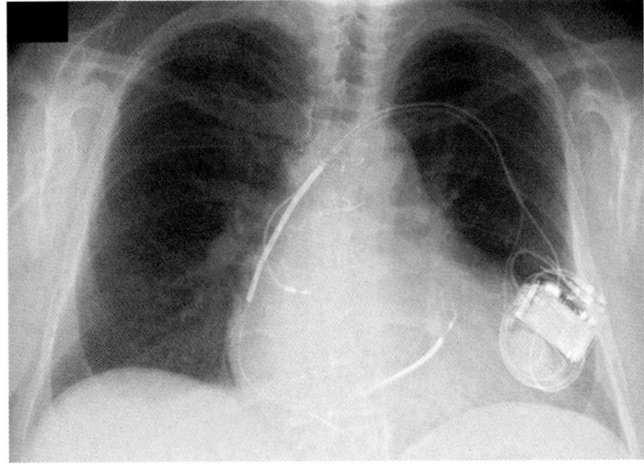

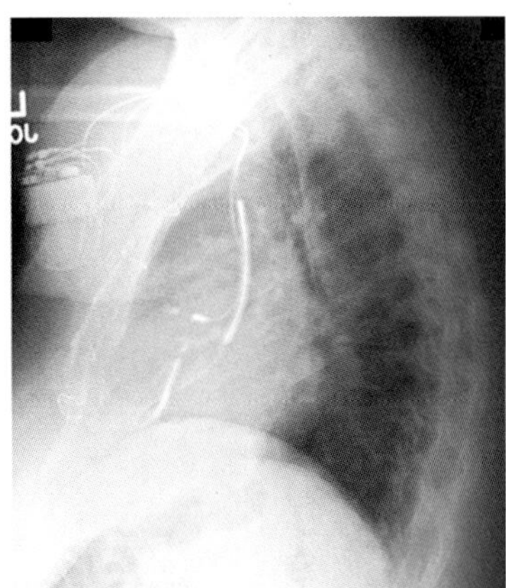

Figure 22-30. Placement of an implantable cardioverter-defibrillator (ICD) lead on the anteroseptal wall of the right ventricular outflow tract.

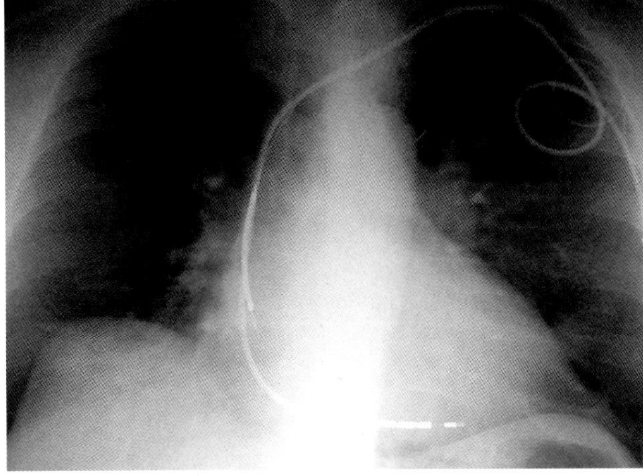

A

Figure 22-31. Transvenous implantable cardioverter-defibrillator (ICD) systems in patients with high defibrillation thresholds. **A,** Posteroanterior (PA) chest radiograph of a transvenous abdominal ICD system with separate right ventricular (RV) and superior vena cava (SVC) leads.

Continued

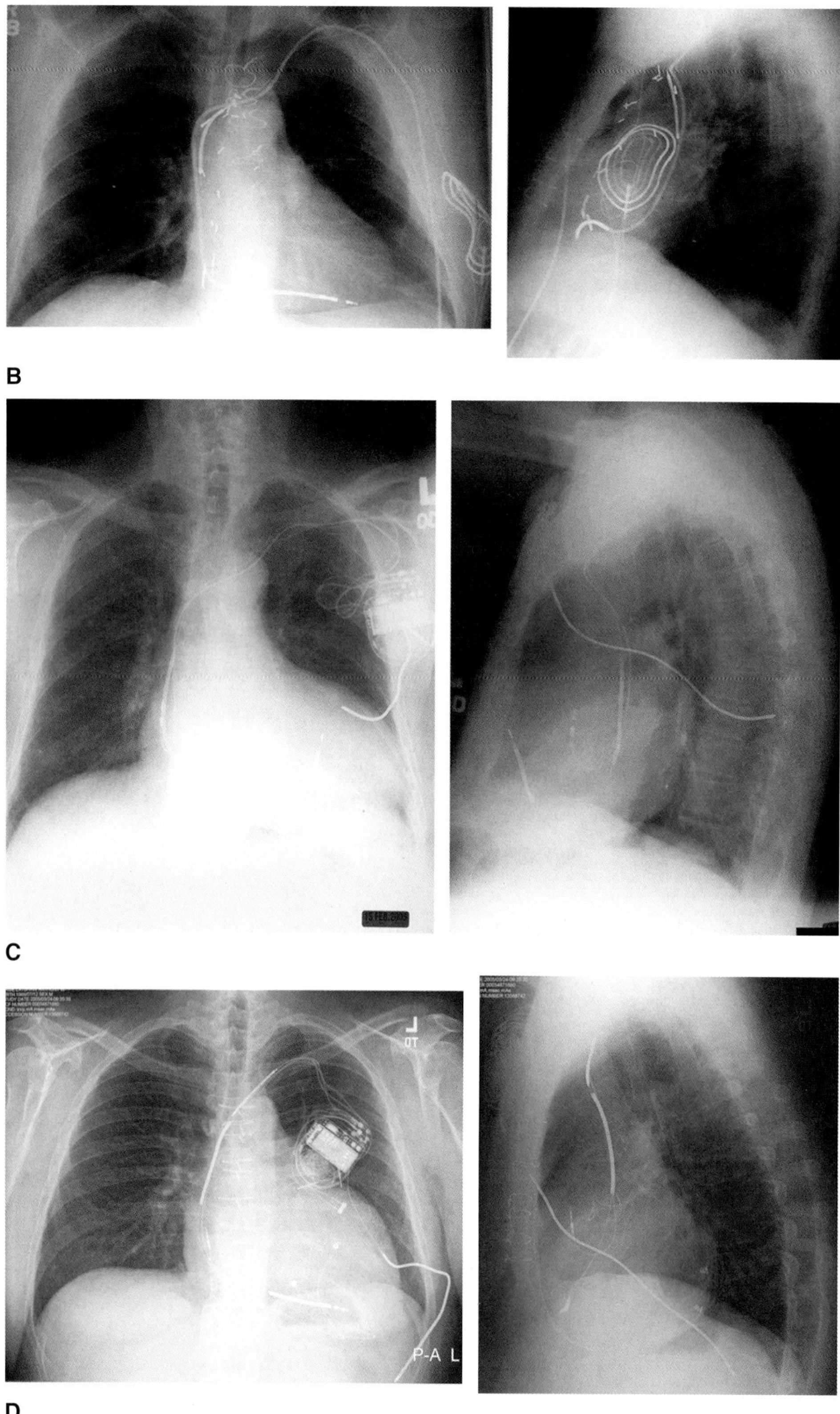

Figure 22-31, cont'd. ***B,*** *PA and lateral chest radiographs of a patient with an abdominal ICD system with separate RV and SVC coils and an axillary patch electrode. The atrial lead has been retracted to the brachiocephalic vein.* ***C,*** *PA and lateral chest radiographs of a left pectoral ICD system with SVC and RV defibrillation coil electrode and a subcutaneous axillary coil electrode.* ***D,*** *PA and lateral chest radiographs of a left pectoral ICD system with an SVC-RV defibrillation coil lead requiring an extra SVC defibrillation lead and a subcutaneous coil implanted along the low lateral posterior chest wall.*

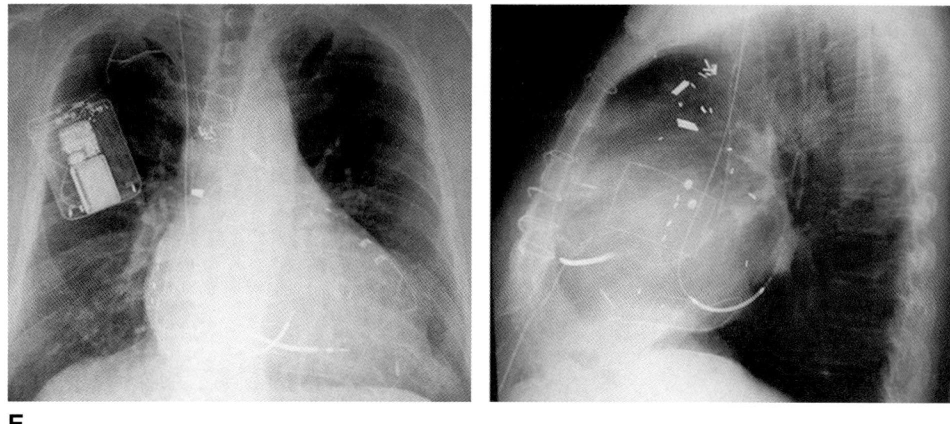

E

Figure 22-31, cont'd. E, *PA and lateral radiographs of a right pectoral ICD lead system with RV defibrillation coil, epicardial patch electrode, and coronary sinus defibrillation coil.*

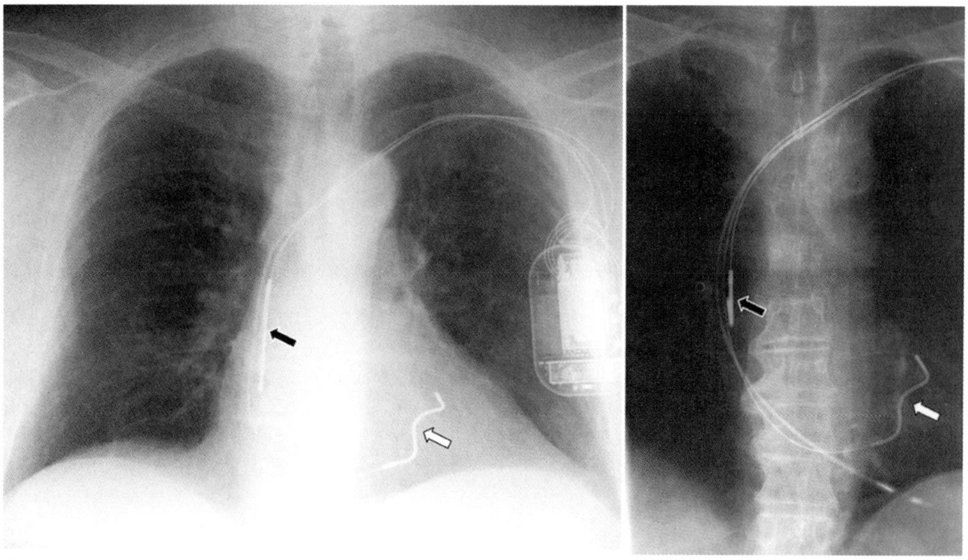

A B 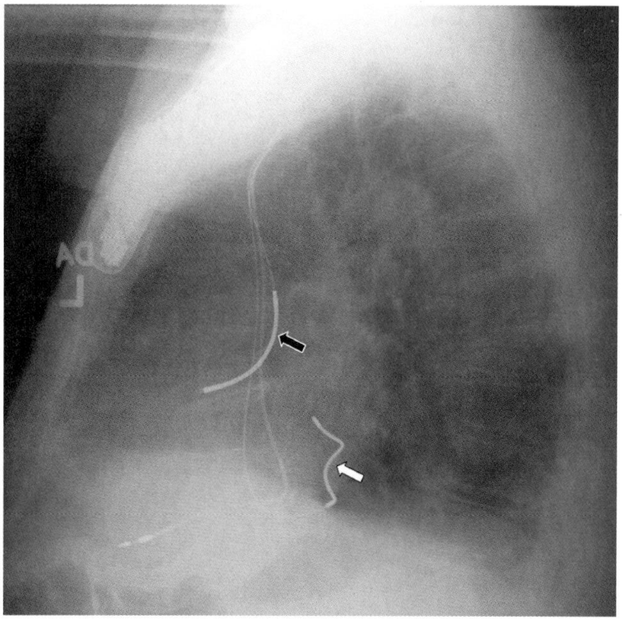 C

Figure 22-32. *Atrial defibrillation lead system. Posteroanterior (PA) (**A**), overpenetrated PA (**B**), and lateral (**C**) chest radiographs demonstrate the InControl, Inc. (Redmond, Wash.) Metrix atrial defibrillator with S-shaped coronary sinus* (white arrows) *and atrial* (black arrows) *defibrillation leads.*

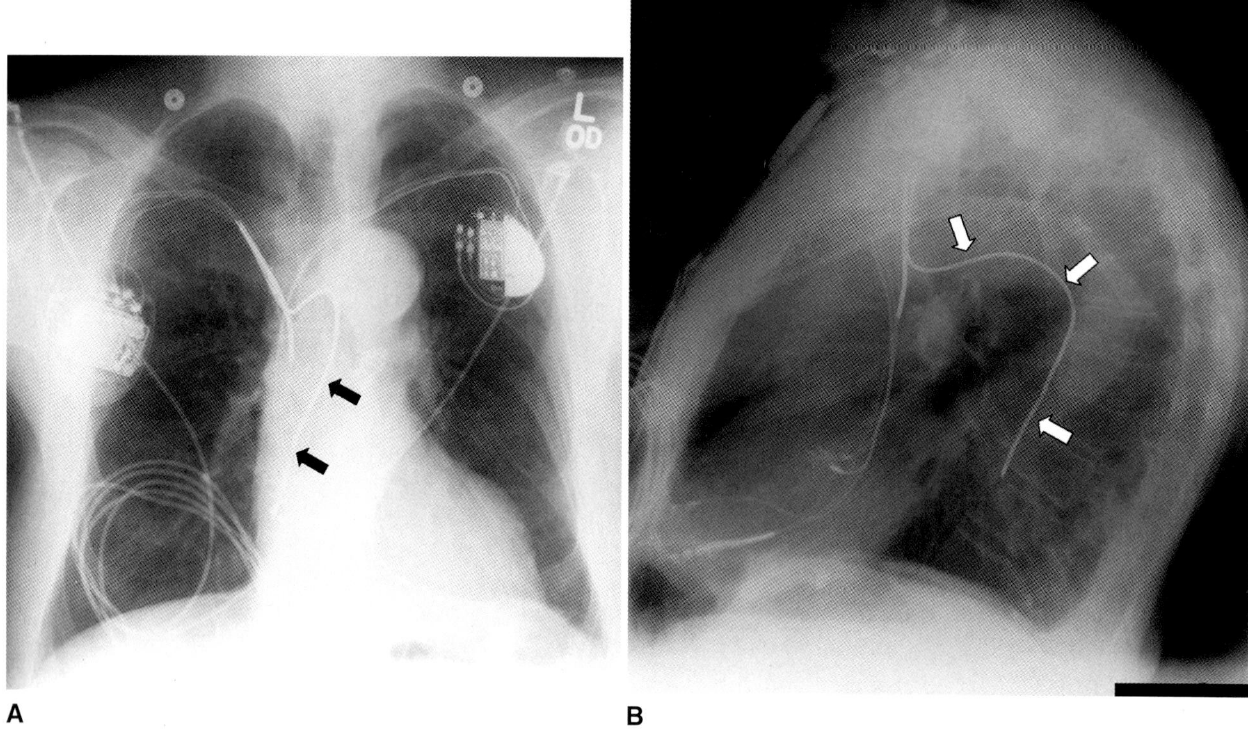

*Figure 22-33. Azygos vein defibrillation lead. Posteroanterior (**A**) and lateral (**B**) chest radiographs of patient from Figure 22-17 in whom high defibrillation thresholds required the addition of an azygos vein defibrillation coil* (arrows). *Note the posterior course from the superior vena cava.*

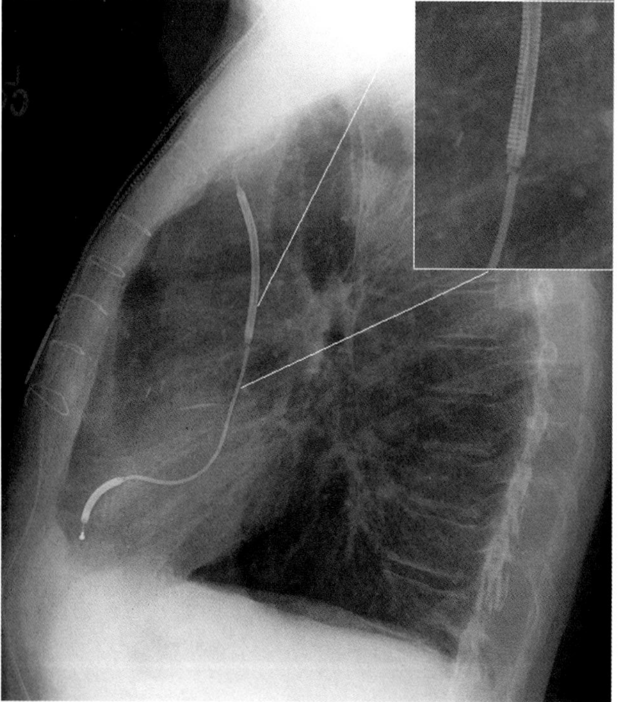

Figure 22-34. Pseudofracture of a Guidant (Boston Scientific, Natick, Mass.) Endotak ICD lead just distal to the proximal high-voltage coil. This pseudo-discontinuity is the normal appearance of this lead.

abdominal and chest radiographs should be obtained in patients with these diagnoses before and after pacemaker or ICD placement.[30,31] It is also important to note cardiac position and mediastinal anatomy on a chest radiograph prior to all device operations, in order to screen for previously undiagnosed congenital cardiovascular anomalies.

Persistent Left-Sided Superior Vena Cava

Occasionally, implantation of leads from the left subclavian or axillary vein results in unexpected inferior passage of the lead on the left side of the chest, before it crosses the midline. This situation typically indicates the presence of a persistent left-sided SVC. From this access, leads placed from the left subclavian vein pass via the left SVC through the CS to the RA or RV (Fig. 22-36). The ventricular lead usually enters the atria posteriorly and loops in the RA before entering the RV (Fig. 22-37). Preoperatively, a persistent left SVC may be suspected from CS dilatation detected on echocardiography, CT, or MRI. In patients with persistent left SVC, placement of transvenous leads from the right axillary/subclavian venous system proceeds normally through the SVC and RA.[32]

Dextrocardia

Dextrocardia should be recognized on the pre-procedure chest radiograph (Fig. 22-38), particularly because its presence may affect on which side an ICD system

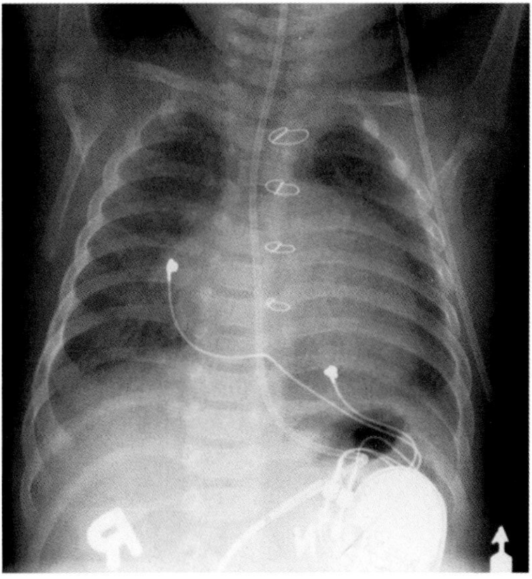
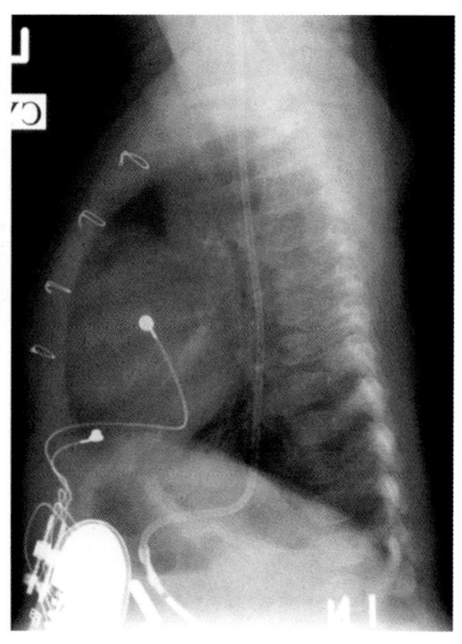

Figure 22-35. *Anteroposterior* (left) *and lateral* (right) *chest and abdominal radiographs of an infant with an epicardial dual-chamber pacemaker system for postoperative complete heart block. The pulse generator in the left upper quadrant of the abdomen is connected to bipolar atrial and ventricular leads.*

Persistent Left Superior Vena Cava

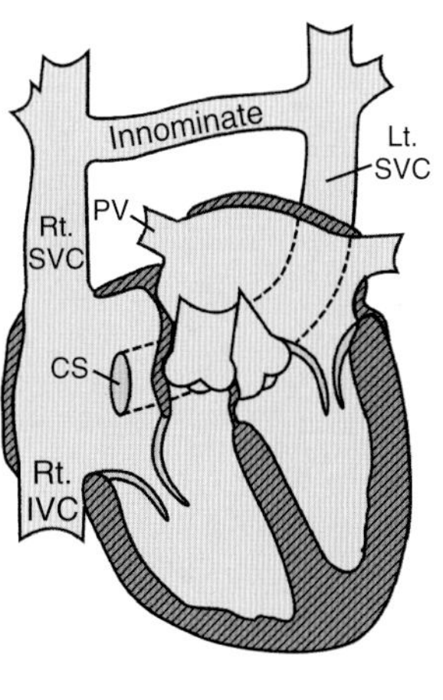

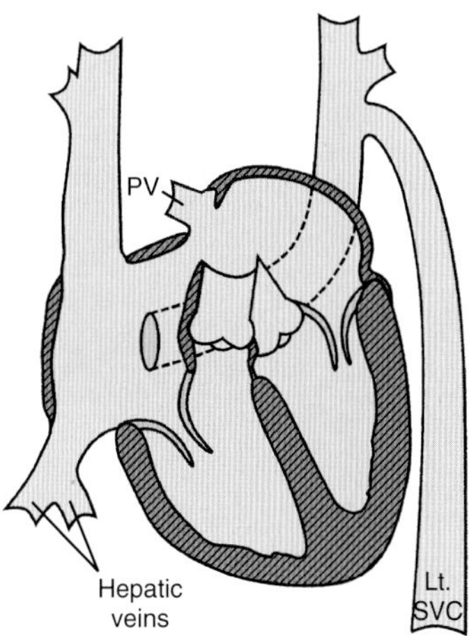

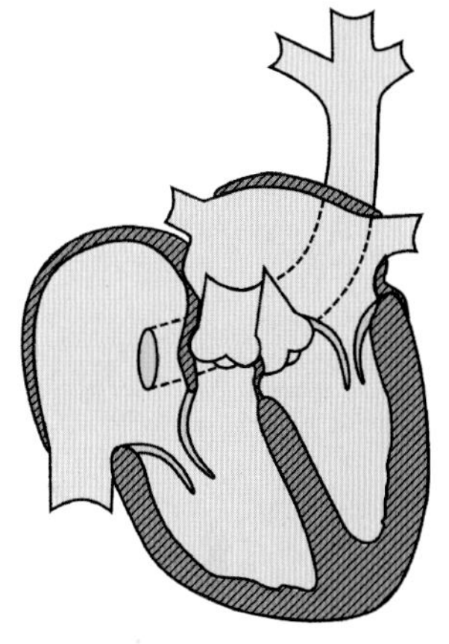

Figure 22-36. *Schematic representation of the three different types of persistent left superior vena cava (SVC) with various insertions of the left SVC into the right heart system. CS, coronary sinus; IVC, inferior vena cava; Lt, left; PV, pulmonary vein; Rt, right; VV, veins. (From Castle LW, Cook S: Pacemaker radiography. In Ellenbogen KA, Kay GN, Wilkoff BL [eds]: Clinical Cardiac Pacing. Philadelphia, WB Saunders, 1995, p 588.)*

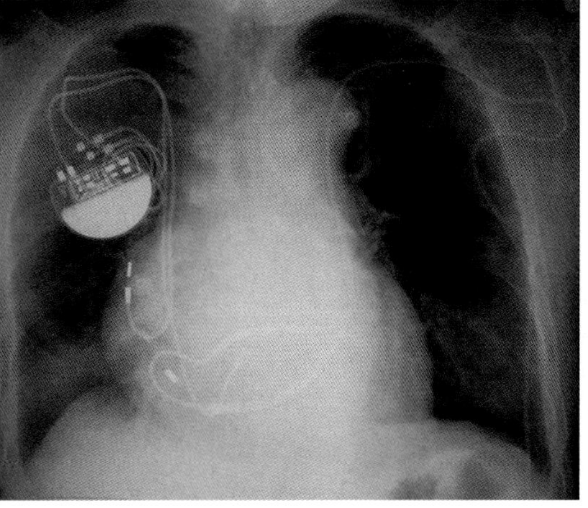
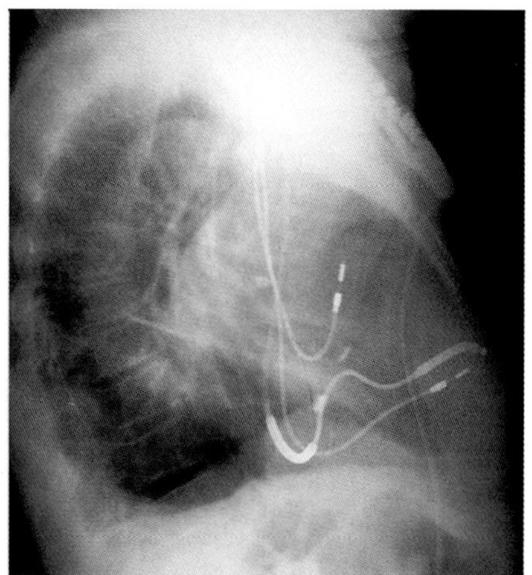

Figure 22-37. *Persistent left superior vena cava (SVC). Posteroanterior* (left) *and lateral* (right) *chest radiographs show an implantable cardioverter-defibrillator (ICD) lead tunneled from the abdomen to the left subclavian vein insertion site, then traversing the left-sided SVC to the distal coronary sinus to the right atrium, and then looping to the right ventricle. A pacemaker from the right pectoral region is also present with atrial and ventricular leads entering via the right subclavian vein.*

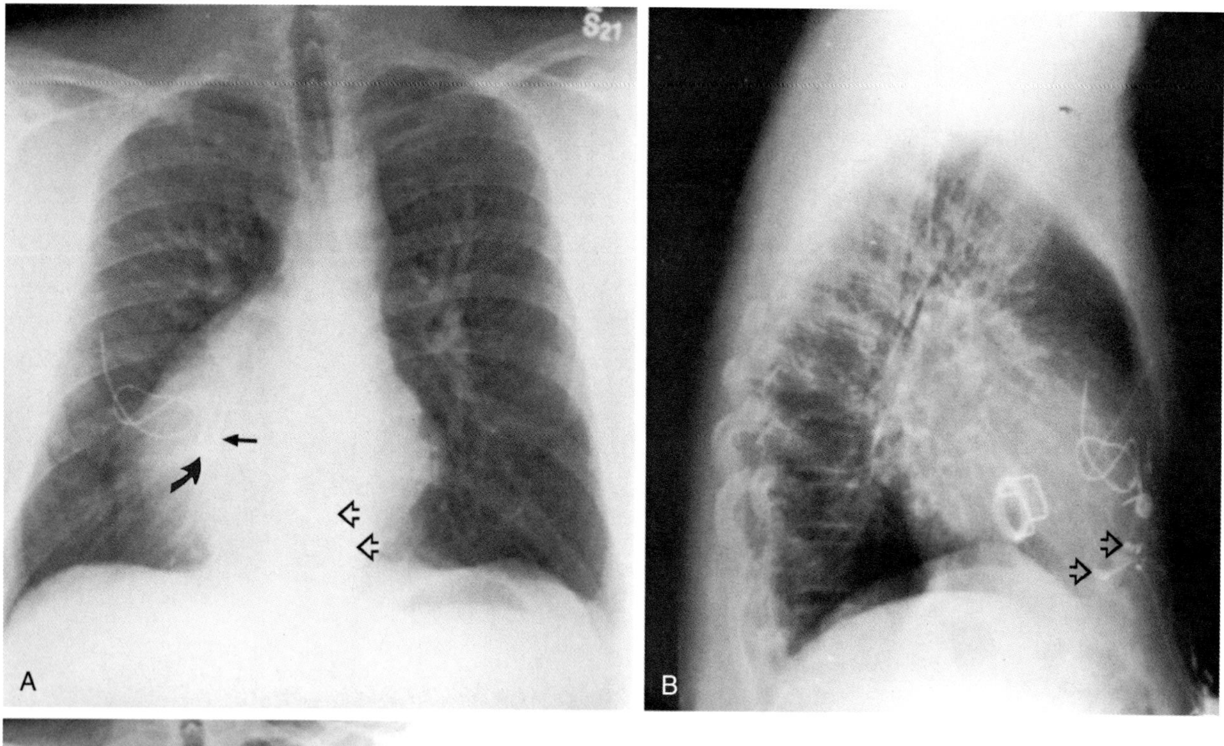

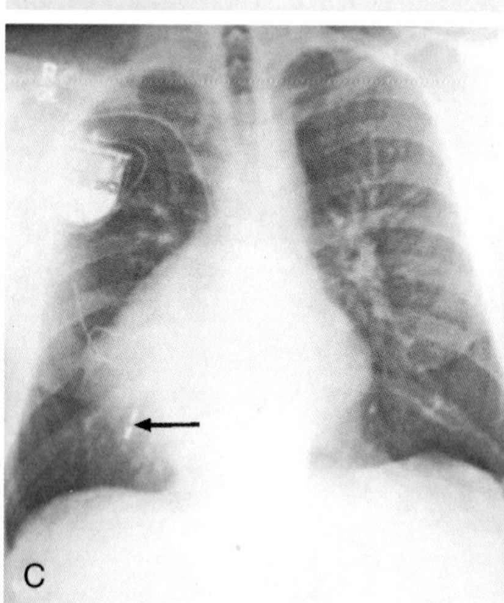

*Figure 22-38. Dextrocardia. **A,** Posteroanterior (PA) chest radiograph obtained in August 1985 demonstrating dextrocardia with a prosthetic mitral valve in place. Remnant stab electrodes can be identified overlying the right precordium (*small curved *and* straight black arrows*). The single-chamber pacing system has two screw-in epicardial leads* (open arrows) *present. **B,** Lateral view of the same patient. **C,** PA chest radiograph dated July 1989 demonstrates abandonment of the previously placed epicardial system. A single-chamber bipolar system is now present with the new transvenous lead near the right ventricular apex* (narrow arrow). *(From Castle LW, Cook S: Pacemaker radiography. In Ellenbogen KA, Kay GN, Wilkoff BL [eds]: Clinical Cardiac Pacing. Philadelphia, WB Saunders, 1995, p 549.)*

may be placed. It is important to note the position of the stomach bubble on the chest radiograph in patients with dextrocardia. In those with situs inversus totalis, in whom the normal right-versus-left position of all organs is completely reversed, the stomach bubble is also right-sided. In those with discordance of cardiac position and abdominal organ position (e.g., dextrocardia with a left-sided stomach bubble), situs inversus totalis is ruled out, and some form of heterotaxy syndrome is present. Patients with heterotaxy syndrome have a high incidence of abnormal systemic venous return and other cardiac anomalies (Fig. 22-39).

Fontan Procedure

A majority of patients with congenital heart disease and functional single-ventricle anatomy undergo staged palliative surgery culminating in a modified Fontan pro-

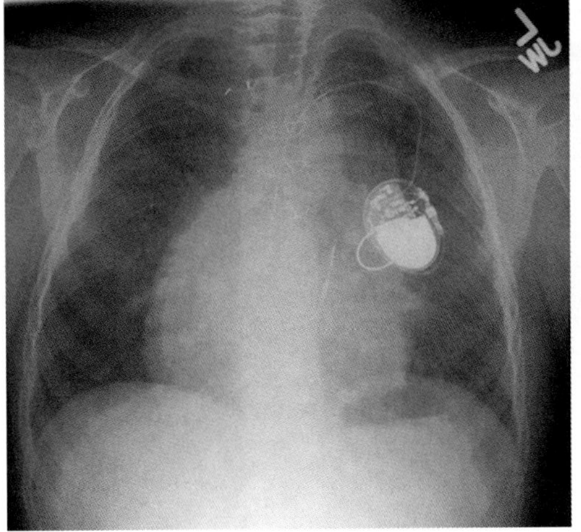
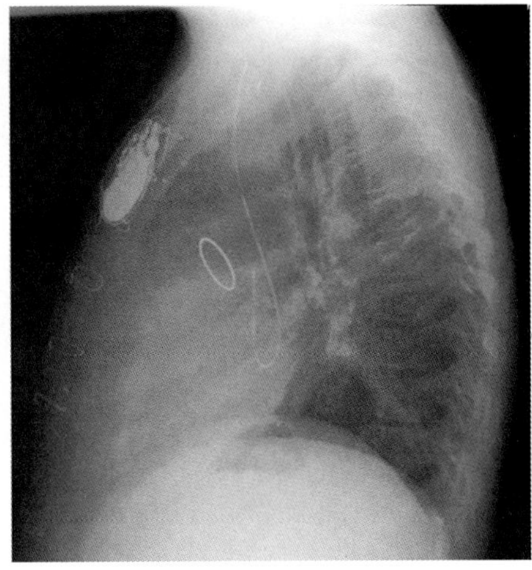

Figure 22-39. *Dextrocardia. Anteroposterior* (left) *and lateral* (right) *chest radiographs in a child with dextrocardia, heterotaxy syndrome, and a single-chamber, transvenous pacing system. The bipolar atrial pacing lead is positioned in the left-sided atrial appendage; the stomach bubble is on the left.*

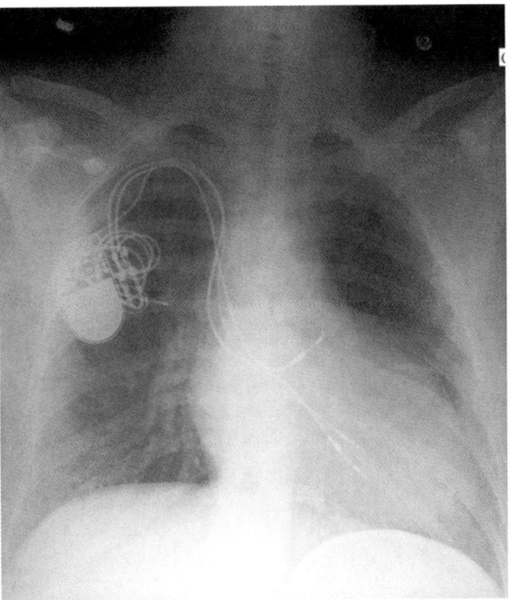
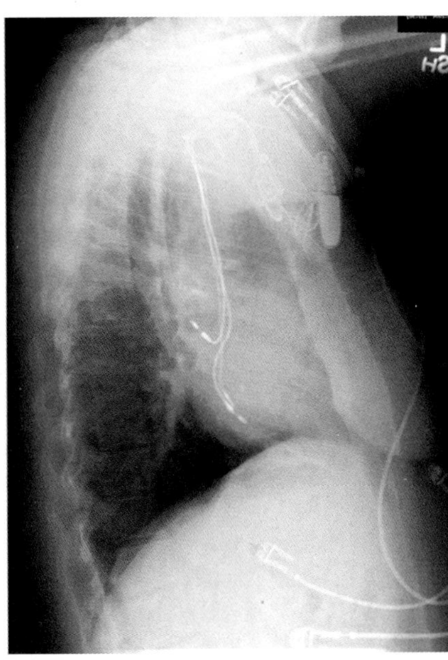

Figure 22-40. *Pacemaker system in D-transposition of the great arteries after a Mustard procedure. Anteroposterior* (left) *and lateral* (right) *chest radiographs show a right-sided pulse generator, a left-sided atrial bipolar lead advanced through the Mustard baffle, a ventricular bipolar lead in the left ventricle, and an abandoned unipolar ventricular lead in the left ventricle.*

cedure. Epicardial systems should be used in such patients because of the high risk for thrombotic complications from endocardial leads.

Senning and Mustard Procedures

Palliative surgery for some congenital heart disease includes creation of intra-atrial baffles that direct systemic venous blood return to the pulmonary ventricle and pulmonary venous return to the systemic ventricle, using either the Senning or Mustard procedure. A majority of patients undergoing palliation with a Senning or Mustard procedure have D- ("uncorrected") or L- ("corrected") transposition of the great arteries. In D-transposition of the great arteries, leads for permanent pacemakers or ICDs are typically placed via the SVC to the morphologic left atrium and LV (Figs. 22-40 to 22-42). In L-transposition of the great arteries, after the "double-switch" procedure (Senning or Mustard and great arterial switch), the leads are placed via the SVC through the intra-atrial baffle to the left-sided atrium and left-sided morphologic RV (Fig. 22-43).

Tetralogy of Fallot

Patients with tetralogy of Fallot have normal AV and ventriculoarterial connections, so the intravenous course of pacing and defibrillation leads is similar to that in patients with normal cardiac anatomy. Patients with this disorder have a higher incidence of persistent left-sided SVC than the general population (Fig. 22-44).

L-Corrected Transposition of the Great Arteries

Patients with unoperated L-transposition of the great arteries have ventricular inversion. Ventricular transvenous pacing leads pass through the SVC to the RA and then to the morphologic, posterior, LV. If advanced through the LV, transvenous leads enter the pulmonary artery. Affected patients have a high likelihood of other associated congenital cardiac anomalies.

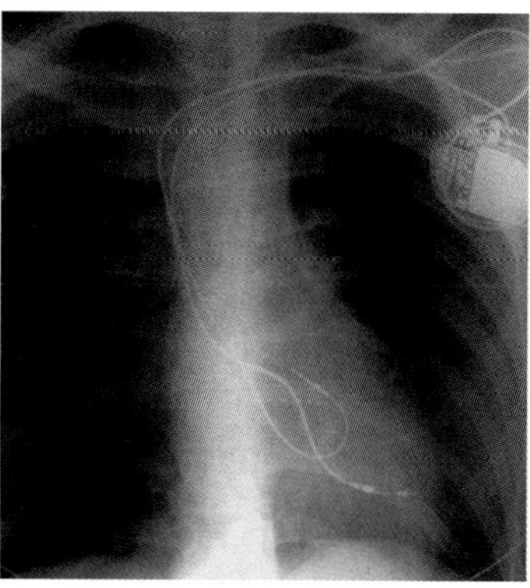

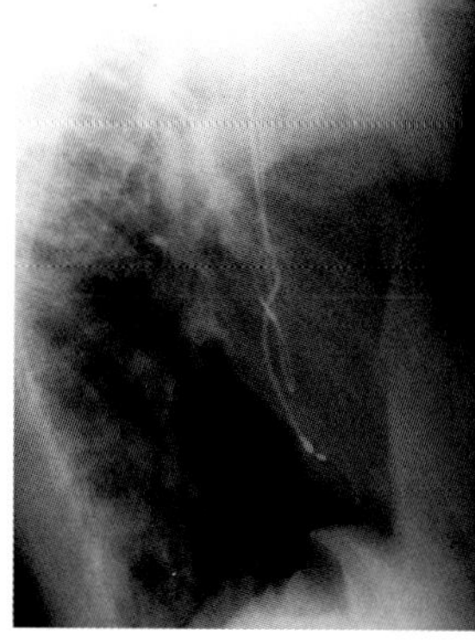

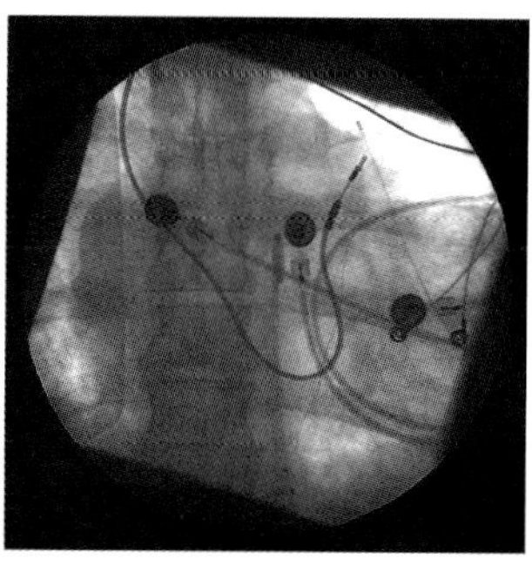

Figure 22-41. Pacemaker system in D-transposition of the great arteries after a Senning procedure. Anteroposterior (AP) (left) *and lateral* (middle) *chest radiographs show the left-sided pulse generator, a bipolar atrial lead advanced through the baffle to the left atrium, and the ventricular bipolar lead tip in the left ventricle. The AP fluoroscopic image* (right) *shows lead placement into the left atrial appendage in a different patient with D-transposition of the great arteries after a Senning procedure.*

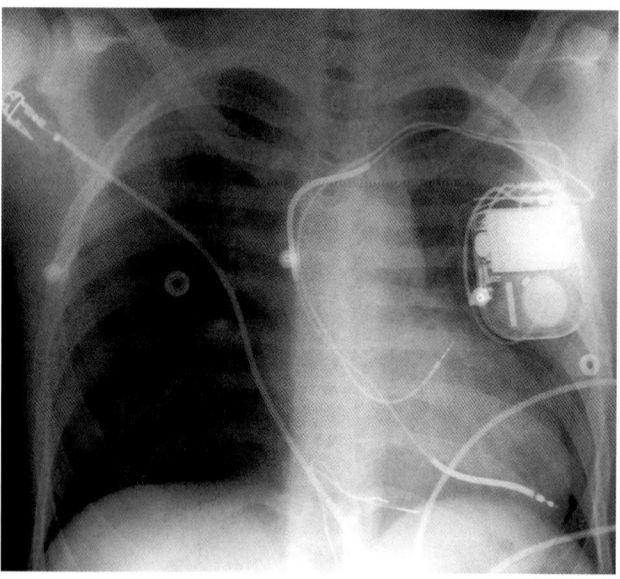

Figure 22-42. Transvenous implantable cardioverter-defibrillator (ICD) system implanted in a pediatric patient after a Senning procedure for D-transposition of the great arteries. Anteroposterior chest radiograph shows a bipolar pacing lead advanced through the atrial baffle with the tip in the left atrial appendage and a dual-coil ICD lead advanced through the atrial baffle with the tip in the left ventricle. Two epicardial temporary pacing wires are present on the surface of the right ventricle.

Implantation Fluoroscopy and Venography

Direct fluoroscopy during the procedure guides the entire lead implantation process. Different radiographic projections can aid delivery of the lead to the most desired sites in the RA, RV, and/or CS.

Transvenous Access Venography

The first and second rib and clavicle serve as the standard landmarks in accessing the axillary/subclavian vein on either the left or the right side. The part of the vein inferolateral to the clavicle and at the lateral border of the first rib is typically considered the axillary vein, and the portion medial to this region, coursing under the clavicle, is the subclavian vein (see Fig. 22-9). Cephalic vein access is usually achieved through venous cutdown under direct visualization, whereas the axillary and subclavian vein access is typically achieved through either a percutaneous puncture using bony landmarks or fluoroscopy to help avoid pneumothorax.

Access via the axillary vein is advantageous to subclavian venous access, in that leads can be inserted more laterally, usually lateral to the subclavius muscle or ligament, potentially reducing the risk of subclavian crush syndrome, as well as the risk of pneumothorax, because access occurs in the extrathoracic portion of the vein. The subclavian/axillary artery lies posterior and cranial to the subclavian/axillary vein. During axillary vein access under PA fluoroscopic guidance, the needle is directed toward the anterolateral first rib with a superficial course until the needle tip is seen to overlie the first rib. The needle is then directed with higher vertical angulation (with more posterior direction) toward the first rib, care being taken to avoid penetration of the needle intrathoracically medial to the medial border of the rib.

In patients with morbid obesity, bony deformities, previous subclavian venous central line access, prior upper extremity deep venous thrombosis, congenital heart disease, or preexisting leads, venous access can be difficult because of stenosis or altered relationships among the venous system, ribs, and clavicle. In these cases, ipsilateral upper extremity venography can be very helpful in defining the course and patency of the axillary/subclavian venous system. Preoperative upper extremity venograms to assess the patency in patients with previously implanted leads (see Fig. 22-9) are also often helpful, although intraoperative fluoroscopic or cineangiographic venography can be performed with simultaneous venous access.[33] Should a left-sided SVC be encountered, this anatomy may also be confirmed with venography.

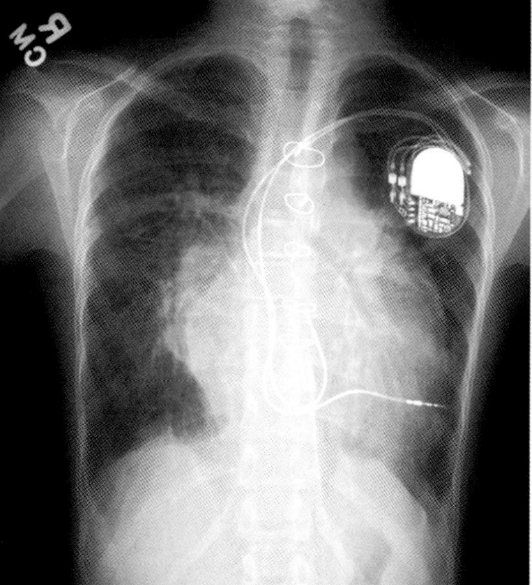
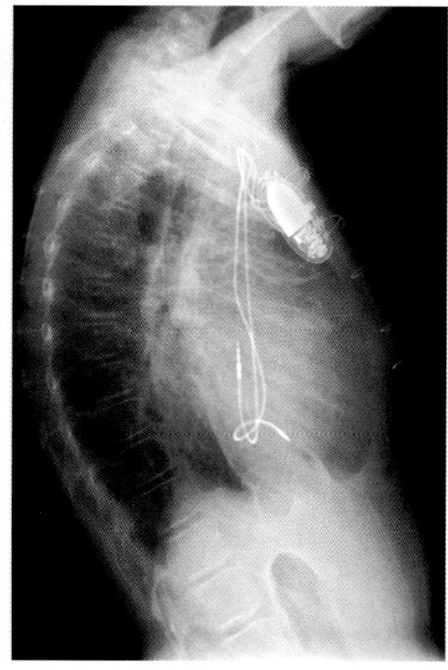

Figure 22-43. Pacemaker system in a patient with L-transposition of the great arteries after Senning and great arterial switch ("double switch") procedures. Anteroposterior (left) *and lateral* (right) *chest radiographs show the left subpectoral pulse generator, the atrial bipolar lead advanced through the atrial baffle into the left atrium, and the ventricular bipolar lead tip in the apex of the left-sided morphologic right ventricle.*

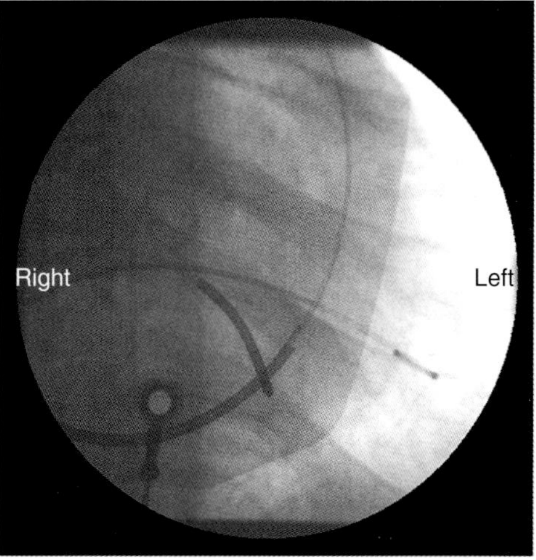

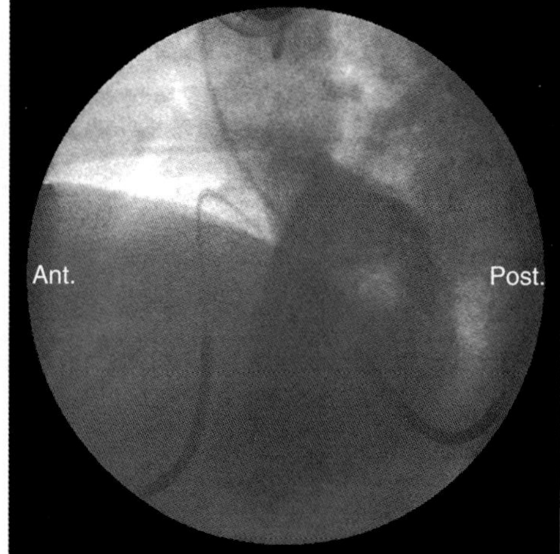

Figure 22-44. Implantable cardioverter-defibrillator (ICD) lead positioning in tetralogy of Fallot with persistent left superior vena cava. Fluoroscopic views show that the ICD proximal defibrillation coil is positioned in the coronary sinus, and the distal coil in the right ventricle. Ant., anterior; Post., posterior. (Courtesy of Gerald Serwer, MD. University of Michigan, Ann Arbor, Mich.).

Traditional Pacing Sites

The RA lead follows the contour of the vascular system without excess redundancy, except in cases of venous tortuosity, but with a J-shaped lead, slack is generally left at the distal portion of the lead. RV leads are generally placed with enough lead slack to allow for lift and closure of the tricuspid valve. Lack of this lifting motion during fluoroscopy may signify a diseased tricuspid valve or tethering of the tricuspid leaflets or chordae by the pacing or ICD lead. In the latter case, repositioning of the lead requires withdrawal of the lead tip back to the RA and fresh entry to the RV between leaflets. Radiographically, a lead positioned at the RVA displays the tip of the lead pointing slightly downward in the AP view and anteriorly on the lateral view; posterior angulation of the lead suggests positioning in the CS. A lead placed onto the RVOT or septum is located more cranially (see Fig. 22-30). A left anterior oblique (LAO) or left lateral view may help to determine septal rather than anterior wall location. Undue tension on leads may result in dislodgment or poor pacing thresholds (Fig. 22-45). In children, greater lead redundancy is desirable to allow for future growth without causing excessive tension on the pacing or ICD lead.[34]

Alternative-Site Pacing

Pacing strategies to suppress atrial arrhythmias have involved selective alternate atrial site or dual atrial site pacing. Pacing the high septum of the RA, near Bachmann's bundle or the ostium of the CS, may shorten intra-atrial conduction and minimize dispersion of refractoriness, thereby perhaps improving atrial fibrillation.[8,9] Fluoroscopically, the RA lead is directed in the LAO view toward the interatrial septum and then withdrawn until the tip begins to straighten, indicating proximity to the RA roof, where it is then fixed to the high septum. The position appears anteriorly directed on the RAO view.[9] The LAO projection is helpful in guiding leads to the low RA septum. The target is the low septum just superior to the ostium of the CS and below the

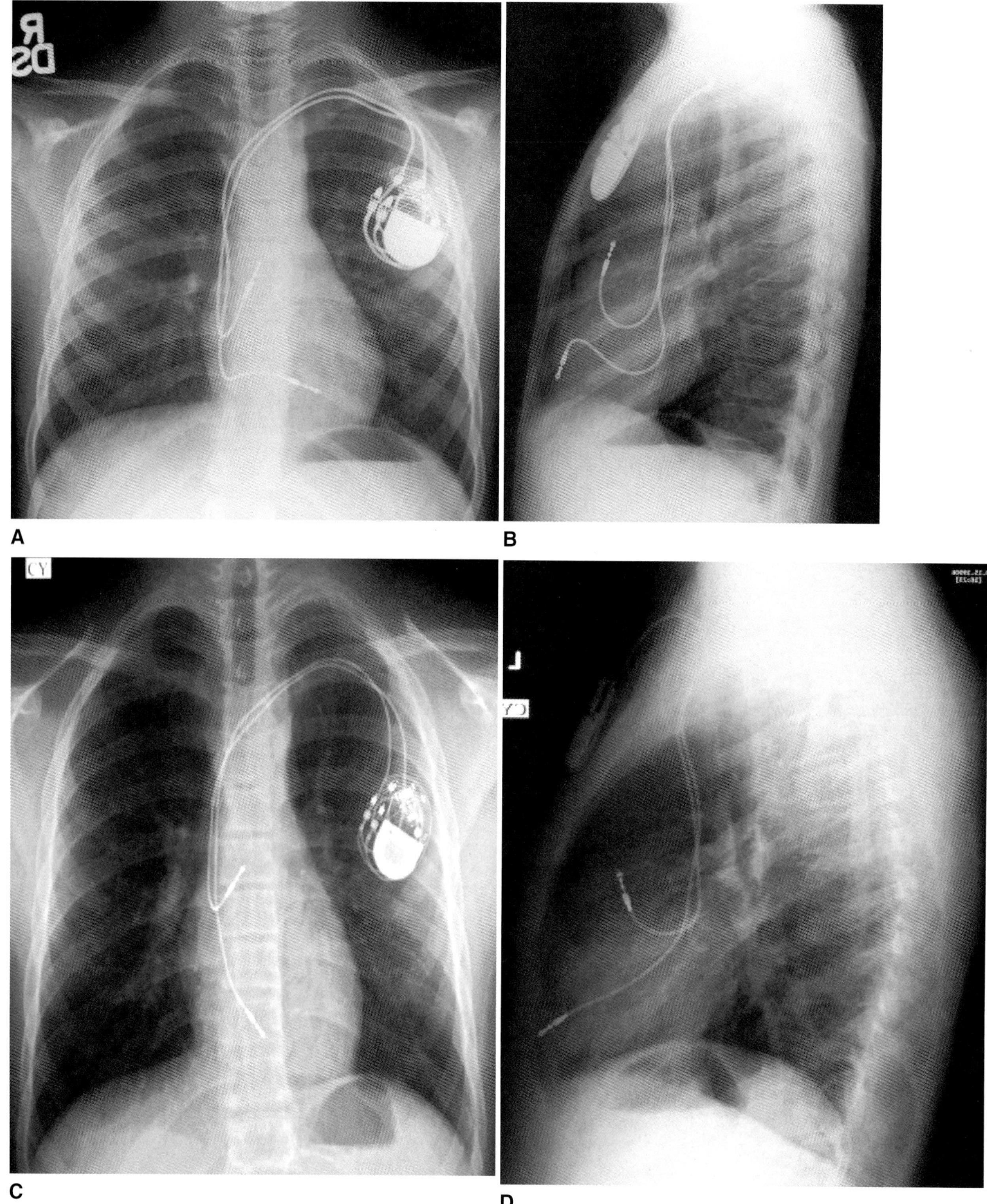

*Figure 22-45. Lead slack. Chest posteroanterior and lateral radiographs of a transvenous dual-chamber pacing system in a child with congenital complete heart block. The atrial and ventricular leads had adequate redundancy after initial system implantation when the patient was 8 years old (**A** and **B**). Six years later, however, both the atrial and ventricular leads have inadequate redundancy (**C** and **D**). Tension on the ventricular lead caused poor pacing and sensing thresholds with intermittent complete loss of capture.*

foramen ovale. Traditional RVA pacing may cause a dyssynchronous LV electrical activation pattern, resulting in dyssynchronous contraction and relaxation that can contribute to heart failure or reduce long-term survival.[35-37]

Therefore, alternative ventricular site pacing has become more conventional. The RVOT or septum has been targeted for RV leads (see Figs. 22-16 and 22-30). These sites may also be used when pacing thresholds are high at the apex or if an ICD lead is present at the apex and separation is required to prevent device-device interactions (see Fig. 22-17).[38] The lead may be placed with use of the AP or RAO view with a gently curved stylet to help advance the lead through the tricuspid valve to the RVOT or pulmonary artery. The lead is then slowly withdrawn with counterclockwise torque to aim the tip toward the RVOT septum, where it can be actively fixed. The LAO view can be used to help determine whether the lead tip is septally or anteriorly directed. His bundle pacing has also been targeted on the RV septum with the goal of maintaining synchronous ventricular activation during ventricular pacing.

Coronary Sinus Venography and Lead Placement

Coronary sinus venography and lead placement are described previously in this chapter and in detail in Chapter 19.

Azygos Venography and Lead Placement

The azygos vein may be a target for ICD defibrillation leads in patients with high defibrillation thresholds (see Figs. 22-11 and 22-33). The azygos vein may be cannulated in the LAO projection and enters the SVC posteriorly just at or below its origin at the confluence of the right and left brachiocephalic veins. The vein often is acutely angled cranially and may require special guiding catheters (e.g., an internal mammary artery [IMA] catheter) to aid in introduction of a guidewire. Venography is often helpful in determining the ostium of the azygos vein and to define its course and branches.

Subcutaneous Patch, Coil, or Array

Defibrillation leads intended for subcutaneous implantation in patients with high defibrillation thresholds have been designed to contain a single coil, a multicoil array, or a patch electrode that can increase the surface area of the defibrillation vector (see Fig. 22-31). These subcutaneous electrodes may be placed across the posterolateral wall of the chest to provide a more posterior vector, or to the left pectoral region in the absence of a left pectoral active-can ICD. The lead system may be best visualized on the lateral chest radiograph or via an RAO or LAO fluoroscopic view.[28]

Lead Extraction

The tip of the telescoping sheath used for lead extraction is radiopaque and is continuously monitored by means of fluoroscopy while being advanced along the course of the lead (Fig. 22-46). Often, the leads are fibrosed and calcified and are clearly visible with fluoroscopy. Also, the dimensions and configuration of the cardiac silhouette and obliteration of the left hemidiaphragm should be followed closely to enable prompt recognition of cardiac tamponade. The details of lead extraction are described elsewhere in this book.

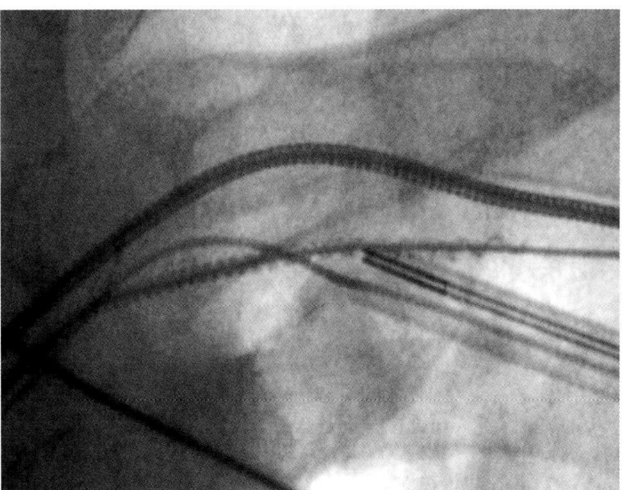

Figure 22-46. Extraction sheath, inserted over the lead targeted for extraction, is guided by means of fluoroscopy.

Detection of Acute Complications

Fluoroscopy may detect development of acute pneumothorax, usually from difficult venous insertion attempts, and may allow immediate follow-up of the stability of the pneumothorax. Enlarging pneumothoraces or hemodynamic compromise usually requires insertion of a chest tube.

In cases of pericardial effusion due to lead perforation, the diagnosis of cardiac tamponade is usually made clinically from a constellation of findings, including hypotension, pulsus paradoxus, and electrical alternans. Cardiac or vascular lacerations or tears are more commonly seen with lead extraction than with traditional lead insertion, but subclinical lead perforations may be more common than suspected. On fluoroscopy, development of a "double shadow" on the cardiac silhouette with visualization of an inner, contracting cardiac border surrounded by a noncontractile pericardial shadow suggests perforation or laceration with pericardial effusion.

Rarely, electromechanical dissociation can occur after defibrillation testing in patients with severe heart failure and severe RA dysfunction. Particularly if prompted by pulse oximetry or blood pressure alarms, a quick fluoroscopic check can help determine the return of mechanical cardiac contractions.

Postimplantation Radiography

A chest radiograph should be obtained after implantation of a pacemaker or ICD system. Postprocedure PA and lateral chest radiographs can confirm the correct and stable position of the generator and leads and assess for complications, such as ipsilateral or contralateral pneumothorax (Fig. 22-47), pleural effusion or hemothorax (Fig. 22-48), and even retained surgical sponges.[39]

Pneumothorax

Pneumothorax is best demonstrated on an upright PA view in full expiration. Pneumothorax is characterized by absence of lung markings over the lung fields (see Fig. 22-47). The border of the lung apex, surrounded by clear air space inside the thoracic cavity, may be visualized. Rare cases have been reported in which the leads have punctured through the SVC, causing a contralateral pneumothorax; this complication is usually associated with contralateral hemothorax.

Hemothorax

Hemothorax is an unusual complication during routine lead placement. Venous tears during lead extraction, however, can be associated with clinically significant hemothorax, which is usually evident during the procedure. Rarely, delayed ooze into the pleural space due to subclavian vein or SVC laceration can result in significant pleural leak (see Fig. 22-48). A hemothorax or pleural effusion is best recognized on upright PA or lateral chest radiograph.

Pericardial Effusion, Cardiac Perforation, and Cardiac Tamponade

Although the cardiac silhouette may be seen to enlarge on chest radiography, particularly on comparison with the pre-implantation chest radiograph, one should not rely on the chest radiograph for a diagnosis of pericardial effusion. If there is clinical suspicion of a pericardial effusion, an echocardiogram should be obtained. Effacement of the left hemidiaphragm with enlarged cardiac silhouette compared with the pre-procedural chest radiograph is usually suggestive of pericardial effusion. An extracardiac location of the tip of the pacing lead suggests cardiac perforation with migration of the lead outside the heart (Fig. 22-49). Unless there is significant migration of the lead tip past the cardiac shadow, the chest radiograph may be insensitive to detection of cardiac perforation, and other imaging modalities, such as echocardiography and cardiac CT, may help determine whether a lead is indeed extracardiac in location.[40]

Lead Dislodgment

Postimplantation chest radiograph helps confirm the position of the lead. Incomplete fixation of the lead screw and insufficient slack due to inadvertent pulls on the lead during suturing of the sleeve can be causes of lead dislodgment. Atrial lead dislodgment may be suspected if the atrial lead hangs straight vertically, if a J shape was seen during implantation (see Fig. 22-49). Dislodgement of the atrial lead into the RV may result in inappropriate ventricular pacing. Ventricular lead dislodgement may be recognized from proximal dis-

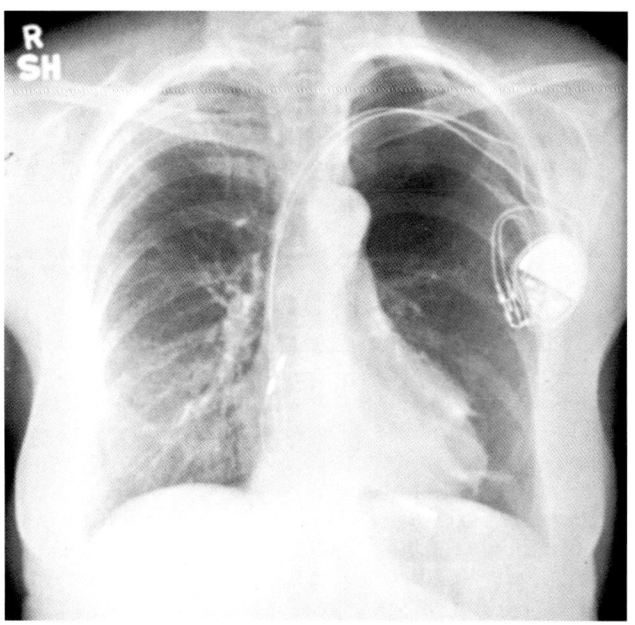

Figure 22-47. Pneumothorax. Posteroanterior chest radiograph demonstrating a dual-chamber pacing system in place with fixed electrodes in both the right atrial appendage and the right ventricular apex. Note the relative radiolucency over the left chest in comparison with the right. There is a moderate-sized pneumothorax on the left, with evidence of subsegmental atelectasis in the lingula and in the left lower lobe. Note the absence of lung markings superiorly. (From Castle LW, Cook S: Pacemaker radiography. In Ellenbogen KA, Kay GN, Wilkoff BL [eds]: Clinical Cardiac Pacing. Philadelphia, WB Saunders, 1995, p 551.)

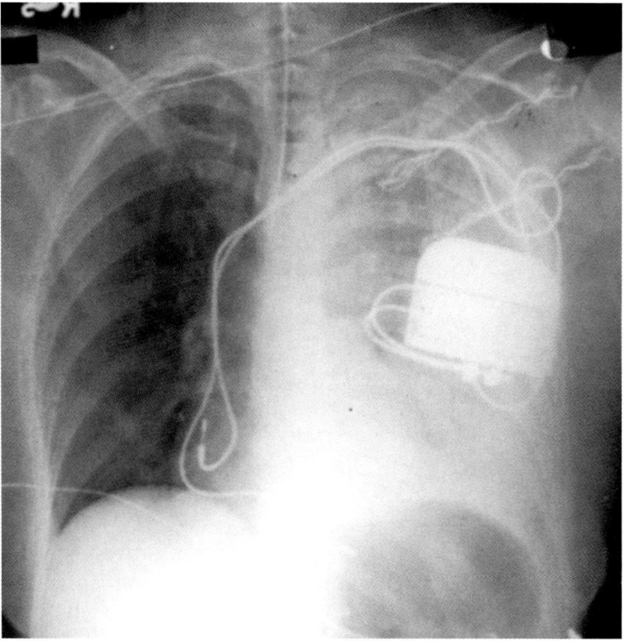

Figure 22-48. Hemothorax. AP portable chest radiograph obtained immediately after pacemaker insertion demonstrates a large hemothorax on the left secondary to perforation of the left subclavian artery. There is almost complete opacification of the left hemithorax. (From Castle LW, Cook S: Pacemaker radiography. In Ellenbogen KA, Kay GN, Wilkoff BL [eds]: Clinical Cardiac Pacing. Philadelphia, WB Saunders, 1995, p 551.)

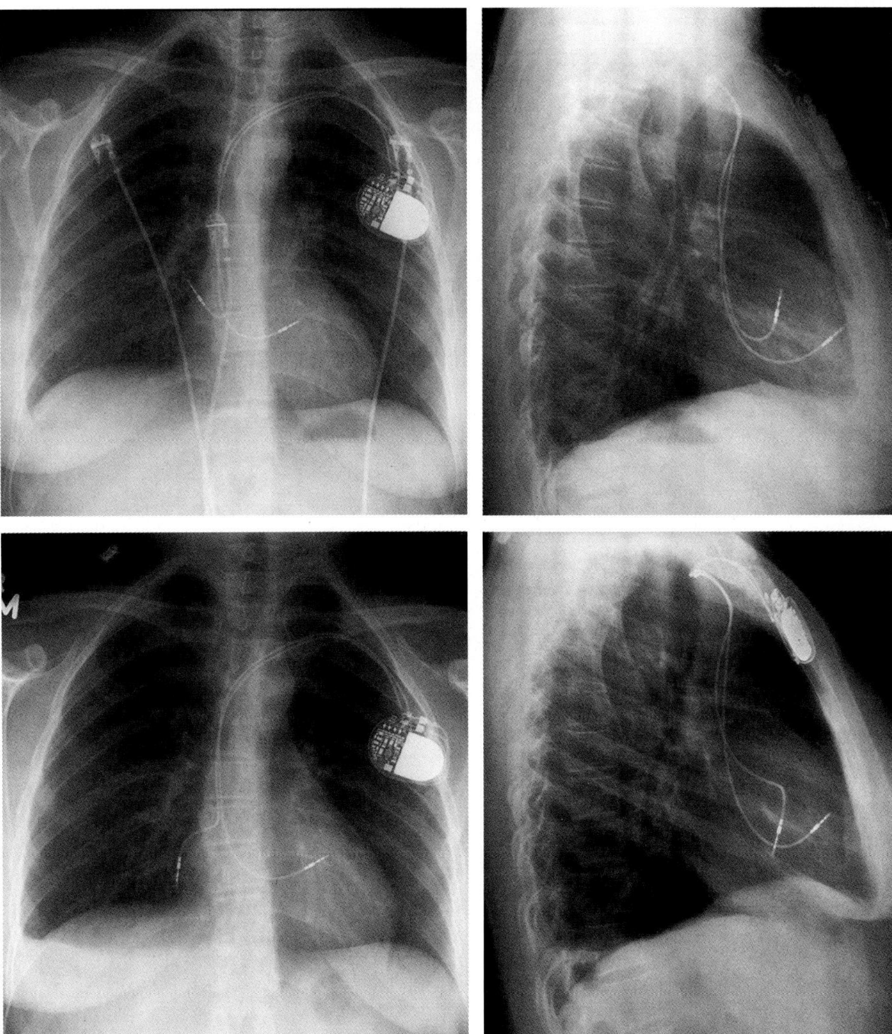

Figure 22-49. Lead dislodgment and perforation. Upper panels, *Posteroanterior (PA) and lateral chest radiographs after atrial and ventricular pacemaker placement. Perforation of the atrial lead past the cardiac border is suspected.* Lower panels, *on follow-up PA and lateral chest radiographs, it is clear that the atrial lead has perforated the cardiac border and become dislodged caudally. (Case reported in Khan MN, Joseph G, Khaykin Y, Ziada KM, Wilkoff BL: Delayed lead perforation: A disturbing trend. PACE 28:251, 2005.)*

lodgments of apically positioned leads or falling of the lead from a higher septal or RVOT location. Similarly, CS lead dislodgment can also be recognized on the AP and lateral chest radiographs.

Lead Conductor Fracture and Insulation Breaks

The lead should be inspected in its entirety. There should be no discontinuity of the coil, nor any sharp angulation or kinking. Such findings suggest lead fracture or the potential for fracture. Pseudofracture due to crimping of insulation from excessive suture ligatures may be found and should indicate a need for close attention to pacing impedance, noise, sensing, and pacing measurements at postimplantation and follow-up device interrogations.

Echocardiography

Echocardiography can play an integral role in diagnostic and therapeutic aspects of pacemaker and defibrillation systems. Echocardiograms can assess LV function, detect and enable guided treatment of pericardial effusion and cardiac tamponade, and detect or follow native or lead vegetations. Echocardiography is also used for optimization of device timing programming (e.g., AV delay optimization) and assessment of RA dyssynchrony in patients receiving or being considered for CRT.

Pericardial Effusion

Echocardiography is the "gold standard" for assessing pericardial effusion after implantation or explantation of pacing or defibrillation systems. A quick bedside echocardiographic assessment to detect pericardial effusion can be performed if clinical suspicion is high. Echocardiography may enable quantification of pericardial effusion as well as help determine whether cardiac tamponade physiology exists. Echocardiography can also be used to monitor effusions, determine the timing of and need for pericardiocentesis, and guide percutaneous pericardiocentesis.

Cardiac Perforation

Echocardiography may detect the presence of a lead artifact in the pericardial space or close to the epicardial

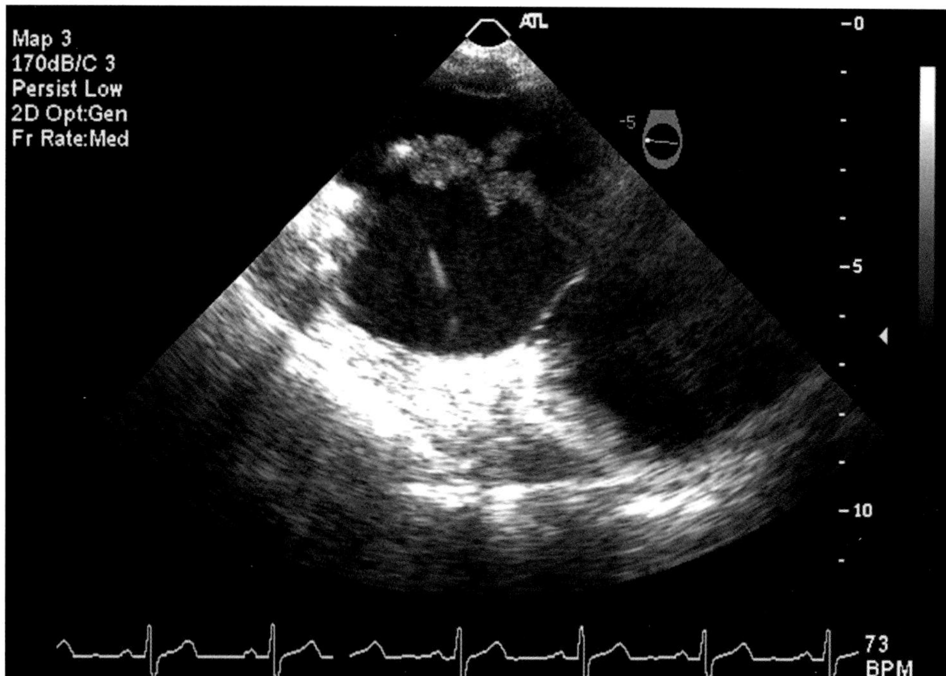

Figure 22-50. Vegetation on a pacing lead demonstrated by transesophageal echocardiography.

surface. This finding may be useful in conjunction with confirmation of the presence of a pericardial effusion and other clinical indicators, such as presence of a pericardial rub, pain, and evidence of cardiac tamponade.

Native/Lead Vegetations

Vegetations may be detected on transthoracic echocardiography but are more commonly defined by transesophageal echocardiography (Fig. 22-50). Distinction between fibrous stranding and infected vegetations may have to be made from clinical history and blood culture results.

Computed Tomography

CT may be useful in certain instances before and after implantation. The modality may clarify the anatomy of congenital or repaired anomalies, thereby greatly aiding in the planning of appropriate approaches to lead implantation. Cardiac CT has also been used in the diagnosis of arrhythmogenic RV dysplasia (ARVD).[41] Postprocedure applications include the assessment of lead tip migration, cardiac perforation, and pericardial effusion. Cardiac CT has been used in the past to assess epicardial ICD patch location and the extent of myocardial coverage as well as relationships to the underlying myocardium. Most commonly, CT may be used as a substitute for MRI in patients with pacemakers and ICDs. Multislice CT is being investigated for assessment of CS anatomy, which may help determine candidacy for transvenous versus epicardial approaches to CRT.[42] Integration of CT with real-time lead positioning is also being explored.

Magnetic Resonance Imaging

Like CT, cardiac MRI may identify important structural details of the heart before device implantation. MRI has been used in the diagnosis of ARVD and of restrictive or hypertrophic cardiomyopathies as well as detection of hibernating myocardium.

Cardiac MRI has generally been contraindicated in patients with implanted pacemakers or ICDs. However, several investigators have studied the safety of noncardiac MRI in patients with implanted pacemakers. Potential risks include heating of leads, rapid or asynchronous pacing, reed switch inhibition, and induction of ventricular fibrillation.[43] Use of noncardiac MRI of varying static magnetic field strengths has been reported in more than 300 patients with implanted pacemakers.[44] Pacing threshold changes, but no adverse patient events have been reported. Studies have generally avoided pacemaker-dependent subjects. Thus, data so far suggest that patients who are not pacemaker dependent may safely undergo noncardiac MRI at specific absorption rates (SARs) of less than 2 W/kg.[44-46] The pacemaker should be interrogated before the procedure to assess pacemaker dependence and inactivate minute ventilation or other rate response features. Outputs may be programmed to subthreshold levels, but this step has not been shown to be essential. The patient should be continuously monitored and personnel familiar with pacemakers should be present in case emergency programming is required. After the procedure, the pacemaker should again be interrogated and a full check performed, including threshold testing.

Currently, MRI is contraindicated in patients with ICDs. Although future generations of ICDs may become MRI safe, there may be a higher risk of current induction via the defibrillation coils, and MRI in patients with these devices has not been well studied.

Summary

Radiography can provide important data about pacing and ICD systems. Preoperative radiographs can yield important anatomic information for the implanting physician. Intraoperative fluoroscopy and venography are invaluable tools, guiding optimal lead placement. Lateral and PA chest radiographs should be obtained after implantation to confirm correct lead placement and to detect potential complications of the implantation procedure. The chest radiograph is an important component of system troubleshooting. During such evaluation, the position and type of generator, the positions and types of all functional and abandoned leads, and the radiographic integrity of components of the system should be determined. Abdominal films may be required if any portion of the pacing or ICD system is in the abdomen. A systematic evaluation of the anatomy and system components is essential.

REFERENCES

1. Hill P: Complications of permanent transvenous cardiac pacing: A 14-year review of all transvenous pacemakers inserted at one community hospital. PACE 10:564, 1987.
2. Filice R: Cardiac pacemaker leads: A radiographic perspective. Can Assoc Radiol J 35:20, 1984.
3. Lappegard K: Pacemaker implantation in patients with persistent left superior vena cava. Heart Vessels 19:153, 2004.
4. Cesario D, Bhargava M, Valderrabano M, et al: Azygos vein lead implantation: A novel adjunctive technique for implantable cardioverter defibrillator placement. J Cardiovasc Electrophysiol 15:780, 2004.
5. Bongiorni MG, Moracchini PV, Nava A, et al: Radiographic assessment of atrial dipole position in single pass lead VDD and DDD pacing. The Multicenter Study Group. PACE 21:2240, 1998.
6. Hertzberg BS, Chiles C, Ravin CE: Right atrial appendage pacing: Radiographic considerations. AJR Am J Roentgenol 145:31, 1985.
7. Daubert C, Gras D, Berder V, et al: [Permanent atrial resynchronization by synchronous bi-atrial pacing in the preventive treatment of atrial flutter associated with high degree interatrial block]. Arch Mal Coeur Vaiss 87(Suppl):1535, 1994.
8. Padeletti L, Michelucci A, Pieragnoli P, et al: Atrial septal pacing: A new approach to prevent atrial fibrillation. PACE 27:850, 2004.
9. Bailin SJ, Adler S, Giudici M: Prevention of chronic atrial fibrillation by pacing in the region of Bachmann's bundle: Results of a multicenter randomized trial. J Cardiovasc Electrophysiol 12:912, 2001.
10. Van Gelder BM, Bracke FA, Oto A, et al: Diagnosis and management of inadvertently placed pacing and ICD leads in the left ventricle: A multicenter experience and review of the literature. PACE 23:877, 2000.
11. Lieberman R, Grenz D, Mond HG, Gammage MD: Selective site pacing: defining and reaching the selected site. PACE 27:883, 2004.
12. Deshmukh PM, Romanyshyn M: Direct His-bundle pacing: Present and future. PACE 27:862, 2004.
13. Kautzner J, Riedlbauchova L, Cihak R, et al: Technical aspects of implantation of LV lead for cardiac resynchronization therapy in chronic heart failure. PACE 27:783, 2004.
14. von Ludinghausen M: The venous drainage of the human myocardium. Adv Anat Embryol Cell Biol 168:I, 2003.
15. Fernandez AL, Garcia-Bengochea JR, Ledo R, et al: Minimally invasive surgical implantation of left ventricular epicardial leads for ventricular resynchronization using video-assisted thoracoscopy. Rev Esp Cardiol 57:313, 2004.
16. Zenati MA, Bonanomi G, Chin AK, Schwartzman D: Left heart pacing lead implantation using subxiphoid videopericardioscopy. J Cardiovasc Electrophysiol 14:949, 2003.
17. Derose JJ Jr, Belsley S, Swistel DG, et al: Robotically assisted left ventricular epicardial lead implantation for biventricular pacing: The posterior approach. Ann Thorac Surg 77:1472, 2004.
18. Roelke M, O'Nunain SS, Osswald S, et al: Subclavian crush syndrome complicating transvenous cardioverter defibrillator systems. PACE 18:973, 1995.
19. Weiner S, Patel J, Jadonath RL: Lead failure due to the subclavian crush syndrome in a patient implanted with both standard and thin bipolar spiral wound leads. PACE 22:975, 1999.
20. Hecht S, Berdoff R, Van Tosh A, Goldberg E: Radiographic pseudofracture of bipolar pacemaker wire. Chest 88:302, 1985.
21. Weissman JL, Kanel KT: Ligature causing pseudofracture of a cardiac pacemaker lead. AJR Am J Roentgenol 166:464, 1996.
22. Fahraeus T, Hoijer CJ: Early pacemaker twiddler syndrome. Europace 5:279, 2003.
23. Carnero-Varo A, Perez-Paredes M, Ruiz-Ros JA, et al: "Reel syndrome": A new form of Twiddler's syndrome? Circulation 100:e45, 1999.
24. Lloyd MA, Hayes DL, Holmes DR Jr: Atrial "J" pacing lead retention wire fracture: Radiographic assessment, incidence of fracture, and clinical management. PACE 18:958, 1995.
25. Daoud EG, Kou W, Davidson T, et al: Evaluation and extraction of the Accufix atrial J lead. Am Heart J 131:266, 1996.
26. Byrd CL, Wilkoff BL, Love CJ, et al: Intravascular extraction of problematic or infected permanent pacemaker leads: 1994-1996. U.S. Extraction Database, MED Institute. PACE, 22:1348, 1999.
27. Stanton MS, Hayes DL, Munger TM, et al: Consistent subcutaneous prepectoral implantation of a new implantable cardioverter defibrillator. Mayo Clin Proc 69:309, 1994.
28. Avitall B, Oza SR, Gonzalez R, Avery R: Subcutaneous array to transvenous proximal coil defibrillation as a solution to high defibrillation thresholds with implantable cardioverter defibrillator distal coil failure. J Cardiovasc Electrophysiol 14:314, 2003.
29. Kratz JM, Schabel S, Leman RM: Pseudo fracture of a defibrillating lead. PACE 18:2225, 1995.
30. Taliercio CP, Vliestra RE, McGon MD, et al: Permanent cardiac pacing after the Fontan procedure. J Thorac Cardiovasc Surg 90:414, 1985.
31. Alexander ME, Cecchin F, Walsh EP, et al: Implications of implantable cardioverter defibrillator therapy in congenital heart disease and pediatrics. J Cardiovasc Electrophysiol 15:72, 2004.
32. Biffi M, Boriani G, Frabetti L, et al: Left superior vena cava persistence in patients undergoing pacemaker or cardioverter-defibrillator implantation: A 10-year experience. Chest 120:139, 2001.
33. Higano ST, Hayes DL, Spittell PC: Facilitation of the subclavian-introducer technique with contrast venography. PACE 13:681, 1990.
34. Gheissari A, Hordof AJ, Spotnitz HM: Transvenous pacemakers in children: Relation of lead length to anticipated growth. Ann Thorac Surg 52:118, 1991.
35. Bedotto JB, Grayburn PA, Black WH, et al: Alterations in left ventricular relaxation during atrioventricular pacing in humans. J Am Coll Cardiol 15:658, 1990.
36. Stojnic BB, Stojanov PL, Angelkov L, et al: Evaluation of asynchronous left ventricular relaxation by Doppler echocardiography during ventricular pacing with AV synchrony (VDD): Comparison with atrial pacing (AAI). PACE 19:940, 1996.

37. Tse HF, Lau CP: Long-term effect of right ventricular pacing on myocardial perfusion and function. J Am Coll Cardiol 29:744, 1997.
38. Epstein AE, Kay GN, Plumb VJ, et al: Combined automatic implantable cardioverter-defibrillator and pacemaker systems: Implantation techniques and follow-up. J Am Coll Cardiol 13:121, 1989.
39. Grier D, Cook PG, Hartnell GG: Chest radiographs after permanent pacing: Are they really necessary? Clin Radiol 42:244, 1990.
40. Sussman SK, Chiles C, Cooper C, Lowe JE: CT demonstration of myocardial perforation by a pacemaker lead. J Comput Assist Tomogr 10:670, 1986.
41. Tandri H, Bomma C, Calkins H, Bluemke DA: Magnetic resonance and computed tomography imaging of arrhythmogenic right ventricular dysplasia. J Magn Reson Imaging 19:848, 2004.
42. Jongbloed MR, Lamb HJ, Box JJ, et al: Noninvasive visualization of the cardiac venous system using multislice computed tomography. J Am Coll Cardiol 45:749, 2005.
43. Sakakibara Y, Mitsui T: Concerns about sources of electromagnetic interference in patients with pacemakers. Jpn Heart J 40:737, 1999.
44. Martin ET: Can cardiac pacemakers and magnetic resonance imaging systems co-exist? Eur Heart J 26:325, 2005.
45. Martin ET, Coman JA, Shelloch FG, et al: Magnetic resonance imaging and cardiac pacemaker safety at 1.5-Tesla. J Am Coll Cardiol 43:1315, 2004.
46. Roguin A, Zviman MM, Meininger GR, et al: Modern pacemaker and implantable cardioverter/defibrillator systems can be magnetic resonance imaging safe: In vitro and in vivo assessment of safety and function at 1.5 T. Circulation 110:475, 2004.

Section Four

Device Electrocardiography

Chapter 23

Timing Cycles of Implantable Devices

PAUL J. WANG • HENRY CHEN • HIDEO OKAMURA • AMIN AL-AHMAD • HENRY H. HSIA

To better understand device behaviors and to optimize management, physicians must be familiar with the timing cycles of implantable pacemakers and their constant interactions with the patient's intrinsic rhythm.[1] Timing cycles refer to the beat-by-beat behavior of implantable devices in response to changes in intrinsic and paced behavior. Although some of the parameters involved in timing cycles are programmable, others are unalterable within the device itself. Each type of device uses timing cycles in a somewhat different way. The purpose of this review is to provide a detailed discussion of the various parameters that affect timing cycles in pacemakers, implantable cardioverter-defibrillators (ICDs), and resynchronization therapy devices.

Revised Pacing System Code

It is necessary to have a basic understanding of the operational modes of the pacemakers. The pacing systems may be single-chamber systems, limited to either atrium or ventricle, or they may be dual-chamber systems. They may sense in one chamber and pace the other, sense one and pace both, or sense and pace both chambers. Their functionality can vary from beat to beat depending on the programmed mode and the underlying rhythm. As a result of a joint approach of the North American Society of Pacing and Electrophysiology (NSAPE) and the British Pacing and Electrophysiology Group (BPEG), a NASPE/BPEG Generic (NBG) Pacemaker Code was developed (Table 23-1). The latest revision, in 2002, incorporated multisite pacing.[2] This is a three- to five-position code used to designate the programmed mode of the device. The first letter designates the chamber or chambers paced. *A* stands for atrium, *V* for ventricle, and *D* for pacing capability in both the atrium and ventricle; *O* is used if the unit is deactivated without pacing. The letter in position II designates the chamber or chambers sensed. *O* stands for asynchronous operation without sensing. The third letter describes the unit's response to a sensed signal. *I* indicates that the pacemaker pacing is inhibited by a sensed event; *T* indicates that a pacing stimulus is triggered by a sensed event; and *D* represents an operating mode in which a stimulus may be triggered by a sensed event in one chamber and inhibited by a sensed event in the other. For example, a *DDD* pacemaker senses an atrial signal that triggers a ventricular pacing output; however, a sensed ventricular signal will inhibit the pacing stimulus in the ventricle. The fourth letter describes the rate-modulation capability. Position V of the revised NBG code is used to denote multisite pacing. Position V represents a change in the NBG code and is represented in Table 23-1 in bold type to emphasize this change. *O* indicates no more than one site in each chamber paced. *A* indicates that more than one pacing site is present in the atrium. *V* indicates that more than one pacing site is present in the ventricle. *D* indicates that more than one pacing site is present in the atrium and ventricle. In the DDDRO mode, there are sensing and pacing at single

TABLE 23-1. The Revised NASPE/BPEG Generic (NBG) Code for Antibradycardia Pacing*

Position	I	II	III	IV	V
Category	Chamber paced O = None A = Atrium V = Ventricle D = Dual (A + V)	Chamber sensed O = None A = Atrium V = Ventricle D = Dual (A + V)	Response to sensing O = None T = Triggered I = Inhibited D = Dual (T + I)	Rate modulation O = None R = Rate adaptive	**Multisite pacing** **O = None** **A = Atrium** **V = Ventricle** **D = Dual (A + V)**
Manufacturer's designation only	S = Single (A or V)	S = Single (A or V)			

*The Code was modified in 2002 and includes multisite pacing.
BPEG, British Pacing and Electrophysiology Group; NASPE, North American Society of Pacing and Electrophysiology.
From Bernstein A, Daubert J, Fletcher R, et al.: The revised NASPE/BPEG generic code for antibradycardia, adaptive-rate, and multisite pacing. PACE 23:260-264, 2002.

sites within the atrium and the ventricle, along with atrial tracking, ventricular inhibition, and rate adaptive pacing. In DDDRV mode, all of the same features are available as in DDDRO, but in addition there is pacing at two sites in the ventricles, such as in the right ventricle (RV) and the left ventricle (LV). Dual-site atrial pacing for atrial fibrillation prevention would be represented as the DDDRA mode.

Single-Chamber Pacing Modes and Timing Cycles

As described earlier, the pacing mode describes the set of basic pacemaker functions. Associated with each pacing mode is a set of rules that govern the timing of events. The beat-to-beat intervals that define when paced events occur in that mode are called timing cycles. The physicians must be familiar with the nomenclature and definition of the timing cycles, as well as the basic rules that govern their behaviors.

Single-Chamber Pacing Modes

SSI Mode

The AAI and VVI modes act in a comparable manner, with pacing and sensing in the same chamber (atrium or ventricle) and the pacing output inhibited by a sensed event in that chamber. For practical purposes, AAI and VVI modes may be considered to be a common SSI mode. In each mode, a pacing output is delivered at the end of the escape interval that corresponds to the programmed lower rate limit (LRL) of the device. If a sensed event (S) occurs, the pacing output is inhibited and the escape interval is reset.

VVI Mode

In the VVI mode, the ventricular inhibited pacing mode, the pacemaker senses and paces in the ventricle. This mode is most appropriate for patients in chronic atrial fibrillation for whom atrial sensing or pacing is not needed. The VVI mode may sometimes be programmed for patients who require infrequent pacing. In the VVI mode, after a sensed intrinsic ventricular activation (R wave) or a paced event (V), the pacemaker waits for the next intrinsic beat. However, if the escape interval elapses before a ventricular signal is sensed, the pacemaker delivers a ventricular pacing stimulus. Any sensed or paced ventricular event initiates the ventricular escape interval. Intrinsic events may occur at intervals shorter than the escape interval, but the longest time between any two ventricular events is the ventricular escape interval (Figs. 23-1 and 23-2). The escape interval defines the LRL (usually expressed in pulses per minute), which may also be called the minimum, basic, or base pacing rate. The timing of ventricular sensed events is initiated when the intrinsic signal reaches the necessary sensing threshold after passing through specific amplifiers and filters. The point in the intrinsic signal that is sensed may be delayed compared with the onset of the ventricular activation of the surface electrocardiogram (ECG). The largest amount of delay in sensing of the intrinsic signal from a right ventricular apical lead occurs in the setting of right bundle branch block.

Refractory Periods/Blanking Periods

To sense and pace within the same chamber, "same-chamber" refractory periods must be included to avoid inappropriate oversensing of the intrinsic event or

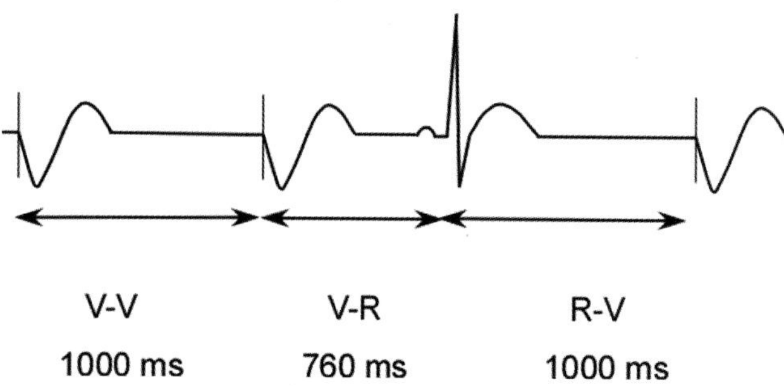

Figure 23-1. VVI mode. The ventricular rate in this example is 1000 msec and is indicated by the V-V interval. The intrinsic R wave comes 760 msec after the second ventricular paced event. The next ventricular paced event occurs 1000 msec after the intrinsic ventricular event. R, ventricular sensed event; V, ventricular paced event.

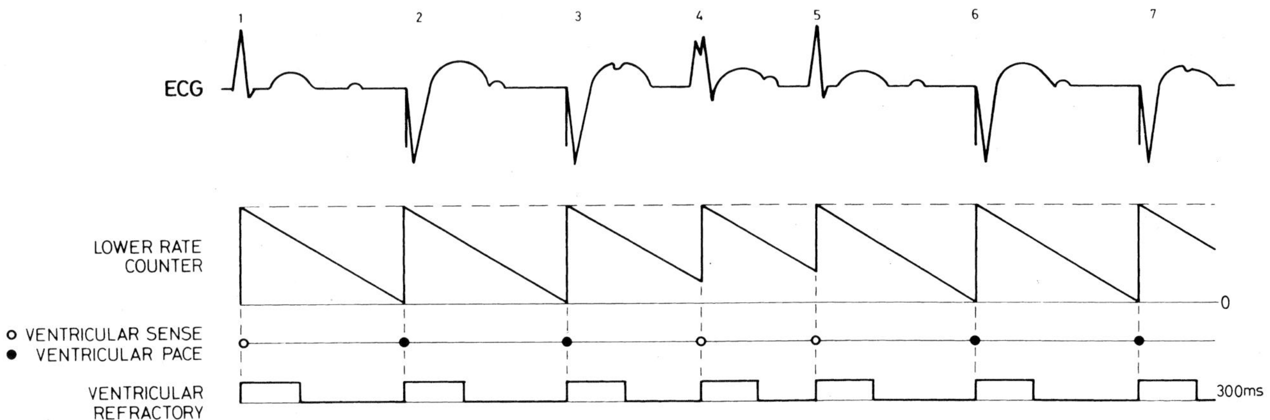

Figure 23-2. *Diagrammatic representation of the VVI mode of pacing (rate = 80 pulses per minute). The QRS marked 1 is sensed. Beats 2 and 3 are paced complexes. A ventricular extrasystole (beat 4) and a normal conducted QRS (beat 5) are sensed. The sixth and seventh beats are paced. The pacemaker ventricular refractory period (300 msec) is shown by a rectangle. Complexes 4 and 5 reset and start the lower rate counter before the zero level has been reached—that is, before completion of the escape or automatic interval. The pacemaker emits its stimulus only from the zero level. ECG, electrocardiogram. (From Lendermans FW: Diagrammatic representation of pacemaker function. In Barold SS [ed]: Modern Cardiac Pacing. Mt. Kisco, NY, Futura, 1985, pp 323-353.)*

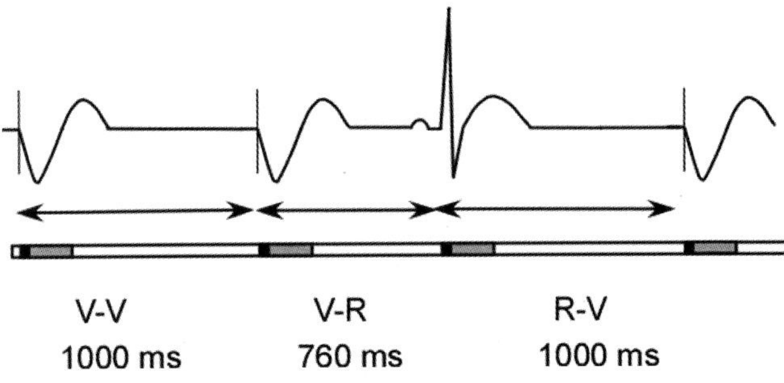

Figure 23-3. *VVI ventricular refractory periods. The black bar indicates the ventricular blanking period, during which events are not sensed. The gray bar indicates the ventricular refractory period, during which ventricular sensed events are not used to reset timing cycles.*

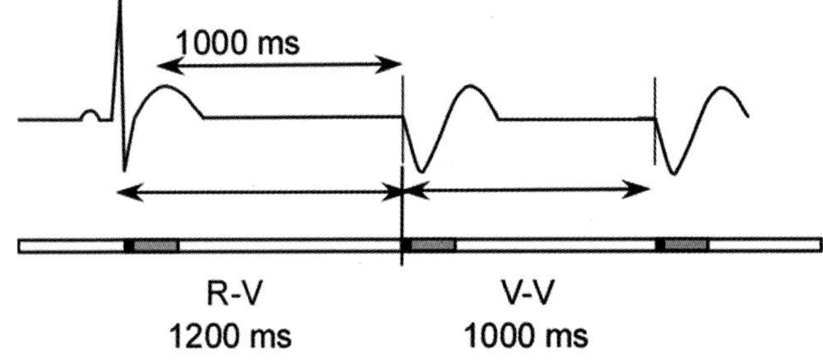

Figure 23-4. *VVI ventricular oversensing. The T wave of the first beat, indicated by the asterisk, is sensed outside the ventricular refractory period. The ventricular escape interval is 1000 msec. Because the T wave of the first beat is sensed, the R-V interval is 1200 msec instead of 1000 msec. The following V-V interval is the expected 1000 msec.*

pacing (Fig. 23-3).[3,4] Immediately after a ventricular paced event, during a ventricular blanking period (VBP) or time interval (ranging from 50 to 100 msec), all ventricular events are "blanked" or not sensed. The VBP is designed to prevent oversensing of the afterpotentials from pacing stimuli. After this period of absolute lack of sensing, there is a ventricular refractory period (VRP), a programmable time window (usually expressed in milliseconds) during which the pacemaker sensing amplifier is active but does not use the ventricular sensed event to reset the timing cycle. Noise sampling may occur during the VRP, and the VRP is used to prevent oversensing due to the paced evoked potentials, the intrinsic ventricular electrogram, or repolarization signals (T wave).

Ventricular Oversensing and Ventricular Undersensing

Ventricular sensing may result in abnormalities in the ventricular timing cycles. The pacemaker senses an event that does not represent ventricular depolarization. Parts of the QRS complex, the T wave,[5] afterdepolarizations,[6] atrial activity,[7,8] noise from lead abnormalities,[9] myopotentials, and electromagnetic interference are possible causes of ventricular oversensing.[10,11] In ventricular oversensing, the additional sensed event resets the ventricular escape interval, resulting in a longer interval than the programmed pacing cycle length (Fig. 23-4). In ventricular undersensing, the pacemaker does not sense an intrinsic ventricular depolarization (R wave). The ventricular escape interval is not reset by this R wave. Instead, the ventricular escape interval is created by the previous sensed or paced event. The pacing interval therefore is shorter than the pacing cycle length (Fig. 23-5).

Hysteresis Rate

Hysteresis provides for a longer escape interval from the last ventricular sensed event to the first ventricular paced event (R-V, called the hysteresis interval) but no

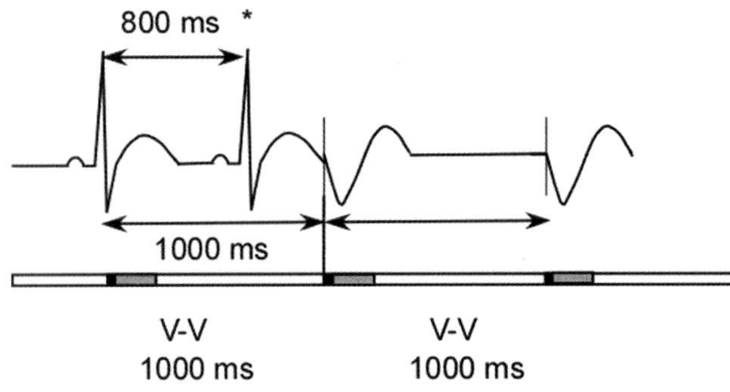

Figure 23-5. VVI ventricular undersensing. The second R wave, indicated by the asterisk, is not sensed. The next event is a ventricular paced event after a ventricular escape interval of 1000 msec. The subsequent V-V interval is also 1000 msec.

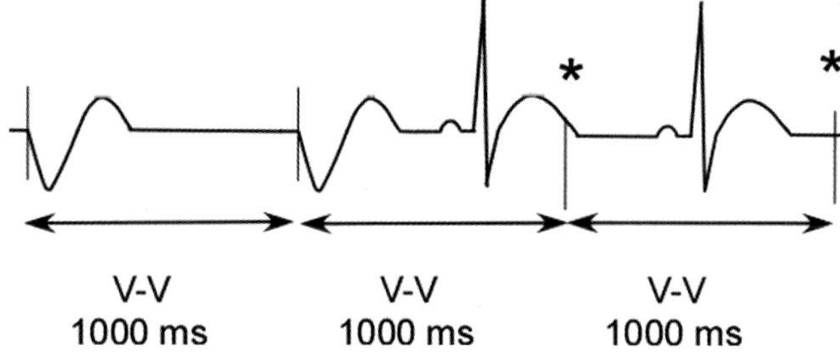

Figure 23-7. VOO mode. In the VOO mode, there are ventricular paced events and no sensing. The first two ventricular events are paced at a V-V interval of 1000 msec. The third event is an intrinsic ventricular event, but it is not sensed in the VOO mode. The next V event, indicated by the asterisk, occurs during the physiologic refractory period of the preceding ventricular event. The final V event, also noted by an asterisk, is also in the physiologic refractory period.

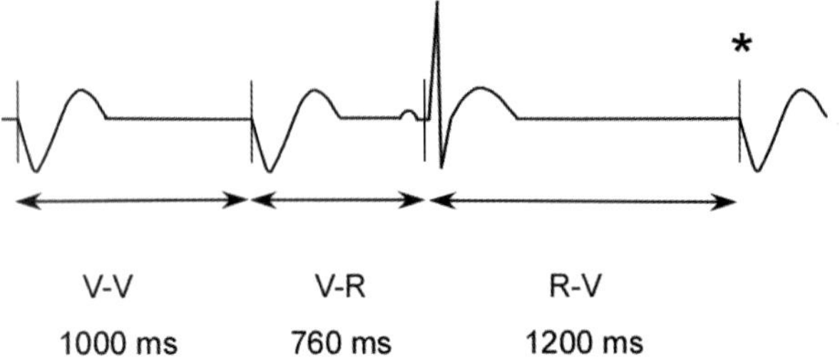

Figure 23-6. VVI ventricular hysteresis. The first and second ventricular events are paced with a V-V interval of 1000 msec. The third event is a ventricular sensed event. The fourth event is a ventricular paced event (indicated by the asterisk) after an R-V interval of 1200 msec. The hysteresis interval is 1200 msec, and the pacing interval is 1000 msec.

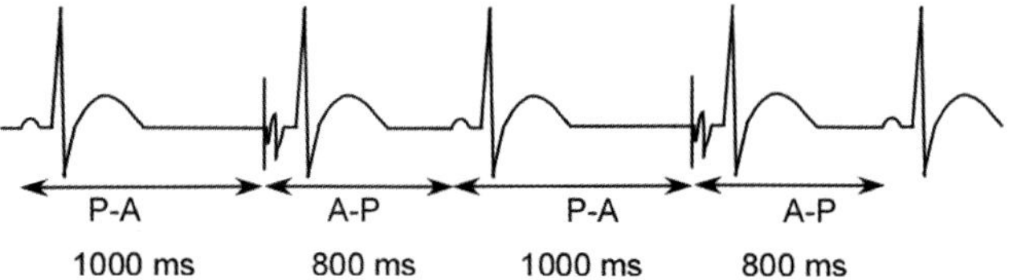

Figure 23-8. AAI mode. The atrial pacing rate in the AAI mode in this example is 1000 msec; it represents the time from either an atrial paced event (A) or an atrial sensed event (P) to the next atrial paced event. Each of the P-A intervals occurs at 1000 msec, whereas the ventricular sensed events may occur earlier than the atrial pacing rate.

change in the time from the last ventricular paced event (Fig. 23-6).[12] Hysteresis allows the intrinsic heart rate to be lower before pacing occurs, but if pacing does occur, it will occur at a faster rate. For example, if the hysteresis pacing rate is 50 beats per minute (bpm) and the base pacing rate is 60 bpm, pacing will not occur if the patient continues to maintain rates faster than 50 bpm. If the heart rate falls below 50 bpm, however, pacing will occur at 60 bpm. This feature favors intrinsic activation and facilitates conduction in the patient with atrial fibrillation or atrioventricular (AV) synchrony in the patient in sinus rhythm. When hysteresis is programmed ON, the maximum V-to-V interval (defined by the lower rate interval) is shorter than the maximum R-to-V interval (defined by the hysteresis interval). Hysteresis is often expressed as an absolute rate (beats per minute) or as an interval (in milliseconds) from the intrinsic R wave to the first ventricular paced event (V). Hysteresis may also be expressed as the difference between the hysteresis rate and the pacing rate or the difference between the hysteresis escape interval (R-V) and the pacing escape interval (V-V). The hysteresis rate may sometimes be expressed as a percentage subtracted from the lower rate. The hysteresis often results in a decreased frequency of pacing, because it allows more time to expire after an intrinsic event. Commonly, the lower rate interval is set to the slowest rate that is desirable hemodynamically. Once pacing occurs, it will continue until the intrinsic ventricular rate exceeds the pacing rate.

VOO Mode

In the VOO mode, ventricular pacing without ventricular sensing is present (Fig. 23-7). No intrinsic events are sensed, and therefore ventricular pacing occurs independently of the intrinsic rhythm. VOO is programmed ON to prevent electromagnetic interference from resulting in ventricular inhibition in the pacemaker-dependent patient.

AAI Mode

In the AAI mode, the atrial inhibited pacing mode, the pacemaker will deliver an atrial pacing stimulus at the end of the atrial LRL, measured from the previous paced or sensed atrial event. If the atrial channel does not sense an intrinsic atrial event and the programmed LRL has expired, the pacemaker will deliver an atrial impulse (Fig. 23-8). Timing is based on sensed intrinsic atrial events (P) or atrial paced events (A). The intervals used in timing can be described as P-P, P-A, A-A, and A-P. Conceptually, the timing intervals in the AAI pacing mode are similar to those of the VVI pacing mode. However, in the AAI mode, only atrial but not ventricular events result in resetting of the timing cycle (Fig. 23-9).

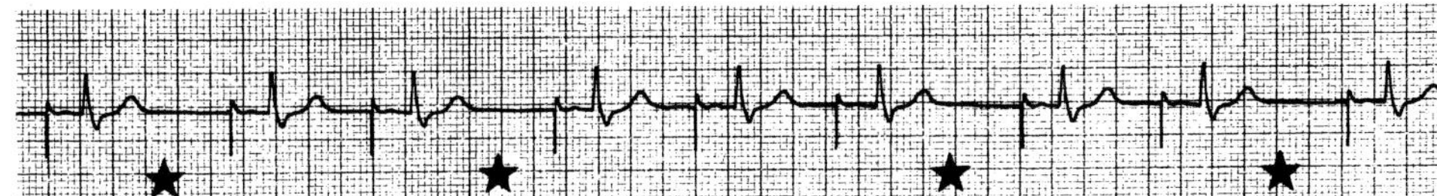

Figure 23-9. AAI pacing. In this example, the pacemaker rate is 70 pulses per minute (ppm), the interval is 857 msec, and the refractory period is 250 msec. There is intermittent prolongation of the interstimulus interval, because the atrial lead senses the far-field QRS complex just beyond the 250-msec pacemaker refractory period. When the refractory period was programmed to 400 msec, the irregularity disappeared, and regular atrial pacing at a rate of 70 ppm was restored. Stars indicate intervals with oversensing. (From Barold SS, Zipes DP: Cardiac pacemakers and antiarrhythmia devices. In Braunwald E [ed]: Heart Disease: A Textbook of Cardiovascular Medicine. Philadelphia, WB Saunders, 1992, pp 726-755.)

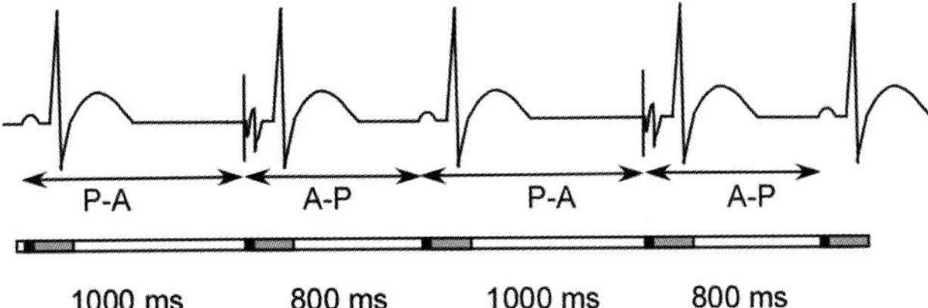

Figure 23-10. AAI mode atrial refractory periods. The atrial pacing rate in the AAI mode in this example is 1000 msec and represents the time from either an atrial paced event (A) or an atrial sensed event (P) to the next atrial paced event. Each of the P-A intervals occurs at 1000 msec, whereas the ventricular sensed events may occur earlier than the atrial pacing rate. The black bar indicates the atrial blanking period, during which events are not sensed. The gray bar indicates the atrial refractory period, during which atrial sensed events are not used to reset timing cycles.

Although individual physician and regional practice variations exist, in general the candidates most suited for the AAI mode are those who are in sinus rhythm and have intact AV conduction. Because this mode does not pace the ventricle, it is not appropriate if compromised AV conduction is suspected.[13] The ability to maintain 1:1 AV conduction during atrial pacing at rates of 120 or 130 bpm or faster during the pacemaker implant procedure is frequently used to determine the absence of significant AV conduction abnormalities. Recent concern about the possible deleterious impact of ventricular pacing has increased the interest in atrial pacing.[14]

The atrial refractory period (ARP) is similar to the VRP and constitutes a time interval after a paced or sensed atrial event in which the pacemaker is refractory to spontaneous atrial signals (Fig. 23-10). It is divided into an atrial blanking period (ABP), often programmable, followed by a refractory period during which noise sampling occurs (Fig. 23-11). The ABP is used primarily to prevent sensing of the afterpotential of the pacing stimulus. The ARP, which ranges from 150 to 500 msec, is used to prevent the atrial lead from oversensing the afterpotential of a paced stimulus, the local evoked potential produced by an atrial pacing stimulus, or "far-field" sensing of the ventricular depolarization.

Atrial hysteresis may also be used in the AAI mode. The P-A interval, called the atrial escape interval (AEI), is longer than the A-A interval (the atrial pacing interval). Atrial hysteresis, similar to ventricular hysteresis, may be used to minimize atrial pacing (Fig. 23-12).

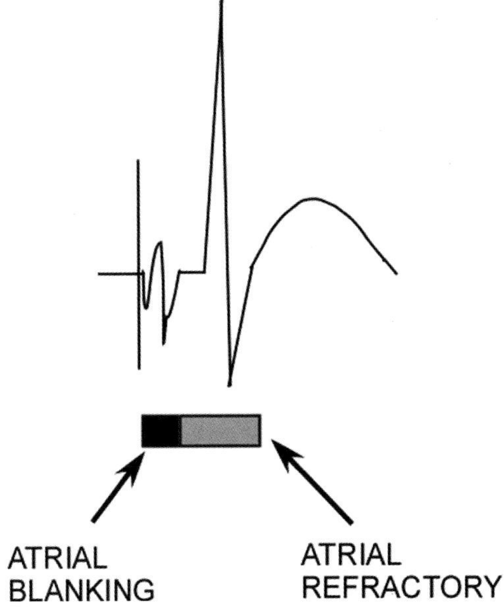

Figure 23-11. AAI blanking period. The black bar indicates the atrial blanking period, during which events are not sensed. The gray bar indicates the atrial refractory period.

Bradycardia Timing Cycles

Dual-Chamber Timing Cycles

Dual-chamber devices in the DDD mode provide a mechanism to combine pacing and/or sensing in either or both chambers.[15-17] These functions include pacing in both the atrium and ventricle, inhibition of pacing by sensed events in the respective chamber, and AV coordinated pacing (Fig. 23-13). A sensed intrinsic atrial event inhibits atrial pacing, and a sensed intrinsic ventricular event inhibits ventricular pacing. An atrial sensed event that occurs before the AEI has "timed out" is "tracked," or followed by a ventricular paced output (see Fig. 23-13). Timing is based on atrial sensed events (P), atrial paced events (A), ventricular sensed events (R), and ventricular paced events (V). Intervals between atrial and ventricular events can be described as A-R, A-V, P-R, and P-V (Fig. 23-14).

Atrioventricular Interval

The atrioventricular interval (AVI) is a programmable parameter that determines the maximum time after an atrial event in which an intrinsic ventricular event can occur before delivery of a ventricular pacing stimulus (see Fig. 23-13). It is initiated after a sensed or a paced atrial event. The AVI is similar to the native P-R interval and hence is programmed to optimize the hemodynamic benefit of AV coordination. The AVI permits atrial contraction, resulting in ventricular filling in end-diastole. The AVI is programmed at rest to maintain coordinated timing of atrial and ventricular contractions, permit intrinsic AV conduction when possible, and conserve generator energy. For patients who do not have coordinated AV contractions due to P-R prolongation, this may result in impaired left ventricular filling, because atrial contraction occurs so much earlier than the ventricular contraction. Recent trials involving patients with both preserved and depressed ventricular function suggest that maintaining intrinsic AV conduction and minimizing right ventricular pacing are also desirable hemodynamically, because improved ventricular contraction and cardiac output are seen with normal ventricular activation. Therefore, a balance must be achieved between permitting a short enough AVI to optimize coordination of atrial contraction and ventricular contraction and prolonging

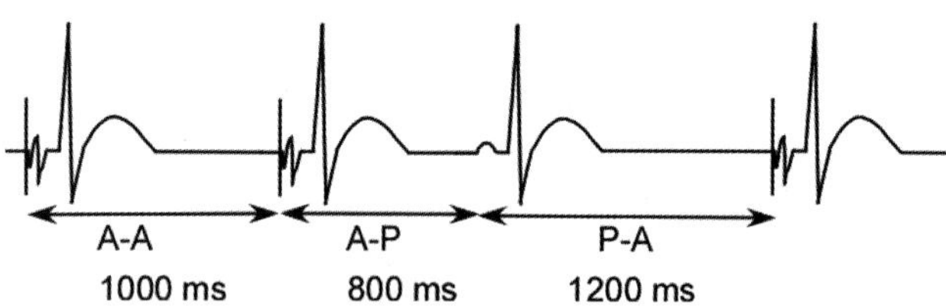

Figure 23-12. AAI atrial hysteresis. The atrial pacing interval in this example is 1000 msec. The atrial hysteresis interval is 1200 msec. The first event is an atrial paced event (A), followed by the second event that is also an atrial paced event 1000 msec later. The third event is an intrinsic atrial event (P) at an interval of 800 msec. The fourth atrial event is a paced event at a hysteresis interval of 1200 msec. The hysteresis interval begins with an intrinsic atrial event and ends with an atrial paced event.

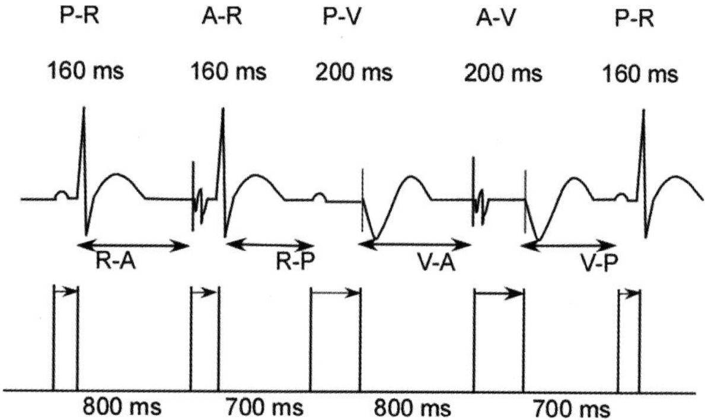

Figure 23-13. DDD mode. The lower rate in this example is 60 beats per minute or 1000 msec. This is an example of ventricular-based timing. The atrial escape interval, or the time from the R-A or V-A, is 800 msec, equal to 1000 msec minus the A-V interval of 200 msec. A, paced atrial event; P, sensed atrial event; R, sensed ventricular event; V, paced ventricular event.

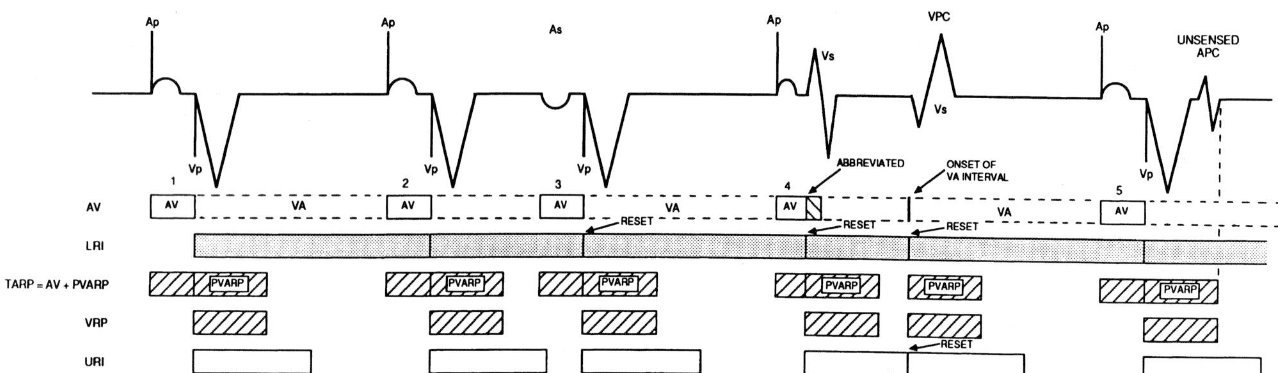

Figure 23-14. Diagrammatic representation of the function of a DDD pacemaker. Hatching indicates refractory periods. Lower rate timing is ventricular based and is controlled by ventricular events (paced or sensed). The four fundamental intervals are as follows: LRI, lower rate interval; VRP, ventricular refractory period; AV, atrioventricular delay; PVARP, postventricular atrial refractory period. The two derived intervals are atrial escape (pacemaker VA) interval, which is equal to LRI – AV, and the total atrial refractory period (TARP), which is equal to AV + PVARP. Reset refers to the termination and reinitiation of a timing cycle before it has "timed out" to its completion according to its programmed duration. Premature termination of the programmed AV delay by Vs is indicated by its abbreviation. The upper rate interval (URI) is equal to TARP. The As (beat 3) initiates an AV interval terminating with Vp; As also aborts the atrial escape interval (AEI) initiated by the second Vp. The third Vp resets the LRI and starts the PVARP, VRP, and URI. The fourth beat consists of an Ap, which terminates the AEI initiated by the third Vp, followed by a sensed conducted QRS (Vs). The AV interval is therefore abbreviated. Vs initiates the AEI, LRI, PVARP, VRP, and URI. Beat 5 is a ventricular extrasystole (ventricular premature contraction), that initiates AIE, PVARP, and VRP and resets the LRI and the URI. The last beat is followed by an atrial extrasystole that is unsensed because it occurs within the PVARP. APC, atrial premature contraction; Ap, atrial paced beat; As, atrial sensed beat; Vp, ventricular paced beat; Vs, ventricular sensed beat. (From Barold SS, Zipes DP: Cardiac pacemakers and antiarrhythmic devices. In Braunwald E [ed]: Heart Disease: A Textbook of Cardiovascular Medicine. Philadelphia, WB Saunders, 1992, pp 725-755.)

A-V conduction for enough time to result in intrinsic ventricular activation. The programmed AVI that results in optimal hemodynamics may vary considerably and may be difficult to predict accurately. Many clinicians select the programmed AVI that permits the P-R interval to be as much as 280 to 300 msec. There may be a role for assessment of interatrial conduction delay in setting the optimal AVI, but data are currently limited.[18] There may be a differential time of ventricular activation, depending on whether the atrium is paced or is activated intrinsically. Usually, the time for a paced electrical impulse to result in atrial activation is longer than the time required for intrinsic atrial activation. A differential AVI may be programmed and is discussed later in this chapter. Finally, to conserve battery energy, the AVI may be extended in patients without AV block, in order to reduce pacing.

Atrioventricular Interval, Crosstalk, and Ventricular Safety Pacing

Crosstalk is the inappropriate sensing of far-field signals from the opposite chamber, causing pacing inhibition or oversensing. One of the most serious manifestations of crosstalk in a dual-chamber pacing system is oversensing of far-field atrial stimuli resulting in ventricular inhibition and asystole in the "pacemaker-dependent" patient. The AVI therefore encompasses multiple refractory and blanking timing intervals on each atrial/ventricular channel, as well as on the "opposite" channel, to prevent crosstalk (Figs. 23-15; see Fig. 23-14).

An atrial pacing output also initiates multiple timing windows on the ventricular channel. Atrial pacing output triggers a VBP at the beginning of the AVI in an attempt to avoid oversensing the atrial stimulus artifact on the ventricular lead (Fig. 23-16). This absolute VBP is usually short, ranging from 20 to 44 msec, and is programmable in certain pacemaker models. Immediately after the VBP, the ventricular sensing amplifier becomes active during the ventricular safety pacing (or crosstalk sensing) window in the second portion of the AVI (up to 80 to 120 msec). Signals sensed during the crosstalk sensing window (<120 msec from the atrial pacing output) are considered "nonphysiologic" due to the close coupling interval and may be caused by oversensing of atrial pacing afterpotentials, spontaneous premature ventricular depolarizations (PVCs), or noise (see Fig. 23-16). Ventricular safety pacing (VSP) is a feature that is designed to prevent inappropriate inhibition of the ventricular pacing caused by crosstalk (Figs. 23-17 and 23-18). After an atrial paced depolarization, if a sensed event occurs during the safety pacing window, the pacemaker, instead of inhibiting ventricular pacing, will deliver a ventricular pacing stimulus at a shortened AVI, typically ranging from 80 to 130 msec. The shortened AVI makes the identification of safety pacing apparent. It also decreases the likelihood of a ventricular paced event occurring during ventricular repolarization, particularly if the baseline AVI is relatively long; this minimizes the risk of ventricular proarrhythmia. Crosstalk in this situation is

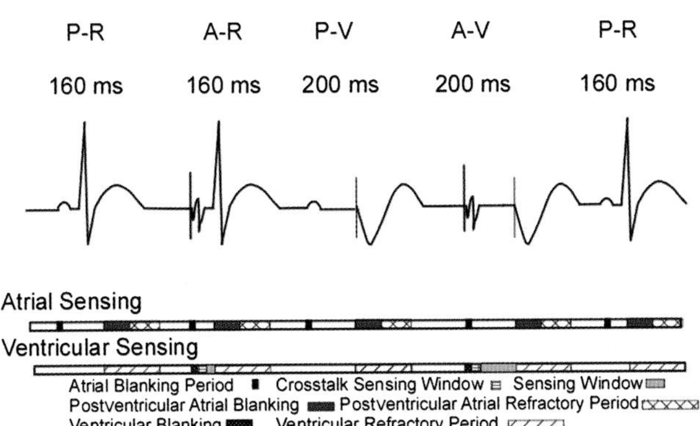

Figure 23-15. DDD refractory periods. The lower rate is 60 beats per minute or 1000 msec. This is an example of ventricular-based timing. The atrial escape interval, or the time from the R-A or V-A, is 800 msec, equal to 1000 msec minus the A-V interval of 200 msec. The refractory periods and sensing windows are given on the atrial and ventricular sensing channels. On the atrial channel, the atrial blanking period occurs after an atrial paced or (usually) an atrial sensed event. After a sensed or paced ventricular event, there may be, on the atrial channel, a postventricular atrial blanking period followed by a postventricular atrial refractory period. On the ventricular channel, the ventricular sensed or paced event creates a ventricular refractory period. On the ventricular channel after an atrial paced event, there is a cross-channel ventricular blanking period, which is usually followed by a crosstalk safety pacing window and an alert period. A, paced atrial event; P, sensed atrial event; R, sensed ventricular event; V, paced ventricular event.

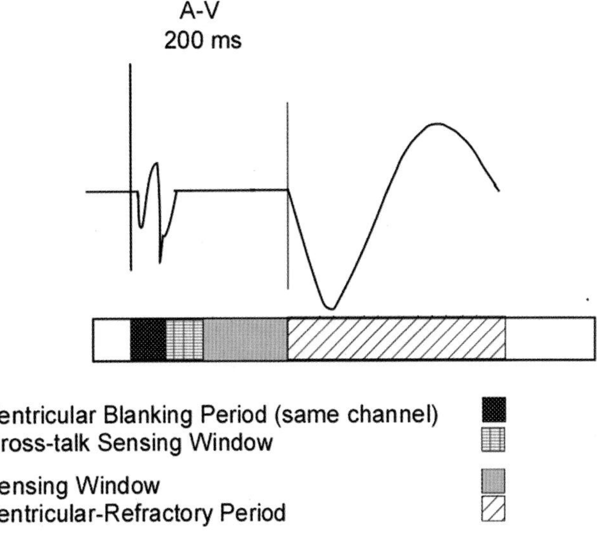

Figure 23-16. DDD safety pacing windows. On the ventricular channel after an atrial paced event, there is a cross-channel ventricular blanking period followed by a crosstalk safety pacing window and an alert period. During the cross-channel ventricular blanking period, no sensing occurs on the ventricular channel. This blanking period prevents the atrial stimulus from inhibiting ventricular output. During the crosstalk safety pacing window, a ventricular sensed event will result in a ventricular paced event at a shorter than usual atrioventricular (A-V) interval, usually 80 to 130 msec. During the sensing window, a sensed ventricular event will result in inhibition of the next ventricular paced event. After the ventricular paced or sensed event, there will be a ventricular refractory period.

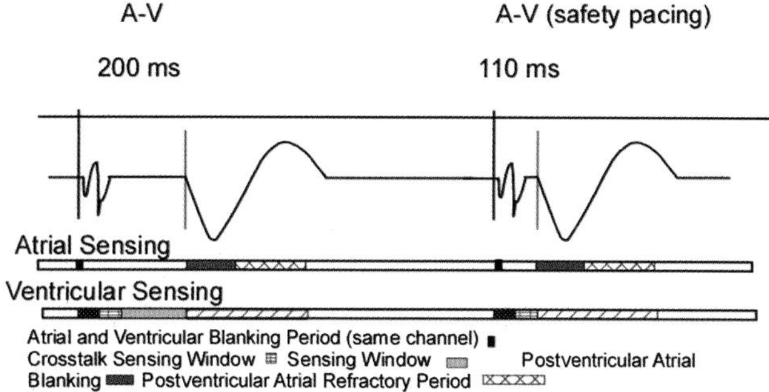

Figure 23-17. Ventricular safety pacing. On the left, there is an atrial paced event (A) and a ventricular paced event (V) separated by an A-V interval of 200 msec. On the right, there is an atrial paced event followed by a ventricular paced event after 110 msec. This represents safety pacing caused by a ventricular sensed event's occurring in the crosstalk safety pacing window

most likely to occur in the presence of high atrial pacing output (e.g., 6 V at 1 msec) along with high ventricular sensitivity (e.g., 2 mV). Safety pacing may also be seen when atrial undersensing occurs and the conducted intrinsic ventricular beat is sensed in the crosstalk safety pacing window (Fig. 23-19).

On the atrial channel, a paced event may result in an absolute atrial blanking period (ABP), preventing sensing of the afterpotential of the pacing stimulus (Fig. 23-20). In some devices, a sensed atrial event also initiates an ABP. After the ABP, sensed atrial events may be used for detection of pathologic atrial tachyarrhythmia for mode-switching, overdrive suppression algorithm, or noise reversion. After a ventricular sensed or paced event, there may be a postventricular ABP (see Fig. 23-20), to prevent the sensing of ventricular paced events or far-field ventricular sensed events on the atrial channel. After a paced or sensed ventricular event, a postventricular atrial refractory period (PVARP) is created (see Fig. 23-20). During the PVARP, atrial events are refractory sensed events and do not affect the timing of events.

Differential Atrioventricular Interval

In some devices, the AVI initiated after a sensed atrial event (SAV) can be different from the AVI initiated after a paced atrial event (PAV). This difference is called a differential AVI. The optimal AVI achieves coordination of the atria and ventricles, particularly the left atrium and the LV. Usually, impulse formation starts first in the sinus node and then travels to the right atrial lead and is on its way to the AV node By the time the event is sensed on the atrial channel, contraction of the atria has already begun, necessitating only relatively short delay until the time that ventricular excitation occurs. There is time that elapses between the initiation of an intrinsic atrial depolarization and the point at which most of the atria are depolarized. This delay is determined by the distance between the initiation point and the location of the lead, as well as the conductive properties of the atrial tissue. In effect, by the time the atrial lead has sensed the intrinsic depolarization, the impulse has already gotten a "head start" to the AV node, compared with an atrial paced event. Programming the AVI after a sensed atrial depolarization (PV) to be shorter than after a PAV (Fig. 23-21) makes the time to ventricular pacing after a PAV similar to that after an SAV. This is an attempt to provide a more physiologic AV synchrony. The SAV may be expressed as a percentage of the PAV or as an absolute difference (up to 100 msec) between the two differential AVIs.

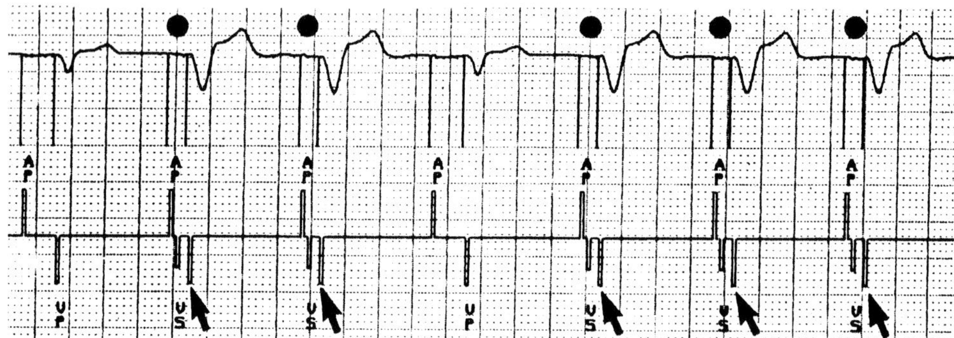

Figure 23-18. Ventricular safety pacing. The top channel is the surface electrocardiogram (ECG). The bottom channel is the marker channel, with the atrial channel on top and the ventricular channel on the bottom. In the absence of crosstalk, the first, fourth, and last atrioventricular (A-V) intervals are equal to the programmed value of 200 msec. Intermittent crosstalk (solid black circles) *leads to activation of the ventricular safety pacing mechanism, so that the A-V interval of the second, third, fifth, and seventh beats is abbreviated to 110 msec. The marker channel below the ECG confirms the presence of crosstalk with ventricular sensing (Vs) of the atrial stimulus (Ap) within the ventricular safety pacing period but beyond the short ventricular blanking period initiated by Ap. The arrows point to Vp triggered at the end of the ventricular safety pacing period (110 msec after the release of Ap). In a DDD pulse generator with ventricular-based lower rate timing, activation of the ventricular safety pacing mechanism by continual crosstalk leads to an increase in the pacing rate even though the atrial escape interval remains constant. (From Barold SS, Zipes DP: Cardiac pacemakers and antiarrhythmic devices. In Braunwald E [ed]: Heart Disease, 5th ed. Philadelphia, WB Saunders, 1997, pp 705-741.)*

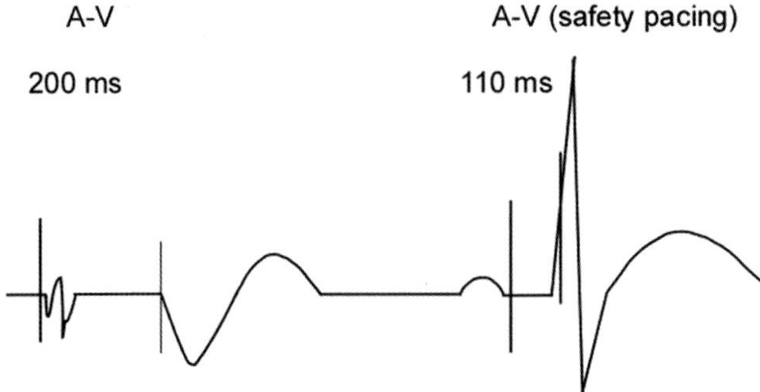

Figure 23-19. Ventricular safety pacing due to atrial undersensing. On the left, there is an atrial paced event and a ventricular paced event, separated by an atrioventricular (A-V) interval of 200 msec. On the right, there is an undersensed intrinsic atrial event, occurring after an atrial pacing stimulus, that is not captured due to physiologic refractoriness. The atrial event conducts to the ventricle. The sensed intrinsic ventricular event falls exactly within the crosstalk safety pacing window, resulting in a ventricular safety pacing.

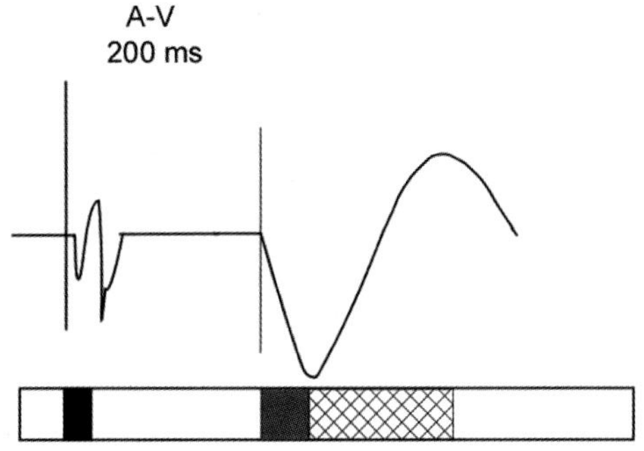

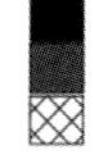

Figure 23-20. DDD mode, atrial blanking period. After an paced or sensed atrial event, there is a blanking period on the atrial channel. After a sensed or paced ventricular event, there may be a postventricular atrial blanking period (PAVB) on the atrial channel, followed by a postventricular atrial refractory period (PVARP). During the PVARP, an atrial sensed event will not be tracked or used to inhibit atrial pacing at the atrial escape interval.

Rate-Adaptive or Dynamic Atrioventricular Delay

The shortening of AVI with exercise provides optimal AV synchrony and is designed to mimic the normal physiologic shortening of the P-R interval. The programmable parameter called rate-adaptive or dynamic AVI permits the modulation of sensed or paced AVIs based on the ventricular rate, either intrinsic or sensor driven. In addition to the hemodynamic benefits of shortening of the AVI, rate-related shortening of AVI decreases the total atrial refractory period (TARP) (see later discussion), permitting a corresponding a higher 2:1 atrial tracking rate. The changes in dynamic AVI may be linear or nonlinear, based on the sensed atrial rate or on the sensor-driven rate, and they are programmed from a baseline AVI to a so-called minimum AVI.

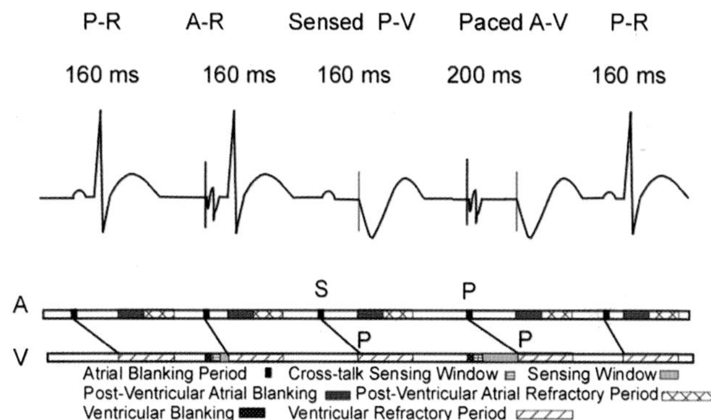

Figure 23-21. Differential atrioventricular interval (AVI). A differential AVI permits a shorter AVI for a sensed atrial event than for a paced atrial event. In the first complex, the sensed atrial event initiates an AVI of 160 msec, but AV conduction occurs within 140 msec. Similarly, in the second complex, the paced atrial event initiates an AVI of 200 msec, but AV conduction is faster than that. In the third complex, the P wave is sensed and initiates a shorter A-V interval of 160 msec, compared with the AVI of 200 msec. In the last complex, the sensed P wave also starts an A-V interval of 160 msec, but AV conduction occurs.

Atrioventricular Interval Hysteresis

The AVI can also be modulated based on the presence or absence of AV conduction with a sensed ventricular event during the AVI, a feature called positive or negative AV/PV hysteresis. The term AV hysteresis is generally used to describe adaptations of either paced or sensed AVIs relative to the patient's intrinsic P-R interval. Similar to heart rate hysteresis, AVI hysteresis is a prolongation of the AVI in response to a ventricular paced event (V), so-called positive AV/PV hysteresis. The longer-than-programmed AVI permits intrinsic AV conduction and minimizes unnecessary ventricular pacing. Positive AV/PV hysteresis is most beneficial to patients who have variable AV conduction. If the intrinsic AV conduction exceeds the AVI hysteresis and no spontaneous R wave is sensed at the end of the AVI (e.g., in AV block), the AVI is shortened to the original programmed value. There is a search function that extends the AVI periodically from the programmed baseline value to the longer AVI hysteresis interval, to promote intrinsic AV conduction and ventricular activation (Figs. 23-22 and 23-23). This function may be termed "search positive AV hysteresis." Alternatively, a negative AV/PV hysteresis is programmed to promote and maintain ventricular pacing and avoid fusion. After an atrial event, if native ventricular conduction is sensed (R wave), then the next AVI will be shortened to promote ventricular pacing and capture (Fig. 23-24). This function may be used to promote ventricular capture, when this is desirable hemodynamically. Such conditions might include pacing for hypertrophic cardiomyopathy or biventricular pacing.

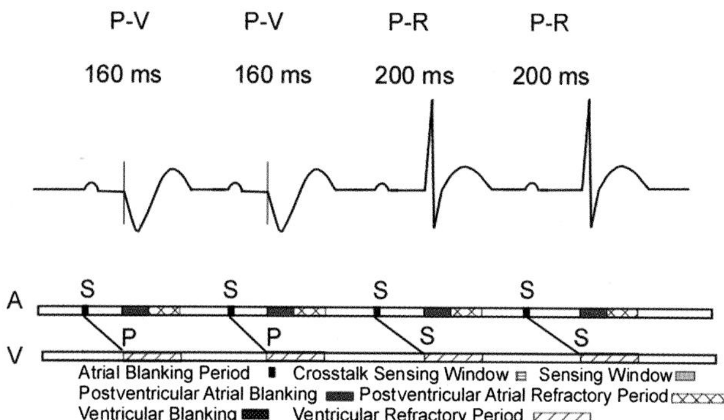

Figure 23-22. Positive atrioventricular (AV) hysteresis. In positive AV hysteresis, the AV interval (AVI) is increased to permit intrinsic AV conduction. If conduction is present, the extended AVI persists. If AV conduction is absent, the AVI is shortened to its previous length.

Postventricular Atrial Refractory Period

After a sensed or paced ventricular event, atrial sensed events do not result in a corresponding AVI for a programmable period of time. This interval, known as the PVARP (Fig. 23-25), is used to prevent sensing of retrograde P waves occurring after a paced or sensed ventricular event. The atrial channel may sense a retrograde atrial signal as an intrinsic event and trigger ventricular pacing, resulting in another ventricular paced event, which also conducts retrograde. This repetitive sequence is known as pacemaker-mediated tachycardia (PMT) (Figs. 23-26 and 23-27), and it may continue in the absence of intervention. PMT may occur at or below the maximum tracking rate (MTR; see later discussion) and is often induced by spontaneous PVCs or loss of atrial capture. The rate of the

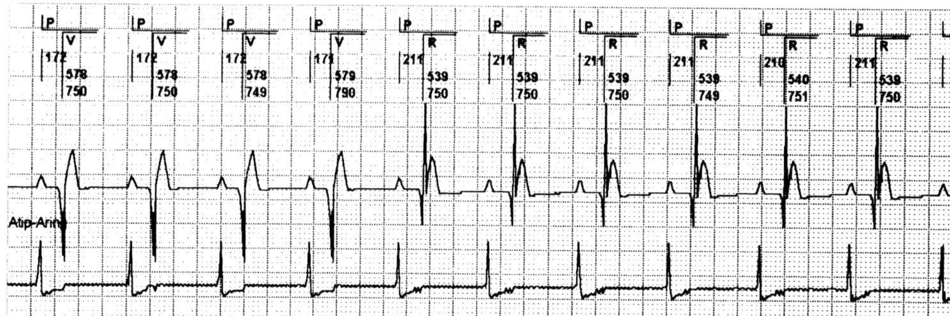

Figure 23-23. Positive atrioventricular (AV) hysteresis. After a period of pacing, a search mechanism is initiated in which the system automatically extends the paced or sensed AV delay. If a native R wave occurs within the extended AV delay, the longer AV delay is maintained, restoring intact AV conduction and allowing for a normal ventricular activation sequence. Although the P-R interval is longer than the P-V interval, there is intact AV conduction. When the AV delay is extended on the 256th cycle, a sensed R wave is seen by the pacemaker, inhibiting the ventricular output and re-establishing the longer AV/PV delay engendered by adding the positive hysteresis interval to the programmed intervals. This results in functional AAI pacing or inhibited pacing, except in the presence of AV block. Although the same result could be accomplished with a fixed long AV or PV delay, if AV block developed, the pacing system would be functioning in a hemodynamically deleterious long AV/PV delay until intact conduction resumed. P, atrial sensed beat; R, ventricular sensed beat; V, ventricular paced beat. (Courtesy of St. Jude Cardiac Rhythm Management Division, Sylmar, Calif.)

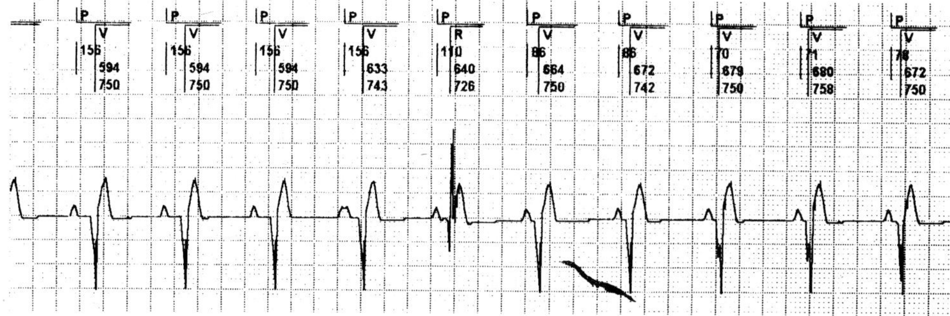

Figure 23-24. Negative AV/PV hysteresis. Stable PV pacing is interrupted by one cycle (110 msec) at a shorter A-Vs interval than the P-V interval (150 msec). This causes shortening of the As-Vp (P-V) interval by the programmed value, restoring PV pacing with full ventricular capture. P, atrial sensed beat (As); R, ventricular sensed beat (Vs); V, ventricular paced beat (Vp). (Courtesy of St. Jude Cardiac Rhythm Management Division, Sylmar, Calif.)

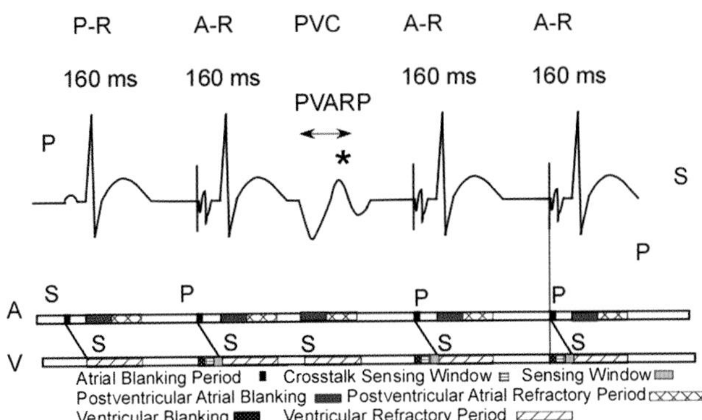

Figure 23-25. Postventricular atrial refractory period (PVARP). A premature ventricular contraction (PVC) results in retrograde conduction, indicated by the asterisk. Because the P wave occurs within the PVARP, it is not tracked and does not initiate a ventricular paced event. Instead, the next atrial paced event occurs after the atrial escape interval has been completed.

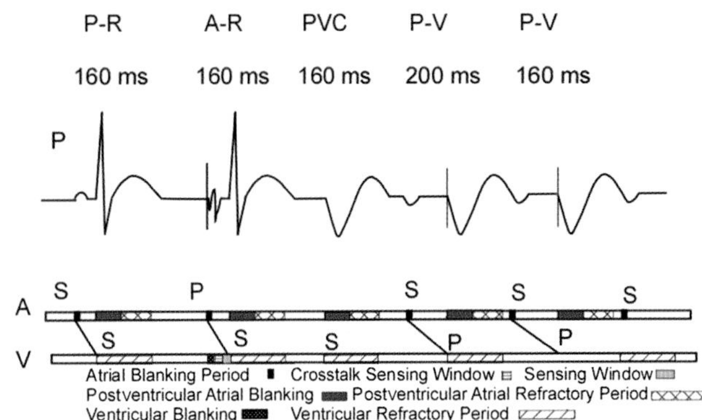

Figure 23-26. Pacemaker-mediated tachycardia (PMT). A premature ventricular contraction (PVC) results in retrograde conduction. Because the retrograde P wave occurs after the postventricular atrial refractory period (PVARP), the P wave is tracked and initiates a ventricular paced event. This ventricular paced event results in another retrograde P wave, which is tracked, resulting in PMT.

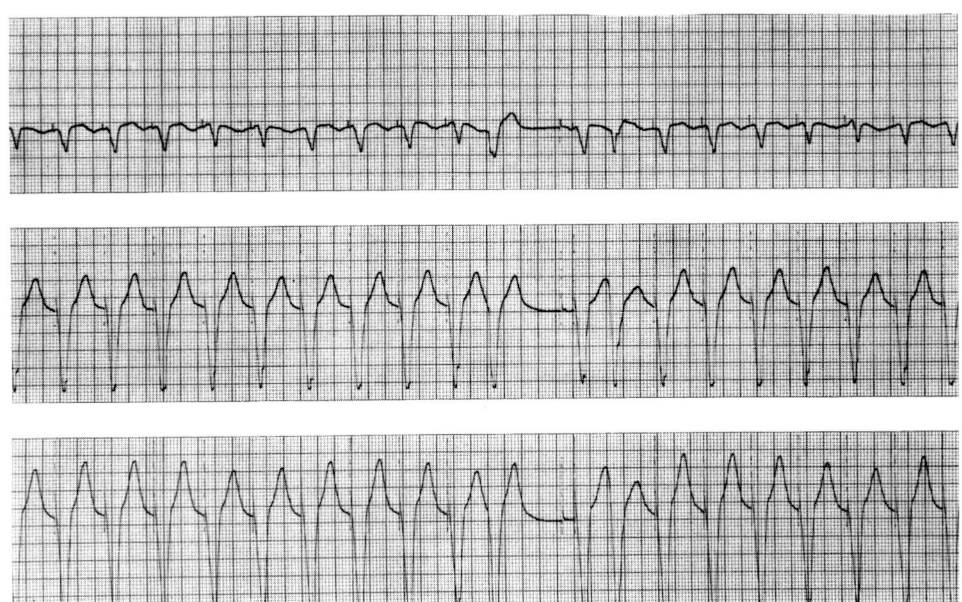

Figure 23-27. Pacemaker-mediated tachycardia terminated and initiated by ventricular extrasystole. The three electrocardiogram (ECG) leads were recorded simultaneously. The upper rate interval (URI) is 500 msec (120 pulses per minute [ppm]); the lower rate interval (LRI) is 857 msec (70 ppm); and the atrioventricular (AV) delay is 150 msec. The cycle length of the tachycardia is longer than the URI. (From Barold SS, Falkoff MD, Ong LS, et al.: Electrocardiography of contemporary DDD pacemakers: A. Basic concepts, upper rate response, retrograde ventriculoatrial conduction, and differential diagnosis of pacemaker tachycardias. In Saksena S, Goldschlager N [eds]: Electrical Therapy for Cardiac Arrhythmias: Pacing, Antitachycardia Devices, Catheter Ablation. Philadelphia, WB Saunders, 1990, pp 225-264.)

PMT depends on the retrograde conduction time, the programmed AVI, and the MTR. Commonly, PMT occurs at the MTR. However, the retrograde conduction time may be long enough to permit tracking of the atrial event with the programmed AVI, so that the rate of the PMT may be less than the MTR. To avoid PMT, the PVARP is usually programmed to be longer than the retrograde conduction time; however, if it is programmed excessively long, the sum of the PVARP and the AVI (the TARP) will determine the rate at which one ventricular paced event occurs for two atrial sensed events, the 2:1 atrial tracking rate (see later discussion). Extension of the PVARP in response to a PVC, the so-called PVC PVARP extension or response, is available in many devices. This algorithm is designed to lengthen the PVARP and to avoid sensing of a retrograde P wave occurring after a PVC that may cause initiation of PMT. Of note, a "PVC" is usually defined by the pacemaker as a spontaneous ventricular depolarization without a preceding atrial paced or sensed event. In some cases,

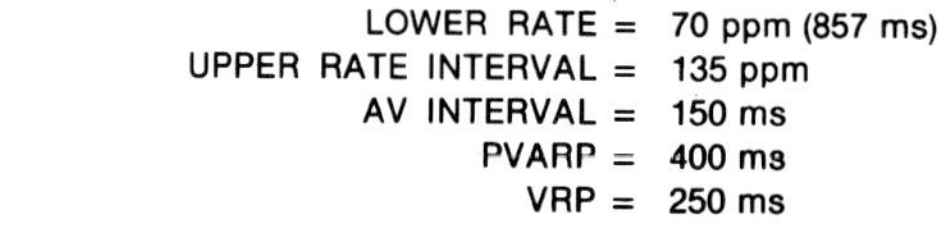

LOWER RATE = 70 ppm (857 ms)
UPPER RATE INTERVAL = 135 ppm
AV INTERVAL = 150 ms
PVARP = 400 ms
VRP = 250 ms

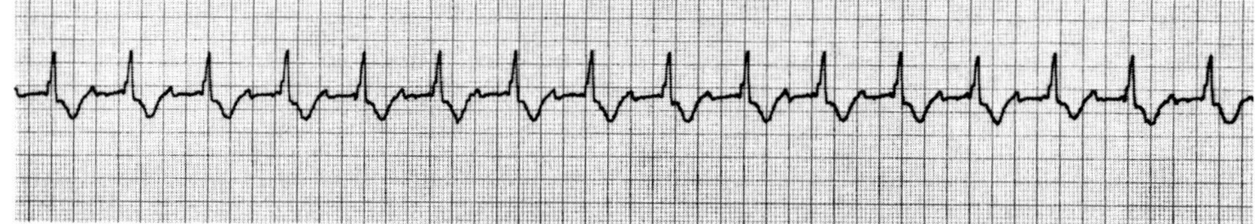

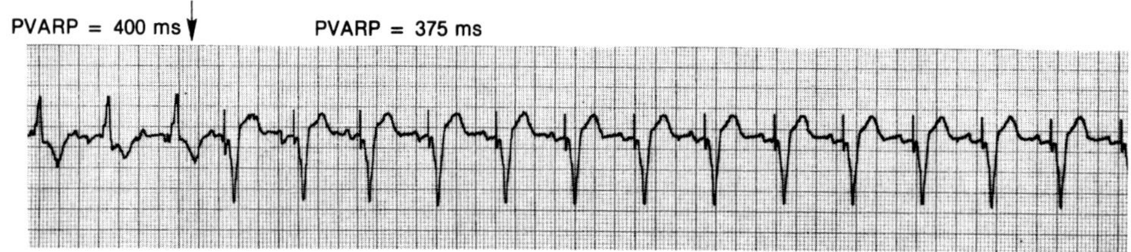

Figure 23-28. Lack of P wave tracking due to a long postventricular atrial refractory period (PVARP), 400 msec. The sinus rate is about 85 beats per minute, and there is a first-degree atrioventricular (AV) block. The P waves fall within the PVARP initiated by the preceding sensed QRS complex. Shortening the PVARP to 375 msec (bottom) *restores 1:1 atrial tracking with the programmed AV interval (150 msec). VRP, ventricular refractory period. (From Barold SS, Falkoff MD, Ong LS, et al.: Timing cycles of DDD pacemakers. In Barold SS, Mugica J [eds]: New Prospectives in Cardiac Pacing. Mt. Kisco, NY, Futura, 1988, pp 69-119.)*

a long PVARP may lead to absence of atrial tracking (Fig. 23-28). Similarly, oversensing of a T wave and programming on the PVC PVARP extension may cause perpetuation of absence of atrial tracking at rates below the LRL (Fig. 23-29). Repetitive functional atrial undersensing may occur in the absence of PVC PVARP extension, particularly if the AV conduction is prolonged and the intrinsic AVI plus the PVARP is longer than the sinus cycle length.[19] Features such as autointrinsic search that cause prolongation of AV conduction may result in PMT by permitting retrograde conduction.[20]

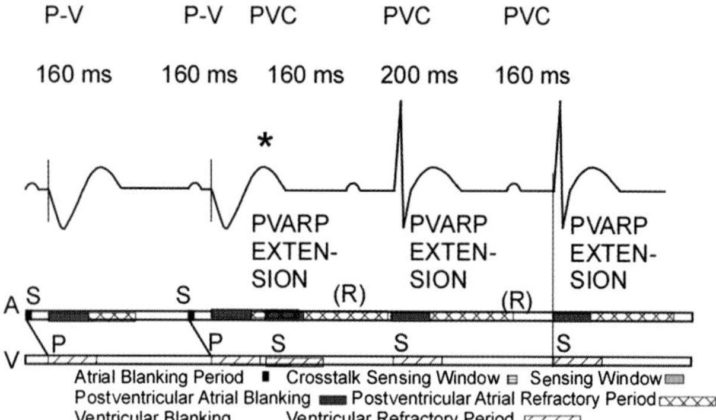

Figure 23-29. Perpetuation of failure to track due to postventricular atrial refractory period (PVARP) extension. T wave oversensing is classified as a premature ventricular complex (PVC). The PVC PVARP extension feature results in the PVARP being extended, which places the subsequent sinus P wave within the PVARP. Because atrioventricular (AV) conduction is present, the next QRS complex is considered a PVC, which again causes PVARP extension.

Upper Rate Behavior

In patients using the DDD, DDDR, VDD, or VDDR modes, one-to-one ventricular tracking of the intrinsic atrial activity is hemodynamically desirable. However, tracking of atrial arrhythmias may result in rapid ventricular pacing and lead to unfavorable hemodynamics. Therefore, these tracking modes have a parameter to limit the fastest rate at which the atrium can be tracked. The fastest rate at which atrial activity can be tracked 1:1 to the ventricle is known as the upper rate or MTR, with a corresponding upper rate interval or maximum tracking interval (Fig. 23-30). In a DDD mode of operation, whether it is atrial based or ventricular based, when the intrinsic atrial activity is faster than the programmed upper rate limit, upper rate behavior will be seen. Atrial rates faster than the MTR can still be sensed and tracked. However, delays in subsequent ventricular-paced beats occur, so the ventricular rate does not exceed the programmed MTR (Fig. 23-31). This effectively prolongs the AVI. The AVI is further extended on repeated cycles, and eventually a subsequent atrial depolarization falls within the PVARP. Because the atrial event occurs within the PVARP, it is not sensed by the atrial channel and does not lead to ventricular pacing. The next atrial event, however, can be tracked and causes ventricular pacing. The pattern that emerges is increasing time between an intrinsic atrial-sensed event and a subsequent ventricular-paced event until an atrial event is not followed by a ventricular-paced beat. Such behavior looks like a Wenckebach pattern during AV conduction and is called pseudo-Wenckebach AV response. The AVI extension is greatest when the P wave occurs just after

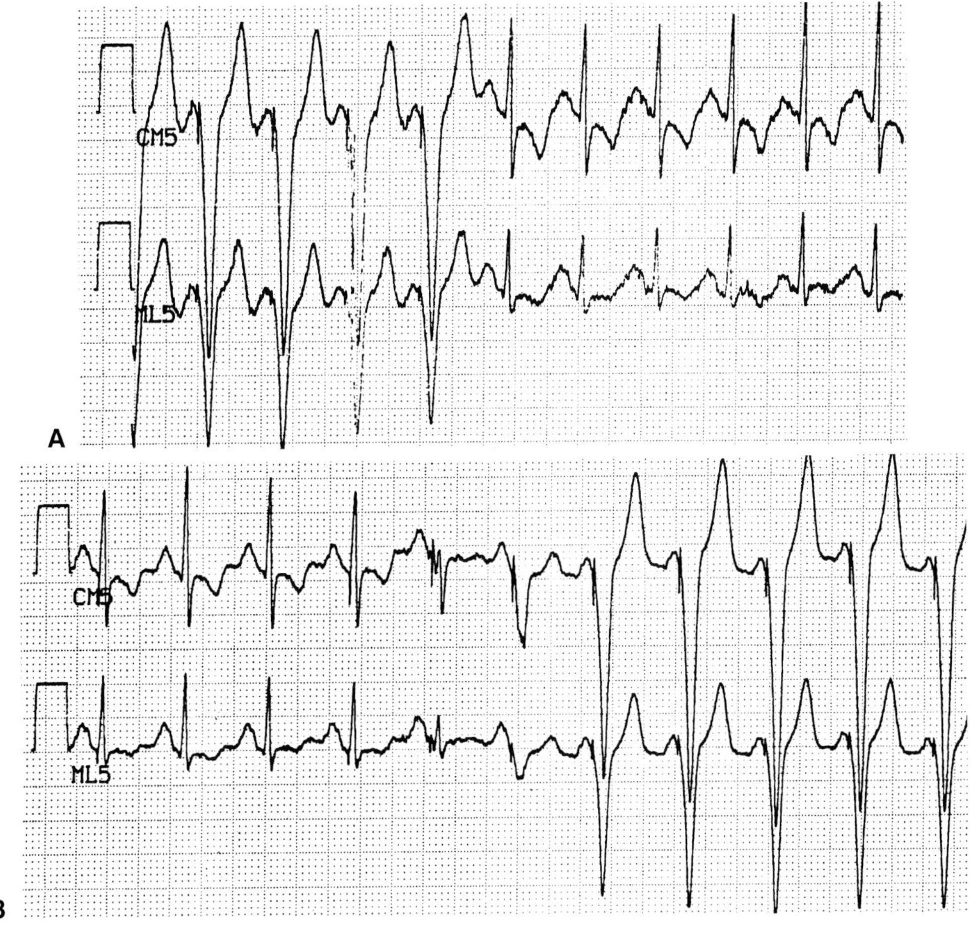

Figure 23-30. Upper rate behavior. ***A,*** *Apparent loss of atrial tracking related to upper rate limitation. The lower rate interval (LRI) is 1000 msec; the upper rate interval is 500 msec; and the atrioventricular interval (AVI) is 75 msec. The electrocardiogram (ECG) was recorded during a treadmill stress test. The P waves on the right are sensed (documented later by markers during repeated exercise,* not shown*) but the pacemaker does not emit a ventricular paced beat because a QRS complex occurs before the termination of the 75-msec AVI, thereby producing a sensed repetitive preempted Wenckebach upper rate response.* ***B,*** *Same patient as* ***A.*** *During the recovery portion of the stress test, as the sinus rate slows, the AVI gradually shortens in a few cycles until it reaches 75 msec. This produces a "reverse Wenckebach" response, with gradually more ventricular captures (fusion beats) until full ventricular capture is reestablished, preceded by a sensed atrial-to-paced ventricular interval of 75 msec. (From Douard H, Barold SS, Broustet JP: Too much protection may be a nuisance. Stimucoeur 25:183-187, 1997.)*

the completion of the preceding PVARP (Fig. 23-32). AVI extension may be seen at constant atrial rates during atrial or sinus tachycardias as well as during atrial premature beats (Fig. 23-33).

If the intrinsic atrial rate continues to increase above the MTR, it will eventually reach the 2:1 AV tracking rate, defined by the TARP, which is the sum of the PVARP and the AVI (Fig. 23-34). The TARP defines the period during which sensing may occur and limits the MTR. TARP determines the rate at which atrial tracking occurs in a 2:1 ratio. At this atrial rate, every other P wave falls into the PVARP and is not sensed. If the intrinsic atrial rate is fast enough, one P wave can fall within the TARP while the next P wave falls outside the TARP and is tracked. If the atrial rate is just a little faster, the first P wave will be tracked and the second P wave will fall just within the PVARP and will not be tracked. As a result, for every two intrinsic atrial events, there is one ventricular-paced beat. Such a phenomenon occurs when the intrinsic atrial rate is faster than the 2:1 AV block rate. The 2:1 AV block rate can be calculated in milliseconds as 60,000 divided by TARP. For example, for an AVI of 150 msec and a PVARP of 250 msec, ventricular pacing may follow atrial sensing 1:1 at a rate of up to 149 bpm. At a sinus rate of 150 bpm, 2:1 atrial tracking occurs and the ventricular rate abruptly drops to 75 bpm.

If a patient has intrinsic AV conduction, the upper rate limit is not needed to permit tracking of rapid sinus rates during exertion. Therefore the upper rate limit, when intrinsic AV conduction is present, may be programmed at a relatively low rate. In patients with complete AV conduction block, however, it is important to permit tracking as the atrial rate rises during exertion. The upper rate limit (MTR) should be programmed high enough to allow 1:1 tracking through maximum

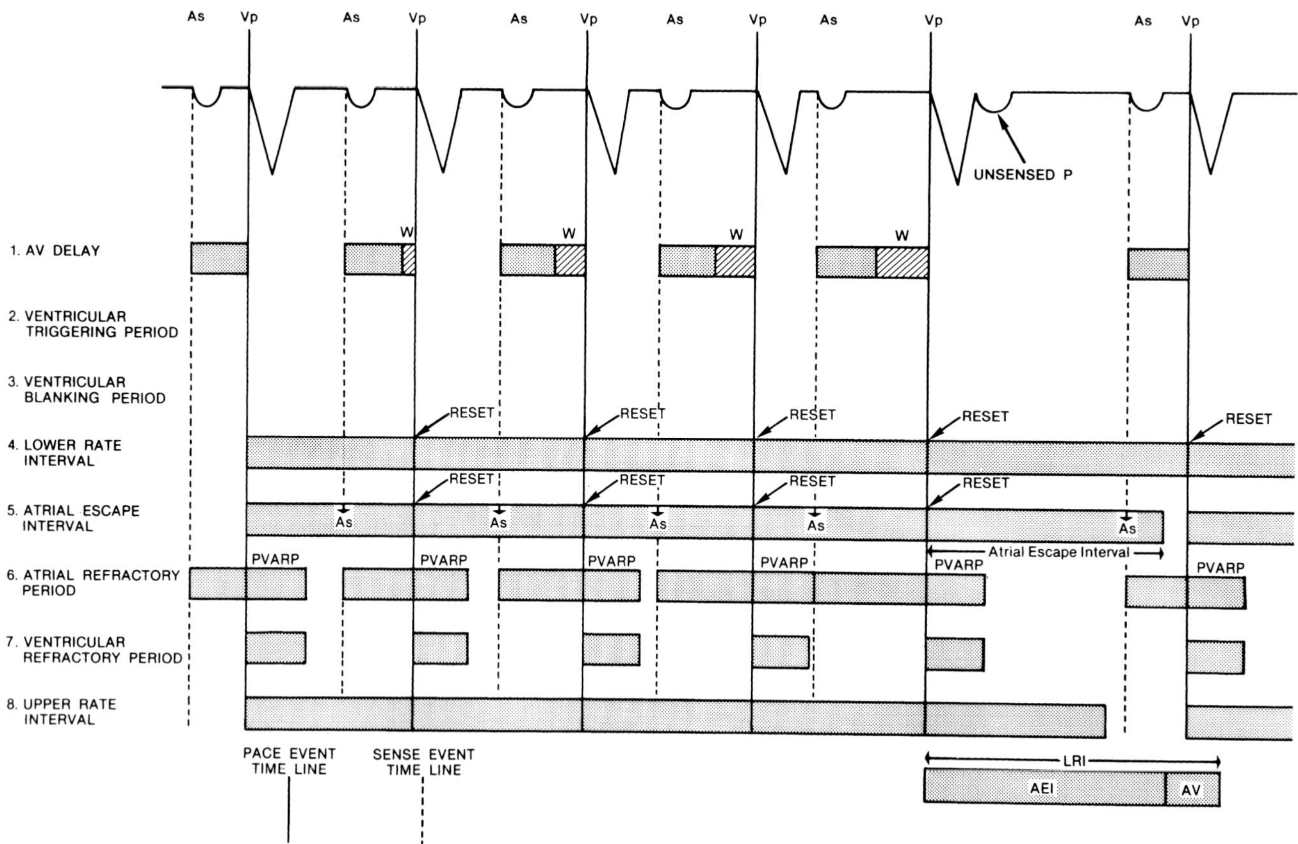

Figure 23-31. *DDD mode upper rate response with pacemaker Wenckebach atrioventricular (AV) block. The upper rate interval (URI) is longer than the programmed total atrial refractory period (TARP). The P-P interval (As-As) is shorter than the URI but longer than the programmed TARP. The As-Vp interval lengthens by a varying period (W) to conform to the URI. During Wenckebach response, the pacemaker synchronizes Vp to As, and because the pacemaker cannot violate its (ventricular) URI, Vp can be released only at the completion of the URI. The AV delay (As-Vp) becomes progressively longer as the ventricular channel waits to deliver its Vp until the URI has timed out. The maximum prolongation of the AV interval represents the difference between the URI and the TARP. The As-Vp interval continues to lengthen as long as the As-As interval (P-P) is longer than the TARP. The sixth P wave falls within the postventricular atrial refractory period (PVARP); therefore, it is unsensed and is not followed by Vp. A pause occurs, and the cycle restarts. In the first four pacing cycles, the intervals between ventricular stimuli (Vp-Vp) are constant and equal to the URI. When the P-P interval becomes shorter than the programmed TARP, Wenckebach pacemaker AV block cannot occur, and fixed-ratio pacemaker AV block (e.g., 2:1) supervenes. AEI, atrial escape interval; As, sensed atrial beat; Vp, paced ventricular beat. (From Barold SS, Falkoff MD, Ong LS, et al.: All dual chamber pacemakers function in the DDD mode. Am Heart J 115:1353, 1988.)*

physiologic atrial rates. However, a 2:1 atrial tracking rate faster than the maximum atrial tracking rate permits a zone of pseudo-Wenckebach behavior before the development of 2:1 block. To accomplish this effect, the TARP (PVARP + AVI) is programmed shorter than the upper rate limit interval.

There may be limitations to minimizing the TARP if retrograde conduction necessitates programming the PVARP to be longer than the retrograde conduction time. To avoid precipitous falls in heart rate, it is preferable to have the 2:1 AV block rate set higher than the MTR, to accommodate high intrinsic sinus rates without sudden AV block. This is achieved by minimizing TARP. There are several common ways to reduce the TARP and thereby raise the 2:1 block rate. The PVARP can be shortened (with consideration of the greater potential for PMT), and the AVI can be programmed to be rate-adaptive and shorten with faster ventricular rates. Rate-adaptive or dynamic PVARP is also available in some models; this shortens PVARP at a faster rate, thereby reducing TARP and raising the 2:1 AV block rate. Caution should be used with rate-adaptive PVARP to confirm that retrograde conduction will not occur at rapid ventricular rates, so that the conduction time does not exceed the PVARP and result in PMT. Alternatively, the pacemaker can be programmed to DDDR mode, relying on the sensor to drive pacing during exertion. If sensor-driven ventricular pacing occurs close to the sinus rate, the ventricular pacing rate will closely follow the sinus rate even though the ventricular pacing rate exceeds the maximum atrial tracking rate. This phenomenon has been termed

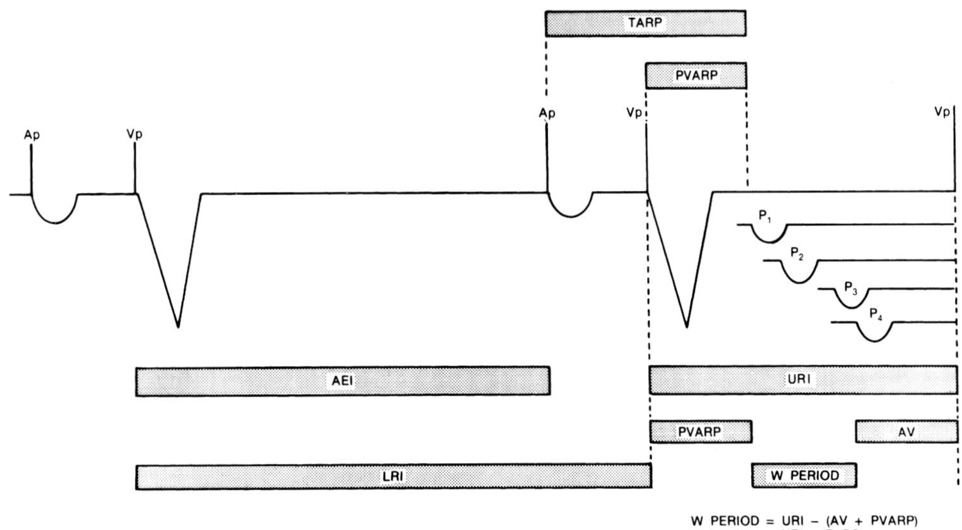

Figure 23-32. *Diagrammatic representation of the mechanism of atrioventricular (AV) interval prolongation in a pulse generator with a separately programmable total atrial refractory period (TARP) and upper rate interval (URI). Lower rate timing is ventricular based. The maximum AV extension, or waiting period (W), is equal to the URI minus the sum of the AV interval and the postventricular atrial refractory period (PVARP), or URI − TARP. A P wave (P1) occurring immediately after the termination of the PVARP exhibits the longest AV interval (i.e., AV + W). A P wave just beyond the W period (P4) initiates an AV interval equal to the programmed value. P waves occurring during the W period (P2 and P3) exhibit varying degrees of AV prolongation to conform to the URI depicted as the shortest interval between two consecutive ventricular paced beats (Vp). If the pacemaker is programmed with As-Vp shorter than Ap-Vp, W becomes URI − (As-Vp) − PVARP; that is, the AV extension becomes longer if the basic As-Vp is shorter than Ap-Vp. However, the maximum As-Vp duration is URI − PVARP, regardless of the programmed AV interval. AEI, atrial escape interval; LRI, lower rate interval: Ap, atrial-paced beat; As, atrial sensed beat. (From Barold SS, Falkoff MD, Ong LS, et al.: Electrocardiography of contemporary DDD pacemakers: A. Basic concepts, upper rate response, retrograde ventriculoatrial conduction, and differential diagnosis of pacemaker tachycardias. In Saksena S, Goldschlager N [eds]: Electrical Therapy for Cardiac Arrhythmias: Pacing, Antitachycardia Devices, Catheter Ablation. Philadelphia, WB Saunders, 1990, pp 225-264.)*

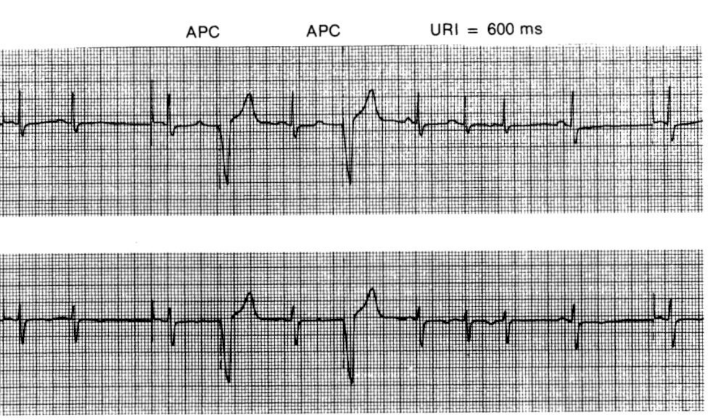

Figure 23-33. *Two-lead electrocardiogram showing DDD pacing (ventricular-based lower rate timing) with sensed atrial premature contractions (APC). The lower rate interval (LRI) is 1000 msec; the atrioventricular interval (AVI) is 200 msec; the upper rate interval (URI) is 600 msec; and the postventricular atrial refractory period (PVARP) is 155 msec. Note the extended AVI generated by the APCs to conform to the URI. This response with single beats should not be called a Wenckebach upper rate response; rather, it is best called an AV extension upper rate response.*

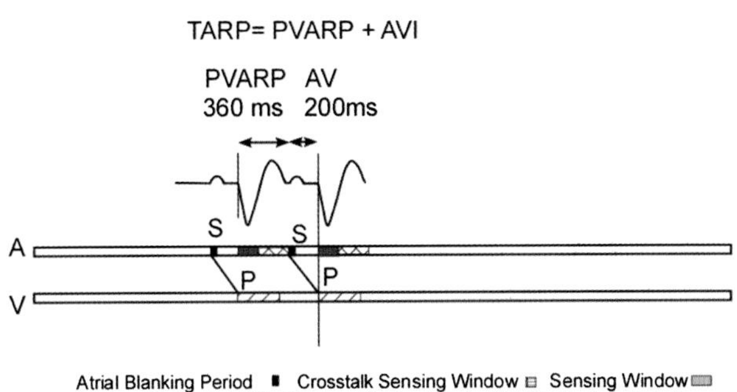

Figure 23-34. *Total atrial refractory period (TARP). The TARP represents the sum of the postventricular atrial refractory period (PVARP) and the atrioventricular interval (AVI). In this case TARP = 360 + 200 = 560 msec. Therefore, 2:1 atrial tracking would occur at an atrial cycle length of 560 msec.*

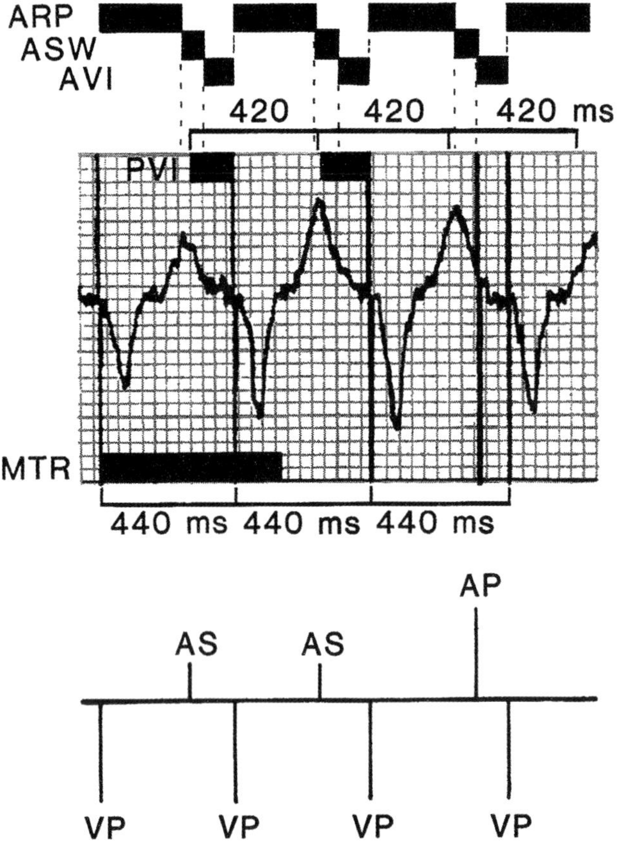

Figure 23-35. *Sensor-driven appearance of atrial tracking. The diagram shows that a P wave may inhibit the sensor-driven atrial stimulus and can resemble P-wave tracking above the maximum tracking rate (MTR) of 100 beats per minute (600 msec). The second and third ventricular complexes are preceded by intrinsic P waves that appear within the atrial sensing window (ASW). Sensing of atrial activity in this window results in inhibition of the atrial stimulus or P-wave tracking above the MTR. The fourth ventricular complex was preceded by an atrial paced event because the intrinsic P wave was within the atrial refractory period. ARP, atrial refractory period; AP, atrial paced event; AS, atrial sensed event; AVI, atrioventricular interval; VP, ventricular paced event. (From Higano ST, Hayes DL: P wave tracking above the maximum tracking rate in a DDDR pacemaker. PACE 12:1044-1048, 1989.)*

sensor-driven rate smoothing (Fig. 23-35), and it resembles tracking above the MTR.[21]

Upper rate behavior may also result in triggering of an apparent failure to sense P waves, because the P wave that falls within the PVARP and the subsequent QRS complex are categorized as a premature ventricular beat. Use of an algorithm to increase the PVARP after a PVC may result in a prolonged period of absence of atrial tracking (Figs. 23-36 and 23-37).[22] Upper rate behavior may also be characterized by intrinsically conducted beats that may preempt the ventricular paced beats at the upper rate. Barold and colleagues[23] reported that a relatively short programmed AVI, a sinus rate faster than the programmed upper rate, a relatively slow programmed upper rate, and relatively normal AV conduction are most likely to be associated with this phenomenon.

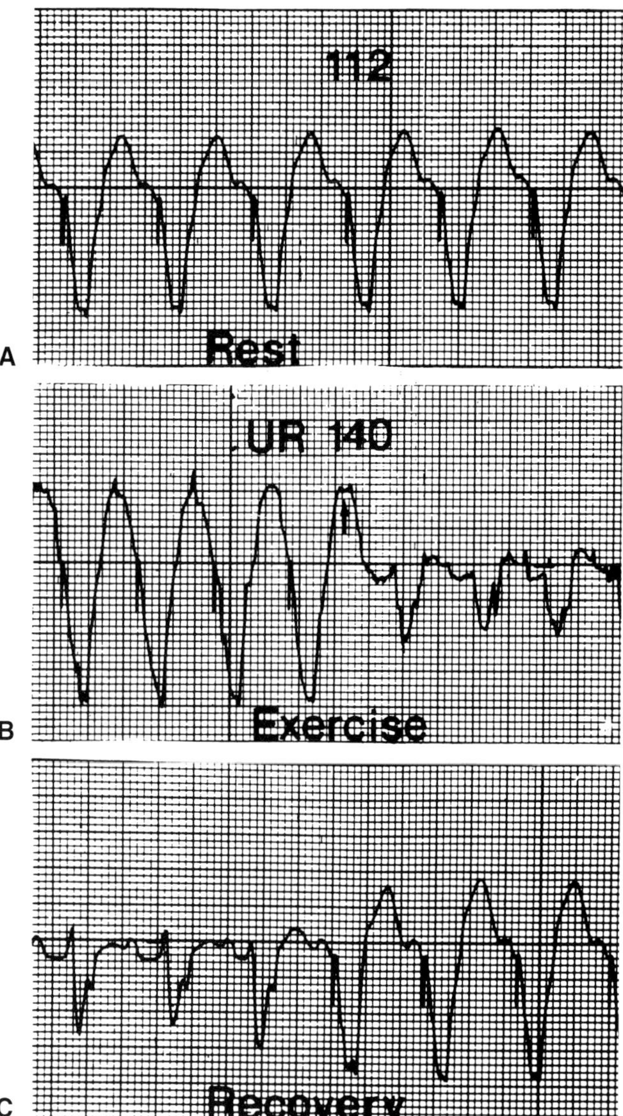

Figure 23-36. *Apparent P wave undersensing. The lower rate is 60 pulses per minute (ppm); the upper rate is 140 ppm; the atrioventricular (AV) delay after P wave sensing is 135 msec (adaptive AV delay with minimum AV delay of 75 msec); the postventricular atrial refractory period (PVARP) is 320 msec; and the automatic PVARP extension is 100 msec.* ***A,*** *At rest, the atrial rate is 112 beats per minute, causing atrial sensing and ventricular pacing with an AV interval of about 100 msec.* ***B,*** *After 1 minute of exercise, Wenckebach upper rate response occurs, and the pacemaker does not sense a P wave* (arrow) *in the PVARP. The P wave in the PVARP allows spontaneous AV conduction with a P-R interval of about 260 msec. The pacemaker interprets the spontaneous QRS as a ventricular premature contraction (VPC) and therefore automatically lengthens the PVARP to 320 + 100 = 420 msec. Subsequent events all are spontaneous; that is, the P wave and conducted QRS complex have a P-R interval longer than the programmed As-Vp interval at that particular atrial rate (apparent lack of atrial tracking). The spontaneous QRS complex continually activates the PVARP extension as the P waves continually fall within the extended PVARP.* ***C,*** *In the recovery phase, the electrocardiogram shows sinus rhythm (P-R interval of 200 msec) and conversion to an atrial synchronous ventricular-paced rhythm with an AV interval of 100 msec. The P-R interval preceding ventricular pacing shows an abrupt shortening of about 40 msec without a change in P-P interval. This results in earlier detection of the conducted QRS complex. The next P wave then falls outside the extended PVARP of 420 msec. As, atrial sensed beat; Vp, ventricular paced beat. (From Van Gelder BM, Van Mechelen R, Den Dulk K, et al.: Apparent P wave undersensing in a DDD pacemaker after exercise. PACE 15:1651, 1992.)*

LOWER RATE = 70 ppm (857 ms)
UPPER RATE INTERVAL = 135 ppm
A-V INTERVAL = 150 ms
PVARP = 400 ms
VRP = 250 ms

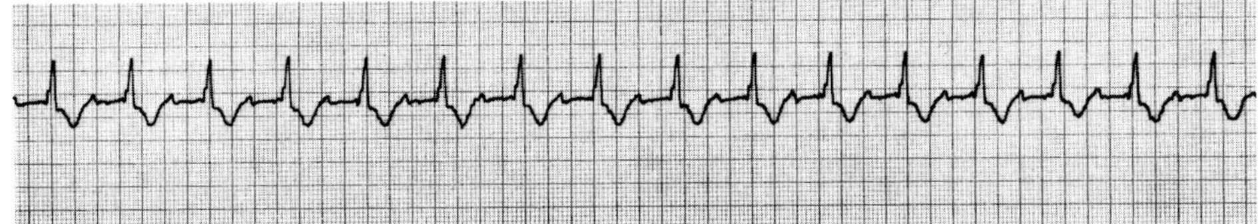

PVARP = 400 ms PVARP = 375 ms

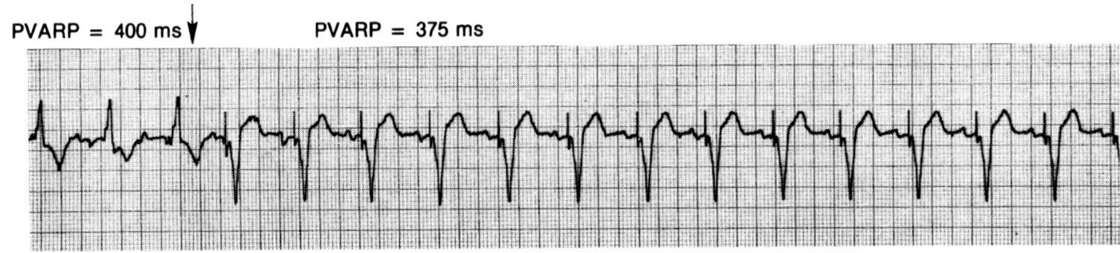

Figure 23-37. Loss of P wave tracking due to long postventricular atrial refractory period (PVARP), 400 msec. The sinus rate is about 85 beats per minute (bpm), and there is first-degree atrioventricular (AV) block. The P waves fall within the PVARP initiated by the preceding sensed QRS complex. Shortening the PVARP to 373 msec (bottom) *restores 1:1 atrial tracking with the programmed AV interval (150 msec). VRP, ventricular refractory period. (From Barold SS, Falkoff MD, Ong LS et al: Timing cycles of DDD pacemakers. In Barold SS, Mugica J [eds]: New Perspectives in Cardiac Pacing. Mt. Kisco, NY, Futura, 1988, pp 69-119.)*

Lower Rate Behavior: Atrial-Based versus Ventricular-Based Timing

LRL timing has already been discussed. The use of atrial- versus[24] ventricular-based timing cycles determines when atrial-paced events occur. With ventricular-based timing, in the DDD mode, an AEI is initiated after a sensed or paced ventricular event (R-A, or V-A) (Fig. 23-38). In ventricular-based timing, the AEI is "fixed." The LRL is the maximum time interval allowed between a ventricular event (either sensed or paced) and the subsequent ventricular pacing stimulus (V-V, or R-V) The LRL is therefore equal to the AEI plus the AVI until the subsequent ventricular pace (R-A-V or V-A-V). The length of the AEI can be determined by subtracting the AVI from the cycle length of the LRL (in microseconds). If another ventricular-sensed event occurs during the AEI, it will reset and initiate a new AEI. If an atrial-sensed event occurs during the AEI (after the PVARP), it will initiate the AVI, with a subsequent ventricular-sensed or paced event within the constraints of the upper rate limit. If the AEI expires sensing any atrial or ventricular event is sensed, the pacemaker will provide an atrial-paced beat.

In ventricular-based timing, it is possible for the effective ventricular rate to be faster than the programmed LRL. This occurs in patients with intact AV conduction and is mainly caused by the difference between the paced AVI and the shorter intrinsic AV conduction (Fig. 23-39). For example, in a pacemaker programmed to an LRL of 60 bpm (1000 msec) that has a programmed AVI of 200 msec, the AEI is 800 msec (LRL – AVI = AEI). If AV conduction is present at 150 msec, the sensed R wave will reset the timing cycle, whereas the AEI is "fixed" at 800 msec. The effective interval between consecutive atrial pacing beats is therefore 950 msec (AEI + A-R), which is approximately 63 bpm (see Figs. 23-38 and 23-39). In patients with intact AV conduction, the effective ventricular rate can be faster than the programmed LRL in a ventricular-based timing system.

Whereas the AEI is fixed in a ventricular-based timing system, the atrial interval (A-A) is fixed in an atrial-based timing system. A sensed R wave occurring during AVI inhibits ventricular output but does not reset the basic A-A interval; therefore, the LRL is not altered. When a R wave is sensed during AEI, the A-A interval is reset, but not the AEI. This results in a longer atrial-to-atrial interval that simulates a physiologic "compensatory" pause. Some pacemaker models deploy a "modified" atrial-based algorithm, such that routine atrial sensed or paced events reset the A-A timing cycle but PVCs reset the AEI or the V-A interval (Fig. 23-40). Early sensing of the ventricular complex on the atrial channel (crosstalk) in a pacemaker with atrial-based timing has been shown to result in prolonged AEIs (Figs. 23-41 and 23-42).[25] In Figure 23-41, at a more sensitive ventricular sensitivity (left panel), there is no evidence of a prolonged AEI, whereas at a less sensitive ventricular sensitivity (right panel), there is significant prolongation of the AEI. Figure 23-42 reveals that the first PVC may be sensed first on the atrial channel, resulting in prolongation of the AEI. In this device, when PVCs are sensed first on the ventricular channel, ventricular-based timing is used to set the AEI. The second PVC in this figure is sensed as a PVC and therefore does not result in prolongation of the AEI.

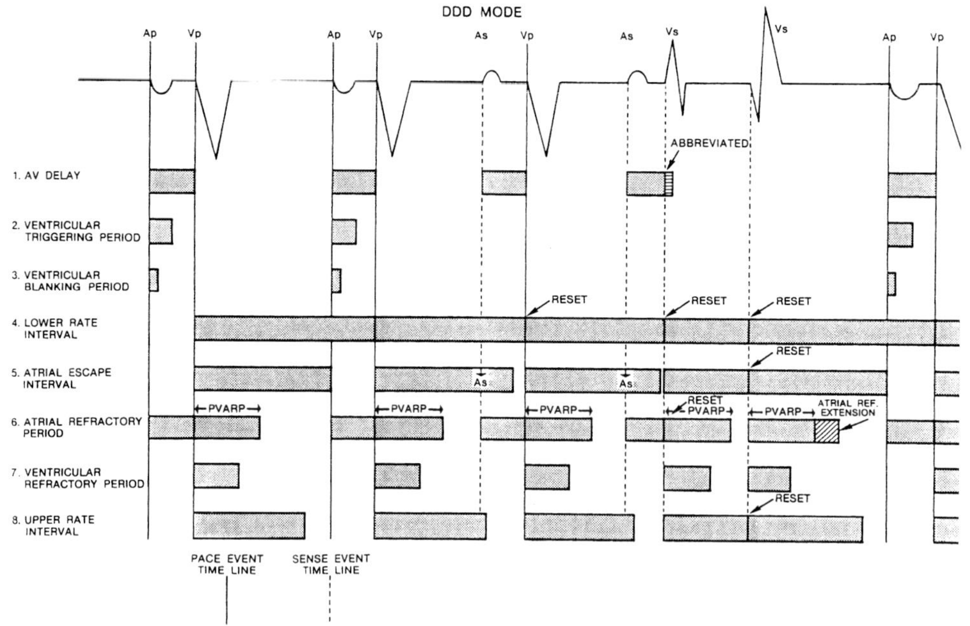

Figure 23-38. *DDD mode with ventricular-based lower rate timing. Diagrammatic representation of timing cycles. The second Vs is a sensed ventricular extrasystole. The fourth atrioventricular interval (AVI), initiated by an As, is abbreviated because the Vs occurs before the AVI has timed out. The postventricular atrial refractory period (PVARP) generated by the ventricular extrasystole is automatically extended by the atrial refractory period extension. This design is based on the concept that most episodes of endless-loop tachycardia (pacemaker macroreentrant tachycardia caused by repetitive sensing of retrograde atrial depolarization) are initiated by ventricular extrasystoles with retrograde ventriculoatrial conduction. Whenever possible, the AVI and the atrial escape (pacemaker V-A) interval (AEI) are depicted in their entirety for the sake of clarity. The arrow pointing down within the AEI indicates that an As has taken place. The As inhibits the release of the atrial stimulus expected at the completion of the AEI. As, atrial sensed event; REF, refractory; ventricular triggering period, ventricular-ventricular safety period; Vs, ventricular sensed event. (From Barold SS, Falkoff MD, Ong LS, et al.: All dual-chamber pacemakers function in the DDD mode. Am Heart J 115:1353, 1988.)*

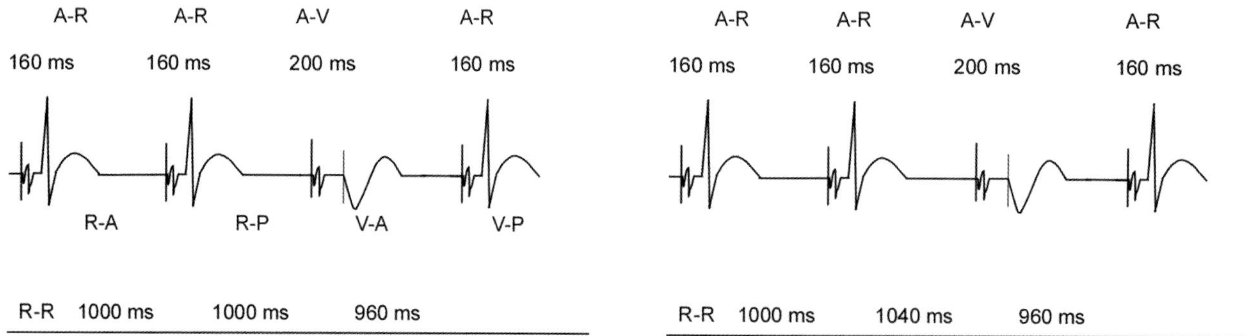

Figure 23-39. *Ventricular-based timing cycles. The lower rate limit is 1000 msec; the atrioventricular (AV) delay is 200 msec; and the atrial escape interval is 800 msec. The R-R intervals are given. Note that the R-R interval is 1000 msec between the first and second beats. Between the second and third beats, the R-R interval is also 1000 msec. Between the third and fourth beats, it is 960 msec because the AV conduction time is less than 200 msec. A, atrial paced event; P, atrial sensed event; R, ventricular sensed event; V, ventricular paced event.*

Figure 23-40. *Atrial-based timing cycles. The lower rate limit is 1000 msec; the atrioventricular (AV) delay is 200 msec; and the atrial escape interval is 800 msec. The R-R intervals are given. Note that the R-R interval is 1000 msec between the first and second beats. Between the second and third beats, the R-R interval is 1040 msec. Between the third and fourth beats, it is 960 msec because the AV conduction time is less than 200 msec. A, atrial paced event; P, atrial sensed event; R, ventricular sensed event; V, ventricular paced event.*

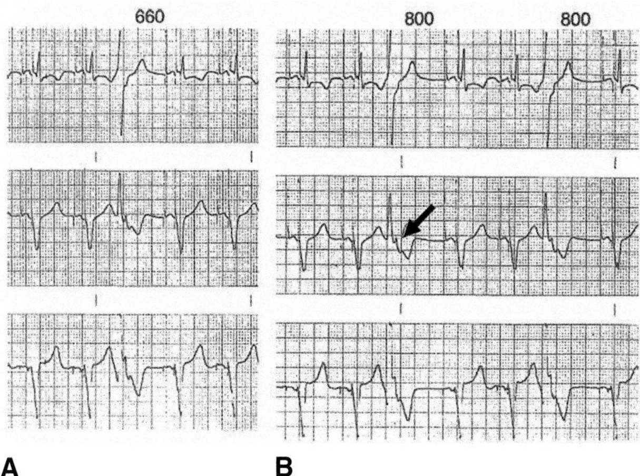

*Figure 23-41. Prolongation of the atrial escape interval (AEI) in an atrial-based timing pacemaker. In the left panel (**A**), the atrial sensitivity was programmed to 0.5 mV and the ventricular sensitivity was 1 mV. The premature ventricular contraction (PVC) resulted in an AEI of 660 msec, corresponding to the programmed AEI of 600 msec. In the right panel (**B**), the atrial sensitivity was still programmed at 0.5 mV, but the ventricular sensitivity was decreased to 4 mV. The PVC* (arrow) *resulted in prolongation of the AEI to 800 msec, corresponding to the programmed lower rate interval of 750 msec. (From Barold SS: Far-field R wave sensing causing prolongation of the atrial escape interval of DDD pacemakers with atrial-based lower rate timing. PACE 26:2188-2191, 2003.)*

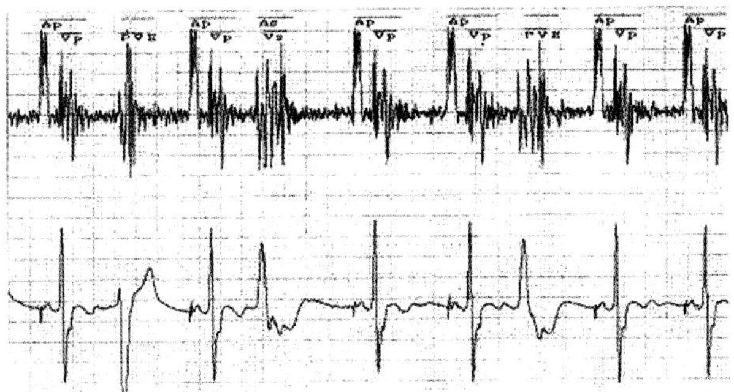

Figure 23-42. Prolongation of the atrial escape interval (AEI) in an atrial-based timing pacemaker caused by far-field R-wave sensing on the atrial channel. The lower rate limit is 800 msec in an atrial-based timing system, except after premature ventricular contractions (PVCs), when ventricular-based timing is present. After the first PVC, the As marker precedes the Vs marker, suggesting early sensing of the R wave on the atrial channel. Early atrial sensing results in prolongation of the AEI, because it is an atrial-based timing system. The second PVC is not sensed first on the atrial channel and therefore is considered to be a PVC, resulting in ventricular-based timing and no prolongation of the AEI. As, atrial sensed event; Vs, ventricular sensed event. (From Barold SS: Far-field R wave sensing causing prolongation of the atrial escape interval of DDD pacemakers with atrial-based lower rate timing. PACE 26:2188-2191, 2003.)

Sensor-Driven or Rate-Adaptive Pacing

Hemodynamics of Exercise and Rate

Since the development of pacemakers in the early 1960s, the goals of pacing therapy have evolved from basic pacing for life support to optimizing physiologic functions. The pacemakers have developed from VOO to DDDR systems. In response to enhanced sympathetic drive during exercise, heart rate (HR) and stroke volume (SV) increase, leading to greater cardiac output ($CO = HR \times SV$). Unlike people who can raise their heart rate considerably during exercise, patients with sinus node or conduction system dysfunction are unable to raise their heart rate adequately. Because heart rate is the predominant determinant of cardiac output compared with stroke volume, the pacemaker must provide rate-adaptive pacing to optimize physiologic response. Impaired heart rate response to increased metabolic demand is known as "chronotropic incompetence." Its definition varies and is sometimes described as inability to achieve 75% of the maximum predicted heart rate for age. Individuals with chronotropic incompetence include patients who have sinus bradycardia with sinus node dysfunction and those in atrial fibrillation with a slow ventricular rate response. Both populations may exhibit blunted heart rate response to stress. Algorithms have been developed to estimate an individual's expected maximum heart rate, as during vigorous exercise. One of the most common estimations is based on patient age (220 − age [years] = maximum heart rate).

Rate-Adaptive Pacing

In order to provide a greater heart rate response with exertion in efforts to support the metabolic demands during exercise, rate-adaptive pacing is essential for patients with chronotropic incompetence. For example, a patient in sinus bradycardia who has sinus node dysfunction could benefit from either an atrial- or a dual-chamber–rate responsive pacemaker in order to achieve a higher heart rate response during exertion than their sinus node can provide. Similarly, patients who have chronic atrial fibrillation and a slow ventricular rate may benefit from a VVIR pacemaker that increases the rate of ventricular pacing with exertion.

Timing Cycles of Sensor-Driven Pacing

Sensor-driven pacing preserves the timing cycles of the basic non–rate-adaptive mode. In the VVIR mode, there is a sensor-indicated rate that serves as the LRL; the ventricular escape interval varies based on the sensor-indicated rate. Similarly, in the DDDR mode, the sensor-indicated rate serves as the LRL. The timing cycles in DDDR are based on the sensor-indicated interval serving as the lower rate interval. The escape interval in a ventricular-based timing device is calculated by subtracting the paced AVI from the sensor-indicated interval.

Rate-Adaptive Algorithms

There are algorithms that attempt to permit more physiologic response to exertion by modulating programmable intervals as rate changes. For example, in some systems the AVI can be shortened when an increased atrial rate is sensed or when the sensor-driven rate increases (rate-adaptive AV delay). This feature attempts to simulate the physiologic narrowing of the AV conduction time (P-R interval) that occurs with exercise. When it is responding to increased intrinsic atrial rates, it also permits a higher MTR. Because the AVI is shortened, the TARP (PVARP + AVI) also shortens, allowing for a higher 2:1 atrial tracking rate (60,000 ÷ TARP in beats per minute). A high 2:1 AV block rate affords a higher MTR to maintain 1:1 AV synchrony. For individuals who cannot tolerate a shortened PVARP because of persistent retrograde conduction, who have impaired A-V conduction, rate-modulation of the AVI can be particularly useful. The AVI also may shorten as the sensor-driven rate increases. This permits the hemodynamic effects of sensor-driven pacing to be optimized with an AVI that shortens with exertion. The PVARP may also be rate-modulated. The rate adaptation is based on the physiologic observation of decreased retrograde conduction time with increased activity seen in normal subjects. When a rate-adaptive PVARP is programmed, the PVARP shortens as the sensor-determined rate increases, which also shortens the TARP (similar to rate-adaptive AVI) and allows for a higher 2:1 tracking rate. However, shortening of the PVARP rests on the assumption that retrograde conduction time will shorten with exertion. Individuals who have retrograde conduction that is slower than that assumed by the algorithms may be at risk for development of PMT.

Noise Response

To minimize electromagnetic interference from lead problems, myopotentials, and environmental noise, noise response algorithms have been developed. Positioned after the VRP, the noise sampling period (usually having a duration of 60 to 200 msec) interprets any sensed events as nonphysiologic noise. This detection results in extension of the VRP or noise sampling period. If the noise is intermittent, inappropriate sensing may result and pacing may be inhibited. With more continuous noise, the pacing can become asynchronous. Depending on the nature of the extrinsic electromagnetic source, the device may "revert" to one of several nominal settings, such as a reset mode, an emergency VVI mode, or the elective replacement indicator settings.

Pacemaker-Mediated Tachycardia Algorithms

Algorithms have been designed to prevent or terminate the phenomenon of PMT in dual-chamber pacemakers. PMT, or endless loop tachycardia (ELT), results from retrograde conduction to the atrium after a ventricular depolarization, which can be sensed and "tracked" by the atrial lead, triggering another ventricular pacing event. The retrograde limb of the PMT is the native conduction system, and the anterograde limb is atrial tracking in the dual-chamber mode. Each ventricular-paced beat results in retrograde conduction and perpetuation of the PMT. PMT is often triggered by a PVC. The uncoupling of AV synchrony, as with failure of atrial capture or a programmed AVI that is excessively long,

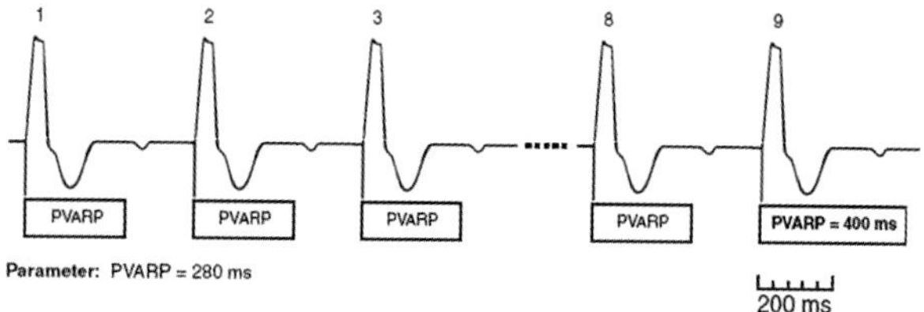

Figure 23-43. Pacemaker-mediated tachycardia (PMT) intervention using extension of the postventricular atrial refractory period (PVARP). PMT is initiated with a premature ventricular beat at the left side of the panel. After eight Vp-As intervals occur in less than 400 msec, the PMT intervention is initiated. The ninth ventricular paced event extends the PVARP to 400 msec for one cycle. Because the next atrial event is not tracked, the PMT terminates. As, atrial sensed event; Vp, ventricular paced event. (From Medtronic Enpulse Device Manual 5-13).

may result in PMT. Some algorithms are designed to prevent the initiation of PMT. The most common PMT-prevention algorithm is PVC-PVARP extension. Without a preceding atrial activation, individuals are especially vulnerable to PMT after a PVC, because retrograde VA conduction occurs relatively easily as the native conduction system is not yet refractory. When the pacemaker senses a ventricular event without a preceding atrial event, it identifies it as a PVC and automatically lengthens the PVARP to protect against potential retrograde conduction. Such a parameter does not require that the PVARP be extended at all times, which would result in an increase in the TARP and a decrease in the 2:1 atrial tracking rate. Algorithms also may detect retrograde conduction when it is present in a sensing window (e.g., the window of atrial rate acceleration detection [WARAD]).

Many algorithms have been developed to detect, terminate, or prevent PMT. Some algorithms may classify an atrial sensed and ventricular paced rhythm as PMT if atrial tracking occurs at a specific rate. The PMT detection rate may be the upper tracking rate or a rate greater than the upper tracking rate. Other algorithms detect PMT if repetitive atrial sensing follows ventricular pacing with a consistent V-to-A interval of less than 400 msec (compatible with retrograde VA conduction). When PMT is detected, different responses can occur. Some devices extend the PVARP, whereas others suspend atrial tracking for one cycle, causing PMT to terminate (Fig. 23-43).

Mode Switching

Automatic mode switching refers to the ability of the pacemaker to automatically switch from one mode of operation to another in response to a sensed atrial tachyarrhythmia[26-29] (Fig. 23-44). When atrial tachyarrhythmias occur, atrial tracking modes such as DDD(R) or VDD(R) can result in rapid ventricular pacing with resultant hemodynamic compromise. Mode-switching algorithms have been developed to detect the presence of atrial tachyarrhythmias and convert the pacemaker to a non–atrial tracking mode such as VVI(R) or DDI(R) (see Fig. 23-44). In some cases, mode switching in DDD

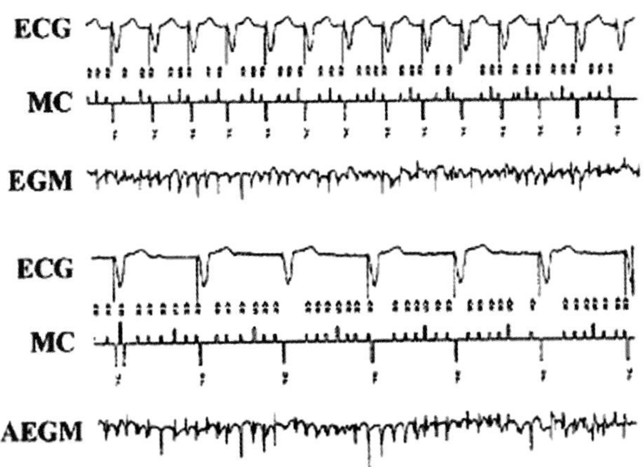

Figure 23-44. Activation of the mode-switching function from DDDR to DDIR. Activation of the mode-switching function results in conversion to the DDIR mode at 60 beats per minute. Mode-switching is seen in the bottom panel. AEGM, atrial electrogram; ECG, surface electrocardiogram; MC, marker channel. (From Lau CP, Leung SK, Tse HF, Barold SS: Automatic mode switching of implantable pacemakers: I. Principles of instrumentation, clinical, and hemodynamic considerations. PACE 25:967-985, 2002.)

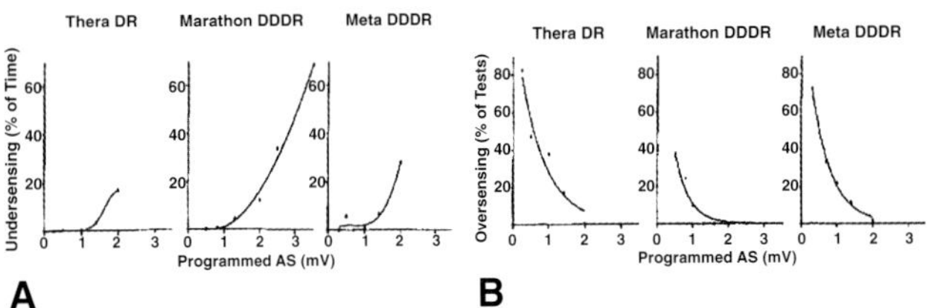

Figure 23-45. Dependence of ability to switch modes based on atrial sensitivity. Atrial undersensing increases as the device is made less sensitive. ***A,*** *At atrial sensitivities greater than 1 mV, atrial undersensing becomes apparent.* ***B,*** *As the atrial sensitivity approaches 2 mV, the degree of oversensing of noise becomes minimal. (From Lau CP, Leung SK, Tse HF, Barold SS: Automatic mode switching of implantable pacemakers: I. Principles of instrumentation, clinical, and hemodynamic considerations. PACE 25:967-985, 2002.)*

may result in either DDI or DDIR. An alternative mode-switching mode is VDI or VDIR. Before mode switching, there may a period of atrial tracking resulting in short paced intervals. Once mode switching is confirmed, the mode changes to the non–atrial tracking mode and the rate gradually decreases to the LRL.

Mode-switching functions are often programmable. The algorithms vary but may be triggered by a specific atrial rate threshold, either an absolute or an averaged atrial rate (in beats per minute). There is usually a requirement for a sustained duration of the high rate (a number of beats or a time duration) before mode switching occurs. Other devices deploy a "running counter" that increases when the atrial rate is faster and decreases when it is slower than a specified rate limit. The pacemaker switches modes only after the counter has reached a predetermined number. This prevents inappropriate mode switching in response to frequent isolated atrial ectopic beats. Some algorithms permit detection of premature atrial beats on a beat-to-beat basis. Lau and colleagues[26] described the perfect mode-switching system as having (1) rapid onset to avoid rapid ventricular pacing during initial detection of atrial tachyarrhythmias, (2) absence of fluctuation in rate or inappropriate response, (3) ability to restore AV synchrony rapidly after termination of atrial tachyarrhythmia, (4) ability to sense atrial tachyarrhythmias at a variety of rates and signal amplitudes, and (5) ability to avoid response to crosstalk, sinus tachycardia, and extraneous noise.

Nonetheless, detection of atrial arrhythmias remains the greatest challenge for mode-switching algorithms.[30-32] Undersensing is possible, because the amplitude of the atrial electrogram may decrease significantly during atrial tachyarrhythmia, compared with sinus rhythm. As the atrial channel becomes more sensitive, fewer undersensed events will occur, but there may be an increase in oversensing of noise or extraneous signals (Fig. 23-45). The ABP does not usually play a significant role in atrial undersensing during atrial fibrillation.[33] Oversensing can also be problematic, as with far-field signals (crosstalk) from ventricular depolarizations, T waves, myopotentials, or environmental noise. In the case of undersensing, mode switching may fail to occur, whereas in oversensing, mode switching may occur inappropriately.

Symptoms are usually minimized during mode switching because of the relative rapidity of the onset of mode switching. Even when mode switching occurs swiftly, however, some patients may remain symptomatic because of the abrupt change in rate. A comparison of three different mode-switching algorithms downloaded into an implanted pacemaker was made[34] (Fig. 23-46). The mean atrial interval was compared with "4 of 7" intervals and with a "1 of 1" interval as a criterion for mode switching. The shorter the criterion, the greater the number of episodes observed. The duration of mode switching decreased with shorter criteria, as expected. The symptoms did not vary significantly.

Atrial Flutter Response

Because atrial flutter may be associated with every other atrial electrogram falling into a blanking period, mode switching during atrial flutter may not reliably occur.[35] A special response may occur when atrial flutter is detected, leading to mode switching and preventing pacing during the atrial vulnerable period.[36] If an atrial event is detected within the PVARP, a programmable interval is created. Subsequent atrial events sensed within this programmable interval are not tracked, and each such event creates another programmable interval. This algorithm permits atrial tracking to be withheld even before mode switching occurs. In addition, atrial pacing does not occur until the programmable interval or PVARP expires. Once this happens, atrial pacing may occur if there are at least 50 msec and no more than the AV delay before the next ventricular paced beat. A related algorithm permits atrial flutter to trigger mode switching. If atrial cycles are sensed at an interval shorter than twice the AV delay plus the postventricular atrial blanking period

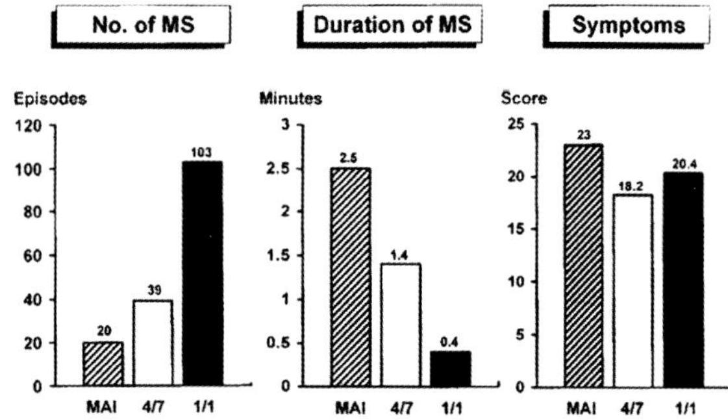

Figure 23-46. Effect of mode-switching criterion on mode switching criteria and frequency. Three different mode switching algorithms were downloaded into an implanted pacemaker. The mean atrial interval (MAI) was compared with 4 of 7 intervals (4/7) and with 1 of 1 interval (1/1) as a criterion for mode switching. The shorter the criterion, the greater the number of episodes observed. The duration of mode switching decreased with shorter criteria, as expected. The symptoms did not vary significantly. (From Marshall HJ, Kay GN, Hess M, et al.: Mode switching in dual chamber pacemakers: Effect of onset criteria on arrhythmia-related symptoms. Europace 1:49-54, 1999.)

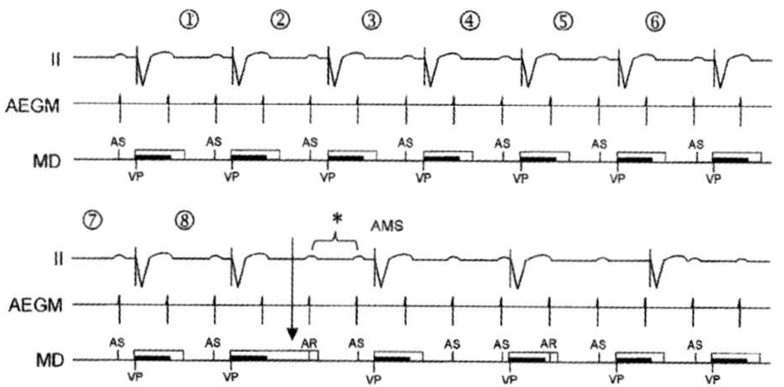

Figure 23-47. Atrial flutter algorithm to trigger mode switching. If atrial cycles are sensed at an interval shorter than twice the atrioventricular (AV) delay plus the postventricular atrial blanking period (PVABP) for eight consecutive cycles (asterisk), *the algorithm extends the PVARP to 400 msec for one cycle* (arrow). *AEGM, atrial electrogram; AMS, automatic mode switching; AR, atrial refractory; AS, atrial sensed; MD, marker diagram; VP, ventricular paced. (From Israel CW, Barold SS: Failure of atrial flutter detection by a pacemaker with a dedicated atrial flutter detection algorithm. PACE 25:1274-1277, 2002.)*

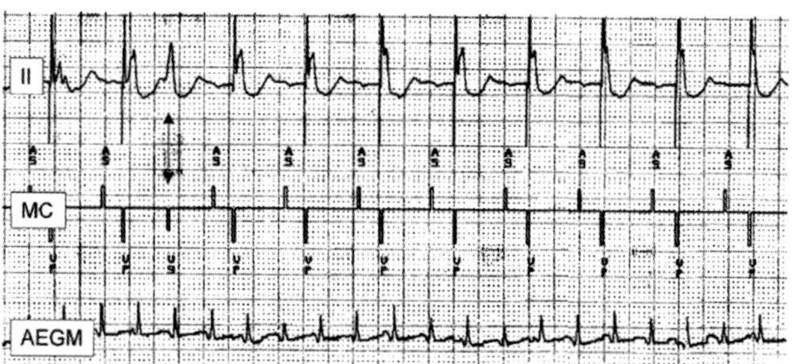

Figure 23-48. Failure of atrial flutter detection algorithm. Atrial flutter has an atrial cycle that places an atrial signal within the postventricular atrial blanking period (PVAB), so that the atrial flutter response never occurs. AEGM, atrial electrogram; MC, marker channel. (From Israel CW, Barold SS: Failure of atrial flutter detection by a pacemaker with a dedicated atrial flutter detection algorithm. PACE 25:1274-1277, 2002.)

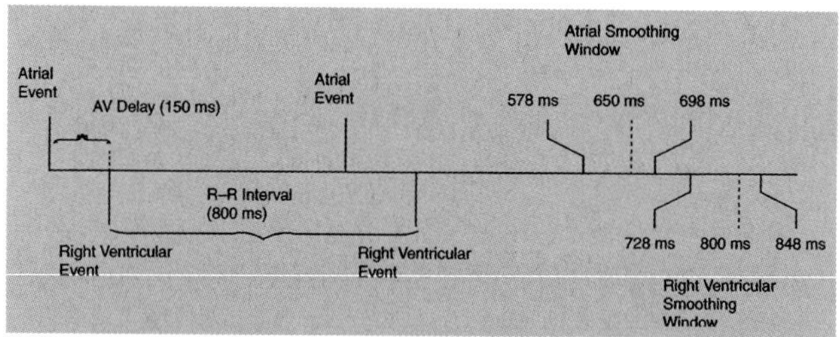

Figure 23-49. Rate-smoothing algorithm. The rate-smoothing algorithm adjusts the intervals of the successive atrial and ventricular events based on the previous cycle length rather than just the programmed atrial escape interval or the upper rate tracking interval. When rates are decreasing, the rate of slowing is constrained by the rate smoothing "down" percentage. In contrast, with increases in rate, such as with rapid atrial tracking, the rate smoothing "up" percentage constrains the rate. In the example, the atrial and ventricular events must occur within the atrial and ventricular smoothing windows.

(PVAB) for eight consecutive cycles, the algorithm extends the PVARP to 400 msec for one cycle (Fig. 23-47). The atrial signal that had been tracked is now refractory and may activate mode switching. Figure 23-48 presents an example of atrial flutter with an atrial cycle that places an atrial signal within the PVAB, so that the atrial flutter response never occurs.

Rate Smoothing

Rate-smoothing algorithms are designed to "smooth" and prevent sudden changes in heart rates accompanied by hemodynamic compromise or symptoms. Sinus arrest may result in an abrupt decrease in heart rate to the escape rate, for example from 80 to 50 bpm. Rate smoothing results in a more gradual decrease in heart rate. The rate of decrease or increase in rate is constrained, respectively, by the programmed rate-smoothing "down" or "up" percentage, usually between 3% and 24%. A rate-smoothing atrial or ventricular window is created, which determines when the next atrial-paced or ventricular-paced event will occur (figure rate smoothing). The ventricular window is created by calculating the previous V-V interval and multiplying it by the rate-smoothing percentage. For example, if the previous cycle length was 1000 msec, the rate-smoothing up percentage was 12%, and the rate smoothing down percentage was 8%, the width of the rate smoothing up window would be 120 msec and that of the rate smoothing down window would be 80 msec. The atrial rate-smoothing window is calculated by subtracting the AV delay from the boundaries of the ventricular rate-smoothing window (Fig. 23-49).

Sudden changes in ventricular rate can also occur in patients with intermittent atrial arrhythmias or atrial fibrillation.[37] Tracking of an atrial arrhythmia that may be too transient or too slow to trigger mode switching can result in palpitations or other symptoms caused by the abrupt increase in heart rate. Rate smoothing up may limit the ventricular rate to reduce the suddenness of the heart rate increase. Mode switching may interact with a variety of other programmed parameters. Ventricular tachycardia prevention algorithms may become inactivated by mode switching.[38]

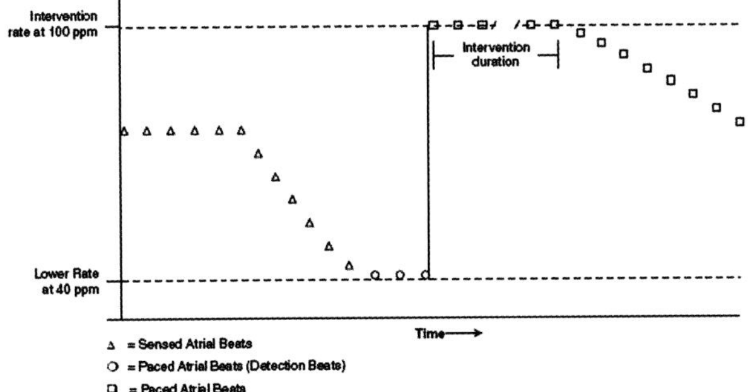

Figure 23-50. Rate drop response. The rate drop response results in pacing at a faster rate (intervention rate) when an abrupt drop in the ventricular rate occurs, defined as a minimum drop in heart rate over a range of detection intervals. A minimum rate for a specific number of intervals alone may be used to trigger this response. The intervention rate is the pacing rate for the programmed period of time. (From Medtronic Enpulse device manual 5-22.)

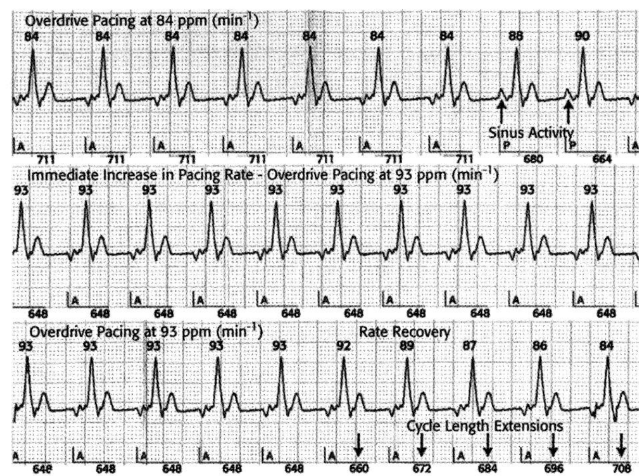

Figure 23-51. Atrial fibrillation pacing suppression algorithm. Atrial fibrillation pacing parameters may be set to stimulate the atrium at rates faster than the intrinsic atrial rate in order to suppress the triggers of atrial fibrillation. When two P waves are detected within a 16-cycle window, the atrial pacing algorithm is initiated. The pacing occurs for a programmable number of pacing cycles. In this example, atrial pacing is already at 84 beats per minute. Because two sinus beats occur, the pacing rate increases. The pacing occurs for a programmable number of intervals, and then the interval is gradually decreased. (From St. Jude Identity device manual.)

Fall Back

The fall back response provides a response very similar to rate smoothing by limiting the rate of the heart rate change.[39] Fall back may occur when the rate decreases from the upper rate limit to the LRL during mode switching or other rate drop response.

Rate Drop Response

Patients who experience neurocardiogenic or vasovagal syncope become symptomatic when the heart rate falls precipitously. The rate drop response (RDR) algorithm is designed to recognize a rapid decline in heart rate using a heart rate–time duration detection window. The degree of rate drop (in beats per minute) within the specified duration (in number of beats) is programmable. The newer algorithm uses an averaged ventricular baseline rate as the reference. Once the RDR is triggered, dual-chamber pacing is initiated at a relatively fast rate, either an absolute rate (100 to 120 bpm) or a relative rate (70% or 80% of the maximum heart rate) (Fig. 23-50). The sudden bradycardia response (SBR) is another example of this type of rate algorithm. This response is initiated by a decline in the atrial rate by more than 10 bpm for a programmed number of beats (1 to 8 beats), with a weighted average serving as the baseline rate. The SBR response consists of pacing at a rate that is 5 to 40 bpm faster than the previous rate.

Prevention of Atrial Fibrillation

There has been considerable interest in using atrial pacing for prevention of atrial fibrillation(AF).[40-44] The Pacemaker Selection Trial for the Elderly (PASE) study and the Canadian Trial of Physiological Pacing (CTOPP)[45] showed that atrial pacing or dual-chamber pacing is associated with a lower occurrence of atrial fibrillation compared with ventricular pacing alone.[40,46,47]

Pacing from sites other than the right atrium, such as the atrial septum or Bachman's bundle, has been shown to decrease the incidence of atrial fibrillation. Atrial pacing at two sites, such as the right atrium and the coronary sinus ostium, has also been examined for its effect on atrial fibrillation. Multisite atrial pacing has also shown varying efficacy in prevention of atrial fibrillation.

There are specific atrial pacing algorithms that have been studied as possible methods of decreasing atrial fibrillation. Prospective randomized trials, such as the Atrial Dynamic Overdrive Pacing Trial (ADOPT) and the Overdrive Atrial Septum Stimulation (OASIS) trial, demonstrated significant reductions in atrial fibrillation burden using the Dynamic Atrial Overdrive (DAO) algorithm (St. Jude Medical, St. Paul, Minn.). Continuous atrial overdrive pacing is maintained by setting the atrial lower rate higher than the intrinsic sinus rate. The atrial pacing rate is adjusted in response to the mean atrial rate or the occurrence of premature atrial beats, or both. Atrial fibrillation pacing parameters may be set to stimulate the atrium at rates faster than the intrinsic atrial rate in order to suppress the triggers of atrial fibrillation (Fig. 23-51). When two P waves are detected within a 16-cycle window, the atrial pacing algorithm is initiated. The pacing occurs for a programmable number of pacing cycles, and then the interval is gradually decreased. Atrial pacing preference (APP) system paces in response to the atrial rate but not to premature atrial beats. In contrast, atrial pacing may specifically respond to atrial sensing in a specific interval. The atrial overdrive in a DDD(R) mode is triggered whenever two spontaneous P waves are sensed in a 16-beat window. The extent of atrial overdrive is a nonprogrammable parameter, determined by the instantaneous atrial rate. Other algorithms that increase atrial pacing include the continuous atrial pacing algorithm, which paces at 30 msec shorter than the intrinsic atrial cycle length, and a double-algorithm

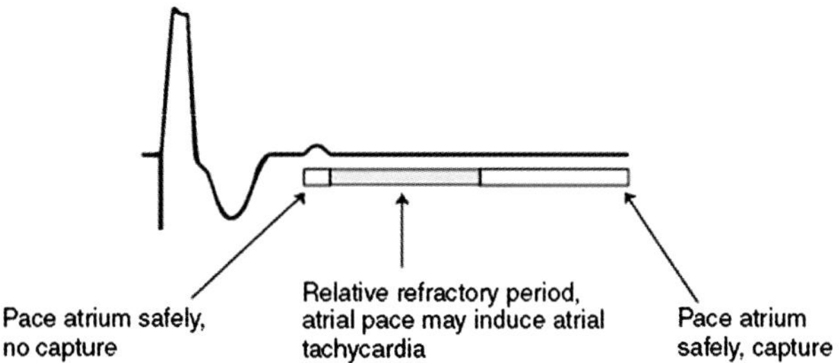

Figure 23-52. *Noncompetitive atrial pacing algorithm. Pacing after a premature atrial beat that occurs during the postventricular atrial refractory period (PVARP) may cause atrial arrhythmias. To prevent so-called competitive pacing, algorithms have been developed. If an atrial event occurs within the PVARP, an additional window, called the noncompetitive atrial pacing (NCAP) period, is created. Atrial pacing is delayed until the end of this period, allowing the atrium additional time to repolarize. (From Medtronic Enpulse device manual 5-10.)*

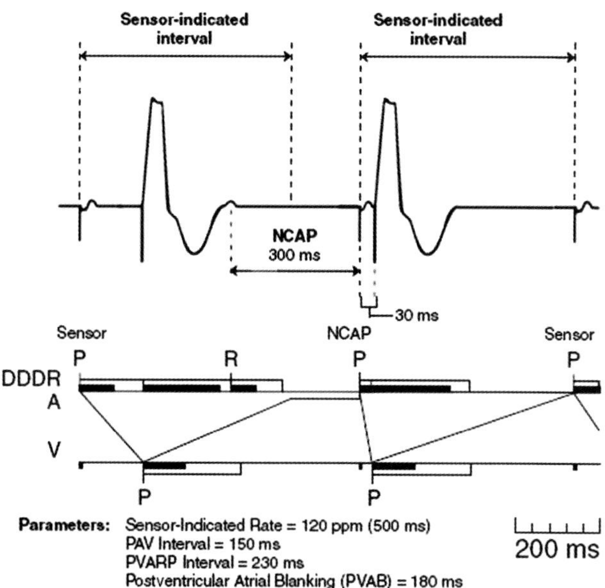

Figure 23-53. *Noncompetitive atrial pacing algorithm and ventricular timing. If an atrial event is sensed during the postventricular atrial refractory period (PVARP), the atrial pacing impulse will be delayed. In order to stabilize the ventricular rate, the atrioventricular (AV) interval may be shortened to a minimum of 30 msec. NCAP, noncompetitive atrial pacing period; PAV, paced A-V interval. (From Medtronic Enpulse device manual 5-10.)*

approach, which alters pacing in response to atrial premature beats (used by the Medtronic AT 500, Medtronic, Minneapolis, Minn.). However, such high-rate overdrive pacing may result in undersensing due to a short atrial sensing window. Rare cases of proarrhythmia have been reported.

Algorithms have also been used to prevent induction of atrial fibrillation caused by atrial pacing after an intrinsic P wave. To prevent so-called competitive pacing, if an atrial event occurs within the PVARP, an additional window, called the noncompetitive atrial pacing (NCAP) period, is created. Atrial pacing is delayed until the end of this period, allowing the atrium additional time to repolarize (Fig. 23-52). In addition, the AV interval may be shortened to a minimum of 30 msec, to stabilize the ventricular rate (Fig. 23-53).

There is a need for greater understanding of the efficacy, technique, and physiology of atrial pacing compared with dual-chamber pacing. In addition to prevention of atrial fibrillation, there is some evidence that atrial overdrive pacing may terminate some atrial arrhythmias that lead to atrial fibrillation.

Noncompetitive Atrial Pacing

In order to prevent atrial pacing after an intrinsic atrial event has occurred during an ARP, or competitive atrial pacing, a noncompetitive atrial pacing feature may be programmed ON. This programmable parameter delays the time at which the atrial pacing stimulus occurs. Atrial sensed events may occur in the PVARP during upper rate behavior, and competitive pacing is most likely to occur when there is sensor-driven atrial pacing (see Fig. 23-52). Shortening the PVARP is another method of preventing competitive pacing, but retrograde conduction may limit this option (see Fig. 23-53).

Managed Ventricular Pacing

Growing evidence in the literature suggests that right ventricular pacing is detrimental to hemodynamics in a number of patient populations. The AAIsafeR algorithm functions in the AAI mode with a conversion to DDD in the event of high-grade AV block.[48] A managed ventricular pacing (MVP) algorithm is designed to minimize unnecessary right ventricular pacing. The MVP algorithm operates in an AAI(R) mode to minimize ventricular pacing; however, ventricular backup pacing is available in a VVI mode if heart block occurs. Backup ventricular pacing is triggered by any A-A interval that occurs without a sensed ventricular event and is delivered at an interval equal to the A-A interval plus 80 msec. MVP automatic switches from an AAI(R) to a DDD(R) mode if no ventricular sensed event occurs in 2 of 4 preceding A-A intervals (multiple heart blocks occur in a 4-beat window) (Fig. 23-54). MVP maintains the dual-chamber DDD(R) mode for 1 minute and then performs an "AV conduction check." The device monitors AV conduction by temporarily switching back to AAI(R) timing during one A-A cycle. The AV conduction check is scheduled at 2 minutes, 4 minutes, 8 minutes, and so on, up to 16 hours after a transition to DDD(R) has occurred. If spontaneous R waves are sensed, the device reverts back to the AAI(R) operation (Fig. 23-55). Significant reduction of ventricular pacing has been demonstrated with the MVP algorithm. A "dynamic atrial refractory period" has been developed to avoid inappropriate switch to DDD(R) mode caused by nonconducted premature atrial ectopy or far-field R-wave oversensing. The net result of MVP is a reduction in the frequency of ventricular pacing.[49]

Ventricular Rate Regularization

Because irregularity of the ventricular rate during atrial fibrillation may be responsible for many of the symp-

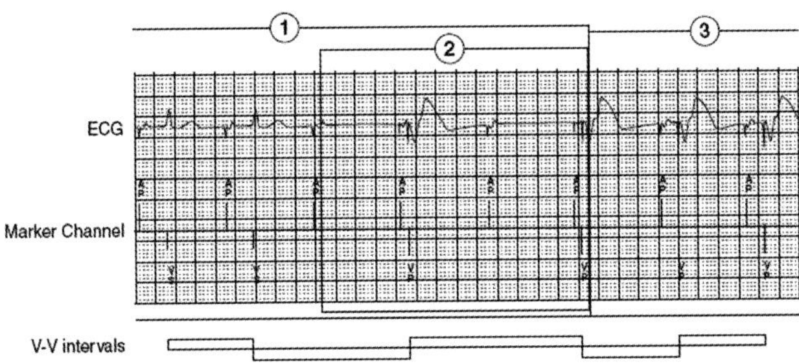

Figure 23-54. *AAIR-to-DDDR mode switching. The managed ventricular pacing algorithm permits the pacemaker to automatically switch from AAIR to DDDR mode and from DDDR to AAIR mode. If transient loss of conduction occurs in the AAIR mode, after an A-A interval without a ventricular sensed event, a ventricular paced event will occur 80 msec after the escape interval. If two of the four most recent A-A intervals are missing a ventricular event, the device will switch from AAIR to DDDR or from AAI to DDD. (1), AAIR mode; (2) AV block results in ventricular backup paced beat; (3) switch to DDDR mode. (From Medtronic Intrinsic 30 7288/7287 reference manual p 169.)*

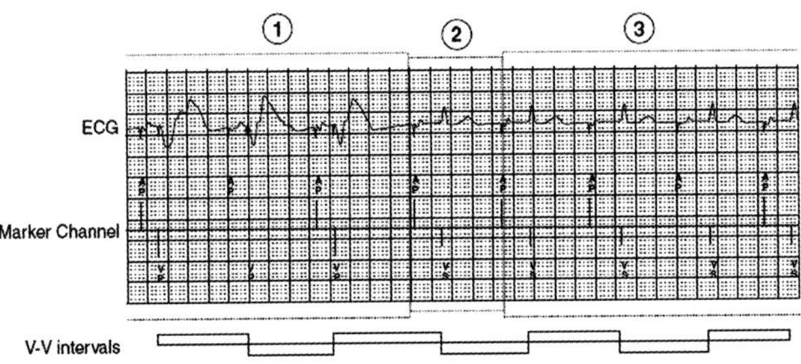

Figure 23-55. *DDDR-to-AAIR mode switching. The managed ventricular pacing algorithm permits the pacemaker to automatically switch from AAIR to DDDR mode and from DDDR to AAIR mode. In the DDDR mode (1), the device periodically checks for atrioventricular (AV) conduction. If AV conduction is present (2), the device switches to the DDDR mode (3). (From Medtronic Intrinsic 30 7288/7287 reference manual, p 169.)*

toms that occur during atrial fibrillation, algorithms may attempt to pace in an effort to regularize the rhythm. These algorithms adjust the presence of pacing in response to the presence of ventricular sensed beats. Algorithms called ventricular response pacing (Fig. 23-56) or ventricular rate regulation (VRR) pace in response to sensed ventricular events.[50] If a ventricular sensed event occurs, the ventricular pacing rate is increased, and if a ventricular paced event occurs, the ventricular pacing rate is decreased. Clinical studies have demonstrated that the variability in ventricular intervals in atrial fibrillation is markedly decreased by this approach (Fig. 23-57).

DDD Hysteresis and Search Hysteresis

Dual-chamber devices are capable of exhibiting hysteresis analogous to ventricular or atrial hysteresis. In dual-chamber hysteresis, the escape interval timed from an intrinsic ventricular event is longer than the escape interval after a paced ventricular event.

In search hysteresis, the LRL is lowered periodically to promote intrinsic activity. After a programmed number of intervals, the device looks for intrinsic activity. During this period, if there is no intrinsic activity, pacing will occur at a rate that is a programmed amount (hysteresis offset) less than the LRL for a specified duration (e.g., eight cycles). If no intrinsic atrial activity is sensed, pacing will resume at the LRL or sensor-indicated rate. Search hysteresis helps to promote intrinsic impulse formation.

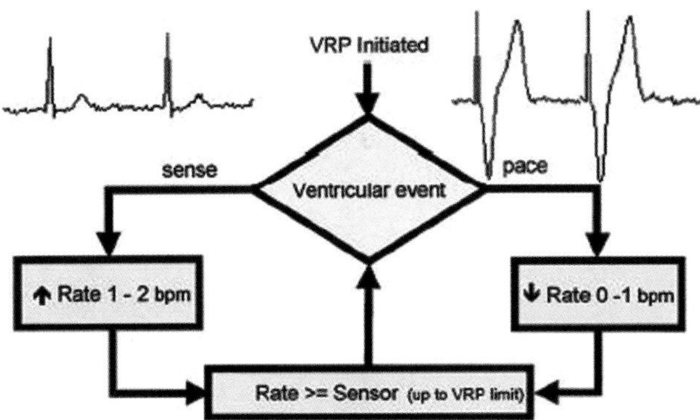

Figure 23-56. *Ventricular response pacing. In response to a ventricular sensed event, the ventricular pacing rate is increased by 0 to 1 beats per minute; in response to a ventricular paced event, the ventricular pacing rate is decreased. VRP, ventricular response pacing. (From Tse HF, Newman D, Ellenbogen KA, et al.: Effects of ventricular rate regularization pacing on quality of life and symptoms in patients with atrial fibrillation. Atrial Fibrillation Symptoms Mediated by Pacing to Mean Rates [AF Symptoms Study]. Am J Cardiol 94:938-941, 2004.)*

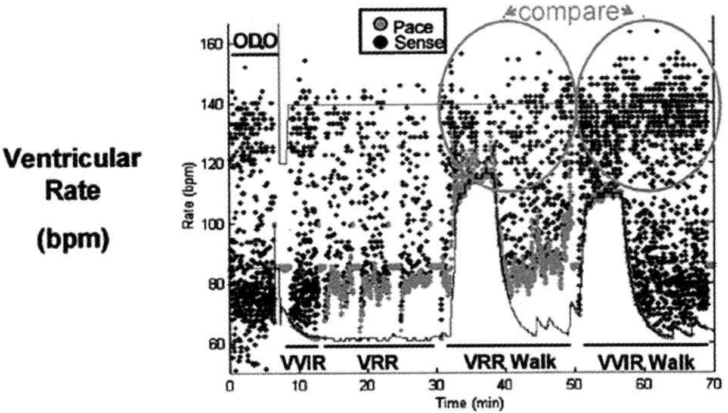

Figure 23-57. *Ventricular response pacing. At rest and during exercise, during VRR (VVIR mode with ventricular response pacing ON), a lower proportion of patients have fast ventricular rates, compared with VVIR only (with ventricular response pacing OFF). VRP, ventricular response pacing; VRR, ventricular response rate. (From Tse HF, Newman D, Ellenbogen KA, et al.: Effects of ventricular rate regularization pacing on quality of life and symptoms in patients with atrial fibrillation. Atrial Fibrillation Symptoms Mediated by Pacing to Mean Rates [AF Symptoms Study]. Am J Cardiol 94:938-941, 2004.)*

Repetitive Ventriculoatrial Synchrony

Competitive atrial pacing may also occur after a premature ventricular complex that conducts retrograde. Unlike in PMT, the P wave falls within the PVARP. However, the next atrial pacing stimulus comes soon

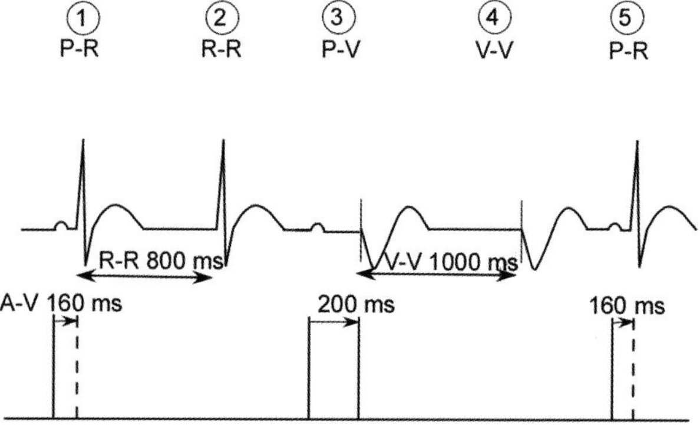

Figure 23-58. *VDD mode. In the VDD mode, atrial sensed events are tracked, initiating an atrioventricular (AV) delay. If the AV delay is not followed by a sensed ventricular event within the programmed AV delay, a ventricular paced event will occur unless the upper rate limit has been reached. In this example, the lower rate is 60 beats per minute (bpm), and the upper rate limit is 120 bpm, with an AV delay of 200 msec. In beat 1, the P wave starts an AV delay, but AV conduction occurs, so that the timing cycle is reset by the ventricular sensed event, the ventricular complex of beat 2. Before the lower rate limit can time out from beat 2 to beat 3, an intrinsic P wave again occurs. In this case, there is no ventricular sensed event by the time the AV interval expires, and so another ventricular paced event occurs in beat 3. The ventricular paced event in beat 3 resets the timing cycle, and a new V-V interval is created. From beat 3 to beat 4, there is no intrinsic P wave or R wave. Therefore, a ventricular paced event at the lower rate limit of 60 bpm (1000 msec) occurs. A new ventricular escape interval is created. Between beat 4 and beat 5, a P wave occurs, which is again tracked, creating a new AV delay. As in beat 1, intrinsic conduction occurs before the new AV delay is completed. A, atrial paced event; P, atrial sensed event; R, ventricular sensed event; V, ventricular paced event.*

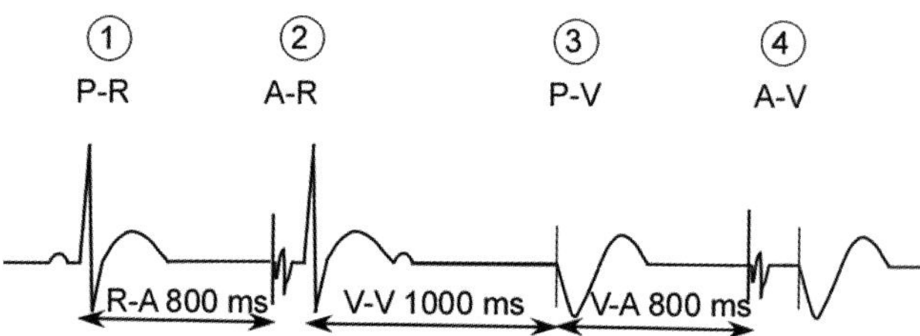

Figure 23-59. *DDI mode. In the DDI mode, atrial sensed events are not tracked but inhibit atrial pacing. If the atrioventricular (AV) delay is not followed by a sensed ventricular event within the programmed AV delay, a ventricular paced event will occur unless the upper rate limit has been reached. In this example, the lower rate is 60 beats per minute (bpm) with an AV delay of 200 msec. In beat 1, the P wave inhibits atrial pacing and the R wave occurs before the lower rate limit times out. In beat 2, atrial pacing occurs at the end of the atrial escape interval, because no spontaneous P wave occurs. The R wave occurs before the lower rate interval of 1000 msec expires. In beat 3, a P wave occurs and results in inhibition of atrial pacing. Atrial pacing occurs at the end of the atrial escape interval of 800 msec, because no atrial sensed event has occurred. Because no sensed ventricular event occurs, a ventricular paced event also occurs. A, atrial paced event; P, atrial sensed event; R, ventricular sensed event; V, ventricular paced event.*

after the P wave and is not captured due to tissue refractoriness. The next ventricular event is paced and conducts retrograde. As a result, the pattern of VA conduction and competitive atrial pacing perpetuates itself. This phenomenon, sometimes been called repetitive non-reentrant VA synchrony, may result in impaired hemodynamics.

Timing Cycles in Other Dual-Chamber Modes

VDD Mode

The VDD mode offers both atrial and ventricular sensing with only ventricular pacing (Fig. 23-58). Tracking of atrial activity occurs similar to the DDD mode. When an atrial event is sensed, the AVI is initiated, and, if a ventricular intrinsic event is not sensed by the end of the interval, a ventricular paced event is triggered. Sensing also occurs in the ventricle, which inhibits ventricular pacing. The VDD mode is not appropriate for individuals who have impaired sinus node function, because there is no atrial pacing. This mode is mostly employed in pacemaker systems in which there is a single lead that paces and senses the ventricle and senses the atrium using a specially designed "floating" atrial electrode.

DDI Mode

AV sequential pacing with dual-chamber sensing, non–P-synchronous DDI mode provides sensing and pacing in the atrium and ventricle but does not track. When atrial events are sensed, atrial pacing is inhibited, but, unlike in the DDD mode, the AVI is not initiated (Fig. 23-59). Ventricular paced events after atrial sensed events will occur at the LRL rather than after the AV delay. Ventricular sensed events result in inhibition of ventricular pacing and resetting of the AEI. Absence of intrinsic atrial events or ventricular events by the end of the LRL results in pacing in the atrium or ventricle, respectively. This mode is best suited for patients who are at risk for atrial tachyarrhythmias, because there is no atrial tracking, resulting in rapid ventricular pacing during atrial tachyarrhythmia. This mode can be useful in cases in which the mode-switching feature is unavailable or does not accurately function. In this mode, the absence of tracking results in the inability of faster intrinsic sinus rates to be followed by ventricular paced beats as the sinus rate increases in response to greater metabolic demands with exertion or exercise. In addition, AV synchrony is lost when the intrinsic sinus rate exceeds the LRL and AV conduction is absent or impaired. The use of DDIR pacing programmed so that sensor-driven pacing predominates will result in maintenance of AV synchrony.

Other Modes

A host of other modes are used less frequently as permanent settings or only in particular circumstances. The asynchronous modes AOO, VOO, and DOO, which pace constantly in the atrium, ventricle, or both chambers, respectively, have been discussed. These modes

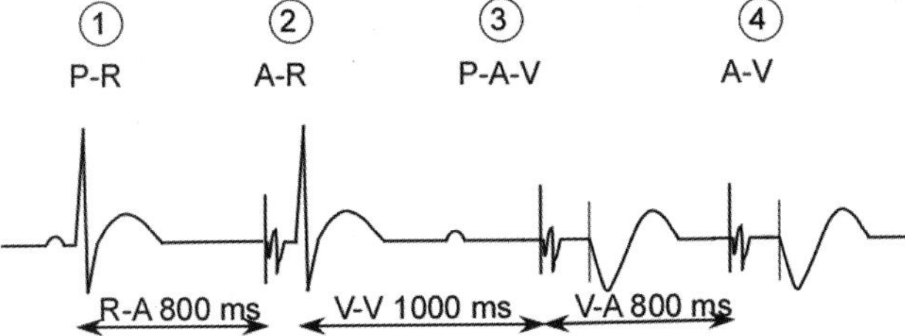

Figure 23-60. DVI mode. In the DVI mode, the atrium and the ventricle are paced, but only the ventricle is sensed. As a result, it is possible that atrial pacing may occur after an intrinsic atrial event. In beat 1, the R wave is sensed and creates a new atrial escape interval of 800 msec. In beat 2, atrial pacing occurs because a ventricular event has not occurred since the last ventricular event. Because there is conduction of the R wave, a ventricular paced event does not occur. In beat 3, a spontaneous P wave occurs, followed by atrial and ventricular pacing. It is possible that the atrial pacing after a spontaneous P wave could result in atrial arrhythmias. In beat 4, atrial and ventricular pacing occurs because no ventricular sensed event has occurred.

are generally used to prevent potential oversensing, such as electromagnetic interferences from electrocautery during surgery. Other sources of possible interference include transcutaneous electric stimulation (TENS), diathermy, and lithotripsy in pacemaker-dependent patients.

There are also triggered modes, VVT and AAT, which deliver an impulse immediately when an event in the respective chamber is sensed. These modes historically were used diagnostically to mark sensed events (in evaluating undersensing or oversensing problems), before the availability of intracardiac electrograms and marker channels. However, triggered modes are not used commonly in current practice.

The VDI mode is used similarly to the VVI mode, in which pacing in the ventricle will occur unless an intrinsic ventricular depolarization is sensed within the LRL. However, atrial sensed events are also sensed, but they do not result in ventricular tracking. Instead, they are recorded for later evaluation, such as evaluation of atrial arrhythmias. Sometimes mode-switching algorithms will initiate the VDI mode if an atrial tachyarrhythmia is sensed.

In the DVI mode (AV sequential, ventricular inhibited), which is the least used mode, the pacemaker provides pacing in both the atrium and ventricle (D), but only events in the ventricle (V) inhibit pacing. An AEI is reset after a sensed or paced ventricular event followed by an asynchronous atrial pacing output. However, a sensed spontaneous ventricular event within the AEI inhibits and resets both atrial and ventricular pacing stimuli. The atrial pacing stimulus is followed by the AVI, and a spontaneous R wave will inhibit the ventricular output. The difference between DVI and DDI is that no atrial sensing is incorporated in the DVI mode, in which constant, competitive atrial pacing may occur (Fig. 23-60). The absence of atrial sensing may result in a paced atrial impulse immediately after an intrinsic atrial event, potentially triggering atrial tachyarrhythmia.

Timing Cycles in Biventricular Pacing

Goals of Biventricular Pacing

The primary goal of bradycardia pacing is to achieve heart rates that are adequate to prevent symptoms and meet metabolic demand.[51,52] To achieve this goal, bradycardia pacing timing cycles are designed to keep the heart rates from being too slow and to maintain appropriate AV synchrony.

Heart failure may be associated with abnormal electrical delay and/or mechanical dyssynchrony. Such depressed and uncoordinated interventricular and intraventricular contraction delays are responsible for the reduced pumping effectiveness. Resynchronization therapy has been shown to improve the functional capacity of patients with wide QRS complexes, left ventricular dysfunction, left ventricular dilatation, and heart failure. Indices such as quality of life, 6-minute walk time, and heart failure class have also been shown to improve with biventricular pacing resynchronization therapy. In addition, randomized studies have demonstrated a decreased mortality rate and improved left ventricular dimensions and function. However, the benefits of resynchronization therapy are based on improved hemodynamics achieved by stimulating the heart in a more coordinated manner and minimizing interventricular and intraventricular dyssynchrony (resynchronization). Therefore, resynchronization requires that consistent pacing be maintained despite the absence of bradycardia. These distinct goals demand a new set of timing cycle rules for biventricular devices.

Timing Cycles: Differences from Dual-Chamber Timing Cycles

Pacing Modes

Pacing modes for resynchronization therapy are similar to those for standard pacemakers, and the general criteria for mode selection are similar. In patients with chronic atrial fibrillation, VVIR pacing is the most commonly used mode, in order to achieve rate responsiveness and to maintain as close as possible to 100% ventricular pacing. In patients without atrial fibrillation, VDI, DDD, and DDDR are the most commonly used modes. VDI is appropriate for patients with normal sinus node function and intact AV conduction. DDDR should be selected for patients with chronotropic incompetence due to relative sinus bradycardia. VDI, DDD, or DDDR mode provides the capability of atrial tracking with AV coordination. The optimal hemodynamics of resynchronization therapy require maintenance of AV synchrony with maximum biventricular pacing and capture. There is no role, therefore, for AAI or other algorithms that promote intrinsic AV conduction. The basic timing cycle during resynchronization therapy relies on an AVI that maintains ventricular capture.

The timing cycles for biventricular pacemakers are potentially complex, depending on which chamber or

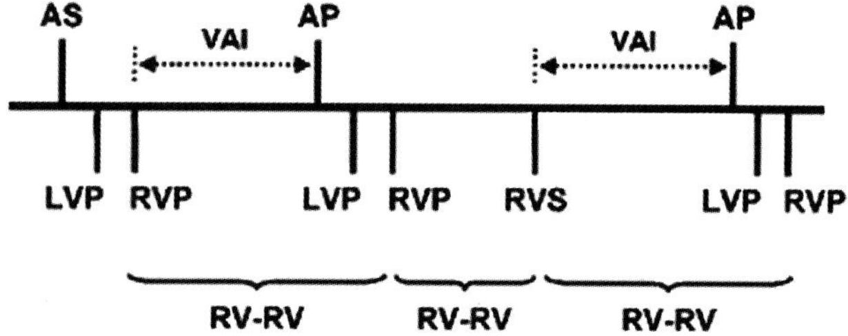

Figure 23-61. Biventricular pacing with right ventricle (RV)–based timing may occur after a sensed or paced atrial event. AP, atrial paced event; AS, atrial sensed event; LVP, paced left ventricular event; RVP, paced right ventricular event; RVS, sensed right ventricular event; RV-RV, interval between RV events; VAI, ventriculoatrial interval. (From Wang P, Kramer A, Estes NA 3rd, Hayes DL: Timing cycles for biventricular pacing. PACE 25:62-75, 2002.)

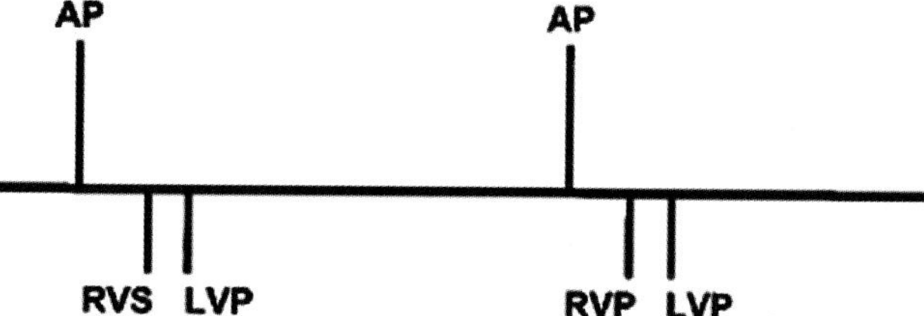

Figure 23-62. Biventricular pacing with right ventricular sensed event (RVS) before left ventricular paced event (LVP). An atrial paced event (AP) starts the atrioventricular (AV) delay. The RVS occurs before the LVP (positive RV-LV interval) in the first cycle. In the next cycle, the AV delay has been shortened so that the right ventricular paced event (RVP) may preempt the RVS. (From Wang P, Kramer A, Estes NA 3rd, Hayes DL: Timing cycles for biventricular pacing. PACE 25:62-75, 2002.)

chambers are sensed, which ventricle or ventricles are paced, the interventricular delay, and the chamber or chambers that reset the escape intervals.[52-56] For most commercially available biventricular devices, the sensing chamber is usually the RV and occasionally both ventricles (for older devices with ventricles connected via a Y-connection). Biventricular pacing activates both ventricular chambers, either simultaneously or sequentially (Fig. 23-61).

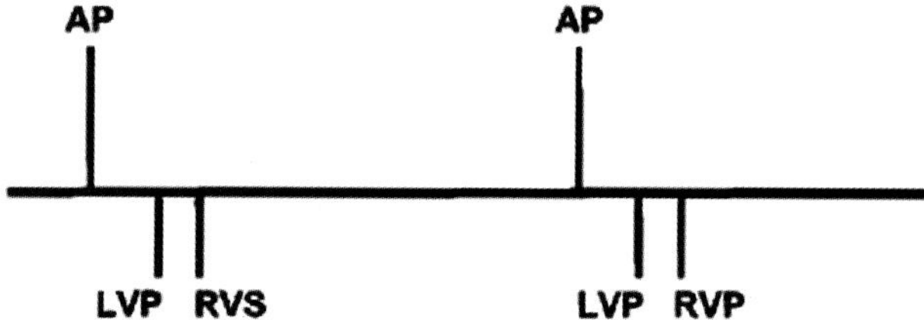

Figure 23-63. Biventricular pacing with left ventricular paced event (LVP) before right ventricular sensed event (RVS). In the first cycle, an LVP occurs before an RVS. In the next cycle, an LVP is followed by a right ventricular paced event (RVP), which may be achieved by shortening the LV-RV interval in response to the sensed RV event. (From Wang P, Kramer A, Estes NA 3rd, Hayes DL: Timing cycles for biventricular pacing. PACE 25:62-75, 2002.)

Atrioventricular Interval in Biventricular Pacing

For biventricular pacing to result in the desired hemodynamic effect, it is necessary for appropriately timed biventricular paced beats to occur after paced or sensed atrial events.[57] Therefore, the AVI must be sufficiently short to ensure biventricular capture and minimize fusion, yet long enough to allow adequate diastolic filling during the atrial contraction. Because the degree of native P-R shortening during exercise may be significant, this can be a particularly challenging task. Similarly, programming an extremely short fixed AV delay that applies to all rates and physiologic conditions is unlikely to be optimal, with ventricular depolarization and contraction occurring too early. In almost all cases, therefore, a form of rate-adaptive AV delay is used in resynchronization devices.

Several algorithms have been designed to maintain biventricular pacing and activation. When there is sensed ventricular activity on one pacing cycle, the AVI is shortened on the next timing cycle. This function is called AV hysteresis. If an atrial event is followed by a sensed right ventricular event, which is then followed by a left ventricular paced event, a right ventricular paced event and a left ventricular paced event may occur on the next cycle by shortening the time from the atrial sensed event to the right ventricular paced event (Fig. 23-62). In addition, if the left ventricular paced event occurs before the right ventricular sensed event, it is possible to shorten the LV-RV timing on subsequent cycles (Fig. 23-63). However, such "negative" AV hysteresis function is often ineffective, because permitting even one cycle with intrinsic conduction can have deleterious consequences. Perpetuation of native AV conduction and absence of biventricular pacing can result, as discussed later. If an intrinsic ventricular event is sensed within the AVI, one option might be to trigger a ventricular paced stimulus from the opposite ventricle, a so-called ventricular sensed response. For example, if a sensed event is detected by the right ventricular lead, a left ventricular pacing output is delivered immediately to maximize left ventricular capture and biventricular activation (Fig. 23-64). However, it is unclear whether there are limits to the benefit of this strategy, particularly with closely timed ventricular premature beats.

Interventricular Timing Delay

Analogous to the AVI in AV delay, there may be delay between pacing in the RV and LV (interventricular delay). There are several permutations of the relationship between the right and left ventricular timing based on the role of biventricular or unipolar sensing. With right ventricular sensing alone, which is predominantly the case in most devices today, the RV-LV interval may be positive, negative, or zero (Fig. 23-65). Several studies have demonstrated clinical or hemodynamic benefits of adjusting interventricular delay in patients who were classified as "nonresponders" to conventional resynchronization therapy. Various echocardio-

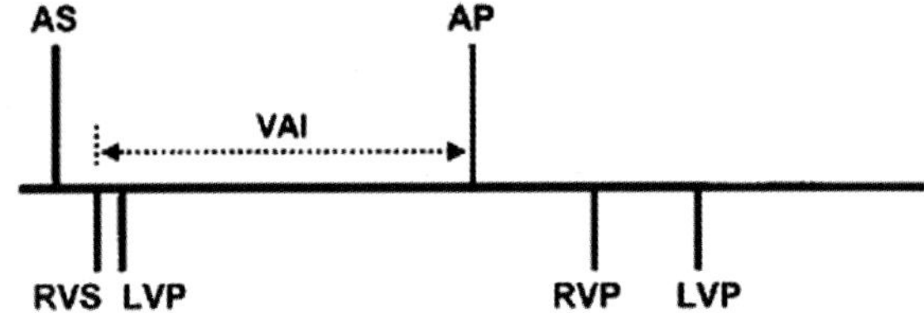

Figure 23-64. Biventricular sense response. If a right ventricular sensed event occurs, one option is for a left ventricular paced event (LVP) to occur almost immediately, to promote biventricular pacing. AS, atrial sensed event; AP, atrial paced event; RVP, paced right ventricular event; RVS, sensed right ventricular event; VAI, ventriculoatrial interval. (From Wang P, Kramer A, Estes NA 3rd, Hayes DL: Timing cycles for biventricular pacing. PACE 25:62-75, 2002.)

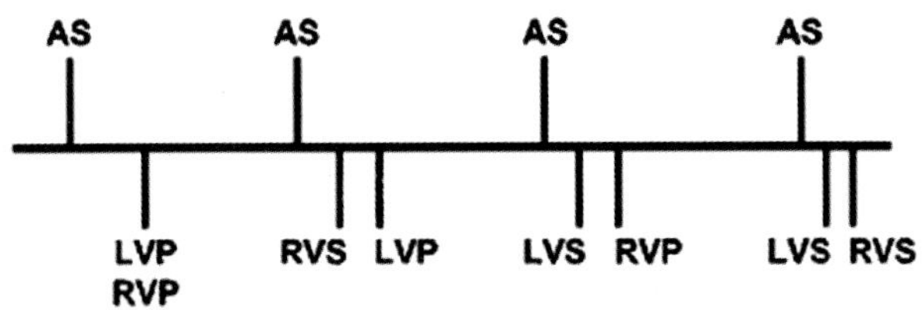

Figure 23-65. Biventricular RV-LV interval. The RV-LV interval may be positive, negative, or zero. AS, atrial sensed event; LVP, paced left ventricular event; RVP, paced right ventricular event;. RVS, sensed right ventricular event. (From Wang P, Kramer A, Estes NA 3rd, Hayes DL: Timing cycles for biventricular pacing. PACE 25:62-75, 2002.)

graphic Doppler parameters and timing intervals have been used to assess interventricular dyssynchrony, and tissue Doppler imaging (TDI) has been used to determine interventricular dyssynchrony for V-V optimization. The interduction of delay raises several theoretical issues. As discussed further in the context of univentricular sensing and biventricular pacing, an interventricular delay may increase the likelihood of induction of ventricular tachycardia due to an unsensed, improperly timed ventricular depolarization.

Lower Rate Behavior

As in dual-chamber pacing, a LRL is established. Atrial pacing will occur if an intrinsic atrial event does not occur at the LRL. There is a combination of events that may initiate ventricular events. In currently available devices, both ventricles may be paced, but timing is based on the RV only. One can theorize that a much larger range of combinations is possible: it is possible to pace both ventricles but to use the RV, LV, or both for ventricular timing.

Univentricular Sensing and Biventricular Pacing

Sensing may occur in one ventricle, as it does in dual-chamber pacing. There is not usually a particular risk of induction of ventricular tachycardia due to competitive pacing. For example, if left ventricular activation occurs before left ventricular pacing would occur, it is unlikely that the left ventricular pacing stimulus would

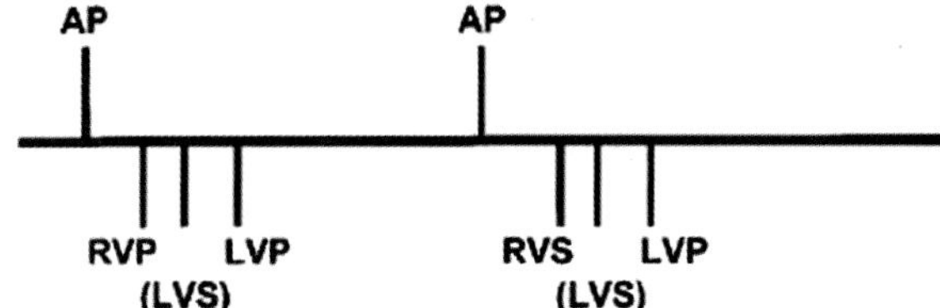

Figure 23-66. Right ventricular sensing only with positive RV-LV intervals. The right ventricle may be the only ventricular chamber sensed. There may be an intrinsic left ventricular event (LVS) that follows the right ventricular paced event (RVP). Because the left ventricular event is not sensed, the left ventricular pacing stimulus (LVP) will still be delivered. Because the LVP occurs after the LVS, the LVP is unlikely to be captured. AP, atrial paced event. (From Wang P, Kramer A, Estes NA 3rd, Hayes DL: Timing cycles for biventricular pacing. PACE 25:62-75, 2002.)

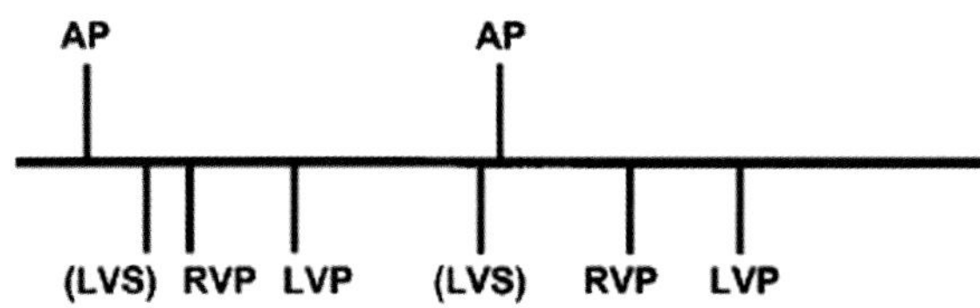

Figure 23-67. Right ventricular sensing only with premature left ventricular extrasystoles. The right ventricle may be the only ventricular chamber sensed. A spontaneous premature ventricular contraction originating in the left ventricle (LVS) will not be sensed if there is a significantly prolonged and negative RV-LV interval. As a consequence, it is possible that the left ventricular pacing stimulus (LVP) combined with the spontaneous LVS may result in ventricular proarrhythmia. There maybe an intrinsic LVS that follows a right ventricular paced event (RVP). Because the LVS is not sensed, the LVP will still be delivered. Because the LVP occurs after the intrinsic LVS, the LVP is unlikely to be captured. AP, atrial paced event. (From Wang P, Kramer A, Estes NA 3rd, Hayes DL: Timing cycles for biventricular pacing. PACE 25:62-75, 2002.)

be captured (Fig. 23-66). However, there may be a set of circumstances that increase the risk of competitive pacing. For example, if the intrinsic LV-RV conduction time is long and a long RV-LV delay is programmed, there are several scenarios that may result in a greater risk of competitive pacing.

In one situation, a left ventricular sensed event occurs before right ventricular and left ventricular pacing occurs. Because there may be a considerable interval between the intrinsic left ventricular event and the left ventricular pacing stimulus, the LV may no longer be refractory, resulting in left ventricular stimulation at a short coupling interval (Fig. 23-67). In another example, an unsensed premature beat that originates in the LV may be followed by an right ventricular paced event and then a left ventricular paced event. In such a case, the right ventricular paced event occurred before conduction from the spontaneous left ventricular PVC to the RV.

Biventricular Sensing and Biventricular Pacing

There are a variety of rules that might be created to determine how, for example, both ventricles could be

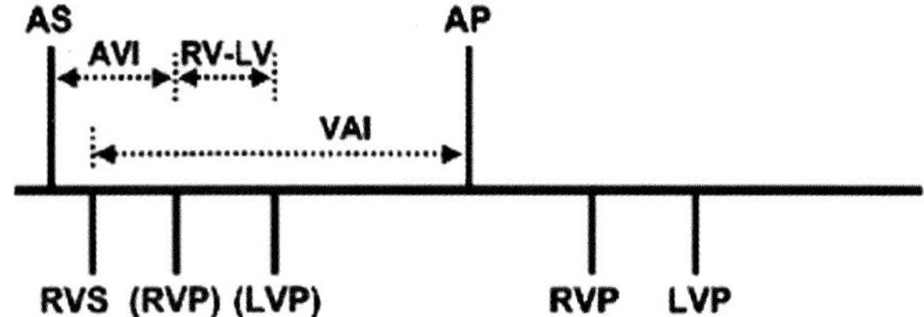

Figure 23-68. Right ventricular sensing only with inhibition of pacing. The right ventricle may be the only ventricular chamber sensed. When a right ventricular event is sensed, the timing cycles may be reset, resulting in inhibition of pacing. AP, atrial paced event; AS, atrial sensed event; AVI, atrioventricular interval; LVP, paced left ventricular event; RVP, paced right ventricular event; RVS, sensed right ventricular event; VAI, ventriculoatrial interval. (From Wang P, Kramer A, Estes NA 3rd, Hayes DL: Timing cycles for biventricular pacing. PACE 25:62-75, 2002.)

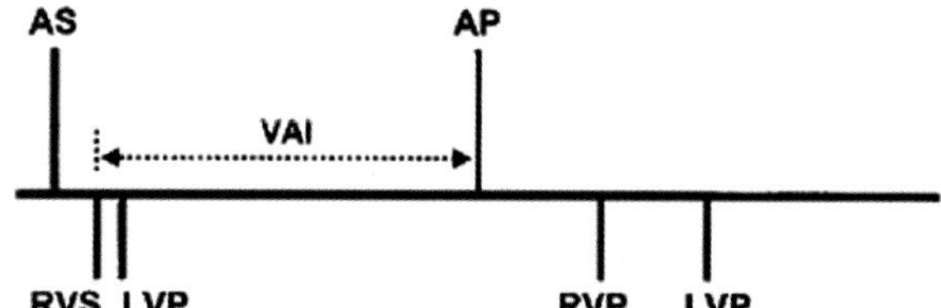

Figure 23-70. Biventricular sensing and pacing. Triggering may be present in devices that sense and pace in both the right ventricle and the left ventricle. If a right ventricular event is sensed, a left ventricular stimulus will be delivered immediately. AS, atrial sensed event; LVP, paced left ventricular event; LVS, sensed left ventricular event; RVP, paced right ventricular event; RVS, sensed right ventricular event; VAI, ventriculoatrial interval. (From Wang P, Kramer A, Estes NA 3rd, Hayes DL: Timing cycles for biventricular pacing. PACE 25:62-75, 2002.)

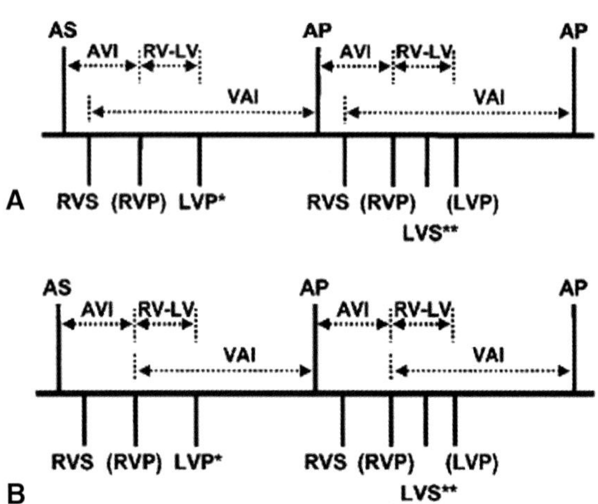

Figure 23-69. ***A,*** *Biventricular sensing and pacing. The right ventricular sensed event (RVS) is used to start the ventriculoatrial interval (VAI).* ***B,*** *The right ventricular pacing interval that would have occurred at the end of the atrioventricular interval (AVI) is used to start the VAI. Parentheses indicated the timing of the paced events that would have occurred if an intrinsic sensed event had not occurred. LVS**, left ventricular sensed event; LVP*, left ventricular paced event. (From Wang P, Kramer A, Estes NA 3rd, Hayes DL: Timing cycles for biventricular pacing. PACE 25:62-75, 2002.)*

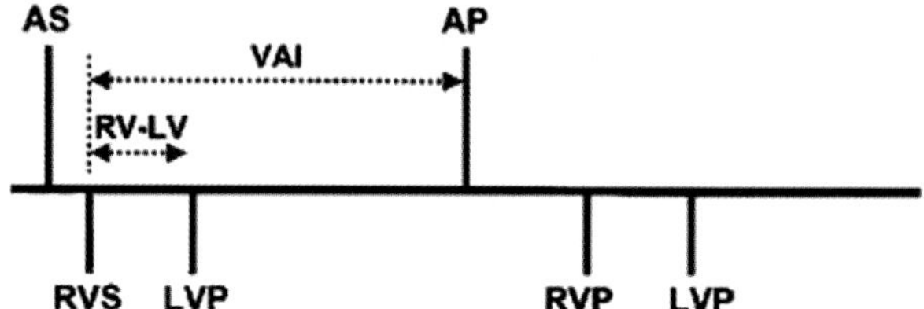

Figure 23-71. Biventricular sensing and pacing. Triggering may be present in devices that sense and pace in both the right ventricle and the left ventricle. If a right ventricular event is sensed, a left ventricular stimulus will be delivered after an RV-LV interval that is positive in value. AS, atrial sensed event; LVP, paced left ventricular event; LVS, sensed left ventricular event; RVP, paced right ventricular event; RVS, sensed right ventricular event; VAI, ventriculoatrial interval. (From Wang P, Kramer A, Estes NA 3rd, Hayes DL: Timing cycles for biventricular pacing. PACE 25:62-75, 2002.)

used for timing. These rules might depend on when the ventricular sensed event occurred. If the sensed event occurred in the AVI, as described earlier, a new V-A interval and timing cycle might be created with no pacing (Fig. 23-68). A variation on this function might be to permit a ventricular paced event from the opposite ventricle to occur (Fig. 23-69). This might be administered immediately after the sensed ventricular event within the AVI (Fig. 23-70) or after the programmed RV-LV delay. The V-A interval might be reset at the point of the right ventricular sensed event within the AVI (see Fig. 23-69A) or at the end of the programmed AVI (see Fig. 23-69B). A right ventricular sensed event may be followed by a left ventricular paced event, after an RV-LV interval of 0 (Fig. 23-70) or after an RV-LV interval that is positive (Fig. 23-71). It is also possible for a ventricular sensed event in the AVI not to trigger a ventricular paced beat from the opposite chamber but to have the AVI time out, with the ventricular paced event occurring at the end of the AVI. In biventricular sensing and pacing, a left ventricular sensed event in the AVI might be followed by a right ventricular sensed event within the programmed AVI (Fig. 23-72). Alternatively, the left ventricular sensed event in the AVI might trigger a right ventricular paced event that would be used to reset the V-A timing cycle (Fig. 23-73). Safety pacing with biventricular pacing might be performed using either both ventricles or only one used as backup pacing.

For sensed events outside the AVI and after the VRP, there are also a variety of responses. A sensed event in the LV or RV might be used interchangeably or might result in a specific pacing response. For example, sensing in either chamber first might be used to trigger a ventricular paced event in the opposite chamber. Alternately, a sensed event in the LV or RV might inhibit pacing in either channel to prevent pacing within the vulnerable period.

A left ventricular sensed event, for example, might inhibit left ventricular pacing, but a right ventricular paced event would occur unless a right ventricular sensed event occurred within the programmed LV-RV delay. If a negative RV-LV were programmed, the right ventricular

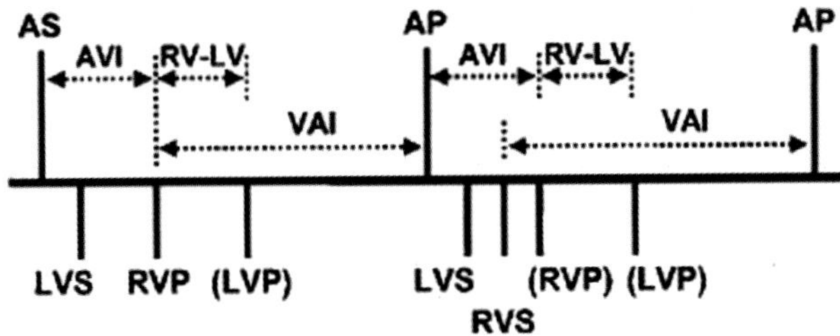

Figure 23-72. Biventricular sensing and pacing. If a left ventricular event is sensed, left ventricular pacing is inhibited. However, a right ventricular stimulus will be delivered. If a right ventricular event is sensed after the left ventricular sensed event, the timing cycles are reset. AS, atrial sensed event; AVI, atrioventricular interval; LVP, paced left ventricular event; LVS, sensed left ventricular event; RVP, paced right ventricular event; RVS, sensed right ventricular event; VAI, ventriculoatrial interval. (From Wang P, Kramer A, Estes NA 3rd, Hayes DL: Timing cycles for biventricular pacing. PACE 25:62-75, 2002.)

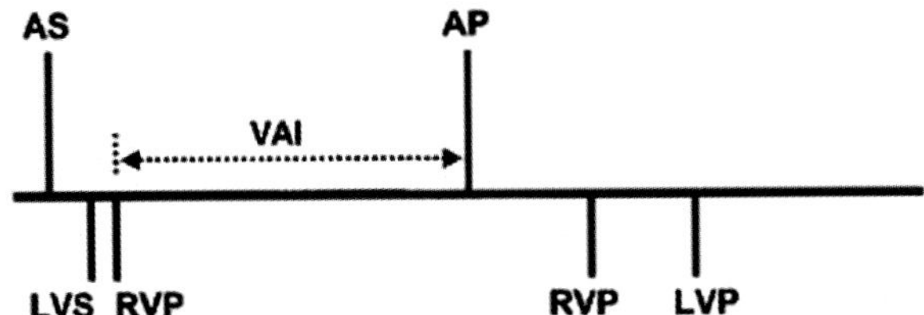

Figure 23-73. Biventricular sensing and pacing. Triggering may be present in devices that sense and pace in both the right ventricle and the left ventricle. If a left ventricular event is sensed, a right ventricular stimulus will be delivered immediately. AP, atrial paced event; AS, atrial sensed event; LVP, paced left ventricular event; LVS, sensed left ventricular event; RVP, paced right ventricular event; VAI, ventriculoatrial interval. (From Wang P, Kramer A, Estes NA 3rd, Hayes DL: Timing cycles for biventricular pacing. PACE 25:62-75, 2002.)

sensed event could result in resetting the timing cycles or in an immediate left ventricular paced event.

Univentricular Pacing

It is possible for a device to be programmed to have univentricular or biventricular sensing but to pace from only one ventricle, such as the LV. In the case of univentricular pacing and sensing, a sensed left ventricular event might result in inhibition of left ventricular pacing and resetting of the V-A timing cycle (Fig. 23-74). If a right ventricular sensed event occurred first, the left ventricular paced event might be inhibited, resetting the timing cycle (Fig. 23-75), or the result might be an immediate left ventricular paced event, to minimize the delay after the right ventricular sensed event (Fig. 23-76).

Biventricular Pacing and Sensing and Premature Beats

Biventricular pacing and sensing may create a particular problem if premature ventricular beats are present. A premature ventricular beat may occur in the A-V interval, resetting the timing cycle. The right ventricular sensed event may inhibit left ventricular pacing (Fig. 23-77) or may trigger a left ventricular paced event.

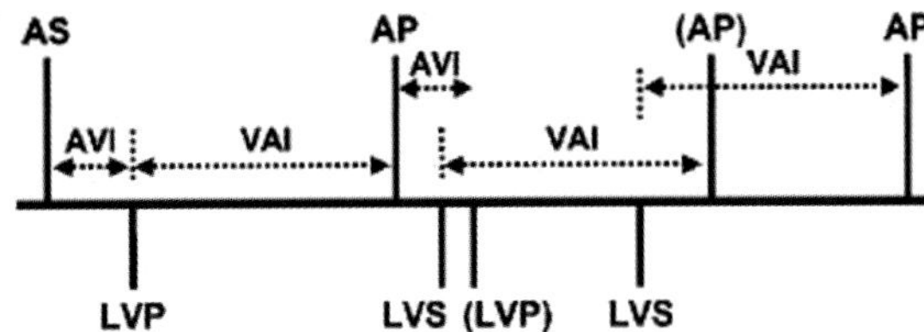

Figure 23-74. Univentricular sensing and pacing. Sensed events in the left ventricle result in inhibition, and reset the timing cycle. AP, atrial paced event; AS, atrial sensed event; AVI, atrioventricular interval; LVP, paced left ventricular event; LVS, sensed left ventricular event; VAI, ventriculoatrial interval. (From Wang P, Kramer A, Estes NA 3rd, Hayes DL: Timing cycles for biventricular pacing. PACE 25:62-75, 2002.)

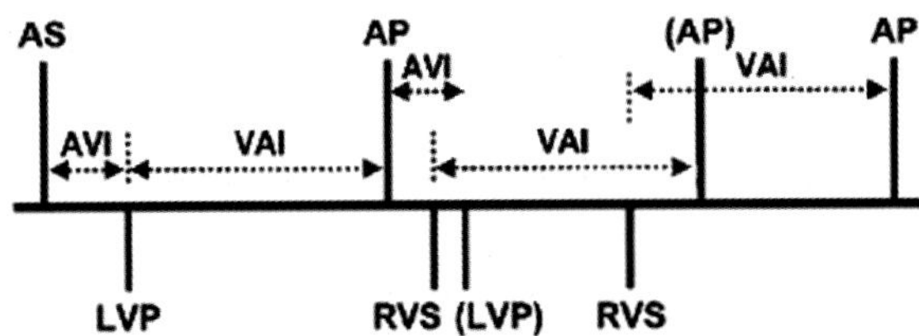

Figure 23-75. Biventricular sensing and univentricular pacing. Left ventricular paced and sensed events reset the timing cycles. Right ventricular sensed events also reset the timing cycle but do not trigger left ventricular pacing. AP, atrial paced event; AS, atrial sensed event; AVI, atrioventricular interval; LVP, inhibited paced left ventricular event; RVS, sensed right ventricular event; VAI, ventriculoatrial interval. (From Wang P, Kramer A, Estes NA 3rd, Hayes DL: Timing cycles for biventricular pacing. PACE 25:62-75, 2002.)

Upper Rate Behavior in Biventricular Pacing

The primary purpose of upper rate behavior in traditional dual-chamber DDD pacing is to prevent rapid atrial tracking during atrial tachycardia. The MTR is a programmable parameter, whereas the 2:1 AV block rate is determined by the TARP (60,000 ÷ TARP). When the MTR is slower than the 2:1 AV block rate, a pseudo-Wenckebach response occurs as the atrial rate increases and exceeds the MTR before the 2:1 AV block develops. When the 2:1 AV block rate is slower than the MTR, a sudden 50% drop in heart rate occurs as the atrial rate exceeds the 2:1 AV block limit.

For biventricular pacemakers, a thorough understanding of the upper rate behavior is crucial in maintaining biventricular pacing. Most patients who need resynchronization therapy have intact AV conduction, so pacemaker-Wenckebach behavior is to be avoided, because extension of the AVI allows sensing inhibition and prevents biventricular pacing. Episodes of high atrial rate are frequently observed in this population, during heart failure exacerbation, exercise with deconditioning, or recurrent atrial arrhythmias. To maintain 100% biventricular pacing, the TARP should be sufficiently short *and* the MTR should be sufficiently high.

Premature Beats and Biventricular Timing Cycles

A premature ventricular beat (PVC) is defined as a ventricular sensed event without a preceding paced or

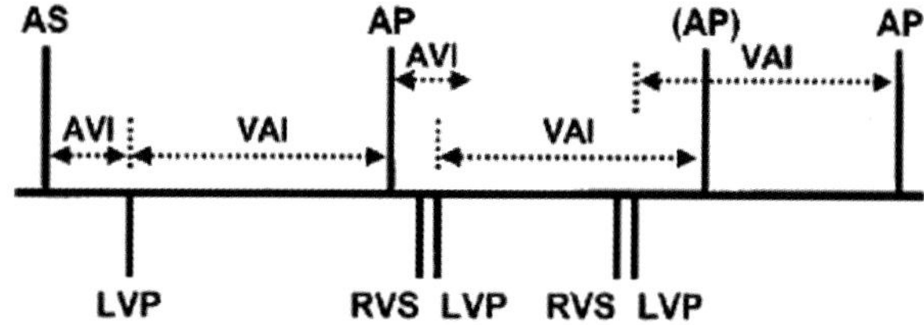

Figure 23-76. Biventricular sensing and univentricular pacing. Left ventricular paced and sensed events reset the timing cycles. Right ventricular sensed events result in triggering. AP, atrial paced event; AS, atrial sensed event; AVI, atrioventricular interval; LVP, paced left ventricular event; RVS, sensed right ventricular event; VAI, ventriculoatrial interval. (From Wang P, Kramer A, Estes NA 3rd, Hayes DL: Timing cycles for biventricular pacing. PACE 25:62-75, 2002.)

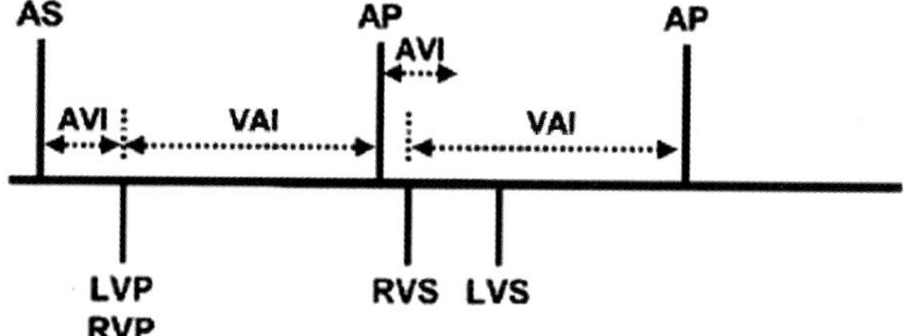

Figure 23-77. Biventricular pacing and sensing and premature beats. A premature ventricular beat occurs within the AVI, with right ventricular sensing first. The left ventricular paced beat is inhibited and left ventricular sensed event results from conduction. Right ventricular–based timing cycles. AP, atrial paced event; AS, atrial sensed event; AVI, atrioventricular interval; LVP, paced left ventricular event; LVS, sensed left ventricular event; RVP, paced right ventricular event; RVS, sensed right ventricular event; VAI, ventriculoatrial interval. (From Wang P, Kramer A, Estes NA 3rd, Hayes DC: Timing cycles for biventricular pacing. PACE 25:62-75, 2002.)

sensed atrial event. In dual-chamber timing cycles, a PVC occurring in the V-A interval would reset the AEI in ventricular-based timing devices. The presence of PVCs provides special challenges in a biventricular system. The PVC-PVARP extension algorithm automatically lengthens the PVARP to protect against potential PMT. However, such PVARP extension can cause subsequent functional atrial undersensing and loss of biventricular pacing. Therefore, the PVC-PVARP extension function should be deactivated in a biventricular system.

In addition, because of the interventricular (RV-LV) conduction delay, which could be considerable in patients with dyssynchrony, a PVC creates ambiguity for the timing cycles. Several possible approaches to this timing issue include a system that uses single-chamber sensing only, a cross-chamber (RV-LV) refractory period after the first ventricular sense, and a ventricular triggering mode in the opposite chamber. In an RV-sense–LV-refractory system, a PVC could have RV sensing occurring in the V-A interval that resets the AEI; the subsequent ventricular pacing (AEI + AVI) can occur "asynchronously" shortly after the delayed, non-sensed LV activation. Such improperly timed pacing stimuli may induce ventricular arrhythmia. A cross-chamber trigger mode on PVC would require an upper rate limit to avoid tightly coupled stimulation that could induce ventricular arrhythmia.

Refractory Periods and Biventricular Pacing

Refractory periods are present after sensed or paced events. In early biventricular devices with RV and LV leads connected in parallel via a Y-connection, a single ventricular depolarization may be sensed by both RV and LV leads. With biventricular sensing, the PVARP could be reset by the second component of the ventricular sensed signal (usually from the LV). In such cases of late left ventricular sensing, the PVARP and TARP are effectively extended by an interval that equals the interventricular sensing delay (RV-LV). Such a prolonged TARP could markedly reduce the atrial sensing window for atrial tracking.

The newer biventricular devices use dedicated right ventricular sensing only with pacing from both the RV and LV. After right or left ventricular pacing, a cross-chamber refractory period may be created. If there is a delay in the LV-RV interval, the total sensed refractory period may be extended. If the device is programmed to a positive LV-RV delay and a new refractory period is created after the RV pacing stimulus, the total VRP may be quite long. This prolonged sensing refractoriness can compromise detection of ventricular tachyarrhythmias.

Loss of Biventricular Pacing

Because the hemodynamic consequences of loss of biventricular pacing can be quite significant, it is important to identify possible causes of loss of biventricular pacing.[58] Biventricular pacing may be lost if the atrial rate increases so that the P wave falls within the PVARP of the preceding ventricular beat. This occurs when the atrial cycle length is equal to the sum of the PVARP and the sensed AV delay (TARP = AVI + PVARP) or greater than the maximum atrial tracking interval. Because the P wave will not be tracked, conduction will occur. Because the resultant QRS complex will initiate a PVARP, the next P wave will fall within the PVARP (Fig. 23-78). In this situation, the programmed AVI is less than the intrinsic P-R interval, so the onset of loss of biventricular pacing requires a faster atrial rate compared with the rate at which biventricular pacing will be restored. Biventricular pacing will not be restored until the atrial cycle length is greater than the sum of the PVARP and the P-R interval, which is called the intrinsic total atrial refractory period (ITARP). In patients with a prolonged P-R interval, ITARP may be significantly longer than TARP. Once atrial undersensing in PVARP occurs during atrial tachycardia, loss of biventricular pacing is perpetuated and may be restored only at much slower atrial rates. Restoration of biventricular pacing will occur when the P wave occurring after the last conducted QRS falls outside the PVARP. Diagrammatically, the relationship between the atrial rate and loss of biventricular pacing may be seen in Figure 23-79. Atrial premature beats with conduction can produce a similar phenomenon by causing atrial undersensing and loss of biventricular pacing.[59] At rapid rates, 2:1 biventricular pacing

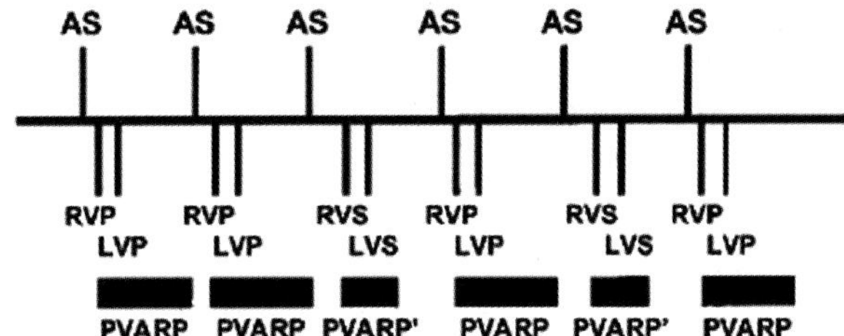

Figure 23-78. *Loss of biventricular pacing with 2:1 biventricular pacing. At rapid atrial rates, every other beat may have biventricular pacing, despite shortening of PVARP. AS, atrial sensed event; LVP, paced left ventricular event; LVS, sensed left ventricular event; PVARP, postventricular atrial refractory period; PVARP, shortening of PVARP after RVS; RVP, paced right ventricular event; RVS, sensed right ventricular event. (From Wang P, Kramer A, Estes NA 3rd, Hayes DL: Timing cycles for biventricular pacing. PACE 25:62–75, 2002.)*

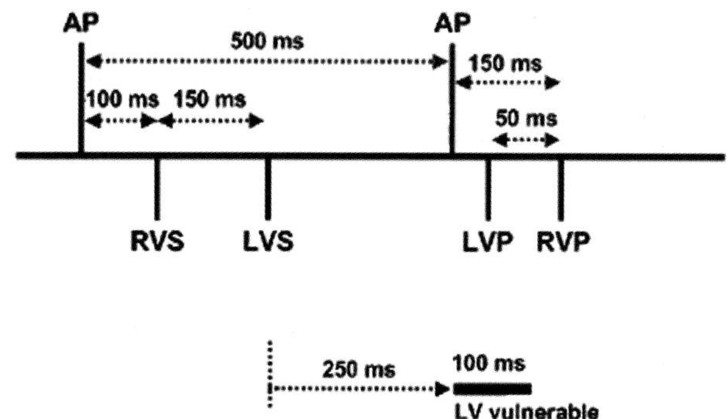

Figure 23-80. *Biventricular pacing with right ventricular–based timing and competitive pacing. The left ventricular paced event (LVP) may occur when the left ventricle is no longer refractory. AP, atrial paced event; LVS, left ventricular sensed event; RVP, right ventricular paced event; RVS, right ventricular sensed event. (From Wang P, Kramer A, Estes NA 3rd, Hayes DL: Timing cycles for biventricular pacing. PACE 25:62-75, 2002.)*

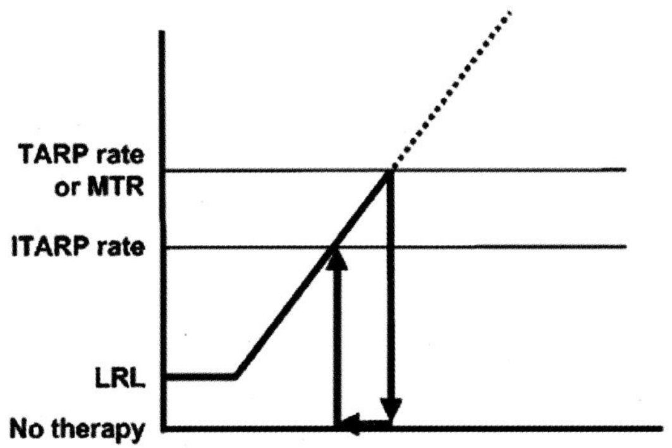

Figure 23-79. *Relationship between atrial rate and the loss of biventricular pacing. As the atrial rate reaches the total atrial refractory period, or TARP (PVARP + A-V interval), biventricular pacing will stop. When the atrial rate falls to the intrinsic total atrial refractory period, or ITARP (PVARP + P-R interval), biventricular pacing resumes. LRL, lower rate limit; MTR, maximum tracking rate; PVARP, postventricular atrial refractory period; x-axis, atrial rate; y-axis, biventricular rate. (From Wang P, Kramer A, Estes NA 3rd, Hayes DL: Timing cycles for biventricular pacing. PACE 25:62-75, 2002.)*

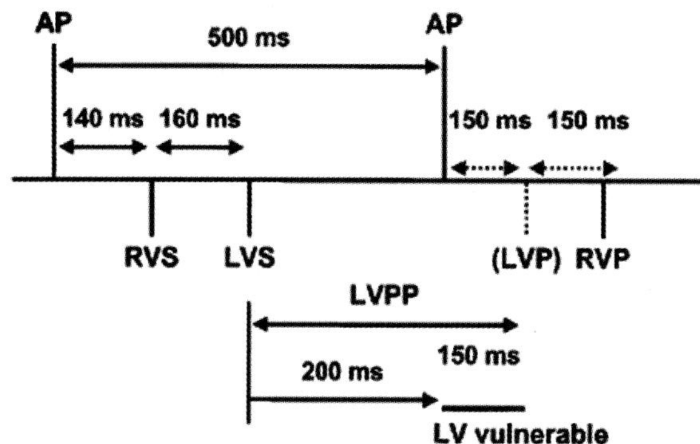

Figure 23-81. *Biventricular pacing with right ventricular–based timing and left ventricular refractory extension. To prevent the possibility of left ventricular pacing (LVP) when the left ventricle is no longer refractory, the LVP may be inhibited if it is occurring too soon after an intrinsic left ventricular event (LVS). AP, atrial paced event; LVPP, left ventricular protection period; RVP, paced right ventricular event; RVS, sensed right ventricular event.*

may occur, even if the PVARP is shortened in response to a right ventricular sensed event (see Fig. 23-79).

Competitive Ventricular Pacing

Biventricular pacing, as described earlier, has introduced a new cause of competitive ventricular pacing, a left ventricular stimulus occurring after left ventricular activation. This occurs because left ventricular sensed events are not used to inhibit ventricular pacing. For example, a conducted ventricular beat with a positive RV sense–LV sense interval due to left bundle branch block may occur and be followed by pacing, with LV pacing occur before RV pacing (Fig. 23-80) because the LV is no longer refractory, potentially inducing a ventricular arrhythmia.

A feature called left ventricular pacing protection (LVPP) has been introduced to prevent left ventricular competitive pacing. After a left ventricular paced or sensed event has occurred, a left ventricular paced event will not occur for the duration of the programmed LVPP (Fig. 23-81).

Another circumstance for competitive ventricular pacing is the occurrence of a left ventricular premature event before conduction can occur to the RV. Particularly if the RV-LV interval is positive, the left ventricular stimulus may find the LV.

Conclusions

As resynchronization therapy has become an important part of the therapy of patients with left ventricular failure and ventricular dyssynchrony, there has been in an increasing recognition of the importance of pacing timing cycles in biventricular pacing. Because biventricular pacing is effective only with constant pacing, the implications of timing cycles for maintenance of biventricular pacing is particularly important. There are unique implications for lower rate and upper rate behavior.

Timing Cycles of Implantable Cardioverter-Defibrillators

Pacing Algorithms in Implantable Cardioverter-Defibrillators

One of the most serious issues involving timing cycles is the interaction between pacing and arrhythmia detection. The basic timing cycles in most ICDs are similar to those of comparable pacemaker devices. Many devices have a number of the following refractory or blanking periods: atrial blanking after ventricular sensed and paced events, ventricular sensed refractory period, ventricular refractory period, postventricular atrial sensed refractory period, atrial blanking after atrial pacing, and ventricular blanking after atrial paced events. Circumstances in which the MTRs and the sensor-driven rates are close to the ventricular tachycardia detection rate are most likely to result in abnormalities in arrhythmia detection. Examples of cases in which the pacing rates are likely to be particularly fast include sensor-driven pacing, tracking at or near the upper rate limit, rate smoothing, rate drop or sudden bradycardia response, ventricular rate regularization, and atrial pacing prevention algorithms. Abnormalities such as atrial oversensing with tracking in the DDD mode may lead to failure to detect ventricular tachycardia. Cases of prolonged undersensing of ventricular tachycardia have been reported during rate smoothing. Cooper and associates[60] observed that ventricular tachycardia remained undetected because the ventricular tachycardia beats occurred within the VBP after atrial paced events. Atrial pacing occurred because rate smoothing had been turned on. Such an interaction is promoted by a slow ventricular tachycardia and rate smoothing algorithm. Shivkumar and colleagues[61] reported a similar case of failure to detect an episode of ventricular tachycardia. Glikson and coworkers[62] conducted a prospective study to examine the role of rate smoothing in preventing ventricular tachycardia detection. During ICD testing in 54 episodes of induced ventricular fibrillation/polymorphic ventricular tachycardia, 3 episodes (5%) of a minimal delay in detection were observed. However, among the 10 monomorphic ventricular tachycardia episodes, 4 had absent detection and 2 had delayed detection. Based on these observations and simulator-based modifications of programmable parameters, these authors observed that long AV delay, high upper rate, and more aggressive rate smoothing increase the risk of ventricular tachycardia underdetection. Figure 23-82 illustrates an

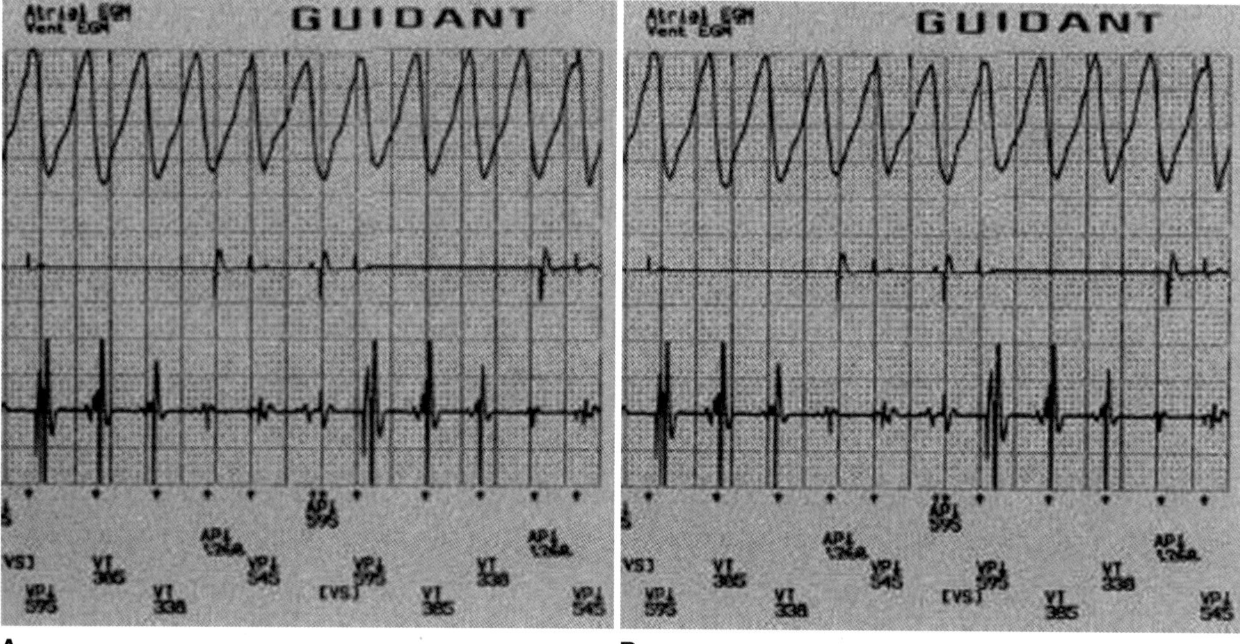

Figure 23-82. Rate smoothing leading to pacing during ventricular tachycardia. Rate smoothing led to atrioventricular (AV) pacing during ventricular tachycardia and the resultant underdetection. ***A** and **B**, Two segments of a recording of sustained monomorphic ventricular tachycardia (VT). VT rate cutoff was 430 ms. Recording channels include* surface ECG *(top),* atrial electrogram *(middle),* ventricular electrogram *(bottom), and event markers. VT beats fall into postatrial pacing (AP) blanking period, resulting in delay in VT detection.* ***C**, Diagram demonstrating failure of detection of VT at 280 ms cycle length. The VT beats fall into blanking period after atrial paced beats. VF, ventricular fibrillation. (From Glikson M, Beeman AL, Luria DM, et al.: Impaired detection of ventricular tachyarrhythmias by a rate-smoothing algorithm in dual-chamber implantable defibrillators: Intradevice interactions. J Cardiovasc Electrophysiol 13:312-318, 2002.)*

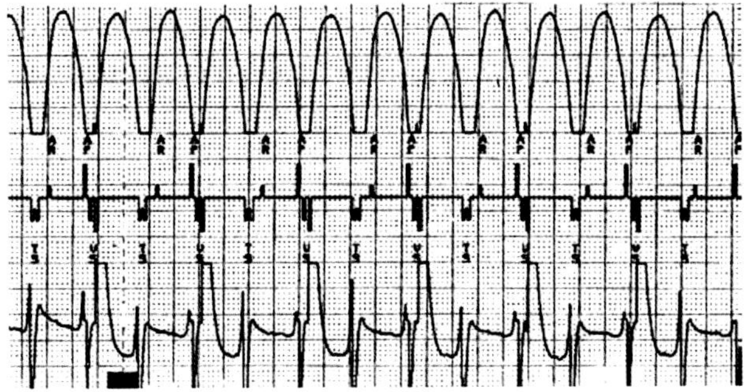

Figure 23-83. Ventricular rate stabilization leading to pacing during ventricular tachycardia. The ventricular rate stabilization algorithm led to pacing during ventricular tachycardia, which led to underdetection. (From Barold SS: Ventricular rate stabilization algorithm of ICD causing dual chamber pacing during ventricular tachycardia. J Interv cardiac Electrophysiol 9:397-400, 2003.)

example of ventricular tachycardia that is underdetected due to a rate-smoothing algorithm. A similar case has been described for the ventricular rate stabilization algorithm (Fig. 23-83).

Rate smoothing has also been proposed as a mechanism for preventing ventricular tachycardia by minimizing abrupt variations in cycle lengths in a short-long-short pattern. Wietholt and colleagues[63] conducted the PREVENT study by randomizing patients in a 3-month crossover design to periods of rate smoothing versus no rate smoothing. Fifty seven (38%) of the 153 patients had 358 ventricular tachycardia episodes with rate smoothing OFF, compared with 145 episodes with rate smoothing ON.

Ventricular sensed events, even ones at a tachyarrhythmic cycle length, are considered sensed for the purpose of bradycardia timing cycles. Therefore, such events result in inhibition of ventricular pacing. Once ventricular tachyarrhythmia detection has occurred, the pacing mode may stay the same or may be altered. In the ventricular tachycardia response (VTR), once ventricular tachycardia detection has occurred, the mode switches to VDI at the ATR/VTR fallback LRL. In some older generators, there is suspension of bradycardia pacing immediately before shock delivery to prevent underdetection of ventricular tachycardia caused by pacing-related refractory periods. In some other generators, the mode may switch from DDD(R) to VVI after charging has ended and during defibrillation therapies.

During shock therapy, there may be specific changes to sensing. After shock therapy and in some devices after charging, there may be a refractory period. After ventricular tachycardia detection and before shock delivery, a number of ICDs nominally suspend pacing for at least 1 to 2 seconds after the shock. After a shock, it is typical that there are changes in the bradycardia parameters. Frequently, the outputs and LRL may be increased for a programmable period of time.

REFERENCES

1. Barold SS: Modern concepts of cardiac pacing. Heart Lung 2:238-252, 1973.
2. Bernstein A, Daubert J, Fletcher R, et al.: The revised NASPE/BPEG generic code for antibradycardia, adaptive-rate, and multisite pacing. PACE 23:260-264, 2002.
3. Barold SS: Clinical significance of pacemaker refractory periods. Am J Cardiol 28:237-239, 1971.
4. Barold SS, Gaidula JJ: Pacemaker refractory periods. N Engl J Med 284:220-221, 1971.
5. Yokoyama M, Wada J, Barold SS: Transient early T wave sensing by implanted programmable demand pulse generator. PACE 4:68-74, 1981.
6. Okreglicki A, Akiyama T, Ocampo C, Flynn D: Polarization potentials causing pacemaker oversensing. Jpn Circ J 62:868-870, 1998.
7. Paraskevaidis S, Mochlas S, Hadjimiltiadis S, Louridas G: Intermittent P wave sensing in a patient with DDD pacemaker. PACE 22(4 Pt 1):689-690, 1999.
8. Frohlig G, Helwani Z, Kusch O, et al.: Bipolar ventricular far-field signals in the atrium. PACE 22:1604-1613, 1999.
9. Rosenheck S, Sharon Z, Leibowitz D: Artifacts recorded through failing bipolar polyurethane insulated permanent pacing leads. Europace 2:60-65, 2000.
10. Barold SS, Falkoff MD, Ong LS, Heinle RA: Oversensing by single-chamber pacemakers: Mechanisms, diagnosis, and treatment. Cardiol Clin 3:565-585, 1985.
11. Tse HF, Lau CP: The current status of single lead dual chamber sensing and pacing. J Interv Card Electrophysiol 2:255-267, 1998.
12. Friedberg HD, Barold SS: On hysteresis in pacing. J Electrocardiol 6:1-2, 1973.
13. Barold SS: Prolonged atrioventricular block during AAI pacing for sick sinus syndrome. J Cardiovasc Electrophysiol 11:1422, 2000.
14. Tripp IG, Armstrong GP, Stewart JT, et al.: Atrial pacing should be used more frequently in sinus node disease. PACE 28:291-294, 2005.
15. Barold SS, Falkoff MD, Ong LS, Heinle RA: Programmability in DDD pacing. PACE 7(6 Pt 2):1159-1164, 1984.
16. Barold SS, Belott PH: Behavior of the ventricular triggering period of DDD pacemakers. PACE 10:1237-1252, 1987.
17. Barold SS, Falkoff MD, Ong LS, Heinle RA: All dual-chamber pacemakers function in the DDD mode. Am Heart J 115:1353-1362, 1988.
18. Parravicini U, Mezzani A, Bielli M, et al.: DDD pacing and interatrial conduction block: Importance of optimal AV interval setting. PACE 23:1448-1450, 2000.
19. Bode F, Wiegand U, Katus HA, Potratz J: Inhibition of ventricular stimulation in patients with dual chamber pacemakers and prolonged AV conduction.[see comment]. PACE 22:1425-1431, 1999.
20. Dennis MJ, Sparks PB: Pacemaker mediated tachycardia as a complication of the autointrinsic conduction search function.[see comment]. PACE 27(6 Pt 1):824-826, 2004.
21. Higans ST, Hayes DL: P wave tracking above the maximum tracking rate in a pacemaker. PACE 12:1044-1048, 1989.
22. Van Gelder BM, Van Mechelen R, Den Dulk K, et al.: Apparent P wave undersensing in a DDD pacemaker after exercise. PACE 15:1651, 1992.
23. Barold SS, Gallardo I, Sayad D: Wenckebach upper rate response of pacemakers implanted for nontraditional indications: The other side of the coin. PACE 25:1283-1284, 2002.
24. Barold SS, Falk off MD, Ong LS, et al.: All dual-chamber procedures function in the DDD mode. Am Heart J 115:1353, 1988.
25. Barold SS: Far-field R wave sensing causing prolongation of the atrial escape interval of DDD pacemakers with atrial-based lower rate timing. PACE 26:2188-2191, 2003.
26. Lau CP, Leung SK, Tse HF, Barold SS: Automatic mode switching of implantable pacemakers: I. Principles of instrumentation, clinical, and hemodynamic considerations. PACE 25:967-983, 2002.

27. Estes NA 3rd: Atrial tachyarrhythmias detected by automatic mode switching: Quo vadis? [comment]. J Cardiovasc Electrophysiol 15:778-779, 2004.
28. Israel CW: Analysis of mode switching algorithms in dual chamber pacemakers. PACE 25:380-393, 2002.
29. Leung SK, Lau CP, Lam CT, et al.: Is automatic mode switching effective for atrial arrhythmias occurring at different rates? A study of the efficacy of automatic mode and rate switching to simulated atrial arrhythmias by chest wall stimulation. PACE 23:824-831, 2000.
30. Passman RS, Weinberg KM, Freher M, et al.: Accuracy of mode switch algorithms for detection of atrial tachyarrhythmias.[see comment]. J Cardiovasc Electrophysiol 15:773-777, 2004.
31. Wood MA, Ellenbogen KA, Dinsmoor D, et al.: Influence of autothreshold sensing and sinus rate on mode switching algorithm behavior [see comment]. PACE 23(10 Pt 1):1473-1478, 2000.
32. Walfridsson H, Aunes M, Capocci M, Edvardsson N: Sensing of atrial fibrillation by a dual chamber pacemaker: How should atrial sensing be programmed to ensure adequate mode shifting? PACE 23:1089-1093, 2000.
33. Nowak B, Kracker S, Rippin G, et al.: Effect of the atrial blanking time on the detection of atrial fibrillation in dual chamber pacing. PACE 24(4 Pt 1):496-499, 2001.
34. Marshall HS, Kay GN, Hess M, et al.: Mode switching in dual chamber procedures: Effects of onset criteria on arrhythmia-related symptoms. Europace 1:49-54, 1999.
35. Irrael CW, Barold SS: Failure of atrial flutter detection by a pacemaker with a dedicated atrial flutter detection algorithm. PACE 25:1274 1277, 2002.
36. Goethals M, Timmermans W, Geelen P, et al.: Mode switching failure during atrial flutter: The "2:1 lock-in" phenomenon. Europace 5:95-102, 2003.
37. Simpson CS, Yee R, Lee JK, et al.: Safety and feasibility of a novel rate-smoothed ventricular pacing algorithm for atrial fibrillation. Am Heart J 142:294-300, 2001.
38. Eguia LE, Pinski SL: Inactivation of a ventricular tachycardia preventive algorithm during automatic mode switching for atrial tachyarrhythmia. PACE 24:252-253, 2001.
39. Barold SS, Mond HG: Fallback responses of dual chamber (DDD and DDDR) pacemakers: A proposed classification. PACE 17: 1160-1165, 1994.
40. Ward KJ, Willett JE, Bucknall C, et al.: Atrial arrhythmia suppression by atrial overdrive pacing: Pacemaker Holter assessment. Europace 3:108-114, 2001.
41. Blommaert D, Gonzalez M, Mucumbitsi J, et al.: Effective prevention of atrial fibrillation by continuous atrial overdrive pacing after coronary artery bypass surgery [see comment]. J Am Coll Cardiol 35:1411-1415, 2000.
42. Levy T, Walker S, Rex S, Paul V: Does atrial overdrive pacing prevent paroxysmal atrial fibrillation in paced patients? Int J Cardiol 75:91-97, 2000.
43. Lam CT, Lau CP, Leung SK, et al.: Efficacy and tolerability of continuous overdrive atrial pacing in atrial fibrillation. Europace 2:286-291, 2000.
44. Attuel P, Danilovic D, Konz KH, et al.: Relationship between selected overdrive parameters and the therapeutic outcome and tolerance of atrial overdrive pacing. PACE 26(1 Pt 2):257-263, 2003.
45. Connolley SJ, Kerr CR, Gent M, et al.: Effects of physiological pacing versus ventricular pacing on the risk of stroke and death due to cardiovascular causes: Canadian Trial of Physiological Pacing Investigators. N Engl J Med 342:1385-1391, 2000.
46. Israel CW, Gronefeld G, Ehrlich JR, et al.: Prevention of immediate reinitiation of atrial tachyarrhythmias by high-rate overdrive pacing: Results from a prospective randomized trial. J Cardiovasc Electrophysiol 14:954-959, 2003.
47. Hakala T, Valtola AJ, Turpeinen AK, et al.: Right atrial overdrive pacing does not prevent atrial fibrillation after coronary artery bypass surgery. Europace 7:170-174, 2005.
48. Savoure A, Frohlig G, Galley D, et al.: A new dual-chamber pacing mode to minimize ventricular pacing. PACE 28(Suppl 1):S43-S46, 2005.
49. Sweeney M, Ellenbogen KA, Casavant D, et al.: Multicenter, prospective, randomized safety and efficacy study of a new atrial-based managed ventricular pacing mode (MVP) in dual chamber ICDs. J Cardiovasc Electrophysiol 16:811-817, 2005.
50. Tse HF, Newman D, Ellenbogen KA, et al.: Atrial Fibrillation SYMPTOMS Investigators: Effects of ventricular rate regularization pacing on quality of life and symptoms in patients with atrial fibrillation (atrial fibrillation symptoms mediated by pacing to mean rates). Am J Cardiol 94:938-941, 2004.
51. Abraham WT: Cardiac resynchronization therapy for the management of chronic heart failure. Am Heart Hosp J 1:55-61, 2003.
52. Barold SS, Herweg B, Giudici M: Electrocardiographic follow-up of biventricular pacemakers. Ann Noninvasive Electrocardiol 10:231-255, 2005.
53. Barold SS, Herweg B: Upper rate response of biventricular pacing devices. J Interv Card Electrophysiol 12:129-136, 2005.
54. Chang KC, Chen JY, Lin JJ, Hung JS: Unexpected loss of atrial tracking caused by interaction between temporary and permanent right ventricular leads during implantation of a biventricular pacemaker. PACE 27:998-1001, 2004.
55. Akiyama M, Kaneko Y, Taniguchi Y, Kurabayashi M: Pacemaker syndrome associated with a biventricular pacing system. J Cardiovasc Electrophysiol 13:1061-1062, 2002.
56. Wang P, Kramer A, Estes NA 3rd, Hayes DL: Timing cycles for biventricular pacing. PACE 25:62-75, 2002.
57. Riedlbauchova L, Kautzner J, Fridl P: Influence of different atrioventricular and interventricular delays on cardiac output during cardiac resynchronization therapy. PACE 28(Suppl 1):S19-S23, 2005.
58. Taieb J, Benchaa T, Foltzer E, et al.: Atrioventricular cross-talk in biventricular pacing: A potential cause of ventricular standstill. PACE 25:929-935, 2002.
59. Lipchenca I, Garrigue S, Glikson M, et al.: Inhibition of biventricular pacemakers by oversensing of far-field atrial depolarization. PACE 25:365-367, 2002.
60. Cooper JM, Sauer WH, Verdino RJ: Absent ventricular tachycardia detection in a biventricular implantable cardioverter-defibrillator due to intradevice interaction with a rate smoothing pacing algorithm. Heart Rhythm 1:728-731, 2004.
61. Shivkumar K, Feliciano Z, Boyle NG, Wiener I: Intradevice interaction in a dual chamber implantable cardioverter-defibrillator preventing ventricular tachyarrhythmia detection [see comment]. J Cardiovasc Electrophysiol 11:1285-1288, 2000.
62. Glikson M, Beeman AL, Luria DM, et al.: Impaired detection of ventricular tachyarrhythmias by a rate-smoothing algorithm in dual-chamber implantable defibrillators: Intradevice interactions. J Cardiovasc Electrophysiol 13:312-318, 2002.
63. Wietholt D, Kuehlkamp V, Meisel E, et al.: Prevention of sustained ventricular tachyarrhythmias in patients with implantable cardioverter-defibrillators: The PREVENT study. J Interv Card Electrophysiol 9:383-389, 2003.
64. Barold SS: Ventricular rate stabilization algorithm of ICD causing dual chamber pacing during ventricular tachycardia. J Interv Card Electrophysiol 9:397-400, 2003.

Chapter 24

Pacemaker Troubleshooting and Follow-up

CHARLES J. LOVE

Pacemakers have advanced from nonprogrammable, single-chamber, asynchronous devices (VOO) to dual-chamber systems with extensive programmability. They now include not only the ability to adjust the pacing rate automatically on the basis of signals that are independent of the intrinsic heart rhythm (DDDR), but also the capability of regulating the stimulation power and sensitivity settings. The analysis of a pacing system was comparatively easy during the early days of pacing, whereas the challenge in evaluating the modern pacemaker has increased to a degree that is concordant with the sophistication of the current devices.

To facilitate these evaluations, manufacturers have incorporated a multitude of diagnostic tools in the pacemaker. These tools have become essential to determine what the pacemaker is doing and why it is doing it. The various diagnostic capabilities commonly either eliminate the need for ancillary testing or provide the direction for additional testing. Occasionally, a given feature provides absolutely unique information that is not readily available by any other technique. These tools, which are integral to the implanted device, can be accessed by the programmer and are the subject of the first part of this chapter. To take advantage of these diagnostic features and to determine the appropriate function of a pacing system, the clinician must have an in-depth knowledge of the system's components, including not only the pulse generator but also the leads, programmed parameters, automatic algorithms, sensors, connectors, and other implanted devices, as well as the patient's physiology. It is crucial that the clinician understand the importance of evaluating the entire system rather than focusing on isolated individual components. The evaluation of malfunctioning pacemaker systems is the subject of the second part of this chapter.

Bidirectional Telemetry

Telemetry is the ability to transmit information or data from one device to another, a capability that was essential to the introduction of pacemaker programmability. This is the ability to noninvasively change the functional and diagnostic parameters of the pacing system by coded commands transmitted to the pacemaker from a programmer.[1-4] The first generation of programmable pacemakers used unidirectional telemetry from the programmer to the pacemaker but was not able to transmit data from the pacemaker to the programmer. This limited the confirmation of a programming change that was electrocardiographically silent (e.g., the sensitivity or refractory period) when a parameter was programmed.

Bidirectional telemetry is communication in two directions. With respect to pacing systems, this means that the pacemaker and programmer can communicate with each other, an essential capability for the development of the multiple diagnostic capabilities that are the subject of this chapter.[5,6] First implemented in rechargeable pacemakers, bidirectional telemetry was developed to confirm the proper alignment of the recharging head with the implanted pacemaker. When the recharging wand was not aligned properly with the pacemaker, there was an audible beep from the charging unit to notify the patient and whoever was in attendance of this condition. When the two devices were properly aligned, the system was silent.

Bidirectional capability was next applied to confirmation of programming. This was particularly valuable for those parameters that did not result in an overt change in pacing system performance and could not be independently identified on an electrocardiographic (ECG) recording. This ability is essential for the DDDR pacemaker and modern implantable cardioverter-defibrillators (ICDs), because these devices can have dozens of independently programmable parameters, most of which are not readily identifiable on the ECG (Fig. 24-1A). Bidirectional telemetry allows interrogation of programmed parameters when the patient is seen during follow-up for routine evaluation or for a suspected pacing system malfunction. Without this feature, there would be no way to determine the current settings of a device for features other than rate and pulse width. It also makes the retrieval of detailed data collected by the pacemaker in its various event counters feasible. Presently, interrogation of pacemaker settings and data can be accomplished remotely. This technique uses a device located in the patient's home, a physician's office, or anywhere an Internet connection or telephone service (wired or cellular) connection is available. Data are retrieved from the device and sent to a central receiving station. The data are made into a report and then can be faxed to the appropriate individual or made available through an Internet web site portal. Although the technology exists to allow programming remotely, this is not currently available due to regulatory issues.

Measured Data

Complementing the interrogation of programmed data is the provision of measured data, including data obtained from the pacemaker detailing information concerning lead and battery function at the time of evaluation. Information regarding demand and asynchronous rates may also be measured (see Fig. 24-1B). Telemetry allows this information to be transferred from the pacemaker to the programmer for evaluation by the clinician.

Battery Status

Although not all systems provide the information in the same manner (some are graphic and others are numeric), data concerning battery function often include a measure of battery voltage, impedance, and current drain.[7-11] All three parameters are interrelated. The battery current drain is a measure of the average current being drawn from the battery, assuming 100% pacing at the programmed rate and output settings. Inhibition or pacing at higher rates, as might occur with intrinsic rhythm or sensor drive, respectively, directly affects the functional battery current drain, as do changes in lead or stimulation impedance. The reported current drain is only an estimate of the actual battery current drain. Newer devices are able to estimate remaining longevity based on true current drain measurements, giving a much more accurate assessment.

The measured current drain of the battery at a known set of parameters can be used to qualitatively assess the effect of programming changes on the longevity of the system. After the rate or output (or both) has been changed, the measured data can be reassessed and the effect of the programming change on longevity estimated. A simple calculation may be used to obtain an estimate of battery longevity when the pacemaker is relatively new. Most manufacturers provide the usable battery capacity reported in ampere-hours (A-hr). For this calculation, the battery's capacity is converted to microampere-hours (μA-hr) and then divided by the measured battery current drain. The result is the anticipated number of hours of normal function at the programmed rate and output. This number, divided by 8760 (the number of hours in 1 year), yields an estimate of the longevity of the system in years. This calculation is best performed with a new system, before there has been significant battery depletion. Many newer pacemakers perform these calculations and display the remaining longevity in years or months, providing a relatively good estimate of remaining longevity.

Virtually every pacemaker incorporates a change in either the magnet or the demand rate (and sometimes in mode or other functions) to signal a level of battery depletion that warrants pulse generator replacement. Most of these changes occur when the battery voltage reaches a predefined level, which is specific for each manufacturer and even for each model of pacemaker. These changes are termed elective replacement time (ERT), recommended replacement time (RRT), or elective replacement indicator (ERI), with further changes in rate or function associated with continued battery depletion being labeled either end of life (EOL) or end of service (EOS). Although these changes may occur abruptly, there is commonly a 3- to 6-month period between activation of the ERT indicator and erratic behavior or device nonfunction caused by continued battery depletion. A marker to determine when to increase the frequency of pacing system surveillance (either transtelephonically or in the office) is included in some systems and is commonly a magnet rate intermediate between a fully functional battery and the ERT indicator. Alternatively, this indication may be given to the clinician during interrogation of the device by a message on the programmer screen or on the programmer report. This is termed an *intensified follow-up indicator,* and it provides an indication of changing battery status before the ERT is reached.

Given the degree of programmability of most current pacemakers, a dual-chamber pacemaker programmed

Basic Parameters

	Initial		Present
Mode	DDDR		DDDR
Base rate	60		60 ppm
Hysteresis rate	Off		Off ppm
Rest rate	45		45 ppm
Max track rate	140	=>	170 ppm
2:1 block rate	175		175 ppm
AV delay	170		170 ms
PV delay	150		150 ms
Rate resp. AV/PV delay	Medium		Medium
Shortest AV/PV delay	70		70 ms
Ventricular refractory	250		250 ms
Atrial refractory	275		275 ms
Ventricular:			
V. AutoCapture	Off		Off
V. Pulse Amplitude	2.00		2.00 V
V. Pulse Width	0.6		0.6 ms
V. Sensitivity	2.0		2.0 mV
V. Pulse Configuration	Bipolar		Bipolar
V. Sense Configuration	Bipolar		Bipolar
Atrial:			
A. Pulse Amplitude	2.00		2.00 V
A. Pulse Width	0.6		0.6 ms
A. Sensitivity	0.2		2.0 mV
A. Pulse Configuration	Bipolar		Bipolar
A. Sense Configuration	Bipolar		Bipolar
Magnet Response	Snapshots+Batt.		Snapshots+Batt.

Extended Parameters

	Initial		Present
AutoIntrinsic Conduction Search™	Off		Off ms
Negative AV/PV Hysteresis/Search	Off		Off ms
Auto Mode Switch	DDIR		DDIR
Atrial Tachycardia Detection Rate	225		225 ppm
Post Vent. Atrial Blanking (PVAB)	100	=>	60 ms
Vent. Safety Standby	On	=>	Off
Vent. Blanking	12		12 ms
PVC Options	Off		Off
PMT Options	Off	=>	Auto Detect
PMT Detection Rate	*	=>	110 bpm

Sensor Parameters

	Initial		Present
Sensor	On		On
Max Sensor Rate	140	=>	160 ppm
Threshold	Auto (+0.0)		Auto (+0.0)
Meas. Average Sensor	2.5		2.5
Slope	8	=>	Auto (+0)
Measured Auto Slope	*	=>	8
Reaction Time	Fast	=>	Slow
Recovery Time	Medium	=>	Fast

* *Not Applicable*
=> *Initial value differs from Present value*
T=> *Temporary programmed value*
— *Unknown/Invalid values*

A

Patient Data

Vent. Lead Type	Unipolar/Bipolar
Atrial Lead Type	Unipolar/Bipolar
Implant Date:	14 Jul 1998 12:06

Patient Information

JOHN Q. PUBLIC ID# 123-45-6789
DOI: 14 JULY, 1998 AT SW MED CNTR
A LEAD: SJM 1388T-46 AB223345
V LEAD: SJM 1388T-52 BC199887
DX:COMPLETE HEART BLOCK, S/P AV
NODE ABLATION, PMKR DEPENDENT
SEVERE PMKR SYNDROME WITH VVI
DR. PAUL A LEVINE 818-493-2900

Measured Data

Date Last Programmed	18 Sep 1998 07:35	
Magnet Rate	98.5	ppm
Ventricular:		
Pulse Amplitude	1.9	V
Pulse Current	3.6	mA
Pulse Energy	3.3	µJ
Pulse Charge	2	µC
Lead Impedance	538	Ω
Atrial:		
Pulse Amplitude	2.0	V
Pulse Current	3.6	mA
Pulse Energy	3.5	µJ
Pulse Charge	2	µC
Lead Impedance	542	Ω
Battery Data	(W.G. 9438-nom. 0.95 Ah)	
Voltage	2.76	V
Current	12	µA
Impedance	<1	kΩ

Test Results

Atrial Capture Threshold	<0.25	V
Atrial Capture Test Pulse Width	0.6	ms
Atrial Capture Test Polarity	Bipolar	
Atrial Capture Safety Margin	>8.0:1@2.00V	
Vent. Capture Threshold	0.50	V
Vent. Capture Test Pulse Width	0.6	ms
Vent. Capture Test Polarity	Bipolar	
Vent. Capture Safety Margin	4.0:1@2.00V	
P-Wave Amplitude	2.5	mV
Atrial Sense Test Polarity	Bipolar	
Atrial Sense Safety Margin	12.5:1@0.20mV	
R-Wave Amplitude	>12.5	mV
Vent. Sense Test Polarity	Bipolar	
Vent. Sense Safety Margin	>6.3:1@2.00mV	

B

Figure 24-1. ***A,*** *Final interrogation of a Pacesetter Affinity DR Model 5330 (St. Jude Medical CRMD, Sylmar, Calif.), showing the programmed parameters and the changes identified since the initial evaluation.* ***B,*** *Measured data telemetry, model, serial number, date and time, patient information entered by the medical staff, and summary of capture and sensing threshold results performed during the evaluation.*

to pace all of the time at maximal output on each channel may last only 2 years. An identical model programmed to outputs of 2.5 V or lower on each channel that are inhibited a significant portion of the time may be anticipated to function properly for 10 years or longer. It would be inappropriate to follow the second unit on a monthly basis beginning 1 year after implantation, whereas it would be equally inappropriate to plan only annual checks on a pacing system programmed with high outputs and 100% pacing. By following some measure of the status of the battery, either directly or indirectly, the clinician can achieve a qualitative assessment about when to increase the frequency of pacing system follow-up.[12]

There are two primary indicators of battery status. One is the battery voltage, which progressively decreases over time. A lithium-iodine power cell is now used in virtually all pulse generators, whereas the power source in an ICD is vanadium pentoxide. The nominal unloaded output voltage of the lithium-iodine cell is 2.8 V, with each manufacturer triggering the RRT indicator at a specified battery voltage based on circuit design considerations. The battery voltage and programmed output voltage are not identical. The programmed output voltage is achieved by modifying the 2.8-V battery output with either voltage multipliers or charge pumps to provide a higher voltage. The battery voltage can also be divided to deliver a voltage lower than 2.8 V. As energy is consumed, the battery voltage progressively decreases due to increased internal impedance. Even with decreasing battery voltage, the device circuitry is designed to maintain the stability of the programmed voltage delivered to the patient. The ability to track the progressive decrease in battery voltage provides an effective guide to the physician regarding the frequency with which the pacing system should be routinely checked for signs of battery depletion. In addition, the measured battery voltage is affected by the battery current drain: the higher the current drain, the lower the battery voltage.

Inversely related to battery voltage is battery impedance. In the lithium-iodine power cell, the release of electrons is generated by the combination of the lithium ion with two iodine atoms. The result of this chemical reaction is the release of two electrons and the formation of lithium iodide. As the lithium iodide accumulates, it forms a resistive barrier between the anode and the cathode. With progressive cell depletion, the increasing amount of lithium iodide results in a rise in the internal impedance of the battery, which some pacemakers can measure and report in the telemetry data. The higher the battery impedance, the lower the cell voltage.

Battery voltage and impedance may be tracked together or individually. If these measurements are provided to the manufacturer's technical service engineers, along with the programmed parameters and an estimate of the percentage of pacing versus inhibition, the remaining longevity of that pacing system can be estimated with reasonable accuracy, assuming that the various parameters remain stable. These calculations have more recently been incorporated into the programmer interface to provide an on-line estimate of longevity in years or months. These estimates are sometimes shown as a range based on the tolerances of the battery measurements (i.e., giving minimum and maximum ranges of longevity), as well as an estimate based on present current drain and actual device use based on data acquired from the event counter diagnostics.

Lead Status

Although many systems provide data concerning lead function, including pulse voltage, current, charge, and energy, the measurement that is used most frequently is that of lead impedance (stimulation resistance). Changes in lead impedance directly affect the other measures of lead function. The terms *resistance* and *impedance*, although technically different, are often used interchangeably by the clinical community. Impedance is a complex concept that reflects a changing environment involving a variety of factors. This results in fluctuations in the moment-to-moment resistance. The resistance to electron flow in a pacing system progressively rises during delivery of the stimulation pulse as a result of polarization at the electrode-myocardium interface and, as a continuously changing variable, it is appropriately termed impedance. Many pulse generators and pacing system analyzers make this measurement at a specific point within the pacing stimulus; this is a resistance. Other devices report the resistance as an average of the impedance throughout the pulse. The actual resistance to current flow imparted by the conductor coil is fixed and represents a small portion of the total stimulation resistance. The polarization at the electrode-myocardium interface, which is related in part to the surface area and geometry of the electrode, and the impedance associated with conduction of the pulse through the body's tissues play a larger role in the overall resistance of the system. All of these factors are incorporated in the single measurement termed *lead impedance* or, more accurately, *stimulation impedance*.

Stimulation impedance is affected by many factors, but primarily by the design of the electrode, including size, configuration, and materials. Manufacturers have designed some electrodes with high impedance values. For any given output, a high-impedance system reduces the overall current drain of the battery and effectively increases the longevity of the device. Other leads have been designed specifically for low polarization to allow for detection of capture with each pace stimulus. Polarization and impedance are not the same phenomenon, although one affects the other. For any given lead model, there is a range of normal impedance values that may be broad; for a specific lead within that model series, however, the impedance should fall within a relatively narrow range.

The clinician can use knowledge of lead impedance to monitor and identify a developing mechanical problem with the lead. This requires baseline and historical data to recognize subtle changes that may reflect conductor fracture or an insulation breach. It is essential to know what device is being used to make these measurements. As noted previously, different devices may obtain these data at different points of the pacing stimulus. Because of these differences, the impedance measurement obtained with a pacing system analyzer at the time of implantation may be significantly different from that obtained by telemetry from the implanted pacemaker moments, if not years, later. This difference does not necessarily imply a problem. Furthermore, impedance may naturally evolve over time, with a fall in impedance occurring during the days to weeks after implantation, followed by a gradual rise toward the initial measurements on a chronic basis. Multiple factors may affect impedance, particularly in a unipolar system. For example, measurements obtained during deep inspiration may significantly differ from those obtained during maximal exhalation. In the same patient, impedance measurements that are based on a single-output pulse have been reported to vary by 100 Ω (or even more) during the same follow-up evaluation, while remaining consistent with normal function. If a marked change in lead impedance from previous measurements (e.g., >200 Ω) is encountered during a routine follow-up evaluation, further evaluation of the pacing system is advisable.[13,14] If the patient has no clinical symptoms and has stable capture and sensing thresholds, operative intervention would be premature, although a more frequent follow-up schedule would be prudent. However, a dramatic change in telemetered lead impedance in the presence of a clinical problem directs the physician toward the likely source of the difficulty (Fig. 24-2).

A dramatic fall in impedance usually reflects a break in the insulation.[15-17] In a unipolar system, an insulation problem provides an alternative pathway for current flow starting closer to the pulse generator, resulting in less energy reaching the heart. An outer insulation break in a bipolar lead tends to result in "unipolarization" of the lead. The amplitude of the stimulus artifact as recorded by an analog ECG is determined by the distance the current travels in the tissues from the cathode (tip electrode) to the anode (ring electrode or housing of the pulse generator). A normally functioning bipolar pacing system in which both active electrodes are inside the heart, separated only 1 to 2 cm, results in a small stimulus artifact. In a unipolar system, the current travels from the tip electrode to the housing of the pulse generator, and therefore the stimulus artifact is large despite equivalent output settings. Some of the newer digital ECG designs result in a marked signal-to-signal variation in amplitude as a result of the digital sampling rate of the recording system. Other recording systems create an artificial uniform amplitude artifact with any high-frequency electrical transient, thereby precluding differentiation of a bipolar from a unipolar pacing system based on the analysis of the ECG recording.

In a previously stable system, a mechanical problem developing with the lead—either a breach in the insulation or a conductor fracture—results in a change in the stimulation impedance, which may be reflected by a change in the ECG-recorded stimulus artifact (Fig. 24-3). In a bipolar pacing system, an insulation defect between the proximal conductor and the tissues of the body is not likely to affect capture thresholds, but it results in a larger stimulus artifact, making it appear unipolar. Depending on the actual location of the insulation failure in either the bipolar or the unipolar lead, stimulation of the extracardiac muscle contiguous to the insulation defect may occur. Insulation failures may also attenuate the electrical signal reaching the pacemaker, possibly resulting in sensing failure.

In a bipolar lead, an insulation defect developing between the proximal and distal conductors can present as a variety of clinical manifestations. Intermittent contact between the two conductors generates a voltage transient that the pacemaker can sense, resulting in inhibition or triggering, depending on the programmed sensing mode and the channel on which the problem has occurred. This small electrical signal is not seen on the surface ECG and is appropriately termed *oversensing*. If the two conductors remain in contact, current flowing down the distal conductor is short-circuited to the proximal conductor and never reaches the electrodes. This may result in a loss of capture and a further reduction in amplitude of the normally diminutive bipolar stimulus artifact on the ECG. In addition, loss of appropriate sensing may occur.

Programming of the output configuration to unipolar (most pacing systems now have this capability) may prevent the loss of capture and possibly undersensing from an internal short circuit. This does not prevent the oversensing behavior associated with make-break electrical transients generated by intermittent contact between the two conductors, as is caused by failed inner insulation. Typically, a bipolar lead with failed internal insulation exhibits a higher impedance when pacing is programmed to the unipolar rather than the

294-03-001024	APR 13 '93	11:46 AM	*
RELAY	TELEMETRY DATA		I
PACING RATE		70 PPM	N
PACING INTERVAL	860 MSec		T
CELL VOLTAGE		2.48 VOLTS	E
CELL IMPEDANCE		< 2.5 KOHMS	R
CELL CURRENT		40.1 UA	M
	ATRIAL (Bi)	VENTRICULAR (Bi)	E
SENSITIVITY	1.3	3.0 MV	D
LEAD IMPEDANCE	501	Low OHMS	I
PULSE AMPLITUDE	3.43	3.13 VOLTS	C
PULSE WIDTH	0.45	0.45 MSEC	S
OUTPUT CURRENT	6.5	HIGH MA	
ENERGY DELIVERED	9.1	HIGH UJ	I
CHARGE DELIVERED	2.94	HIGH UC	N
			C
		RETURN	*

Figure 24-2. Measured data telemetry from a Relay Model 294-03 rate-modulated dual-chamber pacemaker (Sulzer Intermedics, Angleton, Tex.) reporting a low impedance on the ventricular lead as a result of an insulation failure. This also produces an increase in the battery or cell current caused by a higher output current, charge, and energy being delivered by the pacemaker, whether or not it reaches the heart. This system reports extreme values as high or low, whereas other systems report specific numbers.

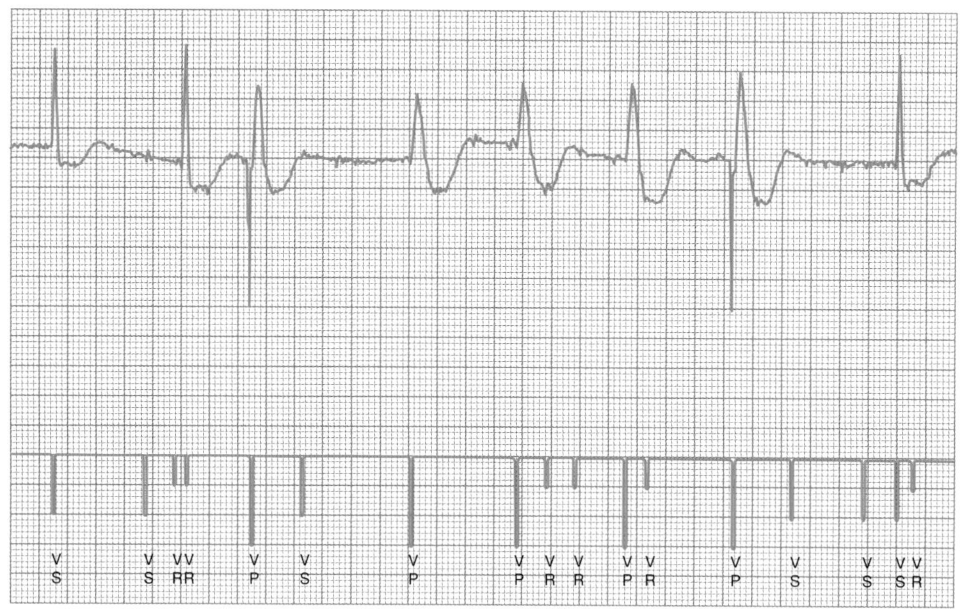

Figure 24-3. Simultaneous electrocardiogram (ECG) and event markers from a Medtronic Activitrax Model 8400 single-chamber, bipolar, rate-modulated pacemaker (Medtronic, Minneapolis, Minn.) with an internal insulation failure of the lead. There are both oversensing (VS and VR) and functional undersensing when the true native complex coincides with the refractory period initiated by the oversensing. During the intervention for lead replacement, the measured lead impedance was 125 Ω. The event markers are both labeled (VP, ventricular pacing; VS, ventricular sensing; VR, sensed event occurring during the refractory period) and identified by different amplitudes of the marker artifacts. The surface ECG should also be examined. This recording system generates a large-amplitude "artifact" to simulate the paced output with any high-frequency transient that is detected independent of the output configuration of the pulse. If no stimulus is detected, no artifact is generated. There are paced QRS complexes identified by the event markers that have no "pacing stimulus" on the ECG, whereas others have a large "unipolar" pacing stimulus visible. The identification of the pacing system malfunction was facilitated by the simultaneous event markers.

bipolar output configuration.[18,19] This is opposite to the expected higher impedance of a bipolar system. Although programming to a unipolar configuration may result in an apparent resolution of a malfunction, it is not a cure and should be considered only as a temporary measure, one that allows the observed problem to be managed on an elective rather than an emergent basis. The malfunctioning lead should be replaced expeditiously.

An increase in lead impedance may be the result of a conductor fracture or a connector problem.[20] When this occurs, the lead impedance often rises to high levels. It is inappropriate, however, to assume that a normal lead impedance is 500 Ω. Leads are available that are designed to have high impedance, with values ranging from 1500 to 2500 Ω. Other leads, at implantation, may have an impedance in the range of 250 to 300 Ω. Therefore, it is essential to look for a trend in serial lead impedance measurements rather than a single measurement. Impedance, taken in conjunction with the stability or changes in capture and sensing thresholds, is the best way to determine the condition of a pacing lead. A mechanical problem with the lead—either a conductor fracture resulting in a high impedance or an insulation failure resulting in a low impedance—eventually results in an overt clinical problem that can be identified by telemetric measurement of the stimulation impedance. If the impedance is sufficiently high, there is no current flow and no effective output. It must be understood that, although the telemetered event markers indicate a pace output, there may by loss of capture. The reduced current flow also results in a fall in the measured current drain of the battery. Note that any problem may be intermittent. This typically occurs when the two broken ends make contact at times but are separated at other times, or, in the case of an insulation failure, when lead movement either opens the compromised area or pushes the edges of the break together, resulting in intermittent normal function.

Before the availability of telemetry for lead impedance measurements, physicians could obtain similar information by oscilloscopic analysis of the pacemaker stimulus. In the 1970s, some manufacturers included a photograph of the pulse wave contour at a variety of different impedance values with the technical manual accompanying each pacemaker. Some computer-based pacemaker ECG follow-up systems are able to record and display the pacemaker pulse at an expanded scale. This allows the pace waveform to be recorded and tracked as a routine part of the periodic pacing system evaluation. Although this feature is available, it is not routinely used, given the ready access to lead impedance measurements provided by the implanted pacing system.

Lead impedance measurements have an indeterminate incidence of false-negative results when the lead problem is only intermittently manifested. The system forces the pacemaker to function asynchronously in an effort to obtain the measurements. The measurements, however, are made over a few cycles. If there is a true lead problem, but it is intermittent and was not present when the measurements were being made, the telemetered lead impedance may be normal. Therefore, if a problem is suspected, repeated measurements should be performed. Use of provocative maneuvers, such as placing manual pressure along the subcutaneous course of the lead or having the patient raise or in other ways manipulate the ipsilateral arm, may be required to unmask a problem.

Some pacemakers are able to report lead impedance measurements on a beat-by-beat basis, allowing the clinician to observe the digital readout of lead impedance on the programmer screen over a protracted number of cycles. Like the oscilloscopic monitoring of the pulse wave morphology, this technique reduces but does not eliminate the incidence of false-negative results. A further enhancement is the automatic periodic monitoring of lead impedance, which results in a graphic display reporting the history of lead impedance performance. Measurements can be obtained continuously or on a daily basis. This increases the frequency of measurement, increasing the likelihood of diagnosing an intermittent lead problem and possibly intervening on an automatic basis (Fig. 24-4). Some devices respond by automatically programming the pacemaker from bipolar polarity to unipolar in the presence of either a marked rise in impedance reflecting a conductor fracture[21] or a marked drop in impedance consistent with an insulation failure.

Event Marker Telemetry

The challenges associated with interpreting the paced ECG have markedly increased with the expanded use of dual-chamber, multisensor, rate-modulated systems. Even with the simplest pacing systems, multiple assumptions had to be made. Most clinicians are comfortable evaluating a surface ECG composed of P waves

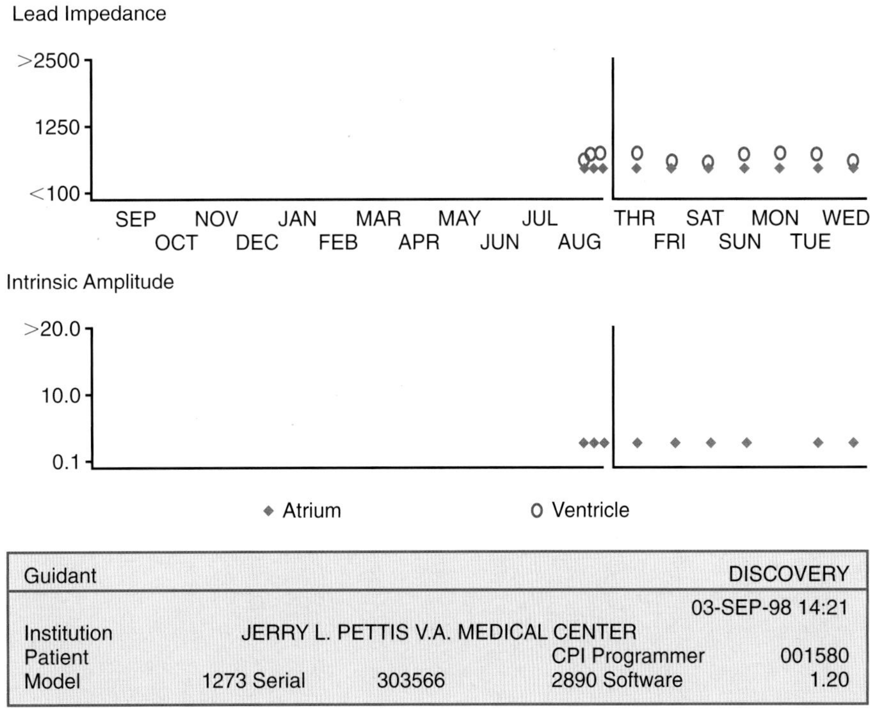

Daily Measurement-Data Table

Date	Atrium Amplitude (mV)	Atrium Impedance (Ω)	Ventricle Amplitude (mV)	Ventricle Impedance (Ω)
02-SEP-98	>3.5	480	PACED	680
01-SEP-98	>3.5	500	PACED	710
31-AUG-98	PACED	500	PACED	710
30-AUG-98	>3.5	480	PACED	710
29-AUG-98	>3.5	500	PACED	680
28-AUG-98	>3.5	470	PACED	670
27-AUG-98	>3.5	470	PACED	710
21-AUG-98	>3.5	480	PACED	710
14-AUG-98	>3.5	480	PACED	720
07-AUG-98	>3.5	480	PACED	680

Figure 24-4. Graphic display and tabular summary of serial automatic atrial and ventricular lead impedance measurements as well as intrinsic signal amplitude from an implanted Guidant Discovery DDDR Model 1273 pacemaker (CPI Guidant, Boston Scientific, Natick, Mass.). This event counter reports measurements made on a daily basis for the past 7 days and the mean weekly measurements before that time, with the potential for extending back a full year. These data were retrieved at a follow-up evaluation.

representing native atrial depolarizations and QRS complexes (or R waves) representing native ventricular depolarizations. The pacemaker does not respond to the P or R wave, but to the intrinsic deflection of the electrical potential inside the heart that occurs as the wave of depolarization passes by the pacing electrode. Although the events inside the heart frequently correspond to events recorded by the ECG, there may be events inside the heart that are not visible on the ECG. In addition, the pacemaker senses and responds to events occurring outside the heart if they are detected by the sense amplifier. Standard ECG recordings may not depict these internal and external electrical events, yet they can affect the behavior of the pacing system. Similarly, standard ECG recordings do not detect the usual sensor signals that may also drive the pacemaker to a variety of different rates and timing settings.

The introduction of dual-chamber pacing significantly increased the level of complexity of the paced rhythm. The interaction between the two channels of the pacing system with the spontaneous rhythms occurring in either the atria or the ventricles added to the potential for confusion. The addition of rate-modulated pacing (i.e., allowing the pacemaker to respond to one or more sensor signals that are invisible on the ECG) further contributed to the challenge of interpreting the paced ECG. Further complexity was added to the pacemaker timing cycles with various atrioventricular (AV)-interval modulation schemes designed to enhance conduction down the patient's AV node, to prevent conduction down the AV node, or simply to enhance the ability to achieve higher pacing rates while maintaining AV synchrony. Various functions that include rate hysteresis and therapeutic pacing rates in response to sudden decreases in native heart rates complicate these systems even further. Most recently, the widespread use of multichamber pacing for cardiac resynchronization and atrial fibrillation suppression has created an even greater degree of complexity.

In the modern pacemaker, interpretation of the paced rhythm requires knowledge of the basic timing intervals. A variety of refractory periods, including the postventricular atrial refractory period (PVARP), the postventricular atrial blanking period, the ventricular refractory period, ventricular blanking period, and paced and sensed AV intervals, must be considered. Some intervals may change depending on the rate, such as the AV interval, atrial escape interval (when under sensor drive or with special features), and the PVARP. The clinician also needs to be aware of a number of device-specific responses to protect the system from a variety of anticipated but undesirable behaviors or clinical events. These include crosstalk, the initiation by a premature ventricular beat of a pacemaker-mediated tachycardia (PMT), mode switching, and multiblock upper rate behavior.

To facilitate interpretation of the paced rhythm, almost all modern pacing systems incorporate the ability to transmit information regarding real-time pacing system behavior to the programmer. These data are displayed on the programmer screen and may also be printed as well. Both paced and sensed events are communicated to the programmer. Displayed as a series of positive or negative marks, with or without alphanumeric annotation, these are generically termed *event markers*. They have the greatest diagnostic value when superimposed above or below a simultaneously recorded surface ECG (Fig. 24-5). Some systems also display the duration of the atrial and ventricular refractory periods and interval measurements. Others show events that are sensed during the refractory period even though they do not play a role in altering the system

ECG Controls

Surface ECG	On	
Position	1	
Gain	0.25	mV/div
Filter	On	
Markers	On	
Position	2	
IEGM	Off	
Position	3	
Gain	5	mV/div
Configuration	--	
Sweep Speed	25	mm/s

Programmed Parameters

Mode	DDDR	
Base Rate	65	ppm
A-V Delay	300	ms
P-V Delay	200	ms
Magnet Response	Temporary Off	
Temporary 30	Off	

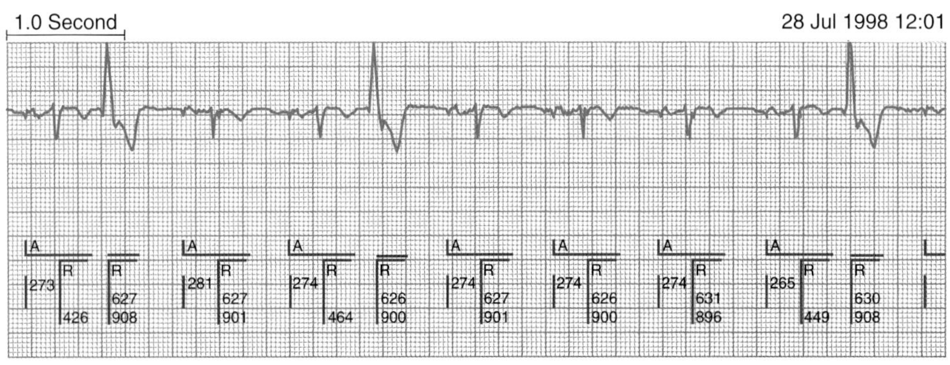

Figure 24-5. Surface electrocardiogram and simultaneous event marker telemetry from a Pacesetter Trilogy DR+ Model 2360 (St. Jude Medical CRMD, Sylmar, Calif.), showing an atrial-paced rhythm with intact atrioventricular nodal conduction and isolated ventricular ectopic beats. Key programmed parameters are shown at the upper right, and recording parameters at the upper left. The numbers refer to the millisecond intervals automatically measured and displayed by the programmer. The horizontal lines that follow the alphabetic label (A, atrial-paced output; R, sensed ventricular event) represent the length of the programmed or functional refractory period.

timing (i.e., they are sensed but not used). Events may be displayed either in a real-time manner or after the tracing has been frozen on the programmer screen by the use of cursors to identify the interval of interest. If the real-time monitor screen method is used to show the rhythm and event markers, the tracing may be frozen and then printed for inclusion in the medical record.

Event markers (also called *marker channels*, *annotated event markers*, and *main timing events* by various manufacturers) are most effectively used when they are displayed with a simultaneously recorded ECG rhythm.[22-25] Without the ECG, the event marker simply reports the behavior of the pacemaker. This information is valuable in showing that an output has been released or that sensing has occurred. What it does not confirm is that the stimulus effectively resulted in capture, or that a sensed event was a true atrial or ventricular depolarization. The presence of an output marker does not confirm that the stimulus even reached the heart. The output marker serves only to confirm that the pacemaker delivered a stimulus from its output circuit. This notation is transmitted directly from the pacemaker to the programmer by way of the telemetry module. An open circuit (e.g., a fractured conductor coil) may preclude the output pulse from reaching the heart, yet the pacemaker would indicate that an output pulse was released. Similarly, a native depolarization may not be sensed, allowing the pacing stimulus to be released at a time when the myocardium is physiologically refractory. If the markers reported that an event was sensed on the atrial channel and was followed by a ventricular output pulse after a preset delay (known as *P-wave synchronous ventricular pacing* or *tracking*), the clinician would know that the pacemaker was capable of sensing in the atria and pacing in the ventricles. Without a simultaneously recorded ECG, it would be impossible to determine whether the pacemaker was responding to inappropriate signals on the atrial channel, whether the ventricular stimulus was effective, or whether a native QRS was present but not sensed. Hence, telemetered event markers are most effective when displayed with a simultaneously recorded ECG.

Event Marker Displays

A variety of different displays have been used over the years. Although not intended for this purpose, the simplest event marker for sensed events was achieved with triggered mode pacing, particularly if the output configuration was unipolar. A sensed event would be marked by the simultaneous release of a pacing stimulus coincident with sensing. This was easily recorded on the ECG, because the stimulus artifact distorted the morphology of the native sensed complex. The next evolutionary step in this technology involved the pacemaker's emitting a series of subthreshold stimuli of varying amplitudes to represent the release of an output pulse, a sensed event, and the end of a refractory period. Both of these systems, the triggered mode and the series of markers, were limited by the fact that the signals required an intact lead system, to allow the pulse to be delivered to the heart through the lead and subsequently recorded for display by the ECG. With a bipolar output pulse, the small artifact might not be readily visible, particularly in the triggered mode, because it would be obscured by the larger native complexes. In addition, if there were an open circuit (most commonly a conductor fracture) or an internal insulation failure involving a bipolar lead, no marker would be visible.

The next improvement was to transmit coded signals representing paced and sensed events from the pacemaker to the programmer. The programmer reconstituted these signals into a series of varying-amplitude pulses or alphanumeric labels representing paced or sensed events. These could be either displayed on a monitor screen or recorded using a printer integral to the programming system, which allowed for the simultaneous recording of a surface ECG acquired by way of a separate set of cables. The simultaneous ECG and markers allowed the clinician to correlate the behavior of the pacemaker directly with the patient's rhythm, to determine whether the system is functioning properly. A calibration signal composed of a series of different amplitude pulses or a legend of the cryptic labels allowed the clinician to interpret the various markers. In an early series of markers, the largest pulse represented a pacing output, the intermediate one indicated a sensed event, and the smallest represented either the end of the refractory period or a sensed complex that occurred during the refractory period. With the advent of dual-chamber pacing systems, a marker pulse extending above the baseline identified atrial events, and ventricular events were labeled with a pulse extending below the baseline.

A further refinement to this system was the addition of alphanumeric annotations, which made the simple (yet cryptic) system just described obsolete. Two common sets of notations have been used and are summarized later. These are not the only possibilities, because some manufacturers use a unique set of symbols to identify paced and sensed events, with the location of the symbol on the recording identifying whether it represents an atrial or a ventricular event. Others have expanded on the set of labels and provide, on command, a detailed explanation.

One method for single-chamber pacing systems with event marker telemetry uses the letter P to reflect a paced event and S to represent a sensed event. This has the potential for causing confusion with other dual-chamber systems in which the letter P reflects a sensed atrial event indicative of a native P wave (with which most medical personnel are familiar, based on their knowledge of the standard ECG). The interpretation of the alphanumeric event markers is often product specific, and the clinic personnel who evaluate the pacing system must take this into account (Fig. 24-6).

In the case of dual-chamber pacing or when the pacemaker knows that it is providing atrial pacing and sensing, a native atrial depolarization may be identified as either the letter P or the combination AS. P is taken from the standard ECG identifier for an atrial

Event Marker Annotation Legend

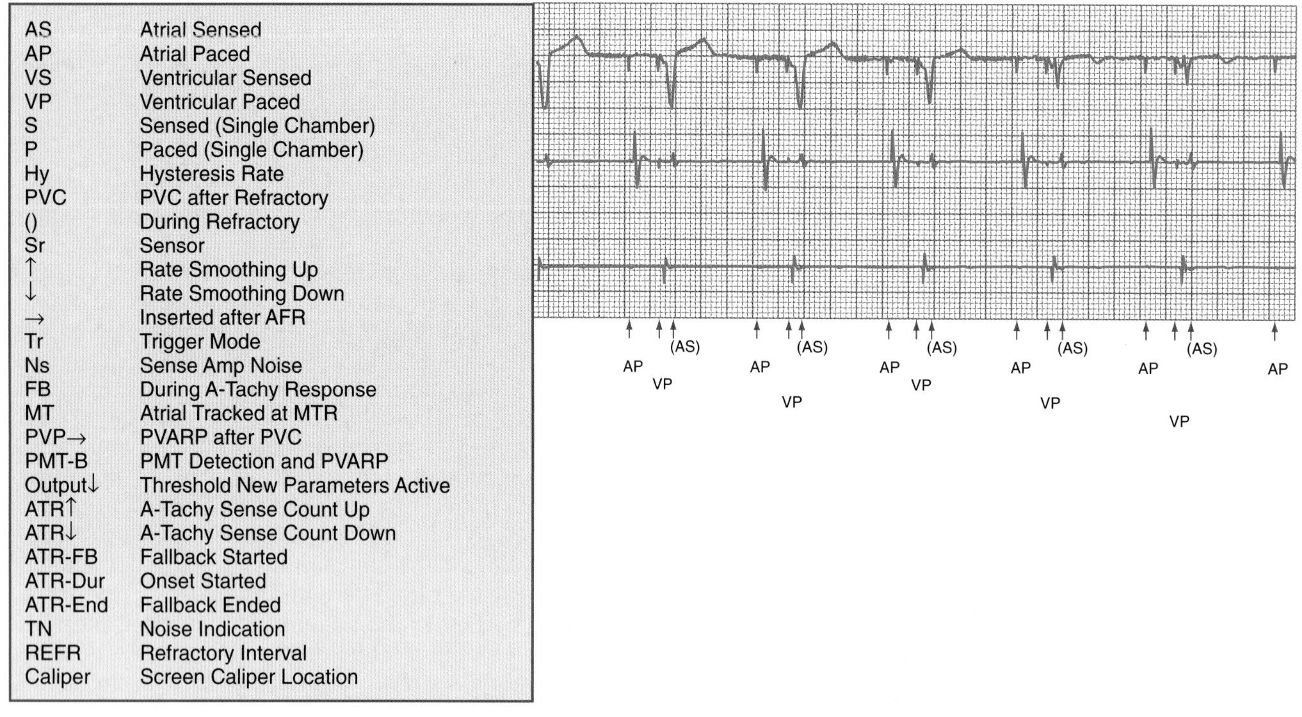

AS Atrial Sensed
AP Atrial Paced
VS Ventricular Sensed
VP Ventricular Paced
S Sensed (Single Chamber)
P Paced (Single Chamber)
Hy Hysteresis Rate
PVC PVC after Refractory
() During Refractory
Sr Sensor
↑ Rate Smoothing Up
↓ Rate Smoothing Down
→ Inserted after AFR
Tr Trigger Mode
Ns Sense Amp Noise
FB During A-Tachy Response
MT Atrial Tracked at MTR
PVP→ PVARP after PVC
PMT-B PMT Detection and PVARP
Output↓ Threshold New Parameters Active
ATR↑ A-Tachy Sense Count Up
ATR↓ A-Tachy Sense Count Down
ATR-FB Fallback Started
ATR-Dur Onset Started
ATR-End Fallback Ended
TN Noise Indication
REFR Refractory Interval
Caliper Screen Caliper Location
(AS) (AS) (AS) (AS) (AS)
AP AP AP AP AP AP
VP VP VP VP VP

End of Report

Figure 24-6. An event marker annotation legend from a Guidant Discovery DDDR Model 1273 pacing system (CPI Guidant, Boston Scientific, Natick, Mass.) is shown on the left. The labels are placed under the simultaneously recorded electrocardiogram (ECG) to identify specific events reflecting the behavior of the pacemaker (right). *Also displayed are simultaneously recorded atrial and ventricular electrograms. AP, atrial-paced event; VP, ventricular-paced event; (AS), atrial-sensed event occurring during atrial refractory period—in this case, it is a far-field R wave that is also visible on the atrial electrogram channel (middle channel on ECG recording).*

depolarization. AS is one abbreviation for an atrial-sensed event. An atrial stimulus may be identified by either the letter A or the combination AP for atrial-paced event.

Analogous lettering is used on the ventricular channel. Again, single-chamber pacing in some systems might still use the letters P to represent a paced event and S to refer to a sensed event. Other systems use R to refer to a native ventricular depolarization, which is generically called an R wave on the standard ECG. This may also be identified by the letter combination VS for a ventricular-sensed event. The letter V in one system might be used to represent a ventricular pacing stimulus, whereas the identical event may be labeled VP (for ventricular pacing) in other systems.

Other symbols may be used for a paced or sensed event, and these symbols are commonly displayed with an identifying key on the resultant printout. Each paced or sensed event may also be identified by a vertical line, going up in the case of atrial events and down for ventricular events. In some cases, a difference in the amplitude of these lines has been retained in conjunction with the alphanumeric lettering. Indeed, as the complexity of the devices increases, the variety of symbols and letters identifying specific events and behaviors is also increasing (see Fig. 24-6).

In many systems, interval measurements between the various events are either calculated automatically and displayed, or measured after cursors are aligned with specific events. There may be a time delay between the actual sensed or paced event and the release of the event marker. This is caused by the finite period that is required for the pacemaker to recognize the event and then transmit the appropriate information to the programmer through the telemetry channel. In most cases, priority is given to the normal function of the pacemaker, with the diagnostic marker feature being delayed. Differences of up to 40 msec between the actual event and the resultant marker have been noted.

Laddergramming

Laddergramming is an advanced adjunct to the interpretation of clinical arrhythmias. It was incorporated in some programming systems by using the known programmed parameters of the pacemaker combined with the event marker information telemetry from the

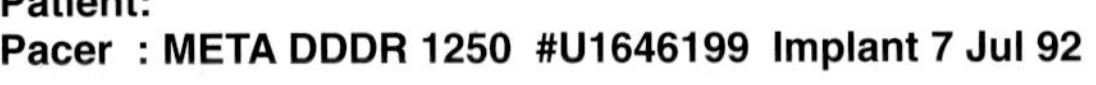

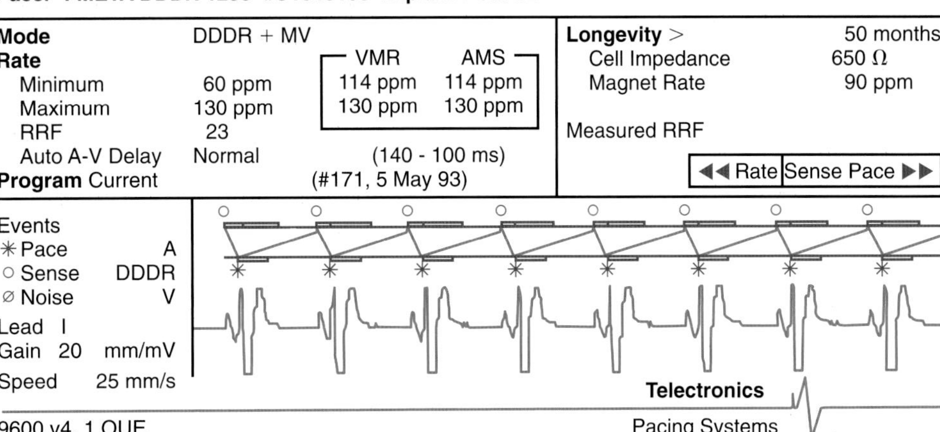

Figure 24-7. Laddergram from a META DDDR Model 1250 rate-modulated dual-chamber pacing system (Telectronics Pacing Systems, now Pacesetter, St. Jude Medical CRMD, Sylmar, Calif.) displayed with a Model 9600 programmer. The event markers are identified by a variety of symbols displayed in a key to the left of the tracing. In addition, battery (cell) impedance and projected longevity are reported in the upper right portion of the tracing, and selected programmed parameters are shown in the upper left quadrant. AV, atrioventricular; RRF, rate response factor.

implanted pacemaker (Fig. 24-7).[23-26] For all the elegance of these graphic interpretations of the pacemaker's behavior, they still require the simultaneously recorded ECG rhythms. Although the pacemaker may be functioning normally, in that it is behaving properly with respect to its programmed parameters, failure to capture or properly sense would not be diagnosed from the various diagrams and markers without the simultaneously recorded surface ECG.[27] Laddergramming has become a teaching tool at this time, because no programmers currently provide this level of graphic description.

Event Marker Limitations

A number of limitations are associated with event marker telemetry. The first is that, by themselves, markers report the behavior of the pacemaker but do not allow the clinician to determine whether this behavior is appropriate for the patient.[27] In this regard, they are analogous to the small hand-held digital counters that report pacing rates and intervals. The counters only detect and report the pacing stimuli, not whether these output pulses are effective in causing a cardiac depolarization or whether native events are properly and consistently sensed. A long interval between consecutive pacing stimuli could reflect normal function because the pacemaker responded appropriately to a native complex, or it could represent a system malfunction with oversensing or no output (e.g., from an intermittent lead fracture). Neither event marker telemetry nor the digital counters should be used independently of a simultaneously monitored ECG rhythm.

The second limitation is that the report of a stimulus output does not mean that there was appropriate capture. Confirmation of capture requires an ECG or concomitant hemodynamic pulse monitoring. In addition, the markers may report that the pacemaker is sensing a signal, but if this signal is not visible on the surface ECG there is cause for concern. Is it an appropriate signal that the pacemaker should be sensing (some intrinsic atrial rhythms may not be visible on the specific lead that is being monitored), or is the system responding to an inappropriate or nonphysiologic signal, such as the make-break potentials associated with a breach of the internal insulation in a coaxial bipolar lead?

Most pacemaker event marker telemetry is limited to real-time recordings. The markers must be telemetered from the pacemaker to the programmer or another display system while the rhythm is being actively monitored. Neither the pacemaker nor the programmer can retrospectively provide markers for a previously recorded rhythm. If the pacemaker is responding to events that are not visible on the surface ECG, the event marker simply confirms this fact but does not identify the specific signal. An evaluation of sensed but otherwise invisible events requires intracardiac electrogram (EGM) telemetry or an invasive procedure to record the signal from the implanted lead. Many premium-level pacemakers have been introduced that have the capability of storing event markers with or without EGMs. These may be stored by the use of a patient trigger such as magnet application,[28] by use of a simple battery-operated radio-frequency transmitter, or on spontaneous activation of specific predefined algorithms or sequences of sensed or paced events.

Electrogram Telemetry

The clinician evaluates a pacing system based on an analysis of the ECG, but the pacemaker does not respond to P waves or QRS complexes. The latter are surface manifestations of the atrial and ventricular depolarizations. The recorded signal that enters the pacemaker's sense amplifier by way of the electrode located within or on the heart is termed an *EGM* or *intracardiac EGM.* The EGM is composed of a number of elements. The portion that is sensed by the pacemaker is termed the *intrinsic deflection;* it reflects the rapid deflection that occurs when the wave of electrical cardiac depolarization passes by the electrode. The intrinsic deflection can be characterized by both amplitude and slew rate. The change in voltage amplitude divided by the time duration of this portion of the signal is the known as the *slew rate*. The unit of measurement for slew rate is volts per second. Most implanted pacemakers require a slew rate of more than 0.5 V/sec for proper sensing. The other portions of the cardiac depolarization, as reflected by the EGM, are termed the *extrinsic deflection*. Although the extrinsic deflection may have an adequate amplitude, the slew rate is usually too low, precluding this portion of the cardiac signal from being sensed by the pacemaker.

At the time of implantation, the amplitude of the EGM is commonly measured with a pacing system analyzer that reports a millivoltage amplitude. The pacing system analyzer uses its own unique set of filters, which may not be identical to those in the pacemaker's sense amplifier. Therefore, the analyzer's reported signal, at best, provides an approximation of what the pacemaker effectively sees. Likewise, the morphology of the EGM observed on a high-fidelity monitor is not identical to the signal as seen by the pacemaker, because filters in the pacemaker's sense amplifier usually have a narrower band-pass and therefore block out some of the frequencies (Fig. 24-8). Examining the EGM recorded with a physiologic recorder or telemetry with a wide band-pass can provide valuable information on the slew rate, splintering of the intrinsic deflection, and other morphologic abnormalities.

Measurements of the peak-to-peak amplitude of the EGM, as recorded at the time of implantation or as telemetered from an already implanted pacemaker, are commonly used to determine the sensing threshold. This approach may be inappropriate if the frequency content of the signal is outside the constraints of the band-pass filter of the sense amplifier. If the clinician wants to determine the sensing threshold for a given patient, the sensitivity of the system should be progressively reduced until the system no longer consistently senses the native signal. The least sensitive setting (usually identified by a millivolt amplitude) at which there is consistent sensing is the sensing threshold. The precision of this measurement is limited by the number and range of programmable sensitivity options in the specific model of pacemaker.[29-31] Almost all modern pacing systems now have the ability to automatically measure the EGM amplitude and report this to the clinician. This measurement is done through the pacemaker's band-pass filter and therefore is a good estimation of the EGM size. The limitation to this method occurs when there is a large beat-to-beat or respiratory variation of the EGM size. The best method available uses this automatic measurement together with a beat-by-beat digital readout of the EGM amplitude. With this approach, the range of actual EGMs can be accurately evaluated.

Other EGMs are obtained after the signal is processed by the pacemaker's sense amplifier. As shown in Figure 24-8, both filtered and unfiltered EGMs may be available. Although the unfiltered telemetered EGM should not be used to determine the sensing threshold, it has many other roles.[32,33] A primary value is in identifying signals that are being sensed but are not visible on the surface ECG. Another role is to facilitate analysis of the timing of the pacing system, because the sensed intrinsic deflection resets one or more timers. The intrinsic deflection at which sensing occurs can best be identified from the EGM; it is only

ECG Controls

Surface ECG	On	
Position	1	
Gain	1	mV/cm
Filter	Off	
Markers	On	
Position	2	
IEGM	On	
Position	3	
Gain	5	mV/cm
Configuration	Vtip-Vring	
Sweep Speed	100	mm/s

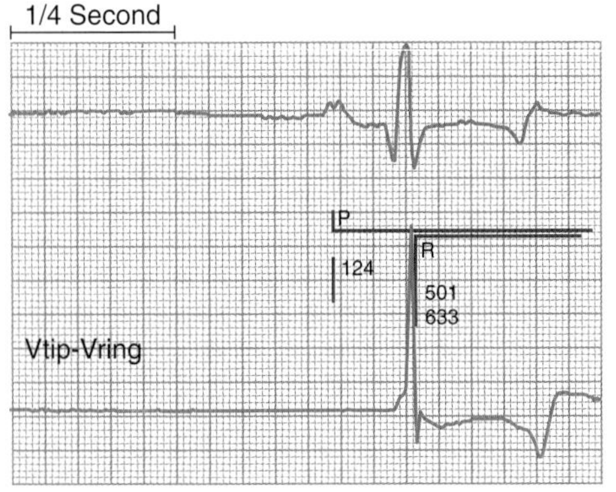

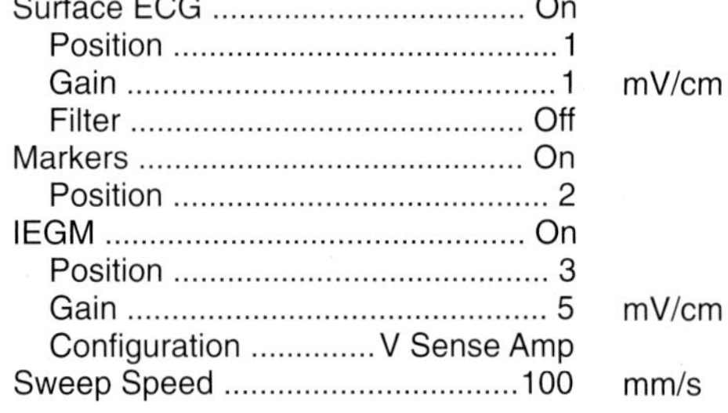

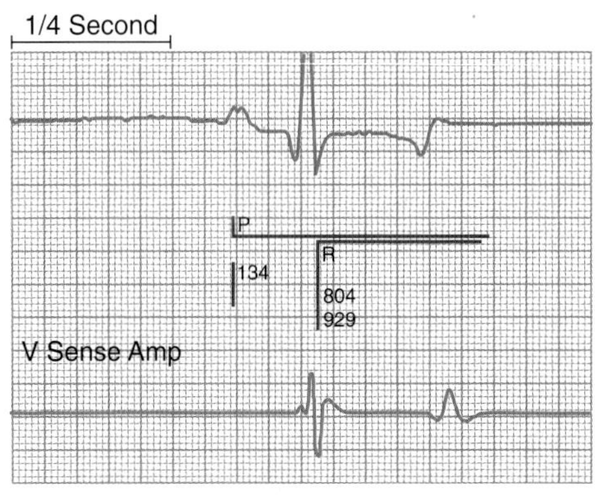

Figure 24-8. *Side-by-side display of telemetered bipolar ventricular electrograms, before being processed by the sense amplifier (Vtip-Vring) on the left and after being processed by the sense amplifier (V Sense Amp) on the right. The simultaneously recorded surface electrocardiogram (ECG) and telemetered event markers are also shown (P, native atrial depolarization; R, native ventricular depolarization), with the horizontal lines representing the atrial* (top) *and ventricular* (bottom) *refractory periods. The circuitry of the sense amplifier has a narrow band-pass filter that modifies the raw signal, which can also be telemetered. These signals were telemetered from a Pacesetter Affinity DR pacemaker, Model 5330 (St. Jude Medical CRMD, Sylmar, Calif.).*

indirectly measured from the surface ECG. In many cases, the telemetered EGM may be used to confirm capture (particularly atrial) when the evoked complex (P-wave or QRS) is not visible in any lead of the surface ECG.[34,35] The evoked EGM may be made more clear through the use of a unique output pulse configuration that can help to cancel the residual polarization artifact, or by recording the signal through electrodes that are not directly involved with the output pulse. The output pulse has a tendency to overload the telemetry or sense amplifier, driving the signal off scale. This is then followed by a refractory period within the telemetry amplifier before anything can again be recognized. However, many of the newer pacing systems have more advanced telemetry systems that are able to blank the output pulse and quickly recover to provide high-quality EGM signals.

The telemetered EGM has been effectively used to diagnose native arrhythmias in which the pacemaker is simply an innocent bystander or to identify retrograde P waves not visible on the surface ECG. The latter ability may facilitate programming of the PVARP to prevent PMTs.[35-43] The telemetered EGM provides clues to why episodes of undersensing may be occurring. Reasons include splintering of the EGM and low slew rates that may place the signal outside the tight constraints of the pacemaker's sense amplifier despite an adequate peak-to-peak amplitude (Fig. 24-9).[44]

The telemetered EGM can also be monitored on a periodic basis to follow the progression of the patient's intrinsic disease process. A decrease in the amplitude of the telemetered EGM was reported to identify early rejection effectively in cardiac transplantation recipients; a return to the baseline amplitude correlated with resolution of the rejection process.[45] Preliminary work on the signal-averaged EGM, either atrial or ventricular, suggests that it may be helpful in identifying disease in the respective chamber that is beyond the resolution of signal-averaging of the surface ECG.[46]

Limitations of Electrogram Telemetry

That the telemetered EGM appears to be of adequate amplitude for sensing does not mean that the pacemaker will sense it. The telemetry amplifier may use filters different from those in the sensing circuit, providing qualitative rather than quantitative data concerning the EGM (see Fig. 24-9). In most pacing systems, telemetered EGMs also suffer from limitations that are similar to those of event markers. They are real-time recordings and cannot be retrospectively provided by the programmer to facilitate the interpretation of an earlier ECG.

Real-time telemetry allows the physician to analyze the behavior of the pacing system when the patient is in the physician's office or clinic while these diagnostics are being accessed with the programmer. This is impractical over a long period. In addition, it does not allow the patient to move around much while these recordings are being obtained. Long-term monitoring of pacing system behavior requires either a Holter monitor, a loop memory recorder, or event counter telemetry, depending on the degree of precision that is desired. Pacemakers with microprocessors and significant random access memory (RAM) can now store select EGMs[47,48] as well as event markers when triggered by the patient or by a predefined set of circumstances. This may markedly reduce the need for Holter

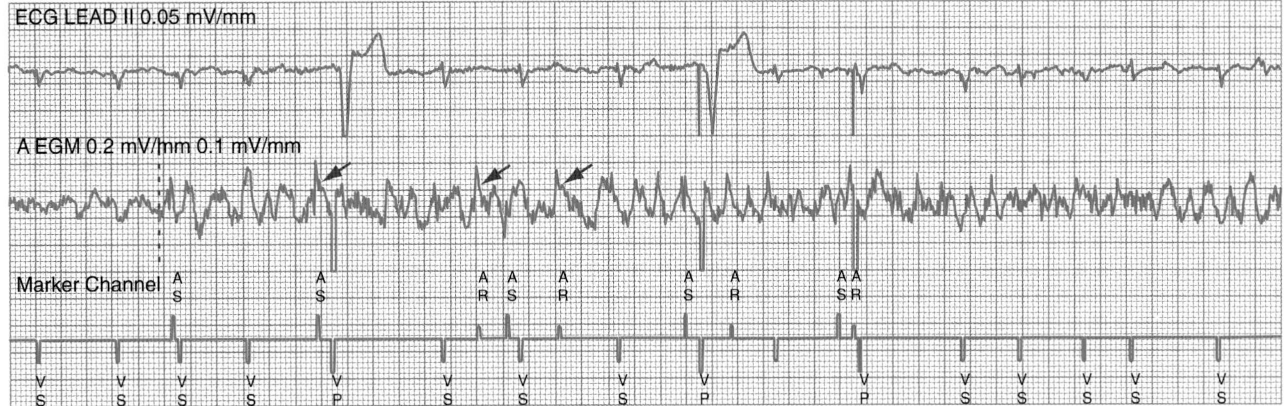

Figure 24-9. Simultaneous surface electrocardiogram (top), *atrial electrogram* (middle), *and event markers* (bottom) *from a patient with a Medtronic Prodigy DR Model 7860 pulse generator (Medtronic, Inc., Minneapolis, Minn.). Although the Automatic Mode Switch algorithm was enabled, this system did not switch modes despite the persistence of atrial fibrillation; the reason is clearly identified from the atrial electrograms, which were telemetered before being processed by the sense amplifier. The atrial fibrillatory signal is a predominantly low-frequency signal identified by the slow-rise deflections, even though the peak-to-peak amplitude was well above the programmed sensitivity and should have been adequate for fibrillation to be sensed. These low-frequency signals were filtered out by the sense amplifier, as demonstrated by the event markers—very few of the fibrillatory signals are sensed (AS or AR); hence, the rhythm never fulfills the rate criteria necessary to initiate mode switching. Note that the signals with a discrete rapid deflection* (arrows) *were properly sensed, whereas those that were not sensed had relatively slow deflections.*

or other monitoring techniques to evaluate intermittent symptoms in patients with pacemakers.

Event Counter Telemetry

Simplistically put, the pacemaker "knows" when it has released an output pulse or responded to a sensed event. The availability of high-density, low-power RAM and read-only memory (ROM) integral to microprocessors that can be incorporated in the pacemaker has given pacemakers the ability to store information about system performance for retrieval at a later date. The objective of the event counters is to facilitate the clinician's ability to analyze and manage the patient's pacing therapy more effectively. Although this may add to the time required for the evaluation, namely to retrieve and interpret these data, the additional time is usually minimal. This technology can provide the clinician with information that is crucial to understanding the performance of the system over time, and consequently to directing the programming of the system and achieving optimal performance. Other techniques, such as standard Holter monitor recordings or repeated exercise tolerance tests, although valuable, are impractical, arduous, and relatively expensive to acquire on a routine or repeated basis.

The first use of stored diagnostic data in cardiac pacemakers was associated with the introduction of multiparameter programmability. Simple data using codes to identify implant indications and medications could be downloaded into the pacemaker for retrieval at subsequent follow-up evaluations. This ability has been expanded, allowing entry of free text (date of implantation, lead model numbers, pharmacologic regimens, and acute implant measurements, including capture and sensing thresholds and lead impedances; see Fig. 24-1B). This information is printed with the programmed parameters each time the pacemaker is interrogated.

Event counters have been expanded since these early efforts. There are now a variety of different diagnostic counters. Some provide information concerning the overall performance of the system, whereas others focus on a specific algorithm or subsystem. Still others provide detailed information on the basis of the time course of events. The number of individual event counters that are currently available from a multiplicity of different devices is too numerous to detail in this chapter. Therefore, select examples are used to illustrate these capabilities.

Total System Performance Counters

The simplest systems keep track of the number of times a pacing stimulus is released or a native complex is sensed. This allows for an assessment of the degree to which the pacemaker was used by calculating the percent pacing in each chamber. A refinement of this ability allows the pacemaker to diagnose bradycardia and, in the dual-chamber modes, to tell whether the bradycardia was the result of sinus node dysfunction or AV block. Event counters with this ability have also been termed *diagnostic data*, *implanted Holter systems*, and *data logging*.[49-55]

With the introduction of dual-chamber pacing (specifically the DDD mode), the potential interactions between the pacemaker and the patient increased from two (pacing or sensing in one chamber) to five (pacing or sensing in the atria or ventricles and sensing ventricular activity without preexisting atrial activity). The situation became even more complex with the introduction of multiple-site ventricular and atrial pacing configurations. Knowledge of how the pacing system has behaved over time, combined with the clinician's knowledge of the patient, provides invaluable information toward assessing the overall performance of the implanted system.

The various annotations described in the event marker section were combined to provide a cryptic description of the different operational states of the DDD mode. These include an atrial-sensed event followed by a ventricular-sensed event (AS-VS or PR), indicating that the pacemaker is inhibited on both channels. Atrial sensing followed by a ventricular-paced event (AS-VP or PV) refers to P-wave synchronous ventricular pacing. Atrial pacing with intact AV nodal conduction or functional single-chamber atrial pacing is indicated by AP-VS or AR. Base-rate pacing in both chambers is represented by AP-VP or AV. A ventricular-sensed event not preceded by atrial activity, either paced or sensed, is a premature ventricular event (PVE), identified by the letter R or the combination VS. Some systems label these events premature ventricular contractions (PVCs).

This information may be collected in conjunction with events occurring in specific rate bins, allowing for a detailed report of heart rate distributions. Additional data that have been collected include the percentage of pacing in the atrium and ventricle, the amount of time at the maximum tracking rate, and the number of episodes in which the pacing system reached the programmed upper rate limit (Fig. 24-10). Additional data may be recorded regarding mode-switching events, PMT termination algorithm use, or the number of times any one of several other special features was activated. The counters are able to continue to accumulate data until one of the pacing state bins is full and cannot accept additional information. At this point, one or more of the counters are frozen. The volume of data that can be stored depends on the memory capacity of the pacemaker that is dedicated to these features.

The following example provides a general idea about the amount of data that can be stored or the quantity of memory. All data are stored in a binary code, represented by a series of 1s and 0s. A binary unit of memory is called a *bit*. Eight bits are a *byte* and result in 256 combinations of 1s and 0s. If each series of combinations represents a single item of data, a total of 256 pieces of information can be stored in a system with eight bits of memory. As the number of bits increases, the amount of data that can be stored increases geometrically. If each pacing state is represented by a single combination of bits, and there are 24 bits in the RAM devoted to these counters, more than 17 million

Mode .... DDD
Sensor .... Passive
Base Rate .... 50 ppm
Max Track Rate .... 145 ppm
Max Sensor Rate .... 135 ppm
A-V Delay .... 250 ms ms
Rate Resp. A-V Delay .... Enable

Note: The above values were obtained when the histogram was interrogated.

Date Read: .... 10 Aug 1998-14:57
Total Time Sampled: 388d 19th 4m 22s
Sampling Rate .... Every Event

Percent of counts paced in atrium 7%
Percent of counts paced in ventricle 19%
Total Time at Max Track Rate 0d 0h 0m 0s

Event Histogram

Event Histogram, Percent of Total Time

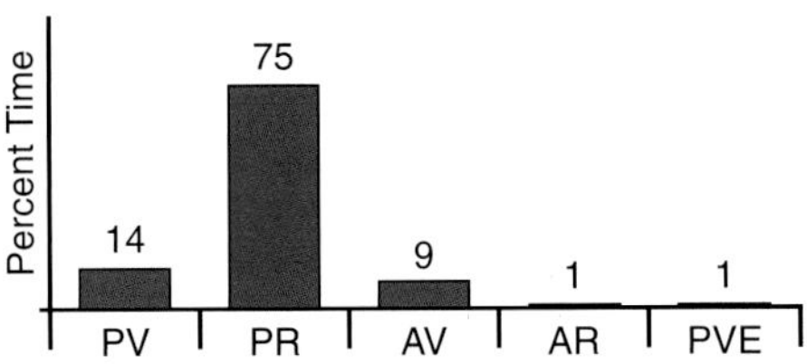

Heart Rate Histogram

Heart Rate Histogram, Percent of Total Time

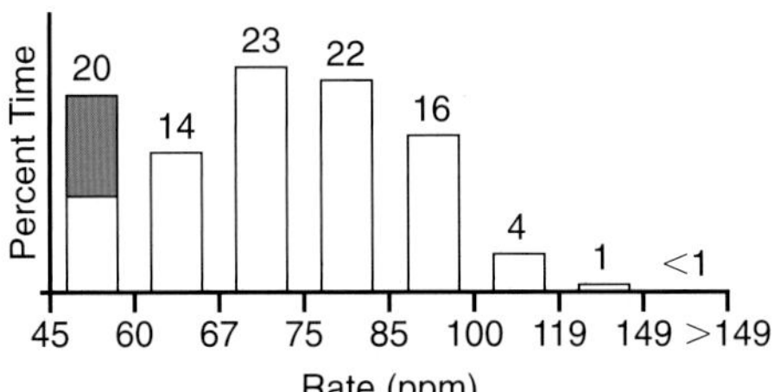

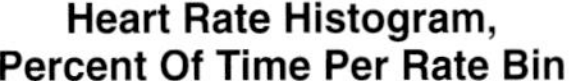

Event Counts

Rate (ppm)	PV	PR	AV	AR	PVE
45-60	997,091	1,888,457	2,621,941	237,669	0
61-67	1,791,645	3,252,366	60	44	553
68-75	1,821,846	7,182,349	0	0	7,330
76-85	410,361	9,349,618	0	0	14,901
86-100	56,251	8,170,791	0	0	87,023
101-119	8,477	2,213,554	0	0	157,939
120-149	214	468,215	0	0	55,365
>149	0	10,675	0	0	1,758
Total:	**5,085,885**	**32,536,025**	**2,622,001**	**237,713**	**324,869**

Total Event Count: 40,806,493

Heart Rate Histogram, Percent Of Time Per Rate Bin

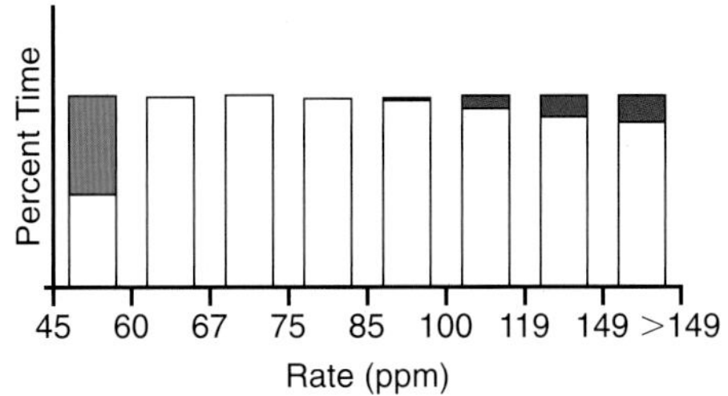

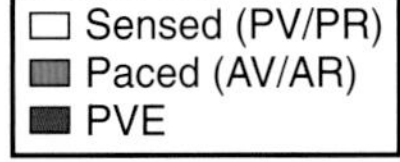

Figure 24-10. Event and heart rate histograms retrieved from a patient with a Pacesetter Synchrony II Model 2022 (St. Jude Medical CRMD, Sylmar, Calif.) programmed to the DDD mode. The key programmed parameters are shown at the upper left, whereas other information is shown at the upper right. These data represent the performance of the pacing system over the preceding 388 days, with monitoring of every event. The event histogram is a graphic display of the relative percentage of events within each of the five basic pacing states, whereas the heart rate histogram is a graphic display of the rate distribution based on atrial-sensed or atrial-paced events. This bimodal distribution reflects normal chronotropic function of the sinus node in this patient, whose pacemaker was placed for intermittent atrioventricular block. The precise number of events in each rate bin and pacing state is shown in the event count table. The percent of time per rate bin represents a normalized display of the relative percentage of atrial-paced or atrial-sensed events and premature ventricular-sensed events in each rate bin during this period of time.

events can be counted and stored in memory for retrieval at the time of routine pacing system follow-up. Reading the counters requires access to the memory banks in the pacemaker through the use of specific coded commands from the programmer. One DDD system introduced in the mid-1980s had sufficient memory to provide a summary of pacing system behavior for a period of about 6 months. As memory capacity has increased and data compression algorithms have evolved, these systems are now able to store much more data for periods in excess of one year.

Storing a simple marker of the pacing state and rate requires relatively little memory compared with storing waveform data representing the rhythm, as depicted by a consecutive series of EGMs. A theoretical 100-Hz bandwidth with 200 samples per cardiac cycle at eight bits of resolution per sample, recording the entire rhythm during a 24-hour period, would require 140,000,000 bits/day, even if the heart rate was a steady 60 bpm.[47] Most implantable defibrillator systems store a series of EGMs preceding and following the delivery of antitachycardia therapy. Premium pacing systems use certain triggers to initiate EGM storage. These triggers may be a high atrial or a high ventricular rate, initiation of mode switching, or activation of any of a number of other specialized algorithms. Storage may also be triggered by application of the magnet or use of a simple transmitter device by the patient when symptoms are present. An older method used to save memory was to provide "snapshots" of representative complexes; the trigger to store these data in an ICD was the delivery of antitachycardia therapy. Extensive storage of cardiac rhythm data within pacemakers became possible with increasingly sophisticated data compression algorithms and more memory than was previously available. Higher-bandwidth data transmission channels are required for this volume of data storage, particularly for long series of rhythms, so that transmission can be accomplished as efficiently and as quickly as possible.

An implanted Holter monitor, complete with stored rhythms, is now available as a stand-alone device, in ICDs, and in high-end pacemakers. Most pacemakers, however, continue to store only data reflecting the total number of times a pacing state was encountered and, in some systems, the distribution of rates or intervals, rate ranges, or mean rates within these pacing states. This information provides the physician with an overview of the function of the system in the patient. Predominant base-rate pacing is expected in patients with marked sinus node dysfunction and in those receiving anti-ischemia medications. On the other hand, predominant base-rate pacing (AP-VP) in patients whose primary indication for pacing was complete heart block suggests either the development of sinus node dysfunction or primary atrial undersensing. In these same patients with high-grade AV block, frequent counts of AS-VS and PVEs, particularly in the absence of known ventricular ectopy, suggests episodes of ventricular oversensing or resolution of the AV block. Large numbers of counts regarding PMTs warrant a reassessment of retrograde conduction and possible adjustment of the programmed PVARP or PMT prevention and termination algorithm. A large number of counts at the maximum tracking rate suggests that the upper rate limit should be reassessed. Event counter telemetry can provide an insight into the overall function of the pacing system; a variation from the clinician's knowledge of the patient may suggest the need for a further evaluation.

When the additional ability to monitor a series of rates and pacing states is added, chronotropic function can be assessed by the distribution of atrial-sensed rates (AS-VS or PR and AS-VP or PV; see Fig. 24-10). Furthermore, atrial pacing at rates above the programmed base rate reflects sensor drive in the DDDR pacing systems, providing an overview of the sensor behavior. The ability to report both rates and pacing states can provide the clinician with a better insight into the cause of PVEs as well as overall pacing system function. True premature ventricular contractions tend to occur at short coupling intervals, which is equivalent to a rapid rate. Large numbers of PVEs might suggest recurrent ventricular arrhythmias.[58,59] If there are large numbers of PVE counts at relatively low rates, the clinician should consider episodes of atrial undersensing or accelerated junctional rhythms, which would also fulfill the pacemaker's criteria for a PVE (i.e., a sensed R wave not preceded by an atrial event).

Subsystem Performance Counters

An increasing number of specific algorithms and capabilities are used either intermittently or potentially independently of the functional performance of the pacing system. An early counter representative of this capability is the sensor-indicated rate histogram, which reports the distribution of pacing rates that would have occurred had the sensor been totally controlling the pacing rates.[56,57] This counter reports the sensor-defined rates, even if the pacemaker was inhibited by a faster native rhythm or the actual functional rate was being controlled by the sensed atrial activity.

Other subsystem performance counters include automatic mode switch histograms, reports of the cumulative length of time for which the system functioned at the maximum tracking rate, the number of times the PMT algorithm was enabled, high atrial or ventricular rate episodes (Fig. 24-11), and sudden rate-drop episodes, among others. These diagnostic counters provide detailed information about the use of a specific algorithm or system behavior that is not activated on a daily basis or is not visible on the ECG, making identification difficult using standard recording techniques such as a Holter monitor.

The principal limitation associated with the two types of counters described to this point is that counts are placed in a bin, either the pacing state alone or the pacing state and rate, which provides a one-dimensional view of the system's behavior. If the period of monitoring is short, as during a casual or brisk walk, the clinician can reasonably assess the behavior of the pacing system. Longer periods of monitoring accumulate and overlap the results of many activities. This precludes an assessment of the pacing system's behavior during a specific activity, or the identification of a symptomatic episode occurring at an earlier time. The ability of the system to store pacing state and rate data with respect to time (i.e., time-based event counters) has been variably termed *event record* or *pacemaker Holter systems*.[60-62] Technically, this is not yet a true Holter monitor, because continuous rhythm recordings are not retained in memory, even though rate data may be available.

Time-based System Performance Counters

Time-based event counters require an extensive amount of memory. Not only are the pacing state and rate stored, but these data must be stored with respect to preceding and subsequent events. The data cannot be simply dumped into a rate or pacing state bin. Each piece of data (i.e., every cardiac event) must have a time reference, which takes significantly more memory than simple histogram-type counters.

Two techniques are available for storing real-time data. One is to continue to accumulate the data until

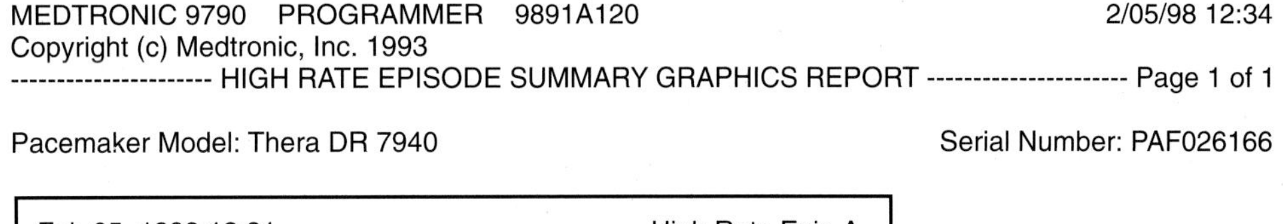
MEDTRONIC 9790 PROGRAMMER 9891A120 2/05/98 12:34
Copyright (c) Medtronic, Inc. 1993
--------------------- HIGH RATE EPISODE SUMMARY GRAPHICS REPORT --------------------- Page 1 of 1

Pacemaker Model: Thera DR 7940 Serial Number: PAF026166

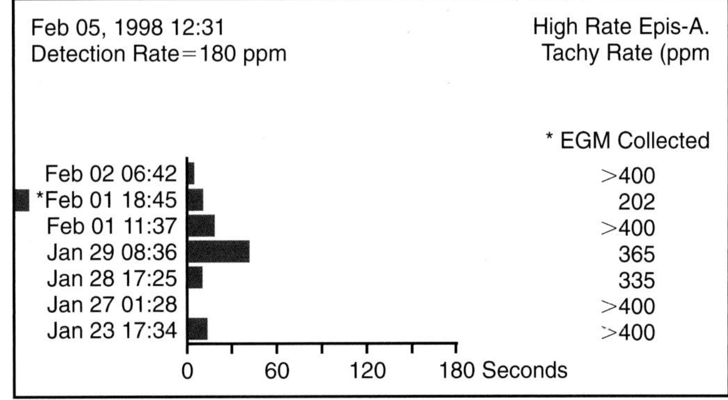

MEDTRONIC 9790 PROGRAMMER 9891A120 2/05/98 12:33
Copyright (c) Medtronic, Inc. 1993
--------------------- HIGH RATE EPISODE SUMMARY GRAPHICS REPORT --------------------- Page 1 of 1

Pacemaker Model: Thera DR 7940 Serial Number: PAF026166

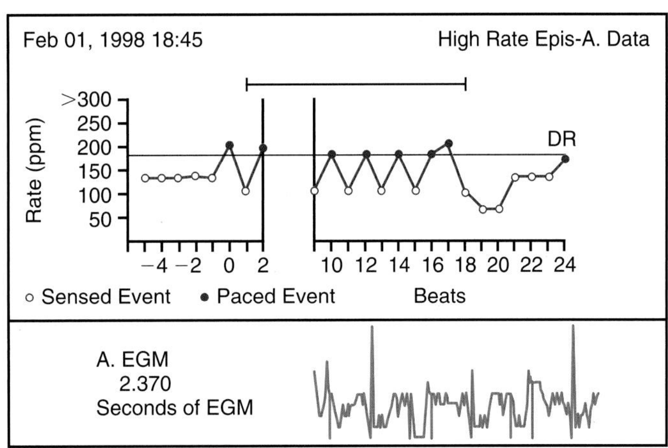

Figure 24-11. High-rate episode summary (top) and high-rate episode graphic with stored atrial electrogram (bottom) from a Medtronic Thera DR Model 7940 (Medtronic, Inc., Minneapolis, Minn.). Such information facilitates the clinician's ability to assess the behavior of the pacing system between office visits. In this case, the specific episode associated with the atrial electrogram reported atrial-paced events occurring above the trigger level for this event counter, which was also above the maximum sensor rate. The electrogram demonstrates atrial pacing with a large far-field R-paced ventricular event; presumably, the labeled high-rate episode was caused by far-field sensing. This knowledge may be helpful in further programming of the pacemaker.

the memory is full and then to freeze the recorded events. Freezing all of the counters at the same time maintains the ratios between the events. A clearing function is usually provided to reset the counters. In some devices, reprogramming of any parameter or specific parameters (e.g., rate or pacing mode) can result in the automatic clearing of these data. This "initial events" or "frozen" recording technique is especially useful for short-term monitoring, as in office-based exercise evaluations. It also allows the system's response to exercise to be evaluated, often without the need for simultaneous ECG monitoring.

The other option is to collect the data continuously. As the counters fill, new data are added at the expense of the oldest data (Fig. 24-12). This has been called "rolling trend," "final trend," or "continuous" data storage and is based on the "first in, first out" (FIFO) principle. When the patient is seen in follow-up, the data acquired over the time immediately preceding the interrogation of the system are available for review. The patient can often recall symptoms and activities during this period. These can be correlated with the behavior of the pacing system at the time of the symptoms. In this manner, the clinical staff caring for the patient may further assess chronotropic function, the behavior of the pacemaker during a variety of special or usual activities, and whether the sensor and other algorithms are behaving appropriately. The clinician may gain insight into the cause of palpitations and other symptoms that may have occurred during this time by correlation of the recorded data and the patient's complaints or activities.[51,58-62]

Sensor-input data have been combined with the actual rates achieved to facilitate reprogramming of the sensor parameters. Once acquired, the data from an exercise session are retained in the memory of the programmer, uploaded to the programmer, and then displayed on a screen. The system's performance is based on a given set of sensor parameters that were in effect at that time. Because the pacemaker has the actual sensor-signal data, it can calculate how the unit would perform in response to a different set of sensor param-

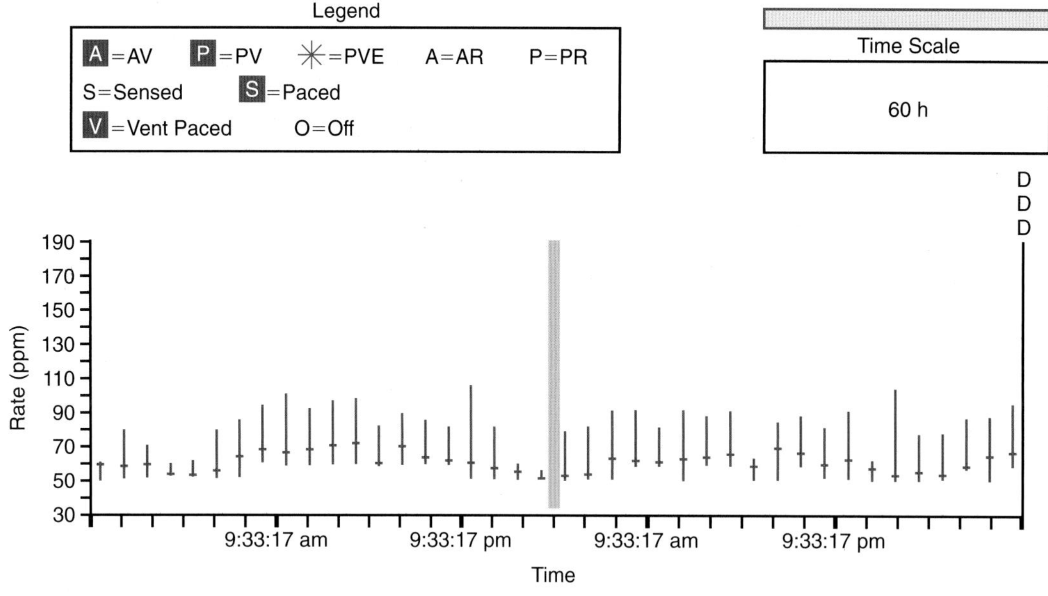

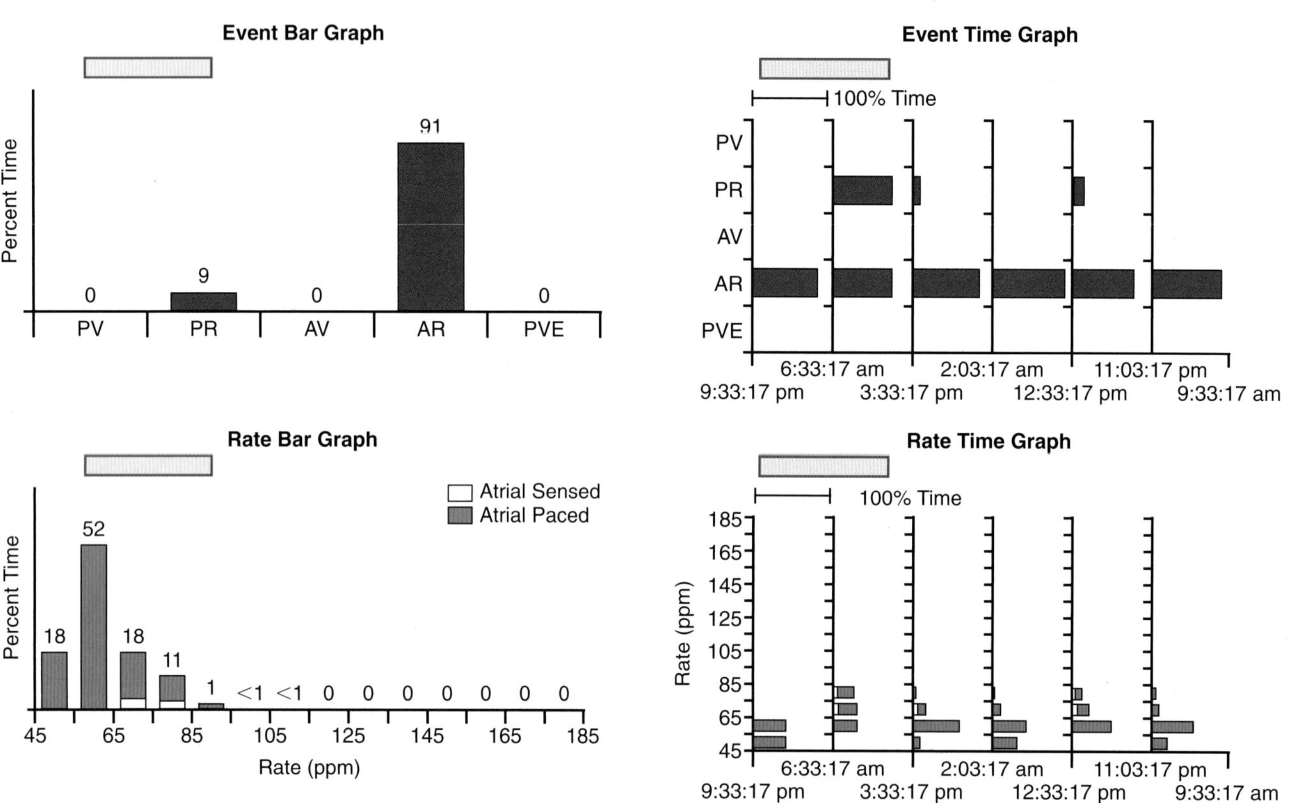

Figure 24-12. Event Record display from a Pacesetter Trilogy DR+ Model 2364 (St. Jude Medical CRMD, Sylmar, Calif.). The sampling interval was 26 seconds, which provides a detailed overview of the behavior of the pacing system for the preceding 60 hours. The top display is an overview of the moment-to-moment behavior of the pacing system, with the vertical lines representing the maximum and minimum rates during each time period (the total displayed interval is divided into 40 equal time segments) and with the cross-bar representing the mean heart rate. The vertical line is displayed if there are two or more complexes in the specific time bin. The display scale can be expanded to display individual events, in which case a specific alphanumeric label is shown consistent with the legend in the upper left. The same data may be displayed as an event bar graph (equivalent to the event histogram) or as a rate bar graph (equivalent to the heart rate histogram). The solid bars represent atrial-paced events; hence, atrial rates greater than the programmed base rate represent sensor drive. Atrial rates lower than the programmed base rate represent "sleep mode" behavior that was also programmed. The time graphs automatically divide the overall monitoring period into six equal segments.

06/11/98 9:25:07 AM
Pacemaker Model: Medtronic Kappa KDR401/403 — Medtronic Vision Software Version 1.3
Serial Number: PER101148 — Copyright (c) Medtronic, Inc. 1996

Exercise Test Report — **Page 1**

Exercise Test Collected: 06/11/98 9:22:20 AM

	During Exercise	Current Values *
Mode	DDDR	DDDR
Lower Rate	60 ppm	60 ppm
ADL Rate	90 ppm	90 ppm
Upper Sensor Rate	115 ppm	125 ppm
Upper Tracking Rate	130 ppm	130 ppm
Optimization	On	On
RR Sensor	Integrated	Integrated
ADL Rate Setpoint	11	11
Upper Sensor Rate Setpoint	15	15

* Note: Current values depicted by Exercise Test Graph

Additional Data

Maximum Achieved Rate	108 bpm
Maximum MV Counts	14
Maximum Activity Counts	5

06/11/98 9:25:18 AM
Pacemaker Model: Medtronic Kappa KDR401/403 — Medtronic Vision Software Version 1.3
Serial Number: PER101148 — Copyright (c) Medtronic, Inc. 1996

Exercise Test Report — **Page 2**

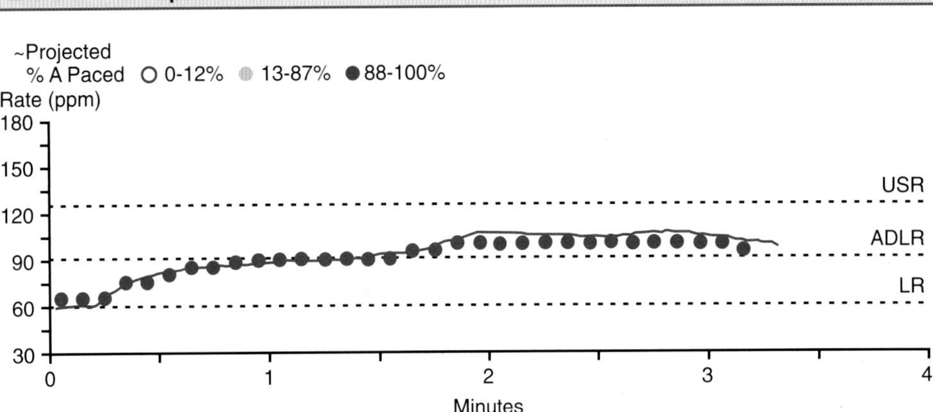

Figure 24-13. *Exercise test report from a patient with a Medtronic Kappa KDR Model 401 (Medtronic, Inc., Minneapolis, Minn.). The circles represent the actual behavior of the pacing system. The thin line represents the behavior of the pacemaker under sensor drive at the current sensor values that had been modeled.*

eters. If a new set of sensor parameters is entered into the programmer, the curves that were based on the original input data are redrawn to display the system's projected behavior in response to the new set of parameters. The clinical staff can then determine which are the best sensor parameters for the individual patient without having the patient perform repeated activities (Fig. 24-13). This feature has been termed *redraw*,[63] *exercise test*, or *prediction model*.[64]

Limitations of Event Counter Telemetry

The major value of event counters is that they provide a review of system performance over time. This is not available from the real-time diagnostic features of measured data and event counter and EGM telemetry. The data, however, are interpretable only after a detailed assessment of the capture and sensing thresholds, in a manner analogous to event marker telemetry. The pacemaker can only store information that it knows about, namely output and sensed events, sensor data, and activation of unique algorithms. If there is a problem with undersensing, the pacemaker releases a pacing pulse, and the counters report a paced rhythm. Similarly, a large number of sensed events may cause the pacemaker to be inhibited on the respective channel. The counter simply reports a large percentage of sensed events, but this may be clinically inappropriate if the cause is oversensing.

With respect to pacing, a rhythm that is predominantly composed of AV- or PV-paced complexes does not necessarily indicate complete heart block. It might result

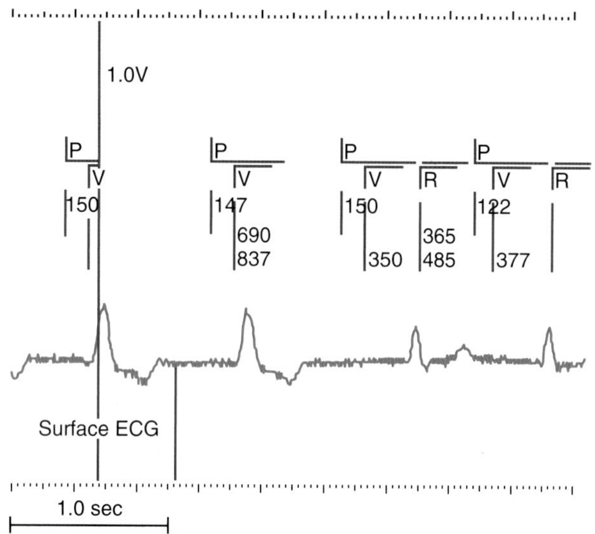

Figure 24-14. Although this printout was obtained during a ventricular capture threshold test in a Pacesetter Synchrony II Model 2022 dual-chamber pacing system (St. Jude Medical CRMD, Sylmar, Calif.), it demonstrates the limitations of some of the telemetry data in the absence of a simultaneously recorded electrocardiogram (ECG). The last two ventricular output pulses were subthreshold, resulting in a loss of capture. The endogenous P wave conducted, but with a marked first-degree atrioventricular (AV) block, placing the R wave outside the ventricular refractory period that was initiated by the subthreshold ventricular output and thereby allowing it to be sensed. Based on event marker and event counter data, this patient would be interpreted as having frequent premature ventricular events (PVEs) interspersed in a stable atrial-sensed, ventricular-paced rhythm; however, in actuality, there was a loss of ventricular capture with intact AV nodal conduction. Key programmed and recording parameters are also included with each printout to facilitate interpretation. EGM, electrogram.

from a programmed AV delay that was not sufficiently long to allow for full conduction through the AV node. Although the ventricular complex could have been fully paced, it could also have been a fusion or pseudofusion beat. The counters cannot differentiate between these complexes, because the native complex had not yet been sensed, the timer had been completed, and an output was delivered. Another situation would be a total loss of ventricular capture with intact AV nodal conduction (Fig. 24-14). The conducted R wave would not have been sensed, because it occurred during the refractory period that followed the ventricular output pulse. An identical result in the counters would occur with intact AV nodal conduction but with ventricular undersensing.

The event counters simply report the system's performance without making any statement or judgment about the appropriateness of this behavior. The information provided by the event counters can be interpreted only after the programmed parameters are known, the pacing and sensing thresholds have been determined, and the status of the native rhythm is known. If the pacemaker is programmed to provide a good margin of safety for both pacing and sensing, the event counters are likely to be an accurate reflection of the patient's clinical rhythms. These data also provide insight into the degree to which the patient requires pacing support at the current programmed parameters, the chronotropic function of the sinus node, and responsiveness of the sensor. Evidence of oversensing or lead dysfunction renders the event counter data suspect with regard to these findings, although a marked change in event counter data can provide the clinician with a clue to a developing problem.

The event counter data cannot be adequately interpreted without knowledge of how these data are collected, the clinical status of the patient, and any unique behavioral performance of the implanted pacemaker. This is illustrated by Figure 24-11, which is an atrial high-rate graphic from a Medtronic Thera DR pacemaker (Medtronic, Inc., Minneapolis, Minn.). The reported rates were greater than 200 bpm, yet the graphic suggests that these were atrial-paced events and that the device is not capable of being programmed to rates this high. It is essential to know how the manufacturer calculates rates. In this case, the device measures the interval between atrial events; if the event preceding the atrial output occurred during the refractory period (labeled AR by the markers), the reported atrial-paced rate would be based on the AR-AP interval. With this knowledge, the graphic report can be understood. If this fact were not known, the graphic would suggest a pacing system malfunction.

Atrial fibrillation (AF) is a major clinical problem that is common in patients who have implanted devices. Management can be improved by knowing whether AF is present, the frequency of AF occurrence, and the duration of the AF episodes. Knowing these data allows the clinician to determine the need for antiarrhythmia therapy, for ventricular rate-slowing medication or interventions, or for anticoagulation. Several diagnostics are available to assist in the management of AF. Figure 24-15 shows examples of these counters. These may consist of the number and duration of the episodes, atrial rates and ventricular rates during the episodes, and specific dates and times so that patient symptoms can be correlated to events.

The one caution in terms of accepting data from these counters is the possibility of oversensing in the atrial channel, which would cause inappropriate assignment of events to these diagnostics. The most common cause of false information is sensing of the far-field QRS by the atrial lead. This leads to double-counting of the heart rate and incorrect classification of the event as atrial high rate. Use of stored EGMs to verify the cause of the high-rate episode is advised whenever possible, to avoid inappropriate treatment for AF that does not really exist.

Mode Switch Episodes				
ID#	**Date/Time**	**A. Max Rate**	**V. Max Rate**	**Duration**
37839	Aug 02, 2005 22:07:37	(Episode in progress)		
37838	Aug 02, 2005 00:19:30	>400 bpm	146 bpm	22 hr
37837	Jul 30, 2005 23:57:31	>400 bpm	94 bpm	48 hr
37836	Jul 22, 2005 03:22:54	>400 bpm	143 bpm	213 hr
37835	Jul 21, 2005 23:35:48	>400 bpm	80 bpm	4 hr
37834	Jul 21, 2005 21:50:57	400 bpm	Paced	2 hr
37833	Jul 21, 2005 01:25:17	>400 bpm	128 bpm	20 hr
37832	Jul 20, 2005 06:24:08	>400 bpm	102 bpm	19 hr
37831	Jul 20, 2005 01:26:59	>400 bpm	80 bpm	5 hr
37830	Jul 20, 2005 00:58:06	375 bpm	Paced	28 min
37829	Jul 19, 2005 05:07:23	>400 bpm	91 bpm	20 hr
37828	Jul 19, 2005 03:04:02	400 bpm	Paced	2 hr
37827	Jul 18, 2005 06:15:20	>400 bpm	95 bpm	21 hr
37826	Jul 18, 2005 04:08:05	>400 bpm	Paced	2 hr
37825	Jul 18, 2005 03:57:48	400 bpm	Paced	10 min
37824	Jul 18, 2005 01:14:07	>400 bpm	Paced	3 hr
37823	Jul 18, 2005 01:01:24	400 bpm	Paced	12 min
37822	Jul 17, 2005 17:24:50	>400 bpm	85 bpm	8 hr
37821	Jul 14, 2005 16:02:06	>400 bpm	154 bpm	73 hr
37820	Jul 14, 2005 00:34:16	>400 bpm	130 bpm	15 hr

A

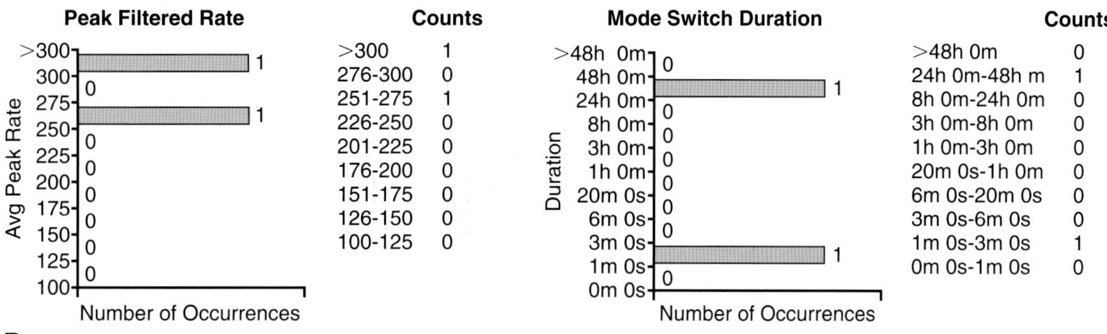

B

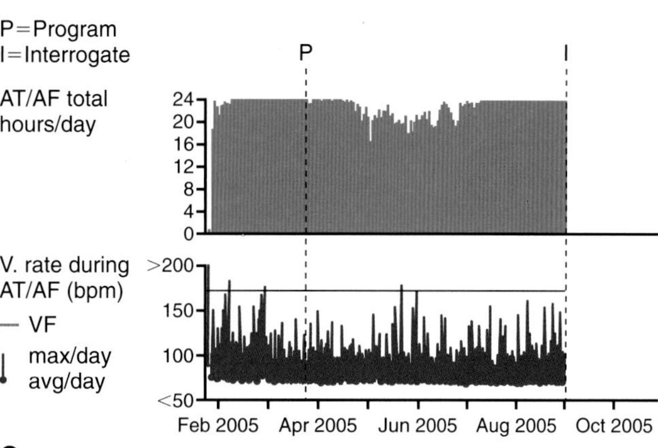

C

Figure 24-15. ***A,*** *Event log from a Medtronic pacemaker with mode switch algorithm showing date, time, and duration of the atrial arrhythmia, presumably atrial fibrillation (AF). Maximum atrial and ventricular rates are also provided.* ***B,*** *Mode switch histogram from a St. Jude pacemaker showing the number of episodes, peak atrial rates, and the duration of the AF episodes.* ***C,*** *Cardiac Compass Report from a Medtronic device implanted into a patient in January of 2005. The patient went into persistent AF 2 weeks after implantation. Note the presence of AF 24 hours/day on the top graph for most of the period monitored. The lower percentage of AF during June and July could have been caused by intermittent sinus rhythm or by undersensing of the atrial fibrillation. The bottom graph shows the average and maximum ventricular rates while the patient was in AF and can be used to determine whether further therapy to control the ventricular response is needed.*

Pacing System Malfunction

Interrogating the pacemaker about programmed parameters and measured data, retrieval of any and all event count data, and the use of the event markers and EGM telemetry capabilities are essential in a routine office-based follow-up evaluation. It is even more important when evaluating a suspected pacing system malfunction. Knowledge of the present programmed settings, combined with the baseline data with which the current results can be compared, is crucial. Many devices have special programming features and idiosyncrasies that may appear to be malfunctions to clinicians who are not completely familiar with the particular system under scrutiny. It is not unusual to hear about devices being explanted and returned to the manufacturer for failure to pace at the programmed rate, only to find that hysteresis had been enabled. The latter is but one of many examples of pseudomalfunctions, which are discussed in greater detail later.[65-69] The remainder of this section focuses on a discussion of pacing system malfunction.

Historical Clues

The first step in the evaluation of the patient with a suspected pacing system problem is to gather as much information about the patient as possible (Table 24-1). This includes the indications for the pacemaker, the operative record of the implantation, the model, and possibly the serial numbers of all portions of the implanted pacing system. In addition, one must obtain the current programmed parameters and all measured data. The programmed parameters and measured data are crucial to the correct evaluation of the device.

Even in the current high-technology environment of cardiac pacing, the history and physical examination continue to be important. The patient should be asked about symptoms relating to potential device malfunction. These include presyncope, syncope, palpitations, slow or fast pulse rates, pain or erythema around the implanted device, fevers, chills, night sweats, and extracardiac stimulation. It is also important to obtain any history of trauma to the area where the device is located, exposure to intense electromagnetic signals (e.g., magnetic resonance imaging), therapeutic radiation, use of electrocautery or defibrillation (internal or external), programming changes by other medical personnel, or exposure to environmental extremes.

Information related to the actual implantation procedure can be important with respect to making clinical decisions. If the implanting physician was unable to obtain an adequate EGM in the atrium for sensing, then atrial undersensing of P waves by the device would be expected. Knowledge of such a situation might prevent a second futile operation for the patient. Another common situation occurs with unusual radiographic findings. What may appear to be a lead dislodgment might actually be the intentional site of placement because of poor sensing or capture thresholds in the "standard" location. In addition, ventricular leads are being implanted with increasing frequency in areas other than the right ventricular (RV) apex. These areas include the RV outflow tract, RV septum, and cardiac veins via the coronary sinus. An otherwise stable and normal system might be interpreted as a potential problem resulting in an inappropriate intervention in the absence of this crucial historical information.

TABLE 24-1. **Evaluation of the Patient with a Potential Pacing System Malfunction**

Know the Patient
Cardiac and noncardiac diagnoses
Exposure to environmental extremes
Exposure to sources of electromagnetic interference
Programming changes performed by others
Know the Pacemaker
Manufacturer
Model and serial number
Alerts or recalls
Current programmed settings
Device idiosyncrasies
Mode and algorithm idiosyncrasies
Know the Leads
Manufacturer
Model and serial number
Alerts or recalls
Connector type
Polarity
Insulation material
Fixation mechanism
Radiographic appearance

The full analysis of a suspected pacing system malfunction is facilitated by access to telemetry and programming information, allowing a detailed noninvasive evaluation. Despite this, an invasive evaluation may sometimes be required (Tables 24-2 and 24-3). The model numbers of the pulse generator and leads should be determined before an invasive evaluation of the system is performed. There may be unique device eccentricities that are known to the manufacturer. In some cases, unique tools or replacement devices may be required. It is therefore wise to contact the manufacturer's technical service group before an operative intervention for an unexpected behavior in an otherwise clinically stable patient.

With respect to a noninvasive system evaluation followed by programming, serious errors may occur in

TABLE 24-2. **Noninvasive Testing**

Office evaluation
Multichannel rhythm strips or 12-lead electrocardiogram
Pulse generator interrogation
Programmed parameters
Measured data—lead and battery function
Event counters
Rhythm monitoring with telemetered electrograms
Event markers
Pacing system evaluation
Capture threshold assessment
Sensing threshold assessment
Sensor evaluation
Special algorithm evaluation
Provocative maneuvers
Ancillary testing
Posteroanterior and lateral chest radiographs
Fluoroscopy
Continuous rhythm monitoring
Telemetry
Holter monitoring
Event or transient arrhythmia monitoring
Transtelephonic or remote monitoring

TABLE 24-3. **Invasive Analysis**

Visual inspection
Connector
Set-screws
Grommets
Insulation
Conductor
Suturing sleeve
Measurements
Capture threshold
Strength–duration curve
Evoked-response amplitude
Polarization amplitude
Sensing threshold
Pacing system analyzer measurement
Peak-to-peak amplitude
Slew rate
Electrogram recording
Stimulation impedance

the absence of full knowledge of the programmed parameters, measured data, and clinical information. Although most patients carry an identification card that identifies the pulse generator model, lead model or models, and serial numbers, this does not provide the current programmed settings. Some patients have more than one device implanted or have noncardiac stimulation devices to treat central nervous system diseases or other diseases. These patients will have multiple identification cards. If the patient has had a device replaced, it is important to determine whether the identification card is the most recent one. Many patients like to keep their old and invalid identification cards as mementos of their previous pacemakers. If chronic leads were reused, the data relating to the leads may or may not be on the new card for the pulse generator, yet a large percentage of pacemaker problems are the result of lead malfunction. Certain leads are less reliable than others, and there have been multiple recalls and alerts regarding leads, making such information vital.

In that the observed system problem may be caused by a lead malfunction, an electrode–tissue interface problem, or the manner in which the pacemaker was programmed for the individual patient, it is prudent to think about the system as a whole. Rather than labeling an observed abnormal behavior as a pacemaker malfunction, it should be termed a *pacing system malfunction*, which expands the focus of the evaluation from the pulse generator to all components of the system.

In the absence of an identification card, model and serial number information may be obtained from the operative report or from adhesive labels (provided with each pulse generator and lead) if they were included in the medical record at the time of implantation. If none of these is available, a radiograph of the patient that includes the area of the pulse generator allows the clinician to match the identification label inside the pulse generator to those in a reference source (Fig. 24-16).[70-72] Although not all pulse generators have these labels, many have a distinct radiographic "skeleton" or radiopaque alphanumeric labels from which the clinician can determine at least the name of the manufacturer, if not the model. All manufacturers provide toll-free numbers that the clinician may call to obtain further information regarding the pulse generator and the leads that are implanted.

Virtually all manufacturers' programmers and devices are capable of automatically identifying the model and serial number of their pacemakers. Unfortunately, only the programmer from the manufacturer of the pacemaker can communicate with that device.

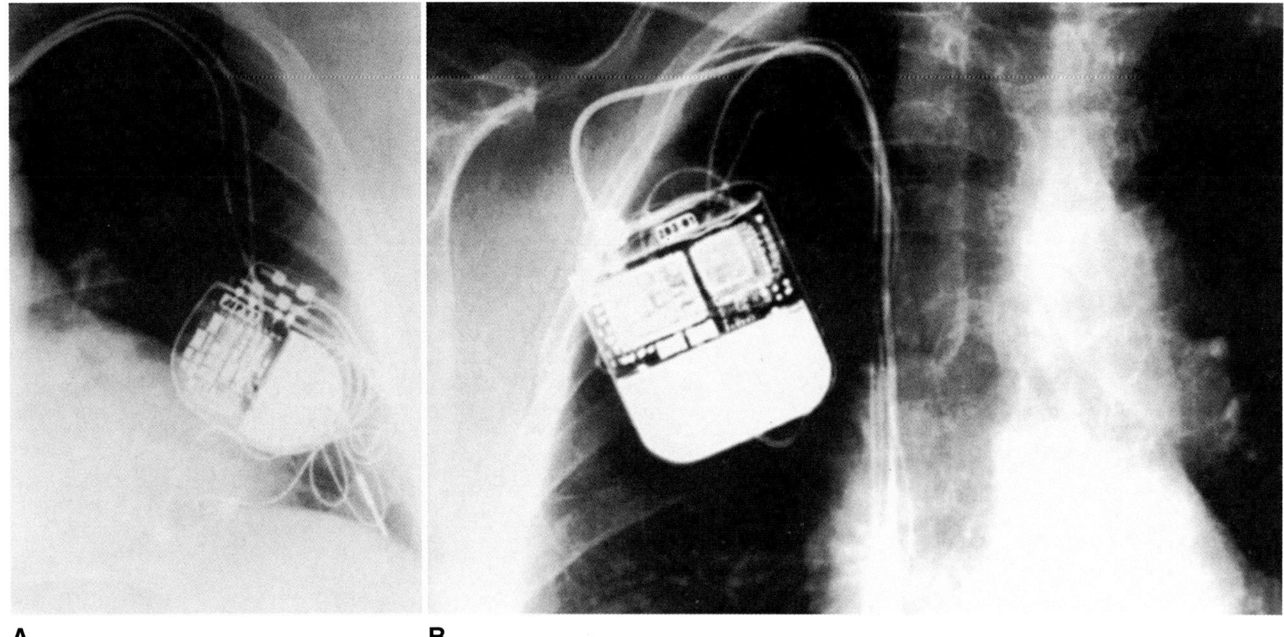

Figure 24-16. ***A*** *and* ***B,*** *Radiographs of two pulse generators showing radiopaque identification tags. Some units do not have this helpful feature, but they can still be identified by the appearance of their unique radiographic "skeletons." Also note that the leads exit the connector block of the pulse generator in a clockwise direction, indicating that the pulse generator is properly situated with the anode facing the subcutaneous tissue. On panel* ***A,*** *also note that the terminal pins of the leads extend through the set-screw connector block, indicating that they are properly and fully inserted into the pulse generator connector. However, it cannot be determined, based on the radiograph, whether the set-screw is fully secured.*

Certain pulse generators are also capable of storing data concerning the patient, implantation date, and lead model (see Fig. 24-1B). These data need to be downloaded into the pacemaker by the clinician or support staff. If the pacemaker and programmer have this capability, the programmer provides much of the data necessary for finding additional patient data. It may be possible to obtain further information from the manufacturer's patient-tracking database. Finally, pulse generators often have a characteristic magnet response signature that can be recorded on an ECG strip, and this may provide clues to the manufacturer or model. The clinician should avoid "blindly" interrogating a device without knowing at least the name of the manufacturer. Unexpected and possibly disastrous reprogramming results have been reported when one manufacturer's programmer was used on another manufacturer's pacemaker, although with current-generation systems this is not very likely.

Knowing the specifics about the implanted pacing system's components is a crucial first step. It is also important to know what, if any, special considerations apply to the device. These might include recalls, alerts, known idiosyncrasies, and the functions of specialized programmable features and rate-modulation sensors.[73-79] Any of these items may affect the observed behavior and guide the further evaluation of the system, as well as any decisions regarding parameter adjustment. For example, a pulse generator that is exhibiting its elective replacement parameters would typically be replaced using the same lead system if the latter had a good capture threshold, a good sensing threshold, and a normal stimulation impedance. If it is known that the lead is under a safety alert or recall, however, the clinician should follow recommended guidelines and, if appropriate, replace the vulnerable lead system at the time of generator replacement. There have been patients who required a second operation to revise another element of the pacing system simply because the implanting physician was unaware of previously reported potential product deficiencies.

Virtually any device could exhibit idiosyncratic behavior that might be mistaken for a malfunction. In addition, functional undersensing as a result of a variety of normal refractory and blanking periods, pauses due to normal hysteresis and sleep rates, and changes in the spontaneous functional behavior of the pacemaker (as with automatic mode switching, rate-drop response, and endless-loop tachycardia [ELT] prevention and termination algorithms) are but a few examples of features that could cause confusion if the clinician is not aware of these capabilities.

Physical Examination and Telemetry

After the history has been obtained and the pacemaker system's specifics are known, the patient should be examined. The implantation site is examined for proper

TABLE 24-4. **Causes of Extracardiac Stimulation**

Improper lead position
Gastric vein
Cardiac vein
Diaphragmatic stimulation
Lead in cardiac vein
Thin right ventricular wall combined with high output
Myocardial perforation
Lead position near phrenic nerve
Active fixation lead—right atrium
Lead withdrawal to innominate, superior vena cava, or subclavian vein
Pacemaker pocket stimulation
Delamination of insulating coating
Device movement (twiddler's syndrome)
Device inserted in pocket upside down
Unipolar output configuration at high output
Irritable skeletal muscles—low stimulation threshold
Breach of lead external insulation

healing or abnormalities such as erosion of suture material, leads, or the generator; erythema; hematoma; seroma; excessive pain on palpation; evidence of trauma; pocket stimulation; device mobility; and generator displacement.

The precordium is inspected for chest wall or diaphragmatic stimulation. The presence of the latter may indicate a number of possible problems (Table 24-4). If the system is unipolar, the pacemaker (if it is coated on one side) may have the anode facing the skeletal muscle or be considered to be upside down in the pocket. The malpositioning of a pacemaker sitting upside down in the pocket may have occurred inadvertently at implantation, may have developed spontaneously (most commonly in conjunction with lax subcutaneous tissues), or may have resulted from the patient's manipulating the pacemaker within the pocket, a condition known as *twiddler's syndrome*.[80-84] Alternatively, the unidirectional insulated coating on the pulse generator or the grommets protecting the setscrews may have been damaged or may have degraded over time. In some situations, pocket stimulation may occur even with the generator in the correct position and the insulation intact.[85] Also note that most pacemakers being produced no longer have coating on one side and therefore are "omnidirectional" with respect to how they are placed into the pocket. High-output settings, placement in or below the pectoral musculature, or high-current delivery as a result of low lead impedance may also be at fault. Outer lead insulation failure may also allow problematic current leakage and local extracardiac muscle stimulation.

The neck veins should be evaluated for distention or the presence of cannon A waves. The latter might indicate an atrial lead problem, inappropriate programming in a dual-chamber system with too long or too short an AV delay assuming otherwise normal electrical function, or pacemaker syndrome in a single-chamber system. Auscultation of the heart for variable-intensity heart sounds, rubs, or gallops may also give clues to the physiology related to the patient–device interaction.[86,87]

Physical maneuvers may be useful to unmask an intermittent symptom or malfunction during an examination. Carotid sinus massage and other vagal maneuvers may slow the intrinsic rhythm so that device function or malfunction becomes evident. Positional changes (sitting or standing up) or having the patient perform in-place exercise or isometric maneuvers may accelerate the heart rate to allow observation for sensing (proper tracking and inhibition). Manipulation of the device and lead may disclose an intermittent lead fracture, loose connection, or insulation failure that was not evident while the patient was lying quietly on the examination table. Other helpful maneuvers include movement of the patient's ipsilateral arm (reaching overhead, across the chest, or behind the back), isometric exercise (pressing the hands together in front of the chest or reaching around the chest to scratch the opposite side), and doing sit-ups (in the case of an abdominal implant) are helpful in identifying an intermittent problem.[88,89] If the patient develops symptoms during the induced abnormal behavior and these symptoms reproduce those that occurred spontaneously, there is a high likelihood that the cause of the symptoms has been identified.

A 12-lead ECG is required to document the pacemaker-evoked morphology of the atrial and ventricular depolarizations at baseline. It may then be helpful to repeat a 12-lead ECG, or at least a multiple-lead ECG, instead of a single-lead rhythm strip, when evaluating a suspected malfunction. A myocardial infarction or progressive cardiomyopathy may have occurred, resulting in a change of capture or sensing thresholds. A change in the paced QRS axis may be a clue to lead dislodgment or malplacement, whereas a change in the intrinsic axis (a new bundle branch block) may be associated with sensing problems. Multiple ECG leads are frequently necessary to recognize the relatively low-amplitude atrial depolarization. In addition, the pacing artifact may not be visible in any given lead, especially if the pacing system is bipolar (Figs. 24-17 and 24-18).[90] Care should be taken in the interpretation of the ECG tracing with regard to the type of recording system used. The older-style analog systems provide a consistent reproduction of the pacing stimulus, varying the relative amplitude of the stimulus with the delivered energy of the system. An unstable paced artifact on an analog ECG is a sign of potential problems. The same cannot be said for digital recording systems, which have generally replaced the older-generation analog

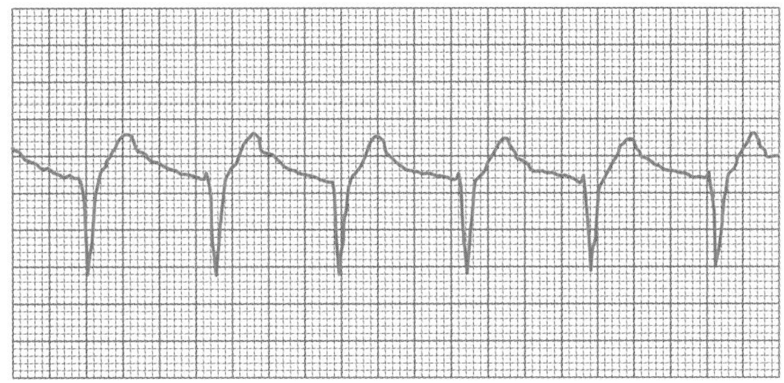

Figure 24-17. An electrocardiographic rhythm strip of a patient with 100% ventricular pacing. The pace artifact is not readily identified because of the small electrical potential generated by the bipolar pacing polarity.

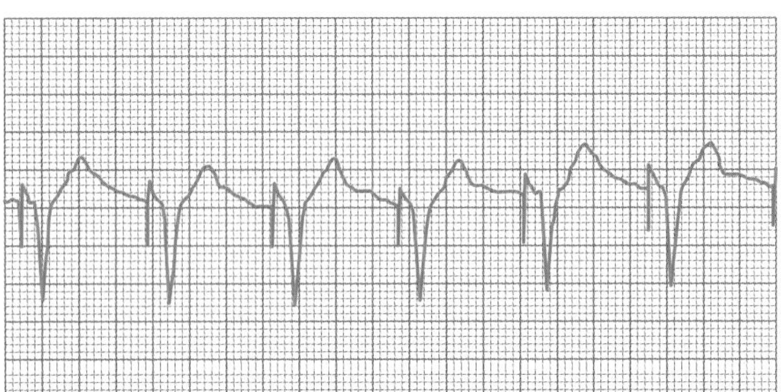

Figure 24-18. Electrocardiographic rhythm strip of a patient with 100% ventricular pacing. The pace artifact is easily identified because of the large electrical potential generated by the unipolar pacing polarity.

systems. Although these allow computer interpretation of the ECG, they can introduce a multiplicity of artifacts and have several idiosyncrasies that have been misinterpreted as a device malfunction when they were actually recording system artifacts (Fig. 24-19).[90-96] In many cases, the pace artifact is not visible in any lead.

After the baseline ECG rhythm strip is obtained, it should be closely inspected for any abnormalities of rate, sensing, loss of capture, or change in paced axis. A tracing with the magnet applied to the pulse generator should also be performed. This provides information about the status of the battery and, if the device is otherwise inhibited, allows for a quick assessment of capture and whether the output is being delivered to the appropriate chamber. If no output is seen during application of the magnet, several possibilities should be considered: the battery may be depleted, the device may be nonfunctional, or an open circuit (e.g., lead fracture) may be present. In some models, the magnet response is programmable (on or off). If the magnet function is disabled, placement of a magnet over it does not result in an overt change in its demand behavior. Alternatively, the magnet may not have been positioned properly, the reed switch may be stuck open, or a magnet with insufficient strength may have been used. The "doughnut" magnet is the strongest type and is preferred over "horseshoe" or "bar" magnets.

The magnet function of each device is unique with regard to the rate and mode of response. The response may differ according to manufacturer, model, and programmed mode of the pacemaker. The magnet response may also be programmable, not only as to whether a response will occur, but also as to the type of response. The clinician should not assume that a DDD device will exhibit a DOO response to application of the magnet. Some dual-chamber devices may pace VOO or may not pace asynchronously. If there are questions about the appropriate response to magnet application, the physician's manual that is supplied with the pacemaker, other reference sources, or the manufacturer should be consulted to determine the expected response.

The initial action should be interrogation and printing of the programmed settings.[97,98] The printout is important because it documents the initial settings and serves as a reference in case the clinician wishes to restore the device to the same settings after the evaluation is complete. Although most programmers have a "return to initial settings" capability, if the programmer is turned off or inadvertently disconnected from the power source, these data will be lost. Virtually all currently implanted pacemakers have the ability to measure and monitor critical system functions. These data should be interrogated and printed. The same recommendation holds for models that have extensive histograms, trend data, or other diagnostic counters. If the settings are routinely retrieved at the beginning of the evaluation, the various programming changes that may be required during the evaluation and that may cause clearing of these counters will not result in loss of critical data. Indeed, on completion of this task, the counters should be cleared so that they reflect the subsequent behavior of the implanted pacing system in response to any changes made by the end of the evaluation.

When reviewing the results of the interrogation, an evaluation of the programmed setting data should be the first step. What are the mode and base rate? Are any special algorithms enabled? Many suspected device malfunctions are eliminated once the programmed parameters become known. These may have been changed by another medical professional since the last evaluation, or they may have been entered incorrectly into the patient's record, accounting for the concern. The former situation has been referred to as *phantom reprogramming*, which most often occurs when another clinician does not notify those responsible for monitoring the patient about the changes made to the pacemaker. Depletion of the battery may also cause a change in the mode, rate, or other parameters. Other causes of mode changes are listed in Table 24-5. Some dual-chamber devices change to a single-chamber mode to conserve power if the battery's voltage drops below a manufacturer-defined value. In other devices, the sensor, data storage, and telemetry may be disabled to slow the rate of battery depletion, in an effort to protect the patient from a no-output state.

In cold climates and high altitudes, new devices that are shipped or transported may cool sufficiently to allow the battery's voltage to drop, triggering the elective replacement behavior even though the device is

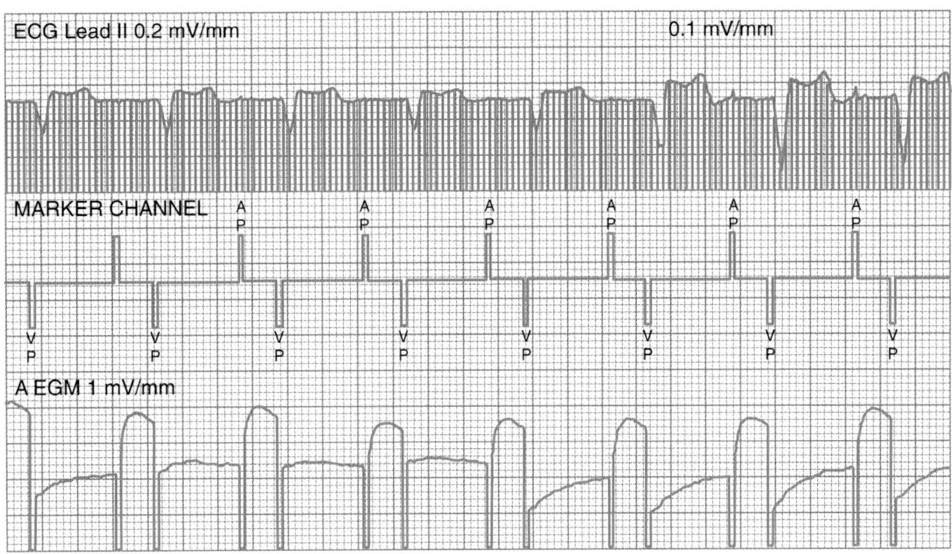

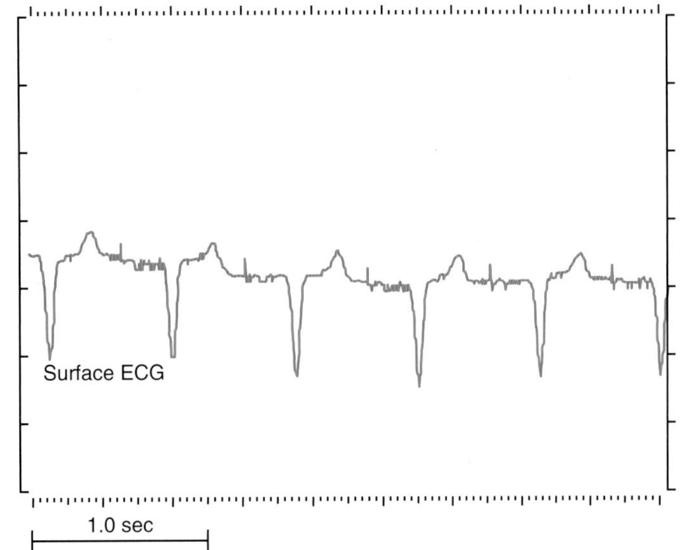

Figure 24-19. Recording of the same rhythm with two different systems. The cause of the high-frequency artifact was never identified but was amplified by the design of the Medtronic 9790 programmer during evaluation of a patient with a Prodigy DR 7860 pacemaker (Medtronic, Inc., Minneapolis, Minn.). The simultaneous event markers identify atrial pacing followed by ventricular pacing. The paced output saturates the telemetry amplifier for the atrial electrogram. The electrocardiogram (ECG) cable was disconnected from the electrodes, and the Pacesetter APS II Model 3003 programmer (St. Jude Medical CRMD, Sylmar, Calif.) was connected to these same electrodes and used as a monitor for the pacing system evaluation. The ECG display in the APS II programmer uses analog recording technology without any artificial amplification of high-frequency transients. Hence, the bipolar outputs are small on the atrial channel and even smaller, such that they are not visualized, on the ventricular channel in this specific lead that was being monitored.

new. Normal function either spontaneously returns or can be reset using the programmer once the device has warmed up to at least room temperature. Attempting to accelerate the warming of the pulse generator by placing it in an oven may damage the pacemaker. Electrocautery and defibrillation can cause mode and polarity changes to occur on some models and may also trigger the elective replacement indicator of the pacemaker. Pacing rate changes may also occur for many other reasons (Table 24-6). Therefore, no assumptions about the expected operating characteristics of a device can be made without the knowledge of the mode and rate.

After the mode and rate have been verified, an evaluation of the remaining programmed parameters is appropriate. The identified output, pulse width, sensitivity, and refractory periods should be reviewed for each channel and correlated with the ECG. The presence and status of any special programmable features should be checked. These include rate-modulation behavior, ELT prevention and termination algorithms, rate and AV-interval hysteresis, time-of-day–dependent or sensor-based rate changes, rate-adaptive AV delay, differential paced and sensed AV delay, rate smoothing, and others. An evaluation of the device's function in relation to all programmed data is performed by comparing the programmed data with ECG and event counter data. In many cases, the event counter diagnostics will minimize if not eliminate the requirement for routine screening Holter monitor studies. The most advanced devices now record high-rate episodes in the atrium and ventricle. Many even record intracardiac electrograms to further document the heart rhythm at the time of the high-rate event, or when triggered by the patient with a magnet or transmitting device.

The measured data are reviewed.[5,44,99] Stimulation impedance for each lead is one of the most important elements of the measured data. Proper interpretation of lead impedance, however, depends on the manufacturer and model of the lead used, the method of measurement, and the historical values of an individual lead's impedance. The other parameters of the lead's

TABLE 24-5. Causes of Apparent Mode and Parameter Changes

Causes
Programming
Special algorithms
Upper rate behavior
Wenckebach
Fixed block
Fallback
Rate smoothing
Base-rate behavior
Sensor drive
Hysteresis
Sudden rate-drop response
Sleep or rest mode
PVARP post–PVE algorithms
Automatic mode switch algorithms
Functional AAI[R] pacing
Autointrinsic conduction search
AV hysteresis search
DDD with mode switch
PMT prevention and termination algorithms
Lead surveillance and configuration change
Battery depletion
Recommended replacement time indicator
End-of-life indicator
Stuck reed switch (DOO, VOO, AOO)
Electromagnetic interference
Electrocautery
Cardioversion and defibrillation
External
Internal
Airport security systems
Electronic article surveillance
Cellular telephone
Magnetic resonance imaging
Cold

PMT, pacemaker-mediated tachycardia; PVARP, postventricular atrial refractory period; PVE, premature ventricular event.

TABLE 24-6. Causes of Rate Change

Causes
Programming
DDD mode with atrial-paced ventricular-sensed complex pacing in ventricular-based timing system
Sensor drive
P-wave tracking modes (DDD, VDD)
Sinus
Atrial tachyarrhythmias
Triggered modes
Special algorithms
Rate hysteresis
Overdrive algorithms
Atrial fibrillation suppression algorithms
Rate smoothing
Circuit failures
Runaway
Recording artifacts
Paper or tape speed errors
Pulse enhancement artifact
Rate slowing
Sensed premature (ectopic) beats
Hysteresis
Oversensing
Open circuit
Battery depletion
Rate acceleration—malfunction
Crosstalk—ventricular based timing
Inappropriate sensor drive
Pressure on piezocrystal sensor
Hyperventilation—minute ventilation sensor
Runaway malfunction

performance, including pulse voltage, pulse charge, pulse energy, and current, should also be correlated with the measured impedance, and internal consistency should be assessed. A marked discrepancy between observed and expected values may identify a telemetry error or measurement error within the pacemaker rather than a primary problem with the lead. It is prudent to repeat the measurements several times if a conflict is noted.[15] Some devices take periodic readings of stimulation impedance and graph these over time (see Fig. 24-4). This is a highly effective tool to spot changes in a lead system.

Another important dataset that may be available measures the battery's status. This can include a measured magnet rate; measured base-rate pacing; projected longevity; elective replacement indicator or status message; and the voltage, impedance, and mean current drain of the battery. The measurements of battery function may be useful to corroborate the measured data from the lead. If the mean current drain remains unchanged despite a major change in the lead's impedance or current, then a telemetry or measurement error should be suspected. Normal mean current drains vary greatly according to generator model, the lead system implanted, and the programmed settings. Once again, tracking these data over time provides the greatest clinical benefit.

After the telemetry and measured data have been obtained and reviewed, a meticulous assessment of the pacing and sensing thresholds is warranted. A complete threshold evaluation should be performed for each lead present. Pacemakers that have automatic algorithms to regulate output should have their diagnostics evaluated for abrupt onset of changes or a large amount of variability (Fig. 24-20). Marked changes in capture or sensing thresholds may imply malfunction of a lead or of the lead-tissue interface when lead impedance values are stable. Other causes of both permanent and transient increases in threshold are discussed later.

If a pacing system problem is suspected, posterior-anterior and lateral chest radiographs should be obtained. It is usually best to request a slightly over-penetrated exposure to visualize the intracardiac segment of the pacing leads for position and integrity. A thoracic spine exposure technique provides optimal penetration for visualization of the pacing leads. The film should be inspected for evidence of conductor disruption; insulation failure as inferred from a deformity in the conductor coil, because the insulation is radiolucent (Fig. 24-21); proper lead placement in the generator connector block, adequate slack in the lead system, electrode perforation, dislodgment or malposition of a lead, generator movement, and proper orientation of the coated side of the can positioned against the muscle (i.e., leads exiting in a clockwise direction, except in devices specifically designed for implantation on the left side of the chest or devices that are not coated; see Fig. 24-16).[100] The latter criterion is especially important when evaluating pocket stimulation in unipolar systems or devices programmed to the unipolar pacing polarity. Given the fact that most new pacemakers and all ICDs are uncoated, leads may exit in either a counterclockwise or clockwise manner, and can be confusing if the construction of the pacemaker

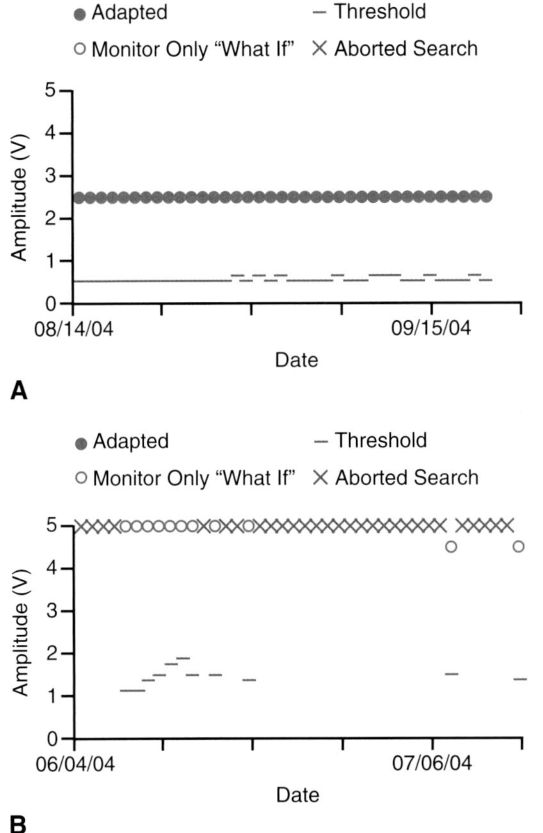

*Figure 24-20. Capture management graphs. Graph **A** is from a patient with a normally functioning capture management algorithm. Note the consistent capture threshold and adapted output. Graph **B** shows a patient in whom the algorithm is not able to identify the threshold. Because the device is not able to determine capture (note the aborted searches), it will be programmed to a high output, resulting in premature battery depletion.*

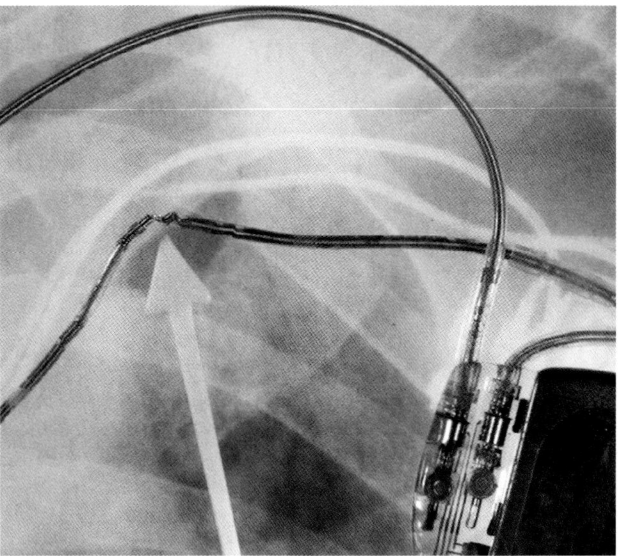

Figure 24-21. Focused view of a posteroanterior chest radiograph showing attenuation of the ventricular lead where it crosses between the clavicle and the first rib. Superimposed on this radiograph is the explanted pulse generator and both atrial and ventricular leads. The attenuation of the conductor coil visualized on the radiograph is associated with a marked disruption of the insulation and conductor coil of the explanted lead at this position (arrow), although the extraction process itself may have contributed to some of the disruption of the lead, exacerbating the abnormality seen on the radiograph. In some cases, overlapping leads or leads overlying other structures make it difficult to visualize a deformity of the conductor coil. If a problem is suspected, multiple views, including oblique and lordotic views, using either standard radiograph techniques or fluoroscopy, may be required.

is not known. Knowledge of the construction of the specific pacemaker, lead, or adapter in question is essential to establishing the proper diagnosis. Close attention should be paid to the infraclavicular area, where pressure from structures around the clavicle and first rib can cause lead failure.[101-115]

On occasion, a fluoroscopic evaluation of the patient may be useful. This shows many of the mechanical or positional problems and defects listed earlier. It also provides a dynamic view of the lead system, facilitating identification of excessive electrode movement consistent with an unstable lead, or it may reveal insufficient slack, with respiratory movement placing traction on the lead and tension at the electrode-tissue interface. Either of these conditions would provide an explanation for an intermittent capture or sensing problem.

Differential Diagnosis of Pacing System Malfunction

Although many pacing system malfunctions are common to single-chamber and dual-chamber devices, the latter present a greater challenge. The section that follows deals with problems seen in both single-chamber and dual-chamber devices. The subsequent section deals with problems unique to dual-chamber devices.

Failure of Output (No Artifact Present)

In the pacemaker-dependent patient, failure to pace represents a potentially catastrophic and lethal situation. The ECG appearance in a single-chamber system is that of no pacing artifact when the intrinsic rate is below the lower rate limit of the device. This may be intermittent or continuous. In a dual-chamber device, the clinician may see an atrial pace alone, ventricular pace alone, or no pacing artifacts at all. Of course, any of the latter may be entirely normal depending on the patient's sinus rate, AV nodal conduction, AV interval settings, enabling of hysteresis or one of its analogs such as sleep mode or rate-drop response, and sensor settings. The causes of a no-output condition are listed in Table 24-7. In evaluating this situation, the clinician must be certain that a malfunction truly exists before taking any corrective action. Remember that the ECG (especially as visualized in a single surface lead) may not display the pacing artifact because of technical factors (Fig. 24-22). This is particularly common in bipolar systems and systems programmed to a lower-than-nominal voltage output. It is important to recognize that the problem may be failure to capture rather than failure to output. Access to telemetered event markers and measured data facilitates the evaluation. Event markers identify the release of an output pulse or recycling resulting from a sensed event, even if this is not visualized on the ECG. If lead impedance is normal (with the previously noted caveat that the problem may be intermittent and multiple measurements should be obtained), this probably reflects a capture problem if there is an output, or an oversensing problem if there is a sensed event. A high impedance suggests an open circuit, whereas a low impedance suggests an insulation failure. Both are probable mechanical problems with the lead, particularly if the lead is coaxial bipolar.

If the markers fail to demonstrate either an ineffective output or an inappropriate sensed event, normal function (e.g., hysteresis) should be considered. At this

TABLE 24-7. Failure to Pace (No Output or Rate Slowing)

Normal system function
Hysteresis
Sleep or rest mode
PVARP extension after premature ventricular contraction
Oversensing
Electromagnetic interference (see Table 24-8)
Inappropriate physiologic signals
Myopotentials
T waves
Afterpotentials
Far-field signals
Make-break signals
Internal insulation failure
Lead chatter
Partial conductor fracture
Crosstalk—in the presence of atrioventricular block
Safety pacing either not available or disabled
Open circuit
Conductor (lead) fracture
Failure to tighten set-screw
Failure to insert lead fully in connector block
Component malfunction
Incompatible lead and pulse generator
Air in pocket—unipolar pulse generator
Pacemaker not in pocket—unipolar pulse generator
Battery depletion
Recording artifact
Isoelectric ectopic beats—properly sensed
Isoelectric paced beats
Rapid recording speed—longer interval between complexes

PVARP, postventricular atrial refractory period.

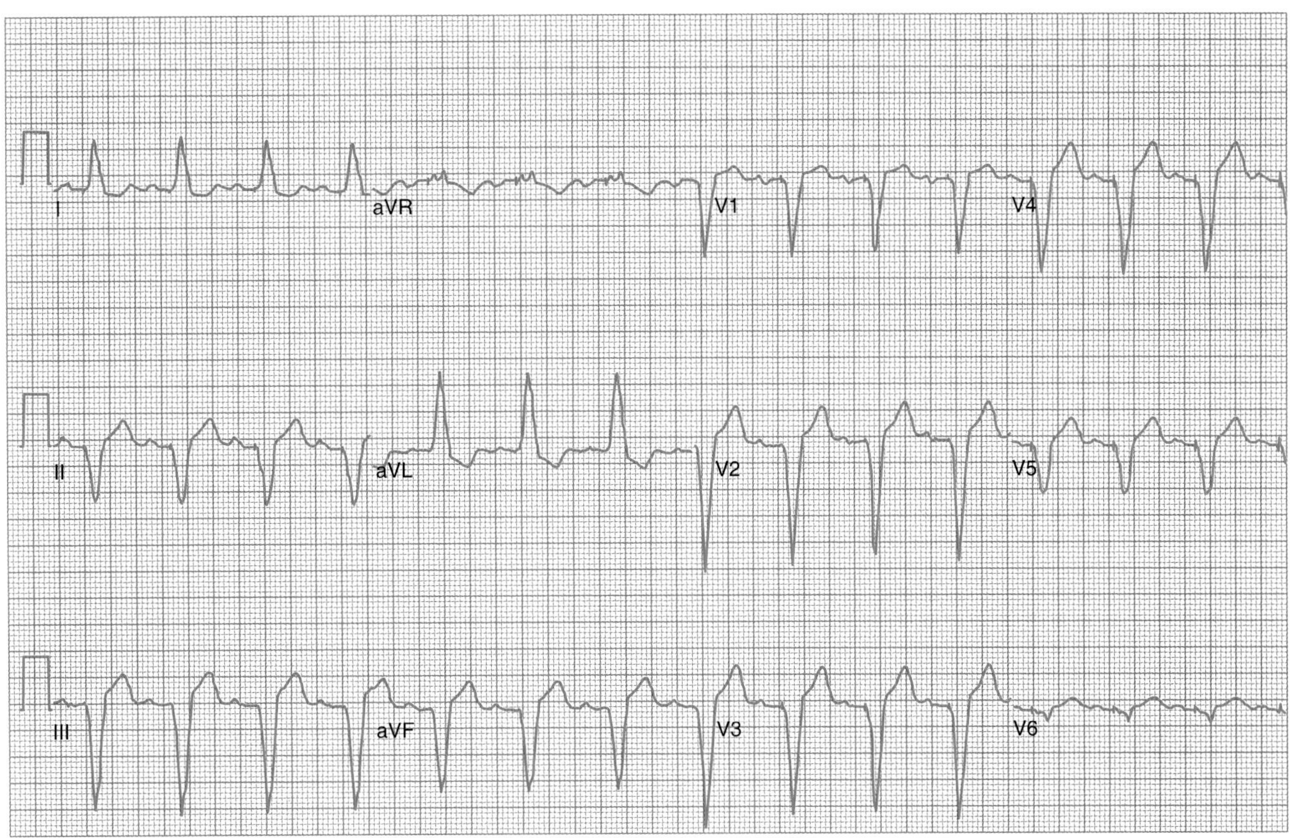

Figure 24-22. *A 12-lead electrocardiogram of a patient with a normally functioning bipolar pacing system. Note that a small pace artifact is seen in lead V4, whereas other leads do not show it at all.*

point, the programmed parameters should be double-checked to determine whether hysteresis or one of its analogs was programmed. Pacemakers have been returned to their manufacturers as defective when hysteresis was enabled. In these cases, the physician was either not aware of the programming or did not understand this feature.[112-114] Other causes of intermittent prolongation of the pacing interval are listed in Table 24-7.

Another source of evaluation error is failure to recognize intrinsic complexes that are present and are properly sensed, causing an appropriate device inhibition. This problem is not uncommon in the hospital's telemetry unit, in which only a single lead is monitored. Premature beats may be present, with the ectopic complexes appearing nearly isoelectric (Fig. 24-23). Although the observer may not recognize the PVC or premature atrial contraction (PAC) on casual observation, the pacemaker senses these events and is appropriately inhibited. The use of multiple leads or a 12-lead ECG recording virtually eliminates this cause of pseudomalfunction.

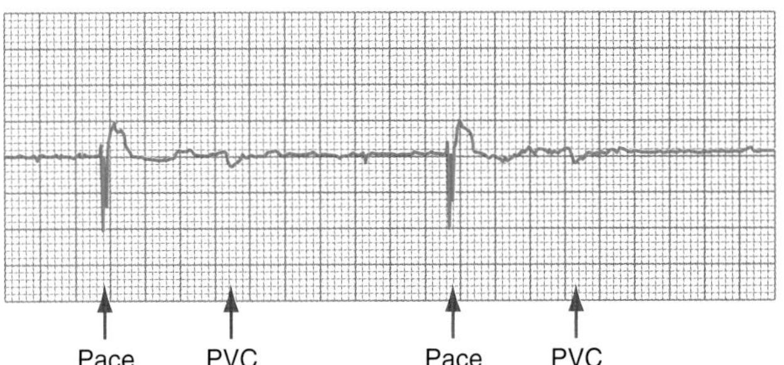

Figure 24-23. *An electrocardiographic rhythm strip of a pacemaker programmed to VVI with a demand rate of 50 bpm. This appears to show an inappropriate bradycardia. Note the low-amplitude waves that map out to the escape interval. These are premature ventricular contractions (PVCs) that appeared almost isoelectric in this lead.*

The lack of an output pulse, most commonly in unipolar systems, is frequently caused by oversensing. The pacemaker, for all its complexity, operates from a relatively simple set of rules. Any event that generates an electrical signal of adequate strength and frequency content (during the alert period) is sensed and resets the timing cycle. Oversensing is the sensing of a physiologically inappropriate or nonphysiologic signal. A cause of intracardiac oversensing in AAI systems is sensing of the far-field QRS complex (Fig. 24-24).[116] This is most common in unipolar systems when the lead is placed in close proximity to the tricuspid valve, with high atrial sensitivity settings, and with short atrial refractory periods. In systems that can deliver antitachycardia pacing therapy, oversensing may result in an inappropriate diagnosis of a tachycardia and therapy delivery.[117] Atrial far-field sensing is also one of

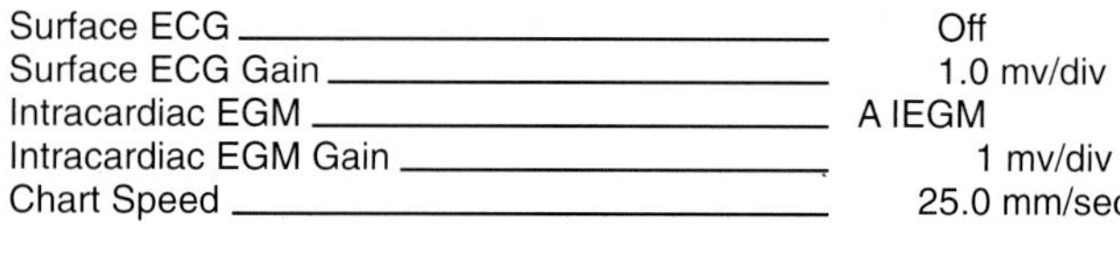

Mode: AAI Rate: 70 ppm
Magnet: TEMPORARY OFF
ECG/IEGM PARAMETERS
Surface ECG Off
Surface ECG Gain 1.0 mv/div
Intracardiac EGM A IEGM
Intracardiac EGM Gain 1 mv/div
Chart Speed 25.0 mm/sec

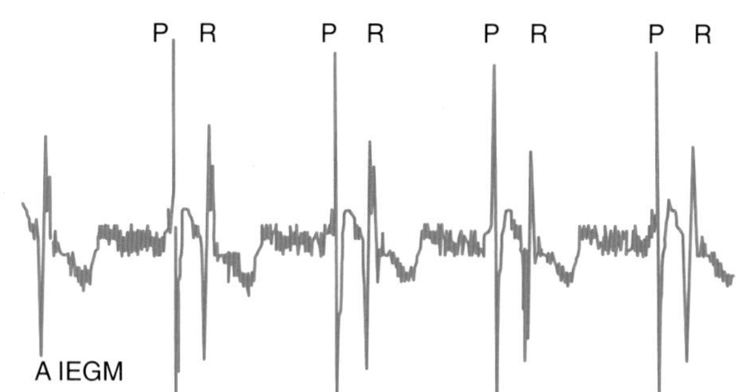

Figure 24-24. An intracardiac electrogram (IEGM) recorded from a unipolar atrial lead. Note the large size of the far-field ventricular electrogram (EGM), labeled R. If the near-field atrial EGM, labeled P were not as large, the device could undersense the atrium, sensing the ventricular EGM in error. ECG, electrocardiogram.

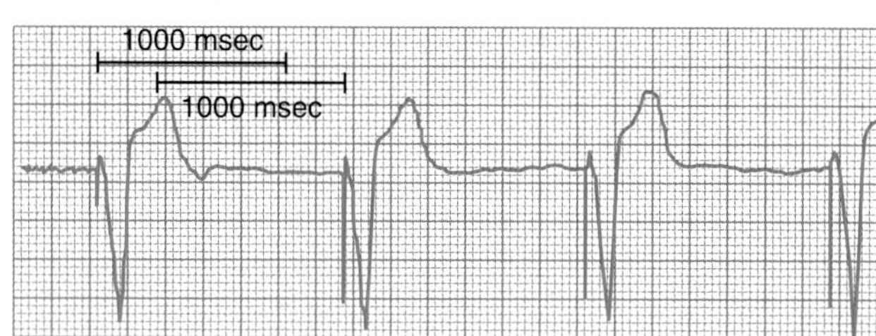

Figure 24-25. Electrocardiographic rhythm strip of a device programmed to VVI at 60 bpm. T-wave oversensing is present. The last sensed event can always be determined by mapping back by the escape interval.

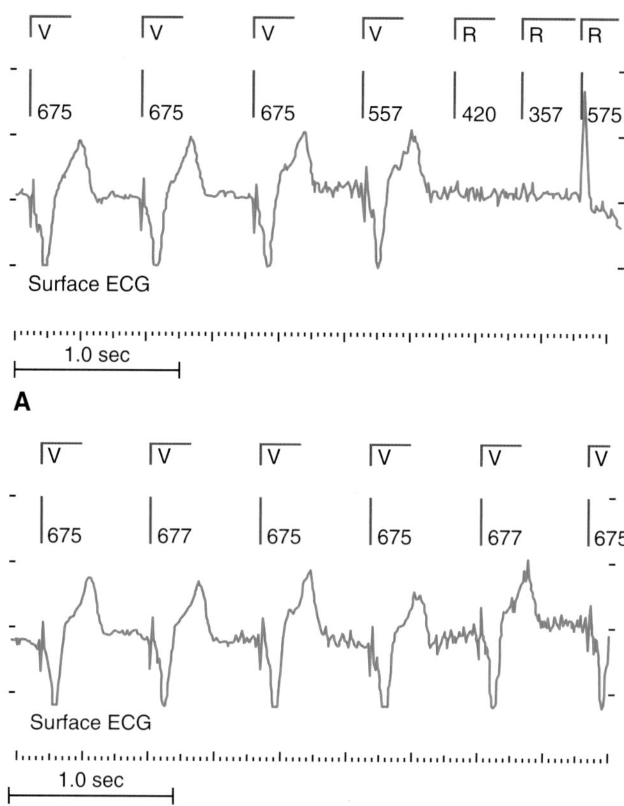

Figure 24-26. ***A,*** *An electrocardiogram (ECG) rhythm strip showing inappropriate inhibition caused by myopotential oversensing.* ***B,*** *An ECG rhythm strip of the same pacing system with a magnet placed over the pulse generator. If a loss of output were still evident with the magnet on, then the problem would not likely be oversensing.*

the most common causes of inappropriate mode switching, because the pacemaker is seeing double the actual heart rate. Far-field sensing is uncommon in VVI systems because of the diminutive size of the P wave, as seen electrically from the ventricle. Although it has been reported, it is usually associated with other problems, such as an insulation abrasion on the atrial portion of the ventricular lead.[15] Sensing of the intracardiac T wave may occur in VVI systems with similar results (Fig. 24-25), although this was a more common problem in the early days of pacing, as was the polarization artifact generated by the output pulse. Other chapters in this text provide a description of polarization and the evoked response. Oversensing of this event occurred with short refractory periods combined with high outputs on certain lead systems. This has also been reported in ICD systems that require short refractory periods and broad band-pass filters in the sense amplifier.

The most common source of a physiologic extracardiac signal that causes oversensing is myopotential inhibition. The pacemaker is capable of sensing muscle depolarizations—not only those of the heart, but also those of noncardiac structures such as the pectoralis, rectus abdominis, and diaphragmatic muscles. Myopotential inhibition of pacemaker output can be seen during arm movements (prepectoral implantation) or when the patient sits up or does a Valsalva maneuver (abdominal implantation; Fig. 24-26). This occurs primarily in unipolar systems, because the anode, the pacemaker's case, remains in close proximity to these muscular structures.[88,89,118-124] Nonphysiologic electrical signals may also cause oversensing. Formerly, electromagnetic interference (EMI) from microwave ovens was a significant problem when pacemakers were encased in plastic or epoxy, with the relatively large antenna created by the discrete components. Newer devices are shielded from EMI by their metal cases and filters. Integrated circuits provide for a smaller antenna, although strong EMI sources can still cause oversensing. A summary of EMI sources and their potential effects is presented in Table 24-8.[125-142]

It has been well documented that intermittent metal-to-metal contact can create electrical signals. These make-break signals may be of sufficient amplitude to

TABLE 24-8. **Causes of Potential Electromagnetic Interference**

Source	Pacer Damage	Total Inhibition	One-best Inhibition	Asynchrony Noise	Rate Increase	Unipolar/ Bipolar
Ablation	Y	Y	N	N	Y	U/B
Antitheft device	N	N	Y	N	N	U
Arc welder	N	Y	Y	Y	N	U/B
Cardiokymography	N	Y	Y	N	Y	U/B
Cardioversion	Y	N	N	N	N	U/B
Citizen's band radio	N	N	Y	N	N	U
Defibrillation	Y	N	N	N	N	U/B
Dental scaler	N	N	Y*	Y*	Y§	U
Diathermy	Y	Y	Y	Y	Y	U/B
Electroconvulsive therapy	N	Y	Y	Y	Y§	U
Electric blanket	N	N	N	Y†	N	U
Electric power tools	N	N	N	Y§	N	U
Electric shaver	N	N	Y§	N	N	U
Electric switch	N	N	Y*	N	N	U
Electric toothbrush	N	N	Y	N	N	U
Electrocautery	N	N	Y*	N	N	U
Electrolysis	Y	Y	Y	Y	Y§	U/B
Electronic article surveillance	N	Y	Y	Y	Y	U/B
Electrotome	N	N	Y	Y	N	U
Ham radio	N	N	Y*	N	N	U
Heating pad	N	N	Y	N	N	U
Lithotripsy	Y§	Y*	Y*	Y*	Y‡	U/B
Magnetic resonance imaging scanner	Y	N	Y	Y	Y‡	U/B
Positron emission tomographic scanner	Y	N	N	N	N	U/B
Powerline (high voltage)	N	N	N	Y	N	U/B
Pulp tester	N	Y*	Y*	Y	N	U
Radar	Y	N	N	N	Y	U/B
Radiotransmission (AM)	N	N	Y*	N	N	U
Radiotransmission (FM)	N	N	Y*	Y*	N	U
Stun gun	N	N	Y	N	N	U/B
Telephone—cellular	N	Y	Y	Y	Y‡	U/B
Telephone—cordless	N	Y	Y	Y	Y‡	U/B
Transcutaneous electrical nerve stimulation	N	Y	N	Y	Y‡	U
Television transmitter	N	Y*	Y*	Y*	N	U
Ultrasound (therapeutic)	Y§	N	Y*	N	N	U
Weapon detector	N	N	Y*	N	N	U

*Remote potential for interference.
†Impedance-based sensors.
‡DDD mode only.
§Piezocrystal-based sensors.
N, no; Y, yes; B, bipolar, U, unipolar.
Data updated from Telectronics (now Pacesetter Inc.), St. Jude Medical, Sylmar, Calif., technical note.

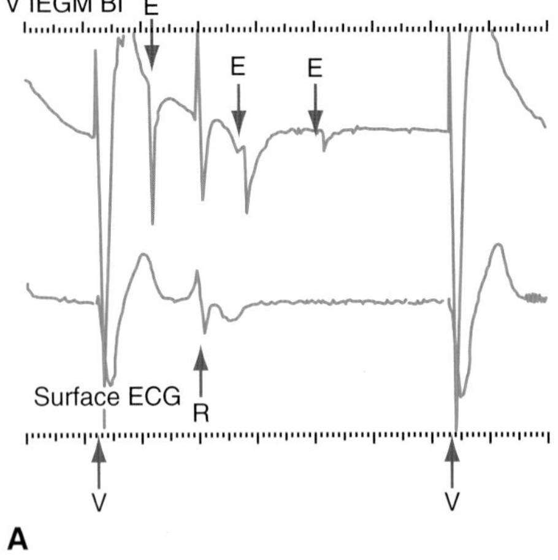

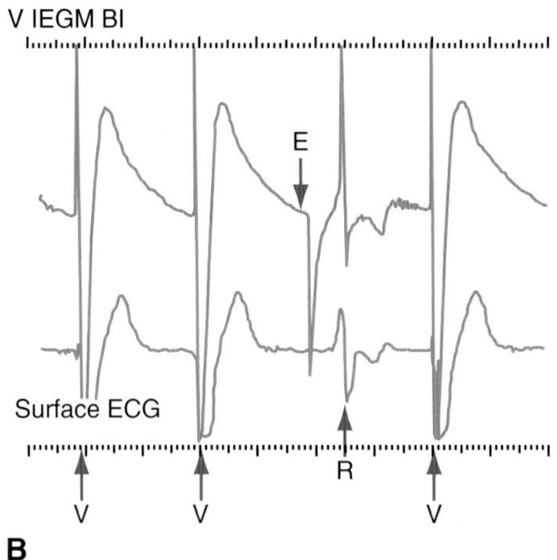

Figure 24-27. ***A*** *and* ***B,*** *Ventricular intracardiac electrograms (IEGMs) as telemetered by a pulse generator, recorded simultaneously with a surface electrocardiogram (ECG). Note the large artifacts (E) on the intracardiac channel seen without ventricular activity (R, native QRS; V, pace output). These were caused by failing inner insulation in a bipolar coaxial lead system. EGM, electrogram.*

be detected by pacing systems. Signals exceeding 25 mV have been recorded in some cases (Fig. 24-27). These large signals present a major problem: the false signal cannot be managed by programming the device to a less sensitive setting, because the nonphysiologic signal is far greater than the physiologic atrial or ventricular depolarization. The sources of these electrical signals include a loose set-screw, fracture of the conductor coil, failed insulation between the anode and cathode conductors in a bipolar system, interaction between active and abandoned pacing electrodes, and a loose retractable fixation screw.[142-150] Other mechanisms can also cause these signals, such as capacitance between the anode and cathode of a coaxial bipolar lead with failing insulation.

Oversensing need not result in pacing system inhibition. In the dual-chamber mode, if oversensing occurs on the atrial channel, it can result in ventricular pacing in response to the false P wave, which, in a patient who is susceptible to retrograde conduction, can precipitate an ELT. If the pacemaker were programmed to the triggered mode (which is one way to manage an oversensing problem that cannot be safely eliminated by programming to a less sensitive value), there would be periods of irregular pacing at a rate exceeding the programmed base rate in the presence of oversensing.

Oversensing can be confirmed by use of the magnet or by reprogramming to an asynchronous mode. If the cause of the pauses or slow rate is oversensing, regular pacing will resume during asynchronous pacing. If a lead failure, open circuit, or other cause exists for the lack of output, then these maneuvers will not result in asynchronous pacing. The use of intracardiac EGMs and event marker telemetry can quickly identify the cause of the pause, whether it is an output pulse that failed to reach the heart or the presence of oversensing. In the case of oversensing, the telemetered EGM may provide a clue to the source of the extraneous signal. As demonstrated in Figure 24-26, this is useful for differentiating the causes of oversensing and deciding on the proper remedy. The normal refractory period timing cycle initiated by the oversensing may give the overt appearance of undersensing, because the native complex that coincides with the electrocardiographically invisible refractory period is not sensed (normal behavior), allowing for time-out of the pacing escape interval and delivery of an output pulse; this is termed *functional undersensing* (see Fig. 24-3). The output pulse, if delivered during a period of physiologic refractoriness initiated by the native cardiac depolarization, may not capture, a phenomenon appropriately termed

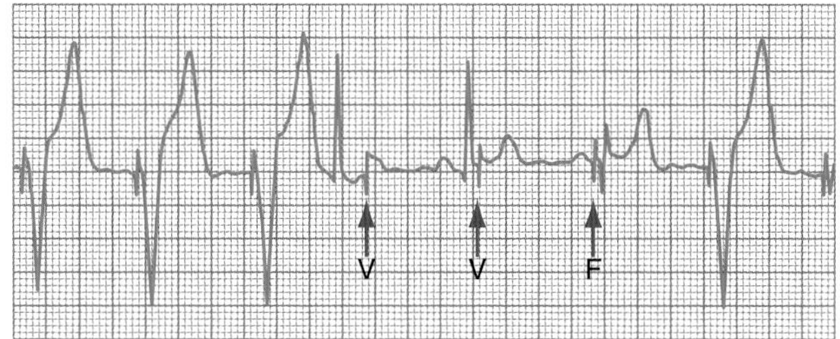

Figure 24-28. Electrocardiogram rhythm strip showing functional noncapture. The problem in this case is the pacing system's failure to sense the QRS. A subsequent pace output (V) occurs during the myocardial refractory period and should not be expected to be captured. The second-to-last QRS represents fusion (F) between the pace artifact and the native QRS.

functional noncapture (Fig. 24-28). The true cause of the observed behavior is readily appreciated with telemetered event markers, but it may be difficult to decipher from the free-standing ECG or rhythm strip.

Primary component failure of the pulse generator circuit is the least common of all the causes of pacing system failure, but it too can result in failure to output (Table 24-9). Patients who have been lost to follow-up may present with complete exhaustion of the power source (battery) and a virtually dead system. As the power source begins to fail, slowing of the pacing rate and erratic behavior may occur (Fig. 24-29). This may also be associated with mode and rate changes with or without sensing problems.

Several problems may be mistaken for pulse generator failure, resulting in a no-output situation. These are generally related to problems at the time of implantation. If the lead is not positioned properly in the connector block of the pacemaker, or if an improper lead is used, the electrical connection may not be complete. This is still an open circuit, but in the presence of a technically normal pulse generator and normal lead. The two are simply not connected appropriately, which is a physician error at the time of implantation. A transient situation has been reported in unipolar systems after wound closure. It is possible for air to be present in the pocket, especially if a large generator is replaced by a smaller one. Air is an effective insulator and prevents contact of the anterior anodal surface of the pacemaker's case with the body's tissues (this applies only to coated pacemakers). The result is an incomplete circuit until the air is absorbed. Subcutaneous emphysema has also been reported to be responsible for loss of anodal contact.[151,152] A similar pseudofailure occurs when a unipolar pulse generator is out of the pocket. If one were able to measure the stimulation impedance in each of these settings, it would be extremely high and well above the standard measurement for the particular lead being used. Event markers would report the release of an output pulse even though the circuit was open, precluding effective pacing.

TABLE 24-9. Causes of Pulse Generator Failure

Battery depletion
Component malfunction
Direct trauma
Loss of hermeticity
Therapeutic radiation
Electrocautery
Defibrillation and cardioversion
Lithotripsy

It is important to keep in mind that virtually all bipolar pacemakers may be programmed to function in the unipolar mode. Failure to output may also be seen with bipolar pacemakers that are connected to a unipolar pacing lead. This is more likely with IS-1 leads because the bipolar and unipolar connectors are similar. Some unipolar leads have a protective metal band where the anodal screw of the pacemaker connector block is located to prevent inadvertent tightening of this screw from damaging the lead. This gives the appearance of a bipolar lead even though no anodal conductor is present and is potentially misleading. Most polarity programmable pulse generators allow the user to designate the lead type as unipolar in a separate field of the programming system. Then, when the standard programmed parameter page is accessed, the bipolar lead option is locked out, minimizing the chance that the device will be accidentally programmed to the bipolar configuration.

In dual-chamber systems, sensing an event on one channel triggers refractory periods on both channels. Oversensing on the ventricular channel initiates both a ventricular refractory period and a PVARP. Depending on its precise timing, the PVARP initiated by the oversensed ventricular event may result in failure to sense a native P wave—yet another example of functional undersensing. A similar phenomenon may be seen in single-chamber systems in the presence of relatively rapid intrinsic rhythms. Oversensing starts a refractory period that may coincide with a native complex. Although this same complex is otherwise perfectly capable of being sensed, the pacemaker's refractory period precludes its being sensed, with the result being apparent undersensing when the true cause of the problem is oversensing. This is most readily identified if the phenomenon occurs while the rhythm is being monitored with the simultaneous display of event markers.

Failure to Capture (Artifact Is Present)

With the advent of the newer ECG recording systems and the use of pulse artifact enhancement, the clinician

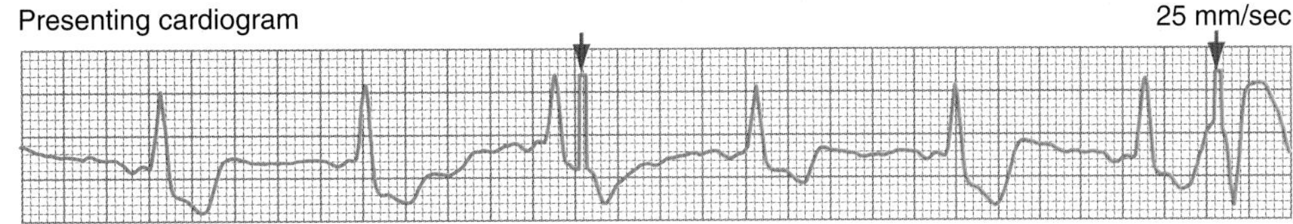

Figure 24-29. Rhythm strip from a patient whose pulse generator is beyond the elective replacement interval. Not only is the pacing rate below the programmed rate of 70 bpm, but the device is not sensing properly. The leads were found to function normally after the device was replaced.

must first be certain that the pace artifact seen is truly from the pacing system. The newer recording and monitoring systems have unique pacemaker pulse detectors that generate a discrete pacemaker pulse artifact in response to any high-frequency transient. There are many extraneous signals that can cause the enhanced ECG, telemetry system, or Holter recorder to place an erroneous pace artifact on the ECG. EMI (including programmer telemetry), loose ECG electrode connections, and subthreshold pulses (as seen with the minute ventilation sensors associated with normal pacemaker function) are examples of situations associated with spurious ECG artifacts (see Fig. 24-19). The use of event marker telemetry and intracardiac EGMs can assist in differentiating the true pacemaker output from a recording system artifact, whereas retrospective analysis of a previously recorded rhythm may prove challenging.

A common cause of functional noncapture is undersensing, with a resultant delivery of the pacemaker impulse during the physiologic refractory period of the myocardium. Although the output does not elicit a depolarization, the problem in this case is related to sensing, not output, and should be evaluated as such (see Fig. 24-28). This is best identified as undersensing, but if one insists on commenting on capture, it is functional noncapture. No matter how high the energy content of the output pulse, the myocardium is physiologically refractory and incapable of being depolarized.

When true noncapture is documented, the patient's safety must be ensured. If the patient is pacemaker dependent or is intolerant of the subsequent bradycardia associated with complete or intermittent loss of capture, the device should be programmed to its highest output. This can often be rapidly achieved by activating emergency VVI mode through the programmer. In most systems, even with a dual-chamber device, this programs the pacemaker to the highest available output in a unipolar output configuration. If consistent capture is still not secured, placement of a temporary pacemaker may be required. Almost all bipolar devices allow programming to the unipolar polarity. This may acutely correct the situation, particularly in the presence of an internal insulation failure, with a resultant short circuit or an open circuit associated with a fracture of the outer (anode) conductor. Although this maneuver eliminates the need for an emergency operative intervention, it is a temporizing measure only, and a lead with a mechanical failure should be replaced.

The causes of noncapture are listed in Table 24-10. The onset of noncapture in relation to implantation of the device and lead system can provide valuable clues to identification of the cause. If loss of capture occurs shortly after lead implantation, dislodgment, malposition, or perforation of the heart by the lead should be high on the list of possible problems. Elevated thresholds that occur during the first several weeks after implantation were more common in the early days of pacing. Although the incidence of this problem has markedly decreased with the introduction of steroid-eluting electrodes and other electrode materials and designs, a significant rise in capture threshold may still occur. The capture threshold rise is attributed to the inflammatory reaction that results from two factors: the pressure and hence trauma applied by the electrode to the endocardium, and a standard foreign-body reaction. The peak of the early threshold rise usually occurs between 2 and 6 weeks after implantation. Use of a higher output during this acute period minimizes the

TABLE 24-10. Causes of Loss of Capture*

Lead dislodgement or malposition
Microinstability
Macrodislodgment
Perforation
Elevated capture thresholds
Lead maturation
Chronic
Progressive cardiac disease
Myocardial infarction
Cardiomyopathy
Metabolic abnormality
Electrolyte abnormality
Drugs
Local damage at electrode–myocardium interface
Electrocautery
Defibrillation and cardioversion
Battery depletion
Circuit failure
Capture management algorithm failure
Inappropriate programming
Too low a safety margin
Evoked response sensitivity setting set to a too sensitive value
Pseudomalfunction
Recording artifacts mimicking a pacing stimulus
Isoelectric evoked potential with visible pacing stimulus
Functional noncapture—delivery of output during physiologic refractory period
Functional noncapture
True undersensing
Functional undersensing

*Pulse artifact present but no evoked potential.

TABLE 24-11. **Metabolic Factors that May Increase Capture Thresholds**

Major changes
Acidosis
Alkalosis
Hypercarbia
Hyperkalemia
Severe hyperglycemia
Hypoxemia
Myxedema
Minor changes
Sleep
Viral infections
Eating

likelihood of noncapture until the threshold improves to its chronic level. A rise in threshold occurring more than 6 weeks after implantation is usually considered to be in the chronic phase of the lead maturation process. The threshold may rise steadily over time until noncapture occurs or until the threshold exceeds the pacemaker's maximum output. This is commonly referred to as *exit block*.[153-159] Older lead models and some epicardial leads are more likely to develop elevated capture threshold levels.[160-163] Some patients demonstrate repeated episodes of this phenomenon and have required multiple lead revisions or replacements. Children with epicardial implants are especially prone to this condition.[153,164] Steroid-eluting leads are useful in minimizing the development of exit block.[166-173] There have been some anecdotal reports proposing the use of high-dose systemic steroids to lower high thresholds, with dosing continued for months and then slowly tapered, but there have been no formal prospective randomized trials to evaluate this pharmacologic intervention.[174-176]

There are many causes of threshold rise in both the acute and chronic phases. Any severe metabolic or electrolyte derangement can lead to acute threshold changes (Table 24-11).[177-188] These are not uncommon in critically ill patients or during and immediately after cardiac arrest. Noncapture may occur secondary to the hypoxemia, acidemia, or hyperkalemia, rather than be the primary event leading to the arrest. In addition, some medications may affect capture thresholds, resulting in significant changes from the patient's baseline (Table 24-12).[189-194] Beat-by-beat capture confirmation and daily capture threshold measurement systems are now in widespread use. These have been reported to identify patients with transient or sustained late rises in capture threshold that would have resulted in loss of capture had the implanted pacemaker been programmed to a standard 2:1 safety margin.[195] As experience continues using systems with these capabilities, understanding of the factors that can affect chronic capture threshold will increase.

TABLE 24-12. **Effects of Specific Drugs on Pacing Thresholds**

Increase threshold
Bretylium
Encainide
Flecainide
Moricizine
Propafenone
Sotalol
Mineralocorticoids
Possibly increase threshold
β-Blockers
Bretylium
Lidocaine
Procainamide
Quinidine
Decrease threshold
Atropine
Epinephrine
Isoproterenol
Glucocorticoids

Although the clinician might expect that fracture of a lead would result in the absence of any visible pacing artifact, this is frequently not the case. The ECG may display a pace artifact with failure to capture, especially in unipolar systems. This occurs because the current passes across the gap in the conductor coil through the fluid in the lead; however, the resistance is high, and the delivered output is likely to be subthreshold. In unipolar systems the anode (i.e., the pulse generator surface) is virtually always intact and provides enough of an electrical transient to trigger the artificial pace artifact circuitry of many monitoring systems. One can also see stimulus artifacts in the setting of a total disruption of both the conductor and the insulating sheath, which allows the output to be delivered to some local tissue, resulting in a stimulus on the ECG even though there is noncapture.[145]

Although modern pulse generators attempt to maintain the programmed voltage output until the battery is exhausted, a reduction in the delivered voltage may occur before the elective replacement indicator is activated. At advanced stages of depletion of the battery, this may result in an ineffective pacing stimulus.

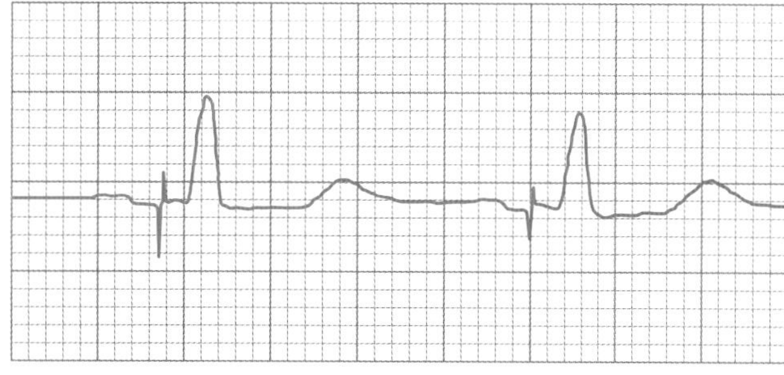

Figure 24-30. Electrocardiogram rhythm strip showing latency. Note the prolonged period from the pace artifact until the evoked QRS. This patient had a serum potassium concentration of 7.1 mEq because of renal failure.

Latency is a finding that may be mistaken for failure to capture. *Latency* is defined as the delay between delivery of the pacing impulse and onset of the evoked potential or electrical systole.[196] Some antiarrhythmic agents or severe electrolyte disturbances, such as hyperkalemia, can cause latency (Fig. 24-30). A Wenckebach type of prolongation, leading to a noncapture and a repeat of the cycle, has also been reported.

Failure to Sense

To comprehend undersensing, it is necessary to understand how the sense amplifier works, where in the cardiac cycle the sensing can occur, and where it cannot occur. A prerequisite for proper sensing is the quality of the EGM; the signal must possess both an adequate amplitude and an adequate frequency content (slew rate) to be sensed properly. A signal of apparently adequate peak-to-peak amplitude may be markedly attenuated by the sense amplifier because of its poor slew rate. The resultant "filtered" signal may be of insufficient size to be recognized as a valid event.[197-202] Table 24-13 lists the causes of sensing failure.

It is often assumed that the pacemaker senses a cardiac event at the beginning of the P wave or QRS complex, as seen on the surface ECG. This is not the case. The surface P wave or QRS is a summation of all electrical events occurring at the cellular level over a period of time (80 to 120 msec or longer). The intracardiac EGM as recorded from a pacing electrode appears as a large-amplitude, relatively rapid deflection (see Fig. 24-8). If one did not know that the recording was an EGM, an atrial signal could be easily mistaken for a QRS complex presumed to have been recorded with a standard surface ECG. It is therefore helpful to record both the atrial and the ventricular EGM simultaneously, the EGM with the simultaneous surface ECG, or telemetered event markers (the newest systems can provide all of these simultaneously). This event, the intrinsic deflection of the QRS or P wave, is generated as the wave of depolarization passes by the electrode. This is the complex that is sensed, even if it occurs well after the onset of the native depolarization. An excellent example of this delayed sensing is in the patient who has right bundle branch block and a pacing electrode in the right ventricle. The native depolarization occurs late in the right ventricle because of the conduction delay. The pacemaker does not sense this event until that depolarization reaches the pacing lead, which is very late in the timing of the surface QRS

TABLE 24-13. Causes of Undersensing

Poor intrinsic signal from implant
Signal amplitude
Slew rate
Deterioration of intrinsic signal over time
Lead maturation
Progression of disease
Cardiomyopathy
New bundle branch block
Myocardial infarction
Respiratory or motion variation
Ectopic complexes not present at implantation
Transient decrease in signal amplitude
Postcardioversion or defibrillation
Metabolic derangement (e.g., hyperkalemia)
Component malfunction
Sensing circuit abnormality
Stuck reed switch
Battery depletion
Mechanical lead dysfunction
Insulation failure
Partial open circuit
Pseudomalfunction
Recording artifact
Normal device function—misinterpreted
Triggered mode
Fusion and pseudofusion beats
Functional undersensing
Long refractory periods
Blanking period
Safety pacing
Oversensing
DVI mode (particularly committed DVI)
Oversensing initiated functional undersensing

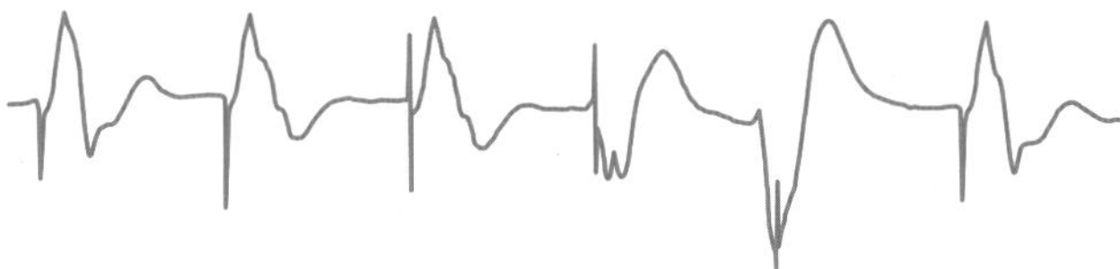

Figure 24-31. Electrocardiogram rhythm strip showing pseudofusion beats. Because the premature ventricular contractions have a right bundle branch block morphology, right ventricular depolarization occurs late within the overall cardiac activation sequence. The QRS complexes cannot be sensed by the pacemaker until late into the surface QRS, resulting in pseudofusion complexes when the escape interval "times out" before the intrinsic deflection has occurred. In these cases, even though the ventricle had started to depolarize, the pacemaker was not yet capable of sensing it.

complex. If it is assumed that sensing occurred earlier, this may be incorrectly labeled *late sensing*. Measurements made from the onset of the QRS complex can misinterpret the timing cycle by more than 100 msec. Therefore, an ECG with a pacing artifact in the QRS (pseudofusion and fusion) can occur in the presence of absolutely normal sensing (Fig. 24-31).[203,204]

The refractory and blanking periods are integral to understanding sensing and whether a native complex is even potentially capable of being sensed. A blanking period is a period of time during which no sensing at all will occur on a given channel. A refractory period is similar to a blanking period, but events occurring during a refractory period may be used for purposes other than resetting escape intervals. These "sensed but not used" events can be used by the device to detect noise on a lead or atrial events for initiation of mode switching. Long programmed refractory and blanking periods can cause undersensing of events occurring within these periods (Fig. 24-32). This might occur in the case of a closely coupled PVC or PAC or very rapid intrinsic rhythms. Although there may be resultant competition, this is not a lead or pulse generator malfunction, in that both are functioning properly and in accord with their design. This is clinically undesirable and reflects inappropriate programmed settings in the pacemaker, a behavior amenable to correction by programming. This is also termed *functional undersensing*, because the pacemaker is not capable of sensing at the time the native signal occurred. On the other hand, the failure to sense the native complex allows the timing period to complete, with the resultant release of an output pulse that may prove to be ineffective because it was delivered at a time of physiologic refractoriness. Functional undersensing commonly results in functional noncapture. A classic example of this phenomenon was the committed DVI pacing system, an early-generation (and now obsolete) AV sequential pacing system that was not capable of sensing on the atrial channel but, with release of an atrial output, was committed to release a ventricular output even in the presence of a native R wave.[203,222]

As in noncapture, the onset of undersensing in relation to implantation of the pacemaker and lead system may direct the clinician to the correct diagnosis of the malfunction. Undersensing that occurs close in time to implantation should lead the physician to suspect dislodgment, malposition, or perforation of the electrode. Problems occurring in chronic systems are frequently caused by mechanical problems with the lead or, if the lead is normal, by programming errors. Occasionally they are attributable to a change in the morphology of the intrinsic cardiac signal associated with disease progression. Inappropriate programmed settings are not uncommon, particularly when sensitivity threshold testing has been performed in a nontemporary manner during follow-up. The clinician may forget to return the sensitivity to the appropriate setting and leave it at or above the threshold setting. Occasionally, the sensing threshold may show a slow decline in the amplitude of the native signal as the lead-tissue interface changes over time.[205-212]

The vector of depolarization can affect the amplitude and slew rate of the intracardiac EGM. Any change in the vector may result in significant changes in the sensing threshold. If a patient with a ventricular pacemaker has a myocardial infarction, develops a bundle branch block, or has PVCs, the intracardiac signal may be insufficient to allow sensing at a previously appropriate setting (Fig. 24-33).[206-208] The same may be seen with atrial implants and PACs. Another cause of vector change is movement of the lead's position associated with respiration. Marked changes in the intracardiac signal can be documented in some patients as the angle of the lead relative to the heart changes with body position or diaphragmatic motion (Fig. 24-34).[209-212] Evaluation of the quality of the intracardiac signal associated with sensing failure is greatly facilitated by access to the telemetered intracardiac EGM.

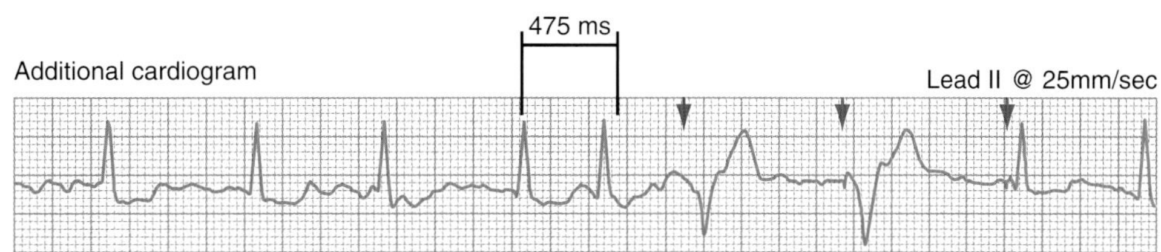

Figure 24-32. Electrocardiogram rhythm strip showing undersensing of the QRS complexes in a patient with atrial fibrillation. The device is programmed to VVI with a demand rate of 70 bpm and a refractory period of 475 msec. Because of a long programmed ventricular refractory period, this does not represent a pacemaker malfunction. The pacemaker will not respond to intrinsic events during the refractory period, a phenomenon termed functional undersensing.

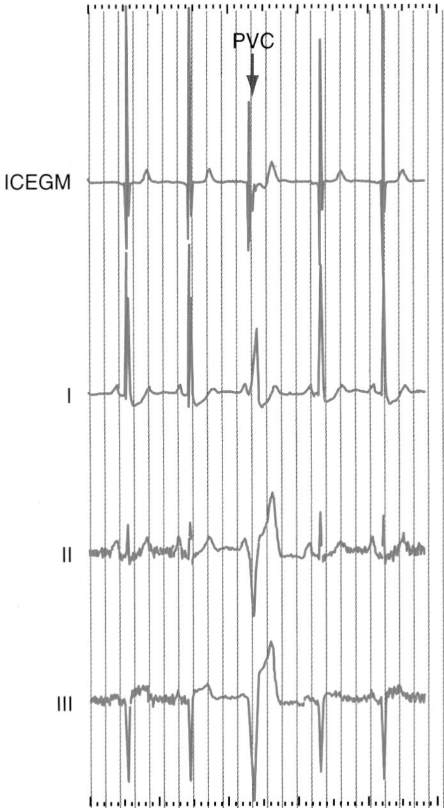

Figure 24-33. The intracardiac electrogram (ICEGM) and surface electrocardiogram (I, II, III) of intrinsic beats and a premature ventricular contraction (PVC). In this example, the PVC electrogram has a peak-to-peak amplitude that is significantly lower than the normal beats and may lead to undersensing.

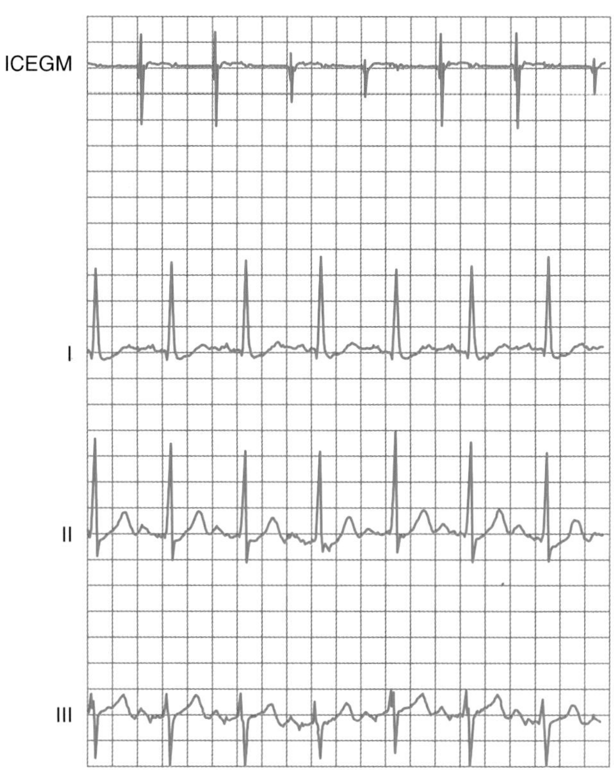

Figure 24-34. Intra-atrial electrogram and surface electrocardiogram. Note the profound variation of the intracardiac signal without apparent change in the surface P-wave morphology. The variation was synchronous with respiratory movements. This situation may be seen in either the atrium or the ventricle. ICEGM, intracardiac electrogram.

As the pacemaker's battery begins to become depleted, erratic behavior may occur, including persistent or intermittent undersensing. Failure of a circuit component may also cause sensing failure. Rarely, the reed switch that activates the magnet mode may stick in the closed position, causing (in most cases) asynchronous pacing. For the same reason, when reviewing a rhythm strip, the clinician must know whether the magnet was over the device when the recording was made. Asynchronous pacing may also be seen during the interference or noise mode function of the device. The latter obligates pacing when the presence of electrical noise is sensed by the pulse generator. Typically, this is defined as multiple sensed events occurring within the terminal portion of the ventricular refractory period. The device then paces asynchronously to protect the pacemaker-dependent patient against inappropriate device inhibition.[142,213]

One frequently misinterpreted reason for failure to sense involves pacemakers that use impedance plethysmography as a rate-modulation sensor. This applies primarily to minute ventilation sensors but now also to "lung wetness" monitoring systems. The system uses the pacemaker's case as the anode for the impedance sensing impulses. Therefore, when the case is out of the pocket, a great deal of electrical noise is generated, because the system is not grounded. This may result in asynchronous pacing until the device is placed into the pocket. If the clinician is not aware of this idiosyncrasy, a malfunction of the pulse generator might be inappropriately diagnosed.

Finally, the use of either external or internal defibrillation can result in temporary or permanent loss of the sensing function. This may be caused by transient saturation of the sensing amplifier pacemaker, circuit damage, or lead-myocardium interface damage. This phenomenon occurs when the large electrical current delivered by the defibrillator is diverted from the pacemaker's circuitry to the pacing lead by way of Zener diodes, which are included in the pacemaker circuitry to protect the pulse generator from large voltage surges. The result may cauterize the myocardium and thereby reduce or eliminate the local EGM. It may also cause a marked elevation in the capture threshold or result in exit block. Capacitive coupling is another mechanism that may allow a current to be induced into the pacing lead, by either a shock or nearby electrocautery use.[214-216]

Dual-chamber Pacemaker Issues

Crosstalk Inhibition

Crosstalk is a potentially catastrophic form of ventricular oversensing that can occur in any dual-chamber mode in which the atrium is paced and the ventricle is sensed and paced. Consider the fact that the common output voltages for the atrial channel range from 2.5 to 5 V. This is the same as 2500 to 5000 mV. The ventricular lead is just several centimeters away from this atrial lead and is "looking" for an electrical event of about 2 mV, which would represent a sensed ventricular depolarization. If the ventricular channel senses the pacing impulse delivered to the atrium, it interprets the event as an R wave. The ventricular output is inhibited, and the patient is left without pacing support. If crosstalk occurs in a patient with complete AV block, ventricular asystole could result in the absence of an escape rhythm with only paced P waves visible.[217-220] Conversely, crosstalk is more difficult to detect when AV nodal conduction is intact. In a system that uses ventricular based timing, it may result in an acceleration of the paced atrial rate with ventricular output inhibition even in the presence of a first-degree AV block that exceeds the programmed AV delay.[220]

As demonstrated in Figure 24-35, crosstalk can be recognized by an acceleration of the atrial-paced rate in a non–sensor-driven dual-chamber system using ventricular-based timing. Note that ventricular sensing occurs virtually simultaneously with atrial output. The AV delay is immediately terminated with ventricular sensing, and the atrial escape interval is started. Therefore, the pacing interval with this type of timing is equal to the atrial escape interval (programmed pacing interval minus AV delay) plus the ventricular blanking period. Rate-modulated pacing systems that use ventricular-based timing have a rate acceleration that is seen at the base pacing rate. Crosstalk may not be readily diagnosed in patients with rate-modulated pacing systems and intact AV nodal conduction if the increased atrial pacing rate is believed to be caused by the sensor.

Pacing systems that use atrial-based timing do not exhibit this rate increase. Although ventricular sensing

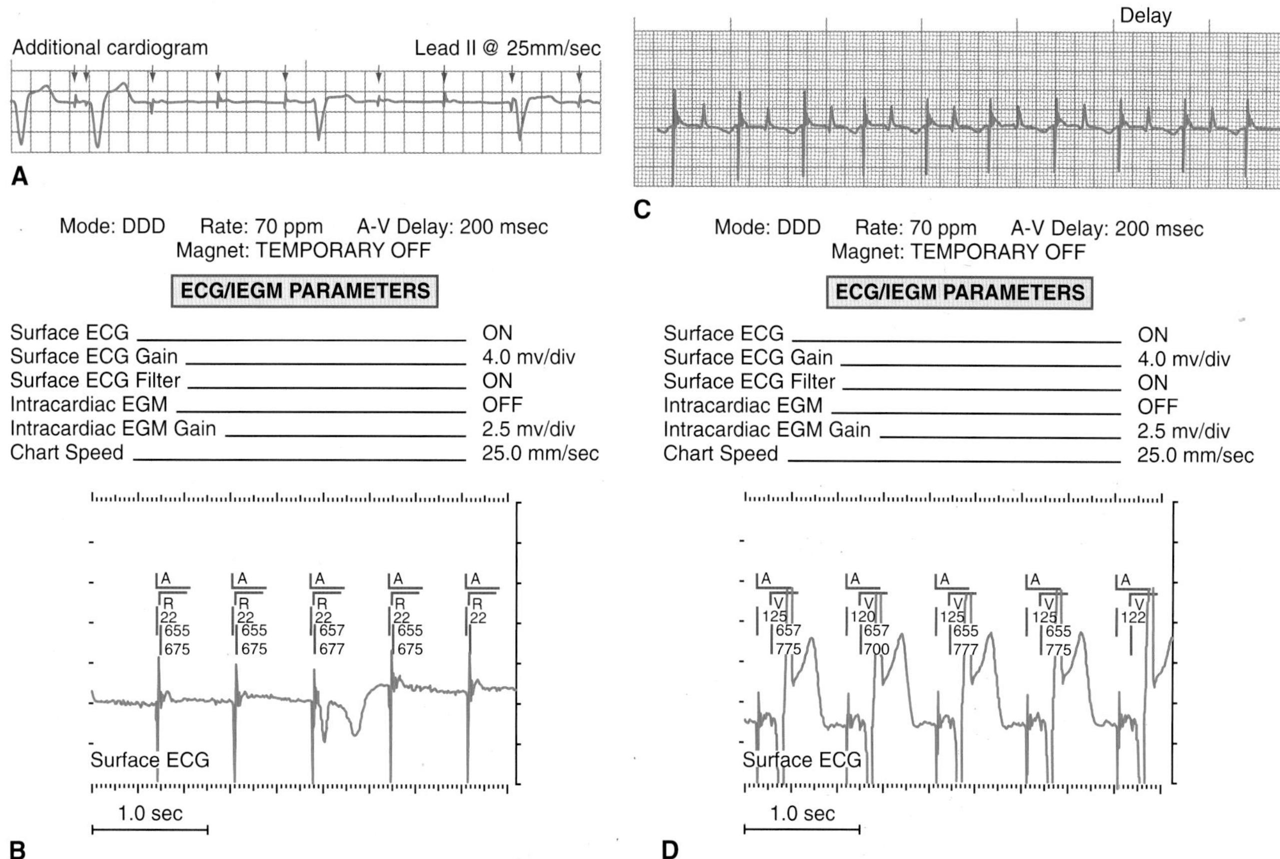

Figure 24-35. ***A,*** *Electrocardiogram (ECG) rhythm strip showing crosstalk in a patient with complete atrioventricular (AV) block, with a ventricular-based pacing system. Note the presence of an atrial output without a ventricular output. A comparison of the interval from the first until the second atrial pulse with that from the second until the third atrial pulse demonstrates that the pacing interval is shortened by the AV interval minus the blanking period (120 msec).* ***B,*** *ECG strip with event markers during crosstalk. Note that the ventricular sensing (R) occurs immediately after the atrial output pulse (A). Safety pacing was turned off.* ***C,*** *ECG rhythm strip showing crosstalk in a patient with intact AV conduction. Because this pacemaker operates with ventricular-based timing, the atrial escape interval resets with each atrial output, elevating the frequency of atrial stimulation.* ***D,*** *ECG rhythm strip and event markers during crosstalk and ventricular safety pacing. Note that, despite the setting of the AV interval to 200 msec, the event markers demonstrate the ventricular stimulus at 125 msec after the atrial output pulses. IEGM, intracardiac electrogram.*

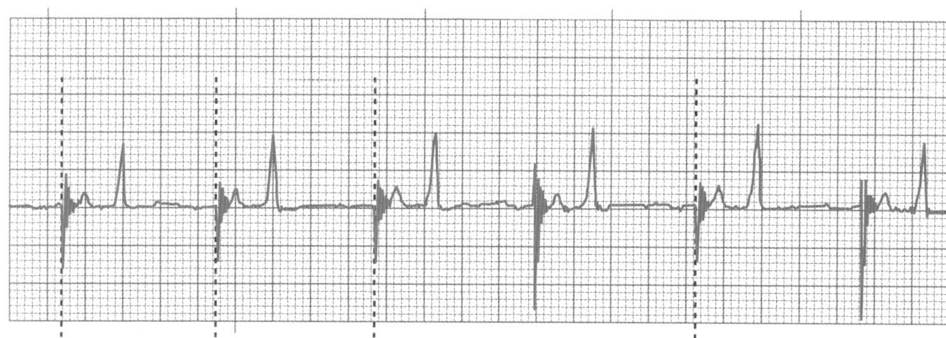

Figure 24-36. Electrocardiogram rhythm strip showing crosstalk with a pacemaker operating with atrial-based timing. Note that the atrial pacing rate remains at the programmed rate of 70 bpm. The atrioventricular interval was programmed to 175 msec.

TABLE 24-14. **Factors Promoting Crosstalk**

High atrial output settings
Pulse amplitude
Pulse width
Pulse current as with low impedance
High ventricular sensitivity setting
Short ventricular blanking period

of the atrial output inhibits the ventricular output, the portion of the AV interval not used is added to the atrial escape interval, maintaining atrial pacing at the programmed interval (Fig. 24-36). Without access to event marker telemetry, ventricular output inhibition due to crosstalk cannot be differentiated from failure to output, as with an open circuit.

Several factors increase the likelihood of crosstalk (Table 24-14). Programmed settings that increase either the ventricular sensitivity or the atrial energy output predispose to this problem. Insulation failure on the atrial lead also increases the chances of crosstalk by increasing the pulse charge and energy. The clinician must be aware that certain pacemaker models are more prone to this phenomenon than are others. This is related to differences in circuit designs and the degree of isolation between the two channels within the pulse generator.[217] Crosstalk may occur within the circuitry of the pulse generator rather than between the pacing leads. Unipolar systems are also significantly more prone to crosstalk because of the larger electrical signal, as sensed by the ventricular channel.[218-223]

There are two approaches to the problem of crosstalk: prevention of crosstalk and prevention of the consequences of crosstalk.

Prevention of Crosstalk. Prevention of crosstalk is approached by proper programming of the device and proper lead placement. Atrial amplitude and pulse width settings that provide an appropriate safety margin without being excessive and ventricular sensitivity settings that are not unnecessarily sensitive are helpful. Newer circuit designs are much more resistant to this problem. Even under ideal circumstances, however, crosstalk may still occur.

The use of an additional ventricular refractory period, known as the *ventricular blanking period* (VBP), is fundamental to prevention.[221] The VBP begins with the atrial output and usually lasts from 12 to 120 msec. In most devices, this is a programmable parameter. During the VBP, nothing (including the atrial output) can be sensed on the ventricular channel. Short VBPs help to prevent the undersensing of intrinsic ventricular activity but may allow crosstalk to occur. Long VBPs virtually ensure the prevention of crosstalk but may cause intrinsic events to not be sensed, a potential problem if the native beat is a late-cycle PVC and the AV interval is programmed to a long length. Functional failure to sense a PVC (because the intrinsic deflection of the PVC coincided with the VBP) may be followed by a ventricular output beyond the myocardial refractory period and on the vulnerable zone of the T wave. This might result in the induction of a ventricular arrhythmia, which could also occur with atrial undersensing if a normally conducted QRS falls into the VBP. The latter event would not be detected, and an unnecessary stimulus would be delivered (Fig. 24-37).

Prevention of Crosstalk Sequelae. The earliest approach to prevention of ventricular output loss as a result of crosstalk was the introduction of the DVI-committed mode (DVI-C). In this version of DVI, ventricular sensing is completely disabled during the AV interval that follows an atrial output pulse. After termination of the AV interval, a ventricular output pulse is committed whether or not an intrinsic ventricular event has occurred. Thus, with DVI-C, there can never be an inhibition of the ventricular output by an atrial output. Although this approach worked, it resulted in confusing ECGs and wasted energy because of the delivery of unnecessary pacing impulses.[203,222] It is also not practical for DDD devices for similar reasons. With the development of the DDD mode, however, manufacturers were able to provide brief refractory periods (blanking periods) starting with the atrial output. Even blanking periods, however, are not a guaranteed prevention for ventricular output inhibition associated with crosstalk.

To ensure patient safety, a unique circuit/algorithm has been integrated into the ventricular channel. The most common approach is the use of a safety output pulse. This is referred to by multiple names, depending on the manufacturer of the device (e.g., safety

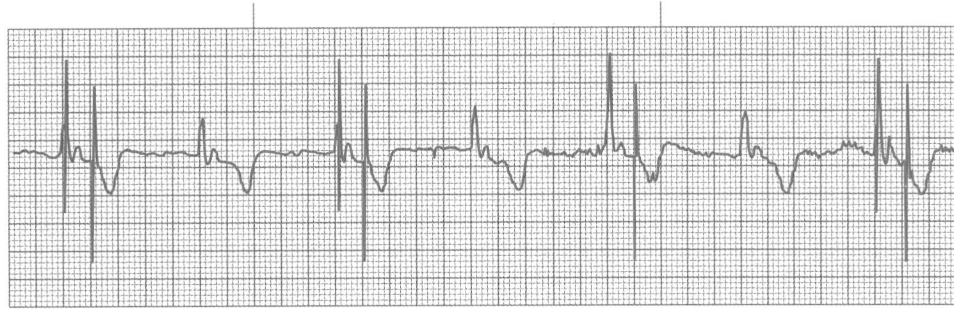

Figure 24-37. Electrocardiogram rhythm strip showing undersensing of native QRS. The device was programmed to the DVI mode, so there is no atrial sensing. When the atrial escape interval expires, the atrial output coincides with the onset of the native QRS. The ventricular blanking period is triggered by the release of the atrial output; this precludes ventricular sensing for 38 msec after the atrial output. If the intrinsic deflection of the native QRS coincides with the ventricular blanking period, it will not be sensed, and a ventricular output will be delivered at the end of the programmed atrioventricular interval.

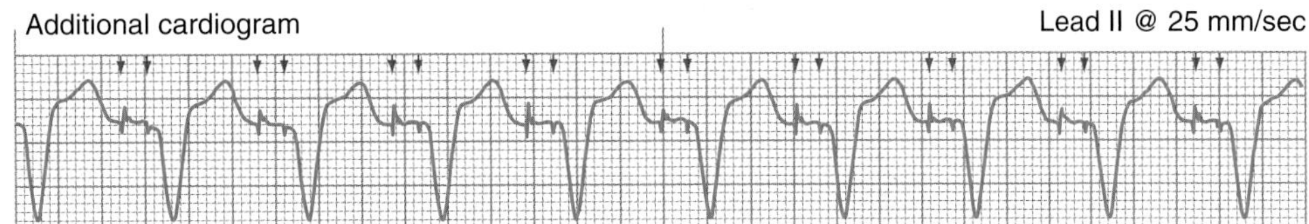

Figure 24-38. Electrocardiogram rhythm strip showing safety pacing. Sensing is occurring on the ventricular channel during the crosstalk sensing window. This causes a ventricular output to be delivered at a shortened atrioventricular (AV) interval. In a ventricular-based timing system, the pacing interval is shortened by the difference between the programmed AV interval and the safety-paced AV interval, because the atrial escape interval is reset by any sensed or paced ventricular event. This results in an AV-paced rate of 93 bpm, even though the device is programmed DDD at 75 bpm and is not capable of rate modulation.

pacing, nonphysiologic AV delay, ventricular safety standby). This method uses a brief sensing period (crosstalk sensing window) after the blanking period. Any electrical event sensed during this crosstalk sensing period is assumed to be crosstalk. A ventricular output is then triggered to be delivered after a shortened AV delay (Fig. 24-38).[223,224] Other events can cause a safety output pulse to occur, including premature ventricular beats, premature junctional beats, and normally conducted ventricular events that occur after undersensed intrinsic atrial beats (see Fig. 24-37). After one of the latter events, if the safety output pulse were to be delivered using a long AV interval, there would be a potential for delivering a tightly coupled and potentially arrhythmogenic stimulus to the ventricle. Therefore, a shortened AV interval is used (typically, between 100 and 120 msec) to deliver the stimulus harmlessly into the depolarizing ventricle while maintaining the ability to rescue the patient in the presence of actual crosstalk. In the presence of a long programmed AV delay and intact AV nodal conduction, crosstalk is signaled by AV pacing at the abbreviated AV delay. Reducing the atrial output, reducing the ventricular sensitivity, or lengthening the VBP should reduce, if not totally eliminate, episodes of crosstalk.

As in crosstalk, delivery of the safety output pulse causes a shortening of the base pacing interval because of the shortened AV interval. If the baseline AV interval is programmed to the same duration as that of the safety output pulse (this has become very common in biventricular devices when treating patients with congestive heart failure), or if a rate-modulated or differential AV interval is present, the presence of safety pacing (i.e., crosstalk) may be difficult or impossible to discern on the standard ECG. The use of event marker telemetry documents the presence of crosstalk or safety output pulses in these situations (see Fig. 24-38).

Finally, delivery of a safety output pulse does not prevent crosstalk. It is designed to prevent the sequelae of crosstalk by preventing ventricular asystole. It is unwise to allow a patient to use this backup mechanism continually. If crosstalk is suspected or documented, the clinician should pursue the potential causes and make the necessary adjustments to terminate this condition. In some situations, such as failure of the lead's insulation, programming changes may not be adequate, and surgical intervention may be required.

Pacemaker-Mediated Tachycardia

Any undesired rapid pacing rate caused by the pulse generator or by an interaction of the pacing system with the patient may be considered PMT. This has classically been associated with the ELT seen in dual-chamber devices. PMT, however, should be assumed to be a more general term. The following are several conditions that are well-documented causes of PMT.

Runaway Pacemaker. The runaway pacemaker is a pacemaker malfunction that may occur in single-chamber or dual-chamber pacing systems. It is usually the result of at least two separate component failures within the pulse generator. The result is the rapid delivery of pacing stimuli to the heart, with the potential for inducing lethal arrhythmias, such as ventricular tachycardia or fibrillation. All modern devices incorporate a runaway protect circuit that prevents stimulation above a preset rate, typically between 180 and 200 bpm. Although extremely rare with modern pacing devices, this represents a medical emergency (Fig. 24-39). Emergent surgical intervention to replace the device or, if all else fails, cut the lead, must be performed. Obviously, a patient who is pacemaker dependent presents a new challenge as soon as the defective pacing system is disabled.[225,226]

Sensor-Driven Tachycardia. Sensor-driven tachycardia is a rapid heart rate occurring in rate-modulated pacemakers. It can occur with any type of sensor-driven pacing system (Table 24-15). Interaction between the patient and external stimuli can cause the rate-modulation system to overreact and pace at a high rate. The most common cause of this PMT type is inappropriate programming of the sensor parameters. In piezoelectric devices, a threshold setting that is too low or a slope setting that is too high results in high pacing rates for low levels of activity. It also exposes the patient to increased pacing rates for nonphysiologic events, such as riding in a car, exposure to loud noise or music, or sleeping on the ipsilateral side to the device implant.[227-237]

One unpublished incident concerned a patient with a bipolar piezoelectric VVIR device. The emergency medical squad had been summoned to treat an unconscious patient. They arrived to find the patient with seizure activity. On viewing the ECG, they found the patient's condition to be wide complex tachycardia at 150 bpm. The patient received repeated direct current cardioversion for this tachycardia without reversion to sinus rhythm. In this case, the seizures were caused by epilepsy, and the vibration-based sensor responded to the seizure by pacing at its upper rate. No spikes had been noted on the ECG because the output configuration was bipolar, which resulted in a diminutive artifact on the monitor (Fig. 24-40).

In the past, pacing systems responsive to central venous temperature changes might have responded to a fever spike with upper rate pacing. This necessitated design of a "nulling" feature, which restores a more appropriate pacing rate after a specified time at the upper rate has occurred. Devices that respond to changes in the evoked QT interval also use this nulling feature, although for different reasons. As the QT interval shortens because of catecholamine increases and

TABLE 24-15. Causes of Sensor-Driven Pacemaker Tachycardia

Vibration sensor—piezocrystal
Pressure on device Patient lying on device, as during sleep, Tapping on device
Submuscular implantation
Loud, low-frequency music
Bumpy ride, as in a tractor, lawn mower, or helicopter
Use of vibration-generating tools
Impedance-based sensors—minute ventilation
Hyperventilation
Electrocautery
Environmental 50- to 60-Hz electrical interference
Evoked QT interval
Rate-dependent QT-shortening spiral
Sympathomimetic drugs

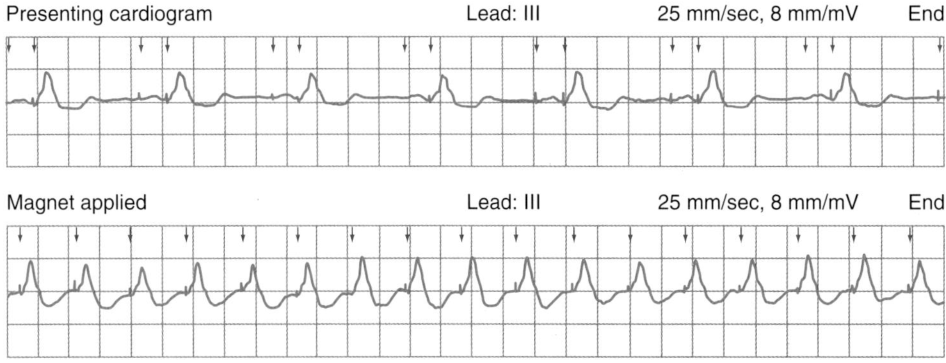

Figure 24-39. Example of a "runaway pacemaker." This device was subjected to direct, unshielded therapeutic irradiation during treatment of a breast carcinoma. The patient presented to the clinic for routine follow-up and had a normal presenting rhythm strip as shown. She had been programmed to DDDR from 70 to 120 bpm. On placement of the magnet over the device, pacing began at the runaway protect rate of 180 bpm. The patient was taken to the operating room, and the device was replaced emergently.

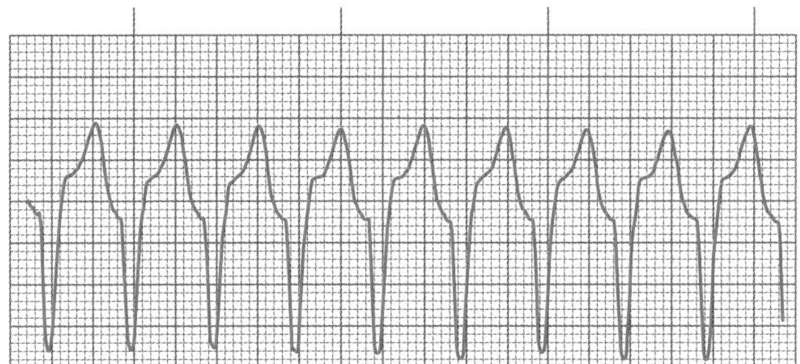

Figure 24-40. Electrocardiogram rhythm strip of pseudoventricular tachycardia caused by rapid ventricular pacing using a bipolar device. Note that the pace artifact is not well seen, leading to this potential misdiagnosis.

changes in the autonomic nervous system, the pacing rate is increased by the device; however, this may cause further shortening of the QT interval by a rate-dependent mechanism. The latter change further increases the pacing rate, which may then spiral to the upper rate limit.

Devices that use thoracic impedance plethysmography to determine changes in minute ventilation may pace at the upper rate during marked hyperventilation, use of electrocautery, hyperventilation during anesthesia induction, and when in close proximity to an electrical power supply. Therefore, it is strongly recommended that this type of rate-modulation feature be disabled before the patient undergoes any surgical procedure (even if electrocautery is not used, because much electrical equipment is present in most operating room suites), treatment with a mechanical ventilator, or treatment in a critical care unit.[236]

Magnetic Resonance Imaging. Exposure to magnetic resonance imaging (MRI) scanners has been reported to cause inappropriately high pacing rates when tested in animals. Some pacemakers have been noted to pace at the radiofrequency (RF) pulse rate of the scanner. This situation resolves immediately with the cessation of the RF output by the scanner.[238-243] MRI may also result in inhibition of the pacing output during the scanning process. Because of these issues, such scanning has been cautioned against by all manufacturers of pacemakers. This is true even though some patients have inadvertently or intentionally undergone MRI without problems. Some physicians have programmed devices in patients who are not pacemaker dependent to the OOO/ODO mode or to a subthreshold voltage output or pulse width, effectively disabling the pacemaker, and pacemaker-dependent patients have had the device programmed to an asynchronous mode. Although this may help, the induced current from having a wire in a moving magnetic field can theoretically stimulate the heart without being connected to the generator. One study that looked at this issue reported that the induced current was subthreshold,[244] even though the potential for stimulation existed. It has also been reported that the capture threshold may rise due to heating at the lead-myocardium interface.

Myopotential Tracking. Myopotential tracking is caused by oversensing of muscle potentials by the atrial channel in a dual-chamber pacing system capable of P-wave tracking. This has become far less common with the use of bipolar sensing, which is preferred by most implanting physicians. It is a greater problem with unipolar dual-chamber systems. A unique sensing modality ("combipolar" sensing, which is sensing between the atrial and ventricular electrodes for a form of wide-dipole bipolar sensing with the entire system restricted to the heart) has the potential to reduce the incidence of atrial myopotential oversensing.[245] Myopotential tracking occurs when the atrial channel senses the electrical activity of the muscle underlying the pulse generator. Those same signals, if sensed on the ventricular channel, would result in myopotential inhibition. The atrial sensitivity setting is usually more sensitive than in the ventricular channel, and myopotential sensing is more likely in the unipolar configuration. When myopotentials are sensed on the atrial channel, the atrial output is inhibited, and a ventricular output is triggered at the end of the AV interval. This pseudo-P wave repeatedly triggers the ventricular output, and ventricular pacing may occur up to the programmed maximum P-wave tracking rate (Fig. 24-41). If the myopotentials are of sufficient amplitude, they may be sensed on the ventricular channel, in which pacing system inhibition may also occur.[88,89,120]

Atrial Arrhythmias. A common cause of rapid pacing in a dual-chamber pacemaker capable of tracking the

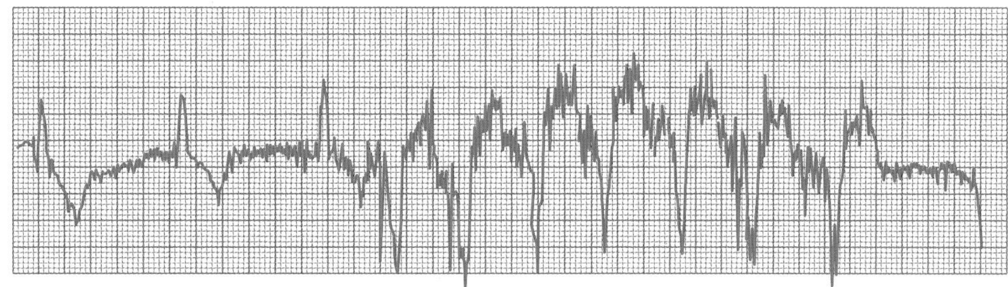

Figure 24-41. Electrocardiogram rhythm strip of myopotential tracking. The electrical activity of the muscle adjacent to the pacemaker case in a unipolar system is sensed by the atrial channel. This causes repeated initiation of the atrioventricular interval up to the maximum tracking rate. Higher-amplitude myopotentials may also cause inhibition of the ventricular channel.

atrium is atrial fibrillation. Any rapid atrial rhythm, such as flutter or ectopic atrial tachycardia, may also cause a similar situation. The pacemaker attempts to track the atrium to the upper rate limit if one of these arrhythmias occurs. This is not a pacemaker malfunction, although it may manifest as rapid ventricular pacing and may be clinically undesirable. Suppression of the arrhythmia with medication or cardioversion may be necessary. Urgently placing a magnet over the pacemaker stops the high-rate tracking. After a programmer is obtained, a nontracking mode may be programmed, or features such as automatic mode switching may be enabled. The latter is most useful in patients with AV block and intermittent atrial arrhythmias. In other cases, modes such as DDI or VVI have proved to be effective. In some cases, mode switching is programmed on but does not activate. This is most likely with poorly sensed atrial fibrillation or with flutter or atrial tachycardia occurring at a rate that causes atrial events to regularly land in the blanking or refractory period. The result may be failure of the pacemaker to see a sufficient number of atrial events to engage the mode-switching algorithm.

Endless-loop Tachycardia. The classic form of PMT is ELT, which can occur in dual-chamber pacemakers that are capable of atrial tracking modes, most commonly DDD or VDD. Only patients who are capable of retrograde ventriculoatrial conduction through the AV node or an AV accessory pathway are capable of sustaining this rhythm. The mechanism is identical to any macroreentrant tachycardia in which two electrical pathways exist between the atria and ventricles. Pacemaker ELT is classically initiated by a PVC. The depolarization is conducted in a retrograde manner to the atria. If the PVARP has ended and the retrograde complex is of sufficient amplitude to be sensed, the atrial channel senses the event and initiates an AV interval. At the end of the AV interval, the pacemaker delivers a stimulus to the ventricle, and the loop is reinitiated (Fig. 24-42). Although PVC is the classic cause of PMT initiation, any situation that results in AV dissociation, allowing a ventricular depolarization to occur without a normally coupled atrial-paced or atrial-sensed event, may begin the loop (Table 24-16). Examples include atrial noncapture, oversensing, and undersensing. In addition, if the programmed AV interval is long (some units allow programming of an interval of up to 350 msec), it may be possible for the AV node to recover in time to conduct the subsequent ventricular-paced event in a retrograde direction, thus initiating another ELT (Fig. 24-43). The absence of anterograde AV nodal conduction does not rule out retrograde conduction over the AV node or a concealed AV accessory pathway. Patients may also exhibit intermittent retrograde conduction or have variations in the retrograde conduction time based on their sympathetic tone and catecholamine status.[246-255]

The rate of ELT depends on the conduction velocity and refractory period of the retrograde AV pathway. If the retrograde AV conduction is the same as or shorter than the upper rate interval (but not shorter than the PVARP), the tachycardia rate is at the programmed upper rate. If the retrograde AV conduction time is slower than the upper rate interval, the tachycardia rate is below the upper programmed rate (Fig. 24-44). Therefore, although the rate of the ELT can never exceed the programmed upper rate of the pacemaker, it may be lower.[254-256] When the rate is lower than the maximum tracking rate, the rhythm has been termed a *balanced* ELT.

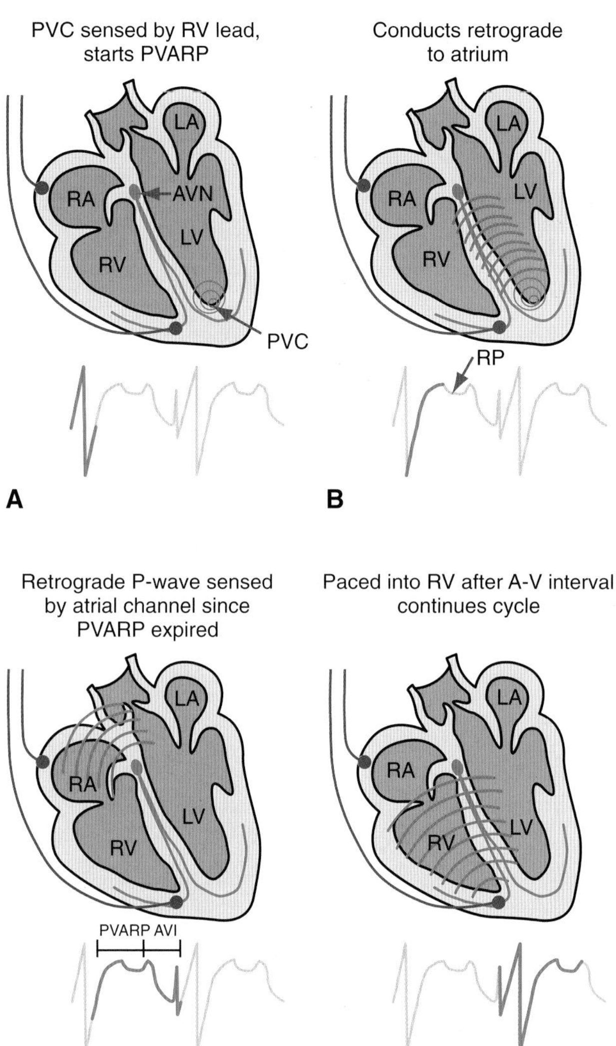

*Figure 24-42. Diagram showing the classic initiation of endless-loop tachycardia by a premature ventricular contraction (PVC) in a patient with retrograde atrioventricular (AV) conduction. **A,** A PVC occurs. **B,** The event is conducted in a retrograde fashion to the atrium, as seen by the inverted (retrograde) P wave (RP). **C,** The retrograde event is sensed by the atrial channel, which causes an AV interval (AVI) to be started. **D,** At the end of the AVI, a stimulus is delivered to the ventricle (if the maximum rate limit is not violated), resulting in retrograde conduction and the perpetuation of this cycle. AVN, atrioventricular node; LA, left atrium; LV, left ventricle; PVARP, postventricular atrial refractory period; RA, right atrium; RV, right ventricle.*

As with crosstalk, there are two approaches to ELT management: prevention of ELT initiation and termination of ELT once it occurs.

TABLE 24-16. **Endless-loop Tachycardia Summary**

Initiation
Premature ventricular ectopic beat
Atrial undersensing
Atrial oversensing
Atrial noncapture
Long programmed AV delay with echo beats
Prevention
PVARP
PVARP extension after ventricular ectopic beat detection
Differential atrial sensing
Rate-responsive AV delay allowing longer PVARP
Adaptive PVARP
High maximum tracking rate—retrograde fatigue
Detection
P tracking at upper rate limit
P tracking at intermediate rate
AV interval modulation
Discrepancy between sensed atrial rate and sensor-indicated rate
Termination
PVARP extension
Withhold of ventricular output
Withhold of ventricular output with early atrial pace

AV, atrioventricular; PVARP, postventricular atrial blanking period.

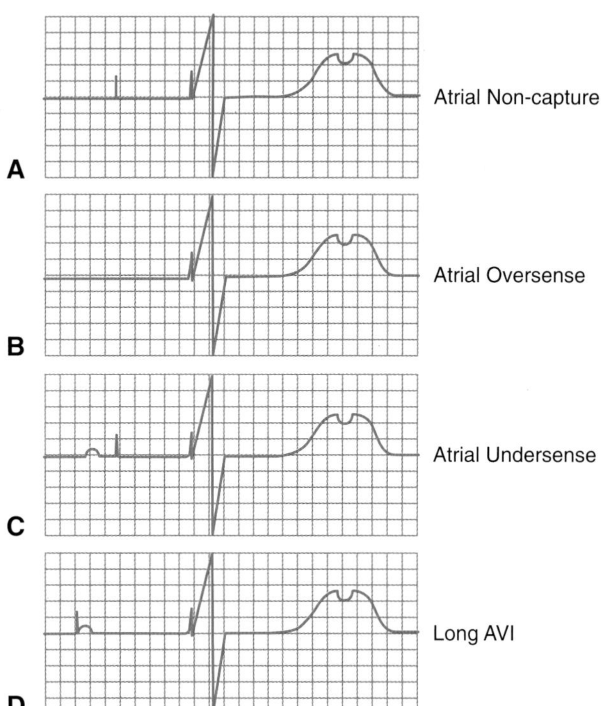

Figure 24-43. Diagram of various initiating events leading to retrograde P-wave conduction and the potential for endless-loop tachycardia. ***A,*** *Atrial noncapture causes ventricular stimulation without the atrioventricular (AV) node being blocked by an anterograde event.* ***B,*** *Atrial oversensing inhibits atrial output and provides just a ventricular output, with the same results as in* ***A. C,*** *Atrial undersensing results in a long AV interval, allowing the AV node time to recover and conduct retrograde.* ***D,*** *A long programmed AV interval may also allow the AV node to recover.*

Prevention of Endless-loop Tachycardia. The main defense against ELT is the use of an appropriate PVARP interval. During the PVARP, the atrial channel cannot sense the retrograde depolarization that would, in a different set of circumstances, initiate the ELT. This is independent of the source of that atrial event. If retrograde conduction is present during implantation or follow-up, it is a simple matter to measure the ventriculoatrial time and program the PVARP to an interval that is longer.[250] Many patients, however, exhibit only intermittent ventriculoatrial conduction, making an accurate assessment difficult. The major limitation of using a long PVARP is that it limits the upper tracking rate of the device (2:1 blocking rate). Some patients in our clinics have ventriculoatrial times in excess of 430 msec. If an PVARP of 450 msec and an AV interval of 150 msec are used, the total atrial refractory period is 600 msec. This causes 2:1 blocking at an atrial rate of 100 bpm, which is far too low for an active patient but may be appropriate for a sedentary patient.

One solution to this problem is the use of ELT prevention algorithms.[257,258] The most common algorithm is PVARP extension on PVE detection. A PVE is defined as a ventricular-sensed event that is not preceded by an atrial-paced or atrial-sensed event. When a PVE is detected, the device prolongs PVARP by a fixed or programmable value for the next cycle. It allows a shorter baseline PVARP to be used, with associated higher 2:1 blocking rates. A variation on this technique is to initiate one DVI cycle after the PVE. This is the ultimate PVARP extension, because the atrial channel remains refractory to sensing throughout the entire atrial escape interval. A problem with most of the PVARP extension algorithms is that functional atrial noncapture may occur. Because there was an atrial output, the system returns to the shorter PVARP, thus allowing for retrograde conduction to be sensed after the AV-paced cycle, simply postponing the ELT for one cycle. In the latter case, the pacemaker does not maintain the long PVARP, because it has delivered an atrial stimulus (albeit ineffective) before a ventricular event. The subsequent ventricular-paced event then leads to ELT (Fig. 24-45). A refinement to the standard PVARP extension algorithm is to add an alert period at the end of the

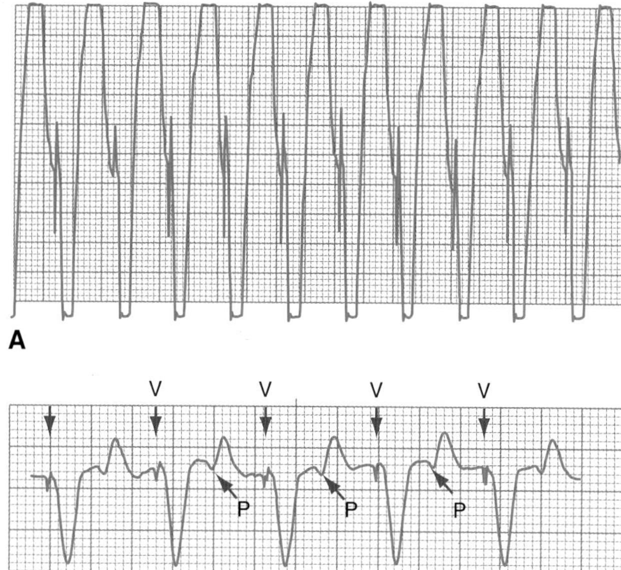

Figure 24-44. ***A,*** *Electrocardiogram (ECG) rhythm strip of endless-loop tachycardia (ELT) with fast ventriculoatrial conduction, which resulted in a rapid ELT at the upper programmed rate of 155 bpm. The lower rate was 60 ppm; the sensed atrioventricular (AV) interval, 150 msec; the postventricular atrial refractory period (PVARP), 275 msec; and the VA time, 300 msec.* ***B,*** *ECG rhythm strip of ELT with slow VA conduction, which resulted in ELT below the programmed upper rate. Because of the slow retrograde conduction, the ELT rate is significantly slower than the programmed upper rate. The lower rate was 60 bpm; the upper rate, 145 bpm; the AV interval, 165 msec; and the PVARP, 250 msec. P, retrograde P wave; V, ventricular output.*

extended PVARP.[246] On release of the atrial output at the end of the alert period, the atrial myocardium will have recovered, allowing for capture, thus precluding retrograde conduction on the next ventricular cycle.

Newer approaches have been made possible by the advent of sensor-driven pacing systems. With a DDDR system, even though the maximum tracking rate may be limited by a long PVARP, faster AV sequentially paced rates may be possible through the sensor. Even though atrial sensing does not occur during the PVARP, sensor-driven atrial pacing may occur. Another alternative in some DDDR pulse generators is to use an adaptive PVARP that is long when the sensor determines that the patient is at rest. When the patient's sensor-indicated rate increases along with the need for higher heart rates, the PVARP is shortened proportionately, allowing higher rates before a 2:1 block upper rate behavior occurs. This approach allows the device to discriminate between early atrial depolarizations at rest (possibly retrograde beats or PACs) and sinus tachycardia with exertion.[259-261] Even in the absence of rate modulation, rate-responsive AV delay algorithms allow a shorter total atrial refractory period and therefore a higher maximum tracking rate, even with a fixed long PVARP.

A comparison of P-wave morphology can allow discrimination between sinus and retrograde atrial depolarizations in some cases; this is referred to as *differential atrial sensing.*[262-266] Mapping of the atrium may allow positioning of the lead at a site that has a large P wave when generated by the sinus node and retrograde P waves that appear small in comparison. The pacemaker sensitivity may be programmed to allow sensing of the anterograde P wave but not the retrograde P wave. Therefore, ELT cannot be initiated or sustained because the loop cannot be completed. Although the retrograde P wave is usually of lower amplitude than the anterograde P wave, this is not always the case; the individual situation needs to be evaluated before any attempt to use atrial sensitivity as a discriminating factor. In addition, the atrial EGM may decrease in amplitude as the sinus rate increases under physiologic stress. Programming a reduced atrial sensitivity to facilitate discrimination between anterograde and retrograde P waves could compromise sensing of rapid intrinsic atrial rhythms.[246]

Another preventive mechanism has been to program a high maximum tracking rate, in the hope of inducing retrograde fatigue and spontaneous termination of any ELT that is allowed to start. Careful assessment of the patient's ability to conduct retrograde should be performed, however, because some patients have superior retrograde conduction (compared with anterograde conduction) and are able to sustain extremely rapid ELTs.[246]

Termination of Endless-loop Tachycardia. The most difficult aspect of applying an ELT termination protocol is having the device determine whether ELT is present (as opposed to a native atrial tachycardia that is being appropriately tracked). This has been approached differently by different manufacturers. Some of the criteria used are simple, and others are more complex. The following are some of the most common techniques for identifying the presence of ELT.

The first criterion is sustained P-wave tracking at the upper rate. This is the most common method of ELT detection. If the pacemaker tracks the P waves at the upper rate for a specific number of intervals, then either the PVARP is prolonged for one cycle, DVI is used for one cycle, or the ventricular output is withheld. The number of events at the upper rate that trigger an ELT termination attempt depends on the particular pulse generator. Some algorithms use a fixed number of beats; in other systems, this is a programmable option. The method of ELT termination may also be programmable (PVARP extension or DVI cycle).[267,268]

The second method used to identify ELT is sustained P-wave tracking at a specific rate that is lower than the upper rate. As previously noted, not all ELTs occur at the upper programmed tracking rate. An ELT rate is always limited by the slowest point in the loop. If the patient has a ventriculoatrial conduction time that is longer than the upper tracking interval, the resulting ELT is slower than the programmed upper tracking rate. This manifestation of ELT is not identified by the sustained upper rate method. Some devices allow initiation of the ELT termination algorithm at a P-wave tracking rate that is lower than the upper tracking rate.

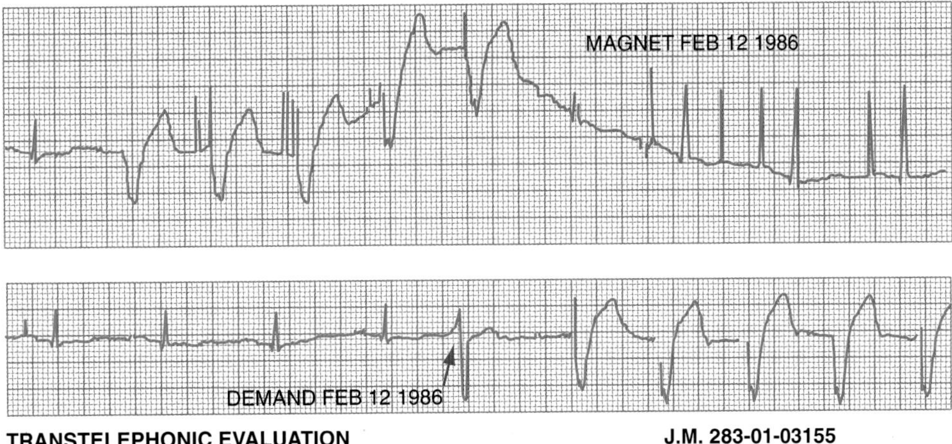

Figure 24-45. Dual-chamber Cosmos (Model 283-01) pulse generator (Sulzer Intermedics, Angleton, Tex. [now Guidant]) programmed with postventricular atrial refractory period (PVARP) extension on premature ventricular event (PVE) detection. Top tracing shows behavior of pacemaker with magnet application. The atrioventricular (AV) delay is programmed to a long value to allow functional single-chamber atrial pacing. Bottom tracing shows demand mode. A ventricular premature contraction occurred (arrow), *causing PVARP extension. The retrograde P wave coincided with the extended PVARP and, appropriately, was not sensed and not tracked. When the atrial output was delivered at the end of the atrial escape interval, it was ineffective (functional noncapture), because the native atrial depolarization had rendered the atrial myocardium physiologically refractory. The delivery of the atrial output caused the pacemaker to shorten the PVARP with the next ventricular paced event, by which time atrial refractoriness had resolved; retrograde conduction followed the paced ventricular complex and initiated an endless-loop tachycardia (ELT). Thus, the PVARP extension simply postponed the initiation of the ELT rather than preventing it. (From Levine PA, Selznick L: Prospective Management of the Patient with Retrograde Ventriculoatrial Conduction: Prevention and Management of Pacemaker Mediated Endless Loop Tachycardias. Sylmar, Calif., Pacesetter Systems, 1990.)*

This lower rate is typically a programmable option, to provide for termination of ELT in this subset of patients.

The third approach to identifying ELT is modulation of the AV interval during sustained P-wave tracking at or above a specific rate. The technique is based on the observation that the ventriculoatrial conduction time in an individual patient is relatively constant. When the device is P-wave tracking at a high rate, the system first assesses the stability of the retrograde interval. The AV interval is then either shortened or lengthened, and the effect on the subsequent retrograde interval is assessed. If an ELT is present and the V-pace to P-sense interval remains constant (i.e., the atrial cycle length is shortened by the shortening of the AV interval), the device confirms ELT and initiates a termination algorithm (Fig. 24-46), either by withholding the ventricular output or by delivering an atrial output after a period of time sufficient to allow for atrial recovery.[260,261] However, if the V-pace to A-sense interval changes by more than a preset amount (i.e., the atrial cycle length is unaffected by the AV interval shortening), ELT is not confirmed, and the device continues to track the atrium normally (see Fig. 24-46).

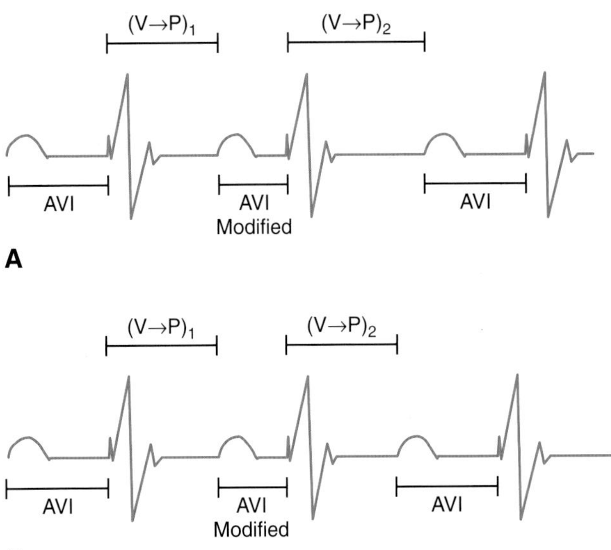

Figure 24-46. Diagram of endless-loop tachycardia (ELT) detection scheme used by ELA Medical (Sorin Group, Milan). ***A,*** *Rapid tracking of sinus tachycardia. The device causes the atrioventricular interval (AVI) to be varied. When the interval is shortened (AVI modified), there is a prolongation of the V-P interval (V-P2 is longer than V-P1) because the sinus node rate is not affected.* ***B,*** *ELT caused by tracking of retrograde P waves. The device again causes the AVI to be varied. In this case, shortening of the AVI has no effect on the next retrograde event (V-P2 is the same as V-P1). This is defined by the device as ELT, and a termination algorithm is activated.*

Cross-stimulation

Cross-stimulation can be defined as stimulation of one cardiac chamber when stimulation of the other is expected (Fig. 24-47). An embarrassing cause of this phenomenon is inadvertent placement of the ventricu-

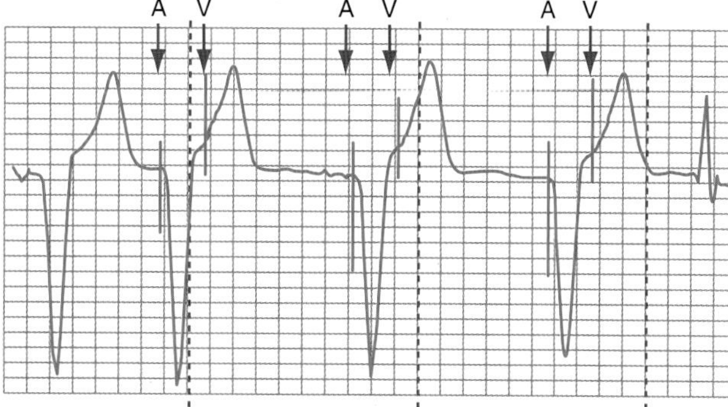

Figure 24-47. Electrocardiogram rhythm strip showing cross-stimulation as a result of lead reversal due to a misconnection at the time of implantation. Although the leads were properly situated in the heart, the atrial lead was placed into the ventricular connector, and the ventricular lead was placed into the atrial connector. Note that the first output delivered stimulated the ventricle, and the second fell into the ST segment when it was delivered into the atrium at the end of the atrioventricular interval, because it was delivered through the atrial lead.

lar lead into the atrial connector and the atrial lead into the ventricular connector of the pulse generator. Dislodgment of either lead into the other chamber may also be a cause. These are both true system malfunctions. Coronary sinus placement of either lead, either intentionally or accidentally, can cause continued or intermittent cross-stimulation. For all of these situations, surgical revision of the pacing system is the only option for correction. There have been several reports of cross-stimulation not related to these situations.[269-272] Internal crossover within the pulse generator circuitry may be the cause. This can be seen in dual unipolar systems with the leads connected but before placement in the pocket, as the current crosses from one electrode to the other and then back to the pulse generator through the other lead. In this case, because the atrial output is first, atrial capture is obscured by ventricular capture. Because the impedance in this system is high, it requires a high output with a very low capture threshold. After the pulse generator is implanted, this phenomenon ceases. There is also a system that has internal energy crossover when a magnet is applied to the pacemaker. Here too, the amount of energy crossover is minimal, and capture can be demonstrated only when the capture threshold is very low. In all cases, crossover resolved after several weeks, and lead maturation resulted in a rise in the capture threshold.

Repetitive Non-reentrant Ventriculoatrial Synchronous Rhythm

The repetitive non-reentrant ventriculoatrial synchronous rhythm is becoming increasingly common with the growth of the DDDR and DDIR modes. It represents a classic example of an adverse interaction between a normally functioning dual-chamber pacemaker and a patient. A prerequisite for this rhythm is intact retrograde conduction. Further, the pacemaker must be programmed with a PVARP that is sufficiently long so that retrograde conduction does not induce ELT. The second prerequisite is a sufficiently high base rate such that there is a relatively short atrial escape interval and an even shorter interval from the retrograde atrial depolarization that renders the atrial tissue physiologically refractory. The retrograde P wave is not sensed because it coincides with the PVARP. This represents functional undersensing. Because of the relatively high rate and the failure to reset the atrial timing cycle (because the retrograde P wave is not sensed), an atrial output is delivered when the atrial myocardium is physiologically refractory. This results in functional atrial noncapture. Hence, after the ineffective atrial output, the AV interval times out, and a ventricular-paced event occurs, by which time the AV node and atrial myocardium have fully recovered, allowing retrograde conduction. The result is an AV-paced rhythm with repeated functional atrial noncapture and functional atrial undersensing, all caused by a coincidence of various key timing intervals. This rhythm is called either *repetitive non-reentrant ventriculoatrial synchrony* or *AV desynchronization arrhythmia*.[273-275] The effect on the patient is the same as that of ventricular pacing with retrograde conduction but in a DDDR/DDIR pacing system. This can lead to symptoms of palpitations, dyspnea, and even syncope. Effectively, the resultant rhythm is a classic rhythm associated with pacemaker syndrome, but unless one recognizes the problem, either normal pacemaker function is diagnosed and the symptoms are unexplained or the disorder is labeled *atrial noncapture* and efforts are directed toward correcting this “malfunction.”

Management requires allowing sufficient time for the atrial tissue to recover. This means either providing a short AV delay at the higher rates or limiting of the specific rates. When AV nodal conduction is intact, the clinician may consider single-chamber AAIR pacing, which would totally avoid this rhythm. If the rhythm is repeatedly triggered by a PVC with retrograde conduction, use of a PVARP extension algorithm that also slows the escape rate, allowing time for the atrium to physiologically recover, is indicated.

It is absolutely essential that the clinician fully understand the interaction between the timing circuits in the pacemaker and those in the heart. The author knows of a patient who was taken back to the operating room for an atrial lead repositioning on two additional occasions after the initial implantation because of this rhythm and the failure by the implanting physician to understand the adverse interaction between the various programmed parameters and the patient's intrinsic rhythms. This was not a lead dislodgment or malposition, although the latter was the working diagnosis. The problem could not be solved by repositioning of the lead, yet that was the diagnosis by the referring physicians because of repeated failure to capture on the atrial channel at the highest outputs that the pacemaker would allow. When evaluated by a

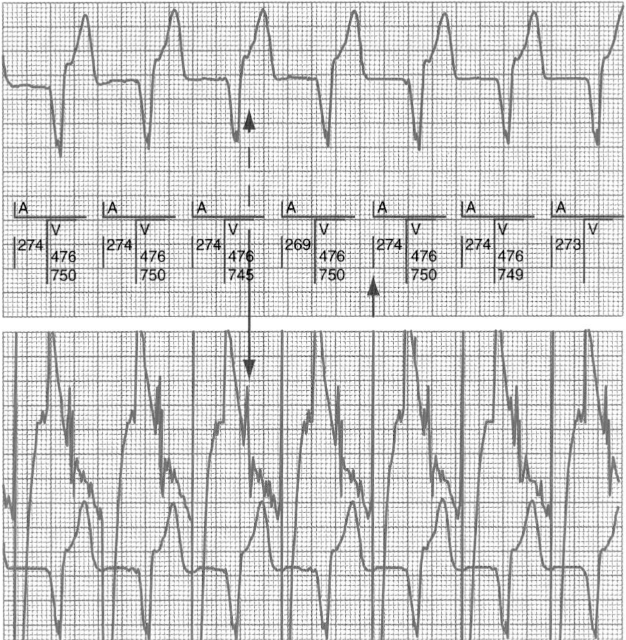

Figure 24-48. Functional atrial noncapture induced during an atrial capture threshold test persisted when the output was returned to the previously effective programmed level. This is an example of repetitive non-reentrant ventriculoatrial synchronous rhythm. The retrograde P wave seen as a negative deflection in the ST segment of the paced QRS complex (long arrow), *as shown on the surface electrocardiogram* (top) *and the rapid deflection on the atrial electrogram* (bottom), *coincides with the atrial refractory period as identified by the event markers. This is consistent with the programmed settings of the pacemaker. Therefore, the failure to sense this P wave is normal, allowing delivery of an atrial output pulse (functional undersensing). The atrial output pulse occurs at a time when the atrial myocardium is still physiologically refractory from the native atrial depolarization; hence, there is failure to capture, but on a functional basis, not as a sign of a malfunction. By the time the ventricular output is delivered, the atrium has recovered, allowing retrograde conduction to again occur. This rhythm persists until the base rate slows or is reduced, allowing the atrium to physiologically recover so that the atrial output effectively captures the atrium.*

knowledgeable physician, this rhythm was suspected because the referring physician described losing atrial capture at 0.5 V and then not being able to regain it at 7.5 V when the base rate was 90 ppm but having absolutely no problems with capture when the base rate was 60 ppm. The referring physician sought advice about where the lead could be positioned (on a fourth operative procedure) to prevent repeated loss of atrial capture. Rather than reoperate, it was advised to leave the rate low and disable the rate modulation. The patient was then sent for a detailed evaluation, at which time it was easy to induce and demonstrate this phenomenon with the aid of the telemetered atrial EGM and event markers (Fig. 24-48). Management was more of a challenge, in that the maximum sensor rate had to be limited to preclude atrial pacing at a high rate, which meant that there would be a relatively short atrial escape interval. This patient's adverse rhythm was triggered by early atrial premature beats.

Follow-up Recommendations

Follow-up of pacing systems has evolved with their increased complexity. The newest devices are able to report automatically determined capture and sensing thresholds. Though these are quite accurate, they are not always reliable. Some capture management algorithms can be foiled by high polarization leads, or frequent fusion beats caused by atrial fibrillation, or programmed AV intervals that allow fusion and pseudofusion. Review of the graph showing the capture thresholds over time will show intermittent high thresholds or many aborted searches (see Fig. 24-20). If this is seen, reprogramming of the AV interval to avoid fusion or turning off the algorithm may be necessary.

If a device is not capable of automatically reporting capture and sensing thresholds, these must be done manually, using the features of the programmer. Capture and sensing thresholds should be determined for each lead implanted. Programming of appropriate safety margins is then performed. After these basic but critical determinations have been made, additional data from the device are evaluated to determine whether arrhythmias have been present (i.e., atrial high rate, ventricular high rate, mode switching). Retrieval of any supporting information, such as EGMs associated with these events, is advised to verify that the counters correctly classified the event and that the event was not caused by oversensing or other extraneous signals as described earlier in this chapter. It is also important to evaluate the sensor indicated rate histogram to determine whether the rate modulation sensor is performing appropriately. A flat response may indicate a sensor programmed to an insensitive setting, or it may reflect an inactive patient. It is therefore important to correlate the sensor findings to the condition of the patient, and then adjust the device accordingly.

The frequency of follow-up visits to the device clinic should be based on the needs of the individual patient and not on how frequently an insurance carrier will pay for these visits. A common standard of practice is to evaluate the patient in the office setting 1 month after implantation, 6 and 12 months after implantation, and then annually thereafter. Additional visits may be necessary if the patient has symptoms or complaints related to the heart rhythm or the implantation site.

Transtelephonic monitoring (TTM) was virtually unchanged for the past 40 years until the recent introduction of home interrogation devices capable of retrieving the same information as the programmer. Classic TTM involves the use of a device that can transmit a rhythm strip over any standard telephone to a receiving station. The receiving station converts the tones sent by the TTM transmitter to an ECG tracing. Using this simple technique, a baseline heart rhythm, magnet strip, and final heart rhythm strip can be recorded. This provides a very basic check of the heart rhythm, whether the device is able to pace, and the condition of the battery as can be determined by the magnet rate. However, because of the limited fidelity of the recording and the single lead that is transmitted, it can be difficult to determine atrial capture and sensing, or even the atrial rhythm. Though many centers do TTM transmission monthly, it has been recommended that a TTM once every 3 months (skipping any time when a clinic visit is due) is adequate until the device begins to show significant wear. At that time, TTMs can be increased to monthly, to determine when the elective replacement indicator has been tripped. In addition, a patient with a pacemaker or lead system that is on alert may warrant more frequent monitoring. Finally, should a patient have a symptomatic event such as palpitations or lightheadedness, a TTM may be done to evaluate the heart rhythm and pacing function. In the United States, Medicare has a guideline for TTM reimbursement that is often used to maximize reimbursement to the entity performing the checks. Note that these guidelines are quite antiquated and do not represent the fact that current generations of pacemakers are far longer lasting and more reliable than the early generations of devices for which the guidelines were developed.

Manufacturers of pacing systems have now introduced interrogation devices that can be placed in the patient's home. These are capable of retrieving all of the programmed settings, telemetry and diagnostic data, and even stored electrograms. These data are then transmitted over a telephone line or Internet connection to a receiving center. The data may be obtained in one of two ways. Currently, most devices require the patient or caregiver to place a wand over the device and initiate the interrogation. However, new devices with long-range telemetry can interrogate the pacemaker from a distance of 20 feet or more. These systems can be set to automatically download data on a regular basis and send it to the receiving center. They can also automatically initiate a transmission if the device has detected an arrhythmia or an out-of-range diagnostic value such as battery depletion or high lead impedance. The receiving center prepares a report that is either faxed or e-mailed to the clinician. Alternatively (or in combination), the report may be viewed via a web portal from any standard web browser. By having access to this detailed information, the pacemaker follow-up center can make much more informed decisions about the nature of a patient's complaints, the status of the pacing system, and the actual rhythms present at that time. At this time, remote programming is not an option. Therefore, should a patient need an adjustment to the device, a trip to the pacemaker center is still necessary. The frequency of monitoring with these more extensive systems is still evolving, although more than quarterly transmissions in asymptomatic patients is probably not warranted. In addition, pacemakers continue to expand their self-diagnostic capabilities and are able to self-determine atrial and ventricular capture and sensing thresholds, They are also able to adjust their sensitivity and output settings automatically. Therefore, the patient may not need to come to the pacemaker center except to reprogram certain parameters or to perform more advanced diagnostic testing.

Summary

Pacing system malfunction, although seemingly difficult to assess, can be categorized in relation to the dysfunction of the leads or the generator and apparent dysfunction related to the idiosyncratic characteristics of the pacemaker's timing algorithms. In contrast to the relative frequency of lead failure as a result of implantation error or deterioration of the lead materials, primary malfunction of the pulse generator is rare. Patient-specific problems or inappropriate program settings are relatively common. Consequently, the keys to understanding unexpected pacemaker behavior are meticulous evaluation of the integrity of the leads, assessment of capture and sensing thresholds, and an understanding of the timing cycles of the specific pacemaker, which is facilitated by access to event marker telemetry.

Clues to the problem and its cause are found in the patient's history, physical examination, and the various diagnostic tests integral to the pacemaker that are retrieved through bidirectional telemetry. With respect to the hardware, the answer is usually lead dysfunction or a behavioral eccentricity detailed in the pacemaker's technical manual. One must always keep the patient's physiology and pathophysiology in mind, because they also affect the function of the pacing system. Furthermore, even if all components of the system are normal, the pacemaker may be programmed to a set of parameters that are no longer optimal for the patient.

When the clinician is presented with a suspected pacing system malfunction, it is essential to proceed in a meticulous and orderly manner, carefully assessing each component of the system, including the pulse generator, the programmed settings, any unique algorithms, the leads, and the patient. If a complete assessment of capture and sensing thresholds, lead impedance, sensor response, and the behavior of any unique algorithms is performed on a periodic basis as part of the routine surveillance of the patient's pacing system, baseline data will be available for comparison with the results of evaluation when and if a problem is suspected.

Acknowledgment

The author would like to acknowledge the previous contribution to this work by Dr. Paul A. Levine, who due to time constraints was not able to participate in the preparation of the current revision of this chapter. His significant work in the past, as well as his friendship and mentoring, remain part of the foundation of the material presented in this chapter.

REFERENCES

1. Furman S: Pacemaker programmability. PACE 1:161, 1978.
2. Furman S, Escher DJW, Fisher JD: Seven-year experience with programmable pulse generators. In Meere C (ed): Cardiac Pacing. Montreal, Pacesymp Publications, 1979, Chapter 19-1.

3. Levine PA: Why Programmability? Indications for and Clinical Utility of Multiparameter Programmability. Sylmar, CA, Pacesetter Systems, 1981.
4. Gold RD, Saulson SH, MacGregor DC: Programmable pacing systems: The medium and the message. PACE 5:777, 1982.
5. Sholder J, Levine PA, Mann BM, Mace RC: Bidirectional telemetry and interrogation in cardiac pacing. In Barold SS, Mugica J (eds): The Third Decade of Cardiac Pacing: Advances in Technology and Clinical Applications. Mt Kisco, NY, Futura, 1982, pp 145-166.
6. Levine PA (ed): Proceedings of the Policy Conference of the North American Society of Pacing and Electrophysiology on Programmability and Pacemaker Follow-up Programs. Clin Prog Pacing Electrophysiol 2:145, 1984.
7. Del Marco CJ, Tyers GFO, Brownlee RR: Lithium pacers with self-contained multiparameter telemetry: First year followup. In Meere C (ed): Cardiac Pacing. Montreal, Pacesymp Publications, 1979, Chapter 28-1.
8. Tanaka S, Nanba T, Harada A, et al: Clinical experience with telemetry pacing systems and long-term followup: Clinical aspects of lead impedance and battery life. PACE 6:A30, 1983.
9. Castellanet MJ, Garza J, Shaner SP, Messenger JC: Telemetry of programmed and measured data in pacing system evaluation and followup. J Electrophysiol 1:360, 1987.
10. Marco D: Pacemaker output settings for lowest current drain and maximum longevity. Reblampa 8:159-162, 1995.
11. Crossley GH, Gayle D, Simmons TW, et al: Reprogramming pacemakers enhances longevity and is cost-effective. Circulation 94(Suppl II):II-245–II-247, 1996.
12. Freedman RA, Marks ML, Chapman P, King C: Telemetered pacemaker battery voltage preceding generator elective replacement time: Use to guide utilization of magnet checks [abstract]. PACE 18:863, 1995.
13. Ben-Zur UM, Platt SB, Gross JN, et al: Direct and telemetered lead impedance. PACE 17:2004-2007, 1994.
14. Danilovic D, Ohm OJ: Pacing impedance variability in tined steroid eluting leads. PACE 21:1356-1363, 1998.
15. Levine PA: Clinical manifestations of lead insulation defects. J Electrophysiol 1:144, 1987.
16. Clarke M, Allen A: Early detection of lead insulation breakdown. PACE 8:775, 1985.
17. Winoker P, Falkenberg E, Gerard G: Lead resistance telemetry: Insulation failure prognosticator. PACE 8:A85, 1985.
18. Phlippin F, O'Hara GE, Gilbert M: Lead impedance measured bipolar vs unipolar: A method to identify lead insulation failure [abstract]. PACE 18:817, 1995.
19. Pickell D, Siegler K, Brewer L, et al: Suspect polyurethane insulated bipolar pacing leads: Clinical management [abstract]. PACE 18:866, 1995.
20. Schmidinger H, Mayer H, Kaliman J, et al: Early detection of lead complications by telemetric measurement of lead impedance. PACE 8:A23, 1985.
21. Mauser JF, Huang SKS, Risser T, et al: A unique pulse generator safety feature for bipolar lead fracture. PACE 16:1368-1372, 1993.
22. Kruse I, Markowitz T, Ryden L: Timing markers showing pacemaker behavior to aid in the follow-up of a physiologic pacemaker. PACE 6:801, 1983.
23. Olson W, McConnell M, Sah R, et al: Pacemaker diagnostic diagrams. PACE 8:691, 1985.
24. Levine PA, Schuller H, Lindgren A: Pacemaker ECG: Utilization of Pulse Generator Telemetry. Solna, Sweden, Siemens Elema AB, 1988.
25. Furman S: The ECG interpretation channel [editorial]. PACE 13:225, 1990.
26. Olson WH, Goldreyer BA, Goldreyer BN: Computer-generated diagnostic diagrams for pacemaker rhythm analysis and pacing system evaluation. J Electrocardiol 1:376, 1987.
27. Levine PA: Pacemaker diagnostic diagrams [letter]. PACE 9:250, 1986.
28. Machado C, Johnson D, Thacker JR, Duncan JL: Pacemaker patient-triggered event recordings: Accuracy, utility and cost for the pacemaker follow-up clinic. PACE 19:1813-1818, 1996.
29. Furman S, Hurzeler P, DeCaprio V: Cardiac pacing and pacemakers. III. Sensing the cardiac electrogram. Am Heart J 93:794, 1977.
30. Levine PA, Klein MD: Discrepant electrocardiographic and pulse analyzer endocardial potentials: A possible source of pacemaker sensing failure. In Meere C (ed): Cardiac Pacing. Montreal, Pacesymp Publications 1979, Chapter 18-1.
31. Levine PA, Podrid PJ, Klein MD, et al: Pacemaker sensing: Comparison of signal amplitudes determined by electrogram telemetry and noninvasively measured sensing thresholds [abstract]. PACE 12:1294, 1989.
32. Levine PA, Sholder J, Duncan JL: Clinical benefits of telemetered electrograms in the assessment of DDD function. PACE 7:1170, 1984.
33. Clarke M, Allen A: Use of telemetered electrograms in the assessment of normal pacemaker function. J Electrophysiol 1:388, 1987.
34. Edery T: Clinical Applications of Pacemaker-telemetered Intracardiac Electrograms. Technical concept paper. Minneapolis, MN, Medtronic, Inc., 1991.
35. Hughes HC, Furman S, Brownlee RR, Del Marco C: Simultaneous atrial and ventricular electrogram transmission via a specialized single-lead system. PACE 7:1195, 1984.
36. Feuer J, Florio J, Shandling AH: Alternate methods for the determination of atrial capture thresholds utilizing the telemetered intracardiac electrogram. PACE 13:1254, 1990.
37. Sarmiento JJ: Clinical utility of telemetered intracardiac electrograms in diagnosing a design dependent lead malfunction. PACE 13:188, 1990.
38. Marco DD, Gallagher D: Noninvasive measurements of retrograde conduction times in pacemaker patients. J Electrophysiol 1:388, 1987.
39. Nalos PC, Nyitray W: Benefits of intracardiac electrograms and programmable sensing polarity in preventing pacemaker inhibition due to spurious screw-in lead signals. PACE 13:1101, 1990.
40. Halperin JL, Camunas JL, Stern EH, et al: Myopotential interference with DDD pacemakers: Endocardial electrographic telemetry in the diagnosis of pacemaker-related arrhythmias. Am J Cardiol 54:97, 1984.
41. Gladstone PJ, Duxbury GB, Berman ND: Arrhythmia diagnosis by electrogram telemetry: Involvement of dual-chamber pacemaker. Chest 91:115, 1987.
42. Hassett JA, Elrod PA, Arciniegas JG, et al: Noninvasive diagnosis and treatment of atrial flutter utilizing previously implanted dual-chamber pacemaker. PACE 11:1662, 1988.
43. Luceri RM, Castellanos A, Thurer RJ: Telemetry of intracardiac electrograms: Applications in spontaneous and induced arrhythmias. J Electrophysiol 1:417, 1987.
44. Levine PA: The complementary role of electrogram, event marker, and measured data telemetry in the assessment of pacing system function. J Electrophysiol 1:404, 1987.
45. Pirolo JS, Tweddel JS, Brunt EM, et al: Influence of activation origin, lead number, and lead configuration on the noninvasive electrophysiologic detection of cardiac allograft rejection. Circulation 84(Suppl III):344, 1991.
46. Berbari EJ, Lander P, Geselowitz DB, et al: Correlating late potentials from the body surface with epicardial electrograms. Eur J Cardiac Pacing Electrophysiol 2:A156, 1992.
47. Barold SS, Bornzin G, Levine P: Development of a true pacemaker Holter. In Vardas PE (ed): Cardiac Arrhythmias, Pacing and Electrophysiology: The Expert View. Dordrecht, The Netherlands, Kluwer Academic, 1998, pp 421-426.

48. Sermasi S, Marconi M: Temporary RAM programming of pacemaker capabilities. In Santini M (ed): Progress in Clinical Pacing 1996. Armonk, NY, Futura, 1997, pp 85-91.
49. Sanders R, Martin R, Frumin H, et al: Data storage and retrieval by implantable pacemakers for diagnostic purposes. PACE 7:1228, 1984.
50. Levine PA, Lindenberg BS: Diagnostic data: An aid to the follow-up and assessment of the pacing system. J Electrocardiol 1:396, 1987.
51. Levine PA: Utility and clinical benefits of extensive event counter telemetry in the follow-up and management of the rate-modulated pacemaker patient. Sylmar, CA, Siemens-Pacesetter, January 1992.
52. Newman D, Dorian P, Downar E, et al: Use of telemetry functions in the assessment of implanted antitachycardia device efficiency. Am J Cardiol 70:616, 1992.
53. Wang PJ, Manolis A, Clyne C, et al: Accuracy of classification using a data log system in implantable cardioverter defibrillators. PACE 14:1911, 1991.
54. Luceri RM, Puchferran RL, Brownstein SL, et al: Improved patient surveillance and data acquisition with a third-generation implantable cardioverter defibrillator. PACE 14:1870, 1991.
55. Stangl K, Sichart U, Wirtsfeld A, et al: Holter functions for the enhancement of the diagnostic and therapeutic capabilities of implantable pacemakers, Vitatext. Dieren, The Netherlands, Vitatron Medical, 1987, pp 1-6.
56. Hayes DL, Higano ST, Eisinger G: Utility of rate histograms in programming and follow-up of a DDDR pacemaker. Mayo Clin Proc 64:495, 1989.
57. Levine PA, Sholder JA, Florio J: Obtaining maximal benefit from a DDDR pacing system: A reliable yet simple method for programming the sensor parameters of Synchrony. Sylmar, CA, Siemens-Pacesetter, 1990.
58. Lascault GR, Frank R, Fontaine G, et al: Ventricular tachycardia using the Holter function of a dual-chamber pacemaker [abstract]. PACE 16:918, 1993.
59. Lascault GR, Frank R, Barnay C, et al: Clinical usefulness of a "diagnostic" dual-chamber pacemaker [abstract]. PACE 16:918, 1993.
60. Levine PA: Holter and pacemaker diagnostics. In Aubert AE, Ector H, Stroobandt R (eds): Cardiac Pacing and Electrophysiology: A Bridge to the 21st Century. Dordrecht, The Netherlands, 1994, pp 309-324.
61. Novak M, Smola M, Kejrova E: Pacemaker built-in Holter counters match up to ambulatory Holter recordings. In Sethi KK (ed): Proceedings of the Sixth Asian-Pacific Symposium on Cardiac Pacing and Electrophysiology. Bologna, Italy, Monduzzi Editore S.P.A., 1997, pp 61-64.
62. Limousin M, Geroux L, Nitzsche R, et al: Value of automatic processing and reliability of stored data in an implanted pacemaker: Initial results in 59 patients. PACE 1997, 20:2893-2898.
63. Intermedics Technical Manual: Relay DDDR Pacing System. Angleton, TX, Intermedics, 1992.
64. Trilogy DR+ 2364L Pulse Generator Technical Manual. Sylmar, CA, Pacesetter, Inc., 1996.
65. Garson A Jr: Stepwise approach to the unknown pacemaker ECG. Am Heart J 119:924, 1990.
66. Furman S: Cardiac pacing and pacemakers. VI. Analysis of pacemaker malfunction. Am Heart J 94:378, 1977.
67. Mond HG: The Cardiac Pacemaker: Function and Malfunction. New York, Grune & Stratton, 1983.
68. Barold SS: Modern Cardiac Pacing. Mt. Kisco, NY, Futura, 1983.
69. Levine PA: Pacing system malfunction. In Ellenbogen KA (ed): Cardiac Pacing. Boston, Blackwell Scientific, 1992, pp 309-382.
70. Morse DP, Steiner RM, Parsonnet V: A Guide to Cardiac Pacemakers. Philadelphia, FA Davis, 1983.
71. Morse DP, Steiner RM, Parsonnet V: A Guide to Cardiac Pacemakers: Supplement 1986-1987. Philadelphia, FA Davis, 1986.
72. Morse DP, Parsonnet V, Gessment LJ, et al: A Guide to Cardiac Pacemaker, Defibrillator and Related Products. Durham, NC, Droege Computing Services, 1991.
73. Van Gelder LM, El Gamal MIH: Myopotential interference inducing pacemaker tachycardia in a DVI programmed pacemaker. PACE 7:970, 1984.
74. Lindenberg BS, Hagan CA, Levine PA: Design dependent loss of telemetry: Uplink telemetry hold. PACE 12:823, 1989.
75. Levine PA, Lindenberg BS: Upper rate limit circuit-induced rate slowing. PACE 10:310, 1987.
76. Levine PA, Lindenberg BS, Mace RC: Analysis of AV universal (DDD) pacemaker rhythms. Clin Prog Pacing Electrophysiol 2:54, 1984.
77. Bertuso J, Kapoor A, Schafer J: A case of ventricular undersensing in the DDI mode: Cause and correction. PACE 9:685, 1986.
78. Erlbacher JA, Stelzer P: Inappropriate ventricular blanking in a DDI pacemaker. PACE 9:519, 1986.
79. Ajiki K, Sagara K, Namiki T, et al: A case of a pseudomalfunction of a DDD pacemaker. PACE 14:1456, 1991.
80. Meyer JA, Fruehan CT, Delmonico JE: The pacemaker twiddler's syndrome: A further note. J Thorac Cardiovasc Surg 67:903, 1974.
81. Veltri EP, Mower MM, Reid PR: Twiddler's syndrome: A new twist. PACE 7:1004, 1984.
82. Lal RB, Avery RD: Aggressive pacemaker twiddler's syndrome: Dislodgment of an active fixation ventricular pacing electrode. Chest 97:756, 1990.
83. Roberts JS, Wenger NK: Pacemaker twiddler's syndrome. Am J Cardiol 63:1013, 1989.
84. Ellis GL: Pacemaker twiddler's syndrome: A case report. Am J Emerg Med 8:48, 1990.
85. Ekbom K, Nilsson BY, Edhag O: Rhythmic shoulder girdle muscle contractions as a complication in pacemaker treatment. Chest 66:599, 1974.
86. Gelleri D: Retrograde (ventriculoatrial) conduction, premature beats, pseudotricuspid regurgitation, systolic atrial sounds, and pacemaker sounds observed together in two patients with ventricular pacing. Acta Med Hung 48:157, 1991.
87. Flickinger AL, Peller PA, Deran BP, et al: Pacemaker-induced friction rub and apical thrill. Chest 102:323, 1992.
88. Jalin P, Kaul U, Wasir HS: Myopotential inhibition of unipolar demand pacemakers: Utility of provocative maneuvers in assessment and management. Int J Cardiol 34:33, 1992.
89. Levine PA, Caplan CH, Klein MD, et al: Myopotential inhibition of unipolar lithium pacemakers. Chest 82:461-465, 1982.
90. Levine PA: Electrocardiography of bipolar single- and dual-chamber pacing systems. Herzschrittmacher 8:86-90, 1988.
91. Cherry R, Sactuary C, Kennedy HL: The question of frequency response. Ambulatory Electrocardiol 1:13, 1977.
92. Sheffield LT, Berson AL, Bragg Remschel D, et al: AHA special report: Recommendation for standards of instrumentation and practice in the use of ambulatory electrocardiography. Circulation 71:626A, 1985.
93. Lesh MD, Langberg JJ, Griffin JC, et al: Pacemaker generator pseudomalfunction: An artifact of Holter monitoring. PACE 14:854-857, 1991.
94. Van Gelder LM, Bracke FALE, El Gamal MIH: Fusion or confusion on Holter recordings. PACE 14:760-763, 1991.
95. Engler RL, Goldberger AL, Bhargava V, Kapelusznik D: Pacemaker spike alternans: An artifact of digital signal processing. PACE 5:748-750, 1982.
96. Slack JP: Identification of recording artefact in a dual chamber (DDD) paced rhythm: Clues from the electrocardiogram. Clin Prog Pacing and Electrophysiol 2:384-387, 1984.
97. Schüller H, Faajhraeus T: Pacemaker EKG: A Clinical Approach. Solna, Sweden, Siemens Elema, 1980.

98. Levine PA, Schüller H, Lindgren A: Pacemaker ECG: An Introduction and Approach to Interpretation. Solna, Sweden, Siemens-Pacesetter, 1986.
99. Wilkoff BL, Firstenberg MS, Moore S, Ching B: Lead impedance velocity as a predictor of pacing lead instability. PACE 16:930, 1993.
100. Karis JP, Ravin CE: Counterclockwise exit of cardiac pacemaker leads: Sign of pulse-generator flip. Radiology 174:711, 1990.
101. Suzuki Y, Fujimori S, Sakai M, et al: A case of pacemaker lead fracture associated with thoracic outlet syndrome. PACE 11:326, 1988.
102. Stokes K, Staffenson D, Lessar J, et al: A possible new complication of subclavian stick: Conductor fracture. PACE 10:748, 1987.
103. Anonymous: Subclavian puncture procedure may result in lead conductor fracture. Medtronic News Winter 16(2):27, 1986/87.
104. Magney JE, Flynn DM, Parsons JA, et al: Anatomical mechanisms explaining damage to pacemaker leads, defibrillator leads, and failure of central venous catheters adjacent to the sternoclavicular joint. PACE 16:445, 1993.
105. Jacobs DM, Fink AS, Miller RP, et al: Anatomical and morphological evaluation of pacemaker lead compression. PACE 16:434, 1993.
106. Arakawa M, Kambara K, Ito HA, et al: Intermittent oversensing due to internal insulation damage of temperature sensing rate-responsive pacemaker lead in subclavian venipuncture method. PACE 12:1312, 1989.
107. Antonelli D, Rosenfeld T, Freedberg NA, et al: Insulation lead failure: Is it a matter of insulation coating, venous approach or both? PACE 21:418-421, 1998.
108. Fyke FE: Simultaneous insulation deterioration associated with side-by-side subclavian placement of two polyurethane leads. PACE 11:1571, 1988.
109. Kranz J, Crystal DK, Wagner CL, et al: Thoracic outlet compression syndrome: The first rib. Northwest Med 68:646, 1969.
110. Witte A: Pseudofracture of pacemaker lead due to securing suture: A case report. PACE 4:716, 1981.
111. Deering JA, Pederson DN: A case of pacemaker lead fracture associated with weightlifting. PACE 15:1354, 1992.
112. Schuger CD, Mittleman R, Habbal B, et al: Ventricular lead transection and atrial lead damage in a young softball player shortly after the insertion of a permanent pacemaker. PACE 15:1236, 1992.
113. Papa LA, Abkar KB, Chung EK: Pacemaker hysteresis. Heart Lung 3:982-984, 1974.
114. Bornzin GA, Arambula ER, Florio J, et al: Adjusting heart rate during sleep using activity variance. PACE 17:1933-1938, 1994.
115. Gammage MD, Hess M, Markowitz T: Initial experience with a rate drop algorithm in malignant vasovagal syndrome. Eur J Cardiac Pacing Electrophysiol 5:45-48, 1995.
116. Brandt J, Fåahraeus T, Schüller H: Far-field QRS complex sensing via the atrial pacemaker lead. I. Mechanism, consequences, differential diagnosis and countermeasures in AAI and VDD/DDD pacing. PACE 11:1432-1438, 1988.
117. Wolpert C, Jung W, Scholl C, et al: Electrical proarrhythmia: Induction of inappropriate atrial therapies due to far-field R wave oversensing in a new dual chamber defibrillator. J Cardiovasc Electrophysiol 9:859-863, 1998.
118. Halperin JL, Camunas JL, Stern EH, et al: Myopotential interference with DDD pacemakers: Endocardial electrographic telemetry in the diagnosis of pacemaker-related arrhythmias. Am J Cardiol 54:97, 1984.
119. Williams DO, Thomas DJ: Muscle potentials simulating pacemaker malfunction. Br Heart J 38:1096, 1976.
120. Ohm OJ, Morkrid L, Hammer E: Amplitude-frequency characteristics of myopotentials and endocardial potentials as seen by a pacemaker system. Scand J Thorac Cardiovasc Surg 22(Suppl):41-46, 1978.
121. Ohm OJ, Bruland H, Pedersen OM, et al: Interference effect of myopotentials on function of unipolar demand pacemakers. Br Heart J 35:77, 1974.
122. Gabry MD, Behrens M, Andrews C, et al: Comparison of myopotential interference in unipolar-bipolar programmable DDD pacemakers. PACE 10:1322, 1987.
123. Gross JN, Platt S, Ritacco R, et al: The clinical relevance of electromyopotential oversensing in current unipolar devices. PACE 15:2023, 1992.
124. Volosin KJ, Rudderow R, Waxman HL: VOOR: Nondemand rate-modulated pacing necessitated by myopotential inhibition. PACE 12:421, 1989.
125. Dodinot B, Godenir JP, Costa AB: Electronic article surveillance: A possible danger for pacemaker patients. PACE 16:46, 1993.
126. Inbar S, Larson J, Burt T, et al: Case report: Nuclear magnetic resonance imaging in a patient with a pacemaker. Am J Med Sci 305:174, 1993.
127. Marco D, Eisinger G, Hayes DL: Testing of work environments for electromagnetic interference. PACE 15:2016, 1992.
128. Toivonen L, Valjus J, Hongisto M, et al: The influence of elevated 50 Hz electric and magnetic fields on implanted pacemakers: The role of the lead configuration and programming of the sensitivity. PACE 14:2114, 1991.
129. Mellenberg DE Jr: A policy for radiotherapy in patients with implanted pacemakers. Med Dosim 16:221, 1991.
130. Mangar D, Atlas GM, Kane PB: Electrocautery-induced pacemaker malfunction during surgery. Can J Anaesth 38:616, 1991.
131. Teskey RJ, Whelan I, Akyurekli Y, et al: Therapeutic irradiation over a permanent pacemaker. PACE 14:143, 1991.
132. Salmi J, Eskola HJ, Pitkanen MA, et al: The influence of electromagnetic interference and ionizing radiation on cardiac pacemakers. Strahlenther Onkol 166:153, 1990.
133. Chin MC, Rosenqvist M, Lee MA, et al: The effect of radiofrequency catheter ablation on permanent pacemakers: An experimental study. PACE 13:23, 1990.
134. McDeller AG, Toff WD, Hobbs RA, et al: The development of a system for the evaluation of electromagnetic interference with pacemaker function: Hazards in the aircraft environment. J Med Eng Technol 13:161, 1989.
135. Godin JF, Petitot JC: STIMAREC report: Pacemaker failures due to electrocautery and external electric shock. PACE 12:1011, 1989.
136. Belott P, Sands S, Warren J, et al: Resetting of DDD pacemakers due to EMI. PACE 7:169, 1984.
137. Erdman S, Levinsky L, Strasberg B, et al: Use of the new Shaw scalpel in pacemaker operations. J Thorac Cardiovasc Surg 89:304, 1985.
138. Gascho JA, Newton MC: Electromagnetic interference in dynamic electrocardiography caused by an electric blanket. Am Heart J 95:408, 1978.
139. Irnich W: Interference in pacemakers. PACE 7:1021, 1984.
140. Kuan P, Kozlowski J, Castellanet MJ, et al: Interference with pacemaker function by cardiographic testing. Am J Cardiol 58:362, 1986.
141. Leeds CJ, Akhtar M, Damato AN, et al: Fluoroscope-generated electromagnetic interference in an external demand pacemaker. Circulation 55:548, 1977.
142. Warnowicz-Papp M: The pacemaker patient and the electromagnetic environment. Clin Prog Pacing Electrophysiol 1:166, 1983.
143. Van Gelder LM, El Gamal MIH: False inhibition of an atrial demand pacemaker caused by insulation defect in a polyurethane lead. PACE 6:834, 1983.
144. Sanford CF: Self-inhibition of an AV sequential demand pulse generator due to polyurethane lead insulation disruption. PACE 6:840, 1983.
145. Salem DN, Bornstein A, Levine PA, et al: Fracture of pacing electrode mimicking failure of pulse generator. Chest 74:673, 1978.

146. Coumel P, Mujica J, Barold SS: Demand pacemaker arrhythmias caused by intermittent incomplete electrode fracture. Am J Cardiol 36:105, 1975.
147. Barold SS, Scovil J, Ong LS, et al: Periodic pacemaker spike attenuation with preservation of capture: An unusual electrocardiographic manifestation of partial pacing electrode fracture. PACE 1:375, 1978.
148. Sarmiento JJ: Clinical utility of telemetered intracardiac electrograms in diagnosing a design dependent lead malfunction. PACE 13:188, 1990.
149. Nalos PC, Nyitray W: Benefits of intracardiac electrograms and programmable sensing polarity in preventing pacemaker inhibition due to spurious screw-in lead signals. PACE 13:1101, 1990.
150. Chew PH, Brinker JA: Oversensing from electrode "chatter" in a bipolar pacing lead: A case report. PACE 13:808, 1990.
151. Santomauro M, Ferraro S, Maddalena G, et al: Pacemaker malfunction due to subcutaneous emphysema: A case report. Angiology 43:873, 1992.
152. Giroud D, Goy JJ: Pacemaker malfunction due to subcutaneous emphysema. Int J Cardiol 26:234, 1990.
153. Shepard RB, Kim J, Colvin HC, et al: Pacing threshold spikes months and years after implant. PACE 14:1835, 1991.
154. Trautwein W: Electrophysiological aspects of cardiac stimulation. In Schaldach M, Furman S (eds): Advances in Pacemaker Technology. New York, Springer-Verlag, 1975, pp 11-23.
155. Siddons H, Sowton E: Threshold for stimulation. In Siddons H, Sowton E (eds.): Cardiac Pacemakers. Springfield, IL, Charles C. Thomas, 1967, pp 145-174.
156. Ohm OJ, Breivik K, Anderssen KS: Strength-duration curves in cardiac pacing. In Meere C (ed): Proceedings of the Sixth World Symposium on Cardiac Pacing. Montreal, January 1979, Chapter 20.
157. Irnich W: The chronaxy time and its practical importance. PACE 3:292, 1980.
158. Davies JG, Sowton E: Electrical threshold of the human heart. Br Heart J 28:231, 1966.
159. Furman S, Hurzeler P, Mehra R: Cardiac pacing and pacemakers. IV. Threshold of cardiac stimulation. Am Heart J 94:115, 1977.
160. Helguera ME, Maloney JD, Woscoboinik JR, et al: Long-term performance of epimyocardial pacing leads in adults: Comparison with endocardial leads. PACE 16:412, 1993.
161. Esperper HD, Mahmoud PO, von der Emde J: Is epicardial dual-chamber pacing a realistic alternative to endocardial DDD pacing? Initial results of a prospective study. PACE 15:155, 1992.
162. Bianconi L, Boccadamo R, Toscano S, et al: Effects of oral propafenone therapy on chronic myocardial pacing threshold. PACE 15:148, 1992.
163. Szabo Z, Solti F: The significance of the tissue reaction around the electrode on the late myocardial threshold. In Schaldach M, Furman S (eds): Advances in Pacemaker Technology. New York, Springer-Verlag, 1975, pp 273-287.
164. DeLeon SY, Ilbawi MN, Backer CL, et al: Exit block in pediatric cardiac pacing: Comparison of the suture-type and fishhook epicardial electrodes. J Thorac Cardiovasc Surg 99:905, 1990.
165. Stojanov P, Djordjevic M, Velimirovic D, et al: Assessment of long-term stability of chronic ventricular pacing thresholds in steroid-eluting electrodes. PACE 15:1417, 1992.
166. Karpawich PP, Hakimi M, Arciniegas E, et al: Improved epicardial pacing in children: Steroid contribution to porous platinized electrodes. PACE 15:1551, 1992.
167. Johns JA, Fish FA, Burger JD, et al: Steroid-eluting epicardial pacing leads in pediatric patients: Encouraging early results. J Am Coll Cardiol 20:395, 1992.
168. Stamato NJ, O'Tolle MF, Petter JG, et al: The safety and efficacy of chronic ventricular pacing at 1.6 volts using a steroid-eluting lead. PACE 15:248, 1992.
169. Hamilton R, Gow R, Bahoric B, et al: Steroid-eluting epicardial leads in pediatrics: Improved epicardial threshold in the first year. PACE 14:2066, 1991.
170. Anderson N, Mathivanar R, Skalsky M, et al: Active fixation leads: Long-term threshold reduction using a drug-infused ceramic collar. PACE 14:1767, 1991.
171. Kruse IM, Terpstra B: Acute and long-term atrial and ventricular stimulation thresholds with a steroid-eluting electrode. PACE 8:45, 1985.
172. Mond H, Stokes K, Helland J, et al: The porous titanium steroid-eluting electrode: A double-blind study assessing the stimulation threshold effects of steroid. PACE 11:214, 1988.
173. Klein HH, Steinberger J, Knake W: Stimulation characteristics of a steroid-eluting electrode compared with three conventional electrodes. PACE 13:134, 1990.
174. Beanlands DS, Akyurekli Y, Keon WJ: Prednisone in the management of exit block. In Meere C (ed): Proceedings of the Sixth World Symposium on Cardiac Pacing. Montreal, January 1979, Chapter 18.
175. Nagatomo Y, Ogawa T, Kumagae H, et al: Pacing failure due to markedly increased stimulation threshold two years after implantation: Successful management with oral prednisolone. A case report. PACE 12:1034, 1989.
176. Preston TA, Judge RD, Lucchesi BR, et al: Myocardial threshold in patients with artificial pacemakers. Am J Cardiol 18:83, 1966.
177. Schlesinger Z, Rosenberg T, Stryjer D, et al: Exit block in myxedema, treated effectively with thyroid hormone therapy. PACE 3:737, 1980.
178. Lee D, Greenspan K, Edmands RE, Fisch C: The effect of electrolyte alteration on stimulus requirement of cardiac pacemakers. Circulation 38:VI124, 1968.
179. Gettes LS, Shabetai R, Downs TA, et al: Effect of changes in potassium and calcium concentrations on diastolic threshold and strength-interval relationships of the human heart. Ann N Y Acad Sci 167:693, 1969.
180. O'Reilly MV, Murnaghan DP, Williams MB: Transvenous pacemaker failure induced by hyperkalemia. JAMA 228:336, 1974.
181. Dohrmann ML, Godschlager N: Metabolic and pharmacologic effects on myocardial stimulation threshold in patients with cardiac pacemakers. In Barold SS (ed): Modern Cardiac Pacing. Mt. Kisco, NY, Futura, 1985, pp 161-170.
182. Sowton E, Barr I: Physiologic changes in threshold. Ann N Y Acad Sci 167:679, 1969.
183. Finfer SR: Pacemaker failure on induction of anaesthesia. Br J Anaesth 66:509, 1991.
184. Hughes JC Jr, Tyers GFO, Torman HA: Effects of acid-base imbalance on myocardial pacing thresholds. J Thorac Cardiovasc Surg 69:743, 1975.
185. Preston TA, Judge RD: Alteration of pacemaker threshold by drug and physiologic factors. Ann N Y Acad Sci 167:686, 1969.
186. Preston TA, Fletcher RD, Lucchesi BR, et al: Changes in myocardial threshold: Physiologic and pharmacologic factors in patients with implanted pacemakers. Am Heart J 74:235, 1967.
187. Emilsson K, Oddsson H, Allared M, Brorson L: An unusual cause of high threshold values at pacemaker implantation. PACE 20:366-367, 1977.
188. Perry GY, Parsonnet V, Werres R, Flowers NC: Transient loss of sensing and capture during coronary angiography in two patients with permanent pacemakers. PACE 18:108-112, 1995.
189. Hellestrand KJ, Burnett PJ, Milne JR, et al: Effect of the antiarrhythmic agent flecainide acetate on acute and chronic pacing thresholds. PACE 6:892, 1983.
190. Levick CE, Mizgala HF, Kerr CR: Failure to pace following high-dose antiarrhythmic therapy: Reversal with isoproterenol. PACE 7:252, 1984.
191. Nielsen AP, Griffin JC, Herre JM, et al: Effect of amiodarone on acute and chronic pacing thresholds. PACE 7:462, 1984.

192. Montefoschi N, Boccadamo R: Propafenone-induced acute variation of chronic atrial pacing threshold: A case report. PACE 13:480, 1990.
193. Salel AF, Seagren SC, Pool PE: Effects of encainide on the function of implanted pacemakers. PACE 12:1439, 1989.
194. Guarnieri T, Datorre SD, Bondke H, et al: Increased pacing threshold after an automatic defibrillatory shock in dogs: Effects of class I and class II antiarrhythmic drugs. PACE 11:1324, 1988.
195. Clarke M, Liu B, Schüller H, et al: Automatic adjustment of pacemaker stimulation output correlated with continuously monitored capture thresholds: A multicenter study. PACE 21:1567-1575, 1998.
196. Grant SC, Bennett DH: Atrial latency in a dual-chambered pacing system causing inappropriate sequence of cardiac chamber activation. PACE 15:116, 1992.
197. Furman S, Hurzeler P, DeCaprio V: Cardiac pacing and pacemakers III: Sensing the cardiac electrogram. Am Heart J 93:794, 1977.
198. Ohm OJ: The interdependence between electrogram, total electrode impedance, and pacemaker input impedance necessary to obtain adequate functioning demand pacemakers. PACE 2:465, 1979.
199. Kleinert M, Elmqvist H, Strandberg H: Spectral properties of atrial and ventricular endocardial signals. PACE 2:11, 1979.
200. Myers GH, Kresh YM, Parsonnet V: Characteristics of intracardiac electrograms. PACE 1:90, 1978.
201. Evans GL, Glasser SP: Intracardiac electrocardiography as a guide to pacemaker positioning. JAMA 216:483, 1971.
202. Levine PA, Klein MD: Discrepant electrocardiographic and pulse analyzer endocardial potentials: A possible source of pacemaker sensing failure. In Meere C (ed): Proceedings of the Sixth World Symposium on Cardiac Pacing. Montreal, January 1979, Chapter 34.
203. Levine PA, Seltzer JP: Fusion, pseudofusion, pseudo-pseudofusion and confusion: Normal rhythms associated with atrioventricular sequential "DVI" pacing. Clin Prog Pacing Electrophysiol 1:70, 1983.
204. Barold SS, Falkoff MD, Ong LS, et al: Characterization of pacemaker arrhythmias due to normally functioning AV demand (DVI) pulse generators. PACE 3:712, 1980.
205. Breivik K, Ohm OJ, Engedal H: Long-term comparison of unipolar and bipolar pacing and sensing, using a new multiprogrammable pacemaker system. PACE 6:592, 1983.
206. Ohm OJ: Demand failures occurring during permanent pacing in patients with serious heart disease. PACE 3:44, 1980.
207. Griffin JC, Finke WL: Analysis of the endocardial electrogram morphology of isolated ventricular beats. PACE 6:315, 1983.
208. Barold SS, Gaidula JJ: Failure of demand pacemaker from low-voltage bipolar ventricular electrograms. JAMA 215:923, 1971.
209. Van Mechelen R, Hart CT, De Boer H: Failure to sense P waves during DDD pacing. PACE 9:498, 1986.
210. Bricker JT, Ward KA, Zinner A, Gillette PC: Decrease in canine endocardial and epicardial electrogram voltage with exercise: Implications for pacemaker sensing. PACE 11:460, 1988.
211. Frohlig G, Schwerdt H, Schieffer H, et al: Atrial signal variations and pacemaker malsensing during exercise: A study in the time and frequency domain. J Am Coll Cardiol 11:806, 1988.
212. van Gelder BM, van Mechelen R, den Dulk, et al: Apparent P-wave undersensing in a DDD pacemaker post exercise. PACE 15:1651, 1992.
213. Sager DP: Current facts on pacemaker electromagnetic interference and their application to clinical care. Heart Lung 16:211, 1987.
214. Lau FYK, Bilitch M, Wintroub HJ: Protection of implanted pacemakers from excessive electrical energy of D.C. shock. Am J Cardiol 23:244, 1969.
215. Levine PA, Barold SS, Fletcher RD, Talbot P: Adverse acute and chronic effects of electrical defibrillation and cardioversion on implanted unipolar cardiac pacing systems. J Am Coll Cardiol 1:14130-1422, 1993.
216. Van Lake P, Levine PA, Mouchawar GA: Effect of implantable nonthoracotomy defibrillation system on permanent pacemakers: An in-vitro analysis with clinical implications. PACE 18:182-187, 1995.
217. De Keyser F, Vanhaecke J, Janssens L, et al: Crosstalk with external bipolar DVI pacing: A case report. PACE 14:1320, 1991.
218. Sweesy MW, Batey RL, Forney RC: Crosstalk during bipolar pacing. PACE 11:1512, 1988.
219. Coombs WJ, Reynolds DW, Sharma AJ, Bennett TD: Crosstalk in bipolar pacemakers. PACE 12:1613-1621, 1989.
220. Levine PA, Venditti FJ, Podrid PJ, Klein MD: Therapeutic and diagnostic benefits of intentional crosstalk mediated ventricular output inhibition. PACE 11:1194-1201, 1988.
221. Batey FL, Calabria DA, Sweesy MW, et al: Crosstalk and blanking periods in a dual-chamber pacemaker. Clin Prog Pacing Electrophysiol 3:314, 1985.
222. Barold SS, Falkoff MD, Ong LS, et al: Interpretation of electrocardiograms produced by a new unipolar multiprogrammable "committed" AV sequential demand (DVI) pacemaker. PACE 4:692, 1981.
223. Levine PA: Normal and abnormal rhythms associated with dual-chamber pacemakers. Cardiol Clin 3:595-616, 1985.
224. Barold SS, Belott PH: Behavior of the ventricular triggering period of DDD pacemakers. PACE 10:1237-1252, 1987.
225. Heller LI: Surgical electrocautery and the runaway pacemaker syndrome. PACE 13:1084, 1990.
226. Mickley H, Andersen C, Nielsen LH: Runaway pacemaker: A still existing complication and therapeutic guidelines. Clin Cardiol 12:412, 1989.
227. Snoeck J, Beerkhof M, Claeys M, et al: External vibration interference of activity based rate-responsive pacemakers. PACE 15:1841, 1992.
228. Lamb LS Jr, Judson EB: Maximal rate response in a permanent pacemaker during chest physiotherapy. Heart Lung 21:390, 1992.
229. Lau CP, Tai YT, Fong PC, et al: Pacemaker-mediated tachycardias in single-chamber rate-responsive pacing. PACE 13:1575, 1990.
230. Madsen GM, Andersen C: Pacemaker-induced tachycardia during general anaesthesia: A case report. Br J Anaesth 63:360, 1989.
231. Fetter J, Patterson D, Aram G, et al: Effects of extracorporeal shock wave lithotripsy on single-chamber rate-response and dual-chamber pacemakers. PACE 12:1494, 1989.
232. Lau CP, Linker NJ, Butrous GS, et al: Myopotential interference in unipolar rate-responsive pacemakers. PACE 12:1324, 1989.
233. French RS, Tillman JG: Pacemaker function during helicopter transport. Ann Emerg Med 18:305, 1989.
234. Volosin KJ, O'Connor WH, Fabiszewski R, et al: Pacemaker-mediated tachycardia from a single-chamber temperature-sensitive pacemaker. PACE 12:1596, 1989.
235. Fearnot NE, Kitoh O, Fujita T, et al: Case studies on the effect of exercise and hot water submersion on intracardiac temperature and the performance of a pacemaker which varies pacing rate based on temperature. Jpn Heart J 30:353, 1989.
236. Seeger W, Kleinert M: An unexpected rate response of a minute ventilation dependent pacemaker [letter]. PACE 12:1707, 1989.
237. Hayes DL: Rate adaptive cardiac pacing: Implications of environmental noise during craniotomy. Anesthesiology 87:1243-1245, 1997.
238. Holmes DR, Hayes DL, Gray JE, Merideth J: The effects of magnetic resonance imaging on implantable pulse generators. PACE 9:360, 1986.
239. Hayes DL, Holmes DR, Gray JE: Effect of 1.5 Telsa nuclear magnetic resonance imaging scanner on implanted permanent pacemakers. J Am Coll Cardiol 10:782, 1987.

240. Erlebacher JA, Cahill PT, Pannizzo F, Knowles RJR: Effect of magnetic resonance imaging on DDD pacemakers. Am J Cardiol 57:347, 1986.
241. Gimbel JR, Johnson D, Levine PA, Wilkoff BL: Safe performance of magnetic resonance imaging on five patients with permanent cardiac pacemakers. PACE 19:913-919, 1996.
242. Achenbach S, Moshage W, Diem B, et al: Effects of magnetic resonance imaging on cardiac pacemakers and electrodes. Am Heart J 134:467-473, 1997.
243. Shellack F, Kanal E: Politics, guidelines and recommendations for MR imaging safety and patient management. J Magn Reson Imaging 11:97-104, 1991.
244. Lauck G, von Smekal A, Wolke S, et al: Effects of nuclear magnetic resonance imaging on cardiac pacemakers. PACE 18:1549-1555, 1995.
245. Schüller H, Binner L, Linde C, et al: Combipolar™ sensing in DDD pacemakers: Do we still need bipolar atrial leads? In Sethi KK (ed): Proceedings of the Sixth Asian Pacific Symposium on Cardiac Pacing and Electrophysiology. Bologna, Italy, Monduzzi Editore S.P.A., 1997, pp 75-79.
246. Levine PA, Selznick L: Prospective Management of the Patient with Retrograde Ventriculoatrial Conduction: Prevention and Management of Pacemaker Mediated Endless Loop Tachycardias. Sylmar, CA, Pacesetter Systems, 1990.
247. Limousin M, Bonnet JL: A multicentric study of 1816 endless loop tachycardia (ELT) responses. PACE 13:555, 1990.
248. Oseran D, Ausubel K, Klementowicz PT, et al: Spontaneous endless loop tachycardia. PACE 9:379, 1986.
249. Rubin JW, Frank MJ, Boineau JP, et al: Current physiologic pacemakers: A serious problem with a new device. Am J Cardiol 52:88, 1983.
250. Levine PA: Postventricular atrial refractory periods and pacemaker-mediated tachycardias. Clin Prog Pacing Electrophysiol 1:394, 1983.
251. Furman S, Fisher JD: Endless loop tachycardia in an AV universal (DDD) pacemaker. PACE 5:486, 1982.
252. Den Dulk K, Lindemans FW, Bar FW, et al: Pacemaker-related tachycardias. PACE 5:476, 1982.
253. Luceri RM, Castellanos A, Zaman L, et al: The arrhythmias of dual-chamber cardiac pacemakers and their management. Ann Intern Med 99:354, 1983.
254. Ausubel K, Gabry MD, Klementowicz PT, et al: Pacemaker-mediated endless loop tachycardia at rates below the upper rate limit. Am J Cardiol 61:465, 1988.
255. Denes P, Wu D, Dhingra R, et al: The effects of cycle length on cardiac refractory periods in man. Circulation 49:32, 1974.
256. Amikam S, Furman S: Programmed upper rate limit dependent endless loop tachycardia. Chest 85:286, 1984.
257. Haffejee C, Murphy J, Gold R, et al: Automatic extension vs. programmability of the atrial refractory period in the prevention of pacemaker-mediated tachycardia. PACE 8:A56, 1985.
258. Den Dulk K, Hamersa M, Wellens HJJ: Role of an adaptable atrial refractory period for DDD pacemakers. PACE 10:425, 1987.
259. Rognoni G, Occhetta E, Perucca A, et al: A new approach to the prevention of endless loop tachycardia in DDD and VDD pacing. PACE 14:1828, 1991.
260. Nitzsche R, Gueunoun M, Lamaison D, et al: Endless-loop tachycardias: Description and first clinical results of a new fully automatic protection algorithm. PACE 13:1711, 1990.
261. Cameron DA, Gentzler RD, Love CJ, et al: Initial clinical experience with a new automatic PMT detection and termination algorithm to discriminate between pacemaker mediated tachycardia due to ventriculo-atrial conduction and normal sinus tachycardia. HeartWeb 2(1), article 96110035, 1996; http://www.webaxis.com/heartweb/1196/pacing0018.htm.
262. Klementowicz PT, Furman S: Selective atrial sensing in dual-chamber pacemakers eliminates endless loop tachycardias. J Am Coll Cardiol 7:590, 1986.
263. Pannizzo F, Amikam S, Bagwell P, et al: Discrimination of antegrade and retrograde atrial depolarization by electrogram analysis. Am Heart J 112:780, 1986.
264. McAlister HF, Klementowicz PT, Calderon EM, et al: Atrial electrogram analysis: Antegrade versus retrograde. PACE 11:1703, 1988.
265. Bernheim C, Markewitz A, Kemkes BM: Can reprogramming of atrial sensitivity avoid endless loop tachycardia? PACE 9:293, 1986.
266. Throne RD, Jenkins JM, Winston SA, et al: Discrimination of retrograde from anterograde atrial activation using intracardiac electrogram waveform analysis. PACE 12:1622, 1989.
267. Van Gelder LM, El Gamal MIH, Sanders RS: Tachycardia-termination algorithm: A valuable feature for interruption of pacemaker-mediated tachycardia. PACE 7:283, 1984.
268. Duncan JL, Clark MF: Prevention and termination of pacemaker-mediated tachycardia in a new DDD pacing system (Siemens-Pacesetter Model 2010T). PACE 11:1679, 1988.
269. Puglisi A, Ricci R, Azzolini P, et al: Ventricular cross stimulation in a dual-chamber pacing system: Phenomenon analysis. PACE 13:993, 1990.
270. Goldschlager N, Francoz R: Ventricular cross stimulation using a pacing system analyzer. PACE 13:986, 1990.
271. Doi Y, Takada K, Nakagaki O, et al: A case of cross stimulation. PACE 12:569, 1989.
272. Levine PA, Rihanek BD, Sanders R, et al: Cross-stimulation: The unexpected stimulation of the unpaced chamber. PACE 8:600, 1985.
273. Van Gelder LM, El Gamal MIH: Ventriculoatrial conduction: A cause of atrial malpacing in AV universal pacemakers: A report of two cases. PACE 8:140-143, 1985.
274. Barold SS: Repetitive non-reentrant ventriculoatrial synchrony in dual chamber pacing. In Santini M, Pistolese M, Alliegro A (eds): Progress in Clinical Pacing 1990. Amsterdam, Exerpta Medica, 1990, p 451.
275. Levine PA: Pacing system malfunction: Evaluation and management. In Podrid PJ, Kowey P (eds): Cardiac Arrhythmia, Mechanisms, Diagnosis and Management. Baltimore, Williams & Wilkins, 1995, pp 582-610.

Chapter 25

Troubleshooting of Implantable Cardioverter-Defibrillators

ANDREW E. EPSTEIN

Since its introduction into clinical practice in the early 1980s, the implantable cardioverter-defibrillator (ICD) has evolved from a treatment of last resort for aborted cardiac arrest to the treatment of choice for the management of resuscitated cardiac arrest and, more recently, for the primary prevention of sudden cardiac death. The original device (AID, Intec Systems, Inc., Pittsburgh) lacked programmability except for turning the device on or off. Its detection rate was fixed, and it had no diagnostic capabilities except to indicate that a charging cycle had been initiated.

With the emergence of additional therapeutic capabilities, including bradycardia and antitachycardia pacing, the need for diagnostic capabilities and features has grown in keeping with the exponential growth in the rate of ICD implantation. The need to recognize and define the initiating events and resulting rhythms at the time of ICD intervention is but one of the reasons that sophisticated telemetry features were developed; other reasons include the need to diagnose ICD malfunction noninvasively and the need to evaluate the performance of the ICD components, including battery and lead integrity.

The purpose of this chapter is to review the available methods for the diagnosis of ICD malfunction using the programmer and noninvasive techniques. Because there is a separate chapter on biventricular devices, only conventional ICDs are discussed here.

Troubleshooting Principles

ICD malfunction is uncommon. The most common reasons for inappropriate therapy or the absence of expected therapy relate to inappropriate programming, lead-related complications, imperfect diagnostic specificity, insufficient understanding of the technical specifications of device function, and drug-device interactions; now only rarely do device-device interactions and true device component malfunctions occur.[1]

Troubleshooting of suspected ICD malfunction follows logically from analysis of the index clinical event, whether it is from a patient report or from device diagnostics. By evaluation of the clinical history, physical examination, radiographic techniques, device memory, and on-line telemetry, the cause of malfunction can usually be determined. The analysis must take into account the specifics of the ICD as well as the sensing and treatment algorithms used to arrive at an accurate diagnosis. Therapy may be delivered or withheld either because of true malfunction of a component or because the device is responding appropriately according to its programming and interaction with the environment (e.g., responses to electromagnetic interference).

Analysis of ICD problems begins with identification of the problem, followed by analysis of its possible cause. Presentation falls into four general areas: multiple shocks, failure to convert ventricular tachycardia (VT) or fibrillation (VF), failure to detect VT or VF, and problems with pacing.[2] Each area is discussed individually.

Initial Evaluation and Tools

Clinical History

As in all other areas of medicine, the keystone to diagnosis is the clinical history. Historical clues suggesting ICD malfunction, although by themselves nondiagnostic, provide the basis for a presumptive diagnosis and suggest further avenues of inquiry. For example, repeated shocks in an asymptomatic patient suggest false signal detection or an atrial arrhythmia. Certain body positions associated with ICD shocks suggest the possibility of lead fracture or lead instability. ICD model, manufacturer, date of implantation, lead type and location, antiarrhythmic drug history, presence or absence of symptoms of heart failure or angina preceding therapy, and other clues are important, because any or all of these factors may have relevance and can be related to ICD therapy. The presence of an implanted pacemaker with an ICD raises the specter of device-device interaction. Therapy during exercise raises the possibility of sinus tachycardia or of atrial fibrillation with a rapid ventricular response. Palpitations may signal either supraventricular tachycardia (SVT) or VT.

Physical Examination

The physical examination may be helpful in pinpointing the exact cause of ICD malfunction. For example, for a patient who reports that certain body positions or movements elicit ICD shocks, reproducing the precise maneuver or the exact circumstances known to elicit the shocks, while simultaneously telemetering the device, may prove the diagnosis of lead failure. Occasionally, patients are reluctant to allow the examiner to do this because the prospect of an ICD shock is psychologically threatening.[3] In such circumstances, the ICD may be placed in a monitor mode, either by programming or with the use of a magnet to suspend tachyarrhythmia detection, while assuring the patient that shock delivery will not occur. The assessment of recordings from the ICD in these situations is discussed later.

Because a common point of lead fracture occurs where transvenous ICD leads pass between the clavicle and first rib,[4,5] manipulation of the device pocket or the lead entry point in the pectoral area may elicit electrical noise artifact, indicating lead conductor fracture.[6,7] Similar artifacts may occur with a loose connection of the set-screw to the lead terminal pin in the ICD pulse generator header. Again, make-break potentials can be demonstrated by noninvasive telemetry, as discussed later.

Other diagnostic clues may be provided by the physical examination, such as detection of an irregular pulse suggestive of atrial fibrillation, which may be readily confirmed by an electrocardiogram. Congestive heart failure is often associated with exacerbation of ventricular arrhythmias.[8-10] Therefore, eliciting symptoms and signs of left ventricular decompensation suggests a possible cause for worsening arrhythmias.

Electrocardiographic Recordings

Objective evidence of the event precipitating ICD therapy, or of an arrhythmia with absence of the expected ICD response, can be extremely helpful and is usually diagnostic (Fig. 25-1). In the days before the availability of stored electrograms (EGMs), such evidence was rarely available unless the patient was hospitalized and monitored at the time of the event. Fortunately, this is now a problem of the past. Nevertheless, even when EGMs are available, they can sometimes be inconclusive or confusing. In addition, if multiple ICD detections have occurred due to any reason including lead failure, SVT, or a VT or VF storm, EGM documentation of the initial event leading to detection may be overwritten due to limited device memory.

Device Telemetry

The advent of device telemetry has revolutionized and greatly simplified analysis of arrhythmias and events suspected of representing ICD malfunction. Early devices (e.g., Ventak, Cardiac Pacemakers [CPI/Guidant], St. Paul, Minn.) were able to emit sounds or beeps synchronous with ventricular EGM detection, enabling identification of oversensing or undersensing. When recorded with a phonocardiogram, a so-called "beep-o-gram" was produced (Fig. 25-2). Although helpful, these crude attempts at telemetry were quickly supplanted by advances that enabled detailed information, such as R-R intervals and ventricular EGMs, to be telemetered (Fig. 25-3).[11] The complexity and sophistication of these diagnostic tools are increasing with the new generation of ICDs. The addition of the atrial channel has greatly simplified analysis of arrhythmic events (Fig. 25-4).

Other diagnostic information is now routinely available from all ICDs, including battery voltage, pacing and sensing lead impedances, charge times, capacitor reformation times, high-voltage lead impedance, and frequency and timing of ventricular events. The finding of a depleted battery, lead impedance out of range (either too high or too low), and R-R intervals can lead to correct diagnoses. The latter is extremely important, because nonphysiologic intervals (short) raise the suspicion of make-brake electrical noise artifact. One

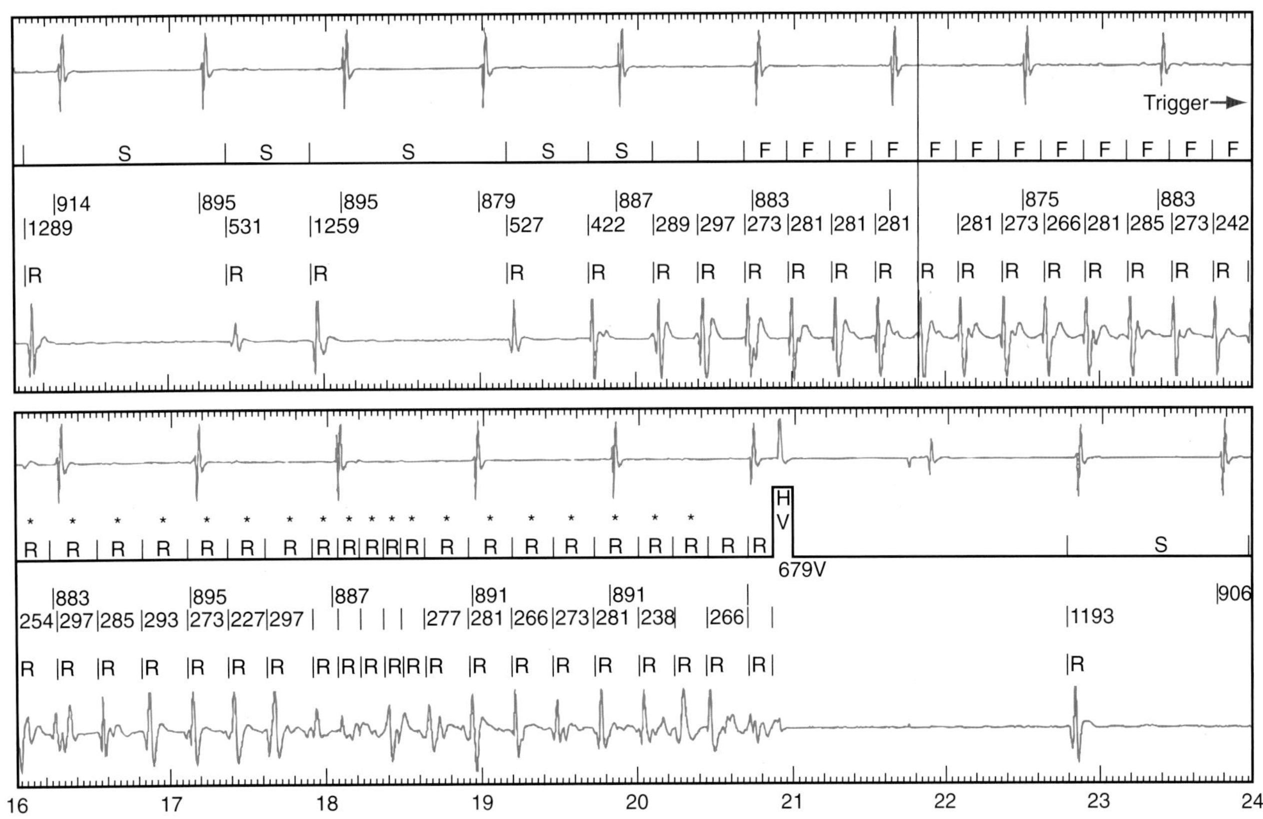

Figure 25-1. The EGM shows sinus rhythm, followed by a rapid, irregular ventricular arrhythmia, followed by a high voltage (HV) shock delivered by a Model 1823 defibrillator (Guidant, Boston Scientific, Natick, Mass.). The three recordings are from the atrial channel, the ventricular pace/sense channel, and the high-voltage ventricular channel. Note that the EGM of the ventricular arrhythmia has a different morphology from that of the preceding sinus rhythm. The first beat is sinus in origin. The second and third beats are premature ventricular depolarizations that do not interrupt the sinus mechanism. They initiate ventricular fibrillation, typified by a rapid, polymorphic EGM.

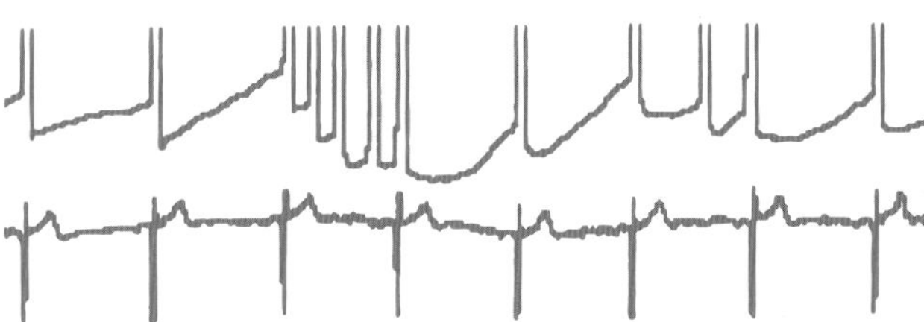

Figure 25-2. This beep-o-gram was recorded from a Ventak ICD (Cardiac Pacemakers, CPI/Guidant, St. Paul, Minn.) that was placed in the test mode by application of a magnet over the device so that shocks could not be delivered. The ICD was programmed to beep synchronously with electrical activity in the sensing channel. The top tracing is a filtered and amplified recording from a microphone responding to ICD beeps that were then converted into an electrical signal. The bottom tracing is a simultaneous surface electrocardiogram. During sinus rhythm (lower tracing) there were extra signals recorded from the microphone (between the third and fourth and between the sixth and seventh sinus beats) that proved to be artifact leading to inappropriate shocks. (From Ballas SL, Rashidi R, McAlister H, et al: The use of beep-o-grams in the assessment of automatic implantable cardioverter defibrillator sensing function. PACE 12:1737-1745, 1989.)

device (Medtronic, Inc., Minneapolis, Minn.) records information regarding both impedance changes (Fig. 25-5) and nonphysiologic R-R intervals.[12]

Radiographic Evidence

Radiographic evidence is helpful if lead malposition, dislodgment, or fracture is suspected (Figs. 25-6 through 25-8).[7] It is recommended, whenever possible, that chest radiographs taken immediately after ICD implantation be compared with radiographs obtained at the time of a problem. Such comparisons may reveal lead malposition and displacement when none is suspected. Radiographs can also be helpful in demonstrating conductor fracture or pin connectors improperly positioned in the header. Examining the radiographic "signature" of the device can help identify the device type when the patient is unaware of the ICD model or type. Knowledge of unique failure modes, such as "migration" of set screws (travel of the right ventricular fixation screw into the channel lumen during shipment) in particular families of ICDs is of course desirable.[13]

Figures 25-6 and 25-7 show examples of lead dislodgment. Because the distal end of the lead is close to

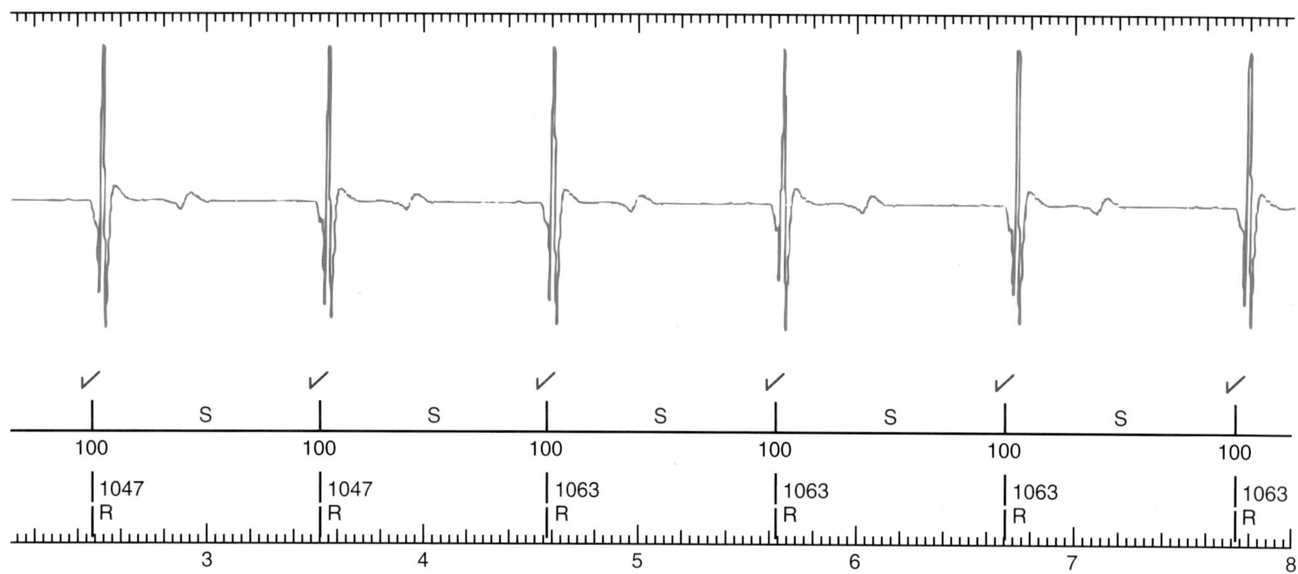

Figure 25-3. The first line of this tracing is an EGM recorded from a St. Jude Medical (Sunnyvale, Calif.) single-chamber Model V193 ICD. This device monitors the heart rate and has the capability of analyzing the EGM morphology. The bottom lines annotate the ICD sensing function. The checks and 100 numbers indicate the degree of matching of the EGM morphology to a sinus rhythm template that can be used to distinguish atrial from ventricular arrhythmias. The 1047 and 1063 numbers indicate cycle length. "S" indicates sinus rhythm, "R" indicates sensed R-waves, and the numbers at the bottom count the seconds of the recording.

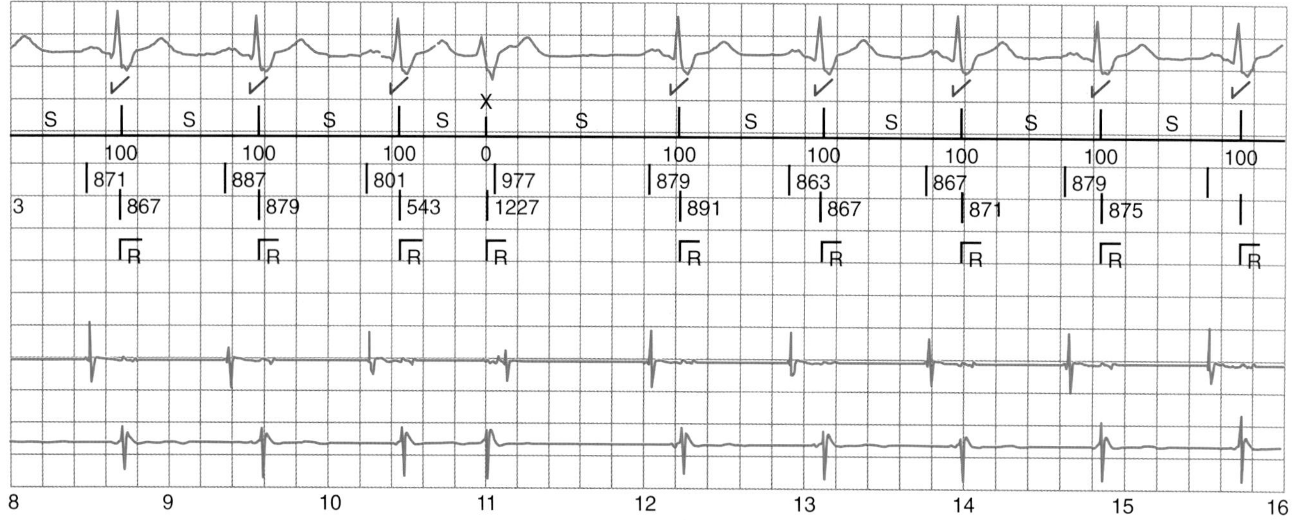

Figure 25-4. As in Figure 25-3, this tracing EGM recorded at a routine clinic follow-up visit shows the ventricular EGM (fourth tracing) as well as an atrial EGM (third tracing) from a dual chamber Model V242 ICD (St. Jude Medical, Sunnyvale, Calif.). The first and second tracings are, respectively, a surface electrocardiogram and a marker channel. In the marker channel, the checks indicate a template match with sinus rhythm (100% registered below the horizontal marker line). The fourth beat, marked "x," is a premature ventricular depolarization with a different morphology than sinus; it is logged as a 0% match. The next two rows of numbers are the P-P and R-R intervals. "S" indicates sinus rhythm as defined by the ICD, as opposed to "T" or "F" if ventricular tachycardia or fibrillation were present, respectively. "R" indicates sensed ventricular activity. The data on atrial and ventricular EGM timing and ventricular EGM morphology allow this device to use discrimination algorithms to differentiate supraventricular from ventricular arrhythmias. In addition it can, of course, function as an atrial, ventricular, or dual-chamber pacemaker.

the tricuspid annulus (see Fig. 25-6A), both atrial and ventricular signals are recorded (see Fig. 25-6B). This leads to "double-counting" such that, for a given heart rate, the ventricular channel registers twice the actual heart rate, satisfying the high rate detection requirement and leading to administration of a shock (see Fig. 25-6B). Figure 25-7 shows a similar example, but the electrical artifacts are more disorganized and irregular, presumably because the lead is more free-floating. Figure 25-8 shows an example of disruption of a transvenous ICD lead as it passes between the clavicle and first rib. Care must be taken to learn the appearance of the welds of the springs, because they can be mistaken for fracture if their usual appearance of being offset from the central axis of the lead is not appreciated (Fig. 25-9).[14] An unusual cause of lead failure, and sometimes failure of telemetry, occurs in "twiddlers"; in these cases, a lead is twisted and fractured (Fig. 25-10) or the ICD is inverted.[15,16]

Presentations

Multiple Shocks

Multiple shocks (Table 25-1) may be the result of incessant VT/VF, repetitive VT/VF, oversensing of T waves, electromagnetic interference, electrical noise artifacts from a fractured conductor or myopotentials in the case of insulation failure, or SVT including sinus tachycardia, atrial fibrillation, atrial flutter, or another mechanism. Sometimes the ICD itself can be proarrhythmic (Table 25-2).

The occurrence of multiple shocks leads to myriad problems. Shocks are poorly tolerated by patients, families, and referring physicians. They can create fear and distrust of that ICD that may be long-lasting and require professional help. Furthermore, they lead to significant

TABLE 25-1. Multiple Shocks

Cause	Management
Usually due to VT or VF	Judicious use of magnet and/or programming ICD off
Supraventricular tachycardia (SVT)	Reprogram, treat arrhythmia, slow ventricular response to AF
Change in substrate	Treat precipitating factor
Ischemia	Revascularize, drug therapy
Drug change	Reprogram or change drug
Sensing malfunction	
Lead failure (conductor or insulation)	Replace lead
Loose connection (e.g., set screw)	Reoperate and reseat screw
T-wave sensing	Reprogram as feasible
P-wave sensing	Reprogram as feasible, but often requires reoperation
External signals	
Electromagnetic interference (EMI)	Avoid cause
Device-device interaction	Reprogram or reoperate

AF, atrial fibrillation; VF, ventricular fibrillation; VT, ventricular tachycardia.

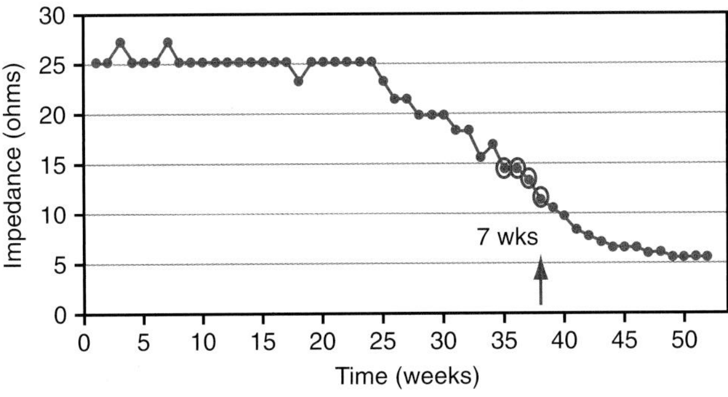

Figure 25-5. The plot shows decreasing ring-coil impedances logged in a GEM ICD (Medtronic, Inc., Minneapolis, Minn.). The first four impedances readings of less than 15 ohms are circled. The arrow indicates that the low-impedance trigger would have provided an alarm 15 weeks before this patient received an inappropriate shock. (From Gunderson BD, Patel AS, et al: An algorithm to predict implantable cardioverter-defibrillator lead failure. J Am Coll Cardiol 44:1898-1902, 2004.)

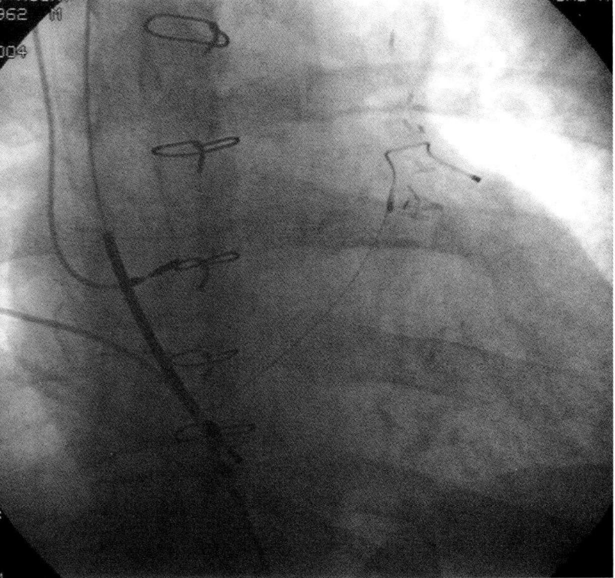

A

Figure 25-6. Panel A shows a biventricular pacing-ICD system (Model V340, St. Jude Medical, Sunnyvale, Calif.) with the right ventricular pacing-sensing-defibrillation lead displaced to the tricuspid annulus.

Continued

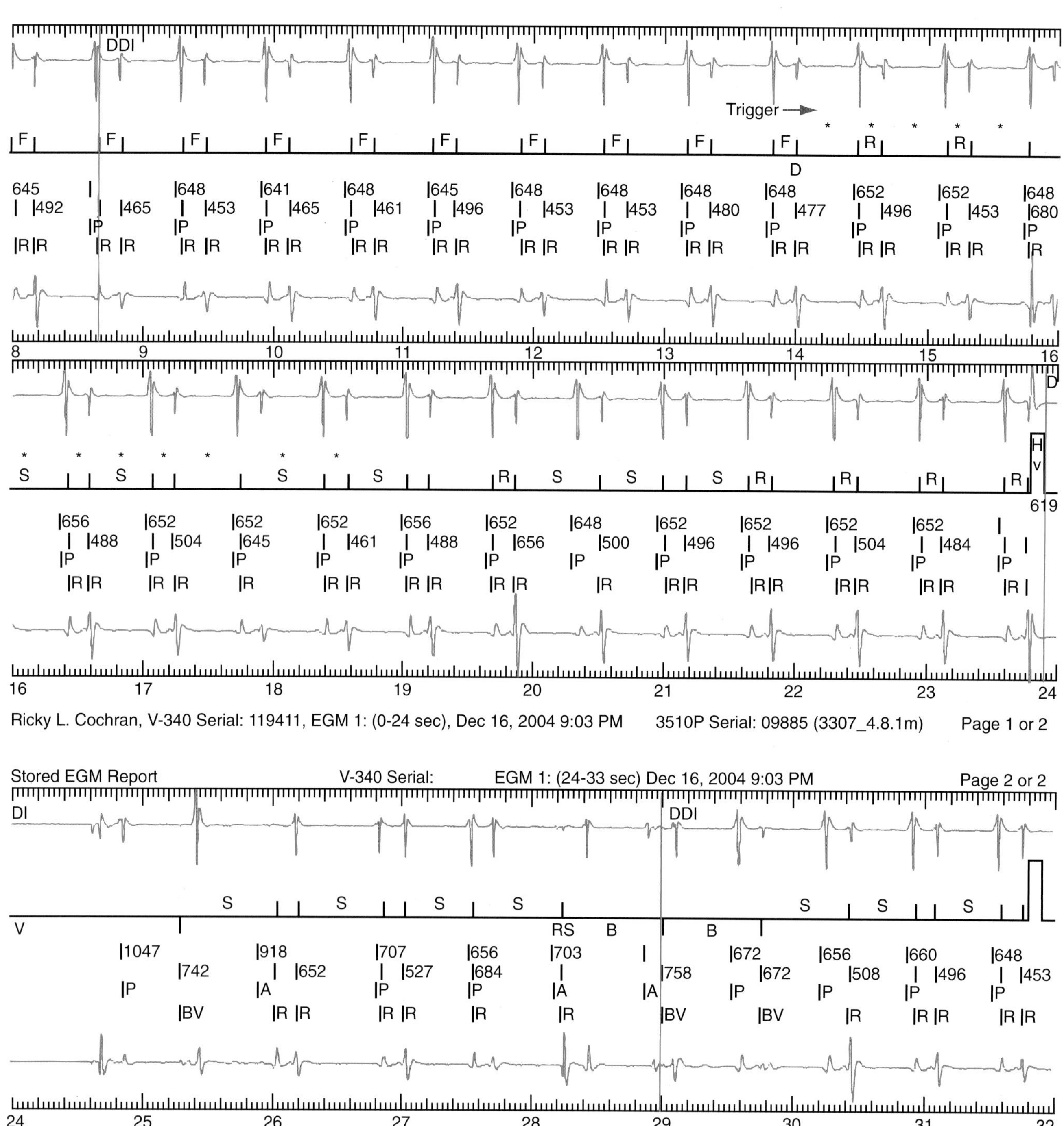

B

Figure 25-6, cont'd. Panel B shows recordings from the ICD. From top to bottom are the atrial EGM, the marker channels, and the ventricular EGM. F indicates fibrillation detection, the numbers are atrial and ventricular cycle lengths, P stands for P wave, and R for R wave. Because the distal end of the lead is close to the tricuspid annulus, both atrial and ventricular signals are recorded in the ventricular channel, such that the ventricular rate counter registers twice the actual heart rate. The R-R labels reflect double-counting from the EGM in the bottom tracing recorded from the right ventricular distal tip. This double-counting satisfied high rate detection, and a shock was delivered (HV).

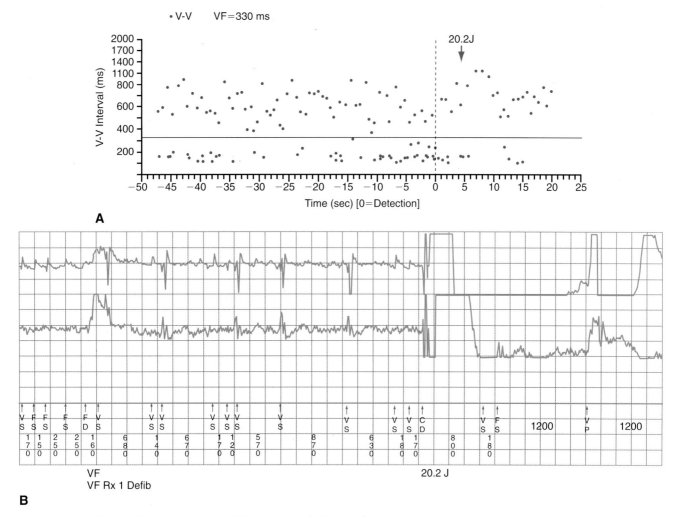

*Figure 25-7. Interval plot **(A)** and stored EGM **(B)** from a patient whose right ventricular defibrillation lead was dislodged to the tricuspid valve. Random electrical signals generated by lead movement in the ventricle provided very rapid and irregular artifacts that were interpreted by the Model 7230 ICD (Medtronic, Inc., Minneapolis, Minn.) as ventricular fibrillation, and a shock was delivered (CD [charge delivered]) on panel **B**.*

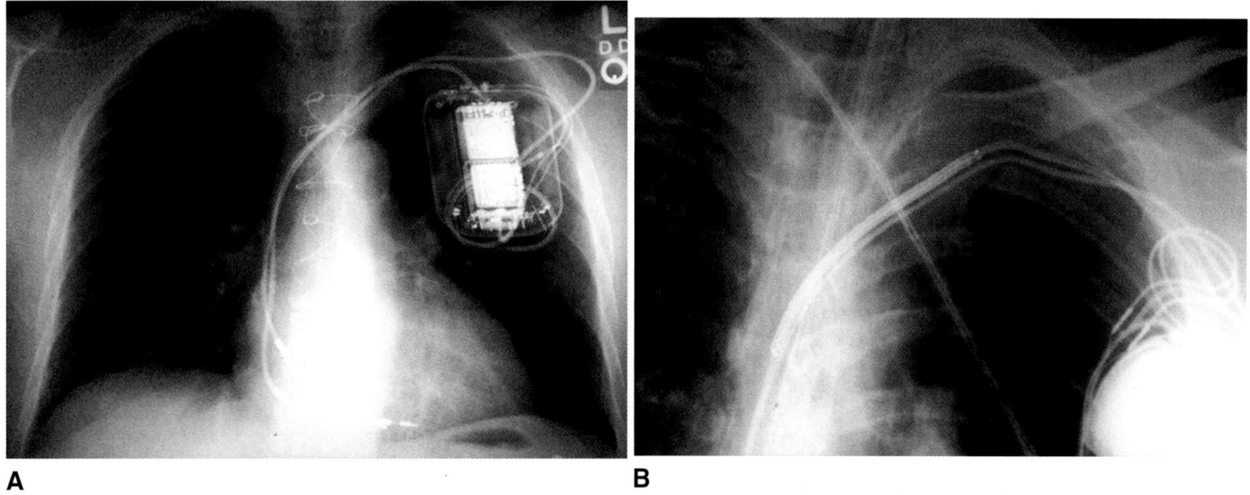

*Figure 25-8. **A,** Posteroanterior chest radiograph of an ICD system from a patient who presented with multiple shocks. The lower lead has a discontinuity where it travels between the clavicle and the first rib. **B,** Close-up view of a different patient with an identical presentation. The fracture again is at the junction between the clavicle and first rib and is easily identified where the superior, high-voltage lead is bent with a discontinuity at the inferior margin. (Courtesy of Dr. Paul A. Levine.)*

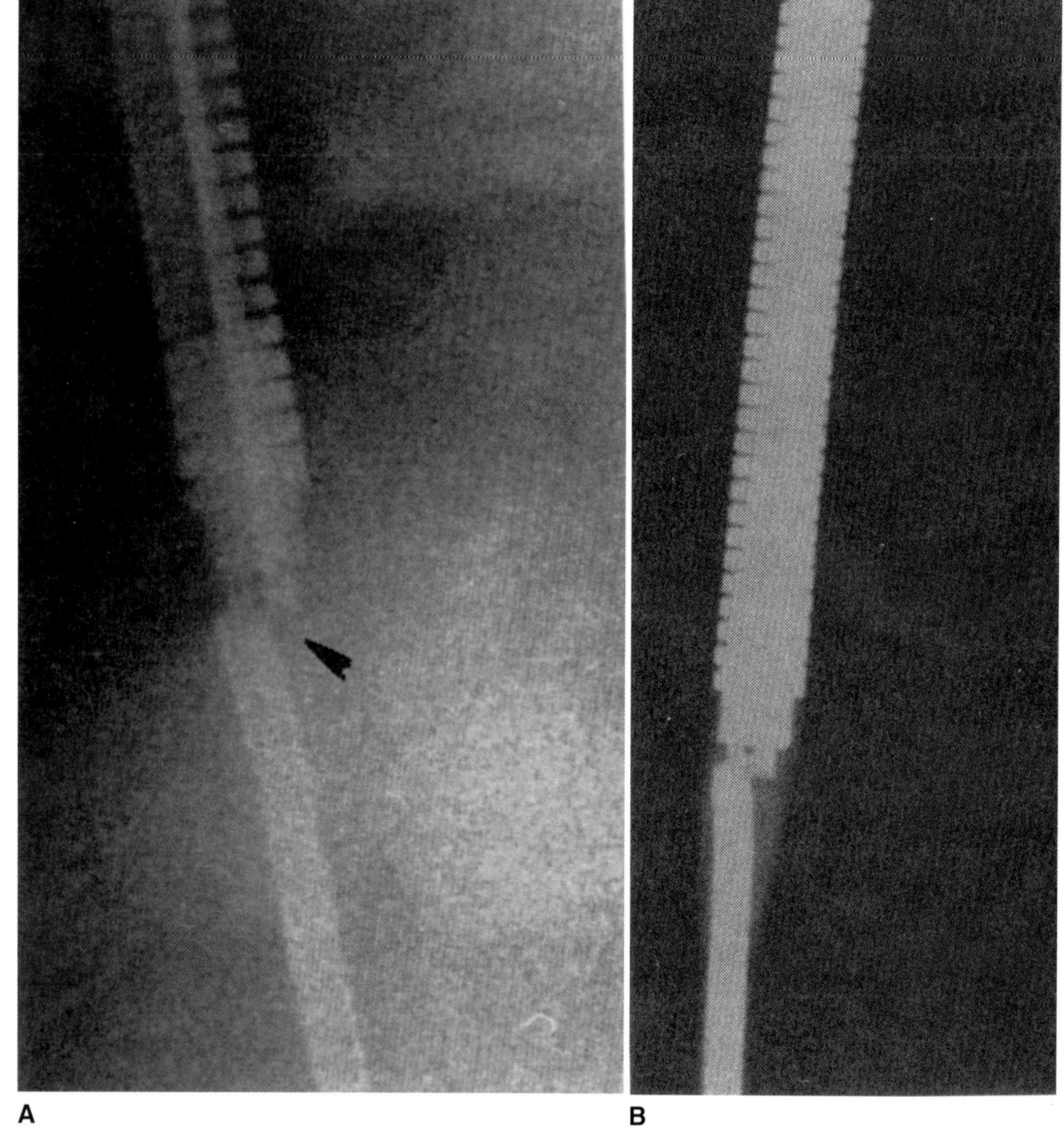

Figure 25-9. ***A,*** *Posteroanterior chest radiograph that was interpreted to show a lead fracture (Endotak, Cardiac Pacemakers, Inc., St. Paul, Minn.). The area is the distal portion of the defibrillation coil with apparent lateral displacement of the electrode* (arrowhead). ***B,*** *Coned-down view of the lead, documenting a continuous metallic connection at the level of the transition from a central electrode to the outer coil. This is the typical appearance of a Guidant Endotak lead, and no fracture is present. (From Kratz JM, Schabel S, Leman RM: Pseudo fracture of a defibrillating lead. PACE 18:2225-2226, 1985.)*

increases in cost of therapy by repeated hospitalizations and testing sessions, and they may jeopardize the doctor-patient relationship. The occurrence of repetitive shocks for whatever reason represents a medical emergency.

The management of multiple ICD shocks must address multiple factors: First, the patient must be comforted, and to do so the underlying rhythm must be determined. Is it sinus, supraventricular, or ventricular? If it is not ventricular, the ICD can be disabled by a magnet or programmer. If it is ventricular, is there a precipitating cause, such as ischemia, heart failure, or lead malfunction? If so, can the shocks be stopped with treatment of the cause, or are antiarrhythmic drugs, β-blockers, or other interventions (e.g., reprogramming, ablation) needed? (These interventions are described later.) Usually, the occurrence of multiple shocks requires admission, because a monitored environment is not only helpful diagnostically but also for patient safety and support.

Perhaps the most difficult causes of multiple shocks to treat are incessant VT and VF. On the one hand, delivered therapy is appropriate; on the other hand, it is not only a horrible experience for patients but also reflects a substrate problem. ICDs do not treat heart disease per se, but only its consequences. Initial

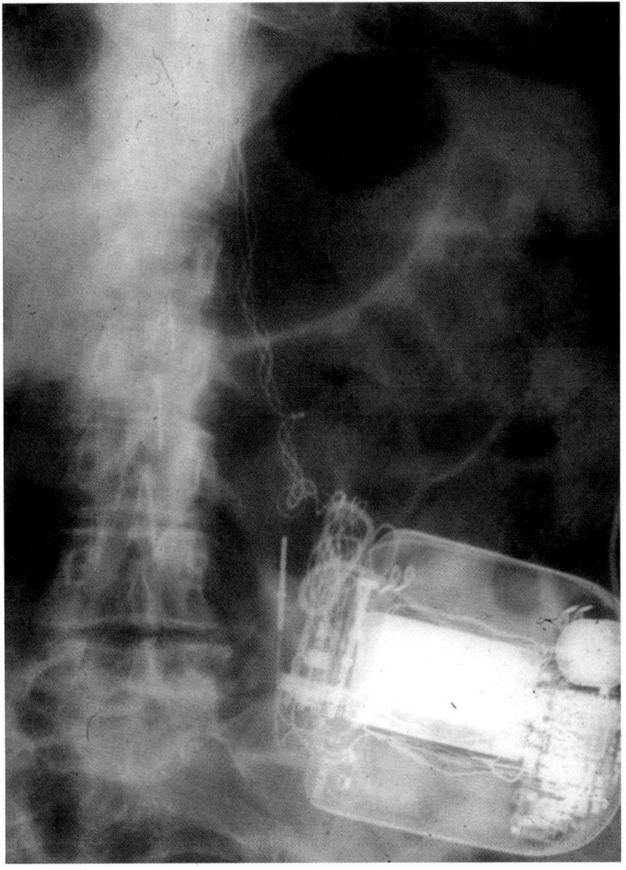

A

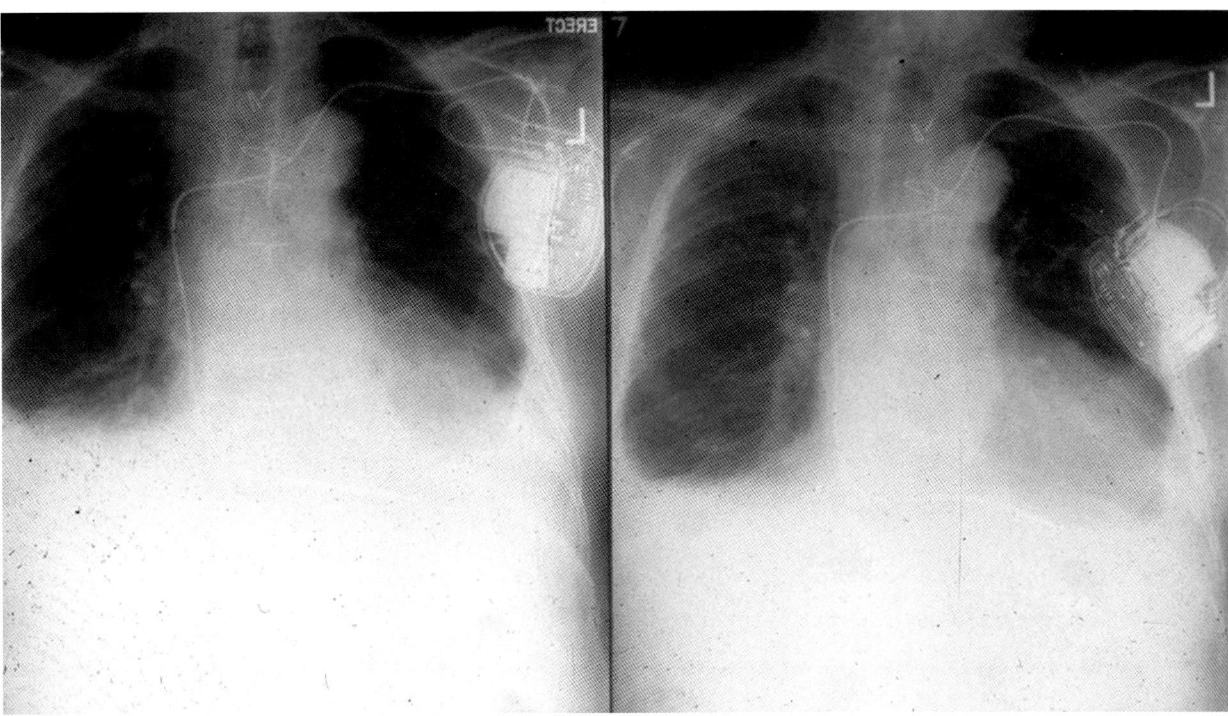

B

*Figure 25-10. Two examples of twiddling. Panel **A** shows a dramatic example of multiple twists of leads in an ICD implanted in the abdomen. Panel **B** shows a more subtle example; the ICD has been rotated 180 degrees. This patient's presentation was one of inability to interrogate the ICD.*

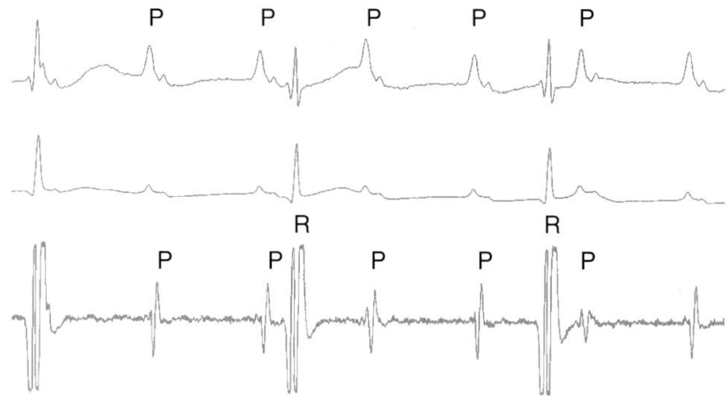

Figure 25-11. Recordings showing counting of both the atrial (P) and ventricular (R) signals from an integrated bipolar ventricular lead (Model RV-1101, Ventritex, Inc., Sunnyvale, Calif.) in a radiographically ideal apical position. Because the patient and her heart were small, the distal spring, used both for defibrillation and as the anode for sensing, came to straddle the tricuspid valve, allowing atrial signals to be recorded.

TABLE 25-2. **Classification of ICD-Induced Proarrhythmia**

ICD-induced tachyarrhythmias
Clinically appropriate therapies, either ATP or shocks leading to:
Acceleration of VT
Deceleration of VT
Induction of supraventricular tachyarrhythmias
Clinically inappropriate therapies
Antitachycardia therapies (ATP, cardioversion, defibrillation) Failure to discriminate between SVT and VT Committed behavior for nonsustained VTs Signal oversensing Electronic noise T or P waves Electromagnetic interference (EMI)
Antibradycardia pacing
Undersensing of spontaneous beats
ICD-induced bradyarrhythmias
Postshock bradyarrhythmias
Postshock increase in pacing threshold leading to noncapture
Postshock reset of a separate pacemaker
Inhibition of antibradycardia pacing due to T-wave oversensing

ATP, antitachycardia pacing; ICD, implantable cardioverter-defibrillator; SVT, supraventricular tachycardia; VT, ventricular tachycardia.
Modified and adapted from Pinski SL, Fahy GJ: The proarrhythmic potential of implantable cardioverter-defibrillators. Circulation 92:1651-1664, 1995.

management centers on the administration of drug therapy,[8,9,17,18] and the ICD usually should be disabled by programming or magnet application. Although antiarrhythmics may be useful, particularly intravenous amiodarone, the judicious use of β-blockers has been found to be extremely beneficial.[9,18] If VT or VF episodes are repetitive or incessant despite drug therapy, it is often advisable to intubate and sedate the patient, disable the ICD, and use an external defibrillator to manage the arrhythmia events. Intra-aortic balloon counter pulsation has been used on occasion with success. With the increased efficacy of radiofrequency ablation, incessant arrhythmias may be treated with the use of this technique.[19]

Oversensing of P waves, T waves, and even atrial flutter may lead to repetitive shocks.[20-22] Atrial oversensing in the ventricle is uncommon; it is usually seen with integrated bipolar leads when the proximal spring is close to or straddling the tricuspid valve, as shown in Figure 25-11.[20,21] P-wave sensing may also be seen when a lead is dislodged to the right atrioventricular junction, as in Figure 25-6. More commonly, T waves are sensed due to their large size relative to the R wave, but sometimes simply because the T wave is huge. Such an example is shown on Figure 25-12 from a patient with hypertrophic cardiomyopathy. Rarely, T-wave oversensing occurs during rate-related bundle branch block,[23] hyperglycemia,[24] and the Brugada syndrome.[25]

First reported in the mid-1990s, myopotentials can also be sensed and interpreted as a ventricular arrhythmia, leading to inappropriate shock therapy. These may arise from the pectoral muscles[26,27] or from the diaphragm.[28,29] The latter has occurred not uncommonly with integrated bipolar leads that presumably lie near the respiratory muscles (Fig. 25-13).

Oversensing can often be rectified by altering the sensitivity or refractory period of the ICD. However, if T waves are large and R waves are small, changing the sensitivity will not suffice. If the sensitivity is decreased, VF may not be identified (Fig. 25-14). Similarly, lockouts imposed by the device to ensure arrhythmia detection limits programming of device refractory periods. One manufacturer provides greater programmability to overcome these problems. Because ICDs, in contrast to pacemakers, vary their sensitivity to identify ventricular activity, altering the amplitude and timing at which sensitivity is adjusted can address this problem.

For the patient with hypertrophic cardiomyopathy, shown on Figure 25-12, the R wave was greater than 25 mV, and the T wave greater than 4 mV. If the sensitivity were decreased significantly, VF might not be reliably sensed. Furthermore, because of prolonged repolarization and sensing of the terminal portion of the T wave, prolonging the ventricular refractory period would not suffice to correct this problem. In this case, avoidance of T-wave oversensing was achieved by altering the threshold start, the decay delay, and the sensitivity. Alternatively, on rare occasions an ICD lead may need to be repositioned or a separate sensing lead placed in a different area of the right ventricle.

In anticipation of T-wave oversensing in the future, one approach that may be useful is to test VF detection

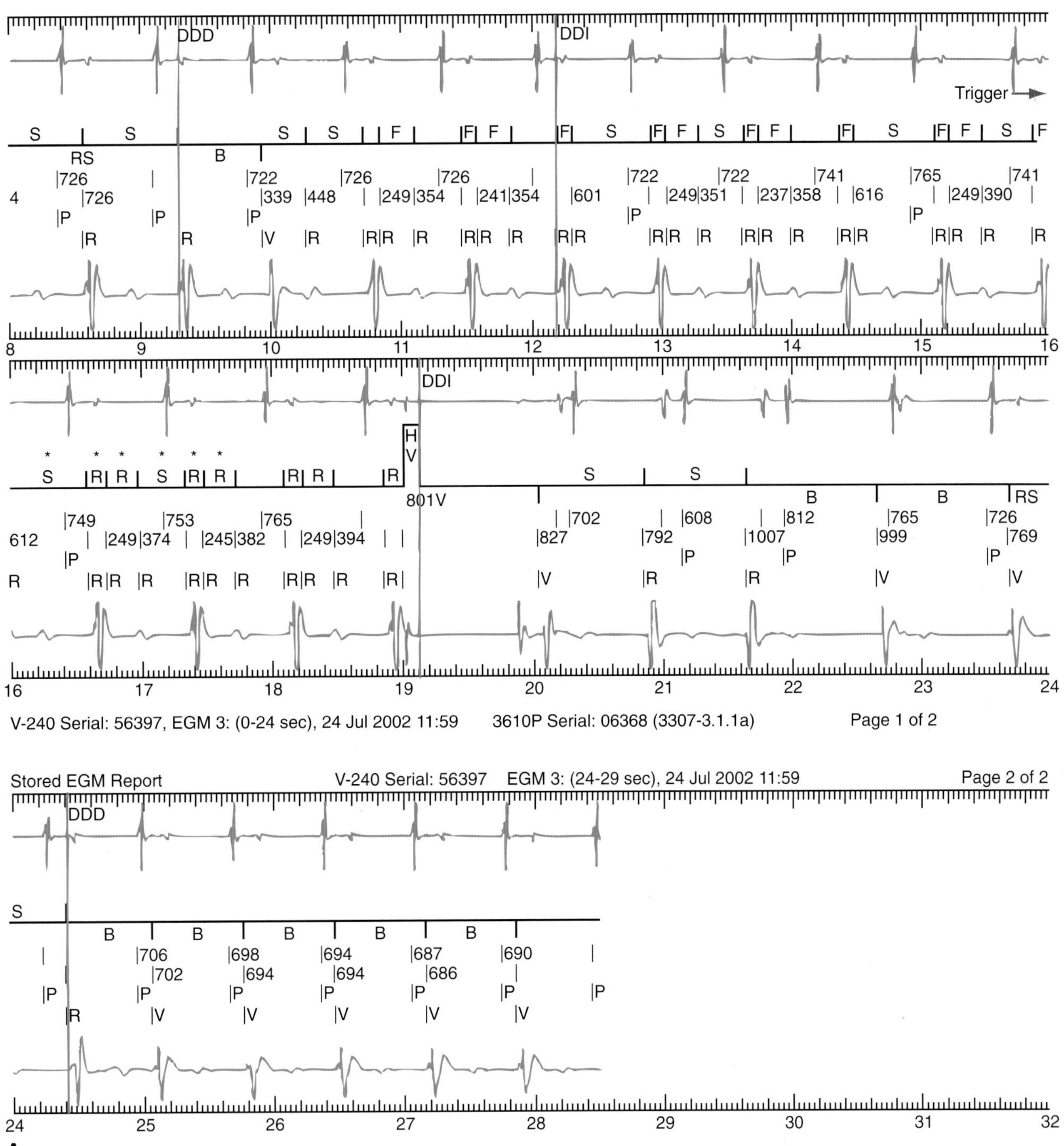

Figure 25-12. Oversensing in a patient with hypertrophic cardiomyopathy. The system comprises a Model V145AC ICD (Ventritex, Inc., Sunnyvale, Calif.), a bipolar atrial lead, and a Model 6936 defibrillation lead (Medtronic, Inc., Minneapolis, Minn.). In Panel **A,** *the tracings from top to bottom show the atrial EGM, the marker channels, and the ventricular EGM. There is both double-counting of the R and T waves (registered as VR in the third beat in the first tracing) and double-counting of multiple components of the R wave itself (registered as RR in both the first and second continuous tracings). In addition, there is triple-counting of both R-wave components and the T wave (registered as RR-R) that leads to fibrillation detection (labeled F) and an ICD shock (labeled HV) in sinus rhythm. The R wave was greater than 25 mV, and the T wave greater than 4 mV. Oversensing was corrected by programming: the threshold start (the signal amplitude at which the sensing sensitivity begins) and the decay delay (the time after a sensed beat when the sensitivity begins to increase) were extended, and the sensitivity was decreased. To ensure proper function, ventricular fibrillation was induced after programming to show that, with more restrictions on sensing, ventricular fibrillation could still be sensed appropriately by the ICD.*

Continued

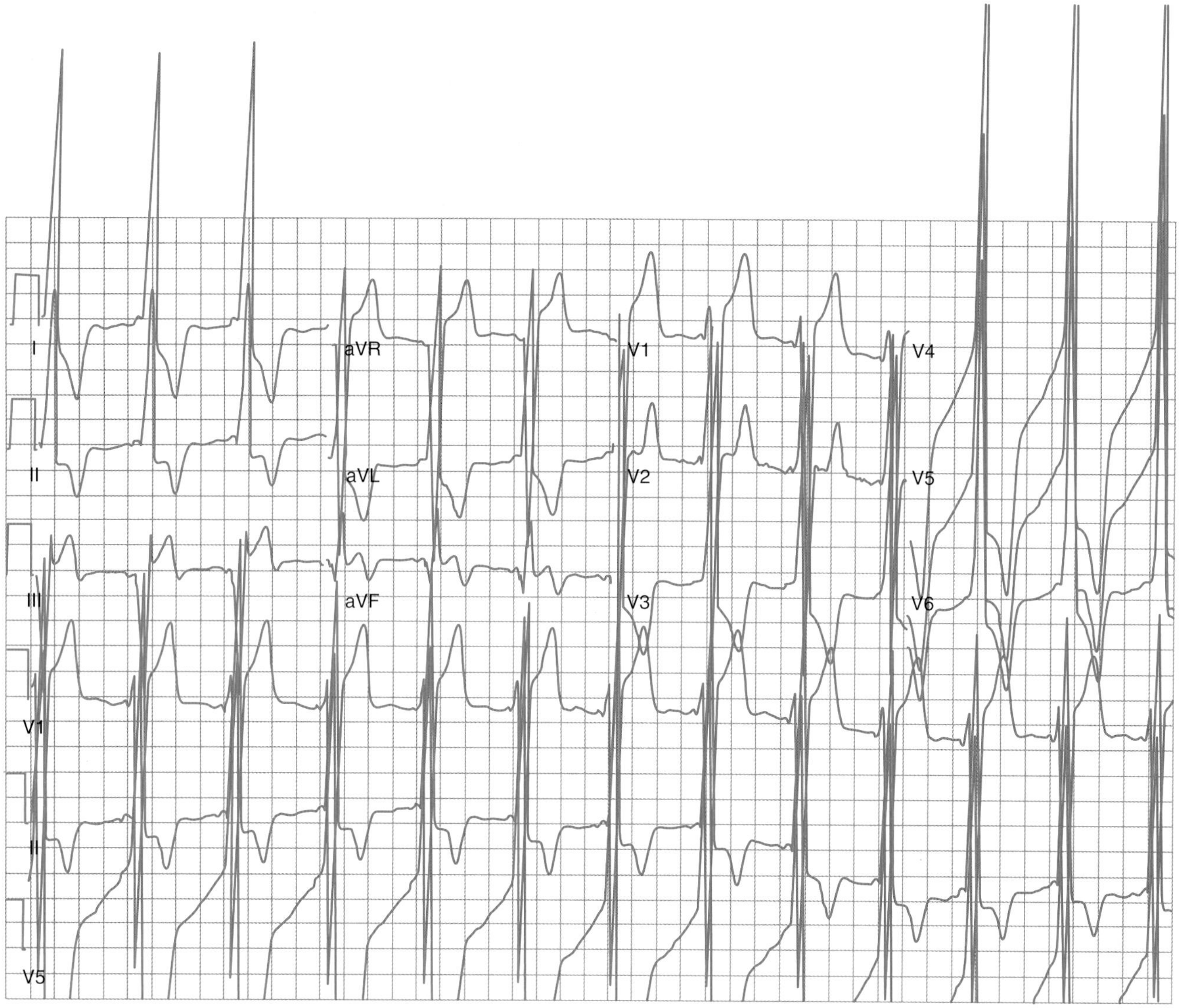

B

Figure 25-12, cont'd. Panel **B** shows the remarkable 12-lead electrocardiogram (ECG) from this patient demonstrating marked left ventricular hypertrophy/voltage.

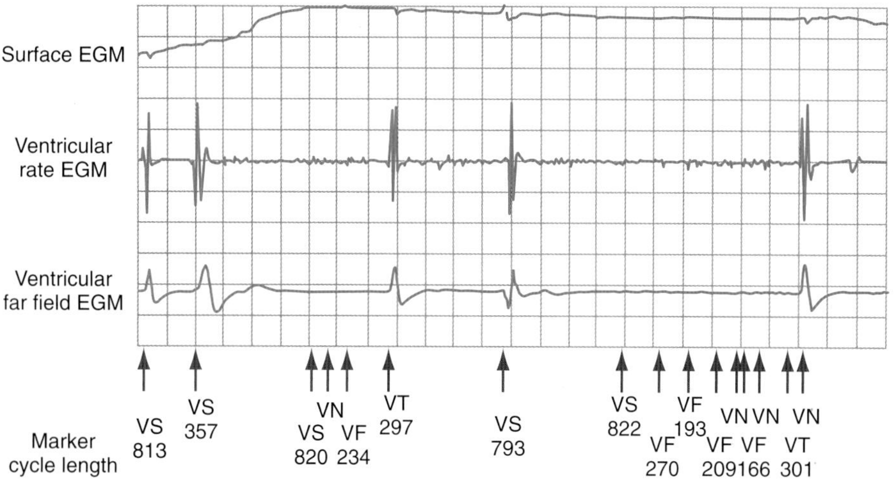

Figure 25-13. Diaphragmatic sensing is demonstrated from a Guidant ICD (Boston Scientific, Natick, Mass.). The three recordings show the surface electrocardiogram (labeled "Surface EGM") the EGM from the sensing lead (labeled "Ventricular rate EGM"), and the EGM from the high-voltage lead (labeled "Ventricular far field EGM"). The marker channel is shown at the bottom. During a Valsalva maneuver, rapid, high-frequency activity is recorded on the sensing channel and is judged by the ICD as ventricular fibrillation (VF). VN, ventricular noise (as defined by the ICD); VS, ventricular sensing. (From Schulte B, Sperzel J, Carlsson J, et al: Inappropriate arrhythmia detection in implantable defibrillator therapy due to oversensing of diaphragmatic myopotentials. J Intervent Cardiac Electrophysiol 5:487-493, 2001.)

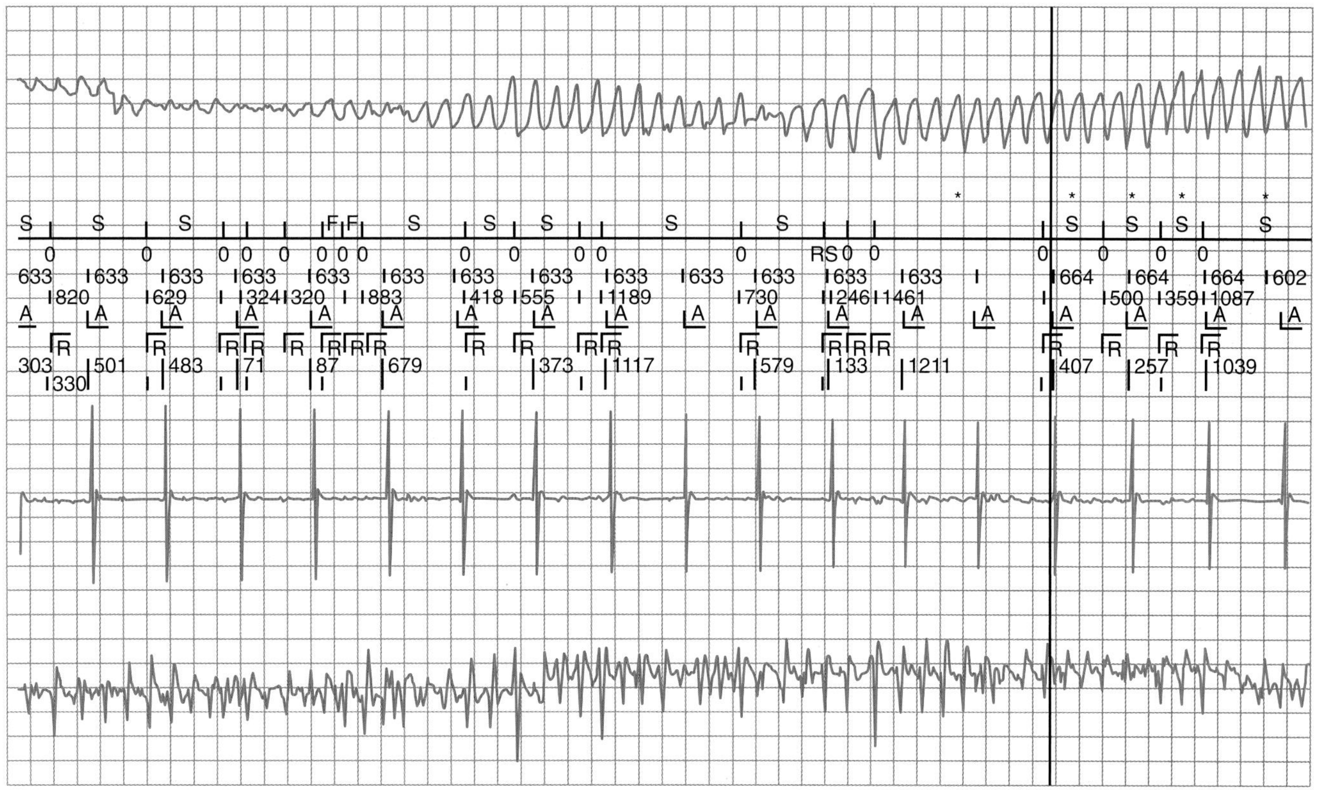

Figure 25-14. *Made during ICD testing, this recording shows ventricular fibrillation that was not detected by a Model V232 ICD (St. Jude Medical, Sunnyvale, Calif.), because the EGM amplitude was below the sensitivity for detection. The tracings show the surface electrocardiogram (ECG), the marker channel, the atrial EGM, and the ventricular EGM. Notice that in the marker channel, only two intervals labeled "F" are shown that signified ventricular fibrillation detection. "S" indicates an EGM interval longer than the tachycardia detection interval. Also note that the zeroes under the marker channel line indicate the absence of a template match with sinus rhythm, but ventricular fibrillation is still not diagnosed, because the cycle length is not short enough as assessed by the ICD sensing circuit. The gain of the ventricular electrogram recording was 6.0 mV/cm, indicating that many of the fibrillation signals were less than 0.5 mV.*

at low sensitivity at the time of implantation. Then, if oversensing occurs in the latter, sensitivity may be decreased without the need for retesting of defibrillation sensing. On the other hand, whenever sensitivity is decreased from a level that has been tested and shown to provide adequate detection of VF, it is imperative to retest VF detection with an electrophysiologic study to demonstrate adequate sensing (see Fig. 25-14).

The sensing of external electrical activity may lead to false detection. In this decade, because of the increased use of ICDs and relatively low lead failure rates, the most common cause (after lead failure, discussed later) is probably electrocautery (Fig. 25-15).[30,31] Other causes include electronic surveillance systems,[30,32] razors,[33] radiofrequency handheld remote controls,[34] ungrounded electrical tools,[30] fluid in a connector port,[35] transcutaneous electrical nerve stimulation (TENS; Fig. 25-16),[36] personal digital assistants (PDAs),[37] and even slot machines[38] and washing machines.[39]

A common cause of multiple shocks is lead failure.[6,17,40-46] When make-break potentials are recorded by the ICD, the rapid electrical activity is interpreted as VF. This is one of the easiest and most characteristic problems encountered. Figure 25-17 shows an example of such recordings. Note the nonphysiologic (extremely rapid) electrical activity that is the signature of this phenomenon. Lead failure may become apparent after shocks.[43]

Although the higher failure rate of ICD leads compared with pacemaker leads is disheartening, it is to be expected, because they are an order of magnitude more complex. In addition, some models have especially high failure rates including both epicardial[41] and endocardial[42,43] leads. In a recently reported case, there was a 37% failure rate (confidence interval, 24% to 54%) at 68.6 months. The study is notable for showing that, not only may failure not become apparent until late follow-up, but also that a "signature" of failure is the occurrence of electrical noise artifact after shock delivery.[43] Failure is not predicted by R-wave changes or changes in pacing characteristics. However, as reported by Gunderson and colleagues,[12] combining the occurrence of an abnormal impedance with a counter showing R-R intervals shorter than 140 msec can identify ICD lead failure with high sensitivity and specificity.

Supraventricular arrhythmias conducting to the ventricles above the ICD detection rate are common causes of multiple shocks.[47] In this instance, device therapy

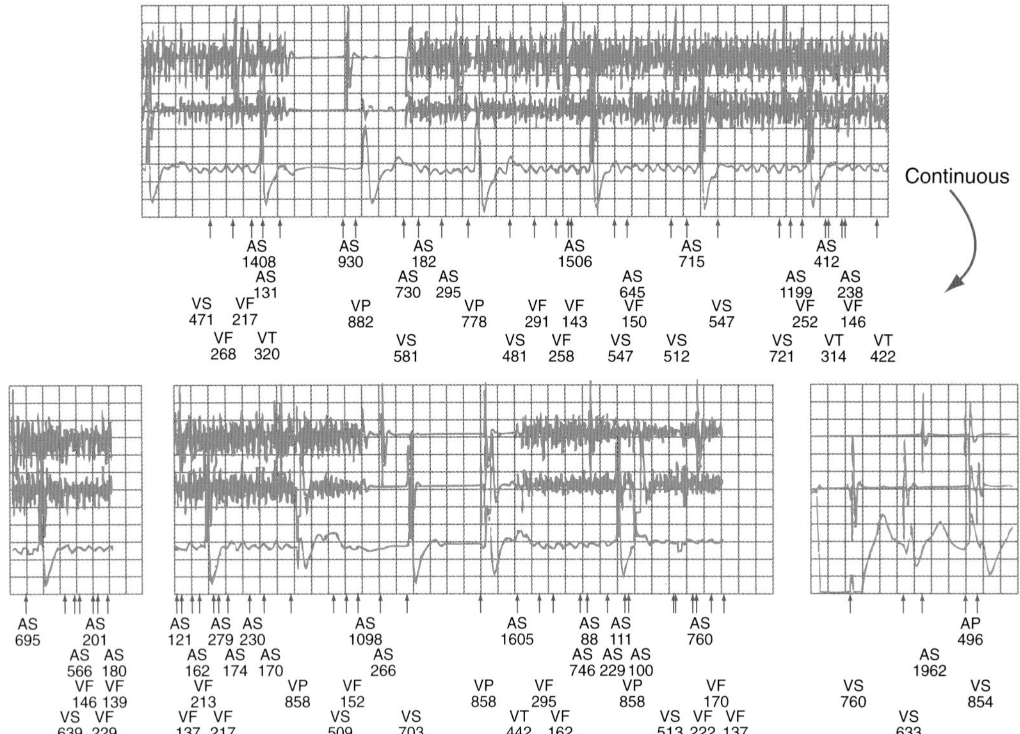

Figure 25-15. This stored EGM was recorded from a Guidant Model 1831 ICD (Boston Scientific, Natick, Mass.) when bipolar cautery was delivered to the patient's ear lobe to remove a skin cancer. Note the electrical noise artifact in the atrial and ventricular sensing-pacing channels (top two EGMs on each tracing, respectively) *but only minimally on the EGM from the high-voltage circuit* (bottom electrograms), *in which sensing does not occur. The atrial and ventricular intrinsic activity can be seen on all channels.*

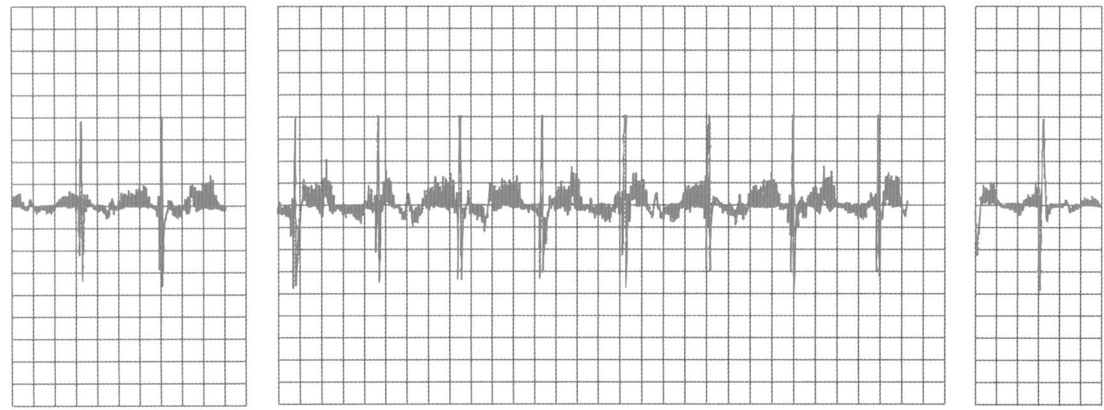

Figure 25-16. The EGM shows electrical noise artifact from a Guidant ICD (Boston Scientific, Natick, Mass.) recorded as the patient applied his spouse's transcutaneous electrical nerve stimulation (TENS) to himself in an attempt to treat muscle aches.

does not reflect malfunction, but rather an appropriate response to tachycardia. The incidence of inappropriate shocks is higher for patients receiving an ICD for primary prevention than those receiving an ICD for secondary prevention.[48,49] In the Sudden Cardiac Death in Heart Failure Trial (SCD-HeFT), 829 patients with class II or III congestive heart failure received an ICD for primary prevention. Of those, 259 (31%) received an ICD shock, and 32% of the shocks were inappropriate. Therefore, 10% of the population receiving a prophylactic ICD received inappropriate shocks.[50]

Atrial fibrillation is the most common cause of multiple shocks in the group of patients undergoing ICD implantation for primary prevention.[49] It can be recognized by its EGM characteristics: the ventricular EGM most often has the same morphology as in sinus rhythm (or atrial fibrillation, if it is the baseline), and it is irregularly irregular (Fig. 25-18). In contrast, polymorphic VT, although irregularly irregular, has varying EGM morphologies (Fig. 25-19).

Detection of atrial arrhythmias may be managed by both drug therapy and device programming. β-Blockers

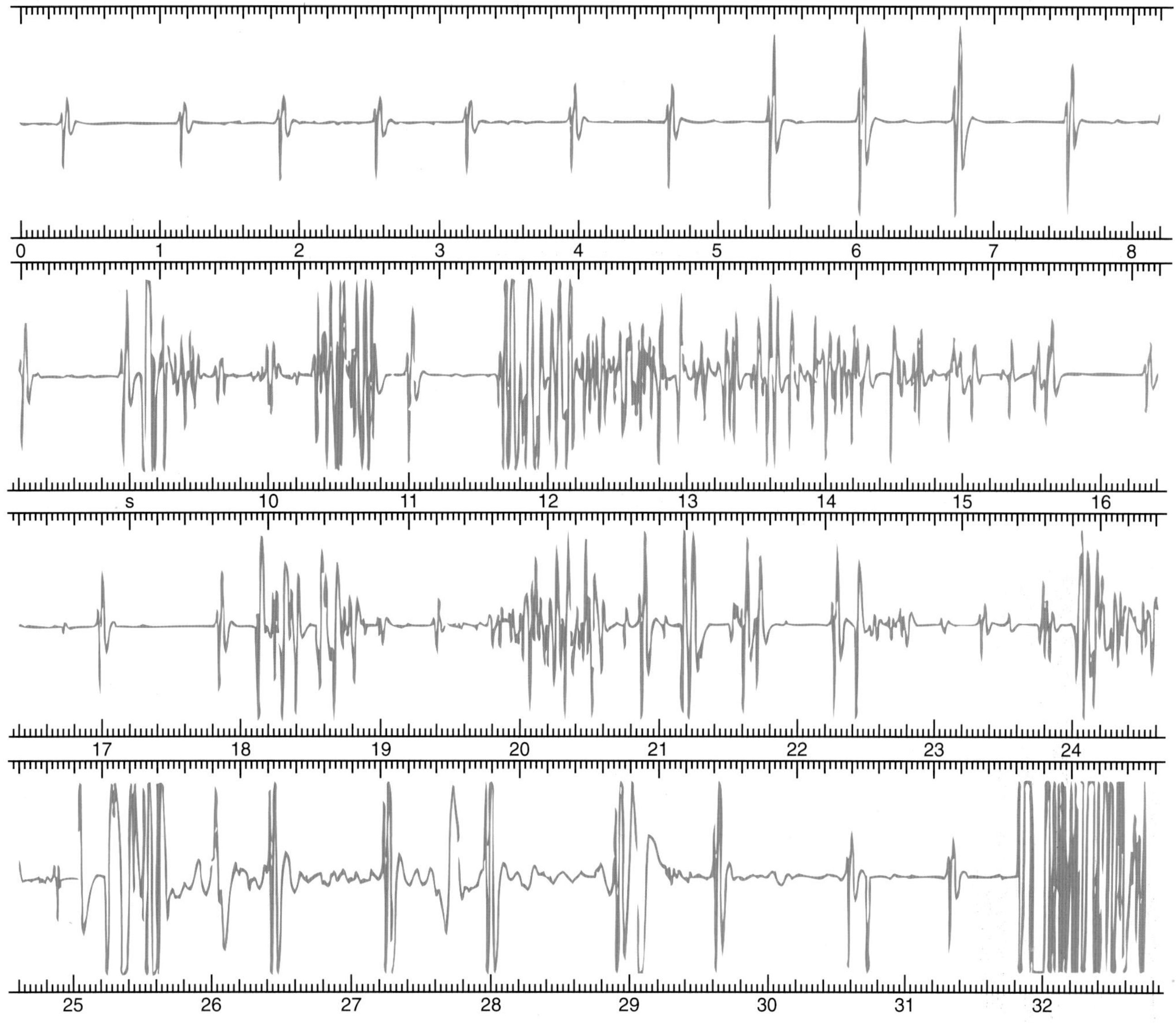

Figure 25-17. The EGM from one of the early devices capable of storing EGMs, a Model V100 ICD (Ventritex, Sunnyvale, Calif. [now part of St. Jude Medical]), shows nonphysiologic, rapid make-break potentials characteristic of conductor fracture.

are a mainstay of therapy to decrease AV conduction, and they are antiarrhythmic themselves. Antiarrhythmic drugs may be prescribed to decrease the frequency of arrhythmia recurrence. Sotalol[51] and azimilide[52] have been efficacious in this regard, and they avoid the organ toxicities associated with amiodarone. ICD programming to avoid inappropriate therapies for supraventricular arrhythmias depend in part on whether a single- or dual-lead system is present.[53-55] For the former, detection enhancements to recognize rate stability and sudden onset are useful. For the latter, these parameters are used in addition to functions that assess AV relationships.

It is controversial whether the addition of an atrial lead improves tachycardia discrimination.[56-58] Multiple reports beginning in the 1990s, when stored EGMs became available, consistently show that the most common cause of inappropriate shocks is SVT.[47] Despite the presence of an atrial lead, the risk of inappropriate shocks from atrial arrhythmias remains about 20% to 30%. In the Antiarrhythmics Versus Implantable Defibrillators (AVID) study, in which single-chamber ICDs were primarily used, the incidence of shocks was 11% for atrial fibrillation and 9% for other SVTs.[48] In a recent randomized trial that compared the incidence of inappropriate therapies from single- with dual-chamber ICDs, 21% of patients in the latter group received inappropriate therapy despite having had detection enhancements enabled.[57] Theuns and associates[58] randomly assigned patients with dual-chamber ICDs to single- or dual-chamber detection. Overall, there was no difference in atrial and ventricular arrhythmia discrimination between the two settings. Figure 25-18 shows an EGM recorded from a patient in whom atrial fibrillation triggered an ICD shock despite a 100% template match with a supraventricular rhythm;

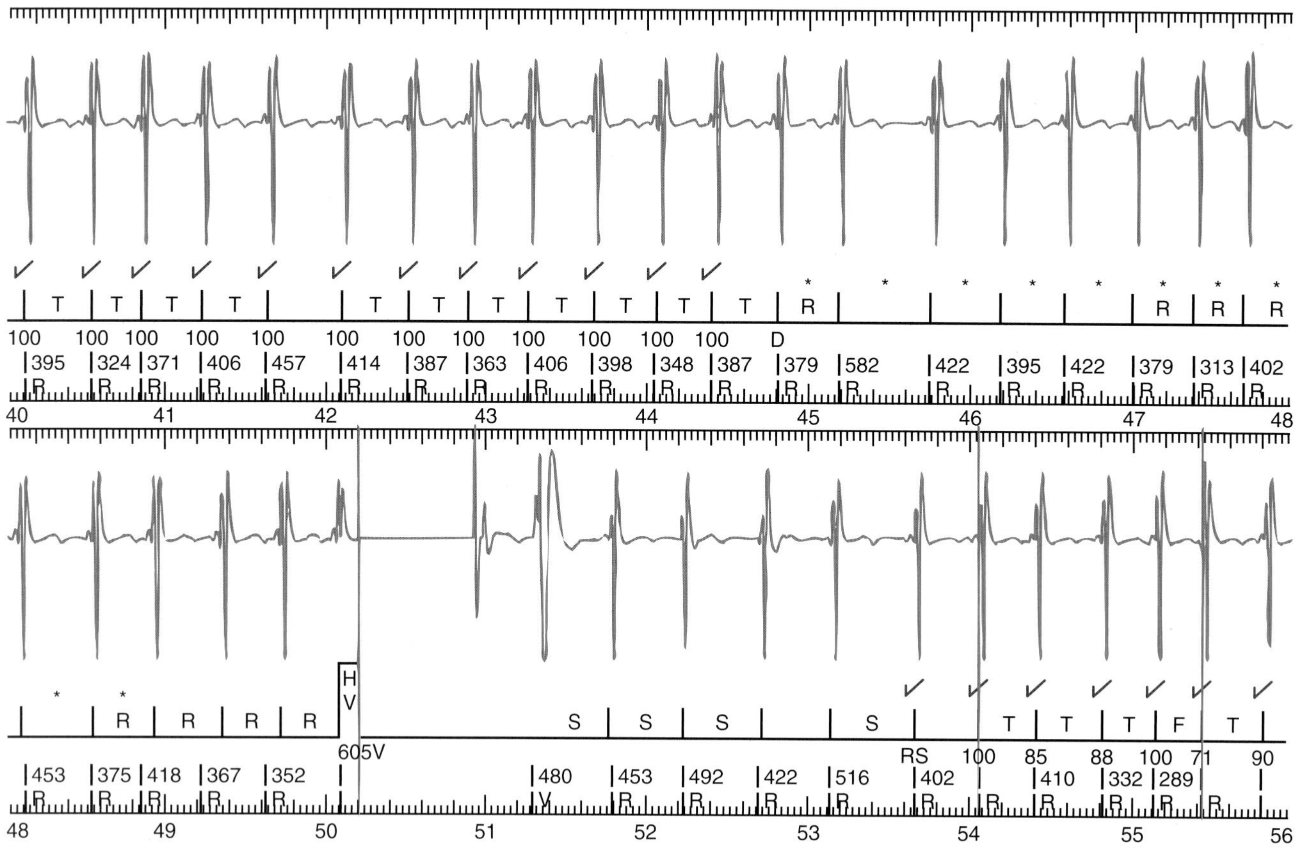

Figure 25-18. *The EGM shows atrial fibrillation above the ventricular tachycardia detection rate leading to an ICD shock (Model V199 ICD, Ventritex, Sunnyvale, Calif. [now part of St. Jude Medical]). The EGM morphology is constant* (top tracing), *and the notations in the marker channel below signify a 100% match to an EGM template of a signal produced by conduction from the atria to the ventricles (i.e., a "sinus beat"). Therapy was delivered because this device has a timer which, when expired, overrides the supraventricular tachycardia discriminator and releases shock therapy as a safety measure so that therapy, if withheld in error, will not be withheld indefinitely.*

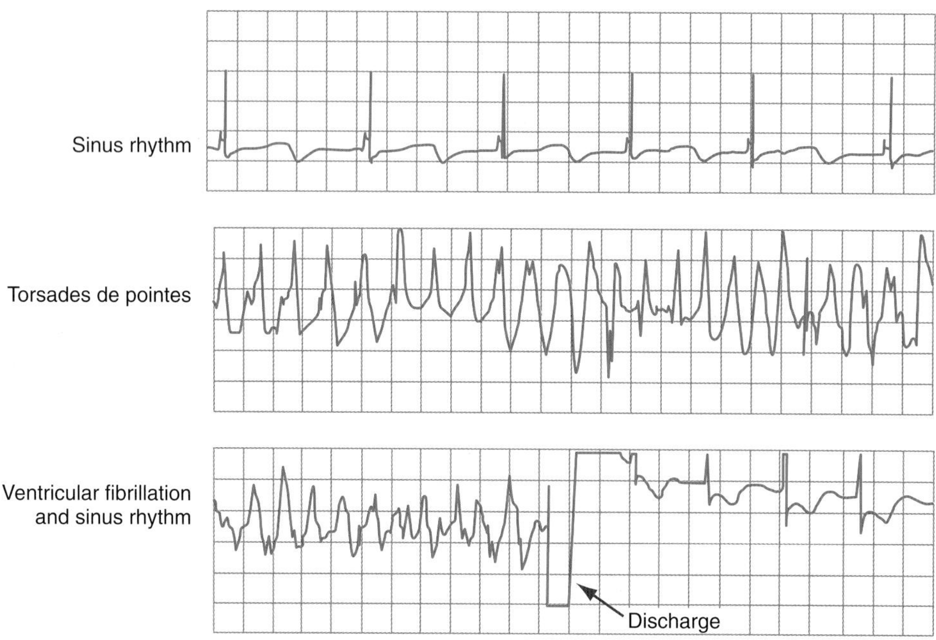

Figure 25-19. *This stored EGM is from a 12-year-old boy with the familial long QT syndrome who had an ICD implanted after resuscitation from a cardiac arrest. After he collapsed in school, ICD interrogation showed sinus rhythm (note the long QT even on the EGM) followed by torsades de pointes ventricular tachycardia, characterized by a polymorphic and constantly changing morphology, and degeneration to ventricular fibrillation (VF). The VF was terminated by a shock, which is labeled on the third tracing. In contrast to the tracing shown in Figure 25-1, there was no monomorphic ventricular tachycardia preceding ventricular fibrillation. (From Moss AJ, Daubert JP: Images in clinical medicine: Internal ventricular defibrillation. N Engl J Med 342:398, 2000.)*

despite the match, the timer withholding therapy expired, overriding the discriminator.

Multiple shocks may also be a proarrhythmic response to drugs or to the ICD itself. Repetitive VT and VF can, of course, be a consequence of antiarrhythmic drug proarrhythmia. In addition, attention to the history may reveal the ingestion of a cardiac stimulant.[59,60] Proarrhythmia may also be caused by the ICD itself.[61-63] Types of device proarrhythmia were reviewed by Pinski and Fahy[62] and are outlined in Table 25-2. A commonly encountered cause of VT induction is undersensing of an ectopic beat followed by a paced beat and subsequent induction of the ventricular arrhythmia (Fig. 25-20). Himmrich and colleagues[63] studied patients with a history of pacemaker-induced tachycardia caused by right ventricular back-up pacing and randomized them to no pacing or to VVI back-up pacing at 60 bpm. No further pacemaker-induced tachycardias occurred in patients in whom pacing was turned off, but they did occur in 5 of 6 patients in whom the pacemaker turned on. The induced arrhythmias were both monomorphic and polymorphic ventricular tachycardias.[63]

A recent development in programmability to decrease the delivery of shock rather than pacing therapy for VT is the option for antitachycardia pacing for very rapid VTs. In the past, it was believed that such an approach would not only be inefficacious but also unsafe. However, Wathen and associates[64,65] showed that, for VTs in the 188 to 250 bpm range, antitachycardia pacing was effective in terminating 81% (72% adjusted). The study was a prospective, randomized trial comparing this treatment strategy with simple shock therapy for fast VTs. The results further showed that empiric antitachycardia pacing was equally safe and was associated with an improved quality of life compared with shock therapy for fast ventricular arrhythmias.[64,65]

Failure to Convert Ventricular Tachycardia or Ventricular Fibrillation

Problems related to the myocardial substrate, ICD programming, or ICD function are the usual reasons for failure to convert an arrhythmia. Changes in substrate are not uncommon and may include ischemia leading to polymorphic ventricular arrhythmias or VF, worsened heart failure that leads to new arrhythmias or conversion to incessant ones, and any combination of events that may increase the pacing, cardioversion, or defibrillation thresholds (Table 25-3).

Problems with therapy most commonly include the programming of ineffective pacing or shock therapies. Antitachycardia pacing may be either underaggressive or overly aggressive, leading to failure of conversion or arrhythmia acceleration.[61-63] If ventricular arrhythmias persist, they may become self-perpetuating due to ischemia and myocardial stretch exacerbated by hemodynamic compromise. These factors, and the arrhythmia duration itself, may also elevate the defibrillation threshold.[66] Other factors that may affect shock efficacy relate not only to the amount of delivered energy but

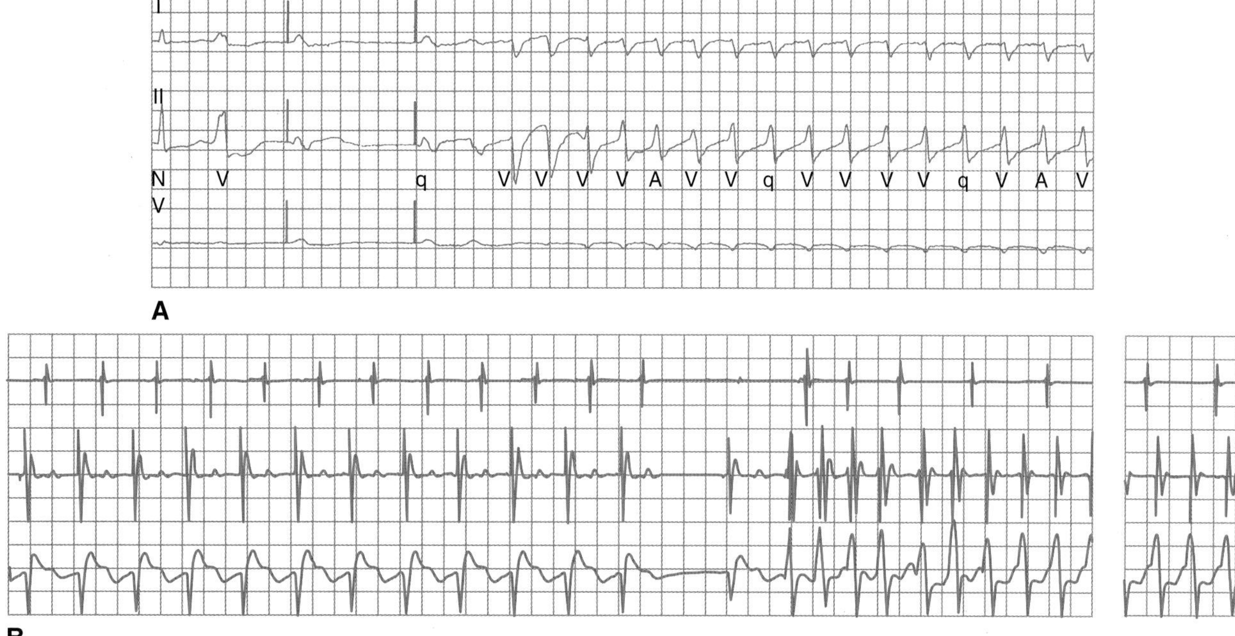

*Figure 25-20. Two examples of pacing-induced ventricular tachycardia are shown. Panel **A** shows telemetry recordings from a hospitalized patient. A premature ventricular contraction (second beat) is not sensed by the ICD; the ICD then delivers two pulses for bradycardia backup pacing, which induce ventricular tachycardia. Panel **B** shows sinus rhythm with a P wave blocked in the atrioventricular conducting system, leading to a pause in the ventricular rhythm. The next ventricular depolarization induces ventricular tachycardia. The three tracings show EGMs from, respectively, the atrial and ventricular pace/sense channels and the high-voltage channel of a dual-chamber ICD (Guidant, Boston Scientific, Natick, Mass.).*

TABLE 25-3. **Nonconversion of Ventricular Tachycardia or Ventricular Fibrillation**

Cause	Management
Problems with VT therapy	*For both VT and VF problems:*
Pacing algorithm	Change therapy prescription
Elevated pacing/ cardioversion threshold	Decrease time to therapy
Incessant VT	Reverse polarity
Problems with VF therapy	Change current path
Elevated defibrillation threshold	Change waveform
Fixed voltage/pulse width	Change drugs that affect rate or DFT
Incessant VF	Treat myocardial substrate
Faulty lead system	
Dislodgment, fracture, loose connector	Revise lead system
ICD failure	Replace ICD
Battery depletion	Replace ICD
ICD-pacemaker interaction	Revise system or reprogram if feasible
Abandoned electrode shunting energy	Extract extra lead

DFT, defibrillation threshold; VF, ventricular fibrillation; VT, ventricular tachycardia.

TABLE 25-4. **Effects of Antiarrhythmic Drugs on Implantable Cardioverter-Defibrillators**

Beneficial
Reduce inappropriate shocks
Suppress sustained VT/SVT
Suppress nonsustained VT/SVT
Enhance antitachycardia pacing
Reduce symptoms by slowing VT rate
Lower DFT (e.g., dofetilide, sotalol)
Adverse
Increase DFT
Increase pacing threshold
Worsen LV function
Proarrhythmia Increase frequency of VT and/or VF Organize atrial fibrillation to atrial flutter with a rapid ventricular response
Sensing interferences Increase tachycardia cycle length such that VT not detected Increase VT cycle length instability so that therapy is inappropriately withheld
Create bradycardia or conduction disturbances leading to: Increased pacing and earlier battery depletion Pacemaker syndrome Worsened CHF by right ventricular pacing-provoked LV dyssynchrony
Cost
Constitutional side effects

CHF, congestive heart failure; DFT, defibrillation threshold; LV, left ventricular; SVT, supraventricular tachycardia; VF, ventricular fibrillation; VT, ventricular tachycardia.

to the shock waveform. For example, efficacy may be improved by altering the tilt of the shock waveform. Evidence indicates that a 50%/50% tilt is more efficacious than the nominal 65%/65% waveform for St. Jude devices.[67] These observations are not transferable to the waveforms of all manufacturers. For Medtronic devices, a randomized comparison of biphasic waveforms with 65%/65% versus 42%/42% tilt found no difference in the defibrillation threshold.[68]

Therapy may also fail if there is component failure of either the ICD or any of its leads. The former is uncommon but has been reported.[1] In the past, defective crystal oscillators led to rapid ventricular pacing, VF, and inability to deliver shock therapy.[69] More recently, electrical overstress (EOS) has led to ICD failure.[70] EOS is the damage to electrical components caused by high voltages or currents that arc within a pulse generator. In addition, there have been recent occurrences of disabling of ICDs, not only electromagnetic interference but also by health care professionals who were unaware that magnet application might permanently inactivate tachycardia detection.[71]

Although interactions between separately implanted pacemakers are less common today, in the past they did interfere with ICD function. Although it was more common for a pacemaker to inhibit detection, by asynchronously pacing during VF (Fig. 25-21), pacing may also reinitiate VT or VF after ICD therapy.[62]

Antiarrhythmic drugs are commonly used in conjunction with ICD therapy (Table 25-4). These agents not only have beneficial effects of decreasing arrhythmia occurrence,[72-74] but they also may affect ICD detection and therapy (Figs. 25-22 and 25-23). Sodium channel blockers and amiodarone may all increase the defibrillation threshold, rendering therapy ineffective.[72-74]

Finally, because until recently remote monitoring has not been available for ICD follow-up[75,76] and warning features (e.g., beeping by the ICD on achievement of the elective replacement indicator),[77] battery depletion may also prevent delivery of effective therapy.

Failure to Detect Ventricular Tachycardia or Ventricular Fibrillation

The first question to ask when an arrhythmia is not detected is whether the ICD system is activated. Is a

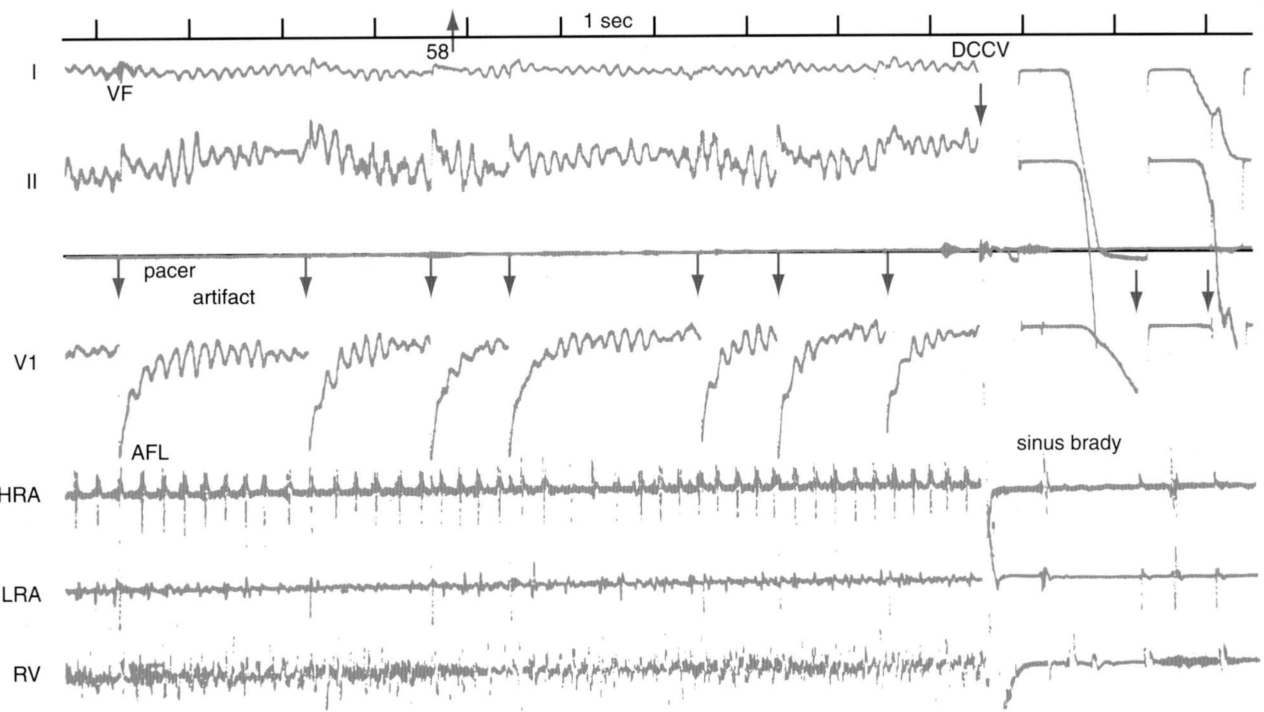

Figure 25-21. The EGM shows the result of intraoperative testing of an ICD implanted with a unipolar pacemaker. The pacemaker was not fully inhibited during ventricular fibrillation (VF), and the large pacemaker artifacts (arrows in lead V1) *were randomly delivered. The ICD failed to recognize VF because it interpreted these large artifacts as a supraventricular rhythm not in the tachycardia detection zone. Sinus rhythm was restored by an external shock (DCCV). (From Kim SG, Furman S, Waspe LE, et al: Unipolar pacer artifacts induced failure of an automatic implantable cardioverter/defibrillator to detect ventricular fibrillation. Am J Cardiol 57:881-882, 1986.)*

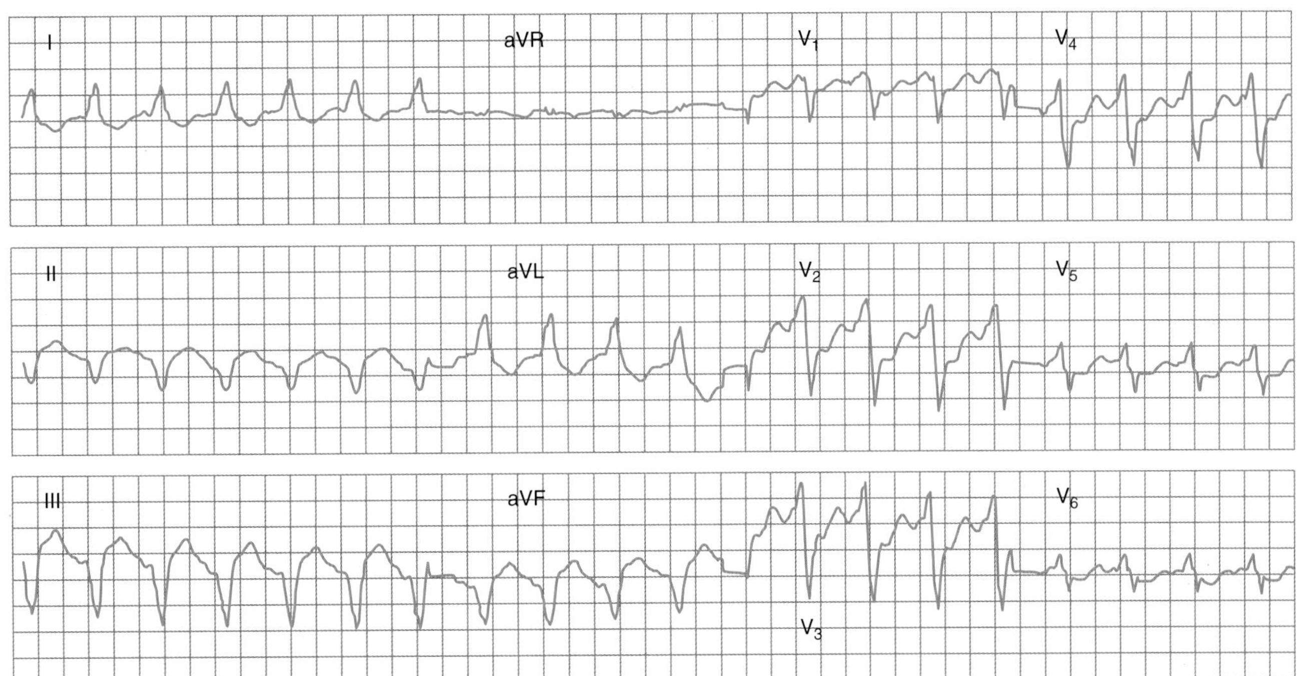

Figure 25-22. This 12-lead electrocardiogram was recorded in the early 1980s, when ICD rate criteria were not programmable. The slow ventricular tachycardia with a rate 113 bpm was well below the ICD detection rate of 156 bpm. Despite symptoms, the patient drove for 4 hours to seek help. Even today, if rate criteria are not satisfied, arrhythmia detection will not occur.

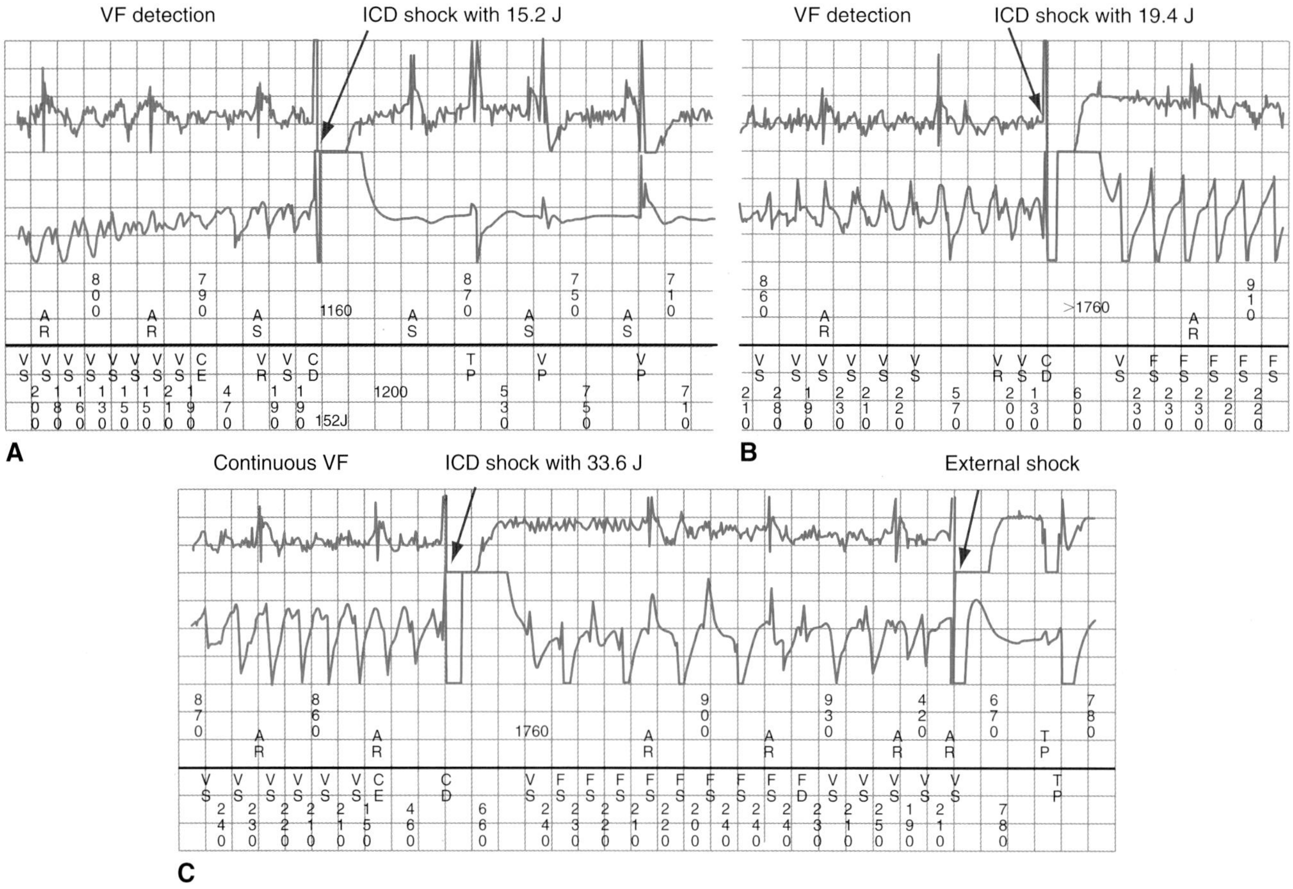

*Figure 25-23. An example of amiodarone increasing the defibrillation threshold. In the absence of amiodarone, the defibrillation threshold was 14 J **(A).** After amiodarone was started for atrial fibrillation, follow-up testing with shocks of 19.4 J **(B)** and 33.6 J **(C)** were ineffective. An external shock was required for restoration of sinus rhythm. The three tracings in all plates show, from top to bottom, the atrial EGM, the ventricular EGM, and the marker channel. (From Rajawat YS, Patel VV, Gerstenfeld EP, et al: Advantages and pitfalls of combining device-based and pharmacologic therapies for the treatment of ventricular arrhythmias: Observations from a tertiary referral center. PACE 27:1670-1681, 2004.)*

magnet over the device, or has one been used to permanently turn it off?[71] Second, if the arrhythmia is ongoing, and is its rate below the ICD detection rate? Has a new drug been started (e.g., amiodarone or a class IC agent) that has slowed the tachycardia rate below the detection rate? (see Fig. 25-22) Has a new drug provoked a new VT, such as torsades de pointes ventricular tachycardia? Is the battery depleted?

The most common reasons for nondetection are inappropriate programming (Table 25-5). Lead dysfunction may also prevent arrhythmia detection. As previously noted, the presence of a second device (e.g., a pacemaker) may lead to detection inhibition if sensing of separate pacemaker stimulus artifacts is interpreted by the ICD as a "normal rhythm." VT and VF may be undersensed (see Fig. 25-14).[78-80] VF nondetection or underdetection is usually due to low-amplitude VF signals (i.e., below the sensitivity of the device). This is more common with integrated bipolar leads than with dedicated bipolar leads.[79]

Detection enhancements have been developed to decrease the frequency of inappropriate shocks due to SVT (Table 25-6). The literature is mixed on the efficacy of detection enhancements to decrease the delivery of inappropriate ICD therapy. On the other hand, the requirement that criteria other than rate must be satisfied before arrhythmia therapy is initiated increases the possibility for falsely failing to detect a ventricular arrhythmia that is present. Swerdlow and coworkers[80] identified six mechanisms of underdetection of VT caused by algorithms to discriminate VT from supraventricular rhythms and nonsustained VT: onset not satisfied (e.g., gradual onset, especially slower ones in the setting of sinus tachycardia), stability not satisfied (e.g., irregular-cycle VT length not satisfying a rate stability criterion to exclude a false diagnosis of atrial fibrillation with a rapid ventricular response as VT or VF), isolated long intervals, VT-VF competition, failure to reconfirm VT, and post-VF suspension of VT detection). Nowadays, another reason for nondetection is morphology of the endocardial EGM similar to that from a supraventricular origin.

A newly recognized cause of underdetection is the application of algorithms to smooth and stabilize the

TABLE 25-5. Nondetection of Ventricular Tachycardia or Ventricular Fibrillation

Cause	Management
Improper/phantom programming (e.g., is system activated?)	Reprogram
VT below detection rate New VT VT slowed by drug(s)	Reprogram detection rate, change drugs
Detection enhancements	Disable, reprogram
Undersensing Deterioration of R wave Oversensing of pacemaker stimulus artifacts	Increase sensitivity Decrease sensitivity, reposition lead
Magnet application	Remove magnet
Battery depletion	Replace device

VT, ventricular tachycardia.

ventricular rate during pacing.[81-84] The common denominator of this mechanism of underdetection is intradevice interaction between pacing parameters and tachycardia detection, which usually leads to the undersensing of ventricular events during blanking periods while pacing. For example, during rate smoothing, to avoid ventricular sensing of atrial stimuli, after each atrial stimulus the ventricular channel is blanked for a fixed interval. In addition, after each ventricular stimulus, the ventricular channel is blanked again. When rate smoothing is activated to decrease symptoms secondary to varying heart rates, ventricular blanking after rapid atrial pacing can lead to nondetection of VT.

Problems with Pacing

Current ICDs provide both bradycardia and antitachycardia pacing therapies. Pacing for either indication may fail because of lead dysfunction or because of a change in the pacing threshold due to a change in substrate or physiologic milieu (e.g., the addition of a drug that increases the pacing threshold, such as flecainide).[74] Radiofrequency ablation may cause not only inappropriate shock therapy but also inhibition of pacing.[85] Although it is theoretically possible that radiofrequency energy may alter the lead-tissue interface and increase the pacing threshold, this has not been observed.[85] However, magnetic resonance imaging (MRI) may increase the pacing threshold and/or alter component function.[86]

As in the case of arrhythmia nondetection, the most common caused of abnormal pacing for bradycardia is inappropriate programming (Table 25-7). Pacing may be inhibited by T-wave[87] and even far-field P-wave sensing in the ventricular channel. As described earlier, oversensing usually leads to inappropriate shock therapy rather than inhibition of pacing.[20-22,88-90] Programming may be both the cause and the remedy for sensing problems.

A most serious and not uncommon cause of abnormal pacing is lead failure, as discussed with regard to the production of electrical noise artifact and inappropriate shocks.[6,17,40-46] ICD leads are complex, with more components than simple pacing leads. This complexity increases the chance for failure. Failure may occur in the conductor, insulation, or connector pins. The fault may be in the header, the yoke, or body of the lead within the vascular system. With subclavian approaches to lead implantation, crush is not uncommon.[4,5] Although the devices are large, "twiddling" may occur (see Fig. 25-10).[15,16] Finally, leads may become dislodged (see Figs. 25-6 and 25-7). Diagnosis of lead failure was discussed in the section on multiple and inappropriate shocks.

Other Issues

Technology has advanced in the field of defibrillation and pacing, as in all fields of medicine, and with progress comes new and unanticipated problems. The use of MRI has expanded, and, although its use is in general contraindicated in patients with an ICD, there is an emerging literature regarding its safety. A completely protected ICD has yet to be developed. Although

TABLE 25-6. Detection Enhancements

Manufacturer	Dual-Chamber Discrimination Enhancements
Biotronik GmbH & Co. (Berlin, Germany)	SMART Detection Algorithm: Ventricular versus atrial rates, P-P and R-R stability, AV relationship and multiplicity, and suddenness of onset
ELA Medical (Sorin Group, Milan)	PARAD Algorithm: R-R stability, P-R association, and ventricular acceleration
Guidant (Boston Scientific, Natick, Mass.)	Suddenness of onset, rate stability, atrial fibrillation rate and stability, and ventricular rate versus atrial rates
Medtronic (Minneapolis, Minn.)	PR Logic Algorithm: Pattern of AV and VA intervals; atrial and ventricular rates; evidence for atrial fibrillation, AV dissociation, and ventricular R-R irregularity; analysis for R-wave sensing in atrial channel; ventricular electrogram morphology
St. Jude Medical (St. Paul, Minn.)	Suddenness of onset, AV association and relation of atrial and ventricular rates, interval stability, and ventricular electrogram morphology

TABLE 25-7. **Problems with Pacing**

Cause	Management
Increased pacing threshold	Reprogram, occasionally replace lead
T-wave sensing inhibits ventricular pacing	Reprogram ventricular refractory period or sensitivity
R-wave sensing inhibits atrial pacing	Reprogram atrial refractory period or sensitivity
Atrial electrical activity inhibits ventricular pacing	Decrease sensitivity or replace lead
Faulty lead system	Revise lead system

some clinicians have suggested that MRI scanning may be safe with newer devices,[86] it is probably premature to make this conclusion. Not only have interactions been reported,[91] series purporting device safety have included only small numbers of patients with relatively few devices. To extrapolate these findings to the more general population would require much greater numbers. Furthermore, even proponents of MRI safety with ICDs acknowledge that "minimal" changes in pacing threshold and battery function may occur.[86] Although a small change in pacing threshold or battery function may be acceptable most of the time, it can be disastrous if safety margins are small, as when batteries are near their end of life or in patients with borderline pacing thresholds.

Rarely, ICD programmers can malfunction. They are slow, and programming is sometimes not intuitive. In the operating room, these issues are frustrating, and malfunction sometimes can be handled only by powering down and rebooting the system or obtaining a new programmer.

Current ICDs are well shielded from external shocks. Nevertheless, it is possible for cardioversion or defibrillation to injure the device. Therefore, whenever external shocks are given, paddles must be placed as far from the ICD as possible. Of course, in an emergency situation, patient resuscitation takes precedence over saving the device. In addition, other medical equipment may injure an ICD, specifically shock wave lithotripsy.[92] The beam should always be aimed away from the ICD if possible.

Finally, psychological issues must be considered when taking care of patients with ICDs, and psychological problems certainly fall into the realm of troubleshooting.[93,94] Among those who have received shocks, imagined shocks, and "phantom shocks," it is not uncommon for the shock to cause concern for patients and their families. Often explanation is satisfactory, but sometimes fear of shocks can be debilitating, akin to a post-traumatic stress disorder. Not only counseling but also drug therapy to decrease anxiety and depression may be warranted. The combination of a benzodiazepine and serotonin reuptake inhibitor is especially useful.

Summary

ICD troubleshooting requires systematic analysis of evidence based on history, physical examination, and analysis of retrieved ICD information. Problems may be approached from the perspective of clinical presentation (failure to detect, failure to convert, problems with pacing) or those of the system components (ICD battery, programming, integrity, and lead integrity and function). With the remarkable diagnostic capabilities of current devices, the reason for an ICD system problem can usually be identified and, in the absence of component failure, remedied by reprogramming.

REFERENCES

1. Hauser RG, Kallinen L: Deaths associated with implantable cardioverter defibrillator failure and deactivation reported in the United States Food and Drug Administration Manufacturer and User Facility Device Experience Database. Heart Rhythm 4:399-405, 2004.
2. Epstein AE: Approach to the patient with suspected implantable cardioverter-defibrillator system malfunction. J Cardiovasc Electrophysiol 2:330-333, 1998.
3. Ballas SL, Rashidi R, McAlister H, et al: The use of beep-o-grams in the assessment of automatic implantable cardioverter defibrillator sensing function. PACE 12:1737-1745, 1989.
4. Magney JE, Parsons JA, Flynn DM, Hunter DW: Pacemaker and defibrillator lead entrapment: Case studies. PACE 18:1509-1517, 1995.
5. Gallik DM, Ben-Sur U, Gross JN, Furman S: Lead fracture in cephalic versus subclavian approach with transvenous implantable cardioverter defibrillator systems. PACE 19:1089-1094, 1996.
6. Lawton JS, Ellenbogen KA, Wood MA, et al: Sensing lead-related complications in patients with transvenous implantable cardioverter-defibrillators. Am J Cardiol 78:647-651, 1996.
7. Gupta A, Zegel HG, Dravid VS, et al: Value of radiography in diagnosing complications of cardioverter defibrillators implanted without thoracotomy in 437 patients. AJR Am J Roentgenol 168:105-108, 1997.
8. Exner DV, Pinski SL, Wyse DG, et al, and the AVID Investigators: Electrical storm presages nonsudden death: The Antiarrhythmics versus Implantable Defibrillators (AVID) Trial. Circulation 103:2066-2071, 2001.
9. Credner SC, Klingenheben T, Mauss O, et al: Electrical storm in patient with transvenous implantable cardioverter-defibrillators: Incidence, management and prognostic implications. J Am Coll Cardiol 32:1909-1915, 1998.
10. Whang W, Mittleman MA, Rich DQ, et al, for the TOVA Investigators: Heart failure and the risk of shocks in patients with implantable cardioverter defibrillators: Results from the Triggers Of Ventricular Arrhythmias (TOVA) Study. Circulation 109:1386-1391, 2004.
11. Marchlinski FE, Callans DJ, Gottlieb CD, et al: Benefits and lessons learned from stored electrogram information in implantable defibrillators. J Cardiovasc Electrophysiol 6:832-851, 1995.
12. Gunderson BD, Patel AS, Bounds CA, et al: An algorithm to predict implantable cardioverter-defibrillator lead failure. J Am Coll Cardiol 44:1898-1902, 2004.
13. Prickett RA, Saavedra P, Ali MF, et al: Implantable cardioverter-defibrillator malfunction due to mechanical failure of the header connection. J Cardiovasc Electrophysiol 14:1095-1099, 2004.
14. Kratz JM, Schabel S, Leman RM: Pseudo fracture of a defibrillating lead. PACE 18:2225-2226, 1985.

15. Beauregard LAM, Russo AM, Heim J, et al: Twiddler's syndrome complicating automatic defibrillator function. PACE 18:735-738, 1995.
16. Boyle NG, Anselme F, Monahan KM, et al: Twiddler's syndrome variants in ICD patients. PACE 21:2685-2687, 1998.
17. Miller JM, Hsia HH: Management of the patient with frequent discharges from implantable cardioverter defibrillator devices. J Cardiovasc Electrophysiol 7:278-285, 1996.
18. Nademanee K, Taylor R, Bailey WE, et al: Treating electrical storm: Sympathetic blockade versus advance cardiac life support-guided therapy. Circulation 102:742-747, 2000.
19. Marchlinski FE, Callans DJ, Gottlieb CD, Zado E: Linear ablation lesions for control of unmappable ventricular tachycardia in patients with ischemic and nonischemic cardiomyopathy. Circulation 101;1288-1296, 2000.
20. Peters W, Kowallik P, Wittenberg G, et al: Inappropriate discharge of an implantable cardioverter defibrillator during atrial flutter and intermittent ventricular antibradycardia pacing. J Cardiovasc Electrophysiol 8:1167-1174, 1997.
21. Scaglione J, Socas AG, De Palma C, Kreutzer E: Inappropriate single chamber ICD discharges due to supraventricular tachycardia with high degree atrioventricular block. J Intervent Cardiac Electrophysiol 11:73-76, 2004.
22. Kelly PA, Mann DE, Damle RS, Reiter MJ: Oversensing during ventricular pacing in patients with a third-generation implantable cardioverter-defibrillator. J Am Coll Cardiol 23:1531-1534, 1994.
23. Coyne RF, Man DC, Sarter BH, et al: Implantable cardioverter defibrillator oversensing during periods of rate-related bundle branch block. J Cardiovasc Electrophysiol 8:807-811, 1997.
24. Krishen A, Shepard RK, Leffler JA, et al: Implantable cardioverter defibrillator T wave oversensing caused by hyperglycemia. PACE 24:1701-1703, 2001.
25. Porres JM, Brugada J, Marco P, et al: T wave oversensing by a cardioverter defibrillator implanted in patient with the Brugada syndrome. PACE 27:1563-1565, 2004.
26. Sandler MJ, Kutalek SP: Inappropriate discharge by an implantable cardioverter defibrillator: Recognition of myopotentials sensing using telemetered intracardiac electrograms. PACE 17:665-671, 1994.
27. Karanam S, John RM: Inappropriate sensing of pectoral myopotentials by an implantable cardioverter defibrillator system. PACE 27:688-689, 2004.
28. Sweeney MO, Ellison KE, Shea JB, Newell JB: Provoked and spontaneous high-frequency, low-amplitude, respirophasic noise transients in patients with implantable cardioverter defibrillators. J Cardiovasc Electrophysiol 12:402-410, 2001.
29. Schulte B, Sperzel J, Carlsson J, et al: Inappropriate arrhythmia detection in implantable defibrillator therapy due to oversensing of diaphragmatic myopotentials. J Intervent Cardiac Electrophysiol 5:487-493, 2001.
30. Pinski SL, Trohman RG: Interference in implanted cardiac devices: Part 1. PACE 25:1367-1381, 2002.
31. Casavant D, Haffajee C, Stevens S, Pacetti P: Aborted implantable cardioverter-defibrillator shock during facial electrosurgery. PACE 21:1325-1326, 1998.
32. Matthew P, Lewis C, Neglia J, et al: Interaction between electronic article surveillance systems and implantable defibrillators: Insights from a fourth generation ICD. PACE 20:2857-2859, 1997.
33. Seifert T, Block M, Borggrefe M, Breithardt G: Erroneous discharge of an implantable cardioveter-defibrillator caused by an electric razor. PACE 18:1592-1594, 1995.
34. Man KC, Davidson T, Langberg JJ, et al: Interference from a hand held radiofrequency remote control causing discharge of an implantable defibrillator. PACE 16:1756-1758, 1993.
35. Heif C, Podczeck A, Krohner K, et al: Cardioverter discharges following sensing of electrical artifact due to fluid penetration in the connector port. PACE 18:1589-1591, 1995.
36. Crevenna R, Stix G, Pleiner J, et al: Electromagnetic interference by transcutaneous neuromuscular electrical stimulation in patients with bipolar sensing implantable cardioverter defibrillators: A pilot safety study. PACE 26:626-629, 2003.
37. Tri JL, Trusty JM, Hayes DL: Potential for personal digital assistant interference with implantable cardiac devices. Mayo Clin Proc 79:1527-1530, 2004.
38. Madrid A, Sánchez A, Bosch E, et al: Dysfunction of implantable defibrillators caused by slot machines. PACE 20:212-214, 1997.
39. Sabaté X, Moure C, Nicholás J, et al: Washing machine associated 50 Hz detected as ventricular fibrillation by an implanted cardioverter defibrillator. PACE 24:1281-1283, 2001.
40. Lawton JS, Wood MA, Gilligan DM, et al: Implantable transvenous cardioverter defibrillator leads: the dark side. PACE 19:1273-1278, 1996.
41. Brady PA, Friedman PA, Trusty JM, et al: High failure rate for an epicardial implantable cardioverter-defibrillator lead: Implications for long-term follow-up of patients with an implantable cardioverter-defibrillator. J Am Coll Cardiol 31:616-622, 1998.
42. Stambler BS, Wood MA, Damiano RJ, et al, and the Guardian ATP 4210 Multicenter Investigators: Sensing/pacing lead complications with a newer generation implantable cardioverter-defibrillator: Worldwide experience from the Guardian ATP 4210 Clinical Trial. J Am Coll Cardiol 23:123-132, 1994.
43. Ellenbogen KA, Wood MA, Shepard RK, et al: Detection and management of an implantable cardioverter defibrillator lead failure: Incidence and clinical implications. J Am Coll Cardiol 41:73-80, 2003.
44. Dorwarth U, Frey B, Dugas M, et al: Transvenous defibrillation leads: High incidence of failure during long-term follow-up. J Cardiovasc Electrophysiol 14:38-43, 2003.
45. Hauser RG, Cannom D, Hayes DL, et al: Long-term structural failure of coaxial polyurethane implantable cardioverter defibrillator leads. PACE 25:879-882, 2002.
46. Kettering K, Mewis C, Dörnberger V, et al: Long-term experience with subcutaneous ICD leads: A comparison among three different types of subcutaneous leads. PACE 27:1355-1361, 2004.
47. Grimm W, Flores BF, Marchlisnski FE: Electrocardiographically documented unnecessary, spontaneous shocks in 241 patients with implantable cardioverter defibrillators. PACE 15:1667-1673, 1992.
48. Klein RC, Raitt MH, Wilkoff BL, et al, and The AVID Investigators: Analysis of implantable cardioverter defibrillator therapy in the Antiarrhythmics versus Implantable Defibrillators (AVID) Trial. J Cardiovasc Electrophysiol 14:940-948, 2003.
49. Daubert JP, Zareba W, Cannom DS, et al: Frequency and mechanism of inappropriate implantable cardioverter defibrillator therapy in MADIT II. J Am Coll Cardiol 43:132A, 2004.
50. Bardy GH, Lee KL, Mark DB, et al, for the Sudden Cardiac Death in Heart Failure Trial (SCD-HeFT) Investigators: Amiodarone or an implantable cardioverter-defibrillator for congestive heart failure. N Engl J Med 352:225-237, 2005.
51. Pacifico A, Hohnloser SH, Williams JH, et al, for the d,l-Sotalol Implantable Cardioverter-Defibrillator Study Group. N Engl J Med 340:1855-1862, 1999.
52. Singer I, Al-Khalidi H, Niazi I, et al: Azimilide decreases recurrent ventricular tachyarrhythmias in patients with implantable cardioverter defibrillators. J Am Coll Cardiol 43:39-43, 2004.
53. Swerdlow CD, Chen PS, Kass RM, et al: Discrimination of ventricular tachycardia from sinus tachycardia and atrial fibrillation in a tiered-therapy cardioverter-defibrillator. J Am Coll Cardiol 23:1342-1355, 1994.
54. Dorian P, Philippon F, Thibault B, et al, for the ASTRID Investigators: Randomized controlled study of detection enhancements versus rate-only detection to prevent inappropriate therapy in a dual-chamber implantable cardioverter-defibrillator. Heart Rhythm 1:540-547, 2004.
55. Hintringer F, Deibl M, Berger T, et al: Comparison of the specificity of implantable dual chamber defibrillator detection algorithms. PACE 27:976-982, 2004.

56. Swerdlow CD: Supraventricular tachycardia-ventricular tachycardia discrimination algorithms in implantable cardioverter defibrillators: State-of-the-art review. J Cardiovasc Electrophysiol 12:606-612, 2001.
57. Deisenhofer I, Kolb C, Ndrepeppa G, et al: Do current dual chamber cardioverter defibrillators have advantages over conventional single chamber cardioverter defibrillators in reducing inappropriate therapies? A randomized, prospective study. J Cardiovasc Electrophysiol 12:134-142, 2001.
58. Theuns DAMJ, Klootwijk APJ, Goedhart DM, Jordaens LJLM: Prevention of inappropriate therapy in implantable cardioverter-defibrillators: Results of a prospective, randomized study of tachyarrhythmia detection algorithms. J Am Coll Cardiol 44; 2362-2367, 2004.
59. Goldstein DS, Epstein AE: A shocking case of pseudoephedrine use. J Intervent Card Electrophysiol 3:343-344, 1999.
60. McBride BF, Guertin D, White CM, Kluger J: Inappropriate implantable cardioverter defibrillator discharge following consumption of a dietary weight loss supplement. PACE 27:1317-1320, 2004.
61. Johnson NJ, Marchlinski FE: Arrhythmias induced by device antitachycardia therapy due to diagnostic nonspecificity. J Am Coll Cardiol 18:1418-1425, 1991.
62. Pinski SL, Fahy GJ: The proarrhythmic potential of implantable cardioverter-defibrillators. Circulation 92:1651-1664, 1995.
63. Himmrich E, Przibille O, Zellerhoff C, et al: Proarrhythmic effect of pacemaker stimulation in patients with implanted cardioverter-defibrillators. Circulation 108:192-197, 2003.
64. Wathen MS, Sweeney MO, GeGroot PJ, et al, for the PainFREE Rx Investigators: Shock reduction using antitachycardia pacing for spontaneous rapid ventricular tachycardia in patients with coronary artery disease. Circulation 104:796-801, 2001.
65. Wathen MS, GeGroot PJ, Sweeney MO, et al, for the PainFREE Rx II Investigators: Prospective randomized multicenter trial of empirical antitachycardia pacing versus shocks for spontaneous rapid ventricular tachycardia in patients with implantable cardioverter-defibrillators: Pacing fast ventricular tachycardia reduces shock therapies (PainFREE Rx II) Trial results. Circulation 110:2591-2596, 2004.
66. Windecker S, Ideker RE, Plumb VJ, et al: The influence of ventricular fibrillation duration on defibrillation efficacy using biphasic waveforms in humans. J Am Coll Cardiol 33:33-38, 1999.
67. Sweeney MO, Natale A, Volosin KJ, et al: Prospective randomized comparison of 50%/50% versus 65%/65% tilt biphasic waveform on defibrillation in humans. PACE 24:60-65, 2001.
68. Shepard RK, DeGroot PJ, Pacifico A, et al: Prospective randomized comparison of 65%/65% versus 42%/42% tilt biphasic waveform on defibrillation thresholds in humans. J Intervent Cardiac Elecrophysiol 8:221-225, 2003.
69. Carpenter CM, Galvin J, Guy M, McGovern BA: Runaway pacemaker in an implantable cardioverter defibrillator. J Cardiovasc Electrophysiol 9:1008-1011, 1998.
70. Hauser R, Hayes DL, Almquist AK, et al: Unexpected ICD pulse generator failure due to electronic circuit damage caused by electrical overstress. PACE 24:1046-1054, 2001.
71. Rasmussen MJ, Friedman PA, Hammill SC, Rea RF: Unintentional deactivation of implantable cardioverter-defibrillators in health care settings. Mayo Clin Proc 77:855-859, 2002.
72. Brode SE, Schwartzman D, Callans DJ, et al: ICD-antiarrhythmic drug and ICD-pacemaker interactions. J Cardiovasc Electrophysiol 8:830-842, 1997.
73. Singer I, Guarnieri T, Kupersmith J: Implanted automatic defibrillators: Effects of drugs and pacemakers. PACE 11:2250-2262, 1988.
74. Rajawat YS, Patel VV, Gerstenfeld EP, et al: Advantages and pitfalls of combining device-based and pharmacologic therapies for the treatment of ventricular arrhythmias: Observations from a tertiary referral center. PACE 27:1670-1681, 2004.
75. Anderson MH, Paul VE, Jones S, et al: Transtelephonic interrogation of the implantable cardioverter defibrillator. PACE 15:1144-1150, 1992.
76. Joseph GK, Wilkoff BL, Dresing T, et al: Remote interrogation and monitoring of implantable cardioverter defibrillators. J Intervent Cardiac Electrophysiol 11:161-166, 2004.
77. Becker R, Ruf-Richter J, Senges-Becker JC, et al: Patient alert in implantable cardioverter defibrillators: Toy or tool? J Am Coll Cardiol 44:95-98, 2004.
78. Sarter BH, Callans DJ, Gottlieb CD, et al: Implantable defibrillator diagnostic storage capabilities: Evolution, current status, and future utilization. PACE 21:1287-1298, 1998.
79. Natale A, Sra J, Axtell K, et al: Undetected ventricular fibrillation in transvenous implantable cardioverter-defibrillators: Prospective comparison of different leads system-device combinations. Circulation 93:91-98, 1996.
80. Swerdlow CD, Ahern T, Chen PS, et al: Underdetection of ventricular tachycardia by algorithms to enhance specificity in a tiered-therapy cardioverter-defibrillator. J Am Coll Cardiol 24: 416-424, 1994.
81. Shivkumar K, Feliciano Z, Boyle NG, Wiener I: Intradevice interaction in a dual chamber implantable cardioverter defibrillator preventing ventricular tachycardia detection. J Cardiovasc Electrophysiol 11:1285-1288, 2000.
82. Glickson M, Beeman AL, Luria DM, et al: Impaired detection of ventricular tachyarrhymias by a rate-smoothing algorithm in dual-chamber implantable defibrillators: Intradevice interactions. J Cardiovasc Electrophysiol 13:312-318, 2002.
83. Wood MA, Ellenbogen KA, Shepard RK, Clemo HS: Atrioventricular sequential pacing by an implantable cardioverter defibrillator during sustained ventricular tachycardia: What is the mechanism? J Cardiovasc Electrophysiol 13:1309-1310, 2002.
84. Grönefeld GC, Israel CW, Padmanabhan V, et al: Ventricular rate stabilization for the prevention of pause dependent ventricular tachyarrhythmias: Results from a prospective study in 309 ICD recipients. PACE 25:1708-1714, 2002.
85. Chin MC, Rosenqvist M, Lee MA, et al: The effect of radiofrequency catheter ablation on permanent pacemakers: An experimental study. PACE 13:23-29, 1990.
86. Martin ET, Coman JA, Shellock FG, et al: Magnetic resonance imaging and cardiac pacemaker safety at 1.5-Tesla. J Am Coll Cardiol 43:1315-1324, 2004.
87. Cossú SF, Hsia HH, Simson MB, et al: Inappropriate pauses during bradycardia pacing in a third-generation implantable cardioverter defibrillator. PACE 20:2271-2274, 1997.
88. Sticherling C, Klingenheben T, Hohnloser SH: An unusual cause of ICD shock. PACE 20:2265-2267, 1997.
89. Hsu SS, Mohib S, Schroeder A, Deger FT: T wave oversensing in implantable cardioverter defibrillators. J Intervent Cardiac Electrophysiol 11:67-72, 2004.
90. Mann DE, Damle RS, Kelly PA, et al: Comparison of oversensing during bradycardia pacing in two types of implantable cardioverter-defibrillator systems. Am Heart J 136:658-663, 1998.
91. Anfinsen OG, Berntsen RF, Aass H, et al: Implantable cardioverter defibrillator dysfunction during and after magnetic resonance imaging. PACE 25:1400-1402, 2002.
92. Vassolas G, Roth RA, Venditti FJ: Effect of extracorporeal shock wave lithotripsy on implantable cardioverter defibrillator. PACE 16:1245-1248, 1993.
93. Sears SF, Conti JB: Quality of life and psychological functioning of ICD patients. Heart 87;488-493, 2002.
94. Schron EB, Exner DV, Yao Q, et al, and the AVID Investigators: Quality of life in the Antiarrhythmics versus Implantable Defibrillators Trial: Impact of therapy and influence of adverse symptoms and defibrillator shocks. Circulation 105:589-594, 2002.

Chapter 26

Programming and Follow-up of Cardiac Resynchronization Devices

MICHAEL O. SWEENEY

Optimal programming of implanted electrical devices for cardiac resynchronization therapy (CRT) requires a sophisticated understanding of the pathophysiologic electrical and mechanical substrates that occur in some patients with symptomatic heart failure due to dilated cardiomyopathy (DCM). Furthermore, optimal CRT programming is an active process that requires sustained vigilance for the remainder of the patient's life and anticipation of the potential for dynamic and related changes in patient condition or device system operation. This is a critically important distinction from conventional pacemakers, which reliably provide bradycardia support with minimal need for periodic programming intervention, particularly with the recent enhancements to automaticity. Similarly, although conventional implantable cardioverter-defibrillators (ICDs) require a slightly higher level of surveillance than pacemakers because of the possibility of clinically silent but important ventricular detections and therapies and several other considerations, they reside primarily in a passive state for the duration of the patient's life. The hybridization of CRT with defibrillation systems (CRTD) therefore invokes all of the complex considerations of optimal CRT and ICD programming. This introduces unique challenges, because the device must simultaneously exist in two fundamentally opposed states of operation: continuous delivery of ventricular pacing and continuous surveillance for ventricular arrhythmia.

Hardware Systems

Non-Independently Programmable Ventricular Polarity Configurations

Transvenous and epicardial left ventricular (LV) pacing leads may be either unipolar or bipolar, although the former dominates current applications. Multiple ventricular pacing polarity configurations are therefore possible. Because programmed polarity settings are common to both ventricular leads but the type of lead (bipolar or unipolar) may not be the same, the following considerations apply.

In a dual bipolar polarity configuration, both lead tips are the active electrodes (cathodes) and the ring or rings are the common (nonstimulating) anode. However, the type of ventricular leads implanted defines the pacing/sensing vector (Figs. 26-1 and 26-2). With two unipolar leads, the bipolar setting results in no pacing or sensing. If both leads are bipolar, both rings act as the common

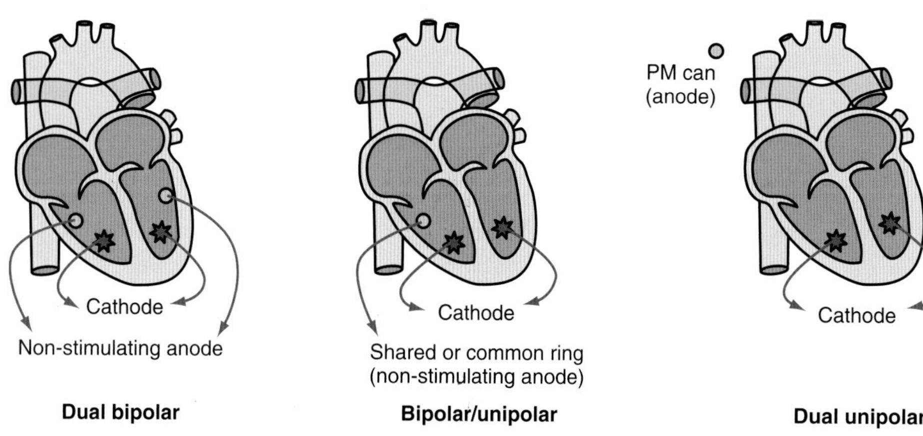

Figure 26-1. Biventricular pacing configurations. PM, pacemaker.

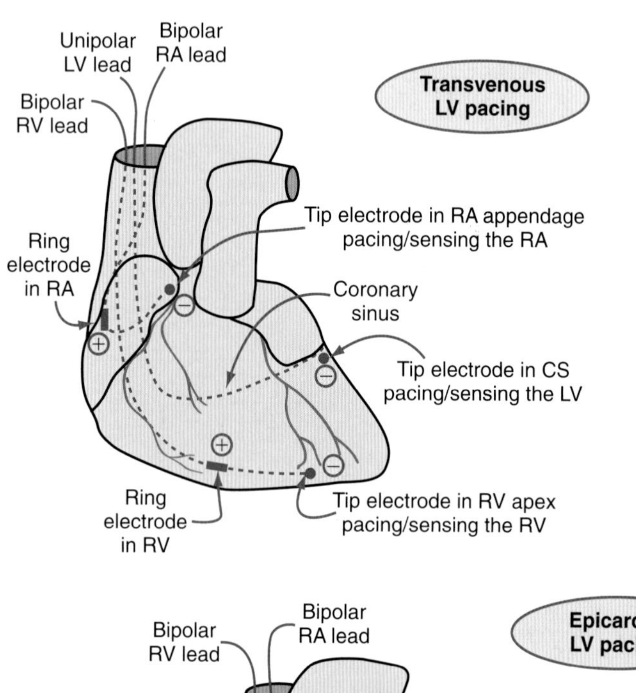

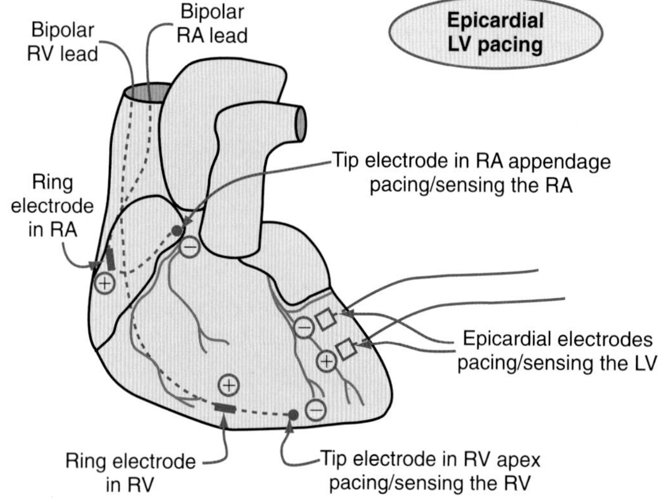

Figure 26-2. Leads and electrodes for biventricular pacing. CS, coronary sinus; LV, left ventricular; RA, right atrial; RV, right ventricular. (Reproduced from Barold SS, Stroobandt R, Sinnaeve A: Cardiac Pacemakers Step by Step: An Illustrated Guide. Malden, MA, Blackwell Publishing, 2003.)

electrode. If one lead is bipolar (typically, the right ventricular [RV] lead) and the other is unipolar (typically the LV lead), the ring on the bipolar lead acts as the common electrode (nonstimulating anode). This configuration results in "shared-ring" bipolar pacing and sensing. This hybrid bipolar/unipolar stimulation configuration ("dual cathodal") is employed in most contemporary CRT pacing systems.

In a dual unipolar polarity configuration, the lead tips are the active electrodes, and the noninsulated device case is the common electrode. This configuration is uncommonly used in CRT pacing systems and is not feasible in CRTD systems because of the concerns regarding ventricular oversensing associated with the unipolar pacing stimulus.

Pulse Generators

Conventional dual-chamber pulse generators or specially designed multisite pacing pulse generators may be used for CRT applications (Fig. 26-3). A conventional dual-chamber pulse generator is well suited for CRT in patients with permanent atrial fibrillation (AF). In this situation, the ventricular port is used for the RV lead and the atrial port is used for the LV lead. This permits programming of independent outputs and ventricular-ventricular timing by manipulation of the atrioventricular (AV) delay. The programming mode can be either DDD/R or DVI/R (see later discussion). A conventional dual-chamber pulse generator can also be used for atrial-synchronous biventricular pacing. The single ventricular output must be divided to provide simultaneous stimulation of the right and left ventricles (dual cathodal system with parallel outputs). This is achieved with a Y-shaped adaptor and results in simultaneous RV and LV sensing, which may result in ventricular double-counting and loss of CRT (see later discussion) or in pacemaker inhibition, in the case of LV lead dislodgment into the coronary sinus with sensing of atrial activity.[1]

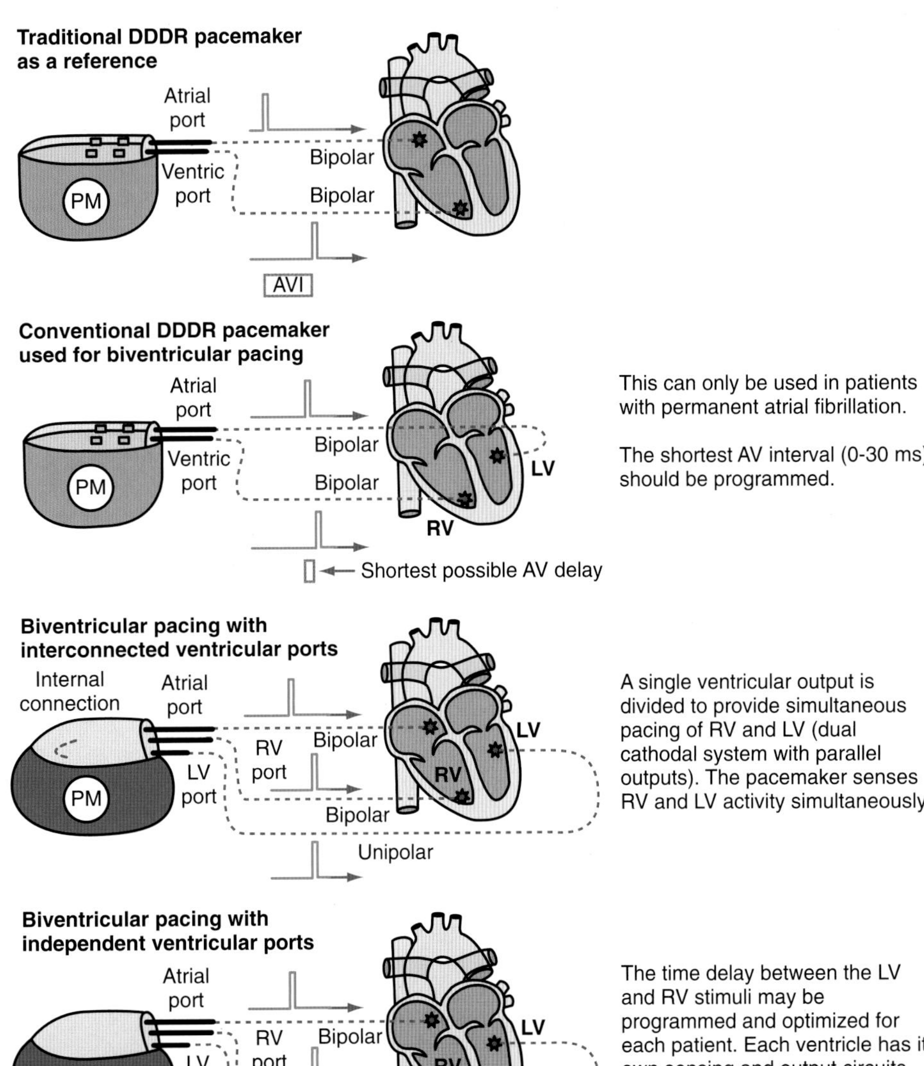

Figure 26-3. Pulse generators for biventricular pacing. AV, atrioventricular; LV, left ventricle; PM, pacemaker; RV, right ventricle. (Reproduced from Barold SS, Stroobandt R, Sinnaeve A: Cardiac Pacemakers Step by Step: An Illustrated Guide. Malden, MA, Blackwell Publishing, 2003.)

First-generation multisite pacing pulse generators similarly provide a single ventricular output for simultaneous RV and LV stimulation; however, two separate ventricular channels internally connect in parallel. This connection is made for both the lead tip and the ring connections and eliminates the need for a Y-adaptor. However, this configuration still provides simultaneous RV and LV sensing with associated limitations.

Second-generation multisite pacing pulse generators have independent ventricular ports. Each ventricular lead therefore has separate sensing and output circuits. This arrangement permits optimal programming of outputs and time delay between RV and LV stimulation for each patient. It also eliminates the potential complications of biventricular sensing.

Programming Considerations for CRT

Pacing Modes

It is axiomatic that for maximal delivery of CRT ventricular pacing must be continuous.

DDD mode guarantees AV synchrony by synchronizing ventricular pacing to all atrial events except during episodes of atrial tachycardia or AF. However, DDD mode increases the probability of atrial pacing (depending on the programmed lower rate limit), which may alter the left-sided AV timing relationship due to interatrial conduction time and atrial pacing latency.

VDD mode guarantees the absence of atrial pacing and synchronizes all atrial events to ventricular pacing at the programmed AV delay. However, if the sinus rate is slower than the lower programmed rate limit, AV synchrony is lost because the VDD mode is operationally VVI.

Although conventional dual-chamber pacemakers are not designed for biventricular pacing and typically do not allow programming of an AV delay of zero or near zero, they are being increasingly used with their shortest AV delay time (0 to 30 msec) for CRT in patients with permanent AF. The advantages include programming flexibility, elimination of the Y-adaptor (required for conventional VVIR devices), protection against far-field sensing of atrial activity (an inherent risk of dual cathodal devices with simultaneous sensing from both ventricles), and cost. When a conventional dual-chamber pacemaker is used for CRT, the LV lead is usually connected to the atrial port and the RV lead to the ventricular port. This provides both for LV stimulation before RV activation (LV preexcitation) and for protection against ventricular asystole related to oversensing of far-field atrial activity if the LV lead becomes dislodged toward the AV groove.

The DVIR mode is ideally suited for this application. The DVIR mode behaves like the VVIR mode, except that there are always two closely coupled independent ventricular stimuli, thereby facilitating comprehensive evaluation of RV and LV pacing and sensing performance. The DVIR mode also provides absolute protection against far-field sensing of atrial activity in case of LV lead dislodgment, because no sensing occurs on the "atrial" (LV) lead in the DVIR mode.

Determining Left Ventricular and Right Ventricular Capture: Importance of Electrocardiography

The 12-lead electrocardiogram (ECG) is essential to ascertain RV and LV capture during follow-up of CRT systems without separately programmable ventricular outputs. It is recognized that six distinct 12-lead ventricular activation patterns may be seen during threshold determination: (1) intrinsic rhythm during loss of RV and LV capture or pacing inhibition (native QRS), (2) isolated RV stimulation, (3) isolated LV stimulation, (4) biventricular stimulation with complete capture, (5) biventricular pacing with fusion between native activation and pacing capture, and (6) biventricular stimulation with anodal capture.

Ventricular pacing thresholds should ideally be performed independently and in the VVI mode, at a rate exceeding the prevailing ventricular rate, so as to obtain continuous ventricular capture without fusion. Alternatively, thresholds can be performed in the VDD or DDD mode at very short AV delays, to ensure full ventricular capture without fusion. In general, it is advisable to initiate threshold determinations at maximum output (voltage and pulse duration), because there is often a significant difference in capture thresholds between RV and LV.

In devices without separately programmable ventricular outputs, RV and LV capture can be determined only by ECG analysis during common ventricular voltage decrement. This requires inspection of a 12-lead ECG to demonstrate a change in electrical axis that confirms independent LV and RV capture.

Pacing from the RV apex produces a negative paced QRS complex in the inferior leads, simply because the activation starts in the inferior part of the heart and travels superiorly, away from the inferior leads (Figs. 26-4 and 26-5). The mean QRS frontal plane axis is superior either in the left or right superior quadrant. Pacing from the RV outflow tract produces a frontal plane axis that is "normal," meaning inferiorly directed (positive QRS in inferior leads) (see Figs. 26-4 and 26-5). Isolated LV pacing produces a rightward axis, similar to maximal ventricular preexcitation over a left-sided accessory pathway (Fig. 26-6). Biventricular pacing (RV + LV) produces a right superior axis as a result of fusion of the RV and LV electrical axes.

A qR or Qr complex in lead I is rare in uncomplicated RV apical pacing. It is present in 90% of cases of biventricular pacing. In biventricular pacing, loss of the q or Q wave in lead I is 100% predictive of loss of LV capture (Fig. 26-7). Examples of the effects of univentricular and biventricular stimulation on the 12-lead ECG are shown in Figure 26-8.

The majority of current CRT systems with pacemaker capability (CRTP) and CRTD systems use a dual cathodal pacing configuration. "Anodal capture" refers

Text continued on p. 1095

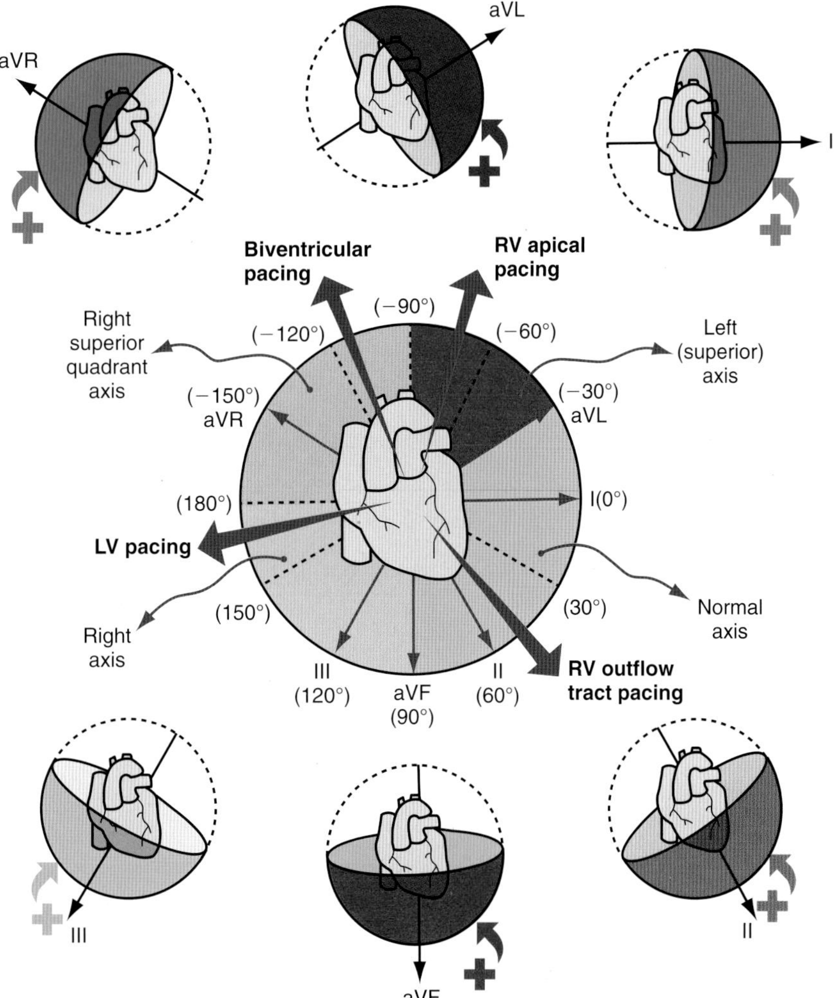

Figure 26-4. Mean QRS axis in the frontal plane during ventricular pacing. LV, left ventricle; RV, right ventricle. (Reproduced from Barold SS, Stroobandt R, Sinnaeve A: Cardiac Pacemakers Step by Step: An Illustrated Guide. Malden, MA, Blackwell Publishing, 2003.)

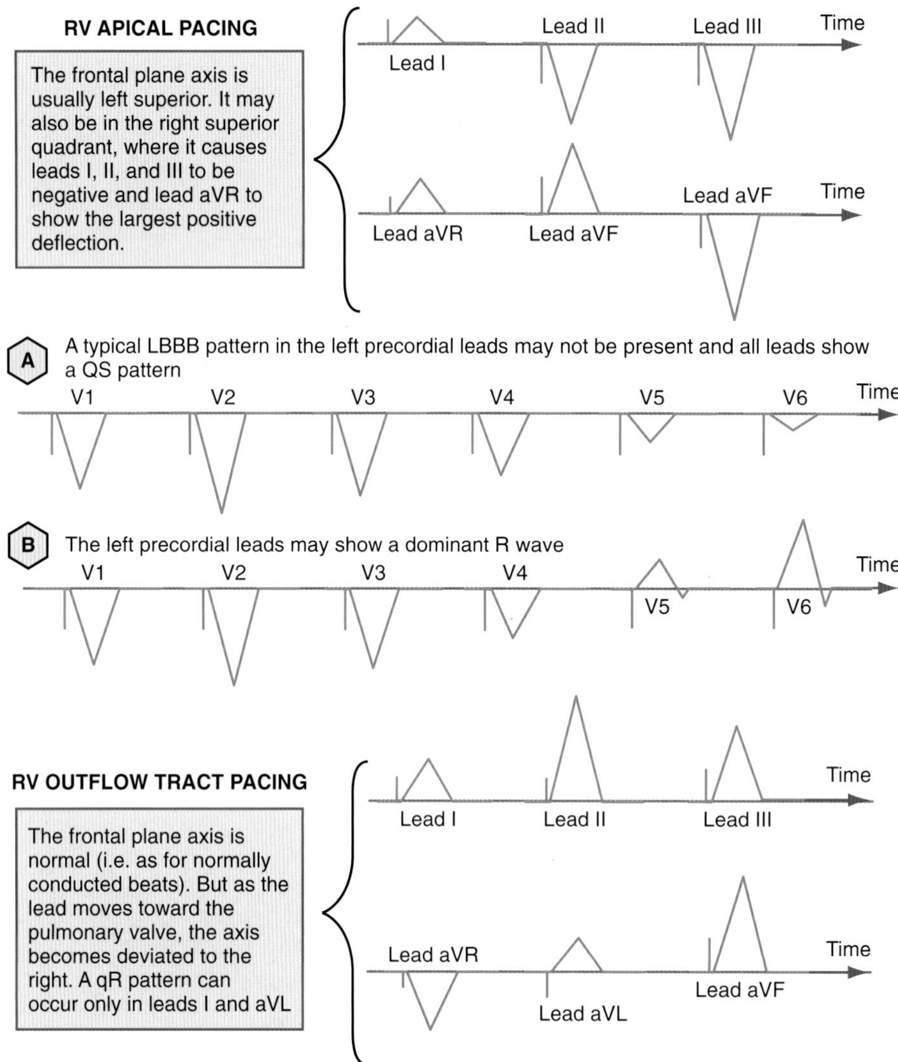
RV APICAL PACING
The frontal plane axis is usually left superior. It may also be in the right superior quadrant, where it causes leads I, II, and III to be negative and lead aVR to show the largest positive deflection.
Lead I
Lead II
Lead III
Time
Lead aVR
Lead aVF
Lead aVF
Time
A
A typical LBBB pattern in the left precordial leads may not be present and all leads show a QS pattern
V1
V2
V3
V4
V5
V6
Time
B
The left precordial leads may show a dominant R wave
V1
V2
V3
V4
V5
V6
Time
RV OUTFLOW TRACT PACING
The frontal plane axis is normal (i.e. as for normally conducted beats). But as the lead moves toward the pulmonary valve, the axis becomes deviated to the right. A qR pattern can occur only in leads I and aVL
Lead I
Lead II
Lead III
Time
Lead aVR
Lead aVL
Lead aVF
Time
The precordial V leads are similar to those with RV apical pacing

Figure 26-5. Electrocardiographic QRS patterns during pacing of the right ventricle (RV) from different sites. LBBB, left bundle branch block. (Reproduced from Barold SS, Stroobandt R, Sinnaeve A: Cardiac Pacemakers Step by Step: An Illustrated Guide. Malden, MA, Blackwell Publishing, 2003.)

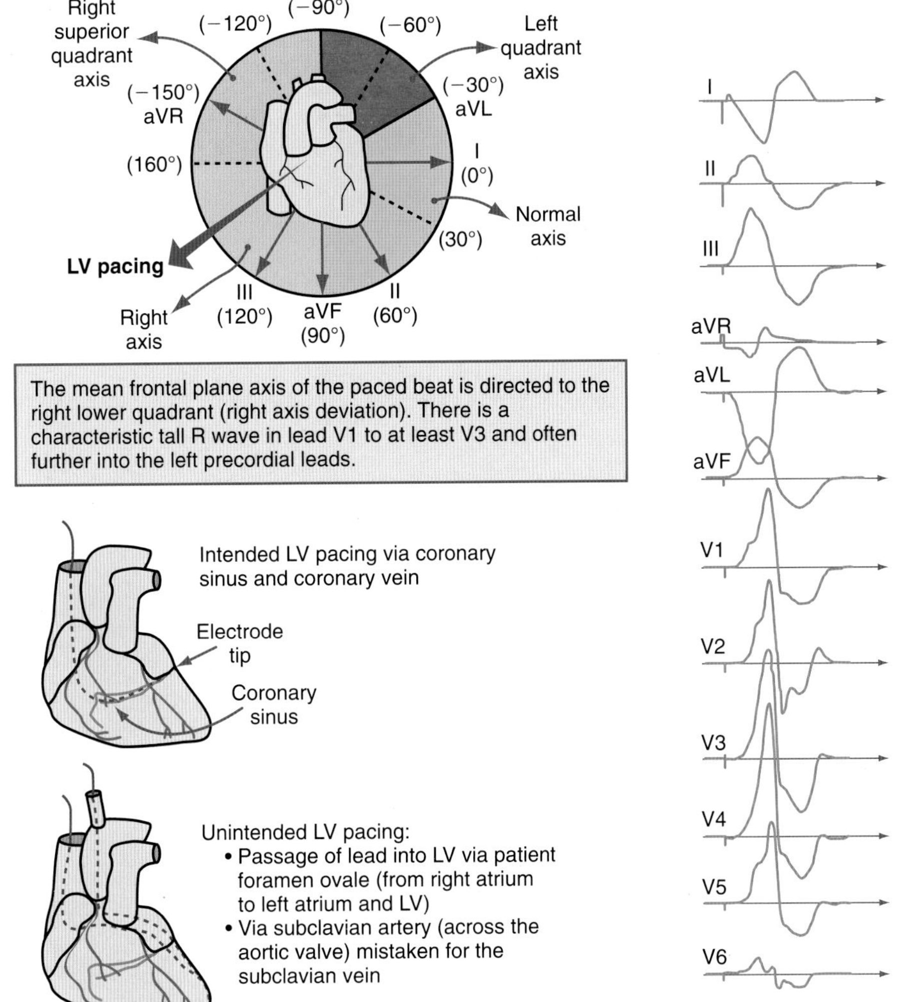
Right superior quadrant axis
(−120°)
(−90°)
(−60°)
Left quadrant axis
(−150°) aVR
(−30°) aVL
(160°)
I (0°)
Normal axis
(30°)
LV pacing
Right axis
III (120°)
aVF (90°)
II (60°)
The mean frontal plane axis of the paced beat is directed to the right lower quadrant (right axis deviation). There is a characteristic tall R wave in lead V1 to at least V3 and often further into the left precordial leads.
Intended LV pacing via coronary sinus and coronary vein
Electrode tip
Coronary sinus
Unintended LV pacing:
• Passage of lead into LV via patient foramen ovale (from right atrium to left atrium and LV)
• Via subclavian artery (across the aortic valve) mistaken for the subclavian vein
I
II
III
aVR
aVL
aVF
V1
V2
V3
V4
V5
V6

Figure 26-6. Electrocardiographic QRS patterns during free wall pacing of the left ventricle (LV). (Reproduced from Barold SS, Stroobandt R, Sinnaeve A: Cardiac Pacemakers Step by Step: An Illustrated Guide. Malden, MA, Blackwell Publishing, 2003.)

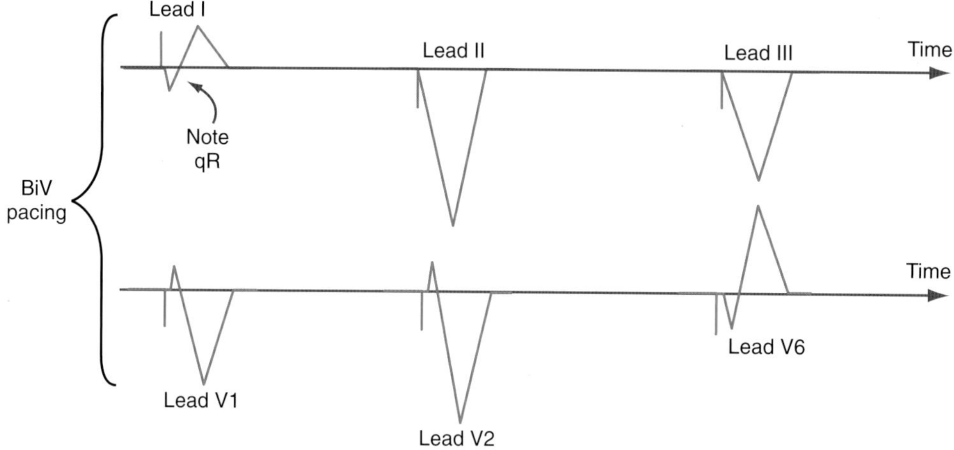

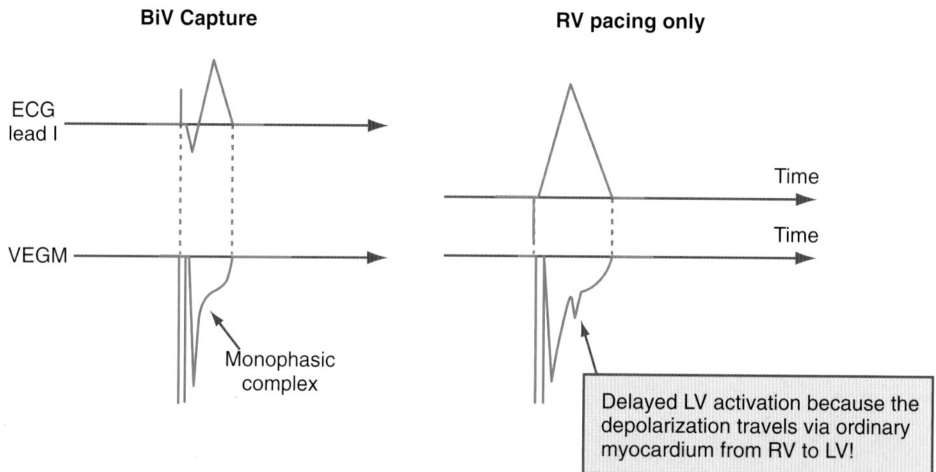

Figure 26-7. Analysis of electrocardiographic (ECG) QRS patterns to ascertain right ventricular (RV) and left ventricular (LV) capture in cardiac resynchronization systems without separately programmable ventricular outputs. BiV, biventricular; VEGM, ventricular electrogram. (Reproduced from Barold SS, Stroobandt R, Sinnaeve A: Cardiac Pacemakers Step by Step: An Illustrated Guide. Malden, MA, Blackwell Publishing, 2003.)

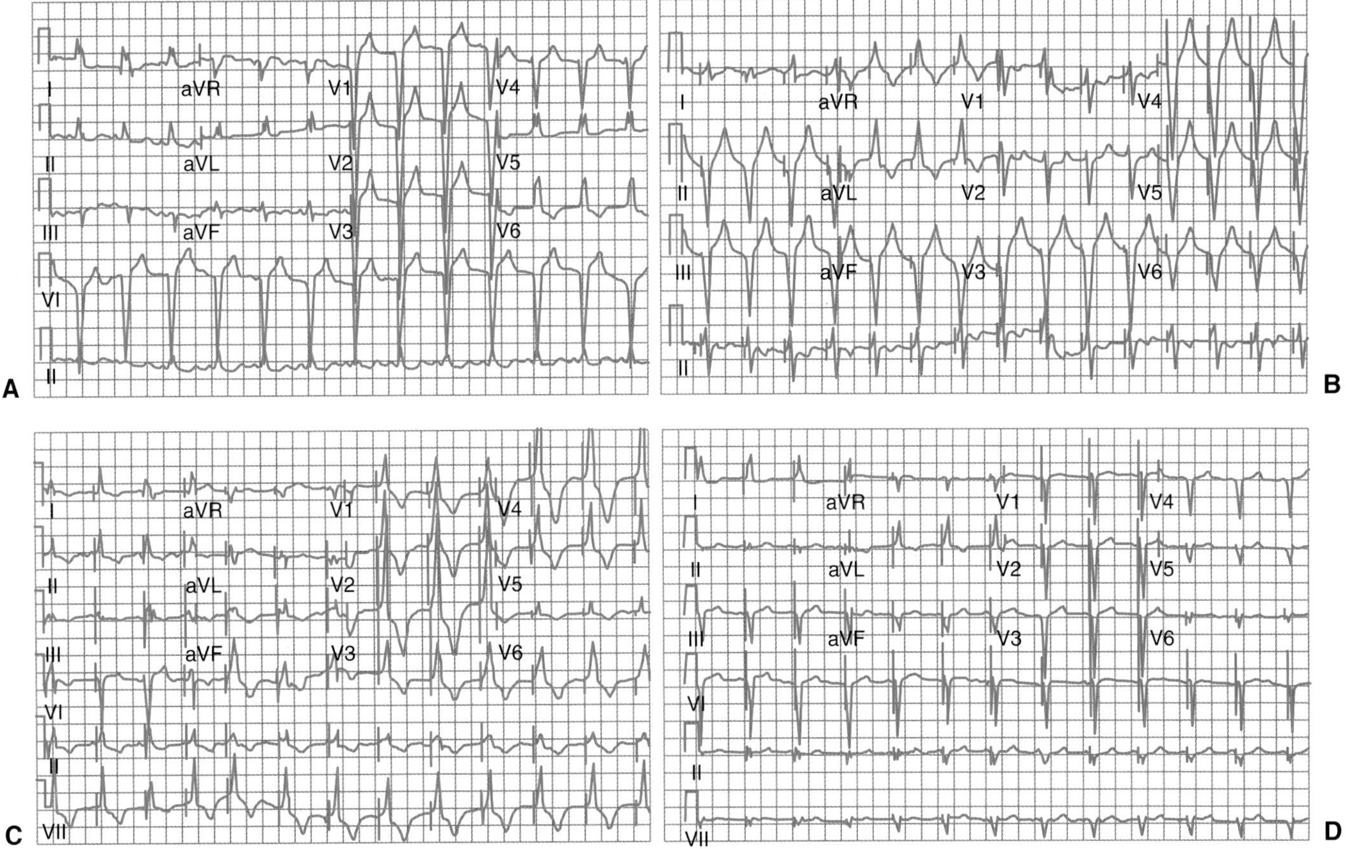

Figure 26-8. QRS morphologies during biventricular stimulation. VVI mode is used to exclude the possibility of fusion with native ventricular activation. ***A,*** *Intrinsic ventricular activation (left bundle branch block).* ***B,*** *RV-only pacing.* ***C,*** *LV-only pacing.* ***D,*** *Biventricular pacing.*

to the situation when myocardial capture occurs at the RV anode. This could theoretically occur in isolation with the LV cathode, but it most commonly occurs with both RV and LV cathodes and is referred to as "triple-site" pacing. Anodal capture is more common at high voltage outputs and with true bipolar RV leads because of the small surface area and higher current density of the ring electrode, as opposed to the larger surface area and lower current density of the coil electrode in integrated bipolar leads.

Anodal capture results in a distinct change in activation pattern, compared with biventricular pacing, that can be appreciated only on the 12-lead ECG (Fig. 26-9). The electrical axis is shifted leftward, and the QRS duration may be shorter as a consequence of increased ventricular fusion. The change in QRS morphology related to loss of anodal capture as voltage output is decremented during a temporary threshold test using a single ECG lead may be misinterpreted as loss of LV capture and result in erroneous overestimation of the LV threshold.

The physiologic consequences of anodal capture are uncertain. One study demonstrated that anodal capture might be advantageous during CRT by counteracting the regional activation delay located at the inferior wall of the LV and improving regional measures of intraventricular dyssynchrony.[2]

Programming Pacing Outputs

It is critically important that the voltage output be adjusted to exceed the ventricular capture threshold for the right and left ventricles in common cathodal devices. Because the capture thresholds in the two chambers are commonly different, this means that the voltage output must exceed capture threshold in the chamber with the higher threshold (usually the LV). Newer pulse generators that permit independent programming of ventricular outputs provide greater flexibility in this regard. Similarly, RV and LV voltage outputs may be separately programmable when a standard DDD device is used to provide RV and LV stimulation in the DVI mode for CRT in cases of permanent AF (see earlier discussion).

Atrioventricular Optimization

AV optimization is important for maximal hemodynamic response to CRT, but it is not essential, because the ventricular pumping function can be improved by CRT even in the presence of permanent AF. Nonetheless, acute hemodynamic studies have consistently demonstrated that AV optimization "re-times" the left atrial-LV relationship and can result in 15% to 40% improvement in indices of LV systolic performance acutely. Furthermore, small changes in AV delay may nullify the hemodynamic benefit of CRT.

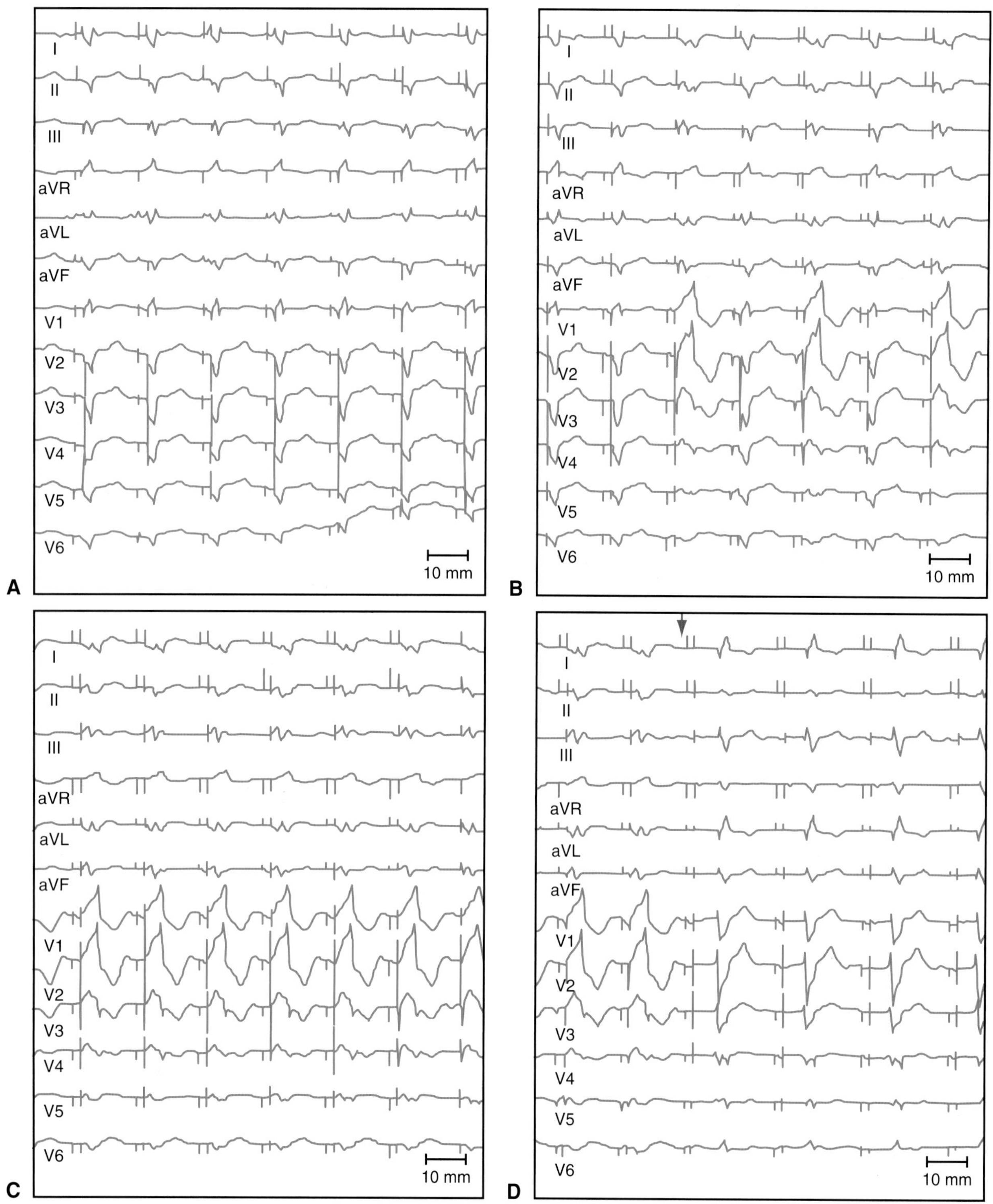

Figure 26-9. 12-lead ECGs recorded at different voltages in order to demonstrate anodal capture. ***A,*** *Constant anodal capture. Note shorter paced QRS duration in lead V1.* ***B,*** *Intermittent loss of anodal capture at lower voltage (beats 3, 5, and 7).* ***C,*** *LV-only capture at lower voltage.* ***D,*** *Total loss of capture. (From Thibault B, Roy D, Guerra PG, et al: Anodal right ventricular capture during left ventricular stimulation in CRT-implantable cardioverter-defibrillators. PACE 28:613-619, 2005.)*

Optimization Using Invasive Hemodynamic Monitoring. Techniques for AV optimization using invasive LV pressure monitoring have been described[3-5] (Fig. 26-10). The optimal AV delay is assumed to be the value that yields at least a 5% increase in aortic pulse pressure, or in LV pressure plus the maximum first derivation of LV pressure (LV + dP/dt_{max}), compared with baseline. These indices are useful because they correlate with stroke volume and global contractile function. However, pulse pressure and LV +dP/dt can be confounded by changes in preload and arterial impedance (afterload). Though this technique is useful for assessing the effects of acute manipulations of AV delay, ventricular stimulation sites, and ventricular sequencing on LV pumping function, it is an impractical approach for routine clinical care. Furthermore, there is some evidence that acute hemodynamic response is not highly correlated with long-term clinical response including reverse ventricular remodeling.

Optimization Using Conventional Echocardiography. Several methods of AV optimization using echo-guided pulsed Doppler analysis of transmitral blood flow velocities to approximate an optimal timing relationship between atrial systole and ventricular filling have been described. The goal is manipulation of the AV delay until the end of the untruncated A wave occurs coincident with mitral valve closure, which represents the onset of ventricular contraction. The common assumption of these methods is that this optimized AV delay will yield the longest diastolic filling time and best acute LV pumping function.

According to the method of Ritter and colleagues,[6,7] optimal sensed AV delay ($SAV_{optimal}$) can be stated algebraically as follows: $SAV_{optimal} = SAV_{short} + [(SAV_{long} + QA_{long}) - (SAV_{short} + QA_{short})]$, where Q is the ventricular pacing stimulus and A is the termination of the A wave. This process is performed in three steps. First, the SAV_{long} and QA_{long} are determined by programming a "long" sensed AV delay (SAV_{long}). The AV delay should be long enough to maintain full ventricular capture but allow spontaneous closure of the mitral valve before aortic outflow occurs (Fig. 26-11). QA_{long} is then measured as the time from the ventricular pacing stimulus

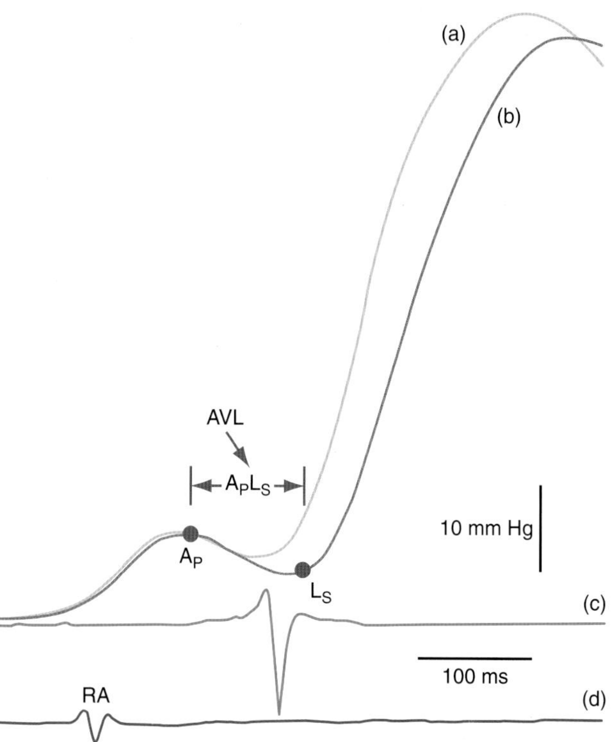

Figure 26-10. Atrioventricular optimization using invasive hemodynamic monitoring. Examples are shown of systolic left ventricular (LV) pressure during pacing (a), intrinsic condition (b), intrinsic LV electrogram (c), and intrinsic right atrial (RA) electrogram (d) recorded from one patient. Also shown here are the presystolic peak (A_P) that results from atrial contraction and the start of pressure development in the LV (L_S), the latter obtained as the point that first attains a slope greater than 10% of the maximum rate of increase of LV pressure. The interval (A_PL_S) between A_P and L_S is defined as atrioventricular mechanical latency (AVL). When the ventricle is preexcited with pacing, the L_S point moves to the left, as shown here in curve a. To show the L_S point in the paced condition, the pacing and intrinsic pressure curves are aligned at the point of electrical activation of the right atrium (RA). Thereafter, the difference between the two curves is obtained. (From Auricchio A, Stellbrink C, Sack S, et al., and Group PTiCHFP-CS: Long-term clinical effect of hemodynamically optimized cardiac resynchronization therapy in patients with heart failure and ventricular conduction delay. J Am Coll Cardiol 39:2026-2033, 2002.)

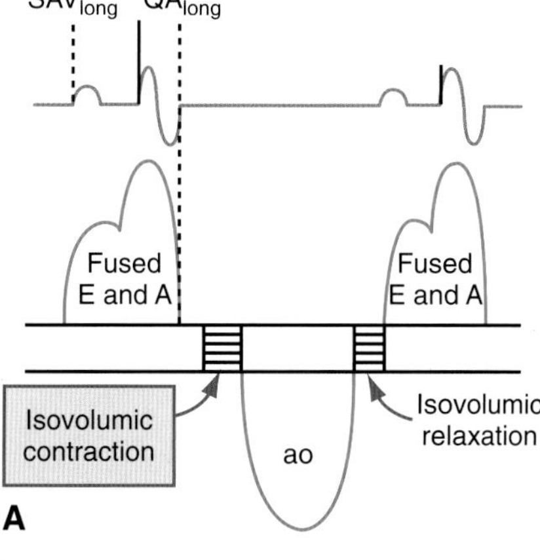

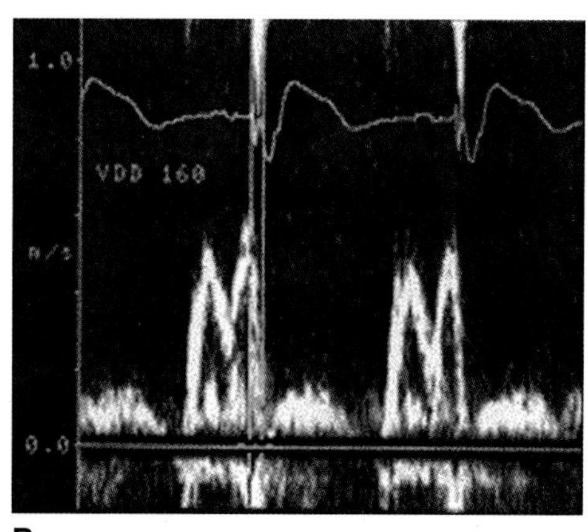

*Figure 26-11. Atrioventricular (AV) optimization using Doppler mitral inflow. Determining SAV_{long} and QA_{long}. **A,** To determine SAV_{long}, a long sensed AV delay that maintains ventricular preexcitation yet allows spontaneous closure of the mitral valve before aortic ejection (e.g., 150 msec) is programmed. Next, the time from V-pace to the end of the A wave is measured. This is QA_{long}, which refers to the QA distance measured when a "long" SAV is programmed. ao, aortic outflow. **B,** Doppler echo of transmitral blood flow with a long AV delay.*

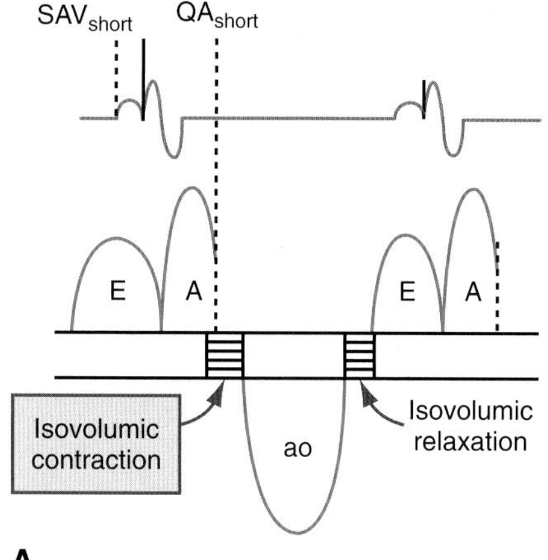

A

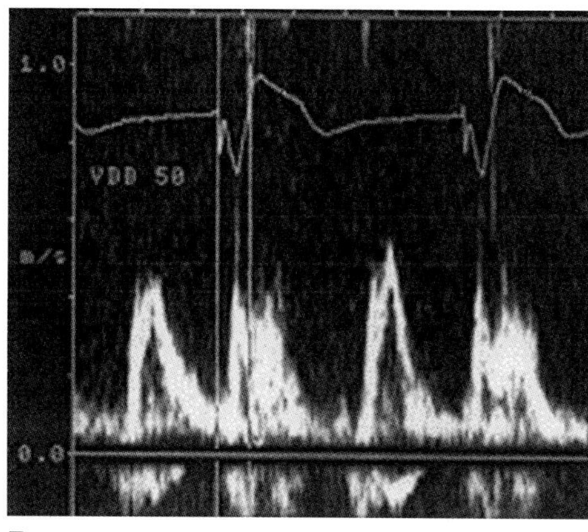

B

*Figure 26-12. Atrioventricular (AV) optimization using Doppler mitral inflow. Determining SAV_{short} and QA_{short}. **A,** To determine SAV_{short}, a short sensed AV delay that results in premature closure of the mitral valve (e.g., 50 msec) is programmed. The time from V-pace to the premature end of the A wave is measured. This is QA_{short}. ao, aortic outflow. **B,** Doppler echo of transmitral blood flow with a short AV delay.*

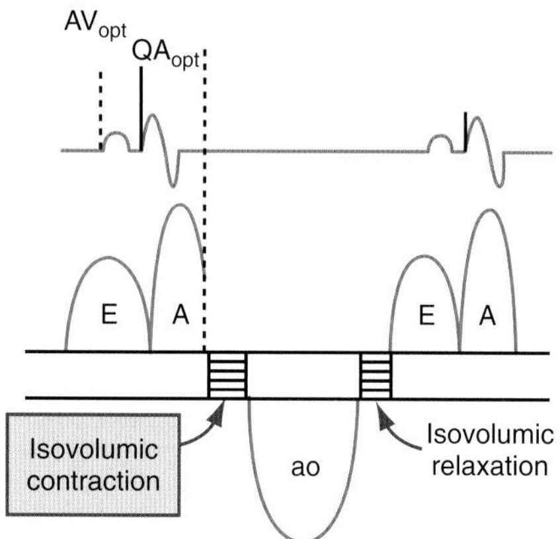

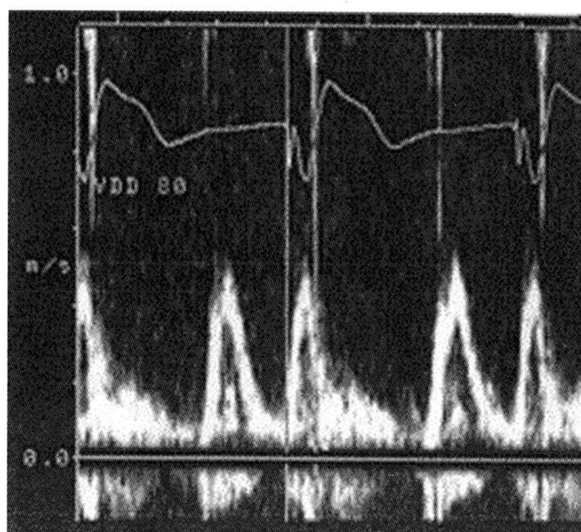

Figure 26-13. Optimized atrioventricular (AV) delay. AV optimization is confirmed by noting the return of normal E- and A-wave separation on Doppler echo of transmitral blood flow. Note the improvement in transmitral blood flow and the increase in left ventricular diastolic filling time, which help increase cardiac output. ao, aortic outflow.

to the end of the A wave. Second, the SAV_{short} and QA_{short} are determined by programming a "short" sensed AV delay (SAV_{short}) that results in forced closure of the mitral valve (Fig. 26-12). QA_{short} is then measured as the time from the ventricular pacing stimulus to the end of the A wave. Caution must be applied not to extrapolate to the end of the A wave but to use the observed end of the A wave. Third, AV optimization is confirmed by noting the return of normal E- and A-wave separation, indicating improved diastolic filling time and optimized AV timing relationship (Fig. 26-13).

This is a rather tedious process and one that is highly operator dependent, because visualization of the terminal portion of the A wave is often difficult and subjective. A potentially more critical limitation is that the basis for the technique was derived from studies of patients with permanent AV block and conventional dual-chamber pacing with RV apical stimulation. This may be physiologically unsound in CRT, where LV pacing modifies the interventricular and intraventricular delay caused by RV-only pacing.

A simplified approach to AV optimization guided by analysis of transmitral blood has been described by Meluzin and coworkers.[8] This approach requires two steps. A "long" AV delay is programmed to achieve full ventricular capture but allow spontaneous closure of the mitral valve before aortic outflow. The time between the end of the A wave (representing the end of the diastolic filling period) and the onset of high-velocity systolic mitral regurgitation (representing the onset of ventricular contraction) is denoted as t1. The optimal AV delay is then calculated as the "long" AV delay minus t1 (in milliseconds). This approach accurately predicted the optimal AV delay based on simultaneous invasive hemodynamic measurements in 78% of patients. Potential limitations include the requirement for at least mild mitral regurgitation and the difficulty in discerning the termination of the A wave and the transition between diastolic and systolic mitral regurgitation.

Optimization Using Intrinsic AV Intervals. Another approach to AV optimization for maximal positive change in LV +dP/dt is derived from the intrinsic AV interval measured from the local right atrial and RV endocardial electrograms (EGMs) using two linear equations[9] (Fig. 26-14). If the native QRS duration (QRSd) is greater than 150 msec, then estimated optimal AV delay (EOAVD) = $(A \times iAVI) + B = (C \times iAVI) + D$, where iAVI is the intrinsic AV interval, $A = 0.7$, $B = -55$ msec, and $D = 0$ msec. (C = constant.) These regression formulas can be very closely approximated by the following simple rules: the programmed EOAVD is 50% of the intrinsic AV interval for patients with a QRSd greater

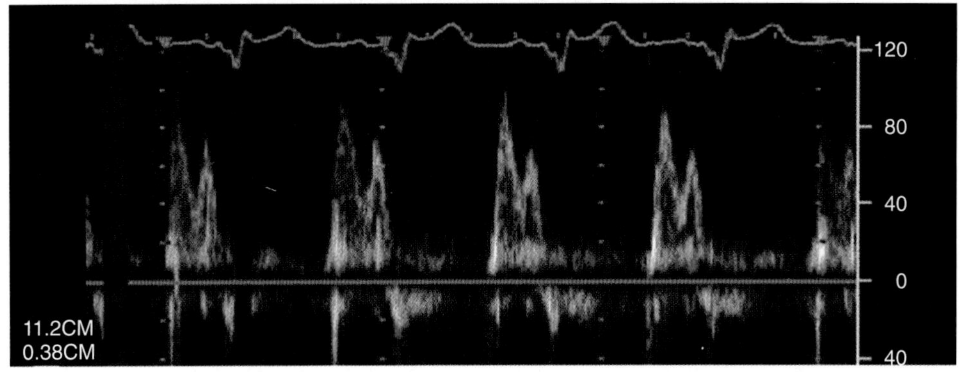

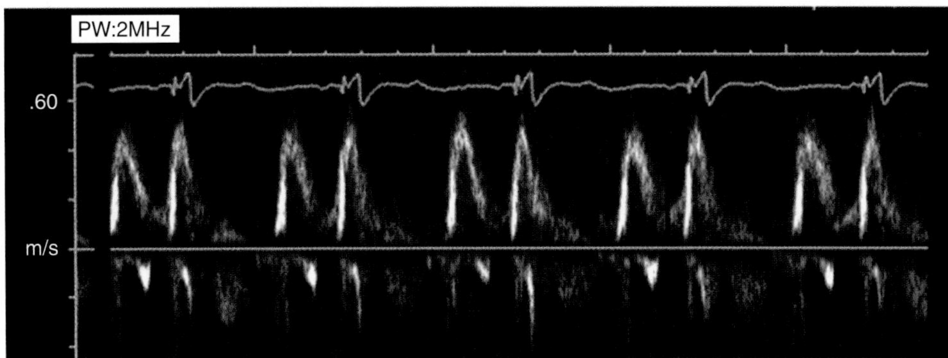

Figure 26-14. Estimated optimal atrioventricular (AV) delay using intrinsic AV intervals. In this example, the intrinsic AV interval (As – Vs) was 200 msec, and the QRSd was 170 msec, therefore estimated optimal AV delay was 100 msec (see text). As, atrial sensed event; Vs, ventricular sensed event.

than 150 msec, and 75% for those with a PR of 120 to 150 msec. This strategy was used in the study design of the Comparison of Medical Therapy, Pacing, and Defibrillation in Heart Failure (COMPANION) trial,[10] which showed significant reductions in mortality and heart failure hospitalizations with CRT at 1 year.

Optimization Using Noninvasive Hemodynamic Monitoring. Recently, finger photoplethysmography (FPPG) has been investigated as a noninvasive tool for hemodynamic optimization of the AV delay during CRT[11] (Fig. 26-15). FPPG correctly identified positive aortic pulse pressure responses with 71% sensitivity and 90% specificity and negative aortic pulse pressure responses with 57% sensitivity and 96% specificity. The magnitude of FPPG changes was well correlated with positive aortic pulse pressure changes ($R^2 = 0.73$). However, the correlation with negative aortic pressure changes was poor ($R^2 = 0.43$). FPPG identified 78% of the patients having positive aortic pulse pressure changes to CRT and also identified the AV delay giving maximum aortic pulse pressure change in all selected patients. This approach has not been clinically validated, but it offers the appeal of a quick, noninvasive measure for correlating changes in AV delay with some meaningful measure of cardiac output.

Clinical Experience with Atrioventricular Optimization. Previous studies have emphasized the importance of a short AV delay during standard dual-chamber pacing in patients with heart failure to optimize the acute hemodynamic response when native AV conduction is prolonged.[12,13] However, in one study, the same benefit could not be documented.[14] It is now recognized that the acute hemodynamic benefit of AV optimization in conventional dual-chamber pacing is negated by the chronic adverse effects of ventricular desynchronization on LV pump function due to RV apical pacing, particularly among patients with systolic heart failure.

Nevertheless, because biventricular pacing overcomes the problem of ventricular desynchronization caused by RV-only pacing, AV optimization has been incorporated into randomized clinical trials (RCTs) of CRT. Using variations on the method of Ritter and colleagues[6] or invasive hemodynamic monitoring, the optimized AV delay in studies of CRT is almost invariably in the range of 80 to 110 msec regardless of other considerations.[3,4,10,15,16] For this reason, some have argued for empiric programming of the AV delay to approximately 100 msec. It is almost certainly true that the optimal AV delay will differ as heart rate and cardiac loading conditions change, so that the optimal AV delay at one point in time may not be optimal under other conditions. Furthermore, the importance of AV delay optimization at rest for chronic clinical and hemodynamic effects remains to be shown. It has also become clear that optimal ventricular synchronization is far more important than AV optimization. The atrial contribution to ventricular filling is probably minimal when the left ventricle is operating at persistently elevated diastolic pressures and atrial mechanical transport is diminished due to myopathic processes.

Recently, Sawhney and colleagues[17] reported a randomized, prospective, single-blind trial of echocardiography-guided AV optimization using the aortic velocity-time integral (VTI) versus an empiric AV delay at 120 msec in 40 CRT patients. Optimal AV delay was

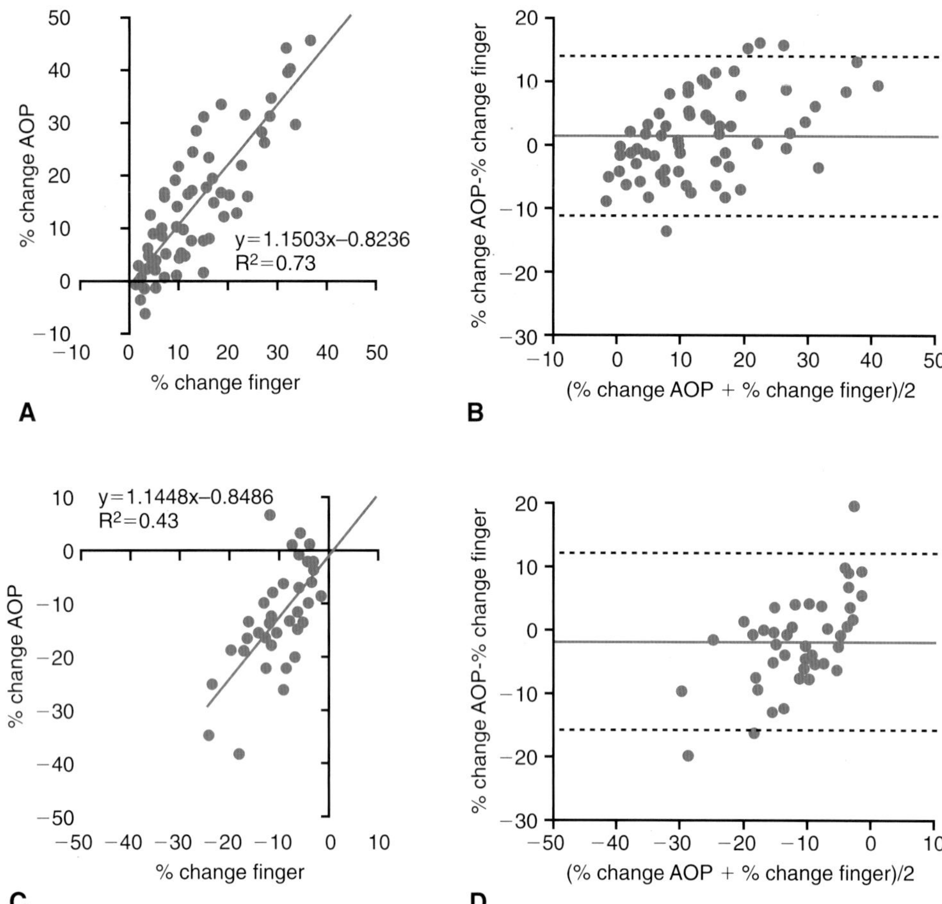

Figure 26-15. *Atrioventricular (AV) optimization using finger plethysmography. Correlation of the change in aortic pulse pressure (AOP) versus finger pulse and the corresponding Bland-Altmann plots.* ***A,*** *Correlation for significantly positive finger responses.* ***B,*** *Bland-Altmann plot for significantly positive finger responses.* ***C,*** *Correlation for significantly negative finger responses.* ***D,*** *Bland-Altmann plot for significantly negative finger responses. (From Butter C, Stellbrink C, Belalcazar A, et al: Cardiac resynchronization therapy optimization by finger plethysmography. Heart Rhythm 1:568-578, 2005.)*

defined as the AV delay that yielded the largest mean aortic VTI at one of eight tested AV intervals (between 60 and 200 msec). A small improvement in ejection fraction was demonstrated in the VTI-optimized group compared with the empiric AV delay group immediately after implementation of CRT. After 3 months, modest improvements in New York Heart Association (NYHA) functional class and standardized quality of life scores were observed in the VTI-optimized group. Not unexpectedly, the mean optimized AV delay program and the empiric AV delay were almost identical (119 and 120 msec, respectively). The authors speculated that individual patient variation accounted for the slight differences in outcome among groups. However, because of the large range of optimal AV delays observed (60 to 200 msec), many patients in the empiric AV delay group had an AV delay that was significantly different from their optimized AV delay. This data, although of interest, is insufficient to recommend AV optimization in all patients who receive CRT.

Interventricular Timing Considerations

First- and second-generation CRTP and CRTD systems deliver simultaneous biventricular stimulation, even when RV and LV stimulation outputs are separately programmable. Simultaneous biventricular stimulation has reproducibly been shown to be effective in the majority of patients in RCTs of CRT. However, despite similar prolongation of the QRS duration and morphology of left bundle branch block (LBBB), considerable heterogeneity in the location of regional mechanical dyssynchrony has been revealed by sophisticated echocardiographic techniques.[18-20] For example, the posterobasal LV most commonly shows the greatest electromechanical delay in LBBB associated with nonischemic dilated cardiomyopathy (NDCMP). However, the greatest electromechanical delay occurs in the interventricular septum (paradoxical septal contraction) in some patients with LBBB and NDCMP. The situation is even more complex in ischemic cardiomyopathy, where regional electromechanical delays are influenced by infarct location. It is therefore reasonable to hypothesize that timed stimulation of different LV regions might be necessary for optimal CRT. In practical application, RV stimulation serves as a surrogate for septal stimulation, but this may be influenced by RV lead position (RV apex versus septum).

Logically, enhancements to biventricular pacing systems might permit tailoring of ventricular stimulation by site and timing to optimally address the diversity of electromechanical phenomena observed among individual patients. In third-generation systems, the relative timing of RV and LV stimulation can be varied. This requires separately programmable RV and LV stimulation outputs and circuitry to permit timing delay between outputs by stimulation site (V-V timing). The goal of V-V timing is site-selective, sequential ventricular stimulation. Theoretically, V-V timing could be achieved with unipolar or dual cathodal electrode configurations. From a practical perspective, unipolar pacing is inapplicable in CRTD, and anodal capture at high outputs with dual cathodal electrode configurations results in unintended biventricular stimulation and could disrupt V-V timing. This is probably relevant only when RV stimulation precedes LV stimulation, because RV capture renders the local myocardium refractory, and anodal capture during high-output LV stimulation will not occur. Accordingly, the use of V-V timing where RV precedes LV stimulation with dual cathodal electrode configurations mandates exclusion of anodal capture by 12-lead electrocardiography at programmed outputs (see earlier discussion). Therefore, V-V timing is optimally delivered with true bipolar (RV and LV) electrode configurations.

Interventricular Timing Operation

Interventricular timing operation in the Medtronic InSync III CRTP system is shown in Figure 26-16. Nominally, selection of biventricular (RV + LV) pacing results in delivery of a pacing stimulus to the other chamber after a 4-msec delay. However, the first chamber paced and the delay interval between paced stimuli to the first and second chambers are separately programmable. The V-V Pace Delay parameter sets the amount of time that elapses between delivery of a stimulus to the first ventricle paced and delivery of a stimulus to the other ventricle. This can be varied between 4 and 80 msec. The V-V Pace Delay parameter necessitates timing interactions to guarantee proper operation of Ventricular Safety Pacing and Ventricular Sense Response. When these are enabled, paces generated in response to a ventricular sense will be delivered at the minimum (4-msec) V-V delay.

Clinical Experience with Sequential Versus Biventricular Stimulation

The long-term clinical experience with sequential biventricular stimulation is limited, and no RCTs have reported on outcomes based on the use of this potential enhancement to CRT. Sogaard and associates[18] used tissue tracking to quantify regions of delayed longitudinal contraction and three-dimensional echocardiography to measure the effects of sequential ventricular stimulation in 21 patients with systolic heart failure and LBBB and QRSd of less than 130 msec. After AV optimization using the Ritter method[6] and simultaneous biventricular pacing, the number of regions displaying delayed longitudinal contraction was reduced and the ejection fraction was increased in all patients. These measurements were then repeated at five different interventricular delay intervals (12, 20, 40, 60, and 80 msec) with either LV or RV preactivation. Optimized sequential ventricular stimulation caused further reductions in regions displaying delayed longitudinal contraction and increases in ejection fraction, which were sustained for at least 3 months. Additionally, sequential ventricular stimulation increased diastolic filling time by about 7% even after AV optimization.

An interesting observation was that the location of myocardial regions displaying delayed longitudinal contraction varied among patients despite similar patterns of LBBB on the surface ECG. In most patients with nonischemic DCM, the delayed regions were located in the posterobasal LV (Fig. 26-17), whereas in ischemic DCM the delayed regions were more frequently in the interventricular septum and inferior wall (Fig. 26-18), although these patterns were not uniformly observed. Correspondingly, optimal sequential ventricular stimulation was achieved with LV preexcitation when the posterobasal region was delayed, and with RV preexcitation when the inferoseptal region was delayed. These beneficial effects were observed over a short range of ventricular timing intervals (±20 msec), and further increases in interventricular delay, or preexcitation of

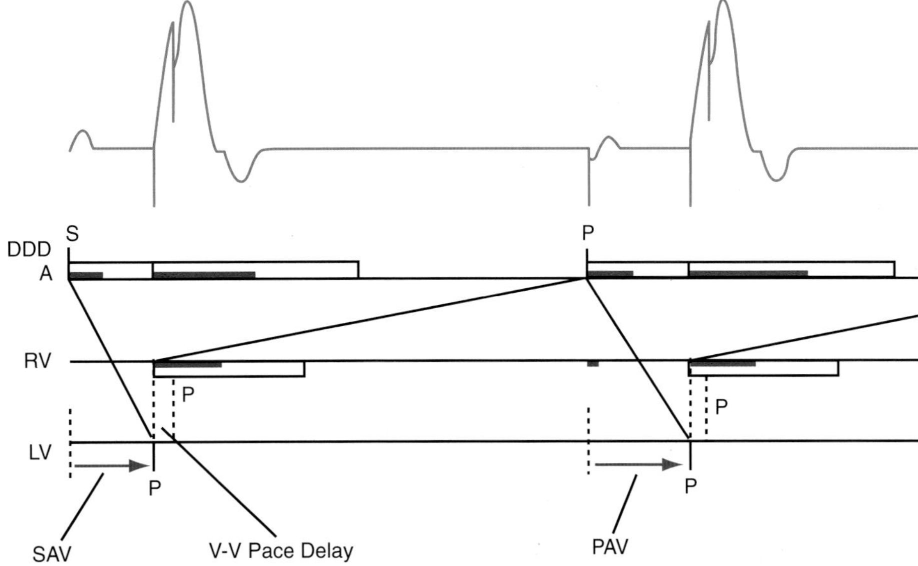

Figure 26-16. Interventricular (V-V) timing operation (Medtronic, Minneapolis, Minn.). A, atrium; LV, left ventricle; P, paced pulse; PAV, paced atrioventricular delay; S, sensed pulse; SAV, sensed atrioventricular delay; RV, right ventricle.

Non-IHD systolic performance at baseline

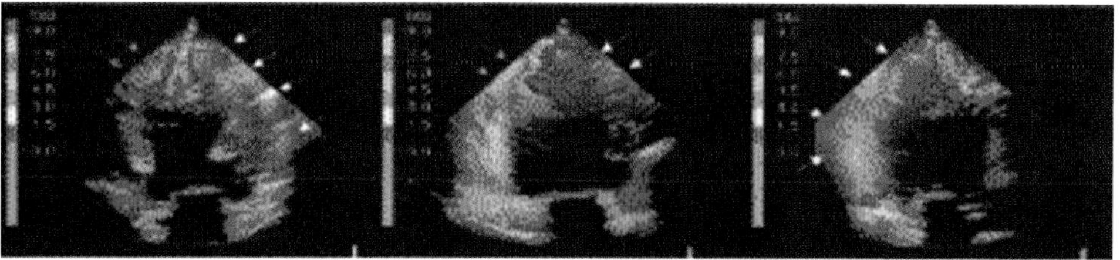

Non-IHD baseline delayed longitudinal contraction

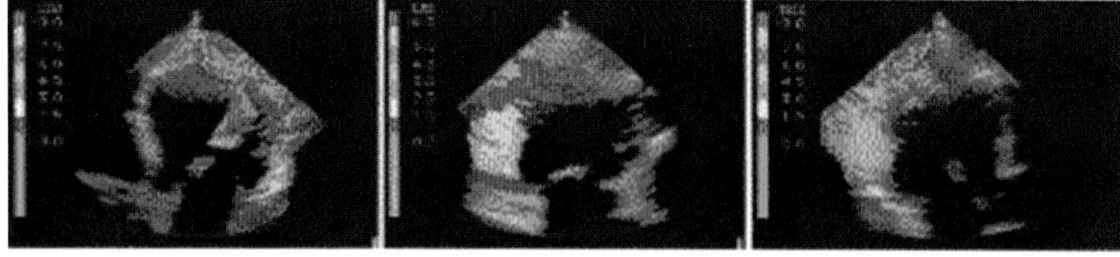

A

Non-IHD systolic performance during CRT (simultaneous)

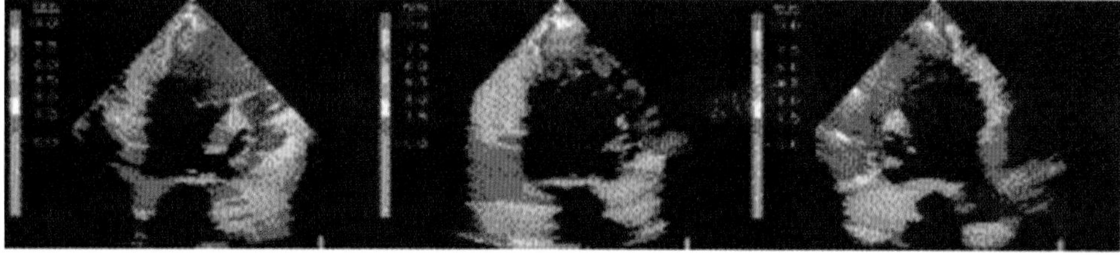

Non-IHD systolic performance during CRT (LV preactivated by 20 ms)

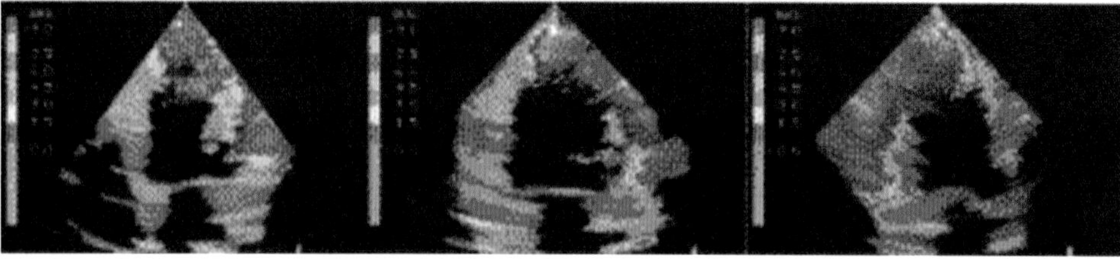

B

Figure 26-17. Effect of sequential ventricular stimulation on left ventricular (LV) systolic shortening. Color-coded scaling at left side of each image indicates regional motion amplitude. ***A,*** Top, left to right: *Baseline tissue tracking images in apical four-chamber, two-chamber, and long-axis views during systole in a patient with idiopathic dilated cardiomyopathy. Note lack of systolic motion in the lateral wall, posterior wall, and distal parts of anterior wall, denoted by gray color and white arrows. Mechanical function of the interventricular septum and inferior walls is abnormal, with greater motion amplitude in segments adjacent to apex* (green arrows). Bottom, left to right: *Extent of myocardium* (colored segments) *with delayed longitudinal contraction in diastole (mitral valve open). Delayed longitudinal contraction is present in lateral, posterior, and inferior walls. Note that the remaining part of the left ventricle (LV) is gray, indicating either no motion or motion toward the base of the heart (relaxation).* ***B,*** *Same patient and views as in panel* ***A*** *(systole).* Top, *Simultaneous cardiac resynchronization therapy (CRT) resulted in contraction of a larger proportion of the lateral wall and posterior wall. In addition, each segment showed improved systolic shortening, as seen from color coding. The abnormal distribution of myocardial motion in the interventricular septum was normalized.* Bottom, *Impact of sequential CRT with activation of the LV 20 msec before the right ventricle. Compared with simultaneous CRT, sequential CRT yielded further improvement in the overall proportion of contracting myocardium in the lateral and posterior walls. In addition, each segment showed further improvement in systolic shortening amplitude. IHD, ischemic heart disease. (From Sogaard P, Egeblad H, Pedersen AK, et al: Sequential versus simultaneous biventricular resynchronization for severe heart failure: Evaluation by tissue Doppler imaging. Circulation 106:2078-2084, 2002.)*

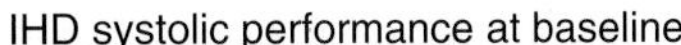

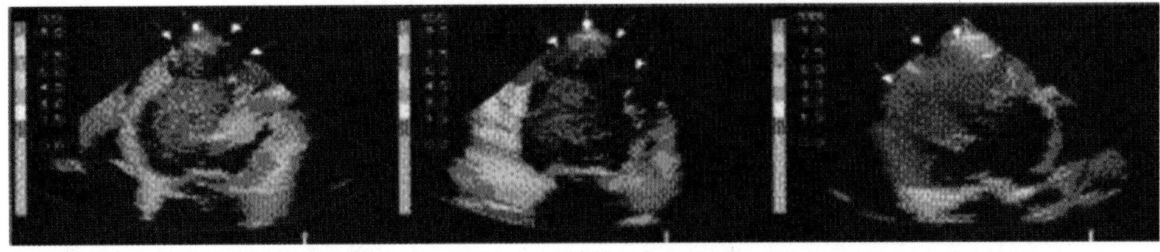

IHD delayed longitudinal contraction at baseline

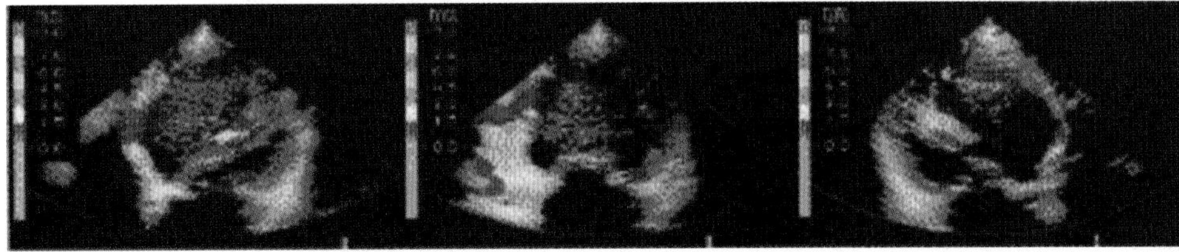

A

IHD systolic performance during CRT (simultaneous)

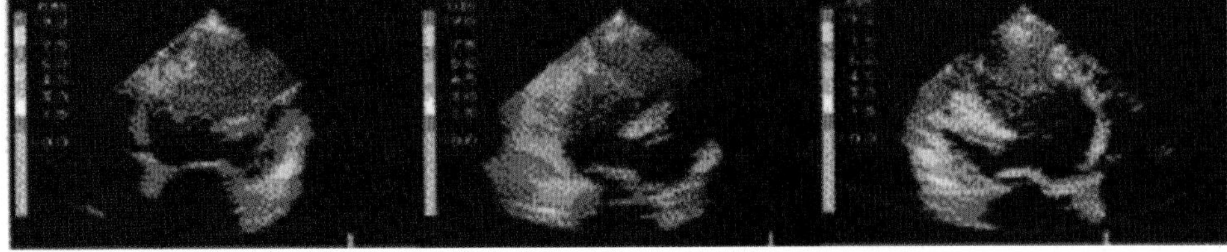

IHD systolic performance during CRT (RV preactivated by 12 ms)

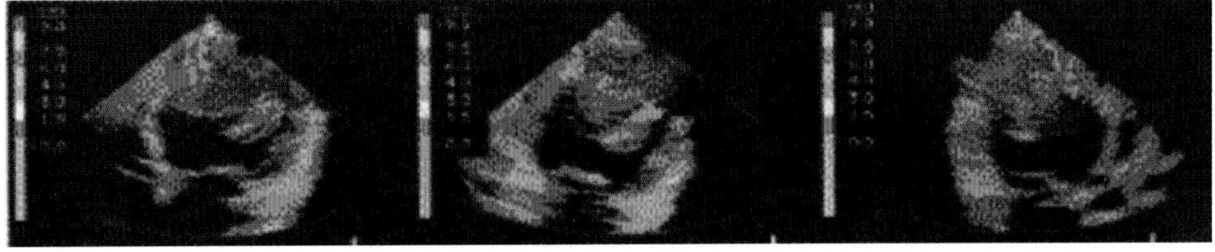

B

Figure 26-18. *Effect of V-V sequential ventricular stimulation on left ventricular (LV) systolic shortening.* ***A,*** Top, left to right: *Baseline tissue tracking images in apical four-chamber, two-chamber, and long-axis views during systole in a patient with idiopathic ischemic cardiomyopathy. Tissue tracking and strain rate analysis indicated apical infarct* (arrows). Bottom, left to right: *Extent of myocardium* (colored segments) *with delayed longitudinal contraction in interventricular septum and anterior and inferior walls (diastole). The extent of myocardium displaying delayed longitudinal contraction is less than that in patients with idiopathic dilated cardiomyopathy.* ***B,*** Top, *In the same patient as in panel* ***A,*** *simultaneous cardiac resynchronization therapy (CRT) resulted in overall improvement in regional systolic shortening.* Bottom, *Impact of sequential CRT with the right ventricular (RV) lead activated 12 msec before the LV lead. Compared with simultaneous CRT, sequential CRT yielded further improvement in systolic contraction amplitude. (From Sogaard P, Egeblad H, Pedersen AK, et al: Sequential versus simultaneous biventricular resynchronization for severe heart failure: Evaluation by tissue Doppler imaging. Circulation 106:2078-2084, 2002.)*

already early activated regions, resulted in worsened mechanical dyssynchrony and reduced pumping function.

Similar benefits of optimized sequential biventricular stimulation were observed by Bordachar and coworkers.[20] Using combined measures of LV diastolic filling time, cardiac output, mitral regurgitant volume and effective regurgitant orifice surface area (Fig. 26-19), systolic dyssynchrony index using tissue Doppler imaging, and extent of myocardium displaying delayed longitudinal contraction (tissue tracking), they found that simultaneous biventricular pacing was the optimal stimulation configuration in only 15% of patients. LV preexcitation was optimal for 61% of patients, with the V-V interval ranging between 12 and 40 msec, whereas RV preexcitation was optimal in 24% patients, with the V-V interval ranging from 12 to 20 msec. All patients demonstrated clinical responsiveness (improved NYHA class, quality of life score, and 6-minute hall walk) and evidence of reverse remodeling (improved ejection fraction, decreased LV end-systolic and end-diastolic volumes) at 3 months.

It is presently unclear what chronic benefit on a population scale, if any, manipulation of interventricular

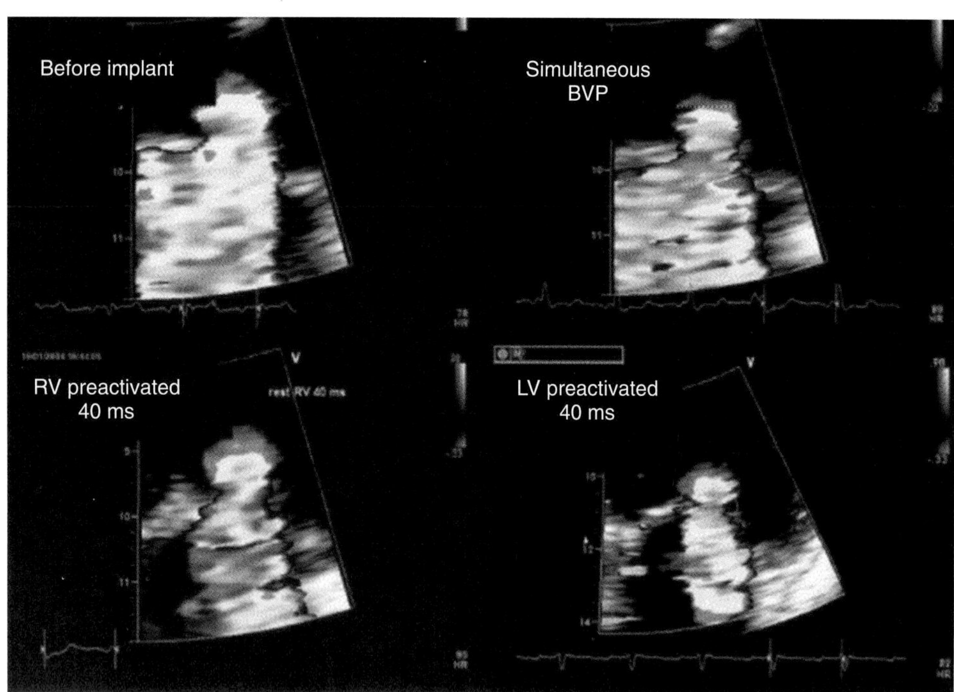

Figure 26-19. Reduction of mitral regurgitation with optimized sequential biventricular pacing (BVP). The preimplantation effective regurgitant orifice area (EROA) was 31 mm²; the simultaneous BVP EROA was 22 mm²; the sequential BVP EROA with right ventricular (RV) preactivation of 40 milliseconds (ms) was 21 mm²; and the optimized sequential BVP EROA with left ventricular (LV) preactivation of 40 ms was 10 mm². (From Bordachar P, Lafitte S, Reuter S, et al: Echocardiographic parameters of ventricular dys-synchrony validation in patients with heart failure using sequential biventricular pacing. J Am Coll Cardiol 44:2157-2165, 2004.)

timing would provide during biventricular pacing. Furthermore, there is emerging evidence that univentricular LV pacing is probably either equivalent or superior to biventricular pacing acutely and chronically (see later discussion).

Right Ventricular, Left Ventricular, or Biventricular Antitachycardia Pacing in CRTD

An interesting recent development in the clinical application of antitachycardia pacing (ATP) is the focus on the stimulation site of origin. It is important to note that the pathophysiologic mechanism of reentrant ventricular tachycardia (VT) is not dependent on, or influenced by, the site of origin of the VT circuit. From a practical perspective, site of origin might be very important, because most VT circuits arise in the left ventricle, and pacing stimuli are conventionally delivered from the RV apex. Because distance and conduction time between the stimulation site and the site of origin affect the ability of pacing stimuli to interact with the reentrant circuit, ATP delivered from the LV pacing lead, or from biventricular pacing leads in CRTD, might improve efficacy compared with RV ATP.

Scientific evidence regarding the relative differences between RV, LV, and biventricular ATP for terminating monomorphic VT is limited. In the Ventak CHF/CONTAK CD study,[21] all ATP among those patients randomly assigned to CRT was delivered simultaneously from the right and left ventricles (biventricular ATP). Monomorphic VT was successfully terminated in 927 (88%) of 1053 episodes. Although this is in alignment with success rates for ATP delivered from the RV apex in other studies,[22-30] no comparison was made between biventricular ATP and RV-only ATP (i.e., patients assigned to no CRT).

The relative efficacy of RV versus biventricular ATP was evaluated in the InSync ICD OUS (Outside United States) Study.[31] ATP termination success was 2.4 times greater with biventricular versus RV ATP and appeared to be associated with fewer accelerations for both slow and fast VT. A similar result was observed in the MIRACLE ICD study, which randomized RV versus biventricular ATP for monomorphic VT induced during implantation. Biventricular ATP had a higher efficacy than RV ATP: 622 (95%) of 658 and 297 (88%) of 336 episodes, respectively ($P < 0.001$). A preliminary report from the VENTAK CHF/CONTAK CD study also showed that biventricular ATP was more successful in patients randomly assigned to CRT pacing therapy.[32] This effect was influenced by LV pacing lead location (improving in lateral locations, worsening in anterior locations) and improved over time in the patients who were receiving CRT.

These data are insufficient to support definitive conclusions regarding the role of ATP at alternative sites for terminating VT. Because of technical limitations, the CRTD ICDs in both studies were capable only of RV or biventricular stimulation and therefore provided no insights on a possible role for isolated LV stimulation. From a theoretical perspective, it is not immediately obvious that LV stimulation should improve ATP success in coronary artery disease, because many reentrant VT circuits arise in the interventricular septum, closer to an RV stimulation site than to an LV free wall stimulation site. Conduction delay out of LV stimulation sites resulting from interposed infarction and fibrosis might modify any advantage related to proximity to the site of VT origin, and this effect may be different in the right ventricle. How these and other factors might influence the relative efficacy of LV ATP is unknown.

Summary of Ventricular Therapy Programming in CRTD

ATP reliably terminates 85% to 90% of slow VT (cycle lengths [CL] <300 to 320 msec) with a low risk of acceleration (1% to 5%). Similar high success and low acceleration rates for fast VT (CLs, 320 to 240 msec) have recently been demonstrated. These results are probably consistent across different substrates (ischemic versus nonischemic DCM) when the common mechanism of VT is reentry. Therefore, ATP should be routinely applied in CRTD regardless of substrate.

Some general recommendations on programming ATP schemes are possible. For VT CLs longer than 300 to 330 msec, burst and ramp pacing are equivalently effective for terminating VT and equivalently low risk for causing acceleration. For VT CLs shorter than 300 to 330 msec, burst pacing is more effective and less likely to result in acceleration than ramp pacing. In either case, the risk of acceleration is inversely related to the VT CL. "Less aggressive" burst stimulation (e.g., 91% versus 81% of VT CL) is more effective and causes less acceleration, especially for fast VT (CL <320 msec).[33] "Tailoring" of ATP to specific induced VTs is not necessary in most situations.

Loss of Cardiac Resynchronization: Causes and Corrective Actions

Optimal CRT operation requires continuous delivery of ventricular pacing. In practical experience, 100% ventricular pacing is difficult to achieve. A reasonable goal is 90% to 95% cumulative ventricular pacing with verified LV capture. A retrospective analysis of the VENTAK CHF/CONTAK CD Biventricular Pacing Study revealed that CRT is interrupted transiently in 36% of patients and permanently in 5% within 2 years of follow-up, and the causes are diverse.[34] Restoration of CRT can usually be accomplished noninvasively and less commonly requires surgical intervention.

Loss of CRT Related to Pacing Operation

Obviously, programming parameters during CRT operation should reflect the goal of continuous ventricular pacing. Therefore, any parameter choice that might reduce the frequency of ventricular pacing should be avoided. The consequence of programmed parameters on continuous delivery of CRT is influenced by the patient's AV conduction status. The majority of patients who receive CRT have reliable AV conduction, and therefore any programming choice that permits the emergence of native ventricular activation will reduce delivery of CRT. In dual-chamber CRT systems, examples include pacing modes that do not synchronize ventricular pacing to atrial activity (e.g., DDI, VVI), inappropriately long AV delays or use of automatic AV interval extension, and any parameter that compromises continuous atrial tracking (true undersensing or pseudoundersensing resulting from a long postventricular atrial refractory period [PVARP], automatic PVARP extensions, or a low upper tracking rate). In single-chamber CRT systems, for patients with permanent AF, the lower rate should be programmed to continuously exceed the spontaneous ventricular rate. The absence of AV conduction renders loss of CRT due to poor programming choices unlikely, because ventricular pacing cannot be inadvertently minimized by competition with native ventricular activation; however, considerations regarding optimal AV delay still apply. Even when these recommendations are implemented, loss of CRT can occur because of the complex interplay between spontaneous electrical activity and inviolable elements of timing cycle operation.

Pseudoatrial Undersensing

A reduction in ventricular pacing due to loss of atrial tracking at high sinus rates ("pseudoatrial undersensing") is common. In this circumstance, high sinus rates and first-degree AV block (which are common in heart failure patients) displace the P wave into the PVARP, resulting in simultaneous loss of atrial tracking and synchronous ventricular pacing. This situation is commonly triggered by automatic PVARP extensions after a premature ventricular contraction (PVC) or other circumstances intended to prevent pacemaker-mediated tachycardia.[35] Spontaneous AV conduction occurs in the form of a preempted upper rate Wenckebach response (Fig. 26-20).

Although it is not required for pseudoatrial undersensing, double-counting of the native ventricular EGM (see later discussion) often participates in the initiation and maintenance of the phenomenon in nondedicated (Y-adaptor) systems or in first-generation dual cathodal CRTP/CRTD systems in which pacing and sensing from the RV and LV occur simultaneously (Fig. 26-21). If spontaneous conduction with LBBB (or any form of ventricular conduction delay) emerges, the LV EGM may be sensed some time after detection of the RV EGM if the LV signal extends beyond the relatively short ventricular blanking period initiated by RV sensing. The LV signal continuously resets the PVARP, resulting in an "implied" total atrial refractory period (iTARP) conflict and maintenance of pseudoatrial undersensing.

Failure to deliver CRT at high sinus rates can be minimized by shortening the PVARP, increasing the upper tracking limit and deactivating the PVC response in the DDD mode. Newer CRT systems minimize ventricular double-counting by employing an interventricular refractory period (IVRP). Ventricular sensed events (i.e., LV sensing) during the IVRP do not reset the PVARP, so the implied TARP conflict is eliminated (Fig. 26-22). Another method for dealing with disruptions to CRT delivery when PVCs cause the following atrial events to fall into the PVARP is the Atrial Tracking Recovery (ATR) system (Medtronic) (Figs. 26-23, 26-24, and 26-25). The ATR system operates in the DDD/R mode when a mode switch episode is not in effect. Under certain conditions, ATR temporarily shortens the PVARP to reduce the intrinsic TARP. The device monitors for eight consecutive

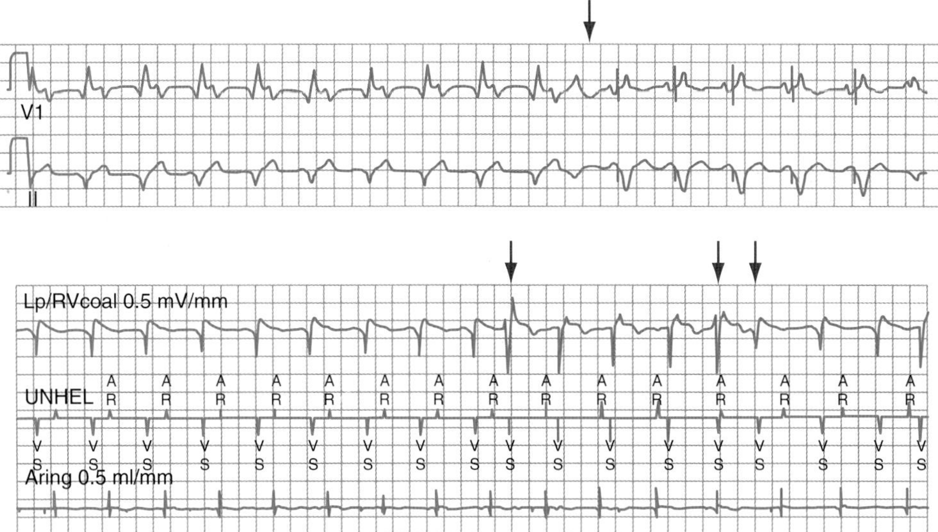

Figure 26-20. Loss of CRT due to pseudoatrial undersensing. Top, Telemetry strip. *Note sinus tachycardia with marked first-degree atrioventricular (AV) block (P-R interval, 400 msec) and loss of atrial synchronous biventricular pacing on left. Atrial synchronous biventricular pacing is restored after premature ventricular contraction* (arrow) *on right. Bottom,* Tracking in same *patient. The sinus rate exceeds the programmed upper rate limit, displacing P waves into the postventricular atrial refractory period (PVARP, marked as AR). Spontaneous AV conduction occurs in the form of a preempted Wenckebach upper-rate response. The first PVC* (first arrow) *resets the PVARP and restores atrial tracking. The second PVC* (second arrow) *occurs coincident with a sinus event, which falls into the postventricular atrial blanking period. The third PVC* (third arrow) *resets the PVARP and reinitiates pseudoatrial undersensing. Atrial tracking is restored when the sinus rate slows slightly at the end of the strip.*

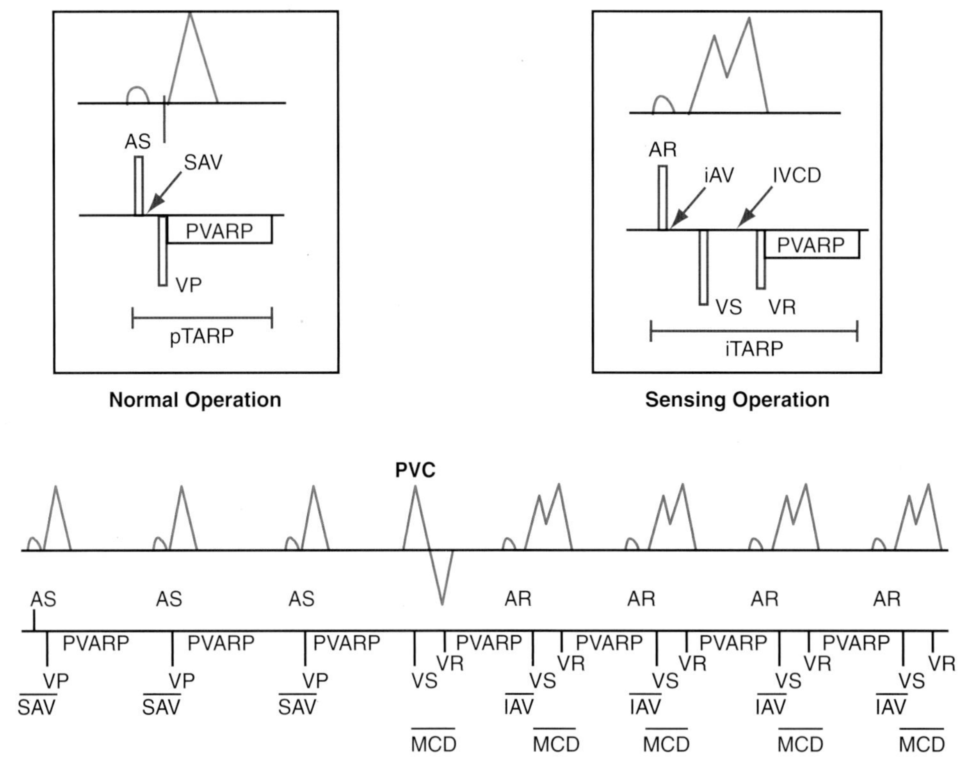

Figure 26-21. Loss of CRT due to pseudoatrial undersensing and ventricular double-counting with implied total atrial refractory period. The premature ventricular contraction (PVC) is double-counted; the second component resets the postventricular atrial refractory period (PVARP), which initiates pseudoatrial sensing. Loss of CRT results in emergence of spontaneous atrioventricular (AV) conduction. Double-counting of the native ventricular electrogram continuously resets the PVARP, perpetuating pseudoatrial sensing. The implied total atrial refractory period (iTARP) is equal to the sensed AV delay (SAV) plus the PVARP plus the interventricular conduction delay (IVCD). AR, atrial refractory event; AS, atrial sensed event; VP, ventricular paced event; VR, ventricular refractory event; VS, ventricular sensed event.

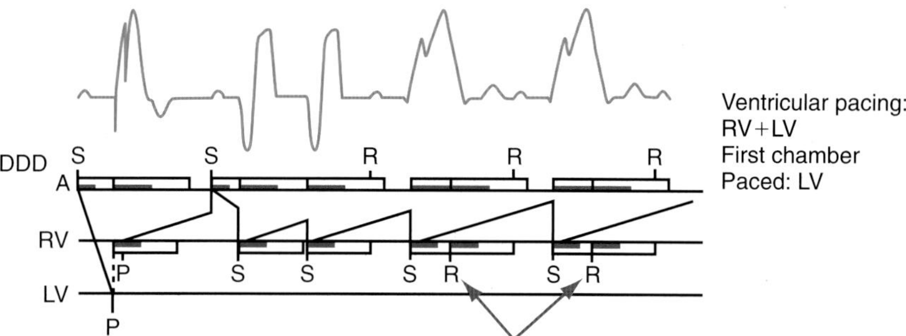

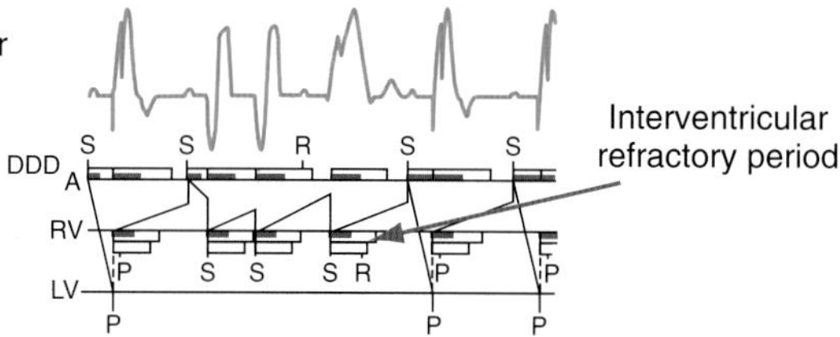

Figure 26-22. Role of interventricular refractory period in eliminating the implied total atrial refractory period and reducing loss of CRT due to pseudoatrial undersensing. A, atrium; LV, left ventricle; P, paced pulse; R, refractory event; RV, right ventricle; S, sensed event.

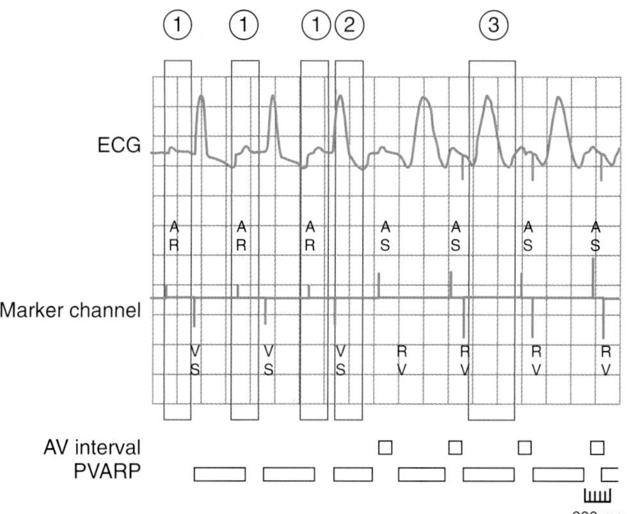

1 Atrial events occur during PVARP and are not tracked.
2 After eight qualifying AR-VS cycles, ATR intervenes to break the pattern. PVARP is shortened.
3 The intervention continues until proper A-V tracking at the programmed SAV value resumes.

Figure 26-23. Atrial Tracking Recovery (ATR) system (Medtronic, Minneapolis, Minn.). AR, atrial refractory event; AV, atrioventricular; ECG, electrocardiogram; PVARP, postventricular atrial refractory period; SAV, sensed atrioventricular delay; VS, ventricular sensed event.

pacing cycles in which all of the following occur: (1) the current ventricular event is sensed, not paced; (2) the last ventricular interval contains exactly one refractory atrial event; (3) the last two atrial intervals vary from each other by less than 50 msec; (4) the last atrial interval is longer than the upper tracking rate interval by at least 50 msec; (5) the last atrial interval is greater than the current SAV plus current PVARP, (6) the last VS-AR interval (from the previous ventricular event to the atrial refractory event) is greater than the postventricular atrial blanking period (PVAB).

To start or continue an ATR intervention, the device sets a temporary truncated PVARP equal to last VS-AR interval minus 50 msec. If this computed value is shorter than the programmed PVAB, then the PVAB value is used. On subsequent pacing cycles during ATR intervention, the device recalculates the temporary PVARP. ATR intervention ends when the ventricular pace occurs at the scheduled SAV interval, or when the computed temporary PVARP is no longer shorter than the otherwise indicated PVARP. If the pacing pattern is interrupted, for example by a ventricular sensed event, the intervention aborts.

Atrial Tracking Preference is a similar but less ornate approach used in Guidant (Boston Scientific, Natick, Mass.) pulse generators (Fig. 26-26). It is designed to maintain atrial-tracked ventricular pacing in DDD(R) and VDD(R) modes at high sinus rates. Tracking Preference temporarily shortens the PVARP to reestablish atrial-tracked ventricular pacing inappropriately lost due to atrial events occurring in PVARP (pseudoatrial undersensing).

Atrial Oversensing

Automatic mode switching is intended to prevent undesirable rapid ventricular pacing due to tracking of atrial tachyarrhythmias during DDD operation. Detection of atrial tachyarrhythmias results in reversion to a nontacking mode (DDI or VDI). Spurious mode switching is a common problem and can result in loss of atrial synchronous ventricular pacing during CRT. The dominant cause of spurious mode switching is oversensing of far-field R-waves.[36-40] This can be recognized on stored marker channels or EGMs by an alternating pattern of atrial cycle lengths with one signal timed close to the ventricular EGM. Less common causes of spurious mode switching include "near-field" or "early" R-wave oversensing (atrial R-wave sensing before arrival of the depolarization wavefront at the ventricular pacing lead position) and oversensing of the paced atrial depolarization during the AV interval.[40,41] Spurious mode switching can usually be eliminated by using bipolar atrial pacing leads, extending the PVAB,

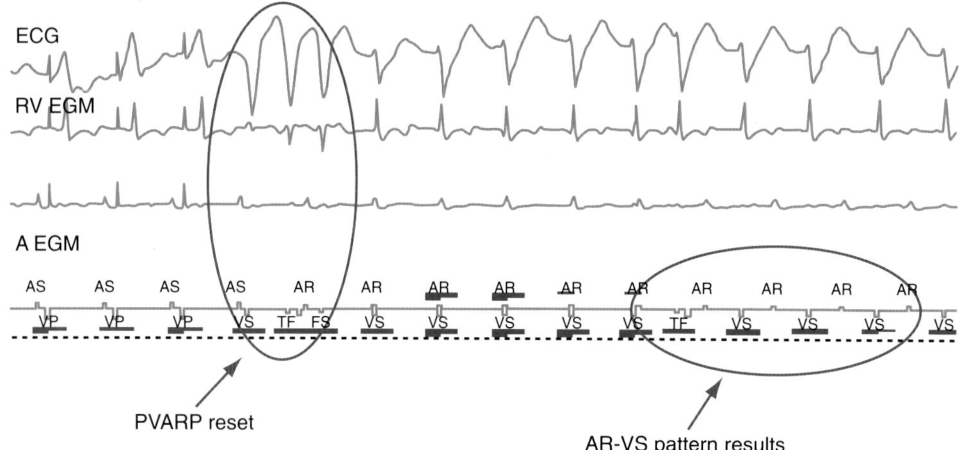

Figure 26-24. Ventricular premature beats cause loss of CRT due to implied total atrial refractory period and pseudo-atrial undersensing. A EGM, atrial electrogram; AR, atrial refractory event; AS, atrial sensed event; ECG, electrocardiogram; PVARP, postventricular atrial refractory period; RV EGM, right ventricular electrogram; VS, ventricular sensed event.

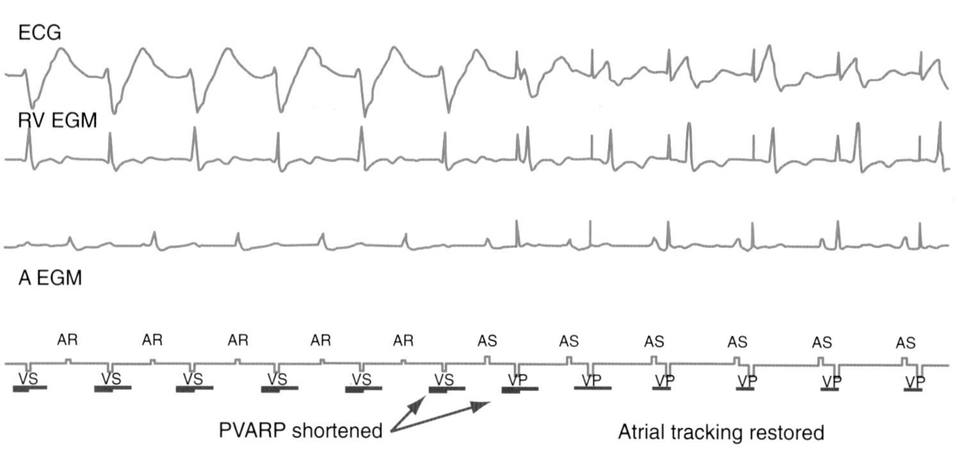

Figure 26-25. Atrial Tracking Recovery operation (Medtronic, Minneapolis, Minn.). A EGM, atrial electrogram; AR, atrial refractory event; AS, atrial sensed event; ECG, electrocardiogram; RV EGM, right ventricular electrogram; VP, ventricular paced event; VS, ventricular sensed event.

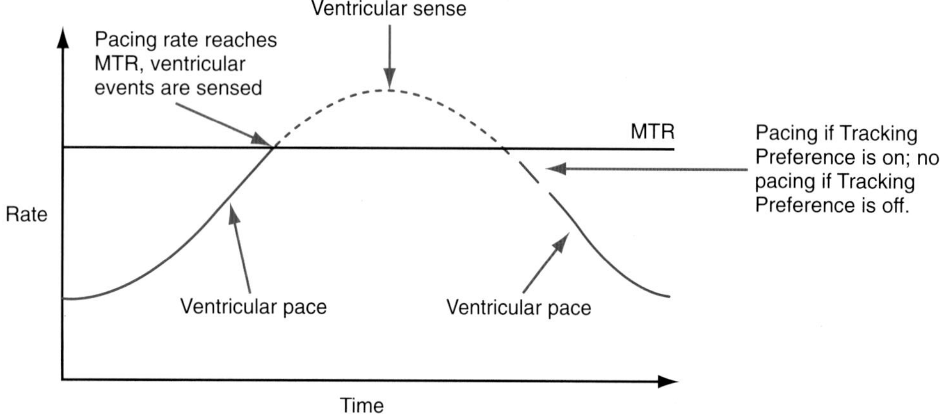

Figure 26-26. Atrial Tracking Preference system (Guidant, Boston Scientific, Natick, Mass.). MTR, maximum tracking rate.

or reducing atrial sensitivity so as to reject far-field signals without compromising atrial sensing.

Loss of CRT due to Prevention of Pacing on the T Wave

Theoretically, conduction delay could prevent a PVC initiated in the left ventricle from reaching the RV electrode (univentricular sensing) and inhibiting the scheduled biventricular pace triggered by a sensed (or paced) atrial event. In this situation, lack of LV sensing could result in competitive ventricular pacing outside the absolute myocardial refractory period. To prevent competitive pacing during the LV vulnerable period (including the T wave), some Guidant CRTD systems incorporate a Left Ventricular Protection Period (LVPP). The LVPP is defined as the period after an LV event, either paced or sensed, during which LV pacing is inhibited; the LVPP is programmable between 300 and 500 msec. The LVPP reduces the maximum LV pacing rate and theoretically could disrupt CRT by preventing LV stimulation when preceded by RV stimulation, depending on the programmed interventricular delay and the conduction time from the RV to LV electrode.

Loss of CRT due to Competition with Native Ventricular Activation

Any situation that permits competition between the delivery of continuous ventricular pacing and native ventricular activation will degrade CRT efficacy. This is far more likely to occur in patients with intact AV conduction.

Atrial Tachyarrhythmias with Rapid Ventricular Conduction. Atrial tachyarrhythmias are a common cause of loss of CRT, accounting for 18% of all therapy interruptions in one study.[34] Paroxysmal AF in patients with dual-chamber CRT systems results in appropriate mode switching and loss of atrial synchronous ventricular pacing (see earlier discussion). In the absence of mode switching, native ventricular activation due to rapidly conducted paroxysmal AF may compete with continuous ventricular pacing (Figs. 26-27 and 26-28).

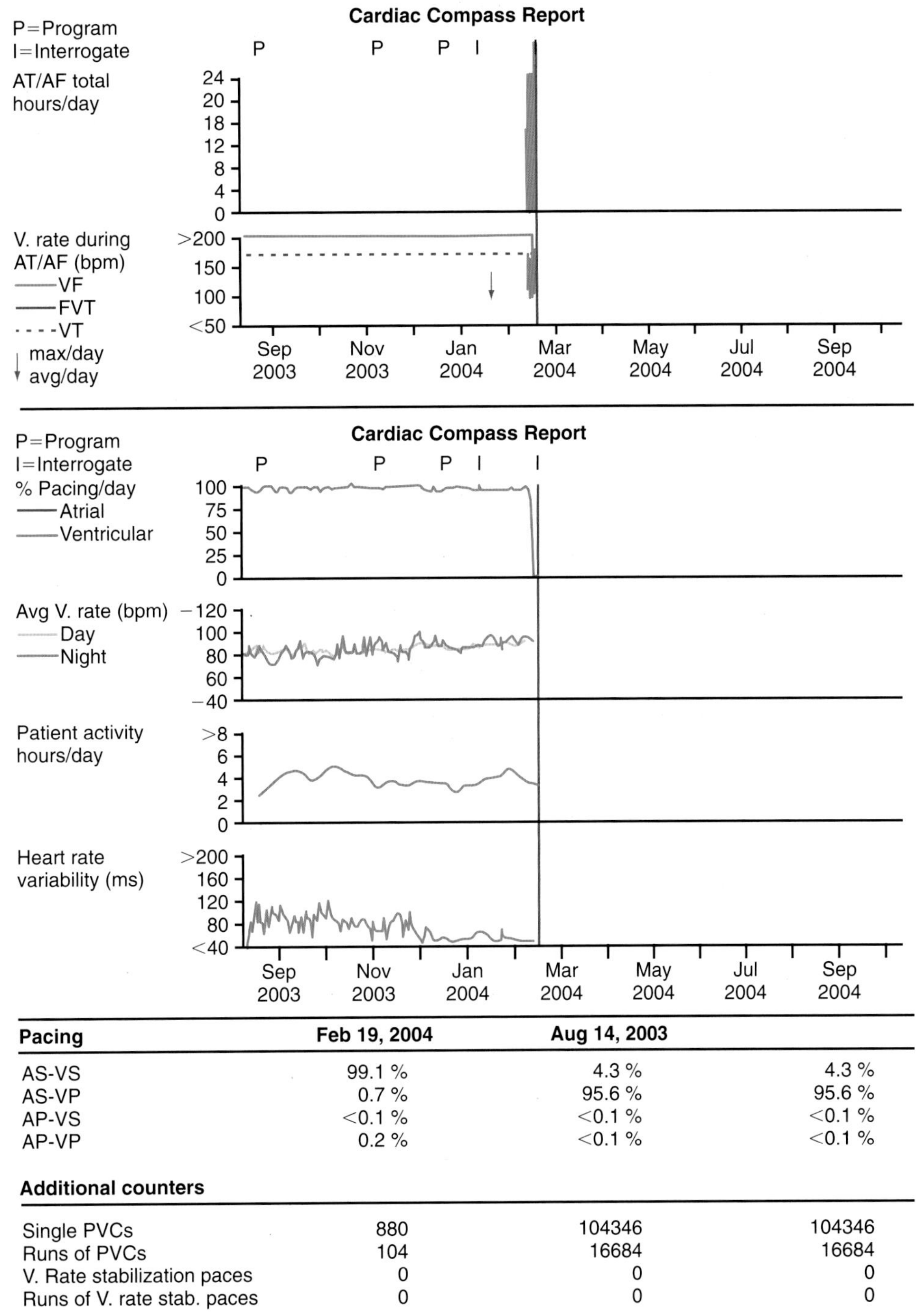

Pacing	Feb 19, 2004	Aug 14, 2003	
AS-VS	99.1 %	4.3 %	4.3 %
AS-VP	0.7 %	95.6 %	95.6 %
AP-VS	<0.1 %	<0.1 %	<0.1 %
AP-VP	0.2 %	<0.1 %	<0.1 %

Additional counters			
Single PVCs	880	104346	104346
Runs of PVCs	104	16684	16684
V. Rate stabilization paces	0	0	0
Runs of V. rate stab. paces	0	0	0

Figure 26-27. Loss of CRT due to atrial fibrillation. Note high percent AS-VP count before onset of atrial fibrillation. Onset of atrial fibrillation with rapid atrioventricular conduction results in sudden loss of CRT, indicated by high percent AS-VS count.

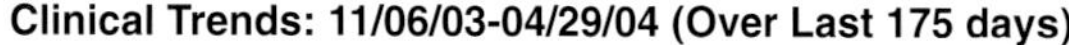

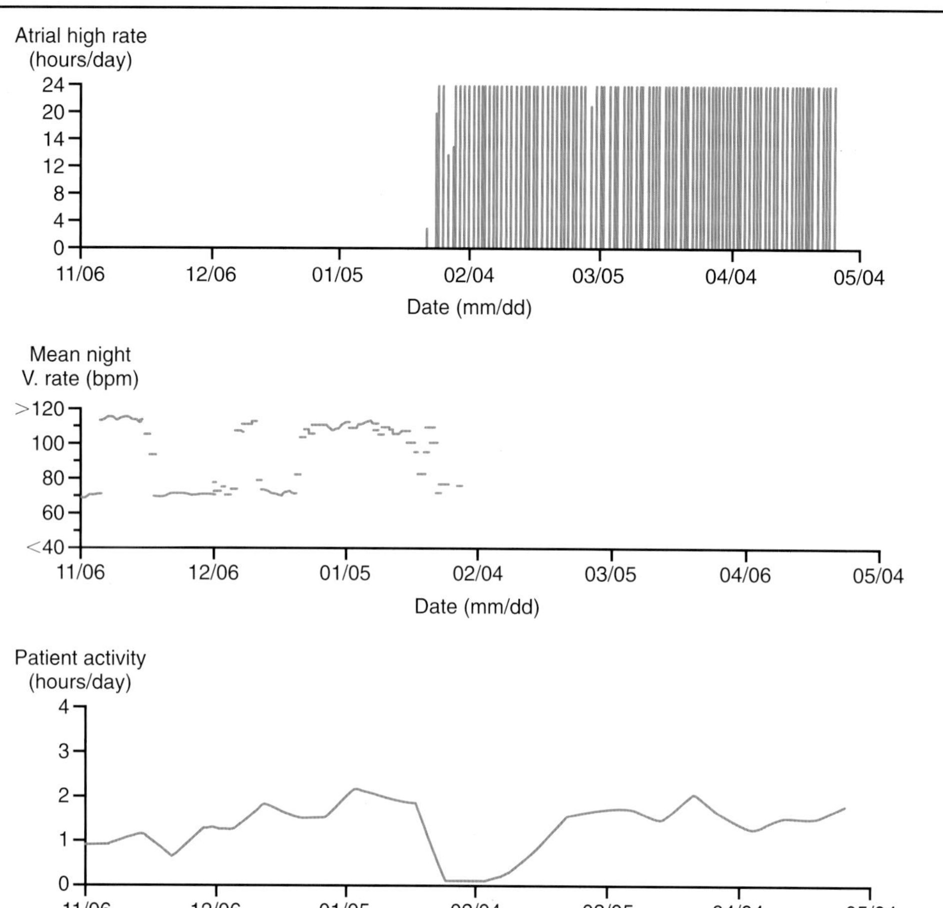

Figure 26-28. Loss of CRT due to atrial fibrillation (AF). Top, *Onset of persistent AF in late January 2004. Note histogram showing AF for 24 hours/day.* Middle, *Increase in mean ventricular rate at night corresponding to onset of AF.* Bottom, *Abrupt decline in patient's activity hours per day corresponding to onset of persistent AF.*

Management should focus on pharmacologic suppression of AF and control of the conducted ventricular response.

Historically, symptoms during AF have been attributed to a combination of loss of AV synchrony and rapid ventricular rate, which may result in significant reductions in cardiac output. More recently, the independent effect of ventricular cycle length irregularity on adverse hemodynamic performance during AF has been recognized.[42-44] One study demonstrated acute improvement in hemodynamic performance and long-term improvements in symptoms and quality of life among patients with chronic AF and a controlled ventricular response after AV junction ablation and VVIR pacemaker implantation.[42]

These benefits were attributed to an independent effect of ventricular rate regularization, because loss of AV synchrony was constant and rapid ventricular rates were excluded by study design. These results contribute to the interpretation of prior studies that reported DDDR pacing with mode switching is preferred to VVIR pacing among patients who have undergone AV junction ablation for uncontrollable ventricular response during paroxysmal AF.[45-48] Such patients are rendered incapable of a rapid ventricular response during paroxysmal AF via mode switching; therefore, the symptomatic benefits are not surprising.

The importance of rate control and regularization of the ventricular response during AF to optimize CRT response should not be underestimated. For example, the relatively neutral effect of biventricular versus RV apex pacing immediately after AV junction ablation in patients with systolic heart failure suggests that the benefits of rate control in AF are so large that they conceal the effect of asynchronous ventricular activation.[49] In patients with permanent AF and single-chamber CRT systems, continuous delivery of ventricular pacing and optimal CRT response may require ablation of the AV junction.

Specific features of pacing operation may increase the percentage of ventricular pacing during rapidly conducted AF and thereby prevent disruptions to CRT. Conducted Atrial Fibrillation Response (CAFR; Medtronic) increases the ventricular pacing rate in alignment with the native conducted ventricular response (Figs. 26-29, 26-30, and 26-31). The intent is to regularize the

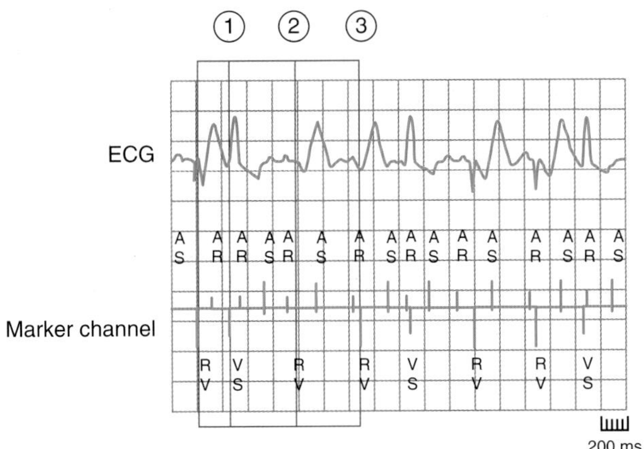

1 BV-AR-VS sequence causes pacing rate to increase by 1 min^{-1}. If Response Level is programmed to Low or Medium.
2 VS-BV sequence causes pacing rate to be unchanged.
3 BV-BV sequence causes pacing rate to decrease by 1 min^{-1}.

Figure 26-29. Conducted Atrial Fibrillation Response (Medtronic, Minneapolis, Minn.). AR, atrial refractory event; BV, biventricular paced event; ECG, electrocardiogram; VS, ventricular sensed event.

ventricular rate by increasing the overall percentage of ventricular pacing while minimizing the increase in overall heart rate. This is achieved by adjusting the pacing escape interval after each ventricular event. The escape interval increases or decreases based on a contextual analysis of the preceding events. For example, a biventricular paced event (BV)–atrial refractory event (AR)–ventricular sensed event (VS) sequence will increment the pacing rate by 1 beat per minute (bpm), whereas a BV-BV sequence will decrement the pacing rate by 1 bpm. The result is a higher percentage of ventricular pacing at an average rate that closely matches the patient's own ventricular response. The maximum rate for CAFR pacing is programmable. The minimum rate derives from the otherwise-indicated (sensor rate, mode switch, or lower rate) pacing interval. When the otherwise-indicated pacing rate is faster than the programmed maximum rate, this feature is suspended and the device operates at the otherwise-indicated pacing rate. The use of CAFR necessitates interactions with other device operations. For example, in DDD and DDDR modes, Ventricular Rate Stabilization and CARF cannot operate at the same time. When both are enabled, Ventricular Rate Stabilization operates only

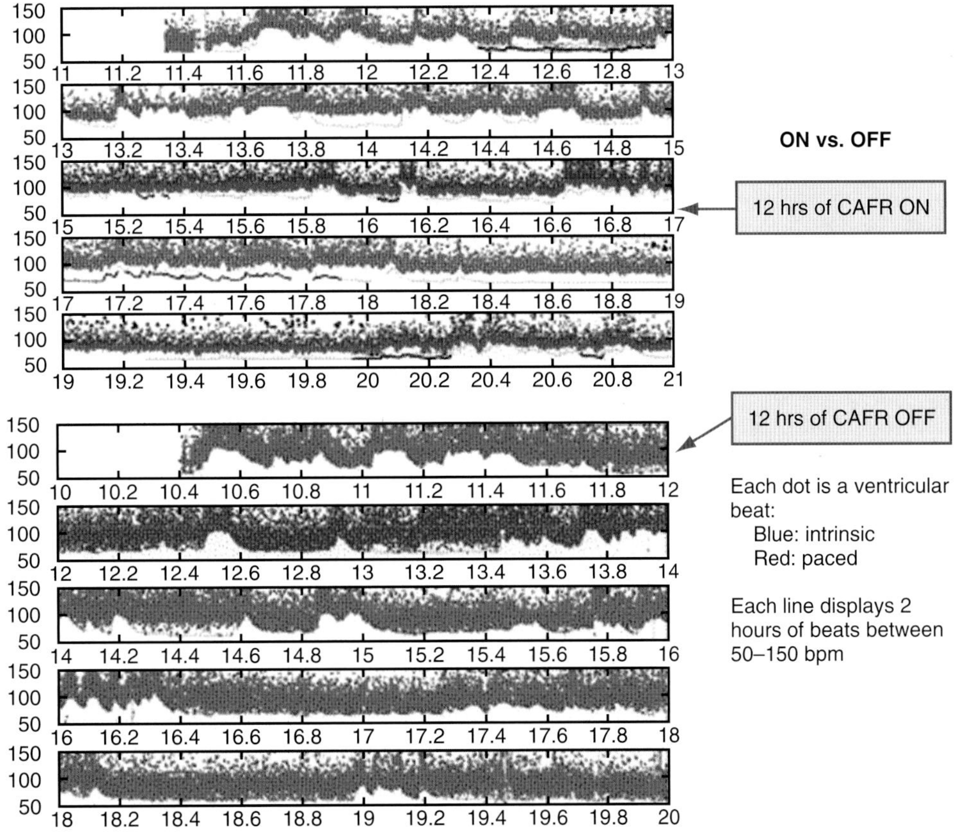

Figure 26-30. Conducted Atrial Fibrillation Response (CAFR, Medtronic, Minneapolis, Minn.). Plot of ventricular beats derived from Holter monitoring of a patient with permanent atrial fibrillation (AF). Top four lines show effect of CAFR therapy; bottom four lines show VVIR pacing (no CAFR therapy). Ventricular paced beats are shown in red, ventricular sensed beats in blue. Note the greater amount (and higher rate) of pacing (red dots) *but also the apparent decrease in fast ventricular beats* (blue dots) *during CAFR operation. (From Yee, et al: Can J Cardiol, 16:133F.)*

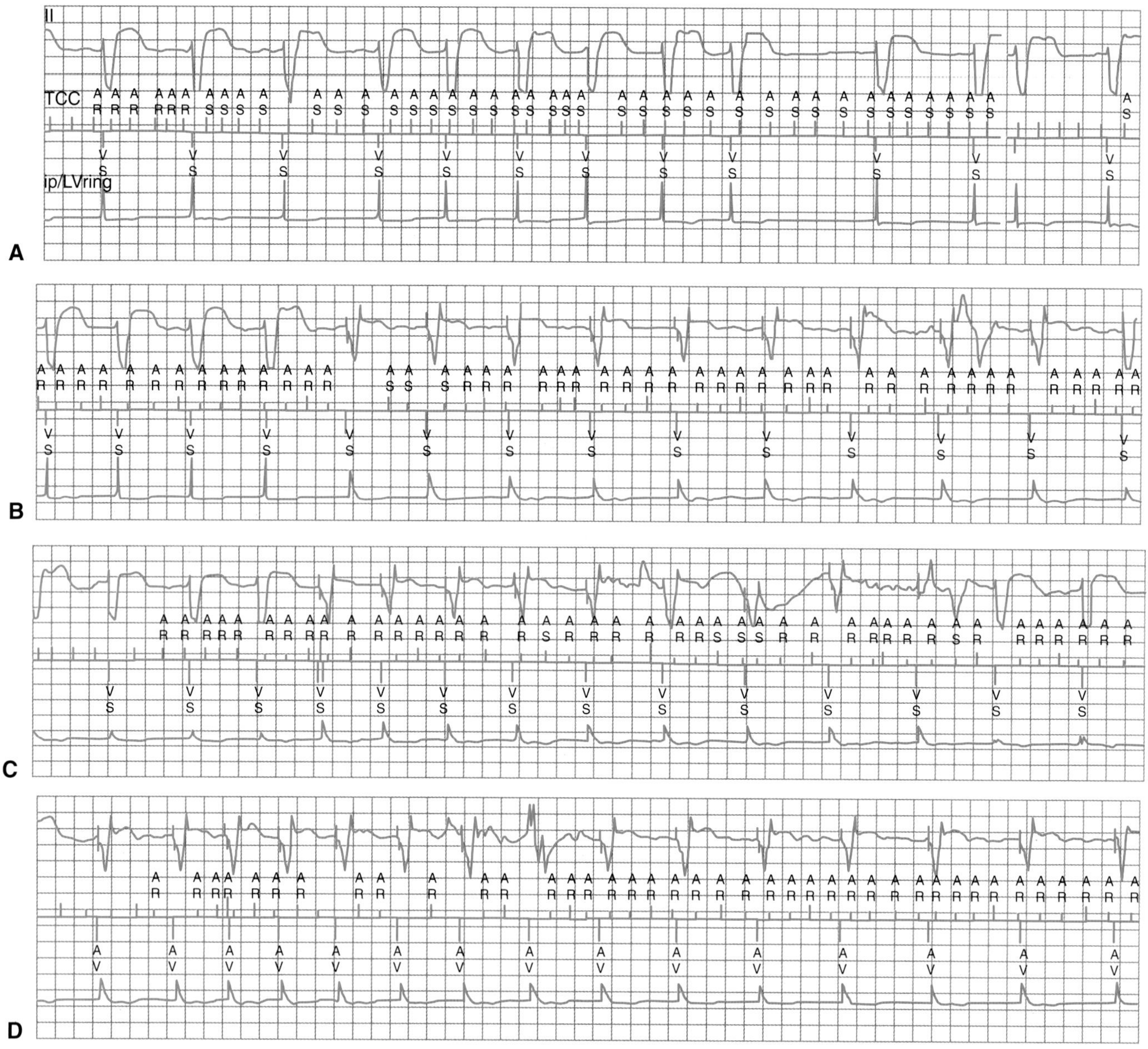

Figure 26-31. Effects of Ventricular Sense Response (VSR) and Conducted Atrial Fibrillation Response (CAFR; Medtronic, Minneapolis, Minn.) on ventricular pacing during atrial fibrillation (AF) with intact atrioventricular (AV) conduction. ***A,*** *Programmed mode is VVI 30 bpm. Note AF with intact AV conduction and absence of ventricular pacing.* ***B,*** *Programmed mode is VVI 30 bpm with VSR ON. Note delivery of biventricular pacing without any increase in ventricular rate.* ***C,*** *Programmed mode is DDD 30 bpm with CAFR ON. Note increase in ventricular pacing rate immediately after mode switch (MS marker) occurs, which initiates CAFR operation.* ***D,*** *Programmed mode is DDD 30 bpm with VSR and CAFR ON. Note increase in ventricular pacing rate immediately after mode switch (MS marker) occurs, which initiates CAFR operation, and also VSR pacing during a premature ventricular contraction (eighth complex from the left).*

when the device is not mode-switched. CAFR operates only in nontracking modes. Therefore, when DDD or DDDR mode is programmed, CAFR operates only during a mode switch. CAFR is suspended during automatic tachyarrhythmia therapies, arrhythmia inductions, manual therapies, and emergency fixed burst, cardioversion, and defibrillation.

Ventricular Rate Regulation (VRR, Guidant) is designed to reduce V-V cycle length variability during conducted atrial arrhythmias by moderating the ventricular pacing rate based on a previous V-V average (Figs. 26-32, 26-33, and 26-34). VRR provides ventricular regulation during conducted atrial arrhythmias, whereas Rate Smoothing (Guidant) is typically more useful for reducing pauses after ventricular premature depolarizations. VRR operates in the DDD/R mode only during an AT/AF mode-switch episode, but it is available all the time in the single-chamber VVI/R modes.

Unlike Rate Smoothing, in which changes are based on the most recent V-V interval, VRR uses a weighted ventricular average based on cycle lengths during the mode-switch episode. This weighted average is made

Figure 26-32. Ventricular Rate Regularization (VRR; Guidant, Boston Scientific, Natick, Mass.). Note reduction in ventricular interval variation but increase in pacing rate during operation with VRR ON (bottom) *versus VRR OFF* (top).

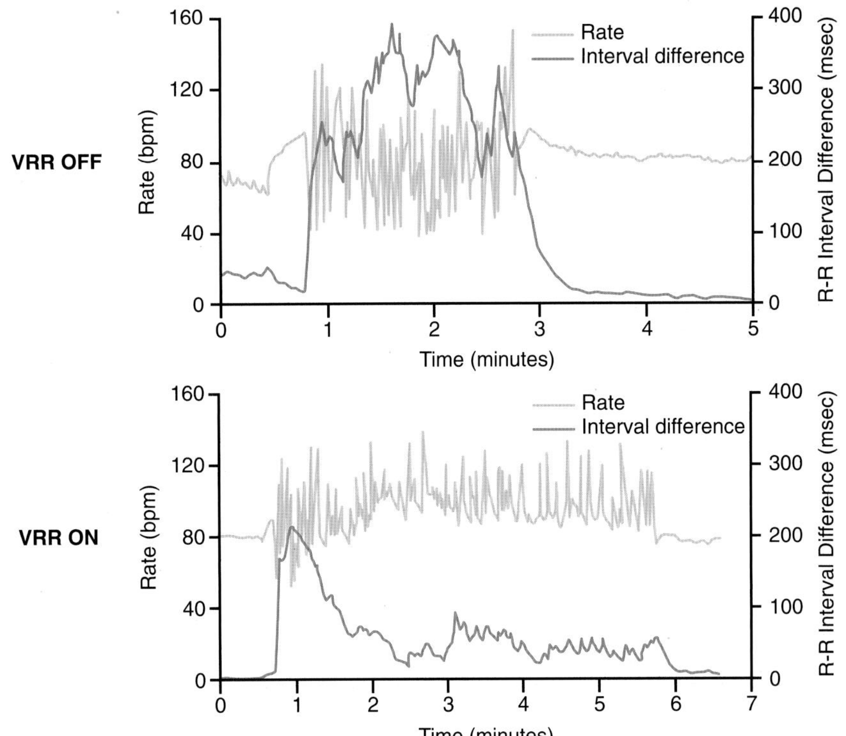

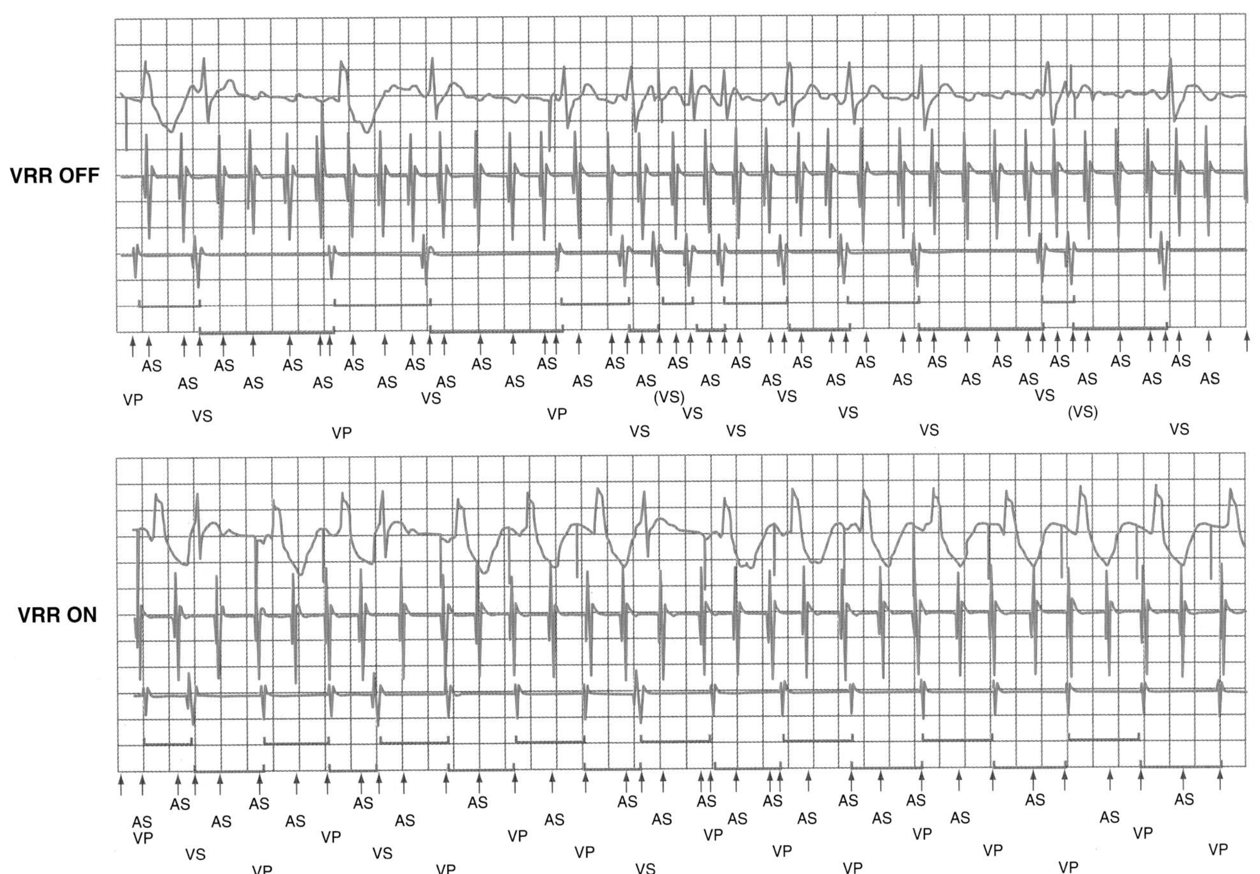

Figure 26-33. Ventricular Rate Regularization (VRR; Guidant, Boston Scientific, Natick, Mass.). Top, VRR OFF. Mean ventricular rate is 167 ± 49 bpm. Note wide ventricular interval variation (horizontal bars). Bottom, *VRR ON. Mean ventricular rate is 138 ± 37 bpm. Note increase in ventricular pacing and reduction in ventricular interval variation* (horizontal bars).

VRR OFF

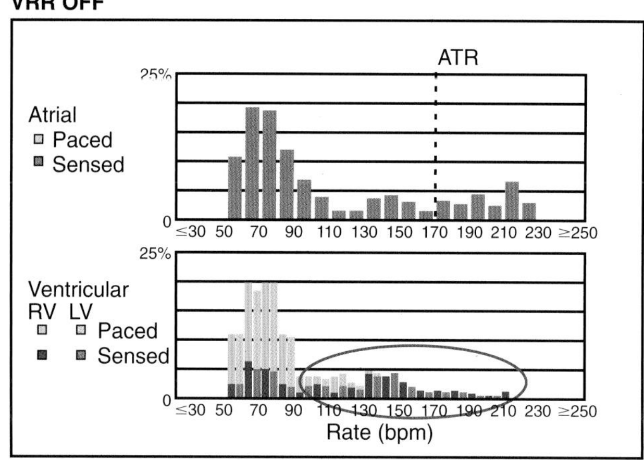

Histograms with VRR OFF

Right Ventricular		
Ventricular Tachy Detections		0
Right Paced	60%	780K
Tracked	63%	491K
Device Determined	37%	289K
Right Sensed	40%	520K
Left Ventricular		
Left Paced	67%	771K
Tracked	65%	501K
Device Determined	35%	270K
Left Sensed	33%	380K

VRR ON

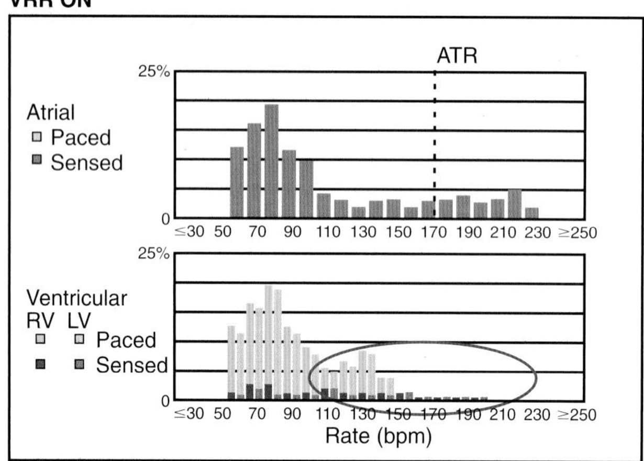

Histograms with VRR ON

Right Ventricular		
Ventricular Tachy Detections		0
Right Paced	83%	605.9K
Tracked	66%	399.9K
Device Determined	34%	206.0K
Right Sensed	17%	124.1K
Left Ventricular		
Left Paced	85%	552.5K
Tracked	67%	370.2K
Device Determined	33%	182.3K
Left Sensed	15%	97.5K

Figure 26-34. Ventricular Rate Regularization (VRR; Guidant, Boston Scientific, Natick, Mass.). Comparison of percent ventricular pacing histograms with VRR OFF (top) *and VRR ON* (bottom). *VRR results in significantly higher frequency of ventricular pacing during atrial fibrillation with rapid ventricular conduction.*

up of two parts: (1) the most recent V-V interval multiplied by 1.1 (if the most recent ventricular event was sensed) or by 1.2 (if the event was paced), which provides 7% of the next calculated VRR pacing rate value, and (2) the calculated VRR interval value just before the most recent ventricular event, which provides 93% of the next calculated VRR pacing rate value. Therefore, the next VRR pacing rate interval = .07 (recent V-V interval × 1.2 or 1.1) + .93 (previous VRR interval calculation). The calculated rate based on the weighted average yields a pacing rate that still adjusts on a cycle-by-cycle basis, but in much smaller increments than during Rate Smoothing. The frequency of VRR pacing is directly related to ventricular cycle length variability (i.e., pacing frequency increases with ventricular cycle length variability).

The use of VRR necessitates interactions with other device operations. The maximum VRR pacing rate is programmable between 60 and 150 bpm.

In dual-chamber modes, Rate Smoothing is temporarily disabled when VRR is active.

Frequent Ventricular Premature Beats. Frequent ventricular premature depolarizations may disrupt CRT. Ventricular Sense Response (VSR, Medtronic) is intended to provide CRT when ventricular sensing occurs. Each RV sensed event triggers a pace in one or both ventricles, as programmed.

When VSR is enabled in a nontracking or single-chamber pacing mode, a sensed ventricular event triggers an immediate ventricular pace. VSR pacing is delivered in one or both ventricles, according to the programmed ventricular pacing pathway. When VSR is enabled in an atrial tracking mode, a sensed ventricular event during the AV interval triggers an immediate pacing output to both ventricles (Fig. 26-35). The triggered output is rendered ineffectual in the chamber where sensing occurred due to ventricular refractoriness. Therefore, the triggered output "resynchronizes" ventricular activation by stimulating the chamber opposite the sensed event.

Some timing rules apply to prevent disruption of normal device operation. VSR pacing stimuli are delivered 1.25 msec after the ventricular sensed event only if the triggered pace does not violate the programmed VSR Maximum Rate. If the ventricular interval measured from the preceding ventricular event is shorter than the VSR Maximum Rate interval, no VSR pacing

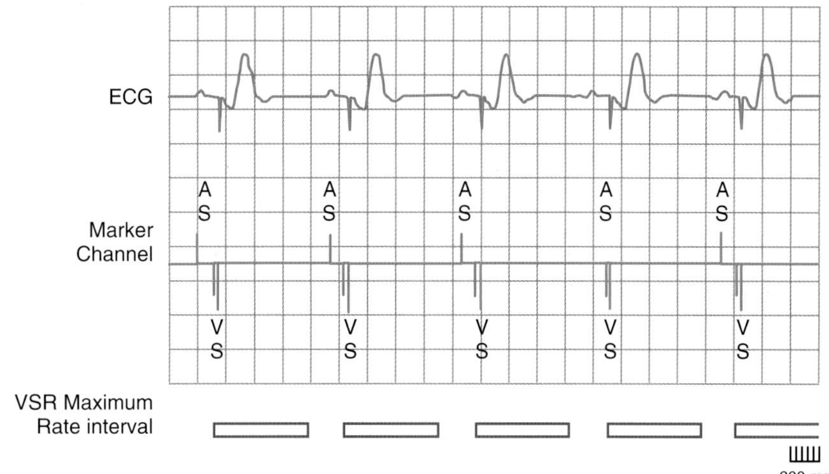

Figure 26-35. Ventricular Sense Response (VSR; Medtronic, Minneapolis, Minn.). Each ventricular event triggers an immediate VSR pace or paces. Because of the close proximity of the Ventricular Sense (VS) and VSR Pace markers, the Biventricular Pace (BV) annotation is not printed on the real-time ECG (electrocardiogram) strip. AS, Atrial sensed event.

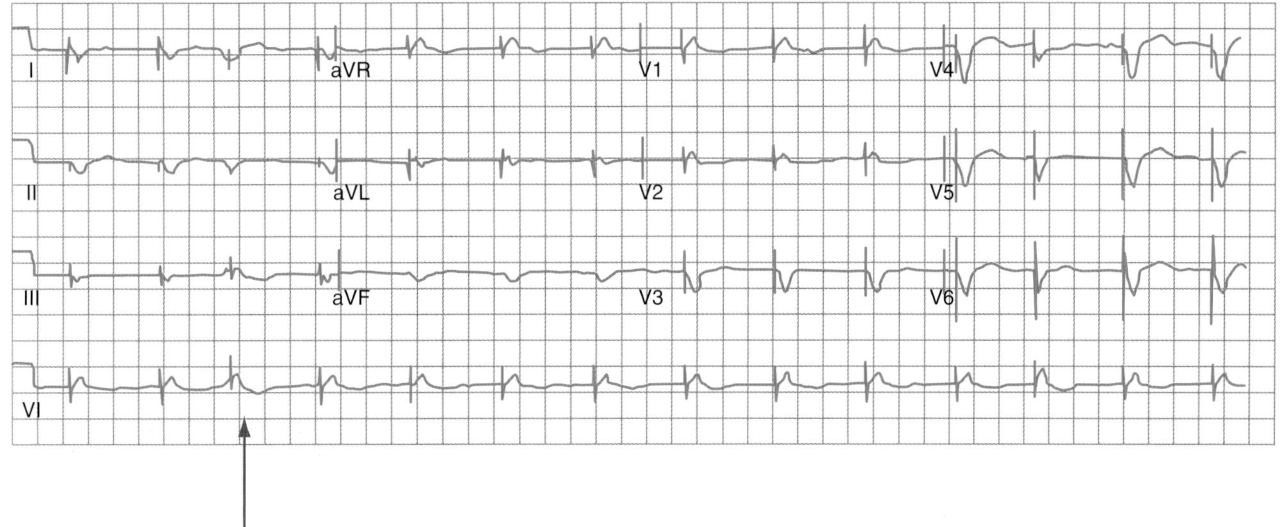

Figure 26-36. Ventricular Sense Response (Medtronic, Minneapolis, Minn.) operation. The third QRS complex (arrow) *is a left ventricular premature contraction (note QS in lead I) that triggers VSR pacing. Note that the ventricular pacing stimulus is delivered almost 100 msec after onset of QRS.*

pulse is delivered. Ventricular sensing for VSR operation occurs via only the RV lead. Operating features of algorithms designed to maximize CRT, such as VSR, may result in pacing that occurs after QRS onset on the surface ECG (Fig. 26-36).

VSR operation necessitates interactions with other device operations. When both VSR and Ventricular Safety Pacing (VSP) are enabled, VSP operation takes precedence during the VSP interval. If a ventricular event is sensed during the VSP interval, the device performs a safety pace at the end of the VSP interval. After the VSP interval expires, VSR remains active for the remainder of the paced AV interval. VSR pacing pulses are not considered in interval calculations for arrhythmia detection or pacing. VSR pacing pulses are not considered in the counts of consecutive sensed and paced events that define the beginning and end of ventricular sensing episodes in storage. VSR operation is suspended during automatic tachyarrhythmia therapies, electrophysiologic study inductions, manual therapies, and emergency fixed burst, cardioversion, and defibrillation.

Loss of CRT due to Differential Left Ventricular Capture Threshold Rise

The principal limitation of the transvenous approach is that the selection of sites for pacing is entirely dictated by navigable coronary venous anatomy. A commonly encountered problem is that an apparently suitable target vein delivers the lead to a site where ventricular capture can be achieved only at very high output voltages or not at all. This presumably relates to the presence of scar on the epicardial surface of the heart underlying the target vein or inadequate contact with the epicardial surface and cannot be anticipated by fluoroscopic examination *a priori*. In some instances, this problem can be overcome by mapping a more proximal or distal site within the same vein, but an alternative lead design may be required to achieve mechanical stability. If this is not successful, surgical placement of LV leads permits more detailed mapping of viable sites in the anatomic region of interest.

There are relatively limited data on long-term pacing thresholds with transvenous or thoracotomy leads for LV pacing. Loss of ventricular capture occurred in 10% of patients in the VENTAK CHF/CONTAK CD study and was the second most common cause of interrupted CRT.[34] Three quarters of these cases were caused by gross dislodgment of the LV lead, and 23% were caused by chronic pacing threshold elevation that was overcome in most cases by increasing the voltage output. A comparison of thoracotomy and transvenous lead system performance in 87 patients who received CRTD systems between 1998 and 2001 reported no significant differences in chronic thresholds, which on average were between 1.5 and 2.0 V up to 30 months after implantation (Fig. 26-37).[50] Similarly, there were no chronic threshold differences between transvenous lead designs (over-the-wire versus preformed shape). An interim progress report of the InSync Registry Post-Approval Study[51] in 903 patients showed similar range and stability of LV thresholds (mean, 1.88 ± 1.44 V) with two different preformed transvenous lead designs at 6 months that were retained at 36 months. In this same report, epicardial voltage thresholds were similarly stable but slightly higher (2.42 ± 0.74 V) at 12 months, although data were available on a much smaller number of patients.

A particularly difficult problem with chronic epicardial leads is exit block, which in some instances results in voltage thresholds that exceed pulse generator output and result in permanent loss of CRT. Although this is infrequent, it is a devastating problem for the patient, because the epicardial approach is usually taken only when the transvenous approach fails. Several factors contribute to this problem relating to lead design and surgical technique. The most commonly used epicardial pacing lead is a fixed helix mechanism without steroid, and chronic doubling of the implantation threshold is common. Furthermore, this situation is made worse by multiple applications of the helix and incautious use of suturing, which increase local tissue trauma and the subsequent inflammatory response.

Loss of CRT due to Phrenic Nerve Stimulation

A second common problem is that the target vein delivers the lead to a site that results in phrenic nerve stimulation and diaphragmatic pacing. This can be difficult to demonstrate during implantation, when the patient is supine and sedated, but it may be immediately evident when the patient is later active and changes body positions, even in the absence of lead dislodgment. Many experienced implanters recognize that once phrenic nerve stimulation is observed acutely (during implantation), it is almost invariably encountered during follow-up despite manipulation of output voltages; therefore, an alternative site for LV pacing is sought. As with high LV capture thresholds, phrenic nerve stimulation can often be overcome by repositioning the LV lead more proximally within the target vein. Occasionally, if there is a significant differential in capture threshold for phrenic nerve stimulation versus LV capture, this can be overcome by manipulation of LV voltage output in CRTP or CRTD systems that permit separate RV and LV outputs. More recently, some LV leads have two or more electrodes, permitting selection of specific LV sites for dual cathodal biventricular stimulation, biventricular stimulation with true bipolar LV stimulation, or true bipolar LV-only univentricular stimulation. It has not been convincingly demonstrated that true bipolar LV stimulation reliably overcomes phrenic stimulation compared with dual cathodal or unipolar LV pacing. On the other hand, selection of alternative LV electrodes for dual cathodal biventricular stimulation may occasionally overcome phrenic stimulation by altering the LV-RV pacing vector. This can be achieved noninvasively using some

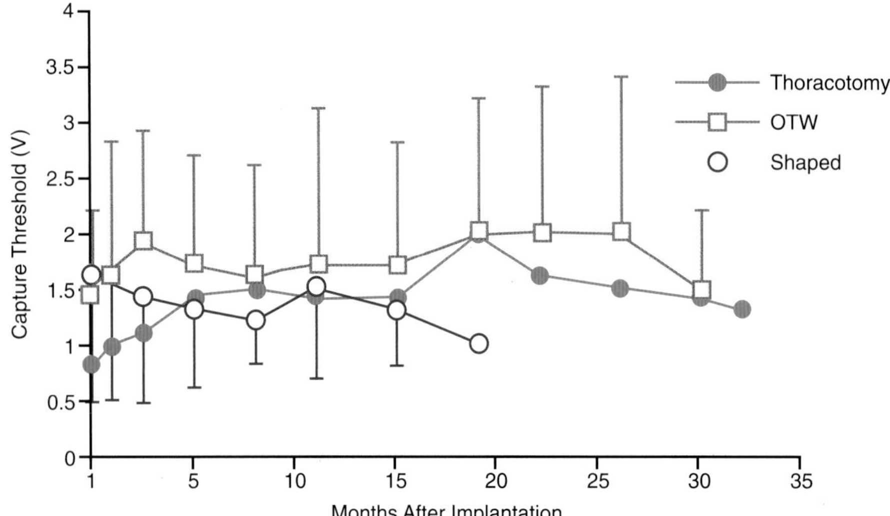

Figure 26-37. Chronic thresholds with various left ventricular lead designs. OTW, over-the-wire design.

Guidant CRTP and CRTD generators and is referred to as "Electronic Repositioning." In either case, the problem of phrenic nerve stimulation is more reliably addressed by LV lead repositioning at implantation. Chronic development of phrenic nerve stimulation results in permanent loss of CRT in about 1% to 2% of patients.[34]

Loss of CRT due to Lead Dislodgment

Acute dislodgment of right atrial and RV electrodes is uncommon, particularly with active fixation leads. The incidence of LV lead dislodgment is considerably higher and has a reported incidence of 5% to 10% in larger studies.[10,15,52] This relates to implanter experience and other technical factors, such as the lack of fixation mechanisms and stresses placed on the proximal portion of the lead at the junction of the right atrium and coronary sinus ostium. Lead dislodgments are readily identified by chest radiography but are usually suspected on the basis of device interrogation that discloses a significant decline in local signal amplitude and/or change in pacing capture threshold. Typically, right atrial leads dislodge onto the floor of the right atrium and RV leads dislodge toward the inflow of the RV. LV leads typically dislodge into the main body of the coronary sinus, and less commonly into the right atrium.

Ventricular Oversensing

Inappropriate Ventricular Therapies and Misclassification of True Ventricular Rhythms due to Ventricular Double-Counting

Conventional pacemaker and ICD generators have been adapted for atrial-synchronous biventricular pacing. The single ventricular output must be divided to provide simultaneous stimulation of the right and left ventricles (dual cathodal system with parallel outputs). First-generation multisite pacing pulse generators similarly provide a single ventricular output for simultaneous RV and LV stimulation; however, two separate ventricular channels internally connect in parallel. This connection is made for both the lead tip and ring connections and eliminates the need for a Y-adaptor. However, this configuration still provides simultaneous RV and LV sensing with associated limitations.

The common consequence of simultaneous RV and LV sensing is double-counting of the prolonged native ventricular EGM.[53,54] During pacing, RV and LV depolarizations are synchronized and refractory periods are prolonged, preventing double-counting. Any situation that inhibits ventricular pacing and permits emergence of the prolonged native ventricular EGM (e.g., ventricular premature beats, loss of atrial tracking during sinus tachycardia, rapidly conducted AF, nonsustained or sustained ventricular tachycardia) can cause ventricular oversensing due to double-counting.

In all of these situations, sensed events in the left and right ventricles are "merged" into a single recording channel in parallel dual cathodal systems. The degree of temporal displacement between sensed RV and LV events depends on the interventricular conduction time and lead position. If the interventricular conduction time during bundle branch block exceeds the relatively short ventricular blanking period initiated by sensing, a single ventricular depolarization may be counted twice. This yields a characteristically oscillating interval plot resulting from cycle-to-cycle variation in the ventricular cycle length. In CRTP systems, this can result in inhibition of ventricular pacing and loss of CRT and spurious high-rate ventricular episodes (Fig. 26-38). In CRTD systems, this may result in inhibition of ventricular pacing and ventricular therapies for sinus tachycardia, rapidly conducted AF, or other supraventricular tachycardias below the programmed VT detection interval, because the double-counting interval exceeds the VT detection interval. The rate of true VT may be overestimated, resulting in misclassification as ventricular fibrillation (VF) and treatment with shocks instead of painless termination by ATP.[55] Similarly, nonsustained VT may satisfy VF detection criteria, resulting in aborted or delivered shocks (Fig. 26-39). Oversensed events due to ventricular double-counting may interfere with dual-chamber detection enhancements.

Pacing inhibition and inappropriate therapies caused by far-field sensing of left atrial activity by the LV lead have also been reported.[56-58] In this situation, ventricular double-counting results from sensing of the far-field atrial and near-field ventricular signals. Ventricular triple-counting can also occur when the far-field atrial signal and both components of the prolonged native ventricular EGM are sensed (Fig. 26-40). Far-field sensing of atrial activity is more likely when the LV lead is close to the AV groove, either due to coronary venous anatomy or because of lead displacement from a more distal position within a venous branch. Rarely, atrial oversensing from a nondisplaced integrated bipolar RV lead causes inhibition of ventricular pacing and double-counting.[59]

Resolving Ventricular Double-Counting

Nondedicated CRTP/D Systems with Y-Adaptors

The options for eliminating ventricular double-counting in nondedicated CRTP and CRTD systems that achieve parallel dual cathodal sensing with a Y-adaptor are limited and mostly unsatisfactory. In one small series, 36% of patients had one or more inappropriate shocks (range, 1 to 64 shocks per patient) as a result of double-counting over a mean follow-up period of 13 ± 7 months.[1] With the exception of misclassification of true VT as VF, double-counting of the native ventricular EGM during conducted supraventricular rhythms caused all inappropriate therapies. This could be overcome only by interrupting AV conduction with catheter ablation or disconnecting the Y-adapted LV lead, because CRTD pulse generators with dedicated univentricular sensing were unavailable.

Medtronic 9790 Programmer 9891A320 7/13/02 10:31
Copyright (c) Medtronic, Inc. 1993
---------------- High rate episode data graphics report ---------------- Page 1 of 1

Stimulator model: InSync 8040 Serial number: PIN633204

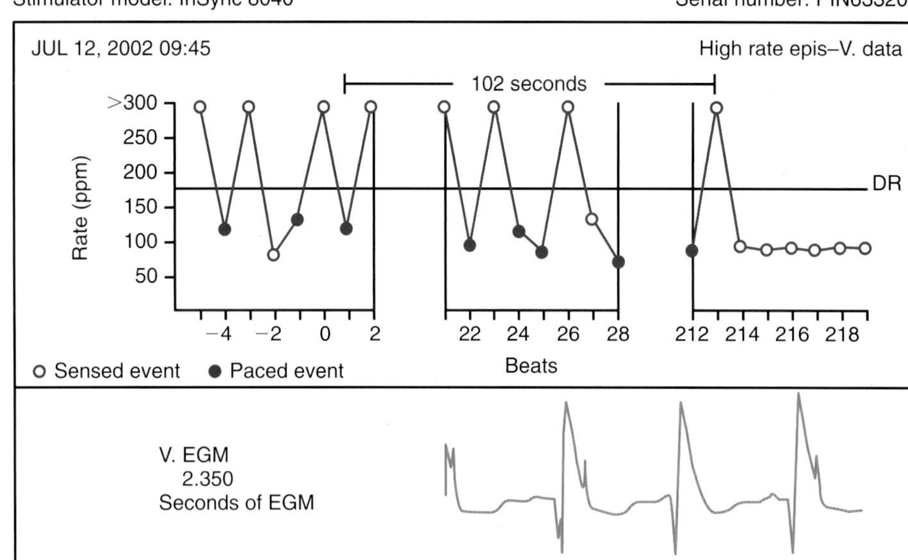

Figure 26-38. Spurious high-rate ventricular episode with stored EGM due to loss of CRT and ventricular double-counting of the native ventricular EGM in a CRT pacemaker. Note the two components of the ventricular EGM; the first deflection is right ventricular activation, and the second deflection is left ventricular activation). Note the characteristic "W" appearance, which results from oscillation of cycle lengths caused by sensing of both components of the prolonged biventricular EGM.

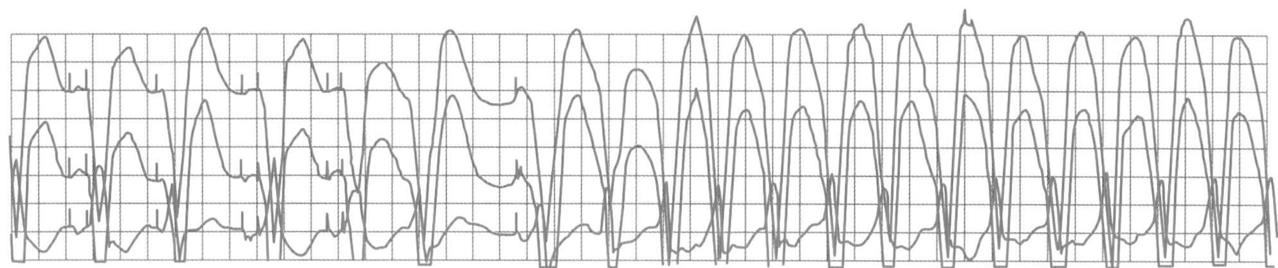

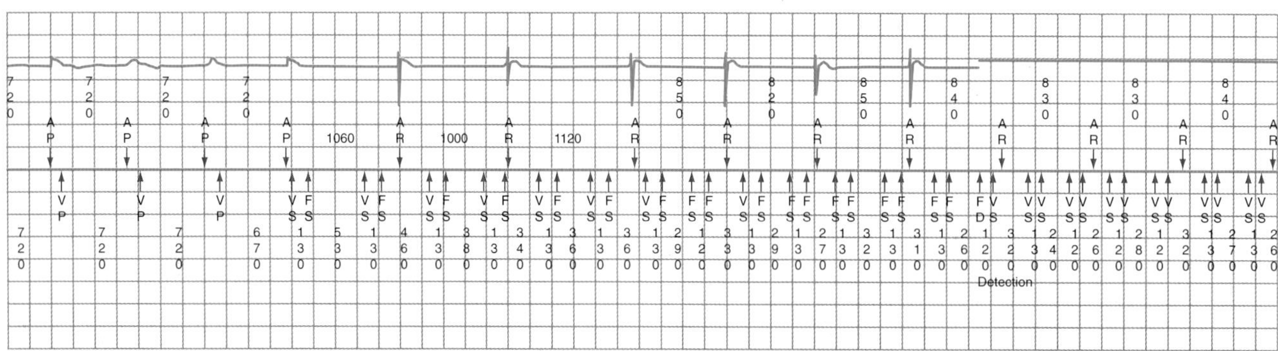

Figure 26-39. Ventricular double-counting during ventricular tachycardia (VT) on a stored EGM in a nondedicated CRT with defibrillation (CRTD) system. Top, *Telemetry strip of nonsustained monomorphic ventricular tachycardia (VT), interrupting biventricular pacing.* Bottom, *Corresponding stored single-channel EGM and marker channel (GEM III AT; Medtronic, Minneapolis, Minn.) for the same event. Note that only the atrial EGM is stored. Double-counting of each VT event (marked as VS-FS or FS-FS) results in misclassification and detection as ventricular fibrillation (VF).*

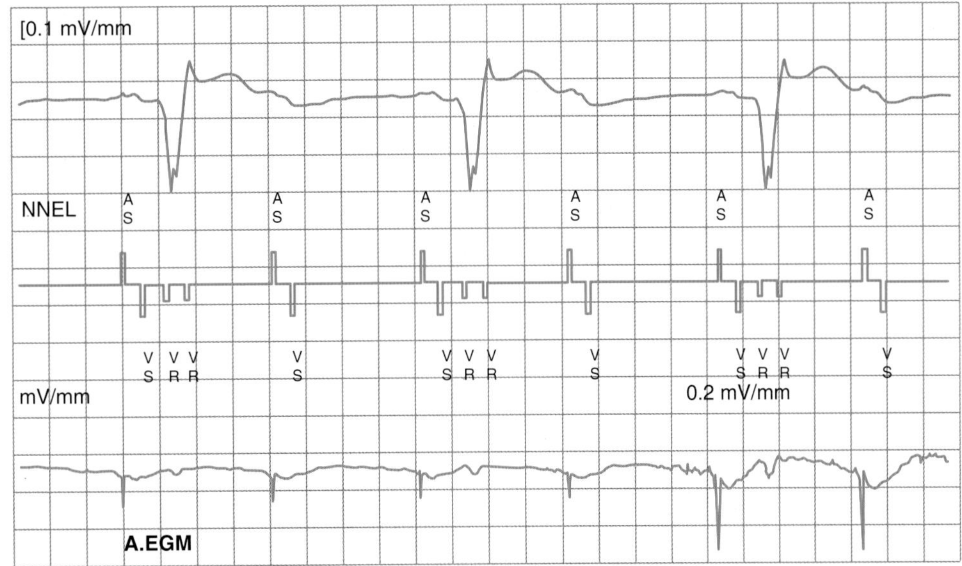

Figure 26-40. Ventricular triple-counting in a nondedicated CRT/pacemaker (CRTP) system. Simultaneous recordings (from top to bottom) of surface electrocardiogram, marker channel, and real-time atrial EGM. The spontaneous rhythm is 2:1 atrioventricular (AV) block. The nondisplaced left ventricular lead senses the late portion of the P wave because of its proximity to the AV groove (note that VS and AS are almost merged), resulting in ventricular pacing inhibition. Alternating P waves conduct, resulting in emergence of the prolonged native ventricular EGM and ventricular double-counting. Thus, there are three ventricular sensed pulses marked for each conducted sinus event: the first (VS) is the far-field atrial signal, and the second (VR) and third (VR) are the two components of the "split" ventricular EGM. (From Lipchenca I, Garrigue S, Glikson M, et al: Inhibition of biventricular pacemakers by oversensing of far-field atrial depolarization. PACE 25:365-367, 2002.)

Theoretically, manipulation of the ventricular blanking period could reduce ventricular double-counting in some situations with nondedicated CRTP or CRTD systems. Manufacturer-specific differences in programmable postventricular sense blanking periods in conventional ICDs may be useful in this regard, but a common concern is failure to detect true VT/VF due to pseudoventricular undersensing when the blanking period is maximally extended.

In some instances, decreasing the programmed ventricular sensitivity may reduce ventricular double-counting if the later of the RV and LV EGMs has significantly lower amplitude than the earlier EGM. This approach mandates validation of VF sensing and detection at the reduced ventricular sensitivity and is generally undesirable.

Second- and third-generation dedicated CRTP and CRTD generators have independent ventricular ports for differential pacing output and timing but restrict ventricular sensing to the RV or LV lead alone, depending on programmability. Removing the Y-adaptor and replacing the generator with one that uses single-site (typically RV) sensing exclusively eliminates the potential complications of biventricular sensing.

Dedicated CRTP and CRTD Systems with Univentricular Sensing

Double-counting of the prolonged native ventricular EGM is eliminated by univentricular sensing, which is either hardwired (RV) or programmable (RV or LV) in dedicated CRTP and CRTD systems. Accordingly, an IVRP (see earlier discussion) is not necessary, although it is provided in some dedicated systems that permit selection of biventricular sensing. However, double-counting of the far-field atrial and near-field ventricular EGM can still occur during (univentricular) LV sensing if the LV lead is in close proximity to the AV groove due to displacement or coronary venous anatomy. In this situation, reprogramming univentricular RV sensing resolves the double-counting problem but does not address LV lead displacement as the cause. Newer bipolar or dual cathodal LV leads will probably not reduce the likelihood of far-field atrial oversensing in nondisplaced leads, because the proximal electrode is closer to the AV groove.

Inhibition of Ventricular Pacing and Inappropriate Therapies due to Ventricular Oversensing of Cardiac Signals

LV lead dislodgment into the coronary sinus may result in inhibition of ventricular pacing in CRTP systems due to atrial oversensing or in simultaneous inappropriate detection of atrial activity as VT/VF in CRTD systems that use RV and LV sensing, even in pacemaker-dependent patients incapable of AV conduction (Fig. 26-41).[56,59,60] In pacemaker-dependent patients, this can result in syncope followed by a high-voltage shock.

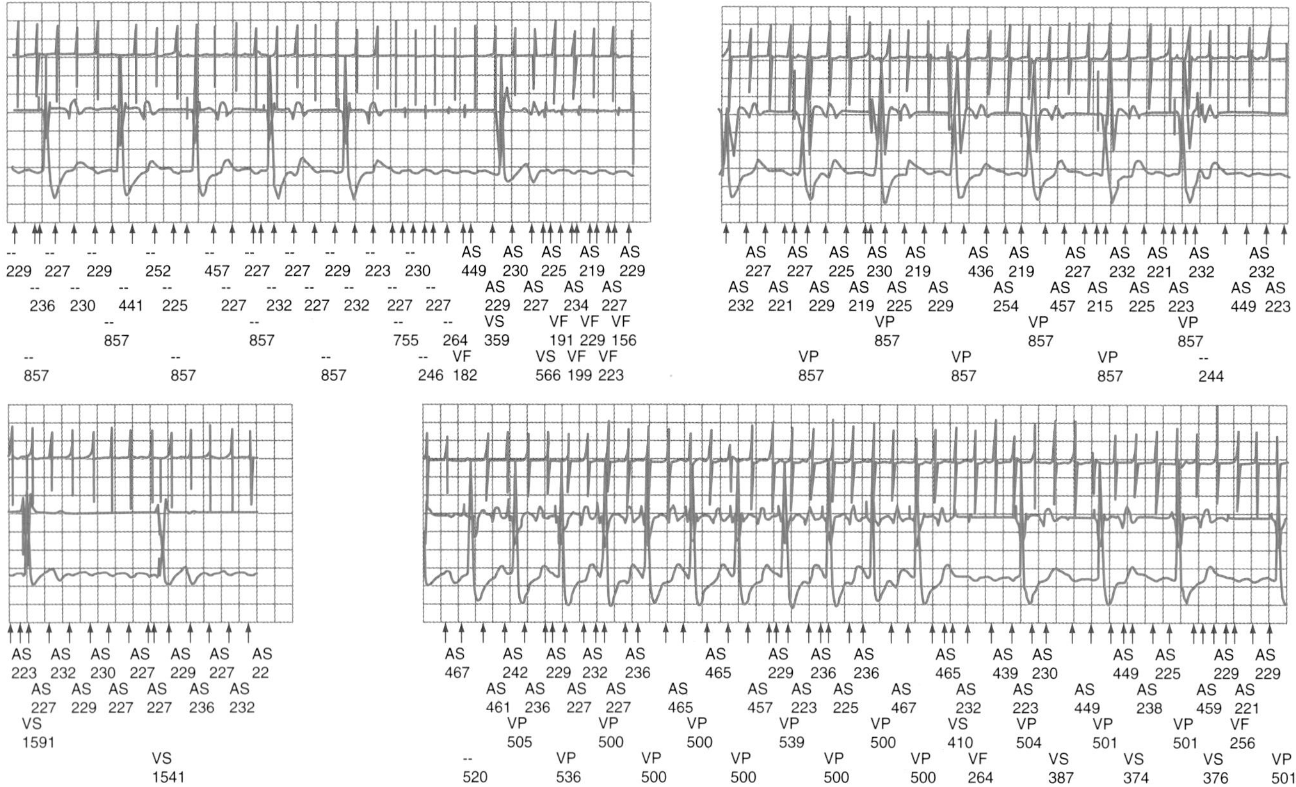

Figure 26-41. Ventricular pacing inhibition and spurious detection of ventricular fibrillation (VF) in a pacemaker-dependent patient caused by dislodgment of the left ventricular (LV) lead in a nondedicated CRT with defibrillation (CRTD) system. Shown are the atrial EGM, near-field ventricular EGM, and far-field ventricular EGM. The LV lead was displaced into the atrioventricular groove, resulting in detection of atrial flutter on the ventricular channel, which inhibited pacing and satisfied VF rate and duration criteria.

Inhibition of Ventricular Pacing and Inappropriate Therapies due to High-Frequency, Low-Amplitude Respirophasic Noise Transients

Respirophasic oversensing is commonly provoked in patients with ICDs during ventricular pacing at maximum or nominal programmable sensitivities and may occur spontaneously, resulting in spurious tachyarrhythmia therapies and pacing inhibition.[61] Differences in the incidence of spontaneous and provoked oversensing between ICD systems appear to be explained on the basis of unique features of their automatic sensing systems and sensing lead design. Spontaneous and provocable oversensing is more common in male patients with ICD systems that use automatic gain control (AGC) sensing and integrated bipolar (IBP) leads. The explanation for the increased relative risk of oversensing with AGC, compared with devices that use automatic adjusting sensitivity (AAS), can be rationalized by considering their respective operations. Under conditions of no pacing or continuous pacing, AGC devices attain maximum sensitivity sooner in the cardiac cycle and maintain it longer than AAS devices do. This difference is most dramatic during conditions of ventricular pacing, where the operational sensitivity of AGC devices is linked to the pacing interval. In contrast, the exponential increase in sensitivity of AAS devices is dissociated from the pacing interval. The large surface area of the coil and wider interelectrode spacing of IBP leads might increase the susceptibility to extraneous far-field signals, analogous to unipolar pacemaker leads. The more narrow interelectrode spacing of true bipolar leads might increase the chance that extraneous far-field signals would arrive at each electrode simultaneously, resulting in signal averaging ("cancellation"). Sensing may therefore be better confined to the local endocardial environment and susceptibility to oversensing reduced, as with conventional bipolar pacing leads. Oversensing can be overcome in more than 50% of patients by programming a reduced sensitivity; however, this requires reconfirmation of the robustness of VF detection. In select cases, persistent oversensing despite reduced sensitivity may require implantation of a separate endocardial rate-sensing lead in the RV outflow tract or use of an ICD pulse generator that does not employ AGC sensing behavior. CRTD patients may be particularly susceptible to respirophasic oversensing due to continuous ventricular pacing (Fig. 26-42).

CRT Proarrhythmia

Small studies have suggested that CRT might reduce the likelihood of inducible or spontaneous ventricular arrhythmia in susceptible patients.[62,63] The VENTAK

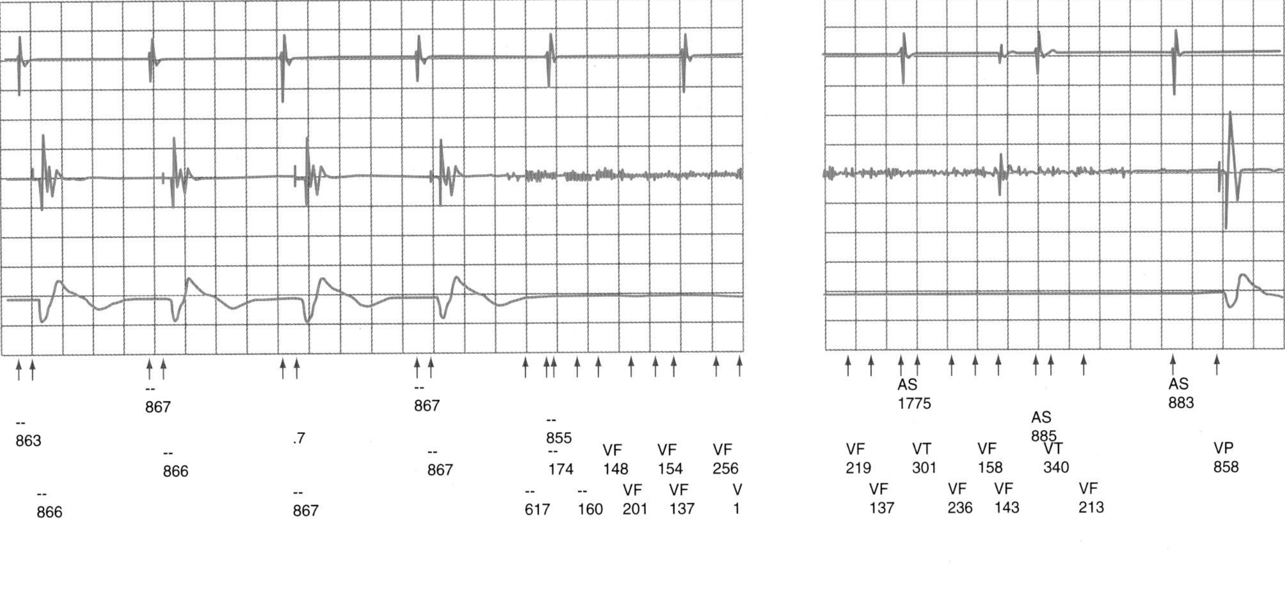

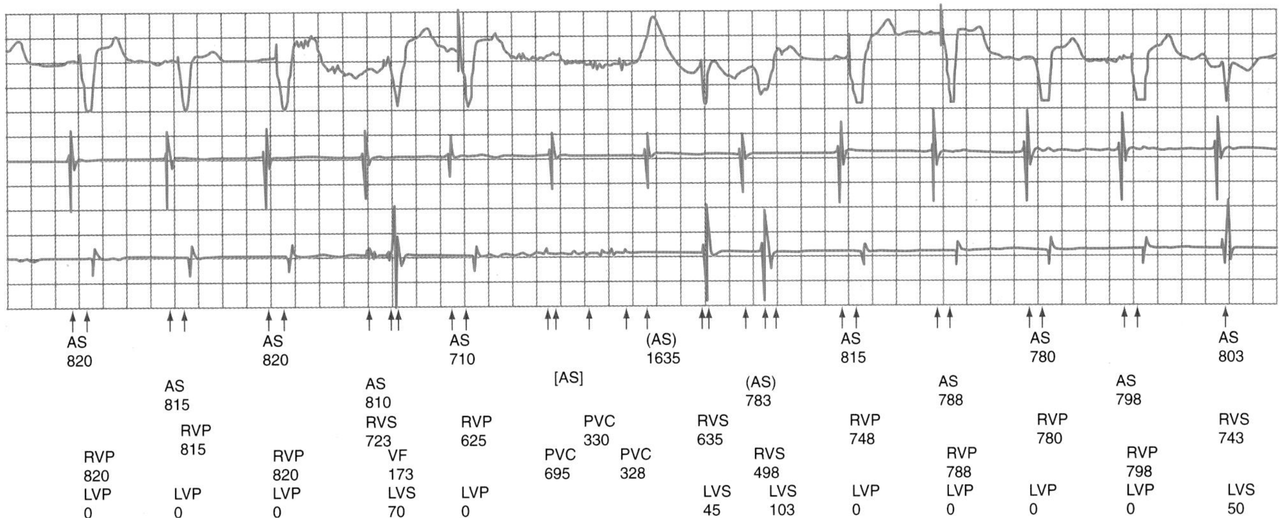

Figure 26-42. *Respirophasic ventricular oversensing resulting in loss of CRT in a pacemaker-dependent patient.* Top, *Spontaneous ventricular oversensing resulting in simultaneous ventricular pacing inhibition, syncope, and spurious detection of ventricular fibrillation denoted by capacitor charging.* Bottom, *Provoked ventricular oversensing during deep breathing at nominal ventricular sensitivity. This was not eliminated by programming a reduced ventricular sensitivity ("Less sensitive").*

CHF study[64] reported a reduction in spontaneous ventricular arrhythmias during 3 months of CRT "On" versus "Off" in 32 patients who served as their own controls. The short duration of follow-up, small number of patients, and stochastic nature of arrhythmia recurrence render these data inconclusive.

This concept has not been confirmed in large RCTs of CRTD, where no significant difference in the incidence or frequency of ventricular tachyarrhythmias between patients randomly assigned to CRT "On" or CRT "Off" was observed.[10,21,52] For example, in the VENTAK CHF/CONTAK CD study, 15% of patients randomized to CRT received appropriate therapies for VT and VF, compared with 16% of patients randomized to no CRT.[21] Excluding patients who had no VT/VF episodes, those patients randomized to CRT had a median of 2.5 episodes, whereas those randomized to no CRT had a median of 2 episodes during the therapy evaluation phase. During the 6-month randomization period in the MIRACLE ICD study, 26% of patients in the control group versus 22% in the CRT group had at least one spontaneous episode of VT or VF (P = .47).[52] Among patients with spontaneous VT or VF, those randomized to CRT had 0.39 VT/VF episodes per month, compared with 0.41 episodes per month among those randomized to no CRT.[52] Additional analysis of MIRACLE ICD data reinforced these observations with regard to overall detection of ventricular arrhythmias.[65] There was no difference by CRT status in the proportion of patients experiencing episodes or in the cycle lengths of the episodes during the randomization period. For primary prevention patients, 18% of those randomized to CRT Off had at least one appropriately detected episode, compared with 14% of patients with CRT On, with average cycle lengths of 285 and 291 msec, respectively. For secondary prevention patients, 28% of those randomized to CRT Off had at least one episode, compared with 27% of those with CRT On, and the average cycle lengths were 352 and 361 msec, respectively.

Nonetheless, an important question is whether pacing site-specific changes in ventricular activation might facilitate the initiation of ventricular arrhythmia under certain conditions. For example, collision of site-specific stimulation wavefronts might create a favorable environment for initiation of scar-related reentry in coronary artery disease. A recent case report described reproducible initiation of monomorphic VT by LV but not RV pacing that could be reliably terminated by RV but not LV ATP.[66] This suggests the possibility that local tissue anisotropy might affect the ability of site-specific stimulation wavefronts to interact with the reentrant VT circuit.

Additionally, the sudden alteration in LV activation sequence from endocardial to epicardial and reversal of wavefront direction from left to right might affect arrhythmogenesis. Recent studies have shown that pacing-site-dependent changes in ventricular activation sequence can alter ventricular repolarization and refractoriness.[67,68]

Medina-Ravell and coworkers[67] demonstrated that LV epicardial and biventricular pacing caused significant increases in the JT and QTc intervals, and LV pacing increased transmural dispersion of repolarization in humans with systolic heart failure (Fig. 26-43). In a small number of patients, LV and biventricular pacing caused frequent R-on-T extrasystoles, leading in one instance to incessant torsades de pointes requiring multiple ICD therapies within hours after institution of biventricular pacing (Figs. 26-44 and 26-45). Despite more modest QTc prolongation, R-on-T extrasystoles and torsades de pointes were completely suppressed by RV endocardial pacing. In rabbit experiments, switching from endocardial to epicardial pacing resulted in prolongation of the QTc and transmural dispersion of repolarization.

These observations were extended by Fish and associates,[68] who used arterially perfused canine LV wedge preparations. The QT interval and transmural dispersion of repolarization increased as pacing was shifted from endocardium to epicardium. In the presence of rapidly activating delayed rectifier potassium current blocker, these changes were accentuated and torsade de pointes arrhythmias could be induced during epicardial, but not endocardial, pacing. The authors concluded that sudden reversal of the direction of activation of the LV wall, as occurs during biventricular pacing, leads to increases in QT and transmural dispersion of repolarization as a result of earlier repolarization of epicardium and delayed activation and repolarization of the midmyocardial M cells. This facilitates the development of torsade de pointes under long-QT conditions.

Other Unusual Complications of CRT

The additional timing cycle complexities of nondedicated and dedicated CRT systems have introduced new forms of "pacemaker-mediated" tachycardias. Barold and colleagues[69] described a "cross-ventricular" endless-loop tachycardia in a conventional dual-chamber pacemaker pulse generator used for CRT during permanent AF with the RV lead in the ventricular port and the LV lead in the atrial port. In the VVIR mode, T-wave oversensing on the LV lead (atrial channel) triggered ventricular pacing on the RV lead (ventricular channel). This could be overcome by reducing atrial channel (LV) sensitivity or by using the DVIR mode, which excludes the possibility of LV sensing (atrial channel). Berruezo and colleagues[70] described an unusual form of pacemaker-mediated tachycardia in a CRT system that was without an atrial

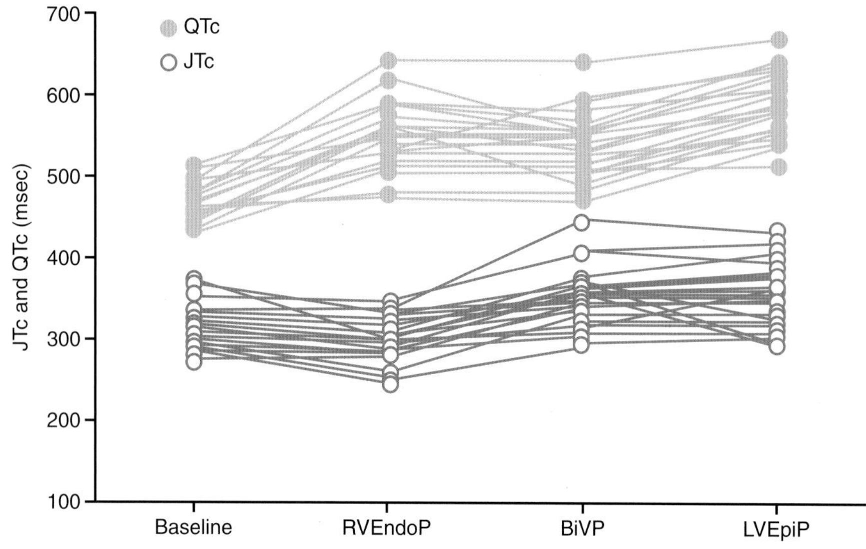

Figure 26-43. Effect of biventricular and left ventricular pacing on QTc interval. BiVP, biventricular pacing; LVEpiP, left ventricular epicardial pacing; RVEndoP, right ventricular endocardial pacing. (From Medina-Ravell VA, Lankipalli RS, Yan GX, et al: Effect of epicardial or biventricular pacing to prolong QT interval and increase transmural dispersion of repolarization. Circulation 107:740-746, 2003.)

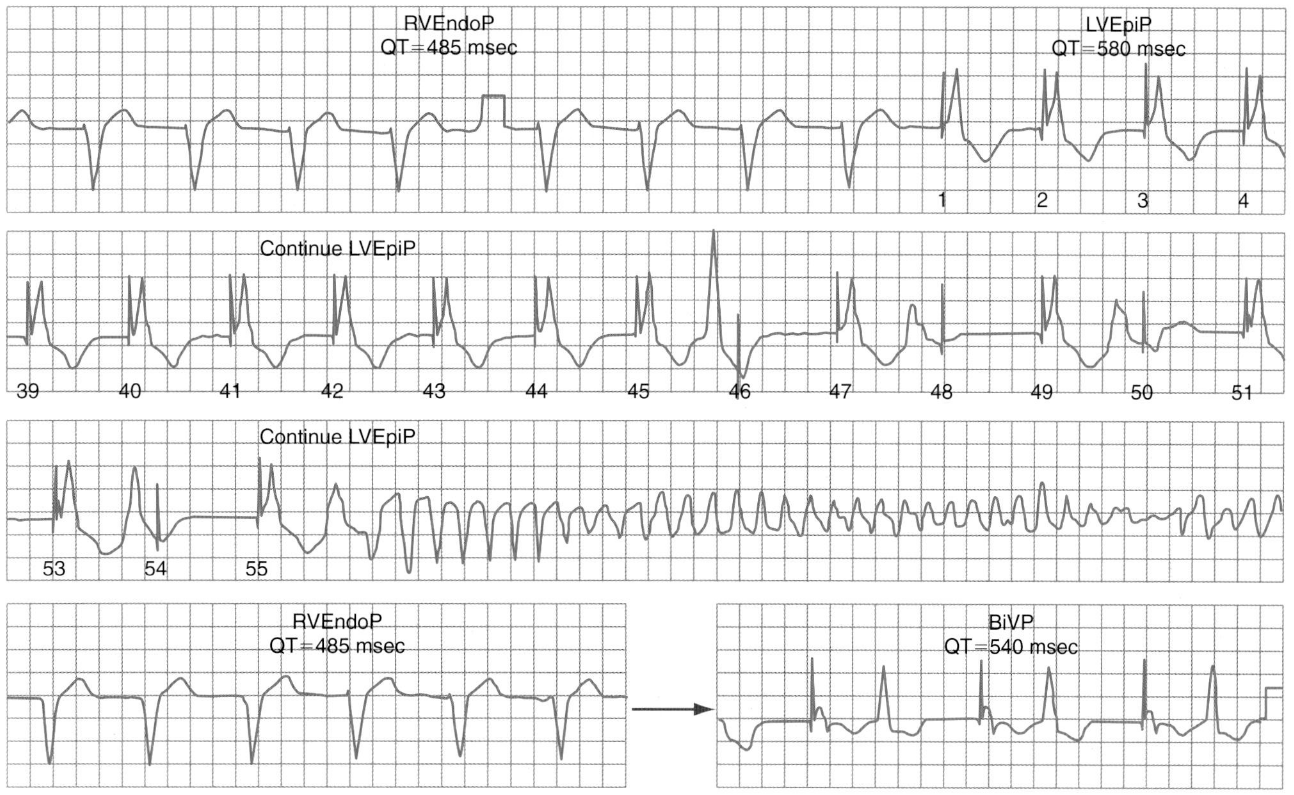

Figure 26-44. Torsades de pointes associated with biventricular pacing. Note that the Q-T interval is 585 msec during left ventricular (LV) pacing and 485 msec during right ventricular (RV) pacing. Polymorphic ventricular tachycardia is initiated by a short-long-short sequence during LV pacing. BiVP, biventricular pacing; LVEpiP, left ventricular epicardial pacing; RVEndoP, right ventricular endocardial pacing. (From Medina-Ravell VA, Lankipalli RS, Yan GX, et al: Effect of epicardial or biventricular pacing to prolong QT interval and increase transmural dispersion of repolarization. Circulation 107:740-746, 2003.)

lead because of "permanent" AF. This was explained by the serendipitous occurrence of spontaneous termination of AF and dislodgment of the LV lead into the coronary sinus, resulting in simultaneous left atrial and LV capture. Because AV conduction was intact, left atrial capture resulted in an RV-sensed event, which triggered the VSR feature (see earlier discussion), resulting in emission of a biventricular pacing stimulus, which perpetuated the phenomenon.

CRT Responders and Nonresponders

Acute response to CRT has been defined on the basis of invasive hemodynamic measurements.[3,4,71] Patients for whom there was an increase in aortic pulse pressure with respect to the intrinsic baseline by more than 5% for any stimulation mode and AV delay combination were characterized as responders. The remaining patients were defined as nonresponders. However, there is some evidence that acute hemodynamic response may not be highly correlated with chronic clinical improvement or reverse remodeling.[72,73] This implies that the lack of an acute hemodynamic response does not preclude clinical CRT response and that the mechanisms of chronic CRT response are more complex than the effects represented by acute hemodynamic measurements.

Accordingly, RCTs of CRT have relied on multiple primary end points (NYHA class, quality-of-life score, and the distance walked in 6 minutes) and secondary end points (peak oxygen consumption [VO_2], time on treadmill, LV ejection fraction and end-diastolic dimension, severity of mitral regurgitation, and a clinical composite response that assigned patients to one of three response groups—improved, worsened, or unchanged[74]). The purpose of the clinical composite score was to combine changes in functional status class with the occurrence of major clinical events, including episodes of clinical deterioration. Clinical deterioration was denoted by death or hospitalization or urgent care for new onset or worsening heart failure.[10] Such clinical composite scores have been shown to be more sensitive than conventional approaches in discriminating active therapy from placebo effect in studies of drugs and electrical device therapy for heart failure.[75]

Using these methods, RCTs have demonstrated that most patients who meet currently accepted implantation criteria[76] respond to CRT. Clinical improvement in

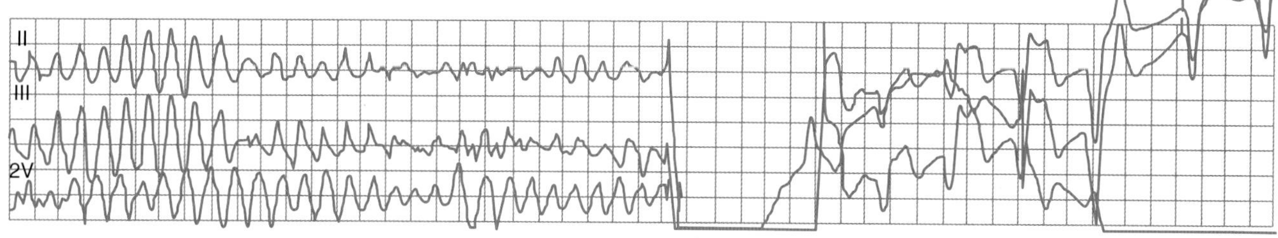

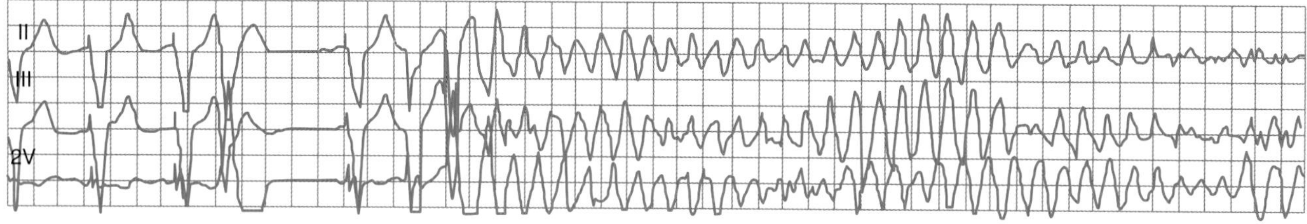

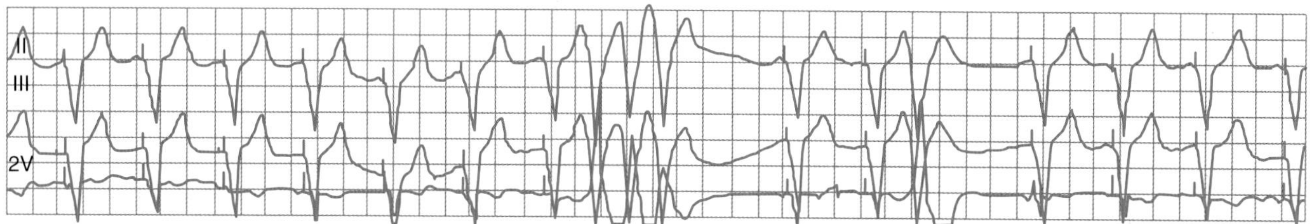

Figure 26-45. *Polymorphic ventricular tachycardia (VT) degenerating to ventricular fibrillation 6 hours after initiation of CRT with defibrillation (CRTD). The patient was a 56-year-old woman with nonischemic dilated cardiomyopathy, left bundle branch block, and no prior history of documented ventricular arrhythmia or syncope. The two sustained events* (top and middle tracings) *occurred within 6 seconds of one another and were terminated by ICD shocks. Note that polymorphic VT was initiated by a short-long-short sequence* (middle tracing). *Note also the salvos of ventricular premature beats in the bottom tracing.*

CRT responders is modest and on average includes a reduction of one or two steps in NYHA class, a 1- to 2-mL/kg/min improvement in peak VO_2, a 50- to 100-m improvement in 6-minute hall walk, reduced heart failure urgent care or hospitalizations, and improved quality of life by standardized measures.

Nonetheless, approximately 20% to 30% of patients fail to respond to CRT.[15,72,77-81] There is no uniform definition of CRT "nonresponse," but it is generally recognized to denote limited or lack of clinical improvement and lack of reverse ventricular remodeling. Although CRT "nonresponse" is most likely a diverse phenomenon, there is emerging consensus that it can be explained on the basis of the interactive consequences of inadequate patient selection and suboptimal LV lead position. The approach to reducing the number of CRT "nonresponders" therefore must include (1) rejection of patients who are destined not to respond (i.e., patients without mechanical dyssynchrony) and (2) maximization of LV stimulation response in patients with mechanical dyssynchrony.

Optimizing Patient Selection to Reduce Nonresponders

Intraventricular dyssynchrony is the pathophysiologic target of CRT. Techniques beyond QRS duration for selecting patients with significant ventricular dyssynchrony who are likely to benefit from CRT are rapidly evolving. The optimal criteria would identify all patients with a high probability of response and reject all patients with a low probability of response.

Clinical Characteristics

Numerous clinical variables have been evaluated for predicting likelihood of CRT responsiveness. Significant AV conduction delay,[82] functional mitral regurgitation,[78] LV end-diastolic dimension greater than 55 mm, and low baseline peak VO_2[83] have been shown to be associated with CRT response in small studies. Baseline contractile function indexed by LV + dP/dt_{max} has been shown to inversely correlate with its subsequent change during LV pacing. Heart failure functional class is positively correlated with CRT response. In several studies, equivalent benefit was observed with CRT in NYHA classes III-IV patients but no significant benefit in Class II.[15,52]

LV ejection fraction has not been shown to reliably correlate with likelihood of CRT response in any study. Sinus rhythm does not appear to be necessary for CRT response. Patients in permanent AF had an acute hemodynamic response similar to that of patients in sinus rhythm in the PATH-CHF study and similar long-term functional improvements in other trials.[15,71,84,85]

The role of the myocardial substrate is an important but unresolved issue in distinguishing CRT responders and nonresponders. Some studies,[78] but not others,[10,15] have suggested that ischemic DCM is less likely to respond to CRT than nonischemic DCM. However, these studies only examined outcomes on the basis of presence or absence of coronary artery disease as the cause of DCM. They did not consider, for example, the more specific possibility that infarct location may influence CRT response. Recently, an analysis of the MIRACLE trial reported that prior anterior infarct accompanying LBBB by ECG criteria predicted a low probability of CRT response.[86] The authors hypothesized that posterior-basal LV stimulation in this situation exaggerates systolic "bulging" of the anterior infarct segment. Another possibility is that slow conduction through a large infarct zone, causing a LBBB pattern, may not reflect intraventricular dyssynchrony and therefore would not be expected to respond to CRT. Infarct location may influence CRT indirectly when epicardial scar results in an inability to achieve pacing capture at the optimal site for LV stimulation (see later discussion).

Baseline QRS Duration

To date, QRSd determined from the surface ECG has been most extensively evaluated as a selection criterion for CRT, on the premise that electrical delay is a reliable marker for spatially dispersed mechanical activation. Numerous studies have reproducibly demonstrated that baseline QRSd is an important predictive factor of acute hemodynamic improvement with CRT. Auricchio and associates[3] showed that there was a positive correlation between the QRSd and the percentage of change in LV + dP/dt and pulse pressure during CRT. This observation was corroborated by Nelson and colleagues.[5]

Baseline QRSd modestly predicted systolic response, as assessed by maximal rate of pressure, defined as percent change in LV $+dP/dt_{max} = 0.61 \times$ QRSd $- 70.2$.

Combining the baseline QRSd and the LV + dP/dt_{max} improved the predictive accuracy for identifying CRT clinical responders. Patients with a baseline QRSd of 155 msec or longer and a baseline LV $+dP/dt_{max}$ of 700 mm Hg/second or less consistently yielded the greatest acute hemodynamic response to CRT (% change LV $+dP/dt_{max} \geq 25\%$).

Prediction curves for contractile function response using baseline QRSd derived from the PATH-CHF and PATH-CHF II studies are shown in Figure 26-46.[87]

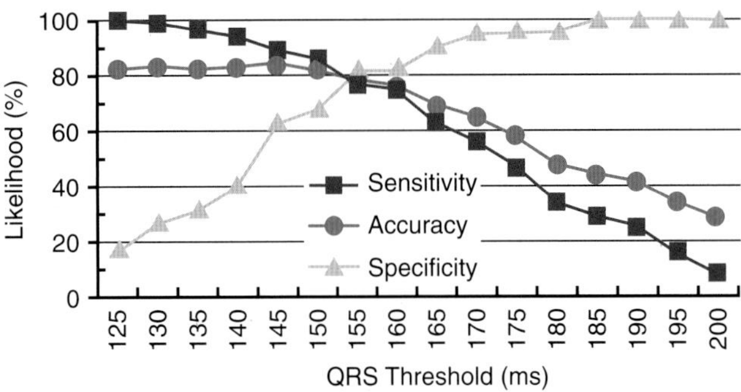

Figure 26-46. Probability of acute hemodynamic response to CRT according to baseline QRSd. (From Kadhiresan V, Vogt J, Auricchio A, et al: Sensitivity and specificity of QRS duration to predict acute benefit in heart failure patients with cardiac resynchronization [abstract]. PACE 23[II]:555, 2000.)

The specificity curve indicates that 80% of CRT nonresponders had a QRSd of less than 150 msec. The sensitivity curve indicates that 80% of CRT responders had a QRSd of greater than 150 msec. The overlap between these QRSd ranges was populated with CRT responders and nonresponders. The predictive accuracy of QRSd to separate responders from nonresponders is fairly constant, at approximately 80%, with a threshold cutoff between 120 and 150 msec. If the QRSd is longer than 150 msec, the likelihood of CRT response is greater. An important qualification is that this analysis is based on acute hemodynamic response to CRT, which, as mentioned previously, may not correlate precisely with chronic clinical improvement or reverse remodeling.[72] However, these observations appear to have been corroborated by the COMPANION trial, in which little or no benefit of CRT or CRTD on death or heart failure hospitalization was observed among patients with a baseline QRSd of less than 150 msec.[10]

In summary, 80% of patients with a QRSd of greater than 150 msec will have a hemodynamic improvement with CRT, and the probability of response is positively correlated with QRSd. Patients with a QRSd of less than 150 msec are less likely to respond to CRT, although this is not uniformly true. Improvements in dyssynchrony seem to be the determinant of the improvements obtained with CRT, and this may be independent of QRSd. Patients with more advanced symptoms of heart failure are more likely to respond to CRT than patients with less severe symptoms.

Pattern of Prolonged QRS Duration

Because RCTs of CRT have specified only prolonged QRS duration and not the pattern of abnormal ventricular conduction as a requirement for enrollment, patients with right bundle branch block (RBBB), LBBB, and "nonspecific" ventricular conduction delay all meet currently accepted implantation indications for CRT.[76] However, only about 10% of patients with advanced systolic heart failure and abnormal ventricular conduction have RBBB.[10,88] Consequently, patients with RBBB have comprised a very small proportion of the enrolled population in RCTs of CRT.

For this reason, only limited data on CRT for RBBB are available. Garrigue and coworkers[89] reported positive clinical response to CRT after 12 months in 9 of 12 patients with RBBB. Only those patients with RBBB and significant electromechanical delay in the left ventricle detected by tissue Doppler imaging responded to CRT. A retrospective analysis of 43 patients with RBBB in the MIRACLE study demonstrated significant improvement only in NYHA functional class with CRT versus no CRT, which led the authors to conclude that patients with RBBB have a similar intermediate-term response to CRT as patients with LBBB.[90] This was not corroborated by the much larger COMPANION study, in which CRT had a neutral effect among patients with RBBB.[10]

A recent study by Egoavil and associates[91] emphasized these uncertainties. The long-term outcomes of CRT in 61 patients with systolic heart failure, prolonged QRSd with RBBB activation pattern, and persistent symptoms (>NYHA class II) despite reasonable medical therapy were pooled from two RCTs (MIRACLE[15] and CONTAK CD[21]). CRT was randomized and assigned to be "On" in 34 patients and "Off" in 27 patients. There was no significant improvement in any outcome variables except for a one-step reduction in NYHA class, which the authors appropriately recognized as a highly subjective parameter. Further, Egoavil and associates[91] seem to have incidentally discovered a flaw in the analysis of Aranda and colleagues[90] that apparently misreported RBBB in 15 of 43 patients.

An important unanswered question in the analysis of Egoavil and associates[91] and others is whether the RBBB pattern was caused by myocardial infarction (see earlier discussion).

There is reason to be circumspect regarding the applicability of biventricular pacing in RBBB. Recent studies have demonstrated that intra-LV dyssynchrony is the most potent predictor of acute and chronic response (including reverse remodeling) to CRT.[19,77,79,82] A significant percentage of patients with LBBB may fail to respond to CRT simply because, despite delayed LV electrical activation, mechanical contraction is not dyssynchronous.[81,92] A similar situation may apply to RBBB but for different reasons. Despite the prolonged QRS duration, proximal RBBB, the most commonly occurring type of chronic RBBB, does not disrupt normal LV activation.[93] Therefore, it is not clear why biventricular pacing would be helpful in chronic proximal RBBB.

However, this may be an oversimplification in patients with systolic heart failure, because abnormalities in electrical activation and mechanical contraction have been incompletely characterized in RBBB compared with LBBB, and preliminary data suggest that important differences may have implications for the application of CRT. A recent study using three-dimensional endocardial activation mapping in a small cohort of patients with RBBB and systolic heart failure demonstrated that LV endocardial activation was similarly delayed in RBBB versus LBBB and that the posterobasal left ventricle was the latest site in either situation.[94] RV endocardial activation was significantly delayed in the anterior and lateral walls in RBBB. This suggests the possibility that RV stimulation in RBBB should target sites other than the apex. This may be an important qualification in the interpretation of limited clinical data on RBBB in randomized trials of CRT, because RV leads were almost uniformly placed at the apex.

There is insufficient clinical evidence to reach definitive conclusions, and this situation will be difficult to overcome because of the under-representation of RBBB in systolic heart failure. This is an important matter in a larger context, because approximately 20% to 30% of patients who meet currently accepted implantation criteria fail to respond to CRT.[15,52,77-80] As discussed earlier, reduction of CRT "nonresponders" must include rejection of patients who are destined not to respond (i.e., patients without mechanical dyssynchrony). Furthermore, LV or biventricular pacing still results in abnormal activation patterns and may worsen ventricular pumping function in hearts without initially abnormal LV contraction patterns.[95] Thus, CRT might actually cause clinical deterioration in patients with systolic heart failure and a prolonged QRSd (regardless of the pattern of abnormal ventricular conduction) but no mechanical dyssynchrony.

Echocardiographic Techniques for Selecting CRT Responders

Recognition of the potential limitations of QRSd for predicting CRT response has stimulated interest in techniques for directly measuring baseline ventricular dyssynchrony. Although preliminary results in small numbers of patients are encouraging, no RCT of CRT has reported on the use of echocardiographic techniques for patient selection.

Sophisticated Echocardiography

Intraventricular synchrony can be assessed echocardiographically from the delay between the maximal posterior displacement of the septum and the maximal displacement of the LV posterior wall measured from an M-mode short-axis view of the LV (septal-posterior wall delay, or SPWD). Pitzalis and coworkers[82] found that the mean SPWD improved from 192 msec to 14 msec after 1 month of CRT, and, among all monitored echocardiographic markers (including interventricular delay, ejection fraction, mitral regurgitant duration, and mitral regurgitant area), it was the only one associated with a favorable response to CRT, defined as an improvement of more than 15% in the LV systolic volume index. The mean SPWD was greater than 130 msec in all responders and was significantly longer in responders versus nonresponders (246 ± 68 versus 110 ± 55 msec).

Tissue Doppler Imaging, Tissue Synchrony Imaging, Tissue Tracking, Strain, and Strain Rate

Another promising echocardiographic technique to identify dyssynchrony and target patients for CRT is myocardial tissue imaging. This technique uses tissue Doppler signals to quantify time to peak systolic velocity or rate of regional myocardial deformation (strain), providing a sensitive estimate of regional myocardial shortening and lengthening that correlates with LV +dP/dt and systolic function in healthy and diseased hearts.[96] In LBBB, Doppler strain imaging demonstrates maximal septal contraction that occurs before aortic valve opening and is accompanied by lateral wall lengthening, consistent with studies in an animal model.[97] The septum then lengthens after aortic valve opening and does not contribute to ejection. Peak lateral wall contraction is observed very late in systole and persists into the postsystolic period. During CRT, systolic contraction can be demonstrated to occur simultaneously in both septal and lateral walls, contributing equally to ejection.[98] The usefulness of this technique in patient selection for CRT remains to be defined in clinical trials, but preliminary results appear encouraging. Ventricular dyssynchrony detected by tissue Doppler imaging has been shown to predict acute and chronic responses (including remodeling) to CRT in several studies.[19,77,99-101]

Limitations of QRS Duration for Selecting CRT Responders: Insights from Echocardiographic Techniques for Assessing Intraventricular Dyssynchrony

There are several reasons why QRSd may not reliably predict CRT response. QRSd reflects both RV and LV activation. In many patients with LBBB, the delay in ventricular activation resides entirely within the left ventricle, as anticipated. However, in some patients with LBBB, delayed RV activation accounts for a significant proportion of electrical delay which manifests on the surface ECG.[102]

More notably, studies with sophisticated echocardiographic techniques have yielded the critically important observation that prolonged QRSd, which is a measure of delayed electrical activation, correlates poorly with mechanical dyssynchrony. This has been convincingly demonstrated using simple[82,103] and sophisticated echocardiographic techniques.[81,92] Yu and colleagues[81] used a dyssynchrony index (Ts-SD), derived from the standard deviation (SD) of the maximal difference in time to peak myocardial systolic contraction (Ts) of 12 LV segments, to assess intraventricular dyssynchrony relative to QRSd. When a dyssynchrony index greater than 32.6 msec (+2 SD of normal controls) was used to define significant intraventricular dyssynchrony, it was present in only 64% of patients with prolonged QRSd (>120 msec). Bleeker and colleagues[92] reported that severe LV dyssynchrony, defined as an electromechanical delay on the tachycardia detection interval between the septal and lateral wall (septal-lateral delay >60 msec), was present in only 60% of patients with LBBB and a QRSd of 120 to 150 msec and in 70% of those with a QRSd greater than 150 msec. Therefore, similar to the observations of Yu and colleagues,[81] about 40% of patients with prolonged QRSd did not have significant intraventricular dyssynchrony. Although the proportion of patients with severe intraventricular dyssynchrony increased with increasing QRSd, linear regression failed to show any significant correlation between QRSd and dyssynchrony.

These observations are critically important and probably explain a significant portion of the CRT nonresponse phenomenon in RCTs, because recent studies have conclusively demonstrated that intraventricular dyssynchrony is the most potent predictor of acute and chronic responses (including reverse remodeling).[19,77,82,99,104] Accordingly, a significant percentage of patients with prolonged QRSd may fail to respond to CRT simply because, despite delayed electrical activation, mechanical contraction is not dyssynchronous. Furthermore, LV or biventricular pacing with an LV lead on the posterior or posterolateral basal LV wall still results in abnormal activation patterns in hearts without initially abnormal mechanical dyssynchrony.[95] LV pacing may worsen the ventricular pumping function if ventricular contraction is not dyssynchronous. For example, CRT might actually cause clinical deterioration in patients with systolic heart failure and a prolonged QRSd but no mechanical dyssynchrony. This may account for the observation that some patients in the MIRACLE trial actually worsened during CRT.

CRT Responders with Normal QRS Duration

Further complicating the matter of patient selection for CRT is the fascinating observation that some patients with DCM and normal or near-normal QRSd have significant mechanical dyssynchrony.[92,105-108] Such patients are systematically excluded from CRT under existing implantation guidelines, but they have been shown to demonstrate similar responses to CRT in terms of clinical improvement and reverse ventricular remodeling as patients with prolonged QRSd and mechanical dyssynchrony.[106,109]

Management in CRT Nonresponders

Once a patient is identified as displaying a limited or absent response to CRT, a systematic search for reversible causes should be undertaken, to guide potentially corrective interventions that may improve outcomes. This search can be partitioned into three interdependent phases: system-related, patient-related, and patient-system interface (Table 26-1).

System-related Causes of CRT Nonresponse

The approach to troubleshooting CRTP and CRTD systems must consider both electrical operation and the effect of various parameter settings on LV pumping function.

The six basic electrical problems of all cardiac pacing systems are (1) undersensing, (2) oversensing, (3) noncapture, (4) loss of output, (5) unanticipated alterations in programmed parameters, and (6) undesirable side effects of programmed parameters. Reprogramming is the most desirable outcome for electrical

TABLE 26-1. **Identifying Correctable Causes of CRT Nonresponse**

Problem	Solution
System-related causes	
Atrial undersensing	
True undersensing	Increase atrial sensitivity, reposition atrial lead
Pseudoundersensing	Shorten PVARP, deactivate PMT and PVC responses, increase upper tracking limit, add interventricular refractory period
Atrial oversensing	
Far-field R waves causing inappropriate switching to nontracking mode	Reduce atrial sensitivity, increase PVAB
Ventricular oversensing	
Inhibition of ventricular pacing	Reduce ventricular sensitivity, reposition RV or LV lead if dislodged, eliminated nondedicated CRT or CRTD system if appropriate
Loss of LV capture	
True loss of capture	Increase voltage output, reposition LV lead
Functional loss of LV capture	Use sequential ventricular stimulation (V-V timing)
Patient-related causes	
Atrial fibrillation	
AV conduction absent	Antiarrhythmic drug for AF suppression
AV conduction present	Antiarrhythmic drug for AF suppression, control ventricular rate with drugs or AV junction ablation, use AF response algorithms
Atrial pacing	
Disruption of optimal left-sided AV coupling	Reduce lower rate, use VDD mode; reevaluate AV delay using echocardiography or other hemodynamic measures
Ventricular conduction delay	Try LV-only or sequential biventricular stimulation
Absence of mechanical dyssynchrony	Abandon CRT, minimize any ventricular pacing if possible
Patient-system interface	
Suboptimal AV coupling	Reevaluate AV delay using echocardiography or other hemodynamic measures
LV lead position	If anterior vein site, reposition LV lead at lateral vein site (cardiac surgical approach if no venous targets or technically insurmountable).

AF, atrial fibrillation; AV, atrioventricular; CRT, cardiac resynchronization therapy; CRTD, cardiac resynchronization with defibrillation system; LV, left ventricular; PVARP, postventricular atrial refractory period; PVC, premature ventricular contraction; PMT, pacemaker mediated tachycardia; PVAB, postventricular atrial blanking period; RV, right ventricular.

problems, because it is painless, risk-free, and inexpensive and spares the patient a potentially morbid procedure.

Atrial Undersensing

Atrial undersensing may result in loss of atrial synchronous ventricular pacing and delivery of CRT. Atrial undersensing can be divided into true undersensing caused by a mismatch between endocardial signal amplitude and programmed sensitivity and functional undersensing caused by atrial events falling in refractory periods (see earlier discussion). This can usually be modified by reprogramming of atrial sensitivity or refractory periods but occasionally requires surgical repositioning of the atrial lead (e.g., in the circumstance of lead dislodgment).

Atrial Oversensing

Atrial oversensing (most commonly due to far-field R-waves) may result in spurious mode-switching (in the DDD/R or VDI/R mode), causing reversion to a nontracking mode (DDI/R or VDI) with loss of atrial synchronous ventricular pacing and CRT (see earlier discussion). Spurious mode-switching can usually be minimized by reducing atrial sensitivity and modifying the PVAB.

Ventricular Oversensing

Ventricular oversensing may cause inhibition of ventricular of ventricular pacing and loss of CRT, as well as spurious detections resulting in misdiagnosis of ventricular tachyarrhythmias. Though this can be addressed by reduction of ventricular sensitivity, caution must be applied to guarantee robustness of VF detection at reduced ventricular sensitivity.

Noncapture

Noncapture is defined as the emission of an atrial or ventricular pacing stimulus without capture. Atrial noncapture results in simultaneous loss of atrial pacing support and AV synchrony in patients with significant sinus bradycardia. In this situation, when AV conduction is intact, biventricular pacing may result in ventriculoatrial synchrony and pacemaker syndrome.

Loss of ventricular capture is the most common reason for a CRT responder to experience a clinical decline after a period of sustained improvement. Ventricular noncapture results in nondelivery of CRT and is more common on the LV lead due to higher chronic pacing thresholds and lead dislodgments. Sudden and complete loss of LV capture is often a dramatic event and is almost always caused by lead dislodgment. Lead dislodgment is readily identified by radiography, although "microdislodgments" resulting in sudden rises in capture threshold are more difficult to discern. Loss of LV capture may be gradual due to exit block. The 12-lead ECG remains a critically important tool for evaluating LV capture even among second- and third-generation devices with separately programmable ventricular outputs for threshold testing. This can be recognized in many instances only by analysis of the ventricular activation pattern on the surface ECG. Noncapture can be successfully overcome by redetermining the single-chamber capture threshold and modifying programmed outputs accordingly in some situations.

Unanticipated Alteration in Programmed Parameters

Unanticipated alteration in programmed parameters refers to device timing cycle operation that is different from that of programmed settings. This situation is most commonly encountered when the pulse generator has reached elective replacement status and the basic pacing mode has been automatically modified (i.e., VVI mode) to conserve battery life until replacement can be achieved. This results in instantaneous and simultaneous loss of AV and ventricular synchrony and may precipitate heart failure decompensation in some CRT patients.

Undesirable Side Effects of Programmed Parameters

Undesirable side effects of programmed parameters refers to a broad range of situations in which programmed settings, despite normal operation, inadvertently impose clinical consequences on the patient. The common example during CRT is phrenic nerve stimulation during LV pacing. Approaches to preventing and overcoming phrenic nerve stimulation were discussed earlier in this chapter.

Patient-Related Causes of CRT Nonresponse

Any interruption of ventricular pacing may reduce CRT response. As noted previously, a reasonable goal is greater than 90% cumulative percent ventricular pacing based on device diagnostics. By far the most common cause of loss of CRT pacing is AF with rapid AV conduction. This results in simultaneous loss of AV synchrony and ventricular synchrony combined with the adverse effects of a rapid, irregular ventricular rate on pumping function. AF and resultant consequences are readily recognized by device diagnostics. The approach here should be aggressive use of drugs to slow AV conduction or restoration of sinus rhythm if possible. Recent evidence suggests that ablation of the AV junction may be necessary to achieve optimal CRT response among patients with permanent AF and intact AV conduction.

Other causes of disruptions to ventricular pacing have already been discussed. Specific device algorithms intended to maximize ventricular pacing during conducted AF, sinus tachycardia with loss of atrial tracking, and high-frequency ventricular premature beats should be exploited.

Patient-System Interface Causes of CRT Nonresponse

The interaction between the patient and the CRT system presents a complex array of potential causes of CRT nonresponse that are often difficult to discern and not easily resolved. Troubleshooting these causes of CRT nonresponse assumes that electrical operation is normal and that patient factors that degrade CRT response independent of electrical operation have been optimized.

Role of Atrial Pacing

A high frequency of atrial pacing can compromise CRT response by disrupting optimal left-sided AV coupling. Programmed paced AV delays (PAV) differ significantly from sensed AV delays (SAV) during sinus rhythm. The reasons are (1) latency in atrial capture and sensing, (2) interatrial conduction delay, (3) latency in ventricular capture, and (4) interventricular conduction delay. The situation is made even more complex because all four elements are influenced by atrial and ventricular lead positions.

Capture latency refers to the delay between emission of the right atrial pacing stimulus and atrial contraction (Fig. 26-47). Sensing latency refers to the delay between the onset of atrial depolarization and the time at which the local endocardial signal is sensed (Fig. 26-48).

Because of latency in atrial capture and sensing, the optimal AV delay for sensed and paced P waves may differ. During sinus rhythm, the programmed SAV begins when the native P wave is sensed, but the physiologic AV interval begins with atrial depolarization and the onset of mechanical contraction. The mean latency between the beginning of atrial depolarization and the time of atrial sensing is 30 to 50 msec. Therefore, the physiologic AV interval is longer than the programmed SAV. The opposite situation occurs during atrial pacing. The programmed AV delay begins with emission of the atrial pacing stimulus, but the physiologic AV interval begins with atrial depolarization and mechanical contraction. The mean latency between atrial output and capture is reported to be 30 to 50 msec; however, it may be greater than 300 msec (Fig. 26-49). The physiologic AV interval is therefore shorter than the programmed PAV. The magnitude of atrial capture and sensing latencies varies among patients and is influenced by many factors, including lead design, sensing circuitry, ampli-

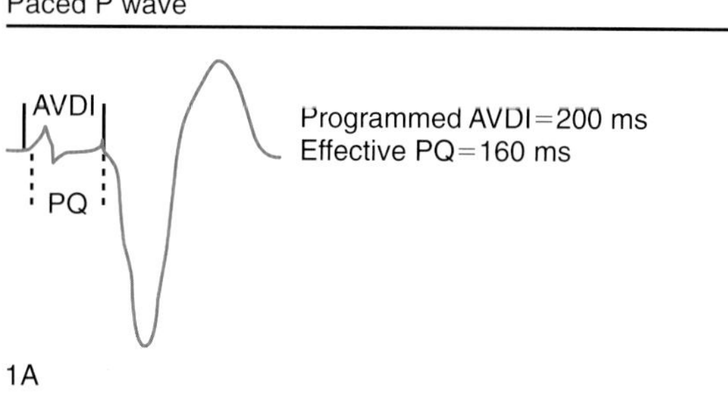

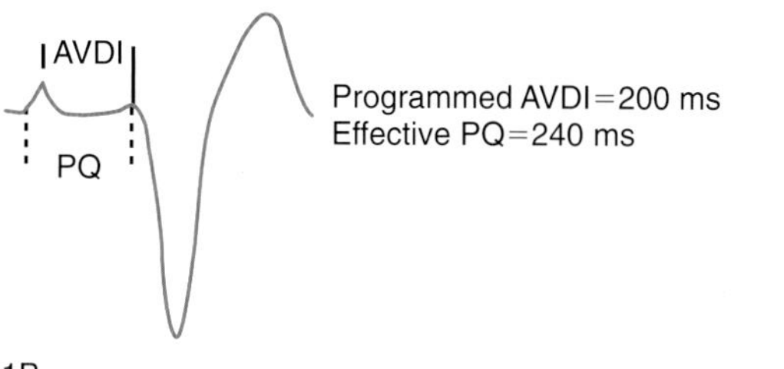

Figure 26-47. Effect of atrial capture and sensing latency on the physiologic atrioventricular (AV) interval. AVDI, atrioventricular delay interval; PQ, PQ interval.

tude and rate of stimulation, and characteristics of the local endocardial atrial EGM.

Further complicating matters is the effect of autonomic innervation of the AV node during atrial pacing. AV intervals during atrial pacing shorten during exercise and lengthen by as much as 150% in the standing or supine position.[110] A mismatch between the lower pacing rate and autonomic balance may contribute to this situation. For example, patients with a relatively high programmed lower rate (i.e., 70 or 80 bpm) often experience significant AV interval extensions during atrial pacing while sleeping because of parasympathetic predominance (Figs. 26-50 and 26-51).

Additionally, significant interatrial conduction delays may arise due to cardiomyopathy and atrial enlargement, antiarrhythmic drugs, and other causes. Interatrial conduction delays are common during right atrial pacing and are influenced by pacing lead position (Figs. 26-52 and 26-53). Right atrial pacing from the regions of Bachmann's bundle, the fossa ovalis, and the coronary sinus ostium result in less-delayed left atrial activation, compared with other common pacing sites such as the right atrial appendage.

The common consequence of these effects is that the optimized AV delay is already in progress before the

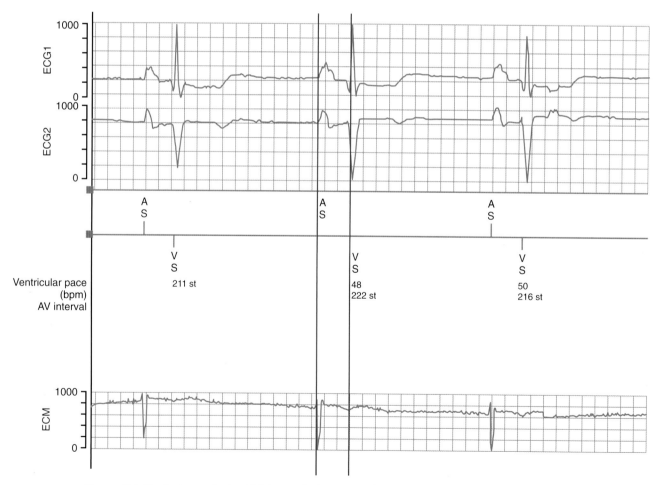

Figure 26-48. Atrioventricular (AV) intervals during atrial sensing. AS and VS occur at the start of the P and R waves, and the AS-VS time of 222 msec corresponds well to the surface electrocardiogram (ECG) P-Q time measured by the cursors. AS, sensed atrial event; VS, sensed ventricular event.

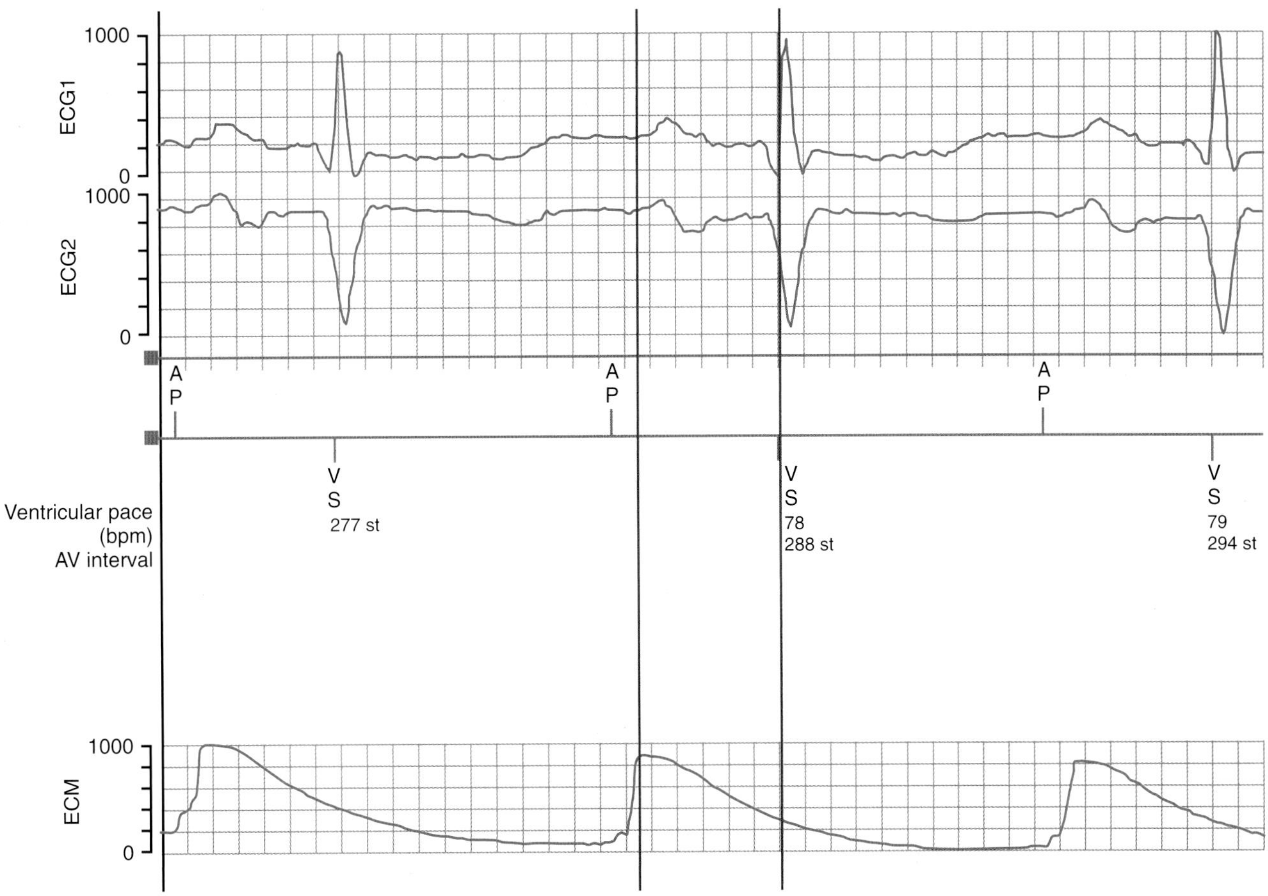

Figure 26-49. Effect of atrial capture latency on atrioventricular (AV) interval during atrial pacing. The AP occurs sooner than the P wave is seen on the surface electrocardiogram (ECG). The AP-VS time is measured at 288 msec, but the time from the start of the P wave to VS time is nearer to 244 msec. Therefore, the AP-VS time is over-reported by the device, compared with the surface ECG. AP, atrial paced event; VS, ventricular sensed event.

left atrial contribution to ventricular filling has begun (Figs. 26-54 and 26-55). In this situation, the optimized AV delay during sinus rhythm may be too short during atrial pacing, with adverse effects on left-sided AV coupling. This can be overcome by increasing the paced AV delay, but the penalty is progressive loss of LV preexcitation (assuming AV nodal conduction is intact), because LV stimulation is excessively delayed. This results in increased intraventricular dyssynchrony compared with LV pacing at shorter AV delays, as was shown by Bernheim and associates.[111] The consequence of this conflict is that an undesirable choice must be made between suboptimal left-sided AV coupling and inadequate LV preexcitation due to fusion. There are two situations in which this situation can be avoided during atrial pacing: (1) AV conduction is absent, thereby excluding progressive fusion; and (2) AV conduction is severely delayed (very long AS-VS time) and left atrial activation is equivalently delayed due to capture latency and interatrial conduction delay.

Atrial pacing should be minimized or avoided altogether if possible. Programming approaches include reducing the lower pacing rate, eliminating sensor-modulated pacing (if active), and choosing an atrial synchronous ventricular pacing mode that does not provide atrial pacing (i.e., VDD at a low programmed rate). If atrial pacing cannot be avoided due to sinus bradycardia, the paced AV delay should be reoptimized using techniques previously described.

Role of Ventricular Conduction Delay

The mere demonstration of ventricular capture on a single-lead ECG strip during pacing of the LV does not guarantee that the ventricular activation sequence has been changed. "Functional" loss of LV capture may occur during synchronous biventricular pacing if there is significant latency from the LV pacing site due to epicardial scar. In this situation, LV activation may be dominated by the electrical wavefront caused by RV pacing, despite an adequately programmed LV output. This phenomenon can be recognized only through the use of a 12-lead ECG. The problem can be overcome by using V-V timing, as previously discussed (Figs. 26-56, 26-57, 26-58, and 26-59).

Whether or not individually optimized sequential biventricular pacing can reduce the number of CRT "nonresponders" is uncertain. Although small studies have shown that sequential ventricular stimulation can

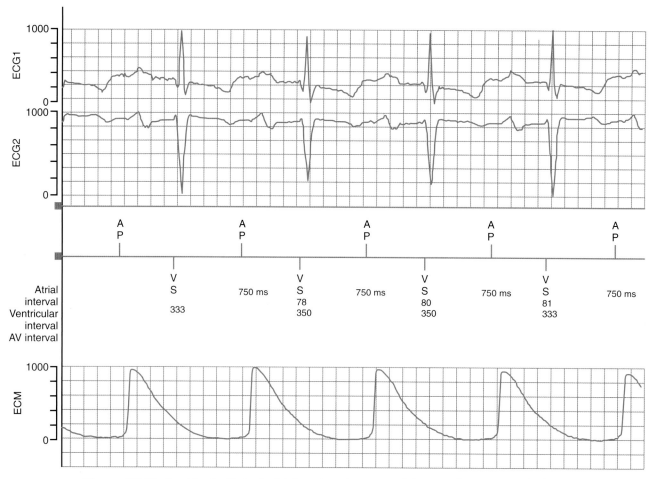

Figure 26-50. Combined effect of atrial capture latency and increased parasympathetic tone during sleep on the atrioventricular (AV) interval during atrial pacing. ECG, electrocardiogram.

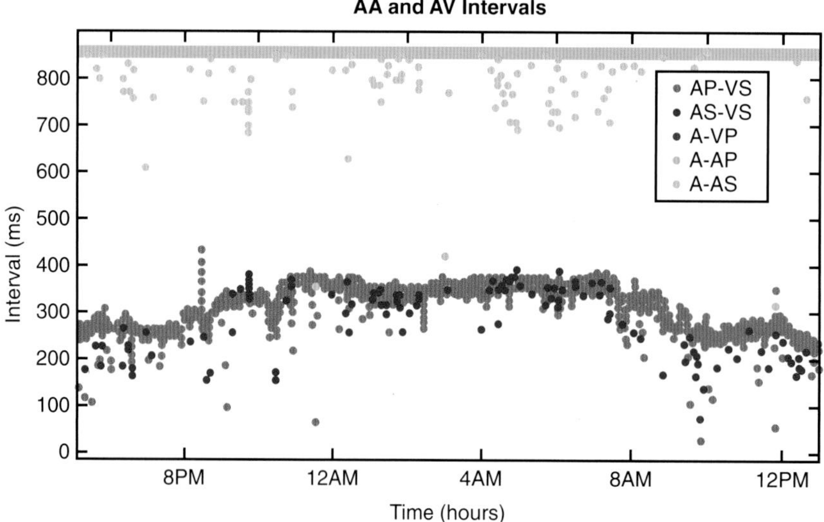

Figure 26-51. Nocturnal response of atrioventricular (AV) conduction during atrial pacing in the same patient as in Figure 26-50. The AP-VS interval is at its longest during sleep, approximately 350 msec. AP-VS, atrial paced–ventricular sensed; AS-VS, atrial sensed–ventricular sensed; A-VP, atrial paced/sensed–ventricular paced; A-AP, atrial paced–atrial paced; A-AS, atrial sensed–atrial sensed.

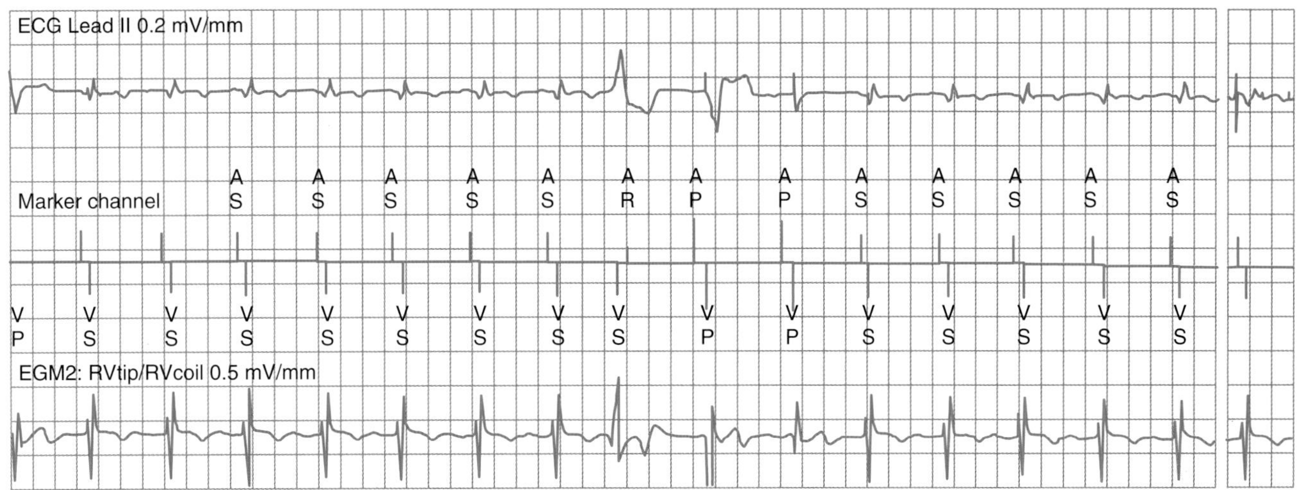

Figure 26-52. Example of significant interatrial conduction delay during pacing from the right atrial appendage and sensing from the left atrial (LA) epicardium. The patient had a single-chamber ICD implanted from the left superior transvenous approach. Antiarrhythmic drug therapy resulted in symptomatic sinus bradycardia. An attempt to add an atrial lead from the left superior approach failed because of an occluded axillary-subclavian vein. A separate single-chamber atrial pacing system was implanted via the right superior transvenous approach. Subsequently, epicardial LA and left ventricular pacing leads were placed for CRT. LA activation is tremendously delayed during sinus rhythm. Note that LA activation (AS) occurs almost simultaneously with the preceding right ventricular (RV) activation (VS), which is delayed due to first-degree atrioventricular (AV) nodal block. As a result, no CRT is delivered. AP, paced atrial event; ECG, electrocardiogram; VP, paced ventricular event.

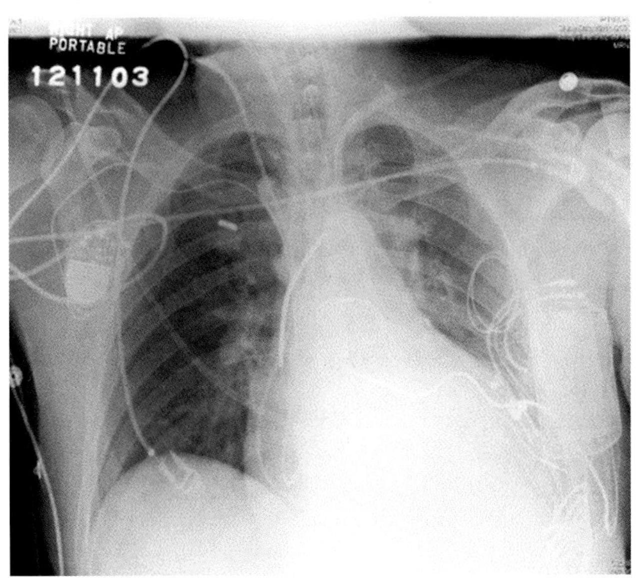

Figure 26-53. Chest radiograph showing right atrial endocardial and left atrial epicardial lead positions in the same patient as in Figure 26-52.

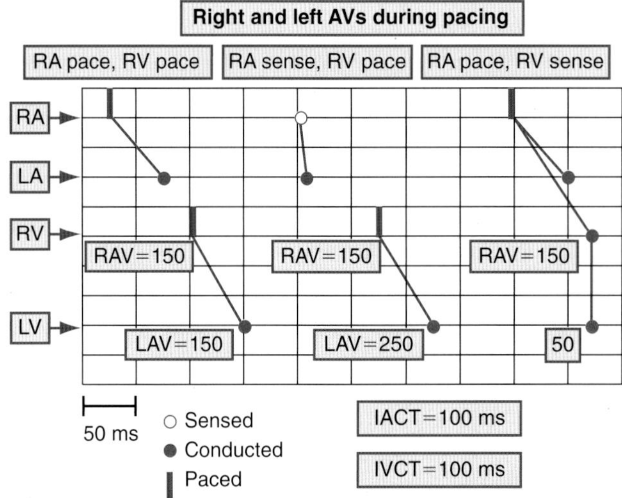

Figure 26-54. Effect of right-sided atrioventricular (AV) delays on left-sided AV coupling during DDD pacing. IACT, interatrial conduction time; IVCT, interventricular conduction time; LA, left atrium; LAV, left-sided AV delay; LV, left ventricle; mS, milliseconds; RA, right atrium; RAV, right-sided AV delay; RV, right ventricle.

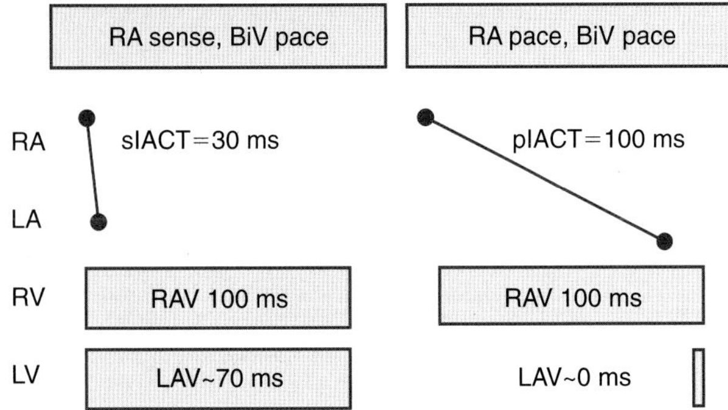

Figure 26-55. Effect of right-sided atrioventricular (AV) delays on left-sided AV coupling during CRT. BiV, biventricular; LA, left atrium; LAV, left-sided AV delay; LV, left ventricle; ms, milliseconds; pIACT, paced interatrial conduction time; RA, right atrium; RAV, right-sided AV delay; RV, right ventricle; sIACT, sensed interatrial conduction time.

reduce intraventricular dyssynchrony,[18] increase diastolic filling time,[18,112] reduce functional mitral regurgitation,[112] and increase LV +dP/dt and cardiac output,[112,113] these findings have not been validated in RCTs. Complicating matters is the consistent observation in all of these studies that the individual response to sequential ventricular stimulation is heterogeneous and unpredictable.

Biventricular or Left Ventricular-Only Stimulation: Is There a Role in CRT Nonresponders?

It is important to note that uncertainty about the requirement of RV stimulation during CRT, uneasiness about long-term LV lead performance, and unavailability of pacing systems with separately programmable ventricular outputs has influenced the use of biventricular pacing, as opposed to left univentricular pacing, in large RCTs. A particular concern is LV lead dislodgment, which has a reported incidence of 5% to 10% in larger studies[10,15,52] and would impose a risk for potentially lethal bradycardia. However, there is some scientific evidence that RV stimulation might not be necessary for optimal CRT response or even that LV pacing alone might be superior to biventricular pacing in some patients.

Left univentricular pacing alone has acute hemodynamic effects that are similar or superior to those achieved with biventricular pacing in some patients.[18,109,114-116] Blanc and coworkers[117] recently extended these observations. Functional capacity (6-minute walk and maximal oxygen uptake), ventricular size and function, and blood norepinephrine levels before and after 12 months of left univentricular pacing were evaluated in 22 patients with DCM, LBBB NYHA class III or IV heart failure. The LV lead was placed in a lateral coronary vein whenever possible, and all patients had

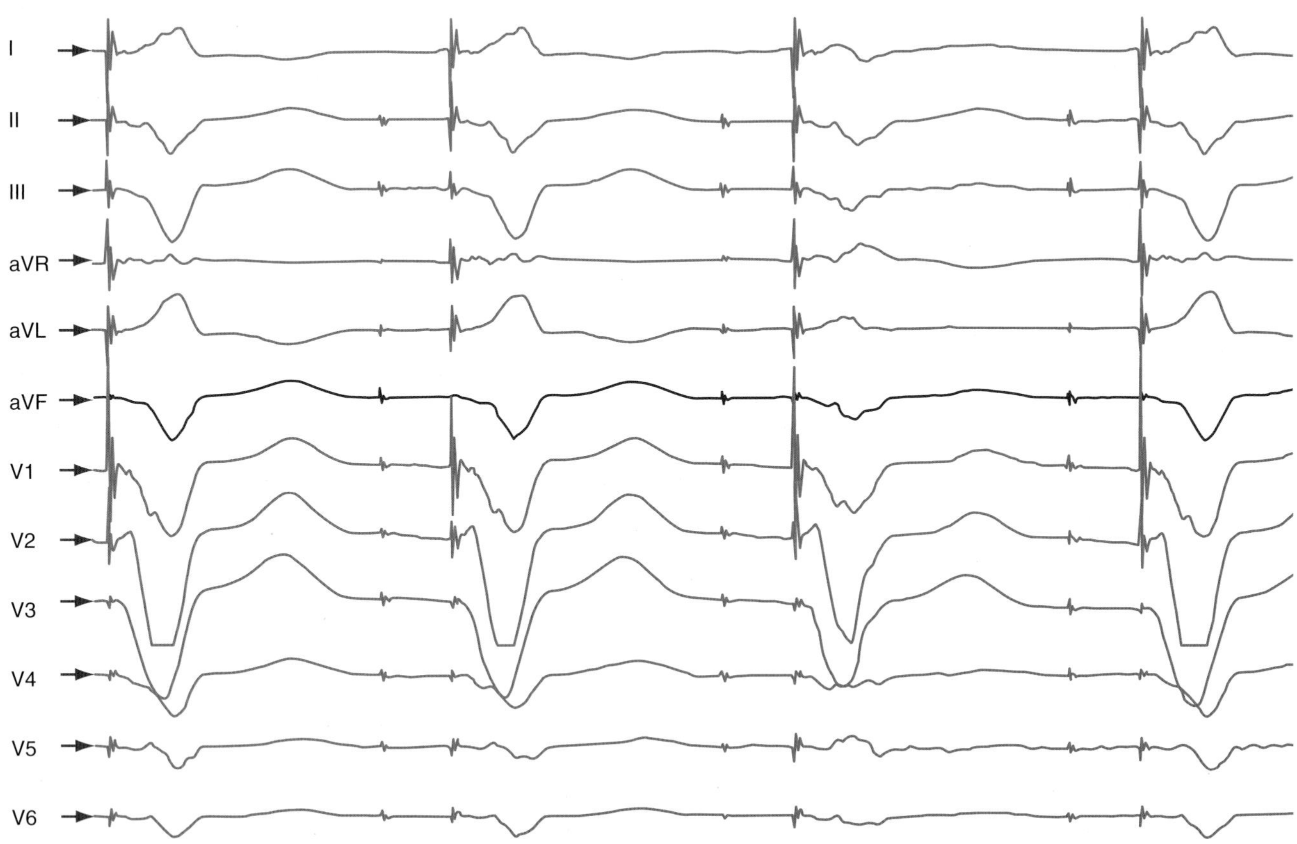

Figure 26-56. Simultaneous biventricular pacing. Note the pattern of right ventricular (RV) apical stimulation; there is no evidence of left ventricular capture based on the paced QRS morphology.

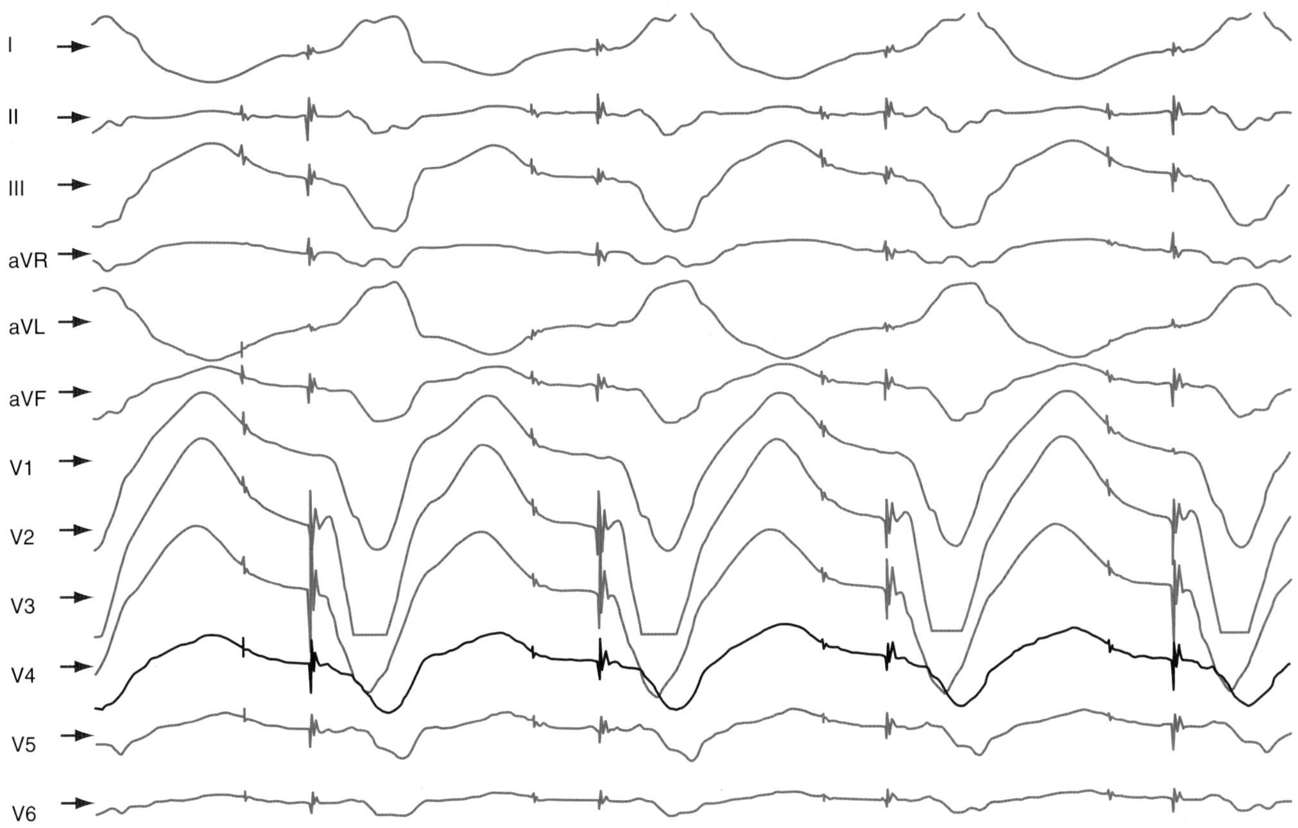

Figure 26-57. *Right ventricular (RV)-only pacing in the same patient as in Figure 26-56. Note the pattern of RV apical stimulation.*

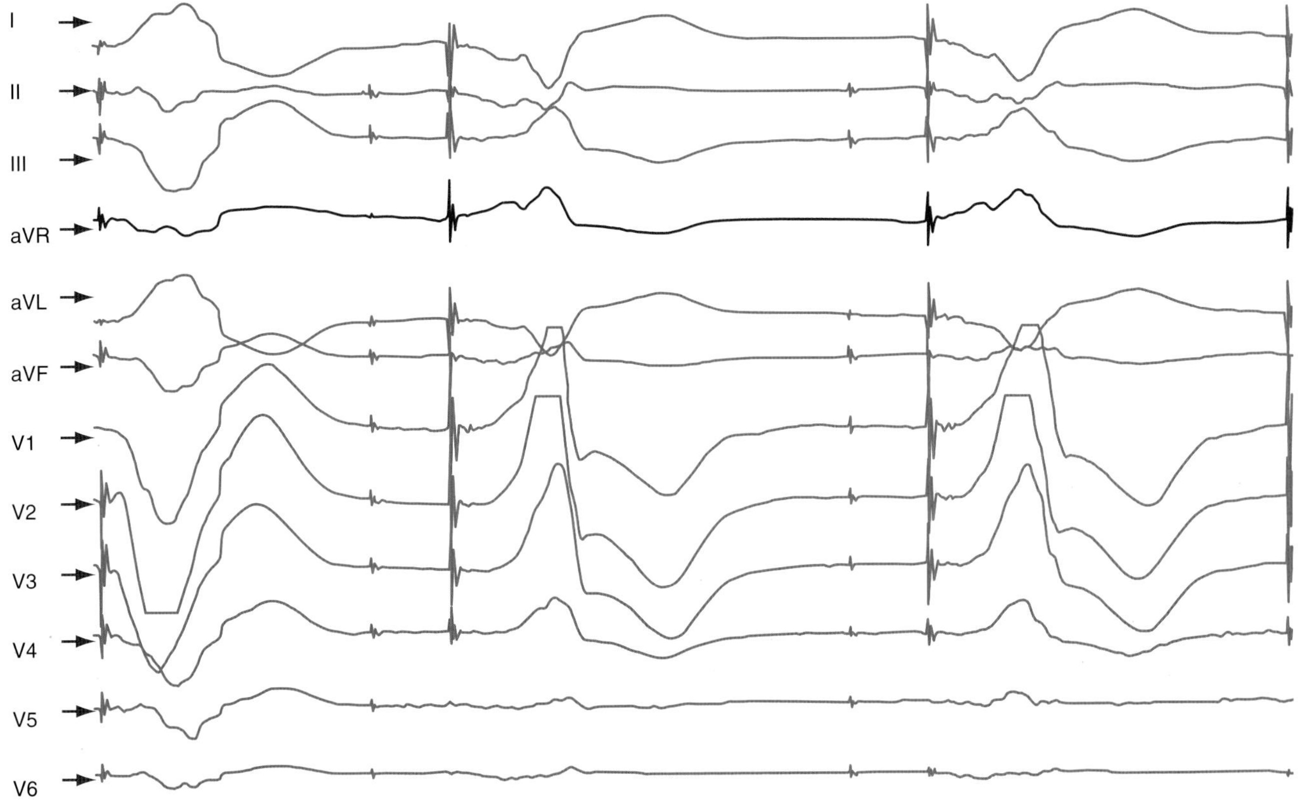

Figure 26-58. *Left ventricular (LV)-only pacing in the same patient. Note the pattern of LV free wall stimulation.*

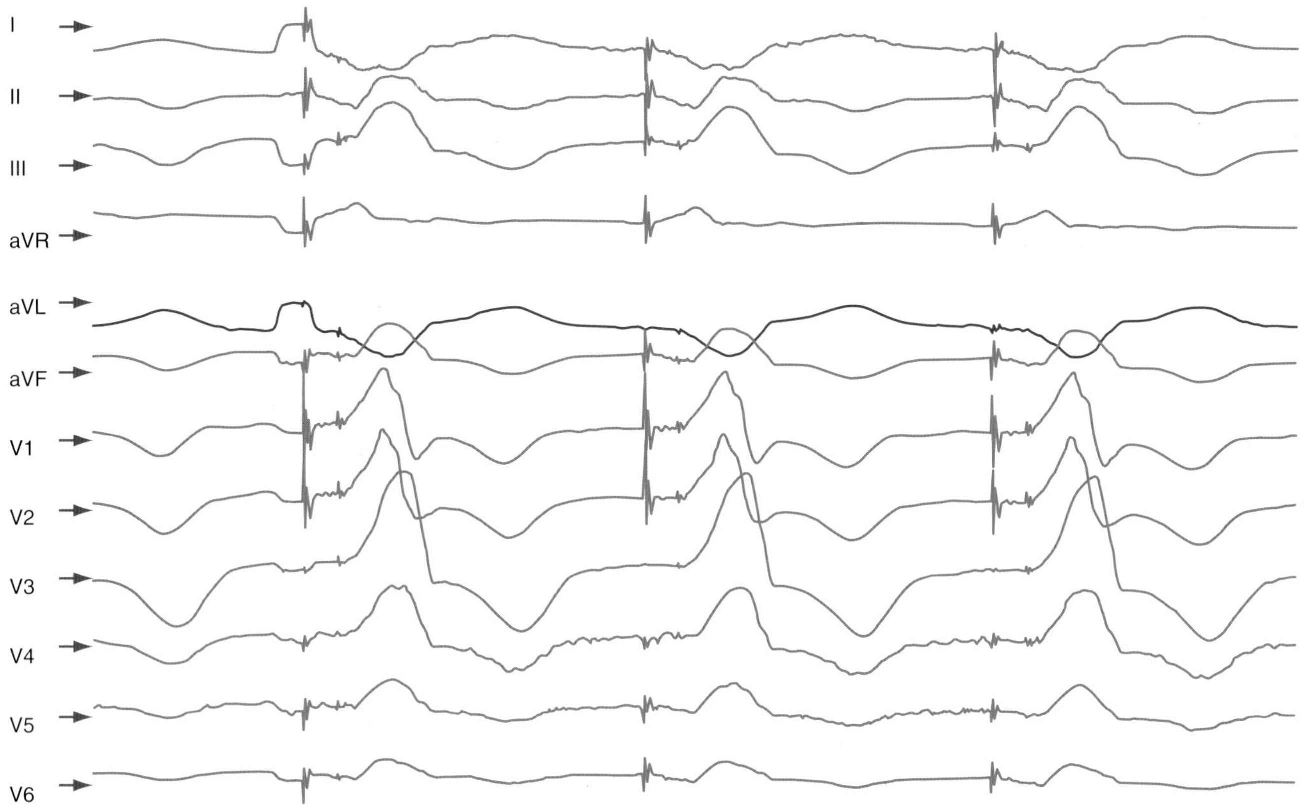

Figure 26-59. Sequential ventricular stimulation with 80-msec offset (LV > RV). Note restoration of biventricular activation.

sinus rhythm to allow atrial synchronous left univentricular pacing with an AV delay initially programmed to 100 msec. Significant improvements in functional capacity, echocardiographic mitral regurgitation, and LV end-diastolic diameter were observed, with a favorable trend toward improvement in LV ejection fraction. These results are encouraging and support persistent benefit (at least to 1 year) of left univentricular pacing in some patients.

Both LV and biventricular pacing synchronize LV contraction. This "re-timing" effect was initially attributed to "preexcitation" of the delayed LV segments. However, insights from tissue Doppler studies have revealed that LV pacing from a late-activated site achieves synchronous contraction by simultaneously delaying all LV segments.[19,112] This is a potentially critical observation, because LV pacing reverses electrical activation and abolishes intraventricular dyssynchrony, but with the result of a marked increase in LV activation time compared with biventricular pacing.[49] The consequences are a greater delay in RV contraction[109] and a shortened diastolic filling time, which may have implications for ventricular pumping function, particularly at higher heart rates.[112,118]

Therefore, it is theoretically possible that LV-only pacing may achieve superior hemodynamic performance compared with biventricular pacing in some patients. For this reason, LV-only pacing should probably be considered in CRT nonresponders initially treated with biventricular pacing. This could be easily achieved noninvasively if a true bipolar LV lead is used with a pulse generator that is capable of separately programmable ventricular outputs. A similar effect could be achieved in the case of a unipolar LV lead (dual cathodal configuration) by programming RV output below the capture threshold. It could not be achieved in a dual cathodal configuration without separately programmable ventricular outputs unless the LV threshold was significantly lower than the RV threshold. In any event, it is not currently possible to identify patients who will respond better to LV alone compared with biventricular pacing.

REFERENCES

1. Kanagaratnam L, Pavia S, Schweikert R, et al: Matching approved "nondedicated" hardware to obtain biventricular pacing and defibrillation: Feasibility and troubleshooting. PACE 25:1066-1071, 2002.
2. Bulava A, Ansalone G, Ricci R, et al: Triple-site pacing in patients with biventricular device: Incidence of the phenomenon and cardiac resynchronization benefit. J Intervent Cardiac Electrophysiol 10:37-45, 2004.
3. Auricchio A, Stellbrink C, Block M, et al: Effect of pacing chamber and atrioventricular delay on acute systolic function of paced patients with congestive heart failure. The Pacing Therapies for Congestive Heart Failure Study Group. The Guidant Congestive Heart Failure Research Group. Circulation 99:2993-3001, 1999.

4. Auricchio A, Stellbrink C, Sack S, et al., and Group PTiCHFP-CS: Long-term clinical effect of hemodynamically optimized cardiac resynchronization therapy in patients with heart failure and ventricular conduction delay. J Am Coll Cardiol 39:2026-2033, 2002.
5. Nelson GS, Curry CW, Wyman BT, et al: Predictors of systolic augmentation from left ventricular preexcitation in patients with dilated cardiomyopathy and intraventricular conduction delay. Circulation 101:2703-2709, 2000.
6. Ritter P, Padeletti L, Gillio-Meina L, et al: Determination of the optimal atrioventricular delay in DDD pacing: Comparison between echo and peak endocardial acceleration measurements. Europace 1:126-130, 1999.
7. Kindermann M, Frölig G, Doerr T, Schieffer H: Optimizing the AV delay in DDD pacemaker patients with high degree AV block: Mitral valve Doppler versus impedance cardiography. PACE 20:2453-2462, 1997.
8. Meluzin J, Novak M, Mullerova J, et al: A fast and simple echocardiographic determination of the optimal atrioventricular delay in patients after biventricular stimulation. PACE 27:58-64, 2004.
9. Auricchio A, Kramer A, Spinelli J, et al: Can the optimum dosage of resynchronization therapy be derived from the intracardiac electrogram? [abstract]. J Am Coll Cardiol 39:124, 2002.
10. Bristow MR, Saxon LA, Boehmer J, et al., and the Comparison of Medical Therapy, Pacing, and Defibrillation in Heart Failure (COMPANION) Investigators: Cardiac-resynchronization therapy with or without an implantable defibrillator in advanced chronic heart failure. N Engl J Med 350:2140-2150, 2004.
11. Butter C, Stellbrink C, Belalcazar A, et al: Cardiac resynchronization therapy optimization by finger plethysmography. Heart Rhythm 1:568-578, 2005.
12. Nishimura RA, Hayes DL, Holmes DR, Tajik AJ: Mechanism of hemodynamic improvement by dual-chamber pacing for severe left ventricular dysfunction: An acute Doppler and catheterization study. J Am Coll Cardiol 25:281-288, 1995.
13. Auricchio A, Sommariva L, Salo RW, et al: Improvement of cardiac function in patients with severe congestive heart failure and coronary artery disease by dual chamber pacing with shortened AV delay. PACE 17:995-997, 1994.
14. Linde-Edelstam C, Nordlander R, Unden A-L, et al: Quality-of-life in patients treated with atrioventricular synchronous pacing compared to rate modulated ventricular pacing: A long-term, double-blind, crossover study. PACE 15:1467-1476, 1992.
15. Abraham WT, Fisher WG, Smith AL, et al., for the MIRACLE Study Group. Cardiac resynchronization in chronic heart failure. N Engl J Med 346:1845-1853, 2002.
16. Cazeau S, Leclercq C, Lavergne T, et al., and The Multisite Stimulation in Cardiomyopathies (MUSTIC) Study Investigators. Effects of multisite biventricular pacing in patients with heart failure and intraventricular conduction delay. N Engl J Med 344:873-880, 2001.
17. Sawhney NS, Waggoner AD, Garhwal S, et al: Randomized prospective trial of atrioventricular delay programming for cardiac resynchronization therapy. Heart Rhythm 1:562-567, 2004.
18. Sogaard P, Egeblad H, Pedersen AK, et al: Sequential versus simultaneous biventricular resynchronization for severe heart failure: Evaluation by tissue Doppler imaging. Circulation 106:2078-2084, 2002.
19. Yu CM, Chau E, Sanderson EJ, et al: Tissue Doppler echocardiographic evidence of reverse remodeling and improved synchronicity by simultaneous delaying regional contraction after biventricular pacing therapy in heart failure. Circulation 105:438-445, 2002.
20. Bordachar P, Lafitte S, Reuter S, et al: Echocardiographic parameters of ventricular dyssynchrony validation in patients with heart failure using sequential biventricular pacing. J Am Coll Cardiol 44:2157-2165, 2004.
21. Higgins SL, Hummel JD, Niazi IK, et al: Cardiac resynchronization therapy for the treatment of heart failure and intraventricular conduction delay and malignant ventricular tachyarrhythmia. J Am Coll Cardiol 42:1454-1459, 2003.
22. Fisher JD, Mehra R, Furman S: Termination of ventricular tachycardia with bursts of rapid ventricular pacing. Am J Cardiol 41:94-102, 1978.
23. Gillis AM, Leitch J, Sheldon RS, et al: A prospective randomized comparison of autodecremental pacing to burst pacing in device therapy for chronic ventricular tachycardia secondary to coronary artery disease. Am J Cardiol 72:1146-1151, 1993.
24. Calkins H, El-Atassi R, Kalbfleisch S, et al: Comparison of fixed burst versus decremental burst pacing for termination of ventricular tachycardia. PACE 16:26-32, 1993.
25. Kantoch MJ, Green MS, Tang AS: Randomized cross-over evaluation of two adaptive pacing algorithms for the termination of ventricular tachycardia. PACE 16:1664-1672, 1993.
26. Hamill SC, Packer DL, Stanton MS, et al., and the Multicenter PCD Investigator Group: Termination and acceleration of ventricular tachycardia with autodecremental pacing, burst pacing, and cardioversion in patients with an implantable cardioverter defibrillator. PACE 18:3-10, 1995.
27. Fisher JD, Zhang Z, Kim SG, et al: Comparison of burst pacing, autodecremental (ramp) pacing, and universal pacing for termination of ventricular tachycardia. Arch Mal Coeur Vaiss 89:135-139, 1996.
28. Newman D, Dorian P, Hardy J: Randomized controlled comparison of antitachycardia pacing algorithms for termination of ventricular tachycardia. J Am Coll Cardiol 21:1413-1418, 1993.
29. Schaumann A, Poppinga A, von zur Muehlen F, Kreuzer H: Antitachycardia pacing for ventricular tachycardias above and below 200 bpm: A prospective study for ramp vs. can mode [abstract]. PACE 20:1108, 1997.
30. Nasir N, Pacifico A, Doyle TK, et al: Spontaneous ventricular tachycardia treated by antitachycardia pacing. Cadence Investigators. Am J Cardiol 79:820-822, 1997.
31. Krater L, Lamp B, Heintze J, et al: Influence of antitachy pacing location on the efficacy of ventricular tachycardia termination. J Am Coll Cardiol 39:124A, 2002.
32. Lozano IF, Higgins S, Hummel J, et al: The efficacy of simultaneous right and left ventricular antitachycardia pacing (BiV ATP) in heart failure patients with an AICD indication improves with time [abstract]. PACE 26:984, 2003.
33. Peinado R, Almendral J, Rius T, et al: Randomized, prospective comparison of four burst pacing algorithms for spontaneous ventricular tachycardia. Am J Cardiol 82:1422-1425, 1998.
34. Knight BP, Desai A, Coman J, et al: Long-term retention of cardiac resynchronization therapy. J Am Coll Cardiol 44:72-77, 2004.
35. Richardson K, Cook K, Wang PJ, Al-Ahmad A: Loss of biventricular pacing: What is the cause? Heart Rhythm 2:110-111, 2005.
36. Brandt J, Fahraeus T, Schuller H: Far-field QRS complex sensing via the atrial pacemaker lead. I. Mechanism, consequences, differential diagnosis and countermeasures in AAI and VDD/DDD pacing. PACE 11:1432-1438, 1988.
37. Brandt J, Fahraeus T, Schuller H: Far-field QRS complex sensing via the atrial pacemaker lead. II. Prevalence, clinical significance and possibility of intraoperative prediction in DDD pacing. PACE 11:1540-1544, 1988.
38. Brandt J, Worzewski W: Far-field QRS complex sensing: Prevalence and timing with bipolar atrial leads. PACE 23:315-320, 2000.
39. Weretka S, Becker R, Hilbel T, et al: Far-field R wave oversensing in new dual chamber ICDs: Incidence, predisposing factors and clinical implications [abstract]. PACE 23:571, 2000.

40. Johnson WB, Bailin SJ, Solinger B, et al: Frequency of inappropriate automatic pacemaker mode switching as assessed 6 to 8 weeks post implantation [abstract]. PACE 19:720, 1996.
41. Frohlig G, Kinderman M, Heisel A, et al: Mode switch without atrial tachyarrhythmias [abstract]. PACE 19:592, 1996.
42. Ueng KC, Tsai TP, Tsai CF, et al: Acute and long-term effects of atrioventricular junction ablation and VVIR pacemaker in symptomatic patients with chronic lone atrial fibrillation and normal ventricular response. J Cardiovasc Electrophysiol 12:303-309, 2001.
43. Daoud EG, Weiss R, Bahu M, et al: Effect of an irregular ventricular rhythm on cardiac output. Am J Cardiol 78:1433-1436, 1996.
44. Clark DM, Plumb VJ, EpsteinAE, Kay GN: Hemodynamic effects of an irregular sequence of ventricular cycle length during atrial fibrillation. J Am Coll Cardiol 30:1039-1045, 1997.
45. Marshall HJ, Harris ZI, Griffith MK, Gammage MD: Atrioventricular nodal ablation and implantation of mode switching dual chamber pacemakers: Effective treatment for drug refractory paroxysmal atrial fibrillation. Heart 79:543-547, 1998.
46. Kamalvand K, Tan K, Kotsakis A, et al: Is mode switching beneficial? A randomized study in patients with paroxysmal atrial tachyarrhythmias. J Am Coll Cardiol 30:496-504, 1997.
47. Brignole M, Gainfranchi L, Menozzi C, et al: Assessment of atrioventricular junction ablation and DDDR mode-swtiching pacemakers versus pharmacological treatment in patients with severely symptomatic paroxysmal atrial fibrillation: A randomized controlled study. Circulation 96:2617-2624, 1997.
48. Marshall HJ, Harris ZI, Griffith MJ, et al: Prospective study of ablation and pacing versus medical therapy for paroxysmal atrial fibrillation: Effects of pacing mode and mode-switch algorithms. Circulation 99:1587-1592, 1999.
49. Leclercq C, Faris O, Runin R, et al: Systolic improvement and mechanical resynchronization does not require electrical synchrony in the dilated failing heart with left bundle-branch block. Circulation 106:1760-1763, 2002.
50. Daoud E, Kalbfleisch FJ, Hummel JD, et al: Implantation techniques and chronic lead parameters of biventricular pacing dual-chamber defibrillators. J Cardiovasc Electrophysiol 13:964-970, 2002.
51. Storm C, Harsch M, DeBus B: InSync Registry: Post Market Study. Progress Report No. 7. Medtronic, Inc., February 2005.
52. Young JB, Abraham WT, Smith AL, et al., and Multicenter InSync ICD Randomized Clinical Evaluation (MIRACLE ICD) Trial Investigators: Combined cardiac resynchronization and implantable cardioversion defibrillation in advanced chronic heart failure: The MIRACLE ICD Trial. JAMA 289:2685-2394, 2003.
53. Barold SS, Herweg B, Gallardo I: Double counting of the ventricular electrogram in biventricular pacemakers and ICDs. PACE 26:1645-1648, 2003.
54. Garcia-Moran E, Mont L, Brugada J: Inappropriate tachycardia detection by a biventricular implantable cardioverter defibrillator. PACE 25:123-124, 2002.
55. Schreieck J, Zrenner B, Kolb C, et al: Inappropriate shock delivery due to ventricular double detection with a biventricular pacing implantable cardioverter defibrillator. PACE 24:1154-1157, 2001.
56. Lipchenca I, Garrigue S, Glikson M, et al: Inhibition of biventricular pacemakers by oversensing of far-field atrial depolarization. PACE 25:365-367, 2002.
57. Taieb J, Benchaa T, Foltzer E, et al: Atrioventricular cross-talk in biventricular pacing: A potential cause of ventricular standstill. PACE 25:929-935, 2002.
58. Oguz E, Akyol A, Okmen E: Inhibition of biventricular pacing by far-field left atrial activity sensing: Case report. PACE 25:1517-1519, 2002.
59. Vollmann D, Luthje L, Gortler G, Unterberg C: Inhibition of bradycardia pacing and detection of ventricular fibrillation due to far-field atrial sensing in a triple chamber implantable cardioverter defibrillator. PACE 25:1513-1516, 2002.
60. Garrigue S, Barold SS, Clementy J: Double jeopardy in an implantable cardioverter defibrillator patient. J Cardiovasc Electrophysiol 14:784, 2003.
61. Sweeney MO, Ellison KE, Shea JB: Provoked and spontaneous high frequency, low amplitude respirophasic noise transients in patients with implantable cardioverter-defibrillators. J Cardiovasc Electrophysiol 12:402-410, 2001.
62. Zagrodzky JD, Ramaswamy K, Page RL, et al: Biventricular pacing decreases the inducibility of ventricular tachycardia in patients with ischemic cardiomyopathy. Am J Cardiol 87:1208-1210, 2001.
63. Walker S, Levy T, Rex S, et al: Usefulness of suppression of ventricular arrhythmia by biventricular pacing in severe congestive cardiac failure. Am J Cardiol 86:231-233, 2000.
64. Higgins SL, Yong P, Scheck D, et al: Biventricular pacing diminishes the need for implantable cardioverter defibrillator therapy. J Am Coll Cardiol 36:824-827, 2000.
65. Wilkoff B, Hess M, Young JD, Abraham WT: Differences in tachyarrhythmia detection and implantable cardioverter defibrillator therapy by primary or secondary prevention indication in cardiac resynchronization therapy patients. J Cardiovasc Electrophysiol 15:1002-1009, 2004.
66. Guerra J, Wu J, Miller JM, Groh WJ: Increase in ventricular tachycardia frequency after biventricular implantable cardioverter defibrillator upgrade. J Cardiovasc Electrophysiol 14:1245-124, 2003.
67. Medina-Ravell VA, Lankipalli RS, Yan GX, et al: Effect of epicardial or biventricular pacing to prolong QT interval and increase transmural dispersion of repolarization. Circulation 107:740-746, 2003.
68. Fish JM, Di Diego JM, Nesterenko V, Antzelevitch C: Epicardial activation of left ventricular wall prolongs QT interval and transmural dispersion of repolarization: Implications for biventricular pacing. Circulation 109:2136-2142, 2004.
69. Barold SS, Byrd CL: Cross-ventricular endless loop tachycardia during biventricular pacing. PACE 24:1821-1823, 2001.
70. Berruezo A, Mont L, Scalise A, Brugada J: Orthodromic pacemaker-mediated tachycardia in a biventricular system without an atrial electrode. J Cardiovasc Electrophysiol 15:1100-1102, 2004.
71. Auricchio A, Stellbrink C, Sack S, et al: Long-term benefit as a result of pacing resynchronization in congestive heart failure: Results of the PATH-CHF Trial. Circulation 102:II-693A, 2000.
72. Stellbrink C, Breithardt OA, Franke A, et al., and PATH-CHF (PAcing THerapies in Congestive Heart Failure) Investigators, CPI Guidant Congestive Heart Failure Research Group. Impact of cardiac resynchronization therapy using hemodynamically optimized pacing on left ventricular remodeling in patients with congestive heart failure and ventricular conduction disturbances. J Am Coll Cardiol 38:1957-1965, 2001.
73. Gorscan J, Kanzaki H, Bazaz R, et al: Usefulness of echocardiographic tissue synchronization imaging to predict acute response to cardiac resynchronization therapy. Am J Cardiol 93:1178-1181, 2004.
74. Abraham WT: Rationale and design of a randomized clinical trial to assess the safety and efficacy of cardiac resynchronization therapy in patients with advanced heart failure: The Multicenter InSync Randomized Clinical Evaluation (MIRACLE). J Card Fail 6:369-380, 2000.
75. Packer M: Proposal for a new clinical end point to evaluate the efficacy of drugs and devices in the treatment of chronic heart failure. J Card Fail 7:176-182, 2001.
76. Gregoratos G, Abrams J, Epstein AE, et al: ACC/AHA/NASPE 2002 Guideline Update for Implantation of Cardiac Pacemakers and Antiarrhythmia Devices: Summary Article. A Report of the American College of Cardiology/American Heart Association

Task Force on Practice Guidelines (ACC/AHA/NASPE Committee to Update the 1998 Pacemaker Guidelines). Circulation 106:2145-2161, 2002.
77. Bax JJ, Mohoek SG, Marwick TJ, et al: Left ventricular dyssynchrony predicts benefit of cardiac resynchronization therapy in patients with end-stage heart failure before pacemaker implantation. Am J Cardiol 92:1238-1240, 2003.
78. Reuter S, Garrigue S, Barold SS, et al: Comparison of characteristics in responders versus nonresponders with biventricular pacing for drug-resistant congestive heart failure. Am J Cardiol 89:346-350, 2002.
79. Yu C-M, Fung W-H, Lin H, et al: Predictors of left ventricular reverse remodeling after cardiac resynchronization therapy for heart failure secondary to idiopathic dilated or ischemic cardiomyopathy. Am J Cardiol 91:684-688, 2003.
80. Yu CM, Fung JWH, Chan CK, et al: Comparison of efficacy of reverse remodeling and clinical improvement for relatively narrow and wide QRS complexes after cardiac resynchronization therapy for heart failure. J Cardiovasc Electrophysiol 15:1058-1065, 2004.
81. Yu CM, Lin H, Zhang Q, Sanderson JE: High prevalence of left ventricular systolic and diastolic asynchrony in patients with congestive heart failure and normal QRS duration. Heart 89:54-60, 2003.
82. Pitzalis MD, Iacoviello M, Romito R, et al: Cardiac resynchronization therapy tailored by echocardiographic evaluation of ventricular asynchrony. J Am Coll Cardiol 40:1615-1622, 2002.
83. Auricchio A, Kloss M, Trautmann SI, et al: Exercise performance following cardiac resynchronization therapy in patients with heart failure and ventricular conduction delay. Am J Cardiol 89:198-203, 2002.
84. Linde C, Leclerc C, Rex S, et al: Long-term benefits of biventricular pacing in congestive heart failure: Results from the Multisite Stimulation in Cardiomyopathy (MUSTIC) Study. J Am Coll Cardiol 40:111-118, 2002.
85. Linde C, Braunschweig F, Gadler F, et al: Long-term improvement in quality of life by biventricular pacing in patients with chronic heart failure: Results from the MUSTIC Study. Am J Cardiol 91:1090-1095, 2003.
86. Reynolds MR, Joventino LP, Josephson ME, and Miracle ICD Investigators: Relationship of baseline electrocardiographic characteristics with the response to cardiac resynchronization therapy for heart failure. PACE 27:1513-1518, 2004.
87. Kadhiresan V, Vogt J, Auricchio A, et al: Sensitivity and specificity of QRS duration to predict acute benefit in heart failure patients with cardiac resynchronization [abstract]. PACE 23(II):555, 2000.
88. Moss AJ, Zareba W, Hall WJ, et al., for the Multicenter Automatic Defibrillator Implantation Trial II Investigators: Prophylactic implantation of a defibrillator in patients with myocardial infarction and reduced ejection fraction. N Engl J Med 346:877-883, 2002.
89. Garrigue S, Reuter S, Labeque J-N, et al: Usefulness of biventricular pacing in patients with congestive heart failure and right bundle branch. Am J Cardiol 88:1436-1441, 2001.
90. Aranda JM, Curtis AB, Conti JB, Stejskal-Peterson S: Do heart failure patients with right bundle branch block benefit from cardiac resynchronization therapy? Analysis of the MIRACLE Study [abstract]. J Am Coll Cardiol 39:96A, 2002.
91. Egoavil CA, Ho RT, Greenspon AJ, Pavri BB: Cardiac resynchronization therapy in patients with right bundle branch block: Analysis of pooled data from MIRACLE and ContakCD trials. Heart Rhythm 2:611-615, 2005.
92. Bleeker GB, Schalij MJ, Molhoek SG, et al: Relationship between QRS duration and left ventricular dyssynchrony in patients with end-stage heart failure. J Cardiovasc Electrophysiol 15:544-549, 2004.
93. Josephson ME: Clinical Cardiac Electrophysiology: Techniques and Interpretations, 3rd ed. Philadelphia, Lippincott, Williams & Wilkins, 2002.
94. Fantoni C, Kawabata M, Massaro R, et al: Right and left ventricular activation sequence in patients with heart failure and right bundle branch block: A detailed analysis using three-dimensional non-fluoroscopic electroanatomic mapping system. J Cardiovasc Electrophysiol 16:112-119, 2005.
95. Wyman BT, Hunter WC, Prinzen FW, et al: Effects of single- and biventricular pacing on temporal and spatial dynamics of ventricular contraction. Am J Physiol 282:H372-H379, 2002.
96. D'Hooge J, Heimdal A, Jamal F, et al: Regional strain and strain rate measurements by cardiac ultrasound: Principles, implementation and limitations. Eur J Echocardiography 1:154-170, 2000.
97. Prinzen FW, Hunter WC, Wyman BT, et al: Mapping of regional myocardial strain and work during ventricular pacing: Experimental study using magnetic resonance imaging tagging. J Am Coll Cardiol 33:1735-1742, 1999.
98. Breithardt OA, Stellbrink C, Herbots L, et al: Cardiac resynchronization therapy can reverse abnormal myocardial strain distribution in patients with heart failure and left bundle branch block. J Am Coll Cardiol 42:486-494, 2003.
99. Sogaard P, Egeblad H, Kim W, et al: Tissue Doppler imaging predicts improved systolic performance and reversed left ventricular remodeling during cardiac resynchronization therapy. J Am Coll Cardiol 40:723-730, 2002.
100. Bax JJ, Molhoek SG, Marwick TH, et al: Usefulness of myocardial tissue Doppler echocardiography to evaluate left ventricular dyssynchrony before and after biventricular pacing in patients with idiopathic dilated cardiomyopathy. Am J Cardiol 91:94-97, 2003.
101. Baxx JJ, Yu C-M, Lin H, et al: Comparison of acute changes in left ventricular volume, systolic and diastolic functions, and intraventricular synchronicity after biventricular pacing and right ventricular pacing for congestive heart failure. Am Heart J 145:G1-G7, 2003.
102. Auricchio A, Fantoni C, Regoli F, et al: Characterization of left ventricular activation in patients with heart failure and left bundle branch block. Circulation 109:1133-1139, 2004.
103. Kerckhoffs RC, Bovendeerd PH, Kotte JC, et al: Homogeneity of cardiac contraction despite physiological asynchrony of depolarization: A model study. Ann Biomed Eng 31:536-547, 2003.
104. Pitzalis MD, Iacoviello M, Romito R, et al: Ventricular asynchrony predicts a better outcome in patients with chronic heart failure receiving cardiac resynchronization therapy. J Am Coll Cardiol 45:65-69, 2005.
105. Yu C-M, Yang H, Lau C-P, et al: Regional left ventricular mechanical asynchrony in patients with heart disease and normal QRS duration. PACE 26:562-570, 2003.
106. Achilli A, Sassara M, Ficili S, et al: Long term effectiveness of cardiac resynchronization therapy in patients with refractory heart failure and "narrow" QRS duration. J Am Coll Cardiol 42:2117-2124, 2003.
107. Kass DM: Predicting cardiac resynchronization response by QRS duration. J Am Coll Cardiol 42:2125-2127, 2003.
108. Gaspirini M, Mantica M, Galimberti P, et al: Beneficial effects of biventricular pacing in patients with a "narrow" QRS duration. PACE 26:169-174, 2003.
109. Turner MS, Bleasdale RA, Dragos Vinereanu D, et al: Electrical and mechanical components of dyssynchrony in heart failure patients with normal QRS duration and left bundle-branch block: Impact of left and biventricular pacing. Circulation 109:2544-2549, 2004.
110. Brandt J, Fahraeus T, Ogawa T, Schuller H: Practical aspects of rate adaptive atrial (AAI,R) pacing: Clinical experiences in 44 patients. PACE 14:1258-1264, 1991.

111. Bernheim A, Ammann P, Sticherling C, et al: Right atrial pacing impairs cardiac function during resynchronization therapy: Acute effects of DDD pacing compared to VDD pacing. J Am Coll Cardiol 45:1482-1487, 2005.
112. Bordachar P, LaFitte S, Reuter S, et al: Biventricular pacing and left ventricular pacing in heart failure: Similar hemodynamic improvement despite marked electromechanical differences. J Cardiovasc Electrophysiol 15:1342-1347, 2004.
113. Perego GB, Chianca R, Facchini M, et al: Simultaneous vs. sequential biventricular pacing in dilated cardiomyopathy: An acute hemodynamic study. Eur J Heart Fail 5:305-313, 2003.
114. Blanc JJ, Etienne Y, Gilard M, et al. Evaluation of different ventricular pacing sites in patients with severe heart failure: Results of an acute hemodynamic study. Circulation 96:3273-3277, 1997.
115. Kass DA, Chen CH, Curry C, et al: Improved left ventricular mechanics from acute VDD pacing in patients with dilated cardiomyopathy and ventricular conduction delay. Circulation 99:1567-1573, 1999.
116. Touiza A, Etienne Y, Gilard M, et al: Long-term left ventricular pacing: Assessment and comparison with biventricular pacing in patients with severe congestive heart failure. J Am Coll Cardiol 38:1966-1970, 2001.
117. Blanc JJ, Bertault-Valls V, Fatemi M, et al: Long-term benefits of left univentricular pacing in patients with congestive heart failure. Circulation 109:1741-1744, 2004.
118. Kass DA: Left ventricular versus biventricular pacing in cardiac resynchronization therapy: The plot thickens in this tale of two modes. J Cardiovasc Electrophysiol 15:1348-1349, 2004.

Chapter 27

Follow-up and Interpretation of Implantable Syncope Monitors

ANDREW D. KRAHN • GEORGE J. KLEIN • LORNE J. GULA • ALLAN C. SKANES • RAYMOND YEE

The advent of prolonged monitoring with implanted loop recorders (ILRs) has revolutionized the quest for detection of elusive infrequent arrhythmias in patients with unexplained syncope. Paroxysmal arrhythmias often result in infrequent and sporadic symptoms that usually resolve before the patient gets to medical attention. The capability of prolonged monitoring has permitted clinicians to obtain a symptom rhythm correlation in most patients with suspected underlying infrequent arrhythmia.

Patients often remain undiagnosed after monitoring with a Holter monitor and an external loop recorder.[1] The outcome in undiagnosed patients is strongly influenced by the presence of underlying heart disease and is not as favorable as in those patients with vasovagal syncope or a diagnosed cause of syncope.[2] Clinicians rely on the initial history, physical examination, and abnormal laboratory results to make a diagnosis by inference in many cases. Ideally, some form of prolonged monitoring captures key physiologic data during the next spontaneous event. External and particularly ILRs are powerful tools for arrhythmia detection.

Implantable Loop Recorders

The ILR (Reveal, Medtronic, Minneapolis, Minn.) has a pair of sensing electrodes 3.7 cm apart on the outer shell that records a single-lead bipolar rhythm strip. The device measures 6.1 × 1.9 × 0.8 cm, weighs 17 g, and has a recommended battery life of 14 months (Fig. 27-1).[3-5] The battery life is typically 18 to 24 months, depending on preimplantation shelf life and patient variability. The recorder is inserted in the left pectoral region using standard sterile technique and local anesthesia in the subcutaneous tissue. It also has been implanted in right parasternal, subcostal, and axillary regions with an adequate albeit lower-amplitude signal.[4] The recorded bipolar electrocardiographic signal is stored in a circular buffer that is capable of storing 21 minutes of uncompressed signal or 42 minutes of compressed signal in one or three divided parts. Because the quality of the compressed signal is negligibly different from that of the uncompressed signal, the compressed form is used most often to maximize the memory capacity of the device. The memory buffer is frozen by means of a handheld activator that is provided to the patient at the time of device implantation. In layman's terms, the device answers the question, "What just happened?" Events stored by the device are downloaded after interrogation with a standard Medtronic 9790 pacemaker programmer (Fig. 27-2).

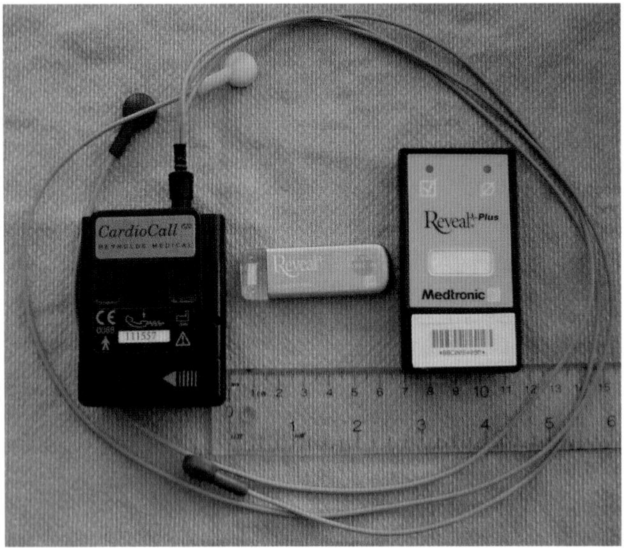

Figure 27-1. Loop recorder technology. From left to right in the photograph, an external loop recorder with cables that attach to electrodes on the patient, the implantable loop recorder, and the patient activator.

The current version of the device (Reveal Plus) has programmable automatic detection of high and low heart rate episodes and pauses (Fig. 27-3). The resultant memory configuration allows for division of multiple 1-minute automatic rhythm strips in addition to one to three manual recordings. This permits automated backup of manual activations to detect prespecified extreme heart rates or pauses (typically <30 bpm, >160 bpm, and pauses >3 seconds); this is often clinically useful in patients who have difficulty activating the device. Three reports have suggested that this feature is more likely than conventional patient activation to detect a borderline or significant arrhythmia.[6,7] Automatic detection also permits detection of asymptomatic heart rate changes that may result in a presumptive diagnosis in the absence of symptomatic recurrence.[7] In a prospective study of 60 patients, automatic detection recorded predetermined "significant" asymptomatic arrhythmias in 15% of patients that led to therapeutic decisions, predominantly pacemaker implantation for bradycardia. Automatic detection has also led to recognition of sensing issues, with transient loss of signal observed in the majority of patients at some point, resulting in automatic detection of pauses (Fig. 27-4).[7-10] Unlike the adjustments of gain and sensitivity that optimize sensing successfully in most patients, this problem appears to stem from transient loss of contact of the sensing electrodes within the device pocket. A relatively tight pocket with adequate anchoring of the device may minimize this problem.

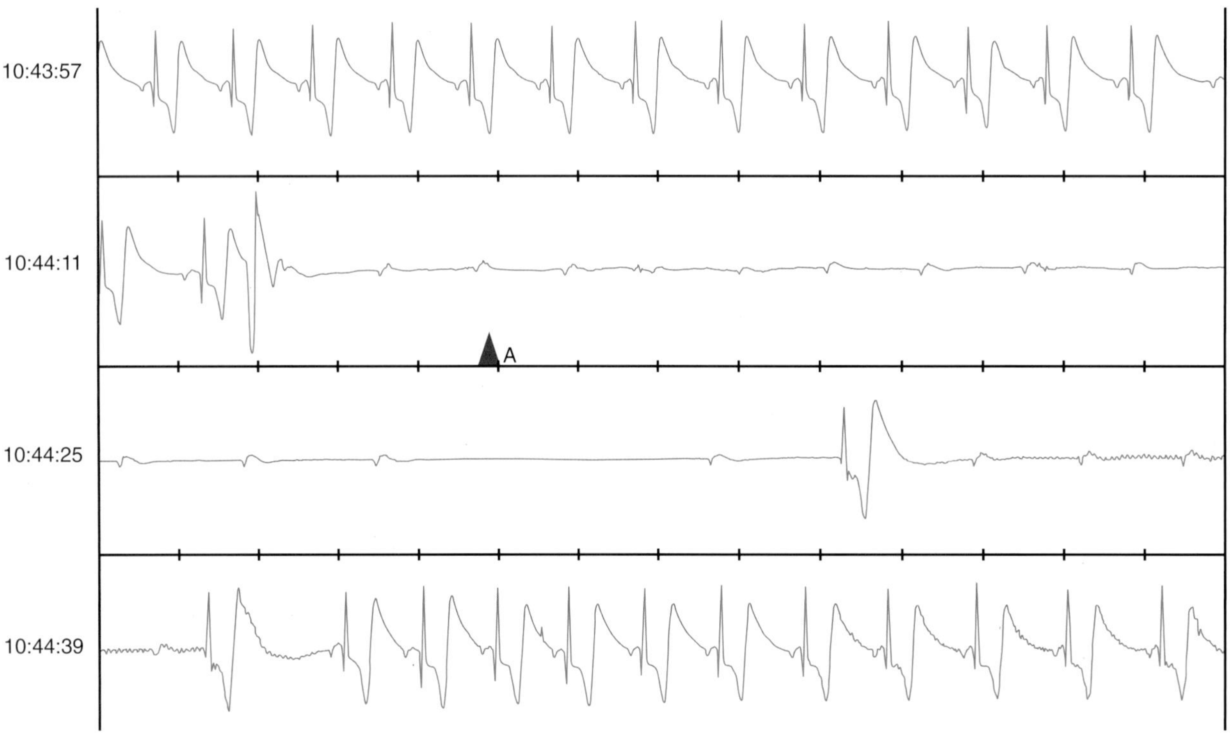

Figure 27-2. Rhythm strip obtained with an implantable loop recorder during syncope in a 73-year-old woman with three syncopal episodes in the previous 2 years. Tilt testing and a trial of an external loop recorder were negative. Each line represents 14 seconds of a single-lead rhythm strip. Note the abrupt onset of complete heart block with visible p waves during a prolonged pause. The arrow and letter A denote automatic activation of the device after detection of a 3-second pause.

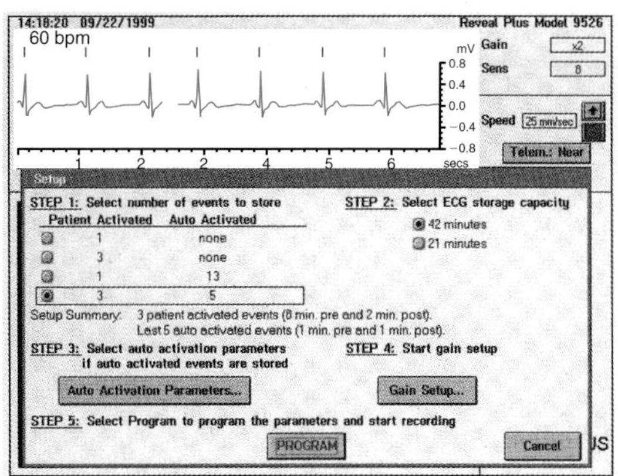

Figure 27-3. Programming interface for the implantable loop recorder. Key elements include use of compressed signal to increase memory capacity, configuration of the memory tailored to the patient's frequency and severity of symptoms, and rate settings for automatic detection. ECG, electrocardiogram.

The implantation procedure is similar to that used for creation of a smaller and more superficial pacemaker pocket. It is typically but not necessarily performed in an electrophysiology or cardiac catheterization laboratory setting. An adequate signal can be obtained anywhere in the left thorax, without the need for cutaneous mapping.[4] Mapping does optimize the sensed signal, and it is recommended for patients in whom automatic detection is desirable to prevent oversensing of T waves and double-counting leading to automatic detection of high-rate episodes. Mapping usually leads to device insertion in a vertical or oblique orientation in the high left parasternal region.[11,12] Right parasternal sites have been used to optimize p-wave amplitude. The patient and a spouse, family member, or friend are instructed in the use of the activator at the time of implantation. Use of prophylactic antibiotics is usually recommended to prevent pocket infection.

After implantation, gain and sensitivity are adjusted according to the manufacturer's specifications. There are no published studies that have systematically identified the optimal method for device setup or follow-up with respect to gain and sensitivity. Chrysostomakis and colleagues[8] suggested that adequate sensing can be obtained in most patients with either an apical or a left parasternal implant position. Boersma and associates[13] implanted one half of their non-autodetect devices in a subcostal position with adequate signal. Experienced device implanters may potentially be misled because the scale for setting gain and sensitivity are the opposite of those conventionally used in pacemakers (although perhaps more logical than the latter). Gain and sensitivity should be adjusted after assessment of the sensed signal during postural changes immediately after implantation, and also during follow-up if there are issues with oversensing or undersensing. A low-amplitude signal resulting in false detection has been noted as a common problem with the device, variably described as oversensing or undersensing.[7-10]

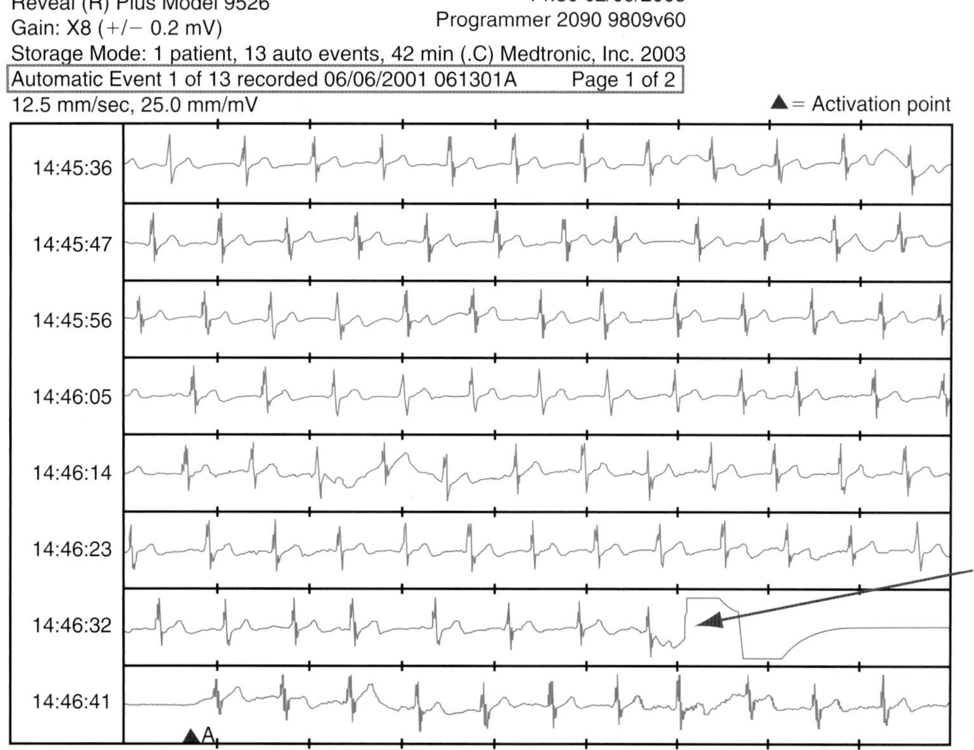

Figure 27-4. Transient loss of signal believed to be caused by loss of tissue electrode contact within the device pocket. Loss of signal (arrow) with amplifier saturation and reacquisition of signal is seen during nonphysiologic recording, which is detected automatically (A) as asystole.

In our recent experience with the Reveal Plus device, 2 (3%) of 60 patients had poor sensing after implantation that resulted in ongoing need for reprogramming with oversensing and undersensing during follow-up.[7,12] Gain and sensitivity required reprogramming in 24 patients (40%) during the first month of follow-up, and in 35 patients (58%) at some point during the 1-year follow-up period. Automatic detection was abandoned in 1 patient in whom sensing could not be improved with reprogramming. Twelve patients (20%) required additional follow-up visits to assess for automatic detection events because of excessive false detection. Undersensing occurred in a single patient with a narrow QRS complex tachycardia that was detected both symptomatically and asymptomatically on several occasions. On one symptomatic occasion, automatic detection did not sense the manually captured tachycardia at 190 bpm. No device-related abnormality could be detected on interrogation.

Early Experience

The first iteration of the ILR was a dual-chamber pacemaker can equipped with a sensing electrode on the lower aspect of the can and a second sensor on a modified leadless header. It was implanted in 24 patients who had recurrent unexplained syncope after negative results with extensive noninvasive and invasive testing, including tilt-table and electrophysiologic (EP) testing.[3] The device was very successful in establishing a symptom-rhythm correlation (88%) in this difficult patient population. These results were validated in a recent study by Boersma and associates[13] with a similar design in 43 patients with unexplained syncope that found a low yield to conventional testing and obtained a symptom-rhythm correlation in 44%. Garcia-Civera and colleagues assessed the selective use of EP testing in combination with tilt testing in 184 patients with unexplained syncope.[14,15] In the subgroup of 15 patients with negative tilt and EP testing, the ILR provided a symptom-rhythm correlation in 47%. These studies suggest that the device has a clear role in patients with ongoing symptoms and negative conventional testing. They also call into question the usefulness of conventional testing in certain patient populations. More recent data suggest that the device may well play a role at an earlier stage in the patient's workup.[16-20]

Further studies have applied the ILR to patients with a lesser burden of syncope and less preimplantation testing, lowering the likelihood of recurrence of syncope after implantation to between 30% and 70%.[6,13,21-24] Several studies have demonstrated the feasibility of the ILR in establishing a symptom-rhythm correlation during long-term monitoring in pediatric and geriatric patients as well as others.[5,6,16,20-23,25-30] The largest of these studies combined data from 206 patients from 3 centers.[22] The majority of patients studied had undergone previous noninvasive testing and selective invasive testing, including tilt testing and EP studies. Symptoms recurred during follow-up in 69% of patients 93 ± 107 days after device implantation. An arrhythmia was detected in 22% of patients, sinus rhythm excluding a primary arrhythmia was seen in 42%, and symptoms resolved without recurrence during prolonged monitoring in 31%. Bradycardia was detected more frequently than tachycardia (17% versus 6%), leading to pacemaker implantation in most patients. Failed activation of the device after spontaneous symptoms occurred in 4% of patients. Devices used in this era did not have the automatic detection capability. Selection bias probably served to withhold the device from patients who were unlikely to activate it, making the activation failure rate in practice higher. In such patients, a symptom-rhythm correlation was not obtained during the monitoring period. As discussed earlier, the automatic detection feature appears to enhance detection in patients who are less likely to successfully activate the device.[6,7,10] No age group had an incidence of bradycardia requiring pacing greater than 30%, suggesting a limited role for empiric pacing in the population with unexplained syncope. Multivariate modeling did not identify any significant preimplantation predictors of subsequent arrhythmia detection other than a weak association with advancing age and bradycardia.

Subsequent Applications of the Implantable Loop Recorder

In the initial application, use of ILRs was focused on the population with recurrent unexplained syncope. Recent trials have focused on other subgroups to obtain symptom-rhythm correlation during spontaneous symptoms. In an investigation of atypical epilepsy, Zaidi and associates studied 74 patients with ongoing seizures despite anticonvulsant therapy or with unexplained recurrent seizures.[31,32] They performed cardiac assessment, including tilt testing and carotid sinus massage, in all patients and implanted ILRs in 10 patients. Tilt testing was positive in 27% of patients, and carotid sinus massage was positive in 10%. Two of the 10 patients who subsequently underwent ILR monitoring demonstrated marked bradycardia preceding seizure activity, one due to heart block and the other due to sinus pauses. This study suggested that seizures that are atypical in presentation or response to therapy may have a cardiovascular cause in as many as 42% of patients and that long-term cardiac monitoring can play a role in select patients with atypical seizures.

The International Study on Syncope of Uncertain Etiology (ISSUE) investigators implanted ILRs in three different populations of patients with syncope to obtain electrocardiographic correlation with spontaneous syncope after conventional testing.[18,19,33] In the first study, tilt testing was performed in 111 patients with a clinical diagnosis of vasovagal syncope, and ILRs were implanted after the tilt test regardless of result. Syncope recurred in 34% of patients in both the tilt-positive and the tilt-negative groups, with marked bradycardia or asystole the most common recorded arrhythmia during follow-up (46% and 62%, respectively). The heart rate response during tilt testing did not predict spontaneous heart rate during episodes, and a much higher incidence of prolonged pauses was observed than was expected based on tilt response, where a marked cardioinhibitory response was uncommon. This study suggests that tilt testing is poorly predictive of rhythm findings during spontaneous syncope and that bradycardia is more common than previously recognized.

The second ISSUE study included 52 patients with syncope and bundle branch block with negative EP testing.[19] Syncope recurred in 22 of the 52 patients during ILR follow-up. Marked bradycardia, mainly attributed to complete atrioventricular (AV) block, was seen in 17 patients, whereas AV block was excluded in 2. Three patients did not properly activate the device after symptoms. Therefore, a significant proportion of this population progressed to complete AV block despite apparent reassurance from the negative EP test results. Syncope may be a clue that conduction system disease is progressive.

The third ISSUE study included 35 patients with syncope and moderate structural heart disease who had negative EP test results.[33] The underlying heart disease was predominantly ischemic heart disease or hypertrophic cardiomyopathy with moderate but not severe left ventricular dysfunction. Although previous studies have suggested that patients with negative EP testing have a better prognosis, there remains concern about the risk of ventricular tachycardia in this group. Importantly, only 2 of the 35 patients had an ejection fraction of less than 30%, which would have made them candidates for primary prevention of sudden death in keeping with the MADIT 2 Trial.[34] Symptoms recurred in 19 (54%) of the 35 patients, with ventricular tachycardia in only 1 patient. In the remaining subjects, bradycardia was detected in 4 and supraventricular tachyarrhythmias in 5. There were no sudden deaths during 16 ± 11 months of follow-up. This study supports a monitoring strategy in patients with left ventricular dysfunction related to ischemic heart disease when EP testing is negative, guided by the ejection fraction and guidelines for primary prevention of sudden death.[35]

Out of the ISSUE studies came a proposed classification[36] of detected rhythm during spontaneous syncope (Table 27-1). This system is very useful in assigning a likely mechanism for the detected rhythm, particularly bradycardia, which may be primary or neurocardiogenic. The classification scheme focuses on sinus rate and AV conduction in assessing the likely state of the autonomic nervous system and its contribution to the underlying hypotension that leads to syncope. This arrangement also permits consistent communication among clinicians and researchers regarding the detected rhythm.

Comparative Studies

Two groups have performed randomized trials comparing the ILR with conventional testing in patients with unexplained syncope. The Randomized Assessment of Syncope Trial (RAST) was a single-center, prospective randomized trial that focused on an initial loop recorder versus conventional testing in patients undergoing a cardiac workup for unexplained syncope[16,17]; patients were crossed over if primary testing was negative. Sixty patients (age 66 ± 14 years, 33 male) with

TABLE 27-1. Electrocardiographic Classification of Detected Rhythm from the Implanted Loop Recorder

Classification	Sinus Rate	AV Node	Comment
Asystole (R-R interval >3 sec)			
1A	Arrest	Normal	Progressive sinus bradycardia until sinus arrest suggests vasovagal
1B	Bradycardia	AV block	AV block with associated sinus bradycardia suggests vasovagal
1C	Normal or tachycardia	AV block	Abrupt AV block without sinus slowing suggests intrinsic AV node disease
Bradycardia			
2A	Decrease >30%	Normal	Suggests vasovagal
2B	HR <40 bpm for >10 sec	Normal	Suggests vasovagal
Minimal HR change			
3A	<10% variation	Normal	Suggests noncardiac cause; unlikely vasovagal
3B	HR increase or decrease 10-30%, not <40 or >120 bpm	Normal	Suggests vasovagal
Tachycardia			
4A	Progressive tachycardia	Normal	Sinus acceleration suggests orthostatic intolerance or noncardiac cause
4B	N/A	Normal	Atrial fibrillation
4C	N/A	Normal	Supraventricular tachycardia
4D	N/A	Normal	Ventricular tachycardia

AV, atrioventricular; HR, heart rate; N/A, not applicable.

Adapted from Brignole M, Moya A, Menozzi C, et al: Proposed electrocardiographic classification of spontaneous syncope documented by an implantable loop recorder. Europace 7:14-18, 2005.

unexplained syncope were randomly assigned to either "conventional" testing with an external loop recorder, tilt testing, and EP testing or immediate monitoring with an ILR with 1 year of monitoring. Patients were offered crossover to the alternative strategy if they remained undiagnosed after their assigned strategy. Patients were excluded if they had a left ventricular ejection fraction of less than 35%.

A diagnosis was obtained in 47% of ILR patients compared with 20% of those undergoing conventional testing (P = .029). Crossover was associated with a diagnosis in 1 of 6 patients undergoing conventional testing, compared with 8 of 21 patients who completed monitoring (17% versus 38%, P = .44). The major difference in diagnostic yield was explained by the detection of bradycardia in 14 patients undergoing monitoring, compared with 3 patients who had conventional testing (40% versus 8%, P = .005). These data illustrate the limitations of conventional diagnostic techniques for detection of arrhythmia, particularly bradycardia. Although there is selection bias in the enrollment of patients referred to an electrophysiologist, this study suggests that tilt testing has a modest yield at best when used as a screening test for all patients undergoing investigation for syncope, and that EP testing is of very limited usefulness in patients with preserved left ventricular function.

Cost modeling and recent cost analysis of the RAST trial suggest that the ILR is cost-effective after noninvasive testing has been performed, comparing favorably with a conventional workup.[17,37,38] Cost analysis suggested that the monitoring strategy had a higher up-front cost but ultimately was more cost-effective because of its higher diagnostic yield, reducing cost per diagnosis by 26%.[17] The cost for a primary monitoring strategy was $5875 ± $1159 per diagnosis, compared with $7891 ± $3193 for a conventional approach first (P = .002). The diagnostic yield after permitting crossover was comparable between the two arms (50% and 47%).

A second randomized trial was published by Farwell and colleagues.[39] They randomly assigned 201 elderly patients (median age 74 years, 54% female) to conventional testing or an ILR.[39] Patients enrolled had recurrent unexplained syncope and negative results on tilt testing and upright carotid sinus massage before randomization. Symptom-rhythm correlation was obtained in 33% of ILR patients but only 4% of conventional patients. After randomization, the ILR patients had fewer hospital days and investigations, which translated into a reduction in cost from £1090 to £379 (P < .05). This cost saving was largely explained by the averting of hospitalization but did not account for the actual device cost, estimated at £809. Nonetheless, it is consistent with the findings from the RAST trial,[17] that the device improves diagnosis without a significant increase in cost. The duration of follow-up in this study was relatively short (mean, 276 ± 134 days). Prolongation of follow-up would have improved the diagnostic yield with the recorder and increased resource use in the conventional arm in patients with recurrent symptoms.

Outcome of Monitoring with the Implantable Loop Recorder

All reports of ILR use have suggested a low incidence of life-threatening arrhythmia or significant morbidity from recurrent syncope during follow-up. This verifies the generally good prognosis of recurrent unexplained syncope in the absence of severe left ventricular dysfunction or when EP testing is negative and the safety of a monitoring approach. Bradycardia is by far the most frequently detected arrhythmia. P waves are often visible in the tracing of interest, shedding light on the likely mechanism of bradycardia.

Although the distinction between primary bradycardia and bradycardia related to neurocardiogenic syncope can be challenging, the mechanism may be inferred from the rhythm at the time of syncope combined with the preceding and recovery rhythms. The cardioinhibitory component of neurocardiogenic syncope is probably responsible for some or much of the detected bradycardia. This is more likely to be the case when there is gradual slowing or oscillation of the heart rate before the index event, as seen during tilt testing. Patient history and demographics also influence the probability of cardioinhibitory syncope as a clinical diagnosis. Of importance, we and other authors have not assigned a diagnosis of bradycardia unless the symptomatic heart rate is less than 40 beats per minute (bpm) or pauses longer than 3 seconds are recorded. Nonetheless, syncope resolves with pacing in the vast majority of patients with ILR-detected bradycardia, regardless of mechanism. We do not turn on rate-drop algorithms in pacemakers that are implanted in this circumstance unless symptoms recur with standard DDD backup pacing at 50 to 60 bpm.

Syncope resolves during long-term monitoring in one third of patients despite frequent episodes before implantation of the ILR. This suggests that syncope has a self-limited cause or reflects a transient physiologic abnormality in these individuals. The alternative explanation is that the device is associated with a placebo effect that protects the patient from recurrence, analogous to that seen in studies of pacing for neurocardiogenic syncope and hypertrophic cardiomyopathy.

The literature supports the role of ILRs in patients with recurrent unexplained syncope for whom noninvasive workup has failed to establish a diagnosis. Based on a defined catchment area, Solano and colleagues estimate that this population represents 5% of patients referred for syncope to a cardiac specialty unit, for an implantation incidence of 34 per 1 million population per year.[24] These patients represent a select group who have been referred for further testing, in whom ongoing symptoms are likely and a symptom-rhythm correlation is a feasible goal. Widespread early use of the ILR is likely to reduce the diagnostic yield as the prevalence of arrhythmias falls, as supported by data from the RAST trial[14-16] and the study by Farwell and colleagues.[40] The diagnostic yield and cost benefit of the device are contingent on the likelihood of recurrent syncope and the usefulness of the information gained from a symptom-rhythm correlation. The device often performs a "rule-out" function by recording sinus rhythm; this information is valuable in eliminating the search for arrhythmia and suggests a vasovagal, psychogenic, or neurologic cause (in that order of likelihood).

The ideal patient for prolonged monitoring with an ILR has symptoms suspicious for arrhythmia; namely, abrupt onset with minimal prodrome, typically brief loss of consciousness, and complete resolution of symptoms within seconds to minutes after onset of the episode. We have historically used a left ventricular ejection fraction of 35% as a cutoff for performing EP testing before employing a prolonged monitoring strategy, as supported by primary and secondary prevention trials using implantable defibrillators. Ideally, patients will have had at least two syncopal episodes in the last 12 months and will have preserved left ventricular function. The inclusion or exclusion of arrhythmia would be useful in redirecting or ending ongoing investigations.

Assar and coworkers[30] examined the baseline characteristics of 167 patients who received an ILR and formulated a risk factor score to predict successful use of the device (Fig. 27-5). Risk factors included age of less than 65 years, absence of structural heart disease, and more than three lifetime syncopal episodes. Based on these variables, patients can be advised regarding the likelihood of successful monitoring. However, this study also illustrated the difficulty in arriving at a diagnosis in elderly patients with infrequent syncope. The authors described the likelihood of recurrence over time in their population. They found that symptoms recurred in 63% of patients, at a mean of 109 ± 120 days after implantation. In those patients who experienced syncope, 31% of syncopal episodes occurred within 30 days, 50% within 2 months, 78% within 6 months, and 93% within 12 months after implantation. Patients who did not experience recurrence while they had their ILR had a 92% syncope-free survival over 24 ± 16 months of follow-up, suggesting that device replacement at the end of battery life is seldom warranted if syncope has not recurred. In a subsequent study, Solano and coworkers[24] compared the outcomes of patients with and without structural heart disease who received an ILR and found an equal incidence of recurrence in the two groups. This may well reflect a difference in study population, including the extent of preimplantation testing, which could select out patients with high or low likelihood of recurrence.

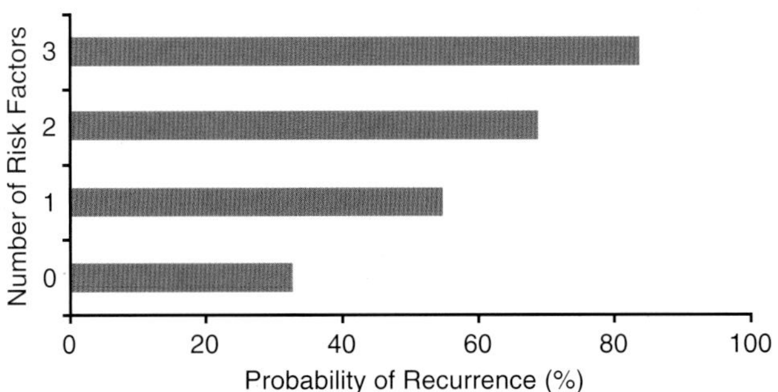

Figure 27-5. Probability of recurrent symptoms during prolonged monitoring based on a simple risk factor score. Risk factors included age less than 65 years, absence of structural heart disease, and more than three lifetime syncopal episodes. The likelihood of syncope during the period of loop recorder implantation was 33% with no risk factors, 55% with one, 69% with two, and 84% with three. (Adapted from Armstrong VL, Lawson J, Kamper AM, et al: The use of an implantable loop recorder in the investigation of unexplained syncope in older people. Age Ageing 32:185-188, 2003.)

Despite the published safety record of prolonged monitoring, there may be a subset of patients who are at excessive risk when considering an ILR. One example might be patients with syncope and underlying heart disease in whom EP testing is falsely negative, such as patients with hypertrophic or dilated cardiomyopathy. We often give strong consideration to empiric use of an implantable cardiac defibrillator in these patients if the history is worrisome for ventricular arrhythmia, even if aggressive EP testing is negative. There also may be a low-risk population in whom implantation of an ILR is not warranted. This group might include patients who are without heart disease and have a relatively low burden of syncope, for whom testing has a low yield and the diagnosis is almost certainly benign.[15]

Other Uses of Implantable Monitors

The current ILR represents only the first expression of an emerging field of long-term physiologic monitoring.[41] Ideally, such a device would monitor a broad range of physiologic functions, including blood pressure, which would provide data invaluable in the evaluation of bradycardia and possible vasovagal syncope. With respect to arrhythmias, ongoing trials are employing ILRs in patients with paroxysmal atrial fibrillation or myotonic dystrophy, after catheter ablation, and for detection of asymptomatic ventricular arrhythmias. The pilot study of the Cardiac Arrhythmias and Risk Stratification After Myocardial Infarction (CARISMA) investigated the feasibility of detecting nonsustained ventricular tachycardia in 30 patients with reduced left ventricular function or after myocardial infarction with the ILR.[42] The device itself would benefit from multivector monitoring on a microprocessor platform to allow more complex signal processing and analysis. Other potential design improvements could include enhanced memory and battery capabilities. With respect to other monitored parameters, sensor development is likely to result in commercial products capable of monitoring blood pressure, glucose concentration, oxygen saturation, brain function, and many other physiologic parameters.[41]

Conclusions

The ILR has significantly improved the ability to obtain symptom-rhythm correlation during infrequent symptoms in patients with unexplained syncope and palpitations. The ILR is especially useful for patients with infrequent unexplained syncope when noninvasive tests are negative. Future development of long-term physiologic monitoring promises to deliver a wide array of useful data to assess and manage chronic and intermittent conditions.

REFERENCES

1. Kapoor WN: Evaluation and outcome of patients with syncope. Medicine (Baltimore) 69:160-175,1990.
2. Soteriades ES, Evans JC, Larson MG, et al: Incidence and prognosis of syncope. N Engl J Med 19:878-885, 2002.
3. Krahn AD, Klein GJ, Norris C, Yee R: The etiology of syncope in patients with negative tilt table and electrophysiological testing. Circulation 92:1819-1824, 1995.
4. Krahn AD, Klein GJ, Yee R, Norris C: Maturation of the sensed electrogram amplitude over time in a new subcutaneous implantable loop recorder. PACE 20:1686-1690, 1997.
5. Krahn AD, Klein GJ, Yee R, Norris C: Final results from a pilot study with an implantable loop recorder to determine the etiology of syncope in patients with negative noninvasive and invasive testing. Am J Cardiol 82:117-119, 1998.
6. Ermis C, Zhu AX, Pham S, et al: Comparison of automatic and patient-activated arrhythmia recordings by implantable loop recorders in the evaluation of syncope. Am J Cardiol 92:815-819, 2003.
7. Krahn AD, Klein GJ, Yee R, Skanes AC: Detection of asymptomatic arrhythmias in unexplained syncope. Am Heart J 148:326-332, 2004.
8. Chrysostomakis SI, Klapsinos NC, Simantirakis EN, et al: Sensing issues related to the clinical use of implantable loop recorders. Europace 5:143-148, 2003.
9. Chrysostomakis SI, Simantirakis EN, Marketou ME, Vardas PE: Implantable loop recorder undersensing mimicking complete heart block. Europace 4:211-213, 2002.
10. Ng E, Stafford PJ, Ng GA: Arrhythmia detection by patient and auto-activation in implantable loop recorders. J Interv Card Electrophysiol 10:147-52, 2004.
11. Himmrich E, Zellerhoff C, Nebeling D, et al: [Where should the implantable ECG event recorder be placed?]. Z Kardiol 89:289-294, 2000.
12. Krahn AD, Klein GJ, Skanes AC, Yee R: Detection of clinically significant asymptomatic arrhythmias with autodetect loop recorders in syncope patients. PACE 26:1070, 2003.
13. Boersma L, Mont L, Sionis A, et al: Value of the implantable loop recorder for the management of patients with unexplained syncope. Europace 6:70-76, 2004.
14. Garcia-Civera R, Ruiz-Granell R, Morell-Cabedo S, et al: Selective use of diagnostic tests inpatients with syncope of unknown cause. J Am Coll Cardiol 41:787-790, 2003.
15. Benditt DG, Brignole M: Syncope: Is a diagnosis a diagnosis? J Am Coll Cardiol 41:791-794, 2003.
16. Krahn AD, Klein GJ, Yee R, Skanes AC: Randomized Assessment of Syncope Trial: Conventional diagnostic testing versus a prolonged mnitoring strategy. Circulation 104:46-51, 2001.
17. Krahn AD, Klein GJ, Yee R, et al: Cost implications of testing strategy in patients with syncope: Randomized assessment of syncope trial. J Am Coll Cardiol 42:495-501, 2003.
18. Moya A, Brignole M, Menozzi C, et al: Mechanism of syncope in patients with isolated syncope and in patients with tilt-positive syncope. Circulation 104:1261-1267, 2001.
19. Brignole M, Menozzi C, Moya A, et al: Mechanism of syncope in patients with bundle branch block and negative electrophysiological test. Circulation 104:2045-2050, 2001.
20. Donateo P, Brignole M, Menozzi C, et al: Mechanism of syncope in patients with positive adenosine triphosphate tests. J Am Coll Cardiol 41:93-98, 2003.
21. Krahn AD, Klein GJ, Yee R, et al: Use of an extended monitoring strategy in patients with problematic syncope. Reveal Investigators. Circulation 99:406-410, 1999.
22. Krahn AD, Klein GJ, Fitzpatrick A, et al: Predicting the outcome of patients with unexplained syncope undergoing prolonged monitoring. PACE 25:37-41, 2002.
23. Nierop PR, van Mechelen R, van Elsacker A, et al: Heart rhythm during syncope and presyncope: Results of implantable loop recorders. PACE 23:1532-1538, 2000.
24. Solano A, Menozzi C, Maggi R, et al: Incidence, diagnostic yield and safety of the implantable loop-recorder to detect the mechanism of syncope in patients with and without structural heart disease. Eur Heart J 25:1116-1119, 2004.
25. Kenny RA, Krahn AD: Implantable loop recorder: Evaluation of unexplained syncope. Heart 81:431-433, 1999.
26. Alboni P, Brignole M, Menozzi C, et al: Diagnostic value of history in patients with syncope with or without heart disease. J Am Coll Cardiol 37:1921-8, 2001.
27. Armstrong VL, Lawson J, Kamper AM, et al: The use of an implantable loop recorder in the investigation of unexplained syncope in older people. Age Ageing 32:185-188, 2003.
28. Mason PK, Wood MA, Reese DB, et al: Usefulness of implantable loop recorders in office-based practice for evaluation of syncope in patients with and without structural heart disease. Am J Cardiol 92:1127-1129, 2003.
29. Rossano J, Bloemers B, Sreeram N, et al: Efficacy of implantable loop recorders in establishing symptom-rhythm correlation in young patients with syncope and palpitations. Pediatrics 112:e228-e233, 2003.
30. Assar MD, Krahn AD, Klein GJ, et al: Optimal duration of monitoring in patients with unexplained syncope. Am J Cardiol 92:1231-1233, 2003.
31. Zaidi A, Clough P, Cooper P, et al: Misdiagnosis of epilepsy: Many seizure-like attacks have a cardiovascular cause. J Am Coll Cardiol 36:181-184, 2000.
32. Zaidi A, Clough P, Mawer G, Fitzpatrick A: Accurate diagnosis of convulsive syncope: Role of an implantable subcutaneous ECG monitor. Seizure 8:184-186, 1999.
33. Menozzi C, Brignole M, Garcia-Civera R, et al: Mechanism of syncope in patients with heart disease and negative electrophysiologic test. Circulation 105:2741-2745, 2002.
34. Moss AJ, Zareba W, Hall WJ, et al: Prophylactic implantation of a defibrillator in patients with myocardial infarction and reduced ejection fraction. N Engl J Med 346:877-883, 2002.
35. Gregoratos G, Abrams J, Epstein AE, et al: ACC/AHA/NASPE 2002 Guideline Update for Implantation of Cardiac Pacemakers and Antiarrhythmia Devices: Summary article. A report of the American College of Cardiology/American Heart Association Task Force on Practice Guidelines (ACC/AHA/NASPE Committee to Update the 1998 Pacemaker Guidelines). J Cardiovasc Electrophysiol 13:1183-1199, 2002.
36. Brignole M, Moya A, Menozzi C, et al: Proposed electrocardiographic classification of spontaneous syncope documented by an implantable loop recorder. Europace 7:14-18, 2005.
37. Krahn AD, Klein GJ, Yee R, Manda V: The high cost of syncope: Cost implications of a new insertable loop recorder in the investigation of recurrent syncope. Am Heart J 137:870-877, 1999.
38. Simpson CS, Krahn AD, Klein GJ, et al: A cost effective approach to the investigation of syncope: Relative merit of different diagnostic strategies. Can J Cardiol 15:579-584, 1999.
39. Farwell DJ, Freemantle N, Sulke AN: Use of implantable loop recorders in the diagnosis and management of syncope. Eur Heart J 25:1257-1263, 2004.
40. Farwell DJ, Sulke AN: Does the use of a syncope diagnostic protocol improve the investigation and management of syncope? Heart 90:52-58, 2004.
41. Klein GJ, Krahn AD, Yee R, Skanes AC: The implantable loop recorder: The herald of a new age of implantable monitors. PACE 23:1456, 2000.
42. Huikuri HV, Mahaux V, Bloch-Thomsen PE: Cardiac arrhythmias and risk stratification after myocardial infarction: Results of the CARISMA pilot study. PACE 26:416-419, 2003.

Chapter 28

Electromagnetic Interference and Implantable Devices

SERGIO L. PINSKI

Sensing of intrinsic cardiac electrical activity is essential for the function of pacemakers and implantable cardioverter-defibrillators (ICDs). Examples of undesired triggering or inhibition of pacemaker output by extraneous signals were identified early after the introduction of demand pacemakers. Hermetic shielding in metal cases, filtering, and interference rejection circuits, together with a preference for bipolar sensing, made contemporary pacemakers and ICDs relatively immune to electromagnetic energy sources in homes and workplaces. Although sources of electromagnetic interference (EMI) remained ubiquitous in the medical environment, they were predictable and avoidable.

New technologies that use more of the electromagnetic spectrum, such as wireless telephony and electronic article surveillance (EAS) devices, have rekindled interest in EMI risks for patients with implanted cardiac devices. Although these technologies do not constitute a major public health threat, adverse interactions can occur. The counterpart to EMI is electromagnetic compatibility, a science aimed at avoiding interference potential by adding shielding or redesigning circuits against specific EMI sources. It is hoped that collaboration among industry, physicians, regulatory agencies, and consumer groups will achieve full compatibility between implanted devices and other technologies. This will require adoption of international standards establishing the upper limit of permissible field intensities for the whole electromagnetic spectrum. Implanted devices should not react to fields below this limit, and more intense fields should be prohibited.

Sources of Electromagnetic Interference

Sources of EMI can be classified according to type and spectral frequency of energy emitted, as well as the environment in which the source is encountered (Table 28-1). For clinical purposes, it is useful to recognize radiated and conducted sources of EMI.

Radiated EMI can result from energy emitted for communication purposes or as an unintended effect of other electrical activity (e.g., motor operation in an electric razor). Electromagnetic fields have both an electric field, measured in volts per meter (V/m), and a magnetic field. The magnetic flux density is measured in milliteslas (mT). Another common way to characterize an electromagnetic field is by the power density, or power per unit area. Power density can be expressed in milliwatts (mW) or microwatts (μW) per square centimeter (cm^2). The unit used to measure how much radiofrequency (RF) energy is actually absorbed by the body is the specific absorption rate (SAR). The SAR is a measure of the rate of absorption of RF energy;

TABLE 28-1. **Documented Sources of Electromagnetic Interference**

Electromagnetic fields
Daily life
Cellular telephones, electronic article surveillance devices, metal detectors, some home appliances (e.g., electric razors), toy remote controls, improperly grounded appliances held in close contact to the body, slot machines
Work and industrial environment
High-voltage power lines, transformers, welders, electric motors, induction furnaces, degaussing coils
Medical environment
MRI scanners, electrosurgery, defibrillation, neurostimulators, TENS units, radiofrequency catheter ablation, therapeutic diathermy
Ionizing radiation
Medical environment
Radiotherapy
Acoustic radiation
Medical environment
Lithotripsy

MRI, magnetic resonance imaging; TENS, transcutaneous electrical nerve stimulation.

it is usually expressed in watts per kilogram (W/kg) or milliwatts per gram (mW/g). Electromagnetic sources can be broadly divided into RF waves, with frequencies between 0.1 Hz and 100 MHz (e.g., electric power, radio and television transmitters, electrosurgical units), and microwaves, between 100 MHz and 12 GHz (e.g., radar transmitters, cellular telephones, microwave ovens) (Fig. 28-1).

The frequency of the EMI determines the efficiency of energy coupling to the device and the resulting effect. The signal may be modulated in amplitude or frequency, and it may occur in bursts or single long pulses. An RF carrier with amplitude modulation induces voltages in the signal processing and detection circuitry of an implanted device that can be misinterpreted as intracardiac signals. The modulation on the carrier is converted (demodulated) to a low-frequency voltage waveform, allowing entry to the signal processing and detection circuitry.[1] If the amplitude modulation has frequency components in the device's physiologic passband, significant interference occurs. Although electromagnetic fields could also mimic RF telemetry and modify programmable parameters in an implanted device, this is very unlikely with current systems. Programming requires access codes to establish the telemetry link, parity checks of transmitted messages, and often simultaneous magnetic reed-switch closure by a steady magnetic field.

Directly conducted galvanic currents (measured in amperes per square meter [$A\text{-}m^2$]) are most commonly introduced into the body therapeutically (e.g., by transcutaneous electrical nerve stimulation [TENS]) but can also result from physical contact with improperly grounded electrical equipment. A wide range of frequencies may affect implanted devices, including the power frequencies of 50 Hz (Europe), 60 Hz (United States), and 400 Hz (aircraft). Pacemakers and ICDs can react to galvanic currents below the perception threshold (~1 mA/cm^2 for moist skin). Clinically, this will result in oversensing in the channel where sensing is occurring.

Static magnetic fields are measured in units of tesla (1 T = 10,000 gauss [G]). The ionizing radiation dose is the amount of energy absorbed per unit mass of material, with units of joules per kilogram (J/kg), or gray (Gy). Radiation found in the environment and near medical imaging equipment has no effect on implanted electronic devices. Therapeutic radiation used in oncology can damage the oxide layers of complementary metal oxide semiconductor-integrated (CMOS) circuits in ICDs and pacemakers, and the effects are cumulative. Acoustic radiation from lithotripsy machines is used to disintegrate kidney and gallbladder stones. About 1500 discharges from a 20-kV spark gap generate pressure shock waves that typically measure 45 megapascals (MPa) at the 12-mm diameter focal area. If pressure waves of this magnitude were applied directly to a pacemaker or ICD, the electronic circuits could be damaged.

Sources of Knowledge Regarding Electromagnetic Interference

Knowledge of EMI effects on implanted devices arises from several sources. Anecdotal reports highlight the possibility of interactions but provide little information regarding overall risk. The interaction may have depended on idiosyncratic programming or device malfunction. In the United States, the Center for Devices and Radiological Health of the Food and Drug Administration (FDA) maintains a database of reported incidents of deleterious interactions (MAUDE) that is searchable on-line.[2] However, reporting is largely voluntary, and documentation is uneven. Case reports published in peer-reviewed journals (especially if they include a rechallenge in a controlled environment) can be most valuable.

Prospective studies can be performed in vitro (i.e., bench testing) or in vivo, using laboratory animals or patient volunteers. In vitro studies are performed with the implantable device submerged in a saline-filled tank (to emulate electrical properties of tissue) and the source of radiated EMI in close proximity. These investigations allow expeditious study of interactions among various EMI sources and devices. Multiple iterations of the experiment permit examination of the effects of distance, position, field strength, and device programming on the frequency and severity of the interaction.

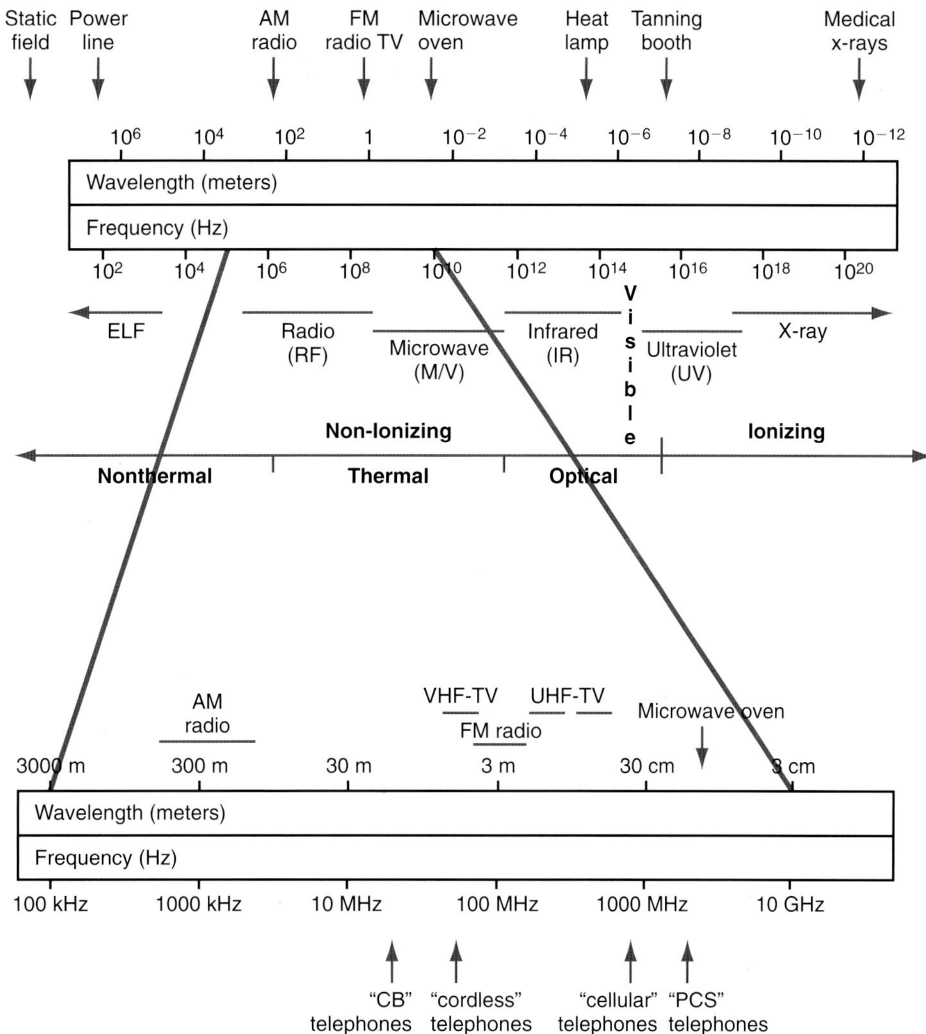

Figure 28-1. Electromagnetic spectrum. Frequencies used for communications in the radio and microwave ranges, 100 kHz to 10 GHz (detailed in the lower bar), can interact with implanted cardiac devices. (Adapted with permission from Moulder JP: Cellular phone antennas and health. Available at http://www.mcw.edu/gcrc/cop/cell-phone-health-FAQ/toc.html)

Although simulation studies predict interference in vivo, they do not match clinical exposures identically. Discrepancies may be related to the inability to replicate the strength and path of induced body fields, body position and movements, and shielding effects of the body. The orientation of the air gap between the source and the saline tank (i.e., perpendicular versus parallel) significantly influences the distance threshold for interaction.[3] Protocols for the testing of interactions between sources of EMI were issued by the American National Standards Institute and the Association for the Advancement of Medical Instrumentation in 2000.[4] A revision is expected in the near future. A novel multichamber heart/trunk simulator allows more realistic in vitro testing of devices.[5] Anatomically based electromagnetic models of the human body allow the use of numerical modeling to quantify the relationship between an external electromagnetic field and the voltage induced in the leads of an implantable device.[6] Such modeling can greatly strengthen the clinical relevance of in vitro simulation studies.

In a few high-risk circumstances (e.g., magnetic resonance imaging [MRI]), in vivo testing is first conducted in laboratory animals implanted with a pacemaker system. More commonly, in vivo simulation studies require controlled patient exposure to potential sources of EMI while the cardiac rhythm is monitored. Patient exposure studies clarify the clinical significance of in vitro interactions. However, because of the time and effort involved, the number of assessed permutations is, by necessity, limited. To avoid inadvertent bias, it is important to recruit patients who are representative of the general population with implanted devices. The fact that many sources of EMI also interfere with real-time or Holter electrocardiographic (ECG) recordings complicates in vivo studies. Bipolar asynchronous pacing pulses that do not elicit a QRS complex are particularly difficult to ascertain. Special recording techniques are often necessary. Furthermore, real-time telemetry between the implanted device and the programmer is often compromised by EMI, even when device function remains otherwise normal. Critical review of the literature suggests that some purported instances of EMI have resulted from this inconsequential phenomenon.[7] Furthermore, the programmer wand placed directly over the device can act as an artificial shield. Analysis of annotated stored electrograms (EGMs), if they are available, is the ideal method to evaluate device behavior during exposure to potential sources of EMI.

In clinical practice, it may be difficult to differentiate EMI from other sources of interference (e.g., myopotentials, lead malfunction, faulty connections) in stored EGMs. EMI typically results in very high-frequency signals of constant amplitude that can be continuous or pulsatile depending on the source and tend to occupy the entire cardiac cycle. EMI is often present in more than one channel; in ICDs, its amplitude is higher in the far-field than in the near-field EGM. Careful history taking usually can retrospectively identify the source of EMI. Diaphragmatic myopotentials typically change in amplitude with the respiratory cycle, and their amplitude is higher in the near-field than in the far-field EGM. Lead fracture or faulty connections inscribe transient, high-amplitude, random signals that saturate the amplifier and occupy only a small fraction of the cardiac cycle. During clinic testing, myopotentials can usually be reproduced by isometric muscle contraction, deep breathing, or the Valsalva maneuver. Oversensing of make-and-break signals can often be reproduced by device manipulation in the pocket. Lead impedances are often abnormal in cases of lead failure or faulty connection.

Pacemaker and ICD Responses to Electromagnetic Interference

The most frequent responses to EMI are inappropriate inhibition or triggering of pacemaker stimuli, reversion to asynchronous pacing, and spurious ICD tachyarrhythmia detection. Reprogramming of operating parameters and permanent damage to the device circuitry or the electrode-tissue interface are much less frequent.

Pacing Inhibition

Sustained pacing inhibition can be catastrophic in pacemaker-dependent patients (Fig. 28-2). Depending on the duration of inhibition and the emergence of escape rhythms, lightheadedness, syncope, or death could result. In pacemakers, protective algorithms make prolonged inhibition uncommon. Patients who are dependent on their ICD for bradycardia pacing may be more vulnerable to severe pacing inhibition from EMI. In ICDs, automatic adjustment of either the gain or the sensing threshold, according to the amplitude of the intrinsic R wave, ensures sensing of low-amplitude ventricular depolarization signals during ventricular fibrillation without oversensing of T waves and extracardiac signals. In the absence of sensed complexes, two potentially life-threatening diagnoses must be considered: asystole (requiring pacing) and fine ventricular fibrillation (requiring amplifier gain adjustments for proper detection). To ensure the detection of ventricular fibrillation, pacing onset triggers an increase in sensitivity in most devices. These very high sensitivity levels (~0.2 to 0.3 mV) can promote oversensing of extracardiac signals. Oversensing perpetuates, because the absence of spontaneous large-amplitude escape beats maintains the high operating sensitivity. Asynchronous pacing may not occur due to lack of reliable ICD noise-reversion modes. Therefore, EMI-induced prolonged inhibition and spurious tachyarrhythmia detection become likely (see later discussion). Simulation studies of the interactions between sources of EMI and ICDs require recreation of a "worst-case scenario" (inducing maximum sensitivity during continuous pacing).

Triggering of Rapid or Premature Pacing

Oversensing of EMI by the atrial channel of a pacemaker or ICD programmed to a tracking mode (DDD, VDD) can trigger ventricular pacing at or near the upper tracking rate limit. Alternatively, automatic mode-switching may occur if this function is enabled (Fig. 28-3). In some pacemakers, detection of noise in the atrial channel can trigger a noise-reversion mode. Preferential detection of EMI is not uncommon, because atrial sensitivity is usually programmed higher

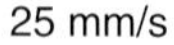

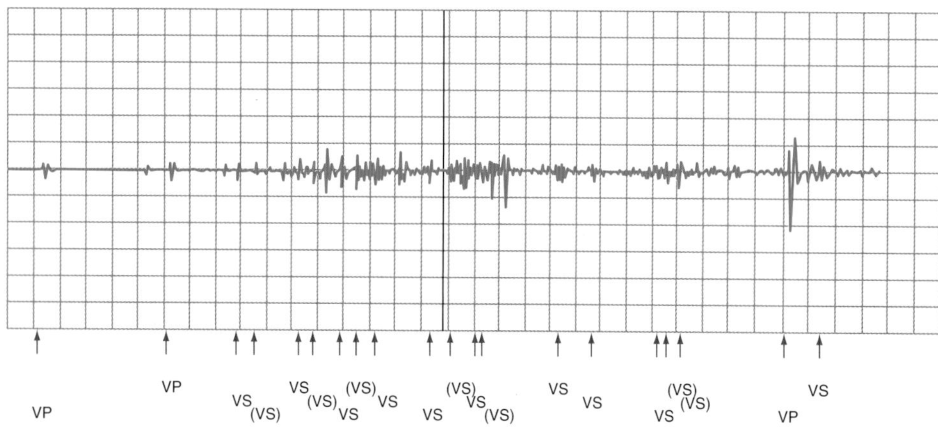

Figure 28-2. Oversensing of electromagnetic interference in a patient with a permanent pacemaker for complete heart block presenting with recurrent syncope. Further inquiry revealed that the interference had occurred during a radiofrequency catheter ablation procedure for atrial tachycardia and could not account for the clinical episodes. Extensive testing (including prolonged monitoring in an epilepsy unit) established malingering and not true episodes of loss of consciousness.

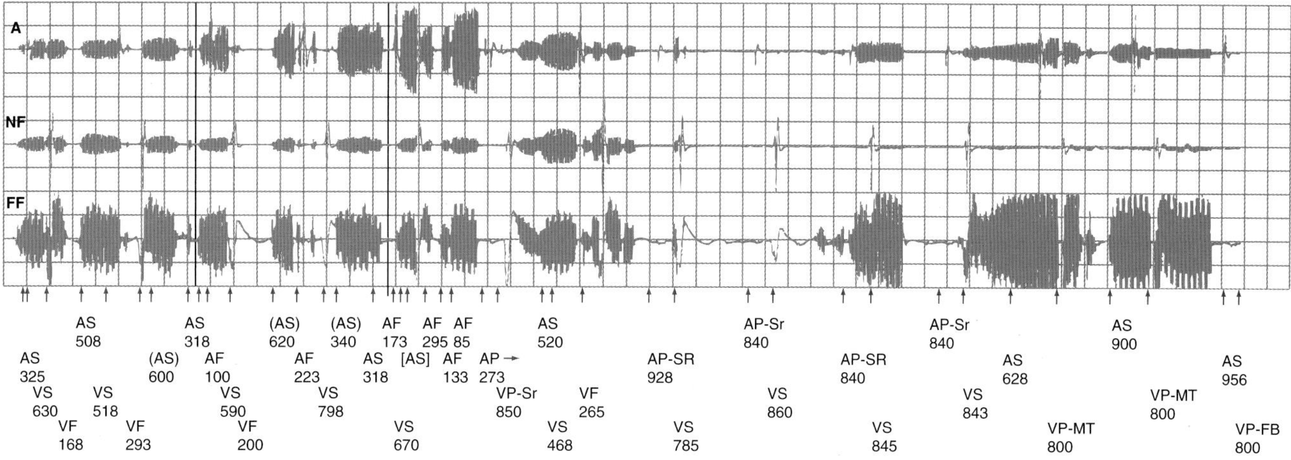

Figure 28-3. Spurious mode-switch due to atrial oversensing of electromagnetic interference (EMI) in a patient with a dual-chamber Guidant ICD. Stored atrial (A), near-field (NF), and far-field (FF) electrograms in a patient who presented for routine ICD follow-up. Nonphysiologic, high-frequency pulsed activity is seen in the three channels, although with higher amplitude in the A and FF traces. Very little ventricular oversensing occurs, so ventricular fibrillation is not detected. However, atrial oversensing results in transient mode switching. The patient could not recall a potential source of EMI.

(more sensitive) than ventricular sensitivity. It is possible to observe rapid pacing due to atrial oversensing as a patient approaches an electromagnetic field, followed by a period of ventricular oversensing (inhibition or mode reversion) as the field becomes stronger. If sustained, inappropriate pacemaker acceleration induced by atrial oversensing can cause palpitation, hypotension, or angina.

Less commonly, EMI can induce rapid pacing via other mechanisms. For example, some sources of EMI can trigger rapid pacing (up to the sensor-triggered upper rate limit) by activating the sensor in minute-ventilation pacemakers. The signal emitted by acoustomagnetic EAS systems is at the same frequency as the pulses used by some minute-ventilation pacemakers to measure transthoracic impedance. Minute-ventilation pacemakers may also erroneously interpret the signals generated by certain monitoring and diagnostic equipment, including cardiac monitors, echocardiography equipment, apnea monitors, and respiration monitors that also use bioelectric impedance measurements.[8,9]

Very strong electromagnetic fields could induce enough voltage in the lead or leads to directly capture the myocardium. For example, 58-kHz acoustomagnetic EAS systems are capable of inducing 3.7 V in pacemaker leads.[10] Isolated premature paced beats (but no sustained rapid pacing) have been observed in patients. In vitro and in vivo animal studies[11] have shown that application of 64-MHz RF power, required to produce MRI scans, can result in rapid pacing at pulsing periods between 200 and 1000 msec. Rapid pacing requires an intact lead connected to a pacemaker. Apparently, energy is coupled to the pacemaker defibrillation protection diodes or to the output circuit, bypassing the runaway protection mechanisms. Very rapid pacing could induce ventricular fibrillation. Irregular rapid pacing at a rate of approximately 100 beats/minute (bpm) temporarily related to RF pulses during MRI was observed in a patient with a VVI pacemaker programmed at subthreshold output.[12]

Spurious Tachyarrhythmia Detection

EMI signals can satisfy ICD tachyarrhythmia detection criteria and lead to spurious ICD discharges (Fig. 28-4). As noted, pacemaker-dependent patients can suffer concomitant inhibition of pacing. In a follow-up study of 341 ICD patients who received education regarding avoidance of sources of EMI, spurious tachyarrhythmia due to EMI occurred five times in four patients.[13] The incidence was 0.75% per patient-year of follow-up. In a study of 200 chronically implanted Medtronic ICDs with detections of ventricular fibrillation, oversensing of EMI was the cause in three patients.[14] Intermittent EMI can result in shock delivery even in noncommitted devices. Many "noncommitted" devices will not abort two consecutive discharges during the same "episode" (i.e., sinus rhythm not redetected in between) and therefore will deliver shocks for repetitive but self-limited EMI.

Noise-Reversion Mode

Pacemakers incorporate protective algorithms against prolonged inhibition from spurious signals (Table 28-2). A common response is transient reversion to asynchronous pacing. These algorithms are based on the fact that rapid frequencies are unlikely to represent myocardial activation. In most pacemakers, a noise-sampling or noise-interrogation window (also known as a relative refractory period) occupies the second part of the ventricular refractory period. Pacemakers do not respond to signals during the initial portion of the ventricular refractory period (i.e., ventricular blanking),

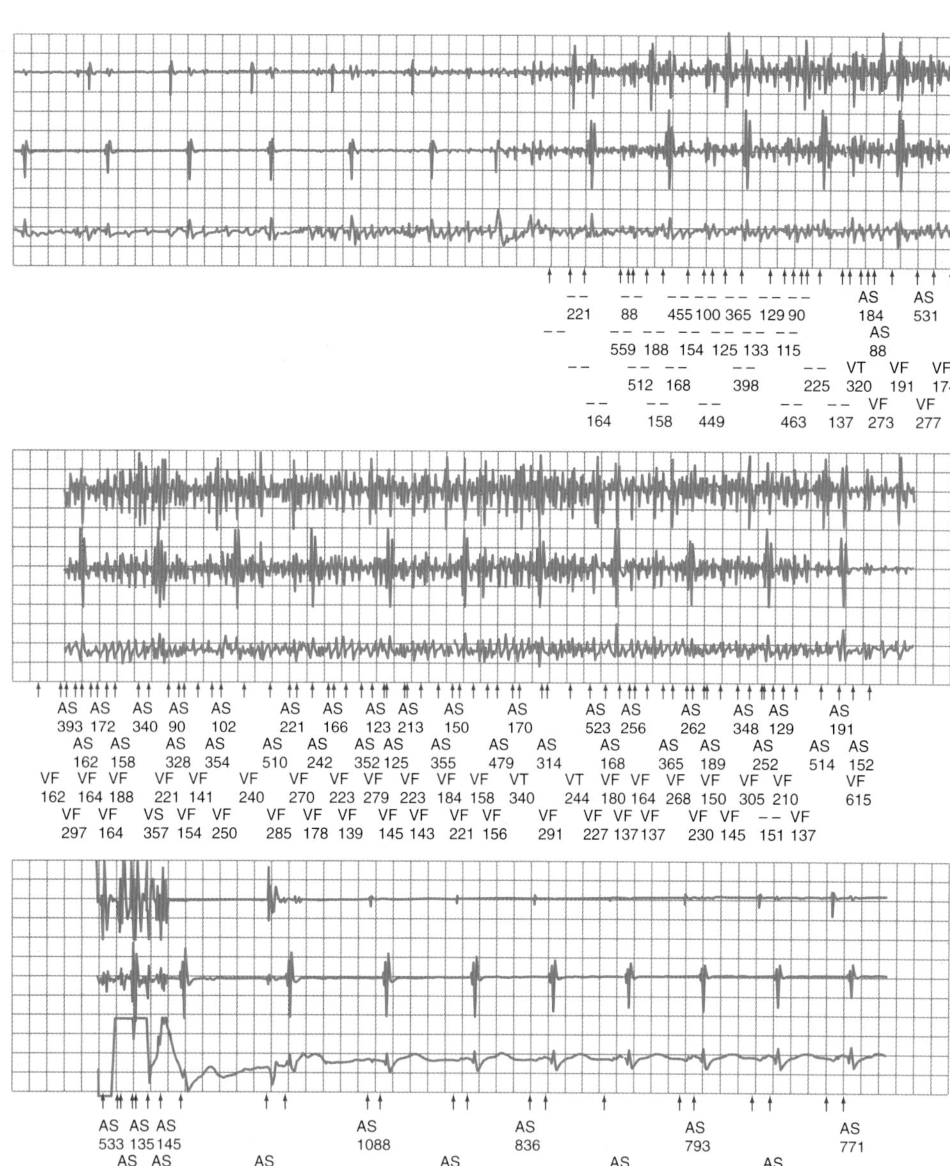

Figure 28-4. *Spurious ICD shock due to electromagnetic (EMI) of unknown cause at home. The stored electrogram was retrieved from the memory of a dual-chamber ICD during a routine checkup in a 60-year-old man. There is simultaneous sudden onset of electrical noise in the three channels (atrial, near field, far field from top to bottom), which is spuriously detected as ventricular fibrillation. There is immediate disappearance of the noise on shock delivery. The episode had occurred several weeks earlier. Similar, shorter episodes with aborted shocks had been stored weeks before. The patient denied having received a shock. Specific questioning did not disclose any potential culprit. The patient had not been subjected to any medical procedure known to induce EMI. The source of the interference remained uncertain. We suspected that the patient had received the shock while using some electrical device at home but did not want to share the information with the medical team. (The immediate disappearance of the interference after the shock suggests that the patient released the device.) Spurious shocks never recurred.*

which is usually nonprogrammable and is fixed or adjusted automatically by the generator based on the strength and duration of the ventricular event. Signals recognized during the noise-sampling window cannot reset the lower rate timer (thus preventing inhibition), but they do affect other timing intervals, most importantly the ventricular refractory period. In some models, a noise-sampling period exists in both the atrial and ventricular channels. The types of responses to signals sensed within the noise-sampling period implemented by different manufacturers include resetting of the entire (retriggerable) refractory period (e.g., Medtronic, Minneapolis, Minn.), resetting of the noise sampling period only (e.g., St. Jude Medical, St. Paul, Minn.), and reversion to asynchronous pacing for one full cycle (e.g., Intermedics [Guidant], Boston Scientific, Natick, Mass.). In the first two types of responses, repetitive triggering of the noise-sampling period eventually leads to asynchronous pacing. During simulation studies, a variable but narrow window of inappropriate pacing or inhibition is frequently observed at field or current strengths just below the reversion thresholds, because of intermittent oversensing. This phenomenon appears to be relatively unimportant during real-life EMI exposure. Occasional inhibition over a range of external field strengths is possible because EMI-induced body currents can fluctuate widely with changes in posture, respiratory phase, and other natural circumstances.[15] Although transient asynchronous pacing is generally safe, it is not completely innocuous. Symptoms secondary to loss of atrioventricular (AV) synchrony and an irregular heartbeat can occur. Competition with the spontaneous rhythm can induce ventricular tachyarrhythmias if the pacing stimulus

TABLE 28-2. Noise-Reversion and Electrical Reset Responses of Contemporary Dual-Chamber Pacemakers Programmed DDDR

Manufacturer	Model	Magnet Response	Full Reset
Biotronik	Phylos/Protos	AUTOMATIC*: DOO at 90 bpm for 10 beats if battery is good; then DDD atprogrammed rate ASYNCHRONOUS: DOO pacing at 90 bpm if battery is good; 80 bpm if ERI SYNCHRONOUS: no effect	VDD, 11% decrease in programmed rate, programmed polarity
Guidant	Insignia	ASYNCHRONOUS:* DOO at 100 bpm if battery is good; 85 bpm if ERI OFF: No change, magnet is ignored EGM mode: No change in pacing mode; magnet application initiates data collection	VVI 65, detected polarity Magnet response is OFF
ELA Medical	Talent/Brio	DOO at 96 bpm gradually declining to 80 bpm at ERI	VVI 70 bpm, unipolar[†]
Medtronic	Sigma Kappa EnPulse AT 500	DOO at 85 bpm if battery is good; DOO 65 bpm if ERI DOO at 85 bpm if battery is good; DOO 65 bpm if ERI or full electrical reset has occurred Disables atrial tachyarrhythmia therapy, no change in pacing.	DDDR 65 bpm, 5 V @ 0.4 msec, programmed polarity[‡] VVI 65 bpm, 5 V at 0.4 msec, detected polarity VVI 65 bpm, 5 V at 0.5 msec, bipolar
St. Jude	Integrity Affinity	Battery test: DOO at 98.6 bpm gradually declining to 86.3 bpm at ERI (if event snapshots enabled, asynchronous pacing starts after 5 sec of magnet application) OFF: no change in pacing	VVI 67.5 bpm, 4 V at 0.6 msec, unipolar
Vitatron	C-60 DR T-60 DR	DOO at 100 bpm at beginning of life, 86 bpm at ERI DOO at 90 bpm indicates that a partial restore has occurred	VVI 65 bpm, unipolar 7.5 V at 0.8 msec

*Nominal.
[†]"Dedicated bipolar" model (Brio DR222) reverts to bipolar.
[‡]In rare circumstances ventricular polarity could reset to unipolar.

captures the ventricle during its vulnerable period. This is extremely uncommon in pacemaker patients, as attested to by the routine use of a magnet during clinic or transtelephonic pacemaker checks.

Implementation of noise-protection algorithms is more difficult in ICDs (Table 28-3). By design, these devices must be able to recognize the rapid rates of ventricular fibrillation. Therefore, long refractory periods after sensed events are not feasible. Furthermore, asynchronous pacing is undesirable in patients who are vulnerable to reentrant ventricular arrhythmias.[16]

ICDs from ELA Medical (Sorin Group, Milan), Guidant, and St. Jude Medical provide programmable noise-reversion modes, but their performance against common sources of EMI is not well documented. Medtronic ICDs lack noise-reversion capabilities.

Electric (Power-on) Reset

Momentarily strong EMI, by inducing very high voltage within device circuits or triggering special microprocessor timers, may reset pacemakers and ICDs to operate in a mode different from the programmed mode. Electrosurgery and external or internal defibrillation are common causes of the reset phenomenon. In the reset mode, the pulse generator functions only with the basic factory preset instructions (pacing mode and parameters) that are stored in the nonvolatile read-only memory (ROM), because communication between the microprocessor and the random-access memory (RAM), which contains the programmable settings, has been interrupted. Most DDD(R) pacemakers reset to the VVI mode (see Table 28-2). The reset mode does not revert back when EMI is discontinued. Resolution of the problem requires a specific programmer command. In some pulse generators, there is no response to magnet application in the reset mode. In some pacemakers, the pacing mode and rate are similar during electrical reset and elective replacement indicator. In others (e.g., St. Jude Medical), strong EMI can trigger a reset mode or ERI. In those cases, clearing the ERI message with the programmer restores normal function. In Medtronic pacemakers, two levels of electrical reset (partial and full) exist. Partial reset tends to occur with less intense interference, preserving the programmed pacing mode and rates. Electrical reset can be differentiated from battery depletion by telemetric assessment of battery voltage and impedance. If reset was caused by EMI, the battery voltage should be normal (approximately 2.8 V), and the battery impedance should be either normal or slightly raised according to battery age.

In ICDs, electrical reset generally results in a "shock-box" configuration, with VVI pacing and maximum energy shocks (see Table 28-3). A special type of reset (called hard-reset by St. Jude Medical, "stand-by" by

TABLE 28-3. **Noise-Reversion, Asynchronous Pacing, and Electrical Reset Responses of Contemporary Implantable Cardioverter-Defibrillators**

Manufacturer	Model	Noise Reversion	Asynchronous Pacing	Electrical Reset
Guidant	Prizm, Prizm II, Vitality AVT	Programmable: AOO, DOO, VOO, Inhibit (nominal XOO)	AOO(R)‡, VOO(R)‡, DOO(R)‡	Non-rate-responsive mode (i.e., DDDR to DDD), lower rate 60 bpm Atrial output 5 V at 1 msec Ventricular output 7.5 V at 1 msec Single zone at 165 bpm, maximum energy × 5
	Ventak Prizm 2/Vitality DS/ Vitality 2	Programmable: AOO, DOO, VOO, Inhibit (nominal XOO)	"Electrocautery" mode Tachyarrhythmia detection disabled, XOO at lower rate limit	Non-rate-responsive mode (i.e., DDDR to DDD), lower rate 60 bpm Atrial output 5 V at 1 msec Ventricular output 7.5 V at 1 msec Single zone at 165 bpm, maximum energy × 5
ELA Medical	Alto 2	Programmable: Inhibit* or not Ventricular sensitivity ↓ until noise (i.e., cycle <63 msec) no longer detected	None	VVI 60 bpm, 4.4 V at 0.37 msec Single zone at 313 msec, 31 J × 4
Medtronic	GEM III, InSync 7272	None	None	VVI 65 bpm, 6 V at 1.6 msec Single zone at 320 msec, 30 J × 6 High-urgency alert sounds every 20 hr until cleared "Severe" reset: tachyarrhythmia therapy OFF, VVI 65 bpm, 6 V at 1.6 msec High-urgency alert sounds every 9 hr
	Marquis VR, DR Maximo VR, DR InSyncII Marquis InSync Maximo InSync Sentry Intrinsic	None	Programmable† DOO, VOO	VVI 65 bpm, 6 V at 1.6 msec Single zone at 320 msec, 30 J × 6 High-urgency alert sounds every 20 hr until cleared "Severe" reset: tachyarrhythmia therapy OFF, VVI 65 bpm, 6 V at 1.6 msec High-urgency alert sounds every 9 hr
St. Jude Medical	Atlas/Epic/ Photon	Programmable: VVI(R): VOO or OFF* DDD(R), DDI(R): VOO, DOO, or OFF* Fixed rate of 50 bpm	Programmable† AOO, VOO, DOO	VVI 60 bpm, 5 V Defib Only: detection rate 146 bpm; maximum available voltage × 3 Hard reset: tachyarrhythmia therapy OFF, VVI at 60 bpm 7.5 V, 0.75 msec, 2.2 mV

(R), Pacing at the sensor-indicated rate if rate-responsive pacing is enabled.
*Nominal.
†Available only when tachyarrhythmia detection is disabled.
‡Requires continuous telemetry link.

Guidant) can occur if there is damage to the ICD microprocessor or memory (e.g., due to radiotherapy). This type of reset is irreversible and cannot be reverted by a programmer command. Prompt generator replacement is usually required.

Closure of the Reed-Switch

Most pacemakers and ICDs contain a magnetic reed-switch that is closed by a 1-mT (Guidant) to 3-mT (Medtronic) static magnetic field. This generally results in temporary asynchronous pacing in pacemakers and temporary suspension of tachyarrhythmia detection and therapy in most ICDs. Normal function returns as soon as the magnetic field dissipates. Older Guidant ICDs were deactivated by continuous application of a magnetic field for 30 seconds or longer. Reactivation required reapplication of the magnet for 30 seconds or longer or a programmer command. Guidant ICDs have been inadvertently deactivated by items that generate inconspicuous strong magnetic fields, such as magnetized screws,[17] stereo speakers,[17] and bingo wands,[18] and also by unadvised magnet application in health care settings.[19] In later devices, this function was programmable and nominally disabled, and it is no longer available in the latest generation of Guidant ICDs.

Transient suspension of antitachycardia pacing due to reed-switch closure may be relatively frequent in daily life. In a study of 46 patients with St. Jude ICDs (which keep a log of magnet reversions), there were nine unexplained inactivations outside the medical environment (10% per patient-year of follow up).[20] Magnet application is being increasingly used to trigger specific behaviors in newer devices, including storage of EGMs and event markers or replay of alert tones. Exposure to a strong magnetic field when these functions are activated can result in eccentric (but clinically inconsequential) device behavior.[21] However, inadvertent asystole can occur when magnet application does not result in asynchronous pacing during electrosurgery.

Damage to the Generator or to the Electrode-Myocardium Interface

In almost all cases, the effects of EMI are temporary, lasting only as long as the device is within range of the source. However, very strong EMI (e.g., electrosurgery, external defibrillation) can cause permanent damage to an implanted device. Circuitry damage (resulting in output failure, pacemaker runaway, and other malfunctions) can occur, requiring generator replacement (at times on an emergency basis). Increases in pacing thresholds secondary to local heat-related injury at the lead-myocardium interface are also possible.

Current devices incorporate elements (Zener diodes, thyristors) that protect the pacing output circuitry and sensing amplifiers by shunting excess energy away from the device. The Zener diode behaves as a short circuit as soon as the voltage exceeds a certain value, such as 10 to 15 V, that is substantially above the output voltage of the pulse generator. Other, less common circuit designs can also limit the current flowing up the lead, but at the expense of inhibition of pacing output during the reception of large voltages.[22] For example, in the Telectronics (St. Jude Medical, Sylmar, Calif.) Meta DDDR 1254 pacemaker, the output circuit switches open to protect the generator if RF current is applied at the same time as the pacing pulse. No pacing output is emitted until the RF energy delivery ceases, although the event markers indicate normal pulse delivery. This behavior results in asystole during RF catheter ablation[23] or application of electrosurgery despite the use of a magnet or reprogramming to the VOO mode.[24]

Clinical Consequences of Electromagnetic Interference

The effects of EMI on pacemakers and ICDs depend on the intensity of the electromagnetic field, the frequency spectrum of the signal, the distance and positioning (angle) of the device relative to the source, the electrode configuration (unipolar or bipolar), nonprogrammable device characteristics, programmed settings, and patient characteristics (Table 28-4).

Transient EMI that produces a one-beat response (e.g., inhibition of a single ventricular pacing pulse) is of no clinical significance. Symptoms can occur with longer exposure. The spatial proximity and orientation of the patient with an implanted device to the potential source of EMI are important. Electrical and magnetic fields decrease inversely with the square of the distance from the source. Devices from different manufacturers differ in susceptibility to various sources of EMI, depending on circuitry design. EMI from digital cellular telephones (cellphones) has largely been suppressed by incorporation of simple RF feedthrough filters to the circuitry. A higher programmed sensitivity level increases device susceptibility to EMI. Unipolar pacemakers are more vulnerable to EMI from sources in the lower range of the frequency spectrum, such as power lines.[25] Left-sided unipolar implanted devices are particularly susceptible because of the larger loop for voltage induction between the lead and the generator. Sensing configuration loses importance at shorter radiation wavelengths. For cellphones, for example, the greatest interaction occurs when the antenna is placed over the device header. Neither the sensing electrodes near the distal tips of the leads, nor the coated lead body, is susceptible.

TABLE 28-4. Factors Influencing Electromagnetic Interference

Intensity of the field
Signal spectrum
Distance and position of the patient
Duration of exposure
Nonprogrammable device characteristics
Lead configuration
Programmed parameters
Sensitivity
Mode (baseline, noise reversion)
Committed versus noncommitted (ICDs)
Patient characteristics
Pacemaker dependency
Susceptibility to asynchronous pacing
Susceptibility to rapid pacing rates

The extent of pacemaker dependency is a main determinant of the clinical sequelae of EMI. Prolonged pacing inhibition does not cause symptoms in a patient with a good escape rhythm, but it could result in catastrophic asystole in a pacemaker-dependent patient.

Sources of Electromagnetic Interference in Daily Life

Cellular Telephones and Other Wireless Communication Devices

By September 2004, there were 1.6 billion subscribers to wireless communications services worldwide. Although cellphones continue to be the most popular wireless communications devices, personal digital assistants, laptop computers, satellite telephones, and other appliances are being increasingly used for wireless voice, data, and video transmission. Assessment of the effects of cellphones on implanted cardiac devices has been complicated by the wide variety of technologies in use.[26] Almost all current wireless telephones operate with digital technologies, although many can fall back to analog operation if their digital mode is not available. The Global System for Mobile Communication (GSM) has become the predominant digital platform worldwide. Other digital technologies in use in the United States and elsewhere include North American Digital Cellular (NADC), also known as Time Division Multiple Access (TDMA-50 Hz); Code Division Multiple Access (CDMA); integrated Dispatch Enhanced Network (iDEN), a cellphone system that also serves as a walkie-talkie platform; and Personal Communication System (PCS). New third-generation (3G) networks with increased speed for data transmission are being deployed. Wireless networks operate in the 820- to 960-MHz or the 1.8- to 2.2-GHz band. The power level used by a wireless telephone (and the consequent emitted electromagnetic field) fluctuates throughout the call, according to distance from the base station and the number of devices being used on the system at the same time. The maximal power of handheld phones is limited to 0.6 W in the United States and 2 W in Europe. Vehicle-mounted units can transmit at higher powers (up to 8 W), but they are not in common use by the general public.

Although isolated case reports have suggested the potential for severe interactions,[27] most research indicates that deleterious interactions are unlikely to happen with normal cellphone use. Large-scale bench-testing studies of the effects of wireless telephones on pacemakers and ICDs have been conducted at the FDA's Center for Devices and Radiological Health,[28,29] the Medical Devices Bureau of Canada,[30] and the University of Oklahoma's Wireless Electromagnetic Compatibility Center.[31,32] These studies encompassed several thousands of runs of telephone-device combinations and provided consistent results. Interference was nonexistent with the now outdated analog telephones. The *pulsed* component of the transmission in digital cellphones was detectable by pacemaker sensing circuitry if the field is strong enough. PCS and similar technologies produced interactions in fewer than 1% of tests, whereas other digital technologies (GSM, TDMA) produced interference in 0% to 25% of tests. In all studies, just a few models were responsible for a disproportionately large number of interactions, and other models were largely immune. An older version of TDMA-11 technology (used only for specialized business applications such as trucking, delivery, and construction in the United States) accounted for most interactions with ICDs. Feedthrough filters, common in modern pacemakers, made devices immune to interference. Almost all interactions occurred at distances of less than 10 cm. Devices always reverted to normal operation when the phone was turned off. In a simulation study, GSM telephones did not induce oversensing or interfere with the detection of simulated ventricular tachyarrhythmias by ICDs.[33]

Systematic investigations of the effects of cellphones in patients with pacemakers and ICDs have documented that severe interactions are improbable with most technologies during regular phone use. In a comprehensive multicenter study, Hayes and colleagues[34] tested 980 patients with implanted pacemakers for potential interference with five types of telephones (one analog and four digital: NADC, TDMA-11, PCS, and CDMA). Telephones were tested in a simulated worst-case scenario; in addition, NADC telephones were tested during transmission to simulate actual use. Patients were monitored while the phones were held at the ipsilateral ear and in a series of maneuvers directly over the pacemaker. The incidence of any type of interference was 20% in the 5533 tests. Tracking of interference sensed in the atrial channel, asynchronous pacing, and ventricular inhibition were the most common reactions observed (14%, 7%, and 6%, respectively). Interference was least frequent with analog (2.5%) and PCS (1.2%) systems. Clinically significant EMI was observed in 7% of tests and was considered severe in 1.7%. *There was no clinically significant EMI episodes when the telephone was placed in the normal position over the ear.* The presence of feedthrough filters in the pacemakers almost abolished the risk of EMI (from 29% to 56% down to <1%).

In a study of 39 pacemakers, EMI was more common with portable 8W GSM telephones than with handheld 2W models (7% versus 3% of tests); oversensing was more frequent at maximal than at nominal sensitivity (6% versus 2% of tests).[35] In a recent study of 100 patients with pacemakers from five manufacturers equipped with feedthrough filters testing a GSM cellphone with maximum power of 2 W in the standby, dialing, and operating mode, only two instances of ventricular inhibition were observed with the phone held directly over the pocket and the ventricular sensitivity programmed unipolar at 0.5 mV or less. Reprogramming of the sensitivity to 1 mV abolished the interaction in both cases.[36] GSM telephones did not induce inappropriate rapid pacing in patients with minute-ventilation pacemakers[37] or atrial oversensing in single-lead VDD pacemakers programmed at maximum atrial sensitivity.[38] In a study of 95 children with a variety of pacemakers programmed to a worst-case scenario, GSM telephones did not induce significant interference.[39] Clinical worst-case scenario testing has not disclosed significant interactions between ICDs and wireless digital telephones.[33,40-43] Digital cellphones do not interfere with the detection of induced ventricular fibrillation in the electrophysiology laboratory.[43] Inconsequential intermittent loss of telemetered EGMs and surface ECGs and inscription of erroneous event markers (i.e., "pseudo-oversensing") recorded via the programmer are common. Limited in vitro and in vivo testing has suggested that 3-W GSM telephones do not interfere with the function of an implantable ECG loop recorder.[44]

Although cellphones can potentially interfere with the function of implanted devices, this interference does not pose a health risk when telephones are placed over the ear. Maintaining an activated cellphone at least 6 inches (15 cm) from the device prevents interactions. The FDA has issued simple recommendations to minimize the risks. Patients should avoid carrying their activated cellphone in a breast or shirt pocket overlying an implanted device. A wireless telephone in use should be held to the ear opposite the side where the device is implanted. A survey of 1567 Japanese patients with implanted pacemakers revealed that, although 94% were right-handed, 41% used the left hand preferentially to hold a wireless telephone.[45] Not-so-obvious reasons for choosing one hand versus the other to hold the phone included hearing loss on one side (10%) and use of the opposite hand for dialing or writing memos (22%). It appears that, at least in some patients, the hand preferentially used to hold the wireless telephone should be considered when selecting the site for pacemaker implantation.

In an in vitro study, personal digital assistants connected to a hospital wireless local area network (WLAN) using the 802.11b protocol did not interfere with a variety of pacemakers and ICDs manufactured by Guidant, Medtronic, or St. Jude Medical.[46] As other wireless communication devices become prevalent, their effects on implanted cardiac devices should be carefully scrutinized.

Electronic Article Surveillance Devices

EAS devices (also known as antitheft devices or antishoplifting gates) are ubiquitous in retail stores, libraries, and office buildings. More than 1 million systems have been installed worldwide. The transmitter in these devices emits an electromagnetic field that is designed to interact with a "tag" in an unpurchased item. As a result of the interaction, the tag emits a signal that is detected by the receiver. Customers are exposed to an electromagnetic field as they walk through the gate, which typically consists of a pair of transmitter and receiver pedestals. EAS systems differ greatly in the frequency and strength of their emitted fields. Available technologies include high-frequency systems (operating beyond 900 MHz), swept RF systems (operating at 2 to 10 MHz), low-frequency acoustomagnetic systems (operating at 30 to 132 kHz), and electromagnetic systems (operating at 20 Hz to 18 kHz). These technologies serve different retailers' needs in terms of area covered, cost, detection, and "false alarm" rate, and they are not strictly interchangeable. The general consumer cannot differentiate these systems by their external appearance. Electromagnetic fields from these devices have the potential to induce interference signals in the sensing circuit of implanted cardiac devices. A sentinel report described a patient with complete heart block and a Ventak (CPI/Guidant) AV ICD in an abdominal pocket who developed multiple shocks and near-fatal inhibition of pacing on exposure to an acoustomagnetic EAS system.[47] Provocative testing with similar equipment in a controlled environment reproduced the interaction. The maximum distance at which ventricular oversensing occurred was 30 cm. When sensitivity was reprogrammed from "nominal" to "least sensitive," the interaction occurred only at closer proximity.

Prospective studies have clarified the incidence, severity, and risk factors for EMI from EAS systems. An in vitro study showed that 20 of 21 pacemaker models reacted to the field of an acoustomagnetic EAS system, and 10 reacted to an electromagnetic system.[48] Responses included inhibition and noise-reversion. Interference occurred when the simulator was within 33 cm of the transmission panel for the acoustomagnetic system, or 18 cm for the electromagnetic system. Mugica and associates[49] exposed 204 patients with pacemakers to two different EAS systems (acoustomagnetic at 58 kHz and electromagnetic at 73 Hz) for up to 30 seconds. Interference occurred in 17% of patients and was twice as likely with the acoustomagnetic system. Atrial tracking, asynchronous pacing, and single-beat inhibition were observed. All of the interactions were transient and were deemed benign. McIvor and coworkers[10] studied the effects of six EASs in 50 patients with pacemakers and 25 patients with ICDs from seven different manufacturers. One exposure protocol mimicked the most common real-life situation, walking at a normal pace midway between the gates. A "worst-case scenario" protocol required the patients to lean against the transmitter gate with the body parallel and then perpendicular to the transmitter. Interactions occurred with 48 pacemakers, almost exclusively with acoustomagnetic systems. No pacemaker reacted to the swept RF systems. Only two patients had transient asynchronous pacing while exposed to an electromagnetic system. The frequency of interactions with the acoustomagnetic system increased with the duration and closeness of the exposure; it was 16% when walking through the gates and 96% when leaning against the pedestal. Transient asynchronous pacing was the most common response, followed by atrial oversensing with tracking, ventricular oversensing with inhibition, and "voltage-induced" paced beats. Changing the sensing configuration from unipolar to bipolar, or programming a lower sensitivity setting, did not abolish the interactions but limited them to closer distances from the center of the gate. There were no instances of false tachyarrhythmia detection, but the ICDs were not programmed to pace during the testing. Groh and colleagues[50] studied the interaction between ICDs and two electromagnetic and one acoustomagnetic EAS devices in 169 patients. No spurious detections occurred during a 10- to 15-second walk through the gates. False ventricular fibrillation detection occurred in three patients during a 2-minute exposure to the acoustomagnetic system. When the 2-minute exposure was repeated during continuous pacing in 126 patients, oversensing was observed in 19 (15%). Oversensing was severe (complete or prolonged pacing inhibition) in 7 patients (6%), including 3 patients who had had spurious tachyarrhythmia detection at baseline and 4 additional patients with Ventritex ICDs who had oversensing during exposure to an electromagnetic system. All of the patients with serious interactions had an abdominal implant; however, by multivariate analysis, diminished R-wave amplitude and a Ventritex ICD were the only predictors of interactions.

In summary, severe interactions between EAS systems and implanted cardiac devices are unlikely when patients walk through the gates at a normal pace. On the other hand, dangerous interactions are likely with prolonged, close exposure to acoustomagnetic or electromagnetic systems. Patients should be instructed not to linger in proximity or lean against theft deterrent gates. Retailers should avoid placing systems where people are required to linger, such as at checkout counters. Merchandise or information (e.g., store floor plans) should not be displayed in close proximity to antitheft systems. The FDA recommends that all manufacturers of electronic antitheft systems develop labeling or signage to post on or near all new and currently installed systems, indicating that an electronic antitheft system is in use. The labeling or signage should be positioned so that it is visible before an individual enters the monitored area.[51]

Metal Detectors

Handheld and walk-through metal detectors are used for security applications. They function by sensing disturbances in electromagnetic fields. Handheld metal detectors typically operate at a frequency of 10 to 100 kHz and produce weak fields (≤4 A/m at a distance of 1 inch). Weapons are detected only within 1 to 4 inches. Walk-through metal detectors have coils on one or both sides of the equipment. They operate in a continuous wave (5 to 10 kHz) or in pulsed mode (200 to 400 Hz). Magnetic fields measured at the chest level inside the arch are less than 2 G.[52] Typically, a person walking through is exposed for 3 seconds. Kolb and coworkers[53] monitored 200 patients with pacemakers and 148 patients with ICDs from a variety of manufacturers for interactions with a standard airport metal detector gate. Pacemakers were reprogrammed to force ventricular pacing and ICDs to maximum sensitivity. Testing included normal walking through the gate and a worst-case scenario in which the chest was as close as possible to the gate and a 360-degree torsion was performed around the body axis. There were no interactions with any system.

The FDA has received one report of a spurious ICD shock triggered by a handheld metal detector in an airport. In several other instances, Guidant ICDs reverted to "monitor-only" mode after being exposed to metal detectors.[2] Current FDA recommendations state that it is safe for patients with implanted cardiac devices to walk through a metal detector gate, although the alarm may be triggered by the generator case. If scanning with a handheld metal detector is needed, patients should ask the security personnel not to hold the detector close to the implanted device longer than is absolutely necessary. A manual personal search can also be requested.[54]

Electric Power

EMI from electric power sources can occur if patients come in proximity to high-voltage overhead power lines (accidentally or by occupation), or it may be caused by electrical appliances that are held close or in direct contact with the chest. Implanted devices are susceptible to interference signals of 50 to 60 Hz, frequencies that lie within the bandwidth sampled for detection of intracardiac signals.

Detrimental effects from incidental exposure to high-voltage lines are unlikely. Even at a distance of 40 m from a 400-kV line, the electric and magnetic field strength is very low. Numerical studies suggested that the thresholds for EMI from magnetic fields at power line frequencies under the worst-case scenario for unipolar pacemakers are 40 μT in the atrium and 140 μT in the ventricle.[55] In vivo studies disclosed that all kinds of responses (inhibition, triggering, noise reversion) could occur, depending on the strength of the field, the generator model, the sensing configuration, and the programmed sensitivity.[25] Trigano and colleagues[56] exposed 250 pacemaker patients to a 50-Hz magnetic field with a flux density of 100 μT (the maximum allowed public exposure by European activities). There were no effects in devices programmed to bipolar sensing. Three patients with unipolar devices had noise-reversion to asynchronous mode; in one, symptomatic pacing inhibition followed. The studies suggest that bipolar sensing protects from EMI in all but the most extreme environmental conditions, such as power-generating stations. With unipolar sensing, inappropriate pacemaker behavior can occur during routine daily exposures.

EMI from household appliances occurs almost exclusively with improper grounding. Washing machines appear to be a frequent offender.[57-59] Anecdotal reports have incriminated slot machines,[60] power drills operated in a wet environmment,[57,61] a current leak from a water boiler (occurring when the hot water faucet was opened),[62] and vibrators.[13] A patient with a normally functioning ICD received spurious shocks due to 60-Hz interference while entering and exiting a public swimming pool; the current leak was otherwise undetectable.[63] Household induction ovens are safe in patients with pacemakers[64] or ICDs.[65]

Two case reports describing patients with spurious ICD discharges due to low-level alternating-current leak are especially illuminating. In a man with spurious ICD discharges caused by use of an electric razor, provocative testing confirmed oversensing of 50-Hz power with the patient's razor and a brand new similar unit. At operative revision, an insulation break was discovered at the ventricular coil of the "integrated" bipolar Endotak (Guidant) lead.[66] A boy with a single-chamber Medtronic ICD with an "integrated" bipolar Sprint lead had spurious detection of ventricular fibrillation due to oversensing of 60-Hz current while swimming in a pool and taking a shower powered by an electrical generator. The proximal and distal coils had been inverted in the device header. Because of the hardwiring in the lead and device header, the generator can had become part of the sensing circuit.[67] Both systems were operating "de facto" in a unipolar sensing mode.

Alternative Medicine Devices

A variety of so-called therapeutic magnets are commercially available for the treatment of arthritis and other musculoskeletal ailments. Despite manufacturers' claims of very strong magnetic field strengths (up to 30,000 G), in vitro testing showed that the magnets were able to close the reed-switch only when placed at less than 1 inch from the generator.[68] Spurious ICD shocks have been reported with unsupervised use of popular battery-operated muscular stimulators for abdominal training.[69] Acupuncture entailing delivery of current to needles inserted in the anterior chest has triggered spurious ICD shocks.[70] The "Zapper" is a battery-powered alternative medicine device that delivers a square-wave output at a constant frequency of 33.3 kHz. These electronic pulse frequencies are applied to both hands. It is marketed "to eliminate cancer, other chronic illnesses, self-diagnosed parasites, and germs." Vendors advise against the use of these devices in patients with pacemakers. Symptomatic pacemaker inhibition due to oversensing has been documented in a patient with heart block during use of the Zapper.[71]

Working Environment Sources of Electromagnetic Interference

Industrial Equipment

The return of the patient with an implanted cardiac device to a work environment suspected of high-level EMI can be challenging. Among the myriad potential EMI sources, arc or spot welders, industrial welding machines, degaussing coils, and electrical motors are frequent causes of concern. Not only do these sources emit energy in the RF spectrum, but their associated magnetic fields could potentially close the reed-switch in pacemakers and ICDs. Static magnetic fields strong enough to close the reed-switch are unlikely to be present in industrial environments. For example, in a petroleum refinery, peak fields of almost 2 mT were measured close to large compressors and in power distribution centers. However, the fields dropped off to less than 0.1 mT at a distance of 4 feet.[72] High levels of electromagnetic radiation exist in the cockpits of general aviation aircraft. However, in vitro testing of five modern pacemakers programmed in a unipolar configuration during flight conditions in single-engine fixed-wing aircraft did not demonstrate EMI.[73] There are no current guidelines regarding certification of air pilots with implanted cardiac rhythm management devices.

Each patient should be evaluated individually, but a few generalizations can be made. Bipolar sensing systems with close-coupled (≤1 cm) electrodes should be used preferentially in patients who may be exposed to high levels of EMI at work. The sensitivity should not be programmed very high in relation to the intrinsic EGM amplitude. Implant testing of ventricular fibrillation detection at the least sensitive setting (e.g., 1.2 mV with Medtronic ICDs) allows estimation of the sensing "safety margin" and appropriate reduction in the chronically programmed sensitivity. It is useful to ask a technical consultant from the device manufacturer to conduct a comprehensive EMI test at the patient's work site. However, this service may not be generally available due to liability issues. There is no professional reimbursement provided for an on-site visit by clinic staff. Testing should include measurement of magnetic fields at various distances from the source and review of telemetered and stored EGMs and event markers while the patient is operating the equipment. (ICDs should be programmed "monitor-only" to avoid spurious shocks).[74] In pacemaker-dependent patients, testing of a device identical to the one implanted coupled to a heart simulator represents a safe, sensitive preliminary step.[75] In patients with Guidant ICDs, a simple screening strategy consisting of listening to QRS-synchronous beep tones (a programmable feature) after extending the detection duration while the patient routinely operates the equipment is safe and effective.[76] In patients with ICDs from St. Jude Medical or Guidant that are exposed to intense magnetic fields at work, inhibition of tachyarrhythmia therapy in response to magnet application can be disabled. Additional general precautions include ensuring appropriate grounding of the equipment and avoiding close contact with the EMI source. Arc welders, for example, should wear nonconductive gloves and should not carry the cables on their shoulder.[77] Accidental grasping of a 60V/30A alternating current power line by a television cable line installer with an ICD triggered a spurious shock due to detection of 60-Hz electrical noise.[78] Patients should be instructed that, if they experience lightheadedness or an ICD shock (see Fig. 28-4), they should stop operating the equipment and contact their physician. Many patients can safely return to work with these precautions.

Medical Sources of Electromagnetic Interference

Patients with implanted cardiac devices (who typically are of advanced age and with severe cardiovascular disease) often require diagnostic and therapeutic procedures that involve strong sources of EMI. Most of these procedures can be performed safely with appropriate planning. Consultation regarding exposure to EMI in the medical environment constitutes a common clinical practice issue for physicians and nurses who are caring for patients with pacemakers and ICDs. The routine use of preprocedural checklists to identify patients with implanted cardiac devices *in advance* is strongly recommended.[79] Likewise, all institutions (especially those with dedicated staff and clinics) should have written policies regarding evaluation and management of patients before, during, and after procedures involving sources of EMI. Continuous education of patients and colleagues in other specialties and avoidance of improvisation will prevent bad outcomes and reduce legal liability.

Magnetic Resonance Imaging

MRI has many advantages compared with x-ray-based diagnostic techniques, including the non-ionizing nature of the radiation and the ability to discriminate among soft tissues without the use of contrast media. In properly operating MRI systems, the hazards associated with direct interactions between their electromagnetic fields and the body are negligible.[80] However, deleterious interactions between these fields and implanted cardiac devices can occur. The FDA database contains several reports of deaths among pacemaker patients during or immediately after MRI.[81] These reports are poorly characterized in terms of type of pacemaker and programming, patients' pacemaker-dependency status, field strength of the MRI unit, imaging sequence, and cardiac rhythm at the time of death. Six deaths during MRI among patients with pacemakers have been reported from Germany.[82] None of these patients was pacemaker dependent. The scans were performed in private radiology practices for orthopedic or neurologic reasons, with 0.5 to 1.5 T scanners and without monitoring. In three cases, ventricular fibrillation was documented. In the other three cases, there was evidence suggesting that asynchronous pacing at 100 bpm, triggered by the magnet, may have induced ventricular fibrillation.

Most older literature regarding interactions between implanted devices and MRI has become obsolete due to the continuous evolution in device construction and function and imaging protocols. However, at most institutions, the presence of an implantable device has remained an absolute contraindication to MRI, precluding a substantial and growing number of patients from the advantages of this imaging modality. In a survey of 1567 Japanese patients with pacemakers, 17% stated that they presented with conditions for which MRI would have been recommended if the device had not been present.[45]

Three types of electromagnetic fields are present in the MRI environment: an "always-on" static magnetic field (with its spatial gradient), a rapidly changing magnetic gradient field, and an RF field (Table 28-5). The last two are pulsed during imaging.[83] Exposure to the static magnetic field (0.2 to 3 T at the center of the magnet bore in current commercially available systems) occurs on entry into the MRI suite. This results in activation of the reed-switch with asynchronous pacing in pacemakers and suspension of tachyarrhythmia detection in most ICDs. Paradoxically, when the MRI static field is perpendicular to the reed-switch axis (i.e., when the patient is inside the gantry of the scanner), the reed-switch may not be activated and demand pacing (as programmed) may persist.[84,85] Even prolonged exposure to static magnetic fields does not result in permanent damage to the reed-switch, telemetric coils, or pacemaker software. The static magnetic field can also impart translational and rotational (torque) forces to a generator containing sufficient ferromagnetic material, which could result in pain and tissue damage. A magnetic force exists only if the magnetic field changes from place to place. Therefore, no magnetic force is measured at the isocenter of the magnet, but it increases rapidly toward the portal of the scanner. On the other hand, magnetic torque is highest at the isocenter of the magnet. In vitro studies

TABLE 28-5. Potential Effects of Magnetic Resonance Imaging on Implanted Cardiac Devices

Static magnetic field
Reed-switch closure
Generator displacement
Radiofrequency field
Alterations of pacing rate (inhibition or triggering)
Spurious tachyarrhythmia detection
Heating
Electrical reset
Time-varying magnetic gradient field
Induction voltage (resulting in pacing)
Heating
Reed-switch closure

have shown that translational attraction and torque levels are mild (i.e., acceleration lower than the gravity of the earth) with current pacemaker and ICD generators exposed at 1.5 T.[86-88] Limited testing suggests that even modern pacemakers can be subjected to potentially dangerous translational attraction with 3.0-T scanners.[87] The metallic parts of the leads are usually composed of MP35N, an alloy of nickel, cobalt, chromium, and molybdenum that is nonferromagnetic. Therefore, leads will not move or dislodge as a result of magnetic attraction.[89]

The RF fields can induce EMI in device circuitry, with resulting inhibition, tachyarrhythmia detection,[90] reset,[91] or rapid pacing. Several mechanisms for rapid pacing have been proposed. Rapid pacing up to the upper track limit can occur in dual-chamber devices if EMI is sensed in the atrial channel. Inhibition and tracking are avoided by programming asynchronous modes. "Runaway" pacing synchronized to the RF pulses (attributed to interference with pacemaker electronics) is the most severe potential complication. Rates up to 300 bpm have been observed in animal studies.[11] Additionally, the time-varying magnetic fields pulsed during imaging can induce voltage in leads (up to 20 V in unipolar leads; much less in bipolar leads) that can pace the heart or interfere with sensing. This could occur when the device is in the OOO mode or when it is programmed to deliver subthreshold pulses.[12] Heating around the lead tip could also result in tachycardia. High-level RF fields can also produce reversible or permanent damage to the device circuitry or memory. MRI has been reported to reprogram[90] or permanently damage ICDs, but not pacemakers. In a patient with a Ventak Mini III single-chamber ICD who inadvertently underwent MRI for a few seconds, the device reverted to an automatic safety mode and had a complete loss of programmability. Postexplantation analysis showed that a major portion of the device memory was corrupt.[92] In in vitro studies, several ICDs manufactured before 2000 were irreversibly damaged by scanning, whereas more current ones were not affected. In 15 dogs with chronically implanted ICDs manufactured after 2000, a 3-to 4-hour MRI scan did not result in device dysfunction, although spurious detection of ventricular tachyarrhythmia was common.[88]

The RF field in an MRI scanner has sufficient energy to cause local heating of long conductive wires, such as pacemaker leads, which could damage the adjacent myocardial tissue. Such thermal changes could result in increased thresholds, or even myocardial perforation. Bench studies have provided varying estimates of the heating at the lead tip, because the cooling effect of circulating blood is difficult to simulate.[88,93] In open-chest dogs with right ventricular pacing or defibrillation leads connected to temperature probes, the maximum recorded heating was only 0.2 °C, even during nonclinical high-SAR imaging protocols.[88] In swine experiments using chronically implanted pacing leads modified by the addition of a thermocouple sensor at the tip, increases in temperature of up to 20 °C were measured during MRI of the heart at 1.5 T and high SAR.[94] Heating peaked within seconds and appeared to depend strongly on the position of the pacing lead within the body-coil of the MRI unit. Maximal heating was observed when the pacemaker and the whole lead were inside the RF field-transmitting body-coil. A significant increase in lead impedance was measured immediately and 2-weeks after scanning. Changes in capture threshold were in general minor, although one right ventricular apical lead showed an acute increase in capture threshold of 2 V that returned to baseline within 2 weeks. There was no release of troponin. Pathologic analysis could not clearly demonstrate heat-induced damage around the lead attachment. In 1 of 15 dogs with chronically implanted ICDs that were subjected to a 4-hour MRI scan, there was immediate failure to capture at maximum output, which resolved after 12 hours. There were no acute or chronic changes in capture threshold in the other animals. Histopathologic analysis revealed no or very limited necrosis or fibrosis around the tip of the lead, which was not different from findings in control animals.

Proponents of the safety of MRI in patients with implanted devices argue that most undesirable clinical events have occurred in patients who were inadvertently subjected to scanning. On the other hand, there were no catastrophic complications in the few reported clinical series of planned MRI in patients. Valhaus and colleagues[84] performed 34 varied MRI examinations with a 0.5-T system in 32 nondependent patients with pacemakers reprogrammed to pace asynchronously above the intrinsic rate. In almost one half of the patients, temporary deactivation of the reed-switch (activated on entering the MRI suite) occurred when the patient was positioned in the gantry of the scanner at the center of the magnetic field. No instance of rapid pacing was seen. Lead impedance and pacing and sensing thresholds did not change. Battery voltage decreased immediately after MRI and recovered within 3 months, without changes in projected longevity. Programmed data and the ability to interrogate, program, or use telemetry were not affected. The authors concluded that MRI at 0.5 T is feasible in select patients with pacemakers and that it does not affect the devices irreversibly.

Martin and coworkers[95] reported results of 62 clinically indicated MRI examinations at 1.5 T in 54 nondependent pacemaker patients. No specific programming was followed. All pacemakers were interrogated immediately before and after MRI scanning. No adverse events occurred. ECG changes and patient symptoms were minor and did not require cessation of MRI. There were significant threshold changes in 10 leads (9.4%). Only 2 (1.9%) of the 107 leads required a change in programmed output. Threshold changes were unrelated to cardiac chamber, anatomic location, peak SAR, or time from lead implantation to the MRI examination. MRI at 2 T was uneventful in 13 nondependent patients with St. Jude Affinity bipolar pacemakers.[96]

Gimbel and associates[97] reported safe MRI of the head and neck in 10 pacemaker-dependent patients. The pacemakers (St. Jude Medical or Medtronic) were reprogrammed DOO or VOO, and MRI pulse sequences were modified to limit the whole-body SAR. There was no significant change in threshold immediately after imaging or 3 months later. There are no clinical series describing the results of MRI in pacemaker-dependent patients. In another study, Gimbel and associates[98] reported 8 MRI scans (7 cranial, 1 lumbar spine) at 1.5 T in 7 patients with ICDs (all but one from Medtronic). Detection was programmed "off," and pacing was set to a subthreshold output during the scan. After MRI, all devices demonstrated no changes in pacing, sensing, impedance, charge time, or battery status. The ICD exposed to the lumbar spine scan reverted to the "power-on-reset" mode, without permanent damage. MRI scanning was safe in 10 patients with Medtronic Reveal implantable loop recorders. In the majority of patients, postscanning device interrogation disclosed artifacts mimicking tachycardia. There was no permanent damage to the devices.[99]

Although recent evidence suggests that, with appropriate planning, select patients with implanted devices could undergo MRI without excessive risk, the presence of such a device should still be considered a *strong relative contraindication* for MRI. Furthermore, as long as manufacturers do not claim their devices to be MR-safe or MR-compatible, physician and institutional liability will continue to preclude wide use of MRI in patients with implantable devices.[100] The following recommendations should be followed if MRI is deemed indispensable for patient care.[101] Scanning of the lower extremities or of the head is less likely to induce severe MRI-induced heating at the lead tip. In nondependent patients, programming of the pacemaker to the OOO mode (if available) or to subthreshold output will avoid most interactions. Rapid pacing secondary to induction voltage is still possible in this mode. Devices in pacemaker-dependent patients should be reprogrammed to asynchronous mode. Low field strengths should be preferred. The patient must be monitored by ECG, pulse oximetry, and direct voice contact during the scan. Resuscitation equipment and the personnel needed to move and resuscitate the patient should be on standby. A professional well-versed in pacemaker function and troubleshooting and the corresponding programmer should be present. Imaging should start with graded scanning sequences (single-slice, low-resolution) and progress to more conventional sequences. Sequences with a high SAR (e.g., turbo spin-echo) are more likely to induce EMI and lead heating and should be avoided if possible. Irnich and colleagues[82] suggested a completely different approach for MRI in non-pacemaker-dependent patients, which includes programming the magnet function "off" (possible with pacemakers from Biotronik [GmbH & Co., Berlin, Germany], Guidant, and St. Jude Medical), reprogramming of the pacemaker to the trigger (i.e., VVT) mode, and triggering of the scanning by the pacemaker artifact, so that scanning is restricted to the myocardial refractory period. A special trigger unit is necessary for this technique. Although the approach is theoretically reasonable, more clinical experience is needed before it can be recommended. Because there is very limited information on MRI in patients with ICDs, this combination should be explored only under investigational circumstances. Tachyarrhythmia detection should be disabled.

Future developments in lead and device design and technology may reduce MRI-induced heating and other forms of interference and make MRI safer.[102,103] Shielding strategies include special coating (i.e., nanomagnetic) and low-pass filtering. A fiberoptic pacing lead (Biophan Technologies, Rochester, N.Y.) has been developed and appears safe in the MRI environment.[104] Coupling of such a lead to a photonic-based implanted pulse generator could in the future produce an MRI-compatible pacing system.

Neurostimulators

Case reports suggest that deep brain stimulators (used to treat Parkinson's disease and other movement disorders) are compatible with pacemakers or ICDs. Two scenarios are possible: the need to implant a cardiac device in a patient with a preexisting neurostimulator[105-107] and the decision to implant neurostimulators in a patient with a cardiac device.[108] Testing protocols and surgical approaches vary accordingly. If possible, testing for interactions should be performed preoperatively with a simulation screener device, intraoperatively, before discharge, and at each programming session. True bipolar sensing should be preferred. Unipolar deep-brain stimulation has not resulted in oversensing by pacemakers or ICDs.[105,107,108] High-energy ICD shocks can reset neurostimulators to the off mode.[105] The programmer wand for Medtronic neurostimulators contains a magnet that will close the reed-switch of a pacemaker or ICD if moved close to the pocket. Transtelephonic monitoring of the pacemaker may require that the neurostimulators be turned off transiently.[108]

Spinal cord stimulation has been used to treat peripheral vascular disease, intractable pain, and refractory angina pectoris. Concomitant use of pacemakers or ICDs and spinal cord stimulators is feasible, but testing is needed to avoid interactions.[109,110] Oversensing of the output of a spinal cord stimulator programmed in a unipolar configuration can result in pacemaker inhibition or noise-reversion. Therefore, only bipolar spinal cord stimulation should be used. If a cardiac device is implanted after a spinal cord stimulator has been placed, bipolar sensing should be preferred. Ekre and associates[111] reported on 18 consecutive patients treated with concomitant spinal cord stimulators for refractory angina and permanent pacemakers. Postimplantation testing consisted of ECG monitoring after programming of the pacemaker to a worst-case scenario (unipolar sensing and high sensitivity) while increasing the bipolar spinal cord stimulator output to the maximally tolerated level. There was no interference during acute testing. During long-term follow-up, there was no clinical evidence of pacemaker malfunction. There is no published experience on the concomitant use of implanted cardiac devices and other stimulators used to treat epilepsy (vagus nerve), fecal incontinence, or neurogenic bladder, but similar testing for interactions appears indicated. Stimulators in which the power source is not implanted but instead is RF-coupled (e.g., Medtronic Mattrix) are contraindicated in patients with pacemakers or ICDs.

Peripheral Nerve and Muscular Stimulation

Peripheral nerve stimulators are used to assess the extent of neuromuscular blockade intraoperatively or in the intensive care unit and to locate nerves for blocks. Frequencies of less than 4Hz (240 bpm) are unlikely to invoke noise-reversion modes. Reproducible inhibition of a unipolar right-sided VVI pacemaker during intraoperative left facial nerve stimulation with the standard train-of-four mode at 2 Hz has been reported.[112] Peripheral nerve stimulators can inhibit the display of pacemaker pulses in modern digital monitors and make the diagnosis of interference difficult.[113] Diagnostic nerve conduction studies with needle electrodes introduced at or distal to elbows or knees are safe in pacemaker patients.[114] Although guidelines suggest that electrodiagnostic studies are safe in patients with ICDs, provided special precautions are taken regarding the duration and frequency of stimulation pulses,[115] experts recommend that tachyarrhythmia detection be turned off during such studies.[116] This topic deserves further study.

TENS is a popular method for the relief of acute and chronic musculoskeletal pain. A TENS unit consists of electrodes that are placed on the skin and connected to a generator that applies 20-μsec rectangular pulses of up to 60 mA at a frequency of 20 to 110 Hz. Output and frequency are adjusted to provide maximum pain relief. Early studies in patients with unipolar pacemakers reported inhibition by TENS, which at times could be eliminated by increasing the sensing threshold.[117] In a study of the effects of TENS (at four sites, in 51 patients with 20 different pacemaker models), there were no instances of interference, inhibition, or reprogramming.[118] It appears that TENS can be used safely in patients with modern implanted bipolar pacemakers and in patients with unipolar pacemakers if sensitivity is reduced. TENS electrodes should not be placed parallel to the lead vector.

There is anecdotal experience with the use of TENS in patients with ICDs. Spurious shocks triggered by TENS application in patients with a variety of lead configurations and sensing algorithms have been documented.[119,120] Ambulatory TENS has triggered ICD shocks in patients in whom acute provocative testing did not show interactions.[121] Therefore, TENS should be avoided in patients with ICDs.

Chronic low-frequency stimulation of thigh muscles with biphasic symmetric pulses of approximately 0.5 msec at frequencies of 15 to 63 Hz is useful in patients with chronic congestive heart failure and muscular weakness, many of whom have pacemakers or ICDs.[122] In a pilot acute study, electrical stimulation of the neck and shoulder and of the thighs induced oversensing in three of eight patients with bipolar ICD systems.[123] In select patients with pacemakers or ICDs in whom acute testing did not demonstrate interaction, long-term stimulation of thigh muscles with two different protocols was safe.[124,125]

Electroconvulsive Therapy

Electroconvulsive therapy (ECT) is useful in major depressive illness, especially in elderly and medically frail patients. Potential concerns are EMI from the ECT shock itself, oversensing of myopotentials during succinylcholine-induced fasciculations or from incomplete muscular paralysis during the induced seizure, and detection of the common but generally benign tachyarrhythmias that occur during the seizure. There are isolated case reports of uncomplicated ECT in patients with pacemakers. The Mayo Clinic has reported on ECT in 26 patients with pacemakers and 3 patients with ICDs, who received a total of 493 treatments.[126] In patients with ICDs, tachyarrhythmia detection was disabled during the procedure. There were no instances of deleterious interference. The authors concluded that ECT was safe in patients with implantable devices; they recommended a consultation and device interrogation before the beginning and at the end of treatments, as well as proper attention to grounding. No special programming appears to be necessary in patients with pacemakers. A nondepolarizing muscle relaxant can be used for patients who demonstrate oversensing of fasciculations. In patients with ICDs, tachyarrhythmia therapy should be disabled before the procedure and re-enabled as soon as the seizure is over.

Video Capsule Endoscopy

PillCam video capsule endoscopy (Given Imaging, Norcross, Ga.), previously marketed as M2A, is useful in the investigation of obscure gastrointestinal bleeding and small-bowel pathology. A miniature camera, equipped with near-focus lenses, acquires video images that are telemetered to a waist belt-mounted receiver at a rate of 2 frames/second at 434 MHz. Once the images have been stored, 8 hours of continuously recorded information is downloaded to a workstation for analysis. The FDA and the device manufacturer consider the presence of a pacemaker or other implanted electrical device a contraindication to video capsule endoscopy. However, case reports and small series suggest that the procedure can be safe in such patients. Among five pacemaker patients who were admitted to the hospital and continuously monitored during capsule endoscopy, there were no instances of interference with pacemaker function, and the quality of the images was good.[127] Dubner and associates[128] challenged 100 patients with a variety of pacemakers with an external video capsule simulator transmitting at the same frequency. In four devices (2 St. Jude, 2 Biotronik), there was noise-reversion operation when the simulator capsule was positioned within 10 cm of the body, close to the generator. The interaction occurred within 10 seconds after capsule activation and was reproducible a week later. During clinical practice, the interaction is likely to occur only during the period in which the capsule descends through the esophagus. The authors recommended that patients with pacemakers undergo initial testing with the external simulator to exclude significant EMI before undergoing the actual procedure with the video-capsule system. In an in vitro study, six ICDs from different manufacturers were exposed to the same external video capsule simulator, for a total of 864 test runs.[129] There was consistent oversensing that resulted in false detection of ventricular fibrillation in the Biotronik Belos ICD. Until more information becomes available, it appears prudent to recommend that patients with ICDs undergo capsule endoscopy only as inpatients and with tachyarrhythmia therapy disabled.

Electrosurgery

Several electrosurgical techniques can generate EMI. The nomenclature of these techniques can be confusing. In Europe, the term "surgical diathermy" is often used to describe electrosurgical techniques, whereas in the United States, diathermy refers to the therapeutic application of current directly to the skin and is used for musculoskeletal ailments. Application of diathermy in heating or nonheating modes can result in excessive heating of tissue around leads and irreversible damage. RF (short-wave) or microwave diathermy is absolutely contraindicated in patients with pacemakers or ICDs.[130]

Some techniques are used in general surgery, and others find their most frequent use in dermatologic surgery.[131] Although the term electrocautery is often used when referring to electrosurgery, in its strict sense electrocautery describes a technique that promotes hemostasis by heating a metal instrument. Because no current is passed in the body, there is little or no risk of EMI. Battery-operated electrocauteries are often used during pacemaker implantation. Electrofulguration and electrodessication are monoterminal techniques that destroy only superficial tissues; they are used mostly in dermatologic surgery. Because there is no dispersive ground electrode, little current is generated in the body away from the lesion being treated. The most common electrosurgery modalities, electrosection (electrocutting) and electrocoagulation, involve passing current through tissue. Coagulation or cutting current is usually delivered in monopolar configuration. Current begins at the active electrode located on the surgical instrument and, after traveling through the body, returns to the electrosurgical generator through a dispersing ground pad. Both cutting and coagulation use high-voltage, low-amperage current with high-frequency radio wave oscillations greater than 100,000 Hz. Pure *cutting* is generated by a continuous signal, rarely in excess of 2000 V. It creates high temperatures, causing cell explosion and evaporation. *Coagulation* is produced by a higher-amplitude signal (up to 10,000 V) that has a very short dwell time. The short intermittent bursts produce heat within the tissue to control bleeding by thermally sealing the end of a blood vessel. Coagulation current is more likely than cutting current to cause interference.[132] A blended current (e.g., 50% of the time on and 50% off) is used most frequently. Few surgeons use pure cutting current unless specifically asked.

In true bipolar electrocoagulation, the current flow is localized across the two poles of an instrument (e.g., coagulation forceps). Because there is little flow of current outside the surgical site and less power is used, it is very unlikely to induce EMI. However, it is useful only for delicate surgical procedures and small vessels. Both monopolar and bipolar configurations are used during therapeutic endoscopic procedures (e.g., polypectomy, bleeding vessel cauterization).[133] Alternative surgical tools that will not produce EMI include the Shaw scalpel[134] (Oximetrix, Mountain View, Calif.), laser scalpels,[135,136] and ultrasound scalpels (Harmonic Scalpel, UltraCision, Smithfield, R.I.).[137] Extensive in vitro testing of a microwave thermotherapeutic device for transurethral ablation of benign prostatic hyperplasia suggests that it does not interact with pacemakers or ICDs.[138]

During electrosurgery in monopolar modes, the electric current spreads out and penetrates the entire body of the patient. This stray current may be interpreted by an implanted device as an intracardiac signal. Pacing inhibition, pacing triggering, automatic mode-switching, noise-reversion, or spurious tachyarrhythmia detection can occur[139] (Fig. 28-5) can occur, depending on the type of device, the programmed settings, the duration of EMI, and the channel in which the current is oversensed. Although some investigators have suggested that electrosurgery is safe in patients with activated ICDs,[140] the risk of spurious tachyarrhythmia detection is clearly present. Electrosurgery can also induce sensor-mediated pacing at the upper rate limit in minute-ventilation pacemakers.[141]

Other types of interaction are more common during electrosurgery than with other sources of EMI. In one study, up to 20% of older pacemakers reverted to the power-on reset mode, especially when the surgical wound was close to the pacemaker pocket.[142] In a more recent prospective study of 45 patients, electrosurgery triggered electrical reset in 7% of the patients.[143] Myocardial electrical burns may occur if there is conductivity between the pacing electrode and the indifferent (return) electrode of the electrosurgical unit. This may be facilitated by a pacing electrode with a small surface area and a higher current density. Furthermore, protective circuitry (i.e., Zener diodes, thyristors) that shunt current away from the device may also contribute to the development of myocardial burns and

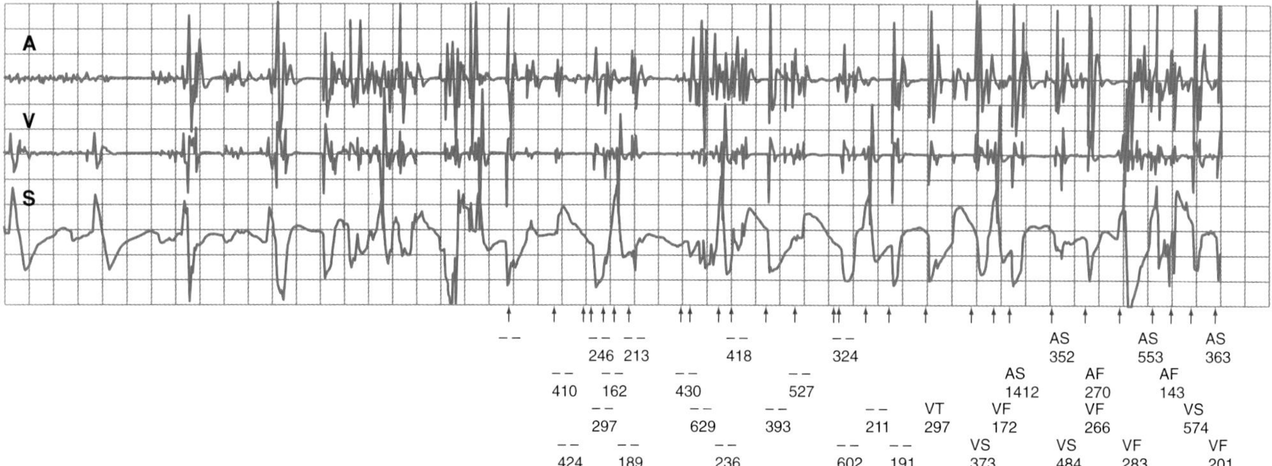

Figure 28-5. Spurious ventricular fibrillation detection due to electrosurgical equipment. Stored atrial (A), ventricular (V), and shocking lead (S) EGMs in a patient with a Ventak atrioventricular Mini III ICD who underwent placement of a Hickman catheter contralateral to the ICD pocket. Nonphysiologic signals are seen in both sensing channels. Tachyarrhythmia therapy was disabled before surgery. The atrial sensitivity was nominal; the ventricular sensitivity was programmed to "less." The device logged-in seven detections during the surgical procedure. (From Pinski SL, Trohman RG: Interference in implanted devices: Part II. PACE 25:1496-1509, 2002, with permission.)

subsequent elevation in pacing thresholds. Severe damage (and even ventricular fibrillation) can occur if the dispersive electrode is disconnected from the circuit, because the pacing electrode becomes the return electrode in the circuit and delivers current to the heart directly.[144] Irreversible generator failure due to damage to internal circuitry can occur, especially when current is applied close to the device pocket. Permanent loss of output or runaway syndrome[145] can be life-threatening. Voltage control oscillator lockout has been identified as a mechanism of sudden output failure after electrosurgery current.[146,147] Irreversible loss of output has been reported after an initial application of electrocoagulation current far away from the pacemaker system (i.e., during hip replacement).[148] Although late recovery of function can occur,[147] the device should not be trusted after initial failure.

Guidelines for the management of patients with implanted devices undergoing electrosurgery have been published (Table 28-6).[149,150] Short notice and scarcity of specialized personnel make compliance with such guidelines difficult, even in a large hospital with a well-staffed pacemaker clinic. Ideally, the patient should be seen before surgery to determine pacemaker dependency and to document pacing and sensing thresholds. Rate-response and tachyarrhythmia detection should be disabled just before surgery. In patients who are not pacemaker dependent, it is best not to change the programmed mode. Pacemaker-dependent patients should be reprogrammed to an asynchronous mode (DOO, VOO, AOO) above the intrinsic rate. Asynchronous pacing modes are not available in many ICDs. Taping of a magnet to the device pocket should be reserved for emergencies. In some pacemakers, magnet application does not result in asynchronous pacing, and in ICDs, magnet application suspends detection but does *not* trigger asynchronous pacing. The SMART magnet safely suspends tachyarrhythmia detection by Medtronic ICDs during surgical procedures without the need for reprogramming.[151] The battery-operated device contains a magnet, an RF transmitter, and light-emitting diodes. A green diode remains lit as long as the magnet is properly placed, indicating that tachyarrhythmia detection and therapy are suspended. Its use facilitates management in non-pacemaker-dependent ICD patients who are undergoing procedures that can produce EMI.

Communication with the operating room personnel, including nurses, anesthesiologists, and surgeons, is very important. Current from the electrosurgical unit distorts the ECG, and it may be impossible to determine whether pacemaker inhibition occurs. Pulse oximeter plethysmography and invasive arterial pressure monitoring are invaluable in this situation. The dispersive pad should be placed as close as possible to the operating site and as far away as possible from the pulse generator and leads, so that the electrical pathway is directed away from the pacing system. For example, during transurethral resection of the prostate, the grounding pad should be on the buttocks or lower leg. Good contact of the pad is mandatory, because with poor contact the pulse generator becomes the

TABLE 28-6. Management of Patients with Implanted Devices Undergoing Electrosurgery

Preoperative
Consider alternative tools (knife and ligatures, ultrasonic scalpel, laser scalpel)
Identify device and determine "reset" mode
Check device (programming, telemetry, thresholds, battery status)
Develop a contingency plan in case arrhythmias or device malfunction occurs during the procedure
In the operating room
Disable tachyarrhythmia therapies
Deactivate rate-responsive features
If the patient is pacemaker-dependent, reprogram device to asynchronous or triggered (with long refractory period) mode.
Remember that asynchronous pacing is not available in most ICDs. In these cases: Decrease the maximum sensitivity If available, program the noise-reversion mode to asynchronous Preapply external transthoracic pacing system Consider insertion of separate transvenous pacing wire
Monitor peripheral pulse or oximeter (ECG is obscured by artifact)
Position the ground pad to keep the active-to-dispersive current pathways as far as possible and perpendicular from the pulse generator-to-electrode pathway. The current should flow away from the pulse generator
Use true electrocautery or bipolar electrocoagulation whenever possible
Limit cutting current to short bursts interrupted by pauses of at least 10 sec
Use the lowest effective cutting or coagulation power output
Do not use probe near device
Reprogram if reset mode is hemodynamically unfavorable
Postoperative
Reactivate ICD tachyarrhythmia therapy as soon as possible
Check device (programming, telemetry, thresholds, battery status)
Reprogram if necessary
Replace generator if circuit damage documented
Replace lead or leads if pacing threshold is too high

anode for the applied current. The patient's body should not come in contact with any grounded electrical device that might provide an alternative pathway for current flow. Proper grounding of all electronic equipment used near the patient is essential.

The monopolar probe should not be used within 15 cm of the pulse generator or lead. Cutting or coagulation time should be as short as possible, using the lowest feasible energy level. If electrosurgery causes inhibition of an implanted pacemaker, it should be used in short bursts so as to produce only one to two dropped beats at a time. If there is no underlying rhythm, current should be applied for less than 1 second at a time, followed by 5- to 10-second periods free from current to allow resumption of rhythm and normal hemodynamics. Ideally, a trained physician and the corresponding programmer should be available within the hospital whenever a patient with an implanted device undergoes electrosurgery. Education, training, and certification of anesthesiologists in perioperative cardiac pacing appear necessary.[152] Because damage to the pacing system may occur, the capability of instituting emergency pacing must be present. An external transcutaneous pulse generator and defibrillator should be available. In case of inadvertent reprogramming that is not hemodynamically tolerated, the pulse generator must be reprogrammed as soon as possible. Magnet application can be attempted as an interim measure (the magnet rate usually varies from 60 to 100 bpm) but is unlikely to help in these cases.

A damaged pulse generator should be replaced expeditiously, especially if runaway syndrome occurs. All devices must be carefully tested after the operation, because malfunction may be inapparent, especially if the spontaneous rhythm is faster than the lower rate of the pulse generator. Ideally, testing should be performed immediately after the operation and repeated 24 to 48 hours later. Endocardial burns should be suspected if the capture and sensing thresholds have increased. Follow-up is then required until stability can be demonstrated. Occasionally, a rise in threshold requires placement of a new pacing lead.

As more surgical procedures are performed outside the hospital (in physicians' offices or in free-standing ambulatory surgery centers), these recommendations become difficult to implement. Although industry-employed allied professionals often participate in the perioperative management of patients with implanted devices in these settings, current guidelines suggest that they should perform technical support tasks only with an appropriately trained and experienced physician in close proximity (i.e., accessible to attend to the patient within a few minutes).[153] It is not clear what precautionary practices are standard in the community. In a survey of 166 cutaneous surgeons[154] performing electrosurgery of epitheliomas in the office setting, many had encountered instances of EMI with pacemakers or ICDs, but very few routinely checked or reprogrammed devices before or after surgery. Most of them restricted current bursts to less than 5 seconds, used minimal power, and avoided electrosurgery around a pacemaker or ICD. The estimated overall incidence of complications was low (0.8 cases per 100 years of surgical practice). The types of interference reported included pacemaker reprogramming, ICD firing, asystole, bradycardia, and premature pacemaker battery depletion. Use of bipolar forceps was not associated with interference.

It is necessary to gather more clinical evidence regarding incidence and severity of EMI with current implantable devices related to various electrosurgical techniques and operations. Current "blanket" recommendations may need to be revised to accommodate different degrees of risk and to allow efficient, cost-effective, high-quality perioperative management in the electrosurgical setting.

Direct Current Cardioversion and Defibrillation

Direct current external cardioversion and defibrillation with paddles (or disposable electrodes) can apply several thousand volts and tens of amperes of current to an implantable device system. Of all sources of EMI, this represents the highest amount of energy delivered in the vicinity of such a device, and it has potential to damage the pulse generator as well as the myocardial tissue in contact with the lead or leads. At times, the backup (reset) mode is activated by the countershock. However, if the protection mechanism is overwhelmed by high-energy input, permanent pulse generator circuitry damage may ensue. Additionally, capacitative coupling or shunting in the pacemaker circuit may induce currents in pacemaker or defibrillator leads sufficient to cause thermal damage (burn) to the electrode-tissue interface, resulting in chronic threshold elevation. In dual-chamber pacemakers, cardioversion energy may be preferentially shunted to the ventricular lead.[155] Even with modern pacemakers, acute exit block can occur. A mild acute initial rise in capture threshold can be followed by exit block a few weeks later.[156]

The risk of damage to the implanted device depends on the amount of energy applied, the characteristics of the device and lead, and the distance between the paddles or pads and the pulse generator and leads. Recommendations for external cardioversion in patients with implanted devices are presented in Table 28-7. In elective situations, the minimum energy that is likely to be successful should be delivered. External cardioversion or defibrillation with a biphasic waveform is more efficient (i.e., requires less energy) than the conventional damped sine wave monophasic shocks and should be preferred in patients with implanted devices. Unipolar pacing systems are more susceptible to damage than bipolar systems. Whenever possible, an anterior-posterior configuration of the shocking electrodes should be employed, because it maximizes the distance between the source and the implanted generator. If an anteroapical position must be used, the electrodes should be at least 10 cm from the pulse generator. However, this may be impossible with devices implanted in a right pectoral pocket, because the anterior paddle will lie directly on top of it. Transient elevations in capture threshold are common after direct-current shocks and should be anticipated. The threshold rise is usually temporary, lasting up to a few minutes, but occasionally the threshold remains elevated permanently, and necessitating lead replacement. Preprocedural and postprocedural interrogation and testing for proper function should follow external direct-current shocks to all implantable devices.

Internal cardioversion is at times attempted in patients who fail external cardioversion of atrial fibrillation. There is limited published experience with this procedure in patients with pacemakers. There were no instances of pacemaker malfunction in seven patients who underwent internal cardioversion of atrial fibrillation, with electrodes in the right atrium and in the coronary sinus or left pulmonary artery, with biphasic shocks of up to 20 J.[157] However, when high-energy endocavitary shocks were used for ablation purposes, pacemaker failure was common.[158]

Radiofrequency Ablation

RF catheter ablation is first-line therapy for a variety of supraventricular and ventricular arrhythmias. Interactions between RF current and implantable devices has been studied most thoroughly during catheter ablation of the AV junction for drug-refractory atrial fibrillation and of monomorphic ventricular tachycardia in patients with ICDs.

RF current (delivered as an unmodulated sine wave at 500 to 1000 kHz) can interact unpredictably with implanted devices. Energy delivery may result in asynchronous pacing, rapid tracking, spurious tachyarrhythmia detection, and electrical reset. Different interactions may be seen (in the same patient) during consecutive energy applications. Interactions are generally transient and terminate with cessation of energy delivery. In vitro and in vivo studies have examined the incidence, mechanisms, and risk factors for these interactions. Dick and colleagues[159] investigated the effects of RF current (55 W; tip temperature 65 to 70 °C) applied to four different pacing or defibrillation leads in a tissue bath model. Photographic and microscopic examination after energy delivery revealed no damage to the target lead. There was no malfunction of the attached pulse generators. The magnitude of induced current measured at the target tip lead was inversely proportional to the distance. Significant current was detected only when the ablation catheter was less than 1 cm from the target lead tip. Chin and associates[160] studied 19 pulse generators implanted in 12 dogs. They found that interactions depended on the proximity of current application to the pacing leads. Interactions were frequent at 1 cm and absent at more than 4 cm. The most dangerous interaction was runaway pacing with possible induction of ventricular fibrillation.

The clinical incidence of acute interaction between RF current application and permanent pacemakers has ranged widely. The incidence and severity of interference depend in part on the protective circuits of the implanted device.[23] The combined incidence of acute pacemaker malfunction during RF current application in three relatively large series involving a total of 125 patients with assorted pacemakers was 44%.[161-163] The most common interaction was asynchronous pacing due to noise reversion, followed by oversensing resulting in refractory period extension and "functional undersensing," pacemaker inhibition, or antitachycardia pacing in special pacemakers. Electrical reset, RF-induced pacemaker tachycardia, erratic behavior, and transient loss of capture were less frequent. In contrast, Proclemer and coworkers[164] did not observe transient or permanent pacemaker dysfunction in 70 consecutive patients with Medtronic Thera and Kappa single- and dual-chamber pacemakers with unipolar leads who underwent AV junction ablation. The pacemakers were implanted before RF ablation in a single-session procedure and were transiently programmed to VVI mode at 30 bpm.

The long-term effects of RF application on permanent pacing systems have been less well studied. Exit block (possibly caused by scar at the lead-tissue interface), lead damage, and chronic generator malfunction (requiring replacement) have been reported.[23,163,165] In two series of patients with pacemakers, changes in lead impedance and pacing and sensing thresholds did not

TABLE 28-7. Management of Patients with Implanted Devices Undergoing External Cardioversion or Defibrillation

Before cardioversion
In patients with ICDs, choose internal cardioversion via the device with commanded shock
Have pacemaker programmer available in the room
Determine (if possible) degree of pacemaker dependency
Program a higher-voltage output
Have transcutaneous external pacemaker available
During cardioversion
Use self-adhesive patches or paddles in an anteroposterior configuration
Keep patches or paddles as far from generator and leads as possible
Use lowest possible energy
Use a biphasic waveform
Respect a time interval of at least 5 min between successive shocks to allow cooling of protective diodes
After cardioversion
Repeat determination of pacing and sensing thresholds immediately, and again 24 hrs later
Consider monitoring for 24 hrs
Consider a higher output for 4 to 6 wks (especially in pacemaker-dependent patients)
Recheck pacemaker in 4 to 6 wks (sooner if there is an acute increase in capture threshold)

appear clinically significant.[23,164] In a study of 59 patients with pre-existent pacemaker (n = 46) or defibrillator (n = 13) leads undergoing AV junction ablation, a significant increase in pacing threshold was present immediately after ablation and became more marked 24 hours later.[166] A twofold increase in pacing threshold was much more likely to occur in patients with defibrillator leads. Two of the ICD patients (15%) and two of the pacemaker patients (4%) had a progressive rise in pacing threshold requiring lead revision. The mechanism of the increased vulnerability of the ICD leads was not clear.

A few simple precautions can minimize adverse outcomes. Complete pacemaker inhibition is dangerous in patients who are without an escape rhythm during ablation of the AV junction. Rate-responsiveness should be disabled. Pacing at the upper rate limit may occur when minute-ventilation pacemakers that measure transthoracic impedance misinterpret RF current.[167] Tachyarrhythmia detection should be disabled in patients with ICDs to prevent spurious therapies. We previously recommended that a temporary transvenous pacemaker (programmed, if necessary, to an asynchronous mode) should *always* be inserted, to avoid asystole.[168] Older pacemakers should not be trusted to provide backup pacing, because loss of output or capture could occur despite programming an asynchronous mode. More recently, we have performed uneventful AV nodal ablation in many patients with modern pacemakers with bipolar leads programmed to the VVI mode at 40 bpm and low sensitivity (4 mV). Ablation should be performed as far as possible from the leads. Pacemakers and ICDs should be checked carefully after RF catheter ablation.

RF energy can be used for ablation of other tissues. Uneventful percutaneous RF trigeminal rhizotomy[169] and intrahepatic RF ablation of liver neoplasms[170] in patients with pacemakers have been reported. With extracardiac RF ablation, the current return pad should be placed as close as possible to the delivery electrodes.[171]

Lithotripsy

Acoustic radiation, from extracorporeal shock wave lithotripsy (ESWL) machines, provides a noninvasive means to disintegrate renal, ureteral, gallbladder, and biliary calculi. With the original device (Dornier HM3, Dornier Medical System, Marietta, Ga.), the patient lies in a water bath and multiple (~1500) hydraulic shocks are generated from an underwater 20-kV spark gap and focused on the calculi by an ellipsoid metal reflector. The shock wave can produce ventricular extrasystoles, so it is synchronized to the R wave. Implanted devices could be subject to electrical interference from the spark gap and mechanical damage from the hydraulic shock wave. Newer units (e.g., Dornier Compact Delta) use an enclosed water cushion for shock wave coupling. Other units use electromagnetic (e.g., Siemens Lithostar, Siemens Medical Systems, Iselin, N.J.) or piezoelectric (e.g., Wolf Piezolith, Richard Eolf GmbH, Knittlingen, Gemany) shock-wave generators.[172] Most information regarding interactions with implanted cardiac devices has been collected with the Dornier HM3 unit.

Several investigators have studied the effects of ESWL on pacemakers in vitro.[173-175] Pacemaker output was not inhibited by properly synchronous shocks, but asynchronous shocks caused inhibition in both unipolar and bipolar devices. During A-V sequential pacing, a shock inappropriately synchronized to the atrial pacing pulse was often sensed by the ventricular channel, with the potential to cause inhibition of the ventricular output. Intermittent reversion to magnet mode can occur because of transient closure of the reed-switch due to the high-energy vibration. Other responses noted during in vitro testing included an increase in pacing rate secondary to tracking of EMI in the atrial channel, noise-reversion, spurious tachyarrhythmia detection,[176] and malfunction of the reed-switch. Activity-sensing pacemakers increased their pacing rate to the upper limit within 1 minute after the shock. ESWL caused no physical damage to the hermetic seal or internal components of the pacemakers tested, except that piezoelectric crystals shattered when an activity-sensing pacemaker was placed at the focal point of the ESWL.[175] In vitro testing of two ICDs with a new-generation lithotripter did not disclose any adverse interactions (even when the generator was placed within the focus of the lithotripter), provided that the shock waves were applied synchronized to the R wave.[177]

Case reports and clinical series suggest that ESWL is safe to use with implantable antiarrhythmic devices as long as the device and target are at least 6 cm apart. Adverse events have been rare and mild, and have occurred mostly with older devices.[178-181] Activity-sensing rate-adaptive devices implanted in the thorax can undergo lithotripsy safely, but the procedure should be avoided if the device is located in the abdomen. Synchronization of the shocks to the R wave is crucial. Activity sensors and tachyarrhythmia detection should be temporarily disabled in all cases. Reprogramming of dual-chamber pacemakers to VVI or VOO (if the patient is pacemaker dependent) avoids ventricular inhibition due to shocks synchronized to the atrial output, irregular pacing rate, tracking of induced supraventricular tachycardia, and triggering of the ventricular output by EMI. Careful follow-up should be performed over the next several months to ensure appropriate function of the reed-switch. In patients with abdominal ICDs, full electrophysiologic testing to confirm satisfactory detection and treatment of induced tachyarrhythmias should be considered. The piezoelectric shock-wave generator does not induce ventricular extrasystoles, and therefore synchronization to the QRS complex is not required. This unit appears especially safe to use in patients with implantable devices.

Dental Equipment

There are multiple potential sources of EMI in the dental office, including sonic and ultrasonic scalers, amalgamators, composite light curing units, x-ray units and view boxes, dental chairs and lights, electronic apex locators, and ultrasonic bath cleaners. Research in this area has been of suboptimal quality. The paucity of reports of severe interactions between modern implantable cardiac devices and dental equipment suggests that this is not a clinical problem. Magnetic fields in the dental office are not strong enough to close the reed-switch.[182] Older reports described pacemaker EMI with magnetorestrictive ultrasonic scalers, but not with piezoelectric ultrasonic scalers.[183] An in vitro study reported pacemaker inhibition by magnetorestrictive ultrasonic scalers up to distances of 37.5 cm.[7] However, review of the published telemetry strips suggests that these were not instances of true pacemaker inhibition, but instead represented interference with the telemetry link. Until further tests are conducted, it is prudent to avoid magnetorestrictive ultrasonic scalers in patients with implanted cardiac devices.[183] Manufacturers of electronic apex locators warn against the use of these devices in patients with pacemakers. In bench testing, four of five electronic apex locators did not interfere with a Biotronik pacemaker.[184] Safe use of an electronic apex locator in a patient with a pacemaker has been reported.[185] Prosthetic dental mini-magnets can activate the reed-switch only if placed very close (1 cm) to the pacemaker and therefore do not represent a risk to patients with pacemaker.[186]

Radiotherapy

Radiotherapy can induce various responses in implanted devices. EMI produced by the radiotherapy machine can result in pacing inhibition, tracking, noise reversion, or inappropriate ICD discharges. Usually, the effects are mild and are observed only while the machine is being switched on or off. Interference may be more severe with betatrons or with linear accelerators that misfire (spark). More important is the risk of permanent generator damage caused by ionizing radiation.[187] Current devices incorporating CMOS technology may incur damage during radiation therapy. Ionizing therapeutic radiation acts on the silicone and silicone oxide insulators within the semiconductors. Two potential mechanisms of damage have been described. Cumulative radiation can result in damage to circuit components, altering transistor parameters or creating electrical shorts that result in premature battery depletion. Failure may manifest as changes in sensitivity, amplitude, or pulse width; loss of telemetry; output failure; or runaway rates. This is uncommon unless the device is directly irradiated. More difficult to predict and avoid is random damage to the device's memory caused by scatter radiation.[188] Modern pacemakers and ICDs include memory error detection and correction schemes in their software programs. As a normal part of daily self-diagnostics, devices locate and correct affected memory locations. However, if the degree of memory alteration is beyond the capability of self-correcting algorithms, the device may invoke a ROM-based operating mode, referred to as "Safety Mode." This ensures that the patient is protected with basic pacing and shock therapy. Physicians should be advised of this possibility and should carefully monitor device operation during and after radiation therapy.

Diagnostic radiology procedures pose no immediate or cumulative effects on pulse generators. The available evidence does not suggest any differences in risk of generator damage for the various available types of therapeutic radiation. It should be remembered that total therapeutic radiation doses may be as high as 140 Gy (14,000 rad) given over several weeks. Until recently, a total absorbed dose of up to 2 Gy was considered safe in permanent pacemakers.[187] Studies with more recent devices suggest that pacemaker susceptibility to radiotherapy is highly variable and that severe malfunction can occur at even lower doses. Mouton and associates[189] irradiated 96 pacemakers in vitro with a high-energy photon beam. One pacemaker suffered severe malfunction at a cumulative dose of 0.15 Gy. At a cumulative dose of 2 Gy, 6% of pacemakers developed severe malfunction. The dose rate also had an effect on the likelihood of failure, and the authors recommended using dose rates lower than the standard of 2 Gy/min. During in vitro testing, 7 of 19 current pacemakers showed prolonged inhibition or changes in frequency during irradiation at 4 Gy/min.[190] Most manufacturers warn that ICDs are more susceptible than pacemakers to damage from radiotherapy. During in vitro irradiation of 11 current ICDs from various manufacturers, oversensing of interference was universal when the generator was in the irradiation field, often resulting in spurious detection of ventricular fibrillation.[191] Four ICDs had complete loss of function at a cumulative dose of 1.5 Gy.[192] Scatter radiation from a linear accelerator has resulted in permanent malfunction of Guidant ICDs in vitro and clinically. ICDs from Medtronic and Biotronik malfunctioned only after direct exposure to more than 50 Gy.[193]

Radiation oncology centers should have protocols for patients with implantable antiarrhythmic devices,[194] but a recent survey reveals wide variations among facilities regarding patient management precautions.[195] Manufacturers offer widely differing guidelines for patient management during radiotherapy, reflecting discrepancies in the perceived mechanism of damage. Vendors agree that the pulse generator should not be situated directly within the radiation field. If that is the case, the generator should be removed and reimplanted away from the field. In many cases, the device can be relocated in an ipsilateral abdominal pocket and the preexistent leads reused with the aid of extenders. Manufacturers also vary as to the total radiation exposure to the generator that should be allowed. For example, Medtronic recommends a limitation of 5 Gy or less for its pacemakers and 1 Gy or less to 5 Gy or less for its ICDs, depending on the model. In contrast, St. Jude Medical recommends a maximal cumulative dose to its pacemakers of 20 to 30 Gy. Guidant offers no guidelines regarding dose limitation, emphasizing the random nature of memory damage by radiation scatter. Guidant recommends maximizing shielding at the machine head but specifically discourages placing a lead apron over the pulse generator during treatment, because of its potential for increasing scatter. In contrast, St. Jude

TABLE 28-8. Management of Patients with Implanted Devices Undergoing Radiotherapy

Before treatments
Avoid betatron
Evaluate device and pacemaker dependency before therapy
Plan radiotherapy to minimize total dose (including scatter) received by generator
Avoid direct irradiation
Consider moving the pulse generator away from the field if the estimated dose is >2 Gy for a pacemaker or >1 Gy for an ICD
During treatments
Disable tachyarrhythmia detection and therapy in ICD patients
Measure actual dose received by the generator during the first treatment, using a thermoluminescent dosimeter or diode to confirm that the planned dose will not be exceeded
Institute appropriate level of monitoring: All patients should be observed by therapists during all treatments and should have their pulse and blood pressure measured before and after each treatment Pacemaker-dependent patients and patients with deactivated ICDs should undergo continuous ECG monitoring during all treatments. Pacemaker-dependent and ICD patients should have weekly device checks
After treatments
All patients should undergo full device check
Consider generator replacement at the earliest evidence of circuitry damage

Medical recommends shielding of the pacemaker with a piece of lead apron. The manufacturers also differ in their recommendations regarding the extent and frequency of patient monitoring during and after radiotherapy.

It is difficult to provide universal guidelines for the management of patients with pacemakers or ICDs who are undergoing radiotherapy. Current official guidelines have not been updated in almost 15 years and do not cover ICDs.[194] Table 28-8 proposes streamlined precautions to consider before, during, and after radiotherapy in patients with implanted cardiac devices.

REFERENCES

1. Barbaro V, Bartolini P, Calcagnini G, et al: On the mechanisms of interference between mobile phones and pacemakers: Parasitic demodulation of GSM signal by sensing amplifier. Phys Med Biol 48:1661, 2003.
2. Center for Devices and Radiological Health: Medical Device Reporting. U.S. Food and Drug Administration. Available at http://www.accessdata.fda.gov/scripts/cdrh/cfdocs/cfMAUDE/search.CFM.
3. Grant FH, Schlegel RE: Effects of an increased air gap on the in vitro interaction of wireless phones with cardiac pacemakers. Bioelectromagnetics 21:485, 2000.
4. American National Standards Institute, Association for the Advancement of Medical Instrumentation: Active Implantable Medical Devices: Electromagnetic Compatibility. EMC Test Protocols for Implantable Cardiac Pacemakers and Implantable Cardioverter Defibrillators. ANSI/AAMI PC69:2000. Washington, DC: American National Standards Institute, 2000.
5. Angeloni A, Barbaro V, Bartolini P, et al: A novel heart/trunk simulator for the study of electromagnetic interference with active implantable devices. Med Biol Eng Comput 41:550, 2003.
6. Dawson TW, Stuchly MA, Caputa K, et al: Pacemaker interference and low-frequency electric induction in humans by external fields and electrodes. IEEE Trans Biomed Eng 47:1211, 2000.
7. Miller CS, Leonelli FM, Latham E: Selective interference with pacemaker activity by electrical dental devices. Oral Surg Oral Med Oral Pathol Oral Radiol Endod 85:33, 1998.
8. Chew EW, Trougher RH, Kuchar DL, et al: Inappropriate rate change in minute ventilation rate responsive pacemakers due to interference by cardiac monitors. Pacing Clin Electrophysiol 20:276, 1997.
9. Southorn PA, Kamath GS, Vasdev GM, et al: Monitoring equipment induced tachycardia in patients with minute ventilation rate-responsive pacemakers. Br J Anaesth 84:508-509, 2000.
10. McIvor ME, Reddinger J, Floden E, et al: Study of Pacemaker and Implantable Cardioverter-Defibrillator Triggering by Electronic Article Surveillance Devices (SPICED TEAS). PACE 21:1847, 1998.
11. Hayes DL, Holmes DR Jr, Gray JE: Effect of 1.5 tesla nuclear magnetic resonance imaging scanner on implanted permanent pacemakers. J Am Coll Cardiol 10:782-786, 1987.
12. Fontaine JM, Mohamed FB, Gottlieb C, et al: Rapid ventricular pacing in a pacemaker patient undergoing magnetic resonance imaging. PACE 21:1336, 1998.
13. Kolb C, Zrenner B, Schmitt C: Incidence of electromagnetic interference in implantable cardioverter-defibrillators. PACE 24:465, 2001.
14. Gunderson BD, Gillberg JM, Swerdlow CD: Importance of oversensing in inappropriate detection of ventricular fibrillation by chronically implanted ICDs. Heart Rhythm 1:S244, 2005.
15. Butrous GS, Male JC, Webber RS, et al: The effect of power frequency high intensity electric fields on implanted cardiac pacemakers. PACE 6:1282-1292, 1983.
16. Saeed M, Link M, Mahapatra S, et al: Analysis of intracardiac electrograms showing monomorphic ventricular tachycardia in patients with implantable cardioverter-defibrillators. Am J Cardiol 85:580-587, 2000.
17. Schmitt C, Brachmann J, Waldecker B, et al: Implantable cardioverter-defibrillator: Possible hazards of electromagnetic interference. PACE 14:982-984, 1991.
18. Ferrick KJ, Johnston D, Kim SG, et al: Inadvertent AICD inactivation while playing bingo. Am Heart J 121:206-207, 1991.
19. Rasmussen MJ, Friedman PA, Hammill SC, et al: Unintentional deactivation of implantable cardioverter-defibrillators in health care settings. Mayo Clin Proc 77:855, 2002.
20. Kolb C, Deisenhofer I, Weyerbrock S, et al: Incidence of antitachycardia therapy suspension due to magnet reversion in implantable cardioverter defibrillators. PACE 27:221, 2004.
21. Levine PA, Moran MJ: Device eccentricity: Postmagnet behavior of DDDR pacemakers with automatic threshold tracking. PACE 23:1570-1572, 2000.
22. Laudon MK: Pulse output. In Webster JC (ed): Design of Cardiac Pacemakers. New York, IEEE Press, 1995, pp 251-276.
23. Ellenbogen KA, Wood MA, Stambler BS, et al: Acute effects of radiofrequency ablation of atrial arrhythmias on implanted permanent pacing systems. PACE 19:1287-1295, 1996.

24. Kleinman B, Hamilton J, Hariman R, et al: Apparent failure of a precordial magnet and pacemaker programmer to convert a DDD pacemaker to VOO mode during the use of the electrosurgical unit. Anesthesiology 86:24, 1997.
25. Toivonen L, Valjus J, Hongisto M, et al: The influence of elevated 50 Hz electric and magnetic fields on implanted cardiac pacemakers: The role of the lead configuration and programming of the sensitivity. PACE 14:2114-2122, 1991.
26. Hayes DL, Carrillo RG, Findlay GK, et al: State of the science: Pacemaker and defibrillator interference from wireless communication devices. PACE 19:1419, 1996.
27. Yesil M, Bayata S, Postaci N, et al: Pacemaker inhibition and asystole in a pacemaker dependent patient. PACE 18:1963, 1995.
28. Ruggera PS, Witters DM, Bassen HI: In vitro testing of pacemakers for digital cellular phone electromagnetic interference. Biomed Instrum Technol 31:358, 1997.
29. Bassen HI, Moore HJ, Ruggera PS: Cellular phone interference testing of implantable cardiac defibrillators in vitro. PACE 21:1709, 1998.
30. Tan KS, Hinberg I: Can wireless communication systems affect implantable cardiac pacemakers? An in vitro laboratory study. Biomed Instrum Technol 32:18, 1998.
31. Schlegel RE, Grant FH, Raman S, et al: Electromagnetic compatibility study of the in-vitro interaction of wireless phones with cardiac pacemakers. Biomed Instrum Technol 32:645, 1998.
32. University of Oklahoma Wireless EMC Center: In Vitro Study of the Interaction of Wireless Phones and Implantable Cardioverter-defibrillators: Executive Summary. Available at http://www.ou.edu/engineering/emc/projects/ICD_X.html.
33. Jiménez A, Hernández Madrid A, Pascual J, et al: Interferencias electromagnéticas entre los desfibriladores automáticos y los teléfonos móviles digitales y analógicos. Rev Esp Cardiol 51:375, 1998.
34. Hayes DL, Wang PJ, Reynolds DW, et al: Interference with cardiac pacemakers by cellular telephones. N Engl J Med 336:1473, 1997.
35. Naegeli B, Osswald S, Deola M, et al: Intermittent pacemaker dysfunction caused by digital mobile telephones. J Am Coll Cardiol 27:1471, 1996.
36. Hekmat K, Salemink B, Lauterbach G, et al: Interference by cellular phones with permanent implanted pacemakers: an update. Europace 6:363, 2004.
37. Sparks PB, Mond HG, Joyner KH, et al: The safety of digital mobile cellular telephones with minute ventilation rate adaptive pacemakers. PACE 19:1451, 1996.
38. Nowak B, Rosocha S, Zellerhoff C, et al: Is there a risk for interaction between mobile phones and single lead VDD pacemakers? PACE 19:1447, 1996.
39. Elshershari H, Celiker A, Ozer S, et al: Influence of D-net (EUROPEAN GSM-standard) cellular telephones on implanted pacemakers in children. PACE 25:1328, 2002.
40. Fetter JG, Ivans V, Benditt DG, et al: Digital cellular telephone interaction with implantable cardioverter-defibrillators. J Am Coll Cardiol 31:623, 1998.
41. Sanmartin M, Fernández Lozano I, Márquez J, et al: Ausencia de interferencia entre teléfonos móviles GSM y desfibriladores implantables: Estudio in-vivo. Rev Esp Cardiol 50:715, 1997.
42. Chiladakis JA, Daviouros P, Agelopoulos G, et al: In-vivo testing of digital cellular telephones in patients with implantable cardioverter-defibrillators. Eur Heart J 22:1337, 2001.
43. Occhetta E, Pelabani L, Bortnick M, et al: Implantable cardioverter-defibrillators and cellular telephones: Is there any interference? PACE 22:981, 1999.
44. de Cock CC, Spruijt HJ, Van Campen LMC, et al: Electromagnetic interference of an implantable loop recorder by commonly encountered electronic devices. PACE 23:1516, 2000.
45. Sakakibara Y, Mitsui T: Concerns about sources of electromagnetic interference in patients with pacemakers. Jpn Heart J 40:737, 1999.
46. Tri JL, Trusty JM, Hayes DL. Potential for Personal Digital Assistant interference with implantable cardiac devices. Mayo Clin Proc 79:1527, 2004.
47. Santucci PA, Haw J, Trohman RG, et al: Interference with an implantable defibrillator by an electronic antitheft-surveillance device. N Engl J Med 339:1371, 1998.
48. Tan KS, Hinberg I: Can electronic article surveillance systems affect implantable cardiac pacemakers and defibrillators? [abstract]. PACE 21:960, 1998.
49. Mugica J, Henry L, Podeur H: Study of interactions between permanent pacemakers and electronic antitheft surveillance systems. PACE 23:333, 2000.
50. Groh W, Boschee S, Engelstein E, et al: Interactions between electronic article surveillance systems and implantable cardioverter-defibrillators. Circulation 100:387, 1999.
51. U.S. Food and Drug Administration, Center for Devices and Radiological Health: Guidance on labeling for electronic anti-theft systems. Available at http://www.fda.gov/cdrh/comp/guidance/1170.pdf.
52. Moss CE: Exposures to electromagnetic fields while operating walk-through and hand-held metal detectors. Appl Occup Environ Hyg 13:501, 1998.
53. Kolb C, Schmieder S, Lehmann G, et al: Do airport metal detectors interfere with implanted pacemakers or cardioverter-defibrillators? J Am Coll Cardiol 41:1386, 2003.
54. Burlington DB: Important information on anti-theft and metal detector systems and pacemakers, ICDs, and spinal cord stimulators. Center for Devices and Radiological Health, Rockville, MD, September 28, 1998. Available at http://www.fda.gov/cdrh/safety/easnote.html.
55. Dawson TW, Caputa K, Stutchly MA, et al: Pacemaker interference by magnetic fields at power line frequencies. IEEE Trans Biom Eng 49:254, 2002.
56. Trigano A, Blandeau O, Souques M, et al: Clinical study of interference with cardiac pacemakers by a magnetic field at power line frequencies. J Am Coll Cardiol 45:896, 2005.
57. Sabate X, Moure C, Nicolas J, et al: Washing machine associated 50 Hz detected as ventricular fibrillation by an implanted cardioverter defibrillator. PACE 24:1281, 2001.
58. Paraskevaidis S, Polymeropoulos KP, Louridas G: Inappropriate ICD therapy due to electrical interference: External alternating current leakage. J Invasive Cardiol 16:339, 2004.
59. Chan NY, Ho LWL: Inappropriate implantable cardioverter defibrillator shock due to external alternating current leak: Report of two cases. Europace 7:193, 2005.
60. Madrid A, Sanchez A, Bosch E, et al: Dysfunction of implantable defibrillators caused by slot machines. PACE 20:212, 1997.
61. Pinski SL, Trohman RG: Interference in implanted devices: Part I. PACE 25:1367, 2002.
62. Manolis AG, Katsivas AG, Vassilopoulos CV, et al: Implantable cardioverter-defibrillator: An unusual case of inappropriate discharge during showering. J Interv Card Electrophysiol 4:265, 2000.
63. Lee SW, Moak JP, Lewis B: Inadvertent detection of 60-Hz alternating current by an implantable cardioverter defibrillator. PACE 25:518, 2002.
64. Rickli H, Facchini M, Brunner H, et al: Induction ovens and electromagnetic interference: What is the risk for patients with implanted pacemakers? PACE 26:1494, 2003.
65. Binggeli C, Rickli H, Ammann P, et al: Induction ovens and electromagnetic interference: What is the risk for patients with implantable cardioverter-defibrillators? J Cardiovasc Electrophysiol 16:399, 2005.

66. Seifert T, Block M, Borggrefe M, et al: Erroneous discharge of an implantable cardioverter-defibrillator caused by an electric razor. PACE 18:1592, 1995.
67. Garg A, Wadhwa M, Brown K, et al: Inappropriate implantable cardioverter defibrillator discharge from sensing of external alternating current leak. J Interv Card Electrophysiol 7:181, 2002.
68. Van Lake P, Mattioni T: The effect of therapeutic magnets on implantable pacemaker and defibrillator devices [abstract]. PACE 23:723, 2000.
69. Wayar L, Mont L, Silva RMFL, et al: Electrical interference from an abdominal muscle stimulator unit on an implantable cardioverter-defibrillator: Report of two consecutive cases. PACE 26:1292, 2003.
70. Lau EW, Birnie DH, Lemery R, et al: Acupunture triggering inappropriate ICD shocks. Europace 7:85, 2005.
71. Furrer M, Naegeli B, Bertel O: Hazards of an alternative medicine device in a patient with a pacemaker [letter]. N Engl J Med 350:16, 2004.
72. Cartwright CE, Breysse PN, Boother L: Magnetic field exposures in a petroleum refinery. Appl Occup Environ Hyg 8:587, 1993.
73. De Rotte AA, Van Der Kemp P: Electromagnetic interference in pacemakers in single-engine fixed-wing aircraft: A European perspective. Aviat Space Environ Med 73:179, 2002.
74. Fetter JG, Benditt DG, Stanton MS: Electromagnetic interference from welding and motors on implantable cardioverter-defibrillators as tested in the electrically hostile work site. J Am Coll Cardiol 28:423, 1996.
75. Marco D, Eisinger G, Hayes DL: Testing of work environments for electromagnetic interference. PACE 15:2016, 1992.
76. Gurevitz O, Fogel RI, Herner M, et al: Patients with an ICD can safely resume work in industrial facilities following simple screening for electromagnetic interference. PACE 26:1675, 2003.
77. Precautions for Electric Arc Welding. St Jude Medical Technical Services. Available at http://www.sjm.com/documents/resources/precautionselectricarcwelding.pdf.
78. Mehdirad A, Love C, Nelson S, et al: Alternating current electrocution detection and termination by an implantable cardioverter-defibrillator. PACE 20:1885, 1997.
79. Sawyer-Glover AM, Shellock FG: Pre-MRI procedure screening: recommendations and safety considerations for biomedical implants and devices. J Magn Reson Imaging 12:510, 2000.
80. Shellock FG, Crues JV: MR procedures: Biologic effects, safety, and patient care. Radiology 232:635, 2004.
81. CDRH Magnetic Resonance Working Group. A Primer on Medical Device Interactions with Magnetic Resonance Imaging Systems. Available at http://www.fda.gov/cdrh/ode/primerf6.html.
82. Irnich W, Irnich B, Bartsch C, et al: Do we need pacemakers resistant to magnetic resonance imaging? Europace 7:353, 2005.
83. Duru F, Luechinger R, Scheidegger MB, et al: Pacing and magnetic resonance imaging environment: Clinical and technical considerations on compatibility. Eur Heart J 22:113, 2001.
84. Valhaus C, Sommer T, Lewalter T, et al: Interference with cardiac pacemakers by magnetic resonance imaging: Are there irreversible changes at 0.5 Tesla? PACE 24:489, 2001.
85. Luechinger R, Duru F, Zeijlemaker VA, et al: Pacemaker reed switch behavior in 0.5, 1.5, and 3.0 Tesla magnetic resonance imaging units: Are reed switches always closed in strong magnetic fields? PACE 25:1419, 2002.
86. Luechinger R, Duru F, Scheidegger MB, et al: Force and torque effects of a 1.5-Tesla MRI scanner on cardiac pacemakers and ICDs. PACE 24:199, 2001.
87. Shellock FG, Tkach JA, Ruggieri PM, Masaryk TJ: Cardiac pacemakers, ICDs, and loop recorder: Evaluation of translational attraction using conventional ("long-bore") and "short-bore" 1.5- and 3.0-Tesla MR systems. J Cardiovasc Magn Reson 5:387, 2003.
88. Roguin A, Zviman MM, Meininger GR, et al: Modern pacemaker and implantable cardioverter/defibrillator systems can be magnetic resonance imaging safe: In vitro and in vivo assessment of safety and function at 1.5 T. Circulation 110:475, 2004.
89. Shellock FG, Morisoli SM: Ex vivo evaluation of ferromagnetism and artifacts of cardiac occluders exposed to a 1.5-T MR system. J Magn Reson Imaging 4:213, 1994.
90. Anfinsen OG, Berntsen RF, Aass H, et al: Implantable cardioverter defibrillator dysfunction during and after magnetic resonance imaging. PACE 25:1400, 2002.
91. Rozner MA, Burton AW, Kumar A: Pacemaker complication during magnetic resonance imaging [letter]. J Am Coll Cardiol 45:161, 2004.
92. Fiek M, Remp T, Reithmann C, et al: Complete loss of ICD programmability after magnetic resonance imaging. PACE 27:1002, 2004.
93. Achenbach S, Moshage W, Diem B, et al: Effects of magnetic resonance imaging on cardiac pacemakers and electrodes. Am Heart J 334:467, 1997.
94. Luechinger R, Zeijlemaker VA, Pedersen EM, et al: In vivo heating of pacemaker leads during magnetic resonance imaging. Eur Heart J 26:376, 2005.
95. Martin ET, Coman JA, Shellock FG, et al. Magnetic resonance imaging and cardiac pacemaker safety at 1.5-Tesla. J Am Coll Cardiol 43:1315, 2004.
96. Leal del Ojo J, Moya F, Villalba J, et al: Is magnetic resonance safe in cardiac pacemaker patients? PACE 28:274, 2005.
97. Gimbel JR, Bailey SM, Tchou PJ, et al: Strategies for the safe magnetic resonance imaging of pacemaker-dependent patients. PACE 28:1041, 2005.
98. Gimbel JR, Kanal E, Schwartz KM, et al: Outcome of magnetic resonance imaging (MRI) in selected patients with implantable cardioverter defibrillators (ICDs). PACE 28:270, 2005.
99. Gimbel JR, Zarghami J, Machado C, et al: Safe scanning, but frequent artifacts mimicking bradycardia and tachycardia during magnetic resonance imaging (MRI) in patients with an implantable loop recorder. Ann Noninvasive Electrocardiol 10:404, 2005.
100. Faris WP, Shein MJ: Government viewpoint: U.S. Food and Drug Administration: Pacemakers, ICDs, and MRI. PACE 28:268, 2005.
101. Gimbel JR, Kanal E: Can patients with implantable pacemakers safely undergo magnetic resonance imaging? J Am Coll Cardiol 43:1325, 2004.
102. Smith JM: Industry viewpoint: Guidant pacemakers, ICDs, and MRI. PACE 28:264, 2005.
103. Stanton MS: Industry viewpoint: Medtronic pacemakers, ICDs, and MRI. PACE 28:265, 2005.
104. Greatbatch W, Miller V, Shellock FG: Magnetic resonance safety testing of a newly developed fiber-optic cardiac pacing lead. J Magn Reson Imaging 16:97, 2002.
105. Tavernier R, Fonteyne W, Vandewalle V, et al: Use of an implantable cardioverter defibrillator in a patient with two implanted neurostimulators for severe Parkinson's disease. PACE 23:1057, 2000.
106. Obwegeser AA, Uitti RJ, Turk MF, et al: Simultaneous thalamic deep brain stimulation and implantable cardioverter-defibrillator. Mayo Clin Proc 76:87, 2001.
107. Rosenow JM, Tarkin H, Zias E, et al: Simultaneous use of bilateral subthalamic nucleus stimulators and an implantable cardioverter defibrillator. J Neurosurg 99:167, 2003.
108. Senatus PB, McClelland S III, Ferris AD, et al: Implantation of bilateral deep brain stimulators in patients with Parkinson disease and preexisting cardiac pacemakers. J Neurosurg 101:1073, 2004.
109. Romano M, Zucco F, Baldini MR, et al: Technical and clinical problems in patients with simultaneous implantation of a cardiac pacemaker and spinal cord stimulator. PACE 16:1639, 1993.
110. Monahan K, Casavant D, Rasmussen C, et al: Combined use of a true-bipolar sensing implantable cardioverter-defibrillator in a

patient having a prior implantable spinal cord stimulator for intractable pain. PACE 21:2669, 1998.
111. Ekre O, Borjesson M, Edvardsson N, et al: Feasibility of spinal cord stimulation in angina pectoris in patients with chronic pacemaker treatment for cardiac arrhythmias. PACE 26:2134, 2003.
112. O'Flaherty D, Wardill M, Adams AP: Inadvertent suppression of a fixed rate ventricular pacemaker using a peripheral nerve stimulator. Anaesthesia 48:687-689, 1993.
113. Rozner MA: Peripheral nerve stimulators can inhibit monitor display of pacemaker pulses. J Clin Anesth 16:117, 2004.
114. LaBan MM, Petty D, Hauser AM, et al. Peripheral nerve conduction stimulation: Its effect on cardiac pacemakers. Arch Phys Med Rehabil 69:358-362, 1988.
115. Nora LM: American Association of Electrodiagnostic Medicine guidelines in electrodiagnostic medicine: Implanted cardioverters and defibrillators. Muscle Nerve 19:1359, 1996.
116. Chémali KR, Tsao B: Electrodiagnostic testing of nerves and muscles: When, why, and how to order. Cleve Clin J Med 72:37, 2005.
117. Chen D, Philip M, Philip PA, et al: Cardiac pacemaker inhibition by transcutaneous electrical nerve stimulation. Arch Phys Med Rehabil 71:27, 1990.
118. Rasmussen MJ, Hayes DL, Vliestra RE, et al: Can transcutaneous electrical nerve stimulation be safely used in patients with permanent pacemakers? Mayo Clin Proc 63:443-445, 1988.
119. Glotzer TV, Gordon M, Sparta M, et al: Electromagnetic interference from a muscle stimulation device causing discharge of an implantable cardioverter-defibrillator: Epicardial bipolar and endocardial bipolar sensing circuits are compared. PACE 21:1996, 1998.
120. Vlay SC: Electromagnetic interference and ICD discharge related to chiropractic treatment. PACE 21:2009, 1998.
121. Pyatt JR, Trenbath D, Chester M, et al: The simultaneous uses of a biventricular implantable cardioverter defibrillator (ICD) and transcutaneous electrical nerve stimulation (TENS) unit: Implications for device interaction. Europace 5:91, 2003.
122. Nuhr MJ, Pette D, Berger R, et al: Beneficial effects of chronic low-frequency stimulation of thigh muscles in patients with advanced chronic heart failure. Eur Heart J. 25:136, 2004.
123. Crevenna R, Stix G, Pleiner J et al: Electromagnetic interference by transcutaneous neuromuscular electrical stimulation in patients with bipolar sensing implantable cardioverter defibrillators: A pilot safety study. PACE 26:626, 2003.
124. Crevenna R, Wolzt M, Fialka-Moser V, et al: Long-term transcutaneous neuromuscular electrical stimulation in patients with bipolar sensing implantable cardioverter defibrillators: A pilot safety study. Artif Organs 28:99, 2004.
125. Crevenna R, Mayr W, Keilani M, et al: Safety of a combined strength and endurance training using neuromuscular electrical stimulation of thigh muscles in patients with heart failure and bipolar sensing cardiac pacemakers. Wien Klin Wochenschr 115:710, 2003.
126. Dolenc TJ, Barnes RX, Hayes DL, et al: Electroconvulsive therapy in patients with cardiac pacemakers and implantable cardioverter defibrillators. PACE 27:1257, 2004.
127. Leighton JA, Sharma VK, Srivasthsan K, et al: Safety of capsule endoscopy in patients with pacemakers. Gastrointest Endosc 4:567, 2004.
128. Dubner S, Dubner Y, Gallino S, et al: Electromagnetic interference with implantable cardiac pacemakers by video capsule. Gastrointest Endosc 61:250, 2005.
129. Dubner Y, Dubner S, Rubio H, et al: Interference from wireless video-capsule endoscopy on implantable cardioverter-defibrillators. Folia Cardiol 12(Suppl C):444, 2005.
130. Feigal DW: FDA Public Health Notification: Diathermy Interactions with Implanted Leads and Implanted Systems with Leads. Available at http://www.fda.gov/cdrh/safety/121902.pdf.
131. LeVasseur JG, Kennard CD, Finley EM, et al: Dermatologic electrosurgery in patients with implantable cardioverter-defibrillators and pacemakers. Dermatol Surg 24:233, 1998.
132. Rozner MA: Review of electrical interference in implanted cardiac devices [letter]. PACE 26:923, 2003.
133. Gruber M, Seebald C, Byrd R, et al: Electrocautery and patients with implanted cardiac devices. Gastroenterol Nurs 18:49, 1995.
134. Erdman S, Levinsky L, Strasberg B, et al: Use of the Shaw scalpel in pacemaker operations. J Thorac Cardiovasc Surg 89:304, 1985.
135. Kott I, Watemberg S, Landau O, et al: The use of CO2 laser for inguinal hernia repair in elderly, pacemaker wearers. J Clin Laser Med Surg 13:335, 1995.
136. Jones SL, Mason RA: Laser surgery in a patient with Romano-Ward (long QT) syndrome and an automatic implantable cardioverter-defibrillator. Anaesthesia 55:362, 2000.
137. Epstein MR, Mayer JE Jr, Duncan BW: Use of an ultrasonic scalpel as an alternative to electrocautery in patients with pacemakers. Ann Thorac Surg 65:1802, 1998.
138. Rasmussen MJ, Rea RF, Tri JL, et al: Use of a transurethral microwave thermotherapeutic device with permanent pacemakers and implantable defibrillators. Mayo Clinical Proc 76:601, 2001.
139. Casavant D, Haffajee C, Stevens S, et al: Aborted implantable cardioverter-defibrillator shock during facial electrosurgery. PACE 21:1325, 1998.
140. Fiek M, Dorwarth U, Durchlaub I, et al: Application of radiofrequency energy in surgical and interventional procedures: Are there interactions with ICDs? PACE 27:293, 2004.
141. Wong DT, Middleton W: Electrocautery-induced tachycardia in rate-adaptive pacemaker. Anesthesiology 94:710, 2001.
142. Lamas GA, Antman EM, Gold JP, et al: Pacemaker backup-mode reversion and injury during cardiac surgery. Ann Thorac Surg 41:155-157, 1986.
143. Roman-Gonzalez J, Hyberger LK, Hayes DL: Is electrocautery still a clinically significant problem with contemporary technology? [abstract] PACE 24:709, 2001.
144. Geddes LA, Tacker WA, Cabler P: A new electrical hazard associated with the electrocautery. Med Instrum 9:112-113, 1975.
145. Heller LI: Surgical electrocautery and the runaway pacemaker syndrome. PACE 13:1084-1085, 1990.
146. Moran MD, Kirchhoffer JB, Cassaver DK, et al: Electromagnetic interference (EMI) caused by electrocautery during surgical procedures [letter]. PACE 19:1009, 1996.
147. Peters RW, Gold MR: Reversible prolonged pacemaker failure due to electrocautery. J Interven Card Electrophysiol 2:343, 1998.
148. Nercessian OA, Wu H, Nazarian D, et al: Intraoperative pacemaker dysfunction caused by the use of electrocautery during a total hip arthoplasty. J Arthoplasy 13:599, 1998.
149. Goldschlager N, Epstein A, Friedman P, et al: Environmental and drug effects on patients with pacemakers and implantable cardioverter/defibrillators: A practical guide to patient treatment. Arch Intern Med 161:649, 2001.
150. Eagle KA, Berger PB, Calkins H, et al: ACC/AHA Guideline Update for Perioperative Cardiovascular Evaluation for Noncardiac Surgery: A Report of the American College of Cardiology/American Heart Association Task Force on Practice Guidelines (Committee to Update the 1996 Guidelines on Perioperative Cardiovascular Evaluation for Noncardiac Surgery). 2002. American College of Cardiology Web site. Available at: http://www.acc.org/clinical/guidelines/perio/clean/perio_index.htm.
151. Technical manual. Smartmagnet 9322. Minneapolis, Minn., Medtronic, Inc., 2001.
152. Rozner M: Pacemaker misinformation in the perioperative period: Programming around the problem. Anesth Analg 99:1582, 2004.
153. Hayes JJ, Juknavorian R, Maloney JD: The role(s) of the industry employed allied professional. PACE 24:398, 2001.

154. El-Gamal HM, Dufresne RG, Saddler K: Electrosurgery, pacemakers and ICDs: A survey of precautions and complications experienced by cutaneous surgeons. Dermatol Surg 27:385, 2001.
155. Das G, Staffanson DB: Selective dysfunction of ventricular electrode-endocardial junction following DC cardioversion in a patient with a dual chamber pacemaker. PACE 20:364, 1997.
156. Waller C, Callies F, Langenfeld H: Adverse effects of direct current cardioversion on cardiac pacemakers and electrodes: Is external cardioversion contraindicated in patients with permanent pacemaker systems? Europace 6:165, 2004.
157. Prakash A, Saksena S, Mathew P, et al: Internal atrial defibrillation: effect on sinus and atrioventricular nodal function and implanted cardiac pacemakers. PACE 20:2434, 1997.
158. Vanerio G, Maloney J, Rashidi R, et al: The effects of percutaneous catheter ablation on preexisting permanent pacemakers. PACE 13:1637, 1990.
159. Dick AJ, Jones DL, Klein GJ: Effects of RF energy delivery to pacing and defibrillation leads [abstract]. PACE 24:658, 2001.
160. Chin MC, Rosenqvist M, Lee MA, et al: The effect of radiofrequency catheter ablation on permanent pacemakers: an experimental study. PACE 13:23, 1990.
161. Chang AC, McAreavey D, Tripodi D, et al: Radiofrequency catheter atrioventricular node ablation in patients with permanent cardiac pacing systems. PACE 17:65, 1994.
162. Pfeiffer D, Tebbenjohanns J, Schumacher B, et al: Pacemaker function during radiofrequency ablation. PACE 18:1037, 1995.
163. Sadoul N, Blankoff I, de Chillou C, et al: Effects of radiofrequency catheter ablation on patients with permanent pacemakers. J Intervent Card Electrophysiol 1:227, 1997.
164. Proclemer A, Facchin D, Pagnutti C, et al: Safety of pacemaker implantation prior to radiofrequency ablation of atrioventricular junction in a single session procedure. PACE 23:998, 2000.
165. Wolfe DA, McCutcheon MJ, Plumb VJ, et al: Radiofrequency current may induce exit block in chronically implanted ventricular leads [abstract]. PACE 1995;18:919.
166. Burke MC, Kopp DE, Alberts M, et al: Effect of radiofrequency current on previously implanted pacemaker and defibrillator ventricular lead systems. J Electrocardiol 34(Suppl):143, 2001.
167. van Gelder BM, Bracke FALE, El Gamal MIH: Upper rate pacing after radiofrequency catheter ablation in a minute ventilation rate adaptive DDDR pacemaker. PACE 17:1437, 1994.
168. Pinski SL, Trohman RG: Interference in implanted devices: Part II. PACE 25:1496, 2002.
169. Sun DA, Martin L, Honey CR: Percutaneous radiofrequency trigeminal rhizotomy in a patient with an implanted cardiac pacemaker. Anesth Analg 99:1585, 2004.
170. Hayes DL, Charboneau JW, Lewis BD, et al: Radiofrequency treatment of hepatic neoplasms in patients with permanent pacemakers. Mayo Clin Proc 76:950, 2001.
171. Rozner MA: Pacemaker and electrocardiographic monitor pseudomalfunction during extracardiac radiofrequency ablation [letter]. Anesthesiology 102:239, 2005.
172. Auge BK, Preminger GM: Update on shock wave lithotripsy technology Curr Opin Urol 12:287, 2002.
173. Langberg J, Abber J, Thuroff JW, et al: The effects of extracorporeal shock wave lithotripsy on pacemaker function. PACE 10:1142-1146, 1987.
174. Fetter J, Patterson D, Aram G, et al: Effects of extracorporeal shock wave lithotripsy on single chamber rate response and dual chamber pacemakers. PACE 12:1494, 1989.
175. Cooper D, Wilkoff B, Masterson M, et al: Effects of extracorporeal shock wave lithotripsy on cardiac pacemakers and its safety in patients with implanted cardiac pacemakers. PACE 11:1607, 1988.
176. Vassolas G, Roth RA, Venditti FJ Jr: Effect of extracorporeal shock wave lithotripsy on implantable cardioverter defibrillator. PACE 16:1245, 1993.
177. Kufer R, Thamasett S, Wolkmer B, et al: New-generation lithotripters for treatment of patients with implantable cardioverter-defibrillator: Experimental approach and review of the literature. J Endourol 15:479, 2001.
178. Drach GW, Weber C, Donovan JM: Treatment of pacemaker patients with extracorporeal shock wave lithotripsy: Experience from 2 continents. J Urol 143:895, 1990.
179. Albers DD, Lybrand III FE, Axton JC, et al: Shockwave lithotripsy and pacemakers: Experience with 20 cases. J Endourol 9:301, 1995.
180. Chung MK, Streem SB, Ching E, et al: Effects of extracorporeal shock wave lithotripsy on tiered therapy implantable cardioverter defibrillators. PACE 22:738, 1999.
181. Vaidyanathan S, Hirst R, Parsons KF, et al: Bilateral extracorporeal shock wave lithotripsy in a spinal cord injury patient with a cardiac pacemaker. Spinal Cord 39:286, 2001.
182. Bohay RN, Bencak J, Kavaliers M, Maclean D: A survey of magnetic fields in the dental operatory. J Can Dent Assoc 60:835, 1994.
183. Trenter SC, Waimsley AD: Ultrasonic dental scaler: Associated hazards. J Clin Periodontol 30:905, 2003.
184. Garofalo R, Ede EN, Dorn SO, et al: Effect of electronic apex locators on cardiac pacemaker function. J Endodontics 28:831, 2002.
185. Beach CW, Bramwell JD, Hutter JW: Use of an electronic apex locator on a cardiac pacemaker patient. J Endodontics 22:182, 1996.
186. Hiller H, Weissberg N, Horowitz G, et al: The safety of dental mini-magnets in patients with permanent cardiac pacemakers. J Prosthet Dent 74:420, 1995.
187. Last A: Radiotherapy in patients with cardiac pacemakers. Br J Radiol 71:4, 1998.
188. Guidant Technical Services Fact Sheet. Impact of Therapeutic Radiation and Guidant ICD/CRT-D/(RT-P/Pacing Systems). Revision Nov. 5, 2004. Available upon request from Guidant Technical Service, St. Paul, Minn.
189. Mouton J, Haug R, Bridier A, et al: Influence of high-energy photon beam irradiation on pacemaker operation. Phys Med Biol 47:2879, 2002.
190. Hurkmans CW, Scheepers E, Springorum BG, et al: Influence of therapeutic irradiation on the latest generation of pacemakers [abstract]. Heart Rhythm 1:S53, 2005.
191. Uiterwall GJ, Hurkmans CW, Springorum BF, et al: Interference signals detection by implantable defibrillators inducted by therapeutic radiation therapy. Heart Rhythm 1:S78, 2005.
192. Uiterwall GJ, Springorum BF, Scheepers E, et al: Influence of therapeutic irradiation on the latest generation of implantable cardioverters/defibrillators. Europace 6(Suppl 1):96, 2004.
193. Hoecht S, Rosenthal P, Sancar D, et al: Implantable cardiac defibrillators may be damaged by radiation therapy [letter]. J Clin Oncol 20:2212, 2002.
194. Marbach JR, Sontag MR, Van Dyk J, et al: Management of radiation oncology patients with implanted cardiac pacemakers: Report of AAPM Task Group No. 34. Med Phys 21:85, 1994.
195. Solan AN, Solan MJ, Bednarz G, et al: Treatment of patients with cardiac pacemakers and implantable cardioverter-defibrillators during radiotherapy. Int J Radiat Oncol Biol Phys 59:897, 2004.

Chapter 29

Pediatric Pacing and Defibrillator Use

GERALD A. SERWER • SARAH S. LEROY

Permanent cardiac pacemakers have been used in children for more than 30 years.[1] Their use has expanded as a result of advances in pacemaker technology that permit greater customization of the pacemaker to the patient and a smaller generator size coupled with increased generator longevity. Although many aspects of pediatric pacing are similar to their counterparts in adult pacing, major differences exist. Not only are children physically smaller than adults, but also their underlying cardiac diseases are different. Their expected longevity, together with the lives that these children lead, are different. As a consequence, differences exist, not only in selection of the optimal pacing system but also in implantation techniques, programming considerations, and follow-up methods.

With advances in medical and surgical therapy for structural heart disease, longevity is increasing. As a consequence, patients with congenital heart disease are reaching adulthood. This chapter, although focused on pediatric pacing, truly deals with the patient of any age who has structural heart disease. Adolescents and adults with structural heart disease, many having undergone surgical repair, present unique problems that are more similar to those of the younger child than to those of an adult with acquired cardiac disease. In our center, we care for patients with devices ranging from newborns through middle adult life. Much of the experience cited here includes such adults, and many of the therapy decisions presented apply to structural congenital disease in all age groups.

Few pacemakers and only a limited number of electrodes are designed specifically with congenital heart patients in mind, and these tend to be "scaled down" versions of existing units. As a consequence, the manner in which devices are used often requires modifications from the standard practice employed in patients with acquired disease. This chapter discusses the unique aspects of this patient group, specifically focusing on pacing indications, electrode and generator selection, implantation techniques, follow-up considerations and methods, and adjustments to the patient's lifestyle, particularly in children, that are necessitated by device implantation. Much of the material presented in other chapters is equally applicable to this group, and therefore this chapter is intended as a supplement rather than a replacement for chapters dealing with similar material.

The expanding use of implantable cardioverter-defibrillators (ICDs), antitachycardia pacing, and resynchronization therapy in patients with congenital heart disease is also discussed in this chapter. Although the use of such devices is limited, they are finding increasing usefulness, especially as their size decreases and newer features are developed. Because of differing causes of tachyarrhythmias and ventricular dysfunction, as well as differing cardiac anatomy, there are differences in the manner of their use that must be considered in congenital heart patients.

Midwest Pediatric Pacemaker Registry

Because the number of congenital heart patients requiring pacemakers is small, one difficulty plaguing research in this area has been the lack of a large experience at any one center. This has led to conclusions based on limited experience that are susceptible to statistical inaccuracies. To address this problem, the Midwest Pediatric Pacemaker Registry (MPPR) was formed as a voluntary project of the members of the Midwest Pediatric Cardiology Society in 1980. Member institutions of this society submit data on patients who require pacemaker implantation, consisting of patient demographics, pacing indication, associated structural cardiac disease, type of generator, type of electrode and threshold data at implantation, and device explantation data. No chronic follow-up data are provided. To promote the submission and validity of the data, annual reports are presented to the Midwest Pediatric Cardiology Society at its annual meeting. Concerns about the types of data collected and the methods of data acquisition are discussed to ensure uniformity among participating institutions.

To date, the Registry contains information on more than 1100 patients who have had implantations of more than 1500 pulse generators and more than 1600 electrodes. These data present a representative sample of current pacing practices among pediatric cardiologists and avoid the bias inherent in data obtained from a single institution. The data are obtained at the time of implantation and at subsequent invasive electrode evaluation (Table 29-1) presents a summary of the data collected. Chronic follow-up data are confined to the date and reason that a generator or electrode was removed from service. Noninvasive electrode threshold data and reprogramming information after implantation are not collected. The Registry collects no ICD data. Throughout this chapter, much of the information presented on pacing indications, device selection, and acute thresholds was obtained from this source.

TABLE 29-1. **Information Collected by the Midwest Pediatric Pacemaker Registry***

Patient demographics
ID number and institution
Date of birth
Date of initial implantation
Pacing indication
Associated structural cardiac disease
Generator information
Manufacturer and model
Implantation date
Programming at implantation
Explantation date
Programming at explantation
Electrode information
Manufacturer and model
Implantation site and route
Pacing thresholds (multiple pulse widths)
Sensing values (RMS amplitude, slew rate)

ID, identification; RMS, mean spontaneous waveform amplitude.
*The data are collected on all new patients entered in the Registry; all generators implanted and explanted; and all electrodes implanted, explanted, or invasively tested.

Indications for Permanent Pacemaker Implantation

Sinus Node Dysfunction

Historically, the most common indication for pacemaker placement was surgically induced heart block. As surgical techniques have improved and the patients have survived longer after cardiac surgery, this has changed. Often occurring many years after surgical repair, the most common indication for cardiac pacing in patients with congenital heart disease is now sinus node dysfunction or sick sinus syndrome. Since 2000, this indication has accounted for 40% to 60% of new implantations, compared with 20% to 25% during the previous decade. Most of these patients have undergone cardiac surgery many years previously, usually involving extensive atrial procedures. The single most common surgical procedure is the atrial switch operation for transposition of the great arteries.[2] The likelihood of needing permanent pacing in this situation increases with the time since surgery.[3] With increased use of the Fontan or right heart bypass procedure, the incidence of sinus node dysfunction is increasing. The indications are similar to those for congenital complete heart block. In addition, the presence of tachyarrhythmias, with the subsequent risk for prolonged asystole after acute termination of the tachycardia, is also an indication for pacemaker implantation (see Fig. 29-3). In patients with sinus node dysfunction after cardiac surgery, our practice is to recommend pacemaker implantation in all of those with a sleeping heart rate of less than 30 beats/min (bpm) even in the absence of symptoms, a decreasing exercise tolerance with inadequate heart rate increase with exercise (see later discussion), or sinus pauses for longer than 3 to 4 seconds. The need for medications known to affect atrioventricular (AV) conduction for the control of tachyarrhythmias in these patients would also necessitate pacemaker placement.[3]

Surgically Induced Heart Block

The next largest indication for pacemaker implantation in children is surgically induced heart block, which

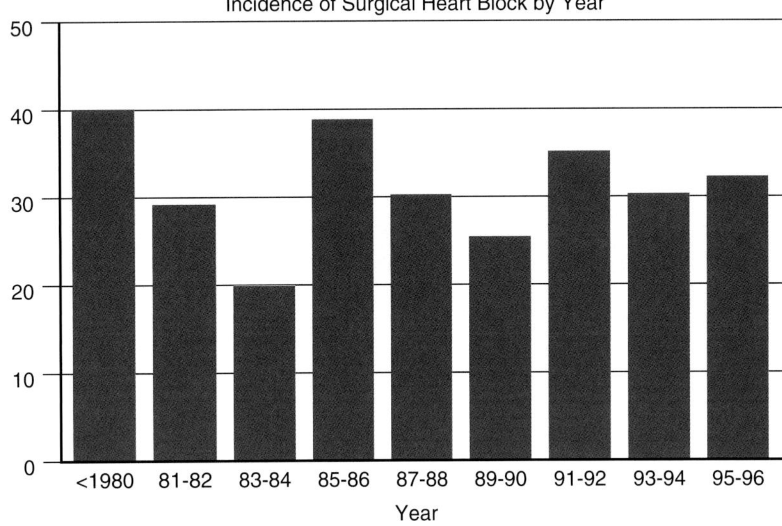

Figure 29-1. The percentage of all children undergoing initial pacemaker implantation in a given period whose indication was surgically induced complete heart block. There has been no significant change in this percentage during the last 16 years. (Data from the Midwest Pediatric Pacemaker Registry.)

classically has accounted for 30% to 40% of children undergoing pacemaker implantation.[4-9] Data from the MPPR show the indication for initial pacemaker placement to be surgically induced heart block in an average of 35% of patients (Fig. 29-1) before 2000. The percentage varies from year to year and reached a low of 20% in 2000. There has been no definite downward trend since 2000, although the underlying structural cardiac diseases in patients with surgically induced heart block have changed dramatically. Since 2000, surgical heart block has accounted for 15% to 30% of initial implantations. Most children acquiring surgical heart block in the last 5 years have had complex disease and have undergone complex surgical repairs. The surgical procedure resulting in the greatest incidence of heart block is the repair of atrioventricular septal defect, which has accounted for 17% of patients with surgical heart block since 1988. The other common diagnoses associated with surgical heart block during the past 5 years are listed in Table 29-2.

Currently, it is unusual for a child with an isolated ventricular septal defect (VSD) to acquire heart block. This was not the case previously. Since 1988, VSD closure has accounted for only 14% of children with surgical complete heart block; atrial switch procedures (Mustard or Senning procedure) for the correction of dextrotransposition of the great arteries have accounted for 12%. Other common lesions associated with surgical heart block are levotransposition of the great arteries, repair of tetralogy of Fallot, and aortic valvular replacement, which usually is associated with the resection of a subaortic obstruction.

Surgical heart block can develop at the time of the initial cardiac repair or at some later point. In addition, the heart block acquired at the time of the repair may be temporary, with return of reliable AV conduction. For this reason, our current practice is to implant only temporary pacing electrodes at the time of the initial surgery and to defer permanent pacemaker implantation for 10 to 14 days in the hope of a return of AV conduction. However, ventricular escape rhythms are unstable, and no child with a permanent surgically acquired complete heart block is discharged without a permanent pacemaker. Even in the hospital, all children are supported with an external pacemaker through temporary pacing wires placed at the time of surgery until consistent AV conduction returns or a permanent pacemaker is inserted. Monitoring should consist of both electrocardiographic (ECG) monitoring and non-ECG monitoring, such as arterial pressure measurements or pulse oximetry. Many ECG monitors detect the pacing artifact and do not recognize the lack of capture with subsequent bradycardia or asystole. This is avoided by the use of a non-ECG method of detecting cardiac ejection, such as pulse oximetry.[10]

TABLE 29-2. Most Prevalent Structural Cardiac Defects Associated with Surgically Induced Complete Heart Block*

Defect	Percentage of Cases
Atrioventricular septal defects	17
Isolated ventricular septal defect	14
Dextrotransposition of the great arteries	12
Levotransposition of the great arteries	12
Tetralogy of Fallot	7
Aortic valve replacement	3

*The most common structural cardiac lesions associated with surgically induced heart block at the time of complete repair for children undergoing initial implantation since 1988.

Data from the Midwest Pediatric Pacemaker Registry.

Congenital Complete Heart Block

The next most common indication for pacemaker implantation is congenital complete heart block. The cause of congenital heart block varies. In many cases, an autoimmune mechanism is implicated, with clinical or laboratory evidence of connective tissue disease in the mother.[11] Congenital heart block is also associated with specific forms of structural disease, particularly those involving abnormalities of the AV junction, such as levotransposition of the great arteries with AV discordance and atrial situs ambiguous.[12] It is common for fetal heart block to "develop" in utero with intact conduction present in the young fetus and heart block developing at 20 to 30 weeks of gestation.

Data from the MPPR indicate that 10% to 25% of patients have congenital heart block as the primary indication for permanent pacing. The age at which the pacing system is implanted varies, ranging from a few hours to more than 20 years. Most children with associated structural cardiac disease who need pacing before 1 year of age have congestive heart failure requiring an increased heart rate for adequate therapy. The mortality rate in such children is also high, with 43% dying by 2 years of age.[13]

For children with structurally normal hearts and congenital heart block, the incidence of pacemaker implantation is lower in younger children but increases with age, associated with a gradually decreasing ventricular rate.[14] The gradual and steady increase in the need for permanent pacing continues with advancing age, reaching 75% by age 20 years (Fig. 29-2). The need for permanent pacing results from the development of syncope, congestive heart failure, or increasing ventricular ectopy, often associated with prolongation of the corrected QT interval (QTc). Death is rare in children with no structural cardiac disease (only 5% by 20 years of age), but it can occur suddenly.

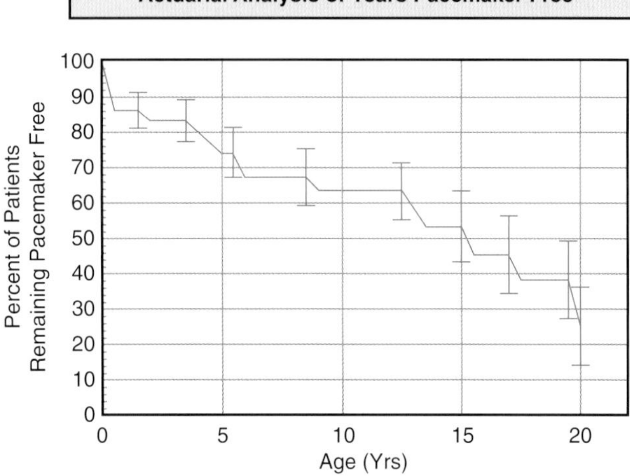

Figure 29-2. Actuarial analysis of months free from pacemaker need for children with congenital complete heart block and structurally normal hearts. By age 20 years, fewer than 30% of patients are pacemaker free. The brackets represent 1 standard error around the mean. (Data from Dorostkar P, Serwer GA, LeRoy S, Dick M II: Long-term course of children and young adults with congenital complete heart block. J Am Coll Cardiol 21:295A, 1993.)

Current recommendations call for the implantation of a permanent pacemaker system whenever congestive heart failure is present. In addition, implantation is recommended if the average heart rate is less than 50 bpm in the awake young infant, if there is a history of a syncopal or presyncopal event, if significant ventricular ectopy is present, or if there is exercise intolerance.[15,16] However, symptoms of exercise intolerance can be difficult to elicit. Many children deny such symptoms, as do their parents, when in fact their exercise tolerance would be improved with permanent pacing. Many parents return after pacemaker implantation to relate that the activity level of their child has markedly increased. They are amazed at this change, because they did not believe that the child was significantly hindered before pacemaker implantation. Exercise testing is often useful as an indicator of the child's exercise capabilities compared with those of a normal child. The physician should also periodically assess the child for increasing cardiac size by chest radiography and for decreasing cardiac function by echocardiography. The presence of either of these conditions should be considered an indication for permanent pacemaker placement.

Finally, some children with congenital complete heart block develop tachydysrhythmias, specifically ventricular tachycardia, which can be controlled only with permanent pacing.[17] The maintenance of a minimal heart rate often suppresses the tendency toward ventricular ectopy, particularly during exercise. The development of tachyarrhythmias with the stress of exercise, even in children with otherwise asymptomatic disease, necessitates pacemaker implantation (Fig. 29-3).

Controversy exists regarding the need for pacing in symptom-free older children with bradycardia of less than 50 bpm while asleep. This is not an absolute indication for pacemaker implantation. However, if bradycardias lower than 50 bpm are present, a detailed history and close follow-up are required to determine the need for pacemaker implantation.

Other Indications

Patients with intermittent complete heart block, either secondary to lesions such as cardiac rhabdomyomas associated with tuberous sclerosis (Fig. 29-4) or idiopathic, and those with long QT syndrome and uncontrollable ventricular tachycardia may also benefit from pacemaker placement.[18] A chronic increase in heart rate shortens the QT interval and decreases the occurrence of ventricular tachycardia. The combined use of pacing and an ICD may be even more efficacious, particularly with the advent of the dual-chamber ICD.

Other indications for pacemaker placement reported in the MPPR include the need for control of atrial tachyarrhythmias unresponsive to pharmacologic therapy, second-degree heart block associated with symptoms, and concern about a sudden loss of AV conduction in patients receiving certain antiarrhythmic therapies known to interfere with AV conduction. Although such indications are rare, the clinician should not restrict pacemaker use to those children with complete heart

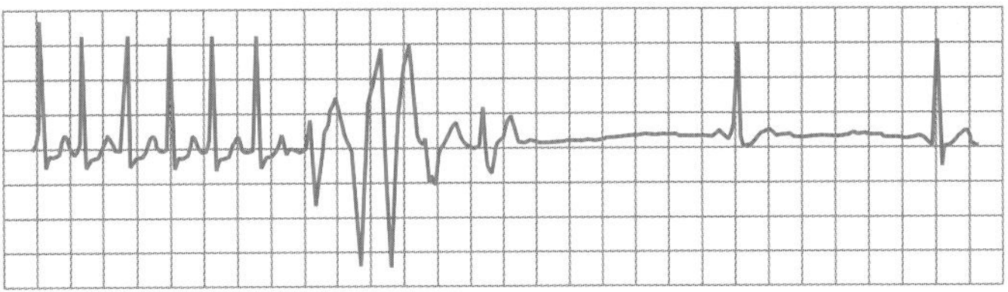

Figure 29-3. Electrocardiogram from a patient with sick sinus syndrome, demonstrating a 1.5-second period of asystole after acute termination of a tachyarrhythmia. Long pauses can result in syncope and are indications for pacemaker implantation. The paper speed is 25 mm/sec.

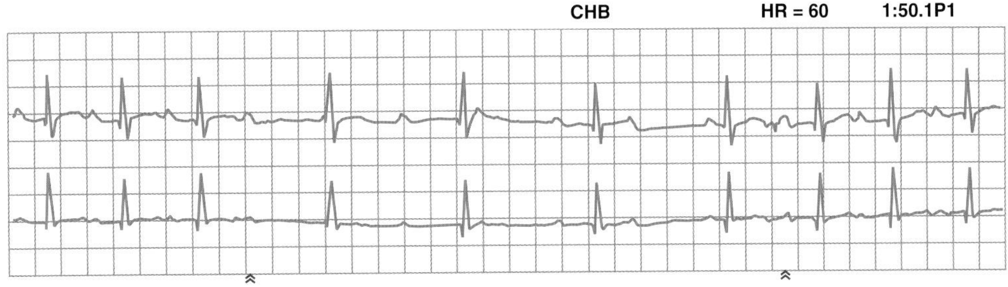

Figure 29-4. Recording from a 24-hour ambulatory electrocardiogram showing a period of complete heart block (CHB) with acute bradycardia (between the arrowheads) in a patient with tuberous sclerosis and cardiac rhabdomyomas. The paper speed is 25 mm/sec. HR, heart rate (in beats per minute).

block. First-degree heart block and trifascicular block with no documented loss of AV conduction are not considered indications for pacemaker implantation.[19]

A relatively controversial indication for pacemaker placement is symptomatic hypertrophic obstructive cardiomyopathy with significant outflow tract obstruction. Although pacemaker placement is not effective in all children with this disorder, both hemodynamic and symptomatic improvements have been observed,[20] with decreases in gradient and measures of diastolic performance. Generators used for this indication must allow programming of relatively short AV intervals and rate-adaptive AV intervals to maximize the QRS width and degree of preexcitation. Younger patients with more rapid heart rates may present insurmountable difficulties.

Categorization of pacing indications is helpful only as a general guide. Each patient must be carefully evaluated to determine the potential benefits from permanent pacing in light of the risks of implantation and the burden placed on the family and child for the subsequent care needed. When all patients in need of pacing are considered together, the indication most often present is sinus node dysfunction. The largest group of patients requiring pacing are those with dextro-transposition of the great arteries, most of whom have undergone an atrial switch procedure (Mustard or Senning procedure) for sinus node dysfunction.

Selection of the Appropriate Pacemaker System

Many factors must be considered in the selection of the most appropriate pacemaker generator and electrode system. Unlike that in the adult patient, the 5-year sur-

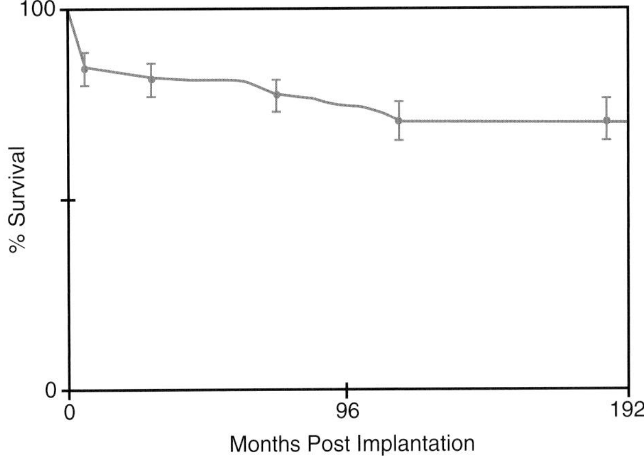

Figure 29-5. Actuarial survival for pediatric patients after pacemaker implantation. Excellent patient longevity is demonstrated. The brackets represent 1 standard error around the estimate. (From Serwer GA, Mericle JM: Evaluation of pacemaker pulse generator and patient longevity in patients aged 1 day to 20 years. Am J Cardiol 59:824, 1987.)

vival rate after pacemaker implantation in children exceeds 70% (Fig. 29-5), and death is usually related to the underlying structural heart defect.[8,21] Therefore, pacing may be needed for more than 50 years in the average child. This affects pacing choices, because the number of replacement generators and electrodes may be high. The average longevity of currently available lithium-powered pulse generators is only 5 years when all children are grouped together (Fig. 29-6). However, when children are divided into those younger and older than 4 years of age at the time of generator implantation, longevity is markedly different (Fig. 29-7). The generator half-life is 5 years for children younger than 4 years of age at implantation and increases to 7 years

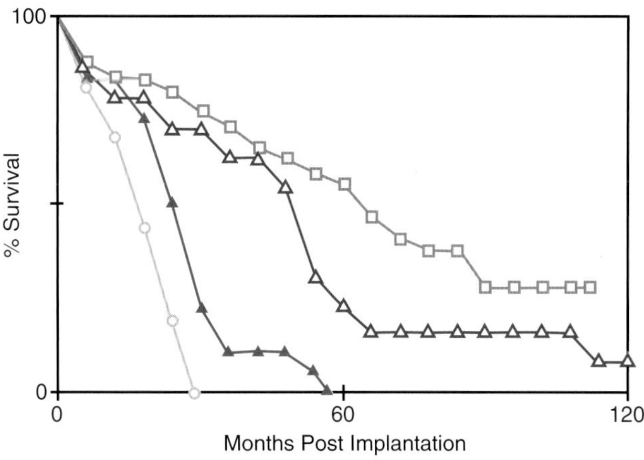

Figure 29-6. Actuarial survival curve for generators using various battery types. Even for lithium-powered generators, only one half last 5 years. Open squares, *current models using lithium batteries;* open triangles, *models using mercury-zinc batteries;* filled triangles, *models using mercury-silver batteries;* open circles, *models using rechargeable batteries. (From Serwer GA, Mericle JM: Evaluation of pacemaker pulse generator and patient longevity in patients aged 1 day to 20 years. Am J Cardiol 59:824, 1987.)*

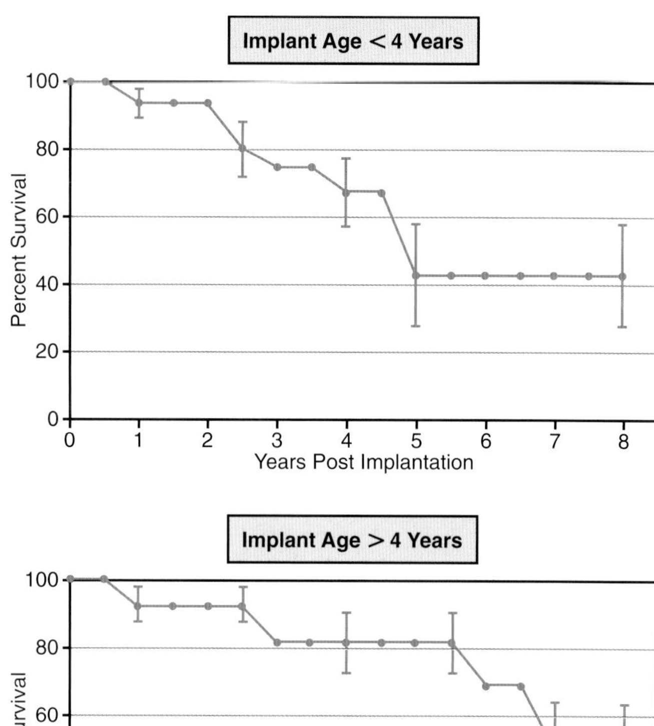

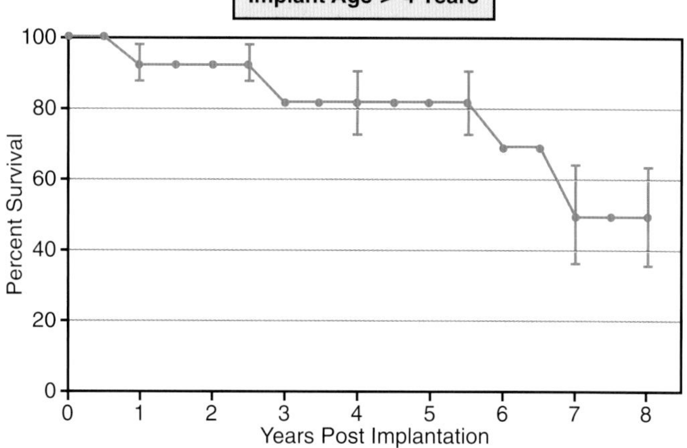

Figure 29-7. DDD generator longevity with the use of epicardial electrodes as a function of patient age at the time of implantation. ***A,*** *Life table analysis of longevity when devices are implanted in children younger than 4 years of age. More than one half require replacement within 5 years.* ***B,*** *Longevity analysis when implant age is greater than 4 years. Half-life has risen to 6.5 years, presumably because of the lower average heart rate in older children.*

for the older children. This is presumably a result of the higher heart rates present in younger patients, when the device is used in dual-chamber mode to track the atrial rate, or of the higher programmed rates used in younger children.

The average epicardial electrode lasts 7 years.[22] With improvements in epicardial electrode design, it is hoped that this will increase. Although the average endocardial electrode's longevity in children is significantly increased, it is still only slightly more than 10 years (Fig. 29-8).[23] For the child undergoing an initial implantation at age 1 year, a minimum of 9 electrode changes and 17 generator changes can be expected. The fact that multiple procedures will be needed and the effects of one procedure on subsequent procedures must be considered.

Generator Selection

The major factors to be considered must be the features of the generator that are of significant benefit to the individual child, battery capacity coupled with projected generator longevity, and the size of the generator. Because newer generators are smaller than earlier ones, size is becoming less of a factor; yet not all generators are the same size. Large generators not only create unsightly protuberances that can have negative psychological consequences but also increase the risk for skin breakdown over the generator due to erosion of the generator or trauma to the skin over the generator, especially in the active child, with a subsequent infection leading to pacing system removal.

Generator Mode Selection

The choices concerning pacing mode are related to single-chamber versus dual-chamber pacing and fixed-rate versus variable-rate pacing. In general, it has been our policy to avoid the use of fixed-rate pacemakers, except in situations in which sinus node and AV node function are intact most of the time, with the pacemaker serving only as a backup for those rare periods when such function is not adequate. This is often the situation when sinoatrial (SA) and AV node function is marginal and antiarrhythmic drugs are required. Even in these cases, generators capable of rate-variable operation are preferable, because the electrophysiologic state may change, and these models allow for a change in mode without replacement of the generator. In addition, should a sudden rate drop occur during exercise, the lower rate of a fixed-rate generator may be inadequate to provide adequate cardiac output. There is no difference in size or capacity of the battery between fixed-rate and rate-variable units. All available generators today have rate-response capabilities.

Although cardiac output increases with exercise, even during fixed-rate pacing (Fig. 29-9), this occurs as

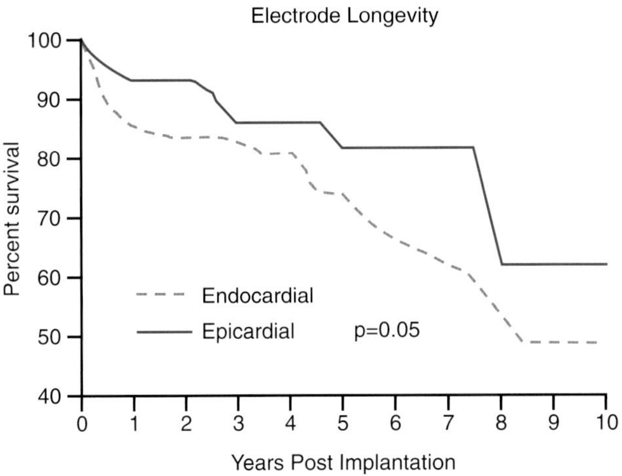

Figure 29-8. Actuarial analysis of endocardial (solid line) *and epicardial* (dashed line) *electrode survival. One half of epicardial electrodes last about 8 years; for endocardial electrodes, the 50% survival time is greater than 10 years. The curves are significantly different (P = .05). (Epicardial electrode data from Serwer GA, Mericle JM, Armstrong BE: Epicardial ventricular pacemaker electrode longevity in children. Am J Cardiol 61:104, 1988; endocardial electrode data from Serwer G, Uzark K, Dick M II: Endocardial pacing and electrode longevity in children. J Am Coll Cardiol 15:212A, 1990.)*

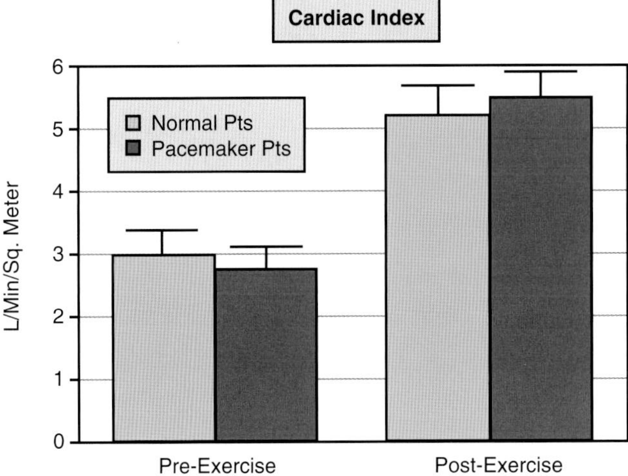

Figure 29-9. Changes in cardiac index as measured by acetylene rebreathing from rest to maximal exercise in normal children and in children with fixed-rate ventricular pacing. The cardiac indices were identical at rest and at maximal exercise. The brackets represent 1 standard error around the mean. Pts, patients. (Data from Serwer G, Dick M II, Eakin B: Cardiac output response to treadmill exercise in children with fixed-rate pacemakers. Circulation 84:II-514, 1991. By permission of the American Heart Association, Inc.)

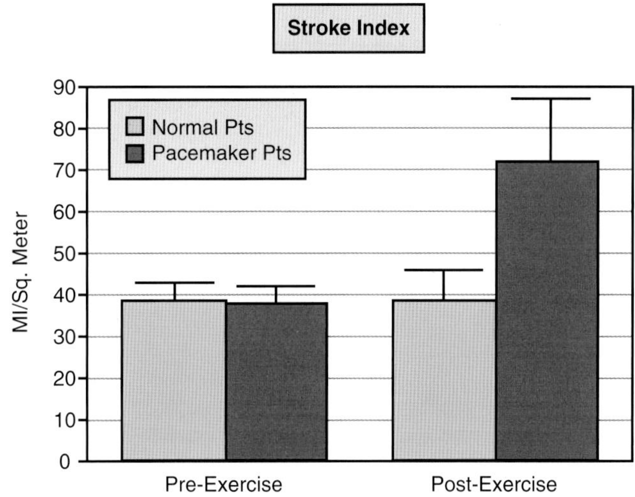

Figure 29-10. Stroke index changes from rest to maximal exercise in normal children and in children with fixed-rate ventricular pacemakers. Pre-exercise values were similar. With exercise, the stroke index increased significantly in the patients with pacemakers to provide an increased output in the face of a fixed heart rate. The brackets represent 1 standard error around the mean. Pts, patients. (Data from Serwer G, Dick M II, Eakin B: Cardiac output response to treadmill exercise in children with fixed-rate pacemakers. Circulation 84:II-514, 1991. By permission of the American Heart Association, Inc.)

a result of a large increase in stroke volume (Fig. 29-10), with presumed increased wall stress and potentially increased myocardial work compared with the same change in cardiac output when a heart rate increase is possible.[24] However, enhanced exercise tolerance is achieved when rate-variable pacing is used.[25] This suggests an advantage to rate-variable pacing in the child who is expected to lead an active life. The rate-responsive mode should always be used unless the patient can demonstrate an adequate intrinsic rate response to exercise by exercise testing or ambulatory ECG.

Single-chamber pacing in either the atrium or the ventricle has been advocated for the treatment of sick sinus syndrome.[15] When atrial pacing is chosen, the presence of normal AV node function must be established by provocative electrophysiologic testing before implantation, especially in the postsurgical patient, because AV nodal disease can accompany SA nodal disease and may not be apparent in the resting, nonprovoked state. AAI(R) pacing has the advantage of preserving the normal ventricular activation sequence with potentially better cardiovascular function. In addition, some evidence in animals points toward the long-term development of myocardial changes when an abnormal pattern of myocardial activation is present.[26] A comparison of cardiac myocyte changes in ventricular free wall pacing versus high septal pacing near the bundle of His, which has a narrower QRS morphology, is striking; the clinical implication of these changes is unknown.[26a]

Atrial electrodes are less reliable than ventricular electrodes, even when they are placed endocardially. Therefore, conditions associated with early atrial electrode failure should serve as a contraindication to AAI pacing. Such conditions include prior extensive atrial surgery in which extensive atrial fibrosis is likely, small atrial size, and prior placement of a large intra-atrial baffle, limiting venous access to viable atrial tissue. After a Fontan procedure (right atrial to pulmonary artery connection), patients also have a low-flow velocity present within the atrium, increasing the risk for venous thrombosis when endocardial electrodes are placed. This is one situation in which long-term anticoagulation may be indicated. In addition, the amount of excitable tissue that can be accessed from a transvenous approach may be limited. Most Fontan procedures today use either a lateral tunnel created along the lateral right atrial wall, limiting this area for pacemaker placement, or an extracardiac conduit, in which case no atrial tissue is accessible.

Single-chamber ventricular pacing, or VVI(R), allows the use of more stable electrode systems and, in the rate-responsive mode, still allows rate variability to be maintained. The importance of atrial systole in the maintenance of cardiac output is debatable and varies from child to child. Because most children have good myocardial function, the atrial contribution is probably minimal. The cardiac output increase with exercise is improved in children with DDD versus VVI pacing. It is unclear, however, whether this increase is the result of atrial synchrony or rate variability. Pacemaker syndrome from VVIR pacing is uncommon but can occur, especially over time. In one series, 19 of 33 patients developed symptoms suggestive of pacemaker syndrome over time (median, 11 years) that resolved with upgrading to dual-chamber pacing.[27] The major factor to be considered in such a choice is the difficulty in placing an adequate atrial electrode. If prior surgery or underlying structural disease precludes atrial electrode placement, single-chamber pacing is an acceptable alternative. However, dual-chamber pacing should be considered for all patients, with single-chamber pacing used only if contraindications to dual-chamber pacing (as discussed later) exist. Even in patients with sinus node dysfunction, dual-chamber pacing should be considered, particularly if AV nodal function is suspect.

We now consider dual-chamber pacing to be the mode of choice in children, and we use single-chamber pacing only if a contraindication to dual-chamber pacing exists and in some small infants in whom cardiac surgery will be needed in the immediate future, with an upgrade to dual-chamber pacing performed at that time. The major contraindications to the use of dual-chamber pacing are (1) persistent atrial tachyarrhythmias; (2) changing AV nodal status, making numerous programming changes necessary; and (3) inability to place reliable atrial and ventricular electrodes. An example of this last contraindication is the small child in whom endocardial pacing is preferred, but the presence of two electrodes in the superior vena cava might present a high risk for thrombosis. Another example is the child who requires epicardial electrode placement in whom atrial electrode placement would necessitate a greatly enhanced surgical procedure. It must be remembered that rate sensors do not function in nonambulatory infants. Therefore, in young infants, single-chamber pacing becomes fixed-rate pacing. The generator's size and functionality are no longer considerations, because dual- and single-chamber pacemakers are comparable in both regards. Table 29-3 relates the most common reasons for not implanting a dual-chamber system.

TABLE 29-3. Contraindications to Dual-Chamber Pacing in Children

Inability to place both an atrial and a ventricular electrode
Small patient size
Limited venous access
Extensive epicardial fibrosis
Persistent atrial tachyarrhythmia
Uncontrolled atrial flutter
Arrhythmia easily triggered by atrial pacing
Pacemaker inability to detect atrial arrhythmia and limit ventricular rate
Changing electrophysiologic status of atrioventricular conduction

Dual-chamber pacing in children has previously been underused. MPPR data show a significant increase in dual-chamber pacing, with 43% of generators implanted in 1991 to 1992 using the DDD or DDDR mode, increasing to a majority (68%) of implantations by 1995 to 1996, and with a further increase, to more than 80%, since 2000. This is in marked contrast to the years before 1983, when fewer than 10% of generators were in the DDD mode (Fig. 29-11). This increase in dual-chamber pacing has been the result of improvements in atrial epicardial electrodes, increased experience with endocardial pacing in children, the smaller size of dual-chamber generators, and a better understanding of the benefits of dual-chamber pacing.

Desirable Generator Features

Current pacemakers permit an almost infinite number of possible programming combinations, allowing far more programming possibilities than will ever be used in any given patient. Because of the diversity of patients with congenital heart disease, however, such programmability is necessary. There are certain features that are more important for children than for adults. This section discusses those programming features considered to be essential, which should influence the choice of the most appropriate pacing generator for a given patient. The discussion begins with those features that are applicable to all generators, both single- and dual-chamber, and then covers features that are unique to rate-responsive pacemakers and dual-chamber pacemakers.

General Characteristics

The most important consideration is related to the range of energy output available, which includes both the pulse width and the pulse amplitude programmability. Although most pacemakers are chronically programmed to have either 2.5 or 5 V of amplitude, the presence of other amplitudes is of key importance. Specifically, when a generator is used with an epicardial electrode, high-output features are mandatory. Although only a minority of children require chronic pacing at outputs greater than 5 V, many children have

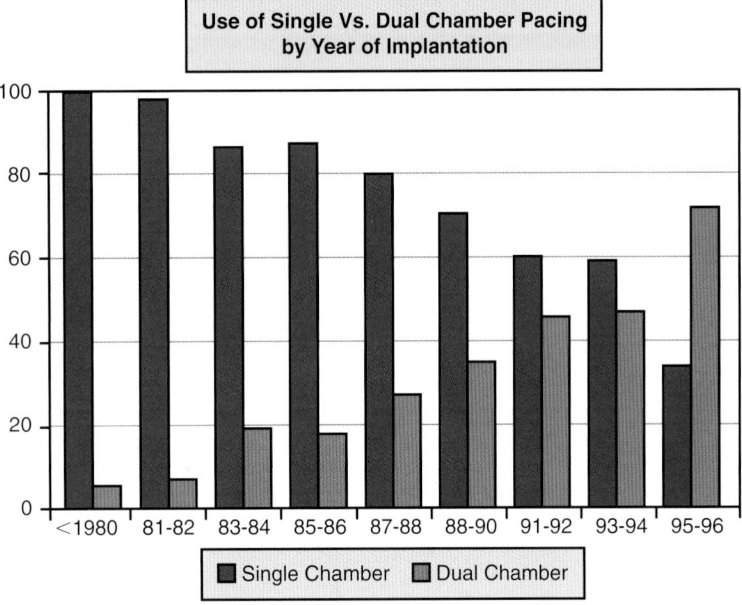

Figure 29-11. Comparison of the percentage of dual-chamber versus single-chamber generators implanted by year. Note the gradual shift from single-chamber to dual-chamber use. (Data from the Midwest Pediatric Pacemaker Registry.)

an initial threshold rise and temporarily require such high outputs. Even with endocardial implants, acute increases in threshold can occur, and the ability to increase the pacemaker amplitude to values greater than 5 V may avert the necessity for emergency electrode replacement. In addition, threshold testing at multiple low-pulse amplitudes allows a more accurate determination of the characteristics of the strength-duration curve. This testing is mandatory to determine the lowest, but still safe, pulse amplitude and width settings. The strength-duration curve characteristics are not constant; they vary not only with time but also in relation to activity and the time of day.[28] Such changes are discussed more fully in the consideration of appropriate follow-up. Knowing where the steep part of the strength-duration curve begins is crucial for appropriate programming, in which the clinician wants to ensure an adequate safety margin but at the same time minimize the energy output, to maximize the generator's longevity. The ability to determine thresholds at a multitude of pulse amplitudes is a necessity.

The same argument also applies to the ability to vary the duration of the pulse width. Again, although the pacemakers in most children are programmed to a relatively small number of pulse durations, the ability to choose from a much larger number of such settings increases the accuracy with which the clinician can characterize the strength-duration curve.

Newer pacemakers now have the ability to automatically determine the voltage threshold, either on a beat-to-beat basis or at predetermined intervals throughout the day, and then adjust the pulse amplitude within a predetermined range to minimize energy drain and potentially increase generator longevity. This is accomplished by looking for an evoked potential after the test pulse, within a predetermined window of time indicating myocardial depolarization. Initially, these pacemakers required special low-polarization electrodes to distinguish true evoked potentials from electrode polarization. Newer designs have improved this discrimination, and now this feature has been expanded to function with most types of electrodes. Some devices still require bipolar electrode systems, and some do not. Both endocardial electrodes[29] and epicardial electrodes[30,31] have been employed with newer devices. Once the voltage threshold has been determined, the amplitude is adjusted to a predetermined amount above the threshold value. Threshold data are saved in the pacemaker, and later interrogation can provide the clinician with the threshold trend over time. Such a feature has been extended to the atrium as well as the ventricle in some devices. Even if the clinician is reticent to allow automatic changes to the output parameters, use of the feature in a "monitor only" mode can provide information as to the long-term changes in threshold and the potential need for programming changes. This feature has the potential to increase generator longevity and decrease the number of pacemaker replacements needed.

The third parameter of key importance to children is the rate. Although the use of fixed-rate pacemakers is becoming less common, the availability of a wide range of both lower and upper pacing rate limits is important in meeting the varying metabolic demands of the patient with congenital heart disease. Programming the upper rate limit of dual-chamber or rate-responsive pacemakers to values of less than 150 bpm is inadequate, particularly in a small child. Even older patients can raise their heart rates well above this value when exercising maximally in the absence of heart block; therefore, pulse generators must provide an upper rate limit of at least 180 bpm, and preferably higher. Newer devices now provide a maximal upper rate of 210 bpm.

The lower rate limit needs are also variable. Immediately after surgery, greater lower rate limits are often necessary to maintain an adequate cardiac output. This

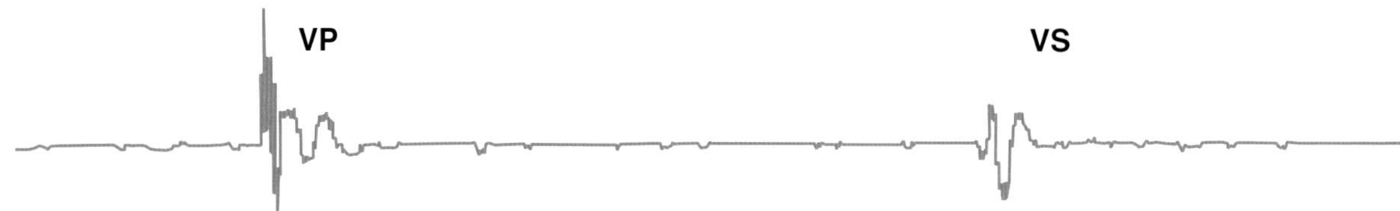

Figure 29-12. Intracardiac EGM from a patient with VVI pacing, showing the duration of the ventricular refractory period (dashed line) *after either ventricular pacing (VP) or sensing (VS). In this example, the ventricular refractory period extends well beyond the termination of electric activity seen by the electrode, to prevent inappropriate T-wave sensing.*

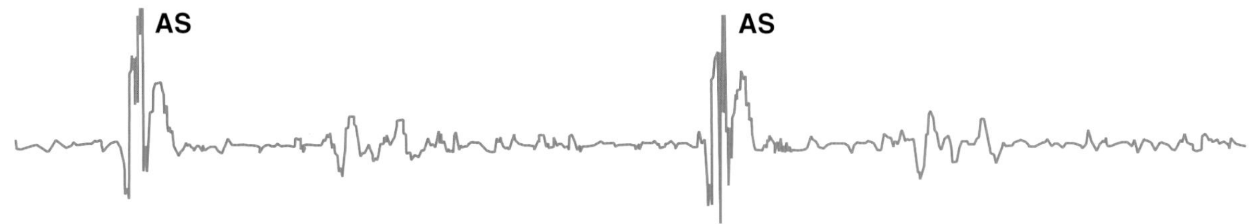

Figure 29-13. Intracardiac atrial EGM recorded from a patient with AAI pacing. The refractory period (dashed line) *must be long enough to prevent sensing of ventricular events by the atrial electrode. Note the marked increase in refractory period required compared with VVI pacing. When AAIR pacing is used, the length of this refractory period may significantly restrict the upper rate limit of the pacemaker.*

is especially important after atrial surgery for patients in whom sinus node function may be impaired. In our opinion, lower rates must be programmable from at least 50 to 120 bpm. Higher lower rates may also be needed to decrease the incidence of tachyarrhythmias.

Another parameter often overlooked is the refractory period. In single-chamber pacing, this is often fixed to an arbitrary value of 325 msec, without much thought being given to whether this value is appropriate. For the ventricular channel, the refractory period must be of sufficient duration to prevent inappropriate T-wave sensing and yet not prevent sensing of spontaneous ventricular depolarizations. The measurement of the pace or sensing point to the T-wave interval from the intracardiac electrogram (EGM) is straightforward (Fig. 29-12). In healthy children, the QT interval decreases with an increasing heart rate. When rate-variable pacing is used, the ventricular refractory period may be appropriate at rest but too long during exercise. Ideally, the period should vary with the pacing rate. Therefore, this value must be long enough to prevent T-wave sensing at the resting heart rate and short enough not to limit appropriate sensing at the upper pacing rate. It is not uncommon for children with complete heart block to have spontaneous ventricular beats during the stress of exercise, which must be appropriately sensed. Appropriate programming is discussed later. Again, the wider the range of available refractory periods that is permitted, the more universally applicable the pacemaker generator is to the entire pediatric population.

For AAI(R) pacing, the refractory period must be long enough to prevent sensing of ventricular events but again must not be too limiting in terms of the upper rate. Recording of the intracardiac EGM shows the extent to which ventricular events are seen by the pacemaker and the minimum value to which the atrial refractory period may be safely programmed (Fig. 29-13). Appropriate programming may be difficult and is a problem with AAI(R) pacing.

Rate-Responsive Pacing

For the single-chamber rate-responsive pacemaker, appropriate settings to mimic the pediatric response to exercise are mandatory. During exercise, the healthy child's heart rate increases in a linear manner with the increasing intensity of the exercise (Fig. 29-14).[32] When healthy children are exercised using the Bruce protocol, the heart rate increases an average of 20 bpm with each increase in exercise stage. This continues throughout the course of the exercise. After an abrupt increase in exercise intensity (i.e., by advancing from stage I to II), the heart rate shows a sudden rapid increase, reaching a plateau value. The child's pacemaker should increase its rate in an appropriate manner with increasing exercise intensity—and this must occur quickly, reaching a plateau value rapidly for that level of intensity. Therefore, not only must the heart rate increase to an appropriate degree, but also it must increase in an appropriate time frame to mimic the normal physiologic response to exercise in the pediatric patient.

After termination of exercise, the heart rate decreases in an exponential fashion (Fig. 29-15). Although there is an initial rapid drop, the heart rate does not reach resting levels for at least 10 minutes. Inappropriate rapid declines in heart rate after exercise termination may not meet the metabolic demands of the body and may result in inadequate cardiac output and a syncopal episode.

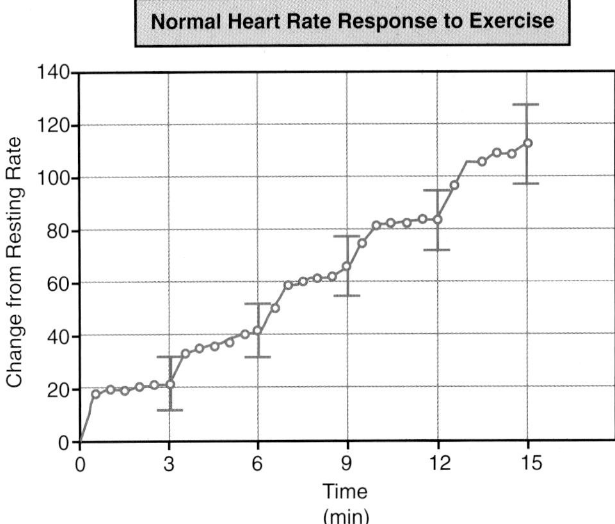

Figure 29-14. Normal heart rate increases from the resting value in normal children exercised using the Bruce treadmill protocol. The brackets represent 1 standard error around the estimate. (Data from Serwer GA, Uzark K, Beckman R, Dick M II: Optimal programming of rate altering parameters in children with rate-responsive pacemakers using graded treadmill exercise testing. PACE 13:542, 1990.)

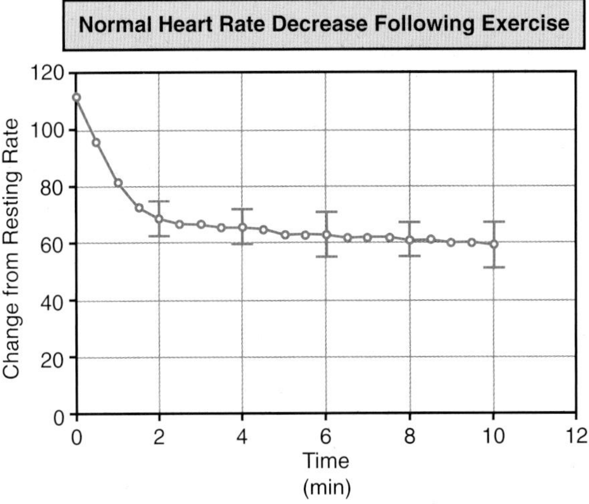

Figure 29-15. Normal heart rate decreases after exercise compared with the pre-exercise value in normal children. Even at 10 minutes after exercise, the heart rate has not yet reached the resting value. The brackets represent 1 standard error around the estimate. (Data from Serwer GA, Uzark K, Beckman R, Dick M II: Optimal programming of rate altering parameters in children with rate-responsive pacemakers using graded treadmill exercise testing. PACE 13:542, 1990.)

With these considerations of the normal heart rate response to exercise in children taken into account, the ideal rate-responsive pediatric pacemaker must have the ability to offer a variety of linear increases in heart rate with increasing exercise intensity (rate-response curves). In addition, it should offer a range of acceleration times (the rate of the heart rate increase with increased exercise intensity), with more rapid acceleration times being preferred. Such increases in heart rate should be independent of resting and maximal rates. After the termination of exercise, the heart rate decline should be exponential but slow enough that the lower rate limit is not reached for a minimum of 10 minutes. Finally, the pacemaker must be able to tailor its detection of increasing exercise levels to the individual patient. Different manufacturers have used several approaches to address this problem, and it is unclear which approach is best. However, all manufacturers allow tailoring of exercise detection to the individual patient, realizing that not all patients produce the same characteristics detectable by the pacemaker in response to the same degrees of exercise. Although simplicity in programming is desirable, the clinician must weigh against it the ability to tailor the pacemaker's settings and optimize its performance for a given patient.

Numerous types of sensors have been used, with the most common being activity (as a function of body vibration), blood temperature, and minute-ventilation. Body vibration sensing is the most useful in children because it does not require special electrodes and is not markedly different in the child than in the adult. Blood temperature and minute-ventilation sensing[33] have been used in children, but to a lesser degree.

Dual-Chamber Pacing

Not only do all the considerations discussed previously apply to dual-chamber pacing, but also additional programmable settings must be considered. The first is the ability to program an appropriate AV interval and to decrease it with increasing atrial rate. Such shortening of the AV interval with increasing atrial rate is clearly desirable in children and should occur with changes in the sensed atrial rate as well as with increases in the paced atrial rate during DDDR pacing. Because this decrease mimics the physiologic response more closely and provides a shorter total atrial refractory period at higher rates, the multiblock rate is higher. This is probably the most important feature of dual-chamber generator selection, because children often reach much higher atrial rates than do adults. If the total atrial refractory period is inappropriately long, multiblock occurs during the course of normal exercise, with a subsequent sudden decline in ventricular rate and the potential for syncope. It is common for children to reach atrial rates in excess of 180 bpm during routine exercise. Should the total atrial refractory period, of which the AV delay is a major part, be abnormally long, problems will occur.

In addition, multiple settings for the postventricular atrial refractory period (PVARP) also are considered desirable, because of its contribution to the total atrial refractory period (TARP) and, ultimately, to the multiblock rate. This parameter must have enough programmability to prevent inappropriate ventricular sensing by the atrial electrode while, at the same time, allowing a multiblock rate of at least 200 bpm (preferably 220 bpm), particularly in younger children. Many newer devices automatically decrease the PVARP with increasing rate to raise the multiblock rate. One should always check the minimal value to be sure it is short enough to provide an adequate multiblock rate. Also, one must be aware of the PVARP value at rest, to be sure it is not inappropriately long.

One closely allied feature that is mandatory is the ability to control the degree of PVARP extension after a spontaneous ventricular depolarization. An automatic extension of the PVARP after spontaneous ventricular depolarization is often used to prevent sensing of retrograde atrial activation, thus avoiding pacemaker-mediated tachycardia. This is not necessarily desirable in children, because the presence of retrograde-only ventriculoatrial conduction is rare and, therefore, the risk for pacemaker-mediated tachycardia is rare. With exercise, spontaneous ventricular depolarizations do occur, and if an inappropriate PVARP extension occurs, normal atrial depolarizations may not be sensed, resulting in a sudden overall decline in the heart rate. The ability to disable this feature must be present for the generator to be appropriate for use in children. This concern is discussed later in regard to the use of exercise testing in follow-up.

Other features that must be considered include the ability to lower the upper rate limit in the presence of atrial tachycardia. The occurrence of such rhythms, especially atrial flutter, is not uncommon, particularly in the postoperative patient. Another feature that may find usefulness is the ability to decrease the lower rate limit based on the time of day. Children, who tend to have a much more predictable schedule than adults, can benefit from having their pacemakers programmed to a lower pacing rate during sleep than during the daytime hours, when a higher heart rate may be needed. This is particularly useful for the child with sinus node disease, because the intrinsic atrial rate cannot be relied on to govern the paced ventricular rate. With an intact sinus node, one can simply set the pacing rate at an appropriately low level for sleep and rest, knowing that it will be at an appropriate rate during waking hours. If sinus node disease is present, however, this may not be the case, and the ability to vary the lower pacing rate with the time of day may be helpful, because this feature can lower the average daily rate and prolong the generator's life. This feature may also be helpful in the single-chamber rate-responsive pacemaker. The final feature now beginning to be introduced is the ability to temporarily extend the AV interval looking for AV conduction. If conduction is found, the AV delay can be lengthened. This is an attempt to promote AV conduction and limit unnecessary ventricular pacing.

Traditional factors that were once important in pediatric pacing, such as the generator's longevity and size, are now less of a concern in the selection of a generator. All generators are much smaller than previous models, and yet longevity has not been sacrificed. This is a consequence of improved circuit efficiency. The difference in size between single-chamber, dual-chamber, and rate-responsive pacemakers is often undetectable. Pediatric patients generally have long life expectancies, and the ability to have a highly programmable pacemaker implanted to meet changing metabolic demands as a consequence of growth, age, or patient desires is indispensable. The difference in cost between a highly programmable unit and one with fewer features is minimal, particularly when the cost is spread over the lifetime of the pacemaker. Table 29-4 summarizes the features that must be considered for the appropriate selection of a generator. The choice of a pacemaker should be based solely on the features it possesses and its ability to meet the demands of the patient.

TABLE 29-4. Desirable Generator Features in Pediatric Pacing

Highly programmable for mode, output, and AV intervals
Rate-responsive mode available
Diagnostic rate counters available
Performance indicators provided (battery voltage, battery current drain, electrode impedance)
Intracardiac electrograms provided
Automatic adjustments to changing status, such as a change in the upper rate limit with the onset of atrial tachyarrhythmias
Variable AV interval with increasing heart rate—either atrial or sensor driven

AV, atrioventricular.

Pacing Electrode Selection

There are many aspects to the choice of an appropriate electrode system in children. The first obvious choice is between the placement of an endocardial or an epicardial system; yet, other choices are often equally important and overlooked. Such choices include the selection of a unipolar versus a bipolar system, the type of electrode fixation to be used, and steroid-eluting versus non-steroid-eluting capabilities.

Endocardial versus Epicardial Pacing

Initially, almost all electrode systems implanted in children were epicardial. This was a consequence of the large size of the endocardial electrodes and pacing generators. With the development of smaller electrodes and generators, this is changing; however, most children still undergo epicardial lead placement as a consequence of small patient size or of other factors that do not permit the placement of an endocardial electrode system. MPPR data show a gradual increase in endocardial electrode use, but one half of all patients still receive epicardial electrodes (Fig. 29-16). Our basic approach is to assume that all children should undergo the placement of an endocardial system; we then evaluate the child for factors that do not allow endocardial electrode use. The major factors to be considered, in addition to patient size, are (1) venous access to the ventricle, (2) the presence of intracardiac right-to-left shunting, (3) the presence of increased pulmonary vascular resistance, (4) the presence of right-sided prosthetic valves, and (5) the presence of severe right ventricular (RV) dysfunction or fibrosis.

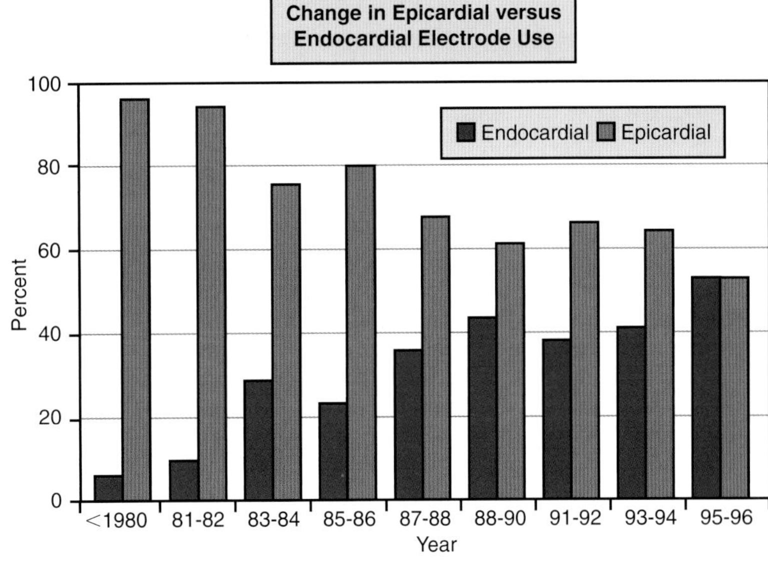

Figure 29-16. Comparison of epicardial with endocardial electrode use in children. Note the gradually increasing use of endocardial electrodes. (Data from the Midwest Pediatric Pacemaker Registry.)

Initially, it was believed that children weighing less than 15 kg and those younger than 4 years of age should not undergo placement of endocardial electrodes.[34] This was based on the beliefs that the subclavian vein and superior vena cava are too small, leading to a high risk for thrombosis, and that the large size of the generators makes implantation in the subclavicular area impractical. With increased experience and smaller generator and electrode sizes, however, many centers now routinely implant endocardial lead systems in children weighing much less than 15 kg.[9,35-37] What the lower range for weight should be is not yet known. From a technical standpoint, children as small as 3 kg can undergo endocardial electrode placement, but the follow-up of such children is too limited to know whether this is in their best interest. A recent study of 39 patients with weights of 2.3 to 10 kg showed that 23% had some pacing system problem related to endocardial electrode placement.[37] Such problems included skin necrosis over the generator, subclavian vein thrombosis, and endocarditis on the electrode. Another 23% required electrode extraction. All except 1 patient had received a single-chamber device.

The risk for vessel thrombosis appears to be less than what was once believed, at least in the short term.[38] Although superior vena caval thrombosis has been reported,[39,40] the true incidence is unknown, because noninvasive methods of detecting thrombosis are not sensitive and angiography is not routinely done unless thrombosis is suspected clinically (Fig. 29-17). Lead displacement secondary to growth remains a concern, although techniques have been proposed to deal with this problem.[9,36] The placement of large electrode loops within the atrium was proposed to allow for growth, but they may not be as effective as originally believed, because they can fibrose to the cardiac wall rather than uncoiling with growth.

The major objection to endocardial electrode use in the small child is related to long-term problems. Because young children can be expected to require numerous electrodes over their lifetime, many more than are needed in adult patients, the clinician must consider how many electrodes can be left in place before problems with vessel obstruction or tricuspid valve dysfunction occur, as well as the difficulty of extraction of old electrodes. Although lead extraction has become more widely used,[41,42] it still represents a significant problem in children, with the potential for damage to the cardiac structures, mainly the tricuspid valve. To commit a child to potentially numerous lead extractions is still a worry. In our institution, current guidelines call for the placement of dual-chamber endocardial systems in children weighing 15 kg or more and the placement of single-chamber endocardial systems, if single-chamber pacing is appropriate, in

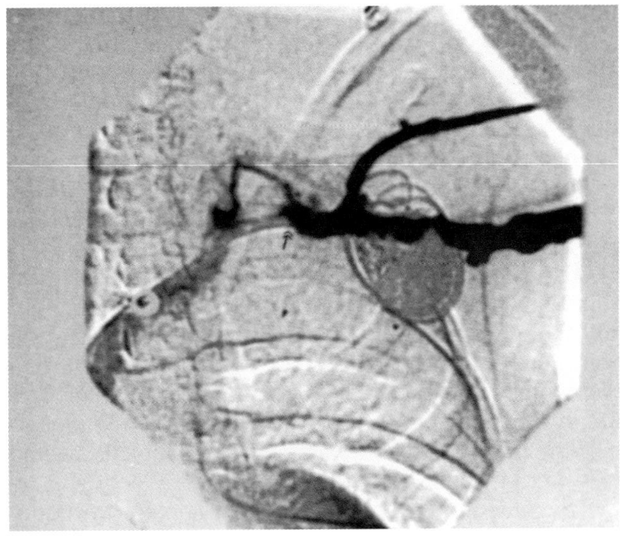

Figure 29-17. Venous angiogram in a patient after endocardial pacemaker implantation through the left subclavian vein. Note the complete obstruction of the subclavian vein at the site of electrode entry (arrow), *with collateral flow around the obstruction.*

children heavier than 8 kg. These guidelines may change as electrode development continues and as data on the long-term follow-up of children with endocardially placed electrodes become available.

The next factor that must be considered is the presence of intracardiac shunting. Electrodes are potential sources of small particulate matter, with the risk for subsequent embolization until endothelialization occurs.[43] Except in the presence of pulmonary vascular disease, this does not tend to be a problem when such particulate matter goes only to the lungs, where it is filtered out of the circulation and eventually absorbed. In the presence of right-to-left shunting, however, the potential for systemic embolization is great. The general recommendation is to avoid such electrodes in patients with documented right-to-left shunting.[34] This also must be considered in patients with the potential for right-to-left shunting, even if their net intracardiac shunt is left to right. Children with atrial septal defects and VSDs can show right-to-left shunting in the setting of elevated RV pressure, even with a net left-to-right shunt.[44,45] The specific hemodynamic situation of the individual child must be considered before endocardial electrode implantation is performed.

The same concerns apply to the child with elevated pulmonary vascular resistance, in whom pulmonary embolization of small matter may further elevate the pulmonary resistance. Whether short-term anticoagulation of such patients until lead endothelialization can occur would preclude such concerns and permit transvenous pacemaker placement has yet to be investigated. If epicardial pacing is not possible, this may be an acceptable alternative, but given the current lack of knowledge concerning the benefit of anticoagulation in this setting, it should not be general practice.

The presence of an artificial tricuspid valve prosthesis negates the ability to use an endocardial pacing system. There have been isolated reports of endocardial electrode placements at the time of open heart surgery through the perivalvular area.[46] This requires cardiopulmonary bypass and can be done only at the time of valvular placement. This technique cannot be used in the usual transvenous implantation; and it prevents lead extraction should that become necessary, except during repeat open heart surgery.

Finally, the physician must consider the state of the right ventricle. Severe RV dysfunction and endocardial fibrosis can occur in children with congenital cardiac disease and may prevent adequate pacing of the right ventricle. This tends to be more prevalent in the older child with long-standing disease. In such children, left ventricular (LV) pacing and, therefore, epicardial pacing may become necessary. In the setting of severe RV dysfunction and dilation, an appropriate endocardial site that permits both adequate sensing and pacing may not be achievable.

The patient who has undergone a Fontan procedure presents a somewhat unique situation. As mentioned previously, controversy exists as to the best approach for electrode placement in these children. If ventricular pacing is required, then the epicardial approach is the only one available. Yet many of these patients have intact AV conduction, require pacing only for sinus node dysfunction, and are best served by atrial-only pacing. The original Fontan procedure connected the right atrial appendage to the pulmonary artery, leaving the entire right atrial chamber available for electrode placement. The more frequently employed technique today either creates a tunnel along the lateral right atrial wall from the inferior vena cava to the pulmonary artery or uses an extracardiac prosthetic conduit. Often a communication exists from the system to the pulmonary atrial chamber, resulting in a right-to-left shunt. Transvenous pacing has been performed in such patients,[47] but electrode placement can be difficult due to the small system venous chamber, and right-to-left embolization with neurologic sequelae has been reported.[47] For these reasons, our approach has been to avoid the transvenous approach unless the epicardial approach is not possible due to extensive fibrosis. Pacing in this group of patients can be extremely challenging regardless of the approach chosen.

In summary, endocardial pacing is generally preferable because of the ease of implantation and the improved longevity of the electrode. Long-term thresholds are as stable as epicardial electrodes and tend to be lower (Fig. 29-18). This permits lower-output programming of the pacing generator, enhancing its longevity. However, there are many situations in which endocardial electrode use is contraindicated (Table 29-5). As such, epicardial electrodes still play a significant role in pediatric pacing, which may be reduced in the future but not be eliminated.

Unipolar versus Bipolar Pacing

The choice between a unipolar and a bipolar electrode configuration used to be an issue only for endocardial implantation. Since the development of bipolar epicar-

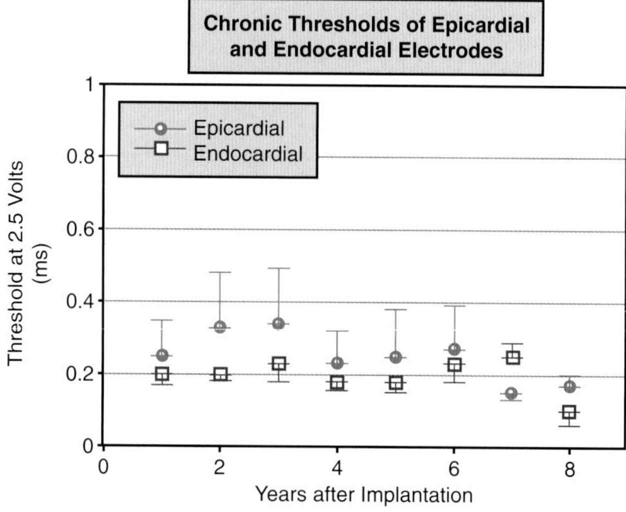

Figure 29-18. Comparison of long-term pulse-width thresholds for endocardial versus epicardial electrodes measured at a pulse amplitude of 2.5 V. Thresholds for both groups show no significant rise, and they do not differ significantly from each other. The brackets represent 1 standard error around the mean.

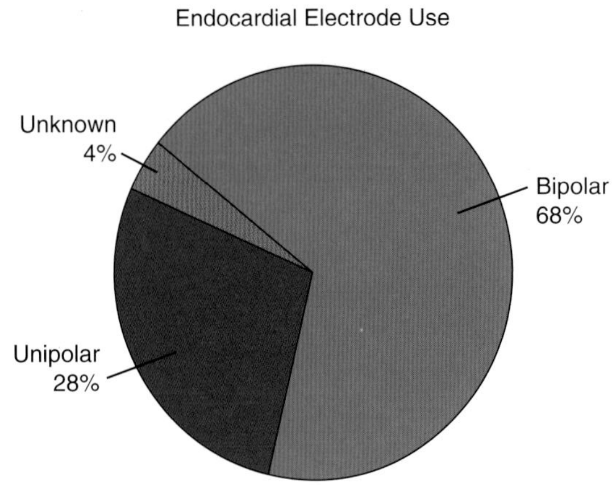

Figure 29-19. Data from the Midwest Pediatric Pacemaker Registry indicating that more than two thirds of endocardial electrode systems use bipolar electrodes.

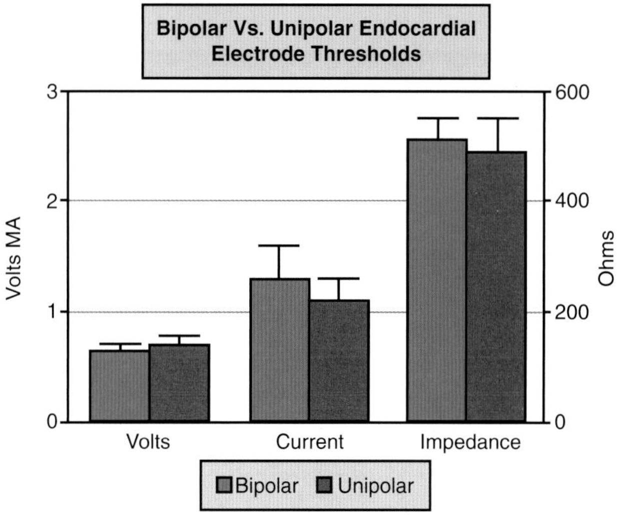

Figure 29-20. Acute implantation thresholds for bipolar versus unipolar endocardial electrodes are not significantly different for voltage, current, or electrode impedance. All were measured at a 0.5-msec pulse width. The brackets represent 1 standard error around the mean. (Data from the Midwest Pediatric Pacemaker Registry.)

TABLE 29-5. Contraindications to Endocardial Pacing

Small patient size (relative)
Presence of intracardiac right-to-left shunting
No venous access
Elevated pulmonary vascular resistance
Prosthetic tricuspid valve
Severe right ventricular dilation or endocardial fibrosis
Presence of hypercoagulable state

dial electrodes, bipolar epicardial pacing is an available option. The data from the MPPR show an increasing trend toward bipolar epicardial pacing. In our institution, more than 90% of all epicardial implants now use bipolar electrodes. The epicardial electrode used is the Model 4968 (Medtronic, Minneapolis, Minn.), which has two electrode heads that are sutured to the epicardial surface. This electrode has thresholds comparable with those of unipolar models but a much higher impedance, often in the 600- to 1200-Ω range, comparable with endocardial electrodes.

For endocardial pacing systems, the choice between unipolar and bipolar pacing becomes more controversial. Again, data from the MPPR show that most endocardial systems are bipolar (Fig. 29-19). Initially, it was believed that unipolar pacing was preferable because of the smaller size of the unipolar pacing electrode.[48] With recent improvements in electrode design, however, this difference in size has become negligible. Electrode body diameters are the important factor in determining the risk for venous thrombosis, and there is a minimal difference. For example, the Model 4057M unipolar screw-in electrode (Medtronic) has a body diameter of 2.2 mm, whereas the 4058M bipolar version has a body diameter of 2.4 mm. This same minimal difference in body size is also seen in passive-fixation electrodes, such as the Model 4023 unipolar steroid-eluting electrode (Medtronic), which has a body diameter of 1.2 mm, compared with 1.9 mm for the bipolar version (Model 4024). Newer electrodes have continued this trend toward small bipolar electrodes. In all cases, the diameter of the electrode's head is smaller for a unipolar electrode, which may make insertion easier, but, once implanted, the size of the head is of little consequence.

A comparison of acute implantation characteristics between unipolar and bipolar electrodes of similar design from the MPPR showed no significant difference for threshold values of voltage, current, or resistance (Fig. 29-20). Long-term thresholds have been believed by some to be improved in unipolar pacing.[48] This has been postulated to be the result of the smaller size of the head and its lower weight, which creates less tension on the endocardial surface, particularly when active-fixation electrodes are used, and therefore leads to less tip fibrosis. However, this appears to be unique only to active-fixation leads and has not been reported to be a problem with passive-fixation tined electrodes.

It was initially believed that sensing using a bipolar electrode was inferior to unipolar sensing because of the close proximity of the two electrodes; however, data from the MPPR show this not to be the case. Acute-implantation R-wave amplitudes and slew rates show no significant difference between unipolar and bipolar electrodes (Fig. 29-21). However, unipolar sensing is more affected by myopotentials and is more prone to oversensing and inappropriate pacemaker inhibition. This has been estimated to be a problem in 31% to 93% of patients, as discussed later. Bipolar sensing is rarely affected by such myopotential inhibition due to the closer proximity of the electrodes. The degree to which such inappropriate inhibition is seen depends on the location of the generator, the provocative tests used,

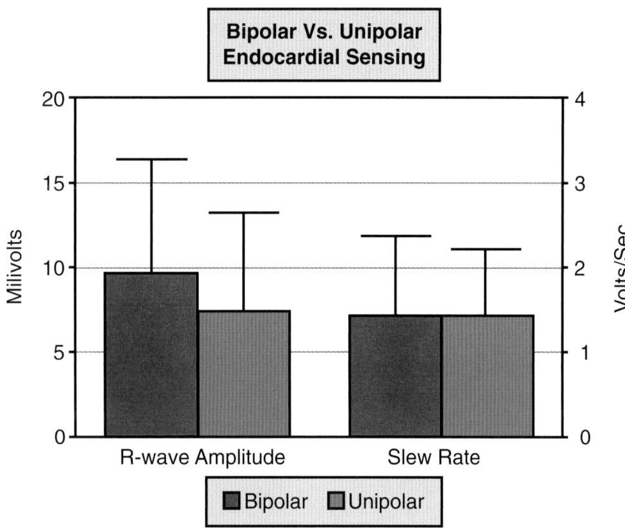

Figure 29-21. Acute implantation electrode sensing for bipolar versus unipolar endocardial electrodes demonstrates no significant difference in either R-wave amplitude (millivolts) or slew rate (volts per second). The brackets indicate 1 standard error around the mean. (Data from the Midwest Pediatric Pacemaker Registry.)

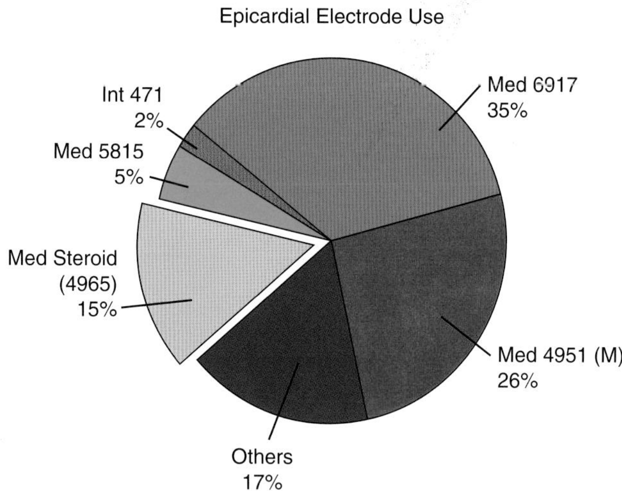

Figure 29-22. Distribution of epicardial electrode types used. The two most common epicardial electrodes are the Medtronic 6917/5069 (screw-in) electrode and the Medtronic 4951(M) (fishhook) electrode. Yet the Medtronic steroid-eluting electrode (exploded slice) has found increasing use in recent years. Med Steroid, epicardial steroid-eluting electrode (Model 4965); Med 5815, myocardial stab-in electrode; Int 471, Intermedics (Guidant, Boston Scientific, Natick, Mass.) screw-in electrode. (Data from the Midwest Pediatric Pacemaker Registry.)

and the generator model implanted. All series, however, report a significant incidence of this problem, which can be a particular concern in active children.

Therefore, it would appear that, in most active children, bipolar pacing is preferred, particularly with the smaller electrode sizes now available. Sensing does not appear to be a problem, and myopotential inhibition is seen less often than in the past. In addition, with bipolar pacing, the risk for extracardiac pacing of the surrounding muscle is minimized, particularly if it is difficult to position the generator in a location where all such stimulation of surrounding muscles can be avoided. This is particularly relevant to implantations with the pocket placed in the subclavicular region. In many children, the lack of significant subcutaneous tissue requires placement of the generator in the subpectoral position, where the risk for extracardiac pacing with a unipolar system increases.

Epicardial Electrode Types

Compared with endocardial electrodes, there are relatively few epicardial electrode types from which to choose. Previously, all electrodes were intramyocardial in type, with the intramyocardial portion being either a corkscrew coil or a single wire with a barbed end (fishhook).[49-51] More recently, a truly epicardial electrode with steroid-eluting capabilities has been developed.[52-54] This is sutured to the epicardial surface and requires direct contact of the electrode with excitable myocardium. It is discussed more fully later in the chapter.

The most widely used electrodes, based on data from the MPPR, are the screw-in corkscrew type, the barbed fishhook type, and the steroid-eluting electrode (Fig. 29-22). The choice of electrode depends on the chamber to be paced and the preference of the implanting physician.

Atrial epicardial implantation requires an electrode that either sits on the epicardial surface or has only a shallow penetration into the atrial myocardium. Should the electrode extend through the chamber wall into the atrial cavity, a low-resistance circuit is established with an inability to pace reliably. Little data can be found concerning the longevity or thresholds of atrial epicardial electrodes. In part, this is related to their limited use and to the fact that constant change in electrode design continues, making long-term comparisons difficult. The most widely used atrial electrode is the fishhook or stab-in electrode, because it does not penetrate deeply into the myocardium, compared with the screw-in or corkscrew type. The newest version (Medtronic Model 4951M), which has a platinized coating, has resulted in slightly improved thresholds at acute implantation (Fig. 29-23). The average threshold at implantation is about 1.05 V and 3.3 mA, measured at a pulse width of 0.5 msec. The average acute electrode impedance is 320 Ω.

The steroid-eluting epimyocardial electrode is receiving increasing use as an atrial epicardial electrode and may become the dominant electrode for atrial epicardial pacing. Although implantation may be slightly more difficult, acute thresholds are comparable. In our institution, this type of electrode is currently used in more than 90% of all atrial epicardial implants. The acute threshold average is 1.0 V at 0.50-msec pulse width, and somewhat higher for the bipolar version. The average impedance is 301 Ω for the unipolar Medtronic Model 4965 and 705 Ω for the bipolar Medtronic 4968 electrode.

More diversity exists in the choice of the electrode for ventricular pacing. A comparison of the original non-

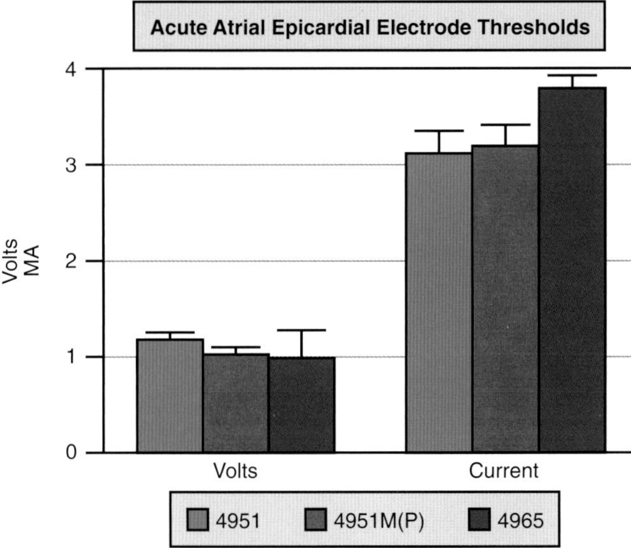

Figure 29-23. Acute implantation voltage and current threshold values measured at a 0.5-msec pulse width for the original fishhook electrode (Medtronic Model 4951) compared with the newer platinized version (Medtronic 4951M) and the steroid-eluting electrode (Medtronic 4965) when implanted on the atrium. Acute thresholds are not statistically different. Current at threshold for the steroid electrode is slightly higher, implying a lower impedance. The brackets represent 1 standard error around the mean. (Data from the Midwest Pediatric Pacemaker Registry.)

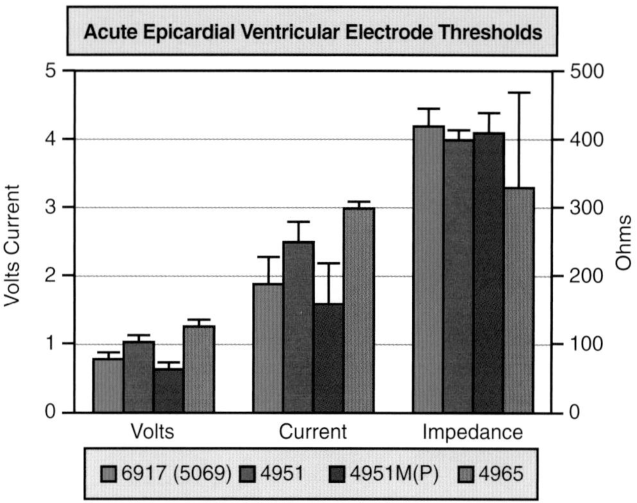

Figure 29-24. Comparison of thresholds for the Medtronic Model 6917 (now known as Model 5069) screw-in electrode, the Medtronic Model 4951 fishhook electrode, the Medtronic Model 4951M(P) platinized fishhook electrode, and the Medtronic steroid-eluting electrode (Model 4965) when implanted on the ventricle shows no significant difference in voltage threshold, but the impedance is slightly lower for the steroid-eluting electrode, similar to findings for atrial use. The brackets represent 1 standard error around the mean. (Data from the Midwest Pediatric Pacemaker Registry.)

platinized fishhook electrode (Medtronic Model 4951) with the screw-in electrode (Medtronic Model 6917 or 5069) reveals essentially no difference in acute implantation thresholds. However, implantation thresholds for the currently available platinized fishhook electrode (Medtronic Model 4951M) are slightly improved (Fig. 29-24). Both steroid-eluting electrodes tended to have slightly higher thresholds. Lead survival appears to be longer for the screw-in electrode than for the fishhook type. Five years after implantation, the lead survival rate of the former was found to be about 84%, whereas that of the fishhook electrode was about 65%.[50] Most failures were caused by exit block. Other studies, however, have found little difference in longevity between these two types of electrodes.[49] Some of this discrepancy between studies is believed to be related to different surgical modes of implantation for the fishhook electrode. Whether or not the lead was stabilized by being sutured to the myocardium was variable. It has been suggested that lack of such stabilization leads to more electrode movement within the myocardium and, therefore, to greater fibrosis and the risk for exit block[50] (see later discussion of implantation techniques).

A recent advance in epicardial pacing, as mentioned earlier, is the steroid-eluting electrode.[52-54] This electrode consists of a platinized flat electrode that sits atop the epicardial surface with a silicone plug impregnated with dexamethasone to allow elution of the dexamethasone onto the area of myocardium being stimulated. About 1 mg of dexamethasone is present within the electrode. Both a unipolar version (Model 4965) and a bipolar version (Model 4968) of this electrode are available from Medtronic. This electrode is affixed to the epicardial surface by sutures, with the active portion of the electrode not extending into the myocardium as with other epicardial electrodes. This is both advantageous and disadvantageous, depending on the patient. For patients whose epicardial surfaces are relatively nonfibrotic, this appears to be an advantage, because there is less myocardial injury to provoke subsequent fibrosis. However, for patients with markedly fibrotic epicardial surfaces, which is often the case after multiple open heart surgical procedures, these electrodes are difficult to use. In such patients, the surgeon must either find an area of myocardium with a limited epicardial fibrotic reaction or strip away a fibrotic reaction to expose the myocardium, which simply leads to further subsequent fibrosis.

Initial experience with this electrode is encouraging. Although acute thresholds appear to be comparable with those of other epicardial electrodes (see Fig. 29-24), the threshold rise is less over the first several months after implantation (Fig. 29-25).[53] In select patients with limited myocardial fibrosis, epicardial electrodes that do not penetrate the myocardium appear to be beneficial; however, care must be taken to choose the most appropriate form of ventricular epicardial electrode to fit the individual patient. All three types of ventricular electrodes in current use have advantages and disadvantages, and no one type is ideally suited to all patients.

Endocardial Electrode Types

As in the adult population, there are several general types of endocardial electrodes in use in children: passive-fixation non-steroid eluting electrodes, passive-

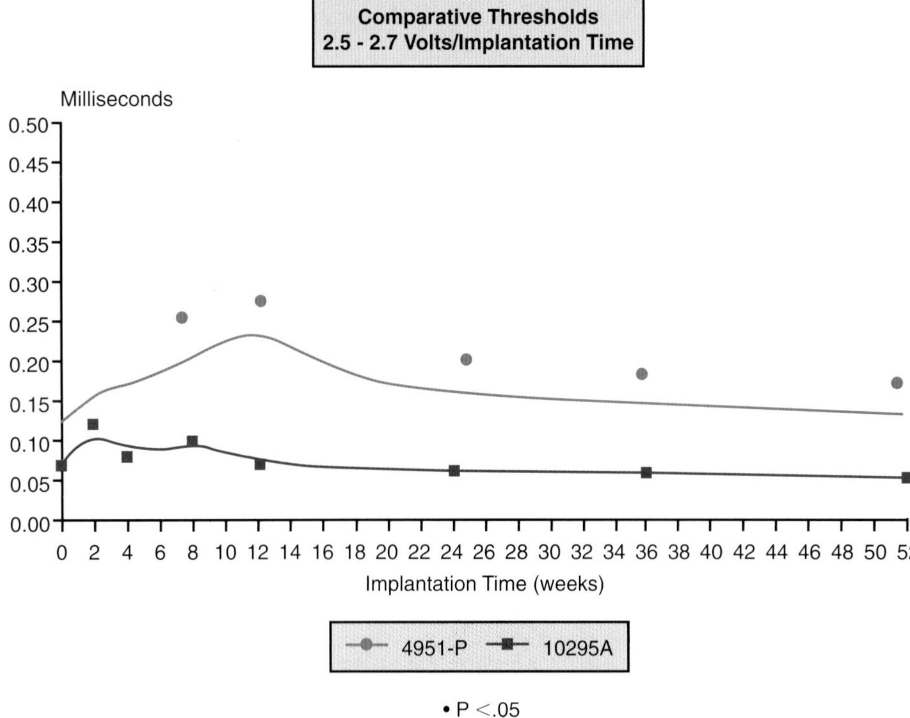

Figure 29-25. Comparative thresholds of the Medtronic Model 4951P platinized fishhook electrode versus the epicardial steroid-eluting electrode (Medtronic Model 10295A, now known as Model 4965) show a lack of significant threshold rise in the first 3 months after implantation for the steroid-eluting epicardial electrode, with threshold improvement at 1 year after implantation. (From Karpawich PP, Harkini M, Arciniegas E, Cavitt DL: Improved chronic epicardial pacing in children: Steroid contribution to porous platinized electrodes. PACE 15:1152, 1992.)

fixation steroid-eluting electrodes, and active-fixation electrodes—both non-steroid-eluting and a recently developed steroid-eluting model. Active electrode data presented here are for the non-steroid-eluting model. The most commonly used endocardial electrode type in children continues to be the active-fixation screw-in electrode (Fig. 29-26). The use of this electrode has been advocated because of its better fixation qualities, given the tremendous range of anatomic variations present in children with congenital heart disease. For implantation within the morphologic left ventricle in a child who has undergone an atrial switch repair for transposition of the great arteries or a child with ventricular inversion, the active-fixation electrode is preferable. Also, in a child whose right ventricle is markedly dilated, such that it is difficult to wedge the electrode into the trabecular recesses of the right ventricle, active-fixation electrodes are preferable.

However, this electrode type is not ideal in all children. A comparison of acute threshold data shows that active-fixation electrodes have the highest acute thresholds (Fig. 29-27). Both non-steroid-eluting passive-fixation electrodes and steroid-eluting passive-fixation electrodes have lower acute thresholds and do not differ from each other. The presence of the steroid does not influence the acute implantation threshold, but with increasing electrode age this is no longer the case. Follow-up data indicate significantly lower electrode thresholds for the steroid-eluting electrode compared with other types.[55] A comparison of steroid-eluting and non-steroid-eluting electrodes showed no difference in chronic thresholds at 5 V of pulse amplitude but did show significant differences at 2.5 and 1.6 V (Fig. 29-28). Therefore, it would appear that the strength-duration curve is significantly shifted leftward for the steroid-eluting electrodes.

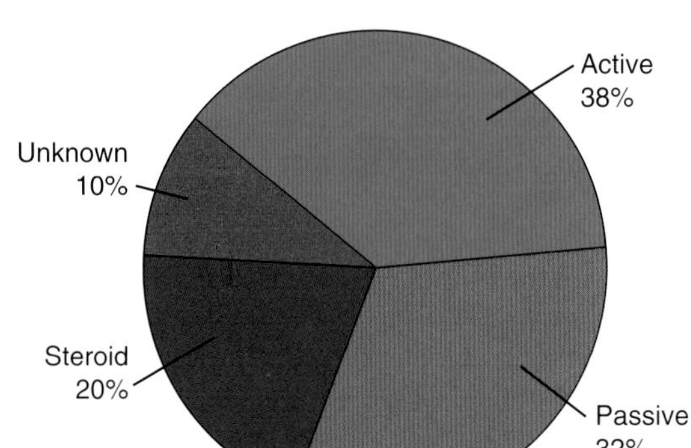

Figure 29-26. Distribution of endocardial electrode types used. Active, active-fixation (screw-in) electrode; passive, passive-fixation (tined) non-steroid-eluting electrode; steroid, passive-fixation steroid-eluting electrode. (Data from the Midwest Pediatric Pacemaker Registry.)

Such changes affect generator programming. In one study,[55] only 33% of generators that used non-steroid-eluting electrodes could be programmed to 2.5 V of pulse amplitude, compared with 77% of generators that used steroid-eluting electrodes. The remainder required a pulse amplitude of 5 V or greater. Therefore, the use of steroid-eluting passive-fixation electrodes allowed chronically lower output settings for the pulse generator, thereby increasing the generator's longevity. The follow-up averaged 3.3 years (median, 3.6 years). There

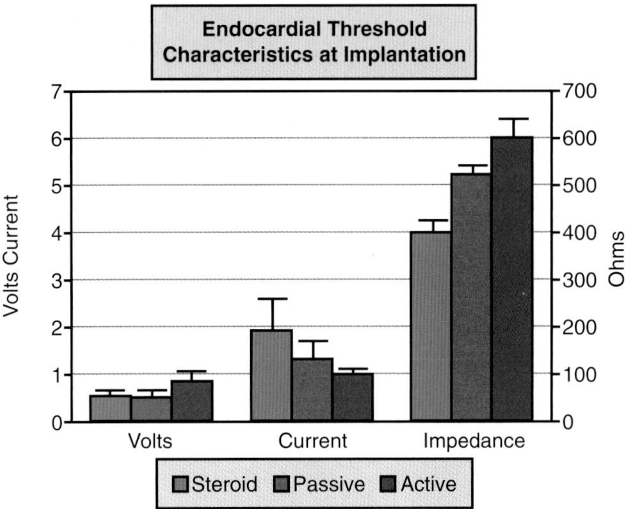

Figure 29-27. Acute thresholds for endocardial electrode types show a tendency toward lower thresholds in the passive-fixation and steroid-eluting electrodes, compared with the active-fixation electrodes. However, the difference in voltage threshold is minimal. The changes become more evident in current and impedance values, with steroid-eluting electrodes having the lowest impedance and the highest current flow. The brackets represent 1 standard error around the mean. (Data from the Midwest Pediatric Pacemaker Registry.)

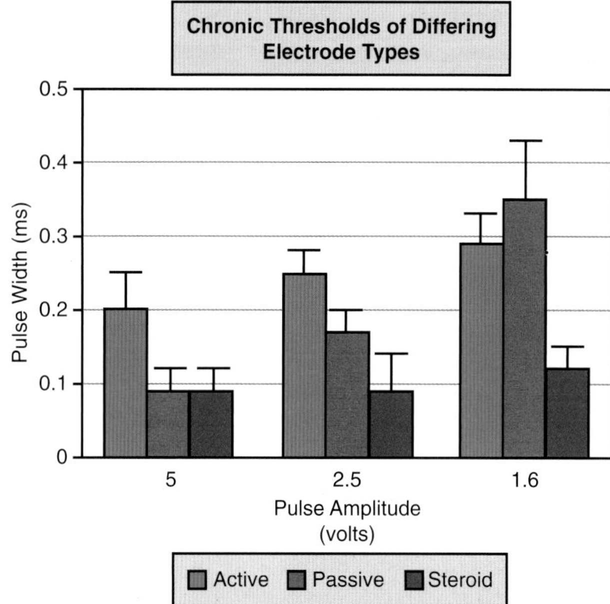

Figure 29-28. Chronic long-term electrode thresholds are significantly higher for active-fixation electrodes than for either passive-fixation or steroid-eluting electrodes. At low pulse amplitudes, steroid-eluting electrodes show significantly lower thresholds than the other types. The brackets represent 1 standard error around the mean. (Data from Serwer GA, Dorostkar PC, LeRoy S, Dick M II: Comparison of chronic thresholds between differing endocardial electrode types in children. Circulation 86:I-43, 1992.)

are insufficient data to compare the newer steroid-eluting active-fixation electrodes with the older types.

Single-lead VDD systems have been employed in children. These systems obviate the need for two electrodes yet maintain AV synchrony[56]; however, problems exist. The major problem is lack of atrial pacing capabilities when sinus node function is inadequate. Also, the spacing of the atrial electrodes from the electrode tip often is too great for use in small children. The electrode must be buckled so that the atrial dipole is within the ventricle (Fig. 29-29), which could lead to ventricular electrode dislodgment. These problems, together with the increased complexity of the electrode construction, with a concomitant potential for increased electrode failure, combine to limit the usefulness of this approach in children, especially smaller children.

In summary, we believe that the ideal pacing system in children is a dual-chamber system with the capacity for rate-responsive pacing, using endocardial atrial and ventricular bipolar electrodes with active-fixation electrodes in the atrium and steroid-eluting passive- or active-fixation electrodes in the ventricle. In situations in which the child's size is marginal or endocardial pacing is contraindicated, we use epicardial pacing. In these situations, the currently preferred electrode is the steroid-eluting electrode for both the atrium and the ventricle or, in the presence of significant epicardial fibrosis, the platinized version of the fishhook electrode for the atrium and the corkscrew electrode for the ventricle. Long-term data are not yet available to show whether the steroid-eluting epicardial electrode performs better in the long term than the intramyocardial electrode.

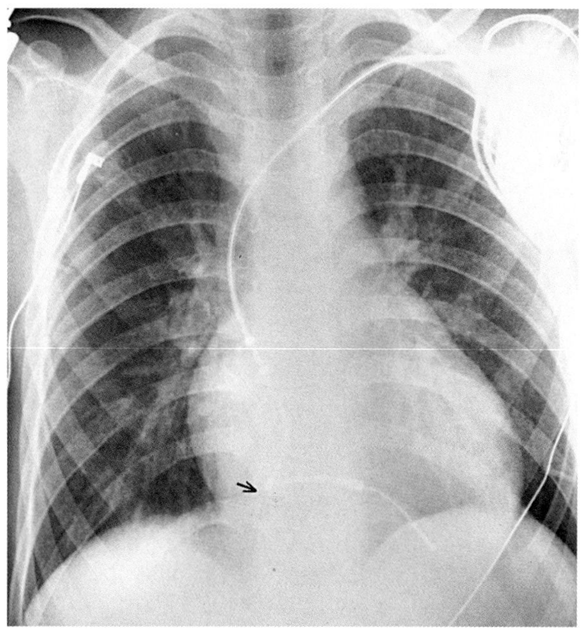

Figure 29-29. Chest radiograph showing placement of a single-pass VDD system. Note the lead buckling in the atrium, which is necessary to place the atrial sensing electrodes (arrow) *within the atrium.*

Implantation Techniques

In many ways, implantation techniques in children are similar to those used in adults, but differences do exist. This section does not attempt to describe again those techniques that are similar but instead focuses on the differences that are important and must be considered.

Epicardial Implantation Techniques

The approach used for the placement of epicardial electrodes is highly variable, depending on the patient's individual circumstances. Approaches to the epicardial surface that have previously been employed include thoracotomy, sternotomy, and subxiphoid incision. The subxiphoid approach requires the smallest incision; through the same incision, both the electrode's implantation on the epicardial surface of the heart and the pacemaker's implantation in the abdomen can be accomplished.[57-59] This approach has been used for both ventricular and atrial epicardial electrode implantation. The disadvantage to this approach is that it exposes only a limited ventricular epicardial or atrial surface, and, in a patient who has extensive epicardial fibrosis as a consequence of prior cardiac surgery, finding a suitable location for implantation of the electrode could be difficult. Such an approach requires a 6- to 7-cm skin incision from the xiphoid tip to a point superior to the umbilicus. The dissection is continued as deep as is believed necessary to provide adequate tissue between the pacemaker and the surface of the skin. Depending on the degree of subcutaneous tissue present, the pacemaker can be implanted above the rectus muscle, below the rectus muscle but above the peritoneum, or, in some circumstances, intraperitoneally, housed in a Silastic pouch sutured to the underside of the peritoneum and anchored to the rectus fascia.[57] The depth to which the incision is carried should be governed solely by the tissue available to cover the pacemaker. When only minimal tissue is present over the pacemaker, not only does an unsightly bulge result, but also the skin is more susceptible to traumatic injury, with a resultant risk for pacemaker erosion and infection.

A left thoracotomy approach is often used in the child who has had prior cardiac surgery in whom the risk for significant epicardial fibrosis is high.[60] This approach affords an increased myocardial surface from which to choose an appropriate pacing site. The generator can be implanted in the abdomen, in the subclavicular region, or, in rare settings, intrathoracically. However, for implantation of a dual-chamber system, this approach affords less exposure of the atrium and requires left atrial pacing. Although this has been accomplished, it introduces complexity into the programming, because the postpace AV interval must be prolonged sufficiently to afford adequate time for RV filling, because of the time necessary for left-to-right atrial excitation spread. The postsense AV interval must be short to avoid an excessive AV interval (Fig. 29-30). For this reason, we believe that right atrial pacing is preferable, but we use left atrial pacing if right atrial pacing is not possible. When the thoracotomy approach is used with an abdominal placement of the generator, the electrode must be passed subcostally to a pocket created in the abdomen through a separate incision. The electrode must not be passed over a rib and must be tunneled from the thoracic cavity to the abdomen as medially as possible, to minimize the risk for traumatic electrode fracture.

Finally, a median sternotomy approach can be used, but this creates the largest and most obvious scar. However, it affords the best exposure of the epicardial surface of both the ventricle and the right atrium. In a patient with significant epicardial scarring and fibrosis, this affords the best likelihood of finding an appropriate pacing site. After the electrode has been implanted, the device can be pulled through the subxiphoid region to the abdominal wall, where, through a separate incision or an extension of the median sternotomy incision, an appropriate pocket can be created.

Regardless of the electrode type chosen, appropriate anchoring of the electrode to the epicardial surface is crucial. Our approach is to insert the electrode into the myocardium and determine the threshold strength-duration curve. If it is acceptable, the electrode is sutured to the epicardial surface, and the thresholds are rechecked. Suturing the electrode to the surface theoretically reduces movement of the electrode tip within the myocardium, with less formation of fibrotic tissue and better long-term performance of the electrode.[50] When the fishhook electrode is used and there is significant epicardial fibrosis, unbending of the barb to permit deeper penetration is often beneficial. There should be several types of myocardial electrodes available during the implantation procedure, to meet whatever situation is encountered.

When the steroid-eluting electrode is used, a suitable position is found by holding the electrode in contact with the epicardial surface and quickly determining the voltage threshold at a single pulse width. If it is acceptable, the electrode is sutured to the epicardial surface, and a complete strength-duration curve is determined. Often, several sites must be tested before a suitable one is found. When using the bipolar version of this electrode, proper orientation of the two heads to each other is mandatory to achieve optimal sensing. For atrial implantation, the interelectrode axis should be perpendicular to the long axis of the ventricle to minimize far-field R-wave sensing. For ventricular use, however, the interelectrode axis should be parallel to the ventricular long axis, to maximize R-wave sensing.

A gentle loop of the electrode should be left in the thoracic cavity to allow for some growth, but excessive loops should be avoided. Instances of entrapment of vascular structures by pacemaker electrodes have been reported.[61,62] The extra length of the electrode is easily coiled and placed within the generator's pocket; even this may allow for some growth, because the electrode wire slowly uncoils with growth of the patient.

The exact placement of the abdominal pocket is generally left to the discretion of the surgeon. However, it should be placed away from the belt line and not in the

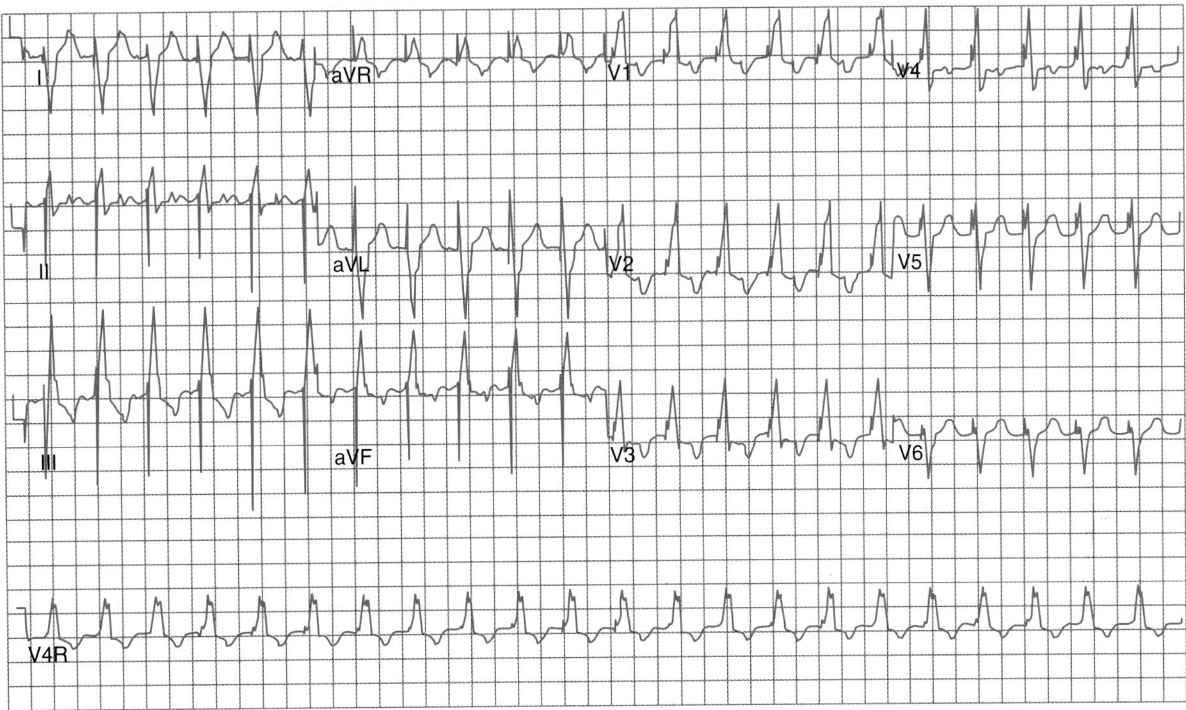

Figure 29-30. Electrocardiogram from a patient with a DDD pacemaker in whom the atrial electrode is on the left atrium. To provide an appropriate time for ventricular filling during both atrial pacing and sensing, either a compromise atrioventricular (AV) interval must be used or the generator must have the ability to alter the AV interval (dynamic AV delay).

upper right quadrant. Placement in the upper right quadrant interferes with subsequent assessment of hepatic size, which may be important in children with structural cardiac disease. The electrodes should be tunneled from the thorax to the abdomen as near the midline as possible, to minimize the risk for electrode fracture.

The placement of unused or redundant electrodes is not recommended. It was once believed that the placement of an unused electrode would provide a "spare" electrode that could be used if the primary electrode failed, thus precluding the need for a second thoracotomy. It was found, however, that if the primary electrode failed, there was a high likelihood that the redundant electrode was also unusable.[15,63] Therefore, the extra electrode provided no benefit to the child.

Endocardial Implantation Techniques

Before endocardial implantation, echocardiography should be performed to make certain no contraindications to endocardial implantation exist—specifically, tricuspid valve dysfunction, right-to-left shunting, interatrial communications, or superior vena caval obstruction. Whether the pacemaker is placed under the left or right clavicle is somewhat arbitrary but may be important for some patients, and the location should be discussed with them. Our general policy is to place the pacemaker on the side opposite the patient's handedness (i.e., if the patient is right-handed, the pacemaker is placed on the left side).

The endocardial approach used for implantation in children is similar to that in adults. Before beginning, transcutaneous pacing electrodes are placed to provide emergency pacing ability. A sudden decrease in intrinsic heart rate caused by the stress of the procedure or the general anesthesia, if administered, is not unusual. Although placement of a temporary transvenous pacing electrode can be done, the stress of this procedure alone can cause bradycardia. In addition, the risk for infection of the permanent system by the temporary electrode must be considered. Transcutaneous pacing electrodes for all sizes of children are now available and function well.

Whether the electrode is introduced into the vascular system by a direct subclavian vein puncture[35,64,65] or by a cephalic vein cutdown procedure[9,36] should be guided by the experience of the implanting physician. In our institution, direct subclavian vein puncture is used exclusively. Our approach is to enter the subclavian vein percutaneously and introduce a guidewire. Using the guidewire's entrance through the skin as the proximal point, an incision is made laterally along the deltopectoral groove. The dissection is then carried down to the pectoralis. At this point, the degree of subcutaneous tissue is examined to determine whether there is sufficient tissue to cover the generator. In many children, this tissue is inadequate, and placement of the generator above the pectoralis results in a significant pacemaker bulge as well as an increased risk for pacemaker erosion and traumatic injury to the tissue covering the pacemaker.[64] This is also psychologically important, because many children are self-conscious about a prominent bulge. If the tissue is believed to be inadequate, the dissection is carried through the pectoralis, using blunt dissection to separate the muscle fibers, and a pocket is created in the subpectoral region. After this pocket is created, a sheath and dilator are introduced into the subclavian vein over the previously positioned guide wire. The electrode is then passed into the right atrium, together with a new guide wire. The sheath is then removed. Retention of the guide wire allows for either the introduction of a second electrode, in the case of a dual-chamber implant, or the option to remove the prior electrode and replace it without having to again puncture the subclavian vein. After the electrodes have been positioned and tested, the guide wire can be removed. The electrodes are then connected to the generator and placed in the pocket. When the subpectoral approach is used, it may be difficult to avoid extracardiac pacing with a unipolar system; for this reason, a bipolar system is preferred.

A third implantation approach is a hybrid of the two methods previously described. In some patients, transvenous implantation would be preferable but there is no venous access; in these cases, the electrode can be inserted into the atrium through an incision in the atrial wall and then advanced into the ventricle across the AV valve.[66] The atrial incision is closed with a purse-string suture after the electrode has been positioned in the ventricle. This provides the advantages of endocardial pacing with improved thresholds when venous access to the ventricle is not available. We have employed this approach in children in whom epicardial electrode thresholds were unacceptable but who had no venous access (Fig. 29-31). This can be especially useful after a right heart bypass (Fontan) procedure, even though anticoagulation is necessary because of implantation within the systemic ventricle.[43]

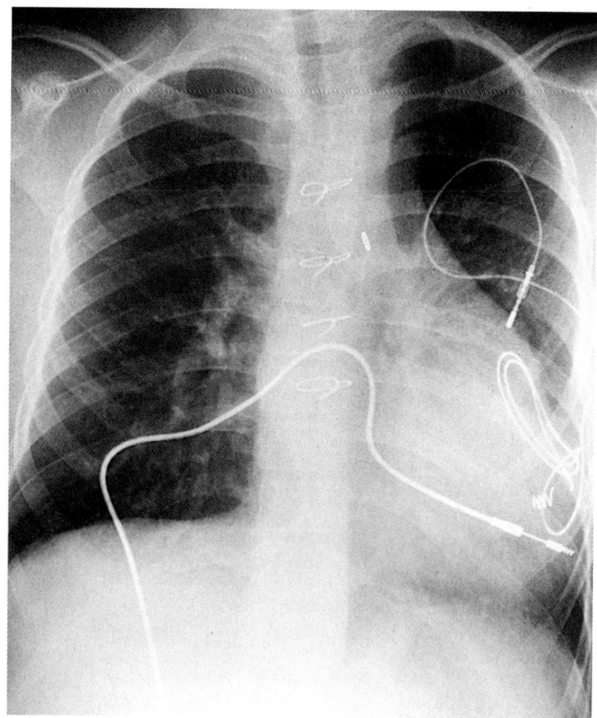

Figure 29-31. Chest radiograph showing placement of an endocardial electrode that has been introduced through the atrial wall, passed through the atrioventricular valve, and secured to the ventricular endocardial surface. The electrode is tunneled to the generator pocket in the abdominal wall.

Recent work has raised the question of the optimal site within the right ventricle for electrode placement. Initially, the RV apex was used, as it affords a stable site. Concern has been raised that the alteration of excitation sequence may lead to altered hemodynamics.[67] Studies have suggested that apical pacing may induce long-term changes in both right and LV performance. Midseptal pacing may be more hemodynamically beneficial, but it is more difficult to achieve a stable electrode position with this approach.[68]

Acute Electrode Evaluation

After placement of the electrode, its electrical characteristics must be determined. For active-fixation or intramyocardial electrodes, 15 minutes should be allowed after placement of the electrode before threshold testing, to permit acute myocardial changes caused by the electrode's entry into the myocardium to subside. All changes do not subside in this amount of time, but this short delay is warranted. Our initial approach is to measure the electrode's impedance and, if possible, the intrinsic EGM amplitudes. The impedance should be between 200 and 600 Ω for an epicardially placed electrode (values up to 1200 Ω can be accepted with the bipolar Medtronic Model 4968 electrode) and between 300 and 700 Ω for an endocardially placed electrode. The amplitude of the EGM should be sufficient to allow appropriate sensing by the generator being implanted. The minimally acceptable signal amplitude varies, depending on the specific generator. If these measurements are found to be acceptable, threshold testing is performed. It is our general practice to set a given pulse width and then determine the minimum pulse amplitude necessary to maintain capture. Multiple threshold determinations at differing pulse widths are performed to define the strength-duration curve adequately. We think it is important to determine the shape of the strength-duration curve, to be certain that the minimum pulse width necessary to pace at any pulse amplitude and the minimum amplitude necessary to pace at any pulse width are sufficiently removed from the proposed generator settings to allow for some movement in the strength-duration curve without risking loss of capture (Fig. 29-32). Data from the MPPR suggest that the minimum voltage necessary to pace the ventricle at a 0.5-msec pulse width is less than 1 V, and for the atrium it is less than 1.5 V. Such threshold guidelines apply to both endocardial and epicardial electrodes.

Before the pulse generator is connected to the electrodes, it is advisable to pace the ventricle at the maximal output of the pacing system analyzer. In children, because of the close proximity of the diaphragm to the electrode, diaphragmatic pacing can occur. If diaphragmatic pacing occurs at the maximal pacing system analyzer output, the electrode must be moved. This is particularly relevant for children with transposition of the great arteries, in whom a ventricular electrode is positioned within the left ventricle. Positioning of the electrode tip at the LV apex puts it in close prox-

Strength-Duration Curve Obtained at Implantation

Current
Volts
Volts MA
Pulse Width (ms)

Figure 29-32. Example of a strength-duration curve determined at implantation. From this curve, the minimum voltage needed to pace at any pulse width and the minimum pulse width needed to pace at any voltage can be determined.

imity to the diaphragm, and there is a high incidence of diaphragmatic pacing. To prevent this, we position the electrode on the midposterior free wall at the approximate level of the papillary muscles (Fig. 29-33). This affords acceptable thresholds with a minimal risk for diaphragmatic pacing. This problem is more often seen in endocardial pacing than in epicardial pacing, but it can occur in either setting.

Follow-up Methods for the Child with a Pacemaker

Proper pacemaker programming and early recognition of inappropriate pacemaker performance require frequent, methodical, and appropriate follow-up. This section discusses the follow-up techniques used and the differences in follow-up routine with increasing time since implantation.

Pacemaker follow-up can be divided into three periods, based on the length of time since implantation. The two most crucial periods are within the first

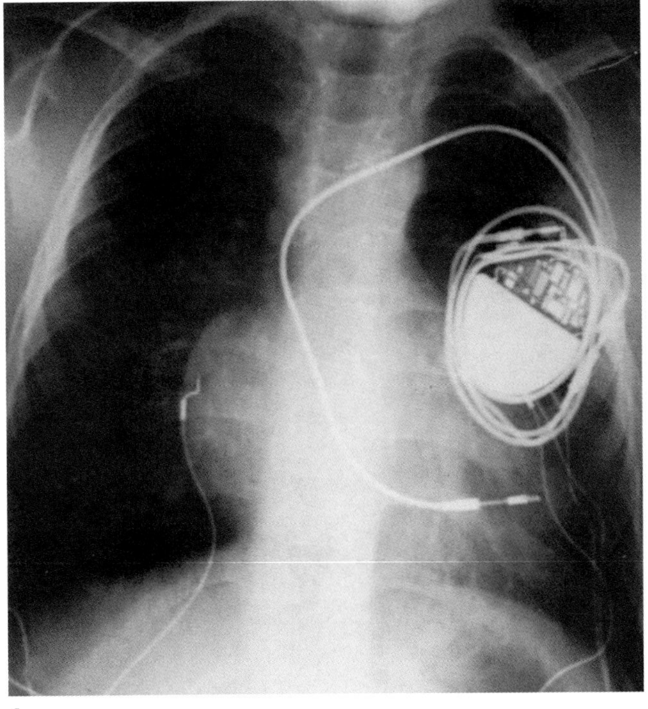
A

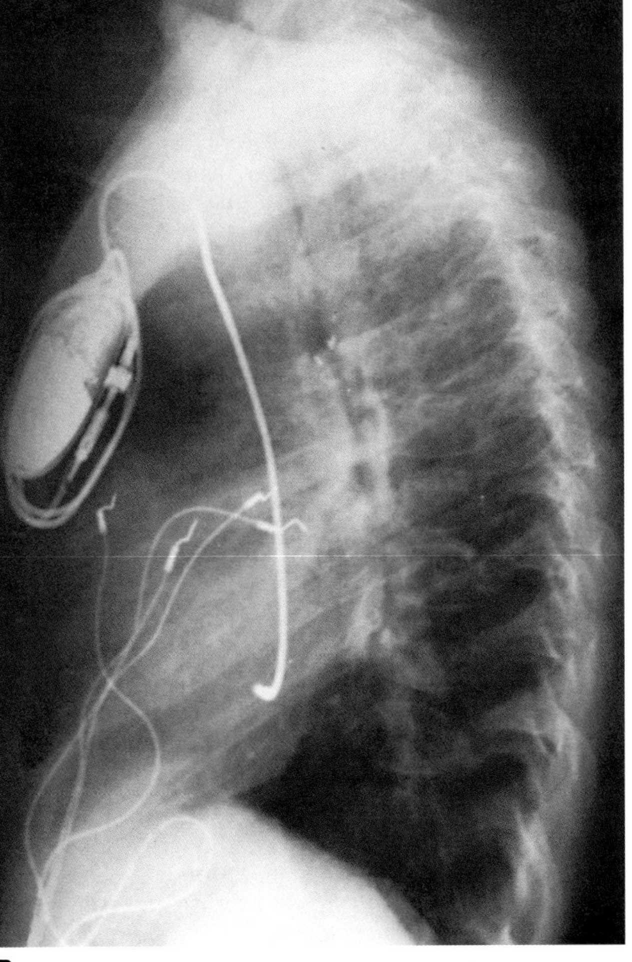
B

*Figure 29-33. Posteroanterior **(A)** and lateral **(B)** chest radiographs from a patient who underwent endocardial electrode implantation after performance of an atrial switch (Senning) procedure for dextrotransposition of the great arteries. Note the electrode position in the left ventricle, away from the ventricular apex and the diaphragm, to avoid diaphragmatic stimulation.*

2 months after implantation (early follow-up) and when the pacemaker approaches its theoretical life expectancy (late follow-up). Between these two periods, the functions of the pacemaker and electrode remain fairly stable, and the generator does not require frequent readjustment. Problems can occur, however, particularly as a result of electrode breakage in the active child. The major components of pacemaker follow-up—pacemaker clinic visit, 24-hour ambulatory ECG recordings, and treadmill exercise testing—are discussed in this section, followed by a description of the differences among the three follow-up periods.

Pacemaker Clinic Visit

During a pacemaker clinic visit, all patients undergo a complete history and physical examination, pacemaker interrogation, threshold testing, evaluation of electrode sensing, and routine ECG testing. When indicated, other tests, such as chest radiography and echocardiography, are also performed. Specific attention must be paid to obtaining a complete history as it relates to potential pacemaker malfunction. Symptoms suggesting pacemaker malfunction include sudden exercise intolerance, dizziness, nausea, and loss of consciousness. In particular, parents often note that their child has "less energy" than previously. One of the more common symptoms in patients with intermittent atrial sensing malfunction is a sudden lack of energy or transient dizziness, which is related to loss of atrial sensing with a resultant acute drop in the pacing rate to the lower rate limit of the pacemaker. This can often be a subtle finding and must be carefully sought, not only in the older child from whom a history can be obtained directly, but also from the parents of the younger child, who must be asked whether they have ever noted sudden changes in the child's activity state or temperament, sudden interruptions of play time, interruptions of eating, or sudden staring episodes suggestive of acute decrease in cardiac output.

The physical examination should relate specifically to complications produced by the presence of pacemaker electrodes, such as AV valve incompetence, the acute appearance of pericardial rubs (suggesting lead perforation), irregular heart rates, pocket infections, or, in unusual situations, stenotic lesions (suggesting extracardiac compression of vessels by the epicardial implanted pacemaker electrodes).

Pacemaker interrogation must consist of interrogation of programmed settings and pacemaker performance data, comprising the electrode's impedance, the generator battery's voltage, the generator's measured pulse amplitude, the electrode's current flow, the energy delivered, the pulse width, and the measured magnet rate. Such parameters can often reveal early signs of electrode dysfunction or approaching generator end-of-service. Impedance changes are of particular usefulness in indicating early exit block (manifested as increasing impedance) and insulation fracture or erosion of the electrode's tip (manifested as a decline in the electrode's impedance).

Next, interrogation of the pacemaker's diagnostic counters is performed to assess the extent to which the pacemaker is being used and the rate variability the patient is experiencing. Information provided by diagnostic counters is variable, depending on the pacemaker model. The most useful data are those collected over many months to assess the degree to which the pacemaker is providing rate variability and to what extent the patient is dependent on the pacemaker. This information is useful in assessing the appropriateness of the lower rate limit in DDD pacing and sinus node function. A high percentage of atrial pacing with a low programmed lower rate limit suggests significant sinus nodal dysfunction (Fig. 29-34).

```
294-03 SN 011821                    APR 28 '93   9:07 AM
   VENTRICULAR RATE HISTOGRAM           DDD

 RANGE (BPM)                           NUMBER OF EVENTS
  70 -                                    ......24405 (1A)
  80 -                                    ......41265 (2A)
 100 -                                    ......34288 (3A)
 120 -                                    ......16113 (4A)
 170 -                                    .........37 (5A)
 300 -
        FILLED BARS - PERCENT ACTUAL EVENTS
```

A

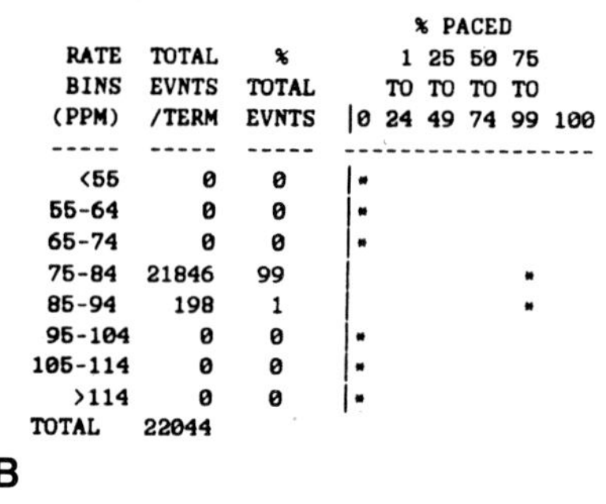

RATE BINS (PPM)	TOTAL EVNTS /TERM	% TOTAL EVNTS	% PACED 0	1 TO 24	25 TO 49	50 TO 74	75 TO 99	100
<55	0	0	•					
55-64	0	0	•					
65-74	0	0	•					
75-84	21846	99					•	
85-94	198	1					•	
95-104	0	0	•					
105-114	0	0	•					
>114	0	0	•					
TOTAL	22044							

B

```
DIAGNOSTIC DATA (CARDIAC CYCLES)          DDD MODE
EVENT COUNTERS LAST CLEARED..SEP  9,   1:50 PM
NUMBER OF:
 PREMATURE VENTRICULAR EVENTS.........57       0 %
 ATRIAL PACE EVENTS FOLLOWED
  BY VENTRICULAR SENSE EVENT..........13       0 %
 ATRIAL PACE EVENTS FOLLOWED
  BY VENTRICULAR PACE EVENT.....648,815        4 %
 ATRIAL SENSE EVENTS FOLLOWED
  BY VENTRICULAR SENSE EVENT ........308       0 %
 ATRIAL SENSE EVENTS FOLLOWED
  BY VENTRICULAR PACE EVENT..16,777,215       96 %

PERCENT PACED - ATRIUM ....................    4 %
PERCENT PACED - VENTRICLE ..................100 %
```

C

*Figure 29-34. Examples of data obtained from generator diagnostic counters showing the number of beats occurring in each rate range. **A,** Data from a patient who had acceptable heart rate variability. **B,** Data from a patient in whom there was minimal heart rate variability; reprogramming was required. **C,** Information about the types of atrial and ventricular beats occurring. This patient had predominantly atrial sensing, followed by ventricular pacing, indicating an appropriate lower rate limit.*

Next, intracardiac EGMs are recorded. The usefulness of such tracings is discussed later. Sensing thresholds are also performed to determine the least sensitive settings that still maintain appropriate sensing.

Finally, threshold determinations from both atrial and ventricular leads are obtained at all pulse amplitudes, producing 100% capture at any pulse width setting. Pulse width thresholds are generally preferred to pulse amplitude thresholds, because most pacemakers have many more pulse width settings than pulse amplitude settings, so more accurate thresholds can be determined by pulse width. All threshold determinations are performed in duplicate. Thresholds are reported as the minimum pulse width that maintains 100% capture at each programmable pulse amplitude. From these data, strength-duration curves are constructed and compared with previously obtained curves to detect shifts. After review of the data, appropriate programming decisions can be made.

Intracardiac Electrogram Determinations

Intracardiac EGMs should be obtained whenever possible. They are obtained both simultaneously with a surface ECG and with telemetered annotation markers that indicate the point during the EGM at which sensing or pacing occurs and the beginning and length of each refractory period. The relationship of programmed refractory periods to the waveform is shown. This is particularly useful for the atrial channel, to ascertain the appropriateness of the programmed settings. For example, if the atrial electrode has been implanted in the left atrium, a determination of the appropriate AV interval can be difficult because the spontaneous P wave on the body surface significantly precedes the time at which atrial sensing occurs (Fig. 29-35). This results in a prolonged PR interval, as determined from the surface ECG recording, that could raise concerns about appropriate generator function.

Recording the annotation markers with the intracardiac EGM also permits minimization of refractory periods, to maximize the multiblock rate and yet not risk oversensing of ventricular depolarization or repolarization by the atrial channel (crosstalk) (Fig. 29-36). This is of even more concern in young children who experience high atrial rates and are at risk for multiblock, with a subsequent sudden decrease in the ventricular rate and a concomitant decrease in cardiac output. This is demonstrated more fully when the results of exercise testing are discussed.

We also find the intracardiac EGM to be helpful in determining decreasing atrial amplitudes over time, with the potential for loss of atrial sensing. With the electrode's aging and fibrosis of the tip, recorded EGM amplitudes may decline, and appropriate changes in atrial sensitivity often need to be made. This is particularly relevant to exercise, during which atrial amplitudes may further decline, as discussed later.

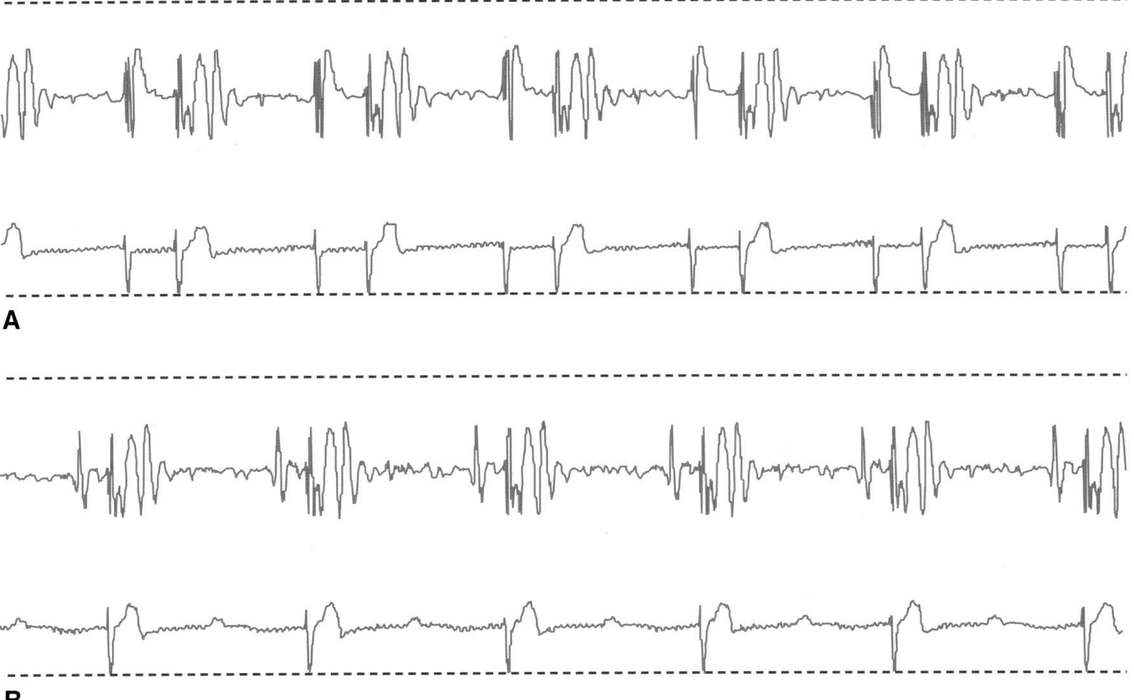

*Figure 29-35. Example of an intracardiac EGM from a patient with left atrial pacing. In both panels, the top recording is the atrial EGM, and the bottom recording is the body surface electrocardiogram. Panel **A** was recorded during atrial pacing. The atrial EGM and the surface P wave occur close to each other. Panel **B** was recorded during atrial sensing. The P wave now precedes the atrial EGM by a considerable time.*

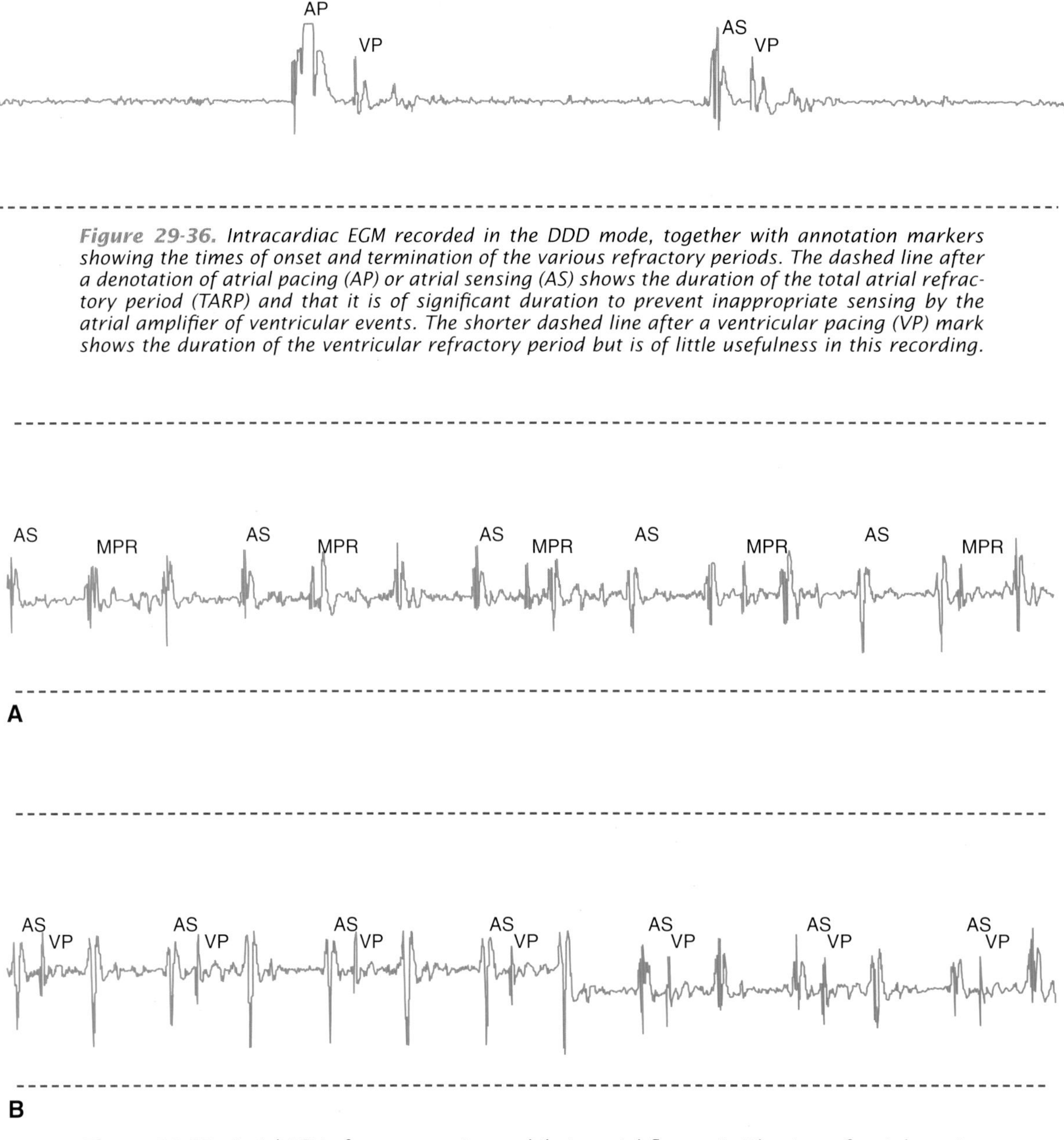

Figure 29-36. Intracardiac EGM recorded in the DDD mode, together with annotation markers showing the times of onset and termination of the various refractory periods. The dashed line after a denotation of atrial pacing (AP) or atrial sensing (AS) shows the duration of the total atrial refractory period (TARP) and that it is of significant duration to prevent inappropriate sensing by the atrial amplifier of ventricular events. The shorter dashed line after a ventricular pacing (VP) mark shows the duration of the ventricular refractory period but is of little usefulness in this recording.

Figure 29-37. Atrial EGMs from two patients while in atrial flutter. ***A,*** *The time of atrial sensing (AS) is variable, as is the atrioventricular interval, because the pacemaker is at the upper rate limit, or maximal paced rate (MPR). Note the changing total atrial refractory period (TARP) as a result of the Wenckebach behavior imposed by the upper rate limit.* ***B,*** *There is a definite 2:1 block, and the pacemaker is not at the upper rate limit. The body surface electrocardiogram was suggestive only of atrial flutter, in that the heart rate was completely regular. VP, ventricular pacing.*

Finally, the intracardiac EGM is also useful in the diagnosis of atrial dysrhythmias. In the active child, the presence of a high-paced rate may not be unusual or may suggest an atrial tachycardia. An example of such a situation is in the presence of atrial flutter (Fig. 29-37). In the first example in the figure, the rapid atrial rate was apparent on the body surface ECG recording, and the pacemaker was at the upper rate limit. In the second example, the body surface ECG recording showed an apparently regular rhythm at a rate below the upper rate limit; the atrial EGM showed atrial flutter.

Exercise Testing

Exercise testing should be an integral part of all pacemaker follow-up in children old enough to undergo treadmill testing. Such testing often pinpoints inappropriate programming, manifested by inappropriate performance. In one series, 43% of patients had clinically significant inappropriate programming while exercising that was not apparent on routine pacemaker testing.[69] Of these patients, 75% showed an inadequate heart rate increase with the stress of exercising. Although most were paced in the VVIR mode, one patient in the DDD mode was shown to have an inadequate exercise response indicative of chronotropic incompetence. All such patients underwent reprogramming with subsequent appropriate heart rate increases. Other patients were shown to have spontaneous beats at maximal exercise, causing an automatic extension of the PVARP and acute multiblock with an acute decline in the heart rate (Fig. 29-38). The development of multiblock was also seen with an acute decline in the heart rate from an inappropriately long total atrial refractory period. The multiblock rate was only slightly above the upper rate limit, causing an abrupt decline in the heart rate (Fig. 29-39). If decreasing the AV interval or the PVARP cannot adequately shorten the TARP, use of the DDDR or VDDR mode may be helpful. When the multiblock rate is reached during either of these pacing modes, the ventricular rate falls to the sensor rate rather than the inappropriately sensed atrial rate, providing a smaller decline in the heart rate. A loss of capture at the maximal heart rate was also observed, even though there had been 100% capture at rest and programming of the pacemaker was believed to be appropriate, based on resting threshold testing (Fig. 29-40).

Changes in pacing thresholds do occur and can either worsen, as the previous example shows, or improve.[26,70] For fixed-rate pacing, thresholds decline after exercise, so that resting thresholds are not necessarily indicative of those present during the stress of exercise (Fig. 29-41). However, these findings may not be applicable to the patient whose pacemaker is in the rate-responsive mode, as the example in the patient who developed loss of capture at maximal exercise showed. This is a potentially serious problem that would not have been apparent had evaluation been performed only while the patient was at rest.

Changes in P-wave amplitude were also documented at maximal exercise.[71-73] A decrease in P-wave amplitude can result in loss of atrial sensing; in the DDD mode, this

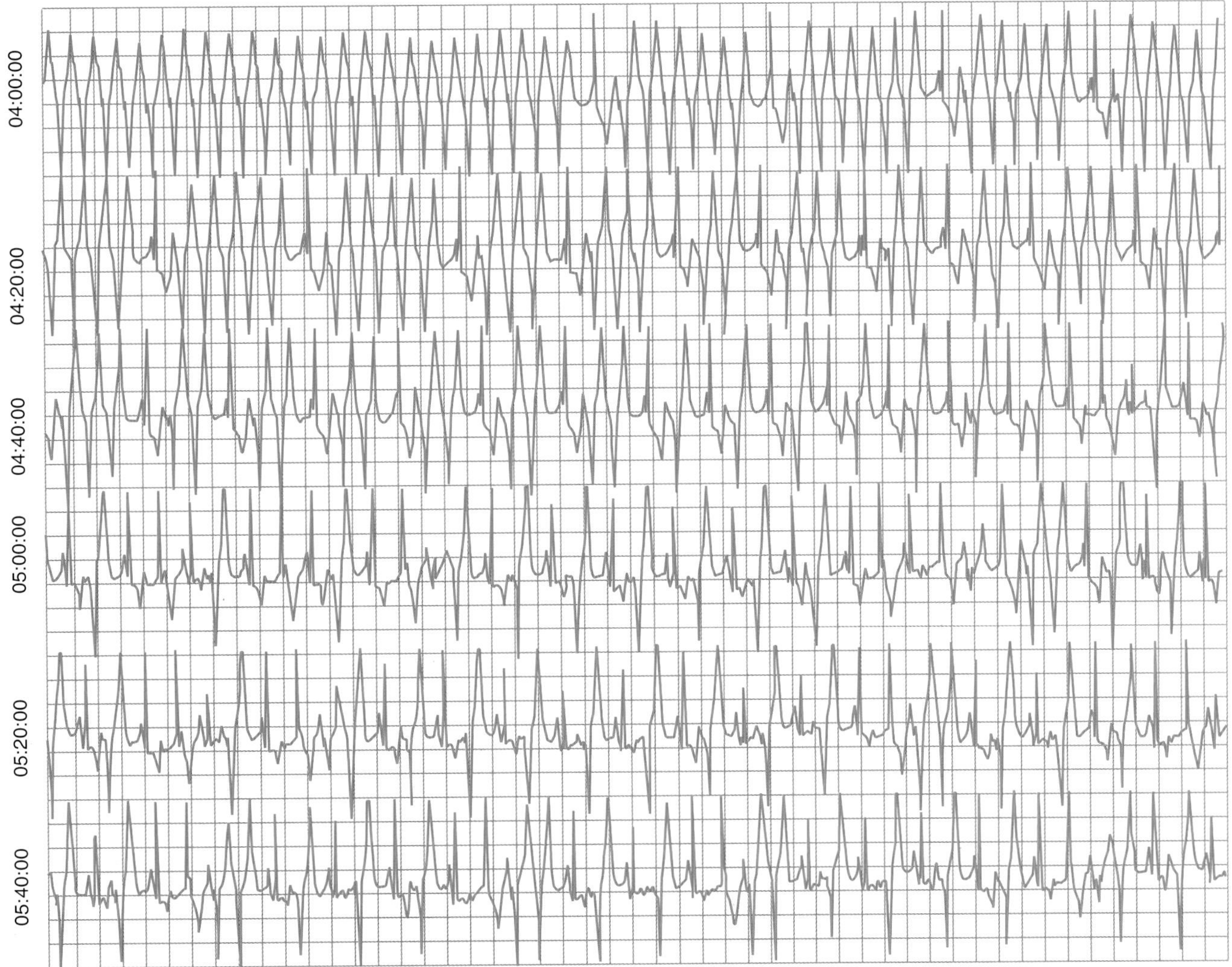

Figure 29-38. Continuous electrocardiographic recording during exercise treadmill testing showing the development of spontaneous beats at maximal exercise. This resulted in automatic extension of the postventricular atrial refractory period (PVARP), with an overall decline in the heart rate from 167 to 141 bpm. This was associated with sudden fatigue and near syncope and was corrected by elimination of the automatic PVARP extension. The paper speed is 12.5 mm/sec, with each row representing 20 seconds. The time since onset of exercise is noted by the numbers in the left margin.

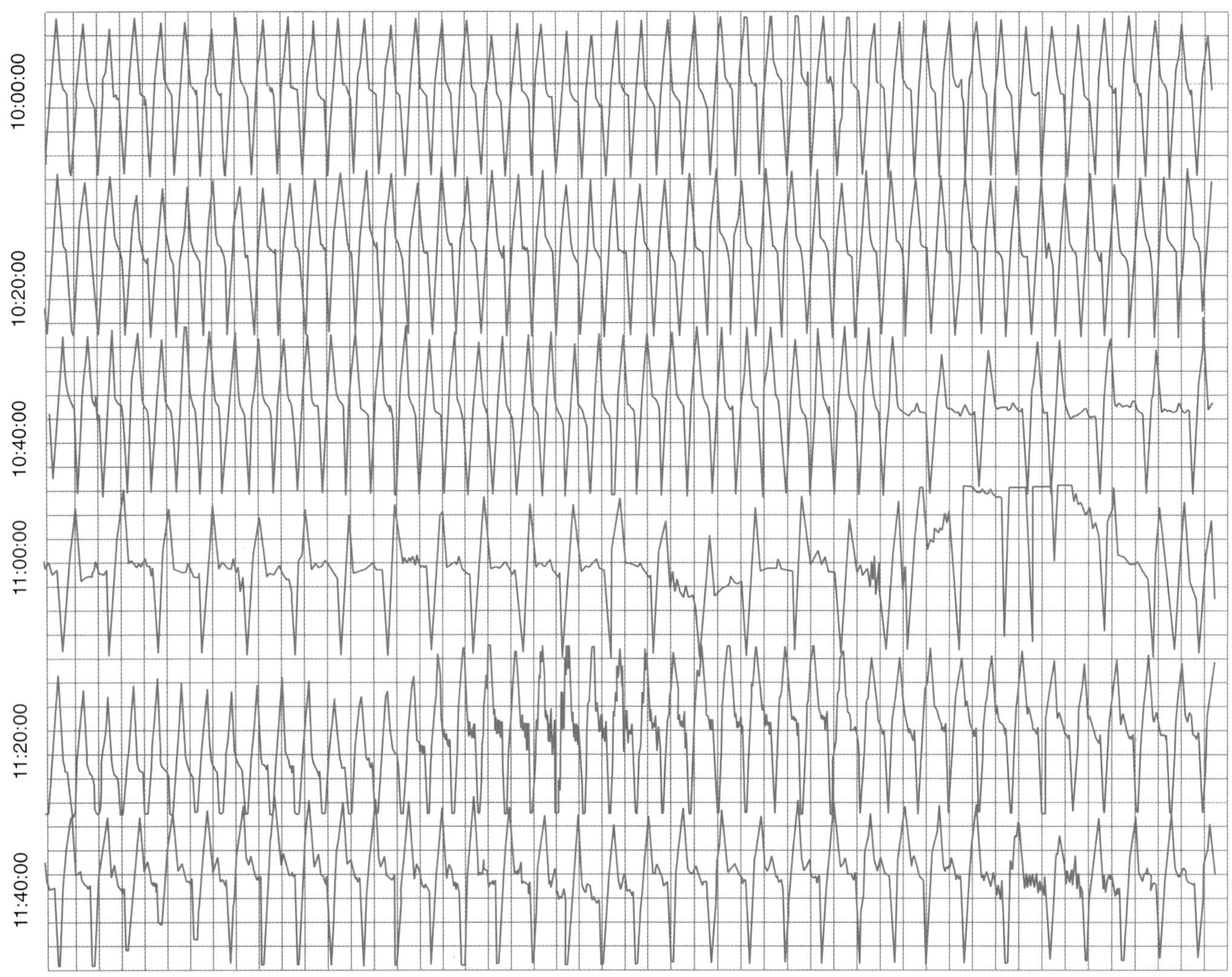

Figure 29-39. Electrocardiographic recording from an exercise test showing the development of multiblock with an acute decline in the heart rate, resulting in syncope. In this example, the patient's upper rate limit was 180 bpm, with a multiblock rate of 187 bpm. This lack of difference between the upper rate limit and the multiblock rate provided no gradual heart rate decline but rather an acute decline in heart rate and cardiac output. The multiblock rate was increased by shortening the postventricular atrial refractory period. The paper speed is 12.5 mm/sec, with each row representing 20 seconds. The time since onset of exercise is noted by the numbers in the left margin.

can cause an immediate drop to the lower rate limit of the pacemaker. The result can be syncope caused by a sudden decrease in cardiac output. Although DDDR pacing can minimize the magnitude of this heart rate drop, the physician should not rely on this mechanism, because the sensor rate may not be the same as the atrial rate, especially during activities, such as swimming or cycling. Myopotential sensing by either channel can have similar effects.[74,75] This is more evident in unipolar systems, but it can occur in bipolar systems.

Ambulatory Electrocardiographic Monitoring

Ambulatory ECG monitoring is also essential in the appropriate follow-up of pediatric patients with pacemakers. This is particularly true for those patients who are unable to exercise, because it may be the only method to evaluate high-rate performance. In many series, 24-hour ambulatory ECG monitoring was the only means by which pacemaker malfunction was detected.[76-78] Such monitoring is particularly valuable in evaluating atrial and ventricular sensing problems and intermittent lack of capture. This is important because myocardial characteristics and, hence, appropriate pacemaker programming may vary, depending on the activity state and time of day.[28] Interactions between the patient's intrinsic rhythm and the pacemaker are also more completely evaluated by ambulatory monitoring, potentially resulting in more optimal programming.

Transtelephonic Pacemaker Monitoring

Transtelephonic pacemaker monitoring also plays an important role in pacemaker follow-up and has undergone major changes recently. Previously, transtele-

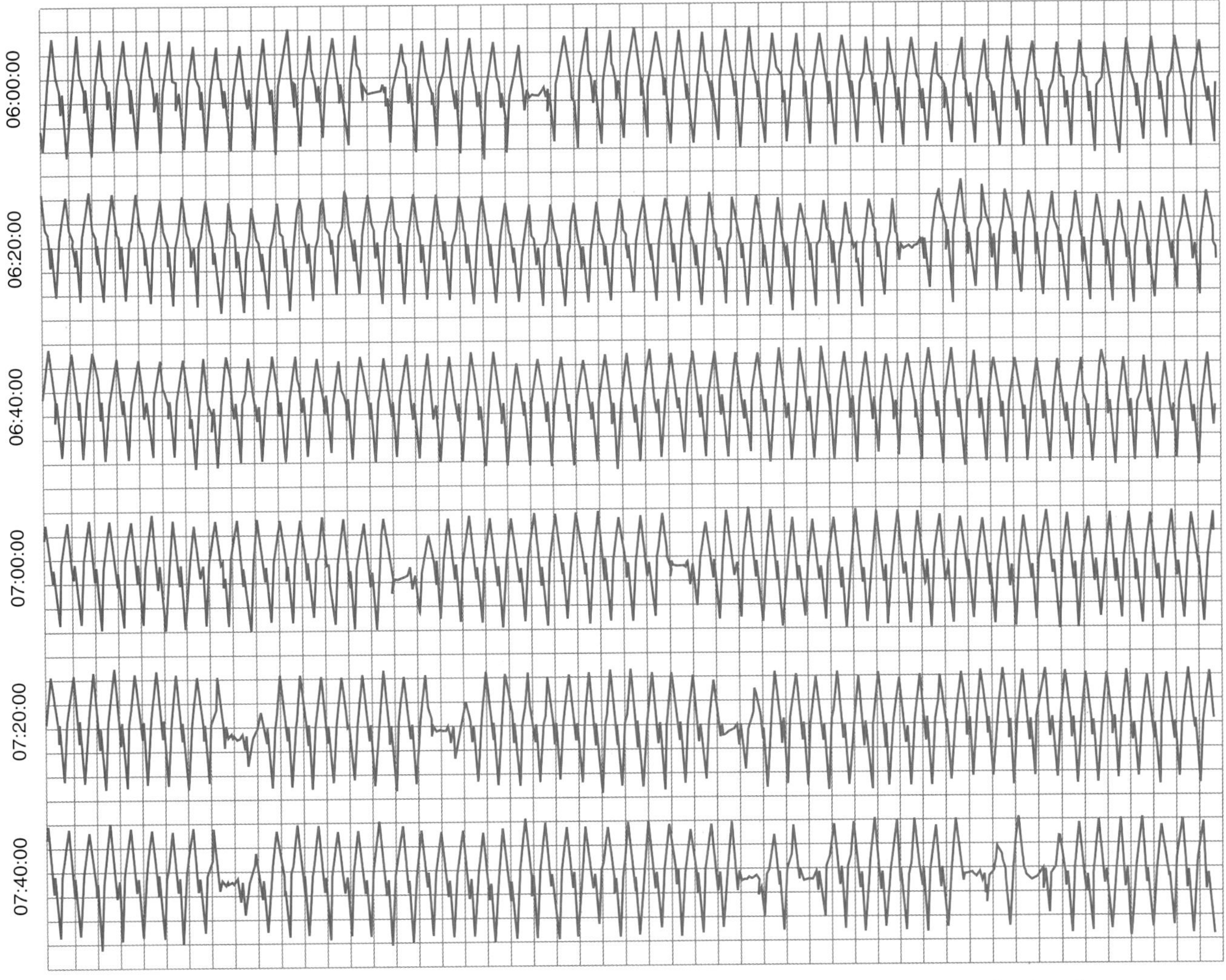

Figure 29-40. Electrocardiographic recording from an exercise test in a patient who developed acute loss of capture at maximal exercise. Threshold testing at rest indicated excellent thresholds, with the minimal pulse width necessary to pace being 0.15 msec at a 5.4-V amplitude. The programmed settings were pulse width 0.5 msec and amplitude 5.4 V. At rest and during early exercise, there was 100% capture; loss of capture occurred only at maximal exercise. The pulse width was subsequently increased to 1.0 msec, with no loss of capture on repeat testing. The paper speed is 12.5 mm/sec, with each row representing 20 seconds. The time since onset of exercise is noted by the numbers in the left margin.

phonic monitoring consisted of only a realtime ECG with and without magnet application. This did provide some information but was often difficult to perform in the uncooperative child. No stored data or trend data were available. Newer systems now permit complete pacemaker interrogation of current and stored information together with trended data and electrode threshold data. If interrogation is interrupted during data retrieval, it is halted until reception is again established and retrieval resumes. This is particularly helpful in the young, uncooperative patient. When interrogation is complete, the data are transmitted in digital form to a central computer, eliminating the need for simultaneous data retrieval and telephone transmission. An example of such a system is the Medtronic CareLink system. At the time of this writing, this and the Biotronik Home Monitoring Service are the only systems available for pacemakers, although others are currently in development.

In our follow-up clinic, the following protocol is used. The patient sends a transmission according to a predetermined schedule, at any time that is convenient. If this is only a routine transmission, nothing further is required from the patient. If there are concerns, the patient calls our clinic and relates the concerns to the pacemaker nurse or technician. Each morning, the system is interrogated and new transmissions are retrieved. If problems are found, the patient is contacted. If the patient has concerns during nonbusiness hours, the on-call physician can be contacted and can retrieve the transmission from any computer. The data are reviewed, and the information is relayed to the patient and the responsible cardiologist. The information provided is summarized on the first page of the

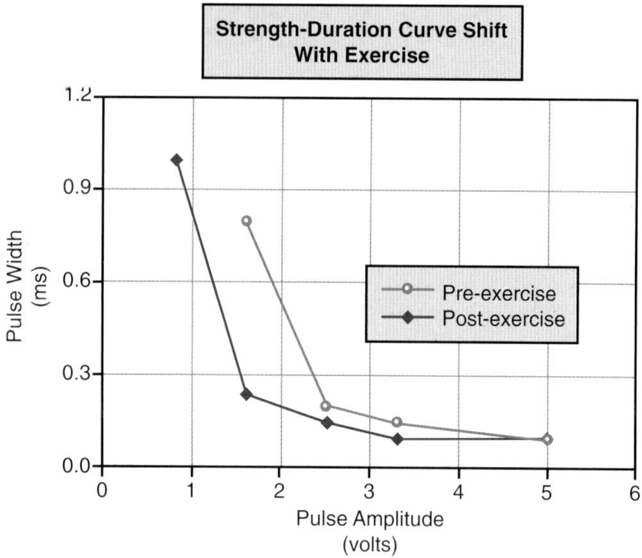

Figure 29-41. Data from a patient with fixed-rate VVI pacing who demonstrated a decrease in thresholds after termination of exercise compared with pre-exercise values. At higher pulse amplitudes, there was a minimal change, but marked changes were noted at lower pulse amplitudes. This denotes a shift of the strength-duration curve leftward, implying an increased excitability of the heart with exercise. (Data from Serwer GA, Kodali R, Eakin B, et al: Changes in pacemaker threshold with exercise in children and young adults. J Am Coll Cardiol 17:207A, 1991.)

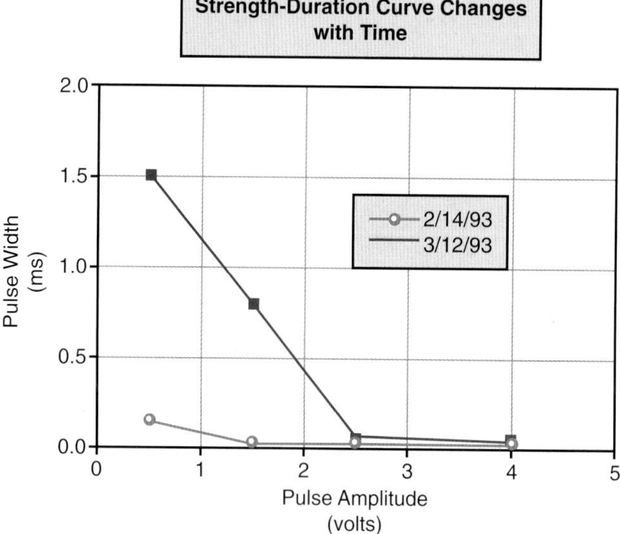

Figure 29-42. Example of change with time in the strength-duration curve. In this patient, the strength-duration curve shows changes that would not have been apparent if thresholds had been determined only at pulse amplitudes greater than 2.5 V.

report. It indicates battery status, electrode thresholds and long-term trends, electrode impedances and long-term trends, counter data (percent paced and sensed in each chamber and number of high-rate episodes), and current programming. Subsequent pages provide a real-time EGM, magnet response, and stored EGMs from high-rate episodes. This information is equivalent to that obtained in a clinic visit. Although the system does not permit reprogramming, it may otherwise obviate the need for a clinic visit if no problems are seen.

For the standard transtelephonic system, longer rhythm strips must be run to assess the pacemaker's function if a motion artifact is present. Routinely, 60-second strips are run to be sure that adequate data are obtained. Both nonmagnet and magnet strips are obtained, as in adult patients. We allow the parents to choose the best time of day to call. They often vary the time at which they call, based on nap or school schedules.

For both systems, reminder notes are sent at the beginning of each month in which a follow-up report is due. The follow-up nurse contacts the patient only if a transmission has not been received within 3 weeks of mailing of the notice.

Transtelephonic monitoring decreases cost by decreasing the number of outpatient visits needed and also provides a method to address parent and child concerns about proper pacemaker function. The capability of the child or the parent to detect pacemaker malfunction is very limited.[79] Use of transtelephonic ECG monitoring not only can confirm pacemaker malfunction but also can reassure the parent and child of proper pacemaker function.

Early Follow-up Period

Follow-up during the crucial early period must be frequent and thorough. This is especially true after a new electrode has been implanted. Our current protocol includes both pacemaker interrogation and noninvasive threshold determination at multiple pulse amplitudes performed at 2 days, 4 weeks, and 8 weeks after implantation. During this period, thresholds often vary, and the generator's output may also need to be reprogrammed to maintain reliable pacing. Exit block, in particular, is common during this period, whereas little to no exit block is noted beyond 3 months after implantation.[78] In another series, there appeared to be a slight increase in threshold after 3 months, but this occurred in only 24% of patients.[80] It is important to determine thresholds at multiple pulse amplitudes, because the strength-duration curve can move only in a horizontal direction, with thresholds at the higher outputs unchanging and thresholds at lower outputs showing marked increases (Fig. 29-42).

In addition, 24-hour ambulatory ECG monitoring is performed within the first week after implantation to assess proper pacemaker function throughout the day, not just for a brief period during pacemaker interrogation. For those children who are old enough to undergo exercise testing, this is performed within the first 2 weeks after implantation. Transtelephonic monitoring is done monthly during this period.

Intermediate Follow-up

During the intermediate follow-up period, defined as 3 months to 5 years after implantation, there tends to be only a small incidence of electrode or generator malfunction. Pacing systems tend to be more stable during this time and do not require as frequent re-evaluation. Our current protocol is to see patients annually for pacemaker interrogation and threshold testing and to obtain 24-hour ambulatory ECG recordings if indicated. Transtelephonic monitoring is done bimonthly unless complicating features are believed to require more frequent monitoring. In addition, patients and their parents are encouraged to send transmissions whenever there is a question about proper pacemaker function. With the newer remote follow-up systems, fewer in-office follow-up visits may be sufficient.

Late Follow-up

During the period between 5 years after implantation and the time for pacemaker replacement, generator failure is more likely than electrode failure. Although electrode failure does occur, the thresholds, in general, tend to be stable, and most electrode failures during this period are a consequence of acute lead fracture and not exit block. There tends to be no warning preceding lead fracture, and no follow-up method currently used has been shown to be useful in predicting such events. However, depletion of the generator's battery can be adequately detected early through the use of monthly transtelephonic ECG monitoring. Ambulatory ECG recordings are still obtained yearly.

Use of Antitachycardia Devices in Children with Congenital Heart Disease

Implantable Defibrillator Use

The use of ICDs in children has been limited by many factors, including uncertainty of the indications for use, device size, and the difficulty initially of implanting the epicardial electrodes. With additional experience in the adult population and a decrease in size of the devices and the electrodes, both epicardial and endocardial, the pediatric use of ICDs is increasing. Silka and colleagues[81] reported on a large multicenter experience with initial use of ICDs in children ranging in age from 1.9 to 20 years. More recently, Hamilton and associates[82] reported on 11 children aged 4 to 16 years in a single-center experience. Kron and coworkers[83] reported on the use of nonthoracotomy electrode systems in 17 children aged 12 to 20 years. A more recent study by Steffanelli and associates[84] reported on the experience at a larger single center with 27 patients. The issues surrounding the use of ICDs in children involve (1) appropriate patient selection, (2) selection of epicardial versus endocardial implantation and the techniques involved, (3) appropriate tachyarrhythmia detection and therapy programming, and (4) appropriate follow-up.

Patient Selection

In all of the series mentioned, all patients had experienced a syncopal or sudden death episode documented to be a ventricular arrhythmia or had an inducible ventricular arrhythmia at electrophysiologic study after their syncopal or sudden death event. In the study of Silka and associates,[81] 76% of children were survivors of a sudden cardiac death episode, whereas 10% had experienced a syncopal episode with inducible sustained ventricular tachycardia; the remainder had drug-refractory ventricular tachycardia. The underlying diagnoses were hypertrophic cardiomyopathy, long QT syndrome, dilated cardiomyopathy, or repaired congenital heart disease. Fewer than one half had depressed ventricular function. In general, any child who has survived a sudden cardiac death episode or has a condition that can result in such an episode should be considered for ICD implantation. Medical therapy should always be employed, but one must decide whether medical therapy alone will completely eliminate the likelihood of a repeat episode. For example, the patient with long QT syndrome who has experienced a sudden death episode should be treated medically and should also undergo ICD placement. Conversely, a child with congenital complete heart block and a documented episode of ventricular fibrillation may require only permanent pacing.

Although cardiomyopathies and primary electrical diseases constitute the most common diagnoses requiring ICD placement, children who have undergone repair of congenital heart disease are beginning to present with malignant ventricular arrhythmias. The most common lesions are tetralogy of Fallot and transposition of the great arteries after Mustard repair.[81] In our experience, 15% of all patients receiving ICDs had undergone prior repair of tetralogy of Fallot. Children with this diagnosis accounted for 22% of patients in the report by Silka and colleagues.[81] Any child who has undergone a ventriculotomy or repair of a coronary artery abnormality is at potential risk for ventricular arrhythmias.

One unresolved issue is whether children who are potentially at risk for a sudden death episode but who have not experienced one should undergo ICD placement (primary prevention). The most recent guidelines[19] list implantation for high-risk patients without syncope as a class IIb indication (class IIb defined as probably useful but less well established by evidence). In our practice, symptom-free children with long QT syndrome and no family history of sudden death are treated medically unless ventricular arrhythmias can be evoked at electrophysiologic study.

Implantation Approaches

Two decisions affect ICD implantation: epicardial versus endocardial electrode placement and subclavicular versus abdominal device placement. Each can be made independently of the other. Initially, only epicardial electrode placement was used in children, owing to the very large size of the transvenous electrode and the inappropriate shocking coil spacing or the need to place a second electrode. Even with transvenous electrode improvements (discussed later), it remains the preferred method for smaller children. The smallest child to receive an endocardial system in the study of Kron and coworkers[83] weighed 32 kg, and the smallest in the study of Hamilton and colleagues[82] weighed 27 kg. In our center, the smallest child has weighed 20 kg. We still use epicardial patches in children who weigh less than 20 kg or in whom there is no venous access to the ventricle.

Patches are usually placed to maximize the distance between them and to maximize exposure of the myocardium to the defibrillation energy. They are sutured to the pericardium rather than the epicardial surface, to minimize growth effects and patch distortion (Fig. 29-43). With time, distortion can develop, but it does not necessarily have an adverse effect on the defibrillatory thresholds. The leads are then tunneled to the abdomen, and the pocket is created, as for implantation of an epicardial pacemaker system. In one case of a child with absent abdominal musculature, the device was placed intrathoracically.

In smaller children, even the small patch electrodes may be too large. In these cases, transvenous coil electrodes, designed to be placed in the superior vena cava, and subcutaneous array electrodes have been placed in the lateral mediastinum. Defibrillatory energy is delivered between these electrodes, traversing the heart in a lateral direction. Such an arrangement has been shown to result in acceptable defibrillatory thresholds, using a multiple coil or a single coil and an active can.[85,86]

With the development of smaller-diameter transvenous electrodes and use of the device can as the second defibrillation electrode, a transvenous system can be used in most children. The currently available electrodes, both single- and dual-coil, can be introduced with a 9F introducer. However, the intercoil spacing in the dual-coil electrode is usually too large to be employed in children. Positioning the second coil properly requires buckling of the electrode within the right atrium (Fig. 29-44), potentially dislodging the electrode tip. Use of the single-coil electrode eliminates this problem. Even with electrode buckling, the superior vena cava coil remains close to the clavicle, placing it at risk for fracture.

Use of a single-coil electrode requires the device can to serve as the second electrode; alternatively, a second intravascular coil or a subcutaneous array can be used as the second electrode. Initially, use of the active can was restricted to implantation of the device under the left clavicle. However, we have implanted the device in an upper left quadrant abdominal pocket with the single-coil, bipolar-pacing, steroid-eluting electrode introduced into the left subclavian vein and tunneled subcutaneously to the device pocket (Fig. 29-45).[87] This technique is similar to the method proposed by Molina and colleagues for transvenous pacemaker implantation in small patients.[88] This approach has been used in children as small as 20 kg in our center. Defibrillatory thresholds have been less than 10 J in all cases, even though the electrode area is reduced.[89] No patient has required an additional electrode, either a subcutaneous array or a second transvenous electrode.

Programming Considerations

The issues of appropriate programming are similar to those in the adult patient. The major concern is the

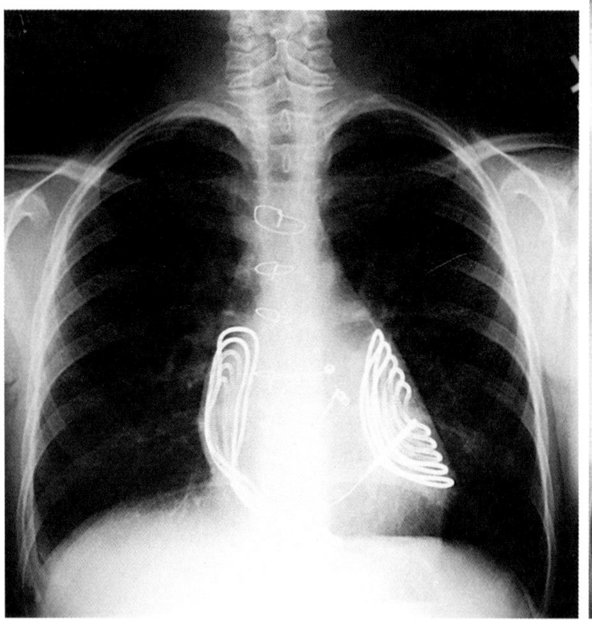

A

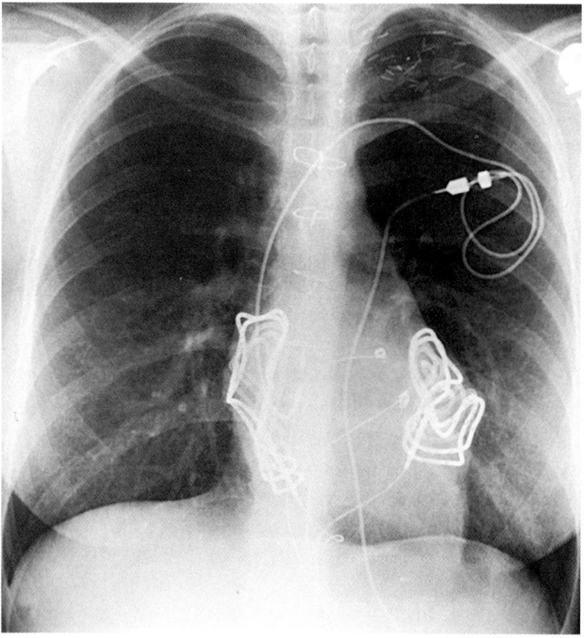

B

Figure 29-43. ***A,*** *Chest radiograph taken after acute placement of epicardial defibrillation patches in a child.* ***B,*** *Chest radiograph in the same child 4 years after implantation, shows buckling of the patches, although the defibrillatory thresholds remain low. Note the placement of a transvenous atrial electrode, which was tunneled to the device in the abdomen using a lead extender because the device had been upgraded to a dual-chamber pacemaker defibrillator. The epicardial ventricular pacing and sensing electrodes placed originally continue to be used.*

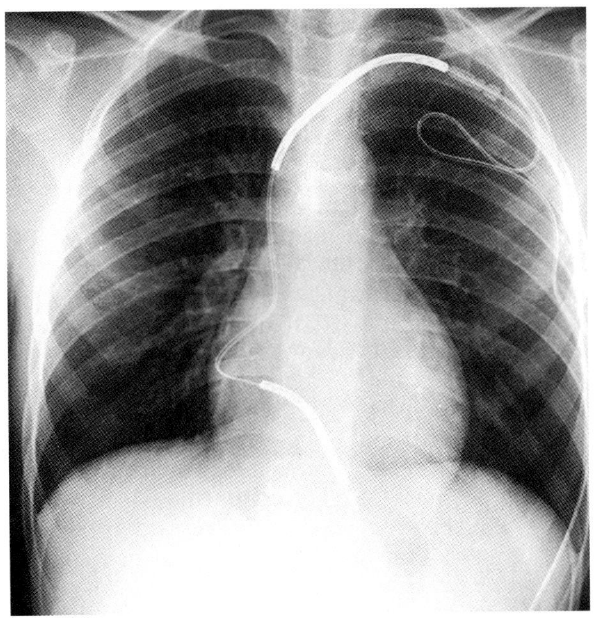

Figure 29-44. Chest radiograph showing placement of a dual-coil single-lead transvenous defibrillator system with the lead tunneled to the abdomen. Note the buckling of the lead within the atrium, which was necessary to place the distal coil properly within the innominate vein. This could potentially dislodge the right ventricular coil and still leaves the distal coil near the clavicle/first rib space.

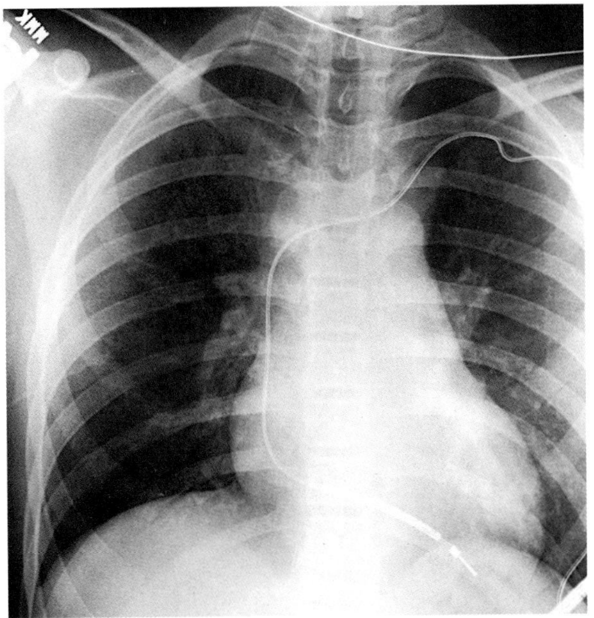

Figure 29-45. Chest radiograph showing placement of a single-coil transvenous defibrillator system with the lead tunneled down the lateral chest wall to the device, which also serves as the second defibrillation electrode and is placed in a left upper quadrant abdominal pocket.

higher sinus rates that can occur in a child. Initially, β-blockers were employed to reduce the maximal sinus rate. However, this approach often resulted in significant exercise intolerance. Although β-blockers may be indicated to treat the underlying disease (i.e., long QT syndrome), their use solely to reduce the maximal sinus rate is no longer necessary. Current devices can now be programmed to very high rates as a criterion of ventricular tachycardia and can also employ other markers, such as increased QRS duration and sudden onset. Yet for most children, use of high rate alone is usually sufficient to detect fibrillation. Also, many children have wide QRS complexes as a consequence of prior cardiac surgery, making this criterion difficult to use. In practice, we program the device to a detection cycle interval that is 50 msec greater than the documented fibrillation cycle interval, consistent with the approach of Hamilton and associates.[82] QRS duration is used only if cycle interval alone has been unable to prevent inappropriate therapy delivery.

Follow-up Procedures

At our center, all children initially underwent induction of ventricular fibrillation 1 week after implantation to ensure that detection and therapy were appropriate. However, if no problems were suspected clinically, defibrillatory thresholds proved to be acceptable in all cases. Determination of thresholds beyond implantation is now reserved for patients in whom there is a suspicion of system malfunction.

At each clinic visit, the device is interrogated, and each recorded event is inspected for cycle length and QRS morphology. Pacing thresholds are also determined, as for pacemaker patients. Recently, transtelephonic systems have been developed to permit interrogation of ICD status remotely. Such systems allow for determination of battery voltage, charge time, electrode impedance, and viewing of event counters, recent events, and real-time EGMs. These systems allow for better and more frequent ICD follow-up without the necessity for repeated clinic visits in otherwise asymptomatic patients.

After each therapy delivery, the child is seen in the clinic and the device is interrogated, or a remote transmission is sent to evaluate the event and to be sure that the therapy was appropriate. This is particularly crucial because inappropriate therapies are not rare. Also, the medical therapy is re-evaluated to ensure that it does not require alteration. Finally, the psychological aspects of the child's reaction to the therapy are evaluated, and support is offered as needed. Assessing the need for long-term support is extremely important and is discussed later.

Antitachycardia Pacing

Pace-termination of atrial arrhythmias is beginning to be used in patients with congenital heart disease.[90] This has become possible with the development of a dual-chamber antitachycardia pacemaker with a rate-response suitable for use in smaller patients. Although it does not have defibrillator capabilities and therefore is not suitable for pace-termination of ventricular tachycardias, the device has proved useful for treatment of atrial flutter, particularly in postoperative patients, in whom atrial flutter is often seen but is difficult to treat with either medication or ablative techniques. The Medtronic AT500 has been used in a series of patients with congenital heart disease and atrial tachycardias.[90] It was shown to successfully terminate the tachycardia in 54% of episodes. Success is influenced by many factors, including proximity of the electrode to the reentrant circuit, atrial size, and the potential for multiple reentrant circuits. It does require placement of both atrial and ventricular electrodes, even if only atrial pacing is anticipated, because ventricular sensing is needed to prevent pacing in 1:1 AV rhythms. In addition, these electrodes must be bipolar in configuration, and close electrode placing is required to minimize far-field oversensing, especially of the atrial electrode. Proper electrode placement and selection are more critical for antitachycardia pacing than for routine pacemaker placement. Proper programming of the tachycardia sensing parameters as well as termination parameters further increases the complexity of their use. Even with this increased complexity, however, these devices provide an important adjunct for patients with drug-resistant atrial tachyarrhythmias, especially when there are indications for bradycardia pacing—a not uncommon situation for this patient group.

Resynchronization Therapy in Patients with Structural Cardiac Disease

Cardiac resynchronization therapy (CRT) has only begun to be used in patients with structural disease. Most patients who might benefit from such therapy have had prior surgery, and they often have RV rather than LV conduction delays. Therefore, implantation criteria developed for patients with ischemic or even nonischemic disease and LV conduction delays have little relevance. Initial studies in the acute postoperative setting have been encouraging for patients with RV failure and RV conduction delay, but experience is limited.[91] Results of limited series looking at the long-term benefits of biventricular pacing also appear promising.[92] Related work using multiple pacing sites simultaneously in the right ventricle in patients with intact AV conduction has also shown acute improvements in cardiac function.[93,94] Nevertheless, unique problems exist in this patient group. LV pacing via a coronary sinus electrode can be problematic due to the small size of the coronary sinus, anatomic variation in its anatomy (especially in the presence of a superior vena cava draining to it), and the possible long-term need for such therapy. Given the coronary sinus electrodes currently available, most LV pacing may need to be accomplished via the epicardial route. Multisite RV pacing is not currently possible from the transvenous route and would require epicardial electrode placement. Proper programming parameters are largely unknown. Acute adjustment with measurement of select hemodynamic parameters may be of some help, but long-term benefits may not be predicted by acute measurements. Although it is anticipated that CRT will prove beneficial, much work remains before it becomes an established therapy for this patient population, especially in those with RV conduction delays.

Prophylactic Medication

There has been significant controversy concerning the need for prophylactic anticoagulants or antibiotic agents for the prevention of subacute bacterial endocarditis in children with pacemakers. The current recommendations of the American Heart Association do *not* suggest the use of antibiotics in children with pacemakers.[95] However, most of these children have other underlying structural diseases that do require the use of antibiotics for prophylaxis. Our current practice is to prescribe antibiotics for prophylaxis of subacute bacterial endocarditis for all children who have endocardial electrodes if there is any AV valve regurgitation present by physical examination or echocardiography. Children with epicardial pacing systems without associated structural cardiac lesions do not require such prophylaxis.

Prophylactic anticoagulation has not been shown to be useful in children who have endocardial pacing systems. Only those children with chronic atrial flutter or fibrillation are routinely anticoagulated. We believe that the risk to the active child from chronic anticoagulation is significant and the benefit derived is minimal.

Psychosocial Adjustments in Children with Pacemakers

Comprehensive care of the child with a pacemaker requires awareness of the psychosocial issues faced by children and families. Although there are issues specific to having a pacemaker, such as dependence on a mechanical device and the certainty of periodic surgeries throughout life, the overall challenges are similar to those faced by children with other types of chronic illness. Treatment goals include facilitation of positive child and family adjustments and prevention of avoidable negative psychosocial outcomes. Important illness-related tasks for parents of children with pacemakers include participating in the treatment plan, preserving emotional well-being for themselves and their children, and preparing for an uncertain future.[96] Children who are at high risk for emotional or behavioral adjustment problems may benefit from early identification and intervention.[97]

Currently, curative therapies are not available for the arrhythmias treated by pacemakers; hence, these children, by definition, have a chronic illness.[98] Because of the underlying disease and the lifelong need for a pacemaker, the children and their families are chronically subjected to stressful experiences, including repeated surgeries, body image changes, and exposure to the possibility of death.[99] Prognoses and disease-imposed physical limitations vary considerably in this population, ranging from the adolescent athlete with congenital complete heart block to the child with severe cardiomyopathy. Although disease severity varies, most patients can anticipate many fruitful adult years, and many are anticipated to have a normal or nearly normal life span.

In one of the few studies examining psychosocial outcomes in this population, no significant differences were found between children with pacemakers and comparison children on standardized measures of trait anxiety, self-competence, and self-esteem.[100] Children with pacemakers were more external in their locus of control orientation than healthy controls but were not significantly different on this measure from children with comparable heart disease who did not have a pacemaker.[100] Interview data from the same study suggest that comparison children were likely to report negative stereotypes about children with pacemakers. These findings are consistent with other studies and indicate that most chronically ill children make positive adjustments, although there is an increased risk for psychosocial problems.[101] The incidence of problems is not insignificant; epidemiologic studies suggest that up to 30% of children with chronic illness demonstrate secondary psychosocial impairment by 15 years of age.[102]

The risk for psychosocial problems in this population can be understood as a response to chronic stress that challenges the adaptive capacities of the children and their families.[103,104] Consistent with this model, negative adjustments are likely to occur when stress exceeds the child's adaptive capacities. Certainly, there is wide variation in children's adaptations, and some children are able to make positive adaptations despite extremely stressful circumstances.[105,106]

Considerable research has aimed to identify the biomedical, age-specific, and social-environmental factors linked with children's adjustments. Many of the factors identified reflect a continuum, with one end representing a protective factor and the other a risk factor. For example, family functioning that is cohesive and adaptable is associated with positive adaptations in children, whereas family functioning that is disengaged and rigid is associated with emotional and behavioral problems in the children.[107]

Disease-related biomedical factors anticipated to affect children's adjustments include diagnosis (disease severity, prognosis, treatment), functional impairment, cognitive abilities, and visibility (physical changes).[108,109] For children with a chronic illness, diagnosis and disease severity are less important predictors of adjustment than are other factors[108]; however, the diagnosis of heart disease during childhood may pose particular challenges, for reasons not well understood.[110] Biomedical factors that may negatively influence psychosocial outcomes for children with heart disease include early mother-infant attachment problems,[111] neuropsychological changes,[112] learning disabilities,[113] and exclusion from competitive sports.[114]

Inherent child factors that may affect adjustment include temperament, developmental stage, and competency.[98,108] For example, an academically gifted child may experience opportunities for self-esteem, socialization, and social recognition that ameliorate the negative effects of having a chronic illness, whereas the child with a learning disability who has a chronic illness is at increased risk for serious adjustment problems.[115]

Social-environmental factors linked with children's adjustments include family environment, mothers' psychological functioning, family economic resources, and children's peer relationships. Families that are adaptive and cohesive and communicate effectively support positive adjustments for children.[116,117] Maternal adjustment may play a particularly important role in children's adjustment,[118,119] and persistent maternal distress (e.g., symptoms of anxiety or depression) warrants intervention.[108] Economic resources appear to be powerful moderators of children's adjustment to stressful life circumstances.[105,106,120] The quality of children's friendships is also important, because positive peer relationships are linked with prosocial behavior, academic achievement, stress resistance, and later, adolescent competence.[121-123] Conversely, negative child peer relationships are associated with academic failure, aggressive behavior,[120,124] and general psychopathology, which persists during adulthood.[125] Social isolation and feelings of loneliness are potential sources of emotional distress for chronically ill children and family members.[98]

Coping methods are the processes used by children and families to accomplish disease-related tasks, maintain normal function, and minimize family disruption. Adaptive parental coping strategies include maintaining family integrity through cooperation and maintenance of an optimistic outlook; maintaining social support, self-esteem, and psychological stability; and understanding the medical situation through communication with other parents and health care providers.[126] Coping is a dynamic process that may promote or hinder positive adjustments.[127] Coping methods can be categorized as problem focused or emotion focused; in general, both methods are used by individuals responding to stress.[127] Problem-focused coping methods involve actions taken to address a stressful situation, whereas emotion-focused methods are those coping methods that change the emotional reaction to an event, such as altering the perception of the experience, blunting, or denial. There are differences in coping strategies employed by fathers and by mothers, and this may be a source of distress within the marriage.[128] Children's coping strategies reflect their developmental stage, and problem-focused strategies precede emotion-focused strategies during childhood.[129]

Implications for Health Care Providers

Knowledge of the factors associated with child and family adjustments, illness-related tasks, and coping methods guide comprehensive treatment for the child with a pacemaker and may be used by providers to clarify what can be realistically influenced within their practices. Comprehensive management of the child with a pacemaker is based on assessments of the child and family, with identification of areas of strength and vulnerability. As described previously, considerable data suggest that key areas to include in the assessment are child functional impairment, school achievement and peer relationships, maternal distress, family functioning, and socioeconomic status. If these factors are favorable, there is a high likelihood that the child will make a positive adjustment to having a pacemaker. Significant problems in any of these areas suggest the need for further assessment, intervention, and possible referral to a mental health professional.

Provider-Family Interactions: Opportunities for Education, Support, and Intervention

Provider-family interactions afford key opportunities for education, support, and intervention aimed at facilitating positive child adjustments. Initial implantation and pacemaker replacement are stressful times for children and families, when many questions and concerns arise. Families are generally more relaxed during routine follow-up visits, making this an optimal time to further the provider-family relationship, explore lifestyle issues, and affirm successes in the child's life. Because questions often arise between visits, it is important to provide ready telephone access to experienced pacemaker professionals.

Communication with providers about the child's prognosis, appropriate activities, and restrictions is necessary for parents and children to adjust to life with a pacemaker. At initial implantation, many parents are unfamiliar with the use of pacemakers in children and may assume that needing a pacemaker means the child's heart is "getting worse" or that the child "won't live long, because only old people get pacemakers." Conversations with the child and family about what the pacemaker means for the child's future are important, because emotional well-being is predicated on a hopeful outlook—one that permits belief in a personal and meaningful future.[130]

As identified previously, feelings of loneliness and social isolation are potential sources of emotional distress for children with pacemakers and family members. Providers can furnish opportunities for social support, both informally, by introducing families in the clinic or hospital, and formally, by sponsoring support groups. Providers can also link families with state and national family support networks and reputable on-line support groups. Children may benefit from meeting other children with pacemakers in the clinic or from having a "pacemaker pen pal." One child who attends our clinic was feeling isolated because he "never met other kids who have pacemakers." A one-time social gathering was arranged with the child, his parents, and three other families who agreed to participate. A pediatric psychologist facilitated the discussion, and the distressed child experienced a more positive mood after the meeting.

Education is necessary so that parents can adhere to monitoring protocols, use medical resources effectively, and provide appropriate activities for their children. Areas to be addressed include the symptoms of pacemaker malfunction, appropriate use of transtelephonic monitoring systems, precautions, activity recommendations, and the need for periodic pacemaker replacement. It is our practice to recommend cardiopulmonary resuscitation (CPR) training for all parents, and parents with pacemaker-dependent children receive CPR training in the hospital before discharge. Education of the child varies based on developmental stage, among other factors. Children who undergo initial pacemaker implantation in infancy or early childhood need ongoing education regarding their disease and treatment to fill in age-related gaps in their understanding. When developing a teaching plan, it is important to remember that children's social networks may include nontraditional family members, school personnel, and extended family members.

Surgery, whether for the initial pacemaker or at the time of replacement, is a stressful time for children and families. Parents often have questions about when to talk to their child about the upcoming surgery and what content they should include. The aim of preoperative education is to facilitate the child's ability to cope with the stress of surgery. The timing, content, and methods used to educate children vary with developmental stage and must be individualized. In general, upcoming surgery should be discussed with young children near in time to the surgery, within 24 to 48 hours. Young children often respond enthusiastically to short play sessions during the preoperative visit, with hospital articles such as anesthesia masks and plastic syringes.

An important functional outcome for children with pacemakers is successful integration into the school community. Although there is realistic concern about negative stereotyping by school personnel,[98] some data suggest that parents believe that school personnel should be informed about their child's illness and that health professionals are the most appropriate people to provide this education.[131] To facilitate school integration, we have used a variety of interventions, including participation in parent-teacher meetings at the child's school, visiting the child's classroom, and making pacemaker models and other materials available to the child for school presentations.

Psychosocial Adjustments in Children with Implantable Cardioverter-Defibrillators

Minimal data are available regarding the adjustments of children and adolescents after ICD implantation. In a study of nine patients, ranging in age from 13 to 49 years, Vitale and Funk[132] reported difficulty sleeping, low energy, and interruptions in planned activities. Problems reported for older patients after ICD implantation include increased anxiety levels, excessive anger, psychological disturbances, sexual abstinence, restricted physical activities, and restricted social activities.[133,134] Some newer studies have emphasized that most older adults appear to make positive adjustments after ICD implantation.[135]

Although the data are lacking, this population would appear to be at risk for the development of psychosocial problems due to disease-related factors, including disease severity, functional impairment, and body image changes. Disease severity is significant, because these children have survived, or are at high risk for, a lethal arrhythmia. Many of the children are survivors of out-of-hospital cardiac arrests, with the fear, drama, and exposure to the possibility of death that such experiences entail. The incidence of anoxic encephalopathy after cardiac arrest is not insignificant; if it does occur, it can be anticipated to affect later adjustment. Visibility is also an issue, because the devices are still large in relation to a child's body mass. The treatment delivered by the device is another source of distress for patients, with ramifications exceeding the pain and potential embarrassment at the time of therapy (see later discussion). Finally, many of the children who require ICD implantation have inherited diseases, such as long QT syndrome, familial dilated cardiomyopathy, or hypertrophic cardiomyopathy. Therefore, health-related concern extends beyond that child to other family members who may be affected. Because of the hereditary nature and severity of these diagnoses, many families have experienced the death of one or more family members, which adds to feelings of grief, anxiety, and guilt.

In our experience, the potential for a life-threatening arrhythmia and receiving a shock are sources of considerable anxiety, particularly for adolescents. Conscious shocks, particularly repeated conscious shocks, can be very traumatic. Three adolescent patients in whom we have implanted ICDs have experienced conscious (appropriate) shocks, and two of them experienced repeated conscious shocks. After these events, all three patients experienced severe anxiety that persisted longer than 1 month. In two patients, school phobias developed. The other patient was home for summer vacation and, very uncharacteristically, would not participate in usual summer activities, preferring to stay at home. One young patient demonstrated classic symptoms of post-traumatic stress disorder, including intrusive re-experiencing of the traumatic event, suicidal thoughts, feelings of detachment, and high levels of anxiety. All three patients required professional counseling, and one was treated with antidepressant medication and biofeedback. All have since returned to school; two are now in college and one in high school. It is important to note that none of these adolescents had a history of psychiatric problems before the ICD implantation.

The body of literature concerning conditioned learning can facilitate our understanding of the effect of unpredictable, conscious shocks on young people. It is known that repeated unpredictable aversive stimuli, in addition to producing fear and avoidance behavior, can have long-term debilitating effects.[136] Many of the experiments done on the effects of aversive conditioning actually used unpredictable electrical shocks as the source of the stimuli. Maier and Seligman[137] proposed that, in such circumstances, people may develop the expectation that their behavior has little effect on their environment, and this expectation may generalize to a wide range of situations. This behavior mode, referred to as *learned helplessness,* has been linked with human depression.[137]

Complicating the situation for patients with tachyarrhythmias is the catecholamine release that occurs secondary to anxiety. The increased heart rate is often perceived as the possible onset of the arrhythmia, leading to increased anxiety and feelings of loss of control. Relaxation under these conditions can present a challenge for young people. Potential therapies, in addition to counseling, include relaxation methods and biofeedback.[138]

Support groups have been shown to be helpful in promoting positive adjustments to chronic illness in a family member.[139] Factors associated with support group participation that may be therapeutic for patients and family members include sharing of information, instilling of hope, universality, altruism, and interpersonal learning.[139] Although this is an effective intervention, the use of support groups by this population so far appears to be limited. Professionals working with these patients report that many younger patients do not participate in ongoing ICD patient support groups, because the groups do not address issues of personal concern, such as work, intimate relations, childbirth, school, friends, and dating. Also, the relatively small numbers of young defibrillator patients in any one geographic area have limited the ability to initiate support groups specifically for this population.

In an attempt to address the needs of this unique population, we have collaborated with the adult electrophysiology service at our hospital on annual "Youth and Young Adult Support Seminars" for ICD patients in their 30s and younger. In addition to educational workshops on topics of interest to young patients, professionally facilitated support groups were provided, according to age, gender, and role (patient, spouse, or parent). It is our belief that the children and adolescents benefited from their interactions with young adult ICD patients, because they could see firsthand that a meaningful future is possible for them. Evaluations revealed that many of the patients had never met another young person with a defibrillator before the conference.

School reentry after ICD implantation has been a source of considerable concern for parents and school professionals. Education of school personnel by clinic staff regarding the child's arrhythmia, how the device works, what to do if therapy is given, and development of an emergency plan for school personnel is routine after implantation. Parental permission is always obtained before the school is contacted, and parents are included as important participants in all school-based meetings. During the meetings, it has been helpful to emphasize the protection afforded by the device and that the purpose of undergoing device implantation is to permit the child to live, as much as possible, a normal life.

The long-term outlook of children requiring either ICD or pacemaker implantation continues to improve. Therefore, a positive attitude must be conveyed to the child, the parents, and the caregivers to allow the child to lead as normal a life as possible.

REFERENCES

1. Moquin PM, Vaysse J, Durand M, et al: Implantation d'un stimulateur interne pour correction d'un bloc auriculo-ventriculo-

ventriculaire chirurgical chez une enfant de 7 ans. Arch Mal Coeur Vaiss 55:241, 1962.
2. Gillette PC, Wampler DG, Shannon C, Oth D: Use of cardiac pacing after the Mustard operation for transposition of the great arteries. J Am Coll Cardiol 7:138, 1986.
3. El-Said G, Rosenberg HS, Mullins LE, et al: Dysrhythmias after Mustard's operation for transposition of the great arteries. Am J Cardiol 30:526, 1972.
4. Shearn RPN, Flemming WH: Fourteen years of implanted pacemakers in children. Ann Thorac Surg 25:144, 1978.
5. Simon AB, Dick M II, Stern AM, et al: Ventricular pacing in children. PACE 5:836, 1982.
6. Walkens JJS: Cardiac pacemakers in infants and children. Pediatr Cardiol 3:337, 1982.
7. Ector H, Dhooghe G, Daenen W, et al: Pacing in children. Br Heart J 53:541, 1985.
8. Serwer GA, Mericle JM: Evaluation of pacemaker pulse generator and patient longevity in patients aged 1 day to 20 years. Am J Cardiol 59:824, 1987.
9. Walsh CA, McAlister HF, Anders CA, et al: Pacemaker implantation in children: A 21-year experience. PACE 11:1940, 1988.
10. Brownlee JR, Serwer GA, Dick M II, et al: Failure of electrocardiographic monitoring to detect cardiac arrest in patients with pacemakers. Am J Dis Child 143:105, 1989.
11. McCue CM, Mantakas ME, Tingelstad JB, Ruddy S: Congenital heart block in newborns of mothers with connective tissue disease. Circulation 56:82, 1977.
12. Kangos JJ, Griffiths SP, Blumenthal S: Congenital complete heart block: A classification and experience with 18 patients. Am J Cardiol 20:632, 1967.
13. Dorostkar P, Serwer GA, LeRoy S, Dick M II: Long-term course of children and young adults with congenital complete heart block. J Am Coll Cardiol 21:295A, 1993.
14. Michaelsson M, Riesenfeld T, Jonzon A: Natural history of congenital complete atrioventricular block. PACE 20: 2098, 1997.
15. Kugler JD, Danford DA: Pacemakers in children: An update. Am Heart J 117:665, 1989.
16. Karpawich PP, Gillette PC, Garrison A, et al: Congenital complete atrioventricular block: Clinical and electrophysiologic predictors of need for pacemaker insertion. Am J Cardiol 48:1098, 1981.
17. Winkler RB, Freed MD, Nadas AS: Exercise-induced ventricular ectopy in children and young adults with complete heart block. Am Heart J 99:87, 1980.
18. Eldor M, Griffin JC, Abbott VA, et al: Permanent cardiac pacing in patients with long QT syndrome. J Am Coll Cardiol 3:600, 1987.
19. Gregoratos G, Cheitlin MD, Conill A, et al: ACC/AHA guidelines for implantation of cardiac pacemakers and antiarrhythmic devices. J Am Coll Cardiol 31:1175, 1998.
20. Rishi F, Hulse LE, Auld DO, et al: Effects of dual-chamber pacing for pediatric patients with hypertrophic obstructive cardiomyopathy. J Am Coll Cardiol 29:734, 1997.
21. McGrath LB, Gonzalez-Lavin L, Morse DP, Levett JM: Pacemaker system failure and other events in children with surgically induced heart block. PACE II:1182, 1988.
22. Serwer GA, Mericle JM, Armstrong BE: Epicardial ventricular pacemaker electrode longevity in children. Am J Cardiol 61:104, 1988.
23. Serwer GA, Uzark K, Dick M II: Endocardial pacing electrode longevity in children. J Am Coll Cardiol 15:212A, 1990.
24. Serwer G, Dick M II, Eakin B: Cardiac output response to treadmill exercise in children with fixed-rate pacemakers. Circulation 84:II-514, 1991.
25. Karpawich PP, Perry BL, Farooki ZQ, et al: Pacing in children and young adults in nonsurgical atrioventricular block: Comparison of single-rate ventricular and dual-chamber modes. Am Heart J 113:316, 1987.
26. Karpawich PP, Justice CD, Cavitt DL, Chang CH: Developmental sequelae of fixed-rate ventricular pacing in the immature canine heart: An electrophysiologic, hemodynamic, and histopathologic evaluation. Am Heart J 119:1077, 1990.
26a. Karpawich PP, Rabah R, Haas JE: Altered cardiac histology following apical right ventricular pacing in patients with congenital atrioventricular block. PACE 22:1372, 1999.
27. Horenstein MS, Karpawich PP: Pacemaker syndrome in the young: Do children need dual chamber as the initial pacing mode? PACE 27:600, 2004.
28. Preston TA, Fletcher RD, Luechesi BR, et al: Changes in myocardial threshold: Physiologic and pharmacologic factors in patients with implanted pacemakers. Am Heart J 74:235, 1967.
29. Lau C, Cameron DA, Nishimura SC, et al: A cardiac evoked response algorithm providing threshold tracking: A North American multicenter study. PACE 23:953, 2000.
30. Cohen MI, Buck K, Tanel RE, et al: Capture management efficacy in children and young adults with endocardial and unipolar epicardial systems. Europace 6:248, 2004.
31. Bauersfeld U, Nowak B, Molinari L, et al: Low-energy epicardial pacing in children: The benefit of autocapture. Ann Thorac Surg 68:1380, 1999.
32. Serwer GA, Uzark K, Beekman R, Dick M II: Optimal programming of rate altering parameters in children with rate-responsive pacemakers using graded treadmill exercise testing. PACE 13:541, 1990.
33. Yabek SM, Wernly J, Check TW, et al: Rate-adaptive cardiac pacing in children using a minute ventilation biosensor. PACE 13:2108, 1990.
34. Gillette PC, Shannon C, Blair H, et al: Transvenous pacing in pediatric patients. Am Heart J 105:843, 1983.
35. Ward DE, Jones S, Shinebourne EA: Long-term transvenous pacing in children weighing ten kilograms or less. Int J Cardiol 15:112, 1982.
36. Spotnitz HM: Transvenous pacing in infants and children with congenital heart disease. Ann Thorac Surg 49:495, 1990.
37. Kammeraad JAE, Rosenthal E, Bostock J, et al: Endocardial pacemaker implantation in infants weighing ≤10 kilograms. PACE 27:1466, 2004.
38. Gillette PC, Zeigler V, Bradhaus GB, Kinsella P: Pediatric transvenous pacing: A concern for venous thrombosis? PACE 11:1935, 1988.
39. Yakvevich V, Alogen D, Papo J, Vidne BA: Fibrotic stenosis of the SVC with widespread thrombotic occlusion of its major tributaries. J Thorac Cardiovasc Surg 85:632, 1983.
40. Sunder SK, Ekong EA, Sevalingram K, Kumar A: SVC thrombosis due to pacing electrodes. Am Heart J 123:790, 1992.
41. Wilkoff BL, Byrd CL, Love CJ, et al: Pacemaker lead extraction with the laser sheath: Results of the pacing lead extraction with the excimer sheath (PLEXES) trial. J Am Coll Cardiol 33:1671, 1999.
42. Kantharia BK, Kutalek SP: Extraction of pacemaker and implantable cardioverter defibrillator leads. Curr Opin Cardiol 14:44, 1999.
43. Sharifi M, Sorkin R, Lakier JB: Left heart pacing and cardioembolic stroke. PACE 17:1691, 1994.
44. Levin AR, Spach MS, Boineau JP, et al: Atrial pressure-flow dynamics in atrial septal defects (secundum type). Circulation 37:476, 1968.
45. Serwer GA, Armstrong BE, Anderson PAW, et al: Use of contrast echocardiography for evaluation of right ventricular hemodynamics in the presence of ventricular septal defects. Circulation 58:327, 1978.
46. Westerman GR, Van Revanter SH: Surgical management of difficult pacing problems in patients with congenital heart disease. J Cardiovasc Surg 2:351, 1987.
47. Shah MJ, Nehgme R, Carboni M, Murphy JD: Endocardial atrial pacing lead implantation and midterm follow-up in young patients with sinus node dysfunction after the Fontan procedure. PACE 27:949, 2004.

48. Moak JP, Friedman RA, Moffat D, et al: Dual-chamber pacing in children: The optimal lead configuration-unipolar or bipolar? J Am Coll Cardiol 17:208A, 1991.
49. Michalik RE, Williams WH, Zorn-Chelten S, Hotches CR: Experience with a new epimyocardial pacing lead in children. PACE 7:83, 1984.
50. Kugler J, Minsour W, Blodgett C, et al: Comparison of two myoepicardial pacemaker leads: Follow-up in 80 children, adolescents, and young adults. PACE 11:2216, 1988.
51. DeLeon SY, Ilbawi MN, Becker CL, et al: Exit block in pediatric cardiac pacing. Thorac Cardiovasc Surg 99:905, 1990.
52. Hamilton R, Gow R, Bahoric B, et al: Steroid-eluting epicardial leads in pediatrics: Improved epicardial thresholds in the first year. PACE 14:2066, 1991.
53. Karpawich PP, Harkini M, Arciniegas E, Cavitt DL: Improved chronic epicardial pacing in children: Steroid contribution to porous platinized electrodes. PACE 15:1151, 1992.
54. Johns JA, Fuh FA, Burger JD, Hammon JW Jr: Steroid-eluting epicardial pacing leads in pediatric patients: Encouraging early results. J Am Coll Cardiol 20:395, 1992.
55. Serwer GA, Dorostkar PC, LeRoy S, Dick M II: Comparison of chronic thresholds between differing endocardial electrode types in children. Circulation 86:I-43, 1992.
56. Rosenthal E, Bostock J: VDD pacing in children with congenital complete heart block: Advantages of a single pass lead. PACE 20:2102, 1997.
57. Robertson JM, Hillel L: A new technique for permanent pacemaker implantation in infants and children. Ann Thorac Surg 44:209, 1987.
58. Ulicny KS Jr, Detterbeck FC, Starek PJK, Wilcox BR: Conjoined subrectus pocket for permanent pacemaker placement in the neonate. Soc Thorac Surg 53:1130, 1992.
59. Ott DA, Gillette PC, Cooley DA: Atrial pacing via the subxiphoid approach. Tex Heart Inst J 9:149, 1982.
60. Lawrie GM, Seale JP, Morris GC Jr, et al: Results of epicardial pacing by the left subcostal approach. Ann Thorac Surg 28:561, 1979.
61. Brenner JI, Gaines S, Cordier J, et al: Cardiac strangulation: Two-dimensional echo recognition of a rare complication of epicardial pacemaker therapy. Am J Cardiol 61:654, 1988.
62. Perry JC, Nihill MR, Ludomirsky A, et al: The pulmonary artery lasso: Epicardial pacing lead causing right ventricular outflow obstruction. PACE 14:1018, 1991.
63. Serwer GA, Dick M II, Uzark K, et al: The value of redundant ventricular epicardial electrode placement in children. PACE 9:531, 1988.
64. Gillette PC, Edgerton J, Kratz J, Zeigler V: The subpectoral pocket: The preferred implant site for pediatric pacemakers. PACE 14:1089, 1991.
65. Hayes DC, Holmes DR Jr, Maloney JD, et al: Permanent endocardial pacing in pediatric patients. J Thorac Cardiovasc Surg 85:618, 1983.
66. Hoyer MH, Beerman LB, Ettedgui JA, et al: Transatrial lead placement for endocardial pacing in children. Ann Thorac Surg 58:97, 1994.
67. Karpawich PP. Chronic right ventricular pacing and cardiac performance: The pediatric perspective. PACE 27: 884, 2004.
68. Karpawich PP, Horenstein MS, Webster P: Site specific right ventricular implant pacing to optimize paced left ventricular function in the young without and without congenital heart disease. PACE 25: 566, 2002.
69. Serwer GA, Dorostkar PC, LeRoy S, et al: Evaluation of rate variable pacemaker function at maximal exertion in children and young adults. PACE 16:899, 1993.
70. Serwer GA, Kodali R, Eakin B, et al: Changes in pacemaker threshold with exercise in children and young adults. J Am Coll Cardiol 17:207A, 1991.
71. Gillette PC, Zinner A, Kratz J, et al: Atrial tracking (synchronous) pacing in a pediatric and young adult population. J Am Coll Cardiol 9:811, 1987.
72. Frohlig G, Blank W, Schwerdt H, et al: Atrial sensing performance of AV universal pacemakers during exercise. PACE 11:47, 1988.
73. Ross BA, Zeigler V, Zinner A, et al: The effect of exercise on the atrial electrogram voltage in young patients. PACE 14:2092, 1991.
74. Bricker JT, Barison A, Traveek MS, et al: The use of exercise testing in children to evaluate abnormalities of pacemaker function not apparent at rest. PACE 8:656, 1985.
75. Jain P, Kaul U, Wasir HS: Myopotential inhibition of unipolar demand pacemakers: Utility of provocative manoeuvres in assessment and management. Int J Cardiol 34:33, 1992.
76. Strathmore NF, Mond HG: Noninvasive monitoring and testing of pacemaker function. PACE 10:1359, 1987.
77. Kerstjens-Frederikse MWS, Bink-Boelkens MTE, de Jongste MJL, Homan van der Heide JN: Permanent cardiac pacing in children: Morbidity and efficacy of follow-up. Int J Cardiol 33:207, 1991.
78. Jarosik DL, Redd RM, Buckingham TA, et al: Utility of ambulatory electrocardiography in detecting pacemaker dysfunction in the early postimplantation period. Am J Cardiol 60:1030, 1987.
79. Vincent JA, Cavitt DL, Karpawich PP: Diagnostic and cost effectiveness of telemonitoring the pediatric pacemaker patient. Pediatr Cardiol 18:86, 1997.
80. Shepard RB, Kam J, Colvin EC, et al: Pacing threshold spikes months and years after implant. PACE 14:1835, 1991.
81. Silka MJ, Kron J, Dunnigan A, Dick M II: Sudden cardiac death and the use of cardioverter-defibrillators in pediatric patients. Circulation 87:800, 1993.
82. Hamilton RM, Dorian P, Gow RM, Williams WG: Five-year experience with implantable defibrillators in children. Am J Cardiol 77:524, 1996.
83. Kron J, Silka MJ, Ohm O-J, et al: Preliminary experience with nonthoracotomy implantable cardioverter defibrillators in young patients. PACE 17:26, 1994.
84. Stefanelli CB, Bradley DJ, Leroy S, et al: Implantable cardioverter defibrillator therapy for life-threatening arrhythmias in young patients. J Intervent Cardiac Electrophysiol 6:235, 2002.
85. Berul CI, Triedman JK, Forbess J, et al: Minimally invasive cardioverter defibrillator implantation for children: An animal model and pediatric case report. PACE 24:1789, 2001.
86. Luedemann M, Hund K, Stertmann W, et al: Implantable cardioverter-defibrillator in a child using a single subcutaneous array lead and an abdominal active can. PACE 27:117, 2004.
87. Fischbach PS, Law IH, Dick M II, et al: Use of a single coil transvenous electrode with an abdominally placed implantable cardioverter defibrillator in children. PACE 23:884, 2000.
88. Molina LE, Dunnigan AC, Crosson JE: Implantation of transvenous pacemakers in infants and small children. Ann Thorac Surg 59:689, 1995.
89. Halperin BD, Reynolds B, Fain ES, et al: The effect of electrode size on transvenous defibrillation energy requirements: A prospective evaluation. PACE 20: 893, 1997.
90. Stephanson EA, Casavant D, Tuzi J, et al., on behalf of the ATTEST Investigators: Efficacy of atrial antitachycardia pacing using the Medtronic AT500 pacemaker in patients with congenital heart disease. Am J Cardiol 92:871, 2003.
91. Dubin AM, Feinstein JA, Reddy M, et al: Electrical resynchronization: A novel therapy for the failing right ventricle. Circulation 107:2287, 2003.
92. Strieper M, Karpawich P, Frias P, et al: Initial experience with cardiac resynchronization therapy for ventricular dysfunction in young patients with surgically operated congenital heart disease. Am J Cardiol 94:1352, 2004.
93. Janousek J, Vojtovic P, Hucin B, et al: Resynchronization pacing is a useful adjunct to the management of acute heart failure after surgery for congenital heart defects. Am J Cardiol 88:145, 2001.

94. Zimmerman FJ, Starr JP, Koenig PR, et al: Acute hemodynamic benefit of multisite ventricular pacing after congenital heart surgery. Ann Thorac Surg 75:1775, 2003.
95. Dajani AS. Taubert KA, Wilson W, et al: Prevention of bacterial endocarditis: Recommendations by the American Heart Association. Circulation 96:358, 1997.
96. Moos RH, Tsu UD: The crisis of physical illness: An overview. In RH Moos (ed): Coping with Physical Illness. New York, Plenum, 1977, p 3.
97. Satin W, LaGreca AM, Zigo MA, Skyler JS: Diabetes in adolescence: Effects of a multifamily group intervention and parent simulation of diabetes. J Pediatr Psychol 14:259, 1989.
98. Eiser C: Growing Up with a Chronic Disease. London, Jessica Kingsley, 1993.
99. Gamble WJ, Owens JP: Pacemaker therapy for conduction defects in the pediatric population. In Roberts N, Gelband H (eds): Cardiac Arrhythmias in the Neonate, Infant, and Child. New York, Appleton-Century-Crofts, 1977, p 469.
100. Alpern D, Uzark K, Dick M II: Psychosocial responses of children to cardiac pacemakers. J Pediatr 114:494, 1989.
101. Wallander JL, Thompson RJ: Psychosocial adjustment of children with chronic physical conditions. In Roberts MC (ed): Handbook of Pediatric Psychology, 2nd ed. New York, Guilford Press, 1995, p 124.
102. Pless IB, Roghmann KJ: Chronic illness and its consequences: Observations based on three epidemiologic surveys. J Pediatr 79:351, 1971.
103. Rolland J: Chronic illness and the life cycle: A conceptual framework. Fam Proc 26:203, 1987.
104. Wallander JL, Varni JW: Adjustment in children with chronic physical disorders: Programmatic research on a disability-stress-coping model. In LaGreca AM, Siegal L, Wallander JL, Walker CE (eds): Stress and Coping With Pediatric Conditions. New York, Guilford Press, 1992, p 279.
105. Garmezy N, Tellegen A: Studies of stress-resistant children: Methods, variables, and preliminary findings. In Morrison F, Lord C, Keating D (eds): Advances in Applied Developmental Psychology, vol 1. New York, Academic Press, 1984, p 231.
106. Werner EE, Smith RS: Vulnerable but invincible: A longitudinal study of resilient children and youth. New York, McGraw-Hill, 1982.
107. Wallander JL, Varni JW, Babani L, et al: Family resources as resistance factors for psychological maladjustment in chronically ill and handicapped children. J Pediatr Psychol 14:157, 1989.
108. Thompson R, Gustafson K: Adaptations to Chronic Childhood Illness. Washington, DC, American Psychological Association, 1996.
109. Stein RE, Jessop DJ: A noncategorical approach to chronic childhood illness. Pub Health Rep 97:354, 1982.
110. Lavigne JV, Faier-Routman J: Psychological adjustment to pediatric physical disorders: A meta-analytic review. J Pediatr Psychol 17:133, 1992.
111. Goldberg S, Simmons RJ, Newman J, et al: Congenital heart disease, parental stress, and infant-mother relationships. J Pediatr 119:661, 1991.
112. Miller G, Tesman JR, Ramer JC, et al: Outcome after open-heart surgery in infants and children. J Child Neurol 11:49, 1996.
113. Wright M, Nolan T: Impact of cyanotic heart disease on school performance. Arch Dis Child 71:64, 1994.
114. Gutgesell HP, Gessner IH, Better VL, et al: Recreational and occupational recommendations for young patients with heart disease. Circulation 74:1195A, 1986.
115. Werner ME, Smith R: Kauai's Children Come of Age. Honolulu, Hawaii, University of Hawaii Press, 1982.
116. Hamlett KW, Pellegrini DS, Katz KS: Childhood chronic illness as a family stressor. J Pediatr Psychol 17:33, 1992.
117. Blechman EA, Delamater AM: Family communication and type 1 diabetes: A window on the social environment of chronically ill children. In Cole RE, Reiss D (eds): How Do Families Cope With Chronic Illness? Hillsdale, NJ, Lawrence Erlbaum, 1993, p 1.
118. Demaso D, Campis L, Wypij D, et al: The impact of maternal perceptions and medical severity on the adjustment of children with congenital heart disease. J Pediatr Psychol 16:137, 1991.
119. Lyons-Ruth K, Zoll D, Conell D, Grunebaum HV: The depressed mother and her one year old infant: Environment, interaction, attachment and infant development. In Field T, Tronick E (eds): Maternal Depression and Infant Disturbance. San Francisco, Jossey-Bass, 1986, p 61.
120. Masten AS, Garmezy N, Tellegen A, et al: Competence and stress in school children: The moderating effects of individual and family qualities. J Child Psychol Psychiatry 29:745, 1988.
121. Green KD, Forehand R, Beck SJ, Vosk B: An assessment of the relationship among measures of children's social competence and children's academic achievement. Child Dev 51:1149, 1980.
122. Masten AS, Morison P, Pellegrini DS: A revised class play method of peer assessment. Dev Psychol 21:523, 1985.
123. Morison P, Masten AS: Peer reputation in middle childhood as a predictor of adaptation in adolescence: A seven year follow-up. Child Dev 62:991, 1991.
124. Pelham WE, Milich R: Peer relationships in children with hyperactivity/attention deficit disorder. J Learn Disabil 17:560, 1984.
125. Cowen EL, Pederson A, Babigian H, et al: Long term follow-up of early detected vulnerable children. J Consult Clin Psychol 41:438, 1973.
126. McCubbin HI, McCubbin MA, Patterson JM, et al: CHIP: Coping-health inventory for parents: An assessment of parental coping patterns in the care of the chronically ill child. J Marr Fam 45:359, 1983.
127. Lazarus RS, Folkman S: Stress, Appraisal, and Coping. New York, Springer, 1984.
128. Affleck G, Tennen H, Rowe J: Mother, fathers, and the crisis of newborn intensive care. Infant Mental Health 11:12, 1990.
129. Compas BE, Worsham NL, Ey S: Conceptual and developmental issues in children's coping with stress. In LaGreca AM, Siegal LJ, Wallander JL, Walker CE (eds): Stress and Coping in Child Health. New York, Guilford Press, 1992, p 7.
130. Yarcheski A, Scoloveno MA, Mahon N: Social support and well-being in adolescents: The mediating role of hopefulness. Nurs Res 43:288, 1994.
131. Andrews SG: Informing schools about children's chronic illness. Pediatrics 88:306, 1991.
132. Vitale MB, Funk M: Quality of life in younger persons with an implantable cardioverter defibrillator. Dimens Crit Care Nurs 14:100, 1995.
133. Cooper DK, Luceri RM, Thurer RJ, et al: The impact of the automatic implantable cardioverter defibrillator on quality of life. Clin Prog Electrophysiol Pacing 4:306, 1986.
134. Kuiper R, Nyamathi A: Stressors and coping strategies of patients with automatic implantable cardioverter defibrillators. J Cardiovasc Nurs 5:65, 1991.
135. Luderitz B, Jung W, Deister A, Manz M: Patient acceptance of implantable cardioverter defibrillator devices: Changing attitudes. Am Heart J 127:1179, 1994.
136. Mazur JE: Learning and Behavior. Upper Saddle River, NJ, Prentice Hall, 1998, p 187.
137. Maier SF, Seligman ME: Learned helplessness: Theory and evidence. J Exp Psychol Gen 105:3, 1976.
138. Stoyva JM, Carlson JG: A coping/rest model of relaxation and stress management. In Goldberger L, Breznitz S (eds): Handbook of Stress: Theoretical and Clinical Aspects. New York, Free Press, 1993, p 724.
139. Teplitz L, Egenes KJ, Brask L: Life after sudden death: The development of a support group for automatic implantable cardioverter-defibrillator patients. J Cardiovasc Nurs 4:20, 1990.

Index

Note: Page numbers followed by f and t refer to figures and tables, respectively.

D

E

U

W